Patricia Car...
1410½ Clay S...
LaPorte, Ind.

Taber's
Cyclopedic Medical Dictionary

INCLUDING

A Digest of Medical Subjects
MEDICINE • SURGERY • NURSING
DIETETICS • PHYSICAL THERAPY
TREATMENTS • DRUGS, ETC.

by

CLARENCE WILBUR TABER

Author, Taber's Dictionary for Nurses, Taber's Condensed
Medical Dictionary, Dictionary of Food and Nutrition,
Dictionary of Gynecology and Obstetrics, etc., etc.

EIGHTH EDITION
Illustrated

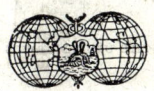

F. A. DAVIS COMPANY • PHILADELPHIA
1958

COPYRIGHT 1940 BY C. W. TABER
COPYRIGHT 1942 BY F. A. DAVIS COMPANY
COPYRIGHT 1945 BY F. A. DAVIS COMPANY
COPYRIGHT 1946 BY F. A. DAVIS COMPANY
COPYRIGHT 1948 BY F. A. DAVIS COMPANY
COPYRIGHT 1949 BY F. A. DAVIS COMPANY
COPYRIGHT 1950 BY F. A. DAVIS COMPANY
COPYRIGHT 1951 BY F. A. DAVIS COMPANY
COPYRIGHT 1952 BY F. A. DAVIS COMPANY
COPYRIGHT 1953 BY F. A. DAVIS COMPANY
COPYRIGHT 1954 BY F. A. DAVIS COMPANY
COPYRIGHT 1955 BY F. A. DAVIS COMPANY
COPYRIGHT 1956 BY F. A. DAVIS COMPANY
COPYRIGHT 1957 BY F. A. DAVIS COMPANY
COPYRIGHT 1958 BY F. A. DAVIS COMPANY

Copyright, Great Britain. All Rights Reserved

58.5

*Library of Congress
Catalog Card No. 58-9211*

PRINTED IN THE UNITED STATES OF AMERICA

Preface to the Eighth Edition

THIS is the eighth edition of this dictionary. A new edition does not fully reveal to the consultant all the changes and improvements that have been made in it. For instance, two to three printings of this dictionary have been made every year, and in each one of these printings many changes and improvements have been made. Now in this eighth edition at least fifty per cent of the material has been revised, rewritten, and reset.

Many obsolescent words have been eliminated to make space for the entry of new and up-to-date terms. The nomenclature of parasitology and allied terms has been standardized by this branch of medicine so that this edition of the dictionary is in complete harmony with the modern textbooks on this subject.

Not only have many new words been introduced, including new subjects, but late developments and new facts pertaining to the various branches of medical science have made it necessary to rewrite, revise, and change the material relating to important subjects such as diseases.

The purpose of this dictionary is to inform as well as to define; to extend information about the things that words symbolize. The dual aim of the work stems from the need of people in medicine and related fields to learn what they have to know quickly and conveniently. The person who wishes to know something about a particular subject is frequently in search of *information*—not words, not a mere definition. Experience shows that such a requirement is met most fittingly by a combined medical dictionary and dictionary of medical subjects. To explain the gratifying popularity of this volume among all classes of medical personnel is to acknowledge the vital part that a dictionary should play in scientific learning. In science, a reader's threshold of exasperation is notoriously and properly low. He expects a dictionary to contribute to his professional performance, and it is a matter of observation that that cannot be done by definitions alone or by the mere herding of scientific facts in alphabetical order. In all these matters, the author of this book has sought to detach it from the commonplace category of dictionaries that deal mostly with terms and spellings. The aim throughout has been to supply voluminous information in the various fields of medical practice, nursing, and allied subjects.

Even though much new matter has been added, the basic material in previous editions which has made this dictionary famous has been retained in this extensive revision.

CLARENCE WILBUR TABER

Publisher's Foreword

THIS is the eighth edition of a dictionary that has long been an indispensable aid to hundreds of thousands of workers in the medical sciences. During its growth in the preceding editions, its authority, scope, and uniqueness of presentation have marked it as vastly more than the usual medical dictionary. In this new edition, as before, its title defines its purpose. *Taber's Cyclopedic Medical Dictionary* stands more than ever as a source of information—a coördinated work of knowledge concerned with every clinical feature of medicine, nursing, and allied sciences.

C. W. Taber, long distinguished for his scholarly contributions to education and lexicography, needs no introduction. For many years, countless educators and students have used his textbooks, in colleges and in secondary and elementary schools from coast to coast. His work as a brilliant and imaginative creator of dictionaries has given him a stature unequaled among present-day medical lexicographers. As the author and compiler of this volume, he has brought to the task not only the keenest erudition, but also the sharpest and liveliest appreciation of his readers' needs.

Long associated with vital trends in medical and nursing activities, the author is widely noted for a host of contributions to these fields. He shares with the late Dr. Nicholas Senn the distinction of having written the first nurses' dictionary ever published. He is the author of more than forty books—both lay and medical—many of them dictionaries in the specialist branches of medicine and nursing. His work as a medical editor is known and revered across the continent. The profession acknowledges not only his scholarly literary output, but also the creative spirit that underlies all his work.

Anatole France has said that the collection of a multitude of facts and principles, arranged in a new and more accessible and understandable form, is as much a piece of creative writing as is fiction or poetry. This dictionary is more than a dictionary for that reason. Its manifold features, visible on almost every page, are creative conceptions, devised to communicate information beyond definitions. Through using the expanded discussions, of etiology, symptoms, diagnosis, treatment, nursing procedures, and the like, the reader learns the author's cyclopedic objective, and obtains authoritative, up-to-the-minute information revealed by no other dictionary.

Reviewers have referred to Mr. Taber as the Webster of the Medical World.

F. A. DAVIS COMPANY

Sources Consulted

THE factual material of this dictionary is supported by the outstanding authorities in medical science. In the early editions, sixteen distinguished medical specialists coöperated with the author in the preparation of the work, resolving the problems in their particular fields. In this eighth edition the book's authority is still further extended by the author's Board of Medical Advisors. In addition, scores of modern reference works and medical and nursing textbooks have been consulted for the verification of facts and for new data. Likewise, the leading medical and nursing periodicals have been freely used for new discoveries and for the latest procedures in the allied medical sciences. To give individual credit to the multitudinous sources consulted would be most difficult.

The data on the content and chemical composition of foods have been largely based upon the findings of Sherman, although other eminent authorities in the field of food and nutrition have been drawn upon. It should, however, be understood that there can be no definite standard of values for any food, and that this accounts for the differences in the findings of various food specialists.

The field covering Bacteriology, Parasitology and similar subjects has been reviewed and brought up to date by an eminent authority. Much new data has also been added to the subjects relating to "blood" by a well-known specialist.

NOTE: "The terms of definitions on physical therapy [contained in this dictionary] have been adopted by the Council on Physical Therapy of the American Medical Association."—H. A. Carter, *Secretary*, Council on Physical Therapy, American Medical Association.

C. W. TABER

Features and Their Use

ONLY a thoroughly trained mechanic would pretend to understand the workings of a complicated piece of machinery with its thousands of parts. Almost any one, however, feels competent to use successfully and to understand a dictionary that in reality represents hundreds of highly specialized subjects. To most persons, a dictionary is a dictionary. Nevertheless, *Taber's Cyclopedic Medical Dictionary* contains many subjects and features never before incorporated in such a reference work.

This work *is a medical dictionary*, but it is more than that. In fact, there is no book with which it may be compared. It is as much a dictionary of medical subject matter as it is a dictionary of medical terms. It is a source book of medical knowledge that will save much time in consulting a great many other works. A few of its more outstanding features are the following:

Pronunciations: Fully 99% of all words are respelled for pronunciation. Long and short vowels are marked diacritically, the primary accent is shown, and frequently the secondary accent. Latin rules cannot be depended upon for the pronunciation of medical words, and authorities do not agree upon any standardized pronunciations. Common usage, however, seems to prevail, and this has been followed as much as feasible in this book. Respellings for pronunciation are accurate and do not distort the actual spelling of the word any more than is necessary to indicate the proper phonetic sound.

Spellings: Diphthongs, for the most part, have been eliminated. Only proper nouns have been capitalized. Words formerly hyphenated, such as gastrointestinal, are now indicated as one word. Proper nouns used as adjectives do not take a capital initial. The letter "k" has been substituted for "c" in such words as leukocytes.

Vocabulary: This is sufficiently extensive to meet the daily needs of the practicing physician, the medical student, and the nurse. Highly specialized topics which belong in separate lexicons, such as botany, and obsolete words have been eliminated. Hundreds of drugs, for instance, that have not been in general use for ten or twenty years, have been weeded out of the vocabulary to make room for the many new drugs not yet appearing in any other medical dictionary. Medical literature has been combed to provide the very latest terms now in good medical standing.

Definitions: These stand out in a paragraph separate and apart from all collateral terms, and apart from additional supplementary matter, thus making it easy to read the definitions. The "See-See" definition has been completely eliminated. Each word has its own complete definition, even at the risk of duplication. No word is defined with a synonym. Supplementary information is often referred to by the word "SEE:" but such material does not pertain to the definition as given. Words marked with an asterisk as they appear in a definition indicate that the word is defined in its proper place.

There probably is no profession in which there is less agreement regarding certain subjects than Medicine. The prevailing opinion of the profession, however, has been given in this dictionary, in so far as this has been available. Unfortunately, this may result in an adverse opinion in some instances, especially if the consultant is not familiar with opposing views, or unduly favorable to a definition other than the one expressed.

Subtopics: Many related words are listed and defined in most dictionaries in the same paragraph, such as the many *acids*, or different forms of the same disease. In this dictionary each of these words has its own vocabulary entrance with its definition separate and apart from other material. These topics are listed in alphabetical order, making access to them easy and quick.

Etymologies: This is the only abridged medical dictionary containing the derivations of words showing their Latin, Greek, and other sources with their meanings. Even the large unabridged medical dictionaries do not contain as many etymologies. These are not merely reproductions from other works, but the result of research which has made possible a great degree of accuracy. Prefixes and Suffixes also appear in alphabetical order the same as words.

Medical Synonyms: For the first time in any abridged medical dictionary, medical synonyms have been incorporated following the definition of a word; that is, when there *are* synonyms for a given term. This is a great aid to medical writers and speakers.

Words Pertaining To: This is another new feature. Following important words will be found a list of other words pertaining to the one defined. In this way, a complete study or cycle of information pertaining to a given term may be acquired by reading the definitions of these words in the text. In many instances, following the definitions will be found a list of related subjects pertaining to the one defined.

First Aid: Practically every form of accident has been listed with first aid treatment. Included among these are poisons and their antidotes, bites and stings of all kinds, fractures, and other accidents, including different forms of unconsciousness.

Diseases: The principal diseases with their various forms are given, together with their diagnosis and symptoms, prognosis, treatment and nursing procedures, including diet.

Dietetics: Practically every food and beverage is listed with all that is known about it. Also mineral content of the human body, and the physiology of digestion, assimilation, and elimination.

Drugs: Many of the terms for drugs have been given their trade-mark names, even though no references to the trade-mark or proprietary nature of the drug is made in the individual listing. These names are in common use by physicians and nurses who may be more familiar with them than with their scientific names.

Nursing Procedures: More of these are given than are usually found in the handbooks of nursing on the market. This dictionary is in fact an epitome of all nursing textbooks.

Tabulations: Many important tabulations will be found in this text, but long tables which interfere with finding words in the dictionary have been grouped in the Appendix.

Only consistent use of this medical dictionary will prove its value and reveal much of its treasures.

Fact-Finding Index

THE user of reference works seldom becomes aware of the many subjects they contain. The following index lists a few of the entries covering such important subjects as *Diagnosis, First Aid, Nursing Procedures,* and *Toxicology.* Many other subjects could be listed in the same manner. They, however, will be found in regular alphabetical order.

Diagnosis
Gait
Gums
Headache
Lips
Mucous membranes
Nail, finger
Nose
Pain
Pulse
Respiration
Skin
Sputum
Stool
Tongue
Unconsciousness
Urine
SEE ALSO: name of each disease

First Aid
Anesthesia
Apoplexy
Asphyxia
Bee sting
Bed bug
Bites
Bleeding
 arterial
 venous
Bot fly
Botulism
Bronchi, foreign body in
Burns
Cat bite
Chiggers
Choking
Clavicle, dislocation of
Concussion of brain
Contusion
Convulsion
Cyanosis
Delirium tremens
Digitalis
Dislocation
Dog bite
Drowning
Drug poison. SEE: name of drug
Ear, foreign bodies in
Elbow, dislocation of
Electric contact and injury
Electric shock
Esophagus, foreign bodies in
Eye, foreign bodies in
Fainting
Femur, fracture of
Fibula, fracture of
Finger, dislocation
Fire emergencies
Fit
Flame, inhalation of
Foreign bodies in ear
Fracture
Freezing
Frost bite
Hair dye poisoning
Heat
 cramps
 exhaustion
 stroke
Hemorrhage
 arterial
 carotid artery
 venous
Hip, dislocation of
Hornet sting
Human bite
Humerus, fracture of
Internal injury
Ivy poisoning
Jaw, dislocation of
Larynx, foreign body in
Neck, dislocation of
Nose, foreign body in
Olecranon, fracture of
Radius, fracture of
Rib, fracture of
Shell shock
Shock
Shoulder, dislocation of
Skull, fracture of
Snake bite
Spider bite
Spine, fracture of
Sprain
 of back
 foot
 riders'
Stomach, foreign bodies in
Strain
Syncope
Tennis elbow
Throat, foreign bodies in
Tibia, fracture of
Tourniquet
Transportation of injured
Unconscious
Unconsciousness
Wounds
 abdominal
 bullet

Nursing Procedures
Addison's disease
Affusion
Agitated depression
Affective psychosis
Allergy
Amebic enteritis
Anemia
Aneurysm
Ankle clonus
Ankylosis
Anthrax
Antistain formulary
Antrum, puncture of
Anuresis
Aperient
Apicolysis
Apoplexy
Arteriosclerosis
Arthritis
Aspiration
Barbiturics
Baths
Bed
Bell's paralysis
Blepharitis
Blister, water
Breath
Bromidrosis
Bronchitis, chronic
Bronchopneumonia
Bronchotomy
Bruise
Bulimia
Burn
 acid
 alkali
 chemical
Bursitis
Byrd-Dew method of resuscitation
Cancer
Cancrum
Carbolic acid solution
Carbuncle
Castor oil
Cataract
Catheter, fever
Catheterization
Celiac disease
Charting
Chilblain
Chill
Chlorine preparations
Cholecystitis
Cholera infantum
Chorea insaniens
Circumcision
Clinical thermometer
Collapse
Colonic irrigation
Colostomy
Colpocystotomy
Colpohysterectomy
Colpoperineoplasty
Coma
Compress
Compression
Containers, handling
Convulsion
Cotton wool sandwiches
Craniectomy
Curettage
Cyclic vomiting
Dead, care of
Death, signs of
Delirium tremens
Dementia
Dementia paralytica
Dermatomyositis
Dermatoplasty
Dextrose
Diabetes
Diarrhea
 acute
 chronic
 infant
 nervous
Diphtheria
Discission
Disinfectant
Diverticulitis
Dorsal (position)
Dorsosacral (position)
Dosage
Douches
Draw sheet
Dressing
Drug action
Drug administration

Fact-Finding Index

Drugs, handling of
Eclampsia
Embolism
Emesis
Emetic
Empyema
Endocarditis
Endocervicitis
Enema
Enteroclysis
Enterocolitis
Enuresis
Epilepsy (diet)
Epistaxis
Esbach's method
Ether bed
Ethylene (precautions)
Excreta, disinfection of
Feeding
Fever, diagnosis of
Flatulence
Flatus
Flesh, examination of
Fomentation
Food requirements
Foot bath, mustard
Foreskin
Fowler's position
Friction
Fumigation
Gait (diagnosis)
Gallstone
Gastric lavage
Gastroenterostomy
Gastrostomy
Genoplasty
Gonorrhea
Gout
Gram's method
Gums (diagnosis)
Gynecology
Hands and skin, sterilization of
Hare lip
Headache
Heat, applications of
Heat cramps
Hemoplegia
Hemoptysis
Hemorrhage
Herniotomy
Hydrotherapy
Hyperthyroidism
Hypnotics
Hypodermoclysis
Hypothyroidism
Hysterectomy
Hysteropexy
Infant, premature feeding
Infection
Infectious diseases
Inflammation
Influenza
Injections
Injury
Insanity
Insect bites and stings
Insomnia
Instruments, care and sharpening
Insulin
  injection
Intubation
Iridotomy
Irrigation, bladder
Kelly pad
Knee, dislocation of
Labor
Laparotomy
Laryngectomy
Laryngoscopy
Larynx

Leech
Leprosy
Leukemia
Lip (diagnosis)
Lithotomy
Lumbar puncture
Lymphangitis
Mastectomy
Mastoidectomy
Measles
Medicine, rectal adm. of
Meningitis
Menorrhagia
Morning care
  sickness
Mouth, care of
Mucous membrane (diagnosis)
Myasthenia gravis
Myocarditis
Myomectomy
Myositis
Nail (diagnosis)
Nasal gavage
Nausea
Needle, care of
Nephrectomy
Nephritis, interstitial
  acute
Nephrotomy
Neptune girdle
Neuritis
Nipple
Nose (diagnosis)
Operation, preparation for, in the home
Ophthalmectomy
Opiate
Orchiectomy
Packs
Pain
  abdominal
  epigastric
  gallbladder
  gastralgia
  head
  thoracic
Palatal paralysis
Palate
Paracentesis
Paranoid violence
Pasteurization
Pediculus
Peptic ulcer
Perineorrhaphy
Perineum, tears of
Phlebitis alba dolens
Plaster casts
Pleurisy
Pneumonia
  hypostatic
Pneumothorax, artificial
Postoperative care
Postpartum hemorrhage
Poultice
Pregnancy
Prenatal care
Preoperative preparation
Preparations given by rectum
Prescription writing
Proctoclysis
Prostatectomy
Pulse
Pyrosis
Quinsy
Resection of rib
Respiration, method of counting
Restraint in bed
Salpingo-oöphorectomy
Salt solution
Schizophrenia

Sedatives
Shock
  shell-
Skin (diagnosis from)
  grafting
Sores
Specimen
Sputum (diagnosis from)
Square knot
Stool (diagnosis from)
Swedish movements
Symptoms
Syncope
Tampons
Tapotement
Teeth (diagnosis from)
Test meal
Thoracentesis
Thrombophlebitis
Thrombosis
  coronary
Thyroidectomy
Tongue (diagnosis from)
Tonsillectomy
Tracheitis
Tracheotomy
Trendelenburg position
Typhoid fever
Unconscious
Unconsciousness
Urine (diagnosis from)
Variola
Vomiting (diagnosis from)
Vomitus (diagnosis from)
Wrist drop

Poisoning

Acetanilid
Acid p.
Aconite
Alkali
Ammonium hydroxide
Antidotes
Antimony
Arsenic
Aspirin
Atropine
Banana oil
Barbital p.
Barbiturics
Barium compounds
Bed bug p.
Belladonna
Benzol p.
Bichloride of mercury
Bismuth
Blue stone
Boracic acid p.
Brass p.
Bromides
Carbon
  dioxide
  monoxide
  tetrachloride
Chloral hydrate
Chromium compounds
Cinchophen
Convulsive poisons
Copper sulfate
Corrosive poisons
Corrosive alkalies
Croton oil
Cyanide poison
Digitalis
Ergot
Fish p.
Formaldehyde
Gasoline
Grain p.
Hemlock
Heroin p.
Hydrochloric acid p.

Fact-Finding Index

Hyoscyamus
Ink p.
Iodine p.
Irritant p.
Lead p.
Manganese
Matches
Meat p.
Mercuric chloride
Mercury
Methyl alcohol
Methyl chloride
Morphine
Narcotism

Nicotine
Nitric acid
Nitromuriatic acid
Opium
Oxalic acid
Paraldehyde
Phenol
Phosphorus p.
Potassium
   chlorate
   chromate
   hydroxide
Ptomaine p.
Rough-on-rats poison

Sedative poisons
Silver nitrate
Soothing syrup
Strychnine
Sulfur dioxide
Sulfuric acid
Tartar emetic
Tellurium
Tin p.
Toadstool poison
Turpentine poison
Verdigris
Vermin killers' poison
Zinc salts

PRONUNCIATION

Diacritics: These are marks over or under vowels to indicate the pronunciations. In this dictionary, only two diacritics are used: The *macron*, showing the name sound or so-called long sound of vowels, as the *a* in rāte, *e* in ēat, *i* in īsle, *o* in ōver, and *u* in ūnite; also *e* as in ĕver, *i* as in ĭt, *o* as in nŏt, *u* as in cŭt.

Accents: These indicate the stress upon certain syllables. A single accent ' is called a *primary* accent. A double accent " is called a *secondary* accent, indicating less stress upon a syllable than that given to a primary accent. Examples are "ob'ject," and "o"ar-i-al'ji-a."

Pronunciations only may be approximately indicated unless all the markings in Webster's New International Dictionary are used which is not practical in an abridged dictionary.

Abbreviations Used in the Text

abbr.	abbreviation	**inf.**	inferior
adm.	administration	**int.**	interior, internal
anat.	anatomy	**K**	potassium, kalium
ant.	anterior	**L.**	Latin
anti.	antidote	**lat.**	lateral
app.	appendix	**LL.**	Late Latin
art.	artery	**m.**	male
AS.	Anglo-Saxon	**ME.**	Middle English
at. wt.	atomic weight	**med.**	medical
bact.	bacteriology	**mg.**	milligram
bet.	between	**Mg**	magnesium
biol.	biology	**N**	nitrogen
BNA	Basle nomina anatomica or Basel anatomical nomenclature	**Na**	sodium, natrium
		neur.	neurology
br.	branch, branches	**NP.**	nursing procedure
C.	Centigrade	**NNR.**	New and Nonofficial Remedies
C	carbon	**nut.**	nutrients
Ca	calcium	**O**	oxygen
Cal.	large Calorie or Calories	**OB.**	obstetrics
cal.	small calorie or calories	**O. Fr.**	Old French
carbo.	carbohydrates	**OPHTH.**	ophthalmology
cc.	cubic centimeter	**opp.**	opposite
cf.	compare	**orig.**	origin
chem.	chemistry	**ORTH.**	orthopedics
Cl	chlorine	**OTO.**	otology
comp.	composition	**ONP**	operating nursing procedure
contra.	contraindication	**p**	page
Cu	copper, cuprum	**P**	phosphorus
der.	derivative	**PATH.**	pathology
dis.	distribution	**pert.**	pertaining
E.	English	**PHARM.**	pharmacy
(e	indicates the word may also be terminated with "e"	**PHYS.**	physiology
		pl.	plural
e.g.	for example	**post.**	posterior
elect.	electricity	**pre.**	prefix
esp.	especially	**pro.**	protein
etiol.	etiology	**prog.**	prognosis
ex.	example	**PSY.**	psychiatry, psychoanalysis, psychology
ext.	exterior, external		
F.	Fahrenheit	**PT.**	physical therapy
Fr.	French	**q.v.**	which see
Fe	iron, ferrum	**rel.**	relating
fem.	female, feminine	**RS.**	related subjects
ff. ind.	fact-finding index	**S**	sulfur
funct.	function	**sing.**	singular
G.	Greek	**sp. gr.**	specific gravity
Ger.	German	**sup.**	superior
Gm.	gram or grams	**SYM.**	symptoms
gr.	grain or grains	**SYMB.**	symbol
gyn.	gynecology	**SYN.**	synonym
H	hydrogen	**USP**	United States Pharmacopoeia
I	iodine	**viz.**	namely
i.e.	that is	*****	denotes more information may be found under the word indicated
ind.	indication		

A

a. Abbr. for *accommodation, anode, anterior,* and *total acidity.*

A. Symb. for *argon.*

Å, or **A. u.** Abbr. for *Angström unit.*

A₂. Abbr. for *aortic second sound.*

A. A. Abbr. for *achievement age.*

āa, āā [Abbr. G. *ana,* a distributive preposition]. Prescription sign denoting the stated amount of each of the substances is to be taken.

a-, an- [G. *alpha,* **p**rivative]. Prefix meaning *without, away from, not,* as *atypical.*

Aaron's sign. Distress in region of heart or stomach upon pressure over McBurney's point* as in *appendicitis.*

ab- [L.]. Prefix meaning *from, away from, negative, absent.*

abacte'rial [G. *a-,* priv. + G. *baktērion,* rod]. Without bacteria.

abactio (ab-ak'shĭ-o) [L. *abactus,* driven away]. Induced abortion.*

abactus venter [" + L. *venter,* belly]. Nonspontaneous abortion.

Abadie's sign (ă-bă-dēz'). 1. In exophthalmic goiter, spasm of the *levator palpebrae superioris.* 2. In tabes dorsalis, insensibility to pressure over *tendo Achillis.*

abaissement (a-bās'mon) [Fr. a lowering]. 1. Depression. 2. Couching. 3. Falling.

abalienated (ab-āl'yen-ā-ted) [L. *abalienare,* to separate from]. Deranged.

abalienatio mentis (ab-al-yen-a'shĭ-o men'-tis). Insanity.

abalienation (ab-āl-yen-ā'shun) [L. *abalienāre,* to separate from]. Physical or mental decay; lunacy or derangement.

abalone (ăb'a-lō-ne) [Origin uncertain]. Large sea snail with flattened shell. Eaten on Pacific Coast. Average serving 100 grams. Pro. 21.7, Fat 0.1, Carbo. 3.7.

abanet (ab'an-et) [Heb. *abnēt,* long scarf]. Girdle or girdlelike bandage. SYN: *abnet.**

abarognosis (ă-bar-og-no'sis) [G. *a-,* priv. + *barys,* weight + *gnosis,* knowledge]. Without sense of weight.

abarthrosis (ab-ar-thro'sis) [L. *ab,* from, + G. *arthron,* joint]. A movable joint or point upon which bones move freely upon each other; diarthrosis.*

abartic'ular [" + *articulus,* joint]. At a distance from a joint.

abarticula'tion. Dislocation of a joint.

abasia (a-ba'zĭ-ă) [G. *a-,* priv. + *basis,* step]. Motor incoördination in walking; astasia. Inability to stand or walk due to loss of coördination; organic disease in such cases usually easily recognized; if not, hysteria is probable.

   a. astasia. Inability to stand or walk.

   a. atactia. Uncertain movements.

   a., choreic. That due to cramps in the limbs similar to movements of chorea.

   a., paralytic. That in which the legs give way from body weight.

   a., paroxysmal trepidant. That caused by trepidation, stiffening legs and making walking impossible.

   a., spastic. Paroxysmal trepidantia.

   a., statica. Uncertainty of movement.

   a., trembling, a. trepidans. That due to trembling of the legs.

abasic (ă-ba'sik). Pert. to abasia.

abate (a-bāt'- [L. *ab,* from + *battere,* to beat]. 1. To lessen or decrease. 2. To cease or cause to cease.

abate'ment. Decrease in severity of pain or symptoms.

abatic (ab-at'ik). Pert. to abasia. SYN: *abasic.**

abaxial (ab-ak'si-al), **abaxile** [L. *ab.,* from + *axis*]. 1. Without the axis of the body. 2. At the opp. end of the axis of a part.

Abbé's catgut ring (ab'bā's). A ring of catgut to reinforce the suture in intestinal anastomosis.

   A.'s condenser. Several nonachromatic lenses to increase illumination under lens of a microscope.

   A.'s operation. 1. For relief of the tic douloureux by resection of the 5th c. nerve. 2. Lateral anastomosis of the intestine.

Abbé-Zeiss apparatus. An instrument for estimating number of blood corpuscles.

Abb'ot's paste. A paste for killing a nerve of a tooth.

Abbott's method. Treatment of lateral curvature of the spine by a series of plaster jackets.

A. B. C. lin'iment. Liniment composed of aconite 40, belladonna 40, chloroform 20.

a.b.c. process. The use of alum, blood, and charcoal in purification of water or sewage or deodorization.

Abderhalden's reaction or **test** (ăb'der-hăl-denz). Creation of ferments in circulation as result of injection of foreign protein, fat, or carbohydrate. Used in testing for pregnancy, acute infections, malignancies, goiter, dementia precox.

abdomen (ab-do'men) [L. *abdomen,* The belly]. The area between the diaphragm and the pelvis.

Contains the stomach with lower part of esophagus, small and large intestines, liver, gallbladder, spleen, pancreas, and bladder. A serous membrane called the *peritoneum* lines this cavity.

   I. DIAG. 1. SKIN: *General discoloration*—jaundice. 2. *Dirty brown*—Addison's disease. 3. *White area*—albinism. 4. *Pale lemon-yellow*—pernicious anemia. 5. *White line (linea albicans)*—ascites, loss of fat, stretching from pregnancy.

   II. RASHES: 1. *Rose-c. spots*—typhoid. 2. *Scaly copper-c. spots*—secondary syphilis. 3. *Lesions with white "mother of pearl" scales*—psoriasis.*

   III. VEINS: *Enlarged, superficial veins*—obstruction of return circulation, abdominal tumors, cirrhosis or abscess of liver.

   IV. PERISTALSIS: *If visible*—colitis, partial internal obstruction. *Reversed p.* Intestinal and pyloric obstruction.

   V. SIZE: *General enlargement*—ascites, peritonitis, tumors, enlarged liver, spleen or both, and gaseous distention; pregnancy. *Boat-shaped* — meningitis, lead color, tumor of brain.

   VI. RETRACTION: Occurs in wasting diseases, inanition due to pyloric or esophageal stenosis, vomiting, purging, cholera, and yellow atrophy of liver.

VII. RIGIDITY: May be caused by appendicitis, inflammation of ovary, psoas abscess, hernia, cholelithiasis, abscess, cysts, sarcoma of adrenals, disease of spleen or kidney, gastric ulcer or carcinoma, peritonitis, intussusception,* etc., according to location affected.

VIII. TENDERNESS, OF THE ABDOMEN: May be due to inflammatory condition of peritoneum or a portion of it over an inflamed viscus. If general, may denote acute or chronic peritonitis, Asiatic cholera, early meningitis, or reflex from chest. Local tenderness depends upon location of tender area.

a., accordion. Nervous pseudotympany.

a., acute. Any acute abdominal condition demanding prompt operation.

a., boat-shaped. SEE: *a., scaphoid.*

a., carinate. SEE: *a., scaphoid.*

a., navicular. SEE: *a., scaphoid.*

a. obstipum. Congenital shortness of the rectus abdominus muscle.

a., pendulous. A relaxed condition of the abdominal wall.

a., scaphoid. Sunken as in emaciation and in meningitis. One whose ant. wall is hollowed.

abdomen, words pert. to: "abdom-" words, alvine, alvus, bythus, carreau, cecopexy, celiac axis, celiagra, "celio-" words, cholecystendisis, cholecystopexy, colica, facies abdominalis, meteorism, ptosis, splanchnic cavity, venter, ventriduct, "ventro-" words, viscera, visceral cavity, visceralgia.

abdominal (ab-dom'i-nal). Pert. to the abdomen, its function and disorders.

a. cavity. Cavity within the peritoneum.

a. gestation. Abdominal pregnancy. Extrauterine pregnancy in belly cavity.

a. reflexes. These consist of muscular contraction of either side of the abdomen, induced by friction on that part.

a. r. I. Pert. to hemiplegia. In such condition reflex is absent on side opposite lesion in transverse myelitis above sixth dorsal, in disseminated sclerosis, and occasionally in cord tumors.

a. r. II. Pert. to pregnancy. With advance toward term, reflex progressively fails in the nulliparous. In the multipara, reflex cannot be elicited after pregnancy.

a. r. III. Pert. to intestinal inflammation. In this condition, reflex is absent. SYN: *Rosenbach's sign # 1.*

a. regions. Nine regions into which the abdomen and its external surface are divided by four imaginary planes, *two horizontal,* one at the level of the ninth costal cartilage (or the lowest point of the costal arch); the other at the level of the highest point of the iliac crest; and *two vertical,* through the centers of the inguinal ligaments (or through the nipples, or through the centers of the clavicles), or curved and coinciding with the lateral borders of the two abdominal recti muscles.

The abdomen may be divided into four quadrants drawing a vertical and a horizontal line through the umbilicus. The contents of each quadrant are:

I. UPPER RIGHT Q: Right lobe of liver, gallbladder, part of transverse colon, part of pylorus, hepatic flexure, right kidney, and duodenum.

II. LOWER RIGHT Q: Cecum, ascending colon, small intestine, appendix, bladder if distended, r. ureter, r. spermatic cord in male, r. ovary and r. tube, and uterus, if enlarged, in female.

III. UPPER LEFT Q: Left lobe of liver, stomach, transverse colon, splenic flexure, pancreas, l. kidney, and spleen.

IV. LOWER LEFT Q: Small intestine, l. ureter, sigmoid flexure, descending colon, bladder if distended, l. spermatic cord in male, uterus, l. ovary, and l. tube in female.

a. rings. The apertures in the abdominal wall, *a.r., external*: An interval in aponeurosis of external oblique, just above and to outer side of crest of os pubis. a.r., triangular: About one inch from base to apex, and half an inch transversely; gives passage to spermatic cord in male, round ligament in female. *a.r., internal or deep*: Situated in the fascia transversalis, midway between the ant. superior spine of ilium and symphysis pubis, half inch above Poupart's ligament; oval form, larger in male. Transmits spermatic cord in male, round ligament in female.

abdominal examination: a. auscultation. Of service in diagnosis of aneurysm, fetal heart sounds and uteroplacental murmur in pregnancy.

a. inspection. Most satisfactorily performed with patient on back with thighs slightly flexed. In health, abdomen is of an oval form, marked by elevations and depressions corresponding to abdominal muscles, umbilicus, and in some degree by form of adjacent viscera. Is larger relatively, to size of chest, in children than in adults; more rotund, and broader inferiorly in females than in males.

Alterations in shape due to disease are *first,* enlargement, which may be general and symmetrical, as in ascites; or partial and irregular, from tumors, hypertrophy of organs, as the liver and spleen, or from tympanitic distention of portions of intestines by gas, as the colon in typhoid fever; *second,* retraction, as in extreme emaciation, and in several forms of cerebral disease, esp..

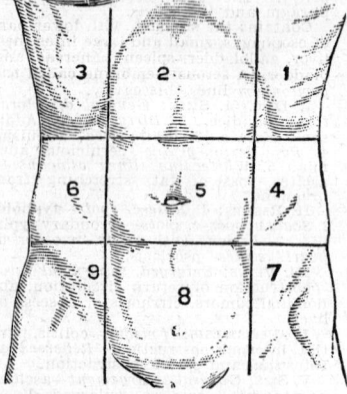

ANATOMIC DIVISION OF ABDOMEN
1. Left hypochondriac region. 2. Epigastric region. 3. Right hypochondriac region. 4. Left lateral abdominal region. 5. Umbilical region. 6. Right lateral abdominal region. 7. Left inguinal (iliac) region. 8. Hypogastric region. 9. Right inguinal (iliac) region. 4, 5, and 6 constitute the mesogastric region.

abdominal palpation   A-3   **aberrant**

noticeable in tuberculous meningitis of children.

The respiratory movements of abdominal walls bear a certain relation to movements of the thorax; are often increased when the latter are arrested and vice versa; thus abdominal movements are increased in pleurisy, pneumonia, pericarditis, etc., but decreased or wholly suspended when disease causes abdominal pain, or in peritonitis.

The superficial abdominal veins are also at times visibly enlarged, indicating an obstruction to the current of blood, either in the portal system as in cirrhosis, or in the inferior vena cava.

a. palpation. May be performed with tips of fingers, whole hand, or both hands; pressure may be slight or forcible, continuous or intermittent. To obtain greatest amount of information, patient should be placed in horizontal position with head slightly raised and thighs flexed. Sometimes necessary to place in standing position or leaning forward.

IND. FURNISHED BY PALPATION: Size and position of viscera; existence of tumors and swellings, whether superficial or deep, large or small, hard or soft, smooth or nodulated, movable or fixed, solid or liquid, and whether they change position with respiration. Also ascertain whether tenderness exists in any portion of the abdominal cavity, and if pain is increased or relieved by firm pressure. Aneurysms of abdominal aorta are usually felt in median line or to left of it, on right side or both sides, and are immovable.

Impulse, if one exists, is systolic and expansive, though when situated high up there also may be a slight diastolic movement. A thrill is rarely perceptible. Surface of tumor, when not ruptured, is rounded and smooth. Effusion of blood into surrounding tissues may produce lobulations.

a. percussion. Patient should be placed in same position as for palpation, and percussion should be for most part mediate. In exploring abdomen by means of percussion, finger should first be placed immediately below the xiphoid cartilage, pressed firmly down, and carried along the median line toward the pubes, striking it all the way, now forcibly, now gently. The *different tones* of stomach, colon, and small intestines will be distinctly heard. Percussion should then be made laterally, alternately to one side, then the other, till whole surface is percussed. *Abdominal aneurysm* gives dullness or flatness over it unless a distended intestine lies above it.

abdominal section. Abdominal incision for any operation on abdominal organs. SEE: *laparotomy.*

abdominoanterior (ab-dom'ĭ-no-an-te'rĭ-or). Position of fetus in utero with belly facing ant. abdominal wall of mother.

abdom"inocar'diac re'flex I. Increased heart consciousness when abdominal sympathetics are stimulated.

a. r. II. Sudden change from recumbent to standing position induces cardiac and vasomotor phenomena in visceroptosis; visceromotor and viscerosensory phenomena in ulcers (gastric, duodenal) and gallbladder disease.

abdominocentesis (ab-dom'ĭ-nō-sen-te'sĭs) [L.*abdomen*, belly, + G. *kentēsis*, puncture]. Abdominal puncture by tapping. SYN: *paracentesis abdominis.*

abdominocys'tic [" + G. *kystis*, bladder]. Pert. to abdomen and bladder.

abdominogen'ital [" + *genitalis*]. Pert. to abdomen and genital organs.

abdom"inohysterec'tomy [" + G. *ystera*, uterus, + *ektomē*, excision]. Removal of uterus through abdominal wall.

abdom"inohysterot'omy [" + " + *tome*, a cutting]. Incision into the uterus through an abdominal opening.

abdom"inoposte'rior. Position of fetus in utero with abdomen toward mother's back.

abdom"inos'copy [L. *abdomen, belly,* + G. *skopein,* to view]. Instrumental examination of abdomen or its viscera.

abdom"inoscro'tal [" + *scrotum*, bag]. Pert. to abdomen and scrotum.

a. muscle. Cremaster m.

abdominothoracic (ab - dom" ĭ - no - tho - ras'ĭk) [" + G. *thōrax*, breastplate]. Pert. to abdomen and thorax.

a. arch. The costal arch, dividing the thorax from the abdomen. [domen.

abdom"inous. Having a prominent ab-

abdom"inouterot'omy [L. *abdomen*, belly, + *uterus*, womb, + G. *tomē*, incision]. Cesarean section. SYN: *abdominohysterotomy.*

abdom"inovag'inal [" + *vagina*, sheath]. Pert. to abdomen and vagina.

abdom"inoves'ical [" + *vesica*, bladder]. Pertaining to the abdomen and the urinary bladder.

a. pouch. Peritoneal fold which includes urachal folds.

abduce (ab-dūs') [L. *abducere*, to draw away]. To draw away.

abducens (ab-dū'senz) [L. drawing away from]. 1. The 6th cranial nerve. 2. The external rectus muscle of the eye, which moves the eyeball outward. 3. Pert. to certain muscles or their nerves drawing from the median line of the body.

a. labiorum. a. oris, *q.v.*

a. nerve. Sixth cranial nerve.* Motor nerve supplying lateral rectus muscle of eye. ORIG: *Fasciculus teres.* SEE: *Cranial nerves, Tables in Appendix.*

a. oculi. BNA. *Musculus rectus lateralis.* Muscle of eye.

a. oris. Muscle of mouth. BNA. *Musculus caninus.*

abdu'cent. Abducting, leading away from.

abduct' [L. *abductus*, past p. *abducere*, to lead away]. To draw away from axis of body or one of its parts.

abduc'tion. Movement away from midline of body, or middle portion of a part as of the arm or thumb.

abduc'tor. A muscle which draws certain parts away from a common center.

Abel's bacillus. One found in nasal secretion in ozena; *Klebsiella ozaenae.*

abenteric (ab-en-ter'ĭk) [L. *ab*, from + G. *enteron*, intestine]. Located in a part outside the intestines, as *a. typhoid.*

abepithymia (ab-ep-ĭ-thī'mĭ-ă) [" + G. *epithymia*, desire]. 1. Perverted desire or longing. 2. Solar plexus paralysis.

Abernethy's fascia (ăb'er-nē-thēz). Superperitoneal areolar tissue separating *ext. iliac art.* from iliac fascia over the psoas.

A.'s sarcoma. A circumscribed fatty tumor occurring principally on the trunk.

aber'rant [L. *ab*, from, + *errare*, to wander]. Wandering from the normal or usual course.

a. pyramidal tract. Several groups of fibers from motor cortex to the cranial nerve nuclei, running apart from the rest of the pyramidal system.

aberratio (ab-er-a'shĭ-o). Aberration.
   a. humorum. Abnormal flow of blood to another tract, as in vicarious menstruation (*a. mensium*).

aberra'tion. 1. Deviation from a normal course. 2. Mental unsoundness, but not insanity. 3. Imperfect refraction.
   a., chromatic. Unequal refraction of different wave lengths of the spectrum producing a blurred image.
   a., diopteric. Spherical a.
   a., distantial. Blurring of a distant object.
   a., mental. Mental unsoundness that may or may not amount to insanity.
   a., spherical. Imperfect focus produced by a convex lens.

aberrom'eter [L. *ab-*, from + *errare*, to wander + G. *metron*, measure]. An instrument for measuring optical error.

abevacuation (ab-ē-vak-u-a'shŭn) [" + *evacuare*, to empty]. Abnormal evacuation either in excess or in deficiency.

abeyance (a-bā'ăns) [Old French]. A temporary suspension of activity, sensation, or pain.

abiochemistry (ab-i-o-kem'is-trĭ) [G. *a-*, priv. + *bios*, life, + *chēmeia*, chemistry]. Inorganic chemistry.

abiogenesis (ab-i-o-jen'e-sis) [" + " + *genesis*, production]. Spontaneous generation.

abiogenet'ic, abio'genous. Pert. to spontaneous generation.

abiological (ab-ī-o-loj'ĭ-kal). Not related to biology or the science of life.

abiology (a-bi-ol'o-jī) [G. *a-*, priv. + *bios*, life, + *logos*, study of]. The study of inanimate things.

abionergy (ab-ī-on'ur-jī) [" + " + *energeia*, action, energy]. Premature degeneration. SYN: *abiotrophy*.

abiosis (ab-i-ō'sis) [G. *a-*, priv. + *bios*, life]. Absence of life.

abiot'ic. Incompatible with life; not viable.

abiotro'phia. Abiotrophy.

abiotrophy (ab-i-ot'ro-fī) [G. *a-*, priv. + *bios*, life + *trophē*, nourishment]. Premature loss of vitality or degeneration of tissues and cells.

abirritant (ab-ir'ĭt-ant) [L. *ab-*, from + *irritare*, to irritate]. Relieving irritation; soothing.

abirrita'tion. 1. Asthenia, or atony. 2. Lowered tissue irritability.

abiuret (a-bi'ū-ret) [G. *a-*, priv. + L. *bis*, double, + urea]. Nonbiuret. Not giving the biuret reaction.

ablactation (ab-lak-ta'shun) [L. *ab*, from + *lac*, milk]. Free of, or cessation of milk secretion; weaning.

ablastem'ic [G. *a-*, priv. + *blastos*, germ, seed]. Not germinal.

ablate' [L. *ablatus*, taken away]. To remove, esp. by excision.

ablatio (ab-la'shĭ-o) [L. *ablatio*, carrying away]. Ablation, removal, detachment.
   a. placentae. Premature detachment of a normally situated placenta.
   ETIOL: Toxemias, anemia, chronic nephritis, syphilis, trauma.
   PATH: Extravasation of blood between placenta and uterine wall, occasionally between muscle fibers of the uterus. The peritoneal coat of uterus may exhibit small linear fissures which allow for free blood to enter the peritoneal cavity. Liver frequently shows marked fatty changes.
   SYM: (a) Hemorrhage, concealed or evident, or a combination of the two. (b) Pain, constant at point of separation of placenta due to blood extruding between muscle fibers. (c) Uterine contraction, constant; occasionally tetanic in nature. (d) Evidences of fetal asphyxia and death, increased fetal movements, and changes in heart-tone rate until final cessation of both. (e) Albuminuria a frequent accompaniment.
   TREATMENT: (a) *Mild cases:* Rest in bed; if near term, induction of labor. (b) *Severe cases:* Shock must first be combated and uterus emptied as rapidly as possible, avoiding accouchement force.* With the child still alive, if the mother's condition allows, a Cesarean section may be indicated. If extensive blood extravasation between muscle fibers we have an apopletic uterus and Porro-Cesarean section is necessary.
   SEE: *placenta.*
   a. retinae. Detachment of retina.

ablation (ab-la'shun) [L. *ab*, from, + *latus*, carried]. Removal of a part, as by cutting. SEE: *ablatio.*

-able; -ible; -ble [L.]. Suffixes: Capable of being; power to be, as *audible.*

ablepsia (ă-blep'sĭ-ă) [G. *a-*, priv. + *blepein*, to see]. 1. Blindness. 2. Dulled perception.

ab'luent [L. *ab*, from, + *luere*, to wash]. An agent possessing cleansing qualities, as a detergent.

ablu'tion. A cleansing or washing. PT: Pouring water out of bucket over body or part. Mechanical effect mild; action depends mainly on temperature.

abmor'tal [L. *ab*, from, + *mors*, death]. Passing from dead or dying to living fiber, as an electric current.

abner'val [" + *nervus*, nerve]. Passing from a nerve to a muscular fiber.

ab'net [Heb. *abnêt*, a long scarf]. A girdle or girdlelike bandage.

abneural (ab-nu'ral) [L. *ab*, from, + G. *neuron*, nerve]. Ventral. Remote from neural or dorsal aspect.

abnor'mal (G. *anomalos*). Not normal. SEE: *chondralloplasia, chondrodysplasia.*

ab'normal'ity. That which is not normal.

abnormity (ab-norm'ĭ-tī). 1. Deformity; abnormality. 2. A monstrosity.

aboiment (ă-bwa-mon') [Fr.]. The making of barking sounds.

aboli'tion [L. *abolescere*, to perish]. Doing away with anything.

aborad (ab-o'rad) [L. *ab*, from, + *oris*, mouth]. Away from the mouth.

abo'ral. Opposite to, or away from, the mouth.

abort' [L. *aboriri*, to perish]. 1. To cause expulsion of an embryo or of the fetus before time of viability. 2. To arrest progress of disease. 3. To arrest growth or development.

aborticide (a-bor'ti-sīd) [" + *caedere*, to kill]. A term etymologically incorrect for an agent causing death of fetus and expulsion from uterus.

abortient (ab-or'shent). 1. Producing abortion. 2. Abortifacient.

abortifacient (a-bor-tĭ-fā'shent) [L. *abortus*, abortion, + *facere*, to make]. A drug which causes an abortion.

abortion (ab-or'shun). 1. The arrest of any physical action or disease. 2. The termination of pregnancy before the term of viability, *i.e.,* before the 28th week, the fetus measuring 35 cm. or less, and weighing less than 3¼ lb. (1500 Gm.). The term *miscarriage* is sometimes applied when occurring after 4th mo. and before 7th mo.; *premature delivery* after 7th mo. and before full term.
   ETIOL: Most common causes in the early months are: (a) diseases of endo-

abortion, accidental   A-5   **abscess, anorectal**

metrium; (b) nephritis; (c) malpositions of uterus; (d) syphilis; (e) defective development of embryo; (f) endocrine disorders esp. of ovaries; (g) toxemias of pregnancy.
SYM: Abdominal cramps and bleeding from vagina.
NP: Send for doctor. Keep patient quiet. Care as for uterine hemorrhage. Save discharges for doctor's inspection. Watch for shock and symptoms of sepsis.
The Catholic Church claims all induced abortions are criminal.

a., accidental. That which occurs spontaneously and accidentally without criminal intent.

a., artificial. When induced or performed purposely, as by a surgeon.

a., criminal. When produced for other than medical purposes.

a., embryonic. Before 4th month.

a., fetal. After 4th month.

a., habitual. When in course of repeated pregnancies with no apparent cause.

a., incomplete. When some of products of conception are retained with continuation of symptoms.

a., induced. When brought on intentionally, criminally or therapeutically.

a., inevitable. That which cannot be stopped or when occurring after the embryo is dead.

a., infected. When accompanied by infection of retained material with resultant febrile reaction. [mother's life.

a., justifiable. When done to save the

a., missed. That in which the fetus died with products of conception retained in uterus.

a., ovular. That which occurs within first three weeks after conception.

a., partial. In multiple pregnancy, aborting of only 1 fetus, or less than the entire number.

a., spontaneous. Occurring naturally without interference.

a., therapeutic. One done when life of mother is endangered by continuation of the pregnancy.

a., threatened. When only earliest signs of abortion are present.

a., tubal. An ectopic (abnormally placed) pregnancy in which the fetus has been expelled through rupture of a uterine tube.

abortionist (a-bor'shun-ist). One who performs a criminal abortion.

abortive (a-bor'tiv). 1. Preventing the completion of. 2. Abortifacient; that which prevents a natural or regular course. 3. Rudimentary.

abortus (a-bor'tus). An abortion.

aboulia (ă-boo'lĭ-ă) [G. *a-*, priv. + *boulē*, will]. Inability to exercise will power. SYN: *abulia, q.v.*

aboulomania (ă-boo'lo-ma'nĭ-ă) [" + " + *mania*, frenzy]. Mental disorder with loss of will power. SYN: *abulomania.*

abrade' [L. *ab*, from + *radere*, to scrape]. 1. To chafe. 2. To roughen or remove by friction.

Abrams' heart reflex. Reduction of area of cardiac dullness resulting from manual friction of precordial and epigastric areas.

A. lung reflex. Following irritation of the skin over the thorax or upper abdominal region, there is an increase in pulmonary area.

abra'sio cor'neae [L. abrasion of cornea]. Removal of corneal excrescences by scraping.

abrasion (ab-ra'shun) [L. *ab*, from, + *radere*, to scrape]. An injury resulting from scraping away of a portion of skin or of a mucous membrane. A brush burn.
Foreign bodies (*q.v.*) may be present.
SYM: Painful, red, denuded surface.
F. A. TREATMENT: Remove any foreign body. Apply mild antiseptic and dressing; may be tannic acid, 5%, gentian violet, 5%, or any bland ointment.
SEE: *avulsion, bruise.*

abra'sive. 1. Producing abrasion. 2. That which abrades.

abreaction (ab-re-ak'shun) [L. *ab*, from, + *rē*, again, + *actus*, acting]. PSY: Reevaluation of an emotion-laden experience during its free discussion with an understanding psychotherapist. Freud calls the process *catharsis.**

abrosia (ab-rō'zĭ-ă) [L. *ab*, from, + *erodere*, to gnaw away]. 1. Fasting; the need for food. 2. A wasting away.

abruptio (ab-rup'shĭ-o) [L. *ab*, from, + *ruptere*, a break]. A tearing away from.

a. placentae. Premature detachment of normally situated placenta. SEE: *ablatio placentae.*

abscess (ab'ses) [L. *abscessus*, a going away]. A localized collection of pus in a cavity; the pus formed by disintegration of tissue. There is an increase of neutrophils in abscesses and active infection.

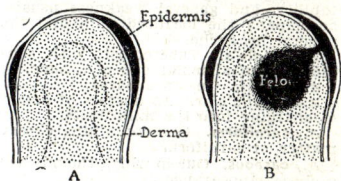

SUBEPITHELIAL ABSCESS
A, Abscesses located at tip of finger lie between dense epidermis and derma; B, Subepithelial abscess developed from felon which perforated derma and spread out beneath epiderma, which is lifted up in a manner analogous to a blister.

a., acute, or warm. One with local symptoms of inflammation, with fluctuation, and pointing; also pressure and constitutional symptoms. Inflammation becomes intensified with increased heat, redness, swelling, and edema. Pain becomes throbbing and greater, with impaired loss of function of the part. An elevation appears, with fluctuation and softening as it reaches the surface, becoming necrotic and yellow, giving way with evacuation of pus. *Pressure symptoms,* according to size and depth. In floor of mouth or neck, swelling may cause dyspnea and dysphagia. *Constitutional symptoms* vary, from slight temperature (fever may be absent in a well walled-off abscess) to high temperature, with rigors and sweats if associated with pyemia and septicemia. Any or all general symptoms may be absent in deep-seated abscesses except loss of weight and strength. If there is active tissue resistance and free absorption of toxin, leukocytosis will occur.

TERMINATION: This may be by pointing, evacuation, and discharge of pus, which may become inspissated, encapsulated, and at times absorbed.

a., alveolar. One of the gum or alveolus.

a., amebic. One containing amebae.

a., anorectal. One in the tissue near the rectum.

a., apical. One at the apex of lung or at extremity of root of a tooth.

a., appendiceal, appendicular. Pus formation about vermiform appendix.

a., arthrifluent. A wandering abscess having origin in a diseased joint.

a., atheromatous. Atheromatous softening in wall of an artery.

a., axillary. One or multiple abscesses in axilla.

a., bartholinian. One affecting Bartholin's gland.

a., Bezold's. A deep abscess in the neck.

a., bicameral. One with two pockets.

a., bilharziasis. One in an intestinal wall caused by *Schistosoma mansoni*.

a., biliary. One of the biliary tract or gallbladder.

a., blind. A dental granuloma.

a., bone. Suppurative periostitis.

a., brain. Seldom primary. May result from suppurative disease of middle ear, mastoid cells, and accessory sinuses. Secondary to lung suppuration, such as lung abscess or bronchiectasis, and following general septicemia. It may be acute, subacute, or chronic. The headache is constant and severe, usually localized over the affected area. Fever, vomiting, vertigo, mental dullness, irritability, and general weakness usually accompany the localized pain and the general headache.

a., Brodie's. Tuberculosis with suppuration of articular end of a bone.

a., bursal. One in a bursa.

a., canalic'ular. An abscess of breast discharging into the milk ducts.

a., carniform. One containing cheesy matter, or carniform.

a., caseous. One in which the pus has a cheesy appearance.

a., cerebral. A brain abscess.

a., cheesy. Caseous abscess.

a., cholangitic. One of the bile duct.

a., chronic, or cold. One with pus but without signs of inflammation; usually of slow development. Formed by liquefaction of tuberculous tissue. May occur anywhere on the body but more frequently in connection with the spine, hips, genitourinary tract, and lymphatic glands. Symptoms may be very mild, pain when present being due to pressure upon surrounding parts. Tenderness often absent. Chronic septic intoxication with hectic fever occurs when there is mixed infection. Amyloid disease usually appears eventually.

a., circumscribed. An abscess limited by exudation of lymph.

a., circumtonsillar. Quinsy.

a., cold. Same as *chronic a.*

a., collar-button. One perforating the palmar fascia into the subcutaneous tissue at the web with superficial accumulations of pus in the palm, connected by a narrow channel with a larger collection of pus in deeper tissues.

a., congestive. One that shows pus at a point distant from where formed.

a., consecutive. A critical abscess.

a., constitutional. One resulting from a general disease.

a., deep. One arising from below the deep fascia.

a., Delpech's. One without fever which develops rapidly, causing great prostration.

a., dental. One about a tooth.

a., dentoalveolar. One at the root of a tooth.

a., diathetic. One caused by a diathesis.

a., diffuse. A collection of pus not circumscribed by a well-defined capsule.

a., Douglas'. One in Douglas' pouch.

a., dry. One that disappears without pointing or breaking.

a., Dubois'. One of the thymus formed in congenital syphilis.

a., embolic. One due to a septic embolus.

a., emphysematous. Same as *tympanitic.*

a., encysted. One with pus circumscribed in a serous cavity.

a., endamebic. Entamebic. Amebic.

a., epiploic. One in the omentum.

a., extradural. One on the dura mater.

a., fecal. A stercoralaceous abscess.

a., filarial. One caused by filaria.

a., fixation. One produced artificially by subcutaneous injection of an irritant.

a., Fochier's. Same as *fixation a.*

a., follicular. One forming in a follicle.

a., frontal. One in the frontal lobe of the brain.

a., fungal. Abscess caused by a fungus.

a., gangrenous. One attended with gangrene of surrounding parts.

a., gas. An abscess containing gas due to *B. aerogenes* or other gas-forming microörganism.

a., gastric. Phlegmonous gastritis.

a., gingival. A parietal one in cemental gingival tissue.

a., glandular. One around a lymph node.

a., gravitation. An abscess in which the pus migrates, sinking to lower depths.

a's., heart. In interstitial myocarditis, multiple small abscesses.

a., helminthic. One caused by a worm.

a., hematic. One due to an extravasated blood clot.

a., hemorrhagic. One containing blood.

a., hepatic. Abscess of the liver.

a., hot. An acute abscess with local inflammation.

a., hypostatic. A wandering abscess.

a., idiopathic. One due to local causes.

a., iliac. One in the iliac region.

a., intramammary. An abscess of the mammary gland.

a., intramastoid. A mastoid process abscess of the temporal bone.

a., ischiorectal. One in the ischiorectal fossa.

a., lacrimal. Suppuration of a lacrimal gland.

a., lacunar. One in the urethral lacunae.

a., lateral, a., lateral alveolar. A periodontal abscess.

a., lumbar. One in the lumbar region.

a., lung. A. occurring in the lung. NP: This may cover a prolonged course. Constitutional treatment is indicated. High caloric diet to build up body tissues and to help overcome infection. Glucose may have to be given intravenously to supply an adequate caloric intake. Bowel hygiene and frequent baths for elimination of toxins. Mouth care essential because of frequent expectoration of pus which has a foul taste and odor. If postural drainage is ordered, the patient's chest should be as nearly straight as possible. The treatment is given for 1 to 2 minutes, but the time is gradually increased to from 15 to 30 minutes twice a day. The patient is encouraged to cough and expectorate. The sputum should be measured, and the amount and character should be recorded. The treatment should not be given just before or after a meal, as it will nauseate the patient.

a., lymphatic. A cold abscess of a lymphatic gland.

a., mammary. One in the female breast.

a., marginal. One near the orifice of the anus.

a., mastoid. Suppuration of the mastoid portion of the temporal bone.

a., mediastinal. Suppuration in the mediastinum.

a., metastatic. A secondary one at a distance from focus of infection.

a., migrating. SEE: *wandering abscess*.

a., miliary. A small embolic abscess. One discharging numerous small collections of pus.

a., milk. A mammary abscess during lactation.

a's., Monro's. Intraepidermal accumulations of cellular debris in the epidermis.

a., mother. A primary abscess giving rise to other abscesses.

a., multiple. A group of abscesses accompanying pyemia.

a., mural. One in tissues of the abdominal wall following celiotomy.

a., nocardial. One caused by *Nocardia*.

a., orbital. Suppuration in the orbit.

a., ossifluent. One dependent on degeneration of bone tissue.

a., Paget's. One recurring about the site of a former abscess.

a., palatal. One in an upper lateral incisor, erupting toward the palate.

a., palmar. A purulent effusion into the tissues of the palm of the hand.

a., parafrenal. One of Tyson's gland.

a., parametric, a., parametritic. One between the folds of the structures adjacent to the uterus.

a., paranephric, a., paranephritic. One in the tissues around the kidney.

a., parapancreatic. One in the pancreatic tissues.

a., parietal. A periodontal abscess arising in the periodontal tissue other than the pulpal foramen.

a., parotid. One of the parotid gland.

a., pelvic. Abscess of the pelvic peritoneum, especially Douglas's pouch.

a., pelvirectal. A deep rectal abscess.

a., periapical. One at the root apex of a tooth. A parietal abscess in the pericemental tissue which is not an extension of a periclasial pocket.

a., peribronchitic. A. in inflamed tissue around the bronchi. SYN: *Faubel's granule*.

a., pericemental. An alveolar abscess not involving apex of a tooth.

a., pericoronal. One around the crown of an unerupted molar tooth.

a., peridental. Periodontal abscess.

a., perinephric. One in tissue about the kidney.

a., periodontal. An alveolar abscess.

a., peripleuritic. One beneath the parietal pleura.

a., periproctic. One in the areolar tissue about the rectum.

a., peritoneal. An encysted mass of exudate in peritonitis.

a., peritonsillar. Quinsy.

a., periurethral. One formed around the urethra. One associated with an inflammation in connective tissues.

a., phlegmonous. An acute abscess.

a., pneumococcic. One due to infection with pneumococci.

a., postcecal. One sometimes occurring in appendicitis.

a., posttyphoid. A chronic abscess following typhoid fever.

a., Pott's. One developing in Pott's disease of the hip.

a., prelacrimal. One of the lacrimal bone.

a., premammary. A small cutaneous abscess on the mammary gland.

a., primary. One originating at point of infection.

a., protozoal. One caused by a protozoan.

a., psoas. One with pus descending in sheath of psoas muscle due to vertebral disease.

a., pulmonary. One of the lungs. Nontuberculous suppuration of lung tissue with one or more localized areas of necrosis resulting in pulmonary cavitation.

a., pulp. 1. A cavity discharging pus formed in the pulp of a tooth. 2. One of the tissues of the pulp of a finger.

a., pyemic. A metastatic one, usually multiple, due to pyogenic organisms.

a., rectal. One in the rectum.

a., residual. One occurring in old inflammatory products.

a., retromammary. One below the mammary gland and within the tissues of the chest wall.

a., retroperitoneal. Same as *subperitoneal a*.

a., retropharyngeal. One of the lymph nodes in the walls of the pharynx. It sometimes simulates diphtheritic pharyngitis. Respiratory obstruction is caused by accumulation of pus behind the posterior pharyngeal wall.

a., root. Dental granuloma. Granulations at root of a tooth.

a., sacrococcygeal. One over the sacrum and coccyx.

a., satellite. A secondary one arising from a primary one situated near it.

a., scrofulous. One due to tuberculous degeneration of bone or lymph nodes.

a., secondary. Embolic abscess.

a., septal. One at the proximal surface of a tooth root.

a., septicemic. One resulting from septicemia.

a's., shirt-stud. Two abscesses communicating by a sinus.

a., spermatic. One of the seminiferous tubules.

a., spinal. One due to necrosis of a vertebra.

a., spirillary. One containing *Spirilla*.

a., splenic. One of the spleen.

a., stercoralaceous. One containing pus and fecal matter.

a., stitch. One formed about a stitch or suture.

a., streptococcal. An abscess caused by streptococci.

a., strumous. A cold abscess of tuberculous causation.

a., subaponeurotic. One beneath an aponeurosis or fascia.

a., subdiaphragmatic. One beneath the diaphragm

a., subepithelial. Infection under the epidermis of the hand with accumulation of pus.

a., submammary. One beneath the mammary gland.

a., subpectoral. One beneath the pectoral muscles.

a., subperitoneal. One between the parietal peritoneum and the abdominal wall.

a., subphrenic. One beneath the diaphragm.

abscess, subscapular   A-8   **absorption**

a., subscapular. One between the serratus anterior and the posterior thoracic wall.

a., subungual. One beneath the distal portion of a finger nail. May follow injuries with pins, needles, or splinters.

a., sudoriparous. One of a sweat gland.

a., superficial. One occurring above the deep fascia.

a., suprahepatic. One in the suspensory ligament between the liver and the diaphragm.

a., sympathetic. One arising some distance from the exciting cause.

a., syphilitic. One occurring in the bones during syphilis.

a., thecal. One in sheath of a tendon.

a., thymus. Dubois' a.

a., tonsillar. Acute suppurative tonsillitis, or quinsy.

a., tooth. Dental abscess.

a., traumatic. One provoked by injury.

a., tropical. An abscess of the liver due to *Endamoeba histolytica*.

a., tympanitic. An abscess that contains air or gas.

a., tympanocervical. One arising in the tympanum and extending to the neck.

a., tympanomastoid. A combined abscess of the tympanum and mastoid.

a., urethral. One of the urethra.

a., urinary. One caused by extravasation of urine.

a., urinous. One which contains pus with urine.

a., verminous. One which contains insect larvae or other animal parasites.

a., von Bezold's. One resulting from mastoiditis by perforation with extension into the digastric fossa, and to tissues of the lateral aspect of the neck. One that burrows in the tissues.

a., wandering. One at a distance from focus of disease with pus along fascial sheaths of muscles.

a., warm. An acute abscess.

a., worm. One caused by or containing worms.

abscession (ab-sesh'un). 1. Metastasis. 2. A critical discharge. 3. An abscess.*

abscission (ab-sĭ'shun) [L. *abscindere*, to cut off]. The removal of a part by excision.

absentia epilep'tica (ab-sen'shĭ-ă). The loss of consciousness in the mild form of epilepsy.

ab'solute al'cohol. A. with no more than 1% of water.

    a. temperature. Temperature reckoned from the absolute zero.

    a. zero. 273.7° below zero Cent. The lowest possible temperature.

absorb' [L. *absorbere*, to suck in]. To suck up as through pores. SEE: *absorbent*.

absorbefacient (ab-sor-be-fā'shent) [" + *facere*, to make]. Causing or that which causes absorption.

absorb'ent. 1. A substance that causes absorption of diseased tissue. 2. Taking up by suction.   [moisture.

    a. cotton. Cotton prepared to absorb

    a. glands. Lymph glands.

absorptiometer (ab-sorp-shĭ-om'e-ter) [L. *absorptio*, absorption + G. *metron*, measure]. An instrument for measuring thickness of liquid drawn by capillary attraction, between glass plates.

absorption (ab-sorp'shun) [L. *absorptio*, from *absorbere*, to suck in]. 1. The taking up of liquids by solids, or of gases by solids or liquids. 2. The taking up of light or of its rays by black or colored rays. 3. The taking up by the body of radiant heat, causing a rise in body temperature. 4. PHYS: The passage of a substance through some surface of the body into body fluids and tissues, as the passage of ether through the respiratory epithelium of lungs into the blood during anesthesia, or passage of oil of wintergreen through the skin, the result of several processes:

Diffusion: Spreading of dissolved substances throughout a solution and through porous or permeable membranes. If a partition has visible openings, passage of liquid occurs and direction of flow is determined by mechanical pressure (such as that due to

Summary of Food Absorption (Final Products of Digestion)

Final Products of Digestion	Absorbable Food Compound	Place of Absorption	Route in Circulation	Food Products Carried by the Blood
Carbohydrates	Monosaccharides	Epithelium of villi of small intestine into capillaries	Blood of portal vein to the liver	Glucose (part of the glucose absorbed and that formed from the fructose and galactose is changed by the liver into glycogen. Other tissues may form glycogen)
Fats	Glycerol and Fatty Acids	Epithelium of villi of small intestine into lacteals	Lacteals to lymphatics, to left thoracic duct, to bloodstream at left subclavian vein	Emulsified fat, the absorbed glycerol, and fatty acids having been reunited in the cells of the mucosa
Proteins	Amino acids	Epithelium of villi of small intestine into capillaries	Blood of the portal vein to the liver	Amino acids
Water		Stomach, small intestine principally in large intestine	Through portal vein and lymphatic vessels	
Mineral Salts		Stomach, small and large intestine	Through portal vein and lymphatic vessels	

gravity), but in physiological absorption the movement of solvent is commonly through membranes having no demonstrable pores and frequently opposite to direction of mechanical pressure.
Filtration: Passage of a fluid through a semipermeable membrane as a result of a difference in hydrostatic pressures.
Osmosis: Passage of a solvent through a membrane separating solutions of unequal concentrations.
RS: *absorbefacient, absorptive, chondrolysis, imbibition, impermeable, osmosis, resorption.*

a., colon. Water (important in the conservation of body fluids) and products of bacterial action are normally absorbed esp. in the ascending colon. Some nutrients and drugs are absorbed by the lower bowel. Cellulose is not digested but passes from the body as residue.
Colonic absorption is facilitated by the following kinds of movement: 1. The ascending colon shows reverse peristalses, which tend to keep the contents packed in the cecum. The food mass remains in the ascending colon for about 24 hours. The alkaline fluid aids bacterial growth, the bacteria setting up the normal process of digestion in the colon. Undigested protein undergoes putrefactive fermentation. 2. The sacculations exhibit "haustral churning." 3. The transverse colon, being suspended like a festoon between the hepatic and splenic flexures, due to the contractions of its longitudinal muscles, shows "pendulum movements" from side to side. 4. Large boli, starting from the transverse colon, can, by mass peristalsis, be moved rapidly down the descending colon and through the sigmoid into the rectum. The activity of the descending colon is such that it is empty most of the time. End products are disposed of in the feces, the elimination of which is aided by gas formed from fermentation. The *Bacillus acidophilus* seems necessary to intestinal processes. The colon excretes calcium, magnesium, and iron salts. 5. From the rectum, masses not promptly evacuated may, by reverse peristalsis, be returned to the transverse colon. SEE: *evacuation.*

a. lines. Dark lines of solar spectrum. SYN: *Fraunhofer's lines.**

a., mouth. Some substances, but no food nutrients, can be absorbed from the mouth; some drugs, esp. alkaloids, can pass through the oral mucosa.

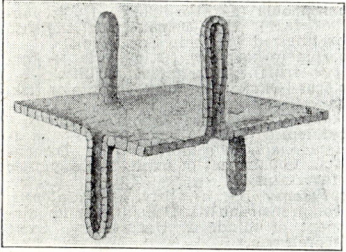

ABSORPTION—INTESTINAL SURFACE
Showing villi and crypts, which greatly increase the number of cells that have access to an epithelial surface.

a., pathological. A. of contents of an excretion or an abnormal product into blood stream.

a. of proteins. In the form of amino acids, produced by digestive hydrolysis, proteins enter the portal vein from the intestinal walls, and through the liver into the general circulation from whence they are absorbed by the tissues. Each tissue synthesizes its own form of protein from the amino acids received from the blood.

a. of radiation. Grotthuss' law states only rays which are absorbed are physiologically active.

a., small intestine. The most important absorption of products of digestion occurs in the small intestines, esp. the ileum. Products of digestion absorbed from the gastrointestinal tract pass into either blood or lymph. The mesenteric veins unite to form the portal vein and carry such blood to the liver; the mesenteric lymphatics are called *lacteals* because during absorption of a fatty meal the lymph which they contain looks milky and is called *chyle.* The lacteals empty into the *cisterna chyli* and are joined by lymphatics from other parts of the body; the mixed lymph is finally emptied into large veins near the heart and is thus mixed with, and becomes part of, the blood.

a. spectrum. A spectrum showing a. lines.

a., stomach. Water, alcohol, and some salts can be absorbed through the gastric mucosa and a small amount of glucose in food.
Substances can also be absorbed from other surfaces of the body such as the skin, the lining of the nose and lungs, the peritoneum and other serous membranes, and the mucosae of the vagina, urinary bladder, and urethra.

absorp′tion co″effi′cient. PT: The ratio of the linear rate of change of intensity of roentgen rays in a given homogeneous material to the intensity at a given point within the same mass.

absorp′tive. Absorbent.

abstergent (ab-stur′jent) [L. *abstergere,* to wipe off]. 1. A cleansing agent. 2. Having cleansing properties. 3. A purgative.

abstersion (ab-ster′shun). Cleansing.

abster′sive. Abstergent. Cleansing.

abstinence (ab′stĭ-nens) [L. *abstinere,* to abstain]. Going without voluntarily.

a. symptoms. Partial collapse resulting from withdrawal of alcohol, stimulants, and some opiates.

ab′stract [L. *abstrahere,* to draw away]. 1. A preparation containing the soluble principles of a drug evaporated and mixed with sugar of milk. 2. *v.* **abstract′.** To remove from. 3. To condense or abbreviate.

abstraction (ab-strak′shun). Bloodletting.
CUPPING: *Dry C.* Employing an exhausted receiver over integument whereby congestion of included skin is effected and sometimes serum effused. *Instruments:* Cupping glasses and suction pump, or small tumblers or wine glasses may be used. *Wet C.* Having congested skin by dry cup, make parallel incisions with lancet or apply spring scarificator. Set to such a depth as to cut only through true skin. Spring the lancets. Set, reapply at right angles, spring again and apply cup. When enough blood has been drawn, wash parts with mild antiseptic solution and cover with dry aseptic or antiseptic compresses.

LEECHING: The American leech is capable of withdrawing one dram of blood; European or Swedish, one ounce. Keep in water one hour before applying. A few drops of blood or little milk smeared on part will induce them to take hold. Eyelids and scrotum should never be leeched and only circumjacent tissues of inflamed areas. If slow in dropping off sprinkle the leech with salt.

PUNCTURE: Passing of a needle, or a narrow scalpel into the cavity filled with pus or into the spinal canal.

SCARIFICATION: Numerous small parallel incisions made in long axis of limb or part.

VENESECTION or PHLEBOTOMY: Opening vein in arm; most advantageous.

abter'minal [L. *ab*, from, + *terminus*, end]. Away from an end toward the center, noting course of.

abulia (a-boo'lĭ-ă) [G. *a-*, priv. + *boule*, will]. Absence of or inability to exercise "will power"; hesitation; indecision. Seen in dementia precox.

abulic (ab-u'lik). Pert. to abulia.

abulomania (a-boo'lo-ma'nĭ-ă) [G. *a-*, priv.+ *boule*, will, + *mania*, frenzy]. A mental disorder accompanied by impaired (or loss of) will power. These are obsolete terms.

abut'ment [Fr. *abouter*, to place end to end]. The tooth to which a bridge is anchored.

A. C. Abbr. for anodal closure.

a. c. Abbr. for L. *ante cibos*, before meals.

a. c. interval. One bet. beginning of auricular and carotid wave; intersystolic period.

acacia (ak-ka'shĭ-a) (Gum Arabic) USP. A dried, gummy exudation from the tree *Acacia senegal*.

USES: Demulcent, and for suspending insoluble substances in water, and for formation of pills and troches.

acalcerosis (ă-kal-ser-o'sis) (G. *a-*, priv. + L. *calx, calcis*, limestone, + *-osis*, condition]. Lack of calcium in the body.

acalculia (a-kal-kŭ'lĭ-ă) [G. *a-*, priv. + L. *calculare*, to reckon]. Inability to solve mathematical problems.

acampsia (a-kamp'sĭ-ă) [" + *kamptein*, to bend]. Inflexibility of a limb; rigidity, ankylosis.

acan'tha [G. *akantha*, thorn]. 1. The spine. 2. A vertebral spinous process.

acanthesthesia (a-kan-thes-the'zĭ-ă) [" + *disthēsis*, sensation]. A sensation as of a prick; a form of paresthesia, q.v.

acan'thion [G. *akanthion*, a thorn]. Tip of ant. nasal spine.

Acanthocephala (ă-kan-tho-sef'ăl-ă) [G. *akantha*, thorn, + *kephalē*, head]. A class of wormlike entozoa related to the Platyhelminthes, including a few species parasitic in man.

acanthocephaliasis (ă-kan"tho-sef-ăl-ĭ'ă-sis). Infestation with Acanthocephala.

acan'thoid [G. *akantha*, thorn, + *eidos*, form]. Thorny; spiny; of a spinous nature.

acanthokeratodermia (ă-kan"tho-ker"ă-to-der'mĭ-ă) [G. *akantha*, thorn, + *keras*, horn, + *derma*, skin]. Hypertrophy of hands and feet. [edema.

  a. adenoides cysticum. Sweat gland
  a. alveolaris. Tumor of epithelium.
  SYN: *epithelioma*.
  a. verrucosa seborrhoica. Warty growths in the senile.

acantholysis (a-kan-thol'is-is) [" + *lysis*, solution]. Any disease of the skin accompanied by atrophy of the prickle-layer.

a. bullosa. A skin condition of large bullae produced by irritation.
SYN: *Epidermolysis bullosa.**

acanthoma (a-kan-tho'ma) [" + *-oma*, tumor]. 1. Papilloma. 2. Cancer of skin.
a. adenoides cysticum. Eruption arising in the rete spinosum of the skin and resembling spiradenoma.

acanthopel'vis [" + *pelyx*, pelvis]. A prominent and sharp pubic spine on a rachitic pelvis.

acanthosis (a-kan-tho'sis) [G. *akantha*, thorn]. Disease of prickle cell layer of skin.

a. nigricans. Chronic inflammatory disease of skin in adult life generally associated with cancer of some internal organ.

ETIOL: Unknown. Hypothetically, disease of the abdominal sympathetic is suggested.

SYM: Symmetrically distributed hard and soft papillary growths accompanied by pigmentation and hyperkeratosis.

PROG: Depends upon presence or absence of underlying carcinomatous factor.

TREATMENT: Empirical and purely symptomatic.

acanthot'ic. Pert. to acanthosis.

acanthulus (a-kan'thu-lus). An instrument for removing thorns or splinters from wounds.

acap'nia [Gr. *akapnos*, smokeless]. The presence of less than normal amount of carbon dioxide in blood and tissues, *e.g.*, after voluntary overbreathing and the condition resulting therefrom.

SYM: Depressed respiration, giddiness, paresthesia, cramps, occasionally convulsions.

acap'nial. Showing or pert. to acapnia.

acar'bia [G. *a-*, priv. + L. *carbo*, coal]. Diminution of carbonate of the blood due to asphyxia.

acariasis (ak-ă-rĭ'a-sis) [L. *acarus*, mite, + G. *-iasis*, condition]. Any disease caused by a mite or *acarus* (*Acaridae*).

acaricide (a-kar'ĭ-sīd) [" + *caedere*, to kill]. 1. An agent that destroys acarids. 2. Destroying a member of order Acarina.

ac'arid, acar'idan. A tick or mite; member of order *Acarina*.

acaridi'asis. Disease caused by a mite. SYN: *acariasis*.

acarinosis (ă-kar-ĭ-no'sis). Disease caused by a mite. SYN: *acariasis*.

acarodermatitis (ak-a-ro-der-mă-tĭ'tis) [L. *acarus*, mite, + G. *derma*, skin, + *-itis*, inflammation]. The itch. Inflammation of skin caused by a mite.

ac'aroid [" + *eidos*, resemblance]. A mite, or resembling one.

acarophobia (a-kar-o-fo'bĭ-ă) [" + *phobos*, fear]. PSY: Delusion that the skin is infested with mites or worms.

acarpia (a-karp'ĭ-a) [G. *a-*, priv. + *karpos*, fruit]. Barrenness; sterility.

ac'arus [G. *akari*, a mite]. A mite or tick.

acaryote (ă-kar'ĭ-ōt) [G. *a-*, priv. + *karyon*, nucleus]. Without a nucleus.

acatalepsia (a-kat-a-lep'sĭ-ă) [" + *katalambanein*, to comprehend]. 1. Dementia. Impairment of mind. 2. Diagnostic uncertainty.

acat'alepsy [G. *a-*, priv. + *katalēpsis*, comprehension]. 1. Dementia or impairment of mind. 2. Uncertainty. SYN: *acatalepsia.**

acatalep'tic. 1. Deficient mentally. 2. Uncertain or doubtful.

acatamathesia (a-kat-a-ma-the'zĭ-ă) [" + *katamathēsis*, understanding]. PSY: 1. Psychic blindness or deafness, or

acataphasia / A-11 / **a.c.e. mixture**

blunting of sensation. 2. Inability to comprehend words, conversation, or signs, due to a brain lesion.

acataphasia (a-kat-a-fa′zĭ-ă) [" + *kataphasis*, affirmation]. Inability to formulate a sentence.

acataposis (ă-kă-tap′o-sĭs) [" + *katapo-sis*, gulping down]. Dysphagia. Difficulty in swallowing.

acatastasia (ă-kat-as-ta′zĭ-ă) [G. *akatastasis*, disorder]. Irregularity or fixed characteristics in the course of a disease or in excretion.

acatharsia (ă-ka-thar′sĭ-ă) [G. *akatharsis*, uncleanness]. Foulness; impurity; lack of purging.

acathectic (ă-ka-thek′tĭk) [G. *a-*, priv. + *kathexis*, holding in]. Inability to retain. Lack of retention.

    a. jaundice. That due to inability of liver cells to prevent bile from passing into lymph and blood.

acathexia (a-ka-theks′ĭ-ă). An inability to retain excretions or secretions.

acathisia (a-ka-thĭz′ĭ-ă) [G. *a-*, priv. + *kathisis*, sitting]. Inability to remain seated.

acaulino′sis [" + L. *caulis*, stalk]. A disease due to a fungus, causing eczematous eruption.

ACC. Abbr. for *anodal closure contraction.*

accelerans (ak-sel′er-ans) [L. pres. part. of *accelerare*, to hasten]. The acceleration heart nerve.

    It increases the rate and force of the heart's action.

accelera′tion [L. *acceleratus*, past p. of *accelerare*, to hasten]. Increasing the motion of, as pulse or respiration.

accelerator (ak-sel′er-a-tor). Anything that increases action or function.

    a. nerve. Nerve increasing heart rate and action. SEE: *accelerans.*

    a. urinae. Bulbocavernosus muscle.

accentua′tion [L. *ad*, to, + *cantus*, a singing]. Marked with a special stress; emphasis.

accept′or [L. *accipere*, to accept]. A substance absorbing nascent hydrogen freed by a reducing enzyme.

    a., hydrogen. Substance which receives h. from a hydrogen donator.

accesso′rius [L. past p. *accedere*, move toward]. Accessory, supplementary, as certain muscles, glands, nerves.

    a. nerve. 11th cranial nerve. Motor nerve made up of a cranial and a spinal part which supplies the trapezius and sternomastoid muscles and pharynx. Accessory portion joins the vagus, to which it supplies its motor and some of its cardio-inhibitory fibers. Afferent fibers carry proprioceptive impulses. ORIG: Medulla and spinal cord.

    a. Willis′ii. Spinal accessory nerve.

acces′sory. Auxiliary; assisting, as accessory glands of the pancreas or Brunner's glands.*

    a. articles of diet. Condiments,* flavors, and stimulants.

ac′cident [L. *accidens*, happening]. 1. An unexpected event. 2. An unforeseen occurrence of an unfortunate nature, a mishap.

    RS: *asphyxia, burn, choking, collapse, coma, dislocations* (under name of bone), *fractures* (the same), *frostbites, fumes, gases, heat cramps and exhaustion, hemorrhages, insect bites, poisons* (name of), *resuscitation, shock, suffocation, sunburn, sunstroke, syncope, unconsciousness, wounds,* etc.

accipiter (ak-sip′it-er) [L. a hawk]. A bandage for the face with clawlike tails.

acclima′tion [F. *à*, to, + *climat*, climate]. To become accustomed to a climate.

acclimatization (a-kli-ma-ti-za′shun). Becoming accustomed to a new climate.

acclimatize (ak-kli′mă-tiz). To make accustomed to a new climate.

accommoda′tion [L. *accomodare*, to suit]. 1. Adjustment. Esp. ant. surface made possible by contraction and relaxation of the ciliary muscles. 2. Adaption. Convergence of eyes brought about by contraction of the extrinsic eye muscles.

    OPHTH: 1. The adjustment of the eye for seeing at different distances. Produced by change in shape of lens, esp. ant. surface. 2. Act of accommodation accompanied by contraction of pupils and convergence of eye, made possible by the contraction and relaxation of the ciliary muscle.

    ANOMALIES: (a) Subnormal accommodation (toxemia). (b) Paralysis (toxins, diphtheria, poisoning, atropine, hematropine, hyoscyamine, scopolamine, syphilis, contusions of eyeball), (c) Spasms (frequently in children and young adults, due to excessive use of eyes). (d) Presbyopia.*

    a., absolute. Accommodation of either eye separately.

    a., amplitude of. SEE: *range of a.*

    a., binocular. Meeting of both eyes at a point in order to carry the object's image to the retina of both.

    a., histologic. Change in cell form and function due to change in surrounding conditions.

    a., mechanism. Method by which curvature of eye lens is changed in order to focus close objects on the retina.

    a., negative. Relaxation by the eye to adjust itself for long distances.

    a., positive. Contraction by the eye to adjust itself for short distances.

    a., range of. Space of vision between its closest and most remote points.

    a. reflex. The normal dilation and contraction of pupil as eye focuses for near and far objects. SEE: *Argyll-Robertson pupil.*

    a., relative. Accommodation produced by the two eyes acting together.

accom′modative iridoplegia. Noncontraction of pupils during accommodation.

accouchée (ak-koo-shay′) [Fr. *accoucher*, to be delivered of child]. One who has been delivered of a child.

accouchement (a-koosh-mon′). The act of delivery in childbirth; parturition.

    a. forcé. Forcible hand delivery.

accoucheur, accoucheuse (ak-koosh-er′, a-koo-shŭz′) (*Fem.*). One who practices obstetrics.

accrementition (a-kre-men-tish′un) [L. *accrescere*, to increase]. Increase of growth by interstitial development from blastema and by reproduction by cellular fission. Gemmation, *q.v.*

accretion (ak-re′shun). 1. Increase by external addition; accumulation. 2. The growing together of parts naturally separate.

accubation (ak-u-ba′shun) [L. *accubare*, to recline near.] 1. Act of taking to one's bed or assuming a reclining posture. 2. Lying in bed with another person.

accum′ulator or storage battery. PT: A vessel containing sulfuric acid diluted until its sp. gr. is 1.200. In this are immersed lead plates.

a.c.e. mixture. An anesthetic for general inhalation made up of one part of *alcohol*, two parts of *chloroform*, and three parts of *ether*. Now seldom used.

acedia (a-sē'dĭ-ă) [G. *a-*, priv. + *kedos*, care]. Indifference. Insensibility. Lack of emotion. SYN: *apathy.*

acenesthesia (a-sen-es-thē'zĭ-ă) [G. *a-*, priv. + *koinos*, common, + *aisthēsis*, sensation]. Absence of a feeling of well-being, present in such disorders as hypochondriasis and neurasthenia.

acen'tric [" + *kentron*, point around which a circle is described]. Not central; peripheral.

aceph'alocyst, acephalocys'tis [G. *akephalos*, headless, + *kystis*, bladder]. An echinococcus cyst; hydatid.
a. racemo'sa. A hydatid uterine mole.

acephalous (ă-sef'al-us). Without a head.

acerbity (a-serb'ĭ-tĭ) [L. *acerbus*, sharp]. Astringency combined with acidity.

acervuline (ă-ser'vu-līn) [L. *acervulus*, a little heap]. Aggregated, occurring in clusters.

acervuloma (ă-ser-vu-lo'mă) [" + *-oma*, tumor]. Intracranial tumor containing brain sand.

acer'vulus [L.]. Sandy, sabulous.
a. cer'ebri. Sabulous matter filling the follicle of the pineal gland; brain sand.

acescence (a-ses'ens) [L. *ascesere*, to become sour]. 1. Slight acidity. 2. Process of souring.

acesent (a-ses'ent). Slightly acid.

acestoma (a-ses-to'mă) [G. *akestos*, curable, + *-oma*]. The fresh granulations which later form a cicatrix. [acetabulum.

acetabular (as-et-ab'u-lar). Pert. to the

acetabulum (as-et-ab'u-lum) [L. a little saucer for vinegar]. The rounded (cotyloid) cavity on the external surface of the innominate bone (*os coxae* or *os innominatum*) which receives head of femur. SEE: *cotyloid cavity*. 2. The ventral sucker of the fluke.

acetanilid (as-et-an'ĭl-id) (antifebrin). USP. A white powder or crystalline substance obtained by interaction of glacial acetic acid and aniline.
INCOMPATIBILITIES: Chloral, antipyrine.
ACTION AND USES: Analgesic and antipyretic. In excessive dose, cardiac depressant. DOSAGE: 3 gr. (0.2 Gm.).
POISONING: SYM: Weakness, sweating, prostration, prolonged cyanosis due to methemoglobin. Depression of cerebral and medullary centers, feeble pulse and respiration. If prolonged, find hematuria, nephritis, and jaundice.
F. A. TREATMENT: Wash out stomach; saline purge; give stimulants; intravenous fluids and blood-transfusion often invaluable.

acetarsone (as-et-ar'sōn). An organic arsenical compound originally introduced as "stovarsol" containing 27.1 to 27.4% arsenic.
ACTION AND USES: In treatment of amebic dysentery and syphilis. Reaction from excessive dose same as arsphenamine.
DOSAGE: Orally: 4 gr. (0.25 Gm.).

acetate (as'e-tāt). A salt of acetic acid.

acetbroman'ilid. Antisepsin, asepsin, an analgesic and hypnotic.

acetic (a-se'tĭk) [L. *acetum*, vinegar]. Pert. to vinegar; sour.
a. acid. Gives vinegar sour taste. CH_3COOH. SEE: *acid, chloracetization.*
a. a. test for albumen. Acetic acid is added to heated urine. If cloudy, albumen present. SEE: *albumen.*
a. fermentation. A continuation of alcoholic fermentation.

aceticoceptor (ă-se"tĭk-o-sep'tor). One of the side chains which have an affinity for the acetic acid radical.

acet'idin. Ethyl acetate.

acetify (a-se'tĭ-fī) [L. *acetum*, vinegar, + *fieri*, to become]. To produce acetic fermentation or vinegar.

acetimeter (ă-se-tim'e-ter) [" + G. *metron*, measure]. An apparatus which determines the acetic acid in fluid.

Acetobac'ter [" + G. *baktērion*, little staff]. A genus of *nitrobacteriaceae*.
A. ace'ti. A form of A., producing vinegar from wine or cider.

acetone (as'e-tōn). Dimethyl ketone $(CH_3)_2CO$, a colorless, volatile, inflammable liquid, miscible with water, useful as a solvent, and having a characteristic irritating odor.
DOSAGE: 5-15 gr. (0.3-1.0 Gm.).
Found in the blood, and in urine in diabetes, faulty metabolism, and after lengthy fasting, produced when the fats are not properly oxidized, due to inability to oxidize glucose in the blood. SEE: *acetonuria, acidosis, ketone, ketosis,* and *tests.*
a. bodies. Certain substances related to acetone. An example is *acetoacetic acid, q.v.* under *acid.*
a. in urine, test for. Take 2 to 3 cc. of urine; acidify with 3 or 4 drops of glacial acetic acid; add a few crystals of sodium nitroprusside, and shake a little. Cover with a layer of strong ammonia. The presence of acetone is indicated by the formation of a purple ring between the layers of liquid.

acetonemia (as-e-to-nē'mĭ-ă) [acetone + G. *aima*, blood]. Large amounts of acetone in blood. SYM: erethism, gradual depression, acidosis.

acetonuria (as-e-to-nu'rĭ-ă) [" + G. *ouron*, urine]. The occurrence of acetone and diacetic bodies in the urine, as in the *ketosis* of diabetes, starvation, etc., which may be due to incomplete oxidation of albuminous substances. SEE: *acetone, acidosis* and *tests.*

acetophenetidin (as-ē-to-fe-net'ĭd-in) (phenacetin) USP. A crystalline substance manufactured from coal tar.
ACTION AND USES: Same as for acetanilid but less depressing.
INCOMPATIBILITIES: Same as for acetanilid.
DOSAGE: 5 to 15 gr. (0.32-1.0 Gm.).

acetous (as'e-tus) [L. *acetum*, vinegar]. 1. Pert. to vinegar. 2. Sour in taste.

acetum (pl. *aceta*) (a-se'tum) [L.]. Vinegar.
The vinegars are solutions of medicinal substances in diluted acetic acid. There is 1 official vinegar. They are seldom prescribed.

acetylcholine (ă-sĕt-ĭl-kō'lēn). A substance found normally in many animal and vegetable tissues. It has been used in the form of its chloride and bromide salts to relax peripheral blood vessels.

acetylsalicylic acid (as'et-il-sal-ĭ-sil'ĭk) (aspirin) USP. A white powder or crystalline substance obtained by action of acetic anhydride on salicylic acid. A substance liberated at the endings of the vagus nerve in the heart, sometimes called "vagal substance". It is a choline ester and is produced at the endings of postganglionic fibers of the parasympathetic division of the autonomic nervous system, in sympathetic ganglia at the synapses between pre- and postganglionic fibers, and at the motor end plates in striated muscles. It is also produced at some sympathetic-nerve endings and along a nerve fiber during the passage of a nerve impulse.

achalasia (ă-kal-a′zĭ-ă) [G. *a-*, priv. + *chalasis*, relaxation]. Failure to relax; said of muscles, such as sphincters, the normal function of which is a persistent contraction with periods of relaxation.

a., pelvirectal. Congenital dilatation of the colon.

a., sphincteral. Intestinal failure of sphincters to relax.

achieve′ment age. Determined by test for proficiency in a subject measured by what average child of that chronological age can do. SEE: *age*.

a. quo′tient (A.Q.). A state of progress in learning ascertained by dividing the achievement age by the mental age.

Achil′les jerk. The motor response to striking tendon of gastrocnemius muscle.

The variations and their significance correspond closely to those of the knee jerk. It is exaggerated in upper motor neuron disease and diminished or absent in lower motor neuron disease. SEE: *reflex*.

Achilles tendon (a-kil′ēz) (*tendo achillis* or *tendo calcaneus*) [Greek warrior, invulnerable except for his heel]. The tendon of the soleus and gastrocnemius muscles, at the back of the heel.

A. t. reflex. Plantar flexion of foot and contraction of calf muscles following blow upon tendon of Achilles. Absent in sciatica.

achillobursitis (a-kil-o-bur-si′tis) [" + L. *bursa*, a pouch + G. *-itis*, inflammation]. Inflammation of the bursa lying over the Achilles tendon.

achillodynia (a-kil-o-din′i-ă) [" + *odyne*, pain]. Pain caused by inflammation bet. the *tendo calcaneus* and the bursa.

achillorrhaphy (a-kil-or′raf-ī) [" + G. *raphē*, sewing]. Suture of *tendo achillis*.

achillotomy (a-kil-ot′o-mĭ) [" + *tomē*, incision]. A division of *tendo achillis*.

achi′lous [G. *a-*, priv. + *cheilos*, lips]. Without lips.

achiria (a-ki′rĭ-ă) [" + *cheir*, hand]. 1. Congenital lack of hands. 2. Loss of sense of possession of one or both hands. 3. Inability to tell on which side of body a stimulus is applied.

achlorhydria (a-klor-hi′drĭ-ă) [" + *chlōros*, green, + *ydōr*, water]. Absence of free hydrochloric acid in the gastric juice.

ETIOL: May be due to gastric carcinoma, pernicious anemia, syphilis of stomach, chronic atrophic gastritis, and neuroses, carcinoma, and in diseases of other organs than the stomach; may be a normal condition in 30% of adults up to 70 yrs. of age, and in 4% of children. SEE: *achylia*.

achloride (ă-klo′rīd). A salt other than a chloride; nonchloride.

achloropsia (ă-klo-rop′se-ă) [G. *a-*, priv. + *chloros*, green, + *opsis*, vision]. Color blindness as regards green.

acholia (ak-o′lĭ-ă) [" + *cholē*, bile]. An absence or want of bile.

acholic (ak-o′lĭk) [" + *cholē*, bile]. Pert. to acholia.

acholuria (a-kol-u′rĭ-ă) [" + " + *ouron*, urine]. In some forms of jaundice, absence of bile pigments in the urine.

achondroplasia (ă-kon-dro-pla′sĭ-ă) [" + *chondros*, cartilage, + *plasis*, a moulding]. Defect in the formation of cartilage at the epiphyses of long bones, producing a form of dwarfism; sometimes seen in rickets.

achor (a′kor) [G. *achōr*, scurf]. 1. Small pustules on hairy parts of body. 2. Pointed pustules. 3. Scabby eruption on scalp and face of infants.

achoresis (ă-ko-re′sis) [G. *a-*, priv. + *chōrein*, to make room]. Contraction of the bladder, stomach, or other hollow viscus, reducing its capacity.

Achorion (ă-ko′rĭ-on). A genus of fungous organisms found in the skin, esp. in hair follicles.

A. schoenleinii. A species of A. in ringworm.

achreocythemia (a-kre-o-sĭ-the′mĭ-ă) [G. *achroios*, colorless, + *kytos*, cell, + *aima*, blood]. Absence of coloring in the blood.

achroacyte (a-krō′a-sīt) [G. *a-*, priv. + *chroa*, color, + *kytos*, cell]. A lymphocyte; a colorless cell.

achroacytosis (a-kro-ă-si-to′sis) [" + " + " + *-osis*, condition]. Many lymphocytes in the peripheral circulation.

achroiocythemia (ă-kroy″o-sĭ-the′mĭ-ă) [G. *achroios*, colorless, + *kytos*, cell, + *aima*, blood]. Deficiency of hemoglobin in red blood cells.

achroma (a-kro′ma) [G. *a-*, priv. + *chrōma*, color]. 1. A form of macula.* 2. An absence of color. Leukoderma. Hereditary, circumscribed skin areas deficient in pigmentation.

achromacyte (ak-ro′mă-sīt) [" + *kytos*, cell]. A decolorized erythrocyte.*

achromasia (ak-ro-ma′zĭ-ă) [G. *achrōmatos*, without color]. 1. Albinism, vitiligo, or leukoderma. 2. Lack of pigment in the skin. 3. Pallor due to poor nutrition.

achromate (ak′rō-māt) [G. *a-*, priv. + *chrōma*, color]. One who is color blind.

achromatic (ak″rō-mat′ĭk) [G. *achrōmatos*, without color]. Colorless.

a. lens. One correcting chromatic aberration.

a. sensation. A descriptive name for visual sensation in white, black and gray, contrasted with the chromatic or colored sensations.

achromatin (ă-krō′mat-ĭn). The basis of a cell nucleus, so-called because it is not readily colored by basic stains.

achro′matism [G. *a-*, priv. + *chroma*, color]. Colorlessness.

achromat′ocyte [" + " + *kytos*, cell]. A decolorized red blood cell.

achromatolysis (ă-kro-mă-tol′is-is) [" + " + *lysis*, loosing]. Dissolution of cell achromatin.

achromatophil (ă-kro-mat′o-fīl) [" + " + *philos*, love]. A cell not stainable the usual way.

achromatopsia (ă-kro-mă-top′sĭ-ă) [G. *achrōmatos*, without color, + *opsis*, vision]. Color blindness; partial or total.

achromatop′sy. Color blindness. SYN: achromatopsia.

achromatosis (a-chro″ma-tō′sis) [G. *achrōmatos*, without color, + *osis*, state]. Condition of being without natural pigmentation. SEE: *achroma*.

achromatous (a-krō′mă-tus). Without color.

achromaturia (ă-krō″mă-tu′rĭ-ă) [G. *achrōmatos*, without color, + *ouron*, urine]. Colorless or nearly colorless urine.

achrom′ia [G. *a-*, priv. + *chroma*, color]. Absence of color. SYN: *achroma*. SEE: *chloranemia*.

a. parasitica. Skin disease causing spotted appearance.

achromic (ă-krō′mĭk). Lacking color.

achromoder′mia [G. *a-*, priv. + *chroma*, color, + *derma*, skin]. Lack of color in skin.

achro′mophil [" + " + *philos*, fond]. Not staining easily.

achromotrich′ia [" + " + *trichia*, condition of the hair]. Lack of color in the hair.

achromycin (ăk-rō-mī′sĭn). An antibiotic effective against Gram-positive and Gram-negative bacteria, rickettsiae, and certain viruses and protozoa.

achroödextrin (ak″ro-o-deks′trĭn) [G. *achroos*, colorless, + *dextrin*]. One of the varieties of dextrin resulting from the first splitting of a polysaccharide molecule, the other being *erythrodextrin*.*

This process is followed by further splitting of the molecules to maltase, a disaccharide, and then to glucose, a monosaccharide. It is not colored by iodine.

achylia (a-kī′lĭ-ă) [G. *a-*, priv. + *chylos*, chyle]. Absence of chyle.

  a. gas′trica. Hypoacidity; a deficiency of hydrochloric acid and of gastric enzymes, present in 40% of adults, in children during febrile diseases and gastroenteritis, during the last months of pregnancy, and in some anemias. Usually secondary to pernicious anemia, carcinoma, chronic appendicitis, cholecystitis, and other conditions. Dilute hydrochloric acid often indicated.

  a. pancreat′ica. Absence or deficiency of pancreatic secretion.

  SYM: Emaciation, fatty stools, impaired nutrition, etc.   [SYN: *achylia*.

achylosis (ă-kī-lo′sis). Absence of chyle.

achylous (ak-ī′lus) [G. *achylos*, without chyle]. 1. Lacking in any digestive secretion. 2. Without chyle.

achymia, achymosis (a-kī′mĭ-ă, a-kī-mo′sis) [G. *a-*, priv. + *chymos*, juice]. Deficiency or absence of chyme.

acicular (a-sĭk′u-lar) [L. *aciculus*, little needle]. Needle-shaped.

a′cid [L. *acidus*, sour]. 1. Any substance containing hydrogen replaceable by metals, yielding hydrogen ions as the only positive ions, when dissolved in water, and affecting indicators in certain ways. SEE: *indicator*. 2. Sour.

  a., acetic, CH_3COOH. It gives the sour taste to vinegar.

  a., adenylic. Assumed to be a vitamin B. It is intimately associated with life processes. A vital metabolic link in energy-transfer mechanisms, muscular contractions, and enzymic reactions; it is involved in fat and carbohydrate metabolism.

  a., a., glacial. A pure anhydrous preparation which melts at 16.7° C. and is consequently crystalline in a cold room.

  a., acetoacetic, $CH_3CO.CH_2COOH$. SYN: *Diacetic acid* (in diabetic urine).

  a., amino. A series of compounds that can be prepared from proteins or made synthetically and which have the general formula $NH_2R.COOH$. Ex: *a., aminoacetic, histidine,* and *tryptophan*.

  a., aminoacetic, $NH_2.CH_2.COOH$. The same as glycine, one of the simplest examples of an amino acid.

  a., ascorbic. Synthetic vitamin C ($C_6H_8O_6$). Similar to natural vitamin in citrus, etc., in comp. and therapeutic value.

  DOSAGE: Infants and children: *prophylactic*, ⅙-¾ gr. (0.01-0.05 Gm.); *curative*, ½ gr. (0.03 Gm.). Adults: *prophylactic*, ¾ gr. (0.05 Gm.); *curative*, ¾-1½ gr. (0.05-0.1 Gm.).

  a., barbituric, $C_4H_4O_3N_2$, Malonyl urea. A heterocyclic compound from which veronal and other hypnotics are derived.

  a., benzoic, C_6H_5COOH. A white crystalline material prepared from coal tar; used in keratolytic ointments.

  a., betaoxybutyric. SYN. for: *a., acetoacetic*.

  a., bile. Any substance occurring in the form of salt in the bile. Ex: *glycocholic* and *a., a., taurocholic*.

  a., boric., H_3BO_3, a., boracic. A white crystalline substance giving very weakly acid solutions, poisonous to plants and animals, and useful as a bacteriostatic. Prepared from interaction of sulfuric acid and borax. USES: Mild antiseptic dusting-powder alone, or diluted with talcum or starch, or as 4% solution to mucous membranes.

  a., butyric, C_3H_7COOH. A liquid having odor of vomitus and rancid butter.

  a., carbolic. Obsolescent name for phenol.

  a., carbonic, H_2CO_3. A weak acid from carbon dioxide dissolved in water.

  a., carboxylic. Any one containing the group COOH. The simplest examples are *formic* and *acetic*.

  a., citric, $C_6H_8O_7.H_2O$. USP. Prepared from lemon or lime juice in form of large white or transparent crystals. USES: As a flavor and in effervescent drinks.

  DOSAGE: 8 gr. (0.5 Gm.).

  a., diacetic. Same as *acetoacetic*.

  a., fatty. One of a series of carboxylic acids which can be combined with *glycerol* to form fats; the simplest members of the series are *formic* and *acetic*; most typical: *stearic* and *oleic*.

  a., formic, HCOOH. The simplest member of the series of fatty acids; a liquid heavier than water and 12 times as strong as acetic acid.

  a., gallic, $C_6H_2(OH)_3COOH$. A crystalline acid that can be prepared from tanbark and plant galls.

  a., glutamic, $COOH.CH_2.CH_2.CHNH_2.COOH$. An important amino acid.

  a., glycocholic, $C_{26}H_{43}NO_6$. Occurs as a sodium salt in bile and can be decomposed into aminoacetic and cholic acids.

  a., glycuronic, $CHO.(CHOH)_4COOH$. Related to the carbohydrates; is found in small quantities in the urine, and occurs among the decomposition products of mucoids.

  a., hydriodic, HI. Used in medicine for its iodine content; its salts are called iodides.

  a., hydrochlor′ic (HCl) (Muriatic acid), USP. An aqueous solution of a gas produced by the interaction of sulfuric acid and sodium chloride. Found naturally (up to 0.4%) in gastric juice; its salts are called *chlorides*. INCOMPATIBILITIES: Alkalies, carbonates and oxides. USES: To check fermentation and putrefaction in stomach by partially restoring necessary hydrochloric acid. DOSAGE: Diluted (10%): 15 ℳ (1 cc.). Taken through a glass tube.

  a., hydrocyanic, HCN. A weak, unstable, poisonous volatile acid which forms salts called cyanides; has a characteristic odor suggesting almonds, and in minute doses stimulates respiration.

  DOSAGE: (Dil.) 1½ gr. (0.1 Gm.).

  a., lactic, $C_3H_6O_3$. Results in nature from the fermentation of lactose (as in sour milk) and when pure is a clear syrupy liquid.

  a., linoleic, $C_{18}H_{32}O_2$. May be prepared from linseed and cottonseed oils and is an example of unsaturated fatty acid.

  a., malic, $C_4H_6O_5$. Found in certain sour fruits as apples and apricots.

a., mineral. Acids prepared from non-organic materials, as sulfuric, hydrochloric, nitric, and phosphoric.

a., muriatic. Obsolescent name for *a., hydrochloric.*

a., nitric, HNO$_3$. A strong corrosive acid prepared from sulfuric acid and a nitrate.

a., oleic, C$_{18}$H$_{34}$O$_2$. An unsaturated fatty acid that can be prepared from various fats and oils.

a., organic. An acid containing the carboxyl radical COOH.

a., oxalic, C$_2$H$_2$O$_4$. A white crystalline solid found in cranberries, rhubarb, and other plants; is poisonous in large quantities, and occurs (as calcium oxalate) in urinary calculi.

a., palmitic, C$_{16}$H$_{32}$O$_2$. A fatty acid prepared from palm oil.

a., pectic. C$_{16}$H$_{22}$O$_{15}$. An acid derived from pectin.

a., phosphoric, H$_3$PO$_4$. Gives rise to salts called phosphates and related compounds widely distributed in nature. DOSAGE: (10%) 15 gr. (1.0 Gm.)

a., phosphorous. H$_3$PO$_3$. A dibasic oxy-acid of phosphorus. It has 1 atom less of oxygen than phosphoric acid.

a., phosphotungstic, P$_2$O$_5$.12WO$_3$42H$_2$O. Used in chemical and histologic technic. Precipitates proteins and alkaloids.

a., picric, C$_6$H$_2$(NO$_2$)$_3$OH. A yellow crystalline substance which reacts with proteins and alkaloids and leaves bright yellow stains.

a., prussic. Obsolescent name for *a., hydrocyanic.*

a., pyrogallic. Same as pyrogallol, C$_6$H$_3$(OH)$_3$. A white crystalline substance which absorbs oxygen rapidly in alkaline solution and is used in gas analysis and photography.

a., pyruvic, CH$_3$CO.COOH. The simplest of the ketonic acids, important in metabolism because of its close relation to *a., lactic.*

a., salicylic, C$_6$H$_4$(OH)COOH. A white, crystalline powder used for its antiseptic and keratolytic actions; its derivatives, the salicylates, are much used as analgesics. USP. A white crystalline powder from oil of wintergreen and sweet birch. INCOMPATIBILITIES: Iron salts, sweet spirit of niter. USES: Externally as antiseptic and irritant. Internally, same as sodium salicylate. DOSAGE: 5-20 gr. (0.3-1.3 Gm.).

a., stearic, C$_{17}$H$_{35}$COOH. A fatty acid prepared from animal fats, esp. beef.

a., sulfonic. Any organic compound of the general formula R.SO$_2$H generally prepared by the action of strong sulfuric acid on benzene or its derivatives.

a., sulfuric, H$_2$SO$_4$. A corrosive, heavy liquid prepared from sulfur and indispensable in the industries.

a., sulfurous, H$_2$SO$_3$. An acid existing in solutions of sulfur dioxide in water and giving rise to salts called sulfites. DOSAGE: (6%) 15-60 gr. (1.0-4.0 Gm.).

a., tannic. A glucoside prepared from oak galls and sumac and yielding gallic acid and glucose on hydrolysis.

a., tartaric. USP. C$_4$H$_6$O$_6$. Occurs free or as tartrates in fruit juices. A light yellow powder, from nut galls, freely soluble in water and glycerin. INCOMPATIBILITIES: Alkalies, alkaloids, and iron salts. USES: Astringent and hemostatic. DOSAGE: 8 gr. (0.5 Gm.).

Acid and Alkaline Reaction of Foods

Foods	Oz. in 100 Calories	Excess of Acid	Excess of Alkali
Almonds	.54	....	1.00
Apples	5.61	....	6.00
Apricots	6.08	....	11.00
Asparagus	15.89	....	3.60
Bacon	.56	.80	....
Bananas	3.58	....	5.60
Barley	.99	2.90	....
Beans—Baked	2.75	....	....
Kidney, dried	1.02	....	5.00
Lima, dried	1.02	....	2.50
String, canned	17.10	....	12.00
Beef—Corned	1.18	2.60	13.00
Dried	1.96	8.30	....
Liver	2.73	7.90	....
Porterhouse	1.30	4.00	....
Round	3.07	10.00	....
Sirloin	1.46	3.90	....
Beets, fresh	7.66	....	23.60
Bread, white	1.34	2.70	....
Buckwheat Flour	1.01	2.00	....
Buttermilk	9.86	....	6.10
Cabbage	11.20	....	18.00
Carrots	7.80	....	24.00
Cauliflower	11.57	....	17.40
Celery	19.07	....	42.40
Chard	9.23	....	41.10
Cheese, Cheddar	.77	1.20	....
Cherries	4.52	....	7.80
Chestnuts	.87	....	3.20
Chicken, Broilers	3.77	10.00	....
Codfish, salt	3.38	12.10	....
Corn, canned	3.60	1.80	....
Cornmeal	.99	1.50	....
Crackers, soda	.85	2.00	....
Cranberries	7.57	....	3.70
Cream	.93	....	.30
Cucumbers	20.28	....	45.50
Dates	1.02	....	3.20

acid, taurocholic   A-16   **acid-base diet**

Acid and Alkaline Reaction of Foods (Continued)

Foods	Oz. in 100 Calories	Excess of Acid	Excess of Alkali
Eggs, whole	2.38	7.50	....
Figs, dried	1.12	....	32.30
Fowls	1.58	4.60	....
Frog's Legs	5.53	12.10	....
Grapes	3.66	....	2.80
Grape Juice	3.53	....	4.00
Haddock	3.71	12.00	....
Halibut	2.93	7.80	....
Ham, smoked	1.32	3.37	....
Lamb, leg	1.57	4.20	....
Lemons	7.96	....	12.00
Lentils	1.01	1.50	....
Lettuce	18.47	....	38.60
Mackerel, fresh	2.54	6.70	....
salt	1.50	2.80	....
Milk, whole	5.10	....	2.60
skimmed	9.61	....	5.00
Molasses	1.23	....	20.80
Mutton, leg	1.85	5.00	....
Oatmeal, rolled	.88	3.00	....
Olives	1.80	....	18.80
Onions	7.24	....	3.10
Oranges	6.86	....	11.00
Orange Juice	8.17	....	14.40
Oysters	7.00	30.00	....
Parsnips	5.43	....	18.30
Peaches, fresh	8.53	....	12.20
canned	7.50	....	10.00
Pears, canned	4.65	....	2.30
Peas, canned	6.37	....	1.50
Pineapple	8.18	....	15.70
Plums	4.18	....	7.30
Pork Chops	1.40	4.00	....
Potatoes	4.23	....	8.60
Prunes	1.17	....	8.00
Pumpkins	13.72	....	5.70
Radishes	12.00	....	9.80
Raisins	1.29	....	6.80
Rhubarb	15.27	....	37.00
Rice	1.01	2.70	....
Salmon	1.80	5.50	....
Sardines	1.31	4.20	....
Sausage	1.50	4.00	....
Shredded Wheat	.97	3.30	....
Spinach	14.76	....	113.00
Squash	7.65	....	6.10
Tomatoes	15.63	....	24.50
Turkey	1.21	3.36	....
Turnips	8.95	....	7.00
Veal, leg	2.89	8.70	....
Walnuts	.50	1.10	....
Watermelons	11.68	....	8.80
Wheat, cracked	.97	3.30	....
Whitefish	2.35	7.60	....

    a., taurocholic. A substance occurring in bile and yielding cholic acid and taurine on hydrolysis.
    a., unsaturated. Organic acid containing less than the maximum possible number of hydrogen atoms. For example, compare unsaturated *oleic* and *linoleic acids* with the saturated *a. stearic*.
    a., uric. A crystalline solid (formula $C_5H_4N_4O_3$) prepared from urine.
    a., valeric, $C_5H_{10}O_2$. Same as valerianic acid, an oily liquid of the fatty acid series, existing in 4 isomeric forms, having a disgusting odor, and prepared from valerian root. ADM: Dilute well with water. Protect teeth by giving through straw or glass tube.
    DOSAGE: 1-8 gr. (0.06-0.5 Gm.).
  acidaminuria (as″id-am″in-u′ri-ă) [L. *acidum*, acid, + amine + G. *ouron*, urine]. Excess of amino acids in voided urine.

acid and alkaline reaction of foods. One of the principles of dietetics is to maintain an equilibrium between the acids and the alkalies in the body, by balancing the ration so that neither an excess of acid-forming or alkali-forming foods is consumed. The following percentages, adapted from Sherman, show both the excess of acid and the excess of alkali in the indicated number of ounces constituting 100 calories. Observe that excess acid foods include: Meats, Fish, Poultry, and Cereals; excess alkali: nearly all vegetables and fruits.

acid-ash diet. Decrease or omit fruits, vegetables, milk. Adjust cals. by increasing neutral or acid-ash foods.

acid-base balance. In metabolism, the balance of acid to base (alkaline ash) necessary to keep the blood neutral (slightly alkaline), between pH 7.35 and pH 7.43.

acid-base diet. One which favors the development of acidosis and which produces a loss of fixed base and water from the tissues; the amount of nitrogen intake compared with the output. Acidosis may be due to increase of ketone* bodies or to excess of acid-ash. This diet is used in rickets, nephritis, and epilepsy, q.v. The value of a balanced acid-base, base-forming diet has not yet been determined.

RS: *acidic effects, acidosis, alkalosis, ash, base, body, ketogenic diet, ketosis;* also names of foods.

acidemia (as-i-de′mĭ-ă) [L. *acidum*, acid, + G. *aima*, blood]. A condition in which uncompensated reduction in alkaline reserve or uncompensated increase in circulating acid substances results in increased acidity of the blood, so that the *p*H drops from a normal range of 7.3-7.5 to more acid values, *e.g.*, 7.0 to 7.3. SEE: *acid-base balance, acidity, acidosis.*

acid-fast. Not decolorized easily when stained by acids. Pertaining to bacteria which after staining are decolorized by a mixture of acid and alcohol. The acid-fast bacteria retain the red dyes, but the surrounding tissues are decolorized.

acidic effects of foods. Proteins, such as meat and eggs, when burned in the body result in a number of end products which are acidic, such as uric acid, sulfuric acid, and phosphoric acid.

They should be neutralized by alkaline substances to form neutral salts, the salts being eliminated by the kidneys. Organic acids, such as benzoic and quinic, may be present following the ingestion of plums, cranberries, and prunes, and may not be burned in the body, the effects being acidic though salts are present. Acidity or its effect in the body is not indicated by its taste or its original acidity.

acid″ifica′tion [L. *acidum*, acid, + *factus*, past p. of *facere*, to make]. Becoming sour; conversion into an acid.

acidifiable (a-sid-ĭ-fī′ă-bl) [" + *fieri*, to be made, + *habilis*, able]. Capable of transformation into an acid.

acidimeter (as-ĭ-dim′ĕ-ter) [" + G. *metron*, measure]. Instrument for testing purity of acids.

acidimetry (as-ĭ-dim′ĭ-trĭ). Determination of an acid's strength, or of the acidity of a fluid.

ac′idism, acidis′mus [L. *acidus*, sour]. Poisoning due to acids introduced from outside.

acidity (a-sid′ĭ-tĭ). Quality of being acid; having an excess of acid; sourness.

In chemistry denoting: (a) the quality of possessing the characteristics of an acid and so, in acids or acid salts, equivalent to basicity; (b) the capacity for saturating an acid evinced by a base; (c) the intensity of an acid reaction, expressed usually in terms of the hydrogen-ion concentration. SEE: *hydrogen ion.*

a. of stomach. Sourness due to fermentation of food in the stomach, or oversecretion of acid. It does not necessarily indicate acidosis.

acidophil(e (as-sid′o-fĭl or fīl) [L. *acidum*, acid, + G. *philos*, love]. Capable of being stained by acid stains such as eosin. Said of cells or parts of cells prepared for microscopic study.

acidophilic (a-sid″o-fĭl′ĭk). Having affinity for acid or pert. to certain tissues and cell granules. SYN: *acidophilous.*

acidophilism (ă-sĭd-of′ĭl-izm). State due to acidophil adenoma of the hypophysis, causing acromegaly.

acidophilous (as-ĭ-dof′ĭ-lus). Capable of being stained by acid stains, said of cells. SYN: *acidophil, q.v.*

a. milk. Milk fermented by *Lactobacillus acidophilus* cultures. USES: To change intestinal flora. Average serving 240 grams. Pro. 8.2, Fat 4.8, Carbo. 3.7. SEE: *milk.*

acidoresis′tant. Acid resisting; said about bacteria.

acido′sic. Having acidosis.

acidosis (as-ĭ-do′sĭs) [L. *acidum*, acid, + G. *-ōsis*, condition]. A disturbance of the acid-base balance of the body. The blood is never acid except in extreme pathological conditions.

It may be caused by an abnormal production of acids in the body and faulty elimination or by abnormal decrease of alkalinity; inability of the body to maintain its normal alkali reserve due to failure of the fatty acids being reduced to their normal end products, the process stopping with the intermediary products such as acetone-bodies. The blood is never acid.

DIAG: In all cases the CO_2 combining power is lowered from 40 to 30 and to 20, showing the degree of acidosis, the normal figures being 55 to 75 cc. per 100 cc. of blood.

Increased ammonia in the urine or sour stomach does not necessarily indicate acidosis, but it is an indication that the body is reacting to prevent this condition.

Acidosis may be determined by the amount of sodium bicarbonate needed to render the urine alkaline. In *compensated* acidosis there is a corresponding reduction of the acids normally found in the blood (*e.g.*, carbonic), so that no actual acidity results.

The *p*H of the blood remains within the normal limits, the alkali defect being small, but in *uncompensated* acidosis the alkali defect is great and therefore the *p*H falls below the lower limit of normal (*p*H below 7.3).

Acetonuria frequently accompanies acidosis but is not identical with it.

Acidosis is secondary to some other disorder. It is common in diabetes, and in some forms of nephritis, in epilepsy, also in diarrhea and in toxemias.

ETIOL: This condition may be produced by a high fat diet with low carbohydrate and protein content. Hunger and starvation, pregnancy, cyclic vomiting and chloroform poisoning are other causes.

SYM: Sickly sweet breath, headache, nausea, vomiting, visual changes, and acetone bodies in urine.

TREATMENT: Administer glucose. Reduce fat in diet. Sodium bicarbonate, 10-20 gr. every 4 hours.

SEE: *acidosic, acidotic, oxyosis.*

acidotic (a-sid-ot′ĭk). Pert. to acidosis.

a′cid pois′oning. Acids have a sour taste and many of them are corrosive or poisonous.

SYM: Burning with disintegration and often discoloration of involved tissues.

F. A. TREATMENT: Dilute and wash with large volumes of water; followed by dilute alkaline substances as baking soda, chalk, soap, milk of magnesia, lime water, weak ammonia, etc. Follow with bland or soothing oils or salves as olive oil, sweet oil, liquid paraffin, cold cream (ung. aq. rosae), lanolin, butter, petroleum jelly, etc. SEE: *name of special acids.*

acid-proof. Acid-fast.

acid-salt. A compound formed when only a part of the hydrogen of an acid is replaced by a metal.

acid'ulate [L. *acidulus*, slightly acid]. To make somewhat sour or acid. [acid.

acidulous (a-sid'u-lus). Slightly sour or

acidum (as'i-dum) [L.]. Acid.

acidu'ric [L. *acidus*, sour, + *durare*, to endure]. Capable of growing in an acid medium, but preferring a slightly alkaline medium, as certain bacteria.

acinesia (as-in-e'si-ă) [G. *a-*, priv. + *kinesis*, movement]. Akinesia. 1. Loss of voluntary motion. 2. Immobility. 3. Interval following the systolic heartbeat.

acinesic (as-in-e'sik). Acinetic, akinetic.

acinetic (as-in-et'ik). 1. Afflicted with akinesia. 2. Lessening muscular action.

aciniform (as-in'i-form) [L. *acinus*, grape, + *forma*, shape]. Resembling grapes.

acinitis (as-in-i'tis). Inflammation of glandular acini.

acinous (as'in-us) [L. *acinus*, grape]. Pert. to glands resembling a bunch of grapes, such as *acini* and *alveolar* glands.

ac'inus (*Pl. acini*) [L.]. Smallest division of a gland; a group of secretory cells surrounding a cavity. It is distinguished from an alveolus by possession of a narrow lumen.

acladio'sis. An ulcerative dermatitis due to the fungus *Acladium castellanii.*

aclasia (ă-kla'si-ă) [G. *a-*, priv. + *klasis*, a breaking away]. Pathologic continuity of structure: chondrodystrophy.

a., diaphyseal. Imperfect formation of cancellous bone in cartilage bet. diaphysis and epiphysis.

aclasis (ak'lă-sis). Pathological continuity of structure. SYN: *aclasia.*

aclas'tic. Not refracting light rays.

acleistocardia (ă-klis-to-kar'di-ă) [G. *akleistos*, not closed, + *kardia*, heart]. Patent foramen ovale.

aclu'sion [G. *a-*, priv. + L. *claudere*, to close]. Imperfect adjustment of opposing tooth surfaces.

acmastic (ak-mas'tik) [G. *akmē*, prime]. Pert. to disease with regular increase of symptoms (*epacmastic*) and decrease (*paracmastic*), or period of decline.

acme (ak'me). 1. The time of greatest intensity of a symptom. 2. Acne.

acne (ak'ne) [corruption of G. *akmē*, point]. Any inflammatory disease of the sebaceous glands.

SEE: *bacchia, bottle nose, stictacne.*

a. albida. Whitish nodules on face. SEE: *milium.*

a. artificialis. A. caused by external disturbance or irritation.

a. atrophica. SEE: *a. varioliformis.*

a. ciliaris. That which affects the edges of the eyelids.

a. decalvans. Quinquad's disease; a purulent folliculitis of the scalp resulting in irregular bald patches.

a. disseminata. SEE: *a. vulgaris.*

a. generalis. A. over the entire body.

a. hypertrophica. Thickening of the lips and sides of nose with *acne rosacea.*

a. indurata. Form of *a. vulgaris* with chronic discolored indurated surfaces.

a. keratosa. Acne in which a horny plug takes the place of the comedo.

a. papulosa. Common acne in which the lesions are papular.

a. punctata. A form with pointed papular lesions the centers of which are black-tipped comedones.

a. rosacea. Called also brandy nose, toper's nose, brandy face, rosy drop; characterized by congestion and telangiectasis; often accompanied by acne and seborrhea of angioneurotic origin.

ETIOL: Result of any disorder giving rise to persistent reflex flushing of the face. Presence of *Demodex folliculorum.* Thyroid and utero-ovarian disturbance in women, dyspepsia, constipation, strong tea or coffee, alcohol, damage in alimentary canal, or local vascular disturbance causing dilatation of cutaneous blood vessels. [underlying cause.

PROG: Depends upon eradication of TREATMENT: Correction of underlying cause, elimination of stimulants, condiments, etc. Radiotherapy and electrolysis; otherwise same as in *acne vulgaris.*

a. simplex. SEE: *a. vulgaris.*

a. tarsi. Acne affecting the sebaceous glands of the eyelids.

a. urticaria (kaposi). A form with itching patches.

a. varioliformis. Variety with pustular eruptions. Contagious. SEE: *molluscum contagiosum.* [plex.

a. vulgaris. Common acne, *acne sim-*

ETIOL: Heritable predisposition possible. Microbic, favored by the oily secretion, and with age, alimentary tract disorders, pelvic irritation, focal infection, as predisposing factors.

SYM: There may be either papules about comedones with black centers, or pustules, or hypertrophied nodules caused by overgrowth of connective tissue. In the indurative type the lesions are deep-seated and cause scarring. Face, neck, shoulders are common sites.

PROG: Curable, though obstinate and recurrent.

TREATMENT: Local in all; systemic when indicated. Locally alternate bathing with hot and cold water; removal of comedones, incision and drainage of abscesses, followed by hot lysol wash, *lotio alba* at night and a sulfur powder by day, then replaced by soothing lotions by day and cold cream at night; or green soap, or resorcin, or mercury bichloride (1:1000) in acute superficial cases. Eliminate rich foods, condiments, and stimulants. Laxatives (*cascara*) and tonics when indicated. Injections of boiled liver extract remarkably successful.

a. bacillus vaccine. Acne bacillus is found mainly in lesions of acne vulgaris. *Staphylococcus albus* is included in the combined acne-staphylococcus vaccine.

DOSAGE: First dose: 25 million acne bacilli, 25 million staphylococci. Doses are gradually increased to 250 million acne bacilli at intervals of 3 days. Subcutaneous route is used mostly. Some favor 0.1 cc. intracutaneously.

acneform (ak'ne-form). Resembling acne.

acneiform (ak-ne'i-form). Acneform.

acnemia (ak-ne'mi-ă) [G. *a-*, priv. + *knēmē*, lower leg]. Wasting of the calves of the legs.

acni'tis [G. *akme*, point, + *-itis*, inflammation]. A papular eruption which becomes pustular, leaving slight scars.

acoin (ak'o-in). A white crystalline powder; bactericide and local anesthetic.

acolasia (ak''o-la'zi-ă) [G. *akolasia*, intemperance]. 1. Lust. 2. Unrestrained self-indulgence. Intemperance.

acom'atol. Pancreatic hormone.

aco'mia [G. *a-*, priv. + *komē*, hair]. Baldness. SYN: *alopecia.*

aconite (ak'o-nit). USP. A poisonous and very powerful alkaloid. The dried tu-

aconuresis A-19 **acrocephalia**

berous root of *Aconitum napellus*. Its action, which is due to the presence of two very potent alkaloids, was well known to the ancients, and believed to have been used as an arrow poison early in Chinese history, and perhaps also by the inhabitants of ancient Gaul.

USES: Cardiac depressant, antipyretic, and diaphoretic. Externally: an irritant.

DOSAGE: Of tincture (10%) 5 to 15 ℳ (0.3-1 cc.).

POISONING: SYM: Slowness and weakness of pupils; coldness of skin, sweating, tingling about face and mouth, burning in throat, sometimes nausea; occasionally cramping in extremities; convulsions; respirations abnormal. Dimness of vision.

TREATMENT: Wash out stomach, and introduce tannic acid, strong, black coffee or strong tea to precipitate the alkaloid; or powdered charcoal to diminish solubility. Strychnine, atropine, artificial* respiration, application of heat.

aconuresis (a-kon″u-re′sis) [G. *akon*, involuntary, + *ouresis*, micturition]. An involuntary voiding of urine.

acoprosis (ă-kop-ro′sis) [G. *a-*, priv. + *kopros*, feces]. Imperfect formation of feces.   [the intestines.

acoprous (ă-kop′rus). Absence of feces in

acor (a′kor) [L. a sour taste]. Acidity.

acoria (a-ko′rĭ-ă) [G. *a-*, priv. + *koros*, satiety]. 1. Lacking in satisfaction after eating but not from hunger. 2. Gluttony. SEE: *bulimia*, *hyperorexia*, *pica*, *parorexia*, *polyphagia*.

acormus (ă-kor′mus). [G. *a-*, priv. + *kormōs*.] 1. Lack of the trunk. 2. A monster without a trunk but with only a head and extremities.

acouesthe′sia [G. *akouein*, to hear, + *aisthēsis*, sensation]. Sense of hearing.

acoumeter (a-kōō′me-ter) [″ + *metron*, measure]. An instrument for determining acuteness of hearing.

acouophonia (ă-koo-o-fo′nĭ-ă) [″ + *phonē*, sound]. Auscultatory percussion.

acouphone (a′koo-fōn). An electric appliance to aid the deaf to hear.

acousia (a-kōō′zĭ-ă) [G. *akousis*, hearing]. The hearing faculty.

acousma (a-kooz′mă) [G. *akousma*, a thing heard]. Nonverbal auditory hallucination.

acousmatagnosis (ă-koos-mă-tag-no′sis) [″ + *agnosia*, ignorance]. Inability to understand what is said, due to mental disorder.

acousmatamnesia (ă-koos-mă-tam-ne′zĭ-ă) [″ + *amnēsia*, forgetfulness]. Loss of memory for sounds.

acoustic (a-koos′tik) [G. *akoustikōs*, rel. to hearing]. Pert. to sound or to the sense of hearing.

a. center. In the temporal lobe of the cerebrum.

a. meatus. The external auditory canal.

a. nerve. (*nervus acusticus*). 8th cranial nerve. FUNCT: Special sense of hearing and equilibrium. ORIG: Two roots, cochlear and vestibular. DIS: Cochlea, vestibule body canals. BR: Cochlear, vestibular. SEE: *cranial nerves*. *Tables in Appendix*.

acous′ticon [G. *akoustikos*, rel. to hearing]. A type of hearing aid.

acoustics (a-koo′stĭks). The science of sounds and their perception.

acquired′ [L. *acquirere*, to get]. Not congenital; gotten after birth.

acraconitine (ak-ra-kon′ĭ-tin). An alkaloid derived from *Aconitum ferox*. SYN: *pseudaconitine*.

acragnosis (ak-rag-no′sis) [G. *akrōn*, extremity, + *gnōsis*, knowledge]. Absence of sensibility in limbs.

a′cral. Pert. to extremities.

acraldehyde (ak-ral′de-hīd). Volatile liquid produced by dry distillation of glycerin. SYN: *acrolein*.

acra′nia [G. *a-*, priv. + *kranion*, skull]. Congenital absence of the cranium, either partial or complete.

acrasia (a-kra′zĭ-ă) [G. *akrasia*, bad mixture]. Without self-control; intemperate.

acratia (a-kra′shĭ-ă) [G. *akrateia*, want of power]. 1. Loss of strength; impotence. 2. Incontinence, or loss of control.

acraturesis (a-krat-u-re′sis) [G. *akratēs*, powerless, + *ouresis*, urination]. 1. Urinary incontinence. 2. Vesicle atony causing feeble urination.

acremonio′sis. A condition marked by fever and development of swellings, due to *Acremonium potronii*.

acribom′eter [G. *acribēs*, exact, + *metron*, measure]. Instrument which measures minute objects.

acrid (ak′rid) [L. *acer*, *acris*, sharp]. Burning, bitter, irritating.

acriflavine (ak′rĭ-fla-vene) USP. A dye manufactured from coal tar.

USES: Antiseptic.

DOSAGE: For irrigations and treatment of wounds, 1 : 4000 to 1 : 1000 solutions in normal saline.

a. neutral. Same as acriflavine but less acid and less irritant.

USES: Urinary antiseptic.

DOSAGE: Orally ½ to 1½ gr. (0.3-0.1 Gm.).

acrimony (ak′rĭ-mō″nĭ) [L. *acrimonia*, pungency]. Quality of being pungent, acrid, irritating.

acrinia (a-krĭn′ĭ-ă) [G. *a-*, priv. + *krinein*, to separate]. Suppression or diminution of an excretion or secretion.

acrisia (a-kris′ĭ-ă) [G. *akrisia*, want of judgment]. Condition of uncertainty in diagnosis and prognosis.

acritical (ak-rit′ik-al) [G. *a-*, priv. + *kritikos*, critical]. Not marked by a crisis.

acritochro′macy [G. *akritos*, not distinguishing, + *chrōma*, color]. Color blindness.

acroagnosis (ak-ro-ag-no′sis) [G. *a-*, priv. + *akron*, extremity, + *gnōsis*, knowledge]. Absence of feeling in a limb.

acroanesthesia (ak″ro-an-es-the′zĭ-ă) [G. *akron*, extremity, + *an-*, priv. + *aisthēsis*, sensation]. 1. Absence of sensation. 2. Lack of sensation in one or more of the extremities.

acroarthritis (ă-kro-ar-thri′tis) [″ + *arthron*, joint, + *-itis*, inflammation]. Arthritis of the hands or feet.

acroasphyx′ia [″ + *asphyxia*, pulse stoppage]. Cold, pale condition of hands and feet; sym. of Raynaud's disease.

acroataxia (a″kro-ă-taks′ĭ-ă) [″ + *ataktos*, out of order]. Ataxia involving, or limited to, the fingers and toes.

ac′roblast [″ + *blastos*, germ]. The outer layer of the mesoblast.*

acrobystiolith (ă-kro-bis′tĭ-o-lith) [G. *akrobystia*, prepuce, + *lithos*, stone]. A calculus of the prepuce.

acrobystitis (ă-kro-bis-ti′tis) [″ + *-itis*, inflammation]. Preputial inflammation.

acrocepha′lia [G. *akron*, tip, + *kephalē*, head]. Pointed condition of the top of the cranium.

acrocephalic (ak″ro-se-fal′ik). A skull with a vertical index above 77; pert. to one with a peaked head.

acrocephaly (ak″-ro-sef′ă-lĭ). A malformed cranial vault having a high or peaked appearance due to premature closure of the coronal, sagittal, and lambdoid sutures.

acrocinesia, acrocinesis (ă-kro-sin-e′sĭ-ă, -sis) [G. *akros*, extreme, + *kinesis*, movement]. Excessive motion.

acrocinetic (a-kro-sin-et′ĭk). Showing acrocinesis.

acrocontrac′ture [G. *akron*, extremity, + L. *contrahere*, to draw together]. Contracture of the hands or feet.

acrocordon (a-kro-kor′dŏn) [" + *chordē*, cord]. A soft pedunculated growth.

acrocyanosis (ak-ro-si-a-no′sis) [" + *kyanōsis*, dark blue color]. Cyanosis of finger tips, and other extremities.

ETIOL: Due to vasomotor disturbances. Seen in catatonia, hysteria, etc.

acrodermatitis (ak″ro-der-ma-ti′tis) [" + *derma*, skin, + *-itis*, inflammation]. Dermatitis of the extremities.

a., continuous. An obstinate eczematous eruption confined to the extremities.

a. hiemalis. A form occurring in winter, affecting the extremities and tending to spontaneous disappearance.

acrodynia (ak-ro-din′ĭ-ă) [" + *odynē*, pain]. 1. Disorder of skin and limbs in children. SEE: *Swift's disease.* 2. Multiple neuritis of digits.

acroesthesia (ak-ro-es-the′zĭ-ă) [" + *aisthēsis*, sensation]. 1. Marked hyperesthesia. 2. Pain in the extremities.

acrogno′sis [" + *gnōsis*, knowledge]. Sensory perception of limbs.

acrohy′pothermy [" + *hypo*, under, + *thermē*, heat]. Abnormal coldness of extremities.

acrokinesia (ak-ro-kin-e′sĭ-ă) [" + *kinesis*, movement]. Excessive motion. SYN: *acrocinesia.*

acrolein (ak-ro′le-ĭn). A volatile liquid produced by dry distillation of glycerin.

acromac′ria. Spider-fingers. SYN: *arachnodactyly.*

acromania (ak-ro-ma′nĭ-ă) [G. *akros*, extreme, + *mania*, frenzy]. Mania accompanied by great motor activity and sometimes by muteness.

acromasti′tis [" + *mastōs*, breast, + *-itis*, inflammation]. Inflammation of the nipple; thelitis.

acromegaly (ak-ro-meg′ă-lĭ), **acromegalia** (ac-ro-me-ga′lĭ-ă) [" + *megas*, megal-, big]. A chronic disease (Marie's disease), characterized by progressive enlargement of the bones of the head, and soft parts of the hands, feet, thorax, and face; often associated with hypertrophy of the pituitary body or with diseases of thyroid gland.

ETIOL: Probably altered function of cerebral hypophysis.

SYM: Anterior fontanelle* often remains open until tenth year. Facial features are enlarged, mandible and malar bones becoming prominent with protrusion of orbital ridge. Teeth become widely separated. Swelling of fingers and toes with redness and pain, vomiting and headache.

acromelalgia (ak-ro-mel-al′jĭ-ă) [" + *melos*, limb, + *algos*, pain]. A disease of the extremities, esp. the feet, with pain upon walking. SYN: *erythromelalgia.*

SYM: Pain, redness, swelling of toes and fingers, headache, and vomiting.

acrometagenesis (ă-kro-mĕt-ă-jen′ĕ-sis) [" + *meta*, beyond, + *genesis*, origin]. Abnormal growth of extremities leading to deformity.

acromial (ak-ro′mĭ-al) [" + *ōmos*, shoulder]. Rel. to the acromion.*

a. angle. The angle at edge of spine of the *scapula* where it ascends to become the *acromion*, q.v.

a. process. The acromion.

a. reflex. Flexion of forearm with internal rotation of hand resulting from quick blow upon acromion. Elicited in hyperkinetic states.

acromicria (ak-ro-mik′rĭ-ă) [" + *mikros*, small]. Congenital shortness or smallness of the extremities.

acromioclavicular joint (a-kro″mĭ-o-klă-vik′u-lar) [" + *ōmos*, shoulder, + L. *clavicula*, small key]. Joint between the acromion (outward extension of spine of the *scapula*, forming part of shoulder) and *clavicle.*

acromiocoracoid (a-kro″mĭ-o-kor′ă-koid) [" + " + *korax*, crow, + *eidos*, resemblance]. Rel. to the acromion and coracoid process.

acro″miohu″meral [" + " + L. *humerus*, shoulder]. Pert. to acromion and humerus.

a. muscle. Deltoid muscle.

acromion (a-kro′mĭ-on) [G. *akron*, tip, + *ōmos*, shoulder]. The lateral, triangular projection of spine of scapula, forming point of the shoulder, and articulating with the clavicle. SEE: *acromiohumeral, acromiothoracic.*

acromiothoracic (a-kro″-mĭ-ō-thō-ras′ĭk) [" + " + *thorax*, breast plate]. Pert. to acromion and thorax.

acromphalus (ak-rom′fal-us) [" + *omphalos*, umbilicus]. 1. Center of navel. 2. Beginning of umbilical hernia, marked by abnormal projection of umbilicus.

acromyle (ak-rŏm′ĭl-e) [G. *akron*, point, + *myle*, patella]. The patella.*

acromyotonia (ak″ro-mĭ-o-to′nĭ-ă) [" + *mys*, muscle, + *tonōs*, tension]. Myotonia of extremities causing spasmodic deformity.

acronarcotic (a-kro-nar-kot′ĭk) [L. *acer, acris*, sharp, + G. *narcosis*, a benumbing]. Having the property of a narcotic and yet irritant in local effects.

acro″neuro′sis [G. *akron*, extremity, + *neuron*, nerve]. Any neurosis, usually vasomotor, in extremities.

acronyx (ak′ro-nĭks) [L. *acer, acris*, sharp, + G. *onyx*, claw]. Ingrowing of a nail.

acropachy (ak′ro-pak-ĭ) [G. *akron*, extremity, + *pachys*, thick]. Thickening of fingers or toes.

acroparal′ysis [" + *paralyein*, to disable at the side]. Paralysis of one or more extremities.

acroparesthesia (ak″ro-par-es-the′zĭ-ă) [" + *para*, beside, + *aisthesis*, sensation]. Extreme paresthesia or morbid sensation of the extremities.

acro″pathol′ogy [" + *pathos*, suffering, + *logos*, science]. Pathology of extremities.

acropathy (ak-rop′ath-ĭ). Any disease of extremities.

acrophobia (ak-ro-fo′bĭ-ă) [G. *akron*, top, + *phobos*, fear]. Morbid fear of high places.

acroposthitis (ak-ro-pos-thi′tis) [G. *akroposthis*, prepuce, + *-itis*, inflammation]. Inflammation of prepuce.

acroscleroderma (ak″ro-skler-o-der′mă) [G. *akron*, extremity, + *sclēros*, hard, + *derma*, skin]. Hard, thickened skin condition. SYN: *scleroderma.*

ac′rose. A substance forming starting point for synthesis of fruit sugars.

acrosinosis (ăk″rō-sĭ-nō′sĭs) [G. *akron*, point, + L. *sinus*, hollow, + G. *-ōsis*, condition]. Condition of having pointed or malformed sinuses.

ac′rosome [G. *akron*, extremity, + *soma*, body]. The ant. end of head of the spermatozoon.

acrosphacelus (ak-ro-sfas′el-us) [" + *sphakelos*, gangrene]. Gangrene of digits. SYN: *Raynaud's disease*.

acroteria (ak-ro-te′ri-ă) [G. *akrotērion*, summit]. The extremities.

acrotic (a-krot′ĭk). 1. [G. *a-*, priv. + *krotos*, striking]. Pert. to failure of or defective beating of the heart. 2. [G. *akrotēs*, an extreme]. Pert. to the surface or glands of the skin.

acrotism (ak′ro-tizm) [G. *a-*, priv. + *krotos*, a striking]. Apparent absence of the pulse.

acrotrophoneurosis (ak-ro-tro″fo-nu-ro′sis) [G. *akron*, extremity, + *trophē*, nourishment, + *neuron*, nerve, + *-osis*, condition]. Trophoneurosis of extremities.

acrylaldehyde (ak-ril-al′de-hīd). A volatile liquid from glycerin. SYN: *acrolein*.

ACS. Abbr. for American Chemical Society. Also antireticular cytotoxic serum.

ACTH. Abbr. for adrenocorticotropic hormone, a pituitary hormone that stimulates the cortex of the adrenal glands. RF. *cortisone*.

act re′flex. Involuntary reflex act immediately following any stimulus.

actin (ăkt′ĭn). One of the proteins in muscle fiber, the other being myosin.

actinic (ak-tin′ĭk) [G. *aktis*, ray]. Pert. to the chemical action of the sun's rays. PT: Pert. to actinism.* Capable of producing chemical changes as applied to radiant energy. Usually applied to radiant energy having this property.
 a. burns. Those caused by ultraviolet or sun rays. F. A. TREATMENT: As for dry heat burns. SEE: *burns*.

actinism (ak′tin-izm). That property of radiant energy which produces chemical changes, as in photography or heliotherapy.

ac″tinochem′istry [G. *aktis*, ray, + *chēmeia*, chemistry]. Action of rays from a luminous source.

actinocutitis. SEE: *actinodermatitis*.

actinodermatitis (ak″tin-o-der-ma-ti′tis) [" + *derma*, skin, + *-itis*, inflammation]. Actinoneuritis. Cutaneous inflammation, acute or chronic, caused by roentgen rays or radium.
 ETIOL: Susceptibility; those with little skin pigment being exceedingly sensitive; failure to use filters when indicated.
 SYM: Varying from reddish erythema, resembling sunburn from single overexposure, to gangrene and sloughing. *Keratoses.* Potentially malignant, may follow in subjects with dry seborrhea of long standing. Ulcers heal slowly if at all.
 TREATMENT: Astringent soothing lotions and boric acid ointment with carbolic acid in mild cases. Radium for x-ray ulcers and keratoses. Surgery in gangrenous forms.

actinogen (ak-tin′o-jen). Any radioactive element.

actinogenesis (ak″tin-o-jen′es-is) [G. *aktis*, ray, + *genesis*, source]. The source or production of actinic rays.

actinogenic (ak″tin-o-jen′ik) [G. *aktis*, *aktin*, ray, + *gennan*, to produce]. Producing rays; radiogenic.

actin′ogram [" + *gramma*, picture]. Roentgen ray photograph.

actin′ograph [" + *graphein*, to write]. A skiagraph. An x-ray picture.

actinol′ogy [" + *logos*, study]. Radiology; science of the chemical effects of light.

actinometer (ak″-tin-om′e-ter) [" + *metron*, meter]. PT: An instrument to measure the intensity of an actinic effect.

Actinomyces (ak-tin-o-mi′sēz) [" + *mykes*, fungus]. A vegetable parasite (*Actinomycetaceae*), causing actinomycosis.

actino″myce′tic. Pert. to Actinomyces.

actinomycetin (ăk″tĭn-ō-mī-sĕt′ĭn). A substance that is antibacterial from *Actinomyces*, effective against some gram-positive and gram-negative organisms.

actinomycin A. (ăk″tĭn-ō-mī′sĭn). An antibacterial substance from *Actinomyces antibioticus*, heat-stable and highly toxic, effective against gram-positive organisms. It is orange-colored, soluble in alcohol and ether.
 a. B. Similar to a. A. but not soluble in alcohol and chemically unsuitable because of its great toxicity.

actino″myco′ma [G. *aktis*, ray, + *mykes*, fungus, + *-oma*, tumor]. A tumor produced by actinomycosis.

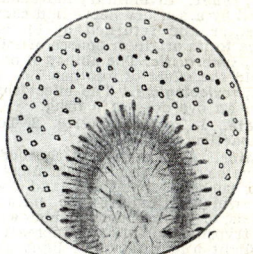

ACTINOMYCOSIS
Part of a "sulfur granule" from discharge. Swollen degenerated ends of ray fungus. The fungus (dark) is surrounded by the lymphocytes (dotted background).

actinomycosis (ak-tin-o-mi-ko′sis) [" + *osis*, condition]. A ray fungus disease in animals, sometimes communicated to man, invading the brain, lungs, gastroenteric tract, or jaw (lumpy jaw).
 ETIOL: *Actinomyces bovis*.
 SYM: Formation of slow growing granulomata, which later break down, discharging viscid pus containing minute yellowish granules. Mouth, tongue, jaw, lungs, and alimentary tract mostly affected. There are thickening of the tract, later suppuration, breaking down of tissues, and discharge of pus through sinuses.
 TREATMENT: Surgical. Incision and drainage, x-ray, and large doses of potassium iodide.

actino″mycot′ic. Pert. to actinomycosis.

actinon (ak′tin-on) [G. *aktis*, *aktin*, ray]. Emanation from actinium, which is one of the radium, actinium, and thorium series.

actino″neuri′tis [" + *neuron*, nerve, + *-itis*, inflammation]. Neuritis due to exposure to radium or x-rays.

actino″prax′is [" + *praxis*, a doing]. Employment of radioactive rays in diagnosis and treatment.

actinoscopy   A-22   **adaptometer**

actinos′copy [" + *skopein*, to write]. Examination of deep structures by x-rays.

actinostereos′copy [" + *stereos*, solid, + "]. Examination by x-ray. SYN: *actinoscopy*.

ac″tinother′apy [" + *therapeia*, healing]. PT: Treatment of disease by rays of light, esp. actinic or chemical light.

ac″tinotoxe′mia [" + *toxikon*, poison, + *aima*, blood]. Blood-poisoning produced by x-ray or radioactivity.

ac′tion [L. *actio*, from *agere*, to do]. Performance of a function, or process; in pathology, a morbid process.

   a., antagonistic. The ability of one drug to antagonize the effect of another.

   a., astringent. One in which the tissue cells are contracted by a chemical combination of drug and tissues, forming an albuminate. If this is not dissolved in fluids surrounding tissues, they are not acted upon further by the drug.

   a. current. PT: Same as *action potential*.

   a. of arrest. Inhibition. [*tion*.

   a., poisonous. SEE: *toxicological ac-*

   a. potential. The momentary difference in electrical potential between active and resting parts of a nerve fiber found when the two parts are connected with a sensitive galvanometer.

   a., reflex. Involuntary movement produced by a sensory nerve and carried to a center and returned by an efferent nerve to its origin or source of stimulus.

   a., synergistic. The ability of one drug to aid the effect of another.

   a., toxicological. The effect resulting from an overdose of a drug.

ac′tivate. 1. To make active. 2. To make radioactive.

ac′tivator. A substance in the body that activates glandular or chemical function, such as cholesterol and cod liver oil, which stimulate the parathyroid glands, or enterokinase* which activates the trypsinogen* of the pancreatic juice. Sunlight and ultraviolet light are also activators. SEE: *antibody*.

ac′tive prin′ciples. The chemical substances in drugs which cause changes in activity of the body; classified as *plant acids, alkaloids, fixed oils, glucosides, essential oils, balsams, oleoresins, saponins, resins, hormones, enzymes or ferments*. q.v. SEE: *drug action*.

ac′tol. Silver lactate, containing 50% silver. Usually employed in solutions from 1: 5000 to 1: 1000 in dentistry as an antiseptic.

actomyosin (ăk-tō-mī′ō-sĭn). The combination of actin and myosin in a muscle.

actual (ak′chu-al) [L. *actus*, past p. of *agere*, to do]. Real, existent.

   a. cautery. Cautery acting by virtue of its heat and not chemically.

acufilopressure (ak-u-fi′lo-presh-ūr) [L. *acus*, needle, + *filum*, thread, + *pressura*, pressure]. Acupressure increased by a ligature.   [*sharpness*.

acu′ity [L. *acuere*, to sharpen]. Clearness,

acu′minate [L. *acuminatus*, sharpened]. Conical or pointed.

acupressure (ak′u-presh″ur) [L. *acus*, needle, + *pressura*, pressure]. Compression of arteries by means of needles.

   a. forceps. Spring-handled forceps for compressing blood vessels.

   a. needles. Elastic needles for same purpose.

▢uncture [" + *punctura*, puncture]. ▢cture with needles for diagnostic and ▢peutic purposes; also in treatment ▢mas of lower limbs.

acus (a′kus) [L. needle]. A surgical needle.

acusection (ak-u-sek′shun) [" + *secare*, to cut]. Section by an electrosurgical needle.

acus′ticus [G. *akoustikos*, hearing]. The auditory or 8th cranial nerve. SEE: *Tables in Appendix*.

acute′ [L. *acutus*, sharp]. 1. Sharp, severe. 2. Having rapid onset, severe symptoms and a short course; not chronic.

acutenaculum (ak″u-ten-ak′u-lum) [L. *acus*, needle, + *tenaculum*, holder]. A needle holder.

acutor′sion [" + *torsio*, twisting]. Twisting of an artery with a needle to control hemorrhage.

acyanoblepsia (a″si-an-o-blep′sĭ-ă) [G. *a-*, priv. + *kyanos*, blue, + *blepsis*, sight]. Inability to discern blue colors. SYN: *acyanopsia*.

acyanopsia (a-si-an-op′sĭ-ă) [G. *a-*, priv. + *kyanos*, something blue, + *opsis*, sight]. Inability to discern blue colors.

acyesis (ă-si-e′sis) [G. *a-*, priv. + *kyēsis*, pregnancy]. 1. Absence of pregnancy. 2. Sterility of the female. 3. Incapability of natural delivery.

acystineuria (ă-sis-tin-u′rĭ-ă) [G. *a-*, priv. + *kystis*, bladder, + *neuron*, nerve]. Inability to control nervous mechanism of the bladder.

ad- [L.]. Prefix. Adherence, increase, toward, as *adduct*.

-ad. [L.]. Suffix. Toward; in direction of.

a. d. [L. *au′ris dex′tra*]. Abbr. *right ear*.

A. D. A. American Dental Association or American Dietetic Association.

ad′alin (Carbromal). USP. A white crystalline powder containing 36% bromine in combination with urea.

   ACTION AND USES: Mildly hypnotic, somewhat analgesic. Used as nerve sedative in neurasthenia, hysteria, and whooping cough.

   DOSAGE: As a sedative, 5 to 10 gr. (0.3-0.6 Gm.) in cold water. As hypnotic, from 10 to 20 gr. (0.6-1.3 Gm.).

adamantine (ad-ă-măn′tin) [G. *adamantinos*, very hard]. Very hard. Pert. to enamel of teeth.

ad″amantino′ma [" + *-oma*, tumor]. A tumor of the jaw, esp. the lower one, arising from the enamel organs.

   It may be partly cystic, partly solid, and may reach a large size; sometimes malignant.

adamantoblast (ad-a-măn′to-blast) [" + *blastos*, germ]. An enamel cell from which tooth enamel is formed.

adamantoblastoma (a-dă-man-to-blas-to′-mă) [" + " + *-oma*, tumor]. Overgrowth of an enamel cell.

adamanto′ma [" + *-oma*, tumor]. An enamel tissue tumor.

Adam's apple [*pomum Adami*]. The laryngeal prominence. SEE: *prominentia laryngea, pomum Adami*.

Adams' operation. Subcutaneous palmar aponeurotomy for Dupuytren's contraction.

   A.'s saw. A saw used in osteotomy.

Adams-Stokes syn′drome. Slow, perhaps irregular pulse, vertigo, syncope, and occasional pseudoepileptic convulsions and Cheyne-Stokes breathing.

adapta′tion [L. *adaptare*, to adjust]. The adjustment of the pupil of the eye to light variations.

adap′ter. A device for joining one part of an apparatus to another part.

adaptom′eter [L. *adaptare*, to fit, + G. *metron*, measure]. Device for measuring time required for ocular adaptation.

addephagia (ad-ef-a'jĭ-ă) [L. *addere*, to add, + G. *phagein*, to eat]. Insatiable hunger.

ad'dict [L. *addictus*, past p. *addicere*, to consent]. 1. To form a habit for the use of a drug. 2. One habituated to the use of a drug.

addiction (ă-dĭk'shun). Enslavement to some habit, esp. the drug habit.

a. state. A condition in which cessation of narcotic or other drug produces definite "symptoms of abstinence." SEE: *alcoholism, narcotism.*

addiment (ad'im-ent) [L. *addimentum*, an increase]. A substance described by Ehrlich, which resembles a ferment in its action and is present in normal serum.

It is destroyed by 56° to 58° C., and when attached to such cells as bacteria or red blood corpuscles by the intermediary body or amboceptor it dissolves or destroys these substances by bacteriolysis or hemolysis. SYN: *complement.*

add'isin. A substance supposed to be present in gastric juice which tends to keep red blood cells and hemoglobin at a normal level through stimulation of bone marrow; named after Thomas Addison, who described pernicious anemia during first half of 19th century.

addisonism (ad'ĭ-sŭn-izm). Symptom complex not due to disease of suprarenal glands, resembling that of Addison's disease.

Addison's disease. One due to deficiency in the secretion of adrenocortical hormones, the result of tuberculous infection of the gland or atrophy of the cortical tissue.

SYM: Bronzing of skin, esp. about the anus and surfaces subject to irritation; pigmentation of mucous membranes, extreme weakness including muscle weakness; asthenia,* moderate anemia of secondary type; marked gastrointestinal disturbances; diarrhea; loss of weight; low blood pressure; faintness or dizziness; nervousness and twitchings; psychic disturbances; white line on pressure of skin which lasts two or three minutes; renal insufficiency and dehydration; pains.

PROG: Formerly fatal within two or three years but now, if diagnosed early enough, it responds to various cortical preparations.

NP: Freedom from anxiety, the prevention of fatigue. The patient should be kept warm and bedsores must be guarded against. Watch the pulse for sudden changes, as fainting and syncope may occur, and patient may die in such an attack. He never should be left alone if confined to the bed. Keep the patient as cheerful as possible.

TREATMENT: Rest, nutritious but easily assimilable diet. A preparation made from the adrenal gland has been successful in some cases. Requires prompt medical attention. SEE: *adrenal, adrenalin, bronzed skin.*

A.'s keloid. Firm, round, discolored patches on skin. SYN: *morphea.* SEE: *scleroderma.*

ad'duct [L. *adductus*, past p. of *adducere*, to bring to]. To draw toward a center.

adduc'tion. 1. Movement of a limb toward the body's center or beyond it. 2. Position assumed by such a movement.

a. of the foot. Its movement around its own axis, or inward rotation around the leg's axis.

adduc'tor [L. a drawer toward]. A muscle which draws toward the medial line of the body or to a common center.

a. reflex. Contraction of adductors of right thigh, indicative of appendicitis, elicited with patient lying completely relaxed and with thighs half flexed. Pressure is exerted outward by a finger on inner side of each knee.

adelomorphous (ad"el-ō-mor'fus) [G. *adelōs*, not seen, + *morphē*, shape]. Having undefined form, as the pepsin glands.

adelphotaxis (ă-del'fō-tăk"sis) [G. *adelphos*, brother, + *taxis*, arrangement]. Grouping of cells in mutual relationships.

adenalgia (ad-en-al'jĭ-ă) [G. *aden*, gland, + *algos*, pain]. Adenodynia.* Pain in a gland.

ad'enase [" + *ase*, enzyme]. Enzyme secreted by the pancreas, spleen, and liver, and which converts *adenine*** into *hypoxanthine.** SEE: *enzymes.*

adenasthenia (ad"en-ăs-the'nĭ-ă) [" + *astheneia*, weakness]. Deficient glandular functional activity.

adendrit'ic [G. *a-*, priv. + *dendritēs*, rel. to a tree]. Without dendrites, as certain cells in spinal ganglia.

adenectomy (ad-en-ek'to-mĭ) [G. *aden*, gland, + *ek*, out, + *temnein*, to cut]. Excision of a gland.

ad"enecto'pia [" + " + *topos*, place]. A gland out of its normal place.

ad"enemphrax'is [" + *emphraxis*, stoppage]. Obstruction to discharge from a gland.

adenia (ad-e'nĭ-ă). Hypertrophy of lymphatic glands with hyperleukocytosis absent.

aden'iform [G. *adēn*, gland, + L. *forma*, shape]. Like a gland in form.

adenin(e (ad'en-in). 6-amino purine, $C_5H_5N_5$, a solid substance of the uric acid group, and derivable from the nucleic acids; e.g., of ox pancreas.

adeni'tis [G. *adēn*, gland, + *-itis*, inflammation]. Inflammation of lymph nodes or a gland.

adeniza'tion. Abnormal change into a glandlike structure.

ad'enoblast [G. *adēn*, gland, + *blastos*, germ]. 1. Any active gland cell. 2. Embryonic cell which forms a gland.

adenocarcinoma (ad-en-o-kar-sin-o'mă) [" + *karkinos*, cancer]. Adenoma* combined with carcinoma.

adenocele (ad'ĕ-no-sēl) [" + *kēlē*, tumor]. A cystic tumor arising from a gland. A tumor of glandular structure.

adenocellulitis (ad"en-o-sel-u-li'tis) [" + L. *cella*, small chamber, + G. *-itis*, inflammation]. Inflammation of a gland and adjacent cellular tissue.

adenochondroma (ad"ĕ-no-kon-dro'mă) [" + *chondros*, cartilage, + *-oma*, tumor]. Adenoma with added characteristics of chondroma.

adenocyst (ad'e-no-sist) [" + *kystis*, sac]. A cystic tumor arising from a gland.

adenocystoma (ad"en-o-sis-to'mă) [" + " + *-oma*, tumor]. Cystic adenoma.

adenodynia (ad"en-o-din'ĭ-ă) [" + *odynē*, pain]. Pain in a gland. SYN: *adenalgia.*

adenofibro'ma [" + L. *fibra*, fiber, + G. *-oma*, tumor]. Fibrous and glandular tissue tumor frequently in uterus.

adenogenous (ad-en-oj'en-us) [" + *gennan*, to produce]. Having origin in glandular tissue.

adenog'raphy [" + *graphein*, to write]. Study of or treatise on glands.

adenohypersthenia (ad"e-no-hi"pers-the'-nĭ-ă) [" + *yper*, excess, + *sthenos*, strength]. Excessive glandular activity.

adenoid   A-24   **adhesion**

adenoid (ad'en-oid) [G. *adēnoeides*, glandular]. A lobulated, lymphoid mass composed of lymphoid tissue similar to the tonsils, and containing masses of lymphocytes* found in tonsils, lymph nodes, spleen, and in the nodules of the intestines. SYN: *pharyngeal tonsil*.

a. tissue. Reticular tissue with lymph cells in the meshes of the network; also called lymphoid tissue.

adenoidectomy (ad-en-oid-ek'to-mĭ) [" + *ektomē*, excision]. Excision of adenoids.

NP: Watch color and pulse for signs of excessive bleeding; children often swallow blood and signs are only as above. SEE: *tonsillectomy*.

adenoids (ăd'ĕn-oids). The pharyngeal tonsils, especially when hypertrophied.

ad″enolipo′ma [G. *adēn*, gland, + *lipos*, fat, + *-oma*, tumor]. A tumor with characteristics of adenoma and lipoma.

adenol′ogy [" + *logos*, study]. Science of the glands.

adenolymphitis (ad-ĕ-no-lim-fī'tis) [" + L. *lympha*, lymph, + G. *-itis*, inflammation]. Inflammation of a lymphatic gland. SYN: *lymphadenitis*.

adenolymphocele (ad″en-o-lim'fo-sēl) [" + L. *lympha*, lymph, + G. *kēlē*, tumor]. Cystic dilatation of a lymph node from obstruction.

adenolymphoma (ad″en-o-lim-fo'mă) [" + " + *-oma*, tumor]. A lymph gland adenoma.

adenoma (ad-en-o'mă) (*Pl. adenomata*) [" + *-oma*, tumor]. A neoplasm of glandular epithelium.

SEE: *chorioadenoma*.

a., acinous. Form with glands having acinous structure.

a., chromophobe. Tumor of pituitary gland composed of cells that do not stain readily.

a., malignant. Adenoma combined with carcinoma. SYN: *adenocarcinoma*.

a., multiglandular. A. containing many small changed glands.

a. sebaceum. Steatadenoma; acanthoma of sebaceous glands. Benign tumorlike growths developing from epithelium of sebaceous glands which undergo fatty but never colloid metamorphosis.

ETIOL: Unknown. Congenital in those mentally below par.

SYM: Pinhead to split-pea size, usually over nose, cheeks, nasolabial folds; yellowish or pinkish.

PROG: Harmless but persistent.

TREATMENT: Electric needle, cutaneous punch, curette.

a. simplex. Form with hyperplastic condition of the glands.

adenomalacia (ad″ĕ-no-mal-a'sĭ-ă) [" + *malakia*, softening]. Glandular softening.

adenomatome (a-dĕ-no'mă-tōm) [" + *tomē*, a cutting down]. Instrument for removing adenoids.

ad″enomato′sis [" + *-oma*, tumor, + *-osis*, increase]. Multiple glandular tissue overgrowths.

adenomatous (ad-ĕ-no'mă-tus). Pert. to adenomas.

adenomere (ad'en-o-mēr) [G. *aden*, gland, + *meros*, part]. The functional part of a gland.

adenomycosis (ad″dĕ-nō-mī-ko'sis) [" + *mykēs*, fungus, + *-osis*, increase]. Disease of the lymph nodes. SYN: *Hodgkin's disease*.

adenomyoma (ad-ĕ-no-mĭ-o'mă) [" + *mys*, muscle, + *-oma*, tumor]. A tumor containing glandular and smooth muscular tissue.

adenomyometritis (ad-en-o-mi-o-me-trī'-tis) [" + " + *metra*, womb, + *-itis*, inflammation]. GYN: A hyperplastic condition of the uterus which is the result of pelvic inflammation and grossly resembles an adenomyoma.

adenomyosis (ad-ĕ-no-mi-o'sis) [" + " + *-osis*, condition]. Ectopic adenomatous growths.

ad″enomyxo′ma [" + *myxa*, mucus, + *-oma*, tumor]. A tumor with adenoma and myxoma characteristics.

ad″enomyx″osarco′ma [" + " + *sarx*, flesh, + *-oma*, tumor]. A tumor with adenoma, myxoma, and sarcoma characteristics.

adenoncus (ad-en-on'kus) [" + *ogkos*, tumor]. A tumor of a gland or its enlargement.

adenopathy (ad-en-op'ă-thĭ) [" + *pathos*, suffering]. Swelling and morbid change in lymph nodes; glandular disease.

ad″enopharyngi′tis [" + *pharygx*, throat, + *-itis*, inflammation]. Inflammation of tonsils and pharyngeal mucous membrane.

adenophlegmon (ad-ĕ-no-fleg'mon) [" + *phlegmonē*, inflammation]. Inflammation (acute) of a gland and its adjacent tissue.

ad″enophthal′mia [" + *ophthalmos*, eye]. Inflammation of the meibomian glands.

ad″enosarco′ma [" + *sarx*, flesh, + *-oma*, tumor]. A tumor with characteristics of adenoma and sarcoma.

adenosclerosis (ad-ĕ-no-skle-ro'sis) [" + *sclērōsis*, hardening]. Glandular induration.

adenosis (ad-en-o'sis) [" + *-osis*, increase]. Any disease of a gland, esp. of a lymphatic gland.

a., syphilitic. Enlarged and indurated lymphatic glands symptomatic of syphilis; most commonly the inguinal, the posterior cervical, and the cubital.

adenotome (ad'en-o-tom) [" + *tomē*, cutting instrument]. An instrument for incision of a gland.

ad″enot′omy [" + *tomē*, a cutting up]. 1. Glandular anatomy. 2. Excision or incision of a gland.

adenotyphus (ad″en-o-ti'fus) [" + *typhos*, stupor]. Abdominal typhus fever.

adeps (ad'eps) [L.]. Lard; omental hogfat.

a. anseri′nus. Goose grease.

a. benzoina′tus. Benzoinated lard.

a. la′nae. Wool fat.

a. ovil′lus, a. ovis. Mutton suet or tallow.

ader′mia [G. *a-*, priv. + *derma*, skin]. Lack of skin, congenital or acquired.

ader″mogen′esis [" + " + *genesis*, production]. Imperfect growth or repair of skin.

adherent (ad-he'rent) [L. *ad*, to, + *haerere*, to stick]. 1. Attached to, as of two surfaces. 2. OB: A placenta that remains attached to the uterine wall after delivery.

adhes′ion. Abnormal joining of parts to each other.

CAUSES OR PREDISPOSING CONDITIONS: 1. Abdominal operations. 2. Congenital bands. 3. Previous intraabdominal; inflammations not treated by operation, as infections of the gallbladder, attacks of appendicitis, and inflammation of the pelvic organs.

SYM: Abdominal pain, nausea, and vomiting; elevation of the pulse without a rise in temperature; intestinal obstruction.

adhesion, primary   A-25   **adnexal**

TREATMENT: Operative at earliest moment. Diathermy* may help through increase of circulation.
PROG: Favorable if early surgical measures are resorted to. SEE: *brisement, cardiosymphysis*.

a., primary. Healing by first intention.

a., secondary. Healing by second intention.

adhesive (ad-he'siv) [F. *adhésif*]. 1. Causing adhesion. 2. Sticky; adhering. 3. That which causes 2 bodies to adhere.

a. inflammation. A serous membrane inflammation exuding fibrinous matter making adhesions possible.

a. plaster [*emplastrum adhaesivum*]. A heavy material, as cloth, coated with gummy sticky materials to remain in place after application. Many varieties are on the market, some are colored, others elastic, and some are waterproofed. Made of resin, rubber, moleskin, soap plaster, or various types of isinglass.
USES: 1. For support as in sprains, strains, etc. 2. Hold dressings in place. 3. Approximate skin edges (narrow strips passed through flame to sterilize) and to make more adhesive. 4. Obliterate cavities. 5. To make pressure. 6. Circular or oval pads to prevent pressure in center. 7. Many other purposes.

adiadochokinesis (a-dī-ad″o-ko-kin-e'sis) [G. *adiadochos*, perpetual, + *kinēsis*, movement]. 1. Inability to make rapid alternating movements. 2. Incessant movement. 3. NEUR: Rapid antagonistic movements which cannot be carried out with accuracy. Seen in cerebellar disease. RS: *asynergia, dysmetria, gait*.

adiaphoresis (ă-di-af-o-re'sis) [G. *a-*, priv. + *diaphoresis*, perspiration]. Deficiency or absence of sweat.

adiapneustia (ad-ī-ap-nŭ'stĭ-ă) [G. *a-*, priv. + *diapneusis*, an exhaling]. Absence of perspiration. SYN: *adiaphoresis*.

adiastole (ă-di-as'to-le) [" + *diastolē*, dilatation]. Imperceptibility of diastole.

adiathermancy (ă-dī-ă-thur'măn-sī) [" + *dia*, through, + *thermē*, heat]. State of being impervious to heat.

adiemorrhysis (ad″i-em-or'i-sis) [" + " + *aima*, blood, + *rysis*, a flowing]. Arrest of capillary circulation.

adip'ic [L. *adeps*, fat]. Relating to fat; fatty.

adipocele (ad'ī-pō-sēl) [" + G. *kēlē*, tumor]. Fat in a hernial sac. Lipocele.

adipocel'lular [" + *cellula*, small storeroom]. Made up of or pert. to fat and connective tissue.

adipocere (ad'ī-pō-sēr) [" + *cera*, wax]. A waxy substance converted from dead tissue.

ad″ipofibro'ma [" + *fibra*, fiber, + G. *-oma*, tumor]. A fibroma and adipoma.

adipogenous (ad-ī-pŏj'en-us) [" + G. *gennan*, to produce]. Inducing the formation of fat.

adipolysis (ad-ī-pŏl'ĭ-sis) [" + *lysis*, setting free]. The hydrolysis of fat.

adipolytic (ad″ip-o-lit'ĭk). Pert. to adipolysis.

adipoma (ad-ip-o'mă) [L. *adeps*, fat, + *oma*, tumor]. Fatty tissue tumor. SYN: *lipoma*.

a″dipopex'is [" + G. *pēxis*, fixation]. The storing of fat.

a'dipose. Fatty, pert. to fat.

a. capsule. Renal fat.

a. fossae. Fatty accumulations on outer mammary surface.

a. tissue. Connective or areolar tissue containing masses of fat cells.

adiposis (ad-ī-po'sis) [L. *adeps*, fat, + G. *-ōsis*, increase]. Abnormal accumulation of fat in the body. SYN: *corpulence, liposis*.

a. doloro'sa. A neurosis, the symptoms of which are nodular formations, chronic bronchitis, and pain.

a. hepat'ica. Fatty degeneration or infiltration of the liver.

a. tuberosa simplex. A disease resembling adiposis dolorosa in which the fat occurs in small circumscribed nodules sensitive or painful to touch. SYN: *Anders' disease*.

adipositis (ad-ĭ-po-si'tis) [L. *adiposa*, fatty tissue, + G. *-itis*, inflammation]. Infiltration of an inflammatory nature in and beneath subcutaneous adipose tissue.

adipos'ity. Excessive fat in the body. SYN: *adiposis*.

adipo″sogen'ital syndrome. Combination of adiposity, impaired development of genital organs, and change in secondary sex characteristics. SEE: *Fröhlich's syndrome*.

adiposuria (ad-ĭ-pō-su'rĭ-ă) [L. *adeps*, fat, + G. *ouron*, urine]. Fat in the urine. SYN: *lipuria*.

adip'sia, ad'ipsy [G. *a-*, priv. + *dipsa*, thirst]. Absence of thirst.

adipsous (ă-dip'sus). Quenching thirst.

ad'itus [L.]. An approach; an entrance.

a. ad antrum. The recess of the tympanic cavity, which lodges head of malleus and greater part of incus.

a. ad aquaeductum Sylvii. The entrance of the sylvian aqueduct, situated at lower posterior angle of third ventricle of brain.

a. ad infundibulum. A small canal leading from the third ventricle into the infundibulum.

a. ad laryngem, a. laryngis. Upper aperture of larynx.

adjuster (ad-jus'ter) [L. *a*, to, + *juste*, just, right]. Device for holding together the ends of the wire forming a suture.

ad'juvant [L. *adjuvans*, pres. p. of *adjuvare*, to aid]. 1. That which assists. 2. MAT. MED: A drug added to a prescription to hasten or increase the action of a principal ingredient; synergist.

Adler's organ-inferiority. A theory that ascribes psychic compensations to structural defects, tending to minimize the importance of psychosexual and other functional inadequacies.

ad lib. Abbr. L. *ad lib'itum*, at pleasure.

admax'illary [L. *ad*, to, + *maxilla*, jaw]. Accessory to the jaw.

a. gland. An occasional accessory salivary gland located near the angle of the jaw excreting through the parotid duct.

adnata (ad-na'tă) [L. *adnatus*, past p. *adnasci*, to grow to]. Layer of conjunctiva touching the eyeball. SEE: *tunica adnata*.

adner'val [L. *ad*, to, + *nervus*, nerve]. Near a nerve.

adneu'ral [" + G. *neuron*, nerve]. Adnerval.

adnex'a [L. *adnectere*, to tie or bind to]. Accessory parts as *a. u'teri*, the oviducts, and ovaries.

a. oculi. Lacrimal glands.

a. uteri. Ovaries and oviducts.

adnex'al [L. *adnexus*, past p. *adnectere*, to tie to]. Adjacent or appending.

adnexi'tis [L. *adnexus* + G. *-itis*, inflammation]. Inflammation of the *adnexa uteri*.

adnexopexy (ad-neks'ō-peks-ē) [" + G. *pexis*, a putting together]. Fixing the fallopian tube and ovary to the abdominal wall.

adolescence (ad-o-les'ens) [L. *adolescens*, pres. p. *adolescere*, to grow up]. The period from the beginning of puberty until adult life. In temperate climates 15 yr. for boys and 13-14 yr. for girls. Recent research proves adolescence is earlier in temperate climates and later in hot and cold regions.

ad"oles'cent. 1. Pert. to adolescence.* 2. Young man or woman not fully grown.

adoral (ad-o'ral) [L. *ad*, to, + *os, oris*, mouth]. Toward or near the mouth.

adosculation (ad-ōs-kû-la'shun) [L. *adosculare*, to kiss]. 1. Impregnation without intromission of the penis. 2. Insertion of one part into the cavity of another.

adrenal (ăd-rēn'ăl) [L. *ad*, to, + *ren*, kidney]. 1. Near the kidney. 2. a. gland. Also called *ad. capsule, ad. body, suprarenal gland, suprarenal capsule*. A triangular shaped body adjacent to and covering the superior surface of each kidney. It is a gland of internal secretion producing hormones essential to life.

EMBRYOLOGY: The adrenal glands are essentially double organs each composed of an outer *cortex* and an inner *medulla*. The cortex arises in the embryo from a region of the mesoderm, which also gives rise to the gonads or sex organs. The medulla arises from ectoderm which also gives rise to the sympathetic nervous system.

ANAT: The entire gland is enclosed in a tough connective tissue capsule from which *traveculae* extend into the cortex. The cortex consists of cells arranged into three zones; the outer *zona glomerulosa*, the middle *zona fasciculata*, and the inner *zona reticularis*. The cells are arranged in a cordlike fashion. The medulla consists of chromaffin cells arranged in groups or anastomosing cords. The two adrenal glands are situated retroperitoneally, each imbedded in perirenal fat above its respective kidney.

The right adrenal measures 4 x 1.3 x .6 cm. (1½ x ½ x ¼ inch), and weighs 2 to 2.5 Gm. (30 to 40 gr). The left adrenal measures 4.5 x 2 x .6 cm. (1¾ x ¾ x ¼ inch), and weighs 2.5 to 3 Gm. (40 to 45 gr.)

PHYS: THE MEDULLA. Secretes the hormone *epinephrine* or *adrenalin* acting on all body structures, innervated by the sympathetic division of the autonomic nervous system. Its effects are similar to those resulting from stimulating sympathetic nerves, namely: elevation of blood pressure resulting from increase in rate and force of heart beat and constriction of arterioles, inhibition of gastrointestinal movements; relaxation of smooth muscles in bronchioles; dilatation of pupils of eyes; liberation of glucose from liver.

The emergency theory or the fright, fight, or flight theory, was advanced by Dr. Cannon of Harvard University to explain the function of the adrenal medulla. According to this theory the medulla secretes very little of its product during ordinary activities, but under the influence of pain, fear, rage, or asphyxia, it secretes a larger amount of its hormone, which enters the blood stream and stimulates body to meet either physical or mental emergencies. The principal secretion of the cortex is corticosterone and other hormones; that of the adrenal medulla, is adrenalin.

Absence or disease of the adrenal cortex may cause Addison's disease, resulting in anemia, tiredness, languor, aching, skin changes, and inability to strain. Poor blood circulation, indigestion, and insomnia. Personality may be altered by an adrenal disorder. One may become morose, self conscious, inhibited, and unhappy. If placid, one may be phlegmatic or with little interest in life. Lack of adrenalin will cause one to react too slowly in an emergency. It has been claimed that professional soldiers, such as Napoleon, exhibit unusual activity as result of adrenalin secretion.

Although the hormone of the adrenal cortex decreases brain excitability, another hormone of the cortex, abbreviated as DOCA, increases it. It is said that disposition may be maintained by the proper balance of these two hormones.

THE CORTEX: Secretes a large number of substances, some twenty-eight crystalline compounds (steroids) of known constitution having been isolated from cortical material. In addition there is an "amorphous" fraction which to date has not been analyzed. Cortical tissue is essential to life. Its removal or destruction results in disturbances in salt balance with loss of sodium and accumulation of potassium. Kidney function is impaired; carbohydrate stores depleted; resistance to stress situations (injury, cold, heat, fatigue, infection) is decreased. SEE: *cortex*.

Among the cortical hormones are *cortisone* (Kendall's compound E), *corticosterone* and its derivatives, among them *desoxycorticosterone* and *17-hydroxycorticosterone* (Kendall's compound F). Cortisone has been shown to have a marked therapeutic value in the treatment of rheumatoid arthritis and other ailments. The secretion of cortical hormones is under the control of the adrenocorticotrophic hormone (ACTH) produced by the hypophysis.

The cortex is also capable of producing androgens and estrogens, the male and female sex hormones.

PATH: *Medulla:* Abnormalities in the function of the medulla are rare. *Hyposecretion* produces few changes of physiological significance. *Hypersecretion* may result from tumors involving the chromophil cells. Symptoms are: paroxysmal hypertension, tachycardia, sweating, dilatation of the pupils, headache.

CORTEX: *Hypersecretion:* This may result from tumors involving the cortex (*primary hypercorticalism*), or from hyperactivity of the anterior lobe of the hypophysis (secondary hypercorticalism). It is accompanied by disturbances involving the sex organs and secondary sexual characteristics (*adrenogenital syndrome*). The symptoms vary with the age of the individual at time of the onset of the disease and the sex of the patient. In fetal life or early childhood, sexual precocity occurs in both sexes and is accompanied by obesity, great muscular development, accelerated growth, and early development of secondary sexual characters. In adult females

there is marked virilism (*masculinization*) and pronounced development of body hair (*hirsutism*); male characters appear, menstruation may cease, mammary glands atrophy. In adult males, the condition is rare and results in feminization; the testes atrophy, mammary glands develop.
  Hyposecretion: Addison's disease. This disease is the result of chronic adrenal cortical insufficiency, which may be brought about by tuberculosis of the glands, cancer, or atrophy. Symptoms are: extreme muscular weakness, fatigue, gastrointestinal disturbances, impaired nervous functioning, reduced basal metabolism, and a characteristic increase in pigmentation of the skin and mucous membrane of the mouth. Various degrees of cortical insufficiency may occur.
  RS: *Addison's disease, adrenalin, adrenalism, asurrenalism, chromaffin, kidney, neurocirculatory asthenia.*

adrenalectomy (ad-rē-nǎl-ek'tō-mǐ) [" + G. *ektomē*, excision]. Excision of an adrenal body.

adren'alin (epinephrin(e). USP. ($C_9H_{13}O_3$-N). Proprietary name for epinephrine. The active principal of the medulla of the adrenal gland. *See: epinephrine.*
  FUNCTION: Thought to be concerned with maintenance of the tonus of blood vessels and heart.
  USES: (a) Heart and circulatory stimulant; (b) raises blood pressure; (c) checks secretions as in rhinitis, asthma, hay fever, etc.; (d) a hemostatic in hemorrhages; (e) for operations on nose, as it renders the tissues bloodless; (f) allays spasm of asthma; (g) contracts the uterus; (h) overcomes local congestions.
  ADM: (a) Locally; (b) hypodermically.
  DOSAGE: *Internally,* 5 to 15 ♏ (0.3-1.0 cc.) of the 1:1000 solution. *Subcut.,* 1/120 ♏ (0.005 cc.). *Locally,* 1:10,000 to 1:1000 solutions. In recent years a solution of 1:100 has been marketed, and recommended for use by inhalation in allergic conditions, particularly asthma.

adrenaline'mia [L. *ad,* to, + *rēn,* kidney, + G. *aima,* blood]. Adrenalin in the blood.

adrenalinu'ria [" + G. *ouron,* urine]. Adrenalin in the urine.

adren'alism. Illness due to overactivity of suprarenal glands.

adrenalitis (ad-re"nǎl-i'tis). Inflammation of the suprarenal gland; adrenitis.

adrener'gic [L. *ad,* to, + *rēn,* kidney, + G. *ergon,* work]. Applied to nerve fibers which when stimulated, release epinephrine (adrenalin) or an epinephrine-like substance at their terminations. The substance has been called *sympathin.* Most postganglionic sympathetic fibers are adrenergic.

adrenin(e (ad-ren'ǐn). A preparation made from the medulla of the suprarenal gland; the adrenal hormone.

adreni'tis. Inflammation of the suprarenal gland. SYN: *adrenalitis.**

adrenop'athy. Suprarenopathy. Any disease of the suprarenal glands.

adren"oster'one. Male sex hormone obtained from urine.

adren'otrope, adrenotrop'ic. One of adrenal type. Pert. to adrenotropism.

adren"otrop'in. Hormone obtained from male urine, controlling islands of Langerhans.

adrenotropism (ad-rĕn-ōt'ro-pizm) [L. *ad,* to, + *rēn,* kidney, + G. *tropē,* turning]. A type dominated by adrenal influence.

adsorp'tion [L. *ad,* to, + *sorbere,* to suck in]. 1. A process whereby a gas or a dissolved substance becomes concentrated at the surface of a solid or at the interfaces of a colloid system. Ex: removal of dyes from solutions by filtration through charcoal. 2. Attachment of one substance to the surface of another.

adster'nal (ad-ster'nal) [L. *ad,* toward + G. *sternon,* chest). In situation, near, or in direction, toward the sternum.

adter'minal [L. *ad,* to, + *terminalis,* end]. Toward extremity of any structure.

adul'terant [L. *adulterare,* to falsify]. That which adulterates or weakens a substance.

adultera'tion. The addition of an impure or weaker substance to another one.

adus'tion [L. *adustus,* past p. *adurere,* to burn]. 1. Being scorched, parched, dry. 2. Application of cauterization.

advancement (ad-vans'ment) [Fr. *avancer,* to set forth]. Operation to remedy strabismus, by which the insertion of an ocular muscle is attached at a point further removed from its origin.
  a., capsular. Attachment of capsule of Tenon in front of its normal position.

adventitia (ad-ven-tish'yǎ) [L. *adventitius,* coming from abroad]. The outermost covering of a structure or organ, such as the *tunica adventitia,* or outer coat of an artery.

adventitious (ad-ven-tish'us). 1. Acquired; accidental. 2. Arising sporadically. 3. Pert. to adventitia.

ad'vitant [L. *ad,* to, + *vita,* life]. A vitamin.

adynamia, adynamy (a-din-am'ǐ-ǎ, -din'-a-mǐ) [G. *a-,* priv. + *dynamis,* strength]. Asthenia,* debility.

adynamic (ad-ī-nam'ik). Weak, feeble, asthenic. Pert. to adynamia.

aegophony (e-gof'o-nǐ) [G. *aix, aigos,* goat, + *phōnē,* voice]. A goatlike bleating sound heard on auscultation of the chest.

aerated (a'er-a-ted) [G. *aer,* air]. Containing air or gas.

aeration (a-er-a'shun). 1. Act of airing. 2. Change of venous into arterial blood in the lungs. 3. Saturating a fluid with gases.

aerendocardia (a-er-en-do-kar'dǐ-ǎ) [G. *aer,* air, + *kardia,* heart]. Bubble of air in the blood within the heart.

aerenterectasia (a"er-en-ter-ek-ta'zǐ-ǎ) [" + *enteron,* intestine, + *ektasis,* stretching out]. Distention of intestine with gas.

aerial (a-e'rǐ-al). Pert. to the air.

aeriferous (a-er-if'er-us) [G. *aer,* air, + L. *ferre,* to bear]. Carrying air.

aeriform (a-er'ǐ-form) [" + L. *forma,* shape]. Airlike; gaseous.

a'erobe [" + *bios,* life]. A microörganism which can live and grow only in the presence of free oxygen.

aerobian (a-er-o'bǐ-an). Aerobiotic; living only in the presence of oxygen.

aerobic (a-er-o'bik). 1. Living only in presence of oxygen. 2. Concerning an organism living only in oxygen.

aero'bion (pl. *aerobia*) [G. *aer,* air, + *bios,* life]. An organism which lives only in presence of oxygen.
  a., facultative. One able to live without oxygen under some conditions, but which normally requires it.
  a., obligate. One which cannot live without air.

aerobiosis (a-er-o-bi-o'sis). Living in an atmosphere containing oxygen.

aerobiotic (a-er-o-bī-ot'ik). Pert. to aerobiosis.

aerocele (a'er-o-sēl) [G. *aer*, air, + *kēlē*, tumor]. Gas within and distending a cavity.

aerocolpos (a"er-o-kol'pos) [" + *kolpos*, vagina]. Distention of the vagina with air.

aerocoly (ă-ĕ-rok'ō-lĭ) [" + *kōlon*, colon]. Distention of colon with gas.

aerocystoscopy (a-ĕr-ō-sis-tos'kō-pĭ) [" + *kystis*, bladder, + *skopein*, to view]. Examination of the bladder, when distended by air, with a cystoscope.

aerodermectasia (a-er-ō-der-mek-ta'zĭ-ă) [" + *derma*, skin, + *ektasis*, stretching out]. Subcutaneous emphysema.

aerodynam'ics [" + *dynamis*, force]. Science of air or gases in motion.

aeroembolism (a-er-ō"em'bō-lizm) [G. *aer*, air, + *embolus*, blood]. A condition in which nitrogen bubbles form in blood and tissues during rapid ascent to high altitudes.

SYM: Boring, gnawing pain in joints, itching of skin and eyelids, unconsciousness, convulsions and paralysis.

Prevention may be secured by becoming supersaturated with oxygen while at high altitude by use of oxygen mask.

aerogen (a'er-o-jen) [" + *gennan*, to produce]. A gas-forming microörganism.

aerogenesis (a-er-o-jen'e-sis) [" + *genesis*, production]. Formation of gas.

aerogenic (a-er-o-jen'ik). Gas-forming.

aerogenous (a-er-oj'en-us). Gas-forming.

aerogoniscope (a-er-og-on'is-kōp) [G. *aer*, air, + *gone*, seed, + *skopein*, to see]. Device for collecting organic dust from the air.

aerohydrop'athy, aerohydrother'apy [G. *aer*, air, + *ydor*, water, + *pathos*, suffering, - + *therapeia*, treatment]. Treatment by application of air and water.

aerometer (a-er-om'e-ter) [" + *metron*, measure]. Device for measuring density of gases.

aeromicrobe (a-er-o-mi'krōb) [" + *mikros*, small, + *bios*, life]. Any aerobic organism.

aeroneurosis (a-er-o-nu-ro'sis) [" + *neuron*, nerve]. A chronic functional nervous disorder affecting aeroplane flyers.

ETIOL: Emotion is the background of their fatigue.

SYM: General irritability, gastric neurosis, insomnia, hyperacidity, and depletion of the high mental center; probably nerve tissue destruction.

aeropathy (a-er-op'ath-ĭ) [" + *pathos*, suffering]. Morbid condition caused by atmospheric pressure, such as *mountain sickness*, and caisson disease.

aeroperito'nia [" + *peritonaiein*, to stretch over]. Distention of peritoneal cavity with gas.

aerophagy (a-er-of'aj-ĭ) [" + *phagein*, to eat]. Swallowing of air.

aerophilous (a-ĕr-of'ĭ-lŭs) [" + *philos*, fond]. Requiring air for development. SYN: *aerobic*.

aerophobia (a-er-o-fo'bĭ-ă) [" + *phobos*, fear]. Morbid fear of a draft or of fresh air.

aerophore (a'er-o-fōr) [" + *phoros*, bearing]. 1. Conducting air. 2. Apparatus for introducing air into lungs of stillborn child.

a'erophyte [" + *phytos*, plant]. An organism or plant that lives upon air.

aeroplethysmograph (a-er-o-ple-thiz'mo-graf) [" + *plethysmos*, enlargement, + *graphein*, to write]. Instrument for recording air respired.

aeropleura (a"er-o-plu'ră) [" + *pleura*, side]. Pneumothorax; air in pleural cavity.

aeroporotomy (a"er-o-po-rot'o-mĭ) [" + *poros*, passage, + *tomē*, cutting]. Operation for admitting air into the air passages.

aeroscope (a'er-o-skōp) [" + *skopein*, to view]. Device for examining air dust.

aerosporin (ā"ĕr-ŏs-pôr'ĭn). An antibiotic from a soil organism similar to *Bacillus aerosporus*.

USES: Said to be more effective than penicillin or streptomycin in typhoid, dysentery, cholera, and other intestinal diseases; also in whooping cough.

ACTION: It attacks gram-negative germs whereas penicillin attacks only gram-positive germs. It does not attack tuberculosis germs as does streptomycin.

aerotaxis (a"er-o-tak'sĭs) [" + *taxis*, arrangement]. Movement of organisms away from or toward air, said of aerobic and anaerobic bacteria.

aerotherapy (a-er-o-ther'a-pĭ) [" + *therapeia*, treatment]. PT: Air-bath therapy.

aerothermotherapy (a"er-o-ther"mo-ther'-ă-pĭ) [" + *thermos*, hot, + *therapeia*, treatment]. Applications of hot air.

aerotonometer (a-er-o-to-nom'e-ter) [" + *tonos*, tension, + *metron*, measure]. Apparatus for measuring tension of gases of the blood.

aerotympanal (a"er-o-tĭm'pă-năl) [" + *tympanum*]. Pert. to air in tympanum.

aerourethroscope (a"er-o-u-reth'ro-skōp) [" + *ourethra*, urethra, + *skopein*, to view]. An apparatus for making urethral examination by electric light, after dilatation by air.

aerourethroscopy (a"er-ō-ū-rē-thros'kō-pĭ). Examination of the urethra when distended with air.

aer"teriver'sion [G. *aēr*, air, + *tērein*, to hold, + L. *vertiō*, a turning]. Eversion of artery ends to stop hemorrhage. SYN: *arterioversion*.

aer"teriver'ter. Instrument for use in aerteriversion. SYN: *arterioverter*.

aesthet'ic moral'ity. Right conduct as an expression of the ego ideal apart from any consideration of prudence or fear of wrongdoing. [Without fever.

afeb'rile [G. *a*-, priv. + L. *febris*, fever].

afen'il. Compound of calcium chloride and urea in aqueous solution.

ACTION AND USES: For calcium deficiency; coagulative.

DOSAGE: 10% solution, 10 cc. intravenously every 2nd or 3rd day.

af'fect [L. *affectus*, past p. *afficere*, to apply oneself to]. PSY: The emotional reactions associated with an experience. SYN: *psychic trauma*.

affection (ăf-fĕk'shŭn) [L. *afficere*, to act upon or affect]. 1. Love, feeling. 2. Disease, physical or mental.

a.. celiac. Intestinal infantilism.

affec'tive [L. *afficere*, to apply oneself to]. Stimulating emotion. [sanity.

a. insanity. Impulsive or emotional in-

a. memory. Memory of a psychic trauma causing recurrence of emotion.

a. psycho'sis. PSY: An emotional one as manic-depressive psychosis.

ETIOL: Possible hereditary predisposition or highly charged emotional environment.

SYM: Occurs most frequently from 18 to 35 yr. of age and more frequently in women. Recurrent attacks common. Overactivity, dehydration, sometimes fever and delirium. Prankish, excited, decorative, abusive, destructive. Flight of ideas, moody, delusions of grandeur.

affective, spasms   A-29   **age of consent**

NP: Don't be oversolicitous, don't bribe, cheat, threaten, be discourteous, lie, or show off patient, or give all they ask. Show no fear. Occupational therapy, exercise, and games. Elimination, packs, and tubs may be indicated.

a. spasms. Attacks of laughing, screaming, or weeping in hysteria.

af′ferent [L. *ad*, to, + *ferre*, to bear]. Carrying impulses toward a center, as when a sensory nerve carries a message toward the brain; also said of certain veins and lymphatics. Opp. of efferent.*

affinity (ă-fĭn′ĭt-ĭ) [L. *affinis*, neighboring]. 1. Common relationship; attraction. 2. Chemical attraction bet. two substances, *i.e.*, oxygen and hemoglobin. SEE: *chemoreceptor.* [of various substances.

a., chemical. Force combining atoms

a. of composition. Tendency to form a compound, without destroying any previously formed compound.

a., elective. Force causing a substance to elect 1 substance rather than another with which to unite.

af′flux [L. *ad*, to, + *fluere*, to flow]. Rush of blood to a part.

affluxion (af-fluk′shŭn). Afflux; congestion.

affu′sion [L. *affusus*, past p. *affundere*, to pour to]. The pouring of water upon, as on the body, for cooling, cleansing, or therapeutic purposes.

IND: Collapse, syncope, shock, asphyxia, and fevers.

CONTRA: Typhoid accompanied by complications, or decompensating heart, or hemorrhagic cases.

NP: Patient may lay on a rubber sheet arranged to direct the water into a pail at bedside. A thin sheet may cover patient. Water can be poured on body through a watering can.

afibrinogenemia (ă-fī-brĭn-ō-jĕn′ē-mĭ-ă). A rare blood disease characterized by the absence of fibrinogen from the blood plasma so that the blood is incoagulable; may be congenital or acquired. Congenital afibrinogenemia is generally transmitted as a Mendelian recessive character by a gene on one of the autosomal chromosomes. The acquired type may occur as a complication of parturition as a result of the entry into the maternal circulation of amniotic fluid or other tissue materials from the placental site.

af′teraction. A term used particularly in connection with nerve centers to designate the fact that they continue to react for some time after the stimulus ceases. In the sensory centers this action gives rise to aftersensations.

af′terbirth. Placenta and membranes expelled after birth of child.

af′terbrain. Section of embryonic brain which develops subsequently into oblongata, auditory nerve and 4th ventricle.
SYN: *metencephalon.*

af′tercat″aract [*Cataracta secundaria*]. Retained portion of lens substance bet. agglutinated layers of capsule; seen after extracapsular cataract extraction.
TREATMENT: Discission or needling.

af′terimage. One that persists subjectively after disappearance of object seen.

If colors are same as object it is called *positive; negative* if complementary colors are seen. In the former case, the image is seen in its natural bright colors without any alteration; in the latter, the bright parts become dark, while dark parts are light.

af′terpains. Uterine cramps due to contraction of uterus, occurring during first few days after confinement (*puerperium*); commonly seen in multiparae.* Pains more severe during nursing.
TREATMENT: Codeine, aspirin, phenacetin, pyramidon, or morphine. The earlier given, the less needed. Ergot for 2 or 3 days postpartum.

af′tersensa′tion. Sensation persisting after stimulus causing it has ceased.

Ag. [L. ab. for argentum]. Chem. symb. of silver.

agalactia (ă-găl-ak′tĭ-ă) [G. *a-*, priv. + *gala, galaktos*, milk]. Absence of milk secretion after childbirth.

agalorrhea (ă-gal-ō-re′ă) [" + " + *roia*, flow]. Arrest of milk flow.

agammaglobulinemia (ă-găm-mă-glō-bŭl-ĭn-ē′mĭ-ă). A rare blood disease characterized by the virtual absence of gamma globulin from the blood plasma with resulting loss of the ability to produce immune antibodies, and the absence of natural blood group isoantibodies from the serum; may be congenital or acquired. The congenital form is inherited like hemophilia as a sex-linked recessive character, and therefore occurs only in male children, being transmitted by females by a gene in the X-chromosomes.

agamogen′esis [G. *a-*, priv. + *gamos*, marriage, + *genesis*, development]. Asexual reproduction.

agar (ăg′ar). 1. Sea weed (alga) belonging to the genus *Gelideum*. The source of agar-agar. 2. A culture medium containing agar-agar, such as bloodagar, used in culturing certain species of bacteria.

agar-agar. A dried mucilaginous product obtained from certain species of algae, especially Gelideum. It is unaffected by bacterial enzymes, hence widely used as a solidifying agent for bacterial culture media; also used as a laxative because of its great increase in bulk upon absorption of water.

AgCl. Silver chloride.

age [Fr. *âge*, L. *aetas*]. The time of existence of anything.

40's and 50's. Prime of maturity but degenerative changes are taking place.

50's and 60's. Symptoms ill defined. May be fatigue, depression, headache, irritability, insomnia, loss of appetite, low-back pain or in bones and joints.

70's and 80's. Endocrine and nutritional deficiency apparent.

SYM: Loss of body mass, skin texture changes, susceptibility to fracture, osteoporosis, arthralgia, senile vaginitis, anemia, emotional instability, mental fatigue, decreased muscular tone, vitamin B and C deficiency.

a., achievement. One determined by a proficiency test in any schoolroom study, measured by the mental ability of the average child of chronological age.

a., chronolog′ical. The years of one's life. SEE: *chronological.*

a., marriageable. One at which the individual is physically suited for marriage. SYN: *nubility.*

a., mental. The age of a person with regard to his mental development; this is determined by a series of mental tests as devised by Binet. Thus, if a woman of 30 can pass only the tests of a child of 12, she is said to have a mental age of 12. SEE: *Binet.*

a. of consent. An arbitrary age fixed by state statutes when a girl is supposed to be responsible for giving her consent to coitus.* It ranges from 10 to 18 years of age. Under that age the

age, words pert. to   A-30   **agglutinogen**

act is legally *rape* even though consented to. In England the age of consent is 13, but between that age and 16, sexual intercourse* is a misdemeanor.

age, words pert. to: adolescence, anility, Binet, cataplasis, climacteric, consenescence, chronological (SEE: *intelligence*), decrepitude, dotage, ecmnesia, geriatrics, gerocomia, geroderma, gerodermia, geromorphism, gerontopia, latency period, longevity, maturation, mental a., old age, puberty, rejuvenescence, senescence, senile, senility, valetudinarian.

-age [L.]. Suffix: put in motion; to do; to move, as *manage*.

agenesia, agenesis (ă-jen-e'sĭ-ă, ă-jen'es-is) [G. *a-*, priv. + *genesis*, production]. 1. Sterility; impotence. 2. Incomplete development.

agenitalism (a-gen'i-tal-ism) [" + L. *genitalis*, genital]. Symptoms resulting from absence of the testicles or ovaries.

agenosomia (ah-jen-o-so'mĭ-ă) [G. *a-*, priv. + *gennan*, to beget, + *soma*, body]. Imperfect development of genitals.

ageusia (ă-gū'sĭ-ă) [" + *geusis*, taste]. Absence of the sense of taste; a partial loss or an impairment of the sense of taste.

ETIOL: It may be due to disease of the chorda tympani on one side, or of the gustatory fibers, or to the excessive use of condiments.

RS: *acoria, anorexia, bulimia, emesis, hiccup, hyperorexia, nausea, parageusia, parorexia, pica, polyphagia, pyrosis, regurgitation, rumination, taste*.

a., gustatory. This is caused by a disordered condition of the taste buds* or of the lingual mucous membrane, or from contact with an irritating substance. It is often associated with acute coryza, and is present when the tongue is heavily furred. It may result from basal meningitis, esp. if tumors are present, or from an injury to the head. Complete loss of taste may result from bilateral disease of the chorda tympani nerve and of the gustatory fibers of the glossopharyngeal nerves.

agger (ăj'er) [L. mound]. ANAT: A mound or pile.   [Ridge of nose.
    a. na'si (BNA). *Crista ethmoidalis*.

agglomerate (ag-lom'er-āt) [L. *agglomeratus*, past p. *agglomerare*, to form into a ball]. To congregate; to form a mass.

agglu'tinable [L. *agglutinare*, to glue a thing]. Capable of agglutination.

agglutinant (a-glu'tin-ant). 1. Anything causing adhesion. 2. Causing to unite or adhere, as healing of a wound.

agglutination (ag-glu-tin-a'shun). 1. Clumping of microörganisms when a specific immune serum is added to a bacterial culture. 2. Clumping of blood corpuscles when incompatible bloods are mixed. 3. Adhesion of surfaces of a wound.

    a., immediate. Healing by first intention.   [tention.
    a., mediate. Healing by second in-

agglu'tinative. Causing or capable of causing agglutination.

agglutinin (ag-lu'tin-in). A specific principle or antibody in blood serum of an animal affected with a microbic disease which is capable of causing the clumping of bacteria peculiar to that disease so that they are more easily engulfed by the white cells. SEE: blood types.

Its antigen* is called an *agglutinogen*.
SEE: *blood grouping, isoagglutinins*.

    a., chief. A. causing immunity in the blood, which has been immunized.
    a., group. A. acting as a specific on 1 species, but which will act on others.
    a., haupt-. SEE: *chief a*.
    a., immune. A. causing immunity, found in the blood either because of recovery from the disease or of having been inoculated with the microörganism.
    a., major. SEE: *chief a*.
    a., minor. A. acting on another organism than the 1 utilized for serum production, in lower dilution.
    a., partial. SEE: *minor a*.

agglutinogen (ag-gloo-tin'o-jen) [L. *agglutinăre*, to glue a thing, + G. *gennan*, to produce]. 1. A substance inherited which agglutinates only the blood of parent and child. It is present on the surface of red cells, identified by certain agglutination reactions with specific diagnostic antisera. 2. A substance causing the formation of agglutinin when introduced into the body.

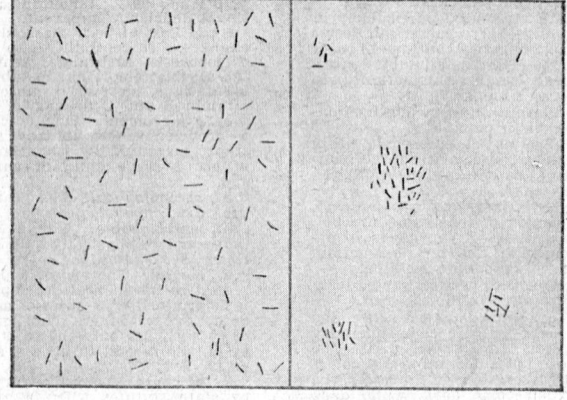

AGGLUTINATION REACTION
Left, negative, with uniform distribution of bacilli; right, positive, with the formation of clumps.

agglutinoid (ă-glu'tĭn-oid) [L. *agglutinare*, to glue a thing, + G. *eidos*, resemblance]. One with the zymotoxic group deficient or absent.

agglutinophilic (a-glu-tĭn-o-fĭl'ĭk) [" + G. *philos*, fond]. Contributing to agglutination.

agglu'tinophore [" + G. *phorein*, to bear). The active agent producing agglutination.

agglutogenic (ag-gloo-to-jen'ĭk) [" + G. *gennan*, to produce]. 1. Pert. to substances from which agglutinins originate. 2. Causing agglutinins.

agglutom'eter [" + G. *metron*, measure]. Device to simplify the agglutination or Widal test.

ag'gregate, ag'gregated [L. *aggregatus*, past p. of *aggregare*, to collect]. 1. Total substances making up a mass. 2. To cluster or come together.

a. glands. Lymphoid follicles found mainly in the ileum. SYN: *Peyer's patches.*

aggres'sin [L. *aggressus*, past p. *aggredi*, to approach]. A supposed substance which renders the action of bacteria more aggressive by lowering the activity of the phagocytes and weakening resisting power.

a'gitated depress'ion. PSY: A psychiatric phase differing from the manic or depressive phases; involution melancholia or a rel. condition.

SYM: Patients are restless, depressed, and agitated, pacing up and down, wringing hands, crying, picking, and rubbing. They have feelings of guilt and ideas of persecution, phobias, and obsessions.

NP: Similar to manic and depressive cases. Prevent patient from hurting self, as from pulling out hairs and tearing skin, etc. Divert patient but do not argue with him. Hydrotherapy indicated. Borax for deodorant.

aglaukopsia (a-glaw-kop'sĭ-ă) [G. *a-*, priv. + *glaukos*, bluish-green, + *opsis*, vision]. Green blindness.

aglobu'lia [" + L. *globulus*, globule]. Marked decrease of red blood cells.

aglutition (ag-lu-tĭsh'un) [" + L. *glutire*, to swallow]. Difficulty in swallowing or inability to swallow.

aglycosu'ric [" + *glykus*, sweet, + *ouron*, urine]. Free from glycosuria.

agmatol'ogy [G. *agma*, fragment, + *logos*, study of]. The study of fractures.

agminate(d (ag'mĭn-āt) [L. *agmen*, a crowd]. Aggregate; grouped in clusters.

a. glands. Lymphoid follicles found mainly in the ileum. SYN: *Peyer's patches.*

ag'nail [AS. *ang*, painful, + *naegel*, nail]. 1. Hangnail. 2. Whitlow.*

agne'a [G. *a-*, priv. + *gnosis*, knowledge]. A condition in which objects are not recognized; agnosis, *q.v.*

agno'sia [G. *ignorance*]. Loss of comprehension of auditory, visual, or other sensations although the sensory sphere is intact; inability to recognize an object.

a., auditory. Deafness of mind.

a., optic. Blindness of the mind.

a., tactile. Inability to distinguish objects by sense of touch.

agomphiasis (ag-ŏm-fĭ'as-ĭs) [G. *agomphios*, toothless, + *iasis*, state]. 1. Looseness of the teeth. 2. Without teeth.

agonad (ă-go'nad) [G. *a-*, priv. + *gonē*, seed]. One without gonads.

agon'adal. Having no gonads.

ag'onal [G. *agōnia*, orig. a contest]. Rel. to the moment of death, or to agony.

agonia (ag-o'nĭ-ă) [G.]. 1. Extreme anguish; mental distress. 2. The death struggle.

ag'onist [G. *agōn*, a contest]. The muscle directly engaged in contraction as distinguished from muscles which have to relax at the same time.

Thus in bending the elbow, the *m. biceps brachii* is the agonist and the triceps the antagonist.

agony (ag'o-nĭ). 1. Extreme suffering, mental or physical. 2. Death struggle.

a. clot, a. thrombus. Clot formed in the heart after long heart failure and when dying.

agoraphobia (ag-o-ra-fo'bĭ-ă) [G. *agora*, market place, + *phobos*, fear]. 1. Morbid dread of open spaces. 2. Dread of crowds of people.

-agra [G. *seizure*]. Suffix: pert. to gout or a gouty affection; loosely, a severe pain; seizure.

agraffe (ă-graf') [F. *agrafer*, to hook, fasten]. An appliance for clamping together edges of a wound.

agrammat'ica [G. *agrammatos*, illiterate]. Agrammatism.

agramm'atism. Inability to form a grammatical or intelligible sentence or to arrange words in grammatical sequence. ETIOL: Cerebral disease.

agranulocyte (ă-gran'u-lō-sīt) [G. *a-*, priv. + L. *granulum*, granule, + G. *kytos*, cell]. A nongranular leukocyte.

agranulocytic (a-gran-ū-lō-sĭt'ĭk). Pert. to agranulocytosis.

agranulocytosis (a-gran"u-lō-sī-tō'sĭs). 1. Condition marked by destructive ulcerative lesions of the throat, *leukopenia.** 2. Marked reduction of polymorphoneuclear leukocytes in the blood and bone marrow.

a., Ludwig's. Purulent inflammation about the floor of the mouth, submaxillary glands, and beneath the jaw.

a., Plaut-Vincent's. An infectious ulceromembranous inflammation of the mucosa caused by *B. fusiformis* associated with a spirillum (*Spironema vincentii*).

agranuloplas'tic [G. *a-*, priv. + L. *granulum*, granule, + G. *plastikos*, formative]. Capable of forming nongranular cells.

agranulo'sis [" + " + *osis*, condition]. Marked reduction of granular leukocytes in blood and bone marrow. SYN: *agranulocytosis.*

agraphia (ah-graf'ĭ-ă) [G. *a-*, priv. + *graphein*, to write]. A loss of ability to express oneself in writing due to a central lesion, or to muscular incoördination.

Copying or writing from dictation may still be possible. It is analogous to or associated with motor aphasia.* SYN: *logographia.* SEE: *anorthography.*

agraph'ic. Pert. to agraphia.

agre'mia [G. *agra*, gout, + *aima*, blood]. Blood condition in gout.

agria (ag'rĭ-ă) [G. *agrios*, wild]. Herpes; malignant pustules or pustular eruption.

agroma'nia [G. *agros*, field, + *mania*, frenzy]. Unreasonable desire for solitude or solitudinous wandering. Morbid desire to live in solitude or in the country.

agrypnia (a-grĭp'nĭ-ă) [G. *agrypnos*, sleepless]. Inability to sleep. SYN: *insomnia;* ahypnia.*

agrypnot'ic. 1. Afflicted with insomnia. 2. That which causes wakefulness.

ague (a'gu) [Fr. *aigu,* sharp, acute]. 1. Intermittent or malarial fever; typified by chills, fever, and sweating. 2. A chill. SEE: *malaria.*

ah. Abbr. for *hypermetropic astigmatism.*

Ahlfeld's sign (ahl'felt). OB: Uterine irregular contractions after the 3rd month of pregnancy.

ahypnia (ah-hip'nĭ-ă) [G. *a-,* priv. + *hypnos,* sleep]. Insomnia or sleeplessness; agrypnia.*

aichmophobia (ăk-mō-fo'bĭ-ă) [G. *aichmē,* point, + *phobos,* fear]. Morbid fear of pointed instruments or of being touched by them or with a finger.

ailurophobia (i'lu-ro-fo'bĭ-ă) [G. *ailuros,* cat, + *phobos,* fear]. PSY: Morbid fear of cats.

A symbolism of psychoneurotic origin.

air (ār) [G. *aer,* air]. The invisible, tasteless, odorless mixture of gases surrounding the earth.

The air, so-called "breath of life," is made up of 21% oxygen, 0.8% argon, 78% nitrogen, aqueous vapor, carbon dioxide, and traces of ammonia, helium, and other rarer gases, but in cities and factories it is polluted. The proportions, esp. of water vapor, are variable. The composition of dry atmospheric air is given approximately in the table below; in the column headed "inspired," the numbers are in volumes per cent.

air cushion. An airtight inflatable cushion. To inflate, a pump like a bicycle pump may be used.

NP: When inflating orally, place layer of gauze over opening and between lips.

air em'bolism. Obstruction of a blood vessel brought about by entrance of air into the blood stream.

It causes blood to froth.

ETIOL: A postoperative possibility, or air may enter during hypodermic injection, if syringe is not properly filled or if during injection a minute vein is punctured. Air should be excluded when giving an intravenous injection.

air hun'ger. Shortness of breath marked by rapid, labored breathing. SYN: *dyspnea.**

Causes the type of respiration similar to that preceding onset of diabetic coma.

ETIOL: Extreme acidosis; seen in excessive loss of blood.

SYM: More complete expiration than normal; increased respiratory rate, 16 to 20 per minute.

air sac. An air vesicle.*

airsickness. Condition similar to seasickness occurring during airplane flight.

air swal'lowing. Oral intake of air either voluntarily or involuntarily. SYN: *aerophagia, q.v.*

Involuntarily, this condition mainly occurs in infants due to improper feed-

	Inspired	Expired	Alveolar*
Oxygen	20.96	16.3	14.2
Nitrogen (including small amounts of argon and other inert gases)	79.00	79.7	80.3
Carbon Dioxide	0.04	4.0	5.5

FUNCTION: 1. Its oxygen is necessary in metabolism, just as it is necessary for combustion. 2. It carries off waste products of metabolism in the form of heat, carbon dioxide, and aqueous vapor.

a., **alveolar.** Air in the alveoli.

a., **complemental.** The amount that may be breathed in over and above the tidal air, by deepest possible inspiration.

a., **minimal.** The small amount of air left in the alveoli by collapse of small bronchi when the supplemental and residual air is driven out when the lungs collapse with the thorax open. This makes it possible for the excised lungs of animals to float, hence the term "lights."

a., **reserve.** Residual air plus supplementary air in the chest after normal expiration. About 5 pt. (2600 cc.).

a., **residual.** The amount remaining in the lungs after the fullest possible expiration. About 1500 cc.

a., **supplemental.** Amount that may be forcibly expired after a quiet expiration. About 1600 cc.

a., **tidal.** The amount that flows in and out of the lungs with each quiet respiration; average of adult male about one pint (500 cc.).

air, words pert. to: "aer-" words, apneumatosis, aspiration, atelectasis, atmos, atmotherapy, atomize, complemental, expiration, inspiration, mephitic, respiration, ventilation.

air bed. Large inflated air cushion used as a mattress. SEE: *air cushion.*

air cell. An air vesicle.*

air conditioning. Adjustment of normal temperature and humidity while insuring adequate ventilation.

ing, in adults in neurasthenia or hysteria or when on a fluid diet.

air vesicle. Pulmonary tissue saccule filling with air during breathing.

air'way. A metallic or rubber instrument inserted into the mouth to keep the air passages of a postanesthetic patient clear until he is conscious.

Aix-Les-Bains (eks-la-băn) **douche massage.*** Water up to 115° F. flowing from a tube on a certain part of body while operator massages that part.

akatamathesia (ah-kăt-ăm-ath-e'zĭ-ă) [G. *a-,* priv. + *katamathesis,* understanding]. Inability to understand.

akathisia (ah-kath-iz'ĭ-ă) [G. *a-,* priv. + *kathisis,* a sitting]. PSY: Inability to remain seated.

Seen in catatonia,* in agitated melancholia, and in some compulsive conditions.

akinesia (ah-kin-e'sĭ-ă) [G. *a-,* priv. + *kinēsis,* movement]. Loss of movement for any reason. Acinesia, *q.v.*

a. **algera.** Form with intense pain caused by any movement.

a. **amnestica.** Form marked by failure of muscular power due to lack of use.

akoas'ma [G. *akouein,* to hear]. Auditory hallucination, consisting of tinnituslike sounds of buzzing, whistling, etc., but also much more complex noises of groans, screams, etc.

akutomy (a-koo'to-mĭ) [L. *acus,* needle, + G. *tomē,* cutting]. PT: The electrical cutting current; acusection.

Al. Chemical symbol for aluminum.

-al [L.]. Suffix: Pert. to, as *abdominal.*

ala (a'la) (*pl. alae*) [L. wing]. 1. An expanded or winglike structure or appendage. 2. Axilla.*

a'lae na'si [L.]. The cartilaginous flap on the outer side of each nostril.

ala'lia [G. *a-*, priv. + *lalia*, talking]. Loss of ability to speak due to defect or paralysis of the vocal organs. Aphasia.
ETIOL: Psychic or due to lesion.
alar (a'lar) [L. *ala*, wing]. 1. Pert. to or like a wing. 2. Axillary.
 a. artery. Small br. of axillary. Supplies tissues of axilla.
 a. cartilage. Lower lateral; one on each side of nose.
 a. vein. The M-shaped arrangement of superficial veins in fold of elbow.
alas'trim [Portuguese, *alastrar*, to spread]. A modified smallpox with pustules not umbilicated and with no secondary rise of temperature.
alate (al'āt) [L. *ala*, wing]. Winged.
al'ba [L. *albus*, white]. 1. White. 2. White substance of the brain.
albar'as [Arabic, white leprosy]. A disease of the skin, forming white anesthetic patches on which the hair turns white.
albedo (al-be'do) [L. from *albus*, white]. Whiteness. Reflection of light from a surface.
 a. ret'inae. Retinal edema.
 a. unguium. White semilunar area at nail root. SEE: *lunula*.
Albee's operation (awl'bez). Removal of upper end of head of femur and corresponding edges of the acetabulum with approximation; artificial ankylosis of the hip.
Albers-Schönberg disease (ăl-bārs-shĕn'-bärg). Abnormal bone calcification giving bones spotted, marblelike appearance and causing them to fracture spontaneously. SYN: *osteosclerosis fragilis; marble bones*.
Al'bert's disease. Achillodynia. Inflammation of the retrocalcanean bursa.
al'bicans (pl. *albicantia*) [L. pres. p. *albicare*, to be white]. 1. White or whitish. 2. One of the *corpora albicantia*. [cortex.
 a., corpus. Whitish body in ovarian
albidum (ăl'bĭ-dŭm) [L.]. White.
albidu'ria [L. *albidus*, whitish, + G. *ouron*, urine]. 1. Passing of white or colorless urine and of low specific gravity. 2. Chyluria.*
Albini's nodules (ăl-bĭ'nĭ). Minute nodules on margins of mitral and tricuspid valves of the heart; sometimes seen in newly born.
albinism (al'bin-ism) [Portuguese from L. *albus*, white]. 1. Abnormal, nonpathological absence of pigment in skin, hair, and eyes, partial or total, frequently accompanied by astigmatism, photophobia, and nystagmus, because the choroid is not sufficiently protected from light because of lack of pigment. 2. A form of macula.* Permanent.
albino (al-bi'no). A person deficient in pigment; one afflicted with albinism.
albinu'ria [L. *albus*, white, + G. *ouron*, urine]. Passing of white or colorless urine of low specific gravity. SYN: *albiduria*.
albocinereous (al-bō-sĭn-e'rē-ŭs) [" + *cinereus*, gray]. Pert. to both white and gray matter of brain and spinal cord.
Albright's disease. Same as Recklinghausen's disease.
albuginea (al-bu-jĭn'ĭ-ă). A layer of firm, white, fibrous tissue forming the investment of an organ or part.
 a. epididymidos. The fibrous coat of the epididymis, resembling the *a. testis*, but with less firmness and strength.
 a. lienis. The white, highly elastic fibrous coat, lying directly beneath the serous investment of the spleen. SYN: *tunica propria of the spleen*.
 a. ovarii. The layer of firm fibrous tissue lying beneath the epithelial ovarian covering.
 a. penis. A strong, very elastic white fibrous coat, forming a sheath common to both corpora cavernosa of the penis.
 a. renis. The fibrous renal capsule.
 a. testiculi, a. testis. The thick, unyielding layer of white fibrous tissue lying under the tunica vaginalis.
albugineotomy (al-bu-jĭn-e-ot'o-mī) [L. *albus*, white, + G. *tomē*, cutting]. Incision of tunica albuginea of the testis.
albuginitis (al-bu-jĭn-i'tis) [" + G. *-itis*, inflammation]. Inflammation of any tunica albuginea.
albu'go [L. whiteness from *albus*]. White opacity of the cornea.
albu'kalin. A substance in leukemic blood.
albu'men [L. *albus*, white]. 1. Egg white; 2. former name for albumin, *q.v.*
 a. water. After removing the specks from 2 eggs, separate the white from the yolk, and then cut the whites across several times, but do not beat. Add ½ pt. of cold boiled water. Stir lightly and add a pinch of salt or a few drops of lemon. For infants the lemon is omitted, and the albumen water must be strained through gauze.
albumimeter (al-bu-mĭm'et-er) [L. *albumen*, + G. *metron*, measure]. An instrument for quantitative estimation of albumin in urine.
albu'min [L. *albumen*, coagulated egg white]. A protein substance found in nearly every animal or plant tissue and fluid.
One per cent of the body consists of albumins. Albumin is found in (a) the blood, as *serum-albumin*; (b) in milk, as *lactalbumin*, and in (c) the white of egg, as *albumen*. It is soluble in cold water; coagulated on heating, then no longer dissolved by cold or hot water. In the stomach coagulated albumin are made soluble by *peptase*, being changed at the same time into albumoses* and peptones.* Vegetable albumin, such as that in cereals, is radically different from animal albumin. The former is harder to digest and to absorb. SEE: "*albumi-*" words, seralbumin, thyroxin.
 a. test. The commonest type of albumin found in urine is serum-albumin. Before testing, certain precautions must be observed: (a) The specimen of urine must be fresh. (b) The specimen must also be clear. To ensure this, the safest way is to filter it through special filter paper (blotting paper makes a good substitute). (c) The urine must be acid. (d) The specimen must be cold.
There are many tests for albumin, but the most usual are the following:
Acetic acid test: Heat the top inch or so of a test-tube filled three parts full of urine over a spirit lamp. A cloudiness will form, which may be due to phosphate or albumin. Add 2 or 3 drops of acetic acid, and if the cloud disappears it is due to phosphates; if it becomes intensified, albumin is present.
Heller's cold test: Take about ½ in. of concentrated nitric acid in a test-tube, and carefully overlay it with the urine, with a pipette. An opaque line appears at the junction of the fluids. This may take a few minutes to develop.
Salicyl-sulfonic acid test: To some urine in a test-tube add 10 to 20 drops of salicyl-sulfonic acid. Alubmin is shown as a white, cloudy precipitate. This may be carried out as a ring test, as in Heller's test. SEE: *Esbach's test*.

albumin, acid   A-34   **alcohol**

Since albuminuria can be caused by many different conditions, the results require careful interpretation.
  SEE: *Esbach's method, Esbach's quantitative estimation.*
  a., acid. Compound resulting from action of acid on a.
  a., alkali. Compound resulting from action of weak alkalies on a.
  a., blood. Serum albumin; one of the blood proteins. Comprises about 60% of the latter.
  a., circulating. A. present in the liquids of the body.
  a., derived. A. changed by chemical action.
  a., egg. Form in egg white.
  a., floating. SEE: *circulating a.*
  a., incipient. Imperfect form of a. found in chyle.
  a., muscle. Form found in muscular tissue.
  a., myosin. A. of meat.
  a., native. Any a. present in an organism normally.
  a., serum. SEE: *blood a.*
  a., soluble. One that has not been altered by chemical action so that it is insoluble in water.
  a., vegetable. Any albumin in or derived from plant tissue.
  a., whey. A. obtained from whey.
albu'minate. Metaprotein, a product of hydrolysis of albumen and globulin.
albuminatu'ria [L. *albumen*, white of egg, + G. *ouron*, urine]. Albuminates in voided urine.
albuminiferous (al-bu-min-if'er-us) [" + *ferre*, to bear]. Producing albumin.
albuminimeter (al-bu-min-im'e-ter) [" + G. *metron*, measure]. Instrument for measuring amount of albumin in urine. SEE: *albumimeter.*
albuminiparous (al-bu-min-ip'ar-us) [" + *parere*, to bear]. Yielding albumin.
albuminogenous (al"bu-min-oj'en-us) [" + G. *gennan*, to produce]. Producing albumin.
albu'minoid [" + G. *eidos*, similarity]. 1. Resembling albumin. 2. Any one of a large class of proteins, such as (a) *collagen** in white fibers of connective tissue, which produces gelatin on boiling; (b) *elastin*, in yellow fibers of connective tissue, and (c) *keratin*,* found in hair, skin, and finger nails; *osseins* in osseous tissue, and *chondrigen* in cartilage.
  They resemble *proteids** in origin and composition of which *albumin* is a type.
albuminolysis (al-bu-min-ol'I-sis) [" + G. *lysis*, solution]. Proteolysis; decomposition of protein.
albu'minone. Noncoagulable protein in blood serum.
albuminoptysis (al-bū-mĭn-op'tĭ-sis) [L. *albumen*, + G. *ptysis*, spitting]. Albumin in sputum.
albuminoreac'tion [" + *rē*, again, + *agere*, to act]. The presence or absence of albumin in the sputum.
  Positive reaction indicates inflammatory condition of lungs.
albuminorrhe'a [" + G. *roia*, flow]. Albumin in urine.
albuminose (al-bu'min-oz). 1. Albumose. 2. Albuminous.
albumino'sis [L. *albumen*, + G. *-osis*, state of]. Abnormal increase of albuminous constituents in blood plasma.
albu'minous. Having the nature of albumen.

albu"minuret'ic [L. *albumen*, + G! *oureti-kos*, causing urine to flow]. Pert. to albuminuria.
albuminuria (al-bu-min-u'rĭ-ă) [" + G. *ouron*, urine]. The presence of albumin in the urine, indicating either a simple mixture of albuminous matters with the urine, or a pathological state of the kidneys.
  It occurs during onset of febrile diseases, and in pneumonia, typhoid, diphtheria. Esp. grave in scarlet fever. Also seen in heart disease.
  SEE: *nephritis, nephrosis.*
  a., cardiac. Caused by disease of the heart valves.
  a., cyclic. Deposit at regular diurnal intervals of small amounts of albumen in the urine, esp. in childhood and youth.
  a., extrarenal or accidental. Due to contamination of urine with pus, chyle, or blood.
  a., functional or transient. One in which the only finding is occasional presence of albuminuria, associated with physical or mental distress or slight emotional excitement. Occurs in some after taking certain foods.
  a. gravidarum. A. developing in pregnant women.
  a., pathological. A. caused by a disease.
  a., physiological. A., in a temporary form, existing without evidence of pathology.
  a., renal. Due to changes in epithelial cells of kidneys, making them pervious to proteins of the blood as in all forms of nephritis.
  a., toxic. Due to toxins generated within the body or by poison from outside source.
albuminu'ric retini'tis. Inflammation of retina characterized by hazy retina, blurred disc margin, distention of retinal arteries, retinal hemorrhages, and white patches in the fundus, esp. the stellate figure at the macula.* SEE: *retinitis.*
albu'moscope [L. *albumen*, + G. *skopein*, to view]. An instrument for determining the presence of albumen in the urine.
al'bumose. The intermediate product produced by enzymes in the splitting of proteins which in the course of digestion becomes peptones.
  Primary albumoses are first formed which in time become "deutero albumoses" or secondary albumoses. They in turn result in peptones or simpler bodies. SEE: *Bence-Jones test for a. in urine.*
albumosemia (al-bu-mo-se'mĭ-ă) [*albumose* + G. *aima*, blood]. Albumose in the blood.
albumosuria (al-bŭ-mō-sū'rĭ-ă) [" + G. *ouron*, urine]. Albumose in the urine.
Alcock's canal. A space in the external fascia of the *ischiorectal fossa*, above the tuberosity of the ischium.*
  It contains the internal pudendal artery, veins, and nerve.
al'cohol [Arabic *al*, the, + *koh'l*, fine antimonial powder]. One of many carbon compounds of the general formula R^1
R^2—COH, where R^1, R^2 and R^3 may be R^3
hydrogen atoms or any organic radicals.
  Examples are methyl alcohol (wood spirits) and ethyl alcohol. Higher alcohols, with more complicated formulae, may be solid and crystalline. Polyhydric alcohols are those containing more than

one OH-group; examples are *glycerol* and *glucose*.
SEE: *"alco-" words, atomicity, cholesterol, delirium tremens, dipsomania.*
a., absolute. Contains 99% alcohol or not more than 1% by weight of water.
a., denatured. Alcohol rendered unfit for use as a beverage or medicine.
a., ethyl. Ordinary or grain alcohol.
ACTION: Externally a rubefacient and astringent used to harden and cleanse the skin. In 70% solution antiseptic. Internally—a narcotic.
USES: One of the most useful of the disinfectants, and sterilizing agents. A good skin-cleanser when used in strength of 50% to 70% and will kill vegetative bacteria in fifteen minutes. The addition of acetone adds to its efficiency both in preoperative and postoperative sterilization of hands and skin. Alcohol is a very useful agent in the sterilization of cutting instruments, for all cutting instruments should be placed in solutions preferably to boiling.
Boiling has a tendency to injure the cutting edges and dull them. Hypodermics and needles are rinsed in alcohol, then in sterile water, to render them clean. Sutures are also sterilized in alcohol. It is not practical to use for large utensils or large bulky equipment as the quantity required would be too much.
a., methyl. Wood spirit.
alcoholase (al'ko-hōl-āz). A ferment converting lactic acid into alcohol.
alcohol'ic. 1. Pertaining to alcohol. 2. One afflicted with alcoholism.
a. fermentation. That which is produced by yeast in bread. RS: *Fermentation, acetic and lactic.*
alcoholism (ăl'kō-hōl-ĭzm) [Arabic *al*, the, + *koh'l*, fine antimonial powder]. Diseased condition due to acute or chronic excessive indulgence in alcoholic liquors.
ETIOL: Unknown. Psychological factors play an important part, a deep-seated neurosis. Subconscious feelings of insecurity and inadequacy, conflicts and frustrations are factors. Vitamin deficiency.
SYM: Edema of brain with serous meningitis in both acute and chronic cases. Thickened *dura* and *pia mater*, some tissue degeneration. Thickening of cerebral blood vessels and some glia cells is found. It acts, at least in part, by inhibiting the ego-ideals and revealing the antisocial. Consequently, a great variety of clinical pictures present themselves, esp. in the acute intoxications; *i. e.*, coma, amnesia,* furor,* automatism. Periodic drinking is a separate type. SEE: *dipsomania.* The persistent heavy drinker develops delirium tremens,* Korsakoff's psychosis,* chronic hallucinosis,* and dementia, *q.v.*
a., acute. Excessive indulgence in a.
SYM: Flushing of face, quickening of pulse, mental exhilaration, followed by incoherent speech, deep respiration, loss of coördination, odor of alcohol on breath, thickened speech, dilated pupils, vomiting, delirium, slow pulse, subnormal temperature, impaired judgment, emotional instability, muscular incoordination, and finally stupor and coma. In coma of alcoholism, patient can be roused by screaming in the ear, or by firm pressure over a sensitive spot, as the supraorbital notch.
TREATMENT: Stomach should be emptied with stomach pump. Douching and flagellation to rouse patient. Large doses of coffee, hot water, saline cathartics, stimulants, massage, sleep, induced perspiration, oxygen inhalation. Glucose and insulin accelerate decrease of alcohol in the blood.
Antibuse causes nausea when alcohol is taken, discouraging chronic drinking. It, however, is toxic. Cortisone prevents the acute stage and hastens recovery, lessening tendency to indulge. Excessive drinking exhausts the adrenals and they are rehabilitated by the adrenal hormone.
a., chronic. Continued use of alcohol.
SYM: Fine tremor, mental impairment, disturbed sleep, injection of conjunctivae, redness of nose, anorexia, coated tongue, nausea, vomiting, constipation alternating with diarrhea. If long continued, atheroma of arteries, cirrhosis of liver, and chronic interstitial nephritis are apt to develop.
This brings mental deterioration in its wake and changes in the central nervous system resulting in impaired memory, failure of judgment, inability to carry on business and lower moral ideals and habits. Natural affection disappears.
TREATMENT: Alcohol should be withdrawn; nutritious diet, graduated physical exercise, constitutional treatment.
SEE: *delirium tremens, intoxication.*
a. psychoses. These include (a) pathological intoxication, (b) delirium tremens,* (c) Korsakoff's psychosis,* (d) acute hallucinosis,* (e) other types.
TREATMENT: Isolation, quiet, sleep, rest; hydrotherapy. Lumbar puncture may be necessary to relieve edema of brain.
a., vitamin treatment. Vitamins B_2 and B_4 help to prevent toxicomania and the proper combustion of the alcohol. A total dosage of 650 cc. of 25% ethyl alcohol, combined with glucose and hepatic extracts given intravenously as follows, has proved successful:
1st day: 180 cc. in two injections (morning and evening).
2nd day: 150 cc. in two injections.
3rd day: 120 cc. in two injections.
4th day: 100 cc. in two injections.
5th and 6th days: 50 cc. in one injection.
alcoholomania (al-ko-hol-o-ma'nĭ-ă) [*alcohol* + G. *mania*, frenzy]. Abnormal craving for intoxicants.
alcoholometer (al-ko-hol-om'et-er) [" + G. *metron*, measure]. An instrument for measuring quantity of alcohol in a fluid.
alcoholophilia (al″ko-hol-o-fĭl'ĭ-ă) [" + G. *philos*, fond]. Morbid craving for alcohol. [hol in the urine.
alcoholu'ria [" + G. *ouron*, urine]. Alco-
alcosol (al'kō-sŏl). A sol using alcohol as the solvent instead of water.
aldehyde (al'de-hĭd) [*al.* abbr. alcohol, + *dehyd*, abbr. dyhydrogenatum, alcohol deprived of hydrogen]. 1. Oxidation product of a primary alcohol. 2. A hydrocarbon wherein hydrogen has been replaced by the —CHO group. 3. Carbon compounds of the general formula $\begin{matrix}H\\R\end{matrix}>CO$; formaldehyde H_2CO, acetaldehyde CH_3CHO, and benzaldehyde C_6H_5-CHO are members of this group. Formaldehyde is a combustible gas but soluble in water; its 40% solution is called formalin. Acetaldehyde and benzaldehyde are liquids.
alembic (al-em'bik) [Arabic *al-inbīq*, the still]. Utensil used for distillation.
alemmal (ă-lĕm'al) [G. *a-*, priv. + *lemma*, husk]. Without a neurilemma, as a nerve fiber.

Aleppo boil   A-36   alienism

Alep'po boil, button, evil, or **sore.** Oriental boil. [*aleuko*- words.

aleuco-. For words beginning thus, see

aleukemia (ă-lū-kē'mĭ-ă) [" + " + G. *aima*, blood]. 1. Deficiency of white blood corpuscles. The existence of leukopenia or aleukocytosis. 2. Pseudoleukemia.

aleukemic (a-lu-ke'mĭk). 1. Marked by aleukemia. 2. Pert. to an early stage of Hodgkin's disease, before blood changes occur.

   a. leukemia. Leukemia in which the total count of white blood corpuscles is normal, regardless of quantitative changes of the blood or leukemic changes in tissues.

aleukia (ă-lu'kĭ-ă) [G. *a*-, priv. + *leukos*, white]. 1. Absence of white blood cells. 2. Absence of blood platelets.

aleukocytosis (a-lu-ko-si-to'sĭs) [" + " + G. *kytos*, cell]. A diminished production of white corpuscles in the blood.

aleuron (al-u'ron) [G. flour]. The protein granules of seeds in which the vitamins* are supposed to be stored.

aleuronat (al-u'ro-năt). Vegetable albumin used for bread for diabetics.

ale'wife [origin uncertain]. Shad-like fish eaten salted in West Indies. Average serving, 230 grams. Pro. 44.6, Fat 11.3.

Alexand'er-Adam's operation. Shortening the round ligaments, suturing their ends to the ext. abdominal ring, for uterine displacements.

alexeteric (ăl-eks-ē-ter'ĭk) [G. *alexētērios*, fit to keep off]. Protective against infection, venom, and poison.

alex'ia [G. *a*-, priv. + *lexis*, speech]. Inability to read, due to a central lesion; word-blindness. A form of aphasia.

   a., musical. Inability to read music. It may be sensory, optical or visual, but not motor. SEE: *anarthria, aphemia*.

alexic (al-ek'sĭk). Defensive, as an alexin.*

alexin (al-ek'sĭn) [G. *alexein*, to ward off]. Defensive substance in normal serum which, in presence of a sensitizer, destroys bacteria and exerts a lytic action on cells. SYN: *complement, q.v.* RS: *immunity, phylaxin, sozin.*

alexin'ic un'it. The lowest amount of alexinic serum required to dissolve a measured quantity of red blood corpuscles in the presence of an excessive amount of hemolytic serum.

alexipharmic (ă-leks-ĭ-far'mĭk) [" + *pharmakon*, poison]. 1. An antidote. 2. Antidotal. Warding off the ill effects of a poison.

alexipyretic (ă-lĕk"-sĭ-pī-ret'ĭk) [" + *pyretos*, fever]. That which lessens fever. SYN: *febrifuge*.

alexocyte (ă-lĕks'o-sit) [" + *kytos*, cell]. A leukocyte supposed to secrete alexin.

alexofixagen (al-ĕks-o-fĭk'sa-jĕn). An antigen stimulating production of complement-fixing antibodies.

aleze (ă-lĕz') [Fr. *alèze*]. A folded cloth to protect the bed from discharges.

algae (al'je) [L. *pl. of alga*]. Any plant belonging to the sub-phylum Algae of the Phylum Thallophyta, the lowest division of the plant kingdom. They are independent plants possessing chlorophyl, having an undifferentiated body and a simple life-history, in size from one-celled microscopic forms to massive seaweeds. They live in salt water or in moist places. Some serve as food or as sources of medicinal products. Examples are Spirogyra, rockweeds, kelps, and Irish moss.

alganesthesia (al-gan-ĕs-the'zĭ-ă) [G. *algos*, pain, + *an*-, priv. + *aisthesis*, sensation]. Absence of normal sense of pain. SYN: *analgesia*.*

algefacient (al-je-fa'shent) [L. *algere*, to be cold, + *faciens*, making]. Cooling, or refrigerant.

algesia (al-je'zĭ-ă) [G. *algēsis*, sense of pain]. Supersensitiveness to pain, hyperesthesia.

algesic (al-je'sĭk). Hyperesthesic; painful.

algesichronometer (al-je"sĭ-kro-nom'et-er) [G. *algēsis*, sense of pain, + *chronos*, time, + *metron*, measure]. An instrument for measuring time taken to feel pain.

algesimeter (al-jes-im'et-er) [G. *algēsis*, sense of pain, + *metron*, measure]. An instrument for measuring sensitiveness of cutaneous surfaces.

algesthesia (al-jes-the'zĭ-ă) [G. *algos*, pain, + *aisthesis*, sensation]. Unusual sensitivity to sensory stimuli, as pain or touch. SYN: *hyperesthesia*.

algetic (al-jet'ĭk). Painful.

-algia [G.]. Suffix signifying *pain*, as in neur*algia*.

algicide (al'jis-īd) [L. *alga*, + *caedere*, to kill]. That which destroys algae.

algid (al'jid) [L. *algidus*, cold]. Cold, chilly.

   a. pernicious fever. A form of malaria with symptoms of collapse.

   a. stage. Cold and cyanotic skin occurring in cholera and some other diseases.

algiomotor (al"jĭ-o-mo'tor) [G. *algos*, pain, + L. *motor*, a mover]. Causing painful contraction of muscles.

algiomus'cular [" + L. *musculus*, muscle]. Causing painful contraction of muscles. SYN: *algiomotor*.

algogenic (al-go-jen'ĭk) [G. *algos*, pain, + *genesis*, production]. 1. Causing neuralgic pain. 2. Lowering body temperature below normal.

algolagnia (al-go-lag'nĭ-ă) [G. *algos*, pain, + *lagneia*, lust]. A sex perversion on part of one who cannot enjoy love or sex when dissociated from some form of pain to the sexual partner, male or female. The subject may be sadist or a masochist. SEE: *masochism, sadism*.

algolagnist (al-go-lag'nist). One who practices algolagnia.*

algom'eter [G. *algos*, pain, + *metron*, measure]. Instrument for testing the sensitiveness to pain.

algophily (al-gŏf'ĭ-lĭ) [" + *philos*, fond]. Sexual pleasure in experiencing bodily pain or inflicting it upon others. Algolagnia.*

algophobia (al-go-fo'bĭ-ă) [" + *phobos*, fear]. Morbid aversion to witnessing or experiencing pain.

algopsychalia (al-go-sī-ka'lĭ-ă) [" + *psychē*, mind]. Hallucinatory depression in which the dread and suicidal trends are ascribed to the hallucinations.

al'gor [L. cold]. 1. A chill. 2. The sensation of cold; cold.

algos (al'gos) [G.]. Pain.

alible (al'ĭ-ble) [L. *alibilis*, from *alere*, to nourish]. Absorbable; nutritive; assimilable.

alices (al'ĭs-ēz) [L.]. The red spots appearing before pustulation in smallpox.

alienation (al-yen-a'shun) [L. *alienare*, to make strange]. Mental disorder, including every form of deviation from the physiological mental activities in conduct. In law, a psychosis varying according to situation involved.

a'lienism. Science of mental diseases.

a'lienist. One who studies disease from an antisocial standpoint; a psychiatrist.

aliform (al'ĭ-form) [L. *ala*, wing, + *forma*, shape]. Having form of a wing.
  a. process. Wing of the sphenoid.

al'iment [L. *alere*, to nourish]. Nutriment, food.

alimen'tary [L. *alimentum*, nourishment]. Of or pertaining to nutrition.
  a. canal or tract. The digestive tube from the mouth to anus, including mouth or buccal cavity, pharynx, esophagus, stomach, small and large intestine and rectum. Drugs administered orally (by mouth) are absorbed in the stomach or intestine by the portal vein and pass through the liver before entering the general circulation, or they may be absorbed into the lacteals and enter the blood-stream by way of the thoracic duct.
  a. duct. The thoracic duct.

alimenta'tion. The general process of nourishing the body; it includes mastication, swallowing, digestion, absorption, and assimilation.
  RS: *anabolism, absorption, catabolism, digestion, metabolism, foods.*
  a., artificial. Feeding of patient unable to take nourishment normally.
  a., forced. 1. Feeding of a patient unwilling to eat. 2. Therapeutic feeding of more nourishment than necessary.
  a., rectal. Injection of food through the rectum. However, little if any nutrients are absorbed through the colon.

alimentotherapy (al-im-en-to-ther'ap-ĭ) [L. *alimentum*, nourishment, + G. *therapeia*, healing]. Treatment employing dietetics. SYN: *dietotherapy.*

alina'sal [L. *ala*, wing, + *nasus*, nose]. Pert. to the *alae nasi* or wings of the nose.

alinement (al-īn'ment) [Fr. *alignement*]. The line along which adjustment of the teeth is made.

aliphatic (al-ĭ-fat'ik) [G. *aleiphar, aleiphatos*, fat, oil]. 1. Belonging to that series of carbon compounds characterized by straight or branching chains of carbon atoms, related to methane and ethane, and including the fats and fatty acids; opposite of *aromatic.* 2. Fatty.

aliquot (al'ĭ-kwot) [L. *alius*, other, + *quot*, how many]. A fractional part divisible into the whole without a remainder.

alisphenoid (al-ĭ-sfe'noyd) [L. *ala*, wing, + G. *sphēn*, wedge, + *eidos*, resemblance]. Pert. to the greater wing of the sphenoid bone.

alkalemia (al-kal-e'mĭ-ă) [Arabic, *al-qili*, ashes of salt wort, + G. *aima*, blood]. An excessive alkalinity of the blood due to a decrease in the *hydrogen ion* concentration or an increase in hydroxyl ions. The blood is normally slightly alkaline (pH 7.4).

alkales'cence. 1. Slight alkalinity. 2. Process of becoming alkaline.

alkales'cent. Alkaline or becoming alkaline.

al'kali [Arabic *al-qili*, ashes of salt wort]. 1. A metallic hydroxide (except ammonia) that has the property of combining with an acid to form a salt, or with an oil to form soap. 2. Any substance which can neutralize acids and affect indicators in certain ways. Ex: *sodium hydroxide*, which turns litmus blue.
  SEE: *"alkal-"* words, *corrosive alkali.*
  a. poisoning (such as *lye, sodium,* or *potassium hydroxide,* etc.). F. A. TREATMENT: Weak acids may be administered; such acids are found in vinegar, orange juice, lemon juice, grapefruit juice, sauerkraut juice, etc. These are to be followed by soothing demulcent substances such as egg white, gelatin, or jelly, crushed bananas, cream or milk, bland oils, starch, water, oatmeal, or barley gruel. Starch water is especially valuable in iodine poisoning. Morphine is useful to allay the pain. Rest, heat, quiet, and adequate fluid intake are imperative. Stimulants are given as necessary.
  CAUTION: Do not give emetics or use a stomach pump if strong alkalies have been taken internally.
  LOCAL: Wash with large amounts of water and apply wet dressings of weak acids such as fruit juices, vinegar, citric or tartaric acids.

alkalimeter (al-kal-im'et-er) [" + G. *metron,* measure]. Device for measuring strength of alkalies.

alkalim'etry. Measurement of degree of alkalinity in a mixture.

al'kaline. Pert. to an alkali or having the reactions of one.

al'kaline ash diet. One consisting of normal amount of protein with moderate salt restriction, adequate in all known essentials. SEE: *basic diet.*

al'kaline effects of foods. Fruits and vegetables contain salts of alkaline metals, such as calcium, magnesium, potassium, and sodium and they exert an alkaline effect in the body. Original acid parts of the salts, and the free acids, such as citric, malic, tartaric, and lactic, are burned in the body to carbonic acid, eliminated by the breath. This makes possible the neutralization of the acidic products from proteins by the alkaline metals. The blood stream and tissues are protected against sudden changes in normal faintly alkaline reaction by the bicarbonates, phosphates, and proteins serving as buffer agents. The body never becomes actually acid in reaction although the alkaline reserve may become depleted. SEE: *acid effects.*

al'kaline reserve. The amount of material in the blood available for neutralizing the acids produced in the course of metabolism,* particularly carbonic acid.
  Is measured indirectly by saturating a sample of *plasma* under special conditions with carbon dioxide, then liberating the gas in a vacuum pump, and measuring the gas. Normally 1 cc. of plasma can carry 0.53 to 0.77 cc. of carbon dioxide; in severe *acidosis* the capacity may be reduced to 0.40 or 0.30.

al'kaline tide. The increase in *alkaline reserve* and occasional occurrence of alkaline urine during gastric digestion, compensating for the simultaneous secretion of acid in the stomach.

alkalin'ity. State of being alkaline. SEE: *antalkaline, hydrogen ion.*

al'kalinize. To make alkaline.

alkalinu'ria [*alkali* + G. *ouron,* urine]. An alkaline urine.

alkalipe'nia [" + G. *penia,* poor]. Low alkali reserve of the body.

alkalitherapy (al-kal-ĭ-ther'ap-ĭ) [" + G. *therapeia,* treatment]. Alkali therapy.

alkaliza'tion. Process of making alkaline.

al'kaloid [*alkali* + G. *eidos,* resemblance]. 1. An active bitter principle that reacts with an acid to form a salt, the latter being used because of its solubility, rather than the alkaloid. 2. An alkaline principle of organic origin; any nitrogenous base, esp. one of vegetable origin having a toxic effect. Ex: *Quinine, morphine, strychnine.*

alkalometry   A-38   **allergy**

INCOMPATIBILITIES: *Tea* (tannin), *coffee* (caffeine).

alkalom'etry [" + G. *metron*, measure]. Dosimetry. Administration of alkaloids.

alkalo'sis [" + G. *-osis*, condition of]. A condition in which the alkalinity of the body tends to increase beyond normal, due to excess of alkalies or withdrawal of acid or chlorides from the blood.

ETIOL: 1. Forced breathing and crying in infants which removes excessive amount of carbonic acid from lungs. 2. Excessive vomiting causing loss of hydrochloric acid and sodium chloride. 3. Excessive use of bicarbonate of soda or other alkalies. 4. Improper diet.

SYM: Irregular breathing, cyanosis, perhaps tetany, tingling of fingers, numbness of extremities, headache, lassitude, nausea, fever, vomiting, mental disturbances, drowsiness, twitching, possible coma, delirium, convulsions.

TREATMENT: Withdraw alkaline foods, drinks, and drugs. Saline and glucose may be necessary, both by rectum and by mouth, if possible.

alkalot'ic. Pert. to alkalosis.

alkaluretic (al-ka-lu-ret'ik) [*alkali* + G. *ouretikos*, a flow of urine]. Causing or that which causes an alkaline urine.

alkap'ton(e [" + G. *aptein*, to possess]. A yellowish-red substance sometimes occurring in urine, the possible result of incomplete oxidation of tyrosin.

alkaptonuria (al-kap-ton-u'rĭ-ă) [*alkapton* + G. *ouron*, urine]. The presence of a yellowish nitrogenous substance in the urine not esp. indicative of disease or a local lesion although found in pulmonary tuberculosis. It turns the urine dark or black. SEE: *brenzkatechinuria*.

alkyl (al'kil) [*al*, abbr. *alcohol*, + G. *ylē*, stuff]. Any univalent alcohol radical.

allachesthesia (al-ă-kes-the'zĭ-ă) [G. *allachē*, elsewhere, + *aisthesis*, sensation]. Tactile sensation remote from point of stimulation.

allantiasis (al-an-tī'ă-sis) [G. *allanto*, sausage]. 1. Sausage-poisoning. 2. Botulism.* SEE: *atriplicism*.

allantochorion (al-lăn-tō-ko'rĭ-ŏn). Fusion of the allantois and chorion into one structure.

allanto'ic. Pert. to the allantois.

allan'toid [G. *allanto*, sausage, + *eidos*, resemblance]. 1. Sausage-shaped. 2. Allantois. 3. Pert. to the allantois.

allan'toin [chemical name, glyoxyldiuride]. A white crystalline powder, considered to be secreted by maggots.

USES: In various forms of indolent ulcers and wounds, by stimulating tissue growth, and inducing granulation.

DOSAGE: ½-2 gr. (0.03-0.12 Gm.). In 0.4% solutions or as an ointment.

allantoinu'ria [*allantoin* + G. *ouron*, urine]. Allantoin in the urine.

allantois (al-an'tois) [G. *allanto*, sausage, + *eidos*, resemblance]. A kind of elongated bladder, between the chorion and amnion of the fetus, which is thrown out from the cauĭel extremity of the embryo, and communicates with the bladder by the urachus. It is very apparent in quadrupeds, but not in the human species. In the lower forms as the allantois is developed, its walls become very vascular, and contain the ramification of what becomes the umbilical artery and vein, which, by the elongation of the allantois, are brought through the villi of the chorion into indirect communication with the vessels of the mother. SEE: *chorion*, *urachus*.

allelic genes (al-lel'ik). Genes which occupy the same locus on a specific pair of chromosomes and control the heredity of a particular characteristic. The heredity of eye color appears to depend on a series of allelic genes; the four A-B-O blood groups are determined by the three allelic genes L^A, L^B, and L^O; the 12 standard Rh-Hr types are transmitted by the eight allelic genes r, r', r'', r^y, R^0, R^1, R^2, and R^z; etc.

allelocatalysis (al-le-lo-kat-ăl'ĭ-sis) [G. *allēlōn*, reciprocally, + *catalysis*, dissolution]. Stimulation of a bacterial culture by the addition of cells of same type.

allelomorph (al-le'lo-morf) [" + *morphē*, shape]. One of a pair of character units, the descendants not showing a mixture of the pair, but one or the other of the unit characters.

allel'otaxis [" + *taxis*, order]. Development of a part from different embryonic structures.

Allen-Doisy unit. Injection in a spayed mouse of the smallest amount of estrus-producing hormone secreted during pregnancy, producing desquamation of vaginal epithelium in the mouse.

Allen's law. The more carbohydrate taken by a diabetic, the less he utilizes.

A.'s treatment. A once popular method of treating diabetes mellitus consisting of a period of absolute fasting followed by a spare diet with little carbohydrate. Then a gradual food increase until 1500 to 2000 calories are reached. Absolute fasting is dangerous in diabetes since it can bring on acidosis and death.

allen'thesis. Introduction of a foreign substance into the body.

allergen (al'er-jen) [G. *allos*, other, + *ergon*, work, + *gennan*, to produce]. A substance supposed to produce symptoms of allergy.*

Allergens include various foods, feathers, dust, pollens, etc.

aller'gic. Pert. to or sensitive to an allergen.

a. extracts. Made from protein of various substances believed to have specific action in producing morbid conditions.

al'lergin [G. *allos*, other, + *gennan*, to produce]. A substance supposed to produce allergy. SYN: *allergen*.

allergiza'tion. Sensitization.

al'lergy [G. *allos*, other, + *ergeia*, work]. 1. Hypersensitivity to a specific substance. 2. A clinical change in the capacity of an organism to react to an infection following a primary one, as in increased susceptibility, or immunity.

EX: An infection of a common cold may render a patient more susceptible to future infection, while an attack of mumps or measles renders the patient less liable; hypersensitiveness of body cells due to proteins such as ferment in the protein molecules, and which causes hay fever or asthma through inhalation, resulting in lesions, or skin eruptions.

Allergic conditions include eczema; allergic rhinitis, or coryza; hay fever; bronchial asthma, and urticaria or hives. Gastrointestinal allergy may appear in children.

NP: *In children:* Avoid extremes of temperature and humidity. Skin must not be chilled and sweating must be prevented. Soap and water must not be used on eczematous parts of the skin. Use pure olive oil or pure mineral oil. An ointment may be ordered which

allergy, food   A-39   **allotropism, allotropy**

should be applied many times during the day in a thin layer, and as often as the child rubs it off. Crude coal tar in equal parts of acetone or alcohol and flexible collodion may be ordered to be painted on the eczematous areas, once each day with a cotton applicator. Brush the skin with dry cotton to remove all loose material.

Woolen clothing and blankets should not be used, or feather stuffed pillows or mattresses. To prevent scratching, cuffs should be used so the child cannot bend the arm at the elbow. Other restraints of arms and legs may be necessary. Elimination diets are indicated.

ETIOL: Heredity, pollen, dust, hair, fur, feathers, scales, or dandruff; also specific foods, such as chocolate, milk, wheat, oranges, nuts, and tomatoes, the most common offenders, and to a lesser extent, eggs.

SYM: Low blood calcium and eosinophilia* frequently present; urticaria, eczema, rash, an acnelike eruption which does not respond to x-ray, asthma, hay fever, migraine, or gastrointestinal disturbances.

TREATMENT: (non-food allergy). Wet packs and an astringent but not oily dressing for relief. Other treatment is in an experimental stage.

RS: *allergen, allergia, anaphylaxis, atopy, autourotherapy, hay fever, hypersensitiveness, immunity.*

a., food. Find the offending food by placing patient for six weeks on a nonallergic diet consisting of tea, coffee, lettuce, carrots, prunes, plums, apricots, veal, lamb, rye crackers, plum jam, olive oil, peppermint candy. If no eruption occurs within a week, add a new food every two weeks until the one causing the trouble expresses itself through appearance of new lesions which then should appear within from two to six hours, and not more than 12 hours. Discontinue use of offending food. Give ultraviolet rays or increase Vitamin D foods. SEE: *anaphylaxis.*

a., heat and cold. Changes of temperature may cause cutaneous reactions such as urticaria and also internal reactions with sensitive persons. Itching, redness of skin, headache, asthmatic symptoms, dyspnea, and shock can follow exposure to cold water. Heat may produce same symptoms.

allesthesia (al-es-the′sĭ-ă) [G. *allos*, other, + *aisthesis*, sensation]. A sensation in one limb which is referred to the other one; allochiria.

alliaceous (al-ĭ-a′se-us) [L. *allium*, garlic]. Tasting like garlic or onions.

allitera′tion [L. *ad*, to, + *littera*, letter]. Dysphrasia, in which words are spoken according to sound.

allo- [G. *allos*, other]. 1. A prefix meaning differentiation from the normal. 2. Indicating a body made stable by heat. 3. CHEM: An isomer, close relative or variety of a compound. Isomerism when there is relative asymmetry.

allochesthe′sia [G. *allache*, elsewhere, + *aisthesis*, sensation]. Tactile sensation remote from point of stimulation. SYN: *allochiria, allesthesia.*

allochezia, allochetia (al-o-ke′zĭ-ă, al-o-ke′shĭ-ă) [G. *allos*, other, + *chezein*, to defecate]. 1. Excretion of nonfecal matter from the bowels. 2. Excretion of feces through an abnormal opening.

allochiria (al-o-ki′rĭ-ă), **allocheiria** [G. " + *cheir*, hand]. Sensation referred to side of body opposite its origin; allesthesia.

Observed in locomotor ataxia and in hysteria.

allochroism (al-ŏk′rō-izm) [" + *chroa*, color]. Change in color.

allochromasia (al-ō-krō-mā′sĭ-ă). Change in color of hair or skin.

allocinesia (al-o-sin-e′sĭ-ă) [G. *allos*, other, + *kinesis*, movement]. Movement on side of body opposite to the one directed. SEE: *allokinesis.*

alloerotism (al-lo-er′ot-ism) [" + *Eros*, god of love]. Gratification of the sexual instinct directed to an external object. Cf. *autoerotism.*

allokinesis (al-o-kin-e′sis) [G. *allos*, other, + *kinesis*, movement]. Movement on side of body opposite to the one directed.

allokinetic (al-o-kin-et′ik) [" + *kinesis*, movement]. Movement caused by external forces.

allola′lia [" + *lalia*, talk]. Speech defect, esp. if due to disease of speech center.

allonal (ăl′o-nol). Registered trade-mark for a compound of allyl-isopropyl-barbituric acid and acetophenetidin; a hypnoanalgesic.

DOSAGE: Average 2 2/3 gr. (0.170 Gm.).

all′opath. A misnomer for a regular medical practitioner.

allopathy (al-lop′a-thĭ). A misnomer for a system of therapeutics administering medicines which produce effects different from those of the disease treated; in principle, the opp. of homeopathy. A term erroneously used for the regular practice of medicine.

allophasis (al-off′as-is) [G. *allos*, other, + *phasis*, speech]. Incoherency, delirium.

alloplasia (al-o-pla′zĭ-ă) [G. *allos*, other, + *plasis*, a molding]. *Heteroplasia.** Replacement of normal cell forms by other cell forms in the tissue.

al′loplasty. Plastic surgery with nonhuman tissue.

allopsychic (al-lo-si′kik) [" + *psyche*, mind]. Ideas not related to the patient's personality, but to the external environment.

allopsycho′sis [" + " + *-osis*, condition]. Derangement of perceptive powers.

allorhythmia (al-o-rith′mĭ-ă) [" + *rythmos*, rhythm]. Irregular cardiac rhythm.

all-or-none law. That a stimulus to a nerve or muscle causes it to respond to its greatest extent or not at all.

allotherm (al′o-therm) [" + *therme*, heat]. An organism whose temperature is directly dependent on its culture medium.

allotox′in [" + *toxikon*, poison]. A substance within the body which protects by destroying toxins inimical to it.

allotriogeustia (al-ot-rĭ-o-just′ĭ-ă) [G. *allotrios*, strange, + *geusis*, taste]. Perverted taste.

allotriophagy (al-o-trĭ-of′ă-jĭ) [" + *phagein*, to eat]. The habit of eating injurious, unusual, and nonedible substances.

allotriuria (al-ot-rĭ-u′rĭ-ă) [" + *ouron*, urine]. Abnormal urine.

allotropic (al-lo-trop′ik) [G. *allos*, other, + *tropos*, direction]. 1. CHEM: Pert. to different forms of the same element without change of chemical composition. 2. Possessing an altered nutritive value.

a. type. One much concerned with what others think, say, or do.

allot′ropism, allot′ropy. Presence of an element in two or more distinct forms with unlike properties.

allox'an [L. *alloxanum*]. A substance obtained by the action of nitric acid or of nascent chlorine upon uric acid.

$$C(OH)_2 < \begin{matrix} CO-NH \\ CO-NH \end{matrix} > CO.$$

It has been found in the intestinal mucus in catarrhal enteritis. It gives a red color to the skin, and has been used as the basis of cosmetic preparations.

allox'in. Any one of a series of *xanthin* bases derived from the splitting of *chromatin*, which on oxidation produces uric acid.

allox'ur bases or bodies [*allox(an)* + *ur(ea)*]. Xanthine bases. Nitrogenous substances formed by splitting of nucleins.

alloxuremia (al-oks-u-re'mĭ-ă) [*alloxur* + G. *aima*, blood]. Xanthine* bases in the blood.

alloxu'ria [" + G. *ouron*, urine]. Xanthine bases in the urine.

al'lyl [L. *allium*, garlic, + G. *ylē*, matter]. A univalent radical. It is present in garlic and mustard.

Almén's tests (ăl-mäns'). Three tests of urine for blood, albumin, and sugar.

almond (ă'mond) [G. *amygdalē*]. COMP: Highly nutritive and rich in nitrogenous components. They surpass cheese and beans by a third in nutrients. Heavy in cellulose. Free from xanthic bodies and purins. They contain considerable albumin.

Average serving, 30 grams. Pro. 6.3, Fat 16.5, Carbo. 5.2, Ca. 0.239, Mg. 0.251, K. 0.741, Na. 0.019, P. 0.465, Cl. 0.037, S. 0.160, Fe. 0.0039. Contains Vit. A. Good source Vit. B and G.

ACTION: Very slow to digest. Should not be eaten in quantities. Laxative due to their oleaginous principles and cellulose content.

alochia (ă-lo'kĭ-ă) [G. *a-*, priv. + *lochios*, pert. to childbirth]. Absence of puerperal* vaginal discharge following childbirth.

aloe (al'o). USP. The inspissated juice of several species of aloe.

ACTION AND USES: A cathartic acting on large intestine; resembling but more irritant than cascara.

DOSAGE: 4 gr. (0.25 Gm.).

alo'gia [G. *a-*, priv. + *logos*, speech]. Inability to express oneself through speech. SYN: *aphasia*.

alopecia (al-o-pe'shĭ-ă) [G. *alopēkia*, fox mange]. Natural or abnormal baldness or deficiency of hair, partial or complete, localized or generalized.

ETIOL: Unknown. Hypothetically, it is of parasitic or neurotic origin.

PROG: Favorable, varying with age of patient and extent of process.

TREATMENT: Prophylactically by personal brush and comb. Massage. Green soap, tar soap, or egg yolk shampoo. Treatment of seborrheic dermatitis if present. Locally, stimulating applications. Systemic tonics, hexamethylenamine, thyroid, internally.

a. **adnati.** Congenital baldness.

a. **areata,** *a.* **Celsi,** *a.* **circumscripta.** Baldness is sharply defined; circumscribed patches which leave the scalp smooth and white, and which are probably due to nervous disturbances or parasites.

a., congenital. Form with absence of hair bulbs at birth.

a. **follicularis.** Inflammation of the hair follicles of the scalp causing loss of hair from affected areas.

a. **furfuracea.** Called also *a. capillitii, pityriasis capitis, seborrhea capillitii,* and *dandruff*. Chronic in course and marked by hyperemia, dandruff and itching, and falling out of hair (exfoliation of scales), which becomes harsh, dry, and lusterless.

a. **localis,** *a.* **neuritica.** Falling of hair in circumscribed spots in area of distribution of scalp nerves.

a. **neurotica.** Baldness following a nervous disease or injury to nervous system, and occurring at site of injury.

a. **pityroides** [G. *pityrôdes*, branny]. Falling of both scalp and body hair, together with abundant bran-like desquamation.

a. **senilis.** Baldness of old age.

a. **simplex.** Baldness prematurely.

a. **symptomatica.** Loss of hair after prolonged fevers or during course of some disease; also may result from changes in internal secretions.

a. **toxica.** Loss of hair thought to be due to toxins of infectious disease.

a. **universalis.** General loss of hair from all parts of body.

al'pha. First letter of Greek alphabet. CHEM: Denotes first in a series of isomeric compounds.

a. **leukocyte.** One that disintegrates during blood coagulation.

a. **test.** A U. S. army test for recruits capable of reading English.

a. **tocopherol** (tō-kŏf'er-ŏl). A tocopherol in vitamin E, the others being *beta, gamma,* and *delta*.

USES: In heart cases including coronary thrombosis a preventive of heart conditions; in Buerger's disease; in hemorrhage.

ACTION: Nontoxic even in large doses. Decreases oxygen requirements of heart muscles 50% or more, increasing blood supply. Decreases excessive capillary permeability, or leakage; reduces blood clot in a thrombus, or prevents its formation and softens scar tissue.

DOSAGE: 300 milligrams daily.

alphus (al'fus) [L.], **al'phos** (G.]. 1. Psoriasis. 2. A pustular, scrofulous affection of the skin accompanied by white crusts.

al'terant [L. *alterare*, to change]. An alterative. That which brings about a favorable change in the body functions.

alterative (awl'ter-a-tiv). A medicine that alters the processes of nutrition and excretion, restoring the normal functions of the system. Ex: *Corrosive mercuric chloride, calomel, arsenic trioxide,* and *potassium iodide*.

al'ternate host [L. *alternare,* do by turns]. A carrier of disease germs, such as the louse, and other insects.

al'ternating cur'rent. PT: An electrical current the direction of which reverses constantly.

al'ternator. PT: So-called sinusoidal alternator; an electromagnetic device consisting of a revolving armature which cuts the lines of force in a magnetic field and which delivers a sinusoidal current from secondary coil of the apparatus.

al'therm, altherm pad. A device containing chemicals applying heat to the eye or a sinus.

altricious (al-trish'us) [L. *altrix*, nourisher]. Slow in developing; requiring long nursing.

al'um [L. *alumen*] (ammonium alum, or potassium alum). USP. Large, colorless

alumen   A-41   **amaurosis, diabetic**

crystals, or white powder, with sweetish, strongly astringent taste.
Its manufacture (which is of great antiquity) is by subjecting alum stone to a roasting process, and treating with sulfuric acid.
DOSAGE: As an astringent, 5 to 15 gr. (0.3-1 Gm.). As an emetic, 1 drachm (4 Gm.).
alu'men [L.]. Alum.
  a. exsiccatum. Alum that has been dried or burnt.
aluminosis (al-ū-min-o'sis) [" + G. -*osis*, condition of]. Chronic catarrhal inflammation of the lungs in alum workers.
alu'minum. A silver-whitish metal. Symb. Al. Atomic weight 26.97.
aluminum acetate (as'et-āt). A salt formed by the reaction between aluminum sulfate and lead acetate. Its aqueous solution, containing 4 to 5%, is known as Burow's Solution.
  USES: Regarded as a valuable local astringent and antiseptic.
  DOSAGE: 5-10 gr. (0.3-0.6 cc.).
alumnol (a-lum'nol). A fine, white, non-hygroscopic powder.
  USES: As a mild antiseptic and, in concentrated solutions, as an irritant and caustic.
  DOSAGE: As surgical antiseptic, in from ½ to 3% solutions; in gynecology, in from 2 to 5%.
alusia (al-u'sĭ-ă) [G. *aluein*, to wander]. Morbidity; hallucination.
alvajel (al-vă-jel'). An ointment made from a tropical plant, of the cactus family, and recommended in x-ray burns.
Alvegniat's pump (al-văn-yats'). Mercurial vacuum pump for removing gases from the blood.
alveobronchi'tis [L. *alveolus*, little tub, + G. *bronchos*, windpipe, + -*itis*, inflammation]. Inflammation of the bronchioles, and pulmonary alveoli; bronchopneumonia.*
alve'olar [L. *alveolus*]. A small depression or pert. to an alveolus.
  SEE: *chilognathopalatoschisis.*
  a. air. The mixture of gases collected by having the subject first execute a normal expiration and then exhale as much additional air (which comes from the alveoli of the lungs) into the collecting device as possible. Its composition is fairly constant at rest. Exercise increases the carbon dioxide above, and voluntary overbreathing decreases it below, 5.5%. For complemental, dead, minimal, reserve, residual, supplemental, and tidal air, SEE: *air, spirometry.*
  a. process. One of four processes which make up each maxillary bone.
alve'olate [L. *alveola*]. Honeycombed; pitted.
alveoli (al-ve'o-li) [L.]. Pl. of alveolus.
  a. dentales (BNA). Tooth sockets.
alveoli'tis [L. *alveolus*, + G. -*itis*, inflammation]. Inflammation of the alveolar processes; pyorrhea.*
alveoloclasia (al-ve-o-lo-kla'zĭ-ă) [" + G. *klasis*, fracture]. Absorption of any part of the alveolar process.
alveolus (al-ve'o-lus) *(Pl. alve'oli)* [L. small hollow or cavity]. 1. A little hollow. 2. The socket of a tooth. 3. Air cell of the lungs. 4. A small depression such as those contained in the honeycomb cells of the gastric mucous membrane. 5. A follicle of a racemose gland.
  a., mucous, of the salivary glands. Those that secrete the ropy material of the saliva, containing mucin.
  a., parietal. An air space in the wall of an alveolar passage in the lung.
  a. pulmoneus. A pulmonary air space.
  a., serous, of the salivary glands. Those that secrete the serous albumin of the saliva, coagulating when heated.
  a., terminal. An air space connected with a pulmonary infundibulum.
alveus (al've-us) [L. a hollow, a cavity]. A canal, tube, duct, or cavity.
  a. ampullascens. Dilation at the receptaculum chyli.
  a. hippocampi. Medullary layer investing the hippocampus major.
alvine (al'vīn) [L. *alvus*, belly]. Pert. to the intestines or abdomen.
  a. concretion. Intestinal stone.
  a. discharge. Stools.
  a. flux. Watery feces.
alvi'nolith [" + G. *lithos*, stone]. An intestinal mass formed from calcareous salts and other matter.
al'vus [L.]. 1. Abdomen and viscera. 2. uterus.
alycin (a-li'sin). A combination of natural salicylates with an alkaline base. Given usually as a powder, or an elixir.
  USES: In rheumatism, arthritis, etc.
  DOSAGE: Average, 1 teaspoonful.
alymphopotent (a-lĭm'fō-pō''těnt) [G. *a*-, priv. + L. *lympha*, lymph, + *potens*, able]. Unable to develop lymphocytes or lymphoid cells.
Alzheimer's disease (ahlts'hi-mer). PSY: Presenile dementia with hyaline degeneration of the smaller blood vessels of the brain.
  ETIOL: Faulty metabolism and imperfect nutrition, with mental enfeeblement.
Am. Symbol for *mixed astigmatism*, or for *ametropic*.
ama (a'mă) [G. *amē*]. Enlargement of a bony canal of labyrinth of the internal ear at the end opposite the ampulla.
A. M. A. Abbr. for American Medical Association.
amaas (ă'măhs). A mild form of smallpox, milk-pox.
am'acrine cell [G. *a*-, priv. + *makros*, long, + *is, inos*, fiber]. Nerve cell without any axis cylinder process.
amal'gam [G. *malagma*, emollient]. Any alloy containing mercury.
amal'gamate. To make an amalgam.
amara (am-a'ră) [L. *amarus*, bitter]. Bitters.
amarthritis (am-ar-thri'tis) [G. *ama*, at same time, + *arthron*, joint, + -*itis*, inflammation]. Polyarthritis. Inflammation of more than one joint at the same time.
amasesis (ă-mas-ē'sis) [G. *a*-, priv. + *masesis*, chewing]. Inability to masticate.
amas'tia [" + *mastos*, breast]. Failure of breast development.
am'ative [L. *amare*, to love]. 1. Expressing sexual desire. 2. Propensity to love.
Amat'o bod'ies. Those seen in leukocytes in scarlet fever.
amaurosis (am-aw-ro'sus) [G. *amauros*, dark, dim, + -*osis*, condition]. Complete loss of vision with no ophthalmoscopic evidence of pathologic conditions within the eye.
  a., albuminuric. A. caused by kidney affection.
  a., amaurotic. A. caused by the atrophying of optic nerve or vision centers.
  a., cerebral. A. caused by brain malady.
  a., congenital. A. from birth on.
  a., diabetic. A. in connection with diabetes.

a., epileptoid. Sudden seizure of blindness, considered to be similar to epilepsy.
a., lead. A. caused by lead poisoning.
a., reflex. A. due to reflex action caused by irritation of a remote part.
a., saburral. A. in conjunction with acute gastritis.
a., tobacco. A. caused by tobacco poisoning.
a., toxic. Blindness from optic neuritis caused by poison. [dition.
a., uremic. A. caused by uremic con-
amaurotic (am-ä-rot'ik). Pert. to one afflicted with amaurosis.
a. family idiocy. Form of idiocy in which the vision is imperfect. SEE: *idiocy, idiot.*
amaxophobia (ä-maks-o-fo'bĭ-ä) [G. *amaxa*, carriage, + *phobos*, fear]. Morbid dread of carriages and wagons or riding in them.
amazia (ä-mā'zĭ-ä) [G. *a-*, priv. + *mazos*, breast]. Congenital lack of the mammary gland.
ambi- [L.]. Prefix: both or both sides; around; about, as *ambidextrous.*
ambidex'trous [" + *dexter*, right]. Ability to work effectively with either hand.
ambilat'eral [" + *latus*, side]. Pert. to both sides.
ambile'vous [" + G. *laevus*, left]. Awkward in use of both hands.
ambio'pia [" + G. *ops*, eye]. Double vision. SYN: *diplopia.**
ambisinis'ter [" + *sinister*, left]. Awkward in use of both hands. SYN: *ambilevous.*
ambiten'dency [" + *tendere*, to stretch]. PSY: The association of diverging impulses to action and opposite trends of thought or emotion with a central idea—an essential mechanism in conflict.
ambivalence (am-biv'ä-lens) [" + *valere*, to be strong]. 1. Possessing ability of equal power or value in two directions. 2. PSY: Linking of opposite or contrary emotional values (love and hate) to the same idea, or toward the same person. The fluctuation from strong like to dislike found in schizophrenia.
ambiv'alency. The condition of being ambivalent.
ambiv'alent. Have equal power or value in both directions.
a. feelings. Two opposite emotions, such as love and hate, for the same person at same time.
ambivert (ăm'bĭ-vĕrt) [L. *ambo*, both, + L. *vertere*, to turn]. One intermediate between an extrovert and an introvert.
ambloma (am-blo'mä) [G. *ambloma*, an abortion]. An aborted fetus.
amblosis (am-blo'sis) [G. *amblosis*, an abortion]. An abortion.
amblyacusia (am"blĭ-ä-koo'sĭ-ä) [G. *amblys*, dull, + *akousis*, hearing]. Dullness of hearing.
amblyaphia (am-ble-af'ĭ-ä) [" + *aphē*, touch]. Dull sense of touch.
amblychromasia (am"blĭ-kro-ma'sĭ-ä) [" + *chromatikos*, pert. to color]. The state in which the cell nucleus stains faintly.
amblychromat'ic. Staining faintly.
amblygeustia (am-blĭ-jus'tĭ-ä) [G. *amblys*, dull, + *geusis*, taste]. Defective or blunted taste.
amblyphonia (ăm-blĭ-fō'nĭ-ä). Impaired hearing. SYN: *amblyacusia.*
amblyopia (ăm-blĭ-o'pĭ-ä) [" + *ōps*, sight]. Reduced or dimness of vision, not dependent upon visible changes in the eye and not refractive (alcoholic, astigmatic, diabetic, *ex anopsia*, malarial, methyl alcohol, quinine, tobacco, toxic, uremic).
a. exanopsia. Dimness of vision resulting from inaccurate focusing on retina due to refractive errors, cataract.
a., postmarital. A. caused by excessive sexual activity.
a. reflex. A. due to irritation of peripheral area.
amblyoscope (am'blĭ-os-kōp) [" + *skopein*, to view]. Instrument for training an amblyopic eye for better vision.
am'bo [G. *ambon*, edge of a dish]. Annular fibrocartilage producing an elevation about a joint cavity, and the elevation itself.
amboceptor (am-bo-sep'tor). So called by Ehrlich. An immune substance or antibody forming a union between an antigen and complement (agent that completes lytic action), as it is assumed it has one affinity for the antigen and one for the complement.
RS: *agglutinins, anaphylaxis, antibody, antigen, immune bodies, opsonins, precipitin, Ehrlich's theory.*
a. unit. Smallest amount of amboceptor required in the presence of which a given quantity of red blood corpuscles will be dissolved by an excess of complement.
ambon (am'bon) [G.]. The ring which surrounds the sockets in which the heads of long bones are received, as the *glenoid cavity.*
am'bos. Incus or anvil bone.
ambrine (am'brĭn) [F. *ambre*, amber]. A preparation of paraffin used in treating extensive burns.
am'bulance [L. *ambulare*, to move about]. Wagon for transportation of the sick and wounded.
am'bulant, ambulatory. Able to walk, not confined to bed.
a. typhoid fever. A mild attack of typhoid fever, in which the patient is not confined to bed. SEE: *typhoid.*
ambustial (am-bus'shal) [L. *amburere*, to scorch]. Pert. to a burn or scald.
ambustion (am-bus'shun). A burn or scald.
ame'ba [G. *amoibe*, change]. A one-celled protozoan minute animal form of life that constantly changes its shape by sending out processes of its protoplasm, by which it moves about and obtains its nourishment.
It is found in great numbers in pools, and in the green slime on the top of the water. It is also found in the mud at the bottom. It possesses an outer translucent substance called the *ectosarc*; but the inner substance is denser, contains a nucleus, and is the *endosarc*. It feeds by surrounding its victim and enclosing it in the so-called *food vacuole*. Oxygen is absorbed from the surrounding water, and CO_2 is eliminated through the plasma membrane. The organism moves by pushing out parts of the cell protoplasm. These projections are called *pseudopodia*, or false legs. Reproduction occurs either by *binary fission* or, more rarely, by a method of *encystment*. There are various types of amebae, but one type is especially well known as being parasitic to man, the *Endamoeba histolytica*, which causes amebic dysentery.
amebiasis (am-e-bi'as-is) [" + *-iasis*, pathologic state]. Infection with amebas, of which *amebic enteritis** is one form. Many forms are not recognized as being due to parasitic infection.

ame′bic. Pert. to or caused by amebas.
  a. carrier state. That in which an individual harbors a form of pathogenic ameba. At least one per cent of the population harbor *E. histolytica*. Often a subacute or chronic form will follow an attack.
  a. dysentery. That caused by *Endameba histolytica*. SEE: *amebiasis*.
  a. enteritis. Intestinal amebic infection. SEE: *a. dysentery*.
  ETIOL: Infection with *Endamoeba histolytica*.
  PATH: Intestinal tissues are penetrated.
  SYM: Diarrhea or dysentery, pain, temperature not high. Presence of the parasite in the feces is only certain diagnosis. May be complicated by liver abscess.
  TREATMENT: Emetine.
  NP: Disinfect stools and linen before washing. Keep patient's utensils separate from others. Protect food from flies.
  a. hepatitis. Abscess of the liver of amebic origin.
  a. proctitis. Infection with amebas affecting the anus and rectum.
ame′bicide [G. *amoibē*, change, + L. *caedere*, to kill]. Destructive to or any agent that kills amebas.
ame′biform [" + L. *forma*, shape]. Formed like an ameba.
amebocyte (a-me′bo-sīt) [" + G. *kytos*, cell]. A cell showing ameboid movements.
ame′boid [" + G. *eidos*, resemblance]. Having the appearance and characteristics of an ameba.
  a. movements. Those possessed by leukocytes which "wander" through capillary walls into surrounding tissues; a process known as diapedesis.
ame′boidism. Ameba-like movements, noting a condition shown by certain nerve cells.
amebula (am-e′bū-lă) [dim. *ameba*]. The ameba-like spore of the malarial parasite.
amebu′ria [G. *amoibē*, change, + *ouron*, urine]. Amebas in the urine.
amelioration (ă-me-lĭ-or-a′shun) [L. *ad*, to, + *meliorare*, to make better]. Improvement; moderation of a condition.
ame′loblast [early English *amel*, enamel, + G. *blastos*, germ]. A cell from which tooth enamel is formed.
ameloden′tinal [" + L. *dens, dent*-, tooth]. Pert. to both enamel and dentine.
Amend's solution (a′mends). An organic iodine preparation, stable, and causing less gastric disturbances than Lugol's solution.
  USES: In conditions where iodine therapy is helpful, as goiter, diseases of upper respiratory tract, and as an alterative.
  DOSAGE: From 10 to 20 drops in glassful of water, ½ to 1 hour before meals.
ame′nia [G. *a*-, priv. + *mēn*, month]. Absence of the menses; amenorrhea.*
amenomania (a-me-no-ma′nĭ-ă) [L. *amaenus*, pleasant, + G. *mania*, frenzy]. Insanity characterized by happiness.
amenorrhea (a-men-o-rē′a) [G. *a*-, priv. + *mēn*, month, + *rein*, to flow]. Absence or suppression of menstruation; normal before puberty, after the menopause, during pregnancy and lactation.
  ETIOL: Some of the more common causes for its suppression at other times are change of climate, febrile diseases, and chronic diseases such as nephritis, tuberculosis, and diabetes. Also ovaritis, discharge from any cavity, endocrine disorders, overwork, emotional excitement, and mental disease.
  SYM: Varied.
  TREATMENT: Good hygiene, proper exercise and constitutional treatment; thyroid extract if there is thyroid deficiency.
  a., partial. Appearing occasionally and at irregular intervals.
  a., physiological. Periods when normally free from menstruation; prepuberty, pregnancy, lactation, postmenopause periods.
  a., primary. *Emansio mensium*. That in which menses have never made their appearance.
  a., secondary. *Suppressio mensium*. That in which, having appeared, they subsequently cease.
amenorrhe′ic. Pert. to amenorrhea.
ament (ă′ment) [L. *ab*, from, + *mens*, mind]. An idiot; one without evidence of mind.
amentia (am-en′shĭ-a). 1. PSY: Intellectual defect of varying degrees.
  The 16 yr. old idiot has intelligence less than that of a normal 4 yr. old; if less than 16 yrs. there is a corresponding grading down in terms of normal. The imbecile's mentality is less than 8 yrs.; the moron's or feebleminded individual's age is not more than 11 (sometimes arbitrarily set at 12). A large percentage of these cases are clearly familial. 2. Feeblemindedness.
ameristic (a-mer-is′tĭk) [G. *a*-, priv. + *meros*, part]. Not segmented.
ametrohemia (ah-mĕt-rō-he′mĭ-ă) [G. *a*-, priv. + *metra*, uterus, + *aima*, blood]. Lack of uterine blood supply.
ametrom′eter [G. *ametros*, disproportionate, + *ōps*, sight, + *metron*, measure]. Instrument for measuring ametropia.
ametropia (a-me-tro′pĭ-ă) [" + *ōps*, vision]. Imperfect refractive powers of eye (hyperopia, myopia, astigmatism), in which the principal focus does not lie on the retina.
amianthinopsy (ăm-ĭ-an′thin-op″sĭ) [G. *a*-, priv. + *ianthinos*, violet, + *opsis*, vision]. Violet blindness.
amicitin (ăm-ĭ-sēt′ĭn) An antibiotic against certain TB Gram-positive bacteria.
amicro′bic [G. *a*-, priv. + *mikros*, small, + *bios*, life]. Not due to microbes.
am′icron(e. A colloid particle unrecognizable through the ultramicroscope.
amicroscop′ic. Too small to be detected through the ultramicroscope.
am′ide. A chemical compound produced by the substitution of an acid radical for one of the hydrogen atoms of ammonia.
am′idin [F. *amidon*, starch]. 1. The part of starch soluble in water. 2. A monacid base. The group C.NH.NH₂.
amido-. A prefix signifying amine, *q.v.*
amid′ulin [Fr. *amidon*, starch]. Soluble starch.
am′igen. See p. A-115.
amimia (a-mim′ĭ-ă) [G. *a*-, priv. + *mimos*, mimic]. Loss of power to express ideas by signs or gestures; inability to comprehend gestures. ETIOL: A brain lesion.
amine (am′in). One of a group of organic compounds containing the amine (NH₂) group, substituted for ammonias, and possessing the general formula RNH₂, characterized by strong pharmacologic activity, and including the ptomaines and alkaloids.

amino- (a-mē′no, am′in-o). Prefix denoting compound containing amine.

amino acid. One of the compounds, of which about 22 different ones are known, derived from the fatty acids by the exchange of a hydrogen atom of the hydrocarbon radical for an amino group. Intermediary products in the catabolism and anabolism of protein. Organic acids in which NH_2 has replaced one of the hydrogen atoms.

In proteins they are the elements combined in units. They contain nitrogen and are found in plant and animal life; in the latter, a product of protein digestion by ferments or bacterial action.

They are the end products of protein digestion; the chief constituents of casein of milk; gluten of flour, and eggs. Proteins are transformed into amino acids in the intestines and are found in the blood stream of the portal circulation and in the intestines. Their presence indicates the progress of digestion and place of same. Tryptophane, cystine, lysine, and histidine are amino acids necessary for tissue repair and growth. Hydroxyaminobutyric acid, isoleucine, leucine, and phenylalanine are other essential amino acids.

All proteins do not contain all the essential amino acids as is the case with milk, cheese, eggs, and meat. Unused amino acids are converted into urea. They pass unchanged through the intestinal wall and portal vein into the blood, then through the liver into the general circulation from which they are absorbed by the tissues according to the specific protein for a specific tissue, each tissue making its own protein from the amino acid, and each deaminizing that which remains unused.

amino compound. Substance containing the group NH_2; same as amines, *q.v.*

amino group. The NH_2 group which characterizes the amines.

RS: *absorption of proteins, aminoacidemia, aminosis, tryptophane, tyrosin.*

aminoacetic acid (am-in′o-ă-sē′tĭk) (glycocoll, glycine). One of the normal constituents of the bile.

It may be prepared by boiling gelatin with hydrochloric acid. A light, white, odorless powder with sweetish taste.

USES: In certain cases of myasthenia gravis, and in progressive muscular atrophy.

DOSAGE: Average, 1½ drams (5 grams) t.i.d.

amino acide′mia (amino acid + G. *aima*, blood). Amino acids in the blood.

aminol′ysis [*amino* + G. *lysis*, a loosing]. Splitting of amines.

aminophyllin(e (a-min″ō-fĭl′ĭn). Mixture of theophylline inducing diuretic action and acting as a myocardial stimulant. SEE: *theophylline.*

DOSAGE: 1½ gr. (0.1 Gm.).

aminopyrine (am″in-o-pi′rĕn) (Pyramidon) USP.

ACTION AND USES: Antipyretic and analgesic similar to antipyrine but with more lasting effects and effective in smaller doses. Same precautions should be used as in other antipyretics.

DOSAGE: 0.3 to 0.4 Gm. (5 to 6 gr.).

INCOMPATIBILITIES: Sweet spirit of niter and tannic acid.

aminosis (am-in-o′sis) [*amino* + G. *-osis*, state]. Production or presence of amino acids in the blood.

aminosuria, aminuria (am-in-o-su′rĭ-ă, -u′rĭ-ă) [" + G. *ouron*, urine]. Amines in voided urine.

amito′sis [G. *a-*, priv. + G. *mitos*, a thread]. Multiplication by division or cleavage of cells. Cell and nucleus division without changes in the nucleus, occurring during regular processes of cell reproduction.

amitotic (ah-mĭt-ot′ĭk). Characterized by amitosis.

am′meter. PT: An instrument calibrated to read in amperes the strength of a current flowing in a circuit.

For medical purposes the ampere is too large a unit; hence, it is divided into a thousand parts or milliamperes. A meter calibrated to read in milliamperes is called a *milliammeter.* SEE: *ampere.*

ammone′mia. Ammonia in the blood due to urea decomposition. SYN: *ammoniemia.*

ammon′ia [*Ammon*, Egyptian deity]. 1. A gas formed by decomposition of nitrogen-containing substances.

Its formula, NH_3, relates it to many poisonous substances (see *amines*) but also to the proteins and to many useful chemicals. Dissolved in water, it neutralizes acids and turns litmus blue.

2. Water charged with the same is called *ammonia water.*

a., aromatic spirit of. A stimulant or an inhalant.

DOSAGE: ½ to 2 drams by mouth.

a. water. Solution of ammonia in water.

DOSAGE: (10%) 15 ℳ (1.0 cc.).

ammo′niac. Ammoniacal.

ammoni′acal. Having the characteristics of or pert. to ammonia.

ammo′niated. Containing ammonia.

ammoniemia (am-mō-nĭ-e′mĭ-ă) [*ammonia* + G. *aima*, blood]. Ammonia in the blood due to decomposition of urea. SYM: Weak pulse, subnormal temperature, gastroenteric disturbances, coma.

ammonium car′bonate (am-o′nĭ-um). Occurs as hard mass with strong odor of ammonia. On exposure to air loses CO_2 and ammonia.

INCOMPATIBILITIES: Acids.

ACTION AND USES: Stimulating expectorant.

DOSAGE: 0.3 Gm. (5 gr.).

a. chlor′ide. White crystalline powder without odor.

INCOMPATIBILITIES: Alkali hydroxides and carbonates.

ACTION AND USES: As an expectorant and diuretic.

DOSAGE: 0.3 Gm. (5 gr.). As a diuretic: 1¼ to 4 drams (5 to 15 Gm.).

INCOMPATIBILITIES: *magnesium sulfate, sodium bicarbonate.*

a. hydrox′ide. This is a solution of ammonia gas in water, used about the house for cleaning purposes, used in artificial ice, and electric refrigerators.

POISONING FROM: Usually results from the effects of gas. SYM: It has irritating effects upon eyes and respiratory tract, burning, choking, increased salivation, painful swelling and vomiting.

F. A. TREATMENT: As in potassium hydroxide poisoning: Weak vinegar, citrus fruit juices followed by oil, milk, and butter.

ammoniuria (am-o-nĭ-u′rĭ-ă) [*ammonia* + G. *ouron*, urine]. An over amount of ammonia in the urine.

amnesia (am-ne′zĭ-ă) [G. forgetfulness]. A loss of memory.

This may be for recent experiences, those subsequent to the disease, and is then termed *anterograde*. When it involves more remote memory stores it is called *retrograde*. Amnesia is often applied to episodes during which the patient forgets his identity, though he may conduct himself properly enough, and following which no memory of the period persists. Such episodes are often hysterical, sometimes epileptic, while trauma, senility, alcoholism, and other organic reaction types account for a smaller number.

PSY: In epilepsy it occurs because of feeble impressions. Partial a. is seen in confusional insanity, lack of retention in senility, and in hysteria there may be lack of recall. SEE: *aphasia, ataxiamnesia, labor*.

a., auditory. Loss of memory as to word meanings.

a., periodic. A. occurring in a period of double consciousness.

a. traumatica. A. caused by injuries.

a., visual. Inability to remember the appearance of objects that have been seen or to be cognizant of printed words.

amnesic (am-ne'sik). Pert. to amnesia.

a. aphasia. Loss of memory. SYN: *amnesia*.

amnestic (am-nes'tik). Amnesic, or causing amnesia.

amniochorial (am″nĭ-o-ko′rĭ-ăl). Rel. to both amnion and chorion.

am″niochorion′ic [G. *amnion*, amnion, + *chorion*, skin]. Rel. to both amnion and chorion. SYN: *amniochorial*.

am″nioclep′sis [*amnion* + *kleptein*, to do secretly]. Gradual unperceived loss of amniotic fluid.

amniog′raphy [" + G. *graphein*, to write]. Radiography of amniotic sac.

am′nion [G. little lamb]. Bag of waters. The inner of the fetal membranes, a thin, transparent sac which holds the fetus suspended in the *liquor amnii*, or amniotic fluid, *q.v.*

This liquid equalizes the pressure about the embryo and keeps it moist. It also acts as a pressure buffer. Premature rupture of the amniotic sac causes a dry birth. SEE: *"amnio-" words; fluid, amniotic; liquor amnii, oligohydramnios*.

amniorrhea (am-ni-or-re′ă) [" + *roia*, flow]. Premature escape of the *liquor amnii*.

amniorrhexis (am-nĭ-o-rek'sis) [" + *rēxis*, rupture]. Rupture of the bag of waters, or amnion.

amnios (am'nĭ-os). The amnion, or the *liquor amnii*.

amniotic (am-ne-ot′ik). Pert. to the amnion.

a. fluid. *Liquor amnii*. The liquid or albuminous fluid contained in the amniotic sac, *q.v.* This fluid is transparent and almost colorless, assuming a milky appearance at full term. It varies from a few ounces to three or four pints. The principal purposes of this fluid are: (a) to protect the fetus from blows, etc., that may be inflicted on the mother; (b) to allow the fetus freedom of motion; (c) to provide the fetus with water; (d) during labor and during each contraction of the uterus, to distend the sac at point of least resistance, which is in the cervical canal, thereby forming a pouch which assists in the dilation of the cervix; (e) when the membranes rupture, this fluid flushes the parturient canal, thereby cleansing, lubricating, and disinfecting it.

a. sac. The bag or sac formed by the amnion.*

am′niotin. Commercial estrogenic hormone product.

amniotitis (am-nĭ-o-ti′tis) [G. *amnion* + *-itis*, inflammation]. Inflammation of the amnion.

amniotome (am′ni-o-tōm) [" + *tomē*, cutting]. Instrument for puncturing fetal membranes.

amnitis (am-ni'tis). Inflammation of the amnion. SYN: *amniotitis*.

amok (am-ok'). [Malay *amoq*, furious]. A state of murderous frenzy.

amor (am'or) [L.]. Love.

a. insanus [L. mad]. Unrestrained libido in the insane. SYN: *erotomania.**

a. lesbicus [L. *Lesbia*, fem. name]. Urningism* as practiced by the female sex. Saphism;* Lesbianism.* It is less common than urningism among males. It is more frequent among prisoners. Intense jealousy and morbid love seem more important to such perverts than does tribadism,* *q.v.*

a. sui [L. self]. Vanity; love of self.

a. veneris [L. Venus]. The clitoris.

amoralia (a-mō-ra′lĭ-ă) [G. *a-*, priv. + L. *moralis*, moral]. Moral imbecility.

amoralis (a-mo-ra′lis). A moral imbecile.

amorphia (a-mor′fĭ-a) [G. *a-*, priv. + *morphē*, form]. Without form. SYN: *amorphism*.

amorphism (a-mor′fizm). State of being without definite form. SYN: *amorphia*.

amorphous (a-mor'fus). Without definite structure.

amotio (am-o′shĭ-o) [L. *amovere*, to move from]. A detachment.

am″pelother′apy [G. *ampelos*, grape vine, + *therapeia*, treatment]. Grape cure.

amperage (ăm-per'ăj). PT: Strength of the electrical current expressed in amperes or milliamperes.

ampere (ăm′pēr). PT: Practical unit of intensity of electric current, which is produced by 1 volt acting through resistance of 1 ohm.

The *international ampere* is practical equivalent of the unvarying current which deposits silver at the rate of 0.001118 Gm. per second, when sent through a standard solution of nitrate of silver in water.

a. meter. Instrument denoting in amperes the strength of a current. SEE: *ammeter*.

amperemeter (am′per-me″ter) [*ampere* + G. *metron*, measure]. Apparatus for measuring amperage of an electric current.

amphet′amine sul′fate. Synthetic white powder employed as a vasomotor stimulant. SYN: *benzedrine sulfate*.

amphi- [G.]. Prefix. On both sides, as *amphibious*. CHEM: Denotes certain positions or configurations.

amphiarthrosis (am-fi-ar-thro′sis) [G. *amphi*, on both sides, + *arthrosis*, joint]. A form of articulation intermediate between diarthrosis and synarthrosis, in which the articulating bony surfaces are separated by an elastic substance to which both are attached, so that the mobility is slight, but may be exerted in all directions. The articulations of the bodies of the vertebrae are examples.

amphiaster (am′fĭ-ăs″ter) [" + *astēr* star]. Double star found during mitosis.*

Amphib′ia [G. *amphibios*, double life]. A class of animals which live on land and in water.

amphiblas′tula [G. *amphi*, both, + *blastula*, little sprout]. A morula formed by unequal segmentation.
amphiblestri′tis [" + *blēstron*, fish net, + *-itis*, inflammation]. Inflammation of retina. SYN: *retinitis*.
amphibo′lia [G. *amphibolos*, doubtful]. The uncertain period of a fever, or disease.
amphibolic (am-fi-bol′ik). Uncertain; ambiguous.
 a. period, or stage. The critical period of a disease when the outcome cannot be certain.
amphib′olous. Changeable; amphibolic.
amphicelous (am-fi-se′lus) [G. *amphi*, both, + *koilos*, hollow]. Concave on each end.
amphicentric (am-fi-sen′trik) [" + *kentron*, center]. Centering at both ends.
amphichroic, amphichromatic (am-fi-kro′ik, -kro-mat′ik) [" + *chroma*, color]. 1. Turning red litmus paper blue, and blue, red. 2. Reacting both as an acid and an alkali.
amphicra′nia [" + *kranion*, skull]. Pain on both sides of head.
am′′phicreat′ine, amphicreat′inine. A leukomaine formed in muscles.
amphicyte (am′fi-sit) [G. *amphi*, both, + *kytos*, cell]. One of the capsule cells enveloping the body of ganglionic neurons.
amphicyt′ula [G. *amphi*, both, + L. *cytula*, little cell]. Impregnated ovum having unequal segmentation of the vitellus.
amphidiarthrosis (am-fi-di-ar-thro′sis) [" + *diarthrosis*, articulation]. An articulation with amphiarthrosis and diarthrosis, such as that of the lower jaw.
amphigas′trula [" + L. *gastrula*, little stomach]. The human ovum in advanced gastrula stage.
amphigony (am-fig′o-ni) [" + *gonos*, begetting]. The sexual process.
amphimixis (am-fi-miks′is) [" + G. *mixis*, mingling]. 1. Sexual reproduction. 2. PSY: Pregenital energies and mechanisms diverted to the genitals during psychosexual maturity.
am′′phimor′ula [" + L. *morula*, little mulberry]. The morula in ovum with unequal composing cells.
amphipyrenin (am′′fi-pi′ren-in) [" + *pyrenos*, stone of a fruit]. The basophile substance of the nuclear membrane of a cell.
amphithe′atre [" + *theatron*, theater]. An operating room with seats arranged around it for students and others.
amphitrichate, amphitrichous (am-fit′ri-kāt, -kus) [" + *thrix*, hair]. Pert. to certain organisms having flagella, or a flagellum at both ends. [*diplopia*.
ampho- [G.]. Prefix: both, as *amphoam′′phodiplo′pia* [G. *amphō*, both, + *diploos*, double, + *ōps*, vision]. Double vision in each eye.
amphojel (am′fō-jěl) [Alumina gel]. A colloidal suspension of hydrated alumina, capable of neutralizing the free hydrochloric acid in not less than 12 volumes of gastric juice of average strength.
 USES: In control of hyperacidity, and as an absorbent.
 DOSAGE: Average, 1 teaspoonful.
am′′phopep′tone. First peptone formed by tryptic digestion of protein.
amphophil, amphophilous (am′fo-fil, am-fof′il-us) [G. *amphō*, both, + *philos*, fond]. Having affinity for either acid or basic dyes.
amphor′ic [L. *amphora*, jar]. Pert. to a sound as that caused by blowing across the mouth of a bottle; a resonance; a cavernous sound heard on percussion of a pulmonary cavity.
amphoric′ity. Producing amphoric sounds.
amphoriloquy (am-fo-ril′ok-wī) [L. *amphora*, jar, + *loqui*, to speak]. Having amphoric sounds in speaking.
amphoroph′ony [" + G. *phōnē*, voice]. Amphoric voice sound.
amphoter′ic, amphot′erous [G. *amphoteros*, both]. Affecting both red and blue litmus.
 a. compounds. Those which may act as a base or an acid, *i. e.*, protein.
 a. reaction. A double reaction of certain liquids which turns red litmus paper blue, and blue, red.
amphoterism (am-fo′ter-izm). Having both acid and basic properties.
amphot′′erodiplo′pia [G. *amphoteros*, both, + *diploos*, double, + *ops*, vision]. Double vision in each eye. SYN: *amphodiplopia*.
amphoton′ic [G. *amphō*, both, + *tonos*, tone]. Pert. to both vagotony and sympathicotony.
amphot′ony [" + *tonos*, tone]. Tonicity of the sympathetic and parasympathetic systems.
amplexatio (am-pleks-a′shĭ-o) [L. *amplexare*, to embrace]. Sexual intercourse, coitus.
ampliation (am-pli-a′shun) [L. *ampliare*, to make wider]. Distention of a part or cavity.
amplifica′tion [L. *amplificare*]. 1. Enlargement of visual area in microscopy. 2. Magnification of sound in telephony.
am′plifier. That which increases magnification of vision or sound.
am′plitude [L. *amplitudo*]. 1. In physics, the distance between extreme limits of an oscillation or vibration. Thus, the a. of vibration of a pendulum is the chord of the arc through which it oscillates; the a. of vibration of a wave is the distance from the crest to the trough of the wave. 2. Of the pulse, its fullness, *i. e.*, the extent of dilatation of the artery at each impulse of the heart.
 a. of accommodation. Total range of eye's accommodative power.
ampoule, ampule (am′pōōl) [L. *ampulla*]. A small glass that can be sealed and its contents sterilized. This is a French invention for containing hypodermic solutions. SEE: *sterule, ampulla*.
ampul′la (pl. *ampullae*) [L. little jar]. 1. Sac-like dilatation of a canal, as the mammary lactiferous ducts, or semicircular canals of the ear. 2. A small, hermetically sealed flask containing a solution for parenteral use; an ampoule.
 a., Lieberkuhn's. Lacteal's blind end in intestinal villi. [the perineal flexure.
 a. of rectum. Portion situated above
 a. of vagina. Upper vaginal area.
 a. of vas deferens. A. underneath bladder near the termination of the vas.
 a. of Vater. Enlargement at gateway of common bile duct and pancreatic duct into the duodenum.
ampulli′tis [" + G. *-itis*, inflammation]. Inflammation of any ampulla, esp. dilated extremity of *vas deferens*.
amputation (am-pu-ta′shun) [L. *ambi*, around, + *putāre*, to trim]. Surgical removal of a diseased member, part, or organ, or operation for correction of a deformity or malformation, or injury, or incision for drainage or treatment.
 a., primary. Before inflammation sets in. [uration.
 a., secondary. During period of sup-

amuck' [Malay *amoq*, furious]. State of murderous frenzy. SYN: *amok*.

amusia (a-mu'sĭ-ă) [G. *amousos*, unmusical]. Music-deafness; inability to produce or comprehend music, as loss of the ability to play a musical instrument. ETIOL: Brain lesion, but cause not clearly understood.

Amussat's operation (am-ŭ-sā's). One for formation of an artificial anus, by lumbar colotomy in ascending colon.

amychophobia (ă-mĭ-ko-fo'bĭ-ă) [G. *amychē*, scratch, + *phobos*, fear]. PSY: Morbid fear of being scratched; fear of the claws of any animal.

amyctic (am-ik'tik) [G. *amyktikos*, mangling]. 1. Irritating, caustic. 2. A caustic or corrosive agent.

amyeloneuria (ă-mi-el-o-nu'rĭ-ă) [G. *a-*, priv. + *myelos*, marrow, + *neuron*, nerve]. Spinal cord paresis.

amyelotrophy (ă-mi-el-ot'ro-fĭ) [G. *a-*, priv. + *myelos*, marrow, + *atrophia*, atrophy]. Spinal cord atrophy.

amygdala (a-mig'da-lă) [L. from G. *amygdalē*, an almond]. 1. Tonsil. 2. A mass of gray matter in the ant. portion of the temporal lobe.

amygdalectomy (a-mig-dal-ek'to-mĭ) [" + G. *ektomē*, excision]. Excision of a tonsil. NP: SEE: *tonsillectomy*.

amygdaline (a-mig'dal-ĭn). 1. Pert. to a tonsil. 2. A bitter tasting glucoside in bitter almonds and cherry laurel leaves.
a. fissure. One on ventral side of temporal lobe, *incisura temporalis*.

amygdalitis (a-mig-dal-i'tis) [L. *amygdala*, almond, + G. *-itis*, inflammation]. Inflammation of a tonsil; tonsillitis.

amygdaloid (a-mig'da-loid) [" + G. *eidos*, resemblance]. Resembling a tonsil or an almond.
a. fossa. A depression for the tonsil.
a. tubercle. A projection from the middle cornu of the lateral ventricle, marking area of the amygdaloid nucleus.

amygdalolith (a-mig'da-lo-lith) [" + G. *lithos*, stone]. Stone in a distended crypt of a tonsil.

amygdalop'athy [" + G. *pathos*, suffering]. Any disease of a tonsil.

amygdalothrypsis (a-mig"dal-o-thrip'sis) [" + G. *thrypsis*, a crushing]. Crushing of a tonsil followed by excision.

amygdalotome (a-mig-dal'o-tom) [" + G. *tomē*, a cutting]. Instrument for excision of a tonsil.

amygdalotomy (a-mig-da-lot'o-mĭ) [" + G. *ektome*, excision]. Removal of a portion of the tonsils.

amyl (am'il) [L. *amylum*, starch, + G. *ylē*, material]. A hypothetical univalent radical, C_5H_{11}, nonexistent in a free state.

amyla'ceous. Starchy.

amylase (am'il-laz) [L. *amylum*, starch, + G. *-asis*, pert. to a colloid enzyme]. A ferment or amylolytic enzyme of the saliva, pancreatic juice and intestinal juice that hydrolyzes starch, producing achroödextrin and maltose.
These products are later acted upon by the maltase of the intestines and converted into dextrose before absorption.
Amylase is more powerful than ptyalin and it acts on uncooked as well as cooked starch. SEE: *antiamylase*.
Examples of amylase are *ptyalin* and *amylopsin*.* SEE: *enzymes*.

amyle'mia [" + G. *aima*, blood]. Hypothetical presence of starch in the blood.

amylin(e (am'il-in). 1. Part of starch soluble in water. 2. A monacid base. The group $C.NH.NH_2$. SYN: *amidin*.

amyl nitrite (am'il ni'trite). A clear yellowish liquid. Ethereal odor.
ACTION AND USES: Vasodilator with quick action but short duration. Used also in bronchial asthma.
DOSAGE: 3 ℳ (0.2 cc.) by inhalation.

amylodex'trin [L. *amylum*, starch, + dextrin]. Soluble substance produced during the change of starch into sugar.

amylodyspep'sia [" + G. *dys*, bad, + *pepsis*, digestion]. Inability to digest starchy foods.

amylogen (am-il'o-jen) [" + G. *gennan*, to produce]. Soluble starch.

amylogenesis (am-i-lo-jen'es-is) [" + G. *genesis*, production]. The production of starch.

amylogenic (am-il-o-jen'ik) [" + G. *gennan*, to produce]. Starch-producing.

am'yloid [" + G. *eidos*, resemblance]. Starch-like, somewhat resembling hyalin. SEE: *chitinous*.
a. kidney. Enlarged, firm, smooth kidney usually associated with amyloid diseases of spleen or liver.
ETIOL: Found in long continued bone suppuration or may be due to syphilis.
SYM: Face pale, waxy skin which may be edematous. Liver and spleen may also be enlarged. Not tender under pressure. Diarrhea if intestines are involved. Albumin, hyaline, and waxy casts in urine. [and organs.

amyloido'sis. Amyloid deposit in tissues

amylolysis (am-il-ol'is-is) [" + G. *lysis*, solution]. Changing of starch into sugar in the process of digestion.

amylolytic (am-il-o-lit'ik). 1. Having the qualities of a hydrolytic enzyme. 2. Pert. to a starch-splitting enzyme converting polysaccharides* into disaccharides* such as ptyalin, *q.v.*
a. enzyme. A ferment that hydrolyzes starch, producing achroödextrin and maltose. SYN: *amylase*.

amylop'sin [L. *amylum*, starch, + G. *opsis*, appearance]. Diastatic enzyme in pancreatic juice which changes starch into achroödextrin and maltose. SEE: *digestion; duodenum; enzymes*.

amylose (am'i-lōz). A group of carbohydrates containing starch, cellulose, and dextrin. SEE: *glycose, saccharose*.

amylosis (am-il-o'sis) [G. *amylon*, starch]. Albuminoid degeneration of the cells.

amylosu'ria [*amylose* + G. *ouron*, urine]. Amylose in the urine.

amylum (am-i'lum) [L.]. Starch.

amylu'ria [L. *amylum*, starch, + G. *ouron*, urine]. Starch in the urine.

amyocardia (ă-mi-o-kar'dĭ-ă) [G. *a-*, priv. + *mys*, muscle, + *kardia*, heart]. Weakness of the heart muscle. SYN: *Myasthenia cordis*.

a'myon [G. *a-*, priv. + *mys*, muscle]. Absence of muscular tissue.

amyostasia (am-i-o-sta'sĭ-ă) [" + " + *stasis*, standing]. Difficulty in standing because of lack of coördination or because of muscular tremors. SEE: *tremor*.

amyosthenia (am-i-os-the'nĭ-ă) [" + " + *sthenos*, strength]. Lack of muscular tone or power.

amyosthen'ic. Pert. to muscular weakness.

amyotaxy (am-i'o-taks-ĭ) [G. *a-*, priv. + *mys*, muscle, + *taxis*, order]. Muscular ataxia.

amyotonia (am-i-o-to'nĭ-ă) [" + " + *tonos*, tone]. Failure of muscular tone.
a. congenita. Thomsen's disease, a disease, usually congenital and hereditary, characterized by tonic spasm and rigidity of certain muscles when an attempt is made to move them after a

amyotrophia | A-48 | **anal canal**

period of rest or when mechanically stimulated. The stiffness disappears as the muscles are used.
amyotrophia (am-i-o-tro'fi-a) [" + " + *trophē*, nourishment]. Muscular wasting. [muscular atrophy.
  a., progressive spinal. Progressive
amyotrophic (am-i-o-trof'ik). Pert. to atrophy.
  a. lateral sclerosis. A progressive muscular atrophy. SYM: Spastic irritability of muscles; increased reflexes.
amyotrophy (am-i-ot'ro-fi). Muscular wasting. SYN: *amyotrophia.**
amyous (ă-mī'ŭs) [G. *a*-, priv. + *mys*, muscle]. 1. Congenitally lacking in muscular tissue. 2. Weak; deficient in muscular strength. 3. Without muscle; fleshless.
amytal (am'it-al). A derivative of barbital.
  ACTION AND USES: Sedative and hypnotic in control of insomnia and as a preliminary to surgical anesthesia.
  DOSAGE: As sedative: 1/3 to 3/4 gr. (0.02 to 0.05 Gm.). Hypnotic: 1½ to 5 gr. (0.1 to 0.3 Gm.).
amyxia (ă-miks'ĭ-ă) [G. *a*-, priv. + *myxa*, mucus]. Deficient mucous secretion.
amyxorrhea (ă-miks-or-rī'ă) [" + " + *roia*, flow]. Lack of normal secretion of mucus.
an- [G.]. Prefix: negative; without or not, as *anemia*.
An. SYMB: Actinon.
A. N. A. Abbr. *American Nurses Association*.
ana (an'ă) [G.]. Meaning "one of each" used in writing prescriptions as āā. SEE: *prescription*.
anab'asis [G. *anabainein*, to go up]. Period of increase in a disease.
anabatic (an-ă-bat'ik). Increased severity; pert. to anabasis.
anabio'sis [G. *ana*, again, + *bios*, life]. Revival of a body which seemed lifeless. SYN: *resuscitation.*
anabiotic (an-ă-bi-ot'ik). Restorative. Any agent that resuscitates or restores.
anabole (an-ab'o-le) [G. a building up]. Vomiting; regurgitation; expectoration.
anabol'ic. Promoting or pert. to anabolism.
  a. nerve. Nerve controlling building processes.
anab'olin. A product of anabolism.
anabolism (an-ab'o-lizm) [G. *anabolē*, a building up]. The building up of the body substance; the constructive or synthetic chemical reactions included in metabolism; a process by which a cell takes from the blood the substance required for repair and growth, building it into a cytoplasm, thus converting a nonliving material into the living cytoplasm of the cell.
  RS: *anabolin, anastate, assimilation, catabolism, metabolism, nutrition, nutritorium, synthesis.*
anabrosis (an-ab-ro'sis) [G. an eating up]. Superficial ulceration.
anacampsis (an-ă-kamp'sis) [G. *anakampsis*, a bending back]. A flexure.
anacamp'tics [G. *anakamptein*, to bend back]. Study of reflection of light or sound.
anacamptometer (an-a-camp-tom'et-er) [" + *metron*, measure]. Device for measuring reflexes.
anacatharsis (an-ak-ath-ar'sis) [G. *anakatharsis*, upward cleansing]. Vomiting; expectoration.
anacathar'tic. That which causes vomiting.

anachlorhydria (an-ă-klor-hīd'rī-ă). Absence of free hydrochloric acid in the gastric juice. SYN: *achlorhydria.**
anacid (an-as'id) [G. *an*, priv., + L. *acidum*, sour]. Subacid, slightly acid; lacking in acidity.
anacidity (an-as-id'it-ī). Abnormal lack or deficiency of acidity.
anaclasim'eter [G. *anaklasis*, refraction, + *metron*, measure]. Instrument for measuring refraction of eyes.
anaclisis (an-ak'lis-is) [G. *anaklisis*, a lying back]. Reclining.
anaclit'ic choice. An early expression of psychosexual development, the opposite of narcissism,* in which the object of one's love is influenced by dependence upon the mother or whoever is responsible for the child's early care, more or less inhibiting other expressions of the sex instinct.
anacroasia (an-ă-kro-a'sī-ă) [G. *an*-, priv. + *akroasis*, hearing]. Inability to understand spoken words.
anacrotic (an-a-krot'ik) [G. *ana*, up, + *krotos*, stroke]. 1. Pert. to a pulse with more than one expansion of the artery. 2. Pert. to two heartbeats traced on the ascending line of a sphygmogram. SEE: *pulse*.
  a. limb. Up-stroke of a pulse wave.
  a. wave. A wave on the up-stroke of a pulse wave.
anac'rotism. Existence of a double beat on ascending line of sphygmogram. SYN: *anadicrotism.**
anacusia, anacu'sis (an-ak-oo'sĭ-ă, -sis) [G. *an*, priv. + *kusis*, hearing]. Complete deafness.
anadenia (an-ad-e'nĭ-ă) [" + *aden*, gland]. 1. Lowered glandular function. 2. Chronic lack of gastric secretion.
anadicrot'ic. 1. Pert. to a pulse with more than one artery expansion. 2. Pert. to two heartbeats traced on the ascending line of a sphygmogram. SYN: *anacrotic*, *q.v.*
anadicrotism (an-ă-dik'ro-tizm) [G. *ana*, up, + *dikrotos*, double beating] Existence of a double beat on ascending line of the sphygmogram.
anadipsia (an-a"dip'se-ă) [G. *ana*, intensive, + *dipsa*, thirst]. Intense thirst.
anadrome (an-ad'ro-me) [G. *anadromos*, a running upward]. 1. Ascending pain. 2. Globus hystericus. 3. Upward determination of the blood.
anaerobe (an-a'er-ōb) [G. *an*, priv. + *aer*, air, + *bios*, life]. A microörganism which thrives best or lives only without oxygen.
anaerob'ic. Having the power to use oxygen for metabolism from oxygen compounds; having the ability to live without air as some microbes.
anaerobiosis (an-a-er-o-bi-o'sis). Life in an oxygen-free atmosphere.
anaerobiotic (an-a-er-o-bi-ot'ik). Able to exist without free oxygen.
anagnosasthenia (an"ag-no-sas-the'nĭ-ă) [G. *anagnōsis*, reading, + *astheneia*, weakness]. Distressing symptoms when trying to read.
anagoge, anagogia (an-ă-go'je, -jī-ă) [G. *anagōgē*, a leading up]. Vomiting.
anakatesthe'sia [G. *ana*, up, + *kata*, down, + *aisthēsis*, sensation]. A sensation as of hovering or bearing down upon one.
anaku'sis. Complete deafness. SYN: *anacusia.**
anal (a'nal) [L. *anus*, a ring]. Rel. to the anus or outer rectal opening.
  a. canal. The terminal portion of the colon, its external aperture being the

anal erotic   A-49   **anaphylaxis**

anus. This is protected by an internal and external sphincter muscle, and remains closed except during defecation. It is about 2.5 to 3.8 cm. (1½ inches) long.

a. erotic (e-rot′ik). Psy: One who indulges in anal erotism,* or that which pertains to it.

a. e. character. One who has persisted in anal erotism after childhood. Sym: Orderliness in all habits, obstinacy, sometimes the manifestation of revenge, spite, and miserliness. See: *erotism.*

a. reflex. Contraction of anal sphincter following irritation of skin about anus. Reflex is lost in lesions of posterior columns of cord and is exaggerated in anal fissures.

analepsis (an-al-ep′sis) [G. *analēpsis*, a taking up]. Gaining strength after an illness. Restoration to health. 2. Epilepsy accompanied by gastric aura. 3. Suspension as in a swing.

analeptic (an-al-lep′tik) [G. *analēptikos*, restorative]. 1. Invigorating. 2. A restorative. 3. That which restores health.

analgesia (an-al-je′zĭ-ă) [G. *an-*, priv. + *algos*, pain]. Absence of normal sense of pain. See: *alganesthesia, labor.*

a. algera, a. dolorosa. Severe pain with loss of sensitivity in a part.

a., paretic. Complete a. of upper limb, in conjunction with partial paralysis.

analgesic (an-al-je′sik). A medicine which relieves pain when given by mouth.

analgetic (an-al-jet′ik). Analgesic; producing freedom from pain, or an agent that lessens pain.

analgia (an-al′jĭ-ă) [G. *an-*, priv. + *algos*, pain]. State of being without pain.

analgic (an-al′jik). Without pain.

analogue (an′al-og) [G. *analogós*, proportionate]. An organ or part similar in function, but differing in structure.

analosis (an-al-o′sis) [G. *analosis*, expenditure]. Wasting away; atrophy.

analysand (an-al′ĭ-zand). Psy: A patient who is being psychoanalyzed.

analysis (ă-năl′ĭ-sĭs) [G. *analysis*, a dissolving]. 1. Separation of anything into its constituent parts. 2. Chem: Determination of, or separation into, its constituent parts of a substance or compound. 3. Psy: Diagnosis and treatment.

a., qualitative. Determining the nature of the elements in a substance.

a., quantitative. Determining the nature and the quantity of elements in a substance.

a., spectrum. Determining the nature of a gas by use of the spectroscope.

analyst (an′ă-list). One who analyzes.

analytic (an-ă-lit′ik). Pert. to any analysis.

analyze (an′al-īz). To make an analysis.

anamnesis (an-am-ne′sis) [G. *anamimnēskein*, to recall to memory]. 1. Recollection; faculty of remembering. 2. That which is remembered. 3. The personal and case history of a patient and his family history. See: *catamnesis.*

anamnestic. 1. Pert. to previous medical history of patient. 2. Assisting the memory.

anamniotic [G. *an-*, priv. + *amnion*]. Without an amnion.

ananabasia (an-an-ab-a′zĭ-ă) [G. *an-*, priv. + *anabasis*, an ascending]. An abulia in which the person seems unable to ascend heights.

ananaphylaxis (an-an-ă-fi-lak′sis) [G. *an*, priv. + *a-*, priv. + *phylaxis*, protection]. That which neutralizes anaphylaxis.*

ananastasia (an-an-as-ta′zĭ-ă) [G. *an-*, priv. + *anastasis*, a rising up]. An abulia in which the person is unable to rise from a sitting position.

anandria (an-an′drĭ-ă) [" + *aner-, andr-*, man]. Impotence; lack in virility.

anangioplasia [" + *aggeion*, vessel, + *plassein*, to form]. Imperfect vascularization of a part.

anangioplastic. Pert. to imperfect development of the vascular system.

anapeiratic (an-ă-pi-rat′ik) [G. *anapeirasthai*, to try again]. Pert. to a nervous affection arising from excessive muscular activity, as an occupational neurosis. [muscular activity.

a. cramp. One arising from excessive

a. c., cyclists. Pain in scrotum, perineum, and thighs from excessive riding.

a. c., occupational. Writer's cramp.

a. c., professional. Spasmodic disorder affecting groups of muscles used in special work or movements.

anaphase (an′a-fāz) [G. *ana*, up, + *phainein*, to appear]. A stage in mitosis when the newly divided chromosomes move towards the opposite poles of the chromatic spindle to form the *diaster*.

anaphia (an-ă′fĭ-ă) [G. *an-*, priv. + *aphē*, touch]. 1. Abnormal sensitiveness to touch. 2. Defective sense of touch. 3. Palpation that reveals no diagnosis.

anaphoresis (an-ă-for-e′sis) [" + *phoresis*, sweating]. 1. Insufficient activity of the sweat glands. 2. Transmission of electropositive bodies into tissues by passage of electric current, the flow toward the positive pole.

anaphoria (an-ă-for′ĭ-ă) [G. *ana*, up, + *phorein*, to carry]. Tendency of eyeballs to turn upward. Syn: *anatropia.*

anaphrodisia (an-af-ro-diz′ĭ-ă) [G. *an-*, priv. + *Aphroditē*, goddess of love]. Diminished or absent sex desire.

anaphrodisiac. An agent that will depress the sexual function. Ex: *bromides, opium, monobromated camphor.*

anaphrodite (an-af′ro-dīt). One with an impairment of sexual desire or with an absence of it.

anaphylactia [G. *an*, again, + *a-*, priv. + *phylaxis*, protection]. Any anaphylactic condition.

anaphylactic (an-ă-fi-lak′tik). Pert. to increasing susceptibility to an infection.

a. shock. Intense symptoms often accompanied by a rash, as the result of a foreign protein injection. See: *shock.*

anaphylactin (an-ă-fi-lak′tin). The substances supposed to produce hypersusceptibility following injection of a foreign protein.

anaphylactogen [G. *an*, again, + *a*, priv. + *phylaxis*, protection, + *gennan*, to produce]. That which produces anaphylaxis or anaphylactin. [ducing anaphylaxis.

anaphylactogenesis. The process of pro-

anaphylactogenic (an-ă-fi-lak-to-jen′ik). Producing anaphylaxis or the agent producing anaphylactic reactions.

anaphylatoxin [*anaphylaxis* + G. *toxikon*, poison]. The poisonous element in anaphylaxis.

anaphylatoxis. Anaphylatoxic reaction.

anaphylaxis (an-a-fil-aks′is) [G. *an*, again, + *a-*, priv. + *phylaxis*, protection]. The opposite of *prophylaxis.** A condition produced artificially and experimentally in lower animals and dependent upon well defined antigen-antibody reaction. A hypersensitive state of the body to a

anaplasia   A-50   **anastomosis, Schmidel's**

foreign protein or a drug, so that the injection of a second dose brings about an acute reaction; known also as *protein sensitization* and *serum sickness*. The term implies symptoms severe enough to produce serious shock.

The reaction does not occur if the initial dose has been administered not more than ten days previously. To prevent anaphylaxis the second dose of serum should be given gradually, *i. e.*, it must be divided into small doses, with a short interval between. Some doctors prefer to give half the dose, and the remainder after half an hour's interval.

Such diseases as asthma, hay fever, urticaria (hives) are thought to be of an anaphylactic nature, being caused by the irritation of a food or by the pollen of some plants and flowers, to which the individual may have become sensitized. Sometimes marked a. following a blood transfusion, esp. if the blood is not transferred immediately after its withdrawal from the donor.

SYM: (a). *Mild a.*: Fever (slight), redness of skin, itching, urticaria. (b) *Severe a.*: Dyspnea, violent cough, chest constriction, cyanosis, fever, skin eruption, pulse variations, collapse.

PROG: Favorable if cause is removed early. Otherwise, may lead to death.

TREATMENT: Hypodermic of some strong heart stimulant such as atropine or adrenalin.

NP: Applications of heat, oxygen inhalations, treatment for shock.

RS: *ananaphylaxis, anaphylactia, anaphylactogen, anaphylactogenesis, anaphylatoxin, anaphylatoxis.*

anapla'sia [G. *ana*, again, + *plasis*, a molding]. 1. Reversion of cells to a more embryonic type. 2. Alteration in cells which produces malignancy.

anaplas'tic. Pert. to anaplasia or restoration of lost part.

anaplasty (an'ă-plas-tĭ) [G. *ana*, again, + *plassein*, to form]. Grafting or restoring lost parts.

anaplero'sis [G. *anaplērōsis*, a filling up]. Transplantation of tissue.

anapnea (an-ap-ne'ă) [G. *anapnein*, to breathe again]. 1. Respiration. 2. Regaining the breath.

anapneic (an-ap-ne'ik). Pert. to anapnea or relieving dyspnea.

anapnograph (an-ap'no-graf) [G. *anapnoē*, respiration, + *graphein*, to write]. An instrument for measuring pressure and speed of respiration.

anapnoic (an-ap-no'ik). 1. Pert. to anapnea. 2. Relieving dyspnea.

anapnom'eter [G. *anapnoē*, respiration, + *metron*, measure]. Instrument for measuring respiratory movements.

anapnother'apy [" + *therapeia*, treatment]. Any gas treatment.

anapophysis (an-ă-pof'ĭ-sis) [G. *ana*, back, + *apophysis*, offshoot]. An accessory spinal process of a vertebra.

anap'tic [G. *an-*, priv. + *aptein*, to touch]. Pert. to anaphia or diminished or lost tactile sense.

anarithmia (an-ă-rith'mĭ-ă) [" + *arithmos*, enumeration]. Inability to count or to use numbers. ETIOL: Brain lesion.

anarthria (an-ar'thrĭ-ă) [" + *arthron*, joint]. 1. Loss of motor power to speak. ETIOL: Motor innervation, of muscular apparatus defect. 2. State of being without vigor. 3. Condition of being without joints.   [partial aphasia.

a. centralis. A central lesion causing

a. literalis. Stammering.

anasarca (an-ă-sar'kă) [G. *ana*, throughout, + *sarx, sarkos*, flesh]. A general dropsical condition.

ETIOL: (a) A chronic heart disease, and cirrhosis of the liver. (b) A local obstruction to circulation by clots within the veins. (c) A compression from without of the veins by a tumor or swelling. (d) A defective metabolism, whereby the water of the body is not excreted, as in nephritis. (e) A severe anemia wherein the quality of the blood is greatly impoverished.

a., acute. With natural color of skin.

anasarcous (an-ă-sar'kus). Dropsical.

anaspadias (an-ă-spa'dĭ-ăs) [G. *ana*, up, + *span*, to draw]. Urethral opening upon upper surface of penis.

anastal'tic [G. *anastaltikos*, checking]. 1. Very astringent. 2. Afferent.

anastasis (an-as'tas-ĭs) [G. a rising up]. 1. Convalescence. 2. Resuscitation. 3. An upward flow of body fluids.

anastate (an'as-tāt). Anything characteristic of an anabolic process.

anastole (an-as'to-le) [G. *anastolē*, laying bare a wound]. Shrinking away or retraction of the lips of a wound.

anastomose (an-as'to-mōs) [G. *anastomōsis*, opening]. 1. Opening of one vessel into another, or the union of one nerve with another. 2. To make such a connection, surgically.

anastomosis (an-as-to-mo'sis) [G. opening]. 1. A communication between two vessels. 2. The surgical or pathologic formation of a passage between any two normally distinct spaces or organs. 3. An end-to-end union or joining together or intercommunication of parts of any network or set of fibers such as nerves, or connective tissue fibers.

a., antiperistaltic. Enterostomy in which the two parts are so joined that the peristaltic wave in each part is in opposite directions.

a., arteriovenous. Anastomosis between an artery and a vein.

a., collateral. A natural one, as that of the arteries at knee joint.

a., crucial. An arterial anastomosis in the proximal part of the thigh, formed by the anastomotic branch of the sciatic, and internal circumflex, the first perforating, and the transverse portion of the external circumflex.

a., Galen's. The anastomosis between the sup. and inf. laryngeal nerves.

a., heterocladic. Anastomosis between branches of different arteries.

a., homocladic. Anastomosis between branches of the same artery.

a., Hyrtl's. An occasional looplike anastomosis bet. right and left hypoglossal nerves in geniohyoid muscle.

a., intestinal. The establishment of a communication between two portions of the intestines.

a., isoperistaltic. Intestinal anastomosis in which the two parts are so joined that the peristaltic wave in each part is in the same direction.

a., Jacobson's. The union of a nerve from the petrous ganglion with the Vidian nerve, or with the tympanic branch of the glossopharyngeal.

a., precapillary. Anastomosis between small arteries just before they become capillaries.

a., Schmidel's. Abnormal communications between the vena cava and the portal system.

a., terminoterminal. Anastomosis between the peripheral end of an artery and the central end of the corresponding vein, and between the central end of the artery and terminal end of vein.
a., ureterotubal. An anastomosis between the ureter and the fallopian tube.
anastomot′ic. Pert. to, or marked by, anastomosis.
anatherapeusis (an-ă-ther″ă-pū′sis) [G. *ana*, up, + *therapeia*, treatment]. Treatment by steadily increasing doses.
anathrepsis (an-ath-rep′sis) [G. *anathrepsis*, a fresh growth]. The regaining of flesh after an illness.
anatomic (an-ă-tom′ik) [G. *anatomnein*, to cut up]. Of or rel. to the anatomy or structure of an organism.
anatomist (an-at′o-mist). A skilled student of anatomy.
anatomy (an-at′o-mī) [G. *ana*, up, + *temnein*, to cut]. The structure or study of structure of organs or a treatise on same.
a., applied. That applied to diagnosis and treatment, esp. surgical treatment.
a., comparative. Comparison of structure of different animals.
a., descriptive. Study of physical structure.
a., gross. Study of structures seen with the naked eye.
a., morbid or pathological. That of abnormal structure.
anat′opism [G. *ana*, without, + *topos*, place]. Inability to conform to social usage.
anatoxic (an-a-toks′ik) [G. *ana*, priv. + *toxikon*, poison]. 1. Pert. to anatoxin. 2. Anaphylactic.
anatoxin (an-a-toks′in) [G. *ana*, priv. + *toxikon*, poison]. A modified toxin retaining the antigenic properties with lessened toxic properties.
anatricrotic pulse (an-a-tri-krot′ik) [G. *ana*, up, + *treis*, three, + *krotos*, stroke]. Three beats on the ascending curve of a pulse wave.
anatripsis (an-at-rip′sis) [G. friction]. 1. A centripetal, or upward movement in massage. 2. Inunction. Rubbing or removing by scraping. 3. Crushing as of a stone.
anatrip′tic (an-at-rip′tik). An agent to be rubbed in.
anatro′pia [G. *ana*, up, + *tropē*, a turning]. Tendency of eyeballs to turn upward; anaphoria.
anaxon(e (an-aks′on) [G. *an-*, priv. + *axon*, axis]. A nerve cell having no neuraxon as those of the retina.
anazoturia (an-az-o-tu′rī-ă) [" + *a-*, priv. + *zōē*, life, + G. *ouron*, urine]. Without urea or nitrogenous substances in the urine.
anchone (ang-ko′nē) [G. *agchein*, to strangle]. Spasm of the throat in hysteria.
anchorage (ang′ko-rāj). 1. Operative fixation of displaced viscus. 2. The part to which anything is fixed, as a tooth to which a bridge is fastened.
ancipital (an-sip′it-al) [L. *anceps*, two-headed]. Two-edged.
anconad (ang′ko-nad) [G. *ankōn*, elbow, + L. *ad*, to]. Toward the elbow.
anconagra (ang-ko-nag′ră) [" + *agra*, a seizure]. Gout of the elbow.
anconal, anconeal (ang′ko-nal, -ne-al). Pert. to the elbow.
a. fossa. Fossa olecrani.
anconeus (an-kon′e-us) [G. *ankōn*, elbow]. Short-extensor muscle of forearm arising from external condyle of the humerus and inserting on olecranon and upper fourth of shaft of ulna.
anconitis (ang-ko-ni′tis) [" + *-itis*, inflammation]. Inflammation of the elbow joint.
ancyroid (an′sir-oid) [G. *ankyra*, anchor, + *eidos*, resemblance]. Shaped like fluke of an anchor.
Andernach's ossicles (ăn′der-năkh). Small bones found in cranial sutures. SYN: *wormian bones.*
Anders' disease. One in which fat occurs in painful nodules. SYN: *adiposis tuberosa simplex.*
An′dersch's ganglion. Ganglion petrosum.
A.'s nerve. Nervus tympanicus.
An′drai's decu′bitus. Lying on sound side during beginning of pleurisy.
andrase (an′drāz) [G. *andrōs*, man, + *ase*]. The hypothetical substance determining male sex. Opp. of *gynase.*
andriat′rics [" + *iatreia*, medical treatment]. Study of diseases of male genitals.
andro- (an′drō) [G. *anēr*, man]. A prefix signifying man.
androgalactozemia (an-dro-gal-ak-to-ze′-mī-ă) [" + *gala*, milk, + *zemia*, loss]. Oozing of milk from male breast.
androgen (ăn′drō-jĕn) [" + *gennan*, to produce]. Substance producing or stimulating male characteristics, as the male hormone.
androgyne (an′dro-jīn) [" + *gynē*, woman]. One possessing genital and sexual characteristics of both sexes. SYN: *hermaphrodite.**
androgynoid (an-droj′ī-noyd) [" + " + *eidos*, resemblance]. A male of hermaphroditic sexual characteristics and tendencies mistaken for a woman.
androgynous (an-droj′in-us) [" + *gynē*, woman]. 1. Resembling or possessing characteristics of both sexes; hermaphroditic. 2. Without definite sexual characteristics.
androg′ynus [" + "]. A hermaphrodite.
android (ăn′droyd) [G. *aner, andr-*, man, + *eidos*, resemblance]. Shaped like that of a man, as a female pelvis.
andrology (an-drol′o-jī) [" + *logos*, study of]. Study of diseases of the male.
andromania (an-dro-ma′nī-ă) [" + *mania*, frenzy]. Abnormal sexual desire in the female. SYN: *nymphomania.**
andromimetic (ăn″drō-mĭm-ĕt′ĭk) [G. *aner, andr-*, man, + *mimētikos*, imitative]. Simulating human processes, as certain types of protozoa.
androp′athy [" + *pathos*, suffering]. Any disease peculiar to the male, as *prostatitis.*
an′drophile [" + *philos*, fond of]. Preferring man, as parasitic organisms.
androphobia (an-dro-fo′bī-ă) [" + *phobos*, fear]. Abnormal fear of the male sex.
androphonomania (an-dro-fo-no-ma′nī-ă) [" + *phonos*, slaying, + *mania*, frenzy]. Psychotic homicidal trends, esp. when violent.
androsterone (ăn-drŏs′ter-ōn). Testicular hormone of male sex, found in urine, which regulates changes taking place at puberty.
It is responsible for development of hair upon face, under arms, and about the pubis, development of sexual organs, voice changes, etc. SYN: *male sex hormone.*
-ane. Indicating a saturated hydrocarbon.
anebous (an-e′bous) [G. *anebos*, immature]. Immature.

aneilema (an-i-le′mă) [G. *ana*, up, + *eileein*, to roll]. 1. Flatulence. 2. Colic.

anelectrotonus (an-el-ek-trot′o-nus) [G. *ana*, up, + *elektron*, electric, + *tonos*, tension]. The state of diminished irritability of a nerve or muscle produced in region near the anode during the passage of an electric current.

Anel's operation (ah-nelz′). Ligation of an artery immediately above and on proximal side of an aneurysm.

A.'s probe. A probe for the lacrimal and nasal ducts.

anemato′sis [G. *an-*, priv. + *aima*, blood, + *-osis*, condition]. 1. General anemia. 2. Pernicious anemia.

anemia (an-e′mĭ-ă) [G. *an-*, priv. + *aima*, blood]. A deficiency of red blood corpuscles, hemoglobin, or both. The total volume of the blood may or may not change. Classified into 3 groups, due to (1) deficiency in materials, (2) disturbed production of red blood cells within bone-marrow, and (3) excessive loss of mature erythrocytes by either hemorrhage or destruction.

ETIOL: Hemorrhage, acute or continuous, following infectious diseases, as scarlet fever or syphilis; from cancer; toxic conditions, as those of pregnancy; jaundice; nephritis, or from absorption of toxins from foci of infection, intestinal obstruction, chemicals, congenital causes, as hemolytic a., due to poor nutrition and iron deficiency. Failure to produce an antianemic factor which is stored in the liver.

When there is a high color index, the anemia is said to be *hyperchromic*, and if low, *hypochromic*.

a., aplastic. This is a form of primary anemia in which bone marrow does not supply enough new red blood corpuscles.

ETIOL: Due to aplasia of bone marrow and destruction of same. SYM: Insidious in onset, profound anemia, may be jaundice and pyrexia. TREATMENT: Repeated blood transfusions.

a., chlorosis (green sickness). Form of anemia in adolescent girls, perhaps due to faulty diet during puberty.

a., drepanocytic. A. in which red blood cells of person assume a sickle shape, legs ulcerate.

a., essential, a., idiopathic. A. caused by pathology of the blood or blood-building organs. SYN: *pernicious a.*

a. lymphatica. A. in conjunction with tumors of the lymph glands. SEE: *Hodgkin's disease.*

a., macrocytic. A. marked by abnormally large erythrocytes.

a., microcytic. A. with abnormally small erythrocytes.

a., myelopathic. A. caused by disruption in bone marrow function.

a., myelophthisic. A. in which blood-building tissues are mechanically displaced.

a., normocytic. A. in which the hemoglobin content remains normal.

a., primary or pernicious. Disease of the blood characterized by severe progressive anemia and achlorhydria. Men are more apt to have it, usually about middle age.

ETIOL: Unknown or failure to produce an antianemic factor, *q.v.* Possible microörganism reaching the bone marrow through the circulation which may cause subacute degeneration of the spinal cord. Possible absence of some hormone in gastric juice that is stored in the liver.

SYM: These are about same as in all anemias: dyspnea, palpitation, malaise, headache, edema of ankles. In this form lemon yellow skin, diarrhea, vomiting, tongue red and sore, mouth dry. Some pyrexia. Remissions and relapses. Progressively worse if untreated. Diminished hydrochloric acid. Diminished red blood cells, some nucleated and some larger than others. Hemoglobin low.

a., secondary. A. which results from an injury or disease.

ETIOL: Result of other diseases or conditions, as large or repeated small hemorrhages, cancer, wasting diseases, acute and chronic infections, nephritis, acute rheumatism and poisoning by arsenic, lead, or mercury.

a., septic. A. due to septic condition in the body.

a., sickle-cell. SEE: *drepanocytic a.*

a., splenic. A. accompanied by an enlarged spleen.

NP: The nursing care of patients with anemia consists of providing adequate rest, taking proper care of the skin, mouth, and teeth, insuring proper elimination, regulating the diet, and administering antianemic medicines which are prescribed by the physician.

Rest: Patients with mild and moderately severe anemias are usually ambulatory, but patients with very severe anemias must be kept in bed and spared all possible exertion. In acute anemia due to blood loss absolute rest is essential; the foot of the bed should be elevated, the patient covered with blankets, and hot water bottles applied to the extremities. Warm, stimulating drinks may be given if the hemorrhage is not from the gastrointestinal tract.

Care of the skin: Daily warm baths and light massage are beneficial. In patients with very severe anemias, special care of the skin of the buttocks and heels may be necessary to prevent the formation of pressure sores. Fresh air and sunshine are indicated, but chilling should be avoided.

Care of the mouth and teeth: Besides ordinary oral hygiene, special care of the mouth is indicated in anemic patients who have soreness of the tongue, mouth, and pharynx. Alkaline mouth-washes are beneficial; if the gums are very sore, pledgets of cotton or gauze may be substituted for a toothbrush for cleaning the teeth.

Elimination: The bowels should be made to act daily; this can be done by regulation of the diet, or by the use of enemas or mild laxatives.

In severe anemias the function of the kidneys may be impaired; for this reason fluids should be given freely to insure an adequate output of urine.

Diet: The nurse's principal function in this regard is to see that the patient takes the diet which has been prescribed for him. This may be a difficult task, since he often has a poor appetite and his mouth and tongue may be sore. Tact and gentle persuasion often necessary.

Medicines: If the patient is taking iron or liver, it is most important that he does not miss a single dose. If he is given a transfusion, the nurse must watch carefully for reaction, and notify the doctor immediately if the patient complains of chilliness, or pain in the chest or back, or shortness of breath, or if his temperature rises. Also tenderness or swelling appears at the site of injection of liver extract.

anemia, words pert. to   A-53   anesthesia

Teaching the patient: Throughout the patient's illness the nurse should never lose the opportunity to impress the patient with the importance of his continuing proper treatment after he leaves the hospital. He should be made to understand that in order to get well and stay well he must continue to follow his diet and to take his medicine. He must also understand that he must revisit his doctor at frequent intervals for checkups and blood counts so that relapse may be prevented.

anemia, words pert. to: anematosis, anemotrophy, anencephalohemia, antianemic, chloranemia, chloremia, chlorosis, ischemia, sickle cell, sura.

anemic (an-e'mik). Pert. to anemia; deficient in red blood cells, or in hemoglobin, or in amount of blood.

   a. factor. Also called hematinic principle.
   A substance obtained from livers which stimulates erythropoiesis. It is produced by the action of vitamin B₁₂. An *intrinsic* factor secreted by stomach glands upon an *extrinsic* factor, present in certain foods. It is stored in the liver.

anemophobia (an-em-o-fo'bĭ-ă) [" + *phobos*, fear]. Abnormal fear of drafts, or of the wind.

anemot'rophy [G. *an*-, priv. + *aima*, blood, + *trophē*, nourishment]. Anemia from deficient formation of blood.

anencephalus (ăn-ĕn-sĕf'ăl-ŭs) [G. *an*-, priv. + *egkephalos*, the brain]. A monstrosity characterized by absence of brain and spinal cord, the cranium being open throughout its whole extent and the vertebral canal converted into a groove.

anepia (an-ep'ĭ-ă) [" + *epos*, word]. Inability to speak.

anergasia (an-er-ga'sĭ-ă) [" + *ergon*, work]. Anergia; functional inactivity.

anergastic reaction (an-er-gas'tik). Disorders involving cerebral lesions, or organic psychoses.
   SYM: *Physical.* Palsy, coma, fits or muscular contractions. [judgment, etc.
   PSY: Loss of memory, impairment of

anergia (an-er'jĭ-ă) [G. *an*-, priv. + *ergon*, work]. Inactivity; sluggishness.

anergic (an-er'jik). Sluggish; inactive. Deficient in energy; listless.
   a. stupor. Acute phase of dementia.

aneroid (an'er-oid) [G. *an*-, priv. + *nēros*, wet, + *eidos*, form]. Operating without a fluid, as air. Ex: *a. barometer.*

aneroplasty (an-er'o-plas-tĭ) [" + *aer*, air, + *plasis*, a molding]. Immersion of a wound to exclude air.

anerythrocyte (an-er-ĭ'thrō-sīt) [" + *erythros*, red, + *kytos*, cell]. A red blood cell without hemoglobin.

anerythroplasia (an-er"ĭ-thrō-plā'zĭ-ă) [" + " + *plasis*, a molding]. Without formation of red blood cells.

anerythroplastic (an-er"ĭ-thrō-plas'tik). Marked by anerythroplasia.

anerythropsia (an-er-ith-rop'sĭ-ă) [G. *an*-, priv. + *erythros*, red, + *opsis*, vision]. Inability to distinguish red clearly.

anesis (an-e'sis) [G. a relaxing]. A lessening of symptoms or of their severity.

anesthecinesia (an"es-the"sĭn-e'sĭ-ă) [G. *an*-, priv. + *aisthesis*, sensation, + *kinesis*, movement]. Combined sensory and motor paralysis.

anesthesia (an-es-the'zĭ-ă). Partial or complete loss of sensation, with or without loss of consciousness, as result of

ANESTHESIA
SCHEMATIC VIEW OF DIFFERENT FORMS OF LOCAL ANESTHESIA

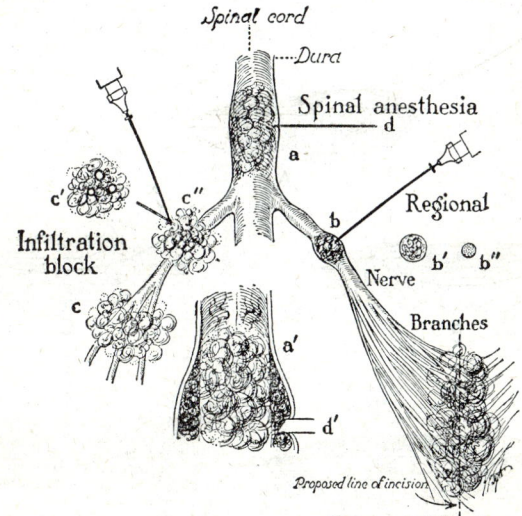

(a) Spinal cord and branches; (b, b', and b") regional anesthesia; (c, c', and c") infiltration block anesthesia; (d) spinal anesthesia; (a' and d') spinal anesthesia (enlarged view). Branches, ultimate arborization of nerve infiltration anesthesia, direct infiltration.

disease, injury, or administration of a drug or gas.

STAGES OF ANESTHESIA: *First stage:* Preliminary excitement, until voluntary control is lost. Hearing is last sense to be lost. Avoid talking in presence of patient.

Second stage: Loss of voluntary control. Corneal reflex still present.

Third stage: Entire relaxation, no rigidity, deep regular breathing, sluggish corneal reflex, and conjunctival reflex lost.

TESTS FOR ANESTHESIA: *Reaction to light:* Exclude light by holding hand over eye, withdraw it quickly, when pupil will reduce in size if anesthesia is complete.

Conjunctival reflex: Place finger at corner of eye on conjunctiva when the eye will attempt to close. This reflex is lost during third stage.

Corneal reflex: If cornea is lightly touched with finger, the eyelid attempts to close. Reflex is brisk during first and second stages, sluggish during third stage, and only lost in deep anesthesia.

Danger signals: If too deep, due to overdose, corneal reflex is lost, pupils widely dilate and cease to react to light. Cardiac and respiratory centers fail, patient ceases to breathe, and heart action stops.

EMERGENCY MEASURES: Artificial respiration by anesthetist; injection of cardiac stimulant, inhalation of carbon dioxide, applications of hot, wet towels over heart, slapping over heart, injection of pure ether into heart muscle.

a., block. That resulting from nerve blocking by injection of alcohol or other substance into or very near to a nerve trunk.

a., bulbar. Pons lesion causing central a.

a., caudal. Spinal anesthesia induced by injection in region of cauda.

a., controlled. Dolitrone. It is injected into the veins and although the patient has no sense of pain he can talk and obey orders but will not remember anything of his experiences while under the drug. Recovery is very prompt. No cumulative effects. It may take the place of sleeping pills.

a., dolorosa. Painfulness of a part with anesthesia of that part, as in thalamic lesions.

a., general. One that is complete and affecting the entire body, with loss of consciousness, when the anesthetic acts upon the brain.

a., Gwathmey's. A. induced by injecting an olive oil and ether solution into the rectum.

a., infiltration. Local anesthesia achieved by injecting a weak cocaine solution.

a., inhalation. General anesthesia achieved by inhaling ether or chloroform vapors, or the like, or nitrous oxide gas.

a., local. One affecting a local area only, the anesthetic acting upon nerves or nerve tracts. SEE: *block anesthesia, infiltration anesthesia.*

a., mental. Failure to recognize sensory stimulations.

a., mixed. Production of general anesthesia by more than one drug, as nitrous oxide gas continued by ether.

a., neural. Injection of an anesthetic into a nerve or immediately around it (*intraneural* and *paraneural*).

a., primary. First stage of anesthesia, *q.v.*

ANESTHESIA
TECHNIC OF SKIN INFILTRATION

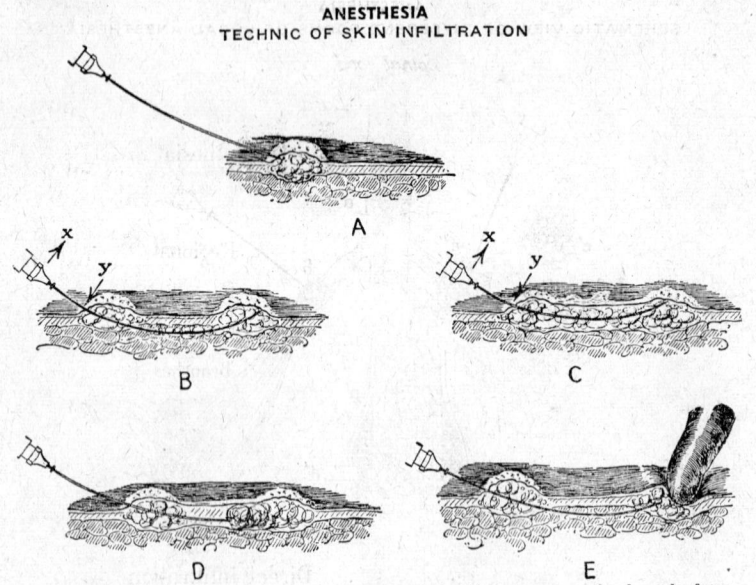

Subdermal painless method. (a) Initial wheal; (b) secondary wheal made from beneath (x and y show direction of force of needle hub); (c) subdermal infiltration made with needle advancing; (d) subdermal infiltration made with needle receding; (e) finger indentation of skin to meet needle point.

a., rectal. General anesthesia produced by introduction of anesthetic agent into rectum.
a., regional. Nerve or field blocking, causing insensibility over a particular area.
a., sexualis. Anaphrodisia or absence of sexual desire.
a., spinal or spinal* puncture. When the injection into the theca is up to level at which nerves of the area enter the spinal cord.
a., surgical. When depth of anesthesia produces relaxation of muscles and loss of sensation and/or consciousness.
a., twilight. State of light anesthesia induced to alleviate labor pains. SEE: *twilight sleep.*
anesthesia, words pert. to: a. c. e. mixture, anesthesiology, anesthesiophore, anesthetic, anesthetist, anesthetization, anesthetize, anesthetizer, apothesine, avertin, barbotage, carbon dioxide, chloracetization, chloroform, chloryl, cocaine, cyclopropane, ether, ethyl chloride, ethylene, general a., labor, local a., neothesin, nitrous oxide, novocain, para-anesthesia, paraldehyde, procaine, rectal a., spinal a., vinethene.
anesthesimeter (an-es-thes-im'et-er) [G. *an-*, priv. + *aisthesis*, sensation, + *metron*, measure]. For measuring anesthetic administered.
anesthesin (ăn-es'thē-sĭn) [G. *an-*, priv. + *aesthēsis*, sensation]. Proprietary local anesthetic.
ACTION AND USES: Nontoxic local anesthetic. May be used as a dusting powder in proportions of from 10 to 20%. Also in form of lozenges for laryngitis and to allay nausea.
DOSAGE: 0.3 cc. (5 gr.).
anesthesiology (an-es-thē-zē-ol'ō-jĭ) [G. *an-*, priv. + *aisthesis*, sensation, + *logos*, science]. Science of anesthesia.
anesthesiophore (an-es-the'zĭ-ō-fōr) [" + " + *phoros*, bearer]. Carrying anesthetic action, as *cocaine.*
anesthetic (an-es-thet'ik). An agent that produces insensibility to pain or touch. According to action, they are subdivided into general and local. SEE: *anesthesia.*
anesthetist (an-es'the-tist). One who administers anesthetics, esp. for general anesthesia.
an″esthetiza′tion. Induction of anesthesia.
anesthetize (an-es'thē-tīz). To place under an anesthetic.
anes′thetizer. One who administers an anesthetic.
anetic (a-net'ik) [G. *anetikos*, relaxing]. 1. Relaxing, soothing. 2. Anodyne.
anetodermia (an-et-ō-der'mĭ-ă) [G. *anetos*, relaxed, + *derma*, skin]. Relaxation of the skin.
an′etus. Any intermittent fever.
aneuria (a-nu′rĭ-ă) [G. *a-*, priv. + *neuron*, nerve]. Defect in or deficiency of nervous energy.
aneur′ic. Pert. to aneuria.
aneurosis (ă-nū-ro′sĭs). 1. Lacking in nervous susceptibility. 2. Deficiency of nerve function.
aneurysm (an'u-rizm) [G. *aneurysma*, a widening]. Arterial dilatation due to pressure of blood on weakened tissues, forming sac of clotted blood.
NP: No exertion permitted. Absolute rest in bed. Later, patient may get up, but warn against vigorous effort. General care in heart conditions should be observed. POSTOPERATIVE CARE: Observe circulation of the affected part. Keep limb warm with an electric pad or blanket, but, as sensation is impaired, apply heat with great care. Inspect affected part every 15 minutes, and adjust limb to help circulation in limb.
SEE: *Berard's a., Cardarelli's sign.*
a., aortic. Affecting any part of the aorta.
a. of arch of aorta. ETIOL: Pressure on trachea, esophagus, veins, or nerves. SYM: Dyspnea, cough, sputum, dysphagia, congestion of head and neck. Inequality in the two radial pulses.
a., arteriovenous. One in which artery and vein become connected by a saccule. ETIOL: Trauma. Weak point, in walls of an artery, due to syphilis, sudden strain, or injury. SYM: Pain, expansile pulsation, bruit. NP: Avoid increasing heart action or raising blood pressure.
a., dissecting. One in which the blood makes its way between the layers of a blood vessel wall, separating them.
a., fusiform. All the walls of the blood vessels dilate more or less equally, creating a tubular swelling.
a., sacculated. One due to the yielding of a weak patch on one side of the vessel and which does not involve the entire circumference; usually due to an injury.
a., varicose. A. forming a blood-filled sac bet. an artery and a vein.

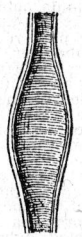

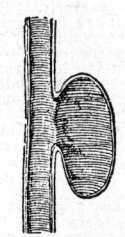

FUSIFORM ANEURYSM   SACCULATED ANEURYSM

aneurysmal (an-ū-riz'măl) [G. *aneurysma*, a widening]. Pert. to aneurysm.
aneurysmectomy (an-u-riz-mek'to-mĭ) [" + *ektomē*, a cutting out]. Extirpation of an aneurysm by removal of its sac.
aneurysmotomy (an-u-riz-mot'o-mĭ) [" + *tomē*, cut]. Incision of the sac of an aneurysm, allowing it to heal by granulation.
anfractuosity (an-frak-tu-os′ĭ-tĭ) [L. *anfractus*, a winding]. A cerebral sulcus.
anfractuous (an-frak-tu'us). Bending; sinuous.
angeitis (an-ge-i'tis) [G. *aggeion*, vessel, + *-itis*, inflammation]. Inflammation of a blood vessel or a lymphatic. SYN: *angiitis.**
an′gel's wing. A very prominent scapula, due to deformity.
Angelucci's syndrome (ăn-jĕ-loot'che). Great excitability, palpitation, and vasomotor disturbance associated with vernal conjunctivitis.
angi (an′gī). Inguinal buboes.
angiasthe′nia [G. *aggeion*, vessel, + *a-*, priv. + *sthenos*, strength]. Loss of vascular tone.
angiectasia, -sis (an-jĭ-ek-ta'zĭ-ă, -tas-is) [" + *ektasis*, stretching]. Enlarged capillaries or abnormal dilation of a vessel.
angiec′tomy [" + *ektomē*, excision]. Excision of section of a blood vessel.

angiectopia (an-ji-ek-to'pĭ-ă) [" + *ektopos*, out of place]. Displacement of a vessel.

angiemphraxis (an-je-em-fraks'is) [" + *emphraxis*, stoppage]. Obstruction of any vessel.

angiitis (an-ji-i'tis) [" + *-itis*, inflammation]. Inflammation of a blood vessel or of a lymphatic.

angina (ăn-ji'na, L. an'jĭ-na) [L. quinsy, from *angere*, to choke]. 1. A sense of suffocation. 2. Disease of the pharynx or fauces.

a., acute. Simple sore throat.

a. cruris. A. due to obstruction of an artery, causing pain and cyanosis of the affected part, with periodic lameness.

a., follicular. A. of the larynx and pharynx from public speaking, excessive drinking of alcoholic liquors.

a. laryngea. Inflammation of the larynx.

a. ludovici, a. ludwigii. Purulent inflammation in the submaxillary region.

a., Ludwig's. Phlegmonous cellulitis of the neck.

a. maligna. Diphtheria.

a., necrotic. Form with gangrenous patches in the mucosa of the air passages, seen in scarlet fever and occasionally in diphtheria.

a. parotidea. Inflammation of the parotid glands. SYN: *mumps.*

a. pectoris. Pain and oppression about the heart; a paroxysmal affection characterized by severe pain radiating from the heart to the shoulder, thence down the left arm, or, rarely, from the heart to the abdomen; apparently dependent upon some lesion of the coronary arteries of the heart, its walls, or valves. Attacks may occur in lesions of the aortic valves. Generally afflicts males of middle age.

SYM: Severe pain in region of the heart; great anxiety, fear of approaching death, and fixation of the body; face pale, ashen, or livid, brow bathed in sweat. Dyspnea often noted; pulse variable, usually tense and quick. Blood pressure is raised during an attack. Attack lasts from a few seconds to several minutes.

PROG: May be grave. Attacks may be intermittent, and with proper rest and care recovery is possible.

TREATMENT: During attack, inhalation of amyl nitrite; nitroglycerin, and hot applications to the precordia. During intervals, absolute rest of body and mind; carefully regulated diet, light but nutritious. General constitutional treatment.

A new method of arresting pain being tried is injection of a local anesthetic just below 3rd rib on left side.

a. simplex. Sore throat. SEE: *acute a.*

a. streptococcus. A. caused by the streptococcus.

a. tonsillans. Quinsy.

a. trachealis. Croup.

a., Vincent's. Ulceration and inflammation of floor of mouth. SEE: *trench mouth.*

anginal (an'jĭ-nal). Pert. to angina.

anginoid (an'jĭ-noid) [L. *angina*, choking, + G. *eidos*, resemblance]. Resembling angina pectoris, or any angina.

anginophobia (an-jĭ-no-fo'bĭ-ă) [" + G. *phobos*, fear]. Intense fear of an attack of angina pectoris.

anginose (an'jĭ-nōs). Pert. to or resembling angina.

an'ginous. Resembling angina. SYN: *anginose.*

angio- (an-gĭ-o) [G. *aggeion*, vessel]. A prefix pert. to a vessel.

an"gioatax'ia [" + G. *ataktōs*, out of order]. Variability in arterial tonus.

angioblast (an'jĭ-o-blast) [" + G. *blastos*, germ]. Embryonic cells from which blood vessels develop.

angiocardiokinet'ic [" + G. *kardia*, heart, + *kinesis*, movement]. Stimulating or that which affects movements of heart and blood vessels.

angiocarditis (an-ji-o-kar'di-tis) [" + " + *-itis*, inflammation]. Inflammation of the heart and large blood vessels. SEE: *carditis.*

angiocav'ernous [" + L. *caverna*, cavern]. Rel. to conditions present in angioma cavernosum.

angiocholecystitis (an"jĭ-ō-kō-lē-sis-ti'tis) [" + *cholē*, bile, + *kystis*, bladder, + *-itis*, inflammation]. Inflammation of gallbladder and bile vessels.

angiocholitis (an-ji-ō-kō-li'tis) [" + " + *-itis*, inflammation]. Inflammation of biliary vessels; cholangitis.

angiocrine (an'jĭ-ō-krĭn) [" + *endon*, within, + *krinein*, to secrete]. Marked by vasomotor disorders resulting from disturbances of the endocrine glands.

angiodermatitis (an"jĭ-ō-der-mă-ti'tis) [" + *derma*, skin, + *-itis*, inflammation]. Inflammation of cutaneous vessels.

angiodystrophia (an-jĭ-ō-dis-tro'fĭ-ă) [" + *dys*, bad, + *trophē*, nourishment]. Faulty nutrition of vessels.

angiofibro'ma (*Pl. a.-fibromata*) [" + L. *fibra*, fiber, + *-oma*, tumor]. An angioma having connective tissue overgrowth.

angiogenesis (an"jĭ-ō-jen'es-is) [" + *genesis*, origin]. Development of blood vessels.

angiogenic (an"jĭ-ō-jen'ik). Pert. to angiogenesis; of vascular origin.

an"gioglio'ma [G. *aggeion*, vessel, + *glia*, glue, + *-ōma*, tumor]. A mixed angioma and glioma.

angiograph (an'jĭ-o-graf) [G. *aggeion*, vessel, + *graphein*, to write]. A variety of sphygmograph.

angiography (an-jĭ-og'ră-fĭ). A description of blood vessels and lymphatics.

angiohyalinosis (an"jĭ-ō-hi"al-in-o'sis) [G. *aggeion*, vessel, + *yalos*, glass, + *-ōsis*, production]. Hyaline or glassy degeneration of the muscular coat of blood vessels.

an"giohyperto'nia [" + *yper*, over, + *tonos*, tension]. Angiospasm; spasmodic contraction of arteries.

an"giohypoto'nia [" + *ypo*, under, + *tonos*, tension]. Angioparalysis; angioparesis; vascular relaxation.

angioid (an'jĭ-oyd) [" + *eidos*, resemblance]. Resembling a blood vessel.

a. streaks. Dark, wavy, anastomosing striae lying beneath retinal vessels.

angiokeratoma (an"jĭ-o-ker-ă-to'mă) [" + *keras*, horn, + *-oma*, tumor]. A skin disease occurring chiefly on feet and legs.

ETIOL: Exciting cause unknown; predisposing cause circulatory weakness with external pressure a concomitant factor in localization.

SYM: Formation of telangiectases or warty growths (in groups), accompanied by thickening of the epidermis along the course of dilated capillaries.

TREATMENT: *Local:* Destruction of lesions by galvanic needle or carbon dioxide snow. *General:* Improvement of general circulation and removal of discoverable venous obstruction to prevent extension.

angiokinet'ic [" + *kinesis*, movement]. Pert. to action of blood vessels.

angioleukasia (an-gĭ-o-lū-ka'sĭ-ă) [" + *leukos*, white, + *asia*, condition]. Dilatation of lymphatics.

angioleukitis (an-jĭ-o-lu-ki'tis) [" + *leukos*, white, + *-itis*, inflammation]. Inflammation of lymphatics.

angiolipo'ma [" + *lipos*, fat, + *-oma*, tumor]. A mixed angioma and lipoma.

angiolith (an'jĭ-o-lith) [" + *lithos*, stone]. 1. A venous calculus. 2. Calcareous deposit in wall of a blood vessel.

angiology (an-jĭ-ol'o-jĭ) [" + *logos*, science]. The science of the blood vessels and lymphatics.

angiolymphitis (an″jĭ-ō-lim-fi'tis) [" + L. *lympha*, lymph, + *-itis*, inflammation]. Inflammation of the lymphatics. SYN: *lymphangitis*.

an″giolympho'ma [" + " + *-oma*, tumor]. Tumor of dilated lymphatics.

angiolysis (an-jĭ-ol'ĭ-sis) [" + *lysis*, destruction]. Obliteration of blood vessels in newly born infants after tying of the cord.

angioma (an-ji-o'mă) [" + *-oma*, tumor]. A growth made up of dilated blood vessels. SEE: "*angio-*" words, *cavernoma*, *chorioangioma*.

  a. cavernosum. Is congenital and appears as an elevated dark red tumor, ranging in size from a pea to that of the hand. It frequently has pulsation; commonly involves the subcutaneous or submucous tissue. TREATMENT: Surgical ligation or electrolysis.

  a. simplex (port wine mark). One that is congenital, made up of capillaries, nonelevated, bright red or purple-red in color; may cover a large surface; usually found on the face, commonly called "Mother's mark." TREATMENT: Electrolysis or application of carbon dioxide snow may be used.

  a., telangiectatic. Is acquired. Appears as bright spot composed of dilated capillaries. Is associated with acne rosacea, gouty predispositions, and exposure to weather.

angiomalacia (an-jĭ-o-ma-la'sĭ-ă) [" + *malakia*, softness]. Softening of blood vessel walls.

angiomatosis (an-jĭ-o-ma-to'sis) [" + *-oma*, tumor, + *-osis*, condition]. Condition of multiple angiomata.

  a. retinae. Primary angioma of retina.

angiomatous (an-jĭ-om'ă-tus). Like an angioma.

angiomeg'aly [G. *aggeion*, vessel, + *megas*, large]. Enlargement of blood vessels, esp. in the eyelid.

angiometer (an-jĭ-om'et-er) [" + *metron*, measure]. Instrument for measuring tension and diameter of vessels.

angiomyocardiac (an-jĭ-o-mi-o-kar'dĭ-ak) [" + *mys*, muscle, + *kardia*, heart]. Pert. to blood vessels and cardiac muscle.

angiomyoma (an″jĭ-o-mĭ-o'mă) [" + " + *-oma*, tumor]. An angioma mixed with a myoma.

angiomyosarco'ma [" + " + *sarx*, flesh, + *-oma*, tumor]. Tumor containing elements of angioma, myoma, and sarcoma.

angioneurectomy (an-jĭ-o-nu-rek'to-mĭ) [" + *neuron*, nerve, + *ektomē*, excision]. Excision of vessels and nerves.

angioneuroedema (an″-jĭ-ō-nu-ro-ē-de'mă) [" + " + *oidema*, swelling]. Acute swelling of subcutaneous or submucous tissue due to vasomotor lesion.

angioneurosis (an-jĭ-o-nū-rō'sis) [" + " + *-osis*, condition]. Spasm or paralysis of blood vessels.

  ETIOL: Disturbance of vasomotor system.

angioneurotic (an-ge-o-nū-rot'ik). Pert. to angioneurosis.

  a. edema. Swelling of submucous or subcutaneous tissues. Sometimes periodic with gastric disturbances. ETIOL: Probably a toxemia.

angioneurotomy (an-jĭ-o-nu-rot'o-mĭ) [G. *aggeion*, vessel, + *neuron*, nerve, + *tomē*, cutting]. Cutting of vessels and nerves.

angionoma (an-jĭ-on-o'mă) [" + *nomē*, ulcer]. Ulceration of a vessel.

angioparal'ysis [" + *paralyein*, loosen, dissolve]. Vasomotor relaxation of blood vessel tone.

angioparesis (an-jĭ-ō-pă'rē-sis) [" + *paresis*, weakness]. Partial paralysis of the vasomotor system.

angiopathol'ogy [" + *pathos*, suffering, + *logos*, science]. Morbid changes of the blood vessels.

angiopathy (an-jĭ-op'a-thĭ) [" + *pathos*, disease]. Any disease of blood vessels or lymphatics.

angioplania (an″jĭ-o-plan'ĭ-ă) [" + *planē*, wandering]. Abnormality or irregularity in course of a blood vessel.

angioplas'ty [" + *plassein*, to form]. Plastic surgery upon blood vessels.

angiopoietic (an″jĭ-ō-poy-et'ik) [" + *poiein*, to make]. Causing the formation of blood vessels, pert. to certain cells.

angiopres'sure. Control of hemorrhage by pressure.

angiorhigosis (an-jĭ-ō-rĭ-go'sis) [G. *aggeion*, vessel, + *rigos*, cold]. Rigidity of vessels.

angiorrhaphy (an-jĭ-or'af-ĭ) [" + *raphē*, seam]. Suture of a vessel or vessels.

angiorrhexis (an-jĭ-or-eks'is) [" + *rēxis*, rupture]. Rupture of a blood vessel.

angiosarco'ma [" + *sarx*, flesh, + *-oma*, tumor]. Mixed sarcoma and angioma.

angiosclero'sis [" + *sklērōsis*, hardening]. Hardening of the walls of the vascular system.

angioscope (an'jĭ-o-skōp [" + *skopein*, to view]. A microscope for studying capillary vessels.

angiosialitis (an″jĭ-ō-si-al-i'tis) [" + *sialon*, saliva, + *-itis*, inflammation]. Inflammation of a salivary duct.

angiosis (an-jĭ-o'sis) [" + *-osis*, condition]. Any disease of the lymphatics or blood vessels.

an'giospasm [" + *spasmos*, tension]. Excessive spasm of vessel tone.

angiospas'tic. Pert. to angiospasm.

angiostaxis (an″jĭ-o-stax'is) [G. *aggeion*, vessel, + *staxis*, trickling]. 1. Hemophilia. 2. Oozing of blood.

angiosteno'sis [" + *stenoein*, to make narrow, + *-osis*, condition]. Contraction of caliber of blood vessels.

angiosteosis (an″jĭ-os-te-o'sis) [" + *osteon*, bone]. Calcareous degeneration of arteries.

angios'tomy [" + *stoma*, mouth]. Artificial fistulous opening into a blood vessel.

angiostrophy (an-jĭ-os'tro-fĭ) [" + *strophē*, twist]. Twisting cut end of a vessel.

angiosynizesis (an″jĭ-ō-sin-ĭ-ze'sis) [" + *synizesis*, contraction]. Collapse of walls of a vessel and their subsequent adhesion.

angiotelectasis (an″jĭ-ō-tel-ek′ta-sis) [" + *telos*, end, + *ektasis*, stretching out]. Dilatation of terminal arterioles.

angiotitis (an-jĭ-ō-tī′tis) [" + *ous*, ear, + -*itis*, inflammation]. Inflammation of blood vessels of the ear.

angiotome (an′jĭ-ō-tōm) [" + *tomē*, cutting]. One of the segments of the vascular tissues of the embryo.

angiotomy (an-jĭ-ot′o-mi) [" + *tomē*, a cutting]. Dissection of blood vessels.

angioton′ic [" + *tonos*, tension]. Pert. to increase of arterial tension.

angiotribe (an′jĭ-ō-trīb) [" + *tribein*, to bruise]. Instrument for crushing the end of an artery to check hemorrhage.

angiotripsy (an′jĭ-ō-trip-sī) [" + *tripsis*, friction]. The use of an angiotribe.

angiotroph′ic [" + *trophē*, nourishment]. Pert. to nutrition of blood vessels.

angi′tis. Inflammation of the blood vessels or lymphatics. SYN: *angiitis*

angle (ang′gl) [L. *angulus*]. A point or corner where two lines meet.

  a., alpha. One found by intersection of visual line with optic axis.

  a., alveolar. Meeting point of the base of the nasal spine and the middle point of the alveolus of the upper jaw.

  a., basilar. Formed by the intersection of a projection line from the nasal point to a line drawn at the base of the nasal spine.

  a., biorbital. Formed by the meeting of the axes of the orbits.

  a., cerebellopontine. Junction of the cerebellum and pons.

  a., costal. Meeting point of the lower border of the false ribs with the axis of the sternum.

  a., craniofacial. The angle formed at the point where the basifacial and basicranial axes join at the midpoint of the sphenoethmoidal sutures.

  a., facial. The angle made by lines from the nasal spine and external auditory meatus meeting between the upper middle incisor teeth.

  a., gamma. Angle formed by line of fixation with optic axis.

  a. of incidence. The angle between a ray incident on a surface and a line drawn perpendicular to the surface at the point of incidence.

  a. of iris. Angle between the cornea and iris at the periphery of the ant. chamber of the eye.

  a. of jaw. The angle at the point where the post. edge of the ramus of the mandible and the lower surface of the body of the mandible join.

  a. of mandible. Angle of the jaw.

  a., metafacial. Angle between the base of the skull and the pterygoid process.

  a., occipital. Formed by the intersection of lines from the basion and from the lower border of the orbit at the opisthion.

  a., ophryospinal. Angle formed by the joining of lines drawn from the auricular point and the glabella at the ant. nasal spine.

  a., parietal. Formed by the meeting of the prolongation of the two lines tangent to the prominent portion of the zygomatic arch and the parietofrontal suture.

  a., pontine. Same as cerebellopontine angle.

  a., pubic. Junction of the rami of the pubes.

  a., sphenoid. Formed by the intersection of lines coming from the nasal point and the tip of the rostrum of the sphenoid, at top of the sella turcica.

  a., sternal. Angle between the manubrium and body of the sternum.

  a., venous. Angle of the internal jugular and subclavian vein.

angophrasia (an-go-fra′zĭ-ă) [G *agchein*, to choke, + *phrasis*, utterance]. Drawling, choking speech in paralytic dementia.

angor (ang′gor) [L. quinsy, anguish]. Violent distress as in angina* pectoris.

Angström's unit (ŏng′strum). PT: An internationally adopted unit of measurement of wave length, one ten-millionth of a millimeter, or one two hundred and fifty-four millionth inch.

Anguil′lula [L. eel]. Genus of nematode worms.

  A. aceti. Vinegar eel.

  A. intestinalis. Parasitic form of nematode infesting intestine in tropics and near tropics.

  A. stercoralis. Free stage of *A. intestinalis*.

anguilluli′asis. Infestation with *Anguillula intestinalis*.

angular [L.]. Having corners or angles.

  a. artery. The artery at the inner canthus of the eye; facial artery.

angulation (ang-gu-la′shun). Formation of angular loops in the intestine.

anhaphia (an-ha′fĭ-ă) [G. *an*-, priv. + *aphē*, touch]. Abnormal or defective sense of touch. SYN: *anaphia*.

anhedonia (an-hed-o′nĭ-ă) [G. *an*-, priv. + *ēdonē*, pleasure]. PSY: Lacking in interest or pleasure; apathy.

anhedonic (an-he-don′ik). Pert. to anhedonia.

anhelation (an-hel-a′shun) [L. *anhelare*, to pant]. Dyspnea, shortness of breath.

anhelitus (an-hel-it′us) [L.]. Asthma; difficult breathing.

anhelose, anhelous (an′hel-ōs, -us) [L.]. Panting.

anhematō′sis [G. *an*, priv. + *aimatoein*, to change into blood]. Defective or insufficient blood formation.

anhemolytic (an-hem-o-lit′ik). Not destructive to the blood cells.

anhepatia (an-he-pa′shĭ-ă) [G. *an*, priv. + *ēpar*, liver]. Failure or lack of liver function.

anhepat′ic. Not produced by the liver.

anhepatogenic (an-hep-at-o-jen′ik) [G. *an*-, priv. + *ēpar*, liver, + *gennan*, to produce]. Not produced by the liver. SYN: *anhepatic*.

anhidrosis (an-hi-dro′sis) [G. *an*-, priv. + *idros*, sweat]. Abnormal deficiency of sweat, general or localized, temporary or permanent, accompanying disease conditions.

  TREATMENT: In symptomatic cases, temporary relief by pilocarpine and hot drinks. Temporary relief only, in generalized forms. Soft, warm clothing, bland, soothing ointments, and lubricants to protect skin.

anhidrotic (an-hi-drot′ik). Checking or anything that checks or prevents perspiration.

anhis′tic, anhis′tous [G. *an*-, priv. + *istos*, tissue]. Seemingly without structure.

anhydra′tion [" + *ydōr*, water]. The state of not being hydrated.

anhydremia (an-hi-dre′mĭ-ă) [" + *aima*, blood]. A lessening of the normal quantity of fluids in the blood.

anhydride (an-hi′drĭd) [G. *anydros*, waterless]. A substance from which the hydrogen and oxygen in the ratio in which they exist in water have been removed.

anhydrochloric — ankle joint

anhydrochlo'ric [" + *chlōros*, green]. Lacking in hydrochloric acid.

anhydromyelia (an-hi-dro-mi-e'lĭ-ă) [" + *myelos*, marrow]. Deficiency in spinal fluid.

anhy'drous. Containing no water.

anhypnia (an-hip'nĭ-ă) [G. *an-*, priv. + *ypnos*, sleep]. Insomnia; sleeplessness; anhypnosis.

anhypno'sis. Insomnia.

anianthinopsy (an-ī-an'thin-op"sĭ) [G. *an-*, priv. + *ianthinos*, violet, + *opsis*, vision]. Inability to recognize violet tints.

anidros (an-id'ros) [G. *anydros*, waterless]. Exhibiting no perspiration.

anidrosis (an-id-ro'sis) [G. *an-*, priv. + *idrōs*, sweat]. Abnormal deficiency of sweat. SYN: *anhidrosis*.

anidrotic (an-i-drot'ik). Pert. to anidrosis. SYN: *anhidrotic*.

anid'rus [G. *anydros*, waterless]. Showing no perspiration. SYN: *anidros*.

anile (an'ĭl) [L. *anus*, an old woman]. Infirm; like an old woman.

aniline (an'ĭ-lĭn) [Ar. *an-nīl*, the indigo plant]. The simplest aromatic amine, $C_6H_5NH_2$, an oily liquid derived from benzene.
DOSAGE: 1 gr. (0.06 Gm.).

anilinophil, anilinophilous (an"ĭ-lin'o-fil, -fĭl-us) [" + G. *philos*, fond]. A structure staining readily with aniline dyes.

anilism (an'il-izm). Chronic aniline poisoning.
SYM: Cardiac and gastric weakness, intermittent pulse, vertigo, muscular depression, cyanosis. [in females.

anil'ity [L. *ănus*, an old woman]. Old age

anima (an'im-ă) [L. air, breath]. The vital principle; breath; air; mind; consciousness.

animalcule (an-i-mal'kule) [L. *animalculum*, little animal]. Unicellular animal organism; protozoan.

anincretinosis (an-in-krē-tĭn-o'sĭs) [G. *an-*, priv. + *incretus* + *-osis*, condition]. A disorder due to failure of some organ of internal secretion.

anion (an'i-on) [G. *ana*, up, + *iōn*, going]. PT: An ion carrying a negative charge. Since unlike forms of electricity attract each other, the ion is attracted by, and travels to, the positive anode. Examples are acid radicals and corresponding radicals of their salts. SEE: *ion*.

anirid'ia [G. *an-*, priv. + *iris*, rainbows]. Congenital absence, complete or partial, of iris; irideremia.*

anischuria (an-is-ku'rĭ-ă) [" + *ischouria*, retention of urine]. Incontinence of urine.

aniseikonia (an-is-ī-ko'nĭ-ă) [G. *anisos*, unequal, + *eikon*, image]. A condition in which the size and shape of the ocular image of one eye differs from that of the other.

anis'ergy [" + *ergon*, work]. Varying degrees of blood pressure in different parts of the system.

aniso- (an'is-o) [G. *anisos*]. Prefix. Unequal, unsymmetrical in combination.

anisochromatic (an-i-so-kro-mat'ik) [G. *anisos*, unequal, + *chrōma*, color]. Not of uniform color.

anisocoria (an-is-o-ko'rĭ-ă) [" + *korē*, pupil]. Inequality of the diameter of the pupil; may be normal or congenital. Often seen in early stages of insanity, each pupil alternating in contraction and dilation. Found in *aneurysms, head trauma, diseases of the nervous system, sclerosis, brain lesion, paresis,* and *locomotor ataxia.*

anisocytosis (an-ĭ-so-si-to'sĭs) [" + *kytos*, cell, + *-osis*, condition]. Inequality in size of cells, esp. erythrocytes. An abnormal condition.

anisog'amy [" + *gamos*, marriage]. Sexual fusion of two gametes of different form and size.

anisognathous (an-ĭ-sog'na-thus) [" + *gnathos*, jaw]. Having upper jaw wider than lower one.

anisohypercytosis (an-is-o-hi-per-si-to'sis) [" + *yper*, above, + *kytos*, cell]. Increase in number of leukocytes with altered proportion of the different varieties. Opposite of *anisohypocytosis*.

anisohypocyto'sis [" + *ypo*, below, + "]. Decrease in number of leukocytes with altered proportion of different varieties. OPP: *anisohypercytosis*.*

anisoiconia (an-i-so-i-ko'nĭ-ă) [" + *eikon*, image]. Failure of retinal images to coalesce.

an"isomas'tia [" + *mastos*, breast]. Breasts unequal in size.

an"isome'lia [" + *melos*, limb]. Inequality between two paired limbs.

anisometrope (an"i-so-me'trōp) [" + *metron*, measure, + *ops*, vision]. One afflicted with anisometropia.

anisometropia (an-i-so-me-tro'pĭ-ă). Inequality in refractive power of the two eyes.

anisometrop'ic. Having unequal refractive power.

anisonormocyto'sis [G. *anisos*, unequal, + L. *norma*, rule, + G. *kytos*, cell]. Abnormal relation in numbers of different forms of leukocytes but with normal number of total leukocytes.

aniso'pia [" + *ops*, vision]. Inequality of visual power of both eyes.

anisopiesis (an-i-so-pi-e'sis) [" + *piesis*, blood pressure]. Apparent inequality of blood pressure in different parts of the body.

anisorhythmia (an"ĭ-sō-rith'mĭ-ă) [" + *rythmos*, rhythm]. Absence of synchronism in rate of the auricles and ventricles or irregular heart action.

anisospore (an'ĭ-so-spōr) [" + *sporos*, seed]. A sexual cell. Opp. of *isospore*.

an"isosthen'ic [" + *sthenos*, strength]. Not of equal muscle strength.

anisotropal (an-is-ot'ro-pal) [" + *tropos*, a turning]. 1. Not equal in every direction. 2. Unequal in power of refraction.

anisotrop'ic. Having different optical properties in different directions, as have certain crystals; double polarizing.

anisotropous (an-ĭ-sot'ro-pus). 1. Not equal in every direction. 2. Unequal in refractive power. SYN: *anisotropal*.

anisuria (an-is-u'rĭ-ă) [G. *anisos*, unequal, + *ouron*, urine]. Alternate polyuria and oliguria, q.v.

ankle (ăng'kl) [A. S. *ancleōw*]. The part between the foot and lower end of leg.
SEE: *astragalus, malleolus*.

a. bone. The astragalus.

a. clonus. A rhythmic extension-flexion of the ankle induced by its sudden dorsiflexion, evidencing upper motor neuron* disease, such as spastic paraplegia, hemiplegia, etc. NP: Keep patient's feet at right angles on a rectangular foot splint. When splint is removed to wash the feet daily, avoid dorsiflexion of foot to prevent movement of ankle clonus or spasm.

a. c. reflex. Succession of rapid contractions and relaxations when foot is pressed dorsally. Occurs in lateral tract disease and disseminated sclerosis.

a. joint. A hinge joint. Lower part of tibia, its *medial malleolus* and *lateral*

ankle, tailor's   A-60   anomalous

malleolus of *fibula* forming socket for the *astragalus*.
    a., tailor's. An abnormal bursa over the head of the fibula in tailors from pressure caused by sitting cross-legged on the floor.
ankyloblepharon (ang-ki-lo-blef'ar-on) [G. *ankylē*, a stiff joint, + *blepharon*, eyelid]. Adhesion of ciliary edges of lids to each other.
ankylochilia (ang-kĭ-lo-ki'lĭ-ă) [" + *cheilos*, lip]. Adhesion of lips to each other.
ankyloglos'sia [" + *glōssa*, tongue]. Tongue-tie.
ankyloproctia (ang-ki-lo-prok'shĭ-ă) [" + *prōktos*, anus]. Stricture or imperforation of the anus.
ankylosed (ang'ki-lozd). Denoting fixation of a joint. Stiffened; held by adhesions.
ankylosis (an-kyl-o'sis) [G. *agkyle*, stiff joint]. Abnormal immobility and consolidation of a joint.
    ETIOL: May be result of disease in which the articular cartilage has been destroyed, the raw bone surfaces coming into contact and bony union taking place. Seen in many joint conditions. May be performed surgically.
    NP: Maintain complete immobility until bone has firmly united, which may be from 6 to 12 weeks. Keep joint in perfect position.
    SEE: *arthrokleisis, arthrolysis*.
    a., artificial. The surgical fixation of a joint.
    a., bony. The abnormal union of the bones of a joint, also called true ankylosis.
    a., extracapsular. That caused by rigidity of parts outside a joint.
    a., false. Spurious ankylosis; that due to rigidity of the surrounding parts.
    a., fibrous. That due to the formation of fibrous bands within a joint only.
    a., intracapsular. That due to the undue rigidity of structure within a joint.
    a., ligamentous. Ankylosis by ligaments or fibrous structures.
    a., true. Same as bony ankylosis.
Ankylos'toma, Ancylostoma [G. *agkylos*, crooked, + *stoma*, mouth]. Old world hookworm, a genus of nematode parasites.
    A. americanum. American hookworm.
    A. duodenale. The hookworm infesting man.
ankylos'toma [G. *agkylē*, stiff joint, + *stoma*, mouth]. Trismus, lockjaw.
ankylostomiasis (ang-kil-o-sto-mi'as-is) [G. *agkylos*, hooked, + *stoma*, mouth, + *-iasis*, infection]. Disease caused by hookworms in the intestine; hence commonly called "hookworm."
    The eggs are discharged in the feces developing into larvae. The infection is gotten through food, water, or the skin of the feet or legs, causing an eruption called "ground itch."
    SYM: Anemia, weakness, and emaciation, increased leukocytes, digestive disorders.
    DIAG: Depends upon finding the eggs or the worm in the stool.
ankylotia (ang-kĭ-lo'shĭ-ă) [G. *agkylos*, crooked, + *ot-*, ear]. Closure or imperforation of external auditory meatus of ear.
ankylotome (ang'kil-o-tōm) [G. *agkylos*, bent, + *tomē*, a cutting]. An instrument for cutting *fraenum linguae*.
ankylurethria (ang-kĭl-ū-re'thrĭ-ă) [" + *ourēthra*, urethra]. Stricture or imperforation of the urethra.

ankyroid (ang'kĭ-royd) [G. *agkyroeides*, anchor-shaped]. Hook-shaped.
    a. cavity. The posterior or descending cornu of lateral ventricle.
anlage (ahn'lăg-ĕ). 1. Rudiments in a developing embryo. 2. The embryonic part in which differentiation first appears.
annatto (an-at'o). Reddish coloring matter obtained from the pulp of *Bixa orellana*, a tropical tree. SYN: *annotto, arnotto*.
annec'tent [L. *annectens*, tying or binding to]. Linking together.
annex'a [L. *annectere*, to tie or bind to]. Accessory parts. SYN: *adnexa*.
annexi'tis [" + G. *-itis*, inflammation]. Inflammation of *adnexa uteri*. SYN: *adnexitis*.
annex'opexy [" + G. *pexis*, putting together]. Fixation of fallopian tubes and ovary to abdominal wall. SYN: *adnexopexy*.
annot'to. Reddish coloring matter obtained from pulp of *Bixa orellana*, a tropical tree. SYN: *annatto, arnotto*.
annuens (an'u-enz) [L. *annuens*, nodding]. *Rectus capitis anterior minor*.
ann'ular [L. *annulus*, ring]. Circular; ring-shaped.
annulorrhaphy (an-u-lor'ă-fī) [" + G. *raphē*, seam]. Closure of a hernial ring by suture.
ann'ulus [L.]. A ring-shaped structure; a ring.
    a. ciliaris. Boundary between choroid and iris.
    a. tympanicus. The tympanic ring.
    a. umbilicalis. Umbilical ring. SEE: *abdominal*.
anoci-association (a-no'sĭ-as-o-sĭ-a'shun). The blocking or exclusion of neuroses, fear, pain and harmful influences or associations to prevent shock, by injection of narcotics hypodermically.
anococcygeal (a-no-kok-sij'e-al) [L. *anus* + G. *kokkyx*]. Rel. to both anus and coccyx.
    a. body. The muscle and fibrous tissue lying between the coccyx and anus.
    a. ligament. A band of fibrous tissue joining the tip of the coccyx with the external sphincter ani.
anod'al [G. *ana*, up, + *odos*, way]. Pert. to the anode.
    a. closure contraction. Contraction of muscles at anode on closure of circuit.
anode (an'ōd) [G.]. The positive pole of an electrical source. Only galvanic (direct current) and static electricity have distinct polarity.
anodinia (an-o-din'ĭ-ă) [G. *an-*, priv. + *dinos*, dizziness]. Absence of vertigo.
anodmia (an-od'mĭ-ă) [" + *odmē*, stench]. The want or absence of the sense of smell; anosmia, *q.v.*
an'odyne [" + *odynē*, pain]. An agent that will relieve pain; milder in form than an analgesic, *q.v.* Ex: *morphine, codeine, acetylsalicylic acid*. SEE: *anetic, apone, antalgesic, antalgic*.
anodyn'ia. 1. Cessation or absence of pain. 2. Loss of sensation.
anoesia (an-o-e'sĭ-ă) [G. *anoēsia*, want of understanding]. Without power of comprehension; anoia,* imbecility, idiocy.
anoetic (an-o-et'ik) [G. *anoētos*, unthinkable]. Rel. to the borderline of consciousness; not fully conscious.
anoia (an-oy'ă) [G. *a-*, priv. + *noos*, understanding]. Anoesia, *q.v.* Idiocy.
anomalous (an-om'al-us) [G. *anōmalos*, uneven]. Irregular. Contrary to the normal.

anom'aly [G. *anomalia*, irregularity]. Anything contrary to general rule.

anomia (an-o'mĭ-ă) [G. *a-*, priv. + *ōnoma*, name]. Inability to remember names of persons and objects.

anonychia (an-o-nik'ĭ-ă) [" + *onyx*, nail]. Absence of the nails.

anonymous (an-on'ĭm-us). Nameless.
 a. artery. Arteria anonyma.
 a. veins. Venae anonymae.

anoopsia (an-o-op'sĭ-ă) [G. *anō*, upward, + *opsis*, vision]. Tendency of one eye to turn upward. SYN: *hyperphoria.**

Anopheles (an-of'el-ēz) [G. *anōphelēs*, harmful, useless]. The mosquito whose bite is responsible for the malaria parasite in man.

anopho'ria [G. *ana*, up, + *phoros*, tending]. Tendency of one eye to turn upward. SYN: *hyperphoria,* *anopia.**

anophthal'mia [G. *an-*, priv. + *ophthalmos*, eye]. Congenital absence of eyes.

anopia (an-o'pĭ-ă) [G. *an-*, priv. + *ops*, eye]. 1. Anophthalmos, lack of one eye or both. 2. Anopsia. 3. Tendency of one eye to turn upward; hyperphoria.

anop'sia [G. *an-*, priv. + *opsis*, sight]. 1. Hyperphoria. 2. Inability to use the vision as in those confined in the dark, or from disuse of an eye in strabismus, or resulting from cataract, or in refractive errors.

anorectal (an-e-rekt'al) [L. *anus* + *rectum*]. Pert. to the anus and rectum.

anorectic, anorectous (an-o-rek'tic, -tus). Having no appetite.

anorexia (an-or-eks'ĭ-ă) [G. *an-*, priv. + *orexis*, appetite]. Loss of appetite.

Seen in malaise, commencement of all fevers and illnesses, also in disorders of alimentary tract, esp. of stomach, and as a result of alcoholic excesses and drug addiction, esp. cocaine. Also result of food fads and faulty feeding.

RS: *acoria, ageusia, bulimia, hyperorexia, nausea, parageusia, parorexia, pica, polyphagia, pyrosis, taste.*
 a. nervo'sa. Loss of appetite for food not explainable by local disease. It may be a part of a psychosis.*

anoria (an-or'ĭ-ă) [G. *anoria*, untimeliness]. Immaturity.

anor'mal [G. *a-*, priv. + L. *normalis*, according to pattern]. Abnormal.

anorrhorrhea (an-or-or-e'ă) [G. *an-*, priv. + *orros*, serum, + *roia*, a flow]. Diminished or imperfect secretion of serous fluid.

anorthography (an-or-thog'ră-fĭ) [G. *an-*, priv. + *orthos*, straight, + *graphein*, to write]. Agraphia,* esp. motor agraphia; loss of power to express oneself in writing. SEE: *agraphia.*

anorthopia (an-or-tho'pĭ-ă) [" + " + *ops*, eye]. 1. Vision in which straight lines do not appear straight; symmetry and parallelism not properly perceived. 2. Squinting.

anorthosis (an-or-tho'sis) [" + " + *osis*, condition]. Absence of or diminished erectility.

anosia (an-o'sĭ-ă) [G. *a-*, priv. + *nosos*, disease]. Normal; without disease.

anosmatic (an-oz-mat'ik) [" + *osmē*, smell]. Deficient sense of smell.

anosmia (an-oz'mĭ-ă). Absence of the sense of smell; anodmia,* anosphrasia.* Frequent in neurasthenia, hysteria, and sometimes in ataxia.

anosmic (an-oz'mik). Lacking in sense of smell.

anos'mous. Anosmic. Pert. to anosmia.

anosodiaphoria (an-o-so-di-af-or'ĭ-ă) [G. *a-*, priv. + *nosos*, disease, + *diaphoria*, difference]. Real or pretended indifference to presence of disease, esp. paralysis.

anosognosia (an-o-sog-no'zĭ-ă) [" + " + *gnosis*, knowledge]. Real or pretended ignorance of the presence of disease, esp. paralysis. Opp. of *pathodixia, q.v.*

anosphrasia (an-os-fra'zĭ-ă) [" + G. *osphrēsis*, smell]. Absence or imperfect sense of smell.

anospi'nal [L. *anus* + *spina*, thorn]. Pert. to center in the spinal cord which controls the contraction of the anal sphincter.

anostosis (an-os-to'sis) [G. *an-*, priv. + *osteon*, bone]. A defective formation or development of bone; failure to ossify.

anotro'pia [G. *ana*, up, + *tropē*, a turning]. Farsightedness. SYN: *hyperopia.**

anoves'ical [L. *anus* + *vesica*, bladder]. Rel. in any way to both anus and urinary bladder.

anov'ular, anov'ulatory [G. *an-*, priv. + L. *ovarium*, ovary]. Not pert. to ovulation. Without ovarian bleeding.

anoxemia (an-oks-e'mĭ-ă) [" + *oxys*, sharp, + *gennan*, to produce, + *aima*, blood]. Lack of oxygen in the blood.

General anoxemia occurs at high altitudes, at reduced pressures, during inhalation of gaseous mixtures low in oxygen, in strangling, and in circulatory failure.

SYM: cyanosis, mental confusion, shock, and sudden collapse. Local anoxemia occurs in passive congestion.

anoxia (an-ox'ĭ-ă) [" + oxygen]. Deficiency of oxygen.
 a., anemic. Deficiency in the oxygen carrying power of the blood.
 a., anoxic. Lessened oxygen tension in arterial blood, but with normal oxygen capacity.

Insufficient supply of oxygen to tissues can result from other causes; hence one distinguishes between the anoxic type of tissue asphyxia on the one hand, and the ischemic (stagnant) and anemic (alteration or destruction of hemoglobin) types on the other hand.
 a., stagnant. Decrease in oxygen from the blood due to insufficiency of circulation.

anox'ic. Pert. to or caused by a general lack of oxygen, and characterized by a generally subnormal oxygen tension of the blood.

an'sa [L. a handle]. Any anatomical structure in the form of a loop.
 a. capitis. The zygomatic arch.
 a. hypoglos'si. Loop of the hypoglossal nerve.
 a. lentic'ular. Fibers entering the lenticular nucleus from the thalamus by way of the thalamic radiation.
 a. of the spinal nerves. Connecting loops of fibers between the ant. spinal nerves.
 a. peduncularis. Fibers passing from the thalamus through the thalamic radiation, under the lenticular nucleus to the cortex of the temporal lobe and insula.
 a. sacralis. Nerve cord connecting the sympathetic trunk with the ganglion impar.
 a. subclavia. Loop of nerve fibers winding around the ant. aspect of the subclavian artery.

anselaphesia (an-sel-af-e'zĭ-ă). Absence of sense of touch or feeling or sensation, esp. of tactile sensibility.

anserine (an'ser-in) [L. *anser*, goose]. Pert. to a goose.

ant-, anti- [G.]. Prefixes: Opposed to; counteracting; against, as *antifebrile*.
antabuse (ăn-tĭ-būz). Tetraethylthiuram. Also called disulfram. Administered to alcoholics to cause violent illness if liquor is taken by patient.
antacid (ant-as'id) [G. *anti*, against, + L. *acidum*, acid]. An agent that will neutralize acidity, esp. in digestive tract. Ex: *magnesium oxide, sodium bicarbonate*.
antag'onism [G. *antagōnizesthai*, to struggle against]. Opposition or contrary action, as bet. muscles or medicines.
antag'onist. That which counteracts the action of anything, as a muscle or drug.
antalge'sic [G. *anti*, against, + *algos*, pain]. Pain-relieving agent. SYN: *anodyne*.
antalgic (ant-al'jik). An anodyne or analgesic.
antalkaline (ant-al'kal-in) [G. *anti*, against, + *alkaline*]. Neutralizing or reducing alkalinity.
antaphrodis'iac [" + *aphrodisiakos*, sexual]. Lessening sexual desire.
antarthritic (ant"ar-thrit'ik) [" + *arthritikos*, gouty]. Remedy for gout.
antasthenic (ant-as-then'ik) [" + *astheneia*, weakness]. 1. Strengthening, invigorating. 2. Agent which invigorates.
antasthmat'ic [" + *asthma*]. 1. An agent that prevents an asthmatic attack. 2. Relieving asthma.
antatrophic (ant-ă-trof'ik) [" + *atrophia*, atrophy]. Preventing or curing atrophy.
ante- [L.]. Prefix: Before, as *antenatal*.
antebrachium (an-te-bra'ke-um) [L. *ante*, before, + *brachium*, arm]. The forearm.
antecurvature (an-te-ker'va-tûr) [" + *curvatura*, bend]. Bending forward abnormally. SYN: *anteflexion*.
an'tedating [L. *ante*, before, + *datus*]. The theory that hereditary defects manifest themselves earlier with each successive generation and often more severely though the clinical picture may change.
antefebrile (an-te-feb'ril) [" + *febris*, fever]. Pert. to the period before a fever.
anteflex'ion [" + *flectere*, to bend]. Abnormal bending forward, *i. e., uterus*, bending forward at its body and cervix.
anteloca'tion [L. *ante*, before, + *locare*, to place]. Forward displacement of an organ or part of the human body.
antemetic (an-tem-et'ik) [G. *anti*, against, + *emetikos*, emetic]. 1. Arresting vomiting. 2. Remedy that controls vomiting and nausea.
ante mor'tem [L.]. Before death.
 a.-m. statement. One made immediately preceding death.
If made with belief that death is approaching, it is held in law as equally binding with a statement made on oath. SYN: *death-bed statement*.
antenatal (ăn"tē-nāt'ăl) [L. *ante*, before, + *natus*, birth]. Occurring before birth.
an'te par'tum [L.]. The time before the onset of labor.
antephialtic (ant-e-fĭ-al'tik [" + *ephialtēs*, nightmare]. Preventing nightmare.
anteposition [L. *ante*, before]. Anterior displacement of the uterus.
anteprostati'tis [L. *ante*, before, + *prostata* + G. *-itis*, inflammation]. Inflammation of glands of Cowper.
antepyret'ic [" + G. *pyretos*, fever]. Before the development of fever; antefebrile. SEE: *antipyretic*.
anteresis (ant-er'e-sĭs) [G. *antereisis*, resistance]. Resistance during reduction of a dislocation.

anterethic (an-ter-eth'ĭk) [L. *anti*, against, + *erethismos*, irritation]. Soothing.
ante'rior [L.]. Before, or in front of.
 a. chamber. Aqueous chamber. Bounded in front by cornea, behind by iris and lens.
antero- [L.]. Prefix: Anterior; front; before, as *anterosuperior*.
anterograde (an"ter-o-grăd) [L. *antero*, anterior, + *gradior*, to step]. Extending frontward.
antero-infe'rior [" + *inferior*, below]. In front and below.
anterolat'eral [" + *latus*, side]. In front and to one side.
anterome'dian [" + *median*]. In front and toward the central line.
anteroposter'ior [" + *posterior*, rear]. Passing from front to rear.
anterosuper'ior [" + *superior*, above]. In front and above.
antever'sion [L. *ante*, before, + *vertere*, to turn]. 1. A tipping or bending forward of an organ. 2. A forward placement of the uterus, the normal position of the healthy uterus. [uterus.
 a. uteri. A forward tipping of the
antevert'ed. Inclined or bent forward; said of uterus.
anthelix (an'the-liks) [G. *anti*, against, + *elix*, coil]. External ear's inner curved ridge. SYN: *antihelix*.
anthelmintic (an-thel-min'tik) [G. *anti*, against, + *elmins*, worm]. An agent used to expel intestinal worms. Ex: *santonin, phenyl salicylate, thymol*.
 a. enema. One given to expel worms. SEE: *enema*.
Anthemis (an'them-is). Chamomile.
anthemorrha'gic [G. *anti*, against, + *aima*, blood, + *rēgnunai*, to discharge]. Agent for preventing or arresting hemorrhage.
anthocy'anin. Pigment of red beet root.
anthocyanine'mia [*anthocyanin* + G. *aima*, blood]. Anthocyanin in the blood.
anthocyaninu'ria [" + G. *ouron*, urine]. Anthocyanin in urine.
Anthomy'ia canicula'ris [G. *anthos*, flower, + *myia*, fly]. A small black horse fly, whose larvae may infest the human intestine, often resulting in alarming gastrointestinal symptoms.
Anthony's fire, St. Name given to erysipelas.
anthopho'bia [G. *anthos*, flower, + *phobos*, fear]. Morbid dislike of flowers.
anthorism, anthorisma (an'thor-izm, -iz'mă) [G. *anti*, against, + *orisma*, a boundary]. A diffuse swelling.
anthracemia (an"thra-se'mĭ-ă) [G. *anthrax*, carbuncle, + *aima*, blood]. Presence in the blood of *B. anthracis*.
anthracia (an-thra'sĭ-ă) [G. carbuncle]. Presence of carbuncles.
anthracoid (an'thra-koid). Like or pert. to anthrax.
anthracoma (an-thrak-o'mă) [G. *anthrax*, carbuncle, + *-oma*, tumor]. Carbuncle.
anthracometer (an-thra-kom'e-ter) [G. *anthrax*, coal, + *metron*, measure]. An instrument for measuring the carbon dioxide in the air.
an"thraconecro'sis [" + *nekrōsis*, deadness]. Necrosis of tissue into dry, black gangrene.
anthraco'sis [" + *-osis*, condition]. 1. Miner's phthisis. A condition of the pulmonary organs due to coal dust inhalation; a pneumoconiosis. 2. A carbuncle, or a corroding ulcer.
anthrax (ăn'thrăks) [G. coal, carbuncle]. 1. A carbuncle. 2. Acute, infectious dis-

anthropo-   A-63   **antibody**

ease caused by *Bacillus anthracis*, usually attacking cattle and sheep.

Man contracts it from animal hair or hides.

ETIOL: *B. anthracis*. Workers in wools, hides, and brushes are commonly affected. The disease may attack the lungs (*woolsorter's disease*), the alimentary tract (*gastrointestinal type*), or the loose cellular tissue, giving rise to *anthrax edema;* more commonly it occurs in the form of a pustule known as an *anthrax boil* or *malignant pustule*. The disease often proves fatal.

TREATMENT: Anti-anthrax serum.

NP: Strict isolation. Old bedding and clothing should be destroyed after use. Other articles adequately disinfected, an hour each for three days by steam; otherwise soak in pure lysol and boil one hour on each successive day. Nurse must keep her hands free from abrasions, and disinfect them after handling patient. She should not attend other patients at same time, esp. surgical or obstetrical cases.

SEE: *anthracoid, Ascoli's reaction, cacanthrax, charbon.*

anthropo- (an'thro-pō) [G.]. Prefix: Pert. to man.

anthropogeny (an-thro-po'je-nī) [G. *anthrōpos*, man, + *gennan*, to produce]. Origin and development of man.

anthropoid (an'thro-poid) [" + *eidos*, resemblance]. 1. Resembling a man. 2. An ape.

anthropol'ogy [" + *logos*, study of]. The science which treats of man.

anthropometry (an-thro-pom'et-rī) [" + *metron*, measure]. Science of measuring the human body and its parts and functional capacities.

Human measurements and types and their relation to psychiatric variants as well as to disease in general is still little understood.

anthropoph'agy [" + *phagein*, to eat]. The eating of human flesh.

an"thropopho'bia [" + *phobos*, fear]. A morbid fear of society or of a particular man.

An early symptom of mental disorder.

anthroposomatology (an"thro-po-so-ma-tol'o-jī) [" + *sōma*, body, + *logos*, study of]. Branch of anthropology dealing with human body.

an"thropotox'in [" + *toxikon*, poison]. Supposed poison exhaled by human lungs.

anthydropic (ant-hi-drop'ik) [G. *anti*, against, + *ydrops*, dropsy]. 1. Correcting dropsy. 2. Agent for relieving dropsy.

anthypnotic (ant-hip-not'ik) [" + *ypnos*, sleep]. 1. Preventing sleep. 2. Agent hindering sleep.

anthysteric (ant-his-ter'ik) [" + *ystera*, womb]. 1. Relieving hysteria. 2. Agent soothing hysteria.

anti- [G.]. Prefix: Against, as *antibody*.

antiagglu'tinin. A specific antibody opposing action of agglutinin.

antial'bumate, antial'buminate. A product resulting from incomplete proteolysis of albumin; parapeptone.

antialbu'min. An albumin constituent; supposed to be source of antialbumose.

antial'bumose. A product formed by peptic digestion of albumin; becomes antipeptone by further hydrolysis.

antialex'in. Anticomplement.

antiam'boceptor. Substance inhibiting action of an amboceptor.

antiam'ylase. Substance neutralizing action of amylase.

antianaphylac'tin. An antibody specific to anaphylactin.

antianaphylax'is. A state of immunity.

antiane'mic [G. *anti*, against, + *an-*, priv. + *aima*, blood]. Curing or preventing anemia.

antian'tibody. An antibody counteracting effect of antitoxin which produced it.

antiapoplec'tic. Relieving or preventing apoplexy.

antiarthritic (an-tī-ar-thrīt'ik) [G. *anti*, against, + *arthritikos*, gouty]. Medicine given to relieve gout.

antibacte'rial. Destroying or stopping the growth of bacteria.

antibacterin (an-tī-bak'ter-in) [G. *anti*, against, + *baktērion*, little rod]. An antibody injected to prevent further germ growth in the body. SEE: *germ theory.*

antibechic (an-tī-bek'ik) [G. *anti*, against, + *bex*, cough]. 1. Relieving cough. 2. A cough remedy.

antibilious (an-tī-bil'yus). Relieving bilious conditions.

antibio'sis [G. *anti*, against, + *bios*, life]. An association of two organisms detrimental to one of them.

antibiotic (ăn-tĭ-bī-ŏt'ĭk). 1. Tending to destroy life. 2. A substance produced by a living organism which has power to inhibit the multiplication of, or to destroy other organisms, especially bacteria. Some affect only gram-positive bacteria; others also the fungi and rickettsiae, and a few affect viruses. Antibiotics are produced by bacteria, molds, and other fungi.

A. *Antibiotics of Bacterial Origin.*
bacitracin ....*Bacillus subtilis*
polymyxins
    Bacillus polymyxa (aerosporus)
subtilin ....*Bacillus subtilis*
tryothricin { *gramicidin* }
            { *tyrocidin* } —*Bacillus brevis*

B. *Antibiotics derived from molds or mold-like organisms.*
achromycin
aureomycin (chlorotetracycline)
    Streptomyces aureofaciens
chloromycetin (chloramphenicol)
    Streptomyces venezuelae
erythromycin
    Streptomyces erythreus
flavicidin (*flavicin*)
    Aspergillus flavus
magnamycin (carbomycin)
    Streptomyces halstedii
neomycin ....*fradieae*
penicillin .....*Penicillium notatum*
streptomycin
    Streptomyces griseus
terramycin (hydroxy-tetracycline)
    Streptomyces rimosus

antiblennorrhagic (an-tī-blen-o-raj'ik) [G. *anti*, against, + *blennos*, mucus, + *rēgnunai*, to burst forth]. 1. Preventing or curing gonorrhea or catarrh. 2. Remedy for these diseases.

an'tibody. A substance in the body which incites immunity (antagonistic to invading bodies) such as the reacting agents in the serum.

Antibodies resemble enzymes in that they are associated with proteins of the serum. Bacteria entering the body stimulate the production of antibodies. Antibodies do not seem to be activating agents except as they accelerate the action of other agents.

They consist of (a) *antitoxins*, which neutralize toxins; (b) *cytolysins* (bacteriolysins) which dissolve cells; (c) *agglutinins*, which cause cells to clump together; (d) *precipitins*, which bring about precipitation of substances; and

(e) *opsonins*, which enhance the phagocytic activity of leukocytes by making bacteria more readily ingested. A substance which induces the production of antibodies is called an *antigen*. Antigen-antibody reaction is generally specific, *i.e.*, an antibody will act only against the antigen which induces its production.

The antibody fighting element is carried by the blood protein, or globulin, of which there are three types: *alpha*, *beta*, and *gamma*. The latter carries the antibodies in pneumonia.

antibody, words pert. to: antianaphylactin, antiantibody, anticutin, anticytost, anticytotoxin, antiricin, antiserum, antitrypsin, autoantibody, autohemolysin, isoagglutinins, lysin, opsonin.

antibrachium (an-te-bra′ki-um) [G. *anti*, against, + *brachion*, arm] (BNA). The forearm.

antibro′mic [" + *brōmos*, smell]. 1. Deodorizing. 2. A deodorant.

antical′culous [" + L. *calculus*, a pebble]. Antilithic.

antican′crin [" + L. *cancrum*, cancer]. Cancroin. Supposed cancer antibody.

anticar′dium [" + *kardia*, heart]. Precordial depression.

anticarious (an-tĭ-ka′re-us) [" + *caries*, decay]. Preventing decay of teeth.

anticathode (an-tĭ-kath′ōd). Portion of vacuum tube opposite cathode. SYN: *target*.

anticheirotonus (an-tĭ-ki-rot′o-nus) [G. *anticheir*, thumb, + *tonos*, tension]. Spasmodic bending inward of thumb in epilepsy or before attack.

anticholagogue (an-tĭ-ko′la-gog) [G. *anti*, against, + *cholē*, bile, + *agōgos*, drawing forth]. Depressing hepatic function.

anticholerin (an-tĭ-kol′er-in) [" + *cholera*]. Substance from cultures of *Spirillum cholerae asiaticae*: employed against cholera.

antic′ipating intermittent. Intermittent with paroxysms recurring earlier each day before the regular time.

an″ticipa′tion. Theory that hereditary defects manifest themselves earlier in each successive generation and often more severely. SYN: *antedating*.

anticli′nal [G. *anti*, against, + *klinein*, to incline]. Leaning in opp. directions.

a. vertebra. Tenth thoracic vertebra.

anticomplement (an-tĭ-kom′ple-ment). A substance combining with and thus neutralizing a complement.

anticonvul′sive [G. *anti*, against, + L. *convulsio*, pulling together]. 1. Relieving convulsions. 2. Agent preventing convulsions.

anticreatinine (an-tĭ-kre-at′in-in). A leukomaine from creatinine.

anti′cus [L. foremost]. (BNA) Anterior. That part nearest the ventral or front surface.

anticu′tin. An antibody neutralizing tuberculin to prevent cutaneous tuberculin reaction. [pyretic drug.

anticyclic acid (an-tĭ-sik′lik). An anti-

anticytol′ysin [G. *anti*, against, + *kytos*, cell, + *lysis*, dissolution]. Antibody inhibiting cytotoxin. SYN: *anticytotoxin*.

anticy′tost. An antibody which gives immunity to cytost; named by Turek.

anticytotox′in [G. *anti*, against, + *kytos*, cell, + *toxikon*, poison]. An antibody specifically inhibiting cytotoxin.

antidiabe′tin. A preparation of saccharine and mannite (a sweetish substance taken from the flowering ash) used as substitute for sugar in diabetes.*

antidiarrhe′ic en′emas. These include the demulcents, astringents, antiseptics, carminative, or sedative enemas, *q.v.*

antidinic (an-tĭ-din′ik) [G. *anti*, against, + *dinos*, dizziness]. 1. Relieving giddiness. 2. Agent preventing vertigo.

antidiphtherin (an-tĭ-dif′ther-in). A substance taken from the culture of diphtheria bacillus and used to prevent the disease.

antidiuretic (an″tĭ-di-u-ret′ik) [G. *anti*, against, + G. *dia*, intensive, + *ourēsis*, urination]. 1. Lessening urine secretion. 2. A drug having such an action.

antido′tal [G. *antidotos*, given against]. Acting as or pert. to an antidote.

antidote (an′tĭ-dōt). A substance which neutralizes poisons or their effects.

Antidotes may be *mechanical*, *chemical*, or *physiological*.

MECHANICAL OR PHYSICAL ANTIDOTES: Those that envelop the poison inside the stomach or coat the mucous membrane of the stomach. These are fats, oils, milk (casein coagulum), whites of eggs, finely divided charcoal, fuller's earth, or mineral oil. (Fats and oils are not desirable in phosphorus, camphor, aspidium, and cantharides p.)

CHEMICAL ANTIDOTES: These act chemically by reacting with the poison to produce an insoluble compound which is inert or less toxic. For example, table salt precipitates silver nitrate and forms an insoluble, harmless silver chloride. Chemical antidotes should be used sparingly and should be removed, as they may produce serious results if allowed to remain in the stomach.

PHYSIOLOGICAL ANTIDOTES: These produce opposite physiological effects or neutralize the effects of the poison, *e. g.*, sedatives are given for convulsives and hypnotics. These should not be given without physician's definite instructions.

UNIVERSAL ANTIDOTES: Many of these have been recommended, the simplest being pulverized charcoal, tannic acid, and magnesium oxide. The charcoal acts physically by *absorption*; the tannic acid *precipitates* metals, alkaloids, and some glucosides; and the magnesia *neutralizes* acids and is an excellent antidote for arsenic. DOSAGE: Mix equal parts and give a teaspoonful well stirred up with water.

antido′tum. An antidote.

antidromic (an-tĭ-drom′ik) [G. *anti*, against, + *dromos*, running]. Running in a direction opposite the usual stream, as when a nervous impulse runs along a sensory fiber in the direction of the sense-organ.

antidyscratic (an-tĭ-dis-krat′ik). Relieving dyscrasia.

antidysenter′ic. 1. Relieving or preventing dysentery. 2. An agent curing dysentery.

antiemet′ic [G. *anti*, against, + *emetikos*, nauseated]. An agent that will prevent or arrest vomiting. Ex: *cocaine, peppermint, bismuth, subnitrate, cerium oxalate*.

antienzyme (an-tĭ-en′zīm). 1. Enzyme neutralizer. 2. An enzyme retarding the activity of another.

antiephial′tic [G. *anti*, against, + *ephialtes*, nightmare]. Hindering nightmare. SYN: *antephialtic*.

an′tifat. An agent which lessens accumulation of fat.

antifeb′rile [G. *anti*, against, + L. *febris*, fever]. 1. A medium reducing fever. 2. Reducing or relieving fever.

antifebrin (an-tĭ-feb′rin). Acetanilid.

DOSAGE: 3 gr. (0.2 Gm.).

antifebrin salicylate *a. salicylate.* Salifebrin.

antifer'ment [G. *anti*, against, + L. *fermentum*, leaven]. Hindering, or an agent which hinders, the action of an enzyme. SYN: *antienzyme.*

antifermen'tative. Preventing the fermentation process. SYN: *antizymotic.*

antigalactagogue (an-ti-gal-ak'tă-gog) [G. *anti*, against, + *gala*, milk, + *agogos*, drawing forth]. An agent that lessens the secretion of milk. Ex: belladonna, probably all *hydragogue* purgatives.

antigalactic (an-tĭ-gal-ak'tic) [" + *gala*, milk]. Diminishing or retarding the secretion of milk.

an'tigen [" + *gennan*, to produce]. A substance which induces the formation of antibodies. An antigen may be introduced into the body or it may be formed within the body. Examples are bacteria, bacterial toxins, foreign blood cells.

a. unit. Smallest quantity of antigen required to fix 1 unit of complement, preventing hemolysis.

antigenic (an-tĭ-jen'ik). Capable of causing the production of an antibody.

antigenophil (an-tĭ-jen'o-fĭl) [" + " + *philos*, fond]. Having an attraction for the antigen. SYN: *antigentophil.*

antigentophil (an-tĭ-jen'to-fĭl). Having affinity for antigen.

antigentother'apy [" + " + *therapeia*, treatment]. Stimulating antibody formation by injecting antigens.

antiglob'ulin. A precipitin which precipitates globulin.

an''tigonorrhe'ic. 1. Curing gonorrhea. 2. An agent relieving gonorrhea.

antihe'lix [G. *anti*, against, + *elix*, coil]. Inner curved ridge of external ear.

antihemicra'nin. A proprietary drug for headache. SYN: *antimigraine.*

antihemol'ysin. A substance which neutralizes hemolysin.

antihidrot'ic [G. *anti*, against, + *hidrotikos*, sweating]. Preventing or checking perspiration. SYN: *anhidrotic.*

antihormone (an-tĭ-hor'mōn). An inhibitory autacoid opposing hormone action.

antihydrop'ic [G. *anti*, against, + *ydrops*, dropsy]. 1. Relieving dropsy. 2. Agent causing disappearance of dropsy.

anti-icter'ic [" + *ikteros*, jaundice]. 1. Relieving icterus. 2. Agent for curing jaundice.

an''ti-immune'. Preventing immunity.

an''ti-isoly'sin. A substance inhibiting action of an isolysin.

antikenotox'in. A substance counteracting fatigue toxins.

antiketogen'esis [G. *anti*, against, + *ketone* + *gennan*, to produce]. Lowering of acidosis through body oxidation of sugar, alcohol, glycerin, and allied substances.

antiketogenet'ic, antiketogen'ic. Pert. to antiketogenesis.

an'tikol. Proprietary antifebrile medicine.

antilac'tase [G. *anti*, against, + *lac*, milk]. An antibody counteracting lactase.

antilemic (an-tĭ-le'mĭk) [" + *loimos*, plague]. 1. Preventing plague. 2. An agent curing the plague.

antilepsis (an-tĭ-lep'sis) [" + *lepsis*, a seizing]. 1. Application of a remedy to a healthy part. 2. An attack or seizure. 3. Taking effect or root. 4. Support of a bandage.

antileptic (an-tĭ-lep'tĭk) [G. *antileptikos*, able to check]. 1. Assisting, supporting. 2. Revulsive.

antilethargic (an-tĭ-leth-ar'jik) [G. *anti*, against, + *lethargos*, forgetfulness]. Preventing sleep.

antilith'ic [" + *lithos*, stone]. An agent that prevents the formation of, or favors the removal of stones or calculi in the urinary or biliary tracts. Ex: *lithium citrate, methenamine, alkaline waters,* and *glycerin.*

antilo'bium [" + *lobos*, ear lobe]. The tragus.

antilogia (an-tĭ-lo'jĭ-ă) [" + *logos*, science]. Contradictory symptoms which render diagnosis uncertain.

antiluetic (an-tĭ-lu-et'ĭk) [" + L. *lues*, pestilence]. Antisyphilitic.

antilysin (an-tĭ-li'sin). A substance neutralizing the lysins of a disease against which an animal has been immunized.

antilysis (an-til'is-is). The result of the action of antilysin.

antilys'sic [G. *anti*, against, + *lyssa*, frenzy]. Preventing or checking rabies. SYN: *antirabic.*

antimalar'ial. An agent that will prevent or relieve malaria. Ex: *quinine.*

antimere (an'tĭ-mēr) [G. *anti*, against, + *meros*, a part]. Any body segment bounded by planes at right angles to the long axis of the body.

antimetro'pia. An ocular disorder in which one eye is hypermetropic, the other myopic.

antimiasmat'ic [G. *anti*, against, + *miasma*, stain]. Preventing or checking malaria. SYN: *antimalarial.*

antimicro'bic [" + *mikros*, small, + *bios*, life]. 1. Not believing in the pathogenicity of microörganisms. 2. Preventing the development or pathogenic action of microbes.

antimicro'bin. Antibody used to prevent further germ growth in the body. SEE: *germ theory.*

antimo'nial. Pert. to or containing antimony.

antimony (an'tĭ-mo''nĭ). SYMB: *Sb.* An element of metallic appearance and crystalline structure. Atomic weight 121.77. Its salts form various poisons and medicinal drugs.

POISONING: SYM: Acrid metallic taste. Cardiac and arterial depressants with additional properties of inducing sweating and vomiting about 30 minutes after injection. In large doses they irritate lining of alimentary tract, resembling arsenic.

F. A. TREATMENT: Vomiting caused by the poison may be sufficient emesis. Wash stomach with strong tea, or dilute tannic acid. Otherwise treat symptomatically. SEE: *tartar emetic.*

antimycotic (an-tĭ-mi-kot'ĭk) [G. *anti*, against, + *mykēs*, fungus]. Checking or destroying bacteria. SYN: *antibacterial.*

antinarcot'ic. Relieving stupor caused by a narcotic.

antinephritic (an-tĭ-nef-rit'ĭk). Serviceable in renal inflammation.

antiner'vin. Bromacetanilid and salicylanilid used as an antineuralgic.

antineuralgic (an-tĭ-nu-ral'jĭk). 1. Relieving neuralgic pain. 2. Agent curing neuralgia.

antineurit'ic. Counteracting nerve inflammation.

antineu'ritin. Antineuritic vitamin or Vitamin B₁.

antin'ion [G. *anti*, against, + *inion*, nape of the neck]. Frontal pole of the skull.

antiop'sonin. A substance that retards opsonin action.

antioxida'tion. Prevention of oxidation.

antiox'ygen. A substance hindering oxidation.

antiparalytic   A-66   **antisialogogue**

antiparalyt'ic. Reputedly relieving paralysis.
antiparasit'ic. 1. Destructive to parasites. 2. Insecticide.*
antiparastati'tis [G. *anti*, against, + *parastates*, testicle, + *-itis*, inflammation]. Inflammation of Cowper's glands.
antipathic (an-tĭ-path'ĭk) [" + *pathein*, to feel]. Opposite; unlike.
antip'athy [" + *pathos*, suffering]. 1. Aversion; disgust; or that which excites repugnance. 2. Chemical incompatibility.
antipepsin (an-tĭ-pep'sin). An antibody counteracting pepsin.
antipeptone (an-tĭ-pep'tōn). Peptone derived from antialbumose through hydrolysis.
antiperiod'ic [G. *anti*, against, + *periodos*, a circle]. Antimalarial; preventing regular recurrences.
antiperistal'sis [" + *peri*, around, + *stalsis*, constriction]. A wave of contraction in the gastrointestinal tract moving towards the oral end.
In the duodenum it is associated with vomiting; in the ascending colon it occurs normally. It may occur in diverticulitis. SEE: *peristalsis*.
antiperistal'tic. 1. Pert. to antiperistalsis.* 2. Impeding peristalsis.*
antiphlogistic (an-ti-phlo-jis'tik) [G. *anti-*, against, + *phlogistos*, on fire]. An agent that tends to relieve inflammation. Ex: *cataplasma of kaolin, ichthyol*.
antiphthisic (an-tĭ-tiz'ĭk) [" + *phthisis*, a wasting]. Checking or relieving phthisis.
antiphthi'sin. Modified tuberculin.
antiplas'tic [G. *anti*, against, + *plastikos*, pert. to molding]. 1. An agent preventing granulation of tissue. 2. One which thins the blood.
antipneumotox'in [" + *pneumon*, lung, + *toxikon*, poison]. An antitoxin opposing pneumotoxin.
antip'odal cell [G. *antipous*, with feet opposite]. One of two nuclear cells at the base of embryo sac in a seed.
antipraxia (an-tĭ-praks'ĭ-ă). Functions or symptoms antagonistic to each other.
antiprostate (an-tĭ-pros'tāt). Cowper's glands.*
antiprostati'tis. Inflammation of Cowper's glands.
antiprothrom'bin [G. *anti*, against, + *prō*, before, + *thrombos*, clot]. Agent preventing formation of thrombin; anticoagulant. SEE: *clotting*.
antiprotozo'al. Destructive to protozoa.
antipruritic (an-tĭ-pru-rit'ĭk) [G. *anti*, against, + L. *prurire*, to itch]. That which relieves itching.
antipsoric (an-tip-so'rik) [" + *psōra*, the itch]. An agent used to prevent or arrest itching. It may be local or general.
antiputrefac'tive. Preventive of putrefaction.
antipyic (an-tĭ-pī'ĭk) [G. *anti*, against, + *pyon*, pus]. Checking suppuration; antipyogenic.
antipyogenic (an″tĭ-pī-o-jen'ĭk) [" + *pyon*, pus]. Preventing or checking pus formation.
antipyre'sis [" + *pyretos*, fever]. Use of antipyretics in fever.
antipyret'ic. An agent that reduces febrile temperatures. Ex: *quinine, antipyrine, acetylsalicylic acid*.
antipyrine (an″tĭ-pī'rĭn) [G. *anti*, against, + *pyr*, fever]. White crystalline powder, odorless and having a slightly bitter taste.
One of the safest coal tar derivatives, which is much less toxic than acetanilid. A. is incompatible with many other drugs and list should be noted.
ACTION: Sedative, analgesic, antipyretic.
USES: Fevers, headache, neuralgia, whooping cough, etc.
DOSAGE: 5 gr. (0.3 Gm.).
INCOMPATIBILITIES: Acids and drugs containing tannic acid; alkalies; salts of iron, mercury, lead and arsenic; iodine and iodides; sodium bicarbonate and salicylate; alum; benzoates; phenol; cinchona alkaloids; resorcin; spirit of ethyl nitrite.
antipyrotic (an-tĭ-pi-rot'ĭk) [G. *anti*, against, + *pyrōtikos*, burning]. That which allays the pain from burns.
antirab'ic. Preventive of, or curing, hydrophobia; antilyssic.
antirachit'ic [G. *anti*, against, + *rachitis*]. 1. Helping to cure rickets. 2. Agent for treating rickets.
   a. vitamin. Vitamin D. SEE: *vitamins*.
antireticular cytotoxic serum. One prepared by Dr. Alexander A. Bogomolets (d. 1946) of Russia. (Abbr., ACS.) A serum made from endothelial cells which line the blood vessels, first tested by Bogomolets. Used successfully in war wounds, treatment after surgery, some types of rheumatism, headaches, insomnia, reducing high blood pressure, and in warding off diseases of the aged, thus prolonging life.
antirheumat'ic. An agent that will prevent or relieve rheumatism. Ex: *sodium salicylate, acetylsalicylic acid, colchicum*.
antiricin (an-tĭ-ri'sin). An antibody to ricin.
antiscabious (an-tĭ-skā'bĭ-us). Preventing or relieving scabies.
antiscorbutic (an-tĭ-skor-bu'tĭk). An agent effective against or a remedy for scurvy. Vitamin C is antiscorbutic. Ex: *citric acid, orange juice, ascorbic acid*.
antisepsin. SEE: *asepsin*.
antisep'sis [G. *anti*, against, + *sepsis*, putrefaction]. The exclusion of putrefactive germs.
antiseptic (an-tĭ-sep'tĭk). An agent that will prevent the growth or arrest the development of microörganisms. Ex: *sodium benzoate, boric acid, carbolic acid, or almost any germicide in diluted form*.
Chemically, antiseptics may be *inorganic*, such as the mercury preparations, or *organic*, such as carbolic acid (phenol). Oxidizing disinfectants liberate oxygen when in contact with pus or organic substances. When in use they should be changed frequently to free them of pus, blood, and other substances. Different types of bacteria require different antiseptics. They are more or less destructive to tissue. They should cause the serum to enter the wound rather than flow from it, and they should prevent absorption of infectious substances.
RS: *asepsis, disinfectant, deodorant, germicide, sterilization*.
antisep'ticism. Therapeutic employment of antiseptic measures.
antiserum (an-tĭ-se'rum). A serum containing an antibody specific in relation to the substance which has produced it through repeated injections.
antisialic (an-tĭ-si-al'ĭk) [G. *anti*, against, + *sialon*, saliva]. Checking or that which checks the secretion of saliva.
antisialogogue (an-tĭ-si-al'o-gog) [" + " + *agogos*, drawing forth]. An agent that lessens or checks the flow of saliva.

Ex: *belladonna, sodium bicarbonate, atropine.*

antispasmod'ic [" + *spasmos,* convulsion]. An agent that will relieve muscular spasm. Ex: *morphine, atropine, asafetida, bromides.* See: *spasm.*

antispas'tic. Agent relieving muscular spasm. Syn: *antispasmodic.*

anti-stain formulary. An anti-stain formulary for removing stains from linens is as follows:

Argyrol: Rinse well while stain is fresh in clear, cold water. For old stain, soak in 1: 1000 bichloride of mercury solution. Rinse in cold water.

Balsam of Peru: Use waste ether to dissolve it before laundering.

Blood: Soak in cold water, then wash. For old stains, use peroxide of hydrogen and ammonia water, persistently.

Chocolate or Cocoa: Use glycerine, then cold water and borax, then boiling water. Soak in these successively while fresh.

Cod Liver Oil: Soak stained fabric in kerosene oil for 1 hour, rubbing lightly occasionally. Then place article in water in which a naphtha soap has been shaved and boil 10 minutes. Rinse in clear water.

Feces: Soak in cold water, rinse, then wash with soap and water (hot). Use a brush to scrub.

Fruit-Stains: Stretch stained article over a basin, pour boiling water directly over the spot until it disappears. If this fails, use Javelle water (a preparation of washing soda and chloride of lime), rinsing bet. each application.

Grass-Stains: Use alcohol, kerosene, or gasoline; afterwards washing soda and hot water. Put in the sun to bleach.

Ink: If fresh, immerse in cold or tepid water, or skimmed milk. Long soaking will bring it out of the goods. Oxalic acid may be applied if care is taken not to leave on too long. It may rot the cloth, though; soak and rinse well. Turpentine may be used on colored fabrics. Old ink-stains respond well to lemon juice, salt and sunlight. Whatever is used, the material should be rinsed and rinsed after using to remove all of the solution.

Iodine: Use alcohol, then rinse well in clear, cold water. Ether or ammonia may be used; rinse well after using.

Iron-Rust: Use lemon juice and salt: expose to the sunlight. For firm fabrics, use strong solution of oxalic acid: Rinse very thoroughly.

Meat-Juices: Soak in clear, cold water.

Medicines: Use alcohol or cold water.

Mercurochrome: Pour hot water through the material. Acid alcohol does very well, or Dakin's Solution and 5% acetic acid (vinegar), equal parts of each. Mix with a stick and when the material has been soaked and the color of the stain removed, wash thoroughly.

Mildew: If fresh, use strong soapsuds and hang in the sunlight. If an old stain, use Javelle water, rinse thoroughly and repeat the washing if indicated.

Nail Polish, Lipstick and Rouge: Ordinary washing or carbon tetrachloride

ANTISEPTICS

Used For	Chemicals	Uses
Hands	Bichloride of mercury (mercuric chloride)	One tablet (7½ grains) in one pint of water makes a 1: 1000 solution, chiefly used to disinfect hands previous to an operation. Continued use irritates skin. Not used to disinfect instruments as it *corrodes the metal.*
Skin	Alcohol (ethyl alcohol)	A 50 to 70 per cent solution will penetrate bacteria, but stronger solutions are not as active. Green soap owes its germicidal action to the alcohol (43 per cent) contained in it.
Skin	Sulfur	Used as ointment to check growth of bacteria and destroy parasites, as in scabies.
Skin	Ichthyol	An antiseptic in various skin diseases to relieve itching and soften skin.
Wounds and Ulcers	Hypochlorite solutions	Dakin's solution contains 45 to 50 per cent sodium hypochlorite. Free chlorine is liberated to combine with NH_2 radical of proteins in tissues to form chloramine; as an antiseptic about 15 times as effective as phenol, besides not being injurious to tissues.
Wounds and Ulcers	Potassium permanganate	An oxidizing disinfectant in 1 to 3 per cent solutions for wounds, and in 1: 1000 to 1 per cent solutions for gargles and douches.
Wounds and Ulcers	Iodoform	Mostly used in gauze soaked with a 5 to 10 per cent solution of iodoform.
Wounds and Ulcers	Picric acid	Used chiefly in treatment of burns or scalds.
Mucous Membranes	Boric acid	A 2 to 5 per cent solution used in eyes, nose or sensitive membranes without any irritation.
Mucous Membranes	Dobell's solution	A 1½ per cent sodium borate, phenol, sodium bicarbonate, glycerine and water solution, mostly used as an alkaline gargle and as an antiseptic nasal douche.
Mucous Membranes	Silver nitrate	A 2 per cent solution in eye of the newborn prevents gonorrheal infection. In strong solutions very destructive to tissues.
Mucous Membranes	Argyrol	As a combination of silver and albumin it is used in 10 to 25 per cent solutions for antiseptic and astringent purposes.

antistalsis   A-68   **antral**

or acetone, followed by a warm chlorine bleach.

PAINTS, VARNISHES: Turpentine, gasoline or benzine applied in the open air. If old stain, soak well in grease to soften, then apply turpentine or the other solutions. Chloroform dissolves lacquer paint stains. Acetone sponged on fabric removes varnish.

PERSPIRATION: Wash in strong soap solution and hang in the sunlight.

PICRIC ACID: Make a solution of one part of boric acid, one part of sodium benzoate, and 98 parts of water. Soak the material in this solution and then rinse well or else boil fabric in strong sodium hydroxide solution for ½ hr. and bleach in Javelle water.

SCORCH: Peroxide of hydrogen applied to the area; then rub well with the material soaked in strong soap solution. Hang in the sunlight.

SILVER NITRATE: Soak in normal saline solution, or soak in a solution of bichloride of mercury 1:1000 to 25 parts of sodium chloride in 2000 cc. of water.

TEA OR COFFEE: If fresh, pour boiling water through it. If old, soak in borax before pouring boiling water over it.

URINE: Soak in boiling water, then pour 5% lysol solution over it.

VASELINE: Wash well with cold water and plenty of mild soap (Ivory). Hot water sets the stain. Use soap freely and rinse thoroughly.

antistal′sis [G. *anti*, against, + *stalsis*, constriction]. Backward movement of bowel contents. Opp. peristalsis, *q.v.*

antistaphylococ′cic. Destructive to staphylococcus.

antistaphylol′ysin. Blood serum substance counteracting staphylolysin.

antistat′ic [G. *anti*, against, + *statikos*, standing]. Counteracting; hostile. SYN: *antagonistic*.   [coccus.

antistreptococ′cic. Destructive to streptococcus.

antistreptococ′cin. The antitoxin of any type streptococcus.

antisu′doral [G. *anti*, against, + *sudor*, sweat]. Checking perspiration. SYN: *antihidrotic*.

antisu′dorin. Commercial name of remedy to correct sweating.

antisyphilit′ic. An agent that will prevent or relieve syphilis. Ex: *mercury, arsenic, bismuth*.

antitabetic (an-tĭ-ta-bet′ĭk). 1. Preventing tabes dorsalis. 2. Agent which mitigates tabetic symptoms.

antithenar (an-tĭ-thē′nar). Placed opposite to the thenar.

antither′mic [G. *anti*, against, + *thermē*, heat]. 1. Reducing temperature. 2. Agent lowering temperature. SYN: *antifebrile, antipyretic*.

antithrombin (an-tĭ-throm′bin). A substance in the blood which prevents or retards coagulation.

antithyroi′din. A serum from sheep's blood after thyroid has been removed.

USES: Exophthalmic goiter and other diseases due to hypersecretion of thyroid gland.

DOSAGE: 0.5 to 1 cc.

antiton′ic. Diminishing tone or tonicity.

antitoxic (an-tĭ-tok′sik) [G. *anti*, against, + *toxikon*, poison]. Neutralizing a poison, specifically an antitoxin.

    a. unit. Sufficient quantity of antitoxin to neutralize 100 toxic units. SYN: *immunizing unit.*

antitox′igen [" + " + *gennan*, to produce]. An antigen stimulating antitoxin production in the blood.

antitox′in. An antibody capable of neutralizing a specific toxin. It is produced by the body cells in response to the presence of a toxin. Examples are *diphtheria antitoxin* and *tetanus antitoxin* which counteract the toxins produced by the diphtheria and tetanus bacteria. Antitoxins are used for prophylactic and therapeutic purposes.

    a. serum. A serum which contains the antitoxin of a disease organism. The serum is obtained from the blood of an animal. It is given in toxic diseases, either (a) subcutaneously, (b) intramuscularly, (c) intravenously.

antitoxin′ogen [G. *anti*, against, + *toxikon*, poison, + *gennan*, to produce]. An antigen promoting production of antitoxin in the blood. SYN: *antitoxigen*.

antitragicus (an-tĭ-traj′ik-us). A small muscle in the pinna of the ear.

antitragus (an-tit-ra′gus). A projection on the ear of the cartilage of the auricle in front of the tail of the helix, post. to the tragus.

antitrismus (an-tĭ-tris′mus). A condition in which the mouth cannot close because of tonic spasm.

antitrope (an′tĭ-trōp) [G. *anti*, against, + *tropē*, a turn]. 1. A symmetrical pair of organs. 2. Antibody.

antitro′pin. An antibody.*

antitryp′sin. An antibody or antiferment inhibiting tryptic action.

antitryp′tic. Counteracting trypsins.

antituberculot′ic. Inhibiting the advance of tuberculosis.

antitu′lase. A serum used in treating for tuberculosis.

antiuratic (an-tĭ-u-rat′ik). Preventing the precipitation of urates.

antivaccina′tion. Opposition to vaccination.

antivaccina′tionist. One who is opposed to vaccination.

antiven′ene. Blood serum of an animal rendered immune to snake bite.

    USES: A specific in treating certain poisonous snake bites.

antivene′real. Preventing or curing venereal diseases.

antivenin (an-tĭ-ven′in). An antigenic substance prepared from immunized animal sera used by injection to overcome the effects of snake bite.

    Special types are used for each variety of snake. Mixed types (polyvalent antivenins) are also available. SYN: *antivenene*.

antiven′om. A snake venom antitoxin.

antiven′omous. Inhibiting venom.

antivi′ral. Inhibiting a virus.

antivi′rus. A bacterial filtrate from a broth medium heated to reduce toxicity; used in the Besredka local immunity method.

antixe′nic. Pert. to living tissue reaction to any foreign substance.

antizymot′ic. An agent that will prevent or arrest fermentation. Ex: *salicylic acid, alcohol.*

antlia (ant′lĭ-ă) [L. a pump]. A pump or syringe.

antodontalgic (ant-o-don-tal′jik) [G. *anti*, against, + *odont*, tooth, + *algos*, pain]. 1. Relieving toothache. 2. Remedy for toothache.

an′tozone. Hydrogen peroxide.

an′tra [L.]. Pl. of antrum.

antracele (an′tra-sēl) [L. *antrum*, cavity, + G. *kēlē*, tumor]. Accumulation of fluid in Highmore's antrum.

antral (an′tral). Pert. to an antrum.

antrec′tomy [L. *antrum* + G. *ektomē*, excision]. Excision of the walls of an antrum.

antritis (an-tri′tis) [" + G. *-itis*, inflammation]. Inflammation of an antrum, esp. that of the a. of Highmore.

antroatticotomy (an-tro-at-ĭ-kot′o-mī) [" + *atticus*, + G. *tomē*, cutting]. Operation to open and remove contents of the antrum and the attic of the tympanum.

antrocele (an′tro-sēl) [" + G. *kēlē*, tumor. Fluid accumulation in Highmore's antrum. SYN: *antracele.**

antrona′sal [" + *nasalis*]. Rel. to the maxillary sinus and nasal fossa.

antrophore (an′tro-fōr) [" + G. *phorein*, to carry]. A medicated bougie for local treatment of any accessible cavity or canal.

antroscope (an′tro-skop) [" + *skopein*, to view]. An instrument for examining the maxillary sinus.

antros′copy. Examination of any cavity by the antroscope.

antros′tomy [L. *antrum*, cavity, + G. *stoma*, mouth]. Operation to open an antrum for drainage.

antrotome (an′tro-tōm) [" + G. *tomē*, incision]. An instrument for cutting open a cavity, esp. in bone.

antrot′omy. Opening an antral wall.

an″trotympan′ic [L. *antrum*, cavity, + G. *tympanon*, drum]. Rel. to the mastoid sinus and the tympanic cavity.

an″trotympani′tis. Chronic inflammation of middle ear and mastoid antrum.

an′trum [*Pl. antra*] [L. from G. *antron*, cavity]. Any nearly closed cavity or chamber in a bone.
   a. auris. External acoustic meatus.
   a. cardiacum. Cardiac portion of the stomach, proximal or superior portion.
   a. mastoideum. Tympanic antrum.
   a., maxillary. The maxillary sinus. SEE: *sinus*.
   a. of Highmore. The air sinus in the maxillary bone.
   a. puncture. Made near floor of nose 1½ inches from external opening. Pus is then drained. NP: Douche antrum 24 hours after puncture. May be necessary for first few days to cocainize nose before passing cannula. Attach syringe to cannula when placed. Teach patient to hold it and to treat self at home.
   a. pyloricum. Bulge in the pyloric portion of the stomach along the greater curvature on distention.
   a. tympanicum. The mastoid antrum.

antu′itrin. Extract of anterior lobe of pituitary body.
   a. G, a. growth. Commercial product derived from the ant. pituitary, containing the growth stimulating element.
   a. gonadotropic. Commercial product derived from the ant. pituitary, containing the gonadotropic hormone.
   a. S. A gonadotropic hormone extracted from the urine of pregnant women.
   a. T, a. thyrotropic. Commercial product derived from the ant. pituitary, containing the thyrotropic element.

anure′sis [G. *an-*, priv. + *ouresis*, urination]. Failure of kidney to secrete sufficient urine, suppression or failure to reach bladder if secreted; found in nephritis (if acute), or congestion, renal abscess, and last stages of chronic nephritis.
   ETIOL: Inhalation of ether; lead, phosphorus, cantharides, or turpentine poisoning; Asiatic cholera; cholera infantum; cholera morbus; gastrointestinal perforation; shock; collapse; typhoid fever; yellow fever; pernicious anemia; hysteria; acute yellow atrophy of the liver. Obstructive suppression is the result of occlusion of one or both ureters.
   NP: Aid action of skin and bowels. Care as in nephritis. Wash skin with hot water, 116° to 120° F., twice a day. Hot drinks. Cover patient well. Prevent chilling and keep out of drafts.

anuret′ic. Pert. to anuresis, *q.v.*

anu′ria [G. *an-*, priv. + *ouron*, urine]. Failure of kidney function. SYN: *anuresis*.

a′nus [L.]. The outlet of the rectum lying in the fold bet. the nates.
   The end of the anal* canal (2.5 to 3 cm.). Fissures of anus in newly born indicative of congenital syphilis.
   a., artificial. Opening of the bowel (usually surgical).
   a., fissure in. A crack in mucosa of rectum.
   a., fistula in. A fistulous connection bet. lumen of rectum and perianal skin.
   a., imperforated. Where the natural opening is closed.
   a., vulvovaginal. An opening into the vulva from the anus.

anvil (an′vil) [A.S. *anfilt*]. Middle ossicle of ear. SYN: *incus*.

anxietas (ang-zi′et-ăs) [L. *angere*, to vex, trouble]. Anxiety, apprehension, restlessness.
   a. tibia′rum. Tiredness, twitching, and unrest in legs when in bed. ETIOL: Increase of the muscular sense.

anxiety neuro′sis. A functional disease in which fear (or the somatic evidences of fear) is the essential part of the picture.
   A symptomatic fear state can be differentiated by recognizing primary disease such as thyrotoxicosis. Fear may exist consciously, or present a group of somatic symptoms not recognized for what they are; in fact, even denied as representing anxiety. Ordinarily, fear as a response to an environmental threat is quite conscious; it may be equally conscious without the patient having the slightest insight as to its causation.
   Fear may be an emotional correlate of organic brain disease; it is outstanding in certain toxic states (notably delirium tremens), may coexist with depression, and occur as night waves.
   Anxiety neurosis is manifested when an intact personality without organic disease, during clear consciousness, complains of palpitation; heart pain; dyspepsia; cold, sweaty, tremulous extremities; constriction of the throat; bandlike pressure about head, among other symptoms. Often these are interpreted as meaning regional disease.
   The real significance is a feeling of inadequacy in meeting some situation, *e. g.*, a tempting situation which is so completely repressed but to be totally unacceptable to the patient as of significance. *Homosexuality** is such a frustrated impulse that may lead not only to an anxiety state but to the much more intense picture of panic—psychotic terror. It is always very important not to rationalize the symptoms as some physical disease, although analysis is not always indicated.

anxious agitated depression. PSY: Depression accompanied by worry, uneasiness, and agitation, esp. rel. to poverty and want, or ruin.
   SYM: Hallucinations may be present but generally they are absent. Delusions

anydremia   A-70   **aortic regurgitation**

that a well-known phenomenon of nature has ceased to exist, such as the day or the night, the sun or the moon, aversion to eating, or the hearing of voices accusing the subject, are other symptoms.

anydremia (an-ĭ-dre'mĭ-ă) [G. *an-*, priv. + *ydōr*, water, + *aima*, blood]. Decrease in normal fluid content of the blood. SYN: anhydremia.*

anypnia (an-ip'nĭ-ă) [G. *an-*, priv. + *ypnos*, sleep]. Condition of sleeplessness.

A. O. C. Abbr. for Anodal Opening Contraction.

aochlesia (a-ok-le'zĭ-ă) [G. *a-*, priv. + *ochlesis*, disturbance]. Tranquillity; rest; catalepsy.

aolan (ā'o-lan). A sterile solution of lactalbumin in colloidal form.

USES: In nonspecific protein therapy, to relieve pain in gonorrheal complications.

DOSAGE: From 5 to 10 cc., at intervals of 5 to 6 days, intramuscularly.

aor'ta [G. *aortē*, aorta]. The main trunk of the arterial system of the body. It is ½ to ¾ inch in diameter at its origin. It arises from the upper surface of the left ventricle, passes upward as the *ascending aorta*, turns backward and to the left (arch of the *aorta*) at about the level of the fourth thoracic vertebra and then passes downward as the *descending aorta*, which is divided into the *thoracic* and *abdominal aorta*. The latter terminates at its division into the two common iliac arteries. At its exit from the ventricle, the aortic orifice is guarded by three semi-lunar valves. The divisions and branches of the aorta are as follows:

THE AORTA
Its 3 Divisions and 58 Branches
Name of Arteries

AORTIC ARCH, 5 *Arteries*
* †
1   2 Coronary (Right and Left) ‡
2   1 Innominate 2
3   1 Carotid (Left Common) .. 2
4   1 Subclavian (Left) 54

THORACIC, 31 *Arteries*
5   3 Bronchial
6   4 Esophageal
7   2 Pericardial
8   20 Intercostal
9   2 Posterior Mediastinal
10   2 Phrenic 2
11   1 Celiac Axis 3
12   1 Superior Mesenteric 5

ABDOMINAL, 22 *Arteries*
13   2 Suprarenal 5
14   2 Renal
15   2 Spermatic and Ovarian
16   1 Inferior Mesenteric 3
17   8 Lumbar 16
18   1 Middle Sacral
19   2 Iliac (R. & L. Com.) 42
    58

(See *Blood* and *Circulation*)

* No. Heads.   † No. Arteries.
‡ Branches.

THE AORTA
Distribution of Branches of the Aorta
Branches of Arteries and Parts Supplied

1 To muscular tissues of heart.
2 Divides into right subclavian and right common carotid.
3 Internal and external, 8 branches each, supplies head.
4 1st Div. { Vertebral, with .... 7 br.
             { Thyroid Axis, with ..... 3 br.
             { Int. Mammary, with ... 8 br.
2nd Div.—Sup. Intercostal, with.. 2 br.
(Head, Up Ext., Arms.)
3rd Div.—Axillary, with .... 7 br.
becomes Brachial, with 7 br.
This divides into
Ulnar, with .... 8 br.
Radial, with ....12 br.
                        54 br.

5 Nutrient of lungs ....
6 To Esophagus, Anastomoses with brs. of inf. Thyroid, Phrenic and Gastric.
7 To Pericardium.
8 To upper and lower border ribs, tissues of sides and back, vertebrae and spinal cord, Anas. br. of Int. Mammary and Axillary.
9 To glands in Mediastinum.
10 Int. and Ext. to Diaphragm, front and sides of Thorax.
11 GASTRIC, to cardiac orifice, end and lesser curvative of stomach.
HEPATIC, to greater curvature, Pancreas, Duodenum, Gallbladder and Liver.
SPLENIC, Greater Curvature, Stomach, Pancreas, Spleen.
12 Pancreas, Duodenum, Mesentery, Ileum, Jejunum, asc. and trans. Colon.
13 To Suprarenal Capsules.
14 To substance of Kidneys, Ureters and capsules.
15 To Testes or Ovaries.
16 To descend. Colon, Sigmoid Flexure, sides of rectum.
17 { Thoracic........to muscles of back.
    { Abdominal....to abdominal muscles.
    { Spinal....................to canal.
18 To Coccyx, anast. with lateral sacral, to rectum.
19 Divides into Int. Iliac, which gives off, Ant. Trunk with 8 br. Post. Trunk with 4 br. These supply Bladder, Prostate Gland, Rectum, Uterus, Ureters, Vagina, Penis, Iliac Bone and Muscle, Hip-joints and Muscles, Cord and Membranes, Sacrum, Glutei muscles. Divides into Ext. Iliac which give off 3 brs., becomes Femoral which gives off 8 brs., becomes Popliteal, gives off 7 brs., divides into Ant. Tibial, gives off 5 brs., and Post. Tibial gives off 7 brs.

aor'tal. Pert. to the aorta.

aortalgia (a-or-tal'jĭ-ă) [G. *aorte*, aorta, + G. *algos*, pain]. Pain due to pathological aortic conditions.

aortarctia (a-or-tark'shĭ-ă) [" + L. *arctare*, to narrow]. Aortic narrowing.

aortectasia (a-ort-ek-ta'zĭ-ă) [" + *ek*, out, + *tasis*, a stretching]. Dilatation of the aorta.

aor'tic. Pert. to aorta or its orifice in the left ventricle of the heart. [disease.
    a. murmur. Symptom of a. valvular
    a. opening. 1. Path through diaphragm for aorta. 2. Post. opening in the diaphragm.
    a. regurgita'tion.* Leakage of the blood from the aorta back into the left ventricle at the recoil of the aorta's elastic walls. ETIOL: Diseases of the heart or aortic valves with defects or weakness of heart muscle.

a. stenosis. Narrowing of *a.* or its orifice due to (1) lesions of the wall with scar formation, (2) infection as in rheumatic fever, or (3) embryonic anomalies. Hypertrophy of the heart is a common result.

a. valves. Three valves in left ventricle at the a. opening.

aortitis (a-or-ti'tis) [G. *aortē*, aorta, + *-itis*, inflammation]. Inflammation of the aorta.

Associated with syphilis in which vascular changes have taken place. A common cause of aortic aneurysm.

SYM: Possible cough, cyanosis, dyspnea, cardiac asthmatic attacks, hemoptysis.

aortocla'sia [" + *klasis*, a breaking]. Aortic rupture.

aortog'raphy [" + G. *graphein*, to write]. Examination of abdominal aorta by x-ray after injection of contrast fluid.

aortolith (a-or'to-lith) [" + G. *lithos*, stone]. Calcareous deposit in the aortic wall.

aortomalacia (a-or-to-mal-a'-sī-ă) [" + G. *malakia*, softness]. Softening of the aorta's walls.

aortop'athy [" + G. *pathos*, disease]. Any aortic disease.

aortopto'sia, aortopto'sis [" + G. *ptosis*, a falling]. Sinking down of abdominal aorta.

aortorrhaphy (a-or-tor'af-ĭ) [" + *raphē*, suture]. Suture of the aorta.

aortosclero'sis [" + *skleros*, hard]. Aortic sclerosis.

aortostenosis (a-or-to-sten-o'sis) [" + G. *stenōsis*, a narrowing]. Narrowing of the aorta.

aortot'omy [" + G. *tomē*, a cutting]. Incision of the aorta.

aos'mic [G. *a-*, priv. + *osmē*, smell]. Without odor.

A. O. T. A. Abbr. *American Occupational Therapy Association.*

apallesthesia (ă-pal"es-the'zĭ-ă) [G. *a-*, priv. + *pallein*, to tremble, + *aisthēsis*, feeling]. Inability to detect vibrations of a tuning fork placed against the body.

apan'dria [G. *apo*, from, + *anēr* (*andr-*), man]. Aversion to males.

apanthropia, apanthropy (a-pan-thro'pi-ă, -ĭ) [" + *anthrōpos*, man]. Morbid aversion to society or to man.

aparalyt'ic [G. *a-*, priv. + *paralyein*, to loosen]. Marked by lack of paralysis.

aparathyrosis (ă-par-ă-thī-ro'sis) [" + *para*, near, + *thyreos*, an oblong shield, + *osis*, denoting increase]. Parathyroid deficiency.

apareunia (a-pa-ru'nĭ-ă) [" + *pareunos*, lying beside]. Impossibility or absence of coitus.

ETIOL: Rudimentary development of vagina, imperforate hymen, stenosis of vagina.

aparthrosis (ap-ar-thro'sis) [G. *apo*, from, + *arthron*, joint, + *osis*, denoting increase]. 1. Diarthrosis. 2. Dislocation.

apastia (ap-as'tĭ-ă) [G. *apastia*, fasting]. Abnormal refusal to eat.

apathetic (ap-ă-thet'ik) [G. *a-*, priv. + *pathos*, disease]. Indifferent; without interest. SYN: *apathic.*

apath'ic. Indifferent. SYN: *apathetic.*

apathism (ap'ath-izm) [G. *a-*, priv. + *pathos*, disease, + *ismos*, condition]. Slow to react; opp. to erethism.*

ap'athy. Indifference; insensibility; without emotion, sluggish, opp. of erethism.*

apectomy (a-pek'to-mĭ) [L. *apex*, tip, + G. *ektomē*, incision]. Eradication of apex of a tooth root. SYN: *apicoectomy.*

ape-hand [A. S. *apa*, ape, + *hand*, hand]. Nerve lesion in which the thumb remains at right angle from hand.

apeidosis (ap-e-i-do'sis) [G. *apo*, away, + *eidos*, form]. Slow disappearance of characteristic form in a disease.

apella (ap·el'ă) [G. *a-*, priv. + L. *pellis*, skin]. 1. A circumcised male. 2. One with a short prepuce.

apellous (ă-pel'us) [G. *a-*, priv. + L. *pellis*, skin]. 1. Without skin. 2. Circumcised.

apenteric (ap-en-ter'ik) [G. *apo*, from, + *enteron*, intestine]. Away from the bowels.

apep'sia [G. *a-*, priv. + *pepsis*, a digesting]. 1. Absence of pepsin in the gastric juice. 2. Imperfect digestion or its cessation.

apepsin'ia. Absence of pepsin in the gastric juice.

apeptous (ă-pep'tus) [G. *a-*, priv. + *peptein*, to digest]. 1. Indigestible; crude. 2. Aeptic.

ape'rient [L. *aperire*, to open]. A very mild purgative, particularly applied to mild purgative waters. Ex: *honey, potassium bitartrate, magnesium oxide.*

NP: Usually given at night on an empty stomach if the drug acts slowly (10 to 12 hours). Saline a. and those having rapid action are given first thing in morning on an empty stomach, half-hour before first drink.

Strong purgatives (castor oil, colocynth, etc.) act in 4 to 6 hours.

Hydragogues (salines and jalap) within 2 hours.

Aperients should not be given in suspected appendicitis, in colic as a rule, in enteritis if diarrhea and vomiting are present.

aperistal'sis [G. *a-*, priv. + *peri*, around, + *stalsis*, constriction]. Absence of peristalsis.

aper'itive [L. *aperire*, to open]. 1. An appetizer. 2. Mild purgative. SYN: *aperient, q.v.*

apertura (ap-er-tu'ră) [L. *apertura*, opening]. An opening.

aperture (ap'er-chure). An orifice or opening.

a'pex (pl. *apices*) [L. *apex*, tip]. The summit or extremity of anything.

a. beat. The point of maximum impulse of the heart against the chest wall felt in the 5th left intercostal space, 3½ inches from middle of sternum about an inch within a line drawn from middle of clavicle parallel with sternum (the mammary line).

Generally may be detected by inspection or palpation; when these fail may be localized by auscultation. In recumbent position apex beat may be elevated an inch or more. When body is inclined to left, beat may be detected in mammary line or even some distance outside. During forced inspiration may become imperceptible or be found below its usual place. During forced expiration, beat becomes more forcible and position elevated. Patient as a rule should be examined in erect or sitting posture, while breathing quietly.

A weak apex beat may be noted: 1. In healthy people. 2. Degeneration or dilatation of the heart. 3. Pericardial effusion. 4. Emphysema. 5. Shock or collapse.

CHANGES IN FORCE AND EXTENT OF: May be increased by: 1. Hypertrophy of heart. 2. Excited action of heart from drugs, reflex irritation, excitement or disease, as exophthalmic goiter. 3. Shrinking of the lungs, as in phthisis.

apex murmur — aphthongia

DISPLACEMENT TO THE LEFT: May result from: 1. Hypertrophy and dilatation of the heart (down and to the left). 2. Pericardial effusion (up and to left). 3. Chronic diseases of left lung and pleura, associated with retraction—as fibroid phthisis and pleural adhesions. 4. Abdominal tumors and effusions (up and to left). 5. The pressure of a pleural effusion on the right side (up and to left).

DISPLACEMENT TO RIGHT: May be caused by: 1. Chronic disease of the right lung or pleura, associated with retraction. 2. Pressure of a pleural effusion on left side.

DISPLACEMENT DOWNWARD: May result from: 1. Hypertrophy and dilatation of heart, chiefly the left ventricle. 2. Pressure of solid growths in upper mediastinum. 3. Aneurysm of aortic arch. 4. Enlargement of liver, causing traction through central tendon of diaphragm. Deformity of chest may cause displacement in any direction.

PRECORDIAL PROMINENCE: May result from: 1. Deformity. 2. Enlargement of heart. 3. Pericardial effusions.

a. murmur. One over the apex of the heart.

a. root. The end of the root of a tooth.

apex'ograph [" + G. *graphein*, to write]. An instrument for determining apex of a tooth root.

A. P. H. A. 1. Abbr. *American Public Health Association.* 2. *American Protestant Hospital Association.*

aphacia (a-fa'sĭ-ă) [G. *a-*, priv. + *phakos*, lentil]. Lack of eye lens.

apha'cic. Pert. to aphacia.

aphagia (a-fa'jĭ-ă) [G. *a-*, priv. + *phagein*, to eat]. Inability to swallow.

aphakia (a-fa'kĭ-ă) [G. *a-*, priv. + *phakos*, lentil]. Absence of eye's crystalline lens. SYN: *aphacia.*

apha'kik. Pert. to aphakia.

aphasia (a-fa'zĭ-ă) [" + *phasis*, speaking]. Inability to express oneself properly through speech, or loss of verbal comprehension.

It is complete or total when both sensory and motor areas are involved. SYN: *loganosia.*

RS: *Agraphia, alalia, anarthria, aphemia, atactic, mind blindness, mind deafness, motor, paraphasia, word blindness.*

a., amnesic. Loss of memory for words.

a., ataxic. Inability to articulate. Similar to *a., motor.*

a., auditory. A. due to pathology of center of hearing.

a. conduction. ETIOL: Due to lesion of conduction path bet. motor and speech centers.

a. gibberish. Utterance of meaningless phrases.

a., motor. Patient knows what he wants to say but cannot say it. Muscles coördinating speech unable to coordinate. May be complete or partial. Broca's area is disordered or diseased.

a., optic. Inability to call name of an object recognized by sight without the aid of sound, taste, or touch; a form of *agnosia.**

a., sensory. Inability to understand spoken words, if word center is involved (auditory a.) or the written word if visual word center is affected (visual a.). If both centers are involved, will not understand spoken or written word.

a., traumatic. A. caused by head injury.

apha'sic, apha'siac. Pert. to aphasia.

aphelotic (af-el-ot'ĭk) [*aphelkein*, to draw away]. Absent minded; given to reverie.

aphelxia (af-elks'ĭ-ă). Absent minded; oblivious of external conditions.

aphemesthesia (ă-fem-es-the'zĭ-ă) [G. *a-*, priv. + *phēmē*, speech, + *aisthesis*, sensation]. Word deafness, or word blindness.

aphemia (a-fe'mĭ-ă) [" + *phēmē*, speech]. Loss of speech due to impairment of the word memory center; amnesic aphasia.* SEE: *alexia, amnesia, anarthria.*

aphephobia (af-e-fo'bĭ-ă) [G. *aphē*, touch, + *phobos*, fear]. Abnormal aversion to being touched by anyone.

aphlogistic (ă-flo-jist'ĭk) [G. *a-*, priv. + *phlogistos*, inflammable]. 1. Not inflammable. 2. Burning without flame.

aphonia (a-fon'ĭ-ă) [" + *phōnē*, voice]. Loss of voice with intact inner speech and not due to central lesion. May occur in chronic laryngitis.

ETIOL: Disease of vocal cords, paralysis of laryngeal nerves, pressure on recurrent laryngeal nerve, or it may be functional due to hysteria or psychiatric causes.

a. clericorum. Clergyman's sore throat.

a. paranoica. The silence of the insane.

aphoresis (ă-for-e'sĭs) [" + *phorēsis*, being transmitted]. 1. Lack of endurance, esp. of pain. 2. Any separation of a part.

aphoria (ă-fo'rĭ-ă) [" + *phoros*, carrier]. Sterility in the female.

aphose (ă'fōz) [" + *phōs*, light]. A subjective perception of darkness, or of a shadow.

aphrasia (a-fra'zĭ-ă) [" + *phrasis*, speech]. Morbid refusal to speak; seen in dementia precox, *q.v.*

a., paralytic. Due to paralysis of the faculty of ideation.

a., superstitious. Avoidance of certain words because of scruples or aversion to their use.

aphrenia (a-fre'nĭ-ă) [" + *phrēn*, mind]. An apparent lack of intellect seen in some forms of dementia.

a. apoplexy. Unconsciousness.

aphrenic, aphrenous (ă-fren'ĭk, -'us). Insane.

aphrodisia (af-ro-dis'ĭ-ă) [G. *aphrodisios*, rel. to *Aphrodite*, goddess of love]. Sexual desire, esp. when morbid, or s. congress.

aphrodisiac (af-ro-diz'ĭ-ak). An agent which stimulates sexual desire.

Alcohol is said to inhibit control of sexual impulses but constant use impairs the sexual powers without lessening desire. Theelin obtained from the urine of pregnant females is being tried for frigidity. Ex: *nux vomica, phosphorus, alcohol,* and *cantharides* are usually classed as aphrodisiacs.

aphronesia (ă-fro-ne'sĭ-ă) [G. *a-*, priv. + *phronēsis*, common sense]. 1. Silliness. 2. Dementia.

aphronia (ă-fro'nĭ-ă) [G. *aphrōn*, foolish]. Mental deficiency; defective functional activity of cerebrum.

aphtha (af'thă) (pl. *aphthae*) [G. small ulcer]. 1. Very small ulcer on a mueous membrane of the mouth. 2. Thrush.

aphthenxia (af-thengks'ĭ-ă) [G. *a-*, priv. + *phthegxis*, utterance]. An aphasia with articulate sounds imperfectly expressed.

aphthongia (af-thon'gĭ-ă) [G. *a-*, priv. + *phthoggos*, voice]. Aphasia due to spasm

aphthous   A-73   **aponeurorrhaphy**

of muscles controlled by the hypoglossal nerve.

aphthous (af'thus) [G. *aphtha*, small ulcer]. Pert. to, or characterized by, ulcers.

aphylac'tic [G. *a-*, priv. + *phylaxis*, a protecting]. Having no immune power.

aphylaxis (ă-fĭ-laks'ĭs). Without immunity against disease.

apical [L. *apex*, tip]. Pert. to the apex.

apices (a'pĭs-ez). Pl. of apex.

apiceotomy (ap'is-e-ot'o-mĭ) [L. *apex*, tip, + G. *tomē*, incision]. Eradication of apex of a tooth root. SYN: *apicoectomy*.

apicitis (ap-ĭ-sī'tĭs) [" + G. *-itis*, inflammation]. Inflammation of any apical structure, esp. apex of lung or tooth root.

apicoectomy (ap-ĭ-ko-ek'to-mĭ) [" + G. *ektomē*, incision]. Amputation of apex of a tooth root.

apicoloca'tor [" + *locare*, to place]. Instrument for locating apex of a tooth root. SYN: *apexograph*.

apicolysis (ap-ĭ-kol'ĭs-ĭs) [" + G. *lysis*, solution]. Artificial collapse of the apex of a lung by making an opening through the anterior chest wall.

NP: Keep patient on affected side and watch for shock and hemorrhage.

apicotomy (ap-ĭ-kot'o-mĭ) [" + G. *tomē*, incision]. Removal of apex of a tooth root. SYN: *apicoectomy*.

apiectomy (ap-ĭ-ek'to-mĭ) [" + G. *ektomē*, incision]. Eradication of apex of a tooth root. SYN: *apicoectomy*.

apinealism (ă-pĭn'e-al-ĭzm) [G. *a-*, priv. + G. *pineus*, pert. to pine, + *ismos*, condition of]. Syndrome due to absence of pineal gland.

ap'inoid [" + *pinos*, filth, + *eidos*, appearance]. Free from dirt; clean.

   a. cancer. Hard cancer.

apiphobia (ă-pĭ-fo'bĭ-ă) [L. *apis*, bee, + G. *phobos*, fear]. Abnormal fear of bees or of insects which buzz like a bee.

apisination (ap-ĭs-ĭn-a'shun) [L. *apis*, bee]. Poisoning from bee stings.

apituitarism (ă-pĭt-u'ĭt-ar-ĭzm) [G. *a-*, priv. + L. *pituita*, phlegm, + *ismos*, condition of]. Condition due to total abeyance of function or removal of pituitary body. Leads to cachexia thyreopriva.*

aplanat'ic lens [" + *planētos*, wandering]. Free from spherical or chromatic aberration. Not wandering.

aplasia (a-pla'zĭ-ă) [" + *plasis*, a developing]. Failure of an organ or part of the body to develop naturally.

aplas'tic [" + *plastikos*, shaped]. Having deficient or arrested development.

apnea (ap-ne'a) [" + *pnoē*, breath]. 1. Temporary absence of respiration following a period of overbreathing or overabundance of oxygen and a decrease of carbon dioxide, a feature of some types of dyspnea.* 2. Asphyxia. 3. Temporary cessation of breathing seen in the Cheyne-Stokes breathing, named after the first two physicians who noticed this type of breathing.

It is a serious symptom esp. in such conditions as arteriosclerosis, meningitis, coma, heart and kidney diseases, and also following an injury to the brain where concussion results. Sometimes this type of breathing is noticed in perfectly healthy children and in the aged during profound sleep.

SYM: It is characterized by a gradual increase in the rate until it ends in a gasp followed by a gradual decrease until the respiration ceases, then it begins again. Another form is sometimes noticed when the respirations gradually increase in force and frequency and then suddenly cease.

apneumato'sis [G. *a-*, priv. + *pneumatoein*, to inflate, + *ōsis*, denoting increase]. Noninflation of air cells.

apo- (ap'o) [G. *apo*, from]. Gr. prefix: From, away, separation, as *apophysis*.

ap'ocain. Local anesthetic, mildly toxic, employed for surface anesthesia and infiltration. SYN: *tutocain*.

apocamnosis (ap-o-kam-no'sis) [G. *apokamnein*, to grow weary]. Weariness, easily induced fatigue.

apocenosis (ap-o-sen-o'sis) [G. *apokenoein*, to drain]. 1. Increased flow of blood or body fluids. 2. Partial evacuation.

apochromat'ic [" + G. *chrōmatikos*, colored]. Without color. SYN: *achromatic*.

apocope (ă-pok'o-pe) [G. *apokopē*, a cutting off]. Amputation.

apocopous (a-pok'o-pus) [G. *apokopos*, cut off]. Castrated.

apocoptic (ap-o-kop'tĭc) [G. *apokoptein*, to cut off]. The effect resulting from the removal of a part.

apocrine (ap'o-krĭn) [G. *apo*, from, + *krinein*, to separate]. Pert. to cells which lose part of their cytoplasm while functioning.

apocrustic (ap-o-krus'tĭk) [G. *apokroustikos*, able to ward off]. 1. Astringent. 2. Repellent. 3. Defensive.

apodemialgia (ap-o-de-mĭ-al'gĭ-ă) [G. *apodemia*, away from home, + *algos*, pain]. 1. An abnormal desire to wander from one's abode or environment; wanderlust. 2. Morbid dislike of a home.

apogee (ap'o-gē) [G. *apo*, from, + *gē*, earth]. Highest stage of a disease.

apokamnosis (ap''o-kam-no'sĭs) [G. *apokamnein*, to grow weary, + *osis*, denoting increase]. Abnormal tendency to fatigue, as in neurasthenia.

apolarthron (ap-o-lar'thrŏn). A natural fish liver oil, of great concentration, each capsule containing 25,000 USP units of Vitamin D, and 30,000 units of Vitamin A.

   DOSAGE: From 2 to not more than 6 capsules per day.

   USES: In any condition where large doses of these vitamins would be indicated, as in arthritis.

apolepsis (ap-o-lep'sĭs) [G. *apolepsis*, a leaving off]. 1. Cessation of a function. 2. Retention or suppression of an excretion or secretion.

apolexis (ap-o-leks'ĭs) [G. *apolexis*, a declining]. 1. The catabolic condition or process. 2. Decline of life.

apomorphine (ap-o-mor'fēn). A morphine derivative prepared from the alkaloid by extraction of one molecule of water.

   a. hydrochloride. A grayish white powder; should not be used if it at once imparts a greenish color when dissolved in 100 parts distilled water.

   ACTION AND USES: Emetic; sometimes valuable in cases of poisoning when stomach pump cannot be employed.

   DOSAGE: 1/12 gr. (0.005 Gm.) *hypodermically*; as *expectorant*, 1/60 gr. (0.001 Gm.).

apomyelin (ap-o-mi'el-ĭn) [G. *apo*, from, + *myelos*, marrow]. A brain substance containing no glycerol.

apone (a'pŏn) [G. *a-*, priv. + *ponos*, pain]. An anodyne.

ap''oneurol'ogy [" + *logos*, word]. The science of aponeuroses.

ap''oneuror'rhaphy [" + *raphē*, suture]. Aponeurotic suture.

aponeurosis (ap-o-nu-ro′sis) [G. *apo*, from, + *neuron*, sinew]. Extension of connective tissue beyond a muscle in round or flattened tendons, or expanded sheets for the attachment of muscular fibers, or means of insertion or origin of a flat muscle, or as a fascia for other muscles.
RS: *aponeurology, aponeurositis, aponeurotic, apophyseal, imbricate, imbrication.*

aponeurositis (ap-on-ū-ro-si′tis) [" + *itis*, inflammation]. Aponeurotic inflammation. [neurosis.

aponeurot′ic. Pert. to, or rel. to, an apo-

aponeurotome (ap-on-ū′ro-tōm) [G. *apo*, from, + *neuron*, sinew, + *tomē*, cutting]. Knife for dividing an aponeurosis.

aponeurotomy (ap-on-u-rot′om-ĭ). Surgical cutting of an aponeurosis.

aponia (a-pon′ĭ-ă) [G. *a-*, priv. + *ponos*, pain]. 1. Abstaining from labor. 2. Absence of pain.

aponic (ap-on′ĭk). Rel. to aponia.

aponoia, aponoea (a-pon-oy′ă, ă-pon-e′ă) [G. *apo*, from, + *nous*, mind]. Amentia.

apophlegmatic (ap-o-fleg-mat′ĭk) [" + *phlegmatikos*, abounding in mucus]. Producing a mucous discharge; expectorant.

apophyseal (ap-o-fiz′e-al) [" + *physis*, growth]. Rel. or pert. to an apophysis.

apoph′ysis. 1. A projection esp. from a bone, an outgrowth without an independent center of ossification.
a. cerebri. The pineal body.
a. of Ingrassias. Smaller wing of sphenoid bone.
a. lenticularis. Temporal bone's orbicular process.
a. of Rau. Long process of malleus.
a. raviana. Gracile process of malleus.

apophysitis (a-pof-ĭ-si′tis) [G. *apo*, from, + *physis*, growth, + *itis*, inflammation]. Inflammation of a bony process which has never been entirely separated from the bone of which it forms a part.

apoplasmia (ap-o-plaz′mĭ-ă) [" + *plasma*, formation]. Deficiency of blood plasma.

apoplectic (ap-o-plek′tĭk) [G. *apoplēktikos*, crippled by stroke]. Pert. to apoplexy.

apoplec′tiform [G. *apoplexia*, stroke, + L. *forma*, appearance]. Like apoplexy.

apoplectig′enous [" + *genos*, origin]. Causing apoplexy.

apoplec′toid [" + *eidos*, form]. Like apoplexy. SYN: *apoplectiform.*

apoplexy (ăp′ō-plĕk-sĭ) [G. *apoplēxia*, a stroke]. 1. Sudden diminution of, or loss of, consciousness and paralysis, due to hemorrhage into brain or spinal cord, or formation of an embolus or thrombus, which occludes an artery. SYN: *stroke.**
2. Condition of an organ marked by a hemorrhage into its substance, as apoplexy of the lung.
SYM: Onset acute. Unconsciousness. Stertorous breathing due to paralysis of portion of the soft palate; expiration puffs out the cheeks and mouth. Pupils sometimes unequal, the larger one being on the side of the hemorrhage. Paralysis usually involves one side of the face, arm and leg of one side, with eyeballs turned away from the side of the body-paralysis, unequal pupils, skin covered with clammy sweat, the surface temperature of which is often subnormal; speech disturbances, onset more gradual if due to a *thrombosis.**
PROG: Depends upon symptoms. Often grave.

NP: As patient recovering from unconsciousness has admitted hearing all that was said in the room, care should be exercised about talking in presence of patient. Complete quiet. Guard against self-inflicted injuries to nonparalyzed side from movements due to irritation. Supine position: Head and body on same plane. Avoid pressure sores by moving patient frequently. Ease breathing by change of position once an hour, turning from paralyzed side to back and reverse. To lie on paralyzed side may require much effort to breathe. Turn body as a whole, not in part, flexing a paralyzed arm across chest, lower extremities flexed. Frequent cleansing of oropharyngeal passages.
External heat if pulse is weak, skin clammy, and temperature lowered. Ice bag if congestion is present, high tension pulse and duskiness of head and face. Avoid blistering or burns by not allowing container to come in contact with surface. Guard against sacral bed sores (not due to pressure; a cutaneous indication of lowered vitality). This is indicated by redness of skin which may be followed by superficial blisters, resulting in a gangrenous ulcer. Constant asepsis and antisepsis if break occurs in skin. Binders to hold dressings; no adhesive plasters.
Use catheter to avoid bed-wetting; enemata instead of purgatives. Avoid pressure of bed clothes by using a bed cradle. Watch for contractures of muscles and avoid by change of position.
Convalescence: Liquid or soft foods; solid ones as patient begins to masticate. Slight elevation of head when feeding which should be done from the paralyzed side unless patient exhibits imperfect sight, when position should be reversed to accommodate.
Feed slowly to avoid stoppage of windpipe. Loss of muscular power of pharynx, of tongue and cheeks must be considered. Frequent bathing; emollients or cocoa butter applied afterward. Watch for danger from heat or cold if loss of sensation is manifested in any part. Systematic massage. No strenuous rubbing. Passive exercises until active movements are possible.
Hemiplegic or chronic state: Careful training of muscles and organs of speech is necessary, later followed perhaps by occupational therapy. Confidence must be inspired, memory trained and emotions controlled by patient. Nurse should teach patient how to sit and how to stand and walk.
F. A. TREATMENT: Keep patient quiet and sitting up or lying down with head and shoulders elevated. Do not give stimulants. Apply cooling applications to head and neck. Do not transport unless absolutely imperative—and then very carefully.
RS: *Aaron's sign, antiapoplectic, aphronia, apoplectic, apoplectiform, apoplectigenous, cataptosis, coma, hemiplegia, ictus.*

apopsychia (ap-op-sik′ĭ-ă) [G. *apo*, away, + *psychē*, mind]. Fainting; syncope.

apoptosis (ap-op-to′sis) [" + *ptōsis*, a falling]. Falling off or out, as a scab or hair.

aporioneurosis (ap-or-ĭ-o-nu-ro′sis) [G. *aporia*, doubt, + *neuron*, nerve, + *osis*, increased]. Anxiety neurosis.

aporrhegma (ap-o-reg′mă) [G. *apo*, away, + *rēgma*, separation]. 1. A biological separation of one substance from another. 2. Any nitrogen-containing substance formed by the removal of carbon dioxide from protein-derivatives, as when histamine, $C_3H_9N_2(CH_2)_2NH_2$, is formed by putrefaction from histidine, $C_3H_3N_2CH_2CH(NH_2)COOH$.

aporrhinosis (ap-or-in-o′sis) [" + *ris*, nose, + *osis*, increased]. Nasal discharge.

aporrhipsis (ap-or-ip′sis) [" + *riptein*, to throw]. Removal of clothing or bed clothes; seen in some psychotic conditions or in delirium.

aposia (a-po′zĭ-ă) [G. *a*-, priv. + *posis*, drink]. Absence of thirst.

apositia (ap-o-sit′ĭ-ă) [G. *apo*, away, + *sitos*, food]. Anorexia* associated with disgust for food.

apos′pory [" + *sporos*, seed]. Absence of spore-producing ability.

apostasis (ap-os′tă-sis) [G. *apostasis*, departure from]. 1. The crisis or end of a disease. Termination by crisis. 2. An abscess. 3. An exfoliation.

apostaxis (ap-o-staks′ĭs) [G. *apo*, from, + *stazein*, to drop]. 1. Epistaxis. 2. Discharge by drops.

apostem (ap′o-stem) [G. *apostēma*, abscess]. An abscess.

apostema (ap-os-te′mă). An abscess.

aposthia (ah-pos′thĭ-ă) [G. *a*-, priv. + *posthē*, foreskin]. Congenital absence of the prepuce.

apothanasia (ă-poth-ă-na′zĭ-ă) [G. *apo*, away, + *thanatos*, death]. Prolongation of life.

apoth′ecaries′ meas′ure. A system of measuring drugs in English speaking countries rapidly being displaced by the metric system, *q.v.*

The scruple and the pound are now seldom used. A portion of a grain is expressed fractionally, as gr. ½, not decimally. The quantity is written in Roman numerals, *q.v.*, with the symbol before it, as gr. v.

Weight

20 grains (gr.)	= 1 scruple (℈)
60 grains (gr.) (3 ℈)	= 1 dram (ʒ)
8 drams (ʒ)	= 1 ounce (ʒ)
12 oz. (ʒ) (5760 gr.)	= 1 pound (lb.)

Volume

60 minims	(♏) = 1 fluidram	(f ʒ)
8 fluidrams	(f ʒ) = 1 fluidounce	(f ʒ)
16 fluidounces	(f ʒ) = 1 pint	(pt.)
2 pints	(pt.) = 1 quart	(qt.)
4 quarts	(qt.) = 1 gallon	(C)

Some points to remember are: The character ʒ represents 60 grains, while f ʒ represents 60 minims. ʒ represents 480 grains only, while f ʒ is necessary to express 480 minims. A minim is not the equivalent of a grain. 480 minims (1 f ʒ) of water weighed at the standard temperature weigh 456.37 grains. This should be remembered for percentage solutions. Specific gravities of liquids vary; a pint of a liquid is not necessarily a pound.

apoth′ecary [G. *apothēkē*, storing place]. A druggist or pharmacist. In England and Ireland one licensed by the Society of Apothecaries as an authorized physician and dispenser of drugs.

ap′othem, ap′otheme [G. *apo*, away, + *thema*, deposit]. The brown precipitate which appears when vegetable decoctions or infusions are exposed to the air, or are boiled a long time.

apothesine (ap-oth′es-in). A local anesthetic of the procaine type (in that it is relatively ineffective when applied to the mucous membrane), but slower in action than procaine. Its toxicity is about equal to that of cocaine, but twice that of procaine.
DOSAGE: 0.08 Gm. (1½ grains).

apothesis (ap-oth′es-is) [G. *apothesis*, a placing back]. Reduction of a fracture or dislocation.

apotheter (a-poth′e-ter) [G. *apothetein*, to stow away]. Navel string repositor.

apotox′in [G. *apo*, away, + *toxikon*, poison]. The anaphylactic substance due to action of toxogenin on injected toxin.

apotrip′sis [G. *apotribein*, to abrade]. Removal of opacity in cornea.

apozem(e (ap′o-zēm) [G. *apo*, away, + *zein*, to boil]. A decoction.

appara′tus [L. *apparare*, to prepare]. 1. A number of parts acting together in the performance of some special function. 2. A mechanical appliance or appliances, used in operations and experiments.

  a., acoustic. Auditory apparatus, the assemblage of parts essential for hearing.

  a., Clover's. A device used in administering ether or chloroform.

  a., Desault's. Desault's bandage.

  a., Fell-O'Dwyer's. An instrument for performing artificial respiration, and for preventing collapse of the lung in chest operations.

  a. ligamentosus colli. The occipito-axoid ligament.

  a. major. Median lithotomy.

  a. minor. Lateral lithotomy.

  a., sound conducting. Those parts of the acoustic apparatus that transmit sound.

  a., sound perceiving. Those central parts of the acoustic apparatus that are essential for the perception of sounds.

  a., vocal. The various organs collectively that subserve phonation.

appendal′gia [L. *appendere*, hang to, + G. *algos*, pain]. Pain in lower right quadrant in region of vermiform appendix.

appendectomy (ap-en-dek′to-mĭ) [L. *ad*, to, + *pendere*, hang, + G. *ektome*, cut out]. Surgical removal of the vermiform appendix.

appen′dical, appendi′ceal. Pert. to an appendix.

  a. reflex. Tenderness at McBurney's point accompanied by rigidity considered a reflex expression by way of sympathetic cerebrospinal arc.

appendicectasis (ap-pen-dis-ek′tă-sis) [L. *appendere*, hang to, + G. *ektasis*, a stretching]. Appendical dilatation.

appendicectomy (ap-en-dis-ek′to-mĭ) [" + G. *ektomē*, a cutting]. Surgical removal of the appendix.

appendices (ap-pen′dĭ-sēz). Plural of appendix.

  a. epiploicae. Pouches of peritoneum, filled with fat and attached to the colon.

appendicial (ap-pen-dis′ĭ-al). Pert. to the appendix. SYN: *appendical*.

appendicitis (ap-pen-di-si′tis) [L. *appendere*, hang to, + G. -*itis*, inflammation]. Inflammation of the vermiform appendix.

It generally occurs between the ages of five and twenty, very rarely before the fifth year or after the fiftieth. It is more common in male adults than in female adults. The disease may be acute, subacute, or chronic.

  a., acute. SYM: (a) Abdominal pain, usually severe and generally throughout the abdomen followed by (b) nausea and vomiting, (c) localization of pain in the right lower quadrant of abdomen

appendicitis, chronic   A-76   **apricot**

with tenderness and rigidity over right rectus muscle or McBurney's point, (d) fever usually rising within several hours, 99° F. to 101° F., (e) pulse increasing with temperature, (f) patient lying on back with right lower extremity frequently flexed to relieve muscle tension, (g) leukocytosis present shortly after onset; (h) in mild cases symptoms begin to subside on the second day, but in more severe cases there may be a cessation of pain indicating that the appendix has ruptured. After a few hours a well defined abscess may be felt in the right iliocecal region showing that nature has walled off the affected area.

TREATMENT: (1) Notify physician as soon as symptoms do not subside. (2) Refrain from giving foods, liquids, cathartics, enemas, and from applying heat. (3) Surgery within 24 hours of onset is safest procedure.

   a., chronic. May follow an acute attack leaving a cicatricial narrowing of the lumen of the appendix, or adhesions. SYM: Gastric indigestion, frequently simulating a gastric ulcer, duodenal ulcer, or gallbladder disease. Tenderness manifested in the right lower abdomen. TREATMENT: Surgical.

   a. obliterans, a., protective. A. with adhesions closing the appendical cavity.

appendico-enterostomy (ap-pen-dik-o-enter-os'to-mĭ) [" + G. *enteron*, intestine, + *stoma*, mouth]. 1. Appendicotomy. 2. The establishment of an anastomosis bet. appendix and intestine.

appendicolithi'asis [" + G. *lithos*, stone]. Formation of calculi in the vermiform appendix.

appendicolysis (ap-pen-dĭ-kol'ĭ-sis) [" + G. *lysis*, a loosening]. Operation which frees appendix from adhesions by a slit in the serosa at its base.

appendicopathy (ap-pen-di-ko'path-ĭ) [" + G. *pathos*, disease]. Any disease of the vermiform appendix.

   a. oxyurica. Lesion of the appendical mucosa supposedly due to oxyurids.*

appendico'sis [" + G. -*osis*, increased]. Noninflammatory state of the appendix. SYM: Dull pain, local soreness, afebrile, but continual discomfort.

appendicostomy (ap-pen-dik-os'to-mĭ) [" + G. *stoma*, mouth]. Operation for irrigating cecum and colon.

appendic'ular. 1. Appendical. 2. Pert. to limbs or that appended to another part.

appen'dix [L.]. An appendage.

   a., auricular. A forward prolongation of the heart-auricle.

   a., ensiform. The third or lowest portion of the sternum.

   a., gangrenous. When inflammation is extreme, blood vessels are blocked in the mesentery, circulation to appendix cut off, and diffuse peritonitis ensues.

   a. vermiformis (*a., vermiform* or *processus vermiformis*). A worm-shaped process projecting from the cecum, whose mucous membrane also lines the appendix, which contains many solitary glands. Its average length is 7.5 cm., and its position is variable. It secretes 1 to 2 cc. of fluid per day.

   SEE: Aaron's sign, appendalgia, "*appendi-*" words, *vermiform*, *voracious*.

appen'dotome [L. *appendere*, hang to, + G. *tomē*, a cutting]. An instrument for excision of appendix.

apperception (ap-per-sep'shun) [L. *ad*, to, + *percipere*, to receive]. The mental process whereby new knowledge is organized and interpreted in the light of past knowledge and experiences.

appercep'tive. Pert. to apperception.

ap'petence(y [L. *appetere*, to strive for]. An appetite or desire.

ap'petite [L. *appetitus*, longing for]. Desire, esp. for food; not necessarily hunger.

   a. juice. Gastric secretion brought about by psychic causes such as sight or odor of food, and by tasting and chewing. It ceases 15 to 20 minutes after mastication is completed.

appetite, words pert. to: Acoria, anorectic, anorectous, anorexia, apositia, appetence(y, appetizer, asitia, avulsion, bulimia, canine a., dysorexia, emesis, hiccup, hyperorexia, malacia, narcomania, nausea, parageusia, parorexia, phagomania, pica, polyphagia, pyrosis, regurgitation, rumination, satiety, taste.

appetition (ăp-pĕ-tĭsh'ŭn) [L. *ad*, toward, + *pe'tere*, to seek]. Desire for some object.

appeti'zer. That which promotes appetite.

applanatio (ap-plan-a'shĭ-o) [L.]. A flattening, as the corneal surface.

   a. cornea. Flattened cornea.

apple (ap'l) [A. S. *aeppel*]. Most widely used of fleshy, many celled fruits having a core from the pome family.

   DRIED: Average serving 60 grams. Pro. 1.0, Fat 1.3, Carbo. 39.7, Ca. 0.032, Mg. 0.037, K. 0.623, Na. 0.050, P. 0.048, Cl. 0.025, Fe. 0.0015. Contains Vitamin A.

   FRESH: Average serving 130 grams. Pro. 0.5, Fat 0.7, Carbo. 16.9, Ca. 0.007, Mg. 0.008, K. 0.127, Na. 0.011, P. 0.012, Cl. 0.005, S. 0.006, Fe. 0.0003. Contains Vitamin A. Good source Vitamins B, C, and G.

ap'ple-head [" + *heăfod*, head]. Dwarf's broad, thick skull.

applicator (ăp'lĭ-kā-tĕr) [L. *applicāre*, to attach]. Device, usually a slender rod of glass or wood, used with a pledget of cotton on the end, to apply medicine to the nose, throat, uterus, or any other body cavity.

apposi'tion [L. *ad*, to, + *ponere*, to place]. 1. Development by accretion. 2. Addition of parts. 3. Fitting together, as the edges of two surfaces.

approximal (ap-proks'im-ăl) [L. *ad*, to, + *proximus*, nearest]. Contiguous; next to.

approximate (ă-proks'ĭm-āt) [L. *ad*, toward, + *proximus*, nearest]. To bring a part toward another, as when bringing the fingers together or an arm toward the body.

apraxia (a-praks'ĭ-ă) [G. *apraxia*, inaction]. 1. Inability to perform certain purposive movements without loss of motor power, sensation, or coördination. 2. Ridiculous and out of the ordinary acts performed by the insane. Inability to understand the meaning of things.

   a. algera. Induction of severe headache by a hysterical attack, thus preventing motion.

   a., ideational. Misuse of objects due to failure to identify them.

   a., motor. Inability to willfully perform acts.

aprication (ap-rĭ-ka'shun) [L. *apricare*, expose to sun]. 1. Sunstroke. 2. Sunbath. Basking in the sun.

apricot (ā'prĭ-kot) [L. *praecoquum*, early ripe]. Fruit resembling small peach in appearance.

   DRIED: Average serving 25 grams. Pro. 1.2, Fat 0.3, Carbo. 15.7, Ca. 0.066, Mg. 0.047, K. 1.157, Na. 1.177, P. 0.117, Cl.

aproctia   A-77   **aqueous chamber**

0.009, Fe. 0.0014. Good source Vitamin A.
FRESH: Average serving 50 grams. Pro. 0.6, Carbø. 6.7, Ca. 0.014, Mg. 0.010, K. 0.248, Na. 0.038, P. 0.025, Cl. 0.002, S. 0.010, Fe. 0.0003. Good source Vitamins A, C, and G.

aproctia (ă-prok'shĭ-ă) [G. *a-*, priv. + *prōktos*, anus]. Imperforation or absence of anus.

aproctous (ă-prok'tus). Having an imperforate anus.

a'pron [O. F. *naperon*, cloth]. Garment to cover front of the body, for protection of clothing during surgical operations, etc.

    a., Hottentot. Hypertrophy of labia minora.

aprosex'ia [G. *aprosexia*, want of attention]. Unintentional inattention, esp. from defective hearing, sight, or mental weakness. Inability to concentrate on anything.

apselaphesia (ap-sel-af-e'zĭ-ă) [G. *a-*, priv. + *pselaphēsis*, feeling]. Absence of tactile sense.

apsithyria, apsithurea (ăp-sith-ĭ'rĭ-ă, -u'-re-ă) [" + *psithyrizein*, to whisper]. Hysterical loss of voice with inability to whisper.

apsychia (ăp-si'kĭ-ă) [" + *psychē*, mind]. Unconsciousness; a faint.

apsychosis (ăp-si-ko'sis) [" + " + *-ōsis*, increased]. Inability to think.

aptyalia, aptyalism (ap-ti-ā'lĭ-ă, -ti'al-izm) [" + *ptyalon*, saliva]. 1. Absence or deficiency of saliva. 2. A condition due to excessive expectoration through loss of oxydases.

apulosis (ap-u-lo'sis) [G. *oulein*, to cicatrize]. A cicatrix.

apyetous (ă-pi'et-us) [G. *a-*, priv. + *pyēsis*, suppuration]. Nonsuppurative, nonpurulent.

apyknomorphous (ă-pik"no-mor'fus) [" + *pyknos*, thick, + *morphē*, form]. Pert. to a cell which stains lightly as its stainable material is scattered.

apyogenous (ă-pi-oj'en-us) [" + *pyon*, pus, + *genos*, origin]. Not due to pus.

apyous (ă-pi'us). Without pus.

apyretic (ă-pi-ret'ik) [G. *a-*, priv. + *pyretos*, fever]. Without fever. SYN: *afebrile.*

apyrexia (ă-pi-reks'ĭ-ă) [" + *pyrexis*, feverishness]. 1. Absence of or intermission of fever. 2. Nonfebrile period of an intermittent fever.

apyrogenetic, apyrogenic (a-pi-ro-jĕ-net'-ĭk, -jen'ĭk) [" + " + *genos*, origin]. Not causing fever.

aqua (ak'wă) (*pl. aquae*) [L. *aqua*, water]. Water.

    a. ammoniae. Water charged with ammonia and stimulants.

    a. chlori. Water charged with chlorine for antisepsis and cleaning.

    a. communis. Faucet water.

    a. destillata. A water obtained by distillation.

    a. fortis. Nitric acid.

    a. labyrinthi. The fluid in the labyrinth of the ear.

    a., medicated (water). An aqueous solution of a volatile substance. Usually contains only a comparatively small percentage of the active drug. Many of them are merely water saturated with a volatile oil. They are used more as vehicles and to give odor and taste to solutions. There are 14 official waters.

    a. menthae piperitae. Peppermint water.

    a. oculi. The fluid (aqueous humor) of the eye.

    a. pura. Purified water.

    a. re'gia. Nitrohydrochloric acid, nitromuriatic acid, *q.v.*, for F. A. Treatment.

    a. rosae. Rosewater, used mainly as a flavor.

    a. sedativa. Sedative lotion containing ammonia water and spirit of camphor.

    a. vitae. Brandy.

aquacapsuli'tis [" + *capsula*, a small box, + G. *-itis*, inflammation]. Serous iritis. SYN: *aquocapsulitis.*

aquaeductus (ak-we-duk'tus) [" + *ductus*, duct]. A channel or canal to convey fluids.

    a. cerebri. Canal lined with ciliated epithelium and going from the third ventricle through the mesencephalon to the fourth ventricle.

    a. cochleae. Canal connecting subarachnoid space and the perilymphatic space of the cochlea.

    a. Fallopii. Canal for facial nerve in petrous part of temporal bone.

    a. Sylvii. a. cerebri.

aquamedin (ak-wa-med'ĭn). A preparation from the isolation of a hormone from the ant. lobe of the pituitary gland which seems to control the water balance in the tissues as insulin controls the balance of sugar in the body.

In diabetes insipidus in which the water balance of the body is upset, aquamedin should be of inestimable benefit.

aquapuncture (ak'wă-pungh'chur) [L. *aqua*, water, + *punctura*, puncture]. 1. Injection of water hypodermically as a placebo. 2. A fine jet of water sprayed on the skin as a counterirritant.

aqueduct (ak'we-dukt) [" + *ductus*, duct]. Canal or passage. SYN: *aquaeductus.*

    a. vestibuli. Small passage reaching from the vestibule to the post. surface of the temporal bone's petrous section.

aqueous (ăk'wē-ŭs) [L. *aqua*, water]. Of the nature of water; watery.

    a. chamber. Ant. chamber of the eye.

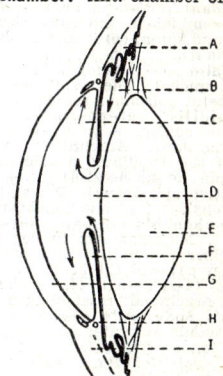

MOVEMENT OF AQUEOUS HUMOR IN THE EYE

Formed by the ciliary body in the posterior chamber, the aqueous humor streams out through the pupil into the anterior chamber and disappears into the sinus venosus sclerae. (Schematic). A, Ciliary body, with ciliary glands; B, posterior chamber; C, anterior chamber; D, pupil; E, lens; F, iris; G, cornea; H, sinus venosus sclerae (canal of Schlemm); I, sclera.

a. humor. Watery liquid, transparent, containing trace of albumin and small amount of salts. Produced by the iris, ciliary body, and cornea. It circulates through the anterior and posterior chambers of the eye and leaves the eye through one of three routes, (a) the posterior route through the zonula, (b) the iris, and (c), the canal of Schlemm. To enter the latter, it passes through the spaces of Fontana to the pectinate villi through which it is filtered.

aquiferous (ak-wif'er-us) [L. *aqua*, water, + *ferre*, to bear]. Carrying water or lymph.

aquocapsuli'tis. Serous iritis.

arabinose (ar'ab-in-ōs). Gum sugar, a pentose, obtained from boiling gum arabic and 0.5 per cent sulfuric acid.

arabinosu'ria [*arabinose* + G. *ouron*, urine]. Arabinose in the urine.

Arachnida (ăr-ăk'nĭ-dă) [G. *arachne*, spider]. A class of the *Arthropoda*, including the spiders, ticks, and mites.

arachnidism (ar-ak'nid-izm) [G. *arachnē*, spider, + *eidos*, form, + *ismos*, condition of]. Systemic poisoning from spider bite.

arachnitis (ar-ak-ni'tis) [" + *itis*, inflammation]. Inflammation of the arachnoid membrane. SYN: *arachnoiditis*, q.v.

arachnodactyly (ar-ak-no-dak'til-I) [" + *dactylos*, finger]. Spider fingers; a state in which fingers and sometimes toes are abnormally long, slender, and curved.

arachnoid (ar-ak'noid) [G. *arachnē*, web, + *eidos*, form]. Resembling a web.

a. cavity. (a) The space between the arachnoid membrane and the dura mater (*cavum subdurale*); (b) the space between the arachnoid membrane and the pia mater (*cavum subarachnoidale* or *subarachnoid space*). The latter contains the cerebrospinal fluid.

a. membrane (*arachnoidea encephali*). The middle (bet. the dura and pia mater) or serous membrane of the brain and spinal cord. SEE: *basiarachnitis*.

arachnoidea (ar-ak-noid'e-ă). A thin, fibrous, middle membrane covering the brain and spinal cord; *a. enceph'ali* and *a. spina'lis.*

arachnoidism (ä-răk-noyd'ĭsm) [G. *arachnē*, spider]. The result produced by the bite of poisonous spiders.

arachnoiditis (ar-ak-noid-i'tis) [G. *arachnē*, spider, + *eidos*, form, + *itis*, inflammation]. Arachnitis; inflammation of the arachnoid membrane.

arachnopia (ar-ak-no'pĭ-ă) [" + L. *pia*, protective membrane]. Pia and arachnoid considered as one membrane.

Aran-Duchenne's disease (ar-ahn-dushens'). Muscular atrophy beginning in the upper extremities and progressing to other parts of the body.

araneous (ă-ra'ne-us) [L. *aranea*, cobweb]. Arachnoid; resembling a cobweb.

Arantius's body, A.'s nodule (ar-an'shĭus). Nodule at center of free border of a semilunar valve leaflet.

A.'s ventricle. Small sac on floor of fourth ventricle.

ar'bor vi'tae [L. *arbor*, tree, + *vita*, life]. ANAT: 1. A tree-like structure; a tree-like outline seen in a section of the cerebellum and the interior fold of the cervix. 2. A series of branching ridges within the cervix of the uterus.

arborescent (ar-bor-es'ent) [L. *arborescere*, to become a tree]. Branching; tree-like.

arborization (ar-bor-i-za'shun) [L. *arbor*, a tree]. Interlacing; ramification; applied to nerve process terminations, fibers and arterioles. SEE: *nerve*.

arc. A curved line; portion of the circumference of a circle.

a. reflex. The path followed by a nerve impulse in a reflex action. The impulse originates in a receptor at the point of stimulation, passes through an afferent neuron or neurons to a reflex center in the brain or spinal cord and from the center out through efferent neurons to the effector organ, a muscle, or gland where the response occurs.

arcade (ar-kād'). Any anatomic structure composed of a series of arches.

a., Flint's. The arteriovenous anastomosis at the base of the pyramid of the kidney. [remedy or nostrum.

arca'num [L. *arcanus*, a secret]. Secret

arcate (ar'kāt) [L. *arcatus*, bow shaped]. Arched, bow shaped.

arch-, archi- [G. *archē*, primitive]. Prefix: First, principal, or chief. Beginning, as *archetype*.

arch, arches [L. *arcus*, a bow]. Any structure or structures of a curved or bow-like outline.

a., abdominothoracic. The lower boundary of the front of the thorax.

a., alveolar. The arch of the alveolar process of either jaw.

a., ant. metatarsal. Formed by the inferior surfaces of the heads of the metatarsal bones of the foot.

a. of the aorta. Proximal curved part of aorta extending to 3rd dorsal v.

a.'s, aortic. 1. Same as arch of the aorta. 2. A series of six pairs of vessels which develop in the embryo. They connect at the truncous arteriosus with the dorsal aortae. During the fifth to seventh weeks, the arches undergo transformation, some persisting as functional vessels, others persisting as rudimentary structures, and some disappearing entirely.

a.'s, branchial. Also called visceral or gill arches. A series of arches which support the gills of fishes. They occur in the human embryo and play an important role in the development of the head and neck. First is the *mandibular*, second, the *hyoid*. The third, fourth and fifth are transitory.

a.'s of Corti. A series of arches made up of the rods of Corti. [ligament.

a., crural. Femoral arch. Poupart's

a., deep crural. A band of fibers arching in front of sheath of femoral vessels.

a., dental. An arch formed by the alveolar process on either jaw, containing teeth and covered by the gums.

a.'s, embryonic. Fetal arches, the aortic, branchial, mandibular, hyoid, pulmonary, and thyrohyoid arches.

a., femoral. Poupart's ligament.

a., hemal. Arch formed by the body and processes of a vertebra, a pair of ribs and the sternum, or other like parts; also the sum of all such arches.

a., hyoid. The second fetal arch which persists in the styloid process, the stylohyoid ligament, and lesser cornu of the hyoid bone.

a., Langer's axillary. A thickened border of fascia forming a bridge across the occipital groove.

a., longitudinal. One of the two anteroposterior arches of the foot; the medial formed by calcaneus, talus, navicular, cuboids, and first three metatarsals; the lateral by the calcaneus, cuboid, and fourth and fifth metatarsals.

a., mandibular. The fetal arch whence

are developed the jawbones, with the malleus and incus.
a., nasal. The arch formed by the nasal bones and by the nasal processes of the superior maxilla.
a., neural. The arch of a vertebra formed by its pedicles and laminae; also the sum of all such arches.
a., palmar. BNA. *arcus volaris.* Deep, an arch formed in the palm by the communicating branch of the ulnar and the radial artery. *Superficial,* an arch in the palm forming the termination of the ulnar artery. [of the fetus.
a.'s, pharyngeal. The branchial arches
a., plantar. BNA. *arcus plantaris.* The arch formed by the external plantar artery and the dorsalis pedis.
a.'s, postaural. The branchial arches.
a., pubic. The portion of the pelvis formed by the rami of the ischia and the ossa pubis on either side.
a., pulmonary. The fifth of the aortic arches on the left side. It becomes the pulmonary artery.
a., stylohyoid. One of the embryonic arches made up of four segments, *viz:* the pharyngobranchial, which develops into the styloid process, the epibranchial, developing into the stylohyoid ligament, the ceratobranchial and hypobranchial which together develop into the lesser cornu of the hyoid bone.
a., supraorbital. A bony arch formed by the prominent margin of the orbit.
a., thyroid. The third fetal arch; its cartilage is represented by the greater cornu of the hyoid bone.
a., transverse. Articulations (metatarsophalangeal) at ball of foot.
a. of a vertebra. The arching portion of a vertebra enclosing the spinal foramen.
a.'s, visceral. The fetal arches.
a., zygomatic. The arch formed by the malar and temporal bones.
archaic type of reaction. An inadequate immature reaction to reality; a reversion to a type once acceptable as normal (*e. g.,* in infancy).
archamphiaster (ark-am'fī-as″ter) [G. *archē,* origin, + *amphi,* around, + *astēr,* star]. Amphiaster formed when polar globules are extruded.
archebiosis (ar-ke-bī-o'sis) [″ + *bios,* life]. Spontaneous generation.
archegenesis (ar-ke-jen'e-sis) [″ + *genesis,* origin]. Generation spontaneously. SYN: *archebiosis.*
archenteron (ark-en'ter-on) [″ + *enteron,* intestine]. Cavity formed by invagination of the blastodermic vesicle.
archeocyte (ar'ke-o-sīt) [G. *archaios,* ancient, + *kytos,* a cell]. A wandering cell.
ar″cheokinet'ic [″ + *kinētikos,* concerning movement]. Pert. to a low and primitive type of motor nerve mechanism as found in the peripheral and ganglionic nervous systems. SEE: *neokinetic, paleokinetic.*
archepyon (ar-ke-pī'on) [G. *archē,* a beginning, + *pyon,* pus]. Unusually thick pus.
ar'chespore, ar″chespo'rium [″ + *spora,* a seed]. Cells giving rise to mother cells of spores.
archetype (ar'ke-tīp) [″ + *typos,* a variety]. Primitive type, from which other forms have developed by differentiation.
archiblast (ar'kĭ-blast) [″ + *blastos,* a germ]. The outer layer which surrounds the germinal vesicle.

archiblas'tic. Derived from, or pert. to, the archiblast.
archiblasto'ma [G. *archē,* origin, + *blastos,* a germ, + *oma,* a tumor]. Tumor of archiblastic tissue.
archigaster (ar-kĭ-gas'ter) [″ + *gastēr,* belly]. The primitive embryonic alimentary canal.
archinephron (ar-kĭ-nef'ron) [″ + *nephros,* kidney]. Primordial kidney, an organ of the embryo. SYN: *mesonephros, wolffian body.*
archineu'ron [″ + *neuron,* sinew]. The central cell of the cerebral cortex, and all its processes.
archipal'lium [″ + L. *pallium,* a cloak]. Olfactory cortex, older than neopallium.
ar'chiplasm [″ + *plasma,* a mold]. The substance of the attraction sphere.
archistome (ar'kis-tōm) [″ + *stoma,* mouth]. Invagination of blastula making little opening into archenteron. SYN: *blastopore.*
architis (ar-kī'tis) [G. *archos,* anus, + *itis,* inflammation]. Inflammation of the anus; proctitis.
archocele (ar'ko-sēl) [″ + *kēlē,* tumor]. Hernia of the rectum.
archocystocolposyrinx (ar-ko-sis-to-kol-po-sir'inks) [″ + *kystis,* bladder, + *kolpos,* vagina, + *syrigx,* fistula]. Fistula of rectum, vagina, and bladder.
archocystosyrinx (ar-ko-sis-to-sir'inks) [″ + ″ + *syrigx,* fistula]. Anovesical fistula.
ar'chon. Poisonous radical of all proteins.
archoptoma (ar-kop-to'mă) [G. *archos,* anus, + *ptōma,* a fall]. Prolapse of the rectum.
archoptosia (ar-kop-to'sĭ-ă) [″ + *ptōsis,* a falling]. Prolapse of rectum.
archoptosis (ar-kop-to'sis). Prolapse of rectum.
archorrhagia (ar-ko-ra'jĭ-ă) [G. *archos,* anus, + *rēgnunai,* to break out]. Hemorrhage from the rectum; archorrhea.
archorrhea (ar-kor-re'ă) [″ + *roia,* flow]. Rectal hemorrhage.
archos (ar'kos) [G.]. The anus.
archostenosis (ar-ko-sten-o'sis) [G. *archos,* anus, + *stenōsis,* a narrowing]. Stricture of the rectum.
arc lamp [L. *arcus,* a bow]. Source of light consisting of gaseous particles from the electrodes of an electric arc which are raised to a temperature of incandescence by an electric current.
arciform (ar'sif-orm) [″ + *forma,* shape]. Bow shaped.
arctation (ark-ta'shun) [L. *arctatiō,* draw close together]. Stricture of any canal opening. [Bowed.
arcuate (ar'ku-āt) [L. *arcuatus,* bowed].
arcuation (ar-ku-a'shun). A bending.
arculus (ar'kŭ-lŭs) [L. *arculus,* a small arch]. Support, in the form of an arch for bedclothes, to protect a part.
ar'cus [L. *arcus,* a bow]. An arc or arch.
a. denta'lis. Dental arch.
a. planta'ris. The plantar arch.
a. seni'lis. Opaque white ring about corneal periphery, seen in aged persons. Due to deposit of fat granules.
a. senilis, false. Has no diagnostic significance. Marked by a sharply delineated ring, yellow or yellowish white. Due to deposit of fat. Keratitis, ulcer, *q.v.*
ardanesthe'sia [L. *ardor,* heat, + G. *an-,* priv. + *aisthēsis,* feeling]. Inability to feel heat.
ardent (ar'dent) [L. *ardens,* burning]. Burning; feverish.
a. spirits. Distilled alcoholic liquors.

ar'dor [L. *ardor*, heat]. Burning; great heat. [urination.
  a. urinae. A burning sensation during
  a. veneris. Sexual desire.
  a. ventriculi. Heart burn; pyrosis.
area (a're-ă) [L. *area*, an open space]. A circumscribed space; one having definite boundaries. SEE: *McBurney's point*.
  a., Broca's. A. in the left hemisphere in post. portion of inferior frontal convolution. Controls speech. In left-handed persons it is in the right hemisphere. [the ovum.
  a. germinativa. A. of germination of
  a., occipital. Portion of brain below the occipital bone. [*area germinativa*.
  a. pellucida. Clear central portion of
  a., rolandic. A. situated in ant. central convolution in front of fissure of Rolando in each hemisphere. Governs motor acts of the body.
areatus (a-re-a'tus). Occurring in circumscribed areas or patches.
arec'oline. Oily anthelmintic and miotic alkaloid derived from betel nut. DOSAGE: 0.05-0.1 gr. (0.003-0.006 Gm.).
areflex'ia [G. *a-*, priv. + L. *reflectere*, bend back]. State without reflexes.
arenaceous (ar-ĕ-na'se-us) [L. *arenaceus*, sandy]. Resembling sand or gravel.
arenation (ar-ē-na'shun) [L. *arena*, sand]. A sand bath or application of hot sand.
arenoid (ar'e-noid) [" + G. *eidos*, form]. Like sand.
are'ola [L. *areola*, a small space]. 1. A cellular, highly fleecy connective tissue, with meshes capable of distention; a tissue occupying the interspaces of the body. 2. A form of macula* showing a hyperemic area about a skin lesion such as that about a boil. 3. A ringlike discoloration as that about the nipple.
  a. papilla'ris. The darkened ring about the female nipple.
  a., secondary. 1. An additional ring surrounding the a. during pregnancy. 2. Any of the large lacunae in ossifying cartilage formed by the absorption of the walls separating the primary areolae.

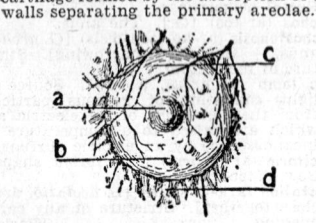

AREOLA
(a) Nipple; (b) Montgomery's gland; (c) primary areola; (d) secondary a.

areolar (ar-e'o-lar). Rel. to the areola.
  a. tissue. Connective tissue which occupies the interspaces of the body.
areoli'tis [L. *areola*, a small space, + G. *itis*, inflammation]. Inflammation of mammary areola.
areometer (a-re-om'e-ter) [G. *araios*, thin, + *metron*, a measure]. Instrument for measuring sp. gr. of fluids.
areosis (ar-e-o'sis) [L. *area*, open place, + G. *osis*, increased]. Dilution; less compact.
arevareva (ar-e"va-ra'va) [Tahitian, skin rash]. Severe skin disease accompanied by decay of vital powers.
  ETIOL: Excessive use of kava.
argamblyopia (ar-gam-bli-o'pi-a) [G. *argos*, idle, + *amblus*, dulled, + *ops*, eye]. Amblyopia due to not using the eye.

Ar'gand burner. Gas or oil lamp having an inner tube by which air is supplied to the flame to increase combustion.
Argas (ar'gas) [G. *argēēis*, shining]. Genus of ticks usually infecting birds, but may attack man, causing severe pain, also fever.
ar'gema [G. *argema*, ulcer]. White corneal ulcer.
argentaffine (ar-jent'af-fin) [L. *argentum*, silver, + *affinis*, associated with]. Taking a silver stain.
argentaffino'ma [" + " + G. *ōma*, tumor]. Growth containing argentaffine elastic fibers.
  May be benign or malignant. Practically without symptoms unless pressing on neighboring structures.
argen'tum. SYMB: Ag. Silver; atomic weight 107.12.
argil'la [G. *argillos*, white clay]. Clay.
argillaceous (ar-jĭ-la'shus). Resembling or composed of clay.
ar'ginase. Enzyme of the liver that splits up arginine and forms urea.
arginine (ar'jĭ-nēn) [L. *argentum*, silver]. Crystalline amino acid, $C_9H_{14}N_4O_2$, obtained from decomposition of vegetable tissues, protamines, proteins and also prepared synthetically.
  It is a guanidine derivative, yielding urea and ornithine on hydrolysis. It is a hexone base.
ar'gol, ar'gols [G. *argos*, white]. Impure cream of tartar formed in wine casks.
ar'gon [G. *argos*, inactive]. An inert gas in the atmosphere. SYMB: A. Atomic weight 39.88.
Argyll-Robertson pupil. More properly the name of a symptom often present in paralysis and locomotor ataxia, in which the light reflex is absent but there is no change in the power of contraction during accommodation.
argyria (ar-jĭ'rĭ-ă) [G. *argyros*, silver]. Bluish discoloration of skin and mucous membranes as a result of the administration of silver.
argyri'asis. Bluish discoloration of skin due to use of silver. SYN: *argyria*.
argyric (ar-jir'ik). Pert. to silver.
argyrism (ar'jir-izm) [G. *argyria*, silver, + *ismos*, condition of]. Bluish discoloration of skin due to use of silver. SYN: *argyria*.
argyrol (ar'jĭ-rol) (silver vitellin). A dark brown, crystalline, protein substance, containing 20% silver.
  USES: As an antiseptic in infections of the eye, nose and throat, and for urethral injections.
  DOSAGE: In strengths of 5% to 50% depending upon the condition.
argyrophil (ar-jĭ'ro-fĭl) [G. *argyria*, silver, + *philos*, fond]. Staining readily or easily impregnated with silver.
argyrosis (ar-jĭ-ro'sis) [" + *osis*, increased]. Bluish discoloration of skin due to use of silver. SYN: *argyria, q.v.*
arhyth'mia. Irregular heart action. SYN: *arrhythmia*.
  a., continuous. Permanent arhythmia.
  a., inotropic. A. caused by disorder of heart muscle's contraction.
  a., perpetual. SEE: *continuous a.*
  a., respiratory. Increase of heart action due to disorder of respiratory movements.
  a., sinus. Disorder of the impulses arising at the sinoauricular node causing heart action to be irregular.
arhythmic (ah-rith'mik) [G. *a-*, priv. + *rythmos*, rhythm]. Pert. to arhythmia. SYN: *arrhythmic.**

ariboflavinosis (ă-rĭ-bō-flā″vĭn-ō′sĭs) [G. *a-*, priv. + riboflavin + G. *-ōsis*, disease]. Condition arising from a deficiency of riboflavin in the diet.
SYM: Lesions on the lips, fissures in the angles of the mouth and seborrhea around the nose.

aridura (ar-ĭd-u′ră) [L. *aridus*, parched]. Dryness, wasting, withering.

aristocar′dia [G. *aristos*, best, + *kardia*, heart]. Cardiac deviation to the right.

aristogen′ics [G. *aristos*, best, + *genea*, race]. Control of factors tending to improve the race. SYN: *eugenics*.

aristol (ă-ris′tol) (thymol-iodide). A reddish brown powder, with faint odor of iodine.
USES: As a mild antiseptic dusting powder, pure, or diluted with equal amount of boric acid.

arithmomania (ar-ĭth-mo-ma′nĭ-ă) [G. *arithmos*, a number, + *mania*, madness]. Repetition of consecutive numbers, unnecessary counting, and insane interest in numbers.

arkyochrome (ar′kĭ-o-krōm) [G. *arkus*, a net, + *chrōma*, a color]. A nerve cell in which the stainable substance is arranged in a network.

arkyostichochrome (ar″kĭ-o-stĭk′o-krōm) [″ + *stichos*, a row, + *chrōma*, a color]. A nerve cell in which the stainable material is arranged both as a network and in parallel lines.

arm [L. *armus*, a shoulder]. The upper extremity from the shoulder to the elbow; also including lower extremity from elbow to the hand.
a. **center.** Center in rolandic area controlling arm motion.
a., **golf.** A form of neurosis seen in golf players after excessive exercise.
a. **hole.** Armpit. SYN: *axilla*.
a., **Saturday-night.** A form of paralysis of the brachial plexus, usually seen in drunkards. ETIOL: Sleeping in a chair, with the arm hanging over the back of the chair while the head rests on the shoulder or arm.

arm, words pert. to: antebrachium, antibrachium, axilla, axillary fossa, brachial, "brachio" words, brachium, cervicobrachial, dislocation, forearm, humerus, radius, skeleton, ulna.

armamentarium (ar-mă-men-ta′rĭ-um) [L. *armamentum*, an implement]. All that a physician or surgeon uses in his practice.

arm′ature [L. *armatura*, equipment]. A part of a dynamo consisting of a coil of insulated wire mounted around a soft iron core.

armil′la (ar-mĭl′lă) [L. *armilla*, bracelet]. The annular ligament of the wrist.

arm′pit [L. *armus*, shoulder, + *puteus*, a well]. Axilla. SEE: *hemorrhages, etc.*

arm-to-arm vaccination. Transferring vaccine virus from one patient to another.

ar′my itch. Chronic itch prevalent during U. S. Civil War.

Arneth's classification of neutrophiles (ar′neth). Based on the number of nuclear lobes which polynuclear neutrophiles contain. The normal are:

Lobes	1	2	3	4	5
%	5	35	41	17	2

A.'s formula. Method of procedure for elaborate differential blood count to estimate number of immature leukocytes. SEE: *formula*.

Ar′nold's canal. Passage in the temporal bone for small superficial petrosal nerve.
A.'s ganglion. Otic ganglion.

A.'s nerve. Auricular branch of vagus nerve.

aro′ma [G. *arōma*, spice]. An agreeable odor.

aromat′ic. 1. Having an agreeable odor. 2. Belonging to that series of carbon compounds in which the carbon atoms form closed rings (as in *benzene*) as distinguished from the *aliphatic* series in which the atoms form straight or branched chains.
a. **compounds.** Ring or cyclic compounds related to benzene, many having a fragrant odor.
a. **spirit of ammonia.** Contains about 35% ammonium carbonate in aromatic dilute alcohol.
ACTION AND USES: Antacid and carminative with uses same as ammonium carbonate.
DOSAGE: 2 cc. (30♏) freely diluted with water.

arrachment (ă-răsh-mon′) [Fr. *arrachement*, a tearing out]. Pulling out the capsule in a membranous cataract, through a corneal incision.

arrec′tor muscles [L. *arrector*, an erector]. Involuntary muscle fibers inserted in the hair follicles on the side toward which the hair slopes. Under the influence of cold or terror they contract, straighten the follicles, and raise the hairs, resulting in "gooseflesh," or *cutis anserina*.

arrecto′res pilo′rum [L.]. Muscles whose contractions cause "gooseflesh." SEE: *arrector muscles*.

arrhea (ar-re′ă) [G. *a-*, priv. + *roia*, a flow]. Suppression or cessation of a discharge.

arrhenoblastoma (a-re-no-blas-to′mă) [G. *arrēn*, male, + *blastos*, germ, + *-oma*, tumor]. An ovarian tumor made up of masculine sex cells and producing virile sex characteristics.

arrhythmia (ar-ĭth′mĭ-ă) [G. *a-*, priv. + *rythmos*, rhythm]. Irregular heart action causing absence of rhythm.
Two or more beats may occur in quick succession, a long pause ensuing, or other irregularities. SEE: *bradycardia* and *tachycardia*.

arrhyth′mic. Signifying loss of rhythm.

arrosion (ar-o′shun) [L. *arrodere*, to gnaw at]. Ulcerous destruction of vessel walls.

ar′senfast. Resistant to the poisonous action of arsenic, esp. spirochetes which acquire immunity after repeated arsenic administration.

arseni′asis [L. *arsenium*, arsenic]. Chronic arsenical poisoning.

arsenic (ar′sen-ĭk) [L. *arsenium*]. SYMB: As. Atomic weight, 74.93; atomic no., 33. A metal of grayish white color, very poisonous, used in the manufacture of dyes and in medicine.
The various compounds are used medicinally as tonics and specifics. Minute traces of arsenic are found in vegetables and animal forms of life. It is a constant element of cell life and is present in eggs, two-thirds being in the yolk, and one-third in the white, the membrane, and the shell.
CUMULATIVE EFFECT: Disorders of alimentary tract, nausea, vomiting, diarrhea, dehydration, neuritis, paralysis of wrist and ankle muscles.
a. **triox′ide.** Used internally in form of Fowler's solution (Solution of Potassium Arsenite) 1%.
USES: Treatment of neuralgia and chorea and certain forms of skin diseases.

DOSAGE: 1/30 ♏ (0.002 cc.). More than a few grains may be fatal.
POISONING: Used as a drug and as a vermin killer.
SYM: *Acute Poisoning*: May appear in a few minutes or when taken with solid food, may not appear for many hours. When the symptoms come on slowly, there are agonizing pain in pit of stomach, sinking sensations, nausea, sore throat, thirst, persistent vomiting, purging, scanty urine which may be bloody, cramps, and collapse.
Chronic Poisoning: Loss of appetite, fainting, abdominal cramps, convulsions, and coma.
TREATMENT, F. A.: Evacuate stomach with emetic. Wash out with stomach tube. Arsenic may be precipitated with iron salts, magnesium oxide (milk of magnesia) in teaspoonful doses.

arsenic, words pert. to: acetarsone, arsenfast, arseniasis, arsenicism, arsenicophagy, arsenionization, "arseno-" words, arsphenamine, bismarsen, mapharsen, neoarsphenamine, neosilver arsphenamine, silver arsphenamine, sulfarsphenamine, tryparsamide.

arsenical (är-sĕn'ĭk-ăl) [L. *arsenica'lis*]. 1. Pertaining to or containing arsenic. 2. A drug containing arsenic.

arsenic-fast. Resistant to toxic action of arsenic. SYN: *arsenfast.*

arsenicism (ar-sen'is-izm) [L. *arsenicum*, arsenic, + G. *ismos*, condition of]. Chronic arsenic poisoning. SYN: *arseniasis.*

arsenicophagy (ar-sen-ĭ-kof'ă-jĭ) [G. *arsenikon*, arsenic, + *phagein*, to eat]. Habitual eating of arsenic.

arsenioniza'tion. Electrolytic diffusion of arsenic ions in tissues.

arse'nium [L.]. Arsenic.

arsen'oblast [G. *arsĕn*, male, + *blastos*, germ]. Male element in nucleus of impregnated ovum; a masculonucleus.

arsenoph'agy [L. *arsenium*, arsenic, + G. *phagein*, to eat]. Habitual eating of arsenic. SYN: *arsenicophagy.**

arsenorelap'sing [" + *re*, back, + *lapsus*, a slipping]. Pert. to syphilitic case which relapses after apparent cure of arsenic.

arsenoresis'tant [" + *resistāre*, to withstand]. Resistant to arsenic compounds.

arsenother'apy [" + G. *therapeia*, treatment]. Treatment with arsenic and its compounds.

ar'senous. Of the nature of, or pert. to, arsenic or its compounds. SYN: *arsenical.*

ar'sin. A very poisonous gas.

arsonvaliza'tion. Application of high frequency current.

arsphenamine (ars-fen-am'ĭn) (salvarsan). A light yellow powder containing about 30% arsenic.
ACTION AND USES: Specific for treatment of syphilis in all stages, particularly in primary stage, usually given in later stages with mercurials. A 25% to 10% solution with glycerin used locally in Vincent's angina. [doses.
DOSAGE: Intravenously, 6 gr. (0.4 Gm.)

ar'tefact [L. *ars*, art, + *factus*, made]. SEE: *artifact.*

arterec'tomy [G. *artēria*, artery, + *ektomē*, excision]. Excising an artery or arteries.

arte'ria (pl. *arteriae*) [G.]. Artery.*
a. den'tis. The small artery supplying dental pulp.

arteriag'ra [" + *agra*, a seizure]. Pain in an artery.

arte'rial. Pert. to one or more arteries.
a. bleeding. Blood is bright red and pumped out. Arrest by pressure on proximal side of vessel (nearest heart).
a. circulation. It is maintained by the pumping of the heart; elasticity and extensibility of arterial walls; peripheral resistance in the areas of small arteries, and by the quantity of blood in the body. SEE: *circulation.*
a. varix. An enlarged and tortuous artery.

arterializa'tion. Aeration of the blood, changing it from venous into arterial.

arteriarctia (ar-te-rĭ-ark'tĭ-ă) [G. *artēria*, artery, + L. *arctus*, bound]. Stenosis or constriction of an artery.

arteriasis (ar-te-rĭ'ăs-is) [" + *iasis*, condition]. Degeneration of an artery.

arteriectasis, arteriectasia (ar-te-rĭ-ek'tas-is, -ta'zĭ-ă) [G. *artēria*, artery, + *ektasis*, a stretching out]. Arterial dilatation. [blood.

ar'terin. Coloring matter of arterial

arterio-at'ony [G. *artēria*, artery, + *atonia*, languor]. Lack of tone in arterial walls.

arteriocap'illary [" + L. *capillus*, like hair]. Pert. to arteries and capillaries.
a. fibrosis. Arteriosclerosis of capillaries and arterioles.

arteriofibro'sis [" + L. *fibra*, fiber, + *osis*, increased. Arteriocapillary fibrosis.

arte'riogram [" + *gramma*, inscription]. Recording of arterial pulse. SYN: *sphygmogram.*

arteriog'raphy [" + *graphein*, to write]. Description of arteries.

arterio'la [L. *arteriola*, small artery]. Small artery.
a. rec'ta. One of the small renal arteries going to the medullary pyramids.

arterioles (ar-te'rĭ-ole). The smallest arteries leading at their distal ends into the capillaries.

arte'riolith [G. *artēria*, artery, + *lithos*, stone]. An arterial calculus.

arteriol'ogy [" + *logos*, study]. Science of arteries, usually combined with study of other vessels, as in angiology.*

arteriosclero'sis [L. *arteriola*, small artery, + G. *sklērōsis*, hardening]. Thickening of the arterial walls with loss of elasticity and contractility.

arteriosclerot'ic. Rel. to arteriolosclerosis.

arteriomala'cia [G. *artēria*, artery, + *malakia*, softening]. Softening of the arteries.

arteriom'eter [" + *metron*, measure]. Instrument measuring variations in the size of a beating artery.

arteriomo'tor [" + L. *movere*, to move]. Causing changes in size of arteries by dilatation and constriction.

arteriomyomatosis (ar-te"rĭ-o-mi-o-mă-to'sis) [" + *mys*, muscle, + *oma*, tumor, + -*osis*, increased]. Thickening of arterial walls due to overgrowth of muscular fibers.

arterio"necro'sis [" + *nekros*, dead, + *osis*, condition]. Arterial necrosis.

arter"iop'athy [" + *pathos*, disease]. Any disease of the arteries.

arterio"pla'nia [" + *planasthai*, to wander]. The presence of an anomalous course in an artery.

arterioplasty (ar-te"rĭ-o-plăs-tĭ) [" + *plassein*, to form]. Repair of an aneurysm, restoring continuity of channel of the artery.

arteriopres'sor [" + L. *pressura*, force]. Causing increased arterial blood pressure.

arteriorrhaphy (ar-te-rĭ-or'af-ĭ) [" + *raphē*, suture]. Arterial suture.

arteriorrhexis (ar-te-rĭ-or-eks'ĭs) [" + *rēxis*, rupture]. Rupture of an artery.

arteriosclerosis [" + *sklērōsis*, a hardening]. A degeneration and hardening of the walls of arteries, capillaries, or veins, due to chronic inflammation and resulting in fibrous tissue formation.

ETIOL: 1. A process of old age as arteries harden, lengthen, and become more tortuous after 50. 2. Due to syphilis. 3. Worry, anxiety, stress, overwork. 4. Alcoholism. 5. Overeating. 6. Lead, arsenic, and intestinal toxins. 7. Focal infections. 8. Kidney diseases. 9. Nervous disturbances. 10. Hereditary when in the young. 11. Deficiency of Vitamins A, B and C. 12. Oversecretion of certain ductless glands.

SYM: Hypertension, pallor, digestive disturbances, fatigue, polyuria, enlarged prostate in the male, myocarditis, angina pectoris, accentuation of second aortic sound, chronic bronchitis, emphysema, dizziness, cerebral anemia, thrombosis, hemorrhage of brain, vasomotor disturbances, cramps in calves and legs, cyanosis of feet. One or more of the foregoing.

NP: Avoid all conditions which induce increase of blood pressure, and excesses of all kinds. Hygienic treatment, normal action of all functions to be maintained. Hot drinks and warmth at extremities and avoidance of being chilled or taking cold. Hot water bottle in bed, flannel underwear in bed, and warm covers. Massage of limbs to avoid cramps and start circulation. Moderation in food, drink and exercise. Avoid indigestion. It is not necessary to remain in bed unless heart is affected by strain, but rest is imperative. A day in bed each week with good sleep at night sufficient. Anxiety should be eliminated. Alcohol omitted and smoking greatly diminished. Avoid all strain upon the heart. Watch for signs of cerebral hemorrhage and guard against cerebral thrombosis by prevention of sudden or continued exertion by the patient.

a. of legs. A form due to failure of circulation in the legs.

SYM: Peculiar sensation in feet and toes, burning pain about arches and ankle, cramps in calf of one or both legs when walking or standing. Worse at end of day.

TREATMENT: Heat to abdomen, rest, care, and cleanliness of feet, oils to keep skin soft, alcohol, theobromine, aminophylline, priscoline. Also, sympathectomy.

arteriosclerotic. Pert. to arteriosclerosis.*

arteriospasm [G. *artēria*, artery, + *spasmos*, pain]. Arterial spasm.

arteriostenosis [" + *stenōsis*, a narrowing]. Contraction of the lumen of an artery, either temporary or permanent.

arteriostosis [" + *osteon*, bone, + *osis*, increased]. Calcification of an artery.

arteriostrepsis [" + *strepsis*, a twisting]. Twisting of divided end of an artery to arrest hemorrhage.

arteriosympathectomy [" + *sympatheia*, suffer with, + *ektomē*, excision]. Removal of arterial sheath containing fibers of sympathetic nerve.

arteriotome (ar-te'rĭ-o-tōm) [" + *tomē*, incision]. Knife for opening an artery.

arteriotomy (ar-te-rĭ-ot'o-mĭ). Surgical division or opening of an artery.

arteriotony (ar-te-rĭ-ot'o-nĭ) [G. *artēria*, artery, + *tonos*, tension]. 1. Blood pressure. 2. Intraarterial blood tension.

arteriovenous [" + L. *vena*, a vein]. Rel. to both arteries and veins.

arterioversion [" + L. *versiō*, a twining]. Everting wall of artery to arrest hemorrhage from open end.

arterioverter (ar-te-rĭ-ov'er-ter). An instrument for everting cut end of an artery for arresting hemorrhage.

arteritis [G. *artēria*, artery, + *-itis*, inflammation]. Inflammation of an artery.

a. deformans. Inflammation of inner coat of an artery. SYN: *chronic endarteritis.**

a. obliterans. Inflammation of intima of artery causing closure of vessel's lumen. SYN: *endarteritis obliterans.**

artery [G. *artēria*]. One of the vessels carrying blood from the heart to the tissues.

Frequently is nearly empty after death. The ancients supposed that air circulated through them; from which supposition they derived their names.

They carry the blood from the right and left ventricles of the heart to all parts of the body. There are two sets, the *pulmonary* and the *systemic*. The pulmonary artery carries the venous blood from the right ventricle to the lungs. The systemic system begins as the *aorta. a.v..* from the left ventricle.

ANAT: They have three coats: The inner, *tunica intima*, or serous; the outer, *tunica adventitia*, or white fibrous, and the middle, *tunica media*, or yellow fibrous. The blood they carry is red. SEE: *Tables in Appendix; Fig. p. A-82*.

artery, words pert. to: adventitia, anacrotism, aneurysm, aneurysmectomy, aneurysmotomy, angina pectoris, arteria, arteriarctia, arteriagra, arteriasis, arteriectasis, arteriomalacia, arteriorrhexis, arteriosclerosis, atheroma, atheromatous, carotid, carotidynia, catadicrotism, circle of Willis, circulation, endarteritis, hypertonia, hypotonia, innominate, lumen, media, mesarteritis, sclerosis, varix, "vas-" words.

arthragra (ar-thra'grä) [G. *arthron*, joint, + *agra*, seizure]. Seizure in the joints. SYN: *gout*.

arthral. Pert. to a joint.

arthralgia (ar-thral'jĭ-ä) [G. *arthron*, joint, + *algos*, pain]. Articular neuralgia. Pain in the joints.

arthrectomy (ar-threk'to-mĭ) [" + *ektomē*, excision]. 1. The operation of opening into a joint cavity with the object of removing dead or diseased tissue. 2. Excision of a joint.

arthredema (ar-thred-e'mä) [" + *oidema*, a swelling]. Edema of a joint.

arthrempyesis (ar-threm-pĭ-e'sĭs) [" + *empyesis*, suppuration]. Suppuration in a joint.

arthresthesia (ar-thres-the'zĭ-ä) [" + *aisthēsis*, sensation]. Joint sensibility; the perception of articular motions.

arthric (ar'thrĭk). Pert. to a joint.

arthrifuge (ar'thrĭ-fūg) [G. *arthron*, joint, + L. *fugāre*, put to flight]. A remedy for gout.

arthritic (ar-thrĭt'ĭk). 1. Gouty. 2. Pert. to arthritis.

arthriticin (ar-thrĭt'ĭs-ĭn). Preparation to aid arthritics.

arthritide (ar'thrĭt-ĭd). A skin eruption assumed to be of gouty origin.

arthritis (ar-thri'tis) [G. *arthron*, joint, + *-itis*, inflammation]. A joint affection characterized by inflammation and other changes varying with type. Two general types: 1. Of infectious origin (rheumatoid a., a. due to rheumatic fever, tuberculous a., gonorrheal a., syphilitic a.). 2. Of noninfectious origin (osteo- a., a. due to metabolic disease, a. due to newgrowths).

TREATMENT: Removal of foci of any infection. Complete rest, mental as well as physical. Build body resistance. Combat anemia and maintain normal level of hemoglobin. Stimulate circulation to overcome capillary destruction, by moderate exercise, food, and massage. *No massage in presence of pain.* Vaccines and baths, medication as indicated. Short-wave diathermy. ACTH and cortisone, especially in rheumatoid a.

NP: Complete rest in bed imperative during acute stage when hands and feet and joints are swollen and painful. Usually, the patient is unable to use them. In order to protect them, complete rest is necessary. Splints may be applied but avoid pressure sores from rubbing. Due to poor circulation and limitation of motion, a daily bath necessary. Bony prominences rubbed with alcohol and well padded. Position should be changed frequently. A cradle may be used to avoid pressure from bedclothes. Apply heat over swollen joints by use of an electric light bulb in a cradle placed directly over the part. Daily elimination essential. May be taken care of with diet aided by a definite time each day for a stool. An enema may be necessary. The mental condition needs special consideration. Strive to keep patient's mind occupied by some form of occupational therapy and if possible, a radio placed in the room will aid in arousing interest.

SEE: *acroarthritis, arthriticin; rheumatism; synovitis, pannous.*

a., acute secondary. One caused by osteitis. SYM: Severe pain, redness, and swelling.

a., a. suppurative. Purulent distention of synovial sac; a serious form.

a., atrophic. One followed by atrophy.

a. deformans. One with deformity. SYM: Begins in fingers; develops progressively. Deformity due to ankylosis, exostosis, and atrophy of soft parts.

a. fungosa. Tuberculosis of a joint.

a., gonorrheal. One due to gonorrheal infection. SYM: Usually attacks knee

ARTERIES OF FACE AND HEAD

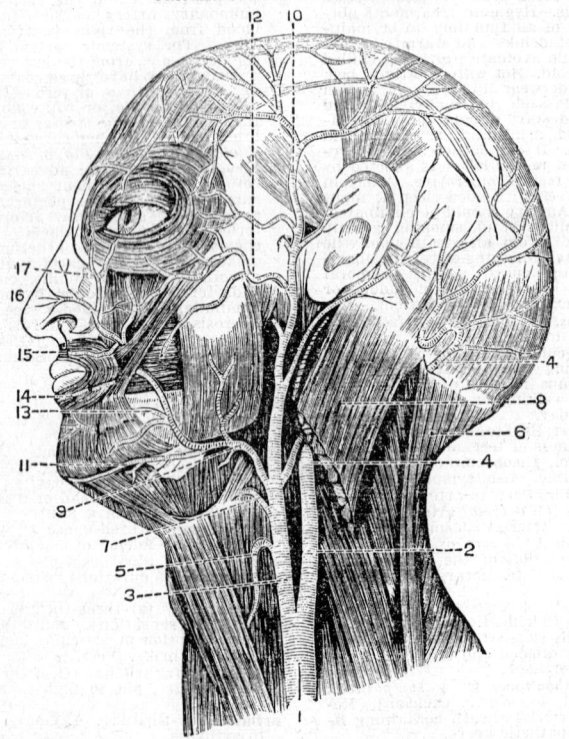

1. Common carotid. 2. Internal carotid. 3. External carotid. 4. Occipital. 5. Superior thyroid. 6. Trapezius muscle. 7. Lingual. 8. Sternocleidomastoid muscle. 9. External maxillary artery. 10. Temporal artery. 11. Submental artery. 12. Transverse facial artery. 13. Inferior labial artery. 14 and 15. Inferior and superior labial arteries. 16. Lateral nasal artery. 17. Angular artery.

joint; during acute stage several joints may be affected.
TREATMENT: Neoprontosil combined with typhoid vaccine relieves pain and effects speedy restoration of joint function.
   a., hypertrophic. Deformed enlargement of the cartilage at the edge of a joint.
   a., osteo-. A form affecting the bones and joints.
   a., pneumococcic. One sometimes appearing as a sequel to lobar pneumonia, affecting one or more joints, and the middle ear.
   a., rheumatoid. A chronic joint disease, with enlarged cartilage and synovial membrane.
   a., syphilitic. One due to acquired or hereditary syphilis. SYM: Enlarged, but not very painful joint.
   a., tuberculous. A. involving epiphyseal cartilage, synovial membrane and joint.
arthritism (ar'thrĭ-tizm) [" + ismos, condition of]. A condition or tendency to inflammation and gouty conditions of the joints and their processes. SEE: oxypathia.
arthro- [G.]. Prefix: Pert. to joints.
arthrobacte'rium [G. arthron, joint, + baktērion, staff]. A bacterium which reproduces by segmentation or fission.
arthrocace (ar-throk'ă-se) [" + kakē, badness]. Caries of a joint.
arthrocele (ar'thro-sēl) [" + kēlē, tumor]. 1. Hernia of a synovial membrane, penetrating the capsule of a joint. 2. Any joint swelling.
arthrochondri'tis [" + chondros, cartilage, + -itis, inflammation]. Inflammation of an articular cartilage.
arthroclasia (ar-thro-kla'sĭ-ă) [" + klasis, a breaking]. Breaking an ankylosed joint.
arthrodesis (ar-throd'es-is) [" + desis, binding]. The surgical fixation of a joint; artificial ankylosis.
arthrodia (ar-thro'dĭ-ă) [G. arthrōdia, a gliding joint]. Gliding joints articulating by surfaces which glide upon each other.
arthrodyn'ia [G. arthron, joint, + odynē, pain]. Pain in a joint.
arthroempye'sis [" + empyēsis, suppuration]. Suppuration in a joint. SYN: arthrempyesis.*
arthroendos'copy [" + endon, with, + skopein, to examine]. Inspection of interior of a joint by endoscope.
arthrog'raphy [" + graphein, to write]. A description of the joints.
arthrogryposis (ar″thro-grĭ-po'sis) [" + grypos, curved, + -osis, increased]. 1. Persistent contracture of a joint. 2. Tetany.
arthrokleisis (ar-thro-kli'sis) [" + kleisis, a closure]. Ankylosis,* both natural and surgical.
ar'throlith [" + lithos, stone]. Calculous deposit in a joint.
arthrology (ar-throl'o-jĭ) [" + logos, study]. The science of joints.
arthrol'ysis [" + lysis, a loosening]. The operation of restoring mobility to an ankylosed joint.
arthromeningi'tis [" + mēninx, membrane, + -itis, inflammation]. Inflammation of a synovial membrane. SYN: synovitis.
arthrom'eter [" + metron, measure]. Instrument for measuring the degree of movement of a joint.
ar'thron. An articulation or joint.

arthron'cus [G. arthron, joint, + ogkos, tumor]. 1. Tumor of a joint. 2. Swelling of a joint.
arthroneural'gia [" + neuron, sinew, + algos, pain]. Pain in a joint.
arthrono'sos [" + nosos, disease]. Joint disease.
   a. defor'mans. Arthritis causing deformity. SYN: arthritis deformans.*
arthropathol'ogy [" + pathos, disease, + logos, study]. Joint disease pathology.
arthropathy (ar-throp'ă-thĭ) [" + pathos, disease]. Any joint disease.
   a., Charcot's. A trophic joint disease with effusion of fluids into a joint, seen in locomotor ataxia and in syringomyelia and sometimes in general paresis.
   a., inflammatory. An inflammatory joint disease; arthritis.
   a., osteopulmonary. Enlargement and swelling of the ends of the long bones following pulmonary disease.
   a., static. A disturbance in a joint of a given extremity secondary to a disturbance in some other joint of the same extremity, as one in the right knee joint secondary to one in the right hip joint.
   a., tabetic. Same as Charcot's arthropathy.
arthrophlysis (ar-throf'lis-is) [" + phlysis, eruption]. An eczematous eruption occurring in rheumatic subjects.
arthrophyma (ar-thro-fī'mă) [" + phyma, swelling]. An articular swelling.
ar'throphyte [" + phyton, growth]. Abnormal growth in joint cavity.
arthroplasty (ar'thro-plas-tĭ) [" + plassein, to form]. Surgical formation or reformation of a joint.
arthropyosis (ar-thro-pĭ-o'sis) [" + pyōsis, suppuration]. Suppuration of a joint.
arthrorheu'matism [" + rheumatismos, flux]. Rheumatism of the joints.
arthrosclero'sis [" + sklērōsis, a hardening]. Stiffening or hardening of the joints, esp. in the aged.
arthro'sis [G. arthron, joint, + -osis, increased]. 1. Joint. 2. Joint affection due to trophic degeneration.
ar'throscope [" + skōpein, to examine]. An endoscope for examining interior of a joint.
arthros'copy. Direct joint visualization by means of an arthroscope.
ar'throspore [" + sporos, a seed]. A bacterial spore formed by segmentation; has greater resistance than an endospore.
arthrosteitis (ar-thros-te-i'tis) [" + osteon, bone, + -itis, inflammation]. Inflammation of the bony structures of a joint.
arthros'tomy [" + stoma, an opening]. The formation of a temporary opening into a joint for drainage purposes.
arthrosynovi'tis [" + G. syn, with, + ōōn, egg, + -itis, inflammation]. Inflammation of synovial membrane of a joint.
arthrotome (ar'thro-tōm) [G. arthron, joint, + temnein, to cut]. Knife for making incisions into a joint.
arthrotomy (arth-rot'o-mĭ) [" + tomē, incision]. Cutting into a joint.
arthrous (ar'thrus). Jointed or pert. to a joint.
arthroxesis (ar-throx-e'sis) [" + xesis, scraping]. Scraping a joint.
ar'tiad [G. artios, even]. CHEM: An element of an even numbered valence. SEE: perissad.
ar'tichoke [Italian articioco]. Perennial plant with edible flowery head.
   a., French, or globe. COMP: Lower

fleshy part nutritious and rich in extractives, manganese present in considerable quantities. Average serving 150 grams. Pro. 4.4, Fat 0.6, Carbo. 17.9. Contains Vitamin B. Good source Vitamins A and G.

ACTION: Slightly irritating to the kidneys. May cause flatulence and griping. The puree is well tolerated by a weak stomach.

a., Jerusalem. Average serving 100 grams. Pro. 2.2, Fat 0.1, Carbo. 17.0. Contains Vitamin C. Good source Vitamin B.

artic'ular [L. *articularis*, joint]. Pert. to articulation.

artic'ulate [L. *articulatus*, jointed]. 1. To join together as a joint. 2. To adjust artificial teeth properly. 3. Clearly spoken. 4. To speak clearly.

artic'ulated. State of articulation or of being jointed. [joints.

articula'tion. The connection of bones; They may be *synarthroses*,* immovable ones, *amphiarthroses*,* slightly movable ones, or *diarthroses*,* freely movable ones. Cartilage, or fibrous or soft tissue lines the opposing surfaces of all joints. 2. The relative position of the tongue and palate necessary to produce a given sound. 3. Speech, clearly enunciated; enunciation.

a., confluent. Speech in which syllables are not clearly enunciated.

artic'ulatory. Rel. to articulation (3.), *q.v.*

artic'ulo mor'tis [L. *articularis*, joint, + *mors*, death]. At the time of death.

articulus (ar-tik'u-lus) [L.]. 1. A knuckle or a joint. 2. A segment.

ar'tifact [L. *ars*, craft, + *facere*, to make]. 1. Anything artificially produced. 2. An apparent structure produced in a cell or tissue by fixation, staining, or other manipulation.

artifi'cial [L. *ars*, art, + *facere*, to make]. Not natural; formed in imitation of nature. SEE: *feeding*.

a. hyperemia. Bringing blood to the superficial tissues by means of "cups," and elastic bandage, or unctions.

a. impregnation. SEE: *insemination.*

a. pneumothorax (nu-mo-thor'aks). Artificial introduction of air into pleural cavity. Oxygen or nitrogen, or filtered atmospheric air is used.

artifi'cial respira'tion. Maintenance of respiratory movements by artificial means.

Call a doctor at once. Laryngeal spasm often blocks air from lungs. Passage of catheter or tube may be necessary to convey air to lungs. Drugs may be needed to counteract spasm and promote circulation. Attempts at a. r., if such a spasm exists, may be useless.

Two USES: (1) in which respiration needs only to be started and maintained artificially for a limited period. Usual combination of Schafer method and inhalation of mixture of CO_2 and O is used as in asphyxia from gases, drowning and electric shock. (2) Cases where artificial respiration must be maintained for days, as in morphine poisoning and infantile paralysis. Apparatus such as respirator is used. More than one hundred methods have been used, including mechanical, electrical and manual types.

SUPPLEMENTARY TREATMENT: Keep warm with blankets; massage with friction; hot water bottles, etc. If possible, head should be directed downhill to aid circulation to brain; it is desirable to turn the mouth toward the wind. Circulation must be maintained by massaging extremities toward the heart. Stimulants such as aromatic spirits of ammonia applied to nostrils intermittently, and injections of drugs, such as epinephrine (adrenalin), ephedrine, ceramine and alphalobeline. Rectal instillations of hot, black coffee. Rhythmical traction of tongue (Laborde) and intermittent dilatation of the external anal sphincter (Pratt) are useful adjuncts. This method should be continued for a prolonged period of time until a physician pronounces patient dead. The use of oxygen or combination of oxygen and carbon dioxide mixtures is highly desirable if they can be obtained. Resuscitation has been necessary from several hours to many days. This method is more satisfactory than the ordinary mechanical device for inducing artificial respiration. It is possible for one operator to perform artificial respiration on two or three patients. Proficiency can be attained only by repeated practice on various types of individuals.

RS: *asphyxia, collapse, coma, drowning, respiration, syncope, shock, unconsciousness, back-pressure arm-lift, Byrd-Dew, Doe, Eve, Fell-O'Dwyer, hip-lift, Howard, Japanese, Laborde, Marmo, Ogata, Prochownick, Schroeder, Schultze, Schafer, Sylvester.*

ar'tisan's cramp. A spasmodic affection of the muscles induced by prolonged work requiring delicate coördination and occurring only in performance of that particular work.

Occupations in which most apt to occur are writing, piano playing, sewing and telegraphing.

artus (ar'tus) [L. *artus*, joint]. A joint or joints; a limb.

aryepiglottic (ar-ĭ-ep-ĭ-glot'ik) [G. *arytaina*, pitcher, + *epi*, upon, + *glōttis*, glottis]. Pert. to the arytenoid cartilage and epiglottis.

ar'yl-. A prefix denoting a radical of the aromatic series.

a. group. In chemistry, a radical group of the aromatic or benzene series.

arylarsonate (ar-ĭ-lar'so-nāt). Salt of arylarsonic acid.

arytenoid (ar-it'en-oid) [G. *arytaina*, ladle, + *eidos*, form]. 1. Resembling a ladle or pitcher-mouth. 2. Relating to the *a. cartilage*, gland, ligament, or muscle.

arytenoidectomy (ar-it″e-noy-dek'to-mī) [" + " + *ektomē*, excision]. Excision of arytenoid cartilage.

arytenoid'itis. Inflammation of arytenoid cartilage.

As. 1. Abbr. for *astigmatism.* 2. SYMB: *arsenic.*

a. s. [L. *auris sinistra*]. Abbr. *left ear.*

asafetida (as-e-fet'id-a) [L. *asa*, gum, + *foetida*, fetid]. USP. A gum resinous substance with characteristic odor and taste.

ACTION AND USES: A carminative and antispasmodic used in hysteria.

DOSAGE: 0.4 Gm. (6 gr.) in pill form or an emulsion as an enema of 1 dram to 100 cc. water.

asaphia (as-af'ĭ-ă) [G. *asapheia*, uncertainty]. Inability to articulate properly due to cleft palate.

asarcia (ă-sar'sĭ-ă) [G. *a-*, priv. + *sarx*, flesh]. Leanness; emaciation.

asbes'tiform [G. *asbestos*, quicklime, + L. *forma*, appearance]. Having structure similar to asbestos.

asbes'tos. Fibrous form of magnesium and calcium silicate.
asbesto'sis [G. *asbestos*, quicklime, + *-osis*, increased]. Lung disease due to protracted inhalation of asbestos particles.
ascariasis (as-kar-i'as-is) [G. *askaris*, pinworm]. Symptoms produced by gastrointestinal worms (*ascarides*, round and thread worms).
ascar'ides. Pl. of *Ascaris*.*
ascaridiasis (as-kar-i-di'ă-sis). Ascarides in intestine and symptoms they cause.
Ascaris (as'kar-is) [Pl. *ascarides*). A genus of nematodes belonging to the superfamily Ascaridoidea which inhabits the intestine of vertebrates.
  A. lumbricoides. A species of *Ascaris* which lives in the human intestine. Eggs are passed with the feces and are transmitted by contaminated water, food, or hands. After swallowing, the eggs containing embryos hatch and the larvae enter the blood stream and pass through the liver and heart, to the lungs where they enter the trachea, are coughed up and swallowed a second time.
  A. lumbricoides var. suum. A variety of *Ascaris* which infests pigs. It is indistinguishable from the human *Ascaris* but eggs from pig *Ascaris* will not develop in man and vice versa.
Aschheim-Zondek test (ash'him-tson'děk). A test for pregnancy. SEE: *test*.
Asch'ner's phenomenon. Slowing of the pulse caused by eyeball pressure.
Aschoff's bodies (ahsh'of). Rheumatic nodules in the myocardium; also in lungs in rheumatic fever complicated by pneumonia.
  A.'s node. Atrioventricular node.
ascia (a'si-ă, as'ki-ă) [L. *ascia*, ax]. Spinal bandage without reverse, each turn overlapping the previous one for a third of its width.
ascites (ă-si'tez) [G. *askitēs*, bag]. Serous fluid in the peritoneal cavity.
  ETIOL: (a) Chronic cardiac disease, (b) chronic renal disease, (c) interference with the portal circulation, (d) tumors of the abdomen, (e) external enlargement of the spleen.
  SYM: Feeling of weight in the abdomen, dyspnea,* edema of the feet, scanty urination, shifting dullness in flanks; fluctuation felt when hand is placed on one side of the abdomen, tapping the opposite side with the tips of the fingers; no aortic pulsation, enlargement more prominent about umbilicus. [cause. SEE: *dropsy*.
  TREATMENT: Directed to the original
  a. chylosus. Chyle in the ascitic fluid.
ascit'ic. Pert. to ascites.
  a. fluid. Sp. gr. 1.005-1.015, clear and pale, straw color with greenish tinge in some cases.
Ascoli's reaction (ahs-ko'lĭs). 1. Precipitation test for anthrax. 2. Miostagmin reaction.*
ascorbic acid (ăs-kor'bĭk) [G. *a-*, priv. + *scorbutus*]. USP. SYN: for synthetic vitamin C.
as'cospore [G. *askos*, bag, + *sporos*, seed]. Spores within an *ascus*,* or sac.
as'cus. A spore case; a sac containing spores.
-ase. A suffix used in forming the name of an enzyme. It is added to the name or a part of the name of the substance upon which it acts. Ex. *lipase* which acts on fats (lipids).
ase'mia, asema'sia [G. *a-*, priv. + *sēmasia*, sign]. Inability to comprehend any type of symbol. SEE: *asymbolia*.

asepsin (ă-sep'sin) [G. *a-*, priv. + *sepsis*, decay]. An antiseptic analgesia, antipyretic drug. SYN: *antisepsin*.
asep'sis. A condition free from germs; free from infection; sterile, free from any form of life. SEE: *antisepsis, antiseptics, sterile, sterilization*.
asep'tic. Rel. to asepsis; free from septic matter.
asep'tic-antisep'tic [G. *a-*, priv. + *sepsis*, decay, + *anti*, against, + *sepsis*]. Both aseptic and antiseptic.
asep'ticize. To make sterile; to free from pathogenic matter.
asex'ual [G. *a-*, priv. + L. *sexualis*, having sex]. Without sex; nonsexual. SEE: *parthenogenesis*.
asexualization (ah-seks-u-al-iz-a'shun). Ablation of the ovaries or testes and in this manner desexing the individual.
ash (ăsh) [A.S. *asce*, ash]. Incombustible, powdery residue of an organic substance that has been burned.
  Residue from food digested in the body is either alkaline or acid.
  The difference in the blood is slight, normally a trifle more alkaline than acid. Mineral elements in food aid in keeping the blood neutral. Some fruits and vegetables which remain acid in the gastrointestinal tract have an alkaline ash when oxidized in the body.
  Acid-producing Foods: All cereals, eggs, meat, fish, cranberries, peanuts, prunes, and quinces. *Alkali-producing Foods:* Most fruits and vegetables, cow's milk, raisins, almonds, chestnuts, currants. SEE: *acid-base balance, acidic effects of foods, acidosis*.
asialia (as-i-a'lĭ-ă) [G. *a-*, priv. + *sialon*, spittle]. Failure to secrete saliva or deficiency of it.
Asiat'ic cholera. An epidemic, acute infectious disease. SEE: *cholera*.
asidero'sis [G. *a-*, priv. + *sidēros*, iron, + *-osis*, condition]. Deficiency of iron in the circulating blood.
asitia (a-sish'ĭ-ă) [G. *a-*, priv. + *sitos*, food]. 1. Aversion to food. SYN: *anorexia*.* 2. The want of food.
asonia (ă-so'nĭ-ă) [G. *a-*, priv. + L. *sonus*, sound]. Tone deafness.
aspar'agus. COMP: Extractive matter high. PURINS: 0.021% or 1.50 gr. per lb. It contains aspargin.
  Av. SERVING (green): 75 grams. Pro. 1.7, Fat 0.2, Carbo. 1.9, Ca. 0.025, Mg. 0.011, K. 0.196, Na. 0.007, P. 0.039, Cl. 0.039, S. 0.041, Fe. 0.0010. VITS: A, variable; B, good; C and G, excellent. Copper 1.4 mg. per Kg. Alkalinity 3.7 cc. per 100 grams, 6.00 per 100 cals. A base-forming food. ACTION: It increases the production of uric acid. It impedes elimination as it is apt to irritate and congest the kidneys.
aspastic (ă-spas'tĭk) [G. *a-*, priv. + *spastikos*, having spasms]. Nonspastic.
as'pect [L. *aspectus*, looking toward]. 1. That part of a surface looking in any designated direction. 2. Appearance, looks.
aspergillosis (ăs-pĕr-jĭl-o'sĭs). Aspergillus in the tissues or on any mucous surface and the condition produced thereby. This condition may develop in the bronchi, lungs, mucous membranes of the eye, nose, or urethra, the aural canal, or the skin. It may even extend through the various viscera, producing mycotic nodules in the lungs, liver, kidney, and other organs.
  a., aural. Otomycosis.

aspergillosis, pulmonary — A-88 — **asphyxiation**

a., pulmonary. Disease of the lungs caused by *Aspergillus fumigatus*.

Aspergillus (ăs-pēr-jĭl'ŭs) [L. *asper'gere*, to sprinkle]. A genus of the *Ascomycetes*, including several species of the molds, some of which are pathogenic.

A. auricula'ris. A species in the external auditory meatus.

A. bar'bae. A species found in mycosis of the head.

A. bonfor'di. A form found in black mycetoma.

A. Bouffardi. Found in black mycetoma.

A. bronchialis. A species in the bronchii of a diabetic patient.

A. concen'tricus. A species once thought to be the cause of *Tinea imbricata* ringworm.

A. fla'vus. A mold found on corn and grain.

A. fumiga'tus. A species that has been found in the ear, nose, and lungs.

A. glau'cus. A bluish mold found on dried fruit, also in the human ear.

A. indulans. The cause of white mycetoma, and of otomycosis.

A. mucuroid'es. A form found in the lungs.

A. nid'ulans. A species causing one form of white mycetoma.

A. ni'ger. A pathogenic form with black spores, frequently present in the external auditory meatus.

A. ocra'ceus. The species which produces the characteristic and desirable odor of coffee.

A. pic'tor. A species found in the patches of pinta.

A. re'pens. A species found in the auditory canal.

aspermat'ic [G. *a-*, priv. + *sperma*, seed]. Pert. to aspermatism.

aspermatism (a-sper'mă-tĭzm) [" + " + *ismos*, condition of]. Lack of formation of spermatozoa due to defective secretion of semen; aspermia.

asper'mia. Lack of or failure to ejaculate semen.

asper'mous. Pert. to aspermia. SYN: *aspermatic*.

as'perous [L. *asper*, rough]. Uneven; having minute elevations.

asper'sion [L. *aspersio*, sprinkling]. Sprinkling an affected part with water; a form of hydrotherapy.*

asphalgesia (as-fal-je'zĭ-ă) [G. *asphi*, own, + *algos*, pain]. A burning sensation and convulsions sometimes felt during hypnosis on touching certain articles.

asphyctic, asphyctous (as-fĭk'tĭk, -tŭs) [G. *a-*, priv. + *sphyxis*, pulse]. 1. Asphyxiated. 2. Without pulse.

asphyxia (ăs-fĭk'sĭ-ă) [" + *sphyxis*, pulse]. 1. Suspended animation in living organisms due to interference with the oxygen supply of the blood. 2. Suspension of the pulse beat. 3. Cyanosis due to interference with circulation. May be general or local.

ETIOL: *Extrinsic Causes:* Choking, gas (illuminating, sewer), exhaust gas (principally carbon monoxide), electric shock, drugs, anesthesia, traumatic asphyxia, crushing injuries of chest, also with compression of chest, injury of respiratory nerves or centers, diminution of oxygenation of environment, drowning. Tumors, such as goiter, pharyngeal and retropharyngeal abscesses. *Intrinsic Causes:* Hemorrhage into lungs or pleural cavity, drowning, foreign bodies in throat, swelling of air passages, diseases of air passages, ruptured aneurysm or abscess, edema of the lung, cardiac deficiency. *Other Causes:* Paralysis of the respiratory center, profound anesthesia, pneumothorax, narcotic drugs and electricity.

SYM: Vary somewhat with etiology. In general, cyanosis, cessation of respiration, pallor, lessened temperature.

F. A. TREATMENT: Artificial respiration, *q.v.*

RS: *acarbia, acroasphyxia, artificial respiration, drowning, gases, resuscitation, suffocation.*

a. carbonica. Suffocation from inhalation of coal or water gas.

a. from chloroform, sulfuric ether, etc. Place body in horizontal position, lower head; open windows; loosen clothing; dash cold water on face; shake chest vigorously. Hold ammonia to nostrils. Introduce piece of ice into rectum. These failing, apply galvanic battery, one pole on throat, other over ensiform process, keeping up current several hours in severe cases, or induce artificial respiration.

a. from cold. Place body in cold room, rub with snow or bathe in ice water till limbs become soft and flexible, then place in dry bed, rub briskly with flannel, use artificial respiration. Soon as signs of returning life give injections of clear coffee and by mouth if patient can swallow.

a. from drowning. a. from hanging or choking. Maintain or reëstablish respiratory movements by artificial means. SEE: *artificial respiration.*

a. livida. When there is difficulty in breathing, but the superficial reflexes are present.

a., local. The congested stage of Raynaud's disease.

a. neonatorum. Imperfect breathing in the new born child.

a. from noxious gases. Carbonic acid, carbonic oxide, fumes of burning charcoal, chlorine or sulfuretted hydrogen gas. Expose at once to fresh air, bathe face and breast with vinegar, and inhale vapor. Give strong coffee, apply cold water to head, warmth to feet. Method used in artificial respiration, or apply positive pole of battery to upper part of spine and negative pole on chest over diaphragm.

F. A. TREATMENT: If unconscious, artificial respiration; soothing substances to lining of respiratory passages, as inhalation; warm, humid air; paraffin spray repeatedly.

a. pallida. When difficulty in breathing is accompanied by weak and thready pulse, pale skin, and absence of superficial reflexes. This is the most serious type.

a. from smoke (suffocation from smoke). SYM: Unconsciousness, dyspnea, also irritation of nose, throat and respiratory passages.

a., traumatic. Discoloration of the head and neck due to compression of the trunk. SYM: Lividity, twitching about the face and limbs; dark color of tongue and lips. TREATMENT: (1) Expose at once to fresh air; (2) bathe face and chest with cold cloth or ice; (3) give strong coffee; (4) cold to head and warmth to feet.

asphyx'ial. Pert. to asphyxia; asphyctic.

asphyx'iant. An agent, especially any gas that will produce asphyxia.

asphyx'iate. To cause asphyxiation, or asphyxia.

asphyx'ia″tion [G. *a-*, priv. + *sphyxis*, pulse]. A state of asphyxia or suffocation. Act of producing asphyxia. SEE: *asphyxia*.

aspidium (as-pid'ĭ-um) (Male fern) USP. The dried root of *filix-mas*, used only in form of oleo-resin.
USE: Against intestinal parasites, esp. tape worm. Care should be taken that it is not administered with an oil, since absorption may occur.
DOSAGE: 4 Gm. once daily according to condition of patient.

as'pirate [L. *ad*, to, + *spirāre*, to breathe]. 1. Aspiration; to remove by suction. 2. A sound like that of the letter *h*.

aspiration (as-pir-a'shun). 1. To draw in or out as by suction. Foreign bodies may be aspirated into the nose, throat, or lungs on inspiration. 2. The withdrawing of a fluid from a cavity by means of suction with an instrument called an aspirator.
Cavities most commonly aspirated are: (a) pericardial c., (b) pleural c., (c) theca (lumbar puncture), (d) abscess c.
OBJECT: (1) To remove fluid from an affected area such as pleural effusion, ascites. (2) To obtain specimens, as blood from a vein or serum from the spinal canal.
NECESSARY ARTICLES: (a) Disinfecting solution for the skin. (b) Local anesthetic. (c) Two aspirating needles with the aspirating apparatus as indicated. (d) Utensil for receiving the fluid, also a sterile receptacle for the specimen. (e) Sterile sponges, towels, basins, etc. (f) Sterile gloves. (g) Sterile forceps. (h) Surgical dressings as the case may require. (i) Stimulant ordered if indication arises.
NP: (a) Place patient in a comfortable position. (b) Drape; be sure patient is warm. (c) Have all equipment in order and in readiness for the use of the physician. SEE: *foreign bodies, lumbar puncture*.

aspirator (as'pir-a-tor). 1. Apparatus for evacuating fluid contents of a cavity.
VARIETIES: Piston Pump A, Compressible Rubber Tube A, Rubber Bulb A, Siphon A, Needles and Trocars.
2. Instrument used in chemical analysis of gases.

aspirin (ăs'per-ĭn). Commercial name for acetylsalicylic acid.
DOSAGE: 5 gr. (0.3 Gm.). In large doses it may cause an acidosis which sometimes is fatal. Severe attacks of asthma may result fatally. It is a strong gastric irritant, and can cause vomiting, nausea, and gastric bleeding. It will not affect a 4-dol* pain. One or two tablets are as effective as five or seven. SEE: *dol*.
POISONING: Due to hypersusceptibility or to large doses.
SYM: Weak and rapid pulse. Extremities cold; face and lips livid or cyanotic. Temperature subnormal. Respirations shallow and labored.
F. A. TREATMENT: Empty stomach, keep patient quiet, stimulate with whisky or strong, hot coffee, large volumes of fluid; epinephrine and ephedrine by injections or instillation in the nose from which they are absorbed.

asporogen'ic [G. *a*-, priv. + *sporos*, seed, + *genos*, origin]. Not reproducing by spores.

asporous (ă-spor'us). Having no spores.

assafet'ida, assafoet'ida [L. *asa*, gum, + *foetida*, fetid]. A resinous substance used as a carminative and antispasmodic in hysteria. SEE: *asafetida*.

assana'tion [L. *ad*, to, + *sanare*, heal]. Improvement of sanitary conditions.

assault', crim'inal. Cohabitation without consent is always legal rape, but even with consent, if the victim is insane, it is legally considered rape.

assident (as'ĭd-ent) [L. *assidere*, to sit by]. Usually associated with a disease, as *assident* symptoms.

assimilable (as-sim'il-a-bl) [L. *assimilāre*, to make like]. Capable of assimilation.

assim'ilate. To absorb digested food.

assimila'tion. The processes whereby the products of digestion are changed to resemble the chemical substances of the body tissues, first passing through the lacteals and blood vessels; transformation of food into living tissue.
The types of chemical reactions involved are chiefly hydrolysis and condensation; also deamination, decarboxylation, desaturation, oxidation, and reduction, *q.v.*
Ex: Esp. some of the chemical reactions going on in the liver during and after absorption, namely, the synthesis of glycogen, the formation of serum proteins, and the alteration of fats. SEE: *assimilable, assimilate, metabolism*.

asso'ciated movements. Synchronous correlation of 2 or more muscles (or muscle groups) which, though apparently not essential for the performance of some function, nevertheless, normally accompany it, as the swinging of arms accompanies normal walking.
Associated movements are lost rather characteristically in cerebellar disease.

asso'ciation ar'eas. Small islands in the brain surrounded by cerebral tissue known as motor and sense areas or association areas, as association fibers connect the motor and sense areas.
They are supposed to be plastic, registering individual experiences in the cerebrum, the organ of *associative memory*.

   a. center. One controlling associated movements.

   a., controlled. An idea suggested by a word uttered by the physician.

   a. of ideas. The linking together in a memory chain of two or more ideas, associated by some similarity, relationship, or by both having been experienced at the same time.

   a. neuron. A neuron which transmits impulses from afferent to efferent neurons.

   a. test. The patient is given a word (*stimulus word*) and he replies immediately with another word (*reaction word*) suggested to him by the first. The words chosen and the time taken in responding (*association time*) may be indicative of the patient's mental condition.

assonance (as'o-nans) [L. *assonare*, to respond to]. Abnormal impulse to use alliteration.

assuetude (as'wĕ-tūd) [L. *assuetudō*, be persuaded to.] 1. Becoming habituated to conditions. 2. Acquiring tolerance of a drug until it loses its effect.

as'surin. Complex substance occurring in brain tissue.

astasia (as-ta'sĭ-ā) [G. *a*-, priv. + *stasis*, stand]. Motor incoördination in standing.

   a. abasia. Combined incoördination for standing or walking. PSY: A mental conflict making it difficult to stand or walk without swerving or swaying.

asteatosis (as'te-ă-to'sis) [G. *a*-, priv. + *stear*, tallow, + -*osis*, condition]. Any disease condition in which there is scantiness or absence of the sebaceous secretion.

   a. cutis. A dry, fissured condition of

the skin together with deficient secretion.

ETIOL: Symptomatic form due to senility, constitutional, or local affections which give rise to trophic changes in the nervous system. Local form may be caused by frequent contact with irritants.

TREATMENT: Removal of underlying cause. Locally, oils and fats.

as'ter [G. *astēr*, star]. The stellate rays forming round the dividing centrosome* during mitosis.*

astereognosis (a-ster-e-og-no'sis) [G. *a-*, priv. + *stereos*, solid, + *gnōsis*, recognition]. Inability to recognize objects or forms by touch.

aste'rion [G. *asterion*, starlike]. A craniometric point at junction of occipital, parietal, and temporal bones.

aster'nal [G. *a-*, priv. + *sternon*, chest]. 1. Not connected with the sternum. 2. Having no sternum.

asteroid (as'ter-oid) [G. *astēr*, star, + *eidos*, shape]. Star shaped.

asthenia (as-the'ni-ă) [G. *a-*, priv. + *sthenos*, strength]. Lack or loss of strength; debility. Any weakness, but one esp. originating in muscular or cerebellar disease.

  a., neurocirculatory. A condition due to excessive stimulation of the adrenal-sympathetic system frequently seen in soldiers.

  ETIOL: Hyperactivity of the adrenal glands.

  SYM: Nervous excitation, palpitation, nerve fatigue, absence of mental or psychic phenomena.

  TREATMENT: Adrenal denervation. SEE: *cerebrasthenia, irritable heart*.

asthenic (as-then'ik). Weak; pert. to asthenia.

  a. body type. A thin, more or less tall person with flat chest, accompanied by inferior muscular development, who centers his interest in his inner self. Usually an introvert.* SEE: *pyknic type*.

asthenometer (as-the-nom'ĕ-ter) [G. *astheneia*, weakness, + *metron*, measure]. An instrument for determining loss of strength.

as'thenope [G. *a-*, priv. + *sthenos*, strength, + *opsis*, power of sight]. One affected with weak sight.

astheno'pia. Weakness or tiring of eyes due to fatigue of ciliary muscle or extra-ocular muscles. Painful vision.

  SYM: Pain in or around eyes; headache, usually aggravated by use of eyes for close work; fatigue; vertigo; reflex symptoms, as nausea, twitching of facial muscles, migraine.

  a., accommodative. Refractive errors such as hyperopia and astigmatism.

  a., muscular. Anomalies of external muscles.

  a., nervous. Hysteria and neurasthenia.

  a., photogenous. Excessive or improper illumination.

  a., reflex. Disease in other organs, as nose, sinuses, teeth.

asthenop'ic. Rel. to asthenopia.

asthenox'ia [G. *a-*, priv. + *sthenos*, strength, + *oxygen*]. Deficient oxygenation of waste products.

asthma (az'mă) [G. *asthma*, panting]. Paroxysmal dyspnea accompanied by the adventitious sounds caused by a spasm of the bronchial tubes or due to swelling of their mucous membrane.

No age is exempt but occurs most frequently in childhood or early adult; in males more frequently than in females.

  TREATMENT: Adrenalin hydrochloride or epinephrine injection, removal of allergen causing attacks, hyposensitization, psychotherapy. A new method being propounded is a slow-acting mixture of gelatin and epinephrine injected into the thigh.

  SEE: *anhelitus, asthmatic, Kopp's asthma*.

  a., cardiac. Dyspnea due to heart disease.

  TREATMENT: Upright position, morphine and venesection, if no anemia is present. When acute pulmonary edema sets in, strophanthin or digitalis.

  a. convulsivum, a., bronchial, a., dyspeptic. Asthma due to a nervous reflex.

  a., hay. Hay fever, *q.v.*

  a., renal. Occurring in Bright's disease.

  a., thymic. Due to enlargement of the thymus. The attacks are sudden and may prove fatal (status lymphaticus).

asthmat'ic [L. *asthmaticus*, panting]. Pert. to or of the nature of asthma.

astigmatic (as-tig-mat'ik) [G. *a-*, priv. + *stigma*, point]. Pert. to or afflicted with astigmatism.

astig'matism [" + " + *ismos*, condition of]. Form of ametropia in which refraction of several meridians of eyeball is different, usually due to change in curvature of cornea and lens.

  ETIOL: Congenital or acquired. Images do not properly focus on retina.

  VARIETIES: Simple, compound, mixed.

astigmat'oscope [" + " + *skopein*, to examine]. Instrument which detects and measures astigmatism.

astigmatos'copy. Use of the astigmatoscope.

astigmometer (ah-stig-mom'ĕ-ter) [G. *a-*, priv. + *stigma*, point, + *metron*, measure]. An instrument for measuring astigmatism.

asto'matous, as'tomous [G. *a-*, priv. + *stoma*, opening]. Without mouth or oral aperture.

astragalar (as-trag'ă-lar) [G. *astragalos*, ankle bone]. Pert. to the astragalus.

astragalectomy (as-trag-al-ek'to-mĭ) [" + *ektomē*, excision]. Excision of astragalus.

astragalus (as-trag'al-us). BNA *Talus*. A bone of the foot which articulates with the tibia and fibula above, and with the calcaneum (os calcis) below. The ankle bone. SEE: *sustentaculum*.

astraphobia (as-tra-fo'bĭ-ă) [G. *astrapē*, lightning, + *phobos*, fear]. Anxiety and terror of thunderstorms.

astrict' [L. *astringere*, to contract]. 1. To contract or *constrict*, as the action of an astringent. To *compress*, as an artery in a hemorrhage. 2. To constipate.

astriction (a-strik'shun). Contraction; compression; constriction.

astring'ent [L. *astringere*, to contract]. 1. Styptic. 2. Agent checking secretion of mucous membranes and which contracts and hardens tissues, limiting secretion of glands. Ex: *Tannic or gallic acid, lead, copper, zinc, bismuth, barium and aluminum salts.* SEE: *stypsis, styptic*.

  a. enema. One given to contract intestinal tissue and to provoke subsequent evacuation of worms. SEE: *enema*.

  a., mineral. They coagulate the albumins when applied to wounds or mucous surfaces, protecting them and making healing possible. They also stop bleeding. In the digestive tract they check secretions and lessen peristalsis, creating constipation. They form albuminates by combining with the albumins. Poisonous effects may result from continued use if deposited in the tissues.

astro- [G.]. Prefix: A star or star-shaped.

as′troblast [G. *astron*, star, + *blastos*, germ]. Primitive nerve cell which develops into an astrocyte.

astroblasto′ma [" + " + *ōma*, tumor]. Tumor composed of astroblasts.

as′trocyte [" + " + *kytos*, cell]. 1. Star-shaped cell forming the neuroglia fibers. 2. Star-shaped bone corpuscle.

astrocyto′ma [" + " + *ōma*, tumor]. Tumor formed from astrocytes.

astrog′lia [" + *glia*, glue]. Astrocytes making up neuroglia tissue.

astrokinet′ic motions [" + *kinesis*, motion]. Movements of centrosome.*

astropho′bia [" + *phobos*, fear]. Morbid fear of stars and celestial space.

astrosphere (as′tro-sfēr) [" + *sphaira*, sphere]. Small body in the cytoplasm considered an independent and indispensable cell constituent.

astrostat′ic [" + *statikos*, standing]. Pert. to astrosphere in its resting condition.

Astu′rian rose. Pellagra; a disease characterized by a rosy rash on the body.

astysia (ă-stiz′ĭ-ă) [G. *a-*, priv. + *stasis*, a standing]. An inability to fully (normally) erect the penis.

asurre′nalism [G. *a-*, priv. + L. *sur*, over, + *ren*, kidney, + G. *ismos*, condition of]. Deficient suprarenal function.

asyllabia (ă-sil-a′bĭ-ă) [G. *a-*, priv. + *syllabos*, a collection]. Recognition of letters but not syllables or words.

asy′lum [L. from G. *asylos*, safe from violence]. An institution for the care of those unable to care for themselves, as the infirm, aged, insane, blind.

  a. ear. Bloody tumor of ear found in the insane. SYN: *hematoma auris.**

asymbo′lia [G. *a-*, priv. + *symbolon*, a sign]. Inability to comprehend words, gestures, or any type of symbol; asemia. Sensory aphasia.

asymmetry (ă-sim′et-rĭ) [" + *symmetria*, symmetry]. Lack of symmetry of parts or organs on opp. sides of body.

asymphytous (ă-sim′fĭt-us) [" + *symphysis*, grow together]. Not grown together.

asymptomat′ic [" + *symptōmatikos*, symptom]. Without symptoms.

asyn′chronism [" + *syn*, together, + *chronos*, time, + *ismos*, condition of]. Lack of concurrence in time.

asynclitism (ah-sin′klit-ism) [" + *synklinein*, to lean together]. GYN: An oblique presentation of the fetal head.
  a., Litzmann's. Where the post. parietal bone of the fetal head presents.
  a., Naegele's. Where the ant. parietal bone of the fetal head presents.

asynergia, asynergy (a-sin-er′jĭ-ă, -jĭ) [" + *syn*, together, + *ergon*, work]. Lack of coördination between muscle groups. Movements are in serial order instead of being made together. Seen in cerebellar diseases.

asynesia (a-sin-e′zĭ-ă) [G. *asynesia*, lack of intelligence]. Stupidness.

asyno′dia (a-sin-o′dĭ-ă) [G. *a-*, priv. + *syn*, with, + *odos*, way]. Failure of simultaneity of orgasm in man and woman in coitus.

asynovia (ă-sin-o′vĭ-ă) [" + *syn*, with, + L. *ovum*, egg]. Lack of or insufficient secretion of synovial fluid of a joint.

asystemat′ic [" + *systēma*, arrangement]. Diffuse; not limited to one system or set of organs.

asystole, asystolia (ä-sis′to-le, -to′lĭ-ă) [G. *a-*, priv. + *systellein*, to draw together]. Faulty contraction of ventricles of the heart.

asystolism (ä-sis′tol-izm) [" + " + *ismos*, condition of]. Retention of contents of the right ventricle of the heart seen in last stages of mitral incompetence.

atabrin(e (at′ă-brin). Commercial preparation used in treatment of malaria. USP. SYN: *quinacrine hydrochloride*.
  DOSAGE: 1½ gr. (0.1 Gm.) three times a day for 3 days. SYN: *atebrin*.

atactic (at-ak′tik) [G. *ataktos*, irregular]. Incoordinate, irregular, as muscular incoördination, esp. in aphasia.

atactiform (ă-tak′tĭ-form) [" + L. *forma*, form]. Similar to ataxia.

atactilia (ă-tak-til′ĭ-ă) [G. *a-*, priv. + L. *tactilis*, pert. to touch]. Inability to recognize tactile impressions.

atarax′ia, a′taraxy [" + *taraktos*, disturbed]. Imperturbability.

atavico′sis [L. *atavus*, ancestor, + G. *-osis*, increased]. Intestinal degeneration from eating highly concentrated foods.

atavism (ăt′ă-vĭzm) [" + G. *ismos*, condition of]. 1. Recurrence of characteristics of a remote ancestor, after remaining latent for 1 or more generations. 2. Reappearance, in a descendant, of a disease or abnormality experienced by a remote ancestor. A reversion to an original type.

atavis′tic. Pert. to atavism.*

ataxaphasia (at-aks-ă-fa′zĭ-ă) [G. *ataxia*, lack of order, + *phasis*, speech]. Inability to arrange words in sentences.

ataxaphemia (at-aks-a-fe′mĭ-ă) [" + *phēmē*, speech]. Lacking in lingual coordination.

ataxia (a-taks′i-a). Motor incoördination manifest during a purposive movement by irregularity and lack of precision.
  SEE: *atactiform, ataxiamnesic, ataxic, ataxoadynamia, ataxodynamia, Brauch-Romberg's sym.*
  a., alcoholic. A. seen in drinkers, caused by peripheral neuritis.
  a., autonomic. Incoördination bet. sympathetic and parasympathetic nervous systems.
  a., Briquet's. Hysteria with skin and leg muscle anesthesia.
  a., cerebellar. Muscular incoördination due to cerebellar disease.
  a., choreic. Lack of muscular coördination seen in persons with chorea.
  a., hereditary cerebellar. Disease of late adolescence. ETIOL: Atrophy of cerebellum. SYM: Ataxic gait, hesitating and explosive speech, nystagmus, and sometimes optic neuritis.
  a., hereditary spinal. Friedreich's disease.* Sclerosis of the post. and lateral columns of spinal cord; occurs in children. SYM: Ataxia in lower extremities, extending to upper; paralysis and contractures follow.
  a., hysterical. Ataxia of leg muscles due to hysteria.
  a., infrapsychic. A state in which emotional expressions appear to have no logical bases or relationship, other than those found in the Unconscious.
  a., locomotor. A sclerosis affecting the post. columns of spinal cord, most commonly due to syphilis.
  SYM: Characterized by incoördination, loss of deep reflexes, disturbances of nutrition, of sensation, and various ocular phenomena, with sometimes loss of sexual power, paralysis of sphincters, epileptiform seizures and dementia. In-

ability to control gait or to touch an article with the hand. SEE: *gait*.
TREATMENT: Best hygienic conditions, rest, nutritious diet, excess of all kinds prohibited, constitutional remedies.

a., Marie's. Hereditary cerebellar ataxia.*

a., motor. Lack of ability for proper coördination of muscles.

a., spinal. Due to spinal cord disease, as in locomotor ataxia.*

a., static. Loss of deep sensibility causing inability to preserve equilibrium in standing.

a., thermal. Condition in which body temperature changes irregularly.

a., vasomotor. Form of autonomic ataxia.* ETIOL: Lack of coördination bet. sympathetic and parasympathetic nervous systems in connection with vasomotor phenomena. SYM: Irregularity in peripheral circulation, alternations of pallor and suffusion, due to spasm of smaller blood vessels.

ataxiadynamia (ă-taks'ĭ-ad-ĭ-nam'ĭ-ă) [G. *ataxia*, lack of order, + *a-*, priv. + *dynamis*, might]. Muscular weakness in combination with incoördination.

atax'iagram [" + *gramma*, writing]. Ataxiagraph record or tracing.

ataxiagraph (ă-taks'ĭ-a-graf) [" + *graphein*, to write]. Instrument measuring swaying in ataxia.

ataxiam'eter [" + *metron*, measure]. Apparatus measuring ataxia.

ataxiamnesia (at-aks'ĭ-am-ne'zĭ-ă) [" + *amnēsia*, forgetfulness]. Suffering from muscular ataxia and amnesia.

atax'ic, atax'ial. Pert. to, or marked by, ataxia.

ataxoadynamia (at-aks-o-ă-dĭ-nam'ĭ-ă) [G. *ataxia*, lack of order, + *a-*, priv. + *dynamis*, might]. Ataxia associated with muscular weakness.

ataxophe'mia [" + *phēmē*, speech]. Incoordination of speech muscles.

ataxopho'bia [" + *phobos*, fear]. Morbid dread of ataxia.

a'taxy [G. *ataxia*, lack of order]. Lack of muscular coördination. SYN: ataxia.

-ate. CHEM: Ternary acids, the names of which end in ic, take the ending *ate* to indicate salts formed from them. SEE: *-ide, -ite.*

atebrin(e (at'ĕ-brin). Proprietary drug used to treat malaria.
DOSAGE: 1½ gr. (0.1 Gm.) three times a day for 3 days. SYN: atabrin.

atelectasis (at-e-lek'tă-sis) [G. *atelēs*, imperfect, + *ektasis*, expansion]. Lack of air in the lungs as in a fetus, or in a portion of an adult lung due to pleural effusion exerting pressure, and blocking the small bronchial tubes.

atelia (at-e'lĭ-ă) [G. *ateleia*, incompleteness]. The retention of childish characteristics in the adult.

atelic (at'el-ik). Without function.

ateliosis (ă-tĕ-lĭ-o'sis) [G. *atelēs*, incomplete, + *-osis*, condition]. A form of infantilism due to pituitary causes in which growth may be arrested without deformity. The voice and face may resemble those of a child.

ateliot'ic. Infantile.

atelo-. Prefix: Imperfect development.

athermic, athermous (ă-ther'mĭk, -mus) [G. *a-*, priv. + *thermē*, heat]. Without fever.

athermosystaltic (ath-er-mo-sis-tal'tĭk) [" + " + *systaltikos*, drawing together]. Not contracting under ordinary temperature variations, said of striated muscle.

atheroma (ath-e-ro'mă) [G. *athērē*, porridge, + *ōma*, tumor]. 1. A sebaceous cyst. 2. Fatty degeneration or thickening of the wall of all the larger arteries. SEE: *arteriosclerosis.*

atheromasia (ath-er-o-ma'zĭ-ă). Atheromatous degeneration.

atheromatosis (ath-er-o-mă-to'sis). Generalized atheromatous condition.

atheromatous (ath-er-o'mă-tus). Pert. to atheroma.

atheronecro'sis [G. *athērē*, porridge, + *nekros*, dead, + *-osis*, condition]. Necrosis or degeneration accompanying arteriosclerosis.

atherosclero'sis [" + *sklērōsis*, hardness]. Senile type of arteriosclerosis characterized by atheromatous degeneration of walls of arteries.

athero'sis [" + *-osis*, condition]. Fatty degeneration of arterial walls.

athetoid (ath'e-toid) [G. *athētos*, not fixed, + *eidos*, resemblance]. 1. Similar to athetosis. 2. Affected with athetosis.

athetosis (ath-ĕ-to'sis) [" + *-osis*, condition]. Slow, repeated, involuntary, purposeless, vermicular, muscular distortion involving part of a limb, toes, and fingers or almost the entire body. ETIOL: Brain lesion, chiefly in children.

ath'lete's foot. Infection of skin of foot by *Tinea microsporon* or *T. megalosporon.* SYM: Cracks, redness, minute vesicles, usually bet. toes, causing itching, pain, disability. SEE: *ringworm.*
TREATMENT: Copper, which is highly fungicidal, is passed through the skin by iontophoresis.* Another remedy: Mix 2 parts phenol and 2 parts camphor; paint bet. toes several times a day. *Precaution:* Do not apply to wet skin. Water causes a breakdown in the preparation, resulting in caustic action.

ath'lete's heart. Incompetence of the aortic valves.

athrepsia, athrepsy (a-threps'ĭ-ă, -ĭ) [G. *a-*, priv. + *threpsis*, nourishment]. Malnutrition, marasmus.*

athreptic (ath-rep'tĭk). Marasmic; pert. to or afflicted with athrepsia.

athrom'bia [G. *a-*, priv. + *thrombos*, a clot]. Defective blood clotting.

athymia (ă-thi'mĭ-ă) [" + *thymos*, animation]. 1. Confusional insanity; amentia. 2. Without emotion. 3. Lack of thymus gland or its secretion.

athymic (ath-i'mĭk). Pert. to athymia.

athy'mism [G. *a-*, priv. + *thymos*, animation, + *ismos*, condition of]. Absence of thymus gland or its secretions. SYN: *athymia* (3).

athyrea (a-thi're-ă) [" + *thyreos*, shield]. A condition due to the absence of the thyroid gland or insufficiency, or suppression of its function resulting in imperfect development of the tissues of the body.

athyreo'sis [" + " + *-osis*, increased]. Condition due to absence of thyroid gland or its secretions, causing imperfect development. SYN: *athyria.*

athyria (a-thi'rĭ-ă) [" + *thyreos*, shield]. Absence of thyroid gland or its secretions, causing imperfect development. SYN: *athyrea.*

athy'roide'mia [" + " + *eidos*, form, + *aima*, blood]. Morbid condition of blood due to absence of thyroid gland or its secretions.

athyroidism (ă-thi'roy-dĭzm) [" + " + *ismos*, condition of]. Suppression of thyroid secretions, or absence of the thyroid gland; athyrea. [the atlas.

atlan'tad [G. *atlas*, a support]. Toward

atlan'tal. Pert. to the atlas.

at'las. The first cervical vertebra by which the head articulates with the occipital bone, so called because of Atlas who was supposed to support the world on his shoulders. SEE: *atlantal, atloaxoid.*

atloaxoid (at-lo-aks'oid) [G. *atlas*, a support, + L. *axis*, a pivot, + G. *eidos*, form]. Pert. to atlas and axis.

atmiat'rics, atmi'atry [G. *atmos*, vapor, + *iatreia*, art of healing]. Treatment of respiratory disease by medicated vapors.

atmic (at'mik). Consisting of or pert. to vapor.

atmo- [G.]. Prefix: Breath, vapor, steam.

atmocau'sis [G. *atmos*, steam, + *kausis*, burning]. Application of superheated steam; substitute for uterine curettage.

atmocautery (at-mo-kaw'ter-ĭ) [G. *atmos*, steam, + *kausis*, burning] Device for cauterization with steam.

atmograph (at'mo-graf) [" + *graphein*, to write]. A spirograph. Device for tracing respiratory movements.

atmometer (at-mom'e-ter) [" + *metron*, measure]. Instrument for measuring exhalations.

at'mos [G. *atmos*, air]. A unit of air pressure; one dyne for one sq. cc.

at'mosphere [" + *sphaira*, sphere]. 1. The gases surrounding the earth to the height of 200 miles. 2. Climatic condition of a locality. 3. PHYSICS: Pressure at sea level of the atmosphere—14.7 lbs. to the sq. in. 4. CHEM: Any gaseous medium around a body.

atmospher'ic. Pert. to the atmosphere.

atmospheriza'tion. Process of transforming venous into arterial blood.

atmother'apy [G. *atmos*, air, + *therapeia*, treatment]. 1. Treatment of disease by medicated vapors. SYN: *atmiatrics.** 2. Treatment by some method of condensing air.

atocia (at-o'sĭ-ă) [G. *a-*, priv. + *tokos*, birth]. Female sterility.

at'om [G. *atomos*, indivisible]. The smallest particle of an element that can exist and take part in a chemical change, retaining its identity, and which cannot further be divided without change of its structure.

Over 90 odd different atoms have been recognized, which in combination with one another or others like themselves make up all the various types of matter that we know. These atoms are themselves composed of still smaller particles called *electrons** and *protons.** Dimensions of atoms are of the order of 10^{-8} centimeters. SEE: *atomic theory, electron theory.*

atom'ic. Pert. to an atom or atoms.

atom'ic the'ory. Formulated by Dalton, who taught that all matter is composed ultimately of atoms.

atom'ic weight. The weight of different atoms as compared with that of *hydrogen*, which is the lightest, and is represented as 1. The heaviest known is that of *uranium*. Oxygen is 16.

atomicity (at-om-is'ĭ-tĭ). 1. Chemical valence or combining power. 2. Number of hydroxyl groups in an alcohol, or in a base.   [of a spray.

atomiza'tion. Converting a fluid into form

a'tomize. To reduce a liquid to the form of a spray or a vapor.

atomizer (at'om-i-zer). Apparatus for changing jet of liquid to a spray.

atonic (a-ton'ik) [G. *a-*, priv. + *tonos*, strength]. Without tension or tone.

atonicity (at-ō-nĭs'ĭ-tĭ). State of being atonic, or without tone.   [mal tone.

atony (at'o-nĭ). Debility; or lack of nor-

a., gastric. Lack of muscle tone in stomach and failure to contract normally, causing slow movement of food out of stomach. Secondary to certain diseases. DIET: Small feedings at frequent intervals; soft foods; little fat. Avoid bulky foods and those requiring much mastication.

at'open [G. *a-*, priv. + *topos*, place]. An allergen, exciting cause of any form of idiosyncrasy or hypersensitiveness.

atophan (ă'to-fan). Analgesic and antipyretic drug. SEE: *cinchophen.*

DOSAGE: 8 gr. (0.5 Gm.).   [placed.

atop'ic. Pert. to atopy.* Displaced; mis-

atopognosis (at-o-pog-nō'sis) [G. *a-*, priv. + *topos*, place, + *gnōsis*, knowledge]. An inhibited sense of touch or feeling, the victim not being able to know where one has touched his skin.

atopomenorrhea (at-op-o-men-or-e'ă) [" + *mēn*, month, + *roia*, flow]. Periodic hemorrhage from any part of the female body other than the uterus; vicarious menstruation.

at'opy. 1. Hereditary allergic disease. 2. The many forms of hypersensitivity or idiosyncrasies.   [Nonpoisonous.

atox'ic [G. *a-*, priv. + *toxikon*, poison].

ATP. Abbr. for *adenosine-5-Triphosphate.* Made up of sugar, adenine, nitrogen, and phosphorus, from which adenylic acid is derived. The breakdown of ATP provides the energy for muscle contraction and possibly many other physiological processes.   [Melancholic.

atrabil'iary [L. *atra*, black, + *bilis*, bile].

a. capsules. Suprarenal capsules.

atremia (at-re'mĭ-ă) [G. *a-*, priv. + *tremein*, to tremble]. Absence of trembling or tremor.

atrepsy (ă'trep-sĭ) [" + *threpsis*, nutrition]. Immunity to tumor cells.

atre'sia [" + *trēsis*, a perforation]. Pathological closure of a normal anatomical opening or congenital absence of the same, esp. that of the esophagus. Term also applied to the retrogression and disappearance of follicles in the mammalian ovary.

atre'sic. Imperforate; pert. to atresia.

atretogastria (ă-tret-o-gas'trĭ-a) [G. *atrētos*, imperforate, + *gaster*, stomach]. Gastric imperforation.

atreturethria (ă-tret-u-re'thrĭ-ă) [" + *ourēthra*, urethra]. Urethral imperforation.

atrichia (ă-trik'ĭ-ă) [G. *a-*, priv. + *thrix*, hair]. Absence of hair.

atrichosis (ă-tri-ko'sis) [" + " + *-osis*, increased]. Having no hair, atrichia.*

atri'chous. Being without flagella.

atrionector (a"trĭ-o-nek'tor) [L. *atrium*, corridor, + *nector*, connector]. Sinoauricular node of Keith.*

at'riotome [" + *tomē*, cutting]. Instrument which cuts connections between the cardiac auricle and ventricle.

atrioventric'ular [" + *ventriculus*, belly]. Pert. to both auricle and ventricle.

atriplicism (ă-trip'lĭ-sizm). Poisoning due to eating one form of spinach, *At'riplex littora'lis.* SEE: *allantiasis.*

a'trium (Pl. *a'tria*) [L. *atrium*, corridor]. A cavity or sinus.

Atrium. A cavity or sinus.

a. ear (of). Portion of the tympanic cavity lying below the malleus; the tympanic cavity proper.

a. heart (of). The upper chamber of each half of the heart. The right atrium receives deoxygenated purple blood from the entire body (except lungs) through the sup. and inf. vena cavae and coronary sinus; the left atrium receives oxygenated red blood from the lungs through the pulmonary veins. Blood passes from the atria to the ventricles through the atrioventricular orifices. In the embryo the atrium is a single chamber which lies between the sinus venosus and the ventricle.

a. infection (of). Site of entrance of bacteria causing an infectious disease.

a. lungs (of). The space at the end of an alveolar duct which opens into the alveoli or air sacs of the lungs.

atro'phia [G.]. Wasting of a part from lack of nutrition. SYN: atrophy.

atrophic (a-tro'fik) [G. *a-*, priv. + *trophē*, nourishment]. Pert. to, or marked by, atrophy. [with atrophy.

atrophied (ă'tro-fēd). Wasted. Afflicted

atrophoderma (ăt-rō-fō-der'mă) [G. *a-*, priv. + *trophē*, nourishment, + *derma*, skin]. Cutaneous atrophy.

a. pigmentosum. Rare skin disease characterized by ulcers, disseminated pigment discolorations, etc. SYN: *xeroderma pigmentosum, q.v.*

atrophodermato'sis [" + " + " + *-osis*, increased]. Any skin disease which has atrophied skin as a sym.

at'rophy. A wasting due to lack of nutrition of any part.

ETIOL: Disuse, disease, injury to trophic nerve centers in spinal cord, or interference with nerve or blood supply.

a., acute yellow. Extensive degeneration of liver cells with jaundice, mental disturbances, and cutaneous hemorrhages.

SYM: Early nervous symptoms before jaundice sets in; slow onset; some fever with nausea and vomiting; black vomit; malaise. Leucine and tyrosine in urine.

NEUR: It obtains in pathologic conditions of the ant. horns of the spinal cord as in destruction of or injury to the peripheral nerves or as in poliomyelitis.* Not common in disease of the cerebrum.

a., Buchwald's. Progressive wasting of the skin. [causing a.

a., compression. Compression of a part

a., correlated. Wasting of a part following destruction of another part.

a., Cruveilhier's. Progressive wasting of the muscles.

a. of disuse. A. from failure to normally use a part.

a., Hoffman's. Progressive muscular wasting, in the legs, hands and forearms.

a., idiopathic muscular. Progressive a. affecting muscle groups and due to muscular changes, developing in early life. SYM: The muscles, esp. those of the face, shoulders, thighs, buttocks, and calves, lose power and waste. In Erb's juvenile type the atrophy begins in shoulders; in Landouzy-Dejerine's type, in the face. PROG: Unfavorable. Incurable but of slow progress.

a., Landouzy-Dejerine. Muscular wasting in face and scapulohumeral area.

a., muscular. Muscular wasting.

a., progressive muscular. Chronic disease marked by progressive wasting of the muscles and paralysis, beginning with the extremities and ultimately causing death from paralysis of muscles of respiration. SYN: *poliomyelitis, chronic anterior; palsy, wasting.*

a., trophoneurotic. Wasting due to disease of the nerves or nerve centers.

a., unilateral facial. Progressive a. of the facial tissues on one side only.

a., white. Wasting of nerve, leaving only white connective tissue.

atrophy, words pert. to: anatrophic, atrophic, auantic, cataplasia, claw-foot, claw-hand, macies, trophoneurosis, wasting palsy.

atrop'ic [G. *a-*, priv. + *tropē*, turn]. Displaced.

a'tropine sul'fate. USP. The salt of an alkaloid obtained from belladonna.

ACTION AND USES: Respiratory and circulatory stimulant, also used to overcome spasm of involuntary muscles, to check secretion, locally for its effects on the eye—externally as local anodyne.

DOSAGE: $1/_{120}$ gr. (0.0005 Gm.)

Atropine is used to dilate pupils before testing eyes for glasses, to relieve muscle spasm, and for many other systemic effects.

POISONING: SYM: Nervousness and excitability. Patient may be delirious. Face flushed, pupils widely dilated, throat dry, great thirst, and difficulty in swallowing, skin flushed and dry, delirium.

F. A. TREATMENT: Empty stomach with stomach pump rather than emetics. Precipitate by introducing tannic acid by the stomach tube, or use a dilute solution of iodine. These must be washed out. Ice caps to the head. Finely divided charcoal should be given to delay its absorption. Pilocarpine is a physiologic antagonist and is sometimes helpful.

In depressant stage, caffeine and artificial respiration should be used. SEE: *atropinism, atropinization, atropinize.*

at'ropinism, at'ropism. Atropine poisoning.

atropiniza'tion. Production of physiologic effect of atropine.

at'ropinize. To bring under the influence of atropine.

atten'tion [L. *attendere*, wait upon]. Power to focus on some phase of consciousness including some aspect of the world of reality.

a. reflex. Change in size of pupil when attention is suddenly fixed. SYN: *Piltz's reflex.*

atten'uant [L. *attenuāre*, to thin]. 1. Diluting, making thin or weak. 2. An agent that thins the blood.

attenuate. To render thin; or make less virulent.

atten'uated. 1. Diluted. 2. Pert. to reduced virulence of pathogenic microorganism.

a. virus. One made less virulent.

attenua'tion. 1. Dilution. 2. Dynamization. 3. Lessening of virulence.

at'tic [G. *attikos*, upper part]. Upper portion of tympanic cavity above tympanic membrane.

a. disease. Chronic suppurative inflammation of attic.

attici'tis [" + *-itis*, inflammation]. Inflammation of tympanic attic.

atticoantrot'omy [" + *antron*, antrum, + *tomē*, cutting]. Operation to remove contents of the attic and mastoid antrum.

atticot'omy [" + *tomē*, a cutting]. Surgical opening of tympanic attic.

at'titude(s [L. *attitūdō*, posture]. Bodily posture(s), esp. the stereotype seen in catatonia* and the theatric expression often seen in hysteria.

a. of combat. The rigid, defensile attitude of the corpse, due to contractions caused by fear, fire, etc.

a., crucifixion. Body rigid with arms at right angles, seen in conditions of hysteroepilepsy.

a., defense. Position automatically assumed to avert pain.
a., forced. Abnormal position due to disease or contractures.
a., frozen. Stiffness of gait, seen in amyotrophic lateral sclerosis.
a., illogical. Peculiar attitudes caused by disease, esp. hysteroepilepsy.
a., passional, a., passionate. Theatric or dramatic gestures and expressions of face and figure assumed by hysteric patients.
a., stereotyped. Position taken and held for a long period, seen frequently in mental diseases.
attol'lens [L. *attolere*, to lift up]. Raising or lifting up.
attrac'tion [L. *attractiō*, to draw toward]. Tendency of particles to approach each other.
a., capillary. The force by which liquids rise in fine tubes, or through pores of loose material.
attrahens (at-ra'hens) [L. *attrahere*, draw toward]. Drawing forward, as a muscle.
attrax'in. Hypothetical substance in solutions supposed to exert chemotactic influence on certain body cells.
attrition (at-rish'un) [L. *attritiō*, a rubbing against]. 1. A chafing or abrasion. 2. Any friction that breaks the skin.
atylosis (at-ĭ-lo'sĭs) [G. *a-*, priv. + *tylōsis*, a callus]. Nontypical tuberculosis.
atyp'ical [" + *typikos*, conformed to a type]. Deviating from the normal.
Au. Symb. for gold (*aurum*).
A. u. or Å. Abbr. for Angström's unit.
auantic (aw-an'tik) [G. *auantikos*, wasted]. Wasted away. SYN: *atrophic*.
au'digram [L. *audire*, to hear, + G. *gramma*, drawing]. Chart of variations of acuteness of hearing.
audile (aw'dil). 1. Pert. to hearing. 2. Ear-minded. 3. PSY: One whose mental images are auditory. SEE: *visile* and *motile*.
audiogram (aw'dĭ-o-gram) [L. *audire*, to hear, + G. *gramma*, drawing]. Record of the audiometer.
audiom'eter [" + G. *metron*, measure]. A delicate instrument for testing hearing, consists of a thermoionic tube circuit in which the tube is placed into oscillation. By varying the electrical constants of the circuit, one may make the emitted tone assume various pitches.
audiom'etry. Testing of the hearing sense.
audiphone (aw'dĭ-fon) [L. *audire* + G. *phōnē*, voice]. Instrument for conveying sound to auditory nerve through the teeth or a bone.
audi'tion [L. *auditiō*, hearing]. Hearing.
a., colored. Color sensation is perceived when certain sounds reach ear.
a., mental. The recollection of a sound based on previous auditory impressions.
a., m. verbal. Mental a., the sounds being words.
auditive (aw'di-tiv). One who is auditory minded, depending upon hearing in learning, or recall.
au"ditogno'sis (aw'dĭtog-no'sis) [L. *auditiō*, hearing, + *gnōsis*, knowledge]. 1. Understanding and interpretation of sounds. 2. Diagnosis by percussion and auscultation.
aud"itooc"ulogy'ric reflex. The sudden turning of the head and eyes in direction of an alarming sound.
aud'itory. Pert. to the sense of hearing.
a. canal (*meatus acusticus externus*). 1. The external canal, about 2.5 cm. from the concha to the tympanic membrane. 2. The internal canal from posterior surface of petrous portion of temporal bone to internal ear.
a. nerve (*n. acusticus*). The 8th pair of cranial nerves; it is a sensory nerve with two sets of fibers: (a) cochlear n. (of hearing), and (b) vestibular n. (of equilibrium), the latter having three branches, the sup., inf., and middle br.
a. reflex. Blinking of the eyes upon the sudden unexpected production of a sound.
a., m. verbal. Mental a., the sounds being words. [cochlea.
a. teeth. Toothlike projections in the
a. tube. Eustachian tube, *q.v.*
aud'itus. The power or the sense of hearing.
Auenbrugger's sign (ow'en-broog-er's). Epigastric prominence due to marked pericardial effusion.
Auerbach's plexus. A plexus of sympathetic nerve fibers situated bet. the longitudinal and circular fibers of the muscular coat of the stomach and intestines. Also called the *plexus myentericus*.
Auer's bodies. Rodlike bodies in lymphocytes in leukemia.
Aufrecht's sign (owf'rekht's). Diminished breathing sound heard above the jugular notch in tracheal stenosis.
augment (aug'ment) [L. *augmentum*, increase]. 1. To add to or increase. 2. The increasing stage of a fever, or of an acute disease.
augmen'tor. Increasing.
a. nerves. Those increasing force and rapidity of the heartbeat.
aula (aw'lă) [G. *aulē*, hall]. Ant. part of third ventricle.
aulatela (aw-lă'tĕ-lă) [" + *tela*, web]. Membrane covering the aula.
auliplex'us [" + L. *plectere*, to twist]. Aulic part of choroid plexus.
aulix (aw'liks) [G. *aulix*, furrow]. Monro's sulcus.
au'ra [L. *aura*, breeze]. The preëpileptic phenomenon.
Visual sensation of fire is rather characteristic but sound, sense of movement of a part, or even dream states known as intellectual aurae, occur. A hysterical "attack" may present a similar phenomenon at its onset.
aural (aw'ral) [L. *auris*, the ear]. 1. Pert. to the ear. 2. Pert. to an aura.
auranti'asis [L. *aurantium*, orange]. Yellowish skin color due to eating large quantities of oranges.
auran'tium [L.]. Orange.
aureomycin. A golden-color antibiotic from the *Actinomycetes*, a species of the genus *Streptomyces*, or *S. aureofaciens*. The best all-round of the mold extracts, except for tuberculosis and typhoid. An effective agent in peritonitis.
USES: Effective on viruses. Lymphogranuloma venereum, psittacosis, typhus, rickettsial pox, spotted fever, external infections of the eye.
auric (aw'rik) [L. *aurum*, gold]. Pert. to gold (*aurum*).
auricle, auricula (aw'rik-l, -u-la) [L. *auricula*, the ear] (BNA). 1. The external ear; pinna or flap. 2. (atrium, BNA).
(1) The protruding portion of the external ear which surrounds the opening of the external acoustic meatus; the pinna. (2) A small conical pouch forming a portion of the right and left atria of the heart. Each projects from the upper anterior portion of each

atrium. (3) A term commonly used erroneously for the atrium.
The right auricle receives the venous (purple) blood from the entire body through the vena cava and the left auricle receives the arterial (red) blood from the lungs through the pulmonary veins.

auric′ular. 1. Rel. to the auricle of the ear. 2. Pert. to the auricles of the heart and its nerves and arteries.
SEE: *polyotia.*

  a. fibrillation. Irregular and rapid contractions of the auricles working independently of the ventricles. Instead of the contraction beginning at the sinoauricular node and being conducted along the bundle of His, to the ventricles, there is a rapid succession of beats at the auricles. Contraction of the auricular muscle causes the waves to pass round and round the auricle. There is no auricular diastole or auricular heartbeat.
  ETIOL: Degeneration of cardiac muscle. Occurs in late stages of mitral disease of heart, after strain of the degenerated cardiac muscle, and in acute rheumatism in children.
  TREATMENT: Digitalis or quinidine.

  a. ventricular tract. A neuromuscular bundle of nerve fibers which pass as the bundle of His* from the right auricle into the ventricle. SEE: *pulse and heart.*

auricula′re (Pl. *auricula′ria*). A craniometric point at center of opening of external auditory canal.

auric″ulocer′vical nerve re′flex. Congestion of ear on same side resulting from stimulation of distal end of divided auriculocervical nerve.

auric″ulopalpe′bral re′flex. Closure of an eye resulting from stimulation by heat or some tactile irritant on the ext. auditory meatus or deeper portions of canal up to the tympanum. SYN: *Kisch's reflex.*

auriculoventric′ular [L. *auricula*, the ear, + *ventriculus*, belly]. Pert. to both auricle and ventricle. SYN: *atrioventricular.*

  a. bundle. A fascicular bundle which forms part of the myocardium, and is made up of the bundle of His,* Tawara's node,* and the Purkinje network.*

auriform (aw′ri-form) [L. *auris*, ear, + *forma*, shape]. Ear shaped.

auriginous (aw-rij′in-us) [L. *auriginosis*, golden]. Pert. to jaundice.

aurilave (au′ri-lāv) [L. *auris*, ear, + *lavāre*, to wash]. An apparatus for cleansing the ear.

auripuncture (aw′ri-punk-tur) [" + *punctura* puncture]. Puncture of tympanic membrane.

auris (aw′ris) [L.]. The ear.

au′riscalp, auriscal′pium [L. *auris*, ear, + *scalpere*, to scrape]. 1. Scraping instrument to remove foreign matter from ear. 2. Earpick.

auriscope (aw′ris-kop) [" + G. *skopein*, to view]. Instrument for making an aural examination.

aurist (aw′rist). Ear specialist. SYN: *otologist.*

auris′tics. Art of treating ear diseases.

auristil′lae [L.]. Ear drops.

aurococcus (aw″ro-kok′us) [L. *aurum*, gold, + G. *kokkos*, berry]. Pyogenic microbe forming golden cultures found in boils, abscesses, carbuncles, pyemia, etc. SYN: *Staphylococcus pyogenes aureus.*

aurometer (aw-rom′et-er) [L. *auris*, ear, + G. *metron*, measure]. Instrument which measures hearing of each ear.

aurother′apy [L. *aurum*, gold, + G. *therapeia*, treatment]. Treatment of disease by adm. of gold salts.

aurum (aw′rum) [L.]. Gold.

auscult′, aus′cultate [L. *auscultāre*, listen to]. To examine by auscultation.

auscultation (aws-kul-ta′shun). Process of listening for sounds produced in some of the body cavities, esp. chest and abdomen, in order to detect or judge some abnormal condition.
  INSTRUMENTS: Stethoscope or phonendoscope.
  PROCEDURE: (Immediate a.): The chest should have some soft, thin covering which will not interfere with the transmission of sound or itself produce sound from the movements of the thoracic walls to which it is applied. A soft towel answers well. When chest is covered with hair moisten later as otherwise it will produce friction sounds, resembling rales. Auscult all over chest anteriorly and posteriorly, on full inspiration, full expiration, and after coughing. In comparing the two sides auscult symmetrical parts. Parts should be in perfect repose. Position of examiner as unrestrained as possible, lest sounds of his own blood vessels be confused with sounds from within the subject.

  a., immediate. When ear is applied directly to bared or thinly covered surface.

  a., mediate. When sounds are conducted from the surface to ear through an instrument.

auscultation, words pert. to: abdominal a., aegophony, auscult, auscultatory, bruissement, bruit, cat's purr, chest, egophony, frolement, heart, lung, percussion, râles, souffle, uterus, vocal resonance.

auscul′tatory. Pert. to auscultation.

  a. percussion. Auscultation at the same time percussion is made.

auscultoplec′trum [L. *auscultāre*, listen to, + G. *plēktron*, hammer]. Instrument used for both auscultation and percussion.

autacoid (aw′ta-koyd) [G. *autos*, self, + *akos*, remedy]. Any chemical substance which is produced normally by chemical reactions within a given tissue, is released into the blood, and affects the activity of some remote tissue whither it is carried.
  Thus during digestion the autacoid *secretin** is formed in the mucosa of the duodenum, is carried in the blood to the pancreas, where it causes secretion. An autacoid (excitatory a.) which can thus excite activity is called a *hormone;** if it depresses activity (inhibitory a.) it is called a *chalone.**

autarcesiology (aw-tar-sē-sī-ol′o-jī) [" + *arkein*, to protect, + *logos*, study]. Branch of immunology pert. to autarcesis.

autarcesis (aw-tar′sē-sis). Resistance to infection through natural immunity.

autarcetic (aw-tar-set′ik). Pert. to autarcesis.

autechoscope (aw-teck′os-kop) [G. *autos*, self, + *echos*, sound, + *skopein*, to inspect]. Instrument for auto-auscultation.

autemesia (aw-tem-e′sī-ă) [" + *emēsis*, vomiting]. Vomiting without apparent cause.

autism (aw'tizm) [" + *ismos*, condition of]. Psy: Mental introversion in which the attention or interest is fastened upon the victim's own ego. A self-centered mental state from which reality tends to be excluded.

autistic (aw-tĭst'ĭk). 1. Self-centered. 2. Daydreaming; phantasy of wish fulfillment.

auto- [G.]. Prefix: Self, as *autoinfection*.

autoactiva'tion [G. *autos*, self, + L. *activus*, acting]. Gland activation by its own secretion.

autoagglutina'tion [" + L. *agglutināre*, adhere to]. Blood corpuscle agglutination of an individual by his own serum.

autoanal'ysis [" + *analyein*, break down]. Patient's own analysis of mental state underlying his mental disorder.

autoan'tibody [" + *anti*, against, + O. E. *bodig*, body]. Antibody acting against products of one in whom it is formed.

autoantitox'in [" + " + *toxikon*, poison]. Antitoxin produced by body itself.

autoau'dible [" + L. *audire*, to hear]. Audible to oneself; pert. to sounds produced in one's own body.

au'toblast [" + *blastos*, germ]. Independent cell, as a bacterium.

autocatalysis (aw-to-kat-al'ĭs-ĭs) [" + *katalyein*, to dissolve]. Production of substances by enzymes which increase their activity.

autocath'eterism [" + *katheterismos*, a letting down into]. Passage of the catheter upon oneself.

autochthonous (aw-tok'tho-nus) [" + *chthōn*, earth]. Found where developed.

a. ideas. Ideas which compel attention, which are not in harmony with one's character, and which arise spontaneously, including auditory hallucinations.

autocinesia, autocinesis (aw-to-sin-e'sĭ-ă, -e'sis) [" + *kinēsis*, motion]. Voluntary movement.

autoclasis (aw'tok'lă-sis) [" + *klasis*, a breaking]. Destruction of a part from internal causes.

autoclave (aw'to-klave) [" + L. *clavis*, a key]. Apparatus for sterilization by steam under 20 lb. per sq. in. at 260° F.

autocondensa'tion [" + L. *con*, together, + *densāre*, to make thick]. A method of applying high frequency currents for therapeutic purposes.

autoconduc'tion [" + L. *con*, together, + *ductere*, lead]. A method, formerly much in vogue in France, of administering high frequency currents.

autocys'toplasty [" + *kystis*, bladder, + *plassein*, to mold]. Plastic repair of bladder with grafts from patient's own body.

autocytolysin (aw-to-sī-tol'ĭ-sin) [" + *kytos*, cell, + *lysis*, dissolution]. Agent destroying erythrocytes. Syn: *autolysin*.

autocytolysis (aw-to-sī-tol'ĭ-sis) [" + " + *lyein*, break down]. Self-digestion or self-destruction of cells.

autoder'mic [" + *derma*, skin]. Pert. to one's own skin, esp. rel. to dermatoplasty,* with patient's own skin.

autodiagno'sis [" + *dia*, through, + *gignoskein*, to know]. Diagnosis of one's own disease.

autodiges'tion [" + L. *dis*, apart, + *gerere*, to carry]. Self digestion. Syn: *autopepsia*.

autodrain'age [" + A. S. *drēhnigean*, strain]. Drainage of a cavity by sending the fluid through a channel made in patient's own tissues.

autoecholalia (aw"to-ek-o-la'lĭ-ā) [" + *echō*, echo, + *lalia*, babble]. Repetition of words of one's own statements.

autoecic (aw-te'sik) [" + *oikos*, house]. Pert. to parasite always infesting the same organism.

autoerot'ic [" + *erōtikos*, relating to love]. Attracted sexually to oneself.

autoerot'icism [" + " + *ismos*, condition of]. Self-love sexually, apart from masturbation. Syn: *autoerotism*.

autoerotism (aw"tō-ĕr-ŏt'izm) [" + " + *ismos*, condition of]. The spontaneous generation of sexual emotion in the absence of an external stimulus, normally or abnormally, and apart from masturbation. See: *eroticism*.

autofundoscope (aw-to-fŭn'do-skōp) [" + L. *fundus*, bottom, + G. *skopein*, to examine]. Apparatus for autoexamination of eye vessels about macular region.

autogenesis (aw-to-jen'ĕ-sis) [" + *genesis*, production]. Abiogenesis; self-production; spontaneous generation.

autogenetic (aw-to-jen-et'ĭk). Pert. to self-production or autogenesis.

autogenic (aw-to-jen'ĭk). Rel. to self production. Syn: *autogenetic*.

autogenous (aw-toj'en-us). 1. Self-producing. 2. Originating within the body. 3. Denoting a vaccine from a culture of bacteria from the patient who is to be inoculated with it.

a. vaccines. Culture infected material from lesion and isolate the organism present in largest numbers. Subculture this. Wash these cultures into a physiological saline solution. Add phenol as preservative. Sterilize.

Dosage: 0.1 cc. initial dose subcutaneously. Increase 0.1 to 0.2 cc. each dose at three-day intervals to 1 to 2 cc. per dose according to the reaction obtained.

au'tograft [G. *autos*, self, + L. *graphium*, knife]. A graft taken from one part of a person's body to fill in another part.

autog'raphism [" + *graphein*, to write]. Nervous state in which tracings made upon the skin leave wheals.

autohem'ic [" + *aima*, blood]. Done with one's own blood.

autohemol'ysin [" + *aima*, blood, + *lysis*, dissolution]. Antibody acting on corpuscles of individual in whose blood it is formed.

autohemol'ysis. Hemolysis of a person's blood corpuscles by his own serum.

autohemother'apy [G. *autos*, self, + *aima*, blood, + *therapeia*, treatment]. Treatment by withdrawal and injection of patient's own blood.

autoimmuniza'tion [" + L. *immunis*, safe]. Immunization produced by an attack of the disease.

autoinfec'tion [" + L. *inficere*, to dye]. Infection by bacteria present within one's own body.

autoinfu'sion [" + L. *in*, into, + *fundere*, to pour]. Forcing blood from extremities to body by applying Esmarch bandages.

autoinocula'tion [" + L. *inoculāre*, to ingraft]. Secondary infection from disease focus already present in body.

au'tointoxica'tion [" + L. *in*, into, + G. *toxikon*, poison]. A condition produced by poisonous products set free within the body. See: *autotyphization*.

Erroneously thought to be poisoning due to faulty digestive processes. See: *food poisoning, intoxication*.

autokinesis (aw-to-kĭn-ē'sis) [" + *kinesis*, motion]. Voluntary action.

autokinet'ic. Being able to move voluntarily.

autolesion (aw-to-le'shun) [G. *autos*, self, + L. *laedere*, to wound]. Injury self-inflicted.

autolysate (aw-tol'ĭ-sāt) [" + *lysis*, solution]. Specific product of autolysis.

autolysin (aw-tol'ĭ-sin). Agent in serum destroying erythrocytes.

autol'ysis. The self-solution or self-digestion which occurs in tissues or cells by ferment in the cells themselves, even after death and in the absence of putrefactive bacteria.

autolyt'ic. Rel. to autolysis. SEE: *enzymes.*

automat'ic [G. *automatos*, self acting]. Spontaneous; involuntary.

autom'atin. Hypothetical heart substance which is supposed to be the natural excitant of the heartbeat.

automatin'ogen [G. *automatos*, self acting, + *gennan*, to produce]. Heart substance which is activated into automatin.

automatism (aw-tom'ă-tizm) [" + *ismos*, condition of]. Automatic actions or behavior without conscious purpose or knowledge.

The subject, though amnesic, appears normal to an observer but the "real" personality is "latent," during a secondary state or period of automatism, usually a hysterical trance. The patient is not responsible for his acts and must not be left for a second. He may carry out complicated acts without any idea of them and any after memory.

automat'ograph [" + *graphein*, to write]. Instrument which records automatic movements.

automysopho'bia [G. *autos*, self, + *mysos*, dirt, + *phobos*, fear]. Morbid dread of personal uncleanliness.

autonephrec'tomy [" + *nephros*, kidney, + *ektomē*, excision]. Ureteral stricture, completely closing it.

autonomic (aw-to-nom'ĭk) [" + *nomos*, law]. Spontaneous, self-controlling.

SEE: *autonomous, autonomy, autopathy.*

a. nervous system. A part of the nervous system which is concerned with control of involuntary bodily functions. It controls function of glands, smooth muscle tissue and the heart. It is commonly defined so as to include the *sympathetic* or *thoracolumbar* division and the *parasympathetic* or *craniosacral* division.

THE SYMPATHETIC SYSTEM, which includes: The paired ganglionated sympathetic trunk, its connections (*rami communicantes*) with the thoracic and lumbar parts of the spinal cord, the large and small splanchnic nerves, and certain ganglia in the abdomen (e. g., the mesenteric ganglia).

THE PARASYMPATHETIC SYSTEM (or autonomic system proper): Certain fibers of some cranial nerves such as the motor fibers of the vagus. Other fibers connected with the sacral part of the spinal cord.

It is best to use the word "autonomic" only in connection with efferent fibers; sensory fibers coming from the viscera and passing through the above named ganglia and trunks to reach the cord may be called "visceral afferents."

GENERAL FUNCTIONS OF THE AUTONOMIC SYSTEM: 1. Stimulating sympathetic fibers usually produces vasoconstriction in the part supplied, general rise in blood pressure, erection of the hairs, gooseflesh, pupillary dilation, secretion of small quantities of thick saliva, depression of gastrointestinal activity, and acceleration of the heart. 2. Stimulating parasympathetic nerves generally produces vasodilation of the part supplied, general fall in blood pressure, contraction of the pupil, copious secretion of thin saliva, increased gastrointestinal activity, and slowing of the heart. SEE: *autonomotropic, nervous system.*

auton'omin. A hormone supposed to correlate endocrine gland activity, inhibiting or stimulating secretions of each according to systemic need.

autonomotrop'ic [G. *autos*, self, + *nomos*, law, + *tropēa*, turning]. Drawn to the autonomic nervous system.

auton'omous. Independent of external influences.

auton'omy. Functional independence.

autop'athy [G. *autos*, self, + *pathos*, disease]. A disease originating without apparent external cause.

autopep'sia [" + *peptein*, to digest]. Digestion by self, as of gastric wall by its own secretion.

autopha'gia, autoph'agy [" + *phagein*, to eat]. Biting oneself.

autophil (aw'to-fĭl) [" + *philein*, to love]. Person having sensitive autonomic nervous system.

autophilia (aw-to-fĭl'ĭ-ă). Narcissism, *q.v.* Self-love.

autophobia (aw-to-fo'bĭ-ă) [G. *autos*, self, + *phobos*, fear]. 1. A psychoneurotic fear of being alone. 2. Abnormal fear of being egotistical.

autophonia (aw-to-fo'nĭ-ă) [" + *phonos*, murder]. Suicide.

autophony (aw-tof'on-ĭ) [" + *phōnē*, voice]. The vibration and echolike reproduction of the patient's own voice, breath sounds, and murmurs.

autoplasmother'apy [" + *plasma*, a thing formed, + *therapeia*, treatment]. Treatment through injecting patient's own blood plasma.

autoplas'tic [" + *plassein*, to form]. PSY: Rel. to psychic modifications in adapting oneself to reality.

autoplasty (aw'to-plas-tĭ) [" + *plassein*, to form]. A grafting of fresh parts taken from the patient's body for the repair of wounds.

autoprecipitin (aw-to-pre-sip'ĭ-tĭn) [" + L. *praecipitāre*, to cast down]. Precipitin active against serum of animal that was injected.

autopsia (aw-top'sĭ-ă) [" + *opsis*, view]. 1. An exploratory incision to determine cause of a disorder or nature of a disease. 2. Autopsy.

autopsy (aw'top-sĭ). Examination of the organs of a dead body to determine cause of death, or pathological conditions.

autopsycho'sis [G. *autos*, self, + *psychē*, the soul]. Mental disease in which patient's ideas about himself are disordered.

autopyother'apy [" + *pyon*, pus, + *therapeia*, treatment]. 1. Treatment of disease by adm. of patient's own pathological excretions. 2. Self-treatment.

autoreinfu'sion [" + L. *re*, back, + *in-*, into, + *fundere*, to pour]. Intravenous injection of patient's blood which has been effused in his body cavities.

autor'rhaphy [" + *raphē*, suture]. Wound closure by tissue taken from edges of the wound.

autosepticē'mia [" + *sēpsis*, decay, + *aima*, blood]. Septicemia from poisons existing within the organism.

autoserodiagno'sis [" + L. *serum*, whey, + G. *dia*, through, + *gnōsis*, knowledge]. Diagnosis through serum from patient's blood.

aut″o-ser″o-sal′var-san [" + " + salvarsan]. Blood serum from patient after salvarsan injection used on the patient himself.

autoserother′apy [" + " + G. *therapeia*, treatment]. Treatment by hypodermic injection of patient's own blood serum.

autose′rous. Pert. to autoserum.

autose′rum. Serum obtained from patient's own blood or cerebrospinal fluid.

autosuggestibil′ity [G. *autos*, self, + L. *suggerere*, to suggest]. Peculiar lack of resistance to any suggestion that may be offered.

autosugges′tion. Acceptance of an idea uninfluenced by others that induces mental or physical action or change.
PSY: 1. Hysteroid aggravation of actual injury. 2. Persistence into normal consciousness of impressions occurring during secondary states. SEE: *hypnotism*.

autosynnoia (aw-to-sĭn-noy′ă) [G. *autos*, self, + *syn*, with, + *nous*, mind]. PSY: Intense concentration to the extent of loss of interest in the outside world; a state of introversion.

autotem′nous [" + *temnein*, to divide]. Pert. to cells propagating by spontaneous division.

autother′apy [" + *therapeia*, treatment]. 1. Spontaneous cure. 2. Treatment of disease by administering patient's own pathological secretions.

autotomy (aw-tot′o-mĭ) [" + *tome*, a cutting]. A surgical operation performed by oneself.

autotopnosia (aw-to-top-no′zĭ-ă) [" + *topos*, place, + *gnōsis*, knowledge]. Inability to orient various parts of body correctly.

autotoxe′mia, autotoxico′sis [" + *toxikon*, poison, + *aima*, blood]. Self-poisoning due to absorption of ferment or poison generated within the body.

autotox′in. Poison generated within the body upon which it acts.

autotransform′er [G. *autos*, self, + L. *trans*, across, + *forma*, form]. A transformer that has part of its turns common to both primary and secondary circuits. SEE: *transformer*.

autotransfusion (aw-to-trans-fu′shun) [" + " + *fundere*, pour]. 1. Bandaging the limbs to force the blood to the vital centers. 2. A method of treating internal hemorrhage by returning the patient's own extravasated blood to the circulation.

The apparatus required is a beaker, glass rod, two cups or small bowls, a funnel, and 250 cc. ampules of 2% sodium citrate; the quantity being used is 10 cc. for each 90 cc. of blood. The apparatus for giving intravenous saline is also prepared, together with some physiological salt solution (0.9%). After opening the abdomen, the blood is allowed to run into the cup, which is then emptied into the beaker containing the sodium citrate.

The mixture is continually stirred by the nurse. After discovering and arresting the cause of the hemorrhage, the rest of the blood is bailed out, and the citrated blood now filtered through several layers of gauze (15-20) over the glass funnel into the saline flask, so that it enters the blood vessel with the saline. CONTRA: (1) Obviously infected blood; (2) stale blood, *i. e.*, when the bleeding has been going on for several days.

autotransplanta′tion [" + " + *plantāre*, to plant]. Transferring a piece of tissue from one part to another in same person.

autotrophic (aw-to-trof′ik) [" + *trophē*, nourishment]. Self nourishing; pert. to green plants and bacteria which form pro. and carbo. from inorganic salts and carbon dioxide.

autotuber′culin [" + L. *tuberculum*, a swelling]. Tuberculin prepared from cultures of patient's own sputum.

autotyphization (aw-to-ti-fĭz-a′shun) [" + *typhos*, fever]. Production of state resembling typhoid fever; due to autointoxication.

autourother′apy [" + *ouron*, urine, + *therapeia*, therapy]. Treatment of various allergic diseases by injections of the patient's own urine.

autovaccina′tion [" + *vacca*, cow]. Vaccination with autovaccine.*

autovac′cine. Vaccine prepared from virus developed in patient's own body.

autoxida′tion [G. *autos*, self, + *oxys*, acid, + *gennan*, to produce]. Spontaneous combining with oxygen.

auxanography (awks-an-og′ră-fĭ) [G. *auxanein*, to increase, + *graphein*, to write]. Determination of most suitable medium for bacterial cultivation.

auxanology (awks-an-ol′o-jĭ) [" + *logos*, study]. Scientific study of growth.

auxesis (awks-e′sis) [G. *auxein*, to increase]. Enlarged in bulk, or size.

auxet′ic. Promoting proliferation in leukocytes and other cells.

auxilytic (awks-ĭ-lit′ik) [G. *auxein*, to increase, + *lyein*, dissolve]. Favoring lysis (2), *q.v.*

auximone (awks′im-ōn) [" + *ormanein*, to excite]. Vitaminlike substance favoring growth in plants.

aux′in. Plant-sprout and human urine hormone promoting growth in plant cells and tissues.

auxocyte (awks′o-sīt) [G. *auxein*, to increase, + *kytos*, cell]. Cell taking part in growth.

auxogluc (awks′ō-glŭk) [" + *glukus*, sweet]. A group of tasteless atoms which combine with gluciphores to form sweet-tasting compounds.

auxol′ogy [" + *logos*, study]. Scientific study of growth of organisms.

auxotroph (awks′ō-trŏf). A mutant or other organism needing a specific factor for growth.

a′va, a′va-ka′va. 1. Intoxicating beverage. 2. Drug used in cystitis, gout and wasting illnesses. SYN: *kava*.

av′alanche theory [F. *avalanche*, descent]. Theory that nervous impulses increase in intensity in passing efferent nerves.

avasculariza′tion [G. *a-*, priv. + L. *vaculāris*, having vessels]. Expulsion of blood, as by use of Esmarch bandage.

Avel′lis′ syndrome. Paralysis of one-half of soft palate, the pharynx, larynx, and loss of pain and heat and cold sensation on opp. side.

averse′ depress′ion. Depression accompanied by defective judgment and rutformation, esp. in the presenile period.

avertin (a-ver′tin). A tribromethanol; is a white, crystalline substance with a melting point at 79° to 80° C. (174° to 176° F.), and is 3½% soluble in water at a temperature of 40° C. Used as a basal narcotic. SYN: *tribomoethanol*.

It is evanescent under steam, and should be protected from light and air. The dissolving of avertin in water must be carried out at a moderate temperature (95° to 104° F.) to prevent it

aviator's disease breaking up, as at a higher temperature hydrobromic acid is split off and dibromacetaldehyde is formed; the latter causes severe injury to the bowel, and must be avoided at all costs. It is prevented by the use of a special test, *viz.*, 5 cc. of a 2½% avertin solution are placed in a clean test tube shortly before the time for the injection, and 1 to 2 drops of an aqueous (1:1000) solution of *Congored* are added. The color must be of a pure orange red. When badly made, the color tends towards blue; such solutions are dangerous to the patient.

The 2½% tested solution is passed into the rectum at body heat 30 minutes before the operation, if possible, in a quiet, dark room. Morphia, 1/6 to 1/3 gr., is given by some authorities, but is not advised as a routine.

The bowel is emptied the previous evening by means of an enema or aperient. It is most important to regulate the dosage to the body weight. This is estimated at 0.08 to 0.1 Gm. (1 1/4 to 1 1/2 gr.) avertin per Kg. body weight in 2½% aqueous solution. In this strength the solution is quickly absorbed by the mucous membrane, becomes detoxicated through chemical action with glycuronic acid, and is excreted in this form through the kidneys in from 6 to 12 hours.

Sleep ensues in from 5-20 minutes after rectal adm. without any stage of excitation, and awakening occurs as from natural sleep. Respiration is slowed, but effect on heart and blood vessels is unimportant with a normal dose. It decreases intraocular pressure with no increase in intracranial pressure.

a'viator's disease. Vasomotor disturbances, headache, and drowsiness seen in aviators.

avidin (av-id′in) [L. *avidus*, greedy]. A proteinlike substance isolated from eggwhite. Said to be an inhibitor of biotin,* a B vitamin named Vit. H.

avirulent (ă-vir′u-lent) [G. *a-* priv. + L. *virus*, poison]. Without virulence.

avitaminosis (a-vi-tă-mĭ-no′sĭs) [" + L. *vita*, life, + *amin*]. Disease due to lack of vitamins in the diet; a deficiency disease. SEE: *avitaminotic, vitamin.*

avitaminotic (ă-vi-tam-in-ot′ĭk). Pert. to or affected with avitaminosis.*

avivement (a-vēv-mon′) [Fr. *avivement*, made alive again]. Refreshing of edges of a wound by operation to hasten healing.

avocado (ăv″o-kă′dō) [Portuguese *abacado*]. Pearshaped, green fruit; alligator pear. Average serving 85 grams. Pro. 1.8, Fat 17.0, Carbo. 5.1 Ca. 0.040, P. 0.050, Fe. 0.006. Contains Vit. C. Good source Vit. A and G, very good source Vit. B.

Avogad′ro's law. Equal volumes of gases contain equal numbers of molecules, pressure and temperature being same.

A.'s number. Number of molecules in one gram-molecular weight of a compound.

avoirdupois′ meas′ure [Fr. *avoir*, to have, + *du*, of the, + *pois*, weight]. A system of weighing or measuring all coarse and heavy articles. 7000 grains equal one pound. Some medicines are bought and sold by avoirdupois weight.

Dry Measure
16 drams (dr.) equal .. 1 ounce (oz.)
16 ounces equal .... 1 pound (lb.)
25 pounds equal .... 1 quarter (qr.)
4 quarters equal ..... 100 weight (cwt.)
20 cwts. equal .... 1 ton (T.)

A-100

Liquid Measure
2 pints equal ..... 1 quart equals 57¾ cubic inches.
4 quarts equal .... 1 gallon equals 231 cubic inches.

To find the capacity of a vessel or space in gallons, divide the contents in cubic inches by 231 for liquid gallons, or by 268.8 for dry gallons.

To reduce gallons to inches, multiply the given number of liquid gallons by 231; then change to higher denominations if required. The dry gallon (halfpeck) contains 268.8 cu. in. Six dry gallons are equal to nearly seven liquid gallons.

The bushel contains 2150.42 cu. in. and is a cylindrical measure 18½ in. in diameter and 8 in. deep. Measures of capacity are all cubic measures. The number of pounds in a bushel depends upon the article contained therein. SEE: *apothecaries' measure, household measures, metric system, Troy weight.*

avulsion (a-vul′shun) [G. *a-*, priv. + L. *avulsio*, a turning away]. 1. A turning away from as in disgust. 2. A tearing away forcibly of a part or structure. If surgical repair is necessary, merely apply a sterile dressing

axanthopsia (aks-an-thop′sĭ-ă) [G. *a-*, priv. + *xanthos*, yellow, + *opsis*, vision]. Yellow blindness. [in or pert. to an axis.

axial (aks′ĭ-al) [L. *axis*, lever]. Situated **a. skeleton.** Head and trunk.

axifugal (aks-if′u-gal) [" + *fugere*, to flee]. Receding from the center. SYN: *centrifugal.**

axilem′ma [L. *axis*, pivot, + G. *lemma*, husk]. Sheath of an axis cylinder.

axil′la (Pl. *axil′lae*) [L. *axilla*, little pivot]. The armpit. [*axillary.*

axillar (aks′ĭ-lar). Pert. to axilla. SYN: **axillary** (aks′ĭ-lar-ĭ). Pert. to the axilla.

ax′ion [G. *axōn*, axis]. Brain and spinal cord. The cerebrospinal axis.

axioplasm (aks′ĭ-o-plazm) [" + *plasma*, a thing formed]. Neuroplasm of an axiscylinder.

ax″ip′etal [L. *axis*, pivot, + *petere*, to seek]. Directed toward the axis. SYN: *axopetal.*

ax′is. The second cervical vertebra* or backbone.
a., basicranial. A. connecting basion and gonion. [to gonion.
a., basifacial. A. from subnasal point
a., binauricular. A. bet. the 2 auricular points.
a., celiac. Celiac artery from abdominal aorta.
a., cerebrospinal. Central nervous system.
a. cylinder. Nerve fiber core. SYN: *axon, neuraxon.*
a., frontal. Imaginary line running transversely through the center of the eyeball.
a., neural. SEE: *cerebrospinal a.*
a., optic. Line of vision.
a., sagittal. Imaginary line running through the eyeball anteroposteriorly.

axis cylinder process. Axon, *q.v.*, or neuraxon. The conducting portion of a nerve fiber. SEE: *axilemma, axioplasm, axite, axofugal, axopetal, axoplasm, axospongium.*

axis traction (ak′sis trak′shun). Traction made on the fetus in the direction of the birth canal.
a. t. forceps. Device used to aid in traction made on the fetus.

axite (aks′īt). Any terminal filament of an axis cylinder.

axo- (aks′o) [G.]. Prefix: Axis.

axodendrite (aks-o-den′drīt) [G. *axōn*, axis, + *dendron*, tree]. Process given off from a nerve cell axon (not an axis cylinder).

axofugal (aks-of′u-gal) [" + L. *fugere*, to flee]. Extending from an axis cylinder process.

axolem′ma [" + *lemma*, husk]. Axis cylinder sheath. SYN: *axilemma*.

axolysis (aks-ol′ĭ-sis) [" + *lyein*, to dissolve]. Destruction of the axis cylinder of a nerve.

ax′on, ax′one [G. *axōn*, axis]. 1. The neuraxon or axis cylinder process, the conducting part of a nerve cell. 2. The cerebrospinal axis. 3. The body axis. SEE: *nerve*.

axoneme (aks′o-nēm) [G. *axōn*, axis, + *nēma*, a thread]. Axial thread of a chromosome.

axoneuron (aks-o-nu′ron) [" + *neuron*, sinew]. A nerve cell of the cerebrospinal system.

axonometer (aks-o-nom′e-ter) [" + *metron*, a measure]. Device for determining the axis of astigmatism.

axopetal (aks-op′et-al) [" + *petere*, to seek]. Directed toward an axis cylinder process.

axophage (aks′o-fāj) [" + *phagein*, to eat]. Glia cell found in myelin excavations in myelitis.

ax′oplasm [" + *plasma*, a thing formed]. Material surrounding fibrils of axis cylinder.

axospongium (aks-o-spon′jĭ-um) [" + *spoggos*, sponge]. The fine fibrillar network of axis cylinder of a nerve cell.

axungia (aks-un′jĭ-ă) [L. *axis*, axis, + *unguere*, to grease]. 1. Lard. 2. Internal body fat.

Ayerza′s disease (ă-yer′să). One characterized by dyspnea, chronic cyanosis, erythemia, enlargement of spleen and liver, and hyperplasia of bone.

Az. Abbr. for *azote*.

aza′lein [L. *azalea*, azalea]. A red dye. SYN: *fuchsin*.

azo-. Prefix indicating substance from a hydrocarbon by replacement by nitrogen of a part of the hydrogen.

azoamyly (az-o-am′ĭ-lĭ) [G. *a-*, priv. + *zōon*, animal, + *amylon*, starch]. Diminution of amount of glycogen stored up in the liver.

azochloramid (ă-zo-klor′ă-mid). A stable, chlorine substance, crystalline and yellow in appearance, soluble in water or triacetin, etc.
USES: As an antiseptic in various infections, including fungi.
DOSAGE: Used in solutions of 1: 500.

azo-compounds. Organic substances of which an example is azobenzene, $C_6H_5N:NC_6H_5$.
They are related to aniline, and include important dyes and indicators. The color changes shown by dimethylaminoazobenzene $C_6H_5N:NC_6H_4N(CH_3)_2$ are given under *"Indicators."*

azoic (az-o′ĭk) [G. *a-*, priv. + *zōē*, life]. Containing no living organisms.

azoospermia (ah-zo-o-sper′mĭ-ă) [" + *zōon*, animal, + *sperma*, seed]. Deficient vitality of the spermatozoa or their absence.

azopro′tein [" + " + *prōtos*, first]. A horse serum protein.

azoru′bin S. A dark red dye excreted in the bile after intravenous injection. Test of hepatic function.

azotation (az-o-ta′shun) [*azote*, nitrogen]. Nitrogen absorption from the air.

az′ote [G. *a-*, priv. + *zōē*, life, so named by Lavoisier because it cannot support life]. Nitrogen.

azotemia (az-o-te′mĭ-ă) [" + *aima*, blood]. Presence of nitrogenous bodies in the blood. SYN: *uremia.**

azotene′sis [" + *enesis*, injection]. Disease due to excess of nitrogen in system. Ex: *scurvy, gangrene*.

azotifica′tion. Atmospheric nitrogen fixation.

azotized (az′ot-īzd). Containing nitrogen.

azotom′eter [*azote*, nitrogen, + *metron*, measure]. Instrument measuring amount of uric acid and urea in urine.

azotorrhea (az-o-to-re′ă) [" + *roia*, flow]. Excess of nitrogenous matter in the feces or urine.

azotu′ria [" + *ouron*, urine]. Increase of urea in the urine.

Az′tec type. Microcephalic idiocy.*

azurophile (azh-u′ro-fĭl) [M. E. *azure*, azure, + G. *philein*, to love]. Staining readily with azure dye.

azurophil′ia. Condition in which some blood cells have azurophil granules.

azygos (az′ĭ-gos) [G. *a-*, priv. + *zygos*, yoke]. Occurring singly, not in pairs.

azygous (az′ĭg-us). Single, not paired.
a. veins. Three unpaired veins of the abdomen and thorax. A. major arises from *vena cava inferior* through the aortic orifice of the diaphragm and the post. mediastinum, ending in the *vena cava superior*.

azymia (a-zi′mĭ-ă) [G. *a-*, priv. + *zymē*, ferment]. State of being without a ferment.

azymic, azymous (ă-zi′mik, -mus). 1. Unfermented or unleavened. 2. Denoting the absence of a ferment.

B

Ba. Symb. barium.
Bab'bitt metal. Antifriction alloy used occasionally in dentistry.
Babcock's test. PSY: The difference between a vocabulary and a nonvocabulary test indicating the degree of mental deterioration.
Ba'bes-Ernst bodies. Metachromatic* bodies seen in bacterial protoplasm.
Babe'sia. A genus of Protozoa belonging to the class Sporozoa which are parasitic in cattle, sheep, horses, dogs and other vertebrates. They infest red blood cells bringing about their destruction with resulting hemoglobinuria. They are transmitted by ticks of the genus *Boophilus*.
  B. bigemina. The causative organism of Texas fever or red-water fever in cattle.
  B. ovis. Causes hemoglobinuria and jaundice in sheep.
babesi'asis. Infection caused by a species of *Babesia*.
Babinski's reflex [L. *reflectere*, to turn back]. Extension of the great toe (extensor plantar) on stroking sole of foot; sometimes a flexion of the other toes when irritation is applied to the sole of the foot. It indicates a lesion of the pyramidal tract and is found in organic hemiplegia,* diseases of nervous system, but not in hysteria.
  B.'s ear-reflex. Inclination of head to diseased side, in middle and internal ear diseases, when galvanic electrode is placed near the ear and when galvanic current is closed.
  B.'s method. Producing reflex contraction of Achilles tendon by tapping it with patient kneeling on a chair.
  B.'s sign. A loss or diminished reflex produced by the Achilles tendon. It is found in sciatica, not in hysteric sciatica.
bacca (bak'ă) [L. berry]. A berry.
Baccelli's sign (băt-chel'ēz). Good conduction of a whisper through nonpurulent effusions. Shows a serous pleuritic exudate.
bacchia (bak'e-ă). Acne rosacea.*
bacciform (bak'sĭ-form) [L. *bacca*, berry, + *forma*, form]. Berry-shaped; coccal.
bacillac (bas'il-ăk) [L. *bacillus*, rod]. Milk preparation soured by *Lactobacillus acidophilus*.
bacillae'mia [" + G. *aima*, blood]. Bacillemia.*
bacillar, bacillary (bas'il-ar, bas'il-ar-ĭ). Pert. to or caused by bacilli or rodlike forms.
  b. layer. Rod-and-cone retinal layer.
bacille'mia [L. *bacillus*, rod, + G. *aima*, blood]. Presence of bacilli in the blood.
bacil'licidal, bacillicid'ic [" + *caedere*, to kill]. Destructive to bacilli.
bacillicide (bas-il'is-īd). An agent destructive to bacilli.
bacil'liculture [L. *bacillus*, rod, + *cultura*, cultivation]. 1. Propagation of bacilli. 2. Culture containing bacilli.
bacil'liform [" + *forma*, form]. Resembling a bacillus in shape.
bacilliparous (ba-sil-ip'ar-us) [" + *parere*, to produce]. Producing bacilli.
bacillogen'ic, bacillogenous (ba-sil-oj'-enus) [" + G. *gennan*, to produce]. 1. Producing bacilli. 2. Originating in bacilli.
bacillopho'bia [" + G. *phobos*, fear]. Morbid fear of bacilli.
bacillo'sis [" + G. -*osis*, infection]. Condition due to infection by bacilli.
bacillum (bas-il'um). 1. Sponge holder. 2. A stick.
bacilluria (bas-il-u'rĭ-ă) [L. *bacillus*, rod, + G. *ouron*, urine]. Bacilli in the urine, though *B. coli* to *Escherichia coli* and *B. typhosus* to *Salmonella typhosus*.
  SYM: *B. coli* reaches urine through the blood stream. Urine contains much mucus but is acid when passed; becomes alkaline on standing. Rise in temperature, malaise, later cystitis and possible pyelitis.
  TREATMENT: Drugs and antiseptics which make urine alternately acid and alkaline. Blood fluids, light, nonstimulating diet, avoid fatigue, rest during day, bed before night meal. Antibiotics.
bacil'lus (pl. *bacilli*). A rod-shaped microörganism belonging to the Schizomycetes.
  b. acid-fast. One very resistant to decoloring effect of acids after staining.
  b. Bordet-Gengou. *Hemophilis pertussis*. Cause of whooping cough.
  b. colon. *Escherichia coli*. A nonpathogenic intestinal form.
  b. butter. *Mycobacterium butyricum*.
  b. comma. *Vibrio comma*. The cause of cholera.
  b. Doderlein's. A large gram-positive bacillus usually present in the vagina. Considered identical with *Lactobacillus acidophilus*. Probably responsible for the acidity of the vagina.
  b. Ducrey's. *Hemophilus ducreyi*. The cause of soft chancre or chancroid infection of the genitalia.
  b. Friedlander's. *Klebsiella pneumoniae*. Cause of lobar pneumonia.
  b. gas gangrene. *Clostridium perfringens*.
  b. Hansen's. *Mycobacterium leprae*. Cause of leprosy.
  b. Kleb's Loeffler. *Corynebacterium diphtheria*. Cause of diphtheria.
  b. Morgan's. *Proteus morganii*. Isolated from patients with summer diarrhea.
  b. Pfeiffer's. *Hematophilus influenzae*.
  b. Schmitz. *Shigella ambigua*. A cause of dysentery.
  b. Shiga. *Shigella dysenteriae*. The first dysentery bacillus described.
Bacillus. A genus of bacteria belonging to the family Bacillaceae. All species of the genus are rod-shaped and produce endospores. Some are motile, others are not. Motile forms bear flagella on all sides (peritrichus). They may occur singly or in chains. Some species develop capsules. All are aerobic and are usually gram-positive. Most are saprophytic; some are pathogenic.
  B. abortus (Bang's b). *Brucella abortus*. The causative organism of contagious abortion in cattle (Bang's disease).
  B. acidi lactici. *Streptococcus lactis*. A non-pathogenic organism occurring naturally in sour milk.

B. acidophilus. *Lactobacillus acidophilus*. A non-pathogenic species found in the intestines of warm blooded animals. Used in the preparation of acidophilus milk which is used therapeutically in the treatment of certain digestive disorders. Considered to be identical with Doderlein's bacillus, *q.v.*
B. aerogenes capsulatus. *Clostridium welchii* (*C. perfringens*). An anaerobic toxin-producing bacillus, considered to be the most important cause of gaseous gangrene. It is a normal inhabitant of the human intestine and is used as an indicator of fecal pollution of water.
B. anthracis. An aerobic, spore-forming bacillus, pathogenic for man and lower animals, being the causative agent of anthrax, *q.v.*
B. botulinus. *Clostridium botulinum*. A saprophytic organism which grows under anaerobic conditions in decaying vegetable matter. In incompletely sterilized cans of food, it produces a potent endotoxin which, when ingested by man, causes botulism, a highly fatal form of food poisoning.
B. enteritidis. *Salmonella* enteritidis, *q.v.*
B. faecalis alcaligenes. *Alcaligenes faecalis*. A non-pathogenic normal inhabitant of the digestive tract.
B. mucosus capsulatus. *Klebsiella pneumoniae* (Friedlander's bacillus). The causative agent of a severe type of pneumonia (lobar pneumonia). Also found frequently in sputa of patients suffering from bronchiectasis.
B. paratyphosus A. *Salmonella* paratyphi A.
B. paratyphosus B. *Salmonella* paratyphi B.
B. paratyphosus C. *Salmonella* paratyphi C.
Causative agents of types of paratyphoid fever.
B. perfringens. *Clostridium welchii.*
B. pertussis. *Hemophilus pertussis*. The causative agent of whooping cough.
B. phlegmonis emphysematosse. *Clostridium welchii.*
B. subtilis. The common hay bacillus.
B. suisepticus. *Pasteurella suiseptica*. The causative agent of swine plague.

bacitracin (băs-ĭ-trā′sĭn). An antibiotic from *Bacillus subtilis* (hay bacillus), obtained from a wound in a patient named Tracy. Active against cocci and anaerobes. It may have an irritant effect upon the kidney. Its use is now confined to local application in skin infections. It does not produce skin sensitization.

back-pressure arm-lift artificial respiration. Place the victim prone (face down) with elbows bent, one hand on the other, head to one side, cheek resting on folded hands. Kneel on one knee—or both, if you achieve better balance—at the victim's head. A. Place your hands on the flat of the victim's back, below the armpit, with your thumbs barely touching, fingers spread outward and downward. B. Rock forward slowly, keeping your elbows straight, until your arms are nearly vertical, thus exerting a steady downward pressure. C. Now rock backward, releasing pressure. Slide your hands outward to grasp the victim's arms just above the elbows. Continue to rock backward. D. As you rock backward, raise and pull the victim's arms toward you until you feel tension in his shoulders. Start over with step A. Repeat the full cycle about 12 times a minute. *Important:* When the victim begins to breathe on his own, synchronize your efforts with his breathing until he breathes strongly. Then stop.

bacteremia (băk-tēr-ē′mĭ-ă) [G. *bakterion*, staff, + *aima*, blood]. Bacteriemia; bacteria in the blood.

Bacteria. Unicellular, plant-like microorganisms, lacking chlorophyll. (*Classification:* See accompanying chart.)

Shape: There are three principal types: (1) the *spherical* or *coccus form*. When appearing singly, they are called *micrococci;* when in pairs, *diplococci;* when in irregular clusters, *staphylococci;* when in chains, *streptococci;* when in regular groups of eight, *sarcinae*. (2) the *rod-shaped form* known as *bacillus*. When the rods are somewhat oval, they are called *coccobacilli;* when attached end to end forming a chain, *streptobaccilli*. (3) *the spiral form*. When the spiral organism is rigid it is called a *spirillum*, when flexible, a *spirochete;* when forming a curved rod, a *vibrio*. (4) involution *forms:* Most bacteria are relatively constant in form in growing cultures, but in old cultures or cultures grown under adverse environmental conditions, aberrant forms such as oversized and Y-shaped individuals appear. These are considered by some to be involution or degenerating forms; by others to be stages in complex life cycles.

Characteristics
Size: An average rod-shaped bacterium measures about 2 microms in length and 0.5 microms in diameter. They vary in size from 0.5 x 0.2 (the influenza bacillus) to 40-60 microms in length by 4-5 microns in width (*B. butschlii*).

Motility: Some bacteria are incapable of movement (all cocci) but most bacilli and spiral forms exhibit independent movement. The power of locomotion depends on the possession of one or more flagella, slender whip-like appendages. Bacteria having no flagella are called *atrichous;* those having a single flagellum at one end, *monotrichous;* those having flagella at each end, *amphitrichous;* those having a tuft at one end, *lophotrichous;* those having flagella protruding from all surfaces of the cell, *peritrichous*.

Capsules: Many bacteria possess a *capsule*, a layer of slimy mucoid substance which surrounds each cell. The presence of a capsule is associated with the virulence of certain pathogenic forms.

Spores: Certain species of the rod-shaped bacteria have the ability to develop an encysted or resting stage known as a *spore* or *endospore*. The size, shape, and position of the spore within the cell are characteristic of particular species. Spores are *terminal*, if formed at the end of a cell; *central*, if formed in the center; *subterminal*, if formed between the center and end. Spore-formation is common among the bacilli but does not occur in the cocci or spiral forms. Bacterial spores are remarkably resistant to heat, drying, and the action of disinfectants. Few pathogenic bacteria form spores, the anthrax and tetanus organisms being exceptions. Unfavorable environmental conditions favor spore-formation.

Reproduction: Binary fission is the usual mode of reproduction. Budding, branching, filamentous growth, and the development of conidia and gonidia also occur.

Colony formation: A group of bacteria growing in one place is called a *colony*. A colony is usually composed of the descendents of a single cell. Colonies differ in shape, size, color, texture, type of margin, and in other characteristics. Each species of bacteria has a characteristic type of colony formation. Sometimes a single species may produce two types of colonies; one the *smooth or S-type*, the other the *rough or R-type*. Sometimes colonies contain clear spots and have a moth-eaten appearance. Such colonies are called *plaques* and are thought to be due to the lytic action of bacteriophage.

Food requirements: Bacteria possess no chlorophyl hence cannot carry on photosynthesis. A few can obtain their energy from inorganic substances. These are termed *autotrophic* and include many of the soil bacteria. The majority derive their nourishment from organic material and are termed *heterotrophic*. If they live on living organisms, they are called *parasites;* if their food is from nonliving organic matter, they are called *saprophytes*. If bacteria produce disease in their host, they are *pathogenic*.

Oxygen requirements: Most bacteria require free or atmospheric oxygen. These are called *aerobes*. Bacteria living in the absence of atmospheric oxygen are called *anaerobes*. Those showing a preference for free oxygen and yet are capable of living in its absence are called *facultative anerobes;* those which grow only in the absence of oxygen are called *obligate anerobes*.

Temperature requirements: Most bacteria grow best at moderate temperatures. These are called *mesophilic*. Cold-living bacteria which thrive in temperatures below 10° C. are called *psychrophilic;* those which thrive in high temperatures even up to 85° C. are called *thermophilic*. The optimum temperature for most saprophytes is around 25° C., for most pathogens, 37° C.

Activities of Bacteria

Enzyme production: Bacteria produce enzymes which act on complex food molecules breaking them down into simpler materials capable of assimilation. *Carbohydrases* act on sugars breaking them down to alcohol and carbon dioxide, a process called *fermentation*. *Proteolytic enzymes* bring about the decomposition of proteins with the formation of ill-smelling products; a process called *putrefaction*. The term *"decay"* is applied to the decomposition of organic substances in the presence of air without the formation of unpleasant odors. *Putrefaction* is the decomposition of organic substances, especially nitrogenous substances, in the absence of air and with resulting unpleasant odors. Bacteria are the principal agents of decay and putrefaction.

Toxin production: Many bacteria produce poisonous substances called *toxins*, which are of two types, (1) *exotoxins* which diffuse from the bacterial cell into the surrounding medium and (2) *endotoxins*, which are liberated only when the bacterial cell dies and disintegrates. Bacteria well known for their toxin production are the diphtheria, tetanus, and botulinus organisms.

Miscellaneous activities: Some bacteria produce *pigments;* some produce light appearing *luminescent* at night. Many chemical substances are produced as a result of bacterial activity, among them acids, gases, alcohol, aldehydes, ammonia, indol. Pathogenic forms produce hemolysins, leucocidins, coagulases, and fibrolysins. Soil bacteria play an important rôle in various phases of the nitrogen cycle (nitrification, nitrogen fixation, and denitrification).

Methods of Studying Bacteria: The principal methods used in the study of bacteria are:

(1) Examination of unstained bacteria in a hanging-drop preparation. Dark-field illumination is necessary to see extremely small forms.

(2) *Staining methods.* General stains, differential stains, stains for special bacteria, and stains for specific parts are employed. Of the differential stains, Gram's method and staining for acid-fast bacteria are the most widely used. Bacteria fall into these groups: *Gram-positive bacteria:* Those which retain the stain. *Gram-negative bacteria:* Those which are decolorized. *Acid-fast bacteria:* Those which, when stained with certain dyes retain the stain even when treated with an acid.

(3) *Cultural methods.* In which the bacteria are grown on various culture media. Media may be *synthetic* or *nonsynthetic*. In the former, the exact composition of the medium is known; in the latter, the constituents are uncertain. Media, on the basis of consistency, may be *liquid* (nutrient broth, milk, blood serum); *liquefiable solid media* which consists of liquid media made solid by addition of gelatin or agar-agar; *nonliquefiable solid media* (potato, carrots, starch paste).

(4) *Animal inoculation.*
(5) *Immunological methods.*
(6) *Sterilization methods.*

Sterilization is the process of rendering any material free of living microörganisms. It may be accomplished by physical or chemical means. The use of chemical agents is usually designated *disinfection*. Physical agents employed are heat, light and filtration. Sterilization may be accomplished in a flame, in a hot-air oven (150°-170° C. for one hour), in streaming steam (100° C. for 20 min. or longer) or by steam under pressure (10-15 lbs.) in an autoclave (121° C. for 20 min.). Ultraviolet light is destructive to bacteria. Filtration is accomplished by the use of cotton or by special filters (Berkefeld, Pasteur, Chamberlain) of unglazed porcelain.

Chemical Agents

Chemical agents which inhibit bacterial growth are called *antiseptics;* those which kill are called *germicides* or *bactericides*. Among disinfectants are strong acids and alkalies, metallic salts (bichlorid of mercury), halogens (chlorine, iodine), oxidizing agents (hydrogen peroxide), organic compounds (phenol, formaldehyde, salicylic acid), and other substances such as boric acid. Substances used in the treatment of germ diseases are called *chemotherapeutic agents*. They include the sulfonamide compounds and the antibiotics.

Bacteriaceae (băk-te-rĭ-ā'se-e). Family of Eubacteriales with rod-shaped cells without endospores.

There are 21 genera, some parasitic and some saprophytic.

Classification of Bacteria
as suggested by the Committee of the Society of American Bacteriologists
Kingdom: Plants. Phylum: Thallophyta. Class: Schizomycetes.

Order	Family	Tribe	Genus
Eubacteriales nonbranching.	Nitrobacteriaceae (nonparasitic).		
	Coccaceae (spherical).	Streptococcaceae (pairs or chains). Neisseriae. Micrococcaeae (single, pairs or clusters).	Diplococcus. Streptococcus. Neisseria. Staphylococcus. Gaffkya (tetrades) Micrococcus. Sarcina.
	Spirillaceae (elongate, curved).		Vibrio (includes V. cholerae). Spirillum.
	Bacteriaceae (rods, form no endospores).		Pseudomonas (incl. b. pyocyaneus). Pasteurella (incl. plague b.). Klebsiella (incl. pneumobacillus). Hemophilus (incl. influenza b.). Escherichia (incl. b. coli). Aerobacter. Proteus. Salmonella (incl. paratyphoid b.). Eberthella (incl. typhoid b.). Shigella (incl. dysentery b.). Brucella (incl. b. of undulant fever) Alcaligenes. Bacteroides.
	Bacillaceae (rods producing spores).		Bacillus. Clostridium (incl. b. of gas gangrene).
Actinomycetales elongated, filamentous form branches related to plants.	Actinomycetaceae.		Leptotricha. Actinomyces.
	Mycobacteriaceae.		Mycobacterium (incl. b. tuberculis). Corynebacterium (incl. b. diphtheriae). Fusiformis.
Chlamydobacteriales sheathed, resemble algae (plants).			
Thiobacteriales, sulfur bacteria from water.			
Myxobacteriales, slimy, found on decay.			
Spirochaetales spirals, related to animal protozoa.	Spirochaetaceae.		Spirochaeta. Saprospira. Cristispira. Borrelia (incl. Sp. of relapsing fever). Treponema (incl. Sp. of syphilis). Leptospira.

bacterial action (in digestive tract). It begins during the first day of birth. Over one hundred million bacteria supposed to be in large intestine of adult.
  B. acidophilus decreases intestinal putrefaction. Lactose, dextrin, fruits, vegetables, and milk favor cultures of intestinal flora and hygiene. Bacteria in the cow's digestive tract have been found to form Vitamins B and G.
  b. digestion. This takes place in the colon in which there are no secreting glands. Fermentive bacteria here change carbohydrates into carbon dioxide, alcohol, and lactic acid. Cellulose only may be acted upon by bacteria. Putrefying bacteria are found in the lower part of the colon where poisonous decomposition-products are produced.
  b. resistance. Development of resistance to a drug by an organism previously susceptible to it. It is much more apt to develop when streptomycin is used.
bactericide (bak-ter′ĭ-sīd) [G. *baktērion*, rod, + L. *caedere*, to kill]. That which destroys bacteria.
bacteriemia (bak-ter-ĭ-e′mĭ-ă) [" + *aima*, blood]. Living bacteria in the blood.
bacterine (bak′ter-en). A bacterial vaccine.
bacterio-. Prefix: Pert. to bacteria.
bacteriogenic (bak-tē-re-ō-jen′ik) [G. *baktērion*, rod, + *gennan*, to produce]. Caused by bacteria.
bacteriolog′ic, bacteriolog′ical [" + *logos*, study]. Pert. to bacteriology.
bacteriol′ogist. One versed in bacteriology.
bacteriol′ogy. Science of microörganisms.
bacteriolysin (bak-te-rĭ-ol′is-in) [G. *baktērion*, rod, + *lysis*, solution]. A substance which is capable of bringing about the dissolution of bacteria. More specifically, an antibody produced within the body of an animal which causes the dissolution or lysis of bacteria. They develop as a result of bacterial infection. The reaction is the result of the interaction of two factors: (1) a thermolabile substance known as *complement* or *alexin* present in blood serum and (2) an *amboceptor* (also called immune body, immune substance, or sensitizer).
bacteriolysis (bak-tē-rē-ŏl′is-is). The disintegration of bacteria generally by a specific antibody.
bacteriolytic (bak-te′′rĭ-o-lit′ik). Pert. to bacteriolysis.
bacterioöpso′nin [G. *baktērion*, rod, + *opsōnein*, to prepare food for]. An opsonin acting on bacteria.
bacteriophage (băk-tē′rĭ-ō-fāj) [" + *phagein*, to eat]. Nonspecific agent destructive to bacteria, normally present in the intestinal tract, esp. of those recovering from a bacterial disease; also found in urine, pus, blood, etc.
  It is assumed by some to be a virus or an ultramicroscopic live agent. The present tendency is to consider it as an enzymelike substance.
  Experimentally being used in dysentery, colon bacillus infection, cholera, and staphylococcus infections, the bacteriophage containing properties virulent for these organisms.
bacteriopha′gia. Destruction of bacteria by lytic agents.
bacterioprecip′itin [" + L. *praecipitāre*, to cast down]. Precipitin occurring in bacteria-treated serum.
bacteriopro′tein [" + *prōtos*, first]. One of the proteins in bacteria bodies.
bacterios′copy. Microscopic examination of bacteria.

bacteriosis (bak-tē-rĭ-o′sis). 1. Infection by bacteria. 2. The action of bacteria in the system.
bacteriosol′vent [G. *baktērion*, rod, + L. *solvens*, dissolving]. Agent causing lysis or solution of bacteria.
bacteriostasis (bak-tē-rĭ-os′tăs-is) [" + *stasis*, a stopping]. The arrest of bacterial growth.
bacte′riostat. An agent inhibiting bacterial growth.
bacteriotox′ic [G. *baktērion*, rod, + *toxikon*, poison]. 1. Toxic to bacteria. 2. Due to bacterial toxins.
bacteriotox′in. Toxin specifically destructive to bacteria.
Bacterium. A genus of bacteria belonging to the family Bacteriaceae. ABBR. *Bact.*
  B. aerogenes. SYN: *Aerobacter aerogenes.* Commonly found in sour milk.
  B. aetrycke. SYN: *Salmonella typhimurium.* Common cause of food poisoning.
  B. ambigua. SYN: *Shigella ambigua* (Schmitz' bacillus).
  B. cholerae-suis. SYN: *Salmonella cholera-suis.* An animal (pig) pathogen.
  B. coli. SYN: *Escherichia coli.* Universally found in the digestive tract of man and higher animals. Nonpathogenic.
  B. dysenteriae. SYN: *Shigella dysenteriae.* (Shiga bacillus.) A cause of bacillary dysentery.
  B. enteritidis. SYN: *Salmonella enteritidis.*
  B. friedlanderi. Friedlander's bacillus.
  B. paradysenteriae. SYN: *Shigella flexneri.* A dysentery bacillus.
  B. paratyphosum A. SYN: *Salmonella paratyphi A.*
  B. paratyphosum B. SYN: *Salmonella paratyphi B.*
  B. pneumoniae. SYN: Friedlander's bacillus *(Klebsiella pneumoniae).*
  B. suipester. SYN: *Salmonella cholerae-suis.*
  B. tularense. SYN: *Pasteurella tularensis.* Causative agent of tularemia.
  B. typhi-murium. SYN: *Salmonella typhimurium.*
  B. typhosum. SYN: *Eberthella typhi.* The typhoid bacillus.
bacteriu′ria [G. *baktērion*, rod, + *ouron*, urine]. Passage of bacteria in the urine.
bacteroid (bak′ter-oid) [" + *eidos*, appearance]. Like a bacterium.
baculiform (bak-u′li-form) [L. *baculum*, rod, + *forma*, shape]. Rod-shaped.
bag, hydrostatic [F. *bague*, sack]. OB: Rubber or silk bag which is inserted into the uterine cavity and then distended with fluid in order to initiate labor and aid in dilatation of cervix.
  The types of bags most frequently used are those of Barnes, Bowman, Champetier, de Ribes, and Voorhees.
  b., Pol′itzer's. Soft rubber bag for middle ear inflation.
bag-of-waters. The amnion.* The membrane enclosing the *liquor amnii* and the fetus.
  It is applied sometimes to that portion of the membrane protruding into the *os uteri.* It is the inner embryonic membrane, the *chorion** being the outer envelope.
baker [A. S. *bacan*, cook by dry heat]. Two or more electric lamps mounted in semicircular containers, called electric light bakers.
baker leg. Knock knee; genu valgum.
Baker's cyst. One containing synovial fluid

baker's dermatitis. Eczematous affection of hand caused by yeast. SEE: *baker's itch.*

baker's itch. Manual eczema from irritation of yeast. SEE: *baker's dermatitis.*

baker's stigmata. Manual callosities from kneading dough.

BAL. Abbr. for British Anti-Lewisite, originally developed for use against lewisite, a poisonous gas of chemical warfare. BAL is administered both by ointment to offset cutaneous burns by lewisite and by intramuscular injection in the treatment of poisoning due to arsenic, mercury, cadmium, or gold.

DOSAGE: 3 mg. per kg. of body weight intramuscularly every 4 hours for 48 hours; then every 6 hours for 24 hours; then every 12 hours for 10 days or until full recovery. SYN: *dimercaprol.*

bal"aneu'tics [G. *balaneuein,* to attend at the bath]. The study of giving baths for therapeutic purposes.

balanic (ba-lan'ik) [G. *balanos,* glans]. Pert. to the *glans clitoris** or *glans penis.**

balanism (bal'an-ism) [" + *ismos,* condition of]. Gynecological treatment by use of pessaries or suppositories.

balanitis (bal-an-i'tis) [" + *-itis,* inflammation]. Inflammation of the glans penis, infectional or gonococcal, and of mucous membrane beneath it with purulent discharge. The prepuce is often affected.

balano- (bal-an-o) [G.]. Prefix: Pert. to the glans penis.

bal"anoblennorrhe'a [G. *balanos,* glans, + *blennos,* mucus, + *roia,* flow]. Gonorrheal inflammation of the external glans penis.

balanoplasty (bal-an-o-plas'tī) [" + *plassein,* to form]. Plastic surgery of glans penis.

balanoposthitis (bal-an-o-pos-thi'tis) [" + *posthē,* prepuce, + *-itis,* inflammation]. Inflammation of the glans penis and prepuce; balanitis.* [prepuce.

balanoprepu'tial. Pert. to glans penis and

balanorrhagia (bal"an-ō-ra'jī-ā) [G. *balanos,* glans, + *rēgnunai,* flow forth]. Hemorrhage from glans penis.

balanorrhea (bal-an-o-re'a) [" + *roia,* flow]. Balanitis with purulent discharge.

baldness [M.E. *balled,* without hair]. Lack of hair on head. RS: *acomia, alopecia.*

Balkan frame. A framework (usually wood) to fit over a bed so that weights may be suspended from it so as to produce the desired continuous traction and yet permit freedom of motion while maintaining immobilization of the desired part being treated.

ball-and-socket joint. Joint in which one rounded bone head fits into cavity of another bone. SYN: *enarthrosis.**

ballism (bal'izm) [G. *ballismos,* jumping about]. 1. Condition characterized by jerking, twisting movements. 2. Paralysis agitans.*

ballis'tics [G. *ballein,* to throw]. Science of curves of projectiles.

ballistopho'bia [" + *phobos,* fear]. Morbid fear of missiles.

balloon'ing [It. *ballone,* great ball]. The distention of a cavity, as vagina, by air or otherwise for examination.

ballot'table [Fr. *balloter,* to toss about]. Capable of showing the ballottement* phenomenon.

ballottement (bal-ot-mon'). The rebound of a fetal extremity when displaced by the examining finger either through abdominal wall or vagina.

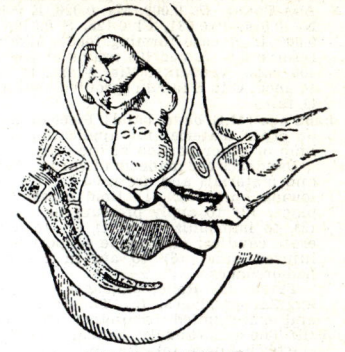

BALLOTTEMENT

ball thrombus. A normal clot in the ante mortem heart. SEE: *thrombus.*

balm [G. *balsamon,* balsam]. 1. A balsam. 2. A soothing or healing ointment.
  b. of Gilead. 1. Mecca balsam from *Commiphora opobalsamum,* probably Biblical myrrh. 2. Balsam fir, source of Canadian balsam. 3. Poplar bud resin.

balneary (bal'ne-ă-rī) [L. *balneum,* bath]. Institution for adm. of balneotherapy.

balneog'raphy [" + G. *graphein,* to write]. Treatise on mineral springs and baths.

balneology (bal-ne-ol'o-jī) [" + G. *logos,* study]. The science of treating disease by baths.

balneotherapeutics (bal"ne-o-ther-ă-pu'-tiks) [" + G. *therapeutikē,* treatment]. Treatment of disease by baths. SYN: *balneotherapy.**

balneotherapy (bal-ne-o-ther'a-pī) [" + G. *therapeia,* treatment]. The treatment of disease by baths. [bath.

bal'neum (pl. *bal'nea*) [L. a bath]. A
  b. are'nae. A sand bath.
  b. lu'teum. A mud bath.

balop'ticon [G. *ballein,* to throw, + *optikos,* pert. to sight]. Apparatus for projecting image of an opaque object on a screen.

bal'sam. Oleoresin or resin containing aromatic acids or essential oils.

balsam of Peru [G. *balsamon,* balsam]. USP. A dark-brown, viscid, resinous liquid. ACTION AND USES: Locally same as benzoin. May be used full strength or in ointment.

DOSAGE: 15 gr. (1.0 Gm.).

balsam'ic. 1. Pert. to balsam. 2. Aromatic.
  b. tincture. Compound tincture of benzoin.

Bal'ser's fatty necrosis. Pancreatitis with fatty necrotic areas in interlobular tissue, and sometimes in pericardial fat and bone marrow.

banana oil, poisoning [Sp. *banana*]. Resulting from amyl acetate used as a vehicle for suspending metals for the purpose of painting with metals, as gilding.

SYM: The effect may not be felt until in the fresh air for several minutes, when victim becomes dizzy, weak, and falls unconscious.

TREATMENT: If unconscious, wrap in a blanket; fan face gently. Give stimulants. Administration of oxygen desirable. Artificial respiration may be desirable.

banana. Comp: Av. Serving: 125 Gm. E. P. Pro. 1.6%, Fat 0.8%, Carbo. 26.2%. Fuel Value: 100 grams give 99 calories. Ash Const: Ca 0.009, Mg. 0.028, K 0.401, Na 0.034, P 0.031, Cl 0.125, S 0.010, Fe 0.00064. A base forming food. Alkaline reserve 5.6 cc. per 100 grams or 5.6 per 100 cals. Vitamins: Vit. A and B, fair to good, C to E fair in sprouted bananas, G fair.

band′age [M.E. *band,* band]. Piece of gauze or other material for application to a limb or other portion of the body.

Bandages are made up of various types and materials and are used for the following purposes: (1) Hold dressing in place; (2) to apply pressure to a part; (3) to immobilize a part; (4) to obliterate cavities; (5) to give support to an injured area; (6) to aid in checking hemorrhages.

Types: (a) Roller bandages. (b) Triangular bandages. (c) The four-tailed and many-tailed (scultetus) bandages. (d) The quadrangular bandage. (e) The elastic bandage (elastic knit, rubber, or combinations). (f) The adhesive. (g) Elastic adhesive. (h) Newer cohesive proprietary bandage under various trade names, such as Sterila Stic, Sanilastic, Bandtex, etc. (i) The impregnated bandages, such as plaster of Paris, water glass (sodium silicate), starch, etc. (j) Rubber bandages. The most important bandages are the following:

b., abdomen (Tri-b.). A single wide cravat or several narrow ones may be used to hold dressing in place, or to exert a moderate pressure. A folded towel or handkerchief should be used to keep it from digging into the flesh.

b., amputation-stump (Tri-b.). This is made in a similar way to the open hand bandage, the limb being laid on the base of the bandage.

b., ankle. One loop is brought around the sole of foot, and the other around the ankle and tied in front or side.

b., axilla. This is a spica-type turn starting under the affected axilla, crossing over the shoulder of the affected side and making the long loop under the opposite armpit.

b., back (Tri-b.). Open Bandage to the Back: This is applied the same as the chest-bandage, the point being placed above the scapula of the injured side.

b., Barton's. For the lower jaw. A double figure of eight b.

b., Borch's. An eye bandage covering both eyes.

b., breasts. (Roller bandages.) Suspensory bandages and compresses for the breasts.

b., buttocks. Use (1) "T" or double "T" binder or (2) open triangle.

b., capeline. A bandage applied to the head or shoulder, or to a stump, like a cap or hood.

b., chalk. A bandage made of immovable stiffening with a mixture of chalk and gum.

b., chest. (Roller bandages.) Figure of eight (spica), many tailed (scultetus), and Tri-b. (open chest) are used.

b., circular. A bandage applied in circular turns about a part.

b., cohesive. Material under various trade names which has an intense power of sticking to itself, but not to other substances. Used to make encircling applications about fingers, extremities, etc., or to build up pads.

b., cravat. Triangular b. folded to form a band around the injured part.

This is done by pulling the point over towards the base, folding the base over the point and then folding again. This makes a bandage wide enough to cover a large knee. When folded a 2nd time, it is wide enough to make the cravat bandage of the elbow. Folded a 3rd time, it could be used in making a figure-of-eight for the foot, ankle, hand, wrist, head, etc. It is an effective bandage in arresting hemorrhages, retaining splints, dressings, and poultices. The center of the cravat should be laid against the affected part, the ends of the cravat carried around the limb and tied over the center of the base. When used to retain splints, it should be tied on the outer side of the limb and against the splint, thus preventing the knot from irritating the skin. When used to retain a dressing in the axilla, the center of the cravat should be placed under the arm and the ends carried upward and crossed over the shoulder and tied in the axillary space of the opposite side, thus forming a figure-of-eight. The cravat can also be used as a sling when only a simple support is needed.

In using cravats for ties or splints, care should be taken so that the knots do not pass over and press unduly on the surface of the limb. Knots should be placed where they are easily found and not subject to pressure, the ends should be neatly tucked in. All knots should be square or reef knots.

b., c., elbow. Bend the elbow about 45 degrees. Place center of bandage over point of elbow. Bring 1 end around forearm, and the other end around upper arm. Pull tight and tie.

b., c., for fist, clenched (or Squire's diagonal figure-of-eight). This is a hand bandage to arrest bleeding or to make pressure. The wrist is laid on the center of the cravat, 1 end is brought around over the fist and back to the starting point, and the same procedure is then repeated with the other end. The 2 ends are pulled tight, twisted, and carried around the fist again so as to make pressure on the flexed fingers.

b., c., for fracture of clavicle. First put a soft pad (2x4 in.) in the forepart of the axilla. A sling made by placing the point of the open bandage on the affected shoulder, the hand and wrist laid on it, are directed toward the opposite shoulder, the point brought over and tucked underneath the wrist and hand. The ends are then lifted and the bandage is laid flat on the chest, the covered hand is carried up on the shoulder, the ends are brought together in the back and tied, the tightness being decided by how high the shoulder should be carried. A cravat bandage is then applied horizontally above the broad part of the elbow, and tied over a pad on the opposite side of the chest. Tightening this cravat pushes out the shoulder.

b., c., sling (for hand and upper arm). This is used for the support of the hand and in fracture of the upper arm. The wrist is laid upon the center of the cravat bandage, the forearm being held at right angle, and the 2 ends are carried around the neck and tied. See: *binder.*

b., crucial. Same as T-bandage.

b., demigauntlet. A bandage that covers the hand, but leaves the fingers uncovered.

b., Desault's (de-sōz'). A special immobilizing bandage of the collarbone or shoulders, using 3 rollers: (1) incorporating arm; (2) incorporating trunk and shoulders, and (3) incorporating forearm and left shoulder.

b., ear. (Roller bandages.) *T-bandage for the Ear:* A piece is sewed across the right angle of the T-bandage large enough to suit the occasion.

b., elastic. Bandages which have the property of stretching and hence making compression when correctly applied. Usually made of special weaves or of rubber to be applied over swollen extremities or joints; or on the chest in empyema; or on fractured ribs; or for supporting varicose veins, etc.

b., von Esmarch's (es'marks). (1) Triangular bandage, *q.v.* (2) Rubber bandage wrapped about an extremity after elevation from its periphery toward the heart to force blood out of the extremity; prior to operation or to increase circulating blood. On removal for surgery, a proximal band is left in place to prevent blood returning to the extremity.

b., eyes. One to retain dressings. The simple roller bandage for one eye or the monocle or crossed b. The binocular or crossed bandage for both eyes. (2 inches by 6 yards.)

b., figure-of-eight. A bandage in which the turns cross each other like the figure 8. To retain dressings or to exert pressure. For joints or to leave joint uncovered; to fix splints for the foot or hand, for the great toe and for sprains or hemorrhage.

b., finger. (Roller bandage.) Oblique fixation at wrist optional at start.

b., foot. *Open bandage of the Foot* (Tri-b.): The foot should be placed on the triangle with the base backward and behind the ankle; the apex is carried upward over the top of the foot. The ends are brought forward, folded once or twice crossed and carried around the foot and tied on top.

b., forearm. (Tri-b.). *Open sling bandage:* For support of the forearm.

b., fourtailed. A strip of cloth with each end split into two. Tails used to cover prominences as elbow, chin, nose, knee, etc.

b., Fricke's. A special immobilizing bandage of the male genitalia.

b., Galen's. A bandage with each end split in three pieces; the middle placed on the crown of the head; the two anterior strips are fastened at the back of the neck, the posterior (two) ones on the forehead, and the two middle ones are tied under the chin.

b., Garretson's. A bandage for the lower jaw, running above the forehead and back again to cross under the occiput and ending under the chin.

b., Genga's. Same as Theden's bandage.

b., Gibson's. A roller or cravat bandage for fracture of the lower jaw.

b., groin. (Special bandage): This bandage is most easily applied with the patient standing or lying on a pelvic rest (an inverted basis is satisfactory). A spica bandage, that is, a figure-of-eight with unequal loop, encircles the trunk and (c) the crossing is either placed anteriorly or lateral-ward. To bandage both groins the double spica is used. Such a double bandage is used principally in applying a plaster cast.

b., Hamilton's. A compound bandage for lower jaw, composed of a leather string with straps of linen webbing.

b., hand. (Roller bandages 1 inch wide.) *Demigauntlet Bandage for the Hand:* To hold a dressing on the back of the hand. For thumb and hand, the ascending spica of the thumb, with spiral of the hand is used. A Tri-bandage for open b. of the hand. A descending spica is used for the thumb and figure-of-eight b. for amputation stump or clenched fist.

b., head. Single recurrent roller capelline or skull cap. *Scalp:* The double roller recurrent bandage for the scalp. *Skull (segmental skull cap):* Any of the quadrants of the skull may be bandaged. *Head (open bandages of):* Use Tri-b., or shawl b. *Tommy head b.:* Place center of narrow cravat under chin, bring ends to top of head and tie single knot. Have patient or an assistant hold ends, and separate knot which forms two loops, place one low on back of head and bring the other forward over forehead, eyes, or chin as necessary; adjust if symmetrical and tie ends on top of head.

b., heel. The Tri-bandage is used.

b., Heliodorus'. A T-bandage.

b., hip. (Tri-b.) *Open Bandage of the Hip:* A cravat bandage or other band is tied around the waist, the point of another bandage is slipped under that and rolled or pinned directly above the position of the wound. The base is rolled up, the ends carried around the thigh, crossed and tied.

b., Hippocrates'. Same as capelline bandage.

b., Hueter's. A spica bandage for the perineum.

b., immovable. A bandage for immobilizing a part.

b., impregnated. Wide meshed bandage. Material impregnated with substances as plaster of Paris, water glass (sodium silicate), starch, etc., which have the power of solidifying after application—used to make molds or immobilize parts of the body.

b., "inacta." Dispersive electrode for surgical diathermy consisting of a fine copper gauze bandage.

b., knee. The knee cravat, the Tri-bandage, and the figure-of-eight are all used.

b., knotted. To exert pressure on a compress or pad over a bleeding wound.

b., Langier's. A many-tailed paper bandage.

b., Larrey's. A many-tailed bandage with edges glued together.

b., leg. Fix the initial end by a circular or oblique fixation at the ankle or with a figure-of-eight of the foot and ankle.

b., Maissonneuve's (ma-zon-nŭv'). A plaster of Paris bandage made of folded cloth held in place by other bandages.

b., many-tailed. For trunk and limbs. A piece of roller to which slips are stitched in an imbricated fashion. One with ends split. SEE: *four-tailed bandage, scultetus bandage, etc.*

b., Martin's. Roller bandage of rubber used to make pressure on an extremity as for varicose veins, etc., and for exsanguination, as Esmarch bandage, *q.v.*

b., neck. (Roller bandages.) *Spica for the Neck:* Bandage, 2½ inches by 8 yards.

Bandage for Use After Operations on the Thyroid Gland: Roller bandage, 2½ inches by 9 yards. *Adhesive Plaster Bandage for Use After Thyroidectomy*: Used to hold dressing on wound in place, and so far has proved more satisfactory. Apply a small dressing to center of strip, and then apply to back of neck. *Special Bandage*: A double loop bandage of the head and neck is made by using a figure-of-eight turn.

b., oblique. A bandage applied obliquely to a limb without reverses.

b., plaster. A bandage stiffened with a paste of plaster of Paris, which sets and becomes very hard.

b., postoperative. (Dressing.) This is a simple divergent or convergent spica of figure-of-eight bandage.

b., pressure. A bandage for applying pressure, usually used to stop hemorrhage.

b., protective. A bandage for the purpose of covering a part or of keeping dressings in place.

b., quadrangular. A towel, large handkerchief, etc., folded variously and applied as a bandage, as of head, chest, breast, abdomen, etc.

b., recurrent. A bandage over the end of a stump.

b., reversed. One applied to a limb in such a way that the roller is inverted or half twisted at each turn, so as to make it fit smoothly.

b., Ribble's. The spica of the instep.

b., Richet's (re-shāz'). A bandage of plaster of Paris to which a little gelatin has been added.

b., roller. A long strip of soft material usually from ½ to 6 inches wide and 2 to 5 yards long rolled on its short axis. When rolled from both ends to meet at center it is called a "double headed roller."

SIZE: More common sizes of roller bandages are as follows:

	Width	Length
Arm	1.5 to 2.5 inches,	8 to 12 yds.
Chest	3 " 4 "	6 " 8 "
Finger	.75 "	1 " 2 "
Foot	2.5 "	4 " 5 "
Hand	1. "	3 " 5 "
Head	2. to 2.5 "	5 " 7 "
Leg	2.5 "	6 " 10 "
Penis	.75 "	2 " 3 "
Shoulder	2.5 "	8 " 12 "
Thigh	3 "	6 " 9 "
Toes	.75 "	1 " 2 "
Trunk	3 to 4 "	8 " 12 "

Bandage Roller: For rolling and re-rolling bandages.

SEE: *bandages of special parts.*

b., rubber. A roller bandage of rubber used for pressure as in swollen parts for immobilization, etc.

b., sanilastic. SEE: *cohesive bandage.*

b., scultetus. Many-tailed bandage. A succession of interlocking, overlapping bands originally used to enclose a rigid support against a fractured extremity, but now used without the splint or impregnated as a supporting bandage of the abdomen or lower extremity.

b., shoulder. (Tri-b.) *Open Bandage of the Shoulder* (Useca): Spica bandage. *Shoulder and Neck*: Shawl bandage of both shoulders and neck. *Special Bandage*: Figure-of-eight bandage is used.

b., silica. A bandage rendered firm by treatment with sodium silicate.

b., spica. When a number of figure-of-eight turns are applied, each a little higher or lower, overlapping a portion of each preceding turn so as to give an imbricated appearance, it is called a spica. For breast, shoulder, limbs, thumb, and great toe. For support, to exert pressure, or to retain dressings. Also for hernia at the groin.

b., spiral reverse. Technic of folding a bandage on itself, during application, to make it fit more uniformly. These reverse folds may be necessary every turn or less depending on contour of part being bandaged.

b., sterilastic. SEE: *cohesive bandage.*

b., suspensory. A bandage for supporting the scrotum.

b., T. One shaped like the letter T. For the perineum and, in certain cases, for the head.

b., tailed. One with ends split.

b., Theden's. A roller bandage applied from below upward over a graduated compress to control hemorrhage.

b., toe. Small bandage should be used, about 2 inches wide.

b., triangular. (von Esmarch bandage.) A 36- to 42-inch square, usually muslin cut diagonally, makes two triangular bandages. Frequently used in First Aid.

b., Velpeau (vel-pōz'). A special immobilizing roller bandage which incorporates the shoulder, arm and forearm.

SEE: *adhesive, binders, cast, cravat, slings.*

band forms [M. E. a band, + L. *forma*, shape]. Neutrophil granular leukocytes with bandlike or horseshoe shaped nuclei. Constitute about 4 per cent of total leukocytes.

Bandl's ring. Line of depression corresponding to site of internal *os uteri*, sometimes felt just above pubis during labor pains.

ban'dy leg. Bowleg. SYN: *genu varum.*

Banti's disease. A syndrome combining anemia, splenic enlargement, hemorrhages, and ultimately cirrhosis of liver.

baptorrhea (bap-tor-e'ă). An infectious discharge from a mucous membrane.

baragnosis (bar-ag-no'sis) [G. *baros*, weight, + *a-*, priv. + *gnōsis*, knowledge]. Inability to estimate weights.

Barba'does leg. Disease marked by hypertrophy of skin and subcutaneous tissue, due to obstruction of circulation in lymphatic or blood vessels. SYN: *elephantiasis, pachydermia.*

barber's itch. Fungous affection of the bearded portions of face and neck. SYN: *Tinea sycosis.*

ETIOL: Due to *Trichophyton tonsurans*.

SYM: Tubercules on hairy parts of face which involve the hair follicles, with suppuration in center of tubercules. Hair dry, brittle, and loose.

b. rash. Barber's itch. SEE: *sycosis.*

barbital (bar'bit-al) [diethylbarbituric acid]. (Veronal). USP. USES: As sedative and hypnotic in simple insomnia, neurasthenia, and sleeplessness of hysteria.

DOSAGE: 5 gr. (0.3 Gm.) in hot water or milk.

POISONING: SYM: Increasing drowsiness, followed by profound sleep and later coma. Respiration and pulse slowed.

F. A. TREATMENT: Evacuate stomach, follow by gastric lavage, with strong, warm, black coffee, leave coffee in stomach; stimulants of all types. Intravenous hypertonic glucose is of very great benefit. Promote perspiration.

b. sodium (soluble barbital, medicinal). USP. Has same properties as barbital but because of greater solubility, more rapidly absorbed. DOSAGE: 5 gr. (0.3 Gm.).

bar′bitalism. Acute or chronic poisoning from use of barbital or its derivatives. SYN: *barbiturism, q.v.*

barbituism (bar-bit′u-izm). Poisoning from use of barbital or its derivatives. SYN: *barbitalism, barbiturism.*

barbit′urate. Barbituric acid salt. Picrotoxin is the best antidote at present.

barbitu′rics. Derivatives of barbituric acid such as *luminal* (phenobarbital), *barbital* (veronal), *dial, amytal, allonal,* and many others. They are narcotics and hypnotics varying from mild sedation to profound sleep. They are not analgesics or anesthetics. They depress respiration rate and volume and, to lesser extent, create circulatory depression with symptoms of shock. May produce excitement and delirium. Used as preanesthetic medication. Dose is according to weight of patient. Adm. by mouth, rectum, or hypodermic injection. Effect minimized by patient's excitement.

NP AFTER CARE: While unconscious, place on side unless an air-way has been inserted, when patient may lie on back. Watch for quiet breathing and gray color of face which should be reported at once to surgeon. Have oxygen ready. Never leave patient while unconscious.

barbiturism (bar′bĭ-tu-rizm). Acute or chronic poisoning from use of veronal, luminal, or any barbituric acid derivatives. SYN: *barbituism.*

SYM: Headache, chills, fever, cutaneous eruption.

barbotage (bar-bo-tăzh′) [Fr. *barboter,* to dabble]. Spinal anesthesia by withdrawal of spinal fluid to which the drug is added before reinjection.

baresthesia (bar-es-the′zĭ-ă) [G. *baros,* weight, + *aisthēsis,* perception]. The pressure sense.

baresthesiometer (bar-es-the-si-om′ĕ-ter) [" + " + *metron,* measure]. Instrument for determining sensibility to pressure in different parts of body.

ba′ric [G. *baros,* weight]. Pert. to barium.

barium (ba′rĭ-um). SYMB: Ba. A metallic element of the alkaline group. Atomic weight 136.4. Barium sulfate is used for taking x-ray pictures of the abdominal tract.

b. compounds. POISONING: Largely used in the paint industries to kill pests; to color fireworks and in the form of soluble barium sulfate to visualize the hollow viscera in x-ray examinations. Poisoning occasionally comes from using the soluble salts in place of the insoluble sulfate.

SYM: Gastrointestinal irritation, pain, vomiting, convulsions, paralyses, and cardiac failures.

F. A. TREATMENT: Precipitate with epsom salts (magnesium sulfate), or Glauber's salts (sodium sulfate). Stimulants. Keep patient warm, increase fluid intake.

bark [Dan. bark]. The outer cover of the woody parts of a plant. Ex: *cascara sagrada, cinchona, wild cherry.*

Barkow's ligaments (bar′kōvs). Ant. and post. ligaments of elbow.

barley [A.S. *baerlic,* barley]. COMP: (pearled b.). AV. SERVING: 30 grams. Pro. 2.6%, Fat 0.3%, Carbo. 23.2%. FUEL VALUE: 100 Gm. give 351 calories. ASH CONST: Rich in minerals. Ca 0.020, Mg 0.070, K 0.241, Na 0.031, P 0.400, Cl 0.016, S 0.120, Fe 0.002. VITAMINS: (whole b.): A and B present, but C practically absent. ACTION: Easy to digest. Laxative due to cellulose content. SEE: *cereals.*

Barlow's disease. Infantile scurvy;* a deficiency disease; occurs in bottle-fed babies who lack other foods.

SYM: Failure to gain weight; tenderness of extremities; hemorrhage of gums, susceptibility to infections, paleness, lack of appetite.

TREATMENT: Vitamin foods in forms assimilable by infants.

barm [A.S. *beorma,* yeast]. Yeast.

Barnes' bag or **dilator.** Rubber bag used to induce premature labor by dilating uterine cervix.

B.'s curve. The segment of a circle whose center is the sacral promontory.

baro- [G.]. Prefix: Weight, heaviness.

barognosis (bar-og-no′sis) [G. *baros,* weight, + *gnōsis,* knowledge]. The ability to estimate weights. OPP: *baragnosis.*

barograph (bar′o-graf) [" + *graphein,* to write]. Self-registering barometer.

baromachrometer (bar-o-ma-krom′et-er) [" + *makros,* long, + *metron,* measure]. Instrument for measuring and weighing infants at time of birth.

bar′oscope [" + *skopein,* to examine]. Instrument noting atmospheric pressure variations, without accurately weighing them.

bar′ospirator [" + *spirāre,* to breathe]. Apparatus producing artificial respiration by means of air pressure variations in a closed chamber.

barotax′is [" + *taxis,* turning]. Protoplasmic reaction to any form of pressure.

barot′ropism [" + *tropē,* turning]. Protoplasmic reaction to any form of pressure. SYN: *barotaxis.*

bar′rel chest. A form of thorax resembling a cylinder.

bar′ren [M.E. *barain,* uncultivated land]. Sterile; incapable of producing offspring.

Bartholin's abscess (bar′to-linz). This develops when B.'s glands* are affected in gonorrhea and when they become occluded in an acute inflammatory process.

B.'s cyst. In chronic inflammation of B.'s glands* cysts are commonly formed. Carcinoma is rare.

B.'s ducts. Large ducts of the sublingual salivary gland. They parallel Wharton's duct* and open with it.

B.'s glands. Two small compound, racemose, mucous glands, pea to bean size, situated beneath the vestibule, one on each side of the vaginal opening and at the base of the labia majora. They lie under the constrictor muscles of the vagina. Their ducts open up on the sides of the vestibule and are 1.5 to 2 cm. in length. They secrete an odoriferous, yellowish, mucous fluid upon the inner surface of the vagina and labia majora, acting as a lubricant for copulation.

bartholinitis (bar-to-lin-i′tis) [Bartholin + G. *-itis,* inflammation]. Inflammation of a vulvovaginal gland.

Baruch's law. Water has a sedative effect when its temperature is the same as that of the skin, and a stimulating effect when it is below or above the skin temperature.

B.'s sign. When rectal temperature remains high after a 15-minute bath in water at 75° F. it points to typhoid fever.

baruria (bar-u'rĭ-ă) [G. *baros*, weight, + *ouron*, urine]. Urine having a high specific gravity.

bary- [G.]. Prefix: Heavy, dull, hard.

baryecoia (bar"ĭ-e-koy'ă) [G. *baryēkoia*, deafness]. Hardness of hearing; deafness.

baryesthesia (bar-ĭ-es-the'zĭ-ă) [G. *barys*, heavy, + *aisthēsis*, feeling]. The pressure sense. SYN: *baresthesia*.

baryglossia (bar-ĭ-glos'ĭ-ă) [" + *glōssa*, tongue]. Having a slow, thick utterance.

barylalia (bar-ĭ-la'lĭ-ă) [" + *lalia*, speech]. Indistinct, husky speech.

baryodmia (bar-ĭ-od'mĭ-ă) [" + *odmē*, stench]. Disagreeable, heavy odor.

baryodynia (bar-ĭ-ō-din'ĭ-ă) [" + *odynē*, pain]. Severe pain.

baryphonia (bar-ĭ-fo'nĭ-ă) [" + *phōnē*, voice]. Difficulty in speaking words.

bary'ta, bary'tes. Barium oxide, BaO; caustic and poisonous.

barythymia (bar-ĭ-thi'mĭ-ă) [G. *barys*, heavy, + *thymos*, mind]. Sullen, gloomy, or melancholy state of mind.

ba'sad [G. *basis*, base]. Denoting the direction toward the base of anything.

ba'sal. 1. Pert. to the base of anything; the base. 2. Of primary importance.
  b. ganglia. The *optic thalamus* and *corpus striatum* located in the floor of the lateral ventricles of the brain.

basal metab'olism [G. *basis*, base, + *metabolē*, change]. The minimal amount of energy or number of calories sufficient to support the basic metabolic processes of a resting individual in the postabsorptive state; the *basal metabolic rate*.
  The metabolic processes are maintenance of respiration, body temperature, peristalsis, circulation, function of glands, etc.
  Zero is used as the normal standard of measurement of basal metabolic rate, above or below, but this varies according to locality, condition of patient, and laboratory technic. Determination of zero point should be verified by determination of 25 normal persons.
  A formula given by Read is pulse rate plus 0.75 pulse pressure minus 72 equals basal metabolic rate. It is measured by amount of oxygen taken from the air or by skin radiation.
  Excess energy above that necessary to sustain the body is called *free energy* or *marginal metabolism*.
  Measured according to surface radiation, the basal metabolic rate drops from 50 calories per hour per sq. meter of surface at 12 years old to at least 40 calories at 17 years old, which rate is maintained until about 35 years old. It slowly decreases until 50 and goes much lower at 60 years of age.
  The brain seems to regulate the expenditure of energy and perhaps its generation through connection with the endocrines. The required brain energy necessary to produce intellectual activity is much less than the amount of physical energy necessary to produce physical activity.
  DIAG: Increased *b. m.* Seen in fevers, pregnancy, leukemia, decompensation, and esp. in hyperthyroidism; from plus 25 to plus 75. Low *b. m.* Indicates hypothyroidism, minus 25 to minus 40; pathological obesity; cachexia; myxedema. RS: *anabolism, catabolism, metabolism*.

bascula'tion [Fr. *basculer*, to swing]. 1. Replacement of a retroverted uterus by swinging it into place. 2. Systolic recoil of the heart.

base [G. *basis*, base]. 1. The lower part of anything. 2. The principal substance in a mixture. 3. (Chem.) A compound containing a metal or the ammonium radical combined with the *hydroxyl* (OH) radical. In general, any substance which will neutralize an acid. SYN: *alkali*. Bases react with acids to form salts, turn red litmus blue, and have a bitter taste. Strong bases feel slippery and are corrosive to human tissues. Ex. Sodium hydroxide (NaOH) (lye or caustic soda); potassium hydroxide (KOH) (caustic potash).
  This includes (a) compounds of metallic elements, as *e. g.*, sodium hydroxide, and (b) various complex nonmetallic substances such as ammonia, the amines,* and the alkaloids. Such substances are detected in solution by the colors they give with *indicators, q.v.*
  b. of heart. Heart surface back and upward, containing pulmonary vein and vena cavae openings.

baseball finger. Results from violent backward dislocation of the terminal phalanx onto the dorsum of the middle phalanx, as when a finger is struck on its tip when extended.

Basedow's disease (baz'e-do). Grave's disease; exophthalmic goiter.
  B.'s syndrome. Flashes of heat, sweating crisis, tachycardia.

basement membrane [G. *basis* + L. *membrana*, membrane]. A thin layer of solid substance underlying the epithelium of mucous surfaces; a part of the corium.* SEE: *membranes*.

base'plate. Plastic material for making dental trial plates.

bas-fond (bah-fawn') [Fr. *bas*, low, + *fond*, bottom]. A fundus.

basi-, basio- [G.]. Prefixes: base.

ba'sial [G. *basis*, base]. Pert. to the basion.

basiarachnitis (ba-sĭ-ar-ak-ni'tis) [" + *arachnē*, spider, + *-itis*, inflammation]. Inflammation of the arachnoid membrane at base of brain.

basiarachnoiditis (ba-sĭ-ar-ak-noy-di'tis) [" + " + *eidos*, form, + *-itis*, inflammation]. Inflammation of the arachnoid membrane at base of brain. SYN: *basiarachnitis*.

basibregmat'ic axis [" + *bregmata*, pl. front of head, + *axis*, pivot]. Vertical line from the basion to junction of coronal and sagittal sutures.

ba'sic. 1. Possessing properties opposite to those of an acid. 2. Fundamental.
  b. diet. Protein 1 Gm. per Kg. ideal body weight. Emphasize milk, all vegetables, all fruits except prunes, plums, cranberries, and possibly grapes. Limit meat, cereals, eggs.
  b. salt. A compound formed when only part of the hydroxide radicals of a base are replaced by the acid radical of an acid.

basicity (ba-sis'ĭ-tĭ). 1. Basic in character. 2. The combining power of an acid; the valence. It is expressed by a number indicating number of hydrogen atoms replaceable by a base.

basicra'nial axis [G. *basis*, foundation, + *kranion*, skull, + *axis*, pivot]. Straight line from the basion to point of angle of mandible.

basifa'cial axis [" + L. *facies*, face, + G. *axis*, pivot]. Straight line from the point of angle of mandible to the subnasal point.

basihyal, basihyoid (ba-sĭ-hi'al, -oyd) [" + *oeidēs*, hyoid]. The body of the hyoid

basilar B-12 **bath, animal**

arch or either of the two bones forming it.
bas′ilar. Basal; pert. to a base.
basilat′eral [G. *basis*, foundation, + L. *lateralis*, pert. to the side]. Both lateral and basilar.
basilem′ma [" + *lemma*, rind]. 1. Basement membrane. 2. Basis supporting framework of nervous tissue of cerebrospinal axis.
basil′ic. Prominent, important.
 b. vein. Large vein on inner side of biceps. Usually chosen for intravenous injection or for withdrawal of blood.
basilysis (bas-il′i-sis) [G. *basis*, base, + *lysis*, loosening]. Crushing the fetal head in labor.
basilyst tractor (ba′sil-ist). Instrument devised by Sir A. R. Simpson consisting of three blades for perforating the fetal head and obtaining a substantial grasp to facilitate delivery of the child.
basioccipital bone (bas-i-ok-sip′it-al) [G. *basis*, base, + L. *occiput*, head, + A.S. *bān*, bone]. Basilar process of occipital bone.
basioglossus (bas-i-o-glos′us) [" + *glossa*, tongue]. Part of hyoglossus muscle attached to base of hyoid bone.
ba′sion. Point at middle border of the foramen magnum.
basiot′ic [G. *basis*, base, + *ous*, ear]. Pert. to base of ear.
basiotribe (ba′si-o-trīb) [" + *tribein*, to crush]. Instrument for crushing the fetal head.
basiotripsy (ba-sī-o-trip′sī). Crushing fetal head.
basiphobia (bas-i-fo′bī-ă) [" + *phobos*, fear]. Fear of walking.
basirrhinal fissure (bas-i-ri′nal) [G. *basis*, + *ris*, nose]. 1. Pert. to base of brain and to the nose. 2. A cerebral fissure at base of olfactory lobe.
basis (ba′sis). Base.
 b. cranii. Base of skull.
basisphenoid (bas-i-sfe′noid) [G. *basis*, base, + *sphēn*, wedge, + *eidos*, form]. Lower portion of sphenoid bone.
basisyl′vian fissure. Transverse basilar portion or stem of sylvian fissure.
basket cell. A multipolar ganglion cell in outermost gray layer of cerebellum.
ba′sograph [G. *basis*, a walking, + *graphein*, to write]. Device for registering abnormalities of gait.
basophil(e (bas′o-fīl or fīl) [G. *basis*, base, + *philein*, to love]. (a) In histology, applied to cells or parts of cells which are readily stained with basic dyes like methylene blue; (b) A type of white blood cell (leukocyte) characterized by possession of coarse granules which stain intensely with basic dyes. Constitute 0.5-1% of leukocytes. Their function is unknown. They increase in certain pathological conditions (Hodgkin's disease, smallpox, chicken pox, myelocytic leukemia); (c) a type of cell found in the ant. lobe of the hypophysis.
basophilia (bas-o-fil′ī-ă). 1. A pathological condition of the blood in which the erythrocytes develop basophile granules. 2. A condition in which many mast cells are present.
basophilic (ba-so-fil′ik). Pert. to method of staining various cells.
basophil′ism. Condition characterized by excessive numbers of basophils.
 b. pituitary. A clinical syndrome (Cushing's disease) characterized by basophilic invasion or adenoma of the pituitary gland. SEE: *Cushing's disease*.
basophobia (bas-ō-fo′bī-ă) [G. *basis*, base,

+ *phobos*, fear]. 1. Emotional inability to stand or walk without muscle impairment. 2. Abnormal fear of walking.
bass deaf′ness. Deafness to bass notes, the higher ones being heard.
Bassini′s operation (bah-sī′nīz). One for inguinal hernia.
bas′tard [O.Fr. *batard*, bastard]. 1. One born out of wedlock. 2. Not legitimate.
Bastedo′s sign (băs-tē′dō) (W. A. Bastedo, physician, New York, born 1873). Tenderness and pain in right iliac fossa on inflation of the colon with air in chronic appendicitis.
 B.'s rule. One for dosage for children from one to twelve years old. For child of x years, adult dose is multiplied by x plus 3.

30

bath [A.S. *baeth*, bath]. The medium and method of cleansing the body or any part of it, or to treat it therapeutically, as with air, light, steam, vapor, water, etc.

Room Temperature   Water Temperature
                              Should Be
Below 76° F..................94-96° F.
Above 76° F......... ....92-94° F.
On hot summer days.. ...... 90° F.
If Rectal Temperature Is   Bath Water
                                Should Be
103° F. ....   90° F.
104° F. ....   86° F.
104.5° F. ....   82° F.
105° F.   ....   76° F.
105.5° F. ....70-60° F.
 Baths May Be Indicated As:
Cold .... 45- 65° F.
Cool .... 65- 75° F.
Tepid .... 75- 85° F.
Warm .... 85- 95° F.
Hot ....95-105° F.
Very Hot ....105-110° F.

The general cleansing bath for a bed patient may be from 110°-115° F. with a room temperature of 75°-82° F.
 THERAPEUTIC EFFECT OF: *Warm and Hot Baths and Applications*: They sooth the cutaneous nerves, and nerves of internal organs in reflex relation with the skin areas to which heat is applied. *Gradually Elevated Hot Tub and Vapor Baths*: They relax all the muscles of the body. *Brief Hot Tub and Shower Baths*: They relieve fatigue but may cause cerebral congestion and wakefulness unless cold compresses are used on the head. *Hot Baths*: They relax tissues, including the capillaries of the skin, drawing blood from the deeper tissues. They also relieve pain. They stimulate the nerves. *Cold Baths and Applications*: They abstract heat and stimulate reaction, especially if followed by frictions and percussion. They contract the small blood vessels when applied locally. *Cold and Hot Applications*: One followed by the other causes revulsion, relieving congestion of internal organs.
 b., acid. 5 oz. hydrochloric acid or 1 gal. vinegar to 30 gal. water.
 b., air. Therapeutic use of air, warmed or vaporized, on the nude body.
 b., alcohol. Use of alcohol on patient, as a stimulant and defervescent, in dilute form.
 b., alkaline. For chronic rheumatism. 1 lb. sodium bicarbonate or washing soda to 30 gal. water.
 b., alum. Use of alum in washing solution, as an astringent.
 b., animal. Therapeutic use of a recently killed animal or its pelt on a patient.

b., antipyretic. SEE: *Brand b.*
b., antiseptic. For irritating, offensive, and parasitic skin diseases. SEE: *carbolic, creosote, sulfur baths.*
b., aromatic. One to which some volatile oil or perfume is added, or some herb.
b., arsenical. Weak solution in tepid bath.
b., arthritic. Alum, ½ lb., to 30 gal. water, or boric acid solution, 2½%, made by adding 2-3 lb. boric acid to 30 gal. water. Tannic acid only as ordered. Amount of any of these baths must be specified by physician and amount checked.
b., astringent. Bathing in liquid containing an astringent.
b., blanket. One in which wet pack and blankets are used.
b., blood. One using fresh animal blood.
b., bog. Peaty mud bath, for therapeutic purposes.
b., borax. Glycerin and borax solution for bathing.
b., box. One in which patient is completely enclosed in box except for his head.
b., bran. 2-3 lb. bran to 30 gal. water, or 3-5 lb. malt or starch to 1 gal. water added to full bath at 95° F. to 96° F., may be used to stop itching.
b., Brand. Full bath of 65° F. combined with strong friction in the water, used in typhoid fever.
b., brine. 7 lb. sea salt to 30 gal. water.
b., bubble. Mechanical production in a bathtub of water of tiny air bubbles by (1) an air distributor which consists of a number of metal tubes through which the air passes to the water, (2) an air pump, and (3) an electric motor that drives the pump.
b., cabinet. Exposure of the skin of the body except the head, to heat from electric lamps, live steam, steam radiators, or electric heaters. Bath cabinets are constructed of wood, marble, or steel.
b., camphor. Bath in air charged with camphor.
b., carbolic. Strength 1-100. Mix 48 oz. pure carbolic in 5 pt. boiling water, putting it into bath before 30 gal. water are added, to make sure of mixing.
b., carbon dioxide. An effervescent saline bath consisting of water, salts, and CO_2. The natural CO_2 baths are known as Nauheim baths, and approach closely CO_2 baths in their therapeutic effects.
b., cold. One used for stimulation, being followed by brisk rub.
b., cold plunge. Tub bath with water at 85-79° F., duration ½ to 3 minutes, with bather using friction while in water.
b., colloid. One containing bran, gelatin, starch, etc., for treatment of dermatitis.
b., continuous. One that is administered for hours, days, weeks, or months. It is a continuous, flowing bath if the prescribed temperature is maintained by keeping a stream of water flowing through the tub.
b., contrasted. Used for hands or feet. Two large basins or pails of sufficient depth, filled with water, one as hot as can be borne, the other as cold as can be borne. Change or add hot and cold water frequently to keep temperatures same as in beginning. Put part to be treated in hot water for 1 minute, then into cold for ½ minute, then again into hot water. Repeat for prescribed length of time, ending with cold water.
b., creosote. 1-2 drams creosote to 30 gal. water, to which 10 oz. glycerine are sometimes added.
b., douche. Large jets of water sprayed on the body.
b., drip sheet. Modified sheet bath.
b., earth. Bathing in warmed earth or sand.
b., electric light. Exposure of the nude body, except the head, to rays from a large number of electric lights placed on the inside walls of a cabinet.
b., electrotherapeutic. An electric current sent through water in which the patient lies, or in which a limb is immersed. Only a faradic current is used for a faradic bath.
b., emollient. Used for irritation and inflammation of skin, and after erysipelas. SEE: *glycerin, linseed, oatmeal, powdered borax, starch baths.*
b., foam. Tub bath to which has been added an extract of a saponin containing vegetable fiber, and through this mixture, O or CO_2 is driven through porous wood or the foam is produced mechanically.
b., foot. Immersion of feet and legs to a depth of 4 inches above ankles in water at 98° F. The temperature of the water is increased.
b., full. The whole body except the head is immersed in water.
b., galvanic. Entire body or one or more limbs immersed in large tub or several smaller basins made of insulating material (porcelain or wood), with electrodes consisting of metal plates in wooden frame to prevent direct contact with patient's body. Motor generators generally preferable to wall plates, or other not ground-free sources of current.
b., glycerin. 10 oz. to 30 gal. water.
b., half. Tub bath with about 18 inches of water; the temperature depends on the case and the desired action.
b., Heller. Form of hydroelectric bath.
b., herb. One to 2 pounds of herbs, such as chamomile, wild thyme, or spearmint, are tied in bag, boiled with 1 gal. of water, and the decoction added to the full bath.
b., hip. SEE: *sitz b.*
b., hot. Tub bath with the water covering the body to a little above the nipples and temperature gradually raised from 98° F. to desired degree (to 108° F.).
b., hot air. Exposure of entire body except head to hot air contained in a bath cabinet.
b., hydroelectric. Application of faradic, galvanic, or sinusoidal current conducted to the patient through water.
b., hyperthermal. One in which the body except head is immersed in water from 105-120° F. for 1 to 2 minutes.
b., immersion. Free tub bath.
b., incandescent light. SEE: *electric light b.*
b., internal. Introduction of large amounts of water into rectum and stomach.
b., kinetotherapeutic. Bath given for underwater exercises of weak or partially paralyzed muscles.
b., linseed. 1-2 lb. to 30 gal. water. Boil emollient in a tied muslin bag, and add the mucilage to the 30 gal. water.
b., lukewarm. Bath in which patient's

whole body except head is submerged in water, temperature, 94-96° F., duration 15-60 minutes.

b., medicated. Bath to which bran, oatmeal, starch, sodium bicarbonate, epsom salts, pine products, tar, sulfur, potassium permanganate, or salt is added.

b., milk. Bath taken in milk, as an emollient or cosmetic.

b., mud. Old form of applying moist heat which depends on availability of certain soils heated by thermal springs or artificially.

b., mustard. For irritant effect, and to draw blood from deeper parts, as in a febrile cold, infantile convulsions, infantile diarrhea, and for shock. A heaping tablespoonful of fresh mustard for each gallon of water. In adults it is used as a hot foot bath.

b., Nauheim (naw′hīm). A bath in which the human body is immersed in warm water and subjected to the action of carbon dioxide gas.

b., neutral. One in which no circulatory or thermic reaction occurs, temperature 92-97° F.

b., neutral sitz. Same as hot sitz bath, except temperature between 92-97° F., and foot bath, 104-110° F., duration 15-60 minutes.

b., oatmeal. 2-3 lb. to 30 gal. water.

b., oxygen. Given by introducing O into the bath through a special device consisting of a metal plate provided with bamboo reeds which are connected to an oxygen tank or by generating the O by chemicals.

b., paraffin. Member is immersed in warm paraffin, 140-150° F., withdrawn, immersed again, withdrawn repeatedly until it is encased. For larger joints, may be applied with paint brush. Apparatus is manufactured in which extremity may remain in bath of paraffin, temperature 130-135° F., equipped with electric heating coils, controlled by a switch and thermostat, lined with insulating material.

b., Peng. A form of foam bath, *q.v.*

b., pine needle. One-half to 1 lb. extract pine needles added to a bath covering the whole body to the chin, temperature 93-98° F., duration 20 minutes.

b., powdered borax. One-half lb. to 30 gal. water; 5 oz. glycerine may be added.

b., reducing. One given to reduce patient's temperature.

b., Russian. Warm vapor bath followed by rubbing and cold plunge.

b., saline. Given in artificial sea water made by dissolving 8 lb. of sea salt, or a mixture of 7 lb. of sodium chloride and ½ lb. of magnesium sulfate in 30 gal. of water.

b., Sandor. A form of foam bath, *q.v.*

b., Schnee. Four cell hydroelectric bath.*

b., seawater or salt. Antipruritic.

b., sedative. A prolonged warm bath. Continuous flow of water may be used. Use air cushion and back rest.

b., sheet. Given by wrapping the patient in a sheet previously dipped in water 80-90° F., and rubbing the whole body with vigorous strokes on the sheet, until all parts of the sheet feel warm.

b., shower. Water sprayed down upon the body from an overhead source.

b., sitz. Immersion of thighs, buttocks, and abdomen below the umbilicus in water. In a hot sitz bath the water is first 92° F. and elevated to 106° F., duration 3 to 10 minutes.

b., sponge. One in which patient's body is moistened with washcloth or sponge.

b., starch. 1 lb. mixed in cold water, pouring boiling water to make starch mucilage, which add to 30 gal. water.

b., steam. Given in a chamber into which steam under low pressure is allowed to escape. Disadvantage is that patient must breathe hot, moist air. Better form of application is that in which subject sits in cabinet or lies in box with head outside.

b., stimulating. One which increases cutaneous effect; used for tonic purposes. SEE: *brine, cold, and mustard baths.* [water.

b., sulfur. 2 or 3 oz. sulfur to 30 gal.

b., sweat. One given to induce perspiration, as in temperature reduction.

b., tonic. One which, through its stimulation of the cutaneous nerves and the response of the autonomic nervous system, quickens the circulation of the blood throughout the body.

b., towel. Given by applying towels dipped in water 70-60° F. to arms, legs, ant. and post. surfaces of trunk successively, removing towel, drying part.

b., vapor. Exposure of skin of body except head to vapor. Sometimes the vapor is impregnated with substances thought to possess therapeutic value, as sulfur, mercury, or camphor.

b., whirlpool. Continuous localized douches for the arm and leg. Water 105-120° F. from a thermostatic mixer is given a swirling motion in special reservoir as it mixes with air forced through an aerator.

b., Ziemssen (tsĕm′sen). Tub bath at 88° F., cold water added slowly until temperature reaches 65° F., patient is rubbed vigorously; duration 20-30 minutes or until chilled.

bathesthe′sia [G. *bathys*, deep, + *aisthēsis*, perception]. Consciousness of joints, muscles, and organs beneath the skin. SYN: *bathyesthesia*.

bath′mic [G. *bathmos*, a step]. Pert. to the vital force controlling nutritional function.

bath′mism [″ + *ismos*, condition of]. Force regulating nutrition and growth.

bathmotrop′ic [″ + *trepein*, to turn]. Promoting excitability of tissues in response to stimuli.

bathopho′bia [G. *bathos*, height, + *phobos*, fear]. A fear of high objects.

bath″yanesthe′sia [G. *bathys*, deep, + *ana-*, priv. + *aisthēsis*, perception]. Loss of deep sensibility.

bathycar′dia [″ + *kardia*, heart]. A fixed abnormally low position of the heart.

bathyesthesia (bath-ĭ-es-thē′zĭ-ă) [″ + *aisthēsis*, sensation]. A consciousness of muscles, joints, and organs under skin.

bathygastry (bath′ĭ-gas-trĭ) [″ + *gastēr*, stomach]. Abnormally low stomach. SYN: *Gastroptosis*.

bathyhyperesthesia (bath-ĭ-hī″per-es-thē′-zĭ-ă) [″ + *yper*, above, + *aisthēsis*, sensation]. Sensitiveness of muscular tissues and deep structures.

batono′ma [G. *batos*, height, + *ōma*, tumor]. A tumor supposed to be caused by vegetable organisms of higher grade than bacteria.

batophobia (bat-ō-fō′bĭ-ă) [″ + *phobos*, fear]. 1. Acrophobia; fear of heights. 2. Dread of anything high.

batrachoplasty (bat′rak-o-plăs-tĭ) [G. *batrachos*, frog, + *plassein*, to form]. Plastic operation for ranula.

battarism (băt′ă-rĭzm). Stuttering.

bat'tery [Fr. *battre*, to beat]. Device for generating galvanic currents by chemical action.

Bat'tey's operation. Excision of healthy ovaries to induce menopause or for other therapeutic purposes.

bauchstiel (bowch'shteel). The abdominal pedicle by which the embryo is attached to the chorionic membrane.

Baudelocque's diameter (bō-dloks'). Distance bet. the depression just beneath the spine of the last lumbar vertebra and the ant. and upper margin of the *symphysis pubis*. The ext. conjugate diameter.

B.'s method. Manipulation to convert a face presentation into one of the vertex.

Bauer qual'imeter. Instrument for measuring intensity and penetrating power of roentgen rays through various metals. SEE: *penetrometer.* [*valvula coli.*

Bauhin's valve (bo-anz'). Ileocecal valve;

baunscheidtism (bown'shīd-izm). Acupuncture for producing counterirritation.

Bava'rian splint. A splint of plaster of Paris between two flannel cloths.

Bayle's disease. A general paresis described in 1822 by Antoine Bayle.

bay'onet leg. Backward dislocation at knee joint of tibia and fibula.

Bazin's disease (bah-zanz'). 1. Buccal psoriasis. Purple or reddish nodules on legs which may ulcerate. 2. Erythema induratum.

B. C. G. Abbr. *Calmette-Guérin bacillus.*

B. C. G. vaccine. (a) Bovine tubercle bacilli are attenuated by long growth over many years with many transfers in a bile-containing artificial medium; (b) a single subcutaneous injection is given to infants who live in a tuberculous environment.

b. d. Abbr. L. *bis die,* twice a day.

bdellometer (del-lom'et-er) [G. *bdella,* leech, + *metron,* measure]. Artificial substitute for a leech.

beaded [A.S. *bed,* prayer]. Referring to disjointed colonies along the inoculation line in a streak or stab.

beads, rachitic. Visible swelling where the ribs join their cartilages, seen in rickets. "Rachitic rosary."

bead test. A method of testing the activity of the digestive process in different parts of the alimentary tract. Beads covered with different types of food are attached by a thread and enclosed in a capsule which the patient swallows after a meal. The time taken for elimination of the beads per rectum is noted, and the remaining food on the beads is carefully examined.

beaker (bē'ker) [O.E. *becke,* beak]. Glass vessel with wide mouth for mixing or holding liquids.

beans [A.S.]. COMP. There are many varieties of beans, but their composition is practically the same. They are heavy in cellulose and have a higher percentage of fats than peas and other lentils, although not so easily digested. All legumes are digested better as a part of a mixed diet.

b., kidney are a good source of B and contain A, but lack in C and G.

b., navy. *Canned:* Vit. C. 5 units per oz., 45 units per 100 cal. Navy b., *dried or canned,* contain Vit. A, and are a good source of Vit. B, but C and G are lacking.

b., string. The carbohydrates of string beans are made up of both nuclein and of inosite which do not produce glucose. They contain 92% water. A good source of Vit. A, C and G and Vit. B, excellent.

bear'ing down. The expulsive effort of a parturient woman, in second stage of labor.

beat [A.S. *bēatan,* to strike]. A pulsation or throb resulting from contraction of the heart, or the passage of blood through a vessel.

b., apex. Stroke of the heart beat felt by the hand when held over the fifth intercostal space on left of chest wall.

b., ectopic. One beginning at a place other than sinoauricular node.

b., forced. Extrasystole brought on by artificial heart stimulation.

b., premature. An extrasystole.

beat knee. A subcutaneous connective tissue inflammation over the patella.

Beccaria's sign (bek-kă'rĭ-ä's). Occipital pulsation in pregnancy.

Constituents of Beans

NUTRIENTS	Pro.	Fat	Carbo.	Cals. per lb.
baked (canned)	6.9%	2.5%	19.6%	583
dried	22.5%	1.8%	59.6%	1565
lima, dried	18.1%	1.5%	65.9%	1586
lima, fresh	7.1%	.7%	22.0%	557
string, fresh	2.3%	.3%	7.4%	184

Ash Constituents

	Ca	Mg	K	Na	P	Cl	S	Fe
dried	.160	.56	1.229	.097	.471	.032	.215	.0079
kidney (dried)	.132	.139	1.144	.041	.475	.041	.227	.0079
lima (dried)	.071	.188	1.741	.249	.338	.026	.161	.0086
lima (fresh)	.028	.070	.613	.088	.133	.009	.057	.0024
string (fresh)	.046	.025	.247	.019	.052	.024	.030	.0010

BASE-FORMING ELEMENTS (alkalinity): *Dried b.* 13.0 cc. per 100 Gm., 5.0 per 100 cal. *String b. fresh.* 5.4 cc. per 100 Gm., 13 per 100 cal. *Lima b. dried.* 41 cc. per 100 Gm., 122 cc. per 100 cal. *Fresh,* 14 cc. per 100 Gm., 12 cc. per 100 cal.

Fuel Value

	Gm.		Cal.	Gm.		Cal.
baked	78	=	100	100	=	128
dried	29	=	100	100	=	345
lima (dried)	28	=	100	100	=	357
lima (fresh)	81	=	100	100	=	123
string (fresh)	248	=	100	100	=	40

bechesthesis (bek-es'thes-is) [G. *bēx*, cough, + *aisthēsis*, feeling]. A feeling in the throat causing one to cough.

bech'ic. 1. Controlling a cough. 2. A cough medicine.

Bechterew-Mendel reflex (bekh'te-rev). A reflex indicating a lesion of the pyramidal tract, and manifested when the cuboid bone is tapped, causing a flexion of the 4 outer toes.

Bechterew's reflex (bĕk'tĕr-ĕv). 1. Contraction of facial muscles due to irritation of nasal mucosa. 2. Dilatation of pupil on exposure to light. 3. Plantar flexion of foot. 4. Flexion of foot in dorsal direction and flexive movement of knee and hip following passive flexion of toes and plantar extension of foot. 5. Contraction of lower abdominal muscles when skin of inner surface of thigh is stroked.

Béclard's hernia (bā-klärs'). Hernia through opening for the saphenous vein.

bed [A.S. *bedd*, bed]. A piece of furniture for rest of body.

"How TO MAKE: *To remake if patient cannot be removed*:
1. Have everything ready before beginning.
2. Untuck all bedclothes.
3. Remove upper bedclothes, fold and place on chair, seeing that they do not touch the floor. Leave a blanket covering the patient.
4. Remove pillows and lay patient flat if possible.
5. Tighten bottom rubber sheet, blanket, and sheet.
6. Turn patient over on to side.
7. Roll draw sheet to middle and brush crumbs, etc., off bottom sheet.
8. Turn patient on to the other side. Remove draw sheet, shake, and place on chair.
9. Brush that side of bottom sheet.
10. Tuck in one end of draw sheet.
11. Make a neat roll of the remainder of draw sheet and put close to patient's back.
12. Turn patient over.
13. The other nurse to take the roll and tuck it under the opposite side so that it is quite taut.
14. Replace pillows.
15. Replace top bedclothes. Loosen them over the patient's feet.
16. Inspect work, seeing that the patient is comfortable and the bed neat.

When possible the bed should be aired.

Changing bottom sheet:
1. Strip bed and remove pillows as in bed making.
2. Tighten rubber sheet and under blanket.
3. Turn patient to one side.
4. Roll the draw sheet and soiled bottom sheet to the middle of bed.
5. Roll one-half of the clean sheet in its place; the middle crease must be placed in the middle of the bed.
6. Tuck in this side.
7. Put in clean draw sheet now, if needed.
8. Roll patient over on to the other side of bed.
9. Second nurse to remove the dirty sheet, unroll clean sheet, pull it tight, and tuck under the mattress.
10. Treat draw sheet in similar manner.

Soiled linen should be placed in a bowl or bucket when removed from the bed, and not thrown on to the floor.

When the patient cannot be rolled, the sheet can be changed from top to bottom, the sheet being rolled widthways instead of lengthways.

The nurse must remember that making the bed is a very tiring procedure for the patient, and therefore all unnecessary exertion should be avoided.

Changing Top Sheet: The clean sheet is opened and placed over the top sheet and the soiled one drawn from top to bottom beneath it."—*Hilda M. Gration, S.R.N.*

b., air. One inflatable with air.

b. blocking. Placing bedblocks under bed to raise it at head or foot.

Foot of b. raised: (a) In shock; (b) bleeding from lower limbs; (c) edema of lower limbs, vulva, or scrotum; (d) some cases of hemorrhoids; (e) to retain enema or aid high colonic injection; (f) when weight is used on lower limbs; (g) in reduction of inguinal hernia.

Head of b. raised: (a) To drain abdomen or pelvis; (b) to aid respiration; (c) in treatment for bleeding from head, neck, or upper chest.

b. case. Hysteria with refusal to leave the bed.

b. fast, b. ridden. Unable or unwilling to leave the bed.

b., fracture. One for patients with fracture.

b., Gatch. One with a jointed bed rest that can be raised into a half-sitting position.

b., hydrostatic. A water bed.

b., metabolic. One arranged to catch the feces and urine.

b. rest. A device for propping up patients in bed.

b., water. A rubber mattress filled with water. USES: Prevention of bed sores.

bedbug (*Cimex lectularius*) [" + M.E. *bugge*, swollen]. An insect which injects an irritating substance causing a purpuric* reaction, or an urticarial* wheal.

TREATMENT: Antipruritic lotions containing phenol, camphor, and menthol. Dusting of guaiacyl powder bet. the sheets is a preventive measure.

b. poison. Usually contains combinations of mercury, nicotine, fluorides, arsenic, or strychnine as principal ingredients, the names of which usually appear on the container.

SYM: Gastrointestinal irritation, abdominal cramping.

F. A. TREATMENT: Wash out stomach and give large quantities of milk and egg whites.

Bed'nar's aph'thae. Minute yellowish patches on either side of the palate of the newly born.

bedpan [A.S. *bedd*, bed, + *panna*, flat vessel]. Device for receiving fecal and urinal discharges from patient confined to the bed.

bedsore [" + O.E. *sāre*, open wound]. Pressure sore. SYN: *decubitus.**

Decubitus consists of ulceration and gangrene of a localized area, usually over the sacrum, due to pressure which limits the nutrition of the affected area by:
1. Inducing a passive congestion in the veins and capillaries surrounding it, thereby restricting the inflow of fresh blood to the part.
2. By squeezing the lymph from its contact with the cells. It is likely to

bedwetting　　　　　　　　　　　B-17　　　　　　**belladonna, atropine poisons**

develop and become serious when spinal cord lesion lowers tissue resistance.
CAUSE: Continued pressure. PREDISPOSING CAUSES: (1) Any factor which interferes with the circulation. (2) Prolonged fever. (3) Emaciation. (4) Obesity. (5) Paralysis. (6) Old age or senility. (7) Poorly made beds. (8) Lack of cleanliness. (9) Bruising. (10) Too infrequent change of positions. (11) Cardiac diseases, nephritis, diabetes, anemia, etc.
LOCATION: The body prominences thinly covered with flesh, as: (1) The end of the spine. (2) The buttocks. (3) The heels. (4) Elbows. (5) Shoulder blades. (6) Back of the head and ears in children.
TREATMENT: (1) Best nursing care, as prevention is easier than a cure. (2) Prophylactic measures in keeping the bed dry and clean. (3) Relieving the pressure as soon as the first signs of redness appear. (4) Report to the attending physician at once. (5) Use the prescribed medication as directed. (6) Keep affected part covered by soft gauze held in place by narrow adhesive straps which will facilitate changing of dressings without further irritating the skin. (7) If nurse is thrown on her own resource for treatment, apply alcohol and massage the surrounding area at least three times a day.
When massaging, keep the fingers or hand still on the part you are massaging and move the tissues. Do not rub the skin as it may break. Zinc oxide may be gently massaged over the affected area. A solution of alum which has been dissolved by alcohol is also very effective. Balsam of Peru is also extensively used. An electric heater may be used to keep the skin warm.
A fresh 5% solution of tannic acid in water may be sprayed on the sore every hour, or gauze saturated in the solution may be applied, keeping the gauze wet with the solution. Discontinue when the sore is covered with a thick tannic layer, which will be in about 12 hours. It may be applied at first showing of redness of skin. The sore should be sterilized, before using tannic acid, if badly infected.

bed'wetting. Name for habit of young children of wetting bed at night. SYN: *enuresis, q.v.*

beef [Fr. *boeuf*, flesh]. COMP: Protein: Nitrogen is the essential characteristic of beef, it being richer in this element than any other food excepting cheese. The fatter the beef the smaller the percentage of nitrogen.

	Gr. per lb.	%
Purins:		
Beef ribs	.113	7.96
Steak	.206	14.45
Sirloin	.130	9.13

CARBO: Very deficient. They are principally in the form of glycogen or animal sugar. FATS: Second only to butter, sugar, bread, rice and pulse. Half its calory value is derived from albumin, an inferior source of energy. MINERALS: Very deficient in salts, although the phosphates are superabundant. Chloride of sodium (salt) is almost nil, and meat may be considered a dechlorated food. NUTRIENTS: Depend upon the amount of fat.
AV. SERVING: 230 Gm.

	Pro. %	Fat %	Cal. per lb.
Porterhouse	21.9	20.4	1230
Sirloin	18.9	18.5	1099
Tenderloin	16.2	24.4	1290

beer [A.S. *bēor*, fermented drink]. Fermented alcoholic beverage from a malt infusion of barley, malt or hops, with aid of brewer's yeast.
Contains about 4% alcohol, 1% sugar, 3% dextrin with small amount of lactic acid, glycerine, and inorganic salts.
ASH CONST. (in grams per 100 cal): Ca 0.008, P 0.061, Fe 0.00217, CaO 0.011, P_2O_5 0.140. CALORIES: 500 per qt.

Beer's operation. Flap operation for cataract or artificial pupil.

bee sting [A.S. *bēo*, bee, + *stingan*, to pierce]. The sting, which is barbed, is usually left in the wound. Plain, mottled redness, and edema result. In the aged, phlebitis, erysipelas, and other septic conditions may occur. The remedy is as stated for insect bites. RS: *apisination.*

beestings (best'ings) [A.S. *bysting*, puffed up]. Colostrum*; first milk after parturition.

beets (red) [L. *beta*, beet]. COMP: Rich in sugar. Calory value less than carrots, turnips, or salsify and less in fat. They contain oxalic acid. NUTRIENTS: Av. SERVING: 100 Gm. Prot. 1.6, Fat 0.1, Carbo 8.8. Vit. A+, B+, C+, G+. FUEL VALUE: 100 Gm.—39 cal. ASH CONST: Ca 0.029, Mg 0.021, K 0.353, Na 0.093, P 0.039, Cl 0.058, S 0.016, Fe 0.0006. *Fresh Beets*: They are base-forming, alkalinity being 10.9 cc. per 100 Gm., or 23.6 per 100 cal. Prot. 2.0, Fat 0.3, Carbo 4.2 per 100 Gm. Vit. A+, B+++, G+++. ACTION: Pickled beets hard to digest. Boiled easier to digest. Slightly laxative. Should be mixed with salads.

beg'ma [G. cough]. 1. A cough. 2. Expectorated matter.

behav'iorism. A theory of conduct which regards normal and abnormal behavior as the result of conditioned reflexes quite apart from the concept of will. It does not apply to conditions resulting from structural disease.

behavior reflex. One acquired as result of training and repetition.

Beh'ring's law. Serum of an immunized person confers immunity on another into whom diphtheria antitoxin is injected.

belch [A.S. *baelcian*, to eructate]. Escape of gas from the stomach through the mouth; to eructate.

belching. Raising of gas from the stomach.
ETIOL: Gastric fermentation; air swallowing; gas-containing foods, foods or drinks taken simultaneously and containing acid and alkaline substances. RS: *eructation, rectus.*

belem'noid [G. *belemnon*, dart, + *eidos*, shape]. Dart shaped; styloid.

belladonna (bel-a-don'a) [It. fair lady] (Deadly Nightshade). USP. The dried leaves and roots of *Atropa belladonna*, the active principle of which is atropine.*
ACTION AND USES: Same as atropine.
DOSAGE: (Leaf) = 1 ℳ (0.06 cc.). (Root) = ¾ ℳ (0.05 cc.).

b. and atropine poisons. These include stramonium, hyoscyamus, scopolamine, belladonna, and atropine.
SYM: Poisoning from them is attended by extreme dryness of mouth and throat, due to paralysis of the chorda tympani nerve which diminishes supply of saliva; huskiness of the voice, redness of tongue, great thirst, difficulty in swallowing, and marked dilatation of the pupils making the eyes prominent, brilliant, staring, and interfering with accommodation of the eye, making near

vision difficult or impossible. Distant vision is unimpaired. Hallucinations, dizziness, vertigo, excitement, and delirium are usually present. The patient may be violent or merely hilarious. Nausea is common, the pulse is at first strong, but later becomes weak and rapid or even imperceptible. Respirations become increased at first, but may be depressed later. The skin is dry and may be hot, and occasionally erythema is present. These symptoms may come on in susceptible patients when these drugs are given in ordinary dosage, but an excessive amount is usually required.

TREATMENT: If drug is swallowed give an emetic or use stomach pump. Morphine usually given as an antidote. Stimulants if necessary; strong, black coffee. Artificial respiration may be required.

Bellini's ducts (bel-lī'nĭ). The excretory tubules of the kidneys.

B.'s ligament. A fasciculus of capsular ligament of the hip reaching the great trochanter.

Bell-Magendie's law. That ant. spinal nerve roots only contain motor fibers and post. roots sensory fibers.

bell'-metal resonance. A metal-like sound heard in pneumothorax.

Belloc's cannula or **sound** (bel-loks'). An instrument for drawing in a plug through nostril and mouth in epistaxis.

bell sound. Bell metal resonance.

Bell's disease. Acute delirious mania; acute periencephalitis.

B.'s law. Post. spinal nerve roots are sensory and ant. ones motor.

B.'s nerves. Internal and external respiratory nerves.

B.'s paralysis. Facial motor lower neuron paralysis affecting 7th cranial nerve.

SYM: Pain or tenderness behind ear and at side of neck followed by complete paralysis of facial muscles. Face expressionless, upper eyelids droop, lower lids sag, as well as corners of mouth. Fluid trickles out of mouth, and tears run down face. Lasts for few weeks to a few months and recovery usually takes place.

NP: Heat to affected side. Bathe eye and keep covered with a pad. Mouth must be kept clean. Light massage as recovery sets in. Teach patient to move facial muscles by frowning, grinning, whistling, etc.

B.'s spasm. Convulsive facial tic.

belly [A.S. *baelg*, bag]. Abdomen; stomach.

b. ache. Colic, gastralgia.

b. button. Umbilicus.

b. of muscle. Nontendinous thick central part of a muscle.

belonepho'bia [G. *belonē*, needle, + *phobos*, fear]. Morbid fear of sharp-pointed objects.

belonoid (bel'o-noid) [G. *belonē*, needle, + *eidos*, shape]. Needle shaped.

belonoskiascopy (bel-o-no-ski-as'ko-pĭ) [" + *skia*, shadow, + *skopein*, to examine]. Subjective retinoscopy by means of shadows and movements to determine refraction.

benadryl (ben'a-dril). A drug effective in common allergies, preventing ill effects of histamine released from body cells during an attack of allergy.

Bence-Jones' albumose. Protein bodies appearing in the urine of persons suffering from disease of the bone marrow.

On heating the urine, a precipitate forms at about 60° C.; this disappears on further heating to the boiling point, and reappears on cooling at 60° C.

Bendien's test. A precipitation test carried out in varying concentrations of blood serum and colloidal vanadic acid, reputed to be of diagnostic value in cancer.

bends [caisson disease]. Pain and weakness caused by increased atmospheric pressure.

This brings about the absorption of atmospheric gases other than oxygen, particularly nitrogen. Release of pressure releases this nitrogen from solution in the blood and causes formation of gas bubbles in the tissues.

TREATMENT: Decompression, or increased pressure reapplied until nitrogen is redissolved in the blood, when gradual cessation of pressure is induced.

beneceptor (be'ne-sep-tor) [L. *bene*, well, + *capere*, to take]. A nerve organ for the reception and transmission of beneficial stimuli.

Benedict's solution. A solution used to test for the presence of glucose. It consists of:

B. test. Place 5 ml. of Benedict's sol. in a test tube and heat to boiling. Add 8-10 drops of urine. Mix and boil vigorously. Let cool slowly. Positive reaction indicated by turbidity of solution due to formation of a precipitate, which is greenish, yellow or brick-red depending on amount of glucose present.

Ben'edikt's syndrome. Hemiplegia with oculomotor paralysis and clonic spasm on opp. side.

benign (be-nin') [L. *benignus*, mild]. 1. Not recurrent. 2. Not malignant. 3. Mild.

b. stupor. A stupor sometimes seen in the depression of manic-depressive psychosis.

benig'nant [L. *benignus*, mild]. 1. Not malignant. 2. Not recurrent. SYN: *benign*.

Benzedrine (ben-ze-drēn'). Trade name for *amphetamine*. A colorless mobile liquid, producing local effects similar to those of ephedrine.

USES: In head colds, by shrinking of the nasal mucosa, sinusitis, hay fever, asthma. Should be used with caution.

CONTRA: Cardiovascular disease.

DOSAGE: As a spray, 1% solution in liquid petrolatum, as an inhalant, one or two inhalations through each nostril at hourly intervals. Continued use should be guarded against, sleeplessness and restlessness may be the result.

b. sulfate. A white, odorless powder, a cerebral stimulant, similar in its action to caffeine.

USES: In the treatment of narcolepsy, and certain depressive psychopathic conditions. Its use should be under the strict supervision of the physician, and the same degree of caution should be exercised as with ephedrine.

DOSAGE: Average, 10 mg.

benzene, or benzol [L. *benzinum*] C_6H_6. A volatile liquid, immiscible with water, able to dissolve fats.

Important theoretically because it is the simplest member of the *aromatic* series of hydrocarbons, and useful practically because, prepared in the distillation of coal tar, it serves in the synthesis of innumerable dyes, drugs, etc. The phenyl *radical*, C_6H_5, will be recognized in the formulae for *phenol*, dimethylaminoazobenzene (which see under *azocompounds*), and *benzoic acid*.

DOSAGE: 2-10 ℳ (0.12-0.6 cc.).

Benzidine test. A test used to determine the presence of blood. Prepare benzidine sol. as follows: to a sat. solution of benzidine in glacial acetic acid, add equal volume of 3% hydrogen peroxide. Appearance of a blue color indicates presence of blood.

benzidin test diet. This consists of milk, crackers and rice.

An iron free diet, its purpose being to free the alimentary tract of any iron; often the stool is tested for iron. Since no iron was in the food, if any is present in the food masses, it must have come from only one source: the hemoglobin of the blood. Such a result is a positive test of bleeding into the intestinal tract, and an evidence of an ulcer. Patients should be watched to be sure that they eat nothing but those foods which are served at the prescribed times.

ben′zoate. Any salt of benzoic acid.

benzocaine (benz-o-kain′). Nontoxic local anesthestic. SEE: *anesthesin*.
DOSAGE: 5 gr. (0.3 Gm.).

benzo′ic acid, USP. May be obtained by sublimation from gum benzoin.
ACTION AND USES: Antiseptic, stimulant and diuretic.
DOSAGE: 5-15 gr. (0.3-1.0 Gm.).

benzoin (ben′zoin, -zo-in) [L. *benzoinum*]. USP. A balsamic resin from styrax b.
ACTION AND USES: A parasiticide; as a protective for ulcers, bedsores, etc.; promotes granulation when applied to wounds. Tr. benzoin comp., which is 10% benzoin, is used for inflamed mucous membrane of the throat and bronchi—by inhalation.

ben′zol [L. *benzinum*]. Same as benzene. Widely used in industry as from coal tar distillation, manufacture of motor fuels, rubber industry, manufacture of cans, lacquer and paint trades.

b. poisoning. SYM: *Acute poisoning from exposure to high concentrations*: Dizziness, weakness, followed by unconsciousness. *Chronic poisoning from prolonged contact*: Leads to aplastic anemia, various hemorrhages from any orifice or into skin, weakness, anorexia, headache.
F. A. TREATMENT: Artificial respiration when indicated; repeated blood transfusions, oxygen inhalations. Otherwise symptomatic treatment.

Bérard's aneurysm (bā-rars′). An arteriovenous aneurysm in the tissues surrounding the injured vein.

Béraud's ligament (ba-rōz′). Pericardial suspensory ligament.

B.'s valve. Krause's* valve. Fold of mucous membrane at beginning of nasal duct.

Ber′covitz test. For pregnancy: Several drops of patient's citrated blood instilled into one eye; if contraction or dilatation of the pupil occurs, sometimes the two eyes alternately, pregnancy is assumed.

Bergeron's chorea (bair-zhĕ-rawn′). A hysterical type of chorea.

Bergmann's incision. One in flank for exposing the kidney.

Beriberi. A clinical syndrome associated with faulty nutrition, endemic in Oriental countries. May be acute or chronic.
ETIOL.: Deficiency in thiamine (vitamin B_1). There is a definite relationship between beriberi and an unbalanced diet, especially one rich in decorticated cereals.
SYM: Multiple neuritis; weakness and wasting of body tissue; palpitation; shortness of breath, dropsy of feet and legs.
TREATMENT: Rest in bed; good hygiene, food rich in Vitamin B, fruit and vegetables. PROG: Good.

Bernard's canal or **duct** (ber-nar′). An accessory pancreatic duct. *Ductus pancreaticus accessorius*. BNA.

B.'s granular layer. Inner layer in cells lining acini of pancreas.

Bernreuter test (bern′rū-ter). A "yes" and "no" test of 125 questions, used to ascertain the attitudes and interest of a patient.

bertillonage (ber′tē-yon-āj). Physical measurement for identification of criminals.

Bertin, Bertini, columns of (ber′tan). Renal cortical columns supporting the blood vessels in the kidneys. The part that separates the medullary pyramids.

B.'s ligament. Iliofemoral ligament.

besoin de respirer (ba-zwan de res-pī-ra′) [Fr. need to breathe]. Sensation inducing act of breathing.

bestiality (bes-tĭ-al′ĭ-tĭ) [L. *bestia*, beast]. Coition with an animal.

beta. Second letter of Greek alphabet. Used as a prefix to chemical words to note isomeric variety or position in compounds of substituted groups.

betanaphthol (be-tă-naf′thol). Occurs as a colorless or buff colored crystalline powder, with faint odor of phenol.
ACTION AND USES: Several times more antiseptic than phenol; irritating to mucous membrane when applied in solution; used externally in ointment 1 to 10%; internally, as intestinal antiseptic, but should be used with caution because of irritating effects on kidneys.
DOSAGE: 4 gr. (0.25 Gm.).

Beta rays. Negatively charged particles emitted by radium; more penetrating than alpha rays. Absorbed by 1 mm. lead or 0.6 mm. platinum.

beta test (ba′ta). An army group intelligence test used with those unable to read English.

be′tacism [G. *bēta*, the letter *b*]. Speech defect giving the *b* sound to other consonants.

betaine hydrochloride (bē-tain′). A colorless crystalline substance, containing 23% hydrochloric acid, and obtained from an alkaloid found in the beet, and other plants.
USES: A convenient method of administering hydrochloric acid, and for the same purpose.
DOSAGE: 8 gr. (0.5 Gm.) dissolved in water, which corresponds to about 18 ℳ dilute hydrochloric acid USP.

betalin S (bā′ta-lin). Synthetic vitamin B_1. 1 mg. contains 400 Sherman units.

betaxin (be-taks′in). Synthetic crystalline vitamin B_1 hydrochloride.
USES: In the various conditions due to deficiency of vitamin B_1, as beriberi, muscular weakness, etc.
DOSAGE: Orally, from 1 to 5 mg. daily. Intramuscularly, from 1 to 10 mg.

Betz cell. A form of giant pyramidal cell in the cortical motor area.

bex (bĕks) [G. *bēx*, cough]. A cough or condition characterized by a cough.

b. convulsiva. Whooping cough.

bezoar (bē-zō′är) (Persian). A concretion from the stomachs and intestines of animals, and also in man as a hair-ball (*trichobezoar*), hair and vegetable fiberball (*trichophytobezoar*), and food-ball (*phytobezoar*).

Bezold's abscess (be′zolt′s). Mastoiditis which involves the tip cell, causing abscess underneath insertion of sternocleidomastoid muscle.

Bi. CHEM: Symb. for bismuth.

bi- [L. *bis*, two]. Prefix: Two, double, twice, as biceps.

biartic′ular [" + *articulus*, joint]. Pert. to two joints; diarthric.

bibasic (bi-ba′sik) [" + G. *basis*, foundation]. Pert. to an acid with two hydrogen atoms replaceable by bases to form salts.

bibulous (bib′u-lus) [L. *bibere*, to drink]. Absorbent.

bicam′eral [L. *bis*, two, + *camera*, a chamber]. Having two cavities or hollows; esp. an abscess divided by a septum.

bicap′sular [" + *capsula*, container]. Having a double capsule.

bicar′bonate [" + carbonate]. A salt resulting from the incomplete neutralization of carbonic *acid*, or from the passing of an excess of carbon dioxide into a solution of a *base*.
Sodium bicarbonate is $NaHCO_3$; calcium bicarbonate is $CaH_2(CO_3)_2$. A carbonate composed of 2 equivalents of carbonic acid and 1 of a base.

  b. blood. That in the blood. An alkali reserve index.

bicarbonatemia (bī-kar-bō-nā-tē-mī-ă). Bicarbonate in the blood.

bicar′diogram [" + G. *kardia*, heart, + *gramma*, a writing]. A cardiogram curve representing the combined effects of the right and left ventricles.

bicellular (bi-sel′u-lar) [" + *cellularis*, little cell]. 1. Composed of two cells. 2. Having two chambers or compartments.

bi′ceps [" + *caput*, head]. Two-headed; in front of humerus and behind femur.

  b. brachii. Muscle of the upper arm, having two heads. Flexes and supinates forearm.

  b. femoris. Muscle of the thigh.

  b. reflex. Biceps muscle contraction when tendon is percussed.

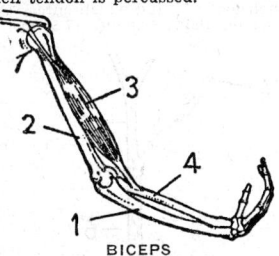

BICEPS
1. Ulna. 2. Humerus. 3. Biceps. 4. Radius.

bicep′tor [" + *capere*, to take]. A receptor having two complementophil groups.

Bichat's canal (bī-shăs′). The subarachnoid canal extending from third ventricle to middle of B.'s fissure carrying the veins of Galen.

  B.'s fat ball or **pad.** Mass of fat behind the buccinator muscle.

  B.'s fissure. The horseshoe fissure separating cerebrum from cerebellum.

  B.'s foramen. Same as B.'s canal.

  B.'s ligament. Lower fasciculus of post. sacroiliac ligament.

  B.'s membrane. *Lamina basalis*.

  B.'s tunic. The tunica intima of the blood vessels.

bichloride of mercury (bī-klo′rīd) (corrosive mercuric chloride). A crystalline salt, Hg Cl_2. SEE: *mercuric chloride*.

POISONING: SYM: Intense burning of throat, mouth, and abdomen; difficulty or inability to swallow; mucous membrane of mouth and throat stained white, resembling boiled meat. Nausea and vomiting, usually bloody. Temperature below normal; collapse ensues.
TREATMENT: Use stomach pump or an emetic. Give white of eggs or milk. Follow with soothing drinks, such as barley water or flour and water. Apply heat to abdomen. Stimulate.

bicho (bē′chō). Epidemic gangrenous proctitis.

biciliate (bi-sil′ĭ-āt) [L. *bis*, two, + G. *kyla*, eyelids]. Having two cilia.

bicip′ital [L. *biceps*, two heads]. 1. Pert. to a biceps muscle. 2. Having two heads.

$Bi_2(CO_3)_3$. Bismuth carbonate.

bicon′cave [L. *bis*, two, + *concavus*, concave]. Concave on each side, as a lens.

bicon′vex [" + *convexus*, rounded raised surface]. Convex on two sides, as a lens.

bicor′nuate, bicornuous [" + *cornutus*, horned]. Having two processes or hornlike projections.

  b. uterus. Anomalous uterus resulting from incomplete union of the mullerian ducts. May be double or single organ with two horns.

bicoro′nial [" + G. *korōnē*, crown]. Pert. to the two coronas.

bicor′porate [" + *corpus*, body]. Having two bodies.

bicus′pid [" + *cuspis*, point]. Having two cusps or prongs.

  b. valves. Valves bet. the left ventricle and left auricle (atrium). SEE: *heart*.

bicuspid (bī-kus′pĭd). One of 2 teeth above and below on each side between the molars and canines.

b. i. d. Abbr. for *bis in die*, twice daily.

Bidder's gang′lion. One of two ganglia or cardiac nerves.

bidermo′ma [L. *bis*, two, + G. *derma*, skin, + -*ōma*, tumor]. A teratoid growth having two germ layers; didermoma.

bidet (bĭ-det′) [Fr. a small horse]. A receptacle with attachments for giving injections, for a hip bath or sitz bath, or for washing the genitals or for douching.

biduous (bid′u-us) [L. *bis*, two, + *diēs*, a day]. Continuing for two days.

Biederman's sign (be′der-mans). Dusky redness of the lower ant. pillars of fauces in certain cases of syphilis.

bier′merin. Hormone in gastric juice. SYN: *addisin*.

Bier's cup (beers). A clear glass cup provided with a pump and bulb named after the inventor.
Its use is to induce hyperemia where there is pronounced external inflammation. These cups vary in size; the smallest ones are used for carbuncles, the largest of such a diameter as will enclose an extremity of the body, as an arm or a foot.

bifa′cial ([L. *bis*, two, + *faciēs*, face]. Having similar opposite surfaces.

bi′fid [" + *findere*, to cleave]. Cleft or split into two parts.

  b. spine. Congenital fissure of vertebral column.

  b. tongue. Cleft tongue.

bifo′cal [" + *focus*, hearth]. Having two foci, as *b. eyeglasses*.

bifo′rate [" + *fora*, opening]. With two openings.

bifurcate (bi-fur′kate) [" + *furca*, fork]. Having two branches or divisions; forked.

bifur′cated. Having two branches; forked.

bifurcation (bī-fūr-kā'shŭn) [L. *bis*, two, + *furca*, fork]. A separation into 2 branches; the point of forking.

Big'elow's ligament. The iliofemoral ligament; Y-ligament.
  B.'s septum. Bony tissue layer under neck of femur. SYN: *calcar femorale*.

bigem'inal [L. *bigeminum*, twin]. Double, paired.
  b. bodies. Either of the two anterior eminences of the corpora quadrigemina.
  b. pulse. Pulse in which beats are in groups of two with pause in between groups. SEE: *pulse, b.*

bigem'inum. A bigeminal body.

bigeminy (bī-jĕm'ĭn-ĭ) [L. *bigeminum*, twin]. Pulse marked by occurrence of 2 beats close together followed by a pause before next pair of beats. SYN: *pulse, bigeminal*.

bilabe (bī'lāb) [L. *bis*, two, + *labium*, lip]. Device used for urethral extraction of vesical calculi.

bilat'eral [" + *latus*, side]. Pert. to, affecting, or rel. to two sides of the body.
  b. symmetry. Symmetry of paired organs. SYN: *bilateralism*.

bilateralism (bī-lat'ĕr-ăl-ĭzm) [" + " + G. *ismos*, condition]. Arrangement on 2 sides; symmetry.

bile (bīl) [L. *bilis*, bile]. A secretion of the liver.

It is a thick, brightly colored, greenish, viscid fluid with a bitter taste which passes into the common bile duct and then into the duodenum as needed. The bile from the liver is straw color, while that from the gallbladder varies from yellow to brown and green. There are more solids in green bile and it is mixed with mucus.

It is also stored in the gallbladder, drawn upon as needed, and discharged into the duodenum. Contraction of the gall bladder brought about by a hormone, cholecystokinin, produced by the duodenum, its secretion being brought about by the entrance of fatty foods (esp. egg yolk and cream) into the duodenum. Added to water, bile decreases surface tension, giving a foamy solution favoring the emulsification of fats and oils; this action is due to the bile salts, mainly sodium glycocholate and taurocholate.

COMP: The bile pigments (principally bilirubin* and biliverdin*) are responsible for the variety of the colors observed. In addition, bile contains cholesterol, lecithin, mucin, and other organic and inorganic substances. The bile does not contain any important enzymes.

FUNCT: Its importance as a digestive juice is due to its emulsifying action which facilitates the digestion of fats in the intestines by pancreatic steapsin, plus a further effect of the bile salts which form compounds with the fatty acids and are necessary for their absorption. Bile also stimulates peristalsis.

Normally the ejection of bile only occurs during duodenal digestion. Bile is both an antiseptic and a purgative. About 1800-2000 cc. are secreted per 24 hr. in the normal adult. SEE: *gallbladder*.

PATH: Interference with the flow of bile produces jaundice, resulting in unabsorbed fats being found in the feces. In such instances, fats should be restricted in the diet. Gallstones also may be produced in the gallbladder when the free flow of bile from the gallbladder is checked, or when pathological conditions impede bile production.

TEST FOR IN URINE: There are several methods of testing for bile in the urine.
1. *Gmelin's Test:* 1 in. of concentrated nitric acid is carefully overlaid with the suspected urine. Bile is present when there is a play of colors at the junction of the fluids. This test can also be carried out by pouring some urine onto blotting or filter paper, and then placing a drop of concentrated nitric acid on the moist paper. From the spreading edge of the drop of acid will develop a ring of various colors in which green predominates and forms the outer band.

2. *Iodine Test:* Take an inch of the suspected urine in a test tube and carefully overlay it with dilute tincture of iodine. A bright green ring will appear at the junction of the fluids, if bile is present.

RS: acholia, acholuria, "bili-" words, cacocholia, calcibilia, "chol-" words, hypercholia, oligocholia, stercobilin, urobilin, urobilinogen.

  b. acids. Complex acids, of which cholic, choleic, glycocholic, and taurocholic acids are examples, and which occur as salts (e. g., sodium taurocholate) in bile. They give bile its foamy character, are important in the digestion of fats in the intestine, and are reabsorbed from the intestine so as to be used again by the liver; this circulation of the bile acids is called the "enterohepatic circulation."

HAY'S TEST FOR: Some urine is placed in a watchglass, and a little powdered sulfur is thrown on the surface. If bile acids are present, the sulfur sinks, due to the lowering of the surface tension by the bile salts.

  b. ducts. Intercellular biliary passages conveying the bile from the liver to the hepatic duct which joins the duct from the gallbladder (cystic duct), to form the common bile duct (ductus choledochus), and which enters the duodenum about 3 inches (7.5 cm.) below

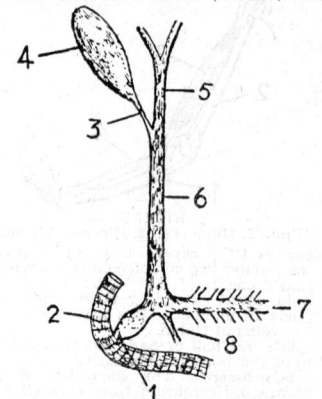

BILE AND PANCREATIC DUCTS
1. Ampulla of Vater. 2. Duodenum. 3. Cystic duct. 4. Gallbladder. 5. Hepatic duct. 6. Common bile duct. 7. Duct of Wirsung. 8. Duct of Santorini.

the pylorus. SEE: *hepatic d., cystic d., common bile d., gallbladder*.

  b. pigments. Complex, highly colored substances found in bile, derived from the red pigment (hemoglobin) of the blood, and imparting the brown color to intestinal contents and feces. Ex: *bilirubin, biliverdin.*

In estimating the concentration of bile pigment in the blood (*Van den Bergh test*), sulfanilic acid is added to the blood serum. If a great excess of bilirubin is present, a purple color is formed. This is called a *direct reaction,* and is said to indicate obstructive jaundice. If the amount of bilirubin is smaller, alcohol must be added to bring out the purple color. This is called an *indirect reaction,* and is said to be indicative of hemolytic jaundice. By comparing the color produced with a standard color, the amount of bilirubin in the blood serum may be estimated; the normal amount is about 2 mg. per 100 cc. of serum.

b. salts. Alkali salts of bile. Sodium glycocholate and sodium taurocholate.

bilharzia (bil-har'zĭ-ă). A parasitic fluke in blood supply of the liver. The eggs are found in great numbers in bladder or rectum.

bili- [L.]. Prefix: Pert. to bile.

biliary (bil'ĭ-ar-ĭ). Pert. to or conveying bile.
RS: *bile, bile ducts, common bile duct, cystic duct, gallbladder, hepatic duct, liver.*

b. calculus. Cholelithiasis. Formation of stone in any of the biliary passages or in the gallbladder.

b. colic. Pain caused by the pressure or passing of gallstones.

b. ducts. Passages conveying bile from liver to hepatic duct. SEE: *bile ducts.*

biliation (bil-ĭ-a'shun). Excretion or secretion of bile.

bilifecia (bil-if-e'sĭ-ă) [L. *bilis,* bile, + *faeces,* excrement]. Presence of bile in the feces.

bilifica'tion [" + *facere,* to make]. The formation of bile.

bilifla'vin [" + *flavus,* yellow]. A yellow pigment derived from biliverdin.

bilifui'vin [" + *fulvus,* tawny]. Biliverdin mixed with other substances.

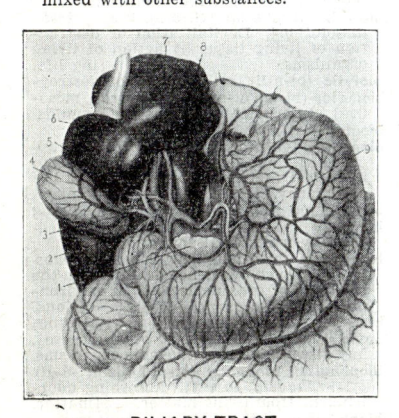

BILIARY TRACT
1. Pancreas. 2. Common bile duct. 3. Cystic duct. 4. Gallbladder. 5. Hepatic duct. 6. Liver. 7. Portal vein. 8. Hepatic artery. 9. Stomach.

bilifuscin (bil-ĭ-fus'in) [" + *fuscus,* brown]. A dark green pigment in gallstones.

biligenesis (bil-ĭ-jen'ĕ-sis) [" + G. *genesis,* origin]. The formation of bile.

biligenet'ic. Forming bile.

biligenic (bil-ĭ-jen'ik). Forming bile. SYN: *biligenetic.*

bilihu'min [L. *bilis,* bile, + *humus,* earth]. A dark residue after applying solvents to bile or gallstones.

bi'lin. Mixture of sodium glycocholate and sodium taurocholate extracted from bile.

bilineurin (bil"ĭ-nū'rin) [L. *bilis,* bile, + G. *neuron,* nerve]. $C_9H_{15}NO_2$. A toxic ptomaine from organic substances; choline.

bil'ious. 1. Pert. to bile. 2. Afflicted with biliousness.
b. fever. Fever with vomiting of bile.
b. remittent. SEE: *b. fever.*

biliousness (bil'yus-nes). 1. A symptom due to disordered condition of the liver causing constipation, headache, loss of appetite, and vomiting of bile. 2. Excess of bile; bilious fever. Fever with vomiting of bile.
TREATMENT: Rest in bed; saline cathartics; light diet, vegetable soup, fish, meat sparingly, no eggs; constitutional remedies.

biliphein (bil-ĭ-fe'in) [L. *bilis,* bile, + G. *phaios,* tawny]. An impure bilirubin.

bilipra'sin [" + G. *prason,* leek-green]. Green pigment similar to bilirubin.

bilipur'pin, bilipurpu'rin [" + *purpur,* purple]. A purple pigment derived from biliverdin.

bilirachia (bil-ĭ-ra'kĭ-ă) [" + G. *rachis,* spine]. Bile in the spinal fluid.

bilirubin (bil-ĭ-ru'bin) [" + *ruber,* red] $(C_{16}H_{18}N_2O_3)$. The orange-colored or yellowish pigment in bile.

It is carried to the liver by the blood, the product of degenerated hemoglobin in bone marrow, in the spleen, and elsewhere. It is chemically changed in the liver and excreted in the bile through the duodenum. As it passes through the intestines it is converted into urobilinogen by the coli bacteria, most of it being excreted through the feces to which it gives their color. If urobilinogen passes into the circulation it is excreted through the urine if the kidneys remain intact.
RS: *bile pigments, cholepyrrhin.*

bilirubinemia (bil-ĭ-roo-bin-e'mĭ-ă) [" + " + G. *aima,* blood]. Bilirubin in blood.

bilirubinu'ria [" + " + G. *ouron,* urine]. Bilirubin in urine.

bil'is [L.]. Bile.
b. bovina, b. bulbata. Oxgall, used as laxative, cholagogue and intestinal antiseptic. SYN: *fel bovis.*

bilither'apy [" + G. *therapeia,* treatment]. Treatment with bile salts.

biliuria (bil-ĭ-u'rĭ-ă) [" + G. *ouron,* urine]. Bile in the urine.

biliverdin (bil-ĭ-ver'din) [" + *viridis,* green]. A greenish pigment in bile formed in oxidation of bilirubin. RS: *bilifulvin, bilipurpin, choleverdin.*

biloc'ular [L. *bis,* two, + *loculus,* cell]. 1. Having two cells. 2. Divided into compartments.

bilron (bil-ron'). Iron bile salts.
USE: In oral management of biliary dysfunction.
DOSAGE: 15 to 60 gr. daily (0.97-3.9 Gm.).

biman'ual [L. *bis,* two, + *manus,* hand]. With both hands; with two hands, as *b. palpation.*

bimax′illary [G. *bios*, life, + L. *maxillaris*, pert. to the jaw]. Pert. to or afflicting both jaws.

binary (bī′nar-ĭ) [L. *binarius*, of two]. 1. Compounded of two elements. 2. Separating into two branches.
  b. acid. One containing hydrogen and one other element.

binau′ral [L. *bini*, two, + *auris*, ear]. Pert. to or having two ears.
  b. arc. The arc from one aural point to another across top of cranium.

binauric′ular [" + *auricula*, little ear]. Pert. to or having two ears. SYN: *binaural*.*

binder [A.S. *bindan*, to tie up]. A broad bandage, most commonly used as an encircling support of abdomen or chest.
  b., abdominal. A wide band fastened snugly about the abdomen for support.
  b., chest. A broad band used for encircling the chest to apply heat, dressings, or pressure, and supporting the breasts. Improved by using shoulder straps to keep from slipping.
  b., double T. A horizontal band about the waist to which two vertical bands are attached in back, brought around leg and again fastened to horizontal band. Holds dressings about perineum or genitalia (esp. male).
  b., obstetrical. A broad bandage encircling entire abdomen from ribs to pelvis, affording support.
  b., T. Two strips of material fastened together, resembling a T, used as a bandage to hold a dressing on perineum of women; or vertex of head, etc.
  b., towel. A towel encircling abdomen or chest with ends pinned or sewed together for support.

bind′web. 1. Connective tissue. 2. Tissue forming framework of brain and spinal cord. SYN: *neuroglia*.

Binet age (bī-nā′). Intellect as measured by the Binet-Simon tests as compared with the age of a normal child. The Binet age of an idiot is 1-2 yr.; the imbecile, 3-9 yr.; the moron, 8-12 yr.

binoc′ular [L. *bini*, two, + *oculus*, eye]. Pert. to both eyes.   [both eyes.
  b. vision. Normal vision and use of

binot′ic [" + G. *ous*, ear]. Pert. to or having two ears. SYN: *binaural*.*

binov′ular [" + *ovum*, egg]. Derived from or pert. to two ova.

binu′clear, binu′cleate [" + L. *nucleus*, kernel]. Having two nuclei.

binucleolate (bi-nū-klē′ō-lāt) [" + *nucleŏlus*, small nut]. Having two nucleoli.

bio- [G.]. Prefix: Life.

bio-assay′ [G. *bios*, life, + O.Fr. *asaier*, to try]. Estimation of strength of a drug.

bi′oblast [" + *blastos*, germ]. A corpuscle that has not yet become a cell; micella.

biocatalyst (bi-o-kat′al-ist) [" + *katalyein*, to dissolve]. An enzyme; a biochemical catalyzer.

biochem′istry [" + *chēmeia*, chemistry]. The chemistry of living things; the science of the chemical changes accompanying the vital functions of plants and animals.

biochemorphic (bi″o-kĕ-mor′fik) [" + " + *morphē*, shape]. Pert. to the relation bet. biologic action of drugs and foods and their chemical constitution.

biochemorphology (bi″o-kĕ-mor-fol′o-jĭ) [" + " + *logos*, study]. Science of chemical structure of substances as related to their action on the body.

bioclimatology (bi″o-kli-ma-tol′o-jĭ) [" + *klima*, climate, + *logos*, study]. Relations of climate to life.

biocolloid (bi-o-kol′oyd) [" + *kollōdēs*, glutinous]. A colloid in animal or vegetable organism.

biocy′toculture [" + *kytos*, cell, + L. *cultura*, cultivation]. A culture made from live leukocyte bearing pus.

biocytoneurology (bi-o-cī-to-nu-rol′o-jĭ) [" + " + *neuron*, nerve, + *logos*, study]. The science of living nerve cells.

biodynam′ics [" + *dynamis*, force]. The science of living force or energy.

biodyne. A group of natural substances secreted by cells and having the function of regulating the growth and metabolism of the cells. They are secreted by cells into the intercellular fluid and act directly on neighboring cells.
  b. ointment. Preparation containing 3% proliferation-stimulating biodynes from liver, 1% respiratory-stimulating biodynes from yeast, and phenyl mercuric nitrate 1:20,000, in a special lanolin-petrolatum base. USES: Externally, for the local treatment of burns and wounds.

biogen (bī′o-jen) [" + *gennan*, to generate]. 1. Protoplasm. 2. Assumed substance of a spiritual body.

biogen′esis [" + *genesis*, origin]. Begetting living things from living things opp. to spontaneous generation.

biogenet′ic. Pert. to biogenesis.

biokinet′ics [G. *bios*, life, + *kinetikos*, moving]. The science of changes in developing organisms. [Pert. to biology.

biolog′ic, biolog′ical [" + *logos*, study].

biolog′icals. 1. Complex substances of organic origin, depending for their action on the processes effecting immunity, used esp. in diagnosis and treatment of disease, as vaccines, serums or antigens. 2. Complex products, of organic or synthetic origin, obtained or standardized by biological methods, as insulin.

biol′ogist. A professional student of or specialist in biology.

biology (bi-ol′o-jĭ) [G. *bios*, life, + *logos*, study]. Science of life and living things. RS: "abio-" words, *genesis*, *orthogenesis*. [living organisms.
  b., dynamic. Science of activities of
  b., static. Science of structures and potentialities of living organisms.

biolysis (bi-ol′ĭs-Is) [G. *bios*, life, + *lysis*, dissolution]. Devitalization or destruction of living tissue by action of living organisms. [ing life.

biolytic (bi-o-lit′ik). Capable of destroy-

biometer (bi-om′et-er) [" + *metron*, measure]. Instrument for measuring sounds.

biomet′rics. Biometry.

biom′etry [G. *bios*, life, + *metron*, measure]. 1. Application of statistics to biological facts. 2. Computation of life expectancy. [organism.

bion (bi′on) [G. *biōn*, living]. Any living

bionergy (bi-on′er-jĭ) [G. *bios*, life, + *ergon*, work]. Vital energy or force.

bionomics (bī″ō-nŏm′ĭks) [" + *nomos*, law]. Branch of science dealing with the relations of organisms to their environment. SYN: *ecology*. [tions.

bion′omy. The science pert. to vital func-

biono′sis [G. *bios*, life, + *nosos*, disease]. Any disease due to pathogenic organisms.

biophagism, biophagy (bi-of′ă-jizm, -ă-jĭ) [" + *phagein*, to eat]. Absorbing nourishment from living matter. [matter.

bioph′agous. Feeding on nonparasitic

biophilia (bi-o-fil′ĭ-ă) [" + *philein*, to love]. Instinct of self-preservation.

biophore (bi′o-fōr) [" + *phoros*, bearing]. The ultimate unit having vital energy.

biophylactic B-24 **bismosol**

biophylac'tic [" + *phylax*, a guard]. Tending to preserve life.
biophysics (bi-o-fiz'iks) [" + *physikos*, natural]. Vital process phenomena.
biophysiol'ogy [" + " + *logos*, study]. Study of morphology and physiology.
bi'oplasm [" + *plasma*, matter]. Protoplasm. Living substance. SEE: *biogen*.
bioplas'mic. Pert. to bioplasm.
bioplas'min [G. *bios*, life, + *plasma*, matter]. A hypothetical substance contained in every living cell, essential to its life.
bioplast (bi'o-plast) [" + *plassein*, to form]. The cellular unit.
bioplas'tic. Pert. to a bioplast.
bi'opsy [G. *bios*, life, + *opsis*, vision]. Excision of a small piece of tissue for microscopic examination.
bios (bi'os) [G.]. Life.
bios'copy [G. *bios*, life, + *skopein*, to examine]. Examination to determine life.
biose (bi'ōs). A saccharide.
biospectrom'etry [G. *bios*, life, + L. *spectrum*, image, + G. *metron*, measure]. Clinical spectrometry to determine presence of foreign matter.
biospectros'copy [" + " + G. *skopein*, to examine]. The clinical spectroscopy of living tissue. [ence of metabolism.
biostat'ics [" + *statikos*, standing]. Sci**biotax'is, bi'otaxy** [G. *bios*, life, + *taxis*, arrangement]. 1. The selecting and arranging activity of living cells. 2. Systematic classification of living organisms. [laws of living organisms.
biot'ics [G. *biōtikos*, living]. Pert. to the
biotin (bi-ot'in) [G. *bios*, life, vital]. A B vitamin named Vit. H. The most powerful life substance known and a great stimulator. It is active in concentrations of one part to four hundred billion parts. It, with avidin,* seems to maintain an equilibrium of vital forces. Lack of this equilibrium may be the cause of disease.
biotomy (bi-ot'o-mĭ) [G. *bios*, life, + *tomē*, incision]. Operation on living animals for pathological or physiological study. SYN: *vivisection*.
biotox'in [" + *toxikon*, poison]. A toxin from living tissues and juices.
biotrip'sis [" + *tripsis*, rubbing]. A condition of the skin seen in old people in which skin wears away.
 May be smooth, pigmented, shiny, esp. on forehead, backs of hands, and shin.
biotropism (bi-ot'ro-pizm) [" + *tropē*, turning]. Increased virulence resulting from therapeutic procedures.
Biot's breathing or respiration (bĭ-ōs'). Rapid breathing with rhythmical pauses. Unfavorable in meningitis.
bio'type [G. *bios*, life, + *typos*, mark]. Fundamental constitution of an organism or those possessing it.
biov'ular twins [L. *bis*, two, + *ovulum*, ovum]. Twins from two separate ova.
bip'ara [L. *bis*, two, + *parĕre*, to give birth]. Woman who has had two labors.
biparasit'ic [L. *bis*, two, + G. *para*, beside, + *sitos*, food]. Pert. to parasite living upon another parasite.
biparen'tal [" + *parĕre*, to bring forth]. Derived from both parents.
bip'arous. Giving birth to two at a time.
bipol'ar [" + *polus*, a pole]. 1. Having 2 poles or processes. 2. Pert. to the use of 2 poles in electrotherapeutic treatments.
 When referring to an alternating current, biterminal should be used.
  b. nerve cell. Cell with 2 processes.
  b. version. Braxton Hicks v.; a combined one. Changing a *cephalic* position into a *podalic* one, or *vice versa*, by placing 1 hand on fundus of uterus and 2 fingers of other hand in cervix.
B. I. P. P. The letters stand for *bismuth, iodoform, paraffin paste*. A paste used during the first World War.
 It is used for deep septic cavities. The wound is first thoroughly irrigated to clear it of pus, and then the cavity is swabbed out quite dry (this last is an important point). The paste is spread on ribbon gauze and packed, not too tightly, into the cavity until it is filled up. Outer dressings of sterile gauze and wool are applied, and these are not removed for two or three days.
biramous (bi-ra'mus) [" + *ramus*, a branch]. Possessing two branches.
Birdsall punch. Modification of the caulk punch for using the cutting current for excision of the prostatic median bar.
birefrac'tive, birefrin'gent [L. *bis*, two, + *refrangere*, to break up]. Splitting a ray of light in two.
birth [M.E. *byrthe*, birth]. Act of being born. Passage of a child from uterus.
  b., complete. The instant of complete separation of the body of the infant from that of the mother, regardless of cord or placenta detached.
  b. control. Any method used to prevent conception, such as artificial devices used by the male or the female.
 Rhythmic control consists of abstention from copulation excepting during a certain period following menstruation, after the descent of the ova and before the next menses. Any change in periodicity necessitates the establishment of a new period of sterility.
  b., cross. With fetus across the uterus.
  b., dry. Birth following premature rupture of the fetal membrane.
  b., live. An infant showing one of the three evidences of life (breathing, heart action, movements of a voluntary muscle) after complete birth. [injury.
  b. mark. Nevus; mark from birth
  b. palsy. Paraplegia or hemiplegia caused by birth injury. Injury to some shoulder muscles may cause Erb's palsy.
  b., premature. One bet. 7th month and term.
  b., still. An infant not exhibiting evidence of life after complete birth.
bisacro'mial [L. *bis*, two, + G. *akron*, point, + *ōmos*, shoulder]. Pert. to both acromial processes.
bisection (bī-sek'shŭn) [" + *sectiō*, a cutting]. Division into 2 parts.
bisex'ual [" + *sexus*, sex]. Hermaphroditic; having imperfect genitalia of both sexes in one person.
bisferious (bis-fer'ĭ-us) [" + *ferire*, to beat]. Having two beats; dicrotic.
bisiliac (bis-il'ĭ-ăk) [" + *ilium*, ilium]. Pert. to the two most distant points of the twoi iliac crests.
bis in d., bis in die [L.]. Twice a day.
bismarsen (bis-mar'sen). A bismuth derivative of arsphenamine containing approximately 13% arsenic and 24% bismuth.
 USES: Same as arsphenamine, but said to be slower in its action.
 DOSAGE: Initial, 0.1 Gm. intramuscularly, succeeding doses, 1½-2 gr. (0.1-0.2 Gm.) at weekly intervals; a few drops of a 2% solution of butyn may be added to lessen the pain on administration.
bismosol (biz'mo-sol). A solution of potassium sodium bismuthotartrate (containing 35% bismuth).
 USES: In treatment of syphilis.
 DOSAGE: Intramuscularly 15 ℳ (1.0 cc.)

every 2 to 7 days for 20 doses; after interval of 1 month a second course may be given.

bismuth (biz'muth) [L. *bismuthum*]. A drug used as a protective for inflamed surfaces, and as an opaque medium for x-ray visualization.

POISONING: SYM: Metallic taste, foul breath, fever, gastrointestinal irritation. Bismuth line at gum margin, ulcerative process of gums and mouth, headache. Albuminuria; resembles lead poisoning with an absence of the blood changes and paralyses.

F. A. TREATMENT: Removal of source of bismuth; gastric lavage; saline cathartic; treat symptomatically.

b. sodium tartrate. Contains 72.7 to 73.9% bismuth. USES: In treatment of syphilis. DOSAGE: ½ gr. (0.03 Gm.) intramuscularly.

b. subcarbonate. USP. USES: As an antacid. SEE: bismuth subnitrate. INCOMPATIBILITIES: Sulfides, acids, acid salts. DOSAGE: 15 gr. (1 Gm.).

b. subgallate (Dermatol). USP. A bright yellow powder without odor or taste. USES: First introduced for treatment of skin diseases. General use—same as bismuth subnitrate. DOSAGE: 15 gr. (1 Gm.).

b. subnitrate. USP. Occurs as heavy white odorless powder. INCOMPATIBILITIES: Acids, tannins, and sulfides. USES: Astringent, protective antiseptic. DOSAGE: 15 gr. (1 Gm.).

bistoury (bis'to-rĭ) [Fr. *bistouri*, surgical knife]. Small surgical knife used in minor operations; special varieties are tenotomes, gum lancets, hernia knives, and lithotomy bistouries.

bite (bīt) [A.S. *bītan*, to bite]. 1. To cut with the teeth. 2. A puncture by an insect. 3. Occlusion of the teeth.

b., close, closed. One in which lower incisors lie behind upper incisors.

b., end-to-end. One in which incisors of both jaws meet along cutting edge when jaw is closed.

b., open. One in which labial teeth cannot come together.

b., over. One in which upper incisors overlap lower ones when jaws are closed.

bitelock. Device for retaining position biterims outside the mouth.

bitem'poral [L. *bis*, two, + *temporalis*, pert. to a temple]. Pert. to both temples or temporal bones.

bite plate. A plate to support a biterim.

biterim. A rim of wax placed on base plate as a guide for inserting artificial teeth.

biter'minal [L. *bis*, two, + *terminalis*, pert. to an end]. Using an alternating current and two poles in electrotherapeutic treatment. SEE: *bipolar*.

bites. Injuries in which body surfaces are torn by insects or animals, resulting in abrasions, punctured, or lacerated wounds.

PREVENTION: Aromatic oils, especially oil of citronella and smoke of all kinds.

SYM: May be evidence of a wound usually surrounded by a zone of redness and swelling, often accompanied by pain, itching, or throbbing. Often become infected and may contain specific noxious materials as bacteria or venom of rabies.

F. A. TREATMENT: If suspected of poison, apply tourniquet first. Induce bleeding to wash out foreign material. Apply antiseptic, sterile dressing.

RS: *bee stings, bedbugs, bot flies, cat bites, chiggers, dog bites, fleas, freezing, frost, hornet, human bites, insects, name of, poisonous fish, scorpions, snakes, spiders, tarantulas, and wasp.*

b., insect. They contain an acid substance resembling formic acid and consequently are relieved by alkalies, as ammonia water, baking soda paste or even soap paste rubbed on.

Others, such as the bee, wasp, and hornet, contain unknown organic substances for which there is no specific antidote. (Remove the "stinger" if one is present.) Poisonous spiders (especially the "black widow"), *q.v.*, scorpions, *q.v.*, tarantulas, *q.v.*, poison fish, *q.v.*, etc., should have the tourniquet applied promptly, incise with any sharp instrument, and cauterize with heat or chemically (nitric acid or silver nitrate). Successive incisions are necessary if swelling progresses. Do not remove tourniquet too soon; use caution in removal.

Bitot's spots. Triangular, shiny, gray spots on the conjunctiva seen in vitamin A deficiency.

bitter (bĭt'er) [A.S. *biter*, strong]. 1. Having a disagreeable taste. 2. Sensation of taste stimulated by strong disagreeable flavor.

bitterling test (for pregnancy). A Japanese carplike fish is placed in a quart of fresh water with 2 teaspoonfuls of a woman's urine. A long tubular oviduct will grow from the fish's belly if the woman is pregnant.

bit'ters [A.S. *biter*, strong]. Herb tonic for stimulating the tone of gastrointestinal mucous membrane.

b., aromatic. Substances having aromatic properties. [digestive mucosa.

b., simple. Those which stimulate the

b., styptic. Those with styptic and astringent properties.

bi'uret" [L. *bis*, two, + *urea*]. A crystalline decomposition derivative of urea.

b. reaction. Rose to violet coloring in an aqueous solution of protein, when dilute solution of copper sulfate and sodium hydroxide are added to it.

b. test. Use of above reaction to detect presence of urea or any soluble protein. SEE: *test, b.*

bivalent (bĭ-vā'lĕnt) [L. *bis*, two, + *valens*, powerful]. 1. Having a valence of 2. 2. BIOL: Double, as a chromosome consisting of 2 joined chromosomes. 3. A bivalent chromosome.

biven'ter [" + *venter*, belly]. A muscle with two bellies; pert. to several muscles.

biven'tral. Digastric; with two bellies.

Bizzozero's corpuscles (bĭt-sŏt'sĕr-ŏs). Nucleated red blood cells, round or elliptical.

Bjerrum screen. Tangent plane for mapping field of vision, esp. central and paracentral scotomata.

B. sign. One seen in glaucoma, a sickle-shaped blind spot usually found in central zone of the visual field. SEE: *sign.*

black (blăk) [A.S. *blaec*, dark]. 1. Devoid of color; reflecting no light. 2. Marked by dark pigmentation.

b. blood. Impure or venous blood.

b. body. PHYS: A body that absorbs all radiation falling upon it.

b. cancer. An abnormal deposit of black matter in various parts of the body in melanosis.

b. death. A contagious, malignant disease, as the bubonic plague.

b. eye. Subcutaneous extravasation of blood into the eye or orbit, usually the result of injury. SYM: Pain, swelling, discoloration. TREATMENT: Cold applications with pressure for 12 to 24 hr.—tends to prevent swelling. Later, apply heat and frequent gentle massage directed toward periphery.

b. head. Comedo.*

b. measles. A severe type of measles in which the eruption is very dark due to hemorrhage under the skin.

b. tongue. Presence of dark patch on back of tongue caused by microphytes. SYN: *glossophytia*.

b. vomit. The vomiting of black matter as in yellow fever.

blackberries [" + *berie*, berry]. NUTRIENTS: A. P. Prot. 1.03, Fat 0.08, Carbo. 6.3 per serving. FUEL VALUE: 100 Gm.—58 cal. ASH CONST: Ca 0.017, Mg 0.021, K 0.169, Na 0.007, P 0.034, Cl 0.010, S 0.020, Fe 0.0006. AV. SERVING: 75 Gm.

blackout. 1. Temporary loss of consciousness. 2. Temporary loss of vision in aviators due to changing course at high speed.

blackwater fever [" + *waeter*, water]. Hemoglobinuria.* A pernicious, fatal, infectious malarial fever due to the destruction of the red blood cells by the malarial organism.

SYM: There is a marked *hematuria;** also jaundice and vomiting. The urine is dark, containing blood.

TREATMENT: Similar to that for typhoid. Keep mouth clean. Guard against suppression of urine. Rectal feeding may be necessary.

black widow [" + A.S. *weoduwe*, widow]. *Lactrodec'tus mac'tans.* A poisonous spider.*

bladder [A.S. *blaedre*, bladder]. 1. A membranous sac or receptacle for a secretion, as the *gallbladder, q.v.* 2. The vesicle which acts as a reservoir for urine. SEE: *urinary b.*

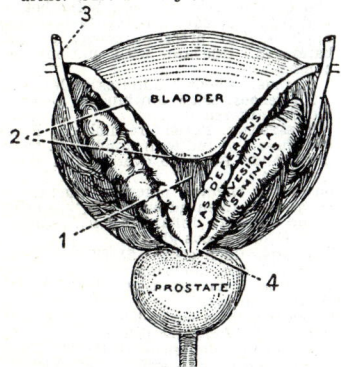

THE MALE BLADDER (rear view)
1. External trigone. 2. Line of reflection of the peritoneum. 3. Left ureter. 4. Ejaculatory duct of right side.

b., atony of. Inability to urinate, due to lack of muscular tone.

b., catarrh of. Cystitis.

b., exstrophy of. The nonclosure of the bladder.

b., irritable. Marked by a constant desire to urinate.

b., nervous. Irritable b. with incomplete urination.

b., stammering of. Interruption of urination.*

b., urinary (*vesica urinaria*). The muscular, membranous, distensible reservoir for the urine, which it receives from the kidneys through the ureters, and which it discharges from the body through the urethra.* It has no function other than that of a reservoir.

ANAT: It is covered with peritoneum and lined with mucous membrane, made up of a vault, two lateral walls, a fundus (the pouch above and behind the trigone*), and a trigone (at the base); the urethral orifice is called the neck.

The bladder is supported by numerous ligaments, supplied by the sup., middle, and inf. vesical arteries, and numerous veins and lymphatics, and innervated with nerves derived from the third and fourth sacral by way of the hypogastric plexus.

It is situated in the ant. part of the pelvic cavity, in front of the ant. wall of the vagina and the uterus, and in the male it lies in front of the rectum. It is about 5x3x5 in. in size and has a storage capacity in health of ½ to 1 pt., although it may be greatly distended.

PHYS: An average of 40 to 50 oz. of urine are secreted within a 24-hr. period. Inability to empty the bladder is known as "retention" and may call for catheterization. Sphincter muscles control retention within the bladder.

PALPATION OF: The bladder cannot be palpated when empty. When full it appears as a tumor in the hypogastric region, which, on palpation, is smooth and oval.

PERCUSSION OF: When containing urine its rounded margin is easily made out by observing the tympanic sound of the intestines on one hand, and dull sound of the bladder on the other.

b.-worm. Larval type of tapeworm.

bland [L. *blandus*, soft]. Soothing, mild.

b. diet. One soothing in flavor and texture; all food which causes chemical, mechanical, or thermal irritation is avoided.

Blandin's glands (blan-dăns'). Glandula lingualis ant. or Nuhn's glands. Glands near tip of tongue.

-blast. A suffix used to designate a cell or a structure which gives rise to a definitive structure. Ex.: *epiblast*, erythroblast, fibroblast.

blast [G. *blastos*, germ]. A nucleated erythrocyte; also called an *erythroblast*. Normally these are not found in the circulating blood, since the red cells lose their nucleus on leaving the bone marrow. In certain blood diseases, such as pernicious anemia, large numbers of nucleated cells may appear in the blood over the period of a few days. This is known as a *blood crisis*.

blast. A violent movement of air such as accompanies the explosion of a shell or bomb; a violent sound as the blast of a horn.

b. injury. A clinical condition which follows severe non-penetrating chest injuries. Effects may vary slight respiratory distress to cessation of respiration.

blaste'ma [G. *blastēma*, sprout]. Immature material from which cells and tissues are formed.

blas'tid, blas'tide [G. *blastos*, germ]. Marking site of the nucleus in the impregnated ovum.

blasto-

blasto- [G.]. Prefix: Germ or bud.

blastocele (blas'to-sēl) [G. *blastos*, germ, + *koilos*, hollow]. The cavity of the blastula, an embryonic stage of development; the segmentation cavity.

blastochyle (blas'to-kīl) [G. *blastos*, germ, + *chylos*, juice]. Blastocelic fluid.

blastocyst (blas'to-sist) [" + *kystis*, bag]. A stage in the development of a mammalian embryo which follows the morula. It consists of an outer layer or trophoblast to which is attached an *inner cell mass*. The enclosed cavity if the *blastocele*. The whole is called *blastodermic vesicle* or *blastocyst*.

blas'tocyte [" + *kytos*, cell]. The morula after change into a cyst.

blas'toderm [" + *derma*, skin]. A disc of cells (*germinal disc*, or *blastodisc*) which develops on the surface of the yolk in an avian or reptilian egg from which the embryo develops; also applied to the *embryonic disc* of mammalian embryos, a disc of cells lying between the yolk sac and the amniotic cavity from which the embryo develops. From the blastoderm, the three germ layers, *ectoderm, mesoderm,* and *endoderm* arise.

blastoderm'ic vesicle. A blastocyst.

blastogen'esis [G. *blastos*, germ, + *genesis*, generation]. 1. Multiplication by budding. 2. Transmission of characteristics from parents to offspring by the germ cells.

blastol'ysis [" + *lysis*, dissolution]. Lysis or destruction of a germ cell.

blasto'ma (pl. *blastomata*) [" + *-ōma*, tumor]. A granular tumor formed by a single type of tissue, including *fibromas* and *chondromas*.

blastomere (blas'to-mere) [" + *meros*, a part]. One of the cells resulting from the cleavage or segmentation of a fertilized ovum.

blastomerot'omy [" + " + *tomē*, incision]. Destruction of blastomeres.

Blastomyces (blăst-ō-mī'sēz) (pl. *blastomyce'tes*) [G. *blastos*, germ, + *mykes*, fungus]. A genus of yeasts with a morphological similarity to the Saccharomyces. Blastomyces refers to those yeasts which are pathogens to man and animals.

B. coccidioi'des (*Coccidioides immitis*). The pathogen of coccidioidal granuloma. Its reproduction in the tissues of infected animals is by endosporulation.

B. dermatit'idis. The pathogen causing in man blastomycetic dermatitis and in some instances generalized blastomycosis.

B. farcimino'sus. The pathogen causing blastomycotic epizootic lymphangitis in horses.

blastomycetes (blas-to-mī-sē'tēs) [" + *mykēs*, fungus]. Saccharomycetes; budding fungi; yeast fungi.

blastomyco'sis [" + *mykēs*, fungus]. A disease caused by budding yeast fungi in the tissues.

blastopore (blas'to-pōr) [" + *poros*, passageway]. The small opening into the archenteron made by invagination of the blastula.

blas'tosphere [" + *sphaira*, circle]. Blastula or germinal vesicle.

blas'tospore [" + *sporos*, seed]. A thallospore formed by budding from a hypha.

blastula (blas'tu-lă). An early stage in the development of an ovum consisting of a hollow sphere of cells enclosing a cavity, the *blastocele*. In large-yolked eggs, the blastocele is reduced to a narrow slit. In mammalian development, the blastocyst or blastodermic vesicle corresponds to the blastula of lower forms.

blas'tular. Pert. to a blastula.

blastulation (blas-tu-la'shun). The formation of the blastula or blastosphere.

Blat'ta orienta'lis [L.]. The common cockroach.

Blaud's pills. Named after a French physician. Contents are sulfate of iron and carbonate of potash. Their use is indicated in anemia,* amenorrhea,* etc.
INCOMPATIBILITIES: *Tea (tannin)*.

bleaching powder (blēsh'ing) [A.S. *blaecan*, to pale]. Chlorinated lime.

blear-eye. Marginal blepharitis. Chronic inflammation of margins of eyelids.

bleb. Elevation of the epidermis, irregularly shaped. A blister or a bulla.
They vary in size from a bean to a goose egg and they contain serous or seropurulent, or bloody fluid. A primary skin lesion. They occur in *dermatitis herpetiformis, pemphigus,* and *syphilis.* SEE: *bulla.*

bleeder [A.S. *bledan*, to bleed]. One who bleeds an abnormal amount. SEE: *hemophilia.*

blee'der's disease. Congenital blood condition marked by inability of blood to coagulate. SYN: *hemophilia.**

bleeding (blēd'ing) [A.S. *bledan*, to bleed]. 1. Emitting blood. 2. Process of emitting blood, as a hemorrhage or operation of letting blood.
The plasma of the blood, when exposed to air, changes its character to fibrin, which entangles the corpuscles and forms a blood clot. For this reason wounds should not be washed with water. Calcium salts are essential to clotting of the blood and they are often given before an operation for this purpose. They contract the cardiac muscles of the heart. SEE: *hemorrhage, blood clotting.*

b., arterial. This is indicated by bleeding in spurts. Color, bright red.
TREATMENT: Pressure with fingers above at nearest pressure point bet. it and heart. Locate drainage artery and apply digital pressure above it until bandaged. Elevate with patient recumbent.

b. time. About 3 minutes or less.

b., venous. Flow continuous. Color of blood, dark red.
TREATMENT: Patient recumbent. Pressure below wound with wound bet. heart and hand. Bandage over wound above and below.

blen'na [G. *blennos*, mucus]. Mucus.

blennadenitis (blen-ad-en-i'tis) [" + *adēn*, gland, + *-itis*, inflammation]. Inflammation of mucous glands.

blennelytria (blen-el-it'rī-ă) [" + *elytron*, vagina]. An abnormal white mucous discharge from vagina or cervical canal. SYN: *leukorrhea.*

blennemesis (blen-em'es-is) [" + *emesis*, vomiting]. Vomiting of mucus.

blenneteritis (blen-en-ter-i'tis) [" + *enteron*, intestine, + *-itis*, inflammation]. Enteritis accompanied by a flow of mucus.

blennisthmia (blen-isth'mĭ-ă) [" + *isthmos*, neck]. Catarrh of the pharynx.

blenno- [G.]. Prefix: Pert. to mucus.

blennocystitis (blen-o-sis-ti'tis) [G. *blennos*, mucus, + *kystis*, bag, + *-itis*, inflammation]. Inflammation of the urinary bladder.

blennogenic, or **blennogenous** (blen-o-jen'ik, or blen-oj'en-us) [" + *gennan*, to produce]. Secreting mucus.

blennoid (blen'oid). Like mucus; mucoid.
blennometritis (blen-o-me-tri'tis) [G. *blennos*, mucus, + *mētra*, womb, + *-itis*, inflammation]. Inflammation of the uterus.
blennophlogisma, blennophlogosis (blen-o-flo-jis'mä, blen-o-flo-jō'sis) [" + *phlox*, flame, + *gennan*, to produce]. Inflammation of a mucous membrane.
blennophthalmia (blen-off-thal'mĭ-ă) [" + *ophthalmos*, eye]. Catarrhal conjunctivitis.
blennoptysis (blen-op'tis-is) [" + *ptyein*, to spit]. Expectoration of mucus from the bronchi.
blennorrhagia (blen-or-a'jĭ-ă) [" + *rēgnunai*, to break forth]. 1. A discharge from mucous membranes, esp. gonorrheal discharges from the genital or urinary tract. 2. Gonorrhea.
  b. of conjunctiva. OPHTH: Adult form: gonorrheal ophthalmia.
  b. of lacrimal sac. A chronic catarrhal inflammation of the mucous membrane lining the lacrimal sac, resulting in retention of the mucous secretion and tears. PROG: Depends upon the degree. TREATMENT: Probe lacrimal apparatus and leave free passage for secretion. Indicated remedies.
  Infantile form: *ophthalmia neonatorum*. TREATMENT: Prophylactic.
blennorrhagic (blen-o-raj'ik). Pert. to blennorrhea; blennorrheal.

blennorrhea (blen-or-ē'ă) [G. *blennos*, mucus, + *roia*, flow]. Discharge from mucous membranes, esp. gonorrheal discharge from genital or urinary tract. SYN: *blennorrhagia*.*
blennorrheal (blen-o-re'ăl). Blennorrhagic; pert. to blennorrhea.
blennorrhinia (blen-or-in'ĭ-ă) [G. *blennos*, mucus, + *ris*, nose]. Coryza. Catarrh of the nasal passages.
blennosis (blen-o'sis). Any disease of a mucous membrane.
blennostasis (blen-os'tas-ĭs) [G. *blennos*, mucus, + *stasis*, a halt]. The checking of any mucous discharge.
blennostat'ic. Diminishing mucous secretion.
blennostrumous (blen-o-stru'mus) [G. *blennos*, mucus, + L. *struma*, scrofula]. Pert. to gonorrhea and scrofula.
blennothorax (blen-o-tho'raks) [" + *thōrax*, chest]. Pulmonary catarrh.
blennotorrhea (blen-ot-or-ē'ă) [" + *ous*, ear, + *roia*, flow]. A discharge of mucus from the ear.
blennurethria (blen-u-rē'thrĭ-ă) [" + *ourēthra*, urethra]. Gonorrhea of the urethra.
blennuria (blen-nu'rĭ-ă) [" + *ouron*, urine]. Excess of mucus in the urine.
blepharadenitis (blef-ar-ad-en-i'tis) [G. *blepharon*, eyelid, + *adēn*, gland, + *-itis*, inflammation]. Inflammation of the meibomian glands. SYN: *blepharoadenitis*.

BLEDING: ARREST OF[1]			
For Wounds of the Face			
Artery	Bone Against Which Pressure Is Applied	Course	Spot to Apply Pressure
Temporal	Temporal bone	Upwards of ½ in. in front of ear	Against bony prominence immediately in front of the ear or on temple
Facial	Low part of lower maxilla	Across the jaw diagonally upward from below	An inch in front of angle of lower jaw on the face
Carotid	Cervical vertebrae	From outer upper edge of sternum to angle of jaw	Deeply down and backwards an inch to the side of the prominence of the windpipe
For Wounds of the Upper Extremity			
Subclavian	First rib behind clavicle	Across middle of first rib to armpit	Deeply down and backwards over center of clavicle against first rib—(depress the shoulder first).
Axillary	Head of humerus	Descends across outer side of armpit to inside of humerus	High up in the armpit against upper part of humerus
Brachial	Shaft of humerus	Along inner side of humerus under edge of biceps muscle	Against shaft of humerus by pulling aside and gripping biceps, pressing deep down tips of fingers against the bone
For Wounds of the Lower Extremity			
(a) Femoral	Brim of pelvis	Down the thigh from the pelvis to the knee from a point midway bet. iliac spine and symphysis pubis to inner side of end of femur at knee joint	Against brim of pelvis, midway bet. iliac spine and symphysis pubis
(b) Femoral	Shaft of femur		High up on the inner side of the thigh, about 3 inches below brim of pelvis, over the line given in the direction of the knee
Posterior Tibial	Inner side of tibia, low down above ankle	Downwards to foot in hollow just behind the prominence of inner ankle	For wounds in the sole of the foot: against the tibia in center of the hollow behind the inner ankle

1. Hilda M. Gration, S.R.N.

blepharal (blef′ar-al). Pert. to an eyelid.

blepharedema (blef-ar-ē-de′mä) [G. *blepharon*, eyelid, + *oidēma*, swelling]. Swelling of the eyelids.

blepharelosis (blef″ar-el-o′sis) [″ + *eilein*, to roll]. Ingrowing eyelashes.

bleph′arism [″ + *ismos*, condition of]. Twitching of the eyelids.

blepharitis (blef-ar-i′tis) [″ + *-itis*, inflammation]. Inflammation of the edges of the lids involving hair follicles and glands opening on surface; ulcerative and nonulcerative.

ETIOL: Astigmatism, excessive use of the eyes, constant exposure to dust, smoke or overbright light, much weeping, etc. Found in conjunctivitis,* measles,* and in catarrhal affections of eye.

SYM: Lids red, tender, and sore, with sticky exudate, ulcers on edges; lids may become inverted, lashes falling out, and epiphoria* occurring. Styes and meibomian cysts are associated with the condition.

NP: Bathe lids with borax and warm water to remove crusts. Ointment to edges. Good food, cod liver oil.

RS: *blear-eye, madarosis*.

b. ciliaris, b. marginalis. Inflammation affecting the ciliary margins of the eyelids.

b. squamosa. B. with scaling.

b. ulcerosa. B. with ulceration.

blepharo- (blef-ar-o) [G.]. Prefix: Pert. to the eyelid.

blepharoadenitis (blef-ar-o-ad-en-i′tis) [G *blepharon*, eyelid, + *adēn*, gland, + *-itis*, inflammation]. Inflammation of meibomian glands.

blepharoadenoma (blef-ar-o-ad-e-no′mä) [″ + ″ + *-ōma*, tumor]. Adenoma or glandular tumor of eyelid.

blepharoatheroma (blef″ar-o-ath-ē-ro′mä) [″ + *athērē*, thick fluid, + *-ōma*, tumor]. Sebaceous cyst of an eyelid.

blepharochalasis (blef-ar-o-kal′as-is) [″ + *chalasis*, relaxation]. Relaxation of skin of eyelid due to loss of elasticity following edematous swellings, such as in recurrent angioneurotic edema of lids.

bleph″arochromidro′sis [″ + *chrōma*, color, + *idrōs*, sweat]. Discolored sweat of the eyelid.

bleph″aroc′lonus [″ + *klonos*, tumult]. Clonic spasm of muscles of the eye.

blepharoconjunctivitis (blef-ar-o-con-junc-ti-vi′tis) [″ + L. *conjunctiva*, + G. *-itis*, inflammation]. Inflammation of eyelids and conjunctiva.

blepharodiastasis (blef-ar-o-di-as′tas-is) [″ + *diastasis*, separation]. Excessive separation of eyelids.

blepharolithiasis (blef-ar-o-lith-i′ăs-īs) [″ + *lithos*, stone]. Concretions within the eyelid.

blepharoncus (blef-ar-on′kus) [G. *blepharon*, eyelid, + *ogkos*, tumor]. Tumor of the eyelid.

blepharon (blef′ar-on). The eyelid; palpebra.

blepharopachynsis (blef″ar-o-pă-kin′sis) [″ + *pachynsis*, thickening]. Thickening of the eyelid.

blepharophimosis (blef-ar-o-fī-mo′sis) [″ + *phimōsis*, narrowing]. Narrowing of slit between eyelids at external angle of eye due to angle being covered by vertical fold of skin.

blepharophryplasty (blef″ă-rof′rī-plas-tĭ) [″ + *ophrys*, eyebrow, + *plassein*, to mold]. Plastic operation for restoration of eyelid and eyebrow.

bleph′aroplast [″ + *plassein*, to form]. A minute mass of chromatin in a cell forming the base of a flagellum.

blepharoplasty (blef′ar-o-plas-tī) [″ + *plassein*, to form]. Plastic operation upon the eyelid.

blepharoplegia (blef-ar-o-ple′jī-ă) [G. *blepharon*, eyelid, + *plēgē*, a stroke]. Paralysis of an eyelid.

blepharoptosis (blef-ar-op-to′sis) [″ + *ptōsis*, a falling]. Dropping of the upper eyelid.

blepharopyorrhea (blef-ăr-o-pī-or-ē′ă) [″ + *pyon*, pus, + *roia*, flow]. Pus flowing from the eyelid.

blepharorrhaphy (blef″ă-ror′răf-ĭ) [″ + *raphē*, seam]. Reducing length of palpebral fissure by stitching margins of eyelids at outer canthus.

blepharorrhea (blef-ăr-ore-ē′ă) [″ + *roia*, flow]. Discharge from the eyelid.

blepharospasm (blef′ar-o-spazm) [″ + *spasmos*, spasm]. A twitching or spasmodic contraction of the orbicularis palpebrarum muscle due to habit spasm, eyestrain or nervous irritability.

blepharosphincterectomy (blef″ar-o-sfink-ter-ĕk′to-mī) [″ + *sphigktēr*, a constrictor, + *ektomē*, excision]. Excision of part of the orbicularis palpebrarum to relieve pressure of eyelid on cornea.

blepharostat (blef′ar-o-stat) [″ + *istanai*, cause to stand]. Device for separating the eyelids during an operation.

blepharostenosis (blef″ar-o-sten-o′sis) [″ + *stenōsis*, a narrowing]. Narrowing of the palpebral slit through inability to open the eye normally.

blepharosynechia (blef″ar-o-si-nek′ī-ă) [″ + *synecheia*, a holding together]. Permanent adhesion of the eyelids.

blepharotomy (blef-ar-ot′o-mī) [″ + *tomē*, a cutting]. Cutting of eyelid.

blepsopathia (blep-so-path′ī-ă) [G. *blepsis*, sight, + *pathos*, disease]. Eyestrain.

Blessig's groove. A mark in the embryonic eye indicating the *ora serrata*, or retinal anterior edge. SEE: *groove*.

blind [A.S. *blind*, unable to see]. Without sight.

blindness [A.S. *blind*, unable to see]. Amaurosis; loss of sight.

b., color. Inability to distinguish one or more primary colors.

b., day. Inability to see in daylight; hemeralopia.

b., letter. Inability to understand the meaning of letters; a form of aphasia.

b., night. Nyctalopia; inability to see at night.

b., psychic. Sight without recognition due to brain lesion.

b., snow. ETIOL: Glare of sunlight upon the snow; temporary.

b., word. Inability to understand written or printed words.

blindness, words pert. to: ablepsia, acatamathesia, achloropsia, "achro-" words, aglaukopsia, amianthinopsy, amaurosis, amaurotic, aphemesthesia, axanthopsia, acritochromacy, blind spot, blindness, chionblepsia, color, hemeralopia, hemiachromatopsia, hemianopia, meropia, mind b., night b., nyctamblyopia, nyctophobia, nyctotyphlosis, tritanopia, typhlology, word b., xanthocyanopia.

blind spot [A.S. *blind*, unable to see, + M.E. *spot*, small bit]. Physiological scotoma situated 15° to outside of fixation point; corresponds to entrance of optic nerve in eye. SYN: optic disc.

blister [M.E. *blester*, a swelling]. 1. A bleb or vesicle containing serum, sometimes caused by a pressure. 2. A collec-

blister, blood   B-30   **blood**

tion of fluid below the epidermis, usually the result of a burn.
TREATMENT: Mild antiseptic, protective dressing if extremely painful due to pressure, may be aseptically punctured and then treated as a wound. SEE: *causes*, as *burn, scald*, etc. An agent producing a bleb. RS: *vesicle, vesicular*.

b., blood. Small subcutaneous or intracutaneous extravasation of blood due to rupture of blood vessels.
TREATMENT: Apply antiseptic and a firm dressing with moderate pressure to aid in stopping extravasation and hasten absorption. Sometimes desirable to puncture aseptically and aspirate.

b., fly. Known as *cantharides* and Spanish fly b., the therapeutic value of which consists in the irritation which it produces, drawing a large amount of blood to an area, thereby relieving the congestion, and improving the circulation.

b., flying. One to be used in more than 1 place.

b., water. One containing water.
NP: Scissors to cut blister must be sterile, as must forceps to handle it and dressings. Absorb fluid with sterile absorbent wool. When removing, snip or cut edges with plaster attached. Catch fluid on cotton wool. See that fluid does not run over skin. Remove raised dead skin and apply dressing. To dress, prepare lint or gauze, spread with zinc or other ointment. Apply and hold with adhesive tape.

bloated (blōt'ĕd) [A.S. *blōtian*, to swell up]. Swollen or distended beyond normal size, as by serum, water, gas, etc.

block [O.Fr. *bloc*, a piece of wood, an obstruction]. 1. To deaden all sensory impressions in a nerve, or in the nerve trunk and roots of the spinal cord through the use of an anesthetic for operative purposes. 2. To obstruct. 3. An obstruction or stoppage.

b., heart. Interferences with the heart's contraction, causing disassociation of the auricular and ventricular rhythms. Due to failure of the contractile impulses to pass through the conductile tissue (atrio-ventricular node and bundle of His).

blocking. 1. Interruption in free association during psychoanalysis as a defense against unpleasant ideas.
2. PSY: A sudden, unaccountable stoppage of speech or thought. May be due to a conflict or painful thought, and exhibited in dementia precox.
3. Process of obstructing or deadening, as a nerve.

Blondlot rays (blon-lō'). Rays of shorter wave length but which resemble light, making certain bodies luminous; also called *n*-rays.

blood [A.S. *blōd*]. The fluid that circulates through the heart, arteries, veins, and capillaries carrying nourishment and oxygen to the tissues and taking away waste matter and carbon dioxide.
FUNCT: (a) Nutrition and respiration of tissues located far from the food and air supplies; (b) transportation of waste from the tissues to the excretory organs; (c) chemical and thermal coordination of the body; (d) defense against infection through the action of antibodies* and phagocytes.*
COMP: Human blood is composed of a fluid part (*plasma**) in which are suspended red and white corpuscles,* platelets* and fat globules. Blood consists of 22% solids and 78% water.
The amount of blood in man, measured in pints, can be computed approximately by dividing the weight in pounds by 14; using the metric system, an adult weighing 70 Kg. has a blood volume of about 5.5 liters. Its *specific gravity* varies from 1.055 to 1.062, the corpuscles being heavier and plasma lighter than this.

Blood			
	Water 78%	Proteins	18.5%
		Glucose	0.1
	Solids 22%	Lipids (fats)	1.4
		Salts (inorganic)	1.5
		Waste products, etc.	0.5

Constituents in Blood

Blood
- Cells
  - Red blood cells (Erythrocytes)
  - White blood cells (Leukocytes)
  - Platelets
- Plasma
  - Water
  - Gases
    - Oxygen
    - Carbon dioxide
    - Nitrogen
  - Foods
    - Carbohydrate (Glucose)
    - Fat (fatty acids)
    - Protein (amino acids)
  - Blood proteins
    - Serum albumin
    - Serum globulin
    - Fibrinogen
  - Salts
    - Chlorides
    - Bicarbonates —— of —— Sodium
    - Sulfates   Calcium
    - Phosphates   Potassium
    -    Magnesium
  - Protective substances:
    - Antitoxin
    - Opsonins
    - Agglutinin
    - Bacteriolysins
  - Autacoids (internal secretions from ductless glands)
  - Waste
    - Urea   Hypoxanthine
    - Uric acid   Guanine
    - Creatinine   Adenine
    - Xanthine   Carnine

blood, chemical analysis — blood, defibrinated

In passing through the lungs the blood gives up carbon dioxide; after leaving the heart it is carried to the tissues as arterial blood, and then returned to the heart. It moves in the principal arteries at the rate of a foot per second and it makes the circuit of the vascular system in about 20 seconds. It constitutes 1/14 of the body weight. SEE: *circulation*.

CHARACTERISTICS: It has a peculiar odor. Arterial blood is bright red or scarlet; the venous blood dark red or crimson.

b., chemical analysis. Specimens should be obtained in the morning before eating or drinking.

If refrigerated they may be kept for a number of days, but samples should be sent to the laboratory as soon as taken. 10 to 20 cc. of venous blood are ordinarily sufficient. 0.25 to 1 cc. of finger blood for micro-Folin blood sugar test. If placed in a container, 2 drops of a 20% solution of potassium oxalate should be added for an ounce of blood. This serves as an anticoagulant. It should then be mixed by shaking. Hemoglobin is low in anemia. Creatinine, urea, and nonprotein nitrogen are high in nephritis, as is uric acid. Blood sugar is high in diabetes. Cholesterol is low in anemia and high in nephrosis.

b., clotting of. The process whereby blood changes into a jellylike, nonfluid mass. Blood plasma normally contains fibrinogen, a protein. When blood is exposed to air, foreign substances, or juices from injured tissues, a new substance, thrombin, appears in it. Thrombin converts fibrinogen into the insoluble fibrin, a stringy, elastic substance that forms a meshwork in which the corpuscles are caught. Calcium deficiency causes tendency to slow clotting.

RS: *athrombia, blood, blood clot, coagulation, c. time test, hemophilia*.

b., constituents. The preceding tables give pertinent data on this subject.

b., defibrinated. If whole blood is stirred in a dish, *e.g.*, with a stick of wood, the stringy, elastic *fibrin* comes out on the stirrer; it can be washed until white. The remaining thick, red blood can no longer clot, and is called defibrinated blood.

If it is centrifuged, the clear liquid which now appears in the upper half of the centrifuged tube is called *serum;* this differs from plasma chiefly in that it contains no more fibrinogen (the parent substance of fibrin). The corpuscles are in the lower half of the tube.

Excess of fibrin in the blood indicates excessive intake, esp. of albuminous foods, a factor in increased coagulation. Excess of urea in the blood frequently found in renal retention such as in Bright's disease. Excess uric acid indicates increased protein metabolism or retention, or both. Uric acid in the blood and urine indicates fermentation of waste products in system and impaired condition of eliminating organs. Hemoglobin is low in anemia. Creatine, urea and nonprotein nitrogen are high in nephritis, as is uric acid. Blood sugar is high in diabetes. Cholesterol is low in anemia and high in nephrosis.

RS: *b. c. casts, b. clot, b. count, b. examination, b. grouping, b. platelets, b.*

Clinically Significant Blood Constituents*

Blood Constituents Tested for Per 100 cc. of Blood	Normal Range	Beginning Pathologic Range Below is indicated by a (—) sign, and above by a (+) sign	Pathologic Range	Significance
Hemoglobin	14-17 Gm.	—12	3-23	Low in anemia
Nonprotein nitrogen (N. P. N.)	25-35 mg.	+35	20-400	High in nephritis
Urea nitrogen	12-15 mg.	+20	5-350	High in nephritis
Creatinine	1-2 mg.	+3.5	to 34	High in nephritis
Uric acid	1-3.5 mg.	+4	to 27	High in nephritis, gout
Blood sugar	70-120 mg.	+150	40-1300	High in diabetes
CO_2 capacity	50-70% by volume	—45	5-130	Low in nephritis, acidosis
Cholesterol	140-170 mg.	—130 +170	60-1000	High in nephritis, low in anemia
Calcium as calcium	9-11 mg.	—8	3-20	Low in tetanus, stages of nephritis
Inorganic phosphorus as phosphorus Adult Children	2.5-4 mg. 4-6 mg.	—4	2.40	Low in rickets. High in stages of nephritis
Chlorides as NaCl: Plasma Whole blood	570-620 mg. 450-520 mg.	—500 —450	300-850 120-700	High in nephritis, with edema, nephritis, eclampsia, low in pneumonia
Icterus index (terms of 1: 10,000 potassium dichromate)	4-6 mg.	+10	10-225	High in hemolytic anemia. Indicates liver disturbances

* Myers: *Jr. Am. Med. Assoc.*, July 21, 1928.

blood, words pert. to

poisoning, b. *pressure, erythrocytes, leukocytes.*

blood, words pert. to: acapnia, acetonemia, acetonuria, achreocythemia, acidemia, adrenalinemia, aeration, afflux, albukalin, albuminosis, albumosemia, aleucemia, -ic, aleukemia, -ic, alexin, alkalemia, aminosis, amylemia, anadrome, anemia, -ic, anhydremia, anoxemia, apocenosis, apoplasmia, apostaxis, anthocyaninemia, atmospherization, blood-attenuant, "auto-" words, avascularization, bacteriemia, basophilia, beat, bends, bilirubinemia, bleeding, buffer, buffer salts, cacemia, calcemia, "carbo-" words, carotenemia, carotenosis, cell-color ratio, chloridemia, chloruremia, "chole-" words, "cine-" words, circulation, clotting, coagulum, coagulation, -time test, coagulin, color index, cosanguinity, diapedesis, differential blood count, dyscrasia, exsanguinate, exsanguine, fibrin, fibrinogen, glycemia, glycosemia, grouping, "hema-" words, "hemo-" words, hydremia, hyperemia, hypoglycemia, icteric index, inemia, inosemia, inosite, lithiasis, melanemia, melitemia, necremia, occult, oligemia, opsonic index, opsonins, oxalemia, oxygenation, oxyhemoglobin, pachemia, plasma, platelet, poikilocytes, -osis, polymorphonuclear, prothrombin, regurgitation, revulsion, sapremia, spanemia, "thromb-" words, transfusion, transudation, revulsion, sapremia, spanemia.

blood bank. Storing place for reserve blood kept for emergency transfusions.
Person donating blood generally bet. 21 and 50 years, with negative history of syphilis, chronic alcoholism and recent illness.
Blood is mixed with sodium citrate, physiological saline solution and glucose, and is then stored at 40° C. Used up to 3 weeks after storage, but preferably should not be older than 5 days. SEE: *blood grouping, blood transfusion, donor.*

blood cell [A.S. *blōd*, blood, + L. *cella*, small chamber]. Minute body in the blood of 2 types; erythrocyte,* or red cell, and leukocyte,* or white cell.
ERYTHROCYTE: SEE: *anisocytosis, normoblasts, poikilocytes, polychromasia.*
LEUKOCYTE: SEE: *eosinophils, lymphocytes, mast cells, myelocytes, transitionals, polymorphonuclear neutrophils; also degenerates.*

b. c. casts. Masses of red cells molded by the renal tubules, the blood originating from the glomeruli. Abnormal microscopic body in the urine composed of coagulated serum covered with red blood cells.

blood cell, words pert. to: achromatocyte, achromatolysis, aglobulia, aleukia, aleukocytosis, anemia, anerythrocyte, anerythroplasia, anerythroplastic, anhematosis, anhemolytic, anisocytosis, Arneth's classification of neutrophils, bioblast, Bizzozero's c., blast, blood cell, cell color ratio, crenation, erythrocytes, erythropenia, "hem-" words, hypercythemia, "leuc-" words, "leuk-" words, megaloblasts, normoblast, oligochromemia, oligocythemia, ozonophore, phagocyte, -osis, polycythemia, spanemia.

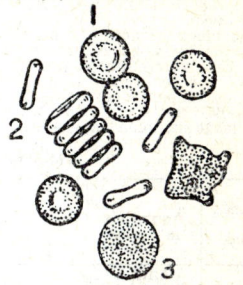

BLOOD CELLS
1. Red blood corpuscles. 2. Red blood corpuscles, side view. 3. White blood corpuscles.

blood clot [" + O.E. *clott*, a mass]. Coagulated mass of blood. SYN: *coagulum*.
It is the result of prothrombin (zymogen, or mother's enzyme), when it forms an enzyme or ferment called *thrombin* by combining with calcium salts in the blood, the thrombin acting on fibrinogen. The latter coagulates on exposure to the air and changes into fibrin. Coagulation Time: Normal, 2 to 8 minutes. SEE: *buffy coat, clotting, coagulation.*

blood corpuscles. The solid and cellular elements in the blood. SEE: *erythrocytes, leukocytes.*

blood count. Enumeration of the red corpuscles and the leukocytes per cubic millimeter.
A blood count shows the variation of the different cells in number per cubic millimeter of blood, and in the character and type of the different cells.
Normally in each cu. mm. of blood there are an average of five million erythrocytes in the male and four and a half million in the female. Altitude increases the number. The leukocytes average five to nine thousand in each cu. mm. varying from day to day.

Tabular Summary of Blood Corpuscles

Cells	Nucleus	Cytoplasm Color	Cytoplasm Granules	Average diameter (Microns)	Number per cmm.
Erythrocytes or red blood corpuscles	Absent	Red	None	7.3	4,500,000 to 5,000,000
Platelets	?	None	None	3	200,000 to 900,000
Leukocytes or white blood corpuscles	Varies with different types	None	Varies with different types	13	5,000 to 9,000

A laboratory technician makes the count, which is done microscopically. A ruled area is used by which the different cells are counted in small squares. The percentage of different cells may be calculated from any number counted, but it is best to count not less than 200. Pathologic cells are also looked for, and platelets, and hemoglobin tests are also made.

A DIFFERENTIAL BLOOD COUNT: This is an examination of the blood by stained specimens to ascertain the characteristic of the red cells and the variety of the white ones.

Some blood diseases, and inflammatory conditions may be recognized in this way. In a differential count, the varieties of the leukocytes and their percentages should be: Polymorphonuclears, 65-70%; small mononuclears, 20-30%; large mononuclears, 4-8%; transitionals, 1/3%; basophils, ¼-½%; eosinophils, ½-2%; platelets, 300,000 per cu.mm.

blood dust. Minute colorless bodies in the blood, particles of the blood corpuscle. SYN: *hemoconia*.

blood examinations. They may be (a) morphological,* (b) chemical, (c) physical, (d) bacteriological, and (e) serological.*

Blood is difficult to study because it so promptly clots unless anticoagulants are added to it. SEE: *b. constituents*.

WHAT THE EXAMINER LOOKS FOR: The number and character of the red blood cells, the percentage of hemoglobin, the coagulation time,* the number and character of white blood cells, the presence of parasites; also the amount of sugar, urea, urea-nitrogen, nonprotein nitrogen, creatinin, and uric acid. Complement fixation tests are made for sus-

Method of Testing Blood Groups

Serum of Group	Agglutinin in Serum	Recipient Red Blood Cells of Group O	A	B	AB	Remarks
O	Anti-A and Anti-B	○	●	●	●	Cells of Group O *not* agglutinated by any sera. Contains no agglutinable substances. *Universal Donors* (45% of adults).
A	Anti-B	○	○	●	●	Cells of Group A agglutinated by sera of Groups O and B (40% adults).
B	Anti-A	○	●	○	●	Cells of Group B agglutinated by sera of Groups O and A (10% adults).
AB	None	○	○	○	○	Cells of Group AB agglutinated by sera of Groups O, A, B. Serum of Group AB contains no isoagglutinins. *Universal recipient* (5% adults).

When recipient is Group O, select Donor from Group O
" " " " A, " " " " O or A
" " " " B, " " " " O or B
" " " " AB, " " " " O, A, B, AB

The Average Blood Pressure of Old Men

Age	Number Examined	Systolic Pressure	Diastolic Pressure	Pulse Pressure
65-69	11	145	81	63
70-74	10	166	91	75
75-79	14	159	89	77
80-84	11	163	84	80
85-89	0	...	..	..
90-94	4	145	81	65

The Average Blood Pressure of Old Women

Age	Number Examined	Systolic Pressure	Diastolic Pressure	Pulse Pressure
65-69	21	154	83	71
70-74	29	158	83	72
75-79	24	170	88	81
80-84	16	183	85	91
85-89	7	170	90	77
90-94	3	137	80	53

pected gonorrhea, and Wassermann for syphilitic infection. Culture should be made if bacteria are suspected.

CHEMICAL FINDINGS: The first figures indicate the normal, the second figures indicate beginning pathology (amount in mg. per 100 cc. of blood): Sugar: 70-100, P., 120; nonprotein nitrogen, 25-35, P., 40; urea nitrogen, 10-15, P., 20; creatinin, 1-2, P., 3; uric acid, 1-3, P., 4; CO_2 combining power, 55-75, P., 45; cholesterol, 150-190, P., 200; sodium chloride, 45-500, P., 400-550 plus.

Whenever blood is to be collected from a vein the following points should be observed:

1. The syringe and needle should be not only sterile, but either dry or washed out with sterile normal saline solution. In particular the syringe should contain no trace of alcohol or ether, and preferably no distilled water.

2. The blood withdrawn is put into test tubes which are sterile and either (a) plain dry or (b) oxalated (*i. e.*, containing a small quantity of sodium or potassium oxalate powder). (a) Plain tubes are required for: Wassermann reaction, Widal and other agglutination reactions, v. d. Bergh reaction, blood calcium. (b) Oxalated tubes are required for: Blood sugar, blood urea, nonprotein nitrogen (N. P. N.), etc.

3. Immediately the blood has been expelled from the syringe, this and the needle should be washed out with normal saline or cold water. In this way "jamming" of the piston is avoided.

blood groups. Scientific findings show that all human bloods fall within four groups, the fourth one being a rare group.

On examining the serum and cells of a number of bloods, Landsteiner (1901) found that the reactions of serum and cells did not occur in a helterskelter manner, but fell into three groups, a fourth one being discovered later. It was also found that the blood group properties were inherited, and that the distribution differs among various races. Prior to these discoveries blood transfusions* were often followed by severe symptoms or death.

In selecting a donor it is essential to know that the donor and the recipient are compatible as to their blood grouping, and a retyping of their blood is made for this purpose. When a donor is used over any extensive period retyping is necessary.

Due to confusion from two classifications (Jansky & Moss), blood groups are now represented by letters indicating their serological characteristics. (See table on B-33.)

INCOMPATIBILITY: This is indicated if there is any clumping or agglutination seen with naked eye.

bloodless. Without blood.
  b. operation. One by which the blood is expelled by compresses from the part which is to be operated upon, or by electrocautery.

blood motes. Minute colorless particles in the blood, bits of blood corpuscles. SYN: *blood dust, hemoconia.*

blood platelets. Small, colorless bodies in circulating blood, averaging about 3 microns in diameter which in shed blood tend to agglutinate into small clusters. They may originate from giant bone-marrow cells (megakaryocytes). They play an important rôle in clotting through release of *thrombokinase* which in presence of calcium reacts with prothrombin to form thrombin.

The normal number in circulating b., is about 250,000 to 300,000 per cmm. Reduction below normal is called *thrombocytopenia*. In certain forms of hemophilia, they are abnormally stable and fail to release thrombokinase, thus increasing coagulation time.

blood poisoning. The entrance of noxious materials, such as bacteria and their toxic products, into the blood stream. SEE: *pyemia, sapremia, septicemia, toxemia.*

blood pressure. As popularly used, the pressure existing in the large arteries at the height of the pulse wave; the systolic intraarterial pressure.

More generally, the pressure exerted by the blood on the wall of any vessel. This pressure reaches its highest values in the left ventricle during systole, it is lower successively in the left arteries, capillaries, and veins, and sinks to subatmospheric values in the large veins during diastole.

The systolic arterial blood pressure itself rises during activity or excitement and falls during sleep. In the normal, relaxed, sitting adult, it is likely to be between 110 and 145 mm. of mercury.

The following findings are considered abnormal: (1) Systolic pressure persistently above 150; (2) diastolic pressure persistently above 100; (3) pulse pressure constantly greater than 50. Blood pressure varies with age, sex, altitude, muscular development, and according to states of worry and fatigue. It is lower in women than in men; low in childhood and high in advancing age as a rule. SEE: *Normal blood pressure.*

  b. p., children's. This is much lower than in adults. Differences in rate of growth varying at different ages are factors in children's blood pressure. Dr. H. G. Richey gives the approximate normal or, perhaps, better said, the average blood pressure at different ages of childhood at the foot of this page.

  b. p., diastolic. Lowest point to which it drops between beats. Average in brachial artery of adult is 60 to 90 mm.

  b. p., normal. Should show a high systolic pressure of about 145 mm. with 10 mm. less for women. Normal diastolic pressure, 60 mm. to 90 mm.; 120 mm. average systolic pressure at the age of 20, and ½ mm. for each year above that age, which would give 135 mm. as normal systolic pressure for a man of about 50. Arterial pressure is not uniform. Most published findings are the results of tests made before the technic of measuring blood pressure was perfected, and before the modern instruments for the purpose existed. Unfortunately, then, such findings cannot be depended upon except in a general way. Life insurance companies have compiled tabulations of blood pressure at different ages. One table presents the above figures.

  b. p., systolic. The highest point caused by the contraction of the heart. 120 to 145 mm.

  RS: *anisergy, anisopiesis, arteriotomy, diastole, hyperpiesia, hypertension, hypotension, pulse pressure, systole.*

blood'shot. Locally congested with blood.
blood smear. Drop of blood spread on a slide for purpose of examination.

blood sugar   B-35   blood test

For the easy recognition of white cells, it is essential that a good smear be made. This is easily done as follows: Cover glasses three-quarters of an inch square must be perfectly clean and lint free. This is accomplished by cleaning them with hydrochloric acid for 24 hr. They are then washed in water and placed in alcohol. A silk cloth is used to dry them. The finger should never come in contact with the flat sides of the glasses.

A small drop of blood the size of the head of a pin is taken on 1 of these cover glasses which in turn is placed upon a second similar film. If they are clean, the blood runs out, covering the entire surfaces in apposition. Just before this movement of the blood stops, the films are gently pulled apart and allowed to dry in the air.

blood sugar. Sugar in the form of about 0.08 to 0.12% dextrose in the blood or about 80-120 mg. per 100 cc. of blood.

It rises after a meal but not more than 160 mg. per 100 cc. of blood but this may vary. Above this amt. sugar enters the urine. Dextrose is half as sweet as cane sugar.

b. s. test. Increased sugar content of the blood, or presence of sugar in the urine indicates faulty metabolism and diabetes. The urine may be free of sugar but the blood sugar may have increased, which necessitates a test being made.

A wound is very slow to heal if there is an excess amt. of blood sugar present. An abnormal amt. in the blood may bring about an occlusion of the blood vessels, thus interfering with nourishment of the tissues which produces gangrene in diabetes and increases susceptibility to infections. Arteriosclerosis also may be induced by an excessive amt. of sugar in the blood.

blood test. To ascertain contents of the blood.

BLOOD UREA: For this test 10 cc. of blood are withdrawn into a sterile test tube containing a few crystals of calcium oxalate.

UREA CONCENTRATION TEST: The patient has a drink at midnight and nothing afterwards. At 6 A. M. the patient passes urine. The amt. is recorded and a specimen put up. 15 Gm. of urea dissolved in 100 cc. of water are taken, and afterwards 4 specimens of urine are obtained at hourly intervals, the whole of each specimen being kept. In the second and third specimens the urine should contain 2% of urea.

UREA CLEARANCE TEST: This test gives more accurate information as to the efficiency of the kidney than the above. It shows the amt. of blood cleared of urea in a given time. It is carried out bet. breakfast and lunch as follows:

The bladder is completely emptied. Exactly one hr. after the bladder is again emptied. The specimen of urine obtained is kept. One hr. after, this is repeated. Blood, for blood urea, is withdrawn at the end of the first hr. No coffee is allowed for breakfast. Tea is sometimes allowed.

BLOOD SUGAR TOLERANCE CURVE: The fasting level of blood sugar is normally 80-120 mg. in 100 cc. If large amts. of carbohydrate are taken the sugar in the blood rises as high as 170 mg. The sugar level falls to fasting level within 2 hr.

TEST: No food or drink after 9 P. M. the evening before. In the morning blood is withdrawn and the amt. of glucose estimated. This represents the fasting level. The patient then empties the bladder completely and drinks a solution of 50 Gm. of glucose in 100 cc. of water flavored with lemon juice. Blood is taken every half hr. for 2½ hr. The bladder is emptied one hr. and 2 hr. after taking the glucose. The urine is tested. In health neither specimen contains sugar. A prolonged curve indicates impaired carbohydrate metabolism.

INTERPRETATION: In a normal person, blood sugar level rises to 170-180 mg.

Normal Blood Pressure

	Systolic Range				Diastolic Range			
Age	Minimum	Average	Maximum		Minimum	Average	Maximum	Pulse Pressure
15-19	105	117	129		73	77	81	40
20-24	108	120	132		75	79	83	41
25-29	109	121	133		76	80	84	41
30-34	110	122	134		77	81	85	41
35-39	110	123	135		78	82	86	41
40-44	112	125	137		79	83	87	42
45-49	115	127	139		80	84	88	43
50-54	116	129	142		81	85	89	44
55-59	118	131	144		82	86	90	45
60-64	121	134	147		83	87	91	47

Boys
5 Years of Age.........About 80
6 Years of Age.........About 85
7 Years of Age.........About 89
8 Years of Age.........About 92
9 Years of Age.........About 95
10 Years of Age.........A Little Over 95
11 Years of Age.........About 96
12 Years of Age.........About 98
13 Years of Age.........About 101
14 Years of Age.........About 106
15 Years of Age.........About 110
16 Years of Age.........About 112
17 Years of Age.........About 112
18 Years of Age.........About 113
19 Years of Age.........About 117

Girls
5 Years of Age.........About 85
6 Years of Age.........About 86
7 Years of Age.........About 89
8 Years of Age.........About 92
9 Years of Age.........About 93
10 Years of Age.........About 96
11 Years of Age.........About 100
12 Years of Age.........About 102
13 Years of Age.........About 103
14 Years of Age.........About 104
15 Years of Age.........About 106
16 Years of Age.........About 107
17 Years of Age.........About 103
18 Years of Age.........About 101
19 Years of Age.........About 105

blood, test for, in urine   B-36   **Boas motor meal**

and then drops to fasting blood level (100 mg. or less) within two to three hours. In a diabetic or a person with impaired sugar tolerance, blood sugar may exceed 180 mg. and appear in urine. The curve is prolonged and drops slowly and tends to remain above fasting blood sugar level. In hyperinsulinism, the curve is lower than normal and blood sugar may fall to low levels (40-60 mg.) four to six hours after administration of glucose.

b., test for, in urine. Take 1 in. of urine in a test tube and add 1 or 2 drops of tincture of guaiacum. Carefully overlay this with ½ in. of ozonic ether. Hold the tube in the hand to warm it for a few minutes. Blood is indicated by the appearance of a blue line at the junction of the fluids.

blood transfusion. The transference of the blood of one person into the blood vessels of another. In direct or immediate transfusion, the blood is transferred without being exposed to air; in *indirect* or *mediate* transfusion, the blood is collected in a receptacle from the donor before transfusion.

b. baby. A child born with a very blue color due to mixture of the venous and arterial blood through a defect in the heart.

b. mass. A compound pill of mercury.

b. ointment. Mercurial ointment. SEE: *mercury.*

b. stone. POISONING: (copper sulfate). SYM: Vomiting which is bluish and which turns darker on addition of ammonia. Pain and cramps in upper part of the abdomen. Convulsions. Pulse first strong and rapid, and later feeble. TREATMENT: Empty stomach by means of a stomach tube or an emetic. Give large quantities of milk or the white of eggs in water. Follow with barley water or gruel or similar demulcent.

b. vitriol. SEE: *copper sulfate.*

blueberries [" + A.S. *berie*, berry]. Av. SERVING: 100 Gm. Pro. 0.6, Fat 0.6, Carbo. 15.1 per serving. ASH CONST: Ca 0.020, Mg 0.007, K 0.051, Na 0.016, P 0.008, Cl 0.008, S 0.011, Fe 0.0009.

bluefish [" + A.S. *fisc*, fish]. NUTRIENTS: A. P. Prot. 19.4, Fat 1.2. FUEL VALUE: 100 Gm.—88 cal.

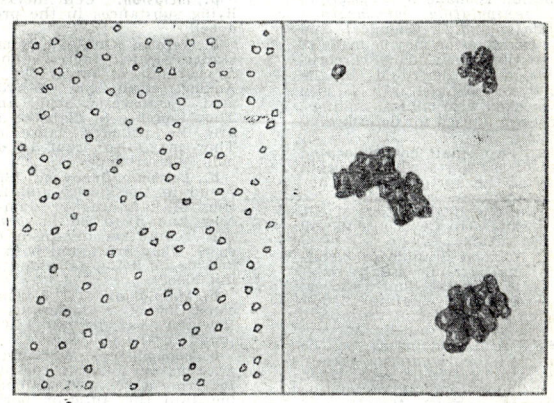

BLOOD TYPING (Direct)

The red blood cells of the donor are mixed with the serum of the recipient. **Left:** Compatibility; no agglutination. **Right:** Incompatibility with formation of clumps. This donor cannot be used.

bloody flux. Dysentery.

bloody sweat. Excretion of blood or blood pigment through the sweat glands. SYN: *hemathidrosis.*

bloody vomit. A result of rupture of the blood vessels of the upper alimentary tract due to injury, disease, or swallowing of blood.

TREATMENT: Do not give stimulants; nothing by mouth. Keep patient quiet and lying down. Cold applications to lower chest and upper abdomen.

bloody weeping. Hemorrhage from conjunctiva.

Blot's perforator (blos). Instrument used to perforate the fetal skull to facilitate its delivery.

blow'fly. Flesh fly that deposits its eggs in flesh; *Musca vomitoria.*

blow'ing respiration. Bellows murmur; bruit de soufflet.

blue [O.Fr. *bleu*, blue]. 1. A primary color of the spectrum; sky color; azure. 2. Cyanotic.

Blumenau's nucleus (bloo'men-ows). Outer part of the cuneate fasciculus.

Blu'menbach's clivus. Sloping part of sphenoid bone behind post. clinoid processes.

blush'ing [A.S. *blyscan*, to be red]. Rush of blood to the face caused by embarrassment or other emotion. SEE: *rubedo.*

B. M. A. Abbr. for *British Medical Association.*

B. M. R. Abbr. for *basal metabolism rate.*

B. M. S. Abbr. for *Bachelor of Medical Science.*

BNA. Abbr. for *Basle nomina anatomica*, an anatomical nomenclature adopted by the German Anatomical Society in 1895, at Basle, Switzerland. It includes some 4500 terms.

Boas motor meal. Test for tonicity of bowels.

If the morning after an Ewald-Boas test meal was given, lavage shows the stomach to be empty, there is normal motility.

B. point. A tender spot left of the 12th dorsal vertebra in cases of gastric ulcer. [drochloric acid in gastric juice.
B. reagent. Formula for testing hy-
B. sign. The presence of lactic acid in the gastric contents.
B. test meal. This is a nonlactic-acid-containing meal. It consists of 30 Gm. of rolled oats boiled in 500 cc. salted water, or two shredded wheat biscuits with 300 cc. of water. This is used as a test of lactic acid. If the patient is to be given the above mentioned test meal, the stomach should be lavaged* the night before.

Bochdalek's ganglion (bok'dal-ek). Ganglion of plexus of dental nerve in the maxilla above the canine tooth.

Bo'do. A genus of protozoan organisms. Some are parasitic in man's intestines.

body [A.S. *bodig*, body]. Soma; corpus. 1. The physical man. 2. The trunk without the head and extremities. 3. The principal part of anything. 4. A small organ or a structure within an organ.
EXAMINATION: The nude body is examined and both sides compared. Physical examination is made by *inspection, palpation, manipulation, mensuration,* and *auscultation, q.v.* Chemical and microscopic examination may be made of the blood, sputum, feces, urine, cerebrospinal fluids, and other fluids of the body. X-ray, or roentgen ray, is also used, and checked with clinical findings. The cardiograph is used for determining heart rhythms.

b., aortic. Two small bodies located in the arch of the aorta which contain the endings of the aortic nerve. They are chemoreceptors responding to changes in the chemical content of the blood esp., changes in CO_2 content and H-ion concentration.

b., basal. A basal granule or blepharoblast. A small granule usually present at the base of a flagellum protozoa.

b., Call-Exner. Darkly staining bodies found in growing follicles of the ovary. Also called vacucles of Call-Exner.

b. carotid. A flat structure at the bifurcation of the common carotid artery. Contains epitheloid cells which serve as chemo receptors, responding to changes in carbon dioxide and oxygen content of the blood and to changes in pH.

b., cavernous. One of three cylindrical bodies of erectile tissue found in the penis. SEE: corpora cavernosum.

b. cavities. The thorax, abdomen, and pelvis.

b. cell. The main portion of a cell, esp. a neuron; the portion that contains the nucleus.

b. cells. Somatic cells. Any cells of the body excepting the reproductive or germinal cells.

b., chromaffin. A number of bodies composed principally of chromaffin cells, *q.v.* which lie serially arranged along both sides of the dorsal aorta. Also called *paraganglionic bodies*. They are ectodermal in origin, having the same origin as cells of the sympathetic ganglia.

b., chromatoid. Darkly staining bodies found in the encysted forms of parasitic amebae. Thought to serve as reserve food. They disappear as cysts grow older.

b., chromophilic. One of the granular bodies in cytoplasm of a nerve cell which stain readily with basic dyes.

b., ciliary. A structure in the eye consisting of the ciliary muscle and ciliary processes. Functions in accommodation.

b., coccygeal. A mass of tissue consisting of one or several small nodules located at tip of coccyx. It contains an arteriovenous anastomosis. Its function is unknown.

b., Donovan's. Organism supposedly causing granuloma inguinale.

b., geniculate, lateral. Two bodies forming elevations on the lateral portion of the posterior part of the thalamus. Each is the termination of afferent fibers from the retina which they receive through the optic nerves and tracts.

b., geniculate, medial. Two bodies lying in the posterior part of the dorsal thalamus, connected by the commissure of Gudden. Each receives fibers from the acoustic center of the medulla and from the inferior colliculus through the brachium.

b., Hassalls. Hassall's corpuscle, found in the medulla of the thymus.

b., Hensen's. A modified Golgi net found in the hair cells of the organ of Corti of the ear.

b., inclusion. Cell inclusions. Nonliving substances in the protoplasm of a cell.

b., ketone. One of a number of substances which increase in the blood as a result of faulty fat metabolism. Among them are B-hydroxybutyric acid, acetoacetic acid, and acetone. They increase in diabetes mellitus and are the primary cause of acidosis. They may also occur in other metabolic disturbances.

b., Leishman-Donovan. Small bodies found in the spleen and liver of victims of kala-azar or dum-dum fever. Now known to be *Leishmania donovani*, causative organism of the disease. They are found both within and outside of living cells and in circulating blood.

b. Malpighian. (1) A renal corpuscle consisting of a glomerulus enclosed in Bowman's capsule; (2) a lymph nodule found in the spleen.

b. mammillary. A rounded body of gray matter found in the diencephalon. It forms a rounded eminence projecting into the anterior portion of the interpeduncular fossa. Their nuclei constitute an important relay station for olfactory impulses.

b., medullary. The deeper white matter of the cerebellum enclosed within the cortex.

b. metachromic. Metachromic granule, *q.v.*

b., Negri. Inclusion bodies found in the cells of the central nervous system of animals infected with rabies. They are acidophilic masses appearing in large ganglion cells or in cells of the brain esp. those of the hippocampus and cerebellum.

b., Nissl. Also called Nissl granules or chromophil substance. Conspicuous structures in nerve cells demonstrated by selective staining. They are absent in the axon and axon-hillock. They show changes under various physiological conditions and in pathological conditions may dissolve and disappear (chromatolysis).

b., Pacchionian. Arachnoid granulation. Numerous small ovoid or villus-like projections of the subarachnoid membrane of the brain. They may project into the superior sagittal sinus as arachnoid villi or they may press against the outer dura and grow into

body, perineal   B-38   **bone**

the inner plate of the cranium forming ovoid depressions.

b., perineal. The mass of tissue which separates the anus from the vestibule and the lower part of the vagina.

b., pineal. The epiphysis, a dorsal outgrowth of the diencephalon. Also called pineal gland.

b., pituitary. The hypophysis; pituitary gland, *q.v.*

b., polar. A small cell produced in cogenesis resulting from the divisions of the primary and secondary oocytes. It has no functional significance.

b., postbranchial. Ultimobranchial bodies. Two bodies which develop from the post. wall of the 4th pharyngeal pouch. They become incorporated into the thyroid gland.

b., psammoma. Laminated calcareous bodies seen in certain types of tumors. Terms also applied to sand-like bodies (brain sand) bound in the pineal body.

b., restiform. The inferior cerebellar peduncles. Two bands of fibers which connect the medulla with the cerebellum.

b., tigroid. The chromophil substance of neurons; Nissl bodies.

b., of vertebra. A short column of bone forming the weight-supporting portion of a vertebra. From its dorsolateral surfaces project the roots of the arch of a vertebra.

b., vitreous. A jelly-like body within the eye which fills the space between the lens and the retina. It is colorless, structureless, and transparent.

b., Wolffian. The mesonephros or middle kidney of the embryo.

body fluids, words pert. to: anastasis, anhydremia, anorrhorrhea, apocenosis, ascites, colliquation, colloid, extravasation, flux, humor, humoral, hydrorrhea, hypoacidity, hypochlorhydria, olighydria, protoplasm, stagnation, succorrhea.

body mechanics. Mechanical correlation of the various systems of the body.

body substances, words pert. to: activator, adenin(e, addisin, agglutinin, aggressin, allergen, allergenic, alloxuremia, alloxurin, antibacterins, antithrombin, apepsinia, ash, aquamedin, autacoid, autotoxin, bacteriolysin, buffer salts, chalone, collagen, collemia, kephalin, ketogenesis, ketonemia, ketones, ketosis, lactacidogen, lecithin, leukomaine, lime, lipacidemia, lipaciduria, lipemia, lysine, melanosis, melanuria, opsonins, oxygenase, parenchymatous, phosphates, purins, trephones, wax, xanthine.

Boeck's sarcoid (beks). A multiple benign one of a superficial nature esp. on arms, face, or shoulders.

boil [A.S. *byl*, a swelling]. A furuncle. An acute circumscribed inflammation of the subcutaneous layers of the skin, gland, or hair follicle.

The deeper tissue inflammation is so severe that blood clots in the vessels and the center dies. This is the cause of the acuteness of the pain; the dead core is ultimately thrown off. Contrary to general opinion, boils do not arise from "bad blood," but are the result of local infection due to an invasion of bacteria from the outside.

TREATMENT: As cold contracts the peripheral vessels, decreasing the amt. of blood in the region and reducing the pain, ice is the first thing to apply. Wet dressing by salt solution should be applied. Clothing should not rub the affected parts. Sunshine, fresh air, exercise out of doors.

Vaccine from pus of one of the boils is sometimes used. Painting with colorless tincture of iodine followed by application of electricity, esp. when abscess on face appears. Collodion with ½ to 2 gr. salicylic acid to the dram is also used over affected area. Injections every day for 6 days, of a pint of dextrose solution.

DIET: A diet of green vegetables, fruit, whole wheat cereals, and milk, little meat; drink plenty of water. SEE: *furuncle, furunculus.*

boiling. Vaporization of a liquid.
1. Boiling water destroys organic impurities. 2. Boiling toughens and hardens albumin in eggs. 3. Boiling toughens fibrin and dissolves tissues in meat. 4. Boiling bursts starch granules. 5. Boiling softens cellulose in cereals and vegetables.

b. point. The degree of heat required to bring a liquid to a boil. It depends upon the liquid. Water boils at 212° F. (100° C.) under ordinary conditions. To kill microörganisms water should be boiled 3-15 minutes. Aeration (pouring from one vessel to another) will overcome the flat taste of boiled water.

bolom'eter [G. *bolē*, a throw, + *metron*, measure]. 1. Device for measuring the force of the heart beat apart from blood pressure. 2. An instrument for gauging minute degrees of radiant heat.

bo'lus [G. *bōlos*, a mass]. A pill-shaped mass.   [food ready to swallow.

b., alimentary. A mass of masticated

bond. A mark or short line bet. atoms to indicate the number and attachments of the valencies of an atom giving a graphic representation of arrangement of the atoms of elements in the molecules of compounds; as, H-Cl.

bone [A.S. *bān*, bone]. The hardest connective tissue that forms the framework of the body. (1) Osseous tissue. A specialized form of dense connective tissue consisting of bone cells (*osteocytes*) embedded in a *matrix* consisting of calcified intercellular substance. (2) An individual unit of the skeleton. Bones give shape to and support the body. They also serve as a storage place for mineral salts and play an important rôle in the formation of blood cells.

It consists of about 50% water, and 50% solid matter, the solids being chiefly cartilage hardened by impregnation with inorganic salts, esp. carbonate and phosphate of lime. The proportion of lime in bone gradually increases and in old age there is such a large proportion that the bones are brittle and break easily.

They surround and protect some vital organs, and give points of attachment for the muscles, serving as levers and making movement possible.

The outer surface is less porous than the inner, and is called the compact tissue; the more porous portion is called cancellous tissue. The compact tissue is tunnelled by a central canal containing marrow, and fine branching canals. In these canals run small blood vessels and lymphatics for the maintenance and repair of bone tissue. This is known as the Haversian system or canals. The exterior covering of the bone, or periosteum, serves to extend the blood supply to the bone. According to their shape, bones are classified as *flat, irregular, long,* and *short.*

bone, ankle   B-39   **borated**

CAVITIES: Depressions, openings, and cavities in bones consist of a *fissure*, a *foramen*, a *meatus* or *canal*, a *sinus* and *antrum*, *groove* or *sulcus*, and a *fossa*.
FORAMEN. Opening for blood vessels or nerves:
fossa. A concavity.
fissure. A slitlike opening.
meatus. A tubelike passage.
sinus. (a) Air cavity within a bone. (b) A groove lodging a blood sinus.
sulcus. A groove.
PROCESSES: Enlargements or protrusions.
crest. A ridge.
condyle. A rounded process for articulation.
head. Rounded end of a bone separated from the body by a constricted region: the neck.
spine. A pointed process.
trocanter. A very large process.
tubercle. A small rounded one.
tuberosity. A large rounded p.
b., ankle. The astragulus or talus.
b., breast. The sternum.
b., carpal. One of the wrist bones (*navicular*).

b., membrane. The intramembranous b.
b., perichondral. One formed beneath the perichondrium.
b., periosteal. One formed by osteoblasts of the periosteum.
b., ping pong. The thin shell of osseous tissue covering a giant cell sarcoma in a bone.
b., replacement. Cartilage b., one which replaces cartilage.
b., sesamoid. One which develops in tendon, as the patella.
b., spongy. Cancellous bone.
b., sutural. A Wormian b.
b., thigh. The femur.
b., Wormian. A small irregularly-shaped b., often found in the sutures of the cranium.
Names of principal bones: SEE: Appendix; also *skeleton*.

bone cell. One in osseous tissue or bone. It may be (a) an osteoblast or bone-forming cell; (b) an osteocyte which lies within a lacuna in bone matrix, or (c) an osteoclast, a giant, mutinucleated cell occupying deep grooves. (Howship's lacunae.)

bone graft. A piece of bone taken either

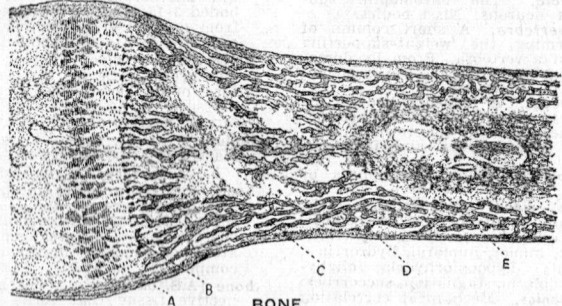

BONE
General view. Longitudinal section of the femur of a six months human fetus.
A. Epiphyseal cartilage. B. Epiphyseal line. C. Bone substance. D. Periosteum. E. Medullary canal.

b., cancellous. A spongy bone in which the matrix forms connecting bars and plates partially enclosing many intercommunicating spaces filled with bone marrow.
b., cartilage. Endochondral bone which develops from cartilage.
b., cavalry. Rider's b. Bony formation in adductor magnus femoris.
b., collar. The clavicle.
b., compact. Dense, hard bone with microscopic spaces.
b., cotyloid. One which during development forms a part of medial portion of the acetabulum. It fuses with the pubis.
b., cranial. A b. of the cranium or brain case.
b., cyst. B. tumor of cystic variety.
b., dermal. A membrane bone.
b., endochondral. Cartilaginous b.
b., epipteric. A small, scalelike b. which occupies the sphenoidal fontanelle.
b., Inca. An incarial b.
b., incarial. The interparietal b., part of the occipital b.
b., incisive. Part of maxilla bearing the incisor teeth.
n., intracartilaginous. Cartilage or endochondral b.
b., innominate. Hip b., composed of the ilium, ischium, and pubis.

from some animal (foreign) or the body of the patient in which it is to be used (autogenous) and placed so as to encourage its growth and union with the bone it is being placed in contact with.
bone grafting. Transplanting a healthy bone to replace missing or defective bone.
bone'let. A small bone.
bone marrow. Medulla or soft tissues in the hollow of long bones and in the extremities of long bones. SEE: *marrow*.
bone reflex. Any result of bone percussion.
bone reflex. A reflex action resulting from tapping or percussion; actually a tendon or muscle reflex.
Bonnet's capsule (bon-nā'). Tenon's capsule.
bo'ny. Resembling or of the nature of bone. SYN: *osseous*.
boopia (bo-op'ĭ-ă) [G. *bous*, ox, + *ōps*, eye]. Ox-eyes observed in hysteria.
booster. A device, consisting essentially of a small induction coil with adjustable core, for increasing the electromotive force of an alternating current circuit, or a device, such as a dynamo, in series to increase the voltage of a direct current circuit.
bo'rate. A basic salt of boric acid.
bo'rated. That to which borax has been added.

borax [L.]. A sodium salt of a form of boric acid.
It is found in some arid regions, and is made by combining a complex boric acid with sodium diborate. Its chief use is as a detergent and water softener; also a weak antiseptic.

borborygmus (bor-bor-ig'mus) (pl. *borborygmi*) [G. *borborygmos*, rumbling in the bowels]. A gurgling, splashing sound heard over the large intestine; intestinal flatus.
PATH: Its absence may denote such obstruction of the bowels as torsion, volvulus, or strangulated hernia. In nervous persons denotes a form of indigestion. Associated with diarrhea and may arise in constipation.

border. The outer part or edge; boundary.
b., brush. A brushlike structure found on the free surface of epithelial cells in the proximal convoluted portion of a renal tubule. It consists of nonmotile hairs.
b., cells. Those in the stomach from which the secretion of acid takes place. They are fewer in number at the cardiac and pyloric ends of the stomach.
b., striated. A modified layer of the surface protoplasm of columnar epithelial cells lining the intestine. It consists of regular, perpendicular striations consisting of minute protoplasmic processes.

Bordet's theory (bor'das). That bacteriolytic sera owe their action to (a) an *antibody* and (b) *alexin*.

boric acid (boric acid, *acidium boricum*). An odorless, white, crystalline powder obtained by condensation and evaporation from certain mineral salts.
In solution it is used as mild antiseptic wash, esp. for the eyes, mouth, and bladder. As an ointment it is valuable in dressing burns, blisters, etc. When large doses are accidentally taken by mouth, as in children, it may be poisonous.
SYM: Nausea, vomiting, diarrhea.
TREATMENT: Wash out stomach. Give saline cathartic and large volumes of water. Stimulants as necessary.

bo'rism. Symptoms caused by internal use of borax or boron compounds.

boroglycerol (bo-ro-glis'er-ōl). A liquid made by heating boroglycerid and glycerin.

borolyptol (bo-ro-lip'tōl). An antiseptic compound of formaldehyde, eucalyptus, myrrh, storax, etc.

bo'ron [L. *borium*]. SYMB: B. At. weight, 11. A nonmetallic element; with oxygen it forms boric acid.

Borrelia (bor-rel'ĭ-ă). A genus of spirochetes including organisms responsible for relapsing fever.
B. vincen'ti. A species found in Vincent's angina.

Borsieri's line (bor-sĭ-a'rī's). In the early stage of scarlet fever, a line drawn on the skin with the finger nail leaves a white mark which quickly turns red and becomes smaller in size. SEE: *scarlatina*.

boss [O.Fr. *boce*, a swelling]. A circumscribed roundish protuberance, as that of a humpback.

bos'selated. Marked by numerous bosses.

bossela'tion. One or more small bosses.

Bossi's dilator (bos'sī). Metal instrument used to dilate the cervix by means of force.

Botal's (Botal'lo's) duct. The ductus arteriosus.

B.'s foramen. Orifice bet. the two atria of the fetal heart.
B.'s ligament. Relic of the ductus arteriosus.

bot flies. Flies belonging to the families *Gastrophilidae, Cuterebridae*, and *Oestridae*. The adults are free-living but the larvae or maggots are parasitic, living on the flesh of their host, producing *myiasis*. The larvae are called *bots*, certain species of which live in the skin forming cystlike lumps called *warbles*. Others form boil-like swellings. Some infest the sinuses of the skull (sheep bot); others the stomach and intestine (horse bot). Human infestation is rare.
TREATMENT: Manually squeezing out the mature "grubs" and application of antiseptics. Grubs can be killed by application of a lanolin ointment (78 ml.), water (9 mil.), benezene hexachloride (9 mil.), rotenone extract (1 ml.), or 5% rotonone extract in linseed oil.

bothrenchyma (both-ren'kĭ-mă) [G. *bothrion*, pit, + *egchyma*, an infusion]. Tissue that is pitted.

botryoid (bot'rĭ-oid) [G. *botrys*, bunch of grapes, + *eidos*, appearance]. Resembling a bunch of grapes.

Botryomyces (bot"rĭ-o-mi'sēz) [" + *mykēs*, fungus]. A genus of fission fungi or bacteria.

bot'tle nose. Acne rosacea of the nose.

botuliform (bot-u'lif-orm) [L. *botulus*, sausage, + *forma*, shape]. Shaped like a sausage. [sausage.

botulin'ic acid. A toxin found in putrid

botulism (bŏt'ū-lĭzm). A severe form of food poisoning from food containing the *botulinus toxin*, produced by *Clostridium botulinum*. This organism is widely found in the soil. Cases of human botulism are usually associated with development of the bacteria under anaerobic conditions in improperly canned foods, esp. meats and nonacid vegetables. The toxin is a powerful exotoxin. It is very thermolabile losing its toxic properties when exposed to temperatures of 75 C-85 C. for 30 m., or boiling for 10 m.
POISONING: The toxin has a selective action on the central nervous system. In fatal cases, cardiac and respiratory failure occur through involvement of the medullary centers. Paralysis may occur, esp. that of the pharyngeal muscles, leading to difficulty in swallowing.
SYM: Intense abdominal cramping, headache, general malaise, difficulty in swallowing, distorted vision, thick speech, nausea, repeated spells of vomiting; later, intense diarrhea, collapse, shock, perhaps unconsciousness. Death may result in from 3 to 7 days.
TREATMENT: Permit vomiting for a while, and give large volumes of fluid bet. attacks, preferably salt water (teaspoonful to a pint), atropine, or belladonna in repeated small doses. Apply heat to abdomen. Stimulants, as hot, sweetened coffee and tea. Cathartics are generally superfluous. Botulinus antitoxin is effective in early stages. A formol toxid (types A and B) provides active immunization.
B.'s coefficient. Proportion of fluid to solids in urine.

Bouchut's method (boo-shus'). Intubation of larynx.
B.'s respiration. Expiration longer than inspiration in children with bronchopneumonia.

B.'s tube. One used for intubation.
bougie (boo-zhē') [F. *bougie*, candle]. Instrument for exploring and dilating canals, esp. the male urethra.
   b., armed. One with caustic attached.
   b., filiform. One of very small size.
   b., obstetrical. GYN: Rubber catheter inserted bet. the fetal membranes and the uterine wall for instituting labor.
bouillon (boo-yawn') [F. *bouillir*, to boil]. Clear beef broth.
   b. culture. Bouillon used as a basis for a bacteriological culture.
boulimia (boo-lim'ĭ-ă) [G. *bous*, ox, + *limos*, hunger]. Abnormal hunger sensation a short time after a meal. SYN: *bulimia, q.v.*
bouquet (boo-kā') [F. nosegay]. 1. The aroma of a wine. 2. A cluster of anything, esp. of blood vessels or nerves.
Bourdin's paste (boor-dans'). A caustic mixture of nitric acid and sublimed sulfur.
Bourdon's test (boor-don'). One administered to determine the alertness of attention, time and accuracy being requisite.
   Certain letters on a printed page are to be crossed out by the subject.
bourdonnement (boor-dŏn-mon') [Fr. a droning]. A humming sound.
boutonnière operation (boo-tŏn-yăr') [F. buttonhole]. 1. Incision through perineum behind an impervious stricture. 2. A buttonhole-like opening in a membrane.
boutons terminaux. Bulblike expansions at the tip of axons which come into synaptic contact with the cell bodies of other neurons.
bo'vine [L. *bovinus*, pert. to a cow]. Pert. to cattle.
   b. lymph. Vaccine virus from a heifer.
bo'vinoid [" + *eidos*, resemblance]. Like that of cattle.
bow'el [O.Fr. *boel*, intestine, from L. *botellus*, little sausage]. The intestine.
   RS: *colon, evacuate, feces, intestines, rectum, sigmoid, stool.*
   b. movement. Evacuation of feces. SYN: *stool, defecation.*
   NUMBER OF: This varies in normal individuals, some having a movement after each meal, others 1 in the morning and 1 at night, and still others only 1 a day. Proper nursing will do much to aid the patient in regular elimination.
bowleg. A bending outward of the lower limb. Bandyleg, genu* varum.
Bowman's capsule. The expanded end of a renal tubule or nephron which invests a glomerulus, the two constituting the renal or Malphigian corpuscle. It consists of a visceral layer closely applied to the glomerulus and an outer parietal layer. It functions as a filter in the formation of urine.
   B's. glands. Branched tobuloalveolar glands located in the lamina propria of the olfactory membrane which serves to keep the olfactory surface moist.
   B. membrane. Thin homogeneous membrane separating corneal epithelium from corneal substance. SEE: *membrane.*
boxnote. A hollow sound heard on percussion in emphysema.
box splint. One for fractures below the knee.
Boyer's bursa (bwă-yas'). One ant. to the thyrohyoid membrane.
   B.'s cyst. A subhyoid cyst.
Boyle's law. The volume of a given mass of gas, at any given temperature, varies inversely as the pressure it bears.

Boze'man-Fritsch catheter. Double-current uterine catheter with several openings at tip.
B. P., B. Ph. Abbr. for *British Pharmacopeia.*
Br. CHEM: SYMB: bromine. BACT: Abbr. for *Brucella.*
bra'chia. Pl. of *brachium*, arm.
brachial (brā'kĭ-al) [G. *brachiōn*, arm]. Pert. to the arm.
   b. artery. Main a. of arm. Continuation of the axillary artery on the inside of the arm.
   b. glands. Lymphatic glands of the arm.
   b. plexus. Network of lower cervical and upper dorsal spinal nerves supplying arm, forearm and hand. SEE: *nerve plexuses.*
   b. veins. Those accompanying the brachial artery.
brachialgia (bra-kĭ-al'jĭ-ă) [" + *algos*, pain]. Intense pain in the arm.
brachio- [G.]. Prefix: Pert. to the brachium.
brachiocephalic (bra-kĭ-ō-sef-al'ĭk) [G. *brachiōn*, arm, + *kephalē*, head]. Pert. to arm and head.
brachiocrural (bra-kĭ-ō-kru'ral) [" + L. *cruralis*, pert. to the leg]. Pert. to arm and leg.
brachiocu'bital [" + L. *cubitus*, forearm]. Pert. to the arm and forearm.
brachiocyllosis (bra-kĭ-o-sil-o'sis) [" + *kyllōsis*, a bending]. Curvature of the arm.
brachiofa'cial [" + L. *facialis*, pert. to face]. Pert. to arm and face.
brachioncus (bra-kĭ-on'kus) [" + *ogkos*, a swelling]. A chronic, hard swelling of the arm.
brachiotomy (bra-kĭ-ot'o-mĭ) [" + *tomē*, a cutting]. Surgical removal or cutting of an arm of the fetus to facilitate delivery.
bra'chium [L. from G. *brachiōn*, arm]. 1. The upper arm from shoulder to elbow. 2. One of the white tracts of the brain.
brachy- [G. *brachys*, short]. Prefix: Short.
brachybasia (brā-kĭ-ba'sĭ-ă) [" + *basis*, walking]. A slow, shuffling gait seen in partial paraplegia. SEE: *gait.*
brachycardia (brak-ĭ-kar'dĭ-ă) [" + *kardia*, heart]. Slowness of heart action. SYN: *bradycardia, q.v.*
brachycephalic, brachycephalous (brak-ĭ-sef-al'ĭk, -al-us) [" + *kephalē*, head]. Having a head disproportionately short.
brachyceph'alism, brachyceph'aly. Shortness of the head.
brachydactylia (brak-ĭ-dak-til'ĭ-ă) [G. *brachys*, short, + *daktylos*, finger]. Shortness of the fingers.
brachygnathia (brak-ĭg-na'thĭ-ă) [" + *gnathos*, jaw]. Abnormal shortness or recession of under jaw.
brachymetropia (brak-ĭ-me-trop'ĭ-ă) [" + *metron*, measure, + *opsis*, sight]. Myopia; nearsightedness.
brachymetropic (brak-ĭ-me-trop'ik). Nearsighted; myopic.
brachyphalan'gia. Shortness of phalanges.
brachypnea (brak-ĭp-ne'ă) [G. *brachys*, short, + *pnoē*, breathing]. Shortness of breath.
brachyuran'ic [" + *ouranos*, roof of mouth]. Having a short palate, or a palatomaxillary index over 115.
bradesthesia (brad-es-the'zĭ-ă) [G. *bradys*, slow, + *aisthēsis*, sensation]. Blunted perception. SYN: *bradyesthesia, q.v.*
Bradford frame. An oblong frame, about 7 x 3, made of 1 in. pipe, covered with canvas strips which run from one side

of the frame to the other and which are movable, thus permitting the patient to urinate and defecate without moving the spine or changing position.

brady- [G. *bradys*, slow]. Prefix: Slow, as *bradycardia*.

bradyacusia (brad-ĭ-ak-oo'sĭ-ă) [" + *akouein*, to hear]. Hardness of hearing.

bradyarthria (brad-ĭ-ar'thrĭ-ă) [" + *arthron*, articulation]. Bradylalia; unusual slowness of articulation of words.

bradycardia (brad-ĭ-kar'dĭ-ă) [" + *kardia*, heart]. Slow heart action. SEE: *arrhythmia, tachycardia*.
 b., sinus. A sinus rhythm with a rate below 60 in an adult, or below 70 in a child.

bradycar'dic. Pert. to bradycardia.

bradycinesia (brad-ĭ-sĭn-e'sĭ-ă) [G. *bradys*, slow, + *kinēsis*, movement]. Extreme slowness of movement. SEE: *bradykinesia*.

bradycrotic (brad-ĭ-krot'ĭk). Pert. to slowness of pulse.

bradydiastole (brad-ĭ-di-as'to-le) [G. *bradys*, slow, + *diastole*, dilatation]. Prolongation of the diastolic pause, as in myocardial lesions.

bradyecoia (brad-ĭ-ek-oi'ă) [G. *bradyēkoos*, hard of hearing]. Hardness of hearing.

bradyesthesia (brad-ĭ-es-the'zĭ-ă) [G. *bradys*, slow, + *aisthēsis*, perception]. Blunted perception.

bradyglossia (brad-ĭ-glos'ĭ-ă) [" + *glōssa*, tongue]. Unusual slowness of speech. SYN: *bradylalia, bradyarthria, bradylogia, bradyphasia, bradyphemia*.

bradykinesia (brad-ĭ-kin-e'sĭ-ă) [" + *kinēsis*, motion]. Extreme slowness of movement.

bradykinetic (brad-ĭ-kin-et'ĭk). Relating to slow movements.
 A slow motion picture exhibiting details very plainly is used for analysis of the patient.

bradylalia (brad-ĭ-la'lĭ-ă) [G. *bradys*, slow, + *lalein*, to talk]. Slowness of utterance. ETIOL: Brain lesion. SEE: *speech*.

bradylexia (brad-ĭ-lex'ĭ-ă) [" + *lexis*, word]. Slowness in reading due to a brain disorder.

bradylogia (brad-ĭ-lo'jĭ-ă) [" + *logos*, speech]. Unusual slowness of speech. SYN: *bradylalia, bradyphasia, bradyphemia*.

bradypepsia (brad-ĭ-pep'sĭ-ă) [" + *pepsis*, digestion]. Slow digestion.

bradyphagia (brad-ĭ-fa'jĭ-ă) [" + *phagein*, to eat]. Slowness in eating.

bradyphasia (brad-ĭ-fa'zĭ-ă) [" + *phasis*, speech]. Extreme slowness of speech. SYN: *bradylalia, bradylogia, bradyphemia*.

bradyphemia (brad-ĭ-fe'mĭ-ă) [" + *phēmē*, speech]. Unusual slowness of utterance of words. SYN: *bradylalia*.

bradyphrasia (brad-ĭ-fra'zĭ-ă) [" + *phrasis*, utterance]. Slowness of speech; seen in some types of mental disease.

bradyphre'nia [" + *phrēn*, mind]. Slowness of mental activity as a result of epidemic encephalitis.

bradypnea (brad-ĭp-ne'ă) [" + *pnoē*, breathing]. Abnormally slow breathing.

bradyspermatism (brad-ĭ-sper'mat-izm) [" + *sperma*, semen]. Abnormally slow emission of semen.

bradysphygmia (brad-ĭ-sfĭg'mĭ-ă) [" + *sphygmos*, pulse]. Abnormally slow pulse.

bradystal'sis [" + *stalsis*, constriction]. Slow peristalsis.

bradytocia (brad-ĭ-to'sĭ-ă) [" + *tokos*, childbirth]. Slow parturition.

bradyuria (brad-ĭ-u'rĭ-ă) [" + *ouron*, urine]. Slowness in passing urine.

braidism (bra'dizm). Hypnotism.

brain [A.S. *braegen*]. A large, soft mass of nerve tissue contained within the cranium; the *encephalon*.
 structure: It is composed of neurons which are nerve cells, and neurologia or supporting cells. The brain consists of gray and white matter. Gray matter is composed principally of nerve-cell bodies and is concentrated in the cerebral cortex and the nuclei and basal ganglia. White matter is composed of nerve-cell processes which form tracts or commissures connecting various parts of the brain with each other.
 It consists of 5 parts: the *cerebrum, cerebellum, pons Varolii, medulla oblongata, q.v.* and *midbrain*.
 The cerebrum represents seven-eighths of the weight of the brain.
 LOBES: 1. Frontal. 2. Parietal. 3. Occipital. 4. Temporal. 5. Insula. 6. Limbic, *q.v.*
 GLANDS: Pineal, pituitary.
 MEMBRANES: Meninges, consisting of the dura mater (external), arachnoid (middle), and pia mater (internal).
 NERVES: Cranial, *q.v.* SEE: Appendix, pages 53, 55.
 The subdivisions of the brain are:
  diencephalon. This includes the epithalmus, thalmus, and hypothalmus (optic chiasma, hypophysis, tuber cinereum, and maxillary bodies).
  mesencephalon. This includes the corpora quadrigemina, tegmentum, and crura cerebri.
  metencephalon. This includes the cerebellum and pons.
  myelencephalon. This includes the medulla oblongata.
  telencephalon. This includes the rhinencephalon, corpora striata, and cerebrun (cerebral cortex).
 ventricles. The cavities of the brain are (a) the *lateral* ventricles (1 and 2) which lie in the cerebral hemispheres; (b) the third ventricle of the diencephalon, and (c) the fourth ventricle of the medulla. The first and second communicate with the third by the interventricular foramina; the third with the fourth by the cerebral canal (aqueduct Sylvius); the fourth with the subarachnoid spaces by the two *foramina of Luschka* and the *foramina of Magendie*. The ventricles are filled with cerebrospinal fluid which is formed by the choroid plexuses in the walls and roofs of the ventricles.
 functions: The brain is the primary center for regulating and coördinating body activities. Sensory impulses are received through afferent nerves; these register as sensations which are the basis for perception. It is the seat of consciousness, thought, memory, reason, judgment, and emotion. Motor impulses are discharged through efferent nerves to muscles and glands initiating activities. Through reflex centers automatic control of body-activities is maintained. The most important reflex centers are the *cardiac, vasomotor*, and *respiratory* centers which regulate circulation and respiration.
 For illustrations of the brain SEE: *Central Nervous System* (C-28) *Cerebrum* (C-32); Nerve Cell Cerebral Corte (N-12).
 The weight of brain and cord is about

1350-1400 Gm., of which total the cord represents 2%. SEE: *spinal cord*.
For picture of brain areas, see diagram under Nervous System, Central.
b., fever. Meningitis.
b. stem. All the brain except the cerebellum and cerebrum. It includes the medulla oblongata, pons, midbrain, and thalamus.
b. sand. Laminated bodies consist-

PATH: General symptoms due to increased intracranial pressure are distinguished from the focal symptoms which vary with the actual structures implicated by the growth. The general symptoms are headache, the change in the retina recognized by ophthalmoscopic examination as "choked disc," and by vomiting (without nausea). Mental changes (esp. dullness), epileptiform

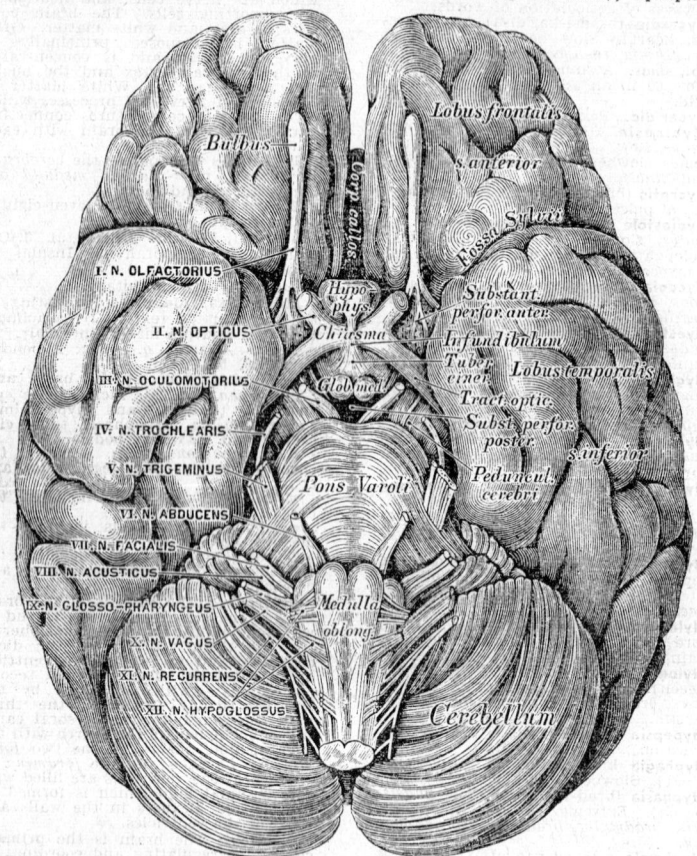

BASE OF THE BRAIN

ing principally of phosphates, and carbonates of calcium, and magnesium found in the pineal body called *corpora arenacea*.
b. tumor. Usually used inexactly to describe any intracranial mass, neoplastic, cystic, inflammatory (abscess), or gummatous. Except the latter, treatment depends on surgery and this on accurate diagnosis, the earlier the better. Here great difficulties may arise due to the inadequate signs of tumor or the simulation of these signs by diffuse diseases such as multiple sclerosis, paresis, internal hydrocephalus, kidney disease, and plumbism.

convulsions, giddiness, are often general but may be localized signs; these latter are very variable. In addition, history and cranial x-ray are of great value. The injection of air into the ventricles prior to x-ray is known as pneumoventriculography.
brains (beef). AV. SERVING: 230 Gm. Pro. 22.1, Fat 21.4, Carbo. 2.5 per serving. Vit. C+. They contain Vit. A. They contain lecithin but are poor in nuclein.
brain storm [A.S. *braegen*, + *storm*, violent weather]. Temporary outburst of mental excitement; often maniacal, esp. in paranoia.

Brain's reflex. Extension of flexed arm on assuming quadripedal posture.
branchial (brang'kĭ-al) [G. *bragchia*, gills]. Pert. to gills.
 b. arches. Five pairs of arched structures which form the lateral and ventral walls of the pharynx of the embryo. They are partially separated from each other externally by the branchial clefts; internally, by the pharyngeal pouches. The fifth arch is rudimentary. They play an important rôle in the formation of structures of the face and neck. The first is the *mandibular arch*, the second the *hyoid arch*. They are also called the visceral arches.
 b. clefts. A series of openings between the branchial arches. They become functional gill slits in fishes.
 b. grooves. A series of furrows separating the branchial arches. They are homologous to the branchial clefts of fishes and amphibians.
 b. muscles. Those which develop in the branchial arches.
branchiogenous (brang-kĭ-oj'en-us) [" + *gennan*, to generate]. Having origin in a branchial cleft.
branchiomeric (brang-kĭ-ō-mĕr'ĭk). Of or pertaining to the branchial arches.
branchiomerism (brang-kĭ-om'er-izm) [" + *meros*, part]. Segmental division of the entoderm.
brandy. Spiritous liquor distilled from wine and containing about 50% alcohol by volume.
branks (brangks) [F. *branques*, pl. branches]. Mumps.
Brasdor's operation (brah-dors'). Ligation of an artery below an aneurysm.
brash [F. *breche*, attack]. 1. A cutaneous eruption. 2. Pyrosis.
 b., water. Acidity of the mouth.
brass founders' ague. Tremors due to zinc poison from inhalation.
brass poisoning. Due to the inhalation of fumes of zinc and zinc oxide with destruction of tissue in respiratory passage.
 SYM: Dryness and burning in respiratory tract; cough; headache; chills; rarely fatal.
 TREATMENT: Entirely symptomatic; inhalations of humidified air make patient more comfortable.
Brauch-Romberg symptom (browkh-rom'-berg). A sign of ataxia; swaying of body when eyes are closed and feet held together.
Braun's hook (browns). Instrument for fracturing clavicle or to assist in decapitation of the fetal head.
Braune's canal (brow'nehs). The parturient canal formed by the uterus, dilated cervix and vulva.
 B.'s ring. A point, supposedly 10 cm. above the margins of the dilated external os. The portion above this ring possesses thin walls, while the remainder forms a thin walled tube.
braw'ny induration. Pathological hardening and thickening of tissues.
Braxton Hicks sign. Intermittent painless uterine contractions observed every 5-15 minutes throughout pregnancy, after uterine body becomes palpable.
Brazil nuts. Av. SERVING: 30 Gm. Prot. 5.0, Fat 20.0, Carbo. 2.0 per serving. FUEL VALUE: 100 Gm.—714 cal.
bread [A.S.]. A food made from flour or meal, yeast, baking powder, etc, by moistening, kneading, and baking.
 COMP: Starch, 40% to 60%, according to method of making. It undergoes carbonic fermentation. Baking the starch in the crumb forms a starchy paste and unites with the gluten, while in the crust, dextrin is produced by heat, with partial caramelization. The gluten forms nitrogen and it is accompanied by cerealin, which peptonizes the nitrogenous matter. Phosphorated lecithin makes up the fats. Potassium and magnesium are well represented. The ash is acid.
 b. paste. Bacterial culture medium.
breakbone fever. Acute epidemic febrile disease. SEE: *dengue*.
breast [A.S. *breōst*]. 1. The upper ant. aspect of the chest. 2. One of the mammary glands. A gland consists of 15-20 lobules divided into smaller ones with cavities or alveoli, the cells of which abstract from the blood the milk-forming substances.
 PATH: Tumors may be benign or malignant. Simplest one is *fibroadenoma*: others are *lipoma* and *cystic adenoma*. Malignant ones are usually *carcinoma*. Early surgery is necessary. A painful breast is usually due to mastitis.*
 CHANGES IN PREGNANCY: 6-12½ weeks, fullness and tenderness, erectile tissues in nipples, nodules felt, pigment deposited around nipple (primary areola), and few drops of fluid may be squeezed out. 16-20½ weeks (secondary areola), small, whitish spots in pigmentation.
 NP: PREVENTIVE CARE: Most complications of the breast during the puerperal period will not occur if proper care is given.
 POINTS TO OBSERVE: 1. Prevent infection of the infant's mouth from improper cleansing and unclean nursing articles. This infection can be carried to the nipples and breasts when the infant nurses.

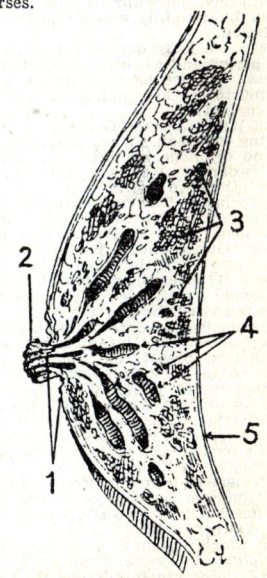

BREAST, SECTION
1. Lactiferous ducts. 2. Papilla or nipple of breast. 3. Lobules of secreting alveoli. 4. Lactiferous sinuses. 5. Pectoral fascia.

2. Care for the breasts aseptically: by proper cleansing of the nipples, the application of sterile dressings, and proper cleansing of the nurse's hands.

3. Early treatment of soreness, cracks and fissures: (a) By the use of sterile nipple shield while the baby nurses, which in most cases is inadequate treatment; (b) by taking the baby off the breast and pumping them at the time the baby would be due to nurse. Pumping should be done under very low pressure and should be repeated until the nipple is well healed. This does away with the danger of infection from the infant's mouth and prevents him from making matters worse by his terrific nursing suction. Antiseptic oil, ointments, etc., may be used to favor the healing process.

4. Limit the nursing period during the first 3 days when no breast milk is available and during the engorgement period when the breasts are extremely sensitive from congestion and distention with milk. The use of the electric pump is stressed during this time.

5. Avoid bruising of the breasts. The use of the electric breast pump in place of brutal manual massage during the extreme sensitive period will prevent this.

6. Keep the nipples soft to avoid cracking. Applications which harden them predispose to cracking.

7. Avoid "caking" of the breasts by the use of the breast pump to remove any excess milk which may plug the ducts. In the home it will be necessary to resort to the hand breast pump or proper manual expression of the milk.

8. Proper support of the breast with a binder which pulls upward and inward. Do not bind tightly enough to restrict circulation.

9. Use ice bags during the engorgement period and when there is any tenderness. The ice bags are particularly soothing to cracked nipples as they relieve congestion.

CARE WHEN ABSCESS OCCURS: 1. Avoid carrying infection. When abscesses occur and drainage has been established, there is danger of carrying infection on your hands to other parts of the mother's body. The nurse must protect the mother, herself, and other patients in the department by the use of proper technic. Gloves should be worn during the dressings and they should be boiled immediately after their removal. Dressings should be disposed of at once and before removing the gloves.

2. Remember the infant's milk supply is endangered. The infant is taken off the affected breast, but sometimes is permitted to nurse the normal breast. At other times pumping of the good breast is ordered during the height of the infection. Nursing orders will, of course, vary with the physician, but the infant's food intake must be kept up if necessary by artificial means.

3. Remember that an abscess may not only impair the function of the breast at this time but may also affect it in subsequent pregnancies.

RS: *Clark's bodies, mamma, mammary glands, mammilla, mammillation, "mast-" words, nipple, scirrhus, sternum.*

b., chicken; b., pigeon. Deformity in which chest is protruding, caused by rickets or obstructed respiration in infancy.

b. milk. Mother's milk. SEE: *colostrum.*

b. pump. One to draw milk from the female breast.

breath (brĕth) [A.S. *braeth*, odor]. The air inhaled and exhaled in act of respiration.

DIAG: Foul odor indicates neglect of mouth or teeth, improper diet, constipation, neglect of exercise, use of drugs, alcohol or tobacco. It also depends upon the food ingested, and may indicate stomatitis, necrosis of jaw, caries of teeth, tonsillitis, diphtheria, gangrene and abscess of the lungs, fetid bronchitis, bronchiectasis, pyothorax, catarrh, diabetes, kidney disease, and other disorders.

Urinous odor: Indicates uremia.

Sweetish odor (that of ripe apples): Found in diabetes mellitus, esp. during coma.

Odor of carnivorous animals: Noted in critical illness, in acidosis and alkalosis.

RS: *air, brachypnea, breathing, bromopnea, bronchi, lungs, oxygen, respiration, ventilation.*

b., rattling and shortness of. Edema; presence of fluids in the air passages.

b., sighing. Air hunger. Occurs in internal hemorrhage.

NP: Watch for after abdominal operations and in typhoid fever.

breathe (brēth) [A.S. *braeth*]. 1. To inhale and exhale air; to respire. 2. To inject by breathing.

breathing (brēth'ing) [A.S. *braeth*, odor]. Act of inhaling and exhaling air. SYN: *respiration.*

This act includes the process of inspiration, or drawing the air into the lungs, and expiration, the forcing out of the air which is caused by the alternate expansion and contraction of the walls of the chest and the lungs.

The normal rate of breathing is: Men, 16-18 per m.; women, 18-20 per m.; children, 20-26 per m.; infants, 30-35 per m. The ratio to pulse in breathing is usually about 1 to 4. In women and children, breathing is largely thoracic or costal; in men and in old of both sexes, it is largely abdominal, or diaphragmatic. Restricted abdominal breathing is observed in pregnancy, in abdominal tumors and effusions; in peritonitis; in diaphragmatic pleurisy; in paralysis of the phrenic nerve from pressure or bulbar disease and occasionally in hysterical abdomen.

SEE: *apnea, asphyxia, Cheyne-Stokes respiration, drowning, dyspnea, orthopnea, stridor, unconsciousness.*

ADVENTITIOUS SOUNDS: Friction sounds produced by the rubbing together of roughened pleural surfaces, may be heard both in inspiration and expiration and often resemble subcrepitant râles, but are more superficial and localized than the latter, and are not modified by cough or deep inspiration.

Metallic tinkling: Silvery bell-like sounds heard at intervals over a pneumohydrothorax or large cavity. Speaking, coughing and deep breathing usually induce them. Must not be confounded with similar sound produced by liquids in the stomach.

Râles: Abnormal bubbling sounds heard in air cells or bronchial tubes, *q.v.*

Succussion-splash or hippocratic succussion: A splashing sound produced by the presence of air and liquid in the chest, may be elicited by gently shaking the patient while auscultating. Nearly always indicates either a hydro- or a pyopneumothorax, although it has been detected over very large cavities. Air and liquid in stomach produce similar sounds. SEE: *respiration, also heart, for auscultation.*

AUSCULTATION OF RESPIRATORY ORGANS: Normal respiration. Vesicular breathing is heard over the body of the lungs and is characterized by a soft, breezy inspiration, and a short, low pitched expiration. Normally, expiration is not more than ½ as long as inspiration. Auscultation over trachea or main bronchi in the interscapula space yields bronchial breathing.

MODIFICATION OF THE RESPIRATORY MURMUR: Amphoric and cavernous breathing. These two are almost identical. Sounds loud, expiration prolonged and hollow. Pitch of amphoric breathing a little higher than cavernous. May be imitated by blowing over the mouth of an empty jar. Heard in: (a) Phthisical or bronchiectatic cavities; (b) pneumothorax, when the opening to the lung is patulous; (c) area of consolidation near a large bronchus; (d) sometimes over lung compressed by a moderate effusion.

b., asthmatic. Harsh breathing with a prolonged wheezing expiration. Is heard all over the chest.

b., bronchial or tubular. Harsh breathing with a prolonged high pitched expiration which has sometimes a tubular quality. Heard over: (1) Phthisical consolidation; (2) pneumonic consolidation; (3) lung which is compressed; (4) rarely over a lung infiltrated with a tumor growth.

b., cogged wheel or jerky. Respiratory murmur not continuous, but broken into waves, not indicative of any special disease, but frequently observed in bronchitis and in incipient phthisis.

b. of emphysema. Weak with prolonged, low pitched or inaudible expiration.

b., exaggerated. Almost same peculiarity as puerile b. Heard over lung that is doing extra work necessitated by some impairment of its fellow.

b., odorous. Due to drugs, alcohol, tobacco, diabetes, kidney disease.

b., puerile. Type heard normally over lungs of children, loud expiration, higher pitched than in vesicular breathing and almost as long as inspiration.

b., rapid. In pneumonia, high fevers, or interference with oxygenation.

b., slow. Found in narcotic poisoning, sleep, or rest, and in cases of brain compression.

b., stertorous. Due to a relaxation of the palate and is characterized by a deep snoring sound on inspiration. It is most always present in apoplexy; the cheeks puff out with each breath on expiration. It is not regarded as a serious symptom, although it may indicate brain or nerve pressure. It is found in deep sleep and in coma.

b., weak or shallow. Noted: (a) When chest walls are thick; (b) in the old and feeble; (c) in emphysema; (d) in pleural effusion; (e) in incipient phthisis; (f) in painful affections of the chest, like pleurodynia and beginning pleurisy; (g) in pulmonary edema.

breath and breathing, words pert. to: anapnea, anapneic, anhelation, anhelitus, anhelose, anima, apnea, asthma, asthmatic, Aufrecht's sign, besoin de respirer, brachypnea, bradypnea, bromopnea, carbonometry, dyspnea, eupnea, exhalation, expiration, halitosis, halitus, hyperpnea, inhalation, inspiration, insufflate, orthopnea, ozostomia, respiration, respiratory center, stertorous.

bredouillement (bra-dwē-mon') [Fr.]. Pronunciation of only part of a word due to rapid utterance.

breech [A.S. brēc, buttocks]. The nates, or buttocks.

b. presentation. The presentation of the buttocks instead of the head in childbirth. Occurs in 1/60 of all fulltime labors.

breeze [Fr. brise, wind]. A movement of air.

b., static. If a dry stick is brought near a patient on an insulated platform receiving a charge from a static machine, the charge will pass gradually to the conductor from the patient in the form of a bluish brush.

bregma (breg'mă) [G. front of head]. That point on the skull where the coronal and sagittal sutures join. The ant. fontanelle in the fetus and young infant.

bregmat'ic. Pert. to the bregma.

breg"mocard'iac reflex. Reduced heart rate following pressure on post. fontanel.

Breisky's disease (bri'skĭs). Atrophy of the vulva. Kraurosis vulvae.

Brenner tumor. A benign fibroepithelioma of the ovary.

brenzkatechinuria (brents"kat'ek-in-u'rĭ-ă) [Ger. brenz, burnt, + catechin, + G. ouron, urine]. Alkaptonuria. Condition in which alkapton is present in urine, causing it to darken on standing.

brick dust. A red deposit of urates in the urine.

bricklayers' cramp. A neurosis with incoordination of muscles of the hand when using the trowel.

b. itch. Eczema from lime mortar.

brickmakers' disease. Hookworm disease. Ankylostomiasis; uncinariasis.

bridge [A.S. brycg]. 1. Narrow band of tissue. 2. Dental plate fastened to a tooth at each end.

b. of nose. The ridge formed by the nasal bones.

bridgework (brij-werk). A partial plate held in place by permanent attachments to other teeth.

b., fixed. Partial plates held by crowns or inlays fastened to the natural teeth.

b., removable. Partial plates held by clasps which permit their removal.

Bright's disease. A generic term for acute and chronic disease of the kidneys. It is usually associated with dropsy and albuminuria. Known also as *nephritis.*

brim [A.S. seashore]. 1. An edge or margin. 2. Brim of pelvis. Superior aperture of the lesser or true pelvis; the inlet. Formed by the iliopectineal line of the innominate bone and the sacral promontory. Oval-shaped in the female; heart-shaped in the male.

brisèment forcé (brēz-mon') [Fr. crushing]. Breaking, by forcible means, of adhesions.

Brissaud's reflex (brĭs-sos'). Contraction of fascial femoris muscle following tickling of sole of foot.

British thermal unit. Amount of heat necessary to raise the temperature of one pound of water 1 degree F. SEE: *calorie.*

broach [A.S. broche]. A dental instrument for enlarging a tooth canal or for removing the pulp.

broad ligament. A transverse fold of peritoneum arising from floor of the pelvic cavity between the bladder and rectum, dividing the minor pelvis into ant. and post. compartments. In its median portion lies the uterus to which it is attached on both sides. Its free superior border contains the uterine tube. A lateral portion of the upper border forms the suspensory ligament of the ovary.

Broadbent's sign. A visible retraction of the left side and back in region of 11th and 12th ribs synchronous with the cardiac systole, in adherent pericardium.

Bro'ca's area. On left side of brain, controlling movements of tongue, lips, vocal cords, or motor speech area. Loss of speech due to hemorrhage from this area. Area parolfactoria.

B.'s convolution. Third left frontal convolution.

B.'s fissure. One surrounding B.'s convolution.

broccoli. Av. Serving: 120 Gm. Pro. 4.0, Fat 0.2, Carbo. 5.0 per serving. Ca 0.122, P 0.059, Fe 0.0001. Vit. A+++, B++, C+, G++.

Brodie's abscess. An abscess of the head of the tibia, or it may be an abscess of any bone.
Etiol: It is usually of tubercular origin or from subacute infection.
Sym: May be aching pains in area, followed by slight swelling and tenderness on movement. Symptoms less acute but similar to osteomyelitis.

brokaw ring. Rubber tubing ring threaded with catgut for intestinal anastomosis.

brom-, bromo- [G. *brōmos*, stench]. Prefixes: Presence of bromine.

bro'melin [L. *bromelia*, pineapple]. Ferment allied to trypsin; found in pineapple juice.
It digests 1500 times its weight of proteins.

bromides (bro'mĭds) [G. *brōmos*, stench]. Salts of bromine.
They are nerve depressants. Adm. by mouth or rectum.
Poisoning: Sym: Fetid breath, mental dullness, depression, weakness, skin eruptions, tremors, headache, vertigo. In large doses exhaustion and cardiac failure.
F. A. Treatment: Evacuate stomach, administer protective mucilaginous drinks, as flour, starch, rice, oatmeal or barley water.

bromidrosiphobia (bro-mid-ros-ĭ-fo'bĭ-ă) [" + *idrōs*, sweat, + *phobos*, fear]. Abnormal fear of personal odors, accompanied by hallucinations.

bromidrosis (brom-ĭ-dro'sis) [" + *idrōs*, sweat]. Fetid or offensive sweat. It occurs mostly on *feet, groins,* and *axillae.*
Etiol: Symptomatic or idiopathic.
Sym: Presence of asafetida, musk, copaiba, urea in sweat. In localized forms, decomposition of sweat after excretion, or as a result of contamination by *B. foetidus*.
NP: Cleanliness, use of an antiseptic, daily change of clothing, deodorant antiseptic powders.
RS: *anhidrosis, chromidrosis, hyperidrosis, ozochrotia, uridrosis.*

bromism, brominism (bro'mĭzm, bro'mĭn-ĭzm) [" + *ismos*, state of]. The results of prolonged use of bromides.*
Sym: Apathy, somnolenee, coldness, headache, feeble heart action, pallor, anorexia, acne, and loss of sexual power.

bro''moder'ma [" + G. *derma*, skin]. Acne-like eruption due to chronic bromide poisoning.

bromo''hyperhidro'sis [" + *yper*, over, + *idrōsis*, perspiration]. Fetid and excessive sweat. See: *bromidrosis*.

bromo''i'odism [" + iodine, + G. *ismos*, state of]. Poisoning from bromoiodides.

bromomania (bro-mo-ma'nĭ-ă) [" + G. *mania*, insanity]. Insanity caused by use of bromides.

bromomenorrhea (bro-mo-men-or-e'ă) [" + *mēnes*, menses, + *roia*, flow]. Offensive and disordered menstruation.

bromopnea (brom-op-ne'ă) [" + *pnoē*, breath]. Offensive breath.

bromo seltzer (bro'mo selt'zer). A proprietary headache powder.
Poisoning: Treatment: Same as for acetanilid, *q.v.*

bromural (brō''mur'al). A white, crystalline substance, α-monobromisovaleryl-urea derived from bromine.
Uses: As a nerve sedative, in mild cases of insomnia, producing sleep of short duration; its action usually ceases after 3 to 5 hours.
Dosage: As nerve sedative, 5 gr. (0.3 Gm.) 3 times a day. As hypnotic, 10 gr. (0.6 Gm.).

bronchadenitis (bronk''ad-en-i'tis) [G. *brogchia*, bronchia, + *adēn*, gland, + *-itis*, inflammation]. Inflammation of bronchial glands.

bronchi (bron'ki) (sing. *bronchus*). The primary divisions of the trachea; divides opp. 3rd dorsal vertebra. The right bronchus is shorter and more vertical than the left one.
They penetrate the lungs, one for the right and the other for the left lung, and terminate in the bronchioles or bronchial tubes.

b., foreign bodies in. May cause various diseases of bronchi, large objects leading to collapse of the lung. Metal bodies, if small, may produce no symptoms. Beans, nuts, seeds, etc., may cause pneumonia, bronchitis or lung abscess.
Sym: Choking and gagging, immediately. Later, symptoms of bronchitis, atelectasis, pneumonia or lung abscess.
Prog: Good, if removed before complications. Better in case of metallic objects than in vegetable bodies.
Treatment: Removal through bronchoscope.

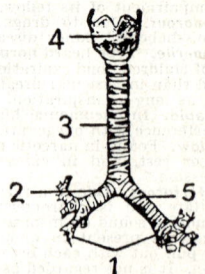

BRONCHI AND TRACHEA
1. Bronchioles. 2. Right bronchus. 3. Trachea. 4. Larynx. 5. Left bronchus.

bronchi, words pert. to: alveobronchitis, bronchadenitis, bronchial tubes, bronchiectasis, bronchioles, bronchitis, bronchocele, bronchopneumonia, bronchorrhea, bronchoscopy, bronchostenosis, bronchotomy, bronchus, "bronch-" words, Charcot-Robin crystals, mesobronchitis, râles.

bronchia (bron'kĭ-ă) [G. *bronchos*]. The divisions of the bronchi.

bronchial (bron'ke-al). Pert. to the bronchi or bronchioles.
  b. crises. Paroxysm of coughing in locomotor ataxia.
  b. glands. Mucous or mixed glands in the bronchi or bronchioles.
  b. tree. Bronchi and bronchial tubes.
  b. tubes. The smaller divisions of the bronchi.
  RS: *bronchi, bronchioli, bronchitis, bronchus.*

bronchiarctia (bron-kĭ-ark'shĭ-ă) [G. *bronchos*, bronchial tubes, + L. *arctare*, to compress]. Bronchial tube stenosis.

bronchiectasis (bron-kĭ-ek'tas-is) [" + *ektasis*, dilatation]. Dilatation of a bronchus or bronchi, usually secreting large amounts of offensive pus.
  ETIOL: Acquired or congenital, on one or both sides of chest. Chronic bronchitis, tuberculosis, whooping cough. Blocking or narrowing of a bronchus, due to pressure or foreign body. A complication of empyema and chronic pulmonary tuberculosis.
  SYM: Cough, dyspnea, expectoration of large amounts of foul smelling secretion, esp. in the morning. Sputum is dark; a pint may be expectorated with first morning attack. When expectorated it settles into 3 layers: (a) Bottom one that is thick and which contains pus cells; (b) a middle layer of brownish fluid; (c) an upper layer of froth.
  NP: Maintain resistance. Position to assist drainage.

bronchiectatic (bron-kĭ-ĕk-tăt'ĭk) [" + *ektasis*, dilation]. Pert. to bronchiectasis.

bronchiloquy (bron-kil'o-kwĭ) [" + L. *loqui*, to speak]. Unusual vocal resonance over a bronchus covered with consolidated lung tissue.

bronchiocele (bron'kĭ-o-sēl) [" + *kēlē*, tumor]. Circumscribed dilatation of a bronchus.

bronchiocrisis (bron-kĭ-o-krī'sis) [" + *krisis*, separation]. Bronchial crisis.

bronchiogenic (bron-kĭ-o-jen'ĭk) [" + *gennan*, to originate]. Having origin in the bronchi.

bronchiolectasis (bron"kĭ-o-lek'ta-sis) [L. *bronchiolus*, air passage, + G. *ektasis*, dilatation]. Dilatation of the bronchioles; capillary bronchiectasis.

bronchioles, bronchioli (bron'kĭ-ols, -o'lĭ) [L. *bronchiolus*, air passage]. The smaller divisions of the bronchi. They lack cartilage.
  Each one terminates in the atrium, an elongated saccule, each of which is covered with alveoli or air cells.
  b., respiratory. The last division of the bronchial tree. They are branches of terminal bronchioles and lead to alveolar ducts leading to the alveoli.
  b., terminal. Next to the last subdivision of a bronchial, leading to the respiratory bronchioles.

bronchiolitis (bron-kĭ-o-lī'tis) [" + G. *-itis*, inflammation]. Inflammation of the bronchioles. [exudation.
  b., exudativa. A form with fibrinous
  b., vesicular. Bronchopneumonia.

bron'chiospasm [G. *bronchos*, + *spasmos*, fit]. Spasmodic narrowing of the lumen of the bronchial tubes.

bronchiosteno'sis [" + *stenōsis*, a narrowing]. Narrowing of the bronchial tubes.
  SYN: *bronchiarctia.*

bronchis'mus [" + *ismos*, state of]. Spasmodic narrowing of the lumen of the bronchial tubes. SYN: *bronchiospasm.*

bronchit'ic. Pert. to bronchitis.

bronchitis (bron-kī'tis) [G. *bronchos*, bronchos, + *itis*, inflammation]. Inflammation of bronchial mucous membrane.
  ETIOL: Usually results from exposure to cold; the inhalation of irritating substances from acute germ diseases.
  SYM: Cough, expectorations, moist and dry râles, fever of 100° F., pain over sternum.
  b., acute catarrhal. Chilliness, malaise. Soreness and constriction behind sternum, increased by coughing; slight fever, 100°-102° F. Cough at first dry and painful, later mucopurulent expectoration which becomes free as inflammation subsides.
  PROG: Favorable. In old, young, and feeble there is danger of its leading to capillary bronchitis or catarrhal pneumonia.
  TREATMENT: *Abortive:* Use hot foot baths, hot drinks, steam inhalations, good nourishment. Internal remedies.
  b., capillary. An inflammation of the smaller bronchi, generally secondary to simple b.
  SYM: Severe spells of coughing; rapid respiration—30 to 80 per minute; dyspnea, high fever—104°-105° F.; weak, rapid pulse. Later lips become blue, extremities cold, mind dull.
  PROG: In young children very grave. May develop into bronchopneumonia.
  TREATMENT: Absolute rest. Temp. of room kept uniformly at 70° or 75° F.—atmosphere kept moist by steam. Internal medication.
  b., chronic. Persistent cough, mucopurulent expectoration. Soreness behind sternum. Fever absent unless disease is severe; dyspnea on exertion.
  NP: Whenever possible it is advisable for an elderly person with chronic bronchitis to move to a dry, warm climate, especially during the winter. The ward or room in the hospital should be kept warm. Bowels should be kept open and constipation avoided. Diet should be nourishing and the doctor may order codliver oil as well as expectorants and respiratory antiseptics.
  b., fetid. Bronchitis with foul-smelling expectoration.
  b., fibrinous. A primary inflammatory disease of the bronchi associated with formation of false membrane.
  SYM: Acute and chronic forms are recognized. Acute is rare, manifests symptoms of acute b., but sputum contains fibrinous casts and there is marked dyspnea. Chronic form characterized by severe cough, dyspnea, and the expectoration of fibrinous plugs. Often lasts a few weeks, then disappears, to return again at definite periods.
  PROG: Guarded; in acute may cause death from suffocation.
  TREATMENT: Moist atmosphere of room during acute attack, and uniformly warm. Internal remedies.
  b., putrid. Chronic form with foul-smelling sputum.
  b., rheumatic. Severe cough in paroxysms, expectoration of scanty, tenacious mucus; aching pains in chest, does not yield to ordinary treatment for bronchitis.

bronchium (brong'kĭ-um) (pl. *bronchia*) [L. bronchus]. A bronchial tube.

broncho- [G. *bronchos*, windpipe]. Prefix: Rel. to the bronchi.

bronchoadenitis   B-49   **bronchus**

bronchoadeni'tis [" + *adēn*, gland, + *-itis*, inflammation]. Inflammation of bronchial glands. SYN: *bronchadenitis*.

broncho″blennorrhe′a [" + *blennos*, mucus, + *roia*, flow]. Copious, thick sputum accompanying chronic bronchitis.

bronchocele (bron′ko-sēl) [" + *kēlē*, tumor]. Goiter, esp. cystic goiter.

bronchoclysis (bron-kok′lĭ-sis) [" + *klysis*, washing]. Introduction of a medicated solution into the bronchi.

bron″choconstric′tion [" + L. *constringere*, to draw together]. Constriction of the lumen of the bronchi.

bron″chodilata′tion [" + L. *dilatāre*, to open]. Dilatation of a bronchus.

bronchoegophony (bron-ko-ĕ-gof′o-nĭ) [" + *aig-*, goat, + *phōnē*, voice]. Egobronchophony; a goatlike sound.

bronchogenic (bron-ko-jen′ĭk) [" + *gennan*, to originate]. Having origin in the bronchi.

bron′chogram [" + *gramma*, a writing]. A roentgenogram of the lungs and bronchi.

bronchog′raphy [" + *graphein*, to write]. Radiography of the bronchi; making a bronchogram.

bronchol′ith (bron′ko-lith) [" + *lithos*, stone]. Calculus in the bronchus or bronchial tube.

broncholithiasis (bron-ko-lith-i′ă-sis) [" + *lithos*, stone]. Calculi in the bronchi.

bronchomoniliasis (bron-ko-mon-il-i′ă-sis) [" + L. *monile*, necklace of chains]. Infection of the bronchial membrane with a species of Monilia.

bronchomo′tor [" + L. *motus*, moving]. 1. Causing change of caliber of the bronchi. 2. An agent causing such a change.

bronchomycosis (bron-ko-mi-ko′sis) [" + *mykēs*, fungus]. Any bronchial disease due to microbes or fungus.

bronchopathy (bron-kop′ath-ĭ) [" + *pathos*, disease]. Any disease of the air passages.

bronchophony (bron-kof′o-nĭ) [" + *phōnē*, voice]. The voice as heard over a normal bronchus.

    b., whispered. Bronchophony when patient whispers.

bronchoplasty (bron′ko-plas-tĭ) [" + *plassein*, to form]. Operation of closing tracheal fistula.

bronchoplegia (bron-ko-ple′jĭ-ă) [" + *plēgē*, stroke]. Paralysis of the bronchial tubes.

bronchopneumonia (bron-ko-nu-mo′ne-a) [" + *pneumōnia*, lung inflammation]. Inflammation of the terminal bronchioles and alveoli.

    ETIOL: Usually a sequel of bronchitis, or resulting from influenza, eruptive fevers of childhood, and other diseases. The pneumococcus is present and, to a lesser degree, the staphylococcus and influenza bacillus. Pneumonic patches around a bronchus which contains gray mucus, and an exudate somewhat like that found in lobar pneumonia fill the air vesicles.

    SYM: Cough and expectoration; respiration short and shallow—from 50 to 75 per minute. Cyanosis may ensue. Nostrils dilate with each inspiration, and in children the temperature reaches 103° or 105° F.; before death, 108° F. Pulse, 140. Vomiting and diarrhea; gradually falling temperature. Duration, 2 to 3 weeks. Improvement may be followed by increased severity as new patches form. In the aged many of these symptoms are absent; slight cough and little sputum; temperature, 100° to 101° F. may or may not be in evidence. Gradually failing strength and increase of dyspnea. The bedridden are susceptible.

    PROG: Depends upon age. Mortality greater in the very young and the very old. Childhood mortality, 30 to 50%.

    NP: Hygienic. Room, 65° to 70° F., moistened with steam. Flannel next to skin. Cold sponge bath, wet pack, and compresses over chest. Stimulation in cyanosis and mustard plaster over chest or back to draw circulation to the surface. Oxygen inhalations. Liquid or semiliquid food. Beware of relapse.

bron″chopul′monary [" + L. *pulmonarius*, pert. to lung]. Pert. to bronchi and lungs.

bronchorrhagia (bron-kor-a′jĭ-ă) [" + *rēgnunai*, to break forth]. Bronchial hemorrhage.

bron″chor′raphy [" + *raphē*, suture]. Suturing of a wound of the bronchus.

bronchorrhea (bron-ko-re′ă) [" + *roia*, flow]. Abnormal secretion from the bronchial mucous membrane, sometimes very offensive (fetid bronchitis*).

bronchorrhoncus (bron-kor-on′kus) [" + *rogchos*, snore]. A bronchial râle.

bronchoscope (bron′ko-skōp) [" + *skopein*, to examine]. An instrument for examining the interior of a bronchus.

bronchoscopy (bron-kos′kō-pĭ). Examination of the bronchi through a bronchoscope.

bronchosinusi′tis [G. *bronchos*, windpipe, + L. *sinus*, a hollow, + G. *-itis*, inflammation]. Infection of bronchi and sinuses at the same time.

bron′chospasm [" + *spasmos*, a spasm]. Spasm of the bronchus.

bronchospirochetosis (bron-ko-spī-rō-kē-to′sis) [" + *speira*, coil, + *chaitē*, wavy hair]. Hemorrhagic bronchitis; bronchopulmonary spirochetosis resulting from spirochetes.

bronchostenosis (bron-ko-sten-o′sis) [" + *stenōsis*, a narrowing]. Narrowing of a bronchus.

bronchos′tomy [" + *stoma*, mouth]. Formation from without of an opening into a bronchus.

bron″chotet′any [" + *tetanos*, tetanus]. Extreme dyspnea due to spasm in the bronchi preventing access of air.

bronchotome (bron′ko-tom) [" + *tomē*, incision]. Instrument for making an incision of the trachea.

bronchotomy (bron-kot′o-mĭ). Incision of a bronchus, the larynx, or trachea.

    NP: Dressing: borosalicylic acid powder. Temperature of room 80° F. and atmosphere saturated with steam.

bron″chotra′cheal [G. *bronchos*, windpipe, + *tracheia*, trachea]. Pert. to both bronchi and trachea.

bron″choty′phoid [" + *typhos*, fever, + *eidos*, resemblance]. Typhoid fever marked by severe bronchitis in initial stage.

bron″choty′phus [" + *typhos*, fever]. Typhus fever accompanied by bronchial catarrh.

bron″chovesic′ular [" + L. *vesicula*, small bladder]. Pert. to bronchial tubes and air passages of the lungs.

bronchus (brŏn′kus) (pl. *bronchi*) [G. *bronchos*]. One of the 2 large branches of the trachea.

    The trachea proper terminates at the level of the 2nd ribs, or 4th dorsal vertebra. The right b. differs considerably from the left b. SEE: *bronchi*.

bronzed skin. A characteristic symptom of Addison's disease which is due to inflammation of the suprarenal capsules.

brood capsule. Cystlike bodies which develop within a hydatid cyst of *Echinococcus granulosus.* Each contains from 3 to 30 scolices.

brossage (brŏs-sazh') [Fr. brushing]. Brushing the averted eyelids with stiff brush, to remove granulations, as in trachoma.

Brouha's test (broo'ăs). A test for pregnancy.
 Daily injection of immature mice of male sex with urine of patient. If, after 10 days, mice have sexual gland secretion, pregnancy of patient is assumed.

brow'ache [A.S. *brū*, brow, + *aken*, to hurt]. Supraorbital neuralgia; migraine.

Brownian movement. BACT: Oscillatory movement distinguished from self motility of living microörganisms.

Brown-Séquard's paralysis (sa-kars'). Reflex flaccid paraplegia occurring during some urinary tract affections.

 B.-S.'s syndrome. Anesthesia of one side of the body and paralysis and hyperesthesia of the other side; found in unilateral compression of the spinal cord.

brow presentation. When the brow or face of the infant comes first on presentation in labor; makes birth almost impossible. Cesarean section indicated.

Brucella (bru-sel'ă). A genus of bacteria, nonmotile, nonsporing, aerobic, gram negative, and pathogenic to man causing undulant fever and contagions and abortion in cattle, hogs, and goats.

brucel'lar. Pert. to Brucella.

brucel'lin. A vaccine made from several species of Brucella.

brucellosis (bru-sel-o'sis) [brucella + *ōsis*]. Infection with Brucella. Undulant fever.

Bruce's septicemia. Malta fever.

Bruch's membrane. A glassy membrane of the uvea of the eye lying between the chorioid membrane and the pigmented epithelium of the retina.

brucine (bru'sin). A poisonous alkaloid from *Strychnos nux vomica* and other *Strychnos* species. Similar to but less powerful than strychnine, *q.v.*

Bruenning electric head-cabinet (bru'ning). Apparatus to apply infrared radiation over face and sinus areas.

bruise [Fr. *bruiser*, to break]. An injury with diffuse effusion into subcutaneous tissue, and in which skin is discolored but not broken.

 b. of head, chest, and abdomen. May be associated with internal injuries.
 SYM: Pain, swelling, tenderness, discoloration. NP: Mild antiseptic if skin is scratched. Cold applications with pressure. Later, heat and massage.

 b. of or contusion of breast. SYM: Pain, swelling, discoloration. NP: Apply cold applications and snug bandage with pressure and elevation. Later, heat and gently massage. SEE: *contusion.*

bruissement (bru-ēs-mon') [Fr. droning noise]. A purring sound heard in auscultation.

bruit (broo'ē) [Fr. noise]. An adventitious sound of venous or arterial origin heard on auscultation.

 b. de craquement. Crackling.

 b. de diable. 1. The venous hum of anemia. 2. Subjective tinnitus of chlorotic patients and a humming hallucination of hearing in the insane.

 b. de frottement. Frictionlike sound.

 b., placental. A purring or blowing noise heard in the pregnant uterus due to fetal circulation of blood, and synchronous with the maternal pulse.

 b. de pot fêlé. Cracked pot sound.

 b. de râpe. Rasping.

 b. de soufflet. Bellows sound.

Brunner's glands. Compound glands of the duodenum and upper jejunum. Also known as duodenal glands.
 They are imbedded in the submucosa tissue, and lined with columnar epithelium. They are similar to the pyloric glands of stomach. They secrete intestinal juice.

brush discharge. In electrotherapeutics, the discharge from a static machine (less commonly from a high frequency apparatus), having a disruptoconvective character and peculiarities that can be produced by the passage of an electrical current through a resistance such as a tube containing glycerine or a damp (or "green") wooden wand. SEE: *static breeze.*

Brussels sprouts. AV. SERVING: 100 Gm. Pro. 4.4, Fat 0.5, Carbo. 7.6 per serving. Ca 0.027, Mg 0.040, K 0.375, Na 0.004, P 0.120, Cl 0.040, S 0.194, Fe 0.0011. Vit. A++, B++, C+++.

bruxism (brŭks'izm). Grinding of the teeth, esp. during sleep; sometimes a manifestation of a neurosis.

Bryce's test. A second vaccination after 5th or 6th day from appearance of vesicles of previous vaccination as a test of latter.

bubo (bu'bo) [G. *boubōn*, groin]. Suppuration of a lymphatic gland, particularly in the axilla or groin, of chanchroidal, tuberculous, gonorrheal or syphilitic origin.
 It is also seen in diseases due to a typhoid poison, or to the absorption of pus by lymphatics which drain into the glands, as in the bubonic plague.
 TREATMENT: *Chanchroidal*: Puncture of suppuration points, pus squeezed out and iodoform emulsion injected. *Tuberculous*: Multiple *small* incisions followed by curettage, ensuing ulceration treated by Bier's cups. Enucleation of infected nodes is contraindicated. Hygienic regimen. *Gonorrheal*: Incision and drainage.

bubonadenitis (bu-bon-ad-en-i'tis) [" + *adēn*, gland, + *-itis*, inflammation]. Inflammation of an inguinal gland.

bubonal'gia [" + *algos*, pain]. Pain in the groin.

bubon d'emblée (bu-boh" dăhm-blă') [Fr.]. Venereal bubo appearing without previous lesion.

bubon'ic plague [" + L. *plāgā*, epidemic]. A very fatal, acute, infectious disease, common in the Orient, esp. India. The Black Death of the Middle Ages.
 ETIOL: Caused by *Pasteurella pestis,* usually carried by rats and fleas, which is imparted to human beings by bite of the rat-flea. It is characterized by enlargement of lymphatic glands, severe toxic symptoms, accompanied by intense adenitis or pneumonia.

bubonocele (bu-bon'o-sēl) [" + *kēlē*, tumor]. Inguinal hernia.

bubononcus (bu-bon-on'kus) [" + *ogchos*, tumor]. A swelling in the inguinal region.

bubonopanus (bu-bon-o-pa'nus) [" + L. *panus,* swelling]. An inguinal bubo.

bucar'dia [G. *bous,* ox, + *kardia,* heart]. Severe hypertrophy of the heart.

bucca (buk'a) [L. mouth, cheek]. 1. The mouth. 2. Hollow part of the cheek.

buc'cal. Pert. to the cheek or mouth.
  b. cavity. The mouth.
  b. glands. Small glands situated in the mucous membranes of the mouth which secrete saliva.
buccella'tion [L. *buccella*, morsel]. Hemostasis by use of a lint pad or compress.
buccinatolabialis (buk-sin-at-o-lā-bĭ-a'lĭs) [L. *buccinator*, trumpeter, + *labialis*, pert. to the lips]. The buccinator and orbicularis oris as one.
buccinator (buk'sin-a-tor) [L. *buccinator*, trumpeter]. The muscle of the cheek. SEE: *muscles*.
buccoversion (buk-o-ver'shun) [L. *bucca*, mouth, + *versiō*, a turning]. Position of part buccal to line of occlusion; said of a tooth.
buccula (buk'ū-lă) [L. a little cheek]. A double chin.
Buck's extension. An apparatus consisting of a weight and pulley for applying extension to a limb.
buckwheat flour. Av. SERVING (cooked): 115 Gm. Pro. 9.4, Fat 1.4, Carbo. 84.4 per serving. Ca 0.039, Mg 0.048, K 0.130, Na 0.027, P 0.226, Cl 0.012, S 0.071, Fe 0.0021.
bucnemia (buk-ne'mĭ-ă) [G. *bous*, ox, + *knēmē*, leg]. Inflammation of the leg; elephantiasis.
budding [M.E. *budde*, to swell]. A form of fission in which the mother cell puts out budlike processes containing their proportion of chromatin, which then separate and become individual cells. SEE: *gemmation*.
Buerger's disease (bur'gers). A disorder affecting the muscles and blood vessels of the legs.
  ETIOL: Thickening and chronic inflammation of blood vessel walls in the leg. Some formation of clots may obtain. Spasm of muscles of blood vessel walls. Allergy as a cause is suspected. Over 80% of cases are tobacco addicts. Many afflicted are susceptible to hay fever and asthma.
  SYM: Cramps in legs but not to be confused with those occurring in the aged. Legs give out, esp. when walking. Gangrene may set in and amputation may be necessary.
  TREATMENT: Hydrotherapy, hot and cold water alternately applied. Heat of various kinds. Discontinue use of tobacco. Make allergy tests; surgery. SEE: *thromboangiitis obliterans*.
buffer (bŭf'ẽr) [Fr. *buffe*, blow]. 1. A substance, esp. a salt of the blood, tending to preserve original hydrogen-ion concentration of its solution, upon adding an acid or base. 2. A substance tending to offset reaction of an agent administered in conjunction with it.
  It is determined by the carbon dioxide which the blood will take. This regulates the balance bet. a condition of normal alkalinity and any tendency toward acidosis.
  b. action. A buffer reaction with the excess acid or alkali bringing about the production of substances less acid or alkaline. As a result there is little or no change in the pH of the solution.
  b. blood. One present in the blood. The principal buffers are: carbonic acid, carbonates and bicarbonates, monobasic and diabasic phosphates, proteins, and alkali protinates. Hemoglobin is an important protein buffer.
  b. food values. The ability of foods to combine with base or acid without changing their reaction.
  Suitable in high gastric acidity, malnutrition, infectious and deficiency diseases, and in low acid content of the stomach. Milk, eggs, and meat have a high buffer value, and cereals, fruits, and vegetables a low buffer value. *Excess acid foods*: Meat, fish, cereals. *Excess alkaline foods*: Most fruits and vegetables, milk and some nuts. *Neutral foods*: Butter, cream, cornstarch, sugar, tapioca, most oils and fats.
  b. salts. Substances in the blood which act as a buffer.
buf'fy coat [Fr. *buffe*, buffalo]. Light stratum of a blood clot when coagulation is delayed.
bug (M.E. *bugge*, swollen). A term applied loosely to any small insect or Arthropod; more specifically a member of the Order, *Heteroptera* which includes the squash bug, chinch bug, and bed bug. They have sucking mouth parts, incomplete metamorphosis, and two pairs of wings, the fore part being half membranous. The following bugs are of medical importance:
  b., assasin. One belonging to the Family, *Triatomidae*. Many are predaceous; others are blood-sucking. *Pantastrongulus*, *Triatoma*, and *Rhodnius* are vectors of trypanosome diseases (Chaga's disease) in man.
  b., bed. A member of the Family *Cimicidae*, esp. those of the *Genus Cimex*.
  b., kissing. Several species of the Family, *Reduviidae*, *Melanolestes picipes* is the common kissing bug, or black corsair.
  b. red. The larvae of mites of the Family *Trombiculidae*, commonly called "chiggers".
buggery (bug'er-ĭ) [Fr. *bougrerie*, heresy]. Unnatural sexual relations through the anus. SYN: *sodomy*.
Buhl's disease (bools). Epidemic hemoglobinuria if associated with acute fatty degeneration. SEE: *Winckel's disease*.
bulb [G. *bolbos*, a bulbous root]. An expansion of a canal, vessel or organ, esp. the medulla oblongata.
  b., aortic. Dilated portion of the truncus arteriosus in the embryo which gives rise to the roots of the aorta and pulmonary arteries.
  b., duodenal. Upper duodenal area just beyond pylorus.
  b. of the eye. The eyeball.
  b., hair. The expanded portion at the lower end of the hair root.
  b., olfactory. The ant. enlargement of the olfactory tract.
  b., terminal of Krause. An encapsulated sensory nerve ending similar in structure to the corpuscles of Pacini. Also called corpuscle of Golgi-Manzoni.
  b. of the urethra. The post. portion of the spongy body.
bul'bar. 1. Pert. to a bulb. 2. Shaped like a bulb. 3. Pert. to the medulla oblongata.
  b. paralysis. Paralysis due to changes in motor centers of the oblongata. SEE: *paralysis*.
bul'biform [G. *bolbos*, bulbous root, + L. *forma*, shape]. Shaped like a bulb.
bulbitis (bul-bi'tis) [" + *-itis*, inflammation]. Inflammation of the urethra in its bulbous portion.
bul'bi vestib'uli (pl.). The glands of Bartholin.
  Two glands an inch long, one on each side of the urogenital space, composed of erectile tissue and veins which, when engorged, narrow the vaginal orifice.

bulbocaverno'sus [G. *bolbos*, + L. *cavernosus*, hollow]. Ejaculator seminis; accelerator urinae, sphincter vaginae muscle.

bulbocav'ernous reflex. Contraction of bulbocavernous muscle on percussing dorsum of penis.

bulbomim'ic reflex. Contraction of facial muscles following pressure on eyeball.

bulbonu'clear [" + L. *nucleus*, kernel]. Pert. to the nuclei in the medulla oblongata.

bulbourethral glands (bul"bo-u-re'thral) [" + *ourēthra*, urethra]. Cowper's glands.

Two small glands about the size of a pea, one on each side of the prostate gland, each with a duct about 1 inch (2.5 cm.) long, terminating in the wall of the urethra. They secrete a viscid fluid forming part of the seminal fluid.

RS: *prostate gland, semen, testicle, urethra.*

bul'bus [G. *balbos*, bulbous root]. SEE: *bulb.*

b. corpus cavernosum. Bulb of the urethra. A bulbous swelling of the corpus cavernosum at base of the penis.

b. vestibuli. Two oval masses of erectile tissue lying beneath the vestibule and resting on the urogenital diaphragm. They are honologous to the bulbus cavernosum urethra of the male.

bulesis (bu-le'sis) [G. *boulēsis*, a willing]. An act of the will; the will.

bulimia (bu-lim'ĭ-ă) [G. *bous*, ox, + *limos*, hunger]. Hunger experienced a short time after a meal; morbid hunger.

Observe if the appetite arises only when presented with food, or if it exists but disappears at sight of food, or after a few mouthfuls have been taken. SEE: *appetite, taste.*

bulim'ic. Pert. to bulimia.

bulla (bul'la) (pl. *bullae*) [L. a bubble]. A large blister or skin vesicle filled with fluid; a bleb, *q.v.*

b. ethmoidal'is. A rounded projection into the middle meatus of the nose underneath the middle turbinated bone, formed by an ant. ethmoid cell.

b. ossea. The dilated portion of the bony external meatus of the ear. SEE: *pompholyx.*

bullate (bul'āt). Said of a surface growth which appears blistered because of convex prominences.

bullation (bul-a'shun) [L. *bulla*, a bubble]. 1. Division into small compartments. 2. Inflation.

Buller's shield. Watch glass securely held in place by adhesive plaster, or junction of skin and plaster sealed with collodion.

Used over nonaffected eye as protection from affected eye.

bullet wound. Puncture wound from a bullet. SEE: *wounds.*

bullous (bul'lus) [L. *bulla*, bubble]. Having the nature of a bulla.

bun'dle. A group of fibers; a fasciculus.

b., Arnold's. The frontopontile tract. It passes from the cerebral cortex of frontal lobe through the internal capsule and cerebral peduncle to the pons.

b., atrioventricular, auriculoventricular. Bundle of His.

b., Brechterew's. The spino-olivary fasciculus or Helweg's bundle.

b. of His. Small bundle of fibers passing from auricle to ventricular musculature and septum.

b., Schultze's. Comma-shaped path of fibers in middle of spinal cord's fasciculus cuneatus.

b., of Turck. The temporopontile tract. Fibers pass from the cerebral cortex of temporal lobe and perminate in the pons.

bundle-branch block. A form of heart block in which the two ventricles contract independently of each other.

bunioid (bun'ĭ-oid) [G. *bounion*, turnip, + *eidos*, resemblance]. Round, as a tumor.

bunion (bun'yun) (*Hallux valgus*) [G. *bounion*, turnip]. Inflammation and thickening of the bursa of the joint of the big toe.

bunogaster (bu-no-gas'ter) [G. *bounos*, mound, + *gastēr*, belly]. Protrusion of the abdomen.

Bunsen burner. A burner named after its inventor.

It has an adjustment by which the air holes at the bottom of the tube can be closed or open and the flame made either luminous or nonluminous. If the holes are closed, the flame burns luminously, *i. e.,* it will give light but a relatively small amount of heat. Its action may be reversed by the opening of the holes.

buphthalmia, buphthalmos (buf-thal'mĭ-ă, -mos) [G. *bous*, ox, + *ophthalmos*, eye]. Condition of infantile glaucoma resulting in uniform enlargement of eye.

Disease may stop spontaneously or continue until it produces blindness.

TREATMENT: Iridectomy, sclerotomy, miotics. SEE: *hydrophthalmos.*

Burdach's tracts. Continuation of dorsolateral column of spinal cord into medulla oblongata. SYN: *cuneate fasciculus.*

buret, burette [Fr. small holder for fluid]. A graduated tube for measuring a reagent.

burn (bŭrn) [A.S. *brinnan*, to burn]. The effect of undue exposure to heat, chemicals or electricity. Burns are classified into three degrees or more according to the extent and depth covered.

b., first degree: This may be more or less superficial, involving only the superficial layers of the skin. It is marked by redness or hyperemia. Shock may occur.

b., second degree: The deeper layers of the skin may be involved. Vesication, the vesicles varying in size. If the corium is not involved and if infection remains absent, scarring will not result.

b., third degree: Destruction of the epidermis and part of corium occurs; the most painful type of burn. Healing requires two to four weeks.

b., fourth degree: This involves the destruction of the entire integument.

b., fifth degree: The muscles are encroached upon, and the scar is deeper, firmer, and immobile. It may break down and ulcerate.

b., sixth degree: The tissues are carbonized; most frequently the fingers and toes.

First degree burns may be fatal if two-thirds of the body surface is involved; *second degree* burns involving one-seventh of the body surface in adults; in a child one-tenth of the body surface may be serious.

The three critical stages are (*a*) the period of irritation (the first twenty-four to forty-eight hours); (*b*) the period of reaction and inflammation (from second day to second week); (*c*) the period of exhaustion and suppuration (from second week to convalescence).

TREATMENT: Old family remedies for burns are now considered useless if not harmful. There are many different treatments for burns, but recent research discards most or all of them. For instance, burns treated with tannic acid may become infected seriously, and liver damage also may occur. Wet or moist dressings hidden from the air may become infected, or healing may be delayed.

In severe burns shock is always present and may cause death. Morphine is administered immediately, followed by intravenous injections of whole blood and of salt solutions to prevent shock. When pain has eased, charred clothing is removed and burned area is gently washed with a detergent. The body or part is then wrapped with thick layers of gauze applied under pressure. More morphine and more salt solution may be necessary and as much as 300,000 units of penicillin. The patient is placed on a clean sheet after bandages are removed, and exposed to the air.

On the second day another injection of penicillin is given, and again on the third day. No applications of any kind are given. Whole blood is better than plasma,* although a plasma extender may be used if whole blood is not available. Deep burns will not heal themselves without skin-grafting. Third degree burns should have grafts within a month; otherwise, infections, chronic anemia, and permanent deformities may result.

For deep third degree burns, a modified form of absorptive pressure dressing, thinner than the original form, and without medication, should be used, under only mild pressure. These now may be had 22 by 18 inches, and 22 by 36 inches.

The open-air exposure causes healing to take place much quicker than with pressure dressings. The fever period is decreased and infection is greatly lessened.

PRECAUTIONS: 1. Never allow a person whose clothing is burning to run. Make him lie down and roll. Wrap him in a rug, blanket, or anything within reach and smother the flames. Be careful not to allow him to inhale the smoke. Cut away the clothing, taking care not to pull any portion of the skin away. 2. Do not open any blisters, as this increases the chance for infections.

COMPLICATIONS (in burns and scalds): Sloughing, gangrene, erysipelas, nephritis, pneumonia, or intestinal disturbances; sudden attacks of rigor, vomiting, rise of temperature or convulsions are all suspicious symptoms. A superficial burn covering a large part of the body is more serious than a small, deep one, unless important nerves and blood vessels are involved. If two-thirds of the skin are destroyed, death may be expected, even in a burn of the first degree. Shock must always be anticipated regardless of degree of burn.

Forms

b., acid. Due to exposure to corrosive acids, as sulfuric, hydrochloric, nitric, etc. F. A. TREATMENT: Wash with large volumes of water; apply dilute alkalies, as baking soda (sodium bicarbonate) paste, soap solution dressing, chalk paste, etc. Follow with a bland oil or ointment.

b., alkali. Due to caustic alkalies, as lye, caustic potash (potassium hydroxide), caustic soda (sodium hydroxide), etc. SYM: Painful lesion of skin often associated with gelatinization of tissue. F. A. TREATMENT: Wash with large volumes of water. Follow by wet dressings of dilute acid, as citron fruit juices, weak vinegar, dilute acetic acid, etc. Later dress with bland ointments or oils, or irrigate with boric acid solution. Follow by instillation of liquid paraffin or other bland oil.

b., brush. A combined burn and abrasion resulting from friction. TREATMENT: Like abrasion, *q.v.*

b., chemical. Injuries due to the action of corrosive or irritating chemicals, as acid burns, *q.v.*, alkali burns, *q.v.*

Burns from chemical acids or alkalies should be treated by flushing the surface with water, thereby removing all traces of the drug. Remember that usually an acid counteracts an alkali, so that weak vinegar, weak ammonia, or a solution of sodium bicarbonate is always safe. A carbolic acid burn is almost always counteracted by alcohol. Never use oil as it helps in the absorption of acid. If lime gets into the eye, flush the eye with water and follow with a solution of weak vinegar.

b., electric. A result of exposure to electricity. The extent of destruction is much greater than that evidenced by initial inspection. TREATMENT: SEE: *electric injuries.*

b. of eye. F. A. TREATMENT: Wash well with warm water and instill bland oil, as sweet oil or paraffin oil. SEE: *lye.*

b., fireworks, from. Such injuries are usually burns, *q.v.*, often with imbedded foreign bodies and a high incidence of infection and tetanus which should be prevented by meticulous care of injury and use of antitetanic serum.

b., flash. Lesion from electric arc.

b., gunpowder, from. Often followed by tetanus which should be prevented by administration of antitetanic serum and meticulous care of injury.

b., heat. From exposure to heat, steam, electric arc, or spark. SEE: *actinic, electric injuries, eschar, heat cramps, heat exhaustion, heat stroke, sunburn.*

Burns' amauro'sis [G. *amauroein*, to darken]. Dimness of sight or blindness following sexual excesses.

bur'rowing. The formation of: (1) A subcutaneous tunnel made by a parasite, or (2) a fistula or sinus containing pus.

bur'sa [G. a leather sac]. A sac or pouch in connective tissue chiefly about joints.

Usually lined with synovial membrane to reduce friction; esp. found bet. tendons and bony prominences, and other places where there is excessive friction. RS: Boyer's b., bursal, bursalis, bursalogy, bursectomy, bursolith, bursopathy, Calori's b.

bur'sal. Pert. to a bursa.

bursa'lis [L. *bursalis*, pert. to a bursa]. Obturator internus muscle.

bursalogy (ber-sal'o-jĭ) [G. *bursa*, leather sac, + *logos*, study]. Anatomy, pathology, and physiology of bursae.

bursectomy (ber-sek'to-mĭ) [" + *ektomē*, excision]. Excision of a bursa.

bursi'tis [" + *-itis*, inflammation]. Inflammation of a bursa.

Inflammation bet. patella and structures over it (prepatellar bursa) is known as "housemaid's knee."

VARIETIES: Simple, suppurative, acute, chronic, and specific due to some known organism.

TREATMENT: Painting skin with iodine. Adenylic acid injections. Application of figure-of-eight bandage. Post. leg splint; otherwise surgery.

bur'solith [" + *lithos*, stone]. A calculus formed in a bursa.

bursop'athy [" + *pathos*, disease]. Any pathological condition of a bursa.

bursula (bur'sū-la) [L. *bursula*, little sac]. A small bursa.

    b. testium. The scrotum.

Burton's line. A blue line along the margin of the gums visible in chronic lead poisoning.

butacaine sulfate (bū'tă-kān). USP syn. for *butyn*.

butane (bū'tan). C_4H_{10}. An anesthetic from petroleum.

butesin (bu'tes-in). A white, crystalline powder, derived from aminobenzoic acid, and having an action similar to anesthesin. SYN: USP, *butyl aminobenzoate*.

    USE: As a local anesthetic.

    DOSAGE: As a dusting powder, pure or diluted; may also be used in form of troches, ointment, or suppository; internally, from 1½ to 3 gr. (0.1-0.2 Gm.).

    b. picrate (pik'rat). A yellow powder combining anesthetic action of butesin and antiseptic effect of picric acid.

    USES: As 1% ointment in treatment of burns and ulcers.

butter [G. *bouturon*]. COMP: It consists largely of butter fat which is made up of stearin. Butyric, palmitic, and oleic acid are the acids found in butter fat. Av. SERVING: 10 Gm. Pro. 0.1, Fat 8.5 per serving. Ca 0.015, Mg 0.001, K 0.014, Na 0.788, P 0.017, Cl 1.212, S 0.010, Fe 0.0002. Vit. A+++, D+, E+.

buttermilk. Av. SERVING: 240 Gm. Pro. 7.9, Fat 9.1, Carbo. 10.8 per serving. Ca 0.105, Mg 0.016, K 0.151, Na 0.064, P 0.097, Cl 0.089, S 0.026, Fe 0.00025. Vit. A+, B++, C+ variable, G+++.

butternuts. Av. SERVING: 20 Gm. Pro. 5.6, Fat 12.2, Carbo. 0.7 per serving. Vit. A+, B++.

buttocks (but'uks) [M.E. *butte*, thick end]. The gluteal prominence, commonly called the "seat" or "rump."

    RS: *breech, clunes, gluteal, nates, rump.*

button anastomosis. One made to unite severed portions of the hollow viscera without suture. Devised by Murphy.

button forceps. Those for holding parts of an anastomosis button while it is being adjusted and placed.

buttonhole. A straight cut through the wall of a cavity.

    b. fracture. Perforation of a bone by a missile.

    b., mitral. Contraction of any orifice to a slit, as that of the heart.

    b. operation. Boutonnière's operation. An artificial slit in a membrane.

button suture. One for preventing a suture from cutting through or into underlying tissue. VARIETIES: Getchell's, lead, Powell's and silver wire. Also perforated shot.

butyl aminobenzoate. USP syn. for *butesin*, q.v.

butylchloral hydrate (bu'til-klo'ral hi'-drāt). A preparation similar in action to chloral, but said to be less depressant and more analgesic.

    USES: Recommended for relief of facial neuralgia.

    DOSAGE: 5 to 20 gr. (0.3 to 1.3 Gm.).

butyn (bu'tin). A colorless, odorless, solid substance derived from coal tar.

    ACTION AND USES: A local anesthetic "proposed" as a substitute for cocaine and novocaine in surface anesthesia, being more promptly absorbed. May be sterilized by boiling.

    DOSAGE: For its anesthetic action in eye, nose, or throat, 1 to 2%.

butyraceous (bu-tĭr-a'shus) [G. *bouturon*, butter]. Containing or resembling butter.

butyrate (bu'tĭr-āt). A salt of butyric acid.

butyr'ic acid. A rancid, viscid acid found in butter and animal excretions.

butyrin (bū'tir-in). A soft, yellowish, semi-liquid fat which gives butter its flavor. It represents 5% of butter fat.

butyroid (bu'tir-oid) [G. *bouturon*, butter, + *eidos*, appearance]. Having the appearance or consistency of butter.

butyrometer (bu-tir-om'e-ter) [" + *metron*, measure]. Device for estimating amt. of butter fat of milk.

butyrous (but'ĭr-us). Of butterlike consistency.

bwamba fever. A So. Amer. disease probably due to a filtrable virus. Onset is sudden; headache, backache, and fever persist for 5-7 days. Nonfatal.

Byrd-Dew method. One for resuscitating newborn child suffering from asphyxia. Operator supports supine child on palms of his hands, allowing head to fall backward. By supination of forearms, operator flexes child's body and effects expiration. By pronation of arms, body is again extended, causing inspiration.

bys'ma [G. plug]. A plug or tampon.

byssa'ceous. Resembling flaxlike threads.

byssino'sis [G. *byssos*, cotton, + *-ōsis*]. Pulmonary condition from inhalation of cotton dust.

byssocausis (bis-o-kaw'sis) [" + *kausis*, burning]. Cauterization by moxa; moxibustion.

bys'soid [" + *eidos*, form]. Consisting of a filamentous fringe, the filaments being of unequal length.

byssophthisis (bis-o-this'is) [" + *phthisis*, a wasting away]. Pulmonary condition caused by inhalation of cotton dust. SYN: *byssinosis*.*

byssus (bis'us) [G. *byssos*, cotton]. The growth of hair on the pubic region.

byth'us [G. *bythus*, depth]. The lower abdominal region.

C

C. Symb: Carbon. Abbr. for congius (gallon), compound, centigrade, Celsius, clonus, closure, etc.
C. Abbr. L. *centum*, one hundred. Also, L. *cum*, without.
C₃ population. Those who are the products of imperfect development, mentally or physically.
Ca. Symb: Calcium; abbr. for cathode.
cabbage [Fr. *cabocher*, to make a swelling]. A leafy vegetable, growing in a head. Raw cabbage: Av. Serving: 85 Gm. Pro. 1.2, Fat 0.2, Carbo. 3.6 per serving. Ca 0.045, Mg 0.015, K 0.247, Na 0.027, P 0.029, Cl 0.024, S 0.066, Fe 0.0011. A base-forming food. Action: Heavy and hard to digest. May cause flatulence. Raw, it serves as an appetizer.
Cabot's ring bodies. Ring shaped bodies sometimes seen in red blood cells in pernicious anemia, lymphatic leukemia, and lead poisoning.
cac- [G.]. Prefix: Bad, as *cachexia*.
CaC₂. Calcium carbide.
cacaerometer (kak-ă-er-om'ĕ-ter) [G. *kakos*, bad, + *aër*, air, + *metron*, measure]. Instrument for testing impurity of air. [Malignant anthrax.
cacan'thrax [" + *anthrax*, carbuncle].
cacao (kă-kā'o) [Mexican from Spanish *cacahuatl*, seed]. Theobroma. Seed used to prepare cacao butter, chocolate, and cocoa. See: *cocoa*.
cacation (kak-a'shun) [L. *cacāre*, to go to stool]. Defecation; going to stool.
cacatory (kak'at-or-ĭ). Accompanied by diarrhea or excessive bowel movements.
cacemia (kas-e'mĭ-a) [G. *kakos*, bad, + *aima*, blood]. A poor condition of the blood.
cacergasia (kas-er-ga'sĭ-ă) [" + *ergasia*, work]. Defective functioning, mentally or physically.
cacesthesia (kak-es-the'zĭ-ă) [" + *aisthēsis*, sensation]. 1. Disorder of sensibility, morbid or otherwise. 2. Malaise.
caché (kash-a') [Fr. covered]. A lead cone covered with paper layers, with mica bottom, used for applying radiotherapy, radium or any radioactive substance.
cachectic (kă-kek'tĭk) [G. *kakos*, ill, + *exis*, habit]. Pert. to cachexia.
cachet (kă-sha') [Fr. a seal]. Two concave pieces of wafer (rice paper) bet. which is placed medicine to be administered, the margins being pressed together so they will adhere.
cachexia (ka-keks'ĭ-ă) [G. *kakos*, ill, + *exis*, habit]. A state of ill health, malnutrition, and wasting.
It occurs in malignancies; advanced pulmonary tuberculosis, when excessive suppuration is present; in chronic cases of certain poisoning; toxemia, and in severe hyperthyroidism.
  c., cancerous. C. caused by cancerous condition.
  c., lymphatic. C. caused by Hodgkin's disease of the lymph nodes.
  c., malarial. C. due to chronic malaria.
  c., pachydermic. C. due to myxedemic condition.
  c., pituitary. Group of symptoms caused by atrophy of pituitary gland, including emaciation, premature aging, atrophy of genitals with loss of secondary sex characteristics and lowering of basal metabolic rate. Syn: *Simmond's disease.*
  c., splenetica. C. caused by disease of the spleen. Syn: *pseudoleukocythemia.*
  c. strumipri'va or **c. thyreopri'va.** Adult type of thyroid activity due to surgical removal of the thyroid gland.
  c., thyroid. Goiter.
cachinna'tion (kak-in-a'shun) [L. *cachinnāre*, to laugh aloud]. Hysteric laughter.
CaCl₂. Calcium chloride; a bleaching powder.
Ca(ClO)₂. Calcium chlorate.
CaCO₃. Calcium carbonate; chalk.
CaC₂O₄. Calcium oxalate.
cacocholia (kak-o-ko'lĭ-ă) [G. *kakos*, bad, + *cholē*, bile]. Abnormal condition of bile.
cacochylia (kak-o-ki'lĭ-ă) [" + *chylos*, chyle]. Impaired digestion.
cacochy'mia [" + *chymos*, chyme]. 1. Disordered metabolism. 2. Cacochylia.
cacocolpia (kak-o-kol'pĭ-ă) [" + *kolpos*, vagina]. 1. Diseased condition of the vagina. 2. Gangrene of the vulva.
cacodontia (kak-o-don'tĭ-ă) [" + *odous, odont-*, tooth]. Bad teeth.
cacoethes (kak-o-e'thes) [" + *ēthos*, character]. 1. Any bad habit, propensity, or disorder. 2. A malignant ulcer.
cacoethic (kak-o-eth'ik). Malignant.
cacogenesis (kak-o-jen'ĕ-sis) [G. *kakos*, bad, + *genesis*, development]. Any abnormal development or growth.
cacogen'ic. Pert. to race degeneration.
cacogen'ics (G. *kakos*, bad, + *gennan*, to produce]. Race degeneration.
cacogeusia (kak-o-gū'sĭ-ă) [" + *geusis*, taste]. A bad taste.
cacoglossia (kak-o-glos'ĭ-ă) [" + *glōssa*, tongue]. Gangrene of tongue.
cacomorphia (kak-o-mor'fĭ-ă) [" + *morphē*, form]. Malformation; deformity.
caconychia (kak-o-nik'ĭ-ă) [" + *onyx*, nail]. Disease of the nails.
cacop'athy [" + *pathos*, disease]. Malignant disease; a severe disorder.
cacophonia (kak-o-fo'nĭ-ă) [" + *phōnē*, voice]. An altered, or abnormal voice.
cacoplasia (kak-o-pla'zĭ-ă) [" + *plassein*, to form]. The formation of diseased structures.
cacoplas'tic [" + *plastikos*, formed]. 1. Pert. to or causing morbid growth. 2. Incapable of normal development or formation.
cacorhythmic (kak-o-rith'mĭk) [" + *rythmos*, rhythm]. Showing irregularity of rhythm.
cacorrhinia (kak-or-in'ĭ-ă) [" + *ris*, nose]. Any disease of the nose.
cacosmia (kă-kos'mĭ-ă) [" + *osmē*, smell]. A form of parosmia.* Imaginary foul odors which do not exist.
cacosphyxia (kak-os-fiks'ĭ-ă) [" + *sphyxis*, pulse]. A disordered pulse.
cacothenics (kă-ko-then'ĭks) [" + *thēnia*, state of being]. Racial degeneration from bad environment.
cacothymia (kak-o-thi'mĭ-ă) [" + *thymos*, spirit]. A disorder of the mind; moral depravity; insane morbidity of temper.
cacotrichia (kak-o-trik'ĭ-ă) [" + *thrix*, hair]. A diseased state of the hair.

cacot'rophy [" + *trophē*, nourishment]. Malnutrition.

cacozyme (kak'o-zīm) [" + *zymē*, leaven]. A ferment capable of inducing a disease.

cacumen (kak-u'men) [L. *cacumina*, summit]. Part of cerebellum below the declivis.

cadaver (kăd-av'er) (pl. *cadav'era*) [L. corpse, from *cadere*, to fall]. A dead body; a corpse. SEE: *cleavage lines*.

cadaveric (kă-dav'er-ĭk). Pert. to a dead body.

cadaverous (kă-dav'er-us). Resembling a corpse.

caduca (kad-dū'kă) [L. *caducus*, falling off]. Thickened membrane of the uterus.

cadu'ceus [L. a herald's wand]. The wand of Hermes or Mercury; used as a symbol of the medical profession.

caducity (kad-u'sĭ-tĭ) [L. *caducus*, falling off]. Feebleness or senility of old age.

cadu'cous membrane. Mucous membrane which develops at conception and envelops the impregnated ovum. SYN: *decidua*.

caffeine, caffeina (kaf'e-in, -ă) [L.]. USP. $C_8H_{10}N_4O_2$. An alkaloid of coffee and tea that is a stimulant and a diuretic.
About 1½ gr. are found in a strong cup of coffee. It is chemically identical with theine found in tea.
ACTION AND USES: Diuretic, cardiac, and respiratory stimulant.
DOSAGE: 1-5 gr. (0.065-0.32 Gm.).
INCOMPATIBILITIES: Alkalies, tannic acid, quinine sulfate.
c. citrated. USP. A mixture of caffeine and citric acid, containing about 52% caffeine. Possesses same properties as caffeine, but more likely to disagree with the digestive functions.
DOSAGE: From 3-8 gr. (0.2-0.5 Gm.).
INCOMPATIBILITIES: Sodium salicylate.
c. with sodium benzoate. USP. A mixture of equal parts of caffeine and sodium benzoate.
ACTION AND USES: Same as caffeine.
DOSAGE: 5 gr. (0.3 Gm.). *Hypoderm.*, 3-7½ gr. (0.2-0.5 cc.). [sodium salicylate.
INCOMPATIBILITIES: Potassium citrate,
c. s. salicylate. NF. A mixture of caffeine with sodium salicylate, containing about 52% caffeine.
DOSAGE: 3 gr. (0.2 Gm.).
USES: Same as caffeine sodium benzoate.

caffeinism (kaf'e-in-ĭzm) [L. *caffeina*]. Chronic effects of excessive use of coffee.
SYM: Sudden flushing of the face, palpitation of the heart, trembling, general depression, anxiety, insomnia, and nervousness.

CaH₂O₂. Calcium hydroxide; slaked lime.

cainotophobia (kī-no-to-fo'bĭ-ă) [G. *kainotēs*, novelty, + *phobos*, fear]. Inability to adapt oneself to a new environment or to anything new. SEE: *nostomania*.

caisson disease (ka'son) [Fr. *caisse*, a box, from L. *capsa*, box]. A condition induced in divers subject to too rapid reduction of air pressure after coming to the surface and after breathing compressed air in caissons.
SYM: Condition may manifest itself on reaching the surface or several hours after. Pains in joints followed by motor and sensory paralysis in lower extremities; bladder and rectum sometimes involved; sometimes hemiplegia instead of paraplegia; gastralgia and vomiting common. In severe cases coma develops and death ensues in a few hours. Ordinarily restored in few days or weeks. SEE: *bends, diver's paralysis, tunnel disease*.

caked breast. A stagnation of milk in the secreting ducts.

Cal. Abbr. of large calory.

cal. Abbr. of small calory.

calage (kal-azh') [Fr. wedging]. Fixation of body in a berth by means of pillows to prevent movement and so to relieve seasickness.

calamine, prepared (kal'a-mīn). A pink powder, containing zinc oxide with small amt. of ferric oxide.
USES: Externally in various skin conditions, as a protective and astringent, as an ointment, or in combination with zinc oxide and lime water, as a lotion.

calca'neal, calca'nean [L. *calcaneus*, heel bone]. Pert. to the calcaneum.

calcaneodynia (kal-ka-ne-o-din'ĭ-ă) [" + G. *odynē*, pain]. Pain in the heel.

calcaneum, calcaneus (kal-ka'ne-um, -us) [L. *calcaneus*, heel bone]. 1. The heel bone, or *os calcis*. It articulates anteriorly with the cuboid bone, and with the astragalus above. 2. Talipes calcaneus, *q.v.*

calcanodynia (kal-kan-o-din'ĭ-ă) [" + *odynē*, pain]. Pain in the heel when standing or walking.

cal'car [L. a spur]. A spurlike process.
c. avis. Hippocampus minor, lower of two elevations on inner wall of post. horn of lateral ventricle of brain.
c. femorale. A bony spur that strengthens the femoral neck.

calca'rea [L. *calx*, lime]. Lime.

calcareous (kal-ka're-us) [L. *calcarius*, pert. to lime]. Of the nature of lime; chalky.

calcarine (kal'kar-ĭn) [L. *calcar*, spur]. Spurshaped.

calcariuria (kal-kar-ĭ-u'rĭ-ă) [L. *calcarius*, pert. to lime, + G. *ouron*, urine]. Calcium salts in the urine.

calcaroid (kal'kar-oid) [" + G. *eidos*, appearance]. Calciumlike deposit in brain tissue.

calcemia (kal-se'mĭ-ă) [" + G. *aima*, blood]. Excess of calcium in the blood.

calcibilia (kal-si-bil'ĭ-ă) [" + *bilis*, bile]. Calcium in the bile.

calcic (kal'sĭk). Pert. to calcium or lime.

calcicosis (kal-si-ko'sis) [L. *calx*, lime, + G. *-osis*, infection]. Pneumoconiosis caused by inhaling dust from limestone, esp. by marblecutters.

calcidin (kal'si-din). A combination of calcium and iodine, containing 15% of the latter.
USES: Has been recommended as an alterative and expectorant in colds and minor irritations of the respiratory tract.
DOSAGE: From 1-3 gr. (0.065-0.2 Gm.) in hot water every 15 to 30 minutes to be effective; larger doses for iodine effect.

calciferous (kal-sif'er-us) [" + *ferre*, to carry]. Containing calcium, chalk, or lime.

calcific (kal-sif'ĭk) [" + *facere*, to make]. Forming lime.

calcification [" + *facere*, to make]. Deposit of lime salts in the tissues; normally in bone.

calcigerous (kal-sij'er-us) [" + *gerere*, to bear]. Containing lime or lime salts.
c. tubes. Dentinal tubules of dentin.

calcigrade (kal'sig-rād) [L. *calcis*, heel, + *gradus*, walking]. Walking on the heels.

calcim'eter [L. *calx*, lime, + G. *metron*, measure]. Device for measuring the calcium in the blood.

calcina'tion [L. *calcināre*, to char]. Expulsion of water and animal matter by heat.

calcine (kal'sīn). To cause calcination.

calcinorrhachia (kal-sin-or-ra'kĭ-ă) [L. *calx*, lime, + *rachis*, spine]. Calcium in the spinal fluid.

calcino'sis [" + G. -*ōsis*, infection]. Deposit of lime salts in tissues.

calcipectic (kal-sĭ-pek'tik) [" + G. *pēgnunai*, to fix]. Pert. to calcipexis.

calcipenia (kal-sĭ-pe'nĭ-ă) [" + G. *penia*, poverty]. Calcium deficiency in body tissues and fluids.

calcipexis, calcipexy (kal-sĭ-pĕk'sis, -pĕks'ĭ) [" + *pēgnunai*, to fix]. The fixation of calcium in body tissues.

calciphilia (kal-sĭ-fĭl'ĭ-ă) [" + *philein*, to love]. Tendency to calcification.

calciprivia (kal-sĭ-priv'ĭ-ă) [" + *privus*, without]. Deficiency or absence of calcium.

calciprivic (kal-sĭ-priv'ĭk). Pert. to deficiency or absence of calcium in the body.

calcis, os [L.]. Heel bone.

cal'cium [L. *calx*, lime]. SYMB: Ca. Atomic weight, 40.09. Silver-white metallic element, the basis of limestone.

Lime is its oxide. Calcium phosphate constitutes 75% of the body ash, and about 85% of mineral matter in bones.

FUNCTION: Calcium must be carried by the blood in solution before being available for bone growth. Unless certain activating substances, such as vitamin D, are present, increased calcium intake does not affect the tissues or blood calcium. The secretions of the parathyroid glands are a factor in the utilization of calcium, making it possible for the blood to carry dissolved calcium. Cholesterol seems to stimulate these glands. Ultraviolet rays upon a cow's diet have raised the amt. of calcium in its milk 25%. Calcium stabilizes tissue cells and seems to affect, if not control, allergy or sensitization.

Quantities of bread, rice, oatmeal, and maize in the diet decrease absorption of calcium and phosphorus, and the alkalinity of the small intestines promotes the formation of insoluble salts.

Calcium is necessary for (a) coagulation of the blood, (b) to give firmness and rigidity to bones and teeth, (c) as a preventive of rickets, (d) as an ion balance, (e) as essential to lactation, (f) for activating enzymes, (g) for the functions of the muscles, nerves, and heart.

Calcium is taken into the body as a constituent of various foods. While much of it may prove insoluble and escape absorption, some of it passes through the intestine into the blood, where it can be found by chemical tests. Its level here is likely to be 9 to 11 mg. per 100 cc. If the calcium in the blood rises above this level, the patient feels depressed and his heart is slow; if the calcium sinks below these figures and approaches, say, 4 mg. per 100 cc. the patient suffers from twitching, spasms and convulsions. Blood deprived of its calcium will not clot, and milk without calcium will not curdle.

Calcium is deposited in the bones, but can be mobilized again to keep the blood level constant when there is a period of insufficient intake. At any given time the body of an adult contains about 700 Gm. of calcium phosphate; of this, 120 Gm. are the element calcium. Ordinarily, an adult takes in more than 0.5 Gm. of calcium per day. In the long run, therefore, one should find a total of 0.5 Gm. of Ca in a combined 24-hour sample of urine and feces.

SOURCES: *Excellent*: Cheese, cream, milks, chard, cauliflower, egg yolk, kale, molasses, beans, rhubarb. *Good*: Almonds, beets, bran, cabbage, celery, carrots, chocolate, dates, figs, kohl-rabi, lettuce, lemons, oatmeal, oranges, pineapples, parsnips, raspberries, spinach, shell fish, turnips, rutabagas, oysters, water cress, walnuts.

SEE: *acalcerosis*, "*calci-*" words.

c. carbonate. $CaCO_3$ (precipitated chalk). USP. A fine, white, tasteless and odorless powder.

ACTION AND USES: An antacid, also antidote to corrosive acid poisoning.

DOSAGE: 15 gr. (1 Gm.).

c. chloride ($CaCl_2$). USP. A very deliquescent salt occurring as translucent crystals having a sharp saline taste.

ACTION AND USES: To raise the calcium content of the blood temporarily and increase coagulation time.

DOSAGE: 15 gr. (1 Gm.).

INCOMPATIBILITIES: Ephedrine.

c. deficiency. SYM: Brittle bones and their poor development, including the teeth, dental caries, rickets, tetany, heart atony, hyperirritability, excessive bleeding.

DIAG: Normal content in blood is 9-10.5 mg. per 100 cc. of blood. It is low in convulsions and in allergic disorders.

c. gluconate. A granular or white powder without odor or taste, containing an equivalent of 8-9% calcium.

ACTION AND USES: Same as calcium chloride; more pleasant to taste, and nonirritating when given hypodermically or intravenously.

DOSAGE: Orally, 75 gr. (5 Gm.); intramuscularly or intravenously, 15 gr. (1 Gm.).

c., high diet. A normal adequate diet including 1½ qt. milk and all other foods high in calcium. Cheese is used frequently instead of meat.

c. lactate. USP. A white, odorless and nearly tasteless powder, less irritating than the chloride.

USES: Same as the chloride.

DOSAGE: 15 gr. (1 Gm.).

c., low diet. Milk, cheese, and other foods high in calcium are avoided.

c. oxide [*calx*, lime]. USP. Occurs as white or grayish-white hard mass.

ACTION AND USES: Germicide and disinfectant; used only in preparation of lime water.

calcium phosphate precipitated. A white, amorphous powder.

USES: As an antacid in treatment of gastric hyperacidity.

DOSAGE: 15 gr. (1 Gm.).

cal'coid [" + G. *eidos*, resemblance]. Neoplasm of the tooth pulp.

calcopherous (kal-kof'er-us) [" + G. *phoros*, bearing]. Containing or producing lime or any salts of calcium.

calcospherite (kal-kos-fe'rĭt) [" + G. *sphaira*, a sphere]. One of many small calcareous bodies found in tumors, nervous tissue, the thyroid, and prostate.

calcreose (kal'kre-oze). A chemical combination of creosote and lime containing approximately 50% creosote.

ACTION AND USES: Same as creosote.

DOSAGE: 15-32 gr. (1.0-2.00 Gm.).

calculary (kal'ku-la-rĭ) [L. *calculus*, pebble]. Pert. to calculus.

cal'culi. Pl. of calculus, q.v.

calculif'ragous [L. *calculus*, pebble, + *frangere*, to break]. Breaking or reducing a stone in the bladder.

calculo'sis [" + G. *-ōsis*, infection]. Having a calculus.

cal'culous (kal'ku-lus). Like a calculus.

calculus (kal'ku-lus) [L. pebble]. (Pl. *calculi*). Commonly called "stone"; any abnormal concretion within the animal body, and usually composed of mineral salts.

Present in kidneys, ureter, bladder, urethra, usually formed of crystalline, urinary salts held together by viscid organic matter, and forming a laminated structure, composed of a nucleus about which are concentric layers of material.

TYPES: *Primary*: Developing in acid urine without antecedent inflammation. *Secondary*: Developing in alkaline urine as a result of inflammation. Commonly composed of urates, oxalate of lime, and uric acid.

ETIOL: *Primary*: Obscure. Hereditary tendency with uric acid diathesis, predisposing cause being crystals in urine. *Secondary*: Infection with cocci that split urea into ammonia and carbon dioxide.

c., biliary. Cholelithiasis*; gallstones. SEE: *gall bladder*.

c., hemic. One formed of coagulated blood.

c., pancreatic. Stone in the pancreas, q.v.

c., renal. Stone in the kidney.

SYM: Urinary retention, sudden and paroxysmal renal colic, ulceration with possibly perforation, ureteral stricture, inflammation of various degrees. If formed *in situ*, symptoms are gradual in character with gleet becoming worse, periurethritis, suppuration, fistulization.

PROG: Serious in uremic stage.

TREATMENT: *Prophylactic*: Relief of retention, low nitrogenous diet, exercise, elimination, dilution of urine by water ingestion. *Palliative*: Pyelotomy* when feasible to drain kidney. *Radical*: Operation.

c., salivary. Stone in salivary duct. Usually affects duct of submaxillary gland.

SYM: Obstructs flow of saliva, causing severe pain and swelling of gland, esp. when eating.

TREATMENT: Removal of stone by surgery.

c., urinary. Stone in the urethra.

SYM: Sudden stoppage of flow of urine with sharp pain if stone comes from bladder, and, if firmly impacted, complete retention or dysuria.*

TREATMENT: Extraction or urethrotomy.*

c., vesical. Stone in the bladder.

SYM: Frequency of urination, pain, diurnal hematuria increased by exercise are suggestive.

PROG: Unless stone is small enough to pass by urethra it will remain with cystitis the result.

TREATMENT: Operation.

calculus, words pert. to: antilithic, aortolith, "calcu-" words, cardiolith, "chol-" words, concretion, gravel, "lith-" words.

calefacient (kal-ē-fa'shent) [L. *calere*, to be warm, + *facere*, to make]. Conveying or that which conveys a sense of warmth when applied to a part of the body.

calf [A.S. cealf]. The swelling on back part of the leg below the knee formed by the gastrocnemius and soleus muscles.

calf's foot jelly. Av. SERVING: 45 Gm. Pro. 1.9, Carbo. 7.8 per serving.

cal'iber [Fr. *calibre*, diameter of bore of gun]. The diameter of any orifice or opening.

calibra'tion [Fr. *calibre*, diameter of bore of gun]. Estimation of the caliber of an opening.

calibrator (kal'ib-ra-tor). Instrument for measuring openings.

c., anastomosis. One for determining size of opening to be united by anastomosis.

c., vaginal. One for determining degree of vaginal relaxation.

calic'ulus [L. *calyculus*, small cup]. A cup-shaped structure.

c. gustato'rius. A taste bud.

c. ophthal'micus. (BNA.) The optic cup.

caliectasis (kal-ĭ-ek'tas-is) [G. *kalix*, cup, + *ektasis*, dilatation]. Dilatation of the renal calyx.

caliga'tion [L. *caligo*, darkness]. Dimness of vision; caligo.

cali'go [L. darkness]. Dimness of vision. SYN: *caligation*.*

caliper(s (kal'ip-er) [corruption from caliber]. 1. Instrument for measuring diameters, as those of chest or pelvis. 2. A mechanical apparatus to aid patients who are suffering from fractures of the legs to walk.

Calliphora vomitoria. Common blowfly sometimes causing myiasis disorders.

callisec'tion [L. *callus*, insensitive, + *sectio*, a cutting]. Vivisection under anesthesia.

Cal'lisen's operation. Lumbar colotomy for an artificial anus.

callomania (kal-lo-ma'nĭ-ă) [G. *kalos*, beautiful, + *mania*, madness]. Belief in one's own beauty; a delusion of the insane.

callo'sal [L. *callus*, tough substance]. Pert. to the *corpus callosum*.

callosity, callositas (kal-os'it-i, -as) [L. *callōsus*, thick-skinned]. Circumscribed thickening and hypertrophy of the horny layer of the skin.

ETIOL: Friction, pressure, or other irritation, oval or elongated, on flexor surfaces of hands and feet, grayish or brownish and slightly elevated, with smooth, burnished surfaces.

TREATMENT: Temporary removal by salicylic acid, caustic potash, or careful shaving. Permanent removal only by removal of cause. SEE: *porosis*.

callosomar'ginal [L. *callus*, tough, + *margo*, margin]. Pert. to the corpus callosum and marginal gyrus, marking sulcus bet. them.

callosum (kal-o'sum) [L. *callōsus*, hard]. The great commissure of the brain bet. the cerebral hemispheres. SYN: *corpus callosum*.

callous (kal'us) [L. *callus*, hard]. Hard; like a callus.

cal'lus. Hypertrophied thickening of circumscribed area of horny layer of skin; *callosity*.* 2. The osseous material thrown out bet. ends of a fractured bone.

c., definitive. Cartilage found bet. 2 ends of a fractured bone.

c., provisional. Temporary deposit bet. ends of a fractured bone.

cal'mant [M.E. *calme*, from G. *kaumē*, noon heat, referring to the hour of siesta]. 1. A soothing or calming medicine; sedative. 2. Of a soothing nature.

calm'ative. 1. Sedative; soothing. 2. An agent that acts as a sedative.

Calmette's reaction (kal-mets'). Slight injection of conjunctiva in one with an

calomel — C-5 — caloripuncture

infective disease upon introduction of toxins of same disease. SYN: *ophthalmic reaction, q.v.*

calomel (kal'o-mel) [G. *kalos*, beautiful, + *melas*, black]. Mercurous chloride, *q.v.*
  DOSAGE: *Laxative* (fractional), 2½ gr. (0.15 Gm.).

calor (ka'lor) [L. heat]. 1. Heat. 2. Moderate heat of fever; with *rubor, tumor, dolor*, it represents the 4 classical signs of inflammation.
  c. anima'lis. Normal heat of the body.

calora'diance [L. *calor*, heat, + *radiāre*, to shine]. Giving out heat rays.

calorescence (kal-or-es'ens). Producing by means of a lens incandescence of a body.

Calori's bursa (kal-o'rēz). One bet. arch of aorta and trachea.

caloric (kal-or'ĭk) [L. *calor*, heat]. 1. Heat. 2. Relating to heat,* or to a calory.*   [of the body.

caloricity (kal-or-ĭs'ĭt-ĭ). Heating power

calorie (kăl'or-ē) [L. *calor*, heat]. A unit of heat. SYN: *calory, q.v.*

calorifacient (kal-or-ĭ-fa'shent) [L. *calor*, heat, + *facere*, to make]. Producing heat.

calorific (kal-or-ĭf'ĭk). Producing heat; calorifacient.*

calorigenet'ic [L. *calor*, heat, + G. *gennan*, to produce]. Pert. to heat production or its increase. SYN: *calorigenic.*

calorigen'ic. Pert. to heat production or its increase.

calorimeter (kal-or-ĭm'e-ter) [L. *calor*, heat, + G. *metron*, measure]. Instrument for determining heat of bodies.

calorimetry (kal-or-ĭm'e-trĭ). A calory measure of heat thrown off by the body under different conditions.

caloripuncture (kal-o''rĭ-punk'tur) [L. *calor*, heat, + *punctura*, a piercing]. Use of heated needles in cauterization by puncture. SYN: *ignipuncture.*

CALORY EQUIVALENTS

	Ergs	Gm.-cm.	Ft.-lb.	Cal.	Kw.-hr.
1 erg	= 1.000	= 1.02×10^{-3}	= 7.37×10^{-8}	= 2.39×10^{-11}	= 2.77×10^{-14}
1 Gm.-cm.	= 9.81×10^{2}	= 1.000	= 7.23×10^{-5}	= 2.34×10^{-8}	= 2.73×10^{-11}
1 ft.-lb.	= 1.36×10^{7}	= 1.38×10^{4}	= 1.000	= 3.23×10^{-4}	= 3.76×10^{-7}
1 calory	= 4.18×10^{10}	= 4.26×10^{7}	= 3.08×10^{3}	= 1.000	= 1.17×10^{-3}
1 kw.-hr.	= 3.61×10^{13}	= 3.66×10^{10}	= 2.66×10^{6}	= 8.58×10^{2}	= 1.000

Calory Needs

ACTIVITY	
Sleeping	0.93
Sitting at rest	1.43
Standing relaxed	1.5
Walking	2.0
Light exercise	2.43
Moderate exercise	4.14

Calories per kilogram per hour

If a day's schedule of activities is recorded the energy expenditure can be estimated. For example, a student nurse might figure her caloric needs as follows:
  Student's weight—120 pounds ÷ 2.2 = 55 kilograms.

Caloric Requirements of Infants and Young Children

They have been estimated as follows:
  1st month .... 20 calories, one at 6, 9, 12, 3, 6, 10, and 2 o'clock
  2nd month .... 35 calories, the same as above
  3rd month and after ... 45 calories, one at 6, 10, 2, 6, and 10 o'clock
  3rd year .... 35 calories for each pound of weight

Calories Required per 24 Hours—Langworthy

Man at very hard muscular work	5,500
Man at moderate muscular work	3,400
Man at moderate to light muscular work	3,050
Man at light muscular work (sedentary)	2,700
Man without muscular work	2,450

Calories Expended

Activity	Kg.		Hours		Per Kg.		Per Hr.		Total
Sleeping	55	x	8	x			0.93	=	410
Sitting in class ...... 2 hr.									
at meals ...... 2 hr.									
studying ...... 1 hr.	55	x	8	x			1.43	=	630
writing ...... 1 hr.									
reading ...... 1 hr.									
Standing	55	x	3	x			1.5	=	250
Walking	55	x	1	x			2.0	=	110
Light exercise	55	x	4	x			2.43	=	535
							Total		1935

The Heat Value of Foods per Gram or 15.43 Troy Grains

One Gm.	Large Cal.	Small Cal.	Physiological Value
Protein	5.7	5,711	4.1
Fat	9.3	9,365	9.3
Carbohydrates	4.1	4.182	4.1

cal'ory, or gram-cal'ory [L. *calor*, heat]. The amount of heat necessary to raise the temperature of one gram of water one degree Centigrade.

In dietetics and metabolimetry a unit 1000 times as large is used; it is called the kilogram-calory, large calory, or simply Calory (capitalized). By the law of conservation of energy, a calory can be converted, under certain conditions, into other forms of energy in definite proportions; the conversion factors for various energy units are given in the above table. SEE: *therm, thermal*.

Calot's solution. Solution of creosote, iodoform, ether, olive oil and guaiacol, used externally on painless granulations of fistulas and in chronic otorrhea. SEE: *solution*.

calva'ria [L. human skull]. Skull cap; cranium, skull.

calvities (kal-vish'ĭ-ēz) [L. *calvus*, bald]. Baldness, alopecia.*

Food Units in Calories Required Daily per Normal Height, Weight and Surface—Boys and Girls

NOTE—First figures for boys; second for girls

Age	Height In.	Weight Lb.	Surface Sq. Ft.	Calories
5	41.57	41.09	7.9	816.2
	41.29	39.66	7.7	784.5
6	43.75	45.17	8.3	855.9
	43.35	43.28	8.1	831.9
7	45.74	49.07	8.8	912.4
	45.52	47.46	8.5	881.7
8	47.76	53.92	9.4	981.1
	47.58	52.04	9.2	957.1
9	49.69	59.23	9.9	1043.7
	49.37	57.07	9.7	1018.5
10	51.58	65.30	10.5	1117.5
	51.34	62.35	10.2	1081.0
11	53.33	70.18	11.0	1178.2
	53.42	68.84	10.7	1148.5
12	55.11	76.92	11.16	1254.8
	55.88	78.31	11.8	1276.8
13	57.21	84.85	12.4	1352.6
14	59.88	94.91	13.4	1471.3

Food Units in Calories Required Daily per Normal Height, Weight and Surface—Men and Women

NOTE—First figures for men; second for women

Height Inches	Weight Lbs.	Surface Sq. Ft.	Proteins	Calories Fats	Calories Carbohydrates	Total
59	....	....	....	....	....	....
	119	14.82	179	537	1074	1790
60	....	....	....	....	....	....
	122	15.03	183	549	1098	1830
61	131	15.92	197	591	1182	1970
	124	15.29	186	558	1116	1860
62	133	16.06	200	600	1200	2000
	127	15.50	191	573	1146	1910
63	136	16.27	204	612	1224	2040
	131	15.92	197	591	1182	1970
64	140	16.55	210	630	1260	2100
	134	16.13	201	603	1206	2010
65	143	16.76	215	645	1290	2150
	139	16.48	209	627	1254	2090
66	147	17.06	221	663	1326	2210
	143	16.76	215	645	1290	2150
67	152	17.40	228	684	1368	2280
	147	17.06	221	663	1326	2210
68	157	17.76	236	708	1416	2360
	151	17.34	227	681	1362	2270
69	162	18.12	243	729	1458	2430
	155	17.64	232	696	1392	2320
70	167	18.48	251	753	1506	2510
	159	17.92	239	717	1434	2390
71	173	18.91	260	780	1560	2600
72	179	19.34	269	807	1614	2690
73	185	19.89	278	834	1668	2780
74	192	20.33	288	864	1728	2880
75	200	20.88	300	900	1800	3000

calx (kalks) [L. lime]. 1. Lime. 2. The heel.
   c. chlorinata. Chlorinated lime. Used as a deodorant and disinfectant.
   c. sulfurata. Sulfurated lime. Used as a depilatory.
   c. usta, c. viva. Burnt lime, quicklime.
calyciform (ka-lis'ĭ-form) [G. *kalix*, cup, + L. *forma*, shape]. Cup-shaped.
calyculus (kal-ik'u-lus) (pl. *calyculi*) [L. little cup]. In anat. a cup- or bud-shaped structure.
   c. gustatorii. Taste bud.
calyx (ka'lix) [G. *kalix*, cup]. Any cuplike division of the kidney pelvis. The minor calyces enclose the tips of the renal pyramids, receiving the urine from the papillary ducts which open at their tips.
   c. major. One of the major subdivisions of the renal pelvis, two or three in number.
   c. minor. A subdivision of a major calyx, each terminating in relation to one to three papillae.
Camerer's law. Two children of same weight but different ages require same amt. of food.
camisole (kam'ĭ-sōl) [Fr. little shirt, from Italian, *camisa*, shirt]. A straitjacket used for restraining violent mental patients.
Cammidge reaction (kam'ij). Urinal reaction in pancreatic disease.
   The result is a light yellow flocculent precipitation in a few hours following test.
cam'phor [G. *kamphora*]. USP. A gum obtained from an evergreen tree native to China and Japan.
   ACTION AND USES: Locally, a mild irritant; internally, a circulatory and respiratory stimulant.
   DOSAGE: 3 ɱ (0.2 cc.) hypodermically; subcutaneously, 3 ɱ (0.2 cc.).
   c. ice. Cosmetic preparation used for mild eruptions and for toilet.
cam'phorated. Combined with or containing camphor.
   c. oil. Liniment containing camphor.
camphoromania (kam-for-o-ma'nĭ-ă) [G. *kamphora*, camphor, + *mania*, madness]. Abnormal craving for camphor.
campimeter (kamp-im'e-ter) [L. *campus*, field, + G. *metron*, measure]. Device for measuring field of vision.
campimetry (kam-pim'et-rĭ). Measurement of field of vision. SYN: *perimetry*.
cam'pospasm [G. *kampē*, a bending, + *spasmos*, spasm]. 1. Abnormal flexing of the body. 2. Static deformity produced in war.
camptocor'mia [G. *kamptos*, bent, + *kormos*, body]. Abnormal flexing of body. SYN: *campospasm*.
camptodactylia (kamp-to-dak-til'ĭ-ă) [" + *dactylos*, finger]. Permanent flexion of fingers or toes.
camp'tospasm [" + *spasmos*, spasm]. Camptocormia; forward trunk flexion seen in soldiers.
canal. A narrow tube, channel, or passageway. SEE also *duct*, *groove*, *space*, *foramen*.
   c. adductor. Hunter's canal; a triangular space lying beneath the sartorius muscle and between the adductor longus and the vastus medialis muscles. It extends from the apex of the femoral triangle to the popliteal space and transmits the femoral vessels and the saphenous nerve.
   c. Alcock's. A canal on the pelvic surface of the obturator internus muscle formed by the obturator fascia. It transmits the pudendal vessels and nerve.
   c. alimentary. The digestive tract from mouth to anus.
   c. alveolar, inferior. A canal located in the mandible for transmitting blood vessels and nerves to the lower teeth.
   c. alveolar, superior. A canal in the maxilla for transmitting blood vessels and nerves to the upper teeth.
   c. anal. The terminal portion of the rectum opening at the anus.
   c. auditory, external. The external auditory meatus; transmits sound waves.
   c. auditory, internal. A canal in the petrous portion of the temporal bone which transmits the acoustic and facial nerves and the acoustic artery.
   c. birth. Parturient canal; passageway through which the fetus passes in parturition, specifically the uterus and vagina.
   c. carotid. A canal in the petrous portion of the temporal bone which transmits int. carotid artery and the int. carotid plexus of sympathetic nerves.
   c. central. A small canal lying in the center of the spinal cord extending from the fourth ventricle to the conus medullaris. Contains cerebrospinal fluid.
   c. cervical. Canal in cervix of uterus extending from internal to external os.
   c. cochlear, spiral. A part of the bony labyrinth of the ear. A spiral tube about 30 mm. long making two and three-quarters turns about a central bony axis, the modiolus. Contains the scala tympani, scala vestibuli, and cochlear duct.
   c. condylar (condyloid). A canal in the occipital bone which transmits emissary vein from the transverse sinus. Opens anterior to the occipital condyle.
   c. craniopharyngeal. A canal in the sphenoid bone of a fetus which contains the stalk of Rathke's pouch.
   c. ethmoid. Two grooves running transversely across the lateral mass of the ethmoid bone to the cribiform plate. Lie between ethmoid and frontal bones. The *anterior ethmoidal canal* transmits the anterior ethmoidal vessels and nerve; the *posterior ethmoidal canal* transmits the posterior ethmoidal vessels and nerve.
   c. facial. A canal in the internal acoustic meatus of the temporal bone which transmits the facial nerve.
   c. femoral. The medial division of the femoral sheath. It is a short compartment about 1.5 cm. long lying behind the inguinal ligament. Contains some lymphatic vessels and a lymph node.
   c. gastric. A longitudinal groove on the inner surface of the stomach following the lesser curvature. Extends from esophagus to pylorus.
   c. Haversian. Minute canals found in compact bone which contain blood and lymph vessels, nerves, and sometimes marrow. Each is surrounded by lamellae of bone comprising a Haversian system. SEE: *bone*.
   c. hyaloid. A canal in the vitreous body of the eye extending from the optic papilla to the post. surface of lens. It serves as a lymph channel. In the fetus it transmits the hyaline artery to the lens.

c. hypoglossal. A canal in the occipital bone which transmits the hypoglossal nerve and a branch of the post. meningeal artery.

c. incisive. A short canal in the maxillary bone leading from incisive fossa in roof of mouth to the floor of nasal cavity. Transmits nasopalatine nerve and branches of the greater palatine arteries to the nasal fossa.

c. infraorbital. A canal in the maxilla lying in the floor of the orbit which transmits the infraorbital nerve and vessels. It terminates anteriorly at the infraorbital foramen.

c. inguinal. A slit in the lower lateral portion of the abdominal wall, extending from the abdominal inguinal ring to the subcutaneous inguinal ring. It is an oblique passageway about 1½ inches long and serves in the male to transmit the spermatic cord and the ilioinguinal nerve and in the female the round ligament of the uterus and the ilionguinal nerve. It forms a channel through which an inguinal hernia descends.

c. intestinal. The alimentary canal from stomach to anus.

c. lacrimal. The lacrimal duct, q.v.

c. mandibular. The inferior alveolar canal, q.v.

c. maxillary. The superior alveolar canal, q.v.

c. medullary. The marrow cavity of a long bone. Contains yellow marrow.

c. membranous semicircular canals. SEE: *semicircular ducts.*

c. nasolacrimal. A canal lying between the lacrimal bone and the inf. nasal conchae. Contains the nasolacrimal duct.

c., Nuck's. In the female, a persistent peritoneal pouch corresponding to the vaginal process of the male.

c., nutritive. An opening on the surface of compact bone through which blood vessels gain access to the medullary cavity of long bones. Also transmits veins.

c., obturator. An opening in the obturator membrane of the hip-bone which transmits the obturator vessels and nerve.

c., pharyngeal. A canal between sphenoid and palatine bones for transmission of branches of sphenopalatine vessels.

c., portal. The connective tissue (continuation of Glissons capsule) and its contained vessels (interlobular branches of hepatic artery, portal vein, and bile duct and lymphatic vessel) located between adjoining liver lobules.

c., pterygoid. A canal of the sphenoid bone transmitting pterygoid vessels and nerve. Also called canal of Vidian.

c., pterygopalatine. A canal lying between maxillary and palatine bones which transmits descending palatine nerves and artery.

c., pulp. The central cavity of a tooth filled with pulp. Contains blood vessels and sensory nerve endings.

c., sacral. Cavity within the sacrum, a continuation of the vertebral canal.

c., Schlemm's. A space or series of spaces at the junction of the sclera and the cornea of the eye into which aqueous humor is drained from the anterior chamber through the pectinate villi.

c., semicircular. The portion of the bony labyrinth of the ear which encloses the three semicircular duct. There are three, the superior, posterior, and lateral which open into the vestibule. They are enclosed within the petrous portion of the temporal bone.

c. spinal. The vertebral canal.

c. spiral cochlear. SEE: *cochlear canal.*

c. spiral (of the modiolus). A series of irregular spaces which follows the course of the attached margin of the osseous spiral lamina to the modiolus. They serve for the transmission of nerves and blood vessels. The spiral ganglion lies in the spiral canal.

c., uterine. The cavity of the uterus.

c. uterocervical. The cavity of the cervix of the uterus.

c. uterovaginal. The combined cavity of the uterus and vagina.

c. vaginal. The cavity of the vagina.

c. vertebral. The cavity formed by the foramina of the vertebral column. Also called spinal canal, neural canal. It contains the spinal cord and its meninges.

c. Volkmann's. Small canals found in bone through which blood vessels pass from the periosteum. They connect with the blood vessels of Haversian canals or the marrow cavity.

c. zygomatico-orbital. A canal in the zygomatic or malar bone that transmits branches of the zygomatic nerve and the lacrimal artery.

canalicular (kan-al-ik'u-lar) [L. *canalicularis*, pert. to a small canal]. Pert. to a canaliculus.

canaliculi (kan-al-ik'u-lī) [L. pl. small channel] (sing. *canaliculus*). Small canals, esp. those opening into the *lacunae* of bones.

canaliculus (kă-nal-ik'u-lus). A small channel or canal.

c. lacrimalis. Lacrimal canal carrying tears from eyes to nose. Extends from puncta to lacrimal sac.

canal'is [L.]. A canal or channel.

c. arteriosus. Blood vessel connecting pulmonary artery and the aorta in the fetus.

c. venosus. Duct connecting the umbilical vein in hepatic region to the ascending vena cava.

canalization (ka-nal-ī-za'shun). Formation of channels in tissue.

can'cellated [L. *cancellus*, lattice]. Reticulated; latticelike.

cancelli (kan-sel'lī) [L. *cancellus*, lattice]. Reticulations forming spongy tissue of bones.

can'cellous [L. *cancellus*, a grating]. Having a reticular or latticework structure, as the spongy tissue of bone.

cancellus (kăn-sĕl'ŭs) [L. a lattice]. An osseous plate of which cancellous bone is composed.

cancer (kan'ser) [L. a crab; ulcer]. 1. A malignant tumor of epithelial origin. 2. Specifically, hyperplasia of epithelial or gland cell with infiltration and destruction of tissue.

ETIOL: Origin unknown. May be caused by various forms of chronic irritation.

SYM: Persistent discharge from a sore that doesn't heal; discharge or bleeding from the nipples; blood in the stools or urine or blood-tinged vaginal discharge; persistent, unexplained indigestion or lack of appetite; persistent pain in the part; a lump esp. in the breast; change in a wart or mole; loss of weight; persistent cough or hoarseness.

TREATMENT: Surgery, radium and x-rays are the only recognized effective methods of treatment for cancer.

Method still in experimental stage is refrigeration in cases of advanced malignant metastases, which has thus far caused alleviation of pain, temporary improvement of the general state of the patients and histological changes in the primary and secondary carcinomatous growths. Also cobra venom injected for pain. A refrigerating blanket is sometimes used in place of cracked ice.

Early diagnosis and application of proper method or combination of methods are necessary for complete cure.

NP: Small pillows and sandbags to relieve strained muscles. Cradles to hold bedclothes away from painful parts. Light bedclothes; 1 wool blanket instead of several cotton ones. Olive oil added to rubbing alcohol prevents chafing and rawness. Bland, neutral soap should be used for bathing.

Destroy odors by using chloride of lime in 1:1000 suspension in bedpans, for dressings, but not for the skin. Apply mixture containing 0.5 Gm. pepsin, 0.2 cc. of diluted hydrochloric acid in 100 cc. of distilled water to cancerous wounds to remove dead tissue and destroy odor.

Cater to individual idiosyncrasies. Do not deny particular foods unless there is a good reason for it. Serve 4 to 6 small meals. Attractively decorated trays stimulate appetite in patient. Diet with minimum of 2000 calories per day.

Keep patient cheerful. Talk and soothe patient out of complaint when possible. Censor talk of visitors so that cheerful attitude will be maintained, and literature as well.

Heat and cold and properly applied splints, to reduce motion and relax muscles, will often relieve pain.

See that bowels function at least every 2 days.

c., adenoid. Malignant variety with tubular cylinders with a lining of epithelium.

c., black. Cancer with dark pigmentation.

c., breast. Scirrhous, hard, and medullary soft.

c. cell. Cell composing cancerous epithelium.

c., hard. C. composed of fibrous tissue.

c., lips. Epithelioma, usually in men, smokers and on lower lip.

c., scirrhous. SEE: *hard c.*

c., stomach. Colloid, epithelial, hard or soft. Usually at pyloric end and lesser curvature. SYM: Pain, dyspepsia; emaciation. Constipation and vomiting.

cancer, words pert. to: adenocarcinoma, apinoid, Bendien's test, "canc-" words, "carcin-" words, carcinoma, cauliflower excrescence, chimney-sweeps' c., colloma, epithelioma, sarcoma, scirrhus.

cancerate (kan'ser-āt). Cancerous; developing into cancer.

cancerigenic (kan-ser-ĭ-jen'ĭk) [L. *cancer*, ulcer, + G. *gennan*, to produce]. Causing or capable of producing cancer.

cancerine (kan'ser-ēn). A ptomaine obtained from urine in uterine carcinoma.

cancerism (kan'ser-izm) [L. *cancer*, ulcer, + G. *ismos*, condition]. Tendency to cancerous formation; cancerous diathesis.

cancerocidal (kan″ser-o-sī'dal) [" + *caedere*, to kill]. Destructive to cancer cells.

canceroderm (kan'ser-o-derm) [" + G. *derma*, skin]. Telangiectasis of skin on chest and abdomen sometimes seen in cancer.

cancerogenic (kan″ser-o-jen'ĭk) [" + G. *gennan*, to produce]. Cancerigenic.* Causing or producing cancer.

cancerology (kan-ser-ol'o-jĭ) [" + G. *logos*, study]. The science of cancer. SYN: *cancrology*.

canceromyces (kan-ser-o-mi'sēz) [" + G. *mykēs*, fungus]. An organism bet. a mycete and a mould considered by Niessen as a cause of cancer.

cancerophobia [" + G. *phobos*, fear]. Morbid fear of cancer.

can'cerous. Pert. to malignant growth.

cancriform (kang'krĭ-form) [L. *cancer*, ulcer, + *forma*, appearance]. Having the appearance of cancer.

cancroid (kan'kroid) [" + G. *eidos*, appearance]. 1. Like a cancer. 2. A type of keloid.* 3. Epithelioma.*

cancrology (kang-krol'o-jĭ) [" + G. *logos*. study]. The study of cancer. SYN: *cancerology*.

cancrum (kang'krum) [L. *cancer*, ulcer]. A rapidly spreading ulcer.

c. na'si. Gangrenous inflammation of nasal membranes.

c. o'ris. Gangrenous stomatitis, noma. NP: Cleanse mouth not less than every 2 hours, the oftener the better. Fluids by mouth, nasal feeding.

c. puden'di. Ulceration of vulva.

Candida. A genus of yeast-like fungi which develop a pseudomycelium and reproduce by budding. They are the primary etiologic agents for many mycotic infections in man.

C. albicans. SYN: *Oidium albicans, Monilia albicans*. A small oval, budding fungus which is the primary etiologic organism of moniliosis (candidiasis).

candidiasis. Infection with any species of *Candida*. SEE: "*Moniliasis*".

candle, international. A unit of luminosity.

c. power. Amt. of light thrown out by a lighted candle, measured in international candles. SEE: *unit, light unit*.

canescent (kan-es'ent) [L. *canus*, gray]. Grayish in color.

cane sugar. Sucrose. Table sugar obtained from sugar cane. SEE: *saccharose*.

ca'nine [L. *caninus*, pert. to a dog]. 1. Pert. to a dog. 2. Pert. to the canine teeth or the 4 teeth known as the eyeteeth (upper and lower) bet. the incisors and molars. 3. A canine tooth.

c. appetite. Abnormal hunger a short time after eating. SYN: *bulimia*.*

c. eminence. Ridge on ant. surface of sup. maxilla.

c. fossa. Depression on sup. maxilla external to the c. eminence.

c. tooth. Tooth situated bet. incisors and 1st premolar t. SEE: *dentition, tooth*.

canities (kan-ish'ĭ-ez) [L. gray hair]. Congenital (rare) or acquired whiteness of the hair.

Acquired form may develop rapidly or slowly, in elderly (*canities senilis*) or in early adult life (*canities praematura*), partial or complete.

ETIOL: Hereditary tendency, prolonged fevers, wasting diseases, worry, overwork, grief, anxiety, nervous shock. In localized type, nerve injury.

canker (kang'ker) [L. *cancer*, ulcer]. Thrush; white spots on mucous membrane of the mouth, aphthae, noma, gangrenous stomatitis.

cannula (kan'u-lă) [L. a small reed]. A tube or sheath enclosing a trocar, the tube allowing the escape of fluid after withdrawal of the trocar.

cantaloupe [I. *cantalupo*]. COMP: Contains considerable cellulose. AV. SERVING: 100 Gm. Pro. 0.6, Fat 0.2, Carbo. 5.7 per serving. Ca 0.017, Mg 0.012, K

Cantani's diet   C-10   **capistration**

0.235, Na 0.061, P 0.015, Cl 0.041, S 0.014, Fe 0.0003. ACTION: May cause flatulence.

Cantani's diet (kăn-tă′nēz). Exclusive meat diet in diabetes mellitus.

can′thal [G. *kanthos,* angle]. Pert. to a canthus.

canthar′idal [G. *kantharos,* beetle, + *eidos,* form]. Pert. to or containing cantharides.

cantharides (kan-thar′id-ēz) [" + *eidos,* form]. USP. Dried insects of the species Cantharis vesicatorin obtained from Spain or Russia. SYN: *Spanish fly.*
    ACTION AND USES: Locally, an irritant; as a vesicant in the form of a plaster. Its use has been almost entirely discontinued.

canthectomy (kan-thek′to-mī) [G. *kanthos,* canthus, + *ektomē,* excision]. Excision of a canthus.

canthitis (kan-thi′tis) [" + *-itis,* inflammation]. Inflammation of a canthus.

cantholysis (kan-thol′ĭs-is) [" + *lysis,* a loosening]. Incision of a canthus to widen palpebral slit.

canthoplasty (kan′tho-plas-tī) [" + *plassein,* to form]. Plastic surgery of canthus of the eye. Enlargement of palpebral fissure by division of the external canthus.

canthorraphy (kan-thor′ă-fī) [" + *raphē,* suture]. Suturing of canthus.

canthotomy (kan-thot′o-mī) [" + *tomē,* a cutting]. Division of canthus.

can′thus [G. *kanthos,* angle]. The angle at either end of the slit bet. the eyelids; *external, internal.* BNA. *Commissura palpebrarum.*

can′tus gal′li [L. cock-crowing]. Children's disease marked by spasm of the larynx followed by noisy inspiration. SYN: *laryngismus stridulus.*

CaO. Calcium oxide, quicklime, calx.

CaOC. Abbr. for cathodal or negative opening contracture.

cap (kăp) [A.S. *caeppe,* hood]. 1. A covering. SYN: *tegmentum.* 2. First part of the duodenum. SYN: *pyloric cap.*
    c., knee-. Bone in front of the knee. SYN: *patella,* q.v.

capac′itance [L. *capacitās,* the taking]. That property of a system of conductors and dielectrics which permits the storage of electric charges. For units of capacitance. SEE: *farad.*

capac′itor. A device used primarily because it possesses the property of capacitance.
    It consists of two conducting surfaces separated by a nonconductor or dielectric.

capac′ity. 1. Capability. 2. Cubic content. 3. Holding power. SEE: *capacitance.*
    c., unit of. Unit of electrical capacity. Capacity of a condenser which, charged with 1 coulomb, gives a potential of 1 volt. SYN: *farad.*

capeline (kap′e-lĭn) [Fr. a hat]. A bandage used for the head, or the stump of an amputated limb.

capiat (ka′pī-at) [L. "let it take"]. An instrument for removing placental remnants, etc., from the uterus.

capillarectasia (kap′ĭ-lar-ek-ta′sĭ-ă) [L. *capillaris,* hairlike, + G. *ektasis,* dilatation]. Dilatation of capillary vessels.

capillaries (kap′ĭl-lă-rēs). 1. Minute blood vessels. 2. Small lymphatic ducts. SEE: *capillary.*

cap′illariomo′tor [L. *capillaris,* hairlike, + *motus,* moving]. Vasomotor, esp. pert. to the capillaries.

capillari′tis [" + G. *-itis,* inflammation]. Inflammation of the capillaries; telangiitis.

capillar′ity. Process by which a liquid's surface, at the point of contact with a solid, is elevated or lowered. SYN: *capillary attraction.*

capillarop′athy [L. *capillaris,* hairlike, + G. *pathos,* disease]. Capillary disorders or disease.

capillaros′copy [" + G. *skopein,* to examine]. Examination of capillaries for diagnostic purposes.

cap′illary [L. *capillaris,* hairlike]. 1. Minute blood vessel, 0.008 mm. in diameter, finer than a hair, carrying blood and forming the capillary system. Capillaries connect the smallest arteries (arterioles) with the smallest veins (venules). 2. One of the small lymphatic ducts which allow passage of nutrient matter and oxygen from the blood to the tissues, and of waste matter from the tissues into the blood. 3. Pert. to a hair; hairlike.
    c., arterial. The very small vessels which are the terminal branches of the arterioles or metarterioles.
    c. attraction. The relative results attending the mutual attraction (cohesion) bet. the molecules of a liquid, and their attraction by a touching solid (adhesion), according to which the fluids rise above or sink away from their level about the sides of the containing vessel, or of capillary tubes or rods or plates immersed in them. When the fluid rises, the phenomenon is known as *attraction,* and cohesion dominates; when it sinks, the phenomenon is styled *repulsion,* and adhesion dominates. (*The Practical Standard Dictionary.*)
    c., bile. Intercellular biliary passageways which convey bile from liver cells to the interlobular bile ducts.
    c., blood. Minute blood vessels which convey blood from the arterioles to the venules. They form an anastomosing network which brings the blood into intimate relationship to the tissue cells. Their wall consists of a single layer of squamous cells called *endothelium* through which blood and oxygen diffuse to the tissue and products of metabolic activity enter the blood stream. They average about 8 microns in diameter.
    c., lymphatic. The smallest lymphatic vessels. They are thin-walled tubes forming a dense network in most tissues of the body. They differ from blood capillaries in that they are generally slightly larger in diameter and end blindly. They collect tissue fluid from the tissues. Lymph capillaries unite to form larger lymphatic vessels.
    c. permeability. The ability of substances to diffuse through capillary walls into the tissue spaces. It is influenced by anoxia, adrenal cortical hormone and the concentration of caions in the blood.
    c. venous. The minute vessels which convey blood from a capillary network into the small veins or venules.

capilliculture (kap-il′ĭ-kul-chur) [L. *capillus,* hair, + *cultura,* cultivation]. Systematic treatment for improvement of the hair.

capillose (kap′ĭl-os). Hairy.

capillus (kap-ĭl′us) [L.]. 1. A hair, esp. of the head. 2. A filament. 3. A hair's breadth; 1/10-1/12 of a line.

capistration (kap-is-tra′shun) [L. *capistrāre,* to halter]. 1. Narrowing of opening of prepuce, so that it cannot be retracted behind the glans penis. SYN: *phimosis.* 2. Lockjaw. SYN: *trismus.*

cap'ital [L. *capitalis*, pert. to the head]. 1. Pert. to the head. 2. Of great importance to life.

cap'itate [L. *caput*, head]. Headshaped; having a rounded extremity.
  c. bone. Third bone in distal row of carpus. Syn: *os capitatum*.

capitatum (kap-ĭ-ta'tum). Third bone in distal row of carpus. Syn: *os magnum*.

capitel'lum [L. dim. of *caput*, head]. BNA. *Capitulum humeri*. The round eminence at lower end of the humerus articulating with radius; its radial head.

capitones (kap'it-ōn-ēz) [L.]. Fetuses with heads too large for normal delivery.

capitular (kă-pit'u-lar) [L. dim. of *caput*, head]. Pert. to a capitulum.

capit'ulum. A small, rounded articular end of a bone.
  c. fibulae. The proximal extremity or head of the fibula; articulates with tibia.
  c. humeri. Rounded prominence at distal end of humerus. Articulates with the radius.
  c. mallei. The head or large rounded extremity of the malleus; bears facet for the incus.
  c. stapedis. The head of the stapes; articulated with lenticular process of incus.

capotement (kă-pōt-mon') [Fr.]. A sound like splashing in the stomach.

cap'reolate, cap'reolary [L. *capreolus*, a tendril]. Spiral or tendril shaped.
  c. vessels. Spermatic vessels.

capric (kap'rik) [L. *caper*, a goat]. 1. Pert. to a goat. 2. Having the odor of a goat.

caprizant (kap'rĭ-zant) [L. *caprizans*, leaping, from *caper*, goat]. Leaping or irregular pulse.

caprokol (cap'ro-kol). A resorcin compound relatively nontoxic, and having a phenol coefficient of over 70.
  c. solution (S. T. 37). A 1: 1000 solution of caprokol.
  Uses: In treatment of ear, nose, and throat, or topically as wet dressing for cuts, burns, or open wounds. Used in either full strength or diluted with 1 or 2 parts warm water.
  Dosage: 2½-3 ℔ (0.15-0.6 Gm.).

capsicum (kap'si-kum). USP. Cayenne pepper; dried, ripe fruit of capsicum.
  Action and Uses: Carminative, stimulant and rubefacient.
  Dosage: 1 ℔ (0.06 cc.).

capsitis (kap-si'tis) [L. *capsa*, small box]. Capsulitis of crystalline lens.

capsot'omy [" + G. *tomē*, a cutting]. Incision through Tenon's capsule.

cap'sula [L. dim. *capsa*, box]. Any capsule, esp. the internal capsule of the brain.
  c. articula'ris. Capsule of a joint.
  c. bul'bi. Tenon's capsule.
  c. fibro'sa hep'atis. Glisson's capsule.
  c. glomer'uli. Bowman's capsule; malpighian capsule.
  c. len'tis. Crystalline lens.

cap'sular. Pert. to a capsule.
  c. ligament. A ligament which surrounds a movable joint.

capsula'tion. Enclosure in a capsule.

cap'sule [L. *capsula*, small box]. 1. A membranous bag or a covering enveloping a part. 2. A gelatinous shell for administering medicine.
  c. auditory. Embryonic cartilaginous capsule which becomes ext. ear.
  c. of Bowman. The glomerular capsule of the kidneys.
  c., brain (external of). A thin layer of white matter which separates the claustrum from the putamen.
  c., brain (internal of). A broad band of fibers white matter which separates the lentiform nucleus on lateral side from the caudate nucleus and thalamus on the medial side.
  c., cartilage. The layer of matrix forms the innermost portion of the wall of a lacuna enclosing a single cell or a group of cartilage cells. It is basophilic.
  c., Glisson's. An outer capsule of fibrous tissue in which is invested the liver, its ducts and vessels.
  c., joint. The fibrous tissues enclosing a joint.
  c., lane. A transparent, structureless membrane which surrounds and encloses the lens of the eye.
  c., nasal; c., optic. Embryonic cartilage developing into nose and eyes.
  c. spinal ganglion cells (of). A thin nucleated sheath investing the cell bodies of sensory neurons in the spinal ganglia. It is continuous with the neurilemma of the associated nerve fiber.
  c. suprarenal or adrenal. "A tough connective tissue capsule which encloses the adrenal gland."
  Function: To supply the vasoconstrictor hormone, called epinephrine.
  Nerve Supply: From the solar and renal plexuses.
  Blood Supply: From branches coming from the renal artery and aorta.
  c. of Tenon. The *fascia bulbi*, a serous sac enveloping the eyeball, forming a socket in which it rotates.

capsulec'tomy [" + G. *ectomē*, excision]. Excision of a capsule.

capsuli'tis [" + G. *-itis*, inflammation]. Inflammation of a capsule.

capsulocil'iary [" + *ciliāris*, pert. to the eyelashes]. Pert. to capsule of lens and ciliary structures.

cap"suloplas'ty [" + G. *plassein*, to mold]. Plastic surgery of a capsule, esp. one of a joint.

capsulorrhaphy (kap-su-lor'ă-fĭ) [" + G. *raphē*, suture]. Suture of a joint capsule or of a tear in a capsule.

capsulotome (kap'su-lo-tōm) [" + G. *temnein*, to cut]. Instrument for incising into capsule of crystalline lens.

capsulotomy (kap-su-lot'o-mĭ) [" + G. *temnein*, to cut]. Cutting of capsule of crystalline lens.

captation (kap-ta'shun) [L. *captātiō*, seizure]. The first stage of hypnosis.

caput (ka'put) (pl. *cap'ita*) [L.]. 1. The head. 2. The upper part of an organ.
  c. coli. Cecum; colonic head.
  c. cornus. Enlarged portion of post. horn of spinal cord's gray matter.
  c. cornus (caput columnae posterioris). "Lies between the apex and cervix."
  c. gallinaginis. Round protuberance on urethral floor. Syn: *verumontanum*.
  c. Medusae. Plexus of veins about the umbilicus in 1 form of cirrhosis of the liver indicating obstruction.
  c. obstipum. Wryneck.
  c. succedaneum. Swelling produced on the presenting part of the fetal head during labor. It may be mistaken for the bag-of-waters.
  Etiol: Effusion of serum into cellular tissue of exposed scalp through venous interference from pressure.

carbamide (kär'bă-mīd). Urea or one of its derivatives. USP. Syn: *urea*.

carbarsone (kar'bar-sōn). A white, crystalline, odorless solid, derived from arsenilic acid; contains about 28% arsenic, having a chemical structure resembling tryparsamide.

USES: In the treatment of amebic dysentery. While it is claimed to be less toxic than acetarsone, reactions common to arsenic compounds may occur. While visual disturbances appear to be rare, the possibility of this occurrence should be kept in mind during the therapeutic use of the drug.

DOSAGE: *Orally* for adults, 3¾ gr. (0.25 Gm.) twice a day for 10 days.

As a retention *enema* for adults, 30 gr. (2 Gm.) dissolved in 200 cc. of warm 2% sodium bicarbonate solution, every other night, for a maximum of 5 doses, if necessary. Oral administration should be interrupted during this interval.

carbohemia (kar-bo-he'mĭ-ă) [L. *carbo*, carbon, + G. *aima*, blood]. Incomplete carbon dioxide elimination from blood.

carbohyd'rates [" + G. *ydōr*, water]. The monosaccharoses, disaccharoses, and polysaccharoses. A class of organic compounds so called because in them the hydrogen and oxygen are in the same ratio as they are in water, so that the group can be represented by the formula CxH_2yOy.

Glucose, $C_6H_{12}O_6$, and sucrose, $C_{12}H_{22}O_{11}$ are typical carbohydrates, but the group also includes the noncrystalline dextrins and starches.

c. foods. These contain only carbon combined with hydrogen and oxygen, such as sugars, starch, and cellulose. 98% of animal carbohydrates is digested. 97% of vegetable carbohydrates is digested.

CLASSIFICATION: (1) Starches—Starch does not remain in the body as starch, but is transformed or converted into sugar. They form fat in the body and produce heat and energy in the body. SEE: *classification of starches*. (2) Sugars—These consist of various kinds, forming: (a) Fat; (b) heat and energy. (3) Glycogen—This may be called animal starch. It is stored as reserve material by the liver and muscles and is readily converted into sugar as needed for the production of heat and energy. (4) Gums—Little is known of the animal gums and they are apparently unimportant. (5) Cellulose—This is the fiber of plants and vegetable cells and not a constituent of the body, but it is usually classified among vegetable food values as a carbohydrate.

CHEMICAL PROPERTIES: (1) Reducing properties; (2) hydrolysis; (3) fermentation; (4) oxidation.

FUNCTION: With the exception of cellulose, to provide energy and heat. Excess is stored in the body as fat, and a small amount as *glycogen* is stored in the liver for future use. They are quickly absorbed. Insulin, a secretion of the pancreas, is necessary for the utilization of carbohydrates by the body.

SEE: *carbohydraturia, cellulose, starches*.

c. high diet. Large amounts of carbohydrate. 0.65 Gm. pro. per Kg. ideal body weight. Bet. meal nourishments.

carbohydratu'ria [" + " + *ouron*, urine]. Sugar in the urine. SYN: *glycosuria*.

carbolic acid [L. *carbo*, coal, + *oleum*, oil] (Phenol C_6H_5-OH). Colorless crystalline coal tar derivative which is a poisonous antiseptic and disinfectant.

Used very freely as an antiseptic and as a dressing for wounds, but it must be considered as a dangerous antiseptic, although not as powerful a one as generally supposed.

DOSAGE: 1 gr. (0.06 Gm.).

It is not (chemically) an acid, but an alcohol. It should not be used on the skin for any length of time, esp. when

Classification of Important Carbohydrates

Classification	Examples	Some Properties
Monosaccharides (monoses) $(C_6H_{10}O_5)_1 \cdot H_2O$ or $C_6H_{12}O_6$	Glucose Fructose	Crystalline, sweet, very soluble. Readily absorbed.
Disaccharides (dioses) $(C_6H_{10}O_5)_2 \cdot H_2O$ or $C_{12}H_{22}O_{11}$ hydrolyzed to simple sugars.	Sucrose Lactose Maltose	Crystalline, sweet, soluble, digestible.
Polysaccharides (polyoses) $(C_6H_{10}O_5)n$ composed of many molecules of simple sugars. (Since the molecular weight is unknown, n refers to an unknown number of these groups, the exact molecular weight being undetermined.)	Starch Dextrin Cellulose Glycogen	Amorphous, with little or no flavor, less soluble. Vary in solubility and digestibility. Form colloidal solutions which cannot be dialyzed.

Digestion of Carbohydrates

Enzyme	Found in	Carbohydrates	End-product
Sucrase (invertase)	Intestine	Sucrose	Glucose and fructose
Maltase	Intestine	Maltose	Glucose
Lactase	Intestine	Lactose	Glucose and galactose
Salivary amylase (ptyalin)	Saliva (mouth)	Starch	Dextrin to maltose
Pancreatic amylase (amylopsin)	Pancreas	Starch	Dextrin to maltose

other antiseptics are available. Its use on skin surfaces may cause capillary destruction, cutting off circulation, and perhaps inducing gangrene. One should be very careful, then, in handling this dangerous antiseptic.

Carbolized petrolatum may produce unfortunate results if continued as an application. Any mixture of carbolic acid with other substances, such as camphor, should be avoided.

Tissue changes may take place as a result of its use without one's immediate knowledge, as carbolic acid produces a local anesthesia. The first indications of its destructive qualities are a whitening or grayish-white and wrinkled appearance of the skin. This becomes darker and the skin may turn black if application is not removed. If the hands or the skin are moistened with the acid it must not be allowed to dry, but it should be washed off immediately. Some are more susceptible to capillary destruction than are others.

Lister employed it as a spray to kill bacteria on the patient's skin and on the doctor's hands, and on surgical instruments. The burning produced by carbolic acid may be neutralized by an application of grain alcohol. SEE: *phenol*.

NP: *Carbolic Acid Solutions, Usual Strengths of*:

STOCK SOLUTION: Equal parts of pure carbolic acid and glycerine.

1 IN 20 SOLUTION: 1 ounce of pure carbolic or 2 ounces of stock solution in 1 pint of water.

1 IN 40 SOLUTION: 1 ounce of pure carbolic or 2 ounces of stock solution in 1 quart of water.

To make a 1 in 20 solution into a 1 in 40 solution add an equal quantity of water.

To make a 1 in 20 solution into a 1 in 60 solution, add 2 parts of water to 1 part of the 1 in 20 solution.

To make a 1 in 20 solution into a 1 in 80 solution, add 3 parts of water to 1 part of the 1 in 20 solution.

carbolism (kar'bo-lizm) [" + " + G. *ismos*, condition]. Poisoning by carbolic acid.

car'bolize [" + *oleum*, oil]. To add or mix with carbolic acid.

carbolu'ria [" + " + G. *ouron*, urine]. Phenol in the urine.

car'bon [L. *carbo*, carbon or coal]. SYMB: C. This nonmetallic element is the characteristic constituent of organic compounds.

A common form is coal. It is found in all living things in its various forms and combinations. It is the basis of all organic matter and makes life possible through a number of combinations with hydrogen, nitrogen, and oxygen. In foods it is a fuel creating animal heat, as fats. The diamond is crystallized carbon. Atomic weight 12. SEE: *arc lamp*.

car'bonate [L. *carbo*, carbon]. A salt of carbonic acid.

c. of soda. Sodium carbonate commercially in crude form, as washing soda. The free alkali present is irritating and in larger concentrations has the effect of sodium hydroxide, *q.v.*

car'bon diox'ide. A colorless, pungent, and acid-tasting gas (CO_2), heavier than air, generally produced in the combustion, decomposition, or fermentation of carbon or its compounds, and found in the air and exhaled by all animals.

The final product of combustion of carbon in food, which the body exhales through the lungs, or eliminates through the kidneys in urine, or in perspiration through the skin.

It is also given off by decomposition of vegetable or animal matter, or formed by alcoholic fermentation, as in rising bread. It is necessary to all plant life and it is absorbed directly from the air.

Although a waste product, in small quantities (up to about 5%) in inspired air, it stimulates respiration; in greater quantities, it produces an uncomfortable degree of hyperpnea with mental confusion.

Although not supposed to be poisonous, it will cause death by suffocation. Over 500,000,000 tons are passed into the air per year, but as it is used by green plants, the air content is kept down to about 0.03%. One sq. yd. of leaf surface can absorb the carbon dioxide from 2500 liters of air in 1 hour. An acre of trees uses 4½ tons a year.

c. d. combining power test. This test, done on blood serum, is a determination of the amount of carbon dioxide which the blood serum can hold in chemical combination.

The blood serum is saturated with carbon dioxide by blowing one's breath into it, removing the carbon dioxide by producing a vacuum, and measuring its volume directly. It is used to detect acidosis or alkalosis and to determine their degree. Carbon dioxide in solution forms a weak acid (H_2CO_3), and the amount of this acid which the blood serum can take up is a measure of its reserve power to prevent the occurrence of acidosis. The normal amount is from 50 to 75 cc. for each 100 cc. of blood (usually expressed as 50-75 volumes %). Values below 50 indicate *acidosis*, above 75 *alkalosis*.

c. d. inhalation. Carbon dioxide mixed with oxygen for inhalation stimulates breathing the same way as increased carbon dioxide production from exercise. Inhalation of oxygen and carbon dioxide is used as an accessory during artificial respiration and as a continuation of resuscitation after spontaneous breathing has returned.

c. d. poisoning. This gas is most commonly used in carbonated drinks and commercially used in dry ice; of itself, it is rarely fatal, unless the patient is in a closed space. It is a profound respiratory stimulant.

SYM: Violent increased breathing; sensation of pressure in the head; ringing in ears, acid taste in mouth; slight burning in nose. Within a short time, respiration almost ceases and patient becomes unconscious.

TREATMENT: Remove to fresh air, administer artificial respiration, inhalation of oxygen.

c. d. test. The alkalinity reserve in the plasma is indicated by the volume percentage of carbon dioxide in the blood. Acidosis shows a percentage below 50, while in coma it is as low as 20. Acidosis indicates faulty metabolism. Diacetic acid is produced as the result of accumulated fatty acids, the product of incomplete oxidation of fats. A test is often made before an operation and the patient treated if acidosis is present, as a mild acidosis might develop into a

carbon dioxide, (solid) therapy

very acute one from the effect of the ether.

c. d. (solid) therapy. Solid carbon dioxide (CO_2 snow) is used for therapeutic refrigeration. Solid CO_2 has a temperature of $-80°$ C. Application to skin 1-2 seconds causes superficial frostbite, 4-5 seconds a blister, 10-15 seconds superficial necrosis, 15-45 seconds ulceration. Now used mostly for certain nevi and warts, occasionally for telangiectasia* and lupus erythematosus.

carbonemia (kar-bo-ne'mĭ-ă) [L. *carbo*, carbon, + G. *aima*, blood]. Excess accumulation of carbonic acid in the blood.

carbon'ic. Pert. to carbon.

c. acid. Acid resulting from mixture of carbon dioxide and water.

c. a. gas. A colorless, pungent, acid-tasting gas, heavier than air, produced in the combustion of carbon or its compounds, and found in the air exhaled by all animals. SEE: *carbon dioxide*.

car'bonize. To char.

car'bon monox'ide. An insidious poisonous gas. It is a colorless, tasteless, odorless gas, gives no warning of its presence, and it is widely distributed as the result of imperfect combustion and oxidation. (CO)

It is found in the exhaust gas from all combustion engines, such as automobiles, airplanes, and gasoline motors which are used extensively on farms. It is likewise present in illuminating gas and it results from the inefficient and incomplete combustion of coal. It is found in sewers, cellars, and mines.

Poisoning may take place even from small amounts inhaled over a long period of time, or from large amounts inhaled over a short time. For example, driving a closed automobile, or parking in an automobile with motor running may result fatally from the inhalation of these noxious fumes, from leaking exhausts and exhaust heaters, or from operating a gasoline motor in an enclosed area, such as a closed garage or basement.

Poisoning from carbon monoxide is produced as a result of a chemical combination of this gas with the hemoglobin of the blood, thus preventing the blood from carrying oxygen to the tissues, and since this combination is a relatively stable one, such a patient may need oxygen administration for prolonged periods in addition to artificial respiration.

SYM: The symptoms of carbon monoxide poisoning are somewhat variable. Respiration is deep and difficult. There may be reddish patches of color about the face and chest. The mucous membrane may have a brighter red hue than normal. The pulse initially may be slowed but it soon becomes increased. There may be pounding of the heart; dizziness is frequent, although the muscular system is often affected so that the extremities may fail. There may be singing in the ear, throbbing in the temples, and faintness and nausea. If the patient is still breathing when found, he usually recovers when brought into the fresh air and given stimulants.

TREATMENT: The administration of 4 to 10% of carbon dioxide gas seems to stimulate respiration effectively in these patients. If breathing has stopped, artificial respiration must be instituted immediately and maintained for a long time. Oxygen should be obtained promptly and used in conjunction with artificial respiration. The intravenous administration of methylene blue is now being used very successfully as an antidote. Moderate doses of x-rays are helpful.

COMPLICATIONS: When such patients recover, they often have some nervous system involvement, including various types of paralysis, blindness, or interference with sensation, or muscular spasms, or twitchings, for an indefinite period of time. Most of these complications disappear in time, but occasionally they remain permanently.

carbonom'etry [L. *carbo*, carbon, + G. *metron*, measure]. Determination of presence and amt. of carbon dioxide exhaled.

car'bon tetrachloride (tet-ra-chlo'rĭd). USP. A clear, colorless liquid, with ethereal odor resembling chloroform; not inflammable. (CCl_4)

USES: Although having narcotic and anesthetic properties resembling chloroform, it is too toxic to be suitable as an anesthetic. Recently came into use as a vermifuge in the treatment of hookworm disease, and other intestinal parasites. Also as a stain remover, type cleaner, etc.

DOSAGE: Adult, single dose 40 ṃ (2.5 cc.), best given in capsule on empty stomach, and followed by a saline purge within 3 hours, or may be given in magnesium sulfate solution. Precaution should be taken in not administering to alcoholics nor to patients low in calcium reserve.

POISONING: Toxic effects due to prolonged inhalation.

SYM: Irritation of eyes, nose, and throat, headache, nausea, anorexia, weakness.

F. A. TREATMENT: Oxygen inhalation, coffee, keep patient warm. Treat symptomatically.

carbonu'ria [L. *carbo*, carbon, + G. *ouron*, urine]. The presence or excretion of carbon dioxide or its compounds in the urine.

carbonyl (kar'bon-ĭl) [" + G. *ylē*, matter]. A characteristic group of aldehydes and ketones: $R-C=O$.
$\quad\quad\quad\quad\quad\quad\quad\quad\quad\quad\quad\;\; |$
$\quad\quad\quad\quad\quad\quad\quad\quad\quad\quad\quad\;\; R$

carboxyl (kar-box'ĭl). The characteristic group of an organic acid: $R-C\langle^O_{OH}$

carboxyhemoglobin (kar-bok"sĭ-hem-o-glo'bĭn) [L. *carbo*, carbon, + G. *oxys*, acid, + *aima*, blood, + L. *globus*, sphere]. Compound formed by carbon monoxide and hemoglobin in poisoning by carbon monoxide.

carboxylase (kar-boks'ĭ-lās). An enzyme which brings about the removal of the carboxyl group (COOH) from amino acids; an enzyme found in brewer's yeast which catalyzes the decarboxylation of pyruvic acid with the production of acetaldehyde and carbon dioxide. In the body this requires the presence of vitamin B_1 (thiamine) which acts as a coenzyme.

carbuncle, carbunculus (kar'bung-kl, -ku-lus) [L. *carbunculus*, little coal]. A circumscribed inflammation of the skin and deeper tissues which terminates in a slough and suppuration and is accompanied by marked constitutional symptoms.

ETIOL: *Staphylococcus pyogenes aureus* most common exciting agent. Predisposing factors the same as in furuncle.* Occurs more frequently in men, and in adults than children. Diabetics are particularly susceptible.

carbuncular   C-15   **cardiac, diet**

SYM: It is characterized by a painful node at first covered by a tight, reddened skin which later becomes thin and perforates, discharging pus through several openings. Most commonly found on nape of neck, on back, or on buttocks.

PROG: Depends upon age and general condition of patient, the young and vigorous recovering promptly. When on the scalp, death usually follows from thrombosis and embolism, and in elderly and debilitated from exhaustion and sepsis.

TREATMENT: General health cared for, elimination free. Autogenous vaccines. Hot, moist dressings (antiseptic) followed by radical cross shaped incision under gas anesthesia when tumor is fluctuant. Pockets to be cleaned out and packed with moist iodoform gauze. X-ray therapy and electrocautery have been employed. Blood sugar should be checked.

NP: Area cleaned and dressed frequently. Strict isolation of utensils, towels, and dishes. If localized areas are not well drained, pyemia may ensue. Infection of deeper veins may occur, or mastoiditis in regions of head and neck.

SEE: *anthracia, anthracoma, anthracosis*, 2, *charbon.*

carbun′cular. Pert. to a carbuncle.

carbunculosis (kar-bun-ku-lo′sis). Appearance of several carbuncles in succession.

Carcasonne's ligament (kar-kă-suns′). The deep perineal fascia. Colles's fascia.

carcinectomy (kar-sin-ek′to-mĭ) [G. *karkinos*, crab cancer, + *ektomē*, excision]. The excision of a cancerous growth.

carcinelcosis (kar-sin-ĕl-ko′sis) [″ + *elkōsis*, ulceration]. An ulcer of a cancerous nature.

carcinogenesis (kar″sin-o-jen′e-sis) [″ + *genesis*, production]. The production or origin of cancer.

carcinogenic (kar″sin-o-jen′ik). Causing cancer.

car′cinoid [G. *karkinos*, cancer, + *eidos*, resemblance]. An epithelial growth resembling a cancer, but having a benign course.

carcinolysis (kar-sin-ol′is-is) [″ + *lysis*, destruction]. Destruction of carcinoma cells.

carcinolytic (kar-sin-o-lit′ik). Destructive to cancer cells.

carcinoma (kar-sin-o′mă) [″ + *-ōma*, tumor]. An epithelial cell new growth or malignant tumor, enclosed in connective tissue, and tending to infiltrate and give rise to metastases. SYN: Cancer.

It may affect almost any organ or part of the body and spread through the blood stream.

ETIOL: Unknown. Irritated surfaces, and extremes of temperature may be held responsible. Sym. absent in early stage.

SYM: *Stomach*. Skin muddy, pale, or slightly jaundiced. Emaciation and loss of weight progressive. Increased resistance over stomach. Inguinal and supraclavicular glands may be palpated. Leukocytosis or relative increase in polynuclear cells. Deficiency of free HCl and presence of lactic acid. Secondary anemic characteristics; blood count not below 1,000,000.

PROG: Favorable if found early.

  c., epithelial. Epithelial cell cancer.

  c., glandular. C. with cells of the secreting variety. SEE: *adenocarcinoma.*

  c., lipomatous. C. with fatty tissue.

  c., melanotic. C. containing melanin.

  c. ossificans, c. osteoid. C. with bony deposit.

  c. sarcomatodes. C. showing transition to sarcomatous type.

  c., scirrhous. C. with firm structural form.

  c., squamous. C. arising from the squamous epithelium.

carcinomatophobia (kar-sin-no″mă-to-fo′-bĭ-ă) [G. *karkinos*, cancer, + *-ōma*, tumor, + *phobos*, fear]. Morbid fear of carcinoma.

carcinomatosis (kar-si-no-ma-to′sis) [″ + ″ *-ōsis*, infection]. The condition giving rise to carcinomata.

carcinomatous (kar-sin-o′mă-tus). Pert. to or affected with cancer.

carcinomec′tomy [G. *karkinos*, cancer, + *-ōma*, tumor, + *ektomē*, excision]. Excision of a cancer.

carcinomelcosis (kar″sin-o-mel-ko′sis) [″ + ″ + *elkōsis*, ulceration]. An ulcerating cancer.

carcinophobia [″ + ″ + *phobos*, fear]. Morbid fear of cancer.

carcinosarco′ma [″ + ″ + *sarx*, flesh, + *-ōma*, tumor]. A mixed tumor of carcinoma and sarcoma.

carcinosectomy (kar-sin-o-sek′to-mĭ) [″ + ″ + *ektomē*, excision]. Excision of a cancer.

carcinosis (kar-sin-o′sis) [″ + ″ + *-ōsis*, infection]. 1. Tendency to the development of malignant disease. 2. A form of carcinoma, beginning generally in the uterus, or the stomach, and spreading to the peritoneum.

carcinous (kar′sin-us). Pert. to or of the nature of carcinoma. SYN: *cancerous.*

car′damom, car′damon [G. *kardamōmon*]. Dried ripe fruit of *Elettaria repens*, used as an aromatic and carminative.

Cardarelli's sign (kar-dă-rel′lis). Tracheal tugging significant of aneurysm of aorta.

cardia (kar′di-a) [G.]. 1. The heart. 2. Upper orifice (esophageal) of stomach connecting with the esophagus. SEE: *heart.*

car′diac [G. *kardia*, heart]. 1. Pert. to the heart or esophageal orifice of the stomach. 2. One afflicted with heart disease. 3. A heart tonic.

  c. arrhythmia. SEE: *arrhythmia.*

  c. atrophy. Fatty degeneration of the heart.

  c. compensation. The ability of the heart through its reserve power to compensate for impaired functioning of its valves.

  c. cycle. The period from the beginning of one beat of the heart to the beginning of the next succeeding beat, including the *systole*, or contraction of the auricles and ventricles propelling the blood onward, and the *diastole*, the period during which the cavities are being refilled with blood.

The auricles contract immediately before the ventricles. The ordinary cycle lasts 8/10 of a second with the heart beating at 72 times per minute. The *auricular systole* lasts 0.1 second; the *ventricular systole*, 0.3 second, and the *diastole*, 0.4 second, thus allowing the heart to rest about 50% of the time. Heart action is also inhibited by the action of the vagus nerve.

RS: *circulation, diastole, heart, systole.*

  c. diet. Variable. Maintenance without labor upon heart.

Avoid gas-producing foods, such as cabbage, onions, turnips, beans, and bulky foods causing distention and pres-

sure upon heart. Fluid intake restricted to 1500 cc. or less. Eliminate salt if edema is present. Small quantities of food at a time. Karrell diet, *q.v.*
c. diet, Smith. A variation of the Karrell diet. Maintenance protein (2/3 to 1 Gm. per Kg.) mostly milk or eggs. The calories made adequate by addition of some cream by the liberal use of carbohydrates. Fluids limited, salt restricted in cases complicated with edema. For the first few days diet is liquid, milk and cream, orange juice and added sugars. After that soft foods are added, pureed vegetables, fruits, toast, cereal, carbohydrate pushed by use of sugars, jelly, honey or sugar candy.
Advantages: An adequate diet; foods may be varied so diet is not so monotonous. The emphasis on carbohydrates is beneficial.
c. hypertrophy. Enlargement of the heart. SEE: *heart, hypertrophy of.*
c. insufficiency. Inadequate cardiac output due to failure of the heart to function properly, as in valvular deficiency.
c. movements. Those caused by the movement of the air in the lungs from the pulsation of the heart.
c. output. The amount of blood discharged from the left (or right) ventricle per minute. Also called *minute volume*. For an average adult with pulse rate of 70, cardiac output is approximately 4 liters.
c. plexus. *Plexus cardiacus.* SEE: *plexuses in Appendix.*
c. reflex. A reflex in which the response is a change in cardiac rate. Stimulation of sensory nerve endings in the wall of the carotid sinus by increased arterial blood pressure reflexly slows the heart (Marey's law); stimulation of vagus fibers in the right side of the heart by increased venous return reflexly increases heart rate (Bainbridge's reflex).
c. reserve. The capacity of the heart to increase cardiac output and raise blood pressure above basal pressure to meet body requirements.
cardiactia (kar-dĭ-ak'tĭ-ă) [G. *kardia*, heart, + L. *actio*, function]. Cardiac stenosis.
cardiagra (kar-dĭ-a'gră) [" + *agra*, seizure]. Serious pains in the chest of a constricting nature. SEE: *angina pectoris.*
cardialgia (kar-dĭ-al'jĭ-ă) [" + *algos*, pain]. Pain at the pit of the stomach or region of the heart, usually occurring in paroxysms.
cardiam'eter [" + *metron*, measure]. Device for marking position of the cardia.
cardiamor'phia [" + *morphē*, form]. Malformation of the heart.
cardianastrophe (kar-dĭ-an-as'tro-fī) [" + *anastrophē*, reversal of position]. Congenital transposition of the heart to the right side. SYN: *dextrocardia.*
cardianesthe'sia [" + *anaisthēsia*, lack of sensation]. Lack of sensation in the heart.
cardianeuria (kar-dĭ-ă-nu'rĭ-ă) [" + *aneuros*, without nerves]. Lack of nerve stimulus to the heart.
cardianeurysma (kar-dĭ-an-u-riz'mă) [" + *aneurysma*, a widening]. Aneurysm of the heart.
cardiant (kar'dĭ-ant). 1. Affecting, or that which affects the heart. 2. A cardiac stimulant.
cardiaortic (kar-dĭ-a-or'tĭk) [G. *kardia*, heart, + *aortē*, aorta]. Pert. to the heart and the aorta.

cardiasthenia (kar-dĭ-as-the'nĭ-ă) [" + *astheneia*, weakness]. Type of neurasthenia with predominance of cardiac symptoms.
cardiasthma (kar-dĭ-az'mă) [" + *asthma*, panting]. Dyspnea due to heart disease.
cardiataxia (kar-dĭ-ă-taks'ĭ-ă) [" + *ataxia*, lack of order]. Incoördination of the heart contractions; very irregular heart action.
cardiatrophia (kar-dĭ-at-ro'fĭ-ă) [" + *atrophia*, lack of nourishment]. Atrophy of the heart.
cardiechema (kar-dĭ-ek-e'mă) [" + *ēchō*, echo]. A heart sound.
cardiectasia, cardiectasis (kar-dĭ-ek-ta'-sĭ-ă, -sis) [" + *ektasis*, dilatation]. Dilatation of the heart.
cardiectomy (kar-dĭ-ek'to-mĭ) [" + *ektomē*, excision]. Excision of the cardiac end of the stomach.
cardielcosis (kar-dĭ-el-ko'sis) [" + *elkōsis*, ulceration]. Ulceration of the heart.
cardiemphraxia (kar-dĭ-em-fraks'ĭ-ă) [" + *emphraxis*, a stoppage]. Obstruction of the blood flow in the heart.
cardiethmoliposis (kar-dĭ-eth-mo-lip-o'sis) [" + *ethmos*, sieve, + *lipos*, fat]. Fat in connective tissue of the heart.
cardieurysma (kar-dĭ-u-riz'mă) [" + *eurys*, wide]. Dilatation of the heart.
cardinal [L. *cardinalis*, important]. Principal, as the cardinal symptoms, temperature, pulse, respiration.
cardio- [G. *kardia*, heart]. Prefix: Pert. to the cardia or heart.
cardioaccel'erator [" + L. *accelerāre*, to hasten]. That which increases the rate of the heart beat.
cardioangiology (kar″dĭ-o-an-jĭ-ol'o-jĭ) [" + *aggeion*, vessel, + *logos*, study]. The science of the heart and blood vessels.
cardioaortic (kar″dĭ-o-ă-or'tĭk) [" + *aortē*, aorta]. Pert. to the heart and the aortic artery.
cardiocele (kar'dĭ-o-sēl) [" + *kēlē*, tumor]. Hernia of the heart.
cardiocentesis (kar-dĭ-o-sen-te'sis) [" + *kentēsis*, puncture]. Surgical puncture of the heart to relieve engorgement of one of its chambers.
cardiocinetic (kar″dĭ-o-sin-et'ĭk) [" + *kinesis*, motion]. Influencing heart action.
cardioclasia (kar-dĭ-o-kla'zĭ-ă) [" + *klasis*, break]. Rupture of the heart.
cardiodemia (kar-dĭ-o-de'mĭ-ă) [" + *dēmos*, fat]. Fatty degeneration of the heart.
cardiodi'lator [" + L. *dilatāre*, to enlarge]. Device for dilating the cardia.
cardiodio'sis [" + *dia*, through, + *-ōsis*, infection]. Dilating the cardiac end of the stomach.
cardiodynia (kar-dĭ-o-din'ĭ-ă) [" + *odynē*, pain]. Pain in the region of the heart.
cardiogen'ic [" + *gennan*, to produce]. Having origin in the heart itself.
car'diogram [" + *gramma*, mark]. A tracing of movements of the heart.
A simple tracing which can be made by placing a thistle tube over the apex of the heart in thin people and connecting it to a tambour, of which the lever writes on moving paper.
cardiograph (kar'dĭ-o-graf) [" + *graphein*, to write]. A device for registering heart pulsations in graphic form.
cardiograph'ic. Pert. to cardiography.
cardiog'raphy. Recording the heart movements.
cardiohepat'ic [G. *kardia*, heart, + *epar*, liver]. Pert. to heart and liver.

cardioinhibitory ["+ L. *inhibere*, to check]. Slowing action of the heart.

cardiokinet'ic ["+ *kinēsis*, motion]. Influencing action of the heart.

car'diolith ["+ *lithos*, stone]. A concretion or calculus in the heart.

cardiol'ogist ["+ *logos*, study]. A specialist in treatment of heart disease.

cardiol'ogy. The science of the heart.

cardiol'ysin [G. *kardia*, heart, + *lysis*, loosening]. A lysin acting on heart muscle.

cardiolysis (kar-dĭ-ol'ĭs-ĭs) ["+ *lysis*, loosening]. Freeing pericardial adhesions to surrounding tissues, involving resection of the ribs and sternum.

cardiomalacia (kar-dĭ-o-mal-a'sĭ-ă) ["+ *malakia*, softening]. Softening of the heart walls.

cardiomegaly (kar-dĭ-o-meg'a-lĭ) ["+ *megas*, large]. Hypertrophy of the heart.

cardiometer (kar-dĭ-om'ĕ-ter) ["+ *metron*, measure]. Device for locating impulse or apex of the heart's beat.

cardiomotil'ity ["+ L. *motilis*, moving]. The ability of the heart to function.

cardiomyoliposis (kar"dĭ-o-mi"o-li-po'sis) ["+ *mys*, muscle, + *lipos*, fat]. Fatty degeneration of the heart.

cardiomyot'omy ["+ " + *tomē*, a cutting]. Severing the constricting muscle of the heart to relieve cardiospasm.

cardioncus (kar-dĭ-on'kus) ["+ *ogkos*, tumor]. Heart aneurysm or a. of the aorta near the heart.

cardionecro'sis ["+ *nekros*, dead]. Necrosis of the heart.

cardionephric (kar-dĭ-o-nef'rĭk) ["+ *nephros*, kidney]. Pert. to heart and kidney.

cardioneu'ral ["+ *neuron*, nerve]. Pert. to nervous control of the heart.

cardioneuro'sis ["+ *neuron*, nerve]. Functional neurosis with cardiac symptoms.

cardiopalmus (kar-dĭ-o-păl'mus) ["+ *palmos*, palpitation]. Palpitation of the heart.

cardiopal'udism ["+ L. *palus*, marsh, + G. *ismos*]. Irregularity of heart action resulting from malaria.

car'diopath ["+ *pathos*, disease]. One with heart disease.

cardiopathy (kar-dĭ-op'ath-ĭ). Any disease of the heart.

cardiopericardi'tis ["+ *peri*, around, + *kardia*, heart, + *-itis*, inflammation]. Inflammation of myocardium and pericardium.

cardiophobia (kar"dĭ-o-fo'bĭ-ă) ["+ *phobos*, fear]. Morbid fear of heart disease.

cardiophone (kar'dĭ-o-fōn) ["+ *phōnē*, voice]. Device for listening to sound of the heart.

cardiophtharsis (kar-dĭ-of-thar'sis) ["+ *phthisis*, wasting]. Destruction of the heart's substance.

cardioplasty (kar-dĭ-o-plas'tĭ) ["+ *plassein*, to form]. Operation of the stomach to relieve cardiospasm.

cardioplegia (kar-dĭ-o-ple'gĭ-ă) ["+ *plēgē*, stroke]. Paralysis of the heart.

cardiopneumat'ic ["+ *pneuma*, breath]. Pert. to the heart and the lungs.

cardiopneumograph (kar-dĭ-o-nu'mo-graf) ["+ " + *graphein*, to write]. Device for recording motion of heart and lungs.

cardioptosis (kar-dĭ-op-to'sis) ["+ *ptōsis*, falling]. Prolapsus of the heart.

cardiopul'monary ["+ L. *pulmō*, lung]. Pert. to both heart and lungs.

car'diopuncture ["+ L. *punctura*, piercing]. Surgical puncture of the heart. SYN: *cardiocentesis*.

cardiopylor'ic ["+ *pyloros*, gatekeeper]. Pert. to the cardiac and pyloric ends of the stomach.

cardiore'nal ["+ L. *rēnalis*, pert. to kidney]. Pert. to both heart and kidneys.

cardiorrhaphy (kar-dĭ-or'af-ĭ) ["+ *raphē*, a suture]. Suturing of the heart muscle.

cardiorrhexis (kar-dĭ-or-reks'is) ["+ *rexis*, rupture]. Heart rupture.

cardiosclerosis (kar-dĭ-o-sklē-ro'sis) ["+ *sklērōsis*, hardening]. Hardening of the cardiac tissues and arteries.

car'dioscope ["+ *skopein*, to examine]. Instrument for listening to heart sounds. SYN: *cardiophone*.

cardiospasm (kar'dĭ-ō-spazm) ["+ *spasmos*, spasm]. 1. Heart spasm. 2. Spasm of the cardiac sphincter of the stomach. The esophagus fails to open properly. Tube dilates from retention of large quantities of food.
ETIOL: Pressure or ulceration with scar formation.
SYM: Regurgitation, esp. at night.
TREATMENT: Dilatation. Also relieved by injection of thiamin chloride.

cardiosphyg'mograph ["+ *sphygmos*, throb, + *graphein*, to write]. Instrument for graphically recording movements of the heart and pulse.

cardiostenosis (kar-dĭ-o-sten-o'sis) ["+ *stenōsis*, narrowing]. Heart constriction and its development.

cardiosym'physis ["+ *symphysis*, growing together]. Destruction of pericardial sac by adhesions.

cardiotachometer (kar"dĭ-o-tak-om'ĕt-er) ["+ *takos*, speed, + *metron*, measure]. An instrument for determining rapidity of heart beat.

cardiother'apy ["+ *therapeia*, treatment]. The treatment of cardiac diseases.

cardiotomy (kar-dĭ-ot'o-mĭ) ["+ *temnein*, to cut]. Incision of the heart.

cardioton'ic ["+ *tonos*, tone]. Increasing tonicity of the heart.

cardiotoxic (kar-dĭ-ō-toks'ĭk) ["+ *toxikon*, poisoning]. Exercising a poisonous effect upon or through the heart.

cardiotromus (kar-dĭ-ot'ro-mŭs) ["+ *tromos*, trembling]. Heart flutterings.

cardiotrophother'apy ["+ *trophē*, nourishment, + *therapeia*, treatment]. Nutritional treatment of heart disorders.

cardiovalvuli'tis ["+ L. *valvula*, valve, + G. *-itis*, inflammation]. Inflammation of valves of the heart. Valvular endocarditis.

cardiovalvulotome (kar-dĭ-o-val'vŭ-lo-tōm) ["+ " + G. *tomē*, cut]. An instrument for excising part of a valve, esp. the mitral valve.

cardiovas'cular ["+ L. *vasculum*, small vessel]. Pert. to the heart and blood vessels.

c. reflex. Sympathetic increase in heart rate when increased pressure in or distention of great veins occurs.

cardiovasology (kar"dĭ-o-vas-ol'o-jĭ) ["+ L. *vas*, vessel, + G. *logos*, study]. Science of the heart and blood vessels. SYN: *cardioangiology*.

cardi'tis ["+ *-itis*, inflammation]. Inflammation of the heart muscles.
ETIOL: Gonococcal, pneumococcal, streptococcal, or due to rheumatism, or to the influenza virus.

Cargile membrane (kar'gĭl). One made from the ox's peritoneum to prevent surgical adhesions.

caribi (kar-ĭ'bĭ). Epidemic gangrenous proctitis.

caricous (kar'ĭk-us) [L. *carica*, fig]. Fig-shaped.

caries (ka′rez) [L. *rottenness*]. Decay and death of a bone or tooth associated with inflammation and the formation of abscesses in the periosteum and surrounding tissues. A progressive decalcification of the enamel and dentine of a tooth, as a result of fermentation of carbohydrates. The etiology is not fully known. Early detection and dental fillings offer the best form of control. Fluorine is assumed to promote resistance to dental caries during the stage of tooth formation. Topical application of sodium fluoride is being tried.

Chronic abscess, tuberculosis, and bacterial invasion of teeth are examples. In caries the bone melts away, while in necrosis large pieces of bone are discharged. Deficiency of vitamins A and G has a direct influence upon caries of the teeth.

   c. fungo′sa. A tuberculosis of bone.

   c., necrotic. Caries with pieces of bone in a suppurative cavity.

   c. sic′ca. Dry tuberculosis of ends of bones and joints unaccompanied by fluid or swelling.

carina (kar-i′nă) [L. *keel of a boat*]. A keel-like structure, esp. the vertebral column of the fetus and the sternum.

carinate (kar′in-āt). Keelshaped; resembling the bottom of a boat.

carious (ka′ri-us) [L. *cariēs*, rottenness]. 1. Affected with or relating to caries. 2. Having pits or perforations. SEE: *caries*.

carmin′ative [L. *carmināre*, to cleanse]. An agent that will remove gases from the gastrointestinal tract. Ex: *asafetida, peppermint, cardamon*.

   c. enema. Given to relieve distention caused by flatulence and also to stimulate peristalsis.

carnal (kar′nal) [L. *caro, carnis*, flesh]. Relating to the flesh. [sexual practices.]

   c. knowledge. Having awareness of

carneous (kar′ne-us) [L. *carneus*, fleshy]. Fleshy.

   c. columns. Columnae carneae. Muscular projections from inner coat of the heart ventricles.

carnification (kar-nĭf-ĭk-a′shun) [L. *caro, carnis*, flesh, + *facere*, to make]. Denoting alteration of tissues, esp. pulmonary tissue.

carniformis (kar-nĭ-form′is) [" + *forma*, appearance]. Fleshlike in appearance.

carnivorous (kar-niv′or-us) [" + *vorāre*, to devour]. Flesh eating.

carnophobia [" + G. *phobos*, fear]. Abnormal aversion to meat.

carnose (kar′nos). Having the consistency of or resembling flesh.

carnosity (kar-nos′it-ĭ) [L. *carnōsitās*, fleshiness]. An excrescence resembling flesh; a fleshy growth.

caro (ka′ro) [L.]. Flesh. [lations.]

   c. luxurians. Excessive spongy granu-

carot′enase [G. *karōton*, carrot]. An enzyme that converts carotene into vitamin A.

carotene (car′o-tēn) (pro-vitamin.) A yellow crystalline pigment present in various plant and animal tissues. It is abundant in yellow vegetables (carrots, squash, corn). It exists in three isomeric forms, alpha, beta, and gamma-carotene which along with cryptoxanthine, are the precursors of vitamin A. Carotene is stored in the liver and kidney and converted to vitamin A in the liver.

carotene′mia [G. *karōton*, carrot, + *aima*, blood]. Carotene in the blood.

caroteno′sis [" + *-ōsis*, infection]. Pigmentation of tissues caused by carotene in the blood.

carotic (kar-ot′ik) [G. *karoun*, to stupefy]. 1. Carotid. 2. Resembling stupor; stupefying. 3. A sleep-producing drug.

carot′id [G. *karōtides*, from *karos*, heavy with sleep, because ancient Greeks believed the carotid arteries caused sleep]. The principal artery of the neck. It divides into the right and left branches.

   c. body. SEE: *carotid*.

   c. sinus. A dilated area at the bifurcation of the common carotid artery which is richly supplied with sensory nerve endings of the sinus branch of the vagus nerve. These when stimulated by distention of the vessel wall brought about by a rise in blood pressure, bring about reflex vasodilation and a slowing of the heart rate.

carotidynia (kar-ot-ĭ-din′ĭ-ă) [" + *odynē*, pain]. Pain elicited by pressure on the common carotid artery.

caro′tin [G. *karōton*, carrot]. A coloring matter in carrots; a lipochrome. Vitamin A is manufactured from this substance by body. It is probably responsible for vitamin in highly colored vegetables, butter, egg yolk. Not found in animal livers. Its chemical structure is unknown. SEE: *carotene*.

car′otinase. A ferment converting carotin into vitamin A. SYN: *carotenase*.*

carotinemia (kă-ro-tĭn-e′mĭ-ă) [G. *karōton*, carrot, + *aima*, blood]. Carotin in excess, causing yellowish skin.

caro′tinoid [" + *eidos*, form]. Having the qualities of carotin.

carpagra (kar-pag′ră) [G. *karpos*, wrist, + *agra*, seizure]. Sudden wrist pain.

car′pal [G. *karpos*, wrist]. Pertaining to the carpus or wrist.

   c. articulation. Wrist joint.

carpale (kar-pa′lē). Any wrist bone.

carpec′tomy [G. *karpos*, wrist, + *ektomē*, excision]. Excision of the carpus or portion of it.

carphologia, carphology (kar-fo-lo′jĭ-ă, -fŏl′ŏ-gĭ) [G. *karphos*, chaff, + *legein*, to pluck]. Involuntary picking at bed clothes, seen esp. in febrile or exhaustive delirium, of the low muttering type.

A grave symptom in cases of extreme exhaustion or approaching death.

carpi′tis [G. *karpos*, wrist, + *-itis*, inflammation]. Inflammation of a carpal joint or joints.

carpo- [G.]. Prefix: Pert. to the carpus.

car′pometacar′pal [G. *karpos*, wrist, + *meta*, beyond, + *karpos*]. Pert. to both carpus and metacarpus.

carpope′dal [" + L. *pēs, ped*, foot]. Pert. to wrist, foot, feet, or hands.

   c. spasm. Spasm of the hands and feet, sometimes seen in laryngismus stridulus, *q.v.*

carpoptosis (kar-pop-to′sis) [" + *ptōsis*, a falling]. Wrist drop.

carpus (kar′pus) [G. *karpos*]. The 8 bones of the wrist.
SEE: *"carpus-" words, pisiform, scaphoid, skeleton, wrist, wrist clonus, wrist drop*.

carreau (kar-ō′) [Fr.]. Tuberculosis and scrofulosis of organs of digestion.

Carrel-Dakin treatment. A method of wound irrigation first utilized by Dr. Alexis Carrel and Dr. Henry Dakin in 1915.

Most suitable for deep septic wounds. A special apparatus is necessary: A glass receptacle for the solution constructed on the principle of a thermos flask for maintaining a constant temperature. From this leads a rubber tube, attached to a glass connection piece, from which are suspended several perforated fine gauge rubber tubes. Each is tied at the lower end, and perforated for about half its length. Any number of tubes can be used, depending on size of wound. The flow is regulated so that a slow dropping occurs continually, thus keeping the wound constantly bathed. A Dakin's special solution of sodium hypochlorite (0.45-0.50%) is used. It decomposes under light. Must be kept in dark bottle and not be older than 36-72 hours.

car'rier [Fr. *carier*, to bear]. 1. One who, or that which carries disease germs. 2. That which carries anything.

One may be immune to a certain germ, such as diphtheria bacilli, and yet be a "carrier" of it to others. In diphtheria, may number 1 to every 75 persons. Carriers spread infantile paralysis, cerebrospinal meningitis, septic sore throat and typhoid, cholera, amebiasis and diphtheria. From 0.5% to 11.6% of typhoid patients become "carriers." (The tsetse fly is a vector of African sleeping sickness; the anopheles mosquitoes are vectors of malaria, and the stegomyia mosquito is a carrier of yellow fever.) Typhoid bacillus can be harbored for years in gall bladder and discharged at intervals through the feces.

SEE: *vector, vection*.

CLASSIFICATION: *Animal Carriers*: Some microörganisms may be carried from an animal to man by *direct contact, indirect transfer,* or by *intermediary hosts*.

Air-borne Infection: Pathogenic organisms in the respiratory tract, discharged from the mouth or nose, may be borne on the air and settle on food, clothing, walls and floors, and if they are of the type which resists drying for a long period they may remain virulent until transmitted to another person. Coughing, sneezing, and expectorating may be responsible for "droplet infection," as may expectorations.

Contact Infection: This is the result of transmission from person to person, as in kissing, coming in contact with those afflicted with communicable diseases, or with utensils handled by one with an infection.

Food-borne Infection: Bacteria may be communicated through food. Root and salad vegetables may carry bacteria from the soil or from manure. Cooking safeguards by destroying microorganisms on food.

Human Carriers: Some parasites may live in or upon the body of those who themselves do not suffer from them, but may be carried by them to others. Carriers may be: (*a*) *Contact* carriers, or those who never show symptoms; (*b*) *incubationary* carriers, or those in whom the infection is starting but has not completed the incubation period, and (*c*) *convalescent* carriers, or those who have recovered but who still harbor the organism causing their disease.

Insect Vectors: An insect may act as a physical carrier, as the housefly, which may transmit the typhoid bacillus, or one that acts as an active intermediate host, such as the Anopheles mosquito, which transmits malaria.

Prenatal Infection: This is the result of the fetus being infected from the mother's blood stream, or from contiguity with the maternal membranes.

Soil-borne Infection: Soil-borne, spore-forming organisms commonly enter the body through wounds, as in tetanus and gas gangrene.

Water-borne Infection: Organisms producing typhoid, dysentery, cholera, and amebic infections may be carried through a water supply, or water in public pools used for bathing. These organisms may pass into the water from the feces of an infected person and be communicated to others.

 c., acute. Patient who is a carrier only during and just subsequent to the convalescent period.

 c., chain saw. Instrument for carrying one end of a thread around a bone to be cut.

 c., chronic. Individual carrying the disease-producing organism for a long period of time or permanently.

 c., drainage tube. Instrument for placing drainage tubes in narrow or deep seated tracts.

 c., ligament. Flat needlelike instrument for drawing ligament through perforations made in the fascia.

 c., ligature. I. for carrying ligatures.

 c., renal. I. for introduction into kidneys. Flexible ones, about 20 in. long.

 c., suppository bladder. I. for depositing suppositories, etc., in the bladder.

 c., temporary. Healthy individual who has not had the disease, but nevertheless carries the organism in his body.

 c., urethral. I. for introductions into ureters. Flexible ones, about 12 in. long.

Carron oil (kar'on) [From Carron Iron Works, England]. A mixture of linseed oil and lime water used as a dressing in treatment of burns.

car'rots [G. *karōton*, carrot]. COMP: Carbohydrates are high. They are principally represented by cane sugar. Carrots are valuable for their salts, 20.7% of their mineral substances escape assimilation. They contain 10% of sugar, 50% of which is lost in cooking, 39% of protein lost in digestion. They are richer in sugar but poorer in starch than potatoes and turnips. AV. SERVING: 120 Gm. Pro. 1.3, Fat 0.5, Carbo. 9.8 in av. serving. Vit. A+++, B++, C++, D+, G++. Ca 0.056, Mg 0.021, K 0.287, Na 0.101, P 0.046, Cl 0.036, S 0.022, Fe 0.00064. ACTION: The nutritive power is small. In large quantities they form a pasty, soft salt. Intestinal absorption is more defective than is the case with potatoes. They should be served with butter or cream to make up some of their deficiencies.

car sickness. Sickness induced by riding in cars. SYM: Similar to seasickness.

cartilage (kar'til-ăj) [L. *cartilagō*, gristle], A type of dense connective tissue consisting of cells embedded in a ground substance or matrix. The matrix is firm and compact rendering it capable of withstanding considerable pressure or tension. Cartilage has a white or gray color, is semiopaque, and is nonvascular. The cells lie in cavities called lacunae. They may be single or in groups of two, three, or four.

Cartilage constitutes a part of the skeleton occurring in the costal cartilages of the ribs, the nasal septum, in the external ear and lining the Eustachian tube, in the wall of the larynx, in the trachea and bronchi, between bodies of the vertebrae, and covering the articular surfaces of bones. It forms the major portion of the embryonic skeleton.

CARTILAGE

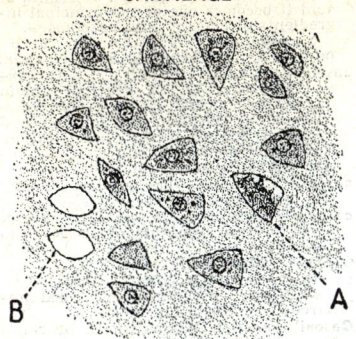

HYALINE CARTILAGE
Section of articular cartilage of the frog. A, Shrunken cartilage cells. B, Lacuna.

c. articular. Hyaline cartilage covering the articular surfaces of bones.
c. hyaline. A bluish-white glassy translucent cartilage. The matrix appears homogeneous although it contains collagenous fibers forming a fine-like network. The walls of the lacunae stain intensely with basic dyes. Hyaline cartilage is flexible and slightly elastic. Its surface is covered by the *perichondrium* except on articular surfaces. Found in articular cartilage, in costal cartilages, in septum of nose, in larynx and trachea.
c., white fibro. Bundles of white fibers pervading the intercellular substance and containing bet. them the cartilage cells. This cartilage joins bones together.
c., yellow or elastic. A network of yellow elastic fibers, holding cartilage cells, and pervading intercellular substance. Found in the epiglottis, the external ear, the auditory tube, strengthening them and maintaining their shape.

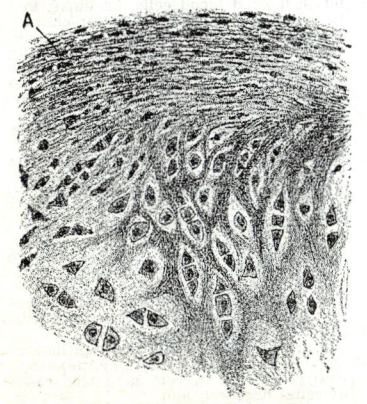

FIBROUS CARTILAGE
Section of intervertebral cartilage, calf's tail. A, Perichondrium.

cartilage, words pert. to: achondroplasia, arthrochondritis, arytenoiditis, "cartilag-" words, "chondr-" words, cricoarytenoid, cricoid, enchondroma, gristle, semilunar, y-cartilage.
cartilagin (kar-til′aj-in) [L. *cartilago*, gristle]. A characteristic principle of hyaline cartilage.
cartilaginification (kar-til-aj-in-if-ik-a′shun) [" + *facere*, to make]. Cartilage formation or chondrification; the development of cartilage from undifferentiated tissue.
cartilaginoid (kar-til-aj′in-oid) [" + G. *eidos*, form]. Resembling cartilage.
cartilaginous (kar-til-aj′in-us). Pert. to or consisting of cartilage.
cartila′go [L.]. Cartilage.
car′uncle [L. *caruncula*, dim. *caro*, flesh]. A small fleshy growth.
c., lacrimal. *Caruncula lacrimalis*. One found on the conjunctiva near the inner canthus. A small, reddish elevation of modified skin.

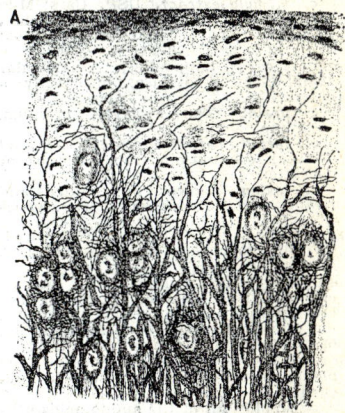

ELASTIC CARTILAGE
External ear, calf. A, Perichondrium.

c., urethral. *Carunculae myrtiformes.* A small, red, papillary growth, highly vascular, sometimes found at the urinary meatus in females. It is characterized by pain on urination and is very sensitive to friction.
caruncula (kar-ung′ku-la) (pl. *carunculae*) [L.]. A tiny, fleshy protuberance. SYN: *caruncle*.
c. myrtiformes. Shreds of the ruptured hymen. SEE: *caruncle*.
carus (ka′rus) [G. *karos*, torpor]. A lethargic, deep sleep.
c. catalep′tica. Catalepsy.
c. ecsta′sis. A trance, or catalepsy.
c. lethar′gus. Lethargy.
caryenchyma (kar-i-en′ki-ma) [G. *karyon*, nucleus, + *en*, in, + *chymos*, juice]. The fluid portion of the protoplasm of a nucleus.
caryocinesia, caryocinesis (kar″ĭ-o-sin-e′-sĭ-ă, -e′sis) [" + *kinēsis*, movement]. Nuclear changes in cell division. SYN: *karyokinesis.*
caryogenesis (kar-ĭ-o-jen′es-is) [" + *genēsis*, production]. The development of a cell nucleus.
caryogenic (kar-ĭ-o-jen′ik) [" + *gennan*, to produce]. Pert. to the cell nucleus.

caryolobic (kar-ĭ-o-lo'bik) [" + L. *lobus*, lobe]. Having a lobeshaped nucleus.

caryolymph (kar'ĭ-o-limf) [" + L. *lympha*, lymph]. The nuclear fluidlike substance.

caryolysis (kar-ĭ-ol'is-is) [" + *lysis*, loosening]. The disappearance of the nucleus of a cell; liquification of the nucleus as occurs in degenerating of irradiated tumor cells.

caryomito'sis. Nuclear changes in cell division. SYN: *caryocinesis.**

cascara sagrada (kas-kar'ă sag-rä'dă). USP. The dried bark of *Rhamnus purshiana*, a small tree grown on western U. S. coast, and in parts of South America. The bark is seldom used, either extract or fluid extract being preferable. DOSAGE: From 15 gr. (1.0 Gm.).

   c. s., *aromatic fluid extract*. USP. DOSAGE: From 20 to 60 ℳ (1.2-4.0 cc.). INCOMPATIBILITIES: Ferric chloride, alkalies, hydrochloric acid, quinine.

   c. s., *extract*. USP. DOSAGE: From 2 to 8 gr. (0.13-0.5 Gm.).

   c. s., *fluid extract*. USP. USES: Mild laxative, less pleasant, but more efficient than the aromatic fluid extract. DOSAGE: From 10 to 30 ℳ (0.6-2 cc.).

case [L. *casus*, happening]. A particular example of a disease; incorrectly a patient.

   c. brain. The calvaria; cranium, skull cap.

   c. fatality rate. Number per thousand of fatal terminations from a disease or operation.

   c. taking. A record of symptoms and history pert. to a patient. SEE: *casuistics*.

caseate (ka'se-at) [L. *caseus*, cheese]. 1. To undergo cheesy degeneration. 2. A lactate.

caseation (ka-se-a'shun) [L. *caseus*, cheese]. 1. Process of converting necrotic tissue into a granular amorphous mass resembling cheese. 2. Precipitation of casein during coagulation of milk.

casein (ka'se-in) [L. *caseus*, cheese]. The principal protein in milk, seen in milk curds.

It supplies all of the amino acids necessary for body tissue. It is a derived albumin. When coagulated by rennin or acid it becomes one of the principal ingredients of cheese. SEE: *caseinogen*.

   c., vegetable. A protein in beans, peas, and other legumes. SYN: *legumin*.

caseinogen (ka-se-in'o-jen) [" + G. *gennan*, to produce]. The principal protein in milk from which casein is derived.

It is the substance in solution and casein* is the result of its precipitation. Its conversion into casein is the essential process in the curdling of milk.

caseose (ka'se-os). The product of gastric digestion of casein.

caseous (ka'se-us). Resembling cheese; pert. to transformation of tissues into a cheesy mass.

CaSO₄. Calcium sulfate.

casoid (ka'soyd) [L. *caseus*, cheese, + G. *eidos*, form]. Bread made of a meal prepared from casein for diabetics.

Casoni's reaction (kă-so'nĭz). Appearance of a white papule on skin at site of an injection of fluid from a hydatid cyst; if it remains and increases after operation, another cyst remains.

cassava (kas-äh'vä) [Sp. *cazabe*, starch]. 1. Tapioca. 2. The manioc plant.

casse'rian ganglion. Ganglion of sensory root of 5th cranial nerve. Term used erroneously for gasserian ganglion. SEE: *gasserian ganglion*.

cast [M.E. *casten*, to carry]. 1. A solid mold of a part, usually applied *in situ* for immobilization, as in fractures, dislocations and other severe injuries.

Most often made of plaster of Paris, sodium silicate, starch, or dextrine which is rubbed into crinoline, then soaked in water, carefully applied to the part and allowed to harden.

2. Plastic or fibrous material thrown off in various pathological conditions, the product of effusion. It is molded to the shape of the part in which it has been accumulated. According to source, casts are classified as bronchial, intestinal, nasal, esophageal, renal, tracheal, urethral and vaginal; as to constituents, classified as bloody, fatty, fibrinous, granular, hyaline, mucous and waxy.

HOW TO RECOGNIZE: They have a limiting membrane enclosing a matrix or substance in which are epithelial cells, pus cells, red blood cells, granules, and fat globules. From these latter characters they take their name as epithelial casts, red blood casts, etc. Casts usually have square ends, their diameter is the same throughout, and usually they do not bend or twist. Their ends are not pointed.

   c., bacterial. Formed from a hyaline matrix filled with these elements. Their presence indicates their origin, the kidneys.

   c., bloody. Same as bacterial casts, *q.v.*

   c., broad. Same as "renal failure" casts, *q.v.*

   c., bronchial. Seen in sputum of cases with asthma and some cases of bronchitis.

   c., epithelial. Contain cells from inner lining of uriniferous tubules. Seen in acute nephritis.

   c., fatty. Those containing epithelium that has undergone degenerative changes, found in very advanced cases of renal degeneration.

   c., fibrinous. Yellowish-brown, sometimes with ragged fractures, and highly refractile.

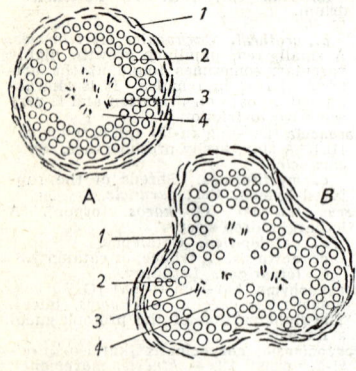

CASEATION

Diagram illustrating: A, Single tubercle; B, Three tubercles running together to produce a large central area of caseation. 1. Fibrous tissue. 2. Inflammatory cells (lymphocytes). 3. Tubercle bacilli. 4. Caseous material.

c., granular. Of varying sizes and made up of albumin and white blood cells, and of serious import in nephritis in its acute and chronic forms.

c., hyaline. Pale cylinders with rounded edges and variable size. Found in irritating conditions of the kidneys, nephritis, and its varying forms.

c., pseudo-. These are epithelial cells swollen and held in groups, resembling casts. Alkaline urine has a tendency to dissolve casts.

c., pus. Found in urine in suppuration of kidney.

c., "renal failure." Those occurring only in last stages of severe renal disease.

c., urinary. Those found in the urine. They may be *hyaline casts.*

c., uterine. Those from the uterus passed in exfoliative endometritis or membranous dysmenorrhea.

c., waxy. Light yellowish, well defined, with tendency to split transversely, found in some cases of amyloid degeneration, and advanced nephritis.

cas′tor oil [Oleum ricini]. A fixed oil expressed from the seed of the plant.

USES: Most valuable and extensively used active purgative in medicine. Esp. desirable in treatment of diarrhea, dysentery, and acute digestive disturbances; often used as a cathartic after parturition and major operations. A somewhat neglected use of this drug is to arrest vomiting due to gastric irritation. The first dose may be vomited, but, if repeated immediately, the second or third dose is almost certain to be retained and have a beneficial effect. Externally, it is used in the treatment of burns, ulcers, and chronic indurative skin diseases, and in such eye conditions as burns and diphtheritic conjunctivitis.

ACTION: Efficient purgative, followed by a tendency to check intestinal activity.

DOSAGE: 4 drams (15 cc.), for adults; 1 dram (4 cc.), for children.

ADM: Give cold with fruit juices, brandy, whiskey, or sodium carbonate.

NP: For adults, a little black coffee just before and after the oil. For children, cover dessert spoon with sugar, pour in oil and powder with sugar. Give drink of milk just before and after.

cas′trate [L. *castrāre*, to prune]. 1. To remove the testicles or ovaries. 2. One who has been castrated. SEE: *spay.*

cas′trated. Desexed; emasculated.

castration (kas-tra′shun) [L. *castrāre*, to prune]. Emasculation; excision of the testicles or ovaries; the analogy of spay.* SEE: *oophorectomy, orchotomy, testectomy.*

c. complex. Morbid fear of castration.

casualty (kaz′u-al-tī) [L. *casualis*, accidental]. 1. Accident causing injury or death. 2. One so disabled, as a soldier.

casuistics (kaz-ū-is′tiks) [L. *casus*, a case]. Study of pathological cases.

cata- [G.]. Prefix: Down or downward; against, or according to, as *catabolism.*

catabasis (kat-ab′a-sis) [G. *kata*, down, + *basis*, going]. The decline of a disease.

catabat′ic. Pert. to catabasis.*

catabiotic (kat″ă-bī-ot′ik) [G. *kata*, down, + *bios*, life.] Used up in the performance of the vital processes.

catabol′ergy [G. *katabolē*, a casting down, + *ergon*, work]. The energy expended by catabolic processes. [olism.

catabolic (kat-a-bol′ik). Pert. to catabcatab′olin. Any product of catabolism.

catabolism (ca-tab′o-lizm) [G. *katabolē*, a casting down]. One of the two metabolic changes, the other being *anabolism.*

Catabolism is the disintegration of living cells into simpler substances, most of which are excreted. Complex molecules are split into smaller ones, others by hydrolysis, with the absorption of water, into simpler ones, and by oxidation. It is the opposite of anabolism, *q.v.* Together they represent metabolism, *q.v.* SEE: *catastate, disintegration.*

catabolite (kat-ab′o-līt). Any catabolism product. SYN: *catabolin.*

cataclasis (kat-ă-clas′is) [G. *kata*, down, + *klasis*, a break]. A fracture.

catacleisis (kat-ak-lī′sis) [" + *kleisis*, closure]. Closure of eyelids by spasm or adhesion.

catacrot′ic [" + *krotos*, beat]. Manifesting the downstroke of a pulse tracing interrupted by an upstroke.

catacrotism (kat-ak′ro-tizm) [" + " + *ismos*]. A pulse with one or more secondary expansions of artery following main beat.

catadicrotic (kat-a-di-krot′ik) [" + *dis*, twice, + *krotos*, beat]. Manifesting 1 or more secondary expansions of a pulse.

catadi′crotism [" + " + " + *ismos*]. Two minor expansions following the main beat of an artery.

catadioptric (kat″ă-dī-op′trik) [" + *diopsesthai*, to see through]. Pert. to refraction and reflection of light.

catadrome (kat′ad-rōm) [" + *dromos*, running]. The onset or the decline of a disease.

catagenesis (kat-ă-jen′es-is) [" + *genesis*, production]. Retrogression or involution.

catagma (kat-ag′mă) [G. *kata*, down, + *agmos*, fracture]. A fracture; a broken bone.

catalase (kat′a-lās). An enzyme present in cells esp. anaerobic bacteria which catalyses the decomposition of hydrogen peroxide to water and oxygen.

catalepsy (kat′al-ep-sī) [G. *kata*, down, + *lēpsis*, seizure]. 1. A neurosis characterized by a loss of sensibility and voluntary movements without any perceptible alteration in circulation. 2. Abnormal condition of muscular rigidity and loss of will, accompanied by hysterical coma. 3. Muscular rigidity occurring under hypnosis.*

Any form of sustained immobility and stupor, esp. the waxy flexibility (*flexibilitas cerea*) seen typically in schizophrenia.*

catalep′tic. Pert. to catalepsy.

cataleptiform (kat-al-ep′tī-form) [G. *kata*, down, + *lēpsis*, seizure, + L. *forma*, shape]. Having the form of catalepsy.

catalep′toid [" + " + *eidos*, resemblance]. Resembling or simulating catalepsy.

catalysis (kat-al′is-is) [G. *katalysis*, dissolution]. Decomposition produced chemically by a substance not affected by the reaction.

catalyst (kat′al-ist) [G. *katalysis*, dissolution]. 1. An agent producing catalysis. 2. An agent employed to speed or maintain a reaction in which it does not participate. SEE: *catalytic, agent.*

catalytic (kat-al-it′ik) [G. *katalysis*, dissolution]. Pert. to catalysis.*

c. agent. A material or substance that, without itself reacting or undergoing change, induces a reaction that cannot take place without its presence.

catalyzer (kat′al-i-zer) [G. *kata*, down, + *lysis*, loosening]. An agent which speeds or maintains a reaction in which it does not take part; a catalyst.*

catamenia (kat-a-me′nĭ-ă) [" + *mēn*, month]. The menses. Periodic menstrual discharge of blood from the uterus.

catame′nial. Pert. to the menses or catamenia.

catamnesis (kat-am-ne′sis) [G. *kata*, down, + *mnēmē*, memory]. A patient's history, after first being seen by physician, including all subsequent examinations. SEE: *anamnesis*.

cataphasia (kat-a-fa′zĭ-ă) [" + *phasis*, speech]. A speech disorder causing an involuntary repetition of the same word.

cataphora (kat-af′o-ră) [G. *kataphora*, lethargy]. Lethargy with short remissions.

cataphoresis (kat-a-for-e′sis) [G. *kata*, down, + *phorēsis*, being carried]. The transmission of electronegative ions or drugs into the body tissues or through a membrane by use of an electric current.

cataphoria (kat-af-o′rĭ-ă) [" + *pherein*, to bear]. Tendency of visual axes to incline below the horizontal plane.

cataphor′ic. Pert. to cataphora or cataphoresis.

cataphre′nia [G. *kata*, down, + *phrēn*, mind]. A dementia type tending to recovery but which shows mental debility.

cataphylaxis (kat-ă-fĭ-laks′is) [" + *phylaxis*, guard]. The process of carrying antibodies, leukocytes, etc., to the site of an infection.

cataplasia (kat-ă-pla′zĭ-ă) [" + *plassein*, to form]. Degenerative change in tissues or cells.

cataplasis (kat-ap′las-is) [" + *plassein*, to form]. 1. The period of decline in life. 2. Application of a coating or a plaster.

cat′aplasm [G. *kataplassein*, to spread over]. A poultice, *q.v.*

The most commonly used are flaxseed, onion, bread and milk, and bran. They are used as counterirritants, drawing the blood to the surface of the body, thereby removing deep seated inflammation.

cataplectic (kat-ă-plek′tĭk) [G. *kata*, down, + *plēxis*, stroke]. Pert. to cataplexy.

cataplexy, cataplexia (kat′a-pleks-ĭ, -pleks′ĭ-a) [" + *plēxis*, stroke]. A form of sudden shock, accompanied by loss of muscular tone, without loss of consciousness, the patient falling to the floor.

ETIOL: May be the result of intense emotion or the sudden onset of a disease or rarely a part of a narcoleptic* attack.

cataptosis (kat-ap-to′sis) [" + *ptōsis*, a falling]. Ptosis; apoplexy, epilepsy, paralysis.

cat′aract [G. *katarraktēs*, a rushing down]. Opacity of lens of eye or its capsule or both.

VARIETIES: Capsular, polar, lamellar, nuclear, cortical, morgagnian (fluid cataract with hard nucleus). Also, congenital, infantile, traumatic, diabetic, and senile, occurring bet. 50-60 years.

STAGES: (a) Incipient stage (spoke-shaped opacities, cloudlike opacities, opacity of cortex or nucleus. (b) Stage of swelling, or immature stage (swollen lens, shallow ant. chamber). (c) Mature stage (lens shrinks due to loss of fluid and becomes opaque, ant. chamber regains its normal depth, no shadow thrown by iris or lens with focal illumination). (d) Hypermature stage (lens becomes either solid and shrunken or soft and liquid).

ETIOL: General diseases (diabetes); occupation (glass blowers); traumatic (concussion, foreign bodies, electric shock); ocular diseases cause complicated or secondary cataracts (iridocyclitis, choroiditis, high myopia, glaucoma).

TREATMENT: A. Extraction, intracapsular, extracapsular. 1. Combined (with iridectomy). 2. Simple (without iridectomy). B. Discission.

c., operation for. NP: *Preoperative*: Shampoo hair if possible, braid in two braids at side of head. *Postoperative*: Avoid turning, jarring, or startling patient. Sand bags at sides of head to prevent turning until permitted. Knee roll and small pillow under small of back to relieve strain. Tie hands loosely with soft bandage at night to prevent patient touching eyes in sleep; explain reason to patient to prevent fright. *Dressing*: A mydriatic, antiseptic lint, petrolatum, antiseptic cotton, narrow flannel roller bandage to keep dressings in place or strip of knitted black yarn 2 inches wide and long enough to cover both eyes.

cataractous (kat-ar-ak′tus). Affected with or of the nature of a cataract.

catarrh (ka-tar′) [G. *katarrein*, to flow down]. Inflammation of mucous membrane.

SEE: *blennorrhinia, coryza, rheum, rhinitis*.

c., dry. Severe spells of coughing with little or no expectoration. Generally seen in the old in association with emphysema or asthma.

SEQUELAE: Emphysema, bronchiectases, and dilation of right ventricle.

PROG: Perfect recovery rarely attainable, but not incompatible with long life.

TREATMENT: Careful regulation of the hygiene. Constitutional.

c., epidemic. Influenza.
c., gastric. Gastritis.
c., intestinal. Enteritis.
c., nasal. Coryza.
c., pulmonary. Bronchitis.
c., uterine. Endometritis.
c., vernal. A chronic form of conjunctivitis occurring usually in spring and summer. Must be differentiated from trachoma and follicular conjunctivitis.
c., vesical. Cystitis.

catarrhal (kat-ă′ral). Of the nature of or pert to catarrh.

catastalsis (kat-as-tal′sis) [G. *kata*, down, + *stalsis*, contraction]. Downward contraction of stomach during digestion; not preceded by a wave of inhibition.

catastaltic (kat-as-tal′tĭk). 1. A nerve impulse passing from above downward. 2. An astringent. 3. A sedative or inhibitory agent. 4. Inhibiting, restraining.

catastasis (kat-as′tas-is) [G. *kata*, down, + *stasis*, halt]. Decline or quieting of symptoms. Restitution of a part.

catastate (kat′as-tāt) [G. *katastatos*, settled down]. One of a succession of catabolic conditions or substances, each being less complex, more stable, and exhibiting less functional activity than its predecessor.

catastat′ic. Pert. to catastasis or a catastate.

cato′nia [G. *kata*, down, + *tonos*, tension]. 1. A phase of schizophrenia in which the patient is unresponsive. The tendency to assume and remain in a

catatonic   C-24   **cathode, dark space**

fixed posture, refusal to move or talk are characteristic of this phase. 2. Stupor.

cataton′ic. Stuporous; pert. to catatonia.

catatricrotic (kat-ă-tri-krot′ĭk) [G. *kata*, down, + *treis*, three, + *krotos*, beat]. Manifesting a third impulse in the descending stroke of the sphygmogram.

catatricrotism (kat-a-tri′kro-tizm) [" + " + *krotos*, beat]. State in which the pulse is catatricrotic.

catatropia (kat-ă-tro′pĭ-ă) [" + *trepein*, to turn]. Having both eyes turned downward.

cat bite. Usually a punctured or lacerated wound, potentially infected with bacteria.

Frequently infected wounds follow even under careful management. If animals are rabid, may lead to hydrophobia.

TREATMENT: Generously applied antiseptic to all parts of bite. Consider cautery and debridement. Antirabies treatment when indicated. Sterile dressings.

RS: *bites, dog bites, galeophilia, galeophobia, human bites, insect bites, insect stings. snake bites.*

cat″electrot′onus [G. *kata*, down, + *ēlektron*, amber, + *tonos*, tension]. The state of increased excitability produced in a nerve or muscle in the region near the cathode during the passage of an electric current.

catenating (kat′en-āt″ing) [L. *catena*, chain]. Linking or connecting, as one disease associated with another.

catenoid (kat′en-oid) [" + G. *eidos*, resemblance]. Chainlike; pert to protozoan colonies whose individuals are joined end-to-end.

cat′gut [A.S. *catta*, to whelp, + *guttas*, to pour]. Sheep's intestine twisted for use as an absorbable ligature.

catharma (kath-ar′mă) [G. *katharein*, to purge]. Product or result of purging.

cathar′sis [G. *katharsis*, purification]. 1. Purgative action of the bowels. 2. The freudian method of freeing the mind by recalling the patient's memory of an event or experience that was the exciting cause of a psychoneurosis; abreaction, *q.v.*

cathar′tic [G. *kathartikos*, purging]. An active purgative, usually producing several evacuations which may or may not be accompanied by pain or tenesmus.

Ex: *Castor oil, calomel, cascara sagrada.* SEE: *purgative.*

cathedral glass. Window glass substitute for transmitting antirachitic rays of sunlight.

catheresis (kath-er′e-sis) [G. *kathairesis*, destruction]. 1. Weakness resulting from medication. 2. Caustic or feebly caustic action.

catheretic (kath-e-re′tik) [G. *kathairesis*, destruction]. 1. Weakening. 2. Slightly caustic.

catherization (kath″e-ri-za′shun) [G. *kathairein*, to destroy]. Act of weakening by medication.

catheter (kath′et-er) [G. *katheter*, a tube placed down into]. A tube for evacuating or injecting fluids through a natural passage. Made of elastic, elastic web, rubber, glass, and metal.

   c., double channel. One providing for inflow and outflow.

   c., elbowed. One which has an acute bend near the beak. USES: Cases of enlarged prostate.

   c., eustachian. One for injection into eustachian tube through nasal passages.

   c., female. One about 5 inches long.

   c., indwelling. One which keeps its position in the ureter.

   c., male. One for bladder evacuation. 12-13 inches long.

   c., prostatic. One designed to pass prostatic obstruction. 15-16 inches long.

   c., self-retaining. One which can be retained at will, effecting bladder drainage.

   c., vertebrated. One in sections to be fitted together, so that it is flexible.

   c., winged. One with little flaps at each side of beak to aid in retaining it in the bladder.

catheter fever. Reactionary rise in temperature from passing of a catheter or urethral bougie.

It usually occurs 24 hours after treatment, or if self-retaining catheter is used, following urination after removal.

SYM: May be rigors and sometimes severe fever, prostration, and suppression of urine.

NP: Light diet, bland drinks, avoid meat, salt, and alcohol for few days. Doctor will keep urine neutral.

catheterization (kath″et-er-i-za′shun) [G. *katheterismos*, an inserting of a catheter]. Introduction of a catheter through the urethra into the bladder for withdrawal of urine.

NP: Treatment should be explained to patient who lies on back with knees drawn up, slightly separated; pillows under head and shoulders to relax abdominal muscles; feet flat on bed. Place screen around bed, tray at right side within reach. Bedclothes arranged so nurse does not touch after scrubbing hands, separating them with elbow. A sterile towel should be placed above and below vulva of female, labia separated with first and second fingers of left hand while nurse swabs vulva with clean hand, using swab on one side only and discarding for clean one. Vestibule should also be swabbed and area about urethral orifice.

Sterile receiver is placed bet. patient's legs. Nurse holds catheter about inch from open end, drains water from it, inspects for flaws, and inserts it into meatus of urethra, being careful not to touch any other part of vulval surface. Insert gently until urine begins to flow, holding it steadily until flow ceases. By withdrawing it slowly more urine may flow. Repeat until catheter is withdrawn.

Place finger over open end, invert over receiver and empty. Dry patient and cover. Report findings and condition of patient, also time. SEE: *autocatheterism.*

catheterize (kath′e-ter-īz). To draw the urine through a catheter.

cathetom′eter [G. *kathetos*, vertical height, + *metron*, meter]. Device to aid in the reading of thermometers.

cathexis (kath-eks′is) [G. *kathexis*, retention]. The emotional or mental energy imparted to an idea.

cath′odal [G. *kathodos*, downward path]. Pert. to the cathode.

cath′ode [G. *kathodos*, from *kata*, down, + *odos*, way]. The negative pole, as opposed to the anode, or positive pole.

   c. dark space. The nonluminous region which envelops and follows the outline of the cathode in a discharge tube at moderately low pressures.

c. stream. Negatively charged electrons, sent out as particles from the cathode in discharges through the vacuum. SEE: *cathode rays.*
cathod'ic. Pert. to a cathode.
cathod'ograph [G. *kathodos,* downward path, + *graphein,* to write]. An x-ray picture; skiagram.
catholicon (ka-thol'ĭ-kŏn) [G. *katholicos,* universal]. A remedy for all diseases; a panacea.
cation (kat'ĭ-on) [G. *kation,* descending]. The name given by Faraday to the element or elements of an electrolyte in electrochemical decomposition appearing at the negative pole, or cathode.
catlin (kat'lin). Surgical knife with double edges.
catochus (kat'o-kus). 1. Coma vigil; catalepsy. 2. A trance; deathlike.
catoptric (kat-op'trik) [G. *katoptrikos,* reflecting]. Pert. to reflected light or mirrors.
catoptrophobia (kat-op-trō-fo'bĭ-ă) [G. *katoptron,* mirror, + *phobos,* fear]. Morbid fear of mirrors or of breaking them. [purgative.
catoteric (kat-o-ter'ĭk). A cathartic or
cat scratch disease. Nonbacterial regional lymphadenitis. Unknown etiology but often follows cat scratches.
cat's-eye pupil. A slitlike pupil.
cat's purr. Purring bruit due to mitral disease.
catulotic (kat-ul-ot'ik) [G. *kata,* down, + *oulē,* scar]. Tending to cause cicatrization.
cat unit. Amount of a drug, per Kg. of animal's weight, required to kill it, when injected intravenously.
cau'da [L. tail]. 1. Tail. The lower part of an anatomical structure. 2. Coccyx. 3. The penis. 4. Insertion of a muscle. 5. The clitoris. [ess. The vermis.
   c. cerebelli. Cerebellar taillike proc-
   c. coccygea. The coccyx. [cord.
   c. equi'na. Termination of spinal
   c. striati. Taillike post. extremity of corpus striatum.
caudad (kaw'dad) [" + *ad,* toward]. Toward the tail; in a post. direction.
caudal (kawd'al) [L. *caudalis,* pert. to a tail]. 1. Pert. to any tail-like structure. 2. Inferior in position.
caudate (kaw'dāt) [L. *caudātus,* having a tail]. Possessing a tail.
caudation (kaw-da'shun) [L. *cauda,* tail]. 1. A lengthened or elongated clitoris. 2. Having a tail or tails.
caudle (kawd'l) [Fr. *caudel,* warm]. A nutritious food made of egg, gruel, sherry, and flavoring.
caul (kawl) [Fr. *cale,* a small cap]. 1. The great omentum. 2. Membranes or portions of the amnion covering head of fetus at birth.
caul'iflower [L. *caulis,* cabbage, + *flos, floris,* flower]. Av. SERVING: 125 Gm. Pro. 2.3, Fat 0.6, Carbo. 3.9 per serving. Ca 0.123, Mg 0.014, K 0.222, Na 0.068, P 0.061, Cl 0.050, S 0.086, Fe 0.0006 per serving. Vit. A+, B++, C+++, G++. A base forming food. Alkaline reserve 5.3 cc. per 100 Gm., 17.5 per 100 cal. ACTION: Laxative.
caul'iflower ear. Malformation of auricle due to injury, as seen in boxers.
   c. excrescence. Condyloma of the cervix uteri.
cauloplegia (kaw-lo-ple'jĭ-ă) [G. *kaulos,* stalk, + *plēgē,* stroke]. Paralysis of the penis.
cauma (kaw'mă) [G. *kauma,* burn]. An inflammatory fever; pyrexia, heat, fever.

c. enteritis. An acute intestinal catarrh.
caumesthesia (kaw-mes-the'zĭ-ă) [" + *aisthēsis,* sensation]. A sense of heat without cause of same.
causalgia (kaw-sal'jĭ-ă) [G. *kausis,* heat, + *algos,* pain]. Intense burning pain with a glossy skin.
cause. That which induces or brings about a particular condition, result, or effect.
   c. constitutional. One that is inherent within the body.
   c. predisposing. One which favors but does not directly induce an effect.
   c. primary. The immediate or precipitating cause.
causoma (kaw-so'mă) [" + *-ōma,* swelling]. A burning; an inflammation of a burning nature.
caustic (kaw'stik) [G. *kaustikos,* capable of burning. 1. Corrosive and burning. 2. An agent that will destroy living tissue. Ex: *silver nitrate, potassium hydroxide, nitric acid.*
   c. potash. Potassium hydroxide, *q.v.*
   c. soda. Sodium hydroxide, *q.v.*
cauterant (kaw'ter-ant) [G. *kautēr,* a burner]. 1. Escharotic; caustic. 2. A caustic agent.
cauterization (kaw-ter-i-za'shun) [G. *kautēriazein,* to burn]. Burning a part; cautery.
   RS: *byssocausis, chemicocautery, electrocautery, galvanocautery, moxibustion, ustion, zestocausis.*
   c., actual. By hot iron. Atmocausis. By steam.
   c., chemical. Cautery by electrolysis. By chemical means.
   c., electrical. By platinum wires heated to incandescence by an electric current; galvanocautery.
   c., potential. By applying a corrosive substance.
cauterize (kaw'ter-iz) [G. *kautēriazein,* to burn]. To burn with a cautery, or to apply one.
caut'erodyne [" + *dynamis,* power]. A radio knife for bloodless surgery.
   It is a small pencillike tube with a wire coil in place of a blade. It seals minor blood vessels. Used for cancer and goiter operations.
cautery (kaw'ter-ĭ) [G. *kautēr,* a burner]. A means of destroying tissue by electricity, heat, or corrosive chemicals. Used in potentially infected wounds; to destroy exuberant granulations (proud flesh) or some neoplasms. Thermocautery consists of red hot or white hot object, usually piece of wire or pointed metallic instrument, heated in a flame or with electricity (electrocautery, galvanocautery).
cava (ka'vah) [L. hollow]. 1. Vena cava. 2. The vulva. 3. Any cavity.
ca'val. Pert. to the vena cava.
cav'alry bone. Rider's bone; bony deposit in the adductor muscles of the thigh.
cavascope (kav'ă-skōp) [L. *cavum,* hollow, + *skopein,* to examine]. Instrument for examining cavities.
cavernil'oquy [L. *caverna,* a hollow, + *loqui,* to speak]. Low pitched sound over pulmonary cavities.
caverni'tis [" + G. *-itis,* inflammation]. Inflammation of the *corpus cavernosum penis.*
caverno'ma [" + G. *-ōma,* tumor]. A cavernous angioma.
cavernosi'tis [L. *cavernosus,* having hollows, + G. *-itis,* inflammation]. Inflammation of the *corpora cavernosa.*

cavernosum (kăv-ĕr-nō'sŭm). One of 2 erectile columns of the dorsum of the penis or clitoris. SYN: *corpus cavernosum.*

cavernous (kăv'ĕr-nŭs) [L. *caverna*, a hollow]. Containing hollow spaces.
 c. angioma. A vascular tumor with many large spaces.
 c. body. Corpus cavernosum.
 c. râle. Bubbling hollow sound.
 c. resonance. Amphoric resonance.
 c. respiration. Hollow sound heard when there is a lung cavity.
 c. rhoncus. A cavernous râle.
 c. sinus. Blood sinus on body of sphenoid bone.
 c. tumor. An angioma.

caviar' (Turkish *khăvyăr*, salted roe]. Av. SERVING: 15 Gm. Pro. 4.5, Fat 3.0, Carbo. 1.1 per serving. Ca 0.137, Mg 0.022, K 0.422, Na 0.874, P 0.176, Cl 1.819.

cav'itary [L. *cavitas*, hollow]. 1. Hollow; having or forming cavities. 2. Any nematode worm.

cavita'tion [L. *cavitas*, a cavity]. Formation of a cavity. Ex: Formation of lung cavity in tuberculosis.

cavitis (ka-vi'tis) [L. *cavum*, hollow, + G. *-itis*, inflammation]. Inflammation of a vena cava.

cavity (kav'it-ĭ) [L. *cavitas*, hollow]. A hollow space, such as a body organ or the hole in a carious tooth.
 c., abdominal. The cavity of the peritoneum bet. the diaphragm and pelvis.
 c., amniotic. That within the amnion.
 c., buccal. The mouth.
 c., cotyloid. The acetabulum.
 c., glenoid. Cavity in head of scapula, which holds the humerus.
 c., pelvic. One containing the bladder and rectum and the uterus in the female.
 c., pulp. One in a tooth containing the dental pulp and nerve termination.
 c., Rosenmüller's. One on either side of openings of eustachian tube.
 c., splanchnic. One of three, the cranial, thoracic, and abdominal, including the pelvic cavity.
 c., visceral. The splanchnic cavity.

cavity, words pert. to: abdominal, achoresis, aerocele, arachnoid, atresia, body, camera, "cav-" words, celom, celoma, celozoic, centesis, cisterna, falling drop, fenestra, introitus, locular, -us, sinus, splanchnic, thoracic, venter.

ca'vum [L. a hollow]. A cavity or a hole.
 c. septi pellucidi. BNA. Cavity of the 5th ventricle of the brain.
 c. tympani. Middle ear cavity.

ca'vus [L. hollow]. Condition of exaggerated height of arch of foot. SYN: *talipes cavus.*

cavus. A hollow or cavity.
 c. talipes. SEE: *talipes cavus.*

Cayenne pepper (kī-ĕn', kă-ĕn'). Capsicum, *q.v.*

Cazenave's lupus (kahz-năv'). 1. Lupus erythematosus. 2. Pemphigus foliaceus.

cc. Abbr: Cubic centimeter; about 16 minims.

CCl₃.CHO. Chloral.

c.cm. Abbr. for cubic centimeter.

Cd. Symb. of cadmium.

Ce. Symb. of cerium.

ceasmic (se-as'mĭk) [G. *keasma*, chip]. Pert. to an abnormal cleavage of parts or to a fissure.

cebione (sē'bĭ-ōn). SEE: *cevitamic acid.*

cecal (se'kal) [L. *caecalis*, pert. to blindness]. 1. Pert. to cecum. 2. Blind, terminating in a closed extremity.

cecectomy (se-sek'to-mĭ) [L. *caecum*, blindness, caecum, + G. *ektomē*, excision]. Removing part of or incision into the cecum.
 NP: Preparation for appendectomy slightly modified.

cecitis (se-si'tis) [" + G. *-itis*, inflammation]. Inflammation of the cecum.

cecoileostomy (se-ko-il-e-os'to-mĭ) [" + *ileum*, ileum, + G. *stoma*, opening]. Making an opening through the abdominal wall into the ileum at the ileocecal valve.

cecopexy (se'ko-peks-ĭ) [" + G. *pēxis*, fixation]. Surgical fixation of the cecum to the abdominal wall.

cecoplica'tion [" + *plica*, fold]. Reduction of a dilated cecum by making a fold in its wall.

cecoptosis (se-kop-to'sis) [" + G. *ptōsis*, a dropping]. Falling displacement of the cecum.

cecosigmoidostomy (se-ko-sig-moid-os'to-mĭ) [" + G. *sigmoeidēs*, shaped like letter S, + *stoma*, opening]. Formation of a communication bet. the cecum and sigmoid.

cecos'tomy [" + G. *stoma*, opening]. Surgical formation of a cecal fistula or artificial anus.

cecot'omy [" + G. *tomē*, a cutting]. Cutting into the cecum.

cecum (se'kum) [L. *caecum*]. A blind pouch at the junction of the small intestines with the ascending colon, and to which the ileum is attached.
 It is slightly below the ileocecal valve and is about 2½ inches (6.3 cm.) deep. The ileocecal valve bet. prevents the backward flow of feces into the intestines. The vermiform appendix is attached to the lower part of the cecum. SEE: "cec-" words.

celarium (se-la'rĭ-um) [G. *koilos*, a hollow]. The epithelium of the celom.

-cele [G. hernia, tumor]. Suffix: A swelling.

celectome (se-lek'tŏm) [G. *kēlē*, tumor, + *tomē*, a cutting]. Instrument for obtaining a piece of tissue from a tumor for examination.

celery [Fr. *celeri*, from G. *selinon*, parsley]. Av. SERVING (raw): 40 Gm. Pro. 0.4, Fat trace, Carbo. 1.3. FUEL VALUE: 100 Gm.—18 cal. Very heavy in cellulose. VITAMINS: A— to +, B++, C++. Ca 0.078, Mg 0.014, K 0.316, Na 0.084, P 0.037, Cl 0.156, S 0.022, Fe 0.0005. Copper, 0.1 mg. per Kg. of fresh celery. A base forming food. Alkalinity, 17.3 cc. units per 100 Gm. 42 cc. per 100 cal. ACTION: It is a stomach and heart stimulant, and is considered to be a nervine, a carminative and a diuretic.

celiac (se'lĭ-ak) [G. *koilia*, belly]. Rel. to the abdominal regions.
 c. artery. The first branch of the abdominal aorta. Branches supply the stomach, liver, spleen, duodenum, and pancreas.
 c. axis. Same as *celiac artery.*
 c. disease. Dilatation of the small and large intestines causing intestinal indigestion, and occurring in children and infants, usually bet. the 9th and 18th months; sometimes bet. the 3rd and 6th years.
 SYM: *First Type:* Porridgelike stools, large in volume. *Second Type:* Diarrhea; foul, large, frothy and acid stools.
 DIET: No carbohydrates, esp. sugar, starches, potatoes, flour, grains, pastries, or puddings. No milk, fats, or cod-liver oil during first days of treatment. Ripe bananas, protein milk. Later frequent

celiac, plexus C-27 **cell**

feedings, meat juice. *Meal for Older Children*: Cottage cheese, egg white, fruits, orange juice, one vegetable at a time but no potatoes. Vitamin D, as viosterol. Maximum diet after 4 to 8 weeks: 80-100 calories per lb. of food. Diet period: One year.

Bread and cereals may be tried in small amounts 3 times a day, one at a time, 3 months apart, but they must be dropped at first signs of relapse.

c. plexus. Sympathetic plexus lying near the origin of celiac artery. SEE: *plexuses*.

celiagra (se-lĭ-ag'ră) [" + *agra*, seizure]. Gouty affection of any abdominal organ.

celial'gia [" + *algos*, pain]. Abdominal pain.

celiectasia (se-lĭ-ek-ta'sĭ-ă) [" + *ektasis*, extension]. Distention of the abdomen.

celiectomy (se-lĭ-ek'to-mĭ) [" + *ektomē*, excision]. Removal of an abdominal organ.

celiocentesis (se-lĭ-o-sen-te'sis) [" + *kentēsis*, puncture]. Puncture of the abdomen. SYN: *paracentesis*.

celiocolpotomy (se"lĭ-o-kol-pot'o-mĭ) [" + *kolpos*, vagina, + *tomē*, incision]. Vaginal opening into the abdomen for removing the products of ectopic pregnancy or of a tumor.

celioelytrotomy (se-lĭ-o-el-ĭ-trot'o-mĭ) [" + *elytron*, sheath, vagina, + *tomē*, incision]. Opening through the vagina into the abdomen.

celioenterotomy (se-lĭ-ō-en-ter-ot'o-mĭ) [" + *enteron*, intestine, + *tomē*, incision]. Incision in the abdominal wall to gain access to the abdomen.

celiogastrostomy (se-lĭ-ō-gas-tros'to-mĭ) [" + *gastēr*, stomach, + *stoma*, opening]. Incision in the abdominal wall for making a gastric fistula.

celiogastrotomy (sel-ĭ-o-gas-trot'o-mĭ) [" + " + *tomē*, incision]. Incision of stomach with abdominal section.

celiohysterectomy (se"lĭ-o-his-ter-ek'to-mĭ) [" + *ystera*, uterus, + *ektomē*, excision]. Removal of uterus through an abdominal incision.

celiohystero-oothecectomy (se-lĭ-o-his-ter--o-o-o-the-sek'to-mĭ) [" + " + *ōon*, ovum, + *thēkē*, box, + *ektomē*, excision]. Removal of the uterus and the ovaries through an abdominal incision.

celiohystero-salpingo-oothecectomy (se-lĭ-o-his-ter-o-sal-pin-go-o-o-the-sek'to-mĭ) [" + " + *salpigx*, tube, + *ōon*, ovum, + *thēkē*, box, + *ektomē*, excision]. Removal of the uterus, fallopian tubes, and ovaries through an abdominal incision.

ce"liohysterot'omy [" + " + *tomē*, incision]. Opening into the uterus through an abdominal incision.

celioma (se-lĭ-o'mă) [" + *-ōma*, tumor]. An abdominal tumor.

celiomyal'gia [" + *mys*, muscle, + *algos*, pain]. Rheumatic pain in muscles of the abdomen.

celiomyomectomy (se-lĭ-o-mī-o-mek'to-mĭ) [" + " + *-ōma*, tumor, + *ektomē*, excision]. Removal of fibroid tumors through an abdominal incision.

celiomyomotomy (se-lĭ-o-mī-o-mot'o-mĭ) [" + " + " + *tomē*, incision]. Incision of muscles of abdomen.

celiomyositis (se-lĭ-o-mi-o-si'tis) [" + " + *-ītis*, inflammation]. Inflammation of muscles of the abdomen.

celioncus (se-lĭ-on'kus) [" + *ogkos*, tumor]. An abdominal tumor.

celioparacentesis (se-lĭ-o-par-ă-sen-te'sis) [" + *para*, beside, + *kentēsis*, puncture]. Puncture of the abdomen.

celiopathy (se-lĭ-op'ath-ĭ) [" + *pathos*, disease]. Any disease of the abdomen.

celiopyosis (se-lĭ-o-pī-o'sis) [" + *pyōsis*, suppuration]. Purulent peritonitis.

celiorrhaphy (se-lĭ-or'af-ĭ) [" + *raphē*, suture]. Suture of wound in the abdominal wall.

celiosalpingectomy (se-lĭ-o-sal-pin-jek'to-mĭ) [" + *salpigx*, tube, + *ektomē*, excision]. Removal of the fallopian tubes through an abdominal incision.

celiosalpingotomy (se-lĭ-o-sal-pin-got'o-mĭ) [" + " + *tomē*, incision]. Opening of the fallopian tube through an abdominal incision.

celioscope (se'lĭ-o-skōp) [" + *skopein*, to examine]. Device for illumination of abdominal cavity.

celioscopy (se-lĭ-os'ko-pĭ) [" + *skopein*, to examine]. Use of the celioscope.

celiotomy (se-lĭ-ot'o-mĭ) [" + *tomē*, incision]. Surgical incision into the abdominal cavity.

c., vaginal. Entering the abdomen through the vagina.

celitis (se-lĭ'tis) [" + *-ītis-* inflammation]. Peritonitis; abdominal inflammation.

cell [L. *cella*, a small chamber]. 1. A small, enclosed or partly enclosed cavity, such as an air cell. 2. A mass of protoplasm containing a nucleus or nuclear material. It is the unit of structure of all animals and plants and is the physical basis of all life processes.

Cells and the products of cells comprise all the tissues of the body. All functional activities of the body are carried on by cells. The structure and form of a cell is closely correlated with its functioning. Cells arise only from preexisting cells, new cells arising by cell division (mitosis or amitosis). Growth and development result from the increase in numbers of cells and the differentiation of cells into different types of tissues. Reproduction is accomplished by specialized germ cells, the spermatozoa and ova, which contain in their nuclei the genes or determiners for hereditary characteristics.

Cell inclusions or paraplastic bodies include (1) *food substances* fat droplets, glycogen and protein granules (2) *chromphil substance* (Nissl bodies). (3) *pigment granules* (melanin) (4) *crystals* of various substances. (5) secretory granules.

Also present in the cytoplasm are submicroscopic bodies called *microsomes*, demonstrated by differential centrifugation. Their exact nature is unknown.

Structure. A typical cell, when killed, fixed and stained, exhibits a centrally located *nucleus* surrounded by *cytoplasm*. (a) *Nucleus*. The nucleus possesses a *nuclear membrane* which encloses a clear *nuclear sap* or *karyoplasm* within which are twisted filaments, *chromonemata*, which contain *chromatin*, a material which stains densely

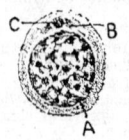

CELL
From testicle of salamander showing: A, Nucleus with chromatin network. B, Centrosome. C, Centriole.

cell, adipose   C-28   **celology**

with basic stains. A network of fine filaments, the *linin net*, supports the chromonemata. Usually present are one or more densely staining bodies, the nucleoli. (b) *Cytoplasm.* This includes the cell protoplasm lying outside the nucleus. Its outermost layer constitutes the *cell membrane* which forms the limiting membrane of the cell. Within the ground substance of the cytoplasm are found cell *organoids,* living components of the cell, and *inclusions* or paraplastic substances which are nonliving. Organoids present in most cells include (1) *chondriosomes* or *mitochondria.* (2) Golgi apparatus. (3) *cell center* or *attraction sphere.* (4) *fibrils* (5) *plastids*, common in plant cells but usually lacking in animal cells.

A cell may produce other cells, and it has the power of exercising the vital processes of life. Cells of one tissue differ from those of other tissues, depending upon the function they perform. Those of one tissue in man are very similar to those of corresponding tissues in all mammals and in fish. The protoplasm of the cell without its nucleus is known as *cytoplasm.**

RS: *amitosis, karyokinesis, mitosis.*

  c., adipose. A fat cell.
  c., blood. An erythrocyte or a leukocyte.
  c. body. Part of the nerve cell or neuron which contains the cell nucleus and cytoplasm. SEE: *nerve.*
  c., daughter. One from a parent cell.
  c., endothelial. A flat c. making up the lining membranes of vessels.
  c., epithelial. One forming epithelial surfaces of membranes and skin.
  c., giant. Large multinucleated cells found in bone marrow; a magakaryocyte. They are thought to give rise to blood platelets.
  c., glia. Spider or mossy cell in neuroglia tissue. SYN: *neuroglia c.*
  c., goblet. Epithelial c. distended with mucus.
  c., interstitial, c., Leydig's. One of many found in connective tissue of the seminiferous tubules of the testes, and such tissues of the ovary which account for their internal secretion.
  c., mother. One which gives rise to 2 or more daughter cells.
  c. mucous. (1) A cell which secretes mucus found in mucus secreting glands. (2) A goblet cell.
  c. neuroglia. Non-nervous cells found in the central nervous system and the retina of the eye. Includes astrocytes oligodendrocytes, and microglia.
  c. plasma. A cell thought to be derived from large lymphocytes. They are found in serous membranes, lymphatic tissues and loose connective tissue.
  c. prickle. A cell possessing spinelike protoplasmic processes which connect with similar processes of adjoining cells. Found in the stratum germinativum of the epidermis.
  c., pus. Pyocyte, pus corpuscle.
  c., pyramidal. A nerve cell of the cerebral cortex.
  c., sickle. An abnormal erythrocyte in anemia.
  c., spider. Star-shaped cell in neuroglia tissue. An astrocyte.
  c., squamous. Flat, scalelike, epithelial cell.

Cellano factor (sĕl'ăn-ō făkt'ŏr). One rarely found lacking in the blood; 99.8 per cent have it. Named for woman by that name who did not have it.

cellase (sel'as). An enzyme acting upon cellose.*
cell-color ratio. The product of dividing the percentage of hemoglobin into the number of red blood cells in a cc.
cellophane (sĕl'ō-fān). Thin, transparent, waterproof sheet of viscose.
  Used as a wound dressing because it does not crack, is singularly free of infection, and wound can be seen without its removal.
cell-organ. A part of certain cells which may perform digestive functions. Ex: *cytosome, plastic.*
cel'lula (pl. *cellulae*) [L. little cell]. 1. A minute cell. 2. A small compartment.
cel'lular. 1. Pert. to, composed of, or derived from cells. 2. Areolar; having interstices.
cellulicidal (sel-ū-lĭ-sī'dal) [" + *caedere,* to kill]. Destructive to cells.
cellulif'ugal [" + *fugere,* to flee]. Extending or moving away from a cell.
cellulin (sel'ū-lin). A carbohydrate forming the basis of vegetable fiber. SYN: *cellulose.*
cellulipetal (sel-ū-lip'et-al) [L. *cellula*, little cell, + *petere,* to seek]. Extending or moving toward a cell.
cellulitis (sel-u-lī'tis) [" + G. *-itis,* inflammation]. Inflammation of cellular or connective tissue, spreading as in erysipelas.
  A deep abscess, in pushing its way to the surface, may result in the formation of a *sinus* leading to an exit on the surface. If the inflammatory fluids are forced into the tissues, rather than being discharged on the surface, and inflammation of tissues results, the condition is known as *cellulitis.*   [pus.
  c., diffuse. That accompanied with
  c., pelvic. Parametritis; inflammation of the parametrium.* Occurs in puerperal fever, or septic conditions of the uterus and appendages.
cellulofi'brous [" + *fibra*, fiber]. Both cellular and fibrous.
celluloneuritis (sel"u-lo-nū-rī'tis) [" + G. *neuron*, nerve, + *-itis,* inflammation]. Inflammation of nerve cells.
  c., acute anterior. Polyneuritis and Landry's paralysis.
cellulose (sel'u-los) [L. *cellula*, little cell]. A fibrous form of carbohydrate constituting the supporting framework of plants; plant fiber.
  It stimulates peristalsis and aids in intestinal elimination. It is not ordinarily chemically changed or absorbed in digestion, remaining a polysaccharide.*
  IND: Atonic constipation due to lax muscular tone.
  CONTRA: Cellulose foods should not be eaten in acute intestinal troubles without the advice of a physician.
  SEE: *cellulin.*
  c. or fiber containing foods. Apples, apricots, asparagus, beans, beets, bran flakes, broccoli, cabbage, celery, mushrooms, oatmeal, onions, oranges, parsnips, prunes, spinach, turnips, wheat flakes, whole grains, whole wheat bread.
  c. high diet. High residue diet, q.v.
cellulotox'ic [" + G. *toxikon*, poison]. 1. Poisonous to cells. 2. Caused by cell toxins.
cel'oglass. Window glass substitute for transmitting antirachitic rays of sunlight.
celol'ogy [G. *kēlē*, hernia, + *logos,* study]. The surgical study of hernias.

celom, celoma (se'lom, se-lo'mä) [G. *koilōma*, a hollow]. The body cavity, esp. of the embryo. The collom.

celonychia (se-lo-nik'ĭ-ä) [G. *koilos*, hollow, + *onyx, onych-*, nail]. Fingernails with concave outer surface.

celoschisis (se-los'kĭ-sis) [G. *koilia*, belly, + *schisis*, fissure]. Congenital fissure of the abdominal wall.

celoscope (se'los-kōp) [G. *koilos*, hollow, + *skopein*, to examine]. Device for throwing light into a cavity.

celosomia (se-lo-so'mĭ-ä) [G. *kēlē*, hernia, + *sōma*, body]. Congenital protrusion of viscera.

celotomy (se-lot'o-mĭ) [" + *tomē*, incision]. A cutting operation for strangulated hernia.

celozo'ic [G. *koilia*, belly, + *zōon*, animal]. Inhabiting any cavity of the body, such as parasitic protozoa.

Cel'sius scale. The reverse of the centigrade scale; a degree Celsius being 1.8 degree Fahrenheit; the boiling point, F. 212°, being zero C., the freezing point, F. 32°, being 100° C.

cementi'tis [L. *caementum*, cement, + G. *-itis*, inflammation]. Inflammation of the dental cementum.

cementoblast (se-men'to-blast) [" + G. *blastos*, germ]. A cell of the inner layer of the dental sac of a developing tooth. They deposit cementum q.v. upon the dentine of the root.

cementocla'sia [" + G. *klasis*, breaking]. Decay of the cementum of a tooth root.

cementoma [" + G. *-ōma*, tumor]. A tumor having its origin in the substantia ossea.

cementum. Thin layer of modified bone formed by cementoblasts and deposited upon the dentine of the root of a tooth; the substantia ossea. To it is attached the alveolar periosteum or peridental membrane which binds the tooth to its socket.

cenesthesia, cenesthesis (sen-es-the'zĭ-ä, -sis) [G. *koinos*, common, + *aisthēsis*, feeling]. 1. A hysterical condition resulting in loss of the consciousness of identity. 2. The sense of pleasurable or painful existence in states of exaltation or depression. 3. The sensing of the normal functioning of the body organs.

cenesthe'sic, cenesthet'ic [" + *aisthēsis*, feeling]. Pert. to cenesthesia.

cenesthopathia (sen-es-tho-path'ĭ-ä) [" + *pathos*, disease]. (1) Malaise or a general feeling of lack of well-being in illness.

cenopho'bia [G. *kenos*, empty, + *phobos*, fear]. Morbid fear of open spaces and of crowds. Syn: *agoraphobia*.

cenopsychic (sen-o-si'kik) [G. *kainos*, new, + *psychē*, mind]. Only recently appearing in mental development.

cenosis (se-no'sis) [G. *kenos*, empty, + *-ōsis*, infection]. 1. Evacuation. 2. Inanition.

cenosite (se'no-sīt) [G. *koinos*, common, + *sitos*, food]. A microörganism not depending for life upon its host, but parasitic in character.

cenotic (se-not'ik) [G. *kenos*, empty]. 1. Purgative; drastic. 2. Pert. to cenosis.

cenotophobia (se-no-to-fo'bĭ-ä) [G.*kainos*, new, + *phobos*, fear]. Morbid aversion to new things and new ideas.

cenotype (sen'o-tīp) [G. *koinos*, common, + *typos*, a type]. An original type.

cen'sor [L. *censere*, to judge]. Psy: A psychic inhibition that prevents abhorrent unconscious thoughts or impulses from seeking objective expression unless in a form unrecognized by consciousness.

center (sen'ter) [G. *kentron*, middle]. 1. Middle point of a body. 2. Nerve cells governing a function.

c., accelerating. One in the medulla accelerating to the heart.

c., arm. One in cerebral cortex controlling arm movements.

c., association. Center controlling associated movements.

c., auditory. One for hearing, in the gyri in sylvian fissure.

c., cardioinhibitory. Medullary center which slows heart action.

c., ciliospinal. One which dilates the pupils.

c., deglutition. One which controls swallowing.

c., diabetic. One in ant. half of floor of fourth ventricle, post. part; glycosuria excited by its puncture.

c., epiotic. Ossification center of mastoid process.

c., erection. Found in lumbar region of spinal cord; controlled from oblongata.

c., gustatory. One in cerebrum which controls taste.

c., leg. One controlling leg movements; located in ascending frontal convolution.

c., motor cortical. Nerve center controlling voluntary movement.

c., nerve. One of many in cerebrospinal or ganglionic nervous systems originating or controlling vital function.

c., ossification. Spot where ossification begins in bones.

c., reflex. Cerebral center transforming sensory impressions into efferent motor ones.

c., respiratory. Medullary center in fourth ventricle controlling breathing.

c., spasm. At junction of medulla and pons; injury causes convulsions.

c., speech. One for articulate speech memories; located in post. part of third left frontal convolution.

c., sweat. Medullary center, subsidiary centers in spinal cord. Controls sweating.

c., temperature. One controlling body temperature.

c., trophic. One of many located in cerebrospinal and sympathetic systems presiding over nutrition.

c., visual. In occipital lobe. Controls sight.

c., word. Cerebral center controlling perception of word meanings.

centesimal (sen-tes'im-al) [L. *centesimus*, hundredth]. Divided into or rel. to hundredths.

centesis (sen-te'sis) [G. *kentēsis*, puncture]. Puncture of a cavity.

centigrade (sen'ti-grād) [L. *centum*, a hundred, + *gradus*, a step]. A thermometer divided into 100° bet. the boiling and freezing point, which is 0 degree. See: *thermometer*.

cen'tigram [" + G. *gramma*, a small weight]. A measure of weight; the hundredth part of a gram; 0.15432 gr. See: *metric measures*.

centiliter (sen'tĭ-le-ter) [" + G. *litra*, measure of wt.]. One hundredth part of a liter; 10 cc.

centimeter (sen'tĭ-me-ter) [" + G. *metron*, measure]. One-hundredth part of a meter; 2/5 of a linear inch (0.3937).

centinormal (sen-tĭ-nor'măl) [" + *norma*, rule]. One-hundredth part of the normal, as the strength of a solution.

centrad (sen'trad) [G. *kentron*, center, + L. *ad*, toward]. Toward the center.

central (sen'tral). Situated at, or rel. to, a center.
  c. bodies. Attraction center of a cell. SYN: *centrosome*.
  c. nervous system. Brain and spinal cord, including their nerves and end organs, controlling voluntary acts. Also called cerebrospinal system, and voluntary nervous system.
  Composed of nerve tissue which forms the brain, spinal cord and the nerves from both. Tissue is made up of gray and white matter. Gray matter is composed of cells of nervous tissue, while the white matter is composed of nerve fibers from the cells. White matter in the brain and cord carries messages or impulses from the body, or outside world, to the cells or gray matter.
  GENERAL FUNCTION OF CENTRAL NERVOUS SYSTEM: Includes: (1) Parts of the brain governing consciousness and mental activities; (2) parts of brain, spinal cord and their sensory and motor nerve fibers controlling skeletal muscles, and (3) end-organs of the body-wall. SEE: *autonomic, parasympathetic, and sympathetic nervous systems*.

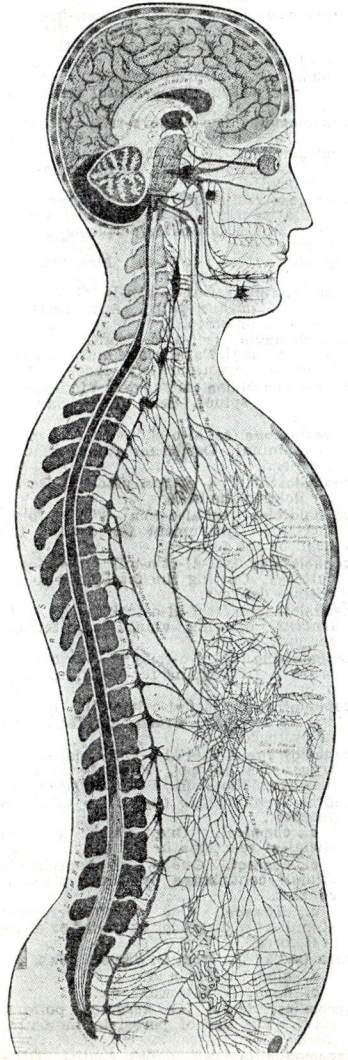

centraphose (sen'tra-fōz) [G. *kentron*, center, + *a-*, priv. + *phōs*, light]. A subjective sensation of a dark spot originating in the optic brain centers. SEE: *centrophose, chromophose*.

cen'tre. Center.

centric (sen'trik). Pert. to a center.

centriciput (sen-tris'ĭ-put) [G. *kentron*, center, + L. *caput*, head]. The central part of upper surface of skull, bet. the occiput and sinciput.

centrifugal (sen-trif'u-gal) [" + L. *fugere*, to flee]. Receding from the center.
  SEE: *axifugal, centrifuge*.
  c. force. The force which impels a thing, or parts of it, outward from the center of rotation.

centrifuge (sen'trĭ-fūj). A machine for the separation of heavier materials from lighter ones, through the employment of centrifugal force.* Used in testing for solids in urine, corpuscles in blood, etc.

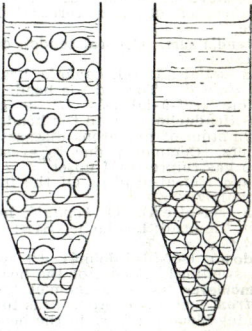

EFFECT OF CENTRIFUGING
Rapidly whirling a tube of blood in a centrifuge hastens sedimentation, and separates corpuscles from plasma. Generally 12 cc. of blood yield 6 cc. of packed corpuscles and 6 cc. of supernatant plasma. (Highly schematic.)

centriole (sĕn'trĭ-ōl). A minute body found in the cell center or attraction sphere of a cell. Preceding mitosis it divides, forming two daughter centrioles (diplosomes). During mitosis the centrioles migrate to opposite poles of the cell and each form the center of the aster to which the spindle fibers are attached. SEE: *mitosis*.

centripetal (sen-trip'e-tal) [G. *kentron*, center, + L. *petere*, to seek]. Toward the center.

centrocinesia (sen″tro-sĭn-e'zĭ-ă) [" + *kinēsis*, movement]. Movement excited from central stimulation.

centrocinetic (sen″tro-sĭn-et'ĭk). Exciting motor action; pert. to centrocinesia.

THE SYMPATHETIC NERVOUS SYSTEM

centrocyte (sen′tro-sīt) [G. *kentron*, center, + *kytos*, cell]. A cell having single and double, hematoxylin stainable, granules of varying size in its protoplasm.

centrodesmus (sen-tro-dez′mus) [" + *desmos*, a band]. The matter connecting the 2 centrosomes in a nucleus during mitosis.

centrolecithal (sen-tro-les′ith-al) [" + *lekithos*, yoke]. "Term applied to ova with yolk centrally located."

centromere. A clear region on a chromosome which marks the junction of its two arms.

centrophose (sĕn′trō-fōz) [" + *phōs*, light]. A subjective sensation of a light spot having its origin in the optic brain centers. SEE: *centraphose*.

centrosclero′sis [" + *sklērōsis*, hardening]. Ossification filling a bone cavity.

cen′trosome [" + *sōma*, body]. The attraction center from which springs the reproductivity of a cell; central body. Structures that are generally double, associated with cell division and other cellular activities. SEE: *astrokinetic motions*, *centrosphere*.

centrosphere (sen′tro-sfēr) [" + *sphaira*, sphere]. The envelope encasing 2 centrosomes.

centrostaltic (sen-tro-stal′tĭk) [" + *stalsis*, contraction]. Pert. to a center of motion.

centrother′apy [" + *therapeia*, therapy]. Any local application that acts upon nerve centers.

centrum (sen′trum) [L. from G. *kentron*, center]. 1. Any center, esp. an anatomical one. 2. Body of a vertebra.

   c. semiova′le. A mass of white matter at center of each cerebral hemisphere.

   c. tendin′eum. Central tendon of the diaphragm.

cephalad (sef′al-ad) [G. *kephalē*, head, + L. *ad*, toward]. Toward the head.

cephalalgia (sef-ă-lal′jĭ-ă) [" + *algos*, pain]. Headache, pain in the head.
A symptom of numerous diseases and disorders. Commonly due to eyestrain and to gastrointestinal upset.

cephalalgic (sef-al-al′jik). Of the nature of cephalalgia.

cephalea (sef-al-e′ă) [G. *kephalē*, head]. Pain in the head; headache. SYN: *cephalalgia*.*

cephaledema (sef-ăl-ĕ-de′mă) [" + *oidēma*, swelling]. Edema of the head.

cephalemometer (sef-ă-lĕ-mom′et-er) [" + *metron*, measure]. Apparatus for determining blood pressure in the head.

cephalhematocele (sef″ăl-hem-at′o-sēl) [" + *aima*, blood, + *kēlē*, tumor]. A bloody tumor communicating with the dural sinuses.

cephalhematoma (sef-al-he-mă-to′mă) [" + *aima*, blood, + *-ōma*, swelling]. A subcutaneous swelling containing blood, often found on the head of a baby several days after birth, when delivery was accompanied by use of forceps. It becomes absorbed within 2-3 months. RS: *caput succedaneum*.

cephal′ic. 1. Cranial; pert. to the head. 2. Superior in position.

   c. version. Turning the fetus during labor so head will present.

cephalin (sef′al-in). A substance resembling lecithin derived from brain substance of an animal. USES: Locally, to arrest hemorrhage.

cephalitis (sef-al-i′tis) [G. *kephalē*, head, + *-itis*, inflammation]. Inflammation of the brain and membranes.

cephalocele (sef-al′o-sēl) [" + *kēlē*, hernia]. Brain hernia.

cephalocentesis (sef-ă-lo-sen-te′sis) [" + *kentēsis*, puncture]. Surgical puncture of cranium.

cephalodynia (sef-al-o-din′ĭ-ă) [" + *odynē*, pain]. Pain in the head; headache, cephalalgia.

cephalohemometer (sef-al-o-hem-om′et-er) [" + *aima*, blood, + *metron*, measure]. Instrument for determining changes in intracranial blood pressure.

cephalo′ma [" + *-ōma*, tumor]. A soft carcinoma.

cephalomenia (sef-ă-lo-me′nĭ-ă) [" + *mēn*, month]. Vicarious menstruation from the nose or head.

cephalomeningitis (sef-ă-lo-men-in-ji′tis) [" + *meninx*, membrane, + *-itis*, inflammation]. Inflammation of the cerebral meninges.

cephalometer (sef-al-om′et-er) [" + *metron*, measure]. Device for measuring the head.

cephalometry (sef-al-om′e-trĭ). Measurement of the head.

cephalomo′tor [G. *kephalē*, head, + L. *motus*, motion]. Pert. to movements of the head.

cephalone (sef′al-ōn) [" + It. *-one*, augmentative particle]. An idiot with a large head and sclerotic hyperplasia of the brain.

cephalonia (sef-a-lo′ni-a). Macrocephaly with hypertrophy.

cephalopathy (sef-al-op′ath-ĭ) [G. *kephalē*, head, + *pathos*, pain]. Any disease of the head or brain.

cephaloplegia (sef-al-o-ple′gĭ-ă) [" + *plēgē*, stroke]. Paralysis of muscles about head, or—less accurately—face.

cephalorhachidian (sef″al-o-ră-kid′ĭ-an) [" + *rachis*, spine]. Pert. to the head and spine.

cephaloscope (sef′al-o-skōp) [" + *skopein*, to examine]. Device for auscultation of the head.

ceph′alostat [" + *statos*, placed]. Device for holding the head.

cephalotome (sef′al-o-tōm) [" + *tomē*, incision]. Instrument for cutting the head of the fetus.

cephalotomy (sef-ăl-ot′o-mĭ) [" + *tomē*, cutting]. Cutting the fetal head to facilitate delivery.

cephalotractor (sef-al-o-trak′tor [" + L. *tractus*, drawing along]. Obstetrical forceps.

cephalotribe (sef′al-o-trīb) [" + *tribein*, to crush]. Instrument for crushing head of fetus.

cephalotripsy (sef′al-o-trip-sĭ) [" + *tribein*, to crush]. Crushing of fetal head in dystocia.

cephalotrypesis (sef′al-o-trip-e′sis) [" + *trypesis*, a boring]. Removing a bone disk from the skull. SYN: *trephination*.

ceptor (sep′tor) [L. *capere*, to take]. A receptor.

   c., chemical. One which initiates chemical reactions in the body.

   c., contact. One which apprehends stimuli contributed by direct physical contact.

   c., distance. One which perceives stimuli at a distance, by aerial or ethereal forces.

cera (se′ra) [L. from G. *kēros*]. Wax.

   c. alba. White wax.

   c. flava. Yellow wax.

ceram′ics, dental [G. *keramos*, potters′ clay]. The use of porcelain in dental work.

ceramodon′tia [" + *odous*, tooth]. Dental ceramics.

ceramuria (ser-am-u'rĭ-ă) [" + *ouron*, urine]. Excessive phosphate excretion in urine. SYN: *phosphaturia*.

cerate (se'rat) [L. *ceratum*, from *cera*, wax]. Unctuous substance of such consistency that it may be spread easily, at ordinary temperature, upon muslin or similar material, with a spatula, and yet not so soft as to liquefy and run when applied to the skin; not often prescribed. Three cerates are official.

ceratocele (ser'ă-to-sēl) [G. *keras*, horn, + *kēlē*, hernia]. Hernia of Descemet's membrane through outer layer of the cornea.

ceratonosus (ser-ă-ton'o-sus) [G. *keras*, cornea, + *nosos*, disease]. A disease of the cornea.

ceratotome (se-rat'o-tōm) [" + *tomē*, incision]. A knife for division of the cornea.

ceratum (se-ra'tum) [L. waxed]. An unctuous solid for application to the skin. SYN: *cerate*.

cercaria (ser-ka'rĭ-ă) [G. *kerkos*, tail]. A free-swimming stage in the development of a fluke or trematode. They develop within sporocysts or redia which parasitize snails or bivalve molluscs. The cercaria emerge from the mollusc and either (1) enter their final host directly or (2) encyst in an intermediate host which is eaten by the final host. In the latter case, the encysted tailless form is known as a *metacercaria*. SEE: *fluke, trematode*.

cerclage (sair-klazh') [Fr. an encircling]. Binding with metal wire of the ends of a fractured bone.

Cercomonas [G. *kerkos*, tail, + *monas*, unit.] A genus of free-living, coprozoic, flagellate protozoa. May be present in stale specimens of feces or urine; Non-pathogenic.

cercomoniasis. Infestation with *Cercomonas intestinalis*. [like structure.

cercus (ser'kus) [G. *kerkos*, tail]. A hair-

cerea flexibilitas (sē'rē-ă fleks-ĭ-bil'ĭ-tas) [L. *cera*, wax, + *flexibilitas*, flexibility]. PSY: A condition in which the limbs can be molded into any desired position.

cereals [L. *Cerealis*, pert. to Ceres, goddess of agriculture]. Edible grains.

COMP: The composition of all cereals is of a similar character. The carbohydrates are in greater proportion than are the other properties. They are mostly in the form of starch (70-80%, oatmeal 67%), and about 10-15% protein.

The albumin is radically different from animal albumin, being a protein requiring a much longer time for the enzymes to digest it. Less of it is absorbed. Nuclein is only in the bran or skin.

Vitamin B abundant in bran. Vitamin E is found in the germ. Sodium chloride small, potash and phosphorus predominate. Magnesium abundant, lime sufficient. Iron found in the germ and outer layer. Water low. The cellulose nearly all lost in grinding and bolting. The whole grain contains about 1% fat.

ABSORPTION OF CEREALS: Proteins, 85%; carbohydrates, 98%; fats, 90%.

Relative Value of the Organic Principles of Cereals

	Protein	Starch	Fats	Minerals
1st	Wheat	Rice	Oats	Barley
2nd	Barley	Corn	Corn	Oats
3rd	Rye	Wheat	Barley	Wheat
4th	Oats	Rye	Rye	Rye
5th	Corn	Oats	Wheat	Corn
6th	Rice	Barley	Rice	Rice

ACTION: Cereals do not seem to generate uric acid. Their reaction is due to lecithin and amylaceous bodies. They are completely and rapidly digested and incite glandular and muscular activity of the stomach and of the pancreatic secretion. They are primarily foods for intestinal digestion. They are antiseptic and prevent putrefaction, retard the absorption of lactose and facilitate the production of lactic acid. They are not irritating to the kidneys because of the absence of xanthic bases and low albumin content. SEE: *name of each*.

cerebellar (ser-e-bel'lar) [L. dim. *cerebrum*, brain]. Pert. to the cerebellum.

cerebellifugal [" + *fugere*, to flee]. Extending or proceeding from the cerebellum.

cerebellipetal [" + *petere*, to seek]. Extending toward the cerebellum.

cerebellitis (ser-ĕ-bel-li'tis) [" + G. *-itis*, inflammation]. Inflammation of the cerebellum.

cerebellospinal (ser-ĕ-bel-lo-spi'nal) [" + *spina*, a thorn]. Pert. to cerebellum and spinal cord.

cerebellum (ser-ĕ-bel'um) [L.]. A portion of the brain forming the largest portion of the rhombencephalon. It lies dorsal to the pons and medulla oblongata, overhanging the latter. It consists of two lateral *cerebellar hemispheres* and a narrow medial portion, the *vermis*. It is connected to the brain stem by three pairs of fiber bundles, the inferior, middle, and superior peduncles. The cerebellum is involved in synergic control of skeletal muscles and plays an important role in the coordination of voluntary muscular movements. It receives afferent impulses and discharges efferent impulse but does not serve as a reflex center in the usual sense, however it may intensify some reflexes and depress others.

cerebral (ser'ĕ-bral, ser-e'bral) [L. *cerebrum*, brain]. Pert. to the cerebrum.

c. hemorrhage. The result of rupture of a sclerosed or diseased blood vessel in brain. Often associated with high blood pressure. RS: *apoplexy, hemiplegia*.

c. cortex reflex (ser-ĕ-bral kor'tĕks). Pupillary contraction of both eyes, when a bright object is brought within field of vision.

cerebralgia (ser-ĕ-bral'jĭ-ă) [" + G. *algos*, pain]. Cephalalgia, headache.

cerebrasthenia (ser"ĕ-bras-the'nĭ-ă) [" + *astheneia*, weakness]. Neurasthenia characterized by feelings of unreality, doubt and anxiety. SYN: *psychasthenia*.

cerebration (ser-ĕ-bra'shun) [L. *cerebratiō*, brain activity]. Mental action of the brain.

cerebriform (sēr-ĕb'rĭ-form). Resembling the brain in form or structure.

cerebrifugal (ser-ĕ-brif'u-gal) [L. *cerebrum*, brain, + *fugere*, to flee]. Away from the brain; pert. to efferent nerve fibers.

cerebrin (ser'ĕ-brin). One of a number of fatty nitrogenous principles from nerve tissue, containing phosphorus.

cerebripetal [L. *cerebrum*, brain, + *petere*, to seek]. Proceeding toward the cerebrum, as nerve fibers or impulses.

cerebritis [" + G. *-itis*, inflammation]. Inflammation of the brain, esp. the cerebrum.

cerebroid (ser'ĕ-broid) [" + G. *eidos*, resemblance]. Cerebriform; resembling the brain substance.

cerebrology (ser-ĕ-brol'o-jĭ) [" + G. *logos*, science]. Science of the brain.

cerebroma (ser-ĕ-bro'mă) [" + G. *-ōma*, tumor]. Brain hernia; any mass in the brain.

cerebromalacia (ser-ĕ-bro-mal-a'sĭ-ă) [" + G. *malakia*, softening]. Softening of the brain, esp. of the cerebrum.

cerebromeningitis (ser-e-bro″men-in-jī'tis) [" + G. *menigx*, membrane, + *-itis*, inflammation]. Inflammation of the cerebrum and its membranes.

cerebrometer (ser-e-brom'et-er) [" + G. *metron*, measure]. Device for registering cerebral impulses.

cerebropathy (ser-e-brop'ath-ĭ) [" + G. *pathos*, disease]. Any disease of the brain, esp. cerebrum.

cerebrophysiology (ser″e-bro-fiz-ĭ-ol'o-jĭ) [" + G. *physis*, nature, + *logos*, study]. Physiology of the brain.

cerebropontile (ser-e-bro-pon'tĭl) [" + *pons, pont-*, bridge]. Pert. to the cerebrum and pons Varolii.

cerebropsychosis (ser-e-bro-sī-ko'sis) [" + *psychōsis*, life]. Any mental disorder due to cerebral lesion.

cer″ebrosclero'sis [" + G. *sklērōsis*, hardening]. Hardening of the brain, esp. of the cerebrum.

cerebroscope (ser-e'bro-skōp) [" + G. *skopein*, to examine]. Instrument for brain diagnosis.

cerebroscopic (ser-e-bro-skop'ĭk). Pert. to cerebroscopy.

cerebroscopy (ser-e-bros'ko-pĭ) [" + G. *skopein*, to examine]. Diagnostic use of the ophthalmoscope as applied to the brain.

cerebrose (ser'e-brōs). $C_6H_{12}O_6$, a compound (brain sugar) derived from brain tissue.

cerebroside (ser'e-bro-sīd). A phosphorous-free class of compounds existing in the brain.

cerebrosis (ser-e-bro'sis) [L. *cerebrum*, brain, + G. *-ōsis*, infection]. Any brain disease. SYN: *encephalosis*.

cerebrospinal (ser″e-bro-spi'nal) [" + *spina*, thorn]. Referring to the brain and spinal cord, as the cerebrospinal axis.

c. fever. Cerebrospinal meningitis. Inflammation of the meninges of the brain and spinal cord; sometimes called "spotted fever" because of rash on the body.

c. fluid. A water cushion protecting the brain and spinal cord from shock.

Shrinking or expanding of the cranial contents is usually quickly balanced by increase or decrease of this fluid. Possibly cell nourishment and the removal of waste are minor functions.

FORMATION OF: The fluid is formed by the choroid plexuses of the lateral and third ventricles, that of the lateral ventricles passing through the foramen of Monro to the third, and through the aqueduct of Sylvius to the fourth ventricle. Here it may escape through the central foramen of Magendie, or the lateral foramen of Luschke into the *cisterna magna*, and so over the brain and cord surfaces, occupying the subarachnoid spaces. It is absorbed by the arachnoid villi and through the perineural lymph spaces of both brain and cord.

CHARACTERISTICS: The fluid is watery, clear and colorless. Normally, the pressure of spinal fluid in a recumbent man (as determined by spinal puncture) is equivalent to 60-120 mm. of water; 200-300 mm. when sitting up. Amt: 100-150 cc. Sp. Gr.: 1.006 to 1.008.

It shows from 1-6 cells per c.mm. (they should be counted at once and not remain in the fluid); not more than 0.03% protein (serum albumen and serum globulin, esp. the latter), and 0.05% of glucose, urea, and salts, varying with the site of puncture. Its concentration and alkaline reserve are similar to that of the blood. It does not clot in standing. Though the choroid plexuses can express certain blood constituents (e. g., iodides), changes in blood sugar, chloride, or urea will manifest themselves quickly in the fluid as well. Otherwise, changes take place largely subsequent to secretion. Turbidity suggests an excessive cell count, if due to red blood cells. Centrifugalization will show a red deposit.

INDICATIONS: Formation of a web after a clear fluid has stood is characteristic of tuberculous meningitis (rarely other inflammatory reactions).

It usually shows a yellowish discoloration due to blood from the subarachnoid spaces (in contrast to blood from trauma of puncture), though for a few days the cells may not be entirely disintegrated. A similar appearance may result from a spinal block above the point of puncture; the yellow to tan or greenish fluid spontaneously coagulating due to an excessive albumen content.

If the blocking is inflammatory (luetic) the cell count is high, but even here 1.0% of albumen is almost diagnostic of block and if the count is low, even a smaller percentage is very suggestive of this so-called "Froin syndrome."

Cell count increases, esp. in inflammatory conditions. In lethargic encephalitis there may be none; in poliomyelitis and polioencephalitis it is often 40-50. The same is true of tabes paresis and syphilitic meningitis. Other types of meningitis show greater reactions and an abscess may show enormous increases. Here polymorphonuclear cells are to be recognized by special straining methods. Occasionally, tumor and other cells may be discovered. SEE: *circulation*.

c. nervous system. Nervous system of brain and spinal cord. SYN: *central nervous system, q.v.*

c. puncture. Surgical puncture, usually at the fourth lumbar interspace, to remove a specimen of the fluid for clinical examination.

RS: *cerebrospinal fluid, cisternal puncture,, spinal puncture*.

cerebrospi'nant. 1. Any agent affecting the brain and spinal cord. 2. Affecting the brain and spinal cord.

cerebrosuria (ser″e-bro-su'rĭ-ă) [L. *cerebrum*, brain, + G. *ouron*, urine]. Cerebrose in the urine.

cer″ebrot'omy [" + G. *tomē*, incision]. 1. Incision of the brain to evacuate an abscess. 2. Dissection of the brain.

cerebrum (ser'e-brum, ser-e'brum) [L.]. The largest part of the brain consisting of two hemispheres separated by a deep longitudinal fissure. They are united by three *commissures*, the corpus callosum and the anterior and posterior hippocampal commissures. The surface of each hemisphere is thrown into numerous fold or convolutions called *gyri* separated by furrows called *fissures* or *sulci*.

c. areas. On the basis of function, several areas have been identified and located. Among them are (a) *Motor projection areas* which give rise to fibers carrying efferent impulses to effector organs, the skeletal muscles. (b) *Sen-*

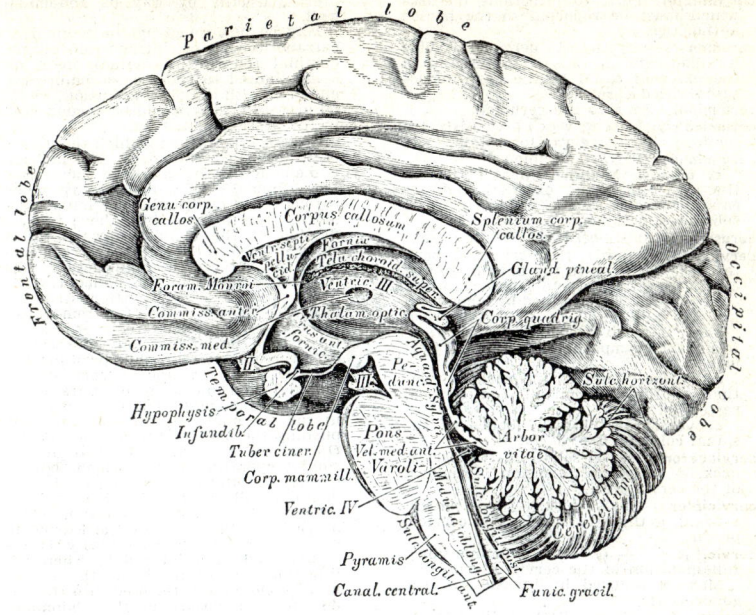

MEDIAN SAGITTAL SECTION OF THE BRAIN.

sory *projection areas* which receive impulses from sense organs or sensory receptors by way of the brain stem. These include the somesthetic, (visual, auditory, gustatory, and olfactory areas), (c) *association areas*, which are concerned with the higher mental faculties.

c. basal ganglia. These are masses of gray matter deeply embedded within each hemisphere. They are the *caudate, lentiform,* and *amygdaloid nuclei* and the *claustrum.*

c. embryology. The cerebrum develops from the telencephalon, the most anterior portion of the prosencephalon or forebrain.

c. fissures and sulci. Lateral cerebral fissure (of Sylvius), central sulcus (of Rolando), parieto-occipital fissure, calcarine fissure, cingulate sulcus, collateral fissure, sulcus circularis, longitudinal cerebral fissure.

c. functions. The cerebrum is concerned with sensations or the interpretation of sensory impulses, and all voluntary muscular activities; it is the seat of consciousness and is the center of the higher mental faculties such as memory, learning, reasoning, judgment, intelligence, and the emotions.

c. gyri. Superior, middle, and inferior frontal gyri; anterior and posterior central gyri; superior, middle and inferior temporal gyri; cingulate, lingual, fusiform, and hippocampal gyri.

c. lobes. The principal lobes: frontal, parietal, occipital, temporal, and central (insula or island of Reil).

c. structure. Each cerebral hemisphere consists of three primary portions, the *rhinencephalon* or olfactory lobe, the *corpus striatum,* and the *pallium* or cerebral cortex. The cortex is a layer of gray matter that covers the surface of each hemisphere. The part covering the rhinencephalon and phylogenetically the oldest is called *archipallium*; the more recent and larger non-olfactory cortex is called *neopallium.*

c. ventricles. Within the cerebrum are two cavities, the lateral ventricles (Nos. 1 & 2) and the rostral portion of the third ventricle.

c. vertebral. The cavity formed by the foramina of the vertebral column. Also called spinal canal, neural canal. It contains the spinal cord and its meninges.

c. Volkmann's. Small canals found in bone through which blood vessels pass from the periosteum. They connect with the blood vessels of Haversian canals or the marrow cavity.

c. white matter. The white matter or medullary substance of each hemisphere consists of three kinds of fibers (1) *commissural fibers* which pass from one hemisphere to the other, (2) *projection fibers* which convey impulses to and from the cortex, and (3) *association fibers* which connect various parts of the cortex within one hemisphere.

c. zygomatico-orbital. A canal in the zygomatic or malar bone that transmits branches of the zygomatic nerve and the lacrimal artery.

ceroma (se-ro'mä) [L. *cera*, wax, + *-ōma*, mass]. A waxy tumor that has undergone amyloid degeneration.

ce′roplasty [L. *cera*, wax, + *plassein*, to mold]. Manufacture of anatomical models and pathological specimens in wax.

cerosis (se-ro′sis) [L. *cera*, wax, + *-ōsis*, infection]. Morbid condition of membranes resembling waxlike scales.

cer'tifiable. Pert. to infectious diseases which must be reported to the health authorities.

cerumen (se-rū'men) [L. *cera*, wax]. The waxlike, soft brown secretion found in the external canal of the ear; inspissated, dried earwax.

ceru'minal. Pert. to the cerumen.

cerumino'sis [L. *cera*, wax, + G. *-ōsis*, infection]. Excessive wax formation.

ceru'minous. Pert. to cerumen.

    c. glands. Modified sweat glands in the skin lining the external auditory canal, which secrete a yellowish brown substance, cerumen.

ceruse (se'rūs) [L. *cerussa*]. White lead.

cervical (ser'vik-al) [L. *cervicalis*, pert. to neck]. 1. Pert. to the neck or to any cervix. 2. GYN: Pert. to the cervix uteri.

    c. plexus. That formed by loops joining the ant. rami of first 4 cervical nerves; it receives communicating rami from the sympathetic ganglia. SEE: *plexus.*

    c. region. That of the neck in relation to the position of the cervical vertebrae.

    c. vertebrae. First 7 bones of the spinal column. SEE: *skeleton.*

cervicectomy (ser-vĭ-sek'to-mī) [L. *cervix*, neck, + G. *ektomē*, excision]. Removal of the cervix uteri.

cerviciplex (ser-vis'ĭ-pleks) [" + *plexus*, a braid, a thing twisted]. The cervical plexus.*

cervicit'is [" + G. *-itis*, inflammation]. Inflammation of the cervix uteri.

May be induced by invasion of the gonococcus.

cervico- [L.]. Prefix: Pert. to the neck.

cervicobra'chial [" + G. *brachion*, arm]. Pert. to the neck and arm.

cervicobuc'cal [" + *bucca*, cheek]. Pert. to the buccal surface of neck of a molar or premolar tooth.

cervicofa'cial [" + *faciēs*, face]. Pert. to the neck and face.

cervicoves'ical [" + *vesica*, bladder]. Pert. to the cervix uteri and bladder.

cervimeter (ser'vĭ-me-ter) [L. *cervix*, neck, + G. *metron*, measure]. Instrument for measurement of cervix uteri.

cervix (ser'viks) [L.]. The neck or a part of an organ resembling a neck. SEE: *"cervico-"* words.

    c., laceration of. There may be: (a) Slight tearing in most primipara; (b) usually heals naturally; (c) deeper tears in manual dilatation and use of forceps; (d) breech presentation may be a cause; (e) balloon bag used if manual dilatation is indicated; (f) prophylactic treatment indicated; (g) many do not make immediate repair of cervix.

    c. uteri. Neck of the uterus. The lower part from the internal os, outward to the external os.

It is rounded and conical in shape, and a portion protrudes into the vagina. It is about 1 in. long, penetrated by the cervical canal through which the fetus and menstrual fluids escape. It is apt to be torn in childbirth, in which case it must be sutured. Laceration may be post., ant., single and bilateral, stellate and incomplete. SEE: *cauliflower excrescence.*

    c. vesicae, c., vesical. Neck of the bladder.

cesarean section (sē-zar'ē-ăn) [L. Caesar, because he was supposed to have been born in this manner]. Removal of the fetus by means of an incision into uterus, usually by way of abdominal wall.

May be performed by the vaginal or extraperitoneal or intraperitoneal abdominal routes, the vaginal operation being limited to those cases before the end of the 7th month of gestation, where no great difficulty would be encountered in the passage of the fetus.

CONSERVATIVE: One in which the uterus is not removed. *Classical:* The incision is made across the fundus of the uterus. *Low Fundal:* The incision is made through the contractile portion of the uterus from a point just above the reflection of the bladder upward for a space of 2-3 inches. *Laparotrachelotomy:* Low cervical cesarean section. The incision is made in the noncontractile lower uterine segment after stripping back the bladder flap. After removal of the fetus and placenta the uterus is sutured and the bladder flap is sewed up over the uterine scar, thus peritonealizing the scar. *Extraperitoneal:* An abdominal incision is made parallel to Poupart's ligament. The incision in the uterus is made extraperitoneally by pushing the bladder to the side. *Portes Operation:* A regular classical or low fundal operation is performed, but in closing the uterus is sutured to the abdominal wall in order that it may drain through the abdominal incision. This operation is employed by the French in cases where the uterine cavity is infected, and at a later date when the infection has disappeared, the uterus may be closed and restored into the abdomen with closure of the abdominal wall.

RADICAL: *Porro:* Cesarean section with removal of the uterus after the fetus has been taken out. This is a supracervical hysterectomy. *Total:* This is a total hysterectomy after the removal of the fetus, used in cases of badly lacerated cervices or in cases of early carcinoma of the cervix.

    c. s., absolute. Where the child cannot be delivered through the natural passages under any circumstances.

IND: (1) Contraction of the bony pelvis with a conjugata vera diameter of less than 5.5 cm. (2) Exostoses of the bony pelvis completely obstructing the birth canal. (3) Tumor masses of the soft parts which hinder the passage of the fetus (fibroid tumors, ovarian cysts). (4) At the present time *placenta praevia centralis* with a living child is considered an absolute indication. (5) Previous cesarean section without an absolute indication but where the postoperative course was stormy and a weakened uterine scar is suspected.

    c. s., relative. Where the child could be delivered through the natural passages, but where such a delivery might jeopardize the life of the mother or the child.

IND: (1) Moderate degrees of contraction of the bony pelvis with a conjugata vera diameter of about 9.5 cm. (2) *Placenta praevia marginalis* or *lateralis* where the life of the child is of great importance. (3) Transverse presentation of the fetus. (4) Oblique presentation of the fetus. (5) A large baby with a moderate degree of disproportion. (6) Habitual death of the fetus during the course of labor. (7) Impacted brow or face presentation where the fetus is alive. (8) Preëclamptic toxemia in patients where a difficult labor is anticipated. (9) Carcinoma of the cervix with rigidity. (10) In cases where hysterectomy is indicated and is to be done in conjunction with the cesarean section. (11) In cases where oophorectomy is indicated. (12) In cases where sterilization is desired, although to allow that patient to deliver normally and sterilize through the vaginal route at a later time is more satisfactory. There are several varieties of cesarean section differing mainly in the technic employed.

cesarotomy (sez-ă-rot′o-mĭ) [Caesar, + G. *tomē*, incision]. Cesarean* section.

Cestoda (ses-tōd′ă). A subclass of the class Cestcidea, phylum Platyhelminthes, which includes the tapeworms. Have a scolex and a chain of segments (proglottids). Ex. *Taenia*. They are intestinal parasites of man and other vertebrates.

cestode (ses′tōd) [G. *kestos*, girdle, + *eidos*, form]. A tapeworm; one of the Cestoda.

ces′toid. Like a tapeworm.

Cestoidea (ses-toi′de-ă). A class of flatworms of the phylum *Platyhelminthes*. Includes the tapeworms.

Cetraria (sē-trā′rĭ-ă). 1. A genus of lichens, chiefly found in northern latitudes. 2. *C. islandica*, or Iceland moss, a lichen used in treating lung and bowel disorders.

cevitamic acid (sev-ĭ-tam′ik). Crystalline vitamin C. This acid was first introduced as ascorbic acid, and is found in abundance in citrus fruits, many vegetables, such as cabbages, tomatoes, paprika, spinach, etc. It may also be prepared from adrenal glands, and from fermentation of certain sugars.

USES: Primarily, for prevention and in treatment of scurvy.

DOSAGE: As a protective in infants, 1/6 gr. (0.01 Gm.), corresponding to about 1 oz. fresh orange juice; adult, 5/6 gr. (0.05 Gm.). Intravenously, 1 1/2 gr. (0.1 Gm.) to 15 gr. (1 Gm.).

INCOMPATIBILITIES: Iron salts, alkalies, and it should be protected from heat and oxidation.

C. G. S. Abbr. for *centimeter-gram-second*, a name given to a system of units for distance, weight and time.

C_2H_4. Ethylene.

CH_4. Methane; marsh gas.

C_2H_2. Acetylene.

C_6H_6. Benzene.

Chaddock's reflexes (chad′dok). 1. Extension of great toe resulting from irritation around ext. malleolus. 2. Flexion of wrist and fanning of fingers when forearm is irritated above and near wrist.

chaeromania (ke-ro-ma′nĭ-ă) [G. *chairein*, to rejoice, + *mania*, madness]. Mania characterized by exaltation and cheerfulness. SYN: *amenomania*.

chain [Fr. *chaine*, from L. *catēna*, chain]. In bacteriology, 3 or more cells attached end to end. In chemistry, atoms held together by one affinity.

c. reflex. One in a consecutive series.

chalarosis (kal-ar-o′sis). Infection with *Chalara*, a fungus producing subcutaneous nodules which break down, forming ulcers.

chalaza (kal-a′ză) [G. sty]. Inflammation of a meibomian gland causing small tumor of eyelid border. SYN: *chalazion*.

chalazion (ka-la′zĭ-on) [G. dim. of *chalaza*, sty]. Small, hard tumor analogous to sebaceous cyst developing on the eyelids, formed by distention of a meibomian gland with secretion. A meibomian cyst. SEE: *chalaza, steatoma*.

chalcosis (kal-ko′sis) [G. *chalkos*, copper, + -*ōsis*, infection]. 1. Chronic poisoning from copper. 2. Copper deposits in lungs and tissues.

chalice cell (tshal′is) [G. *kalix*, cup]. Crateriform shell remaining after mucus has been discharged from an epithelial cell. SYN: *goblet cells*.

chalicosis (kal-ĭ-ko′sis) [G. *chalix*, limestone, + -*ōsis*, infection]. Lung disorder due to inhalation of stone particles. SYN: *pneumoconiosis, q.v.*

chalinoplasty (kal-in′o-plas-tĭ) [G. *chalinos*, corner of mouth, + *plassein*, to mold]. Plastic surgery of the mouth and lips, esp. of corners of mouth.

chalone (kal′on) [G. *chaloun*, to relax]. An autacoid that inhibits the action of a hormone* or which diminishes cellular activity. SEE: *autacoid*.

chalybeate (kal-ib′e-āt) [L. *chalybs*, from G. *chalyps*, steel]. 1. Pert. to or composed of iron; ferruginous. 2. Agent containing iron.

Chamberland filter (sham-ber-län). An unglazed porcelain filter through which water can be forced under pressure. Intercepts all but ultramicroscopic microorganisms.

chamber (chăm′ber) [G. *kamara*, vault]. Compartment or closed space.

c., anterior. The space bet. the cornea and iris.

c., aqueous. Ant. and post. chambers of the eye, containing the aqueous humor.

c., posterior. Space behind the iris, ant. to the lens.

c., vitreous. Cavity behind the lens in the eye containing the vitreous humor.

chamomile (kam′o-mĭl) [G. *chamaimelon*, earth apple, so called from smell of its flowers]. Flowers of the *Anthemis* yielding a bluish volatile oil and a bitter infusion.

chancre (shang′ker) [Fr. anything that consumes, from L. *cancer*, ulcer]. A hard, syphilitic, primary ulcer. The first sign of syphilis.

INCUBATION: Two to 3 weeks.

SYM: Begins as erosion or papule which ulcerates superficially. Generally single; sometimes multiple. Has a scooped out appearance due to level or sloping edges which are adherent. It has a shining red or raw floor with some deposit. Induration constant. No pain. Slightly purulent secretion. Heals without leaving scar. May appear on the penis, urethra, eyelid, conjunctiva, and elsewhere. SEE: *dualism, 2*.

c., hard; c., hunterian. Primary lesion of syphilis. SEE: *chancre*.

c., simple; c., soft. A nonsyphilitic venereal ulcer. SYN: *chancroid*.

c., true. SEE: *hard c*.

chancroid (shang′kroyd) [" + G. *eidos*, form]. A nonsyphilitic venereal ulcer, highly infectious; a simple or soft chancre.

INCUBATION: Two to 3 days.

SYM: Begins with pustule or ulcer; multiple; abrupt edges; rough floor; yellow exudate; purulent secretion; sensitive and inflamed. Scar remains. Rapid progress. May affect the penis, urethra, vulva, or anus.

chancrous (shang′krus). Pert. to or of the nature of chancre.

change of life. The menopause;* climacteric.*

charbon (shar-bon′) [Fr. coal]. Infection with *B. anthracis*. SYN: *anthrax*.

charcoal (shăr'kōl) [M.E. *charken*, to creak, + *coal*]. Wood charcoal. USP. Very fine powder prepared from soft charred wood.
ACTION AND USES: Internally for absorption of gas.
DOSAGE: Activated 15 gr. (1.0 Gm.), purified animal 5 gr. (0.3 Gm.).
c. fumes. SEE: *carbon monoxide*.

Charcot-Leyden crystals (shar-ko'-li'den). Elongated, double pyramid shaped crystals made up of spermine and found in the sputum of bronchial asthma.

Charcot-Robin crystals (shar-co'-ro-ban'). Tiny crystals found in blood in leukemia.

Charcot's arthropathy (shar-ko'). Joint effusion seen in locomotor ataxia.
C.'s disease. Multiple cerebrospinal sclerosis with locomotor ataxia.
C.'s joint. Result of disease of the sympathetic innervation, producing atrophic disorder of a joint.
SYM: Lightninglike pains, swelling and effusion of liquid into the joint. Marked instability of joint, destruction of bone, and dislocation.

chard [Fr. *carde*, from L. *carduus*, artichoke]. AV. SERVING: 100 Gm. Pro. 2.6, Fat 0.4, Carbo. 4.8 per serving. Vit. A+++, B+ to ++. FUEL VALUE: 100 Gm. equal 38 cal. Ca 0.150, Mg 0.071, K 0.318, Na 0.086, P 0.040, Cl 0.039, S 0.124, Fe 0.0025. A base forming food; alkalinity 5.8 cc. per 100 Gm., 41 per 100 cal.

charlatan (shar'lă-tăn) [Italian *ciarratano*, seller of papal indulgences]. A boasting pretender to special knowledge or ability, as in medicine. SYN: *quack*.

charlatanry (shar'lă-tăn-rĭ) [Italian *ciarlataneria*]. Undue pretension to knowledge or skill or an instance of it. SYN: *quackery*.

Charles' law. All gases on heating expand equally, and on cooling contract equally, according to temperature relation. Same as GAY-LUSSAC's law.

charley horse [slang]. An athletic injury, usually a bruised or a torn muscle associated with cramping in the muscles.
F. A. TREATMENT: Cold applications.

charpie (shar'pĭ) [Fr.]. Shreds of linen for dressing wounds.

charta (kar'ta) [G. *chartēs*, piece of paper]. Preparation intended principally for external application, made either by saturating paper with medicinal substances or by applying the latter to the surface of the paper by the addition of some adhesive liquid.
It should not be confounded with *chartula*, meaning "a little paper," folded so as to form a receptacle containing a dose of medicinal substance. There is no official paper.

chart'ing. The making of a tabulated record of the progress of a disease; a clinical record.
ITEMS TO RECORD: Information about the patient and his treatment that may be gathered only by the nurse who is in constant attendance. The doctor may not sit at the bedside of the patient day and night, so he deputizes the nurse to gather the information he needs. Your notes then aid the doctor in making his diagnosis, and upon these notes of the patient's reactions and progress he bases his treatment. The nurse's responsibility for supplying this information is very great. Verbal reports are not sufficient; they take time, and make mistakes possible.
Record the following:
General: BATHS AND PACKS: Record an accurate description of medicinal baths and packs, also reaction to same. Under treatments, chart hot and cold applications. [marks."
BLOOD PRESSURE: Record under "Re-
COUNTERIRRITATION: Chart under treatment. State length of *time* applied and to *what part* of the body.
DIET: If patient is on regular diet, it is sufficient to chart *Breakfast, Dinner, and Supper*, but when on any other diet, chart exactly what the patient takes. The *amount* of liquids taken should be charted, not "Water P. R. N." 1. Hours of giving. 2. Kind: full, light, soft, liquid, special. 3. Appetite: good, poor, special likes and dislikes.
DISCHARGE OR DEATH: Chart discharge or death of patient, with *hour* and *date* of same.
DRESSING ROOM: The Dressing Room Nurse is responsible for the charting of anything out of the ordinary done in the dressing room, such as a hypodermic injection, the removal of sutures, insertion or removal of a drain, or the application or removal of plaster casts.
DRESSINGS: Chart the *change* of dressings on wounds and the *amount* and *character* of *drainage*; remark "Specimen Saved" if this has been done. 1. Hour. 2. By whom done. 3. Stitches or drains removed. 4. Patient's reaction if pained or shocked by dressing.
DRUGS: Any unfavorable reaction from drugs or treatments should be charted. Chart *time* when drugs or treatments are administered. All medicines, treatments, preparation, etc., are to be charted by the nurse who administers same, whether she has charge of the patient or not. Confine name of medicine and dose to the prescribed column. When administering soluble salts, dispensed in solution, state *number of grains* administered, *not the amount of solution*. The administration of medicines other than by mouth should be indicated, as *per hypodermic, per injection, per inunction*, or *per rectum*. Any prominent or unusual therapeutic action or idiosyncrasy resulting from a drug should be recorded as a "Remark." A special prescription is written in full in the medication column the first time it is given. After that, chart ℞ Medicine or ℞ Capsule, as the case may be. After first charting, chart the name of principal ingredient, adding the word "Compound." Note discontinuance of medicine or treatment as a "Remark."
EYE: When the eye is treated for the first time, or when treatment is changed, chart the *exact medication* in detail; afterwards the remark "Eye treated" may be used.
FLUIDS: 1. Hours of giving. 2. Kind. 3. Amount. The amount should be totaled and the total charted every 12 hours.
HEAT: Chart by *whose* order heat is applied to an unconscious patient, and *who executed* the order.
INFANT FEEDING: The *formula* should be charted the *first time*; afterwards, *amount* given, and if regurgitated, approximate the *amount*.
LABORATORY: 1. Hour. 2. Kind of specimen. 3. By whom taken. 4. By whom ordered (not necessary in case of routine urine specimen on admission).
MEDICATIONS: 1. Hour of giving. 2. Kind; name of drug and preparation. 3. Amount. 4. By whom given. 5. Manner of giving: mouth, hypo, rectum, intravenous, etc. 6. Patient's reaction.

Charting, Latin Abbr. Which May Be Used in, and Their Meanings

Abbr.	Phrase	Meaning
a or āā	ana	of each
abs. feb.	absente febre	when there is no fever
a.c.	ante cibos	before eating
ad	ad	to, up to
ad effect.	ad effectum	until effectual
ad gr. acid.	ad gratam aciditatem	to an agreeable acidity
ad gr. gust.	ad gratum gustum	to an agreeable taste
ad lib.	ad libitum	at pleasure; as much as is needed
ad neut.	ad neutralizandum	to neutralization
ad sat.	ad saturandum	to saturation
adst. feb.	adstante febre	when fever is present
ad us.	ad usum	according to custom
ad us. ext.	ad usum externum	for external use
aeq.	aequales	equal
ag. feb.	aggrediente febre	when the fever increases
agit. ante sum.	agita ante sumendum	shake before taking
alt. dieb.	alternis diebus	every other day
alt. hor.	alternis horis	alternate hours
alt. noc.	alternis nocta	every other night
aq.	aqua	water
aq. bull.	aqua bulliens	boiling water
aq. cal.	aqua calida	warm water
aq. dest.	aqua destillata	distilled water
aq. ferv.	aqua fervens	hot water
aq. frig.	aqua frigida	cold water
aq. menth. pip.	aqua menthae piperitae	peppermint water
aq. pur.	aqua pura	pure water
arg.	argentum	silver
bal.	balneum	bath
bal. sin.	balneum sinapis	mustard bath
bib.	bibe	drink
b. i. d.	bis in die	twice daily
bis.	bis	twice
bis in 7d.	bis in septem diebus	twice a week
b.p.		blood pressure; boiling point
bull.	bulliat	let it boil
C.		Centigrade carbon calory
c.	cum	with
cap.	capsula	a capsule
cat.	cataplasma	a poultice
cc.		cubic centimeter
chart.	charta	paper
cito disp.	cito dispensetur	let it be dispensed quickly
c.m.	cras mane	tomorrow morning
c.m.s.	cras mane sumendus	to be taken tomorrow morning
c.n.	cras nocte	tomorrow night
cochl. amp.	cochleare amplum	tablespoonful
cochl. infant.	cochleare infantis	teaspoonful
coch. mag.	cochleare magnum	a tablespoonful
coch. med.	cochleare medium	a dessertspoonful
coch. parv.	cochleare parvum	a teaspoonful
comp.	compositus	compounded of
cong.	congius	a gallon
contra	contra	against
cont. rem.	continuantur remedia	let the medicines be continued
c.v.	cras vespere	tomorrow night
cyath.	cyathus	glassful
cyath. vinos.	cyathus vinosus	wineglassful
D.	dosis	dose
d.	da	give
d. d. in d.	de die in diem	from day to day
decub.	decubitus	lying down
det.	detur	let it be given
dieb. alt.	diebus alternis	on alternate days
dil.	dilue	dilute
dim.	dimidius	half
div.	divide	divide
div. in p. aeq.	divide in partes aequales	divide into equal parts
don.	donec	until
emp.	emplastrum	a plaster
en.		enema
exhib.	exhibeatur	let it be given
ext.	extractum	extract
ext. liq.	extractum liquidum	liquid extract
Fahr.		Fahrenheit (temperature scale)
Fe.	ferrum	iron
f.h.	fiat haustus	make a draught
f.m.	fiat mistura	make a mixture
f.p.	fiat pilula	make a pill

Charting, Latin Abbr. Which May Be Used in, and Their Meanings *(Continued)*

Abbr.	Phrase	Meaning
ft.	fiat	let it be made
Gm.		gram
gr.	granum	grain
gtt.	gutta	a drop
h. n.	hac noc'te	tonight
hor. som. or h. s.	hora somni	at bedtime
ind.	indies	daily
inf.	infusum	an infusion
inj.	injectio	an injection
liq.	liquor, oris	a liquor
m.	misce	mix
mod. praes.	modo praescripto	as prescribed
mor. dict.	more dicto	in the manner directed
mor. sol.	more solito	in the usual manner
n. b.	no'ta be'ne	note well
noct.	noc'te	night
non rep.	non repetatur	do not repeat
O.	octarius	a pint
o. d.	oculus dexter	right eye
ol.	oleum	oil
o.m.	omni mane	every morning
omn. bid.	omnibus bidendis	every 2 days
omn. bih.	omni bihoris	every 2 hours
omn. hor.	omni hora	every hour
omn. noct.	omni nocte	every night
o. s.	oculus sinister	left eye
p.a.a.	parti affectae applicetur	let it be applied to the affected region
part aeq.	partes aequales	equal parts
post. cib. or p. c.	post cibos	after eating
p.r.	per rectum	by the rectum
p. r. n.	pro re nata	as needed
pulv.	pulvis	a powder
p.v.	per vaginam	by the vagina
q. i. d.	qua'ter in di'e	four times a day
q.l.	quantum libet	as much as is wanted
q. s.	quantum sufficiat	a sufficient quantity
q.v.	quantum volueris	at will
℞	recipe	take (thou)
rep.	repetatur	let it be repeated
rep. sem.	repetatur semel	let it be repeated once only
s.a.	secundum artem	by skill
sig.	signetur	let it be labeled
sing.	singulorum	of each
s. o. s.	si o'pus sit	if necessary
ss.	semi	one-half
stat.	statim	at once
sum.	sumat or sumendum	let him take, or let it be taken
s.v.	spiritus vini	spirits of wine
s. v. gall.	spiritus vini gallici	brandy
T.		temperature
tab.	tabella, tabellae	a tablet, tablets
t. i. d.	ter in die	thrice daily
tinct. or tr.	tinctura	tincture
ung.	unguentum	ointment
ur.		urine

MENSTRUATION: Note on nurse's notes. Note in red on temp. graph, using term "catamenia."

NURSING CARE: 1. Hour. 2. Baths: shampoos; larkspur cap. 3. Alcohol rubs; decubitus dressing. 4. Special mouth care. 5. Sitting up for first time. 6. Out of bed for first time. 7. Walking for first time. (Treatments are also charted, but as treatments.)

OPERATING ROOM: Before taking chart from hall to operating room, the nurse is to assure herself that all laboratory reports are in the chart. She records second preparation for operation, and any other treatment given at that time. Record the *name of interne* or *orderly* who performs male catheterism.

OPERATIONS: 1. Name of operation. 2. Preparation for operation. 3. Preliminary anesthetic if given by nurse or on ward. 4. Hour of going to O. R. 5. Hour of return from O. R. 6. Condition on return. 7. Hour of recovery from anesthetic. 8. Condition every half hour for next 3 or 4 hours, depending on state patient is in and severity of operation.

PHYSICIAN: Record his visit. Doctor's orders must be recorded and time when they are carried out.

PHYSIOTHERAPY: Occupational Therapy: 1. Hour of going for treatment. 2. Hour of return. 3. Condition of patient.

POSTOPERATIVE: *Changing position* of postoperative patients should be recorded under "Remarks."

SPECIMENS: Record the taking of *specimens* of bloods, of exudates, transudates, etc., for examination. The result will be shown by the report of the pathologist.

SURGICAL PREPARATIONS: The nurse who does surgical preparations will sign her name after "Preliminary preparation of field of operation." Also observe the same rule for narcotics.

SYMPTOMS: Record accurate descriptions of all symptoms, such as *character of pulse* and *respiration, psychic condition, description of pain,* and *nature of any discharge,* etc. The remarks should be appropriate and well chosen. *Subjective* as well as *objective symptoms* should be recorded.

TIME: Everything relating to the patient's progress should be charted as it occurs. Record the *hour* with all statements on charts. Record on the first line of the sheet the *day* and *date of admission,* whether the patient *walked in,* or was admitted *per ambulance,* and *condition* of patient. Four-hour graphic charts are kept for all surgical and obstetrical cases the first 3 days (time 8-12-4); and for all patients whose temperature is above normal. The T. P. R. of all other patients are charted at 6 A. M. and 4 P. M.

TREATMENTS: 1. Hour of giving. 2. Nature of treatment. 3. By whom given. 4. Patient's reaction.

VISITS OF CLERGYMAN (specially important in case of Roman Catholic patients): 1. Hour. 2. Name of clergyman. 3. Rite performed.

X-RAY: 1. Hour. 2. To x-ray room, or portable at bedside. 3. Return from x-ray room. 4. Condition of patient.

MISCELLANEOUS: Any sudden or marked change in patient's condition. Notification of patient's relatives and clergyman. Special charts are also provided for certain purposes, such as the temperature, pulse and respiration chart; an anesthesia chart, generally kept by the anesthetist; blood-pressure chart, used in conditions apt to affect the blood pressure; intake and output charts used in nephritis, and laboratory records usually filed with the patient's chart. If any laboratory records have been made and not filed with the chart, their existence should be noted on the clinical chart at the time made and also upon the final page of the chart.

Physical Symptoms: 1. APPETITE: Good. Poor. Special likes or dislikes.

2. CONVULSIONS: Type. Duration. Consciousness lost. Aura.

3. DEFECATION: SEE: *Excretions and Feces.*

4. DIAPHORESIS: State whether slight, moderate, or profuse.

5. EMESIS: State the *amount, color, odor, consistency* of the vomitus, and *manner of ejecting.* (SEE: Nausea.)

6. ENEMAS: Results and *unusual appearances,* distention before or after; describe *results* fully. Note whether or not flatus was expelled with the return of the enema. Chart the *solution,* the *strength,* and *amount* used. Also for douches and irrigations.

7. EXCRETIONS: Chart *time, character,* and *other facts.*

8. FECES: Enema or natural movement. Amount. Consistency. Abnormal constituents. Defecation accompanied by pain or tenesmus. [Rash.

9. GENERAL APPEARANCE: Color. Posture.

10. HEMORRHAGES, DISCHARGES, ETC.: Chart a *description,* etc. When unusual, *save specimens* for examination.

11. NAUSEA: Accompanied by vomiting. Following certain foods, drugs or treatments.

12. NERVES: All nervous symptoms, excitability, etc.

13. PAIN: Location. Time of onset. Character: Sharp, dull, burning, grinding, throbbing. Duration: Constant, for how long. Intermittent, intervals.

14. PATHOLOGICAL CONDITIONS: *Vomiting, convulsions,* etc. Record *time, duration, severity, general appearance* of patient before, during, and after the attack. *T. P. R.* immediately after, and *what was done* to relieve condition. Chart explanation as to the cause.

15. PULSE: Rate: beats per minute. Character: full, bounding, weak, thready, faint. Rhythm: regular, irregular, intermittent.

16. RESPIRATION: Rate per minute. Character: deep, shallow, difficult, easy, labored, quiet, stertorous, Cheyne-Stokes. Rhythm: regular, irregular, gasping.

17. SLEEP: Record should be made of the *hours of sleeping* during the day, as well as at night. If impossible to estimate same accurately, approximate it. *Time* and *amount* of sleep obtained by the patient should be noted, if possible.

18. TEMPERATURE: If for some legitimate reason temperature is omitted, write *hour* in designated space, leave temperature space unmarked. When recording next temperature, bring line across this space to the adjoining and record the next temperature. By mouth, rectum or axilla. Degree. Following chill, or treatment.

19. T. P. R.: Temperature, pulse and respiration taken as ordered. The nurse charts the T. P. R. and general condition of the patient before going to the operating room, and the pulse and respiration with general condition upon return from the operating room.

20. UNCONSCIOUSNESS OR COMA: Time of onset. Duration.

21. UNUSUAL CONDITIONS: Chart these, such as appearance of blood, twitching, convulsions, coma, drowsiness, lethargy, unconsciousness.

22. URINE: State *time* of voiding, the *amount, color* and *appearance,* whether voided or per catheter. Note time of beginning 24-hour specimen; when bladder is emptied for the purpose, this specimen is sent to laboratory for qualitative test. Remark the *ending* of 24-hour specimen. Note *amount* on chart and on laboratory label. Send specimen to the laboratory for all patients remaining in the hospital over night. At 7 P. M. and 7 A. M., day and night nurses remark whether or not very ill patients voided during the day or night. Immediately upon admission begin 24-hour specimen of urine for all diabetic patients. Check may be used in the urine column: (a) When patient uses lavatory. (b) When he voids with defecation. At all other times the amount of urine is to be charted (totaled every 12 hours and *total* charted also). Accompanied by pain or burning. Any abnormal appearance. Specimen to laboratory.

23. VOMITING: Cause. Forcible or projectile. Vomitus: Amount. Color. Odor. Consistency. Any unusual constituents.

Mental Symptoms: 1. Calmness. 2. Cheerfulness. 3. Delirium: Kind. 4. Depression: Degree. Apparent effect of visitors, etc., on. 5. Delusions, on what special subjects. 6. Hallucinations. 7. Illusions, on what special subjects. 8. Temper fits. 9. Willingness to coöperate. 10. Worry.

chartula (kar'tu-lă) [L. dim. of *charta*, piece of paper]. A paper containing a medicinal powder.

chaude-pisse (shōd-pēs'). The burning sensation during urination in acute gonorrhea.

chauffage (sho-fazh') [Fr. *chauffer*, to heat]. A heated cautery at low temperature applied over a part about ¼ in. from it.

Chauffard's syndrome (sho-fars'). Peculiar symptoms of polyarticular joint disease with splenic and glandular enlargement in young children.

chaulmoogra, chaulmugra, chaulmaugra (tschawl-moo'gră, tschawl-mū'gră, tschawl-maw'gră). A vegetable oil used in treatment of leprosy, arthritis, and some chronic forms of dermatoses.

Chaussier's areola (sho-sĭ-ăs'). Indurated tissue around the lesion of a malignant pustule.

check. 1. To slow down or arrest the course of. 2. To verify.

 c. bite. Impression of teeth on plastic material to check articulation.

 c. experiment. Control experiment, or one checked against another.

cheek [A.S. *ceáce*, check]. Side of face forming lateral wall of mouth below eye. SEE: *bucca, buccal, buccinator, gena, malar bone, melitis, meloncus.* [*icum.*

 c. bone. The malar bone, *os zygomat-*
 c. muscle. Buccinator.
 c. retractor. Device for enclosing cheek at the mouth's angle for properly exposing operating field.

cheese [A.S. *cēse*, from L. *caseus*, cheese]. The compressed casein of milk, flavored and altered by bacterial action.

 COMP. (American): Pro. 28.8, Fat 35.9, Carbo. 0.3.

 FUEL VALUE: 100 Gm. equal 434 cal. Amer. red cheese has a little greater food value than has pineapple cheese. Other classes are lower in food values.

 ASH CONST: Ca 0.931, Mg 0.037, K 0.089, Na 0.606, P 0.683, Cl 0.880, S 0.263, Fe 0.0013.

 VITAMINS: Vit. A: A very good source in whole milk cheese, 700 units per oz. or 560 per 100 cal. Cottage cheese contains the vitamins A, B, C, but G is lacking in all cheese.

 ACTION: Cheese is slow to digest, but it is completely digested. Length of time in the cooking of cheese prolongs its digestion, but does not affect its digestibility. Over 97% of cheese is digested. SEE: *tyrogenous, tyroid, tyroma.*

cheilitis (ki-li'tĭs) [G. *cheilos*, lip, + -*ītis*, inflammation]. Inflammation of the lip.

 c. exfoliativa. Seborrheic dermatitis of the lips. SYM: Formation of slight, dry, adherent scales and crusts. Chronic. Exacerbates and improves at intervals. PROG: Obstinate and recurrent. TREATMENT: Ointments, lotions, x-rays.

cheilognathopalatoschisis (kī-lŏg″năth-ō-pāl-ă-tŏs′kĭ-sĭs) [" + *gnathos*, jaw, + L. *palatum*, palate, + G. *schisis*, cleft]. Malformation in which there is a cleft in the hard and soft palate, upper jaw and in the lip.

cheiloplasty (kil'o-plăs-tī) [" + *plassein*, to form]. Plastic operation upon the lips.

cheilosis (kī-lō′sĭs) [G. *cheilos*, lip, + -*ōsis*, disease]. Morbid condition of lips with reddened appearance and fissures at the angles, seen frequently in vitamin B deficiency, ariboflavinosis.*

cheilostomatoplasty (kil-os-to′măt-o-plas-tī) [" + *stoma*, mouth, + *plassein*, to form]. Plastic building up of mouth.

cheilotomy, chilotomy (ki-lŏt′o-mĭ) [" + *tomē*, incision]. Excision of part of the lip.

cheloid (ke′loid) [G. *chēlē*, claw, + *eidos*, form]. Keloid skin disease with fibrous growths at site of a scar.

chem′ic, chem′ical [G. *chēmeia*, chemistry.]. Pert. to chemistry.

 c. balance of the body. Foods burned within the body may produce either an alkaline or an acid ash.

 Foods, then, may be either acid or base forming. As the blood and tissues are slightly alkaline, foods should be base forming in order to produce an alkaline reserve. All cereals, meat, fish and eggs are acid producing, as are most nuts, cranberries, and rice. Alkali producing foods include most vegetables and fruits; also almonds and milk. SEE: *acidosis, alkalosis, ash, body.*

 c. change. A change in which a substance breaks up or combines with other substances to make new substances with new properties or characteristics. Ex: Oxygen and hydrogen combine together to form *water*. Sodium (a metal) and chlorine (a gas) combine together to form *sodium chloride*, or common salt. Oxygen combines with hemoglobin when the hemoglobin in the blood comes into contact with the oxygen in the air in the alveoli of the lungs to form *oxyhemoglobin*. The difference can be seen by comparing the bright scarlet of the arterial blood containing oxyhemoglobin with the bluish color of the venous blood containing hemoglobin.

 c. compound. (1) A substance consisting of two or more chemical elements in definite proportions and in chemical combination and for which a chemical formula can be written. Ex: *water* (H₂O), *salt* (NaCl). (2) A substance which can be separated by chemical means into simpler substances.

 c. elements. Common gases are oxygen, carbon dioxide, and nitrogen. SEE: *element.*

 c. elements (in the human body):

Oxygen	65.	%
Carbon	18.	%
Hydrogen	10.	%
Nitrogen	3.0	%
Calcium	1.5	%
Phosphorus	1.0	%
Potassium	0.35	%
Sulfur	0.15	%
Chlorine	0.15	%
Magnesium	0.05	%
Iron	0.004	%
Iodine	0.00004	%

 Also traces of copper, zinc, manganese, silicon, fluorine, and perhaps arsenic, nickel, cobalt, and aluminum. These elements must be supplied daily in the food. Traces of other minerals and of gases in the body are *arsenic, copper, iodine,* and *manganese*. Gases are *carbon dioxide, carbon monoxide,* and *methane, q.v.* SEE: *acid base balance, body, mineral elements, name of each element.*

 c. reflex. Any reflex action initiated by a chemical stimulus.

chemicocautery (kem-ik-o-kaw′ter-ĭ) [G. *chēmeia*, chemistry, + *kautērion*, branding iron]. Cauterization by chemical agents.

chemicogen′esis [" + *genesis*, production]. Chemical fertilization of an ovum.

cheminosis C-42 **chemosis**

Chemical Elements and Composition of the Human Body
These elements are supplied to the body day by day in the food provided by nature, or in air or water; natural foods supply them in about the proper proportion to maintain perfect health.

			Lb.	Oz.	Gr.
1	O¶	Oxygen—A gas, will fill a space of 750 cubic feet	111	0	0
2	C¶	Carbon—Constitutes fat, used for fuel to create animal heat	21	0	0
3	H†	Hydrogen—A gas, will fill a space of 3000 cubic feet	14	0	0
4	N¶	Nitrogen—Basis of muscles and solid tissues, supplied by nitrates	3	8	0
5	Ca†	Calcium—The metallic base of lime, the bone base	2	0	0
6	P¶	Phosphorus—All phosphates contain phosphorus	1	12	190
7	S¶	Sulfur—All sulfates contain sulfur	0	2	210
8	Na†	Natrium (Sodium)—The base of all the salts of soda	0	2	116
9	Cl¶	Chlorine—Constitutes with sodium, common salt	0	2	47
10	F†¶	Fluorine—Found combined in the bones	0	2	0
11	K†	Kalium (Potassium)—The base of all salts of potash	0	0	290
12	Fe†	Ferrum (Iron)—	0	0	100
13	Mg†	Magnesium—The base of magnesia and magn. salts	0	0	12
14	Si¶	Silicon—The base of silex, found in hair, teeth, nails	0	0	2
		The elements of a person weighing	152 lbs.		

† Positive (Alkali)
¶ Negative (Acid)

C—All things that have life contain carbon.
O—½ of earth's crust, 8/9 of water, 1/5 of air.
H—1/9 of water. N—4/5 of air.

The organic acids in the body combined with potassium undergo oxidation and are transformed into alkaline carbonates which render the urine and blood alkaline. They are found much more abundantly in vegetables than in animal food.

Compounds of the Human Body
The 17 combinations of these 14, or 16 elements, are all being used and consumed in the body continuously, and it is therefore necessary that they be supplied in proper food, or in pure air, or pure water.

			Lb.	Oz.	Gr.
1	H_2O	Water, composed of oxygen and hydrogen	111	0	0
2	Gelatin	Many tissues are composed of this	15	0	0
3	Fat, CHO	Constitutes the adipose tissue	12	0	0
4	Ca_3PO_4	Phosphate of lime, part of earthy matter of bones	5	13	0
5	Fibrin	Forms the blood clot	4	4	3
6	Albumin	Found in the blood and almost every organ	4	3	0
7	$CaCO_3$	Carbonate of lime, also a part of the bones	1	0	0
8	$Fe_2O_2 2HO$	Hemoglobin furnishes the coloring matter of the blood	0	9	150
9	CaF_2	Fluoride of Calcium, found in bones	0	3	0
10	Na_2SO_4	Sulfate of Soda, found in blood	0	1	170
11	Na_2CO_3	Carbonate of Soda, found in blood and bones	0	1	72
12	K_2SO_4	Sulfate of Potash, found in the blood	0	0	400
13	Na_3PO_4	Phosphate of Soda } In brain and nerves	0	0	400
14	K_3PO_4	Phosphate of Potash }	0	0	100
15	NaCl	Chloride of Sodium (common salt) in the blood	0	0	376
16	$Mg_3 2PO_4$	Phosphate of Magnesia, in the bones with phosphate of lime	0	0	75
17	SiO_2	Silica, found in the hair, teeth and nails	0	0	3
		The proximate principles in a person weighing	152 lbs.		

cheminosis (kem-in-o'sis) [" + -*ōsis*, infection]. Any disease caused by chemical agents.

chemiotaxis (kem-i-o-taks'is) [" + *taxis*, arrangement]. Cellular repulsion and attraction.

chemise (she-mēz') [Fr. shirt]. Surgical dressing to prevent hemorrhage after surgery upon bladder or rectum.

chem'ism [G. *chēmeia*, chemistry, + *ismos*, condition]. Chemical energy.

chemist (kem'ist). One trained in chemistry.

chem'istry [G. *chēmeia*, chemistry]. The science that treats of the molecular and atomic structure of matter.

chemokine'sis [" + *kinēsis*, movement]. Increased energy incited by a chemical substance.

chemolysis (kem-ol'is-is) [" + *lysis*, dissolution]. Chemical decomposition or decay.

chemomorphosis (kem-o-mor-fo'sis) [" + *morphē*, form]. Change of form as the result of chemical action.

chemopallidectomy (kĕm-ō-păl-ĭ-dĕk'tō-mī) Chemical injection of absolute alcohol in the brain to destroy the globus pallidus in Parkinson's disease.

chemophysiol'ogy [" + *physis*, nature, + *logos*, understanding]. Physiologic chemistry.

chemorecep'tor [" + L. *receptor*, receiver]. (1) Side chain in a living cell having an affinity for chemical substances and fixing them. (2) A sense organ or sensory nerve ending which is stimulated by a chemical substance.

chemore'flex [" + L. *reflectere*, to bend back]. Reflex resulting from chemical stimulus.

chemosis (ke-mo'sis) [G. *chēmē*, cockleshell, + -*ōsis*, infection]. Swelling of conjunctiva about the cornea.

chemotactic (kem-o-tak'tĭk) [G. *chēmeia*, chemistry, + *taxikos*, arranging]. Pert. to chemotaxis.

chemotaxis (kem-o-tak'sĭs) [" + *taxis*, arrangement]. Attraction and repulsion of living protoplasm to a chemical stimulus.

chemotherapy (kem-o-ther'a-pĭ) [" + *therapeia*, treatment]. Application of chemical reagents in treatment of disease, that have a specific and toxic effect on microörganism causing the disease, without harming the patient.

chemotic (ke-mot'ĭk). Pert. to chemosis.

chemotropism (kem-ot'ro-pizm) [G. *chēmeia*, chemistry, + *tropos*, direction]. Ability or impulse to progress or turn in a certain direction due to the influence of certain chemical stimuli. SYN: *chemotaxis*.

chenopodium oil (ken-o-po'dĭ-um). USP. Oil of American wormseed. Colorless, a pale yellow volatile oil with pungent, irritating odor.

ACTION AND USES: Anthelmintic against hookworm.

DOSAGE: From 5 to 15 ℳ (0.3-1 cc.).

cherophobia (ker-o-fo'bĭ-ă) [G. *chairein*, to rejoice, + *phobos*, fear]. Morbid fear of and aversion to gaiety.

cherries [G. *kerasion*, the fruit]. COMP: Contain much cellulose. They contain citric and malic acids. AV. SERVING: 75 Gm. Pro. 0.8, Fat 0.6, Carbo. 12.5 per serving. Vit. A++, B+, C++. Ca 0.019, Mg 0.016, K 0.213, Na 0.023, P 0.031, Cl 0.014, S 0.011, Fe 0.0004. ACTION: A drink made of cherry stems will act as a diuretic within an hour of its consumption. Cherries change uric acid into hippuric acid, and for this reason they are used in gout, but intestinal trouble may result from too free use.

chest [A.S. *cest*, a box]. The thorax.

MENSURATION: *Object*: First, to ascertain the comparative bulk of the 2 sides; second, to ascertain amt. of expansion and retraction accompanying inspiration and expiration of the 2 sides.

The points of measurement are the spinous processes behind and the median line in front on the level of the 6th costosternal articulation. The right side is from half an inch to an inch larger than the left.

When a pleural cavity is distended with air or fluid the measurement of the affected side may exceed that of the healthy side by 2 or 3 inches; after removal of the fluid there may be an equal diminution in the measurement of the affected side, as compared with the healthy one. In emphysema the total difference bet. the fullest inspiration and fullest expiration on the affected side will scarcely exceed 1/16 of an inch, while on the other side there may be a difference of 2 or 3 inches. The list of affections in which variations in expansion are to be estimated by measure is the same as that referred to under INSPECTION.

PALPATION: Serves to detect any thoracic tenderness, edema, friction fremitus or râles, and to determine the vocal fremitus and amt. of expansion. Edema of chest walls is recognized by "pitting" when pressure is made with finger. It may be observed in empyema, after the application of a blister, and in general dropsy.

The friction sound of pleurisy and harsh, sonorous râles can sometimes be detected by palpation. Thoracic tenderness is observed in pleurisy; in phthisis and pneumonia from being associated with pleurisy; in pleurodynia, in intercostal neuralgia (confined to certain spots); and in surgical affections like caries, and fracture of the ribs; and in contusion and inflammation of the parietes.

PERCUSSION: *Precautions*: Place finger being used as a pleximeter firmly against chest and preferably parallel to ribs. Make finger which is used as plessor strike the one on chest perpendicularly, fix forearm, and use no more force than can be obtained from a gentle swing of the wrist. Percuss all parts of chest anteriorly and posteriorly, both in inspiration and expiration. In comparing sides be sure to percuss corresponding parts.

Normal Resonance: On the right side pulmonary resonance extends from half an inch to an inch above the clavicle, downward to upper border of 6th rib in front, and to a line drawn through the 10th spinous process posteriorly. On left side pulmonary resonance extends from a half inch to an inch above the clavicle downward, within the mammary line to the 10th rib and posteriorly to a line drawn through the 10th spinous process.

Cracked Pot Sound: Modified tympany, can be simulated by percussing over the cheek when mouth is partially open. May be normally heard over the chest of a crying infant. In the adult it usually indicates a cavity which has a free communication with a bronchus. Best detected by keeping ear near open mouth of patient while percussing.

Dullness or flatness is recognized in: (1) Phthisical condition; (2) pneumonic consolidation; (3) pleural effusions of all kinds, except air; (4) collapse of lung; (5) congestion and edema of lung; (6) enlargement of liver or spleen (at base); (7) morbid growths in the lung.

Hyperresonance is observed in: (1) Pneumothorax; (2) cavities, tuberculous or bronchiectatic; (3) emphysema; (4) lowered pulmonary tension in the initial stage of pneumonia, and above a pleural effusion (Skoda's resonance); (5) flatulent distention of the stomach or colon frequently observed over the left base. A *tympanitic note* is a hollow, drumlike sound, like that which is normally obtained by percussing the larynx or empty stomach. The above conditions are also capable of producing tympany.

Pitch: Depends largely upon the volume of air, tension of walls of cavity, and upon size of opening that communicates with the cavity. The less the air the greater the tension, and the smaller the opening the higher will be the pitch of the note. In beginning phthisical consolidation, the note over the affected apex is higher pitched. It must be remembered that normally the note over the right apex is higher pitched than that over the left.

Resistance: The greater the dullness the greater will be the resistance; therefore, there is always more resistance over a large pleural effusion than over a pneumonic or phthisical consolidation.

RS: *barrel chest, breathing, Cheyne-Stokes respiration, fremitus, hydrothorax, pectoral, pectoralis, pectoriloquy, resonance, respiration, "thoraco-" words*.

c., emphysematous. In advanced emphysema thorax is short and round; anterior-posterior diameter is often as long as the transverse diameter; ribs are horizontal; angle formed by divergence of the costal margin from the sternum is very obtuse or quite obliterated. Often termed "barrel shaped."

c. prominences and depressions. An unnatural prominence or depression is often observed over the lower part of the sternum and is generally congenital. The term "funnel" breast or "shoemaker's" breast (because it may result from pressure of tools) has been applied to the sternal depression.

A unilateral or local depression may be due to: (a) Phthisical consolidation; (b) cavity; (c) pleurisy with fibrous adhesions.

A unilateral or local prominence may be due to: (a) Pleurisy with effusion; (b) pneumothorax, hydrothorax, haemothorax; (c) aneurysm or tumor; (d) compensatory emphysema, resulting from impairment of the opposite lung; (e) cardiac enlargements (left side); (f) enlargements of abdominal organs, esp. liver and spleen.

c., phthinoid. Ant. post. diameter is short, thorax long and flat, ribs oblique. Scapula prominent; spaces above and below clavicles are depressed. Angle formed by divergence of the costal margins from the sternum is very acute.

c., rachitic. May resemble phthinoid, but usually sides are considerably flattened and sternum prominent, so term pigeon breast has been applied. The sternal ends of the ribs are enlarged or "beaded" and this characteristic has given rise to the term "rachitic rosary." Is often a circular construction of the thorax at level of the xiphoid cartilage. SEE: *circulatory system.*

c. regions. Ant., post., and lateral. *Ant. Divisions* (R. and L.): Clavicular, infra- and supraclavicular, mammary and inframammary, upper and lower sternal. *Post. Divisions* (R. and L.): Scapular, infrasuper- and interscapular. *Lateral Divisions*: Axillary and infraaxillary.

chest expansion, normal. In the male, 2 in.; in the female, 2½ in. *Capacity*: Normal male, 22 yr. old, 5.8 ft., 230 to 240 cu. in. Normal female, 19 yr. old, 5.25 ft., 145 to 150 cu. in. Expansion denotes capacity of air taken into lungs and is estimated to average about 2.3 cu. in. for each in. of height. This varies with age, the young adult having a greater capacity than the aged. Those given to exercise or physical work have a greater lung capacity than others.

chestnut [M. E. *chesten*, from G. *kastanon*, chestnut]. AV. SERVING (Roasted): 50 Gm. Pro 2.6, Fat 2.3, Carbo. 17.7 per serving. FUEL VALUE: 100 Gm. equal 244 cal. VITAMINS: B+, G+. Ca 0.034, Mg 0.051, K 0.560, Na 0.065, P 0.093, Cl 0.006, S 0.068, Fe 0.0007.

Cheyne-Stokes reflex (chān-stōks). Rhythmic acceleration, deepening, and stopping of breathing movements.

Cheyne-Stokes respiration. An irregular type of arrhythmic breathing occurring in certain acute diseases of the central nervous system, heart, lungs, and in intoxications.

At first it is slow and shallow, then it increases in rapidity and depth until it reaches a maximum. Then it decreases gradually until it stops for 10 to 20 seconds, then repeating in the same manner. It frequently occurs before death. Associated with cerebral, cardiac, renal, and pulmonary affections.

chiasm, chiasma (kī'azm, ki-az'ma) [G. from *chiazen*, to mark with letter X]. 1. A crossing. 2. An incomplete crossing of the optic fibers (the outer fibers not crossing each other); the point of crossing of the fibers of the optic nerves.

chiastometer (ki-as-tom'et-er) [G. *chiastos*, crossed, + *metron*, measure]. Instrument for measurement of deviation of optic axes.

chicken [A.S. *cicen*]. The flesh of domestic fowl cooked and served as food. Av. SERVING: 230 Gm. Pro 49.6, Fat 5.8 per serving. Ca 0.058, Mg 0.118, K 1.694, Na 0.421, P 1.518, Cl 0.378, S 1.146, Fe 0.0150. Vit. A− to +, B+, G+. FUEL VALUE: 100 Gm. equal 109 cal.

c. breast. Abnormal prominence of the sternum. SYN: *pectus carinatum.*

c. fat clot. A yellowish blood clot.

chickenpox. A mild, contagious, infectious disease, marked by an eruption of vesicles on skin and mucous membranes. SEE: *varicella.*

chickory [G. *kichora*]. COMP: Low in mineral values. AV. SERVING: 16 Gm. Pro 0.3, Fat 0.1, Carbo. 0.05 per serving. ACTION: An aperient and stimulant. SEE: *condiments.*

chig´gers. (1) The chigoe, jigger, or sand flea (*Tunga penetrans*). (2) Redbugs. The six-legged larvae of mites of the family Thrombiculidae, order Acarina of the class Arachnida. Also called rougets, harvest mites, scrub mites. They are parasitic on insects, various vertebrates, and man. Eggs are laid on the ground and hatch in about 12 days, after which they attach to host at first opportunity. The redbugs attach themselves to the surface of the skin and inject a salivary secretion which dissolves the surrounding tissues. A tubular structure, a *stylostome*, is developed which is used in ingesting the semi-digested tissue debris. The mites do not feed on blood. The most common species attacking humans in N. America is *Eutrombicula alfreddugesi*. The irritation is the result of sensitization to the injected saliva.

Treatment. Alcohol or camphor allays itching. Bathing with baking soda or ammonia gives relief. Protection against redbugs can be obtained by rubbing dibutyl phthalate or benzyl benzoate or a 50-50 mixture of the two in clothing.

chignon fungoid (shēn-yon´). A bacterial invasion of the hair.

chigo, chigre (chē´go, chē´grä) [Sp.]. A jigger or sand flea.

chilblains (chil´blāns) [A.S. *cele*, cold, + *blegen*, to boil]. Inflammation and swelling of the feet, toes, or fingers caused by cold.

SYM: Reddish, violaceous plaques or patches on hands and feet, occasionally the ears. Persistent, giving rise to smarting, burning, itching, esp. when parts become warm. In severe types frostbite corresponds to second degree burns, showing vesicles, bullae, ulcer, and necrosis. TREATMENT: Stimulants followed by iron tonics.

NP: If circulation is not restored rub parts with warm hands; place patient in a cold room, give warm, nutritious drinks (no alcohol).

CHRONIC FORM: Warm, dry, woolen stockings should be worn, and thick, loose shoes. Wash the hands and feet daily in very hot water, drying quickly. Avoid sitting too close to a fire. For the itching, paint with tinct. iodine, or apply spirits of wine as a lotion, gently rubbed in. If broken, keep clean and covered with some soothing ointment, such as calamine, lanolin, or pure vaseline, spread on lint. The administration of calcium lactate is found to be of benefit in some cases.

To relieve inflammation and itching dissolve 3 drams of bicarbonate of soda in very hot water, then, holding a swab of wool in forceps, dab freely on and off the part for 10 minutes twice a day. Follow by rubbing in stainless iodine ointment.

child [A.S. *cild*]. A young person of either sex, bet. infancy and youth. SEE: *pediatrics, pedophilia, puerile, puerilism, quadruplets, quintuplets, sibling, triplets, twins.*

child'bed. Puerperium. Period during and immediately subsequent to parturition.

  c. b. fever. Puerperal fever.
  Recently, vaccine has been injected into both sufferers from childbed fever and expectant mothers with excellent results. [child; parturition. SEE: *labor.*

childbirth. The process of bringing forth a

child crowing. Spasmodic closure of glottis, of brief duration, and succeeded by noisy inspiration. SYN: *laryngismus stridulus.*

chilectro'pion [G. *cheilos*, lip, + *ektropos*, turning out]. Eversion of the lip.

chilitis (ki-li'tis) [" + -*itis*, inflammation]. Inflammation of the lips. SEE: *cheilitis.*

chill (chǐl) [A.S. *cele*, cold]. A disturbance of the heat regulating mechanism of the body, accompanied by shivering and fall of temperature.

Chills accompany various diseases, esp. malaria, and are coarse or fine, diffuse, trembling, etc.

ETIOL: (a) Onset of an exanthema. (b) Formation of pus somewhere in the body. (c) Onset of diseases such as pneumonia. (d) Puerperal infection, when following 2 or 3 days after childbirth. (e) Postoperative chill indicative of complications or infection.

SYM: A real chill is ushered in by extreme chilly sensation, chattering of the teeth and, in extreme cases, a marked tremor of the entire body and a rapidly rising temperature.

NP: (a) Make patient comfortable by supplying external heat and extra blanket. (b) Give hot drink when permitted or tolerated. (c) Give patient moral support. (d) Take temperature as soon as possible, then again about 20 minutes after chill subsides. (e) Chart a report to attending physician, length of duration, degree of severity, and temperature. SEE: *ague.*

  c., nervous. Accompanied by a chilly sensation but not with fever. It may follow severe pain or extreme nervousness. It usually passes quickly and is seldom serious.

chiloangioscopy (ki-lo-an-jĭ-os'ko-pĭ) [G. *cheilos*, lip, + *aggeion*, vessel, + *skopein*, to examine]. Microscopical examination of the circulation in the lip.

chilognathopalatoschisis (kĭ-log″nath-o-pal-at-os'kis-is) [" + *gnathos*, jaw, + L. *palatum*, palate, + G. *schisis*, fissure]. Fissure of the lip, palate, and alveolar process.

Chilomas'tix mesnil'i. A species of Mastigophora that is parasitic in the intestines. [+ *schisis*, fissure]. Harelip.

chiloschisis (ki-los'kis-is) [G. *cheilos*, lip,

chilostomatoplasty (kĭ-los-to″mă-to-plas″tĭ) [" + *stoma*, mouth, + *plassein*, to form]. Plastic operation for harelip.

chilot'omy [" + *tomē*, incision]. 1. Surgical removal of a portion of the lip for excision of a growth. 2. Cutting of an overgrowth at the articular end of a long bone to free its movement.

chim'ney-sweeps' cancer. Epithelioma of the scrotum.

chin [AS. *cin*, chin]. Point of the lower jaw; mentum; region below lower lip.

  c. cough. Whooping cough, q.v.
  c. jerk. Reflex contraction of muscles of mastication on suddenly depressing the jaw.
  c. reflex. Clonic movement resulting from percussing or stroking lower jaw.

chiniofon (kin'ĭ-o-fŏn). USP. A derivative of sulfonic acid, containing approximately 27% iodine.

USES: In treatment of amebic dysentery, and as a substitute for iodoform in surgical dusting powders.

DOSAGE: Orally, for adults, from 4-15 gr. (0.25-1 Gm.) 3 times a day; rectally, 15-75 gr. (5 Gm.) dissolved in 200 cc. water. Treatment combining both has been used in acute cases, and serious chronic ones, and course of treatment requiring from 7 to 14 days.

INCOMPATIBILITIES: Moisture, mineral acids, ferric chloride, and oxidizing agents.

chionablepsia (kĭ-on-ab-lep'sĭ-ă) [G. *chiōn*, snow, + *ablepsia*, blindness]. Snow blindness.

chirapsia (kĭ-răp'sĭ-ă) [G. *cheirapsia*, a touching with the hands]. Friction; massage.

chirognostic (kĭ-rog-nos'tĭk) [G. *cheir*, hand, + *gnōstikos*, knowing]. Having the ability to distinguish the right from the left.

chirokinesthesia (kĭ-ro-kin-es-the'sĭ-ă) [" + *kinēsis*, movement, + *aisthēsis*, sensation]. Subjective perception of motions of the hand.

chiromeg'aly [" + *megas*, large]. Enlargement of the hands, wrists, or ankles.

chi'roplasty [" + *plassein*, to form]. A plastic operation on the hand.

chiropodalgia (kĭ-ro-pod-al'jĭ-ă) [" + *pous*, foot, + *algos*, pain]. Pain in hands and feet. SYN: *acrodynia.*

chiropodist (ki-rop'o-dist) [" + *pous*, foot]. One who practices chiropody.

chiropody (ki-rop'od-ĭ) [" + *pous*, foot]. Treatment of minor disorders of the feet.

chiropompholyx (ki-ro-pom'fo-liks) [" + *pompholyx*, a bubble]. Inflammatory disease of skin confined to hands and feet. SYN: *pompholyx*, q.v.

SYM: Peculiar blebs or vesicles in groups.

chiropractic (ki-ro-prak'tik) [" + L. *practos*, done with the hand]. A system of manipulative treatment which teaches that all diseases are caused by impingement on spinal nerves and can be corrected by spinal adjustments.

chiropractor (ki-ro-prak'tor). One who practices chiropractic methods.

chirospasm (ki'ro-spazm) [" + *spasmos*, spasm]. Spasmodic affection of muscles of hand, or writers' cramp.

chirurgery (ki-rur'je-rĭ) [" + *ergon*, work]. Surgery.

chirurgia (ki-rur'jĭ-ă). Surgery.

chirurgical (ki-rur'jĭk-al). Surgical.

chitinous (ki'tin-us) [G. *chitōn*, a tunic]. Pertaining to or composed of chitin.
 c. degeneration. Amyloid degeneration.

chloasma (klo-az'mă) [G. *chloazein*, to be green]. Pigmentary skin discolorations, usually those occurring in yellowish brown patches or spots.
 ETIOL: Ordinarily nonpathological. In symptomatic types there may be abnormal physiology function.
 SYM: Areas rounded or oval with ill-defined margins, light yellow to black. In those due to external factors pigmentation develops only at sight of irritation or beyond. In symptomatic forms constitutional cause underlies.
 TREATMENT: Constitutional when indicated.
 c. gravida'rum. Same as c. uterinum, *q.v.*
 c. hepaticum. So-called "liver spot" following dyspepsia.
 c., idiopathic. C. caused by external agents, such as sun, heat, mechanical means, x-rays, etc.
 c., symptomatic. C. caused by various diseases, as syphilis or cancer.
 c. traumaticum. Skin discolorations from traumatic agencies.
 c. uteri'num. Brown discolorations of skin in pregnancy.

chloracetization (klo-ras-ĕt-iz a'shun). Production of local anesthesia by chloroform and glacial acetic acid.

chloralamide (klo″răl-ăm′id). A hypnotic safer than chloral.
 DOSAGE: 15-45 gr. (1.0-3.0 Gm.).

chloral hydrate (klo'ral). USP. Colorless, transparent crystals having aromatic, slightly acrid odor, and caustic, faintly bitter taste; soluble in alcohol and water.
 ACTION AND USES: As a hypnotic in insomnia due to nervous excitation.
 DOSAGE: From 10-30 gr. (0.65-2.0 Gm.).
 INCOMPATIBILITIES: In aqueous solution, acetanilid, alkaloids, borax, sodium bicarbonate, aromatic spirits of ammonia.
 POISONING: *Sym:* Depresses and eventually paralyzes the central nervous system. There may be nausea and vomiting due to gastric irritation. Pulse is feeble, respirations are shallow and irregular, lassitude, weakness, dizziness, sleep.
 F. A. TREATMENT: Dilute, then wash out stomach. Emetics do not work. Stimulants, esp. coffee, caffeine, or tea should be given in large doses. Keep patient warm. Administer artificial respiration.

chloramphenicol (klor-ăm-phĕn'i-cŏl). USP syn for *chloromycetin, q.v.*

chloranemia (klor-an-e'mĭ-ă) [G. *chlōros*, green, + *a-*, priv. + *aima*, blood]. An anemia resembling that of chlorosis occurring in some diseases, such as cancer and tuberculosis.

chlorate (klo'rāt). A salt of chloric acid. SEE: *potassium chlorate.*

chlorbu'tanol. Colorless crystals, with taste and odor resembling camphor.

chlorbu'tol. Colorless crystals, with odor and taste resembling camphor. SEE: *chlorobutanol.*

chlorcosane (klor-co-sān') (chlorinated paraffin). Used as a solvent for dichloramine T, *q.v.*

chloremia (klo-re'mĭ-ă) [G. *chlōros*, green, + *aima*, blood]. Anemia with diminution of hemoglobin and decrease in number of red corpuscles.

chlorephidrosis (klor-ef-ĭ-dro'sis) [" + *ephidrōsis*, perspiration]. Greenish perspiration.

chloretone (klo'rĕ-tōn). Colorless crystals, resembling camphor in odor and taste. SEE: *chlorobutanol.*

chlorhydria (klor-hi'drĭ-ă) [" + *ydōr*, water]. Excess of hydrochloric acid in stomach.

chloride (klo'rīd) [G. *chlōros*, green]. A binary compound of chlorine; a salt of hydrochloric acid. Normal whole blood contains 450-500 mg. per 100 cc. of blood, principally in the form of sodium chloride. Chlorides are increased in nephritis, eclampsia, anemia, and cardiac disease; decreased in fevers, diabetes, and pneumonia.
 Test for is determined on whole blood as a rule. Normal value for whole blood is 450-500 mg; for blood plasma, 570-620 mg.; for blood serum 350-390 mg.
 c., test for in urine. To a test tube half filled with urine is added a drop or 2 of nitric acid, which holds the phosphates in solution. Then a 3% solution of silver nitrate is added to the specimen, drop by drop, till about 6 drops have passed. This forms a white, curdy precipitate at once. The test should be compared with a known normal specimen of urine. *Diminished chlorides* are found in chronic nephritis, early stages of pneumonia, malignant disease, and in gastritis. Chlorides are increased in a diet rich in salt, in rickets, and hepatic cirrhosis.

chloridemia (klor-ĭ-de'mĭ-ă) [" + *aima*, blood]. Chlorides in the blood.

chloridim'eter [" + *metron*, measure]. An instrument for estimating amt. of chlorides in a fluid.

chloridimetry (klor-ĭ-dim'e-trĭ). Determination of amt. of chlorides in the body fluids.

chloridrom'eter. Device for estimating amt. of chlorides in urine.

chloriduria (klor-id-u'rĭ-ă) [G. *chlōros*, green, + *ouron*, urine]. Presence or excess of chlorides in urine.

chlorinated (klor'in-ă-ted) [G. *chlōros*, green]. Impregnated with chlorine.
 c. lime. Calcium hypochlorite widely used in solution as a bleach, as an antiseptic, and as a ringworm preventive.

chlorina'tion. Treatment of water by addition of chlorine and its compounds for the killing of bacteria. 0.15 to 0.7 parts are used for million gallons of water.

chlorine (klo'rēn) [G. *chlōros*, green].
 SYMB: Cl. A highly irritating gas and destructive to the mucous membranes of the respiratory passage-ways. It is very poisonous and excessive inhalation may cause death. Carefully inhaling ammonia or alcohol will counteract the effects of chlorine inhalation. Chlorine is an active bleaching agent and germicide. Both of these effects are due to its oxidizing powers. It is used extensively in the purification of water supplies and for disinfection. It is a chemical element with an atomic weight of 35.4.
 FUNCTIONS: Chlorine is found combined with sodium in the blood and exercises some influence upon metabolism, and helps to maintain osmotic pressure, and aids in the regulation and stimulation of muscular action. The body fluids contain 0.85% salt solution. The inorganic salts keep in solution the proteins of the blood, milk, and other secretions. Chlorine is present in the hydrochloric acid of the gastric juice. It aids digestion, activates enzymes, and is essential to normal gastric secretion.

chlorine, preparations

EXCRETION: The excretion of chlorine during a 31-day fast measured from 3.77 Gm. on the first day to 0.13 Gm. on the last day of the fast. It leaves the body in the form of chloride ions.

DEFICIENCY SYM: (a) Hunger for salt, (b) loss of weight, (c) achlorhydria, (d) disturbances of digestion, (e) miner's cramps, (f) incomplete water retention.

c. preparations. Those used for disinfecting.

Chlorazene, or Dakin's solution, and other chlorine disinfectants are very effective in their germicidal power. As a disinfecting agent in washing dishes and utensils used by infected patients, 1/10 of 1% solution should be used; the dishes should then be washed well in soap and hot water and rinsed well, or boiled and then washed well after the boiling.

STOOLS: For disinfection of the stools of patients, 5% or even stronger solutions may be used for one-half hour or longer. The utensil is set aside and covered while the solution functions. Dakin's solution is nonirritating and is used as a wound disinfectant, but it must be carefully prepared daily by the laboratory and used only when fresh.

chlorite (klō'rīt). A salt of chlorous acid; used as a disinfectant and bleaching agent.

chloroanemia (klor-o-a-ne'mĭ-ă) [G. *chlōros*, green, + *a-*, priv. + *aima*, blood]. Anemia occurring in cachectic conditions. SYN: *chlorosis*.

chloroazodin (klŏr-ō-ăz'ō-dĭn). USP. Syn. for *azochloramine*, a germicidal preparation of chlorine.

chlorobutanol (klō-ro-bū'tan-ol). USP. (Chlorbutol, chloretone.) Colorless crystals, with camphor odor and taste.

USES: Antiseptic and local anesthetic, useful in relief of vomiting, and as a preservative in many pharmaceuticals.

DOSAGE: From 10 gr. (0.6 Gm.), preferably in capsule.

INCOMPATIBILITIES: Decomposed by alkalies, and should not be mixed with borax, carbonates, etc. Liquefies with menthol and phenol.

chlor'oform [L. *chloroformum*]. $CHCl_3$. USP. A heavy, clear, colorless liquid with strong ethereal odor, formed by the action of chlorinated lime on methyl alcohol.

ACTION AND USES: A general anesthetic, more dangerous than ether. Locally an irritant used in liniments. Internally a carminative and anodyne.

DOSAGE: 5 ℳ (0.3 cc.).

c. anesthesia. For some time chloroform anesthesia was more popular than ether. It is 6 times as strong, but it was found to be more harmful.

When employed, the chloroform is well diluted with air. It is not inflammable except when mixed with alcohol, although volatile at low temperatures. It tends to decompose and to form hydrochloric acid and carbonyl chloride and the latter substance is supposed to cause after-sickness. Chloroform should be kept in dark bottles in a dark, cool place.

ADVANTAGES: The period of excitement following anesthesia is relatively short. It does not irritate the mucous membranes and it produces excellent muscular relaxation. Neither does it cause excessive secretion of the respiratory mucous membrane. It has a pleasant odor and it acts more agreeably than some other anesthetics.

PHYSIOLOGICAL ACTION: When inhaled it is promptly absorbed through the mucous membranes of the respiratory tract. After being eliminated by the lungs it seems to remain unchanged.

DANGERS: Dangerous symptoms may develop very suddenly. Circulatory depression may develop with cardiac arrest. It is a severe cardiac and respiratory depressant. It lowers chemical body pressure and body temperature; also blood pressure. It produces toxic changes in body chemistry, and is very detrimental to the bladder and kidney functioning. It should never be given without plenty of oxygen, in the proportion of 95% of air and 5% of chloroform. This form of anesthesia should not be used for a patient with a cardiac disease. Because it is not inflammable it may be used when work is to be done with a cautery, diathermy, or when the x-ray is used around the head or mouth. It also may be used in acute pulmonary pathology.

GENERAL REACTIONS: These include headache, nausea, vomiting, bronchial irritation and hysterical symptoms, but to a lesser extent than as a result of other anesthetics. Milk and lime water may allay vomiting and nausea, or lavage with a lukewarm solution of carbonate of soda. In stubborn cases a hypodermic injection of morphine, ¼ gr. (0.016 Gm.), may be ordered. SEE: *chloracetization, chloroformin, chloroformism.*

chlorofor'min. A toxin extracted by chloroform from the tubercle bacilli.

chloroformism (klo'ro-form-izm). The habit of inhaling chloroform and the resulting symptoms.

chloroleukemia (klo-ro-lū-ke'mĭ-ă) [G. *chlōros*, green, + *leukos*, white, + *aima*, blood]. Leukemia with chlorosis.

chloroma (klo-ro'mă) [" + *-ōma*, growth]. A greenish sarcoma of the periosteum of cranial bones; "green cancer."

chloromycetin (klor-ō-mī-sē'tĭn). An antibiotic from a South American mold (*Streptomyces venezuelae*). Effective against epidemic typhus, Rocky Mountain spotted fever, undulant fever, urinary infections, bacillary dysenteries, whooping cough, psittacosis, virus pneumonia, scrub and murine typhus, rickettsialpox, and lymphogranuloma virus, and typhoid.

chloromyeloma (klo-ro-mī-el-o'mă) [" + *myelos*, marrow, + *-ōma*, growth]. Chloroma accompanied by multiple growths in bone marrow.

chloropenia (klo-ro-pe'nĭ-ă) [" + *penēs*, poor]. Deficiency in chlorine; hypochloremia.

chloropenic (klo-ro-pēn'ik). Deficient in chlorine.

chlorophane (klo'ro-fān) [G. *chlōros*, green, + *phainein*, to show]. A green-yellow pigment in the retina.

chlorophyl, chlorophyll (klo'ro-fĭl) [" + *phyllon*, leaf]. The green coloring matter in plants consisting of chlorophyll-a and chlorophyll-b. It acts as a catalytic agent in the process of photosynthesis in which carbon dioxide from the air reacts with water from the soil to form simple carbohydrates, which are used for energy or converted into more complex substances and stored.

chloro'pia [" + *opsis*, vision]. Vision in which all things appear green.

chloroplast. Small round green bodies found in the cells of leaves and stem of plants which are important in the process of photosynthesis. They possess a stroma and contain four pigments: chlorophyll-a, chlorophyll-b, carotin, and xanthophyll.

chloroplas'tid [" + *plastos*, form]. A chlorophyl granule.

chloroprivic (klor-o-priv'ĭk) [" + L. *privāre*, to deprive of]. Lack of, or due to loss of, chlorides.

chlorop'sia [" + *opsis*, vision]. Vision in which all things seem green. SYN: *chloropia*.

chlorosarco'ma [" + *sarx*, flesh, + *-ōma*, tumor]. Sarcomatous form of chloroma.

chloro'sis [" + *-ōsis*, infection]. A form of anemia* in adolescent girls, perhaps due to faulty diet during puberty. Green sickness.

chlorotic (klo-rot'ĭk). Of the nature of or afflicted with chlorosis.

chloroxyl (klō-roks'ĭl). Cinchophen hydrochloride.

USES AND DOSAGE: Same as cinchophen

chlorpromazine. SEE: *thorazene*, p. T-66.

chlorum (klo'rum) [L.]. Official name of chlorine.

chloruremia (klor-ŭ-re'mĭ-ă) [G. *chlōros*, green, + *ouron*, urine, + *aima*, blood]. Urinary chlorides retained in the blood.

chloru'ria [" + *ouron*, urine]. Chlorides in the urine.

chlo'ryl. Anesthetic mixture of ethyl and methyl chlorides.

Ch.M. Abbr. for *Chirur'giae magis'ter*, Master of Surgery.

choana na'rium (ko-a'na) [G. *choanē*, funnel]. Post. nares or opening into the nasopharynx of the nasal fossa on both sides.

choanoid (ko'an-oyd) [" + *eidos*, shape]. Shaped like a funnel.

chocolate [Sp. from Mexican *choco*, cacao, + *latl*, water]. 1. Preparation made by grinding roasted cacao or theobroma seeds. 2. Beverage prepared by dissolving in water or milk. SEE: *cocoa*.

choked disk. Inflammation of the optic disk. Also called papillitis or optic neuritis. SEE: *disk*.

choking [A.S. *aceocian*, to suffocate]. Obstruction within respiratory passage or constriction about the neck, interfering with breathing and circulation of brain.

SYM: Face purple, eyes protrude, arms thrown about, coughing. Constriction and injury about neck, cyanosis, dizziness, unconsciousness.

TREATMENT: Remove constriction. Artificial respiration. Slap violently on back. Severe blow bet. shoulders. With children, compress chest with the hands squeezing suddenly and vigorously. If foreign body in throat, such as meat, insert thumb and forefinger and try to grasp it. If child, grasp by legs and reverse head for a moment. If the article is swallowed, do not give purgative. If sharp or angular, give plenty of rye or other bread, potatoes, and cheese. If lodged in throat and breathing is possible, interference should be limited until professional aid is at hand. SEE: *foreign bodies (in throat)*.

cholago'gia [G. *cholē*, bile, + *agein*, to lead forth]. Excretion of bile from gallbladder.

cholagogue (ko'lă-gog) [" + *agein*, to lead forth]. A purgative that stimulates the flow of bile. Ex: *Calomel, inspissated oxgall, sodium glycocholate, and sodium taurocholate.*

cholangiogastrostomy (ko-lan″jĭ-o-gas-tros′to-mĭ) [" + *aggeion*, vessel, + *gastēr*, stomach, + *stoma*, mouth]. Formation of a communication bet. a bile duct and the stomach.

cholangiography (ko-lan-jĭ-og'ră-fĭ) [" + " + *graphein*, to write]. X-ray or skiagraphic examination of the bile ducts.

cholangioma (ko-lan-jĭ-o'mă) [" + " + *-ōma*, tumor]. A tumor of the biliary ducts.

cholangiostomy (kol-an-jĭ-os'to-mĭ) [" + " + *stoma*, mouth]. The surgical formation of a fistula into the gallbladder.

cholangiotomy (kol-an-jĭ-ot'o-mĭ) [" + " + *tomē*, incision]. Incision of an intrahepatic bile duct for removal of gallstones.

cholangitis (ko-lan-ji'tis) [" + " + *-ītis*, inflammation]. Inflammation of the gall or bile duct. May be obstructive or catarrhal.

cholascos (ko-las'kos) [" + *askos*, bag]. Escape of bile into the peritoneal cavity.

cholecyst (kol'e-sist) [" + *kystis*, cyst]. A pearshaped sac on the undersurface of the right lobe of the liver, the reservoir for the bile. SYN: *gallbladder, vesica fellea*.

cholecystalgia (ko-le-sis-tal'jĭ-ă) [" + " + *algos*, pain]. Biliary colic.

cholecystectasia (ko-le-sis-tek-ta'zĭ-ă) [" + " + *ektasis*, dilatation]. Dilatation of the gallbladder.

cholecystectomy (ko-le-sis-tekt'o-mĭ) [" + " + *ektomē*, excision]. Excision of a gallbladder.

cholecystendysis (ko-le-sis-ten'dĭ-sis) [" + " + *endysis*, entrance]. Removal of a gallstone by incision, suturing wound in gallbladder and abdominal wall.

cholecystenterorrhaphy (ko-le-sist-en-ter-or'ă-fĭ) [" + " + *enteron*, intestine, + *raphē*, suture]. Suture of gallbladder to intestinal wall.

cholecystenterostomy (ko-le-sist-en-ter-os'to-mĭ) [" + " + " + *stoma*, opening]. Suturing of gallbladder to intestine.

cholecystic (ko-le-sis'tĭk) [" + *kystis*, cyst]. Pert. to the gallbladder.

cholecystitis (ko-lĕ-sis-ti'tis) [" + " + *-ītis*, inflammation]. Inflammation of the gallbladder. It may be acute or chronic.

ETIOL: Gallstones, bacteria, parasites, organic or inorganic substances. Extension of inflammation or growths from adjacent organs.

SYM: Distention through thickening of bile may give rise to pain and tenderness on palpation. Suppuration, ulceration, or gangrene may ensue. Jaundice appears when obstruction occurs.

TREATMENT: Principally dietetic, for which see *gallbladder*. Half teaspoonful Epsom salts in warm water on rising help to empty gallbladder. Fats in diet should be strictly limited. Surgery may be indicated.

NP: *Postoperative*: Fowler's position to aid drainage. Watch for shock and symptoms of pneumonia. Sodium bicarbonate solution if needed to prevent vomiting. Stomach may have to be washed out. Flatus tube or carminative* enema, to relieve abdominal distention. An aperient 1st night, a saline aperient 3rd morning. Fluids in abundance and light diet after bowels have acted. Change soiled dressings. Remove drainage tube when it ceases to function. Prevent infection.

cholecystnephrostomy (ko″le-sist-nef-ros′-to-mī) [" + " + *nephros*, kidney, + *stoma*, mouth]. Making an anastomosis of gallbladder into renal pelvis.

cholecystocolostomy (ko-le-sis-to-ko-los′-to-mī) [" + " + *kolon*, colon, + *stoma*, mouth]. Making a passage from gallbladder to colon.

cholecystocolotomy (ko-le-sis-to-ko-lot′o-mī) [" + " + *tomē*, incision]. Incision into gallbladder and colon.

cholecystoduodenostomy (kol-e-sis-to-du-o-den-os′to-mī) [" + " + L. *duodeni*, twelve, + G. *stoma*, mouth]. Surgical formation of a passage from gallbladder to duodenum.

cholecystogastrostomy (ko-le-sis-to-gas′tros′to-mī) [" + " + *gastēr*, belly, + *stoma*, mouth]. Surgical formation of a passage from the gallbladder to the stomach.

cholecys′togram [" + " + *gramma*, mark]. An x-ray picture of the gallbladder.

cholecystography (ko-le-sis-tog′rā-fī) [" + " + *graphein*, to write]. Examination of the gallbladder by x-ray.

cholecystoileostomy (ko-le-sis-to-il-e-os′-to-mī) [" + " + L. *ileum* + G. *stoma*, mouth]. Forming a communication bet. the gallbladder and ileum.

cholecystojejunostomy (ko-le-sis-to-je-ju-nos′to-mī) [" + " + L. *jejunum*, empty, + *stoma*, mouth]. Forming a communication bet. the gallbladder and jejunum.

cholecystokinin (ko″le-sĭs″tō-kī′nĭn) [" + " + *kinein*, to move]. A hormone supposed to stimulate action of the gallbladder.

cholecystolithiasis (ko-le-sis-to-lith-i′ā-sis) [" + " + *lithos*, stone]. Gallstones in the gallbladder.

cholecystolithotripsy (ko-le-sis-to-lith′o-trip-sī) [" + " + " + *tripsis*, a crushing]. Crushing of a gallstone in the unopened gallbladder.

cholecys′tomy [" + " + *tomē*, incision]. Cutting into the gallbladder. SYN: *cholecystotomy*.

cholecystopathy (ko-le-sis-top′ă-thī) (" + " + *pathos*, disease]. Any gallbladder affection.

cholecystopexy (ko-le-sis′to-pek-sī) [" + " + *pexis*, fixation]. Suturing the gallbladder to the abdominal wall.

cholecystoptosis (ko-le-sis-top-to′sis) [" + " + *ptōsis*, fall]. Displacement of the gallbladder downward.

cholecystorrhaphy (kō-lē-sis-tor′ă-fī) [" + " + *raphē*, suture]. Suturing of the gallbladder.

cholecystostomy (kol-e-sis-tos′to-mī) [" + " + *stoma*, opening]. Surgical formation of a permanent opening into gallbladder through abdominal wall.

cholecystotomy (ko-le-sis-tot′o-mī) [" + " + *tomē*, incision]. Incision of gallbladder through the abdominal walls for removal of gallstones.

choledochectasia (ko-led-o-kek-ta′zī-ă) [G. *choledochos*, common bile duct, + *ektasis*, distention]. Distention of the common bile duct or *ductus choledochus*.

choledochitis (ko-led-o-ki′tis) [" + -*itis*, inflammation]. Inflammation of common bile duct.

choledochoduodenostomy (ko-led″o-ko-du-o-den-os′to-mī) [" + L. *duodeni*, twelve, + G. *stoma*, opening]. Surgical communication bet. the common bile duct and duodenum.

choledochoenterostomy (ko-led″o-ko-en-ter-os′to-mī) [" + *enteron*, intestine, + *stoma*, opening]. Surgical passage bet. common bile duct and intestine.

choledocholithiasis (ko-led″o-ko-lith-i′ā-sis) [" + *lithos*, stone]. Calculi in the common bile duct.

choledocholithotomy (ko-le-do-ko-lith-ot′-o-mī) [" + " + *tomē*, incision]. Removal of a gallstone through an incision of the bile duct.

choledocholithotripsy (ko-led-o-ko-lith′o-trip-sī) [" + " + *tripsis*, a crushing]. Crushing of a gallstone in the common bile duct.

choledochoplasty (kol-e-do′ko-plas″tī) [" + *plassein*, to form]. Operation for repair of common bile duct.

choledochorrhaphy (ko-led-o-kor′ră-fī) [" + *raphē*, suture]. Suturing the severed ends of the common bile duct.

choledochostomy (kol-ed-o-kos′to-mī) [" + *stoma*, mouth]. Surgical formation of an opening into common bile duct through abdominal wall.

choledochotomy (kol-ed-o-kot′o-mī) [" + *tomē*, incision]. Surgical incision of the common bile duct.

choledochus (ko-led′o-kus) [G. *cholē*, bile, + *dechesthai*, to receive]. The common bile duct. SYN: *ductus choledochus*.

cholehemia (ko-le-he′mī-ă) [" + *aima*, blood]. Bile in the blood. SYN: *cholemia*.

choleic (ko-le′ĭk). Cholic; pert. to the bile.

chol′elith [G. *cholē*, bile, + *lithos*, stone]. A bile stone.

cholelithiasis (kol-e-lith-i′as-is) [" + *lithos*, stone]. Formation of, or presence of calculi or bilestones in the gallbladder or gallduct.

They may remain dormant or be responsible for few symptoms.

SYM: Digestive disturbances; heaviness in right hypochondrium, tenderness on pressure over gallbladder. Gallstone colic when passing through bile duct if obstructed. Pain may radiate to back and right shoulder. Colic usually manifest when stomach is empty. Jaundice if flow of bile is obstructed. Pain may be associated with vomiting, acidity, and sweating. Gallbladder may be palpated if distended. [necessary.

TREATMENT: If colic is severe, surgery

cholelithic (ko-le-lith′ĭk). Pert. to or caused by biliary calculus.

cholelithotomy (kol-e-lith-ot′o-mī) [G. *cholē*, bile, + *lithos*, stone, + *tomē*, incision]. Removal of gallstones through a surgical incision.

cholelithotrity (ko-le-lī-thot′rĭ-tī) [" + " + L. *tritus*, crushing]. Crushing of a biliary calculus.

cholemesis (kol-em′e-sis) [" + *emein*, to vomit]. Bile in the vomitus.

cholemia (ko-le′mī-ă) [" + *aima*, blood]. Bile salts in the blood.

cholepathia (ko-le-path′ī-ă) [" + *pathos*, disease]. Faulty contractions of bile ducts.

c. spas′tica. Spasmodic contraction of biliary ducts.

choleperitoneum (ko-le-per-ĭ-to-ne′um) [" + *peri*, around, + *teinein*, to stretch]. Bile in the peritoneum.

cholepyrrhin (ko-le-pir′ĭn) [" + *pyrros*, flame colored]. Impure bilirubin. SYN: *biliphein*.

chol′era [" + *rein*, to flow]. An acute, specific, infectious disease characterized by diarrhea, painful cramps of muscles, and tendency to collapse. Also called *Asiatic c., Indian c., algid c., asphyctic c., epidemic c., malignant c.*, and *pestilential c.*

ETIOL: Causative organism, Vibrio cholera (also called Vibrio coma, Spilillum cholerae asiaticae, Spirillum chol-

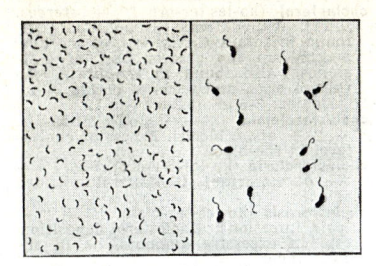

CHOLERA VIBRIO
Left, smear from young culture; right (higher magnification), stain for flagella.

erae, comma bacillus) which is found in the stools. Transmission may be through water supply, foods, immune carriers, or from man to man, either direct or indirect. The only portal of infection is the alimentary tract.
INCUBATION: A few hours to 4 to 5 days.
SYM: Four stages are usually described as follows:
Invasion: At the conclusion of the incubation period there is malaise, headache, diarrhea, and anorexia. Headache and slight fever are present. May last a few days, and then subside. Under such circumstances, may be termed cholerine. Sometimes this stage is lacking entirely.
Evacuation: Purging, violent, vomiting, and muscular cramps. Stools loose, copious, and watery, and present a typical rice water appearance. Sometimes there are particles of blood, as well as mucus. Vomiting severe and persistent; material expelled may also resemble rice water. Muscular cramps commonly start in extremities, involve calves of legs, and later even hands, hands, feet, and trunk. Thirst unquenchable and hiccough sometimes develops. Signs of depression soon terminate in collapse. Duration of stage, 2 to 12 hours; seldom more.
Stage of Collapse: Almost complete arrest of circulation, eyes sunken, cheeks hollow, nose pinched, skin dry and wrinkled, body surface cold, covered with clammy sweat, breath cool, temperature in axilla 85-95° F., while in the rectum it may be 103° F. or more. Respirations quickened, pulse weak, systolic blood pressure from 50 to 60, urine suppressed; evacuation and cramps may continue. Mind usually clear until toward the close when coma develops. Stage lasts from few hours to 1 or 2 days, and generally ends in death.
Stage of Reaction: Sometimes, even when death seems imminent, surface temperature begins to rise, vomiting ceases, bowel evacuations become less frequent, more feculent* and convalescence is established. Complete recovery may ensue in from 1 to 2 weeks. Occasionally, typhoid symptoms set in, temperature goes from 106-107° F. and outcome is fatal. Sometimes in this stage, an erythemal eruption or one of the urticarial type appears, particularly on extremities. Such eruptions have no special significance.
SEE: *anticholerin, "choler-" words*.
c. infantum. An acute disease of childhood, accompanied by vomiting, purging, and collapse.

ETIOL: Inflammation of the gastrointestinal tract and possible disturbance of the sympathetic ganglia.
SYM: Onset gradual or abrupt. Diarrhea usually initial symptom. Stools thin, serous, musty odor, and alkaline reaction. Vomiting, everything rejected, thirst intense. Temperature 105-108° F., pulse rapid, feeble, urine scanty. Collapse follows and is indicated by pinched features, hollow eyes, sunken fontanelles, and cold body surface. Dehydration marked. Reaction may set in or death result from exhaustion. End may be characterized by symptoms of spurious hydrocephalus, restlessness, convulsions, irregular pupils, and coma, probably toxemic, as there is no cerebral lesion.
PROG: Grave.
TREATMENT: Change of surroundings advisable. Fresh air and good hygienic surroundings most advantageous. Careful regulation of diet, which may be temporarily limited to barley water. If mother's health permits, breast feeding is preferable. Otherwise, utmost care and cleanliness are necessary in connection with artificial feeding.
c. morbus. An acute, sporadic disease, resembling cholera, but not excited by the comma bacillus of Koch.
SYM: Intense cramps in stomach, vomiting and purging of bilious material, moderate fever, and great prostration. In severe cases, discharges become serous and symptoms of collapse develop.
PROG: Favorable; death rarely occurs.
DURATION: Twenty-four to 48 hours.
TREATMENT: Hot applications to abdomen. Internal remedies, such as tincture of camphorated opium, are frequently helpful.
c. sicca. A term sometimes applied to a fulminating variety of cholera which occurs without vomiting or purging.
After death, intestines are found to contain rice water fluid not discharged during life on account of paralysis of muscular coat of the bowel.
COMPLICATIONS: Anuria, hyperpepsia, bronchopneumonia, parotitis, conjunctive keratitis, iritis, and gangrene of extremities.
DIFFERENTIAL DIAG: Cholera morbus, bacillary dysentery, food and metallic poisonings. Sometimes, cultural tests are necessary for definite diagnosis.
PROG: Most unfavorable in the old, young, and those suffering from chronic disease. Early collapse, cyanosis, and anuria are bad omens. Mortality averages about 50%.
TREATMENT: *Prophylactic*: Quarantine, which should provide for screened enclosures. Protection of water supply, disinfection of stools and vomits, as well as contaminated articles. Personal cleanliness, esp. of hands, and avoidance of uncooked foods.
Active: Absolute rest in bed and adequate warmth. Diet consists largely of barley water or whey. Use of cathartics inadvisable. Morphine of questionable value. Anticholera serum has met with little success. Atropine in doses of 0.01 gr., morning and night, seems helpful. In cases of collapse, normal salt solution at temperature of 98° in quantities of 500 cc. to 1000 cc., intravenously, should be given. Caffeine, sodium benzoate, camphor, and pituitary extract are also used.
IMMUNIZATION: Has been undertaken by a vaccine made from heat killed

cultures. It is administered subcutaneously in from 2 to 3 doses, beginning with 0.5 cc. and then 0.1 cc., each dose containing about 8,000,000 organisms per cc. The protection afforded usually lasts for at least 3 months.

choleraic (kol-ē-ra'ĭk). Pert. to cholera.

cholerase (kol'er-ās). The special bacteriolytic enzyme of cholera vibrio.

choleresis (kol-er-e'sis) [G. *chole*, bile, + *eresis*, removal]. The excretion of bile by the liver.

choleretic (kol-er-et'ĭk). Pert. to choleresis, or any agent that increases excretion of bile by the liver.

choleric (kol'er-ik). Irritable; quick-tempered without apparent cause.

choleriform (kol-er'ĭ-form) [G. *chole*, bile, + *rein*, to flow, + L. *forma*, shape]. Appearing like cholera.

cholerigenous (kol-er-ij'en-us) [" + " + *gennan*, to produce]. Giving rise to cholera.

cholerine (kol'er-ēn). A mild form or initial stages of Asiatic cholera.

cholerization (kol-er-ĭ-za'shun) [G. *chole*, bile, + *rein*, to flow]. Inoculation against cholera.

cholerophobia (kol-er-o-fo'be-a) [" + " + *phobos*, fear]. Morbid fear of acquiring cholera.

cholerrhagia (kol-er-ra'jĭ-ă) [" + *regnunai*, to burst forth]. A flow of bile.

cholerythrin (kol-er'ĭ-thrin) [" + *erythros*, red]. 1. Cholera-red. 2. Pigment in urine of tropical residents.

cholesta'sia [" + *stasis*, stoppage]. Arrest of the bile excretion.

chol"estat'ic. Caused by arrest of biliary excretion.

cholesteatoma (kol-es-te-ă-to'ma) [G. *chole*, bile, + *stear*, fat, + -*oma*, tumor]. 1. (Primary.) A pearl tumor or pearly nodules in brain. 2. (Secondary.) One of suppurative otitic origin in presence of marginal perforations. Fatty degeneration of epithelium containing cholesterin crystals caused by nature's effort to arrest suppuration. Chloroform test to determine green ring.

choles'terase [" + *stereos*, solid]. A cholesterol ferment.

cholesteremia (ko-les-ter-e'mĭ-ă) [" + " + *aima*, blood]. Cholesterol in the blood.

cholesterin (ko-les'ter-in) [" + *stereos*, solid]. Sterol; solid alcohol combined with fatty acids, forming a crystalline fat from bile and nerve tissue.
It is held in solution in bile by the bile salts and is insoluble in water. It is deposited in the urine in the form of irregular flat platelets. It occurs in nearly every living tissue and makes it possible for the cells to hold large quantities of water. It checks the fat splitting enzymes and regulates fat metabolism, and absorption. The bile acids are derived from its mother substance. It also makes possible immunization from snake venom and neutralizes it.
DOSAGE: 3-5 gr. (0.2-0.3 Gm.).
DIAG: Normal content in blood is 150-170 mg. per each 100 cc. of blood. It increases after heavy, fatty meals, in diabetes, in some degenerative disorders, in pregnancy, arteriosclerosis, and obstructive jaundice. SEE: "*cholest-*" words.

cholesterinemia (ko-les-ter-in-e'mĭ-ă) [" + " + *aima*, blood]. Presence of cholesterol in the blood. SYN: *cholesterolemia*.

cholesterinuria (ko-les-ter-ĭn-u'rĭ-ă) [" + " + *ouron*, urine]. Passing of cholesterin in the urine.

cholesterol (ko-les'ter-ol) [" + *stereos*, solid]. A monatomic alcohol, $C_{27}H_{45}OH$, found in fats and oils, esp. in the bile, making up the greater part of gallstones. Also found in the brain, the yolk of eggs, and seeds of plants.
DOSAGE: 3-5 gr. (0.2-0.3 Gm.).

cholesterolemia (ko-les-ter-ol-e'mĭ-ă) [" + " + *aima*, blood]. Excess of cholesterol in the blood.

cholesteroluria (ko-les-ter-ol-u'rĭ-ă) [" + " + *ouron*, urine]. Cholesterol in voided urine.

cholesterosis (ko-les-ter-o'sis) [" + " + -*osis*, infection]. Cholesterol deposition, esp. in excessive amounts, as in the gallbladder.

choletelin (ko-let'el-in) [" + *telos*, end]. Yellow coloring derived from bilirubin.

choletherapy (ko-le-ther'ă-pĭ) [" + *therapeia*, treatment]. Use of oxgall as a medicine. [urine]. Bile in urine.

choleuria (ko-le-u'rĭ-ă) [" + *ouron*,

choleverdin (ko-le-ver'din) [" + L. *viridis*, green]. Green pigment appearing in gallstones and in urine in jaundice. SYN: *biliverdin.*

choline (kŏl'ēn) [G. *chole*, bile]. A ptomaine found in bile and suprarenal extract; a decomposition product of lecithin essential for functioning of the liver. Claimed to be a Vit. B. complex.

cholinergic. Term applied to nerve endings which liberate acetylcholine.
  c. fibers. They include all preganglionic fibers (2) all postganglionic parasympathetic fibers (3) postganglionic sympathetic fibers to sweat glands (4) efferent fibers to skeletal muscle.

cholochrome (ko'lo-krōm) [" + *chroma*, color]. Any bile pigment.

cholohemothorax (ko-lo-hĕm-o-tho'raks) [" + *aima*, blood, + *thorax*, chest]. Bile and blood in the thorax.

chololith (kol'o-lith) [" + *lithos*, stone]. A gallstone; biliary calculus.

chololithiasis (kol"o-lith-l'ăs-is). Presence of concretions in the gallbladder. SYN: *cholelithiasis.*

cholorrhea (kol-or-re'ă) [G. *chole*, bile, + *roia*, flow]. Excessive secretion of bile.

choloscopy (ko-los'ko-pĭ) [" + *skopein*, to examine]. Testing the biliary function.

cholosis (ko-lo'sis) [" + -*osis*, infection]. A perversion of bile secretion.

choluria (ko-lu'rĭ-a) [" + *ouron*, urine]. Bile salts in the urine.

chondral (kon'dral) [G. *chondros*, cartilage]. Pert. to cartilage.

chondralgia (kon-dral'jĭ-ă) [" + *algos*, pain]. Pain in or around a cartilage.

chondralloplasia (kon"dral-o-pla'zĭ-ă) [" + *allos*, other, + *plassein*, to form]. Presence of cartilage in abnormal places.

chondrectomy (kon-drek'to-mĭ) [" + *ektome*, excision]. Surgical excision of a cartilage.

chondric (kon'drik) [G. *chondros*, cartilage]. Pert. to cartilage.

chondrification (kon-drĭ-fĭ-ka'shun) [" + L. *facere*, to make]. Conversion into cartilage.

chon'drigen [" + *gennan*, to produce]. Basal substance of cartilage, which turns into chondrin on boiling. SYN: *chondrogen.*

chondrin (kon'drĭn) [G. *chondros*, cartilage]. Gelatinlike matter obtained by boiling cartilage.

chondriosome (kon'drĭ-o-sōm) [" + *soma*, body]. A constituent of cytoplasm in the protoplasm of a cell. May be concerned in the production of germ cells.

chondritis (kon-dri'tis) [" + -*itis*, inflammation]. Inflammation of cartilage.

chon″droadeno'ma [" + *aden*, gland, + -*oma*, tumor]. Cartilaginous tissue in an adenoma.

chon″droangio'ma [" + *aggeion*, vessel, + -*oma*, tumor]. Cartilaginous elements in an angioma.

chondroblast (kon'dro-blast) [" + *blastos*, germ]. Cell of primitive cartilage in the embryo.

chondroclast (kon'dro-klast) [" + *klastos*, broken into bits]. A cell concerned in the absorption of cartilage.

chondroconia (kon-dro-ko'ni-ă) [" + *konis*, dust]. Reddish granules in myelocytes.

chondrocostal (kon-dro-kos'tal) [" + L. *costa*, rib]. Pert. to costal cartilages.

chondrocranium (kon-dro-kra'ni-um) [" + *kranion*, head]. The cartilaginous embryonic cranium before ossification.

chondrocyte (kon'dro-sīt) [" + *kytos*, cell]. A cartilage cell.

chondrodynia (kon-dro-din'ĭ-ă) [" + *odynē*, pain]. Pain in or about a cartilage.

chondrodysplasia (kon″dro-dis-pla'zĭ-ă) [" + *dys*, bad, + *plassein*, to form]. Abnormal cartilage growth.

chondrodystrophy (kon-dro-dis'tro-fī) [" + *dys*, difficult, + *trophē*, nourishment]. Defect in cartilage formation at epiphyses of long bones.

chondrofibroma (kon-dro-fĭ-bro'mă) [" + L. *fibra*, fiber, + G. -*oma*, tumor]. A mixed tumor with elements of chondroma and fibroma.

chondrogen (kon'dro-jen) [" + *gennan*, to produce]. The cement substance of cartilage.

chondrogenesis (kon-dro-jen'es-is) [" + *genesis*, production]. Formation of cartilage.

chondroid (kon'droid) [" + *eidos*, resemblance]. Resembling cartilage; cartilaginous.

chondroituria (kon-dro-ĭ-tu'rĭ-ă) [" + *ouron*, urine]. Chondroitic acid in urine.

chondrolipoma (kon-dro-lip-o'mă) [" + *lipos*, fat, + -*oma*, tumor]. Cartilaginous and fatty tissue tumor.

chondrology (kon-drol'o-jī) [" + *logos*, study]. The science of cartilages.

chondrolysis (kon-drol'ĭ-sis) [" + *lysis*, dissolution]. The breaking down and absorption of cartilage.

chondro'ma [" + -*oma*, tumor]. A cartilaginous tumor of slow growth.
It may occur any place where there is cartilage. It causes no pain.

chondromalacia (kon-drō-mal-a'sĭ-ă) [" + *malakia*, softening]. Softness of any cartilage.

chondromalacosis (kon-drō-mal-ă-ko'sis) [" + " + -*ōsis*, infection]. Cartilage softening. SYN: *chondromalacia*.*

chondromatous (kon-dro'mă-tus) [" + -*oma*, tumor]. Pert. to chondroma, or tumor of a cartilage.

chondromucoid (kon-dro-mu'koid) [" + L. *mucus*, mucus, + G. *eidos*, form]. Mucin in cartilage.

chondromyoma (kon-dro-mi-o'mă) [" + *mys*, muscle, + -*oma*, tumor]. Myoma and cartilaginous neoplasm combined.

chondromyxoma (kon-dro-mĭk-sō'mă) [" + *myxa*, mucus, + -*oma*, tumor]. Chondroma with myxomatous elements.

chondromyxosarcoma (kon-dro-mĭk″sō-sar-kō'mă) [" + " + *sarx*, flesh, + -*oma*-tumor]. A cartilaginous and sarcomatous tumor.

chondropathology (kon-dro-path'ol-o-jī) [" + *pathos*, disease, + *logos*, study of]. Pathology of cartilages.

chondropathy (kon-drop'ath-ī) [" + *pathos*, disease]. Any disease of cartilage.

chondrophyte (kon'dro-fīt) [" + *phyton*, a growth]. A growth from articular cartilage.

chondroplast (kon'dro-plast) [" + *plassein*, to mold]. Cell of primitive cartilage in the embryo. SYN: *chondroblast*.

chondroplas'tic. Pert. to plastic operations on cartilage.

chondroplasty (kon'dro-plas-tī) [G. *chondros*, cartilage, + *plassein*, to mold]. Plastic or reparative surgery on cartilage.

chondroporosis (kon-dro-po-ro'sis) [" + *poros*, passage]. The porous condition of cartilage, pathological or normal, during ossification.

chondroproteins (kon-dro-pro'te-ins) [" + *prōtos*, first]. A group of glucoproteins found in cartilage, tendons, and connective tissue.

chondrosarcoma (kon-dro-sar-ko'mă) [" + *sarx*, flesh, + -*ōma*, tumor]. Cartilaginous sarcoma.

chondro'sis [" + -*ōsis*, infection]. The development of cartilage.

chon″droster'nal [" + *sternon*, chest]. Pert. to sternal cartilage.

chondrotome (kon'dro-tōm) [" + *tomē*, a cutting]. Device for dissection of cartilage.

chondrotomy (kon-drot'o-mī) [" + *tomē*, incision]. Dissection or surgical division of cartilage.

chondroxiphoid (kon-dro-zi'foid) [" + *xiphos*, sword, + *eidos*, form]. Pert. to the ensiform cartilage or xiphoid.

chondrus (kon'drus) [G. *chondros*]. Cartilage.

Chopart's amputation (sho-pars'). Disarticulation at the midtarsal joint.

chor'da [G. *chordē*, cord]. A string or tendon.
  c. dorsalis. The notochord.
  c. gubernaculi. An embryonic structure forming a part of the gubernaculum testis in the male and the round ligament in the female.
  c. obliqua. The oblique ligament, an oblique cord which connects the shafts of the radius and ulna. Extends from lateral side of tubercle of ulna to a point just below radial tuberosity.
  c. tendinea. A small tendinous cord which connects the free edge of an atrioventricular valve to a papillary muscle.
  c. tympani. A branch of the facial nerve which leaves the cranium through the stylomastoid foramen, transverses the tympanic cavity and joins a branch of the lingual nerve. Efferent fibers innervate the submaxillary and sublingual glands; afferent fibers convey taste impulses from ant. two thirds of the tongue.
  c. umbilicalis. Umbilical cord connecting fetus and placenta.
  c. Willisii. One of several fibrous cords across the superior longitudinal sinus.

chordal (kor'dal). Pert. to a chorda, esp. the notochord.

chordée (kor-de') [Fr. corded]. Downward, painful curvature of the penis on erection in gonorrhea caused by inflammatory infiltration of the corpus spongiosum which interferes with its distensibility.

A common occurrence in gonorrhea as the result of trauma.

chorditis (kor-di'tis) [G. *chordē*, cord, + *-itis*, inflammation]. Inflammation of a cord, esp. the spermatic, or a vocal cord.

c. nodo'sa. Formation of small, whitish nodules on one or both vocal cords.

SYM: Hoarseness, inability of singers to register tones properly.

TREATMENT: Vocal hygiene. Surgical removal of nodules if they do not respond to conservative therapy.

chordoskeleton (kor-do-skel'et-on) [" + *skeleton*, a dried-up body]. That part of the skeleton in the embryo formed about the primitive spinal cord.

chordot'omy [" + *tomē*, dissection]. Division of any cord to relieve pain.

chorea (ko-re'ă) [G. *choreia*, dance]. A nervous affection marked by muscular twitching.

c. Sydenham's. St. Vitus' dance. Occurs mostly in children.

SYM: Lasts 6 to 8 weeks. Often accompanied with irritability, constipation, anemia, and loss of appetite; infectious. Movements of the head are irregular, and muscles of arms and face may be involved. Has a definite relation to scarlet fever, rheumatism and other infections.

PROG: Usually recover in course of 2 or 3 months. Relapses not infrequent. Rare complication is death from heart disease. Among possible sequelae are imbecility and chronic chorea.

TREATMENT: Rest of body and mind, remove child from school; place under most favorable hygienic conditions. Careful search should be made for reflex irritation as adherent prepuce, intestinal parasites, eyestrain, etc. All excitement avoided. Keep out of doors. Internal remedies.

SEE: *Bergeron's chorea, jactitation.*

c., electric. Progressively fatal spasmodic disorder.

ETIOL: Possibly of malarial origin. Occurs usually in Italy. SYN: *Dubini's disease.*

c., epidemic. Religious emotional neurosis, manifest in the 14th century in Europe, exhibited in form of dancing mania. SYN: *dancing mania.*

c. gravidum. A form seen in some pregnant women, usually in those who have had chorea before, esp. in their first pregnancy.

c., Huntington's. A hereditary and chronic form manifested in adult life.

c., hyoscine. Movements simulating chorea, and sometimes accompanied by delirium, seen in acute hyoscine intoxication.

c., insaniens. Movements so violent patient is unable to walk, eat or even lie down.

SYM: Fever develops, mind becomes delirious. Death frequently results from exhaustion. This form usually observed in adults, and esp. in primipara.

PROG: Frequently terminates fatally through exhaustion.

TREATMENT: Quiet, hygienic life. Forced feeding. Severe cases complicating pregnancy will call for induction of premature labor. Constitutional remedies.

NP: Rest in bed. Sides of crib should be padded. Light bed clothes, soft and free from wrinkles to avoid dermatitis. Isolation necessary. Visitors restricted; esp. no children. If possible tub baths prolonged as sedative; warm water and hot sponging. Rhythmic breathing and rhythmic exercises as improvement sets in. Quietness. If violent, make bed on floor surrounded by bolsters. Rubber under sheets, soft blanket. Nourishing diet. Food in small pieces, as patient may not masticate. No glass utensils. Feed slowly. Precautions against bed sores. Mouth hygiene. Water bet. meals. Bowels should be active. Measure and test urine for albumin. No exertion.

c., major. C. with violent hysterical muscular action.

c., mimetic. C. due to imitative movements.

c., minor. Ordinary form of chorea.

c., posthemiplegic; c., postparalytic. Involuntary movements of patients subsequent to a hemiplegic attack.

c., rhythmic. C. with movements at regulated times.

c., senile. C. developing in senility.

choreal (ko-re'al). Pert. to chorea.

choreic (ko-re'ik). Pert. to or of nature of chorea.

choreiform (ko-re'ĭ-form) [G. *choreia*, dance, + L. *forma*, form]. Of the nature of chorea.

choreomania (ko-re-o-ma'nĭ-ă) [" + *mania*, madness]. Epidemic chorea, as the dancing mania of the middle ages.

chorioadenoma (ko-rĭ-o-ad-en-o'mă) [G. *chorion*, skin, + *adēn*, gland, + *-ōma*, tumor]. Adenoma of the chorion.

chorioangioma (ko-rĭ-o-an-jĭ-o'mă) [" + *aggeion*, vessel, + *-ōma*, tumor]. A vascular tumor of the chorion.

choriocapillaris (ko-rĭ-o-kap-il-la'ris) [" + L. *capillaris*, hairlike]. Capillary layer of choroid.

choriocele (ko'rĭ-o-sēl) [" + *kēlē*, hernia]. A protrusion of the chorioid coat of the eye through a defective sclera.

chorioepithelioma (ko-ri-o-ep-ĭ-the-lĭ-o'mă) [" + *epi*, upon, + *thēlē*, nipple, + *-ōma*, tumor]. Excessive proliferation of chorionic epithelium. SYN: *syncytioma malignum.*

chorioid (ko'rĭ-oid). Vascular coat of eye bet. sclera and retina. SYN: *choroid, q.v.*

chorioma (ko-rĭ-o'mă) (pl. *chorio'mata*) [" + *-ōma*, tumor]. A tumor of the chorion.

choriomeningitis (ko-rĭ-o-men-in-jĭ'tis) [" + *meninx*, membrane, + *-itis*, inflammation]. Cerebral meningitis with cellular infiltration of the meninges.

c., acute lymphocytic. Disease resembling epidemic encephalitis, ant. poliomyelitis, and meningitis.

chorion (ko'rĭ-on) [G.]. Membrane developed from the external epiblastic layer and an internal mesoblastic layer which together form the wall of the primitive blastocyst.

It lies bet. the amnion and decidua reflexa and it envelops, protects, and supplies nourishment to the embryo. The epiblastic epithelium is the trophoblast.

This layer is rapidly differentiated into 2 layers, the cytotrophoblast which immediately surrounds the ovum (cells of Langhans), and the plasmoditrophoblast which is undifferentiated protoplasm (syncytium), the cells of which erode the mucous membrane. The irregular trophoblastic buds are penetrated by mesoblastic tissue carrying with it fetal blood vessels and thus converting the buds into chorionic villi.

The cells of the villi are arranged in layers covering the vascular core of

CHORION

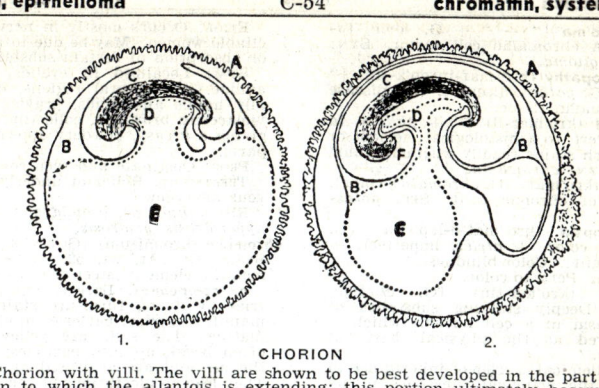

A, Chorion with villi. The villi are shown to be best developed in the part of the chorion to which the allantois is extending; this portion ultimately becomes the placenta. B, Extra-embryonic coelom. C, Amniotic cavity. D, Primitive gut or embryonic intestine. E, Yolk sac or umbilical vesicle.

mesoblast. (a) Layer of Langhans, inner layer of discrete cells. (b) Syncytium, outer layer of undifferentiated multinucleated protoplasm.

During the first few weeks of pregnancy, the entire surface of the ovum is covered with branching villi. The villi in contact with the decidua basalis rapidly multiply to form the *chorion frondosum*. Over the rest of the ovum the villi grow less rapidly and finally atrophy to disappear completely about the 4th month; this layer is called the *chorion laeve*.
SEE: *"chorio-"* words.
c. epithelioma. Very malignant tumor of uterus occurring most commonly after a vesicular mole and sometimes after an abortion.
chorionic (ko-rĭ-on'ĭk). Pert. to the chorion.
c. villi. The vascular projections from the chorion.
chorionitis (ko-rĭ-on-i'tis) [G. *chorion*, skin, + *-itis*, inflammation]. 1. Inflammation of the chorion. 2. Inflammation of the true skin, or corium.
chorioretinitis (ko-rĭ-o-ret"ĭn-i'tis) [" + L. *rete*, network, + G. *-itis*, inflammation]. Inflammation of choroid and retina.
chorista (ko-ris'tă) [G. *chōristos*, separated]. An error of development showing separation from the rudiments in a developing embryo.
choristoma (ko-ris-to'mă) [" + *-ōma*, tumor]. A neoplasm due to overdevelopment of embryonic rudiments.
choroid (ko'roid) [G. *chorioeidēs*, skinlike]. Dark brown, vascular coat of eye bet. sclera and retina, extending from *ora serrata* to optic nerve.

Consists of blood vessels, united by connective tissue containing pigmented cells, and is made up of 5 layers: (1) suprachoroid; (2) layer of large vessels; (3) layer of medium sized vessels; (4) layer of capillaries; (5) *lamina vitrea* (homogeneous membrane placed next to pigmentary layer of retina).

FUNCTION: Nutrient organ for retina, vitreous, lens. SEE: *auliplexus,* "*choroid-*" words.
choroideremia (ko-roy-der-e'mĭ-ă) [G. *chorioeidēs*, skinlike, + *erēmia*, destitution]. Absence of the choroid coat of the eye.
choroiditis (ko-roid-i'tis) [" + *-itis*, inflammation]. Inflammation of choroid.

c., anterior. When outlets of exudation are at the choroidal periphery.
c., areolar. In which inflammation spreads from around the macula lutea.
c., central. Exudation is limited to the macula.
c., diffuse or disseminated. When the fundus is covered with spots.
c., exudative. When covered with patches of inflammation.
c., metastatic. When due to embolism.
c. serosa. Increase of fluids in eyeball raising intraocular pressure, resulting in atrophy of optic nerve and blindness. SYN: *glaucoma.**
c., suppurative. When suppuration occurs.
choroidocycli'tis [" + *kyklos*, a circle, + *-itis*, inflammation]. Inflammation of the choroid coat and ciliary processes.
choroidoiritis (ko-royd-o-i-ri'tis) [" + *iris*, iris, + *-itis*, inflammation]. Inflammation of the choroid coat and iris.
choroidoretinitis (ko-royd-o-ret-in-i'tis) (" + L. *rete*, network, + G. *-itis*, inflammation]. Inflammation of choroid and retina.
choromania (ko-ro-mā'nĭ-ă) [G. *choros*, dance, + *mania*, madness]. Epidemic dancing mania; choreomania.
Christian Science. A religion and system of healing disease of mind and body which teaches that all cause and effect is mental, and that sin, sickness, and death will be destroyed by a full understanding of the Divine Principle of Jesus' teachings and healing. (Webster's *New Int. Dictionary*, 2nd ed.)
Chris'tison's formula. To estimate solids in urine per 1000 parts, multiply last 2 figures of specific gravity by 2.33.
Chrobak pelvis (kro'bak). A deformed pelvis caused by hip joint disease.
chromaffin (krō-măf'ĭn) [G. *chrōma*, color, + L. *affinis*, having affinity for]. 1. Staining readily with chromium salts. 2. Noting pigmented cells forming medulla of the suprarenal glands and the paraganglia.
c. system, c. tissue. The mass of tissue forming paraganglia and medulla of suprarenal glands, which secretes adrenalin and stains readily with chromium salts.

Same kind of tissue is also found along abdominal aorta and in sympathetic nerves or ganglia. SEE: *suprarenal glands*.

chromaffino'ma [" + " + G. -ōma, tumor]. A chromaffin cell tumor. SYN: *paraganglioma*.

chromaffinopathy (kro-maf-in-op'ă-thĭ) [" + " + G. *pathos*, disease]. Any disease of chromaffin tissue.

chromaphil (kro'maf-ĭl) [" + *philein*, to love]. Pert. to a histological element or cell which stains readily with chromium salts. SYN: *chromaffin*.

chromate (kro'māt) [G. *chrōmatos*, color]. A salt of chromic acid. SEE: *potassium c.*

chromatelopsia (kro"mat-ĕ-lop'sĭ-ă) [G. *chrōma*, color, + *atelēs*, imperfect, + *opsis*, sight]. Color blindness.

chromat'ic. Pert. to color.

chromatin (krō'mă-tĭn) [G. *chrōma*, color]. Deeply staining substance of protoplasm in a cell nucleus which is considered as the physical basis of heredity.

The chemical carrier of inheritance in a cell; the principal substance in its nucleus; it determines the nature of daughter cells, *q.v.* SEE: *"chrom-" words*.

chromatinolysis (kro"mă-tin-ol'ĭ-sis) [" + *lysis*, dissolution]. 1. Destruction of chromatin. 2. The emptying of a cell, bacterial or other, by lysis.

chromatinorrhexis (kro"mă-tin-or-rek'sis) [" + *rēxis*, rupture]. Splitting of chromatin.

chromatism (kro'mă-tĭzm) [" + *ismos*]. 1. Unnatural pigmentation. 2. Chromatic aberration.

chromatodysopia (kro-mă-to-dis-o'pĭ-ă) [" + *dys*, ill, + *opsis*, sight]. Color blindness.

chromatogenous (kro-mă-toj'en-us) [" + *gennan*, to produce]. Causing pigmentation or color.

chromatolysis (kro-mă-tol'ĭ-sis) [" + *lysis*, dissolution]. Tigrolysis; the disintegration and disappearance of the chromophil granules of a cell, esp. that occurring in neurons as a result of injury to the cell body or its axon.

chromatometer (kro-ma-tom'et-er) [" + *metron*, measure]. A scale of colors for testing color perception.

chromatopathy (kro-ma-top'ă-thĭ) [" + *pathos*, disease]. Any skin disease that is marked by pigmentation.

chromat'ophil, chromatophil'ic [" + *philein*, to love]. Staining easily.

chromatophore (kro-mat'o-fōr) [" + *pherein*, to bear]. A pigment bearing cell.

chromatopsia (kro-mă-top'sĭ-ă) [" + *opsis*, vision]. Abnormally colored vision.

chromatoptometry (kro-mat-op-tom'e-trĭ) [" + *optein*, to see, + *metron*, measure]. Measurement of color perception.

chromatosis (kro-mă-to'sis). Pigmentation.

chromaturia (kro-mă-tu'rĭ-ă) [" + *ouron*, urine]. Abnormal color of the urine.

chro'micized. Mixed with a chromium salt.

chromidiosis (kro-mid-ĭ-o'sis) [G. *chrōma*, color]. Overflow of chromatin and nuclear substance into cell protoplasm.

chromid'ium (pl. *chromidia*) [" + *-idion*, a dim. termination]. Central chromatic body of a blood platelet.

chromidrosis (kro-mĭ-dro'sis) [" + *idrōs*, sweat]. Excretion of colored sweat.

(a) It may be *black*. This may be present in hysteria due to indican in the sweat, and associated with constipation. (b) *Red sweat*. It may be due to an exudation of blood into the sweat glands, or to microörganisms in those glands.

ETIOL: Occurs mostly in nervous, excitable women. May be due to ingestion or absorption of certain substances.

SYM: Localized in eyelids, breasts, axillae, genitocrural regions, occasionally hands and limbs, grayish, bluish, violaceous, brownish, collecting on skin, giving a greasy, powdery appearance to parts.

PROG: Obstinate and recurrent.

TREATMENT: Relief of underlying nervous affection.

RS: *anhidrosis, bromidrosis, hidrosis, hyperidrosis, uridrosis.*

chromium (kro'mĭ-um) [G. *chrōma*, color]. SYMB: Cr. At. wt. 52. A very hard, metallic element, steel gray in color.

c. compounds. Largely used in industries by dyers, furniture stainers and manufacturers of batteries in chromium plating. The salts are yellowish and often break up into particles; float in the air and are aspirated by patients. They lead to ulcerations of the nose and respiratory passages.

POISONING: SYM: A disagreeable taste in the mouth, pain, diarrhea, collapse and cramping.

TREATMENT: Chalk, magnesia, and other weak alkalies to neutralize its acid effects. Wash out stomach and give soothing drinks.

chro'moblast [" + *blastos*, germ]. An embryonic cell that becomes a pigment cell.

chromocholoscopy (kro-mo-ko-los'ko-pĭ) [" + *cholē*, bile, + *skopein*, to examine]. Examination of the biliary function by a pigment extraction test.

chromocrinia (kro-mo-krin'ĭ-ă) [" + *krinein*, to separate]. The secretion or excretion of pigmented matter.

chromocystoscopy (kro-mo-sis-tos'ko-pĭ) [" + *kystis*, cyst, + *skopein*, to examine]. Determination of functional activity of kidneys by use of dyes.

chromocyte (kro'mo-sĭt) [" + *kytos*, cell]. Any colored cell.

chromocytometer (kro-mo-sĭ-tom'et-er) [" + " + *metron*, measure]. Instrument for determining the hemoglobin in red blood corpuscles.

chromodermatosis (kro-mo-der-mă-to'sis) [" + *derma*, skin, + *-ōsis*, infection]. Any pigmented skin disease.

chro"modiagno'sis [" + *dia*, through, + *gnōsis*, knowledge]. Diagnosis by change of color of the serum.

chromogen (kro'mo-jen) [" + *gennan*, to produce]. Any principle that may be changed into coloring matter.

chromogen'esis [" + *genesis*, production]. Production of pigment.

chromogen'ic. Pigment producing.

chromolipoid (kro-mo-lip'oid) [G. *chrōma*, color, + *lipos*, fat, + *eidos*, appearance]. Any lipoid, such as carotin, that is pigmented. SYN: *lipochrome*.

chromolume (kro'mo-lŭm) [" + L. *lumen*, light]. Device for producing colored light rays.

chromolysis (kro-mol'is-is) [" + *lysis*, dissolution]. 1. Destruction of chromatin. 2. Lysis of a cell. SYN: *chromatolysis*.

chromo'ma [" + *-ōma*, tumor]. Neoplasm assumed to be derived from chromatophore cells.

chromomere (kro'mo-mēr) [" + *meros*, part]. (1) One of a series of chromatin granules found in a chromosome. (2) A highly refractile purple granule which forms the central portion of a blood platelet.

chromometer (kro-mom'e-ter) [" + *metron*, measure]. Device for determining the pigment in a substance.

chromometry (kro-mom'et-rĭ). The estimation of coloring matter.

chromopar'ic [G. *chrōma*, color, + L. *parēre*, produce]. Producing color; chromogenic.

chromopex'ic [" + *pēxis*, fixation]. Fixing coloring matter, as the liver.

chromophage (kro'mo-fāj) [" + *phagein*, to eat]. A phagocyte that destroys pigment believed to be present in the blanching of hair. SYN: *pigmentophage*.

chromophane (kro'mo-fān) [" + *phainein*, to show]. Retinal pigment.

chromophil(e (kro'mo-fĭl) [" + *philein*, to love]. 1. Any structure that stains easily. 2. Staining readily.

chromophilic (kro-mo-fĭl'ĭk). Staining readily; chromophilous.

chromophilous (kro-mof'ĭl-us). Chromophilic.

chromophobe (krō'mō-fōb) [G. *chrōma*, color, + *phobos*, fear]. Resistant to stain or a cell which does not stain.

chromophor'ic [G. *chrōma*, color, + *pherein*, to bear]. Pert. to or bearing color.

chromophose (kro'mo-fōz) [" + *phōs*, light]. A subjective sensation of a spot of color in the eye. SEE: *centraphose, centrophose*.

chromophytosis (kro-mo-fi-to'sis) [" + *phyton*, plant, + -*ōsis*, infection]. Pigmentation of skin due to a vegetable parasite. Tinea, or pityriasis versicolor.

chro'moplasm [" + *plasma*, matter]. The network of a cell nucleus.

chromoplas'tid [" + *plastos*, formed]. A pigment granule in protoplasm.

chromoprotein (kro-mo-pro'te-in) [" + *prōtos*, first]. A pigmented conjugated protein made up of pigment and a simple protein, as hemoglobin.

chromop'sia [" + *opsis*, vision]. Chromatopsia; colored vision.

chromoptometer (kro-mop-tom'e-ter) [" + *optein*, to see, + *metron*, measure]. Instrument for determining keenness of color vision.

chro"moradiom'eter [" + L. *radius*, ray, + G. *metron*, measure]. An instrument for measuring penetrative power of roentgen rays.

chromoscope (krō-mō-skōp) [" + *skopein*, to examine]. Instrument for determining color perception.

chromoscopy (krō-mos'kō-pĭ) [" + *skopein*, to examine]. 1. Examination for color vision. 2. Administration of dyes to stain the urine and in this manner make a diagnosis of kidney function.

chromosome (kro'mō-sōm) [G. *chrōma*, color, + *sōma*, body]. A microscopic rod, J- or V-shaped body which develops from the nuclear material of a cell and is especially conspicuous during mitosis. They stain deeply with basic dyes. They contain the genes or hereditary determiners.

The V-shaped, threadlike bodies formed by the breaking up of the chromatin network in the nucleus of a cell during mitotic division. From the network stage the chromatin assumes a tangled skein appearance, which again breaks into short, V-shaped lengths known as *chromosomes*. The number of chromosomes is constant for each species of animal. In man they number 48 or in 24 pairs, one derived from each parent. The germ cells, sperm and ova contain only one chromosome of each pair. Their function is said to be concerned with the transmission of hereditary traits from the parents to their offspring, carrying the genes like beads on a string.
2. The unit of chromatin in the nucleus of a cell.
SEE: *allosome, axoneme, heredity*.

c., accessory. An unpaired monosome, which does not divide, but goes into only 1 of the daughter cells. SYN: *allosome, heterochromosome*.

c., bivalent. Two chromosomes united temporarily.

c., sex. An accessory c., so named because it is thought to transmit sexual characteristics.

c., X. The sex chromosome. Females possess two X-chromosomes in all somatic cells. The mature ovum contains one X-chromosome. In somatic cells of the male, the X-chromosome has a diminutive mate, the Y-chromosome. Half of the mature sperm contain the X-chromosome, half the Y-chromosome. Zygotes are either XX or XY. XX zygotes developing into females. XY zygotes developing into males. The x-chromosomes contain the genes for sex-linked characters.

c., Y. The Y-chromosome is usually devoid of genes and is absent in the male of certain animals (some insects and nematodes).

chro"mother'apy [" + *therapeia*, treatment]. The use of colored light in the treatment of disease.

chromotox'ic [" + *toxikon*, poison]. Caused by toxic action on the hemoglobin.

chromoureteroscopy (kro-mo-u-ret-er-os'-ko-pĭ) [" + *ourētēr*, ureter, + *skopein*, to examine]. Inspecting orifices of ureters after giving a substance to dye the urine.

chronaxia (kron-ak'sĭ-ă) [G. *chronos*, time, + *axia*, value]. Time intensity relation of electrical stimuli.

chronaximeter (kron-aks-im'et-er) [" + " + *metron*, measure]. Device for measuring chronaxia.

chronaxy (kro'nak-sĭ) [" + *axia*, value]. A number expressing the sensitiveness of a nerve to electrical stimulation.

It is the minimum duration, measured in seconds, during which a current of prescribed strength must pass through a motor nerve in order to cause contraction in the associated muscle; the strength of direct current (the rheobasic voltage) which will just suffice if given an indefinite time is first determined, and exactly double this strength is taken for the final determinations.

chron'ic [G. *chronos*, duration]. Long drawn out; applied to a disease that is not acute.

chronicity (kro-nis'it-ĭ). State of being chronic.

chronobiol'ogy [G. *chronos*, time, + *bios*, life, + *logos*, study of]. Science of duration of life, and methods of prolonging it.

chronograph (kron'o-graf) [" + *graphein*, to write]. Device for recording short intervals of time.

chronological (krŏn"ō-lŏj'ĭ-kăl) [G. *chronos*, time, + *logos*, understanding]. Occurring in natural sequence according to time.

c. age. The number of years of one's life.
By educators, for those 16 and over, assumed to be 16 years, no matter how much greater it may be; determined by the results of intelligence tests. SEE: *age, intelligence quotient*.

chron'oscope [G. *chronos*, time, + *skopein*, to examine]. Device for measuring extremely short intervals of time.

chronotrop'ic [" + *trepein*, to turn]. Pert. to all that modifies periodically recurring action, such as the heart beat.
  c. fibers. Those which control contraction of the heart.

chronot'ropism [" + " + *ismos*, condition of]. Modification of periodical movements through external causes.

chrysarobin (kris-ar-o'bin) (goa powder). USP. A mixture of neutral principles obtained from a substance deposited in the wood of *Araroba*, a leguminous tree grown in South America.
  ACTION AND USES: Antiparasitic and an irritant. Employed in the treatment of fungous diseases of the skin in a 2 to 20% ointment.
  INCOMPATIBILITIES: Turns brown on exposure to air; turns red in ammonia water; deep brown with nitric acid.

chthonophagia (thon-o-fa'jĭ-ă) [G. *chthōn*, earth, + *phagein*, to eat]. Eating clay or dirt; geophagy.

Chvostek's sign (shvos'teks). Local spasm following a tap on one side of face.

chylangioma (ki-lan-jĭ-o'mă) [G. *chylos*, chyle, + *aggeion*, vessel, + *-ōma*, tumor]. 1. Tumor of intestinal lymph vessels containing chyle. 2. Retention of chyle in lymphatic vessels with dilatation.

chyle (kīl) [G. *chylos*]. The milklike contents of the lacteals and lymphatic vessels of the intestine consisting of the products of digestion and principally absorbed fats. It is carried by the lymphatic vessels to the cisterna chyli and then by way of the thoracic duct to the left subclavian vein where it enters the blood stream. Four to 5 pounds are formed in 24 hours. Sp. gr. 1.015. Reaction is alkaline.
  RS: *achylia*, *achylosis*, *achymia*, *achymosis*, "chyl-" words, *cisterna chyli*, *oligochylia*, *receptaculum chyli*, *secretion*.

chylemia (ki-le'mĭ-ă) [" + *aima*, blood]. Chyle in the peripheral circulation.

chylidrosis (ki-li-dro'sis) [" + *idrōs*, sweat]. A milklike sweat resembling chyle.

chylifacient (ki-li-fa'shent) [" + L. *facere*, to make]. Forming chyle.

chylifaction (ki-li-fak'shun) [" + L. *facere*, to make]. The formation of chyle.

chylifactive (ki-lif-ak'tiv). Forming chyle; chilifacient.

chyliferous (ki-lif'er-us) [G. *chylos*, chyle, + L. *ferre*, to carry]. Carrying chyle.

chylification (ki-lĭ-fĭ-ka'shun) [" + *facere*, to make]. Formation of chyle.

chylocele (ki'lo-sēl) [" + *kēlē*, tumor]. Infused chyle in *tunica vaginalis testis*.

chyloderma (ki-lo-der'mă) [" + *derma*, skin]. Lymph accumulated in the enlarged lymphatic vessels and thickened skin of the scrotum; lymph scrotum; scrotal elephantiasis.

chylology (ki-lol'o-jĭ) [" + *logos*, study of]. The study of chyle.

chylomediastinum (ki-lo"me-dĭ-as-tī'num) [" + L. *mediastinum*, being in the middle]. Chyle in the mediastinum.

chylomicron (ki-lo-mi'kron) [" + *mikros*, small]. Small particle of fat in the blood after digestion and absorption of fat in the food, and perceptible under a microscope.

chylopericardium (ki-lo-per-ĭ-kar'dĭ-um) [" + *peri*, around, + *kardia*, heart]. Chyle in the pericardium.

chyloperitone'um [" + " + *teinein*, to stretch]. Effused chyle in peritoneal cavity.

chylophoric (ki-lo-for'ĭk) [" + *phoros*, bearing]. Conveying chyle; chyliferous.

chylopoiesis (ki-lo-poi-e'sis) [" + *poiēsis*, production]. Formation of chyle and absorption by lacteals in the intestines. SYN: *chylification*.

chylopoietic (ki-lo-poi-et'ĭk) [" + *poiēsis*, production]. Pert. to formation of chyle.

chylosis (ki-lo'sis) [" + *-ōsis*, infection]. Formation of chyle. SYN: *chylifaction, q.v.*

chylotho'rax [" + *thōrax*, chest]. Chyle in pleural cavities.

chylous (kī'lus) [G. *chylos*]. Pert. to or of the nature of chyle.

chyluria (ki-lu'rĭ-ă) [" + *ouron*, urine]. Chyle or fat globules in the urine.

chyme (kīm) [G. *chymos*, juice]. The mixture of partly digested food and digestive secretions found in the stomach and small intestine during digestion of a meal; it is a varicolored, thick, but nearly liquid mass. SEE: "chym-" words, *enchyma*, *oligochymia*.

chymifica'tion [" + L. *facere*, to make]. 1. Formation of food into chyme. 2. Gastric digestion.

chymosin (ki'mo-sin) [G. *chymos*, juice]. Milk curdling enzyme found chiefly in gastric juice. SYN: *rennet*, *rennin*.

chymosinogen (kī-mo-sin'o-jen) [" + *gennan*, to produce]. A substance from which chymosin is formed.

C. I. Abbr. for color index.

cibisitome (si-bis'it-ōm) [G. *kibisis*, pouch, + *tomē*, a cut]. Instrument for incision of capsule of the lens.

cicatricial (sik-ă-trish'al) [L. *cicatrix*, scar]. Pert. to a cicatrix.

cicatricotomy (sik-ă-trik-ot'o-mĭ) [" + G. *tomē*, incision]. Incision of a cicatrix or scar.

cicatrix (sik'a-triks, sik-a'triks) [L.]. A scar left by a healed wound.
  Lack of color is due to absence of pigmentation. Cicatricial tissue is less elastic than normal tissue, hence it usually presents a contracted appearance.
  TREATMENT: Skin graft, carbon dioxide snow, x-rays, or radium.

cicatrizant (sik-kat'riz-ant) [L. *cicatrix*, scar]. Favoring or causing cicatrization.

cicatrization (sik-at-ri-za'shun) [L. *cicatrix*, scar]. Healing by scar formation. SEE: *intention*.

cic'atrize [L. *cicatrix*, scar]. To heal by scar tissue.

cid'er [G. *sikera*, strong drink, from Hebrew *shēkār*]. Apple juice. AV. SERVING: 120 Gm. Pro. 1.0, Carbo. 15.0 per serving. ASH CONST: Ca 0.008, Mg 0.011, K 0.095, Na 0.020, P 0.009, Cl 0.006, S 0.002, Fe 0.0002. RS: *beer*, *vinegar*, *wine*.

cilia (sil'ĭ-ă) (sing. *cil'ium*) [L. pl.]. 1. Eyelashes. 2. Hairlike processes projecting from epithelial cells, as in the bronchi, which wave mucus, pus, and dust particles upward. SEE: *biciliate*.

ciliariscope (sil-i-a'ri-skōp) [L. *ciliaris*, pert. to eyelash, + G. *skopein*, to examine]. Instrument for examination of the ciliary region of the eye.

ciliarotomy (sil-ĭ-ar-ot'o-mĭ) [" + G. *tomē*, incision]. Surgical section of the ciliary zone in glaucoma.

cil'iary [L. *ciliaris*, pert. to eyelash]. 1. Pert. to any hairlike processes. 2. An eyelid, and eyelash.
  c. arteries. Branches of the ophthalmic artery which supply the choroid layer.

c. body. Extends from base of iris to ant. part of choroid; consists of ciliary processes and ciliary muscle.

c. ganglion. A ganglion lying in the posterior part of the orbit. Receives preganglionic fibers through the oculomotor nerve from the nucleus of Edinger-Westphal of the midbrain. From it six short ciliary nerves pass to the eyeball. Postganglionic fibers innervate the ciliary muscle, sphincter of the iris, and the smooth muscles of blood vessels of these structures and the cornea.

c. glands. Glands of Moll, a form of sweat glands of the eyelid.

c. muscle. Accommodation muscle of eye.

c. processes. Consist of about 70 folds arranged meridionally so as to form a circle, have same structure as rest of choroid and secrete nutrient fluids which nourish neighboring parts, as cornea, lens, vitreous body. They also serve as points of attachment for the suspensory ligament of the lens.

c. reflex. Normal movement of pupil in accommodation of eye.

cil'iate [L. *cilia*, eyelashes]. Having hairlike projections resembling cilia.

ciliated (sil'ĭ-a-ted). Possessing cilia.

c. epithelium. Epithelium with hairlike processes on surface. They waft only in one direction and line the respiratory tract and fallopian tubes.

ciliectomy (sil-ĭ-ek'to-mĭ) [L. *cilium*, eyelash, + G. *ektomē*, excision]. Excision of portion of ciliary muscle, body, or border of eyelid.

ciliospinal (sil-ĭ-o-spi'nal) [" + *spina*, thorn]. Pert. to the ciliary body and spinal cord.

c. center. Spinal cord center which controls dilatation of the pupil.

c. reflex. Dilation of pupil following stimulation of the skin of the neck by pinching or scratching the skin.

ciliotomy (sil-ĭ-ot'o-mĭ) [" + G. *tomē*, incision]. Section of the ciliary nerves.

cilium (sil-ĭ-um) [L.]. 1. An eyelash. 2. Hairlike process of certain cells.

cillosis (sil-o'sis) [L.]. Twitching of an eyelid, spasmodically.

cimbia (sim'be-ă) [L.]. Slender band of white fibers crossing the ventral surface of a cerebral peduncle.

Cimex lectularius (si'meks lek-tū-la'rĭ-us). The bedbug.

cinchona (sin-ko'nă) [Sp. *cinchon*, from Countess of Cinchon who was cured by bark in 1638]. (Peruvian bark.) USP. The dried bark of the tree cinchona, the source of quinine. Its preparation, the tincture and compound tincture, useful as a bitter tonic.
DOSAGE: 1 dram (4 cc.).

cinchonism (sin'kon-izm) [" + G. *ismos*, condition of]. Poisoning from cinchona or its alkaloids.

cinchonize (sin'ko-nīz) [Sp. *cinchon*]. To bring under the influence of cinchona or its alkaloids, esp. quinine.

cinchophen (sin'ko-fen) (atophan). USP. Light yellow powder with slightly bitter taste; a dangerous drug to use.
ACTION AND USES: An analgesic in gout and acute arthritis; an antipyretic. Often toxic.
DOSAGE: 15 ♏ (1.0 cc.).

c. poisoning. Out of 117 cases of poisoning reported there were 61 deaths.
SYM: Gastric irritation, nausea, vomiting, belching, heartburn, vertigo, weakness, diarrhea, itching, rash, jaundice, stupor. When chronic it is often associated with profound liver damage. Those with gallbladder disease, inflammation, or cirrhosis of liver, the undernourished and those suffering from alcoholism are esp. susceptible.
F. A. TREATMENT: Largely symptomatic. Wash out stomach; give large quantities of fluids and saline catharsis. Sugars, glucose, intravenously. Insulin if sugar appears in the urine.

cinclisis (sin'klis-is) [G. *kigklisis*, a wagging]. Rapid winking, or quick, spasmodic movements of any part of the body.

cincture sensation (sink'tŭr) [L. *cinctura*, from *cingere*, *cinctum*, to gird]. Sensation of a tight girdle about the waist.
SYN: *zonesthesia*.

cinemat'ics [G. *kinema*, motion]. Science of motion; kinematics.

cinematoradiography (sin-e-mat″o-rā-dĭ-og'ra-fĭ) [" + L. *radius*, ray, + G. *graphein*, to write]. Radiography of an organ in motion.

cineplas'tics [G. *kinein*, to move, + *plastikos*, formed]. Formation after amputation of muscles of a stump, so that it is possible to impart motion and direction to an artificial limb.

cineraceous (sin-e-ra'shus) [L. *cinis*, *ciner-*, ash]. Like ashes.

cinerea (sin-e're-ă) [L. *cinerius*, ashenhued]. The gray matter of the brain and nervous system.

cine'real. Pert. to gray matter of the nervous system.

cineritious (sin-er-ish'us) [L. *cineritius*, ashen]. Ashen, as the gray matter.

cinesalgia (sin-es-al'jĭ-ă) [G. *kinēsis*, motion, + *algos*, pain]. Pain caused by movement of muscles.

cinesi- [G. *kinēsis*, motion]. Prefix: Motion. See also *kinesi-*.

cinesia (sin-e'sĭ-ă) [G. *kinēsis*, motion]. Motion sickness, as car sickness, seasickness.

cinesthesia (sin-es-the'zĭ-ă) [" + *aisthēsis*, sensation]. 1. The sense of motion. 2. The false sense of moving in space.

cinetocytopenia (si-net″o-si-to-pe'nĭ-ă) [" + " + *penia*, poverty]. Having an abnormally small number of cinetocytes in the blood.

cingulum (pl. *cin'gula*) (sin'gu-lum) [L. girdle]. (1) A band of association fibers in the cingulate gyrus extending from anterior perforated substance posteriorly to the hippocanal gyrus. (2) An eminence on the lingual surface of the incisor teeth especially the upper ones. It is situated near the gum. Also called *basal ridge*.

cion (si'ŏn) [G. *kiōn*, uvula]. The uvula.

cioni'tis [" + *-itis*, inflammation]. Inflammation of the uvula.

cionoptosis (si-on-op-to'sĭ-ă) [" + *ptōsis*, a falling]. A lengthened uvula.

cionotome (si-on'o-tōm) [" + *tomē*, incision]. Instrument for excision of the uvula.

cionotomy (si-on-ot'o-mĭ) [" + *tomē*, incision]. Excision of uvula.

circa (sir'kă) [L.]. Prefix: About.

circinate (sŭr'si-nat) [L. *circinatus*, made round]. Circular.

cir'cle [L. *circulus*, dim. of *circus*, a ring]. Any ringshaped structure.

c. of diffusion. One or more on projection plane of an image not in focus of the lens.

c. of Willis. Union of the ant. and post. cerebral arteries (branches of the

circle, vascular   C-59   **circulation, fetal**

carotid) forming an anastomosis at base of the brain.

    c., vascular. One around the mouth formed by inf. and sup. coronary arteries.

cir′cuit [L. *circuire*, to go around]. Course or path of an electric current.

    c. breaker. A safety device for opening an electrical circuit; a switch.

    c., closed. A circuit through which electricity is passing or can pass.

    c., electric. The path through conductors by which an electric current passes.

    c., ground. Ground or earth as part of electric circuit.

    c., high frequency. A spark gap, condenser, and the oscillatory transformer or resonator.

    c., magnetic. The closed path of magnetic lines; *e. g.*, the magnetic circuit of a transformer.

    c., open. A circuit having some break in it so that current is not passing or cannot pass. This break may be intentional, as an open switch, or accidental, as a blown fuse, a loose connection, or a broken wire.

    c., short. An accidental overflow of current due to the establishment of a low resistance bypass.

cir′cular [L. *circularis*, pert. to a ring]. 1. Shaped like a circle. 2. Recurrent.

    c. insanity. That in which manic and depressive attacks follow one another without intervals of lucidity.

circula′tion [L. *circulatio*, movement in a circle]. Movement in a circular course.

    c. of the aqueous humor of the eye. SEE: *aqueous*.

    c. of bile salts. The sodium glycocholate and taurocholate found in hepatic bile pass with it into the intestine, where they are absorbed along with the fats. They therefore pass with the blood of the portal vein back to the liver, where they are again used in making fresh bile.

    c. of the blood. The blood leaving the left ventricle enters the aorta, from which it escapes into the various large arteries. It thus reaches the coronary arteries of the heart itself and the arteries of the head, body wall, abdominal viscera, and extremities. Passing through the various capillary systems, it is gathered into veins, of which there are 2 systems. (1) Most veins empty their blood into the *venae cavae superior* and *inferior*. (2) The veins from the stomach, pancreas, spleen, and intestine unite to form the *vena portae*, which runs to the liver. Here it breaks up into a new capillary system, which drains through the hepatic veins into the *vena cava inferior*. The combined blood of the *venae cavae* and the coronary veins enters the right atrium, passes through the right ventricle, and is forced out into the pulmonary artery. The pulmonary capillary system drains by way of the pulmonary veins into the left atrium and thence into the left ventricle.

    c. of the cerebrospinal fluid. SEE: *cerebrospinal*.

    c., collateral. C. through small vessels which enlarge to compensate for an obstruction in the large vessels.

    c. coronary. Circulation through the muscular tissue of the heart. Blood leaves the aorta through the r. and l. coronary arteries which supply the myocardium. Blood passes through capillaries and is collected in veins most of which empty into the coronary sinus which opens into the right atrium. A few of the small veins open directly into the atria and ventricles.

    c., enterohepatic. SEE: *c. of bile salts*.

    c. fetal. Circulation through the fetus. Blood, oxygenated in the placenta passes through the umbilical vein and ductus venosus to the inferior vena cava and thence to the right atrium from which it may follow one of two courses (1) through the *foramen ovale* to the left atrium and thence through the aorta to the tissues or (2) through the right ventricle, pulmonary artery, and ductus arteriosus to the aorta, and thence to the tissues. In either case the blood bypasses the lungs which are not functioning before birth. Blood is returned to the placenta through the umbilical arteries which are continuations of the hypogastric arteries. At

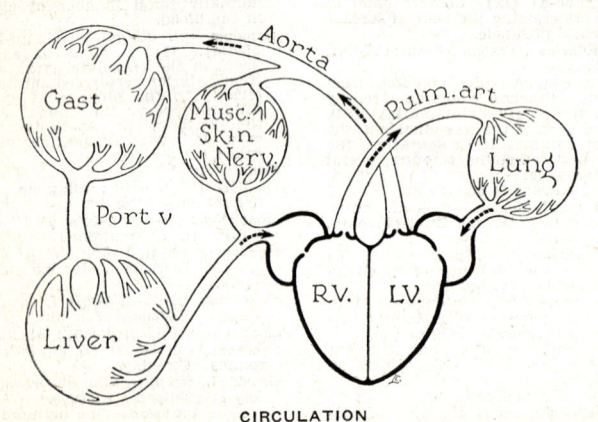

CIRCULATION

General scheme of the circulation of blood in man. Beginning with the lung, the abbreviations follow in this order: **LV**, left ventricle; **Gast**, gastrointestinal organs; **Port. v.**, portal vein; **Musc.**, System of voluntary muscles; **Nerv.**, Nervous system; **RV.**, right ventricle; **Pulm. art.**, pulmonary artery.

circulation, of the lymph

birth or shortly after, the ductus arteriosus and the foramen ovale close establishing normal circulation. Failure of either to occur gives rise to a "blue baby".

c. of the lymph. Lymph is formed from the tissue fluid which fills the tissue spaces of the body. It is collected into lymph capillaries which carry the lymph to the larger lymph vessels. These converge to form one of two main trunks, the right lymphatic duct and the thoracic duct. The rt. lymphatic duct drains the right side of the head, neck, and trunk and right upper extremity; the thoracic duct drains all the remaining portion of the body. The latter has its origin at the cisterna chyli which receives the lymphatics from the abdominal organs. It courses upward through the diaphragm and thorax and empties into the left subclavian artery near its junction with the l. int. jugular vein. The rt. lymphatic duct empties into the rt. subclavian vein. Lymph vessels have along their course lymph nodes which function as filtering structures filtering out bacteria and particulate substance preventing their entrance into the blood stream. Lymph flow is maintained by difference in pressure at the two ends of the system. Important accessory factors aiding the flow of lymph are breathing movements and muscular activities.

c., portal. Veins from the pancreas, spleen, stomach, intestines unite behind the pancreas and form the portal tube or vein. This takes blood, rich in the products of digestion, to the liver, where it breaks up into smaller vessels and capillaries.

c., pulmonary. The venous blood which is received into the right auricle passes through the tricuspid valve into the right ventricle. From there into the pulmonary artery, which divides into 2 branches, 1 going to each lung. (This is the only instance when an artery contains venous or dark blood deficient in oxygen.) The artery breaks up in the lung into capillaries, and here, by means of the hemoglobin in the red corpuscles, takes up oxygen from the inspired air. Red arterial blood returns to the heart by the 4 pulmonary veins, 2 from each lung entering the left auricle. (This is the only instance where veins contain oxygenated blood.)

c. rate. The minute volume or output of the heart per minute. In an average size adult with a pulse rate of 70, the amount is approximately 4 liters.

c., systemic. General circulation through the whole body except the lungs.

c., venous. C. of the blood via the veins.

circulation, words pert. to: adiemorrhysis, anangioplastic, angioneurosis, arterial c., arteries, chiloangioscopy, circulatory, enterohepatic (SEE: *bile acids*), fetal, fuliginous, heart, hyposphyxia, infarct.

circulation time. The time required by a particle of blood to make the complete circuit of both the systemic and pulmonary systems. Circulation time is determined by injecting a substance into a vein and timing its reappearance in arteries at the point of injection or some other point in the body. Such would necessitate the blood with the contained substance passing through veins to the heart and through the right atrium and ventricle, through the pulmonary circuit to the lungs and back through the left atrium and ventricle, and then out through the aorta and arteries to the place where detected. Dyes such as florescein, methylene blue or substances such as potassium ferrocyanide or histamine have been used as tracers. Ave. circulation time is 18 to 24 seconds. Circulation time is reduced in anemia and hyperthyroidism; increased in hypertension, myxoderma, and cardiac failure.

c. time, pulmonary. The time required for blood to pass through the lungs. Ave. time 11 seconds.

c. time test. Saccharin may be injected into a vein at the elbow. The patient says "sweet" the instant a sweet taste is detected in the mouth. The time, measured with a stop watch, bet. the injection and detection of the sweet taste is the time required for the blood to flow from the arm through the right auricle and ventricle, the lungs, back to the left side of the heart, and up to the capillaries of the tongue. This is the "arm to tongue" circulation time which normally is 10-15 seconds.

cir'culatory. Pert. to circulation.

c. system, inspection of. Inspection detects any abnormal centers of pulsation,* the apex* beat and its position, force, and extent, and any unnatural prominence over the precordial region. SEE: *abdomen, apex beat, chest, heart, lungs, pulsation*.

circum- [L.]. Prefix: Around, as *circumduction*.

circumarticular (sĭr″kŭm-ar-tĭk'ū-lar) [L. *circum*, around, + *articulus*, a joint]. Surrounding a joint. SYN: periarthric.

circumcision (ser-kum-sī'shun) [L. *circumcisio*, a cutting around]. Removal of the end of the prepuce by a circular incision.

NP: The foreskin is often tight after birth. It should be pulled back gently at the first bath to see that the meatus is clear, and then left alone for 8 days. After this, if still tight, it should be picked up in the thumb and finger and gently coaxed backwards twice a day. If it is inclined to bleed, smear it with an antiseptic ointment, such as yellow oxide of mercury. Care must be taken not to strip it backwards too far or constriction of the glans (paraphimosis) may occur. If tightness still persists or there is any difficulty in passing urine, a doctor should be consulted. Often the gentle passage of a probe by the doctor, underneath the skin of the prepuce, will obviate any need to circumcise. Strict asepsis must be maintained in the dressing of a circumcision. Pemphigoid skin rashes sometimes occur as a result of the infection of the wound.

PREPARATION FOR: Dorsal position. Screen. The patients are painted with alcohol (7%), picric acid, or mercurochrome. Iodine is not used in genitourinary surgery. Drape in a lithotomy sheet and 4 towels. SEE: *apellous, posthetomy*.

circumclusion (ser-kum-klu'zhun) [L. *circumcludere*, to shut in]. Acupressure by use of a pin under an artery and a wire loop over it, attached to each end of the pin.

circumcor'neal [L. *circum*, around, + *corneus*, horny]. Around the cornea.

circumcres'cent [" + *crescere*, to grow]. Developing around or over a part.

circumduction (sir-kum-duk'shun) [" + *ducere*, to lead]. 1. The action or swing of a limb, such as the arm, in such a manner that it describes a coneshaped

circumflex

figure, the apex of the cone being formed by the joint at the proximal end, while the complete circle is formed by the free distal end of the limb. 2. Circular movement of the eye.

circumflex (sir'kum-fleks) [" + *flectere*, to bend]. Winding around, as a vessel.

circum'sular [" + *insula*, island]. Surrounding the island of Reil.

circumintes'tinal [" + *intestinālis*, pert. to intestine]. Around the intestine.

circumlen'tal [" + *lens*, lens]. Situated around the lens.

circumnu'clear [" + *nucleus*, kernel]. Surrounding the nucleus.

circumoc'ular [" + *oculus*, eye]. Surrounding the eye.

  c. core. A nucleus.

circumor'al [" + *os, or-*, mouth]. Encircling the mouth.

  c. pallor. White area around the mouth contrasting vividly with color of face, esp. seen in scarlet fever.

circumorbital (sĕr″kŭm-or'bĭt-ăl) [" + *orbita*, orbit]. Around an orbit.

circumpolariza'tion [" + *polaris*, polar]. The rotation of a ray of polarized light.

circumre'nal [" + *rēnalis*, pert. to kidney]. Around or about the kidney.

cir'cumscribed [" + *scrībere*, to write]. Limited in space.

cir″cumstantial'ity [L. *circumstantia*, a standing around]. The mention of irrelevant facts and details in conversation.

circumval'late [L. *circum*, around, + *vallāre*, to wall]. Surrounded by a wall or raised structure.

  c. papillae. V-shaped row of papillae at base of tongue.

circus movements (ser'kus). "Contraction or excitation wave traveling continuously in circular fashion around a ring of muscle or through the wall of the heart." (*Lewis.*)

cirrhonosus (sir-ron'o-sus) [G. *kirros*, tawny, + *nosos*, disease]. Disease of the fetus marked by a golden yellow color of the pleura and peritoneum.

cirrhosis (sir-ro'sis) [G. *kirros*, yellow, + *-ōsis*, infection]. An interstitial inflammation with hardening, granulation, and contraction of the tissues of an organ, more esp. the liver.

  ETIOL: Deposits of connective tissue about the blood vessels causing, through contraction, an obstruction of the portal circulation.

  c., alcoholic. That of the liver due to alcoholism.

  c., atrophic. One marked by atrophy of the liver. SYM: Early enlargement of liver. Tongue coated, anorexia, fullness and distress after eating; vomiting of frothy mucus, flatulence, constipation, and dark urine. Gradual shrinking of the organ, with ascites, hypertension, hemorrhoids. As obstruction becomes greater portal blood finds new channels, and the superficial abdominal veins enlarge, notably about the umbilicus, forming the so-called *caput medusae*. PROG: Unfavorable except in early stages.

  c., biliary. Affecting the liver and gallbladder. ETIOL: Chronic retention of bile. SYM: Jaundice, hypochondriac fullness, urine dark and bile stained; stools, clay colored. Loss of strength, indigestion, fever irregularly. DIET: No special diet. Prohibit all alcoholic liquors.

  c., fatty. C. with fatty infiltration of the liver cells.

cisternal, puncture

  c., hypertrophic. In which the connective tissue hyperplasia starts from the periphery of the capillary bile ducts instead of from ramifications of portal vein as in atrophic form.

  SYM: Jaundice marked, liver large, yellow, and surface smooth or finely granular, spleen swollen. Disease may last 1 or 2 years, but abrupt termination may occur at any time in convulsions and coma.

  TREATMENT: Constitutional.

  c. of liver. A chronic disease characterized anatomically by a hyperplasia of the connective tissue and destruction of the secreting cells shown chiefly by symptoms of portal obstruction. SEE: *c., atrophic.*

  c. of lung. A chronic disease of the lung, characterized by an overgrowth of fibrous tissue.

  SYM: Moderate dyspnea and chronic cough—expectoration may be slight but is often profuse and fetid from having been retained in bronchiectatic cavities—no fever, and general health may be preserved for many years.

  PROG: Incurable—duration from 10 to 20 years.

  TREATMENT: Palliative — consists in good hygiene and use of remedies directed to the bronchiectasis.

  c., portal. C. with inflammation and ensuing obstruction to portal circulation.

cirrhotic (sir-rot'ĭk). Pert. to or affected with cirrhosis.

cirsectomy (sir-sek'to-mĭ) [G. *kirsos*, varix, + *ektomē*, excision]. Excision of a portion of a varicose vein.

cirsenchysis (sir-sen'kĭ-sis) [" + *enchysis*, a pouring in]. Injection of varicose veins.

cirsocele (sir'so-sēl) [" + *kēlē*, hernia]. Dilation of veins of spermatic cord. SYN: *varicocele.*

cirsodesis (sir-sod'ĕ-sis) [" + *desis*, ligation]. Ligation of varicose veins.

cirsoid (sir'soid) [" + *eidos*, resemblance]. Resembling a varix. SYN: *varicose.*

cirsomphalos (sir-som'fā-los) [" + *omphalos*, navel]. Varicose veins around the navel.

cirsotome (sir'so-tōm) [" + *tomē*, incision]. Instrument for cutting varicose veins.

cirsotomy (sir-sot'o-mĭ) [" + *tomē*, incision]. Treatment of a varicosity by multiple incisions.

cister'na, cis'tern [L. a vessel]. Any reservoir cavity.

  c. chy'li. BNA. *Receptaculum chyli.* A dilated sac into which is emptied the intestinal, 2 lumbar, and 2 descending lymphatic trunks; the origin of the thoracic duct.

  c. subarachnoid. Wide spaces in the cranial cavity between the arachnoid and the pia mater. Contains cerebral spinal fluid.

cisternal (sĭs-ter'năl). Concerning a cavity filled with fluid.

  c. puncture. A spinal puncture with a hollow needle bet. the cervical vertebrae, through the dura mater into the cisterna at base of brain.

  PURPOSE: (a) To inject a drug or a serum as in cerebral meningitis or cerebral syphilis, or (b) to remove excess spinal fluid and consequent pressure which inhibits the flow of spinal fluid to the lumbar region, esp. when the fluid cannot be obtained by lumbar puncture. SEE: *cerebrospinal fluid, spinal puncture.*

Citelli's syndrome. Poor memory, mental backwardness, insomnia or drowsiness, and lack of concentration in those with adenoids or sphenoid sinusitis.

citochol reaction (sī'to-kol). The use of concentrated cholesterolized extract of heart muscle as the antigen for a rapid flocculation test. [and a base.

citrate (sit'rāt). Compound of citric acid
   c. solution. Used to prevent clotting of blood that has been shed.

citrin (sit'rin). Vitamin P. Antiscorbutic in action and found in lemon juice.

citron [L. *citrus*, juniper fruit] (candied). AV. SERVING: 75 Gm. Pro. 1.1, Fat 1.1, Carbo. 58.6 per serving. Ca 0.121, Mg 0.018, K 0.210, Na 0.011, P 0.033, Cl 0.003, S 0.020. No iron. A base forming food; alkalinity 9.8 cc. per 100 Gm.; 3.0 per 100 cal.

Cl. Symb. of chlorine.

cladosporiosis (klad″o-spo-rī-o'sis) [G. *klados*, branch, + *sporos*, seed, + *-ōsis*, infection]. Infection with *Cladosporium*, a fungus, marked by appearance of gummatous nodules.

cladothricosis (klad-o-thrī-ko'sis) [″ + *thrix*, hair, + *-ōsis*, infection]. Infection with *Cladothrix*.

clam. A bivalve belonging to the phylum Mollusca. AV. SERVING (round): 90 Gm. Pro. 9.5, Fat 0.9, Carbo. 4.7. AV. SERVING (long): 60 Gm. Pro. 8.1, Fat 1.0, Carbo. 1.7. ASH CONST. (round): Ca 0.106, Mg 0.098, K 0.131, Na 0.705, P 0.046, Cl 1.220, S 0.224. ASH CONST. (long): Ca 0.124, Mg 0.079, K 0.212, Na 0.500, P 0.122, Cl 0.910, S 0.213.

clamp (klamp) [Danish, *klamp*, hook]. Device for compression of vessels.

clang [L. *clangere*, to peal]. A loud, metallic sound.
   c. tint. A delicate tone.

clap [A.S. *claeppan*, to throb]. Popular term for gonorrhea.
   c. threads. Slimy threads of mucus and pus in urine during gonorrhea.

clapotage, clapotement (klă-po-tazh′, klă-pot-mon′) [Fr.]. Any splashing sound in succussion of a dilated stomach.

Clap'ton's lines. Green lines on dental margin of gums in copper poisoning.

clar'et stain or **cheek** [L. *clarētum*, light red]. Capillary nevus of cheek. SYN: *nevus flammeus*.

clarificant (klar-if'ik-ant) [L. *clarus*, clear, + *facere*, to make]. Any agent that clears the turbidity of a liquid.

Clarke's bodies. Alveolar sarcomatous intranuclear bodies of breast.
   C.'s column. Gray matter, the trophic center for the direct cerebellar tract; the vesicular column.

clasmatoblast (klaz-mat′o-blast) [G. *klasma*, fragment, + *blastos*, germ]. A mast cell.

clasmatocyte (klaz-mat′o-sīt) [″ + *kytos*, cell]. A large, wandering, uninucleated cell, with many branches.

A fixed macrophage of loose connective tissue. They are capable of ingesting particulate material and have the property of electively storing certain dyes in colloidal solution. In inflammatory conditions they become actively ameboid.

clasmatocytosis (klaz-mat-o-sī-to'sis) [″ + ″ + *-ōsis*, infection]. Breaking up of clasmatocytes and islands of granules formed from their débris.

clasmatodendro'sis [″ + *dendron*, tree, + *-ōsis*, infection]. A breaking up of astrocytic protoplasmic expansions.

clasmato'sis [″ + *-ōsis*, infection]. Crumbling into small bits; fragmentation, as of cells. [joint in cerebral palsies.

clasp-knife rigidity. Spastic action in a

clastic (klas'tik) [G. *klastos*, broken, from *klaein*, to break]. Causing division into parts.

clastothrix (klas'to-thriks) [″ + *thrix*, hair]. Brittleness of the hair. SYN: *trichorrhexis*.

claudication (klaw-di-ka'shun) [L. *claudicāre*, to limp]. 1. Limping. 2. Loss of function, temporarily due to spasm (arterial) in brain or heart. 3. An obstruction.
   c., intermittent. Arterial spasm with subsequent painful cramping of the legs and lameness.

Claudius' cells (klaw'dĭ-us). Large columnar cells external to the organ of Corti.
   C.'s fossa. Small depression in post. part of pelvis, on either side, in which lies the ovary.

claustrophilia (klaws-tro-fil'ĭ-ă) [L. *claustrum*, a closed space, + G. *philein*, to love]. Dread of being in an open space, as in neurasthenia or a morbid desire to be shut in with doors and windows closed.

claustrophobia (klaws-tro-fo'bĭ-ă) [″ + *phobos*, fear]. PSY: Fear of being confined in any space, as in a locked room. Opp. of *agoraphobia.**

claustrum (klaws'trum) [L. A closed space]. 1. A barrier. 2. Thin layer of gray matter separating the ext. capsule from the island of Reil.

clausura (klaws-su'ră) [L. closure]. Atresia of a passage, closure.

clava (kla'vă) (pl. *clavae*) [L. club]. Enlarged extremity of the *funiculus gracilis* in post. portion of medulla oblongata. *Tuberculum gracile*. [Clubshaped.

cla'vate [L. *clavatus*, pert. to a club].
   c. nucleus. Collection of nerve cells within the clava.

clav'icle [L. *clavicula*, dim. of *clavis*, key]. The collarbone; a bone curved like the letter f, which articulates with the sternum and the scapula.
   c., dislocation of. Forward. Sternal end. TREATMENT: (a) Knee placed against spine. (b) Draw shoulders back. (c) Apply clavicle bandage with pad on dislocated end of bone.

Outer Extremity: Bone upon upper surface of acromion, or upon ant. part of spine of the scapula. SYM: (a) Prominence upon surface of acromion which disappears when arm is raised. (b) Shoulders flattened, arm hanging close to trunk. TREATMENT: (a) Raise shoulder, draw backward. (b) Place pad in axilla, bringing elbow close to side. (c) Secure arm and forearm to chest with pad in axilla. (d) Pressure by pad and gutta percha plate on projecting clavicle strapped in place. SEE: *jugulum*.

   c., fracture of. SYM: (1) Swelling, pain, protuberance with sharp depression over the injured bone. (2) Patient supports arm at the elbow, arm useless.

F. A. TREATMENT: (a) Place ball of cloth, 1 or 2 handkerchiefs, tightly rolled, under armpit. (b) Apply arm sling. Bandage elbow to side, hand and forearm extending across the chest. (c) Or, lay patient on back, on the floor, with blanket beneath until medical aid arrives. This position keeps shoulders back and prevents broken ends of bone from rubbing.

TREATMENT (medical): (a) Have assistant draw arms and shoulders backward. (b) Raise shoulders and support in upward, backward, and outward direction. (c) Cover parts with adhesive plaster and bandage.

clavicular (kla-vik'u-lar). Pert. to the clavicle.

cla'vus [L. nail]. 1. A corn or callosity. 2. A sharp head pain like the driving of a nail into the head.

clawfoot (klaw'fut). Muscular wasting with distortion, giving foot appearance of a claw. SYN: *pes cavus*.

clawhand. Muscular atrophy and clawlike flexion of fingers.

clear'ing agent. One that makes microscopical objects more transparent.

cleavage (kle'vej) [A.S. *cleofian*, to adhere]. 1. Splitting a complex molecule into 2 or more simpler ones. 2. Cell division following the fertilization of an egg. SYN: *segmentation*.
  c. cell. The blastomere.
  c., hydrolytic. Hydrolysis.
  c. lines. Those appearing in linear direction when a pin punctures a cadaver.

cleft [M.E. *clyft*, crevice]. A fissure.
  c. palate. A congenital palatine fissure forming 1 cavity for the nose and mouth.
  c. sternum. A congenital fissure of the breastbone.
  c. tongue. One with furrows.

cleido- (kli'do) [G. *kleis*, clavicle]. Prefix: Pert. to the clavicle.

cleidorrhexis (kli-do-rek'sis) [G. *kleis*, clavicle, + *rēxis*, rupture]. Fracture or bending the clavicles of the fetus for delivery.

cleidotomy (kli-dot'o-mǐ) [" + *tomē*, a cutting]. Dividing a fetal clavicle to facilitate delivery.

cleptoma'nia [G. *kleptein*, to steal, + *mania*, madness]. Impulsive stealing, the intrinsic value of the article not being the motive. SYN: *kleptomania, q.v.*

clergyman's sore throat. A form of granular pharyngitis.

Clev'enger's fissure. *Sulcus temporalis inferior* bet. 2nd and 3rd occipital convolutions.

climacteric (kli-mak'ter-ǐk, kli-mak'ter'-ǐk) [G. *klimaktēr*, a round of a ladder]. That period that marks the cessation of a woman's reproductive period.
  Usually takes place bet. the ages of 44 and 48. Seldom before or after. SEE: *change of life, menopause*.
  c., grand. The 63rd year.

climatol'ogy [G. *klima*, climate, + *logos*, study of]. Branch of meteorology which is the study of climate and its relation to disease. SEE: *bioclimatology*.

climatotherapy (kli-mat-ō-ther'ap-ǐ) [" + *therapeia*, treatment]. Change of climate as a treatment of a disease.

cli'max [G. *klimax*, ladder]. Period of greatest intensity.

cli'mograph [G. *klima*, climate, + *graphein*, to write]. A graph of the effect of climate on health.

clinic (klin'ǐk) [G. *klinikos*, pert. to a bed]. 1. Bedside examination. 2. A center for physical examination and treatment of ambulant patients living at home or who are not hospitalized.

clin'ical. 1. Pert. to the course of a disease, or the symptoms as opposed to anatomical changes. 2. Pert. to a clinic.
  c. thermometer. One which measures body temperature.

They may be sterilized for practical purposes by first wiping them carefully to remove adherent mucus, then immersing in 5% formalin solution, where they remain until wanted again. A thorough rinsing in water is then necessary to remove the formalin.
  For pocket use, 10% formalin solution put daily in metallic case, with washing before and after insertion of thermometer, will keep it free from risk of transmission of pathogenic organisms. Five per cent phenol or 50% alcohol solutions are also frequently used for this purpose. SEE: *thermometer*.
  c. unit. In biochemistry, a measure of the acidity of gastric juice. Thus, if it takes 24 cc. of N/10 NaOH to neutralize 100 cc. of gastric juice, the juice is said to contain 24 clinical units; 100 clinical units = 0.3634% HCl.

clinician (klin-ish'an) [G. *klinikos*, pert. to a bed]. A practicing physician; clinicist.

clinoid (kli'noid) [G. *klinē*, bed, + *eidos*, appearance]. Resembling a bed in shape.
  c. processes. Three pairs of prominences on upper surface of sphenoid bone.

clinom'eter [G. *klinein*, to decline, + *metron*, measure]. Instrument for estimation of power of rotation of ocular muscles.

cli'noscope [" + *skopein*, to examine]. Instrument for measuring the weakness of ocular muscles.

clinostat'ic [G. *klinē*, bed, + *stasis*, position]. Caused by assuming a recumbent position.

clinostat'ism. The recumbent position.

cliseometer (klis-e-om'et-er) [G. *klisis*, inclination, + *metron*, measure]. Device for measuring the female pelvic inclination.

clithrophobia (klith-ro-fo'bǐ-ă) [G. *kleithria*, keyhole, + *phobos*, fear]. Morbid fear of being locked in.

clition (klit'ǐ-on) [G. *klitus*, slope]. A craniometric point in center of highest part of the clivus on the sphenoid bone.

clitoridauxe (klit-or-id-awk'sē) [G. *kleitoris*, clitoris, + *auxē*, increase]. Hypertrophy of the clitoris.

clitoridectomy (klit-or-ǐ-dek'to-mǐ) [" + *ektomē*, excision]. Excision of clitoris.

clitoriditis (klit-or-id-i'tis) [" + *-itis*, inflammation]. Inflammation of the clitoris.

clitoridotomy (klit-tor-ǐ-dot'ō-mǐ) [" + *tomē*, incision]. Incision of the clitoris.

clitoris (kli'tor-is) [G. *kleitoris*]. One of the organs of the female genitalia. It is an erectile structure located beneath the anterior labial commissure and partially hidden by the anterior ends of the labia minora. It is homologous to the penis of the male.
  Structure. It consists of three parts: a body, two crura, and a glans. (a) The body, about an inch in length, consists of two fused corpora cavernosa. It extends from the pubic arch above to the glans below. (b) The two *crura* are continuations of the corpora cavernosa and serve to attach them to the inferior rami of the pubic bones. They are covered by the ischiocavernosus muscles. (c) The *glans* which forms the free distal end is a small rounded tubercle composed of erectile tissue. It is highly sensitive. The glans is usually covered by a hood-like prepuce and its ventral surface is attached to the frenulum of the labia.

c. crises. Recurring crises of involuntary excess of sexual feeling culminating in a true orgasm with spasm of the clitoris followed by lancinating pains in the genital organs lasting for hours. Rare. ETIOL: *Tabes dorsalis.*

clitoris, words pert to: anorthosis, balanic, caudation, clitorism, corpora cavernosa, erectile, -ion, -or, frenulum, smegma.

clitorism (klit'or-izm) [G. *kleitoris*, + *ismos*]. The counterpart of priapism. A long continued, painful condition in the female with recurring erection of the clitoris with an occasional orgasm.

ETIOL: Intense masturbation, hysteria, nymphomania, or excessive coitus.

clitoritis (klit-o-ri'tis) [" + -*itis*, inflammation]. Inflammation of the clitoris. SYN: *clitoriditis.*

cli'vus [L. a slope]. A surface that slopes, as the sphenoid bone.
  c. blumenbach'ii. The slope at base of skull.

cloaca (klo-a'ka) [L. a sewer]. 1. Cavity lined with endoderm at the posterior end of the body which serves as a common passageway for urinary, digestive and reproductive ducts. Present in adults of birds, reptiles and amphibia and in the embryos of all vertebrates. 2. An opening in the sheath covering necrosed bone.

clonic (klon'ik) [G. *klonos*, turmoil]. Pert. to alternate contraction and relaxation of muscles.
  c. spasm. One marked by muscular contraction and relaxation. Occurs in 2nd stage of epilepsy.

clonicity (klon-is'ĭ-tĭ) [G. *klonos*, turmoil]. Being clonic.

clonicotonic (klon-I-ko-ton'ĭk) [" + *tonikos*, tone]. Both clonic and tonic, as some forms of muscular spasm.

clon'ism, clonis'mus [" + *ismos*, condition of]. Condition of being affected with clonic spasms, or a succession of them.

clon'ograph [" + *graphein*, to write]. An instrument for registering spasmodic movements.

clon'ospasm [" + *spasmos*, spasm]. Rapid alternation of muscular contraction and relaxation.
  The rate is much slower than a tremor. In upper motor neurone paralysis, sharp flexion of ankle often produces ankle clonus.

clon'us [G. *klonos*, turmoil]. Spasmodic alternation of contraction and relaxation; opposite of *tonus*. SEE: *wrist clonus.*

Cloquet's canal (klo-kās'). An irregular passage (hyaloid) through center of the vitreous body in the fetus.

closed core transformer. A transformer having a continuous core of magnetic material (usually iron) without any air gap.

Clostrid'ium. A genus of bacteria belonging to the family Bacillaceae. They are anerobic, spore-forming rods and are widely distributed in nature. They are common in the soil and in the intestinal tract of man and animals, and are frequently found in wound infections. Several are pathogenic in man, being the primary causative agents for gaseous gangrene.
  Important species are:
  Cl. botulinum. Grows in improperly processed food. Produces a powerful exotoxin, the cause of botulism, q.v.
  Cl. chauvei. Cause of backleg Iquarter evil, symptomatic anthrax) in cattle.
  Cl. histolyticum. A proteolytic organism found in wounds. Has a liquifying effect on human tissues.
  Cl. novyi. Found in cases of gaseous gangrene. Produces a strong, soluble exotoxin.
  Cl. perfringens. SYN: *Cl. welchii.*
  Cl. septicum. Found in cases of gangrene in man, cattle, hogs, and other domestic animals.
  ....Cl. sporogenes. Frequently associated with other organisms in mixed gangrenous infections.
  Cl. tetani. The causative organism of tetanus or lockjaw. Produces a powerful exotoxin, a portion of which affects nerve tissue, another portion is hemolytic.
  Cl. welchii. The most important cause of gas gangrene in wound infections. Produces a number of distinct toxins.

clot (klŏt) [A.S. *clott*]. 1. To coagulate. 2. A thrombus; a coagulum, as of blood or lymph.
  SEE: *blood, clotting of.*
  c., agony. One formed in the heart when death ensues from prolonged heart failure.
  c., antemortem. One formed in the heart or its cavities before death.
  c., blood. A coagulum formed of blood.
  c., chicken fat. A yellow-colored blood clot.
  c., currant jelly. A clot of fibrin of reddish color and jellylike consistency.
  c., distal. One formed in a vessel on distal side of a ligature.
  c., external. One formed outside a blood vessel.
  c., heart. A thrombus within the heart. [tion of clot.
  c., internal. One formed by solidifica-
  c., laminated. One formed in a succession of layers filling an aneurysm.
  c., muscle. One formed in coagulation of muscle plasma.
  c., passive. One formed in the sac of an aneurysm.
  c., plastic. One formed from the intima of an artery at the point of ligation.
  c., postmortem. One formed in the heart or in a large blood vessel after death. [imal side of a ligature.
  c., proximal. One formed on the prox-
  c., stratified. Thrombus consisting of layers of different colors.

clothes louse. *Pediculus corporis;* a body louse.

cloth'ing [A.S. *clāthian*, to clothe]. Clothes prevent use of too much fuel, a greater amt. of carbon dioxide being given off when light clothing is worn.
  Air spaces in a fabric conserve heat. It is texture, not the material, that makes for warmth. Woolen fabrics lose in warmth when the material is matted down and the air spaces are destroyed. Wool and silk absorb more moisture than other fabrics but silk loses it more readily. Cotton and linen come next but linen loses moisture quicker than cotton. Open mesh is necessary to prevent chill from evaporation. Knitted fabrics absorb and dry more readily than woven fabrics of the same material. Temperature inside a hat worn by a man varies from 13° to 20° hotter than outside temperature. Body heat increased when moisture from wet garments cannot escape.

clouding of consciousness. PSY: A state of mental confusion characterized by insufficiency of perception and impaired attention, and resulting in loss of orienta-

cloudy swelling   C-65   **coagulation**

tion of time and place, amnesia and ill-adjusted reactions. Occurs in toxic, febrile, and other deliria. SEE: *consciousness*.

clou′dy swelling. Degeneration in which the tissues swell and become turbid.

clove-hitch. A knot consisting of 2 contiguous loops which are placed around an object, the ends of the cord being toward each other; used for making traction on a part for the reduction of dislocations or for restraining mental or delirious patients.

clove, oil of. USP. A volatile oil distilled from the dried flower buds of the clove tree. SYN: *Caryophyllus*.
ACTION AND USES: Antiseptic and aromatic. Useful also as an anodyne in dental practice.

clo′ven spine. Spina bifida. Congenital defect of spinal canal walls caused by lack of union bet. laminae of the vertebrae.

clown′ism. Grotesque actions and attitudes.

clubbed fingers. Rounding of ends and swelling of fingers in children with congenital heart disease and in older children and adults with long standing pulmonary disease.

clubfoot. Nontraumatic foot deviation. SEE: *kyllosis, talipes*.

clubhand. Deformity of the hand resembling clubfoot.

clumping [A.S. *clympre*, a lump]. 1. Adhesion of wound surfaces. 2. Clumping of microörganisms in a culture when specific immune serum is added. SYN: *agglutination*.

clu′nes [L. pl.]. The buttocks; nates.

clupeine (klū′pē-ēn) [L. *clupea*, herring]. A protamine from the spermatozoa of the herring.

clysis (klī′sis) [G. *klyzein*, to cleanse]. Injection of fluid for washing out the blood in a cavity.

clysma (klis′mä) [G.]. An enema.*

cly′ster [G. *klystēr*, enema]. Rectal injection or enema; a clysma.

C. M. Abbr. for *chirurgiae magister*, Master in Surgery.

cm. Abbr. for *centimeter*.

cnemial (ne′mī-al) [G. *knēmis*, leg]. Pert. to the leg, esp. the shin.

cnemis (ne′mis) [G. *knēmis*, leg]. Shin, lower leg, tibia.

cnemitis (ne-mī′tis) [" + -*itis*, inflammation]. Inflammation of the tibia.

CO₂. SYMB: Carbon dioxide.
    CO₂ therapy. Therapeutic application of low temperatures with solid carbon dioxide. SEE: *refrigeration*.

co″activ′ity [L. *coactāre*, to force]. Action that aids an enzyme to function, as the action of bile salts upon lipase, but not the same as that incited by an activator.
    Dialysis will remove the bile salts, whereas an active enzyme cannot be transformed back to an inactive zymogen, proving the difference bet. coactivity and *activation*.

coadunation (ko-ad-u-na′shun) [L. *co*, together, + *ad*, to, + *unus*, one]. Union or junction of dissimilar substances in 1 mass.

coagglutina′tion [" + *agglutinans*, gluing]. Clumping by an antigen and the homologous antibody of the corpuscles of another organism.

coagglu′tinin. An antibody that is effective on 2 or more organisms.

coag′ula [L. pl. a blood clot]. Plural of *coagulum*.

coagulable (ko-ag′u-lă-bl) [L. *coagulum*, blood clot]. Capable of clotting; apt to clot.

coagulant (ko-ag′u-lant) [L. *coagulans*, congealing]. 1. That which causes a fluid to coagulate. 2. Causing coagulation.

coagulase (ko-ag′u-lāz) [L. *coagulum*, blood clot]. Any enzyme, such as thrombin, which causes coagulation. SEE: *coagulin, coagulum*.

coag′ulate [L. *coagulāre*, to congeal]. To lessen the properties of fluidity.

coag′ulated. Clotted or curdled.
    c. proteins. Derived proteins (insoluble), resulting from the action of alcohol on protein, or heat on p. solutions.

coagula′tion [L. *coagulatiō*]. The process of clotting.
    Coagulation depends upon the presence of five substances (1) prothrombin, (2) thrombin, (3) thrombophastin (thrombokinase), (4) calcium in ionic form, and (5) fibrinogen. Prothrombin is converted to thrombin by the action of thromboplastin in the presence of calcium ions. Thrombin then acts on the soluble fibrinogen of the plasma

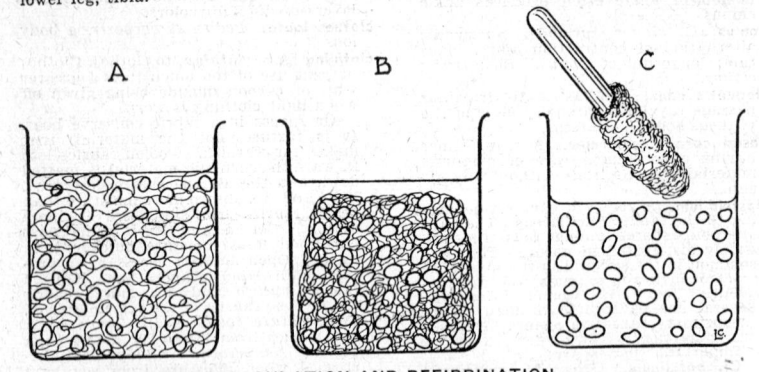

COAGULATION AND DEFIBRINATION
A, A fresh clot contains fibrin threads, corpuscles, and serum. B, On standing, the fibrin contracts, retaining most of the corpuscles, but releasing some of the serum. C, If blood is stirred before and during the process of coagulation, the fibrin clings to the stirring rod and leaves the mixture of corpuscles and serum called defibrinated blood.

converting it to insoluble fibrin. The fibrin forms a meshwork of fibers in which the corpuscles of the blood become entangled thus forming a clot. Shrinkage of the fibrin causes the exudation of plasma minus fibrinogen which constitutes blood serum. When blood is shed through an injured vessel, thromboplastin is liberated from the injured tissues and from degenerating blood platelets. This initiates the clotting mechanism.

In schematic form, the clotting process is as follows: *prothrombin* + *thromboplastin* + *calcium ions* → *thrombin*
Thrombin + fibrinogen → **fibrin**.

Clotting is retarded by (1) cold, (2) smooth surfaces, (3) decalcifying substances such as citrates and oxalates, (4) neutral salts such as magnesium or sodium sulfate, (5) certain substances of biological origin such as hirudin, heparin, snake venoms, cysteine, and dicoumarol.

Clotting is hastened by (1) warming, (2) providing a rough surface, (3) use of chemical substance such as adrenalin, thrombin, thromboplastin.

coagulation time. "The time it takes for blood to clot when exposed to the air." This can be determined by (1) collecting blood in a small test tube and noting elapsed time from moment blood is shed to time it coagulates or (2) collecting blood in a small capillary tube and breaking off small pieces of the tube at 30 sec. intervals. Coagulation is indicated by the appearance of fine threads of fibrin between the broken ends of the tube.

coag'ulative. Causing coagulation.

coag'ulin [L. *coagulāre*, to congeal]. A specific substance, produced in the body of an animal by an injection of a substance, which will cause quickened coagulation in that of another. SEE: *coagulase*.

coagulinoid (ko-ag'u-lin-oid) [" + G. *eidos*, form]. A coagulin whose function has been destroyed by heating to 65°-70° C.

coagulometer (ko-ag-u-lom'et-er) [" + G. *metron*, measure]. Device for measuring the blood's coagulability.

coaguloviscom'eter [" + *viscosis*, gummy, + G. *metron*, measure]. An instrument for determining the rapidity of the coagulation of the blood.

coag'ulum [L.]. 1. A blood clot. 2. A curd.

coalesce (ko-al-es') [L. *coalēscere*, to grow together]. To fuse; run or grow together.

coales'cence [L. *coalēscere*, to grow together]. Fusion or growing together of 2 or more parts of bodies.

coal tar. A tar that is produced in the destructive distillation of bituminous coal, as crude creosol.

coapta'tion [L. *coaptāre*, to fit together]. The adjustment of separate parts to each other, as the edges of fractures.

coarctate (ko-ark'tāt) [L. *coarctāre*, to tighten]. To press or pressed together.
  c. retina. Funnelshaped retina.

coarcta'tion [L. *coarctatio*, a tightening]. 1. Compression of the walls of a vessel. 2. Shriveling. 3. A stricture.

coarctotomy (ko-ark-tot'o-mī) [" + G. *tomē*, incision]. Cutting or division of a stricture.

cobra venom solution (kō'brä věn'ūm). Minute quantities of the secretion of the cobra in sterile physiological salt solution, and standardized so that 1 cc. is equivalent to 5 mouse units.

Recommended to be effective in relieving severe pains of inoperable tumors, and other intractable pains.

Its action is said to be slower than that of morphine, but of longer duration, and does not produce addiction.

DOSAGE: Intramuscularly, 0.5 cc. for first dose, the next day 1 cc., and this dose be administered for 2 or 3 successive days until definite relief is noted, after which 1 cc. every other day, or at longer intervals, according to the judgment of the physician.

cocaine hydrochlor'ide (ko-kān'). USP. The hydrochloride of an alkaloid obtained from erythroxylin cocoa.

CHIEF USES: Local anesthetic. A habit-forming drug. [(0.015 Gm.).

DOSAGE: Topical application of ¼ gr.

POISONING: SYM: Initially, a stimulation of the nervous system, with excitement, incoherent talking, restlessness, hallucinations, etc., followed by profound depression, nausea, dizziness, tingling of hands and feet, alterations of pulse, increased respirations, dilated pupils; occasionally convulsions, collapse, and death.

TREATMENT: When taken by mouth, evacuate stomach. Administer tannic acid, strong, black coffee, or strong tea to dilute the poison and act as a stimulant. Apply external heat. Slapping or moving the patient valuable, but should not be overdone. Artificial respiration and injection of adrenalin.

cocainism (ko-kān'izm) [L. *cocaina*, + G. *ismos*, condition of]. The habitual use of cocaine; more rare than morphinism.

Cocaine is often used with morphine, or as a substitute.

SYM: Slight headache and dizziness, followed by a feeling of well being and increased mental activity, which does not endure; no sensation of hunger or fatigue. The addict is witty and active, with vivid illusions and hallucinations, usually of the pleasing and wishful type. When the effect wears off, activity diminishes and mood fluctuates from well being to irritability, morosenose, and suspicion. Patient becomes neglectful of home, work, and social obligations; will associate with other habitués, or prostitutes; exhibit pervertism; and may commit sexual crimes.

PROG: Usually die of cardiac failure, paralysis, or intercurrent disease due to debility. Abstinence produces gastric disturbances, and fearful hallucinations.

cocainization (ko-kān-ī-za'shun). Inducing analgesia by use of cocaine.

cocainize (ko-kān'īz). To put under the influence of cocaine.

cocainomania (ko-kān-o-ma'ne-ă) [L. *cocaina*, + G. *mania*, madness]. Intense desire for cocaine and its results.

Coccidia (kō-sĭd'ĭ-ă). An order of protozoa belonging to the class Sperozoa. All are intracellular parasites usually infecting epithelial cells of the intestine and associated glands. They are principally parasites of lower animals causing great economic loss among domestic and game animals. Practically all domestic animals suffer from coccidial disease. Only one species, Isopora hominis infects humans and the area of infestation is largely confined to the far East.

coccidioidomycosis (kŏk-sĭd-ĭ-ō-ĭd-ō-mī-kō'sĭs). A coccidiodial granuloma. SYN: "valley fever," desert rheumatism," "San Joaquin Valley fever."

Exists in two forms (1) *primary coccidioidomycosis* which is an acute, self-limiting disease involving only the respiratory organs and (2) *progressive coccidioidomycosis*, a chronic, diffuse, malignant disease that may involve almost any part of the body.

ETIOL. Caused by a pathogenic fungus, *Coccidiodes immitis*.

PROG. For the primary type, favorable; for the progressive type, grave, often fatal.

coccidiosis (kok-sid-ĭ-o'sis) [G. dim. of *kokkos*, berry, + *-ōsis*, infection]. Nodular formations scattered over the body due to infestation with Coccidium and resulting symptoms.

coccobaccili (kŏk-ō-bă-sĭl'ĭ-ă). Bacilli which are short and thick and somewhat ovoid in form.

coccogenous (kok-oj'en-us) [" + *gennan*, to produce]. Produced by cocci.

coccoid (kok'oid) [" + *eidos*, appearance]. Resembling a micrococcus.

coccus (kok'us) (pl. *cocci*) [G. *kokkos*, berry]. A type of bacteria which is spherical or ovoid in form. When they appear singly they are designated *micrococci*; in pairs, *diplococci*; in clusters like buches of grapes, *staphylococci*; in chains, *streptococci*; in cubical packets of eight, *sarcinae*. Many are pathogenic causing such diseases as septic sore throat, erysipelas, scarlet fever, rheumatic fever, pneumonia, gonorrhea, meningitis, and puerperal fever. SEE: *Bacteria*.

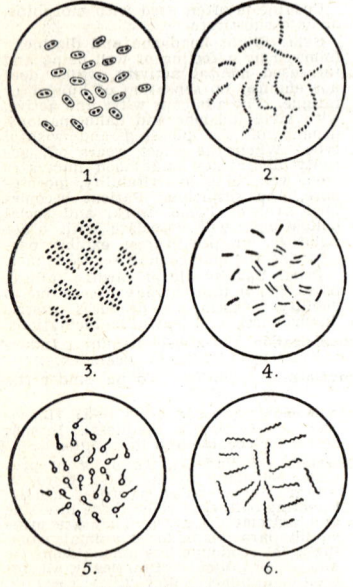

TYPES OF BACTERIA
1. Diplococci. 2. Streptococci. 3. Staphylococci. 4. Bacilli. 5. Bacilli with spores. 6. Spirilla.

coccyalgia (kok-sĭ-al'jĭ-ă). [G. *kokkyx*, coccyx, + *algos*, pain]. Pain in the coccyx.

coccydynia (kok-sĭ-din'ĭ-ă) [" + *odyne*, pain]. Pain in or around the coccyx; coccyalgia.

ETIOL: (a) Injury to bone of coccyx; (b) to soft parts around it; (c) disease of either; (d) hemorrhoids.

coccygeal (kok-sij'ē-al). Pert. to the coccyx.

coccygectomy (kok-sij-ek'to-mĭ). Excision of the coccyx.

coccygodynia (kok-sĭ-go-din'ĭ-ă) [" + *odyne*, pain]. Pain in the coccygeal region; coccyalgia.

coccyodynia (kok-sĭ-o-din'ĭ-ă) [" + *odyne*, pain]. Pain in region of coccyx. SYN: *coccygodynia*.

coccyx (kok'siks) [G. *kokkyx*]. Last 4 bones of the spine. Usually ankylosed and articulating with the sacrum above.

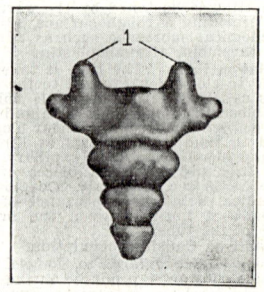

Coccyx, posterior surface. **1. Cornu.**

cochineal (koch'in-ēl) [L. *coccinella*]. Dried female insect, used as carmine coloring matter for pharmaceutical products, and as a dye in laboratory work.

Antispasmodic and anodyne, used in whooping cough and nervous affections.

cochlea (kok'lē-ă) [G. *kochliās*, a spiral]. A winding cone-shaped tube forming a portion of the inner ear. It contains the *organ or Corti*, the receptor for hearing.

The chochlea is coiled resembling a snail shell, winding two and three-quarters turns about a central bony axis, the *modiolus*. Projecting outward from the modiolus is a thin bony plate, the *spiral lamina* which partially divides the cochlear canal into an upper passageway, the *scala vestibuli* and a lower one, the *scala tympani*. Lying between the two scales is the *cochlear duct*, in the floor of which lies the *spiral organ* (of Corti). The base of the cochlea adjoins the vestibule; at the cupulo or tip, the two scalae are joined at the *helicotrema*.

cochlear (kok'le-ar). Pert. to the cochlea.
  c. nerve. One supplying the cochlea.
cochleare (kok-le-a're) [G. *kochliarion*]. Spoonful.
cochleariform (kok-le-ar'ĭ-form) [" + L. *forma*, shape]. Spoonshaped.
cochleitis (kok-le-i'tis) [G. *kochliās*, spiral, + *-itis*, inflammation]. Inflammation of the cochlea. SYN: *cochlitis*.
cochleoörbicular reflex (kok-le-o-or-bik'u-lar). Contraction of orbicularis palpebrarum muscle resulting from sudden noise being produced near ear.

cochleopalpebral reflex (kok-lē-ō-pal'pē-bral). Contraction of orbicularis palpebrarum muscle resulting from sudden noise being produced near ear.

cochleovestibular (kok-le-o-ves-tib'u-lar) [G. *kochliās*, spiral, + L. *vestibulum*, from *vestis*, garment]. Pert. to the cochlea and vestibule of the ear.

cochlitis (kok-li'tis) [" + *-itis*, inflammation]. Inflammation of the cochlea.

cock'roach [Sp. *cucaracha*]. *Blatta orientalis*. A common insect belonging to the order Orthoptera, which infests homes and eating places. They are swift-running omnivorous insects averaging about 2 cm. in length. Through their dual contact with filth and food, they may transmit mechanically, bacteria, protozoan cysts, and helminth ova. Common genera are *Blatta*, *Blatella* and *Periplaneta*.

COCL. Abbr. for cathodal opening clonus.

co'coa [Sp. *coco*, from G. *kokkos*, berry].
1. A substance prepared from the seed of cacao or theobroma, with all possible fat expressed. 2. The beverage made from 1.

COMP: A nerve food of real nutritive value. Contains albumin, fats, and carbohydrates. Much of the fat of cocoa butter is removed in making powdered chocolate and cocoa. Cane sugar represents the carbohydrates. Oxalates abound and phosphate and sulfate of potassium and of magnesium are found in the ash. Theobromine dimethylxanthine is the active principle but is heavier in chocolate than in cocoa. Its reaction is about the same as caffeine. Sugar is higher in chocolate. A cup of cocoa made of 10 Gm., and one of chocolate made of 15 Gm. contains:

	Cal.	Theobromine	Oxalates
Cocoa	74	0.13	0.045
Chocolate	74	0.19	0.012

Av. SERVING (cocoa): 5 Gm. Pro. 1.1, Fat 1.4, Carbo. 1.9 per serving. Av. SERVING (chocolate): 30 Gm. Pro. 3.9, Fat 14.6, Carbo. 9.1 per serving. ASH CONST. (cocoa): Ca 0.112, Mg 0.420, K 0.900, Na 0.059, P 0.709, Cl 0.051, S 0.203, Fe 0.0027. ASH CONST. (chocolate): Ca 0.092, Mg 0.293, K 0.563, Na 0.012, P 0.455, Cl 0.051, S 0.045, Fe 0.0027.

cocoa butter (oil of theobroma). USP. The fat obtained from the roasted seed of theobroma or cacao. USES: Suppositories and in toilet preparations as a lubricant.

co'comalt. A trade product in powder form to be mixed with milk as a beverage.

COMP: Pro. 13.06%, Carbo. 78.31%, Fat 3.68%, Fiber 0.74,% Ash 3.33%. ASH CONST: Ca 0.30, P 0.33, Fe 0.02. In 1 oz: Ca 0.09, P 0.09, Fe 0.005 Gm. VITAMINS: D, 81 USP. Units per oz. A, B, G present in the beverage. FUEL VALUE: Adds 115.5 cal. to a glass of milk, making a total of 73% caloric value. It increases in a glass of milk Ca 37.5%, P 52.9%, Pro. 46.7%, Carbo. 201.5% and Fats 12.2%.

cocon'sciousness [L. *co*, together, + *conscius*, aware]. A conscious objective state in which subconscious impressions rise to the surface.

In dual* personality, one character (only) may be cognizant of the other.

cocontraction (kō-kon-trak'shun) [" + *contractio*, a drawing together]. Adjustment of 2 muscles during contraction, said of antagonist muscles in co-ordination.

co'conut [fruit of *Cocos nucifera*]. Considerable cellulose. Av. SERVING (dried): 100 Gm. Pro. 4.3, Fat 41.0, Carbo. 44.5 per serving. Av. SERVING (fresh): 50 Gm. Pro. 2.9, Fat 25.0, Carbo. 14.0. Dried: Ca 0.059, Mg 0.059, K 0.597, Na 0.073, P 0.155, Cl 0.239, S 0.056. Fresh: Ca 0.024, Mg 0.020, K 0.300, Na 0.036, P 0.074, Cl 0.120, S 0.056. Vit. (in both) : A+, B++, G++.

coconut milk. ASH CONST: Ca 0.020, Mg 0.009, K 0.144, P 0.010, S 0.008. No sodium, chlorine or iron.

coctolabile (kok-to-la'bĭl) [L. *coctus*, cooked, + *labilis*, perishable]. Incapable of remaining unaltered when subject to boiling water.

coctoprecipitin (kok-to-pre-sip'it-in) [" + *praecipitāre*, to cast down]. A precipitin produced by injecting a serum that has been boiled.

coctostabile (kok-to-stab'il) [" + *stabilis*, resisting]. Incapable of being altered or destroyed by boiling water.

cod (salt) [A.S. *codd*, small bag]. Av. SERVING: 60 Gm. Pro. 15.8, Fat 0.2 per serving. Vit. B++. 100 Gm. equal 104 cal.

codeine (ko'de-ĭn) [L. *codina*, from G. *kōdeia*, poppyhead]. USP. An alkaloid obtained from opium.

ACTION AND USES: Analgesic, hypnotic sedative with effects resembling morphine.

DOSAGE: ¼ to 2 gr. (0.015-0.13 Gm).

POISONING: SYM: Depression of central nervous system to the point of sleep.

TREATMENT: Similar to morphine.

INCOMPATIBILITIES: Ferrous iodide, Lugol's solution.

c. phosphate. USP. Phosphate of the alkaloid codeine with a preference because of its free solubility in water.

DOSAGE: Same as codeine.

c. sulfate. USP. The sulfate of the alkaloid codeine. ACTION AND USES: Same as codeine. DOSAGE: Same as codeine.

Codivilla's extension (ko-di-vil'lă). One for fractures made by weight pulling on a nail passed through the lower end of the bone.

cod liver oil (oleum morrhuae). USP. A fixed oil obtained from the fresh livers of the cod fish. The official oil is standardized for its vitamin A and D content.

ACTION AND USES: Certain conditions of nutritive deficiency.

DOSAGE: 2½ drams (10 cc.).

INCOMPATIBILITIES: Light and air, both being contributing factors toward rancidity.

coefficient (ko-ef-fish'ent) [L. *con*, together, + *efficere*, to produce]. A figure put before a chemical formula to express amt. or degree of normal change in a substance under stated conditions.

c. of absorption. Volume of gas absorbed by a unit volume of a liquid at 0° C. and a pressure of 760 mm.

c., Baumann's. Ratio of ethereal sulfates to all sulfates in urine.

c., biological. Amt. of potential energy used by body at rest.

c., Bouchard's. Ratio bet. amt. of urine and total solids of the urine.

c., Falta's. Percentage of ingested sugar eliminated from the system.

c., isotonic. Number showing the amt. of salt to be added to distilled water to prevent the destruction of erythrocytes when it is added to blood.

c., lethal. Concentration of disinfectant that will kill bacteria in the shortest length of time at 20-25° C.

c., urotoxic. Number showing toxicity of the urine: *i. e.*: amt. of toxic matter produced by 1 Kg. of the poison in 24 hours.

coelom. The cavity in an embryo between the split layers of lateral mesoderm. In mammals it develops into the pleural, peritoneal, and pericardial cavities.

c. extra-embryonic. In man, the cavity in the developing blastocyst which lies between the mesoderm of the chorion and the mesoderm covering the amniotic cavity and yolk sac.

coenocyte. A multinucleated mass of protoplasm; a mass of protoplasm in which cell membranes are between the nuclei, as in striated muscle cells; a syncytium.

coen'zyme [L. *co*, together, + G. *en*, with, + *zymē*, leaven]. Enzyme activators. SEE: *coactivity*. A diffusible, heat stable substance of low molecular weight which when combined with an inactive protein, called *apoenzyme* forms an active compound or a complete enzyme called *holoenzyme*. Examples are adenylic acid, riboflavin, and coenzymes I and II.

coetaneous (ko-e-ta'ne-us) [" + *aetās*, age]. Having the same age or date.

coexcitation (ko-ek-sī-ta'shun) [" + *excitāre*, to arouse]. Simultaneous excitation of 2 parts or bodies.

coferment (ko-fer'ment) [" + *fermentātiō*, ferment]. A coenzyme.

cof'fee [L. *caffea*]. Seed of the berry of *Coffea arabica*.

COMP: Coffee has no nutritive value unless it be as a nerve food, but it is the most powerful stimulant that can be safely taken into the system. It contains some nitrogenous material, cellulose, aromatic oils, and fatty substances; sugar and dextrin, potassium phosphate, and a few mineral substances. Caffeine is its essential principle and this is combined with caffeotannic acid, making it slightly antiseptic.

A cup of coffee contains 1½ gr. of caffeine. This principle is a trimethyl xanthine and it is related to the purin bodies, so that coffee increases the production of urinary uric acid. Coffee sometimes causes mild but enduring cardiac pain which disappears if the beverage is withdrawn. The purins amount to 2%.

AV. SERVING: 240 gr. Pro. 0.5, Carbo. 3.4. Milk adds to its nutritive power and lowers the stimulating effect.

ACTION: *Stomach*: Action is light and aids digestion. Cold coffee with plenty of water does not fatigue the stomach. Even with dyspepsia strong coffee does not always prove baneful.

Circulation: Raises the tension of the vascular and nervous systems. Raises the temperature, modifies the heart beats. Relieves fatigue, stimulates activity, esp. cerebral and muscular activity. Prevents sleep through increased cerebral stimulation. Whether it diminishes the consumption of albumin is a debatable question. While it increases the power of production it does so as a stimulant, which must be compensated for by rest and sleep.

Kidneys: It is a diuretic, producing uric acid and taxing the suprarenal capsules. Overdoses are toxic, causing caffeinism, *q.v.*

IND: Use where a quick stimulation is necessary. As an antidote for morphine and opium, in acute alcoholism, and where it is necessary to keep one awake. It is being used in Europe for low blood pressure.

CONTRA: Do not use in affections of the heart; in angina; hypertension; scleroma; neurasthenia; dyspepsia; acne rosacea; psoriasis; uremia; gout; arthritis; liver complaints, and congestion of the visual organs, or when alkaloids or quinine sulfate are being administered. SEE: *chocolate, cocoa, tea*.

c.-ground vomit. Vomit similar to coffee in pigment and consistency, occurring in cancer of the stomach.

coffeurin (kof-e-u'rin) [" + G. *ouron*, urine]. A principle said to exist in urine after excess use of coffee.

The urine then becomes brownish, deep brown, or red, and has the odor of coffee.

cogni'tion [L. *cognōscere*, to know]. Awareness, having perception and memory.

cog'wheel respira'tion. A sudden, brief halt in inspiration and expiration.

cohabita'tion [L. *cohabitāre*, to dwell together]. 1. Sexual intercourse. 2. State of monogamy.

coherent (kō-hēr'ĕnt). 1. Sticking together, as parts of bodies or fluids. 2. Consistent; making a logical whole.

cohe'sion [L. *cohaerere*, to adhere]. The property of adhering.

cohe'sive. Adhesive; sticky.

Cohnheim's fields. Irregular groups of fibrile seen in a cross section of a striated muscle fiber. Also called *Cohnheim's areas*.

Cohnheim's theory (kŏn'hīmz). Theory that tumors result from embryonal cells not utilized for fetal development.

coil [L. *colligere*, to gather together]. 1. A spiral formed by winding some substance. 2. A coil of wire for passage of electric impulses.

c., Bris'tow. Small, portable faradic coil operated on 2 dry cells and the simple device of an iron core sliding in and out of the primary coil which allows a flexible regulation of the secondary current. It is used for muscle stimulation in weak but not paralyzed muscles.

c., choke. Coil of wire which may or may not be provided with a movable laminated iron core, used to limit the flow of current in alternating current circuits. An electrical device using the inductive properties of the alternating current to limit or retard the current entering or leaving an apparatus.

c., faradic. Device for the production of an induced current from a direct current source. Its essential parts are (1) a primary coil consisting of a few turns of insulated thick wire around a soft iron core, (2) a secondary coil consisting of many turns of insulated fine wire, (3) an interrupting device.

c., gland. Sweat gland.

c., induction. Large faradic coil.

c., Oudin (oo-dan'). A coil of fine wire with a large number of turns which increases voltage to such an extent that when the high frequency machine runs at full power there will be a corona discharge to the air from the Oudin (monoterminal) outlet.

c., primary. SEE: *faradic c.*

c., Ruhmkorff (rūm'korf). An apparatus consisting of 2 insulated coils, the primary made up of a few turns of coarse wire, the secondary consisting of many turns of fine wire, enclosing a core of soft iron wires. The primary coil is connected with current supply and an interrupter. Induction coil in which

secondary coil is not movable but is fixed at point of maximum intensity.
c., secondary. See: *faradic c. or high frequency.*
c., spark. Specially designed faradic coil for graduated muscular contraction by electrical muscle stimulation.
c., Tesla. Coil in a modern diathermy apparatus magnetically coupled to the first coil, and the 2 together are known as the resonator.
coiled posture. A natural position with some, but esp. assumed in cerebral diseases, in hepatic, intestinal, or renal colic. See: *posture, illustration,* below.
coilonychia (koy-lo-nik′ĭ-ă) [G. *koilos,* hollow, + *onyx, onych-,* nail]. Nails that have a concave outer surface.
coin counting. A sliding movement of tips of thumb and index finger over each other in paralysis agitans.
c. test. A metal-like sound heard in pneumothorax. Syn: *bell metal resonance, q.v.*
coital (ko′ĭ-tal). Pert. to coition.
coition (ko-ish′un) [L. *coïtus,* a uniting]. Cohabitation. Sexual intercourse* bet. man and woman. *Copulation, coitus, concubitus, q.v.*
coitophobia (ko-i-to-fo′bĭ-ă) [″ + G. *phobos,* fear]. Morbid fear of the sexual act.
coitus (ko′i-tus) [L. a uniting]. Coition, copulation, *q.v.* Sexual intercourse bet. man and woman.
c., à la vache. C. with woman in knee-chest position.
c. interrup′tus. Withdrawal of the penis from the vagina before the seminal emission occurs.
The practice leaves the ejection centers still hyperemic and the seminal vesicles not completely emptied, inducing an earlier return of the libido. Chronic congestion of the prostate may also ensue. The tissues of the female genitalia are not deplethorized for some time which may induce chronic congestion. The psychic reaction in both sexes is unfavorable and may lead to a more or less permanent conflict.
c. reservatus. 1. Same as *c. interruptus.* 2. Onanism.*
colal′gia [G. *kōlon,* + *algos,* pain]. Pain in the colon.
colation (ko-la′shun) [L. *colatiō,* from *colāre,* to strain]. Straining, filtering.
colauxe (kol-awks′e) [G. *kōlon,* + *auxē,* increase]. Distention of the colon.
colchicum (kol′chik-um) [G. *kolchikon*]. Colchicum seed, USP. The seed of a plant of the same name.
Action and Uses: An antineuralgic and analgesic, sometimes used in acute gout.
Dosage: From 3 ℳ (0.2 cc.).
cold [A.S. *cold, ceald*]. 1. A catarrhal affection of the respiratory mucous membranes known as the common cold. 2. The opposite of heat, *q.v.*
cold, common. An acute catarrhal inflammation of the upper respiratory tract. Also called *coryza, rhinitis.*
Etiology: Filterable virus or allergic and metabolic disturbances.
Symptoms: Congestion of nasal mucosa with partial or complete occlusion of nostrils; continuous watery discharge with more or less continuous sniffing and blowing of nose. Headaches and dull pains in the face and head are common. Constitutional symptoms may appear, such as fever, body aches, easy fatigability.
Treatment: Treatment is mainly for the relief of symptoms. Spraying with ephedrine hydrochloride or inhalation of benzedrine or menthol relieves congestion. Coal-tar derivatives relieve malaise and aching. Anti-histamines are sometimes effective. Codeine and papaverine in combination give relief in a high percentage of cases.
c., asphyxia. Place body in cold room, rub with snow or ice water, use artificial respiration. See: *artificial respiration, asphyxia fr. cold, respiration.*
c., chest. Bronchitis.* Inflammation of the bronchial mucous membranes.

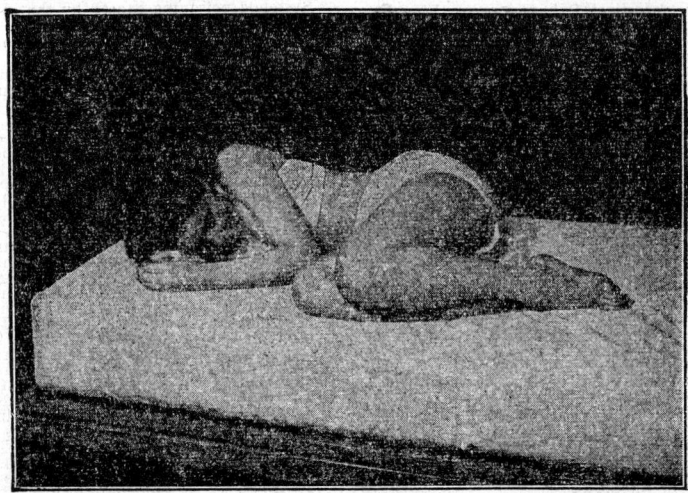

Posed by professional model *Photo by Whitaker*
COILED POSTURE

c. cream. USP. White flavored ointment used mainly as a cosmetic and for chapped skin, minor excoriations of the face, and herpes labialis.

c., head. Coryza,* rhinitis.* Acute catarrhal inflammation of the nasal mucous membranes.
TREATMENT: Vitamin A does not prevent or reduce severity. Codeine and opium derivatives in combination have given relief in 71% of patients. Teaspoonful of salt in glass of water has been effective in preventing colds.

c. pack. Used to reduce temperature.

c. sore. Fever blister. Eruption of vesicles on an inflammatory base. SEE: *herpes.*

colectomy (ko-lek'to-mi) [G. *kōlon*, + *ektomē*, excision]. Excision of part of the colon.

coleocele (ko'le-o-sēl) [G. *koleos*, sheath, vagina, + *kēlē*, hernia]. A vaginal hernia.

coleocystitis (ko-le-o-sĭs-ti'tĭs) [" + *kystis*, bladder, + -*itis*, inflammation]. Inflammation of the vagina and bladder.

coleot'omy [" + *tomē*, incision]. Incision into the pericardium or into the vagina.

colibacellemia (ko-lĭ-bas-ĭl-le'mĭ-ă) [G. *kōlon*, colon, + L. *bacillus*, little rod, + G. *aima*, blood]. Colon bacillus in the blood.

colibacillo'sis [" + " + G. -*ōsis*, infection]. Infection with the colon bacillus.

colibacilluria (ko-lĭ-bas-ĭl-u'rĭ-ă) [" + " + G. *ouron*, urine]. Colon bacillus in the urine.

colibacil'lus [" + L. *bacillus*, little rod]. The *Bacillus coli.*

colic (kol'ĭk) [G. *kōlikos*, pert. to the colon]. 1. Spasm in any hollow or tubular soft organ accompanied with pain. 2. Pert. to the colon.
SEE: *cholecystalgia, tormina.*

c., biliary. In bile ducts usually associated with a gallstone.

c., infantile. Occurring in infants, principally first few months. SYM: Extremities cold, abdomen distended and hard.

c., intestinal. Pain may occur throughout the abdomen and is frequently due to errors of diet.

c., lead. Associated with lead poisoning, occupational, painters, etc. Severe abdominal colic. Lead line may be found on gums and basic stippling in red blood cells.

c., menstrual. Abdominal pain during menses due to some uterine disorder.

c., renal. In region of one of the kidneys and toward the thigh. Pain radiates from kidney region around over abdomen into the groin. It accompanies the passage of calculus. Rigors pronounced.

c., uterine. Painful menstruation. SYN: *dysmenorrhea.*

col'ica [L.]. 1. Abdominal colic. 2. Colic artery.

c. pictonum. Painter's colic.

c. scortorum. Abdominal pain in prostitutes.

colicoli'tis [G. *kōlon*, colon, + -*itis*, inflammation]. Colon inflammation due to *B. coli.*

colicople'gia [" + *plēgē*, stroke]. Lead poisoning with colic and lead paralysis.

colicystitis (ko″lĭ-sis-ti'tĭs) [G. *kōlon*, colon bacillus, + *kystis*, bladder, + -*itis*, inflammation]. Inflammation of bladder. ETIOL: *Bacillus coli.*

colicystopyelitis (ko″lĭ-sis″to-pi-ĕ-li'tis) [" + " + *pyelos*, pus, + -*itis*, inflammation]. Inflammation of bladder and pelvis of kidney. ETIOL: *Bacillus coli.*

col'iform [L. *colum*, sieve, + *forma*, form]. 1. Sieve form; cribriform. 2. Pert. to microörganisms resembling the *Bacillus coli communis.*

co'li infection. Infection with *Bacillus coli communis.*

colilysin (ko-lil'ĭ-sin) [G. *kōlon*, colon bacillus, + *lysis*, dissolution]. A hemolysin formed by *Bacillus coli communis.*

colinephri'tis [" + *nephros*, kidney, + -*itis*, inflammation]. Nephritis caused by the colon bacillus.

coliplication (ko-lĭ-pli-ka'shun) [" + L. *plica*, fold]. Operation for correcting a dilated colon.

colipuncture (ko-lĭ-punk'tŭr) [" + L. *punctura*, a piercing]. Puncture of the colon to relieve distention. SYN: *colocentesis.*

colipyuria (ko-lĭ-pī-u'rĭ-ă) [" + *pyon*, pus, + *ouron*, urine]. Pus in urine due to *Bacillus coli.*

colisep'sis [" + *sepsis*, putrefaction]. Infection caused by the colon bacillus.

coli'tis [" + -*itis*, inflammation]. Inflammation of the colon.

c., mucous. Colitis accompanied by large quantities of mucus. More common in women than in men and among nervous types. A secretory neurosis of the large intestine.
SYM: Attacks occur paroxysmally accompanied by constipation. Spastic, colicky pain in midabdomen. Tenacious, gelatinous mucus and shreds of mucous membrane may be passed.

c., ulcerative. Ulceration of inner lining of colon with dilatation.
SYM: Passage of watery, offensive stools with mucus and pus. Abdominal pain, tenderness, or colic. Maybe temperature, intermittent or irregular fever. Hemorrhage and perforation may occur.

colitoxemia (ko-lĭ-toks-e'mĭ-ă) [" + *toxikon*, poison, + *aima*, blood]. Toxemia caused by the colon bacillus.

colitoxico'sis [" + " + -*ōsis*, infection]. Systemic poisoning caused by the colon bacillus.

colitox'in [" + *toxikon*, poison]. A toxin generated by the colon bacillus.

coliuria (ko-lĭ-u'rĭ-ă) [" + *ouron*, urine]. Presence of *Bacillus coli* in the urine. SYN: *colibacilluria.*

collagen (kol'aj-en) [G. *kolla*, glue, + *gennan*, to produce]. 1. A substance existing in the various tissues of the body, as in the white fibers of connective tissue. 2. A protein which can be prepared from connective tissue (tendons, etc.) and from which gelatin can be made.

collagen disease. So called because all connective tissues are involved which may have a common origin in cell malformation, such as hardening of arteries, arthritis, rheumatic fever, and certain serious maladies, although symptoms and actions in each are different. Connective-tissue fibers have conspicuous alterations in each of these diseases, although the collagen diseases may result from the same cell dysfunction in each case. Disturbance in nuclei acid metabolism of the collagen-producing cells may be one of the factors in these changes.

collapse' [L. *collapsus*, fallen to pieces]. 1. An abnormal retraction of the walls of an organ. 2. A sudden failure of vital power due to reflex inhibition of the heart and respiratory system, or to loss

collapse, of lung   C-72   **colloid**

of blood, low metabolism, or undue lowering of the blood pressure.
The term collapse designates a profound degree of shock, q.v., induced by functional inhibition of the vasomotor center, to distinguish it from the shock of exhaustion of the same center resulting from physical violence or impressions of fear. Intense fear may induce a complete collapse, as is sometimes seen in a victim about to be executed.
SYM: Similar to those of hemorrhage. The peripheral arteries are depleted of blood, and the veins, esp. in the splanchnic region, are congested; apathy; extreme pallor; cold, clammy perspiration; thin, rapid pulse; fall of blood pressure; unconsciousness.
NP: The head of bed, or head and shoulders of patient should be lowered. Hot blankets and hot water bottles may be placed about the patient's body. The arms and lower extremities may be bandaged in critical cases. The heart needs sugar. The doctor may administer adrenalin into the circulation. A physician should be called in all cases of collapse. Raise blood pressure.
   c. of lung. Artificially induced by: (a) Artificial pneumothorax; (b) thoracoplasty, or (c) avulsion of phrenic nerve.

collap'sing. Falling into extreme and sudden prostration resembling shock.
   c. pulse. Pulse of aortic insufficiency or regurgitation; water-hammer pulse. SYN: *Corrigan's pulse.*

collapsother'apy [L. *collapsus*, fallen to pieces, + G. *therapeia*, treatment]. Treatment of pulmonary affections by unilateral pneumothorax and immobilization of affected lung.

collar (kol'ar) [L. *collum*, neck]. 1. A band worn round the neck. 2. Structure or marking formed like a neckband.
   c. of Venus, c., venereal. Mottled appearance of the skin of the neck occasionally seen in syphilis. SYN: *melanoleukoderma colli.*

col'larbone. The clavicle, q.v. SEE: *jugulum.*

collat'eral [L. *con*, together, + *lateralis*, pert. to a side]. 1. Accompanying, as side by side. 2. Subordinate or secondary. 3. Not related lineally. 4. An accessory nerve or blood vessel. 5. A minute side branch of the axon or axis cylinder of a neuron which passes outward at right angles to the axon.
   c. circulation. That of small anastomosing vessels, esp. when a main artery is obstructed.
   c. eminence. An elevation in the floor of the lateral ventricle.
   c. fissure. A fissure on the median surface of the cerebral hemisphere.
   c. ganglia. Ganglia of the sympathetic division of the autonomic nervous system, located near origins of the celiac and mesenteric arteries. Include the celiac and mesenteric ganglia. Also called *prevertebral ganglia.*
   c. trigone. The angle between the diverging inferior and posterior horns of the lateral ventricle.

collat'erals [L. *con*, together, + *lateralis*, pert. to a side]. Minute side branches of processes of axone or axis cylinder processes.

collect'ing plates. The electronegative element of a galvanic battery.

collecting tubules. Small ducts which receive urine from several renal tubules and discharge it into papillary ducts which open into a renal calyx at the tip of a papilla.

collemia (kol-e'mĭ-ă) [G. *kolla*, glue, + *aima*, blood]. A colloidal form of matter in the blood causing capillary obstruction.

Colles' fascia (kol'ēz). Inner layer of superficial fascia of perineum.
   C.'s fracture. The transverse fracture of the distal end of radius (just above wrist) with displacement of hand backward and outward.
   C.'s law. A theory, long accepted (since the advent of the Wassermann test), that a syphilitic child may be born of a mother who is not affected by the nursing child who may affect others. Later in life it has been demonstrated that the mother may show signs of late tertiary syphilis, although her Wassermann was negative at the birth of child.

colliculectomy (kol-lik″u-lek'to-mĭ) [L. *colliculus*, mound, + G. *ektomē*, excision]. Removal of the *colliculus seminalis.*

colliculi'tis [″ + G. *-itis*, inflammation]. Inflammation of the *colliculus seminalis.*

collic'ulus [L. mound]. A little eminence.
   c. anterior. The more forward eminence on the lamina quadrigemina.
   c. bulbi, c. bulbi intermedius. Erectile tissue encircling the male urethra at the entrance to the bulb.
   c. cervicalis (*urethrae muliebris*). The crest on the posterior wall of the female urethra.
   c. inferior. One of two elevations forming the lower portion of the corpora quadrigemina of the midbrain.
   c. seminalis. An oval enlargement on the crista urethralis, an elevation in the floor of the prostatic portion of the urethra. On its sides are the openings of the ejaculatory ducts and numerous ducts of the prostate gland.
   c. superior. One of two elevations forming the upper portion of the corpora quadrigemina of the midbrain.
   c. urethralis. C. seminalis.

col'lier's lung. Pulmonary disease due to inhalation of coal dust. SYN: *anthracosis.*

Colling's elec'trotome [G. *elektron*, amber, friction of which produces electricity, + *tomē*, incision]. Apparatus for using cutting current to relieve fibrous obstruction of neck of bladder in prostatic hypertrophy by endovesical or transurethral operation.

Collip unit. Dosage unit of parathyroid extract. One-one hundredth of the quantity necessary to increase by 5 mg. the amount of calcium in 100 cc. of blood after 15 hours in a dog weighing 20 Kg.

colliquation (kol-ĭ-kwa'shun) [L. *con*, together, + *liquāre*, to melt]. 1. Abnormal discharge of a body fluid. 2. Softening of tissues due to liquefaction. 3. A wasting.

colliquative (ko-lik'wă-tiv). Pert. to a liquid and excessive discharge, as a *c. diarrhea.*

collo'dium, collo'dion [L. from G. *kollōdēs*, glutinous]. Preparation intended for external use (protective for surgical dressings), having for its base a solution of pyroxylin or gun cotton, in a mixture of ether and alcohol. Two are official.
   c., flexible. USP. A more elastic preparation of collodium, containing camphor and castor oil.

colloid (kol'oid) [G. *kollōdēs*, glutinous]. 1. Gelatinous; like glue; opposite of crystalloid.* 2. A particle invisible to the naked eye, which instead of dissolving, is held in a state of suspension.

colloid, cancer   C-73   **colonitis**

3. Gelatinous substance developing in colloid degeneration and carcinoma. Colloids are insoluble, incapable of crystallization, and not diffusible through animal membranes.

A lessened amount of colloids results in increase of kidney stones. Acute physical distress depresses body-level of protective colloids, as do undersupply of Vitamin A or oversupply of Vitamin D, or a diet too rich in calcium, nitrogen, phosphates or alkali. SEE: *kidney stone.*

c. cancer. One in which the tumor cells have a gluelike appearance.

c. chemistry. This deals with such systems and substances, and with the problems of emulsions, mists, foams, and suspensions. [liquid.

c. cyst. A sac containing a jellylike

c. degeneration. A mucoid degeneration seen in the protoplasm of epithelial cells. [skin.

c. millium. Colloid degeneration of the

c., suspension. A mixture holding particles in suspension, the forms of which change with the forces acting upon them, such as milk, fat, etc.

c. thyroid. Semi-fluid, jelly-like substance filling the follicles of the thyroid gland. It contains the thyroid hormone.

colloidal (kol-loyd´ăl). Pert. to a colloid.

colloidal dispersion. A mixture containing colloid particles which fail to settle out and are held in suspension. They are common in animal and plant tissues, the protoplasm of cells being a colloidal mixture. Particles of colloidal dispersions are too large to pass through cell membranes and such dispersions usually appear cloudy.

colloidin (kol-loi´din). A jellylike substance seen in colloid degeneration.

colloidoclasia (kol-oid-o-kla´sĭ-ă) [G. *kollōdēs,* glutinous, + *klasis,* fracture]. A rupture of the body's colloid equilibrium.

colloidopexy (kol-oid´o-pek-sĭ) [" + *pēxis,* fixation]. Fixation of colloids during metabolism.

collo´ma [G. *kolla,* glue, + *-ōma,* tumor]. 1. A colloid degeneration of a cancer. 2. A cyst containing a gelatinous substance.

collonema (kol-o-ne´mă) [" + *nēma,* yarn]. Tumor of mucoid tissue. SYN: *myxoma, myxosarcoma.*

collopexia (kol-o-peks´ĭ-ă) [L. *collum,* neck, + G. *pēxis,* fixation]. Fixation of the *cervix uteri.*

col´lum [L. neck]. 1. The necklike part of an organ. 2. The neck.

collutory (kol´lu-to-rī) [L. *colluĕre,* to rinse]. A gargle or mouth wash.

collyrium (kol-lir´ĭ-um) [G. *kollyrion,* an eyesalve]. An eyewash.

colobo´ma [G. *kolobōma,* a mutilation]. A congenital fissure of the choroid iris, or eyelids.

colocentesis (ko-lo-sen-te´sis) [G. *kŏlon,* colon, + *kentēsis,* puncture]. Surgical puncture of the colon to relieve distention.

colocholecystostomy (ko-lo-kol-e-sis-tos´to-mĭ) [" + *cholē,* bile, + *kystis,* bladder, + *stoma,* opening]. Surgical formation of a communication bet. colon and gallbladder. SYN: *cholecystocolostomy.*

colocleisis (ko-lo-klī´sis) [" + *kleisis,* closure]. Occlusion of the colon.

coloclysis (ko-lok´lĭ-sis) [" + *klysis,* washing]. A colonic enema.

coloclyster (ko-lo-klis´ter) [" + *klyzein,* to cleanse]. A colonic enema.

colocolostomy (ko-lo-kol-os´to-mĭ) [" + *kŏlon,* colon, + *stoma,* mouth]. Formation of a connection bet. 2 portions of the colon.

colocynth (kol´o-sinth) [G. *kolokynthē,* fruit of *Citrullus colocynthis*]. USP. Dried pulp of unripe colocynth fruit.

ACTION AND USES: A drastic hydragogue cathartic. DOSAGE: 2 gr. (0.12 Gm.)

coloenteritis (ko-lo-en-ter-i´tis) [G. *kŏlon,* colon, + *enteron,* intestine, + *-itis,* inflammation]. Inflammation of mucous membrane of small and large intestines.

colofixa´tion [" + L. *fĭxātĭō,* fixation]. Suspension of the colon in ptosis.

co´lon [G. *kōlon*]. The large intestine from the cecum to the rectum, 4 to 6 feet long, and divided into the *ascending,* the *transverse,* and the *descending colon.*

Beginning at the cecum, a pouch bet. the small intestines and the ascending colon, it passes the right kidney under the concave surface of the liver and lower part of the stomach to the spleen, descending past the left kidney to the sigmoid flexure.

c. bacteria. *Bacillus coli communis* is the most commonly found. Whatever digestion takes place in the colon is due to bacteria. A large number of fermentative bacteria are found in the middle portion of the colon. They change carbohydrates into carbon dioxide, alcohol, and lactic acid. This is the only way cellulose may be acted upon in the body. Putrefying bacteria are found in the lower part of the colon. These produce decomposition products which may be absorbed with toxic effect.

c. digestion. *Mechanical:* Antiperistaltic waves move the food mass in the ascending colon back toward the cecum, which aids in further mixing it.

Chemical: No digestive enzymes are secreted in the colon, but an alkaline fluid aids in the completion of digestion begun in the small intestines. Those products of bacterial action which are absorbed into the blood stream are carried by the portal circulation to the liver before they get into the general circulation. There is also a great deal of water absorbed in the colon rather than in the small intestines. The fluids of the body are conserved in this way, and in spite of the large volumes of secretions (saliva, etc.) added to the food during its progress through the alimentary canal, the contents of the colon are gradually dehydrated until they assume the consistency of normal feces or even become quite hard.

SEE: *absorption; colon; defecation.*

colon, words pert. to: anus, appendices epiploicae, cecum, cholecystocolostomy, -otomy, colalgia, colitis, "colo-" words, diverticulitis, -ulum, haustra, -al, jejunum, pendulum movements, peristalsis, rectum, small intestines, vermiform appendix.

colonalgia (ko-lon-al´jĭ-a) [G. *kŏlon,* colon, + *algos,* pain]. Pain in the colon.

colonic (ko-lon´ik). Pert. to the colon.

c. irrigation. Injection into the colon of a large amt. of fluid which is intended to fill colon and flush it.

Administered not to induce defecation but to wash out material situated above the defecation area and to lave the wall of the bowel as high as the water can be made to reach. Two primary methods: 1 tube, involving filling colon to capacity through a single tube and allowing liquid to run out through the same tube, and, 2-tube method, employing separate inflow and outflow tubes.

colonitis (ko-lon-i´tis) [G. *kŏlon,* colon, + *-itis,* inflammation]. Inflammation of the colon. SYN: *colitis.*

colonom'eter [L. *colonia,* colony, + G. *metron,* measure]. Device for estimating colonies of bacteria on a culture plate.

colonopexy (ko″lon-o-pek-sĭ) [G. *kōlon,* colon, + *pēxis,* fixation]. Process of attaching part of colon to abdominal wall.

colonorrhagia (ko″lon-or-ra′jĭ-ă) [" + *regnunai,* to burst forth]. Hemorrhage from the colon.

colonorrhea (ko″lon-or-re′ă) [" + *roia,* flow]. Mucous colitis.

colonoscope (ko-lon′o-skōp) [" + *skopein,* to examine]. Instrument for examination of the colon.

colonos'copy. Examination of upper portion of rectum with an elongated speculum.

col′ony [L. *colonia*]. A collection of microorganisms in a culture.

colopexos'tomy [G. *kōlon,* colon, + *pēxis,* fixation, + *stoma,* mouth]. Resection of the colon and fixation to abdominal wall to establish an artificial anus.

colopexotomy (ko-lo-peks-ot′o-mĭ) [" + " + *tome,* incision]. Incision and fixation of colon.

colopexy, colopexia (ko′lo-pek-sĭ, ko-lo-peks′ĭ-ă) [" + *pēxis,* fixation]. Fixation of the sigmoid or cecum to the abdominal wall by suture.

coloplication (ko-lo-pli-ka′shun) [" + L. *plica,* fold]. Making a fold in the colon to reduce its lumen.

coloprocti'tis [" + *prōktos,* anus, + *-itis,* inflammation]. Colonic and rectal inflammation.

coloproctostomy (ko-lo-prok-tos′to-mĭ) [" + " + *stoma,* opening]. Making a communication bet. a segment of colon and the rectum.

coloptosia (ko-lop-to′sĭ-ă) [" + *ptōsis,* dropping]. Prolapsus of the colon, esp. of the transverse c.

coloptosis (ko-lop-to′sĭs) [" + *ptōsis,* dropping]. A downward displacement of the colon.

colopuncture (ko′lo-punk-chur) [" + L. *punctura,* piercing]. Puncturing the colon.

col′or [L.]. A visible quality, distinct from form, and light and shade.

  c. blindness. Inability to identify 1 or more of the primary colors. Daltonism.

  c. hearing. A sense of color caused by a sound.

  c. index. The hemoglobin content of red blood cells compared with the normal, found by dividing the percentage of hemoglobin by that of erythrocytes.*

  It is an expression of the average amount of hemoglobin contained in each red cell. Normally this index is about 1; indices below 1 indicate that the red cells are abnormally small; above 1, that they are abnormally large. SEE: *volume index.*

color, words pert. to: achromate, -tic, -topsia, -tosis, achromodermia, "acro-" words, alba, albedo, albicans, allochroism, allochromasia, aneryhtropsia, anisochromatic, aurantiasis, -ium, auric, canescent, carotene, "chrom-" words, flavescent, isochromatic, melanin, nigrescent, pigmentation, pigment-producing rays, rubescent, rubiginous, rubor, rufous, vermilion, versicolor, xanthic.

colorectitis (ko-lo-rek-ti′tĭs) [G. *kōlon,* colon, + L. *rectum,* + G. *-itis,* inflammation]. Inflammation of colon and rectum. SYN: *coloproctitis.*

colorectostomy (ko-lo-rek-tos′to-mĭ) [" + " + G. *stoma,* opening]. Formation of passage bet. colon and rectum.

colorim′eter [L. *color,* color, + G. *metron,* measure]. Instrument for measuring amt. of pigments.

colostomy (ko-los′to-mĭ) [G. *kōlon,* colon, + *stoma,* mouth]. Incision of the colon for purpose of making a more or less permanent fistula in treatment of carcinomatous stenosis of lower portion of colon, and in cases of inoperable carcinoma of rectum.

  c. diet. A low residue diet.*

  c., inguinal. Incision of colon to form artificial anus.

  NP: Change dressings *p.r.n.* Protect skin around opening from discharge by covering with sterile zinc oxide ointment. Remove ointment when cleaning with sterile sweet oil. Chart amt. and nature of discharge. Prevent impaction, watch diet orders, irrigate through upper *or* lower loop *as ordered.*

colostra'tion [L. *colostrum*]. Infant diarrhea assumed to be caused by colostrum.

colostrorrhea (ko-los-tror-re′ă) [" + G. *roia,* flow]. Abnormal secretion of colostrum.

colos′trum [L.]. Secretion from the lactiferous glands before the onset of true lactation 2 or 3 days after delivery.

  The secretion contains, mainly, serum and white blood corpuscles. So-called "first milk." Av. amt. sugar 3%, fat 6%, salts 6.4%.

colotomy (ko-lot′o-mĭ) [G. *kōlon,* colon, + *tome,* incision]. Incision of colon. SEE: *Callisen's operation.*

coloty′phoid [" + *typhos,* fever, + *eidos,* resemblance]. Typhoid fever with ulceration of colon.

colpalgia (kol-pal′jĭ-ă) [G. *kolpos,* vagina, + *algos,* pain]. Vaginal pain.

colpatresia (kol-pat-re′zĭ-ă) [" + *a-,* priv. + *trēsis,* a perforation]. Occlusion or pathological closure of the vagina.

colpectasia (kol-pek-ta′sĭ-ă) [" + *ektasis,* distention]. Dilatation of the vagina.

colpec′tomy [" + *ektomē,* excision]. Cutting out part of the vagina.

colpeurynter (kol-pu-rin′ter) [" + *eurynein,* to dilate]. A bag for dilatation of the vagina sometimes used instead of the intracervical hydrostatic bag for the induction of labor.

colpeurysis (kol-pu′rĭs-ĭs) [" + *eurynein,* to widen]. Enlarging of the vagina by surgery.

colpitis (kol-pi′tĭs) [" + *-itis,* inflammation]. Vaginitis. Inflammation of the vagina.

  ETIOL: Most often produced by bacterial invasion, particularly by the gonococcus. May be caused by chemical irritation through the use of too strong chemicals for douching, and from a highly acid urine. Foreign bodies in the vagina (pessaries, etc.) may produce colpitis when there is poor sex hygiene.

  SYM: Free, purulent vaginal discharge, sometimes offensive and occasionally stained with blood. There is irritation of the vulva, frequency of micturition, and smarting pain on the passage of urine. The vaginal mucous membrane is reddened and there may be superficial ulceration.

  TREATMENT: In general, colpitis is relieved by the use of cleansing douches after removing the etiological factors.
  SEE: *vaginitis.*

  c. emphysematosa. Air bleb formation in the vagina as seen in *B. welchii* infection.

  c. mycotica. That due to the presence of yeasts and molds.

colpitis, senilis   C-75   **column, of Clarke**

c. senilis. That accompanied by atrophy of the mucous membrane with the formation of highly vascular papillae. Seen in elderly women who have passed the menopause.
   c., trichomonas. That due to the *Trichomonas vaginalis.* Characterized by punctate hemorrhagic spots in the vagina and a frothy yellowish leukorrhea.

colpocele (kol'po-sēl) [" + *kēlē*, hernia]. Hernia into the vagina.

colpoceliotomy (kol'po-se-lĭ-ot'o-mĭ) [" + *koilia*, belly, + *tomē*, a cut]. Entering the abdomen surgically through the vagina.

colpocleisis (kol-po-klī'sis) [" + *kleisis*, a closure]. Operation of occluding the vagina

colpocystitis (kol-po-sis-tī'tis) [" + *kystis*, bladder, + *-itis*, inflammation]. Inflammation of vagina and bladder.

colpocystocele (kol-po-sis'to-sēl) [" + " + *kēlē*, hernia]. Prolapse of the bladder into the vagina.

colpocys'toplasty [" + " + *plassein*, to form]. Treatment of vesicovaginal fistula.

colpocystosyrinx (kol"po-sis-to-sir'inks) [" + " + *syrigx*, fistula]. Fistula bet. bladder and vagina.

colpocystotomy (kol-po-sis-tot'o-mĭ) [" + " + *tomē*, incision]. Cutting into the bladder through the vagina.
   NP: Prevent bladder distention. Record intake and output. If retention catheter is present, irrigate twice daily with solution ordered and be sure catheter is kept draining. If female patient, keep clean and comfortable with external irrigations over the vulva.

colpocystoureterocystotomy (kol"po-sis"-to-u-re"ter-o-sis-tot'o-mĭ) [" + " + *ourētēr*, ureter, + *kystis*, bladder, + *tomē*, incision]. Incision into the ureter through the walls of the bladder and vagina.

colpodesmorrhaphia (kol-po-des-mor-a'fĭ-ă) [" + *desmos*, band, + *raphē*, suture]. Repair of the vaginal sphincter.

colpodynia (kol-po-din'ĭ-ă) [" + *odynē*, pain]. Pain in the vagina. SYN: *colpalgia*.

colpohyperplasia (kol-po-hi-per-pla'zĭ-ă) [" + *yper*, over, + *plasis*, a forming]. Excessive growth of mucous membrane of the vagina.
   c. cystica. Infectious inflammation of the vaginal walls which is characterized by the production of small blebs.

colpo"hysterec'tomy [" + *ystera*, uterus, + *ektomē*, excision]. Removal of the uterus through the vagina.
   NP: Watch for vaginal packs and remove as ordered. Watch for retention catheters and care for per routine orders.

colpohysteropexy (kol-po-his'ter-o-pek-sĭ) [" + *pēxis*, fixation]. Fixation of uterus through the vagina.

colpohysterot'omy [" + " + *tomē*, incision]. Incision through the vagina into the uterus, as for excision of a fibroma.

colpomyomectomy (kol-po-mi-o-mek'to-mĭ) [" + *mys*, muscle, + *-ōma*, tumor, + *ektomē*, excision]. Removal of a fibroid tumor of the uterus through the vagina.

colpomyomotomy (-mot'o-mĭ) [" + " + " + *tomē*, incision]. Incision of uterus through the vagina for removal of tumor.

colpopathy (kol-pop'ă-thĭ) [" + *pathos*, disease]. Any pathology of the vagina.

colpoperineoplasty (kol-po-per-ĭn-ē'o-plas-tĭ) [" + *perinaion*, perineum, + *plassein*, to form]. Plastic operation on vagina and perineum.
   NP: Irrigate perineum with warm sterile water b.i.d. and after bedpan. Warm glycerine dressings are often applied to relieve pain and discomfort. If leg holders are not convenient, fold a sheet in triangular shape, roll towards point, place under knees of patient, drawing them up, bring one end over shoulder and under opposite arm, and tie. After operation, a towel should be pinned around limbs to hold in position. Light diet for few days.

colpoperineorrhaphy (kol-po-per-in"e-or'raf-ĭ) [" + " + *raphē*, suture]. Operation for mending perineal tears in vagina. SYN: *colpoperineoplasty.*

col'popexy [" + *pēxis*, fixation]. Suture of a relaxed and prolapsed vagina to the abdominal wall.

colpoplasty (kol'po-plas-tĭ) [" + *plassein*, to form]. Plastic operation upon vagina.

colpoptosis (kol-pop-to'sis) [" + *ptōsis*, a falling]. Prolapse of the vagina.

colporrhagia (kol-po-ra'jĭ-ă) [" + *rēgnunai*, to burst forth]. Excessive vaginal discharge. Vaginal hemorrhage.

colporrhaphy (kol-por'ă-fĭ) [" + *raphē*, suture]. Suture of vagina.

colporrhexis (kol-por-reks'is) [" + *rēxis*, rupture]. Operative repair of defective vaginal floor.

colposcope (kol'po-skōp) [" + *skopein*, to examine]. An instrument for examining the fornices of the vagina and *cervix uteri.*

col'pospasm, colpospas'mus [" + *spasmos*, spasm]. Spasm of the vagina. SYN: *vaginismus.*

col'postat [" + L. *stāre*, to stand]. Device for holding a radium applicator in the vagina.

colpostenosis (kol-po-sten-o'sis) [" + *stenōsis*, narrowing]. Stenosis or narrowing of the vagina.

colpostenotomy (kol-po-sten-ot'o-mĭ) [" + " + *tomē*, incision]. A cutting operation for dilating the lumen in stricture of the vagina.

colpotherm (kol'po-thurm) [" + *thermē*, heat]. Electrical device introduced into the vagina to convey heat.

colpotomy (kol-pot'o-mĭ) [" + *tomē*, incision]. An incision of the vagina.

colpoureterocystotomy (kol-po-u-re"ter-o-sis-tot'o-mĭ) [" + *ourētēr*, ureter, + *kystis*, + *tomē*, incision]. Exposure of the ureteral orifices by incision through the walls of the vagina and bladder.

colpoureterot'omy [" + " + *tomē*, incision]. Incision of the ureter through the vagina.

colpoxerosis (kol-po-zē-rō'sis) [" + *xērōsis*, dryness]. Abnormal dryness of the vulva and vagina.

columella (kol-ū-mel'lă) [L. dim. of *columna*, column]. 1. A column. 2. BACT: Portion of the sporangiophore upon which are borne the spores.
   c. na'si. The ant. part of the septum of nose; *concha nasalis,* a turbinate bone.

column (kol'um) [L. *columna,* pillar]. A supporting anatomical part resembling a cylinder.
   c., anterior. Ant. portion of gray columns on either side of the spinal column.
   c. of Clarke. A group of column cells in the cervix of the post. gray column of the spinal cord.

column, direct cerebellar   C-76   **coma**

c., *direct cerebellar.* A bandlike tract of ascending white fibers immediately in front of the line of entrance of the post. nerve roots on the posterolateral surface of the spinal cord.
c. *of Goll.* Inner division of the white column of the spinal cord; contains sensory fibers.
c. *of Gowers.* Tract of ascending fibers ant. to the direct cerebellar column, and on the lateral surface of the spinal cord.
c., *lateral.* Lateral white column of the spinal cord bet. lines of entrance and exit of ant. and post. nerve roots.
c. *of Morgagni.* One of several vertical ridges in mucous membrane at junction of anus and rectum.
c., *posterior.* Post. portion of gray columns of spinal cord.
c., *posterovesicular.* Same as column of Clarke.
c., *respiratory.* Longitudinal fibrous bundle starting at upper portion of medulla and running down to the 4th cervical nerve.
c., *Sertoli's.* A columnar figure in testicle formed by collections of Sertoli's cells.
c., *spinal.* The line of vertebrae from the head to the pelvis, making up the bony flexible case for the spinal cord.
c. *of Turck.* A subdivision of the white column of the spinal cord.
c., *vesicular.* Line of ganglion cells on inner side of post. column.
columna (ko-lum'na) (pl. *columnae*) [L.]. A column or pillar.
c. *adiposa.* Fat column.
c. *bertini.* Interpyramidal extension or renal column supporting renal blood vessels.
c. *carnea.* A muscular projection within the cardiac ventricles.
c. *nasi.* Nasal septum.
c. *rugarum vaginae.* Fold of mucous membrane of the vagina which is arranged in a columnar fashion.
colum'nar layer. Retinal rod-and-cone layer.
columning (kol'um-ing). Introduction of tampons in vagina to support the prolapsed uterus.
colyone (ko'lĭ-ōn) [G. *kōlyein*, to hinder]. An autacoid which inhibits hormone or cellular activity. SYN: *chalone.*
colypeptic (ko-lĭ-pep'tĭk) [" + *peptikos*, peptic]. Slowing up digestive processes.

colyphrenia (kol-ĭ-fre'nĭ-ă) [" + *phrēnē*, mind]. Abnormal tendency to mental inhibition.
colyseptic (ko-lĭ-sep'tĭk) [" + *sepsis*, putrefaction]. Antiseptic.
colytic (ko-lit'ĭk) [G. *kōlyein*, to hinder]. Inhibitory.
co'ma [G. *kōma*, a deep sleep]. An abnormal deep stupor occurring in illness, or as a result of it, or it may be due to an injury. The patient cannot be aroused by external stimuli.
   ETIOL: May be due to alcoholism, to hysteria, epilepsy, narcotics, poisons, gases, sunstroke, heat exhaustion, uremia, or injury. More than 50% of cases are due to trauma to the head or circulatory accidents in the brain due to hypertension, sclerosis, thrombosis, tumor or abscess formation. The chief causes of coma are: (a) Trauma, as in accidents, hemorrhage, and shock; (b) vascular disease; (c) organic disease of the central nervous system; (d) metabolic disorders; (e) acute infections of the brain or meninges; (f) acute infections and bacterial intoxications, as in fevers, botulism, and other diseases; (g) parasites; (h) the effects of drugs; alcohol, atropine, chloral, chloroform, cyanides, carbon dioxide, carbon monoxide, hyosine, phenols, paraldehyde, trional, sulphonal, veronal, ether, gases and various fumes; (i) extreme temperatures; (j) excessive loss of blood; (k) neurotic causes, as in malingering.
   GENERAL TREATMENT: First aid treatment should be strictly limited; patient should not be moved other than to slightly raise the head. Movement without aid of a physician is dangerous. The collar should be loosened. Cold compresses to head and hot ones to the spine and abdomen may be indicated. Stomach pump in case of poisoning indicated. Insulin injection for diabetic coma may be given unless the coma is due to too much insulin. Sugar may be administered if it can be taken. Urine should be examined for albumin, and dropsy looked for in pregnant women. In uremic coma, stimulate elimination. Lumbar puncture or bleeding may be necessary. Induce sweating. In hysteric coma no treatment is needed. The patient revives if ignored.
   NP: Test urine for cause, and for retention. Regulate bowels. Clean mouth; glycerine and borax may be used. Keep

Diagnosis of Diabetic and Hypoglycemic Coma[1]

	Diabetic Coma	**Hypoglycemic Coma**
Onset	Gradual.	Often sudden.
History	Often of acute infection in a diabetic or no previous history of diabetes.	Recent insulin injection, or inadequate meal or excessive exercise after insulin.
Skin	Flushed, dry.	Pale, sweating.
Tongue	Dry.	Moist.
Breath	Smell of acetone.	No acetone.
Respiration	Deep (air hunger).	Shallow.
Pulse	Rapid, feeble.	Normal or bounding.
Eyeball Tension	Low.	Normal or raised.
Urine	Sugar and acetone.	None, unless bladder has not been emptied for some hours.
Blood Sugar	Raised [over 200].	Subnormal [40-70].
Blood Pressure	Low.	Normal.
Abdominal Pain	Common and often acute.	Sometimes sense of constriction.

[1] Sears. *Medicine for Nurses.*

coma, alcoholic   C-77   **commutator**

water out of trachea. Keep eyes cleansed. Apply an ointment to prevent lids from sticking together. Guard against bed sores. May have to be fed artificially. SEE: *catochus, narcoma.*

c., alcoholic. Due to alcohol.

c., apoplectic. Due to cerebral hemorrhage or apoplexy; one side of body, or the extremities, 1 or more, will be paralyzed. No fever at first but 1 pupil may be larger than the other. Coma indicates pressure on the brain in most instances. SEE: *apoplexy.*

c., diabetic. Occurring in diabetes, due to presence of diacetic acid in system and to acidosis. Paralysis not present. SYM: Sweet breath; showers of short granular casts may appear in urine when diabetic coma is threatened by acidosis. Hyperglycemia is present, and softening of eyeballs may occur.

TREATMENT: Insulin has prevented diabetic coma to a large extent but an overdose may induce it. It must not be given if coma is due to insulin. An initial dose of 30-60 units may be given (½ intravenously, ½ subcutaneously), followed by ½-3 hr. intervals by doses of 20 units or more subcutaneously. Examine urine hourly for dextrose; if urine is sugar-free, more dextrose must be given. More than 150 units in 12 hr. rarely needed. Young children usually require smaller doses and seldom more than 80 units in 12 hr. SEE: *insulin.*

c., uremic. The result of disturbed kidney metabolism, causing autointoxication through the retention of unknown substances in the blood and producing acidosis. Seen in nephritis as a result of lack of elimination of kidney toxins.

SYM: In general, respiration stertorous, face livid, skin dry, hard and rapid pulse, blood pressure raised, sphincters relaxed according to cause; urinous odor on breath, urine scanty and containing many casts and albumin. Complete retention may occur.

c. vigil. Delirious lethargy with open eyes and partial consciousness.

co'matose. In a condition of coma.

comedo (kom'e-do) [pl. *comedon'es*) [L. a glutton]. Blackhead; fleshworm. Discolored dried sebum plugging an excretory duct of the skin.

ETIOL: Reflex or local disturbance causing increased activity of sebaceous glands. Constipation, dyspepsia, chlorosis, menstrual derangements are contributory factors. Also caused by the follicle or face mite. *Demodex folliculorum* which lives in the hair follicles and sebaceous glands of various mammals.

SYM: Commonly affects the face, back, and ears; chronic, frequently associated with seborrheic dermatitis, or acne, usually during convalescence.

PROG: Obstinate and persistent, but amenable to treatment.

TREATMENT: Aside from removal of plugs, treatment is essentially that of acne, *q.v.*

comes (ko'mēz) (pl. *com'ites*) [L. companion]. A blood vessel which accompanies a nerve or another blood vessel.

com'mon bacillus [named from shape]. The causative organism of Asiatic cholera, *Vibrio cholerae asiaticae.*

com'ma tract. A longitudinal bundle of descending fibers in the *fasciculus cuneatus* of the spinal cord. Schultze's bundle.

commen'sal [L. *com*, together, + *mensa*, table]. One of two organisms which live in an intimate, non-parasitic relationship, one to the other.

commensalism. The symbiotic relationship of two organisms of different species in which neither is harmful to the other and one gains some benefit such as protection or nourishment. Ex: Nonpathogenic bacteria in human intestine.

comminute (kom'in-ūt) [" + *minuĕre*, to crumble]. To break into pieces.

com'minuted fracture. A crushed bone.

comminution (kom-in-u'shun) [L. *comminutiō*, crumbling]. Reducing a solid body to varying sizes by grating, pulverizing, slicing, granulating, and by other processes. SEE: *attenuation, dynamization.*

commissu'ra (pl. *commissurae*) [L. a joining together]. A commissure.

c. anterior alba. A narrow band of white substance near ant. median fissure of the spinal cord.

c. anterior cerebri. White bundle crossing from side to side in the ant. wall of the 3rd ventricle.

c. anterior grisea. Part of gray commissure in front of and bet. the *commissura anterior alba.*

c. brevis. Post. portion of inferior cerebellar vermiform process.

c. hippocampi. A little triangular space bet. the diverging crura of the fornix.

c. magna. Corpus callosum.*

c. simplex. Lobule on superior vermiform process of the cerebellum.

commissu'ral. Pert. to a commissure.

commissure (kŏm'ĭ-shūr) [L. *commissura*, a joining together]. 1. A transverse band of nerve fibers passing over the midline in the central nervous system. 2. A suture of the skull. 3. The coming together of two structures, as the lips, eyelids, or nymphae.

In gynecology the ant. and post. commissures of the vulva are used to denote its 2 ends. The ant. commissure passes immediately above the clitoris, the post. constitutes the ant. edge of the perineum.

common bile duct. Duct carrying bile to the duodenum and receiving it from the cystic and hepatic ducts. SYN: *ductus choledochus.* SEE: *bile.*

commu'nicable disease. A disease which may be transmitted directly or indirectly from one invidiual to another.

communicable disease, words pert. to: alternate host, carriers, contagion, -ious, -ium, cowpox, endemic, epidemic, epidemiology, immune, -ity, immunologic diseases, immunology, incubation, infection, isolation, lues, microbe, micrococcus, microörganism, quarantine, transmissible, vection, vector.

commu'nicans [L. *communicare*, to connect with]. One of a number of communicating nerves or arteries.

c. hypoglossi. The descending branch of the 12th cranial nerve.

c. peronei. Fibular connecting nerve.

c. poplitei. Lateral sural cutaneous nerve.

c. Willisi. Transverse artery at back of arterial ring at base of brain; posterior and communicating artery.

com'mutator [L. *commutāre*, to change]. Device for reversing electric current direction, usually segmental ring attached to dynamo on which brushes slide. Also similar hand operated devices.

Method of Transfer of Some Common Communicable Diseases

Disease	How the Bacteria Leave the Bodies of the Sick	How They May Be Transferred	How They May Enter the Bodies of the Well
Typhoid.	Feces and urine.	Direct contact. Hands of nurse or attendant. Linen and all articles used by and about patient. Hands of "carriers" soiled by their own feces. Water polluted by excreta. Food grown in or washed with such water. Milk diluted or milk cans washed with such water. Flies.	Through mouth in infected food or water and thence to intestinal tract.
Diphtheria.	Sputum and discharges from nose and throat.	Direct contact. "Droplet infection" from patient coughing. Hands of nurse. Articles used by and about patient.	Through mouth to throat or nose to throat.
Scarlet fever.	Discharges from nose and throat.	Direct contact. Hands of nurse. Articles used by and about patient.	Through mouth and nose.
Pneumonia.	Sputum and discharges from nose and throat.	Direct contact. Hands of nurse. Articles used by and about patient.	Through mouth and nose to lungs.
Influenza.	As pneumonia.	As pneumonia.	As pneumonia.
Smallpox.	Discharges from nose and throat. Skin lesions.	Direct contact. Hands of nurse. Articles used by and about patient.	Thought to be through mucous membrane of respiratory tract.
Syphilis.	Infected tissues. Lesions.	Direct contact. May be by kissing or by sexual intercourse. Dishes, food, toilets, towels, bathtubs, drinking cups, etc.	Directly into blood and tissues through breaks in skin or membrane.
Tetanus.	Excreta from infected herbivorous animals and man.	Soil, especially that with manure or feces in it. Dust, etc. Articles used about stables.	Directly into blood stream through wounds. (Is anaerobe and prefers deep, incised wound.)
Tuberculosis, Human.	Sputum. Lesions. Feces.	Direct contact, such as kissing. "Droplet infection" from person coughing with mouth uncovered. Sputum from mouth to fingers, thence to food and other things. Soiled dressings.	Through mouth to lungs and intestines. From intestines *via* lymph channels to lymph vessels and to tissues.
Tuberculosis, Bovine.		Milk.	Same as Tuberculosis, Human.
Cholera.	Excreta from intestinal tract.	As in typhoid, through feces.	As in typhoid, through mouth to intestinal tract.

Method of Transfer of Some Common Communicable Diseases (Continued)

Disease	How the Bacteria Leave the Bodies of the Sick	How They May Be Transferred	How They May Enter the Bodies of the Well
Dysentery.	As above.	As above.	As above.
Hookworm.	Feces.	Direct contact with soil polluted with feces. Eggs in feces hatch in sandy soil. Feces may also contaminate food.	Larvae enter through breaks in skin, specially skin of feet, and, after devious passage through the body, settle in the intestine.
Meningitis.	Discharges from nose and throat.	Direct contact. Hands of nurse or attendant. Articles used by and about patient. Flies.	Mouth and nose.
Infantile paralysis.	Discharges from nose and throat.	Direct contact. Hands of nurse or attendant.	Through mouth and nose.
Gonorrhea.	Lesions. Discharges from infected mucous membranes.	Direct contact, as in sexual intercourse. Towels, bathtubs, toilets, etc. Hands of infected persons soiled with their own discharges. Hands of attendant.	Directly onto mucous membrane. Through breaks in membrane.
Ophthalmia neonatorum (gonorrheal infection of eyes of newborn).	Pus discharges from eye.	Direct contact with infected areas, as vagina of infected mother during birth. Other infected babies. Hands of doctor or nurse. Linens, etc.	Directly on the conjunctiva.
Whooping cough.	Discharges from respiratory tract.	Direct contact with persons affected.	Mouth and nose.
Mumps.	Discharges from infected glands and mouth.	Direct contact with persons affected.	Mouth and nose.
Measles.	Like scarlet fever.	Like scarlet fever.	Like scarlet fever.
Trachoma.	Discharges from infected eyes.	Direct contact. Hands, towels, handkerchiefs, possibly clothing.	Directly on conjunctiva.
Leprosy.	Uncertain, may be from lesions. Bacilli found in nodules which may break down, forming lesions.	Uncertain.	Uncertain.

Comolli's sign (ko-mol'lĭs). A triangular swelling corresponding to the outline of the scapula when fractured.

comose (kō'mōs) [L. *comōsus*, hairy]. Hairy. Having much hair.

compact' [L. *compactus*, joined together]. Dense, packed, solid.

 c. bone. Hard or dense bone which forms the superficial layer of all bones, in contrast to spongy or cancellous bone found chiefly in the ends of long bones.

compar'ative anat'omy. Human anatomy compared with that of animals.

compatibil'ity [L. *con*, with, + *pati*, to suffer, + *habilis*, to fit]. State of suitability to be mixed or taken together without unfavorable results, as drugs.

compat'ible. Not opposed to; able to mix with another substance without destructive changes.

com'pensating. Making up for a deficiency.

 c. operation. Tenotomy of the associated antagonists in diplopia.

compensa'tion [L. *cum*, with, + *pensāre*, to weigh]. Making up for a defect, as cardiac circulation competent to meet

compensation, failure of

demands made upon it, regardless of valvular defect.

PSY: A far reaching psychic mechanism, best described by an example. The individual handicapped by a physical deformity or variation, or by a character defect, may escape the consciousness or revelation of the inferiority, by accomplishment resulting from compensatory ambition. More simple, the short man struts or the incompetent brags.

Sublimation* is often similar, but varies in the sense that the substitution of a higher (social goal) gratifies the infrasocial drive by replacement—rather than the going to the opposite extreme in a merely camouflaging manner.

c., failure of. Inability of heart muscle to cope with cardiac defect with ensuing muscle exhaustion. It indicates a diseased heart muscle.

ETIOL: Diseased myocardium; back pressure, due to mitral regurgitation, mitral or aortic stenosis, or aortic regurgitation.

comp'lement [L. *complēre*, to complete]. A substance or body producing bacteriolysis or hemolysis which, by means of an amboceptor, is connected with a bacterial or animal cell.

It is present in all sera. Strictly speaking, c. is not an antibody, but a natural property of blood.

RS: *albumin antialexin, antialbumate, antialbumin, anticomplement, Ehrlich's theory.*

c. unit. Smallest quantity of complement required for hemolysis of a given amount of red blood corpuscles with 1 amboceptor unit present.

complement'al, complement'ary. Supplying something that is lacking.

c. air. Amt. of air (1600 cc. or 3 pt.) that can be inspired over and above the tidal air by the deepest inspiration. SEE: *air.*

c. colors. Any 2 primary colors which, when blended, produce white light.

complemen'toid [L. *complēre*, to complete, + G. *eidos*, form]. A complement, the lysis-causing power of which has been destroyed.

complementophil (kom-ple-ment'o-fĭl) [" + G. *philein*, to love]. Having the power to combine with a complement.

com'plex [L. *complexus*, woven together]. 1. PSY: A subconscious idea (or group of ideas) which have become associated with a repressed wish or emotional experience and which may influence behavior although the person may not have any appreciation of the connection between the repressed desire and his thoughts or actions. 2. All the ideas, feelings, and sensations connected with a subject. 3. Intricate.

In Freudian psychology a grouping of ideas with an emotional background. These may be harmless, and the individual fully aware of them, *e. g.*, an artist sees every object with a view to a possible picture, and is said to have established a complex for art. Often, however, the complex is aroused by some painful emotional reaction, such as fright or excessive grief, which, instead of being allowed a natural outlet, becomes unconsciously repressed, and later manifests itself in some abnormality of mind or behavior. According to Freud, the best method of determining the complex is through the medium of psychoanalysis. Jung and Rivers, however, suggest finding out the complex by a series of time and reaction tests. SEE: *Oedipus and Electra c.*

RS: *castration complex, inferiority c., Jocasta c., superiority c.*

c., castration. Morbid fear of being castrated.

c., inferiority. A repressed state of mind in which one feels himself inferior to others.

c., superiority. Exaggerated conviction of one's own superiority; also pretense of being superior to compensate for a supposed inferiority.

complex'us [L.]. 1. The total indications or phenomena of a morbid state. 2. Semispinalis capitis muscle.

complica'tion [L. *cum*, with, + *plicāre*, to fold]. An added difficulty; a complex state. A disease or accident superimposed upon another without being specially related, yet affecting or modifying the prognosis of the original disease, *e. g.*, pneumonia is a complication of measles, and is the cause of many deaths from that disease.

component. A constituent part of.

com'pos men'tis [L.]. Of sound mind; sane.

com'pound [L. *componere*, to place together]. A substance composed of two or more elements combined in definite proportions by weight and having specific properties of its own.

Compounds are formed in plants and animals and are of two types, *organic* and *inorganic.*

c. astigmatism. Myopia of both vertical and horizontal meridians.

c. cathartic pills. Ones composed of calomel, colocynth, gamboge, and jalap.

c. fracture. One having an open wound into seat of fracture.

c., inorganic. One of many compounds which, in general, contain no carbon.

c. microscope. One consisting of 2 or more lenses.

c. organic. A compound containing carbon. Examples are carbohydrates, proteins, and fats.

compress (kom'pres) [L. *compressus*, squeezed together]. 1. Cloth, wet or dry, folded and applied firmly to a part to prevent hemorrhage or to relieve inflammation; made of cotton, oakum, marine lint, jute, etc. 2. (kŏm-prĕs'). To press together into smaller space. 3. To close by squeezing together, as a wound.

c., abdominal. Three folds of linen reaching from sternum to pubis, overlapping sides of abdomen, wrung out of the water at 70° F., held in place by flannel binder little wider than linen, long enough to reach around the body.

c., chest. Application of 2 pieces of old linen of sufficient size to fit the entire chest from the clavicles down to the umbilicus, wrung out of water at 60° F., and covered with flannel.

c., cold. Linen cloth, several layers dipped in cold water, slightly wrung out, applied to given part. To secure constant temperature, compress is frequently renewed, ice bag or aluminum coil through which ice water is circulating is placed on it. Duration, 30-60 minutes.

c., forehead. A soft towel wrung out of water below 60° F. renewed at least every 2 minutes.

c., hot. Linen cloth folded into several layers, dipped in hot water (107-115° F.) slightly wrung out and placed on part to be treated, covered with a piece of flannel, large enough to overlap the linen slightly. Temperature is maintained at constant level by renewing compress or by coil through which hot water (107-115° F.) is circulating.

c., neck. Application of a soft towel wrung out of water bet. 42-60° F.

c., precordial. Pad of 4 layers of linen cloth, moistened in water 60-65° F., is applied over the heart region. On this is placed a coil through which water at 60-65° F. is circulating. This water temperature is reduced until ice water is used. Duration, 10-45 minutes. Twice daily.

c., Priessnitz. Cold wet compress.

c., spinal. Usually the application of a soft cloth wrung out of ice water, renewed every 2-3 minutes. Applied to cervical region for meningitis, cerebral congestion and nervous asthenia; dorsal region for hysterical vomiting and to lumbar region for renal and uterine hemorrhage.

c., throat. Application of 2 strips of linen 3 inches wide and long enough to reach from beneath 1 ear under the chin to the opposite ear, wrung out of water at 60° F., a piece of flannel ¼ inch wider covers it and overlaps at top of head.

c., trunk. Consists of 3 folds of linen from axilla to pubis and reaching around the trunk, wrung out of water 60-75° F., covering with flannel bandage secured by pins. Changed every hour.

c., wet. Application of 2 or more folds of old linen wrung out of water at prescribed temperatures and covered with flannel.

compres'sion [L. *compressio*, a compression]. A squeezing together; state of being pressed together.

c. atrophy. That in a part due to steady compression.

c. of the brain. Same as cerebral compression, *q.v.*

c., cerebral. Pressure on the brain produced by increased intercranial fluids, embolism, thrombosis, tumors, and skull fractures. More serious than concussion.*

SYM: Deep unconsciousness; full, bounding pulse; deep, stertorous, slow respiration; flushed face; high blood pressure; pupils varying in size. Temperature may rise and there may be retention or incontinence of urine and feces. *Danger Signals:* Cheyne-Stokes respiration, rise in temperature, quickening of pulse.

NP: Watch for change of symptoms; pulse, respiration, color, urine, and bed sores; also convulsions, bleeding from ears and nose, and oozing at back of throat, or for cerebrospinal fluid from ears, which may indicate fracture. Constant care of mouth and eyes. SEE: *circumclusion.*

c., digital. Arterial compression by means of the fingers.

c., myelitis. That due to pressure on the spinal cord, often due to a tumor.

compres'sor. 1. Instrument for making pressure on a part. 2. Contraction of a muscle, causing compression of another structure.

compul'sion [L. *compulsiō*, an urging]. Act performed to relieve fear connected with obsession; dictation by the patient's subconscious, arising against the subject's wishes and, if denied, causing uneasiness. Impulsive actions, on the contrary, often seem to express the personality.

c. neurosis. Obsession or psychoneurosis urging one to perform an absurd act or to say something silly.

compul'sive. Exercising or applying compulsion.

c. ideas. PSY: An idea that continues to suggest against one's will the commitment of an overt act, such as murder or suicide.

compul'sory. Compelling action against one's will.

c. movements. Movements caused by injury to a nerve center.

con- [L.]. Prefix: Together with, as *congenital.*

conarium (ko-na'rĭ-um) [G. *konarion*, a little cone]. The pineal gland. *Corpus pineale* (BNA).

conation (ko-na'shun) [L. *conatio*, an attempt]. Any desire or impulse compelling action.

concassation (kon-kas-a'shun) [L. *con*, with, + *quassere*, to crush]. 1. Shaking of a precipitate in a bottle or pulverizing by beating. 2. Mental distress.

Concato's disease (kon-kä'tōs). Progressive inflammation of serous membranes. ETIOL: Tuberculosis.

concave (kon'kāv) [L. *con*, with, + *cavus*, hollow]. Having a spherically depressed or hollow surface.

concav'ity [" + *cavitas*, a hollow]. A hollowed surface, with curved, bowl-like sides.

conca"vocon'cave [" + *cavus*, hollow, + *con*, with, + *cavus*, hollow]. Concave on opposing sides.

concavocon'vex [" + " + *convexus*, vaulted]. Concave on 1 side and convex on opp. surface.

concentration (kon-sen-tra'shun) [L. *concentratiō*, in the center]. 1. Increase in strength of a fluid by evaporation. 2. Medicine strengthened by evaporation. 3. Fixation of mind on 1 subject to exclusion of all other thoughts.

con'cept [L. *conceptum*, something devised]. An idea.

concep'tion [L. *conceptiō*, a conceiving]. The union of the male sperm and the ovum of the female; fertilization.

With a cycle of 28 days, menstruation normally lasts 5 days followed by a period of repair and proliferation of 9 days. During this time a woman is usually sterile as ovulation has not occurred. Conception is most likely to occur during the 14-18th days of the cycle. During this period, the ovum is discharged from the follicle and makes its way through the Fallopian tube to the uterus. If fertilization does not occur during this time the ovum disintegrates and for the remaining portion of the menstrual cycle (the ten days preceding menstruation) conception is very unlikely to occur.

concha (kong'kä) [G. *kogchē*, shell]. 1. The outer ear or the pinna. 2. The inferior turbinated bone. 3. Patella. 4. Vulva.

c. auriculae. A concavity on the median surface of the auricle of the ear, divided by a ridge into the upper *cymba conchae* and a lower *cavum conchae*. The latter leads to the ext. auditory meatus.

c. bullosa. Turbinated bone expansion, during chronic rhinitis.

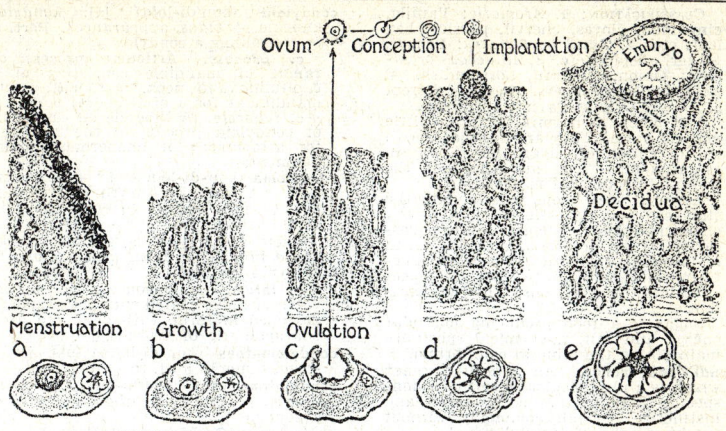

MENSTRUATION, CONCEPTION, AND IMPLANTATION
(a) Menstruation. (b) Growth. (c) Ovulation, ovum becomes impregnated. (d) Ovum in morula stage becomes implanted. Endometrium in pregravid stage. corpus luteum of pregnancy developing. (e) Endometrium has become decidua and ovum is growing between D. Capsularis and D. Basalis.

c. nasal. One of the three scroll-like bones which project medially from the lateral wall of the nasal cavity; a turbinate bone. The superior and middle conchae are processes of lateral mass of the ethmoid bone; the inferior concha is a face bone. Each overlies a meatus.

c. Santorini. C. nasalis suprema.

c. sphenoidalis. One of two curved plates located on anterior portion of body of sphenoid bone. Forms part of roof of nasal cavity.

conchitis (kong-ki'tis) [" + -itis, inflammation]. Inflammation of any concha.

conchoidal (kong-koi'dal) [" + eidos, shape]. Having the shape of a shell.

conchoscope (kong'ko-scōp) [" + skopein, to examine]. Instrument for examination of the nasal cavity.

conchotome (kong'ko-tōm) [" + tomē, incision]. Device for excision of middle turbinated bone.

concoc'tion [L. con, with, + coquere, to cook]. The boiling of 2 or more substances together.

concom'itant [L. cum, together, + comēs, companion]. Accessory; taking place at the same time.

concrement. A concretion as of protein and other substances. If infiltrated with calcium salts, such is termed a calculus.

concrescence (kon-kres'ens) [L. con, together, + crescere, to grow]. The union of separate parts; coalescence.

concrete (kon'krēt) [L. concretus, solid]. Condensed, hardened, or solidified.

concre'tion [L. con, with, + crescere, to grow]. 1. A calculus. 2. Solidification of a fluid substance.

concub'itus [L. concumbere, to lie together]. Copulation, coition, sexual intercourse.

concus'sion [L. concussus, shaken violently]. "Shaking" from impaction against an object.

c. of the brain. Cerebral concussion. A common result of a blow to the head, or fall on the end of spine with transmitted force, usually causing unconsciousness, either temporary or prolonged. Return of consciousness may be gradual. Patient may suddenly draw up knees and vomit. Resembles result of skull fracture.

SYM: Vary with location and extent of injury from transient dizziness to various paralyses, or unconsciousness; unequal pupils, shock. If uncomplicated, patient comes round within several hours. *Period of reaction* accompanied by vomiting, temperature 99° or 100° F., rapid pulse, flushed face, restlessness, headache, cerebral irritation 12-24 hours afterwards.

F. A. TREATMENT: Keep patient quietly lying down with head and shoulders slightly elevated. *Do not* give stimulants. Transportation should be delayed if possible. Sedatives only if patient is hyperexcited. Cool applications to head and neck are soothing. Reassure patient if conscious. Heat to extremities if cold. Report any adverse symptoms, such as bleeding, at once. Darkened room best. SEE: *contusion, transportation of injured.*

c. of labyrinth. Deafness resulting from a blow to the head or ear.

c., spinal. Lesion of spinal cord due to injury or jarring.

condensa'tion [L. con, with, + densāre, to make thick]. 1. Making more solid. 2. Changing a liquid to a solid or a gas to a liquid. 3. PSY: The union of ideas to form a new mental pattern.

CHEM: A type of reaction in which 2 or more molecules of the same substance react with each other and form a new substance with higher molecular weight and different chemical properties.

conden'ser [" + densāre, to make thick]. Device for solidifying vapors and liquids. SEE: *capacitor*.

c., electrical. Device for storing of electricity by using 2 conducting surfaces and a nonconductor.

con'diment [L. condere, to pickle]. Appetizing ingredient added to food.

CLASSIFICATION: 1. *Aromatic*: Vanilla, cinnamon, cloves, chervil, parsley, bay leaf, etc. 2. *Acrid or Peppery*: Pepper, ginger, allspice, etc. 3. *Alliaceous or Allylic*: Onion, mustard, horseradish. 4. *Acid*: Vinegar, capers, gherkins, citron. 5. *Animal Origin*: Caviar, anchovies.

Too much is harmful and too little may do harm. They are not foods, with the exception of sugar. Some contain essential oils. They are helpful in the assimilation of food material.

ACTION: They seem to stimulate the stomach and intestines, perhaps by chemical action although this is questioned. They do irritate, esp. if taken in too large quantities. They are appetizers and through psychic influences stimulate the secretions. They are antiseptic.

Sugar is a food producing muscular energy and salt, a chemical substance maintaining the mineral equilibrium.

condi'tional reflex. An inherited reflex which is a physiological result of a non-specific stimulus that is automatic and instinctive, though commonly without the knowledge of the individual.

condi'tioned reflex. One acquired as result of training and repetition.

con'dom [L. *condus*, a receptacle]. A rubber or fish skin sheath worn over the penis during coition to avoid conception by retention of the semen within this artificial sac, or to prevent infection; the opp. of pessary.

conduc'tance [L. *conducere*, to lead]. The conducting ability of a body or a circuit for electricity.

The best conductor is that which offers the least resistance. Examples of good conductors are gold, silver, and copper. When expressed in figures, conductance is the reciprocal of resistance. The unit is the ohm.

conduc'tion [L. *conducere*, to read]. PHYS: The process whereby a state of excitation affects successive portions of a tissue or cell, so that the disturbance is transmitted to remote points.

Conduction occurs not only in the fibers of the nervous system, but also in muscle fibers.

c., bone. Sound conduction through cranial bones.

conductiv'ity. The specific electric conducting ability of a substance.

Numerically, conductivity is the reciprocal of unit resistance, or resistivity. The unit is the ohm per cm. Specific conductivity is sometimes expressed as a percentage. In such cases the conductivity is given as a percentage of the conductivity of pure copper under certain standard conditions.

conductor (kon-duk'tor) [L. *conducere*, to lead]. 1. Medium transmitting a force. 2. A guide directing a surgical knife.

condylar (kon'dĭ-lar) [G. *kondylos*, knuckle]. Pert. to a condyle.

condylarthrosis (kon-dil-ar-thro'sis) [" + *arthrōsis*, a joint]. A form of diarthrosis;* an ovoid head in an elliptical cavity.

condyle, condylus (kon'dīl, -lus) [G. *kondylos*, knuckle]. A rounded protuberance at the end of a bone forming an articulation.

condylectomy (kon-dĭ-lek'to-mī) [" + *ektomē*, excision]. Excision of a condyle.

condylion (kon-dil'ĭ-on) [G. *kondylion*, knob]. Point on lateral (outer) surface of the mandibular condyle.

condyloid (kon'dĭ-loid) [G. *kondylos*, knuckle, + *eidos*, appearance]. Pert. to or resembling a condyle.

c. process. Articular process on ramus of mandible consisting of a capitulum and neck. Articulates with mandibular fossa of temporal bone.

c. tubercle. A tubercle on capitulum of condyloid process of the mandible for attachment of temporomandibular ligament.

condyloma (kŏn-dĭ-lō'mă) [" + -ōma, tumor]. A wartlike growth of the skin, usually seen on the external genitalia or near the anus.

There are 2 types, a pointed variety, and a broad, flat form which is usually of syphilitic origin.

c. latum. A mucous patch on the vulva or anus, coated with gray exudate, flattened in form, with delimited area, characteristic of syphilis.

condylomatous (kon-dĭ-lo'mat-us) [" + -ōma, tumor]. Pert. to a condyloma.

condylotomy (kon-dĭ-lot'o-mī) [" + *tomē*, incision]. Division without removal of a condyle.

cone (kōn) [G. *kōnos*, cone]. 1. A shape with circular base with sides sloping to a point above. 2. Retinal flask-shaped figure in layer of rods and cones. 3. A receptor cell concerned with color vision.

c. of light. Triangular light areas on the membrana tympani extending downward from the umbo.

c. ocular. Cone of light in int. of eyeball.

confabula'tion [L. *confabulārī*, to talk together]. PSY: The relation of imaginary experiences to fill in gaps in the memory.

confec'tio, confec'tion [L. *con*, with, + *facere*, to make]. Sugarlike soft solids in which 1 or more medicinal substances are incorporated with the object of affording an agreeable form for their administration and a convenient method for their preservation. Not often prescribed, and not official.

confinement (kon-fīn'ment) [Fr. *confīner*, to restrain in a place]. The puerperal state or period of childbirth.

con'flict [L. *con*, with, + *flīgere*, to strike]. 1. Opposing action of incompatibles. 2. PSY: The conscious or unconscious struggle bet. two opposing desires or courses of action. A technical term applied to a state in which social goals dictate behavior contrary to more primitive (often subconscious) desires.

confluence of sinuses. The union of the sagittal sinus with the transverse sinuses; torcular Herophili.

con'fluent [L. *confluere*, to run together]. Running together, as when the pustules in smallpox merge.

conformator (kon'for-ma"tor) [L. *con*, with, + *forma*, form]. Apparatus for establishing cranial outlines.

confrontation (kon-frun-ta'shun) [" + *frons*, face]. The examination of 2 patients together, 1 with a disease and the other from whom the disease was supposed to be contracted.

congelation (kon-je-la'shun) [L. *congelāre*, to freeze]. Freezing, or a frostbite.

congenerous (kon-jen'er-us) [L. *con*, with, + *genus*, race]. Possessing the same function, as synergistic muscles.

congen'ital [L. *congenitus*, born together]. Occurring during fetal life; not hereditary. RS: *etiology, pathology, predisposition*.

congested (kon-jes'ted) [L. *congerere*, to heap together]. Hyperemic; containing an abnormal amt. of blood.

conges'tion [L. *congerere*, to heap together]. A localized inflammation which may or may not be accompanied by infection, such as a felon, a boil, a carbuncle. SEE: *affluxion, hyperemia*.
  c. active. Congestion resulting from increased flow of blood to a part or dilatation of blood vessels.
  c. passive. Hyperemia resulting from interference with flow of blood from capillaries into venules. May also result from myocardial insufficiency.

congestive (kon-jes'tiv). Pertaining to congestion.
  c. fever. Malarial fever.

congius (kon'jĭ-us) (pl. *con'gii*) [L.]. A gallon.

conglo'bate [L. *con*, with + *glōbāre*, to make round]. In 1 mass, as lymph glands.

congloba'tion [" + *globus*, a ball]. Aggregation of particles in a mass.

conglom'erate [" + *glomerāre*, to heap]. 1. An aggregation in one mass. 2. Clustered; heaped together.
  c. gland. A gland with several lobes.

conglutin (kon-glu'tin) [L. *conglutināre*, to glue together]. A protein resembling casein found in peas, beans, and almonds.

conglu'tinant. Promoting adhesion, as of the edges of a wound.

conglu'tinate [L. *conglutinātiō*, an adhering]. Having the quality of adhesiveness.

conglutination (kon-glu-tin-a'shun) [L. *conglutinātiō*, an adhering]. 1. Coalescence, adhesion. 2. Reaction, such as agglutination.

coniasis (kon-i'ă-sis) [G. *konis*, dust]. Dustlike calculi in gallbladder and bile ducts.

conidia (ko-nid'ĭ-ă) (pl. of *conidium*) [G. *konidion*, a particle of dust]. Asexual spores of fungi.

conidiophore (kon-id'ĭ-o-for) [" + *phoros*, bearing]. The stalk supporting conidia.

coniol'ogy [G. *konis*, dust, + *logos*, study of]. The study of dust and its effects.

conio'sis [" + *-ōsis*, infection]. Any condition caused by inhalation of dust.

coniza'tion [G. *kōnos*, cone]. Coring and removal of the mucous lining of cervical canal and its glands by the cutting high frequency current for treatment of chronic endocervicitis.

conjuga'ta [L.]. Diameter of pelvis, measured from center of the promontory of the sacrum to the back of the symphysis pubis.
  c. vera. Sometimes written *c.v*. Same as conjugata, *q.v.*

conjugate (kon'jŭ-gāt) [L. *con*, with, + *jugum*, yoke]. 1. Paired or joined. 2. An important diameter of the pelvis, measured from the center of the promontory of the sacrum to the back of the symphysis pubis.
  c. deviation. Deviation of both eyes to either side.
  c., diagonal. Measured from the lower edge of the symphysis to the sacrum, and can be determined during life, whereas the true conjugate cannot, except immediately after labor. It is about ¼-¾ in. longer than the true conjugate, or about 5 in.
  c. diameter. Same as conjugate (2).
  c., external. Measured from the spine of the last lumbar vertebra to the front of the pubes (this can be done only with calipers), and is normally about 8 in.
  c., true. Same as conjugate (2). It should measure not less than 4¼ in. and is sometimes as large as 4½ or 4¾ in. If less than 4¼ in., the pelvis is a deformed one.

conjuga'tion [" + *jugum*, yoke]. A coupling together. In biology, the union of two unicellular organisms accompanied by an interchange of nuclear material as in *Paramecium*.

conjuncti'va [" + *jungere*, to join]. Mucous membrane which lines eyelids and is reflected onto eyeball.
  DIVISIONS: (1) Palpebral, covering under surface of lids; (2) bulbar, coating ant. portion of eyeball; (3) fornix, transition portion forming fold bet. lid and globe.
  INSPECTION: Palpebral and ocular portions should be examined. Color and degree of moisture and presence of foreign bodies should be observed; also petechial hemorrhages and inflammation.
  PATH. CONDITIONS: Trachoma and pannus as well as discoloration. *Yellowish discoloration*: Seen in jaundice, certain fevers, and hemolysis. May be due to fatty deposits. *Bluish-white or pearly discoloration*: Seen in anemia, nephritis, and phthisis. Sky-blue coloring is noted in whooping cough. *Pale conjunctivae*: Observed in anemias.
  SEE: *Calmette's reaction; catarrh, vernal; Krause's gland; limbus*.

conjunctival reflex (kon-junk-ti'val). Closure of eyelids when conjunctiva is touched or threatened.

conjunctivitis (kon-junk-tĭ-vi'tis) [L. *con*, with, + *jungere*, to join, + G. *-itis*, inflammation]. Inflammation of conjunctiva.
  TREATMENT: Directed against the specific type of infection.
  c., acute contagious. Pink eye. ETIOL: Koch-Weeks bacillus.
  c., catarrhal. One due to irritation or cold.
  c., follicular. Type characterized by pinkish round bodies in retrotarsal fold.
  c., gonorrheal. Acute c. due to contact with the gonococcus.
  c., granular. Acute, contagious, inflammatory c. with granular elevations on the lids which ulcerate and cicatrize. SYN: *trachoma*.
  c., membranous. Acute conjunctivitis characterized by a false membrane; with or without infiltration.
  c., phlyctenular. Circumscribed type characterized by lymphoid tissue in small red nodules.
  c., purulent. That characterized by abundant purulent discharge. ETIOL: Gonorrhea. Ex: *Ophthalmia neonatorum*.
  c., vernal. One beginning in the spring and disappearing when cold weather begins.

conjunctivo'ma [" + " + G. *-ōma*, tumor]. A tumor of the conjunctiva.

conjunctivoplasty (kon-junk-tĭ'vo-plas-tĭ) [" + " + G. *plassein*, to form]. Removal of part of cornea, but replacing with flaps from the conjunctiva.

connec'tive [L. *connectere*, to bind]. That which connects or binds together.
  c. tissue. One of the four main tissues of the body. It includes an embryonic connective tissue (mesenchyme and mucous) and (b) adult connective tissue. The latter is subdivided into

four general groups (1) vascular tissues (blood, lymph), (2) connective tissue proper (areolar, white fibrous, yellow fibrous, reticular, adipose), (3) cartilage and (4) bone. Connective tissues are concerned primarily with supporting bodily structures and binding parts together. They also are involved in other functions such as food storage, blood formation, and defensive mechanisms of the body.

co′noid [G. *kônos*, cone, + *eidos*, shape]. Resembling a cone; conical.

c. ligament. Lower and inner portion of coracoclavicular ligament.

c. tubercle. Eminence on inf. surface of clavicle to which is attached the conoid ligament.

conomyoidin (ko-no-mi-oid′in) [" + *mys*, muscle, + *eidos*, form]. Contractile protoplasm in cones of the retina.

consanguinity (kon-san-gwin′it-I) [L. *consanguinitās*, kinship]. Relationship by blood.

conscious (kon′shus) [L. *conscius*, aware]. Being aware and having perception.

con′sciousness [L. *conscius*, aware]. PSY: A state of awareness.

It implies an orientation to time, place, and person; *i. e.*, the individual knows approximately the date, the nature of his environment, his name and other pertinent personal data.

The content of consciousness is a composite of memories and the comprehension of external reality; the emotional status and the individual's goals also enter. It is then a large part of that described as "personality" in its largest sense.

Consciousness varies its intensity and extent from minute to minute. In crises, vivid ideational association may lead to an exaggerated state of awareness. In states of relaxed contentment, it lessens, to disappear completely in sleep. This differs from the pathologic condition of coma in which the patient cannot be aroused.

In so-called pathologic sleep (*e. g.*, encephalitis lethargica) and in stupor, though aroused, the patient is unable to postpone again lapsing into dullness; normal sleep can be adequately combated by the demands of reality. Stupor is produced largely by the factors resulting in coma; the personality is relatively intact but "hazy." In contrast there are conditions in which a real personality change manifests itself. Clouding of consciousness may simulate the dullness but usually not the other characteristics of stupor. On the contrary, such patients may impress one as relatively alert.

The loss of orientation to time and place but not to person constitutes delirium. A quiet delirium may not easily reveal itself even in certain states of automatism in which one finds evidence of the "real personality"; there may appear on casual examination little to arouse suspicion, yet brutal acts, total absence of memory, reveal these as major abnormalities (SEE: *epilepsy*). The "clouded" patient with obvious emotionalism (fear) and violent hallucinations is obviously psychotic.

Clouding of consciousness may be diagnosed from the appearance of the patient in catatonic stupor and it may be difficult to realize the patient is quite lucid and that experiences are being registered accurately and can be later recalled. In true clouding, stimuli usually fail to register.

Again, in some ambulistic states, experiences may register but cannot be recalled after return to a normal state. During a later secondary state, it is apparent that the failure of memory is only a repression and not its absence. Consciousness, on the other hand, may erroneously appear to be present in so-called "coma vigil" because the eyes are open and expression may be alert.

c., clouding of. A phase of delirium in which the patient's consciousness is cloudy or not clear.

consciousness, words pert. to: absentia epileptica, anoetic, apperception, apraxia, attention, bathyesthesia, cacesthesia, cenesthopathia, coconsciousness, liminal, subconscious, threshold of, unconsciousness.

consenescence (kon-sen-es′ens) [L. *consenescere*, to grow old]. The state of growing old.

consen′sual [L. *con*, with, + *sentire*, to feel]. Reflex stimulation from another part.

c. light reflex. Contraction of unexposed pupil in sympathy with exposed pupil.

c. reflex. Any reflex occurring on opposite side of body from point of stimulation.

consolidation (kon-sol-id-a′shun) [L. *consolidāre*, to make firm]. The act of becoming solid. Esp. used in connection with the solidification of the lungs due to engorgement of the lung tissues, as occurs in acute pneumonia.

constella′tion [L. *con*, with, + *stella*, star]. Ideas arising from unrepressed emotions.

constipation (kon-sti-pa′shun) [L. *constipāre*, to press together]. A sluggish action of the bowels.

PREDISPOSING CAUSES: No habitual bowel movement from childhood; worry, anxiety, fear, sedentary life.

DIRECT CAUSES: Failure to establish regular and definite time for bowel movement, improper diet, lack of physical exercise, ingestion of too much sugar, and a lack of bulk in the diet. It also may be due to atonic or spastic peristalsis, to reverse peristalsis, and to obstruction.

GENERAL CORRECTIVE MEASURES: Plenty of fresh vegetables, fruits, milk, and an abundance of water. Limit coffee, tea, white sugar, meats, fish, and pastries. Cut down starches. Plenty of physical exercise, avoid all that worries, establish regular habit time for bowel movement, and do not eat when under the influence of strong emotion. Do not hurry defecation or read at the time, or go to stool when excited and greatly worried.

RS: *colon, defecation, diet, feces, in testine, stool.*

c., atonic. Lack of muscle tone due to lack of exercise of abdominal muscles, and to abdominal ptosis.*

TREATMENT: Exercise and diet of fruits and vegetables, bulky residue in the absence of colitis; massage, abdominal belt if ptosis of the abdomen exists; vitamin B, fats and water.

c., obstructive. Due to an obstruction in the intestines. Surgical aid needed. Preoperative diet should contain low residue and no gas forming foods.

c., spastic. Constipation accompanied by intestinal spasms.

constitution

Etiol: Excessive use of laxatives, nervousness, too much tobacco, alcohol, condiments, sugar, and irritants; also may be due to the presence of diverticula, or diverticulitis.
Treatment: Avoid irritating foods; atropine for the spasms.

constitu′tion [L. *constituere*, to establish]. The physical makeup and functional habits of the body.

constitu′tional. Pert. to the body as a whole.
  c., disease. One which affects the entire body.
  c., psychosis. Functional psychosis; not of organic origin.

constric′tion [L. *con*, with, + *stringere*, to draw]. 1. A binding or squeezing of a part. 2. The narrowing of the caliber of a vessel by pressure.

constric′tor [" + *stringere*, to draw]. 1. That which binds or restricts a part. 2. A muscle, such as a sphincter, which can narrow or close a canal.

construct′ive metabolism. The binding up or anabolic process.

consult′ant [L. *consultāre*, to counsel]. A consulting physician or surgeon who acts only in an advisory capacity.

consulta′tion [L. *consultātiō*]. Diagnosis and proposed treatment by 2 or more physicians at one time.

consumption (kon-sump′shun) [L. *consumere*, to waste away]. 1. Tuberculosis.* 2. Wasting. 3. The using up of anything.

consump′tive. Pert. to or afflicted with tuberculosis.

con′tact [L. *con*, with, + *tangere*, to touch]. 1. Mutual touching or apposition of 2 bodies. 2. Closing of an electric current. 3. One who has been exposed to contagion.
  c., complete. When entire surface of 1 tooth touches entire surface of an adjoining tooth, proximally.
  c., direct. Communication of a contagious disease through a healthy person touching an infected body.
  c., immediate. Same as direct contact.
  c., indirect. The spread of a contagious disease by some medium other than direct touch of the sick person.
  c., lens. A thin bowl-shaped shell of glass made to fit over the cornea.
  c., mediate. Same as indirect contact.
  c., proximal or **proximate.** Touching of teeth on their adjacent surfaces.
  c., surface. Proximal surface of a tooth.

con′tact breaker. Device for breaking a galvanic current.

conta′gion [L. *contangere*, to touch]. The process of transferring a specific disease either by direct or indirect contact.
See: *virulent, virus*.

contagios′ity [L. *contagiōsus*, contagion]. The state of being contagious.

conta′gious. That which is transmissible by contact, as "communicable diseases."
All contagious diseases are infectious, but not all infectious diseases are contagious.
Not communicable through the air.
See: *eruptive*.

contagium (kon-ta′ji-um) [L.]. The agent causing infection or contagion.

containers, care and handling of. As contamination of the container in which a specimen is to be placed may render the results of the examination futile, and so interfere with the doctor's diagnosis based upon it, extreme care must be observed by the nurse in handling all such articles.

1. See that they are perfectly clean, inside and outside, and that the surfaces are intact. Cracked and broken containers must not be used. The containers never must be completely filled.

2. If the presence of bacteria is suspected, the container must first be sterilized, unless this has already been done by the laboratory.
To clean glassware: (a) Using very little soap-powder, boil in water. (b) Brush well under running water. (c) Rinse well in running water. (d) Place potassium in bichromate solution for 20 minutes. (e) Rinse well in running water. (f) Rinse in distilled water. (g) Rinse again in distilled water. (h) Invert in basket and drain dry.
Sterilization of glassware: This is accomplished by hot air or dry heat, boiling water, flowing steam, steam under pressure, and the use of germicidal* chemicals.

3. *Labels:* All containers should be labeled, when used, with the name of the patient and his room number; also the name of the attending physician. "Request forms," sometimes used as labels, are made up to suit the individual laboratory or hospital. Provision is made for recording necessary data as indicated, including date when specimen was taken, and under what circumstances, and for what substances the examination is to be done, together with other information desired.

4. *Time:* If the required specimen cannot be furnished at once, make a note of what is needed, inform the patient, the supervisor, and any other nurse who may attend to the patient in your absence.

5. *Charting:* Note on the chart all specimens sent to the laboratory, when sent, and any other data that seem pertinent.

6. *Care of specimen:* Cover immediately after depositing in the container; check label or "request form," and see that the container is intact, and that there is no danger of spilling while in transit.

contiguity (kon-tĭ-gū′ĭ-tĭ) [L. *contiguus*, touching]. Contact or proximity without continuity.
  c., amputation in. Amputation through a joint.
  c., law of. If 2 ideas occur in association they are apt to be repeated.
  c., solution of. Dislocation or displacement of 2 normally contiguous parts.

con′tinence [L. *continere*, to hold back]. Self restraint, used esp. in connection with refraining from sexual indulgence.

continuity (kon-tĭ-nū′ĭt-ĭ) [L. *continuus*, continued]. The state of being continuous or intimately united.
  c., amputation in. Amputation through a long bone.
  c., solution of. Division of normally continuous parts by fracture, rupture, laceration, incision.

contin′uous [L. *continere*, to hold together]. Without break, cessation, or interruption.
  c. spec′trum. An unbroken series of wave lengths, either visible or invisible. Such a spectrum is produced by light from incandescent solids, liquids, or gases under high pressure passed through a prism. Also an unbroken range of radiations of different wave

lengths in any portion of the invisible spectrum.

contor′tion. A twisting into an unusual shape.

contour (kon′toor) [L. *con*, with, + *tornāre*, to turn around]. Outline or surface configuration of a part.

contoured (kon′toord). Having an irregular, smooth, undulating surface resembling a relief map. [*contraindication*.

contra- [L.]. Prefix: Opposite; against, as

contra-ap′erture [L. *contra*, against, + *apertura*, opening]. A 2nd opening made in an abscess.

contraception (kon-tra-sep′shun) [" + *conceptiō*, a conceiving]. The prevention of conception.

contracep′tive. Any agent or device used to prevent conception, such as condoms,* pessaries,* or medication. None can be guaranteed to prevent conception.

contract′ [L. *contrahere*, to draw together]. To draw together, reduce in size, or shorten.

contrac′tile. Able to contract or shorten.

contractil′ity [L. *contrahere*, to draw together]. Having the ability to contract or shorten.

contrac′tion [L. *contractio*, a drawing up]. A shortening, as that of a muscle, or a reduction in size; a shrinking. SEE: *cholepathia spastica, chronotropism.*

contracture (kon-trak′chur) [L. *contractura*]. Permanent contraction of a muscle due to spasm or paralysis.

  c., functional. Decrease of a contracture during anesthesia or sleep.

contrafissura (kon″trä-fĭ-shu′rä) [L. *contra*, against, + *fissura*, fissure]. A fracture at a point opp. from where the blow was received.

contraindication (kŏn″trä-ĭn-dĭ-kā′shŭn) [" + *indicāre*, to point out]. Any symptom or circumstance indicating the inappropriateness of a form of treatment, otherwise advisable.

contralat′eral [" + *latus*, side]. Originating in, or affecting, the opposite side of the body. ANTO: *ipsilateral*.

  c. reflexes. 1. Passive flexion of 1 part following flexion of another. 2. Passive flexion of 1 leg causing similar movement of opposite leg.

con′trast sprays. Those administered by sitting on side of bathtub, spraying feet and legs with warm water for 1 minute and cold water for 1 minute. Alternate for 10 minutes twice daily.

contravolit′ional [L. *contra*, against, + *velle*, to wish]. In opp. to or without the will; involuntary.

contrecoup (kaun″tra-kōō) [Fr. counterblow.] Occurring on the opposite side.

  c. injury. An injury to parts of the brain located on the side opposite that of the primary injury, as when the frontal and temporal lobes of the brain are forced against the irregular bones of the anterior portion of the cranial vault as a result of a blow on the back of the head.

contrectation (kon-trek-ta′shun) [L. *contrectāre*, to handle]. 1. Examination by palpation. 2. Manipulation. 3. Impulse to embrace, caress or sexually dally with one of the opposite sex; spooning.

control (kon-trōl′) [L. *contra*, against, + *rotulus*, catalogue]. 1. To regulate or maintain. 2. A standard against which observations or conclusions may be checked in order to establish their validity, as a control animal or a control experiment.

  c. animal. An animal subjected to the same conditions as the experimental animal except for the specific factor being tested.

  c. experiment. An experiment in which all the factors or conditions are the same except for the one factor being tested. Used to check the validity of the conclusions drawn from the test experiment.

  c. experiment. Same as control (2).

contrude (kon-trŭd′) [L. *con*, with, + *trūdere*, to thrust]. 1. Abnormal lingual curve or line of dental arch. 2. To crowd together, as the teeth.

contru′sion. Having the teeth crowded.

contuse (kon-tuz′) [L. *contundere*, to bruise]. To bruise.

contusion (kon-tu′zhun) [L. *contusiō*, a bruise]. An injury in which the skin is not broken.

  SYM: Pain, swelling and discoloration.

  F. A. TREATMENT: Apply cold applications. Follow with firm bandage to prevent swelling. Twenty-four to 48 hours later, heat is desirable followed by massage. SEE: *concussion*.

co′nus [G. *kōnos*]. 1. A cone. 2. Post. staphyloma of myopic eye.

  c. arteriosus. Right cardiac ventricle's upper rounded ant. angle, where pulmonary artery arises.

  c. medullaris. Conical portion of lower spinal cord.

convalescence (kon-val-es′ens) [L. *convalescere*, to become strong]. The period of recovery after the termination of a disease or an operation.

convales′cent. 1. Getting well. 2. One who is recovering from a disease or operation.

  c. diet. A soft diet.

convection (kon-vek′shun) [L. *convehere*, to convey]. The transference of heat by means of currents in liquids or gases which result from changes in density.

convec′tive discharge. Discharge from a high potential source in the form of visible or invisible stream of electrical energy passing through the air to the patient.

convergence (kon-ver′jens) [L. *con*, with, + *vergere*, to incline]. 1. Visual lines directed to a nearby point. 2. The moving of 2 or more objects toward the same point. SEE: *Illustration*, next page.

convergent (kon-ver′jent). Tending toward a common point.

conver′sion [L. *convertere*, to turn round]. Change from one state to another.

  c. symptom. PSY: A term for a repressed emotion that becomes manifested through a physical symptom; seen in hysteria.

converter, rotary. Apparatus used to convert a direct current into an alternating one or vice versa.

  It consists essentially of a dynamo which, by varying the arrangement of its collecting mechanism, allows the collection of either a direct or alternating current at the other end.

con′vex [L. *convexus*, vaulted, arched]. Curved evenly; the segment of a sphere.

convex″ocon′cave [" + *con*, with, + *cavus*, hollow]. Concave on 1 side and convex on opp. surface. SYN: *concavoconvex*.

convexocon′vex [L. *convexus*, arched]. Convex on 2 opp. faces.

convolute (kon′vo-lūt) [L. *convolvere*, to roll together]. Rolled, as a scroll.

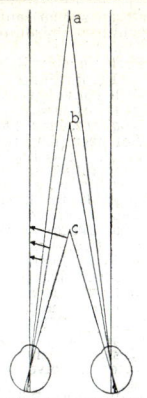

CONVERGENCE
When an object is brought from a distant position (a) to a near position (b), the eyes are rotated medially to make the lines of vision meet at the object. The closer the object, the greater the degree of convergence as measured by the angles indicated by arrows.

con′voluted. Convolute, rolled.
  c. tubule. The proximal convoluted tubule lies between Bowman's capsule and the loop of Henle; the distal convoluted tubule lies between the loop of Henle and the collecting duct.
convolution (kŏn″vō-lū′shŭn) [L. *convolvere*, to roll together]. 1. A winding motion. 2. A turn or fold. 3. ANAT: A coil of tissue on the brain surface, separated by fissures. 4. A gyrus.
  c., angular. A gyrus forming post. portion of inf. parietal lobule.
  c.'s, annectant. The 4 gyri connecting the c.'s on upper surface of occipital lobe with parietal and temporosphenoidal lobes.
  c., ant. central. SEE: *ascending frontal c.*
  c., ant. choroid. *Gyrus choroides.*
  c., anteroparietal. SEE: *ascending frontal c.*
  c., ant. orbital. One which lies in front of the orbital sulcus.
  c., Arnold's. *Gyri posteriores inferiores.*
  c., ascending frontal. One forming ant. boundary of fissure of Rolando.
  c., ascending parietal. One parallel with ascending frontal c. separated from it by fissure of Rolando, except at extremities, where they are generally united.
  c.'s, Broca's. The inf., or 3rd, frontal c.
  c., callosal, callosomarginal. *Gyrus fornicatus.*
  c.'s, cerebral. Those of the cerebrum.
  c. of the corpus callosum. *Gyrus fornicatus.*
  c., cuneate. *Gyral isthmus.*
  c., dentate. A small, notched gyrus rudimentary in man, situated in dentate fissure, below tenia hippocampi.
  c., ext. olfactory. Small projections forming outer boundary of the olfactory grooves.
  c., hippocampal. *Uncinate gyrus.*
  c., inf. frontal. The lower and outer part of frontal lobe.
  c., inf. occipital. A small one lying bet. middle and inf. occipital fissures.
  c., inframarginal. *Superior temporosphenoidal c.*
  c., insular. One of a group of small c.'s forming the island of Reil, entirely concealed by the operculum.
  c., int. orbital. The gyrus next outside of the gyrus rectus.
  c.'s, intestinal. The coils of the intestines.
  c., marginal. One beginning in front of locus perforatus anterior and bounding longitudinal fissure on mesial aspect of the hemisphere.
  c., middle frontal. One continuous post. with ascending frontal c. and extending forward over ant. end of hemisphere to its orbital surface.
  c., middle occipital. One bet. 1st and 3rd occipital c.'s.
  c., middle temporosphenoidal. A small gyrus continuous with the middle occipital or angular gyrus.
  c., occipitotemporal. Two small c.'s on lower surface of temporosphenoidal lobe.
  c., olfactory. *Olfactory lobe.*
  c.'s, orbital. Small gyri on orbital surface of frontal lobe.
  c.'s, parietal. *Ascending parietal c.* and *superior parietal c.*
  c., post. orbital. A small one on post. and outer side of orbital sulcus, and continuous with inf. frontal c.
  c., second (or middle) frontal. One continuous post. with ascending frontal c.
  c., sup. frontal. One which bounds great longitudinal fissure, arising post. from upper end of ascending frontal c.
  c., sup. occipital. Upper of the 3 c.'s on sup. surface of occipital lobe.
  c., sup. parietal. Portion of parietal lobe limited ant. by upper part of the fissure of Rolando, post. by ext. parietooccipital fissure, and inf. by intraparietal sulcus.
  c., sup. temporosphenoidal. Upper of 3 c.'s forming temporosphenoidal lobe. It lies just below and is parallel with sylvian fissure.
  c., supramarginal. The ant. portion of inf. parietal lobule behind inf. extremity of intraparietal fissure (sulcus), below which it joins the ascending parietal c.
  c. of the sylvian fissure. The c. that bounds the fissure of Sylvius.
  c., transverse orbital. The gyrus occupying post. portion of inf. surface of frontal lobe, at ant. extremity of fissure of Sylvius.
  c., uncinate. One extending from near post. extremity of occipital lobe to apex of temporosphenoidal.
convul′sant [L. *convulsio*, a pulling together]. 1. An agent which produces a convulsion. 2. Causing onset of a convulsion.
  c. poisons. The common ones are strychnine and other drugs of the nux vomica groups, and various, special, infrequently used drugs, such as brucine, ignatia, picrotoxin.
  SYM: These produce a sense of suffocation, dyspnea, and then muscular rigidity; there are powerful tetanic contractions which may be very painful. These spasms may be brought on by trivial stimuli, such as touching the patient or they may come on at vary-

convulsion C-89 **copper**

ing intervals of from 3 to 30 minutes and may last from 1 to 5 minutes. Trismus, cyanosis, and tachycardia are frequent accompaniments. Death results from asphyxia or exhaustion.

TREATMENT: Dilute the contents of the stomach with milk, water, boiled tea, etc., and induce emesis by titillating the uvula; then administer a teaspoonful of pulverized charcoal, dilute tannic acid, or dilute potassium permanganate solution and again induce vomiting. Sedatives may be ordered by the physician. Oxygen and artificial respiration may be indicated.

convul′sion [L. *convulsio*, a pulling together]. Paroxysms of involuntary muscular contractions and relaxations generally in children.

Convulsions due to tetanus and hydrophobia are easily distinguished and for the most part involve a small portion of the voluntary musculature. On the contrary, strychnine poisoning convulsions involve the entire body. The word is accurately applied to unilateral attacks as seen in jacksonian epilepsy and, less likely, in hysteria. They are usually accompanied by unconsciousness. This is not the case in strychnine poisoning, hysteria, or in jacksonian epileptic attacks until the 2nd side is involved.

ETIOL: *In General*: Epilepsy, eclampsia, meningitis, tetanus, uremia. Poisoning from aspidium, brucine, camphor, cyanides, strychnine, santonin. In *children* the cause is often dietary; other causes, rickets, neuropathic tendency, spasmophilia, syphilis, malnutrition, malaria, acute infectious disease, cervical disease, toxemias, or unknown. Calcium is low. Guanidine should be considered. In *adults*, due to epilepsy, heat cramps, strychnine, or food poisoning.

TREATMENT: If an infant, put him in a bath of 95° F. or mustard and water at 85° F. Cold applied to head. Cause must first be found or injury may result from bath. If cause is undetermined, keep patient from injuring self. Soft pad bet. teeth to avoid biting tongue or cheeks. Warm bath, with cold to head; if fever is present, tepid or cool bath. Sedatives or anesthesia may be advised by physician. *After Care*: Rest in bed, absolute quiet, careful diagnosis without unduly disturbing patient.

Recent successful method of therapy has been the injection, in 1 large dose, of 600,000 international units of Vitamin D.

c., clonic. One having intermittent contractions, muscles being alternately contracted and relaxed.

c., epileptiform. One accompanied by unconsciousness.

c., hysterical. C. caused by hysteria.

c., puerperal. Eclamptic c. in pregnant or puerperal woman.

c., salaam. Spasm of sternomastoid muscles causing bowing motions of the body.

c., tonic. One in which the contractions are maintained for a time, as in tetany.

c., toxic. C. caused by action of a toxin on nervous system.

c., uremic. C. caused by uremic condition.

convulsion, words pert. to: anticonvulsive, athetosis, chill, chorea, epilepsy, hydrophobia, hysteria, ictus, jactitation, mimetic, paroxysm, spasm center, spasmophilia, strychnine poisoning, tetanus, tic, tremor.

convul′sive. Pert. to convulsions.

c. reflex. Incoördinate contraction of muscles in a convulsive manner.

c. tic. Spasm of face.

cook′ing [L. *coquere, coctum*, to cook]. The process of preparing foods for eating. *Purpose* . . . cooking makes most foods more palatable, easier to masticate, improves their digestibility, and destroys or inactivates harmful organisms or toxins which may be present.

PURPOSE AND EFFECT OF: *Action on Cellulose*: The fibers of cellulose that consist of walls enclosing starch granules swell through absorption of water, and heat with water causes them to break. In chewing cooked food these small particles of cellulose are mixed with other parts and are thus made easier to digest. Too much cooking or too much water dissolves out minerals and vitamins.

Action on Protein: Soluble proteins become coagulated and their loss is thus prevented. The loss in steaming is 1% less than in boiling.

Action on Soluble Substances: These are often lost in boiling, and even sugars, mineral substances and starches, though insoluble to a certain extent, suffer a certain loss in this process.

Action on Starch: The starch granules now swell and are changed from insoluble (raw) starch to soluble starch capable of being converted into sugar in the process of digestion and of being assimilated in the system.

Cooking releases the aromatic substances and extractives that contribute odors and taste to foods. These stimulate the appetite and make the food more palatable.

Most microörganisms are destroyed in the ordinary processes of cooking, but some require a higher degree of heat and longer cooking to effect this result, as pork.

Coo′lidge tube. An x-ray tube whose cathode consists of a spiral tungsten wire surrounded by a molybdenum tube.

coördinated reflexes (ko-or′dĭn-at-ed). The reverse of convulsive reflexes in that action occurs coördinately.

coördination (ko-or-din-a′shun) [L. *con*, with, + *ordināre*, to arrange]. The working together of various muscles for the production of a certain movement.

More generally, the working together of different systems of the body in a given process as the coördination bet. the system of glands and involuntary muscles in digestion.

copiopia (ko-pĭ-o′pĭ-ă) [G. *kopos*, fatigue, + *opsis*, sight]. Eyestrain causing fatigue.

copodyskinesia (ko-po-dis-kĭn-e′sĭ-ă) [" + *dys*, difficult, + *kinēsis*, motion]. Occupational neurosis.

cop′per (cuprum) [G. *kupros*]. SYMB: *Cu*. At. wt. 63.57. A metal, small quantities of which are utilized by the body. Its salts are an irritant poison.

FUNCTION AND USES: It functions with iron in its transformation into such substances as hemoglobin, and it seems to be an activating principle when used in the treatment of blood dyscrasias. Salts of copper are used to color peas and other vegetables and fruits. The small consumption of it in this way seems harmless and it appears to be re-

tained by the liver. It aids tissue respiration and the synthesis of cytochrome. It is present in the liver at all times and is excreted by the kidneys.
 DEFICIENCY SYM: Anemia, weakness, impaired respiration and growth, and poor utilization of iron.
 SOURCES: Found in many vegetable and animal tissues. SEE: *chalcosis,* *Clapton's lines,* names of foods.
copperas (kop'er-ăs). Green vitriol. Pale bluish-green crystals. SEE: *ferrous sulfate.*
cop'per sul'fate (blue vitriol). USP. Deep blue, shiny crystals or granular powder.
 ACTION AND USES: Stimulant, astringent, and powerful emetic.
 DOSAGE: As an astringent, ¼ gr. (0.016 Gm.); as an emetic, 5 gr. (0.3 Gm.).
 POISONING: SYM: A disagreeable, coppery, metallic taste, with tightness in the throat, nausea and vomiting, thirst; abdominal pains, cramps, and suppression of urine.
 F. A. TREATMENT: Wash out stomach, give egg whites raw or beaten. Give demulcent drinks.
coprecip'itin [L. *con,* together, + *praecipitāre,* to cast down]. One which acts on 2 or more organisms.
copre'mia [G. *kopros,* feces, + *aima,* blood]. Intestinal autointoxication, so called, caused by waste products in the blood.
coprohematol'ogy [" + " + *logos,* study of]. Study of the blood in the feces.
coprolagnia (kop-ro-lag'nĭ-ă) [" + *lagneia,* lust]. An erotic satisfaction at the sight or odor of excreta.
coprolalia (kop-ro-la'lĭ-ă) [" + *lalia,* babble]. PSY: A morbid desire to use sacrilegious or obscene words in ordinary conversation. Seen in obsessional neurosis or dementia precox.
coprolith (kop'ro-lith) [" + *lithos,* stone]. Hard, inspissated feces.
coprology (kop-rol'o-jĭ) [" + *logos,* study of]. Examination of the feces. SYN: *scatology.*
coproma (ko-pro'mă) [" + *-ōma,* tumor]. Accumulation of feces in the rectum. SYN: *fecaloma, scotoma, stercoroma.*
coprophagy (ko-prof'ă-jĭ) [" + *phagein,* to eat]. The eating of excrement.
coprophilia (kop-ro-fĭl'ĭ-ă) [" + *philein,* to love]. Abnormal interest in feces; a perversion in adults.
coprophobia (kop-ro-fo'bĭ-ă) [" + *phobos,* fear]. A morbid disgust at the sight of filth of any kind.
coprostasis (kop-ros'tas-ĭs) [" + *stasis,* a stoppage]. The scybalous impaction of feces; constipation.
coprozo'a [" + *zōon,* animal]. Protozoa in fecal matter outside of the intestine.
coprozo'ic. Pert. to coprozoa; found in feces or fecal matter.
copula (kop'u-lă) [L. *copulāre,* to bind together]. 1. An immune body. 2. Sexual intercourse. 3. A narrow part bet. 2 structures.
copulation (kop-u-la'shun) [L. *copulātĭō*]. Sexual intercourse bet. the sexes. SYN: *coition,* coitus,* cohabitation, concubitus.*
cor, cordis (kōr) [L.]. The heart.
 c. adiposum. Fatty degenerative tissue in the heart.
 c. bovinum. Hypertrophied heart.
 c. hirsutum. Shaggy heart surface appearance.
 c. juvenum. Heart disorder combined with orthostatic albuminuria.
 c. tomentosum, c. villosum. SEE: *c. hirsutum.*
coraco-acromial (kor"ă-ko-ă-kro'mĭ-ăl) [G. *korax,* raven, + *akron,* point, + *ōmos,* shoulder]. Pert. to acromial and coracoid processes.
cor'acoid [" + *eidos,* appearance]. Formed like the beak of a crow.
 c. ligament. Ligament in upper region of shoulder blade.
 c. notch. Notch in upper portion of scapula.
 c. process. Projection from the shoulder blade.
coramine (cō'ra-mēn). A 25% aqueous solution of pyridine-beta-carboxydiethylamide.
 USES: As a circulatory and respiratory stimulant.
 DOSAGE: Orally, hypodermically, intramuscularly, or intravenously, from 15 to 30 ɱ (1.0-2.0 cc.), increased as condition demands.
Corbus' disease. Balanitis with gangrene.
corbus thermophore (kor'bus therm'o-fōr). Small round instrument with tapering metal tip 2 inches long carrying a thermometer in center for insertion in cervix or urethra for application of medical diathermy.
cord [G. *chordē*]. A stringlike structure.
 c. bladder. Distention of the bladder without discomfort. Tending to void frequently and dribbling after urination.
 ETIOL: Lesion affecting the post. roots of the spinal column.
 c. spermatic. Cord by which the testis is suspended to the abdominal inguinal ring. It consists of the ductus deferens, blood vessels, lymphatics, and nerves supplying the testis and epididymis. These are enclosed in the cremasteric fascia which forms an investing sheath.
 c., spinal (*medulla spinalis*). That portion of the central nervous system contained in the spinal canal. The center of the cord consists of gray matter, which is composed of nerve cells, dendrites, and their processes. The white matter is arranged in tracts outside the gray matter. It consists of medullated nerve fibers which are (a) going to and from the brain, (b) connecting various layers of gray matter in the cord, (c) leaving and entering the spinal column. The cord serves as a center for the transmission of impulses to and from the brain. It is the center of reflex acts. SEE: *"chord-"* words.
 c., umbilical. One which connects the umbilicus of the fetus to the placenta.
cor'date. Shaped like a heart.
cor'diform [L. *cor,* heart, + *forma,* shape]. Shaped like a heart.
cordi'tis [" + G. *-itis,* inflammation]. Inflammation of a spermatic cord; funiculitis.
cor'dopexy [G. *chordē,* cord, + *pēxis,* fixation]. Operative fixation of an anatomical cord, esp. the vocal cords.
cordot'omy [" + *tomē,* incision]. Spinal cord section of lateral pathways to relieve pain. SYN: *chordotomy.*
coreclisis (kor-e-klī'sis) [G. *korē,* pupil, + *kleisis,* closure]. Occlusion of the pupil.
corectasia, corectasis (kor-ek-ta'zĭ-ă, -ta-sis) [" + *ektasis,* dilatation]. Dilatation of the pupil of the eye; corediastasis.
corectome (ko-rek'tōm) [" + *ektomē,* excision]. Instrument used for cutting or removing the iris. SYN: *iridectome.*

corectomedialysis (kor-ek″to-me-dī-al'ĭ-sis) [" + " + *dialyein*, to set free]. Separating outer border of iris from its ciliary attachment.

corectomy (ko-rek'to-mĭ) [" + *ektomē*, excision]. Surgical removal of the iris. Syn: *iridectomy*.

corectopia (kor-ek-to'pĭ-ă) [" + *ek*, out of, + *topos*, place]. Having the pupil to one side of center of iris.

cored carbon. Electrode with carbon shell and core of metal or metal salt. See: *impregnated carbon*.

coredialysis (ko-re-dī-al'is-is) [G. *korē*, pupil, + *dialysis*, separation]. Separation of iris' outer border from its ciliary attachment. Syn: *corectomedialysis.**

corediastasis (kor-ed-ĭ-as'ta-sis) [" + *diastasis*, a standing apart]. Dilatation of pupil. Syn: *corectasia.**

corelysis (kor-e-li'sis) [" + *lysis*, destruction]. Obliteration of pupil because of adhesions of iris to cornea.

coremorphosis (kor-e-mor-fo'sis) [" + *morphē*, form, + -*ōsis*, infection]. Establishment of an artificial pupil.

corencleisis (kor-en-kli'sis) [" + *egklein*, to enclose]. Formation of an artificial pupil by ligating the iris through a corneal incision.

coreometer (ko-re-om'e-ter) [" + *metron*, measure]. Instrument for measurement of the pupil.

coreom'etry [" + *metron*, measure]. Measurement of the pupil of the eye.

coreoncion (kor-e-on'sĭ-on) [" + *ogkos*, hook]. Double hooked iris forceps.

coreoplasty (ko're-o-plas-tĭ) [" + *plassein*, to form]. Any operation for forming an artificial pupil.

corestenoma (kor-e-sten-o'mă) [" + *stenōma*, contraction]. Narrowing of pupil.

c. congen'itum. Partial congenital obliteration of pupil by excrescences.

coretomedialysis (kor-et-o-mē-dī-al'is-is) [" + *temnein*, to cut, + *dialysis*, division]. Making of an artificial pupil through the iris.

coretomy (ko-ret'o-mĭ) [" + *tomē*, incision]. Any cutting of the iris.

Corex-D glass. Window glass which transmits the solar ultraviolet rays more fully than any other glasses except quartz.

corium (ko'rĭ-um) [G. *chorion*, skin]. The layer of the skin lying immediately under the epidermis, the dermis, or true skin. Consists of two layers, papillary and reticular. It is composed of loose connective tissue in which are numerous capillaries, lymphatics, and nerve endings. In it lie hair follicles, sebaceous glands, sweat glands and their ducts and smooth muscle fibers.

corm [G. *kormos*, a stem]. A short, solid, underground stem. Ex: *Colchicum*.

corn [A.S.]. Indian corn or maize. Av. Serving (sweet): 100 Gm. Pro. 3.1, Fat 1.0, Carbo. 19.2 per serving. Vit. A+, B++, E+, G+. Ash Const. (sweet corn): Ca 0.006, Mg 0.033, K 0.113, Na 0.040, P 0.103, Cl 0.014, S 0.046, Fe 0.0008. Ash Const. (corn meal): Ca 0.018, Mg 0.084, K 0.213, Na 0.039, P 0.190, Cl 0.146, S 0.111, Fe 0.0009.

corn [L. *cornu*, horn]. Horny induration and thickening of the skin, hard or soft, according to location. Syn: *clavus*.

Etiol: Pressure or friction or both from ill-fitting shoes.

Sym: Hard corns on exposed surfaces have a horny core of conical shape extending down into the derma, causing pain and irritation. Soft corns occur bet. the toes, kept soft by moisture and maceration, and may lead to inflammation beneath the corn. Infection with pyogenic organisms results in suppuration.

Treatment: Remove cause. Properly fitting shoes of soft leather and proper shape. Astringents or caustics, or dissection under local block anesthesia followed by painting with iodine or thymol iodide. Excision in suppurative cases followed by iodine or immersion in warm aqueous lysol solution. Soft corns dissected similarly with cotton pad protection to prevent maceration.

cor'nea [L. *corneus*, horny]. Clear, transparent, ant., glasslike portion of coat of eyeball. It is pearly white in health. Curvature is greater than rest of eyeball.

Composed of 5 layers: (1) Layer of epithelium; (2) Bowman's membrane (ant. limiting membrane); (3) substantia propria; (4) Descemets' membrane; (5) layer of endothelium.

cornea, words pert. to: abrasio corneae, albugo, anterior chamber, applanatio c., arcus senilis, argema, "cera-" words, chemosis, circumcorneal, "kerat-" words, leukoma, macula corneae, megalocornea, microcornea, nebula, obfuscation, pannus, peritomy, phlyctenula, rhytidosis, rutidosus, staphyloma, synechia.

cor'neal. Pert. to the cornea.

c. reflex. Closure of eyelids resulting from direct corneal irritation.

corneitis (kor-ne-i'tis) [L. *corneus*, horny, + G. -*itis*, inflammation]. Inflammation of the cornea. Syn: *keratitis*.

corneoiri'tis [" + G. *iris*, iris, + -*itis*, inflammation]. Inflammation of iris and cornea.

corneomandibular reflex (kor-ne-o-man-dĭb'u-lar). Deflexion of mandible toward opposite side when cornea is irritated while mouth is open and relaxed.

corneosclera (kor-ne-o-skle'ră) [" + *sklēros*, hard]. The cornea and sclera considered together. [hornlike.

corneous (kor'ne-us) [L. *corneus*]. Horny;

c. layer. Horny outer layer of the epidermis. Syn: *stratum corneum*.

c. tissue. Substance of the nails.

cornic'ulum [L. *cornu*, horn]. A small, hornlike process.

c. laryn'gis. Small, hornlike nodule on arytenoid cartilage.

cornifica'tion [L. *cornu*, horn, + *facere*, to make]. The process of becoming hard.

Corning-glass. Window glass substitute for transmitting the antirachitic rays of sunlight.

cor'nu [L. horn]. Any excrescence like a horn.

c. ammo'nis. Hippocampus major of [brain.

c. cuta'neum, c. huma'num. Hornlike excrescence on skin.

cor'nual. Pert. to a cornu.

c. myeli'tis. Myelitis of ant. cornua of spinal cord.

coro'na [G. *korōnē*, crown]. Any structure resembling a crown.

c. capi'tis. Crown of head.

c. cilia'ris. Circular figure on inner surface of ciliary body.

c. den'tis. Crown of a tooth. [penis.

c. glan'dis. Post. border of *glans*

c. radia'ta. 1. Radiating fibers from optic thalamus. 2. Layer of cells placed radially about the ovum.

c. veneris. Blotches on forehead parallel to hairline. A lenticular syphilide.
co′ronal. Pert. to a corona.
  c. suture. One which joins the parietal and frontal bones of the cranium.
coronary (kor′o-na-rĭ) [L. *coronarius*, pert. to a crown or circle]. 1. A term applied to blood vessels of the heart which supply blood to its walls. 2. Encircling, surrounding.
  c. arteries. Those of the heart supplying the heart muscle. There are also a right and left c. artery of the stomach. Narrowing and spasm of the c. heart arteries produce angina pectoris.
cor′oner [L. *corōnātor*, crown officer]. County officer who investigates and holds inquests over those dead from unknown or violent causes.
cor′onoid [G. *korōnē*, crow or crown, + *eidos*, appearance]. Shaped like a crow's beak or crown.
  c. fossa. An oval depression on ant. surface of distal end of humerus. Receives coronoid process of ulna.
  c. process. 1. A process on proximal end of ulna. Forms ant. portion of semilunar notch. 2. A process on the ramus of the mandible which serves for attachment of the temporalis muscle.
coroparelcysis (kor′′o-par-el′si-sis) [G. *korē*, pupil, + *parelkein*, to draw aside]. Bringing the pupil to one side in central corneal opacity.
coroscopy (ko-ros′ko-pĭ) [′′ + *skopein*, to examine]. Shadow test to determine refractive error of an eye. Syn: *skiascopy*.
corot′omy [′′ + *tomē*, incision]. Any cutting of the cornea.
cor′pora (sing. *corpus* [L.]. Bodies.
  c. cavernosa penis. Two columns of erectile tissue on dorsum of the penis.
  c. olivaria. Two oval masses behind pyramids of the oblongata.
  c. quadrigemina. Four rounded bodies of gray matter in the midbrain making up the lamina quadrigemina. The ant. pair is called the *nates;* the post., the *testes*.
corpulence (kor′pū-lĕns) [L. *corpulentia*]. Fatness of the body. Syn: *obesity*.
corpulent (kor′pū-lĕnt) [L. *corpulentus*]. Fat; obese.
cor pulmonale (kor pŭl′mŏn-āl-ĭ). A serious condition caused by air polution in presence of any respiratory infection. See: *lung-heart disease.* L-47.
cor′pus [L. body]. (pl. corpora). The principal part of any organ; any mass or body.
  c. albicans. A mass of fibrous tissue which replaces the regressing corpus following rupture of the graffian follicle. It forms a white scar which gradually decreases in size and eventually disappears.
  c. amylaceum. Mass having an irregular, laminated structure like a starch grain, found in the prostate, neuroglia, etc.
  c. annulare. Pons Varolii.
  c. aranacea. Brain sand; psammona bodies found in the pineal body.
  c. Arantii. Tubercle found in center of semilunar valves.
  c. bigeminum. Optic lobe.
  c. callosum. The great commissure of the brain bet. the cerebral hemispheres.
  c. cavernosum. Any erectile tissue, esp. the erectile bodies of the penis, clitoris, male or female urethra, bulb of the vestibule, or the nasal conchae.
  c. ciliare. Ciliary body.
  c. dentale, c. dentatum. Gray layer in white substance of the cerebellum.
  c. fimbriatum. White layer edging the lower cornu of the lateral ventricle.
  c. flavum. A waxy body seen in the central nervous system.
  c. geniculate. The medial or lateral geniculate body, 2.v.; a mass of gray matter lying in the thalamus.
  c. hemorrhagicum. Blood clot formed in the cavity left by rupture of the graafian follicle.
  c. highmorianum. Mediastinum testis.
  c. interpedunculare. Gray matter bet. peduncles before the pons Varolii.
  c. luteum. If pregnancy does not occur, the yellow body is known as the *corpus luteum or menstruation* or false corpus luteum. It reaches full size in about 10 days and then regresses rapidly being replaced by the *corpus albicans*. If conception occurs, the *corpus luteum* of pregnancy or the true corpus luteum continues to grow until about the 13th week when it reaches its full size (about 3 mm. in diam.), after which it slowly regresses. *Function:* the corpus luteum is an endocrine organ producing a hormone, *progesterone*, which acts synergistically with estrogens to bring about changes in the uterine mucosa during the second half of the menstrual cycle. It sensitizes the uterine mucosa inducing normal implantation of the blastocyst and the development of decidual membranes. In the absence of conception, regression of the corpus luteum with resulting diminution of hormone secretion brings about a shedding of the uterine endometrium or menstruation.
  c. mammillare. A mammillary body; a rounded body in the anterior part of the interpeduncular fossa.
  c. pampiniforme. Parovarium.
  c. pyramidale. 1. Pyramid of the oblongata. 2. A lobe of the epididymus.
  c. quadrigeminae. The anterior pair are called *superior colliculi;* the posterior or inferior pair, *inferior colliculu*.
  c. restiforme. The restiform body or inferior cerebellar peduncle. A band of fibers, principally ascending, in the medulla oblongata which connects the spinal cord below with the cerebellum.
  c. rhomboidale. See: *c. dentatum*.
  c. spongiosum. Erectile tissue surrounding the urethra.
  c. striatum. A structure in the cerebral hemispheres consisting of two basal ganglia (the caudate and lentiform nuclei), and the fibers of the internal capsule which separate them.
  c. subthalamicum. The subthalamic nucleus (corpus Luysii), lying in the ventral thalamus.
  c. vitreum. Vitreous portion of eye.
  c. wolffianum. Wolffian body.
cor′puscle [L. *corpusculum*, little body]. 1. A minute particle or corpusculum. 2. A small body. 3. A blood cell. There are 2 varieties, red and white, found in the blood.
  c., amniotic; c., amylaceous. Starchlike rounded body found in tissue, usually nervous, showing degeneration.
  c., axile; c., axis. The center of a tactile c.
  c., Bennett's. See: *Drysdale's c.*
  c., Bizzozero's. Blood platelet.
  c., blood. An erythrocyte or leukocyte.
  c., bone. A bone cell.
  c., Burckhardt's. Yellowish particles found in secretion of trachoma.

c., calcareous. A lime-containing cell found in dentine of a tooth.

c's., cancroid. Characteristic nodule in cutaneous epithelioma.

c., cartilage. A cell characteristic of cartilage.

c's., chorea. Hyaline bodies found in the corpora striata in chorea.

c., chromophil. Tiny body found in cytoplasm of a nerve cell. SYN: *Nissl's body.*

c's., chyle. C. seen in chyle.

c., colloid. SEE: *c., amniotic.*

c., colostrum. Large c. found in colostrum.

c's., corneal. Connective tissue c's. found in fibrous tissue of cornea.

c. of Donne. SEE: *colostrum c's.*

c's., Drysdale's. Elements found in the fluid of ovarian cysts.

c., educated. A cell derived from a mother cell which has overcome the toxic effects of bacteria of a disease.

c's., genital. Nerve terminals in the external genitalia.

c's., Gierke's. Particles seen in the nervous system.

c's., Gluge's. Particles seen in diseased nervous tissue.

c's., Golgi-Mazzoni. Tactile c's. with extensively branched nerve fibers and with few lamellae, found in subcutaneous tissue of the fingertips.

c's., Hassall's. C's. found in the thymus gland.

c's., Krause's. Nerve endings in mucosa of genitalia, mouth, nose and eyes.

c's., lymph. Leukocytes found in blood and lymph.

c's., malpighian. C's. found in the spleen and kidney.

c's., Mazzoni's. Nerve endings resembling Krause's c's.

c's., Meissner's. SEE: *tactile c's.*

c's., Norris'. Invisible disks in blood serum.

c's., pacinian. Largest of the end organs of the skin, found in the subcutaneous tissues.

c., phantom. A red blood corpuscle which has lost its coloring matter.

c., tactile. A rounded nerve ending found in the papillae of the corium, esp. of the fingers and toes.

c., terminal. A nerve ending. SEE: *nerve.*

c., touch. SEE: *tactile c.*

c's., Wagner's. SEE: *tactile c's.*

corpus'cular. Pert. to corpuscles.

corpus'culum [L. little body]. Corpuscle.

c. renis. Malpighian corpuscle and its capillaries in the kidneys, where secretion of the water in urine occurs.

correc'tant, correc'tive [L. *corrigere,* to correct]. 1. A drug that modifies action of another. 2. Pert. to such a drug.

Corrigan's disease. An abnormal condition caused by aortic regurgitation, and recognized by visible pulsation in the main arteries.

C.'s pulse. A full bounding pulse, which appears to be completely empty bet. beats; is associated with aortic insufficiency. SYN: *water-hammer pulse.*

corro'sion [L. *con,* with, + *rodere,* to gnaw]. Disintegration, esp. carious disintegration of a tooth.

corro'sive. Disintegrating, as eating away.

c. alkalies. These are corrosive hydroxides most commonly of sodium, ammonium, and potassium, as well as carbonates. Because of their great combining power with water, and their action on the fatty tissues they cause rapid deep destruction. They have a tendency to gelatinize tissue with a somewhat grayish color forming a soapy, slippery surface, accompanied by pain and burning.

TREATMENT: First, dilute the poison before giving any emetic and apply weak acids for prolonged periods.

Such dilution always delays absorption somewhat and makes it easier to induce vomiting. Second, remove the poison; this is best done by making the patient vomit. Emesis is more easily produced in a distended stomach. Titillate the uvula or pharynx with the finger, and again give the patient more fluid, repeating the process until the fluid returns clear. Among the most useful diluents and emetics for this purpose are (a) tepid water, (b) soapy water, (c) salty water, (d) baking soda (sodium bicarbonate) water (*do not use washing soda*), (e) milk. A useful and widely available first aid emetic of this type is warm, soapy, greasy dish water. Any of these emetics should be used in generous amounts in all ordinary cases. (About 4 to 7 glassfuls may be used).

Where the corrosives, such as lye or mineral acids, have been in the stomach for some time, there may be danger of perforating the stomach. In such cases there is excruciating abdominal pain, muscular rigidity, and often collapse. Following the washing of the stomach, the appropriate antidote may be administered if it is available.

c. poisons. These include (a) strong acids, alkalies, strong antiseptics, including bichloride of mercury, carbolic acid (phenol), lysol, cresol compounds, tincture of iodine, and arsenic compounds. They are destructive and have a disintegrating effect upon tissues similar to burns, and may result in death. If swallowed, any part of alimentary canal may be affected. Tissues involved are altered, easily perforated, or destroyed. Death comes very shortly from shock, or swelling of throat and pharynx, which causes choking; or by closure of esophagus, causing slow starvation.

SYM: Intense burning about mouth, throat, pharynx, and abdomen; abdominal cramping, retching, nausea, vomiting, and often collapse. There may be bloody vomitus (hematemesis) and diarrhea, the stools being watery, mucoid, bloody, and possibly stained with the poison or its products, resulting from its action on the contents of the alimentary tract. Stains about the lips, cheeks, tongue, mouth, or pharynx are often characteristic brown; violaceous or black stain on mucous membranes, which appear dry or parched. Carbolic acid or phenol leaves a white or gray stain resembling boiled meat; hydrochloric acid stains are grayish; nitric acid leaves a yellow stain; sulfuric acid leaves tan or dark burns.

cor'tex [L. rind]. (*Pl. cortices.*) 1. The outer layers of an organ as distinguished from its inner substance. 2. Outer layer of a bone or of the skull.

c. cerebri. The cortex of the brain, composed mainly of gray or cineritious substance. SEE: *arm center.*

c. renis. The cortical substance of the kidney, made up of urinary tubes and blood vessels, supported by a stroma or matrix.

cortical. Of or pertaining to the cortex of an organ.

Corti's arches (kor'tēz). Arches formed by junction of Corti's rods. [of C.

　C.'s canal. Spinal canal in organ C.
　C.'s cells. Hair cells of organ of C.
　C.'s membrane. One that covers Corti's organ.
　C.'s organ. Prominence on inner portion of basal membrane in cochlear duct and containing terminal auditory apparatus. [gan of C.
　C.'s rods. Supporting pillars of or-
　C.'s teeth. Huschke's* teeth; tiny toothlike protuberances at edge of cochlear labium vestibulare.
　C.'s tunnel. Corti's canal.

cortiadrenal (kor-tĭ-ad-re'nal) [" + ad, toward, + rēn, kidney]. Pert. to cortex of adrenal gland.

cor'tical. Pert. to the cortex.

corticifugal (kor-tĭ-sĭf'u-gal) [L. cortex, rind, + fugere, to flee]. Passing from the cerebral cortex.

corticipetal (kor-tĭ-sĭp'e-tal) [" + petere, to seek]. Passing toward cerebral cortex.

corticoadre'nal [" + ad, toward, + rēn, kidney]. Pert. to cortex of adrenal gland.

corticoaf'ferent [" + adferre, to bear to]. Passing toward the cerebral cortex. SYN: corticipetal.*

corticoef'ferent [" + efferre, to bring out of]. Passing from the cerebral cortex. SYN: corticifugal.*

corticopedun'cular [" + pedunculus, little foot]. Pert. to cortex and cerebral peduncles.

corticopleuritis (kor-tĭ-ko-plŭ-ri'tis) [" + G. pleura, rib, + -itis, inflammation]. Inflammation of the outer parts of the pleura.

corticospi'nal [" + spina, thorn]. Pert. to cerebral cortex and spinal cord.

corticosterone. A hormone secreted by the adrenal cortex which influences carbohydrate metabolism. It is essential for normal absorption of glucose, the formation of glycogen in the liver and tissues, and the normal utilization of carbohydrates by the tissues.

corticotro'pic. Pert. to corticotropin.

corticotro'pin. The adrenotropic factor or principle in the ant. lobe of the pituitary gland. Stimulates adrenal cortex in secreting steroid hormones. SYN: ACTH, q.v.

cor'tin [L. cortex, rind]. An assumed hormone of cortex of suprarenal gland.

cortisone (kort'ĭ-sōn). Abbr. for 17-hydroxy-II-dehydrocortico-sterone. A hormone from the cortex of the adrenal glands. Also known as Compound E. It relieves symptoms of rheumatoid arthritis, restores to normal abnormal brainwave patterns in Addison's disease and possibly in epilepsy. It influences rate of utilization of sugars, fat and proteins and mineral balance and most of the vital life processes. RF. ACTH.

corusation. The subjective sensation of flashes of light.

coryleur (kor-il-er') [Fr.]. Coryl sprayer.

Cory"nebacte'rium diphthe'riae. The diphtheria bacillus.

coryza (ko-ri'za) [G. koryza]. Cold in the head; an acute catarrhal inflammation of the nasal mucous membrane.
　c. spasmod'ica. Hay fever.

cosen'sitize [L. con, with, + sensitīvus, sensitive]. To sensitize to more than one infection.

cosmesis (kŏs-me'sĭs). A regard for the appearance of a patient.

cosmetic (koz-met'ik) [G. kosmētikos, pert. to adornment]. Powder or cream for improving complexion.
　c. operation. One for correcting an unsightly skin formation or structural conformation of face. [tilage.

cos'ta (pl. costae) [L.]. Rib. SEE: carcos'tal. Pert. to a rib.
　c. cartilage. Cartilaginous part of a rib articulating with the sternum.

costal'gia [L. costa, rib, + G. algos, pain]. Pain in the region of a rib; pleuralgia.

costectomy (kos-tek'to-mĭ) [" + G. ektomē, excision]. Excision of a rib.

cos'tive [L. contraction, from constipāre, to press together]. Constipated.

cos'tiveness [L. contraction, from constipāre, to press together]. Constipation.

costochon'dral [L. costa, rib, + G. chondros, cartilage]. Pert. to a rib and its cartilage.

costoclavic'ular [L. costa, rib, + clavicula, a little key]. Pert. to ribs and clavicle.

costocor'acoid [" + G. korax, crow, + eidos, form]. Pert. to ribs and coracoid process of scapula.

costogenic (kos-to-jen'ĭk) [" + G. gennan, to produce]. Pert. to defect arising from bone marrow of ribs.

costopneumopexy (kos"to-nu'mo-pek-sī) [" + G. pneumōn, lung, + pexis, fixation]. Anchoring a lung to a rib.

costoster'nal [" + G. sternon, chest]. Pert. to a rib and the sternum.

costotome (kos'to-tōm) [" + G. tomē, incision]. Knife or shears for cuttting through a rib or cartilage.

costotomy (kos-tot'o-mĭ) [" + tomē, incision]. Excision of a rib or part of one. SYN: costectomy, q.v.

costo"transverse' [" + transvertere, to turn aside]. Pert. to the ribs and transverse processes of articulating vertebrae.

costover'tebral [" + vertebra, joint]. Pert. to a rib and a vertebra.

cot'ton [M.E. coton, from Ar. qutun, cotton]. Fluffy covering of the plant Gossypium.
　c., absorbent. Cotton prepared to absorb liquids.
　c., styptic. Cotton impregnated with an astringent.
　c. wool sandwiches. These are used when a sharp pointed foreign body, such as a pin, has been swallowed.
　Wisps of finely separated cotton wool are placed bet. bread. Bread and butter may be used, but cotton wool is rather apt to collect into a pasty mass in the mouth with butter; therefore it is better to use only bread or bread and jam, or any jam containing pips which, mingling with the cotton wool, prevent its rolling up into a ball.
　To prepare, cut thin pieces of bread, spread fine wisps of cotton wool onto it, and smear a little jam over it to make it stick to the bread. Care should be taken to arrange the cotton wool so that pieces will not be pulled out when the sandwich is bitten.
　Several small sandwiches should be given at each meal until the pin has been passed in the feces.

cotyledon (kot-ĭ-le'don) [G. kotylēdōn, hollow of a cup]. 1. Mass of villi on chorionic surface of the placenta. 2. Any of rounded portions into which the placenta's uterine surface is divided. 3. Seed leaf of a plant embryo.

cotyloid (kot'ĭl-oid) [G. kotyloeidēs, cup shaped]. Shaped like a cup.
　c. cavity. The acetabulum or socket receiving the head of the femur.

couching (kow'ching) [Fr. *coucher*, to lay down]. Displacement of the lens downward in cataract.

cough [M.E. *coughen*]. A violent expiratory effort preceded by a preliminary inspiration. The glottis is partially closed, the accessory muscles of expiration are brought into action, and the air is noisily expelled.
SEE: *antibechic, bechesthesis, bechic, begma, bex, convulsive, laryngismus stridulus, pertussis.*

c., aneurysmal. Brassy and clanging, heard in patients suffering from aneurysm.

c., asthmatic. More like an attack of dyspnea than a cough.

c., brassy. Met with in cases where there is pressure on the left recurrent laryngeal nerve, as in aortic aneurysm.

c., bronchial. Heard in cases of bronchiectasis.* May be provoked by change of posture, as in getting up in morning. SPUTUM: Fetid odor and copious. Dirty gray. That heard in bronchitis,* in earlier stages, is hacking and irritating; in later stages, looser and easier. SPUTUM: Thin, frothy mucus.

c., diphtherial. Heard in laryngeal diphtheria; noisy and brassy, with stridulous breathing.

c., dry. One unaccompanied by moisture.

c., effective. When sputum is brought up.

c., hacking. A series of repeated efforts, as occurs in the early stages of pulmonary tuberculosis.

c., harsh. A metallic cough occurring in laryngitis.

c., hiccough. Singultus. Seen in forms of hysteria, unfavorable if seen toward end of acute disease.

c., hysterical. Incessant and barking.

c., ineffective. When there is no sputum.

c., laryngeal. Seen in laryngitis.* Shrill and husky. SPUTUM: Small plugs of mucus.

c., loud. Hysterical cough, q.v.

c., moist. A loose cough accompanied by moisture.

c., painful. The suppressed cough of the early stages of pleurisy and pneumonia.

c., paroxysmal. That occurring in whooping cough and bronchiectasis. Also described as spasmodic.

c., pulmonary. Hard and painful in pneumonia. SPUTUM: 1. *Scanty*, very tenacious, rusty colored from being tinged with blood. In early stages of tuberculosis, hacking and irritating; in later stages, frequent and paroxysmal. 2. *Purulent*, greenish-yellow; may be streaked with blood. In later stages, nummular or coinshaped.

c., reflex. Due to irritation from the middle ear, pharynx, stomach, or intestine. It may occur singly or coupled, or it may be hacking in character.

c., short. A dry cough seen in the early stages of a common cold or catarrhal influenza.

c., whooping. Seen in pertussis.* Convulsive, short, followed by a whoop. SPUTUM: Tough mucus, followed by vomiting.

coulomb (koo-lom'). Unit of electrical quantity. It is the quantity of electricity transferred by 1 ampere in 1 second.

count. The number obtained by determining the number of units of the object being counted per unit of volume, as bacteria count, red cell count, platelet count, reticulocyte count, differential count, parasite count, etc.

counter'act. To act against or in opposition to.

counter'action. That action of a drug or chemical agent having an action opposing that of another agent.

counterextension (kown-ter-eks-ten'shun) [L. *contra*, against, + *extendere*, to extend]. Back pull or resistance to extension on a limb.

counterir'ritant [" + *irritāre*, to excite]. An agent that is applied locally to produce inflammatory reaction with the object of affecting some other part, usually adjacent to or underlying the surface irritated. Ex: *Mustard, chloroform, cantharides.*

There are 3 degrees of irritation produced by the following agents: *rubefacients*, which redden the skin, the 1st degree; *vesicants*,* which produce a blister or vesicle, the 2nd degree, and *escharotics*,* which form an eschar or slough or death of tissue, the 3rd degree. SEE: *aquapuncture (2), seton.*

counterirrita'tion [" + *irritāre*, to excite]. Superficial irritation, or agent producing it, which relieves some other irritation of deeper structures.

countero'pening [" + A.S. *open*]. A 2nd opening, as in an abscess, not draining satisfactorily from 1st incision.

coun'terpressure instrument. To provide counter-retraction to offset that exerted by exit of needle.

coun'terpuncture [L. *contra*, against, + *punctura*, puncture]. Counteropening.* An additional opening made to help drainage, as an abscess.

coup de soleil (koo-da-sŏ-lay') [Fr.]. Sunstroke.

coup'ling [L. *copula*, bond]. Slow pulse, heart beats alternately strong or weak; seen in digitalis poisoning.

courses (kōr'siz) [L. *cursus*, a flowing]. Menses; catamenia.

Coutard's method or **technic.** A method of x-ray irradiation consisting of 10 equal applications.

couveuse (koo-vuz') [Fr. a brooder]. Infant incubator.

cover cell (kŭv'ér). A cell which serves to protect another cell of specialized function. SEE: *cell.*

cov'erglass. Thin glass disc to cover a mounted object to be microscopically examined.

cowperi'tis [Cowper + G. -*itis*, inflammation]. Inflammation of Cowper's glands.

Cowper's glands. The bulbo-urethral glands. A pair of compound tubular glands about the size of a pea beneath the bulb of the male urethra, and emptying a mucous secretion into it. Discovered by Wm. Cowper, an English anatomist (1666-1709). They are small round bodies, yellow in color. They correspond to the Bartholin* glands in the female. SEE: *antiprostate, antiprostatitis.*

cowpox (kow'pox). Vaccinia; pustular eruption on teats and bag of a cow in form of bluish vesicles, containing a virus which may produce smallpox in a human being; also claimed to render a subject permanently immune from the disease.

cox'a [L. haunch]. 1. The *os innominatum*. 2. The hip joint.

c. valga. Opp. of *c. vara*. Deformity produced when angle of head of femur with the shaft is increased above 120°.

c. vara. A deformity produced by decrease in angle made by head of femur with the shaft. Normally it should be 120°; but in c. vara it may be 80-90.° It occurs in rickets or may be due to bone injury.

coxal'gia [" + G. *algos*, pain]. 1. Pain in the hip. SYN: *coxodynia*. 2. Hip joint disease. SYN: *coxitis*.

coxi'tis [" + G. *-itis*, inflammation]. Hip joint disease.

coxodyn'ia [" + G. *odynē*, pain]. Pain in the hip joint. SYN: *coxalgia*.

coxofem'oral [" + *femur*, thigh]. Pert. to the hip and femur.

coxo″tuberculo'sis [" + *tuberculum*, a little swelling]. Tuberculous condition of the hip joint.

c. p. Abbr. Chemically pure.

Cr. SYMB: Chromium.

crab louse. *Phthirius inguinalis*. One that infests the pubic region.

crachotement (krā-shŏt-mon(g)') [Fr.]. Inability to spit, even with a strong desire to do so; usually accompanied by syncope following utero-ovarian operation.

cracked pot sound. Percussion sound resembling that heard when striking a cracked pot, indicative of a pulmonary cavity.

cra'dle [A.S. *cradel*]. Frame for keeping bedclothes from pressing on a wound or fractured part.

craigi'asis. Infection with Craigia microorganism causing symptoms peculiar to dysentery.

cramp [M.E. *crampe*]. A spasmodic, esp. a tonic, contraction of 1 or many muscles, usually painful.

In certain occupations, the attempted use of muscle groups habitually employed may lead to a so-called "professional cramp," though other motor formulae are easily executed by the affected muscles. In writer's cramp, the attempt to write induces painful spasm of the hand muscles (similarly telegrapher's, watchmaker's, seamstress' cramp, etc.).

SYM: Excruciating pain, hard and contracted lumps of muscle.

TREATMENT. Depends upon cause and location. In muscular cramps try to extend muscle, compress it and apply heat and massage.

SEE: *bricklayer's cramp, heat cramp, systremma, writer's cramp*.

c., clonic. Wryneck caused by rheumatism. SYN: *rheumatic torticollis.**

cran'berries. A bright red, acid berry of the plant *Oxycoccus*.

They contain benzoic acid but have an excess of base. They increase acidity of urine because the benzoic acid is converted into hippuric acid. The same is true of plums and prunes. Av. SERVING: 130 Gm. Pro. 0.5, Fat 0.8, Carbo. 0.109 per serving. Vit. A+, C++. Ca 0.018, Mg 0.007, K 0.077, Na 0.010, P 0.013, Cl 0.009, S 0.007, Fe 0.0006.

cra'nial [G. *kranion*, skull]. Pert. to the cranium.

SEE: *motor, trifacial, trigeminus, trochlear, Weber's syndrome, cranial nerves in Appendix*.

c. bones. Those that comprise the cranium or brain case.

c. nerves. Also nerves #3, 4, 6, 11, and 12 are now considered to be mixed nerves as it is rather firmly established that they carry afferent proprioceptive impulses. These have their origin in the brain, 12 in number. Name, number and functions of cranial nerves are as follows:

1st Pair—Olfactory. Special sense of smell.

2nd Pair—Optic. Special sense of sight.

3rd Pair—Oculomotor or *Motor Oculi*. Great motor of eye, supplies 5 of the 7 eye muscles.

4th Pair—Patheticus or *Trochlear*, Motor of superior oblique muscle of eye.

5th Pair—Trigeminus or *Trifacial*. Great sensory nerve of head and face; divides into 3 portions, viz., 1st Ophthalmic, Sensory; 2nd Sup. Max., Sensory; 3rd Inf. Max., Sensory, Motor and a lingual nerve of the sense of taste. Most difficult of all the cranial nerves to trace.

6th Pair—Abducens. Motor of external rectus of eye.

7th Pair—Facial or *Portio Dura*. Great motor nerve of face muscles; exclusively motor at its origin, but it subsequently receives fibers from the (5th) Trigeminus, which give it some sensory function.

8th Pair—Acoustic or *Auditory*, or *Portio Mollis of 7th*. Special sense of hearing.

9th Pair—Glossopharyngeal. In part a special nerve of taste, nerve of sensation, and also contains motor fibers.

10th Pair—Pneumogastric Vagus or *Par Vagum* (a mixed nerve). At its origin it is exclusively sensory, but lower down it is also motor and capable of providing both for sensation and motion in organs to which distributed.

11th Pair—Spinal Accessory. Considered to be exclusively motor, but some authorities claim for it sensory fibers. Accessory portion joins the vagus, to which it supplies its motor and some of its cardioinhibitory fibers. Spinal portion supplies the trapezius and sternomastoid muscles.

12th Pair—Hypoglossal. Exclusively motor. SEE: *Appendix*.

LESIONS OF THE CRANIAL NERVES GIVE RISE TO THE FOLLOWING MANIFESTATIONS:

First (Olfactory) : Loss or disturbance of the sense of smell.

Second (Optic) : Blindness, of various types depending upon the exact location of the lesion.

Third (Oculomotor) : Ptosis (drooping) of the eyelid, deviation of the eyeball outward, dilatation of the pupil, double vision.

Fourth (Trochlear) : Rotation of the eyeball upward and outward, double vision.

Fifth (Trigeminus) : *Sensory root*: Pain or loss of sensation in face, forehead, temple and eye. *Motor root*: Deviation of the jaw toward paralyzed side, difficulty in chewing.

Sixth (Abducens) : Deviation of the eye inward, double vision.

Seventh (Facial) : Paralysis of all the muscles on 1 side of the face; inability to wrinkle the forehead, to close the eye, to whistle; deviation of the mouth toward the sound side.

Eighth (Auditory and Vestibular) : Deafness or ringing in the ears; dizziness; nausea and vomiting; reeling.

Ninth (Glossopharyngeal) : Disturbance of taste; difficulty in swallowing.

Tenth (Vagus) : Disease of the vagus nerve is usually limited to 1 or more of its divisions. Paralysis of the main trunk on 1 side causes difficulty in swallowing and talking, and hoarseness. The commonest disease of the vagus is of its left recurrent branch (see above) which causes hoarseness as its principal manifestation.

Eleventh (Spinal Accessory): Drooping of the shoulder; inability to rotate the head away from affected side.

Twelfth (Hypoglossal): Paralysis of 1 side of the tongue; deviation of tongue toward paralyzed side; "thick" speech.

craniectomy (kra-nĭ-ek'to-mĭ) [" + *ektome*, excision]. Opening of skull for cerebral hemorrhage, tumor of brain, fracture of skull, or epilepsy.

NP: Take blood pressure every 15 minutes for first 12 hours, every half hour for second 12 hours, and then as ordered until discontinued. Do not leave patient alone for first 24 hours. Watch for and report at once any changes in blood pressure, pulse, respiration, temperature, and any evidence of paralysis.

craniocele (kra'nĭ-o-sēl) [" + *kēlē*, hernia]. Protrusion of the brain from the skull.

craniocer'ebral [" + L. *cerebrum*, brain]. Rel. to skull and brain.

cranioclast (kra'nĭ-o-klast) [" + *klastos*, broken]. Instrument for crushing fetal skull in delivery.

cra'nioclasty [" + *klastos*, broken]. Crushing of fetal head in dystocia.

craniocleidodysostosis (kra"nĭ-o-kli"do-dis-os-to'sĭs) [" + *kleis*, clavicle, + *dys*, bad, + *osteon*, bone, + *-ōsis*, infection]. Defective ossification of bones of head, face and clavicles; a congenital condition.

cra'niograph [" + *graphein*, to write]. Device for making graphs of the skull.

craniol'ogy [" + *logos*, study of]. The study of the skull, its size, and shape, esp. in reference to different races.

craniomalacia (kra-nĭ-o-mal-a'sĭ-ă) [" + *malakia*, softening]. Softening of the skull bones.

craniometer (kra-nĭ-om'et-er) [" + *metron*, measure]. Instrument for taking cranial measurements.

craniomet'ric points. Any prominences or marks on skull for defining the configuration of the cranium; for use in craniometry.

craniom'etry [G. *kranion*, skull, + *metron*, measure]. Study of the skull and measurement of it without its soft parts.

craniopharyngeal (kra"nĭ-o-far-in'je-al) [" + *pharyx*, the pharynx]. Pert. to cranium and pharynx.

craniopharyngioma (kra-nĭ-o-far-in-jĭ-o'mă) [" + " + *-ōma*, tumor]. Tumor of portion of the *hypophysis cerebri*.

cranioplasty (kra'ne-o-plas-tĭ) [" + *plassein*, to form]. Plastic operation on skull.

cra'niopuncture [" + L. *punctura*, puncture]. Puncture of the skull.

craniorhachischisis (kra-nĭ-o-rak-is'kis-is) [" + *rachis*, spine, + *schizein*, to split]. Congenital fissure of skull and spine.

craniostosis (kra-nĭ-os-to'sĭs) [" + *osteon*, bone]. Congenital ossification of cranial sutures.

craniotabes (kra-nĭ-o-ta'bēz) [" + L. *tabes*, a wasting]. Atrophy in infancy of cranial bones.

ETIOL: Marasmus, rickets, or syphilis.

craniotome (kra'nĭ-o-tōm) [" + *tome*, incision]. Device for forcible reduction of fetal skull in labor.

craniotomy (kra-nĭ-ot'o-mĭ) [" + *tome*, incision]. Breaking up fetal skull to facilitate delivery in difficult parturition.

craniotonos'copy [" + *tonos*, tone, + *skopein*, to examine]. Auscultatory percussion of cranium.

craniotympan'ic [" + *tympanon*, kettledrum]. Pert. to skull and middle ear.

cra'nium [L. from G. *kranion*]. That portion of the skull which encloses the brain; consists of single frontal, occipital, sphenoid, and ethmoid bones and the paired temporal and parietal bones.

SEE: *skeleton*.

RS: *acrocephalia, antinion, craniology, craniomalacia, occipital, parietal bone, skeleton, vitreous, zygoma, zygomatic arch.*

crap'ulent, crap'ulous [L. *crapula*, excessive drinking]. Intoxicated.

crassamen'tum [L. *crassare*, to make thick]. Coagulum, blood clot.

crater'iform [G. *kratēr*, bowl, + L. *forma*, shape]. Saucer-shaped, craterlike, or goblet-shaped.

cravat' ban'dage [Fr. *cravate*, a Croatian]. Triangular b. folded to form a band around the injured part. SEE: *bandage*.

cream [L. *cremor*, thick juice]. The rich, yellowish part of milk.

Av. SERVING (medium, 1 oz.): 25 Gm. Pro. 0.6, Fat 7.5, Carbo. 0.9 per av. serving. Ca 0.086, Mg 0.010, K 0.126, Na 0.035, P 0.067, Cl 0.080, S 0.030, Fe 0.00022. Slightly alkaline reserve. Vit. A+++, B++, C+ variable.

cream of tartar. Potassium bitartrate, $KHC_4H_4O_6$. An aperient and diuretic.

DOSAGE: 1-4 Gm. Usually given in hot water with lemon juice to flavor. SEE: *argol*. [produced by a fold.

crease (krēs) [L. *crista*, tuft]. A line c., *gluteofemoral*, c., *ileofemoral*. The crease that bounds the buttocks below.

creatinase (kre-at'in-ās) [G. *kreas*, flesh, + *ase*, enzyme]. An enzyme that decomposes creatinine.

creatine (kre'at-in) [G. *kreas*, flesh]. Methylglycocyamine, $NH:C(NH_2)N-(CH_3).CH_2.COOH + H_2O$, a colorless, crystalline substance that can be isolated from various animal organs and body fluids.

DOSAGE: 1-2 gr. (0.06-0.12 Gm.).

Found esp. in muscle juice and in blood. Not normally found in urine of adult men, but in women it obtains during menstruation, pregnancy, and in puerperium. It is constantly found in the urine of children and is present in fevers and during starvation. As it loses water it turns into creatinine before it is excreted in the urine.

creatinemia (kre-a-tĭn-e'me-ă) [" + *aima*, blood]. Excess of creatine in circulating blood.

creatinine (kre-at'in-in) [G. *kreas*, flesh]. Methylglycocyamidine, $C_4H_7ON_3$.

It can also be isolated as colorless crystals from animal material. It is one of the nonprotein constituents of blood, and increased quantities of it are found in advanced stages of renal disease. It is a normal and an alkaline constituent of urine and blood. About 0.02 Gm. per Kg. of body weight is excreted by the kidneys per day. It generally represents 3 to 7% of urine nitrogen content.

DOSAGE: 1-2 gr. (0.06-0.12 Gm.).

creatinuria (kre-ă-tĭn-u'rĭ-ă) [" + *ouron*, urine]. Creatinine in urine.

creatorrhea (kre-ă-tor-re'ă) [" + *roia*, flow]. The presence of muscle fibers in

creatotoxism   C-98   **crevice, gingival**

the feces, seen in some cases of pancreatic disease.

creatotoxism (krē″ă-to-toks′izm) [" + *toxikon*, poisoning]. Meat poisoning.

crèche (krāsh) [Fr.]. A day nursery for children.

Credé's method (krā′day). 1. The means whereby the placenta is expelled by downward pressure on the uterus through the abdominal wall with the thumb on the post. surface of the fundus uteri and the flat of the hand on the ant. surface, the pressure being applied in the direction of the birth canal. 2. For treatment of the eyes of the newborn, the use of 1% silver nitrate solution instilled into the eyes immediately after birth for the prevention of *ophthalmia neonatorum* (gonorrheal ophthalmia).

cremas′ter [G. *kreman*, to suspend]. One of the fascialike muscles suspending and enveloping the testicles and spermatic cord.

cremaster′ic [G. *kremastos*, hanging]. Pert. to the cremaster muscle.

   c. fascia. One of the coverings of the spermatic cord.

   c. reflex. Retraction of testis when skin is stroked on front inner side of thigh.

cremation (kre-ma′shun) [L. *crematio*, a burning]. Reduction of bodies of the dead by heat as a substitute for burying.

cre′mor [L.]. Cream.

   c. tar′tari. Cream of tartar.

crenate (krē′nat) [L. *crena*, a notch]. Notched or scalloped, as crenated condition of blood corpuscles.

crena′tion [L. *crena*, a notch]. The conversion of normally round red corpuscles into shrunken, knobbed, starry forms, as when blood is mixed with salt solution of, say, 5% strength. SEE: *plasmolysis.*

creosote (krē′o-sōt) [G. *kreas*, flesh, + *sōzein*, to preserve]. USP. A mixture of phenols obtained from wood tar.

   ACTION AND USES: Locally, antiseptic and anesthetic. Internally, gastrointestinal antiseptic and as a stimulating expectorant in chronic bronchitis and tuberculosis.

   DOSAGE: 4 ℥ (0.25 cc.).

crepitant (krĕp′ĭ-tănt) [L. *crepitare*, to crackle]. Crackling; having or making a crackling sound.

crepitation (krĕp-ĭ-tā′shŭn) [L. *crepitare*, to crackle]. 1. A crackling sound heard in certain diseases, as the râle heard in pneumonia. 2. A grating sound heard on movement of ends of a broken bone.

crep′itus [L. *crepitare*, to crackle]. 1. The noise of gas discharged from the intestines. 2. Crepitation.*

   c. redux. Râle indicating approaching recovery in pneumonia.

crepuscular (kre-pus′ku-lar) [L. *crepusculum*, twilight]. Pert. to twilight.

cres′cent [L. *crescere*, to grow]. Shaped like a sickle or the new moon.

   c. of Gianuzzi (jăn-noot′tse). A crescent shaped group of serous cells lying at the base of or along the side of a mucous alveolus of a salivary gland, also called demilune of Heidenhein.

   c., myopic. Grayish patch in fundus of eye due to atrophy of choroid.

crescentic (kres-en′tik). Sickleshaped.

cresol (krē′sol). USP. Yellowish brown liquid obtained from coal tar, having 4 times germicidal properties of phenol.

   USE: A surgical disinfectant in ¼ to 1% solution. Cresols possess distinct advantage as disinfectants. In practice they are diluted, but they are far from being nonpoisonous. One disadvantage is their disagreeable odor. A compound solution of cresol has about twice the germicidal power of pure phenol. On account of its saponaceous character, it is much used for disinfection of the skin, for lubricating the hands, and for vaginal douches in the form of aqueous solutions containing from 1-5%.

   DOSAGE: 1 gr. (0.06 Gm.).

cresomania (kres-o-ma′nĭ-ă) [*Croesus*, wealthy king of Lydia, 6th Century B. C., + G. *mania*, madness]. Hallucination of possessing great wealth.

cress, water. One of the plants of the mustard family.

   Rich in iodide, and it has a high allyl content. Its mineral value is higher than nearly all the herbaceous vegetables. Av. SERVING: 20 Gm. Pro. 0.2, Fat 0.2, Carbo. 0.8 per av. serving.

   VITAMINS: A+++, B++, C+++, G++ to +++. Ca 0.187, Mg 0.034, K 0.287, Na 0.099, P 0.005, Cl 0.061, S 0.167, Fe 0.00297.

crest [L. *crista*, tuft]. The ridge or part surrounding a process esp. on a bone.

cre′tin [Fr.]. One afflicted with congenital myxedema; an idiotic dwarf.

   A cretin is characterized by lack of stature and of mental development; rarely if ever exceeds the mental age of 10.

   The skin is rough and dry, and the hair coarse, dry, and brittle. Teeth erupt slowly and are of poor quality and irregularly placed. The tongue is large and apt to protrude from a mouth which constantly drools saliva. A cretin child is potbellied, swaybacked, and prone to umbilical hernia. Adult cretin is myxedematous.

   TREATMENT: Desiccated thyroid* or thyroxin.

   PROG: Cannot be entirely overcome.

cretinism (krē′tin-izm) [" + G. *ismos*, condition]. Congenital affection, characterized by a lack of physical and mental development.

   ETIOL: A congenital deficiency in secretion of the thyroid hormones.

   SYM: An abnormal condition of the thyroid gland, myxedema and idiocy or imbecility.

   c., endemic. SYM: Stature short (3 or 4 feet); head large, flat anteroposteriorly and broad laterally; eyes wide apart; nose flat; lips thick; tongue large and may protrude; chest narrow; abdomen prominent; fingers short; genitalia not developed; subcutaneous tissues at root of neck are thickened from mucoid or fatty deposits; thyroid gland frequently enlarged; mental condition that of idiocy. Found in the Alps and Pyrenees.

   c., sporadic cases of. Present the same features but the thyroid instead of being larger is smaller. Found in various parts of world. SEE: *cretin.*

cretinoid (cre′ti-noid) [" + G. *eidos*, resemblance]. Having the symptoms of cretinism, or resembling a cretin, due to a congenital condition.

cre′tinous. Pert. to a cretin or to cretinism.

crevice (krev′is) [Fr. *crever*, to break, from L. *crepāre*, to break]. A small fissure, or crack.

   c., gin′gival. The fissure produced by the marginal gingiva with the tooth surface.

crevicular (krev-ik′u-lar). Pert. to the gingival crevice.

crib′rate [L. *cribrum*, a sieve]. Profusely pitted or perforated like a sieve.

cribra′tion [L. *cribrum*, a sieve]. The state of being perforated.

crib′riform [" + *forma*, form]. Sievelike.
 c. fascia. Inner superficial fascia of thigh.
 c. plate. The thin, perforated, medial portion of the horizontal plate of the ethmoid bone.

cricoarytenoid (krī-ko-ă-rit′en-oid) [G. *krikos*, ring, + *arytaina*, pitcher, + *eidos*, form]. Extending bet. the cricoid and arytenoid cartilages.

cricoderma (krī-ko-der′mă) [" + *derma*, skin]. Ringshaped infiltrations in center of indurations on the skin.

cricoid (krī′koid) [" + *eidos*, form]. Ringlike.
 c. cartilage. A ringlike cartilage forming the lower back part of the larynx.

cricoidectomy (krī-koid-ek′to-mī) [" + *ektomē*, excision]. Excision of cricoid cartilage.

cricoidynia (krī-koi-din′ĭ-ă) [" + " + *odynē*, pain]. Pain in cricoid cartilage.

cricopharyn′geal [" + *pharygx*, gullet]. Pert. to the cricoid cartilage and pharynx.

cricothyreotomy (krī-ko-thi-re-ot′o-mī) [" + *thyreos*, shield, + *tomē*, a cut]. Division of the cricoid and thyroid cartilage.

cricothyroid (krī-ko-thī′roid) [" + " + *eidos*, form]. Pert. to the thyroid and cricoid cartilages.

cricot′omy [" + *tomē*, incision]. Division of the cricoid cartilage.

cricotracheot′omy [" + *tracheia*, windpipe, + *tomē*, incision]. Division of the cricoid cartilage and upper trachea in closure of the glottis.

crinogenic (krin-o-jen′ĭk) [G. *krinein*, to secrete, + *gennan*, to produce]. Producing or stimulating secretion.

crisis (krī′sis) [G. *krisis*]. 1. The turning point of a disease; a very critical period often marked by a long sleep and profuse perspiration. 2. The term used for the sudden descent of a high temperature to normal or below; generally occurs within 24 hours. 3. Sharp paroxysms of pain occurring over the course of a few days in certain diseases, e. g., gastric c., vesical c., Dietl's c., laryngeal c., etc. SEE: *lysis*.
 c., blood. The appearance in the blood of large numbers of nucleated erythrocytes over the course of a few days.
 c., Dietl's. In cases of floating kidney, the ureter becomes kinked and urine is obstructed, producing symptoms of renal colic.
 c., false. When temperature falls and the pulse rate remains high, suggesting that later on the temperature may rise again.
 c., true. One accompanied by a fall in the pulse rate.

crista [L.]. A crest or ridge.
 c. ampullaris. A localized thickening of the membrane lining the ampullae of the semicircular canals; it is covered with neuroepithelium containing auditory cells.
 c. galli. A ridge on the ethmoid bone to which the *falx cerebri* is attached. [crest.
 c. lacrimalis posterior. The lacrimal
 c. spiralis. A ridge on the spiral lamina of the cochlea.*

critical (krit′ik-al) [G. *krinein*, to judge]. 1. Pert. to a crisis. 2. Dangerous.
 c. reflex. Abnormal tension of an area resulting from direct stimulation of that area.

Crookes' dark space. Nonluminous region enveloping outline of the cathode in a discharge tube. SEE: *cathode, dark space.*
 C. tube. An early form of vacuum discharge tube devised by Sir William Crookes and used by him for the study of cathode rays.

cross birth. Presentation of the fetus where the long axis of the fetus is at right angles to that of the mother and requiring version.

crossed reflexes (krŏst). 1. Passive flexion of 1 part following flexion of another. 2. Passive flexion of 1 leg causing similar movement of opposite leg.

cross eye. Manifest deviation of one eye when looking at an object. SYN: *strabismus,** squint.

crossing over. The process in which a group exchanges place wtih a similar group of genes on a homologous chromosome. It occurs during synapsis in meiosis.

cross knee. Knock knee. SYN: *genu valgum.*

crotaphion (kro-tă′fĭ-on) [G. *krotaphos*, the temple]. Tip of greater wing of sphenoid bone.

crotchet (krotch′et) [Fr. *crochet*, small hook]. Sharp hook for extracting fetus after craniotomy.

croton oil (kro′ton) [G. *krotōn*, shrub]. (*oleum tiglii*). USP. A fixed oil expressed from the seed of the croton plant.
 ACTION AND USES: Drastic cathartic, externally as a rubefacient.
 DOSAGE: 1 ℳ (0.06 cc.) diluted with sugar or olive oil.
 POISONING: SYM: Severe abdominal pains, vomiting, marked diarrhea, and shock. Skin cold and clammy; face pinched; pulse rapid and small; collapse follows.
 TREATMENT: Stomach pump or an emetic. Give soothing drinks, such as milk, barley water, or whites of eggs.

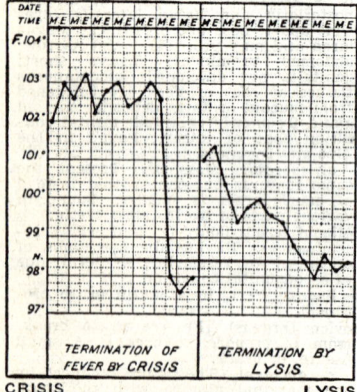

TERMINATION OF FEVER BY CRISIS — CRISIS

TERMINATION BY LYSIS — LYSIS

After Sears.

crounotherapy

Stimulate; apply external heat. Atropine, belladonna, or morphine to relieve cramping.

crounotherapy (kroo″no-ther′ă-pē) [G. *krounos*, spring, + *therapeia*, treatment]. Use of mineral waters for therapeutic purposes.

croup (crōōp) [Fr. *coupe*]. Disease characterized by suffocative and difficult breathing, laryngeal spasm, and sometimes by the formation of a membrane.

 c., catarrhal. Acute catarrhal laryngitis.

 c., membranous. Croupous laryngitis or true croup. Inflammation of larynx with exudation forming a false membrane. SYM: Those of laryngitis; loss of voice; noisy, difficult, and stridulous breathing; weak, rapid pulse; livid surface, fever moderate. PROG: *Grave*. Death may come in 36 hours. TREATMENT: Similar to that for diphtheria, *q.v.* Hot water to throat, emetics, and medicated inhalations. Produce vomiting. SEE: *carpopedal spasm, steam tent*.

 c., spasmodic or **false.** Catarrhal laryngitis without formation of false membrane, but with spasm of the glottis. Occurs in children. SYM: Difficult breathing, metallic cough, swollen membrane with tenacious mucus. PROG: Favorable. TREATMENT: Hot foot bath, emetic, inhalation of steam.

croupous (kroo′pus). Pert. to croup or having a fibrinous exudation.

 c. membrane. False membranous formation found in croup.

 c. pneumonia. Lobar pneumonia.

crown′ing [L. *corōna*, crown]. Stage in delivery when fetal head presents at the vulva.

crownwork [L. *corōna*, crown]. Artificial crown for a tooth.

crucial (krŭ′shal) [L. *crucialis*, from *crux*, cross]. 1. Cross shaped. 2. Decisive.

cru′cible [L. *crucibulum*]. A vessel for melting substances with great heat.

cru′ciform [L. *crux*, cross, + *forma*, shape]. Shaped like a cross.

crude (krŭd) [L. *crudus*, unripe; raw]. Raw, unrefined, or in a natural state.

cru′ra (sing. *crus*) [L. pl. legs]. A pair of elongated masses or diverging bands, resembling legs.

 c. cerebel′li. Cerebellar peduncles.

 c. cer′ebri. Pair of bands joining cerebellum to medulla and pons.

 c. of diaphragm. Two pillars connecting spinal column and diaphragm.

 c. of the fornix. Arches made by division of the fornicate extremities.

crural (kru′ral) [L. *cruralis*, pert. to the leg]. Pert. to the leg or thigh; femoral.

 c. arch. Femoral arch.

 c. hernia. Femoral hernia.

crus (pl. *cru′ra*) [L.]. 1. The leg. 2. Any structure resembling the leg.

 c. cerebri. Either of the 2 peduncles connecting the cerebrum with the pons.

crust, crust′a [L. *crusta*]. 1. A scab. A secondary lesion; dry serous or seropurulent, brown, yellow, red or green exudations on a free surface. 2. An outer covering or coat.

Seen in eczema, seborrhea, syphilis, impetigo, favus and *tinea tonsurans*, or scalp ringworm.

 c. lactea. Seborrhea of scalp in nursing infants. SEE: *galactophlysis*.

cryalgesia (kri-al-je′zĭ-ă) [G. *kryos*, cold, + *algos*, pain]. Pain from the cold. SYN: *crymodynia*.

cryanesthesia (kri-an-es-th... *an-*, priv. + *aisthēsis*, sensat... of sense of cold.

cryesthesia (kri-es-the′zĭ-ă) [″ + *aisth... sis*, sensation]. Sensitiveness to th... cold.

crymodynia (kri-mo-din′ĭ-ă) [G. *krymos*, cold, + *odynē*, pain]. Pain from cold. SYN: *cryalgesia*.

crymophilic (kri-mo-fil′ĭk) [″ + *philein*, to love]. Showing preference for cold, as certain microörganisms.

crymophylactic (kri-mo-fĭ-lak′tĭk) [″ + *phylaxis*, guarding against]. Resistant to cold.

crymother′apy [″ + *therapeia*, treatment]. The use of cold in treating disease.

cryo-aerotherapy (kri-o-a-er-o-ther′ă-pī) [G. *kryos*, cold, + *aēr*, air, + *therapeia*, treatment]. Cold air bath in which, by degrees, the patient is accustomed to freezing temperature.

cryocautery (kri-o-kaw′ter-ĭ) [″ + *kauter*, a burner]. Device for collection and application of solid carbon dioxide.

cry′ogen [″ + *gennan*, to produce]. Mixture of carbon dioxide snow at - 176° F.

cryogenic (kri-o-jen′ĭk). Producing or pert. to low temperatures.

cryom′eter [G. *kryos*, cold, + *metron*, measure]. A thermometer for measuring very low temperature.

cryophil′ic [″ + *philein*, to love]. Preferring low temperatures.

cryoscope (kri′o-skōp) [″ + *skopein*, to examine]. Device for performing cryoscopy.

cryoscopy (kri-os′ko-pē). Comparison of freezing point of blood, urine, and other fluids with that of distilled water.

cryotherapy (kri-o-ther′ă-pī) [G. *kryos*, cold, + *therapeia*, treatment]. The therapeutic use of cold.

cryotol′erant [″ + L. *tolerāre*, to bear]. Able to tolerate very low temperatures.

crypt (kript) [G. *kryptein*, to hide]. A tubule; follicle or pit.

 c. of Lieberkühn. Intestinal glands; tubular depressions in the intestinal mucous membrane. They are lined with columnar epithelium and have circular apertures opening upon the surface.

 c's., Morgagni′s. Recessions or pockets in rectal mucosa.

 c., synovial. Pouch in a joint's synovial membrane.

cryptamnesia (kript-an-am-ne′zĭ-ă) [″ + *an-*, priv. + *amnēsia*, forgetfulness]. Subconscious memory.

cryptectomy (krip-tek′to-mĭ) [″ + *ektomē*, excision]. Excision of a crypt.

crypthesthesia (krip-tes-the′zĭ-ă) [″ + *aisthesis*, perception]. Intuition.

cryptic (krip′tĭk) [G. *kryptikos*, hidden]. Having a hidden meaning; occult.

cryptitis (krip-ti′tis) [G. *kryptein*, to hide, + *-itis*, inflammation]. Inflammation of a crypt or follicle.

cryptococcosis. (European blastomycosis, Torulosis, Busse-Buschke's disease). A sub-acute or chronic infection which may involve any organ of the body, lungs, skin, but having a marked predilection for the brain and its meninges.

ETIOL: SYN: *Torula histolytica*, *Cryptococcus hominis*. A fungus, *Cryptococcus neoformans*.

SYMPTOMS: Development of single or multiple abscesses. In the cerebral type, headache, dizziness, vertigo, stiffness

muscles; in final stages coma spiratory failure. Often mistaken orain tumor.
PROG: Grave; in cerebral form usually fatal.

Cryptococcus. SYN: *Torula*. A genus of pathogenic yeast-like fungi which is the causative agent of European blastomycosis (Cryptococcosis).

cryptodidymus (krĭp-to-dĭd'ĭ-mus) [" + *didymos*, twin]. One fetus concealed within another.

cryptogenetic (krĭp-to-jen-et'ĭk) [" + *gennan*, to produce]. Of unknown or indeterminate origin.

   c. infection. The invasion of bacteria without outward evidence of entry into the body. SEE: *infection*.

cryptoglio'ma [" + *glia*, glue, + *-ōma*, tumor]. A glioma that has not yet revealed itself.

cryptolith (krĭp'to-lith) [" + *lithos*, stone]. A concretion in a glandular follicle.

cryptomenorrhea (krĭp-to-men-o-re'ă) [" + *mēn*, month, + *roia*, flow]. Monthly subjective symptoms of menses without flow of blood.

cryptomerorachischisis (krĭp"to-mer"o-rak-ĭs'kĭs-ĭs) [" + *meros*, part, + *rachis*, spine, + *schisis*, cleavage]. Spina bifida occulta without a tumor but with bony deficiency.

cryptomnesia (krĭp-tom-ne'zĭ-ă) [" + *mnēsis*, memory]. Subconscious memory.

cryptophthal'mus [" + *ophthalmos*, eye]. Complete congenital adhesion of eyelids to globe of eye.

cryptoplas'mic [" + *plasma*, matter]. Having existence in a concealed form.

cryptopodia (krĭp-to-po'dĭ-ă) [" + *pous*, foot]. Fibromata of feet so diffuse as to resemble pads.

cryptopyic (krĭp-to-pi'ĭk) [" + *pyon*, pus]. Having concealed suppuration, as a pyemia without apparent etiology.

cryptoradiom'eter [" + L. *radius*, ray, + G. *metron*, measure]. Device for estimating penetrative power of x-rays.

cryptorchid (kript-or'kĭd) [" + *orchis*, testis]. One with testicles which have not descended into the scrotum.

cryptorchidectomy (kript-or-kĭ-dek'to-mĭ) [" + " + *ektomē*, excision]. Operation for an undescended testicle.

cryptorchidism (kript-or'kĭd-izm) [" + " + *ismos*, condition of]. Failure of testicles to descend into scrotum.
Pregnant mare's gonadotropic hormone found in its urine causes descent and growth of testicles.

cryptorchis (kript-or'kĭs) [" + *orchis*, testis]. One with undescended testicles. SYN: *cryptorchid*.*

cryptorrhea (krĭp-to-re'ă) [" + *roia*, flow]. Excessive secretion of a ductless gland.

cryptorrheic (krĭp-to-re'ĭk) [" + *roia*, flow]. Pert. to internal secretions. SYN: *cryptorrhetic*.*

cryptorrhet'ic [" + *roia*, flow]. Pert. to the internal secretions.

cryptoscope (krĭp'to-skōp) [" + *skopein*, to examine]. Fluoroscope.

cryptotox'ic [" + *toxikon*, poison]. Having unknown toxic properties.

cry reflex (kri). Sudden painful response cry during sleep.

crys'tal [G. *krystallos*, clear ice]. A symmetrical shape produced by chemical compounds, certain salts, and by frost.

   c., blood. One composed of hematoidin.

   c., Böttcher's. SEE: *c., spermin*.

   c., Charcot-Leyden. Found in asthmatic sputum, leukemic blood, etc. Octahedral and composed of a phosphate.

   c., Charcot-Neumann. Spermin crystals found in semen and some animal tissues.

   c., Charcot-Robin. A type formed in blood in leukemia.

   c. hemin. Yellowish or brown crystals which appear when dried blood or hemoglobin is heated with a few drops of acetic acid and salt. They are crystals of hemin, the hydrochloride of heme. Their presence constitutes a delicate and reliable test for blood.

   c., spermin. Composed of spermine phosphate and seen in prostatic fluid on addition of a drop of ammonium phosphate solution.

crystallin (krĭs'tăl-ĭn). Globulin of the crystalline lens.

crys'talline. Resembling crystal.

   c. deposits. ACID GROUP: Includes the urates, oxalates, carbonates, and sulfates. ALKALINE GROUP: Includes the phosphates, cholesterin, systine, ammonium urate.

   c. lens. The lens of the eye in the capsule behind the pupil. It separates the *aqueous* from the *vitreous* humor. It is transparent and refracts the rays of light, impinging them upon the surface to bring them to a focus on the retina.

crystalliza'tion [G. *krystallos*, clear ice]. The formation of crystals.

crys'talloid [" + *eidos*, form]. 1. Like a crystal. 2. Opposite of *colloid;* a substance capable of crystallization, which in solution can be diffused through animal membranes, and is readily soluble, e. g., salt, sugar.

crystalloiditis (kris-tal-oid-i'tis) [" + " + *-itis*, inflammation]. Inflammation of crystalline lens.

crystaliopho'bia [" + *phobos*, fear]. Abnormal fear of glass or objects made of glass.

crys'tallose. A sweetening agent (saccharinate of sodium) said to be many times sweeter than sugar and to be used as a substitute for it.

crystallur'ia. The appearance of crystals in the urine. May occur following the administration of sulfonamides. Their formation can be prevented by administration of adequate amounts of alkali.

crystalluridrosis (krist-al-ū-rĭd-ro'sis) [G. *krystallos*, clear ice, + *ouron*, urine, + *idrōs*, sweat]. Crystallization of urinary elements on the skin.

Cs. Sym. for cesium, a metallic element.

Ctenocephalides (tĕn-ō-sĕf'ă-lĭds). A genus of fleas belonging to the order Siphonaptera. Common species are *Ct. canis* and *Ct. felis*, the dog flea and cat flea. The adults feed on their hosts while larvae live on dried blood and feces of adult fleas. Adults may attack man and other animals. They serve as intermediate host of the dog tapeworm, *Dipylidium caninum*, and may transmit other helminth and protozoan infections.

Cu. Symb. for *copper* (*cuprum*).

cubic measure. 1728 cubic inches (cu. in.) = 1 cubic foot (cu. ft.). 27 cubic feet = 1 cubic yard (cu. yd.).

cu'bital [G. *kubiton*, the elbow]. Pert. to the ulna, or to the forearm.

cu'bitus [L. from G. *kubiton*]. Elbow; forearm; ulna.
   c. valgus. An abnormal curvature of the humeral diaphysis; congenital or due to rickets.
   c. varus. Deformity due to fracture of either condyle of the humerus, the extended forearm deviating out from the axis of the arm; gunstock deformity; congenital.

cu'boid [G. *kubos*, cube, + *eidos*, resemblance]. Like a cube.
   c. bone. *Os cuboideum*. Outer bone of tarsal or instep bones.

cucumbers. Fruit of *Cucumis saturis* vine. Av. Serving: 75 Gm. Pro. 0.6, Fat 0.2, Carbo. 1.3 per av. serving. Ca 0.016, Mg 0.009, K 0.140, Na 0.010, P 0.033, Cl 0.030, S 0.020, Fe 0.0002. Vit. A – to +. Vit. B+. Vit. G++ to +++.

cucurbit (ku-ker'bit) [L. *cucurbita*, gourd]. Cupping glass.

cul-de-sac [Fr. *cul*, bottom, + *de*, of, + *sac*, bag]. A narrow cavity or vessel open only at 1 end, as of the eye.
   c., Douglas'. The peritoneal pouch bet. the ant. wall of the rectum and the post. wall of the uterus.

-cule, -cle [L.]. Suffix: Little, as *molecule*, *corpuscle*.

Cu'lex. A genus of small to medium sized mosquitoes of cosmopolitan distribution. Some species are vectors of disease organisms.
   C. pipiens. The common house mosquito. Serves as a vector of *Wucheria bancrofti*, the causative agent of filariasis.
   C. quinquefasciatus. Common in the tropics and sub-tropics; the most important intermediate host of *Wucheria bancrofti*.

Culicidae (kū-lĭs'ĭ-dē). A family of insects belonging to the order Diptera. Includes the mosquitoes.

culicifuge (ku-lĭs'ĭf-ŭj) [L. *culex*, gnat, + *fugere*, to flee]. An agent to prevent mosquito attacks.

cul'men [L. summit]. Top or summit of a thing.
   c. cerebelli. Most prominent part of the vermis sup. near its ant. extremity.

cultiva'tion [L. *cultivāre*, to cultivate]. Growing microörganisms in an artificial medium.

cultural (kul'tu-ral) [L. *cultura*, tillage]. Pert. to cultures of microörganisms.

cul'ture [L. *cultura*]. Bact: A mass of microörganisms growing in laboratory culture media.
   c., blood. Used in the diagnosis of specific infectious diseases. Test consists of withdrawing blood from a vein, under sterile precautions, placing it in or upon suitable culture media, and determining whether or not germs grow in the media. If organisms do grow, they are identified by bacteriologic methods.
   c., gelatin. A c. of bacteria on gelatin.
   c., hanging block. A thin slice of agar seeded on its surface with bacteria, and then inverted on a cover slip and sealed in the concavity of a hollow glass slide. This method is used to study the mode of cell division.
   c., hanging drop. A c. accomplished by inoculating the bacterium into a drop on a cover glass, and mounting it in the depression on a concave slide.
   c. medium. A substance on which microörganisms may grow. Those most commonly used are broths, gelatin, and agar, which contain the same basic ingredients. Salt should be used in media if blood is added to them to prevent the blood from hemolyzing.
   c., negative. A c. made from suspected matter which fails to reveal the suspected organism.
   c., physical. The training of the body by means of gymnastics.
   c., positive. A c. which reveals the suspected organism.
   c., pure. The c. of a single form of microörganism uncontaminated by other organisms.
   c., stab. A bacterial c. made by thrusting into the c. medium a point inoculated with the matter under examination.
   c., stock. A permanent c. from which transfers may be made.
   c. tissue. The growing to tissue cells in artificial nutrient fluids.

cu.mm. Abbr. for cubic millimeter.

cumulative (ku'mu-la-tiv) [L. *cumulus*, a heap]. Increasing in effect.
   c. drugs. Those which, after being received into the body in small doses, often repeated, are not immediately eliminated, but tend to accumulate in the system and suddenly produce symptoms of poisoning. Carbolic acid and mercurial preparations are examples of drugs which act in this way.

cum'ulus. A raised place; a heap of cells.
   c. cophorus. A mass of follicle cells which surrounds the ovum. It projects into the antrum of the Graafian follicle. Also called *discus proligerus*.

cuneate (ku'ne-āt) [L. *cuneus*, wedge]. Wedgeshaped.
   c. fasciculus, c. funiculus. Continuation of posteroexternal column of cord into the medulla.
   c. nucleus. Gray matter at end of cuneate fasciculus.

cuneiform (ku-ne'ĭ-form) [L. *cuneus*, wedge, + *forma*, shape]. Wedge-shaped.
   c. bones. Those of the tarsus, internal, middle, and external.
   c. cartilage. One of two small pieces of yellow elastic cartilage which lies in the aryepiglottic fold of the larynx immediately anterior to the arytenoid cartilage.
   c. hysterectomy. Excision of a wedge of uterine tissue.

cuneo- [L.]. Prefix: A wedge.

cu"neocu'boid [L. *cuneus*, wedge, + G. *kubos*, cube, + *eidos*, shape]. Pert. to cuboid and cuneiform bones.

cuneohysterectomy (ku-ne-o-his-ter-ek'-to-mi) [" + *ystera*, uterus, + *ektomē*, excision]. Excision of a wedge of tissue from the post. surface of the *cervix uteri* to correct abnormal anteflexion.

cu'neus [L.]. Wedgeshaped lobule of brain on mesial surface of occipital lobe.

cunic'ulus [L. an underground passage]. Burrow in epidermis made by the itch mite.

cunnilingus (kun-nĭ-lĭn'gus) [L. *cunnus*, pudenda, + *lingua*, tongue]. Application of tongue or mouth to the cunnus, *q.v.*, a practice not peculiar to either sex and also observed among various animals.

cun'nus [L.]. 1. The vulva,* pudenda.* 2. Vagina.

cup [G. *kupe*, hollow]. 1. Small drinking vessel. 2. A cupping glass.
   c., favus. Depression around a hair.
   c., glaucomatous. "Pressure excavation" of optic dish in glaucoma.

c. optic. In the embryo a double layered cuplike structure connected to the diencephalon by a tubular optic stalk. It gives rise to the sensory and pigmented layers of the retina.

c. physiologic. A slight concavity in the center of the optic disk.

cu'pola [L. *cūpula*, little tub]. The little dome at apex of cochlea and of spiral canal.

c. space. Tympanic attic.

cupping. Application of glass vessel from which the air has been exhausted by heat or a special suction apparatus to the skin in order to draw blood to the surface.

SEE: *leech.*

c., dry. Used to relieve kidney and in pneumonia to relieve congestion and pain, or to stimulate the kidneys; also to induce hyperemia in infected areas. DURATION: 10-20 minutes.

c., wet. Application of cupping after incision of the skin. Seldom now used. The area for both forms of cupping should first be shaved and sterilized.

cu'prum [L.]. Abbr. Cu. Copper, *q.v.*

curare, curari (kū-räh'rē) [Spanish *curaré*, he, to whom it comes, falls]. Toxic extract of *Strychnos* plant family used to paralyze motor nerve endings.

DOSAGE: 1/12 gr. (0.005 Gm.).

curarization (kū"räh-ri-zā'shŭn) [Spanish *curaré*, he, to whom it comes, falls]. Condition following introduction of curare: eyelids heavy, nystagmus, husky voice, weak jaw and throat muscles, inability to raise head, arms and legs.

Employed to lessen severity of convulsions produced by metrazol shock therapy and relaxation of muscles as in tetanus, etc. C. sets in with dosage in ratio of 1 cc., or 10 mg. per 15-20 pounds body weight with males and older patients slightly more. Effects noted in 15 minutes.

curd [M.E.]. Milk coagulum. Milk coagulated in the stomach forming what is known as a "curd."

cure [L. *cura*, care]. 1. Course of treatment of patients. 2. Restoration to health.

curet, curette (ku-ret') [Fr. *curette*, a cleanser]. Scraping instrument for removing foreign matter from a cavity.

curettage (ku-ret'aj) [Fr.]. Scraping of a cavity.

c., uterine. Scraping with a curette to remove impregnated ovum or its remnants clinging to uterine wall.

NP: 1. It is essential that the patient's buttocks are not pulled down below edge of table. If this is done when legs are elevated in leg rests or stirrups, an undue strain is apt to result in sacroiliac trouble. There is at least 1 case on record where gangrene of the foot followed prolonged pressure by stirrups.

2. The exterior surfaces are either scrubbed and irrigated with sterile water or painted, using either iodine or mercurochrome. The vaginal surfaces are included, as is also the cervix. The patient has already been placed on a Kelly pad, on which a sterile towel has been placed. A sterile towel is now placed across the pubes. Another is now placed crosswise across the buttocks. The "floating" nurse takes a strip of narrow adhesive plaster, about 18 in. long, holding it by the ends, well away from her. The "sterile" nurse then throws over the middle of the tape a sterile towel so that tape holds towel in middle fold. The "floating" nurse places edges of tape around patient's hips so that sterile towel is stretched tightly across rectum. Sterile leggings are now pulled over patient's legs and a lithotomy sheet draped down on the perineum.

3. Uterine packing should be ready. This form of packing is usually of gauze 1½ in. wide and 18 in. long.

curettement (ku-ret'ment) [Fr.]. The scraping of a part by means of a curette.

curie (ku-re'). The standard unit of quantity of radon, being the amt. in equilibrium with 1 Gm. of radium element.

cu'riegram [*Curie* + G. *gramma*, writing]. A radium photograph.

curietherapy (kū-rī-ther'ă-pī) [" + G. *therapeia*, treatment]. Radium therapy.

curled. BACT: Said of parallel chains in wavy strands, such as in anthrax colonies.

cur'rant. A small, seedless raisin.

Av. SERVING (fresh): 50 Gm. Pro. 0.8, Fat 0.2, Carbo. 6.4 per serving. Vit. C+++. Av. SERVING (dried): 50 Gm. Pro. 1.2, Fat 0.9, Carbo. 32.1 per serving. ASH CONST. (fresh): Ca 0.026, Mg 0.017, K 0.211, Na 0.007, P 0.038, Cl 0.006, S 0.14, Fe 0.0005. ASH CONST. (dried): Ca 0.082, Mg 0.044, K 0.873, Na 0.081, P 0.195, Cl 0.060, S 0.044, Fe 0.0025.

cur'rant jelly clot. Postmortem, soft, red clot in heart and vessels.

cur'rent [L. *currere*, to run]. A flow, as of water, or the transference of electrical impulses.

c., alternating. A current which periodically flows in opposite directions. Alternating current waves may be either sinusoidal or nonsinusoidal. The alternating current wave used most commonly therapeutically is the sinusoidal. Its variations in strength in either direction are the same; *i. e.*, starting from zero it rises with a gradual increase in voltage and amperage until a certain maximum is reached, when, without any pause or break, it decreases in the same gradual manner until the zero line is again attained; then, still without pause, the same process is repeated with equal intensity but in the opposite direction. This constitutes 1 cycle; 1 cycle equals 2 alternations. Furthermore, the cycle follows a definite law, the intensity of the current at any point being proportional to the sine of the angular displacement.

c., constant. SEE: *direct current.*

c., continuous. SEE: *direct current.*

c., cutting. Needle point or blade connected to 1 terminal of a high frequency machine producing current of undamped oscillations; large dispersive electrode is connected to other terminal. With appropriate strength of current, the needle or blade will cause rapid dissection due to molecular disruption along the line of application.

c., damped. An oscillating current of electricity in which the amplitude of successive alternations becomes less and less until it finally dies away.

c., d'Arsonval direct. SEE: *diathermy.*

c., De Watt'eville. Combined use of galvanic and faradic current made possible by use of special switch known as De Watteville switch.

c., direct. A current that flows in 1 direction only. When used medically it is called the "galvanic" current. This current has distinct and important constant polarity and marked secondary chemical effects. SEE: *electrolysis*.

c., direct vacuum tube. A current obtained from a d.c. source by applying to the part to be treated a vacuum electrode connected to 1 terminal of the machine, the other terminal being grounded.

c., electric cutting. SEE: *cutting current*.

c., farad'ic. An intermittent, alternating current induced in the secondary winding of an induction coil.

c., Frimandeau (frim-an'dō). Interrupted galvanic current obtained by use of Frimandeau coil. Is an unidirectional current.

c., galvan'ic. A steady unidirectional current produced by chemical action in a single or multiple dry or wet cell, or obtained from a direct current lighting or power circuit ("main"), or from an alternating current circuit by the introduction of (a) motor generator, (b) rectifier, and (c) "B Battery" eliminator. Galvanic and so-called static currents are the only unidirectional currents and the only ones possessing constant polarity.

c., grounded. Ground on earth, a part of an electric circuit.

c., high frequency. A current having a frequency of interruption or change of direction sufficiently high so that tetanic contractions are not set up when it is passed through living contractile tissues.

c., induced. An electric current generated in an adjacent coil by varying the magnetic field or by means of a moving magnetic field, or by motion of the coil in a fixed field.

c., interrupted. A current which is frequently opened and closed. SEE: *interrupter*.

c., inverse. A term used to describe current flowing through a tube in the wrong direction as a result of imperfect rectification of alternating current or of current from an induction coil. The unused half of the voltage cycle in half-wave rectification of alternating voltage.

c., Lapicque. Interrupted current of low frequency, unidirectional. Apparatus is a source of galvanic current, a metronome to interrupt the current, and 15 condensers of 2 microfarad capacity wired in parallel with a selector.

c., leakage. SEE: *grounded current*.

c., low frequency. An alternating current whose frequency in cycles per second is low in reference to a particular standard, such as the pitch frequency of "middle C" or, in some cases, the common frequency limit of audition. In general, low frequency currents are attended by tetanic contraction when passed through the body.

c., low tension. Same as low frequency currents.

c., Morton wave. An interrupted current obtained from a static machine by applying to the part to be treated a flexible metal electrode connected to the positive terminal of the machine, the negative terminal being grounded, and a suitable spark gap being employed bet. the terminals.

c., os'cillating. A current alternating in direction, and of either constant or gradually decreasing amplitude. An oscillating current of constant amplitude is called an undamped current; one of gradually decreasing amplitude, a damped current.

c., pulsating. A current pulsating regularly in magnitude. As ordinarily used, applies to a unidirectional current.

c., sinusoidal (si'nus-oid-al). SEE: *alternating current*. An alternating current following the sine law and of such frequency as to afford the opportunity of separate (clonic) muscular contractions.

c., static. Electricity produced by friction.

c., surging. Interrupted or alternating current in which the strength attained during each period of flow gradually increases to a maximum and then gradually decreases to zero.

c., undamped. An alternating current of electricity in which the amplitude of successive alternations is maintained.

c., unit of. Ampere, *q.v.*

c., Watteville. A faradic current reinforced by a constant current flowing through the secondary of the coil in the same direction as the current of break.

c., wave-o. Type of static current.

curriculum (kur-rik'u-lum) [L. a course]. A course of study.

Curschmann's spirals (koorsh'mahnz). Coiled spirals of mucus seen in sputum of asthma, etc. SEE: *sputum*.

curtasal (kur-ta-säl'). An odorless, white, crystalline substance, composed of sodium and calcium formate, with a small amt. of magnesium citrate.

USE: As a substitute for table salt, for salt-free diet in cardiac and renal diseases, etc.

DOSAGE: To suit the taste, as a rule requiring twice the amt. of table salt.

curvature (kŭr'vă-chŭr) [L. *curvatura*, a slope]. A bending or sloping away from a rectilinear surface, either normal or abnormal; a curve.

A flexure of the spine, caused by disease or relaxation of muscles and ligaments.

SEE: *kyphosis, lordosis, scoliosis*.

curve [L. *curvus*]. A bend.

c. of Carus. An arc corresponding with the pelvic axis. [curved.

curvi- [L.]. Combining form, meaning

Cus'co's spec'ulum. A duckbill vaginal speculum manipulated by a screw.

Cushing's disease. Adrenal cortical hyperfunction.

C's syndrome. Pituitary basophilism due to the presence of a hypophysial adenoma. The disease is rare occurring most commonly in young women. Symptoms are: adiposity of face, neck, and trunk; kyphosis; sexual dystrophy with amenorrhea in females, impotence in males; hypertrichosis of face and trunk; dusky appearance of skin with purple striae; vascular hypertension.

cusp (kusp) [L. *cuspis*, a point]. 1. Point of the crown of a tooth. 2. Central part of free edge of the leaflet of a valve of the heart.

cuspid (kus'pid) [L. *cuspis*, a point]. The 4 teeth with conic crowns (canine).

cuspidate (kus'pi-dāt) [L. *cuspis*, point]. Having cusps.

cuta'neous [L. *cutis*, skin]. Pert. to the skin.

c. respiration. The transpiration of gases through the skin.

c. pupillary reflex. Especially the back of the neck.

c. reflex. Common gooseflesh.

cu'ticle [L. *cuticula,* dim. of *cutis,* skin].
1. A layer of solid or semisolid substance which covers the free surface of a layer of epithelial cells. It may be of a horny or chitinous consistency; sometimes it is calcified. Examples of a tooth, capsule of lens of eye. 2. The epidermis of the skin.

c. hair (of). A single layer of clear cells which forms the outer layer of a hair.

c. inner root sheath (of). A layer of scalelike cells which forms innermost layer of the root sheath. Lies next to the cuticle of the hair.

cuticula (ku-tĭk'u-lă) [L. dim. of *cutis,*
cuticulariza'tion. Growth of epidermis over a sore or wound.

cutis (ku'tĭs) [L]. The skin.

c. anserina. "Gooseflesh" caused by erection of skin papillae, as from cold or shock.

c. laxa. Dermatolysis, or hypertrophy of the skin and subcutaneous tissue.

c. pendula. Flabby skin.

c. vera. The corium*; deep layer of skin.

c. verticis gyrata. Looseness and hypertrophy of the skin which may hang in folds.

cutisector (ku-tis-ek'tor) [L. *cutis,* skin, + *sector,* a cutter]. Device for excision of skin.

cutitis (ku-ti'tis) [" + G. *-itis,* inflammation]. Inflammation of skin. SYN: *dermatitis.*

cutization (kū-tĭ-za'shun) [L. *cutis,* skin]. Skinlike condition of a mucous membrane as result of continued exposure.

cut throat. Injury depends upon position in which it was caused.
NP: *First Aid:* Send for doctor. Have subject lying down, head and shoulders raised. Press head on chest. If trachea is severed, keep open and free from clot. Compress bleeding points with clean, wet cloths. Reassure patient, keep lips moist, do not leave him for an instant. Artificial respiration if necessary.

cyanemia (si-an-e'mĭ-ă) [G. *kyanos,* dark blue, + *aima,* blood]. Blue color of blood.

cyanephidrosis (si-ăn-ef-ĭ-dro'sis) [" + *ephidrōsis,* sweating]. Bluish sweat.

cyanhidrosis (si-ăn-hĭ-dro'sis) [" + *idrōsis,* sweat]. Exuding bluish sweat.

cyan"hemoglob'in. A compound of hydrocyanic acid and hemoglobin which gives blood a bright red color. Present in hydrocyanic acid poisoning.

cyanide (si'ăn-ĭd). A compound containing the radical —CN, as potassium cyanide (KCN) sodium cyanide (NaCN).

c. poisoning. Cyanides are among the most common and most deadly poisons known. They stop cellular respiration by inhibiting the action of cytochrome oxidase, carbonic anhydrase, and other enzyme systems.
SYM: Start within a few seconds, rarely longer than 2 minutes. The patient utters a cry and falls insensible. Respiration is first rapid and convulsive, later slow and gasping. Death usually comes within 5 minutes. When smaller doses are taken, there is an acrid taste, a choking feeling, anxiety, dizziness, confusion, and headache. Convulsions with frothing of the mouth. Often incontinence. Pulse rapid, feeble, and irregular.
F. A. TREATMENT: Must be very prompt. Empty stomach. Wash it out extensively. Mouth administration and intravenous injection of sodium thiosulfate sometimes helpful. Artificial respiration and cardiac stimulants should be tried. Methylene blue injections are sometimes of value.

cyano- [G.]. Combining form, meaning *dark blue.*

cyanochroia (si-an-o-kroi'ă) [G. *kyanos,* dark blue, + *chroia,* color]. Cyanosis.

cyanoder'ma [" + *derma,* skin]. Blue discoloration of skin. SYN: *cyanosis.*

cyan'ogen. (1) The radical CN; (2) A poisonous gas, CN-CN.

cyanomycosis (si"an-o-mi-ko'sis) [G. *kyanos,* dark blue, + *mykēs,* fungus]. Development of blue pus due to *Micrococcus pyocyaneus.*

cyanopathy (si-an-op'ă-thĭ) [" + *pathos,* disease]. Blue discoloration of skin. SYN: *cyanosis.*

cyanophil (si-an'o-fĭl) [" + *philein,* to love]. Blue staining substance of plants and animals.

cyanophilous (si-an-of'ĭl-us). Having an affinity for blue dyes.

cyanopia, cyanopsia (si-an-op'ĭ-ă, -si-a) [G. *kyanos,* dark blue, + *opsis,* vision]. Vision in which all objects appear to be blue.

cy'anosed. Affected with cyanosis.

cyanosis (si-an-o'sis) [G. *kyanos,* dark blue, + *-ōsis,* infection]. Slightly bluish, grayish, slatelike, or dark purple discoloration of the skin.
When entire body is affected the color is dusky leaden.
ETIOL: Deficiency of oxygen and excess of carbon dioxide in blood caused by gas or any condition interfering with entrance of air in the respiratory tract; also by overdoses of certain drugs, or any form of asphyxiation.
TREATMENT: Remove cause. Artificial respiration together with oxygen inhalation or oxygen plus carbon dioxide. Stimulants; heat and massage are valuable adjuncts. SEE: *asphyxia, unconsciousness.*

c., congenital. Usually associated with stenosis of the pulmonary orifice, an imperfect ventricular septum, or a *patulous foramen ovale.*

c., enterog'enous. Induced by intestinal absorption of toxins.

c., false. Due to abnormal pigment in the blood.

c. retinae. Bluish appearance of retina seen in congenital heart disease, polycythemia, and in certain poisonings, as dinitrobenzol.

cyanotic (si-an-ot'ik). Of the nature of, affected with, or pert. to, cyanosis.

cyasma (si-az'mă) [G. *kyēsis,* pregnancy]. Lenticular pigmentation of skin of pregnant women.

cyclarthrosis (si-klar-thro'sis) [G. *kyklos,* circle, + *arthron,* joint, + *-ōsis,* infection]. A lateral ginglymus or pivot joint which makes possible rotation.

cycle (si'kl) [G. *kyklos,* circle]. A series of movements or events; a sequence.

c., cardiac. The series of consecutive movements through which the heart passes in performing 1 heart beat; it includes contraction or *systole,* relaxation or *diastole,* and a short rest pause, the *diastasis;* a complete cycle corresponds to 1 pulse beat, which takes 0.8 of a second.

cyclectomy (si-klek'to-mĭ) [" + *ektomē,* excision]. Excision of a portion of the ciliary body or muscle or ciliary border of eyelids.

cy'clic. Periodic.

c. insanity. Manic depressive psychosis; a form in which mania, melancholia, and sanity succeed each other at intervals; circular insanity.

cy'clical vomiting. Periodical and recurring attacks of vomiting met with in those of a nervous temperament. The condition is usually associated with acidosis.

SYM: Dizziness, loss of appetite, headache, nausea may occur. Patient then vomits about every ½ hr. for 1-2 days. Great thirst, slight rise of temperature, rapid pulse, prostration.

NP: At first glucose, barley sugar, or easily assimilated carbohydrate. Nothing during attacks. Keep warm in bed; mouth washes.

SEE: *nausea, vomiting*.

cyclicot'omy [G. *kyklikos*, circular, + *tomē*, incision]. Cutting of the ciliary muscle.

cycli'tis [G. *kyklos*, circle, + *-itis*, inflammation]. Inflammation of ciliary body.

SYM: Tenderness in ciliary region, swelling of upper lid, circumcorneal injection, deposits on Descemet's membrane, reduced or hazy vision, increased or decreased tension. Pain in or about the eye, worse at night, and on pressure. Its course is rapid, progressively unfavorable.

COMPLICATIONS: Iritis, choroiditis, scleritis, glaucoma.

TREATMENT: Local (atropine, heat, dionin, protection from light); general (salicylates, diaphoresis, rest; treat underlying cause if possible).

c., plastic. Ciliary body inflammation accompanied by that of entire uveal tract, giving rise to a fibrinous exudate in ant. chamber and vitreous.

c., purulent. Suppurative inflammation of ciliary body and iris. [out iritis.

c., serous. Simple inflammation without iritis.

cyclo-. G. A. combining form meaning (1) circular or pertaining to a cycle; (2) pertaining to the ciliary body of the eye.

cycloceratitis (si-klo-ser-a-ti'tis) [G. *kyklos*, circle, + *keras*, cornea, + *-itis*, inflammation]. Inflammation of cornea and ciliary body.

cyclochoroiditis (si-klo-ko-roi-di'tis) [" + *chorioeidēs*, skinlike, + *-itis*, inflammation]. Inflammation of ciliary body and choroid coat of eye.

cyclodial'ysis [" + *dialysis*, dissolution]. Operation performed in certain types of glaucoma to produce communication bet. ant. chamber and suprachoroidal space for the escape of aqueous humor.

cycloduc'tion. [" + L. *ducere*, to lead]. Movement of a part, as the eyeball, produced by the oblique muscle.

cycloid (si'kloid) [" + *eidos*, form]. Extreme variations of mood from elation to melancholia.

cyclokerati'tis [" + *keras*, cornea, + *-itis*, inflammation]. Inflammation of cornea and ciliary body.

cyclomastopathy (si"klo-mas-top'ă-thĭ) [" + *mastos*, breast, + *pathos*, suffering]. Excessive tissue proliferation of the breast.

cyclophoria (si-klo-fo'rĭ-ă) [" + *phoros*, bearing]. Rotation of eyeball due to insufficiency of oblique muscles.

cyclople'gia [" + *plēgē*, a stroke]. Paralysis of ciliary muscle.

cycloplegic (si-klo-ple'jik). Producing cycloplegia.

cyclople'gios [G. *kyklos*, circle, + *plēgē*, a stroke]. Agents which cause paralysis of ciliary muscle.

cyclopro'pane (C_3H_6). A gaseous anesthetic agent, colorless, slightly heavier than air, with a not unpleasant odor. Administered with 70 to 95% oxygen it produces unconsciousness in 1 to 2 minutes. Fire and explosion must be guarded against.

cycloserine (sī-klō-sēr'ĭn [L. *cyclo*, round, + *serine*]. An amino acid and antibiotic from a fungus. It blocks nutrients essential to the life of the tubercle bacillus; also effective in infections of the genitourinary tract.

cyclo'sis [G. *kyklōsis*, circulation]. A streaming movement of protoplasm such as is seen in certain plant and animal cells.

cyclothymia (si-klo-thi'mĭ-ă) [G. *kyklos*, circle, + *thymos*, mind]. PSY: Cyclic insanity.

cyclothy'mic. Pert. to cyclothymia.

c. personality. PSY: One in which periods of elation and sadness alternate. SYN: *syntonic*.

cyesedema (si-e-se-de'mă) [G. *kyēsis*, pregnancy, + *oidēma*, swelling]. Thickening of cutis; bloating in pregnancy.

cyesiology (si-e-si-ol'o-gĭ) [" + *logos*, study of]. The study of pregnancy.

cyesis (si-e'sis) [G. *kyēsis*]. Pregnancy.

cyetic (si-et'ĭk). Pert. to pregnancy.

cylicotomy (sil-ik-ot'o-mĭ) [G. *kylix*, cup, + *tomē*, incision]. To cut ciliary muscle. SYN: *cyclotomy*.

cylin"droadeno'ma [G. *kylindros*, cylinder, + *adēn*, gland, + *-ōma*, tumor]. An adenoma containing cylindrical masses of hyaline material.

cylindroid (sil-in'droid) [" + *eidos*, shape]. 1. Cylinder shaped. 2. A mucous, spurious cast in urine.

HOW TO RECOGNIZE: They have twists and turns, varying markedly in diameter in different places, most frequently pointed at the ends and frequently crossing an entire field. They do not usually have cellular intrusions.

cylindro'ma [" + *-ōma*, tumor]. Malignant tumor containing a collection of cells forming cylinders.

cylindrosarco'ma [" + *sarx*, flesh, + *-ōma*, tumor]. A tumor containing properties of cylindroma and sarcoma.

cylindruria (sil-in-dru'rĭ-ă) [" + *ouron*, urine]. Cylindroids in the urine.

cyllosis (sil-o'sis) [G. *kyllōsis*]. Clubfoot.

cymbocephalic (sim-bo-sef-al'ĭk) [G. *kymbē*, boat, + *kephalē*, head]. Having a boatshaped head.

cynanche (sin-ang'ke) [G. *kyōn*, dog, + *agchein*, to choke]. Severe sore throat.

c. malig'na. Gangrenous sore throat.

c. tonsilla'ris. Tonsillitis, quinsy.

cynan'thropy [" + *anthrōpos*, man]. Insanity in which the patient behaves like a dog.

cyn'ic spasm [G. *kynikos*, doglike]. Spasm of face muscles causing a grin or snarl like a dog.

cynobex (sin'o-beks) [G. *kyōn*, dog, + *bēx*, cough]. Dry, barking cough.

cynophobia (sin-o-fo'bĭ-ă) [" + *phobos*, fear]. Unreasonable fear of dogs. SYN: *lyssophobia*.

cynorex'ia [" + *orexis*, appetite]. Morbid appetite, bulimia.*

Cyon's experiment (si'onz). A stimulus to an intact ant. spinal nerve root resulting in a stronger muscle contraction than the same stimulus to the peripheral end of a divided nerve root.

C.'s nerve. A filament of the vagus; depressor nerve of heart.
cyophoria (si-o-for'ĭ-ă) [G. *kyos*, fetus, + *phoros*, bearing]. Pregnancy.
cyopho'ric. Pert. to pregnancy.
cyotrophy (si-ot'ro-fĭ) [G. *kyos*, fetus, + *trophē*, nutrition]. Nourishment of the fetus.
cypridopathy (sĭ"prĭ-dop'ă-thĭ) [G. *Kypris*, Venus, + *pathos*, disease]. Any venereal disease.
cypridophobia (sĭ"prĭ-do-fo'bĭ-ă) [" + *phobos*, fear]. 1. Morbid fear of venereal disease. 2. Abnormal fear of the sexual act. 3. False belief of having a venereal disease.
cypriphobia (sip-rĭ-fo'bĭ-ă) [" + *phobos*, fear]. Morbid aversion to and fear of coitus.
cyrtometer (sir-tom'et-er) [G. *kyrtos*, bent, + *metron*, measure]. Instrument for measuring circumference of chest and comparison of chest curves.
cyrtosis (sir-to'sis) [" + *-ōsis*, infection]. Having any abnormal curvature of the spine.
cyst (sist) [G. *kystis*, bladder, sac]. 1. A bladder. 2. Any sac containing a liquid.
 c., adventitious. C. formation around a foreign body.
 c., blood. Bloody tumor. SYN: *hematoma*.
 c., Boyer's. Subhyoid bursal cyst.
 c., chocolate. Ovarian c. with darkly pigmented gelatinous content.
 c., colloid. C. with gelatinous contents.
 c., daughter. C. growing out of the walls of another cyst.
 c., dentigerous. One containing teeth. SYN: *follicular odontoma*.
 c., dermoid. One containing elements of hair, teeth, or skin.
 c., extravasation. C. arising from hemorrhage into tissues.
 c., follicular. C. arising from occlusion of small follicle or gland.
 c., Gaertner's. Cyst of the remnants of the Wolffian duct.
 c., intraligamentary. Cystic formation bet. the leaves of the broad ligament.
 c., mucous. Retention cyst composed of mucus.
 c., nabothian. Cystic formation caused by closure of the ducts of the nabothian glands in the cervix uteri by the healing of an erosion.
 c., ovarian. Cystic formation in the ovary. SEE: *ovary*.
 c., paraovarian. Cystic formation of the paraovarium.
 c., piliferous. Same as dermoid cyst. Tumors made up of all 3 primary germ layers and containing hair, teeth, bone, sebaceous material, and skin.
 c., retention. One retaining the secretion of a gland, as in a mucous or sebaceous cyst.
 c., sebaceous. One of a sebaceous gland.
 c., seminal. C. composed of semen.
 c., unilocular. C. containing only 1 cavity.
 c., vaginal. Cystic formation in the vagina.
cyst, words pert. to: acephalocyst, atheroma, dermoid, echinococcus, encysted, endocyst, hydatid, hydrocyst, hydroma, mucocele, nabothian, retention c., sac, saccate, saccule, steatoma.
cystadenoma (sist-ad-en-o'mă) [G. *kystis*, bladder, + *adēn*, gland, + *-ōma*, tumor]. An adenoma containing cysts. Cystoma blended with adenoma.

cystalgia (sis-tal'jĭ-ă) [" + *algos*, pain]. Paroxysms of pain in the bladder.
cystatro'phia [" + *atrophia*, atrophy]. Atrophy of bladder.
cystauchenotomy (sis-taw-ken-ot'o-mĭ) [" + *auchēn*, neck, + *tomē*, incision]. Incision into the neck of bladder.
cystectasy (sis-tek'tă-sĭ) [" + *ektasis*, dilatation]. 1. An operation for extracting calculus from the bladder by dividing the membranous portion of the urethra, and then dilating neck of bladder. 2. Dilatation of bladder.
cystectomy (sis-tek'to-mĭ) [" + *ektomē*, excision]. Excision of cystic duct.
cysteine (sist'e-in). A sulfur-containing amino acid, beta-thio alpha-amino propionic acid, $C_3H_7NSO_2$, found among the decomposition products of proteins.
cyster'ethism [G. *kystis*, bladder, + *erethismos*, irritation]. Irritability of the bladder; vesical irritation.
cysthitis (sis-thi'tis) [G. *kysthos*, vulva, + *-itis*, inflammation]. Inflammation of the vulva.
cysthus (sis'thus) [G. *kysthos*, vulva]. 1. Vulva. 2. Anus.
cysthypersarcosis (sist-hi-per-sar-ko'sis) [G. *kystis*, bladder, + *yper*, over, + *sarkōsis*, growth of flesh]. Hypertrophy of muscular coat of the bladder.
cys'tic. Pert. to a cyst, or to the urinary bladder.
 c. duct. The duct of the gallbladder which unites with the hepatic duct from the liver to form the common bile duct.
 c. tumor. Tumor composed of cysts.
cysticercosis (sis-tĭ-ser-ko'sis) [G. *kystis*, bladder, + *kerkos*, tail, + *-ōsis*, infection]. Infestation by larva *Taenia solium*.
cysticercus (sis-tis-er'kus) [" + *kerkos*, tail]. Encysted larvae of tapeworms.
cysticolithectomy (sis"tĭ-ko-lĭ-thek'to-mĭ) [" + *lithos*, stone, + *ektomē*, excision]. Removal of an impacted stone from the cystic duct.
cysticorrhaphy (sis-tĭ-kor'ră-fĭ) [" + *raphē*, suture]. Suture of the cystic duct.
cysticotomy (sis-tĭ-kot'o-mĭ) [" + *tomē*, incision]. Incision of cystic bile duct. SYN: *choledochotomy*.
cystidolaparotomy (sis"tĭ-do-lap"ar-ot'o-mĭ) [" + *lapara*, flank, + *tomē*, incision]. Incision into bladder through abdomen after abdominal section.
cystidotrachelotomy (sis"tĭ-do-tra"ke-lot'o-mĭ) [" + *trachēlos*, neck, + *tomē*, incision]. Incision into neck of bladder. SYN: *cystauchenotomy*.*
cystifelleotomy (sis"tĭ-fel-e-ot'o-mĭ) [" + L. *fel*, bile, + G. *tomē*, incision]. Incision of gallbladder through abdominal walls. SYN: *cholecystotomy*.
cys'tiform [" + L. *forma*, form]. Having the form of a cyst; cystic; cystoid.
cystigerous (sis-tij'er-us) [" + L. *gerere*, to bear]. Containing cysts.
cystin(e ($C_6H_{12}N_2S_2O_4$) [G. *kystis*, bladder]. A sulfur-containing amino acid, which can be obtained by oxidation from cysteine and which is likewise obtained from proteins.
 It is needed for tissue repair and growth. SEE: *histidine, lysine, tryptophan*.
cystinuria (sis-tĭn-u'rĭ-ă) [" + *ouron*, urine]. Cystine in the urine, seen in jaundice and hepatic disease.
cystistax'ia [" + *staxis*, dripping]. Blood oozing from the mucous membrane of the bladder.

cystitis (sis-ti′tis) [" + -*itis*, inflammation]. Inflammation of the bladder of 2 types: Nonbacterial (trauma, chemicals), and bacterial (acute or chronic, superficial, interstitial, or complicated by pericystitis).
SYM: *Acute*: Frequent and painful strangury, diurnal and nocturnal, with possibly bacteria and blood in urine. *Chronic*: Secondary to some other lesion with possibly pyuria as only symptom.
c. cystica and **granulosa.** *Chronic*: Slight frequency of urination. Leukoplakia: Chronic pyuria and painful irritation, perhaps hematuria. TREATMENT: Treatment of its cause, after which it cures itself. Relief of irritation by instillations and irrigations. DIET: Milk diet, bland, unirritating foods, barley water, soda water; later, eggnog, eggs, milk pudding, fish, and fowls in this order.

c., ulcerative. Aside from tuberculosis, carcinoma, syphilis, there are elusive ulcer (violent chronic irritation of bladder without gross evidence of cystitis), solitary ulcer, incrusted ulceration (bacterial, causing intense cystitis).

cystitome (sis′tĭ-tōm) [" + *tomē*, incision]. Instrument for incision into sac of crystalline lens.

cystit′omy [" + *tomē*, incision]. 1. Incision of capsule of crystalline lens. 2. Incision into the gallbladder.

cysto- [G.]. Prefix: Pert. to the urinary bladder or a cyst.

cystoadenoma (sis″to-ad-en-o′mă) [G. *kystis*, bladder, + *adēn*, gland, + -*ōma*, tumor]. A tumor containing cystic and adenomatous elements.

cystobubonocele (sis″to-bu-bo′no-sēl) [" + *boubon*, groin, + *kēlē*, hernia]. Hernia involving the bladder.

cystocarcino′ma [" + *karkinos*, ulcer, + -*ōma*, tumor]. Glandular tumor distended with fluid secretion of the gland.

cystocele (sis′to-sēl) [" + *kēlē*, hernia]. A bladder hernia.
Injury to the vesicovaginal fascia during delivery may allow the bladder to pouch into the vagina causing a cystocele.

cystocolos′tomy [" + *kolon*, colon, + *stoma*, mouth]. Formation of communication bet. the gallbladder and colon.

cystodiaphanoscopy (sis″to-di-ă-fan-os′ko-pī) [" + *dia*, through, + *phanein*, to shine, + *skopein*, to examine]. Transillumination of abdomen by an electric light in bladder.

cystodyn′ia [" + *odynē*, pain]. Paroxysmal pains in the bladder. SYN: *cystalgia*.

cystoelytroplasty (sis″to-el′ĭ-tro-plas-tī) [" + *elytron*, vagina, + *plassein*, to form]. Repair of a vesicovaginal fistula.

cystoepiplocele (sis″to-ē-pip′lo-sēl) [" + *epiploon*, omentum, + *kēlē*, hernia]. Protrusion of a portion of the bladder and the omentum.

cystoepithelio′ma [" + *epi*, upon, + *thēlē*, nipple, + -*ōma*, tumor]. Epithelioma in stage of cystic degeneration.

cystofelleotomy (sis-to-fel-e-ot′o-mī) [" + L. *fel*, bile, + G. *tomē*, incision]. Incision of gallbladder through abdominal wall. SEE: *cholecystotomy*.

cystofibro′ma [" + L. *fibra*, fiber, + G. -*ōma*, tumor]. Fibrous tumor containing cysts.

cystogram (sis′to-gram) [" + *gramma*, mark]. A radiographic film of the bladder.

cystography (sis-tog′ră-fī) [" + *graphein*, to write]. Making radiographs of the bladder.

cys′toid [" + *eidos*, appearance]. Bladderlike.

cystolith (sis′to-lith) [" + *lithos*, stone]. A vesical calculus.

cystolithectomy (sis-to-lith-ek′to-mī) [" + *ektomē*, excision]. Excision of a stone from the bladder.

cystolithiasis (sis-to-lĭ-thī′ă-sis) [" + *lithos*, stone]. Calculi in the bladder.

cystolith′ic. Pert. to a vesical calculus.

cystolutein (sis-to-lu′te-in) [G. *kystis*, cyst, + L. *luteus*, yellow]. Yellow coloring matter in cysts.

cysto′ma (pl. *cysto′mata*, *cysto′mas*) [" + -*ōma*, tumor]. A cystic tumor; a growth containing cysts.

cystom′eter [" + *metron*, measure]. Device for estimating the capacity of the bladder and its pressure reactions.

cystomor′phous [" + *morphē*, form]. Cystlike; cystoid.

cystomyxoadenoma (sis″to-mik″so-ad-en-o′mă) [" + *myxa*, mucus, + *adēn*, gland, + -*ōma*, tumor]. Myxoma and adenoma with cystic degeneration.

cystomyxo′ma [" + " + -*ōma*, tumor]. Myxoma with cystic formation.

cystonephro′sis [" + *nephros*, kidney]. Cystiform dilatation of kidney tubules.

cystoneural′gia [" + *neuron*, nerve, + *algos*, pain]. Neuralgia of the bladder or pain without apparent cause; cystalgia.

cystoparaly′sis [" + *paralysis*, a loosening from the side]. Paralysis of bladder.

cys′topexy [" + *pēxis*, fixation]. Surgical fixation of bladder to wall of abdomen.

cystophotog′raphy [" + *phōs*, light, + *graphein*, to write]. Taking pictures of interior of bladder.

cystoplasty (sis′to-plas-tī) [" + *plassein*, to form]. Plastic operation upon the bladder.

cystoplegia (sis-to-ple′jī-ă) [" + *plēgē*, stroke]. Paralysis of the bladder.

cystopto′sia, cystopto′sis [" + *ptōsis*, a dropping]. Prolapse into the urethra of the vesical mucous membrane.

cystopyelitis (sis-to-pi-e-li′tis) [" + *pyelos*, pelvis, + -*itis*, inflammation]. Cystitis with pyelitis.

cystopyelonephritis (sis-to-pi-e-lo-nef-ri′tis) [" + " + *nephros*, kidney, + -*itis*, inflammation]. Inflammation of urinary bladder, kidney, and pelvis of kidney.

cystoradiog′raphy [" + L. *radius*, ray, + G. *graphein*, to write]. Radiography of the gall- or urinary bladder.

cystorectostomy (sis-to-rek-tos′to-mī) [" + L. *rectum*, + G. *stoma*, opening]. Making a surgical communication bet. the bladder and rectum.

cystorrha′gia [" + *rēgnunai*, to burst forth]. Hemorrhage from the urinary bladder.

cystorrhaphy (sist-or′ă-fī) [" + *raphē*, suture]. Suture of bladder.

cystorrhe′a [" + *roia*, flow]. A discharge of mucus from the urinary bladder.

cystosarco′ma [" + *sarx*, flesh, + -*ōma*, tumor]. Sarcoma containing cysts.

cystoscope (sist′o-skōp) [" + *skopein*, to examine]. Instrument for interior examination of bladder.

cystoscopy (sis-tos′ko-pī) [" + *skopein*, to examine]. Examination of the bladder with the cystoscope.

cys′tospasm [" + *spasmos*, spasm]. Spasmodic contractions of the urinary bladder.

cystospermitis (sis-to-sperm-i'tis) [" + *sperma*, semen, + *-itis*, inflammation]. Inflammation of seminal vesicles.

cystos'tomy [" + *stoma*, opening]. Surgical incision into the bladder.

cystotome (sist'o-tōm) [" + *tomē*, incision]. Knife for incision of bladder.

cystotomy (sist-ot'o-mī) [" + *tomē*, incision]. Incision of bladder.

cystotrachelotomy (sis-to-trak-e-lot'o-mī) [" + *trachelos*, neck, + *tomē*, incision]. Incision into neck of bladder. SYN: *cystauchenotomy*.

cystoureteritis (sis-to-u-re-ter-i'tis) [" + *ourētēr*, ureter, + *-itis*, inflammation]. Inflammation of ureter and urinary bladder.

cystoureterogram (sĭst″ō-ū-rē'tĕr-ō-grăm) [" + " + *gramma*, mark]. A picture of the bladder and ureter.

cystoure'throscope [" + *ourēthra*, urethra, + *skopein*, to examine]. Device for examining the post. urethra and urinary bladder.

cytarrhagia (sit-ar-ra'jī-ă) [G. *kytos*, hollow, cell, + *rēgnunai*, to burst forth]. Hemorrhage from socket of a tooth.

cytase (si'tās) [" + *ase*, enzyme]. A ferment in phagocytes.

cyto- [G.]. Indicating the cell.

cytoarchitectonic (si″to-ark-ĭ-tek-ton'ĭk) [G. *kytos*, cell, + *architektonikē*, architecture]. Pert. to structure and arrangement of cells.

cytobiology (si-to-bi-ol'o-jī) [" + *bios*, life, + *logos*, study of]. Biology of cells.

cytobiotax'is [" + " + *taxis*, arrangement]. Grouping and apparent coöperation bet. embryonic cells. SYN: *cytoclesis*. [nucleus. SEE: *cyton*.

cy'toblast [" + *blastos*, germ]. A cell

cytocentrum (si-to-sen'trum) [" + *kentron*, center]. Sphere of attraction.

cytoceras'tic [" + *kerastos*, mixed]. Pert. to cells changing to a higher form.

cytochemism (si-to-kem'izm) [" + *chemeia*, chemistry, + *ismos*, condition of]. Reaction of body cells to chemical agents or the injections of antitoxin.

cytochem'istry [" + *chemeia*, chemistry]. The chemistry of the living cell.

cytochrome (si'to-krōm) [" + *chrōma*, color]. A heme compound widely distributed in animals and plants. It plays an important role in cellular respiration. It is a mixture of three hemochromogens, designated cytochromes A, B and C.

cytochylema (si-to-ki-le'mă) [" + *chylos*, juice]. The more fluid constituent of cell protoplasm.

cytoci'dal. Destructive of living cells.

cytocide (si'to-sīd) [G. *kytos*, cell, + L. *caedere*, to kill]. That which destroys cells.

cytoclas'tic [" + *klasis*, destruction]. Destructive to cells.

cytoclesis (si-to-kle'sis) [" + *klēsis*, a call]. The apparent coöperation of cells with each other. SYN: *cytobiotaxis*.

cytocyst (si'to-sist) [" + *kystis*, a cyst]. The remains of a cell enclosing a mature schizont.

cytoden'drite [" + *dendron*, tree]. A dendrite given off from the body of a nerve cell.

cytodiagno'sis [" + *dia*, through, + *gignoskein*, to know]. Diagnosis by examination of the contents of an exudating cell.

cytodieresis (si-to-di-er'e-sis) [" + *diairesis*, division]. Cell division, amitosis or mitosis.

cytodistal (si-to-dis'tal) [" + *distāre*, to be distant]. Pert. to a neoplasm remote from the cell of origin.

cytofin (si'to-fin) [G. *kytos*, cell]. An alloxur body allied to a purine formed by thymic acid.

cytogenesis (si-to-jen'es-is) [" + *genesis*, origin]. Origin and development of the cell.

cytogenous (si-toj'en-us) [" + *gennan*, to produce]. Cell forming, esp. those of connective tissue.

cytoglobin (si-to-glo'bĭn) [" + L. *globus*, sphere]. A globin from lymphocytes and leukocytes.

cytoglycopenia (si-to-gli-ko-pe'nĭ-ă) [" + *glukos*, sweet, + *penia*, poverty]. Deficient glucose of blood cells.

cytog'ony [" + *gonē*, seed]. The formation of the cell.

cytohistogen'esis [" + *istos*, web, + *genesis*, origin]. The structural development of cells.

cytohyaloplasm (si-to-hi'al-o-plazm) [" + *yalos*, transparent, + *plasma*, matter]. Reticular network of protoplasm.

cytoid (si'toid) [" + *eidos*, form]. Resembling a cell.

cytoinhibition (si″to-in-hi-bish'un) [" + L. *inhibere*, to restrain]. Phagocytic cell action in preventing the lysis of bacteria.

cytokeras'tic [" + *kerastos*, mixed]. Pert. to cellular development.

cytokine'sis [" + *kinēsis*, movement]. Changes in cellular protoplasm outside of the nucleus during mitosis.

cytology (si-tol'o-gī) [" + *logos*, study of]. The science of cell life and cell formation.

cytolymph [" + L. *lympha*]. Matrix of cytoplasm of cells.

cytolysin (si-tol'ĭs-in) [" + *lysis*, dissolution]. An antibody which produces disintegration of cells.

cytol'ysis [" + *lysis*, destruction]. Dissolution of cells by specific amboceptors and complements. *Hemolysis* is the term used in case of red blood corpuscles, and *bacteriolysis* for bacteria.

cytomachia (si-to-mak'ī-ă) [" + *machē*, fight]. Cellular activities and resistance during infection by microörganisms.

cytometaplasia (si″to-met-ă-pla'zī-a) [" + *metaplasis*, change]. Change of form or function of cells.

cytometer (si-tom'et-er) [" + *metron*, measure]. Instrument for estimating the number of cells.

cytom'etry [" + *metron*, measure]. The counting and measuring of cells.

cytomicrosome (si-to-mik'ro-sōm) [" + *mikros*, small, + *sōma*, body]. Minute granules in the protoplasm (cytoplasm) of the cell.

cytom'itome [" + *mitos*, thread]. Any part of the network of the cytoplasm.

cytomorphol'ogy [" + *morphē*, form, + *logos*, study of]. The study of the structure of cells.

cytomorphosis (si-to-mor-fo'sis) [" + " + *-ōsis*, infection]. The cellular transformations resulting from senescence or senile changes.

cyton (si'ton) [G. *kytos*]. 1. A cell. 2. The body of a nerve cell; also called perikaryon.

cytopathology (sī″tō-păth-ŏl'ō-jī) [" + *pathos*, disease, + *logos*, study]. Study of the cellular changes in disease.

cytope'nia [" + *penia*, lack]. Diminution in cellular elements of blood.

cytophagocytosis C-110 **Czerny operation**

cytophagocyto′sis [" + *phagein*, to eat, + *kytos* + *-ōsis*, infection]. Destruction of other cells by phagocytes.
cytophagous (si-tof′ag-us). Devouring or destructive of cells.
cytophagy (si-tof′aj-ĭ) [G. *kytos*, cell, + *phagein*, to eat]. Cell destruction by phagocytes. SYN: *cytophagocytosis.*
cytophil(e (si′to-fĭl) [" + *philein*, to love]. Having an affinity for or attracted by cells.
cytophylaxis (si-to-fi-lak′sis) [" + *phylaxis*, guarding against]. The protection of cells against lysis.
cytophylet′ic [" + *phylē*, tribe]. Pert. to genealogy of cells.
cytophys′ics [" + *physikē*, study of nature]. The physics of cellular activity.
cytophysiol′ogy [" + *physis*, nature, + *logos*, study]. Physiology of the cell.
cytoplasm, cytoplasma (si′to-plazm, -plaz′-ma) [" + *plasma*, matter]. 1. Protoplasm. 2. Cell plasm not including the nucleus.
cytoplas′tin [G. *kytos*, cell]. The plastin substance of the cytoplasm.
cytoproximal (si-to-proks′im-al) [" + L. *proximus*, nearest]. Pert. to a nerve fibril or axis cylinder nearest to the cell of origin.
cytoreticulum (si-to-ret-ik′u-lum) [" + L. *reticulum*, network]. The fibrillar network supporting fluid of protoplasm.
cytoscopy (si-tos′kop-ĭ) [" + *skopein*, to examine]. Microscopic examination of cells.
cytosome (si′to-sōm) [" + *sōma*, body]. The cell body which surrounds its nucleus.
cytospongium (si-to-spun′jĭ-um) [" + *spoggos*, sponge]. The network of a cell containing the fluid portion of protoplasm.
cytost (si′tost) [G. *kytos*, cell]. A specific toxin from an injured cell.
cytostasis (si-tos′tă-sis) [" + *stasis*, stoppage]. Stasis of white blood corpuscles, as in incipient stage of inflammation.
cytostromatic (si-to-stro-mat′ĭk) [" + *strōma*, coverlet]. Pert. to the cellular stroma.
cytotactic (si-to-tak′tik). Pert. to cytotaxia.
cytotax′ia, cytotax′is [G. *kytos*, cell, + *taxis*, arrangement]. Attraction or repulsion of cells for each other.
cytother′apy [" + *therapeia*, treatment]. Treatment by use of glandular extracts; organotherapy.
cytoth′esis [" + *thesis*, a placing]. Restoration or repair of injured cells.
cytotoxin (si-to-toks′in) [" + *toxikon*, poison]. An exotoxin that attacks different organs and tissues, produced by injection of foreign cells.
  SEE: *endotoxin, erythrotoxin, exotoxin, leukocidin, lysis, neurotoxin.*
cytotrophoblast (sī-tro′fo-blast) [" + *trophē*, nourishment, + *blastos*, germ]. The thin inner layer of the trophoblast composed of cuboidal cells, the outer layer being the syntrophoblast; also called layer of Langhans.
cytotropic (si-to-trop′ik) [" + *tropē*, a turn]. Having an affinity for cells.
cytozo′ic [" + *zōon*, animal]. Living within or attached to a cell, as certain protozoa.
cytozyme (si′to-zīm) [" + *zymē*, ferment]. A supposed substance which produces thrombokinase.
cytula (si′tū-lă) [L. dim. of G. *kytos*, cell]. The impregnated ovum.
cyturia (si-tu′rĭ-ă) [G. *kytos*, cell, + *ouron*, urine]. Presence of any kind of cells in the urine.
Czermak's spaces (chăr′măks). The interglobular spaces in dentine because of failure of calcification.
Czerny-Lembert suture (chăr-nĭ-lam-bār′). An intestinal suture in 2 rows.
Czerny operation (chăr′nĭ). A radical hernia operation.

D

D. Abbr. for *da, detur,* let there be given; for *dexter,* right; in optics, for *diopter;* in dentistry, for *deciduous.* SYMB: For Vitamin D potency.

Da Costa's disease. Retrocedent gout.

dacrocystitis (dak″ro-sis-ti′tis) [G. *dakry,* tear, + *kystis,* bladder, + *-itis,* inflammation]. Inflammation of the lacrimal (tear) sac.

dacryadenal′gia [" + *adēn,* gland, + *algos,* pain]. Pain in a lacrimal gland.

dacryadeni′tis [" + " + *-itis,* inflammation]. Inflammation of a lacrimal gland.

dacryadenoscirrhus (dak-rĭ-ad-en-o-skir′-us) [" + " + *skirros,* hardening]. Induration of a lacrimal gland.

dacryagogatresia (dak″rĭ-a-gog-ă-tre′sĭ-ă) [" + *agōgos,* leading, + *a-,* priv. + *trēsis,* perforate]. Occlusion of a tear duct.

dacryagogue (dak′rĭ-ă-gog) [" + *agōgos,* leading]. That which stimulates the secretion of tears.

dacrycystal′gia [" + *kystis,* cyst, + *algos,* pain]. Pain in a lacrimal gland; dacryocystalgia.

dacryelcosis (dak-rĭ-el-ko′sis) [" + *elkōsis,* ulceration]. Ulceration of the lacrimal apparatus.

dacryoadenal′gia [G. *dakryon,* tear, + *adēn,* gland, + *algos,* pain]. Dacryadenalgia; pain in a lacrimal gland.

dacryoadenitis (dak-rĭ-o-ad-en-i′tis) [" + " + *-itis,* inflammation]. Inflammation of lacrimal gland.

Rare; seen as complication in epidemic parotitis (mumps of lacrimal gland); also present in Mikulicz's disease; may be acute or chronic. Neoplasms.

SYM: Redness, swelling of lid over it, febrile symptoms; pain.

COMPLICATIONS: Abscess.

PROG: Can abort, if seen early; otherwise guarded. Fistula through integument or into conjunctival sac. Apt to be obstinate.

TREATMENT: Quiet. Internal remedies. Better to open through conjunctival sac, instead of integument. Sometimes has a chronic form.

dacryoblennorrhe′a [" + *blenna,* mucus, + *roia,* flow]. Discharge of mucus from a lacrimal sac, and chronic inflammation of the sac.

dacryocele (dak′rĭ-o-sēl) [" + *kēlē,* hernia]. Protrusion of a lacrimal sac.

dacryocyst (dak′rĭ-o-sist) [" + *kystis,* cyst]. The lacrimal (tear) sac.

dacryocystalgia (dak-rĭ-o-sis-tal′jĭ-ă) [" + " + *algos,* pain]. Pain in the lacrimal sac.

dacryocystec′tomy [" + " + *ektomē,* excision]. The excision of membranes of the lacrimal sac.

dacryocystitis (dak-rĭ-o-sis-ti′tis) [" + " + *-itis,* inflammation]. Inflammation of the tear sac involving mucous membrane of the lacrimal sac, together with submucous membrane, which later extends to connective tissue surrounding it, terminating in phlegmonous inflammation.

May be chronic, syphilitic, trachomatous, and tuberculous.

SYM: Epiphora, redness and swelling in area of sac which may also extend to lids and conjunctiva; pain, esp. on pressure over the lacrimal sac; overflow of tears.

TREATMENT: Hot compresses, incision, and drainage if fluctuant; attempt to restore permeability of duct with probe when acute symptoms have subsided; in chronic cases extirpate sac or do intranasal operation (dacryocystorrhinostomy).

PROG: Guard against abscess and lacrimal fistula at side of nose.

dacryocystoblennorrhea (dak-rĭ-o-sis″to-blen-or-re′ă) [" + " + *blenna,* mucus, + *roia,* flow). Chronic blennorrhea of the lacrimal sac.

dacryocystocele (dak-rĭ-o-sis′to-sēl) [" + " + *kēlē,* hernia]. Protrusion of lacrimal sac.

dacryocystopto′sis [" + " + *ptōsis,* a falling]. Prolapse of the lacrimal (tear) sac.

dacryocystorrhinostomy (dak-rĭ-o-sis-tor-rin-os′to-mĭ) [" + " + *ris,* nose, + *stoma,* opening]. Lumen of tear sac brought into direct communication with nasal cavity.

dacryocystosyringotomy (dak″rĭ-o-sis″to-sĭr-in-jot′ō-mĭ) [" + " + *syrigx,* tube, + *tomē,* incision]. Making an opening bet. the lacrimal sac and the nasal cavity.

dacryocystotome (dak-rĭ-o-sis′to-tōm) [" + " + *tomē,* incision]. Device for incision of lacrimal sac.

dacryocystot′omy [" + " + *tomē,* incision]. Incision of the lacrimal sac.

dacryohemorrhea (dak″rĭ-o-hem-o-re′ă) [" + *aima,* blood, + *roia,* flow]. Shedding of bloody tears.

dac′ryolin [G. *dakryon,* tear]. An albuminous matter in tears.

dac′ryolite, dac′ryolith [" + *lithos,* stone]. Concretion in lacrimal passages.

dacryoma (dak-rĭ-o′mă) [" + *-ōma,* tumor]. 1. A lacrimal tumor. 2. Obstruction of lacrimal puncta producing epiphora.

dacryon (dak′rĭ-on) [G. *dakryon*]. The lacrimal point of juncture of the lacrimal, frontal, and upper maxillary bones.

dacryops (dak′rĭ-ops) [G. *dakry,* tear, + *ops,* eye]. Constant flow of tears; dacryorrhea.

dacryopyorrhea (dak″rĭ-o-pi-o-re′a) [" + *pyon,* pus, + *roia,* discharge]. Discharge of pus from lacrimal duct.

dacryopyo′sis [" + *pyōsis,* suppuration]. Suppuration in the lacrimal sac or duct.

dacryorrhe′a [" + *roia,* flow]. Excessive flow of tears.

dacryosolenitis (dak″-rĭ-o-so-len-i′tis) [" + *sōlēn,* duct, + *-itis,* inflammation]. Inflammation of a lacrimal or nasal duct.

dacryosteno′sis [" + *stenōsis,* narrowing]. Stricture of a lacrimal or nasal duct.

dacryosyr′inx [" + *syrigx,* tube]. A lacrimal fistula.

dactyl (dak′til) [G. *daktylos,* finger]. A finger or toe; a digit of the hand or foot.

dactyl′ion [G. *daktylos,* finger]. Adhesions bet. or union of fingers or toes.

dactylitis [" + *-itis*, inflammation]. Chronic disease of bones of fingers and toes in very young children.
ETIOL: Usually tuberculous.
SYM: Bones enlarged, painful, chronically inflamed; pus may form and skin break, with abscess.

dactylocampsodynia (dak"tĭ-lo-kamp"so-dĭn'ĭ-ă) [" + *kampsis*, bend, + *odynē*, pain]. Painful contraction of 1 or more fingers.

dactyl'ogram [" + *gramma*, a mark]. A fingerprint.

dactylog'raphy [" + *graphein*, to write]. 1. The study of fingerprints. 2. The act of using a machine for blind deaf mutes to convey by touch the signs of speech.

dactylogryposis (dak"tĭ-lo-grĭ-po'sĭs) [" + *gryposis*, curve]. Permanent contraction of the fingers.

dactylology (dak-til-ol'o-jĭ) [" + *logos*, study]. Representing words by signs made with the fingers.

dactylomeg'aly [" + *megas*, large]. Abnormal size of fingers and toes.

dactylos'copy [" + *skopein*, to examine]. Examination of fingerprints for purpose of identification.

dactylospasm (dak'tĭl-o-spazm) [" + *spasmos*, spasm]. Cramp of a finger or toe.

dactylus (dak'tĭ-lus) [G. *daktylos*]. A toe or finger.

Dakin's solution. A solution for cleansing wounds.
It is prepared from washing soda (sodium carbonate) and chloride of lime and it makes a weak alkaline solution (0.4 to 0.5%) of sodium hypochlorite. SEE: *chlorine preparations.*

daltonism (dawl'ton-izm). Color blindness.

dam. A thin sheet of rubber to protect cavities or the field of dental operation from fluids.

damp (damp). 1. Moist, humid. 2. A noxious gas.
  d., after-. Air with large per cent of carbon dioxide.
  d., black, choke. A gas formed by oxygen and the giving off of carbon dioxide by the coal.
  d., cold. Vapor charged with carbon dioxide.
  d., fire. Methane, CH_4, found in coal mines.
  d., stink. Hydrogen sulfide.
  d., white. Carbon monoxide.

damped oscilla'tion. A current alternating in direction and of gradually decreasing amplitude. SEE: *current, oscillating.*

damping. The steady diminution of the amplitude of successive vibrations, as of an electric wave or current.

dance, St. Vitus'. A disease characterized by involuntary and irregular jerkings and movements in diverse groups of muscles. SEE: *chorea.*

Dan'ce's sign. Slight retraction in the right iliac region in some cases of intussusception.

dan'cing disease. Epidemic dancing mania of Italy, supposed to have been caused by the bite of the tarantula. SEE: *tarantism.*
  d. mania. Epidemic chorea.

dandelion greens. Those of a well-known plant which grows both as a weed and cultivated. They are bitter and tonic, and are eaten like spinach.
COMP: NUTRIENTS: AV. SERVING: 50 Gm. Pro. 1.2, Fat 0.5, Carbo. 5.3 per serving. ASH CONST: Ca 0.105, Mg 0.036, K 0.461, Na 0.168, P 0.072, Cl 0.099, S 0.017, Fe 0.0027. Vit. A+++, B++, C+, D+, E+, G++.

dan'druff (*dermatitis seborrheica*). Exfoliation of the epidermis of the scalp in the form of dry, white scales which fall. Scalp scurvy. Sometimes due to seborrhea.*
TREATMENT: Salicylic acid, 1 dram; mercury chloride, 4 gr.; methylated spirit, 6 oz.

dandy fever (dan'dĭ). Dengue. An acute, epidemic, febrile disease occurring in southern U. S. and East and West Indies, characterized by swelling and stiffness of the joints, severe pain, gastric disturbance, and a dermal exanthem. SEE: *dengue.*

Danielssen's disease. Anesthetic leprosy.

d'Arsonvalism (ar-son-val'izm). Obsolete term indicating the employment of d'Arsonval current therapeutically.

d'Arsonvalization (ar-son-val-iz-a'shun). The employment of the d'Arsonval current in the form of autocondensation, autoconduction, or the direct biterminal method. SEE: *diathermy.*

dartoid (dar'toid) [G. *dartos*, skinned, + *eidos*, form]. Resembling the *tunica dartos* in its slow, involuntary contractions.

dar'tos [G.]. The muscular, contractile tissue beneath the skin of the scrotum.*
  d. muscle reflex. Wormlike contraction of dartos muscle following sudden cold application to perineum.

dartre (dar'tr) [Fr.]. Any chronic skin disease.

dar'trous [G. *dartos*, skinned]. Of the nature of herpes; herpetic.

darwin'ian ear. Congenital deformity of the ear in which the helix is absent at upper angle.
  d. tubercle. A blunt point projecting from upper part of the helix.

dasetherapy (das-e-ther'ă-pĭ) [G. *dasos*, forest, + *therapeia*, treatment]. Treatment of disease by residence in a region of pine and spruce trees.

dasym'eter [" + *metron*, measure]. Device for estimating density of gases.

date. The fruit of the palm; an oblong berry with a grooved seed.
COMP: NUTRIENTS (dried, E. P.): AV. SERVING: 13 Gm. Pro. 0.3, Fat 0.4, Carbo. 10.2 per serving. Ca 0.065, Mg 0.069, K 0.611, Na 0.055, P 0.056, Cl 0.228, S 0.070, Fe 0.0030. Vit. A+, B++, G+. A base-forming food. Alkaline reserve 11.0 cc. per 100 Gm., 3.2 per 100 cal.

daturine (da-tu'rĭn). The active principle of stramonium. A poisonous alkaloid.
USES: Manias, epilepsy, as a hypnotic in insanity, etc. Action resembles atropine, *q.v.*

daughter cell. One formed by the division of a mother cell.
  d. cyst. A small c. growing out of the walls of a large c.
  d. nucleus. Formation of a new n. by a diaster.

Davidson's sign. The lessening of pupillary illumination when an electric light is held in the closed mouth. Indicates presence of a tumor or fluid in the maxillary sinus.

Davis' law: "Ligaments or any soft tissue, when put under even a moderate degree of tension, if that tension is unremitting, will elongate by the addition of new material; on the contrary, when ligaments, or other soft tissues, remain uninterruptedly in a loose or lax state they will gradually shorten, as the effete material is removed, until they come to maintain the same relationship to the bony structures with which they are united that they did before their shortening. Nature never wastes her time and material maintaining a muscle or a ligament at its original length when the distance between their points of origin and insertion is for any considerable time, without interruption, shortened."

day blind′ness. Inability to see well in a bright light.

de- [L.]. Prefix: Down or from.

deacidifica′tion [L. *de*, from, + *acidus*, sour, + *facere*, to make]. Neutralization of acidity.

deactiva′tion [" + *activus*, acting]. The process of becoming inactive.

dead [A.S. *dēad*]. Deprived of life.

When death has occurred in a public institution the patient's name, hour of death, and name of the ward should be written on a piece of paper and pinned to the front of the nightdress, or identified according to the custom of the institution. It is important that the "laying out" be completed before the commencement of rigor mortis. If the doctor is not present at the time of death immediate steps must be taken to inform him, since no preparation of the body may be begun until the doctor has officially pronounced the patient dead. It will sometimes happen that the private duty nurse will be asked to stay until after the funeral, but, in any case, she will not hurry away until assured everything in the room is in order, and that she can be of no further service. See: *death*.

d., care of. About 8 hours after death a change takes place in the body. The muscles gradually become stiff and rigid. To this change is given the name "rigor mortis," or cadaveric spasm.

Beginning in the muscles of the lower jaw and the back of the neck, the stiffness spreads to the muscles of the chest, the upper limbs, and the trunk, the lower limbs being the last part affected. Rigor disappears in the same order as it appeared, lasting, as a rule, about 4 or 5 days, depending on cause of death and the surrounding temperature.

As soon as death has been declared official, and friends have withdrawn, the nurse closes the eyes, keeping the lids in contact by pads of wet wool or lint. The lower jaw is prevented from falling back by passing a bandage round the point of the chin and over the head. A four-tailed bandage with a slit to receive the point of the chin may be used. After rigor mortis is well established, the bandage may be removed. Arms are crossed over chest and the wrists tied. Head and shoulders should be elevated. This aids in preventing discoloration of exposed portions of the body. Next, the limbs are straightened, and within 1 hour the body should be "laid out." After washing, the orifices are plugged with cotton wool, the legs are tied together, any wound or wounds are dressed, the hair is brushed; rings and earrings are removed (unless it is the special wish of the relatives that such be left), artificial dentures are inserted, and a clean nightdress is put on. A clean sheet is now placed over the corpse up to the level of the chin and the face is covered with a clean handkerchief.

When the patient is of Hebrew faith, the above procedure is carried out, except for the following: The body is not washed, no pins may be used, the hair is not combed, the hands are not crossed, but are tied with arms at full length and the finger or toe-nails are not cut.

deaf mute. A deaf and dumb person.

deaf-mut′ism. The state of being both deaf and dumb.

deafness [A.S.]. Loss of ability to hear, complete or partial.

ETIOL: May occur from several causes, such as (1) injury or disease of that part of the *cortex* controlling the center for hearing; (2) may be due to *hysteria*, without any abnormality of the ear or brain; (3) may be due to injury of the ear from *loud noises*, such as the firing of a gun at close range; (4) disease of the labyrinth of the internal ear; (5) an abnormal mental state may produce auditory aphasia or *psychic d.*, *q.v.*

Prostigmin has proved effective in relieving both acute and chronic deafness.

D. caused by pressure by eardrum on small mid-ear bones is helped by drilling hole behind ear through mastoid connecting with eardrum from behind. Progressive d. with roaring in ears helped by drilling hole into outermost semicircular canal and construct permanently open tiny window in ear.

RS: *anacusia, anacusis, aphemesthesia, asonia, baryecoia, bass deafness, mind deafness*.

d., bass. Inability to hear some of the low tones.

d. central. Deafness resulting from lesions of auditory tracts of the brain or auditory centers of the cerebral cortex.

d., cerebral. Due to brain lesion.

d. conduction. Deafness resulting from any condition which prevents sound waves from being transmitted to the auditory receptors. May be due to (a) wax obstructing ext. auditory meatus; (b) inflammation of the middle ear; (c) ankylosis of ear bones; (d) fixation of footplate of stirrup.

d., cortical. D. due to disease of the cortical centers.

d., mind. See: *psychic d.*

d., occupational. That which is caused by working in places where noise is very deafening.

d. perception or nerve deafness. Deafness resulting from lesions involving sensory receptors of cochlea or fibers of the acoustic nerve.

d., psychic. Condition in which auditory sensations persist, but due to lesions in auditory centers the sounds are not comprehended.

d., simulated. Malingering.

d., tone. Inability to distinguish musical sounds.

d., word. See: *psychic d.*

dealbation (de-al-ba′shun) [L. *dē*, from, + *albāre*, to whiten]. Bleaching.

deamidiza′tion [" + Fr. *amidon*, starch]. The decomposition of amino acids.

deam′inase. An enzyme which causes deaminigation.

de′′amina′tion. Removing of amino group — NH_2 from an amino-acid. SYN: *deaminization*, *q.v.*

deaminization (de-am-in-i-za′shun). A chemical decomposition whereby substances like the amino acids and alkaloids lose their amino groups and form ammonia.

Alanine can be deaminized to give ammonia and pyruvic acid: $CH_3.CH(NH_2)$-$COOH + O = CH_3.CO.COOH + NH_3$. Each tissue is supposed to deaminize its amino acids. Deamination may be simple, oxidative, or hydrolytic. Oxidizing en-

deanesthesiant — **D-4** — **decant**

zymes are called deaminizing enzymes, when the oxidation is accompanied by splitting off of amino groups.

deanesthe'siant [L. *dē*, from, + G. *an-*, priv. + *aisthēsis*, sensation]. That which will overcome anesthesia.

deaquation (de-ä-kwa'shun) [" + *aqua*, water]. Removal of water from anything; dehydration.

dearterializa'tion [" + G. *artēria*, artery]. Changing character of arterial into venous blood; deoxygenation.

death [A.S. *deadth*]. Permanent cessation of all vital functions. SEE: *dead*.

d., black. A term given to death from the plague.

d., causes. (a) Gradual wearing out of tissue and loss of energy with cessation of function without disease, as in *old age;* (b) as the result of disease represented by (1) the culmination of its ravages in the ordinary progress of the affection, or (2) as sudden death; also as the result of (c) injury from *accidents*. Injury is considered the major cause of death, although there is scarcely a disease known that may not be a cause of *sudden* death. Sudden death may be result of (a) circulatory failure, (b) cerebral causes, (c) respiratory causes, (d) neuroendocrinohumeral causes, (e) shock, (f) intoxications, (g) obstetrical causes, (h) infantile causes. In 10% of cases of sudden death no disease has been discovered.

d., local. Gangrene or necrosis of a part.

d., molar. SEE: *local d*.

d., molecular. That of cell life.

d. rate. This is the number of deaths occurring per 1000 of the population in a given area within a specified time.

d. rattle. Sound heard in the throat of the dying.

d., signs of. The principal one is (a) cessation of the heart's action. Other indications are (b) opaqueness of the cornea; (c) the absence of reflexes; (d) manifestations of *rigor mortis;* (e) a mottled discoloration of the body, esp. over all parts where there is pressure. Many cases of death have been reported only to find after 24 hours that the person was not dead. For such reasons more or less elaborate tests have sometimes been used to determine without doubt whether life is or is not extinct. The signs mentioned usually are sufficient to confirm one's opinion that death has taken place.

d., somatic. That of the entire organism.

d. tests. (a) A drop of ether is instilled into the conjunctival sac of 1 eye, the other being used as control. A reddening of the conjunctiva proves that life is present. (b) Sometimes the physician may pass a stylet through a small incision in the first intercostal spaces to the heart. Any movement of the heart will be communicated through the stylet. Removing the stylet may induce cardiac movement which may be augmented by artificial respiration. (c) A piece of litmus paper has been used under the eyelid, an acid reaction being shown by contact with the tears, the blood, or the organ in contact with the paper if death has taken place. (d) If a blister on the skin caused by application of a flame contains fluid, death is said to only be apparent, but if the blister fills with air and bursts with a crackling noise, leaving a dry skin, the person is dead. (e) Moisture appearing upon the face of a mirror held over the mouth and nostrils is indicative of the fact that life is not extinct.

d., to determine how long since it occurred. (a) The leg is divided from the ankle to the knee into 3 parts. (b) Beginning with the kneepan as a 4th part, the limb to the thigh is further divided into 6 parts, or 10 in all for the entire limb. If Section 1 is colder than Section 2, the body is assumed to have been dead for 1 hour; if Section 2 is colder than Section 3, the body has been dead 2 hours, and so on. Experiments conducted in temperatures bet. 40° and 80° F. proved fairly accurate in over 100 examinations. In an emergency, the usual symptoms of death are often found to be unreliable. Attempts at revivification should continue to be made indefinitely. No harm can be done in attempting to resuscitate one who seems to be deceased. Successes are numerous.

death, words pert. to: agonal, agonia, ante mortem, articulo mortis, autophonia, autopsia, autopsy, demise, euthanasia, in articulo mortis, in extremis, lethal, mors, mortuary, "necr-" words, posthumous, post mortem, putrefaction, putrescence, putrid, rigor mortis, rutidosus, suicide, thanatophobia.

death-bed state'ment. A declaration made at the time immediately preceding death. Such a statement, if made with the consciousness and belief that death is impending, is held in law as equally binding with a s. made under oath. SYN: *ante-mortem statement*.

debil'itant [L. *debilis*, weak]. A remedy used to reduce excitement. 2. That which weakens.

debil'itate [L. *debilis*, weak]. To produce weakness or debility.

debil'ity [L. *debilis*, weak]. Weakness of tonicity in functions or organs of the body. SEE: *cataphrenia*.

debouchement (da-boosh-mon') [Fr.]. Opening or emptying into another part.

Debove's membrane (de-bōvz'). Layer of connective tissue cells bet. the epithelium and basement tissue of mucous membranes of air passages and intestinal mucosa.

débridement (da-bred-mon') [Fr.]. 1. Enlargement of a wound in operating. 2. Slitting a constricting band of tissue.

deca-, dec- [G. *deka*]. Prefix: Ten.

decagram (dek'a-gram) [G. *deka*, ten, + *gramma*, weight]. A weight of 10 Gm. or 154.34 gr.

decalcification (dē-kăl-sĭ-fī-kā'shŭn) [L. *dē*, down, + *calx*, lime, + *facere*, to make]. The removal of or the withdrawal of lime salts from bone.

decal'cify [" + *calx*, lime]. To soften bone by removal of calcium or its salts by acids.

decaliter (dek'a-le-ter) [G. *deka*, ten, + Fr. *litre*]. A measure of 10 liters; 610.28 cu. in.

decaivant (de-kal'vant) [L. *dēcalvāre*, to make bald]. Destroying hair or making bald.

decameter (dek'am-e-eter) [G. *deka*, ten, + *metron*, measure). A measure of 10 meters; 393.71 in.

decanormal (dek-ă-nor'mal) [" + L. *norma*, rule]. Pert. to a solution 10 times as strong as a normal one.

decant' [L. *dē*, from, + *canthus*, corner]. To pour off liquid so the sediment remains in the bottom of the container.

de″canta′tion [" + *canthus*, corner]. The gentle pouring off of a liquid from its sediment.

decapita′tion (dē-kăp-ĭ-tā′shŭn) [" + *caput*, head]. SYN: *decollation*. (1) The separation of the head from the body; beheading. (2) In obstetrics, the separation of the head of the fetus from the body to facilitate delivery. (3) Separating the head from the shaft of a bone.

decapsula′tion [" + *capsula*, little box]. Removal of a capsule of an organ.

decarboxylation, decarboxylization (de-kar-boks-il-a′shun, -i-za′shun). A chemical decomposition whereby substances like the amino acids lose their carboxyl (COOH) groups; the example of histidine is given under *aporrhegma*.

decay′ [L. *dē*, down, + *cadere*, to fall]. Decomposition of organic matter by the action of microorganisms in the presence of air and without the production of unpleasant odors.
SEE: *cementoclasia, chemicolysis*.

decerebra′tion [" + *cerebrum*, brain]. Removal of the brain.

dechlorina′tion [" + G. *chloros*, green]. SYN: *dechlorization*. Reduction in the amount of chlorides in the body by reduction of or withdrawal of salt in the diet; dechloridation.

dechlorura′tion [" + " + *ouron*, urine]. Decrease in chlorates excreted in the urine produced by diet. SYN: *dechlorization*.

decholesterolization (de-ko-les-ter-o-li-za′-shun) [" + G. *cholē*, bile, + *stereos*, solid]. Reducing cholesterol from the system.

decholin (dek′o-lin). An oxidation product of cholic acid, derived from ox bile. Recommended to be used in chronic cholecystitis and as a diuretic.
DOSAGE: 3¾-7½ gr. (0.25-0.5 Gm.).

deci- [L.]. Prefix: *Decimus*, tenth.

decibel (des′ĭ-bel) [L. *deci*, + *bel*, unit of sound]. The unit of intensity and volume of sound.

decidua (de-sid′u-ă) [L. *deciduus*, falling off]. The name given to the endometrium or mucous membrane when conception occurs and which envelops the impregnated ovum.
This may be seen in both the uterine and ectopic pregnancies. The gland structures of the endometrium and the interstitial cells undergo marked hypertrophy. The decidua divides itself into an outer, or compact layer, and an inner spongy layer.
    d. basalis (*serotina*). That part of the decidua which unites with the chorion to form the placenta.
    d. capsularis (*reflexa*). That part of the decidua which surrounds the chorionic sac.
    d. graviditatis. The pregnancy decidua.
    d. menstrualis. The layer of the uterine endometrium that is shed during menstruation.
    d. parietalis. The nonplacental lining of the uterus; the decidua.
    d. reflexa. Same as capsularis.
    d. serotina. Part of the internal wall to which the ovum is attached.
    d. vera. The true decidua that is present throughout the entire endometrium during gestation. SEE: *caducous membrane*.

decidual (de-sid′u-al). Pert. to or resembling the decidua.

decidualitis (de-sid-u-al-i′tis) [L. *deciduus*, falling off, + G. -*itis*, inflammation]. A bacterial infection of the decidua.

deciduation (de-sid-u-a′shun) [L. *deciduus*, falling off]. The loss of the decidua during menstruation.

deciduitis (de-sid-u-i′tis) [" + G. -*itis*, inflammation]. Inflammation of the decidua.

deciduoma (de-sid-u-o′ma) [" + G. -*ōma*, tumor.] A uterine tumor containing decidual tissue. Thought to arise from portions of decidua retained within the uterus following an abortion.
    d., benign. The more or less normal invasion of the uterine musculature by the syncytium which disappears after the gestation is completed.
    d. Loeb's. Decidual tissue produced within the uterus of experimental animals as a result of mechanical or chemical stimulation.
    d., malignant. A tumor consisting of syncitial and Langhans cells which have a tendency to invade the general system by means of the blood stream, and having a high mortality.
    ETIOL: This tumor arises following a full term pregnancy, an ectopic pregnancy, an abortion, a miscarriage, and particularly a vesicular mole.
    DIAG: May be made by histologic study, aided by the symptoms and the Aschheim-Zondek test which remains strongly positive during the presence of this type of tumor.
    TREATMENT: The treatment is the surgical removal of the uterus, and adnexae, and any local growths that may be accessible. This should be followed by deep x-ray therapy over the pelvis and the secondary growths.

deciduomatosis (de-sid-u-o-mă-to′sis) [" + " + -*ōsis*, infection]. Excessive and irregular formation of decidual tissue in the nonpregnant state.

deciduosarco′ma [" + G. *sarx*, flesh, + -*ōma*, tumor]. Chorioma malignum; a tumor of the chorion.

deciduous (de-sid′u-us) [L. *deciduus*, falling off]. Falling off.
    d. teeth. The milk teeth or temporary teeth, 10 in each jaw: 4 incisors, 2 canines, and 4 molars. They usually appear at 6 months and fall out at the end of 6 years. Those of the lower jaw appear before the upper ones, as follows: *Lower central incisors*, at 6-9 months. *Upper incisors*, at 8-10 months. *Lower lateral incisors and first molars*, at 15-21 months. *Canines*, at 16-20 months. *Second molars*, at 20-24 months. SEE: *dentition*.

decigram (des′ig-ram) [L. *deci*, ten, + G. *gramma*, weight]. One-tenth of a gram, about 1.54 gr.

deciliter (des′ĭ-lĭ-ter) [" + Fr. *litre*]. One-tenth of a liter; 6.1 cu. in.

decimeter (des′im-e-ter) [" + G. *metron*, measure]. One-tenth of a meter; 3.93 in.

decinor′mal [" + *norma*, rule]. Having one-tenth the standard strength.

declinator (dek′lin-a-tor) [L. *declināre*, to turn aside]. Instrument used during trephining for holding apart the dura mater.

decline (de-klīn′) [L. *declināre*, to turn aside]. 1. Progressive decrease. 2. Declining period of a disease.

decli′vis cerebel′li. Sloping post. portion of the monticulus of the sup. vermis of the cerebellum.

decoc′tion [L. *dē*, down, + *coquere*, to boil]. A liquid preparation made by boiling vegetable substances with water.

When the strength and method of preparation are not otherwise specified, it is made by boiling 5 parts of the coarsely comminuted drug for 15 minutes with enough water to make 100 parts. There are no official decoctions. SEE: *apothem, apozeme.*

decollation (de″kol-a′shun) [" + *collum,* neck]. Fetal decapitation. SYN: *detruncation.*

decollator (de′kol-ă-ter). Device for decapitation of the fetus.

décollement (de-kol-mon′) [Fr. ungluing]. Separation of 2 normally adherent structures.

decompensa′tion [L. *dē + compensāre,* to make good again]. Failure of compensation, as in circulation of the heart.

decom′plementize. To take away the complement from.

decomposition (de-com-po-zish′un) [" + *componere,* to put together]. 1. The putrefactive process; decay. 2. Reducing a compound body to its simpler constituents. SEE: *fermentation, resolution.*

 d., double. A chemical change in which the molecules of 2 interacting compounds exchange a portion of their constituents.

 d., hydrolytic. 1. Chemical change in substances due to addition of 1 molecule of water.

 d., simple. A chemical change by which a molecule of a single compound breaks into its simpler constituents or substitutes the entire molecule of another body for 1 of these constituents.

decompres′sion [" + *compressio,* a squeezing together]. 1. The removal of pressure, as from gas in the intestinal tract. SEE: *Wangensteen's method.* 2. The slow reduction or removal of pressure on deep-sea divers and caisson workers to prevent development of bends, q. v.

 d. explosive. In aviators, decompression resulting from an extremely rapid rate of descent. Causes violent expansion of involved gases.

 d. illness or sickness. Caisson disease, or bends, q. v., compressed air illness.

de″contamina′tion. The process of rendering an object, person, or area free of a contaminating substance such as a poison-gas or radioactive substance.

de″cortica′tion [" + *cortex,* bark]. The removal of the surface layer of an organ or structure, as the removal of a portion of the cortex of the brain from the underlying white portion.

 d. pulmonary. Removal of the pleura of the lung, or a portion of the surface lung-tissue.

 d. renal. Removal of capsule of the kidney.

dec′rement [L. *decrementum,* decrease]. Declining period of a disease.

decrep′itate [L. *decrepitāre,* to crackle]. To cause decrepitation or a crackling noise.

decrepita′tion [L. *decrepitāre,* to crackle]. A crackling noise.

decrepitude (de-krep′ĭ-tud) [L. *decrepitāre,* to rattle]. Senile breaking down.

decubation (de-ku-ba′shun) [L. *dē,* down, + *cumbere,* to lie]. 1. The act of lying down. 2. The recovery stage of an infectious disease.

decu′bital [" + *cumbere,* to lie]. Pert. to a bed sore.

decubitus (de-ku′bi-tus) [L. a lying down]. 1. A bed sore.* 2. A patient's position in bed. SEE: *Andral's decubitus.*

 d., acute. Bedsore due to presence of cerebral lesions.

decussate (de-kus′at) [L. *decussāre,* to cross, as an x]. To cross, or crossed, as in the form of the letter *x.* Interlacing or crossing of parts.

decussa′tion. 1. A crossing of structures in form of an x. 2. The place of crossing; chiasma.

 d. of the pyramids. Crossing of fibers of pyramids of the medulla oblongata from 1 pyramid to the other.

 d. optic. The crossing of the fibers of the optic nerves; the optic chiasma.

decussorium (de-kus-o′rĭ-um) [L. *decussāre,* to cross, as an x]. Instrument for depression of the dura following trephining.

D-D-T. Dichloro-diphenyl-trichloroethane (2, 2-bis (parachlorophenyl) 1, 1, 1-trichloroethane). An insecticide effective against more varieties of insects than any other medium, esp. the flea, fly, louse, mosquito, bedbug, cockroach, Japanese beetle and European corn borer.

 toxicity. When ingested orally may cause acute poisoning. Symptoms are vomiting, numbness and partial paralysis of limbs, anorexia, tremors, depression and death.

deep reflexes (dēp). Opposite of superficial or skin reflexes; reflexes within, or fractional stretch reflexes.

Deer fly. A biting fly belonging to the genus *Chrysops* which carries *Bacterium tularense* to man.

 d. f. malady. Fever transmitted to man from rodents bitten by fly or other insects, or by direct contact. SYN: *tularemia.**

defat′ted [" + A.S. *fǣlt,* to fatten]. Deprived of fat.

defecalgesiophobia (def″e-kal-je-sī-o-fo′bī-ă) [L. *defaecāre,* to remove dregs, + G. *algēsis,* pain, + *phobos,* fear]. Fear of defecating because of pain.

defecation (def-e-ka′shun) [L. *defaecāre,* to remove the dregs]. Evacuation of the bowels.

The bulk of the feces depends upon the amt. of cellulose in the diet. 170 Gm. is the average weight of the feces in 24 hr., if the diet has been a mixed one. A vegetable diet will raise this to 400-500 Gm.

The food residues, reaching the rectum, cause a sensation referred to as a "call to stool," or the urge to defecate. The sensation is related to periodic increase of pressure within the rectum and contracture of its musculature.

The expulsion of a fecal mass is accompanied by coördinated action of the following mechanisms: (1) Involuntary contraction of the circular muscle of the rectum behind the mass, followed by contraction of the longitudinal muscle; (2) relaxation of the internal (involuntary) and external (voluntary) sphincter ani; (3) voluntary closure of the glottis, fixation of the chest, and contraction of the abdominal muscles, causing intraäbdominal pressure. SEE: *cacation, cacatory, constipation, feces, stool.*

defec′tive [L. *defectus,* a failure]. 1. Not perfect. 2. A person deficient in 1 or more physical, mental, or moral powers.

defensive protein. An antibody, *q.v.*

 d. reflex. Retraction or tension in defense against an action or threatened action.

def′erens [L. carrying away]. Ductus or *vas deferens.*

deferent (def′er-ent) [L. *deferre,* to carry away]. Away from or downward. SEE: *afferent, efferent.*

d. duct. Vas deferens.

deferentectomy (def-er-en-tek'to-mĭ) [" + G. *ektome*, excision]. Cutting of the *vas deferens*.

deferential (def-er-en'shal) [L. *deferre*, to carry away]. Pert. to or accompanying the ductus deferens.

deferentitis (def-er-en-ti'tis) [" + G. *-itis*, inflammation]. Inflammation of the *vas deferens*.

deferred' shock. Delayed onset of symptoms of shock.

deferves'cence [L. *defervescere*, to become calm]. The period that marks the subsidence of fever to normal temperature.

defibrina'tion, defibriniza'tion [L. *dē*, from, + *fibra*, fiber]. Process of being deprived of fibrin. SEE: *coagulation*.

defi'ciency [L. *deficere*, to lack]. A lack, something missing.

   d. disease. One due to a deficiency of a substance essential in body metabolism.

   The deficiency may be due to inadequate intake, inadequate digestion, inadequate absorption, inadequate utilization, or excessive loss through excretory channels.

   EXAMPLES . . . Night blindness and keratomalacia due to lack of vitamin A; beriberi, polyneuritis, due to lack of thiamine; pellagra due to lack of niacin; ariboflavinosis due to lack of riboflavin; scurvy due to lack of vitamin C; rickets and osteomalacia due to lack of vitamin D; pernicious anemia due to lack of folic acid and vitamin B$_{12}$.

defin'itive. Clear and final; without question.

deflagra'tion [L. *deflagrāre*, to burn furiously]. Sudden, sharp combustion usually with a crackling sound.

defloration (def-lo-ra'shun) [L. *dē*, from, + *flos, flor-*, flower]. The destruction of the hymen, either during coitus, by accident, or vaginal examination. As a rule the tear is in the post. edge.

deflores'cence. Disappearance of an eruption of the skin.

defluvium (dē-flu'vĭ-um) [L. *defluere*, to flow down]. Falling out or loss of the hair.

   d. capilorum. Falling out of the hair.
   d. unguium. Falling of or loss of nails.

defluxion (de-fluk'shun) [L. *defluxio*, a down flowing]. A flowing down; copious discharge or loss of any kind.

deforma'tion [L. *dē*, from, + *forma*, form]. The act of deforming; a disfiguration.

deform'ities. If present after injury, usually imply presence of fracture or dislocation, or both. May be due to extensive swelling, extravasation of blood, rupture of muscles, etc.

deform'ity. An unnatural alteration in the form of a part or organ. Distortion of any part or general disfigurement of the body. It may be acquired or congenital.
RS: *cardiamorphia, cat's ear, chilochisis, Chrobak pelvis, orthomorphia, redressement.*

   d., anterior. Abnormal ant. convexity of the spine. SYN: *lordosis.**

   d., gunstock. One in which the forearm when extended makes an angle with the arm, because of displacement of axis of the extended arm. ETIOL: Condylar fracture at elbow.

   d., Madelung's. Distortion of the radius at its lower end, with ulnar displacement backward.

   d., seal fin. Outward deflection of the fingers in rheumatoid arthritis.

   d., silver-fork. The peculiar deformity seen in Colles' fracture.

   d., Sprengel's. Congenital upward displacement of the scapula.

   d., Velpeau's. Silver-fork deformity, *q.v.*

   d., Volkmann's. Congenital tibiotarsal dislocation.

defunda'tion [L. *dē*, from, + *fundus*]. Excision of the uterine fundus.

defurfura'tion [" + *furfur*, bran]. Shedding of epidermis in scales; branny desquamation.

Deg. Abbr. for *degeneration* or *degree*.

degan'glionate [L. *dē*, from, + G. *ganglion*, tumor]. To deprive of ganglia.

degen'erate [" + *genus*, race]. 1. A sexual pervert; loosely applied to a low mental or moral type. 2. To deteriorate.

degen'erates [L. *degenerāre*, to degenerate]. A term used to include all cellular masses whose staining reactions, form, size, etc., do not admit of classification. Although the number of these cells is determined in each differential they do not enter into the per cents of the differential.

degenera'tion. Deterioration or impairment of an organ or part in structure of cells and the substances of which they are a part.

   ETIOL: Due to changes in size (decrease or increase) and other changes.

   d., Abercrombie's. SEE: *amyloid d.*
   d., adipose. SEE: *fatty d.*
   d., albuminoid. SEE: *amyloid d.*
   d., amyloid. Starch infiltration of tissue in various organs or parts, forcing the cells apart; a condition usually accompanied by pus and suppuration.

   d., ascending. Nerve fiber d. progressing to the center from the periphery.

   d., bacony. SEE: *amyloid d.*
   d., calcareous. Deposits of lime salts in tissues and parts.

   d., caseous. Cheesy alteration in tissues seen in tuberculosis of same.

   d., cloudy swelling. A condition in which protein substances in cells become cloudy, the cells increasing in size, with minute droplets of protein substances. Occurs in infectious diseases, and in those of the kidneys, liver, the heart and its muscles, and in the glands.

   d., colloid. Jellylike disorganization of a part.

   d., cystic. Cyst formation accompanying degeneration.

   d., descending. Nerve fiber d. progressing toward the periphery from the original lesion.

   d., fatty. Disturbance of fat metabolism changing a part into an oily substance.

   d., fibroid. Change of membranous tissue into that of a fibrous nature.

   d., gray. Gray d. in nerve tissue due to chronic inflammation.

   d., hyaline. Caused by hyaline deposits, replacing musculoelastic elements of blood vessels with a firm, transparent substance which causes loss of elasticity. It is responsible for hardening of the arteries and is often followed by calcification or deposit of lime salts in dead tissue. Calcification also may result in concretions.

   d., lardaceous. SEE: *amyloid d.*
   d., mucoid. Disorganization of mucous cells.

   d., myxomatous. SEE: *mucoid d.*

d., parenchymatous. SEE: *cloudy swelling d.*

d., secondary. SEE: *wallerian d.*

d., senile. Bodily and mental changes of the aged.

d., vitreous. SEE: *hyaline d.*

d., wallerian. Nerve fiber d. after separation from its nutritive center.

d., waxy. Amyloid or lardaceous degeneration.

d., Zenker's. Amyloid d. in muscular tissue.

degeneration, words pert. to: amylosis, "ather-" words, athetoid, atrophic, cacogenic, cacothenics, cardiomyoliposis, caseate, -tion, catalysis, cataplasia, ceroma, cerosis, chitinous d., colloid, heart, pythogenesis, sarcomatosis, scirrhous, steatosis, swelling, vitreous.

degen′erative. Pert. to or accompanied by degeneration.

deglu′tible [L. *deglutīre*, to swallow]. Capable of being swallowed.

deglutition (deg-lu-tish′un) [L. *deglutīre*, to swallow]. The act of swallowing.

deglu′titive. Pert. to deglutition.

degusta′tion [L. *degustāre*, to taste]. The sense of taste.

dehiscence (de-his′ens) [L. *dehiscere*, to gape]. A bursting open, as of a graafian follicle.

dehy′drate [L. *dē*, from, + G. *ydōr*, water]. CHEM. to deprive of or lose, or to become free of water.
 MED. To deprive the body or tissues of water.

dehydration (dē-hī-drā′shŭn) [" + G. *ydōr*, water]. The process of dehydrating. Occurs when output of water exceeds water intake. May result from deprivation of water, excessive loss of water, reduction in total quantity of electrolytes, or injection of hypertonic solutions.

dehydroandrosterone (dē-hī-drō-drŏs′tĕr-ōn). SYN: *dehydroisoandrosterone*. An androgenic substance $C_{19}H_{28}O_2$ present in urine with about one-fifth the potency of androsterone.

dehydrocorticosterone (dē-hī-drō-kôrt-ĭ-kŏ-stĕr-ōn). 11-dehydrocorticosterone (Kendall's compound A). $C_{21}H_{28}O_4$. A physiologically active steroid isolated from the adrenal cortex. It is important in water and salt metabolism.

dehydrogenase (dē-hī-drog′ĕn-ās). An enzyme which catalyzes the oxidation of a specific substance causing it to give up its hydrogen.

dehydroisoandrosterone (dē′′hī′drō-ĭ-sō-ăn-drŏs′′ter-ōn). A 17-ketosteroid excreted in normal male urine. It possesses androgenic activity.

Deiters's cells (dī′terz). 1. Supporting cells in organ of Corti. 2. Spider cells of the neuroglia. 3. Neuro cells, the neuraxons of which become the axis cylinders of nerve fibers. SEE: *cell.*

D.'s nucleus. Collection of cells back of the acoustic nucleus.

D.'s process. Axis-cylinder process or neuraxon.

dejecta (de-jek′tă) [L. *dejicere*, to cast down]. Feces; intestinal waste.

dejection, dejecture (de-jek′shun, -ŭr) [L. *dejicere*, to cast down]. 1. A cast down feeling, or mental depression. 2. Defecation or act of defecation.

Dejerine's disease (da-zhĕ-rēns′). Interstitial neuritis of infants.

D.'s syndrome. S. with deep sensitivity repressed but with normal tactile sense, caused by lesion of long root fibers of post. column.

dekanormal (dek-ă-nor′mal) [G. *deka*, ten, + L. *norma*, rule]. Having 10 times the strength of normal, as a solution.

de Kraft blue pencil. Vulcanite fiber tube tightly packed with asbestos powder, metal cap at 1 end for attachment of ground chain, and blue metal tip covers end toward patient. Used for static brush discharge.

delacrima′tion [" + *lacrimāre*, to shed tears]. Epiphora; more or less constant overflow of tears.

delactation (de-lak-ta′shun) [" + *lactāre*, to suckle]. Weaning or cessation of lactation.

delamina′tion [" + *lamina*, plate]. The division into laminae, esp. that of a blastoderm into 2 layers, epiblast and hypoblast.

delayed reflex (dē-lād′). Any in which the response is abnormally delayed.

d. symptoms. Delayed onset of symptoms, as of shock.

delectatio morosa [L.]. Dallying with voluptuous thoughts.

deligation (de-lĭ-ga′shun) [L. *deligāre*, to tie up]. The application of ligatures.

delimita′tion [L. *dē*, down, + *limitāre*, to limit]. Determination of limits of an area or organ in diagnosis.

deliquesce′. To cause liquefication.

deliquescence (del-ik-wes′ens) [L. *deliquescere*, to grow moist]. The process of becoming liquefied as result of absorption of water from the air.

deliquescent (del-ik-wes′ent). Pert. to a substance which absorbs water from the atmosphere.

delire de toucher (de-lĭr-dĕ too-shā′) [Fr.]. An abnormal desire to touch things.

delir′iant [L. *delirāre*, to be out of one's head]. An agent that will produce delirium. Ex: *atropine, hyoscine.*

delirifacient (de-lir′ĭ-fa′shĭ-ent) [" + *facere*, to make]. A drug causing delirium. SYN: *deliriant.*

delirium (de-lĭr′ĭ-um) [L.]. Disorientation for time and place, usually with illusions and hallucinations. A state of mental confusion and excitement.
 The mind wanders and speech is incoherent, and the patient is in a state of continual, aimless physical activity. There are many forms of delirium, depending mainly upon the cause, but 2 main types are generally recognized:
 RS: *alcoholism; carphologia; consciousness, clouding of; dipsomania; fever delirium; mussitation; potomania; restraints.*

d., acute. One developing suddenly and speedily, resulting in recovery or death.

d., alcoholic. SEE: *delirium tremens.*

d., chronic. D. of chronic psychoses, without febrile characteristics.

d. constantium. D. of patients with reiteration of same fixed idea.

d. cordis. Violent heart beat.

d. epilepticum. D. either following an epileptic attack or appearing instead of an attack.

d. e potu. SEE: *d. tremens.*

d. ex inanitione. D. in cases of anemia, occurring usually when fever subsides.

d., febrile. D. occurring with fever.

d. of grandeur. Condition in which patient exaggerates his own power and importance.

d. hystericum. Delirium of hysteria.

d., lingual. Form where meaningless sounds are muttered constantly.

d., maniacal. Often associated with high temperature and acute illness. The low muttering type accompanied by great physical exhaustion, as seen in cases of typhoid fever. Poisoning from certain drugs may induce delirium.

d. metabolicum. Form in which patient feels he is not using his own name and objects and people about him are not in their real characters and that they are spying upon him.

d. mussitans. Excitement causing lingual d.

d. of negation. Form in which patient thinks parts of his body are missing.

d., partial. D. reacting on only a portion of the mental faculties, causing only some of the patient's actions to be unreasonable.

d. of persecution. D. in which patient feels he is being persecuted by those about him.

d., toxic. D. produced by presence of toxins in the body.

d., traumatic. D. following injury or shock.

d. tremens. A psychic disorder involving hallucinations, both visual and auditory, found in habitual users of alcoholic beverages.

The lack of nicotinic acid is a factor in the development of d. t.

SYM: Hallucinations, as seeing snakes or monsters, hearing noises. Patient is excited and usually talking or yelling incoherently.

F. A. TREATMENT: Sedatives, esp. paraldehyde and bromides. Treat for shock if present. Glucose and fluids in large quantities. Induce free perspiration. Restraints may be necessary. Hypodermics of apomorphine hydrochloride may be sedative in the maniacal individual.

NP: The patient must never be left alone for an instant, since attempts at suicide are frequent in such cases. The nursing of delirium needs endless patience, tact, and understanding. Restraint should be avoided if possible.

d., violent. Feverish d. with exaltation and great strength.

delitescence (del-it-es'ens) [L. *delitescere*, to be hidden]. An unusually complete and speedy resolution of an inflammation.

deliver [Fr. *delivrer*, to free]. To aid in childbirth by removal of a fetus or placenta.

delivery [Fr. *delivrer*, to free]. Expulsion of the child at birth with placenta and membranes from the mother. SEE: labor.

d., abdominal. Removal of the child by Cesarean section.

d., forceps. Delivery of the child by the use of tractor instruments.

d., postmortem. Delivery of the child after death of the mother either by the abdominal or vaginal route.

d., precipitate. A precipitate delivery is one that occurs under nonaseptic conditions and when the physician is not present. In the true sense it is one which follows a precipitate labor regardless of who is present.

TO PREVENT A PRECIPITATE DELIVERY: *Watch the patient carefully.*

A multipara needs more careful watching against this predicament than a primipara. However, this should not be taken as an excuse because it is possible for it to occur in a primipara.

Do not wait for the head to be visible in a multipara if she is having frequent hard pains, particularly if they are bearing down in type, but have her seen by the physician immediately. In a primipara it is fairly safe to wait, in the majority of cases, until a small portion of the head is seen at the vaginal orifice during a pain before putting the patient up for delivery.

Remember to watch both the primipara and multipara who has received an analgesia, since precipitation can occur with little or no warning. This means watching for bulging of the perineum during the pains by viewing the vulva and not taking it for granted that because the patient is fairly quiet no progress is being made.

Encourage the patient to breathe through her mouth during each pain so that she does not bear down.

Administer drop ether if local custom permits. If pushed properly it can effectively stop contractions and may be employed safely for a reasonable time to prevent sudden expulsion of the child.

d. premature. Delivery of a fetus after the twenty-eighth week but before full term.

d., spontaneous. Delivery of the child without external aid.

delomorphous (del-o-mor'fus) [G. *dēlos*, evident, + *morphē*, form]. Having definite form and shape.

d. cells. Granular cells which stain easily; found next to basement membrane in stomach; glands in cardiac region.

delousing (de-lows'ing) [L. *dē*, from, + A.S. *lūs*]. Ridding of lice by their destruction.

del'ta for'nicis [L.]. A triangular surface on lower side of fornix; *commissura hippocampi*.

del'toid [G. *delta*, letter d, + *eidos*, resemblance]. Shaped like the Greek letter Δ.

d. ligament. Internal lateral l. of ankle joint.

d. muscle. The *musculus deltoideus*, which covers the shoulder prominence.

d. ridge. Ridge on humerus where deltoid muscle is attached.

de lunat'ico inquiren'do [L.]. Legal process to determine alleged incompetence of a person.

delusion (de-lu'shun) [L. *deludere*, to cheat]. A false belief, as that the individual is Napoleon. Differs from hallucination which involves the false excitation of one or more of the senses.

MOST IMPORTANT DELUSIONS: Those which cause the patient to harm others, or himself, such as: (a) Fear of being poisoned, causing the patient to refuse food; (b) those leading to suicide, or inflicting injury upon self; (c) false beliefs, such as having been guilty of the unpardonable sin; (d) those of persecution.

d., depressive. One causing a saddened state.

d., expansive. Conviction of one's own fineness, power or importance.

d., fixed. Those that remain unaltered.

d., fleeting. These come and go.

d. of grandeur. A false sense of possessing wealth or power.

d. of negation. SEE: nihilistic d.

d., nihilistic (ni-hil-is'tik). One that causes the victim to believe that everything has ceased to exist.

d. of persecution. D. in which patient feels everyone about him is against him.

d., reference. One that causes the victim to read a meaning not intended in the acts or words of others, usually an interpretation of slight or ridicule.

d., systematized. Logical correlation with false reasoning and deduction.

d., unsystematized. D. without any correlation between ideas and surroundings.

delu′sional [L. *deludere*, to cheat]. Pert. to a delusion.

dement′ [L. *de*, from, + *mens*, mind]. One who has lost his sanity.

demented (de-men′ted). Of unsound mind.

dementia (de-men′shi-ä) [L. *de*, from, + *mens*, mind]. Irrecoverable deteriorative mental state, the common end result of many entities.

SEE: *cataphrenia; table*, p. D-10.

d., alcoholic. D. in terminal portion of chronic alcoholic state.

d., apathetic. D. with diminished sensitivity, occurring in the last stages of disease, usually.

d., apoplectic. Form following cerebral hemorrhage or tumors.

d., catatonic. A form of d. precox.

d., chronic. An incurable form occurring at any time of life.

d., epileptic. That accompanied by mental deterioration, and due to long continued epilepsy.

d. naturalis. Congenital form; idiocy.

d., organic. D. caused by lesions of nerve centers.

d. paralytica. Paresis or general paralysis of the insane. A paretic form of neurosyphilis occurring in syphilitics, characterized by progressive dementia and a diffuse generalized paralysis. Generally terminates in death if untreated. ETIOL: Antecedent syphilitic infection. DURATION: Several months to 3 or 4 years.

IN GENERAL: (1) Often seen in the young who have inherited syphilis, usually 10 or 20 years later. (2) If not treated, lead to deterioration, physical and mental, eventually fatal. (3) Sometimes classified into 3 common types, spoken of as the *deluded*, the *depressed*, and the *demented*. (4) Without treatment, the disease may pass through 3 stages of development.

THE DELUDED TYPE: *The First Stage*: (1) Memory defective. (2) Very excitable. (3) Hallucinations of hearing. (4) Judgment defect. (5) Weaken self control. (6) Acute excitement may occur. (7) Peculiar "in and out" movement of tongue. "Trombone tremor." (8) Slurred, hesitating speech with drawling. (9) Ankle and knee jerks absent, increased, or floppy. (10) Restlessness and irritability. (11) Pleased with self. (12) Delusions of grandeur. (13) Feels unusually well. (14) Feels able to work when not fit. (15) Mental weakness steadily progresses. (16) Tremors of tongue, face, and hands. (17) Unsteady gait. (18) Loss of facial expression due to muscular weakness. (19) Irregular, unequal pupils without reflex to light. (20) Difficult urination.

The Second Stage: (1) About beginning of 2nd year. (2) Delusions may be repeated but gradually forgotten. (3) Dull, stupid; shows no emotion. (4) Seizures occur. (5) Patient becomes dull and flushed, then unconscious. (6) Unconsciousness may last few minutes to an hour. (7) Seizures resemble epilepsy but less severe. (8) Seizures followed by hemiplegia or monoplegia. (9) Congestive attacks. (10) Rise of temperature before seizure. (11) Physical signs more marked. (12) Muscular weakness shown in gait, handwriting and in speech. (13) Often becomes fat.

The Third Stage: (1) Little interest shown except in food. (2) Evidence of mind disappears. (3) Grinding of teeth. (4) Becomes wasted. (5) Unable to control excretions. (6) Becomes bedridden. (7) Seizures may continue.

THE DEPRESSED TYPE: (1) Remissions not so common. (2) Depression. (3) Physical signs same as the deluded type. (4) Runs longer course. (5) Delusions of unworthiness or persecution. (6) Delusions are of much greater magnitude.

THE DEMENTED TYPE: (1) All become demented but not noticeable from the start. (2) Run a prolonged course. (3) Delusions do not occur. (4) Dull, forgetful, unable to work. (5) Commonest type in females.

TREATMENT: Most effective treatment is artificial fever therapy for not less than 50 hr., at 105° F. in 10-15 sessions, combined with chemotherapy.

NURSING OF GENERAL PARALYTICS: (1) Patient must be under constant observation. (2) Their bones are fragile, hence they should be handled carefully. (3)

Main Differential Diagnosis of Schizophrenia and Manic Depressive Psychoses

Findings in Mental Examination	Schizophrenia	Manic Reaction	Depressive Reaction
1. General behavior and activity.	Odd, incongruous, silliness, irrelevance, and incoherence of stream of thought.	Pressure of talk and activity. Flight of ideas and distractability.	Slowness of thought and activity. Depressed facies.
2. Affective disorder present.	Loss of affect or inadequate affect.	A frank elation or quick oscillations.	A frank depression.
3. Trend reactions.	Delusions of various types, ideas of reference, ideas of influence, paranoid ideas. Hallucinations usually prominent.	Expansive ideas to fit in with elation. No hallucinations.	Self-condemnation and self-recrimination to fit in with depressive affect. Hallucinations rare.
4. Sensorium changes.	Sensorium generally clear. Insight usually absent.	May be clouded. Insight may be present.	Often clouded. Insight often present.

Prevent decubitus. (4) Artificial fever is sometimes induced. (5) Must be kept warm during rigors. (6) If patient has convulsions, he must be watched carefully to prevent him from injuring himself. (7) Watch for distended bladder. (8) Check on elimination. (9) Avoid all quarreling. (10) Patients have a tendency to eat greedily and may have difficulty in swallowing. Care must be exercised to prevent choking. (11) Watch for possible collapse. (12) Death may occur during a seizure. [noid tendencies.

d. paranoides. D. precox with para-
d., paretic. Paralytic dementia, q.v.
d., postfebrile. D. following severe cases of infectious diseases.
d. precox. Though a disease entity, it is best replaced by the term "schizophrenia,"* since it is not always associated with dementia nor always occurring in the young. It has been characterized as a "dream state," a psychosis represented by a dreaming mind in a sleeping body, the latter being easily aroused but not the former. Twenty per cent of the patients in the hospitals of the U. S. are afflicted with this psychosis.
d., presenile. One beginning in the 5th decade. SYM: Apathy, loss of memory, disturbances of speech and gait.
d., secondary. D. occurring after a primary mental disease, such as mania.
d., senile. That occurring in the aged. SYM: Progressive mental deterioration with loss of memory, esp. for recent events, with occasional intercurrent attacks of excitement. [syphilis.
d., syphilitic. D. caused by lesion of
d., terminal. D. following another form of mental disease. SEE: secondary d. [use of some drug.
d., toxic. That due to the excessive

demerol (dĕm'er-ŏl). A white, colorless, crystalline compound, soluble in water, having a neutral reaction and an analgesic effect similar to morphine.

demi- [L.]. Prefix: Half.

demilune cells (dem'ĭ-lūn) [L. demi, half, + luna, moon]. Collection of marginal cells in form of a half moon in submaxillary gland.

demineraliza'tion [L. de, from, + minare, to mine]. Loss of salts by excessive secretion and excretion. [Death.

demise' [L. demittere, to send from].

Dem'odex. Genus of mites and ticks of the class Arachnida and order Acarina.
D. folliculo'rum. The pimple mite, which often infests hair sacs and sebaceous follicles.

demog'raphy [G. demos, the people, + graphein, to write]. Statistical study of births, marriages, and deaths, and physical, moral, and intellectual development.

demonoma'nia [G. daimon, devil, + mania, madness]. Obsolete term for psychotic belief that one is possessed by demons.

demonop'athy [" + pathos, disease]. A mania in which one is convinced of being possessed of devils. SYN: demonomania.

Demours' membrane (de-moorz'). A fine membrane bet. the endothelial layer of the cornea and the substantia propria. SYN: Descemet's membrane, lamina elastica posterior.

demucosa'tion [L. dē, from, + mucus]. Excision of mucosa of any part of body.

demul'cent [L. demulcere, to stroke softly]. An agent that will soothe the part or soften the skin to which applied. The term is usually restricted to agents acting on mucous membrane. Ex: Glycerin, honey, lanolin, milk, mucilage of acacia, mucilage of tragacanth, olive oil.

demutiza'tion [L. dē, down, + mutus, mute]. Overcoming mutism by teaching the patient to speak or to use the sign language.

dena'tured [" + natura, nature]. Subject to having the nature of a substance changed, or to render unfit for consumption, as alcohol, q.v.

dendraxon (den-drak'son) [G. dendron, tree, + axōn, axle]. The terminal filaments of the neuraxon of a nerve cell.

den'dric. Pert. to or possessing a dendron.

dendriform (den'drĭ-form) [G. dendron, tree, + L. forma, shape]. Branching or like a tree in shape.

den'drite [G. dendrĭtēs, pert. to a tree]. A branched protoplasmic process of a neuron which conducts impulses to the cell body. There are usually several to a cell. They form synaptic connections with other neurons.
d. extracapsular. Dendrites of neurons of autonomic ganglia which pierce the capsule surrounding the cell and which extend for considerable distances from the cell body.
d. intracapsular. Dendrites of neurons of autonomic ganglia which ramify beneath the capsule forming a network about the cell body.

dendrit'ic. Treelike in form.
d. calculus. A renal stone molded in the form of the pelvis and calyces.

dendroid (den'droid) [G. dendron, tree, + eidos, form]. 1. Dendriform, pert. to dendrites. 2. Arborescent, treelike.

dendron (den'dron) [G. tree]. A dendrite. A protoplasmic branch from a nerve cell.

dendrophagocytosis (den″dro-fag-o-sī-to'-sis) [" + phagein, to eat, + kytos, cell, + -ōsis, infection]. The absorption of portions of astrocytes by microglia cells.

dener'vated [L. dē, from, + G. neuron, nerve]. 1. Excision, incision, or blocking of a nerve supply. 2. A condition in which the nerve supply is blocked or cut off.

dengue (deng'ga) [Sp]. Acute, epidemic, febrile disease lasting 8 days, seldom fatal.
ETIOL: A virus transmitted by the mosquito, Aedes aegyoti.
SYM: Two fever periods with intermissions; eruptions similar to measles; severe pain in muscles and joints. SEE: breakbone fever.

denidation (den-id-a'shun) [L. dē, from, + nidus, nest]. Removal during menstruation of the nidus of a fertilized ovum.

dens (pl. dentes) [L.]. 1. A tooth. 2. The odontoid process of the axis. A process on the body of the axis which serves as a pivot for the rotation of the atlas.
d. bicuspidus. The bicuspid tooth, d. premolaris. BNA.
d. caninus. BNA. The canine tooth.
d. deciduus. BNA. Milk tooth, first tooth.
d. incisivus. BNA. Incisor tooth.
d. molaris. BNA. Molar tooth, grinder.
d. permanens. BNA. One of the 32 teeth making up the permanent denture.
d. sapientiae. Late tooth, wisdom tooth. d. serotinus. BNA.

densimeter (den-sim'e-ter) [L. densus, thick, + G. metron, measure]. Instrument for measuring densities.

densitom'eter [" + G. metron, measure]. A special densimeter for measuring bac-

density   D-12   **dentinosteoid**

terial growth and effect upon it of antiseptics and bacteriophages.

den′sity [L. *densitās*, thickness]. 1. Relative weight of a substance compared with some other substance of equal bulk. 2. The quality of being dense.

dentag′ra [L. *dens*, tooth, + G. *agra*, seizure]. Toothache.

den′tal. Pert. to the teeth.

   d. **arch.** The arch formed by the cutting and chewing surfaces of the teeth.

   d. **caries.** Decay of the teeth. SEE: caries.

   d. **curve.** The curve or bow of the line of the teeth in the jaw. The different portions of the curve are described as follows: *Alignment c.* The line passing through the center of the teeth from the middle line through the last molar. *Buccal c.* The curve extending from the cuspid to the 3rd molar. *Compensating c.* The occlusal line of bicuspids and molars. *Labial c.* The curve extending from cuspid to cuspid.

   d. **disk.** A thin, circular piece of paper, or cloth, or other substance charged with abrasive powder for cutting or polishing teeth and fillings.

   d. **engine.** A machine operated with foot power, or by an electric or a water motor, to give a swift rotary motion to drills, burs, and burnishers.

   d. **formula.** A method of expressing briefly the dentition of mammals in which the numbers of the teeth are given in the form of a fraction, the numbers of the upper teeth forming the denominator, those of the lower teeth the numerator.

The dental formula of man is:

i. $\frac{2-2}{2-2}$ c. $\frac{1-1}{1-1}$ b. or pm. $\frac{2-2}{2-2}$ m $\frac{3-3}{3-3}$ 32.

dentalgia (den-tal′ji-ă) [L. *dens*, tooth, + G. *algos*, pain]. Toothache.

dentaphone (den′tă-fōn) [" + G. *phōnē*, sound]. Device for conveying sound through the teeth.

dentate (den′tāt) [L. *dentātus*, toothed]. Notched; having short triangular divisions of the margin; toothed.

den′tes [L.]. Teeth; plural of *dens*, q.v.

dentibuc′cal [L. *dens*, tooth, + *bucca*, cheek]. Pert. to both the cheek and teeth.

dent′icle. A small toothlike projection.

dentic′ulate [L. *denticulatus*, small toothed]. Finely toothed.

   d. **body.** Corpus dentatum.

dentifica′tion [L. *dens*, tooth, + *facere*, to make]. Conversion into dental structure.

dentifrice (den′tif-ris) [" + *fricāre*, to rub]. A powder or other substance for cleaning teeth.

dentigerous (den-tij′er-us) [" + *gerere*, to bear]. Having or containing teeth.

dentila′bial [" + *labium*, lip]. Pert. to both teeth and lips.

dentilin′gual [" + *lingua*, tongue]. Pert. to both teeth and tongue.

dentim′eter [" + G. *metron*, measure]. Device for measuring teeth.

den′tinal. Pert. to dentine.

dentine, dentin (den′tēn, den′tin) [L. *dens*, tooth]. The osseous tissues of a tooth, enclosing the pulp cavity.

dentinifica′tion [" + *facere*, to make]. Formation of dentine.

dentini′tis [" + G. *-itis*, inflammation]. Inflammation of dentine.

dentinogenesis (děn-tĭn-ō-jěn′ĕ-sis). Formation of dentine in development of a tooth.

   d. **imperfecta.** Aplasia or hypoplasia of the enamel and dentine of a tooth.

   d. **nucleus.** A mass of gray matter in the medulla of each cerebellar hemisphere.

den′tinoid [" + G. *eidos*, form]. 1. Resembling dentine. 2. A tumor arising from dentine.

dentino′ma [" + G. *-ōma*, tumor]. A dentine tumor.

dentinos′teoid [" + G. *osteon*, bone, + *eidos*, form]. Small tumor arising from dentine. SYN: *dentinoid*.

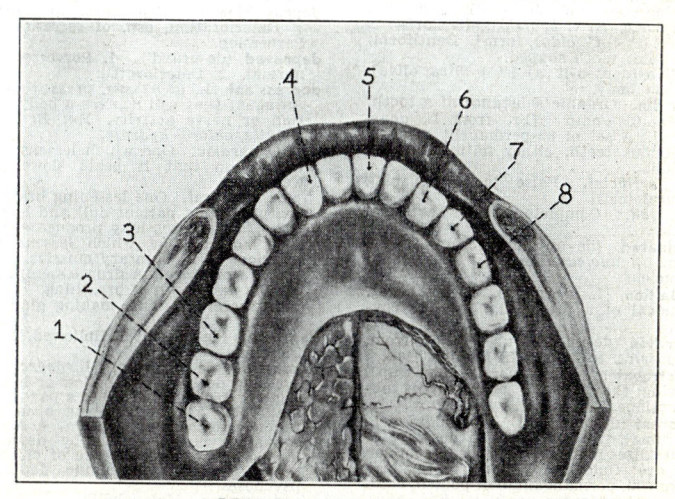

DENTITION—TEETH IN SITU
1. Third molar. 2. Second molar. 3. First molar. 4. Lateral incisor. 5. Central incisor. 6. Canine. 7. First premolar. 8. Second premolar.

dentist   D-13   **depression, cardiac**

den'tist [L. *dens*, tooth]. A practitioner of dentistry.

dent'istry. That branch of medicine which deals with the care of the teeth and associated structures. It is concerned with the prevention, diagnosis, and treatment of diseases of the teeth, and gums. 2. The art or profession of a dentist.
   d. esthetic. Repair and restoration or replacement of carious or broken teeth.
   d., operative. Phase dealing with dental operations on mouth as contrasted with dental laboratory work.
   d. prosthodontia (prŏs-thō-dŏn'shĭ-ă). The art of replacing defective or missing teeth through the use of artificial appliances such as bridges, crowns, artificial dentures, etc.

denti'tion [L. *dentitiō*]. The process and time of teething. SEE: p. D-12.
   d., primary. Eruption of 20 deciduous, or milk teeth. ORDER OF ERUPTION: Two central incisors, lower; 7th month. Four central and lateral incisors, upper, 8th and 10th months. Two lateral incisors, lower, 12th to 14th month. Four frontal molars, 12th to 14th month. Four canines, 18th to 20th month. Four post. molars, 24th to 30th month.
   d., secondary (32 teeth). The eruption of the permanent teeth, beginning at about the age of six. Completed by the 15th year with the exception of the "wisdom" teeth, which appear bet. the 18th and 25th years. ORDER OF ERUPTION: The incisors and canines are followed by the same teeth. The frontal molars are followed by 1st bicuspids. The post. molars are followed by 2nd bicuspids, then the 1st, 2nd and 3rd molars follow. SEE: *teeth*.
   SYN: *odontiasis, teething*.

dentoalve'olar [L. *dens*, tooth, + *alveolus*, small hollow]. Pert. to alveolus of a tooth.

dentoalveoli'tis [" + " + G. *-itis*, inflammation]. A purulent inflammation of the tooth socket linings, characterized by looseness of the teeth and gum shrinkage. SYN: *pyorrhea alveolaris*.

den'toid [" + G. *eidos*, form]. Dentiform; odontoid; tooth shaped.

dentoliva (dent-o-li'va) [" + *oliva*, olive]. Olivary body.

dentor'din. Organic substance of a tooth.

denture (den'chur) [Fr. from L. *dens*, tooth]. A set of 32 permanent or of 20 deciduous teeth, either natural or artificial.
   d., artificial. False teeth replacing natural teeth.
   d., full. Complete set of artificial teeth.

denucleated (de-nu'kle-āt-ed) [L. *dē*, from, + *nucleus*, kernel]. Deprived of a nucleus.

denuda'tion [L. *denudāre*, to lay bare]. Removal of a protecting layer or covering.

denutrition (de-nu-trish'un) [L. *dē*, from, + *nutrīre*, to nourish]. Malnutrition.

deob'struent [" + *obstruere*, to block up]. Having the property of removing obstructions.

deodorant (de-ō'dor-ant) [" + *odorāre*, to perfume]. An agent which destroys or neutralizes foul odors. Those in common use are: Chloride of lime, creolin, izal, iodoform, permanganate of potash, chlorine and hydrogen peroxide. SEE: *odor*.

deodorize (de-o'dor-īz) [" + *odor*, odor]. To remove foul odor.

deodorizer (de-o'dor-ī-zer) [" + *odor*, odor]. That which deodorizes.

deontology (de-on-tol'o-jĭ) [G. *deonta*, things to be done, + *logos*, study of]. Medical ethics.

deoppila'tion [L. *dē*, from, + *oppilāre*, to stop up]. The doing away with obstructions.

deor'sum [L.]. Downward or turning downward.
   d. ver'gens. Turning downward.

deorsumduction (de-or"sum-duk'shun) [L. *deorsum*, downward, + *ducere*, to lead]. Bending downward.

deos'sification (dē-ŏs-ĭ-fĭ-kā'shŭn) [L. *dē*, from, + *os*, bone, + *facere*, to make]. Loss of or the removal of mineral matter from bone or osseous tissue.

deox'idate [" + G. *oxys*, sharp]. To deprive a chemical of oxygen.

deoxida'tion [" + *oxys*, sharp]. Process of depriving of oxygen.

deoxidizer (de-ok'sĭ-di-zer) [" + *oxys*, sharp]. A deoxidizing substance.

depersonaliza'tion [" + L. *persona*, person]. A sense of being someone else; a lessened sense of one's own identity.

depilate (dep'il-ate) [L. *depilāre*, to pluck out hair]. To strip of hair.

depilation (dep-il-a'shun) [L. *de* + *pilus*, hair]. The process of hair removal. SEE: *epilation*.

depil'atory [" + *pilus*, hair]. An agent used for the removal of hair.

deplete (de-plēt') [" + *plēre*, to fill]. To empty, as in blood letting; to produce depletion.

depletion (de-ple'shun) [" + *plēre*, to fill]. Withdrawal of fluid, esp. the blood.

deplumation (de-plu-ma'shun) [" + *pluma*, down]. Falling of eyelashes as result of disease.

depolariza'tion (dē-pō"lăr-ĭ-zā'shŭn) [" + *polus*, pole]. The process of reducing to a nonpolarized condition; destruction of polarity.

deposit (de-poz'it) [" + *ponere*, to place]. 1. Sediment. 2. Matter collected in any part of an organism, normal or otherwise.

deprava'tion [L. *depravāre*, to impair]. 1. Deterioration, esp. of secretions. 2. Perversion.

depraved (de-prāvd'). 1. Perverted; abnormal. 2. Deteriorated.

depress'ant [L. *depressus*, pressed down]. An agent that will depress a body function or nerve activity. Ex: Bromides, aconite, chloral hydrate.
   d., cardiac. One which lessens heart action, so that it beats slower and weaker.
   d., cerebral. One lessening brain activity, making patient dull and less active. Large doses may produce sleep.
   d., motor. One which lessens contractions of involuntary muscles.
   d., respiratory. A drug lessening frequency and depth of breathing.
   d., secretory. One making gland secretions less.

depressed (de-prest'). 1. Hollowed. 2. Low in spirits.

depression (de-presh'un) [L. *depressiō*, a pressing down]. 1. A hollow or lowered region. 2. The lowering of a part as the mandible. 3. The lowering of a vital function such as respiration. 4. A mental state characterized by dejection, lack of hope, and absence of cheerfulness. Observed in manic depressive psychoses.
   d., averse. Melancholia.
   d., cardiac. Notch in ant. margin of left lung for the cardiac apex.

depressomotor [" + *motor*, mover]. A drug which diminishes muscular movements by lessening the impulses for motion sent from the brain or spinal cord.

depressor (de-pres'or) [L.]. Instrument for depressing a part.
  d. nerve. A nerve, the stimulation of which brings about a fall in blood pressure through reflex vasodilation and slowing of heart beat.
  d. reflex. More or less transient stimulation of depressor fibers.
  d., tongue. Device used to flatten tongue for throat examinations.

dep'rimens oc'uli [L.]. *Musculus rectus inferior*.

depri'val [L. *dē*, from, + *privāre*, to remove]. Deprived of or without organs, parts, or functions.

depriva'tion [" + *privāre*, to remove]. Deprival.

deprive'ment [" + *privāre*, to remove]. Being without function, parts or organs. Syn: *deprival*.

depuliza'tion [" + *pulex*, flea]. Destruction of fleas which carry the plague bacillus.

dep'urant [L. *depurāre*, to purify]. A medicine that purifies through the removal of *excreta*.

depura'tion [L. *depurāre*, to purify]. Process of freeing from impurities.

dep'urative. Cleansing.

depura'tor [L. *dē* + *purus*, pure]. 1. That which purifies. 2. An emunctory.

deradenitis (der-a-den-ī'tis) [G. *derē*, neck, + *adēn*, gland]. Inflammation of a lymph gland of the neck.

deradenoncus (der-ad"e-non'kus) [" + *ogkos*, tumor]. Swelling or tumor of a neck gland.

derangement (de-rānj'ment) [Fr. disorder]. Disorder of the mental functions, especially those involving the intellect.

deratization (de-rat"i-za'shun) [L. *dē*, from, + *rattus*, rat]. Extermination of rats.

Derbyshire neck (dar'be-shĕr). Goiter.

Dercum's disease (der'kŭm). Dystrophy of subcutaneous connective tissue; painful. Syn: *adiposis dolorosa, paratrophy*.

dereistic (de-re-is'tik). Pert. to overexercise of the imagination to the extent of ignoring reality, as seen in day dreaming.

der'ic (der'ik) [G. *deros*, skin]. Pertaining to the skin or surface of the body as distinguished from enteric.

derivation (der-iv-a'shun) [L. *derivāre*, to draw off]. Diversion of fluids from 1 to another part.

deriv'ative [L. *derivāre*, to draw off]. 1. That which is not original or fundamental. 2. Anything derived from another body or substance. 3. That which produces derivation. 4. In embryology that which develops from a preceding structure as the derivatives of the germ layers.

derm, derma [G. *derma*, skin]. The *cutis vera*, or true skin.

Dermacentor (dĕr-mă-sĕnt'or). A genus of ticks belonging to the order Acarina, family Ixodidae.
  D. andersoni. The wood tick, a species of ticks which is parasitic on man or other mammals during some part of their life cycle. May transmit causative agents of Rocky Mountain spotted fever, tularemia, anaplasmosis, brucellosis, Q fever, and several forms of virus encephalomyelitis, also causes tick paralysis.
  D. variabilis. A species of ticks similar to *D. andersoni*. The larvae infest rodents; adults, principally dogs, but may infest man. May transmit same diseases as *D. andersoni*.

der'mad [G. *derma*, skin, + L. *ad*, toward]. Toward the skin; externally.

dermagra (der-mag'rā). [" + *agra*, seizure]. A deficiency disease. Syn: Debility, gastrointestinal disturbance, erythema, convulsions, and nervous and mental disorders. Syn: *Pellagra*.

dermal. Relating to the skin or derma.

dermalax'ia [G. *derma*, skin, + *malaxis*, softening]. Morbid relaxation or softness of the skin.

dermalgia (der-mal'jĭ-ă) [" + *algos*, pain]. Pain in the skin.

dermametropathism (der"mă-mĕ-trŏp'ă-thizm) [" + *metron*, measure, + *pathos*, disease]. Diagnosis of skin disease by observing the markings made by drawing a blunt pencil across the skin.

dermamyiasis (der-mă-mī-i'ă-sis) [" + *myia*, fly]. Skin disease caused by invasion of larva of dipterous insects.

dermanaplasty (derm-an'ă-plas-tī) [" + *anaplassein*, to reform]. Skin grafting.

dermapos'tasis [" + *apostasis*, a falling away]. Abscess formation accompanying a disease of the skin.

dermat-, dermato- [G.]. Prefixes: Skin.

dermatagra (derm-ă-tag'rā) [G. *derma*, skin, + *agra*, seizure]. 1. Pellagra. 2. Dermatalgia. 3. Gouty affection of the skin.

dermatalgia (derm-ă-tal'jĭ-ă) [" + *algos*, pain]. Paresthesia with localized pain in the skin. Syn: *dermalgia*.

dermatatrophia (derm-at-ă-tro'fī-ă) [" + *atrophia*, atrophy]. Atrophy of the skin.

dermatauxe (der-mă-tawk'sē) [" + *auxē*, increase]. Hypertrophy of the skin.

dermatitis (der-mat-i'tis) [" + *-itis*, inflammation]. Inflammation of skin evidenced by itching, redness and various skin lesions.
  Etiol.: Lack of Vitamin G, skin irritants, as poison ivy, corrosives, acids, alkalies or hypersusceptibility on part of patient.
  Treatment: Remove irritant by washing with soap and water, then by alcohol and ether. Dress with calamine lotion or bland oils or ointment.
  d. aestivalis [L. *aestiva*, summer]. Hot weather dermatitis.
  d. calorica [L. *calor*, heat]. That due to heat or cold, as sunburn, etc.
  d. cercarial. Dermatitis resulting from infestation with the cercaria of blood flukes belonging to the genus *Schistosoma*; Achistosome dermatitis or swimmer's itch.
  d. congelationis [L. *congelatio*, cold]. Frostbite, chilblain. See: *chilblain*.
  d. exfoliativa. Acute or subacute inflammation of the skin commonly involving whole surface and characterized by redness and abundant flaky desquamation.
  Etiol: Unknown.
  Sym: May be primary with constitutional symptoms (fever, debility, and gastrointestinal upset), with sudden eruption, pink turning dark red, followed by thin, flaky, loosely adherent, grayish or brownish scales, tender skin, tension and stiffness. In secondary type it follows certain scaly diseases of the skin (eczema, seborrheic dermatitis, psoriasis); pigmentation (slate or mahogany color) is frequent.
  Prog: Guarded. Recurrences are frequent and sometimes death follows.

TREATMENT: Attention to general health (drugs, tonics internally). Locally, soothing oily applications. SYN: *pityriasis rubra.*

d. gangraenosa. Skin inflammation of gangrenous form.

d. herpetiformis. Chronic, inflammatory disease characterized by erythematous, papular, vesicular, bullous, or pustular lesions with tendency to grouping and with itching and burning.
ETIOL: Direct cause unknown. Occurs mostly in adult males though no age is exempt.
SYM: Slight; constitutional. Lesions develop suddenly and spread peripherally. Disease is variable and erratic and attack may be prolonged for weeks or months. Secondary infection may follow from trauma.
PROG: Amelioration of attack, but permanent relief cannot be promised.
TREATMENT: Removal of sources of reflex irritation. Arsenic, sodium cacodylate, thyroid (with circumspection), quinine. Soothing mixtures externally. Excoriated areas to be protected by mild antiseptics.

d. hiemalis [L. *hiems*, winter]. Dermatitis occurring in cold weather.

d. infectiosa eczematoides. Pustular eruption during or following a pyogenic disease. SYN: *Engman's disease.*

d. medicamentosa. Drug eruption.
ETIOL: Idiosyncrasy or sensitization to the drug in question. Most probably anaphylactoid, not true anaphylactic reaction. Cosmetics, arsenic (wallpaper, etc.), butyn, phenobarbital, etc., are some of the 50 drugs reported.
SYM: With exception of bromine and iodine, the eruption is not characteristic and may resemble almost any condition or disease.
TREATMENT: Removal of cause, saline cathartics, and alkaline diuretics.

d. multiformis. Form with lesions of a pustular nature.

d. papillaris capillitii. Formation on scalp and neck of surface elevations interspersed with pustules and ending in scarlike elevations resembling keloids.

d. repens. Inflammatory disease of the skin following injury.
ETIOL: Uncertain. One theory is of peripheral neuritis with secondary parasitic invasion. *Staphylococcus albus* may be present.
SYM: Serous undermining of upper layers of epidermis with formation of numerous white abscesses in adjacent rete. Begins as localized redness with vesiculation or pustulation, spreading until central patch of glazed, denuded rete is surrounded by ragged border of slightly elevated, serously undermined horny epidermis. Denuded areas may be entirely healed before peripheral extension takes place.
PROG: Rebellious to treatment.
TREATMENT: Removal of material for bacteriologic examination and autogenous vaccine. Locally Ruggles' mixture (salicylic acid, tannic acid, alcohol), or potassium permanganate, and boric acid, formalin, silver nitrate.

d. seborrheica. Acute or subacute inflammatory skin disease beginning on the scalp, characterized by rounded, irregular, or circinate lesions covered with yellowish or brownish-gray greasy scales.
ETIOL: Lowered vitality, indigestion, excessive amounts of certain foods (fats) are predisposing factors. Probably mildly infectious though not yet definitely proved.
SYM: On the scalp it may be dry with abundant grayish branny scales, or oozing and crusted, constituting eczema capitis,* and may spread to forehead and postauricular regions. On the forehead it shows scaly and infiltrated lesions with dark red bases, some itching, localized loss of hair; on eyebrows and eyelashes dry, dirty white scales, itching; on nasolabial folds or vermilion border of lips (SEE: *Cheilitis exfoliativa*); on sternal region, greasy and unctuous to the touch; in interscapular, axillary, and genitocrural regions.
TREATMENT: Care to general health, restricted diet eliminating fatty foods. For inflamed areas: Soothing ointments. For cleansing: Benzine followed by sweet or olive oil. No soap or water. Silver nitrate, sulfur, resorcin, ammoniated mercury, or salicylic acid.
SYN: *alopecia furfuracea, pityriasis capitis, seborrhea corporis, seborrhea sicca.*

d. venenata. Any inflammation caused by local action of various animal, vegetable, or mineral substances on the surface of the skin. Commonly called ivy poisoning.
ETIOL: Drugs, acids, alkalies, plants. Runs an acute course with recurrence.
SYM: Vary from simple hyperemia to gangrene and sloughing. Majority are erythematous, limited to part touched by irritant, becoming papular, vesicular, or pustular with burning or itching.
TREATMENT: Incision and drainage of bullae followed by alcohol sponge and preceded by soap and water to remove toxicodendron (poison ivy) oil. Locally aluminum acetate, lead acetate or lead lactate, or lead and opium water freely on gauze. When dry and scaly, calamine ointment by day and carbolized zinc oil by night. No soap and water until lesions heal. In ivy poisoning internal administration of rhus toxicodendron in minute doses cautiously increased. SEE: *skin.*

d. verrucosa. SYN: *Chromoblastomycosis q. v.* A dermatitis characterized by the formation of wartlike nodules on the skin. These may enlarge and form papillomatous structures which sometimes ulcerate.
ETIOL: A fungus, *Hormodendrum pedrosoi.*

d., x-ray. Skin inflammation due to overdose of x-ray.

dermatoautoplasty (der″mat-o-aw′to-plas-tĭ) [" + *autos*, self, + *plassein*, to form]. Grafting of skin taken from some portion of the patient's own body.

Dermatobia (dĕr-mă-tō′bĭ-a). A genus of bot-flies belonging to the order *diptera*, family *Cuterebridae.*

D. hominis. A species of bot-flies found in parts of tropical America whose larvae infest man and cattle. The eggs are transported by mosquitoes of the genus *Psorphora.*

dermatobia′sis (der-mat-o-bī′as-is) [" + *bios*, life]. Infestation by the larvae of *Dermatobia hominis.* The larvae live in the skin forming marblelike boils.

dermatocele (der′mă-to-sēl) [" + *kēlē*, hernia]. Tendency of hypertrophied skin and subcutaneous tissue to hang loosely in folds. SYN: *dermatolysis.*

d. lipomato′sis. A pedunculated lipoma with cystic degeneration.

dermatocelidosis (der-mat-o-kel-i-do'sis) [G. *derma*, skin, + *kēlis*, spot, + *-ōsis*]. Freckles; a macular eruption.

dermatocellulitis (der-mat-o-sel-u-li'tis) [" + L. *cellula*, little cell, + G. *-itis*, inflammation]. Inflammation of subcutaneous connective tissue.

dermatoconiosis (der-mat-o-kon-i-o'sis) [" + *konia*, dust]. Occupational dermatitis caused by the irritation of dust.

dermatocyst (der'mat-o-sist) [" + *kystis*, cyst]. A skin cyst.

dermatodynia [" + *odynē*, pain]. Pain in the skin; dermatalgia.*

dermatofibroma [" + L. *fibra*, fiber, + G. *-ōma*, tumor]. A skin fibroma.

dermatogen (der-mat'o-jen) [" + *gennan*, to form]. Antigen from a skin disease.

dermatogenous [" + *gennan*, to produce]. Of the nature of or producing skin or disease of skin.

dermatoglyphics (der-mă-to-glif'ĭks) [" + *glyphē*, a carving]. Study of surface markings of the skin, esp. those of hands and feet.

dermat'ograph [" + *graphein*, to write]. 1. A device for marking the body for diagnosis. 2. A wheal made on the skin in dermatography.

dermatographia, dermatog'raphy [" + *graphein*, to write]. 1. A treatise on the skin. 2. A form of urticaria in which wheals are made by pressure.

der"matohet'eroplasty [" + *eteros*, other, + *plassein*, to mold]. Grafting with grafts from another's skin.

dermatoid (der'mă-toid) [" + *eidos*, form]. Resembling skin.

dermatokelidosis (der-mat-o-kē-li-do'sis) [" + *kēlidoun*, to stain]. A macular eruption; freckle.

dermatol'ogist [" + *logos*, understanding]. A skin specialist.

dermatol'ogy [" + *logos*, understanding]. The science of the skin and its diseases.

dermatolysis (der-mă-tol'is-is) [" + *lysis*, a loosening]. Tendency of hypertrophied skin and subcutaneous tissue to hang in folds. Loose skin. SYN: *cutis laxa, cutis pendula.*

dermatoma (G. *derma*, skin, + *-ōma*, growth]. Circumscribed thickening of skin.

dermatome (der'ma-tōm) [" + *tomē*, incision]. 1. Instrument for incising the skin or for cutting thin transplants of skin. 2. A segmental skin area innervated by various spinal cord segments. 3. The lateral portion of the somite of an embryo which gives rise to the dermis of the skin; the cutis plate.

dermatomere (der'mă-to-mēr) [" + *meros*, part]. A segment of embryonic integument.

dermatomucosomyositis (der"ma-to-mŭ-ko"so-mi-o-si'tis) [" + L. *mucosa*, mucous membrane, + G. *mys*, muscle, + *-itis*, inflammation]. Inflammation of the skin, involving mucosa and muscles.

dermatomycosis (der"mat-o-mi-ko'sis) [" + *mykēs*, fungus, + *-ōsis*]. A disease of the skin due to a mycosis.

dermatomyoma [" + *mys*, muscle, + *-ōma*, tumor]. Myoma of the skin.

dermatomyositis (der"ma-to"mi-o-si'tis) [" + " + *-itis*, inflammation]. Inflammation of the skin and muscles.

NP: Rest in bed with skillful turning is essential. Mouth lesions should be irrigated frequently with hot boric acid or saline solution. Hot baths and hot fomentations help stiffness. Measures to promote free sweating every second day have been recommended. Hot, dry, flannel bandages and baking half an hour 3 times daily have also been applied. Avoid fatigue and chilling. Massage, graduated exercise and electrotherapy are helpful in preventing or treating muscular atrophy and contractures.

dermatoneurosis [" + *neuron*, nerve, + *-ōsis*]. Skin disease of nervous origin.

dermatopath'ia [" + *pathos*, disease]. Any disease of the skin.

dermatopathol'ogy [" + " + *logos*, study of]. Study of diseases of the skin.

dermatop'athy [" + *pathos*, disease]. Any skin disease. SYN: *dermatopathia.*

dermatopho'bia [" + *phobos*, fear]. Abnormal fear of having a skin disease.

dermatophyte (dĕr'mă-tō-fīt) [" + *phyton*, plant]. A plant parasite which grows in or on the skin. They rarely penetrate deeper than the epidermis or its derivatives, hair, and nails. They cause such skin diseases as favus, tinea, or ringworm, eczema, erythrasma. Important dermatophytes include the genera *Achorion, Microsporon, Trichophyton,* and *Epidermophyton.* All are fungi.

dermatophytide (der-mă-tof'ĭ-tēd) [" + *phyton*, plant]. A toxic rash or eruption occurring in dermatomycosis.

dermatoplas'tic [" + *plassein*, to form]. Pert. to skin grafting.

dermatoplasty (der"mat-o-plas-tĭ). Transplanting living skin to cover cutaneous defects caused by injury, operation, or disease.

There are 4 methods. First, *Reverdin's*: Small grafts of cuticle only. Second, *Thiersch's*: Larger grafts including entire thickness of true skin. Third, *Wolfe's*: Large grafts of skin devoid of subcutaneous fat. Fourth, *Krause's*: Large grafts with underlying fat tissue.

NP: Carefully disinfect the skin from which grafts are to be taken. The wound to which the grafts are applied should be dressed with narrow strips of gutta-percha tissue, rendered aseptic by washing with soap and water, rinsing thoroughly in sterilized water, immersing in 2% formalin solution for 1 hour; again rinsing in sterilized water, placing in physiologic solution until needed.

DRESSING: Safety pins. Gauze, cotton, roller bandage. Great care must be taken in adjusting bandage. If too much pressure is put on grafts they will die. These wounds are sometimes dressed with a light compress of sterilized gauze, saturated with a warm physiologic solution.

dermatorrhagia (der"mă-tor-ra'jĭ-ă) [G. *derma*, skin, + *rēgnunai*, to burst forth]. Hemorrhage into or from the skin.

dermatorrhea (der"mă-tor-re'ă) [" + *roia*, flow]. Excessive secretion of sebaceous glands.

dermatosclerosis (dĕr-mă-tō-skl-rō'sĭs). Scleroderma, q. v.

dermatoscopy (der-mă-tos'ko-pĭ) [" + *skopein*, to examine]. Examination of the skin with a high powered lens.

dermatosiophobe (der-mă-to'sĭ-o-fōb) [" + *-ōsis* + *phobos*, fear]. One having a morbid fear of acquiring a skin disease.

dermatosiophobia (der-mă-to"sĭ-o-fō'bĭ-ă). Dread of skin disease.

dermatosis (der-mat-o'sĭs) [G. *derma*, skin, + *-ōsis*]. Any disease of the skin.

dermatosome (der'ma-to-sōm) [" + *sōma*, body]. Section of equatorial plate in mitosis.

der"matother'apy [" + *therapeia*, treatment]. Treatment of skin diseases.

dermatothlasia (der″mă-to-thla′zĭ-ă) [" + *thlasis*, a bruising]. An uncontrollable tic or impetus to pinch the skin.

dermatotome (der′mă-to-tōm) [" + *tomē*, incision]. 1. One of the fetal skin segments. 2. A knife for incising the skin or small lesions.

dermatotropic (der-mă-to-trop′ĭk) [" + *tropē*, a turning]. Acting esp. on the skin.

dermatoxerasia (der″mă-to-ze-ra′sĭ-ă) [" + *xērasia*, dryness]. Roughening of skin. SYN: *xeroderma*.

dermatozo′on [" + *zōon*, animal]. Animal parasite of the skin.

dermatrophia (der-ma-tro′fĭ-ă) [" + *atrophia*, atrophy]. Atrophy of the skin.

dermic (der′mĭk) [G. *derma*, skin]. Pert. to the skin.

dermis (der′mis) [L.]. The skin; *cutis vera* or true skin.

dermi′tis [G. *derma*, skin, + *-itis*, inflammation]. Inflammation of skin.

der′moblast [" + *blastos*, germ]. Part of mesoblastic layer, developing into the corium.

dermographia, dermography (der-mo-graf′ĭ-ă, -mog′raf-ĭ) [" + *graphein*, to write]. The appearance of elevated red marks on the skin as the result of pressure or stroking its surface; seen in vasomotor ataxia.

der′moid [" + *eidos*, form]. 1. Resembling the skin. 2. A dermoid cyst.

d. cyst. A nonmalignant cystic tumor in which are found elements derived from the ectoderm, such as hair, teeth, or skin. They occur frequently in the ovary but may develop in other organs such as the lungs. 2. An ovarian teratoma.

dermoidec′tomy [" + " + *ektomē*, excision]. Excision of a dermoid cyst.

dermol′ysin [" + *lysis*, loosening]. A substance in the blood supposed to be capable of dissolving the skin.

dermol′ysis [" + *lysis*, loosening]. A rare destructive disease of the skin.

dermomyco′sis [" + *mykēs*, fungus, + *-ōsis*]. A skin disease produced by a vegetable parasite. SYN: *dermatomycosis*.

dermonosol′ogy [" + *nosos*, disease, + *logos*, study of]. The pathology of skin affections.

dermopathy (der-mop′ath-ĭ) [" + *pathos*, disease]. Any skin disease.

dermophlebitis (der-mo-fle-bi′tis) [" + *phleps*, vein, + *-itis*, inflammation]. Inflammation of superficial veins and surrounding skin.

dermophylax′is [" + *phylax*, a guard]. The protective function of the skin in warding off infections.

dermophyte (der′mo-fīt) [" + *phyton*, plant]. A vegetable skin parasite. SYN: *dermatophyte*.

dermorrha′gia [" + *rēgnunai*, to burst forth]. Hemorrhage from or into the skin. SYN: *dermatorrhagia*.

dermoskel′eton [" + *skeleton*, skeleton]. The skin, teeth, hair, and nails.

dermostenosis (der-mo-sten-o-′sis) [" + *stenōsis*, narrowing]. A tightening of the skin. SEE: *scleroderma*.

dermosynovitis (dĕr-mō-sĭn-ō-vī′tĭs) [" + *syn*, with, + L. *ovum*, egg, + G. *-itis*, inflammation]. Inflammation of the synovial sheaths and the adjacent skin.

dermosyphilop′athy [" + *syn*, together, + *philein*, to love, + *pathos*, disease]. Any syphilitic disease of the skin.

dermotrop′ic [" + *tropē*, a turning]. Acting esp. on the skin.

dermovac′cine [" + L. *vaccinus*, pert. to a cow]. A vaccine for skin inoculation.

desanimania (des-an-ĭ-ma′nĭ-ă) [L. *dēs*, without, + *animus*, mind, + G. *mania*, frenzy]. Amentia; dementia.

desatura′tion [L. *dē*, from, + *saturāre*, to fill]. A process whereby a saturated organic compound is converted into an unsaturated one, as when stearic acid, $CH_3 \cdot (CH_2)_{16}COOH$, is changed into oleic acid, $C_{17}H_{33}COOH$. The product is likely to differ in other ways as well.

Desault's appara′tus or **ban′dage** (de-sōz′). Bandage used for fracture of clavicle. SEE: *bandage*.

descemetitis (des-em-et-i′tis) [G. *-itis*, inflammation]. Inflammation of Descemet's membrane on the corneal post. surface; serous cyclitis.

Descemet's membrane (des′māz). A fine membrane bet. the endothelial layer of the cornea and the substantia propia; *lamina elastica posterior*. SEE: *Demours' membrane*.

descemetocele (des-se-met′o-sēl) [G. *kēlē*, hernia]. Protrusion of Descemet's membrane.

descendens (de-sen′dens) [L. *dē*, from, + *scandere*, to climb]. Descending; a descending structure.

d. hypoglossi, d. noni. A branch of the hypoglossal nerve given off at the point where it curves around the occipital artery, which passes down obliquely across the sheath of the carotid vessels (sometimes within it) to form a loop just below the middle of the neck with branches of the 2d and 3rd cervical nerves.

descensus (de-sen′sus) [L. a falling]. Falling, descent. SYN: *ptosis*.

d. testis. BNA. Passage of the testicle down into the scrotum. SYN: *migration of testicle*.

d. uteri. Defective pelvic floor allowing the uterus or part of the uterus to protrude out of the vagina.

VARIETIES: *First Degree*: Where the cervix uteri reaches down to the vaginal introitus. *Second Degree*: Where the cervix uteri protrudes out of the vagina. *Third Degree*: Where the entire uterus lies outside of the vagina. This is the condition known as procidentia uteri.

ETIOL: This condition may be congenital or acquired, although it is most usually acquired. The etiological factors are congenital weakness of the uterine supports, as in the virginal types of prolapsus; injury to the pelvic floor or uterine supports during childbirth.

SYM: The condition is most often seen following instrumental deliveries, or where the patient has been allowed to bear down before the cervix is fully dilated. With it there is frequently associated a prolapsus of the ant. and post. vaginal walls, as seen in cystocele and rectocele. In the early stages there are dragging sensations in the lower abdomen, backache while standing and on exertion, sensation of weight and bearing down in the perineum, frequency of urination and incontinence of urine in cases associated with cystocele. In the later stages a protrusion or a swelling at the vulva is noticed on standing or straining, and leukorrhea. In procidentia there is frequently pain on walking, inability to urinate unless the mass is reduced, and quite commonly a cystitis.

TREATMENT: The treatment depends upon the age of the patient, the degree

of prolapsus, and the associated pathology. In general, there is orthopedic, postural, or surgical treatment. Where conservation is desired the use of the pessary is clearly indicated, or conservative surgery (round ligament shortening and pelvic floor repair) may be practiced. In the elderly patient where the uterus is pathological, a hysterectomy (abdominal or vaginal) accompanied by vaginal plastic work is indicated, depending upon the preferences of the operator. In the presence of large cystocele the interposition operation may be of value. In the old patient who may be a poor surgical risk, colpocleisis (surgical closure) is of value.
SYN: *prolapsus uteri.*

desensitiza'tion. Term applied to the condition when sensitized animals on recovering from an anaphylactic shock do not react to a subsequent injection of the antigen within a reasonable period.

desen'sitize [L. *de*, from, + *sentire*, to perceive]. 1. To deprive of or lessen sensitivity by nerve section or blocking. 2. To abate anaphylactic sensitiveness.

desex'ualize [" + *sexus*, sex]. To castrate, or to perform ovariotomy or testectomy.

deshydre'mia [" + *ydōr*, water, + *aima*, blood]. Lack of fluid elements of the blood.

desiccant (des'ĭk-ant). Causing desiccation or dryness.

des'iccate [L. *desiccāre*, to dry up]. To dry.

desicca'tion [L. *desiccāre*, to dry up]. The process of drying up. SEE: *electrodesiccation.*

 d., electric. Electric therapy to cure a lesion.

desiccative (des'ĭk-a″tĭv, des-sik'ă-tiv). Causing to dry up.

desmalgia (dez-mal'jĭ-ă) [G. *desmos*, band, + *algos*, pain]. Pain in a ligament.

desmectasia, desmectasis (des-mek-ta'sĭ-ă, -tă-sis) [" + *ektasis*, dilatation]. The stretching of a tendon.

desmepithelium (des-mep-ith-e'lĭ-um) [" + *epi*, upon, + *thēlē*, nipple]. The epithelial lining of vessels and synovial cavities.

desmitis (des-mi'tis) [" + *-ītis*, inflammation]. Inflammation of a ligament.

desmo- [G. *desmos*. Prefix: A bond, a ligature.

desmobacte'ria [" + *baktērion*, little rod]. Group of bacteria of a filiform shape; similar to genus Bacilli.

desmocyte (dez'mo-sīt) [" + *kytos*, cell]. A supporting tissue cell. SYN: *fibroblast, fibrocyte.*

desmocytoma (dez-mo-sĭ-to'ma) [" + " + *ōma*, tumor]. A tumor formed of desmocytes; a sarcoma.

desmodyn'ia [" + *odynē*, pain]. Pain in a ligament.

desmo'enzyme. An enzyme which is bound to the protoplasm of cells and incapable of being extracted by present known methods, in contrast to *lyoenzymes* which can be readily extracted.

desmogenous (des-moj'en-us) [" + *gennan*, to produce]. Of connective tissue origin.

desmo'glycogen. A poorly soluble form of glycogen. Differs from the more soluble form (lyoglycogen) in that it is composed of polymers of greater molecular weight.

desmog'raphy [" + *graphein*, to write]. A description of or treatise on ligaments.

des'moid [" + *eidos*, form]. 1. Tendonlike; fibroid. 2. A very tough and firm fibroma.

desmology (des-mol'o-jĭ) [" + *logos*, science]. Science of tendons and ligaments.

desmo'ma [" + *-ōma*, tumor]. A tumor of the connective tissue.

desmoneoplasm (dez-mo-ne'o-plazm) [" + *neos*, new, + *plasma*, matter]. A connective tissue tumor.

desmopathy (des-mop'ă-thĭ) [" + *pathos*, disease]. Any ligament disease.

desmopexia (des-mo-peks'ĭ-ă) [" + *pēxis*, fixation]. Fixation of round ligaments to the abdominal wall for the correction of uterine displacement.

desmoplas'tic [" + *plassein*, to form]. Causing or forming adhesions.

desmopyknosis (dez-mo-pik-no'sis) [" + *pyknōsis*, a condensation]. Dudley's operation. Shortening of round ligaments by attaching them by loops to the ant. uterine wall.

desmorrhexis (des-mor-reks'is) [" + *rēxis*, rupture]. Rupture of a ligament.

desmosis (des-mo'sis) [" + *-ōsis*]. Any disease of the connective tissue, esp. of the skin.

desmosome (des'mo-sōm) [" + *sōma*, body]. A small thickening in an intercellular bridge.

desmotomy (des-mot'o-mĭ) [" + *tomē*, incision]. Dissection of ligament.

desoxy. Prefix meaning *deoxidized* or a *reduced form of.*

desoxycholic acid. 3, 12 dihydrocholanic acid ($C_{24}H_{40}O_4$), an acid found in bile.

desoxycortico sterone (dĕs-ŏk-ĭ-kôr-tĭkŏs'tĕr-ŏn). An active steroid hormone produced by the adrenal cortex. It plays an important role in the regulation of water and salt metabolism.

 d. acetate. An acetate ester of desoxycorticosterone and the form in which the hormone is usually administered in its therapeutic use. It may be injected intramuscularly or implanted as pellets subcutaneously.

desoxyephedrine (dĕs-ŏk-ĭ-ĕf'ĕd-rĭn). A synthetic compound, related to amphetamine and ephedrine, which acts as a cerebral stimulant and vasoconstrictor. Usually used in the form of dextrodesoxyephedrine hydrochloride for the relief of fatigue, to overcome sleepiness or drowsiness, and to counteract a depressed mood.

desoxyribose (dĕs-ŏk-ĭ-rīb-ōs). A phosphoric ester of a pentose present in nucleic acid. Occurs in the nuclei of all cells.

desox'yribonuclease. An enzyme produced by certain streptococci which hydrolyzes desoxyribonucleoprotein of the nuclei of cells. It is utilized in surgery for the liquifying of thick pus thus facilitating drainage.

desox'yribonucleic acid. Thymonucleic acid or desoxypentosenucleic acid. A compound originally extracted from the thymus gland and later found to be universally present in the nuclei of all cells. One of two principle classes of nucleic acids; contains desoxyribose.

desoycholaneresis. Increased amount of desoxycholic acid in the bile.

despumation (de-spu-ma'shun) [L. *de*, from, + *spuma*, froth]. Separation of froth or scum from a liquid.

des'quamate [" + *squamāre*, to scale off]. To shred or scale off the surface epithelium.

desquamation (des-kwa-ma'shun) [" + *squama*, scale]. Scaling of the skin or cuticle.

desquamative (des-kwam'ă-tiv) [" + *squamāre*, to scale off]. Of the nature of desquamation or pert. to, or causing it.

desquamous (des-kwam'us) [" + *squamāre*, to scale off]. Scaling or falling off, as the skin.

dessertspoon. One holding about 2 fluid drams. Spoons are not all uniform in capacity.

desudation (de-su-da'shun) [L. *dē*, from, + *sudāre*, to perspire]. Excessive sweating often followed by slight pustular eruption.

detelec'tasis [" + *ektasis*, dilatation]. Lack of normal inflation; collapse of an organ.

deter'gent [L. *detergere*, to cleanse]. A medicine that purges or cleanses; cleansing.

deteriora'tion [L. *deteriorāre*, to deteriorate]. Retrogression; said of impairment of mental or physical functions.

determina'tion [L. *determināre*, to limit]. 1. A tendency in a definite direction, as of blood, to a part. 2. A quantitative analysis.

deter'miners [L. *determināre*, to limit]. Genes* or the element in chromosomes* supposed to be responsible for inherited traits.

determinism (de-term'in-izm) [" + G. *ismos*, condition of]. The theory that all human action is the result of innate urges although they may not be conscious ones.

deter'sive [L. *detergere*, to cleanse]. Detergent; cleansing or purging.

dethy'roidism [L. *dē*, away, + G. *thyreoeides*, like a shield]. Condition resulting from removal of the thyroid.

dethy'roidized [" + G. *thyreoeides*, like a shield]. Without a thyroid gland.

de'tonating chamber. A muffler surrounding the discharging balls of a static machine or resonator to deaden the sound of a spark discharge.

detona'tion [L. *detonāre*, to thunder loudly]. A violent noise caused by an explosive combustion.

detox'icate [L. *dē*, from, + G. *toxikon*, poison]. To remove the toxic principle of a substance. SYN: *detoxify*.

detoxify (de-toks'ĭ-fī) [" + " + L. *facere*, to make]. To remove the toxic quality of a substance. SYN: *detoxicate*.

detrition (de-trish'un) [" + *terere*, to wear]. The wearing away of a part, esp. through friction, as that of the teeth.

detritus (de-trī'tus) [" + *terere*, to wear]. Any broken down or degenerative tissue or carious matter.

detruncation (de-trun-ka'shun) [" + *truncus*, trunk]. Decapitation, esp. of a fetus. SYN: *decollation*.

detru'sor uri'nae [L.]. Ext. longitudinal layer of muscular coat of bladder.

detumes'cence [L. *dē*, down, + *tumescere*, to swell]. 1. Subsidence of a swelling. 2. Subsidence of erectile tissue of genital organs (penis and clitoris) following erection.

deutencephalon (dūt-en-sef'ă-lon) [G. *deuteros*, second, + *egkephalos*, brain]. The interbrain. SYN: *thalamencephalon*.

deuteranopia, deuteranopsia (du-ter-an-o'pĭ-a, -op'sĭ-ă) [" + *anopia*, blindness]. Green blindness, so named because green is the 2nd of the primary colors. SEE: *protanopia, tritanopia*.

deuterium (dū-te'rĭ-um) [G. *deuteros*, second]. Heavy hydrogen; the mass 2 isotope of hydrogen, symbol H^2 or D.
    d. oxide. Heavy water.

deuteroal'bumose [" + L. *albumen*, white of egg]. An albumose formed in peptic digestion of proteins.

deuteroelas'tose [" + L. *elasticus*, elastic]. A deuteroalbumose formed in the peptic digestion of elastin.

deuteromyosinose (du-ter-o-mī-o'sĭn-ōz) [" + G. *mys*, muscle]. A product of myosin digestion.

deuteropathi'a, deuterop'athy [" + *pathos*, disease]. A disease caused by a preceding disease.

deu'teroplasm [" + *plasma*, matter]. SYN: *paraplasm*. Inclusion bodies.

deutoscolex (du-to-sko'lex) [" + *skolex*, intestinal worm]. Secondary daughter cysts which develop on the inner wall of a hydatid cyst.

devasa'tion [L. *dē*, away, + *vasa*, vessel]. Destruction of blood vessels.

devasculariza'tion [" + *vascularis*, pert. to a vessel]. Loss or draining of blood from a part.

devel'opment [Fr. *de'velopper*, to unwrap]. Growth to full size or maturity. Progress of an egg to the adult state. Evolution.

development, words pert. to: anoria, aplasia, aplastic, apposition, ateliosis, ateliotic, auxanology, auxology, cacogenesis, caryogenesis, cavalry bone, cenopsychic, chondrification, chondrosis, chorista, choristoma.

developmental (de-vel-op-men'tal) [Fr. *développer*, to unwrap]. Pert. to development.

deviation (de-vĭ-a'shun) [L. *dē*, from, + *via*, way]. Going out of the way; departure from normal.
    d., conjugate. Deviation of face and eyes to the same side in paralytics.
    d., minimum. The smallest deviation that a prism can produce.
    d. of complement. Incapable of hemolysis.

deviom'eter [" + " + G. *metron*, measure]. Device for estimating degree of strabismus.

devisceration (de-vis-er-a'shun) [" + *viscus, viscer-*, internal organ]. Removal of viscera. SYN: *evisceration*.

devitaliza'tion [" + *vita*, life]. 1. Destruction or loss of vitality. 2. Anesthetizing sensitive pulp of a tooth; known as "killing the nerve."

devolu'tion [L. *devolvere*, to roll down]. Catabolism; degeneration.

dew cure. Walking with bare feet in grass wet with dew. SYN: *kneippism*.
    d. point. Temperature at which dew begins to form.

dexiocar'dia [G. *dexios*, right, + *kardia*, heart]. Displacement of heart on right side of the body.

dexter (deks'ter) [L. *dexter*, right]. On the right side.

dextrad (dex'trad) [L. *dexter*, right, + *ad*, toward]. Toward the right side.

dextral (dex'tral). Pert. to the right side.

dex'tran [L. *dexter*, right]. $C_6H_{10}O_5$. A monodextrin.

dex'trase [L. *dexter*, right]. An enzyme that splits dextrose and converts it into lactic acid.

dex'trin [L. *dexter*, right]. A yellowish-white powder which forms mucilaginous solutions in water and can be prepared by the action of heat or acid on starch. It is a carbohydrate of the formula $(C_6H_{10}O_5)n$. In digestion it is soluble or gummy matter into which starch is converted by diastase and is the result of the 1st chemical change in the digestion of starch.

dextrinuria (deks-trin-u'rĭ-ă) [" + G. *ouron*, urine]. Dextrin in the urine.

dextro- [L. *dexter, dextr-*]. Prefix: To the right.

dextrocardia (deks-tro-kar'dĭ-ă) [" + G. *kardia*, heart]. Having the heart on the right side of body.

dextrocar'diogram [" + " + *gramma*, a writing]. A cardiogram representing action of the right ventricle.

dextroc'ular [" + *oculus*, eye]. Having a stronger right eye than the left one.

dextrocularity (deks-trok-ū-lar'ĭ-tĭ) [" + *oculus*, eye]. The condition of having the right eye stronger than the left.

dextroduc'tion [" + *ducere*, to lead]. The movement of visual axis to the right.

dextrogas'tria [" + G. *gaster*, belly]. Having the stomach on right side of body.

dextrogyrate. To turn to the right Bending of light rays to the right.

dextrogyre (deks'tro-jīr) [" + *gyrāre*, to turn]. A substance turning to the right.

dextroman'ual [" + *manus*, hand]. Right-handed.

dextrop'edal [" + *pēs, ped-*, foot]. Having greater dexterity in using the right leg than the left one.

dextropho'bia [" + G. *phobos*, fear]. Abnormal aversion to objects on right side of body.

dextrorotatory (deks-tro-ro'tă-tor-ĭ) [" + *rotāre*, to turn]. Turning rays of light to the right.

dextrose (deks'troz) [" + *ose*, chemical name for sugar]. A simple sugar of the monosaccharose* group; also known as glucose, or grape sugar. $C_6H_{12}O_6$, a crystalline solid which can be made by the action of acids on starches and occurs naturally in the juices of plants and the body fluids of animals.

It is very soluble in water, is an important constituent of corn syrup and honey, and is an example of the *carbohydrates*, q.v. The most important of the monosaccharide group. It is usually associated with levulose. Its presence in the urine in large amounts is symptomatic of diabetes. This may also obtain in brain injuries, cirrhosis of the liver, in normal pregnancies, and as a result of the administration of adrenalin or thyroxin. It is formed in the digestive tract by the action of enzymes on carbohydrates. It occurs naturally.

DOSAGE: 6 oz. (180.0 Gm.) daily.

NP: For rectal or subcutaneous injection 5% watery solutions are used: 1 oz. of glucose to 1 pt. of water, or added to normal saline.

USP: SEE: *disaccharose, glucose*.

RS: See *diabetes, glycosuria, glycuresis, hyperglycemia, hypoglycemia*.

dextrosinistral (deks-tro-sin-is'trăl) [" + *sinister*, left]. From right to left.

dextrosuria (deks-trōs-ū'rĭ-ă) [*dextrose* + G. *ouron*, urine]. Dextrose in the urine.

dextrotrop'ic, dextrot'ropous [L. *dexter*, right, + G. *tropos*, a turning]. Turning to the right.

dextrover'sion [" + *vertere*, to turn]. Turned toward the right.

dezymotize (de-zi'mo-tīz) [L. *dē*, from, + G. *zymē*, leaven]. To free of ferments or germs.

dho'bie itch. Tropical name for form of *Tinea cruris* that is more intense than that of temperate zone.

di- [G.]. Prefix: Twice.

diabetes (di-a-be'tēz) [G. *dia*, through, + *bainein*, to go].

d. bronze. hemochromatosis. A disease of metabolism characterized by deposition of pigment in various organs of the body, cirrhosis of the liver and pancreas, and diabetes.

d. descipiens. D. mellitus minus polyuria.

d., gouty. D. in people leading a life of too much food and too little exercise.

d. hepatogenes. D. mellitus caused by liver disease.

d., hysterical. Polyuria induced by a hysterical attack or state.

d. insipidus. Polyuria.* SYM: Enormous amounts of urine, pale and watery. Sp. gr. 1.002-5. No sugar or albumin. More common in the young. Thirst, weakness, dry skin. ETIOL: Tumors of pituitary, head injury, etc. PROG: Essentially chronic. TREAT: Pitressin jelly in nostrils for polyuria. Surgery.

d. melli'tus. A disease of metabolism.

ETIOL: Perhaps a result of overactivity of the adrenal and pituitary gland, or a lesion in the pancreas, the result of the destruction of certain cells in the islands of Langerhans. May be caused by temporary but severe overactivity of the ant. pituitary lobe rather than malfunction of islets of Langerhans, which may be secondary though direct cause.

SYM: Inability to utilize glucose because of the failure of the pancreas to secrete insulin in sufficient quantity to take care of the glucose in the normal diet. An abnormal discharge of urine is another characteristic.

Urine sp. gr. 1.020-40; sugar excessive; urine shows diacetic acid, betaoxybutyric acid, acetone in last stages. Constitutional and more common in men and after the age of 40. Increased thirst, frequent urination, 3 to 10 qt. a day; itching, frequently about the genitals. Fasting blood sugar raised above normal range of 90 to 120 mg. per 100 cc. of blood; boils and carbuncles; loss of weight, emaciation, weakness, and debility. Coma ensues with weakness, and sweet odor of breath; nausea, headache, vomiting, dyspnea, sense of intoxication, delirium, deep coma, and death.

COMPLICATIONS: Very little resistance to infections; cellulitis and gangrene may set in as a result of injury to the skin. Albuminuria and pulmonary tuberculosis not uncommon.

PROG: Younger the age, the more unfavorable. Life may be prolonged although no cure has as yet been found.

TREATMENT: X-ray applied to the adrenals and pituitary glands is being tried, rather successfully. This relieves the necessity for frequent hypodermic injections of insulin. Measured, balanced diet; reduction of carbohydrates and foods containing them; at least until sugar in urine is greatly lowered, or disappears, and without an increase of sugar in the blood. Quantitative 24 hr. examination for sugar in urine to determine carbohydrate tolerance. When normal caloric food requirements are met, and sugar excretion continues, with an excess of sugar in the blood, insulin may be necessary. Its use is not required in every case and may be dangerous if not properly given. Avoid excitement and worry. Regular, quiet living, and outdoor mild exercise.

DIET: Some would treat with low carbohydrate intake and smaller or no insulin intake, in which case the ketogenic-antiketogenic ratio should never exceed 2 to 1, or if a larger carbohydrate intake is permitted and increased insulin intake is necessary, in this case any

diabetes, mellitus

foods are given except those containing sugar. The first objective is to make the urine sugar free and acetone free. A small amt. of fat is permitted to overcome the acetone condition. The first diet should be below maintenance requirements.

Give large quantities of water, tea, or clear broth, until excess glucose is eliminated and the urine is sugar free. The diet may now be increased in P., C. and F., until the glucose tolerance has been reached. Fat may be increased if diet is below energy requirements, ½ to twice the amt. of glucose in the diet. Authorities differ on diet. Glucose may have to be added if the glucose tolerance is too low, but insulin may be necessary to care for excess glucose. Low blood sugar is called *hypoglycemia,* which may cause insulin shock and result in death. This may be overcome by feeding carbohydrates such as orange juice, or administering glucose, but it must be done quickly. All food should be weighed to meet estimate of C., P. and F. necessities. Too much glucose will cause *glycosuria.** Vitamins, minerals, and bulk must also be considered in the diet. Three meals per day; carbohydrate in dilute form, as found in 5% and 10% fruits and vegetables, although cereals may be allowed for breakfast but a lower percentage of vegetables and fruits for the other 2 meals.

No gluten flours, as most of them contain starch excepting diabetic flours or similar preparations containing no starch or sugar. Washed bran may be added to such flours, or combined with agar, to make wafers. They merely add bulk.

Individualized diet for each patient, according to grains of C., P. and F. ordered by a physician, is the safest.

PHYS: The total glucose in any diet is equal to all the carbohydrates plus 58% of the proteins, plus 10% of the fat. Glucose is necessary in the utilization of carbohydrates as well as proteins and fats. The carbohydrates are reduced to monosaccharides, principally glucose, the proteins to amino acids which are deaminized in the liver and changed to glucose and fatty acid and then oxidized. (Fifty-eight per cent of the protein molecule is converted into glucose and 45% to fatty acids.) Ninety per cent of fats are changed to fatty acids and 10% to glucose. Glucose is necessary to complete the oxidation of the fatty acids. Incomplete oxidation of fatty acids produces acetone bodies which, if accumulated, result in acidosis,* the cause of diabetic coma.

Most authorities use a ratio of Fat: Acid 1.5 to 1 of glucose, or 2 to 1. Normal range of glucose is 0.07% to 12%, the average 10%. In diabetes this may be raised to 0.15%, to 2% or 3%, or higher. High blood sugar is known as *hyperglycemia.** It is the excess sugar that renders diabetics susceptible to infections.

Globin insulin for cases not controlled by protamine zinc insulin. Impaired vision with retinal bleeding helped by large doses of vitamin B and C.

NP: The nursing care of the patient with diabetes includes general hygienic care, giving insulin, collecting specimens, preventing and treating complications, serving the prescribed diet, and teaching how to take care of himself.

General hygienic care: Care of the skin and feet. The skin must be kept scrupulously clean. Daily warm baths are essential. Irritation or bruises should be promptly attended to, as any break in the skin heals with difficulty, and diabetics are susceptible to bedsores, infection and gangrene. Because of the poor circulation in the feet they should have special care. They should be kept clean and dry, especially between the toes. Care should be taken in trimming the toenails, as the slightest abrasion of the skin may become infected. Olive oil or lanolin to keep the feet soft and smooth. Tight shoes must be avoided. The care of the mouth and teeth is most important. The teeth should be brushed well at least 3 times a day and a mouthwash should be used before and after eating. The patient should be encouraged to see his dentist regularly. The bowels should be kept open by regulation of the diet, if possible, or by laxatives or enemas. Constipation should be guarded against as it predisposes to coma.

Administration of Insulin: The dosage and frequency in which insulin is given will depend on the individual patient and the physician prescribing it. In administering the drug, precautions necessary in giving hypodermic injections should be observed. Care taken not to inject the drug repeatedly in the same area and trauma should be avoided. Every diabetic patient should be taught to give himself insulin or if he is unable to give it to himself, some member of the family should be taught the full particulars.

Collecting Specimens: Both single and 24-hour specimens may be collected in 24 hours. They are usually examined daily. It is especially important that the specimens are accurately collected, labeled, and sent to the laboratory on time. The diagnosis and treatment is based mostly upon the results of the urine examination. Specimens of blood may be collected by the physician, for blood chemistry. The specimen is taken early in the morning before the patient has his breakfast.

Prevention of Complications: Close observation of the patient is necessary. Shock may be avoided if the patient is closely watched or if the patient has been taught that when he has the slightest symptom of insulin reaction to call the nurse. He may be instructed to eat a lump or 2 of sugar to keep a chocolate bar within his reach.

Acidosis and coma may also be prevented by the recognition of first symptoms and prompt treatment. The chief symptoms of acidosis are pain in the abdomen, nausea, vomiting, drowsiness, and difficult breathing. The doctor should be notified when the first symptoms appear. The patient kept warm with blankets and hot water bottles. He should not be left alone. His pulse should be closely watched. Heart stimulants are given if necessary.

The Diet: The diet is the most important factor in treatment. While the nurse may not be directly responsible for the preparation of the food, she should know how to prepare and calculate a diabetic diet. She should be able to teach the patients their foods, their caloric value, and methods of preparing them. It is her responsibility to see that the patient eats his diet. She should see that it is prepared and served as palatable and attractive as possible. Food left on the tray should be carefully measured or weighed. The quantity actually eaten should be recorded.

Teaching the Patient: There is perhaps no other disease in which it is as important that the patient is taught all the factors involved in the management and treatment. The patient should understand that he will have to continue treatment all his life and that he must abide strictly by everything taught him in the hospital. His mouth and teeth should be kept in good condition. It is necessary to pay particular attention to his feet. His diet must be followed. He should also understand the complications that may arise and the measures he may take to prevent them. He is taught to take his insulin and examine his urine. He should be taught importance of reporting to physician for frequent check-ups.

RS: *aleuronat; Cantani's diet; casoid; coma, diabetic; hyperglycemia; insulin; insulin shock; melituria.*

d., pancreatic. D. associated with disease of the pancreas.
d., phlorizin. Glycosuria caused by administration of phlorizin.
d., puncture. SEE: *artificial d.*
d. renal. Renal glycosuria. Condition characterized by a low renal threshold for sugar. Glucose tolerance is normal and diabetic symptoms are lacking.
d., true. SEE: *d. mellitus.*
diabetic (di-ab-et′ik). Pert. to diabetes.
d. center. Area in the floor of the fourth ventricle.
d. ear. Otitis media diabetica.
d. neuritis. Multiple neuritis of diabetes.
d. sugar. Glucose in the sugar of the urine of diabetics.
d. tabes. Diabetes with neuritic pains in leg and loss of knee jerk.
diabetide (di-ab-e′tīd). A cutaneous form of diabetes.
diabetin (di-ă-be′tin) [G. *dia*, through, + *bainein*, to go]. Pure crystallized levulose used as a substitute for cane sugar in diabetes.
diabetogenic (di-ab-et-o-jen′ik) [" + *gennan*, to produce]. Causing diabetes.
diabetogenous (di-ab-e-toj′en-us) [" + *gennan*, to produce]. Diabetogenic*; caused by diabetes.
diabetometer (di-ab-et-om′e-ter) [" + *metron*, a measure]. A device for measuring sugar in diabetic urine.
diab″olep′tic [G. *diabolos*, devil, + *lepsis*, a seizure]. One professing to have supernatural communication, esp. with the devil.
diabro′sis [G. *diabrōsis*, an eating through]. A corrosion causing perforation.
diabrot′ic [G. *diabrōsis*, an eating through]. 1. Corrosive. 2. An escharotic or corrosive.
diacele (di′as-ēl) [G. *dia*, between, + *koilia*, a hollow]. The 3rd ventricle of the brain.
diacetate (di-as′et-āt). A salt of diacetic acid.
diacetemia (di-as-et-e′mĭ-ă) [diacetic acid + G. *aima*, blood]. Diacetic acid in the blood.
diace′tic acid. Acetoacetic acid, found in acidosis and in the urine of the diabetic. It is similar to acetone and is found in serious diabetes and in persistent vomiting after anesthesia.
d. TEST FOR IN URINE: Half fill a test tube with freshly voided urine. Then add, drop by drop, some ferric chloride solution, which will cause a deposit of iron phosphate to form. Now filter the mixture and add a few more drops of ferric chloride. If diacetic acid is present a port wine color develops. The specimen is now divided into 2, 1 being used as a control. One-half is boiled, when the color will quickly disappear if it is due to diacetic acid.
diacetonu′ria [diacetic acid + G. *ouron*, urine]. Diacetic acid in urine; diaceturia.
diaceturia (di-as-ĕ-tu′rĭ-ă) [" + G. *ouron*, urine]. Diacetonuria; diacetic acid in urine.
diac′id [G. *dis*, twice, + L. *acidus*, soured]. Having 2 atoms of hydrogen replaceable with a base.
diaclasia (di-ak-la′sĭ-ă) [G. *dia*, through, + *klan*, to break]. A fracture, esp. breaking a bone before surgery.
diaclast (di′ă-klăst) [" + *klan*, to break]. Device for perforating the fetal skull.
diacrinous (di-ăk′rin-us) [G. *diakrinein*, to separate]. Pert. to cells which secrete outwardly; exocrine.*
diacrisis (di-ăk′ri-sis) [G. *diakrisis*, separation]. 1. A change in the character of a secretion. 2. Any disease having an altered secretion. 3. A critical discharge.
diacrit′ic, diacrit′ical [G. *dia*, apart, + *krinein*, to judge]. Diagnostic; said of symptoms.
diad (di′ad) [G. *dis*, twice]. An element or radical having an atomicity of 2; a bivalent.
di′aderm. Blastoderm composed of ectoderm and entoderm, and containing bet. them the segmentation cavity.
diadochokinesia (di-ă-dok″o-ki-ne′sĭ-a) [G. *diadokos*, succeeding, + *kinesis*, motion]. Ability to make antagonistic movements, as pronation and supination, in quick succession.
di′agnose [G. *dia*, through, + *gignoskein*, to know]. To determine the cause and nature of a pathological condition; to recognize a disease.
diagnosis (di-ag-no′sis) (pl. *diagnoses*) [" + *gnōsis*, knowledge]. Recognition of disease states from symptoms, auscultation, inspection, palpation, percussion, posture, reflexes, general appearances, abnormalities and abnormal attitudes and habits, microscopic and chemical examinations, x-ray, mechanical, and other means.
d., clinical. One determined by symptoms alone; they may be *objective* (visible symptoms); *subjective* (those of internal or mental origin), and *cardinal* (those pert. to respiration, pulse, and temperature). Symptoms may be *local* or conditions may be pathological. Each disease seems to have some symptom or symptoms in common with some other disease.
d. cytological. D. based on cells present in body tissues or exudates.
d., differential. Comparison of symptoms of 2 similar diseases to determine from which the patient is suffering. SEE: *differential diagnosis.*
d. by exclusion. True d. by elimination of all others.
d. pathological. D. based on structural lesions present.
d., physical. D. by external examination only.

diagnosis, roentgen

 d. roentgen. D. based on roentgenograms.
 d., serum. D. by means of serum and its effects.
diagnosis, words pert. to: abdomen; acatalepsia; anaphia; appetite; auscultation; autoserodiagnosis; blood; breathing; cerebroscopy; chest; chromodiagnosis; chromoscopy; colic; coma; constipation; convulsion; cough; diffusion; ear; examination, physical; eyeball; eye; face; fatigue; feces; fever; food poisoning; gait; gums; head, examination of; headache; hunger, inspection; infection; inflammation; nail; nausea; organ, see name of; pain; palate; pallor; palpation; palpitation; percussion; perspiration; position; posture; pulse; pupil; pus; reflexes; respiration; skin; sputum; syncope; teeth; temperature; tongue; unconsciousness; urine; vertigo; vomiting.
diagnos'tic. Pert. to a diagnosis.
diagnosti'cian, di'agnost [G. *dia*, through, + *gignoskein*, to know]. One skilled in diagnosis.
diagraph (di'ă-graf) [" + *graphein*, to write]. Device for recording outlines, esp. of the cranium.
dial. A derivative of barbital,* but more active.
 Uses: Sedative and hypnotic.
 Dosage: ½-1½ gr. (0.01 Gm.). See: *barbital.*
dialectrol'ysis [G. *dia*, through, + *ēlecktron*, amber, + *lysis*, loosening]. Treatment by ionization.
Dialis'ter pneumosin'tes. A bacterium found in the nasal secretion at beginning of influenza.
dialy- [G.]. Prefix: To separate.
dialysate (di-al'is-āt) [G. *dia*, through, + *lyein*, to loosen]. A liquid that has been dialyzed.
dialysis (di-al'is-is) [" + *lysis*, loosening]. 1. The passage of a solute through a membrane. 2. A process in which a liquid to be purified or studied is enclosed in a thin, membranous sack and exposed to water or any other solvent which continually circulates or changes outside the sack.
 Diffusible substances pass through the membrane, but colloidal material does not. See: *absorption, diffusion, osmosis.*
dialyt'ic. Belonging to or resembling the process of dialysis.
di'alyze [G. *dia*, through, + *lyein*, to loosen]. To make a dialysis or to have made one.
dialyzable (di-al-iz'ă-bl). Capable of dialysis.
dialyzer (di'al-īz-er) [G. *dia*, through, + *lyein*, to loosen]. Membrane used in performing dialysis.
diamagnet'ic [" + *magnēs*, magnet]. Repulsion by the magnet.
diameter (di-am'et-er) [" + *metron*, a measure]. The distance from any point on the periphery of a surface, body, or space to the opposite point.
 d., anterior transverse, of the fetal head. See: *temporal d.*
 d., anteroposterior, of the pelvic cavity. The distance bet. middle of symphysis pubis and upper border of 3rd sacral vertebra.
 d., a., of the p. inlet. The distance from upper part of symphysis pubis to promontory of sacrum.
 d., a., of skull. The distance in a straight line bet. the metopic point and the most remote point upon the external surface of the tabular portion of the occipital bone, or bet. most prominent

diameter, internal biorbital

point of the glabella and the most prominent point upon the external surface of the occipital bone.
 d., basilobregmatic. Distance in a straight line bet. basilon and bregma.
 d., Baudeloque's. See: *external conjugate d. of pelvis.*
 d., biauricular. 1. Distance in a straight line bet. 2 points on a line passing over the vertex and uniting the 2 auricular points, each immediately above the ridge which continues the zygomatic arch backward. 2. Transverse distance bet. the centers of external auditory meatuses, or bet. middle point of the upper margins of each external auditory meatus.
 d., biglenoid. Distance bet. the center of 1 glenoid cavity of the temporal bone and that of the other.
 d., bigoniac. Distance bet. the 2 gonions.
 d., bijugal. Horizontal distance bet. 2 malar points.
 d., bijugular. Transverse distance bet. 2 jugular points.
 d., bimalar. The transverse distance bet. 2 malar points.
 d., bimandibular. Transverse distance bet. tubercles on the inferior borders of the inferior maxilla.
 d., bimastoid. Transverse distance bet. 2 mastoid processes of the temporal bone.
 d., biparietal. Transverse distance bet. parietal eminences on each side.
 d., bisacromial. Transverse distance bet. 2 acromial processes.
 d., bisiliac. Transverse distance bet. most distant points of the crests of the 2 ilia. Syn: *intercristal d.*
 d., bisischiadic. See: *transverse d. of pelvis.*
 d., bitemporal. Distance bet. 2 most distant points of the coronal suture.
 d., bitrochanteric. Distance bet. the highest point of 1 trochanter major and that of the other. Syn: *intertrochanteric d.*
 d., bizygomatic. Greatest transverse distance bet. most prominent points of the zygomatic arches.
 d., cervicobregmatic. Distance bet. anterior fontanel and junction of the neck with floor of the mouth.
 d., diagonal conjugate, of the pelvis. The distance from the upper part of the symphysis pubis to the most distant part of the brim of the pelvis.
 d., external biorbital. Greatest transverse distance bet. outer borders of external orbital apophyses of the frontal bone.
 d., external conjugate, of the pelvis. Anteroposterior d. of the pelvic inlet measured externally; distance from the skin over the upper part of symphysis pubis to the skin over a point corresponding to the sacral promontory.
 d. of fetal skull. Important diameters at full term are: Suboccipitobregmatic, 3¾ in.; cervicobregmatic, 3¾ in.; frontomental, 3 1/5 in.; occipitomental, 5 in.; supraoccipitomental, 5½ in.; occipitofrontal, 4½ in.; suboccipitofrontal, 4 in.; biparietal, 3¾ in.; bitemporal, 3 1/5 in.
 d., frontomental. Distance from top of forehead to point of chin.
 d., inial. Distance in a straight line, in median line of skull, bet. most prominent points of the inion and the glabella.
 d., internal biorbital. Greatest transverse distance bet. inner borders of the

diameter, interspinous   D-24   **diaphragm**

external orbital apophyses of the frontal bone.

d., interspinous. Distance bet. 2 anterior superior spines of the ilia.

d., maximum anteroposterior, of the skull. Distance, in the median line. bet. the most prominent part of the glabella and the most prominent point in the middle line upon the tabular portion of the occipital bone.

d., m. frontal. Distance bet. 2 stephanions.

d., m. occipital. Distance in a straight line bet. 2 asterions.

d., m. transverse, of the skull. Longest horizontal transverse line that can be drawn within the cranium.

d., mentobregmatic. Distance from chin to middle of anterior fontanel.

d., minimum frontal. Distance bet. 2 extremities of supraorbital line.

d., occipitofrontal. That extending from root of the nose to most distant point of the occiput.

d., occipitomental. Greatest distance bet. occiput and chin.

d. of pelvis. OBST: *Anteroposterior*: the distance bet. the sacrovertebral angle and the symphysis pubis. *Bi-ischial*: Bet. the ischial spines. *Conjugata diagonalis*: Bet. the sacrovertebral angle and the symphysis pubis. *Conjugata vera*: The true conjugate. Bet. the sacrovertebral angle and the middle of the post. aspect of the symphysis pubis (about 1.5 cm. less than the diagonal conjugate). *Deventer's Oblique*: Bet. the sacroiliac synchondrosis on 1 side and the ileopectineal eminence on the other side. *Intercristus*: Bet. the crests of the ilium. *Interspinous*: Bet. the spines of the ilium. *Intertrochanteric*: Bet. the greater trochanters when the hips are extended and the legs are held together. *Internal conjugate*: Bet. the promontory of the sacrum and the upper edge of the symphysis pubis. *Pelvic*: Any diameter of the pelvis found by measuring a straight line bet. any 2 points. *Transverse d. of the inlet*: Bet. the 2 most widely separated points of the linea terminalis, at right angles to the *conjugata vera*. *Transverse d. of the pelvic outlet*: Bet. the tuberosities of the ischium. SEE: *pelvis*.

d., sacrosubpubic. Distance bet. middle of promontory of sacrum and middle of lower border of the triangular ligament of pubic symphysis.

d., sagittal. SEE: *basilobregmatic d.*

d., sternovertebral. Distance from sternum to vertebral column, measured externally.

d., suboccipitobregmatic. That extending from middle of ant. fontanel to lowest accessible point of the occiput.

d., suboccipitofrontal. Greatest distance bet. forehead and junction of occiput with the neck.

d., subtemporal. Distance bet. point upon sphenotemporal suture which is crossed by the ridge upon the inferior surface on the greater wing of the sphenoid bone of 1 side and a similar point on the other side.

d., temporal. Greatest horizontal distance bet. 2 opposite points upon the line passing over the vertex and uniting the 2 auricular points, on surface of the temporal bones.

d., trachelobregmatic. D. bet. ant. fontanel and meeting point of neck with floor of mouth.

d., vertical, of fetal head. That extending from highest point of head to ant. margin of foramen magnum.

diamid(e (di-am'id) [L. *di*, two, + *amide*]. A double amide. SEE: *hydrazine*.

diamine (di-am'in) [" + *amine*]. A chemical compound with 2 NH$_2$ radicals.

diaminu'ria [" + " + " G. *ouron*, urine]. Diamines in the urine.

diapason (dī-ă-dă-pa'sun) [G. *dia*, through, + *pasōn*, all]. A diagnostic tuning fork used in diseases of the ear.

diapedesis (di-ă-ped-e'sis) [" + *pēdan*, to leap]. Passage of blood cells, esp. leucocytes by ameboid movement through the unruptured wall of a capillary vessel.

diaphane (di'ă-fān) [" + *phainein*, to appear]. 1. The investing membrane of a cell. 2. A very small electric light utilized in transillumination.

diaphanometer (di"ă-fan-om'et-er) [" + " + *metron*, a measure]. A device estimating amt. of solids in a fluid by its transparency.

diaphanom'etry [" + " + *metron*, measure]. Determination of translucency of a fluid, as the urine.

diaphanoscope (di-ă-fan'o-skōp) [" + " + *skopein*, to examine]. Device for electric examination of body cavities.

diaphanos'copy [" + " + *skopein*, to examine]. Examination of fluids by the diaphanoscope.

diaphemetric (dī"ă-fe-met'rĭk) [" + *aphē*, touch, + *metron*, measure]. Pert. to degree of tactile sensibility.

diaphoresis (di-ă-for-e'sis) [" + *pherein*, to carry]. Profuse sweating.

diaphoretic (di-ă-for-et'ic) [" + *pherein*, to carry]. A sudorific or an agent which increases perspiration. The term sudorific is usually confined to those active agents that cause drops of perspiration to collect on the skin. Ex: *camphor*, *opium*, *pilocarpine*. Heat may also be included as such an agent.

d. drugs. These produce their effects either by stimulation, or general applications, or both.

d., nauseating. One, such as warm drinks or sweat baths, which dilates superficial capillaries and causes relaxation.

d., refrigerant. One that acts on sweat centers in the spinal cord and medulla, and reduces circulation, *i. e.*, lobelia, tobacco.

d., simple. One that stimulates sudoriferous glands, such as sulfur.

diaphragm (di'ă-fram) [" + *phragma*, wall]. 1. Thin membrane such as one used for dialysis; 2. In microscopy, an apparatus located beneath the opening in the stage by means of which the amount of light passing through the object can be regulated; 3. A rubber or plastic cup which fits over the cervix uteri and used for contraceptive purposes; 4. A musculomembranous wall separating the abdomen from the thoracic cavity with its convexity upward.

It contracts with each inspiration, flattening out downward, permitting the descent of the bases of the lungs. It relaxes with each expiration, elevating it and restoring its inverted basinshape. The deeper the inspiration the lower the descent of the diaphragm; the greater the expiration, the higher does it rise.

Its origin is at a level with the 6th ribs or intercostal spaces ant., and the 11th or 12th ribs post. The right half rises higher than the left. The lower surface is in relation to the suprarenal

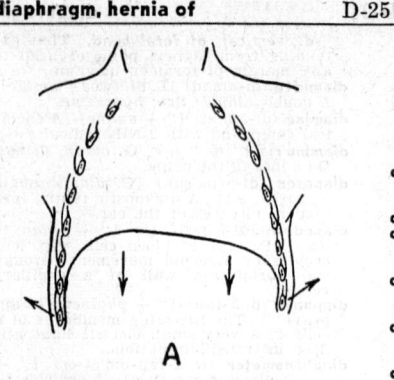

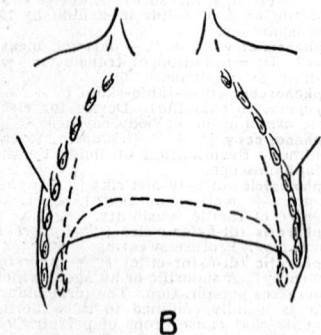

ACTION OF THE DIAPHRAGM
A. Expiration
B. Inspiration

bodies of the kidney, the liver, spleen, and cardiac end of the stomach. It aids in defecation and parturition. It becomes spasmodic in hiccoughs and sneezing.

SEE: *midriff, phrenic, "phren-" words, tendineum centeum.*

  d., hernia of. Protrusion of abdominal contents through the diaphragm. ETIOL: Congenital or through injury.

  d., pelvic. The musculofascial layer forming the lower boundary of the abdominopelvic cavity.

It is funnelshaped, and is pierced in the midline by the urethra, vagina, and rectum. Consists of a muscular layer made up of the paired levator ani and coccygeus muscles. The fascial layer consists of 2 portions, the parietal and visceral layers, the former being made up of the peritoneum continuous with the connective tissue sheaths of the psoas and iliac muscles; the visceral layer is split from the parietal layer at the white line passing downwards and inwards to form the upper sheath of the levator ani muscles; the ant. part of this layer unites the bladder to the post. wall of the pubes.

The middle portion splits into 3 parts: (a) The vesical layer investing bladder and urethra; (b) rectovaginal layer forming the rectovaginal septum; (c) the rectal layer investing the rectum; the post. part is the base of the broad ligament where it sheaths the uterine arteries and supports the cervix.

  d. urogenital. Urogenital trigone, or triangular ligament. A musculofascial sheath which lies between the ischiopubic rami. It lies superficial to the pelvic diaphragm and in the male surrounds the membranous urethra, in the female it surrounds the vagina.

diaphragmal'gia [G. *dia*, through, + *phragma*, wall, + *algos*, pain]. Pain in the diaphragm.

diaphragmat'ic. Pert. to the diaphragm.

diaphragmati'tis [G. *dia*, through, + *phragma*, wall, + *-itis*, inflammation]. Inflammation of the diaphragm.

diaphragmatocele (di″ă-frag-mat′o-sēl) [" + " + *kēlē*, hernia]. Hernia of the diaphragm.

di″aphragmi'tis [" + " + *-itis*, inflammation]. Inflammation of the diaphragm. SYN: *diaphragmatitis.*

di″aphragmodyn'ia [" + " + *odynē*, pain]. Pain in the diaphragm.

diaph'ysary [" + *phyein*, to grow]. Pert. to or affecting the shaft of a bone.

diaphysec'tomy [" + " + *ektomē*, excision]. Removal of part of the shaft of a long bone.

diaphysis (di-af′ĭ-sis) [" + *plassein*, to grow]. The shaft or middle part of a long cylindrical bone. SEE: *apophysis, epiphysis.*

diaphysitis (di-ă-fĭ-si′tis) [" + " + *-itis*, inflammation]. Inflammation of shaft of a long bone.

diaplasis (di-ap′la-sis) [" + *plassein*, to form]. Reduction of a fracture or dislocation. SYN: *diorthosis.*

di'aplex [" + L. *plexus*]. Choroid plexus of 3rd ventricle.

diaplex'al. Pert. to the diaplex.

diaplex'us [G. *dia*, through, + L. *plexus*, braid]. Choroid plexus of 3rd ventricle.

diapnoic (di-ap-no′ik) [G. *dia*, through, + *pnein*, to breathe]. 1. Pert. to or causing perspiration, esp. insensible p. 2. A mild sudorific.

diapoph'ysis [" + *apophysis*, outgrowth]. An upper articular surface of transverse process of a vertebra.

diapyesis (di-ap-i-e′sis) [" + *pyon*, pus]. Suppuration.

diapyetic (di-ă-pi-et′ik). Pert. to or causing suppuration.

diarrhea (di-ă-re′ă) [G. *dia*, through, + *rein*, to flow]. Morbid frequency of bowel evacuation, the stools having a more or less fluid consistency. It is a frequent symptom of gastrointestinal disturbances and is primarily the result of increased peristalsis.

ETIOL: Diet, inflammation or irritatation of the mucosa of the intestines, gastrointestinal infections, certain drugs, psychogenic factors.

  d., acid. Green, broken stools with sour odor.

  d., acute. TREATMENT: Barley water, lime water, whey, albumin water, isinglass, rice milk, arrowroot, corn flour, white of eggs; brandy or sherry. Gradual return to ordinary diet.

  d., bilious. Bile in the stools.

  d., catarrhal. D. caused by degeneration in the intestines.

  d., choleraic. D. accompanying cholera in severe form with vomiting and collapse.

  d., chronic. TREATMENT: (a) Light food; lean meat, white fish, white of eggs, tongue, scraped meat, potted meat, poultry; spinach, vegetable marrow, puree of potato; milk puddings, arrowroot, corn flour; jelly; cooked apples;

diarrhea, colliquative   D-26   diathermy

toast, cereals, but not whole wheat; cake; dry toast, rusk; whey, buttermilk, sour milk; tea, coffee, or cocoa (in moderation); red wine, whortleberry wine. Avoid oatmeal, all fibrous foods and causes of intestinal fermentation, meat extracts, strong soups, much sugar, and fat.

(b) Pure milk diet; fresh milk, sour milk.

(c) If very persistent, try protein diet: Raw meat, sandwiches, eggs on toast, chicken, fish, sweetbread, custard, junket, jelly; with small allowance of zwieback, rusk, or toast; butter, sour milk, alum, whey; red wines.

(d) Any food which has been passed through a fine hair sieve.

d., colliquative. Variety causing collapse, due to frequency of evacuation.

d., congestive. Form caused by congestion of alimentary tract.

d., critical. D. causing a crisis, or occurring at the time of a crisis.

d., dry. Variety in which stools are exceptionally small, but can cause death.

d., dysenteric. D. with mucus and bloody discharge.

d., emotional. Form caused by emotional stress.

d., fatty. D. with stools containing undigested fat particles.

d., infantile. In children under 2 years. Dysentery, q.v. SYM: Skin dry, temperature, high; thirst, pains, increase of stools with change of color and consistency. TREATMENT: Water, woolen clothing, no food, warm baths, hot applications or mustard plaster, emetic enemas, cleanliness, fresh air.

d., inflammatory. Type caused by increased vascularity of intestinal mucosa.

d., intermittent. D. recurring, due possibly to malarial poisoning.

d., lienteric. Watery stools with undigested food particles.

d., membranous. D. with passage of pieces of intestinal mucosa.

d., nervous. Nervous increase of peristalsis. TREATMENT: In general, heat externally, rest, enemas and cathartics if resulting from constipation; sedatives if of nervous origin. DIET: Starvation diet of broth, and hot water for a day or 2.

d., mucous. D. with mucus in stools.

d., puerperal. Form occurring in puerperas, caused by septicemia or indigestion.

d., purulent. Presence in stools of pus, due to intestinal ulceration.

d., serous. Water stools.

d., simple. Variety in which stools contain only normal excreta.

d summer. D. occurring during summer heat and due usually to pathogenic bacteria present in contaminated food.

d., ulcerative. Severe d. with ulceration of mucosa of intestines.

diarthric (di-ar'thrik). Pert. to 2 or more joints.

diarthrosis (di-ar-thro'sis) [G. *dia*, through, + *arthrōsis*, a joining]. An articulation in which opposing bones move freely; a hinge joint.

diartic'ular [G. *dis*, two, + L. *articulus*, joint]. Pert. to 2 joints.

diaschisis (di-as'ki-sis) [G. *dia*, apart, + *schizein*, to split]. Disturbance or injury to 1 part of central nervous system may cause alteration in function of some distant part.

diascope (di'as-kōp) [" + *skopein*, to examine]. A glass held against the skin for ascertaining noncongestive changes.

diastal'sis [" + *stalsis*, contraction]. Ability to distinguish 1 thing from another.

diastal'tic. Denoting reflex action.

diastase (di'as-tas) [G. *diastanai*, to separate]. A specific enzyme or ferment in plant cells, such as in sprouting grains and malt, and in the digestive juice which converts starch into sugar.

d. index. Normal index in urine bet. 6.6 and 30. Lower if kidney is diseased. In acute disease of pancreas may be 200 or more, due to pancreatic obstruction.

diastasis (di-as'ta-sis) [G. a separation]. 1. In surgery, injury to a bone involving separation of an epiphysis. 2. In cardiac physiology, the last part of diastole.

It follows the period of most rapid diastolic filling of the ventricles, consists of a period of retarded inflow of blood from auricles into ventricles, lasts (in man under average conditions) about 0.2 seconds, and is immediately followed by auricular systole.

d. recti. A separation lateralward of the 2 halves of the *m. rectus abdominis*.

diaste'ma [G. an interval or space]. 1. A fissure. 2. A space bet. 2 teeth.

diastematocrania (di-as″tem-at-o-kra'nĭ-ă) [" + *kranion*, cranium]. Congenital sagittal fissure of the skull.

diastematomyelia (di-as″tem-at-o-mī-e'lĭ-ă) [" + *myelos*, marrow]. Congenital splitting of the spinal cord.

diastematopye'lia [" + *pyelos*, pelvis]. Median slit of the pelvis; congenital.

dias'ter [G. *dis*, twice, + *astēr*, star]. SYN: *amphiaster, q. v.* In mitosis the achromatic figure consisting of two asters connected by spindle fibers. 1. Daughter star. 2. Figure formed by 2 aster-shaped masses of chromatin in a maturing ovum.

dias'tole [G. *diastellein*, to expand]. PHYS: The normal period in the heart cycle during which the muscle fibers lengthen, the heart dilates, and the cavities fill with blood, the atria before the ventricles; roughly, the period of relaxation alternating with systole or contraction, thus constituting the pulsation of the heart. SEE: *heart, murmurs, pulse, systole*.

diastol'ic. Pert. to diastole.

d. pressure. This is the point of the greatest cardiac relaxation.

If the diastolic pressure does not drop in proportion to the systolic pressure this is known as a sign of danger.

RS: *blood pressure, diastole, pulse, pulse p., systolic p.*

diastrephia (di-as-tref'ĭ-ă) [G. *diastrephein*, to pervert]. Psychosis exhibiting extreme cruelty.

diatax'ia [G. *dis*, two, + *ataxia*, lack of order]. Ataxia of both sides of body.

d. cerebra'lis infanti'lis. Birth palsy.

diatela, diatele (di-ă-te'lă, -lē) [G. *dia*, between, + L. *tela*, web]. Membranous roof of 3rd ventricle.

diater'ma [" + *terma*, end]. Portion of the floor of 3rd ventricle.

diathermal (di-a-ther'mal) [" + *thermē*, heat]. Permeable by radiant heat.

diather'manous [" + *thermainein*, to heat]. Diathermal*; permeable by heat.

diather'mia [" + *thermē*, heat]. An inferior term for diathermy. SEE: *diathermy*.

diather'mic. Of the nature of diathermy or of its results.

diathermy (di'ă-ther″mĭ) [G. *dia*, through, + *thermē*, heat]. The therapeutic use

of a high frequency current to generate heat within some part of the body.
The frequency is greater than the maximum frequency for neuromuscular response, and ranges from several hundred thousand to millions of cycles per second.

d., medical. The generation of heat within the body by the application of high frequency oscillatory current for medical purposes.

d., short wave. Treatment by patient's being placed in the path of diathermic rays, but not in contact with either electrode.

d., surgical. D. of high degree for electrocoagulation, cauterization, etc.

diathesis (di-ath'e-sis) [G. *diathenai*, to dispose]. Constitutional predisposition to disease.

diathet'ic. Pert. to diathesis, or predisposition.

di'atom [G. *dis*, twice, + *atomos*, atom]. One of a group of unicellular microscopical plants belonging to the Algae. They possess a siliceous cell wall.

diatom'ic. 1. Containing 2 atoms; said of molecules. 2. Bivalent.

diato'ric [G. *diatoros*, bored through]. Artificial teeth attached with vulcanized rubber to their bases.

diax'on, diax'one [G. *dis*, twice, + *axōn*, axis]. A neuron having 2 axons.

diazo-. A formative of names of compounds derived from 2 aromatic hydrocarbons, containing 2 atoms of nitrogen with phenyl.

d. reaction. A deep red color in urine. SEE: *Ehrlich's d. r.*

diba'sic [G. *dis*, twice, + *basis*, base]. Containing in each molecule 2 atoms of hydrogen replaceable by a base; said of acids.

diblas'tula [" + *blastos*, sprout]. A blastule containing the ectoderm and entoderm.

Dibothriocephalus (di-both"rĭ-o-sef'al-us) [" + *bothrion*, pit, + *kephalē*, head]. SYN: *Diphyllobothrium*, q. v.

dical'cic [" + L. *calx*, lime]. Containing 2 atoms of calcium in a molecule.

d. orthophosphate. CaHPO₄. A salt, often found in the urine.

dicalcium
d. orthophosphate. 2H₂O to formula. Used therapeutically for calcium and phosphorus deficiencies.

dichloramine-T (di-klor'a-mēn). USP. White powder containing about 28% chlorine.
ACTION AND USES: Germicide and disinfectant.

dichloro-hexyl-resorcinol (dī-klō"rō-hek"-sĭl-rē-sor'sĭn-ōl). An antiseptic effective against streptococcus, staphylococcus and *B. pyocyaneus*.

dichot'omy, dichotomiza'tion [G. *dicha*, twofold, + *tomē*, a cut]. 1. Division into 2 parts, as bifurcation of the embryo. 2. Sharing of fees between practitioner and consultant.

dichroic (di-kro'ĭk). Pert. to dichroism.

dichroism (di'kro-izm) [G. *dis*, twice, + *chroa*, color]. Property of a substance appearing to be 1 color by direct light and another by transmitted light.

dichro'masy [" + *chrōma*, color]. Able to see only 2 colors.

dichromat'ic. Being able to see only 2 colors.

dichromatopsia (di-kro-mat-op'sĭ-ă) [G. *dis*, twice, + *chrōma*, color, + *opsis*, sight]. Ability to distinguish only 2 primary colors.

dichro'mic. 1. Containing 2 atoms of chromium. 2. Seeing only 2 colors.

dichro'mophil [G. *dis*, twice, + *chrōma*, color, + *philein*, to love]. Double staining with both acid and basic dyes.

dichromophilism (di-kro-mof'il-izm) [" + " + *ismos*, condition of]. Having the capacity for double staining.

Dick method. A toxin-antitoxin injection for the prevention of scarlet fever.

D. test. *Negative Reaction*: Some slight inflammatory changes due to irritation by proteins in fluid administered. SEE: *Schick method; Schick test.*
In a manner somewhat similar to the Schick testing for diphtheria, a person's susceptibility to scarlet fever may be ascertained by the injection of a standardized toxin of the *Streptococcus hemolyticus*. A positive reaction in the shape of erythema appears in about 12 to 24 hours. Patients convalescent from scarlet fever invariably give a negative reaction. Susceptible persons can subsequently be actively immunized by graded doses of a specific toxin, or passively immunized by the administration of scarlet fever antitoxic serum.

dicliditis (dik-lĭ-di'tis) [G. *diklides*, valve, + *-itis*, inflammation]. Inflammation of a cardiac or other valve.

diclidostosis (di-klid-os-to'sis) [" + *osteon*, bone]. Ossification of the venous valves.

diclidot'omy [" + *tomē*, incision]. Cutting a valve, esp. a rectal one.

dico'ria [G. *dis*, double, + *korē*, pupil]. Double pupil in each eye.

dicrotic (di-krot'ĭk) [G. *dikrotos*, beating double]. One heartbeat for 2 arterial pulsations; rel. to a double pulse.

d. notch. In a pulse tracing, a notch on the descending limb.

d. wave. A positive wave following the dicrotic notch.

dicrotism (di'krot-izm) [" + *ismos*, condition of]. The state of being dicrotic.

dictyoma (dik-tĭ-o'ma) [G. *diktyon*, net, + *-ōma*, tumor]. A retinal tumor.

dicumarol (dī-cū'mă-rōl). A trade name for *bishydroxycoumarin* USP, an anticoagulant that decreases activity of prothrombin in the blood plasma and hence increases prothrombin time.

USES: In prophylaxis and treatment of intravascular clotting, in postoperative thrombophlebitis, pulmonary embolism, acute peripheral embolism and thrombosis, and recurrent idiopathic thrombophlebitis. Used also in management of acute coronary thrombosis. Frequently an adjunct to *heparin*, q.v. RS: *heparin, menadione sodium bisulfite, vitamin K*.

CONTRAINDICATIONS: Subacute bacterial endocarditis, recent brain and spinal surgery, purpura and blood dyscrasias, and in absence of prothrombin determination.

DOSAGE: Original dose, 200–300 mg. orally. Succeeding doses (with prothrombin activity over 25 per cent), 100–200 mg. daily.

didac'tylism [G. *dis*, twice, + *daktylos*, finger]. The congenital condition of having only 2 digits on a hand or foot.

didial (di'di-ăl). Proprietary hypnotic.

didymalgia (did-im-al'jĭ-ă) [G. *didymos*, testis, + *algos*, pain]. Pain in a testicle.

didymitis (did-ĭ-mi'tis) [" + *-itis*, inflammation]. Inflammation of a testicle. SYN: *orchitis*.

didymodynia (did"ĭ-mo-din'ĭ-ă) [" + *odynē*, pain]. Pain in a testicle.

didymus (did'ĭ-mus) [G. *didymos*, twin, testis]. 1. A twin. 2. A double monstrosity. 3. A testicle.

diechoscope (di-ek'o-skōp) [G. *dis*, twice, + *echo*, echo, + *skopein*, to examine]. A stethoscope that gives 2 sounds in 2 different parts at the same time.

di''elec'tric [G. *dia*, through, + *elektron*, amber]. An insulating substance offering great resistance to passage of electricity by conduction through which electric force may act by induction.

dielectrolysis (di''e-lek-trol'ĭ-sis) [" + " + *lysis*, loosening]. The forcing of a drug or medicinal compound to a particular part of the body by osmosis brought about or accelerated with an electric current.

diencephalon (di-en-sef'ă-lon) [" + *egkephalos*, brain]. SYN: *thalamencephalon, interbetween brain, 'tweenbrain*. Second portion of the brain or that lying between the telencephalon and mesencephalon. It includes the epithalamus, thalamus, metathalamus and hypothalamus.

Dientamoeba (dī-ěn-tă-mē'bă). A genus of parasitic protozoa characterized by possession of two similar nuclei. They belong to the class *Sarcodina*, order *Amebidae*.

D. fragilis. A species of parasitic amebae inhabiting the intestine of man. There is strong evidence that it may sometimes be pathogenic producing symptoms such as intestinal colic, diarrhea, and lowered vitality.

dieresis (di-er'e-sis) [G. *dia*, + *airein*, to take]. 1. Breaking up or dispersion of things normally joined, as by an ulcer. 2. Mechanical separation of parts by surgical means.

dieret'ic. Dissolvable, or separable.

diet [G. *diaita*]. 1. Food substances, liquid and solid, regularly consumed in the course of normal living. 2. A prescribed allowance of food adapted for a particular state of health, as a diabetic diet. 3. To cause to eat or drink sparingly in accordance with prescribed rules.

 d. balanced. (a) One adequate in energy-providing substances (carbohydrates and fats), (b) Tissue-building substances (proteins), (c) Inorganic substances (water and mineral salts), (d) Regulating substances (vitamins), (e) Substances for certain physiological processes such as bulk for promoting peristalic movements of the digestive tract.

diet, words pert. to: acid ash d.; acid base d.; alkaline ash d.; basic d.; bland d.; calcium high and low d.; carbohydrate high d.; cardiac d.; cardiac d., Smith; cellulose high d.; colostomy d.; elimination d.; Evans-Strang d.; fat low d.; feeding; fluid d.; general or house d.; iron high d.; Karrell d.; ketogenic d.; light d.; liquid full d.; liquid high caloric d.; liquid or fluid d. without milk; liquid restricted d.; liquid surgical d.; residue d. high and low; roughage d.; saltfree d.; salt low d.; salt poor d.; Schmidt's intestinal d.; Schmidt-Strassburger d.; Sippy d.; soft d.; tube feeding; Van Noorden's d.; vitamin d.; water balance d.

dietary (di'ĕ-ta-rĭ). A regulated diet.

dietetic (dī-ĕ-tet'ik). Pert. to diet.

dietet'ics [G. *diaitētikos*]. The science of the use of foods in health and disease. Some fundamental principles and facts of this science will be summarized here.

CONSERVATION OF ENERGY: There must be as much chemical energy in the food as will equal the amt. of work done by the subject or patient plus the heat which he constantly loses. The number of calories in his daily food must in the long run equal his *basal metabolic rate* plus his additional metabolism due to muscular work and added heat losses. Thus a subject whose basal rate is 1700 calories per 24 hours may during the day do work and lose heat adding, say, 2000 calories to his output; he must, therefore, somehow get 3700 calories from his diet.

1 Gm. of fat gives about 9.3 cal.
1 Gm. of carbohydrate 4.0 cal.
1 Gm. of protein 4.0 cal.

CONSERVATION OF MATTER: Everything that leaves the body, whether exhaled as carbon dioxide and water, or excreted as urea and minerals, must be replaced in the food and can be accounted for by chemical analysis. Thus if a man excretes 10 Gm. of nitrogen daily he must receive 10 Gm. of it in his diet, for the element can neither be created nor destroyed. Accordingly, he would receive 60 Gm. of protein.

DIFFICULTY OF SOME ORGANIC SYNTHESES: The power of the body to build tissue is limited, and for a given purpose only certain raw materials can be used. Thus proteins are "made up" of carbon, hydrogen, oxygen, and nitrogen; but eating charcoal and inhaling the gases would not enable one to make tissue protein. For instance, hemoglobin cannot be synthesized unless the body is supplied with proteins containing the pyrrole ring. This group occurs in the amino acids, tryptophane, prolin, and oxyprolin; proteins which do not contain these amino acids therefore are insufficient for needs of the body.

SUMMARY: A diet should contain: (a) Water, (b) carbohydrates, (c) fats, (d) proteins, (e) minerals, (f) roughage (indigestible residue), (g) vitamins and other accessories.

diethyl stilbestrol (dī''eth''ĭl stil''bĕs'trŏl). SYN: *stilbesterol*. A synthetic preparation possessing estrogenic properties. It is several times more effective than natural estrogens and may be given orally. It is used therapeutically in the treatment of menopausal disturbances and other disorders due to estrogen deficiencies.

DOSAGE: 1/10 to ½ mg., orally, per day.

dietitian (di-ĕ-tish'an) [G. *diaita*, diet]. One scientifically trained in dietetics (which includes nutrition) and who is in charge of the diet of an institution.

Dietl's crisis (de'tlz). Renal colic; accompanied by scanty, bloodstained urine.

Dieulafoy's triad. Tenderness, muscular contraction, and skin hyperesthesia in acute appendicitis at McBurney's point.

differen'tial [L. *dis*, apart, + *ferre*, to bear]. Marked by differences.

 d. blood count. Determination of the number of each variety of leukocytes in a cubic millimeter of blood.

 d. diagnosis. Diagnosis based on comparison of symptoms of 2 or more similar diseases to determine which the patient is suffering from. SEE: *blood count, diagnosis*.

differentia'tion [" + *ferre*, to bear]. Acquirement of functions different from those of the original type.

diffrac'tion. The change which occurs in light when it passes through crystals, prisms, or parallel bars in a grating in which the rays appear to be turned aside

diffusate   D-29   **digestibility of foods**

producing dark or colored bands or lines, or other phenomena. Term is also applied to similar phenomena in sound and electricity.

diffusate (dif'fu-sāt) [" + *fundere*, to pour]. In the process of dialysis, that portion of a liquid which passes through a membrane and which contains crystalloid matter in solution. SYN: *dialysate*.

diffuse (dif-fūs') [" + *fundere*, to pour]. Spreading, scattered, spread.

    d. inflammation. One not localized.

diffusible (dif-fu'zib-l). Capable of being diffused.

diffu'sion [L. *dis*, apart, + *fundere*, to pour]. 1. Absorption of a liquid such as the absorption, by cells, of water from lymph when the percentage of salt is less in lymph than in the cells.

When the percentage is greater in the lymph than in the cells water is withdrawn from the latter. SEE: *osmosis*.

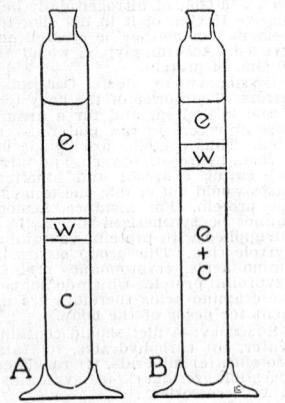

DIFFUSION

The experiment begins in A with a thin layer of water, w, separating a large volume of ether, e, above from an equal volume of the much heavier carbon tetrachloride, c, below. B. Three weeks later the layers are still distinct, but the lowest layer has visibly increased in volume at the expense of the uppermost layer. Ether has passed through the water into the carbon tetrachloride.

    2. A process whereby different gases interpenetrate and become mixed, due to the incessant motion of their molecules. Similarly, if aqueous solutions of different materials stand in contact, mixing occurs on standing, even if the solutions be separated by thin membranes.

    3. The tendency of molecules of a substance (gaseous, liquid, or solid) to move from a region of high concentration to one of lower concentration.

digastric (di-gas'trĭk) [G. *dis*, double, + *gastēr*, belly]. Having 2 bellies; said of certain muscles.

Digenea (dī-jĕn-ē'ă). An order of parasitic flatworms belonging to the class Trematoda and characterized by having an asexual generation, living usually in molluscs, alternating with a sexual generation living in vertebrates as their final host. It includes all the flukes parasitic in man. These include four groups of flukes, *q.v.*

digen'esis [" + *genesis*, production]. Reproduction in which alternate generations are asexual.

digest' [L. *dis*, apart, + *gerere*, to carry]. 1. To undergo digestion. 2. To make a condensation of a subject.

diges'tant [" + *gerere*, to carry]. 1. An agent that will digest food or aid in digestion. Ex: *pepsin, pancreatin*. 2. A preparation made from the digestive glands or lining membrane of the stomach, classified according to the foods it digests, such as *carbohydrate* or *protein*.

digestibility of foods. The following substances normally leave the stomach in from 1 to 2 hours:

200 grams		1. Beer
100-200	"	2. Boiled milk
200	"	3. Broth, with no ingredients
200	"	4. Cocoa, plain
200	"	5. Coffee, plain
200	"	6. Eggs (soft)
200	"	7. Light wines
200	"	8. Peptones, all kinds with water
200	"	9. Tea, plain
200	"	10. Water, carbonated
100-200	"	11. Water, pure (30 Gm.— 1 ounce)

The following foods leave the stomach in 2 to 3 hours:

150 grams		1. Asparagus
100	"	2. Beef sausage
300-500	"	3. Beer
300-500	"	4. Boiled milk
50	"	5. Cakes
200	"	6. Carp
150	"	7. Cauliflower, boiled or as a salad
150	"	8. Cherries, stewed or raw
200	"	9. Cocoa with milk
200	"	10. Coffee and cream
100	"	11. Eggs, raw or scrambled, hard boiled or omelette
200	"	12. Malaga wine
150	"	13. Potatoes, boiled or mashed
200	"	14. Sweetbreads (boiled)
200	"	15. Veal brains
300-500	"	16. Water
70	"	17. White bread, fresh or old, dry or with tea
70	"	18. Zwieback, fresh and old, dry or with tea

The following foods leave the stomach in 3 to 4 hours:

150 grams		1. Apples
250	"	2. Beef, raw or boiled
100	"	3. Beefsteak, chopped
100	"	4. Beefsteak, roasted, warm or cold, lean
250	"	5. Calves' feet, boiled
150	"	6. Cakes
150	"	7. Carrots
150	"	8. Cucumber salad
160	"	9. Ham, boiled
150	"	10. Potatoes, boiled
150	"	11. Radishes (raw)
200	"	12. Salmon, boiled
200	"	13. Smoked fish
150	"	14. Spinach
230	"	15. Spring chicken, boiled
150	"	16. Turnips
100	"	17. Veal, roasted, warm or cold
150	"	18. Rye bread
260	"	19. Squab, boiled
195	"	20. Squab, roasted
150	"	21. White bread

digestible   D-30   **digestion, intestinal**

The following foods leave the stomach in 4 to 5 hours:

250 grams	1.	Duck, roasted
250 "	2.	Goose, roasted
200 "	3.	Herrings
240 "	4.	Partridges, roasted
200 "	5.	Peas (mashed)
210 "	6.	Pigeon, roasted
100 "	7.	Smoked meats
250 "	8.	Smoked tongue
150 "	9.	String beans (boiled)
250 "	10.	Tenderloin beefsteak, roasted

Individual, pathological conditions, and the manner of cooking, the amt. of food ingested, must all be considered in reference to digestibility.

diges'tible. Pert. to that which may be digested.

diges'tion [L. *digestio*, a taking apart]. The process by which food is broken down, mechanically and chemically, in the gastrointestinal tract and is converted into absorbable forms.

Salt, the simplest sugars (such as glucose), crystalloids in general, and water can be absorbed unchanged; but starches, fats, and proteins for the most part are not absorbable until disintegrated by the digestive fluids, and even the sugar sucrose (a disaccharose*) must first undergo inversion.

The chemical actions are chiefly hydrolytic; they are brought about by a variety of enzymes, each of which acts in an acid or alkaline or neutral juice according to its peculiar properties.

The higher carbohydrates are converted into monosaccharoses*; proteins (through successive stages of peptones and polypeptides) ultimately into amino acids, and fats into fatty acids and glycerine. In the stomach the soluble casein of milk is converted into insoluble paracasein resulting in its coagulation or clotting. This is brought about by the enzyme pepsin. The *rennin* and *acid* are responsible for the clotting of milk, which normally occurs in the stomach. An enzyme lipase is able to attack fats in emulsified form. It liberates, for instance, butyric acid from the fats in milk, and thus causes the characteristic odor of vomitus. The chemical actions are facilitated by the churning, wavelike motions of the stomach walls. When the chyme is ready to leave the stomach, the pylorus opens from time to time and the chyme is spurted into the duodenum.

d., artificial. D. outside the living organism by a ferment. [cecum.

d., cecal. Digestive process in the

d., duodenal. The acid chyme is now made alkaline, and the fats it contains are emulsified by the action of bile. A fresh set of enzymes adapted to these new conditions are supplied by the pancreatic juice which enters by 2 ducts and by the intestinal juice which comes from small glands in the wall of the intestine itself. The hydrolysis of starches, fats, and proteins is carried to its physiological completion here, and in the remainder of the small intestine.

d., extracellular. That occurring outside the body of the cell.

d., gastric. Portion of the digestive process taking place in the stomach.

d., intestinal. Hydrolytic processes continue here, and absorption of the products is active. SEE: *absorption.* From the ileum the food residues pass in a nearly liquid state through a small opening into the ascending colon. A sphincter muscle prevents backflow. True digestive processes in the colon are slight, but there is normally much bacterial action (the products of which are mostly absorbed) and reabsorption of water. The remaining substances, now colored by pigments which entered with bile and changed to a firm consistency by the loss of water, pass on through the transverse colon, the descending colon, and the sigmoid flexure into the rectum. They are retained in the rectum by the action of sphincters until there is an opportunity for defecation.

DIGESTIVE JUICES: ACTION OF
On Proteins, Fats, and Carbohydrates

Digestive Juice	Proteins	Fats	Carbohydrates
Saliva			Changes cooked starch into maltose.
Gastric Juice	1. Curdles milk. 2. Changes proteins into peptones.		
Pancreatic Juice	Changes peptones to simpler substances.	Changes fats to fatty acids and Glycerol.	Changes sugars into simpler forms.
Bile		Emulsifies fats.	
Intestinal Juice	Complete the change of peptones into amino acids.		Completes the change of all sugars into the simplest form, glucose.

On Foods

Food	Ferment or Enzyme	Digestive Juice	Where Juice Acts
Protein	Pepsin.	Gastric juice, acid.	Stomach.
	Trypsin.	Pancreatic juice, alkaline.	Small intestine.
	Erepsin.	Succus Entericus, alkaline.	Small intestine.
Fats	Lipase.	Pancreatic juice.	Small intestine.
Carbohydrates	Ptyalin.	Saliva, alkaline.	Mouth and in stomach.
	Amylopsin.	Pancreatic juice, alkaline.	Small intestine.
	Invertase.	Succus Entericus.	Small intestine.

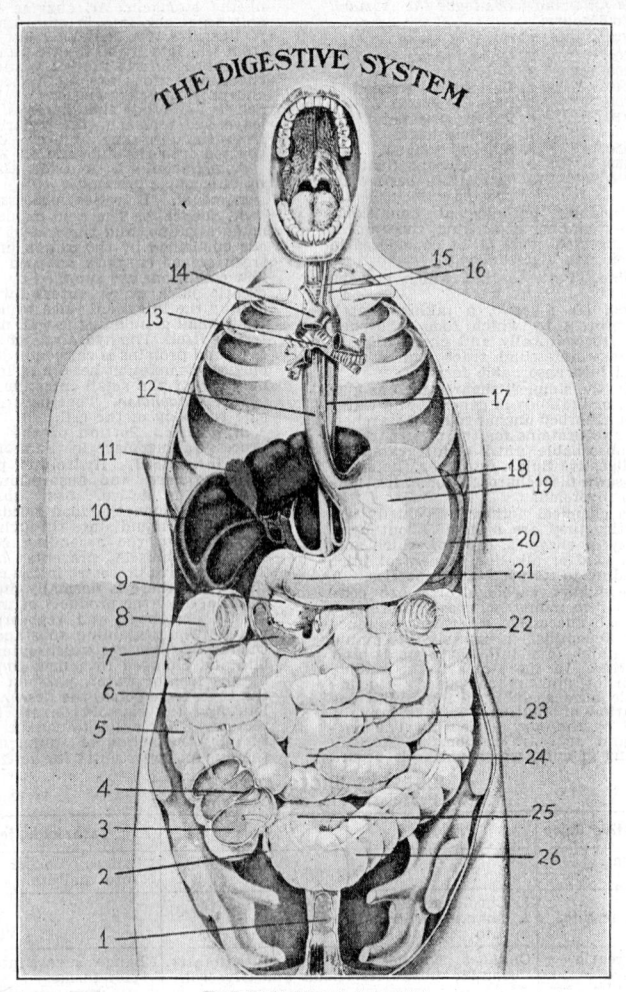

digestion, intracellular   D-31   **digestion, words pert. to**

THE DIGESTIVE SYSTEM
1. Rectum. 2. Appendix. 3. Cecum. 4. Ileocecal valve. 5. Ascending colon. 6. Small intestines. 7. Duodenum. 8. Transverse colon. 9. Pancreas. 10. Liver. 11. Gallbladder. 12. Esophagus. 13. Trachea. 14. Aorta. 15. Carotid artery. 16. Subclavian artery. 17. Aorta. 18. Cardiac orifice. 19. Stomach. 20. Spleen. 21. Pyloric orifice. 22. Transverse colon. 23. Jejunum. 24. Ileum. 25. Sigmoid flexure. 26. Descending colon.

d., intracellular. Digestion within the cell body.
d., oral. Portion of the digestive process taking place in the mouth.
d., pancreatic. Portion of digestive process influenced by pancreatic juice.
d., peptic. SEE: *gastric d.*
d., primary. D. by gastrointestinal tract.
d., salivary. Digestive action by the saliva. SEE: *salivary digestion.*
d., secondary. Cellular assimilation of nutritive material.
d., tryptic. SEE: *pancreatic d.*

digestion, words pert. to: absorption, achylia, achylosis, achylous, alible, amylodyspepsia, aneilema, antialbumate, antialbumin, antialbumose, antipeptone, apepsia, apepsinia, assimilable, assimilate, -tion, autopepsia, bacterial d., bloat, bradypepsia, cacochylia, caseose, catastalsis, cell-organ, chyle, chylifaction, chyme, chymification, colon, colypeptic, dietetics, digestants, duodenal, dyspepsia, ereptic d., eructation, eupepsia, gastric, heart burn, indigestion, intestinal d., lipolytic, lysin, metabolism, "pept-" words, predigestion, regurgitation, saliva, salivary d., salivary glands, succorrhea, succus.

digestive (di-jes'tiv). Pert. to digestion.
   d. juice. One of several secretions which aid in processes of digestion.

dig'it (pl. dig'iti) [L. *digitus*, finger]. A finger or toe.

digital (dij'it-al) [L. *digitus*, finger]. Pert. to or resembling a finger or toe.
   d. reflex. Sudden flexion of terminal phalanx of a finger or thumb when nail is suddenly tapped.

digitalis (dij-it-a'lis) [L. *digitus*, finger, because of its fingershaped corolla]. USP. Foxglove. The dried leaves of *Digitalis purpurea*.
   ACTION AND USES: Heart stimulant, indirectly diuretic.
   DOSAGE: 1½ gr. (0.1 Gm.). Infusion of digitalis: 1½ fluid dram (6 cc.). Tincture digitalis: 15 ℳ (1 cc.).
   POISONING: A valuable drug widely used in treatment of cardiac and other chronic diseases. May be acute or chronic from its cumulative effect.
   SYM: Digestive disturbances, as nausea, and vomiting. Frequently distressing headache. Cardiac irregularities are common, esp. slowing of heart with ventricular extra systoles or partial heart block.
   F. A. TREATMENT: Evacuate stomach, administer diffusible stimulants; cathartics and sedatives are desirable. These patients are chronically ill or digitalis would not be used. Esp. care necessary in their management.

digitalism (dij'it-al-izm) [" + G. *ismos*, condition of]. The poisonous effects produced by digitalis.

digitalization (dij-it-al-iz-a'shun). Subjection of an organism to the action of digitalis.

dig'itate [L. *digitus*, finger]. Having fingerlike impressions or processes.

digitation (dij-it-a'shun) [L. *digitus*, finger]. A fingerlike process.

dig'itus [L.]. A finger or toe.

diglossia (di-glos'si-ă) [G. *dis*, double, + *glōssa*, tongue]. Having a double tongue.

dihydromorphinone hydrochloride (di-hī-drō-morf'in-ōn). USP syn for *dilaudid hydrochloride*.

dihydrostreptomycin (di-hī''drō-strĕp-tō-mī'sin). Derivative of *streptomycin* and originally thought to be less toxic. Uses and dosage same as with parent drug.

dihydrotachysterol (di-hī''drō-tăk-ĭ-ster'-ōl). A hydrogenated tachysterol obtained by irradiation of ergosterol.
   In hypoparathyroidism aids absorption of calcium from digestive tract.

dihydrotheelin (di-hī''drō-thē'ĕl-ĭn). Commercial hormone preparation obtained from hogs' ovaries and urine of pregnant mares or synthetically from estrone. SYN: *estradiol*.

dihysteria (di-his-ter'ĭ-ă) [G. *dis*, double, + *ystera*, the uterus]. State of having a double uterus.

diktyo'ma [G. *diktyon*, net, + *-ōma*, tumor]. A ciliary epithelium tumor.

dilaceration (di''las-er-a'shun) [L. *dilacerāre*, to tear apart]. A tearing apart.

dilantin sodium (di'lăn-tĭn). *Sodium diphenyl hydantoinate*. It is related to the barbiturates. A derivative of glyceryl urea. An anticonvulsant used especially in the treatment of epilepsy.

dila'tant [L. *dilatāre*, to enlarge]. Anything that causes dilation.

dilatation (di-la-ta'shun) [L. *dilatāre*, to expand]. 1. Expansion of an organ or vessel. 2. Expansion of an orifice with a dilator.
   d. digital. Dilatation of an opening or a cavity by use of the fingers.
   d. heart (of the). Abnormal increase in the size of the cavities of the heart, a common result of valvular disease or hypertension.
   d. stomach (of the). Condition in which the stomach is extremely dilated. Acute d. of the stomach or acute gastromesenteric ileus may occur as a postoperative or postpartum condition and usually results from obstruction of the duodenum.

dilatation, words pert. to: capotement, cardiectasia, cardiodiosis, cecoplication, choledochectasia, ciliospinal, ciliospinal center, vasodilator and vasomotor center.

dila'tion. 1. Expansion of an orifice with a dilator. 2. Expansion of an organ or vessel. SYN: *dilatation*.

dilator (di-lā'tor) [L. *dilatāre*, to expand]. Instrument for dilating muscles, stretching cavities or openings.
   RS: *anal, aural, esophageal, lacrimal, laryngeal, meatus, nasal, rectal, sinus, tracheotomy, urethral, uterine, vaginal*.
   d., Barnes. Rubber bag that is filled with fluid.
   d., Bossi. A multiple pronged instrument that dilates by separation of the prongs.
   d., Goodell. Similar to the Bossi except that it has but 3 prongs.
   d., gyn. An instrument for dilating the cervix uteri.
   d., Hegar's. Graduated metal sounds that are inserted into the cervical canal and cause a graded dilatation.
   d., Tent's. Small cones made of seaweed, sponge, or tree roots which are inserted into the uterine canal dry and, on absorbing moisture, expand to cause a slow dilatation.

dilaudid hydrochloride (di-law'did) (dihydromorphinone hydrochloride). A white crystalline powder, odorless, and freely soluble in water. USP. SYN: *dihydromorphinone h*.
   USES: As a narcotic and sedative instead of morphine, over which it is claimed to have an advantage in producing less nausea, and in having less hypnotic properties.
   DOSAGE: As sedative or relief of pain, 1/24 gr. (0.0025 Gm.) orally; subcutaneously: 1/32 gr. (0.002 Gm.) being equivalent to 1/6 gr. (0.01 Gm.) morphine. [dilutes.

dil'uent [L. *diluere*, to dilute]. That which

dilution (di-lu'shun) [L. *diluere*, to dilute]. 1. Process of rendering a substance attenuated or diluted. 2. A diluted substance.

dimercaprol (di-mer-kăp'rŏl). USP syn. for *BAL, q.v.*

dimetria (di-me'trĭ-ă) [G. *dis*, double, + *mētra*, uterus]. A double uterus.

dimorphous (di-mor'fus) [" + *morphē*, form]. Occurring in 2 different forms.

dimp'ling. The formation of a dimple or dimples due to retraction of the subcutaneous tissue. Occurs in certain carcinomas.

dineuric (di-nu'rik) [" + *neuron*, nerve]. Having 2 axis-cylinder processes.

dinical (din'ĭ-kal) [G. *dinos*, vertigo]. Pert. to giddiness or vertigo.

dioner (di-ŏn-er). An assistant to a mortician.

dionin (di'o-nin) (ethylmorphine hydrochloride). USP. A white, slightly bitter powder.

USES: As a sedative, analgesic, and antispasmodic; externally, in iritis and other affections of the eye.
DOSAGE: Internally: ¼ gr. (0.015 Gm.).

diopsimeter (dĭ-op-sim′et-er) [G. *diopsis*, vision, + *metron*, measure]. Device for exploring the visual field.

diop′ter [G. *dioptron*, something that can be seen through]. Refractive power of lens with focal distance of 1 meter, used as unit of measurement in refraction.

dioptometer (di-op-tom′et-er) [" + *metron*, measure]. Device for measuring ocular refraction.

dioptom′etry [" + *metron*, measure]. The determination of refraction and accommodation of the eye.

dioptral (di-op′tral) [G. *dioptron*, something that can be seen through]. Pert. to a diopter.

dioptric (di-op′trik). 1. Dioptral; pert. to refraction of light. 2. A diopter.

diop′trics [G. *dioptron*, something that can be seen through]. The science of refraction of light.

diorthosis (di-or-tho′sis) [G. *dia*, through, + *orthos*, straight]. Reduction of a fracture or dislocation. SYN: *diaplasis*.

diosmosis (di-oz-mo′sis) [" + *ōsmos*, a pushing]. Passage of a fluid through a membrane. SEE: *dialysis, osmosis*.

dioxid(e (di-oks′ĭd) [G. *dis*, twice, + *oxys*, sharp]. 1. A compound having 2 oxygen atoms to 1 of another element. 2. A gas given off by the lungs. Extraneous gases inhaled may be exhaled also.

dipeptid(e) (di-pep′tid) [" + *peptein*, to digest]. A derived protein obtained by hydrolysis of proteins or condensation of amino acids.

dipeptidase (dī-pĕp′tĭd-ās). An enzyme that hydrolyzes dipeptids to amino acids.

diphallus (dī-făl′ŭs). A condition in which there is either a complete or incomplete doubling of the penis or clitoris.

dipha′sic [" + *phasis*, a phase]. Having 2 phases.

diphonia (di-fō′nĭ-ă) [" + *phōnē*, voice]. Simultaneous production of 2 different voice tones.

diphtheria (dif-the′ri-a) [G. *diphthera*, a skin]. An acute infectious disease characterized by the formation of a false membrane on any mucous surface, and accompanied by great prostration.
ETIOL: Causative organism, the Klebs-Loeffler bacillus. The disease is rare under 1 year of age. The vast majority of cases occur before the age of 10, but older children and adults are not exempt. Both sexes equally susceptible. Esp. prevalent in fall and winter months. Transmission through direct contact with a human carrier, or as a result of exposure through contact with articles that have been contaminated by the diphtheria patient. INCUBATION: Two to 8 days.
SYM: Onset gradual. Usually slight headache; often backache. Temperature 100° F. to 103° F., and sore throat with presence of yellowish-white membrane adherent to tonsils or pharyngeal walls. Cervical adenitis may develop early in severe types. In nasal diphtheria, fever is a much more evident symptom. Adenitis often severe, serous discharge from nostrils which may be blood tinged; strong fetid odor common.
d. antitoxin. The antibody which counteracts the diphtheria toxin; the blood serum of a horse or some other animal which has been immunized against diphtheria toxin.
d. carrier. A person harboring in his body the Klebs-Loeffler bacillus without manifest symptoms, thus acting as a distributor of the infection.
There are few things that have not been used for the treatment of diphtheria carriers. Various dyes, and antiseptics of all descriptions have been tried, as well as the application of ultraviolet rays. Complete removal of the tonsils and adenoids will afford more satisfactory results in freeing the individual of diphtheria organisms than any other procedure that may be undertaken. When dealing with a chronic carrier, it is sometimes well to determine through animal inoculation whether or not the organism is virulent, a nonvirulent organism making it unnecessary to restrain the patient by quarantine measures.
d., laryngeal. In this type, croupy cough, aphonia, stridulous respiration due to narrowing of glottic opening are early evidences of the disease. Restlessness, anxious expression, retractions of the supraclavicular and intercostal spaces evident on inspiration. In this type of infection, the danger from asphyxiation due to mechanical obstruction is far greater than any serious results from toxemia. Diphtheria of the conjunctiva, external auditory canal, lips, or genitalia is sometimes seen. Also, diphtheritic infections of postoperative wounds sometimes occur.
COMPLICATIONS: Postdiphtheritic paralysis, associated with loss of voice, regurgitation of fluids through the nostrils, as well as weakness of lower extremities. Acute myocarditis very common. Nephritis not rare. Cervical adenitis, profuse epistaxis in nasal cases, otitis media, or mastoiditis may develop. In the laryngeal form, bronchopneumonia and chronic laryngeal stenosis are the chief complications seen when the membrane is found only below the glottis.
d. toxin. An exotoxin produced by the diphtheria bacillus. A thermolabile substance capable of producing in susceptible animals the same symptoms brought about by inoculation with the living organism.
d. toxin-antitoxin. A mixture of diphtheria toxin and antitoxin. Used in the treatment of diphtheria to produce active immunity. It has been replaced by d. toxoid.
d. toxoid. Diphtheria toxin which has been detoxified. Used to produce active immunity against diphtheria.
DIFFERENTIAL DIAGNOSIS: Tonsillitis, scarlet fever, acute pharyngitis, streptococcus sore throat, peritonsillar abscess, and Vincent's angina may frequently require consideration. Examination of a smear from infected area is advisable, but cultures should be obtained in every instance for the purpose of confirming the diagnosis. In the laryngeal type, edema of the glottis, foreign bodies, retropharyngeal abscess, and catarrhal croup may require consideration.
PROG: Favorable when antitoxin in sufficient amounts is administered within 3 days from time of onset. If given on 1st day, death should hardly ever occur. In laryngeal diphtheria, intubation or, rarely, tracheotomy, is usually necessary, as well as an adequate dose of diphtheria antitoxin. Restless-

diphtheria, toxoid   D-34   **diphtheritis**

ness, abdominal pain, and vomiting are prognostic signs that commonly foretell a fatal end.

ACTIVE IMMUNIZATION: Since all individuals are not susceptible to diphtheria, and because this doubtful factor may be determined by means of the Schick test, it is usually advisable to make use of this test in adults before administering either toxin-antitoxin or toxoid. In children under 5 years, the Schick test may commonly be dispensed with on the assumption that a majority are susceptible. Toxin-antitoxin when used is administered in 1 cc. doses, subcutaneously, at intervals of 1 week; from 3 to 4 months must elapse after such treatment in order to allow time for the required immunity to become established. Generally, there is less likely to be an unpleasant reaction when toxin-antitoxin is used in adults than if toxoid were chosen for those who have passed the age of 15. Toxoid, which is a detoxified diphtheria toxin, is esp. advantageous for immunizing the very young. Usually given in 3 doses subcutaneously, the 1st injection consisting of ½ cc. and 2nd and 3rd of 1 cc. each. With this material, the interval bet. each of the 3 injections is 1 week, and immunity is established earlier than with the use of toxin-antitoxin and is also more enduring. Necessary arrangements must first be made for isolation. The second thought will concern diphtheria antitoxin. The quantity to be administered depends upon site of infection and duration of disease. According to Hoyne's table, the dosage below will serve as a guide.

It must be remembered that the cause of death in laryngeal diphtheria is usually asphyxiation or bronchopneumonia, and it is this type of the disease in which intubation is commonly essential to the saving of life. Concerning the foregoing, it should be borne in mind that more than 1 site of infection may exist. Consequently, a corresponding increase in dosage may be necessary, but more than 50,000 units of diphtheria antitoxin will seldom be a factor in bringing about recovery.

Having decided upon the dosage, it is usually well to administer the total amt. determined upon at once. This may be given in a number of ways, the subcutaneous, intramuscular, and intravenous routes being those that are the most popular. For all practical purposes, the intramuscular route is the one for selection.

SITE OF INJECTION: The outer muscles of the thigh are preferable to administration in the buttock. If the antitoxin has been recently removed from an icebox, it should be slightly warmed before administration. Under no circumstances, however, should the temperature be allowed to exceed 98°; otherwise, deterioration, as well as coagulation, of the antitoxin may result. All customary aseptic precautions must be taken when antitoxin is administered.

In this type, surgical interference is generally a necessity. Intubation is always to be preferred to tracheotomy, provided an experienced operator is available, and furthermore, that the patient is safeguarded by hospitalization which will make possible any attention required within a moment's notice.

GENERAL MEASURES: Ten days should be minimum period for any diphtheria patient to remain in bed, regardless of the lightness of attack. In cases with myocardial involvement, prolonged rest in bed may be as important as the early administration of diphtheria antitoxin.

TREATMENT: No interference with the diphtheria membrane is advisable. Gargles should not be used, although cleansing mouthwashes are permissible. On the other hand, the use of suction in nasal cases is sometimes of distinct advantage. Early in an attack of the ordinary type of diphtheria, a liquid diet, consisting of plenty of water, fruit juices, and nourishing broths, may be required. Where the membrane is not extensive, a soft diet can soon be adopted, not neglecting the free use of vegetables. In the acute stage, stimulants of any description are rarely necessary. In fact, they are more likely to do harm than good. During convalescence, small doses of strychnine as a tonic may be of value, and at times epinephrine chloride 1: 1000 in doses of 5 ℳ subcutaneously is sometimes helpful. However, next to the use of diphtheria antitoxin, absolute rest in bed is the most valuable agent.

In laryngeal diphtheria, surgical interference is generally a necessity. Intubation is always to be preferred to tracheotomy, provided an experienced operator is available, and furthermore that the patient is safeguarded by hospitalization which will make possible any attention required within a moment's notice.

SEE: *anatoxin, antitoxin, diphtheria carrier, Klebs-Loeffler bacillus, Schick test.*

d., surgical or **wound.** Diphtheric membrane formation on wounds.
diphthe′rial. Pert. to diphtheria.
diphtheriaphor (dif-the′rĭ-ă-for) [G. *diphthera*, a skin, + *phorein*, to carry]. A diphtheria carrier or vector.
diphtheric (dif-the′rĭk). Pert. to diphtheria.
diphtherin (dif′the-rin) [G. *diphthera*, a skin]. The toxin of diphtheria, from *Corynebacterium.*
diphtheritic (dif-ther-it′ĭk). Pert. to diphtheria.
diphtheritis (dif-ther-i′tis) [G. *diphthera*, a skin, + *-itis*, inflammation]. Another name for diphtheria.

Name	Description	Dosage in units
Tonsillar diphtheria	Membrane is limited to 1 or both tonsils.	5,000-15,000
Pharyngeal diphtheria	Membrane has extended beyond the tonsils.	15,000-25,000
Nasal or nasopharyngeal diphtheria	Membrane extends into the nasal passages.	20,000-40,000
Laryngeal diphtheria	Membrane in larynx, causing dangerous stenosis.	15,000-30,000

diph'theroid (dif'the-roid) [" + *eidos*, appearance]. 1. Resembling diphtheria or the bacteria which cause diphtheria. 2. The formation of a false or pseudomembrane not due to the diphtheria bacillus.

diphtherotox'in [" + *toxikon*, poison]. The specific toxin of the diphtheria bacillus.

diphthongia (dif-thon'jĭ-ă) [G. *dis*, double, + *phthoggos*, voice]. The simultaneous utterance of 2 vocal sounds of different pitch in pathological conditions of the larynx.

Diphyllobothˈrium [" + *phyllon*, leaf, + *bothrion*, pit]. A genus of tapeworms belonging to the order Pseudophyllidea and characterized by possession of a scolex possessing two slit-like grooves or bothria. Formerly called *Dibothriocephalus*.

D. cordatum. The heart-headed tapeworm, a small species infesting carnivors in Greenland, formerly known as *D. mansoni*. The plerocercoids are occasionally found in man.

D. erinacei. A species infesting dogs, cats, and other carnivors. Larval stages are occasionally found in man.

D. latum. The broad or "fish" tapeworm. The adult lives in the intestine of fish-eating mammals and man. It is the largest human tapeworm and may reach a length of 50 to 60 feet (ave. 20 ft.). The eggs develop into ciliated larvae called *coracidia* which are eaten by certain species of copepods in which each becomes an *onchosphere* which develops into a *procercoid*. Further development occurs in a fish where it develops into a worm-like *plerocercoid* or *sparganum* larva. Infection of the final host occurs following eating improperly cooked fish. Pathological effects are abdominal pain, loss of weight, digestive disorders, progressive weakness, and a severe type of anemia.

diphyodont (dif'ĭ-o-dont) [" + *phyein*, to produce, + *odous*, tooth]. Having 2 sets of teeth; as man.

diplacusis (dip-lă-ku'sis) [G. *diploos*, double, + *akousis*, hearing]. Variety of disturbed perception of pitch characterized by hearing 2 tones for every sound produced.

diplegia (di-ple'jĭ-ă) [G. *dis*, twice, + *plēgē*, a stroke]. Paralysis of similar parts on both sides of the body. SYN: *double hemiplegia*.

diplegic (dip-le'jik). Pert. to diplegia.

diploalbuminuˈria [G. *diploos*, double, + L. *albumen*, white of egg, + G. *ouron*, urine]. Coexistence of physiologic and pathologic albuminuria.

diplobacilˈlus [" + L. *bacillus*, a little stick]. A double bacillus, 2 being linked end to end.

diplobacteˈrium [" + *baktērion*, little rod]. An organism made up of 2 adherent bacteria.

diploblastic (dip-lo-blas'tĭk) [" + *blastos*, germ]. The ectoderm and endoderm having 2 germ layers.

diplocarˈdia [" + *kardia*, heart]. Having a double heart.

diplococcemia (dipˈlo-kok-se'mĭ-ă) [" + *kokkos*, berry, + *aima*, blood]. Diplococci in the blood.

Diplococˈcus (dĭp-lō-kok'us) [" + *kokkos*, berry]. A genus of bacteria belonging to the family Lactobacteriaceae. They are gram positive organisms occurring in pairs.

D. gonorrhoeae. *Neisseria gonorrhoeae* causative organism of gonorrhea.

D. pneumoniae. SYN: *pneumococcus*, *D. lanceolatus*, *Micrococcus pneumoniae*, *Micrococcus lanceolatus*, *Streptococcus pneumoniae*. A species of bacteria, oval or spherical in shape, gram-positive, nonmotile. They possess a capsule. The species is made up of a number of distinct strains of which some 33 different serological types have been isolated. Many others have been described. It is the causative agent of certain types of pneumonia esp. lobar pneumonia and is associated with other infectious diseases such as cerebrospinal meningitis, otitis media, and septicemia.

diploe (dip'lo-e) [G. *diploē*, fold]. Cancellated tissue bet. the tables of the skull.

diploetˈic, diploˈic [G. *diploē*, fold]. Pert. to the diploe or cancellated tissue bet. cranial tables.

diplogenˈesis [G. *diploos*, double, + *genesis*, production]. Having 2 parts or producing 2 substances.

diploid (dĭp'loyd). Having double the haploid number of chromosomes. Said of somatic cells which contain twice the number of chromosomes present in the egg or sperm.

diplokaryon (dĭp-lo-kar'ĭ-ŏn). A nucleus containing twice the diploid number of chromosomes.

diplomellituria (dĭp-lō-měl'ĭ-tur'ĭ-ă) [" + *meli*, honey, + *ouron*, urine]. Condition in which diabetic and nondiabetic glycosuria occur either simultaneously or alternately in the same individual.

diplomyelia (dĭp-lō-mī-ēl'ĭ-ă) [" + *myelos*, marrow]. Condition in certain types of spina bifida in which the spinal cord is doubled.

diploneuˈral [" + *neuron*, nerve]. Having 2 nerves from different origins, as certain muscles.

diplophonia (dip-lo-fo'nĭ-ă) [" + *phōnē*, voice]. Having 2 different voice tones at the same time. SYN: *diphonia*.

diplopia (dip-lo'pĭ-ă) [" + *opsis*, sight]. Double vision; monocular (astigmatism, subluxated lens, incipient cataract); binocular (due to derangement of extra-ocular muscles).

d., binocular. Double vision occurs when both eyes are used but not in focus. Seen in disease of the eyeballs, cranial-nerve affections, disease of the cerebellum, cerebrum, and meninges. The more distantly appearing object is the true one.

d., crossed. Binocular vision in which the images are reversed.

d., direct. SEE: *homonymous d.*

d., heteronymous. SEE: *crossed d.*

d., homonymous. Double vision in which right-hand image appears on right side and left-hand image on left side. OPP: *crossed d.*

d., monocular. Double vision with 1 eye.

d., unocular. SEE: *monocular d.*

d., vertical. D. with 1 of 2 images higher than the other.

diplopiometer (dip-lo-pĭ-om'et-er) [" + " + *metron*, measure]. Device for estimating double vision.

dipˈloscope [" + *skopein*, to examine]. Device for study of binocular vision.

diplosomaˈtia [" + *sōma*, body]. Twins joined at 1 or more points. SYN: *diplosomia*.

diplosoˈmia [" + *sōma*, body]. Twins joined together. SYN: *diplosomatia*.

dipp'ing. 1. Palpation of the liver by a quick depression of the abdomen. 2. The act of immersing an object in a solution; esp., applied to the dipping of cattle for the control of cattle ticks.

diprosopus (dĭp-rō-sōp'ŭs). A fetal monster characterized by possession of a double face.

dipsomania (dip-so-ma'nĭ-ă) [G. *dipsa*, thirst, + *mania*, mania]. PSY: A morbid and uncontrollable craving for alcoholic beverages. SEE: *alcoholism*.

dipsopathy (dip-sop'ă-thĭ) [" + *pathos*, disease]. 1. Dipsomania. 2. Limitation of intoxicants for purposes of cure.

dipsophobia (dĭp-sō-fĭ'bĭ-ă). Morbid fear of drinking.

dipsosis (dip-so'sis) [" + -*ōsis*]. Abnormal thirst.

dipsotherapy (dip-so-ther'ă-pĭ) [" + *therapeia*, treatment]. Limitation of water to be drunk as a cure.

Diptera (dĭp'ter-ă). An order of insects characterized by having sucking or piercing mouth parts, one pair of wings, and complete metamorphosis. It includes the flies, gnats, midges, and mosquitoes. It contains many species involved in the transmission of pathogenic organisms.

dipterous (dĭp'ter-ŭs). Having two wings; characteristic of the order Diptera.

dipylidiasis dī-fĭl'ĭd-ĭ-ās-ĭs). Infestation with the tapeworm, *Dipylidium caninum*.

Dipylidium (dī-fĭl-ĭd'ĭ-ŭm). A genus of tapeworms belonging to the family *Dipyliidae* which infests dogs and cats.
D. caninum. A species of Dipylidium, a common parasite of dogs and cats. Occasionally human infestation may occur through the accidental ingestion of lice or fleas which serve as the intermediate host.

direct'. Immediate, uninterrupted.
d. current. One flowing in 1 direction only. SEE: *current*.
d. light reflex. One in which response occurs in same side as the stimulus.
d. murmur. That due to stenosis of cardiac orifices.
d. reflex. Prompt contraction of sphincter of iris when light entering through pupil strikes retina of eye.

director (dī-rek'tor) [L. *dirigere*, to lay straight]. Grooved device for guiding a knife.

direc'toscope [" + G. *skopein*, to examine]. Device for examination of the larynx.

dir'igomo'tor [" + *motor*, mover]. Controlling or directing muscular activity.

dis- [L.]. Prefix: Free of, undo, as *disable*.

disaccharid(e (di-sak'ĭ-rĭd) [G. *dis*, two, + *sakcharon*, sugar]. A member of the disaccharose* group of carbohydrates. SEE: *carbohydrates*.

disac'charose [G. *dis*, two, + *sakcharon*, sugar]. A *complex* sugar that may be split into 2 molecules of monosaccharids. The 2 monosaccharoses resulting from the decomposition may be different or identical. Thus the disaccharose *maltose*, $C_{12}H_{22}O_{11}$, for each molecule yields 2 molecules of glucose, $C_9H_{12}O_6$, while the disaccharose sucrose, $C_{12}H_{22}O_{11}$, yields a molecule each of glucose and fructose.

The disaccharoses consist of the following:

LEVULOSE: The same as *fructose*. In the body this is formed in the digestion of sucrose. It is found in fruits, plants, and in honey.

MALTOSE: Malt sugar. This is found in malt and malt products, and in germinating seeds. It is acted upon in the intestines by maltase, resulting in dextrose as an end product. It is a reducing sugar.

SUCROSE: Cane sugar or table sugar. A nonreducing sugar. It comes from sugar cane, sorghum, maple sugar, sugar beets, and honey. An increase in temperature while heating sucrose results in caramel. It is acted upon in the intestines by *sucrase*, and enzyme converting it into dextrose and levulose as end products.

Some sugars undergo fermentation by yeasts, or decomposition is brought about by bacteria or molds. They oxidize sugars into carbon dioxide and water. Alcohol is produced when dextrose ferments.

Most of the sugar on the market consists of beet and cane sugar. Ripe fruits, and vegetables to a lesser degree, contain sucrose. The starch of green fruits is changed to a mixture of sucrose, glucose, and levulose. Sucrose gives the sweet flavor to ripe fruits. It has the following chemical characteristics:
1. Extremely soluble. Cold water will hold in solution almost twice its weight of sucrose. Hot water will dissolve even more.
2. It crystallizes very easily.
3. It melts at about 160° C., changing to an amber hue and growing darker, becoming less sweet and acquiring a bitter flavor called "caramel."

SEE: *carbohydrates, monosaccharoses, polysaccharoses.*

disarticula'tion [L. *dis*, apart, + *articulus*, joint]. Amputation through a joint.

disassimila'tion [" + *ad*, to, + *similāre*, to make like]. Changing assimilated material into less complex compounds, freeing potential energy.

dis"asso"cia'tion [" + *associāre*, to unite with]. A mental condition in which ideas are split from the consciousness and which are no longer amenable to objective control such as amnesial somnambulism,* catalepsy,* dual personality,* fugues,* and trances.

disc [G. *diskos*, a flat dish]. A round, flat, platelike structure. SEE: *disk*.

discharge (dis-charj') [M.E. *dischargen*, an oozing out]. 1. The escape (especially by violence) of pent up or accumulated energy or of explosive material. 2. The flowing away of a secretion or excretion of pus, feces, urine, etc. 3. The material ejected by discharge (2nd def.).

SEE: *abscession (2), arrhea, cenosis.*

d., brush. That from a static machine having a disruptoconvective character.

d., cerebral cortical. The violent action of a diseased portion of the cerebral cortex that gives rise to an epileptic paroxysm.

d., convective. One from a high potential source in the form of electrical energy passing through the air to the patient.

d., disruptive. A passage of current through an insulating medium due to the breakdown of the medium under electrostatic stress.

d., disruptoconductive. The static brush discharge simulating both the convective and the disruptive or spark discharge.

d., electric. A slow or instantaneous bringing back to a neutral electric condition, by which every highly electrified body loses its surplus electricity, giving it up to surrounding bodies less highly electrified.

d., lochial. Uterine excretion following childbirth. SEE: *lochia*.

d., silent. The gradual loss of electricity by even isolated bodies, owing to the conductibility of air and its contained vapors, together with that of the isolating bodies themselves.

discharge tube. A vessel of insulating material (usually glass) provided with metal electrodes, which is exhausted to a low gas pressure and permits the passage of electricity through the residual gas when a moderately high voltage is applied to the electrodes.

discharg'ing. The emission of or the flowing out of material as the discharge of pus from a lesion. Excreting.
 d. lesion. A lesion of nerve center in brain suddenly discharging motor impulses.

dischrona'tion [L. *dis*, apart, + G. *chronos*, time]. Failure of relativity in the consciousness of time.

discission (dĭ-sish'un) [" + *scindere*, to cut]. Rupture of the capsule of the crystalline lens in operation for cataract. NP: Mild antiseptic or aseptic dressing; mydriatic; bandage, 2 inches wide, 5 to 7 yards long.

discitis (dis-kī'tis) [G. *diskos*, disk, + -*itis*, inflammation]. Inflammation of any disk, esp, an interarticular cartilage. SYN: *meniscitis*.

discoblas'tic [" + *blastos*, germ]. Pert. to discoid segmentation of yolk in an impregnated ovum.

discoblastula (dĭs-kō-blăst-ūl'ă). A modified blastula found in highly telolecithal eggs as in birds in which the blastomeres form a cellular cap (germinal disc or blastoderm) which is separated from the yolk by a space, the blastocoele.

dis'coid [" + *eidos*, form]. Like a disc.

discoplacen'ta [" + *plakous*, a flat cake]. A disklike placenta.

discre'te [L. *discretus*, separated]. Separate; opposed to confluent.* Said of certain eruptions on the skin.

discrimi'nation. The process of distinguishing or differentiating.
 d. one-point. The ability to locate specifically a point of pressure on the surface of the skin.
 d. tonal. The ability to distinguish one tone from another. This is dependent upon the integrity of the transverse fibers of the basilar membrane of the organ of Corti.
 d. two-point. The ability to localize two points of pressure on the surface of the skin, and to identify them as discrete sensations. Also called tactile discrimination.

dis'cus. A disk.
 d. articularis. An interarticular fibrocartilage; an articular disk.
 d. proligerus. The cumulus oophorus, *q.v.*

discuss' [L. *discutere*, to dissipate]. To disperse, scatter, or cause to disappear.

discussion (dis-kush'un) [L. *discutere*, to dissipate]. Dispersal of a tumor or swelling.

discutient (dis-kū'shent) [L. *discutere*, to dissipate]. Agent which disperses a lesion or tumor.

disdiaclast (dis-dī'ă-klast) [G. *dis*, two, + *diaklan*, to break through]. A doubly refracting element in the tissues of striated muscles.

disease' [L. *dis*, apart, + Fr. *aise*, ease]. Literally the lack of ease: a pathological condition of the body that presents a group of symptoms peculiar to it and which sets the condition apart as an abnormal entity differing from other normal or pathological body states.
 d. acute. D. having a rapid onset and of relatively short duration.
 d. chronic. One having a slow onset and lasting for a long period of time.
 d. communicable. D. the causative organism of which is transmissible from one person to another, either directly or indirectly through a carrier or vector.
 d. congenital. D. which is present at birth. May be due to hereditary factors, or prenatal infection.
 d. constitutional. (1) D. due to an individual's hereditary make-up. (2) A disease involving the body as a whole in contrast to one involving specific organs.
 d. contagious. An infectious disease readily transmitted from one person to another.
 d. deficiency. A disease resulting from inadequate intake or absorption of essential dietary factors such as vitamins or minerals.
 d. degenerative. A disease resulting from degenerative changes that occur in tissues and organs, characteristic of old age.
 e. endemic. A disease which is present more or less continuously in a community.
 d. epidemic. D. which attacks a large number of individuals in a community at the same time.
 d. familial. A d. which occurs in several individuals of the same family.
 d. functional. A d. in which no anatomical changes can be observed to account for the symptoms present.
 d. hereditary. D. due to hereditary factors transmitted from parent to offspring.
 d. idiopathic. D. for which no causative factor can be recognized.
 d. infectious. D. resulting from the presence in the body of a pathogenic organism.
 d. malignant. (1) Cancer, q. v. (2) D. in which the progress is extremely rapid generally threatening or resulting in death within a short time.
 d. occupational. D. resulting from factors associated with the occupation engaged in by the patient.
 d. organic. D. resulting from recognizable anatomical changes in an organ, or tissue of the body.
 d. pandemic. An epidemic disease which is extremely widespread involving an entire country, continent, or possibly the entire world.
 d. parasitic. D. resulting from the growth and development of parasitic organisms (plants or animals) in, or upon the body.
 d. periodic. Disease that occurs at more or less regular intervals or at the same time each year.
 d. psychosomatic. D. which structural changes in or malfunctioning of organs are due to the mind, esp., the emotions.
 d. sporadic. D. in which only occasional cases occur; not epidemic or endemic.
 d. subacute. D. in which symptoms are less pronounced but more prolonged than in an acute disease; intermediate between acute and chronic disease.
 d. venereal. Abr. V. D. includes syphilis, gonorrhea, and chancroid. Disease usually acquired through sexual relations.

disengage'ment [Fr. désengagement]. GYN: The displacement of the fetal head from within the maternal pelvis.

disequilibrium   D-38   **disinfection, of field of operation**

disequilib′rium [L. *dis*, apart, + *aequus*, equal, + *libra*, balance]. On unequal and unstable equilibrium.

disinfect (dis-in-fekt′) [" + *inficere*, to corrupt]. To free from infection by physical or chemical means.

disinfec′tant [" +*inficere*, to corrupt]. A chemical which kills bacteria. SYN: germicide, bactericide. Common disinfectants are (1) the halogens-chlorine, fluorine, (2) salts of heavy-metals-mercuric chloride (bichloride of mercury), silver nitrate, (3) acids—sulphurous acid, (4) alkalies—chloride of lime, (5) organic compounds—formaldahyde, alcohol 70%, iodoform, organic acids, phenol (carbolic acid), cresols, benzoic and salicylic acids and their sodium salts, (6) Misc., substances—thymol, hydrogen peroxide, potassium permanganate, boric acid. An agent that frees from infection. Term is usually applied to a chemical agent which kills bacteria or other micro-örganisms.

disinfecting agents. SEE: *alcohol, borax, boric acid, chlorine preparations, cresols, formaldehyde, hydrogen dioxide, kreseptol, mercuric chloride, nitric acid, phenol, potassium permanganate, sulfur, urotropin.*

disinfec′tion [L. *dis*, apart, + *inficere*, to corrupt]. The application of disinfectants. It is not possible to insure a 100% disinfection of a room. Disinfestation, or the killing of vermin by chemicals and their vapors, however, is possible.

   d. of blankets and woolens: May be steam disinfected, or soaked for 2 hours in 5% carbolic and then washed. Cotton goods may also be so treated, or boiled before washing.

   d. of excreta. Should be soaked in 5% carbolic solution for 1 hour before disposal. All infected excreta should be burned, but sputum may be treated as excreta if impossible to burn.

   d. of field of operation. A safe rule is to make the disinfection, if anything, too extensive. Thus, in operations of any magnitude upon scalp and large wounds of this structure, and all operations on the skull and its contents the entire scalp must be shaved and disinfected.

In operations upon the breast, the axilla and half of the chest must be prepared, and if glands of neck are involved the entire neck must be included in field of operation.

In amputation of foot and lower third of leg the disinfection must extend as far as knee, and in all higher amputations it should include the whole limb and corresponding side of pelvis.

In all abdominal operations below the umbilicus the pubis must be shaved, and the surface disinfection must include the whole ant. surface and both sides as far as the breasts.

In operations on the stomach, liver, and bile ducts the field extends from the pubis to the breasts. A general warm bath, liberal use of potash soap and a scrubbing brush must precede disinfection of the field of operation in all abdominal and pelvic operations, including hernia and varicocele.

In operations upon parts of the body difficult to disinfect, as scalp, palm of

DISINFECTANTS

Used For	Chemicals	Uses
Purifying the air and certain solutions.	Formaldehyde.	A 40 per cent solution of formaldehyde gas is called formalin. A 4 per cent solution preserves tissues, a 1 to 2 per cent solution disinfects instruments.
	Sulfur dioxide.	Formed by burning sulfur. Disinfects but will bleach colored fabrics.
	Chlorine.	This gas in presence of moisture is a powerful disinfectant; used mostly as chlorinated lime to disinfect stools and urine, also to remove odors. Used commercially to purify drinking water.
Sinks, etc.	Phenol (carbolic acid).	Two to 5 per cent solutions fatal to all bacteria. Concentrated solutions are corrosive.
	Cresols.	Generally prepared as emulsions or soapy solutions under trade name of Lysol; more powerful than phenol.
Skin.	Iodine.	A 3 per cent solution of iodine in alcohol is used to disinfect the skin before an operation.
Wounds.	Mercurochrome.	Two per cent solution is used for surface wounds and infections.
Urethral irrigation. Cervix uteri.	Acriflavine.	Maintains its high antiseptic power in the presence of serum. Used as a 1 per cent solution for painting the cervix, as a 1 in 2000 solution for urethral irrigation, or a 1 in 1000 solution as a lotion.
Bedpans and other articles.	Lysol.	Disinfectant and antiseptic. A 1 in 100 solution often used instead of 1 in 20 carbolic for disinfecting articles such as bedpans. A soapy preparation which cleanses as well as disinfects. Can be used as an antiseptic, half a dram to 1 pint for douching and swabbing.
Mouthwash.	Permanganate of potash.	Antiseptic and disinfectant. Diluted with water to a pink color, it is useful as a mouthwash or gargle.

disinfection, of field of operation

hand, and sole of foot, it is advisable to apply for 2 or 3 hours a potash soap poultice for sake of macerating the thick epithelial layers of the epidermis, preparatory to the chemical disinfection of the surface; scrub with hot water and potash soap, then rinse; then use alcohol, ether, spirits of turpentine or benzine. Alcohol is universally useful in hand and surface disinfection.

The mucous membranes are active, absorbing surfaces so that the use of solutions of carbolic acid, mercuric bichloride, and other potent antiseptics is fraught with danger. The free use of any of these agents in the vagina, uterus, or rectum has frequently resulted in serious poisoning, and in some instances death.

Disinfection of the mouth should invariably precede the use of a general anesthetic, as in doing so the danger of inflammatory complications of the air passages following anesthetization is greatly diminished. For this purpose and to prepare the mouth for operation, the safest, most efficient and agreeable solution consists of a saturated solution of boric acid with the addition of a teaspoonful of listerine to each ounce. The solution is applied with a soft tooth brush or swab of cotton.

In grave operations, such as excision of superior or inferior maxilla, and amputation of tongue, the employment of the solution is preceded by thorough cleansing of the teeth and the mucous membrane is swabbed with peroxide of hydrogen.

In operations upon the rectum, a brisk cathartic, and high rectal enema are given, followed by irrigation and swabbing with Thiersch's solution (salicylic acid, ½ dram; boric acid, 3 drams; sterilized water, 1 qt.).

Vaginal disinfection is more satisfactory. After a thorough scrubbing with hot water and potash soap, peroxide of hydrogen and pure alcohol are relied upon in the chemical disinfection of the mucosa. The vaginal disinfection is preceded by shaving and disinfection of the external genitals.

Catheterization should always be preceded by disinfection of the meatus with alcohol and 1:1000 solution of mercuric bichloride.

The ear should be mechanically cleansed of wax, dirt, blood clot, etc., and then be carefully disinfected by a stream of warm sublimate solution, 1: 2000 or hydrogen peroxide, till it is absolutely clean. Nose cleansed and thoroughly sprayed with boric acid solution.

disinfestation (dis-in-fes-ta'shun) [" + *infestāre*, to strike at]. The process of killing infesting insects or parasites.

disintegra'tion [" + *integer*, entire]. The product of catabolism; the falling apart of the constituents of a substance.

disjoint'. To disarticulate or to separate bones from their natural positions in a joint.

disk [G. *diskos*, a disk]. A round, flat, platelike structure.

d. anisotropic. A dark, shining, highly refractile disc forming a part of the striation of the myofibril of a striated muscle fiber. Also called A or Q stripe.

d. articular. A disc of dense fibrous tissue or fibrocartilage found in the structure of certain joints, esp., the temporo-mandibular joint.

dislocation, divergent

d., blood. A red blood corpuscle.

d., Bowman's. Segment of a muscle fiber.

d., choked. Inflammation of the optic disk. SYN: *papillitis*.

d. diameter. Optic disk diameter.

d. embryonic. An oval disc of cells in the blastocyst of a mammal from which the embryo proper develops. Its lower layer, the endoderm forms the roof of the yolk sac, its upper layer the ectoderm forms the floor of the amniotic cavity. The primitive streak develops on the upper surface of the disc.

d., epiphyseal. Disklike epiphysis at vertebral centrum's ends.

d. germinal. A disc of cells on the surface of the yolk of the eggs of reptiles and birds from which the embryo develops; the blastoderm.

d. Hensen's. A pale disc occurring in the middle of the anisotropic or a disc during contraction of a myofibril.

d. holder. Microscope joint to enable mobility in every direction.

d. intercalated. A highly refractive band which extends transversely across the fiber of cardiac muscle. They are bounded on each side by Z plates.

d., intermediate. Myofibrils. Also called Z line or Krause's membrane.

d., interpubic. Disk of cartilage bet. the pubic bones at their symphysis.

d., intervertebral. A fibrocartilage substance bet. vertebral surfaces.

It may rupture but it does not slip. It serves as a shock absorber. The gelatinous mass in the center is called the *nucleus pulposus*. When this slips out because of injury to the surrounding ring it is called herniation or a slipped disk. The cervical or the lower lumbar region may be injured causing pressure on nerve roots if in the lumbar region, with back and leg pains. Sneezing, spinal injury, and the ageing process may cause the trouble.

d., isotropic. A disc lying between the A discs of a striated muscle myofibril. Also called I or J. disc. It extends across the entire muscle fiber.

d. M. A thin line lying in the center of Hensen's disc.

d., Merkel's. A disclike expansion found at the end of sensory nerve fibers in the epidermis. It is a touch receptor. Also called *tactile disc*.

d., optic. Area of the retina where optic nerve enters it.

d. proligerous. SEE: *germinal d.*

d. Q. The anistropic or A disc of a striated muscle myofibril.

d. tactile. Merkel's disc, *q.v.*

d., Thorington's. Device used for retinoscopy.

d. Z. The intermediate disc of a striated muscle fiber, *q.v.*

dis″loca′tion [L. *dis*, apart, + *locāre*, to place]. The displacement of any part, more esp. the removal temporarily of a bone out of its normal position in a joint.

d., closed. Simple dislocation, *q.v.*

d., complete. One which completely separates the surfaces of a joint.

d., complicated. One which is associated with other important injuries.

d., compound. One in which the joint communicates with the external air.

d., congenital. One which exists from or before birth.

d., consecutive. One in which the luxated bone has changed its position since its first displacement.

d., divergent. One in which the ulna and radius are dislocated separately.

d., habitual. One which often recurs after replacement. [displacement].

d., incomplete. A subluxation; a slight

d., intrauterine. One which occurs to the fetus in the utero. [finger.

d., metacarpophalangeal joint. D. of This is usually complicated by an interposition of tendons or other structures, and if reduced tends to slip out immediately. In many instances manipulating of this region only tends to make it more difficult for a subsequent reduction; therefore, immobilize* the disturbed area with well placed and padded splints of hand and wrist. Send patient to doctor, promptly.

d., Monteggia's. Dislocation of hip joint in which head of femur is near anterosuperior spine of the ilium.

d., Nelaton's. Dislocation of the ankle in which the astragalus is formed up bet. the end of the tibia and the fibula.

d., old. A dislocation in which no reduction has been accomplished, even after many days, weeks, or months.

d., partial. Same as incomplete.

d., pathologic. One which results from paralysis or disease of joint or supporting tissues.

d., primitive. One in which the bones remain as originally displaced.

d., recent. One in which there is no complicating inflammation.

d., simple. One in which the joint is not penetrated by a wound.

d., subastragalar. Separation of the calcaneum and the scaphoid from the astragalus.

d., thyroid. Displacement of the head of the femur into the thyroid foramen.

d., traumatic. One due to injury or violence. SEE: *Names of bones in alphabetical order.*

dismemb'er. To remove an extremity or a portion of it.

disorganiza'tion [" + G. *organon*, a unified organ]. Alteration in an organic part, causing it to lose most or all of its distinctive characteristics.

diso'ma. A monster possessing two trunks.

disorientation (dis-o-ri-en-ta'shun) [" + Fr. *orienter*, to face the east]. Inability to estimate direction or location, or to be cognizant of time or of persons.

disparate points (dis'par-at) [L. *disparare*, to separate]. Points on the 2 retinas which are not corresponding or identical, causing objects to appear double.

dispareunia (dis-par-ū'nĭ-ă) [G. *dyspareunos*, badly mated]. Pain in the female during coitus.

dispen'sary [L. *dispensare*, to give out]. Place or clinic for free dispensation of medicines and treatment.

dispense (dis-pens') [L. *dis*, out, + *pensare*, to weigh]. To prepare or deliver medicines.

dispereme (dis-per-em') [G. *dis*, two, + *speirēma*, coil]. Stage that succeeds the diaster and precedes division of cell body, when threads of daughter cell are convoluted.

disperse (dis-pers') [" + *spergere*, to scatter]. To scatter, esp. applied to the scattering of light rays.

disper'sion. 1. Act of dispersing. 2. That which is dispersed.

d., coarse. Mechanical suspension.

d., colloidal. Colloid solution.

d. me'dium. Liquid in which a colloid is dispersed.

d., molec'ular. A true solution.

d. particles. Colloid particles in a colloid system.

d. system. A colloid solution.

displace'ment [Fr. *déplacer*, to lay aside]. 1. Removal from the normal or usual position or place. SEE: *cardianastrophe*. 2. Adding to a fluid one of greater density causing the first fluid to be dispersed. 3. Attachment of emotion from repressed conflict to some apparently indifferent idea.

PSY: The transfer of an emotion pert. to 1 set of ideas to an inappropriate idea; although properly thus associated in the unconscious.

disposi'tion. A natural tendency or aptitude exhibited by an individual or group of individuals. This may be manifested toward acquiring a certain disease, presumably due to hereditary factors.

dissect (dis-sekt') [L. *dissecāre*, to cut up]. To separate tissues and parts of a cadaver for anatomical study.

dissection (dis-sek'shun) [L. *dissecāre*, to cut up]. The cutting of parts for purpose of separation and studying of the same.

dissem'inated. Scattered or disturbed over a considerable area, esp., applied to disease organisms; scattered throughout an organ or the body.

d. sclerosis. A degenerative disease of the nervous system; insular sclerosis.

dissipa'tion (dis-ĭ-pa'shun) [L. *dissipāre*, to scatter]. Dispersion of matter. Act of being wasteful and living a dissolute life, esp., drinking to excess.

dissociation (dis-so-sĭ-a'shun) [L. *dis*, apart, + *sociatiō*, union]. Separation, as the separation by heat of a complex compound into simpler molecules.

d., microbic. Substrains arising from pure strains.

d. of personality. Split in consciousness resulting in 2 different phases of personality, neither being aware of the words, acts, and feelings of the other. SEE: *dual personality, multiple personality.*

d., psychological. Disunion of mind of which the person is not aware. Dual personalities, fugues, somnambulism, are so classified. May be result of trying to find a solution or substitution for a repressed complex.

d. symptoms. Anesthesia to heat, cold, and pain, without loss of muscular sense or tactile sensibility.

dissolu'tion [L. *dissolvere*, to dissolve]. Death; pathological resolution or breaking up of the integrity of an anatomical element.

dissolve (di-zolv') [L. *dissolvere*, to dissolve]. To cause absorption of a solid in and by a liquid.

dissolvent (diz-ol'vent) [L. *dissolvens*, dissolving]. 1. Having the power to dissolve. 2. That which is capable of disintegrating.

dissol'ving. To cause to enter into a solution.

distad (dis'tad) [L. *distāre*, to be distant, + *ad*, toward]. Away from the center.

distal (dis'tal) [L. *distāre*, to be distant]. Farthest from the center, from a medial line, or from the trunk. Opposite of *proximal.*

distend' [L. *distendere*, to stretch out]. 1. To stretch out. 2. To become inflated.

disten'tion [L. *distendere*, to stretch out]. The state of being distended. SEE: *goblet cell, Wangensteen's method.*

distichiasis (dis-tĭ-kī'a-sis) [G. *dis*, two, + *stichos*, row]. Two rows of eyelashes, the post. of which is directed inward toward the eye.

distil' [L. *destillāre*, to drop from]. To vaporize by heat, condensing and collecting the volatilized products.

dis'tillate [L. *destillāre*, to drop from]. The portion of a substance subject to distillation which passes in the form of a vapor and condenses.

distilla'tion [L. *destillāre*, to drop from]. Condensation of a liquid, heated to a volatilization point, as the condensation of steam from boiling water.
  It is used for the purification of water, and other purposes. Distilled water should not be exposed as it readily takes up impurities from the atmosphere.
  d., destructive. The process of decomposing complex organic compounds by heat in the absence of air, and condensing the vapor of the liquid products.
  d., dry. D. of solids without liquids.
  d., fractional. Separation of liquids based upon the difference in their boiling points.

distinctom'eter [L. *distinguere*, to mark out, + G. *metron*, measure]. Device for palpation of abdomen along its borders.

distobuccal (dis-to-buk'al [L. *distāre*, to be distant, + *bucca*, cheek]. Pert. to the distal and buccal walls of bicuspid and molar teeth.

Dis'toma, Dis'tomum (dis'to-ma, -mum) [G. *distomios*, double mouthed]. Former name of genus of trematods worms. Its members have been placed in many new genera.

Dis'tomata. A suborder of the Class Trematoda (flukes).

dis'tome. A fluke with two suckers; an oral and a ventral sucker or *acetabulum*.

distomiasis (dĭs-tō-mī-ās'ĭs). Infestation with flukes, which flukes may infest the intestine, liver, bile ducts, gallbladder, blood vessels, or lungs.

distor'tion. 1. A twisting or bending out of regular shape. 2. A writhing or twisting movement as of the muscles of the face. 3. A deformity in which the part or structure is altered in shape. 4. In psychiatry, adapting an idea to conform with a patient's wishes.

distractibil'ity [L. *dis*, apart, + *tractio*, a drawing]. PSY: A condition of mental wandering in which the thoughts are attracted by extraneous conditions or influenced by a disassociation of consciousness.

districhiasis (dis-trik-i'as-is) [G. *dis*, double, + *thrix*, hair]. Two hairs growing from the same hair follicle.

distrix (dis'triks). The splitting of ends of the hairs.

dito'cia, dito'kia [G. *dis*, double, + *tokos*, birth]. Twin birth.

ditokous (dit'o-kus). Giving birth to twins.

Dittrich's plugs (dit'ricks). Small particles in fetid sputum composed of pus, detritus, bacteria, and fat crystals.

diuresis (di-u-re'sĭs) [G. *dia*, through, + *ourein*, to urinate]. Abnormal secretion of urine.
  This occurs in diabetes mellitus, and also in hysteria, as an early symptom of chronic interstitial nephritis, as the result of fear or anxiety, from drinking large quantities of fluid, and in diabetes insipidus, when 200-300 oz. per day may be passed. SYN: *polyuria*. SEE: *antidiuresis, antidiuretic*.

diuretic (di-u-ret'ik). Increasing or an agent which increases the secretion of urine.
  Diuretics act in two ways (1) by increasing glomerular filtration or (2) by decreasing reabsorption from the tubules. An increase in blood flow in the renal vessels increases urine formation by increasing glomerular filtration-pressure and by increasing the number of glomeruli functioning.
  Diuretics act on the kidney cells, increasing permeability, and also on the circulation to the kidneys. Alcohol dilates the blood vessels of the kidneys and thus increases circulation to them.
  Cold applications have a diuretic action by contracting superficial vessels and raising blood pressure. SEE: *diuresis*.
  d., alterative. One eliminated by the kidney which aids diseased urinary tract surfaces.
  d., hydragogue. One increasing renal flow.
  d., refrigerant. One which alleviates irritation from urine.

diuretin (dĭ-u-re'tin) [G. *dia*, through, + *ourein*, to urinate]. A white, odorless powder, original soluble sodium salicylate salt of theobromine.
  USES: Diuretic; myocardial stimulant.
  DOSAGE: Average, 15 gr. (1 Gm.).
  INCOMPATIBILITIES: Acids, ferric salts, lime water, etc.

diur'nal [L. *diēs*, day]. 1. Daily. 2. Happening in the daytime, or pert. to it; opposed to *nocturnal*.

divagation (div-a-ga'shun) [L. *divagari*, to wander about]. Disconnected and incoherent speech.

divergence (di-ver'jens) [L. *divergere*, to tend apart]. Separation from a common center, esp. that of the eyes.

diver'gent [L. *divergere*, to tend apart]. Radiating in different directions.

diver's paralysis. Occupational disease due to returning too suddenly to normal atmosphere after working under high air pressure. SYN: *bends, caisson disease, tunnel disease*.

divertic'ula [L. *diverticulāre*, to turn aside]. Plural of *diverticulum, q.v.*

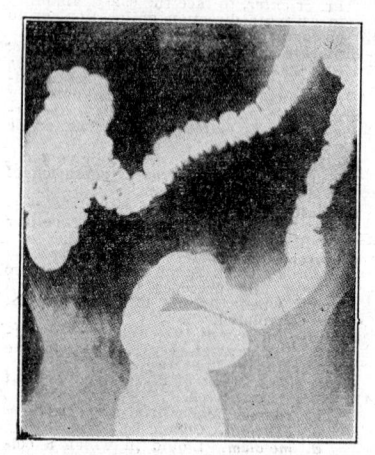

MULTIPLE DIVERTICULA
OF THE COLON

diverticula, hernia

d. hernia. Hernia containing part of the intestine.

diverticulec'tomy [" + G. *ektomē*, excision]. Surgical removal of a diverticulum.

diverticuli'tis [" + G. *-itis*, inflammation]. Inflammation of a diverticulum or of diverticula in the colon, causing stagnation of feces in little distended sacs of the colon (diverticula).

d., acute. SYM: Similar to appendicitis; inflammation of peritoneum, formation of an abscess, and finally gangrene accompanied by perforation may ensue. Symptoms are felt on left side.

d., chronic. SYM: Constipation growing worse, mucus in stools, griping abdominal pains at intervals. Wall of bowels may thicken, which may produce chronic intestinal obstruction. TREATMENT: Olive oil enemas, colonic lavage, liquid paraffin.

diverticulo'sis [" + G. *-ōsis*]. Diverticula of the colon.

diverticulum (di-ver-tik'u-lum) (pl. *diverticula*) [L. *diverticulāre*, to turn aside]. A sac or pouch in the walls of a canal or organ, esp. the colon.

d., Meckel's. Vestiges of the vitelline duct sometimes appearing as an extended pouch at the lower portion of the ileum.

divulsor (di-vul'sor) [L. *dis*, apart, + *vellere*, to pluck]. Device for dilatation of a part.

d., pterygium. Instrument for separating corneal portion of the pterygium.

d., tendon. Device for separating tendon from surrounding tissue.

dizygotic twins (di-zi-got'ik) [G. *dis*, two, + *zygon*, yoke]. Twins who are the product of 2 ova and who are dissimilar in most ways. [vertigo.

diz'ziness [A.S. *dyzig*, foolish]. Giddiness,

Dobell's solution (do'belz). Carbolic acid, borax, sodium bicarbonate, glycerine, and water in solution.

Dobie's globule (dō'bē's). A very tiny spherical body in a striated muscle fiber's light band.

DOCA *Desoxycorticosterone.* SEE: *STH*.

dochmiasis, dochmiosis (dok-mi'as-is, -mi-o'sis) [*Dochmius*, a nematode parasite]. Hookworm disease. SYN: *ankylostomiasis, uncinariasis*.

Dochmius (dok'mi-us). A species of parasite. SYN: *ankylostoma*.

Dock's test meal. Shredded wheat biscuit and 9-12 oz. water. SEE: *Ewald's t. m.*

dodecadactylitis (do-dek-a-dak-til-i'tis) [G. *dōdeka*, twelve, + *daktylos*, finger, + *-itis*, inflammation]. Inflammation of duodenum.

dodecadactylon (do-dek-a-dak'til-on) [" + *daktylos*, finger]. The duodenum.

Doe's method (Orlando Witherspoon Doe, American physician, 1843-1890). To resuscitate a stillborn infant; enclosed in an air-tight box with only the mouth and nose exposed, inspiration is produced by exhausting the air in the box, expiration by forcing in warm air.

dog bite. Lacerated wound by a dog. SEE: *rabies.*

Preserve the dog alive if possible to determine the presence of rabies. Rabies may result from the bite of many animals, including man. The virus is unknown but it has an affinity for the central nervous system.

INCUBATION PERIOD: Seven or 8 weeks, never less than 3 weeks, before the beginning symptoms appear. Rabies has been known to develop a year after the bite.

SYM: (1) The incubation period; (2) a premonitory stage; (3) a phase of excitement; (4) a short terminal period. No symptoms are manifest during the incubation period, with possible exception of numbness about the wound. There may be a slight rise in temperature, malaise, and irritability.

The 3rd period brings dysphagia,* dysarthria* and dyspnea,* a husky voice, and excitement. The patient becomes increasingly restless with abnormal sensitivity to sounds, sights, odors, and all stimuli. Spasms of the diaphragm, larynx, and pharynx follow with inability to take water without localized convulsions. Temperature rises, but seldom exceeds 102° F. Vomiting, sweating, and pallor may be in evidence. The pupils sometimes are unequal and there is a spasm of the jaw causing a clicking sound, and a husky voice. Terror and delusion, and excitement may be followed by depression. The jaw relaxes; death occurs on 5th or 6th day following this period.

TREATMENT: Cauterize wound with strong tincture of iodine or silver nitrate, or, if the dog is known to be rabid, cauterize with strong nitric acid or use actual cautery. A saturated solution of sodium bicarbonate should be applied to wash off excess acid. If nitric acid is not available, a strong solution of phenol may be employed which should later be washed off with alcohol. The wound must be kept open and the flow of blood may be induced or maintained by suction. Pasteur treatment should be given as quickly as possible. With this treatment only 0.3% develop hydrophobia. This is esp. important if the bite is about the head or neck. SEE: *hydrophobia, rabies.*

dol. Symbol for degree of pain registered on the dolorimeter. Each degree covers 2 gradations on the 21 gradations of this device. A headache producing a 2-dol pain may cease after taking aspirin, but a 4-dol pain will not be reduced to a 2-dol pain by taking aspirin. Increasing dosage will not help.

dolichocephalic (dol″ĭk-o-se-fal'ĭk) [G. *dolichos*, long, + *kephalē*, head]. Having a skull with a long ant. post. diameter.

dolichohieric (dol-ĭk-o-hi-er'ĭk) [" + *ieros*, sacred]. Having a slender sacrum.

dolichopellic, dolichopelvic (dol-ĭk-o-pel'-ĭk, -pel'vĭk) [" + *pellis*, pelvis]. Having an abnormally long or narrow pelvis.

dolichosigmoid (dol-ĭk-o-sig'moid) [" + *sigma*, the letter S, + *eidos*, form]. Having an abnormally long sigmoid flexure.

doll's head anesthesia. Anesthesia affecting the head, neck, and upper thorax.

dolor (do'lor) [L.]. Physical or mental pain. SEE: *calor, rubor, tumor.*

d. cap'itis. Headache.

dolorific (dol-o-rif'ik) [L. *dolor*, pain]. Causing pain.

dolorimeter (dŏl-ŏr-ĭm'et-er). *Symb.* dol (L. *dolor*, pain, + *meter*, measure). Device for measuring degree of pain that may be felt. Twenty-one gradations have been recorded. The threshold, or zero, represents 220 millicalories of heat; and the ceiling, 480 millicalories.

dolorogen'ic [" + G. *gennan*, to produce]. Causing pain.

domatophobia (do-mat-o-fo'bĭ-ă) [G. *dōma*, house, + *phobos*, fear]. A form of claustrophobia; abnormal aversion to being in a house.

domicil'iary [L. *domis*, house]. Pert. to a house, as treatment.

dom'inant [L. *dominans*, ruling]. That which is inherited from 1 parent developing to the exclusion of a contrasting character from the opp. parent. One who or that which gives something.

 d., hydrogen. A substance which gives up hydrogen to another substance. SEE: *hydrogen acceptor*.

donee (dō-nē') [L. *donāre*, to give]. One who receives blood transfused from another, the donor.

Donné's corpuscles (don-nāz'). Bodies in colostrum having ameboid movements.

 D.'s test. To determine pus in urine, mix with 10% solution of potassium hydrate. Pus is present if a lumpy hyaline mass with air bubbles rising slowly is formed when mixture is shaken.

do'nor [L. *donāre*, to give]. One who furnishes blood for transfusion.

 d., universal. One whose blood is of Group O, and whose blood is not agglutinated by the blood of anyone.

Don'ovan body. Supposed causative agent of lymphogranuloma inguinale, *q.v.*

doraphobia (do-ră-fo'bĭ-ă) [G. *dora*, hide, + *phobos*, fear]. Abnormal aversion to touching the hair or fur of animals.

Dorel'lo's canal. A bony canal in tip of temporal bone enclosing abducens nerve.

Dorendorf's sign. A filling up or fullness of the supraclavicular groove in aneurysm of the aortic arch.

dormison (dor'mĭ-sŏn). Trade name (Schering) for *methylparafynol*, a sleep-inducing drug. Said to be nontoxic, free of barbituric derivatives, or after-effects.

dorsabdom'inal [L. *dorsum*, back, + *abdere*, to hide]. Pert. to the back and abdomen.

dorsad (dor'sad) [" + *ad*, toward]. Toward the back.

dor'sal [L. *dorsum*, back]. Thoracic. Pert. to the back.

 d. elevated position. Patient is on the back, head and shoulders elevated at an angle of 30° or more. Employed for digital examination of genitalia, and in bimanual examination.

 d. inertia posture. In which patient rests on the back showing tendency to turn to either side or to slip down in bed. This may be seen in great weakness, in acute infectious diseases such as typhoid, mental apathy, and in muscular weakness. SEE: *Illustration below*.

 d. nerves. Nerves emerging from the dorsal vertebrae.*

 d. recumbent position. Same as dorsal elevated, except extremities are moderately flexed and rotated outward, the soles of the feet resting upon bed or table, or legs may be extended. With legs not flexed it is used for examination of chest, abdomen, and lower limbs. With legs flexed, it is used in giving douches, for bathing, for catheterizing, and for applying abdominal compresses. The patient may be placed in this position for bimanual palpation, or for vaginal examinations and repair of lesions following parturition.

 d. reflex. Irritation of the skin over the erector spinal muscles, causing contraction of muscles of the back.

 d. rigid posture. One in which both legs (or the right one) are drawn up; observed in peritonitis, meningitis, ascites, and tympanites. The right leg is drawn up in appendicitis, in pelvic inflammation, renal calculus, in right ureter, in psoas abscess or in peritonitis on the right side. SEE: Next page.

 d. vertebrae. Twelve bones of the spinal column bet. the cervical and lumbar vertebrae. SEE: *position, posture*.

dorsalgia (dor-sal'jĭ-ă) [" + G. *algos*, pain]. Pain in the back. SYN: *notalgia, rachialgia*.

dorsi-, dorso-, dors- [L.]. Combining form for *dorsum*, back.

dorsiduct (dor'sĭ-dukt) [L. *dorsum*, back, + *ducere*, to lead]. To draw toward the back or backward.

dorsiduc'tion [" + *ducere*, to lead]. Drawing toward the back.

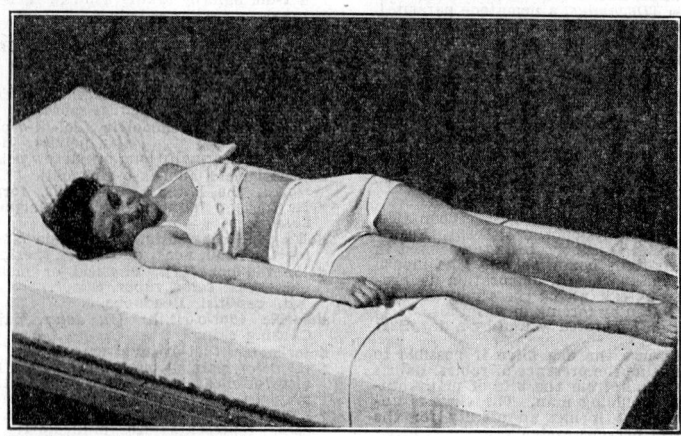

Posed by professional model   *Photo by Whitaker*
DORSAL INERTIA POSTURE
Showing weak patient slipping down into bed.

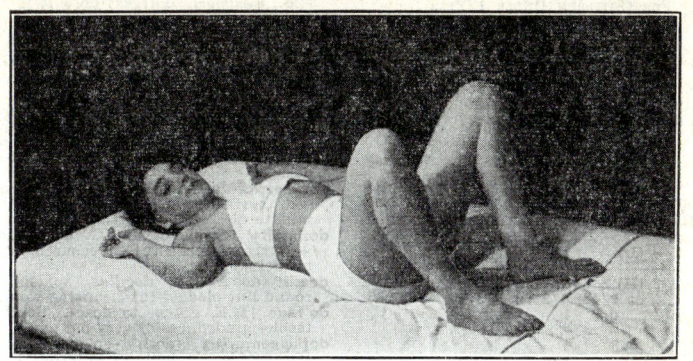

Posed by professional model *Photo by Whitaker*
DORSAL RECUMBENT POSITION

dorsiflect (dor′sĭ-flekt) [" + *flectere*, to bend]. Bending backward.

dorsiflex′ion [" + *flectere*, to bend]. The act of bending or flexion toward the dorsum, or rear; opposite of plantar-flexion. Also applied to straightening or extending the toes.

dorsim′esad [" + G. *mesos*, middle, + L. *ad-*, toward]. In the direction of the dorsimeson.

dorsim′eson [" + G. *mesos*, middle]. The median plane of the back.

dorsispinal (dor″sĭ-spi′nal) [" + *spina*, thorn]. Pert. to the back and spine.
 d. veins. Veins around the vertebrae.

dorsoceph′alad [" + G. *kephalē*, head, + L. *ad*, toward]. Situated toward the back of the head.

dorsodynia (dor-so-din′ĭ-ă) [" + G. *odynē*, pain]. Rheumatism in the muscles of upper part of back.

dorsosa′cral [" + *sacrum*, sacred, "sacred bone"]. Pert. to lower back.
 d. position. Patient lies upon the back, same as in the dorsal recumbent position,* excepting that thighs are flexed upon abdomen and legs upon thighs which are abducted. Leg holders are used to support legs in position.
 Used for gynecological examinations and treatments, in plastic operations on genital tract, in vaginal hysterectomy, and in diagnosis and treatment of diseases of urethra and bladder. SYN: *lithotomy position*.

dor′sum [L.]. The back or post. surface of a part.

dos′age [G. *dosis*, dose]. The amt. of medicine to be administered to a patient at one time.
 d. from tablets (usually hypodermic): Young's rule for children:

FOR CHILDREN FROM 1-12 YEARS
Formula:

$$\frac{\text{Age in yr.}}{\text{Age} + 12} \times \text{Adult dose} = \text{child's dose.}$$

Example 1: The adult dose of sodium bicarbonate is gr. xx. How much should a 4-year-old child receive?

$$\frac{4}{4 + 12} \times 20 = 5$$

∴ the child should receive gr. v.

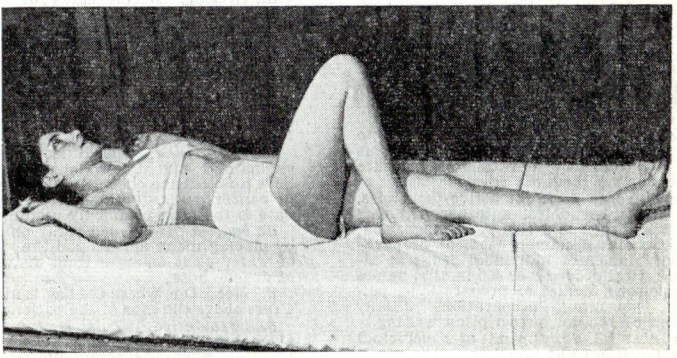

Posed by professional model *Photo by Whitaker*
DORSAL RIGID POSTURE
With right leg drawn up.

dosage, from tablets   D-45   **douche, intrauterine**

FOR CHILDREN UNDER 1 YEAR
FREID'S RULE
Formula:

$$\frac{\text{Age in mo.}}{150} \times \text{Adult dose} = \text{child's dose.}$$

Example II: The adult dose of morphine sulfate is gr. 1/4. How much should an 8-month-old child receive?

$$\frac{8}{150} \times \frac{1}{4} = \frac{1}{75}$$

∴ the child receives 1/75 gr. of drug.

WHEN THE STRENGTH OF THE TABLET ON HAND IS GREATER THAN THAT DESIRED
Give:

$$\frac{1/4 \ (D)}{1/3 \ (H)} = \frac{q}{1 \text{ tablet } (Q)} \quad q = \frac{3}{4}$$

or 1/4 : 1/3 :: Q : 1

$$\frac{q}{3} = \frac{1}{4}, \quad q = \frac{3}{4}$$

Give 3/4 of a 1/3 gr. tablet. To prepare: Dissolve the 1/3 gr. tablet in the number of ♏ indicated by the denominator, give the number of ♏ indicated by the numerator.

Note: Dilutions must range bet. 6 and 16. If the number indicated by the numerator or denominator is less than 6, multiply both numerator and denominator by the same number, then prepare the drug.

To prepare 3/4 of a tablet: 3/4 × 3/3 = 9/12. Dissolve tablet in 12 ♏ of water and give 9 ♏.

WHEN THE TABLET ON HAND IS OF WEAKER STRENGTH THAN THE DOSE WANTED
Give morphine gr. 1/6 from 1/8 gr. tablets.

Since 1/6 is greater than 1/8 it will be necessary to take 2 tablets or 1/4. Find relation bet. what is desired and what you have.

$$\frac{1/6 \ (D)}{2/8 \ (H)} = \frac{q}{1 \text{ tablet } (Q)} \quad q = \frac{8}{12}$$

or 1/6 : 1/4 :: q : 1

$$\frac{2}{8} \cdot q = \frac{1}{6} \quad Jq = \frac{8}{12}$$

Dissolve two 1/8 gr. tablets in 12 ♏ of water and give 8 ♏.

The proportionate dose for any age under 20 may also be found by taking 1/20 of the full therapeutic dose, and multiplying the result by the age in years.

Old people often require smaller doses. When given per rectum the dose is usually rather larger than when given by the mouth; if given hypodermically the dose is generally smaller.

d. meter. An instrument designed to estimate the quantity of radiation, so as to determine the duration of exposure when using roentgen rays.

dosage, words pert. to: active principles, alkaloids, antidotes, autotherapy, drug action, drugs and their administration, drugs with 2 names, medical preparations, names of individual drugs in alphabetical order (over 400 in all), names of poisons, names of preparations, poison, poisoning, preparations usually given by rectum, prescription writing.

dose (dōs) [G. *dosis*]. Amt. of a medicinal preparation to be taken at 1 time.

    d., divided. Fractional portions adm. at short intervals.

    d., lethal. A fatal dose.

    d., maximum. Largest dose it is safe to adm.

    d., minimum. Smallest dose that will be effective.

dosimeter (do-sim'e-ter) [" + *metron*, measure]. Device for measuring very small doses.

    d., Mecapion. Instrument registering 180 roentgens to determine x-ray dosage.

    d., Victoreen'. Apparatus which registers 256 roentgens to measure x-ray dosage.

dosimetric (do-sĭ-met'rik). Pert. to dosage.

    d. system. One of regular or determinate dosage.

dosimetry (do-sim'et-rĭ) [G. *dosis*, dose, + *metron*, measure]. Measurement of medicinal doses.

dossil (dos'ĭl) [L. *docillus*, spigot]. A round lint pledget for cleansing wounds.

do'tage [M.E. *doten*, to doze]. Senility; feeble-mindedness of very old age.

dothienenteritis (doth-i-en-en-ter-i'tis) [G. *dothien*, a boil, + *enteron*, intestine, + *-itis*, inflammation]. Inflammation of Peyer's patches. SYN: *typhoid fever.*

double (dŭb'l) [L. *duplus*, twofold]. Combining 2 things or qualities.

    d. consciousness. Expression of 2 phases of personality.

    d. personality. A split in consciousness, neither personality being aware of acts and words of other. SEE: *dual personality, multiple personality.*

    d. touch. Exploration with a finger in 1 cavity and thumb in another.

    d. uterus. State of having a double uterus. SYN: *dihysteria.*

    d. vision. Seeing 2 images of an object at the same time. SYN: *diplopia.*

douche (doosh) [Fr. *doucher*, to pour]. A current of vapor or stream of water, hot or cold, directed against a part.

Douches may be made up of plain water or water that is medicated. The douche may be for the purpose of personal hygiene or for the treatment of a local condition. In hemorrhage, temperature, 120° F.; in inflammation, 115° F. Usual quantity, 4 qt.

    d., air. Air current directed on body for therapeutic purposes.

    d., alternating. SEE: *Scotch d.*

    d., astringent. One containing substances for shrinking the mucous membrane, such as alum or zinc sulfate.

    d., circular. Needle spray or application of water to body through horizontal jets size of a needle from number of small rose sprays so placed that the water is projected against the skin of bather from 4 directions simultaneously.

    d., cleansing. One used for purposes of personal cleanliness; usually contains an alkaline substance. Temperature, 105° F.

    d., deodorizing. One to deodorize the vagina and vaginal secretions when they have an offensive odor. Used most often in cancer cases. Potassium permanganate is the most commonly used agent.

    d., fan. A fan-shaped spray obtained by placing index finger upon the stream of water as it emerges from distal end of douche hose.

    d., high. One where the bag is at least 4 feet above the hips of the patient.

    d., intrauterine. This is sometimes given immediately postpartum or postabortum when the cervix uteri is still patent. Hot water alone or water containing vinegar is used for the control of postpartum hemorrhage.

The intrauterine douche tube is a very useful, though dangerous, instrument in hands of an unskilled nurse. PREPARATION AND USE: Boil the tube 15 minutes in soda solution, expel air by allowing solution to run freely before inserting. Do not insert beyond the shield. Hold in position while using; use no force; attach a rubber tube to back flow, and provide a basin for the escaping fluid.

NP: (1) It is essential that the patient's buttocks are not pulled down below edge of table. If this is done when legs are elevated in leg rests or stirrups, an undue strain is apt to result in sacroiliac trouble. There is at least 1 case on record where gangrene of the foot followed prolonged pressure by stirrups. (2) The exterior surfaces are either scrubbed and irrigated with sterile water or painted, using either iodine or mercurochrome. The vaginal surfaces are included, as is also the cervix. The patient has already been placed on a Kelly pad, on which a sterile towel has been placed. A sterile towel is now placed across the pubes. Another is now placed crosswise across the buttocks. The "floating" nurse takes a strip of narrow adhesive plaster, about 18 in. long, holding it by the ends, well away from her. The "sterile" nurse then throws over the middle of the tape a sterile towel so that tape holds towel in middle fold. The "floating" nurse places edges of tape around patient's hips so that sterile towel is stretched tightly across rectum. Sterile leggings are now pulled over patient's legs and a lithotomy sheet draped down on the perineum. (3) Uterine packing should be ready. This form of packing is usually of gauze 1½ in. wide and 18 in. long.

d., jet. A solid stream from the douche hose.

d., low. One where the bag is 1-1½ feet above the hips of the patient.

d., medicated. One containing a medicinal substance for the treatment of local conditions. Lysol, tincture of iodine, and bichloride of mercury are the most commonly used.

d., neutral. Douche given at average surface temperature of body—90°-97° F.

d., pail. General affusion with pails of water at 3 temperatures dashed over the patient in quick succession. Temperatures of 1st bath, 100°, 96° and 90° F., reduced 2 degrees each, given once or twice weekly.

d., perineal. One projected upward from a bidet* placed just above floor; patient sits in armchair, crescent-shaped seat, and receives douche upon perineum.

d., rain. Overhead shower.

d., Scotch. Alternating of hot and cold jets of water against local area of skin.

d. solutions. *Alum*: ½ to 1%. *Bichloride of Mercury*: 1:3000-1:10,000. *Boracic Acid*: 2%. *Carbolic Acid*: ⅛ to 1%. *Green Soap*: 1%. *Lysol*: ⅛ to ½%. *Potassium Permanganate*: 1/10 to 1%. *Silver Nitrate*: 1/10%. *Sodium Bicarbonate*: 2%.

d., stimulating. The use of copious amt. of hot or cold water in case of pelvic congestion.

d. temperatures. For a *cleansing douche*, 105° F. For a *hemorrhage douche*, 120° F. For an *inflammation douche*, 115° F. For a *neutral douche*, 92° to 97° F. For a *vaginal douche*, 98° to 115° F.

d., vaginal. Long warm douche, 20 to 30 minutes, flowing slowly from height not greater than 15 in. above patient's pelvis, temperature from 98° to 115° F., from 3 qt. to 5 gal. daily.
SEE: *Elliott's treatment.*

d., vapor. Stream of vapor projected from the douche hose, given with or without intervening flannel clothes.

Douglas' cul-de-sac. Peritoneal sac which lies behind uterus and in front of rectum.

D.'s pouch. Same as D.'s *cul-de-sac.*

douglasitis (dug-las-i'tis) [G. *-itis*, inflammation]. Inflammation of the *cul-de-sac* of Douglas.

dow'el [Fr. *douille*, socket, from L. *ductus*, leading]. Metal pin for fastening an artificial crown to a tooth root.

Dowell test. Injection of ant. pituitary in flexor surface of arm, which causes an erythema at point of injection in a pregnant woman.

Doyère's eminence (dwah-yair'). Elevation where a nerve filament enters a muscle.

D. P. Abbr. for Doctor of Pharmacy.

dr. Abbr. for dram or drachm.

D. R. Abbr. for reaction of degeneration.

drachm (dram) [G. *drachmē*, a weight]. A unit of weight in apothecaries' system. SYMB: ʒ. SYN: *dram.*

dracontiasis (drā-kŏn-tĭ-ā-sĭs) [G. *drakontian*, little dragon]. SYN: dracunculosis, *q.v.*

dracunculiasis (drā-kŭn-kū-lī-ās-ĭs). Infestation with the nematode, *Dracunculus medinensis.*

dracunculosis (drā-kŭn-kū-lō-sĭs). The condition of being infested with the guinea worm.

Dracunculus (drā-kŭn-kŭl'ŭs). A genus of parasitic nematodes belonging to the suborder *Camallanata.*

D. medinensis. The guinea worm or "fiery serpent". A species of nematode which is a common human parasite esp., in parts of Asia and Africa. The adult gravid female lives in subcutaneous tissues and may reach a length of 3 or 4 ft. Embryos are deposited in a blister formed on the skin which breaks liberating embryos into water. Intermediate host is a species of *Cyclops.* Human infestation results from drinking water containing infested Cyclops.

drain (drain) [A.S. *drehnigean*, to draw off]. 1. Exit or tube for discharge of morbid matter. 2. To draw off a fluid.

d., absorbable. One taken up by lymphatic and venous system.

d., capillary. Drawing off by capillary attraction. Never use in suppuration, etc.

d., nonabsorbable. One made from horsehair, gauze, rubber, glass, or metal. TYPES: *abdominal, antrum, perineal, suprapubic,* etc.

d., tubular. One prepared from bone. Absorbed 8-10 days.

drainage (dra'nāj) [A.S. *drehnigean*, to draw off]. The free flow or withdrawal of fluids, as pus from a cavity or wound. SEE: *autodrainage, drain.*

d., capil'lary. D. by method of capillary attraction.

d., funnel. D. with glass funnels.

d., postural. D. for draining nasal area and the sinuses.
The patient lies on his back on a bed with shoulders over the side and head hanging down.

drainage, tube   D-47   **dromotropic**

d. tube. Device for allowing escape of pus, serum, blood, or other fluids from a wound, abscess, etc.

d. t. carrier. Device for placing drainage tube in position.

d. t. trocar. Device to introduce drainage tube without making a large incision.

dram [G. *drachmē*, a weight]. Sixty gr. or 1/8 oz. apothecary weight; 3.888 Gm., 27.34 gr. or 1/16 oz., avoirdupois.

d., fluid. A teaspoonful or 1/8 of a fluid ounce or 57.1 gr. of distilled water, the equivalent of 3.70 cc. In Great Britain 54.8 gr. of distilled water or 3.50 cc.

dram′atism [G. *drama*, acting, + *ismos*, state of]. Dramatic behavior and lofty speech in insanity.

drapetomania (drap-et-o-ma′nĭ-ă) [G. *drapetēs*, runaway, + *mania*, madness]. Insane impulse to wander from home.

dras′tic [G. *drastikos*, effective]. 1. Acting strongly. 2. A very active purgative, usually producing many evacuations, and accompanied by pain and tenesmus. Ex: croton oil, elaterin.

draught (draft) [A.S. *dragan*, to draw]. 1. A drink. 2. Drawing liquid into the mouth.

draw sheet. One so arranged that it can be removed easily from under a patient.

NP: In cases where patients are unconscious, draw sheets should be placed under them; these are sheets of soft cotton material of double thickness, 3 feet wide and about 3 yards long, to cover the bed under the buttocks and thighs. Just enough of the folded sheet should be passed under the patient to cross the bed, the rest being rolled up and the roll is tucked firmly under the mattress: any soiled portion may from time to time be drawn away from under, the patient sponged clean, and a dry length of the rolled up part pulled under him.

drepanocyte (dre-pan′o-sīt) [G. *drepanē*, sickle, + *kytos*, cell]. Sickle or crescent cell.

drepanocytemia (dre-pan-o-si-te′mĭ-ă) [" + " + *aima*, blood]. Sickle cell anemia.

drepanocytic (dre-pan-o-sit′ĭk) [" + *kytos*, cell]. Pert. to or resembling a sickle cell.

dressing [Fr. *dresser*, to treat a wound]. Covering, protective, or support for diseased or injured parts.

NP: Before beginning to do anything to a wound, however slight, the following rules must be known and carried out:

1. Have everything ready before preparing patient.
2. Lift sterile towel, wool, gauze and instruments needed for the dressing with sterile forceps into a sterile receptacle.
3. Fold down bedclothes, remove bandage, and arrange mackintosh to protect bedclothes.
4. *Preparation of Hands*:
    (a) Nails must always be kept short and clean.
    (b) Scrub up to the elbows with brush and soap under running water for 3 minutes by the clock.
    (c) Rinse off all soap.
    (d) Soak in perchloride of mercury (1 in 2000) for 2 minutes.
    (e) If nurse is to wear gloves, dry on sterile towel or dehydrate with methylated spirit. A nurse sometimes has difficulty in putting on wet sterile rubber gloves. This difficulty will be overcome if she lathers her hands with soap, or rinses them in spirit after she has "scrubbed up."
    (f) The hands must be clasped in front, not touching apron, etc., while returning to the bed.
5. Arrange sterile towel in position.
6. Nothing coming in contact with wound must be touched by fingers. Use forceps for removing dressing, holding swabs while cleaning the wound, and for applying fresh dressing.
7. Keep wound covered while cleaning surrounding parts.
8. Never use a soiled bandage, or fasten the knot or pin over the wound.
9. If the discharge comes through the dressings at any time it must either be done again or a thick pad of cotton wool be placed over and round it, fastened on with a bandage.
10. Leave the patient dry, comfortable, and warm.
11. After the dressing, wash everything with soap and water, and put away. Scrub instruments with brush in cold water, then soap and water, taking special care with serrated edges, etc. Sterilize and put away.

RS: *adhesive plaster, bandages, compresses, cravats, protectives.*

d., absorbent. Gauze, sterilized gauze, absorbent cotton, lint, lint cloth, paper lint, absorbent wool, wood wool, moose pappe, spongiopilin.

d., hot moist. Most common form is saturated hot boric solution, heated to as hot as can be borne by bare forearm of nurse. Sterile towel unfolded, gauze dressings dropped into it, immersed in solution at middle, wrung out by turning dry ends in opposite directions. Dressing is then applied, with sterile forceps, directly to the wound and a dry, sterile towel is sometimes used over it, to keep dressing in place. Heat is best maintained by infrared generator.

Dreyer's tuberculin or **vaccine** (dri′erz). A tuberculosis vaccine prepared by removing the lipoid material from tubercle germs.

Drinker respirator. Apparatus in which alternating positive and negative air pressure upon the patient creates artificial respiration. Commonly called the "iron lung".

drip [A.S. *dryppan*, to drip]. 1. To fall in drops. 2. To instill drop by drop.

d., intravenous. Slow injection of glucose and saline solution, a drop at a time, intravenously.

d., Murphy. Slow rectal instillation of a fluid drop by drop.   [*drip sheet*.

drip sheet. Modified sheet bath. SEE: bath

drisdol (dris-dol′). Crystalline vitamin D, in solution of propylene glycol.

USES: In vitamin D deficiency, as rickets, tetany, etc.

dromomania (dro-mo-ma′nĭ-ă) [G. *dromos*, a running, + *mania*, madness]. Insane impulse to wander.

dromotrop′ic [" + *trepein*, to turn]. Pert. to supposed fibers in cardiac nerves which influence conductivity of muscles.

drop [A.S. *dropa*] [L. *gutta*]. 1. A minute spherical mass of liquid. 2. Falling of a part from paralysis or injury.

d., ague. Fowler's solution.

d., black. Vinegar of opium.

d. culture. A bacterial culture in a drop of culture media.

d. finger. Baseball finger.

d. foot. Toes dragging in walking with falling of foot due to paralysis of dorsal flexor muscles.

d., knockout. A drug to cause unconsciousness; usually adm. for criminal purposes.

d. wrist. Paralysis of extensor muscles causing hand to hang down from forearm.

droplet. Very small drop.

d. infection. That conveyed by means of infective particles, as when carried in a spray from the nose or mouth. Usual mode of infection from common cold.

dropsy (drop'sĭ) [contraction L. *hydrops*, dropsy, from G. *ydōr*, water]. A condition rather than a disease. Morbid accumulation of water in the tissues and cavities; hydrops.

ETIOL: Heart disease, kidney disease, cirrhosis of the liver, and other causes. The kidneys have little to do with retention of tissue fluids, but the body chemistry is more at fault in Bright's disease.

DIET: Sufficient proteins, carbohydrates, fats, vitamins, and iron, reducing the sodium intake: a salt free diet with an acid base. Potassium or other salt substitutes may be used.

d. of amnion. OB: Abnormal increase in amt. of amniotic fluid. SYN: *polyhydramnios*.

d. of the belly. Ascites.

d. of brain. Hydrocephalus. [ease.

d., cardiac. That due to cardiac dis-

d. of chest. Hydrothorax.

d. of peritoneum. Hydroperitoneum.

d., ovarian. A collection of fluid in the ovary forming a crust.

d., tubal. A collection of fluid in the fallopian tube. SYN: *hydrosalpinx*.

d., uterine. A collection of fluid in the uterine cavity. SYN: *hydrometra*.

Drosoph′ila. A genus of flies belonging to the order Diptera. Includes the common fruit flies.

D. melanogaster. A genus of fruit flies used extensively in the study of genetics. The development of the chromosome theory of heredity was largely the outcome of research on this species.

drowning [A.S. *druncnian*, to drown]. A special type of asphyxia resulting from the body being submerged in water or some other field. External respiration is blocked by a spasm of the larynx or the filling of the lungs with fluid.

SYM: Unconsciousness, cessation of respiration, cyanosis, etc., depending upon duration of submersion. Due to action of the epiglottis, there is very little, if any, water in the lung.

F. A. TREATMENT: Artificial respiration at once. Do not waste time trying to get water out of lungs. Apply external heat, massage extremities, use oxygen or oxygen-carbon dioxide mixtures with resuscitation. May have to be kept up for several hours.

RS: *artificial respiration, asphyxia, shock, syncope, unconsciousness.*

drug [Fr. *drogue*]. A medicinal substance, used in the treatment of disease.

drug action. LOCAL: When the drug is applied locally or direct to a tissue or organ it combines to form an albuminate with the cells' albumins. This action may be: 1. *Astringent a*: When the drug cannot act because the albuminate does not dissolve. 2. *Corrosive a*: When the drug is strong enough to destroy cells. 3. *Irritating a*: When too much of the drug combines with cells to impair them.

GENERAL OR SYSTEMIC ACTION: When the drug enters the blood stream by absorption or direct injection affecting tissues and organs not near the site of entry. Systemic action may be: 1. *Specific*: When specific in the cure of a certain disease. 2. *Substitutive*: When it supplies substances deficient in the body. 3. *Physical*: When some of the constituents of a cell are dissolved by the action of the drug in the blood stream. 4. *Chemical*: When the drug or some of its principles combine with the constituents of cells or organs to form a new chemical combination. 5. *Salt Action*: Osmosis* caused by dilution of salt (also acids, sugars, and alkalies) in the stomach or intestines by fluid withdrawn from the blood and tissues, or diffusion* when water is absorbed by cells from the lymph. 6. *Selective*: Action produced by drugs which only affect certain tissues or organs. 7. *Synergistic*: The stimulating of the action of one drug by another drug. 8. *Antagonistic*: Counteraction of one drug by another one. 9. *Physiological*: The effect of a drug on a normal animal body. 10. *Therapeutic*: The effect upon diseased organs or tissues. 11. *Side Action*: Creating an effect not desired. 12. *Empiric*: An effect produced but not proved by laboratory experiment. 13. *Toxicological*: A poisonous effect generally from result of an overdose.

CUMULATIVE: The effect of drugs too slowly excreted or absorbed so that an accumulation of the drug in the body produces a poisonous effect. Such drugs should not be administered continuously.

d. a., incompatible. Ill effects produced by 2 or more drugs antagonistic to each other.

drug action, words pert. to: active principles, alkaloids, antidotes, dosage, drugs and their administration, drugs with 2 names, medical preparations, names of individual drugs in alphabetical order (over 400 in all), names of poisons, names of preparations, poison, poisoning, preparations usually given by rectum, prescription writing.

drug addiction. A condition caused by excessive or continued use of habit-forming drugs. SYN: The symptom-pattern may be changed according to the drug used. In general there may be a change in personality, loss of appetite, or the appetite is dulled; disturbance in normal sleep-rhythm, generally a weight loss. The addict may be dull, sleepy, and incoördinated in movement having the appearance of intoxication. The eyes often tearing, and bloodshot; a watery fluid at times dripping from the nose. When intramuscular or intravenous injection is used there may be scars, hardening and swelling of the arm tissues.

drug rashes: Drugs of which large doses are liable to produce a rash are: Arsenic, belladonna, bromides, chloral, iodides, opium, phenacetin, quinine, sera, sodium salicylate, turpentine (the nurse may notice the rash on the buttocks after a

drugs, administration of

turpentine enema has been given), and the application of cyanide gauze to a wound (in this latter case the rash is confined to the area of the wound, which is surrounded by "sores").

Antipyrin: Papular, erythematous rash, sometimes accompanies by edema and much irritation.

Arsenic: Papular or erythematous rash, sometimes urticarial. Prolonged use may produce pigmentation of skin.

Belladonna: Erythematous rash, usually accompanied by intense itching.

Bromides: Usually like acne vulgaris. Sometimes erythema.

Chloral: Papular erythema.

Enemata (soap) may cause erythema or urticaria if hard soap is used.

Iodides: Usually papular erythema, sometimes with acnelike pustules.

Phenolphthalein: Macular rash, sometimes purpuric.

Quinine: Very irritable erythema or urticaria.

Salicylate: Erythematous rash, possibly morbilliform.

Serum: Usually urticaria.

Sulfonal: Erythematous or urticarial rash.

drugs (special) **and their administration.**
ACIDS: When acids are administered they should be given well diluted through a glass tube, because they are corrosive to the enamel and the dentine of the teeth. They should be given with much water and the drinking tube should be placed well back in the mouth to prevent the fluid coming in contact with the teeth before passing into the throat. Hydrochloric acid is one preparation that should always be given with the above thought in mind.

ARTIFICIAL TEETH: A solution for artificial teeth. Plain normal salt solution or boric acid solution diluted one-half may be used.

BARBITAL DERIVATIVES: All such preparations should be crushed and dissolved in hot milk before given. The potion should be given from one-half to one hour before sleep is desired. All procedures should be taken care of before the medicament is given in order that nothing shall disturb the patient after the drug is administered.

CALOMEL: This drug should always be followed by a saline purgative. Unless the intestine is emptied of calomel within a reasonable time it may continue to be absorbed and produce poisonous symptoms.

ELIXIR OF IRON, QUININE AND STRYCHNINE: When administering these drugs they should be given well diluted with much water, through a glass tube. A bitter effect will be produced if given before meals.

FOWLER'S SOLUTION: When a nurse is giving a patient Fowler's solution or *Liquor potassii arsenitis* the dosage must be started at the minimum and increased gradually until the maximum is reached, then decreased in the same manner. This is to prevent cumulative action.

HABIT FORMING DRUGS: Whenever the use of habit forming remedies is indicated, the nurse should use them only after exhausting every art of her profession to relieve pain, discomfort, or insomnia. If these efforts fail, she may then give the dose ordered; but the patient should never be informed of the nature of the remedy given.

INSULIN: When this is administered, it should be given hypodermically, 2 or 3 times per day according to the instructions of the attending physician, and 15 minutes to one-half hour before a meal.

IODINE: When iodine is applied to the skin and there is a burning from the application, alcohol should be used to wash away the accumulation and prevent further burning, or any caustic effect.

LAXATIVES: These are best given in the evening, because it usually takes 6 or 8 hours for them to produce an effect. The saline purgatives are usually given well diluted on an empty stomach, in the morning. The other purgatives are also usually given in the morning, or as ordered and needed.

MOUTHWASH: Stock solutions used for mouthwash should be diluted one-half or more before being given to the patient. The special solutions, such as S.T. 37, or Dobell's solution, should be diluted according to instructions from the attending physician. Only enough for the immediate mouth washing should be used at a particular time. To take into the patient's room a glass or cupful, when the patient will only use about one-half of the amt., is not an economic procedure.

HORSE SERUM: When it is to be administered, information should be obtained as to whether the patient has had serum recently, as a reaction is liable to occur if not sufficient time has elapsed bet. the inoculations. If uncertain, a test should be made by injecting a few drops of the horse serum hypodermically, and within a short time a reaction will occur. A small spot appears at the site of the injection if the patient has a tendency to susceptibility.

OXYGEN: The most commonly used method for the administration of oxygen consists of inserting a catheter into a nostril, or into each nostril. Oxygen may also be given from a tank by means of a mask over the patient's nose and mouth, or the patient may be placed in an oxygen tank, or an oxygen chamber or room. The last 2 methods are very dangerous and must be used very cautiously, as the danger from fire hazard is very great. These 2 methods are very expensive.

SALINE PURGATIVES: Should always be given to the patient when the stomach is empty, preferably in the morning.

SIEDLITZ POWDERS: These should be mixed or dissolved in about one-fourth glass of water; a separate glass for each powder, the white and the blue. At the bedside, the one glass of mixture is poured into the other and the patient drinks this mixture before it effervesces.

TYPHOID VACCINE: This should be administered by hypodermic injection. The 1st or initial dose should be 0.5 cc., and 2nd and 3rd doses should consist of 1 cc. of solution in each dose. The container should be well shaken before the dosage is withdrawn. The injections should be 7 days apart. When giving the injection the insertion should be made bet. the musculature of the upper arm or distal or outer part.

drugs and their administration, words pert. to: active principles, alkaloids, antidotes, dosage, drug action, drugs with 2 names, medical preparations, names of individual drugs in alphabetical order

Drugs and Their Common Names

CHEMICAL NAMES	COMMON NAMES
Nitric Acid	Aqua Fortis
Nitro-Hydrochloric Acid	Aqua Regia
Copper Sulfate	Blue Vitriol
Potassium Bitartrate	Cream of Tartar
Mercury Subchloride	Calomel
Calcium Carbonate	Chalk
Potassium Carbonate	Salt of Tartar
Potassium Hydroxide	Caustic Potash
Sodium Chloride	Common Salt
Iron Sulfate	Copperas, or Green Vitriol
Mercury Perchloride	Corrosive Sublimate
Aluminum and Potassium Sulfate	Dry Alum
Magnesium Sulfate	Epsom Salts
Light Carburetted Hydrogen	Fire Damp
Lead Sulfide	Galena
Sodium Sulfate	Glauber's Salts
Glucose	Grape Sugar
Lead Lotion	Goulard Water
Iron Bisulfide	Iron Pyrites
Tin Oxide	Jewelers' Putty
Nitrogen Protoxide	Laughing Gas
Calcium Oxide	Lime
Silver Nitrate	Lunar Caustic
Calcium Chloride	Muriate of Lime
Potassium Nitrate	Niter or Saltpeter
Sulfuric Acid	Oil of Vitriol
Arsenic Sulfide	Realgar
Lead Oxide	Red Lead
Iron Oxide	Rust of Iron
Ammonium Chloride	Sal Ammoniac
Calcium Hydroxide	Slaked Lime
Sodium Carbonate	Soda
Ammonia	Spirits of Hartshorn
Hydrochloric Acid	Spirits of Salt
Calcium Sulfate	Stucco, or Plaster of Paris
Lead Acetate	Sugar of Lead
Basic Copper Acetate	Verdigris
Mercury Sulfide	Vermilion
Acetic Acid (Diluted)	Vinegar
Ammonia	Volatile Alkali
Hydrogen Oxide	Water
Ammoniated Mercury	White Precipitate
Zinc Sulfate	White Vitriol

(over 500), names of poisons, names of preparations, poison, poisoning, preparations usually given by rectum, prescription writing.

drugs, handling of. Read the label or other printed instruction issued with medicine carefully; measure out accurately the doses (quantities) ordered, and never guess.

A measuring glass or spoon should be employed, marked either in drams and ounces only, or with the words teaspoon, dessertspoon, and tablespoon also.

One drop equals 1 minim. Symbol, ♏. One teaspoonful equals 1 dram. Symbol, ʒ. Two teaspoonfuls equal 2 drams or 1 dessertspoonful. Four teaspoonfuls equal ½ ounce or 1 tablespoonful. Two tablespoonfuls equal 1 ounce. Symbol, ʒ.

Important Points: (1) The cork must never be left out of the bottle, as a necessary property may evaporate or the drug may become a dangerous concentration. (2) The drug compartment must be kept locked.

To Give a Dose of Medicine: Make quite sure: (a) To whom it has to be given; (b) what has to be given; (c) when it has to be given; (d) the amt. to be given.

Shake the bottle, measure the dose, again note label. Give to patient and see that it is swallowed. A small drink of water will take away unpleasant taste or medicine may be taken through a straw. As in feeding, the patient's head and shoulders should be well raised before the dose of mixture is given to him.

drugs, words pert. to: absorbent, alkaloids, alterative, ampule, analeptic, analgesic, anesthetic, anodyne, antacid, antagonistic action, anthelmintic, antiarthritic, antidiuretic, antiemetic, antilithic, antiperiodic, antipyretic, antiseptic, antisialagogue, antispasmodic, antizymotic, aperient, aromatic, astringent, a. action, balsam, biochemorphic, bitters, cachet, calmant, capsule, cardiac depressant or stimulant, carminative, cathartic, caustic, cerate, cerebral depressant or stimulant, cholagogue, confection, convulsant, correctant, corrosive, counterirritant, decoction, delirifacient, demulcent, deodorant, depilatory, depressant, depressomotor, depurant, detergent, diaphoretic, digestant, disinfectant, diuretic, drug administration, ecbolic, elixir, emetic, emmenagogue, emollient, emulsion, enzyme, epispastic, errhines, escharotic, evacuant, excitomotors, expectorant, extract, febrifuge, ferment, fluidextract, galactogogue, glandular therapy, glucosides, glycerite, hematinic, hemostatic, hormone, hydragogue, hypnotic, idiosyncrasy, infusion, irritation, lamella, laxative, liniment, local remedy, lozenge, mixture, motor depressant or stimulant, mucilage, mydriatic, myotic, oil, ointment, oleate, oleoresin, organotherapy, oxytocics, paper, pharmacognosy, pharmacology, pill, plant acids, plaster, poisonous action, powder, prophylactic, protein shock therapy, purgative, refrigerant, resins, respiratory depressant or stimulant, revulsant, rubefacient, saline purgative, saponins, secretory depressant or stimulant, sedative, sensitization, serum therapy, sialogogue, solution, somnifacient, soporific, specific, spirit, sterule, stimulant, stomachic, styptic, sudorific, suppository, synergistic action, systemic remedies, tablet, tannins, teniacide, tincture, tonic, toxicological action, vaccine therapy, vasoconstrictor, vasodilator, vermicide, vermifuge, vescette, vesicant, vinegar, vulneraries, water, wine. SEE: *names of drugs (over 500) in alphabetical order.*

drum [A.S. *drumme*]. The ear drum or tympanic cavity; the tympanum or cavity of the middle ear.

drunkenness [A.S. *drincan*, to drink]. Alcoholic intoxication.

druse (drūs) [Ger. "a rock cavity lined with crystals"]. 1. Rupture of tissues with no lesion of surface. 2. Small, hyaline, globular pathological growths formed on optic papilla.

dry cells. A zinc container lined with thin blotting paper which serves as the negative electrode, carbon rod in center as positive electrode, a paste of ammonium chloride, zinc chloride, manganese dioxide, and granulated carbon fills space bet. electrodes, preventing polarization.

dry diet. A temporary high carbohydrate diet with measured liquid given bet. meals only.

dry ice. Solidified carbon dioxide used for commercial refrigeration.

dry measure. A measure of volume for dry commodities, as follows:
  2 pints (pt.) = 1 quart (qt.)
  8 quarts = 1 peck (pk.)
  4 pecks = 1 bushel (bu.)

Drys'dale's corpuscles. Non-nucleated, granular cells present in the fluid of certain ovarian cysts.

du'alism [L. *dualis*, pert. to two]. 1. The condition of being double or two-fold. 2. The theory that the human body consists of two entities, mind and matter, which are independent of each other. 3. The theory that blood corpuscles arise from two types of stem cells; myeloblasts giving rise to the myeloid elements and lymphoblasts giving rise to the lymphoid elements.

dual personality. A split in consciousness which results in the expression of 2 different phases of personality at various intervals, neither personality, as a rule, being aware of the words, acts, and feelings of the other. When this does rarely occur it has been called "co-consciousness."

SEE: *co-consciousness, dissociation of personality, multiple personality, vigilambulism.*

Dubini's disease (doo-be'nēz). Rhythmic, rapid contractions of a group or groups of muscles. SYN: *electric chorea, spasmus Dubini.*

duboisine (du-boi'sin). Alkaloid derivative of plant *Duboisea myoporoides.*
  USES: Its sulfate is used as a hypnotic, and to treat paralysis agitans.
  DOSAGE: 0.0008-0.0015 Gm. (1/80-1/40 gr.).

d., poisoning from. Resembles atropine, *q.v.*

Duchenne's disease (du-shen'). 1. Bulbar paralysis. 2. Tabes dorsalis.

Ducrey's bacillus (du-kray') *Hemophillus ducreyi*. The cause of soft sore, or chancroid; small, rod-shaped organism found in pairs.

duct [L. *ducere*, to lead]. 1. A narrow tubular vessel or channel, especially one serving to convey secretions from a gland. 2. A narrow enclosed channel containing a fluid, as the semicircular duct of the ear.

d., accessory pancreatic. D. of the pancreas, leading into pancreatic d. or the duodenum near the mouth of the common bile d.

d., alimentary. SEE: *thoracic d.*

d. alveolar. A branch of a respiratory bronchiole which leads to the alveolar sacs of the lungs.

d. Bartholin's. The major duct of the sublingual gland proper.

d's biliary. The canals which carry bile. The intrahepatic ducts include the bile canaliculi and interlobular ducts; the extrahepatic ducts include the hepatic duct, cystic duct, and common bile duct.

d., Botallo's. Fetal blood vessel connecting the pulmonary artery and aorta. The *ductus arteriosus.*

d., cochlear. Canal of the cochlea.

d. common bile. Duct formed by the confluence of the hepatic and cystic ducts. It conveys bile to the duodenum opening at the ampulla of Vater.

d. Cuvier's. One of a pair of fetal veins (the common cardinal veins) which convey blood from the pre- and posterior cardinal veins to the sinus-venosus of the heart. The right one becomes the sup. vena cava.

d., cystic (*d. cys'ticus*). Excretory d. of gallbladder. SEE: *gallduct.*

d. efferent. Any duct conveying secretion from a gland.

d., ejaculatory (*d. ejaculatorius*). Conveys semen into urethra.

d. endolymph. In the embryo a tubular projection of the otocyst ending in a blind extremity, the endolymph sac; in the adult it connects the endolymphatic sac with the utricle and saccule.

d. excretory. Any duct which conveys a product from an organ, as the excretory duct of a salivary gland.

d., galactophorous. Duct carrying milk in mammary glands' lobes.

d., Gartner's. A remnant of the wolffian duct extending from the parovarium through the broad ligament into the vagina.

d., hepatic (*d. hepat'icus*). Receives bile from liver. SEE: *gallduct.*

d's., intralobular bile. SEE: *biliary d.*

d. lacrimal. One of two short ducts, inferior and superior, which conveys tears from the lacrimal lake to the lacrimal sac. Their openings are on the margins of the upper and lower eyelids.

d. lactiferous. One of fifteen to twenty ducts which drain the lobes of the mammary gland. Each opens in a slight depression on the tip of the nipple.

d., Leydig's. SEE: *wolffian d.*

d. lymphatic. One of two main ducts conveying lymph to the blood stream. The left lymphatic duct (thoracic duct) drains the left side of the body above the diaphragm and all of the body below the diaphragm; the right is a smaller duct draining the right side of the body above the diaphragm. Both enter into the subclavian veins near their junctions with the int. jugular veins.

d. mammary. SEE: lactiferous duct.

d., mesonephric. SEE: *wolffian d.*

d. mesonephric. The cut which in the embryo connects the mesonephros with the cloaca. In the male it develops into the ductus deferens. Also called Wolffian duct.

d., metanephric. Ureter.
d., milk (*d. lactiferus*). A mammary duct entering the nipple.
d., Müller's. Bilateral ducts in the embryo that go to form the uterus, vagina, and fallopian tubes.
d. nasolacrimal. The duct which conveys tears from the lacrimal sac to the nasal cavity. It opens beneath the inferior nasal concha.
d. omphalomesenteric. The vitelline duct, *q.v.*
d., pancreat'ic (*d. pancreaticus*). Conveys pancreatic juice to the duodenum. Also called the d. of Wirsung.
d. paraurethral. Skene's duct, *q.v.*
d., parotid (*d. parotide'us*). Discharges parotid secretions into mouth.
d., prostatic (*d. prostat'ica*). One of 20 ducts which discharge prostatic secretion into the urethra.
d., right lymphatic. D. carrying lymph near liver on right side of body.
d. s of Rivinus. Five to fifteen ducts (the minor sublingual ducts) which drain the posterior portion of the sublingual gland.
d. salivary. Any of the ducts which drain a salivary gland.
d. of Santorini. The accessory pancreatic duct.
d., secretory. A gland's smaller canals.
d., segmental. A pair of embryonic tubes, located bet. visceral and parietal layers of mesoblast on each side of body.
d. s semicircular. Three membranous tubes forming a part of the membranous labyrinth of the inner ear. They lie within the semicircular canals and bear corresponding names, superior, posterior, and lateral.
d. seminal. Any of the ducts which convey semen, specifically the ductus deferens and the ejaculatory duct.
d. Skene's. Paraurethral duct. One of two slender ducts which open on either side of the urethral orifice in the female.
d., spermatic. Vas deferens.
d., Stenson's, Steno's. Parotid gland d.
d., sublingual. SEE: *Rivini's and Bartholin's d's.*
d., submaxillary. SEE: *Wharton's d.*
d., sudorif'erous. Sweat duct.
d. tear. Any that convey tears, inc. excretory ducts of lacrimal glands, lacrimal ducts, and nasolacrimal ducts.
d., testicular. Vas deferens.
d., thoracic (*d. thorac'ius*). Discharging into subclavian vein.
d., umbilical. Embryonic d. bet. cavity of intestines and umbilical vesicle. The vitelline duct, *q.v.*
d. utriculosaccular. A short one connecting the utricle and saccule of inner ear.
d., vitelline. The narrow duct which in the embryo connects the yolk sac (umbilical vesicle) with the mid gut. Also called yolk stalk, umbilical d.
d. (of) Wirsung. The major pancreatic d.
d. Wolffian. The mesonephric duct.
duct'less [" + A.S. *læssa*]. Having no duct, secreting only internally.
d. glands. Ductless glands secrete internally one or more hormones which have a specific action upon the body. SEE: *endocrine, endocrinology, exocrine.*
ductule (duk'tūl) [L. *ducere*, to lead]. A very small duct.
d. aberrant. One of a group of small tubules associated with the epididymis. They are blindly ending, representing the vestigial remains of the caudal group of mesonephric tubules.
ductus. Latin for duct. Used in BNA.
d. arteriosus. A channel of communication bet. main pulmonary artery of the fetus and aorta.
d. choledochus. The common bile duct.
d. cochlearis. The cochlear duct *q.v.* Also called *scala media.*
d. communis. One about 3 in. long formed by union of cystic and hepatic d.'s; carries the bile to the intestine.
d. deferens. Excretory duct of the testicle. Conveys sperm from the epididymis to the ejaculatory duct. SYN: *vas deferens.*
d. efferent. One of a group of 12-14 small tubes which constitute the efferent ducts of the testis. They lie within the epididymis and connect the rete testis with the ductus epididymis. Their coiled portions constitute the lobulus epididymis.
d. hemithoracicus. Ascending branch of thoracic opening either into right lymphatic duct or close to angle of union of right subclavian and right internal jugular veins.
d. hepaticus dexter. One issuing from the right lobe of the liver, uniting with the d. hepaticus sinister and forming the hepatic duct.
d. hepaticus medius. An occasional branch of the hepatic duct conveying bile from the quadrate lobe.
d. hepaticus sinister. One issuing with d. hepaticus dexter to form hepatic duct.
d. prostatici. Ducts for secretion of prostate into the urethra.
d. sacculo-utricularis. Small tube connecting saccule of internal ear with utricle.
d. venosus. Smaller, shorter, and post. of 2 branches into which umbilical vein divides after entering the abdomen; empties into the inf. vena cava.
Duhrssen's incisions of the cervix uteri. Incisions made in the undilated cervix in order to allow for completion of the delivery of the fetus.

They are made at 4-hour intervals in order that if there is any extension of the incision at the time of the passage of the fetus, this extension will not go into the broad ligaments and the uterine arteries.

duipara (dū-ip'ăr-ă) [L. *duo*, two, + *parēre*, to bear]. A female pregnant for the 2nd time.

dulcin (dul'sin) [L. *dulcis,* sweet]. A toxic substance, 200 times sweeter than sugar. SYN: *sucrol, dulcite.*

dulcite. A sugar ($C_6H_{11}O_6$) found in certain plants. Also called *dulcitol* or *dulcose.*

dull [A.S. *dol*]. 1. Not resonant on percussion. 2. Not mentally alert.

dullness, dulness (dul'nes) [A.S. *dol*]. 1. Lack of normal resonance on percussion. 2. State of being dull.

dumb [A.S.]. Mute. Unable to speak.
d. ague. Latent malaria not expressed by ordinary signs.

dumb'bell crystals. Crystals shaped like a dumbbell.

dumb'ness [A.S.]. Muteness.

duode'nal [L. *duodeni,* twelve]. Pert. to the duodenum.
d. activities. The entry of acid chyme into the duodenum brings about discharge of bile from the gallbladder and the secretion of pancreatic juice by the pancreas. These enter through the

common bile duct. Bile salts alkalinize the chyme and emulsify the fats. Through the action of pancreatic enzymes, the following changes occur: *stealsin* (pancreatic lipase), hydrolyzes neutral fats to fatty acids and glycerol; *amylopsin* (pancreatic amylase) hydrolyzes starch to maltose; *maltose* hydrolyzes maltose to glucose. Three proteolytic enzymes: *trypsin, chymotrypsin*, and *carboxypeptidase* act on proteins hydrolyzing them to proteoaes, peptones, and amino acids.

d. bulb. Area of duodenum just beyond the pylorus.

SECRETORY PHENOMENA: One of these substances, secretin,* excites the pancreas to increased production of its juice; the other, cholecystokinin, causes the gallbladder to contract and force its contents through the ductus choledochus into the duodenum. In addition, nervous mechanisms contribute to the co-ordination which exists here, regulating the rate of discharge of chyme from the stomach, varying both quality and quantity of the various secretions, and determining the rate of passage through the duodenum. For the action of particular juices: SEE: *bile; digestion; enzyme; functions of pancreas; juice gastric; juice, pancreas; succus entericus.*

MOTOR PHENOMENA: (a) First part of duodenum (*pars superior, duodenal cap, d. bulb*) is the small portion immediately following the pylorus. It is regularly full of material and consequently visible in roentgenograms as a spade-shaped shadow. (b) The next part (*pars descendens*) is that into which the common bile duct (*ductus choledochus*) and pancreatic ducts open. Movement through it and through (c) the pars inferior and (d) the pars ascendens is rapid, so that they are normally inconspicuous by x-ray. Throughout the duodenum the mucosa is thrown into folds (*plicae circulares*) and shows the active projections called villi. The folds are permanent and inactive. The villi, which stud the surface of the folds as well as the spaces bet. them, exhibit waving and thrusting movements.

d. delay. Delay in the movement of food through the duodenum due to conditions such as inflammation of lower portion on the intestine which reflexly inhibits duodenal movements. d. papilla major. Slight elevation in descending portion of the duodenum bearing openings of the common bile duct and main pancreatic duct. d. papilla minor. Slight elevation about 2 cm. above the p. major bearing opening of the accessory pancreatic duct.

d. ulcer. Broken mucous membrane, usually accompanied by suppuration and perhaps a sore is present which bleeds with more or less danger of perforation. It heals slowly due to constant passage of irritating fluids and food over it, distention of stomach and contraction and relaxation of gastric muscles, acids of foods, bile and gastric juice, condiments and concentrated sugar solution.

TREATMENT: Mucin; metaphen* used successfully, 1:500 solution, a teaspoonful after each meal.

DIET: Same as for peptic ulcer. SEE: *peptic ulcer.*

d. papilla. Raised surface near entrance of ductus choledochus communis into duodenum.

duodenectasis (dū-ō-děn-ěk'tă-sĭs). Chronic dilatation of the duodenum.

duodenectomy (du-o-den-ek'to-mĭ) [" + G. *ektomē*, excision]. Excision of part or all of the duodenum.

duodeni′tis [L. *duodeni*, twelve, + G. *-itis*, inflammation]. Inflammation of the duodenum.

duodenocholecystostomy (dū-od-en″o-kol-e-sis-tos'to-mĭ) [" + G. *cholē*, bile, + *kystis*, bladder, + *stōma*, mouth]. Formation by surgical means of a fistula bet. duodenum and gallbladder.

duodenocholedochotomy (du-od-en″o-koled-o-kot'o-mĭ) [" + G. *choledochos*, bile duct, + *tome*, incision]. Surgical incision of the duodenum to reach the gallbladder.

duodenocystostomy (du-od-en″o-sist-os'to-mĭ) [" + G. *kystis*, bladder, + *tome*, incision]. Formation of a passage bet. the duodenum and the bladder.

duodenoenterostomy (du-od-en″o-en-ter-os'to-mĭ) [" + G. *enteron*, intestine, + *stōma*, opening]. Formation of passage bet. the duodenum and intestine.

duodenogram (du-o-de′no-gram) [" + G. *gramma*, a writing]. A roentgenogram of the duodenum.

duodenohepatic (du-o-den-o-he-pat′ik) [" + G. *ēpar, epat-*, liver]. Pert. to duodenum and liver.

duodenojejunostomy (du-o-den-o-jej-u-nos'to-mĭ) [" + *jejunum*, empty, + G. *stōma*, opening]. Making a passage bet. the duodenum and jejunum.

duodenos′copy [" + G. *skopein*, to examine]. Inspection of the duodenum with an endoscope.

duodenostenostomy (du-o-den-o-sten-os'-to-mĭ) [" + G. *stenos*, narrow, + *stōma*, opening]. The making of an opening through the abdomen into the duodenum.

duodenostomy (du-o-den-os'to-me) [" + G. *stoma*, opening]. Operation of making a permanent opening into the duodenum through the wall of the abdomen.

duodenotomy (du-o-den-ot'o-me) [" + G. *tome*, incision]. An incision into the duodenum.

duodenum (du-o-de′num) [L. *duodeni*, twelve]. The first part of the small intestines connecting with the pylorus of the stomach and extending to the jejunum.

It receives the hepatic and pancreatic secretions through the same duct. It is 8 to 11 inches long. Brunner's glands

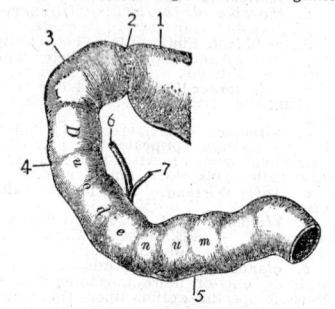

THE DUODENUM

1. Pyloric end of the stomach. 2. Pyloric valvule. 3. Upper transverse part. 4. Descending part. 5. Lower transverse part. 6. Choledochus duct. 7. Pancreatic duct.

duplication, duplicature   D-54   **dynamoscopy**

are found in the duodenum, and the chyle is formed here. Lieberkühn's glands are also found here.

It is a crucial section of the alimentary canal, since in it occurs the mixing of (1) the acid chyme from the stomach, (2) the bile from the liver and gallbladder, (3) the pancreatic juice entering by way of 2 ducts, and (4) the intestinal juices secreted by the glands of Brunner and the crypts of Lieberkühn.

NERVE SUPPLY: Pancreatico-duodenal plexus and the vagus.

BLOOD SUPPLY: Pancreatico-duodenal and gastroduodenal arteries.

RS: *Brunner's glands, choledochoduodenostomy, duodenal digestion, duodenal ulcer, gallbladder, glands, intestines, Lieberkühn's glands, liver, pancreas.*

duplica'tion, du'plicature [L. *duplicāre*, to double]. A doubling or folding, or state of being folded.

duplica'tus. Fetal monstrosity in which the cephalic or the pelvic end is doubled or both.

dupp (dŭp) [imitative origin]. Word denoting 2nd sound at cardiac apex heard in auscultation. It is due to the closing of the pulmonary and aortic semilunar valves.

The 1st sound is longer and pitched lower. SEE: *heart, auscultation of; lubb; lubb-dupp.*

Dupuytren's contraction (du-pwē-trănz'). Contraction of palmar fascia causing ring and little fingers to bend into palm so that they cannot be extended.

du'ra [L. *durus*, hard]. Dura mater.

   d. mater [L. hard mother]. The outer membrane covering the spinal cord (*d. m. spina'lis*) and brain (*d. m. cer'ebri* or *enceph'ali*). SEE: *pia mater, tentorium.*

dural (du'ral) [L. *durus*, hard]. Pert. to the dura.

durama'tral [" + *mater*, mother]. Pert. to the dura. SYN: *dural.*

du'raplasty [" + G. *plassein*, to form]. Plastic repair of the dura mater.

durematoma (du-rem-at-o'mă) [" + G. *aima*, blood, + *ōma*, tumor]. Accumulation of blood bet. arachnoid and dura.

duritis (du-ri'tis) [" + G. *-itis*, inflammation]. Inflammation of the dura. SYN: *pachymeningitis.*

duroarachnitis (du-ro-ar-ak-ni'tis) [" + G. *arachnē*, cobweb, + *-itis*, inflammation]. Inflammation of dura and arachnoid membrane.

durocaine (du'ro-kān). Spinal anesthetic. Procaine hydrochloride in pseudohypobaric solution.

Duroziez's murmur (du-ro-zī-ez'). Double murmur over femoral artery on pressure.

dust. Minute, fine particles of earth; any powder.

   d. blood. Hemoconia.

   d. cells. Reticulo-endothelial cells in the walls of the alveoli of the lungs which ingest or destroy dust particles.

   d., ear. Fine calcareous bodies found in the gelatinous substance of the otolithic membrane of the ear; otoconia, or otoliths.

dust'ing powder. Any fine powder for dusting on skin. [vovaginal gland.

Duverney's gland (doo-ver-nas'). The vul-

dwarf. An abnormally short or undersized person; a pigmy.

   d. achodroplastic. One with normal trunk but possessing shortened extremities, with a large head, and protruding buttocks.

   d. asexual. One with deficient sexual development.

   d. cretin. One resulting from deficient development of the thyroid gland.

   d., diabetic. One due to diabetes.

   d., hypophysical. One due to hypofunction of ant. lobe of the hypophysis.

   d., infantile. One showing marked physical, mental and sexual underdevelopment.

   d., micromelic. One with very small limbs.

   d., ovarian. An undersized female due to absence or underdevelopment of the ovaries.

   d., phocomelic. One with abnormally short diaphyses.

   d., physiologic. A normal dwarf.

   d., pituitary. A hypophysical one.

   d., rachitic. One due to rickets.

   d., renal. One due to renal osteodystrophy.

   d., sexual. One showing normal sexual development.

dwarfism. Condition of being abnormally small. May be hereditary, or a result of endocrine dysfunction, deficiency diseases, renal insufficiency, diseases of the skeleton or other causes.

dy'ad. 1. A pair. 2. A pair of chromosomes formed by the division of a tetrad in miosis. A dyad represents a single chromosome split precociously for a subsequent division. 3. In *Chem.* A bivalent element or radical.

dynamia (dī-nam'ĭ-ă) [G. *dynamis*, power]. Vital energy or ability to combat disease.

dynamic (di-nam'ik) [G. *dynamis*, power]. Pert. to vital force or inherent power, opp. of *static.* [is inherent in mind.

   d. psychology. A theory that energy

dynam'ics [G. *dynamis*, power]. The science of bodies in motion and their forces.

dynamization (di-nam-iz-a'shun) [G. *dynamis*, power]. The attempt to add to the potency of medicines by agitation or comminution.* SEE: *attenuation.*

dy'namo [G. *dynamis*, power]. Apparatus for conversion of mechanical energy into electrical power.

Chief parts are (1) magnetic field produced by electromagnets, (2) armature which is coil of insulated wire mounted around a soft iron core, (3) collecting device, (4) mechanical power which keeps either the armature or electromagnet moving in relation to another.

dynamogen'esis [" + *genesis*, growth]. The capacity to call forth increased energy.

dynamogen'ic [" + *gennan*, to produce]. Pert. to, or caused by, an increase of energy.

dynamograph (di-nam'o-graf) [" + *graphein*, to write]. Device for recording muscular strength.

dynamometer (di-nam-om'e-ter) [" + *metron*, measure]. 1. A device for measuring muscular strength. Simple dynamometer is spring scales bet. segment to be examined and examiner's hand. 2. A device for giving the magnifying power of a lens.

dynamoneure (di-nam'o-nūr) [" + *neuron*, nerve]. A motor, spinal nerve cell.

dynamoscope (di-nam'o-skōp) [" + *skopein*, to examine]. Instrument for auscultation of muscles.

dynamoscopy (di-nam-os'ko-pī) [" + *skopein*, to examine]. Auscultation of muscles.

dyne (dīn) [G. *dynamis*, power]. A unit of force which would propel a mass of weight of 1 gram with a velocity of 1 cm. in a second.
dys- [G.]. Prefix meaning bad, difficult, painful.
dysacous'ia, dysacous'ma [G. *dys*, bad, + *akousis*, hearing]. Discomfort caused by loud noises.
dysacusia (dis-a-ku'si-a) [" + *akousis*, hearing]. Abnormal discomfort from noises; *dysacousma*.
dysadrenia (dis-ă-dre'nĭ-ă) [" + L. *ad* toward, + *rēn*, kidney]. Functional disorder of the kidneys.
dyse'mia [" + *aima*, blood]. Blood deterioration.
dysalbumose (dis-al'bū-mōs) [" + L. *albumen*, white of egg]. A variety of albumose insoluble in water or hydrochloric acid.
dysantigraphia (dis-an-tĭ-gra'fĭ-ă) [" + *anti*, against, + *graphein*, to write]. Inability to copy writing or printed letters.
dysaphia (dis-af'ĭ-ă) [" + *aphē*, touch]. Dullness of the sense of touch.
dysarhythmia (dis-a-rĭth'mĭ-ă). Abnormal rhythm.
   d. cerebral. Abnormal rhythm in brain waves indicated by the electroencephalogram. Characteristic of epilepsy.
dysarteriotony (dis″ar-te-rĭ-ot'o-nĭ) [" + *artēria*, artery, + *tonos*, tension]. Abnormal blood pressure, either too low or too high.
dysarthria (dis-ar'thrĭ-ă) [" + *arthron*, articulation]. 1. Difficulty in articulation of joints, as in amyostasia. 2. Incorrectly applied to imperfect speech; stammering.
dysarthro'sis [" + *arthrōsis*, joint]. Joint malformation.
dysbasia (dis-ba'zĭ-ă) [" + *basis*, a step]. Difficulty in walking, esp. when due to disease of the brain or spinal cord.
dys'bolism [" + *bolē*, a throwing]. Disordered metabolism.
dysbulia (dis-bu'lĭ-ă) [" + *boulē*, will]. 1. Inability to fix the attention; difficulty experienced in thinking; mind weariness. 2. Weak and uncertain will power.
dyschezia (dis-ke'zĭ-ă) [" + *chezein*, go to defecate]. Constipation due to habitual neglect to respond to stimulus to defecate.
dyschiria (dis-ki'rĭ-ă) [" + *cheir*, hand]. Inability to tell which side of the body has been touched.
   If referred to the wrong side it is called *allochiria*;* to both sides, *synchiria*.* SYN: *achiria*.
dyscholia (dis-ko'lĭ-ă) [G. *dys*, bad, + *cholē*, bile]. Morbid condition of the bile.
dyschondroplasia (dĭs-kŏn-drō-plā'zĭ-a). Disease, usually hereditary, resulting in disordered growth. Characterized by multiple exostoses of growth of the epiphyses, esp. of the long bones, metacarpals, and phalanges. Also called multiple cartilaginous exostoses, diaphyseak aclasis, etc.
dyschroa, dyschroia (dĭs-krō-ă, dĭs-krō'ĭ-ă). Discolored skin, esp. of the face; poor or bad complexion.
dyschromatopsia (dis-kro-mat-op'sĭ-ă) [" + *chrōma*, color, + *opsis*, vision]. Imperfect color vision.
dyschro'mia [" + *chrōma*, color]. Discoloration, as of the skin.
dyscinesia (dis-sin-e'zĭ-ă) [" + *kinēsis*, movement]. Impairment of voluntary movements.
dyscoimesis (dis-koy-me'sis) [" + *koimēsis*, a sleeping]. Delay in falling asleep.

dysco'ria [" + *korē*, pupil]. Abnormal form of the pupil.
dyscrasia (dis-kra'sĭ-ă) [" + *krasis*, mixture]. Morbid condition supposed to be caused by toxins in the blood.
dyscrasic dis-kra'sik) [" + *krasis*, mixture]. Pert. to dyscrasia.
dyscri'nism [" + *krinein*, to secrete, + *ismos*, condition of]. Any disorder of secretions, esp. of an endocrine gland.
dysdiadochokinesia (dis″dĭ-ă-do″-ko-kin-e'sĭ-ă) [" + *diadochos*, succeeding, + *kinesis*, movement]. Inability to quickly substitute antagonistic motor impulses.
dysdiemorrhysis (dis-di-em-or'ĭ-sis) [" + *dia*, through, + *aima*, blood, + *rysis*, a flowing]. Sluggish circulation of capillaries.
dyse'mia [" + *aima*, blood]. Any blood disease.
dysendocriniasis (dis-en-do-krin-i'a-sis) [" + *endon*, within, + *krinein*, to secrete]. Faulty function of the endocrine glands.
dysendoc'rinism [" + " + " + *ismos*, state of]. Faulty function of the endocrine glands; dysendocriniasis.
dysendocrisi'asis [" + " + *krinein*, to secrete]. Faulty function of the endocrine glands; dysendocriniasis.
dysenteric (dis-en-ter'ĭk) [" + *enteron*, intestine]. Pert. to dysentery.
dysentery (dis'en-ter-e) [" + *enteron*, intestine]. A term applied to a number of intestinal disorders, esp. the colon, characterized by inflammation of the mucous membrane.
   ETIOL: Bacterial or viral infection, infestation by protozoa or parasitic worms, or chemical irritants.
   SYM: Abdominal pain, tenesmus, diarrhea with passage of mucus or blood.
   d., amebic. Due to amebas. SYM: Similar to catarrhal d. with intermissions. TREATMENT; SEE: Amebiasis.
   d. bacillary. An acute infectious disease caused by bacteria of the genus Shigella, esp. *Sh. dysenteriae, Sh. paradysenteriae,* and *Sh. sonnei.* It may occur sporadically or in epidemics. In addition to intestinal symptoms, a severe toxemia may occur due to exo- and endotoxins produced by the organisms. In epidemics the fatality rate may be 20% or more.
   d. balantidial. B. caused by ciliate protozoan, Balantidium coli.
   d., catarrhal. Due to change of weather, diet, or water. SYM: Diarrhea, vomiting, abdominal pain, desire to stool, and fever. Increasing stool: bloody. TREATMENT: Liquid diet. Rest in bed. Irrigation of colon.
   d., diphtheric. Epidemic intestinal affection, caused by vegetable organism in drinking water. SYM: Intensified catarrhal d. symptoms. TREATMENT: Dietetic, same as other forms of the disease. Milk alone, 4 to 5 pt., lean meat, only.
   d., malignant. A form in which symptoms are very pronounced and progress rapidly, usually terminating fatally.
   d. viral. D. caused by virus.
dysergasia (dis-er-ga'sĭ-ă) [" + *ergon*, work]. Inability to function properly. SYN: *neurasthenia*. In Psy., a behavior disorder characterized by disorientation, hallucinations, dreamstates, and delirium. Possibly due to toxic conditions such as uremia, or alcohol intoxication.
dysergastic (dis-er-gas'tik). Pert. to dysergasia.
   d. reaction. Hallucinations, fears, disorientation, dream states, and other mental disorders resulting from poor circulation and nutrition of the brain.

dysergia (dis-er'jĭ-ă) [G. *dys*, bad, + *ergon*, work]. Lack of co-ordination in muscular voluntary movements.

dysesthesia (dis-es-the'zĭ-ă) [" + *aisthesis*, sensation]. 1. Sensations, as of the pricks of pins and needles, or of crawling. SYN: *formication*. 2. Failing sensitivity, esp. of touch. 3. Painfulness of any sensation which is not normally painful.

d., auditory. Abnormal discomfort from loud noises. SYN: *dysacusia*.

dysfunction (dis-funk'shun) [" + L. *fungi*, to be busy]. Absence of complete normal function.

dysgalac'tia [" + *gala*, milk]. Defective milk secretion.

dysgenesia, dysgenesis (dis-jen-e'sĭ-ă, -sis) [" + *genesis*, procreation]. Impairment or loss of procreative powers. SYN: *sterility*.

dysgen'ic [" + *gennan*, to produce]. Causing racial deterioration.

dysgen'italism [" + L. *genitalis*, pert. to genitals, + G. *ismos*, state of]. Condition caused by abnormal genital development.

dysgerminoma (dis-jer-min-o'mă) [" + L. *germen*, a sprout, + G. *-ōma*, tumor]. A neoplasm in sex cells in hermaphrodites and in undescended testicles or undeveloped ovaries.

dysgeusia (dis-gu'sĭ-ă) [" + *geusis*, taste]. Perversion or impairment of sense of taste.

dysglan'dular [" + L. *glans*, gland-, acorn]. Abnormal functioning of glands, esp. those of internal secretion.

dysglycemia (dis-gli-se'mĭ-ă) [" + *glykus*, sweet, + *aima*, blood]. Faulty blood sugar metabolism.

dysgno'sia [" + *gnōsis*, knowledge]. Any anomaly of intellect. SYN: *dysthymia*.

dysgone'sis [" + *gonē*, seed). 1. Functional disorder of the genital organs. 2. Poor growth of bacterial culture.

dysgon'ic [" + *gonē*, seed]. Bacterial cultures of sparse growth.

dysgraph'ia (dĭs-grăf'ĭ-ă) [" + *graphein*, to write]. 1. Inability to write properly. Usually the result of a brain lesion. 2. Writer's cramp.

dyshematopoiesia (dis-hem"ă-to-poy-e'-sĭ-ă) [" + *aima*, blood, + *poiēsis*, making]. Imperfect blood formation.

dyshidria (dis-hid'rĭ-ă) [" + *idrōs*, sweat]. 1. Retention of contents of the sweat follicles. 2. Milk perspiration.

dyshor'monal [" + *orman*, to excite]. Caused by endocrine disturbance.

dyshor'monism [" + " + *ismos*, state of]. Deficiency or excessive production of hormones or any internal secretions.

dysidrosis (dis-id-ro'sis) [" + *idrōs*, sweat, + *-ōsis*]. Disorder of the perspiratory apparatus. Never appears in the aged or children. SYN: *dyshidria*. SEE: *pompholyx*.

dysin'sulinism [" + L. *insula*, island, + G. *ismos*, state of]. Imperfect secretion of insulin.

dyskerato'sis [" + *keras*, horn, + *-ōsis*]. Epithelial alterations in which a certain number of isolated malpighian cells become differentiated. Any alteration in the keratinization of the epithelial cells of the epidermis. Characteristic of many skin disorders.

dyskine'sia [" + *kinēsis*, movement]. Defect in voluntary movement.

d. al'gera. Condition in which active movement is painful.

d. intermit'tens. Limb disability occurring intermittently.

d., uterine. Pain in the uterus on movement.

dyskinet'ic [G. *dys*, bad, + *kinēsis*, movement]. Having disordered normal movement.

dyskoimesis (dis-koy-me'sis) [" + *koimēsis*, sleeping]. Difficulty in going to sleep.

dyslalia (dis-lal'ĭ-ă) [" + *lalein*, to talk]. Impairment of speech due to defect of speech organs.

dyslexia (dis-leks'ĭ-ă) [" + *lexis*, diction]. Difficulty in reading as result of brain lesion. Visual confusion by which similarly shaped letters, such as o, e, c, b, p, h, or n, cause the victim to transpose letters in reading, seeing such a word as "pot" for "top." The number so afflicted are more than those who are blind. Eight to 25% of all children have such reading difficulties, boys being affected more than girls by four to one.

dyslochia (dis-lo'kĭ-ă) [" + *lochia*, lochia]. Disordered lochial discharge, or premature cessation.

dyslogia (dis-lo'jĭ-ă) [" + *logos*, understanding]. Difficulty in expression of ideas.

dysmasesis (dis-mas-e'sis) [" + *masēsis*, mastication]. Difficulty in masticating. SYN: *dysmastesis*.

dysmegalop'sia [" + *megas*, size, + *opsis*, vision]. Inability to visualize correctly the size and shape of things.

dysmenorrhea (dis-men-or-e'ă) [" + *mēn*, month, + *rein*, to flow]. Painful or difficult menstruation, either primary or secondary.

Adm. of testosterone propionate has proved effective in a number of cases. Vaginal smears should be taken twice a week to indicate overdosage, the average tolerance level being 500 mg.

d., congestive. Condition caused by pelvic congestion.

d., inflammatory. Condition caused by pelvic inflammation.

d., mechanic. SEE: *obstructive d.*

d., membranous. A severe spasmodic dysmenorrhea which is accompanied by the passage of a cast of the uterine cavity. Treated by curettage, and if not relieved, hysterectomy.

d., neurotic. Form caused by neurosis.

d., obstructive. D. caused by obstruction of menstrual flow.

d., primary. Difficult menstruation starting from the first period and usually a result of maldevelopment of the uterus.

ETIOL: Malposition of uterus; infantile uterus; sharply anteflexed uterus; pinpoint external os of the cervix; individuals with a low threshold for pain.

OPERATIVE TREATMENT: Dilatation or cervical hysterotomy.

d., secondary. When periods were, at the outset, normal, but, because of the development of some pathological state in the pelvis, there is a disturbance of menstruation.

ETIOL: *Cervix*: Diseases of the cervix; lacerations with scar formation; acute, subacute, and chronic endocervicitis. *Body of the Uterus*: Chronic endometritis; hyperplastic endometrium; fibroids, particularly the submucous and intramural types of fibroids; chronic metritis; acquired malposition of the uterus. *Tubal Conditions*: Acute, subacute, and chronic salpingitis. *Ovarian Conditions*: Cystic oöphoritis, endometrial cysts of the ovary, ovarian tumors of marked size. *Parametrium*: Uterosacral and broad ligament parametritis.

GENERAL HYGIENE: A healthy outdoor life, correct action of the bowels, and adequate sleep and relaxation.

OPERATIVE TREATMENT: Correction of any pathology in the pelvis.

MEDICAL TREATMENT: In general, this consists in a free use of anodyne coal tar products accompanied by antispasmodics (tincture of belladonna, nux vomica, cannabis indica), and depressants (bromides, barbituric acid derivatives).

    d., spasmodic. D. caused by uterine contractions of spasmodic form.

dysmetria (dĭs-me'trĭ-ă) [" + *metron*, measure]. An inability to fix the range of a movement.

Rapid and brusk movements made with more force than necessary. Seen in cerebellar affections. RS: *adiadochokinesis, asynergia, gait.*

dysmetrop′sia [" + " + *opsis*, vision]. Inability to visualize correctly the size and shape of things. SYN: *dysmegalopsia.*

dysmimia (dĭs-mĭm′ĭ-ă) [" + *mimeisthai*, to imitate]. 1. Inability to express oneself by gestures or signs. 2. Inability to imitate.

dysmnesia (dĭs-ne′zĭ-ă) [G. *dys*, bad, + *mnēmē*, memory]. Any impairment of memory.

dysmorphophobia (dĭs-morf-o-fo′bĭ-ă) [" + *morphē*, form, + *phobos*, fear]. Morbid fear of deformity; a form of paranoia.

dysmorphosis (dĭs-mor-fo′sĭs) [" + " + *-ōsis*]. Not normal in form.

dysmyoto′nia [" + *mys*, muscle, + *tonos*, tone]. 1. Muscle atony. 2. Excessive muscle tonicity. SYN: *myotonia.*

dysneuria (dĭs-nu′rĭ-ă) [" + *neuron*, nerve]. Impairment of the nervous function.

dysodontiasis (dĭs-o-don-tī′as-ĭs) [" + *odous*, tooth]. Painful or difficult dentition.

dysontogenesis (dīs-ŏn-tō-jĕn′ĕ-sĭs) [" + *ōn*, being, + *genesis*, development]. Defective development of an organism.

dysontogenet′ic [" + " + *gennan*, to produce]. Pert. to defective development.

dysopia (dĭs-o′pĭ-ă) [" + *opsis*, vision]. Defective or painful vision.

dysop′sia [" + *opsis*, vision]. Defective vision. SYN: *dysopia.*

dysorexia (dĭs-o-rek′sĭ-ă) [" + *orēxis*, appetite]. Perverted or lessened appetite.

dysosmia (dĭs-oz′mĭ-ă) [" + *osmē*, smell]. Impairment of the sense of smell.

dysostosis (dĭs-os-to′sĭs) [" + *osteon*, bone]. Defective bone formation.

    d., cleidocranial. A congenital ossification of the skull with partial atrophy of clavicles.

dysovarism (dĭs-o′var-ĭzm) [" + L. *ovarium*, ovary, + G. *ismos*, condition]. An abnormality due to disturbance in the ovarian internal secretion.

dysox′idizable [" + *oxys*, sour]. Not easy to oxidize.

dyspan′creatism [" + *pagkreas*, pancreas, + *ismos*, condition of]. Impaired pancreatic function.

dyspareunia (dĭs-pa-ru′nĭ-ă) [G. *dyspareunos*, unhappily mated as bedfellows]. Painful coitus.

ETIOL: Most often brought about by a resistant hymen, ulceration of the fourchette, urethritis, vaginitis, and inflammatory conditions in the pelvis; often the result of psychoneurotic rather than a physical condition.

dyspepsia (dĭs-pep′sĭ-ă) [G. *dys*, bad, + *peptein*, to digest]. Imperfect digestion. Not a disease in itself, but symptomatic of other diseases or disorders.

    d., acid. With excessive acid.

    d., alcoholic. Caused by excessive use of alcoholic beverages.

    d. atonic. Due to lack of muscular tone in the digestive organs.

    d., biliary, bilious. Form in which there is insufficient quantity or quality of bile secretion.

    d., cardiac. Form occurring during heart disease.

    d., catarrhal. Due to inflammation of the stomach.

    d. fermentative. D. caused by excessive fermentation of food and characterized by frequent eructation of gas; also called "gaseous" or "flatulent" d.

    d., gastric. D. caused by faulty stomach function.

    d., gastrointestinal. D. caused by faulty function of stomach and intestines.

    d., hepatic. D. caused by liver disease.

    d., hysterical. D. present during hysterical attacks.

    d., intestinal. Due to abnormal state of pancreatic, biliary, and intestinal secretions.

    d., nervous. Indicated by gastric pain and palpitation due to a lesion of nerves innervating the digestive tract, or to emotional states.

dyspeptic (dĭs-pep′tĭk) [" + *peptein*, to digest]. 1. Affected with or pert. to dyspepsia. 2. One afflicted with dyspepsia.

dyspeptone (dĭs-pep′tōn) [" + *peptein*, to digest]. An insoluble product of gastric digestion.

dysperma′sia [" + *sperma*, seed]. Difficult or painful orgasm during coitus.

dysper′matism [" + " + *ismos*, condition]. Difficult or painful orgasm during coitus. SYN: *dyspermasia.*

dysper′mia [" + *sperma*, seed]. Difficult or painful orgasm during coitus. SYN: *dyspermasia.*

dysphagia, dysphagy (dĭs-fa′jĭ-ă, -jĭ) [" + *phagein*, to eat]. Inability to swallow as a result of spasm of the esophagus, seen in hysteria.

    d. constriricta. D. due to narrowing of the pharynx or esophagus.

    d. globosa. Globus hystericus, *q.v.*

    d. lusoria. D. caused by pressure exerted on the esophagus by an anomalous right subclavian artery.

    d. paralytica. D. due to paralysis of muscles of deglutition.

    d. spastica. D. resulting from a spasm of pharyngeal or esophageal muscles.

dysphasia (dĭs-fa′zĭ-ă) [" + *phasis*, speech]. Impairment of speech.

dysphemia (dĭs-fe′mĭ-ă) [" + *phēmē*, speech]. Stammering.

dysphonia (dĭs-fo′nĭ-ă) [" + *phōnē*, voice]. Difficulty in speaking; hoarseness.

    d. clerico′rum. Clergyman's sore throat.

    d. pu′berum. Change of voice in boys during puberty.

dysphoria (dis-fo'rĭ-ă) [" + *pherein*, to bear]. Exaggerated feeling of depression and unrest without apparent cause.

dysphrasia (dis-fra'zĭ-ă) [" + *phrasis*, a speech. Impairment of speech. SYN: *dysphasia*.

dysphrenia (dis-fre'nĭ-ă) [" + *phrēn*, mind]. Functional or constitutional psychosis; the opp. of the organic type.

dysphylaxia (dis-fĭ-laks'ĭ-ă) [" + *phylaxis*, watching]. Waking too early from sleep.

dyspinealism (dis-pĭn'e-al-ism) [" + L. *pinealis*, pert. to a pine cone, + G. *ismos*, condition of]. Functional impairment of pineal gland.

dyspitu'itarism [" + L. *pituita*, mucus]. Condition due to disorder of the pituitary body in which both hyperpituitarism and hypopituitarism are present at the same time.

dyspla'sia [" + *plassein*, to form]. Abnormal development of tissue. SYN: *alloplasia heteroplasia*.

dyspnea (disp-ne'a) [" + *pnoē*, breathing]. Labored or difficult breathing usually accompanied by pain.
ETIOL: Insufficient oxygenation of the blood resulting from disturbances in the lungs, low oxygen pressure of air, circulatory disturbances, hemoglobin deficiency, and other causes may be: acidosis, excessive CO_2 content of blood, excessive muscular activity, lesions of the respiratory center, emotional excitation, hyperexcitability of Hering-Breuer reflex, cardiac asthma, and orthopnea.
SYM: Audible, labored breathing, distressed, anxious expression, dilated nostrils, protrusion of abdomen and expanded chest; gasping; marked cyanosis.
d. cardia. D. due to cardiac insufficiency.
d., expiratory. As in asthma and bronchitis; wheezing and painful expiration. Secretions in respiratory tract cause of sound.
POISONS: May be induced by cyanides, carbon monoxide, strychnine during convulsions.
d. inspiratory. D. due to interference in passage of air to the lungs.
d. renal. D. due to kidney disorder.

dyspneic (disp-ne'ĭk) [G. *dys*, bad, + *pnoē*, breathing]. Affected with or due to dyspnea.

dyspra'gia [" + *pragein*, to do]. Difficulty in functioning.

dysraphism (dĭs-rüf'ĭsm). In the embryo, failure of raphe-formation, or failure of fusion of parts which normally fuse.
d. spinal. A general term applied to failure of fusion of parts along the dorsal midline. May involve any of the following structures: skin, vertebrae, skull, meninges, brain and spinal cord.

dyspraх'ia [" + *prassein*, to perform]. Painful functioning.

dyssta'sia [" + *stasis*, standing]. Difficulty in standing.

dysstat'ic [" + *stasis*, standing]. Showing difficulty in standing.

dyssyner'gia [" + *syn*, with, + *ergon*, work]. Failure of muscular co-ordination. SYN: *ataxia*.

dyssystole (dis-sis'to-lĭ) [" + *systolē*, contraction]. Dilatation with cardiac insufficiency. Asystole; incomplete systole.

dysta'sia [" + *stasis*, a standing]. Difficulty in standing.

dystaxia (dis-tax'ĭ-ă) [" + *taxis*, arrangement]. Partial ataxia.

dysteleology (dis-te-le-ol'o-jĭ) [" + *teleos*, complete, + *logos*, knowledge]. The study of rudimentary organs.

dysthymia (dis-thĭm'ĭ-ă) [" + *thymos*, mind]. 1. Mental perversion; melancholia. 2. Condition resulting from malfunctioning of the thymus gland during childhood.

dysthyreosis (dis-thĭ-re-o'sis) [" + *thyreos*, shield, + *-ōsis*]. Impaired functional activity of thyroid gland. SYN: *dysthyroidism*.

dysthyroidism (dis-thĭ'roi-dizm) [" + " + *eidos*, form, + *ismos*, state of]. Imperfect development and function of the thyroid gland.

dystith'ia [" + *tithēnia*, nursing]. Difficulty or inability to nurse at breast.

dystocia (dis-to'sĭ-ă) [" + *tokos*, birth]. Difficult labor. May be produced by either the passenger (the fetus) or the passage (the pelvis of the mother).
FETAL CAUSES: (a) Usually large babies; (b) malpositions of the fetus (transverse presentation, face, brow, breech, or compound presentations); (c) abnormalities of the fetus (hydrocephalus, tumors of the neck or abdomen, hydrops of the fetus); (d) multiple pregnancy (interlocked twins).
MATERNAL CAUSES: *Uterus*: (a) Primary and secondary uterine inertia; (b) congenital anomalies of the uterus (bicornuate uterus); (c) tumors of the uterus (fibroids, carcinoma of the cervix); (d) abnormal fixation of the uterus by previous operation.
Bony Pelvis: Contracted pelves, the commoner clinical types of which are (a) flat pelvis, rachitic and nonrachitic, (b) generally contracted pelvis; (c) flat and generally contracted pelvis; (d) funnel pelvis; (e) exostoses of the pelvic bones; (f) tumors of the pelvic bones.
Cervix Uteri: (a) Bandl's contraction ring; (b) rigid cervix that will not dilate; (c) stenosis and stricture preventing dilatation.
Ovary: Ovarian cysts that block the pelvis.
Vagina and Vulva: (a) Cysts; (b) tumors; (c) atresias and stenoses.
DIAG: Can generally be made before the patient goes into labor by vaginal examination and external pelvimetry.
TREATMENT: Varies according to the condition present that causes the dystocia. In general it aims toward the correction of the abnormality in order to allow the fetus to pass. If this is not possible, operative delivery must be resorted to. SEE: *cephalotripsy*.

dystonia (dis-to'nĭ-ă) [G. *dys*, bad, + *tonos*, tone]. Impairment of tonicity.

dyston'ic [" + *tonos*, tone]. Pert. to distonia or hyper- or hypotonicity of tissues.

dysto'pia [" + *topos*, place]. Malposition; displacement of any organ.

dystopic (dis-top'ĭk) [" + *topos*, place]. Not in place.

dys'topy [" + *topos*, place]. Malposition of an organ. SYN: *dystopia*.

dystro'phia [" + *trephein*, to nourish]. Progressive weakening of a muscle. SYN: *dystrophy*.
d. adiposogenitalis. Disease of the anterior pituitary gland showing genital atrophy and obesity, Fröhlich's syndrome.
d. Landousy-Djerine. A form of d., in which there is marked atrophy of facial muscles, shoulder girdle and arm. Facial atrophy produces a peculiar expression called *myopathic facies*.

d., progressive muscular. Progressive atrophy of muscles beginning in terminals of motor nerves. ETIOL: Nutritional disorder.

d. pseudohypertrophic muscular. An hereditary disease usually beginning in childhood in which muscular ability is lost. At first certain muscles atrophy followed by atrophy. Also called Erb's paralysis.

dystrophic (dis-trof'ik) [" + *trephein*, to nourish]. Pert. to dystrophia.

dystrophodex'trin [" + " + L. *dexter*, right]. A starchy material in normal blood but slightly soluble.

dystrophoneurosis (dis-trof″o-nu-ro′sis) [" + " + *neuron*, nerve, + *-osis*]. Defective nutrition accompanied by a nervous disease.

dystrophy (dis′tro-fī). Dystrophia, *q.v.*

dystrypsia (dis-trip′sĭ-ă) [" + *tripsis*, digestion]. Impaired secretion of pancreas.

dysuria (dis-u′rĭ-ă) [" + *ouron*, urine]. Painful or difficult urination, symptomatic of numerous conditions. Vesical tenesmus.

There is a persistent desire to urinate, and there may be a condition of strangury, the urine being passed drop by drop accompanied by pain. This may be indicative of cystitis, neuralgia of the bladder, urethritis; urethral stricture; hypertrophied, cancerous, ulcerated prostate in the male; prolapsus of uterus in the female; pelvic peritonitis and abscess; metritis; cancer of the cervix, or dysmenorrhea. Pain and burning may also be caused by concentrated acid urine.

dysu'riac [" + *ouron*, urine]. One affected with dysuria.

dyszooamylia (dis-zo″o-am-il′ĭ-ă) [" + *zōon*, animal, + *amylon*, starch]. Failure to transform dextrose into glycogen.

dyszoosper'mia [" + " + *sperma*, seed]. Imperfect formation of spermatozoa.

E

E. Abbr. for *electromotive force, emmetropia,* and *eye;* also symb. for *voltage.*

Eales' disease (ēlz). Repeated hemorrhages into the retina and vitreous.

ear [A.S. *eáre*]. Organ of hearing. Consisting of external, middle, and internal ear.

e., blood supply of. Ant. and post. auricular, stylomastoid, petrosal, and int. auricular arteries.

e. bones. Bonelets of tympanic cavity. SYN: *ossicles.*

e. cauliflower. A deformity consisting of a thickening of the external ear resulting from repeated blows. Commonly seen in prize-fighters.

e. drum. The tympanum, or cavity in middle ear.

e. dust. Calcareous concretions in membranous labyrinth. SYN: *otoconia, otolith.*

e., examination of. Watch test for hearing, color, size, and shape, discharge from middle or inner ear, tenderness upon pressure in front or back of ear; inflammation or bulging, perforations, or scars of or in drum.

Acute hearing sometimes precedes delirium. *Deafness* indicates want of attention, wax in external ear passage, paralysis of auditory nerve or effect of

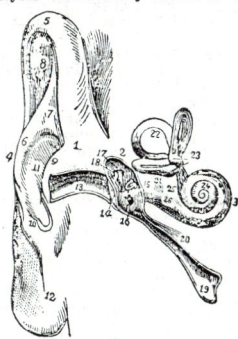

THE EAR
1. External ear; 2. Middle ear; 3. Internal ear; 4. Pinna; 5. Helix; 6. Antihelix; 7. Scaphoid fossa; 8. Fossa helicis; 9. Tragus; 10. Antitragus; 11. Concha; 12. Lobe; 13. External Auditory meatus; 14. Tympanic membrane; 15. Tympanic promontory; 16. Foramen rotundum; 17. Posterior wall of the tympanum; 18. Auditory ossicles; 19. Eustachian tube; 20. Facial canal; 21. Vestibule; 22. Semicircular canals: superior, inferior, horizontal; 23. Ampulla; 24. Cochlea; 25. Prominentia spiralis; 26. Scala tympani.

quinine or other drugs. *Pallor of ears, tongue, and gums* indicates loss of blood or poverty of blood. *Ringing in ears* is noted in nervous debility, cerebral hyperemia and anemia, in disease of ear, Ménière's disease, and after use of certain drugs like quinine and salicylic acid.

e., external. Comprises auricle and external auditory canal; is separated from middle ear by tympanic* membrane or drum.

e., foreign bodies in. These are usually insects, pebbles, beans, or peas. Insects in the ear cannot be attracted from the ear by a bright light inasmuch as they crawl in head first and usually do not see the light.

SYM: Pain, ringing or buzzing in the ear, and, if an insect, there is a great noise.

TREATMENT: Drop in bland oil and so float insect out of ear. Warm water may be used though it does not work quite as well. In case of a solid foreign body, oil or water should not be used, inasmuch as it may cause the body to be pushed further in the ear or may cause it to swell and become firmly embedded. Such foreign bodies in the ear do not constitute an emergency and should be left untreated until seen by a physician. If no physician is available within a reasonable period, it is sometimes possible to remove foreign body by placing a large drop of glue or soft, sticky chewing gum on the end of a match and gently introducing it until it touches the foreign body. Leave it in contact for a moment to allow it to adhere and then withdraw it.

Swimmers sometimes find that water enters the ear and will not flow out spontaneously. This may occasionally be dislodged by a sudden tap on the side of the head above the ear, or by introducing a long wisp of cotton which will draw out the water by capillarity.* Occasionally this sensation of water in the ear is not due to water, but to the swelling of the cerumen* that is usually present. In such instances, the above methods will not work. These patients should seek relief by repeatedly irrigating the ear with warm oil or water.

e., internal. Consists of the cochlea containing the sensory receptors for hearing and the vestibule and semicircular canals which contain the receptors for equilibrium and the sense of position. Innervated by the cochlear and vestibular branches of the auditory nerve.

e., middle. An irregular cavity in temporal bone. In front it communicates with eustachian tube which forms an open channel bet. middle ear and cavity of nasopharynx. Behind, middle ear opens into mastoid antrum, and this in turn communicates with the mastoid cells. There are two openings into the inner ear, both of which are covered with membrane. A string of tiny bones, joined together, extends from the tympanum to the *foramen ovale* of the internal ear. These are: (1) malleus, (2) incus, (3) stapes.

e. nerve supply of. *External:* 5th, 7th, 10th cranial nerves and branches from cervical plexus. *Middle:* 7th and 9th cranial nerves and sympathetic fibers. *Internal:* 8th cranial nerve.

e., swelling in front or behind. ETIOL: Mumps, mastoid disease, scurvy, anthrax, or gangrenous stomatitis.

e.-wax. Wax in the ear. SYN: *cerumen.*

ear, words pert. to: acoustic meatus, aditus, angiotitis, ankylotia, annulus, antihelix, antilobium, antitragicus, antitragus, antrotympanitis, asylum ear, auricle, auriculare, "auris-" words, binaural, blennotorrhea, bulla ossea, cavum tympani, cerumen, cochlea, concha, crista ampullaris, cupola, deafness, endolymph, epitympanum, eustachian, foreign bodies, helix, hydrotis, incus, labyrinth, labyrinthitis, macrotia, malleus, microtia, ossicles, "ot-" words, pinna, politerization, scala tympani, suprameatal, tinnitus aurium, tympanum, "utri-" words, vestibule, vitreous, wax.

earache. Aural pain. SYN: *otalgia*.

earth eating. Eating clay or dirt. Sometimes done by children who lack lime; also by the insane. SYN: *chthonophagia, geophagism, geotragia.*

ear trumpet. A tubular device to aid the deaf in hearing.

eat [A.S. *etan*]. 1. To devour as food. 2. To take solid food. 3. To corrode.

eating, words pert. to: abrosia, acataposis, acoria, allotriophagy, amasesis, apastia, appetite, bradyphagia, bulimia, chthonophagia, dysphagia, esculent, fastidium, fasting, geophagia, hunger, hyperorexia, mastication, parorexia, pica, polyphagia.

Eberthel'la. A genus of *Bacteriaceae* causing intestinal inflammation.
  E. typhosa. SYN: *E. typhosi, Salmonella typhosa.*

eberthe'mia [Eberth + G. *aima*, blood]. The presence of typhoid bacilli (*Bacillus typhi abdominalis*, or Eberth's bacilli) in the blood.

eber'thian. Pert. to or caused by Eberth's bacillus.

Eb'ner's glands. Serous glands of the tongue usually found in the vicinity of the circumvallate papillae.

ebona'tion [L. *e*, out, + A.S. *ban*, bone]. Removal of bony fragments from a wound.

Ebstein's diet. One used in the treatment of obesity. Very little carbohydrate is permitted.
  Breakfast: Tea ½ pint, no milk or sugar; bread or toast 2 ounces, plenty of butter. *Dinner*: Clear soup, meat 4 or 6 ounces, fat gravy, boiled vegetables, fresh fruit. *Afternoon*: Like breakfast. *Supper*: One egg; fat roast meat, ham, or fish; bread 1 ounce, butter, cheese, and fruit.
  E.'s disease or lesion. Epithelial necrosis and hyaline degeneration of the renal tubules in diabetes mellitus.
  E.'s leukemia. A rapidly progressing form of leukemia.

ebullition (eb-u-lish'un) [L. *ebullire*, to boil]. 1. Boiling. 2. Effervescence.

eburnation (e-bur-nā'shun) [L. *eburnus*, made of ivory]. Changes in bone causing them to become dense like ivory and hardened.

eburneous (e-bur'ne-us) [L. *eburnus*, made of ivory]. Resembling ivory; ivory-colored.

ecaudate (e-kaw'dāt) [L. *e*, without, + *cauda*, tail]. Without a tail.

ecbolic (ek-bol'ik) [G. *ekbolikos*, throwing out]. 1. Hastening labor by toning up uterine muscles. 2. Causing abortion. 3. Any agent producing or hastening labor or abortion. Ex: *cotton root, ergot, tansy*. SYN: *abortifacient.*

eccentric (ek-sen'trik) [G. *ekkentros*, from the center]. 1. Peculiar, abnormal in action or ideas. 2. Proceeding away from a center. 3. Peripheral.

e. atrophy. Atrophy with dilatation.

e. convulsion. One caused by peripheral irritation.

e. hypertrophy. Hypertrophy of a hollow organ with dilation.

e. limitation. Having smaller visual field than normal.

eccentro-osteochondrodysplasia. A pathological condition of bones due to imperfect bone formation. Ossification occurs in several centers instead of one common center. Also called *Morquio's disease.*

eccentropiesis (ek-sen"tro-pi-e'sis) [" + *piēsis*, pressure]. Pressure from within exerted outward for treatment of anal fistula.

ecchondroma, ecchondrosis (ek-on-dro'mă, -dro'sis) [G. *ek*, out, + *chondros*, cartilage, + *-ōma*, tumor]. A chondroma or cartilaginous tumor.

ecchondrotome (ek-on'dro-tōm) [" + " + *tomē*, incision]. Knife for excision of cartilage.

ecchymoma (ek-ĭ-mo'mă) [" + *chymos*, juice, + *ōma*, tumor]. An extravasated blood tumor. A swelling due to the accumulation of blood in subcutaneous tissues such as occurs following a bruise.

ecchymosis (ek-ĭ-mo'sis) (pl. *-ses*) [" + " + *ōsis*]. A form of macula appearing in large irregularly-formed hemorrhagic areas of the skin. The color is red, changing to blue, greenish brown, or yellow.
  ETIOL: Extravasation of blood into areolar tissue.

ecchymotic (ek-i-mot'ĭk) [" + *chymos*, juice]. Resembling or rel. to an ecchymosis.

eccrinology (ek-rin-ol'o-jĭ) [" + *krinein*, to secrete, + *logos*, study of]. The science of secretions.

eccrisis (ek'kris-is) [" + *krisis*, separation]. The expulsion of morbid or waste products. SYN: *excretion.*

eccrit'ic [" + *krinein*, to secrete]. Promoting or that which promotes excretion.

eccyclomastopathy (ek-si"clo-mas-top'ă-thĭ) [" + *kyklos*, circle, + *mastos*, breast, + *pathos*, disease]. A mass of lesions of the breast made up of connective tissue and/or epithelial cells. SYN: *cyclomastopathy.*

eccyesis (ek-si-e'sis) [" + *kyēsis*, pregnancy]. Extrauterine or ectopic pregnancy.

ecdem'ic [G. *ekdēmos*, foreign]. Not endemic nor epidemic, as a disease carried to a region from without.

ecdemomania (ek-de-mo-ma'nĭ-ă) [" + *mania*, madness]. Wanderlust; abnormal desire to wander. SYN: *drapetomania, dromomania, vagabondage.*

ecderon (ek'dĕ-ron) [G. *ek*, out, + *deros*, skin]. Epidermis, or outer portion of skin, as distinguished from *enderon*,* or inner portion.

ecdysis (ĕk-dĭs'ĭs). 1. The shedding or sloughing off of the epidermis of the skin; desquamation. 2. The shedding of the outer covering of the body as occurs in certain animals such as insects, crustaceans, and snakes; molting.

ECG. (ecg). Abv. for electrocardiogram.

echidnase. An enzyme present in snake venom which produces inflammation.

echidnin (ĕ-kĭd'nĭn). 1. The venom of poisonous snakes. 2. The active principle present in snake venom.

Echidnophaga (ĕ-kĭd'nō-fāj). A genus of fleas belonging to the family Pulicidae.

E. gallinacea. The sticktight flea which is the most important flea pest of poultry. It collects in clusters on the heads of poultry and in the ears of mammals. It may infest humans, esp., children.

echinate (ek'ĭ-nāt) [G. *echinos*, hedgehog]. 1. Spiny. 2. In agar streak, a growth with pitted or toothed margins along the inoculation line; in stab cultures, coiled growth with pointed outgrowths.

echinococcosis (ĕ-kin-o-kok-ko'sis) [" + *kokkos*, berry]. Infestation with echinococcus.

echinococcotomy (ĕ-kin-o-kok-ot'o-mĭ) [" + " + *tome*, incision]. Operation for evacuation of an echinococcus cyst.

Echinococcous (e-kin-o-kok'us) (pl. *Echinococci* [" + *kokkos*, berry]. A genus of tapeworms. They are minute forms consisting of a scolex and three or four proglottids.
   e. cyst. A cyst resulting from the development of the larva of the dog tapeworm.
   e. cysticus. Disease resulting from a single hydatid cyst occurring in the liver.
   e. disease. Infestation with the larva of Echinococcous which causes the formation of hydatid cysts.
   e. granulosus. A species of tapeworms which infests dogs and other carnivors. Its larva called a hydatid develops in other mammals including man and causes the formation of hydatid cysts.
   e. hydatidosus. Variety of E. characterized by development of daughter cysts from the mother cyst.

Echinorhynchus (ĕ-kin-o-rin'kus) [" + *rygchos*, beak]. Formerly considered a genus of parasitic worms belonging to the Acanthocephala. It has been divided into many sub-groups.
   E. gigas. Macracanthorhynchus hirudinaceus, a worm commonly parasitic in pigs, but occasionally found in man.

echinosis (ĕ-kin-o'sis) [" + *-ōsis*]. Blood corpuscles appearing like a sea urchin, having lost their smooth outlines. Crenation of red blood cells.

Echinostoma (ĕ-kĕn-ŏs'tō-mă). A genus of flukes characterized by a spiny body and the presence of a collar of spines near the anterior end. They are found in the intestines of many vertebrates, esp. aquatic birds. They occasionally occur as accidental parasites in man.

echinulate (ĕ-kin'u-lāt) [G. *echinos*, hedgehog]. A bacterial growth having lateral spines. Seen along line of inoculation.

echo (ĕk'ō) [G. *echō*, echo]. A reverberating sound.
   e. acou'sia. Subjective echoes of sounds just normally heard.
   e., amphor'ic. Amphoric sound sometimes heard in auscultation of chest. SEE: *chest, percussion of.*
   e. sign. Repetition of closing word of a sentence, a sign of epilepsy or other brain conditions.
   e. speech. Involuntary repetition of a sentence or word spoken by another. SYN: *echolalia.*

echokinesia (ek-o-kin-e'sĭ-ă) [" + *kinēsis*, movement]. Involuntary repetition of another's gestures.

echolalia (ek-o-la'lĭ-ă) [" + *lalia*, babble]. An involuntary, parrotlike repetition of words spoken by others, often accompanied by twitching of muscles, as seen in schizophrenia.

echomatism (ĕ-ko'mă-tizm) [" + *ismos*, condition of]. Automatic repetition of another's actions.

echomimia (ĕ-ko-mim'ĭ-a) [" + *mimēsis*, imitation]. The imitation of the actions of others without meaning as seen in dementia precox.

echomotism (ĕ-ko-mo'tizm) [" + L. *motus*, moving]. Imitation of movements.

echopathy (ĕ-kop'ă-thĭ) [" + *pathos*, disease]. Imitation of another's actions and repetitions of his words; a neurosis.

echophotony (ĕ-ko-fot'o-nĭ) [" + *phos*, light, + *tonos*, tone]. Production of color sensations by stimulus of sounds heard.

echophra'sia [" + *phrasis*, speech]. Patient's meaningless repeating of words spoken to him. May be accompanied by muscle twitching; seen in dementia precox.

echopraxia (ĕ-ko-praks'ĭ-ă) [" + *prassein*, to perform]. Imitation, without meaning, of motions made by others. SYN: *echoprax'is* [" + *prassein*, to perform]. Senseless repetition by the patient of movements made by the physician in treatment.

eclabium (ek-la'bĭ-um) [G. *ek*, out, + L. *labium*, lip]. Eversion of a lip.

eclampsia (ĕ-klamp'sĭ-ă) [" + *lampein*, to flash]. 1. A sudden attack of convulsions or an epileptiform seizure not of central origin. 2. A major toxemia of pregnancy accompanied by high blood pressure, albuminuria, oliguria, tonic and clonic convulsions, and coma. May occur pre-, intra-, or postpartum.
   ETIOL: Unknown. Occurs more often in primiparae, in multiple pregnancy, in hydramnios, in hydatidiform mole, in patients with severe anemia, and in the undernourished.
   PATH: Seen most frequently in the kidney, liver, brain, heart, and placenta. The kidney shows degenerated tubal nephritis, the tubal epithelium showing cloudy swelling, fatty degeneration, and coagulation necrosis. The liver is enlarged and mottled, there are periportal thrombosis and degeneration of the periphery of the lobules with subcapsular hemorrhages. The brain shows edema, hyperemia, thrombosis, and hemorrhages. The heart shows cloudy swelling and degenerative myocarditis. The placenta shows infarcts, thromboses, and hemorrhages.
   SYM: Edema of the legs and feet, puffiness of the face, hyperpiesis,* and albuminuria.* Severe headaches, dizziness, spots before the eyes, epigastric pain, convulsions (beginning with fixation of the eyeballs, rolling of the eyes, twitchings of the face, arms, and hands; the paroxysms then involve the entire body), blueness of face, protrusion of the tongue, frothing at the mouth, and coma. There may be one or many convulsions. The pulse is rapid and bounding, the temperature usually rises to 103° or 104° F., and the blood pressure varies bet. 140 and 200 mm. Hg systolic. The patient may continue in coma until death.
   TREATMENT: *Prophylactic:* The most important. Good prenatal care, with careful watching of the patient's blood pressure, urine, and weight; instituting medical management as soon as any abnormal findings are presented, and terminating labor if unsuccessful in reducing the signs of danger.
   The Attack: Prevent the patient from doing herself bodily harm (tie her in bed, protect the tongue by keeping the teeth separated). In general, promote elimination by subcutaneous injection of

eclampsia, albuminuric

salt solution, lavage of the stomach, saline catharsis, and the use of hypertonic glucose solution intravenously. Reduce the irritation of the nervous system by Strogonoff treatment with morphine and scopolamine, by the use of large doses of chloral hydrate and bromides by rectal instillation, or by the use of any of the barbiturates. If necessary to control a long sustained convulsion, ether may be used. The blood pressure may be reduced by venesection, or by the use of veratrone.

Delivery: This should not be instituted until the general condition of the patient has improved unless the patient is in active labor, in which case the labor should be aided by the use of forceps as soon as is possible. Cesarean section should not be done unless there is some other obstetrical reason. If medical management shows no improvement, then labor must be instituted by one of the recognized methods, because only the removal of the pregnancy will allow for improvement in the condition of the mother.

PRECAUTIONS IN (during a convulsion): (a) The patient *must not* be left alone. (b) Restrain only enough to keep her in bed. Side boards or some type of restraint must be used after the convulsion to make certain the patient will not fall out of bed during the coma, delirium, and restless stage. (c) Use mouth gag to keep patient from biting her tongue. (d) See that the physician is notified immediately. (e) See that the physician's orders are carried out. (When a nurse is cognizant of a physician's routine in these cases she will be given more authority and responsibility in anticipating his desires before his arrival.) (f) Have the fetal heart checked frequently, in cases of convulsion before delivery, because the fetal circulation is interfered with and the infant may register signs of distress.

e., albuminuric. E. caused by presence of albuminuria.

e. gravidum. E. in women during pregnancy.

e. infantile. A convulsion occurring in children. It is of reflex origin being associated with teething, acute digestive disorders, worm infestation, or cerebral congestion.

e. nutans. SYN: *nodding spasm, sallam convulsion.* E. characterized by nodding movements.

e. puerperal. A convulsion occurring near the end of pregnancy, during labor, or immediately following labor.

e. uremic. E. resulting from uremia due to suppressed urine formation.

eclampsism (e-klamp'sizm) [" + " + *ismos*, condition of]. Puerperal eclampsia without convulsive seizures.

eclamp'tic [" + *lampein*, to flash]. Rel. to, or of the nature of, eclampsia.

eclamptism (ē-klamp'tizm) [" + " + *ismos*, state of]. Condition due to autointoxication incident to pregnancy.

eclamptogen'ic [" + " + *gennan*, to produce]. Causing convulsions.

eclamptogenus (ek-lamp-toj'en-us) [" + " + *gennan*, to produce]. Producing convulsions. SYN: *eclamptogenic.*

eclectic (ek-lek'tik) [G. *eklektikos*, selecting]. Selecting from various sources what seems to be the best.

e. school of medicine. One employing indigenous plants or "specifics" according to patient's symptoms.

eclecticism (ek-lek'ti-sizm) [" + *ismos*,

E-4

ecthyma

state of]. A system of medicine treating disease through specific remedies for individual pathological conditions, rather than by treating body as a whole. Remedies, principally botanical.

eclysis (ek-lī'sis). A mild syncope.

ecmnesia (ek-ne'zī-ā) [G. *ek*, out, + *mnēsis*, memory]. Inability to remember recent events as seen in senility. The memory of before and after events not affected.

ecoid (e'koid) [G. *oikos*, house, + *eidos*, resemblance]. The framework of a red blood corpuscle.

ecology (e-kol'o-gī) [" + *logos*, study of]. The physiology of organisms as affected by their environment. SYN: *bionomics.*

ecomania (e-ko-ma'nī-ā) [" + *mania*, madness]. An extreme humbleness manifested before those in authority but a dominating, irritable attitude towards members of the family. Manifested in chronic alcoholism.

écouvillonage (a-koo-vī-yon-ahzh') [Fr.]. The cleansing and application of remedies to a cavity by means of a brush or swab.

ecphoria (ek-fôr'ī-ā). An engram, or the reestablishment of a memory trace or engram.

ecphyadectomy (ek-fī-ā-dek'to-mī) [G. *ekphyas*, appendix, + *ektomē*, excision]. Removal of vermiform appendix. SEE: *appendectomy.*

ecphyaditis (ek-fī-ad'ī-tis) [" + *-itis*, inflammation]. Inflammation of vermiform appendix. SYN: *appendicitis.*

ecphylactic (ek-fī-lak'tīk) [G. *ek*, out, + *phylaxis*, guarding]. Pert. to ecphylaxis.

ecphylax'is [" + *phylaxis*, protection]. Impotent antibodies or phylactic agents in the blood.

ecphyma (ek-fī'mā) [" + *phyma*, growth]. An outgrowth or excrescence, as a wart.

écrasement (ā-krăz-mon') [Fr. *ecraser*, to crush]. Excision by means of an écraseur.

écraseur (ā-krā-zer') [Fr. *ecraser*, to crush]. A wire loop used for excisions.

ecstasy (ek'sta-sī) [G. *ekstasis*, a standing out]. An exhilarated, trancelike, or exalted state.

ecstrophy (ek'stro-fī) [G. *ekstrophe*, a turning out]. Turning an organ inside out. SYN: *exstrophy.*

ec'tad [G. *ektos*, without]. Toward the surface; outward; externally.

ec'tal [G. *ektos*, without]. External, outer, on the surface.

ectasia, ectasis (ek-ta'sī-ā, -sis) [G. *ek*, out, + *teinein*, to stretch]. Dilatation of any tubular vessel.

e. ventriculi paradoxa. Hourglass stomach.

ectasin (ek'tas-in) [" + *teinein*, to stretch]. A tuberculin-derived substance causing vasomotor dilation.

ectat'ic [" + *teinein*, to stretch]. Distensible or capable of being stretched.

ecten'tal [G. *ektos*, without, + *entos*, within]. Pert. to entoderm and ectoderm.

e. line. Point of entodermal and ectodermal junction.

ectethmoid (ekt-eth'moid) [" + *ēthmos*, sieve, + *eidos*, form]. Lateral mass of the ethmoid bone.

ecthyma (ek-thī'mā) [G. *ek*, out, + *thyein*, to rush]. An acute, noncontagious, inflammatory, pustular, cutaneous eruption on a hardened base which may be followed by slight scarring or temporary pigmentation.

ecthyma, scrofulosum   E-5   **ectopic, gestation**

ETIOL: Lowered resistance to common pathogenic organisms (particularly *Staphylococcus aureus*), uncleanliness, poor hygienic surroundings, general debility. Slightly infectious and autoinoculable.

SYM: Circular or irregularly oval lesions, the bases excoriated, raw and sensitive to pressure, until the crusts drop off, leaving scars or pigmented spots.

PATH: Epidermal, originating in upper prickle-cell layer.

PROG: As a rule favorable, but depending to some extent upon patient's general condition.

TREATMENT: Tonics and simple nourishing diet. Crusts to be removed by starch poultices, etc., lesions cleansed, and mild antiseptic applied. If sluggish, paint with silver nitrate, balsam of Peru, gentian violet, or mercurochrome.

   e. scrofulosum. Form seen in scrofula.

   e. syphiliticum. Pustular eruption occurring in tertiary syphilis.

ecthyreosis (ek-thī-rē-o'sis) [" + *thyreos*, shield, + *-ōsis*]. Loss of thyroid gland function.

ectiris (ek-ti'ris) [G. *ektos*, without, + *iris*, iris]. The external portion of the iris.

ecto- [G. *ekto*]. Prefix: Outside.

ectoan'tigen [G. *ektos*, out, + *anti*, against, + *gennan*, to produce]. 1. Any toxin or stimulator of antibody formation. 2. An antigen assumed to have its origin in ectoplasm of bacterial cells or one loosely attached to the surface of bacteria and capable of being separated from the bacterial cell.

ec'toblast [" + *blastos*, germ]. Old term for the ectoderm or epiblast of an embryo.

ectocardia (ek-to-kar'dī-ă) [" + *kardia*, heart]. Having the heart out of normal position.

ectochoroidea (ek"to-ko-roy'de-ă) [" + *chorioides*, choroid]. Outer layer of choroid coat of the eye.

ectocinerea (ek-to-sin-e're-ă) [" + L. *cinereus*, ashen]. The outer gray matter of the brain.

ectocolos'tomy [G. *ektos*, outside, + *kōlon*, colon, + *stōma*, opening]. Formation through the abdominal wall of an opening into the colon.

ectocon'dyle [" + *kondylos*, knuckle]. The outer condyle of the bone.

ectocornea (ek-to-kor'ne-ă) [" + L. *corneus*, horny]. External layer of the cornea.

ectocu'neiform [" + L. *cuneus*, wedge, + *forma*, form]. External cuneiform bone.

ectocytic (ek-to-si'tĭk) [" + *kytos*, cell]. Outside of the cell.

ectodac'tylism [" + *daktylos*, finger, + *ismos*, state of]. Lack of a digit or digits.

ectoderm (ek'to-derm) [" + *derma*, skin]. The outer layer of cells in a developing embryo.

From it are developed skin structures, the nervous system, organs of special sense, the pineal and part of pituitary and suprarenal glands. SYN: *epiblast.*
SEE: *entoderm*.

ectoder'mal [" + *derma*, skin]. Rel. to the ectoderm.

ectodermatosis (ek-to-der-mă-to'sis) [" + " + *-ōsis*]. Disorder due to faulty development of the ectoderm.

ectoder'mic [" + *derma*, skin]. Pert. to the ectoderm. SYN: *ectodermal*.

ectodermoi'dal [" + " + *eidos*, resemblance]. Pert. to or resembling the ectoderm.

ectodermo'sis [" + " + *-ōsis*]. Illness resulting from congenital maldevelopment of ectodermal structures. SYN: *ectodermatosis*.

   e. erosiva pluriorificialis. SYN: *dermatostomatitis*. A form of erythema multiforme characterized by fever, chills, profuse salivation, and the development of vesicles on the lips, tongue, and cheeks and later erythematous lesions on the hands. The disease is rare, occurring in children and young persons.

ectoen'tad [" + *entos*, within]. From without inward.

ectoen'zyme [" + *en*, in, + *zymē*, leaven]. An extra-cellular enzyme or one that acts outside of the cell that secretes it.

ectogenous (ek-toj'en-us) [" + *gennan*, to produce]. Having its origin outside of a body or structure, as infection.

ectoglia (ek-tog'lī-ă) [G. *ektos*, outside, + *glia*, glue]. Superficial embryonic layer in beginning of stratification of the medullary tube.

ectoglob'ular [" + L. *globulus*, globule]. Not within blood cells or globular bodies.

ectog'ony [" + *gonos*, seed]. Influences on the mother's body and metabolism from the developing zygote.

ectokelostomy (ek-to-ke-los'to-mī) [" + *kēlē*, hernia, + *stōma*, opening]. Making an external opening into a hernial sac to prepare for a radical operation.

ectolecithal (ek-to-les'ith-al) [" + *lekithos*, yolk]. Pert. to ovum having food yolk placed near the surface.

ectol'ysis [" + *lysis*, dissolution]. Ectoplasmic lysis.

ectomere (ek'to-mēr) [" + *meros*, part]. One of the blastomeres forming the ectoderm.

ectome'soblast [" + " + *blastos*, germ]. Cells from which will be developed the ectoblast and mesoblast.

ectomy (ek'to-mī) [G. *ektomē*]. Excision of any organ or gland.

ectonu'clear [G. *ektos*, outside, + L. *nucleus*, kernel]. Occurring outside a cell nucleus.

ectopagus (ĕk-tō-fāg'ŭs). An abnormal detus consisting of twins fused at the thorax.

ectopar'asite. A parasite that lives on the outer surface of the body.

ectoperitoni'tis [" + *peritonaion*, peritoneum, + *-itis*, inflammation]. Inflammation of the parietal layer of peritoneum (layer lining the abdominal wall).

ectopia (ek-to'pī-ă) [G. *ek*, out, + *topos*, place]. Malposition or displacement of an organ or structure esp. if congenital.

   e. cordis. Malposition of the heart in which heart lies outside of the thoracic cavity.

   e. lentis. Displacement of the crystalline lens of the eye.

   e. pupillae. SYN: *corectopia*. Displacement of the pupil.

   e. renis. Displacement of the kidney.

   e. testis. Displacement of the testis.

   e. vesicae. Displacement of the bladder, esp. exstrophy of the bladder.

   e. visceral. An umbilical hernia.

ectopic (ek-top'ĭk) [" + *topos*, place]. In an abnormal position; said of a fetus.

   e. beat. Cardiac beat beginning at a point other than sinoauricular node.

   e. gestation or pregnancy. Implantation of the fertilized ovum outside of the uterine cavity. There is usually a decidual reaction in the uterus, but the decidua is poorly developed and the decidua reflex is absent. The tubal decidual reaction is meager.

LOCATIONS: *Abdominal*: In the free abdominal cavity and attached to one of the abdominal viscera, usually secondary to tubal. *Interstitial*: In the interstitial portion of the tube. *Ovarian*: In the ovary. The ovarian and primary abdominal types are very rare. *Tubal*: In the fallopian tube, the most frequently encountered. The pregnancy may be situated in the interstitial, ampullar, or isthmic portion of the tube, the isthmic type being the most common.

ETIOL: Most commonly associated with inflammatory conditions of the tube and other conditions which mechanically interfere with the downward passage of the ovum, such as diverticula, polypi in the tubal lumen, peritoneal adhesions, and a large migrating ovum. Any variety of pregnancy or any combination of varieties may occur (uterine plus ectopic, bilateral ectopic, etc.).

SYM: (a) Missed menstruation; (b) tenderness, soreness, pain on affected side; (c) pallor, weak pulse, signs of shock or hemorrhage; (d) pain may be reflected to shoulder; (e) perhaps bluish discoloration of umbilicus.

Unruptured: Amenorrhea may or may not be present; vague pains in the abdomen usually on one side; irregular hemorrhage. The diagnosis at this stage can be made only by the absence of definite signs of uterine pregnancy, and colpotomy incision with an inspection of the internal genitalia.

Ruptured: *Without a severe hemorrhage*: Severe pain in the lower abdomen with fainting spells which occur repeatedly. Diagnosis made by puncture which reveals the free blood in the abdominal cavity.

Tragic, with overwhelming hemorrhage: Sudden collapse with cold, clammy sweat, rapid pulse, Cullen's sign in women with thin abdominal walls, lowering blood pressure, gaseous distention of the abdomen, desire to defecate with no relief of the pressure on defecation (due to bloody distention of the cul-de-sac), shock, air hunger, and other signs of severe hemorrhage. Diagnosis is confirmed by the return of free blood on post. puncture. After several attacks there is a leukocytosis of 12 to 15,000, and the hemoglobin is lowered.

DIFFERENTIAL DIAGNOSIS: Ectopic must be differentiated from uterine pregnancy, acute salpingitis, twisting of the pedicle of an ovarian cyst or pedunculated fibroid tumor, and hemorrhage from a ruptured graafian follicle or corpus luteum cyst.

TREATMENT: Once the diagnosis of ectopic pregnancy is made, operative treatment is indicated. In those cases where there is profound shock from hemorrhage, the patient should be supported by blood transfusion and saline infusions before major surgery is attempted. SEE: celiocolpotomy.

e. rhythm. Any cardiac rhythm that is abnormal or irregular.

ec'toplasm [G. *ektos*, outer, + *plasma*, a thing formed]. The outermost layer of cell protoplasm.

ec"toplas'mic [" + *plasma*, a thing formed]. Pert. to ectoplasm.

ectoplas'tic [" + *plassein*, to form]. Formed at the periphery; ectoplasmic.

ectopotomy (ek-to-pot'o-mĭ) [G. *ek*, out, + *topos*, place, + *tomē*, incision]. Removal of the fetus in ectopic pregnancy.

ectopterygoid (ek"to-ter'ĭ-goyd) [G. *ektos*, outside, + *pteryx*, wing, + *eidos*, form]. *Musculus pterygoideus externus*.

ectopy (ek'to-pĭ) [G. *ek*, out, + *topos*, place]. Displacement. SYN: *ectopia*.

ectoret'ina [G. *ektos*, outside, + L. *rete*, net]. Outer layer of retina.

ectos'copy [" + *skopein*, to examine]. Diagnosis by study of thoracic movements when patient speaks, or by abdominal movements.

ectostosis (ekt-os-to'sĭs) [" + *osteon*, bone, + -*ōsis*]. Formation of bone beneath the periosteum.

ectotoxe'mia [" + *toxikon*, poison, + *aima*, blood]. Toxemia from introduction of a toxin into the body.

Ectotrichophyton (ĕk-tō-trī-kŏf'ĭ-tŏn). Term applied to Trichophyton ectothrix, a genus of parasitic fungi, attaching hair follicles and hair.

ectozoon (ek-to-zo'on) [" + *zōon*, animal]. Parasitic animal that infests the outer integument of the body.

ectrodactylism (ek-tro-dak'til-izm) [G. *ektrōma*, abortion, + *daktylos*, finger, + *ismos*, state of]. Congenital absence of 1 or more fingers or toes.

ectropic (ek-tro'pĭk) [G. *ek*, out, + *trepein*, to turn]. Pert. to complete or partial eversion of a part, generally the eyelid.

ectropion (ek-tro'pĭ-on) [" + *trepein*, to turn]. OPHTH: Eversion, as the edge of an eyelid.

ETIOL: Old age; relaxation of skin; cicatrix following trauma; infection; palsy of facial nerve.

e. of the cervix uteri. GYN: A turning out of the edges of the cervix following laceration.

ectro'pionize [" + *trepein*, to turn]. To evert, or cause an eversion.

eczema (ek'zĕ-mă) [G. *ekzein*, to boil out]. Cutaneous inflammatory condition, acute or chronic, with erythema, papules, vesicles, pustules, scales, crusts, or scabs alone or in combination, dry, or with watery discharge, and with thickening or infiltration and more or less itching or burning. More a symptom than a disease. SYN: *dermatitis*.

ETIOL: Essential cause unknown. No class, age, or sex is exempt, but those with thin, dry skins are more susceptible. Not infectious. Two classes of causes: (1) External or exciting (parasitic, irritation, occupational and non-occupational, chemicals, etc.). (2) Constitutional or predisposing (nerve strain and reflex irritation, anaphylactic reactions, hyperglycemia, etc.).

SYM: Primary type characterized by erythematous, papular, vesicular, or pustular lesions. In secondary type, the lesions evolve from primary variety. Invasion by pathogenic organisms may cause suppuration.

e. capitis. That on the head. Oozing dermatitis seborrheica.*

e., erythematous. Dry, pinkish, ill-defined patches with itching and burning, slight swelling with tendency to spread and coalesce, branny scaling, roughness and dryness of skin. May become generalized.

e. fissum. Form of e. with painful openings in the joint regions.

e., hypertrophicum. E. with a permanent enlargement of papillae of the skin, or skin growths.

e., lichenoid. E. with a thickened condition of the skin.

e. madidans. Variety with raw, erythematous points exuding moisture.

e., Marginum, tinea cruris. E. caused by ringworm.

e., papular. Pin-point to pinhead-sized reddish, pinkish, or violaceous papules with rounded or acuminate thin-walled vesicles which, when ruptured, become covered with thin yellowish crust of dried sebum or inspissated pus interspersed with raw areas of denuded epithelium. Skin as a result of irritation and chronic congestion becomes thick and infiltrated and dark red.

e., pustular. Includes many forms: Follicular, impetiginous or consecutive types, including *eczema rubrum* (red, glazed surface with little oozing); *eczema madidans* (raw, red, and covered with moisture); *eczema crustosum* (more or less crusting with exudate); *eczema fissum* (thick, dry, inelastic skin with cracks and fissures); *squamous eczema* (chronic, on soles, legs, scalp; multiple, circumscribed infiltrated patches with thin, dry scales); *eczema sclerosum* (marked thickening, elephantiasislike papillary hypertrophy resulting in rough, horny, verrucose patches on legs, soles, and palms with fissuring); *furrowed eczema* (slightly erythematous skin, harsh and dry, with innumerable cracks on outer epidermal layer).

PROG: Chronic, amenable to treatment but prone to relapse and recurrence.

TREATMENT: *Internal*: Simple diet, elimination of highly seasoned foods and pastries, condiments and stimulants. Free elimination and water drinking. Opium to be avoided as it increases itching. In gouty and rheumatic, colchicum, salicylate and salines. Pilocarpine, particularly in the dry skinned. X-rays and light exposures. Counterirritation to spinal areas. Removal of focal infections. Avoidance of foreign proteins. *External*: No soap and water. Removal of crusts and scales by oils or cold cream. In acute stage, in moist types, lotions by day and carbolized zinc oxide ointment at night. Carbolic acid for itching or in dry types, boric acid bath or compress, 10 to 15 minutes a day to relieve irritation, or cupful of baking soda in bathtub of water at 98°. Put 3 cups of boiled oatmeal in cheesecloth bag and squeeze in water until cloudy.

Skin tests should be made to find cause of any irritation. Salves alone or alternated with lotions. In advanced and subacute stage with infiltration use stimulating applications with calamine lotion and zinc oil. Tar in subacute and chronic types. In circumscribed types with thickening, salicylic acid in ointment or plaster together with green soap shampoo. Potassium permanganate for pruritus and healing. SEE: *allergy, patch-test, tetter.*

e. rubrum. SEE: *e. madidans.*

e., seborrheic. Form marked by excessive secretion from the sebaceous glands. SYN: *seborrhea.*

e. squamosum. E. with scaly formation.

e., vesicular. Formation of vesicles on the scalp in eczema.

eczem'atous [G. *ekzein*, to boil out]. Marked by or resembling eczema.

Edebohl's position (ed'e-bōl). The dorsal recumbent position with the buttocks resting upon end of table, the lower limbs flexed backward toward the abdomen sufficiently to permit holding the position with legs supported from ankles in a support attached to 2 straight uprights extending 1 on each side at end of table.

ede'ma [G. *oidēma*, swelling]. A condition in which the body tissues contain an excessive amount of tissue fluid. It may be local or general. Generalized edema is called dropsy, or anasarca.

ETIOL: Edema may result from increased permeability of the capillary walls; increased capillary pressure due to venous obstruction or heart failure; lymphatic obstruction; disturbances in renal functioning; reduction of plasma proteins; inflammatory conditions; chemical substances such as bacterial toxins, venoms, caustic substances, and histamine.

May occur by diffusion,* osmosis,* or dialysis.* Acid in the tissue, such as resulting from a sting, produces absorption of water which causes local edema.

TREATMENT OF GENERAL EDEMA: Bed rest desirable. Salt intake restricted. This may be moderate or severe restriction, depending upon degree of edema. Fluid intake restricted; may be as low as 600 cc. in 24 hours. This proscription may be relaxed when free diuresis has been attained. Diuretics are effective when renal function is good, edema mild, and when underlying abnormality of cardiac function, capillary pressure, or colloid osmotic pressure are being corrected, simultaneously. Diuretics contraindicated in the true nephritic edema of acute diffuse glomerulonephritis. They are often useless in cardiac edema associated with advanced renal insufficiency. Useful diuretics are urea, theobromine, theophylline, potassium nitrate, chloride, or acetate, ammonium chloride, or nitrate, and the mercurial diuretics, salyrgan, mercupurin (both given intravenously), and mercurin suppositories. The diet in edema should be adequate in protein, high in calories, rich in vitamins, and low in salt. When diuresis appears, the diet may become normal.

e., acute circumscribed. Form with separated swellings on the body, but usually on the face. [motor disorder.

e., angioneurotic. E. caused by vaso-

e., blue. Hysteric paralysis inducing a swollen, bluish condition of a limb.

e. bullosum vesicae. Form affecting the bladder.

e. of glottis. An infiltration of the submucosa of the larynx, with cough, loss of voice and feeling of suffocation.

e., inflammatory. E. of inflamed tissues.

e., malignant. E. characterized by a rapid course, and speedy destruction of tissue. [infiltration.

e., purulent. E. caused by purulent

e., salt. Form caused by increase of salt in the diet.

edema, words pert. to: angioneuroedema, cephaledema, chemosis, lung, nephritis, phlegmasia alba dolens.

edematous (e-dem'at-us) [G. *oidēma*, swelling]. Pert. to, or affected with, edema.

edible (ĕd'ĭ-bl) [L. *edere*, to eat]. Suitable for food. [sweeten]. Sweetening.

edul'corant [L. *ē*, out, + *dulcorāre*, to

edulcorate (e-dul'ko-rāt) [" + *dulcorāre*, to sweeten]. 1. To sweeten. 2. To wash out salts or acids.

EEG. Abbr. for *electroencephalogram.*

effect'or [L. *effectus*, accomplishing, from *efficere*]. One of the nerve endings having the efferent process end in a gland or muscle cell. The terminal arborizations of efferent or motor nerves. Also applied to effector organs (muscles and glands).

e. organ. A structure which when stimulated produces an effect, specifically muscles and glands.

ef'ferent [L. *ex*, out, + *ferre*, to carry]. Carrying away from as efferent nerves which conduct impulses from the brain or spinal cord to the periphery, efferent lymph vessels which convey lymph from lymph nodes, and efferent arterioles which carry blood from glomeruli of the kidney.

e. nerves. Motor nerves. They can carry impulses having the following effects: (1) Motor, causing contraction of muscles; (2) secretory, causing glands to secrete, and (3) inhibitory, causing some organ to become quiescent.

effervesce (ef-er-ves′) [L. *effervescere*, to boil up]. To boil, or form bubbles on the surface of a liquid.

effervescence (ef-er-ves′ense) [L. *effervescere*, to boil up]. Formation of bubbles of gas coming up to surface of fluid.

efferves'cent. Bubbling. Rising in little bubbles of gas.

effleurage (ef-flūr-ahzh′) [Fr. *effleurer*, to touch lightly]. In massage, deep or superficial stroking.

efflorescence (ef-flor-es′ens) [L. *efflorescere*, to bloom]. A rash; a redness of the skin. SYN: *exanthem.*

efflorescent (ef-flor-es′ent) [L. *efflorescere*, to bloom]. Becoming powdery or drying from loss of water of crystallization.

effluve [L. *e*, out, + *fluere*, to flow]. A conductive discharge of a high potential current through a dielectric.

effluvium (ef-lu′vĭ-um) (pl. *effluvia*) [L. a flowing out]. An invisible emanation or exhalation. SYN: *odor, vapor.*

effuse' [L. *ex*, out, + *fundere*, to pour]. Thin, widely spreading. Applied to a bacterial growth which forms a very delicate film over a surface.

effu'sion [" + *fundere*, to pour]. Escape of fluid into a part, as the pleural cavity, such as empyema, or pyothorax (pus), hydrothorax (serum), hemothorax (blood), chylothorax (lymph), pneumothorax (air), hydropneumothorax (serum and air), and pyopneumothorax (pus and air).

egersis (ē-ger′sĭs). Extreme or abnormal wakefulness; extremely alert.

egesta (e-jes′tă) [" + *gerere*, to bear]. Waste matter eliminated from the body.

egg [A.S. *aeg*]. 1. The female sex cell or ovum applied especially to an ovum which after fertilization is passed from the body and develops outside as in fowls. 2. The mammalian ovum.

e. albumen. The white of an egg. SEE: *vitellin, vitellus, yellow sac.*

egg'plant [A.S. *aeg*, + L. *planta*, sprout]. COMP: NUTRIENTS: 250 Gm. Pro. 3.00, Fat 0.8, Carbo. 10.8 per av. serving. Vit. A+, B+, C+, G++. Ca 0.011, Mg 0.015, K 0.140, Na 0.010, P 0.034, Cl 0.024, S 0.016, Fe 0.0005.

ego (e′go) [G. *egō*, I]. PSY: That part of the unconscious that has been influenced by the senses and which has taken on consciousness in its contacts with reality. A sum total of the innate endowments, environmental impressions, and the reactive tendencies arising out of the conflict between them.

E-8 Ehrlich's side-chain theory

NUTRITIVE VALUE OF CHICKEN EGG

		Whole Egg	Egg White	Egg Yolk
Av. SERVING		50 Gm.	35 Gm.	15 Gm.
"	Pro.	6.7%	4.3%	2.4%
"	Fat	5.2%	0.1%	5.0%
MINERALS				
"	Ca	.067	.015	.137
"	Mg	.011	.010	.160
"	K	.140	.160	.115
"	Na	.145	.156	.075
"	P	.180	.014	.524
"	Cl	.106	.155	.094
"	S	.195	.216	1.66
"	Fe	.0030	.0001	.0086
VITAMINS	A	+++	—	+++
"	B	+ to ++	—	++
"	D	++	—	+++
"	G	+++	++	+++

e. ideal. The unconscious perfection of an individual's pattern or standard of character, usually identified with one greatly admired.

The social standards of the individual in contrast to his instinctive unsocial desires. While undoubtedly there is an inherent difference in the child's capacity to attain an ego ideal as definitely as to attain mature intelligence, much of its formulation depends upon teaching and example in the early years.

Organic disease modifies its evolution, and even more definitely may effect its involution. The later experiences of life, each in turn, add some little modification. It constitutes one phase of "conflict." Overdevelopment or compensatory overemphasis may lead to manifestations neither desirable from the social nor personal viewpoints.

e. instincts. All instincts not of a sexual nature.

e. libido. One concentrated in and upon the ego and not manifested toward external objects. Manifested in narcissistic disorders.

e., super. An inner censor (outside of the field of consciousness) of the ego.

egobronchophony (e″go-bron-kof′o-nĭ) [G. *aix, aig-*, goat, + *brogchos* + *phōnē*, voice]. A bleating sound with bronchophony. SEE: *egophony.*

egocen'tric [G. *ego*, I, + *kentron*, center]. Pert. to a withdrawal from external world with concentration upon inner self.

egoma'nia [" + *mania*, madness]. Abnormal self-esteem and self-interest.

egophony (eg-of′o-nĭ) [G. *aix, aig-*, goat, + *phōnē*, voice]. A nasal sound somewhat like the bleat of a goat heard in auscultation when the subject speaks in a normal tone.

egotrop'ic [G. *ego*, I, + *tropos*, a turning]. Interested chiefly in oneself; self-centered. [glion.

Eh'renritter's ganglion. The jugular gan-

Ehrlich's side-chain theory (air′lik). So named because the protoplasmic cell is said to possess the certain receptors or "side-chains" which are capable of becoming fixed to certain protein groups with which they have a chemical affinity. This "fixation" is of value to the cell in that it enables it to attach the various food substances which it needs for nourishment. The molecules of a toxin, according to this theory, contain 2 groups for attachment to the cell.

HAPTOPHORE GROUP: It becomes fixed to a suitable cell receptor. When this happens, the receptor detaches from the cell and floats off in the blood stream. The cell responds to this loss by producing more effectors, which are again liberated into the blood, where they combine with toxins and thereby render them inert, and so form free antitoxin.

TOXOPHORE GROUP: Toxicity results when this becomes attached to certain receptors of the cell called toxiphiles, and this union is prevented by rendering the haptophore group inert. SEE: *immunity.*

E.'s theory of immunity. A theory which attempts to explain the formation of antitoxin in the blood. Also known as E.'s side-chain theory, *q.v.*

Ehrlich-Hata "606." A specific for syphilis. SYN: *salvarsan.*

Eichhorst's corpuscles (īk′horst). Spherical, small blood corpuscles found in pernicious anemia.

E.'s neuritis. Neuritis involving nerve sheath and interstitial muscular tissues.

eidoptometry (i-dop-tom′et-rī) [G. *eidos,* form, + *optein,* to see, + *metron,* measure]. Determination of visual acuteness.

eighth cranial nerve. Acoustic nerve, *q.v.*

eikonom′etry [G. *eikon,* image, + *metron,* measure]. Determination of distance of an object by measuring the image produced by a lens of known focus.

eiloid (i′loid) [G. *eilein,* to coil, + *eidos,* appearance]. Having a coil-like structure.

Eimeria (i-me′rĭ-ă). A genus of sporozoan parasites belonging to the class Telosporidea, subclass Coccidiida. They are intracellular parasites living in the epithelial cells of vertebrates and invertebrates. They rarely are parasitic to man.

E. hominis. A species in the pleural exudate of man.

eisodic (i-sod′ik) [G. *eis,* into, + *odos,* way]. Centripetal or afferent, as nerve fibers of a reflex arc.

eiweissmilch (i′vĭs-milk). Milk with curd broken up and whey removed, mixed with malt sugar, and boiled buttermilk for infant feeding.

ejacula′tio (e-jak-u-la′she-o) [L.]. Sudden expelling, as of semen.

e. precox (pre′kox) [L.]. Premature ejaculation. Inability to prevent ejaculation of semen at the beginning of copulation, or prior to it.

ejaculation (e-jak-u-la′shun) [L. *ejaculari,* to throw out]. Ejection of the seminal fluids from the male urethra, or of the secretions of the vaginal glands, esp. Bartholin's glands, in the female.

e. mechanism of. Ejaculation consists of two phases, (1) the passage of spermatozoa and the secretions of the accessory organs (*bulbo-urethral* and prostate glands and seminal vesicles) into the urethra, and (2) the expulsion of the seminal fluid from the urethra. The former is brought about by contraction of the smooth muscle of the vas deferens, and the increased secretory activity of the glands; the latter by the rhythmical contractions of the bulbocavernous and ischiocavernous muscles and the levator ani.

Ejaculation is a reflex phenomenon. Afferent impulses arising principally from stimulation of the glans penis pass to the spinal cord by way of the internal pudendal nerves. Efferent impulses arising from a reflex center located in the upper lumbar region of the cord pass through sympathetic fibers in the hypogastric nerves and plexus to the vas deferens and seminal vesicles. Other impulses arising from the 3rd and 4th sacral segments pass through the internal pudendal nerves to the ischocavernous and bulbocavernous muscles.

Erection of the penis usually precedes ejaculation. Ejaculation occurs normally during copulation or it may occur as a nocturnal emission. The amount of seminal fluid discharged contains up to 300,000,000 spermatozoa.

RS: *coitus, coitus interruptus, excitation, orgasm, semen.*

ejac′ulatory. Pert. to ejaculation.
 e. duct. The terminal portion of the seminal duct formed by the union of the ductus deferens and the excretory duct of the seminal vesicle.

ejecta (e-jek′tă) [L. *ejaculari,* to throw out]. Matter thrown off by the body. SYN: *dejecta, egesta.*

EK, EKG. Abbr. for *electrocardiogram.*

ekphorize (ek′fo-riz) [G. *ek,* out, + *phorein,* to bear]. A bringing back of the effect of a psychic experience in an attempt to reëxperience it in memory. SEE: *engram.*

elaiop′athy [G. *elaion,* oil, + *pathos,* disease]. Swelling of joints due to contusion, followed by fatty deposits. SYN: *eleopathy.*

elastic (e-las′tik) [G. *elastikos,* elastic]. Capable of being stretched and returning to its original state; having elasticity. [stretched.
 e. bandage. One which can be
 e. cartilage. Yellow cartilage such as is found in the epiglottis, pharynx, external ears, and auditory tube.
 e. lamina. Descemet's membrane.
 e. skin. Rare condition in which there is unusual elastic state of the skin.
 e. stocking. One worn to place pressure on surface of the foot, or portion of the leg.
 e. tissue. Connective tissue supplied with elastic fibers as found in the middle coat of arteries.

elasticity (e-las-tis′it-ī) [G. *elastikos,* elastic]. The quality of returning to original size and shape after compression or stretching.

elastin (e-las′tin) [G. *elastikos,* elastic]. 1. An albuminoid substance forming the principal constituent of yellow elastic tissue, comprising about 30% of this tissue. 2. A protein which can be prepared from various connective tissues. SEE: *albumnoid.*

elas′tinase [G. *elastikos,* elastic]. A ferment that dissolves elastin.

elas′toid [G. *elastikos,* elastic, + *eidos,* form]. Pert. to a substance formed by hyaline degeneration.
 e. degeneration. Hyaline d. of elastic fibers of an artery.

elasto′ma [" + *-ōma,* tumor]. A chronic disease of the skin; pseudoxanthoma.

elastometer (e-las-tŏm′et-er) [" + *metron,* measure]. Device for measuring elasticity.

elastom′etry [" + *metron,* measure]. The measurement of elasticity of tissues.

elas′tose. A peptone resulting from gastric digestion of elastin.

elaterin (e-lăt′er-in) [G. *elatērios,* driving]. The neutral principle obtained from *elaterium,* a plant grown in the Mediterranean region.   [tic.

ACTION AND USES: Hydragogue cathar-
DOSAGE: 1/20 gr.

ela′tion [L. *elatus,* borne out of]. PSY: Joyful emotion. It is pathologic when out of accord with patient's actual circumstances.

el'bow [A.S. *eln*, forearm, + *boga*, bend]. Joint of arm and forearm.

e., dislocation, ant. TREATMENT: Reduction by direct pressure with moderate extension.

e. jerk. Striking tendon of biceps or triceps muscle causes involuntary bending or jerk of elbow.

e. joint. Joint between arm and the forearm. Includes the humeroulnar, humeroradial, and proximal radioulnar articulations.

e., d., lateral. Frequently accompanied with fracture of condyle. TREATMENT: Reduction under anesthesia; hyperextension; lateral pressure; traction, and flexion. Arthrotomy if irreducible. Dressing, bandage, and sling, or 2 lateral angular splints.

e., d., post. SYM: Olecranon projects. Arm flexed. Lower end of humerus felt at bend. Elastic fixation of elbow. Distance increased bet. olecranon and condyles. TREATMENT: Reduce by hyperextension of forearm. Ant. angular splint for 2 weeks. Frequent dressings, massage, and movements.

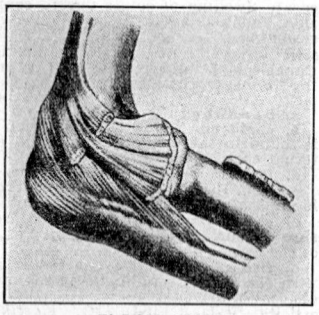

ELBOW JOINT

e. reflex. Sharp extension of forearm resulting from tapping of triceps tendon while arm is held loosely in bent position.

elbow, words pert. to: anconad, anconagra, anconal, anconeal, anconeus, anconitis, tennis elbow.

elcosis (el-ko'sis) [G. *elkōsis*, ulceration]. Fetid ulceration.

Electra complex [G. *Elektra*, Agamemnon's daughter, who helped assassinate her mother, because of love for her father, whom the former had slain]. PSY: A group of symptoms due to suppressed sexual love of daughter for father. OPP: *Oedipus complex, q.v.*

elec'tric [G. *ēlektron*, amber]. Pert. to, caused by, or resembling electricity.

e. baker. Device for placing intense heat on a part, as in arthritis. SEE: *baker.*

e. contacts and injuries. Injuries from electricity vary with type and strength of current, length of contact, location of contact, such as legs, arms, etc., and hence vary from trivial burns to complete charring; or unconsciousness from either paralysis of the respiratory center, fibrillation of the heart, or both.

Direct currents of less than 300 volts are seldom fatal, but alternating currents of 15 to 60 cycles may be fatal, even when below 100 volts. Ordinary household or office currents vary from 30 to 220 volts.

INSULATION: Protection against such currents may be made with dry nonconductors, such as folded newspapers, magazines, cardboard, wood, rubber, clothing, etc. These may be used to move patient from the contact or to remove wire from patient. It is always preferable to turn off the current if possible. If patient is in water, remember that it is electrically charged and special precautions must be taken. On a humid or rainy day ordinary insulators may contain sufficient moisture to conduct electricity. Make sure insulators are dry.

High tension currents, such as those used about the x-ray or in conducting currents for long distances or for special industrial locations cannot be insulated by such means. Such currents may jump through rubber, paper, or strips of wood. A safe procedure is to ascertain the source of current and have it shut off, otherwise multiple tragedies result. TREATMENT: SEE: *electric shock.*

e. field. Field exerting force of one dyne on unit positive charge. SEE: *intensity of electric field.*

e. muscle stimulation. Two types of current, faradic used for stimulation of nerve to the muscle, and galvanic used for stimulation of nerve and muscle. Contraction of muscle with galvanic occurs only at *make* or if strong enough at *break.* Used for diagnosis and treatment in neuromuscular diseases.

e. shock. SYM: Burns, with loss of consciousness; contact or proximity to source of current are principal symptoms.

F. A. TREATMENT: Carefully free victim from source of current with nonconductors such as dry wood, paper, rubber, etc., or shut off current. Prolonged artificial respiration may be necessary. SEE: *shock.*

e. valve. A vacuum tube having for one electrode a hot filament. Often used in rectifying alternating to direct current, as in roentgen generators.

electri'city [G. *ēlektron*, amber]. "A form of energy which, when in motion, exhibits magnetic, chemical, mechanical and thermal effects, and when at rest or in motion exerts a force on other electricity. Recent investigations indicate that it is discrete and granular in nature. Electricity may be of 2 kinds, namely, positive and negative."—Sheldon.

e., atmospheric. E. existing in the atmosphere.

e., faradic. SEE: *induced e.*

e., franklinic. SEE: *static e.*

e., frictional. Generation of static e. by rubbing 2 articles together.

e., galvanic. E. generated by chemical action.

e., induced. E. generated in a body from another body close by, without contact.

e., magnetic. E. induced by means of a magnetic device.

e., medical. Generation of e. by a device which can be adjusted for treating medical cases.

e., negative. Electric charge caused by an excess of electrons negatively charged.

e., positive. Electric charge caused by loss of negative electrons.

e., static. E. generated by friction.

e., unit of. SEE: *ampere, coulomb, farad, ohm, volt, watt.*

elec′trify [" + L. *facere*, to make]. To charge a body with electricity.

electriza′tion [G. *ēlektron*, amber]. The act of charging the body with electricity.

electroanesthesia [" + *a*-, priv. + *aisthēsis*, sensation]. Local anesthesia induced by an anesthetizing substance injected into tissues by electricity.

electrobiol′ogy [" + *bios*, life, + *logos*, study of]. Science of electric phenomena in the living body.

electrobios′copy [" + " + *skopein*, to examine]. Electric test to determine if life is extinct.

electro″car′diogram [" + *kardia*, heart, + *gramma*, writing]. A typical record of normal heart action shows certain waves called P, Q, R, S, and T waves. Sometimes a U wave is seen. The first or P wave is caused by contraction of the atria. The Q, R, S, and T waves are related to contraction of the ventricles. The cause of the U wave is unknown. The electrocardiogram gives important information concerning the spread of excitation to the different chambers of the heart and it is of value in the diagnosis of cases of abnormal cardiac rhythm and myocardial damage.

electrocar′diograph [" + " + *graphein*, to write]. Device for recording variations in action of heart muscles.

electro″car′diography [" + " + *graphein*, to write]. The making of and study of graphic records electrocardiograms produced by electrical currents originating in the heart.

elec″trocar″diopho′nograph [" + " + *phone*, voice, + *graphein*, to write]. Device for recording heart sounds.

elec″trocatal′ysis [" + *kata*, down, + *lysis*, loosening]. Chemical decomposition produced by electricity.

electro″cau′tery [" + *kauter*, burner]. Cauterization by means of an apparatus consisting of a holder containing a wire, which may be heated to a red or white heat by a current of electricity, either direct or alternating.

electrochem′istry [" + *chēmeia*, chemistry]. Science of chemical changes produced by electricity.

elec′trochemy [" + *chēmeia*, chemistry]. Therapy concerned with physical applications, such as electricity, which produce chemical effects in the tissues.

electrocis′ion [" + L. *caedare*, to cut]. Excision by electric current.

elec″trocoagula′tion [" + L. *coagulare*, to thicken]. Coagulation of tissue by means of a high frequency electric current. The heat producing the coagulation is generated within the tissue to be destroyed.

electrocontractility (e-lek″tro-kon-trak-tĭl′ĭ-tĭ) [" + L. *contrahere*, to contract]. Contraction of muscular tissue by electrical stimulation.

electrocryptectomy (e-lek″tro-krip-tek′to-mī) [" + *kryptos*, concealed, + *ektomē*, excision]. Destruction of tonsillar crypts by diathermy.

electrocu′tion [G. *ēlektron*, amber, + L. *secutus*, following]. The destruction of life by means of electric current.

electrocystoscopy (e-lek″tro-sis-tos′ko-pī) [" + *kystis*, bladder, + *skopein*, to examine]. The use of electric light to see the interior of the bladder.

elec′trode [" + *odos*, way]. A medium intervening bet. an electric conductor and the object to which the current is to be applied. In electrotherapy an electrode is an instrument with a point or a surface from which to discharge current to the body of a patient.

 e., active. SEE: *therapeutic e.*
 e., brush. A wire brush used to apply electricity to a part of the body.
 e., cataphoric. E. devised so that the current passes from the positive pole to the body through a medicated solution.
 e., Cherry's. Vaginal electrodes for medical diathermy treatments of pelvic infections.
 e., depolarizing. E. with greater resistance than the part of the body in the circuit.
 e. diffusion. SEE: *cataphoric e.*
 e., dispersive. When electrodes may be applied in pairs dissimilar in size and shape, then the smaller electrode is called the active, and the larger, the dispersive, indifferent, or inactive electrode.
 e., exciting. SEE: *therapeutic e.*
 e., franklinic. Form used for the application of static discharge.
 e., Guttman. Electrode for intramural electrocoagulation of the inferior turbinate.
 e., Hyam's. Special cutting current instrument for "conization" by high frequency current in treatment of chronic endocervicitis.
 e., hydrogen. Form absorbing hydrogen gas.
 e., impregnated. SEE: *therapeutic e.*
 e., indifferent. SEE: *e., dispersive.*
 e., multiple point. Several sets of terminals providing for the use of several electrodes. SEE: *multiterminal.*
 e., negative. Cathode.
 e., non-polarizable. E. constructed to prevent polarization.
 e., normal. E. with constant cross section of 10 square centimeters.
 e., point. An electrode with an insulating handle at one end and a metallic point at the other for use in applying static sparks.
 e., positive. Anode.
 e., prescription. Therapeutic e. made according to a physician's prescription.
 e., Roblee. Pelvic diathermy electrode introduced by Roblee, consisting of hard rubber vaginal speculum.
 e., roller. Form of e. made like a roller.
 e., silent. SEE: *dispersive e.*
 e., spark ball or point. An insulating handle having on one end a metallic ball or point. Used in giving static sparks.
 e., therapeutic. E. devised so the carbon is impregnated with medicinal preparations.
 e., vacuum. Hollow glass tubes or bulbs from which the air has been exhausted to varying degrees and to which the current is conveyed by a wire passing through one end or by a metal collar surrounding the stem without any internal connection. Used for high frequency and static currents.
 e., vaginal. SEE: *Cherry's electrode.*
 e., Zener's. Cervicovaginal diathermy electrode with 4 blades closing about cervix concentrating heat in cervical canal and immediate parametrium.
 e., zinc. Used connected to positive pole of galvanic machine for ionic medication.

elec″trodesicca′tion [" + L. *desiccāre*, to dry up]. The destructive drying of cells and tissue by means of short high frequency electric sparks, in contradistinction to fulguration, which is the destruction of tissue by means of long high frequency electric sparks.

elec″trodiagno′sis [" + *dia*, through, + *gnōsis*, knowledge]. The determination of the functional states of various organs and tissues according to their response to electrical stimulation.

electro″dial′ysis. A method of separating electrolytes from colloids by passing a current through a solution containing both.

electrodynamometer (e-lek-tro-di-nam-om′et-er) [" + *dynamis*, power, + *metron*, measure]. An instrument to measure the strength of an electric current either alternating or direct, as by means of the interaction of 2 wire coils carrying the current.

electroencephalogram (ē-lĕk-trō-ĕn-sĕf′ă-lō-grăm) [G. *ēlektron*, amber, + *kephalos*, brain, + *gramma*, a writing]. A tracing on an electroencephalograph.

electroencephalograph (ē-lĕk-trō-ĕn-sĕf′ă-lō-grăf) [G. *ēlektron*, amber, + *kephalos*, brain, + *graphein*, to write]. An instrument for recording electrical fluctuations of the brain after amplification of more than a billion times.

Experiments show a direct connection between the brain records and intelligence of the subjects tested. Brain waves are designated as Alpha rhythm with a frequency of about 10 waves a second; the Beta rhythm 25 per second, and the Delta waves 1/6 second and more.

electrog′raphy [G. *ēlektron*, amber, + *graphein*, to write]. Making of an x-ray picture. SYN: *skiagraphy*.

electro″hemos′tasis. The arrest of blood by means of a high-frequency current.

electrolithotrity (ē-lĕk-trō-lĭ-thŏt′rĭ-tĭ). The destruction of a calculus by means of an electric current.

electrol′ogy [" + *logos*, science]. The branch of science that deals with the phenomena and properties of electricity.

electrolysis (e-lek-trol′ĭ-sis) [" + *lysis*, a dissolution].

Ex: The passage of an electric current through hydrochloric acid (HCl) results in its decomposition, hydrogen ʋas being produced at the cathode and chlorine gas at the anode.

electrolyte (e-lek′tro-līt) [" + *lytos*, solution]. 1. A solution which is a conductor of electricity. 2. A substance which, in solution, conducts an electric current and is decomposed by the passage of an electric current.

Ex: Acids, bases, and salts are common electrolytes.

 e., amphoteric. One which produces both hydrogen (H-) and hydroxyl (OH-) ions.

electrolytic (e-lek-tro-lĭt′ĭk) [" + *lytos*, solution]. Caused by or rel. to electrolysis.

 e. conduction. In metals the electrical charges are carried by the electrons of inappreciable mass.

In solutions the electrical charges are carried by electrolytic ions, each one of a mass several thousand times as great as the electron. When a direct current passes through an electrolytic solution bet. metallic electrodes immersed in it, the positive ions move to the cathode, the negative ions to the anode.

elec′trolyzer [" + *lysis*, solution]. Instrument for reducing stricture with electricity.

electromag′net [" + *magnes*, magnet]. A magnet consisting of a length of insulated wire wound around soft iron core.

electromagnet′ic [" + *magnes*, magnet]. Pert. to an electromagnet.

 e. induc′tion. Generation of an electromotive force in an insulated conductor moving in an electromagnetic field, or in a fixed conductor in a moving magnetic field.

electromag′netism [" + " + *ismos*, state of]. Science of mutual relations of electricity and magnetism.

electromassage [" + *massein*, to knead]. Massage combined with application of electrization.

electrom′eter [" + *metron*, measure]. An instrument for measuring pressure quantity and intensity of electricity, i. e., differences in electric potential.

electromo′tive [" + L. *motor*, motion]. Pert. to passage of electricity in a current, or motion produced by it.

 e. force (abbreviation, E. M. F.). That effect of difference of potential which, on the closing of a circuit, causes a flow of electricity from one place to another, giving rise to an electric current. The strength of an electric current is directly proportional to the impressed electromotive force, and inversely proportional to the resistance in the case of direct current and to the impedance in the case of alternating current. Electromotive force is measured in volts or in some convenient multiple or fraction of a volt. Microvolt, millivolt and kilovolt are, respectively, one-millionth volt, one-thousandth volt and 1000 volts.

electro″my′ogram. A graphic record of the contraction of a muscle as a result of electrical stimulation.

electro″myog′raphy. The preparation, study of, and interpretation of electromyograms.

elec′tron [G. *elektron*, amber]. An extremely minute corpuscle or charge of negative electricity which revolves about the central core or nucleus of an atom. They are the smallest known particles that exist, their mass being 1/1845 that of a hydrogen atom. When emitted from radioactive substances known as *beta particles* or rays.

electro″narco′sis. The induction of narcosis by the application of electricity to the body. Used in the treatment of schizophrenia.

electro″neg′ative [" + L. *negāre*, to deny]. Condition of being charged with negative electricity which results in the attraction of bodies positively charged and the repulsion of bodies negatively charged.

electron′ic [G. *ēlektron*, amber]. Pert. to electrons.

electroniza′tion [G. *ēlektron*, amber]. The use of radiation to restore electrical equilibrium.

elec′tropath [" + *pathos*, disease]. One skilled in practice of electrotherapy.

electropathol′ogy [" + " + *logos*, study of]. Determining electrical reaction of muscles and nerves as means of diagnosis.

electro″phore′sis (e-lek-tro-for-e′sis [" + *phorein*, to bear]. Diathermy or ionto-phoresis. SEE: *phoresis*. The movement of charged colloidal particles through the medium in which they are dispersed as a result of changes in electrical potential. Electrophoretic methods are useful in the analysis of protein mixtures as protein particles move with different velocities dependent principally on the number of charges carried by the particle.

electrophorus (e-lek-trŏf′ŏr-ūs) [" + *phorein*, to bear]. An instrument for

electrophototherapy   E-13   **elephantiasis**

obtaining static electricity by means of induction.

electrophother′apy [" + *phōs*, light, + *therapeia*, treatment]. Treatment by means of electric light.

electro″phre′nic. Pertaining to stimulation of the phrenic nerve by electricity.

electropos′itive [" + L. *positivus*, emphatic]. The condition of being subject to repulsion by bodies positively electrified, and to attraction by bodies negatively electrified.

electro″physiol′ogy [" + *physis*, nature, + *logos*, study of]. A branch of physiology which deals with the relations of body functions to electrical phenomena such as the effects of electrical stimulation upon the tissues, the production of electrical currents by organs and tissues, the therapeutic use of electric currents, etc.

electropneumatotherapy (e-lek″tro-nu″-mă-to-ther′ă-pĭ) [" + *pneuma*, air, + *therapeia*, treatment]. Treatment of voice by faradic current into the larynx.

electroprogno′sis [" + *prognōsis*, foreknowledge]. Prognosis by means of electrical reactions.

elec′tropuncture [" + L. *punctura*, a piercing]. Piercing tissues with an electric needle.

electropyrexia (e-lek″tro-pi-reks′ĭ-ă) [" + *pyressein*, to be feverish]. Elevation of temperature by electricity.

electroradiometer (e-lek″tro-ră-dĭ-om′e-ter) [" + L. *radius*, ray, + G. *metron*, measure]. An electroscope for differentiation of radiant energy.

electro″retin′ogram. A record of the action currents of the retina made by placing one electrode upon the cornea and the other on the optic nerve or the posterior pole of the darkened eyeball.

electroscission (e-lek″trō-sĭ′shŭn) [G. *ēlektron*, amber, + L. *scindere*, to cut]. Division of tissues by electrocautery.

electroscope (e-lek′tro-skōp) [" + *skopein*, to see]. An instrument which detects positive or negative static electricity.

electro′shock. Shock produced by an electric current.

   e. s. therapy. The induction of convulsive seizures by the passing of an electric current through the brain. Used in the treatment of certain types of psychoses.

electrostat′ic [" + *statikos*, causing to stand]. Pert. to static electricity.

   e. generator. A device that generates static electricity. SEE: *influence machine*.

   e. unit. Any unit of electrical measurement based on the attraction or repulsion of a static charge, as distinguished from an electromagnetic unit, which is defined in terms of the attraction or repulsion of magnetic poles.

electrosur′gery [" + *cheir*, hand, + *ergon*, work†]. Surgery accomplished by electricity.

electro″tax′is [" + *taxis*, arrangement]. The movement of a cell or an organism toward or away from an electrical stimulus.

electro″thana′sia. Death resulting from electric shock; electrocution.

electrotherapeutics (e-lek″tro-ther-ă-pu′-tĭks) [" + *therapeutikē*, treatment]. The use of electricity in the treatment of disease.

electrotherapist (e-lek″tro-ther′a-pĭst) [" + *therapeia*, treatment]. A medical graduate who has had special training and has acquired skill in the therapeutic use of electricity. The term is sometimes used incorrectly to designate any one who administers electrical treatments.

elec″trother′apy [" + *therapeia*, treatment]. Use of electricity in treating disease. SYN: *electrotherapeutics*.

elec′trotherm. An electrical apparatus for the therapeutic application of heat to the surface of the body. Used for relief of pain.

electrothermotherapy (e-lek″tro-ther″mother′a-pĭ) [" + *thermē*, heat, + *therapeia*, treatment]. The production of heat within the living tissues for therapeutic purposes by means of bodily resistance to the passing of an electric current.

elec′trotome. An electrocautery device used for surgical procedures.

electroton′ic [" + *tonos*, tone]. Of or pert. to electrotonus.

electroto′nus [" + *tonos*, tone]. The change in the irritability of a nerve or muscle during the passage of an electric current.

electrotropism (e-lek-trot′ro-pĭzm) [" + *tropē*, a turning, + *ismos*, condition of]. Reaction of cells to an electrical current.

electuary (e-lek′tu-a-rĭ) [G. *ekleichein*, to lick up]. Medicinal substance mixed with saccharine matter to form pasty mass.

eleidin (ĕ-lē′ĭd-ĭn) [G. *elaion*, oil]. An acidophil substance present in the stratum lucidum of the epidermis.

el′ement [L. *elementum*, a rudiment]. In modern chemistry, a substance which cannot be separated from itself by ordinary chemical processes. They exist in a free and in a combined state. Over 90 have been identified. SEE: *Appendix for table of Chemical Elements*.

element, words pert. to: atom, body, chemical e., mineral e., monad, name of each element, oxidation, oxide, radicle.

eleoma (el-e-o′mă) [G. *elaion*, oil, + *ōma*, tumor]. A neoplasm sometimes following injection of oil into the tissues.

eleometer (el-e-om′et-er) [" + *metron*, measure]. Instrument for determining quality and spec. gravity of oils.

eleomyenchysis (el″e-o-mi-en′kis-is) [" + *mys*, muscle, + *egchysis*, infusion]. 1. The intramuscular injection of oils for chronic local spasms. 2. Prosthesis* by paraffin injection.

eleop′athy [" + *pathos*, disease]. Swelling of joints due to fatty deposits. SYN: *elaiopathy*.

eleoptene (el-e-op′tēn) [" + *ptēnos*, fleeting]. The fluid part of a volatile oil.

eleosaccharum (e″le-o-sak′ar-um) [" + *sakcharon*, sugar]. A mixture of powdered sugar with a volatile oil.

eleotherapy (el-e-o-ther′ă-pĭ) [" + *therapeia*, treatment]. The use of oil for therapeutic purposes.

eleotho′rax [" + *thōrax*, chest]. The injection of oil into the pleural cavity to compress a tuberculous lung.

elephantiasis (el-ē-fan-tī′as-is) [G. *elephas*, elephant]. SYN: *lymphedema, filariasis*. A chronic condition characterized by pronounced hypertrophy of the skin and subcutaneous tissues resulting from obstruction of the lymphatic vessels. The lower extremities and the scrotum are parts most frequently involved.

   ETIOL: E. may be congenital (Milroy's disease), or the result of metastatic invasion of the lymph nodes by tumor cells; inflammatory E. results from filariasis or local infection of the lymph nodes. Elephantiasis is most common

Elements Having Medicinal Uses

Element	Compound Form	Some Medicinal Uses
Aluminum (Al)	Alum	Astringent to contract mucous membranes, as a gargle and a douche.
	Aluminum acetate	Astringent and antiseptic in surgical dressings.
Arsenic (As)	Arsenic trioxide Potassium arsenite	Hematinic, i.e., in minute doses, it increases the amount of red corpuscles in the blood, thereby acting as a tonic to improve the appetite and digestion.
Barium (Ba)	Barium sulfate	Coats the stomach and intestines for taking x-ray pictures.
Bismuth (Bi)	Bismuth subnitrate Bismuth subcarbonate	Insoluble compounds used as dusting powders on the skin; astringents, and antiseptics for ulcerations of the stomach.
Boron (B)	Boric acid (boracic acid)	Mild antiseptic, nonirritating, particularly used for an eyewash.
Bromine (Br)	Sodium and Potassium Bromide	Nerve sedatives.
Calcium (Ca)	Calcium chloride Calcium lactate	Assists in clotting of the blood. Calcium compounds are used for the treatment of tetany in children. Calcium salts are necessary for the growth of bones and teeth, for regulating muscular, nervous, and glandular activity.
Chlorine (Cl)	Sodium chloride Chlorinated lime	Disinfectant for urinals and excreta. A deodorant.
Copper (Cu)	Copper sulfate (blue vitriol)	Removes granulations on the eyelids in trachoma. Produces vomiting. Used as an astringent.
Hydrogen (H)	All acids, e. g., hydrochloric	Dilute solutions extract water from the tissues, and in the stomach aid digestion.
	Hydrogen peroxide	Antiseptic.
Iodine (I)	Iodine tincture	Antiseptic.
	Potassium iodide	Treatment of syphilis, to increase secretions, and as treatment in hyperthyroidism.
Iron (Fe)	Iron chloride	Hematinic as in cases of anemia. Astringent.
Lead (Pb)	Lead acetate	Astringent. Contracts tissues in ulcers and wounds.
Magnesium (Mg)	Magnesium citrate "Milk of Magnesia"	Purgative. Cathartic, neutralizes acidity of the stomach.
	Magnesium sulfate (Epsom salt)	Purgative. Allays inflammations.
Mercury (Hg)	Mercuric chloride (bichloride of mercury)	Local antiseptic.
	Mercurous chloride (calomel)	Cathartic.
	Mercuric salicylate	Intramuscular injection in syphilis.
Nitrogen (N)	Nitrous oxide (laughing gas)	Anesthetic.
	Ammonia water	Cleanser, heart stimulant.
Oxygen (O)		Used in resuscitation in anoxemia, and in basal metabolism.
Phosphorus (P)	Sodium phosphate	Saline purgative. Reduces accumulation of fluid in the tissues, as in edema.
Potassium (K)	Potassium acetate	Diuretic.
	Potassium permanganate	Antiseptic for wounds.
	Potassium sodium tartrate	Saline purgative.
Radium (Ra)	Radium bromide	Treatment for cancer.
Silver (Ag)	Silver nitrate	Antiseptic to contract mucous membranes of eye, to cauterize, and for nose and throat inflammations.
Sodium (Na)	Sodium bicarbonate (baking soda)	Acidosis treatment.
Sulfur (S)		Used in ointments for skin diseases. May be used as a laxative.
Zinc (Zn)	Zinc oxide	Astringent.
	Zinc stearate	Dusting powder (irritating if inhaled).
	Zinc sulfate	Produces vomiting.

in tropical countries and is caused by infestation by *Wucheria bancrofti*, a filarial worm.
  e. arabum. SYN: *elephantiasis*.
  e. graecorum. Leprosy.
  e. telangiectodes. E. with blood vessel enlargement.
el'evator [L. *elevāre*, to lift]. 1. Curved retractor for holding lid away from the globe of the eye. 2. One for raising depressed bones by levers or screws.
eleventh cranial nerve. Accessorius nerve, *q.v.*
eliminant (ē-lim'ĭ-nant) [L. *ē*, out, + *limen*, threshold]. 1. Effecting evacuation. 2. Agent aiding in elimination.
eliminate (ē-lim'ĭ-nāte) [" + *limen*, threshold]. To expel; to rid the body of waste material.
elimina'tion [" + *limen*, threshold]. Excretion of waste body products by the skin, kidneys, and intestines.
  e. diet. Based on patient's history of food sensitiveness and results of skin tests. The "elimination diet" found to relieve the patient's symptoms is increased by gradual addition of foods to which patient has been found to be non-sensitive, until in so far as possible all the essentials of an adequate diet are included.
elimination, words pert. to: constipation, costive, defecation, dejecta, egesta, ejecta, evacuate, feces, names of excretions, nisus.
elinguation (ē-lĭn-gwā'shun) [L. *ē*, out, + *lingua*, tongue]. The operation of removing the tongue from the oral cavity.
elixir [Arabic *alexir*, philosopher's stone]. A sweetened, aromatic, hydro-alcoholic liquid used in the compounding of medicines. Elixirs constitute one of the most commonly used classes of preparations, and contribute largely toward the possibility of pleasant medication. The National Formulary contains many of the more popular formulae, but only 2 elixirs are official.
El'liott treat'ment. Treatment given by means of rubber bag that distends vagina when attached to machine delivering water at temperature of 115° to 128° F. maintained for 45 to 60 minutes; used in pelvic inflammatory disease.
elutriation (e-lū-trĭ-a'shun) [L. *elutriāre*, to cleanse]. The separation of insoluble particles from finer ones by decanting the fluid.
elytritis (el-ĭ-trī'tis) [G. *elytron*, vagina, + *itis*, inflammation]. Inflammation of the vagina.
elytrocele (el'ĭ-tro-sēl) [" + *kēlē*, hernia]. Hernia into the vagina. SYN: *colpocele*.
elytroclasia (el"ĭ-tro-kla'sĭ-a) [" + *klasis*, rupture]. Rupture of the vagina.
elytrocleisis (el"ĭ-tro-klī'sis) [" + *kleisis*, closure]. Closure of the vagina.
elytronitis (el-ĭ-tro-nī'tis) [" + *itis*, inflammation]. Inflammation of the vagina.
elytroplasty (el'it-ro-plas"tĭ) [" + *plassein*, to form]. Plastic operation upon the vagina.
elytroptosis (ĕl"ĭ-trŏp-tō'sĭs) [" + *ptōsis*, a dropping]. Prolapse of the vagina.
elytrorrhaphy (el-ĭ-trŏr'ră-fī) [" + *raphē*, suture]. Suture of vaginal wall.
elytrostenosis (el"ĭ-tro-sten-o'sis) [" + *stenōsis*, narrowing]. Narrowing of the vagina.
elytrotomy (el-ĭ-trŏt'o-mĭ) [" + *tomē*, incision]. Incision of vaginal wall.
emaciate (e-mā-sĭ-āt) [L. *ēmaciāre*, to grow thin]. To cause to become excessively lean.

ema'ciated. Excessively lean.
emacia'tion [L. *ēmaciāre*, to grow thin]. Wasting of the flesh; state of being extremely lean.
  ETIOL: Malnutrition; diseases of gastrointestinal canal. If rapid: Marasmus, Addison's d., tuberculosis, cancer, diabetes, suppuration, hyperthyroidism, chronic diarrhea, stricture of esophagus, pyloric obstruction; parasites; loss of sleep, exophthalmic goiter, starvation.
  SEE: *lean, tabes, wasting*.
emaculation (em-ak-u-la'shun) [L. *ēmaculāre*, to remove spots]. Removal of spots from the skin.
emailloid (em-a'loid) [Fr. *émail*, enamel, + G. *eidos*, form]. Tumor having its origin in tooth enamel.
emana'tion [L. *ē*, out, + *manāre*, to flow]. 1. Something given off; radiation; emission. 2. A disintegration product.
  e., actinium. One given off by actinium. SYN: *actinon*.
  e., radium. A radioactive gas given off by radium. SYN: *niton*.
  e., thorium. One given off by thorium. SYN: *thoron*.
emansio mensium (em-an'sĭ-o men'sĭ-um) [L.]. Amenorrhea in which menstruation has never occurred.
emasculation (e-mas-ku-la'shun) [L. *ēmasculāre*, to castrate]. Castration;* excision of the testicles. RS: *spay*.
emballometer (ĕm-băl-ŏm'ĕt-ĕr) [G. *emballein*, to throw, + *metron*, a measure]. Device employed in connection with a stethoscope.
embalming (em-bahm'ing) [L. *in*, in, + *balsāmum*, balsam]. Preservation of a dead body against putrefaction.
embed'ding [" + A.S. *bedd*, to bed]. In histology, the process by which a piece of tissue is placed in a firm medium such as paraffin or celloidin in order to support it and keep it intact during the subsequent cutting into thin sections for microscopic examination.
embola'lia [G. *embolos*, thrown in, + *lalia*, babble]. Meaningless language of the insane. SYN: *embolophrasia*.
embole (em'bo-lē) [G. a throwing in]. 1. Reduction of a dislocation. 2. Formation of the gastrula by invagination. 3. Enarthrosis. SYN: *emboly*.
embol'ic. Pert. to or caused by embolism.
embol'iform [G. *embolos*, thrown in, + L. *forma*, form]. 1. Resembling a nucleus. 2. Wedge-shaped, as the *nucleus emboliformis*.
embolism (em'bo-lizm) [G. *embolē*, a throwing in, + *ismos*, condition]. Obstruction of a blood vessel by foreign substance or a blood clot. RS: *embolus, thrombosis, thrombus*.
  Diagnosis depends upon the factors predisposing. Arteriosclerosis favors a diagnosis of thrombosis, while auricular fibrillation, bacterial endocarditis, or thrombophlebitis points to embolism. Nearly always embolism is due to bacterial endocarditis.
  e., air. One caused by air bubble. SEE: *air embolism*.
  e., fat. Globules of fat obstructing blood vessels.
  e., pyemic. E. caused by purulent matter.
embolophrasia (em"bol-o-fra'zĭ-ă) [" + *phrasis*, utterance]. Meaningless speech. SYN: *embolalia*.
em'bolus (pl. *emboli*) [G. *embolos*, plug]. A mass of undissolved matter present in a blood or lymphatic vessel brought there by the blood or lymph current. Emboli may be solid, liquid, or gaseous.

embolus, air   E-16   **embryulcus**

Other emboli may consist of bits of tissue, tumor cells, globules of fat, air bubbles, clumps of bacteria, and foreign bodies such as bullets. Emboli may arise within the body or they may gain entrance from without. Occlusion of vessels from emboli usually results in the development of infarcts, q.v. SEE: *thrombus, thrombosis*.
NP: Postoperative cases must be handled with great care. Sudden sitting up or turning over, esp. from 5th to 9th day, may displace an embolus into the circulation and cause sudden death. Fat embolism is not uncommon in bone injuries and fractures, and bacterial emboli may be present in blood "poisoning." SEE: *embolism*.
   e., air. An air bubble in the veins, the right atrium, or ventricle, or in the capillaries. SEE: *air embolism*.
   e., coronary. May be complication of arteriosclerosis and cause angina pectoris. SYM: Similar to pulmonary e.
   e., pulmonary. The commonest embolus met with. SYM: Face gray, eyes staring and wild, look of distress, gasping for breath; sudden death.
em'boly [G. *embolē*, a throwing in]. Formation of the gastrula from invagination. SYN: *embole*.
embrace reflex (em-brās') [L. *brachium*, arm]. A variety of defensive reflex. The throwing out of the arms in an attitude of embrace, in fearful response.
embrasure (em-bra'shur) [Fr. *embrasér*, to widen an opening]. An opening widening outwardly or inwardly.
   e., buccal. Opening spreading toward the buccal aspect.
   e., labial. Embrasure opening toward the labial aspect.
   e., lingual. One spreading to the lingual aspect.
   e., occlusal. Space mesially and distally bet. marginal ridges of approximating teeth.
embroca'tion [G. *embrochē*, fomentation]. 1. Fomentation, such as the application of heat and moisture; a stupe. 2. A drug rubbed into the skin.
embryectomy (em-brĭ-ek'to-mĭ) [G. *embryon*, embryo, + *ektomē*, excision]. Removal of an extrauterine embryo.
embryo (em'brĭ-o) [G. *embryon*]. 1. The young of any organism in an early stage of development. 2. Stage in prenatal development of a mammal between the ovum and the fetus. In humans, stage of development between the second and eight weeks, inclusive.
STAGES OF DEVELOPMENT: Following fertilization, cells multiply (cleavage) resulting in formation of a *morula* which develops into a *blastocyst*, consisting of a trophoblast and inner cell mass. Two cavities (amniotic cavity and yolk sac) arise within the *inner cell mass*. These are separated by the *embryonic disc* which gives rise to the three germ layers (*ectoderm, mesoderm, and endoderm*) which develop into the *embryo proper;* the blastocyst wall or *trophoblast* gives rise to auxillary structures.
During the period of the embryo (3rd to 8th weeks) the germ layers of the embryonic disc give rise to the principal organ systems and the body acquires a somewhat human form. After the second month, the developing young is called a *fetus*.
   e. development of. 1. *Period of the ovum;* (first two weeks) Blastocyst forms. embryo enters uterus and implantation occurs. 2. *Period of the embryo* (3rd to 8th weeks). Embryo increases in length from about 1.5 mm. to 23 mm. Organ systems arise and embryo acquires human form. 3. *Period of the fetus* (3rd to 9th month) (a) 3rd month, 4 in. long.
The alimentary canal, liver, pancreas, and lungs develop from *endoderm;* muscle, all connective tissues, blood, lymphatic tissue and the epithelium of blood vessels, body cavities, kidney, gonads, and suprarenal cortex develop from *mesoderm;* the epidermis nervous tissue, hypophysis, and the epithelium of the organs, nasal cavity, mouth, salivary glands, bladder, and urethra develop from *ectoderm*.
embryocardia (em-brĭ-o-kar'dĭ-ă) [G. *embryon*, embryo, + *kardia*, heart]. Heart action in which first and second pause are equal, and resembling the fetal heart sounds. Another variety is an undue lengthening of the first sound followed by a long pause.
ETIOL: Overworked heart; digitalis poisoning.
embryoctony (em-brĭ-ok'to-nĭ) [" + *kteinein*, to kill]. Destroying the fetus in utero, as in cases where delivery is impossible, or for abortion. SEE: *craniotomy*.
embryogenet'ic, embryogen'ic [" + *gennan*, to originate]. Pert. to or giving rise to an embryo.
embryog'eny [" + *gennan*, to develop]. The growth and development of an embryo.
embryol'raphy [" + *graphein*, to write]. A treatise on the embryo.
embryol'ogy [" + *logos*, study]. The science which deals with the origin and development of an individual organism.
embryo'ma (em-brĭ-o'mă) [" + *ōma*, tumor]. A tumor consisting of derivatives of the embryonic germ layers but lacking in organization; a dermoid cyst.
embry'onal [G. *embryon*, embryo]. Pert. to or resembling an embryo.
embryonic (em-brĭ-on'ĭk) [G. *embryon*, embryo]. Pert. to or in condition of an embryo.
embryoniza'tion [G. *embryon*, embryo]. Reversion of a cell or tissue to an embryonic structure.
embryonoid (em'brĭ-on-oyd) [" + *eidos*, form]. Having the appearance of an embryo.
embryoplas'tic [" + *plassein*, to form]. Having a part in the formation of an embryo; said of cells.
embryotocia (em'brĭ-o-to'sĭ-ă) [" + *tokos*, birth]. An abortion; delivery of an embryo.
embryotome (em'brĭ-o-tōm) [" + *tomē*, incision]. Instrument used in dismemberment of fetus in utero.
embryotomy (em-brĭ-ot'o-mĭ) [" + *tomē*, incision]. The dissection of a fetus to aid its delivery.
embryotoxon (em-brĭ-o-tox'on) [" + *toxon*, bow]. Congenital marginal opacity of the cornea.
embryotroph (em'brĭ-o-trof) [" + *trophē*, nourishment]. A fluid resulting from the enzyme action of the trophoblasts upon the neighboring maternal tissue and which nourishes the embryo from the time of implantation into the uterus.
embryotrophy (em-brĭ-ot'ro-fĭ) [" + *trophē*, nourishment]. Nutrition of the fetus.
embryulcia (em-brĭ-ul'sĭ-ă) [" + *elkein*, to draw]. Forcible removal of the fetus as by embryotomy or taking a dead fetus with instruments.
embryulcus (em-brĭ-ul'kus) [G. *embryoulkos*]. Instrument for extracting a fetus.

emedullate (e-med'ul-āt) [L. ē, out, + medulla, marrow]. To remove the marrow from a bone.

emer'gency [L. emergere, to raise up]. An unexpected serious happening, demanding immediate action.

e. light reflex. Marked pupillary contraction, frowning, and closure of eyelids, resulting from sudden powerful light stimulus of retina.

e. theory. Formulated by Cannon: Adrenal secretion is stimulated by sympathetic nervous system activity to meet bodily emergencies, as emotional excitement, pain, etc.

emergency, words pert. to: asphyxia, asphyxiation, bites, choking, convulsion, dislocation, drowning, fainting, fire emergencies, foreign bodies, fumes, gases, poisoning, shock, stings, unconsciousness.

emer'gent [L. emergere, to raise up]. 1. Growing from a cavity or other part. 2. Sudden, unforeseen.

emesis (em'e-is) [G. emein, to vomit]. Vomiting.

May be gastric, systemic, nervous, reflex, or irritation of vomiting center.

NP: The relation of vomiting to eating is important, and the nurse should determine how it is affected by pain, by soft or solid foods, by liquids, by odors before or after eating or drinking, and its character and color. SEE: *anacathartic, antemetic, emetic, vomit, vomitus*.

e., gastric. In gastric ulcer, gastric carcinoma, acute gastritis, chronic gastritis, gastrectasis, gastric hyperesthesia, hyperacidity and hypersecretion, Asiatic cholera, pressure upon stomach.

e., irritation. Drugs, uremia, nephritis, some brain tumors, chloroform, ether.

TREATMENT: Depends upon the cause. After vomiting, patient may be given a small dose of baking soda in warm water, and then nothing by mouth for some time. Hot applications to the abdomen are helpful.

e., nervous. Tumor or abscess of brain, sea sickness, acute myelitis, meningitis, anemia and hyperemia of brain, concussion and contusion of brain, fracture of skull, Ménière's disease, migraine, paresis, sclerosis.

e., reflex. Irritation of fauces and pharynx; coughing, removal of viscous secretion from nasopharynx, eyestrain, unpleasant odors and sights, shock, nervousness, anticipation, anxiety, hysteria, morning sickness, gastric crisis of tabes, various heart troubles, hiccough.

e., systemic. Pulmonary tuberculosis, whooping cough, peritonitis, irritations of bowels, acute obstruction of bowels, renal or biliary colic, Addison's disease.

emetic (e-met'ik) [G. emein, to vomit]. Medicine that produces vomiting. Ex: *apomorphine, a. hydrochloride, ipecac, mustard, sodium chloride.*

e., direct. Those acting directly on gastric nerves, e. g., mustard.

e., indirect. Those acting on vomiting center of brain, as apomorphine.

e., local. Those which act through nerve irritation, such as salt.

e., systemic. Those acting through the circulation, irritating vomiting centers by stimulation, such as mustard, soapy water, syrup of ipecac.

One tablespoonful of mustard in ½ pint of water; or 2 of common salt with sufficient water to be swallowed.

Dilute contents of stomach before giving any emetic. Emetics may be dangerous because of their own toxic effect, as in severe heart or blood vessel diseases, tuberculosis, advanced pregnancy, rupture, ulcers of the stomach, or corrosive poisoning. For these reasons chemical emetics are omitted from the nurse's treatment of poisoning.

TREATMENT: Vomiting may be induced by generous amounts of warm water, preferably warm soapy water and by titillating the uvula or posterior pharynx. Gastric lavage is preferable to emetics in poisoning. Emetics may induce vomiting by their local effect, as copper sulfate or zinc sulfate, mustard, ipecac, etc., in small doses diluted in water; or by their effect on the central nervous system, such as apomorphine hydrochloride which works by hypodermic injection. Emesis is much more likely to take place when the stomach is distended.

em'etine [G. emein, to vomit]. Powdered, white alkaloid obtained from ipecac, q.v.

emetine bismuth iodide (em'e-tin biz'muth i'o-dīd). A combination of emetine and bismuth containing about 25% emetine and 20% bismuth.

ACTION AND USES: Same as emetine.
DOSAGE: 1-3 gr. (0.06-0.2 Gm.).

e. hydrochloride. USP. The hydrochloride of an alkaloid obtained from ipecac. [dysentery.]
ACTION AND USES: Chiefly in amebic
AVERAGE DOSAGE: Parenterally, 1 gr. (0.06-0.2 Gm.).

em'etism [G. emein, to vomit, + ismos, condition of]. Poisoning from overdose of ipecac.

SYM: Acute inflammation of pylorus, hyperemesis, diarrhea, and perhaps coughing and suffocation.

emetocathar'tic [" + katharsis, a purging]. Producing both emesis and catharsis.

emetol'ogy [" + logos, understanding]. Study of emetics and their action.

E. M. F. Abbr. for *electromotive force*.

emiction (e-mik'shun) [L. ē + mingere, to urinate]. The act of urination.

emigra'tion [" + migrāre, to move]. Passage of white blood corpuscles through the walls of capillaries and veins during inflammation.

em'inence [" + minere, to hang on]. A prominence or projection, esp. of a bone.

e., arcuate. A rounded eminence on upper surface of petrous portion of temporal bone. SYN: *jugum petrosum*.

e., articular, of the temporal bone. A rounded e. forming ant. boundary of the glenoid fossa.

e., auditory. A collection of gray matter on floor of 4th ventricle of brain at its lower part, forming the deep origin of the auditory nerve.

e., bicipital. A tuberosity for insertion of biceps muscle on radius.

e., blastodermic. An elevated mass of cells of a developing ovum forming the blastoderm.

e., canine. A vertical ridge on the external surface of the superior maxilla.

e., collateral. One bet. middle and post. horns in lat. ventricle of brain.

e. of Doyère. Slight elevation of muscular fiber corresponding to entrance of a nerve fiber.

e. of the aquaeductus Fallopii. A ridge which traverses the inner wall of the tympanum above the fenestra ovalis.

e., frontal. A rounded prominence on either side of median line, a little below center of frontal bone (B. N. A., *tuber frontale*).
e., germinal. The *discus proligerus*.
e., hypothenar. One on ulnar side of palm, formed by muscles of little finger.
e., iliopectineal, e., iliopubic. E. on upper aspect of pubic bone above the acetabulum, marking the junction of bone with the ilium (B. N. A., *eminentia iliopectinea*).
e. intercondyloid. A process on the head of the tibia lying between the two condyles.
e., mamillary. Projection of inner pillars of fornix.
e., median. Ant. bodies of medulla oblongata separated by ant. median fissure.
e., nasal. A prominence on vertical portion of frontal bone above the nasal notch and bet. the 2 superciliary ridges.
e., occipital. Protuberance on occipital bone.
e., olivary. Oval projection at upper part of medulla o., above extremity of lateral column.
e., parietal. The marked convexity on outer surface of parietal bone (B. N. A., *tuber parietale*).
e.'s, portal. The small median lobes on lower surface of liver.
e. pyramidal. An elevation on the mastoid wall of the tympanic cavity. It contains a cavity in which lies the stapedius muscle.
e., thenar. The ball of the thumb.
eminentia (em-in-en'shǐ-ā) (L.). An eminence.
e. alveolaris. Bony prominence on mandible 1½ in. ant. and sup. to the tonsil; corresponds to the location of the last molar tooth.
e. articularis. Prominence on temporal bone.
e. collateralis. Prominence on inferior horn of the lateral ventricle.
em'issary [L. *ē*, out, + *mittere*, to send]. 1. Providing an outlet. 2. An outlet.
e. veins. Small veins piercing the skull, carrying blood from the sinuses within to the veins without the skull.
emissio (e-mis'sǐ-o) [L.]. A discharge; emission.*
e. seminis. Discharge of semen.
emission (e-mish'un) [L. *ē*, out, + *mittere*, to send]. The discharge, esp. involuntary, of semen by the male, particularly during sleep. SYN: *pollution*. SEE: *ejaculation*.
emmenagogue (em-en'ă-gog) [G. *emmēna*, menses + *agein*, to lead]. An agent that stimulates the menstrual function. Ex: *ergot, preparations of iron, manganese dioxide, viburnum*.
e., direct. E. directly affecting the organs involved.
e., indirect. E. effective in alleviating the causative disorder, such as anemia.
emmenia (em-me'nǐ-ă) [G. *emmēna*]. The menstrual flow.
emmen'ic. Pert. to the menses.
em'menin [G. *emmēna*, menses]. A placental hormone causing precocious maturity.
emmeniopathy (em-me-nǐ-o'path-ǐ) [" + *pathos* disease]. Any disorder of the menstruation.
emmenol'ogy [" + *logos*, science]. Science of menstruation.
emmetrope (em'met-rōp) [G. *emmetros*, in due measure, + *opsis*, sight]. One endowed with normal vision.

emmetropia (em-me-tro'pǐ-ă) [" + *opsis*, sight]. Normal condition of eye in refraction; with eye at rest parallel rays are focused on retina; ability to focus on the retina a luminous point from 3.9 to 4.7 in. from the eye.
emmetrop'ic. Normal in vision. SEE: *hypermetropic, myopic*.

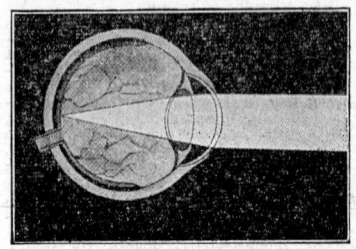

EMMETROPIC EYE
Parallel light rays brought to a focus upon retina, with lens at rest.
SEE: *hyperopia, myopia*.

Em'met's operation. 1. Uterine trachelorrhaphy. 2. Suturing of a lacerated perineum. 3. Converting a sessile submucous tumor of the uterus into a pedunculated one. 4. Operation for procidentia uteri.
emol'lient [L. *ē*, out, + *mollīre*, to soften]. An agent that will soften and soothe the part when applied locally. The term is usually confined to agents affecting the surface of the body. Ex: *ointment of rose water, olive oil, petrolatum*. SEE: *demulcent*.
e. enema. One for the purpose of coating membranes and allaying local pain and irritation, in order to soften and protect tissues.
emotion (e-mo'shun) [*ēmovēre*, to disturb]. 1 A mental state or strong feeling affect usually accompanied by physical changes in the body such as alteration in heart rate and respiratory activity, vasomotor reactions, and changes in muscle tone. 2. A mental state or feeling such as fear, hate, love, anger, grief, joy. These constitute the "drive" which brings about the motor adjustment necessary to satisfy instinctive needs.

Frustration is normally associated with displeasure and the intensifying of need; the process of gratification is accompanied by pleasurable feeling tone which persists for a variable period in less intense form. Somatic (e. g., postural) changes precede and immediately follow the emotion; at least the two are inseparable and the recognition of "affect" (apart from one's subjection sense) is dependent upon the presence of its appropriate physical correlates.

Anxiety, or fear, arises when one doubts his ability adequately to meet a situation; neutralization consists of "flight" from the danger, and a struggle (fight) to remove the threat. The physical changes are those favorable to success and phylogenetically may well have antedated the psychic phase of the fear. Often a partial syndrome of fear may exist with this latter phase apparently absent (and denied), and then the condition may be considered heart disease, stomach trouble, toxic goiter, etc. Other physical affect reactions may

emotion, disorders of. An emotion is not felt in the same way by healthy persons as by one suffering from schizophrenia. In the latter, there is a decrease of pleasure, hate, love, and other emotions. There is a loss of affection for relatives and a lack of interest in things. The emotions he does show are not in harmony with his ideas; for example, he may smile while describing tortures and terrors.

be similarly confusing. Civilized man may find an instinctive goal unattainable because his conditioned (moral) reactions regard the goal as socially objectionable (or even deny the goal entirely). Here arise the conflict and the starting point of psychogenic disease.

Unhappiness is marked in manic depressive psychosis. It varies in degree and may lead to suicide. In the excited stage undue happiness is marked. Depressions and elations have no apparent cause.

Emotions are easily aroused in aged persons and in alcoholics.

Depressed patients are so wrapped up in their own misery they take no notice of anything else. Excited patients cannot concentrate their attention. Confused ones may not realize they are not in the proper place for their actions. Hallucinated patients are influenced by imaginary voices. Deluded ones have unreasonable fears.

emotion, words pert. to: affective, agonia, alusia, amor, amor sui, athymia, cathexis, manias, noci association, parapathia, psychiatry, sex.

emo′tional [L. ēmovere, to disturb]. Relating to any of the emotions.
  e. attitudes. Those which express any of the emotions, such as joy, sorrow, etc. Seen in hysteroepilepsy.
  e. instability. Psy: Pert. to a psychopathic personality given to easy rage, brooding, and vastly fluctuating moods.

emotivity (e-mo-tiv′ĭ-tĭ) [L. ē, out, + motus, moving]. One's capability for emotional response.

em′pasm. A powder, usually perfumed, for external application to the body.

empathema (em-path-e′ma) (pl. empathemata) [G. en, in, + pathos, suffering]. Ungovernable or dominant passion.
  e. atonicum. Hypochondriasis.
  e. entonicum. An active mania.
  e., inane. Passion and excitement without cause or purpose.

empath′ic. Pert. to, or characterized by, emotions.

empathy (em′pa-thĭ) [G. en, in, + pathos, feeling]. 1. Sympathetically trying to identify one's feelings with those of another. 2. Consciousness of coidentification in a social group of two or more members.

emphlysis (em′flis-is) (pl. emphlyses) [" + phlysis, an eruption]. Any vesicular or exanthematous eruption.

emphractic (em-frak′tik) [G. emphraxis, an obstruction]. 1. Obstructive, as clogging of pores of skin. 2. Anything that obstructs a function.

emphraxis (ĕm-frăk′ĭs). A stoppage, or obstruction; an infarction.

emphysatherapy (em-fiz-ă-ther′ă-pī) [G. emphysan, to inflate, + therapeia, treatment]. Injection of gas into a cavity for therapeutic purposes.

emphysema (em-fi-se′mă) [G. emphysan, to inflate]. 1. Distention of tissues by gas or air in the interstices. 2. A condition in which the alveoli of the lungs become distended or ruptured. Usually the result of an interference with expiration, or loss of elasticity of the lung.
  e. atrophic. Syn: senile e.
  e. chronic hypertrophic. E. accompanied with bony changes resulting in the so-called "barrel chest".
  e. compensatory. E. which results from overstretching of a functional part of the lung when another portion fails to function. A secondary condition seen in tuberculosis, or pneumonia. Also called complemental e.
  e. cutaneous. Subcutaneous e.
  e., gangrenous. Malignant variety of edema caused by a microbe.
  e., interstitial. Rupture of air cells from overdistention, and escape of air into interlobular tissue.
  e. pulmonary. "E. vesicular".
  e. subcutaneous. Presence of air or gas in subcutaneous tissues, with consequent distention. Often caused by infection by gas-producing organisms, esp., Bacillus aerogenes.
  e., surgical. Cutaneous emphysema due to operation, esp. after wounds of respiratory tract.
  e., vesicular. Overdistention of alveoli and smaller bronchial tubes with air. Sym: Dyspnea upon exertion; accelerated pulse, cough, and expectoration of whitish mucus. Short inspiration, prolonged expiration. Treatment: Tonics, stimulants, rest.

emphysematous (em-fi-sem′at-us) [G. emphysan, to inflate]. Affected with or pert. to emphysema.

empir′ic [G. empeirikos, experimental]. One who relies solely upon experience.

empirical (em-pir′ĭk-al) [G. empeirikos, skilled]. 1. Pert. to or based on experience. 2. Pert. to an empiric.

empiricism (em-pir′is-izm) [" + ismos, condition of]. 1. Experience, not theory, as basis of medical science. 2. Quackery.

emplastic (em-plas′tik) [G. emplastikos, clogging]. 1. A constipating medicine. 2. Fit to be used as a plaster in one.

emplas′trum (pl. emplastra) [G. emplastron, a plaster]. Preparation for external application, and of such consistency that it requires heat to spread it, and adheres to the skin when applied. Not often prescribed. Four are official. Syn: plaster.

emprosthotonos (em-pros-thot′o-nos) [G. emprosthen, forward, + tonos, tension]. Lying with body incurved and resting upon forehead and feet with face downward. See: Illustration, p. E-18.

Sometimes seen in tetanus and strychnine poisoning. The reverse of opisthotonos. See: posture.

emptysis (ĕmp′tĭ-sĭs) [G. a spitting]. Expectoration of blood or blood stained mucus; hemoptysis.

empyema (em-pi-e′ma) [G. en, within, + pyon, pus]. Pus in a body cavity, esp. in the pleural cavity.
  Sym: Chills, fever, and sweating. Skin is gray, malar flush, appetite poor, marked malaise, pain in side, cough, emaciation. Dyspnea may ensue.
  Treatment: Aspiration; open operation. Constant irrigation of pleural cavity by regular suction is an effective treatment.
  NP: Postoperative: Patient should sit up inclined to affected side to facilitate drainage, then to opp. side to aid expansion of lung. See: resection.
  e. encapsulated. Collection of pus walled off by adhesions.
  e., interlobular. Form with pus bet. lobes of lung.

empyema, necessitatis   E-20   encelialgia

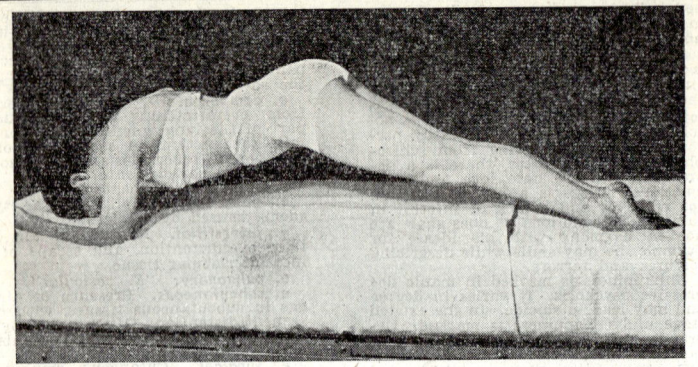

Posed by professional model   *Photo by Whitaker*
EMPROSTHOTONOS.

e. necessitatis. Form in which pus can escape spontaneously.

e., pulsating. Form with cardiac beats causing pulsation of chest wall.

empyesis (em-pī-e'sis) [G. *empyein*, to suppurate]. A pustular eruption on the skin.

empyocele (ĕm'pī-ō-sēl) [" + *kēlē*, tumor]. A collection of pus in a sacculated cavity, especially in the scrotum; a suppurating hydrocele.

emul'gent [L. *ēmulgere*, to drain out]. Extracting or draining.

e. vessel. Blood vessel of the kidney.

emulsifica'tion [L. *emulsio*, emulsion, + *facere*, to make]. 1. Process of making an emulsion. 2. The breaking down of large fat globules in the intestine to smaller, uniformly, distributed particles, accomplished largely through the action of bile acids which lower surface tension.

emul'sifier [" + *facere*, to make]. Anything used to make an emulsion.

emulsify (e-mul'sĭ-fī) [" + *facere*, to make]. To form into an emulsion.

emul'sion [L. *emulsiō*]. A mixture of 2 liquids not mutually soluble.
If they are thoroughly shaken, one will divide into globules and is called the *discontinuous* or *dispersed* phase; the other is then the *continuous* phase. Milk is an emulsion in which butter fat is the discontinuous and water the continuous phase.

emul'soid (ē-mŭl'soyd) [" + G. *eidos*, form]. A colloid in an aqueous solution in which the colloid has a marked attraction for water to the extent that the dispersoid contains large quantities of water. Also called hydrophilic or lyophilic colloids. Protoplasm, starch, soap, gelatin, and egg white are common examples.

emulsum (e-mul'sum) [L.]. A fluid in which oil or resin is suspended by means of a mucilaginous substance.

emunctory (e-munk'to-rī) [L. *ēmungere*, to cleanse]. 1. Pert. to organ or duct having an excretory function. 2. An excretory duct, *i. e.*, pores of skin.

enamel (en-am'el) [A.S. *en*, on, + *amaile*, ivory]. SYN: *substantia adamantina*. It is the hardest substance in the body. The hard, white, dense substance forming a covering for the crown of the teeth.

e. mottled. Condition in which the enamel acquires a mottled appearance as a result of the ingestion of excessive amounts of fluorides in water or foods.

e. organ. A cup-shaped structure which forms on the dental lamina of an embryo. It produces the enamel and serves as a mold for the remainder of the tooth.

enanthem, enanthema (en-an'them, -the'- mă) [G. *en*, in, + *anthēma*, blossoming]. Eruption of mucous membrane. Ex: Koplik's spots. SEE: *rash*. OPP: *exanthem*.

enanthematous (en-an-them'at-us) [G. *en.* + *anthēma*, a blossoming]. Of the nature of an enanthema.

enanthesis (en-an-the'sis) [" + *anthein*, to bloom]. A skin eruption due to internal disease.

enanthrope (en'an-thrōp) [" + *anthrōpos*, man]. The source of a disease originating internally.

enantiobiosis (en-an-tī-o-bī-o'sis) [G. *enantios*, opposite, + *bios*, life]. The condition in which associated organisms are antagonistic to each other. SEE: *symbiosis*.

enantiopathy (en-an-tī-op'ath-ī) [" + *pathos*, disease]. Treatment of one disease by another disease antagonistic to it, as malaria in general paresis.

enarkyochrome (en-ar'kī-o-krōm) [G. *en*, in, + *arkus*, network, + *chrōma*, color]. A nerve cell arranged like a network, taking a stain best in the cell body.

enarthri'tis [" + *arthron*, joint, + *itis*, inflammation]. Inflammation of a ball- and-socket joint.

enarthrosis (en-ar-thro'sis) (Pl. *enarthroses*) [" + *arthrōsis*, joint]. A ball-and- socket joint; a form of diarthrosis.
RS: *amphiarthrosis, condylarthrosis, diarthrosis, synarthrosis, synchrondrosis*.

encan'this [G. *en*, in, + *kanthos*, angle of the eye]. An excrescence or new growth at the inner angle of the eye.

encapsula'tion [L. *en*, in, + *capsula*, a little box]. 1. Inclosure in a sheath not normal to the part. 2. The process of the formation of a capsule or a sheath about a structure.

encatarrhaphy (en-kat-ar'raf-ī) [G. *egkatarraptein*, to sew in]. Insertion of an organ or tissue into a part where it is not normally found.

enceinte (on-sant') [Fr.]. Pregnant.

encelial'gia [G. *en*, in, + *koilia*, belly, + *algos*, pain]. Abdominal pain.

encephalalgia (en-sef-al-al'ji-ă) [G. *egkephalos*, brain, + *algos*, pain]. Deep-seated head pain. SYN: *cephalalgia*.

encephalasthenia (en-sef"al-as-the'nĭ-ă) [" + *asthenia*, weakness]. Deficiency in brain power.

encephalatrophy (en-sef-al-at'rof-ĭ) [" + *a-*, priv. + *trophē*, nourishment]. Cerebral atrophy.

encephalic (en-sef-al'ĭk) [G. *egkephalos*, brain]. Pert. to the brain or its cavity.

encephalin (en-sef'al-in) [G. *egkephalos*, brain]. A nitrogenous glucoside obtained from brain tissue by boiling.

encephalitis (en-sef-ă-li'tis) [" + *itis*, inflammation]. Inflammation of the brain.
ETIOL: It may be a specific disease entity due to a virus, or it may occur as a sequella of influenza, measles, German measles, chicken pox, smallpox, vaccinia, or several other diseases.
  e., cortical. E. of brain cortex only.
  e., epidemic. SEE: *e. lethargica*.
  e., hemorrhagic. Hemorrhage in brain inflammation.
  e. hyperplastica. Acute encephalitis without suppuration.
  e., infantile. Brain inflammation in the young causing cerebral palsy.
  e., influenzal. SEE: *e. lethargica*.
  e. lethargica (leth-ar'jĭ-ka). Epidemic neurotaxis, epidemic stupor, Type A encephalitis (Japan), Economo's disease. An infective disease of virus origin which first appeared pandemically in 1916-1917. It appeared epidemically in various regions of the world up to 1925 usually following epidemics of influenza. Occurs usually in winter months. Since that time, it has occurred sporadically.
  SYM: Stupor, ocular paralyses, tremor, nocturnal wakefulness. The face becomes expressionless and grave. Moral changes may result. The symptoms vary in different individuals. The disease is notifiable. SYN: *sleeping sickness*.
  e., meningo-. E. combined with meningitis.
  e. neonatorum. A form occurring in the newly born. ETIOL: Fatty cells in the brain.
  e. periaxialis. Inflammation of the white matter of the cerebrum, occurring mainly in the young.
  e., purulent. E. characterized by abscesses in the brain.
  e., pyemic, e., pyogenic. SEE: *purulent e.*
  e. St. Louis type. A virus disease which first occurred epidemically in the summer of 1933 in and around St. Louis. Now endemic in America. Occurs most frequently during summer months.

encephalocele (en-sef'al-o-sēl) [L. *en*, in + *kēlē*, hernia]. Protrusion of the brain through a cranial fissure.

encephalocystocele (en-sef-al-o-sis'to-sēl) [" + *kystis*, a bladder, + *kēlē*, hernia]. Protrusion of brain distended by herniated sac containing fluid.

encephalodialysis (en-sef"al-o-di-al'is-is) [" + *dialysis*, loosening]. Softening of the brain.

encephalogram (en-sef'al-o-gram) [" + *gramma*, a writing]. A roentgen ray picture of the brain.

encephalography (en-sef-al-og'ra-fĭ) [" + *graphein*, to write]. 1. Examination of head following the introduction of air into the subarachnoid space as a means of diagnosis. 2. Roentgenography.

encephaloid (en-sef'ă-loid) [" + *eidos*, form]. 1. Resembling the cerebral substance. 2. A malignant neoplasm of brainlike texture.
  e. cancer. Malignant brainlike tumor. SYN: *encephaloma*.

encephalolith (en-sef'al-o-lith) [L. *en*, in, + G. *egkephalos*, brain, + *lithos*, stone]. A calculus of the brain.

encephalology (ĕn-sĕf-ă-lŏ'lĕj-ĭ). [L. *en*, in + " + *logos*, study of]. That division of medical science which deals with the structure, function, and pathology of the brain.

encephalo'ma [" + *ōma*, tumor]. 1. Tumor of the brain. 2. Brain cancer.

encephalomalacia (en-sef-al-o-mal-a'sĭ-ă) [" + *malakia*, softening]. Brain softening.

encephalomeningi'tis [" + *mēningx*, membrane, + *itis*, inflammation]. Inflammation of the brain and its membranes.

encephalomeningocele (en-sef-al-o-men-in'go-sēl) [" + " + *kēlē*, hernia]. Protrusion through the cranium of membranes and brain substance.

encephalomere (en-sef'al-o-mēr) [L. *en*, in + *meros*, part]. A primitive segment of the embryonic brain; a neuromere.

encephalometer (en-sef-al-om'e-ter) [" + *metron*, measure]. An instrument for measuring the cranium and locating brain regions.

encephalomyelitis (en-sef-al-o"mĭ-el-i'tis) [" + *myelos*, marrow, + *itis*, inflammation]. Encephalitis with myelitis.

encephalomyelopathy (en-sef-al-o-mĭ-el-op'a-thĭ) [" + " + *pathos*, disease]. Any disease of brain and spinal cord.

encephalon (en-sef'ă-lon) [G. *egkephalos*, brain]. The brain, including the cerebrum, cerebellum, medulla oblongata, and pons, diencephalon and mid-brain.

encephalop'athy [" + *pathos*, disease]. Any dysfunction of the brain.

enceph'alopuncture [" + L. *punctura*, a piercing]. Puncture into the brain substance.

encephalopyosis (en-sef-al-o-pi-o'sis) [" + *pyōsis*, suppuration]. Abscess of the brain.

encephalorrhagia (en-sef-al-or-a'jĭ-a) [" + *rēgnunai*, to burst forth]. Hemorrhage of the brain.

encephalosclerosis (en-sef"al-o-skle-ro'sis) [" + *sklērōsis*, hardening]. Brain hardening.

encephalo'sis [" + *osis*]. A degenerative process of the brain.

encephalospi'nal [" + L. *spina*, thorn]. Pert. to brain and spinal cord.
  e. axis. Cerebrospinal axis.

encephalothlipsis (ĕn-sĕf"ă-lō-thlĭp'sĭs). Compression of the brain.

encephalotome (en-sef'al-o-tōm) [" + *tomē*, incision]. Instrument for incising brain tissue.

encephalotomy (ĕn-sĕf"ă-lŏt'ŏ-mĭ) [" + *tomē*, a cutting]. 1. Brain dissection. 2. Surgical destruction of the brain of a fetus to facilitate delivery.

enchondroma (en-kon-dro'mă) [G. *en*, in, + *chondros*, cartilage, + *ōma*, tumor]. A cartilaginous tumor occurring generally where cartilage is absent or within a bone where it expands the diaphysis.

enchondrosarcoma (en-kon"dro-sar-ko'-mă) [" + " + *sarx*, flesh, + *ōma*, tumor]. Sarcoma made up of cartilaginous tissue.

enchondrosis (ĕn-kŏn-drō'sĭs). A cartilaginous outgrowth from bone or cartilaginous tissue; an enchondroma.

enchylema (en-ki-le'mă) [" + *chylos*, juice]. Fluid granular matter in interstices of cell body and nucleus. SYN: *cytochylema*.

enchyma (en'ki-mă) [" + *chymos*, juice]. A fluid formed from chyme which elaborates and repairs tissues and cells.

enclave (ĕn-klăv') [Fr. *enclavér*, to surround]. A mass of tissue which becomes enclosed by a tissue of enother kind.

enclavement (en-klăv'ment) [Fr.]. GYN: An impaction of the fetus in the pelvic strait.

enclitic (en-klit'ik) [G. *egklinein*, to incline]. Having the planes of the fetal head inclined to those of the maternal pelvis.

encolpism (en-kol'pizm) [G. *en*, in, + *kolpos*, vagina, + *ismos*, condition]. Medication by vaginal suppositories and injections.

encolpitis (en-kol-pi'tis) [" + *kolpos*, vagina, + *itis*, inflammation]. SYN: *endocolpitis*. Inflamed condition of the vaginal mucosa.

encra'nial [" + *kranion*, cranium]. Intracranial or within the cranium.

encyesis (en-si-e'sis) [" + *kyēsis*, pregnancy]. Normal uterine pregnancy.

encyopyelitis (en-si-o-pi-e-li'tis) [" + " + *pyelos*, pelvis, + *itis*, inflammation]. Inflammation of the renal pelvis occurring in normal pregnancy.

encysted (en-sist'ed) [" + *kystis*, cyst]. Surrounded by membrane; encapsulated.

end [A.S. *ende*]. A termination; extremity.
 e. artery. An artery which does not anastomose directly or indirectly with other arteries, *e. g.*, in kidney and spleen, etc.
 e. body. Substance that kills bacteria in immunity to typhoid. SYN: *complement*.
 e. brain. The telencephalon.
 e. bud, e. bulb, e. capsule. The terminal of a sensory nerve.
 e. end-bulb of Krause. An encapsulated nerve-ending found in the skin and conjunctiva; mediates sense of cold.
 e. organ. An encapsulated sensory nerve-ending.
 e. organ, neuromuscular. Spindle-shaped bundle of specialized muscle fibers in which sensory nerve fibers terminate in muscles; muscle spindle.
 e. organ neurotendinous. Specialized tendon fasciculi in which sensory nerve fibers terminate in tendons; a tendon spindle.
 e. result. The ultimate or final result.

Endamoeba (ĕn''dăm-ē'bă). A genus of parasitic cyst-forming amebae infesting hosts other than humans. Sometimes confused with Entamoeba, *q.v.*

endangeitis, endangitis (end-an-je-i'tis, -ji'tis) [G. *endon*, within, + *aggeion*, vessel, + *itis*, inflammation]. Inflammation of the endangium.

endangium (en-dan'ji-um) [" + *aggeion*, vessel]. Inmost coat or intima of blood vessels.

endaortitis (end''a-or-ti'tis) [" + *aortē*, aorta, + *itis*, inflammation]. Inflammation of inner coat of the aorta.

endarterial (end-ar-ter'i-al) [" + *artēria*, artery]. 1. Pert. to the inner portion of an artery. 2. Within an artery.

endarteritis (end-ar-ter-i'tis) [" + " + *itis*, inflammation]. Inflammation of innermost coat or intima of an artery resulting from syphilis, trauma, pyogenic bacteria, or infective thrombi.
 e., acute. Of large arteries. Rare.
 e., chronic. Degeneration of arterial coats in the aged. SYN: *atheroma*.
 e. deformans. Thickening of intima or replacement with atheromatous or calcareous deposits.
 e. obliterans. Chronic progressive thickening of intima leading to stenosis or obstruction of lumen.

endeictic (en-dī'tĭk). Symptomatic.

endem'ic [G. *en*, in, + *dēmos*, people].
 e. disease. A disease which is present more or less continuously in a community. Used in contrast to sporadic or epidemic.
 e. neuritis. A form of polyneuritis. SYN: *beriberi*.

ende''moepidem'ic [" + " + *epi*, on, + *dēmos*, people]. Endemic, but becoming epidemic periodically.

endermat'ic, enderm'ic [" + *derma*, skin]. Administering medicine through the skin.

endermo'sis [" + " + *ōsis*]. 1. Administration of medicines through the skin. 2. Herpetic affection of any mucous membrane.

en'deron [" + *deros*, skin]. The dermis or corium; the portion of a mucous membrane underlying the epithelial layer.

en'dive. ASH CONST: Ca 0.104, Mg 0.013, K 0.380, Na 0.109, P 0.038, Cl 0.167, S 0.035, Fe 0.00123. AV. SERVING: 15 gr. Pro 0.2, Fat trace, Carbo. 0.6. Vit. A+, C + to ++.

endoaneurysmorrhaphy (en''do-an-ū-ris-mor'af-I) [G. *endon*, within, + *aneurysma*, aneurysm, + *raphē*, suture]. Opening an aneurysmal sac and suturing its orifice.

endoangiitis (en''do-an-ji-i'tis) [" + *aggeion*, vessel, + *itis*, inflammation]. Inflammation of the coat of blood vessels. SYN: *endoarteritis, endophlebitis*.

en''doantitox'in [" + *anti*, against, + *toxikon*, poison]. An antitoxin within a cell.

en''doappendici'tis [" + L. *appendere*, to hang, + G. *itis*, inflammation]. Inflammation of mucosa of the vermiform appendix.

endoarteritis (ĕn''dō-ăr-tĕr-ī'tĭs) [G. *endon*, with, + *arteria*, artery, + *-itis*, inflammation]. Endarteritis, *q.v.*

en''doausculta'tion [" + L. *auscultāre*, to listen to]. Auscultation by esophageal tube passed into the stomach.

endoblast (en'do-blast) [" + *blastos*, germ]. 1. The nucleus cell. 2. Inner layer of the blastoderm. SYN: *endoderm, hypoblast*.

endobronchi'tis [" + *brogchos*, windpipe, + *itis*, inflammation]. Inflammation of bronchial mucosa.

endocar'diac, endocar'dial [" + *kardia*, heart]. Within the heart or arising from the endocardium.

endocarditis (en-do-kar-di'tis) [" + " + *itis*, inflammation]. Inflammation of the lining membrane of the heart or *endocardium*.

It is usually confined to the external lining of the valve, sometimes to the lining membrane of its chambers. Generally of bacterial origin.

NP: Practically the same as that for pericarditis and other heart conditions. Rest in bed essential, but during symptoms of dyspnea patient should be propped up in bed and supported by pillows with arms resting on pillows. All bodily activities should be kept at a minimum. Patient should not reach for

endocarditis, chronic

anything. Pulse should be taken before and after any exertion and if it does not return to original pulse within 2 minutes after the effort it indicates strain as a result. Normal bowel action essential; no stimulating drinks, esp. in the evening.
TREATMENT: Antibiotic therapy for at least one month. Procaine penicillin in large doses is usually employed, although streptomycin, aureomycin, terramycin, and chloramphenicol are sometimes effective.

e., chronic. SEE: *ulcerative endocarditis.*

e., exudative. Begins as an acute affection. Rheumatism chief cause. SYM: Auscultation may give only indication—a prolongation of heart sound. PROG: Guarded. TREATMENT: Absolute rest.

e., malignant. Usually secondary to suppurative inflammation elsewhere. SEE: *ulcerative endocarditis.*

e., subacute bacterial. A condition caused by lodgment of the *Streptococcus viridans* in an abnormal heart or in valves damaged by rheumatic fever.

e., ulcerative. A rapidly destructive form, characterized by necrosis or ulceration of the valves and the deposition of colonies of micrococci.
SYM: High fever; chills; profuse sweats; great prostration; often delirium and stupor; hurried breathing; rapid, irregular pulse; brown, fissured tongue; jaundice and diarrhea frequently present.
PROG: Almost invariably fatal. Duration few days to several weeks.
TREATMENT: Ice bags to heart. Light, nutritious diet. Stimulants.

e., vegetative. Fibrinous clots on ulcerated valvular surfaces. SEE: *exudative endocarditis.*

endocar'dium [" + *kardia,* heart]. Lining (serous) membrane of inner surface and cavities of the heart.
It is continuous with the intima or int. coat of arteries.

endocervical (en-do-ser'vĭ-kal) [" + L. *cervix,* neck]. Pert. to the endocervix.

endocervicitis (en-dō-ser-vĭ-si'tis) [" + " + G. *itis,* inflammation]. Inflammation of mucous lining of the cervix uteri.
Usually chronic and due to infection, and accompanied by erosion.
SYM: Opaque, whitish-yellow, often thick and lumpy vaginal discharge, esp. preceding menstruation.
TREATMENT: *General:* Patient should be kept as quiet as possible, food generous, and bowels active. *Local:* Hot vaginal douches 3 times a day, first of Lugol's solution, later as acute stage subsides, an astringent douche.
Another method is the Cherry treatment which employs bipolar electrode to coagulate membrane and glands, via the vaginal orifice.

endocervix (en-do-ser'vĭks) [G. *endon,* within, + L. *cervix,* neck]. The lining of the canal of the cervix uteri.

endochondral (en-do-kon'dral) [" + *chondros,* cartilage]. Within a cartilage.

endochorion (en-do-ko'rĭ-on) [" + *chorion,* chorion]. The inner chorion; vascular layer of allantois.

endochrome (en'do-krōm) [" + *chrōma,* color]. The coloring matter (not green) of a cell's endoplasm.

endocoli'tis [" + *kōlon,* colon, + *itis,* inflammation]. Inflammation of the mucosa of colon. SEE: *colitis.*

endocolpitis (en-do-kol-pi'tis) [" + *colpos,* vagina, + *itis,* inflammation]. Inflammation of the vaginal mucosa. SYN: *encolpitis.*

endocom'plement [" + L. *complēre,* to fill]. An intracellular complement or one contained within the erythrocyte.

endocorpus'cular [" + L. *corpusculum,* corpuscle]. Within a corpuscle.

endocra'nial [" + *kranion,* cranium]. 1. Intracranial or within the cranium. 2. Pert. to the endocranium.

endocrani'tis [" + " + *itis,* inflammation]. Inflammation of endocranium. SYN: *pachymeningitis, external.*

endocra'nium [" + *kranion,* cranium]. The dura mater of the brain which forms the lining membrane of the cranium.

endocrinasthenia (en"do-krin-as-the'nĭ-ă) [" + *krinein,* to secrete, + *astheneia,* weakness]. Neurasthenia due to dysfunction of the endocrines.

endocrine (ĕn'dō-krīn, -krĭn) [" + *krinein,* to secrete]. 1. An internal secretion. 2. Endocrinous. 3. Pertaining to a gland that produces an internal secretion.

e. gland. A ductless gland; a gland which produces an internal secretion discharged into the blood and lymph and circulated to all parts of the body. The active principles of the glands called *hormones* produce effects on tissues more or less remote from their place of origin. Some endocrine glands produce both an internal and external secretion (Ex: pancreas, testes).
The endocrine glands include: *hypophysis cerebri* (pituitary gland), thyroid gland (the thymus and pineal body have not been shown to produce any hormones), parathyroid glands, adrenal (suprarenal) glands, islands of Langerhans of the pancreas, and the gonads (ovaries and testes). Other structures such as the gastrointestinal mucosa and the placenta have an endocrine function.
The hormones secreted by the ductless glands may have a specific effect on an organ or tissue, or in some cases the effect is general affecting the entire body as in the case of the thyroid hormone which affects the rate of metabolism. Hormones may have an *excitatory* or stimulating effect, or a *retarding* or inhibiting effect. Hormones are effective in extremely minute amounts. They are not stored in the body but are destroyed or excreted. Among the physiological processes affected by hormones are: rate of metabolism and the metabolism of specific substances such as carbohydrates and calcium; growth and developmental processes; the secretory activity of other endocrine glands; the development and functioning of the reproductive organs; psychic sexual characteristics and libido; the development of personality and higher nervous functions; the ability of the body to meet conditions of stress; resistance to disease.
Endocrine dysfunction may result from (a) *hyposecretion* in which an inadequate amount of the hormone(s) is secreted or (b) *hypersecretion* in which excessive amounts of hormones are produced. Secretion of endocrine glands may be under nervous control, or it may be controlled by chemical substances in the blood; in some cases, other hormones. Many pathological conditions are the result of, or associated with, the malfunctioning of the endocrine glands.

endocrinism E-24 **Endodermophyton**

endoc′rinism [" + " + *ismos*, condition]. Disease due to malfunction of one or more of the endocrine glands. SYN: *endocrinopathy*.

endocrinology (en-do-krin-ol′o-gĭ) [" + " + *logos*, science]. The science of the endocrines, or ductless glands, and their functions.

endocrinopath (en″do-krin′o-path) [" + " + *pathos*, disease]. One affected by a disorder of one or more glands of internal secretion.

endocrinopathic (en″do-krin-o-path′ĭk) [" + " + *pathos*, disease]. Of the nature of endocrinopathy.

endocrinopathy (en″do-krin-op′ă-thĭ) [" + " + *pathos*, disease]. A disease due to disorder of an endocrine gland or glands.

endocrinosis (en″do-krin-o′sĭs) [" + " + *ōsis*]. Condition resulting from dysfunction of an endocrine gland.

endocrinotherapy (en″do-krin-o-ther′ă-pĭ) [" + " + *therapeia*, treatment]. Treatment with endocrine preparations.

endocrinous (en-dok′rin-us) [" + *krinein*, to secrete]. Pert. to internal secretions or endocrine glands.

endocrit′ic [G. *endon*, within + *krinein*, to secrete]. Referring to internal secretions.

en′docyst [" + *kystis*, cyst]. The innermost layer of any hydatid cyst.

endocystitis (en-do-sis-ti′tis) [" + " + *itis*, inflammation]. Inflammation of membrane of bladder.

endoderm (en′do-derm) [" + *derma*, skin]. Inner layer of cells of an embryo. SYN: *hypoblast*. The entoderm, *q.v.*

Endodermophyton (ĕn-dō-dĕrm″ō-fī′tŏn). Former name of a genus of parasitic fungi growing in the epidermis of the skin. Now included in the genus *Trichophyton*, *q.v.*

The Principal Endocrine Glands:

Name	Position	Function	Diseases Connected With It
The Thyroid Gland	Two lobes in neck joined by a narrow band called the isthmus.	Influences growth and nutrition through its hormone thyroxin.	1. Goiter — an enlargement of the gland. 2. Cretinism. 3. Myxedema. 4. Exophthalmic goiter.
The Parathyroid Glands	Four tiny glands, 2 on each side, in the neighborhood of the thyroid.	Influence nutrition of muscle tissue.	Tetany. A disease in which painful spasms of the hands and feet occur. Chiefly seen in the muscles of children.
The Suprarenal (or adrenal) Capsules	One lies above each kidney. Each has an outer layer, the cortex (bark), and an inner layer, the medulla (pith).	Hormone of cortex influences growth and sexual development. Hormone of medulla is called adrenaline, affects blood pressure, keeps up muscle tone, has some effect on the coloring matter in the skin.	Addison's disease: SYM: Muscular weakness. Low blood pressure. A darkening of the skin. Vomiting.
The Pituitary Gland	About the size of a pea, lying in the floor of the skull. It is in 2 lobes, an anterior and posterior.	Anterior lobe influences growth, especially of bones. Posterior. Has an action somewhat like that of adrenalin.	Acromegaly. A disease in which there is enlargement of the bones of the hands, feet, and head.
The Thymus Gland	Found just beneath the sternum. Weighs about half an ounce at birth, develops up to puberty, after which it atrophies.	—	—
The Pineal Gland	About the size of a small cherry stone, connected with the upper surface of the brain.	—	—
The Testicles and Ovaries	—	Cause the development of the secondary sexual characters such as the growth of hair and deepening of the voice in the male.	Dementia precox.

Note that of the 7, 2 are found in the brain, 2 small pairs and 1 large single one in the neck, 1 pair in the abdomen and 1 in the thorax.

Table Showing the Important Results of Disease of the Endocrine Glands[1]

Gland	Name of Hormone	Hypersecretion In Children	Hypersecretion In Adults	Hyposecretion In Children	Hyposecretion In Adults
Thyroid	Thyroxin	Hyperthyroidism (exophthalmic goiter).		Cretinism.	Myxedema.
Parathyroid	Parathormone	Generalized osteitis fibrosa, with high blood calcium.		Tetany, with low blood calcium.	
Suprarenal (cortex)	Cortin or Eucortone	Sexual precocity.	Obesity, increased hairiness.	Addison's disease.	
(mendulla)	Adrenalin	—		—	
Pituitary (anterior lobe)	—	Gigantism	Acromegaly.	Infantilism.	?
(posterior lobe)	Pituitrin	? Disorder of carbohydrate metabolism.		Diabetes insipidus.	

[1] Sears, *Medicine for Nurses* (Modified).

endodiascopy (en-do-di-as'kō-pĭ) [" + *dia*, through, + *skopein*, to examine]. X-ray examination of a cavity.

endodontitis (en"do-don-ti'tis) [" + *odous, odont-*, tooth, + *itis*, inflammation]. Inflammation of the dental pulp.

en"doenteri'tis [" + *enteron*, intestine, + *itis*, inflammation]. Inflammation of lining membrane of intestines.

endoen'zyme [" + *en*, in, + *zymē*, leaven]. An intracellular enzyme.

endogastrectomy (en-do-gas-trek'to-mĭ) [" + *gastēr*, belly, + *ektome*, excision]. Excision of the gastric mucosa.

endogastric (en-do-gas'trik) [" + *gastēr*, stomach]. Pert. to the stomach's interior.

endogastritis (en-do-gas-tri'tis) [" + " + *itis*, inflammation]. Inflammation of the lining membrane of the stomach.

endogen'ic [" + *gennan*, to produce]. Having origin within the organism. SYN: *endogenous*.

endogenous (en-doj'en-us) [" + *gennan*, to produce]. 1. Produced within a cell or organism. 2. Concerning spore formation within the bacterial cell. SYN: *endogenic*.

endoglob'ular [" + L. *globulus*, a globule]. Within the blood corpuscles, as malarial germs.

endointoxica'tion [" + L. *in*, into, + G. *toxikon*, poison]. Poisoning due to an endogenous toxin.

endolabyrinthitis (en"do-lab-ĭ-rin-thi'tis) [" + *labyrinthos*, labyrinth, + *itis*, inflammation]. Inflamed condition of the membranous labyrinth.

endolaryn'geal [" + *larygx*, larynx]. Within the larynx.

Endolimax na'na (en-do-li'maks) [" + *leimax*, meadow]. A minute species of ameba inhabiting the intestine of man, monkeys, and other mammals. It is a nonpathogenic organism living as commensually within its host.

endolum'bar [" + L. *lumbus*, loin]. In the lumbar portion of the spinal cord.

endolymph (en'do-limf) [" + L. *lympha*]. Pale, limpid fluid within the labyrinth of the ear.

endolymphat'ic [" + L. *lympha*]. Rel. to the endolymph.

    e. duct. A slender duct extending from post. surface of the saccule of the inner ear. It ends blindly in the petrous portion of temporal bone as a dilated pouch, the endolymphatic sac, endomastoididitis, mastoid antrum.

endolysin (en-dol'is-in) [" + *lysis*, a loosening]. Bacterial substance within a leukocyte which destroys bacteria.

endol'ysis [G. *endon*, within, + *lysis*, a dissolution]. Disintegration of cell cytoplasm.

endomastoiditis (en"do-mas-toy-di'tis) [" + *mastos*, breast, + *eidos*, form, + *itis*, inflammation]. Inflammation of mucosa lining the mastoid cavity and cells.

endometrectomy (en"do-me-trek'to-mĭ) [" + *mētra*, uterus, + *ektome*, excision]. Excision of uterine mucosa. SEE: *curettage*.

endometrial (en-do-me'trĭ-al) [" + *mētra*, uterus]. Pert. to the lining mucosa of the uterus.

    e. cyst. An ovarian cyst or tumor that bleeds, which may develop dense and extensive adhesions.

endometrioma (en-do-me-trĭ-o'mä) [" + " + *ōma*, tumor]. A tumor containing shreds of ectopic endometrium; found most frequently in the ovary, cul-de-sac, rectovaginal septum, and the peritoneal surface of the post. portion of the uterus.

endometriosis (en-do-me-trĭ-o'sis) [" + " + *ōsis*]. Ectopic endometrium located in various sites throughout the pelvis or in the abdominal wall.

endometritis (en-do-me-tri'tis) [" + " + *itis*, inflammation]. Inflammation of the endometrium, the inner mucous lining of the uterus.

    ETIOL: Produced by bacterial invasion. May be acute, subacute, or chronic, the acute cases most commonly resulting from gonococcal infection or following abortion or full term pregnancy. The subacute type is the result of repeated acute attacks as is the chronic type. Occasionally the chronic type may be a tuberculous infection. There are many other conditions which are labeled as endometritis but which are of either vascular or endocrine origin. Some of these misnomered conditions are senile endometritis, hyperplastic endometritis, hypertrophic endometritis, etc.

    SYM: There are no specific symptoms of this condition, in acute cases the symptoms resembling those of acute pelvic peritonitis. In the chronic cases, menorrhagia is common, but a positive

endometritis, cervical   E-26   **endosteum**

diagnosis cannot be made without a curettage and a histological study of the recovered material. SEE: *cervix uteri, endometrium, uterus.*

   e., cervical. Inflammation of the inner portion of the cervix uteri.

   e. decidual. Inflammation of the mucous membrane of a gravid uterus.

   e. dissecans. E. accompanied by development of ulcers and shedding of the mucous membrane.

   e., fungous. Endometrial enlargement with bleeding and granulations.

   e., septic. Form caused by septic poisoning.

   e., simple. Catarrhal inflammatory condition of the endometrium.

endometrium (en-do-me'trĭ-um) [" + *mētra*, uterus]. The mucous membrane lining the inner surface of the uterus. Histologically, it consists of a surface epithelium made up of a single layer of columnar cells, a few of which bear cilia. Invaginations of the epithelium form simple, branched tubular glands which extend to the myometrium. The glands are separated by connective tissue resembling mesenchyme which forms the *stroma*. There is no submucosa; the mucosa lying closely attached to the myometrium.

The endometrium is supplied by two types of arteries; *straight arteries* which supply the deeper third or basal layer of the endometrium and *spiral arteries* which supply the spongy and compact layers. They penetrate between the glands and form a subepithelial capillary plexus. These arteries show marked changes in response to hormonal stimulation during the menstrual cycle.

Between puberty and the menopause, the uterine endometrium passes through cyclic changes which constitute the menstrual cycle, *q.v.* These changes are related to the development and maturation of the Graffian follicle, the discharge of the ovum, and the subsequent development of the corpus luteum in the ovary.

Following fertilization of the ovum, the endometrium serves as nesting place and implantation occurs. The endometrium fuses with the developing chorion of the embryo and at birth there is a splitting off and shedding of the uterine lining or *decidua*. During pregnancy, the *decidua basalis*, the endometrium lying between the chorionic vesicle and the myometrium, develops into the maternal portion of the placenta, *q.v.*

endom'etry [" + *metron*, measure]. Measurement of the interior of a cavity or organ.

endomix'is [G. *endon*, within + *mixis*, mixture]. Mixture of the cell nuclear and cytoplasmic substance.

endomyocarditis (en"do-mī-o-kar-dī'tis) [" + *mys*, muscle, + *kardia*, heart, + *itis*, inflammation]. Inflammation of the endocardium and myocardium.

endomysium (ĕn-dō-mĭz'ĭ-ŭm) . A thin sheath of connective tissue consisting principally of reticular fibers which invests each striated muscle fiber and binds the fibers together within a fasciculus.

endoneuri'tis [" + *neuron*, nerve, + *itis*, inflammation]. Inflammation of the endoneurium.

endoneurium (ĕn-dō-nū'rĭ-ŭm) [" + *neuron*, nerve]. Henle's sheath. A delicate connective tissue sheath which surrounds nerve fibers within a fasciculus.

endoparasite (en-do-par'as-īt) [" + *parasitos*, parasite]. Any parasite living within its host.

endopathy (en-dop'ath-ĭ) [" + *pathos*, disease]. Any endogenous disease.

endopelvic (en-do-pel'vic) [" + L. *pelvis*, basin]. Within the pelvis.

   e. fasciae. The downward continuation of the parietal peritoneum of the abdomen to form the pelvic fasciae which have a very important part in the support of the pelvic viscera.

endopericarditis (en"do-per"ĭ-kar-dī'tis) [" + *peri*, around, + *kardia*, heart, + *itis*, inflammation]. Endocarditis complicated by pericarditis.

endoperimyocarditis (en"do-per-ĭ-mī"o-kar-dī'tis) [" + " + *mys*, muscle, + *kardia*, heart, + *itis*, inflammation]. Inflammation of the pericardium, myocardium, and endocardium.

endoperitonitis (en"do-per-ĭ-to-nī'tis) [" + *peritonaion*, peritoneum, + *itis*, inflammation]. . Superficial inflammation of the peritoneum.

endophlebitis (en"do-fle-bi'tis) [" + *phleps*, vein, + *itis*, inflammation]. Inflammation of inner coat of a vein.

   e. obliterans. E. causing obliteration of a vein.   [tal vein.

   e. portalis. Inflammation of the portal vein.

en'doplasm [" + *plasma*, matter formed]. The internal, more fluid protoplasm of a cell which lies within the ectoplasm which forms the peripheral layer.

endoplast (en'do-plast) [" + *plassein*, to form]. A cellular nucleus.

end-organ. The expanded end of a nerve fiber in a peripheral structure.

   e. sensory. An encapsulated termination of a nerve fiber which serves as a receptor.

endorrhachis (en-do-rā'kis) [G. *endon*, within, + *rachis*, spine]. Membrane lining; the spinal dura mater.

endorrhinitis (en-do-ri-ni'tis) [" + *ris*, *rin-*, nose, + *itis*, inflammation]. Inflammation of the mucous membranes of the nose. SYN: *coryza*.

endosalpingitis (en"do-sal-pin-jī'tis) [" + *salpigx*, tube, + *itis*, inflammation]. Inflammation of lining of fallopian tubes.

endoscope (en'do-skōp) [" + *skopein*, to examine]. Metal, rubber, or glass tube for examining cavities through natural openings.

endoscopy (en-dos'ko-pĭ) [" + *skopein*, to examine]. Inspection of cavities by use of the endoscope.

endosep'sis [" + *sēpsis*, decay]. Septicemia having its origin within the body.

endoskel'eton [" + *skeleton*, skeleton]. Internal bony framework of the body. SEE: *exoskeleton*.

endosmometer (en-dos-mom'et-er) [" + *ōsmos*, a thrusting, + *metron*, measure]. Device for estimating inward passage of liquid through a septum.

endosmose, endosmosis (en'dŏs-mōs, -mō'sis) [" + *ōsmos*, a thrusting, + *ōsis*]. Osmosis in which flow of water is from the outside liquid to the solution within a membranous cell.

en'dospore [" + *sporos*, a seed]. BIOL: Thick walled spore within the bacterium.

endosteitis (en"dos-te-i'tis) [" + *osteon*, bone, + *itis*, inflammation]. Inflammation of the endosteum or of medullary cavity of a bone.

endosteo'ma [" + " + *ōma*, tumor]. A tumor in the medullary cavity of a bone.

endos'teum [" + *osteon*, bone]. Membrane lining bone in the medullary cavity.

endostitis (en″dos-tī′tis) [" + " + itis, inflammation]. Inflammation of the endosteum or the medullary cavity of a bone.

endostoma (en-dos-to′mă) [" + " + ōma, tumor]. Osseous tumor within a bone.

endostosis (en-dos-to′sis) [" + " + ōsis]. The development of an endostoma.

endothelial (en-do-the′lī-al) [" + thēlē, nipple]. Pert. to or consisting of endothelium.

endotheliocyte (en″do-the′lī-ō-sīt) [" + kytos, cell]. Large, phagocytic, wandering cell found in circulating blood and in tissue.

endotheliocytosis (en″do-the″lī-o-si-to′sis) [" + " + kytos, cell, + ōsis]. Abnormal increase in endothelial cells.

en″dothe″lioino′ma [" + " + is, in-, fiber, + ōma, tumor]. Tumorous growth arising from endothelium containing fibrous substance.

endotheliolysin (en″do-the-lī-ol′is-in) [" + " + lysis, dissolution]. An antibody found in snake venom which dissolves endothelial cells.

endotheliolytic (en″do-thē-lī-o-lit′ĭk) [" + " + lysis, dissolution]. Capable of destroying endothelial tissue.

endothelioma (en″do-the-lī-o′mă) [" + " + ōma, tumor]. Malignant growth of lining cells of the blood vessels.

endotheliomyoma (en″do-the″lī-o-mi-o′-mă) [" + " + mys, muscle, + ōma, tumor]. Muscular tumor with elements of endothelium.

endotheliomyxoma (en″do-the″lī-o-miks-o′-mă) [" + " + myxa, mucus, + ōma, tumor]. Myxoma with element from endothelium.

endotheliotoxin (en″do-the-lī-o-toks′in) [" + " + toxikon, poison]. A specific toxin which acts on endothelial capillary cells, causing hemorrhages.

endothe′lium [" + " + thēlē, nipple]. A form of squamous epithelium consisting of flat cells which line the blood and lymphatic vessels and the heart. It is derived from mesoderm.

end′otherm knife. A knife devised for using a high frequency current.

endother′mal [G. endon, within, + thermē, heat]. 1. Pert. to production of heat within an organism. 2. Pert. to absorption of heat during formation of chemical compounds. SYN: endothermic.

endother′mic [" + thermē, heat]. 1. Storing up potential energy or heat. 2. Absorbing heat. 3. Accompanied by heat absorption.

endothermy (en′do-ther″mī) [" + thermē, heat]. A term used as a synonym for surgical diathermy.

en′dothrix [" + thrix, hair]. The parasite causing tinea tonsurans.

endothyreopexy (en-do-thī′re-o-peks″ī) [" + thyreos, shield, + pēxis, fixation]. Displacing the thyroid gland and fixing it to the side of the neck.

endothyroidopexy (en″do-thī″royd-o-peks′ī) [" + " + eidos, form, + pēxis, fixation]. Operative displacement of the thyroid gland and fixing it to the side of the neck. SYN: endothyreopexy.

endotoscope (en-do′to-skōp) [" + ous, ot-, ear, + skopein, to examine]. An ear speculum. SYN: otoscope.

en″dotoxico′sis [" + toxikon, poison, + -ōsis]. Poisoning due to an endotoxin.

en′dotoxin [" + toxikon, poison]. Bacterial toxin confined within the body of a bacterium, freed only when the bacterium is broken down.

SEE: cytotoxin, erythrotoxin, exotoxin, leukotoxin, neurotoxin.

endotracheitis (en-do-tra-ke-i′tis) [" + tracheia, trachea, + itis, inflammation]. Inflammation of the tracheal mucosa.

endotrachelitis (en″do-tra-kel-i′tis) [" + trachēlos, neck, + itis, inflammation]. Inflammation of the endocervical tissues. SYN: endocervicitis.

en″dovasculi′tis [" + L. vasculum, vessel, + G. itis, inflammation]. Inflammation of the endangium or inner coat of a blood vessel. SYN: endangeitis.

endove′nous [" + L. vēna, vein]. Within a vein. SYN: intravenous.

end plate. The terminal mass of a nerve fiber ending on a muscle cell.

end-plate, motor. An ending in a striated muscle fiber; a myoneural junction.

end product. The final waste or excretory product of digestion that passes from the system.

endyma (en′dĭm-ă). Membranous lining of cerebral ventricles. SYN: ependyma.

en′ema (pl. enemas or enema′ta) [G.]. Injection of water, either plain or containing various drugs, etc., into the rectum and colon to empty the lower intestine, or to introduce food or medicine for therapeutic purposes.

  e., analeptic. One with ½ teaspoonful of salt to a pint of tepid water; a "thirst" enema.

  e., anthelmintic. One given to expel worms. Some thread worms will be carried away with a soapsuds enema with turpentine. When given, the results should be scrutinized very closely to see if worms have been expelled. It may be necessary to send a specimen to the laboratory for microscopic or macroscopic examination. If so, the specimen must be sent immediately and while warm. Thermos bottles may be provided for such purposes. If so, the nurse should have the bottle warmed so that no time will be lost in getting the specimen to the laboratory.

  USES: Quassia is used as an infusion for rectal injection in the treatment of pin or thread worms. To 1 dram of quassia chips add 8 ounces of cold water and let it stand for 2 or 3 hours. Strain and use for a single injection. [rhea.

  e., antidiarrheic. One given for diar-
  e., antiseptic. One for the destruction of microörganisms. [spasms.
  e., antispasmodic. One to counteract
  e., astringent. One given to contract intestinal tissue and to provoke subsequent evacuation of worms. Those given for anthelmintic* purposes are also useful when an astringent is needed. The following astringents are credited with inhibiting worms by dehydration, and with reducing the intestinal mucosa which harbors them:

  Alum in a 1 to 250 parts solution, mixed with water.

  Calumba as ordered by the physician.

  Limewater in a saturated strength solution.

  Phenol (carbolic acid) in a one-fourth of 1% solution, to a one-half of a 1% solution.

  Quinine bisulfate in a 1 to 2000 parts solution, or a 1 to 500 solution. Also used in amebic colitis for an irrigation.

  Sodium chloride in a hypertonic solution. This in double strength or 1 tablespoonful to the quart.

  Tannic acid solution, 1 to 2500 parts of water.

  Vinegar in a one-half dilution.

  e., blind. The insertion of a rubber tube to cause expulsion of gas or flatus. SEE: carminative enema.

e., carminative. One given to relieve distention caused by flatus and to stimulate peristalsis.

It calls for an examination of the patient's abdomen both before and after administering the enema. Special attention must be paid to the exclusion of flatus and of fecal matter. Often there is a high degree of distention, and it is vastly important to know of the relief from flatulence and accumulated feces. A very detailed description must be given after a careful examination has been made of the returns.

The carminative enema should be sufficiently warm, as it is to reach more of the intestinal tissues than the general cleansing enema, and as it also causes a greater hyperemia. It should penetrate farther than most enemas.

The temperature may be 115° F. Hot normal saline solution, 110° F., to the amt. of 500 cc., to which 1 dram, or 4 cc., of spirits of peppermint or tincture of asafetida has been added, may be used in relieving a patient of flatulence. The amt. of the solution may be increased to 1000 cc., which will give good results.

e., cleansing. One to empty the lower intestine or the colon.

PROCEDURE: 1. Bring all equipment to bedside. 2. Screen bed. 3. Turn patient on left side, with right leg flexed, in as comfortable a position as possible. 4. Place small rubber sheet covered with large towel under buttocks. 5. Cover shoulders with 1 bath blanket folded crosswise. Cover legs with other bath blanket, fan-folding upper bedding to foot of bed, and having blankets lap a few inches over patient's buttocks. 6. Hang enema can on stand, having it about 2 feet above patient (not more), and see that stopcock is working properly. 7. See that solution is the proper temperature. 8. Lubricate rectal, or enema, tube for about 2 inches at end. 9. Run a little of the solution through tube into bedpan to warm tube. Close stopcock. 10. Insert tube into rectum. If you meet with resistance wait a few seconds, then proceed. 11. Open stopcock and let fluid run in. If it seems to be flowing too fast pinch the tube with your finger and thumb. 12. If patient complains of sharp pain, or is unable to retain fluid, stop flow for a minute. 13. When all fluid has been run in slowly remove tube and place bedpan. 14. Detach enema, or rectal, tube and lay in emesis basin. *Do not put it into the can.* 15. See that patient is comfortable on pan, covered with the bath blankets and the signal within reach. 16. Remove and care for enema tray. 17. When patient has finished expelling enema remove pan and do perineal toilet as usual. 18. Remove bath blankets and replace upper bedding. 19. If patient has used toilet paper himself provide soap and water for his hands. 20. Chart enema as directed.

e., demulcent. SEE: *emollient enema.*

e., Dobell's. One for nutritive purposes.

e., egg and ether. Used as a last resort in the relief of distention.

It consists of magnesium sulfate, 1 ounce of ether, and the whites of 2 eggs. Water enough is added to make 1 pint of fluid. Mix the egg whites with the ether and beat until the mixture bubbles, then add the magnesium sulfate which has been dissolved in hot water; lastly, add the remaining warm water. All should be ready before the final water is added.

CHARTING: The results of a carminative enema for flatulence should be noted and charted. The abdomen should be examined both before and afterward to be sure of the results obtained. If hard and distended before giving the enema, and soft and flat afterwards it is evident good results have been obtained. Do not rely entirely upon the patient's word. If there should be any amt. of foam in the bedpan this indicates relief from the flatulence has been obtained.

e., emollient. One given to soften and protect tissues by making a coating over membranes, allaying local pain and irritation, and to act as a vehicle for the rectal administration of drugs.

It should be given at a temperature of about 105° F., or in a severe case at about 100° F. After giving the record must show if the patient felt relieved, and to what extent; also if the solution was retained in its entirety.

1. Mix *amylum* 2 drams with 1 ounce of cold water, then add 5 ounces of boiling water. Boil mixture 1 or 2 minutes to the consistency of mucilage. Now cool to about 105° F., and give slowly with a large catheter. If too small a catheter is used the solution will not pass through, if of a pastelike consistiency. A bulb or piston syringe attached to a rectal tube may be used. From 10 to 30 minims of laudanum are often used in this enema as prescribed by the attending physician. It is best given by means of a small hand syringe, the solution being injected rather than flowing by gravity. The results are also better given in this manner.

2. *Olive oil or cottonseed oil* will also act as an emollient when injected. The tissues in this way are prevented from coming in contact with irritating substances, thus relieving the pain of inflammations through protecting the delicate membrane.

3. *Mucilage of acacia* is used as an emollient, 1 ounce to 5 ounces of water, or a thin, strained tea from boiled flaxseed, 4 or 5 ounces, also acts as a good emollient. This, of course, is only used on a doctor's order.

4. *The bismuth enema* may be given for its emollient effect. This also must be prescribed by the physician. Four or 5 ounces of water are used in which to dissolve the bismuth. Too large an amt. of enema may not be retained, in which case the effect desired is lost; the water will be absorbed and the bismuth will form a coating over the intestinal mucosa.

5. *Thin, strained gruel*, 4 ounces, may be given for emollient effect, and it may be absorbed as a nutrient.

e., evacuating. SEE: *cleansing enema.*

e., Ewald's. A nutritive enema containing red wine, 20% grape sugar solution with wheat flour boiled in it, mixed with eggs.

e., flatus. One to relieve gas pressure. Contains 1 dram of glycerine and ½ ounce of magnesium sulfate in 4 ounces of water.

e., high. One to reach the colon. Insertion of rubber tube into rectum to carry water as far as possible. Too frequent irrigation, esp. with hot water, may cause diverticula.

e., lubricating. Administered after an operation for hemorrhoids, and in order to soften the feces and lubricate the passage or anal canal to the external orifice or anus. When there is an impaction of feces, a lubricating enema may be given, followed in 2 hours by a cleansing enema.

OLIVE OIL, 4 to 6 ounces, warmed, may be given, or cottonseed oil warmed in quantities of from 4 to 6 ounces in the evening. The patient should remain in a prone position with hips elevated for half an hour following the enema in order to help retain the oil and thus aiding it in passing higher in the colon.

WARM SWEET OIL, 4 ounces, injected into the rectum with a bulb or piston syringe, will serve the purpose better than the usual enema apparatus. The hips should be elevated, and a cotton pad held against the anal region for a few minutes in order to help retention.

e., m. and m. Eight ounces of milk, and 8 ounces of molasses. The mixture may also be in proportions of 6 to 6. This is esp. efficient, as the sugar of the molasses with the milk forms gases which distend the bowels, causing frequent copious bowel movements. Starch water may be added to a 6 to 6 mixture to the extent of 4 ounces.

e., Mayo. Granulated sugar, 2 ounces, 1 ounce of sodium bicarbonate, and 8 ounces of water.

The sodium bicarbonate is added to the sugar and water mixture at the bedside, just before the solution is ready to be given. The combination of the sugar with the acid content of the intestine coming in contact with the bicarbonate causes a fermentation and production of gases. The bowels thus become inflated, causing a hyperdistention which produces bowel action.

e., medicinal. An enema to which some drug or medication has been added on order of attending physician. It is necessary that this enema be retained and absorbed. It may be given to medicate diseased conditions of the rectum, sigmoid, or colon, or for absorption for its general effects. Although substances (other than fluids) are not absorbed in the large intestine as extensively as in the small intestine, the chemical changes that may occur must be very simple if any absorption may be expected. SEE: *preparations usually given by rectum*.

e., Noble's. One dram of turpentine mixed well with glycerine, 2 ounces; mix 3 ounces of magnesium sulfate with 4 ounces of water, and pour the 2 mixtures together.

e., nutrient or nutritive. One to give sustenance to a patient unable to be fed otherwise.

It may consist of peptonized milk, glucose, and other solutions. The temperature must be about body heat, and whatever food material is used should never be boiled.

The various prescriptions usually ordered are: (1) Foods most apt to be absorbed; (2) concentrated, easily digested and assimilable substances; (3) predigested foods; those that have been peptonized, such as milk, eggs, and meat broth.

Alcohol, brandy, and whisky produce energy but they do not feed the tissues. The energy produced reduces the tax upon the body's tissues for energy, and conserves the proteins as nourishing factors. Alcohol, however, should be restricted as too much is destructive to the tissues. Dextrose is irritating although otherwise nutritive and absorbable.

TEMPERATURE OF SOLUTION: This should be 105° F. The attending physician prescribes the diet and the time of feeding. Much depends upon the condition of the patient and the diet prescribed.

GLUCOSE: If glucose is prescribed, 3 ounces of 5-10% solution may be used. A very good nutritive enema is prepared by peptonized milk, 4 ounces, liquid beef preparation, ½ ounce, the white of 1 egg stirred into the mixture, and about 15 grains of salt. To this 15 cc. of *spiritus frumenti* may be added. This serves a double purpose because it is both nutritive as well as stimulating. Another formula is malted milk, 15 grams; somatose, 4 grams; water, 4 ounces; sodium chloride, 15 grains; white of egg and peptonized milk, 1 ounce. Another is peptonized milk, 5 ounces, with white of 1 egg, alcohol, 1 dram, and 15 grains of salt. These solutions are best heated by setting in a pan of hot water.

PROCEDURE: An evacuating enema of normal saline solution is usually given every 24 hours as an aid to absorption and to remove any mucus. The feedings may be given at 4 A. M. and at 8 A. M., followed at 12 noon with the cleansing enema, and a feeding at 4 P. M. and 8 P. M. The feedings should not consist of more than 4 to 8 ounces. The cleansing enema, however, is preferably given in the morning at about 6 o'clock, then the feeding may be given at 7 o'clock. This interval gives time to recover from any peristaltic irritation.

Not too much should be given at one time, and not at too frequent intervals. Every 2 hours should be sufficient *if only 2 or 3 ounces are given* at a time. The nurse should endeavor to estimate the amt. absorbed in a given time. Some feedings are ordered every 3 hours during the day, or every hour to 6 hours. If given every 4 hours during the day, the feeding at 4 or 6 o'clock in the morning may be omitted because the cleansing enema is usually given early in the morning to prepare the intestinal tract for the day's feedings.

The injections are given with a catheter which should be lubricated. Glycerine should not be used, as it activates peristalsis. At least 15 to 20 or 30 minutes should be taken for giving a nutritive enema, as the slower the feeding is given, the better are the chances of retention.

If patient cannot lie on left side for injection, hips should be elevated on a pillow (rubber covered). No air should be introduced through the rectal tube while giving the enema, as there may be a tendency to expel the solution.

PRECAUTION: Avoid anything that incites peristalsis. Be sure that the cleansing enema is administered before beginning a series of feedings as indicated. Every precaution should be taken to prevent the expulsion of the feeding, as the patient depends on this feeding for sustenance. Any expulsion of the feeding would defeat the purpose of the treatment.

e., olive oil. Mix 4 ounces of olive oil with 1 dram of turpentine, beating the mixture well so as to break the oil globules. This will cause sufficient peristalsis to move the bowels.

e., one-two-three. Magnesium sulfate, 1 ounce; glycerine, 2 ounces, and hot water, 3 ounces (115° F.).

This mixture must be given with a small tube because of the small quantity, and the action desired. The results following the injection are more satisfactory if given very carefully with assistance to help the patient retain it.

One or 2 drams of turpentine may be added to the one-two-three enema. In adding turpentine, the glycerine and turpentine must be beaten well together and added to the magnesium sulfate and water. The turpentine must be mixed well with the oil to prevent irritation of the mucous lining of the bowel, otherwise it may be absorbed and cause kidney irritation. All ingredients must be well mixed together before giving to the patient.

e., pancreatic. One containing pancreatin.

e., physiological salt solution. One teaspoonful of salt to a pint of water is a normal salt solution. It may be abbreviated as N. S. Sol. The distention made by this enema excites peristalsis and evacuation. There is no harm in retaining this enema. Often ordered when there is dehydration.

e., purgative. This produces action when other enemas fail; it should be a *high enema*. The rectal tube should be inserted at least 6 inches. The ingredients are 1 pint soapsuds, ½ ounce of magnesium sulfate crystals, 1 ounce glycerine, and ½ ounce oil of turpentine. Beat the glycerine and oil of turpentine into an emulsion and add the other ingredients.

Another purgative enema is ordinary soapsuds to which is added 15 grains of powdered ox-gall. This usually produces drastic results.

2. Ox-gall, 60 grains, with 4 ounces of castor oil may be used with the whites of 2 eggs stirred into the mixture. To this add 1 pint of very warm water at about 115° F.

3. One-half ounce of ox-gall may be added to 1 quart of plain water, or one-half of this mixture may be used with desired results.

e., quantity of. For retention, 3-8 ounces. Cleansing: For a child: ½-1½ pints; infants: ½-2 ounces; adults: 2-4 pints.

e., quassia. SEE: *quassia*.

e., retention. This is one to retain. It may be used to provide nourishment, to medicate a diseased mucous membrane, or for absorption purposes, or for general, local, or systemic action. This enema must be of constituents which will not stimulate the nerve endings and reflexly promote peristalsis. It necessarily must consist of a small amt. of solution. The rectum and lower bowel must first be well cleansed, and all irritation resulting from evacuation must subside before giving, or the purpose will be defeated. The patient should be placed on left side with knees flexed, and the rectal tube inserted high; 6 inches or more. Allow the fluid to flow through the tube before inserting to expel air. Pressure on tube should be made with fingers to prevent loss of liquid. Lubricate tube before inserting, and introduce with a twisting motion, slowly pushing it in so as not to bring discomfort to the patient. Unless absolutely necessary, the tube should not be slipped forward or backward to make the solution flow. Pushing may stimulate peristalsis. If the fluid does not readily flow, grasp tube in one hand, squeezing, compressing, and relaxing, so that suction will cause solution to flow. Allow fluid to run very slowly, stopping occasionally to aid retention. If the least desire to expel is manifested fluid should be stopped until the desire to evacuate has passed. Upon withdrawal of tube, which should be done quickly, pressure with a pad of cotton should be made over anus for a minute or two to prevent evacuation. The patient should be informed of the purpose of this enema so that coöperation may be secured. Enemata classed in the retention group may include the following: *emollient, lubricating, medicinal, nutritive, sedative, stimulating,* q.v.

e., Rosenheim's. A nutrient one, containing cod liver oil, sugar, and peptone in a 3% soda solution.

e., saline. One with solution of magnesium sulfate in warm water.

e., sedative. Retention enema given for its soothing action and to allay irritability. The temperature should be about 100°-105° F. Before and after it has been administered, the condition of the patient must be noted and recorded. Watch for untoward effects.

Paraldehyde may be ordered in delirium tremens, and this should be dissolved in thin, boiled starch solution. In water it dissolves in the proportion of 1 to 8. It must be injected with a small catheter. Paraldehyde is also sometimes ordered in epilepsy, manias, and various nervous irritations. The dosage varies in different institutions and among different physicians.

Chloral Hydrate: This may be administered as a sedative but only on a doctor's order. There are dangers attendant upon the administration of the drug in almost any form. The usual dosage for an enema is 20 grains dissolved in 3 ounces of olive oil or 3 ounces of hot milk, or boiled cornstarch. It should be given at a temperature of 105° F. and administered with a small catheter as a *high* enema. The higher, the better the absorption.

Luminal Sodium, Veronal, or *Trional*: These are hypnotics. Three to 6 ounces may be dissolved in 3 ounces of thin starch water. If the drug is dissolved in a small amt. of plain hot water, and the mixture stirred into the starch water it will be a better solution.

Sodium Bromide: Fifteen to 60 grains may be dissolved in 3 ounces of warm milk, as ordered by a physician.

Paregoric: The tincture may be given per rectum if added to at least 2 ounces of thin starch water. The mixture should contain at least 2 ounces but not more than 4 ounces. It is prescribed for some specific result desired and given only on a physician's order.

Laudanum: This is sometimes given, 10 to 30 grains to 3 ounces of starch water for absorption.

e., shock. One to ward off shock.

e., simple mixed. A soapsuds enema to which is added 1 dram of salt and ½ ounce of molasses.

e., soapsuds. The soapsuds are either ready prepared, or may be made by placing soap particles in a shaker and agitating the water until the right constituency is obtained. The foam is not removed. If liquid soap is used, 1 ounce to 1 quart of water is the right propor-

enema, s. s. & p.   E-31   **enolase**

tion. A milky solution is of sufficient strength. Strong soapsuds should not be used, as there is danger of injuring the intestinal mucosa. The mild soaps, such as castile, are best for suds.
INCOMPATIBILITIES: *Magnesium sulfate.*
  e., s. s. & p. A mixture of 1 dram of peppermint added to a soapsuds solution. The peppermint may be added to a plain water solution, 1 dram to 16 ounces; a good enema to relieve flatulence.
  e., s. s. & t. A mixture of thick liquid soap; green soap is best. Add ¼ ounce or 1 dram of turpentine and beat the 2 ingredients thoroughly together. The emulsion of this mixture is stirred into 1 quart of water at 115° F.
  e., stimulating. This may be grouped with the medicated and the retention enemas. It is supposed to cause irritation. Should be given at 115° F. It is intended to excite activity and ordered when the patient is in shock, or in some unconscious state, as from narcotic poisoning. The patient's condition must be compared both before and after giving. Ingredients used are the following:
COFFEE: Eight ounces black coffee with 1 of *spiritus frumenti* given in 4-ounce doses and repeated in 2 hours if absorption has taken place. Otherwise, 4 ounces every 4 to 6 hours. Black coffee and warm saline solution, the coffee being cooked in the solution. A cup of coffee made from 1 tablespoonful of ground coffee to 1 cup of water gives the equivalent of 0.1 to 0.2 gram or 1½ to 3 grains of caffeine.
SALINE SOLUTION: Hot normal saline solution, 4 ounces, with ½ to 1 ounce of *spiritus frumenti.*
DIGITALIS: Tincture of digitalis or an infusion of digitalis mixed with black coffee and normal saline solution.
LUGOL'S SOLUTION: This solution with normal saline solution may be given per rectum as ordered.
  e., temperature of. Carminative, stimulating, and for inflammations, 115° F. For hemorrhage, 120° F. For others, 105° F.
  e., thirst. Analeptic enema, *q.v.*
  e., yeast. One quart of warm water and ½ cake of yeast, thoroughly mixed and given very warm.
enema, words pert. to: cococlyster, colonic irrigation, clyster, enteroclysis, medicine, rectal administration of.
enepidermic (en-ep-ĭ-der'mĭk) [G. *en,* in, + *epi,* upon, + *derma,* skin]. Pert. to drugs applied without friction. SEE: *inunction.* Applied to or placed upon the surface of the skin. A term used in connection with application of medicinal agents to the skin without fraction.
energometer (en-er-gom'e-ter) [" + *ergon,* work, + *metron,* measure]. An instrument for measuring blood pressure. Especially one used in studying pulse pressure.
en'ergy [" + *ergon,* work]. The capacity of a system for doing work or its equivalent in the strict physical sense.
  Energy is manifested in various forms: Motion (kinetic e.), position (potential e.), light, heat, sound, and so on. These forms are mutually interchangeable according to certain laws. Thus, the chemical energy residing in 1 gram of glucose can be liberated in the form of heat, so that if complete oxidation (to carbon dioxide and water) is carried out at 20° C. and atmospheric pressure one obtains 3.74 calories of heat. This fact is fundamental in the science of dietetics.
  For a table showing the relative magnitudes of the various units in which energy is measured, see *Calorie.*
  e. changes. These may be physical or chemical, or both. Movement of a part of the body, as the arm, shortens and thickens the muscles involved and changes the position and size of cells, temporarily, but the intake of oxygen in the blood, combining with sugar and fat, creates a chemical change, producing heat, and waste products within the cells, which in turn produce fatigue if not eliminated.
  e., conservation of. The theory that no energy in the universe can be lost, but that it may be transformed into other forms.
  e., latent. That which exists but which is not being used.
  e., potential. SEE: *latent e.*
  e., radiant. That form of energy which is transmitted through space without the support of a sensible medium. Radio waves, infrared waves, visible rays, ultraviolet rays, x-rays, gamma rays and the recently discovered cosmic rays are energy in this form.
  e., static. SEE: *latent e.*
energy, words pert. to: chemism, chemokinesis, dietetics, kinetic, metabolism, physical agents, radiant, synergic, unit, vril.
enerva'tion [L. *enervatio,* to weaken, + *nervus,* nerve]. Weakness; failure of nerve energy.
engagement. In obs. the entrance of the fetal head or the part being presented into the superior pelvic strait.
En'gelmann's disc. A narrow zone of transparent material lying on each side of the intermediate disc in the isotropic or I disc of a striated muscle fiber.
englobe' [G. *en,* in, + L. *globus,* a ball]. To absorb within a spherical body, as the ingestion of bacteria by the phagocytes.
Engman's disease. Pustular eruption resembling eczema, which often occurs simultaneously with a pyogenic process. SYN: *dermatitis infectiosa eczematoides.*
engorged (en-gorjd') [Fr. *engorger,* to obstruct, to devour]. Distended, as with blood.
engorge'ment [Fr. *engórger,* to obstruct, to devour]. Vascular congestion; distention.
engram (en'gram) [G. *en,* in, + *gramma,* mark]. 1. Supposititious traces on protoplasm made by irritants or stimuli which, when repeated, form a habit after the stimulus ceases; the mnemic hypothesis. 2. The result of a psychic experience supposed to have established a pattern in memory. SEE: *ekphorize, mnemic theory.*
engraphia (en-gra'fĭ-ă) [" + *graphein,* to write]. The process of making engrams, *q.v.*
enhem'atospore [" + *aima,* blood, + *sporos,* spore]. A spore of the malarial parasite. SYN: *enhemospore, merozoite.*
enhemospore (en-hem'o-spōr) [" + " + *sporos,* spore]. A spore of the malarial parasite. SYN: *enhematospore, merozoite.*
enkatarrhaphy (en-kat-ar'af-ĭ) [G. *egkatarrhaptein,* to sew in]. Artificial implantation of a structure where it does not normally occur.
enolase (ē'nō-lās). An enzyme present in muscle tissue which converts phosphoglyceric acid to phosphopyruvic acid.

enomania (e″no-ma′nĭ-ă) [G. *oinos*, wine, + *mania*, madness]. Craving for alcohol; delirium tremens.

enophthalmus (en-of-thal′mus) [G. *en*, in, + *ophthalmos*, eye]. Recession of eyeball into orbit.

enosto′sis [″ + *osteon*, bone, + *ōsis*]. An osseous tumor within the cavity of a bone.

ensiform (en′sĭ-form) [L. *ensis*, sword, + *forma*, form]. Swordlike structure.
  e. cartilage. Lower part of sternum, below the gladiolus. SYN: *xiphoid cartilage or process*. SEE: *chondroxiphoid, xiphodynia*.

enosimania (ĕn-ō-sĭ-mā′nĭ-ă). A mental state characterized by excessive and irrational terror.

ensisternum (en-sĭ-ster′num) [″ + G. *sternon*, sternum]. The tip of the sternum; ensiform or xiphoid appendix. SYN: *metasternum*.

enstrophe (en′stro-fe) [G. *en*, in, + *strephein*, to turn]. Inversion; a turning inward, esp. of eyelids.

en′tad [″ + L. *ad*, toward]. Toward the inside; inwardly.

en′tal [G. *entos*, within]. Pert. to the interior; inside, central.

entamebiasis (ent-am-e-bi′as-is) [″ + *amoibē*, change]. Infestation with Entameba.

Entameba (ent-am-e′ba) [″ + *amoibē*, change]. A genus of ameba several of which live in the intestine of man. Some are parasitic. Characterized by the presence of 4 or 8 nuclei in their cysts.
  E. buccalis. E. gingivalis, q.v.
  E. coli. Found normally in the upper intestinal tract. Nonparasitic.
  E. gingivalis. Non-pathogenic species which inhabits the mouth.
  E. histolytica. A parasitic form of ameba, the cause of amebic dysentery and tropical abscess.
  E. kartul′isi. Found in the pus of necrotic bone abscesses.
  E. tetrage′na. Now considered identical with E. histolytica.
  E. un′dulans. A species found in the intestine.

entasia (en-ta′sĭ-ă) [G. *entasis*, a straining]. Spasmodic muscular contraction.

entelechy (en-tel′e-kĭ) [G. *entelecheia*, actuality]. 1. Complete development. 2. The activating cause of everything.

enteradeni′tis [G. *enteron*, intestine, + *adēn*, gland, + *-itis*, inflammation]. Inflammation of intestinal glands.

en′teral [G. *enteron*, intestine]. Within the intestine as distinguished from *parenteral*.

enteralgia (en-ter-al′jĭ-ă) [″ + *algos*, pain]. Neuralgia or pain in the intestines. Intestinal cramps or colic.

enterectasia (en-ter-ĕk-tā′sĭ-ă) [″ + *ektasis*, dilatation]. Dilatation of the small intestines.

enterectomy (en-ter-ek′to-mĭ) [″ + *ektomē*, excision]. Excision of a portion of the intestines.

enterelcosis (en-ter-el-ko′sis) [″ + *elkōsis*, ulceration]. Intestinal ulceration.

enterepiplocele (en-ter-ep-ip′lo-sēl) [″ + *epiploon*, omentum, + *kēlē*, hernia]. Hernia involving the bowel and omentum.

enteric (en-ter′ik) [G. *enteron*, intestine]. Pert. to the intestinal tract.
  e. fever. Typhoid fever.
  e. pills. Those which will not dissolve until they reach the intestines.

enter′icoid [″ + *eidos*, resemblance]. Resembling typhoid fever.

enteritis (en-ter-i′tis) [″ + *-ītis*, inflammation]. Inflammation of the intestines, more particularly of the mucous and submucous tissues, usually of the small intestines.
  e., acute catarrhal. Acute inflammation of ileum and colon with diarrhea and intestinal catarrh. SYM: Frequent, watery, light colored stools, abdominal colic, flatus. Attack short. TREATMENT: Liquid diet, laxatives, milk purgatives; complete rest.
  e., chronic catarrhal. Chronic inflammation of intestines and colon with chronic diarrhea. SYM: Less severe than acute catarrhal enteritis. TREATMENT: Diet restricted to milk, soups, cooked fruits, and vegetables. Rest.
  e., croupous. Diphtheritic. A sequel of typhoid fever and other diseases. Often characterized by formation of false membrane. TREATMENT: SEE: *chronic c. e.*
  e., mucous. A condition involving the intestinal mucosa characterized by excessive secretion of mucus and passage in the stools of shreds of pseudomembranous material. Usually accompanied by constipation or diarrhea or both alternating; intestinal myxoneurosis.

entero- [G. *enteron*, intestine]. Prefix: Noting some relation to the intestines.

enteroanastomosis (en″ter-o-an-as″to-mo′sĭs) [″ + *ana*, up, + *stomōsis*, a mouth]. Intestinal anastomosis.

enteroan′tigen [″ + *anti*, against, + *gennan*, to form]. An antigen derived from the feces.

enteroapokleisis (en″ter-o-ap-o-kli′sis) [″ + *apokleisis*, a shutting out]. Operation for exclusion of a part of the intestine.

enterobacteriotherapy (ĕn″tĕr-ō-băk-tē″-rĭ-o-ther′ă-pī) [″ + *baktērion*, little rod, + *therapeia*, treatment]. Use of vaccines containing intestinal bacteria.

enterobi′asis [″ + *bios*, life]. Infestation with pin worms (*Enterobius vermicularis*).

enterobil′iary [″ + L. *bilis*, bile]. Pert. to the intestines and the bile passages.

Enterobius (ĕn-tĕr-ō′bĭ-ŭs). A genus of parasitic nematode worms, formerly *Oxyuris*.
  E. vermicularis. A species or nematode worms which inhabits the cecum, appendix, and neighboring regions of the intestine. In females, the genital organs and bladder may become infected. Female worms average 8 to 13 mm. in length, males, 2 to 5 mm. Distribution is world wide. Infestations characterized by irritation of the anal region and allergic reaction of the neighboring skin, accompanied by intense itching which may result in loss of sleep, excessive irritability, and sometimes sexual disorders.

enterobro′sia [″ + *brōsis*, an eating]. Perforation of the intestine.

enterocele (en′ter-o-sēl) [″ + *kēlē*, hernia]. 1. A hernia of the intestine. 2. Post. vaginal hernia.

enterocentesis (en″ter-o-sen-te′sis) [″ + *kentēsis*, puncture]. Puncture of intestine to withdraw gas or fluids.

enterochirurgia (en″ter-o-ki-rur′jĭ-ă) [″ + *cheir*, hand, + *ergon*, work]. Intestinal surgery.

enterocholecystostomy (en″ter-o-ko″le-sis-tos′to-mī) [″ + *cholē*, bile, + *kystis*, a bladder, + *stōma*, opening]. Making an opening bet. the gallbladder and small intestine. SYN: *cholecystenterostomy*.

enterocholecystotomy (en″ter-o-ko″le-sis-tot′o-mĭ) [" + " + tomē, incision]. Incision of both gallbladder and intestine.

enterocinesia (en″ter-o-sin-e′sĭ-ă) [" + kinēsis, movement]. Intestinal movement. SYN: peristalsis.

enterocinetic (en″ter-o-sin-et′ik) [" + kinēsis, movement]. Pert. to or promoting peristalsis.

enteroclysis (en-ter-ok′li-sis) [" + klysis, injection]. 1. Injection of a nutrient or medicinal liquid into bowel. 2. Irrigation of colon with large amt. of fluid intended to fill the colon completely and flush it. SEE: proctoclysis.

PREPARATIONS USED: 1. Bicarbonate of soda, 1 teaspoonful of soda to a pint or quart of normal saline solution. 2. Boiled water with boric acid, ½ to 1 dram to a quart. 3. Powdered alum, 1 teaspoonful to a quart of water, may be used. 4. Flaxseed-tea, made very thin. 5. Normal salt solution, 1 teaspoonful of salt to 1 pint of water. This need not be sterile, unless indicated by rectal operation or condition. 6. Oil of peppermint or cinnamon, 5 to 15 drops to a pint of saline solution or plain water. 7. Potassium permanganate, 3 to 10 grains to 2 quarts of water. 8. Silver nitrate, 10 to 20 grains to a quart of water. Normal saline solution should be used after the silver nitrate treatment. 9. Solution of tannic acid, 1 to 2%. 10. Witch hazel solution.

CHARTING: Note all symptoms of the patient; the amount of the solution given; its nature; time of administering; length of treatment; results obtained and the reaction of the patient as to relief, discomfort, or untoward symptoms.

en′teroclysm [G. enteron, intestine, + klysmos, an injection]. A high enema. SYN: enteroclysis.

enterococcus. Any species of streptococcus inhabiting the intestine.

enterocoele (en″ter-o-se′le) [" + koilia, hollow]. The abdominal cavity.

enterocolitis (en″ter-o-ko-li′tis) [" + kōlon, colon, + itis, inflammation]. Inflammation of intestines and colon, a disease of teething, principally during summer, bet. 6 and 18 months and often later.

SYM: Abdomen swollen, diarrhea, pain, rising temperature. Stools frequent, often 1 an hour. Contain mucus or blood. Urine scanty. Convulsions. The more common types are the catarrhal, tuberculous, and ulcerative.

TREATMENT: Dietetic, anodynes, cold water. DIET: Stop all food; give plenty of water by mouth or rectum. After 24 or 48 hours begin with lemon water, white of egg, whey or buttermilk. In a few days add cream to buttermilk or whey. Institute correct diet for infant feeding.

enterocrinin (ĕn-tĕr-ok′rĭn-ĭn) [G. enteron, intestine, + krinein, to separate]. Hormone from animal intestines, which aids digestion by stimulating the secretion of intestinal juice by the intestinal glands.

enterocyst (en′ter-o-sist) [" + kystis, cyst]. A cyst of the intestinal wall.

enterocystocele (en″ter-o-sis′to-sēl) [" + " + kēlē, hernia]. Hernia of the bladder wall and intestine.

enterocysto′ma [" + " + ōma, tumor]. Cystic tumor of the intestinal wall. SYN: enterocyst.

enterodyn′ia [" + odynē, pain]. Pain in the intestine. SYN: enteralgia.

en″teroenteros′tomy [" + enteron + stōma, opening]. Formation of a communication bet. 2 segments (not continuous) of the intestine.

enteroepiplocele (en″ter-o-e-pip′lo-sēl) [" + epiplōon, omentum, + kēlē, hernia]. Hernia of small intestine and omentum.

en″terogastri′tis [" + gastēr, belly, + itis, inflammation]. Inflammation of stomach (gastritis) and of the intestines (enteritis).

enterogastrone (en″tĕr-ō-gas′trōn) [" + gastēr, belly]. A hormone secreted by the intestinal mucosa which depresses gastric motility and secretion.

enterogenous (en-ter-oj′en-us) [" + gennan, to produce]. Originating in the intestines.

en′terogram [" + gramma, mark]. Tracing or graph of intestinal movements.

enterog′raphy [" + graphein, to write]. 1. A description of the intestines. 2. Making of an enterogram.

en″terohepat′ic [" + ēpar, ēpat-, liver]. Pert. to intestines and the liver.

en″terohepati′tis [" + " + itis, inflammation]. Inflamed condition of both intestine and liver.

enterohydrocele (en″ter-o-hi′dro-sēl) [" + ydōr, water, + kēlē, hernia]. Hydrocele with loop of intestine in the sac.

enteroidea (en-ter-oyd′e-a) [" + eidos, form]. The intestinal fevers; those caused by intestinal bacilli including enteric and parenteric fevers.

enterokinase (en-ter-o-kin′āz) [" + kinēsis, movement]. A substance or hormone occurring in the mucosa of the duodenum, necessary for the activation of the trypsinogen of the pancreatic juice which is converted into trypsin. One of the enzymes of the succus entericus. It has no fat-splitting properties.
RS: enzyme, prosecretin, trypsin, trypsinogen.

en′terolite [" + lithos, stone]. Intestinal calculus.

enterolith (en′ter-o-lith) [" + lithos, stone]. An intestinal concretion.

enterolithiasis (en″ter-o-li-thi′ă-sis) [" + lithos, stone]. The formation or existence of enterolites.

enterol′ogy [" + logos, study]. The study of the intestinal tract.

en″teromega′lia, en″teromeg′aly [" + megas, large]. Abnormal enlargement of the intestines. SYN: megacolon, megaloenteron.

Enteromonas hominis (ĕn-tĕr-ŏm′ō-năs). A minute flagellated, protozoan parasite which lives in the intestine of man. It is rare and considered nonpathogenic.

enteromyiasis (ĕn-tĕr-ō-mĭ-ă′sĭs). Disease due to the presence of maggots (the larvae of flies), in the intestines.

enteromyco′sis [" + mykēs, fungus, + ōsis]. Disease of intestine due to bacteria. May include bacterial diseases.

enteron (en′ter-on) [G.]. The intestine.

enteroneuri′tis [G. enteron, intestine, + neuron, nerve, + itis, inflammation]. Neuritis of the intestine.

enteronitis (en-ter-on-i′tis) [" + itis, inflammation]. Inflammation of the small intestine. SYN: enteritis.

enteroparesis (en-ter-o-par′e-sis) [" + paresis, relaxation]. Flaccidity of the intestinal walls with diminished peristalsis.

enteropathy (en-ter-op′a-thĭ) [" + pathos, disease]. Any intestinal disease.

enteropexy (en′ter-o-peks-ĭ) [" + pēxis, fixation]. Fixation of the intestine to the abdominal wall.

enteroplasty (en'ter-o-plas-tĭ) [" + *plassein*, to form]. Plastic operation on intestines. NP: Watch diet and fluid orders. Care of mouth. SEE: *laparotomy*.

enterople'gia [" + *plēgē*, stroke]. Paralysis of the bowels.

enteroplex (en'ter-o-pleks) [" + *plexis*, a weaving]. Instrument for joining cut edges of intestines.

en'teroplexy [" + *plexis*, a weaving]. Union of divided parts of the intestine.

enteroptosis (en-ter-op-to'sis) [" + *ptōsis*, a dropping]. Prolapse of the intestine or abdominal organs.

enterorrhagia (en"ter-or-ra'jĭ-ă) [" + *rēgnunai*, to burst forth]. Hemorrhage from the intestines.

enterorrhaphy (en-ter-or'ră-fī) [" + *raphē*, suture]. The stitching of the lips of an intestinal wound, or of the intestines to some other structure.

enterorrhexis (en-ter-or-reks'is) [" + *rēxis*, rupture]. Rupture of the intestine.

enteroscope (en'ter-o-skōp) [" + *skopein*, to examine]. Device for examination of intestines.

enterosep'sis [" + *sēpsis*, decay]. Intestinal toxemia; sepsis developed from the intestinal contents.

enterospasm (en'ter-o-spazm) [" + *spasmos*, spasm]. Painful peristalsis.

enterosta'sis [" + *stasis*, a standing]. Intestinal stasis. Cessation of or delay in the passage of food through the intestine.

enterosteno'sis [" + *stēnōsis*, a narrowing]. Narrowing or stricture of the intestine.

enterostomy (en-ter-os'to-mĭ) [" + *stoma*, opening]. Surgical formation of a permanent opening into the intestine through the abdominal wall.

enterotome (en'ter-o-tōm) [" + *tomē*, incision]. Instrument for incision of intestines.

enterotomy (en-ter-ot'o-mĭ) [" + *tomē*, a cutting]. Incision or dissection of the intestines.

en"terotox'in. A toxin produced by certain species of bacteria which produces symptoms characteristic of food poisoning.

enterotox'ism [" + *toxikon*, poison, + *ismos*, condition]. Absorption of intestinal toxins. SYN: *enterosepsis*.

enterotrop'ic [" + *tropē*, a turning]. Affecting or attracted by the intestines.

enterovac'cine [" + L. *vacca*, a cow]. A vaccine composed of fecal bacteria.

enterozo'ic [" + *zōon*, animal]. Pert. to parasites inhabiting the intestines.

enterozo'on [" + *zōon*, animal]. Any intestinal animal parasite.

entheomania (en-the-o-ma'nĭ-ă) [G. *entheos*, inspired, + *mania*, madness]. Religious insanity.

enther'mic [G. *en*, in, + *thermē*, heat]. Promoting or pert. to warmth.

enthesis (ĕn'thĕ-sĭs) [G. a putting in). The use of metallic or other inorganic substances to substitute for or replace lost tissue.

enthetic (en-thet'ĭk) [" + *tithenai*, to place]. Introduced from outside. SYN: *exogenous*.

ento- [G.]. Prefix, *entos*, within, inside.

en'toblast [G. *entos*, within, + *blastos*, germ]. The endoderm or hypoblast.

entocele (en'to-sēl) [" + *kēlē*, hernia]. 1. Internal hernia. 2. Displacement of a part, inward.

entochondrostosis (en"to-kon-dro-sto'sis) [" + *chondros*, cartilage, + *ōsis*]. The development of bone within cartilage.

entochoroidea (en"to-ko-roy'de-ă) [" + *chorioeidēs*, choroid]. The inner layer of the choroid; coat of the eye.

entocineria (en-to-sin-e'rĭ-ă) [" + L. *cinereus*, ashen]. The internal gray matter of nerve centers, esp. of the brain.

entocone (en'to-kōn) [" + *kōnos*, cone]. The inner post. cusp of an upper molar tooth.

entocor'nea [" + L. *corneus*, horny]. Post. or inner lining membrane of cornea. SYN: *Descemet's membrane*.

entocyte (en'to-sīt) [" + *kytos*, cell]. Int. part of a cell within the ectoplasm. SYN: *endoplasm*.

entoderm (en'to-derm) [" + *derma*, skin]. SYN: *endoderm*, *hypoblast*. The inner layer of cells in the blastoderm.* The innermost of the three primary germ layers of a developing embryo. It gives rise to the epithelium of the digestive tract and its associated glands, the respiratory organs, bladder, vagina and urethra.

entoectad (en-to-ek'tad) [" + *ektos*, without, + L. *ad*, toward]. From within outward.

entome (en'tōm) [G. *en*, in, + *tomē*, a cut]. Knife for division of urethral stricture.

entomion (en-to'mĭ-on) [G. *entomē*, notch]. The tip of mastoid angle of the parietal bone.

entomol'ogy [G. *entomon*, insect, + *logos*, science]. The study of insects.
  e. medical. That branch of entomology which deals with insects and their relationship to disease.

entophyte (en'to-fīt) [G. *entos*, within, + *phyton*, plant]. Any vegetable parasite within the body.

entophyton (en-tof'ĭt-on) [" + *phyton*, plant]. Vegetable parasite in the body. SYN: *entophyte*.*

entopic (en-top'ĭk) [G. *en*, in, + *topos*, place]. Normally situated; in a normal place.

entoptic (en-top'tĭk) [G. *entos*, within, + *optikos*, seeing]. Situated in the eyeball.

entoptoscopy (en"top-tos'ko-pī) [" + *ōps*, eye, + *skopein*, to examine]. Inspection of intraocular shadows.

entoral (en-to'răl) [" + L. *os*, or-, mouth]. An oral respiratory vaccine.
  USES: For immunization against colds.

entoret'ina [" + L. *rete*, a net]. Internal layer of the retina.

entorrhagia (en-tor-a'jĭ-ă) [" + *rēgnunai*, to burst forth]. Internal hemorrhage. SEE: *enterorrhagia*.

entos'thoblast [G. *entosthe*, from within, + *blastos*, germ]. Hypothetical nucleus of the nucleolus. SYN: *entoblast*.

entotic (en-to'tĭk) [G. *entos*, within, + *ous*, *ot*-, ear]. Pert. to int. of ear or to perception of sound due to condition of the auditory apparatus.

entozoon (en-to-zo'on) [" + *zōon*, animal]. Any animal parasite in any internal org⊕n.

en'trails [L. *interaneus*, interior]. The intestines.

entrophia (en-tro'fĭ-ă) [G. *en*, in, + *trophē*, nourishment]. Normal growth and nourishment.

entrophy (ĕn-trō'fī). That portion of energy within a system which cannot be utilized for mechanical work.

entro'pion [" + *trepein*, to turn]. Inward curling of eyelid, esp. lower lid, with lashes.
  ETIOL: Spastic contraction of muscular fibers or of a cicatrix.

entropion, citatricial   E-35   **enzyme**

    e. citatricial. A resulting from scar tissue on the inner surface of the lid.
    e. spastic. A resulting from a spasm of the orbicularis oculi muscles.

entro′pionize [" + *trepein*, to turn]. To invert or correct by turning in.

entro′pium [" + *trepein*, to turn]. Inward curling of eyelids. SYN: *entropion*.

en′typy. A turning inward.

enucleate (e-nu′kle-āt) [L. *enucleāre*, to remove the kernel of]. 1. To remove a tumor or a structure from the body without rupturing; to remove a part entire. 2. To destroy or take out the nucleus of a cell.

enucleation (e-nu-kle-a′shun) [L. *enucleāre*, to remove the kernel of]. 1. Removal of a tumor from its capsule. 2. Act of unfolding.

enu′cleator [L. *enucleāre*, to remove the kernel of]. Instrument for separating a tumor mass, as a myoma.

enuresis (en-u-re′sis) [G. *enourein*, to void urine]. Incontinence. Involuntary discharge of urine, complete or partial, diurnal or nocturnal, dependent upon pathologic or functional causes, although it may be voluntary as representative of a behavior pattern.

    A child, for instance, may feel neglected, or feel a desire for attention, and attempt to center attention upon himself by deliberately wetting his bed. Urinary control, however, is generally established after the second year, although incontinence may be reëstablished as a pathological manifestation after the fourth or not later than the eighth year.

    Condition in adults abolished by administration of A. P. L., commercial gonadotropic preparation from placenta, in large doses of 4000 international units.

    e., diurnal. Urinary incontinence during the day and its etiology is of a pathological nature. It may be caused by muscular contractions brought about by laughing, coughing, or crying, and it often persists for long periods of time, esp. after protracted illness, but more frequently in the female.

    ETIOL: Enuresis may result from urethral irritation, and fecal incontinence is sometimes associated with it. Excessive water drinking. There may be deficiency of the cord due to injury, cystitis may be present, and it may be associated with various diseases, such as diabetes insipidus and mellitus, epilepsy, or mental deficiency.

    Children suffering from enuresis may be shy and sensitive; sometimes gloomy. These nervous manifestations may result from the reaction to the condition, or they may be a part of the behavior pattern of which the enuresis is a symptom. Parents should be taught to differentiate between physiological and mental causes of enuresis, as the child who is suffering from pathological symptoms should not be reproached or punished for that which is beyond his control.

    TREATMENT: Examine the urine as soon as possible, esp. to ascertain the presence of white cells which are indicative of abnormality of the urinary tract. Great concern or censure should be avoided as it adds to apprehensiveness on part of child. If the result of a behavior pattern, the condition should be ignored as much as possible, but the cause of the behavior difficulty needs to be found and corrected.

    Fluid should be restricted late in day, and diurnal voidings should be spaced at more than ordinary intervals. The child may be awakened once or twice in the night and when fully awake, robed and walked to the bathroom. As improvement is noticed the number of awakenings may be lessened. The foot of the bed may also be elevated.

    e., nocturnal. Urinary incontinence during the night. Wetting is irregular, and unaccompanied by urgency or frequency. Incontinence may cease for several weeks only to return. This type is more common in boys than in girls.

envi′ronment [L. *in*, in, + *virer*, to turn]. The surroundings, conditions, or influences which affect an organism, or the cells within an organism.

    e. external. Those influences which are outside the body.
    e. internal. Those influences within the body. Specifically, the tissue fluid constitutes the internal environment.

enzygotic (en-zi-got′ĭk) [G. *en*, in, + *zygon*, yoke]. Developed from the same ovum.

    e. twins. Identical twins; those developed from one ovum. SEE: *dizygotic*.

enzyme (en′zim) [" + *zymē*, leaven]. An organic catalyst produced by living cells but capable of acting independently of the cells producing them. They are complex colloidal substances which are capable of inducing chemical changes in other substances without themselves being changed in the process. Many enzymes have been isolated in pure crystalline form and all have proved to be protein in nature.

    Enzymes are found particularly in digestive juices, acting upon food substances causing them to break down into simpler compounds. They are capable of accelerating greatly the speed of chemical reactions.

    The reactions affected by the digestive enzymes are chiefly decompositions of a hydrolytic nature, but enzymes are equally important in the synthetic reactions of assimilation.

    Each hydrolytic enzyme has been given a name which indicates the substance upon which it acts with the addition of the suffix *ase*. As an example, *lipases* indicate fat-splitting enzymes; *amylases*, starch-splitting ones, and *proteases*, protein-splitting enzymes. Some of them take a qualifying adjective, as salivary or pancreatic enzymes. Exceptions are the enzymes rennin, pepsin, and trypsin.

    The substance acted upon by an enzyme is called the *substrate*. Zymogen is the name given to the inactive enzyme within a cell. The more common groups of enzymes are: (a) Hydrolytic e., fat, protein, starch, and sugar-splitting e's. (b) Coagulating e's or those which cause clotting. (c) Oxidases or oxydizing e's, deaminizing e's. Those destroying aminos or amino groups during oxidation. (d) Reductases or reducing e's. (e) Those producing carbon dioxide without the use of free oxygen. (f) Those which produce the breakdown of a larger molecule into a smaller one without change of composition. (g) Mutases, those which bring about chemical rearrangement without change of the molecules in size.

    Enzymes are specific in their action, *i. e.*, they will act only upon a certain substance or a group of chemically closely related substances and no other; each enzyme has an optimum temperature at which it acts with greatest efficiency; each enzyme is influenced by the reaction of the medium in which it acts, there being an optimum degree of acidity or alkalinity.

Enzyme activity can be retarded or inhibited by (a) low temperatures, (b) high temperatures, (c) presence of salts of heavy metals (copper, mercury), (d) dehydration, (e) ultraviolet radiation.

Enzymes sometimes require the presence of additional substances in order to make them active. Nonspecific substances which activate enzymes are called *activators* (Ex: HCl for pepsin); specific substances which act selectively with certain enzymes only are called *coenzymes* (Ex: enterokinase for trypsinogen).

e., amylolytic. E. changing starch to sugar.

e., autolytic. E. producing autolysis, or cell digestion.

e., bacterial. E. developed by bacteria.

e. coagulating. E. converting soluble proteins into insoluble ones. Ex: rennin. A coagulase.

e., deamidizing. E. dividing amino acids into ammonia compounds.

e. decarboxylating. E. which separates CO_2 from organic acids. (Ex: *carboxylase*).

e. digestive. E. which is involved in digestive processes in the alimentary canal.

e. extracellular. E. which produces its effects outside the cell that produces it.

e. of fermentation. E. produced by bacteria or yeasts which bring about the fermentation of substances esp., carbohydrates.

e., glycolytic. E. oxidizing sugar.

e. hydrolytic. E. which decomposes a substance by the addition of water.

e., inorganic. A metallic colloidal solution, acting somewhat like an e.

e. intracellular. An enzyme that acts within the cell which produces it.

Summary of the Main Enzymatic Processes in Digestion*

Site	Secretion	Enzyme	Substrate	Degree of Digestion	Products of Digestion
Mouth.	Saliva.	Ptyalin.	Starch.	Slight.	Dextrins, maltose.
		Maltase (?).	Maltose.	Very slight.	Glucose.
Stomach.	Gastric juice.	Pepsin.	Protein.	Incomplete.	Proteoses, peptones.
		Lipase.	Emulsified fats.	Very slight.	Fatty acids, glycerol.
Intestine.	Pancreatic juice.	Trypsin.	Proteins. Proteoses. Polypeptides.	Nearly complete.	Peptides, amino acids.
		Steapsin.	Fats.	Nearly complete.	Fatty acids, glycerol.
		Amylopsin.	Starch.	Nearly complete.	Dextrins, maltose.
		Maltase.	Maltose.	Fairly complete.	Glucose.
		Lactase.	Lactose.	Fairly complete.	Glucose, galactose.
		Invertase (?)	Sucrose.	Fairly complete.	Glucose, fructose.
		Rennin.	Casein.	Complete.	Paracasein.
		Erepsin.	Ordinary peptides.	Nearly complete.	Amino acids.
Intestine.	Intestinal juice and intestinal mucosa.	Erepsin.	Ordinary peptides.	Nearly complete.	Amino acids.
		Amylase.	Starch.	Nearly complete.	Dextrins, maltose.
		Rennin.	Casein.	Generally complete.	Paracasein.
		Enterokinase.	Activates trypsin.		
		Lipase.	Fat.	Nearly complete.	Fatty acids, glycerol.
		Maltase.	Maltose.	Complete.	Glucose.
		Lactase.	Lactose.	Complete.	Glucose, galactose.
		Invertase.	Sucrose.	Usually complete.	Glucose, fructose.
		Nucleinases.	Nucleic acids.	Usually complete.	Mononucleotides.
		Nucleotidases.	Mononucleotides.	Usually complete.	Nucleosides phosphoric acid.
		Nucleosidases (in mucosa).	Nucleosides.	Usually complete.	Purine bases, carbohydrates.

* Harry M. Vars, Ph.D., *Cyclopedia of Medicine, Surgery and Specialties.*

e. inverting. E. that converts a double sugar (sucrose) into simple sugars.
e. lipolytic. E. that acts on fats hydrolyzing them to glycerol and fatty acids; a lipase.
e., oxidation. SEE: *deamidizing e.*
e. oxidizing. E. that catalyzes oxidative reactions; an oxidase or dehydrogenase.
e., polypeptolytic. E. having a hydrolytic action on the polypeptids.
e., proteolysis. E. changing proteins into peptones.
e., reducing. Reductase. One that withdraws oxygen.
e. respiratory. E. that acts within tissue cells catalyzing oxidative reactions with the release of energy. Ex: *flavoproteins, cytochromes.*
e., steatolytic. SEE: *lipolytic e.*
e., sucrolastic. E. dividing or decomposing sugar.
e., uricolytic. E. converting uric acid into urea.
e. Warburg's yellow. An oxidative enzyme isolated from yeast cells.
e. yellow. A flavoprotein. One of a group of enzymes involved in cellular oxidations.
enzymolysis (en-zim-ol'ĭ-sis) [G. *en*, in, + *zymē*, leaven, + *lysis*, dissolution]. Chemical change caused by an enzyme. SYN: *enzymosis.*
enzymo'sis [" + " + *ōsis*]. Fermentation due to an enzyme. SYN: *enzymolysis.*
enzymu'ria [" + " + *ouron*, urine]. Enzymes in the urine.
eonism (e'on-izm). Desire to dress in the clothing of the opposite sex; a sexual perversion. SYN: *transvestitism.*
eosin(e (e'ō-sĭn, -sēn) [G. *eōs*, dawn (rose colored)]. ($C_{20}H_8Br_4O_5$.) 1. A dye derived from action of bromine on fluorescein. An acid dye much used for diagnostic purposes.
Brownish-red crystals used in microscopy as a stain. SYN: *tetrabromfluorescein.*
2. Any of several similar dyes.
3. Rosy-red; dawn colored.
eosin'oblast [G. *eōs*, dawn, + *blastos*, germ]. A bone marrow cell which develops into a myelocyte. SYN: *myeloblast.*
eosinopenia (e″o-sin-o-pe'nĭ-ă) [" + *penia*, poverty]. Abnormally small number of eosinophil cells in the peripheral blood.
eosinophil(e (e-o-sin'o-fĭl, or -fĭl) [" + *philein*, to love]. A cell or cellular structure that stains readily with the acid stain, *eosin*; specifically an eosinophile leucocyte.
Eosinophils are present in small numbers under normal conditions. Supposed to originate in bone marrow.
They are large, slightly irregular cells with very distinct, bright pink granules. These granules cover the protoplasm, often making it invisible. Occasionally there are vacuoles scattered about through the granules. The nucleus is of a polymorphonuclear type. They make up from ½ to 2% of the white cells of normal man. SEE: *oxyphil.*
e. leucocytes. Spherical cells found in blood and sometimes in connective tissues having a diameter of 9 to 14 microms. The nucleus is polymorphic usually having two lobes connected by a thin strand. The cytoplasm contains numerous coarse, highly refractile granules which stain intensely with eosin or other acid stains. They constitute 2 to 4 per cent of the white cell count.

Eosinophil leucocytes originate in the red bone marrow. Their function is not well established. They are ameboid but do not exhibit phagocytic activity. They increase in number in certain diseases such as asthma and in certain infestations with animal parasites. They decrease in number in circulating blood following the administration of ACTH or cortisone.
eosinophilia (e″o-sin-o-fĭl'ĭ-ă) [" + *philein*, to love]. 1. Accumulation of unusual number of eosinophil cells in the blood. 2. Condition of being eosinophilic.
eosinophilic (e″o-sin-o-fĭl'ĭk) [" + *philein*, to love]. Readily stainable with eosin.
eosinoph'ilous [" + *philein*, to love]. 1. Easily stainable with eosin. 2. Having eosinophilia.
eosinotactic (e-o-sin-o-tak'tĭk) [" + *taktikos*, arranged]. Attraction or repulsion of eosinophil cells.
epacmastic (ep-ak-mas'tĭk) [G. *epi*, upon, + *akmē*, prime]. Denoting increase of symptoms. RS: *acmastic, paracmastic.*
epac'tal [G. *epaktos*, added to]. Supernumerary.
e. bone. Wormian bone.
eparsalgia (ep-ar-sal'jĭ-ă) [G. *epairein*, to lift, + *algos*, pain]. Any disorder due to overstrain of a part. SYN: *epersalgia.*
eparter'ial. Located over or above an artery.
epaxial (ep-ak'sĭ-al) [G. *epi*, upon, + L. *axis*, axis]. Situated above or behind any axis.
epencephalon (ep-en-sef'al-on) [" + *egkephalos*, brain]. The metencephalon; the anterior portion of the embryonic hind brain (rhombencephalon) from which arise the pons and cerebellum.
ependyma (ep-en'dim-ă) [G. *ependyma*, wrap]. Membrane lining the cerebral ventricles and central canal of spinal cord.
e. medullae spinalis. The spinal portion of the e.
e. ventriculorum cerebri. The ventricular portion of the e.
epen'dym'al. Pertaining to the ependyma.
e. cells. Cells of the developing neural tube which give rise to the ependyma. They arise from spongioblasts derived from the neural epithelium.
e. layer. The innermost of three layers which form the neural tube of an embryo.
ependymitis (ep″en-dim-i'tis) [" + -*itis*, inflammation]. Inflammation of the ependyma.
ependymoblast (ep-en'dĭ-mo-blast [" + *blastos*, germ]. An embryonic ependymal cell or ependymocyte.
ependymocyte (ep-en'dĭ-mo-sīt) [" + *kytos*, cell]. A cell of the ependymal region.
ependymo'ma [" + *ōma*, tumor]. A tumor arising from fetal inclusion of ependymal elements.
epersal'gia [G. *epairein*, to lift, + *algos*, pain]. Pain and soreness due to overuse or unaccustomed use of a part.
ephebic (ef-e'bik) [G. *ephēbikos*, pert. to puberty]. Pert. to adolescence.
ephebology (e-fe-bol'o-jī) [G. *ephēbos*, puberty]. The study of puberty and its changes.
ephedrine (ef'ed-rin). An alkaloid obtained from *Ma huang*, a species of *Ephedra*; first isolated by Nagai in 1887. *Ma huang* had a reputation in ancient

ephedrine, hydrochloride   E-38   **epidermization**

Chinese medicine as a diaphoretic and antipyretic. It was not until recent times, however, that its action was studied and its valuable therapeutic properties made known.
ACTION: Similar to that of adrenalin. Its effects, although less powerful, are more prolonged, and it exerts an action when given orally, whereas adrenalin is effective only by injection. Ephedrine orally (or by injection) dilates the bronchial muscles, contracts the nasal mucosa, and raises the blood pressure. Chiefly used for its bronchodilator effect in asthma, and for its constricting effects on the nasal mucosa in hay fever.
DOSAGE: From 1/4-5/6 gr. (0.015-0.05 Gm.). Some patients need carefully regulated doses. The least dose which will give the specific desired effect is desirable.
INCOMPATIBILITIES: *Calcium chloride, iodine, tannic acid.*
e. hydrochloride. USP. A more soluble salt of the alkaloid, containing about 80% ephedrine.
DOSAGE: ⅜ gr. (0.025 Gm.); locally, in from ½ to 3%.
INCOMPATIBILITIES: *Sodium bicarbonate.*
e. sulfate. This contains about 75% ephedrine; dosage and uses same as *e. hydrochloride,* but believed by some to be more irritant.
ephelis (ef-e'lis) [G. *ephēlis,* freckle]. Freckle, lentigo.*
ephemeral (e-fem'er-al) [G. *epi,* upon, + *ēmera,* day]. Of brief duration.
ephidrosis (ef-ĭ-dro'sis) [G. *ephidrōsis,* a sweating]. Abnormal amt. of sweating.
e. cruenta. Sweat containing blood.
e. saccharata. Diabetic condition in which sugar is present in sweat.
e. tincta. Colored sweat. SYN: *chromidrosis.*
epi-, ep- [G.]. Prefix meaning upon, at, in addition to.
epiallopregnanolone (ĕp″ĭ-al″o-prĕg-nan'ō-lōn). Male sex hormone in urine of pregnant women, which helps to form male sex characteristics.
epiblast [G. *epi,* upon, + *blastos,* germ]. SYN: *Ectoderm, q.v.* Outer layer of cells of the blastoderm. SEE: *hypoblast.*
epiblastic (ep-ĭ-blas'tĭk) [" + *blastos,* germ]. Pert. to the epiblast.
epibole, epiboly (ĕ-pĭb'o-lĭ) [G. *epibolē,* cover]. Inclusion of the hypoblast within the epiblast, due to swifter growth of the latter. SEE: *emboly.*
epibular (ĕp-ĭ-būl'ar). Lying upon the bulb of any structure; more specifically, located upon the eyeball.
epican'thus [G. *epi,* upon, + *kanthos,* canthus]. A fold of skin extending from the root of the nose to the median end of the eyebrow, covering the inner canthus and caruncle. It is a characteristic of the Mongolian race and may occur as a congenital anomaly in Caucasiana.
epicardia (ĕp-ĭ-kărd'ĭ-ă). [" + *kardia,* heart]. The abdominal portion of the esophagus extending from the diaphragm to the stomach, about 2 cm. in length.
epicar'dium [" + *kardia,* heart]. The inner or visceral layer of the pericardium,* which forms a serous membrane forming the outermost layer of the wall of the heart.
epicele, epicoelia (ep'ĭs-ēl, -ĭ-coy'lĭ-a) [" + *koilia,* hollow]. The fourth ventricle of the brain.

epichordal (ĕp-ĭ-kôrd'ăl). Located dorsad to the notochord.
epicomus (ĕp-ĭ-kōm'ŭs). A monster with a parasitic twin, or head attached to the summit or vertex of the skull.
epicondylalgia (ĕp-ĭ-kŏnd-ĭ-lăl'jĭ-ă). [" + *kondylos,* condyle, + *algos,* pain]. Pain in the elbow joint in the region of the epicondyles.
epicon'dyle [" + *kondylos,* condyle]. The eminence at the articular end of a bone above a condyle.
epicra'nium [" + *kranion,* cranium]. Soft parts covering the cranium.
epicranius (ep-ĭ-kra'nĭ-us) [" + *kranion,* cranium]. Occipitofrontal muscle and scalp.
epicri'sis [" + *krisis,* crisis]. A supplementary or secondary crisis following a return of morbid symptoms.
epicritic (ep-ĭ-krĭt'ĭk) [G. *epikritikos,* judging]. Pert. to extreme sensibility, such as that of the skin when it discriminates between degrees of sensation caused by touch or temperature.
epicysti'tis [G. *epi,* upon, + *kystis,* bladder, + *itis,* inflammation]. Inflammation of cellular tissue above the bladder.
epicystot'omy [" + " + *tomē,* incision]. Opening above the symphysis pubis into the bladder.
epicyte (ep'ĭ-sīt) [" + *kytos,* cell]. 1. An epithelial cell. 2. A cell membrane.
epidem'ic [" + *dēmos,* people]. Appearance of an infectious disease not of local origin which attacks many people at the same time in the same area. SEE: *Winckel's disease.*
e. jaundice. Infectious or spirochetal jaundice; Weil's disease. An infectious disease caused by a spirochete, *Leptospira, icterohaemorrhagiae.* SYM: Onset of sudden fever, in a few days followed by jaundice, hemorrhage into skin, and anemia. SEE: *caribi, endemic, pandemic.*
epidemiog'raphy [" + " + *graphein,* to write]. Study of epidemic diseases.
epidemiologic (ep″ĭ-dem'ĭ-o-loj'ĭk) [" + " + *logos,* study]. Pert. to the study of epidemics.
epidemiologist (ep″ĭ-dem-ĭ-ol'o-jist) [" + " + *logos,* study]. One who specializes in epidemic diseases.
epidemiology (ep-ĭ-dem-ĭ-ol'o-jĭ) [" + " + *logos,* study]. The science of epidemic diseases.
epider'mal, epider'mic [" + *derma,* skin]. Pert. to the epidermis.
epidermatoplasty (ep-ĭ-der-mat'o-plas-tī) [" + " + *plassein,* to mould]. Grafting with pieces of epidermis with the underlying layer of the corium.
epidermic (ep-ĭ-der'mĭk) [" + *derma,* skin]. Pert. to the external layer of the skin or epidermis.
epidermidol'ysis [" + " + *lysis,* loosening]. Loosening of the epidermis. SYN: *epidermolysis.*
epidermido'sis [" + " + *ōsis*]. Any disease of the skin. SYN: *epidermosis.*
epider'mis [" + *derma,* skin]. Cuticle, or outer layer of skin; scarf-skin.
It consists of four layers; (1) stratum germinativum (stratum mucosum, stratum Malpighi) which is the innermost; (2) stratum granulosum; (3) stratum lucidum; and (4) stratum corneum, the outermost.
epidermi'tis [" + " + *itis,* inflammation]. Inflammation of the superficial layers of the skin.
epidermization (ep-e-der-mĭ-za'shun) [" + *derma,* skin]. Skin grafting. Conversion of deeper germinative layer of cells into outer and horny layer of epidermis.

epidermoid (ep-ĭ-der'moyd) [" + " + *eidos*, form]. 1. Resembling or pert. to the epidermis. 2. A tumor arising from aberrant epidermal cells. SYN: *cholesteatoma*.

epidermolysis (ep-ĭ-der-mol'ĭs-is) [" + " + *lysis*, loosening]. Loosening of the epidermis.

  e. bullosa. A form characterized by formation of deep seated bullae appearing after irritation or rubbing of a part.

epidermo'ma [" + " + *ōma*, growth]. An excrescence on the skin.

epidermomycosis (ep-ĭ-der"mo-mĭ-ko'sis) [" + " + *mykēs*, fungus, + *ōsis*]. Skin disease caused by a fungus.

Epidermophyton (ep-ĭ-der-mof'ĭ-ton) [" + " + *phyton*, plant]. A genus of fungi causing tinea cruris or Dhobie itch, *q.v.*

  E. floccosum. The causative agent of certain types of tinea, esp., *tinea pedis* (athlete's foot), *tinea cruris*, and others.

epidermophytosis (ep-ĭ-der-mo-fĭ-to'sis) [" + " + " + *ōsis*]. Infection by a species of Epidermophyton. SYN: *Dhobie itch, washerwoman's itch, tinea cruris, tinea inguinalis.*

epidermo'sis [" + " + *ōsis*]. Any disease affecting the skin esp., the epidermis.

epidi'ascope [" + *dia*, through, + *skopein*, to examine]. Lantern used for projection of images on a screen. SYN: *episcope.*

epididymectomy (ep-ĭ-did-ĭ-mek'to-mĭ) [G. *epi*, upon, + *didymos*, testis, + *ektomē*, excision]. Removal of the epididymus.

epididymis (ep-ĭ-did'ĭ-mis) (Pl. *epididymidēs*) [" + *didymos*, testis]. A small, oblong body resting upon and beside the post. surface of the testes, consisting of a convoluted tube 18-20 ft. long, enveloped in the tunica vaginalis, ending in the vas deferens.

  It consists of (1) the *head* caput or globus major which contains 12 to 14 efferent ducts of the testis, (2) the *body*, and (3) the *tail* (cauda or globus minor). It constitutes the first part of the excretory duct of each testis. The epididymis is supplied by the internal spermatic, deferential, and external spermatic arteries; it is drained by corresponding veins.

epididymitis (ep-ĭ-did-im-i'tis) [" + " + *itis*, inflammation]. Inflammation of the epididymus.

  ETIOL: Inflammation of internal genitals traveling up urethra. SEE: *epididymus.*

  e., gonorrheal. In third to eighth week of gonorrhea, symptoms either acute (swelling increasing rapidly involving testes, scrotum, etc.) or subacute (moderate swelling developing slowly), with pain.

  TREATMENT: Rest in bed, immobilization of testes, local applications, ice pack.

  e., nongonorrheal. Resembles gonorrheal but often terminates in gross suppuration. TREATMENT: Prophylactic, by gentleness in treatment of urethritis. Suspensory bandage, hygienic regimen. Operation if palliative measures fail.

  e. nonspecific. E. resulting from invasion of the epididymus by pyogenic organisms. May occur in connection with urethral stricture, cystitis, or prostatitis.

  e., relapsing. Any acute form that becomes chronic.

  e. specific. E. resulting from the organisms of gonorrhea, syphilis, pneumonia, meningitis, or other diseases.

  e. traumatic. E. which occurs in the absence of a demonstrable causative factor.

epididymodeferentectomy (ep-ĭ-did-ĭ-mo-def"er-en-tek'to-mĭ) [" + " + L. *deferens*, carrying away, + G. *ektomē*, excision]. Excision of epididymis and vas deferens.

epididymodeferen'tial [" + " + L. *deferens*, carrying away]. Concerning both the epididymis and vas deferens.

epididymoörchitis (ep-ĭ-did-im-o-or-ki'tis) [" + " + *orchis*, testis, + *itis*, inflammation]. Epididymitis with orchitis.*

epididymot'omy [" + " + *tomē*, incision]. Incision into the epididymis.

epididymovasotomy (ep-ĭ-did"im-o-vas-os'to-mĭ) [" + " + L. *vas*, vessel, + *tomē*, incision]. Making an anastomosis bet. the epididymis and the vas.

epidu'ral [" + L. *durus*, hard]. Located over or upon the dura.

  e. space. Space outside of dura mater of brain and spinal cord.

epifascial. On or upon a fascia.

epifolliculitis (ep-ĭ-fol-lik-u-li'tis) [" + L. *folliculus*, follicle, + G. *itis*, inflammation]. Inflammation of hair follicles of the scalp.

epigas'ter [" + *gastēr*, belly]. Embryonic structure which develops into the large intestine. SYN: *hindgut.*

ep"igastral'gia [" + " + *algos*, pain]. Pain in the epigastrium.

epigas'tric [" + *gastēr*, belly]. Pert. to the epigastrium. SEE: *precordia.*

  e. reflex. Contraction of the upper portion of the rectus abdominis muscle when skin of the epigastric region is scratched.

epigastrium (ep-ĭ-gas'trĭ-um) [" + *gastēr*, belly]. Region over the pit of the stomach. SEE: *Auenbrugger's sign.*

epigastrocele (ep-ĭ-gas'tro-sēl) [" + " + *kēlē*, hernia]. Hernia in the epigastrium.

epigastrorrhaphy (ep-ĭ-gas-tror'ă-fĭ) [" + " + *raphē*, suture]. Suture of an abdominal wound in the epigastric area.

epigenesis (ep-ĭ-jen'es-is) [" + *genesis*, formation]. In embryology, the theory that parts of an organism arise by a process of progressive development from simple to complex structures through the utilization of cells as building units; in contrast to preformation which holds that parts exist in the ovum performed.

epiglottid'ean [" + *glottis*, glottis]. Pert. to the epiglottis.

epiglottidectomy (ep"ĭ-glot-id-ek'to-mĭ) [" + " + *ektomē*, excision]. Excision of the epiglottis.

epiglottiditis (ep'ĭ-glot-tid-i'tis) [" + " + *itis*, inflammation]. Inflammation of the epiglottis. SYN: *epiglottitis.*

epiglot'tis (pl. *epiglottidēs*) [" + *glottis*, glottis]. A thin leaf-shaped structure located immediately posterior to the root of the tongue which covers the entrance of the larynx when swallowing. It consists of the epiglottic cartilage, an impaired laryngeal cartilage, and is covered with mucous membrane.

epiglottitis (ep'ĭ-glot-ti'tis) [" + " + *itis*, inflammation]. Inflammation of the epiglottis. SYN: *epiglottiditis.*

epihy'al [" + *uoeidēs*, U-shaped]. Pert. to the arch of the hyoid.

  e. bone. Ossified stylohyoid ligament.

epilate (ep'ĭ-lāt) [L. *ē*, out, + *pilus*, hair]. To extract the hair by the roots.

ep'ilating [" + *pilus*, hair]. Depilating; extracting a hair.

e. dose. The quantity of roentgen rays or radium necessary to cause temporary loss of hair.
e. forceps. Tweezers for pulling out hairs.
epilation (ep-i-la′shun) [" + *pilus*, hair]. Extraction of hair. SYN: *depilation*.
epilatory (e-pil′a-tor-ĭ) [" + *pilus*, hair]. Pert. to removal of hairs, or that which removes them. SYN: *depilatory*.
epilemma (ep-ĭ-lem′ă) [G. *epi*, upon, + *lemma*, husk]. Neurilemma of small branches of nerve filaments.
ep′′ilep′sy [G. *epilēpsia*, seizure]. An episodic disturbance of consciousness during which generalized convulsions may occur.

ETIOL: Unknown; however, electroencephalographic studies reveal a direct relationship between changes in electrical brain potentials and the occurrence of seizures. Heredity plays an important role.

SYM: Often a peculiar sensation or feeling (the aura) precedes loss of consciousness. The patient falls during the attack, often injuring himself; he may bite his tongue, pass urine, and awake to realize something has happened because of muscular soreness.

There is a tendency to sleep following the attack; indeed attacks may occur only during sleep. The convulsion may be replaced by a so-called equivalent—during the unconsciousness, violent, antisocial or unnatural conduct may occur (automatism), which may have vast medicolegal significance.

On recovery, amnesia is complete and so no precautions to hide the antisocial acts are taken; this in itself is significant, esp. if associated with postautomatism, sleep, and a particularly vicious type of crime. The epileptic may gradually deteriorate, and in some cases finally become completely demented.

TREATMENT: Do not attempt to stop attack. During attack arrange head so as to facilitate breathing. Prevent tongue from being bitten, or from obstructing windpipe. Place pad between teeth during attack. Afterward allow patient to sleep. Dilantin is used as an anticonvulsant without depressive action, but toxicity must be guarded against.

DIET: Ketogenic diet, *q.v.* One rich in fat has been successful in some cases due to the fact that it produces acidosis. An acid condition of the system seems to improve such patients. Fasting causes ketosis, or a mild acidosis, but a high-fat, low-carbohydrate diet produces the same condition. (a) Very little meat; no salt; milk, 2 pints, and 2 eggs daily; white fish sometimes; bread and butter; plenty of vegetables. (b) Lactovegetarian diet. (c) Salt-free diet. (d) Bread made with sodium bromide. Avoid overeating; tea, coffee, alcohol, strong soups, etc.

GRAND MAL: Often preceded by a peculiar sensation known as an aura, beginning in finger or toe and rising until head is involved, when patient gives shrill cry and falls unconscious; tonic spasm followed by clonic movements; face cyanosed; frothing at mouth; coma.

PROG: Unfavorable, although not fatal.

PETIT MAL: Seizure consists of momentary unconsciousness.
e. abortive. Petit mal.
e., cardiac. E. causing severe interference with heart action.
e., cortical. SEE: Jacksonian e.
e. focal. SYN: *cortical e., Jacksonian e. symptomatic e.* E. due to a local injury or lesion of the motor areas of the cerebral cortex.
e., hemiplegic. SEE: *cortical e.*
e., idiopathic. Presence of epilepsy without known cause.
e. Jacksonian. E. in which convulsions tend to be restricted to certain groups of muscles, or limited to one side of the body, due to disease involving the cortex. Also called cortical or symptomatic e.
e., menstrual. Form in which attacks coincide with menstruation.
e. myoclonic. E. in which clonic contractions of muscles, esp., those of the extremities, occur between seizures. SEE: myoclinia.
e., nocturnal. Occurs only during sleep. Symptoms similar to grand mal. PROG: Favorable.
e., partial. SEE: *cortical e.*
e. reflex. E. in which attacks are induced by peripheral irritation.
e., sleep. Spasmodic uncontrollable desire to sleep. SYN: *narcolepsy.*
e., spinal. E. due to lateral sclerosis of the spinal cord.
e. symptomatic. Cortical, focal, or Jacksonian e. Epilepsy due to an identifiable lesion of the brain.
e., syphilitic. E. present in syphilis.
e., thalamic. Form with lesion of the thalamus, causing hallucinations.
e. toxemic. E. due to presence of toxic substances in the blood.
e., traumatic. E. caused by trauma, particularly of the cranial vertex.
e. uncinate. E. due to a lesion of the uncinate gyrus of the temporal lobe.
epilepsy, words pert. to: absentia epileptica, analepsis, aura, cataptosis, fit, furor epilepticus, haut mal, ictus, status epilepticus.
epilep′tic [G. *epilēptikos*, pert. to a seizure]. 1. Concerning epilepsy. 2. Individual suffering from epileptic attacks.
epilep′tiform [G. *epilēpsia*, seizure, + L. *forma*, form]. Having the form of epilepsy.
epileptogen′ic, epileptog′enous [" + *gennan*, to produce]. Giving rise to epileptoid convulsions.
e. zone. Certain motor areas in cerebral cortex, irritation of which gives rise to an epileptic seizure.
epilep′toid [" + *eidos*, resemblance]. Resembling epilepsy. SYN: *epileptiform.*
epileptol′ogy [" + *logos*, study]. Study of epilepsy.
epileptosis (ep-ĭ-lep-to′sis) [" + *ōsis*]. Any mental disease due to epilepsy.
epiloia (ep-il-oi′ă). SYN: *tuberous sclerosis, tuberose gliosis, hypertrophic nodular gliosis.* A syndrome consisting of mental deficiency, adenoma sebaceum, epileptic fits, hypertrophic sclerosis of the brain, tumors in the kidneys, and nodules on floor of lateral ventricle.
epimandibular (ep′′ĭ-man-dib′u-lar) [G. *epi*, upon, + L. *mandibulum*, jaw]. Above or upon the lower jaw.
epimenorrhagia (ep-ĭ-men-o-ra′jĭ-ă) [" + *mēn*, month, + *rēgnunai*, to burst forth]. Profuse menstruation.
epimenorrhea (ep-ĭ-men-o-re′ă) [" + " + *roia*, flow]. Too frequent menstruation.
epimerite (ep-ĭ-mer′ĭt) [" + *meros*, part]. An organ of certain protozoa by which they attach themselves to epithelial cells.
epimysium (ep-ĭ-mis′ĭ-um) [" + *mys*, muscle]. Outermost sheath of connective tissue which surrounds a skeletal muscle. Consists of irregularly dis-

epinasty E-41 **episiostenosis**

tributed collagenous, reticular, and elastic fibers, connective tissue cells, and fat cells.

ep'inasty [" + *nastos*, pressed close]. More vigorous growth on the upper than on the under surface, leading to a downward curvature of an organ.

epinephrectomy (ep-ĭ-ne-frek'to-mĭ) [" + *nephros*, kidney, + *ektomē*, excision]. Excision of the suprarenal gland. SYN: *adrenalectomy*.

epinephrine (adrenalin) (ep-ĭ-nef'rĭn) [G. *epi*, upon, + *nephros*, kidney]. ($C_9H_{13}NO_3$). SYN: *adrenalin, adrenine, suprarenalin, suprarenin*. USP. The active principle of the medulla of the adrenal gland, occurring as a white or light brown powder, darkening on exposure to the air. It has been prepared synthetically. It is employed therapeutically as a vasoconstrictor, cardiac stimulant, to induce uterine contractions and to relax bronchioles. Its effects are similar to those brought about by stimulation of the sympathetic division of the autonomic nervous system.
DOSAGE (1:1000 solut.): *Subcut.*, 1/120 gr. (0.0005 Gm.)
e. hydrochloride solution. USP. A 1:1000 solution of the drug.
USES: To check local hemorrhage, to relieve asthmatic paroxysms, shock, etc. Also to prolong action of local anesthetics by constricting blood vessels, which prevents rapid absorption.
AVERAGE DOSAGE: Hypodermically, 8 ℳ (0.5 cc.).
INCOMPATIBILITIES: Light, heat, and air, iron salts, and alkalies.

epinephrinemia (ep''ĭ-nef''rĭ-ne'mĭ-ă) [" + " + *aima*, blood]. Epinephrine in the blood.

epinephritis (ĕp''ĭ-nef-ri'tis) [G. *epi*, upon, + *nephros*, kidney, + *itis*, inflammation]. Inflammation of an adrenal gland.

epinephro'ma [" + " + *ōma*, tumor]. A lipomatous tumor of the kidney. SYN: *Grawitz's tumor, hypernephroma*.

epineural (ep-ĭ-nū'ral) [" + *neuron*, nerve]. Located upon a neural arch.

epineurium (ep''ĭ-nu'rĭ-um) [" + *neuron*, nerve]. The general connective tissue sheath of a nerve. SEE: *nerve*.

ep'iot'ic [" + *ous*, *ot-*, ear]. Located above the ear.
e. center. Ossification center of temporal bone forming upper and post. part of the auditory capsule.

epipas'tic [" + *passein*, to sprinkle]. Resembling a dusting powder.

epipharynx (ep-i-far'inks) [" + *pharygx*, pharynx]. Nasal portion of pharynx. SYN: *rhinopharynx*.

epiphenom'enon [" + *phainomenon*, phenomenon]. An exceptional and extraneous phenomenon in a disease.

epiphora (e-pif'o-ra) [G. downpour]. Abnormal overflow of tears down the cheek.

epiphylac'tic [G. *epi*, upon, + *phylaxis*, protection]. Pert. to epiphylaxis.

epiphylax'is [" + *phylaxis*, protection]. Increase of defensive powers of the body.

epiphyseal (ep-ĭ-fĭz'e-al) [G. *epiphysis*, a growing upon]. Pert. to or of the nature of an epiphysis.

epiphyseolysis (ep''ĭ-fĭz-e-ol'is-is) [" + *lysis*, loosening]. Separation of an epiphysis.

epiphyseopathy (ep''i-fĭz-e-op'ă-thĭ) [" + *pathos*, disease]. Any disease of an epiphysis or of the pineal gland.

epiphysial (ep-ĭ-fĭz'a-al) [G. *epiphysis*, a growing upon]. Of the nature of or concerning an epiphysis.*

epiphysis (ep-if'is-is) (pl. *epiphysēs*) [G. a growing upon]. 1. A juvenile piece of bone separated from a parent bone in early life by cartilage, but later becoming a part of the larger (or parent) bone; a center for ossification at each extremity of long bones. SEE: *diaphysis*.
e. cerebri. The pineal body.

epiphysitis (ep''ĭ-fĭz-i'tis) [" + *-ītis*, inflammation]. Inflammation of an epiphysis, esp. that at the hip, knee, and shoulder in infants.

epipial (ep-ĭ-pi'al) [G. *epi*, upon, + L. *pia*, tender]. Situated above or upon the pia mater.

epiplocele (ep-ip'lo-sēl) [G. *epiploon*, omentum, + *kēlē*, hernia]. Hernia containing omentum.

epiploenterocele (e-pip''lo-en'ter-o-sēl) [" + *enteron*, intestine, + *kēlē*, hernia]. Hernia consisting of omentum and intestine.

epiploic (ep-ĭ-plo'ĭk) [G. *epiploon*, omentum]. Pert. to the omentum.
e. foramen. The opening between the greater and lesser peritoneal cavities.

epiploitis (e-pi-plo-i'tis) [" + *-ītis*, inflammation]. Inflammation of the omentum.

epiplomerocele (ep-ip-lo-mer'o-sēl) [" + *mēros*, thigh, + *kēlē*, hernia]. Femoral hernia containing omentum.

epiplomphalocele (ep-ip-lom'fal-o-sēl) [" + *omphalos*, navel, + *kēlē*, hernia]. Umbilical hernia with omentum protruding.

epiploon (ep-ip'lo-on) [G. omentum]. The omentum*; esp. the great omentum.

epiplopexy (ep-ip'lo-peks-ĭ) [" + *pēxis*, fixation]. Suturing of omentum to the ant. abdominal wall.

epiplosarcomphalocele (ep-ip''lo-sar-kom'-fal-o-sēl) [" + *sarx*, flesh, + *omphalos*, navel, + *kēlē*, hernia]. An umbilical hernia with protruding omentum. SYN: *epiplomphalocele*.

epiploscheocele (ep-ip-los'ke-o-sēl) [" + *oscheon*, scrotum, + *kēlē*, hernia]. Omental hernia into the scrotum.

episclera (ep-ĭ-skle'ră) [G. *epi*, upon, + *sklēros*, hard]. Loose connective tissue between sclera and conjunctiva.

episcleral (ep-ĭ-skle'răl) [" + *sklēros*, hard]. Overlying the sclera of the eye.

episcleritis (ep-ĭ-skle-ri'tis) [" + " + *-itis*, inflammation]. Inflammation of the subconjunctival layers of the sclera.

ep'iscope [" + *skopein*, to examine]. Projection lantern for examination of an object on a screen. SYN: *epidiascope*.

episioclisia (ep-iz''ĭ-o-klis'ĭ-ă) [G. *episeion*, pudenda, + *kleisis*, closure]. Surgical closure of the vulva.

episioelytrorrhaphy (ĕ-pis''ĭ-o-el-ĭ-tror'ră-fĭ) [" + *elytron*, vagina, + *raphē*, suture]. Narrowing of vagina and vulva.

episioperineorrhaphy (e-pis''ĭ-o-per-in-e-or'ă-fĭ) [" + *perinaion*, perineum, + *raphē*, suture]. Suturing of the vulva and perineum for the support for a prolapse of the uterus.
NP: Prevent necessity for straining on defecation, routine perineal care.

episioplasty (e-pĭ'si-o-plas'tĭ) [" + *plassein*, to form]. Plastic surgery on the vulva.

episiorrhaphy (e-pis''ĭ-or'ră-fĭ) [" + *raphē*, suture]. Sewing of a lacerated perineum.

episiostenosis (ĕ-pis''ĭ-o-stĕ-no'sĭs) [" + *stenōsis*, narrowing]. Narrowing of the vulvar slit.

episiotomy (e-pis″ĭ-ot′o-mĭ) [" + *tomē*, incision]. Incision of perineum at end of second stage of labor to avoid laceration of perineum.

episol (ep′is-ol). A preparation of sodium morrhuate.
Uses: For obliteration of varicose veins.
Dosage: From ½ to 1 cc. by injection.

epispadias (ep-ĭ-spa′dĭ-as) [G. *epi*, upon, + *span*, to tear away]. Congenital opening of urethra on dorsum of penis, and in the female, opening by separation of the labia minora and a fissure of the clitoris.

epispas′tic [" + *span*, to draw]. An agent that, applied locally, will produce a serous or puriform discharge by exciting inflammation.

episplenitis (ep″ĭ-sple-ni′tis) [" + *splēn*, spleen, + *-itis*, inflammation]. Inflammation of the splenic capsule.

epistasis (e-pis′ta-sis) [" + *stasis*, standing]. 1. A substance rising to the surface instead of sinking; scum, as on the urine. In heredity a condition in which the presence of a gene or determiner prevents another gene not allelomorphic to it from expressing itself. 2. The checking of any discharge. See: *hypostasis*.

epistax′is [G. *epistaxein*, to bleed from nose]. Hemorrhage from nose.
Etiol: Trauma, picking the nose with finger, direct blow, postoperative, foreign bodies; diseases (local and general, violent exertion, basilar skull fracture, menstrual suppression, vicarious menstruation, and high altitudes.
Treatment: Lie quietly propped up in bed, cold compresses, adrenalin locally, followed by cautery of bleeding vessel, packing, radium. Simple nose bleed may be stopped ordinarily by elevating head of patient and pinching nostrils. Refrain from breathing through or blowing nose. Pressure across upper lip or cold cloths placed over nose and on back of neck are beneficial.
NP: In severe nose bleeding, if necessary, pack entire nose or upper pharynx (retrograde packing). Occasionally epinephrine, styptics, or astringents may be used. However, for most First Aid purposes, these are unsatisfactory.

episternal (ep-ĭ-ster′nal) [G. *epi*, upon, + *sternon*, chest]. Situated above the sternum.

epister′num [" + *sternon*, chest]. Upper portion of the sternum. Syn: *manubrium*.

epistropheus (ep-ĭ-stro′fe-us) (pl. *epistrophei*) [" + *strephein*, to turn]. BNA. Second cervical vertebra. Syn: *axis*.

epitendineum (ep-ĭ-ten-din′e-um) [" + *tenōn*, tendon]. The fibrous sheath enveloping a tendon.

epitenon (ĕp-ĭt′ĕ-non) [" + *tenōn*, tendon]. The connective tissue holding a tendon within its sheaths. Syn: *epitendineum*.

epithalamus (ep-ĭ-thal′ă-mus) [" + *thalamos*, chamber]. The uppermost portion of the diencephalon. It includes the pineal body, trigonum habenulae, striae medullares thalami, and the posterior commissure.

epithalaxia (ep-ĭ-thal-aks′ĭ-ă) [" + *thēlē*, nipple, + *allaxis*, falling]. Desquamation of epithelial cells, esp. of lining of the intestine.

epithe′lia [" + *thēlē*, nipple]. Epithelial layer or cells.

epithelial (ep-ĭ-the′lĭ-al) [" + *thēlē*, nipple]. Pert. to or composed of epithelium.

e. cancer. Carcinoma composed of epithelial cells. Syn: *epithelioma*.

e. casts. Aggregations of renal epithelium, with cells filled with granules or fat droplets. They often preserve their original form in the epithelial tubes.

e. cells. Cells which are irregular in shape, having a single nucleus. Frequently 2 or 3 are joined together. May be hyaline or granular.

e. tissue. Those cells which form the outer surface of the body, and line the body cavities and the principal tubes and passageways leading to the exterior. They form the secreting portions of glands and their ducts, and important parts of certain sense organs. The cells of epithelial tissues lies closely approximated to each other and contain very little intercellular substance. They are arranged in one or a few layers and are devoid of blood vessels. See: *tissue, epithelial*.

epithe″lioblasto′ma [" + " + *blastos*, germ, + *ōma*, tumor]. Epithelial cell tumor.

epitheliogenic, epitheliogenetic (ep-ĭ-the″-lĭ-o-jen′ik, -jen-et′ĭk) [" + " + *gennan*, to produce]. Caused by epithelial proliferation.

epithelioid (ep-ĭ-the′lĭ-oyd) [" + " + *eidos*, form]. Resembling epithelium.

epitheliolysis (ep-i-the-lĭ-ol′ĭ-sis) [" + " + *lysis*, dissolution]. Death of epithelial tissue. The destruction or desolving of epithelial cells by an epitheliolysin.

epithelioma (ep-ĭ-the-lĭ-o′mă) [" + " + *ōma*, tumor]. A malignant tumor consisting principally of epithelial cells; a carcinoma. A tumor originating in the epidermis of the skin or in a mucous membrane.

e. adamantine. An adamantinoma, *q.v.*

e. adenoides cysticum. A basal-cell carcinoma of low malignancy, occurring on the surface of the body, esp., the face. Characterized by formation of cysts.

e. basal cell. Syn: *e. adenoides cysticum, rodent ulcer*. One derived from cells in the basal layer of the epidermis (stratum germinativum).

e., deep seated. Involving lymphatic glands; irregular rounded ulcers, occurring after several months.

e. molluscum. Molluscum epitheliale, *q.v.*

e., papillary. Malignant, more often occurring in men and after middle life. Attacks genitals, nose, eyelids, or lower lip, etc.

e., superficial. Papules, yellowish or brownish, degenerating and forming ulcers, secreting a yellowish fluid.

epitheliomatous (ep″ĭ-thē-lĭ-ō′măt-ŭs) [" + " + *ōma*, tumor]. Pert. to epithelioma.

epitheliosis (ep-ĭ-thē-lĭ-o′sis) [" + " + *ōsis*]. Trachomalike proliferation of the conjunctival epithelium.

epithelium (ep-ĭ-the′lĭ-um) (pl. *epithelia*) [" + *thēlē*, nipple]. The layer of cells forming the epidermis of the skin and the surface layer of mucous and serous membranes. The cells rest on a basement membrane and lie closely approximated to each other with little intercellular material between them. Epithelium may be *simple*, consisting of a single layer, or *stratified*, consisting of several layers. Cells comprising epithelium may be flat (squamous), cube-shaped (cuboidal) or cylindrical (columnar). Modified forms of epithelium include: ciliated, pseudostratified, glandular, and neuroepithelium. Epithelium may include *goblet cells*, which secrete mucous. Squamous epithelium is differentiated into *endothelium*, which lines the blood vessels and the heart, and *mesothelium*, which lines the serous cavities. Epithelium serves the general functions of protection, absorption, secretion, and specialized functions such as movement of substances through ducts, production of germ cells, and reception of stimuli. Its ability to regenerate is high.

e., ciliated. E. with cilia at the free ends of the cells.

e., columnar. E. composed of cells shaped like pillars.

e. cuboidal. E. consisting of cube-shaped or prismatic cells with height approximately equal to width.

e., cylindrical. SEE: *columnar e*.

e. germinal. The e. which covers the surface of the genital ridge of the urogenital folds of an embryo. It gives rise to seminiferous tubules of the testes and the surface layer of the ovary. It is thought to give rise to the germ cells (spermatozoa and ova).

e. glandular. E. consisting of cells which secrete.

e. laminated. Stratified epithelium.

e., maternal. Uterine e. contrasted with that of the embryo.

e. mesenchymal. E. of the squamous type which lines the subarachnoid and subdural cavities, the chambers of the eye, and the perilymphatic spaces of the ear.

e., neuro-. E. terminating the nerves of special sense.

e., pavement. E. of flat, platelike cells.

e. pigmented. E. consisting of cells containing pigment granules.

e. pseudostratified. E. in which the bases of cells rest on the basement membrane but the distal ends of some do not reach the surface. Nuclei of the cells lies at different levels giving the appearance of stratification.

e., squamous. SEE: *pavement e*.

e., stratified. E. with the cells in layers.

e. transitional. A form of stratified epithelium in which the cells have the ability of adjusting themselves to mechanical changes such as stretching and contracting. Found only in the urinary system (pelvis of kidney, ureter, bladder, and a part of the urethra).

epithem (ep'ĭthem) [G. *epithēma*, a cover]. Any external application, as a poultice.

epitonic (ep-ĭ-ton'ik) [G. *epitonos* strained]. Increased tonus.

epitox'oid [G. *epi*, upon, + *toxikon*, poison, + *eidos*, form]. Any toxoid which has less affinity for an antitoxin than is possessed by the toxin. SYN: *toxon*.

epitrichium (ep-ĭ-trik'ĭ-um) [" + *trichion*, hair]. Superficial layer of the epidermis of the fetus.

epitrochlea (ep-ĭ-trok'lē-ă) [" + *trochalia*, pulley]. The inner condyle of the humerus.

epitrochlear (ep-ĭ-trok'lē-ar) [" + *trochalia*, pulley]. Pert. to the inner condyle of the humerus.

epituberculo'sis [" + L. *tuberculum*, tubercle, + G. *ōsis*]. Resembling tuberculosis but without tubercle bacilli. SYN: *paratuberculosis*.

epitur'binate [" + L. *turbo*, top]. The tissue upon or covering the turbinate bone.

epitympanum (ep-ĭ-tim'pan-um) [" + *tympanon*, drum]. The attic of middle ear; area above the drum membrane.

epityphlitis (ep"ĭ-tif-li'tis) [" + *typhlon*, cecum, + *-itis*, inflammation]. Appendicitis.

epizoic (ep-ĭ-zo'ik) [" + *zōon*, animal]. Parasitic on the epidermis.

epizoicide (ep-e-zo'is-ĭd) [" + " + L. *caedere*, to kill]. That which destroys epizoa. SEE: *epizoon*.

epizoon (ep-ĭ-zo'on) (pl. *epizoa*) [" + *zōon*, animal]. An animal organism externally parasitic.

épluchage (ā-plü-shazh') [Fr. cleaning]. Wound excision for removing contaminated tissues.

eponychium (ep-o-nik'ĭ-um) [G. *epi*, upon, + *onyx, onych-*, nail]. The horny embryonic structure from which the nail develops.

ep'onym [G. *epōnymos*, named after]. A name for anything (diseases, organs, functions, places) adapted from the name of a particular person.

eponym'ic [G. *epōnymos*, named after]. Pert. to eponym. SYN: *eponymous*.

epon'ymous [G. *epōnymos*, named after]. Named after a person.

epoöphorectomy (ep"o-o-fo-rek'to-mĭ) [G. *epi*, upon, + *ōophoron*, ovary, + *ektomē*, excision]. Removal of the parovarium.

epoophoron (ĕp-ō-ŏf'ŏr-ŏn) [G. *epi*, upon, + *oophoron*, ovary]. SYN: *parovarium, organ of Rosenmuller*. A rudimentary structure located in the mesosalpinx consisting of a longitudinal duct (duct of Gartner) and ten to fifteen transverse ducts. It is the remains of the upper portion of the mesonephros and is the homolog of the head of the epididymis in the male.

epsom salt (ep'sŭm). USP. SEE: *magnesium sulfate*.

epulis (ep-u'lis) [G. *epoulis*, a gumboil]. A fibrous, sarcomatous tumor having its origin in the periosteum of the lower jaw.

e., malignant. Jaw sarcoma made up of giant cells.

epuloid (ep'u-loid) [" + *eidos*, form]. 1. Like an epulis. 2. Tumor of the jaw or gum appearing like an epulis.

epulosis (e-pu-lo'sis) [" + *-ōsis*]. Cicatrization; a cicatrix.

epulot'ic [G. *epoulis*, gumboil]. Promoting cicatrization.

equa'tion [L. *aequāre*, to make equal]. 1. State of being equal. 2. In chem. a symbolic representation of a chemical reaction.

equa'tor. Line encircling a round body and equidistant from both poles.

e. of a cell. The boundary of a plane through which the division of a cell occurs.

e. of crystalline lens. Line which marks the junction of the anterior and posterior surfaces; the aequator lentis. To it are attached the fibers of the suspensory ligament.

e. oculi. An imaginary line encircling the bulb of the eye midway between ant. and post. poles.

equato'rial [L. *aequāre*, to make equal]. Pert. to an equator.

e. plate. Mass of chromosomes at equator of the nuclear spindle during karyokinesis.

equi- [L.]. Prefix meaning *equal*.

equilibrating (e-kwil'ĭ-brāt-ing). Maintaining equilibrium.

equilibrating, operation

e. operation. Section of the antagonist of a paralyzed ocular muscle. SEE: *tenotomy.*

equilib'rium [L. *aequus*, equal, + *libra*, balance]. Equipoise. Condition in which contending forces are equal.

e., nitrogenous. Having amt. of nitrogen in egesta equal to that of ingesta.

e., physiological. Having egesta equal to the ingesta.

equilin(e (ek'wĭl-ĭn) [L. *equus*, horse]. Crystalline estrogenic hormone derived from pregnant mares' urine, which affects growth of female sex organs. SYN: *theelin.*

equina'tion [L. *equinus*, equine]. Inoculation with virus of horsepox.

equinia (e-kwĭn'ĭ-ă) [L. *equus*, horse]. Infectious disease of horses which can also affect man. SYN: *glanders.*

equinovarus (e-kwī"no-va'rus) [L. *equinus*, equine, + *varus*, bent inward]. A form of clubfoot with a combination pes equinus and pes varus.

equivalence (e-kwĭv'al-ens) [L. *aequis*, equal, + *valere*, to be worth]. 1. Quality of being equivalent. 2. Condition in which 2 radicals reacting are of the same valence and 1 displaces the other in a compound.

equivalent (e-kwĭv'a-lent) [" + *valere*, to be worth]. 1. Equal in power, force, or value. 2. Amount of weight of any element needed to replace a fixed weight of another body.

Er. or **E.** Symbol for *erbium.*

E.R. Symbol for external resistance.

erasion (e-ra'zhun) [L. *ē*, out, + *radere*, to scrape]. 1. Laying open a diseased part and scraping away diseased tissue. 2. Scraping away morbid products.

Erben's reflex (erb'ens). Retardation of pulse when head and trunk are forcibly bent forward.

er'bium. A rare metallic element. SYMB: Er. Atomic weight, 166.

Erb's paralysis or palsy. Paralysis of group of muscles of shoulder and upper arm involving cervical roots of 5th and 6th spinal nerves.

The arm hangs limp, the hand rotates inwards and normal movements are lost. SEE: *paralysis.*

erec'tile [L. *erigere*, to erect]. Able to become erect.

e. center. A reflex center located in the lumbosacral region of the spinal cord. Cutaneous stimuli applied to the genitalia or neighboring parts are the most frequent cause of erection. When the penis is stimulated, afferent impulses pass over the dorsal nerve of the penis, a branch of the internal pudendal nerve to the center; efferent impulses pass over the nervi erigentes to the blood vessels of the penis bringing about vasodilatation. Other stimuli such as visual, olfactory, auditory, and psychic conditions may induce erection.

e. tissue. Vascular tissue which, when filled with blood, becomes erect or rigid, as the clitoris or penis.

erec'tion [L. *erigere*, to erect]. The state of swelling, hardness, and stiffness observed in the penis and to a lesser extent in the clitoris of the female, generally during sexual excitement.

Due to engorgement with blood of the *corpora cavernosa* and the *corpus spongiosum* of the penis and the *c. cavernosa clitoridis* of the female.

It is necessary in the male for the intromission of the penis into the vagina of the female and for the emission of semen. After ejaculation the blood withdraws from the penis and the erection is reduced. Erection of the penis also occurs normally under other special conditions. Abnormal, persistent erection of the penis is called priapism.*

RS: *clitoris, coition, coitus, copulation, ejaculation, emission, excitation, penis, sexual intercourse.*

e. center. This is in lumbar and sacral region; responds to organic and psychic stimuli and with the genitalia responding to peripheral irritation of the sensory nerves. This center is not directly under control of the will. The *nervi erigentes* in the first 3 sacral nerves under excitation convey their impulse to the *corpora cavernosa.* Reflex stimuli also affect it.

erec'tor [L. *erigere*, to erect]. A muscle that raises a part.

e. spinae reflex. Irritation of the skin over the erector spinae muscles causing contraction of muscles of the back.

erect posi'tion. One having the occiput and heels in line with nose, groin, and great toes in same relative plane.

Employed in the practice of ballottement, in differentiation of tumors, cystic and solid hernias, and examination of pelvic joints.

eremacausis (er"em-ak-aw'sis) [G. *ērema*, slowly, + *kausis*, burning]. Slow oxidation of organic matter exposed to heat.

eremophobia (er-em-o-fo'bĭ-ă) [G. *erēmos*, solitude, + *phobos*, fear]. Dread of being alone.

erep'sin. Term applied to a peptid-splitting enzyme found in the *succus entericus* (intestinal juice). The peptid-splitting action is now known to be due to the action of several peptidases which act on peptids which have escaped pancreatic digestion transforming them to amino acids.

erethin (er'e-thin) [G. *erethizein*, to irritate]. The principle of tuberculin which causes fevers.

erethism (er'e-thizm) [G. *erethisma*, stimulation]. Abnormal excitement or irritation which may be combined with collapse.

erethis'mic [G. *erethisma*, stimulation]. Pert. to or causing erethism. SYN: *erethitic.*

erethisophrenia (er-e-thĭ-so-fre'nĭ-ă) [G. *erethizein*, to irritate, + *phrēn*, mind]. Unusual mental excitability.

erethistic (er-e-this'tik) [G. *erethisma*, stimulation]. Erethismic, exciting.

erethitic (er-ĕ-thĭt'ĭk) [G. *erethisma*, stimulation]. Causing erethism; irritable, excited.

ereuthrophobia (er"u-thro-fo'bĭ-ă) [G. *erythros*, red, + *phobos*, fear]. Pathological fear of blushing. SYN: *erythrophobia.*

erg [G. *ergon*, work]. In physics, the amount of work done when a force of 1 dyne acts through a distance of 1 centimeter.

One erg is roughly 1/980 gram-centimeter; that is, to raise a load of 1 gram against gravity the distance of 1 centimeter requires that a force of 980 dynes operate through a distance of 1 centimeter and hence that 980 ergs of work be done. SEE: *unit, work.*

ergasia (er-ga'sĭ-ă) [G. *ergasia*, work]. Functions of the mind and behavior resulting therefrom in contrast to those depending upon physiological functions.

ergasiodermatosis (er-gas″ĭ-o-der-mă-to′-sis) [" + *derma*, skin, + *-ōsis*]. Dermatosis due to occupational cause.

ergasiomania (er-gas″ĭ-o-ma′nĭ-ă) [" + *mania*, madness]. Active interest in a task without completing it, seen in certain phases of manic excitement.

ergasiophobia (er″gas-ĭ-o-fo′bĭ-ă) [" + *phobos*, fear]. Abnormal dislike for assuming responsibility or for work of any kind.

ergasthenia (er-gas-the′nĭ-ă) [G. *ergon*, work, + *astheneia*, weakness]. Overwork and debility caused therefrom.

ergas′tic [G. *ergon*, work]. Possessing potential energy.

ergastoplasm (er-gas′to-plazm) [" + *plasma*, a thing formed]. Cytoplasm with higher power than ordinary plasma. SYN: *kinoplasm*.

er′gin [G. *ergon*, work]. Substance presumed to be present in blood or tissue fluids which upon uniting with an allergen produces the symptoms of allergy.

ergograph (er′go-graf) [" + *graphein*, to write]. An apparatus for recording the contractions of muscles and measuring the amount of work done.

ergom′eter [" + *metron*, measure]. An apparatus for measuring the amount of work done by a human or animal subject.

ergopho′bia [" + *phobos*, fear]. Morbid dread of working.

ergophore (er′go-fōr) [" + *pherein*, to bear]. That part of an antigen on which the specific properties of the substance depend. SYN: *toxophore*.

er′goplasm [G. *ergon*, work, + *plasma*, a thing formed]. SYN: *kinoplasm, archoplasm*. Protoplasm peculiar to the centrosome, and composing the attraction sphere.

er′gostat [" + *statos*, standing]. A machine for measuring work done by a contracting muscle.

ergos′terin, ergos′terol. A substance derived from yeast, ergot, and other fungi, and resembling cholesterol in composition.

  e. irradiated. E. subjected to ultraviolet radiation which develops vitamin D₂ potency. A remedy for rickets. It is believed that it activates some gland, perhaps the parathyroid, making possible better use of calcium and phosphorus. It is said to be present in skin and tissue. SYN: *viosterol*.

ergot (er′got) [L. *ergota*]. A drug obtained from *claviceps purpurea*, a fungus which grows parasitically on rye. It is a mixture of several alkaloids.
  USP. ACTION AND USES: As a uterine stimulant, and hemostatic.
  DOSAGE: 30 gr. (2 Gm.). Fluid extract: 30 ℳ (2 cc.).

  e. poisoning. May come from eating bread made with diseased grain or by taking overdoses of the drug.
  SYM: Appear several hours after administration. Vomiting, burning, and cramping in abdomen, great thirst, profound weakness, diarrhea; slow, weak pulse; anesthesia, tingling and twitching in extremities; occasionally convulsions, anuria; if patient survives may develop gangrene of fingers, toes or limited areas of skin.
  F. A. TREATMENT: Gastric lavage, cathartics, warm baths, increase fluid intake, stimulants as coffee, caffeine, and tea in large doses.

ergotamine (ĕr-gŏt′ăm-ēn). A crystalline alkaloid (C₃₃H₃₅O₅N₅) derived from ergot.

  e. tartrate. SYN: *gynergen*. A white crystalline substance which stimulates smooth muscle of blood vessels and the uterus inducing vasoconstriction and uterine contractions. Used in the treatment of migraine.

ergotherapy (er-go-ther′ă-pĭ) [G. *ergon*, work, + *therapeia*, treatment]. Work used as a treatment of disease.

  e., passive. Generalized muscular exercise excited by faradic current.

ergotism (er′go-tizm) [L. *ergota*, ergot, + G. *ismos*, condition]. Poisoning resulting from excessive use of ergot or from eating food made from rye or wheat infected with the fungus *claviceps purpurea*. May be acute or chronic.

ergotrate (er′go-trāt). An active principle isolated from ergot.
  USES: Same as ergot.
  DOSAGE: 1/320 gr. (0.2 mg.) orally, intramuscularly, or intravenously.

ergotrop′ic [G. *ergon*, work, + *tropos*, a turning]. Pert. to ergotropy.*

ergotropy (er-got′ro-pĭ) [" + *tropos*, a turning]. Injection of nonspecific proteins to increase body resistance.

Erichsen's disease (ĕr′ĭk-sĕn). SYN: *railway spine*. A group of symptoms following injury to the spine.

eriom′eter [G. *erion*, wool, + *metron*, measure]. Device for measuring minute particles.

Eristalis. A genus of flies belonging to the family Syrphidae. The larva, called rat-tailed maggot, may cause intestinal myiasis in man.

erode (e-rōd′) [L. *erodere*, to gnaw away]. 1. To wear away. 2. To eat away by ulceration.

erogenous (e-roj′en-us) [G. *erōs*, love, + *gennan*, to produce]. Causing sexual excitement. SYN: *erotogenic*.*

  e. zone. Any part of the body which, by touching or stroking, causes sexual excitement. Ex: The penis, the perineum, the nipples, labia, or clitoris.

erosion (e-ro′shun) [L. *erodere*, to gnaw away]. An eating away of tissue; destruction of a surface layer, either external or internal, by physical or inflammatory processes.

  e. of the cervix uteri. The alteration of the epithelium on a portion of the cervix as a result of irritation by infection.
  SYM: In the early stages, the epithelium shows necrosis which nature tries to heal by a down growth of epithelium from the endocervical canal. If this is accomplished by a single layer of tissue, having a grossly granular appearance, it is called a simple granular erosion. If the down growth is excessive, and shows papillary tufts, it is called a papillary erosion.
  Histologically, the papillary erosion shows many glands of the branching racemose type whose epithelium is the mucus-bearing cell with the nucleus at the base. In the healing process, squamous epithelium grows over the eroded area with the following results: the squamous cells take the place of the tissue beneath it completely, giving a complete healing, or the glands fill with squamous plugs and remain in that state, or the mouths of the glands are occluded by the squamous cells and cysts are formed (nabothian cysts). In the congenital type of erosion the portio is covered by high columnar epithelium.
  TREATMENT: Prophylaxis, proper care of the cervix following delivery, proper hygiene by means of douches, and cau-

erosion, dental   E-46   **erysipelotoxin**

terization of the early erosion with the electrocautery is usually curative. In cases of erosion in association with a badly lacerated cervix amputation of the cervix is indicated.

e. dental. The wearing away of the surface layer (enamel) of a tooth.

erosive (e-ro′siv) [G. *erodere*, to gnaw away]. 1. Able to produce erosion. 2. An agent that erodes anything.

erotic (e-rot′ik) [G. *erōtikos*, pert. to love]. Pert. to sexual passion. SYN: *lustful.*

erot′icism [" + *ismos*, condition of]. Excessive or morbid libido; also intense but normal sex desire.

   e., al′lo. Eroticism directed to an external object rather than to self. SEE: *eroticism, erotomania.*

   e., anal. Sensations of pleasure experienced by the child through defecation, which later are inhibited.

   e., oral. Sensation of pleasure experienced when nursing at the breast, modified and sublimated but continuing into adult life through normal contacts of the lips, mouth, and throat.

   e., auto-. 1. Self-gratification of the sexual instinct. 2. Self-admiration combined with sexual emotion, such as that obtained from viewing one's naked body, or one's genitals. SEE: *erotomania, zones, erotogenic.*

e′rotism [" + *ismos*, condition of]. PSY: eroticism.

erotogenic (er″o-to-jen′ik) [G. *erōs*, love, + *gennan*, to produce]. Producing sexual excitement. SEE: *erotic zones.*

erotology (er-o-tol′o-ji) [" + *logos*, study]. The study of love and its manifestations.

erotomania (e-rot-o-ma′ni-ă) [" + *mania*, madness]. Unrestrained libido in the insane. SEE: *eroticism, zones, erotogenic.*

erotopathia (er-o-to-path′i-ă) [" + *pathos*, disease]. Any abnormal or perverted sex impulse.

erotophobia (er-o-to-fo′bi-ă) [" + *phobos*, fear]. Aversion to sexual love or its manifestations.

erotopsychic (er-o-to-si′kik) [" + *psychē*, mind]. Mental perversion of the sexual impulse.

errat′ic [L. *errāre*, to wander]. Wandering, as from one part of the body to another part; roving, odd. SYN: *eccentric.*

errhine (er′in) [G. *en*, in, + *ris*, rin-, nose]. An agent that will increase the secretion of the mucous membrane lining the nose. SYN: *sternutatory.* Ex: *quillaja, salicylic acid.*

erubes′cence [L. *erubēscere*, to grow red]. Reddening of the skin; a blush.

eructa′tion [L. *eructāre*, to belch]. Raising of gas or acid fluid from the stomach; belching. SYN: *oxyrygmia.*

eruption (e-rup′shun) [L. *eruptio*, a breaking out]. 1. A breaking out, esp., applied to the appearance of a skin lesion or rash accompanying a disease such as measles or scarlet fever. 2. The appearance of a lesion such as redness or spotting on the skin or mucous membrane. 3. The breaking through of a tooth through the gum; the cutting of a tooth.

   e. creeping. A skin lesion characterized by a tortuous elevated red line which progresses at one end while fading out at the other. It is caused by the migration of the larvae of certain nematodes, esp. *Ancylostoma braziliense* and other cat and dog nematodes which occur as accidental invaders of man. The larvae of certain species of flies (*Gasterophilus, Hypoderma*) may produce similar effects (*dermamyiasis linearis migrans oestrosa*).

   e. drug. Dermatitis medicamentosa; skin reaction resulting from the ingestion of certain drugs, such as iodides.

   e., primary. Blebs, macules, papules, pustules, tubercules, tumors, vesicles, wheals or phomphi, *q.v.*

   e., secondary. Crusts, excoriations, fissures, pigmentations, scales, scars, ulcers, *q.v.*

   e. serum. E. caused by the injection of a serum.

erup′tive [L. *eruptio*, a breaking out]. Breaking out, as with a rash.

erysipelas (er-is-ip′el-as) [G. *erythros*, red, + *pella*, skin]. Acute, febrile disease with localized inflammation and swelling of skin and subcutaneous tissue accompanied by systemic disturbance of variable degree. SYN: *St. Anthony's fire.*

ETIOL: *Streptococcus erysipelatus.*

PATH: The skin of the face is most commonly infected. Lesion involves skin and subcutaneous tissues.

SYM: Eruption begins on first or second day as minute erythematous patch, spreading peripherally, affected skin becoming swollen, painful, burning, itching, red with glazed, shining surface. Eruption begins to fade about 4th day.

PROG: Favorable generally in idiopathic types but sometimes fatal in traumatic and phlegmonous (scalp, puerperal women) and in gangrenous always so.

TREATMENT: Symptomatic (constitutional) with mercurial purge followed by salines at outset. Antistreptococcus serum, convalescent serum, whole blood transfusions, ultraviolet and x-ray therapy, sulfanilamide.

DIET: Milk and other fluids; no alcohol.

   e., ambulant. E. which disappears from one part of the body and reappears in another.

   e., erythematous. E. in a mild form.

   e., facial. Form found mainly on the face.

   e., idiopathic. E. which does not develop subsequent to trauma or injury.

   e., migrans. Widely spread form of e.

   e., phlegmonous. Purulent form of e.

   e., surgical. E. developing in a wound.

   e., traumatic. SEE: *surgical e.*

erysipelatous (er″i-si-pel′a-tus) [" + *pella*, skin]. Of the nature of or pert. to erysipelas.

erysipeloid. Erythema migrane or serpens (er-is-ip′e-loid [" + " + *eidos*, form]. An infective dermatitis resembling erysipelas usually limited to the hands and characterized by hyperemia, edema, and occasionally systemic complications.

ETIOL: It is caused by *Erysipelothrix rhusiopathiae*, usually acquired by contact with pork or fish products.

Erysipelothrix (ĕr-ĭ-sĭ-pĕl′ō-thriks). A genus of bacteria belonging to the family Corynebacteriaceae. They are branching filamentous, rod-shaped, non-motile organisms.

   E. rhusiopathiae. The causative agent of swine erysipelas and erysipeloid in man.

   E. erysipelatus suis. Causative agent of swine erysipelas.

erysip′elotox′in. The toxin produced by *Streptococcus erysipelatos*, the causative agent of erysipelas.

Eruptive, Infective, and Contagious Diseases

Name	Period of Incubation	Time of Eruption	Duration of Eruption	Period of Quarantine
1 Scarlet Fever	2- 5 days	12-24 hr. after onset	4-5 days	21 days.
2 Smallpox	8-12 days	3rd day of fever	14 to 21 days	21 days.
3 Measles	10 days	4th day of fever	5 to 10 days	14 days.
4 Roetheln	5-21 days	2nd day of fever	3 days	5 days.
5 Mumps	14 to 21 days			Until all swellings have subsided.
6 Whooping Cough	7-10 days			28 days.
7 Chickenpox	4-27 days	2nd day of fever	7 days	7 days.
8 Diphtheria	5 days			7 days, and until 2 successive nose and throat cultures, 24 hr. apart, are negative.
9 Typhus Fever	12 days	5th or 6th day of fever	14 days	14 days.
10 Typhoid Fever	14 days	4th day of fever	20 days	Release after 2 successive negative cultures of urine and feces not less than 24 hr. apart.
11 Erysipelas	3- 7 days	2nd day of fever	4 days	

SEE: *quarantine.*

erythema (er-ith-e′mă) [G. redness]. A form of macula showing diffused redness over the skin.
ETIOL: Caused by capillary congestion, usually due to dilatation of the superficial capillaries as a result of (1) some nervous mechanism within the body, (2) inflammation, (3) as a result of some external influence, such as heat, sunburn, etc.
    e. annulare. E. with rounded, raised marginal lesions.
    e. circinatum. In red circles.
    e. congestivum. E. with congestive state of skin.
    e., diffuse. Widely spread over body.
    e. dose. The amount of radiant energy sufficient to evoke perceptible redness of the skin.
    e., hyperaemicum. Caused by heat or cold (erythema caloricum, chilblain), sun (erythema solare), artificial heat, as from hot water bottle or electric pad (erythema ab igne).
    e. infectiosum. Contagious form with rose-colored eruption.
    e. intertrigo. Chafing of opposing surfaces, with erythema and often with maceration and abrasion.
    e. multiforme. A macular eruption with dark red papules or tubercles. Usually on extremities appearing in successive eruptions of short duration. No itching, burning or rheumatic pains. May appear in separate rings, concentric rings, in disk-shaped patches, in distributed elevations, and figured arrangements.
    e. nodosum. Red and painful nodules on legs associated with rheumatism. Also caused by certain drugs and food poisoning.
    e., punctate. In minute points, as scarlet fever rash.

    e. symptomaticum. Hyperemia of the skin with level patches.
    e. venenatum. Form caused by an irritation from minerals, poisons, etc.
erythemat′ic, erythem′atous [G. *erythēma*, redness]. Pert. to or marked by erythema.
erythemogen′ic [" + *gennan*, to produce]. Pert. to erythema.
erythemomegalal′gia [" + *megas*, great, + *algos*, pain]. Painful redness of skin. SYN: *erythromelalgia.*
erythralgia (er-ĭ-thral′jĭ-ă) [G. *erythros*, red, + *algos*, pain]. A condition of painful redness of the skin. SYN: *erythromelalgia.*
erythrasma (er-ĭ-thraz′mă) [G. *erythros*, red]. Reddish-brown eruption in patches in the axillae and groins due to a fungus.
erythredema (ĕ-rĭth″rĕ-de′mă) [" + *oidēma*, swelling]. SYN: *acrodynis, Swift's disease, dermatopolyneuritis, pink disease.* A disease occurring in infants characterized by lesions of the skin on the hands and feet, swelling of the extremities, digestive disturbances. It is frequently followed by multiple arthritis. Its cause is unknown.
erythre′mia [" + *aima*, blood]. Excessive increase of red blood corpuscles with cyanosis. SYN: *polycythemia rubra.*
er′ythrism [" + *ismos*, condition of]. Redness of the hair and beard with ruddy complexion.
erythristic (er-ĭ-thris′tĭk) [G. *erythros*, red]. Ruddy complexion. Having reddish hair.
erythro. Prefix meaning "red."
erythroblast (er-ith-ro′blast) [" + *blastos*, germ]. The youngest erythroblasts are called basophilic erythroblasts or proerythroblasts. Successive stages are polychromatophil erythroblasts or megablasts, and normoblasts. Erythro-

blasts possess hemoglobin. In the embryo they are found in blood islands of the yolk sac, body mesenchyma, liver, spleen, and lymph nodes; after the third month they are restricted to the bone marrow.
e. fetalis. A hemolytic disease of the new born characterized by anemia, jaundice, and enlargement of the liver and spleen, generalized edema (hydrops fetalis). ETIOL: It is due to the development in an Rh negative mother of antibodies against an Rh positive fetus. This occurs following a preceding pregnancy in which the fetus was Rh positive or following transfusion of Rh positive blood.

erythroblaste′mia [" + " + *aima*, blood]. An excessive number of erythroblasts in the blood.

erythroblas′tic [" + *blastos*, germ]. Pert. to erythroblasts.

erythroblasto′ma [" + " + *ōma*, tumor]. A tumor (myeloma) with cells resembling megaloblasts.

erythroblasto′sis [" + " + *ōsis*]. A condition marked by many erythroblasts in the blood.

erythrochloropia (er″ĭ-thro-klo-ro′pĭ-ă) [" + *chlōros*, green, + *ōps*, eye]. Partial color blindness with ability to see only red and green.

erythrochromia (er″ĭ-thro-kro′mĭ-ă) [" + *chrōma*, color]. Hemorrhagic red pigmentation of the spinal fluid.

erythroclas′tic [" + *klan*, to break]. Destructive to red blood cells.

eryth′roconte [G. *erythros*, red]. An abnormal rod-shaped structure found in erythrocytes in cases of pernicious anemia.

erythrocyano′sis [" + *kyanos*, blue, + *ōsis*]. Red or bluish discoloration on the skin with swelling, itching, and burning.

erythrocyte (e-rith′ro-sīt) [" + *kytos*, cell]. Red blood corpuscle.
Each is a non-nucleated, biconcave disc averaging 7.7 microns in diameter. The body of the cell consists of a spongelike *stroma* containing a respiratory pigment, *hemoglobin* enclosed in a cell membrane of proteins in combination with lipoid substances. Hemoglobin is a conjugated protein consisting of a colored iron-containing portion, *hematin* and a simple protein, *globin*. It combines readily with oxygen to form an unstable, compound, *oxyhemoglobin*.
NUMBER. In a normal person, the number of erythrocytes average about 5,000,000 per cu. millimeter. (5,500,000 for males, 4,500,000 for females.) The total number in an average sized person is about thirty five trillion. The number per cubic millimeter varies with (1) *age*, being higher in infants, (2) *time of day*, being lower during sleep, (3) *activity* and *environmental temperature*, increasing in both conditions, and (4) *altitude*. Persons living at altitudes of 10,000 ft. or more may have a red cell count of 8,000,000 or more.
FUNCTIONS: The primary function of the red blood cells is to carry oxygen and carbon dioxide. They also play a role in the regulation of the acid-base balance of the blood and in the formation of bile pigments which are derived from decomposition products of hemoglobin.
ORIGIN: Red cell formation (*erythropoiesis*) in the adult takes place in the red bone-marrow, principally in the vertebrae, ribs, sternum, diploe of cranial bones, and proximal ends of the humerus and femur. They arise from large nucleated stem-cells (*proerythroblasts*) which give rise to *erythroblasts* in which hemoglobin appears. These give rise to *normoblasts* which extrude their nuclei. Red cells at this stage possess a fine reticular network and are known as *reticulocytes*. This reticular structure is lost before the cells enter circulation as *mature erythrocytes*.
The proper formation of erythrocytes depends upon several factors among them: (a) healthy condition of the bone marrow; (b) dietary substances such as iron, cobalt, and copper, all essential for the formation of hemoglobin; essential amino acids, and certain vitamins, esp., B_{12} and folic acid (pteroylglutamic acid); (c) an *antianemic factor* stored in the liver.
LIFE HISTORY AND FATE . . . The average length of life of a red blood cell is estimated to be about 120 days. Cells are continuously dying and disintegrating. The cellular debris is picked up by the cells of the reticulo-endothelial system esp., those of the spleen, liver, and bone marrow. Hemoglobin is broken down, and proteins and iron are stored and utilized in the formation of new erythrocytes. The iron-containing portion, *hematin*, gives rise to *bilirubin*, which is excreted in the bile as one of the bile pigments.
VARIATIONS: On microscopic examination, erythrocytes may reveal variations in the following respects (1) *Size anisocytosis*, (2) *Shape* (poikilcytosis), (3) *Staining reaction* (achromia, hypochromia, hyperchromia, polychromomatophilia), (4) *Structure* (possession of bodies such as Cabot's rings, Howell-Jolly bodies, a reticular network, or nuclei), (5) *Number* (anemia, polycythemia).

e. achromatic. A phantom corpuscle or one from which the hemoglobin has been dissolved; a colorless corpuscle.

e. basophilic. E. in which cytoplasm stains blue indicating the presence of basophilic material. May be diffuse (basophilic material uniformly distributed) or punctate (material appearing as pin point dots).

e. crenated. E. with a serrated or indented edge usually the result of withdrawal of water from the cell as occurs when cells are placed in hypertonic solutions.

e. immature. An erythroblast.

e. orthrochromatic. E. that stains with acid stains only, cytoplasm appearing pink.

e. polychromatic. E. that does not stain uniformly.

erythrocythemia (er″ĭth″ro-si-the′mĭ-ă) [" + " + *aima*, blood]. Enormous increase in red blood cells. SYN: *erythremia, polycythemia*.

erythrocytolysis (er-ĭth″ro-si-tol′ĭ-sis) [" + " + *lysis*, dissolution]. Dissolution of red blood corpuscles with the escape of hemoglobin; hemolysis.

erythrocytom′eter [" + " + *metron*, measure]. Instrument for counting red blood corpuscles.

erythrocytoöpso′nin [" + " + *opsōnein*, to prepare food for]. A substance opsonic for red corpuscles.

erythrocytorrhexis (er-ĭ-thro-si-tor-reks′-is) [" + " + *rēxis*, rupture]. The breaking up of red blood cells with particles or fragments of the cell escaping into the plasma; plasmorrhexis.

erythrocytoschisis (er-ĭ-thro-si-tos′kis-is) [" + " + *schisis*, division]. The break-

erythrocytosis (ĕr-ĭth-rō-sī-tōs'ĭs). Abnormal increase in the number of red blood cells in circulation; polycythemia, erythemia erythrocytothemia.

erythroderma (er"-ĭth-rō-derm'ă). Erythema, erythrodermia, *q.v.*
  e. desquamativum. A disease in infants characterized by redness of skin and development of scales; Leiner's disease.
  e. ichthyosiforme congenitum. A congenital condition characterized by thickening and redness of the skin; may resemble ichthyosis or lichen.
  e. maculopapular. A condition of the skin characterized by redness and eruption of macules and papules.
  e. squamosum. An eruption of the skin consisting of groups of papules covered by scales; parapsoriasis.

erythrodermia (er-ĭ-thro-der'mĭ-ă) [" + *derma*, skin]. Abnormal redness in the skin. SYN: *erythema*.

erythrodextrin (er-ĭth-ro-dex'trĭn) [" + L. *dexter*, right]. Form of dextrin from splitting of a polysaccharide molecule. SEE: *achroodextrin*.

erythrogen'esis [" + *genesis*, development]. The development of red blood corpuscles.

erythrokatalysis (er-ĭ-thro-ka-tal'ĭ-sis) [" + *katalysis*, dissolution]. Ingestion and digestion of red blood corpuscles.

erythrol tetranitrate (er'ĭth-rol tet-ra-nī'trāt). A white crystalline mass with explosive properties like nitroglycerine, but used in medicine as a dilute powder or in tablets.
  USES: As an antispasmodic and vasodilator, with action similar to nitroglycerine.
  DOSAGE: ¼ to ½ gr. (0.015-0.03 Gm.).
  INCOMPATIBILITIES: Especially alcohol, and should not be rubbed with other substances.

erythroleukemia (er-ĭ-thro-lu-ke'mĭ-ă) [G. *erythros*, red, + *leukos*, white, + *aima*, blood]. Many immature cells in the blood causing anemia.

erythroleukosis (er-ĭ-thro-lu-ko'sis) [" + " + *ōsis*]. Abnormal increase of red cells and granulocytes.

erythrol'ysin [" + *lysis*, dissolution]. An agent causing erythrolysis. SYN: *hemolysin, erythrocytolysin*. SEE: *lysin*.

erythrol'ysis [" + *lysis*, dissolution]. Dissolution of red blood corpuscles. SYN: *erythrocytolysis*.

erythromelalgia (er-ĭ-thro-mel-al'jĭ-ă) [" + *melos*, limb, + *algos*, pain]. A skin neurosis accompanied by burning and throbbing which come and go, affecting any one of the extremities, esp. the feet.

erythrome'lia [" + *melos*, limb]. Erythema of extensor surfaces of extremities but without pain.

erythron (er'ĭ-thrŏn). Capillaries in red marrow in which erythrocytes are formed.

erythroneocytosis (er"ĭ-thro-ne"o-sī-to'sis) [" + *neos*, new, + *kytos*, cell, + *ōsis*]. Regenerative forms of red blood cells in the blood.

erythronoclastic (er-ĭ-thron-o-klas'tĭk) [" + *klan*, to break]. Destructive to erythrons.

erythropar'asite [" + *parasitos*, parasite]. A red blood corpuscle parasite.

erythrop'athy [" + *pathos*, disease]. Disease of the red blood corpuscles.

erythropenia (er"ĭ-thro-pe'nĭ-ă) [" + *penia*, poverty]. Deficiency of red blood corpuscles.

erythrophage (er-ĭth'ro-fāj) [" + *phagein*, to eat]. A phagocyte which destroys red corpuscles.

erythropha'gia [" + *phagein*, to eat]. Destruction of red blood cells by phagocytes.

eryth'rophile, erythroph'ilous [" + *philein*, to love]. Readily staining red.

erythrophobia (e-rith"ro-fo'bĭ-ă) [" + *phobos*, fear]. 1. Abnormal dread of blushing or fear of being diffident or of being embarrased. 2. A morbid fear of, or aversion to, anything colored red.

erythrophose (e-rith'ro-fōs) [" + *phōs*, light]. Any red subjective perception of a bright spot. SEE: *phose*.

erythrophthi'sis [" + *phthisis*, wasting]. Serious damage to the restorative power of the red corpuscles.

erythrophthor'ic [" + *phtheirein*, to destroy]. 1. Rapid destruction of erythrocytes. 2. By any means other than hemolysis.

erythrop'ia, erythrop'sia [" + *opsis*, vision]. Condition in which objects appear to be red.

erythroplasia (er-ĭth-rō-plā'sĭ-ă). A condition considered to be precancerous characterized by the appearance of erythematous lesions involving the junctions of the epithelium of the skin and mucous membranes at the mouth, anus, penis, and vulva.

erythropoiesis (e-rith"ro-poy-e'sĭs) [" + *poiēsis*, making]. The formation of red blood corpuscles.

erythropoietic (er"ĭth"ro-poy-et'ĭk) [" + *poiēsis*, making]. Pert. to red blood cells.

erythroprosopalgia (er"ĭth"ro-pros-o-pal'jĭ-ă) [" + *prosōpon*, face, + *algos*, pain]. A neurosis marked by redness and pain in the face.

erythropsia (er-ĭ-throp'sĭ-ă) [" + *opsis*, vision]. Perversion of color vision in which all objects look red.

erythrop'sin [" + *opsis*, vision]. Pigment in the external portion of the rods of the retina. SYN: *rhodopsin, visual purple*.

erythropykno'sis [" + *pyknos*, dense, + *ōsis*]. Alteration of red blood cells by malarial parasites; "brassy bodies." SYN: *pyknosis*.

erythrorrhex'is [" + *rēxis*, rupture]. Rupture of a cell and escape of its plasma. SYN: *erythrocytorrhexis, plasmorrhexis*.

erythro'sis [" + *ōsis*]. A reddish-purple discoloration of the skin and mucous membranes in polycythemia.

er"ythrothrom"bomono'blasto'sis. A disorder characterized by appearance in the blood of excessive numbers of erythroblasts, thrombocytes, and immature monocytes. Other symptoms include enlargement of the spleen, increase in basal metabolism, and bone atrophy.

erythrotoxin (er-ĭth"ro-toks'in) [" + *toxikon*, poison]. An exotoxin that attacks red blood cells. SEE: *leukotoxin*.

erythruria (er-ĭ-thru/rĭ-ă) [" + *ouron*, urine]. Red color of the urine.

Esbach's method (es'baks). A method of estimating quantity of albumin in urine. The urine is collected for 24 hours, and after stirring well, a specimen is taken.
  The specific gravity is read and, if necessary, urine is diluted until it shows a reading of 1.010 or below. It should be slightly acid. It is poured into a special Esbach's test tube, which is marked off in grams, until the letter U (urine) is reached. Then Esbach's reagent is poured in up to the mark R.

E.'s method, estimation of albumen

The tube is tightly corked and gently inverted once or twice, care being taken to prevent bubbles forming.

The tube is now set aside, upright, for 12 hours. It must not be disturbed, and the temperature of the room should be kept constant. The albumin is seen as a precipitate at the bottom of the tube, and is read off in grams per liter. If grains per ounce are required, multiply the result by 0.4. Esbach's reagent contains picric acid and citric acid. RS: *albumen*.

E.'s quantitative estimation of albumen. Apparatus required:

(*a*) An Esbach's albuminometer. This is a large test tube marked with a scale for reading off the precipitate in grams per liter. Above this is the letter U, and about 2 in. higher is the letter R.

(*b*) Esbach's reagent. Consists of: Picric acid, 10 Gm.; citric acid, 20 Gm.; water, 1 liter.

The following points should be noted before carrying out the test:
1. The urine must be acid.
2. Its specific gravity must be 1.010 or below. If above this the urine must be diluted with an equal quantity of water, the final result being multiplied by 2.
3. The urine should be cold.
4. Keep the specimen in a room with a constant temperature.

Technic: Pour some of the urine into the Esbach's tube up to the letter U. Then add reagent up to the letter R. Cork, and then gently invert the tube 2 or 3 times, taking care not to form bubbles. The tube is now set aside in an upright position and the precipitate allowed to settle for 12 hours. It is then read off on the scale as grams per liter. If it is desired in grains per ounce the number of grams is multiplied by 0.4, *e. g.*, if the precipitate reaches the figure 4 it means that there is present 4 Gm. of dried albumen to 1 liter of water. To bring this to grains per ounce $4 \times .4 = 1.6$ gr. per ounce. RS: *albumen*.

escape mechanism. In psychiatry, the reaction of a person in adjusting temporarily to difficult, unpleasant, or intolerable situations by unconsciously employing another means which is less difficult or more pleasant.

escape, vagal. Occurrence of a ventricular contraction when the normal rhythmical beat of the heart has been stopped or inhibited by stimulation of the vagus nerve. Also called "escape from inhibition", "escape of the heart", or "vagus escape."

escape, ventricular. Occurrence of single or repeated ventricular contractions from impulses arising in the atrioventricular node. Also called nodal extrasystole.

eschar (es′kar) [G. *eschara*, scab]. A slough, esp. one following a cauterization or burn. SEE: *escharotic*.

escharotic (es-kar-ot′ik) [G. *eschara*, scab]. Agent used to destroy tissue and to cause sloughing which produces what is known as an *eschar*. The third degree of counterirritation.

They are caustics, the mild ones being used in the treatment of skin diseases; the stronger being employed to destroy infected tissue, and to counteract the bites of animals and insects; caustic soda and antimonial ointment being applied for this purpose. Silver nitrate is used by some physicians as a solution to be painted around the *meatus urinarius* for incontinence of the urine. They may be acids, alkalies, metallic salts, phenol or carbolic acid, carbon dioxide, or the cautery; epispastics, *q.v.*

eschatin (es′kă-tin). An extract of suprarenal cortex.
  USES: Specific in Addison's disease.
  DOSAGE: Average, 1-5 cc. subcutaneously.

Escherichia (esh-er-ik′ĭ-ă). A genus of bacteria belonging to the family Enterobacteriaceae, tribe Eschericheae. They are common inhabitants of the alimentary canal of man and other animals.
  E. coli. SYN: *Bacterium coli communis*. The colon bacillus. A short, plump, gram-negative, nonsporeforming motile bacillus almost constantly present in the alimentary canal of humans and some animals. They are normally non-pathogenic but may cause inflammatory condition of the gall bladder, urinary bladder and the peritoneal cavity. Their presence in milk or water is an indicator of fecal contamination.

Escherich's reflex (esk′ĕr′ĭk). Pursing or muscular contraction of lips resulting from irritation of mucosa of lips.

eschrolalia (es-kro-lal′ĭ-ă) [G. *aischros*, indecent, + *lalia*, babble]. Utterance without meaning of obscene words. SYN: *coprolalia*.

Escudero's test. A test for gout.

es′culent [L. *esculentus*, eatable]. Suitable to be eaten.

escutcheon (es-kutch′un) [Fr. *escuchon*, shield, from L. *scutum*, shield]. The coarse pubic hair in the adult.

eserine (es′er-ĭn). USP. SEE: *physostigmine*.

Es′march's bandage. A rubber bandage for controlling bleeding. Before operation commences, bandage is applied tightly to limb, commencing at distal end and reaching above site of operation, where a rubber tourniquet is firmly applied. The bandage is then removed. This renders operative area absolutely bloodless. SEE: *bandage*.

esodic (es-od′ik) [G. *esō*, within, + *odos*, way]. Centripetal or afferent; pert. to sensory nerves conducting impulses toward the brain and spinal cord.

esoenteritis (es′′o-en-ter-i′tis) [″ + *enteron*, intestine, + *-itis*, inflammation]. Inflammation of the mucous membrane of the intestine.

esoethmoiditis (es-o-eth-moy-di′tis) [″ + *ēthmos*, sieve, + *eidos*, form, + *-itis*, inflammation]. Inflammation of membrane of ethmoid cells.

esogastri′tis [″ + *gastēr*, belly, + *-itis*, inflammation]. Catarrhal inflammation of the gastric mucous membranes.

esophagalgia (ĕs-ō-făj-ăl′jĭ-ă). Pain in the esophagus.

esophageal (e-sof-ă′je-al) [G. *oisophagos*, esophagus]. Pert. to the esophagus.

esophagectasia, esophagectasis (ĕ-sŏf-ă-jĕk-tă′sĭ-ă). Dilatation of the esophagus.

esophagec′tomy [″ + *ektomē*, excision]. Excision of a part of the esophagus.

esophagismus (e-sof-aj-is′mus) [″ + *ismos*, condition of]. Esophageal spasm.

esophagitis (e-sof-a-ji′tis) [″ + *-itis*, inflammation]. Inflammation of the esophagus.

esophagocele (e-sof′a-go-sēl) [″ + *kēlē*, hernia]. Hernia of the esophagus.

esophagodyn′ia [″ + *odynē*, pain]. Pain in the esophagus.

esophagoenterostomy (e-sof″a-go-en-ter-os′to-mĭ) [" + *enteron*, intestine, + *stoma*, mouth]. Formation of communication bet. the esophagus and intestine with excision of stomach.

esophagogastros′copy [" + *gastēr*, belly, + *skopein*, to examine]. Inspection of esophagus and stomach through an illuminated instrument.

esophagogastrostomy (e-sof″ă-go-gas-tros′to-mĭ) [" + " + *stoma*, mouth]. Formation of a communication bet. the esophagus and stomach.

esophagomalacia (e-sof″ă-go-măl-a′sĭ-ă) [" + *malakia*, softness]. Softening of the esophageal walls.

esophagomycosis (e-sof″a-go-mi-ko′sis) [" + *mykēs*, fungus, + *ōsis*]. Bacterial or fungous disease of esophagus.

esophagoplasty (e-sof″ă-go-plas′tĭ) [" + *plassein*, to form]. Repair of the esophagus by a plastic operation.

esophagoplication (e-sof″ă-go-plĭ-ka′shun) [" + L. *plicāre*, to fold]. Reduction of dilation of the esophagus by taking tucks in its walls.

esophagopto′sia, esophagopto′sis [" + *ptōsis*, a falling]. Relaxation and prolapse of the esophagus.

esophagoscope (e-sof′ag-o-skōp) [" + *skopein*, to examine]. Device for examination of esophagus.

esoph′agospasm [" + *spasmos*, spasm]. Spasm of walls of the esophagus.

esophagostenosis (e-sof″a-go-stē-no′sis) [" + *stenōsis*, contraction]. Stricture or narrowing of the esophagus.

esophagostomy (e-sof-ag-os′to-mĭ) [" + *stoma*, opening]. Formation of esophageal fistula.

esophagotome (e-sof′a-go-tōm) [" + *tomē*, incision]. Instrument for forming an esophageal fistula.

esophagotomy (e-sof-ag-ot′o-mĭ) [" + *tomē*, incision]. Making of an incision in esophagus, so as to remove foreign substance.

esophagus (e-sof′a-gus) (pl. *esophagī*) [G. *oisophagos*]. A musculomembranous canal extending from the pharynx to the stomach. Length about 9 inches. RS: *epicardia, epicardium, gullet*.
  e., foreign bodies in the. F. A. TREATMENT: The patient may complain of pain or an uncomfortable feeling deep in the chest. The article often can be dislodged by making the patient vomit by wiggling the finger in the back part of the throat, or it may be displaced downwards by giving thick materials to the patient to swallow.
  Such foods as mashed or boiled potatoes, oatmeal, gruel, soft bread, etc., usually adhere to the object, prevent its irritation on the wall of the esophagus and aid in carrying it to the stomach.
  A physician should always be called. Foreign bodies in the stomach are ordinarily not dangerous and usually pass through the alimentary tract in a few days without danger. However, it may be dangerous to give cathartics or enemas. These patients should always be under the care of a physician.

esophoria (es-o-fo′rĭ-ă) [G. *esō*, inward, + *pherein*, to bear]. OPTH: Tendency of visual lines to converge. SEE: *exophoria*.

esophylac′tic [" + *phylaxis*, protection]. That which is phylactic or protective.

esophylaxis (es″o-fĭ-laks′is) [" + *phylaxis*, protection]. The protective biological action against disease exercised by the fluids and cells of the body. SEE: *exophylaxis*.

esosphenoiditis (es″o-sfen-oy-di′tis) [" + *sphēn*, wedge, + *eidos*, form, + *itis*, inflammation]. Osteomyelitis of the sphenoid bone.

esoteric (es-o-ter′ik) [G. *esōteros*, within]. Coming from within the organism.

esotropia (es-o-tro′pĭ-ă) [G. *esō*, inward, + *trepein*, to turn]. Marked turning inward of eye, crossed eyes.

-ess [Fr.]. Suffix noting female sex.

es′sence [L. *essentia*, being or quality]. 1. The spirit or principle of anything. 2. An alcoholic solution of volatile oil.

essen′tial [L. *essentia*, being or quality]. 1. Pert. to an essence. 2. Indispensable. 3. Specific; independent of a local morbid condition. SYN: *idiopathic*.
  e. amino acid. One of the ten amino acids necessary for normal growth. SEE: *amino acid*.
  e. oil. Any volatile oil of vegetable or animal origin.

es′ter. In organic chemistry, a compound formed by the combination of an organic acid with an alcohol.
  Ex: Ethyl acetate is an ester formed by combining acetic acid with ethyl alcohol. Esters are commonly liquids with characteristic fruity or flowery odors.

esterase (es′ter-ās). Generic term for an enzyme that catalyzes the hydrolysis of esters.
  e. acetylcholine. Cholinesterase, an enzyme that quickly hydrolyzes acetylcholine to acetic acid and choline.

es′terize. To convert into an ester.

esterol (es′ter-ol). Known also as benzyl succinate; a white, odorless powder.
  USES: As an antispasmodic.
  DOSAGE: 5 gr. (0.3 Gm.).

es″thematol′ogy [G. *aisthēma*, sensation, + *logos*, science]. Science of the sense organs and their function.

esthesia (es-the′zĭ-ă) [G. *aisthēsis*, sensation]. 1. Perception, feeling, sensation. 2. Any disease that affects the senses or perceptions. It forms the termination of many medical words.

esthe′sioblast [" + *blastos*, germ]. An embryonic ganglion cell. SYN: *ganglioblast*.

esthesiol′ogy [" + *logos*, science]. Science of sensory phenomena. SYN: *esthematology*.

esthesiomania (es-thez″ĭ-o-mă′nĭ-ă) [" + *mania*, madness]. Insanity with sensory hallucinations and perverted moral sensibilities.

esthesiometer (es-the-zĭ-om′et-er) [" + *metron*, measure]. Device for measuring tactile sensibility.

esthesioneurosis (es-the′zĭ-o-nu-ro′sis) [" + *neuron*, nerve, + *ōsis*]. A loss of feeling without any apparent organic lesion.

esthe″siophysiol′ogy [" + *physis*, nature, + *logos*, study]. Physiology of the sense organs.

esthesioscopy (es-the′zĭ-os′ko-pĭ) [" + *skopein*, to examine]. Testing tactile and other forms of sensibility.

estheticokinetic (es-thet″ĭ-ko-kin-et′ĭk) [" + *kinēsis*, motion]. Being both sensory and motor.

esthiomene (es-thĭ-om′en-e) [G. *esthiomenos*, eating]. A chronic hypertrophic ulcerative vulvovaginitis of unknown origin.

esthiomenus (es-the-om′e-nus) [G. *esthiomenos*, eating]. Swelling and ulceration of perianal region and vulva.

es′tival [L. *aestivus*, pert. to summer]. Relating to or occurring in summer.

estivo-autumnal [" + *autumnalis*, pert. to autumn]. 1. Pert. to summer and autumn. 2. A term applied to form of malarial fever.

Est'lander's operation. Resection of a part of 1 or more ribs and excision of diseased pleura in chronic empyema.

estradiol (ĕs-trā'dĭ-ŏl). SYN: *dihydrotheelin*. Dihydroxyestrin, $C_{18}H_{24}O_2$, a crystalline steroid possessing estrogenic properties found in the ovary, the follicular fluid, corpus luteum, placenta, and adrenal gland. Large quantities are found in the urine of pregnant women and mares and in the urine of stallions; the latter two serving as sources of the commercial product. In the body it is converted to estrone and estriol. It is believed to be the true estrogenic hormone.

e. dipropionate. An estrogen very effective in menopause.

es'triol. Hormone found in urine of pregnancy. SYN: *theelol*.

es'trogen. Any substance, natural or artificial, which induces estrogenic activity; more specifically the estrogenic hormone produced by the ovarian follicle and other structures; the female sex hormone. Estrogens are responsible for the development of secondary sexual characteristics, cyclic changes in the vaginal epithelium (and the endothelium) of the uterus. They are used in the treatment of menopausal symptoms. Natural estrogens include estradiol, estrone, and estriol. Synthetic estrogens used clinically are dihydroethylstilbesterol (hexestrol) and dienestrol.

estrogenic (es-tro-jen'ĭk) [G. *oistros*, mad desire, + *gennan*, to produce]. Causing estrus.

es'trone. Theelin, $C_{18}H_{22}O_2$; an estrogenic hormone found in the ovary, the urine of pregnant women and mares, the placenta, the urine and testes of stallions and in certain vegetable compounds (palm oil). Used in the treatment of estrogen deficiencies. It is less active than estradiol, but more active than estriol. Also called folliculin, follicular hormone.

es'trual [G. *oistros*, mad desire]. Pert. to the rutting of animals.

estrua'tion [G. *oistros*, mad desire]. Rutting of animals during heat period.

es'trum, es'trus [G. *oistros*, mad desire]. In mammals other than primates, the recurrent period of sexual activity called "heat", characterized by congestion of and secretion by the uterine mucosa, proliferation of vaginal epithelium, swelling of the vulva, ovulation, and acceptance of the male by the female.

e. cycle. The cycle from the beginning of one estrus period to the beginning of the next. Includes proestrus, estrus, and metestrus followed by a short period of quiescence called *diestrus*.

estua'rium [L. *aistus*, heat]. Vapor bath.

état mamelonné (ā-tä' mă-mĕ-lon-nā') [Fr. knobby state]. Condition of gastric mucosa in chronic inflammation with nodular projections.

e'ther [G. *aithēr*, air]. 1. Hypothetic substance once regarded as permeating all space and capable of transmitting electromagnetic vibrations. 2. Any organic compound in which an oxygen atom links together 2 carbon chains.

DOSAGE: 15 gr. (1.0 Gm.)

The general formula is R'OR''. The ether used for anesthesia is diethyl ether, $C_2H_5OC_2H_5$, and was formerly called sulfuric ether because it can be prepared from ethyl alcohol and sulfuric acid. As an anesthetic it is nauseating and it affects the kidneys.

e. anesthetic. Ethyl oxide, or diethyl ether $(C_2H_5)_2O$, the common ether used in anesthesia. It is a thin, colorless, highly volatile, and highly inflammable liquid with a specific gravity at 25° of 0.713-0.716. It was formerly called sulfuric ether because it was prepared from ethyl alcohol and sulfuric acid. It is widely used for general anesthesia. The action of ether is slower than other general anesthetics and the margin of safety is greater.

PHYS. ACTION: Ether stimulates the respiratory mucous membranes and the respiratory center in the medulla oblongata. It stimulates and accelerates the action of the heart. It lowers body temperature and raises blood pressure unless given in large doses or continued over a long period, when it lowers blood pressure. It produces fair muscular relaxation and increases mucus and other secretions. It produces slight changes in body chemistry. It is usually chosen for most brain surgery and is the best anesthetic if properly administered.

CONTRA: Its use is avoided in acute respiratory infections, in pulmonary tuberculosis, renal diseases, diabetes, brain tumors, and conditions in which congestion may be present or caused in the brain. It acts as an irritant upon the kidneys and inhibits urinary secretion and elimination. It is also irritating to the muscular glands.

AFTER EFFECTS: Excitement with desire to talk follows ether anesthesia, the patient perspires freely, and exhibits signs of nausea and begins to vomit, all before the return to consciousness, which may not be regained for several hours. Upon awakening he feels dizzy, complains of headache and thirst. These effects may last for hours. The flow of saliva and the secretion of mucus may be increased. It is usually excreted from the body within 24 hr. Pneumonia is the most common complication following ether anesthesia. Gas pains may give trouble. Sodium bicarbonate in water sipped slowly, or small pieces of ice held in the mouth may relieve nausea and vomiting. Warm or cold water; the quantity permitted to relieve thirst depends upon the surgeon. The head should be turned to one side when vomiting, to prevent vomitus from passing into the trachea. Cold compresses may be placed to head and a rectal irrigation may be given to relieve gas pressure, or a rectal tube may be inserted for the purpose. SEE: *chloroform a., ethylene a.*

e. asphyxia. Suffocation during ether anesthetization. SEE: *e. anesthesia, gases, resuscitation.*

e. bed. One prepared to prevent patient from injuring self, to keep patient warm, and to protect bedding.

ARTICLES NECESSARY: Bedding for making an ordinary closed bed. Two small rubber sheets. Two draw sheets (or special "ether sheets"). Two bath blankets. Two pieces of bandage about 3 in. wide. Two towels. Two emesis basins. Pad and pencil. Small pieces of gauze or paper wipes. Paper bags. Safety pins. Shock blocks. Rubber pillow case. Hot water bottles filled and covered (if they are to be used).

ether, drunkenness — **ethyl, chloride**

PROCEDURE: 1. Make up bottom part of bed as usual. 2. Place 1 small rubber where region of operation will come. 3. Place another across head of mattress where patient's head will lie. 4. Cover each with a draw sheet, tucking it firmly under mattress. 5. Spread the 2 bath blankets 1 over the other, with tops 6 in. from top of mattress. Hot water bottles to be placed between these. Tuck lower blanket in at sides. 6. Place top bedding as usual but do not tuck in. 7. Fold top sheet over bed blanket to protect it. Fold all top bedding together, including the top bath blanket, even with mattress edge all around, then fold toward side of bed away from the door, or where the stretcher will be placed, until it lies in a neat fold. 8. Tie 1 pillow upright on its side against bars at top of bed with bandage. 9. Put rubber pillow case on other pillow and have it ready to put under patient's knees if needed. 10. Place shock blocks at foot of bed on each side ready for instant pushing into position. 11. Place pad, pencil, emesis basin, wipes and 1 towel on bedside table, other towels over headbar of bed. 12. Place chairs and table out of way of the stretcher.

 e. drunkenness. Intoxication produced by imbibing ether.
ethereal (e-the′re-al) [G. *aithēr*, air]. Pert. to or made with ether.
 e. oil. A volatile oil.
etherin (e′ther-in) [G. *aithēr*, air]. A tuberculous toxin extracted by ether. SYN: *etherobacillin*.
etherion (e-the′ri-on) [G. *aithēr*, air]. A gas of extreme tenuity in the atmosphere.
etherization (e″ther-ĭ-za′shun) [G. *aithēr*, air]. Administering ether to induce anesthesia.
e′therize [G. *aithēr*, air]. To anesthetize by use of ether.
e″therobacil′lin [" + L. *bacillus*, rod]. Poison extracted from tuberculosis bacilli.
etheromania (e″ther-o-ma′nĭ-ă) [" + *mania*, madness]. Addiction to use of ether.
ethics. A system of moral principles or standards governing conduct.
 e. medical. A system of principles governing medical conduct. It deals with the relationship of a physician to the patient, the patient's family, his fellow physicians, and society at large.
 e. nursing. A system of principles governing conduct of a nurse. It deals with the relationship of a nurse to the patient, the patient's family, her associates and fellow nurses, and society at large.
ethiopifica′tion [G. *Aithiops*, an Ethiopian, + L. *facere*, to make]. Pathological blackening of skin or production of argyria.*
ethmo- [G.]. Prefix denoting "connected with or pert. to the ethmoid bone."
ethmocardi′tis [G. *ēthmos*, sieve, + *kardia*, heart]. Chronic inflammation and proliferation of cardiac connective tissue. SYN: *cardiosclerosis*.
eth′moid [" + *eidos*, form]. Sievelike, cribriform.
 e. bone. Sievelike spongy bone which forms a roof for the nasal fossae and part of floor of ant. fossa of skull, and containing air sinuses.
 e. sinus. Air cells or space inside ethmoid bone.
ethmoi′dal [" + *eidos*, form]. Pert. to the ethmoid bone or sinuses.

ethmoidectomy (eth-moy-dek′to-mī) [" + " + *ektome*, excision]. Excision of ethmoid cells.
 NP: Patient in sitting position, ice packs to nose often ordered.
ethmoidi′tis [" + " + *-itis*, inflammation]. Inflammation of ethmoidal cells. May be acute or chronic. SYM: Headache, acute pain bet. eyes, nasal discharge.

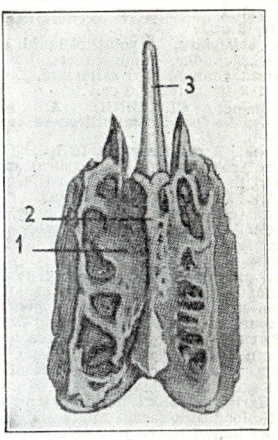

ETHMOID BONE
1. Cribriform plate. 2. Crista galli. 3. Perpendicular plate.

ethmyphitis (eth-mif-i′tis [" + *yphē*, tissue, + *-itis*, inflammation]. Diffuse inflammation of cellular tissue. SYN: *cellulitis*.
ethnog′raphy [G. *ethnos*, race, + *graphein*, to write]. The description of the human race.
ethnol′ogy [" + *logos*, science]. The science of human races.
ethyl (eth′il) [G. *aithēr*, air, + *ylē*, matter]. In organic chemistry, the radical C_2H_5 which enters into the constitution of many compounds such as ethyl ether, ethyl alcohol, and ethyl acetate.
 e. acetate. $CH_3CO.OCH_2CH_3$, acetic ether. A colorless liquid used as a solvent.
 e. alcohol. CH_3CH_2OH Grain alcohol. SEE: *alcohol, ethyl*, Transparent, colorless, volatile liquid of characteristic odor and a burning taste. The most important poison in medical and legal professions. It is the active principle of alcoholic beverages, and many proprietary preparations. SEE: *alcohol*.
 e. aminobenzoate. Same as benzocain.
 e. bromide. CH_3CH_2Br, hydrobromic ether. Used for local anesthesia.
 e. carbamate. $C_2H_5OCONH_2$ urethane. Used to induce sleep and in the treatment of myeloid and lymphatic leukemia.
 e. chaulmoograte. The ethyl esters of the fatty acids of chaulmoogra oil. Used in the treatment of leprosy.
 e. chloride. CH_3CH_2OH, hydrochloric ether. USP. A very volatile liquid with a pleasant odor. USES: Local anesthetic in minor surgery, or used in much the same way as chloroform. It produces muscular spasms and, if not given cautiously, may result in sudden respira-

ethyl, formate — E-54 — **euchlorhydria**

tory paralysis. It is used only for a very short anesthesia.

e. formate. HCOOC₂H₅, formic ether; a volatile antispasmodic and anesthetic.

e. iodide. CH₃CH₂I, hydriodic ether; used in treatment of asthma.

e. nitrite, spirit of. Commonly known as sweet spirit of niter. USP. Oily liquid. ACTION AND USES: Diuretic and for relief of arterial spasm. DOSAGE: 30 ㎖ (2 cc.).

e. salicylate. A volatile liquid, characteristic odor, same effects, but less irritant than methyl salicylate. DOSAGE: From 5-10 ㎖ (0.3-0.6 cc.).

e'thylamine. CH₃CH₂NH₂. An amine formed in the decomposition of certain proteins.

e'thylene. A colorless gas (CH₂CH₂) prepared from alcohol by dehydration and found in illuminating gas to the extent of 4%. It is colorless, and has a sweetish taste but a pungent, foul odor. It is lighter than air and diffusable when liberated. It is inflammable and explosive.

e. anesthesia. Since ethylene is a rather weak anesthetic, it usually is given in a combination of oxygen 20%, cyclopropane 10%, and ethylene 70%.

PHYS. EFFECTS: It causes less alteration in the blood gases than does nitrous oxide. The CO₂ content is not altered. Full muscular relaxation and slight irregularity in heart action, respiration, and blood pressure. Analgesia results before loss of hearing or before complete unconsciousness. Nausea and vomiting seldom persist as long as 24 hr., but it generally disappears before consciousness has returned.

ADVANTAGES: Slightly stimulating to cardiac and respiratory systems. It lowers body temperature; less toxic than any known anesthetics. It is not irritating to mucous glands and kidneys. It has a short period of induction and makes possible a very rapid recovery. There is an absence of cyanosis, and a minimum of emesis. The difference between ethylene and any other anesthetic known today is that there is a less marked effect on all the systems of the body. It is the choice anesthetic for old patients and for poor surgical risks, and when moderate anesthesia is desired or where complete relaxation is not required.

DISADVANTAGES: Has an objectionable smell; is highly inflammable and explosive; increases capillary bleeding; the relaxation is not so complete or as perfect as from the use of ether anesthetics.

PRECAUTIONS: *Many lives have been lost because someone was careless and a spark was emitted from some immediate source. Ethylene should be stored where there is plenty of air. The administration must be done away from fire or electric appliances or x-ray apparatus. All lights should be turned on before bringing the tanks into the room to prevent sparking from the plug or lighting fixture. Furniture should never be dragged into the room or rolled into the room while the anesthetic is being given. The humidity of the room should be checked during the administration of this anesthetic. Not even the exit lights should be burning during the giving of this anesthetic.*

Ethylene does not combine with air as do other anesthetics but floats around as clouds; as the vapor rises in a cloud-like form any gust of air may carry it out of the room and should someone be on the outside smoking or the elevator cause a sparking, an explosion would result with the destruction of life in a most devastating manner. Ethylene always comes in red tanks. Oxygen is stored in green tanks. Nitrous oxide is stored in blue tanks. Carbon dioxide is stored in gray tanks. SEE: *chloroform a., ether a.*

etiolate (e'tĭ-o-lat) [Fr. *étioler*, to blanch]. Pale or sickly from lack of light or long continued illness.

etiologic, etiological (e″tĭ-o-loj'ik, e-tĭ-o-loj'ik-ăl) [G. *aitia*, cause, + *logos*, study]. Pert. to causes.

etiology (e-tĭ-ol'o-jĭ) [″ + *logos*, study]. The study of the causes of disease which result from an abnormal state producing pathological conditions.

CONGENITAL: Embryonic malformations and conditions occurring during fetal life, such as abnormalities, anomalies, and monstrosities.

e″tiotrop'ic. Directed toward the cause of a disease, said of a drug or treatment which destroys or inactivates the causal agent of a disease; opposite of nosotropic, *q.v.*

etrohysterectomy (e″trō-hĭs-tĕr-ĕk'tō-mĭ). Excision of the uterus through the abdominal wall in the hypogastric region.

etymology (et-ĭ-mol'o-jĭ) [G. *etymon*, true meaning of a word, + *logos*, science]. The science of the derivation of words.

Most medical words are derived from the Latin and Greek, but many of those from the Greek have reached us through the Latin, being modified by that language. When 2 Greek words are used to form 1 word, they generally are connected by the letter "o."

Many medical words have been formed from 1 or more *roots*, forms used or adapted from the Latin or Greek, and many of them are modified either by a *prefix* or a *suffix*, or both. A knowledge of important Latin or Greek roots, and of prefixes will reveal the meaning of a great many other words.

Eubacteriales (ū-băk-tē-rĭ-a'lēs) [G. *eu*, well, + *baktērion*, little rod]. The true bacteria. Includes the simplest and least differentiated forms. SEE: *bacteria, classification of.*

eubiotics (u-bi-ot'ĭks) [G. *eu*, well, + *bios*, life]. Hygienic living.

eu'bolism [″ + (*meta*)*bolē*, change, + *ismos*, condition]. Normal metabolism.

eucaine hydrochloride (ū-kān'hy-dro-chlō'rĭd). USP. White, crystalline powder.

USES: Local anesthetic. [2 to 5%. DOSAGE: Topically, in strengths from INCOMPATIBILITY: Salicylates.

eucalyptol. USP. A substance obtained from oil of eucalyptus.

DOSAGE: 5 gr. (0.3 Gm.).

eucalyptus, oil of (u-kal-ĭp'tŭs) [G. *eu*, well, + *kalyptein*, to cover]. USP. Oil distilled from fresh leaves of the plant.

ACTION AND USES: As an expectorant and antiseptic.

DOSAGE: 8 ㎖ (0.5 cc.).

eucapnia (ū-kăp'nĭ-ă). Presence of normal amounts of carbon dioxide in the blood.

euchlorhydria (ū-klōr″hī-drĭ'ă). Presence of the normal amount of free hydrochloric acid in the gastric juice.

eucholia (ū-kō'lĭ-ă). Normal condition of bile as regards its constituents and amount secreted.

euchylia (ū-kī'lĭ-ă) [" + *chylos*, chyle]. Normal condition of the chyle.

eucrasia (ū-krā'sĭ-ă). Condition of normal health; state of the body in which all activities are in normal balance.

eudiaphoresis (ū-dī"ă-fo-re'sis) [" + *dia*, through, + *pherein*, to carry]. Normal secretion of perspiration.

eudiemorrhysis (u"dī-em-or'ĭ-sis) [" + " + *aima*, blood, + *rysis*, flow]. The normal blood flow through the capillaries.

eudiom'eter [G. *eudia*, good weather, + *metron*, measure]. An instrument for testing purity of air and analysis of gases.

euesthesia (u-es-the'sĭ-ă) [G. *eu*, well, + *aisthēsis*, sensation]. Having normal senses.

eugenics (u-jen'iks) [" + *gennan*, to produce]. The science which deals with the physical, moral, and intellectual improvement of the human race by careful and judicious mating. It is also concerned with (1) the sterilization of mental defectives; (2) intermarriages; (3) restriction of marriage bet. persons physically unfit; (4) birth control and allied problems. SEE: *aristogenics*.
  e. negative. Those measures which seek to restrict the numbers of offspring of undesirable types.
  e. positive. Those measures which seek to bring about an increase in the numbers of offspring of families of the better types.

eugenism (u'jen-ism) [" + " + *ismos*, condition]. The circumstances of environment and heredity which tend to bring about happy and healthy existence.

euglobulin (eū-glŏb'ŭl-ĭn). A true globulin, or one soluble in distilled water and dilute salt solution. SEE: *pseudoglobulin*.

eugon'ic [" + *gonē*, seed]. Pertaining to a luxuriant growth of bacteria.

eukinesia (u-kin-e'sĭ-ă) [" + *kinēsis*, motion]. Normal power of movement.

eumenorrhea (eu-mĕn-or-rē'ă). Normal menstruation.

eunoia (u-noy'ă) [" + *nous*, mind]. Soundness of mind.

eunuch (ū'nuk) [G. *eunē*, bed, + *echein*, to hold]. Castrated male; one who has had his testicles removed.
  The absence of the testicular secretions produces certain symptoms, such as a female type of voice and loss of hair on the face.

eunuchism (ū'nŭk-ism). Condition resulting from complete androgen deficiency such as occurs following castration.

eunuchoid. Having the characteristics of a eunuch, such as retarded development of external and accessory sex organs, absence of beard and bodily hair, high-pitched voice, and striking lack of muscular development.
  e. pituitary. E. Due to failure of the ant. lobe of the pituitary to secrete gonadotrophic hormones; secondary hypogonadism.

eunuchoidism (ū-nŭk-oyd-ism). Condition resulting from androgen deficiency of the testes regardless of etiology.

eupancreatism (u-pan'kre-ă-tizm) [G. *eu*, well, + *pagkreas*, pancreas, + *ismos*, condition]. Normal condition of the pancreas.

eupep'sia [" + *pepsis*, digestion]. Normal digestion, as distinguished from dyspepsia.

eupep'tic [" + *pepsis*, digestion]. Possessed of a good digestion.

euphonia (ū-fōn'ĭ-ă). Having a normal, clear voice.

euphoria (ū-fo'rĭ-ă) [" + *pherein*, to bear]. 1. A condition of good health. 2. PSY: A feeling of well being; mild elation.* [ing quickly and well.

euplas'tic [" + *plassein*, to form]. Heal-

eupnea (up-ne'ă) [" + *pnein*, to breathe]. Normal breathing, as distinguished from dyspnea and apnea.

eupraxia (ū-prak'sĭ-ă) [" + *prassein*, to do]. Normal capacity to execute a motor pattern. SEE: *paralysis*.

eupraxic (ū-prak'sik) [" + *prassein*, to do]. Contributing to proper functioning.

euquinine (ū-kwī'nĭn) (quinine ethyl carbonate). USP. Nearly tasteless, light, fleecy crystals.
  DOSAGE: Same as for quinine, but may be given in larger doses.
  USES: Same as for quinine.

euresol (u're-sol). A trade name for resorcinol monacetate.
  ACTION AND USES: Antiseptic, largely used for scalp lotions, in alcoholic solutions 3 to 5%.

Euro'fium. A genus of molds.
  E. malig'num. A species causing inflammation in ext. auditory meatus.

euryon (u're-on) [G. *eurys*, broad]. Either end of bilateral diameter of head.

euryosomic, eurysomatic (ū"rĭ-ō-sōm'ĭk, -rĭ-sōm-at'ĭk) [" + *sōma*, body]. Having a thick, squat body.

eu'rythrol. Extract of ox spleen; used in chlorosis and anemia.
  DOSAGE: 60-120 ℥ (3.75-7.5 cc.).

eustachian (u-sta'kĭ-an). After Eustachio, an Italian anatomist. Pert. to the auditory tube. [*rinx.*
  RS: *salpingemphraxis*, *syringitis*, *sy-*
  e. catheter. Instrument for introducing medicated vapor into the eustachian tube.
  e. tube. The auditory tube (from the middle ear to the pharynx, 3-4 cm. long and lined with mucous membrane).
  e. valve. At the entrance of the inf. vena cava. SYN: *valvula venae cavae inferioris*.

eustachitis (u-sta-kī'tĭs). Inflammation of the eustachian tube.

eusystole (u-sis'to-lĭ) [G. *eu*, well, + *systellein*, to draw together]. A state of the systole of the heart that is normal in time and force.

eutectic (u-tek'tĭk) [" + *tēktos*, melting]. Easily melted.
  e. mixture. A mixture of two or more substances which has a melting point lower than that of any of its constituents.

euthanasia (u-than-a'zĭ-ă) [" + *thanatos*, death]. 1. An easy death. 2. The proposed practice of ending a life in case of incurable disease.

euthenics (ū-then'ĭks) [G. *euthēnia*, well-being]. The science of improvement of the race through modification of the environment; in contrast to eugenics, *q.v.*

eutocia (u-to'sĭ-ă) [G. *eu*, well, + *tokos*, birth]. Normal or natural labor and childbirth.

eutonon (u'tō-non) [" + *tonos*, tension]. Proprietary liver extract, possibly a hormone, suggested for use in treating vascular diseases.

evacuant (e-văk'ŭ-ant) [L. *evacuans*, making empty]. Drug which moves the bowels.

evac'uate [L. *evacuāre*, to empty]. To discharge, esp. from the bowels.

evacuation (e-vak-u-a'shun) [L. *evacuāre*, to empty]. 1. Emptying, esp. the bowels. 2. The material discharged from the bowels; stool. 3. Removal of air from a closed container; the production of a vacuum. RS: *absorption, feces, stool*.

evacuator (e-vak'u-a-tor) [L. *evacuāre*, to empty]. Device for emptying, as of the bowels or for irrigating the bladder and removing calculi.

evag'inate [L. *ē*, out, + *vagina*, sheath]. Pert. to protrusion of some part or organ from its normal place.

evagination (e-vaj-in-a'shun) [" + *vagina*, sheath]. 1. Emergence from a sheath. 2. Protrusion of an organ or part. SEE: *invagination*.

evanes'cent [L. *evanescere*, to vanish]. Not permanent; of brief duration; passing gradually.

Evans-Strang diet, modified. SEE: *reduction diet*.

evapora'tion [L. *ē*, out, + *vaporāre*, to steam]. 1. Change from liquid form to vapor. 2. Loss in volume due to conversion of a liquid into a vapor.

Eve's method (F. C. Eve, physician, Hull, England) (resuscitation in drowning). Place the victim downward on a stretcher with ankles and wrists tied to handles, arms extending away from the body beyond the head. Support stretcher on a trestle about 34 inches high. Hold head of stretcher down to a tilt of about 45 degrees, and keep it there until no more water drains from the mouth. Then start rocking for a few minutes; then reduce tilt about 30 degrees each way with ten double rockings a minute. This introduces twenty times as much air as does the Schafer method. Remove wet clothing as the rocking proceeds, rub the body, and place hot-water bottle at back of neck, adding warm blankets about the patient. Paralysis of the diaphragm is thus prevented. SEE: *resuscitaion, artificial respiration*.

evec'tics [L. *evehere*, to carry up]. Acquiring of bodily energy.

eventra'tion [L. *ē*, out, + *venter*, belly]. 1. Partial protrusion of the abdominal contents through an opening in the abdominal wall. 2. Removal of contents of the abdominal cavity.

    e. of the diaphragm. Elevation of the diaphragmatic dome into the thoracic cavity.

eversion (e-ver'shun) [" + *vertere*, to turn]. Turning outward. SEE: *chilectropion*.

    e. of the cervix. A turning out of the cervical edges subsequent to laceration. SYN: *ectropion of cervix*.

évidement (ā-vēd-mòn') [Fr. a scooping out]. Scraping away morbid tissue.

evipal (e'vī-pal). A derivative of urea, occurring as a white powder.

    USES: As a hypnotic of short duration but of rapid action; nervous insomnia and in labor.

    DOSAGE: 4 gr. (0.259 Gm.) to be used cautiously in liver damage.

    e., soluble. USES: In short surgical operations as an anesthetic, given intravenously.

eviration (e-vī-ra'shun) [L. *ē*, out, + *vir*, man]. 1. Castration. 2. Effemination or defemination, or transformations of psychical personality due to the development of contrary sexual instincts.

evisceration (e-vis-er-a'shun) [" + *viscera*, viscera]. 1. Removal of the viscera. 2. Removal of the contents of a cavity. 3. Protrusion of the viscera.

    e. obstetrical. Removal of the thoracic and abdominal contents of a fetus to facilitate delivery.

evis''ceroneurot'omy [" + " + G. *neuron*, nerve, + *tomē*, incision]. Scleral evisceration of the eye with division of optic nerve.

evolu'tion [" + *volvere*, to roll]. A process of orderly and gradual change or development.

More generally, any orderly and gradual process of modification whereby a system, whether physical, chemical, social, or even intellectual, becomes more highly organized.

    e. doctrine of. The view that all present day species of plants and animals, including man, have come into existence by gradual, continuous change from earlier pre-existing forms. It considers that life first came into existence as a simple primordial mass of protoplasm from which, through a series of progressive changes, the highly complex, specialized forms of today arose.

    e., spontaneous. Spontaneus birth of a child in transverse presentation.

evul'sion [" + *vellere*, to pluck]. 1. Tearing away of a part or new growth. 2. Forcible extraction, as of teeth.

Ewald's test dinner. Chopped meat, 165 Gm.; stale bread, 35 Gm., with a small portion of butter. This content is withdrawn in 3 hours. In this test, further action is desired than just 1 hour's effect could produce.

    E.'s t. meal. White bread or rolls (no crust), 40 Gm., and water or clear tea, 400 cc. No butter, sugar, milk, or cream taken with this portion. One hour after giving, the contents of the stomach are expressed. Time plays a very important part in the carrying out of the treatment.

ex- [L.]. Prefix: *Out, away from*.

exacerbation (eks''as-er-ba'shun) [L. *ex*, over, + *acerbus*, harsh]. Aggravation of symptoms or increase in the severity of a disease.

exacrinous (eks-ak'rin-us) [G. *ex*, outside, + *krinein*, to secrete]. Concerning a gland's external secretion.

exaltation. A mental state characterized by feelings of grandeur, excessive joy, elation, and optimism; an abnormal feeling of personal well-being or self-importance.

examina'tion, phys'ical [L. *examināre*, to examine]. The act or process of examining the body and its products as to fitness or for symptoms of a disease.

Local examination includes specific parts and organs. Laboratory examination includes urinalysis, tests, cultures, basal metabolism, etc.

Terms employed indicating type of examination are: physical, bimanual, digital, oral, rectal, O.B. (obstetrical), roentgen, cystoscopic.

    e. physical. Examination of the body for detection of symptoms of disease. Four procedures utilized are *inspection, palpation, percussion,* and *auscultation*.

exangia (eks-an'jī-ă) [G. *ex*, out, + *aggeion*, vessel]. Any dilatation of a blood vessel. Ex: *aneurysm, varix*.

exanthem, exanthema (eks-an'them, -an-the'mă) (pl. *exanthem'ta*) [G. *exanthēma*, eruption]. Any eruption of the skin, accompanied by inflammation, *e. g.*, measles, scarlatina, erysipelas, *q.v.*

exanthematous (eks-an-them'ă-tus) [G. *exanthēma*, eruption]. Pert. to an exanthem, eruption or rash.

exanthrope (eks'an-thrōp) [G. *ex*, out, + *anthrōpos*, man]. A cause or source of a disease originating outside the body.
  e. dental. The preparation of a cavity in a tooth prior to filling.
  e. of the optic nerve. A slight depression in the center of the optic papilla or disk from which retinal vessels emerge. It is more pronounced in glaucoma.
  e. recto-uterine. The recto-uterine pouch or pouch of Douglas.

exarteritis (eks-ar-ter-i'tis) [" + *artēria*, artery, + *itis*, inflammation]. Inflammation of the outer coat of an artery.

exarticula'tion [L. *ex*, out, + *articulus*, joint]. Amputation of a limb through a joint.

excava'tion [" + *cavus*, hollow]. 1. A hollow or depression. 2. Formation of a cavity.
  e. of optic nerve. A cupping of the optic disk.

excen'tric [G. *ex*, out, + *kentron*, center]. Away from; efferent.

excerebration (eks-ser-e-bra'shun) [L. *ex*, out, + *cerebrum*, brain]. Removal of brain.

excernant (eks-ser'nant) [L. *excernere*, to excrete]. Bringing about an evacuation or excretion. SYN: *excretory*.

excip'ient [L. *excipiens*, from *ex*, out, + *capere*, to take]. Any substance added to a medicine to give it form and consistency. SYN: *vehicle*.

excis'ion [L. *excisiō*, from *ex*, out, + *caedere*, to cut]. An act of cutting away or taking out.

excitabil'ity [L. *excitāre*, to rouse]. Sensitiveness to being stimulated.
  e., independent. Power of a muscle to respond to a stimulus without intervention of motor nerves.
  e., reflex. Sensitiveness to reflex irritation.

excit'ant [L. *excitāre*, to rouse]. An agent that will excite a special function of the body; subdivided, according to action, as *motor*, *cerebral*, etc. Ex: *alcohol*, *cocaine*, *strychnine*.

excita'tion [L. *excitāre*, to rouse]. 1. The act of exciting. 2. Condition of being stimulated or excited. The entire vasomotor system of nerves is involved.
  SYM: (Of sex impulse.) Eyes prominent, pupils dilated, conjunctiva injected, cardiac palpitation, turgescence of genitalia with erection of penis or clitoris. Sensory stimulation of the genitals causes ejaculation of the semen through the *ductus ejaculatorius* in the male, and of the vaginal glands in the female.
  The 3rd and 4th sacral nerves acting upon the *bulbocavernosus* muscles are responsible for ejaculation in the male. In the female, friction of the vaginal membranes incites a series of stimuli to the *thalamus* and from there to the cerebral cortex from which centrifugal impulses are sent to the erection and ejaculation centers of the spinal cord, flowing out to the periphery, causing erection of the clitoris and stimulating circulation to the genitals and the muscles to rhythmic action and causing glandular ejaculation, esp. of the glands of Bartholin.
  RS: *clitoris, copulation, coition, coitus, ejaculation, emission, erection, penis, sexual intercourse*.
  e. direct. Stimulation of a muscle with an electrode.
  e. indirect. Stimulation of a muscle *via* its nerve.

  e. wave. The wave of irritability originating in the atrioventricular node which sweeps over the conductile tissue of the heart and induces contraction of the atria and ventricles.

excit'ing [L. *excitāre*, to rouse]. Causing excitement.
  e. cause. Acting immediately as a cause of disease.

excitoglan'dular [" + *glans*, gland-, kernel]. Increasing glandular function.

excitometabol'ic [" + G. *metabolē*, change]. Increasing metabolic changes.

excitomo'tor [" + *motor*, moving]. Increasing rapidity of muscular activity.

excitomus'cular [" + G. *mys*, muscle]. Causing muscular activity.

excitonu'trient [" + *nutrire*, to nourish]. Stimulating nutrition.

exci'tor [L. *excitāre*, to rouse]. That which incites to greater activity. SYN: *stimulant*.

excitosecre'tory [" + *secretiō*, a hiding]. Tending to bring about secretion.

excitovas'cular [" + *vasculāris*, pert. to a vessel]. Increasing circulation.

exclave (eks'klāv) [L. *ex*, out, + *clavis*, key]. Detached part of an organ.

excochleation (eks-kok-le-a'shun) [" + *cochlea*, spoon]. Curettage of a cavity.

excoriation (eks-ko-rī-a'shun) [" + *corium*, skin]. Abrasion of the epidermis or of the coating of any organ of the body by trauma, chemicals, burns, or other causes.

excrement (eks'krē-ment) [L. *excernere*, to take away]. The feces, excreta, dejecta. SEE: *excretion*.
  e., menstruum. Menstrual discharge.

excrementitious (eks-kre-men-tish'us) [L. *excernere*, to take away]. Of the nature of excrement.

excrescence (eks-kres'ens) [L. *ex*, out, + *crescere*, to grow]. An outgrowth from the surface of a part. RS: *eruption, macula, nodule*.

excre'ta [L. from *excernere*, to take away]. Waste intestinal matter; dejecta; feces. Waste material cast off by the body.
  e., disinfection of. CARBOLIC ACID: A 5% solution to be used in quantity at least equal to the amount of the material to be disinfected.
  CAUSTIC LIME: In the form of freshly prepared milk lime—this should contain about 1 part by weight of hydrate of lime mixed with 8 parts of water, to be used in an amount equal to that of the excreta to be disinfected.
  CHLORIDE OF LIME: Dissolve in the proportion of 4 ounces to 1 gallon of water. One quart of this solution for disinfection of each liquid discharge. For solid fecal matter a stronger solution or a larger quantity of above solution will be required.
  It will be prudent to use a large quantity of the standard solution recommended for a copious liquid discharge. With a spatula the formed material should be broken up and covered with chlorinated lime. The container should be set aside and the feces or urine, with the coating of lime, covered with a lid or newspapers. Let the mixture stand for 1 hour, stirring the lime into the contents from time to time, then it may be emptied into the sewer.
  CUPRIC SULFATE: Is used as chloride of lime but in a 4% solution.
  INVOLUNTARY DISCHARGES: These should be cared for by placing oakum pads under the patient. The pads should be thoroughly wrapped in strong paper after being soiled to prevent scattering

of the feces. In handling all infected discharges, the nurse should wear rubber gloves.

e., kinds of. (1) Carbon and oxygen. Both given off as carbon dioxide from the lungs. (2) Hydrogen and oxygen. Both forming water and given off as: (a) Vapor from the lungs; (b) perspiration from the skin; (c) in urine from the kidneys. (3) Nitrogen: Given off in urine from the kidneys. (4) Intestinal excreta: (a) Waste mineral matter; (b) foreign matter; (c) unassimilated food material; (d) water and liquids.

excrete (eks-krēt') [L. *excernere*, to separate]. To separate and expel useless matter not utilized by the body.

excre'tin. A crystalline substance found in the feces. A fraction of the hormone, secretin, which stimulates pancreatic secretion.

excre'tion [L. *excernere*, to separate]. 1. Waste matter, excreta. 2. The elimination of waste products from the body.

 e., organs of. INTESTINES: Indigestible residue, water and bacteria.

 KIDNEYS: Filter from the blood water, nitrogenous substances (urea, uric acid, creatin, creatinine) mineral salts.

 RESPIRATORY SYSTEM: Carbon dioxide, water vapor, and probably gases.

 SKIN: Small amt. through perspiration of water, salts, minute quantities of urea. Its excretory function is stimulated by kidney inactivity. Diaphoretics, hot packs, and warm blankets stimulate skin and aid kidneys, thus helping to avoid uremic coma.

excretion, words pert. to: acatastasia, acathectic, acathexia, acoprosis, acrinia, allochezia, apocenosis, apolepsis, cholagogia, cholestasia, defecation, dejecta, elimination, emunctory, excrement, excreta, expectoration, feces, hydragogue, ichor, incontinence, lung, perspiration, pore, respiration, sanies, semen, skin, sputum, sweat, urination, urine, void.

ex'cretory [L. *excernere*, to separate]. Pert. to or bringing about excretion.

excur'sion [L. *ex*, out, + *currere*, to run]. 1. Wandering from the usual course. 2. Extent of movement of the eyes from a central position.

excurva'tion [" + *curvus*, bend]. A curvature outward. SYN: kyphosis.

excystation (eks"sis-ta'shŭn) [G. *ex*, out, + *kystis*, cyst]. Pertaining esp. to the escape of certain organisms (parasitic worms, protozoa) from an enclosing cyst wall or envelope. Process which occurs in the life cycle of an intestinal parasite after encysted form is ingested.

exemia (eks-e'mĭ-ă) [" + *aima*, blood]. Loss of blood from circulation, though accumulation in a part.

exencephalia (eks-en-sef-al'ĭ-ă). A term for encephalocele, hydrencephalocele, meningocele, and synencephalocele.

exenteration (eks-en-ter-a'shŭn) [" + *enteron*, intestine]. 1. Evisceration. 2. Removal of viscera of fetus in embryotomy.

exercise [L. *exercitātiō*, training the body]. Functional activity of the muscles, voluntary or otherwise.

 e., active. A form of bodily movement which the patient performs with or without the personal supervision of the operator.

 e., assistive. A form of bodily movement which the patient performs assisted by the operator or some mechanical means such as a pulley or weight.

 e., blowing. One in which water is blown from 1 bottle to another, thus increasing intrabronchial pressure which tends to aid in expansion of the lung. It is by this means that an empyema* cavity is obliterated.

 e., Buerger's postural (bur'gers). Used for circulatory disturbances of the extremities.

 e., Brandt's. Exercises for pelvic lesions. Fallen into disuse due to the attendant dangers.

 e., crawling. Devised for treatment of scoliosis,* essentially for children.

 e., free. Form of bodily movement which is carried through by patient against least possible resistance.

 e., Frenkel's. Used to teach tabetics to walk.

 e., Krida knee. In intertrochanteric fractures of femur, remove post. half of plaster cast from the knee to the toes; anterior portion of leg cast remains attached to spica, and maintains position of hip. When patient is face down, this permits knee to be flexed and extended and ankle exercised.

 e., Lewin circulatory. Passive exercise for leg for circulatory disturbance of extremity. (1) Patient lying supine, limb is elevated 60°, allowed to rest on support 30 seconds to 3 minutes. (2) Leg is then lowered to hang over side of bed 2-5 minutes. (3) Limb is then placed horizontal and heat applied 3-5 minutes.

 e., Master's. Ascending and descending 2 steps a variable number of times. Used as a tolerance test for circulatory efficiency and as an exercise in heart disease.

 e., Mosher's. For dysmenorrhea. Lie on back on floor with knees bent, feet on floor. Raise abdomen, relax it, contract it forcibly and relax. Repeat 10 times.

 e., passive. Form of bodily movement which is carried through by the operator without the assistance or resistance of the patient. Same as relaxed movement.

 e., resistive. Form of supervised bodily movement, with or without apparatus, which offers resistance to muscle action.

 e., rhythm. Used in obstetrical paralysis. Exercise to song or music.

 e., Schott's. Named after the Dr. Schott of Nauheim, who first scientifically administered Nauheim baths. It consists of slowly and evenly executed exercises with slight resistance, for cardiac diseases.

 e., sling suspension. Method of supporting arm or leg to be exercised in a sling suspended from overhead, thus eliminating the weight of the extremity as a hindrance during movement.

 e., static. Alternate contraction and relaxation of a muscle or group of muscles without movement of the joint. Also known as muscle setting.

 e., Stokes-Oertel (er'tel). For arteriosclerosis. A system in which walking and hill climbing are combined with restrictions of fluids.

 e., therapeutic. Scientific supervision of bodily movement, with or without apparatus, for purpose of restoring normal function to diseased or injured tissues.

 e., water. Hydrogymnastics.

ex'ercise bone. Bony growth developing in a muscle due to overexercise.

exeresis (eks-er'es-is) [G. *ex*, out, + *eiresis*, taking]. Excision of any part.

exfetation (eks-fe-ta'shŭn) [L. *ex*, out, + *foetus*, fetus]. Ectopic gestation.

exflagella'tion [" + *flagellum*, a switch]. The formation of microgametes (flagellated bodies) from the microgametocytes. Occurs in the malarial organism (Plasmodium) in the stomach of a mosquito.

exfolia'tion [" + *folium*, leaf]. The scaling off of dead tissue. RS: *apostasis*.

exhala'tion [" + *halāre*, to breathe]. The process of breathing outward; the opposite of inhalation; emanation of a gas or vapor.

exhaus'ter [" + *haurīre*, to drain]. A cataract evacuator for removal of loosened or fluid matter by vacuum pressure through a hollow needle.

exhaus'tion [" + *haurīre*, to drain]. 1. State of being exhausted, extreme fatigue, or weariness; loss of vital powers; inability to respond to stimuli; 2. Process of removing the contents of or using up a supply of anything; 3. To draw or let out.
  e. heat. Heat prostration; a condition resulting from exposure to high temperatures. Characterized by drowsy state of mind, rapid breathing, paleness, cold, sweaty skin, and normal or below normal temperature.

exhib'it [L. *exhibere*, to display]. 1. To show. 2. To administer a drug. 3. Collection of objects for public inspection.

exhibi'tionism [L. *exhibere*, to display, + G. *ismos*, condition]. 1. An abnormal impulse that causes one to expose the genitals to one of the opposite sex, seen in paretic and senile dementia, epilepsy, and other mental defects. 2. Tendency to attract attention in other ways.

exhibitionist (eks-i-bi'shun-ist) [L. *exhibere*, to display]. 1. One with an abnormal desire to attract attention. 2. One who yields to an impulse to expose the genitals to the view of one of the opposite sex.

exhilarant (eks-il'ă-rănt) [L. *exhilāre*, to gladden]. That which is mentally stimulating.

exhuma'tion [L. *ex*, out, + *humus*, earth]. Disinterment of a corpse.

Ex'ner's nerve. One from the pharyngeal plexus to the cricothyroid membranes.
  E. plexus. A plexus of nerve fibers forming a layer near the surface of the cerebral cortex.

exo- [G.]. Prefix: Without; outside of.

exocar'dia [G. *exō*, out, + *kardia*, heart]. Congenitally abnormal position of the heart.

exocar'dial [" + *kardia*, heart]. Occurring outside of the heart.

exocataphoria (eks-o-kat-ă-for'ĭ-ă) [" + *kata*, down, + *pherein*, to bear]. A downward and outward turning of the visual axes.

exocoli'tis [" + *kōlon*, colon, + *itis*, inflammation]. Inflammation of the peritoneal coat of the colon.

exocrine (eks'o-krēn) [" + *krinein*, to separate]. 1. The external secretion of a gland, opp. of endocrine. 2. Term applied to glands whose secretion reaches an epithelial surface either directly or through a duct.

exocystis (eks-o-sist'is) [" + *kystis*, bladder]. Prolapse of the urinary bladder.

exodic (eks-od'ik) [" + *odos*, way]. Efferent, centrifugal. Transmitting impressions outward from the central nervous system.

exodontia (eks-o-don'shĭ-ă) [" + *odous*, *odont-*, tooth]. 1. Extraction of a tooth. 2. Protrusion of teeth forward.

exodontol'ogy [" + " + *logos*, science]. Branch of dentistry concerned with extraction of teeth.

exoen'zyme [" + *en*, in, + *zymē*, leaven]. One that does not function within the cells from which it is secreted.

exogamy (eks-og'am-ĭ) [" + *gamos*, marriage]. 1. Marriage outside of same family; outbreeding. 2. BIOL: Conjugation bet. gametes of different ancestry, as in some protozoans. SEE: *heterosexuality*.

exogastri'tis [" + *gastēr*, belly, + *itis*, inflammation]. Inflammation of the peritoneal coat of stomach.

exogenous (eks-oj'en-us) [" + *gennan*, to produce]. Originating outside of an organ or part.

exohemophylaxis (eks"o-hem"o-fĭ-laks'is) [" + *aima*, blood, + *phylaxis*, protection]. Injection of one's own blood mingled with arsphenamine.

exohysteropexy (eks-o-his-ter-o-peks'sĭ) [" + *ystera*, uterus, + *pēxis*, fixation]. Fixation of the uterus by implanting the fundus into the abdominal wall.

exometritis (eks-o-me-tri'tis) [" + *mētra*, womb, + *itis*, inflammation]. Inflammation of the peritoneal coat of the uterus.

exomphalos (eks-om'fă-los) [G. *ex*, out, + *omphalos*, navel]. 1. Umbilical protrusion. 2. Umbilical hernia. SYN: *exumbilication*.

exopath'ic [G. *exō*, out, + *pathos*, disease]. Pert. to a disease originating outside of the body.

exophoria (eks-o-fo'rĭ-ă) [" + *pherein*, to bear]. OPHTH: Tendency of visual axes to diverge outward. SEE: *esophoria*.

exophthal'mia [G. *ex*, out, + *ophthalmos*, eye]. Abnormal protrusion of the eyeball. SYN: *exophthalmos*.
  e. cachectica. Exophthalmic goiter.
  e. fungosa. Late stage of glioma retinae.

exophthalmic (eks-of-thal'mik) [" + *ophthalmos*, eye]. Pert. to protrusion of the eyeball.
  e. goiter. A goiter marked by protrusion of the eyeballs, increased heart action, and enlargement of the thyroid gland. Graves disease.

exophthal'mos, exophthal'mus [" + *ophthalmos*, eye]. Abnormal protrusion of eyeball. May be due to thyrotoxicosis, tumor of the orbit, orbital cellulitis, leukemia, or aneurysm.
  e. pulsating. E. accompanied by pulsation and bruit due to an aneurysm behind the eye.

exophylac'tic [G. *exō*, out, + *phylaxis*, guarding]. Pert. to exophylaxis.

ex"ophylax'is [" + *phylaxis*, guarding]. Protection from disease originating outside the body, as by the skin.

ex'oplasm [" + *plasma*, matter]. Outer protoplasm of a cell. SYN: *ectoplasm*.

exorbitism (eks-or'bĭ-tizm) [L. *ex*, out, + *orbita*, eye]. Protrusion of eyeball. SYN: *exophthalmos*.

exormia (eks-or'mĭ-ă) [G. *ex*, out, + *ormē*, rash]. Any papular skin disease.

exosep'sis [G. *exō*, out, + *sēpsis*, decay]. Septic poison of external origin.

exoserosis (eks-o-ser-o'sis) [L. *ex*, out, + *serum*, whey, + G. *ōsis*]. An oozing of serum or discharging of an exudate.

exoskel'eton [G. *exō*, out, + *skeleton*, skeleton]. 1. The hard outer covering of certain invertebrates such as the molluscs and arthropods. Composed of chitin or calcareous material or both. 2. In vertebrates, the hard outer covering such as the shell of a turtle, or more specifically, the hard parts of the body surface derived principally from the ectoderm. These include such structures as hair, nails, feathers, scales, etc.

exosmo'sis [G. *ex*, out, + *ōsmos*, a thrusting, + *ōsis*]. Diffusion of a fluid from within outward, as from a blood vessel.

exosplenopexy (eks-o-sple'no-peks-ĭ) [G. *exō*, out, + *splēn*, spleen, + *pēxis*, fixation]. Suturing the spleen to opening in the abdominal wall.

exostosis (eks-os-tō'sĭs) [G. *ex*, out, + *osteon*, bone]. A bony growth which arises from the surface of a bone, often times involving the ossification of muscular attachments.
  e. bursata. An e. arising from the epiphysis of a bone and covered with cartilage and a synovial sac.
  e. cartilaginea. E. consisting of cartilage underlying the periosteum.
  e. dental. E. on the root of a tooth.
  e. multiple osteocartilaginous. SYN: *hereditary deforming chondroplasia; dyschondroplasia; diaphyseal aclasis.* A disorder of growth characterized by the development of multiple exostoses, usually located on the diaphyses of long bones near the epiphyseal lines. Results in irregularities of growth of the epiphyses and often times secondary deformities.
  ETIOL: Unknown; tends to be hereditary occurring more frequently in males than females.

exoter'ic [G. *exōterikos*, outer]. Pert. to causes developing outside the body. SYN: *exopathic*.

exother'mal, exother'mic [G. *exō*, out, + *thermē*, heat]. Chemical reaction with production of heat.

exothy'mopexy [" + *thymos*, thymus, + *pēxis*, fixation]. Suturing of an enlarged thymus gland to the sternum.

exothyreopexy (eks-o-thī're-o-peks-ĭ) [" + *thyreos*, shield, + *pēxis*, fixation]. Suture of the thyroid and external fixation to induce atrophy.

exothy'ropexy [" + " + *pēxis*, fixation]. Suture of the thyroid and external fixation to induce atrophy. SYN: *exothyreopexy*.

exotoxin (eks-o-toks'ĭn) [" + *toxikon*, poison]. A toxin produced by a microorganism and excreted into its surrounding medium. It can usually be recovered from the liquid medium in which the toxin-producing organisms have developed. Exotoxins are usually unstable being sensitive to the effects of chemicals, light, and heat. Exotoxins are produced by the diphtheria and tetanus organisms.
The exotoxins differ with regard to the particular tissues of the host that may be affected.
  RS: *cytotoxin, endotoxin, erythrotoxin, leukocidin, leukotoxin, neurotoxin*.

exotro'pia [" + *tropē*, a turning]. Divergent strabismus; abnormal turning of one or both eyes outward.

expansion (eks-pan'shŭn) [L. *expandere*, to spread out]. Increase of volume; spreading out.
  e., coefficient of. Increase in length or in volume when temperature is raised 1° C. from zero.
  e. muscle. Degree a muscle may be stretched by an attached weight.

expansive delusion. Belief in one's power and wealth, accompanied by a feeling of well-being.

expec'tant [L. *ex*, out, + *spectāre*, to watch]. Waiting.
  e. treatment. Treatment of symptoms as they arise.

expecta'tion. Hoping, anticipation.

  e. of life. Probable duration of life after a given age.

expec'torant [L. *ex*, out, + *pectus, pector-*, breast]. An agent that facilitates the removal of the secretions of the bronchopulmonary mucous membrane.
Expectorants are sometimes classed as *sedative* expectorants and *stimulating* expectorants.
  Ex: *Ammonium carbonate, ammonium chloride, ipecac*.

expectoration (eks-pek'to-ra'shŭn) [" + *pectus, pector-*, breast]. Expulsion of mucus or phlegm from the throat or lungs.
May be mucous, mucopurulent, serous, or frothy.
It is viscid and tenacious in *pneumonia*, sticks to anything, and is rusty in appearance. It is frothy, often streaked with blood, and greenish-yellow in character from pus in *bronchitis*. In *tuberculosis* it varies from small amt. of frothy fluid to abundant greenish-yellow, offensive sputum often streaked with blood.
  SEE: *anabole, anacatharsis, apophlegmatic, sputum, vomica*.

expel' [L. *expellere*, to drive out]. To drive out.

expira'tion [L. *ex*, out, + *spirāre*, to breathe]. The expulsion of air from the lungs in breathing. Its sound is the shortest breath sound heard.
Any longer sound will be pathological. In emphysema it is longer than the inspiration.
Muscles used in expiration are the *int. intercostal muscles, m. rectus abdominis, m. transversus abdominis, the triangularis sterni* and possibly the *iliocostalis, serratus post. inf.*, and *quadratus lumborum*. SEE: *inspiration, respiration*.
  e. active. Expiration accomplished as a result of muscular activity, as in forced respiration. The muscles used in respiration are: the muscles of the abdominal wall (ext. and int. oblique, rectus, and transverse abdominus); the internal intercostals, serratus posticus inferior, and quadratus lumborum.
  e. passive. E. during quiet respiration in which no muscular effort is required. It is brought about by the elasticity of the lung, recoil of the elastic tissues of the chest, such as the costal cartilages, and the weight of the thoracic wall.

expiratory (eks-pī'ră-tor-ĭ) [" + *spirāre*, to breathe]. Pert. to expiration.
  e. center. The part of the respiratory center in the medulla controlling e. movements.

expire. 1. to breathe out or exhale. 2. To die.

explant' [" + *planta*, sprout]. To remove a piece of living tissue from the body and transfer to an artificial culture medium for growth as in tissue culture. Opp. of implantation, *q.v.*

explora'tion [L. *explorāre*, to search out]. Examination by various means of an organ or part.

explo'ratory [L. *explorāre*, to search out]. Pert. to an exploration.

explo'sive speech. Sudden and explosive utterance. SEE: *speech*.

express' [L. *expressus*, from *expremere*, to press out]. To squeeze out.

expres'sion [L. *expressus*, from *expremere*, to press out]. 1. Expelling anything by pressure. 2. Facial disclosure of feeling or emotion. SYN: *facies*. SEE: *face*.

expul'sive [L. *ex*, out, + *pellere*, to drive]. Having a tendency to expel.
  e. pains. Labor pains which are effective, contracting the uterine muscle.
exsanguinate (eks-san'gwin-āt) [" + *sanguis*, blood]. 1. To deprive of blood. 2. Bloodless.
exsanguination (eks-san-gwin-a'shun) [" + *sanguis*, blood]. The process of expressing blood from a part.
exsanguine (ek-sang'win) [" + *sanguis*, blood]. Anemic; bloodless.
exsec'tion [" + *secāre*, to cut]. Excision.
exsiccant (ek-sik'ant) [" + *siccāre*, to dry]. 1. Absorbing or drying up a discharge. 2. An agent that absorbs moisture. 3. A dusting or drying powder.
exsicca'tion [" + *siccāre*, to dry]. The act of drying by heat. SYN: *desiccation*.
exsic'cative [" + *siccāre*, to dry]. Causing to dry up or that which drys. SYN: *desiccative*.
exso'matize [G. *ex*, out, + *sōma*, body]. To remove from the body.
exstrophy (eks'strof-ī) [" + *strephein*, to turn]. Eversion; turning inside out of a part.
  e. of the bladder. A congenital malformation in which the lower portion of the abdominal wall and anterior wall of the bladder are lacking and the bladder is everted through the opening; ectopia vesicae.
ext. Abbr. of L. *extractum*, extract.
extempora'neous [L. *extemporaneus*, without time]. Not prepared according to formula but devised for the occasion.
  e. mixture. A preparation to be taken at once because of tendency to deteriorate.
extension (eks-ten'shun) [L. *extendere*, to stretch out]. 1. The movement by which the 2 ends of any part are pulled asunder. A movement which brings the members of a limb into or toward a straight condition. 2. The opposite of flexion. 3. The application of a pull (traction) to a fractured or dislocated limb.
  e., Buck's. A method of producing traction by applying adhesive tape or moleskin to the skin and keeping it in smooth close contact by means of circular bandaging of the part to which it is applied. The adhesive strips are placed longitudinally to the member, the superior ends being about 1 in. from fracture site. Weights sufficient to produce the required extension are fastened to the inferior end of the adhesive strips, by means of a rope which is run over a pulley to permit of free motion.
exten'sor [L. *extendere*, to stretch out]. A muscle that extends a part.
exte'rior [L.]. Outside of; external.
exte'riorize. 1. In surg. to temporarily expose a part; marsupialization, *q.v.* 2. In Psych. the process of turning one's interests outward.
extern(e (ek'sturn) [L. *externus*, outside]. A recently advanced medical student living outside of a hospital who assists in the medical and surgical care of patients. SEE: *intern*.
external [L. *externus*, outside]. Exterior; lateral; opp. of medial or internal.
externa'lia [L. *externus*, outside]. External genitalia.
exteroceptive (eks"ter-o-sept'iv) [" + *ceptus*, from *capere*, to take]. Pert. to end organs receiving impressions from without.
exteroceptor (eks-ter-o-sep'tor) [" + *ceptus*, from *capere*, to take]. A sense organ adapted for the reception of stimuli from outside the body. Ex: The eye.
exterofec'tive [" + *facere*, to make]. Pertaining to responses to stimuli mediated by the central nervous system and somatic nerves in contrast to those mediated through the autonomic nervous system.
ex'tima [L. outermost]. The outer layer of a blood vessel; the tunica adventitia.
extinction. 1. The process of extinguishing or putting out. 2. The complete inhibition of a conditioned reflex as a result of failure to reinforce it.
  e. of mercury. Causing the disappearance of mercury by rubbing with lard or some other agent.
extirpation (eks-tir-pa'shun) [L. *extirpāre*, to root out]. Excision of a part—taking out by the roots.
extor'sion [L. *ex*, out, + *torquire*, to twist]. Rotation of an organ or limb, outward.
extra- [L.]. Prefix: Outside of, in addition to.
extraärtic'ular [L. *extra*, outside, + *articulus*, joint]. Outside a joint.
ex'tract [L. *extractum*, from *extrahere*, to draw out]. 1. A solid or semisolid preparation made by extracting the solubles with water or alcohol and evaporating the solution. 2. Active principle of a drug obtained by distillation or chemical processes.
  e., alcoholic. One in which alcohol acts as the solvent.
  e., aqueous. One in which water is the solvent.
  e., aromatic fluid. E. made from an aromatic powder.
  e., compound. E. prepared from more than 1 drug.
  e., ethereal. E. using ether as the menstruum.
  e., fluid. One made into a solution from a vegetable drug, which contains medicinal components.
  e., powdered. A crushed, dried extract.
  e., soft. E. of the consistency of honey.
  e., solid. E. made by evaporating the fluid part of a solution.
extrac'tion [L. *extractum*, a drawing out]. 1. Pulling out, as a tooth. 2. The removing of the active portion of a drug.
extract'or [L. *extractum*, a drawing out]. Instrument for removing foreign bodies. VARIETIES: Esophageal, throat, shot, tympanum, tissue, etc.
  e., tissue. Needles, trocars or pointed instruments with a form of barb for extracting soft tissue for examination.
  e., tube. Device for removing an intubation tube from trachea.
extrac'tum (ext.) [L. a drawing out]. Solid or semi-solid preparations produced by evaporating solutions of vegetable principles.
  The official extracts are either powders or soft solids. The majority can be obtained in powdered form and many prefer them that way. Extracts are usually about 5 times the strength of the crude drug. Fourteen are official.
extracys'tic [L. *extra*, beyond, + G. *kystis*, bladder]. Outside of or unrelated to a bladder or cystic tumor.
extradu'ral [" + *durus*, hard]. 1. On outer side of the dura mater. 2. Unconnected with the dura mater.
extragenital (eks-trä-jen'ī-tal) [" + *genitalis*, genital]. Outside of or unrelated to the genital organs.

extrahep´atic [" + G. *êpar, êpat-*, liver]. Outside of or unrelated to the liver.

extraligamen´tous [" + *ligāre*, to bind]. Outside of or unrelated to a ligament.

extramalle´olus [" + *malleōlus*, little hammer]. The external or lateral malleolus.

extramar´ginal [" + *margō*, margin]. Pert. to subliminal consciousness.

extramastoiditis (eks-trā-mas-toy-dī´tis) [" + G. *mastos*, breast, + *eidos*, form, + *-itis*, inflammation]. Inflammation of outside tissues contiguous to the mastoid process.

extramedul´lary [" + *medulla*, marrow]. Outside of or unrelated to any medulla, esp. the m. oblongata.

extraneous (eks-tra´ne-us) [L. *extraneus*, external]. Outside and unrelated to an organism.

extranu´clear [L. *extra*, beyond, + *nucleus*, kernel]. Outside of a nucleus.

extrapo´lar [" + *polus*, pole]. Outside instead of bet. poles, as the electrodes of a battery.

extrasensory. Pertaining to forms of perception not dependent upon the five primary senses; e. g., thought transference. Abb. ESP.

extrasys´tole [" + G. *systellein*, to contract]. Premature contraction of one of the parts of the heart, which may be induced experimentally by stimulating the heart at any time except during the absolute refractory period. In humans it is the result of some factor that initiates an impulse in the impulse-conducting system. It may occur either in the presence or absence of organic heart disease. It may be of reflex origin being initiated by stimuli from almost any part of the body or it may be of central origin. It usually results in abnormal heart rhythm.
 e. auricular. Premature contraction of the atrium at some point outside the S-A. node.
 e. nodal. E. occurring as a result of the origin of an impulse in the A-V node.
 e. ventricular. E. which occurs after the normal contraction of the ventricle has ceased. Usually followed by a long "compensary pause".

extrau´terine [" + *uterus*, womb]. Outside the uterus.

extravag´inal [" + *vagina*, vagina]. Outside the vagina.

extravasate (ek-strav´a-sāt) [" + *vas*, vessel]. 1. To escape from a vessel into the tissues, said of serum, blood, or lymph. 2. Exudate so escaping.

extravasation (eks-tra-va-sa´shun) [" + *vas*, vessel]. The escape of fluids into the surrounding tissue.

extravas´cular [" + *vasculum*, vessel]. Outside a vessel.

extraventric´ular [" + *ventriculus*, little belly]. Outside of any ventricle, esp. one of the heart.

extrem´ital [L. *extrēmus*, last]. Pert. to an extremity. SYN: *distal*.

extrem´ity [L. *extrēmus*, last]. 1. The terminal part of anything. 2. An arm or leg.
 RS: *acanthokeratodermia, "acro-" words, dactyl, dactylus.*
 e. lower. The lower limb, including the hip, thigh, leg, ankle, and foot.
 e. upper. The upper limb, including the shoulder, arm, forearm, wrist and hand.

extrin´sic [L. *extrinsecus*, from *extra*, outside, + *secus*, otherwise]. From or coming from without.
 e. muscles. Those partly attached to the trunk and partly to a limb.

extroversion (ek-stro-ver´shun) [L. *extra*, out, + *vertere*, to turn]. 1. Eversion; turning inside out. 2. PSY: The direction of energy to objects in the environment.

ex´trovert [" + *vertere*, to turn]. A personality-reaction type; one who is interested mainly in ext. objects and actions.
 The extreme pathologic extrovert reaction is seen in manic depressive insanity. OPP: *introvert, q.v.*

extrude (eks-trūd´) [L. *extrudere*, to squeeze out]. To push out of a normal position or situation.

extru´sion [L. *extrudere*, to squeeze out]. 1. Occupying an abnormal external position. 2. Position of a tooth pushed forward from line of occlusion.

extubation (eks-tu-ba´shun) [L. *ex*, out, + *tuba*, tube]. Removal of a tube, as the laryngeal tube.

exudate (eks´u-dāt) [" + *sudāre*, to sweat]. 1. Accumulation of a fluid in a cavity, or matter that penetrates through vessel walls into adjoining tissue, or the passing out of pus or serum, or the matter so passed.
 They may be classified as *catarrhal, fibrinous, hemorrhagic, diphtheritic, purulent*, and *serous*, the fluids being different in various affections. A fibrinous exudate may wall off a cavity, resulting in adhesions following an operation, as in empyema* and appendicitis. Inflammatory processes tend to wall off the injured area to localize the inflammation and to prevent its spread. 2. An inflammatory product withdrawn through a membrane for exploratory purposes. SEE: *exudation, infection, inflammation, pus, resorption*.

exuda´tion [" + *sudāre*, to sweat]. Morbid oozing of fluids, usually the result of inflammatory conditions. SEE: *ant. choroiditis, central choroiditis, exudate, exudative choroiditis.*

ex´udative [" + *sudāre*, to sweat]. Having the property of exudation.

exude´ [" + *sudāre*, to sweat]. To pass off slowly through the tissues; said of a semisolid or fluid.

exumbilica´tion [" + *umbilicus*, navel]. Protrusion of navel. SYN: *exomphalos*.

exuviae (eks-u´vī-e) [L. *exuere*, to strip]. Cast-off parts, as desquamated epidermis; a slough.

eye [A.S. *ēáge*]. Organ of vision; composed of 3 coats: (a) *Retina*, sensory for light; (b) *uvea* (choroid, ciliary body, and iris), nutritional; (c) *sclera* and *cornea*, serve to protect delicate retina.
 These layers enclose two cavities, the more anterior or *ocular chamber* being the space lying in front of the lens. It is divided by the *iris* into an *anterior chamber* and a *posterior chamber*, both of which are filled with a watery *aqueous humor*. The cavity behind the lens is much larger and filled with a jelly-like *vitreous body*. The lens is suspended behind the iris by the ciliary zonule. Anteriorly, the cornea is covered by the *conjunctiva* which continues and forms the inner layer of the eyelids.
 e. aphacia (a-fas-i-a). An eye from which the crystalline lens has been removed.
 e. black. Ecchymosis of the tissues surrounding the eye.
 e. closure reflex. Contraction of orbicularis palpebrarum with closure of lids resulting from percussion above supraorbital nerve.
 e., cold compresses: PURPOSE: (a) To relieve congestion of eyelids; (b) to

eye, cross   E-63   **eye, muscles**

control intraocular hemorrhage; (c) occasionally for conjunctivitis and early lid injuries to prevent hemorrhage into tissues.

PROCEDURES: Scrub hands: (a) Wring compresses out of boric acid solution with forceps and place on ice to chill; (b) place over lids and extend over cheek; (c) change every 30 seconds.

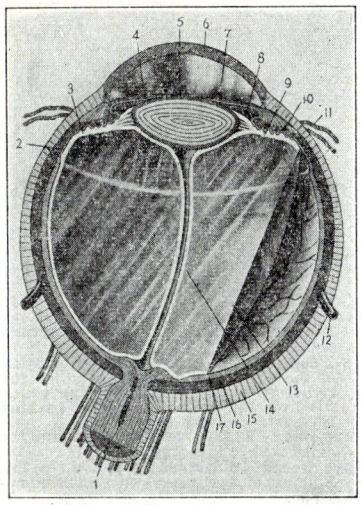

THE EYE

1. Optic nerve. 2. Ciliary part of retina. 3. Ciliary zonule. 4. Iris. 5. Capsule of lens. 6. Cornea. 7. Anterior chamber. 8. Posterior chamber. 9. Suspensory ligament of lens. 10. Ciliary muscle. 11. Anterior ciliary arteries. 12. Vena vorticosa. 13. Vitreous. 14. Hyaloid canal. 15. Sclera. 16. Choroid. 17. Retina.

Each compress may be used over and over if there is no pus. When pus is present, may be used only once.

e. cross. Strabismus, *q.v.*

e. dark adapted. An eye which has become adjusted for viewing objects in dim light; one adapted for scotopic or rod vision. Depends upon the regeneration of a light sensitive substance, visual purple.

e. dominant. The eye which a person unconsciously gives preference to as a source of stimuli for visual sensations.

e., examinations and diagnosis. The diagnosis of disease which the physician makes from an examination depends largely upon symptoms manifested by the pupils of the eyes.

CONTRACTED PUPILS: They may denote irritative lesions of the 3rd nerve (in early stages of anesthesia from chloroform, or during alcoholic excitement) or they may result from opium poisoning. Contraction of *one* pupil indicates irritative lesion of the opposite side of the brain, situated at the 3rd nerve nuclei, or a paralysis of the sympathetic nerve fibers due to a lesion somewhere in their course.

DILATED PUPILS: They may result from belladonna or atropine or from irritating of the sympathetic, or they may occur during the attacks of dyspnea, in the last stages of anesthesia. Dilation of one pupil indicates a paralysis of the 3rd nerve from some brain lesion, or an irritation of the cervical sympathetic.

FLOATING SPECKS: They may indicate the want of transparency in the humors of the eye, or they may be due to some form of dyspepsia, migraine, excessive eyestrain, or severe falls.

SQUINTING: In the course of a brain disease, this is an unfavorable symptom.

e. exciting. In sympathetic ophthalmia, the damaged eye which is the source of sympathogenic influences.

e. fixing. In strabismus, the eye that is directed toward the object of vision.

e., foreign body in. Manifested by pain, lacrimation, spasm of the eye; later there is redness, swelling and occasionally headache.

F. A. TREATMENT: Tearing itself often washes dust from the eye. Bringing the upper lid over the lower and directing patient to roll eye, often deposits dust on the margin of the lower lid.

Great care is necessary in removing larger particles, and should be done in a quiet place with excellent illumination. Follow by instillation of 1 or 2 drops of a bland oil into the eye. A mild antiseptic, as 5%-10% mild silver proteinate, is desirable. If inflamed, use repeated hot compresses.

If for any reason patient cannot be taken care of at once, the eye should be bandaged to keep it closed and thus avoid scratching the lid. There should be no delay in having the speck removed, as serious injury to the eyeball or to the vision may result. The longer the foreign body remains in the eye the deeper it becomes embedded.

Infection may be carried into the eye, resulting in an ulcer of the cornea. Metal produces a chemical effect, as it disintegrates, which affects the eyeball. The x-ray is sometimes used to detect any tiny particles of metal, and the electromagnet to remove them. Sympathetic ophthalmia,* the transference of inflammation from an injury to the normal eye, may be produced by wounds which pierce the eyeball. Loss of vision in both eyes may result.

e. hare's. Lagophthalmos; condition in which the eye cannot be completely closed.

e., hot compresses: PURPOSE: (a) To increase the blood supply to the eyelids and eyeballs; (b) to relieve pain.

PROCEDURES: Scrub hands: (a) Apply vaseline to area to which compresses are to be applied; (b) wring compresses dry with forceps and test on wrist and apply as hot as patient can tolerate; (c) to increase blood supply to eyelids, place compresses over lids and extend over cheek; to increase blood supply to eyeballs, place compresses over lids and extend over brow; (d) use new compresses for each application if pus is present; (e) when last compress is removed, dry the eyelid.

e. light adapted. An eye that has become adjusted to viewing objects in bright light; one adapted for phototic or cone vision. One in which visual purple has been bleached.

e. muscles. Movements of the eye ball are brought about by six muscles: the superior, inferior, medial and external rectus muscles and the superior and inferior oblique muscles.

e. nerve supply of. 2nd. or optic nerve; *eye muscles*, 3rd. or oculomotor, 4th. or trochlear, and 6th. or abducens; *lid muscles*, facial to orbicularis oculi and oculomotor to levator palpebrae. Sensory fibers to orbit furnished by ophthalmic and maxillary fibers of the 5th or trigeminal. Sympathetic post-ganglionic fibers are derived from the carotid plexus, their cell bodies lying in the superior cervical ganglion. They supply the dilator muscle of the iris, lacrimal gland, and smooth muscle fibers in the eyelid; parasympathetic, fibers from the ciliary ganglion pass to the ciliary muscle and constrictor muscles of the iris.

e. pink. Acute epidemic conjunctivitis.

e. refracting media of. Aqueous humor, lens, and vitreous body.

e. refracting surfaces of. Cornea and anterior and post surfaces of the lens.

e. squint. Strabismus, *q.v.*

e. squinting. The eye affected in strabismus.

e. sympathizing. In sympathetic ophthalmia, the uninjured eye which responds to sympathogenic influences.

e. vision. Light entering the eye passes through the cornea, then through the *pupil*, an opening in the iris, and on through the crystalline lens and the vitreous body to the retina. The aqueous humor, lens and vitreous body constitute the refracting media of the eye. Through changes in the curvature of the lens brought about by its elasticity and contraction of the ciliary muscles, light rays are focused on the retina where they stimulate the rods and cones, the sensory receptors. The cones are concerned with color vision; rods with vision in dim light. Sensory impulses are conveyed over the optic nerve to the brain where, in the visual area of the cerebral cortex located in the occipital lobe, they register as visual sensations. The amount of light entering the eye is regulated by the pupil, its size being controlled by the dilator and constrictor muscles of the iris.

e. watery. Epiphora; abnormal secretion of tears.

eyeball [A.S. *ēage* + M. E. *bal*]. The body of the eye.

It has 3 humors: Aqueous, lens or crystalline, and vitreous. Tension and position in relation to orbit should be noted.

PATH: *Exophthalmos*, or protrusion. If bilateral may be due to goiter. Eyeball may appear to protrude in fright, asthma, and spasmodic croup. It is noted in thrombosis of sup. longitudinal sinus, cardiac atrophy, laryngeal stenosis and paralysis of ocular movements. One or both may be affected due to hemorrhage in orbit, to aneurysm, exostosis, or tumor of orbit, or enlarged lacrimal glands. *Enophthalmos*: Bilateral or unilateral recession of eyeball.

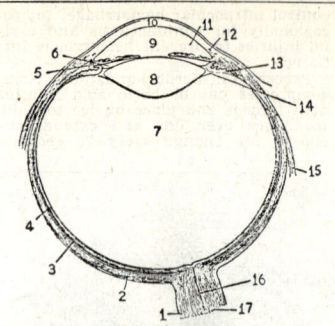

THE EYEBALL
1. Nerve sheath. 2. Sclerotic coat. 3. Choroid coat. 4. Retina. 5. Ciliary body. 6. Posterior chamber. 7. Corpus vitreum. 8. Crystalline lens. 9. Anterior chamber. 10. Cornea. 11. Iris. 12. Sinus venosus sclerae. 13. Ciliary processes. 14. Spatia zonularia. 15. M. rectus medialis. 16. Canal for central artery. 17. Optic nerve.

eye′brow [A.S. *ēage*, eye, + *braew*, brow]. The arch over the eye; also its covering, esp. the hairs.

eye′cup. 1. The optic vesicle, evagination of the embryonic brain from which the retina develops. 2. A small cup which fits over the eye and used for bathing the surface of the eye.

eye′glass. A glass lens used to aid the defective eye in seeing.

eye′ground [A.S. *ēage* + *grund*, earth]. Fundus of eye, seen with ophthalmoscope.

eye′lash [" + *lasche*, a thin whip]. Cilium.* A stiff hair on the margin of the eyelid. SEE: *capsulociliary*, "*cili-*" words, *phalangosis, trichiasis*.

eye′lid (*palpebra*) [" + *hlīdan*, to cover]. One of two movable protective folds which when closed, cover the anterior surface of the eyeball. They are separated by the *palpebral fissure*. The upper (palpebrae superior) is the larger and more movable. It is raised by contraction of the levator palpebral superioris muscle. Angles formed by the lids at inner and outer ends are known as the *canthi*. The cilia, or eyelashes, are attached. The post. surface is lined by the *conjunctiva*, a mucous membrane.

e. dropping. Ptosis.

e. fused. A congenital anomaly resulting from failure of the fetal eyelids to separate.

eyestrain. Tiredness of the eye due to overuse or uncorrected defect. SYN: *asthenopia*.

eyetooth. A cuspid or upper canine tooth.

eye worm, African. *Loa Loa*, a genus of nematode which frequently infests the eye.

F

F. 1. Abbr. of *Fahrenheit, field of vision, formula, Fusiformis.* 2. Symbol for *fluorine.*

F₁. In genetics the first filial generation, the offspring of a cross between two unlike individuals.

F₂. The second filial generation or the offspring of a cross between two individuals of the F₁ generation.

FA. Abbr. for *fatty acid.*

F. A. Abbr. for *field ambulance.*

F. and R. Abbr. for *force and rhythm.*

fabel'la [L. little bean]. Fibrocartilages or bones which sometimes develop in the head of the gastrocnemius muscle.

fabrication (fab-ri-ka'shun) [L. *fabricāre,* to forge]. Recital of that which is not true, seen in Korsakow's syndrome.

F. A. C. D. Abbr. *Fellow of the American College of Dentists.*

face [L. *facies*]. Anterior part of the head from forehead to chin and extending laterally to but not including the ears; the visage or countenance.

ANAT: *Arteries of Face and Head:* Left common carotid with ext. and int. branches. Right common carotid with ext. and int. branches and circle of Willis. *Bones of:* The face has 14 bones. SEE: *skeleton. Veins of Face and Neck:* Ext. and int. jugular.

COLORING: *Brownish-yellow spots:* Liver spots. Seen in pregnancy, malignancies of liver or uterus, and in exophthalmic goiter. Cosmetics and facial irritants, sunburn and exposure to weather also factors. Occurs in many diseases including Addison's disease, diabetes, hemochromatosis, pellagra, acanthosis nigricans, and others. Also occurs in arsenic poisoning.

Yellowish discoloration: Jaundice due to presence of excess of bile pigments in the blood.

Cyanosis: May be due to acquired or congenital malformations of the heart,

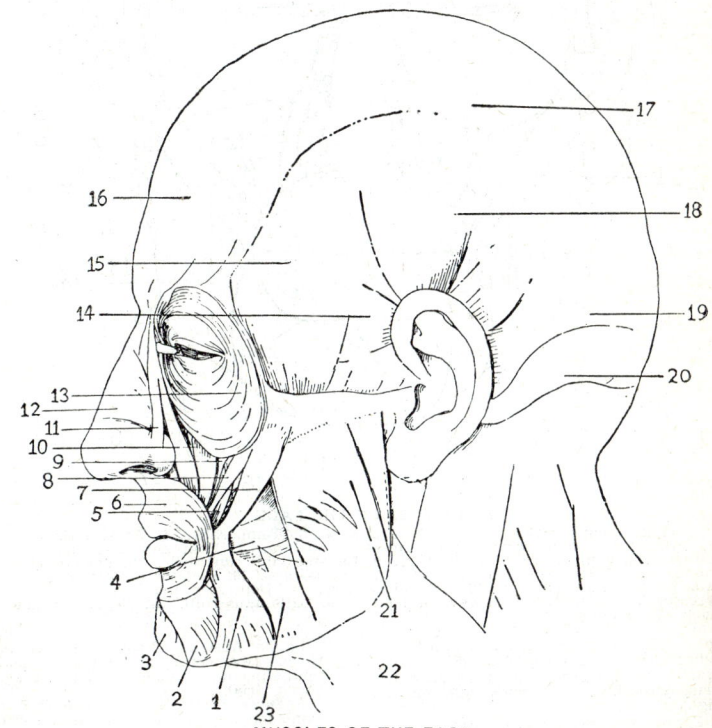

MUSCLES OF THE FACE
1. Depressor anguli oris. 2. Depressor labii inferioris. 3. Levator menti. 4. Buccinator. 5. Levator anguli oris. 6. Orbicularis oris. 7. Zygomaticus major. 8. Zygomaticus minor. 9. Depressor alae nasi. 10. Levator labii superioris. 11. Levator labii superioris alae que nasi. 12. Compressor narium. 13. Orbicularis palpebrarum. 14. Auricularis anterior. 15. Temporalis. 16. Frontalis. 17. Galea aponeurotica. 18. Attollens aurem. 19. Auricularis posterior. 20. Occipitalis. 21. Masseter. 22. Latissimus colli. 23. Risorius.

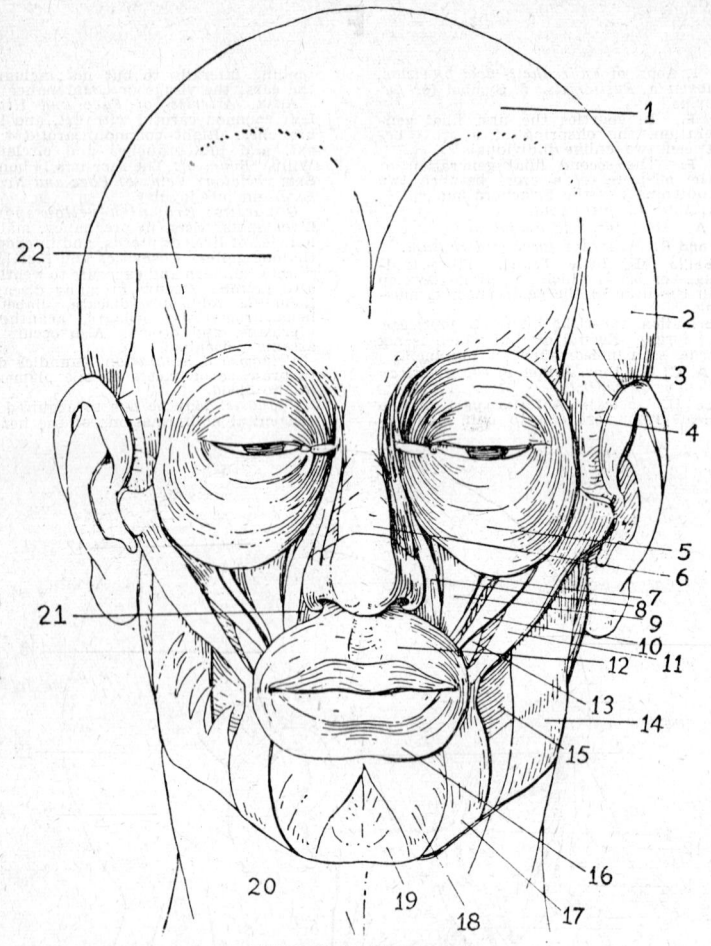

MUSCLES OF THE FACE

1. Galea aponeurotica. 2. Attollens aurem. 3. Temporalis. 4. Auricularis ant. 5. Orbicularis palpebrarum. 6. Compressor narium. 7. Depressor alae nasi. 8. Levator labii superioris alae que nasi. 9. Levator labii superioris. 10. Zygomaticus minor. 11. Zygomaticus major. 12. Orbicularis oris. 13. Levator anguli oris. 14. Masseter. 15. Buccinator. 16. Orbicularis oris. 17. Depressor anguli oris. 18. Depressor labii inferioris. 19. Levator menti. 20. Latissimus colli. 21. Depressor alae nasi. 22. Frontalis.

to asthma, whooping cough, pulmonary tuberculosis, croup, obstruction of trachea, aneurysm, tumor, asphyxia, drug poisoning, emphysema, dilation of right side of the heart. SEE: *cyanosis.*

Expression. Absence of expression: Myasthenia gravis, paralysis agitans.

Flushing (hyperemia): May be permanent or evanescent. Produced by the emotions if temporary. Permanent flushing may be due to febrile diseases, pulmonary tuberculosis, convulsions, alcoholism, ovarian tumors, goiter, plethora-hypertrophy of the heart.

Pallor: Absence of color. May be due to excessive confinement indoors, malnourishment, anemia, hemorrhage, shock, fright.

Redness, alternating with pallor: Emotion such as anger, cerebrospinal meningitis, typhoid, menopause, and general vasomotor disturbances.

Sallowness: Cachexia, cancer, lead poisoning, chronic gallbladder disease, some anemias, Addison's disease, arthritis deformans, constipation, hepatic, pancreatic, and enteric diseases.

DIAGNOSIS BY: The following conditions affect the features: Mouth breathing, chronic alcoholism, drug habits, abdominal diseases, facial hemiplegia, insular sclerosis, cretinism, myxedema, congenital syphilis, exophthalmic goiter, myopathic and myasthenic conditions, paralysis agitans, encephalitis lethargica, locomotor ataxia, acromegaly, mongolian idiocy, acute diffuse peritonitis, dyspnea, hysteria, late stages of pulmonary tuberculosis, lobar pneumonia, renal diseases, typhoid fever, hippocratic facies.

EDEMA: Swelling of the face from edema is noted in cardiac, renal, and blood diseases, pneumothorax, mediastinal tumors, and aneurysm. It may be localized and evanescent due to urticaria, angioneurotic edema, or anaphylaxis. Seen in thrombosis of sup. longitudinal sinus, and in glanders.

EXPRESSION: *Absence of expression from half the face downward, drawn and distorted*: Indicates facial paralysis of opposite side. *Anxious or pinched look*: Forerunner of unfavorable conditions. *Hippocratic facies*: A cadaverous appearance seen in cholera and acute general peritonitis. *Risus sardonicus*: A sardonic smile caused by contraction of mouth muscles which indicates abdominal affections, such as spasms and peritonitis. *Sudden lack of expression*: Apathy and immobility, generally bad symptoms, except in mental weakness and hysteria.

f. presentation. Fetal face presentation in childbirth.

f., spasms of. May be intermittent, continuous, bilateral or unilateral.

May be due to teeth, disorders of skin, nose, eyes, or constitutional nervous disorders. May be *mimic* or *habit* spasms; choreic, winking spasms, convulsive tic, blepharospasm. Closure of eyelids caused by spasm of orbicular muscles, due to affection of the nerve supply, the eye muscles, or to eye diseases. Clonic unilateral spasm due to epilepsy. Spasm of eyelids, chin, upper lips, or muscles of face seen in early stages of meningitis. Tonic spasms due to tetanus, spasms following paralysis, hysteria, and tic douloureux.

facet, facette (fas'et) [Fr. *facette*, small face]. A small, smooth area on a bone or other hard surface.

fa′cial [L. *facies*, face]. Pert. to the face.

f. center. Brain center causing facial movements.

f. nerve. Seventh cranial nerve, a mixed nerve consisting of efferent fibers supplying the facial muscles, the platysma muscle, the submaxillary and sublingual glands; afferent fibers from taste buds of the ant. two thirds of the tongue and from the muscles. ORIG. afferent fibers from geniculate ganglion; motor and secretory fibers from nuclei in pons. DIS: Ear, face, palate, tongue. BR: Tympanic, chorda tympani, post. auricular, digastric, stylohyoid, temporal, malar, infraorbital, buccal, supramaxillary, inframaxillary. SEE: *cranial nerves*.

f. paralysis. Affecting the muscles of the face. The 7th cranial nerve is involved.

f. reflex. Contraction of facial muscles following pressure on eyeball.

f. spasm. Tic. SEE: *cranial nerves, face, facies, paralysis, tic*.

facies (fash′i-ez) [L.]. 1. Face. 2. Countenance. 3. Surface.

f. abdomina′lis. Pinched, anxious, shrunken and drawn expression seen in abdominal troubles.

f. adenoid. Stupid appearance with open mouth.

f. aor′tica. Expression seen in aortic valve insufficiency, bluish sclera, cheeks sunken, face sallow.

f. hepat′ica. Seen in liver affections: Skin sallow, conjunctivae yellow, and eyeballs sunken.

f. hippocrat′ica. Seen in those dying from long continued illness or from cholera; cheeks and temples hollow, eyes sunken, complexion leaden, and lips relaxed.

f. mitra′lis. Seen in mitral insufficiency. Capillaries more or less visible, cheeks pink, more or less cyanosis.

f., myopath′ic. Due to muscular weakness, esp. that of the face, lids drop and lips protrude.

f. ovari′na. Seen in women with ovarian tumor; face drawn and pinched.

f. tetanica. Senile appearance due to wrinkling in tetanus.

f., typhoid. Dusky complexion, injected conjunctivae and dull expression.

facilitation (fas-il″it-a′shun) [L. *facilis*, easy]. Making an action or process easier, the energy of an impulse being added to that of other impulses activated at the same time.

fa′cing [L. *faciēs*, face]. An inlay to form the outer surface of a tooth.

faciobrachial (fa-shi-o-bra′ki-al) [" + G. *brachion*, arm]. Pert. to the face and arm, esp. to juvenile muscular dystrophy.

faciocer′vical [" + *cervix*, neck]. Pert. to the face and neck, esp. to progressive dystrophy of facial muscles.

faciolin′gual [" + *lingua*, tongue]. Pert. to the face and the tongue, esp. a paralysis of them.

fa′cioplasty [" + G. *plassein*, to form]. Plastic surgery of the face.

facioplegia (fa″shĭ-o-ple′jĭ-ă) [" + G. *plēgē*, stroke]. Facial paralysis. SYN: *prosopoplegia*.

facioscapulohumeral (fa″shĭ-o-skap″u-lo-hu′mer-al) [" + *scapula*, shoulder blade, + *humerus*, shoulder]. Pert. to the face, the scapula, and the upper arm.

F. A. C. P. Abbr. for *Fellow of the American College of Physicians*.

F. A. C. S. Abbr. for *Fellow of the American College of Surgeons*.

factitious (fak-tish′us) [L. *factitius*, made by art]. Not natural; esp. of certain skin lesions.

factor. A condition, element, influence, or circumstance that contributes to a result.

f. accessory food. A substance in food which does not serve as a source of energy but is essential for normal growth and development or normal metabolic activities; a vitamin, *q.v.*

f. antianemic. A substance stored in the liver, essential for the normal development of red blood cells in the bone marrow. It is formed in the stomach and intestine by the interaction of an *extrinsic factor* present in certain foods, esp. those rich in the B-complex vitamins and an *intrinsic factor* present in gastric juice. Also called *antianemic principle, hematinic principle, erythrocyte maturation factor (EMF)*. It is used in the treatment of pernicious anemia.

f. hereditary. A gene.

f. lethal. A gene which when homozygous, causes the death of an individual before development is complete.

f. milk. A substance present in certain strains of mice which is transferred to offspring through milk from the mammary glands, and is capable of inducing the development of mammary cancer.
f. Rh. SEE: *Rh blood factor.*
fac′ulta″tive [L. *facere*, to do]. BIOL: 1. Able to live under conditions of temperature or oxygen supply which vary. 2. Able to do something not compulsory; voluntary.
fac′ulty [L. *facultās*, function]. 1. A mental attribute or sense. 2. Ability to function.
f., affective. Capacity for expressing emotions.
f., germinative. Power of a germ to develop.
fagopyrism (fag-ō-pīr′izm) [L. *fagopyrum*, buckwheat]. Buckwheat poisoning.
Fahr. Abbr. for *Fahrenheit.*
Fahraeus' test. A measuring of the speed at which red blood corpuscles settle.
Fahrenheit scale. The one used in the U. S. A., and England. The freezing point of water is 32° and the boiling point 212°. Indicated by capital letter F.
SEE: *thermometer.*

Fahrenheit and Centigrade Scales					
F.	C.	F.	C.	F.	C.
500°	260°	248°	120°	95°	35°
401	205	239	115	86	30
392	200	230	110	77	25
383	195	212	100	68	20
374	190	203	95	50	10
356	180	194	90	41	5
347	175	176	80	32	0
338	170	167	75	23	— 5
329	165	140	60	14	—10
320	160	122	50	+ 5	—15
311	155	113	45	— 4	—20
302	150	105	40.54	—13	—25
284	140	104	40	—22	—30
275	135	100	37.8	—40	—40
266	130	98.5	36.9	—76	—60
		1 deg. F.	= .54°	C.	
		1.8 "	= 1°	C.	
		3.6 "	= 2°	C.	
		4.5 "	= 2.5°	C.	
		5.4 "	= 3°	C	

faint [O.F. *faindre*, to feign]. 1. To feel weak, as though about to lose consciousness. 2. Weak. 3. Syncope. SEE: *fainting.*
fainting (fānt′ing) [O.F. *faindre*, to feign]. Loss of consciousness due to cerebral anemia or insufficient blood to the brain.
SYM: Prior to onset, patient may be pale, weak, dizzy, cold perspiration, uncomfortable abdominal sensation, and may fall on the ground unconscious. Pulse is usually weak, rapid, often irregular.
F. A. TREATMENT: If patient is sitting, lower head between the knees, or preferably have patient lie down with the head lower than the body. Elevate lower extremities. Apply heat. Rub extremities toward the heart. Stimulate by administering spirits of ammonia to the nostrils at intervals. When able to swallow, give hot black coffee, strong tea, or other hot drinks.
Twenty drops of aromatic spirits of ammonia in hot water may likewise be used by mouth.
RS: *apoplexy, asphyxia, coma, shock, swoon, syncope, unconsciousness.*
faint′ness [O.F. *faindre*, to feign]. 1. A sensation of impending loss of consciousness. 2. A sensation due to lack of food.
SEE: *lipothymia.*

falcate (fal′kăt) [L. *falx*, sickle]. Sickle-shaped.
falcial (fal′sĭ-ăl) [L. *falx*, sickle]. Pert. to the falx.
fal′ciform [" + *forma*, form]. Sickle-shaped.
f. ligament. The triangular ligament attached to sides of the sacrum and coccyx by its base. SYN: *great sacro-ischiadic l.*
f. process. Process of the dura that divides the hemispheres of the cerebrum. SYN: *falx cerebri.*
fal′cula [L. little sickle]. The falx cerebelli.
fal′cular [L. *falcula*, little sickle]. 1. Sickle-shaped. 2. Pertaining to the *falx cerebelli.*
fallec′tomy [G. *ektomē*, excision]. Cutting away part of the fallopian tube.
falling drop. 1. A metallic tinkle heard over the normal stomach and bowel when inflated. 2. The same sound heard over large cavities containing fluid and air, as observed in hydropneumothorax.
f. sickness. Epileptic condition.
f. of the womb. Dropping of the uterus, so that it protrudes into vagina. SYN: *descensus uteri.*
fallo′pian. Pert. to parts named for the Italian anatomist Fallopius.
f. canal. C. in petrous bone for *nervus facialis.*
f. ligament. Round ligament of the uterus.
f. tube. SYN: *uterine tube, oviduct.* The tube or duct which extends laterally from the lateral angle of the uterus, terminating near the ovary. It serves to convey the ovum from the ovary to the uterus and spermatozoa from the uterus toward the ovary. Medially each tube opens into the uterus; distally each opens into the peritoneal cavity. Each lies in the superior border of the broad ligament.
BLOOD SUPPLY: Derived from branches of the uterine and ovarian arteries.
NERVE SUPPLY: Pelvic, ovarian, and uterine nerve plexuses send fibers to the tubes.
ANAT. The narrow region near the uterus, the isthmus continues laterally as a wider *ampulla*. The latter expands to form the terminal funnel-shaped *infundibulum*, at the bottom of which lies a small opening, the *ostium*, through which the ovum enters the oviduct. Surrounding each ostium are a number of fingerlike processes called *fimbria*, one of which the *fimbria ovarica* is considerably longer than the others, extending towards the ovary. Each tube averages about 4½ in. in length and ¼ in. in diameter. Its wall consists of three layers: mucosa, muscular layer, and serosa. The epithelium of the mucosa consists of ciliated and non-ciliated cells. Ciliary action aids in the movement of the ovum towards the uterus. The muscular layer consists of an inner circular and an outer longitudinal layer of smooth muscle. The serosa consists of connective tissue underlying the outermost layer of peritoneum.
fallostomy (fal-os′to-mī) [G. *stoma*, opening]. Surgical opening of the fallopian tube.
fallot′omy. Division of the fallopian tubes. SYN: *salpingotomy.**
Fallot, tetratology of. A congenital condition characterized by defect in the interventricular septum, stenosis of the pulmonary artery, dextroposition of

false ribs   F-5   **fasciculus, gracilis**

the aorta, and hypertrophy of the right ventricle. The defects are sometimes carried into adult life.

false ribs. The lower 5 pairs of ribs. SEE: *ribs, vertebrae.*

falx [L.]. Any sickle-shaped structure.

   f. cerebelli. A fold of the dura mater which forms a vertical partition between the hemispheres of the cerebellum.

   f. cerebri. A fold of the dura mater which lies in the longitudinal fissure and separates the two cerebral hemispheres.

   f. inguinalis. BNA. The conjoined or conjoint tendon which forms the origin of the transversus abdominis and internal oblique muscles.

   f. ligamento'sa. The broad ligament of the liver. SYN: *falciform ligament.*

F. A. M. A. Abbr. for *Fellow of the American Medical Association.*

famil'ial [L. *familiā*, family]. Pert. to or common to the same family, as *f. symptoms.*

family (fam'il-e) [L. *familiā*, family]. 1. A group consisting of parents and their children. 2. In biological classification, the division bet. the *order* and *genus.*

   f., degenerate. One that produces offspring of low or subnormal mentality.

   f., Jukes. A family whose history covers 5 generations of degeneracy.

   f., Kallikak. An American family with 1 branch mentally unfit and another of average intelligence.

fam'ine fever. Relapsing fever.

fang [A.S. *fōn*, to seize]. 1. A sharp-pointed tooth. 2. The root of a tooth.

   f.'s, poison. Two teeth in upper jaw of poisonous reptiles adjacent to their poison glands.

far'ad. A unit of electrical capacity. The capacity of a condenser which, charged with 1 coulomb, gives a difference of potential of 1 volt.

This unit is so large that one-millionth part of it has been adopted as a practical unit called a microfarad.

farad'ic. Pert. to induced electricity.

   f. contrac'tion, graduated. Produced by Smart or Bristow coils.

far'adism. The therapeutic use of an interrupted current to stimulate muscles and nerves. Such a current is derived from the secondary or induction coil.

faradiza'tion. The treatment of nerves or muscles with the faradic current; the condition of nerves or muscles so treated.

faradother'apy [G. *therapeia*, treatment]. Treatment of disease by the faradic current.

farastan (far'a-stan). A combination of iodine and cinchophen.

USES: As an analgesic and antipyretic.
DOSAGE: 3¾ gr. (0.25 Gm.) with same caution as with cinchophen.

far'cy [L. *farcīre*, to stuff]. A form of glanders.

   f. bud. A glanderous tumor.

   f., button. Farcy marked by dermal tubercular nodules.

farina (far-i'nă) [L.]. Wheat ground to pass a #20 sieve with only small siftings.

farina'ceous [L. *farina*, flour]. 1. Starchy. 2. Pert. to flour.

far-point. The farthest point of vision at which objects can be distinctly seen with eyes in complete relaxation.

Farre's tubercles (fars). Carcinomatous masses on surface of the liver.

far-sight'ed. Pert. to far-sightedness. SYN: *hypermetropic, hyperopic.*

far-sight'edness. An error of refraction in which, with accommodation completely relaxed, parallel rays come to a focus behind the retina. SYN: *hypermetropia, hyperopia.*

fascia (fash'i-a) (pl. *fasciae*) [L. a band]. 1. A fibrous membrane covering, supporting, and separating muscles. 2. A bandage. They also unite the skin to underlying tissue.

Fascia may be *superficial*, a nearly subcutaneous covering permitting free movement of the skin, and *deep*, enveloping and binding muscles.

   f., anal. F. of connective tissue covering levator ani muscle from the perineal aspect.

   f., Buck's. A fascial covering of the penis, derived from Colles' fascia.

   f., cervical, deep. Fascia of the neck covering the muscles, vessels and nerves.

   f., c., superficial. Fascia of the neck just inside the skin.

   f., Cloquet's. Femoral fascia.

   f., Colles'. Inner layer of the perineal fascia.

   f., cremasteric. F. covering the cremaster muscle of the spermatic cord.

   f., cribriform. The fascia of the thigh covering the saphenous opening.

   f., dentata. Gray matter in the cerebral dentate convolution.

   f., infundibuliform. Funnel-shaped f., derived from interior abdominal wall, encasing the spermatic cord and testis.

   f., intercolumnar. F. derived from external abdominal ring sheathing the spermatic cord and testis.

   f., ischiorectal. SEE: *anal f.*

   f. lata. Wide covering encasing thigh muscles.

   f., lumbodorsal. Deep investing membrane covering deep muscles of the trunk and back.

   f., pectineal. Pubic section of f. lata.

   f., pelvic. Fascial tissues of extreme importance in the maintenance of normal strength in the pelvic floor. SEE: *pelvic diaphragm* under *"diaphragm."*

   f., thyrolaryngeal. F. covering thyroid gland.

   f., transversalis. F. located between perineum and transversalis muscle.

fascial (fash'e-al) [L. *fascia*, band]. Pert. to or of the nature of fascia.

   f. reflex. Muscular contraction resulting from percussing facial fascia.

fasciaplasty (fash'ĭ-ă-plas"tĭ) [" + G. *plassein*, to form]. Plastic surgery of fascia.

fascicle (făs-sĭk'le). A fasciculus.

fascicular (fas-sĭk'u-lar) [L. *fasciculus*, little bundle]. 1. Arranged like a bundle of rods. 2. Pert. to a fasciculus.

fasciculus (fa-sĭk'u-lus) (pl. *fasciculi*) [L. a little bundle]. A bundle of nerve or muscle fibers. More specifically a division of a funiculus of the spinal cord consisting of fibers of one or more tracts. Sometimes the term is used as a synonym for "tract". SYN: *fasciola.*

   f. cuneatus. A triangular shaped bundle of nerve fibers lying in the dorsal funiculus of the spinal cord. Its fibers enter the cord through the dorsal roots of spinal nerves and terminate in the medulla. Also called tract of Burdach.

   f., fundamental. Portion of ant. column of spinal cord continuing into medulla oblongata.

   f. gracilis. A bundle of nerve fibers lying in the dorsal funiculus of the spinal cord medial to the f. cuneatus. Conducts sensory impulses from the periphery to the medulla.

f. longitudinal. *Inferior longitudinal fasciculus.* A bundle of association fibers connecting the occipital and temporal lobes of the brain; *medial longitudinal fasciculus,* a bundle of fibers running from the spinal cord to the upper portion of the midbrain; superior or dorsal longitudinal *fasciculus,* a bundle of association fibers connecting the frontal lobe with the occipital and temporal lobes.

f., posterior longitudinal. Nerve fiber bundle running bet. corpora quadrigemina and nuclei of 4th and 6th nerves.

f. teres. Column on both sides of median furrow on 4th ventricle's floor.

f. unciformis. Fibers within sylvian fissure connecting frontal and temporosphenoid lobes. SYN: Unciformis.

fasciectomy (fă-shĭ-ek'to-mĭ) [L. *fascia,* band, + G. *ektomē,* excision]. Excision of strips of fascia.

fasciod'esis [" + G. *desis,* binding]. Operation of attaching a fascia to a tendon or another fascia.

fasciola (fă-se'o-lă) [L. little band]. A bundle of nerve or muscle fibers. SYN: *fasciculus, q.v.* [dentata.

f. cinerea. Upper portion of fascia

Fasci'ola [L. *fascia,* band]. A genus of flukes belonging to the class Trematoda.

F. hepatica. A species of flukes infesting the liver and bile ducts of cattle, sheep, and other herbivors; the common liver fluke. An occasional parasite of man. Intermediate hosts are snails belonging to the genus Limneus. Formerly called *Distomum hepaticum.*

fasci'olar [L. *fasciola,* little band]. Pert. to the fasciola cinerea.

fascioliasis (fas-she-o-li'as-is) [L. *fascia,* band]. Infection of the body with a genus of trematode worms. SYN: *distomiasis.*

fas'cioplasty [" + G. *plassein,* to form]. Plastic operation on a fascia.

fasciorrhaphy (fash-ĭ-or'af-ĭ) [" + *raphē,* suture]. Suturing a fascia.

fasciotomy (fash-ĭ-ot'o-mĭ) [" + G. *tomē,* incision]. Surgical incision and division of a fascia.

fascitis (fash-i'tis) [" + G. *itis,* inflammation]. Inflamed condition of a fascia.

fast [A.S. *faest,* fixed]. 1. Resistant to the effects or action of a chemical substance. 2. Fasting.

f. acid. Term applied to bacteria esp. the tuberculosis group which after staining are not decolorized when treated with acid.

f. drug. Term applied to bacteria or other organisms which become resistant to drugs such as penicillin.

fastidium (fas-tid'ĭ-um) [L. aversion]. Aversion to food or to eating. Sometimes seen in hysteria but not as the result of delusions.

fastigatum (fas-tĭ-ga'tum) [L. pointed]. The gray matter on both sides of the inf. vermiform process of the cerebellum. SYN: *nucleus fastigii.*

fastigium (fas-tij'ĭ-um) [L. ridge]. 1. The highest point. The full period of development of acute, infectious diseases when the temperature reaches the maximum or *stadium* and all symptoms have developed. 2. The most posterior portion of the 4th ventricle formed by the junction of the ant., and post., medullary vela projecting into the medullary substance of the cerebellum.

fast'ing [A.S. *faest,* firm]. Going without food for a stated period.

It has been used successfully in treatment of various disorders, esp. epilepsy.

Energy requirements of body metabolism during fasting are supplied by the oxidization of fats which, if glucose is not supplied, results in the products of incomplete fat combustion, such as fatty acids, diacetic acid, and acetones, producing ketosis or a mild acidosis. This condition occurs quickly in children and they have little glycogen reserve. SEE: *jejunitas.*

fast'ness [A.S. *faest,* firm]. Resistance to stains or destructive agents.

fat. 1. Adipose, obese, corpulent. 2. Greasy, oily. 3. CHEM. A triglyceride ester of fatty acids; one of a group of organic compounds closely associated in nature with the phosphatides, cerebrosides, sterols. The term *lipids* or *lipides, q.v.,* is applied in general to fats or fatlike substances. Fats are insoluble in water but soluble in ether, chloroform, benzene and other fat solvents. Upon hydrolysis, fats break down into fatty acids and glycerol (an alcohol). Fats are hydrolyzed by the action of acids, alkalies, lipases (fat-splitting enzymes) and superheated steam.

Chem. structure. In the fat molecule, one molecule of glycerol in combined with three of fatty acids. Three fatty acids, oleic acid ($C_{18}H_{34}O_2$), stearic acid ($C_{18}H_{36}O_2$), and palmitic acid ($C_{18}H_{32}O_2$) comprise the bulk of the fatty acids present in the neutral fats found in body tissues. According to the fatty acid with which the glycerol is combined, corresponding fats are *triolein, tristearin,* and *tripalmitin.* These three fats are the principal fats present in foods.

Physiologic functions of: 1. Fats serve as a source of energy. 2. Subcutaneous fats form an insulating layer which prevents loss of heat. 3. Fat acts to support and protect certain organs such as the eye and kidney. 4. It provides a concentrated reserve of food. 5. It provides essential fatty acids necessary for normal growth and well-being. 6. It is a vehicle for natural fat-soluble vitamins. 7. In conjunction with carbohydrates, fats serve as protein sparers. 8. They are an important constituent of cell structure forming an integral part of the cell membrane. 9. When properly distributed, fat gives a pleasing contour to the body.

Digestion and absorption of fats. In the stomach, emulsified fats such as cream or egg yolk are acted on by gastric lipase; however, most fats undergo digestion in the intestine where they are acted on by a pancreatic lipase, *steapsin,* which hydrolyzes them to fatty acids and glycerol. Although containing no lipolytic enzymes bile is essential for the digestion of fats. Bile aids in the emulsification of fats and also has a hydrotropic action, *i. e.,* renders substances such as fatty acids, which are normally insoluble in water, readily soluble in the fluids of the intestine. Bile salts also act as specific activators of the pancreatic lipase. Bile salts react with fatty acids forming water-soluble, diffusible, soaps which facilitate the emulsification of fats. Glycerol and fatty acids enter the epithelial cells where they recom-

fat metabolism

bine to form neutral fats most of which enters the lacteals. The fats are carried by the lymph through lymph vessels to the thoracic duct from which they enter the blood stream. After a meal rich in fats the mesenteric lymph vessels are filled with a milklike fluid, the *chyle,* containing finely emulsified fat particles, called *chylomicrons.*

Metabolism of fats. Absorbed fats are utilized in the following ways: (a) oxidized with the release of energy, (b) deposited in adipose tissue as storage fat, (c) incorporated in the cells of tissues as an integral part of the protoplasm, (d) desaturated and stored in the liver, (e) excreted in the secretions of the mammary and sweat glands, and in the feces.

Sources of body fats. In addition to fat being absorbed from the intestine, body fat may arise from the conversion of carbohydrates (glucose) or proteins into fat. Fat may possibly be converted into carbohydrates but this occurs only to a limited extent.

Intermediary metabolism of fats. In the oxidation of fat to carbon dioxide and water, several intermediary substances (ketones) are formed. The principal ones are acetoacetic acid, beta-hydroxybutyric acid, and acetone. Excessive production of ketone bodies which occurs when fats are incompletely oxidized is called ketosis. This especially occurs when there is an interference in carbohydrate metabolism, as in diabetes. Ketosis also occurs in certain fevers, in toxemias of pregnancy, and hyperthyroidism. Ketosis results in acidosis.

Fat nutrition. Fats have a high caloric value yielding 9.3 Cal. per gram. as compared with 4.0 and 4.1 Cal. for carbohydrates and proteins respectively. The average diet of 3000 Cal. should contain 30 to 40 per cent of its caloric value in fats. The average diet contains from 50 to 130 grams of fat. Quantities in excess of 150 grams are repulsive and difficult to digest. In addition to their nutritive values, fats improve the taste and odor of foods, provide a feeling of satiety, are absorbed slowly prolonging their nutritive effects, and because of their high caloric content, are of especial importance in high-caloric diets.

Contra. Fat intake should be reduced in diseases of the gall bladder and liver.

RS: bile, gall bladder, liver, fatty acids, lipases, ketones, glycerol.

f. depot. Accumulations of fat in certain regions of the body such as the buttocks or abdominal wall.

f. low diet. Approximately 40 to 50 Gm. fat daily. SEE: *reduction diet.*

f. neutral. Compounds of the higher fatty acids (palmitic, stearic, and oleic) with glycerol. They are the common fats of animal and plant tissues.

f. and protein-free diet. 1. Carbohydrates. 2. Honey. 3. Fruit juices. 4. Juicy fruits. 5. Melons. 6. Cucumbers. 7. Marmalades and jellies. 8. Rhubarb. 9. Fresh tomatoes.

fat, words pert. to: absorption, acid, "adip-" words, calory, chondrolipoma, chromolipoid, digestion, fatty acids, fatty casts, fuel value, hydrogenation, ketogenic diet, "lip-" words, obesity, palmitic acid, palmitin, steariform, stearin, steatolysis, tissue.

fatigue (fă-tēg') [L. *fatigare,* to tire]. 1. A feeling of tiredness or weariness resulting from continued activity. 2. The state or condition of an organ or tissue in which its response to stimulation is reduced or lost as a result of overactivity. 3. To bring about a condition of fatigue.

Fatigue may be the result of: (a) excessive activity which results in the accumulation of metabolic waste products such as lactic acid, (b) malnutrition (deficiency of carbohydrates, proteins, minerals, or vitamins), (c) circulatory disturbances such as heart disease, or anemia which interfere with the supply of oxygen and energy materials to tissues, (d) respiratory disturbances which interferes with the supply of oxygen to tissues, (e) infectious diseases in which toxic products are produced or body metabolism altered, (f) endocrine disturbances such as occur in diabetes, hyperinsulinism, and menopause, (g) psychogenic factors such as emotional conflicts, frustration, worry, boredom, (h) physical factors such as incorrect posture, flat feet, (i) miscellaneous factors, such as eye strain.

f. acute. Fatigue with sudden onset such as occurs following excessive exertion relieved by rest.

f. chronic. Long-continued fatigue not relieved by rest. Indicative of disease such as tuberculosis or diabetes or other conditions of altered body metabolism.

RS: bradyphrenia, glycogen, narcotic, stimulant, sleep.

f. muscular. The reduced capacity of a muscle to perform work as a result of repeated contractions. Fatigue may be partial or complete.

f. reaction. In tuberculosis, an elevation of temperature following exertion.

f. stance. Fatigue resulting from standing for long periods of time.

f. syndrome. Neurasthenia, *q.v.*

fatty. Of or pertaining to fats or fatty substances; adipose.

f. casts. Mass of fat droplets arranged frequently in groups and probably remains of a true epithelial cast.

f. degeneration. A change involving the deposition of fat in the cytoplasm. SEE: *fat, heart.*

fatty acid. A hydrocarbon in which one of the hydrogen atoms has been replaced by a carboxyl (COCH) group; a monobasic aliphatic acid made up of an alkyl radical attached to a carboxyl group.

The digestion and absorption of fats in foods.

The saturated fatty acids include: acetic, butyric, caproic, caprylic, capric, lauric, formic, myristic, palmitic, and stearic acids all of which contain an even number of carbon atoms. All are homologues of formic acid.

The unsaturated fatty acids include: Those of (a) the *oleic series:* oleic, tiglic, hypogeic, palmitoleic, and physetoleic acids and (b) the *linoleic* or *linolic series:* linoleic, linolenic, clupanodonic, arachidonic, hydrocarpic, and chaulmoogric acids. The latter two are used in the treatment of leprosy.

f. a., essential. The unsaturated fatty acids, *q.v.* In certain animals, the absence of these fatty acids in their diet leads to loss of weight, eczematous condition of the skin, and kidney disorders.

By boiling with alkalies, esp. in alcoholic solutions, also by the action of many ferments, as the steapsin of the pancreatic juice, fats are split up into glycerine and free fatty acids.

fauces   F-8   **feces**

The fatty acids unite with the alkalies present, forming salts of fatty acids, the soaps (sodium soap, or hard soap, and potassium soap, or soft soap). If fats contain free fatty acid (rancid fats) they can, on melting, form an emulsion with water and a little soda; in this process of emulsion the fats are finely divided, forming a milky fluid.

As emulsification is dependent upon the presence of soap, formed by the union of fatty acid and alkali, a purely neutral fat cannot be emulsified. Emulsification is an important process in the absorption of fats in foods.

fauces (faw'ses) [L. the throat]. The aperture leading from the mouth into the pharynx, or cavity of the throat.

The ant. pillars of the fauces are known as the *glossopalatine arch*, and the post. pillars, as the *pharyngopalatine arch*. SEE: *fossa*.

fau'cial [L. fauces, the throat]. Pert. to the fauces.

  f. reflex. Gagging or vomiting resulting from irritation of fauces.

faucitis (faw-si'tis) [" + G. *-itis*, inflammation]. Inflammation of the fauces.

faveolate (fav-e'o-lāt) [L. *faveōlus*, little honeycomb]. Honeycombed. SYN: *alveolate*.

fave'olus [L. little honeycomb]. A depression or small pit, esp. on the skin.

favism. A condition common in Sicily and Sardinia resulting from sensitivity to a species of bean, *Vicia faba*. It is characterized by fever, anemia, abdominal pain, and may lead to prostration and coma. It is caused by ingestion of the beans, or inhalation of the pollen.

favus (fa'vus) [L. honeycomb]. Contagious skin disease characterized by pinhead to pea-sized, saucer-shaped, yellowish crust usually over hair follicles and accompanied by musty odor and itching. It may spread all over the body.

ETIOL: Fungus, *Achorion schönleinlii*.
SYM: As stated.
PATH: Invasion of hair shafts and epidermis.
PROG: Good.
TREATMENT: X-rays for hair surfaces. Ointments containing sulfur, oleate of mercury, ammoniated mercury, chrysarobin, iodine.
SYN: *crusted* or *honeycomb ringworm*, *tinea favosa*.

F. C. S. Abbr. for *Fellow of the Chemical Society*.

F.D. Abbr. for local distance.

Fe. Chem. symb. for iron (*ferrum*).

fear [A.S. *faer*]. PSY: Primitively, the emotional reaction to an environmental threat, it now also presents itself frequently as an indicator of inner problems; fright, dread.

A partial fear reaction may be considered the expression of somatic disease. Fear is met with clinically, esp. in anxiety neuroses, anxious psychotic pictures (*e. g.*, depression), and in toxic deliria (*e. g.*, delirium tremens). At the somatic level, hyperthyroidism and hyperadrenalism may strongly simulate the fear state. SEE: *emotion*.

febricide (feb'-rĭ-sīd) [L. *febris*, fever, + *caedere*, to kill]. Destructive to fever. SYN: *antipyretic*.

febric'ula [L. little fever]. Mild fever of short duration without other pathology.

febrifacient (feb-rĭ-fa'sĭ-ent) [L. *febris*, fever, + *facere*, to make]. Producing fever.

febrific (fĕ-brĭf'ĭk) [" + *facere*, to make]. Producing or conveying fever.

febrifugal (feb-rĭf'u-gal) [" + *fugāre*, to put to flight]. Reducing fever.

febrifuge (feb'rĭ-fūj) [" + *fugāre*, to put to flight]. That which lessens fever. SYN: *antipyretic*.

feb'rile [L. *febris*, fever]. Feverish; pert. to a fever. SEE: *fever*.

  f. state. A term used to describe constitutional symptoms which accompany a rise in temperature. Pulse and respiration usually rise with headache, pains, malaise, loss of appetite, concentrated and diminished urine, constipation, restlessness, hot dry skin, insomnia, irritability.

febripho'bia [" + G. *phobos*, fear]. Anxiety or fear induced by a rise in body temperature.

febris (fe'bris) [L.]. Fever.
  f. acmastica. Continued fever.
  f. castrensis. Typhus and remittent fever.
  f. enterica. Typhoid fever.
  f. flava. Yellow fever.
  f. lactea. Milk fever.
  f. remittens. Remittent fever.
  f. undulans. Malta fever.
  f. variolosa. A form of smallpox.

fe'cal [L. *faeces*, feces]. Pert. to, or of the nature of, feces.
  f. vomit. Feces in vomitus.
ETIOL: Strangulated hernia or intestinal obstruction preventing anal outlet.

fecalith (fe'kal-ith) [" + G. *lithos*, stone]. A fecal concretion. SYN: *coprolith*.

fecaloid (fe'kal-oid) [" + G. *eidos*, form]. Resembling feces.

fecaloma (fe-kal-o'mă) [" + G. *ōma*, tumor]. [L. *faeces*, feces]. SYN: *Coproma, scatoma, stercoroma*. A large mass of accumulated feces in the rectum resembling a tumor.

fecalu'ria [" + G. *ouron*, urine]. Fecal matter in the urine.

feces (fe'sez) [L. *faeces*]. Stools; excreta; dejecta; excrement. Body waste, such as food residue, bacteria, epithelium, and mucus, discharged from the bowels by way of the anus.

AMOUNT OF: Twenty-five to fifty Gm. of solid, or 100-200 Gm. of moist substance on a mixed diet, per day. From 0.5-0.9 Gm. per day of nitrogen is excreted on a non-nitrogenous diet.

COLOR OF: The color of the feces may be indicative of various disorders as shown by the following: *Black*: May follow intestinal hemorrhage, or the use of drugs such as bismuth, iron, tannin, manganese, or charcoal. *Bloody*: May indicate hemorrhoids, cancer of the rectum, ulcers, fissures, abraded rectal membrane from dry feces, eroded rectal polypus, acute proctitis, foreign bodies, colitis, and intussusception or strangulated hernia in children. May also result from cancer of the colon, rupture of abdominal aneurysm, typhoid fever, phosphorus poisoning, jaundice, yellow fever, dengue, septicemia and yellow atrophy of the liver. *Clay-colored*: May denote impaired bile formation or obstruction, phosphorus poisoning or yellow atrophy of the liver. Rarely indicates tumor or movable kidney. *Green*: Seen as the result of increased flow of bile, the use of calomel, and, commonly, diarrheas in young children. In the latter cases, may be due to bacterial growth.

COMPOSITION: Residue of food, water, products of secretions, of bacterial de-

feces, sheep F-9 **feeding tube**

composition, indol, skatol, cholesterol, mucous and epithelial cells, purin bases, pigment, microörganisms, inorganic salts, and sometimes foreign substances.

DIAGNOSIS BY: The reducing effect of the intestinal flora upon the feces is considered an index of intestinal conditions, the less reduction indicating the best condition. Low reduction may be caused by green vegetables, fruits, and milk; while meat and egg protein result in the opposite condition.

FORM AND CONSISTENCY: (a) Normally, soft and formed; (b) hard, nodular, or scybalous in constipation; (c) fluid or mushy in diarrhea; (d) flattened or ribbonlike in rectal obstruction or spastic colitis; (e) frothy in fermentative conditions; (f) greasy in jaundice, etc.

INSPECTION OF: This should include the *color,* the *formation,* their *odor,* and the presence of any observable *foreign substances,* including *calculi.*

MUCUS: Always important, and should be reported. Normally, none seen. May occur: (a) As superficial gelatinous streaks or blobs; (b) mixed with the stool, and only apparent on making a thin paste with water; (c) mixed with blood, as in dysentery; (d) composing almost the entire stool, sometimes as firm bands or cords.

ODOR: This varies much with disease and dietary differences. It is most marked on a meat diet, and almost absent on a milk diet. Variations, such as sour, pungent, putrid, etc., occur in different diseases. *Offensive:* Obtain in jaundice, acute indigestion, enteritis, erysipelas, typhoid fever, rachitis, and occasionally in constipation. *Putrid:* May be the result of syphilitic or carcinomatous ulceration of the rectum or gangrenous dysentery. *Sour:* Normal stools of infants.

PARASITES: The presence of various intestinal parasites can be determined by examination of the feces. Gross examination may reveal the presence of nematodes or tapeworms; however, microscopic examination is necessary to determine the presence of protozoa, helminth ova, or larvae. In examination of feces, stools are collected in clean, dry, containers. For microscopic examination, representative bits of feces, or mucus are emulsified in saline solution on a clean slide, then spread evenly, and covered with a coverglass. Enterbiasis is best diagnosed by examination of scrapings from the anal and perianal regions.

REACTION: The normal reaction is neutral or slightly alkaline. An acid reaction usually indicates some fermentation in the gut or an excess of vegetables in the diet. The stools of infants are usually acid.

f., sheep. Small masses broken off from stonelike feces remaining in colon too long.

feces, words pert. to: acoprosis, acoprous, anus, bilifecia, colon, constipation, defecation, dejecta, elimination, excreta, excretion, hypostasis, impaction, intestine, meconium, melanorrhea, melena, rectum, scatacratia, scybalum, sigmoid, skatol, steatorrhea, stercoraceous, stercoremia, stool.

Fe(C$_3$H$_5$O$_3$)$_2$. Ferrous lactate; lactate of iron.

Fe(C$_6$H$_5$O$_7$). Citrate of iron.

Fechner's law (fek'nerz). The magnitudes of sensation produced by given stimuli form an arithmetical progression, the stimuli forming a geometrical progression. SYN: *psychophysical law.*

FeCl$_2$. Ferrous chloride.
FeCl$_3$. Ferric chloride.
FeCO$_3$. Ferrous carbonate; c. of iron.

fec'ula [L. *faecula,* dregs]. 1. Sediment. 2. Starch.

feculent (fek'u-lent) [L. *faecula,* dregs]. Having sediment.

fecundate (fe'kun-dāt) [L. *fecundāre,* to bear fruit]. To fertilize or impregnate or render fertile.

fecundation (fe-kun-da'shun) [L. *fecundāre,* to bear fruit]. Impregnation; fertilization.

f., artificial. Impregnation by injecting the seminal fluid into the uterus by mechanical means.

fecundity (fe-kun'dit-I) [L. *fecundāre,* to bear fruit]. Ability to produce offspring; fertility.

feeblemind'edness [L. *flebilis,* tearful, + A.S. *gemynd,* to think]. Arrested mental development as distinguished from temperamental abnormality. Amentia. On the basis of intelligence tests, feebleminded individuals are classified into three groups; *morons* (I.Q. 50-70), *imbeciles* (I.Q. 20-50), *idiots* (I.Q. below 20).

feed'ing [A.S. *fedan,* to give food to]. Taking or giving nourishment, esp. extra-orally.

The latter is sometimes necessary because the patient either refuses or is unable to eat.

f., artificial. This is accomplished through the *nostrils,* the *esophagus,* and the *rectum;* also through *gastrostomy* or *duodenostomy.*

f., colonic. Less useful with psychotic than with physically sick patients but at times it can be utilized. It is now somewhat questionable owing to the limited ability for absorption in the colon.

f., esophageal. Used after operations on tongue or jaw, diseases of mouth, in mental cases, and forcible feedings. Mouth gag needed in last 2 cases. Also used for test meals.

f., forcible. This is by way of esophagus or rectum.

f., nasal. Largely used for children, and when unable to take nourishment normally, such as in delirium, coma, and stupor, diseases of mouth and pharynx. Any strained liquid food that will pass through catheter can be used. Temperature of feeding, 100° F. Olive oil and swabs needed for cleaning nostrils.

f., rectal. Commonest form used although it is admitted that little nourishment can be absorbed through colon. Normal saline often used with glucose, making a 5-10% solution by adding ½ to 1 oz. of glucose to 10 oz. of normal saline. Rectal washout should be given once in 24 hr. from 10 to 11 A. M.

f., tube. Done through the mouth or nostril, the latter requiring a much smaller tube and a little more dexterity, but less likely to be successfully resisted. With patient lying, arms bound to body by encircling sheets, the lubricated (glycerine) tube is gently passed into pharynx and, avoiding the larynx, it is projected into the stomach. Entry into the larynx produces struggling and cyanosis. Sugar, eggs, cereals, whiskey, etc., are added to milk and then slowly introduced.

feeling

feel'ing [A.S. *fēlan*, to feel]. The conscious phase of nervous activity. The (a) emotions or centrally stimulated f.'s and (b) those sensations peripherally produced by excitation of peripheral nerves including those of the special senses.

feet (pl. of *foot*) [A.S. *fēt*]. The pedal extremities of the legs.
RS: *carpopedal spasm, chilblain, chiropodalgia, chiropodist, chiropody, extremity, foot.*

Fehl'ing's solution. A solution used for detecting the presence of sugar in urine. It consists of equal parts of Solutions A and B prepared as follows: Solution A—dissolve 34.65 Gm. of copper sulfate in water and make up to 500 cc. Solution B—dissolve 125 Gm. of potassium hydroxide and 173 Gm. of potassium sodium tartrate (Rochelle salt) in water and make up to 500 cc. Mix equal portions of solutions A and B immediately before using.

fel [L.]. Bile.
f. bo'vis. Ox gall. USP. Dried fresh bile of the ox, used principally in form of an extract.
ACTION AND USES: A laxative, intestinal antiseptic, chologogue.
DOSAGE: 6 gr. (0.4 Gm.).
SYN: *bilis bovina.*

fellatio (fel-a'shi-o). A form of sex perversion in which gratification is accomplished by buccal intromission of the penis; buccal coitus.

Fell-O'Dwyer's method (George E. Fell, Buffalo physician, born 1850; Joseph O'Dwyer, New York physician, 1841-1898). Artificial respiration by means of a bellows, forcing air through an intubation tube into the lungs.

fel'on [A.S. *feloun*, malignant]. Suppuration of terminal joint of a finger. SYN: *paronychia,* runround, whitlow.*

felt'work [Ger. *falzen*, to join, + A.S. *worc*, to make]. 1. Fibrous network. 2. A plexus of nerve fibrils. SYN: *neuropilem.*

fe'male [L. *femella*, little woman]. 1. A woman or girl-child. 2. Pert. to a woman. SEE: *genitalia, female.*
f. sex hormone. H. secreted by the ova which develops the uterus, vagina, and breasts at puberty, aids in regeneration of mucosa following menstruation, stimulates uterine contraction. SYN: *estrin, estrogen.*

fem'inism [L. *femina*, woman]. 1. The female character. 2. Possession of female characteristics by the male. 3. Social movement for female independence.

feminiza'tion [L. *femina*, woman]. Acquiring or adoption of female characteristics.

fem'oral [L. *femur, femor-*, thigh]. Pert. to the thigh bone or femur.
f. artery. One beginning at *ext. iliac a.*, terminating behind the knee as the popliteal a., on inner side of femur.
f. reflex. Extension of knee and flexion of foot resulting from irritation of skin over upper ant. third of thigh.
f. vein. Continuation of the popliteal vein upward toward the *ext. iliac vein.* SYN: *crural vein.*

fem'orocele [L. *femur*, thigh, + G. *kēlē*, hernia]. Femoral hernia.

femorotib'ial [" + *tibia*, pipe]. Rel. to the femur and tibia.

fe'mur [L.]. The thigh bone.
It extends from the hip to the knee and is the longest and strongest bone in the skeleton.

RS: *calcar femorale, cavalry bone, cotyloid cavity, femoral, trochanter.*

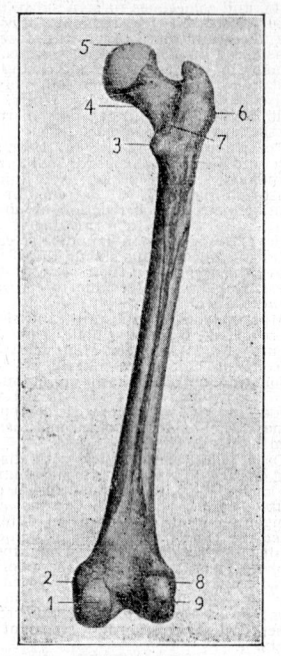

THE FEMUR
1. Internal condyle. 2. Internal tuberosity. 3. Lesser trochanter. 4. Neck of femur. 5. Head. 6. Greater trochanter. 7. Intertrochanteric line. 8. External tuberosity. 9. External condyle.

fenes'tra (pl. *fenestrae*) [L. window]. 1. An aperture frequently closed by a membrane. 2. An open area, as in the blade of a forceps.
f. ovalis. An oval opening on the inner wall of the middle ear or tympanum leading to the vestibule, into which the base of the stapes fits. Also called *fenestra vestibuli.*
f. rotunda. Leading into the cochlea. It is closed by a membrane, the secondary tympani membrane. Also called *fenestra cochleae.*

fen'estrated [L. *fenestra*, window]. Having openings.
f. membrane of Henle. Elastic tissue layer in intima of larger arteries.

fenestra'tion [L. *fenestra*, window]. 1. Condition of having fenestra. 2. An operation in which an artificial opening is made into the labyrinth of the ear. Resorted to in cases of otosclerosis.

ferment' [L. *fermentum*, from *fervere*, to ferment]. 1. To decompose. 2. (fer'-ment). A substance capable of producing fermentation in other substances. 3. A catalytic agent which is capable of inducing fermentation in substances with which it comes in contact. SYN: *enzyme, q.v.*

fermentation   F-11   **fertilization**

RS: *bromelin, cacozyme, chymase, cholesterase, enzyme, hydrolyst, myopsin, pancreatin, steapsin, trypsin, trypsinogen, tyrosinase, yeast.*

fermenta′tion [L. *fermentum*, leaven]. The oxidative decomposition of complex substances through the action of enzymes or ferments, produced by microorganisms. Bacteria, molds, and yeasts are the principal groups of organisms involved in fermentation. Fermentations of economic importance are those involved in the production of alcohol, lactic and butyric acids, and the baking of bread.

RS: *acid, acetic f., alcohol, autolysis, autolytic, azymic, digestion, enzyme, ferment.*

f. acetic. The production of acetic acid by the bacterial oxidation of ethyl alcohol under aerobic conditions.

f. alcoholic. The production of ethyl alcohol from carbohydrates usually through the action of yeasts.

f., amylolyt′ic. The process of hydrolyzation of starch with the formation of sugar.

f., autolyt′ic. One in the tissues which disintegrates them after death.

f. butyric. Formation of butyric acid from bacterial action on carbohydrates under anaerobic conditions.

f. citric acid. Formation of citric acid from action of molds on carbohydrates.

f., invertin. One that converts cane sugar into dextrose and levulose by invertin.

f., lactic. That which sours milk.

f. lactic acid. Formation of lactic acid from carbohydrates by action of lactic acid bacteria. The genera *Streptococcus* and *Lactobacillus* are the forms usually involved. Lactic acid is responsible for the souring of milk.

f. oxalic acid. Formation of oxalic acid from carbohydrates from the action of certain molds, esp., *Aspergillus.*

f. proprionic acid. Formation of proprionic acid from carbohydrates from action of certain bacteria.

f. test. A confirmation test for sugar in the urine. Gas forms in the fermentation tube if sugar is present.

f., viscous. Production of gelatinous material by different forms of bacilli.

fermen′toid [" + G. *eidos*, form]. A ferment without fermentive power.

fermentum (fer-men′tum) [L.]. Yeast; a ferment.

fern. A plant belonging to the class Filicinae, of the division Tracheophyta (formerly phylum Pteridophyta.

f. male. *Aspidium filix-mas*, from the rhizomes and stipes of which is obtained oleoresin, a polyhydric phenol, the most commonly used anthelminthic for all species of tapeworms.

-ferous [L.]. Suffix meaning producing.

ferrated. Combined with iron or containing iron.

ferri-, ferro- [L. *ferrum*, iron]. Prefix used to indicate *presence of iron.*

fer′ric [L. *ferrum*, iron]. SYN: *ferruginous.* 1. Pertaining to or containing iron. 2. Denoting a compound containing iron in its trivalent form.

fer′ric ammo′nium cit′rate. USP. Thin, garnet-red crystals, containing about 17% of iron.

USES: As a pleasant chalybeate, given in solution.

DOSAGE: 10-30 gr. (0.6-2 Gm.).

f. amm. cit. virides. USP. Thin green scales or granules, containing approximately 15% iron.

USES: Intramuscularly, in anemia.

DOSAGE: ¼-1½ gr. (0.015-0.1 Gm.).

INCOMPATIBILITIES: Mineral acids, vegetable astringents, fixed alkalies.

f. chlor′ide (FeCl₃). USP. Used principally in form of tincture.

ACTION AND USES: An astringent, used in application of throat, also as a hematinic.

DOSAGE: 10 ♏ (0.6 cc.) freely diluted.

INCOMPATIBILITIES: Tea (tannin), magnesium sulfate, sodium bromide.

ferricyanide. A salt of hydroferricyanic acid.

ferrihemoglobin. Methemoglobin, a reduced form of hemoglobin.

fer′rin. An iron-containing compound isolated from liver tissue.

ferrit′in. An iron-phosphorus-protein complex containing about 23% iron. It is formed in the intestinal mucosa by the union of ferric iron with a protein, *apoferritin.* Ferritin is the form in which iron is stored in the tissues, principally in the reticulo-endothelial cells of the liver, spleen and bone marrow.

ferrom′eter [L. *ferrum*, iron, + G. *metron*, measure]. Device for estimating proportion of iron in the blood.

ferropectic (fer-o-pek′tik) [" + G. *pēxis*, fixation]. Pert. to fixing iron.

ferropexia (fer-o-pek′sĭ-ă) [" + G. *pēxis*, fixation]. Iron fixation.

ferroprotein. A protein combined with an iron-containing radical. Ferroproteins are important oxygen-transferring enzymes. e.g. Warburg's enzyme cytochrome oxidase) *q.v.*

ferrous (fer′ous) [L. *ferrum*, iron]. SYN: *ferruginous.* 1. Pertaining to iron. 2. Denoting a compound containing iron of a lower valence than three.

fer′rous car′bonate (FeCO₃). Iron carbonate, used chiefly in form of Blaud's pills.

ACTION AND USES: To increase number of red blood cells, indicated in anemia.

DOSAGE: 5-10 gr.

f. i′odide (FeI₂). USP. An unstable preparation of iron used in form of syrup. Should be transparent, pale or yellowish-green liquid.

ACTION AND USES: Same properties as iron and iodide.

DOSAGE: 15 ♏ (1 cc.).

INCOMPATIBILITIES: Codeine, quinine.

f. sulfate (FeSO₄). USP. Green vitriol. Pale, bluish-green crystals.

ACTION AND USES: Internally, same as other preparations of iron, also in preparation of Blaud's pills.

DOSAGE: 2-5 gr. (0.13-0.32 Gm.).

INCOMPATIBILITIES: Alkalies, chlorides, tannic acid, and oxidizing agents.

ferruginous (fĕr-rū′jĭn-ŭs) [L. *ferrugo*, iron rust]. SYN: *chalybeate.* 1. Pertaining to or containing iron. 2. Of the color of iron rust.

fer′rule [L. *viriola*, little bracelet]. A band or ring of metal applied to the end of root or crown of a tooth to strengthen it.

fer′rum [L. iron]. SYMB: Fe. Iron.

fer′tile [L. *fertilis*, from *ferre*, to bear]. 1. Impregnated. 2. Capable of reproduction.

fertility (fŭr-tĭl′ĭ-tĭ) [L. *fertilis*, from *ferre*, to bear]. Quality of being productive or fertile.

fertiliza′tion [L. *fertilis*, from *ferre*, to bear]. 1. Fecundation; impregnation of an ovum with the spermatozoon of the male, the male sex cell being carried in the seminal discharge.

This usually takes place in the fallopian tube. Spermatozoa have been found in the tube alive 48 hours after

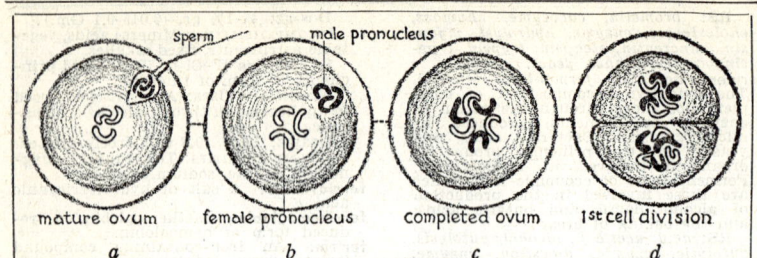

fertilizin F-12 **fetometry**

FERTILIZATION
(Diagrammatic): a. Sperm enters mature ovum. b. Sperm loses its tail and becomes male pronucleus. c. Male and female pronuclei fuse to form complete nucleus containing half male and half female chromosomes. d. Complete nucleus divides, each new nucleus containing half male and half female chromosomes.

the last coitus. On meeting the ovum the head of the spermatozoon penetrates it and its tail drops off. Cell division begins and the fertilized ovum enters the uterus.
2. BOT: The union of the male and female gametes. In higher plants, when the pollen tube enters the ovule, two gametes emerge, one uniting with the egg to form the zygote, from which the embryo develops; the other uniting with two endosperm nuclei to form a primary endosperm cell from which the endosperm (reserve food) develops.
RS: *chemicogenesis, coitus, conception, impregnation, ovum, spermatozoa, sterile, sterility.*

fertilizin. A substance, possibly a glycoprotein extracted from eggs which when added to a suspension of sperms causes agglutination of the sperms. It probably aids in fertilization by fixing sperm to the egg membrane. It is complementary to *antifertilizin*, a substance extracted from sperm which agglutinates eggs.

fervescence (fer-ves′ens) [L. *fervescere*, to grow hot]. Increase of fever.

fes′ter [L. *fistula*, ulcer]. To become inflamed and suppurate.

festina′tion [L. *festināre*, to hasten]. Morbid acceleration of gait seen in some nervous afflictions such as paralysis agitans.

festoon (fes-tōōn′) [L. *festum*, decoration]. The wreathlike curvature of the gums around the necks of the teeth.

fe′tal [L. *foetus*, fetus]. Pert. to a fetus.
f. circulation. The course of the flow of blood in a fetus. Significant differences between fetal and postnatal circulation are the presence in the fetus of (a) *umbilical arteries* and *vein* which carry blood to and from the placenta, (b) *foramen ovale*, an opening in the interatrial septum, and (c) *ductus arteriosus*, a vessel connecting the pulmonary artery with the aorta. The latter two enable the blood to by-pass the lungs which are nonfunctional in the fetus. SEE: Fig. of fetal circulation p. F-13.

fetalism (fē′tal-izm) [" + G. *ismos*, condition]. Retention of fetal structures after birth.

feta′tion [L. *foetus*, fetus]. Pregnancy.

feticide (fē′ti-sīd) [" + *caedere*, to kill]. Intentional destruction of fetal life.

fet′id [L. *fetere*, to stink]. Rank or foul in odor.

fetish, fetich (fē′tish) [Portug. *feitico*, from L. *factitius*, artificial]. That which attracts one of the opposite sex to another, or which excites the libido.
It may be the hair, the lips, or the dress. Undue value set upon such a fetish is called "fetishism," *q.v.* Religious fetishism sees divine attributes in its idols and holy images. The fetish becomes a symbol. SEE: *libido.*

fe′tishism [" + G. *ismos*, state]. 1. Belief in some object as possessing power, or being capable of inspiring a stimulus. 2. Substitution for a normal love object (a person) of parts or possessions of such a one. Libido gratification from contact with articles of dress, braid of hair, etc.
A form of masochism which finds a sex stimulus at the sight of a woman's shoe or glove, or other article of apparel, or of some part of the body such as the hair, esp. the pubic hair. To the masochist,* all such symbols are indicative of the woman's domination.

fetom′etry [L. *foetus*, fetus, + G. *metron*, measure]. Estimation of size of the fetus or its head before delivery.

Development of Fetal Tissue

Ectoderm
1. Epidermis.
2. Epithelium of:
External and internal ear.
Nasal cavity.
Mouth.
Anus.
Amnion, chorion.
Distal part of male urethra.
3. Nervous tissue.

Mesoderm
1. Connective tissues.
2. Male and female reproductive tracts.
3. Blood vessels, lymphatics.
4. Kidneys, ureters, trigone of bladder.
5. Pleura, peritoneum, pericardium.
6. Muscles.

Entoderm
1. Respiratory tract except nose.
2. Digestive tract except mouth and anus.
3. Bladder except trigone.
4. Male urethra, proximal portion.
5. Female urethra.

fetoplacen'tal [" + *placenta*, a flat cake, from G. *plakous*]. Pert. to the fetus and its placenta.

fe'tor [L. *fetere*, to stink]. Stench; an offensive odor.

    f. ex. ore. Offensive breath, halitosis.

    f. oris. Halitosis.

fe'tus [L. *foetus*]. The child *in utero* after the 3rd month of development.

fetus. 1. The latter stages of the developing young of an animal within the uterus or within an egg. 2. In humans, the child in utero from the third month to birth.

    f. amorphus. A shapeless fetal monster; one scarcely recognizable as a fetus.

    f. calcified. A lithopedion, *q.v.*

    f. compressus. A f. papyraceous, *q.v.*

    f. in feto. Condition in which a small imperfect fetus called *parasite*, is contained with the body of another fetus, the *autosite*.

    f. mummified. A dead fetus which was assumed a mummified form upon failure of resorption to occur.

    f. paper doll . . . f. papyraceous, *q.v.*

    f. papyraceous. In twin pregnancy, the dead fetus pressed flat by the development of the living twin.

    RS: *ambloma, amnion, amniotic sac, bag-of-waters, capitones, cephalotripsy, cirrhonosus, fixity, lanugo, vernix caseosa, viable.*

fe'ver [A.S. *fēfer*, from L. *fervere*, to grow warm]. 1. Pyrexia, or elevation of temperature above normal, 98.6° F. 2. A disease which is characterized by an elevation of body temperature, such as typhoid fever, yellow fever.

    CLASSIFICATION (Wunderlich): (a) Subfebrile, 99.5°-100.4°; (b) slightly febrile,

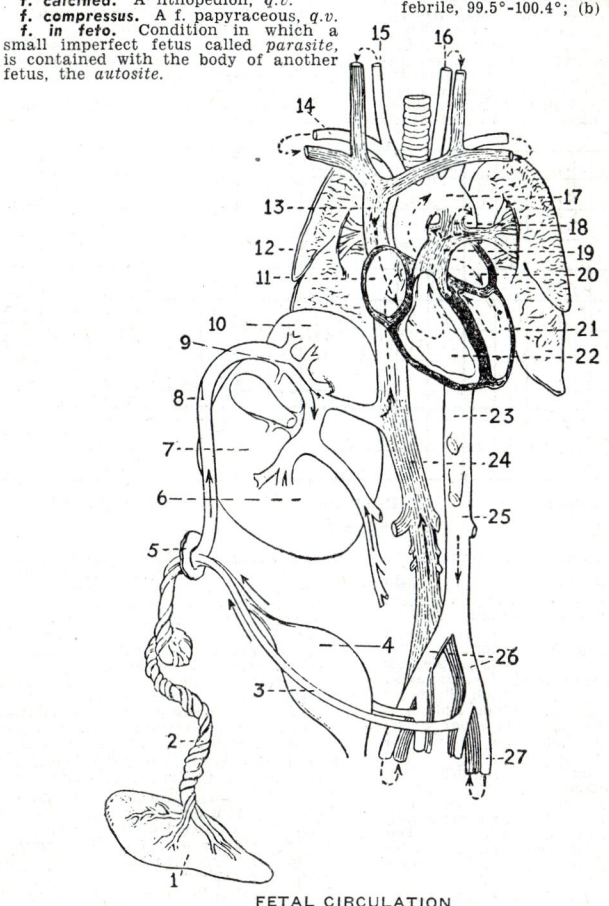

FETAL CIRCULATION
1. Placenta. 2. Umbilical cord. 3. Left hypogastric artery. 4. Bladder. 5. Umbilicus. 6. Right lobe of liver. 7. Liver. 8. Umbilical vein. 9. Ductus venosus. 10. Left lobe of liver. 11. Right atrium. 12. Right lung. 13. Superior vena cava. 14. Right subclavian artery. 15. Right common carotid. 16. Left common carotid. 17. Arch of the aorta. 18. Aorta. 19. Pulmonary artery. 20. Auricle or left atrium. 21. Left ventricle. 22. Right ventricle. 23. Aorta. 24. Inferior vena cava. 25. Aorta. 26. Common iliac arteries. 27. External iliac artery.

100.4°-101.3°; (c) moderately febrile, 101.3°-103.1°; (d) decidedly febrile, 103.1°-104°; (e) highly febrile, 103.1° A. M., 104.9° P. M.; (f) hyperpyretic, above 106°.

ETIOL: In the young, moderate increase in body temperature may result from minor causes and is of less significance than in the adult. After childhood, fevers may be caused by: (a) a hot environment or the generation of body heat by physical means, (b) neurogenic factors such as injury to the diencephalon or mid-brain. The diencephalon contains reflex centers regulating heat loss. (c) dehydration such as occurs after excessive diuresis, (d) chemical substances such as caffeine or cocaine when injected into the blood stream, (d) the injection of proteins or their products, or the breakdown of necrotic tissue. These are the *aseptic fevers* such as follow surgery or coronary occlusion. (e) infectious diseases or inflammation. Fever is the result of the breakdown of bacterial proteins or toxins liberated by the disease organisms which affect the heat-regulating centers. (f) severe hemorrhage.

PERIODS: *Invasion or onset of fever*: While temperature is rising and until maximum is reached, gradual, as in typhoid, or sudden, as in scarlet fever. *Fastigium or stadium*: When the fever is more or less stationary with possible variations often reaching the maximum. *Defervescence*: During which the fever declines until normal. When sudden it is known as *crisis, as in lobar pneumonia;* when gradual, *lysis,* as in measles.

SYM: Face flushed; hot, dry skin; anorexia; headache; nausea and sometimes vomiting; constipation and sometimes diarrhea; aching all over; scant, highly-colored urine; tissue waste. Delirium possible if temperature is over 105° F. or with some, less. Convulsions may follow, esp. in children; coma.

f., childbed. Puerperal sepsis. An infection of the genital tract following childbirth. SEE: *puerperium.*

f., continuous. As in scarlet fever, typhus, or pneumonia, in which there is a slight diurnal variation.

f. delirium. It corresponds to (a) the degree of temperature, (b) to the activity of the toxin giving rise to the fever, (c) to the rapidity of tissue change, (d) to the extent of circulatory disturbance, and (e) to the previous habits of the individual.

f., induced. That artificially produced to favorably modify the course of a disease, notably paresis. Sustained fever of 105° F., or even higher, maintained for 6 to 8 or 10 hours may be induced by the use of medical diathermy, etc. The production of malaria, and of rat-bite fever permit of a series of fever-reactions of fairly long duration, while protein injections are capable of arousing only acute and, at times, dangerous febrile reactions.

f., intermittent. As in malaria and Malta fever with minimum normal or subnormal temperature, and with marked diurnal variation.

f., remittent. As in typhoid fever, septic fever, or remittent fever, with minimum temperature above normal, and with marked diurnal variation.

f., septic. One due to septic matter in the body.

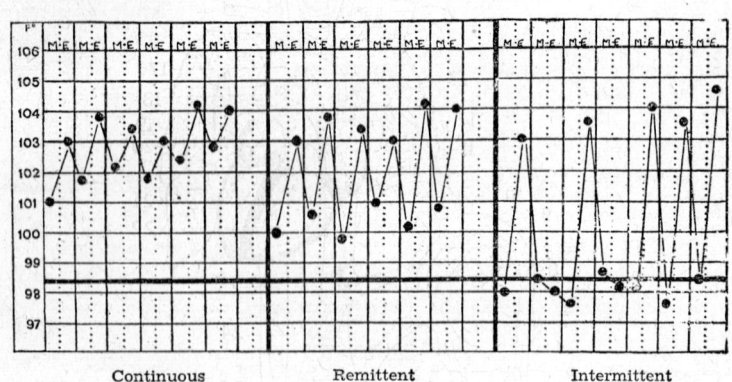

Continuous   Remittent   Intermittent
FEVER

fever, words pert. to: adustion; afebrile; ague; alexipyretic; algid, pernicious; amphibolia; anetus; antepyretic; antifebrile; antipyresis; apyretic; apyrexia; apyrogenetic; athermic; athermous; Baruch's sign; cauma; crisis; defervescence; dengue; febricula; febrifacient; febrifuge; fervescence; food f.; gastric f.; hectic; hectic flush; intermittent f.; lysis; marasmopyra; name of fever; pulse; "pyr-" words; quartan; quintan; quotidian; respiration; subsultus; synochus; temperature; vesicular; worm.

fi'at (pl. fi'ant) [L.]. "Let there be made," a term used in writing prescriptions.

fi'ber [L. *fibra*]. Threadlike or filmlike element, as a nerve fiber. A neurone or the axonal portion of a neurone.

RS: *chondrofibroma, cilia, cimbria, cingula, "fibr-" words, filament, filamentous, filiform, filum.*

f., accelerator. One causing increased heart pulsations.

f., afferent. One carrying incoming impulses to nerve cells.

f., efferent. One carrying outgoing impulses.

f., epicritic. One carrying sensations of heat and cold, making possible tac-

fiber, inhibitory   F-15   **fibroblast**

tile discrimination and light pressure sensation, each according to its separate fibers.

f., inhibitory. One causing slower heart action.

f., medullated; f., myelinated. Nerve fiber in which axis cylinder is sheathed in myelin.

f., nonmedullated; f., unmyelinated. Nerve fiber in which there is no myelin sheath bet. axis cylinder and neurilemma.

f., nerve. The part of a nerve cell which carries impulses. SEE: *nerve*.

f., protopathic. One causing sensation of heat, cold, or pain.

fi'bra [L.]. A fiber.

fibralbu'min [" + *albumen*, white of egg]. Globulin.

fibremia (fi-bre'mĭ-ă) [" + G. *aima*, blood]. Fibrin formed in the blood, causing embolism or thrombosis. SYN: *inosemia*.

fi'bril [L. *fibrilla*, little fiber]. A small fiber. A very small filamentous structure, oftentimes the component of a cell or a fiber.

f. muscle. A myofibril; an extremely minute fibril found within the cytoplasm of smooth muscle cells and in the sarcoplasm of striated and cardiac muscle fibers.

f. nerve. A neurofibril; delicate fibrils found in the cell body and processes of a neuron.

fibril'la (pl. *fibrillae*) [L.]. A fibril or small fiber.

fibril'lar, fib'rillary [L. *fibrilla*, little fiber]. Pert. to, or consisting of, fibrils.

fib'rillated [L. *fibrilla*, little fiber]. Composed of minute fibers. SYN: *fibrillar, fibrous*.

fibrillation (fi-bril-a'shun) [L. *fibrilla*, little fiber]. 1. The formation of fibrils. 2. Quivering of muscular fibers. 3. Tremor or rapid action of the heart.

f. auricular. Extremely rapid, incomplete, contractions of the atria resulting in fine, rapid, irregular, and uncoordinated movements. Also called *atrial f.*

f. ventricular. A condition similar to auricular fibrillation resulting in rapid, tremulous, and ineffectual contractions of the ventricles. May result from (a) mechanical, injury to the heart, (b) occlusion of coronary vessels, (c) effects of certain drugs such as excess of digitalis or chloroform, and (d) electrical stimuli.

fibrillolysis (fi-bril-ol'is-is) [" + G. *lysis*, dissolution]. Dissolution of fibrils.

fibrillolyt'ic [" + *lysis*, dissolution]. Dissolving fibrils.

fibrin [L. *fibra*, fiber]. A whitish, filamentous protein formed by the action of thrombin on fibrinogen. The conversion of fibrinogen, a hydrosol, into fibrin, a hydrogel is the basis for the clotting of the blood. The fibrin is deposited as fine interlacing filaments in which are entangled red and white cells and platelets, the whole forming a coagulum or clot.
RS: *blood clot, clotting, fibrinogen, prothrombin, thrombin*.

f. ferment. The substance in shed blood that converts fibrinogen to fibrin. SYN: *thrombin*.

f. film. A pliable, elastic, film prepared from fibrin isolated from human blood plasma. Used in neurosurgery as a substitute for the dura mater.

f. foam. A spongelike substance prepared from human fibrin. When impregnated with thrombin it is used in surgery as a hemostatic agent. Especially useful in neurosurgery and in injuries to parenchymatous organs. It is slowly absorbed.

fibrination (fib-rin-a'shun) [L. *fibra*, fiber]. Abnormal amt. of fibrin in the blood.

fibrinemia (fi-brin-e'mĭ-ă) [" + G. *aima*, blood]. Presence of fibrin in the blood. SYN: *fibremia*.

fibrinogen (fi-brin'o-jen) [" + G. *gennan*, to produce]. A protein present in the blood plasma which through the action of thrombin in the presence of calcium ions is converted into fibrin; this brings about the clotting of the blood.
SEE: *blood, clotting of, coagulation*.

fibrinogen'ic, fibrinog'enus [" + G. *gennan*, to produce]. Producing fibrin.

fibrin'ogenopen'ia. Reduction in the amount of fibrinogen in the blood usually the result of a liver disorder.

fi'brinoid [" + G. *eidos*, form]. Resembling fibrin.

f. material. A fibrinous substance which develops in the placenta, increasing in quantity as the placenta becomes older. Its origin is attributed to the degenerating decidua and trophoblast. Its forms an incomplete layer in the chorion and decidua basalis and also occurs in the form of small irregular patches on the surface of the chorionic villi. In late pregnancy, the material may have a striated or canalized appearance to which the term *canalized fibrinoid* is applied.

fibrinolysin (fi-brin-ol'is-in) [" + G. *lysis*, dissolution]. A substance formed in the blood by pathogenic streptococci which dissolves fibrin.

fibrinol'ysis [" + *lysis*, dissolution]. Due to the action of a proteolytic enzyme which converts insoluble fibrin into soluble substances.

fibrinolyt'ic [" + *lysis*, dissolution]. Pert. to the splitting up of fibrin.

fibrinope'nia [" + G. *penia*, poverty]. Fibrin and fibrinogen deficiency in the blood.

fibrinoplas'tic [" + G. *plassein*, to form]. Of the nature of fibrinoplastin.

fibrinopu'rulent [" + *purulentus*, festering]. Consisting of pus and fibrin.

fibrinos'copy [" + G. *skopein*, to examine]. Physical and chemical examination of the fibrin of blood clots and exudates. SYN: *inoscopy*.

fibrino'sis [" + G. *ōsis*]. Excess of fibrin in the blood.

fibrinous (fi'brin-us) [L. *fibra*, fiber]. Pert. to, of the nature of, or containing, fibrin.

fibrinuria (fi-brin-u'rĭ-ă) [" + G. *ouron*, urine]. Passage of fibrin in the urine.

fibro- [L.]. Prefix: Relation to fibers or fibrous tissues.

fibroadenia (fi-bro-a-de'nĭ-ă) [L. *fibra*, fiber, + *adēn*, gland]. Fibrous degeneration of glandular tissue.

fibroadenoma (fi-bro-ad-e-no'mă) [" + " + *ōma*, tumor]. Adenoma with fibrous tissue forming a dense stroma.

fibroad'ipose [" + *adeps, adip-*, fat]. Being fibrous and fatty.

fibroangio'ma [" + G. *aggeion*, vessel, + *ōma*, tumor]. A fibrous tissue angioma.

fibroareolar (fi-bro-ar-e-o'lar) [" + *areola*, little space]. With fibrous tissue and areolar arrangement.

fi'broblast [" + G. *blastos*, germ]. Any cell or corpuscle from which connective tissue is developed. SYN: *desmocyte, fibrocyte*.

fibroblast F-16 **fibromyitis**

fibroblast. SYN: *fibrocyte, desmocyte*. A type of cell found in nearly all forms of connective tissues. Connective tissue fibers are formed either within fibroblasts or from material outside of but close to and under the influence of fibroblasts.

fibroblastoma (fi-bro-blas-to'mă) [" + " + *ōma*, tumor]. Tumor of connective tissue or fibroplastic cells.

fibrobronchi'tis [" + G. *brogchia*, air tubes, + *itis*, inflammation]. Croupous bronchitis.

fibrocarcino'ma [" + G. *karkinos*, cancer, + *ōma*, tumor]. A carcinoma in which the trabeculae are resistant and thickened with granular degeneration of the cells.

f. cysticum. A f. with enclosed cysts.

fibrocar'tilage [" + *cartilagō*, gristle]. A type of cartilage in which the matrix contains thick bundles of white or collagenous fibers. Found in the intervertebral discs.

fibrocel'lular [" + *cellula*, little cell]. Both fibrous and cellular. SYN: *fibroareolar*.

fibrochondritis (fi"bro-kon-drī'tis) [" + G. *chondros*, cartilage, + -*itis*, inflammation]. Inflammation of fibrocartilage.

fibrochondro'ma [" + " + *ōma*, tumor]. Tumor of fibrous tissue and cartilage.

fi'brocyst [" + G. *kystis*, cyst]. A fibrous tumor that has undergone cystic degeneration or one which has accumulated fluid in the interspaces.

fibrocystic (fi-bro-sis'tik) [" + G. *kystis*, cyst]. 1. Consisting of fibrocysts. 2. Fibrous with cystic degeneration.

fibrocysto'ma [" + " + *ōma*, tumor] Fibroma combined with cystoma.

fibrocyte (fī'bro-sīt) [" + *kytos*, cell]. A fibrous tissue cell. SYN: *desmocyte, fibroblast*.

fibroelas'tic [" + G. *elastikos*, elastic]. Pertaining to connective tissue containing both white, nonelastic, collagenous fibers and yellow elastic fibers.

fibroenchondroma (fi-bro-en-kon-dro'mă) (pl. *fibroenchondromata*) [" + G. *en*, in + *chondros*, cartilage, + *ōma*, tumor]. An enchondroma containing fibrous elements.

fibrofat'ty [" + A.S. *faet*, fat]. Consisting of both fibrous and adipose tissue.

fibroglio'ma [" + " + *ōma*, tumor]. A fibroma partly glioma.

fi'broid [" + G. *eidos*, form]. 1. Containing or resembling fibers. SEE: *degeneration*. 2. A colloquial term for fibroma, esp. fibroma of the uterus. SYN: *fibroma*.

f., interstitial. Tumor in muscular wall of uterus which may grow inward and form a *polypoid fibroid*, or outward and become a *subperitoneal fibroid*.

f., uterine. The cause is unknown as is the case of other tumors.

Testosterone propionate and progesterone have inhibited their development, experimentally.

fibroidectomy (fi-broi-dek'to-mĭ) [" + " + *ektomē*, excision]. Surgical removal of a fibroid tumor.

fibrolipo'ma [" + G. *lipos*, fat, + *ōma*, tumor]. A lipoma having much fibrous tissue.

fibro'ma (pl. *fibromata*) [" + G. *ōma*, tumor]. A fibrous, encapsulated, connective tissue tumor.

A fibroma is irregular in shape and slow in growth. Consistency, firm. Painless except by pressure or cystic degeneration. May be found in the periosteum. May affect the jaws, the occiput, pelvis, vertebrae, ribs, long bones and sternum.

f. of breast. A benign tumor, nonulcerative and painless.

f., intramural. Located in muscle tissue of uterus bet. peritoneal coat and endometrium.

f. molluscum pedunculum of vulva. A pedunculated fibroid tumor of the vulva.

f., submucous. Encroaching upon endometrial cavity; sessile or pedunculated.

f., subserous. Lying beneath peritoneal coat of uterus, often pedunculated.

f., uterine. A fibroid tumor of the uterus.

PATH: A benign tumor varying in size from a millet seed to a size large enough to fill the entire abdominal cavity. May be single or multiple. These tumors are completely encapsulated by a fibrous connective tissue capsule in which the blood vessels that supply the tumor are found. They are subjected to numerous benign degenerations, such as necrobiotic changes (red and gray degeneration), hyaline changes, telangiectatic and lymphangiectatic changes, calcareous degeneration, fatty degeneration, and infection. Occasionally, a fibroid will show sarcomatous degeneration.

SYM: In the white race, fibromata rarely cause symptoms before the age of 30, but in the colored they may appear at any time during the active sex life. Although the cardinal symptoms of fibroid tumors are supposed to be dysmenorrhea, menorrhagia, and leukorrhea, these symptoms are found only infrequently and the symptomatology is directly related to the location of the tumors in the uterus. Following this contention, tumors that encroach upon the bladder region cause frequency and dysuria;* those pressing on the rectum cause a rectal tenesmus;* those that encroach upon the endometrium cause menorrhagia* and dysmenorrhea,* and very large subserous growths may be absolutely symptomless.

TREATMENT: Fibromata producing no symptoms should be left in place and the patient kept under observation. If unusually rapid growth is evidenced, they should be removed. Tumors that produce symptoms need intervention. The type of treatment depends upon age of patient, location, and size of tumor, and symptoms present. In general, wherever possible, conservation of the menstrual function should be considered. Tumors larger than a fetal head are better treated by surgical removal than by radiotherapy. Fibromectomy is clearly indicated in patients who hope subsequently to become pregnant.

SEE: *fibrosis uteri*.

fibromatosis (fi"bro-mă-to'sis) [L. *fibra*, fiber, + G. *ōma*, tumor, + *ōsis*]. SYN: *fibrosis*. The development simultaneously of many fibromas.

fibromatous (fī-brō'mă-tŭs) [" + G. *ōma*, tumor]. Pert. to, or of the nature of, a fibroma.

fibromectomy (fi-bro-mek'to-mĭ) [" + " + *ektomē*, excision]. Removal of a fibroid tumor.

fibromem'branous [" + *membrana*, web]. Having both fibrous and membranous tissue.

fibromus'cular [" + *musculus*, muscle]. Consisting of muscle and connective tissue.

fibromyi'tis [" + G. *mys, my-*, muscle, + -*itis*, inflammation]. Inflammation of

fibromyoma F-17 Filaria

the muscular system followed by fibrous degeneration of muscular fibers and atrophy.

fibromyoma (fi-bro-mi-o'mă) [" + " + ōma, tumor]. 1. Fibrous tissue myoma. 2. GYN: A fibroid tumor of the uterus that contains more fibrous than muscle tissue.

fibromyomectomy (fi-bro-mi-o-mek'to-mĭ) [" + " + ektomē, excision]. Removal of a fibromyoma from the uterus, leaving that organ in place.

fibromyosi'tis [" + " + -itis, inflammation]. Chronic muscular inflammation with hyperplasia of connective tissue. SYN: *inomyositis.*

fibromyotomy (fi-bro-mi-ot'o-mĭ) [" + " + tomē, incision]. Opening of a fibroid tumor.

fibromyxoma (fi-bro-miks-o'mă) [" + G. *myxa*, mucus, + *-ōma*, tumor]. A fibroma that has partially undergone myxomatous degeneration.

fibromyxosarco'ma [" + " + *sarx*, flesh, + *ōma*, tumor]. 1. A sarcoma containing fibrous and myxoid tissue. 2. A mucoid degenerated sarcoma.

fibroneuroma (fi″bro-nu-ro'mă) [" + G. *neuron*, nerve, + *ōma*, tumor]. A mixed neuroma and fibroma. SYN: *inoneuroma.*

fibroösteoma (fi″brō-ŏs-tē-ō'mă) [" + G. *osteon*, bone, + *-ōma*, tumor]. Tumor containing bony and fibrous elements.

fibropapilloma (fi″bro-pă-pĭ-lo'mă) [" + *papilla*, nipple, + G. *ōma*, tumor]. A mixed fibroma and papilloma sometimes occurring in the bladder.

fibropericardi'tis [" + G. *peri*, around, + *kardia*, heart, + *-itis*, inflammation]. Fibrinous pericarditis.

fibropla'sia [L. *fibra*, fiber, + G. *plasis*, a molding]. The development of fibrous tissue, as in wounds.

fibroplas'tic [" + G. *plassein*, to form]. Giving formation to fibrous tissue.
 f. tumor. Small spindle-celled sarcoma.

fibroplastin (fi-bro-plas'tin) [" + G. *plassein*, to form]. A globulin in blood serum and other body fluids. SYN: *fibrinoplastin, paraglobulin.*

fibropsammo'ma [" + G. *psammos*, sand, + *ōma*, tumor]. A tumor containing fibromatous and psammomatous tissue.

fibropu'rulent [" + *purulentus*, festering]. Pus containing flakes of fibrous tissue.

fibrosarco'ma [" + G. *sarx*, flesh, + *ōma*, tumor]. A spindle-celled sarcoma containing much connective tissue.

fibrosis (fi-bro'sis) [" + G. *ōsis*]. Abnormal formation of fibrous tissue.
 f., arteriocapillary. Arteriolar and capillary fibroid degeneration.
 f. of lungs. Formation of scar tissue in connective tissue framework of lungs following inflammation, pneumonia, and in pulmonary tuberculosis.
 f. uteri. A condition of the uterus manifested by excess of fibrous tissue, predominating symptom being menorrhagia.*
 The uterus may be large or small. The endometrium* may be normal, atrophic, or in the larger number show hyperplastic and hypertrophic glandular and interstitial endometritis of vascular origin.
 ETIOL: Not definitely known, but it is seen in patients with syphilis, those who have had a number of pregnancies, and in conditions where venous stasis has been present over a long period, such as in chronic retroversion with or without infection and procidentia.

TREATMENT: May be surgical or by means of x-ray or radium.

fibrositis (fi-bro-si'tis) [" + G. *itis*, inflammation]. Nonsuppurative inflammation of white fibrous connective tissue anywhere in the body.
 f. bursal. F. of a bursa, bursitis.
 f. intramuscular. F. of fibrous sheaths of muscles; muscular rheumatism; interstitial myositis.
 f. periarticular. F. of the fibrous tissue of the articular capsule.
 f. perineural. F. of the fibrous sheath surrounding nerves, esp., the sciatic nerve; sciatica.
 f. subcutaneous. F. of the subcutaneous tissue; panniculitis.

fibrous (fi'brus) [L. *fibra*, fiber]. Composed of or containing fibers; as in contradistinction to (osseous) bony composition.

fibrot'ic [L. *fibra*, fiber]. Marked by or pert. to fibrosis.

fib'ula [L. pin]. BNA. Calf bone (*peroneal bone*). One of the longest and thinnest bones of the body. The outer and smaller bone of the leg from the ankle to the knee, articulating above with the tibia, and below with the tibia and astragalus. SEE: *peroneal, peroneus, tibia.*

fib'ular [L. *fibula*, pin]. Rel. to the fibula.

fibulocalcaneal (fib″u-lo-kal-ka'ne-al) [" + *calcaneus*, pert. to the heel]. Pert. to the fibula and calcaneus, or *os calcis.*

field [A.S. *feld*]. A specific area in relation to an object.
 f., au'ditory. The space or distance within the limit of hearing.
 f. of vision. That portion of space which the fixed eye can see.

fifth cranial nerve. Trigeminus or trifacial n., q.v.
 f. ventricle. Space separating layers of septum lucidum.

fig [L. *ficus*, fig]. A fruit of *Ficus carica.* AV. SERVING (dried): 45 Gm. Pro. 1.8, Fat 0.1, Carbo. 33.4. Vit. A+, B+, G+. (Fresh): 75 Gm. Pro. 1.1, Carbo. 14.1. Vit. A+ to ++, B+, C variable, G+. ASH CONST. (dried): Ca 0.162, Mg 0.071, K 0.964, Na 0.046, P 0.116, Cl 0.043, S 0.056, Fe 0.0030. ASH CONST. (fresh): Ca 0.053, Mg 0.022, K 0.303, Na 0.012, P 0.036, Cl 0.014, S 0.010. SEE: *dates, fruits.*

fig'ure A body; form, shape, or outline.
 f. achromatic. In mitosis or meiosis, the spindle fibers and the asters.
 f. chromatic. The chromosomes or the chromatin material.

fila (fi'lă) [L. *filum*, thread]. Plural of *filum*, q.v.
 f. coronaria. A fibrous band extending from the base of the medial cusp of the tricuspid valve to the aortic annulus.
 f. olfactoria. Groups of fibers consisting of the axons of olfactory cells which form the olfactory nerves. These pass from the olfactory epithelium through the cribriform plate and terminate in the olfactory bulb.

filaceous (fil-a'she-us) [L. *filum*, thread]. Composed of filaments. SYN: *filamentous.*

fil'ament [L. *filum*, thread].
 f. axial. A fine filament forming the central axis of the tail of a spermatozoan.

filamen'tous [L. *filum*, thread]. BIOL: Made up of long, interwoven or irregularly placed filaments.

Filaria (fil-a'rī-ă) [L. *filum*, thread]. Term formerly applied to a genus of nematodes belonging to the superfamily Filarioidea.

F. bancrofti. Wucheria bancrofti, q.v.
F. loa. Loa loa, q.v.
F. medinensis. Dracunculus medinensis, q.v.
F. sanguinis hominis. Wucheria bancrofti, q.v.

filaria. A long filiform nematode belonging to the superfamily Filarioidea. The adults live in vertebrates including man, inhabiting man, being found in the lymphatic vessels and lymphatic organs, circulatory system, connective tissues, esp., subcutaneous tissues, and serous cavities. Typically, the female produces larvae called *microfilariae* which may be sheathed or sheathless. These reach the peripheral blood or lymphatic vessels where they may be ingested by a blood sucking arthropod (mosquitos, gnats, flies). In the intermediate host, they transform into a *rhabditoid larva*, which metamorphoses into an infective filifariform larvae. These migrate to the proboscis and are deposited in or on the skin of the vertebrate host. The species of filaria which are parasitic in man all belong to the family Acanthocheilonematidae.

fila′rial [L. *filum*, thread]. Pert. to or caused by Filariae.

filariasis (fil-ar-i′as-is) [L. *filum*, thread]. A chronic disease due to one of the filariae.

filarici′dal [" + *caedere*, to kill]. Pert. to that which is destructive to Filaria.

Filatov's disease. An exanthematous affection resembling scarlatina analogous to German measles.

F.'s spots. Koplik's spots.

fil′bert. A small nut. Av. Serving: 35 Gm. Pro. 5.5, Fat 22.9, Carbo. 4.5. Ca 0.287, Mg 0.140, K 0.618, Na 0.019, P 0.354, Cl 0.067, S 0.198, Fe 0.0041. Vit. B++, G++. A and C lacking. Fuel Value: 15 Gm. = 100 cal.; 1 lb. = 3040 cal.; 100 Gm. = 667 cal.

fil′iform [L. *filum*, thread, + *forma*, form]. 1. Biol: Pert. to a growth that is uniform along the inoculation line in stab or streak cultures. 2. Hairlike, filamentous.

f. papillae. Smallest tongue papillae.

fil′ipuncture [" + *punctura*, a piercing]. Insertion of a slender wire or thread in an aneurysm to induce coagulation.

fil′let [L. *filum*, thread]. 1. A bandage shaped like a loop. 2. Two bundles of sensory fibers in the medulla, pons, and brain. Syn: *lemniscus*.

f. of corpus callosum. Fibers forming white substance of the gyrus fornicatus.

f., olivary. Nerve fasciculus surrounding olivary body.

filling (fĭl′ing) [A.S. *fyllan*, to fill]. 1. The material for insertion in a tooth cavity; usually gold, amalgam, or cement. 2. The operation of filling tooth cavities.

film. 1. A thin skin, membrane, or covering. 2. A thin sheet of material, usually cellulose, coated with a light sensitive emulsion used in taking pictures. 3. In microscopy, a thin layer of blood or other material spread on a slide or cover slip.

fil′opressure [L. *filum*, thread, + *pressura*, pressure]. Pressure on a blood vessel caused by a ligature.

filovaricosis (fi′lo-var-ik-o′sis) [" + *varix*, a dilated vein, + G. *ōsis*]. Dilatation or thickening of the axis-cylinder of a nerve fiber.

filter [L. *filtrare*, to strain through]. 1. To pass a liquid through any porous substance which holds solid particles. 2. Device for filtering liquids, light rays, or radiations. See: *absorption, osmosis.*

f. bed. Large scale filter to purify the water supply.

f., Berkefeld. One of diatomaceous earth which will not pass bacteria.

f., infrared. Cell of water and red glass which confines radiation to spectral region from 600 to 1400 mu, red glass alone from 600 to 4000 mu.

f., Kitasato's. Suction variety of filter, using porcelain dilator.

f., Pasteur-Chamberlain. Filters of unglazed porcelain capable of retaining bacteria and some viruses; a force either pressure or suction is required to force or draw the liquid through the filter.

f. paper. Coarse form of paper used in filtering solutions.

fil′ters [L. *filtrare*, to strain through]. In radiation therapy, screens or various substances which permit passage of some wave lengths while absorbing others.

fil′trable [L. *filtrare*, to strain through]. Capable of passing through the pores of a porcelain filter, through which bacteria cannot pass.

fil′trate [L. *filtrare*, to strain through]. The fluid which has been passed through a filter. The residue is the *precipitate*.

f. glomerular. The fluid which passes from the blood through the capillary walls of the glomeruli of the kidney. It is a protein-free plasma from which urine is formed.

filtra′tion [L. *filtrare*, to strain through]. The process of straining through a filter. See: *absorption, filter.*

f. of roentgen rays. The absorption of some of the relatively longer wave lengths of roentgen radiation by placing in the path of the rays some absorbing medium, such as aluminum, copper, or zinc.

filtratometer (fil-tra-tom′et-er) [" + G. *metron*, measure]. Device for measuring gastric filtrates.

fil′trum [L.]. A filter.

fi′lum [L.]. A threadlike structure.

f. terminale. A long, slender filament forming end of spinal cord.

fimbria (fim′brĭ-ă) (Pl. *fimbriae*) [L. fringe]. Any structure resembling fringe.

f. ova′rica. The longest fringelike extremity of the fallopian tubes; extending from the infundibulum close to the ovary.

f. tubae. Fringelike portion at abdominal end of the fallopian tubes.

fimbriate (fim′brĭ-āt) [L. *fimbria*, fringe]. 1. Biol: Having fingerlike projections. 2. Fringed.

f. body. Corpus fimbriatum.

fim′briated [L. *fimbria*, fringe]. Fringed.

fimbria′tum [L. fringed]. 1. Outer end of the oviduct. 2. White band on edge of the cornu inferius of lateral ventricle of the brain. Syn: *corpus fimbriatum.*

fimbriocele (fim′brĭ-o-sēl) [L. *fimbria*, fringe, + G. *kēlē*, hernia]. Hernia including the fimbriated portion of the oviduct.

fin′ger [A.S.]. A digit of the hand.

f., dislocation of the. First, be certain that there is no fracture. Dislocations occur only at a joint. If there has been a crushing injury, assume that a fracture is present until an x-ray has been made. Dislocations of a finger are usually easily diagnosed and quite easily reduced. They may be caused by blows, falls, and similar causes.

If there is no fracture, it may be treated by asking the patient to steady and support his own wrist (or getting somebody else to do so) for countertraction. Then take hold of the finger beyond the dislocated muscles and tendons, and with the other (free) hand slip the dislocated bone into place.

This is to be followed by an application of a splint from the tip of the finger well into the palm of the hand. This may be made of cigar box wood, wire, tongue depressors, heavy cardboard, etc.

Do not under any circumstances attempt to reduce a dislocation of the thumb joint nearest to the palm of the hand.

f. print. An imprint made by the cutaneous ridges of the fleshy portion of the distal end of a finger. Finger prints are used for purposes of identification.

f. stall. A finger cot.

finger, words pert. to: acroataxia, acrodynia, arachnodactyly, baseball f., camptodactylia, dactyl, dactylus, digit, digitate, nail, phalanges, phalanx.

Finsen light. Blue and violet light with heat waves excluded. Used in treatment of lupus and other skin affections.

fire [A.S. *fyr*]. Flame producing heat.

f. emergencies. If a person's clothing catches fire, he should be rolled in a rug or blanket to smother flames. It may be necessary to trip him to prevent his running about, as this only fans the flames.

If patient is trapped in a burning building, this particular room should have doors closed to prevent cross breezes from increasing the fire. The window should be opened if patient is to be rescued by lowering him, using any appropriate carry. Do not open any door more than a few inches to ascertain possibility of escape. A burst of flame or hot air may push door in and asphyxiate anyone in the room. Wet cloths or towels should be held over mouth and nostrils to keep out smoke and gases. SEE: *burn, flame, gases, transportation.*

f., St. Anthony's. Erysipelas. Also called *St. Francis' fire.*

first aid. The administration of emergency assistance to individuals who have been injured or otherwise disabled, prior to the arrival of a doctor, or transportation to a hospital or doctor's office. In no sense assume to be the substitution for medical care.

first aid, words pert. to: antidote, apoplexy, artificial respiration, asphyxia, bites, burn, coma, dislocation, drowning, emetic, fainting, flames, food poisoning, foreign bodies, fracture, freezing, frost bite, fumes, gases, insect bites, laceration, name of poison, poison, shock, snake bite, unconsciousness.

first cranial nerve. Olfactory n., *q.v.*

fish poisoning. A form of food poisoning caused by eating poisonous fish. Some fish are inherently poisonous, others become poisonous through decomposition, infection, by feeding on other poisonous forms, or by poisonous metabolic substances produced during the spawning season.

The symptoms are very similar to those of meat poisoning, but perhaps more intense. Headache, vertigo, thirst, indigestion, vomiting, cramps, diarrhea and skin eruptions. Convulsions may occur.

SHELL FISH: The onset is very rapid, but seldom are there gastrointestinal symptoms. Collapse may ensue and death occur in a few hours. Other fish poisonings only differ in degree in gastrointestinal symptoms from meat poisoning.

TREATMENT: Emetics, purgatives, and stimulants. Medical treatment for convulsions. Follow treatment with oatmeal or barley water, esp. if nauseated; later, water with a pinch of salt. SEE: *food poisoning, meat poisoning.*

fish skin. A condom made of a fish bladder.

f. s. disease. A disease of the skin characterized by increase of the horny layer and deficiency of the skin secretions. SYN: *ichthyosis, q.v.*

fission (fish'un) [L. *fissio*, from *findere*, to cleave]. 1. Splitting into 2 or more parts. 2. A method of asexual reproduction seen in bacteria, protozoa, and other lower forms of life in which the cell or the body divides into two or more parts each of which develops into a complete individual.

fissip'arous [L. *fissio-, findere,* to cleave, + *parere,* to bring forth]. Reproducing by fission.

fissura (fis-u'rǎ) (pl. *fissurae*) [L.]. Fissure. SYN: *cleft, sulcus.*

fis'sural [L. *fissura,* fissure]. Pertaining to a fissure.

fissure (fish'ur) [L. *fissura*]. 1. A groove or natural division, cleft or slit, deep furrow in the brain, liver, spinal cord, and other organs. 2. Ulcer or cracklike sore. 3. A break in the enamel of a tooth.

f. anal. A linear ulcer on the margin of the anus.

f., auricular. F. of petrous portion of the temporal bone.

f. of Bichat. A fissure below the corpus callosum in the cerebellum.

f., Broca's. Fissure encircling the 3rd left frontal convolution.

f., Burdach's. F. connecting lateral surface of insula and inner surface of operculum.

f., calcarine. F. extending from the cerebrum's occipital end to the occipital f.

f. callosomarginal. A conspicuous sulcus in mesial surface of cerebral hemisphere running above and concentric with the curved upper surface of the corpus callosum.

f., central. SEE: *Rolando's f.*

f. Clevenger's. F. the inferior occipital fissure.

f. collateral. F. on inferior surface of cerebral hemisphere separating subcalcarine and subcollateral gyri.

f.'s, Henle's. Connective tissue areas bet. the muscular fibers of heart.

f., hippocampal. F. of brain extending from post. part of corpus callosum to the tip of temporal lobe.

f. inferior orbital. A fissure at the apex of the orbit through which pass the infraorbital blood vessels and maxillary branch of the trigeminal nerve; the sphenomaxillary fissure.

f., interparietal. F. separating parietal convolutions of the brain.

f. longitudinal. A fissure on the lower surface of the liver.

f., occipitoparietal. The fissure bet. the occipital and parietal lobes of the brain.   [upper and lower eyelids.

f., palpebral. Opening separating the

f., portal. The opening into the liver on its under surface; continues into the liver as the portal canal.

f., Rolando's. F. separating frontal and parietal lobes.
f., sphenoidal. F. separating the wings and body of the sphenoid.
f. of Sylvius. The lateral cerebral fissure. A f. separating the frontal and parietal lobes from the temporal lobe of the brain.
f. transverse. 1. The fissure bet. the cerebellum and cerebrum of the brain. 2. A f. on lower surface of the liver which serves as the hilum transmitting vessels and ducts to the liver.
f. umbilical. Ant. portion of liver's longitudinal fissure which contains the round ligament, the obliterated umbilical vein.
f., Wernicke's. F. dividing the temporal and parietal lobes from the occipital lobe.

fistula (fis'tu-la) [L. a pipe]. An abnormal tubelike passage from a normal cavity or tube to a free surface or to another cavity. May be congenital due to incomplete closure of parts or may result from abscesses, injuries, or inflammatory processes.
f., anal. F. near the anus.
f., biliary. One through which bile is discharged after a biliary operation.
f., blind. One open at only 1 end.
f., cervical. 1. An abnormal opening into the cervix uteri. 2. An opening in the neck leading to the pharynx, resulting from incomplete closure of the brachial clefts.
f., cervicovaginalis laqueatica. Fistula in the vaginal portion of the cervix uteri bet. the uterine canal and the vagina.
f., complete. F. with both external and internal opening.
f., enterovaginal. One bet. the bowel and vagina.
f., fecal. One in which there is a discharge of feces through the opening.
f., metroperitoneal. F. between uterine and peritoneal cavities.
f., parotid. One through which there is an abnormal leakage of saliva onto ext. surface of cheek.
f., perineovaginal. Opening from vagina through the perineum.
f., rectovaginal. Opening bet. rectum and vagina.
f., ureterovaginal. Opening bet. ureter and vagina.
f., vesicouterine. Opening bet. uterus and bladder.
f., vesicovaginal. Opening from bladder into the vagina.

fistulatome (fis'tu-la-tōm) [" + G. *tomē*, incision]. Instrument for incising a fistula.
fistulectomy (fis-tu-lek'to-mĭ) [" + G. *ektomē*, excision]. Excision of a fistula.
fistulization (fis"tu-li-za'shun) [L. *fistula*, pipe]. Becoming fistulous.
fistuloenterostomy (fis"tu-lo-en-ter-os'to-mĭ) [" + G. *enteron*, intestine, + *stoma*, opening]. Operative closure of a biliary fistula and formation of new passage of bile into the intestine.
fistulous (fis'tu-lus) [L. *fistula*, pipe]. Pert. to, or containing, a fistula.
fit (fĭt) [A.S. *fitt*]. A sudden attack, convulsion or paroxysm.
F. A. TREATMENT: Do not try to stop attack. Prevent patient from hurting or injuring self. Place a pad between teeth to prevent biting tongue or cheeks. Allow patient to sleep. SEE: *catalepsy, cataleptiform, epilepsy.*
fixa'tion [L. *fixus*, from *figere*, to fasten]. 1. The act of holding or fastening in a fixed position. The condition of being fixed. Immobilizing, making rigid. 2. PSYCH: A phase of psychosexual development in which the libido is arrested at an inferior or presexual level. For example father or mother fixation.
f. of complement. The action of a complement, a constituent of fresh blood serum, on an antigen, which, in turn, has been acted on by its antibody. During the uniting of antigen, antibody, and complement, the complement is rendered inactive or destroyed, and this process is known as f. of complement. The basis of the Wassermann and Kolmer tests for syphilis and other tests for infectious diseases.
f. forceps. Forceps for holding a part.
f. point. Point of clearest vision, for which eye accommodation is focused.
fixation of eyes. The movement of the eyes for the most acute vision in which they are directed toward an object so that the visual axes meet and the image of the object falls on corresponding points of each retina.
f., field of. The widest limits of vision in all directions within which the eyes can fixate.
f. point. The fovea or the point on the retina where the visual axes (fixation lines) meet the point of clearest vision.

fix'ative [L. *fixus*, from *figere*, to fasten]. 1. A substance that serves to make firm or fixed. 2. One used to harden and preserve pathological specimens.
fix'ing [L. *fixus*, from *figere*, to fasten]. Rapid killing of tissue elements so that their normal living form is preserved.
fix'ity [L. *fixus*, from *figere*, to fasten]. OB: The stage when the head of the fetus enters the mother's pelvis.
Fl. ABBR. for fluid. *Symb.* of fluorine.
flabel'lum [L. fan]. White fibers in form of a fan-shaped bundle in corpus striatum.
flaccid (flak'sid) [L. *flaccidus*, flabby]. Relaxed, flabby, having defective or absent muscular tone.
fla'gellant [L. *flagellum*, whip]. 1. Pert. to flagella. 2. Pert. to stroking in massage. 3. One who practices flagellation.
flagellate (flaj'el-āt) [L. *flagellum*, whip]. 1. With 1 or more flagella. 2. A protozoon with 1 or more flagella.
f. cell. One with long cilia for propulsion.
flagella'tion [L. *flagellum*, whip]. 1. Flogging. 2. Massage by strokes. 3. Applying electricity by tapping the body. 4. A form of sexual perversion through which the libido is stimulated by striking the gluteal region with a whip or lashes.
It was practiced during the 13th and 15th centuries as an atonement, and to kill the desires of the flesh, but instead it stimulated sensuality and so it was discontinued.
Spanking children should be avoided, as the first excitation of the sex instinct is sometimes aroused as a result. It is practiced by masochists on the opposite sex. The pervert sometimes subjects himself to this form of castigation to stimulate the libido.
flagellum (fla-jel'um) (pl. *flagella*) [L. whip]. A hairlike, motile process on the extremity of a bacterium or protozoon. The locomotor organ of sperm cells.
flail joint. A joint with excessive mobility after resection.
flames, inhalation of. SYM: Intense irritation of nose, throat, pharynx, windpipe and lungs; with choking, coughing, interference with respiration; intense

swelling of throat; breathing is markedly limited. Shock.
TREATMENT: Administration of oxygen; occasionally tracheotomy necessary. Pain relieved by spraying nose and throat with a local anesthetic of low toxicity. Follow with oil sprays. Steam inhalations are very soothing, and may have to be kept up for long periods of time. SEE: *burn, fire, gases.*

flank [Fr. *flanc*, side]. The part bet. ribs and upper border of ilium. SEE: *latus*. Also loosely used to refer to the outer side of the thigh, hip, and buttock.

flap [Dutch *flappen*, to strike]. A mass of partly detached tissue attached at the base after resection.

   f. amputation. A flap covering the end of a part left after an amputation.

   f. extraction. Removal of cataract so as to make a flap in the cornea.

flare. A flush or spreading area of redness which surrounds a line made by drawing a pointed instrument across the skin. It is the second reaction in the "triple response" *q.v.* and due to dilatation of the arterioles.

flarim'eter. A modified spirometer for estimating vital capacity, blood pressure, heart rate, etc.

flash method. Means of pasteurizing milk by rapidly raising temperature of milk to 178° F., maintaining it there for a few minutes and letting it fall to 40° F.

   f. point. The temperature at which a substance will burst into flame.

flatfoot. Abnormal flatness of sole and arch of foot.

The inner longitudinal and ant. transverse metatarsal arches are those that may be depressed. It may be *acute, subacute,* or *chronic.* SYN: *pes planus, splayfoot.*

   f., spasmodic. The foot is held everted by spasmodic contraction of the peroneal muscle.

flat'ness. Resonance heard on percussing over solid organs, or fluid in the thoracic cavity.

flatulence (flat'u-lens) [L. *flatulentia*, a blowing]. Gas in the digestive tract due to fermentation or decomposition.
NP: *If of the stomach,* sit patient upright, apply heat to epigastrium or a counterirritant. Give sodium bicarbonate in hot water to be sipped slowly, or peppermint water or ginger tea.
If in intestines, have patient lying down for ½ hr. before and after meals. No fluids with meals but hot water may be sipped afterwards. Give carminatives, carminative enema if needed, or pass a flatus tube. See that bowels are regular. SEE: *distention, gastrointestinal decompression, Wangensteen method.*

flatulent (flat'u-lent) [L. *flatulentia*, a blowing]. Affected with or caused by gas in the alimentary tract.

fla'tus [L. a blowing]. 1. Gas in digestive tract. 2. Expiration of air; eructation. SEE: *borborygmus.*

   f. tube. A rectal tube to procure expulsion of flatus in distention and before a saline enema.
NP: It may be passed 6-8 inches, but a long tube is preferable. It may be left in position for 20-30 minutes. Patient on back or side. Lubricate tube and insert gently. Lower end of tube is placed in a deodorant solution in vessel beside the bed.

   f. vaginalis. GYN: Expulsion of air from a voluminous vagina.

flave'do [L. *flavus*, yellow]. Yellowness, as of the skin; sallowness; jaundice.

flavescent (fla-ves'ent) [L. *flavus*, yellow]. Yellowish.

flav'icin, falv'acin, falvo'cin. An antibiotic substance obtained from certain fungi, esp., *Aspergillus flavus.*

flav'in. One of a group of natural water-soluble pigments occurring in milk, yeasts, bacteria, and some plants. All contain the flavin or isoalloxazine nucleus and are yellow in color. Present in riboflavin and in Warburg's yellow enzyme.

fla'vism [" + G. *ismos,* condition]. Having a yellow tinge to the hair.

flavo- [L. *flavus,* yellow]. Prefix: yellow.

Flavo"bacter'ium. A genus of rod-shaped bacteria belonging to the Achromobacteriaceae. They are found in soil and water and produce an orange-yellow pigment in cultures.

flavo"pro'tein. One of a group of conjugated proteins which constitute the yellow enzymes essential in cellular respiration.

flax'seed. Seed of *Linum usitatis simum.* SYN: linseed.

   f. poultice. A soft, usually hot and moist paste for external application, such as a flaxseed poultice, linseed meal, bran, flour, or hops boiled with water and wrapped in cheesecloth or other fabrics.
PURPOSE: (a) Action is mainly through heat; (b) counterirritant effect is slight; (c) used for inflammations, abscesses, relief of pain, and pulmonary congestion.
PROPORTIONS: One part flaxseed meal and 1½ parts boiling water. One cup of meal and 1½ cups of water make a poultice approximately 6 x 4 x 1.
ARTICLES NEEDED: (a) Flaxseed meal; (b) boiling water; (c) saucepan; (d) large spoon; (e) one teaspoonful of soda bicarbonate powder; (f) old muslin, size in proportion to that of affected area; (g) bandage or binder; (h) hot water bottle and cover or flannel protector; (i) cup for measuring.
PROCEDURE: (a) Put the required amount of water on to boil. (b) Collect the necessary articles. Fill the hot water bottle, 125° F. (c) Spread the muslin on the table. (d) When the water is boiling briskly, add flaxseed gradually and stir vigorously. Cook until it drops from the spoon. When removed from the stove, add one teaspoonful of soda bicarbonate powder. (e) Beat well to incorporate air. (f) Spread it on the old muslin about 1 inch thick and fold the muslin in envelope fashion. Fill the saucepan with water. (g) Obtain the hot water bottle and carry the poultice to the patient between the folds of the hot water bottle. (h) Test the temperature of the poulice by applying it to the back of the wrist. Apply the poultice to the area slowly and lay the hot water bottle over it. (i) Secure poultice with binder or bandage. If previous poultices have been applied and the hot water bottle is over the area, remove it, place the poultice, and refill and replace the bottle.
When the treatment is discontinued, remove the poultice, dry the part, and place the hot water bottle or flannel over the area for 2 or 3 hours.

fl. dr. Abbr. of *fluidram.*

flea (flē) [A.S. *flēa*]. Fleas of the genus *Xenopsylla* transmit the bacillus of plague *(Pasteurella pestis)* from rats to humans. Fleas may transmit other

diseases such as tularemia, endemic typhus, and brucellosis, and they serve as intermediate hosts for the cat and dog tapeworms.
SEE: *Ctenocephalides.*
f. bites. Hemorrhagic puncta* surrounded by erythematous* and urticarial patches, as the result of the injection of their saliva.
PREVENTION: Dust the skin with powdered camphor or naphthalene.
f. cat. *Ctenophalides felis.*
f. chigger. *Tungra penetrans.* Also called chigger, jigger, and sand fleas.
f. dog. *Ctenophalides canis.*
f. human. *Pulex irritans.*
f., rat. *Xenopsylla cheopis.*

fleam (flem) [Fr. *flieme,* from G. *phleps,* vein]. Lancet used in venesection.

Flechsig's areas (flekh'zig). Ant., lateral, and post. areas of each lateral half of the medulla.

fleece of Stilling. Meshwork of white fibers that surrounds the dentate nucleus of the cerebellum.

flesh [A.S. *flaesc*]. The soft tissues of the animal body, esp. the muscles. SEE: *carnivorous, carnophobia, meat, meat poisoning.*
f., examination of animal. *General rule:* Examine for (1) Color; (2) consistency; (3) proportion of fat; (4) odor; (5) taste.
COLOR: *Yellow*—May be produced by food. In disease due to biliary compounds. *Brown*—Rare, except in old meat undergoing decomposition. *Dark Purple*—May indicate animal has died a natural death, suffered from acute fever, tuberculosis, or rinderpest. Avoid. *Dark Reddish-Brown*—May indicate animal has been hunted or overdriven, poisoned, drowned or suffocated. Avoid. *Scarlet*—Rare. Indicates arsenic or monoxide poisoning. *Diffused redness*—Indicates that animal may have been poisoned, or the meat frozen. *Green or Violet*—Indicates the beginning of putrefaction. Dangerous. *Saffron*—Indicates artificial coloring or smoked pork. *Brilliant Red*—Due to poisonous bacteria. *Gray*—Usually in sausages. Due to bacteria. *Phosphorescent Flesh*—Not due to putrefaction. Usually found in fish and shellfish. Sometimes in meat, esp. veal. Due to bacteria and generally transmitted from fish kept in the same place with meat. Increased by warmth. *White*—Rare, except in calves. Found in certain diseases. Avoid.
GENERAL TEST: *Color* — Neither very pale nor dark purple. *Appearance*—Marbled. *Consistency* — Firm and elastic. Not flabby or sodden. Should hardly moisten the finger. *Odor*—Free from odors.
f. goose. *Cutis anserina, q.v.*
f., proud. 1. Fungous growth. 2. Excessive granular tissue in a wound or ulcer.

fletch'erism. Taking small amounts of food at a time with excessive mastication.

flex [L. *flexus,* from *flectere,* to bend]. To bend upon itself, as a muscle; flexion; bending.

flexibilitas cerea (fleks-ĭ-bil'it-as se're-a) [L.]. A cataleptic state in which a subject maintains the limbs in the position in which they are placed. Characteristic of catatonic patients.

flexibil'ity [L. *flexus,* from *flectere,* to bend]. Quality of being bent without breaking; adaptability. SYN: *pliability.*

flex'ible [L. *flexus,* from *flectere,* to bend]. Capable of being bent without breaking.
flexile (fleks'il) [L. *flexus,* bent]. Pliant; flexible.
flexion (flek'shun) [L. *flexus,* bent]. The act of bending or condition of being bent, in contrast to extending. SEE: *antecurvature, clawfoot, clawhand.*
flex'oglass. Window glass substitute for transmitting antirachitic rays of sunlight.
flex'or [L. *flectere,* to bend]. A muscle that bends a part, in a generally proximal direction; as opposed to an extensor.
flex'ure, flex'ura [L. *flexura,* a bending]. A bend.
f., duodenojejunal. Curve at meeting point of jejunum and duodenum.
f., hepatic. The bend on right side forming junction of the ascending with the transverse colon.
f., sigmoid. The s-like loop (in *left iliac fossa*) of the descending colon as it meets the rectum. SEE: *colon.*
f., splenic. Bend at junction of transverse with descending colon.
flick'er. The sensation of alternating intervals of brightness caused by interruptions in light stimuli.
flight of ideas. PSY: Continuous but fragmentary stream of talk.
Connection can be followed but direction is frequently changed, often by chance stimuli from the environment.
flint disease. Deposit of fine particles in the lungs. SYN: *chalicosis.*
floating [A.S. *flota,* a raft]. Moving about. Out of normal location.
f. kidney. One movable from its normal bed of fat.
ETIOL: A blow, a sudden movement, laxity of the peritoneum complicated by inflammation, kinking of ureter and damming of urine.
SYM: Dragging pain in loin, chronic indigestion, albuminuria, painful urination, urine scanty and frequent. Neurasthenic complaints.
TREATMENT: Rest in bed. Diet to increase weight. A kidney pad may be ordered. If so, adjust before getting out of bed. Patient should not be told nature of condition. *Nephropexy* may be indicated if kidney is healthy; otherwise, possible *nephrectomy.*
f. ribs. The 11th and 12th ribs which do not articulate with the sternum.
floats [A.S. *flota,* a raft]. Glass capsules containing labels to float in an exposed liquid to designate its nature.
floccillation, floccitation (flok-sĭ-la'shun, -ta'shun) [L. *flocculus,* little tuft]. Semiconscious pricking at bedclothes in fevers and stupors. SYN: *carphologia, carphology.*
floccose (flok'os) [L. *floccōsus,* full of wool tufts]. BIOL: Pert. to a growth made up of short and densely but irregularly interwoven filaments.
floc'cular [L. *flocculus,* little tuft]. Pert. to the flocculus of the cerebellum.
floc'culence [L. *flocculus,* little tuft]. State of being flocculent or resembling shreds or tufts of cotton.
flocculent (flok'u-lent) [L. *flocculus,* little tuft]. Resembling the white portion of "floating island" or a fluid or culture containing whitish shreds of mucus.
flocculoreac'tion [" + *re,* again, + *agere,* to act]. Flocculation of a serum reaction.
floc'ulus (pl. *flocculi*) [L. tuft]. 1. A lobe below and behind the middle peduncle of the cerebrum on each side of the

flocculus, retinae   F-23   **fluke, intestinal**

median fissure. 2. A small tuft of wool-like fibers.
    f. retinae. Ciliary process of retina.
flooding (flūd'ing) [A.S. *flōd*]. Profuse uterine bleeding.
Flood's ligament. A band of ligaments attached to lower part of lesser tuberosity of the humerus.
floor. The surface which forms the lower limit of a cavity or space, as the floor of the cranial cavity, fourth ventricle, mouth, nasal fossa, or pelvis.
flora (flō'ra) [L. *flos, flor-*, flower]. 1. Plant life as distinguished from animal life.
    2. Plant life occurring or adapted for living in a specific environment.
flour [A.S. flower of meal, from L. *flos, flor-*, flower]. Finely ground meal obtained from wheat, or other grain; any soft fine powder. SEE: *bread, cereal.*
Flourens' theory (floo-ronz'). That thought is a process dependent upon the entire cerebrum.
flow [A.S. *flōwan*, to flow]. 1. Action of flowing; said of liquids. 2. The menstrual discharge. Bleeding from the uterus, but not as profusely as in flooding. SEE: *cholerrhagia, cholorrhea, osmosis.*
flower [L. *flōs, flor-*, flower]. That part of a plant which comprises the organs of reproduction. Ex: *anthemis, arnica, matricaria.* A complete flower includes a calyx, corolla, stamens, which produce pollen, and a pistil which produces the ovule.
flucticuli (fluk-tik'ū-lī) (sing. *flucticulus*) [L. "little waves"]. Wavelike markings on lateral wall of 3rd ventricle.
fluctua'tion [L. *fluctuāre*, to flow in waves]. A wavy impulse felt in palpation and produced by vibration of body fluid.
    DIAG: If felt over lower bowel ascites usually is present. May be caused by peritoneal hemorrhage. If confined to limited portion of abdomen tuberculous peritonitis is indicated; over central portion, bladder distention. In lower abdomen in women, an ovarian cyst or pregnancy. In right hypochondria, a hydatid cyst; abscess of liver, distended gallbladder; over left hypochondria, cysts or abscess. Above umbilicus, dilated colon or stomach partly filled with fluid and gas.
flu'id [L. *fluidus*]. A nonsolid, liquid, or gaseous substance.
    f., amniotic. GYN: The fluid that fills the fetal membranes in pregnancy. A clear, yellowish fluid. Spec. grav., 1.006. It is composed of albumin, salts (chiefly urea), and water, and suspended in it are lanugo, epidermal cells, *vernix caseosa*, and meconium.* It is derived from the cells of the amnion, although some claim it comes from the fetal urine and others that it is derived from the maternal circulation. Its chief function is protection for the fetus. SEE: *amnion.*
    f. cerebrospinal. That found in central canal of spinal cord and in the ventricles of the brain, also in the subarachnoid space about the brain and spinal cord. It is formed by the choroid plexuses of the ventricles.
    f. diet. One for postoperative cases for the first 2 days following an operation, carbonated water, ginger ale, tea, albumin, water, beef tea, broth, coffee. Raw fruit juices and milk should not be given unless ordered. SEE: *liquid diet.*
    f. extracellular. The tissue fluid or the fluid occupying spaces between the tissue cells; interstitial fluid.

    f. extravascular. All the body fluids outside the blood vessels; includes tissue fluid, fluids within the serous and synovial cavities, the cerebrospinal fluid, and lymph.
    f. interstitial. The tissue fluid.
    f. intracellular. The fluid contained within cells, and comprising about 50% of body weight.
    f. intraocular. The fluid within the ant. and post. chambers of the eye.
    f. retention. Failure to expel fluids of the body normally. OPP: *fluid balance.* It occurs in nephritis with massive albuminuria. When protein content of plasma falls below 4% fluid cannot be attracted back into the blood stream and edema occurs. This is why a high protein diet was indicated by Epstein in chronic parenchymatous nephritis. Fluid is retained in congestive heart failure. It should be detected by decreased urinary output. Retention of salt is another cause of fluid retention. Salt retention attracts fluid to maintain the isotonic concentration. A salt-free diet is indicated in fluid retention.
    f. serous. A fluid in the serous cavities.
    f. synovial. Pl. *synovia.* The fluid contained within synovial cavities, bursae, and tendon sheaths.
    f. tissue. The interstitial or extracellular fluid.
    f. water balance. Regulation of amount of water in the body by its controlling mechanism. The balance is upset when fluids are lost by vomiting, bleeding, or when dehydration occurs. When vital reflexes are disorganized, as in shock, collapse, septicemia, and toxemias, dehydration ensues. Increased fluid intake is indicated, but vitality may be so low fluid may pool in stomach, or if given rectally may lie in colon and not be absorbed. Intravenous, subcutaneous, and intraperitoneal injections may then be indicated.
fluidextract, fluidextractum (flext.) [L. *fluidus* + *extractum*, extract]. Solution of the soluble constituents of organic drugs of such strength that each cc. represents 1 Gm. of the drug.
    The majority contain a comparatively large percentage of alcohol and many of these give precipitates with water. Most of them contain tannic acid and should not be used with agents incompatible with that drug. Twenty-five fluidextracts are official.
flu'idounce. Eight fluidrams. SYMB: f ℥.
flu'idram. Measure of capacity equal to 57.1 gr. of distilled water; equal to 3.70 cc. SYMB: f ʒ.
fluke (flook) [A.S. *flōc*, flatfish]. A parasitic worm belonging to the class Trematoda, phylum Platyhelminthes. Those parasitic in man belong to the order Digenea. Most flukes have complex life cycles which include asexual generations that live in a mollusc (snail or bivalve). Stages of a typical fluke include adult, egg, miracidium, sporocyst, redia, cercaria, and metacercaria.
    f. blood. A schistosome. Flukes of the genus Schistosoma, *S. haematobium, S. mansoni,* and *S. japonicum.* Adults live principally in the mesenteric and pelvic veins. They cause schistosomiasis and schistosome dermatitis (swimmer's itch).
    f. intestinal. Species of intestinal flukes infesting man include: *Gastrodiscoides hominis, Fasciolopsis buski, Heterophyes heterophyes, Metagonimus yokogawai.*

fluke, liver   F-24   **folia**

f. liver. Flukes which live in the liver and bile ducts. Species infesting man include: *Clonorchis sinensis, Fasciola hepatica, Dicrocoelium dendriticum,* and *Opisthrochis felineus.*

f. lung. Only one species is common in man, namely *Paragonimus westermani.*

flu'mina pilo'rum [L. rivers of hair]. The curved lines along which the hairs of the body are arranged, esp. in the fetus.

flu'or al'bus [L. white flow]. White discharge from the uterus or vagina. SYN: *leukorrhea.*

fluorescein (flū-or-es'ein). A red crystalline powder.

USES: Chiefly in diagnostic purposes, detecting foreign bodies in the eye, or corneal lesions.

DOSAGE: Two per cent solution in sodium bicarbonate solution.

fluorescence (flu-or-es'ens) [L. *fluere,* to flow]. Luminescence of a substance when acted on by short wave radiation.

Usually ultraviolet, first noted in fluospar; caused by absorption of certain wave lengths and simultaneous emission of a longer wave length, which terminates simultaneously with the cessation of the incident exciting radiation.

fluorescent (flu-or-es'ent) [L. *fluere,* to flow]. 1. BIOL: Having 1 color by transmitted light and another by reflected light. 2. Luminous when exposed to other rays.

f. screen. 1. A sheet of cardboard, paper, or glass coated with a material which fluoresces visibly, such as calcium tungstate, used as the chief part of a fluoroscope when roentgen rays, radium rays, or electrons impinge upon it; a substitute for a fluoroscope in a darkened room. 2. A sheet of cardboard, paper, or glass, coated with anthracene or other fluorescing materials, to observe ultraviolet radiations.

fluoridation (flū-ôr-ĭ-dā'shŭn). The addition of fluorides to a water supply as a means of preventing dental caries.

fluoride (flu'or-īd) [L. *fluere,* to flow]. A compound of fluorine with a radicle; a salt of hydrofluoric acid.

fluorine (flu'or-en) [L. *fluere,* to flow]. Gaseous, chemical element. SYMB: F. Atomic weight, 19.

This is found in the soil in combination with calcium. It seems absolutely necessary to plant life and in animal life it helps to form the bones and teeth. Unsoluble mineral elements must be absorbed by plant life and taken into the animal body as food before they can be assimilated, but f. was liquefied by Moissan and Dewar in 1897. It is found in cow's milk, yolk of egg, and brain.

fluorometer (flu-o-rom'et-er) [" + G. *metron,* to measure]. Device for adjusting the shadow in skiagraphy.

fluoroscope (flu'or-ō-skōp or flu-or'o-skōp) [" + G. *skopein,* to examine]. A device consisting of a fluorescent screen suitably mounted, either separately or in conjunction with a roentgen tube, by means of which the shadows of objects interposed between the tube and the screen are made visible.

fluoros'copy [" + G. *skopein,* to examine]. The use of a fluoroscope for medical diagnosis or for testing various materials by roentgen rays.

fluorosis (flu-or-o'sis) [" + G. *ōsis*]. Chronic fluorine poisoning, sometimes marked by mottling of tooth enamel. Often results from too much fluoride in drinking water.

flush [A.S. *fluschen,* to fly up]. Sudden redness of the skin.

f., hec'tic. Redness of the cheeks seen in some chronic affections, such as pulmonary tuberculosis, and due to rise of temperature.

f., hot. One accompanied with sensation of heat; common in neuroses and psychoneuroses and during menopause.

flut'ter [A.S. *floterian,* to fly about]. A tremulous movement, esp. of the heart as auricular and ventricular flutter.

f. auricular. Condition in which contractions of the atrium become extremely rapid (200-400 per min.). In *pure flutter,* a regular rhythm is maintained, in *impure flutter,* the rhythm is irregular.

flux [L. *fluxus,* a flow]. 1. An excessive flow or discharge from an organ or cavity of the body; diarrhea. 2. Discharge from the bowels.

f., bloody. Dysentery.

fly [A.S. *flēoge*]. An insect belonging to the order Diptera, characterized by possessing sucking mouth parts, one pair of wings, and incomplete metamorphosis. Term is sometimes applied to insects belonging to other orders (ex. May fly, dragon fly). SEE: *Diptera.*

f. black. *Simulium, q.v.*

f., blow. Flies of the family *Calliphoridae.* They breed in dung or the flesh of dead animals. Also called *bluebottle flies.* SEE: *Calliphora vomitoria.*

f., bot. Botfly, *q.v.*

f. flesh. The *Sarcophagidae, q.v.*

f., house. *Musca domestica, q.v.*

f. sand. *Phlebotomus, q.v.*

f. screwworm. A fly belonging to the families *Calliphoridae* and *Sarcophagidae, q.v.*

f., tsetse. *Glossina palpalis.* One which transmits African sleeping sickness or trypanosomiasis.

SEE: *blister.*

f. warble. The *Oestridae, q.v.*

foam. A mixture of finely divided gas bubbles interspersed in a liquid.

F. M. (fi'at mistu'ra) [L.]. Abbr. for "let a mixture be made."

fo'cal [L. *focus,* hearth]. Pert. to a focus.

f. infection. One occurring near a focus, such as the cavity of a tooth.

f. lesion. A limited central lesion.

fo'cus (pl. *foci*) [L. the hearth]. The point of convergence of light rays or waves of sound.

f., real. Point at which convergent rays intersect.

f., virtual. The point at which divergent rays would intersect if prolonged backward.

fog'ging, fog'ging sys'tem. A method of testing vision, used particularly in testing astigmatism, and in postcycloplegic examination.

fold [A.S. *foltan,* to fold]. A ridge; a doubling back. SYN: *plica.*

f., amniotic. Folded edge of the amniotic membrane where it rises over and finally encloses the embryo of birds, reptiles and some mammals.

f., genital. Fold of skin in the embryo on each side of the genital tubercle which develops into the labia minora in the female.

f., mesouterine. Fold of peritoneum supporting the uterus.

fo'lia (pl. of *folium*) [L.]. 1. A leaf or leaflike structure. 2. One of the folds

foliaceous   F-25   **fontanel, fontanelle**

or gyri seen on the surface of the cerebellum.

foliaceous (fo-li-a'she-us) [L. *folia*, leaves]. Resembling or pert. to a leaf.

folic acid (fō'lik). Pteroylglutamic acid. Found in liver, yeast, and green leaves. Used in treating pernicious anemia, macrocytic anemia, celiac syndrome, and sprue.

folie (fol-e') [Fr. foolish, mad]. Mania; psychosis.
   f. circulaire. SYN: *circular insanity*. Frequent repetition of excited and depressed phases of manic-depressive psychosis.
   f. du doute (fol-e' du doot). Abnormal doubts about ordinary acts and beliefs; inability to decide upon definite standards of conduct.

folium (pl. *folia*) [L. leaf]. Thin, broad, leaflike structure.
   f. vermis, f. cacuminis. A fold on the posterior part of the upper surface of the vermis of the cerebellum.

foll'icle [L. *folliculus*, little bag]. 1. A small secretory sac or cavity. 2. A lymphatic nodule, (obs).
   f. aggregated. Peyer's patch, *q.v.*
   f. atretic. An ovarian follicle that has undergone degeneration or involution.
   f., graafian. GYN: Small excretory organ in the cortex of the ovary. The complete development of the primary oocyte to the stage where the ovum is fully developed. SEE: *ovary*.
   f. growing. A developing follicle of the ovary.
   f. hair. An invagination of the epidermis from which a hair develops.
   f., nabothian. Dilated cyst of the glands of the cervix uteri.
   f. ovarian. A spherical structure in the cortex of the ovary consisting of an oogonium, or an oocyte and its surrounding epithelial (follicular) cells. Follicles are of three types: 1. *Primary*, consisting of an oogonium and a single layer of follicular cells. 2. *Growing*, in which the follicle cells proliferate forming several layers and the first maturation division occurs. 3. *Vesicular*, or *Graafian* follicle which possesses a cavity *(antrum)* containing the follicular fluid *(liquor folliculi)*. The oocyte lies in the *cumulus oophorus*, a mass of cells on the inner surface. The cells lining the follicle constitute the *stratum granulosum*. The follicle is a secretory structure producing estrogens.
   f., sebaceous. Oil gland of the skin.
   f. solitary. A single lymph nodule of the intestine.
   f. thyroid. Spherical or ovoid structure found in the thyroid gland lined with a single layer of cuboidal epithelial cells which secrete the thyroid hormone. The follicles are filled with *colloid*, a viscid substance rich in iodine.
   f. vesicular. One containing a cavity; a mature ovarian or Graafian follicle.

folliclis (fol'ik-lis) [L. *folliculus*, little bag]. Indolent papulonecrotic lesion, esp. on the extremities and possibly the face.

follic'ular [L. *folliculus*, little bag]. Pert. to a follicle or follicles.
   f. tonsillitis. Inflammation of follicles on surface of the tonsil which become filled with pus.
   f. tumor. A sebaceous cyst.

follic'ulin [L. *folliculus*, little bag]. An internal secretion of the ovary which, with lutein and ovulin, forms the oophorin hormone. SEE: *estrin*.

folliculitis (fol-ik-u-li'tis) [" + G. *-itis*, inflammation]. Inflammation of a follicle or follicles.
   f. barbae. Inflammation of the follicles of the bearded parts. SEE: *sycosis vulgaris*.
   f. decalvans. Purulent follicular inflammation of the scalp resulting in irregular alopecia and scarring. SYN: *acne decalvans, Quinquad's disease*.
   ETIOL: Essential cause unknown. Affects mostly males between 2nd and 4th decades.
   SYM: Initial inflammatory papule or pustule at mouth of follicle pierced by a hair is followed by crusting and desiccation, when it drops off along with loosened hair. Bald patches, with slight depressed whitish center surrounded by inflamed margin. Extends peripherally.
   PATH: Perivascular, particularly lower half of follicle sheaths; sebaceous gland atrophy and flattened papillae.
   PROG: Baldness is permanent, though extension may be arrested.
   TREATMENT: Tonics internally. Externally, ointments, frequent shampoos, and daily antiseptic.
   f. sebacea. Inflammation of the sebaceous glands, with accumulation of secretion. SYN: *acne*.

folliculoma (fol-ik-u-lo'mă) [" + G. *ōma*, tumor]. A tumor of the ovary originating in a graafian follicle, in which the cells resemble the cells of the *stratum granulosum*.

folliculose (fol-ik'u-lōs) [L. *folliculus*, little bag]. Composed of follicles.

folliculo'sis [" + G. *-ōsis*]. Presence of an abnormal quantity of lymph follicles.

folliculus (fŏ-lik'u-lus) (pl. *fol'liculi*) [L. little bag]. A follicle.
   f. oophorus vesiculosus. A graafian follicle, *q.v.*

fomentation (fo-men-tā'shun) [L. *fomentāre*, to apply a poultice]. A hot, wet application for the relief of pain or inflammation. SEE: *stupe*.
   f., boracic. This may be prepared with boracic lint, which is already impregnated with boracic acid, and is colored pink as a distinguishing mark; or boracic acid may be added to lint, either in form of powder or crystals, and then wrung out of boiling water as before.
   f., medical. Instead of lint, 2 or 3 thicknesses of flannel are used, and the fomentation is applied to unbroken skin, otherwise procedure is same as for a surgical fomentation; it is unnecessary to boil it; flannel is used because it retains the heat better than lint. This fomentation is also called a *stupe*, *q.v.*
   f., surgical. SEE: *hot moist dressing*.

fom'es (pl. *fomites*) [L. tinder]. Any substance that absorbs and transmits infectious material.

fom'ites (sing. *fomes*) [L. *fomes*, tinder]. Plural of *fomes* and transmitting infectious material.

Fontan'a's spaces. Spaces bet. the processes of ligamentum pectinatum of the iris. These convey the aqueous humor sinus venosus sclerae.

fontanel, fontanelle (fon-tan-el') [Fr. *fontanelle*, little fountain']. An unossified space or "soft spot" lying between the cranial bones of the skull of a fetus. They include the frontal anterior or greater occipital posterior or lesser sphenoidal ant. lateral and mastoid post. lateral fontanels the last two being paired.

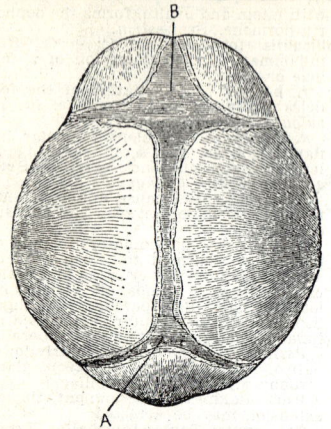

THE FONTANELS
B. Anterior fontanel.
A. Posterior fontanel.

  f., anterior. At the junction of the coronal, frontal, and sagittal sutures.
  f., posterior. At the junction of the sagittal and lambdoid sutures.
fonticulus (fon-tik'u-lus) [L. little fountain]. SYN: *fontanel*.
food. Sing. of *foods, q.v.*
food accessories. Nutrient substances which do not provide energy but furnish substances essential for the growth and well-being of the body. Includes water, mineral salts, and vitamins.
food allergies. Allergic reactions resulting from ingestion of foods to which a person has become sensitized. One may become sensitive to almost any food but shellfish, pork, eggs, milk, spinach, lettuce, strawberries and tomatoes are the most common offenders.
  SYM: Urticaria (hives), certain exzemas, nausea, vomiting, diarrhea, and intestinal cramps. A syndrome (angioneurotic edema) characterized by a transient swelling of various parts of the body and spasm of the intestine may result.
food ball. Gastric stone made up of fruit and vegetable skins, seeds and fibers. SYN: *phytobezoar*.
  f. course of (through the alimentary canal). Foods enter the mouth and in the buccal area reduced to a pulp or semifluid mass through the processes of mastication and insalivation (the mixing of food with saliva). Swallowing or deglutition then occurs. In swallowing, the food mass or *bolus* passes into the *pharynx* and then through the *esophagus* to the *stomach*, the entrance of which is guarded by the cardiac sphincter.
  Stomach. In the stomach the food is stored and mixed with gastric juice. After it attains a certain fluid consistency, it passes through the *pyloric* sphincter into the small intestine.
  Small intestine. In the first portion or *duodenum* the intestinal contents, now called *chyme* is mixed wtih bile, secreted by the liver, and the pancreatic juice, both of which enter through the opening of the common bile duct. In the next two portions, the *jejunum* and *ileum*, the chyme is mixed with the intestinal juice secreted by the intestinal glands or crypts of Liebekuhn. In the small intestine, digestion is completed and the end products of digestion (simple sugars, amino acids, fatty acids and glycerol) are absorbed into the capillaries and lacteals of the intestinal mucosa.
  Large intestine. Undigestible material passes from the small intestine into the large intestine (colon) through the *ileocecal valve* located at the junction of the ascending colon and the cecum, a blind pouch which terminates in the vermiform appendix. The material continues through the colon (ascending, transverse, descending and sigmoid) to the *rectum* from which it is discharged through the *anal canal* as the feces, at the anus or anal orifice. In the large intestine, the major portion of the water of the intestinal contents is absorbed. Digestive changes are limited to the action of bacteria which bring about putrefaction and fermentation of incompletely digested foods. No enzymes are secreted by the glands of the large intestine.
f. enriched. F. to which have been added vitamins or minerals removed in refining and processing; foods in which the vitamin and (or) mineral content has been increased either by addition or by irradiation.
food fever. Sudden rise in temperature accompanying digestive disturbances in children, supposed to be result of intestinal autointoxication. Lasts from 3 or 4 days to several weeks.
food infections. Illness resulting from infectious organisms which enter the body in food or drink. Among the organisms which may be ingested are (1) bacteria, esp., those of the salmonella group and certain staphylococci and streptococci, typhoid, paratyphoid, and dysentery bacilli, (2) the eggs, encysted forms or larvae of animal parasites such as *Trichinella*, tapeworms, and other parasitic worms.
food. Nutrient substances; substances which in the body serve as a source of energy or provide materials for the growth and repair of tissue. Foods are organic substances (proteins, carbohydrates, fats) present in animal and plant tissues. Nutrient substances which do not provide energy are called *food accessories, q.v.* The term "foods" is commonly used to refer to any substance taken into the body which serves a nutrient function.
food poisoning. An attack of illness or a digestive disorder resulting from the ingestion of foods containing poisonous substances. True food poisoning includes mushroom poisoning, shellfish poisoning, poisoning resulting from foods contaminated with poisonous insecticides or other poisons, milk sickness (due to milk from cows that have fed on certain poisonous plants); and occasionally poisoning resulting from eating foods that have undergone putrefaction or decomposition. It may also be due to bacteria, especially paratyphoid bacilli and staphylococci ingested in food.
f. protective. Foods which are the richest sources of basic nutritional needs (water, proteins, vitamins, essential fatty acids, inorganic salts). These include milk, milk products, eggs, fruits, and leafy vegetables.
f. rashes. In those with an idiosyncrasy to some protein certain rashes may be

ORGANIC

Proteins

Elements	Symbol	Per Cent	End Products
1. Carbon	C	.53 %	Urea, uric acid, H_2SO_4, CO_2, H_2O.
2. Hydrogen	H	.07 %	Salts set free.
3. Oxygen	O	.22 %	Proteins are tissue, muscle, nerve and
4. Nitrogen	N	.16 %	brain builders and also furnish heat and
5. Sulfur	S	.015%	energy.
6. Phosphorus	P	.005%	
7. Other Minerals			
		1.00 %	

Classification of Proteins

Albumen	Casein	Gluten	Myosin
Eggs	Milk	Cereals	Fowls
Meat	Cheese	Beans	
		Peas	
		Lentils	
		Nuts	

Carbohydrates $(C_x(H_2O)_y)$

Elements	Symbol	Per Cent	End Products
1. Carbon	C	76%	Salts set free
2. Hydrogen	H	12%	CO_2 and H_2O
3. Oxygen	O	12%	
		100%	

Classification of Carbohydrates

Glucose	Cane Sugar	Cellulose
$C_6H_{12}O_6$	$C_{12}H_{23}O_{11}$	$C_6H_{10}O_5$

Carbohydrates as well as fats are heat and energy producers, but neither can take the place of proteins, as they contain no nitrogen. They consist principally of the sugars, starch, cellulose and fibers.

Fats

Elements	Symbol	Per Cent	End Products
1. Carbon	C	45%	CO_2 and H_2O
2. Hydrogen	H	06%	Fats are heat and energy producers and
3. Oxygen	O	49%	not tissue or cell builders.
		100%	

Classification of Fats

Fats	Oils	Nuts	Olives
Butter, Lard			

Food Accessories
Water, Minerals, Vitamins

TEMPERATURE BEST SUITED FOR STORAGE OF FOODS

Fruits

	Degrees F.
Apples	31-32
Bananas	34-36
Berries	34-36
Cantaloupe	32
Cranberries	33-34
Dried Fruits	35-40
Fresh Fruits	33-40
Lemons	36
Oranges	36
Watermelons	32

Vegetables

Fresh	33-35

Meats and Fish

	Degrees F.
Brined Meats	35-40
Beef, Fresh	37-39
Fish, Fresh	25-30
Fish, Frozen	25
Fish, Dried	25
Ham	30-35
Lard	34-35
Mutton	32-36
Oysters	33-40
Oysters in Shell	40
Oysters in Tubs	35
Pork	30-33
Poultry	29
Poultry, Frozen	5-10
Veal	32-36
Milk	50-60

the only symptom of toxemia. They may be in form of *urticaria, erythema,* or *papules,* or a combination of these.

"It is ordinarily assumed that an average man in health performing light to moderate muscular work requires per day about 0.25 pound protein and 3050 calories of energy, the latter being supplied in small part by protein, but mostly by fat and carbohydrates. Men in professional life, by performing less muscular work, require smaller amounts.

"The commonly accepted American dietary standard for such men calls for 0.22 pound protein and 2700 calories of energy in the daily food. The amount of mineral matter required is not stated, since there is little accurate information available on this point.

"A diet made up of ordinary foods and supplying the necessary amounts of protein and energy would undoubtedly supply an abundance of mineral matter. It has been found that women and children consume somewhat less food than men. The assumption is usually made that, provided a woman is engaged in some moderately active occupation, she requires about eight-tenths as much as a man with a similar amount of work.

"In calculating the results of dietary studies (which may be most conveniently expressed in amounts for 1 man for 1 day), it is further assumed that a boy 13-14 years old and a girl 15-16 years old also require about eight-tenths as much food as a man at moderately active muscular labor; a boy of 12 and a girl 13-14 years old, about seven-tenths; a boy 10-11 and a girl 10-12 years old, about six-tenths; a child 6-9 years old, about five-tenths; one 2-5, about four-tenths, and an infant under 2 years, about three-tenths."—*U. S. Dept. Agriculture.*

food requirements (showing daily quantities of the principal foods for a patient weighing about 132 lb.):

Salad and Vegetable .... 200 Gm.
Raw Vegetable .... 100 Gm.
Fruit .... 375 Gm.
Fat (butter, oil, etc.) ..... 100 Gm.
Milk .... 1250 Gm.
Cream .... 100 Gm.
Egg .... One to one-and-a-half
Meat, Viscera, Fish .... 70 Gm.
Potatoes .... 125 Gm.
Bread .... 60 Gm.
Zwieback or Cookie .... 20 Gm.
Starch (flour, rice, farina,
  oatmeal, etc.) .... 30 Gm.
Sugar or Honey .... 30 Gm.

Contain about 90 Gm. protein, 164 Gm. fat, 244 Gm. carbohydrate, with total calories 2886 and about 3.4 Gm. sodium chloride.

BY THE AVERAGE HEALTHY
ADULT MAN AT MODERATE WORK
Proteins ..100 Gm. 12-15% caloric value
Fats ...... 100 Gm. 20-30% caloric value
Carb. ... 500 Gm. 50-70% caloric value
Water .. 3000 c.c.
Minerals as follows: calcium 0.8 Gm., phosphorus 1.5 Gm., sodium 3 to 6 Gm., potassium 2 to 4 Gm., sodium chloride 5 to 15 Gm. and vitamins, *q.v.*

Seven Basic Food Groups as recommended by the U. S. Dept. of Agriculture are: 1. Leafy Green and Yellow Vegetables, 2. Citrus fruit, tomatoes, raw cabbage, 3. Potatoes and other vegetables and fruits, 4. Milk, cheese, ice cream, 5. Meat, poultry, fish, eggs, dried peas, beans, 6. Bread, flour, cereals, whole grain or enriched, 7. Butter and fortified margarine.

foods [A.S. *fōda*]. Nutritive substances necessary to nourish, protect, and maintain the body.
SEE: *names of condiments, drinks, and foods, according to alphabetical order.*

foot [A.S. *fōt*]. *(pes).* The terminal portion of the lower extremity. The bones of the foot include the *tarsus, metatarsus,* and *phalanges.* SEE: *skeleton.*

f. arches. Four arches: (a) Int. longitudinal; (b) outer l., and (c) 2 transverse ones.

f. athlete's. SEE: *athlete's foot.*

f. bath, mustard. AIM: To aid action of hot water in relieving congestion in some distant part of the body.

ARTICLES NEEDED: Bath blanket. Small rubber sheet and large bath towel. Foot tub with water at 110° F. and bath thermometer which is left in tub during treatment. Mustard. Old muslin about 6 in. square. Tablespoon. Hot water bottle filled and covered. Pitcher of extra very hot water.

PROCEDURE: 1. Measure mustard in the proportion of 1 tablespoonful to 1 gallon of water and tie in the square of muslin. 2. Put in tub and add water. Rub mustard bag between fingers to dissolve mustard and allow it to diffuse through the water. 3. Loosen upper bedding at foot of bed and turn back to patient's knees. 4. Flex knees. 5. Place rubber sheet covered with bath towel across bed under patient's feet. 6. Put tub on towel and place feet in tub, arranging patient as comfortably as possible. 7. Cover knees, feet and tub with bath blanket, tucking under tub so it does not drop into water. 8. Lay upper bedding down over blanket and tub but do not tuck in. 9. Continue treatment 20 minutes unless patient complains of burning sensation. In that case stop it at once. 10. As bath cools add hot water from pitcher. Lift feet out before doing this. Check temperature with thermometer. 11. Watch patient and if she feels faint stop treatment at once. The swift withdrawal of blood from head to feet may cause syncope. 12. At end of treatment lift feet, draw tub toward you and put feet down on towel. Remove tub. Dry feet well. 13. Put hot water bottle at foot of bed if desired and permitted. Arrange bedding and make patient comfortable. 14. Clean and replace equipment. 15. Record treatment.

f. cleft. Condition in which a cleft extends between the digits to the metatarsal region, usually due to a missing digit.

f. contracted. Clawfoot or *pes cavus, q.v.*

f. flat. Flatfoot *q.v.; pes planus.*

f. immersion. Condition resulting from prolonged immersion of the feet in water.

f., Madura. Bone hypertrophy and degeneration, frequently followed by suppuration or gangrene.

foot candle. Amt. of light radiated 1 ft. from a standard candle. SYN: *light u.*

footdrop. A falling or dragging of the foot from paralysis of the flexors of the ankle.

foot'ling presentation. Presentation of feet foremost in labor.

foot plate. Base of the stapes; an ossicle of the tympanum. It fits into, and closes, the *fenestra vestibuli* (oval window).

foot pound. Amt. of energy required to raise 1 pound 1 foot from a level.

foot print. An impression of the foot, esp., an ink impression used for identification of infants.

  f. splay. Flatfoot accompanied by extreme eversion of the foot.

  f. weak. Condition resulting from weakened muscles, or from faulty walking habits. Results in chronic eversion of the foot.

forage (for-azh') [Fr. boring]. Cutting a channel by diathermy through an enlarged prostate.

foramen (for-a'men) (pl. *foram'ina*) [L. an opening]. A passage or opening; an orifice, a communication between 2 cavities of an organ, or a hole in a bone for passage of vessels or nerves.

  f., intervertebral. Opening bet. every 2 articulated vertebrae for passage of nerves to and from spinal cord.

  f. magnum. It pierces the occipital bone through which passes the spinal cord from the brain. [lateral ventricles.

  f. of Monro. Opening bet. 3rd and

  f. obturator. Large oval f. below acetabulum bounded by the pubis and ischium. SEE: *Magendie's f.*

  f. ova'le. 1. Opening at lower post. of septum in fetus, bet. 2 cardiac auricles. 2. Oval opening in post. margin of great sphenoidal wing, for inf. maxillary nerve and small meningeal artery.

force, unit of. Amount of force necessary to move a weight of 1 Gm. 1 cm. in 1 second. SYN: *dyne*.

forceps (for'seps) [L. a pair of tongs]. Pincers for holding, seizing or extracting. There are at least 100 distinct varieties of forceps, varying according to the operation for which they are intended.

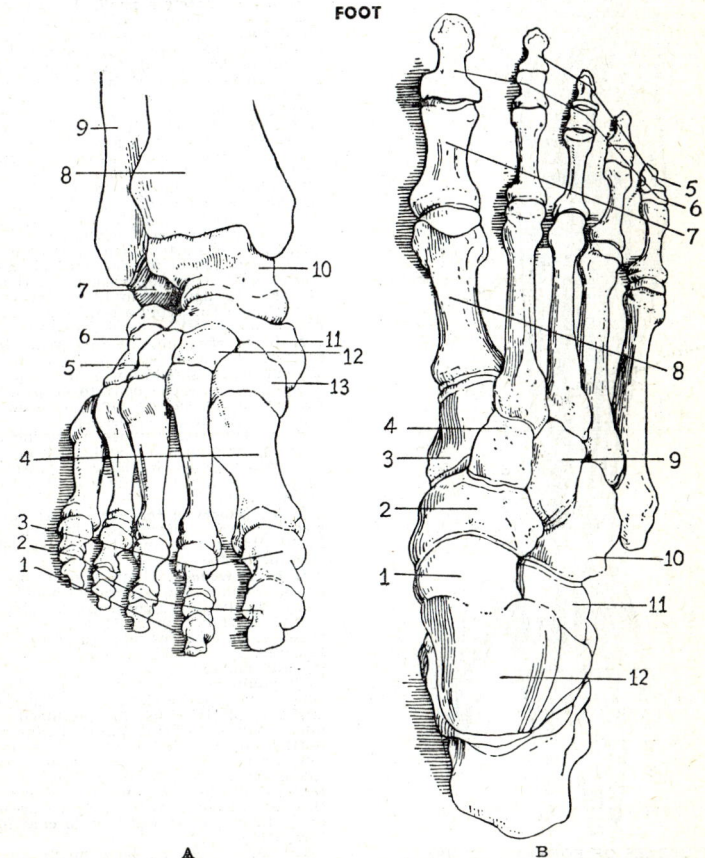

FOOT

A **B**

TARSAL AND METATARSAL BONES AND PHALANGES

1. 3rd Phalanges. 2. 2nd Phalanges. 3. 1st Phalanges. 4. Metatarsals. 5. External Cuneiform. 6. Cuboid. 7. Os Calcis. 8. Tibia. 9. Fibula. 10. Astragalus. 11. Scaphoid. 12. Middle Cuneiform. 13. Internal Cuneiform.

1. Astragalus. 2. Scaphoid. 3. Internal Cuneiform. 4. Middle Cuneiform. 5. 3rd Phalanges. 6. 2nd Phalanges. 7. 1st Phalanges. 8. Metatarsals. 9. External Cuneiform. 10. Cuboid. 11. Os Calcis. 12. Astragulus (talus).

forcipate (for'sip-āt) [L. *forceps, forcip-,* tongs]. Forceps shaped.

for'cipressure [" + *pressura,* pressure]. Arresting hemorrhage by pressure on an artery with forceps.

fore- [O.Eng.]. Prefix meaning *before* or *in front of.*

forearm (fōr'arm) [A.S. *fore,* in front, + *arm,* arm]. The part of arm between elbow and wrist.

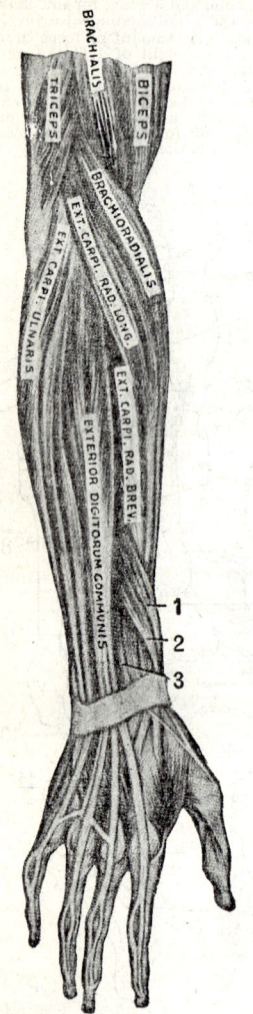

MUSCLES OF FOREARM, WRIST, AND HAND

forebrain (fōr'brān) [" + *bregen,* brain]. Ant. portion of the brain of the embryo. SYN: *prosencephalon.*

fore'finger [" + *finger,* finger]. The first or index finger.

fore'gut [" + *gut,* a pouring]. First part of the embryonic digestive tube whence pharynx, esophagus, stomach, and duodenum are formed. SYN: *protogaster.*

forehead (fōr'ed) [" + *heāfod,* head]. The brow. SYN: *frons, metopon.*

for'eign bod'ies. Slivers, cinders, dirt, or small objects in the skin, ears, eyes, nose and internally frequently lead to infection, and if not removed lead to unsightly marks or tattooing of the skin and inflammation of the organ involved.

F. A. TREATMENT: Carefully asepticize the areas involved. Foreign material can be carefully removed piece by piece, or by vigorous swabbing with gauze or brush, using a soapy solution. Follow with an antiseptic dressing.

SEE: *ear, esophagus, eye, nose, stomach, throat.*

f. b., extracting a small. In attempting to remove a small foreign body, first cover area with an antiseptic; sterilize a clean needle by heating it to a dull or bright red heat in a flame. This can be done with a single match; inasmuch as both ends of the needle get hot it is wise to hold the far end in a nonconductor of heat, such as folds of paper, sticking it in a cork, or in the edge of a small book; allow it to cool and disregard black deposit on the needle which is sterile carbon and will not interfere with procedure. Then introduce the needle at right angles to the direction of sliver and lift it out.

Most persons attempt to stick the needle in direction of the foreign body and consequently have to thrust many times before they manage to lift sliver out. When removed, apply an antiseptic and cover wound with a sterile dressing.

f. b. in the ear. If any vegetable matter, such as a bean, pea, etc., is in the ear, water should not be introduced, as it may cause the body to be pushed further in the ear or cause it to swell and become firmly embedded.

F. A. TREATMENT: Place a globule of glue on the end of a match stick or an applicator; gently introduce it until it touches the foreign body and then remove gently.

f. b.; insects in the ear. SYM: Loud buzzing, pain, dizziness. TREATMENT: Flood ear with warm oil or water, letting insect float out.

f. b. in wounds. They are often present in wounds and generally should be left undisturbed if a surgeon is available within a short time. If small, as a sliver, it may be desirable to remove it. If large, it may be very dangerous to try any method of removing, inasmuch as it might be embedded in large blood vessels, muscles, etc., and removing it might result in much loss of blood or might cause breaking off of splinters, particles of rust, dirt, etc.; within a very few moments tissue juices, blood, and the natural reaction of swelling would tend to fill in the wounds and cover this foreign material, making it exceedingly difficult for the doctor to care for the patient.

In such instances, it is much wiser when possible, to leave the large foreign body in position, and obtain the services of a doctor promptly.

forensic (for-en'sik) [L. *forensis,* pert. to a forum]. Pert. to the law; legal.

f. medicine. Legal medicine or medicine in relation to the law.

forepleasure

fore'pleasure [A.S. *fore*, before, + L. *placere*, to please]. That derived from any action that induces or intensifies sexual desire, such as kissing or stimulating any erogenous zone in the female, esp., before cohabitation.

fore'skin [" + *skinn*, skin]. Prepuce* or loose skin at and covering the end of the penis.
Excision of the prepuce constitutes circumcision. *Smegma* praeputii* is secreted by Tyson's glands and collects under the foreskin. SEE: *circumcision*.
NP: In infant cases the nurse must see that the prepuce is not adherent or interfering with urination. Abnormalities must be reported to the doctor.

-form [L. *forma*]. Suffix meaning *having the form of*.

formaldehyde (for-mal'de-hīd). USP. A colorless, pungent, irritant gas commonly made by oxidation of methyl alcohol; the simplest member of the group of aldehydes.* It is used in medicinal form of a solution of 40% formaldehyde or formalin HCHO.
ACTION AND USES: A germicide, and disinfectant; also a preservative and fumigant. A 10% solution is useful as an astringent.
A 1% or 2% solution used for cleansing dishes, instruments, or fabrics. Formaldehyde is a powerful germicide, esp. in the form of gas, because of its penetrating power, but it is active only in the presence of an abundance of moisture. The solution is germicidal in the strength of from 1% to 2%, but the action may be delayed from 20-30 minutes. It hardens tissues and is often used in histology for this purpose. It has a similar hardening effect on the living skin; it is very irritating to mucous membranes and produces reddening, inflammation, and necrosis, if applied repeatedly or continuously. It is sometimes used in soap for disinfection of the hands. A 10% solution is used for sterilizing feces, urine, and sputum; 5% to 10% for clothing and towels. SEE: *fumigation*.
POISONING: SYM: Local irritation of eyes, nose, mouth, throat; respiratory and gastrointestinal tracts and central nervous system; causing vertigo, stupor, abdominal pain, convulsions, unconsciousness, renal damage.
F. A. TREATMENT: Administration of dilute aromatic spirits of ammonia, very dilute ammonia water, as ammonium acetate which seems to combine with the formaldehyde, forming nonpoisonous methenamine. Otherwise symptomatic treatment.
 f., casein. Antiseptic product.
 f., gelatin. Antiseptic wound dressing.

for'malin. Wood alcohol with a 40% content of formaldehyde. SEE: *aldehyde*.

formate (for'māt). A salt of formic acid.

formatio (for-ma'shī-ō) [L. formation]. A structure with definite arrangement and shape. [dulla oblongata.
 f. reticula'ris. Dorsal part of the me-

forma'tion. 1. A structure, shape, or figure. 2. The giving of form or shape to, or the development of a structure.
 f. reticular. SYN: *formatia reticularis, substantia reticularis*. A reticular structure formed of gray matter and interlacing fibers of white matter found in the medulla oblongata between the pyramids and the floor of the 4th ventricle. It is also present in the spinal cord, midbrain, and pons.

fornix

forme fruste (form früst) [Fr. from L. *forma*, form, + *frustra*, without effect]. An aborted form of disease arrested before running its course.

for'mic [L. *formica*, ant]. Pert. to ants and to formic acid.

for'mic acid. H.COOH, a clear, pungent, liquid obtained from the oxidation of formaldehyde or wood alcohol. It was originally obtained from the distillation of the bodies of red ants, and is probably the cause of the pain and swelling resulting from the bites or stings of certain insects or the irritation from nettles.
 f. aldehyde. Formaldehyde.
 f. ether. Volatile anesthetic liquid ethyl formate.

formica'tion [L. *formica*, ant]. A sensation as of ants creeping upon the body; a form of paresthesia.

formiciasis (for-mis-i'as-is) [L. *formica*, ant]. Symptoms caused by ant bites.

formilase (for'mil-ās). A ferment which converts acetic acid into formic acid.

formin (for'min). SEE: *methenamine*.

for'mula [L. a little form]. 1. A rule prescribing ingredients with proportions for the preparation of a compound. 2. CHEM: An expression by symbols of the constitution of a molecule consisting of letters, each denoting 1 atom of 1 elementary substance, with figures denoting the number of atoms present.
Collections of atoms which constitute a group by themselves (radical) are often separated by periods or parentheses, and in this case figures prefixed or appended to the parentheses or placed before an expression contained within periods apply to all the symbols embraced by the parentheses or periods.
In all other cases, a figure prefixed to a symbolical expression for a molecule, like a coefficient in an algebraical f., is understood to be a multiplier of all the symbols following.
 f., Arneth's. Method of estimating number of immature leukocytes by means of an elaborate differential blood count.
 f. dental. F. showing the number and arrangement of the teeth. For the permanent teeth,

$$i\frac{2}{2}, \ c\frac{1}{1}, \ pm\frac{2}{2}, \ m\frac{3}{3} = \frac{8}{8} \times 2 \ 32.$$

 f. empirical. The f. of a compound which shows the atoms and their numbers in a molecule, as H_2O.
 f., official. One in a pharmacopeia.
 f. structural. The formula of a compound which shows the relations of the atoms to each other in a molecule. The atoms are shown joined by valence bonds, for example: H-O-H.

form'ulary [L. *formula*, a little form]. A book of formulas.
 f., national. One issued by the *American Pharmaceutical Association*.

formyl. The radical of formic acid, HCO.

for'nicate [L. *fornix*, arch; brothel]. 1. Arched or vaultlike. 2. To indulge in unlawful cohabitation.

fornica'tion [L. *fornix*, brothel]. The act of illicit sexual intercourse.

for'nicolumn [L. *fornix*, arch, + *columna*, column]. The ant. pillar of the fornix.

fornicommissure (for-nĭ-kom'is-ūr) [" + *commissura*, a joining together]. The commissure or body of the fornix uteri.

for'nix (pl. *fornices*) [L. arch]. 1. A fibrous vaulted band connecting the cerebral lobes. 2. Any body with vaultlike or arched shape.

f. conjunctivae. OPHTH: Loose fold connecting palpebral and bulbar conjunctivae.

f. uteri. Ant. and post. spaces into which the upper vagina is divided. These recesses are formed by protrusion of the cervix uteri into the vagina.

f. vaginae. The f. uteri, *q.v.*

fortifica'tion spectrum. Appearance of dark patch with zigzag outline in visual field. SYN: *scintillating scotoma, teichopsia.* [ment of tularemia.

Foshay's serum. One used in the treat-

fossa (fos'a) (pl. *fossae*) [L. ditch]. A furrow or shallow depression.

f., axillary. The armpit.

f., Claudius'. Triangular area harboring the ovary.

f., iliac. One of the concavities of the iliac bones of pelvis. The right one contains the appendix.

f. lacrimalis. Hollow of frontal bone holding the lacrimal gland.

f. navicularis. One bet. the hymen and fourchette.

f. ovalis. 1. BNA. Opening in thigh for large saphenous vein. 2. Remnant of embryonic foramen ovale in right cardiac auricle.

f., Rosenmuller's. Depression in pharynx posterior to opening of eustachian tube.

f. supratonsillaris. Space bet. anterior and posterior pillars of the fauces above the tonsil.

fossette (fos-et') [Fr. a little ditch]. 1. A small depression or fossa. 2. A small but deep corneal ulcer.

foulage (foo-lazh') [Fr. impression]. Kneading with pressure of the muscles.

fourchet, fourchette (foor-shet') [Fr. *fourchette*, a fork]. A tense band or transverse fold of mucous membrane at the post. commissure of the vagina, connecting the post. ends of the labia minora.

The *fossa navicularis*, a more or less deep *cul-de-sac* anterior to the fourchette, separates it from the hymen. It disappears after defloration or parturition, leaving a more open vulva below and behind. SYN: *frenulum labiorum pudendi.*

fourth cranial nerve. Trochlear n., *q.v.*

fovea (fo've-ă) [L. pit]. A pit or cuplike depression. SEE: *fossa*.

f. centralis. Pit in the middle of macula lutea.

foveate (fo'vē-āt) [L. *fovea*, pit]. Pitted; having depressions.

foveation (fo-ve-a'shun) [L. *fovea*, pit]. Pitting, as in smallpox.

foveola (fo-ve'o-la) [L. little pit]. A minute pit or depression.

Fowler-Murphy method. Elevation of head of bed with tube through an incision in right iliac fossa for drainage in diffuse suppurative peritonitis. Continuous rectal irrigation with a physiological salt solution accompanies the treatment.

Fow'ler's position. This places the patient in a semi-sitting position.

The head of bed may be raised on blocks, pins, or other support, or the back rest may be elevated, or patient may rest upon 4 or 5 pillows. It is more easily maintained if the patient sits in a swing or hammock, made by folding a bedsheet lengthwise, placing center of sheet tightly across the buttocks, with 1 end on each side. The ends are fastened securely at head of the bed, or as high as ends will reach.

This position may be ordered if patient is suffering from dyspnea,* after a thyroid, or an abdominal operation and where there is drainage expected. Some pneumonia cases are placed in this position. In many instances it is contraindicated.

F.'s solution. One containing 1% arsenic trioxide.

USES: Largely in chorea, as an alterative; in malaria, etc.

DOSAGE: Average, 3 ℳ (0.2 cc.).

INCOMPATIBILITIES: Alkaloidal salts, iodides, tannic acid, iron salts, quinine, etc.

fraction. One or more of the separable parts of a substance.

fractional. Pertaining to a fraction or a portion of a whole.

fractional test meal. *"Fractional examination of stomach contents."* A method for the collection and examination of stomach contents as follows. First the residual contents are removed and then the test meal given. After the meal, samples are removed every 15 min. for two hours, examined and submitted to chemical tests.

Free hydrochloric acid, bile, blood, starch, mucus, and the total of acids are looked for. Free hydrochloric and total acids are normally small in amt.

In peptic ulcers there is a high acid curve, and a low one in carcinoma, and an absence of acid in pernicious anemia.

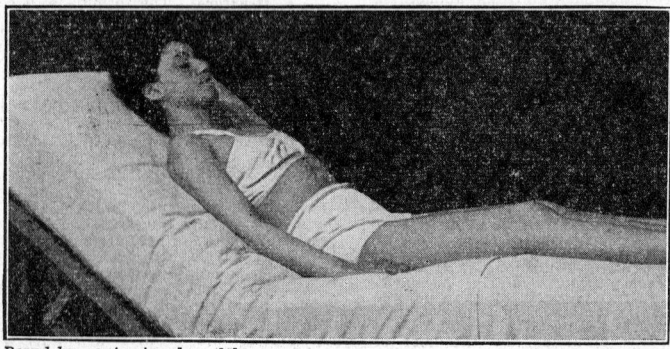

Posed by professional model   *Photo by Whitaker*

FOWLER'S POSITION

fracture (frak'tūr) [L. *fractura, frangere*, to break]. 1. A sudden breaking of a bone. 2. A broken bone.
RS: *agmatology, buttonhole f., cerclage, extension, green stick f., Lucas-Championnière's method, malunion, name of bone fractured, splint, thrypsis*.

f., cause of:
1. *By direct violence*, when the bone is broken directly at the spot where the force was applied, as in fracture of the tibia by being run over.
2. *By indirect violence*, where the bone is fractured by a force applied at a distance from the site of fracture and transmitted to the fractured bone, as in a clavicle fractured by falling on the outstretched hand.
3. *By muscular contraction*, when the bone is broken by a sudden violent contraction of the muscles. The patella is the bone most frequently fractured in this way.

In certain diseases and conditions bones break easily with scarcely any violence, *e. g.*, osteomalacia, syphilis, osteomyelitis, etc.

f., varieties of:
1. *Simple*: The bone is broken, but there is no external wound.
2. *Compound*: The bone is broken, and there is an external wound leading down to the site of fracture.
3. *Complicated*: The bone is broken, and has injured some internal organ, *e. g.*, a broken rib piercing a lung.
4. *Comminuted*: The bone is broken or splintered into pieces.
5. *Impacted*: The bone is broken, and one end is wedged into the interior of the other.
6. *Incomplete*: The line of fracture does not include the whole bone.
7. *Green Stick*: The bone is partially bent and partially broken, as when a green stick breaks. It occurs in children, especially in those with rickets.
8. *Depressed*: When a piece of the skull is broken and driven inwards.
9. *Separation of an epiphysis* takes place between the shaft of a bone and its growing end, and occurs only in young patients.

f., signs of:
(a) Loss of power of movement.
(b) Pain with acute tenderness over the site of fracture.
(c) Swelling and bruising.
(d) Deformity and possible shortening.
(e) Unnatural mobility. The nurse should never try to obtain this sign.
(f) Crepitus or grating which is heard when the ends of the bone rub together. The nurse should never try to obtain this sign.

To find out the kind of fracture and its exact position the x-rays are used. By this means a skiagraph of the bone is taken, showing the fracture and its extent.

f., treatment of:
1. FIRST AID TREATMENT: In simple fractures the limb or part must be kept immovable by means of splints, such as folded newspapers or umbrellas, or proper wooden splints if they are at hand. The clothing should not be removed unless there is dangerous hemorrhage.

If it is an upper extremity it should be supported in a sling, and the patient may then walk. If a lower limb is injured the patient should remain lying, and no attempt to walk should be made.
2. LATER TREATMENT:
(a) Reducing the fracture, *i. e.*, placing the fragments in proper position.
(b) Keeping the bone in position by means of splints until union has taken place.
(c) Restoring the limb's former functions under instruction.

In compound fractures, before treating the fracture any bleeding must be arrested, the wound is then washed and cleaned with some antiseptic lotion, and when quite clean a sterilized dressing is put on and secured by a bandage. Splints are then applied as in simple fractures.

fragilitas (fra-jil'i-tas) [L. brittleness]. Fragility.
f. crin'ium. Brittleness, as of the hair, showing splitting and breaking of the shaft. Cause unknown.
TREATMENT: Scalp cleanliness with occasional petrolatum rub. Clipping may retard splitting of distal ends. Singeing is harmful.
f. oss'ium. Brittleness of bones. SYN: *osteopsathyrosis*.
f. sanguinis. Blood fragility.

fragil'ity [L. *fragilitās*, brittleness]. State of brittleness.
f. capillary. Breaking down of capillaries due to changes in saline content of the blood.
SYM: May be oozing of blood through skin of the legs.
f. of the blood. Tendency of blood corpuscles to divide up or dissolve.
f. test. If red blood cells are placed in distilled water, they rapidly swell and burst, since they normally are suspended in a solution of much greater osmotic pressure. This phenomenon is called *hemolysis*. If they are suspended in a solution of normal saline, the cells retain their normal shape and do not burst. If they are placed in successively weaker solutions of saline, a point is reached at which some of the cells burst and liberate their hemoglobin within a given length of time, while others do not (*partial hemolysis*). Finally, at a given dilution, all of the cells have burst within the alloted time, which is usually 2 hours. The cells of normal blood begin to hemolyze in about 0.44%, and complete hemolysis occurs in about 0.35% saline. If the cells are abnormally "fragile," hemolysis occurs in stronger solutions of saline.

fragmenta'tion [L. *fragmentum, frangere*, to break]. Breaking up into fragments.
frambe'sia [L. *framboesia*, raspberry]. Infectious tropical disease. SYN: *yaws*.
frambesioma (fram-be-zĭ-o'mă) [" + G. *ōma*, swelling]. Primary lesion of yaws.
Frankenhäuser's ganglion (frang'ken-hoy-zerz). A nerve ganglion sometimes found in lateral walls of the cervix uteri.
Frank'lin glasses. Bifocal spectacles.
franklin'ic electric'ity. Electricity produced by friction. SEE: *electricity, static*.
Fraunhofer's lines (frown'hō-fer). Absorption bands or lines seen in a spectrum, caused by the absorption of groups of light rays in their passage through solids, liquids, or gases.
freckle (frek'l) [Old Norse *frecken*, a freckle]. Small local pigmentation, brownish or yellowish, of the skin.
ETIOL: Exposure to sun in majority. Universal types are probably symptomatic (anemia, abdominal disorders, etc.).

free association   F-34   **Freud, Sigmund**

SYM: Minute circumscribed brownish pigmentary macules appearing chiefly on face and dorsal surfaces of hands, more marked in spring and summer. In *lentigo senilis* the forearms are affected in individuals showing other senile skin changes.
TREATMENT: Protection from the sun. Locally, mercuric chloride-alcohol-water with circumspection, symptoms of dermatitis to be controlled by calamine lotion or cold cream. SYN: *lentigines, lentigo, ephalis.*

free associa′tion. 1. Uncontrolled ideas when not under mental restraint or direction. 2. PSY: The procedure which requires the patient to speak aloud his thought flow, word for word, without censorship.

freez′ing [A.S. *frēosan*, to freeze]. Frigidity of a limb due to cold.
Most common in the debilitated, the exhausted, and those accustomed to alcoholic beverages.
SYM: Paleness, cyanosis, coldness. Unconsciousness usually develops.
F. A. TREATMENT: Vigorous massage, application of dry heat with gradual increase in temperature. Sudden applications of heat undesirable. Hot drinks and stimulants but no alcohol. SEE: *frostbite.*
   f. microtome. One for cutting frozen objects.
   f. mixtures (for ice bags). 5 oz. sal ammoniac, 5 oz. niter and 1 part of water.
Equal parts of sal ammoniac, salt, and niter.
   f. point. Temperature at which liquids freeze.

Frei′s disease. Venereal disease affecting the inguinal area, chiefly, with formation of buboes. SYN: *lymphogranuloma inguinale* or *venerea*, *Nicolas - Favre disease.*
   F.'s test. Test given to confirm diagnosis of lymphogranuloma inguinale.
Consists of injecting an extract from the lymph nodes of a patient with lymphogranuloma into the skin. Positive reaction is evidenced by marked reddening and thickening of the skin about the site of the injection.

fremitus (frem′it-us) [L. a clashing]. Vibratory tremors felt by palpation through the chest wall.
VARIETIES: Vocal or tactile, friction, hydatid, rhonchal or bronchial, cavernous or succussion, pleural, pericardial, tussive, thrills. SEE: *palpation.*
   f. vocal. Vibrations of the voice transmitted to the ear on auscultation of the chest of a person speaking. In determining the vocal fremitus observe following precautions: Palpate symmetrical parts of chest; make firm pressure; when comparing use the same pressure on the 2 sides; apply hands as nearly parallel to ribs as possible; remember the fremitus is normally increased over the right apex. Is decreased in (1) Pleural effusions—air, pus, blood, serum, or lymph; (2) emphysema; (3) pulmonary collapse from an obstructed bronchus; (4) pulmonary edema; (5) morbid growths of the lung.

fre′nal [L. *fraenum*, bridle]. Pert. to the frenum.

frenose′cretory [" + *secernere*, to secrete]. Exercising an inhibitory power over the secretions.

frenotomy (fre-not′o-mĭ) [" + G. *tomē*, incision]. Division of any frenum, esp. for tongue-tie.

frenulum (pl. *frenula*). [L. a little bridle.]
SYN: *vinculum.* 1. A small frenum.
2. A small fold of white matter on the upper surface of the anterior medullary velum extending to the corpora quadrigemina.
   f. clitoridis. The union of inner parts of the labia minora on undersurface of the clitoris, *q.v.*
   f. labiorum pudendi. Fold of membrane connecting post. ends of labia minora.
   f. linguae. A fold of mucous membrane which extends from the floor of the mouth to the inferior surface of the tongue along its midline.
   f. praepu′tii. One that unites the foreskin (prepuce) to the glans penis.
   f. of tongue. One attaching lower side of tongue to the gum.

frenum (fre′num) (pl. *frena*) [L. *fraenum*, bridle]. A fold of mucous membrane which connects two parts, one more or less movable and which serves to check the movement of this part. SEE: *frenulum.*
   f. clitoridis. A stringlike structure at lower border of the 2 layers of the 2 labia minora forming the *praeputium clitoridis.*
   f. glandis. Median folds connecting lower surface of glans penis with skin of the body of penis.
   f. linguae. Fold on lower side of tongue attached to the gum.
   f. pudendi. The fourchette, *q.v.*

frenzy. A state of violent mental agitation; maniacal excitement.

fre′quency [L. *frequens*, often, constant].
1. The number of repetitions of a phenomenon in a certain period of time as the f. of heart beat, f. of sound vibrations. 2. In biometry, the ratio of the number of individuals falling into a single group to the total number of individuals classified. 3. The rate of oscillation or alternation in an alternating current circuit, in contradistinction to periodicity in the interruptions or regular variations of current in a direct current circuit.
The frequency is computed on the basis of a complete cycle, a complete cycle being one in which the current rises from zero to a maximum, returns to zero, and rises to an opposite maximum and returns to zero.

Freud, Sigmund (froyd). A famous Austrian psychoanalyst, whose teachings stress the theory:

1. Of the existence of a subconscious mind.

2. That psychical processes are never accidental or due to chance, but are determined by laws, as are physical events.

3. That emotional processes have the attributes of quantity, and can be displaced from one idea to another.

4. That the sex instinct does not develop at puberty, but that the child experiences a rich sexual life, and from this is derived the later stages of *narcissism* or self-love, *homosexuality* or attraction to the same sex, *heterosexuality*, which is the normal attraction to the opposite sex. SEE: *Œdipus complex.*

5. That dreams are fulfillments of wishes which find no realization in waking hours; theories are also formulated with regard to the importance of sex in dreams.

6. Freud also suggests that forgetting, misplacing articles, and slips of the tongue or pen are the outward mani-

festation of repression. SEE: *abreaction, psychoanalysis, etc.*

freudian (froy'di-an). Pert. to Sigmund Freud or his theories of unconscious or repressed libido or past sex experiences or desires as the cause of various neuroses, the cure for which is the restoration of such conditions to consciousness through psychoanalysis.

Freund's operation (froyndz). Total abdominal hysterectomy for cancer of uterus. SYN: *laparohysterectomy.*

fri'able [L. *friāre*, to crumble]. Easily broken or pulverized.

fric'tion (in massage) [L. *fricare*, to rub]. Strong, circular manipulations always followed by centripetal stroking.
Given with the thumb or the tips of the fingers. The aim is to squeeze pathologically changed parts, and by carrying the diseased tissues into the healthy substances, expose them to a firm stroking, so as to have them absorbed by the lymphatics. In hydrotherapy, friction is used in drying patients after tonic baths, shampoos, salt glows, wet mitten friction and drip sheet rubs.
 f., dry. F. using no liquid.
 f., moist. F. using a liquid or oil.
 f. murmur, f. sound. A frictional sound heard in pleurisy.

fric'tional electric'ity. Electricity produced by friction. SEE: *electricity, static.*

Friedländer's bacillus (frēd'len-derz). *Bacterium pneumoniae.*
 F.'s disease. Extreme degree of fibrous tissue in the intima closing the lumen. SYN: *endarteritis obliterans.*

Fried'man's test. The injection, in 4 cc. doses twice a day for 2 days, of the urine of a woman suspected of pregnancy into an unmated female rabbit will cause the formation of corpora lutea and corpora hemorrhagica in the rabbit at the end of 2 days if the woman is pregnant.

Fried'mann's disease. Relapsing infantile spastic spinal paralysis.

Fried'reich's ataxia (freed'rix). Rare disease resembling locomotor ataxia occurring in the children of a family, esp. girls. SYN: *family ataxia, hereditary ataxia.*
 F.'s disease. SEE: *F.'s ataxia.*
 F.'s sign. Sudden collapse of the cervical veins previously distended, at each diastole, caused by an adherent pericardium. The lowering of the pitch of the percussion note during inspiration which occurs over an area of cavitation.

fright [A.S. *fryhto*, fear]. Extreme sudden fear.
 f. neuroses. Traumatic hysteria.
 f. precordial. Anxiety felt before melancholic frenzy.

frigid (frij'id) [L. *frigor*, cold]. 1. Cold. 2. Irresponsive to emotion, applied esp. to the inability to feel sex desire on the part of a woman.

frigid'ity [L. *frigor*, cold]. In the female, absence of sexual desire. Inability to have an orgasm. TREAT: Massage or exercise of the pubococcygeus muscle.

frigolabile (frī-go-la'bl) [L. *frigor*, cold, + *labilis*, unstable]. Capable of being destroyed by low temperature.

frigorific (frig-o-rif'ik) [" + *facere*, to make]. Generating cold.

frig'orism [" + G. *ismos*, condition]. A condition due to long exposure to cold.

frigostabile (fri-go-sta'bl) [" + *stabilis*, firm]. Incapable of being destroyed by low temperature.

frigotherapy (frig-o-ther'ă-pī) [" + G. *therapeia*, treatment]. The use of cold in treatment of disease.

Frisch's bacillus. *Klebsiella rhinoscleromatis,* a gram-negative encapsulated bacillus found in the lesions of rhinoscleroma.

frit [Fr. *fritte, frire,* to fry]. 1. The material from which glass or the glazed portion of pottery is made. 2. A similar material for making the glaze of artificial teeth.

frog'belly. Flaccid abdomen in children afflicted by rickets, and atony of abdominal cells resulting from dyspepsia, accompanied by flatulence.
 f. face. Flatness of face resulting from intranasal disease.

Fröhde's reagent (freh'dez). A test for alkaloids; 1 part of sodium molybdate in 1000 parts of strong sulfuric acid.

Frohlich's syndrome (frā'liks). Dystrophia adiposogenitalis; a condition characterized by adiposity of the female type, atrophy or hypoplasia of the gonads, and altered secondary sex characteristics. Due to lesions of the hypothalamus and hypophysis.

Froin's syndrome (fro-wans'). Yellow cerebrospinal fluid which rapidly coagulates. It contains an excess of lymphocytes, and also globulin.

frolement (frol-mon') [Fr.]. 1. Very light friction with the hand in massage.* 2. A sound resembling rustling heard in auscultation.

Frommann's lines (from'mahnz). Transverse lines in the axis-cylinder of medullated nerve fibers after being stained by silver nitrate.

frons (fronz) [L.]. The forehead.

fron'tad [L. *frons, front-,* brow, + *ad,* toward]. Toward the frontal aspect.

frontal (fron'tal) [L. *frons, front-,* brow]. 1. Anterior. 2. Pertaining to the forehead bone.
 f. bone. Forehead bone.
 f. lobe (of the cerebrum). Four main convolutions in front of the central *sulcus.*
 f. plane. A plane parallel with the long axis of the body and at right angles to the median sagittal plane.
 f. sinuses. A pair of hollow spaces in the frontal bone lying above the orbits. They are lined with mucous membrane, contain air, and communicate with the middle nasal meatus by means of the nasofrontal duct.

fronto- [L. *frons, front-,* brow]. Prefix: Ant. position, or relationship with the forehead.

frontoma'lar [" + *mala,* cheek]. Rel. to the frontal and malar bones.

frontomax'illary [" + *maxilla,* jaw]. Rel. to the frontal bone and maxillary bones.

frontoparietal (fron"to-pă-ri'ē-tăl) [" + *parietalis,* pert. to a wall]. Pert. to the frontal and parietal bones.

frontotem'poral [" + *tempora,* the temples]. Pert. to frontal and temporal bones.

front-tap reflex. Contraction of gastrocnemius muscles resulting from percussing stretched muscles of extended leg.

frost'bite. Freezing or effect of freezing of a part of the body.
The nose, fingers, and toes are usually the parts affected.
 SYM: Tingling, redness, followed by paleness and numbness of affected area.

It is of 3 degrees: (a) Transitory hyperemia following numbness; (b) formation of vesicles, and (c) gangrene.

F. A. TREATMENT: The Red Cross now advises rapid warming of frostbitten parts of the body of persons who have suffered prolonged exposures to cold. Stimulate with tea, coffee, beef tea. Artificial respiration if unconscious. Cases have been known to recover when parts were black and all hope had been given up, except amputation.

f.-itch. Itching skin disease in cold climates. SYN: *pruritus hiemalis*.

frottage (fro-tazh') [Fr. rubbing]. 1. A condition of *hyperesthesia sexualis* often associated with lowered virility inducing an irresistible impulse of pressing up behind women in crowds, thus producing an orgasm. 2. Massage technic using rubbing.

trotteur (fro-ter') [Fr. *frottage*, rubbing]. One who practices frottage.

frozen sleep. Hypothermia, *q.v.*

fruc'tose [L. *fructus*, fruit]. Levulose. Fruit sugar.

A monosaccharose and a hexose, having the same empirical formula as glucose, $C_6H_{12}O_6$, and found in corn syrup, honey, fruit juices, and in the syrup resulting from the inversion of sucrose; an invert sugar. It produces glycogen and maintains normal content of glucose in the blood. In the liver, it may be converted into glycogen which, in turn, may be converted into glucose. SEE: *disaccharose*.

fructosuria (fruk"to-sū'rĭ-ă) [" + G. *ouron*, urine]. Fructose in the urine.

fruit [L. *fructus*, fruit]. BOT: A ripened ovary consisting of a seed or seeds and the surrounding tissue. Ex: *pod of a bean, nut, grain, pome*, or *berry*. The edible product of a plant consisting of ripened seeds and the enveloping tissue.

COMP: Carbohydrates in the form of fruit sugar form the chief nutritive value of fruits. Seventy-five per cent of it is a mixture of dextrose and levulose. Proteins and energy factors are variable. Good source of vitamins and mineral elements. Iodine content, 6 to 120 parts per billion. *Pectose bodies*: The principle in fruits that causes them to jelly. *Pectose*, found in unripe fruit. *Pectin*, found in ripe fruit. *Pectosic acid*, from pectose, in cooked fruit. *Pectic acid*, from pectin, in fruit cooked a long time.

PRINCIPAL ACIDS IN FRUITS AND OTHER FOODS: 1. Acetic, in wine and vinegar. 2. Citric, in lemons, oranges, limes, citron, etc. 3. Malic, in apples, pears, apricots, peaches, currants, gooseberries, etc. 4. Tannic, in gallnuts. 5. Oxalic, in rhubarb, sorrel, cranberries, etc. 6. Tartaric, in grapes, pineapples and tamarinds. 7. Salicylic, in currants, cranberries, cherries, plums, grapes, crabapples and berries. *Combined acids*: (a) Citric; (b) malic, in raspberries, strawberries, gooseberries, cherries, etc. (a) Citric, (b) malic, (c) oxalic in cranberries. They contain iron and other mineral substances. Some of the fruit acids, esp., citric and malic acids, when oxidized in the body leave an alkaline residue and thus have an alkalizing effect.

ONE CLASSIFICATION OF FRUITS: 1. Watery, acidulated fruits. 2. Sugar-containing fruits. 3. Amylaceous or oil fruits. The water of fruits possesses special properties similar to mineral spring water.

fruit sugar. Fructose, levulose, *q.v.*

frumentaceous (fru-men-ta'she-us) [L. *frumentum*, grain]. Resembling or belonging to grain.

frumenti, spiritus [L. essence of grain]. Whisky.

frumentum (fru-men'tum) [L. grain]. Wheat or other grain.

frustration [L. *frustrā*, in vain]. 1. The failure of libido to find adequate outlet. 2. The condition which results from the thwarting or prevention of acts which if performed would bring satisfaction or gratification of physical or personality needs.

FSH. The follicle stimulating hormone secreted by the ant. lobe of the hypophysis.

Ft. Abbr. of L. *fiat*, or *fiant*, let there be made. Also for *florentium*.

fuel value. Energy to be produced by oxidation of edible foods after eating. SEE: *calory, energy, food requirements*.

-fuge [L.]. Suffix meaning *to expel*.

fugitive (fu'jit-iv) [L. *fugitivus*, wandering]. 1. Temporary, transient. 2. Wandering; pert. to inconstant symptoms.

fugue (fūg) [L. *fuga*, flight]. 1. Flight automatism. Leaving home or surroundings on a hysterical impulse generally with loss of memory as to identity and the past. 2. PSY: A form of consciousness similar to that produced by dual or multiple personality, purpose and direction of conduct and action being retained.

Fuld's test. A test for the antipyretic power of the blood serum.

fulgurant (ful'gu-rant) [L. *fulgurāre*, to lighten]. Severe and sudden, as a *f. pain*.

ful'gurating [L. *fulgurāre*, to lighten]. Pert. to fulguration. SYN: *fulgurant*.

fulguration (ful-gu-ra'shun) [L. *fulgurāre*, to lighten]. Destruction of tissue by means of long high frequency electric sparks. SEE: *electrodesiccation*.

fuliginous (fu-lij'in-us) [L. *fuligō*, spot]. Resembling soot, esp. in color.

full'ing [A.S. *fullian*, to fill]. A movement in massage; kneading.

Palms hold a limb bet. them, the fingers extended, the limb being rolled backward and forward.

full term. Normal end of pregnancy, when the fetus is 20-21 in. long, has finger and toenails reaching to end of digits, and, if a boy, with both testicles descended. It should weigh from 7 lb. upward and have been nourished in the womb for not less than 40 weeks.

ful'minant [L. *fulmināre*, to lighten]. Fulgurant. Coming in lightninglike flashes of pain, as in tabes dorsalis.

ful'minating [L. *fulmināre*, to lighten]. Fulgurant; occurring with very great rapidity, said of certain pains.

fumes [L. *fumus*, smoke]. Vapors, esp. those having irritating qualities.

f., nitric acid. Used in various chemical processes.

SYM: Choking, gasping, swelling of mucous membranes, tightness in chest, cough and shock. Symptoms may last for 1 week or more.

TREATMENT: Allow patient to inhale aromatic spirits of ammonia, followed by steam inhalations at intervals and oily spray repeatedly. Oxygen may be necessary because of limited space for air exchange.

fumig'ant. An agent used in fumigation. Common fumigants are hydrocyanic acid, calcium cyanids, methyl bromide, sulfur dioxide, naphthalene, and ortho- and paradichlorobenzene.

fumiga'tion [L. *fumigāre*, to fumigate].
1. The use of poisonous fumes or gases to destroy living organisms, esp., rats, mice, insects, and other vermin. Fumigants are relatively ineffective against bacteria and viruses, consequently the practice of terminal disinfection of the sick room, formerly a common practice, has been discontinued. 2. The disinfecting of rooms by gases.

fu'ming [L. *fumus*, smoke]. Having a visible vapor.

function (fŭng'shŭn) [L. *functia, fungi,* to perform]. 1. The action performed by any structure. In a living organism this may pertain to a cell or a part of a cell, tissue, organ, or system of organs. 2. The act of carrying on or performing a special activity. Normal function is the normal action of an organ. Abnormal functioning or the failure of an organ to perform its function are the bases of disease or disease processes. Structural changes in an organ constitute pathological changes and are common cause of malfunctioning although an organ may function abnormally in the absence of observable structural changes.

function, words pert. to: absorption, anabolism, analogue, assimilation, atelic, cacergasia, catabolism, catabiotic, choloscopy, digestion, excretion, metabolism, secretion, syzygiology.

func'tional [L. *functio, fungi,* to perform]. 1. Pertaining to function. 2. A word applied to disturbances of function in a variety of ways.
The disturbance of function of one organ by structural change in another is at times termed functional, but incorrectly, as it represents organic change. Disturbances of function resulting from unfortunate conditioning of the organism to an external situation may more suitably be called functional, though this "conditioning" may be purely structural.
   f. disease. One not organic, or in which changes of an organ are not in evidence; a disturbance of any organ's functions.
   f. psychosis. One exhibited in psychosis, in which no pathology of the central nervous system is apparent.

funda (fŭn'dă) [L. a sling]. A four-tailed bandage.

fundal (fŭn'dal) [L. *fundus*, base]. Pert. to a fundus.

fund'ament [L. *fundamentum*, foundation]. 1. A foundation. 2. The anus.

fund'ic. Pertaining to a fundus.

fun'diform [L. *fundus,* sling, + *forma,* shape]. Sling-shaped or looped.

fun'dus (pl. *fundi*) [L. base]. 1. The larger part, base, or body of a hollow organ. 2. The portion of an organ most remote from its opening.
   f. glands. Minute tubelike glands of the gastric mucosa in the cardiac section.
   f. uteri. The body of the uterus from the internal os of the cervix upward above the fallopian tubes.
   f. oculi. Post. inner part of eye as seen with ophthalmoscope.

fundusectomy (fun-dus-ek'to-mĭ) [" + G. *ektomē*, excision]. Excision of the fundus of the stomach. SYN: *cardiectomy*.

fun'gate [L. *fungus*, mushroom]. To grow like a fungus.

fungating (fŭn'gāt-ing) [L. *fungus*, mushroom]. Growing rapidly like a fungus, applied to certain tumors.

fungi (fŭn'jī) [L. *fungus,* mushroom]. 1. Plural of fungus. 2. A division of plants which includes the bacteria, slime molds, algalike fungi, sac fungi, club fungi, and imperfect fungi. They were formerly considered as a subdivision of the Thallophytes. Fungi are simple dependent plants lacking chlorophyll. Their bodies show little differentiation and they have relatively simple life cycles. They include the molds, rusts, mushrooms, toadstools, lichens, and yeasts. Many forms are pathogenic to plants and animals.
   f. fission. The bacteria or Schizomycetes.
   f. imperfect. The Fungi Imperfects (Class *Deuteromycetes*). A group of fungi so-called because their life cycles are only partly known, the sexual stage being absent. Many species are parasitic causing disease.
   f. slime. The slime molds (*Myxomycetes*).
   f. true. Fungi with a plant body composed of hyphae. Include the algal fungi (*Phycomycetes*), sac fungi (*Ascomycetes*), club fungi (*Basidiomycetes*) and imperfect fungi (*Fungi Imperfecta*).

fungicide (fun'ji-sīd) [" + *caedere*, to kill]. Bactericide; that which destroys bacteria or fungi.

fung'icid'in. An antibiotic obtained from *Streptomycetes griseus* which possesses fungistatic and fungicidal properties. It is not antibacterial.

fungiform (fŭn'jif-orm) [" + *forma,* shape]. Fungus-shaped.
   f. papillae. Small, rounded eminences on middle and ant. parts of dorsum and esp. along sides of tongue.

fungista'sis [" + G. *stasis*, a halting]. A condition in which the growth of fungi is inhibited. SEE: *fungicide.*

fun'gistat [" + G. *statikos,* standing]. That which inhibits the growth of fungi.

fungistat'ic [" + G. *statikos,* standing]. Inhibiting the growth of fungi.

fungoid (fŭn'goid) [" + G. *eidos,* form]. Having the appearance of a fungus.
   f., chignon. Bacterial growth of the hair. SEE: *chignon f.*

fungosity (fun-gos'it-ĭ) [L. *fungus*, mushroom]. A soft excrescence.

fungous (fŭn'gus) [L. *fungus*, mushroom]. 1. Fungoid, *q.v.* 2. Swiftly growing, as a soft excrescence.

fungus (fŭn'gus) [L. *mushroom*]. 1. A vegetable cellular organism that subsists on organic matter, such as bacteria and molds. 2. A plant belonging to the division Fungi. 3. A sponge-like morbid excrescence on the body resembling fungus. SEE: *actinomycosis, cladosporiosis.*
   f. haematodes. Malignant bleeding growth.

fu'nic [L. *funis*, cord]. Pert. to the umbilical cord.
   f. souffle. SYM: The purring sound heard over the pregnant uterus, and having the same rate as the fetal heart beat.

fu'nicle [L. *funiculus*, little cord]. A small, threadlike structure. SYN: *funiculus.*

funicular (fū-nik'ŭ-lar) [L. *funiculus,* little cord]. Pert. to the spermatic, or umbilical cord.
   f. process. That part of the tunica vaginalis that covers the spermatic cord.

funiculitis (fu-nik-u-li'tis) [" + G. *-itis,* inflammation]. Inflammation of the spermatic cord.

funiculopexy (fū-nik'ŭ-lo-peks-ĭ) [" + G. *pēxis,* fixation]. Suturing the spermatic cord to the tissues in cases of undescended testicle.

funiculus (fu-nik'u-lus) (pl. *funiculi*) [L. little cord]. 1. Any small structure resembling a cord. 2. A division of the white matter of the spinal cord consisting of fasciculi or fiber tracts lying peripherally to the gray matter. Differentiated into dorsal, lateral, and ventral funiculi. 3. Old term for the umbilical cord or the spermatic cord. 4. Formerly a synonym for *fasciculus*, q.v.

fu'niform [L. *funis*, cord, + *forma*, shape]. Cordlike.

fu'nis [L. cord]. 1. A cordlike structure. 2. The umbilical cord.

fun'nel [L. *fundere*, to pour]. Conical, wide, open-mouthed device for pouring through its open tube at end into another vessel.
   f. drainage. Drainage by funnels.
   f. breast. Sternal depression of chest walls resembling a funnel.

funny bone. The internal condyle of the humerus.

fur [Fr. *forre*, covering]. A deposit forming on the tongue, q.v.

furacin. Trade name for *nitrofurazone*, q.v.

fur'cal [L. *furca*, fork]. Forked.

furcula. The hypobranchial eminence, an elevation in the floor of the embryonic pharynx at the level of the 3rd and 4th branchial arches. It gives rise to the epiglottis and the aryepiglottic folds.

furfur (fur'fur) [L. bran]. Scurf; dandruff.

furfuraceous (fur-fu-ra'shus) [L. *furfur*, bran]. Scaly, or resembling scales.

furibund (fū'rĭ-bund) [L. *furibundus*, *furere*, to rage]. Maniacal; raging, as in certain types of insanity.

fu'ror [L. rage]. PSY: Extremely violent outbursts of anger, often without provocation.
   f. amatorius. Insatiable sexual desire.
   f. epilepticus. Epileptic insanity, or sudden anger as expressed by epileptics.
   f. femininus. Nymphomania.*
   f. genitalis. Erotomania.*
   f. uterinus. SEE: *f. femininus*.

furuncle (fū'rung-kl) [L. *furunculus*, a boil]. A boil. SYN: *furunculus*.

furunc'ular [L. *furunculus*, a boil]. Pert. to a boil.

furunculoid (fū-rung'kŭ-loid) [" + G. *eidos*, form]. Resembling a furuncle or boil. SYN: *furunculous*.

furunculosis (fū-rung-kŭ-lo'sis) [" + G. *ōsis*]. A condition resulting from boils.

furunc'ulous [L. *furunculus*, boil]. Pert. to or of the nature of a boil or boils.

furun'culus (fu-rung'ku-lus) [L. a boil]. Boil, furuncle. Acute, deep-seated phlegmonous inflammation formed in the skin usually ending in suppuration and necrosis.
   ETIOL: Bacterial, promoted by lessened resistance to microbic invasion, trauma, irritation (chemical), excessive sweating, focal infection.
   SYM: Neck, axillae, face, buttocks and legs are sites of predilection, beginning in hair follicle or sudoriparous gland as subcutaneous swelling or acuminate pustule around hair shaft, skin smooth and shining, with pain and tenderness. Lesion may come to head, or become boggy and fluctuant, or regression may take place before suppuration, resulting in disappearance by absorption (blind boil). Lesion ruptures on maturity, discharging core, necrotic tissue, and pus; healing follows.
   TREATMENT: Eradication of systemic disease. Yeast, autogenous vaccines, sodium citrate. Locally, hot, moist, antiseptic dressings to hasten maturity followed by radical incision when lesion is walled off. Soft poultices to be avoided. Alpine sun lamp, x-rays, calf liver diet, insulin in presence of blood sugar.

Fusarium (fū-za'rĭ-um) [L. *fusus*, a spindle]. A genus of fungus.

fuscin. A brown pigment, a melanin, present in the outermost layer (pigmented epithelium) of the retina.

fuse [L. *fusus*, *fundere*, to pour]. A safety device comprising a strip of wire of easily fusible metal, the conductance of which is predetermined. The metal fuses and breaks circuit when excess of current passes through. Convenient forms mounted in plugs, bet. hard metal ends under screwheads.

fu'sible [L. *fusus*, a thing poured]. Capable of being melted.

fu'siform [L. *fusus*, spindle, + *forma*, shape]. 1. Tapering at both ends. Spindle-shaped. 2. BIOL: Pert. to gelatin which liquefies in parsnip form.

Fusifor'mis [" + *forma*, shape]. A genus of *Mycobacteriaceae* containing spindle-shaped organisms.
   F. ac'nes. *Corynebacterium acnes*.
   F. den'tium. Long spindle-shaped organisms associated with *Borrelia vincenti* in ulcerative stomatitis.

fusion (fu'shun) [L. *fundere*, to pour]. Meeting and joining together through liquefaction by heat. The process of fusing or uniting.
   f. faculty. Blending of the images of binocular vision into a single perception having the quality of depth.
   f. spinal. The fusion of two or more vertebrae, an operation resorted to in the treatment of certain deformities of the spine.

Fus'obacter'ium. A genus of nonspore forming, nonencapsulated, nonmotile, gram-negative bacteria usually found in necrotic lesions, associated with spirochaetes.
   F. plauti-vincenti. A species found in lesion of the buccal cavity.

fusocel'lular [L. *fusus*, spindle, + *cellulus*, little cell]. Spindle celled.

fusospirillosis (fū"so-spir-il-o'sis) [" + *spirillum*, coil, + G. *-ōsis*]. Vincent's angina.

fusospirochetal (fū"zo-spi-ro-ke'tăl) [" + G. *speira*, coil, + *chaitē*, hair]. Pert. to fusiform bacilli and spirochetes such as found in Vincent's angina.

fusospirocheto'sis [" + " + " + *-ōsis*]. Infection with fusiform bacilli and spirochetes.

fusostreptococcosis (fū"so-strep"to-kok-ko'sis) [" + G. *streptos*, twisted, + *kokkos*, berry, + *-ōsis*]. Infection with fusiform bacteria and streptococcus.

fustiga'tion [L. *fustigare*, to beat with a rod]. In massage, beating with light rods.

fututio (fū-tū'shĭ-o). Sexual intercourse.

fututrix (fū-tū'triks). A girl or woman who practices tribadism, q.v.

G

G. 1. A constant in Newton's law of gravitation. 2. In aviation physiology, G. is a unit of force resulting from acceleration or centrifugal motion.

Ga. Chemical symb. for *gallium*.

gad'fly. An insect which lays eggs under the skin of its victim, which cause swellings simulating a boil. Multiple furuncles appear with hatching of larva. A fly belonging to the family Tabanidae, *q.v.* Includes horseflies, deerflies, and other bloodsucking flies.
TREATMENT: Evacuate larva and apply antiseptics of benzoin and carbolic acid type. SEE: *botfly*.

gadolinium (gad-o-lin'ĭ-um). SYMB: Gd. A very rare element; at. wt., 157.3.

Gaffkya (gaf'kĭ-ă). A genus of bacteria of the family *Micrococcaceae*.
G. tetrag'ena. SYN: *Micrococcus tetragenus*. Found associated with the tubercle bacillus and present in lesions of the respiratory passageways, in the blood and spinal fluid. Of low pathogenicity.

gag [imitative]. 1. Device for keeping the jaws open or forcibly opening the mouth. 2. To retch or cause to retch.
g. reflex. Gagging and vomiting resulting from irritation of fauces.

gait (gāt) [A.S. *geat*, gate, door]. Manner of walking.
CHARACTERISTIC: 1. Body leans backward and feet are widely separated in pregnancy, obesity, ascites, and large abdominal tumors. 2. Limping or hobbling gait is seen in rheumatism, sciatica, hip or knee joint disease or injury, metatarsal neuralgia, and affections of lower extremities. 3. When standing with feet close together in locomotor ataxia, aural vertigo, disease of middle cerebellar lobe, patient sways extremely and may fall. 4. Gait is slovenly in the weak, anemic, and apathetic, and in chronic mental or physical defects.
SEE: *asynergia, adiadochokinesis, brachybasia, dysmetria, steppage, walking*.
g., ataxic. Raising foot high, striking ground suddenly with entire sole.
g., brachybasic. Shuffling gait of partial paraplegia.
g., cerebellar. A staggering movement.
g., cow. Swaying due to knock-knees.
g., equine. Raising foot by flexing thigh on abdomen. Characteristic of peroneal paralysis. Slow, awkward.
g., festinating. Body bent forward and rigid. Walks on toes as though pushed. Starts slowly, increases and does not stop until patient meets an obstruction. Seen in paralysis agitans.
g., flat-footed. Toes everted, legs often bowed.
g., frog. That of infantile paralysis: hopping.
g., hemiplegic. Patient abducts paralyzed limb, swings it around and brings it forward so foot comes to ground in front of him.
g., Huntington's chorea. A few normal paces, a long slow one, and then one or two hops.
g., multiple neuritis. That of a high-stepping horse. Steppage gait, *q.v.*
g., paralysis agitans. Tendency to begin slowly, then rapidly, falling forward.
g., paralytic. Feet dragged with slow movements. Stumbles easily. Seen in chronic myelitis.
g., scissor. One in which legs cross in walking.
g., spastic. A stiff movement, toes seeming to catch and drag, legs held together, hips and knee joints slightly flexed. Seen in spastic paraplegia, sclerosis of lateral pyramidal columns of cord. Also in tumor of spinal cord and arachnoiditis.
g., steppage. Foot and toes lifted high, heel brought down first. Seen in peripheral neuritis, late stages of diabetes, alcoholism, chronic arsenical poisoning.
g., waddling. Feet wide apart and walk resembling that of a duck. Seen in coxa vera and double congenital displacement of hip when lordosis is present.

galact-, galacto- [G.]. Combining forms, pert. to *milk*.

galactacrasia (gal-ak-tă-krā'zĭ-ă) [G. *gala*, milk, + *krasis*, mixture]. An abnormal composition of milk.

galactan (gal-ak'tan) [G. *gala*, milk]. A complex carbohydrate forming galactose upon hydrolysis.

galac'tase [G. *gala*, milk]. An enzyme or proteolytic ferment of milk.

galacte'mia, galacthemia (gal-ak-the'mĭ-ă) [" + *aima*, blood]. Milky condition of the blood.

galactic (gal-ăk'tĭk) [G. *gala*, milk]. Pert. to flow of milk.

galactidrosis (gal-ak-tĭ-drō'sĭs) [" + *idrōs*, sweat]. A milklike sweat.

galactin (ga-lak'tin) [G. *gala*, milk]. A basic amorphous substance in milk. SYN: *prolactin*.

galactischia (găl-ăk'tĭs-kĭ-ăh). SYN: *galactoschesis*. Suppression of the secretion and flow of milk.

galactoblast (gal-ak'to-blast) [" + *blastos*, germ]. Body found in mammary acini; contains fat globules.

galactocele (gal-ak'to-sēl) [" + *kēlē*, hernia]. 1. A tumor caused by the retention of fluid in a milk duct. 2. Hydrocele containing a milklike liquid.

galactogogue (gal-ak'to-gog) [" + *agōgos*, leading]. Agent that promotes the flow of milk.

galact'oid. Resembling milk.

galact'olip'in. A phosphorus-free nitrogenous combined with galactose; a cerebroside.

galactoma (gal-ak-to'ma) [" + *ōma*, tumor]. Cystic tumor of female breast. SYN: *galactocele*, 1.

galactom'eter [" + *metron*, measure].

Device for measuring amt. of cream in milk by its specific gravity and degree of opacity. SYN: *lactometer.*

galactop'athy [" + *pathos,* disease]. 1. Treatment of nursing infants by drugs administered to the mother. 2. Therapeutic use of milk.

galactopex'ic [G. *gala,* milk, + *pēxis,* fixation]. Making galactose permanent.

galac'topexy [" + *pēxis,* fixation]. The fixation of galactose.

galactophagous (gal-ak-tof'ag-us) [" + *phagein,* to eat]. Feeding upon milk.

galactophlysis (gal-ak-tof'lis-is) [" + *phlysis,* eruption]. 1. Eruption of vesicles containing milklike contents. 2. Infantile seborrhea of scalp. SYN: *crusta lactea.*

galac'tophore [" + *pherein,* to bear]. A milk duct.

galactophoritis (gal-ak-tof-or-i'tis) [" + " + *-itis,* inflammation]. Inflammation of a milk duct.

galactophorous (gal-ak-tof'or-us) [" + *pherein,* to bear]. Giving milk.
  g. ducts. Excretory ducts of the mammae.

galactophthisis (gal-ak-tof'this-is) [" + *phthisis,* wasting]. Debility and emaciation as result of excessive milk secretion.

galactophygous (gal-ak-tof'ig-us) [" + *phygē,* flight]. Arresting flow of milk.

galactoplania (gal-ak-top-la'nĭ-ă) [" + *planē,* wandering]. Secretion of milk in some abnormal part due to suppression of normal lactation.

galactopoietic (gal-ak"to-poy-et'ĭk) [" + *poiein,* to make]. Having to do with the production of milk.

galactopyra (gal-ak-to-pi'ră) [" + *pyr,* fire]. Milk fever.

galactorrhea (gal-ak-tor-e'ă) [" + *roia,* flow]. 1. Continuation of lactation, or flow of milk at intervals after cessation of nursing. 2. Excessive flow of milk.

galactoschesia, galactoschesis (gal-ak-tos-ke'sĭ-ă, -tos'ke-sis) [" + *schesis,* suppression]. A stopping of the milk secretion.

galactoscope (gal-ak'to-skōp) [" + *skopein,* to examine]. Device for measuring quality of milk. SYN: *galactometer, lactoscope.*

galactose (găl-ăk'tōs) [G. *gala,* milk]. $C_6H_{12}O_6$ a monosaccharide or simple hexose sugar.
  Galactose is an isomer of glucose and is formed along with glucose, in the hydrolysis of lactose. It is dextrorotatory and reduces alkaline copper solutions such as Fehling's solution. It is a component of cerebrosides. In the digestive tract, galactose is readily absorbed; in the liver it is converted into glycogen.
  g. tolerance test. Patient fasts overnight and then empties bladder. 40 Gm. of galactose in 500 cc. of water are taken orally, then specimens of urine are collected hourly for five hours and the amount of galactose excreted determined. A normal person will excrete up to 3 Gm. in this period. Amounts esp. above 6 Gm. in excess of this indicate impairment of liver function.

galactosis (gal-ak-to'sis) [" + *ōsis*]. The secretion of milk.

galactostasis (gal-ak-tos'ta-sis) [" + *stasis,* a stopping]. Cessation or checking of milk secretion. SYN: *galactoschesia.*

galactosu'ria [" + *ouron,* urine]. Galactose in the urine.

galactotherapy (gal-ak-to-ther'ă-pĭ) [" + *therapeia,* treatment]. Treatment of a nursing infant by drugs administered to the mother. SYN: *galactopathy.*

galactotoxin (gal-ak"to-toks'in) [" + *toxikon,* poison]. A poison in milk produced by bacteria.

galactotox'ism [" + " + *ismos,* state of]. Milk poisoning.

galactotrophy (gal-ak-tot'ro-fĭ) [" + *trophē,* nourishment]. Feeding with nothing but milk.

galactoxism (gal-ak-toks'izm) [" + *toxikon,* poison, + *ismos,* state of]. Poisoning by milk. SYN: *galactotoxism.*

galactozymase (gal-ak-to-zi'mās) [" + *zymē,* leaven]. A starch hydrolyzing ferment in milk.

galactu'ria [" + *ouron,* urine]. The passing of milky urine. SYN: *chyluria.*

ga'lea [L. helmet]. The epicranial aponeurosis which connects the bellies of the occipitofrontal muscle.

galeanthropy (ga-le-an'thro-pĭ) [G. *galē,* cat, + *anthrōpos,* man]. A delusion that one has become transformed into a cat.

Ga'len, Claudius. (130-200?) A noted Greek physician and medical writer, born in Mysia and later residing in Rome. Recognized as the "authority" on medicine until the Middle Ages. Called the father of experimental physiology.

galen'ic. Pertaining to Galen or his teachings.

galenicals, galenics (gă-lĕn'ĭ-kăls, -ĭks). 1. Herb and vegetable medicines. 2. Crude drugs and medicinals as distinguished from pure active principles contained in them. 3. A medicine prepared according to an official formula.

Ga'len's veins. The veins running through the tela chorioidea formed by the joining of the terminal and choroid veins, and forming the v. cerebri magna which empties into the straight sinus.

galeophilia (gal-e-o-fĭl'ĭ-ă) [G. *galē,* cat, + *philein,* to love]. Fondness for cats.

galeophobia (gal-e-o-fo'bĭ-ă) [" + *phobos,* fear]. Abnormal aversion to cats.

galeropia, galeropsia (gal-er-o'pĭ-ă, -rop'-sĭ-ă) [G. *galeros,* cheerful, + *opsis,* vision]. Unusual clearness of vision.

gall [A.S. *galla*]. 1. An excoriation. 2. The bitter secretion of the liver stored in the gallbladder bile.
  It has no ferments and it assists in the emulsifying of fats. It also stimulates intestinal action and multiplies the action of the pancreatic juice threefold. It is discharged through the cystic duct into the duodenum.
  RS: *words; bile duct; calculus; "chol-" words; colic, biliary; cystic duct; vesica fellea.*

gall'bladder [A.S. *galla* + *blaeddre,* bladder, blister]. Pear-shaped sac on undersurface of right lobe of liver holding bile from the liver until discharged through cystic duct; ¾ in. long, 1 in. greatest diameter; capacity 50-75 cc. concentrated bile equivalent to 1½ pt. liver bile.
  DIET IN DISEASES OF: In decreased flow, low fat diet using emulsified fats. In distress aggravated by peristalsis, use a low residue diet. Five small meals a day for all disorders of gallbladder. Eggs have a tendency to empty the gallbladder. Avoid chocolate, fats, ice cream, and foods containing them. No condi-

ments or strong coffee, small amount of salt allowable, no strongly flavored vegetables. No fried foods.
Syn: *vesica fellea*.

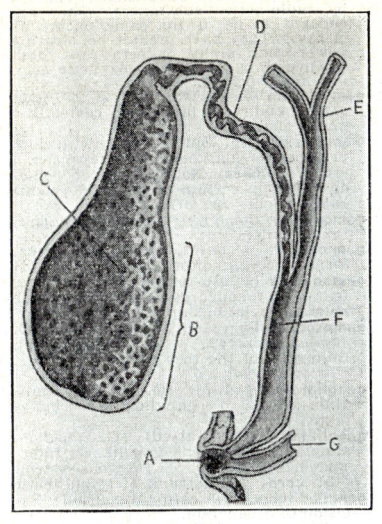

GALLBLADDER
A. Ampulla in duodenal wall into which both ducts open. B. Fundus. C. Gallbladder. D. Cystic duct. E. Common hepatic duct. F. Bile duct. G. Pancreatic duct.

gall'duct [" + L. *ductus*, a passage]. Tube carrying bile from the liver and gallbladder.

gal'lon. Four quarts; 231 cubic inches.

gall'stone [A.S. *galla*, bile, + *stān*, stone]. Concretion formed in the gallbladder or bile ducts generally after 35th year.
  Gallstones may be classified as (1) *pure*, consisting of either cholesterol, calcium bilirubin, or calcium carbonate, or (2) *mixed*, consisting of cholesterol in combination with one or more of the other constituents. In addition to the substances named, gallstones may contain albuminates, cellular debris, or foreign substances such as bacteria, esp., typhoid bacilli. So called "soft" stones (those consisting principally of cholesterol) can be visualized by x-ray only under optimal conditions by cholecystography.
  Sym: Stone may remain dormant and give little distress unless inflammation and distention of the gallbladder take place or unless it enters and is unable to pass through the biliary ducts, when colic ensues. The pain may radiate to the back and right shoulder, usually several hours after eating and when the stomach is empty; flatulence, jaundice usually absent.
  Treatment: Hot turpentine fomentation over region of gallbladder; hypodermic of morphine under physician's directions; surgical aid. Surgery.
  NP (postoperative): Position, propped up in bed to prevent pneumonia, to permit free drainage, and relieve pressure on diaphragm. Lavage if vomiting is persistent. Only liquids in small amt.

given. Note character of drainage and stools for color and nature of contents, and for proper discharge of bile. Protect drainage from all areas. Use cradle if no dressing is permitted, and absorbent pad at side for discharge. Syn: *biliary calculus*.
  RS: *bilifuscin, biliphein, biliprasin, calculus, cholecystendisis, cholelithiasis*.

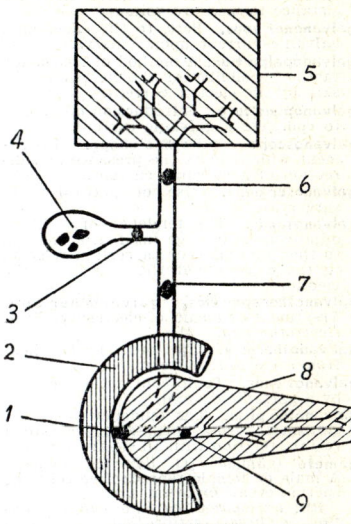

GALLSTONES
(After Sears)
Diagram showing the positions in which gallstones may be found. 1. Gallstone impacted at entrance of bile duct into duodenum. 2. Duodenum. 3. Cystic duct. 4. Gallbladder with stones. 5. Liver. 6. Hepatic duct. 7. Common bile duct. 8. Pancreas. 9. Pancreatic duct with pancreatic calculus.

Gal'ton's whistle. A whistle with which a note may be changed, used to test the hearing.

galvan'ic. Pert. to galvanism.
  g. battery. A series of cells, giving a combined effect of all the units, and generating electricity by chemical reaction.
  g. cell. One of a series of cells generating electricity through chemical reaction.

gal'vanism. Therapeutic use of direct current of electricity.

galvanization (gal-van-i-za'shun). Employment of a galvanic current.

galvanocau'tery. Cauterization of tissue by means of an electric current. See: *electrocautery*.

galvanocontractil'ity. Capability of a muscle of contracting under a galvanic stimulation.

galvanofaradiza'tion. Combined use of galvanic and faradic current made possible by use of a De Watteville switch.

galvanom'eter. An instrument that measures current by electromagnetic action.
  It may consist of a magnetic needle delicately suspended in the center of a permanent coil of wire, or a suspended coil between the poles of a fixed mag-

net. When the current is applied to the coil, the needle is deflected over a calibrated scale.

Galvanometers detect current and enable one to determine its direction, amperage, and voltage. The d'Arsonval form is more common, in which a coil moves in a permanent magnetic field. The instrument is called a voltmeter when used in series with a high resistance to measure voltage.

galvanoner′vous. Pert. to the effect of a galvanic current upon a nerve.

galvanopalpa′tion. A method of measuring tactile sensibility of the nerves of the skin by the electric current.

galvanopunc′ture. Introduction of needles to complete a galvanic current.

galvanoscope (gal-van′o-skop). Instrument which shows the presence and direction of a galvanic current.

galvanosur′gery. Use of galvanism in surgery.

galvanotax′is. The tendency of a living organism to arrange itself in a medium so that its axis bears a certain relation to the direction of the current in the medium.

galvanotherapeu′tics, galvanother′apy. Treatment by means of electricity. SYN: *electrotherapy.*

gal′vanotherm″y. Treatment by the heat from a galvanic battery.

galvanot′onus. Tonic contractions caused by a galvanic current.

galvanotro′pism. The tendency of an organism to grow, turn, or move into a certain relation with an electric current.

gamete (gam′ēt) [G. *gametēs,* spouse]. A male or female reproductive cell; the spermatozoon or ovum, *q.v.*

RS: *anisogamy, chromosome, conception, embryo, fertilization, gene, maturation, ovum, spermatozoon.*

The ovum (1/125 in. in diameter) and the spermatozoon (1/500 in. in length). Each mature human germ cell has 48 chromosomes or 24 pairs which are reduced to one-half the number during maturation.

gamet′ic (G. *gametēs,* spouse]. Pert. to gametes.

gametocide (gam′et-o-sīd) [" + L. *caedere,* to kill]. An agent destructive to malarial gametocytes.

gametocyte (gam′et-o-sīt) [" + *kytos,* cell]. The sexual cell forming the gamete. An oocyte or spermatocyte.

gametogen′esis. For formation of gametes: oogenesis or spermatogenesis. SEE: *maturation.*

gametog′ony. The phase in the life cycle of the malarial parasite (*Plasmodium*) in which male and female gametocytes, which infect the mosquito, are formed.

gamet′ophyte. In plants, the sexual or gamete-producing generation which alternates with the asexual or spore-producing generation.

Gam′gee tissue. A dressing made of a thick layer of absorbent cotton between 2 layers of absorbent gauze; used for surgical dressing.

gam′ic. Sexual; esp. as applied to eggs which develop only after fertilization in contrast to those which develop parthenogenetically.

gam′ma (G. letter g.). 1. Third letter of the Greek alphabet. 2. In Chem., used to designate the third of a series, as the third carbon atom in an aliphatic chain. 3. One microgram, or one thousandth of a milligram (0.001 mg.); one millionth of a gram.

g. globin. A protein formed in the blood. Ability to resist infection is related to concentration of such proteins.

g. rays. Electro-magnetic waves of extremely short wave-length emitted by radio-active substances. They are thought to be of the same nature as X-rays. They have greater penetrating power than alpha or beta rays, and, when passing through a magnetic field, are not deflected. SEE: *rays.*

gam′macism [G. *gamma,* g, + *ismos,* state of]. Inability to pronounce correctly *g* and *k* sounds.

Gamna's disease. Splenomegaly with slow, progressive enlargement of the spleen.

G's. nodules. Nodules stained yellow or brown in certain varieties of splenic enlargement. SEE: *G's. disease.*

gamo- [G.]. Combining form from *gamos,* sexual union.

gam′ont [" + *ontos,* being]. A sexual form of certain protozoans.

gamophobia (gam-o-fo′bĭ-ă) [" + *phobos,* fear]. Psychoneurotic aversion to the marriage relationship.

gampsodactylia (gamp″so-dak-til′ĭ-ă) [G. *gampsos,* curved, + *daktylos,* finger]. Deformity of the toes resembling claws. SYN: *clawfoot.*

ganglial (gang′glĭ-ăl) [G. *gagglion,* ganglion]. Pert. to a ganglion. SYN: *ganglionic.*

gangliated (gang′lĭ-at-ed) [G. *gagglion,* ganglion]. 1. Having ganglia. 2. Intermixed. [nervous system.

g. cord. Main trunk of sympathetic

gangliec′tomy [" + *ektomē,* excision]. Excision of a ganglion.

gangliform (gang′lĭ-form) [" + L. *forma,* shape]. Formed like a ganglion.

ganglioform (gang′lĭ-o-form) [" + L. *forma,* shape]. Shaped like a ganglion. SYN: *gangliform.*

ganglioglio′ma [" + *glia,* glue, + *ōma,* tumor]. A ganglion cell glioma.

ganglioglioneuroma (gang″glĭ-o-glī″o-nŭ-ro′mă) [" + " + *neuron,* nerve, + *ōma,* tumor]. Ganglion cells, glia cells, and nerve fibers in a nerve tumor.

ganglioma (gang-lĭ-o′mă) [" + *ōma,* tumor]. 1. Tumor of a lymphatic gland. 2. A swelling of lymphoid tissue.

ganglion (gang′lĭ-ŏn) (pl. *ganglia*) (G. *gagglion,* ganglion). 1. A mass of nervous tissue composed principally of nerve-cell bodies and lying outside the brain or spinal cord; e.g. the chain of ganglia which form the main sympathetic trunks; the dorsal root ganglion of a spinal nerve. 2. Cystic tumors developing on a tendon or aponeurosis; sometimes occur on the back of the wrist due to strain, such as excessive practice on the piano.

g., abdominal. Any one of the abdominal ganglia.

g., ant. cerebral. Corpus striatum. Corpus striatum and corpus lenticulare together.

g., aorticor′enal. A g. lying near to the lower border of the celiac g. It is located near the origin of the renal artery.

g., Arnold's auricular. Tiny g. located beneath foramen ovale. SYN: *otic g., otoganglion.*

g., auricular. SEE: *Arnold's auricular g.*

g., autonomic. A ganglion of the autonomic division of the nervous system.

g., basal. Mass of gray matter beneath 3rd ventricle. Consisting of the caudate, lentiform, and amygdaloid nuclei and the claustrum.

g., basal optic. Mass of gray matter beneath 3rd ventricle.

g., cardiac. SYN: *ganglion of Wrisburg.* Tiny g. toward which converge the fibers of superficial cardiac plexus. It lies on the right side of the ligamentum arteriosus.

g., carotid. G. formed by filamentous threads from the carotid plexus beneath the carotid artery.

g., celiac. SYN: *semilunar g.* One of a pair of prevertebral or collateral ganglia located near the origin of the celiac artery. They form a part of the celiac plexus.

g., cerebral. Main cerebral nerve centers.

g., cervical. Three pairs of ganglia (superior, middle, inferior) located in the neck region. They are the ganglia of the cervical portion of the sympathetic trunk.

g., cervic-uterine. SYN: *Frankenhauser's ganglion.* G. of uterine cervix.

g., cervicouterine. G. of uterine cervix.

g., ciliary. Tiny g. located in the rear portion of the orbit.

g., coccygeal. A g. located in the coccygeal plexus and forming the lower termination of the two sympathetic trunks; sometimes absent.

g., collateral. A prevertebral ganglion, *q.v.*

g., dorsal root. SYN: *posterior root g.; spinal g.* A g. located on the dorsal root of a spinal nerve. Contains the cell bodies of sensory neurons.

g., Gasserian. SYN: *semilunar g.* It lies on the sensory root of the trigeminal nerve and from it arise the three branches (ophthalmic, maxillary, mandibular.)

g., geniculate. A ganglion on the pars intermedia, the sensory root of the facial nerve. It lies in the ant., border of the ant., geniculum of the facial nerve.

g., inf. mesentric. A prevertebral sympathetic ganglion located in the inf., mesenteric plexus near the origin of the inf., mesenteric artery.

g., interpeduncular. SEE: *nucleus, interpeduncular.*

g., intervertebral. A spinal ganglion, *q.v.*

g., jugular. A g. located on the root of the vagus nerve and lying in upper portion of jugular foramen.

g., lateral. One of a chain of ganglia forming the main sympathetic trunk; also called vertebral ganglion.

g., lenticular. SEE: *ciliary g.*

g., lumbar. G. usually four in number in the lumbar portion of the sympathetic trunk.

g., Meckel's. SEE: *sphenopalatine ganglion.*

g., nodosum. G. of the trunk of the vagus nerve. Located immediately below jugular ganglion. It makes connections with the spinal accessory nerve, hypoglossal nerve, and the sup. cervical ganglion of the sympathetic trunk.

g., ophthalmic, g., optic. SEE: *ciliary g.*

g., otic. SYN: *Arnold's g.* A small ganglion located deep in the zygomatic fossa immediately below the foramen ovale. It lies medial to the mandibular nerve. It supplies postganglionic parasympathetic fibers to the parotid gland.

g., petrous. G. located on lower margin of temporal bone's petrous portion.

g., pharyngeal. G. in contact with the glossopharyngeal nerve.

g., phrenic. One of a group of ganglia joining the phrenic plexus.

g., renal. One of a group of ganglia joining the renal plexus.

g., sacral. Four small ganglia located in the sacral portion of the sympathetic trunk. They lie on the anterior surface of the sacrum and are connected to the spinal nerves by gray rami.

g., semilunar. 1. The Gasserian g. *q.v.* 2. The celiac g. *q.v.*

g., sphenopalatine. A g. associated with the great superficial petrosal nerve (branch of facial) and the maxillary nerve. It transmits both sympathetic and parasympathetic fibers to the nasal mucosa, palate, pharynx and orbit.

g., spinal. SYN: *dorsal root g.; post. root g.* Ganglionic enlargement of spinal nerves' dorsal roots.

g., spiral. A long coiled ganglion in the cochlea of the ear. It contains bipolar cells, the peripheral processes of which terminate in the organ of Corti. The central processes form the cochlear portion of the acoustic nerve and terminate in the cochlear nuclei of the medulla.

g., submaxillary. A g. lying between the nylohyoideus and hyoglossus muscles and suspended to the lingual nerve by two small branches. Peripheral fibers pass to the submaxillary and sublingual glands and the mucous membrane of floor of mouth.

g., superior mesenteric. A prevertebral ganglion of the sympathetic nervous system which lies close to the celiac ganglion and with it forms a part of the celiac (solar) plexus. It lies close to the base of the sup., mesenteric artery.

g., suprarenal. G. situated in the suprarenal plexus.

g., sympathetic. Those of the thoracolumbar (sympathetic) division of the autonomic nervous system. Include vertebral or lateral ganglia (those forming the sympathetic trunk) and prevertebral or collateral ganglia, more peripherally located.

g., temporal. Tiny g. joining the ant. branches of sup. cervical g.

g., terminal. A ganglion of the autonomic division of the nervous system which lies close to or within the organ innervated.

g., thoracic. One of 12 ganglia of thoracic area of sympathetic nerve.

g., tympanic. On tympanic portion of the glossopharyngeal nerve.

g., vestibular. SYN: *Scarpa's ganglion.* A bilobed g. located on the vestibular branch of the acoustic nerve at the bottom of the int., acoustic meatus. Its peripheral fibers arise in the maculae of the sacculus and utriculus and the cristae of the ampullae of the semicircular ducts.

gang'lionated (G. *gagglion*, ganglion). SYN: gangliated. Having or consisting of ganglia.

ganglionectomy (gang-lĭ-o-nek'to-mĭ) [" + *ektomē*, excision]. Excision of a ganglion.

ganglioneuroma (gang″glĭ-o-nū-ro'mă) [" + " + *ōma*, tumor]. A neuroma containing ganglion cells.

ganglionic (gang-lĭ-on'ik) [G. *gagglion*, ganglion]. Pert. to or of the nature of a ganglion.

ganglionitis (gang-lĭ-on-i'tis) [" + *-itis*, inflammation]. Inflamed condition of a ganglion.

gang'lioside. A cerebroside present in the brain and containing neuraminic acid, a particular type of fatty acid.

gangosa. A lesion of the nose and hard palate, regarded as a late stage of yaws; rhinopharyngitis mutilans.

gangrene (gan'grĕn) [G. *gaggraina*, an eating sore]. The putrefaction of soft tissue; a form of necrosis. SYN: *mortification*.

ETIOL: Usually results from cutting off of blood supply to an organ or tissue, which may result from inflammatory processes, injury, or degenerative changes such as arteriosclerosis. It is commonly a sequela of boils, frostbite, crushing injuries, or diseases such as diabetes, tuberculosis, syphilis, and Raynaud's disease. The part that dies is known as a *slough*, if the soft tissues are involved, or a *sequestrum*, if it is a bone that dies. It must be removed before healing can take place.

g., anemic. G. resulting from an obstructed circulation in the part.

g., angioneurotic. State resulting from thrombotic arteries and veins.

g., diabetic. Moist gangrenous condition arising in some diabetics.

g., dry. This results when the part that dies has little blood and when it remains aseptic. The arteries but not the veins are obstructed. The tissues dry and drop off, the process continuing for weeks or months. SYM: Pain in early stages. The part is cold and black and begins to wither. The toes are generally first affected spreading to the knee. Usually seen in advanced diabetes and arteriosclerosis.

g., embolic. Gangrenous condition arising subsequent to an embolic obstruction.

g., gas. This is gangrene in a wound infected by the gas bacillus (*bacillus Welchii*), a microörganism.

It is an anaerobe* and Gram-positive. It has no motility. It forms spores and the gas produced ferments sugars and it also forms a toxin. It is found in the intestines and may be carried in soiled clothing and dressings. A specially prepared antitoxin is used for treatment.

Most recent method of treatment to prevent amputation has been the combined use of antiserum, sulfanilamide or sulfapyridine, and irradiation. Inhalations of concentrated oxygen have also been somewhat successful.

g., humid. SEE: *moist g.*

g., idiopathic. When the cause is unknown.

g., infective. Due to infection, as in carbuncle necrosis, cancrum oris and cancrum noma.

g., moist. This occurs after a crushing injury, usually at distal part of an extremity, or when dry gangrene is infected with putrefactive bacteria, and when the part is full of blood. SYM: The part is hot, red, later cold and bluish, commencing to slough. It spreads rapidly and there is an offensive odor. The process is known to the layman as "mortification." Death may result in a few days.

g., primary. G. developing in a part without previous inflammation.

g., secondary. G. developing subsequent to local inflammation.

g., senile. G. developing in the limbs of the senile. Supposed to be due to arteriosclerosis.

g., symmetric. G. on opposite sides of the body in corresponding parts. Usually the result of vasomotor disturbances. Characteristic of Raynaud's and Buerger's disease.

g., traumatic. Result of extensive injuries.

g., white. Moist gangrene developing in patients with anemia and lymphatic obstruction.

gangrenosis (gang-gren-o'sis) [" + *-ōsis*]. Condition of mortification or gangrene.

gan'grenous [G. *gaggraina*, an eating sore]. Of the nature of gangrene.

gan'oblast [G. *ganos*, brightness, + *blastos*, cell]. An enamel cell. SYN: *ameloblast*.

Ganser's syndrome (gan'zerz sin'drōm). "Nonsense syndrome." Absurd acts and speech seen in prison psychosis, hysteria, and other states.

gap. An opening or a break; an interruption in continuity.

g., auscultatory. A period of silence which occurs in the determination of blood pressure by the auscultatory method. Exact cause unknown.

g., cranial. A congenital fissure in the skull.

g., silent. A silent period noted in blood pressure determination by the auscultatory method although no interruption is noted in palpation at the wrist.

gargarism (gar'gar-izm) [G. *gargarisma*, a gargle]. A gargle or throat wash.

gargle (gar'gl) [L. *gurgulio*, windpipe]. 1. A wash for the throat. 2. To wash out the throat with a throat wash.

gargoylism. SYN: *lipochondrodystrophy, Hurler's disease*. A condition usually congenital characterized by dwarfism, kyphosis, and other skeletal abnormalities, disturbances in lipoid metabolism, and usually mental deficiency.

garlic [A.S. *gar*, spear, + *leak*, the leek]. An edible, strongly flavored bulb, of *Allium Sativum* used mainly for seasoning. COMP: The active principle of garlic is sulfide of allyl.

ACTION: It is a gastric stimulant and an intestinal antiseptic. Slightly diuretic and an irritant for the kidneys, stimulating them as well as the circulation and the nerves.

INDICATIONS: Its sulfurated essence is anticatarrhal.

gar'rot [Fr. *garroter*, to tie fast]. A form of tourniquet.

Gart'ner's duct. A small duct, the mesosalpinx lying parallel to the uterine tube. It is a vestigial structure representing the persistent mesonephric duct. Also called duct of the epoophoron; ductus epoophori longitudinalis.

gas. 1. A fluid substance which not only takes the shape of the containing vessel but expands and fills the vessel no matter what its volume. 2. An airlike fluid subject to expansion and convertible into a liquid by cooling or compression.

Among the common important gases are oxygen; illuminating gas; exhaust gas; sewer gas, which contains carbon monoxide (*q.v.*), carbon dioxide (*q.v.*); the anesthetic gases (SEE: *anesthesia*); ammonia (*q.v.*); the poison war gases, etc. Liquids and solids when heated often give off fumes which may be poisonous; among the more common are the mineral acids, ammonia water, mercury and its compounds, cyanides, zinc-containing metals, etc. SEE: *gases*.

g. bacillus. SEE: *gangrene*.

g. (in the) blood. The principle gases found in the blood are oxygen, nitrogen, and carbon dioxide. They may be dissolved in the plasma or they may exist in loose chemical combination with other compounds, as oxygen combined with hemoglobin.

g., digestive tract. Among the gases in the digestive tract are: oxygen, nitrogen, hydrogen, carbon dioxide, methane, and in decomposition of proteins, hydrogen sulfide, indol, skatol, ammonia, etc.

g., distention. Abdominal distention is result of abnormal gaseous, fluid, or solid accumulation in abdominal cavity. It may be: (a) acute; (b) chronic; (c) local, or (d) general. The abdominal wall, the cavity, or the intraäbdominal viscera may be involved. *Postoperative*: Result of complication following an operation. Limited to lower part of small, and all of large intestines. Careless administration of anesthesia may be a cause, as is degree of peritonitis. *Preoperative*: Enema is a preventive. TREATMENT: No cold fluids, change of posture, insertion of rectal tube, enemata only as advised by surgeon.

g. excretions. Oxidation produces carbon dioxide or carbonic acid gas, from one-half to two-thirds of a cubic ft. per hr. being produced by an adult male of average weight. Activity increases the amount. Ordinarily only water vapor and carbon dioxide are given off.

g. gangrene. That caused by the gas bacillus. SEE: *gangrene*.

g., illuminating. This is a mixture of various combustible gases including hydrogen and carbon monoxide. Its poisonous effects are largely due to carbon monoxide, *q.v.* TREATMENT: Resuscitation, *q.v.*

g. in the blood. Dissolved gases are found in the blood in the form of oxygen, nitrogen, and a small portion of carbon dioxide, with carbonic acid from the tissues.

g., laughing. Nitrous oxide.

g., marsh. Methane.

g., mustard. Poisonous gas used in warfare (dichlorethyl sulfide).

g., refrigerant. A number of these gases are used in ordinary household mechanical refrigerators. Poisoning due to leaks, faulty connections or breakage, and gas dissipated into the atmosphere. Among these gases are methyl chloride, ammonia, sulfur dioxide and more than 20 other gases. Most of these are toxic. Careful researches are now being carried on to develop nontoxic gases. Warning agents mixed with these gases are not a guarantee of protection to infants, children, hospital patients, firemen and refrigerator workers; therefore, instead of merely adding a protective agent, it would be wiser to have a nontoxic refrigerant. *Methyl chloride* is responsible for more poisoning than other refrigerant gases. *Sulfur dioxide*: As this is a respiratory irritant it is easily detected, so serious poisoning is not likely to occur.

g., tear. A gas that irritates the conjunctiva and which produces a flow of tears.

gas'ator. Device for adm. chlorine gas for respiratory infections.

gaseous (gas'e-us). Of the nature or form of gas.

gases, war. Any chemical substances whether solid, liquid, or vapor, used to produce poisonous or irritant effects. They can be classified as *lacrimators, sternutators, lung irritants, vesicants*, and those that act as a systemic poison. Some gases have multiple effects.

They are known as persistent or nonpersistent, *i. e.*, those which diffuse and are dispersed fairly rapidly, and those which linger and evaporate slowly. They can be classified as suffocating gases, irritating gases, vesicants, and general poisons or toxic gases.

It is of the greatest importance that those rendering first aid should avoid becoming casualties; precautions must be taken, masks worn, as well as being applied to the patients. Strict discipline must be maintained during gas raids in order to avoid panic. If gas training has been thorough and if organization is good, much may be done to lessen the effect, and maintain a good morale.

Decontamination centers are essential and nurses must understand that thorough decontamination of clothing, boots, ambulances, etc., is vitally necessary, and they should make themselves familiar with the necessary detail.

g., lewisite. Contains arsenic and smells of geraniums.

SYM: Similar to those of vesicant gas, *q.v.*, but come on at once and as a rule are not so severe. Arsenic can be recovered from the serum of the blisters and symptoms of arsenic poisoning may occur.

TREATMENT: Similar to that for vesicant gas, *q.v.*

g., lung irritant. Ex: *Chlorine and phosgene*.

SYM: Burning sensation of the eyes, nose, and throat, bronchitis and pneumonia, sometimes followed by edema of the lungs and probably death.

TREATMENT: Remove patient from exposure, apply respirator; if there has been exposure to phosgene (smells like musty hay) the symptoms may be delayed and the patient may collapse later. It is important, therefore, to provide complete rest, remove patient on a stretcher, and provide warmth; oxygen may be required in large quantities over a fairly long period.

g., mustard. Dichlorethyl sulfide. SEE: *g., vesicant*.

g., nose irritant. Diphenylchloroarsine. An irritant smoke.

SYM: Intense pain in the nose, throat, and air passages and sneezing followed by headache and aching in teeth and jaws, acute mental depression, and sometimes vomiting.

TREATMENT: Casualties must be reassured that no permanent harm is done and should be warned against removing respirator in spite of the fact the symptoms may get worse after donning it. This is a gas likely to lead to "panic." Nasal douching with warm sodium bicarbonate is helpful.

g., suffocating. Made from chlorine compounds.

g., tear. Substance which, when dispersed into the air, causes the eyes to be blinded by tears. Ex: *Bromoacetone*.

SYM: Causes much inconvenience. Irritation of the nose and eyes, and free lacrimation so that it is impossible to see.

TREATMENT: As a rule, none is necessary, for upon removal from the infected area, the symptoms tend gradually to subside.

g., toxic. Hydrocyanic acid type.

g., vesicant. Attack every part of body; clothing and boots are infected and a source of danger.

Ex: mustard g., lewisite.

SYM: Do not appear at once; may be 6 hr. or longer before the patient is aware of anything wrong. Pain in the eyes, lacrimation, and discharge may be the first evidence, the eyelids swelling and the patient being unable to see;

there is a diffuse redness of the skin, followed by blistering and ulceration.

PROG: Healing is very slow, but generally follows if treatment is prompt and efficient.

TREATMENT: Decontamination is essential and must be thorough. Bathe eyes freely with normal saline or plain water; a drop or 2 of castor oil will prevent lids sticking; no bandage should be worn. The patient should be scrubbed, if possible, under a hot or warm shower for 10 minutes. Bleach cream or powder, if ordered, should be applied first, and left in contact with the skin for 5 minutes. If, in spite of these precautionary measures, blisters arise, they may be successfully treated with tannic acid.

g., vomiting. That induces emesis, specifically chloropicrin.

gas′oline″. A product of the destructive distillation of petroleum.

Most motor fuel contains ethyl lead, ethyl antimony or ethyl arsenic combinations which increase the toxicity markedly. Slightly antiseptic if free from these compounds, and may be used to wash grease out of wounds, although ether is better.

SYM. OF POISONING: Giddiness, headache, intoxication, nervous disturbance, muscular tremors, difficulty in respiration, paralyses, convulsions, cyanosis, unconsciousness, pulmonary hemorrhage. Usually no local disturbance of stomach.

F. A. TREATMENT: Fresh air, inhalation of oxygen and carbon dioxide; artificial respiration when necessary. Otherwise treat symptoms.

gasomet′ric. Pert. to measurement of gases.

gasometry (gas-om′et-rĭ) [G. *metron*, measure]. Estimation of amount of gas present in a mixture.

gasp. To catch the breath; to inhale and exhale with quick, difficult breaths; the act of gasping.

gasserectomy (gas-er-ek′to-mĭ) [G. *ektome*, excision]. Excision of the gasserian ganglion.

gasse′rian arteries. A branch from the int. carotid a. and one of the middle meningeal a. to the gasserian ganglion. SEE: *ganglion*.

gas′sing. The use of war gases, *q.v.*

gaster-, gastero-, gastro. Combining forms meaning "pertaining to the stomach or the region of the stomach."

gasteral′gia [G. *gaster*, belly, + *algos*, pain]. Pain in the stomach.

gasterangiemphraxis (gas″ter-an″jĭ-em-fraks′is) [" + *aggeion*, vessel, + *emphraxis*, obstruction]. 1. Congestion of blood vessels of stomach. 2. Pyloric obstruction.

gasterasthenia (gas-ter-as-the′nĭ-ă) [" + *astheneia*, weakness]. Debility of the stomach. SYN: *gastrasthenia*.

gasterhysterotomy (gas″ter-his-ter-ot′o-mĭ) [" + *ystera*, uterus, + *tome*, incision]. Incision of uterus through abdomen. SEE: *cesarean operation*.

gastorrhagia (gas-tor-a′jĭ-ă) [" + *regnunai*, a bursting forth]. Hemorrhage from the stomach.

gastradenitis (gas-trad-en-i′tis) [" + *aden*, gland, + *-itis*, inflammation]. Inflammation of the stomach glands.

gastralgia (gas-tral′jĭ-ă) [" + *algos*, pain]. Paroxysmal epigastric pain without gastric lesion.

SYM: Pain radiates to the back when stomach is empty. Warm foods and drinks, and pressure over painful area relieve pain. Not to be confused with other gastric disturbances. Dilatation never present. Hyperacidity obtains in certain forms; hematemesis absent. In females, it is most frequent near the menopause.

gastralgocenosis (găs-trăl″gō-sĕn-ōs′ĭs) Gastric pain due to emptiness of stomach; hunger pangs due to hunger contractions, powerful peristaltic contractions which sweep over the stomach.

gastralgokenosis (gas-tral-go-ken-o′sis) [" + " + *kenosis*, emptiness]. A sensory neurosis of the stomach.

gastraneuria (gas-tra-nū′rĭ-ă) [" + *neuron*, nerve]. Defective action of nerves of the stomach.

gastrasthe′nia [" + *astheneia*, weakness]. Debility of the stomach. SYN: *gasterasthenia*.

gastratrophia (gas-tra-tro′fĭ-ă) [" + *atropheia*, atrophy]. Atrophy of the stomach.

gastrecta′sia, gastrec′tasis [" + *ektasis*, dilatation]. Dilatation of the stomach. May be acute or chronic.

ETIOL: Obstruction of pylorus; atony, overeating, congenital weakness, imperfect peristalsis, omental hernia, periduodenal adhesions, gastroptosis.

SYM: *Chronic*: Vomiting of food taken several days before, vomitus sour, contains fatty acids, mucus, bacteria. *Acute*: Severe, sudden pain accompanied by collapse. Small, rapid pulse, temperature subnormal, upper abdominal pain resembling angina pectoris. Distended and tympanic abdomen. Vomiting of fluids and eructation of gas.

gastrectomy (găs-trĕk′tō-mĭ) [G. *gaster*, belly, + *ek-tome*, excision]. Surgical removal of a part or the whole of the stomach.

gas′tric [G. *gaster*, stomach]. Pert. to the stomach.

g. analysis. Determines quality of secretion, amount of free and combined hydrochloric acid, absence or presence of blood, bile, bacteria, fatty acids. Esp. necessary if gastric ulcer or carcinoma is suspected.

g. digestion. 1. As food passes through the cardiac orifice into the stomach, it tends to accumulate in the lowest part of the major curvature. 2. Successive portions of food are added to this, tending to accumulate in the innermost portion of the mass. The walls of the stomach gradually relax receptive relaxation adapting themselves to the amount of the contents. This is the result of a *gastric feeding reflex* which also inhibits peristalsis in the remaining portion of the stomach. 3. Within the mass, salivary digestion continues for a short time, but in those portions touching the stomach wall, the salivary ptyalin is destroyed by the acid.

CHEMICAL ASPECTS: During the meal, nervous impulses from the brain are carried to the stomach by way of the vagi; they result from the sensations of sight, smell, and taste. In addition, the stretching of the stomach wall excites the gastric glands by local nervous mechanisms, and chemical substances initially present in the food (preformed secretagogues) or produced during the digestion of the food (derived secretagogues) are absorbed and further stimulate the gastric glands.

The following changes occur in the food while in the stomach. Pepsin acts on proteins of high molecular weight hydrolyzing them to proteoses and peptones. Pepsin also coagulates milk. Hydrochloric acid is essential for the activity of pepsin. It also dissolves collagen, disintegrates nucleoproteins, hydrolyzes double sugars, and is responsible for the antiseptic action of the gastric juice. Gastric lipase acts on emulsified fats reducing them to fatty acids and glycerol but its action is limited.

MOTOR ASPECTS: After the initial relaxation, the stomach increases its pressure upon its contents. The cardiac sphincter closes firmly to prevent regurgitation into the esophagus. The pyloric part of the stomach begins to exhibit wavelets of contraction which run toward the pylorus. They become deeper, and their focus of origin shifts in the direction of the cardia.

At first the pylorus, like the cardia, remains firmly closed, and the wavelets result only in mixing and in facilitating the chemical comminution and solution. Now the pylorus begins to open occasionally, allowing the acid chyme to spurt at intervals into the duodenum. The further course of the chyme is described under *duodenal digestion*.

g. fever. Fever accompanied by gastric disturbances.

g. glands. Cardiac, fundic or oxyntic, and pyloric glands of the stomach.

These are tubular glands lying in the mucosa of the wall, and the gastric juice exudes from them just as sweat drips from one's forehead. The general result of gastric digestion is the reduction of the ingested mass to a mushy, gray mixture called "acid chyme."

They contain (a) chief, zymogenic, or peptic cells which secrete pepsinogen, the inactive form of pepsin; (b) parietal border, or oxyntic cells which secrete hydrochloric acid, and (c) mucous cells found in the neck of the gland, which secrete mucin.

g. juice. The digestive juice of the gastric glands of the stomach. It contains pepsin, hydrochloric acid, mucin, small quantities of inorganic salts, and the "intrinsic factor" of the antianemic principle. It is strongly acid having a pH of 0.9 to 1.5. It is a thin colorless fluid, its total acidity being 0.45-0.60% and free HCl, 0.40-0.50%. It has a specific gravity of 1.002-1.004. The amount secreted in 24 hours varies greatly. In a fasting stomach secretion occurs at a rate of 8 to 15 cc. per hour.

The mixture of acid and pepsin has effects which neither substance has alone, and dissolves some proteins with remarkable speed. Rennin is the cause of the normal clotting of milk in the stomach. There is also a lipase which can release butyric fat from butter fat, and thus gives the characteristic odor to vomitus.

DIAG. (findings): *Carcinoma*: Lactic acid, blood, Boas-Oppler bacilli, sarcinae, and sometimes tumor cells are present; frequently no hydrochloric acid is found. *Hyperacidity*: May indicate gastric ulcer. *Lactic Acid*: Present in carcinoma. *Pus Cells*: Indicate severe damage to stomach. *Red Cells*: Same significance as pus cells.

RS: *gastric analysis, hydrochloric acid, hyper- and hypochlorhydria, stomach, digestion in.*

g. lavage. Washing out of the stomach.

USES: 1. To empty stomach when contents are irritating, as in prolonged postanesthetic vomiting, and in some cases of regurgitant vomiting in acute intestinal obstruction. 2. To clean cavity before an operation is performed upon it. 3. To remove poison in cases in which this method of treatment is indicated. 4. For removal of a test meal.

METHOD: If possible patient is propped up in bed; a rubber sheet and towel are placed around neck and arranged to protect clothing in front. The apparatus required is: An esophageal tube, with glass connection; a length of rubber tubing and a funnel; several pints of solution and a solution thermometer; glycerine to lubricate tube; a towel and receiver for vomit, which patient may be allowed to hold; a pint measure and pail for returned fluid; a receiver for stomach contents, and sodium bicarbonate solution, a dram to the pint. Condy's fluid, 1-10,000; normal saline solution, or other solution may be used, which should be prepared at a temperature of 100° F.

The procedure is explained to the patient if he is capable of understanding. His mouth is cleaned and he is asked to swallow the lubricated tube which is placed in his mouth. He is encouraged to try and control the desire to retch. As the tube is swallowed the nurse will gently help to pass it along. When a special mark on the tube is on a level with the patient's lips the tube may be expected to be in the stomach, and the funnel is then inverted to empty the stomach of its contents; if nothing is seen, the tube should be passed farther in until it is found to be in the stomach.

If possible collect stomach contents in receiver provided. Then pinch the tube below funnel and fill the funnel with solution, expel air from the tube by pinching and rubbing it upwards towards the funnel. Let fluid run in very slowly, using from ½ to 1 pint at a time; invert funnel and let this run out, repeat until all fluid has been used or until it returns clear. When the treatment is finished, pinch tube and withdraw it quickly, giving patient a mouthwash immediately, and then place soiled tube in a basin of tepid water.

The siphoned gastric contents should be examined, and the amount of returned solution measured and inspected for blood, bile, and mucus. If necessary, it should be saved for the doctor's inspection.

g. motor meals. These meals are used to test the motor activity of the stomach and intestines. SEE: *Boas motor m., test m., Von Leube m.*

g. mucin (mu'sin). A fine, straw-colored powder, prepared from hog stomach.

USES: As a protective in peptic ulcer.

DOSAGE: Varies according to the severity, from 1 teaspoonful to 1 tablespoonful in warm water or milk ½ hour before meals.

g. ulcer. An ulcer of the stomach. SYN: *peptic ulcer, q.v.*

gastricism (gas'tris-izm) [G. *gastēr*, belly, + *ismos*, state]. Any gastric disorder.

gas'trin [G. *gastēr*, belly]. A hormone that stimulates secretion of the glands in the cardiac end of the stomach. It is formed at the pyloric end of the stomach.

gastritis (gas-trī'tis) [" + -*itis*, inflammation]. Inflammation of the stomach.

Characterized by epigastric pain or tenderness, thirst, nausea, vomiting, and diarrhea. The mucosa may be atrophic or hypertrophic.

ETIOL: Generally unknown. May result from infection, excessive indul-

gastritis, acute   G-10   **gastroesophagitis**

gence in alcoholic beverages, dietary indiscretions. Pain in the region of the stomach may be due to causes other than gastritis, such as cancer. Gastritis may be due to an excess or a deficiency of hydrochloric acid, and a remedy suitable for one would not be proper for the other condition. The type must first be determined before medication.

g., acute. SYM: Moderate fever; anorexia, coated tongue; intense pain in epigastrium, persistent vomiting, thirst; prostration. PROG: Good. TREATMENT: Absolute rest. In severe cases no food by mouth till stomach becomes retentive. Thirst allayed with cracked ice.

g., atrophic. Chronic g. with atrophied mucosa and glands.

g., chronic. SYM: Weight and distress after eating; often tenderness on palpation. Eructations of gas and some liquid, nausea and vomiting frequently, constipation. PROG: Good. TREATMENT: Hygienic conditions, regulated diet.

g., excess acid (hyperchlorhydria). SYM: Pain more intense than in acid deficiency. Good appetite. TREATMENT: Milk, water, and eggs for 2 weeks; olive oil; baking soda; alkaline foods and water.

g., hypertrophic. G. combined with glandular hypertrophy and infiltration.

g., phlegmonous. Acute g. with suppuration of the mucosa and submucosa.

g., polypous. G. characterized by knoblike projections on the surface.

g., pseudomembranous. G. marked by membranous patch formation.

gastro- [G. *gastēr*, stomach]. Used in compounds to denote the *stomach*.

gastroanastomosis (gas″tro-an-as″to-mo′sis) [" + *ana*, up, + *stoma*, mouth, + *-ōsis*]. Formation of passage bet. 2 pouches of stomach for relief of hourglass contraction.

gastroblennorrhea (gas-tro-blen-or-e′ă) [" + *blennos*, mucus, + *roia*, flow]. Excessive secretion of gastric mucus.

gastrobrosis (gas-tro-bro′sis) [" + *brōsis*, eating]. Perforating ulcer of the stomach.

gastrocele (gas′tro-sēl) [" + *kēlē*, hernia]. Hernia of the stomach.

gastrochronorrhea (gas-tro-kron-or-re′ă) [" + *chronos*, time, + *roia*, flow]. Chronic gastric disease marked by permanent hypersecretion with dilatation and thickening of stomach walls and hypertrophy of glands. SYN: *Reichmann's disease.*

gastrocnemius (gas-trok-ne′mĭ-us) [" + *knēmē*, leg]. The large muscle of the leg. Extends foot and helps to flex knee upon thigh.

gastrocol′ic [" + *kōlon*, colon]. Pert. to stomach and colon.

g. omentum. The great omentum. SYN: *epiploon.*

g. reflex. Peristaltic wave in colon induced by entrance of food into fasting stomach.

gastrocoli′tis [" + " + *-itis*, inflammation]. Inflammation of stomach and colon.

gastrocoloptosis (gas-tro-kol-op-to′sis) [" + " + *ptōsis*, dropping]. Downward prolapse of stomach and colon.

gastrocolostomy (gas-tro-kol-os′to-mĭ) [" + " + *stoma*, opening]. Establishment of permanent passage bet. stomach and colon.

gastrocolotomy (gas-tro-ko-lot′o-mĭ) [" + " + *tomē*, incision]. Incision into stomach and colon.

gastrocolpotomy (gas-tro-kol-pot′o-mĭ) [G. *gastēr*, belly, + *kolpos*, vagina, + *tomē*, incision]. An incision of abdomen into upper part of vagina.

gastrodiaphane (gas-tro-di′af-ān) [" + *dia*, through, + *phainein*, to show]. Device for electrically illuminating stomach interior, making visible its outlines through the abdomen.

gastrodiaphanos′copy, gastrodiaph′any [" + " + " + *skopein*, to examine]. Examination of interior of the stomach by rendering its walls translucent by an electric light introduced into the organ.

gastrodisciasis (gas-trō-dĭs-kē-ās′ĭs). Infestation by a fluke, *Gastrodiscoides hominis.*

gastrodiscoides (gas-trō-dĭs-kē-ĭd′-ăs). A genus of flukes belonging to family Gastrodiscidae, sub-order Amphistomata.

g. hominis. A species of flukes commonly infesting hogs but occasionally found in man.

gastroduodenitis (gas″tro-dū-od-en-i′tis) [" + L. *duodenum*, duodenum, + G. *-itis*, inflammation]. Inflammation of stomach and duodenum.

gastroduodenostomy (gas″tro-du-o-den-os′to-mĭ) [" + " + G. *stoma*, mouth]. Formation of an artificial opening between the stomach and duodenum.

gastrodynia (gas-tro-din′ĭ-ă) [" + *odynē*, pain]. Pain in the stomach. SYN: *gastralgia.*

gastroelytrotomy (gas-tro-el-ĭt-rot′o-mĭ) [" + *elytron*, vagina, + *tomē*, incision]. Cesarean section through linea alba into upper portion of vagina. SYN: *gastrocolpotomy.*

gastroenteralgia (gas″tro-en-ter-al′jĭ-ă) [" + *enteron*, intestine, + *algos*, pain]. Pain in stomach and intestines.

gastroenter′ic [" + *enteron*, intestine]. Pert. to stomach and intestines or to a condition involving them both.

gastroenteritis (gas-tro-en-ter-i′tis) [" + " + *-itis*, inflammation]. Inflammation of the stomach and intestines.

gastroenterocolitis (gas″tro-en″ter-o-kol-i′tis) [" + " + *kōlon*, colon, + *-itis*, inflammation]. Inflammation of stomach, small intestine, and colon.

gastroenterocolostomy (gas-tro-en-ter-o-ko-los′to-mĭ) [" + " + " + *stoma*, opening]. Creation of a passage bet. the stomach, small intestine, and colon.

gastroenterol′ogy [" + " + *logos*, study]. The pathology of the stomach and intestine.

gastroenteroptosis (gas″tro-en-ter-op-to′sis) [" + " + *ptōsis*, a dropping]. Prolapse of stomach and intestines.

gastroenterostomy (gas-tro-en-ter-os′to-mĭ) [" + " + *stoma*, opening]. Surgical anastomosis between the stomach and small bowel.

This operation is required for patients who are suffering from carcinoma or cicatricial stricture of pyloric orifice of the stomach.

NP: The procedure of preparation is the same as for appendectomy up to the stage of exposure of the viscera.

gas″troenterot′omy [" + " + *tomē*, incision]. Incision of stomach and intestine through abdominal wall.

gas″troepiplo′ic [G. *gastēr*, belly, + *epiplōon*, omentum]. Pert. to stomach and great omentum.

gastroesophagitis (gas-tro-e-sof-aj-i′tis) [" + *oisophagos*, gullet, + *-itis*, inflammation]. Inflammation of stomach and esophagus.

gastroesophagostomy (gas″tro-es-o-fa-gos′to-mī) [" + " + *tomē*, incision]. Formation of passage from the esophagus into the stomach.

gastrogastrostomy (gas-tro-gas-tros′to-mī) [" + *gastēr*, belly, + *stoma*, opening]. Formation of passage in hourglass contraction bet. the 2 gastric pouches. SYN: *gastroanastomosis*.

gastrogavage (gas-tro-ga-vazh′) [" + Fr. *gaver*, to gorge fowls]. Artificial feeding through an opening into the stomach.

gastrogen′ic [" + *gennan*, to produce]. Having its origin in the stomach.

gastrograph (gas′tro-graf) [" + *graphein*, to write]. Device for determining the stomach's mechanical action.

gastrohelcosis (gas″tro-hel-ko′sis) [" + *elkōsis*, ulceration]. Ulcer of the stomach.

gas′trohepat′ic [" + *ēpar*, *ēpat*-, liver]. Pert. to stomach and liver.

gastrohepatitis (gas-tro-hep-ă-ti′tis) [" + " + -*itis*, inflammation]. Combination of gastritis and hepatitis at same time.

gastrohydrorrhea (gas-tro-hi-dro-re′ă) [" + *ydōr*, water, + *roia*, flow]. Excretion of much watery fluid, other than gastric juice, into the stomach.

gastrohysterectomy (gas-tro-his-ter-ek′-to-mī) [" + *ystera*, uterus, + *ektomē*, excision]. Removal of the uterus through an abdominal incision.

gastrohysteropexy (gas″tro-his″ter-o-peks′ī) [" + " + *pēxis*, fixation]. Ventrofixation of the uterus.

gastrohysterorrhaphy (gas-tro-his-ter-or′-af-ī) [" + " + *raphē*, suture]. Fixation of uterus to the abdominal wall. SYN: *gastrohysteropexy*.

gastrohysterotomy (gas-tro-his-ter-ot′o-mī) [" + " + *tomē*, incision]. Incision of uterus through abdomen. SYN: *gasterhysterotomy*.

gastroiliac (gas-trō-īl′ī-ak) [" + L. *iliacus*]. Pert. to stomach and ileum.

g. reflex. Physiologic relaxation of ileocecal valve resulting from food in stomach.

gastrointes′tinal [" + L. *intestinum*, intestine]. Pert. to stomach and intestine.

g. decompression. Drainage of gases from the body cavities and tissues by use of suction through a tube inserted through the nostrils and into the digestive tract. SEE: *Wangensteen method*.

gastrojejunostomy (gas-tro-je-ju-nos′to-mī) [" + L. *jejunus*, empty, + G. *stoma*, opening]. Surgical anastomosis between the stomach and jejunum.

gastrolith (gas′tro-lith) [G. *gastēr*, belly, + *lithos*, stone]. A concretion in the stomach.

gastrolithiasis (gas″tro-lith-i′ă-sis) [" + *lithos*, stone]. Formation of calculi in the stomach.

gastrology (gas-trol′o-jī) [" + *logos*, study]. Study of function and diseases of the stomach.

gastrol′ysis [" + *lysis*, loosening]. Breaking adhesions bet. stomach and adjoining structures.

gastromalacia (gas-tro-mal-a′sī-ă) [" + *malakia*, softening]. Softening of the stomach walls.

gastromegaly (gas-tro-meg′ă-lī) [" + *megas*, *megal*-, large]. Enlargement of the stomach.

gastromenia (gas-tro-me′nī-ă) [" + *mēn*, month]. A form of vicarious menstruation through the stomach.

gastromycosis (gas-tro-mi-ko′sis) [" + *mykēs*, fungus, + -*ōsis*]. Disease of the stomach due to fungi.

gastromyotomy (gas-tro-mi-ot′o-mī) [" + *mys*, muscle, + *tomē*, incision]. Incision of circular muscular fibers of stomach.

gastromyxorrhea (gas-tro-miks-or-e′ă) [" + *myxa*, mucus, + *roia*, flow]. Excessive secretion of gastric mucus.

gastronephritis (gas-tro-nef-ri′tis) [" + *nephros*, kidney, + -*itis*, inflammation]. Inflammation of the stomach and kidney at same time.

gastronesteostomy (gas-tro-nes-te-os′to-mī) [" + *nēstis*, jejunum, + *stoma*, opening]. Formation of communication bet. jejunum and stomach. SYN: *gastrojejunostomy*.

gastropancreatitis (gas″tro-pan″kre-ă-ti′-tis) [" + *pagkreas*, pancreas, + -*itis*, inflammation]. Inflammation of the stomach and pancreas at same time.

gastroparalysis (gas″tro-par-al′is-is) [" + *paralyein*, to loose from sides]. Paralysis of the stomach.

gastroparesis (gas″tro-par′e-sis) [" + *paresis*, paralysis]. Mild form of gastroparalysis.

gastropathy (gas-trop′ă-thī) [G. *gastēr*, belly, + *pathos*, disease]. Any disorder of the stomach.

gastroperiodynia (gas″tro-per″ī-o-din′ī-ă) [" + *periodos*, period, + *odynē*, pain]. Periodic pain in the stomach. SYN: *gastralgia*.

gastropexy, gastropexis (gas-tro-peks′e, -is) [" + *pēxis*, fixation]. Suture of the stomach to the abdominal walls for correction of displacement.

Gastrophilus (găs-trŏf′ĭl-us). A genus of botflies belonging to the family Oestridae, order of Diptera. The larvae infest horses and occasionally man.

G. hemorrhoidalis. In which eggs are laid on lower lip and jaws of equines.

G. intestinalis. In which eggs laid on inner side of legs and abdomen. Moisture from tongue stimulates hatching of eggs, larvae then being transferred to the mouth from which they migrate to stomach and intestines. In man, larvae enter the skin and infest subcutaneous regions causing a creeping eruption (larva migrans) *q.v.*

G. nasalis. The chin fly. Eggs are laid on shafts of hairs on lower lip and jaw.

gastrophrenic (gas-tro-fren′ĭk) [" + *phrēn*, diaphragm]. Rel. to the stomach and diaphragm.

gastroplasty (gas′tro-plas″tī) [" + *plassein*, to form]. Plastic operation on the stomach.

gastroplegia (gas-tro-ple′jī-ă) [" + *plēgē*, stroke]. Paralysis of the stomach.

gastroplication (gas-tro-pli-ka′shun) [" + L. *plicāre*, to fold]. Stitching the walls of the stomach to reduce dilatation.

gastroptosia, gastroptosis (gas-trop-to′-sī-ă, -sis) [" + *ptōsis*, a dropping]. Abnormal falling of the stomach, Glénard's disease.

Usually accompanied by the displacement of other organs, the abdomen being pendulous. SEE: *bathygastry*.

gastroptyxis, gastroptyxy (gas-trop-tiks′-is, -ī) [" + *ptyxis*, a folding]. Reduction of a dilated stomach. SYN: *gastroplication*.

gastropylorectomy (gas-tro-pi-lor-ek′to-mī) [" + *pylōros*, pylorus, + *ektomē*, excision]. Excision of stomach at pyloric end.

gastropylor′ic [" + *pylōros*, pylorus]. Rel. to stomach and pylorus.

gastroradiculitis (gas-tro-rad-ik-ū-li′tis) [" + L. *radix*, root, + G. -*itis*, inflammation]. Inflammation of the post. spi-

gastrorrhagia   G-12   **gavage**

nal nerve roots, the sensory fibers of which supply the stomach.

gastrorrhagia (gas-tror-ra'jĭ-ă) [" + *rēgnunai*, to burst forth]. Hemorrhage from stomach.

gastrorrhaphy (gas-tror'ă-fĭ) [G. *gastēr*, belly, + *raphē*, suture]. Suture of a stomach wall.

gastrorrhea (gas-tror-rē'ă) [" + *roia*, flow]. An excessive secretion of gastric juice.

gastrosalpingotomy (gas-tro-sal-pin-got'o-mĭ) [" + *salpigx*, tube, + *tomē*, incision]. Incision of the oviduct by abdominal section.

gastroschisis (gas-tros'kis-is) [" + *schisis*, cleft]. A congenital fissure in wall of abdomen which remains open.

gastroscope (gas'tro-skōp) [" + *skopein*, to examine]. Device for inspecting stomach's interior.

gastros'copy [" + *skopein*, to examine]. Examination of the stomach and abdominal cavity.

gastro'sia [G. *gastēr*, belly]. Excessive hydrochloric acid in the stomach. SYN: *gastroxia*.

    g. fungo'sa. Gastrosia in which fungi in the stomach give rise to organic acids.

gastro'sis [" + *-ōsis*, disease]. Any disease of the stomach.

gas'trospasm [" + *spasmos*, spasm]. A gastric spasm.

gastrosplen'ic [" + *splēn*, spleen]. Of or pert. to stomach and spleen.

gastrostaxis (gas-tro-staks'is) [" + *staxis*, trickling]. Hemorrhage of blood from membrane of the stomach.

gastrostenosis (gas-tro-sten-o'sis) [" + *stēnōsis*, narrowing]. Contracted state of the stomach.

    g. cardiaca. Stenosis of cardiac orifice.

    g. pylorica. Stenosis of pylorus.

gastrostogavage (gas-tros"to-gă-vazh') [" + *stoma*, opening, + Fr. *gaver*, to gorge fowls]. Injection through a gastric fistula, of food.

Peptonized milk, albumen water, or eggnog during first week, soft diet the second week with more liberal diet with improvement. TEMPERATURE: 100° F. SEE: *gavage*.

gastros'toma [G. *gastēr*, belly, + *stoma*, opening]. A fistula of the stomach.

gastros'tomize [" + *stoma*, opening]. To perform a gastrostomy.

gastrostomy (gas-tros'to-mĭ) [" + *stoma*, opening]. Surgical creation of a gastric fistula through the abdominal wall.

It is necessary in carcinoma, and in some cases of cicatricial stricture of the esophagus; made for purpose of introducing food into stomach.

NP: Teach patient to care for self after hospitalization. Help patient to make mental adjustment. Care of mouth.

gastrosuccorrhea (gas-tro-suk-or-e'ă) [" + L. *succus*, juice, + G. *roia*, flow]. An excessive secretion of gastric juice with increased acidity; hypersecretion.

gastrother'apy [" + *therapeia*, treatment]. 1. Treatment of gastric diseases. 2. Treatment with extract of gastric mucosa; used esp. in pernicious anemia.

gastrotome (gas'tro-tōm) [" + *tomē*, incision]. Instrument for incising stomach or abdomen.

gastrotomy (gas-trot'o-mĭ) [" + *tomē*, incision]. Gastric or abdominal incision.

gastrotonometer (gas-tro-to-nom'e-ter) [" + *tonos*, tension, + *metron*, measure]. Instrument for measuring intragastric pressure by insufflation of air or carbonic acid gas.

gastrotrachelotomy (gas-tro-tra-kel-ot'o-mĭ) [" + *trachelos*, neck, + *tomē*, incision]. Cesarean section in which the uterus is opened by a transverse incision across the cervix.

gastrotrop'ic [" + *tropikos*, turning]. Attracted to or affecting the stomach.

gastrotubotomy (gas-tro-tu-bot'o-mĭ) [" + L. *tuba*, tube, + G. *tomē*, incision]. Incision into fallopian tube through abdomen. SYN: *gastrosalpingotomy*.

gastrotympanites (gas"tro-tim-pan-i'tes) [" + *tympanon*, drum]. Gaseous distention of the stomach.

gastrox'ia [" + *oxys*, sour]. Abnormal acidity of contents of stomach.

gastroxynsis (găs-trŏks-ĭn'sĭs) [" + *oxynein*, to sharpen]. Excessive hydrochloric acid secretion by stomach. SYN: *hyperchlorhydria*.

gastrula (gas'tru-lă) [L. dim. G. *gastēr*, belly]. Stage in embryonic development following the blastula in which the embryo assumes a two-layered condition. The outer layer being the *ectoderm* or *epiblast;* the inner layer, the *endoderm* or *hypoblast*. The latter lines a cavity, the *gastrocoel* or *archenteron* which opens to the outside through an opening, the *blastopore*.

gastrula'tion [L. *gastrula*, little belly]. The development of the gastrula.

Gatch bed. A bed in which the patient can be raised and held into a half-sitting position.

gath'ering [A.S. *gaderian*, to collect]. An abscess or swelling.

ga'tism [Fr. *gater*, to spoil]. Vesical or rectal incontinence.

gatophilia (gat-o-fil'ĭ-ă) [G. *gatos*, cat, + *philein*, to love]. Abnormal love for cats.

gatophobia (gat-o-fo'bĭ-ă) [" + *phobos*, fear]. Aversion to cats. SYN: *ailurophobia, galeophobia*.

Gaucher's disease (go-shāz'). Primary epithelioma of the spleen or splenic anemia.

gauge (gāj) [Fr. a measuring rod]. Device for measuring size, capacity, amount or power of an object or substance; a standard of measurement.

English, French and American systems of measurement. English now little used as standard. French number may be found by multiplying diameter in millimeters by 3. The American by multiplying by 2.

Gault's reflex (galt). Contraction of orbicularis palpebrarum muscle resulting from sudden noise being produced near ear.

gauntlet (gawnt'let). A glovelike bandage which fits the hand and fingers.

gauss (gaws). The unit of intensity of a magnetic flux.

Gauss' sign (gaws). Unusual mobility of the uterus in the early weeks of pregnancy.

gauze (gawz) [Fr. *gaze*, gauze]. Thin, transparent fabric used in surgery.

    g., absorbent. G. from which oily matter and sizing has been removed.

    g., antiseptic. G. containing antiseptic material.

    g., aseptic. 1. A gauze sterilized and packaged in an aseptic container and ready for surgical use. 2. A gauze rendered free of microörganisms.

gavage (ga-vazh') [Fr. *gaver*, to gorge fowls]. Feeding with a stomach tube, or with a tube passed through the nares, pharynx, and esophagus into the stomach; the food is in liquid or semiliquid form at a temperature of about 100° F. SEE: *gastrostogavage.*

Gavard's muscle (ga-varz'). The oblique muscular fibers of the stomach's coat.

Gawalowski's test (gav-al-ov'skĭ). Test for sugar made by use of ammonium molybdate and indicated by a blue color.

Gayet's disease (gā-yas'). A lethargic sleep resembling sleeping sickness. It is rare and fatal.

Gay-Lussac's' law. All gases on heating expand equally and on cooling contract equally, according to temperature relation. SEE: *Charles' law.*

Geigel's reflex (gī'gel). Reflex in females resembling cremasteric reflex* in males.

Geisböck's disease or **syndrome** (gĭs'-beck). Abnormal number of red corpuscles in blood with cardiac hypertrophy and elevated blood pressure, without splenic enlargement. SYN: *polycythemia hypertonica.*

Geissler tube (gīs'ler). The original discharge tube for showing the luminous effects of discharges through rarefied gases. The density of the gas in the tube is roughly one-thousandth that of atmospheric pressure.

gel (jel) [L. *gelāre,* to congeal]. 1. A semisolid condition of a precipitated or coagulated colloid. Jelly. A jellylike colloid. 2. Coagulum of a sol.

gelatin (jĕl'ă-tĭn) [L. *gelatina,* gelatin]. A derived protein obtained by the hydrolysis of collagen present in the connective tissues of the skin, bones, and joints of animals.
  USES: It is used as a food, in the preparation of pharmaceuticals, as a medium for the culture of bacteria, and as an agent to speed up coagulation of the blood.
  INCOMPATIBILITIES: Tea (tannin).
  g. culture. Gelatinous base for bacterial growth.
  g. disk. G. circlet for eye therapy.
  g. peptone. Digestive product of gelatin.
  g., nutrient. SEE: *g. culture.*

gelat'inase [L. *gelatina,* gelatin]. An enzyme that liquefies gelatin.

gelatiniferous (jel-at-in-if'er-us) [" + *ferre,* to bear]. Producing gelatin.

gelatiniza'tion [L. *gelatina,* gelatin]. Transformation into a gelatinous mass.

gelatinize (je-lat'in-īz) [L. *gelatina,* gelatin]. To convert into gelatin.

gelatinoid (jel-at'in-oyd) [" + G. *eidos,* resemblance]. Resembling a gelatin; colloid.

gelatinolytic (jel-at"in-o-lit'ĭk) [" + G. *lysis,* dissolution]. Dissolution or splitting up of gelatin.

gelat'inotho'rax [" + G. *thōrax,* chest]. Injection of gelatin solution intrapleurally.

gelatinous (jel-at'in-us) [L. *gelatina,* gelatin]. Containing or of the consistency of gelatin.

gelation (jel-a'shun) [L. *gelāre,* to congeal]. The transformation of a colloid from a sol into a gel.

Gellé's test (zhel-ā'). A tuning fork is connected with a rubber tube inserted in the ear. Pressure is produced by an attached bulb and, if ear is normal, vibrations are felt. SEE: *test.*

gelodiagno'sis [L. *gelāre,* to congeal, + G. *dia,* through, + *gnōsis,* knowledge]. Identification of bacteria by means of a gelose culture medium.

gelose (jĕ'lōs) [L. *gelāre,* to congeal]. 1. Gelatinous element of agar, $C_6H_{10}O_5$. 2. Bacterial culture medium.

gelosis (jel-o'sis) [" + G. *ōsis*]. A hard lump appearing to be frozen.

gelotherapy (jel-o-ther'ă-pĭ) [G. *gelōs,* laughter, + *therapeia,* treatment]. Inducing hilarity in treatment of certain morbid states of the mind.

gelotripsy (jel'o-trip-sĭ) [L. *gelāre,* to congeal, + G. *tripsis,* a rubbing]. The massaging away of indurated swellings.

-gels. A termination to indicate colloids in a solid state.

Gély's suture (zhā-lē'). One for closing intestinal wounds employing cross stitches. SYN: *cobbler's suture.*

gemellus (jem-el'us) [L. twin]. Either of 2 muscles inserted in the obturator internus tendon.

geminate (jem'i-nāt) [L. *geminātus,* paired]. In pairs.

gemination. Development of two teeth within a single alveolus.

gem'ma. 1. A small budlike, reproductive structure, produced by lower forms of life. 2. Any small budlike structure such as a tastebud or end-bulb.

gemmation (jem-ma'shun) [L. *gemmāre,* to bud]. Fission by budding.
  Budlike processes or daughter cells, each containing chromatin, separate from the mother cell from which the bud is projected.

gemmule (jem'ul) [L. *gemmula,* little bud]. 1. A gemma, q.v. 2. One of numerous minute processes present on the dendrites of a neuron.

gena (je'na) [L. *gena,* cheek]. The side of the face or cheek.

genal (je'nal) [L. *gena,* cheek]. Pert. to the cheek. SYN: *buccal.*

gene (jēn) [G. *gennan,* to produce]. SYN: *gen,* q.v. 1. An hereditary determiner. 2. A factor present in the gametes which is responsible for the transmission of hereditary characteristics to the offspring. Genes are self-reproducing ultramicroscopic particles found within cells and located at definite points on chromosomes. They are capable under certain circumstances of giving rise to a new character, such a change being called a mutation.
  g., epistatic. One of a pair of factors which masks the expression of another pair.
  g., holandric. A gene located in the nonhomologous portion of the Y-chromosome.
  g., inhibiting. A gene which prevents the expression of another gene.
  g., lethal. A gene which when in a homozygous condition brings about an effect which results in the death of an individual.
  g., modifying. A gene which influences or alters the effect of another gene.
  g., multiple. A group of genes which have more or less equal and cumulative effects upon the same character.
  g., sex-linked. A gene contained within the X-or sex chromosome.

gen'era. Plural of genus.

general or **house diet.** A diet supplying the normal nutritive requirements of an ambulatory patient with no restriction of food articles.

gen'eralize [L. *genus,* race]. 1. To become or render general. 2. To become systemic, as a local disease.

gen'erating plate. That plate which is chemically acted upon in an electric cell.

generation (jen-er-a'shun) [L. *generāre,* to beget]. 1. An act of forming a new organism. 2. A group of animals or plants the same distance removed from an ancestor, as the first filial (F_1) generation. 3. The average span between one generation and the next, for hu-

generation, alternation of   G-14   **genes**

mans, approximately thirty-three years. 4. The production of an electric current.

g's., alternation of. A mode of reproduction in which a sexual generation alternates with an asexual generation, characteristic of all plants above the Thallophytes. It also occurs in some of the lower animals such as the Coelenterates.

g., asexual. Reproduction which occurs without the union of sexual elements or gametes, such as reproduction by fission, or spore production.

g., F$_1$. The first filial generation; the offspring of a given mating or cross.

g., sexual. Reproduction by the union of male and female cells.

g., spontaneous. SYN: *abiogenesis*. The theory that living things can originate from nonliving matter.

g., viviparous. Normal method of g. among higher animals, of bringing forth live offspring.

generative (jen'er-a-tiv) [L. *generāre*, to beget]. Concerned in reproduction of or affecting the species.

generic (jen-er'ik) [L. *genus*, *gener-*, kind]. 1. General. 2. Pert. to a genus. 3. Distinctive or characteristic of a genus.

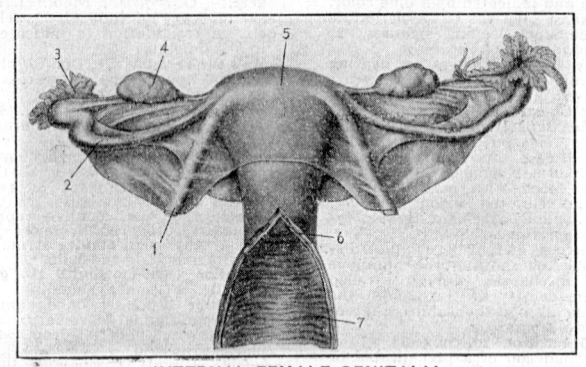

genes (sing. *gene*) (jēns) [G. *gennan*, to produce]. The hypothetical units controlling heredity which are believed to be situated in the chromosomes. There are specific points on the chromosomes for genes governing each characteristic. Genes on different chromosomes are transmitted independently; genes on the same chromosome are said to be linked. The genes occur in pairs, corresponding to the pairing of the chromosomes, one derived from each parent, and each pair of genes determines the individual's genotype for the trait in question. Defective genes cause the body to create abnormal molecules resulting in phenylketonuria, *q.v.*

One-half of these determiners are supposed to represent each parent. SEE: *chromosome, heredity.*

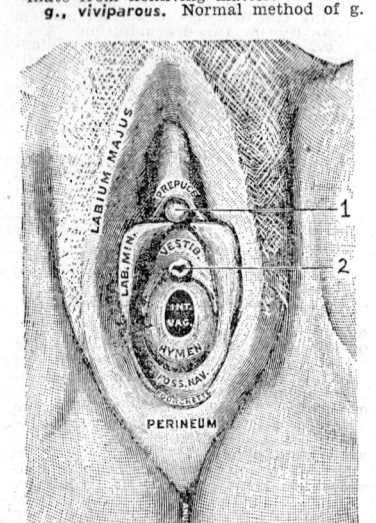

INTERNAL FEMALE GENITALIA
1. Round ligament. 2. Tube. 3. Fimbria. 4. Ovary. 5. Uterus. 6. Cervix uteri. 7. Vagina.

EXTERNAL FEMALE GENITALIA
1. Clitoris. 2. Meatus urinarius.

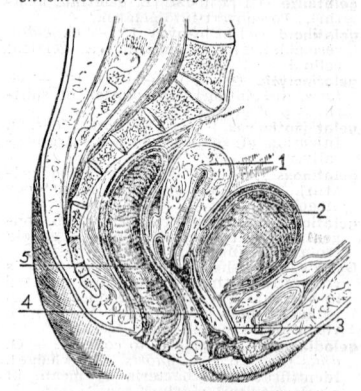

SECTION OF FEMALE GENITALIA
1. Uterus. 2. Bladder. 3. Urethra. 4. Vagina. 5. Rectum.

gene'sial, genes'ic [G. *genesis*, origin]. Pert. to generation.

genesiology (jen-e-sĭ-ol'o-jĭ) [" + *logos*, science]. The science of reproduction.

genesis (jen'es-is) [G. origin]. 1. Act of reproducing; generation. 2. The origin of anything.

genetic (jen-et'ik) [G. *genesis*, origin]. Pert. to generation.

geneticist (jen-et'ĭ-sist) [G. *gennan*, to produce]. One who specializes in genetics.

genet'ics [G. *gennan*, to produce]. The science that accounts for natural differences and resemblances among organisms related by descent. 2. The study of heredity and its variation. SEE: *eugenics*.

genetopathy (je-ne-top'ath-ĭ) [G. *genesis*, origin, + *pathos*, disease]. Disease affecting the generative function.

genetous (jen'et-us) [G. *genesis*, origin]. From birth. SYN: *congenital, q.v.*

Geneva Convention. An international agreement made in Geneva, Switzerland, in 1864 and 1906 safeguarding the wounded and those engaged in aiding them in warfare, resulting in establishing of the Red Cross Society.

genial (je'nĭ-al) [G. *geneion*, chin]. Rel. to the chin.

   g. tubercle. A nodule on the lower

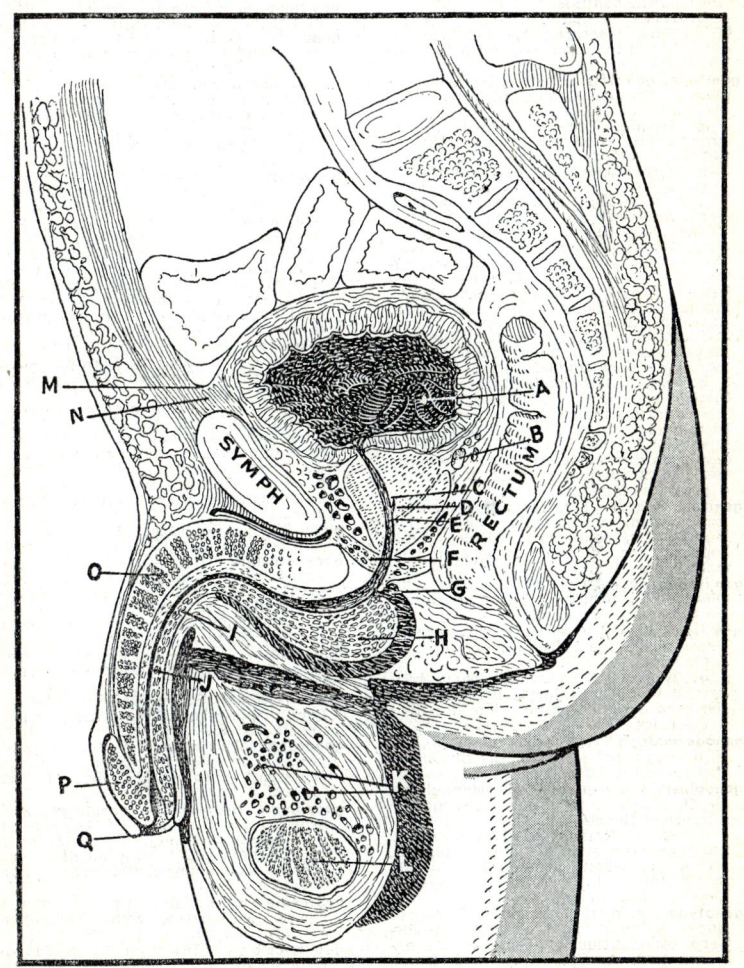

MALE GENITALIA
A. Ureteral orifice. B. Seminal vesicle. C. Colliculus seminalis or verumontanum. D. Prostatic utricle. E. Orifice of ejaculatory duct. F. Suspensory ligament. G. Cowper's gland. H. Bulb of corpus spongiosum. I. Corpus spongiosum. J. Urethra. K. Seminal plexus. L. Testicle. M. Peritoneal fold. N. Space of Retzius. O. Corpus cavernosum. P. Glans penis. Q. Prepuce.

jawbone on either side of the symphysis.
geniculate (jen-ik′u-lāt) [G. *geniculāre*, to bend the knee]. 1. Kneed. 2. Bent as a knee. 3. Pert. to the ganglion or geniculum of the facial nerve.
    g. otalgia. Pain transmitted from the facial nerve to the ear.
geniculum (jen-ik′u-lum) [L. little knee]. A structure resembling a knot, or a knee.
genion (je′nĭ-on) [G. *geneion*, chin]. Apex of the spina mentalis.
genioplasty (je′nĭ-o-plas″tĭ) [" + *plassein*, to form]. Plastic surgery of the chin or cheek.
genital (jen′ĭ-tal) [L. *genitalis*, genital]. Pert. to the genitals.
    g. reflex. Functional nervous manifestations, masturbation, and convulsions, resulting from any form of genital irritation.
genitalia, gen′itals (jen-it-al′ĭ-ă) [L. *genitalis*, genital]. Organs of generation; reproductive organs.
    g., female. Those concerned with reproduction. With the hymen acting as line of boundary, the female generative organs are divided into external and internal.
    The *external* genitalia consist of those structures ext. to the hymeneal ring. Collectively, they are termed the vulva or *pudendum* and include the mons veneris, labia majora, labia minora, clitoris, fourchet, fossa navicularis, vestibule, vestibular bulb, Skene's glands, glands of Bartholin, hymen and vaginal introitus, and perineum.
    Internal are the 2 ovaries, the fallopian tubes, the uterus, and vagina. SEE: *mammary glands.*
    g., male. Two bulbourethral (Cowper's) glands, 2 ejaculatory ducts, 2 glandular organs producing spermatozoa (the testes or gonads), 1 penis with urethra, 2 seminal ducts (vasa deferentes or ductus deferentes), 2 seminal vesicles, 2 spermatic cords, 1 scrotum, 1 prostate gland, *q.v.*
genitals, words pert. to: adiposogenital, agenitalism, agenosomia, andriatrics, andropathy, condyloma, edeology, fallopian tube, female, hypogenitalism, male, pudendum.
gen′itoplas″ty [L. *genitalis*, genital, + G. *plassein*, to form]. Reparative surgery on the genital organs.
gen′itou′rinary [" + G. *ouron*, urine]. Pert. to the genitals and the urinary organs.
    g. system. Organs and parts concerned with the kidneys, urinary bladder, and organs of generation and their accessories.
genodermatosis (jen″o-der-mă-to′sis) [" + *derma*, skin, + *-ōsis*]. Any congenital disease of the skin.
genoplasty (jen′o-plas-tĭ) [L. *gena*, cheek, + G. *plassein*, to form]. Any plastic surgery of the cheek.
    DRESSING: Narrow strip of sterilized gauze, narrow strip of adhesive plaster, cotton, collodion, camel's hair brush, safety pins, inch roller bandage, 6 towels, gauze sponges.
genotype (jen′o-tīp) [G. *gennan*, to produce, + *typos*, type]. 1. Basic hereditary combination of genes of an organism. 2. A type species. 3. Group marked by same hereditary characteristics. The hereditary make-up of an individual as determined by his genes. Each pair of genes determines the genotype for a different characteristic. For example, certain genotypes determine the various blood groups, other genotypes determine the eye color, etc.
genotypic (jĕn-o-tip′ik) [G. *gennan*, to produce, + *typos* type]. Pertaining to a genotype.
Gensoul's disease (zhahn′soolz). A phlegmonous inflammation of the mouth floor and the subcutaneous and intermuscular tissue of the submaxillary region. SYN: *Ludwig's angina.*
gentian (jĕn′shĭ-ăn). USP. Dried rhizome roots of the plant. *Gentiana lutea.*
    g., violet. A dye derived from coal tar. Used in indelible pencils and in 5% solution in treatment of burns and indolent ulcers. Widely used as a stain in histology, cytology, and bacteriology.
gen″tianophil(e, gen″tianoph′ilous. Easily and readily staining with gentian violet.
genu (je′nu) [L. knee]. 1. The knee. 2. Any structure of angular form resembling a bent knee.
    g. extrorsum. SEE: *g. varum.*
    g. introrsum. SEE: *g. valgum.*
    g. recurvatum. Hyperextension at the knee joint.
    g. val′gum. Knock-knee.
    g. va′rum. Bowleg.
genuclast (jen′u-klăst) [" + G. *klan*, to break]. Instrument for breaking knee joint adhesions.
genucu′bital [" + *cubitus*, elbow]. Pert. to the elbows and knees, esp. the knee-elbow position.
    g. position (knee-elbow). One with the patient on the knees, thighs upright, body resting on elbows, head down on hands, employed when not possible to use the knee-chest position.
genupectoral (jen″u-pek′to-ral) [" + *pectus*, breast]. Pert. to the chest and knees.
    g. position. Knee-chest position, *q.v.* for illustration.
    A position assumed by the female patient in which the patient is supported upon her knees and chest, and when the vaginal lips are open the vagina fills with air. This position is used for purposes of examination, treatment, and as an orthopedic aid in retroversion of uterus.
ge′nus [G. *genos*, race]. BIOL: The division between the species and the family.
genyantralgia (jen″ĭ-an-tral′jĭ-ă) [G. *genys*, jaw, + *antron*, cave, + *algos*, pain]. Pain in the antrum of Highmore.
genyantritis (jen″ĭ-an-tri′tis) [" + " + *-ītis*, inflammation]. Inflammation of the antrum of Highmore.
genyoplasty (jen′ĭ-o-plas-tĭ) [" + *plassein*, to form]. Any plastic operation on the chin.
geode (je′ōd) [G. *geōdēs*, earthlike]. A lymph space connected with the lymphatic system.
geograph′ical tongue. Numerous scaly patches on dorsal surface of tongue coalescing into gyrate figures. SEE: *tongue.*
geophagia, geophagism, geophagy (je-o-fa′jĭ-ă, -of′a-jĭzm, -of′a-jĭ) [G. *gē*, earth, + *phagein*, to eat]. A condition in which the patient eats unedible substances, as chalk or earth. SYN: *chthonophagia.*
geotragia (je-o-tra′jĭ-ă) [" + *trōgein*, to chew]. Earth eating. SYN: *chthonophagia, geophagism.*
geo″trich′o′sis. Infection by a fungus, *Geotrichum* which usually attacks the lungs. Symptoms resemble those of chronic bronchitis or tuberculosis. May also infect the mouth or intestine.
Geot′richum. A genus of fungi belonging to the family Eremascaceae; the causative agent of geotrichosis, *q.v.*

gephyrophobia (jef-ĭ-rō-fo′bĭ-ă) [G. *gephyra*, bridge, + *phobos*, fear]. Aversion to bodies of water, or to crossing over bridges over water, or to traveling on boats.

geratic (je-rat′ik) [G. *gēras*, old age]. Rel. to old age.

geratology (jer-ă-tol′o-jī) [" + *logos*, study]. The study of old age. SYN: *gereology*.

Gerdy's fibers (zher′dēz). The superficial transverse ligament of the fingers.

gereology (je-re-ol′o-jī) [G. *gēras*, old age, + *logos*, study]. The science of old age.

geriatrics (jer-ĭ-at′riks) [" + *iatrikē*, medical treatment]. Study and treatment of the diseases of old age.

Gerlach's valve. An inconstant valve present at the opening of the vermiform process (appendix) into the cecum.

Gerlier's disease (zher-le-āz′). Paralyzing vertigo.
SYM: Pains in head and neck, disturbance of vision, vertigo, ptosis, weakness of muscles of the neck and of extremities.

germ [L. *germen*, a microbe]. 1. The first rudiment of an organism, or organ. 2. An ovum. 3. A microörganism, esp., one that causes disease.
 g. cell. An ovum or spermatozoon.
 g., dental. The rudimentary structure from which a tooth develops; includes the dental papilla and the enamel organ. Also called *tooth germ*.
 g., disease. A disease which is caused by a microörganism. Germ diseases are infectious or transmissible.
 g. epithelium, g. ridge. Ridge of epithelium in the embryo from which develops the sexual portions of the body.
 g., hair. The rudimentary structure from which a hair develops. Consists of an ingrowth of epidermal cells called *hair peg* which pushes into the corium.
 g. layers. Three primary layers of cells in an embryo from which the organs and tissues develop. They are the *ectoderm*, *mesoderm*, and *endoderm*, *q.v.*
 g. plasm. The reproductive tissues in contrast to the non-reproductive tissues which constitute the *soma*.
 g. theory. (of disease). The hypothesis that disease is the result of the presence of microörganisms or their products in the body.

German measles. Acute contagious disease with rash of short duration, resembling measles and scarlet fever. SYN: *rötheln, rubella*.

germicidal (jerm-ĭ-si′dal) [L. *germen*, microbe, + *caedere*, to kill]. 1. Destructive to germs. 2. Pert. to an agent destructive to germs.

germicide (jer′mis-īd) [" + *caedere*, to kill]. A substance that destroys germs. Germicides are chemical preparations designed to kill bacteria, the most common being carbolic acid, 1: 1000; bichloride of mercury, 1: 2000; potassium permanganate, 1: 800; boric acid, chloride of lime, cresol, formaldehyde, hexylresorcinol, hydrogen peroxide, iodine, iodoform, mercurochrome, and silver nitrate.
Bacteria and spores may be killed by boiling for 30 minutes, by dry heat at 160° to 170° F. for an hour, by steam at 121° C. for 20 minutes.

germ′inal [L. *germen*, microbe]. Pertaining to a germ or reproductive cells, egg or sperm, or to germination.
 g. center. A light area of lymphocytopoietic cells which occupies the center of lymphatic nodules of the spleen, tonsils, and lymph nodes.
 g. disc. A disc of cells on the surface of the yolk of a teloblastic egg from which the embryo develops; the blastoderm.
 g. epithelium. 1. The epithelium which covers the surface of the genital ridge of an embryo. 2. The epithelium which covers the surface of a mature mammalian ovary.
 g. vesicle. Nucleus of oocyte, *q.v.*

germina′tion [L. *germināre*, to sprout]. 1. Development of an impregnated ovum into an embryo. 2. The sprouting of the spore or seed of a plant.

ger′minative [L. *germināre*, to sprout]. Pert. to germination. SYN: *germinal*.

gerocomia (jer-o-ko′mĭ-ă) [G. *gerōn*, old man, + *komein*, to care for]. The hygiene of old age, or old men.

geroder′ma, gerodermia (je-ro-der′mĭ-ă) [" + *derma*, skin]. An appearance of senility brought about by premature loss of hair, wrinkling of the skin, and general atrophy.

geromaras′mus. Emaciation which accompanies extreme old age.

geromorphism (je-ro-mor′fĭzm) [" + *morphē*, form, + *ismos*, state of]. Appearance of age in youth.

gerontal (jĕ-ron′tal) [G. *gerōn*, old man]. Pert. to an old man or to the aged. SYN: *senile*.

gerontology (je-ron-tol′o-jī) [" + *logos*, study of]. The study of the phenomena of old age. SYN: *geriatrics*.

gerontophil′ia. Fondness or love for old people.

gerontopia (jer-on-to′pĭ-ă) [" + *ops*, vision]. Second sight due to change in the refractive power of the lens. SYN: *senopia*.

gerontoxon (jĕ-ron-toks′on) [" + *toxon*, bow]. Degenerative circle about corneal ext. surface seen in the aged. SYN: *arcus senilis*.

Gerota's capsule. The perirenal fascia.

gestal′tism. The theory that the objects of mind come as wholes which cannot be split up into parts and which are unanalyzable.

gestation (jes-ta′shun) [L. *gestāre*, to bear]. Period of intrauterine fetal development. SYN: *fetation, gravidity, pregnancy*.
RS: *amnion, amniotic fluid, pregnancy, parturition*.
 g., abdominal. Ectopic g. in which the product of conception is lodged in the peritoneal cavity.
 g., cervical. The temporary retention of the ovum within canal of cervix uteri after its expulsion from the uterus in abortion.
 g., cornual. G. in an ill-developed cornu of a bicornuate uterus.
 g., ectopic. Conception outside the uterus.
 g., interstitial. Tubal g. in which the ovum is developed in that portion of oviduct that traverses wall of uterus.
 g., ovarian. A form of ectopic g. in the ovary.
 g., plural. G. with more than 1 embryo.
 g., prolonged, g., protracted. G. prolonged beyond the usual period.
 g. sac. The amnion and its contents.
 g., secondary abdominal. Extrauterine g. in which the fetus, originally situated in oviduct or elsewhere, has become lodged in abdominal cavity because of the rupture of the fetal sac.
 g., secondary. The ovum becomes dislodged from original seat of implanta-

g., tubal, g., tubarian. Ectopic g. in which the product of conception is lodged in the oviduct.

g., tuboabdominal. Extrauterine g. in which fetal sac is formed partly of the abdominal extremity of the oviduct and partly of plastic exudation in the neighborhood.

g., tuboövarian. Extrauterine g. in which the fetal sac is made up of the ovary and the abdominal end of the oviduct.

g., uterotubal. G. in which the ovum is developed partly in uterine portion of oviduct and partly within cavity of uterus.

gestosis (jes-to'sis) [L. *gestāre*, to bear, + G. *ōsis*]. Any disorder of pregnancy.

gher'kin. A form of pickle. COMP: It is more of a condiment than a vegetable or a food.
ACTION: An appetizer and probably a gastric stimulant to a small degree.

Ghon's primary lesion. A bean-shaped shadow in the x-ray of the lung seen in certain cases of pulmonary tuberculosis in children.

ghost corpuscle. Depigmented red blood corpuscle. SYN: *phantom corpuscle*.

giant cell. One of large size with several nuclei, appearing to be made up of many cells, but not clearly outlined, found in both kinds of marrow, esp. in red marrow and spleen; a megakaryocyte.

g. c. tumor. Rare, benign, encapsulated tumor in lower jaw or on alveolar process of upper jaw in the young.

giantism (ji'an-tizm) [G. *gigas, gigant-*, giant]. Abnormal development of the body or its parts. SYN: *gigantism*.

Gianuzzi's cells or **crescents** (jan-oot'sez). Crescent-shaped groups of serous cells found in the mixed salivary glands. They appear as darkly-staining cells forming a caplike structure on the alveoli. Also called *demilumes of Heidenhain*.

Giardia (gī-ar'dī-ă). A genus of protozoa possessing flagella which inhabit the small intestine of man and other animals. They are pear-shaped, possess two nuclei and four pairs of flagella. They attach themselves to the cells of the intestinal mucosa, from which they absorb their nourishment.

G. enterica, G. intestinalis, G. lamblia. Form with 4 pairs of flagella and a sucking disk, with a shape like a pear. SYN: *Cercomonas intestinalis, Lamblia intestinalis*.

G. intestinalis, G. lamblia. Species of Giardia found in man. They were formerly considered nonpathogenic but evidence indicates that they interfere with the absorption of fats, their presence being connected with recurring attacks of diarrhea and the passage of stools containing large amounts of unabsorbed fats and quantities of yellow mucus. They form cysts intermittently.

giardiasis (gī-ar-dī'as-is). Infection with *Giardia lamblia*. SYN: *lambliasis*.

Gibbon's hydrocele (gĭb'ŏn). A hydrocele and large hernia combined.

gibbos'ity [L. *gibbōsus*, humped]. 1. Condition of having a humpback. 2. A hump or gibbus, as the deformity of Pott's disease.

gibbous (gĭb'bus) [L. *gibbus*, humped]. Humped; protuberant or humpbacked.

gid'diness. State of dizziness. SYN: *vertigo*.

Giemsa's stain (gĕm'zah). A stain for staining blood smears. Used for differential leucocyte counts and for the detection of parasitic microörganisms.

Gifford's reflex (gĭf'ford). Pupillary contraction resulting from endeavoring forcibly to close eyelids which are held apart.

gigan'tism [G. *gigas, gigant-*, + *ismos*, state of]. Abnormal development of the body or of a part. SYN: *giantism*.

g., acromegalic. G. in which acromegalic features (overgrowth of the bones of the hands, feet, and face) are present. Due to excessive production of the growth hormone after full skeletal growth has been attained.

g., eunuchnoid. G. accompanied by eunuchoid features and sexual insufficiency.

g., normal. G. of the body in which the bodily proportions and functional activities are normal. Usually the result of hypersecretion of the growth.

gigan'toblast [" + *blastos*, germ]. A very large nucleated red corpuscle.

gigantocyte (ji-gan'to-sīt) [" + *kytos*, cell]. 1. A giant cell. 2. A very large red blood corpuscle.

gigantosoma (ji-gan-to-so'mă) [" + *sōma*, body]. Abnormal size of the body. SYN: *giantism, gigantism*.

Gimbernat's ligament (zham-băr-nahz'). Ligamentum lacunare.

gin'ger. USP. Dried rhizome of the plant Zingiber officinale.
ACTION AND USES: A carminative, aromatic and stimulant. Chiefly in form of tincture.
DOSAGE: 10 m (0.6 cc.).

gingiva (jin-jī'vă) [L. gum]. The gum; the tissues which surrounds the necks of the teeth and covers the alveolar processes of the maxilla and mandible.

g., labial. G. covering labial surfaces of the teeth.

g., lingual. G. covering lingual surface of the teeth. [to the gums.

gingival (jĭn'jiv-al) [L. *gingiva*, gum]. Rel.

gingival'gia [" + G. *algos*, pain]. Pain in the gums. [gums.

gingiv'ally [L. *gingiva*, gum]. Toward the

gingivectomy (jĭn"jĭ-vek'to-mĭ) [" + G. *ektomē*, excision]. Excision of gum tissue in pyorrhea. SYN: *ulectomy*.

gingivitis (jĭn-jĭ-vī'tis) [L. *gingiva*, gum, + G. *-itis*, inflammation]. Inflammation of the gums, characterized by redness, swelling, and tendency to bleed. SYN: *ulitis*.
ETIOL: May be local due to improper dental hygiene, poorly fitting dentures, or appliances, poor occlusion, or it may accompany generalized stomatitis associated with mouth and upper respiratory infections. May also occur in deficiency diseases such as scurvy, blood dyscrasias, or metallic poisoning.

g., expulsive. Osteoperiosteitis of a tooth in which the tooth is expelled from its socket.

g., gravidum. Gingivitis of pregnancy. Characterized by generalized hypertrophy of the gums which may progress to the state of tumor-formation.

g., interstitial. Inflammation of the gums and alveolar processes which precede pyorrhea.

g., phagedenic. A rapidly spreading ulceration of the gums accompanied by extensive ulceration and sloughing of tissue.

gingivoglossitis (jĭn"jĭ-vo-glos-sī'tis) [" + G. *glōssa*, tongue, + *-itis*, inflammation]. Inflammation of the gums and tongue. SYN: *stomatitis*.

ginglyform (jĭn'glĭ-form) [G. *gigglymos*, hinge, + L. *forma*, shape]. In the form of a hinge. SYN: *ginglymoid*.

ginglymoarthrodial

gin'glymo-arthro'dial [" + *arthrōdia*, gliding joint]. Pert. to a joint that is both hinged and arthrodial. SEE: *arthrodia*.

ginglymoid (jing'lĭ-moyd) [" + *eidos*, form]. Pert. to or shaped like a hinged joint.

ginglymus (jing'lĭ-mus) [G. *gigglymos*, hinge]. A hinge joint; diarthrosis.* SEE: *joint*.

Giraldès' organ (zhir-al-dās'). A vestige of the wolffian body at post. side of the testicle. SYN: *paradidymis*.

girdle (gir'del) [A.S. *gyrdel*]. 1. A zone or belt; cingulum, the waist. 2. A structure which resembles a circular belt or band.
 g. anesthesia. A portion around the body without sensation.
 g., Neptune. Stimulating or heating compress of linen covered by flannel encircling trunk from lower end of sternum to pubes.
 g. pain. Painful sensation around the body.
 g., pelvic. The portion of the lower extremities to which the lower limbs are attached. Composed of the two innominate or hip bones.
 g. sensation. Same as g. pain.
 g., shoulder. The portion of the upper extremities to which the upper limbs are attached. Composed of the two clavicles and two scapulae.
 g. symptom. A symptom in tabes as of a tight girdle, such as a feeling of constriction about the chest; also found in compression of the cord due to collapse of the vertebrae as in Pott's disease.

glabel'la [L. *glaber*, smooth]. The smooth surface of the frontal bone lying between the superciliary arches; the portion directly above the root of the nose.

gla'brate [L. *glaber*, smooth]. 1. Bald. 2. Smooth.

glabrificin (glab-rif-is'in) [" + *facere*, to make]. A variety of antibody which exposes a capsulated bacterium to the action of lysin.

gla'brous [L. *glaber*, smooth]. 1. Bald. 2. Smooth. SYN: *glabrate*.

glacial (gla'shal) [L. *glacialis*, icy]. Glassy; resembling ice.

glad'iate [L. *gladius*, sword]. Sword-shaped. SYN: *ensiform, xiphoid*.

gladi'oline. An alkaloid from tissue of the brain.

gladiolus (glad-i'o-lus) [L. *gladiolus*, little sword]. The intermediate and principal segment of the sternum, *q.v.*

glairin (glār'in) [L. *glair*, mucus]. Gelatinous substance in water of some sulfur springs.

glair'y [L. *glair*, mucus]. Viscous, mucoid.

gland [L. *glans, gland-*, kernel]. 1. A secretory organ or structure. 2. A cell or a group of cells which has the ability to manufacture a substance (secretion) which is discharged and used in some other part of the body or is excreted.
 On the basis of complexity of structure, glands may be *simple* (consisting of one or a few secreting units) or *compound* (consisting of many secreting units whose secreting leave the gland by a common duct). Simple tubular glands may be *straight, coiled,* or *branched*.
 Glands consisting of one cell are called *unicellular*; those of more than one cell, *multicellular*.
 On the basis of their secretion, glands are *mucous* (those producing a viscous, slimy secretion), *serous* (those producing a clear watery secretion) or *mixed* (those producing both).

G-19 **gland, Blandin's, Blandin-Nuhn's**

On the basis of the presence or absence of ducts, glands are *exocrine* (those which possess ducts which carry the secretions to an epithelial surface) and *endocrine* (those without ducts and whose secretions enter the blood or lymph).
 On the basis of the shape of the secreting units, glands are *tubular* (secreting portion elongated with a narrow lumen) or *saccular* (secreting portion in the form of a sac or flask). If the lumen of the secreting portion is wide, it is termed an *alveolus*, if narrow, an *acinus*. Glands composed of these types of units are termed *alveolar* and *acinar*, respectively.
 On the basis of the manner by which secretion is accomplished, glands are *merocrine* (secretion forms within cells and is passed through cell membranes into excretory ducts), *apocrine* (secretion forms in apical ends of cells which break off and form a part of the secretion). Ex: *mammary gland*.
 Holocrine (entire cell with its contents is extruded as the secretion. Ex: *sebaceous glands*.
 Glands may be *simple* (tubular or saccular), opening by a single duct upon a surface, or *compound*, consisting of many tubular or saccular cavities. The secretory glands are of 2 kinds: (a) Ductless or endocrine; (b) having ducts. In those without a duct, the secretion leaves the duct by way of the lymph or blood. They are: The *gonads* or sex glands, the *pineal, pituitary, thyroid, parathyroid, thymus,* and *adrenal glands*.
 GLANDS PECULIAR TO THE FEMALE: Bartholin's g., Duverney's g., nabothian g., ovaries, Skene's g., uterine g., glans clitoridis, mammary g.
 GLANDS PECULIAR TO THE MALE: Cowper's g., seminal g., prostate g., Tyson's gland.
 g., absorbent. Any one of the lymphatic glands.
 g., accessory. Gland functioning as an accessory to another gland.
 g., acinotubular. A gland structurally midway bet. an acinous and a tubular g.
 g., acinous. A g. whose secreting units are composed of saclike structures each possessing a narrow lumen.
 g., adrenal. An endocrine gland lying above each kidney. SEE: *adrenal glands*.
 g's., aggregate. Lymphatic glands in patch formation found mainly in ileum. SYN: *Peyer's patches*.
 g's., agminated. SEE: aggregate g's.
 g's., albuminous. Digestive tract glands secreting a fluid containing albumin.
 g., anal. Glands in the region of the anus.
 g., apocrine. A gland whose cells lose some of their cytoplasmic contents in the formation of the secretion. Ex: *mammary gland, some sweat glands*.
 g., areolar. SYN: *glands of Montgomery*. Large sebaceous and rudimentary milk glands present in the areola surrounding the nipple of the female breast.
 g's., auricular. External otic lymph nodes.
 g's., axillary. Axillary lymph nodes.
 g's., Bartholin's. SYN: *major vestibular glands*. Numerous glands which open into the vestibule of the female. Homologous to bulbourethral glands of the male.
 g's., Blandin's; g's., Blandin - Nuhn's. Tiny racemose g's. secreting mucus and saliva, near the tip of the tongue on the undersurface.

g.'s, Bowman's. Simple, branched, tubular glands present in the olfactory mucosa of the nasal cavity.

g.'s, brachial. Glands in the arm and forearm.

g.'s, bronchial. Mixed glands lying in the submucosa of the bronchi and bronchial tubes.

g.'s, Bruch's. Conjunctival lymph nodes in lower lids.

g.'s, Brunner's. Glands in the duodenal submucosa secreting intestinal juice.

g.'s, buccal. Acinous glands in the cheek tissue.

g., bulbourethral. Cowper's gland. Two small glands above the bulb of corpus spongiosum, whose secretion forms part of seminal fluid.

g., cardiac. Glands of the stomach near the cardiac orifice of the esophagus.

g., carotid. Tiny gland at fork of carotid artery.

g.'s, cecal. Cecal lymph nodes.

g.'s, ceruminous. Glands in auditory canal excreting cerumen.

g.'s, cervical. Lymph glands situated in the neck.

g., ciliary. SEE: *Moll's g's.*

g., circumanal. The anal glands, *q.v.*

g.'s, Cobelli's. Glands in the esophageal mucosa.

g., coccygeal. SEE: *Luschka's glands.*

g., compound. A g. consisting of a number of branching duct systems which open into the main excretory duct.

g., compound tubular. G. composed of numerous minute tabules leading to a lone duct.

g., conglobate. Lymphatic gland.

g., conglomerate. SEE: *acinous gland.*

g., Cowper's. SEE: *bulbourethral g.*

g., cutaneous. Glands of the skin, esp., the sebaceous and sudoriferous glands. Also includes modified forms such as the ciliary, ceruminous, anal, preputial, areolar, tarsal glands.

g., cytogenic. A gland whose product is living cells, such as the testis or ovary.

g.'s, decidual. Glands possessing no secretory duct.

g., ductless. A gland which lacks an excretory duct; an endocrine gland, *q.v.*

g.'s, duodenal. SEE: *Brunner's g's.*

g.'s, Duverney's. SEE: *Bartholin's g's.*

g., Ebner's (g. of von Ebner). Serous glands of the tongue located in the region of the vallate papillae, their ducts opening into the furrows surrounding the papillae.

g., endocrine. An organ or structure which secretes a hormone that is absorbed into the blood or lymph; a ductless gland. The principal endocrine glands are the hypophysis, thyroid, and testes, *q.v.* SEE: *endocrine glands.*

g.'s, Frankel's. Tiny glands located below the margin of the vocal cords.

g., fundic. Glands of the body and fundus of the stomach; gastric glands which secrete gastric juice.

g.'s, Gay's. Multiple sweat glands developed to a great extent.

g., genal. Gland in buccal submucosa.

g.'s, genital. SEE: *sexual g's.*

g.'s, gingival. Glands at gum margins.

g.'s, hair. Sebaceous glands opening into each hair follicle.

g.'s, haversian. Glands secreting synovial fluid.

g.'s, hematopoietic. Glands participating in blood production.

g.'s, hemolymph. Modified glands containing blood and lymph sinuses, which probably participate in the formation of the leukocytes and the destruction of red blood corpuscles.

g.'s, hepatic. Lymph nodes located in front of the portal vein.

g.'s, inguinal. Lymph nodes in the inguinal region.

g., interscapular. Embryonic lymphatic tissue.

g., interstitial. G. in connective tissue of seminiferous tubules of testes and which produce internal secretions. SYN: *interstitial or Leydig's cells.*

g.'s, intestinal. Simple or branched tubular glands of the intestine which secrete the succus entericus. Include Brunner's glands, and crypts of Lieberkühn.

g.'s, jugular. SEE: *cervical g.*

g. (of) Krause's. Small glands in the conjunctiva of the eyelids, also called accessory lacrimal glands.

g.'s, labial. Multiple acinous glands bet. the mucosa of the lips and the opening on the inner lip.

g., lacrimal. A compound tubuloalveolar gland, located in the roof of the orbit which secretes tears.

g., lactiferous. SEE: *mammary glands.*

g.'s, Lieberkühn's. Tiny tubular glands on the intestinal mucosa.

g., lingual. Glands of the tongue, includes the ant. lingual glands (g's. of Nuhn), post. lingual glands (g's. of von Ebner) and mucous glands at the root of the tongue.

g.'s, Littre's. Tiny mucous glands in the urethral mucosa in the cavernous portion.

g.'s, lumbar. Lymphatics located behind the peritoneal region and the lower section of the diaphragmatic post. part.

g., Luschka's. G. located near the coccygeal tip.

g., lymph, g., lymphatic. Nodule of lymphatic tissue, found along the path of a lymphatic vessel.

g., mammary. A compound alveolar gland which secretes milk.

g., mandibular. The submaxillary gland, *q.v.*

g.'s, Meibobian. Glands situated in the eyelid secreting sebaceous substance which keeps the lids from adhering. Tarsal glands.

g., merocrine. A gland in which the cells remain intact in the process of the elaboration and discharge of their secretion.

g.'s, Mery's. SEE: *Cowper's g's.*

g.'s, Moll's. Modified sweat glands in the eyelid.

g.'s, Montgomery's. Areolar glands, *q.v.*

g.'s, Morgagni's. SEE: *Littré's g's.*

g.'s, muciparous, g.'s, mucous. G.'s. secreting mucus.

g.'s, nabothian. Dilated mucous glands in the uterine cervix.

g.'s, odoriferous. G. exuding odoriferous materials, as those around the prepuce or anus.

g.'s, oxyntic. Gastric glands usually found in the abdominal cardiac region.

g.'s, pacchionian. Small masses along the surface of the dura mater in the cranium.

g.'s, palatine. Mucous glands in the tissue of the palate.

g., parathyroid. SEE: *parathyroid.*

g.'s, paraurethral. Small rudimentary glands which open on either side of the posterior portion of the urethral orifice in the female; Skene's glands.

g., parotid. Largest salivary gland located in front of the ear. It is a compound tubuloacinous, serous gland.

g's., Peyer's. SEE: *aggregate glands.*
g., pineal. Tiny glandular body of conical shape located bet. 2 sup. quadrigeminal bodies, connected with the thalamus, but not a part of the brain.
g., pituitary. The hypophysis cerebri, *q.v.* Also see *pituitary.*
g's., preputial. SEE: *Tyson's gland.*
g., prostate. G. surrounding male bladder neck and urethra. SEE: *prostate.*
g's., pulmonary. Glands in lung tissue.
g's., pyloric. Gastric glands near the pylorus secreting gastric juice.
g., racemose. SEE: *acinous g.*
g's., Rivini's. SEE: *sublingual g's.*
g., saccular. An alveolar gland.
g., salivary. Any gland secreting saliva, as parotid, sublingual and submaxillary. SEE: *salivary glands.*
g., sebaceous. A simple or branched alveolar gland which secretes sebum. They are found in the skin. Their ducts usually opening into hair follicles.
g's., seminal. Testicles.
g's., serous. SEE: *albuminous g's.*
g., sex. Old term for a gonad, the ovary, or testis.
g's., Skene's. The paraurethral glands, *q.v.*
g's., solitary. SEE: *intestinal g's.*
g's., sublingual. Tiny salivary glands situated on either side of the tongue.
g's., submaxillary. Tiny salivary glands on either side of the tongue in the submaxillary triangles.
g's., sudoriferous. g's., sudoriparous. Glands secreting perspiration situated in the skin. Sweat glands, *q.v.*
g., suprarenal. The adrenal gland, *g.v.*
g's., sweat. SEE: *sudoriferous q.v.*
g., tarsal. Meibomian glands, *q.v.*
g., thymus. The thymus body or thymus, *q.v.*
g., thyroid. Ductless g. situated in the neck in front of the trachea.
g's., tracheal. Acinous g's. of the tracheal mucosa.
g., tubular. A g. whose terminal secreting portions are narrow tubes.
g's., Tyson's. Tiny sebaceous glands found on the inner surface of the prepuce and on the glans of the penis.
g's., urethral. SEE: *Littre's g's.*
g's., vaginal. Acinous g's. in the vaginal mucosa. These are found only in uppermost portion near the cervix. The major portion of the vaginal mucosa is devoid of glands.
g's., vestibular. G's. of the vaginal vestibule. They include the *minor vestibular glands* and the *major vestibular glands* (glands of Bartholin).
g's., vulvovaginal. SEE: *Bartholin's g's.*
g's., Waldeyer's. G's. in the eyelid.
g's., Weber's. G's. in the tongue mucosa.
g's. of Zeis. Large sebaceous glands found in the eyelids. They are associated with the follicles of the eyelashes.
g., Zuckerkandl's. Tiny tawny lobe occasionally seen bet. geniohyoid muscles.
gland, words pert. to: acinous, "aden-" words, admaxillary, "adreno-" words, anadenia, apophysis, autoactivation, blennadenitis, bubonoadenitis, bubononcus, bubonopanua, bulbivestibuli, bulbourethral, chondroadenoma, chorioadenoma, deradenitis, endocrine, fibroadenia, gastric, glans, holocrine, name of each gland, pituitrin, seborrhea, sebum, semen, "sial-" words.

glanders (glan'derz) [L. *glans, gland-,* kernel]. SYN: *farcy, equinia.* Contagious infection of *Malleomyces mallei* in horses and mules, communicable to man.

SYM: Fever, inflammation of the skin and mucous membranes esp., those of the nasal cavity, with formation of ulcers and abscesses. Small subcutaneous nodules (farcy buds) develop which break down giving rise to ulcers. Beginning as small areas, these tend to spread and coalesce involving large areas and giving rise to a viscid, mucopurulent discharge with a foul odor. May occur in acute or chronic form. In the acute form, prognosis is grave, the disease often ending fatally.

glandula (glan'du-la) (pl. *glandulae*) [L. little kernel]. A small gland. SYN: *glandule.*

glan'dular [L. *glandula,* little kernel]. Pert. to or of nature of a gland.
g. therapy. Treatment of disease with endocrine glands or their extracts. SYN: *organotherapy.*

glandule (glan'dŭl) [L. *glandula,* little kernel]. A small gland. SYN: *glandula.*

glans [L. kernel]. 1. A gland. 2. Goiter. 3. A nut.
g. clitoridis. The head of the clitoris.
g. penis, g. phalli. Bulbous end of the penis. SEE: *clitoris, penis.*

glare [M.E. *glaren,* to glow]. Temporary blurring of vision, with possible permanent injury to retina from intense light (visible radiation) emanating from highly reflecting objects, such as sunlight reflected from water or snow, or projected by automobile headlight, or by a therapeutic lamp.

glase'rian artery. SYN: *tympanic artery.* A branch of internal maxillary artery; goes to tympanum.
g. fissure. A fissure in the temporal

glass, polarized. A medium that permits the exiting light waves to vibrate in only one direction.
g., swallowing. F. A. TREATMENT: SEE: *cotton-wool sandwiches.*
g., ultraviolet transmitting. Glass designed to admit ultraviolet radiation through it.

The best transmits from 50 to 60% of the solar radiation, between 290 and 320 millimicrons. With age the transparency to these rays drops off 50%.

glass'es [A.S. *glaes,* glass]. 1. Transparent refractive device worn to correct eye defects. 2. Device worn to protect eyes from glare. Federal specifications are "shade No. 3 filter lens."
g., bifocal. Those in which the refracting power of the lower portion differs from that in the upper portion, the lower portion being used for viewing near objects, or reading the upper portion for distant objects.

glas'sy [A.S. *glaes,* glass]. Hyaline; vitreous; like glass, smooth and shiny.

Glau'ber's salt. Crystalline salt used as a hydragogue purgative.

glauco'ma [G. *glaukos,* green, + *oma,* swelling]. Disease of eye characterized by increase in intraocular pressure which results in atrophy of optic nerve and blindness of 2 general types, *primary,* which sets in without known cause, and *secondary,* in which there is an increase in intraocular pressure due to other eye disease. The acute type often attended by acute pain. The chronic type has an insidious onset. Normal tonometer reading is 13 to 22. ETIOL: Closing of the canal of Schlemn.

glaucoma absolutum   G-22   **globulin, antihemophiliac**

TREATMENT: *Nonoperative*: Miotics (eserine, pilocarpine), phospholine iodide, massage, heat, sedatives, elimination.
Operative: Paracentesis of cornea, iridectomy (broad peripheral), cyclodialysis, ant. sclerotomy, sclerotomy with inclusion of iris as iridotasis or iridocleisis, sclerectomy, Elliott's trephine or Lagrange enucleation.
SEE: *ciliarotomy*.

g. absolutum. Eye completely blind, cornea insensitive, ant. chamber shallow, excavated optic disc, eye as hard as stone, extremely painful.

g., chronic. Pressure up to 45-50, enlargement of ant. ciliary veins, cornea clear, dilated pupil, pain, poor vision during attacks, field may be normal, no cupping early.

g., infantile. Buphthalmos resulting in uniform enlargement of eye with increased pressure.

g. simplex. Pressure not high, contracted field, glaucomatous cupping, blindness, no acute attacks. TREATMENT: Prostigmine.

glaucomatous (glaw-ko'ma-tus) [" + *ōma*, swelling]. Pert. to glaucoma.

gleet [Fr. *glette*, slime]. A mucous discharge from the urethra in chronic gonorrhea.

Glénard's disease (gla-narz'). Prolapse of 1 or more of the internal organs. SYN: *enteroptosis, splanchnoptosis*.

glenohumeral (gle-no-hu'mer-al). Pert. to the humerus and the glenoid cavity.

g. ligaments. Three ligaments in shoulder.

gle'noid [G. *glēnē*, cavity, + *eidos*, form]. Having the appearance of a socket.

g. cavity. The socket which receives the head of the humerus, below the acromium at the junction of the superior and axillary borders.

g. fossa. The mandibular fossa, which receives the capitulum of the mandible.

gli'a [G. glue]. The neuroglia, *q.v.*; the non-nervous or supporting tissue of the brain and spinal cord.

g. cells. Neuroglia cells, includes astrocytes, oligodendroglia (oligoglia), and microglia. SEE: *cell, neuroglia*.

gliacyte (gli'as-īt) [" + *kytos*, cell]. A neuroglia cell.

gli'adin [G. *glia*, glue]. A protein separable from the gluten of wheat. It is deficient in lysine. It contains 94.11% amino acid.

glial (gli'al) [G. *glia*, glue]. Concerning glia or neuroglia.

gliarase (gli'ar-ās) [G. *glia*, glue]. Astrocytic mass with fission of cytoplasm.

gliobacte'ria [" + *baktērion*, little rod]. A zooglear mass containing bacilli.

glioblasto'ma [" + *blastos*, germ, + *ōma*, tumor]. A neuroglia cell tumor. SYN: *glioma*.

g. multiforme. A neoplasm of the central nervous system, esp., the cerebrum, consisting of a variety of cellular types.

Gliocladium, Aspergillus, and **Penicillium.** It is highly bacteriostatic towards Gram-positive bacteria and is effective against certain plant pathogens.

gliococ'cus [" + *kokkos*, berry]. A micrococcus in a mass of zooglea.

gliocyte (gli'o-sīt) [" + *kytos*, cell]. A neuroglia cell. SYN: *gliacyte*.

gliocyto'ma [" + " + *ōma*, tumor]. A neuroglia cell tumor.

gliogenous (gli-oj'en-us) [" + *gennan*, to produce]. Of the nature of neuroglia.

glio'ma (pl. *glio'mata*) [" + *ōma*, tumor]. 1. A sarcoma of neurogliar origin. 2. Neoplasm or a tumor composed of neuroglia cells.

g. retinae. Malignant tumor of retina; occurs in children under 5 years of age; metastasizes late. SEE: *pseudoglioma*.

gliomatosis (gli-o-mat-o'sis) [" + " + *ōsis*]. Formation of a glioma.

gliomatous (gli-o'mă-tus) [G. *glia*, glue, + *ōma*, tumor]. Affected with or of the nature of a glioma.

gliomyoma (gli-o-mī-o'mă) [" + *mys, myo-*, muscle, + *ōma*, tumor]. A mixed glioma and myoma.

glioneuroma (gli-o-nŭ-ro'mă) [" + *neuron*, nerve, + *ōma*, tumor]. A tumor having the characteristics of glioma and neuroma.

gliosarco'ma [" + *sarx*, flesh, + *ōma*, tumor]. Glioma combined with fusiform cells of sarcoma.

gliosis (G. *glia*, glue, + *-osis*). Proliferation of neuroglial tissue in the central nervous system.

gliosome (gli'o-sōm) [" + *sōma*, body]. One of the rounded bodies seen in neuroglia cells.

gliotoxin. An antibiotic obtained from several different fungi, esp. *Trichoderma*.

glischrin (glĭs'krĭn) [G. *glischros*, gluey]. Mucinous substance formed in urine by *Bacillus glischrogenes*.

glischruria (glis-kru'rĭ-ă) [" + *ouron*, urine]. Glischrin in the urine.

glisso'nian cirrhosis. Inflammation of peritoneal coat of the liver. SYN: *perihepatitis*.

glissoni'tis [G. *-itis*, inflammation]. Inflammation of Glisson's capsule.

Glisson's capsule (glĭs'uns). The outer capsule of fibrous tissue investing the liver. SYN: *capsula fibrosa hepatis*.

glo'bin [L. *globus*, globe]. A protein constituent of hemoglobin. It is a histone and yields histidine upon hydrolysis.

g. insulin. SEE: *insulin, globin*.

globinom'eter [" + G. *metron*, measure]. Device for estimating the number of blood corpuscles in a given amount of blood. SYN: *cytometer*.

glo'boid [" + G. *eidos*, form]. Spheroid; resembling a globe.

g. bodies. Minute ultramicroscopical microörganisms such as pathogens of poliomyelitis.

globular (glob'u-lar) [L. *globus*, a globe]. Resembling a globe or globule; spherical.

globule (glob'ūl) [L. *globulus*, globule]. Any small rounded body.

globulicidal (glob"u-lis-i'dal) [" + *caedere*, to kill]. Destructive to red blood corpuscles.

globulim'eter [" + G. *metron*, measure]. Device for determining relative proportions of hemoglobin.

globulin (glŏb'ū-lĭn). [G. *globulus*, globule]. One of a group of simple proteins insoluble in pure water but soluble in neutral solutions of salts of strong acids with strong bases.
Ex: *serum, globulin, fibrinogen, myosinogen, lactoglobulin legumin*.

g., Ac—Accelerator globulin; a globulin present in blood serum which speeds up the conversion of prothrombin to thrombin in the presence of thromboplastin and calcium ions.

g., antihemophiliac. SYN: *Thromboplastinogen; thrombocytolytic factor*. A clotting component present in the plasma which is essential for the normal agglutination and disintegration of blood platelets. It is deficient in the blood of hemophiliacs.

g. gamma. That fraction of serum globulin with which most of the immune antibodies are associated. Most of the antibodies to viruses, bacterial agglutinogens, exotoxins, and injected foreign proteins are contained in the gamma globulin fraction. They are thought to arise from plasma cells.

g., human immune. A preparation of globulins antibodies obtained from the human placenta. It contains the antibodies or immune factors against measles and is used in the prevention, modification, and treatment of measles.

g., serum. Globulins present in blood plasma or serum; the fraction of the blood serum which antibodies are associated. By electrophoresis, they can be separated into alpha-, beta-, and gamma-globulins, which differ in their isoelectric points.

glob'ulism [" + G. *ismos*, state]. 1. Abnormal amt. of red corpuscles in the blood. 2. Administration of medicine in globules.

globulolysis (glob-u-lol'is-is) [" + G. *lysis*, dissolution]. Red blood corpuscle destruction. SYN: *hematolysis*.

globulolytic (glob-u-lol-it'ik) [" + G. *lysis*, dissolution]. Capable of destroying red blood corpuscles.

globulose (glob'u-lōs) [L. *globulus*, globule]. Albumose or proteid produced by the digestion of globulins.

globu'lysis [L. *globus*, globe, + G. *lysis*, destruction]. Destruction of red blood corpuscles. SYN: *globulolysis, hemolysis*.

globus [L.]. A globe or sphere.

g. hystericus. A lump in the throat in hysteria and other neuroses.

ETIOL: Probably due to functional disturbance of the 9th cranial nerve, and spasm of the pharyngeal muscles.

g. major. Head of epididymus.
g. minor. Lower end of epididymus.
g. pallidus. Pale section within the lenticular nucleus. SEE: *paleostriatum*.

glomangioma (glŏm"ăn-jĭ-ō'mă). A benign tumor which develops from an arteriovenous glomus of the skin.

glom'erate [L. *glomerāre*, to wind into a ball]. Conglomerate, clustered, grouped.

glomer'ular [L. *glomerulus*, little skein]. Clustered. Pert. to a glomerulus.

glomerule (glom'er-ul) [L. *glomerulus*, little skein]. A glomerulus.

glomer'uli (sing. *glomerulus*) [L. *glomerulus*, little skein]. 1. Small structures in the malpighian body of the kidney made up of capillary blood vessels in a cluster and enveloped in a thin wall, giving off uriniferous tubules. 2. Plexuses of capillaries. Twisted secretory parts of sweat glands.

glomerulitis (glom-er-ū-li'tis) [" + G. *-itis*, inflammation]. Inflammation of glomeruli, esp. of the renal glomeruli. SYN: *glomerulonephritis*.

glomerulonephritis (L. *glomerulus*, little skein, + G. *nephros*, kidney, + *-itis*, inflammation). SYN: *glomerulitis*. A form of nephritis in which the lesions involve primarily the glomeruli. May be acute, subacute, or chronic. Etiology is unknown but it frequently follows other infections, esp., those of the upper respiratory tract. Characterized by hematuria, edema, hypertension, and in severe cases, dyspnea, delirium, convulsions, and coma.

glomerulus (*pl. glomeruli*) (L. little skein). 1. A small rounded mass or spherical structure. 2. A small tuft of capillary loops enclosed within Bowman's capsule, the expanded end of a renal tubule, and two comprising a Malpighian body or renal corpuscle. It serves as a filtering structure in the formation of urine.

g., olfactory. A rounded body found in the olfactory bulb formed by the numerous terminal branches of the dendrites of a mitral cell intertwining with the terminal fibers of several olfactory receptor cells.

glomus (glo'mus) [L.]. A small, round swelling made up of tiny blood vessels and found in a stroma containing many nerve fibers.

g., caroticum. The carotid body. *q.v.*
g., choroideum. An enlargement of the choroid plexus at its entrance into the inferior corum of the lateral ventricle.
g., coccygeum. The coccygeal body, *q.v.*

glos'sa [G. tongue]. The tongue.

glos'sal [G. *glōssa*, tongue]. Rel. to the tongue.

glossalgia (glos-sal'jĭ-ă) [" + *algos*, pain]. Pain in the tongue. SYN: *glossodynia*.

glossectomy (glos"ek'to-mĭ) [" + *ektome*, excision]. Partial or complete excision of tongue. SYN: *elinguation, Kocher's operation*.

Glossina. A genus of flies called tsetse flies. Includes about 20 species of bloodsucking flies which are confined principally to central and southern Africa. They transmit the trypanosomes (*Trypanosoma gambiense, T. rhodesiense*) the causative agents of sleeping sickness in man and other trypanosomes which infect wild and domestic animals. Important species are *Glossina palpalis, G. morsitans, G. tachinoides,* and *G. swynnertoni.* SEE: *Trypanosoma, sleeping sickness.*

glossi'tis [" + *-itis*, inflammation]. Inflammation of the tongue.

g., acute. Associated with stomatitis, *q.v.* The tongue is covered with ulcers and is tender and painful. Another form affects the parenchyma of tongue and is characterized by edema, which may spread to surrounding structures, producing asphyxia and necessitating tracheotomy operation.

SYM: Tongue is painful; saliva thick and viscid, rendering swallowing difficult. Marked malaise, and often a rise in temperature.

TREATMENT: Oral cleanliness by frequent use of antiseptic mouthwashes. Potassium chlorate orally because it is excreted by the salivary glands and acts as a salivary antiseptic. Fluid food, to avoid discomfort and pain. Bowels kept open by using saline aperients.

g. areata exfoliativa. Geographical tongue.

g., chronic. Sometimes while suffering from chronic ill health, chronic dyspepsia, and septic teeth, this condition arises.

SYM: Tongue is large, pale, and flabby, and shows indentation marks from teeth pressure. Mouth is uncomfortable and there may be an unpleasant taste or foul odor.

TREATMENT: Improvement of the general health, relief of constipation, careful attention to oral hygiene.

g. desic'cans. A painful, raw, and fissured tongue.

g. median rhomboidal. An inflammatory area, somewhat diamond shaped, found on the dorsum of the tongue anterior to the vallate papillae.

g. Moeller's. Glossodynia exfoliativa, *q.v.*

g. parasit'ica. Black tongue. SYN: *glossophytia*.

glosso- [G. *glōssa*, tongue]. Prefix: Signifies pert. to the tongue.

glossocele (glos'so-sēl) [G. *glōssa*, tongue, + *kēlē*, swelling]. Swelling and protrusion of the tongue due to disease or malformation.

glossodynamometer (glos″so-din-a-mom'e-ter) [" + *dynamis*, power, + *metron*, measure]. Device for measuring contractile power of the tongue muscles.

glossodynia (glos-o-din'ĭ-ă) [" + *odynē*, pain]. Pain in the tongue. SYN: *glossalgia*.

   g. exfoliativa. Moeller's glossitis. A chronic superficial inflammation of the tongue characterized by burning or pain and increased sensitivity to hot and spicy foods.

glos″soepiglot'tic [" + *epi*, upon, + *glōttis*, back of tongue]. Pert. to the ligament bet. base of tongue and epiglottis.

glossoepiglottidean (glos″o-ep-I-glŏ-tid'e-an) [" + " + *glōttis*, back of tongue]. Rel. to the tongue and epiglottis.

   g. folds. Three mucous membrane folds from base of tongue to the epiglottis. SYN: *plicae epiglotticae*.

   g. ligament. Elastic band from base of tongue to the epiglottis in middle g. fold.

glossograph (glos'o-graf) [" + *graphein*, to write]. A graph for showing the tongue's movements in speaking.

glossohyal (glos-o-hi'al) [" + *yoeidēs*, U-shaped]. Rel. to tongue and hyoid bone. SYN: *hyoglossal*.

glosso″kin'esthet'ic. Pertaining to movements of the tongue, esp., those in speech.

glosso″la'bi'al. Pertaining to the tongue and lips.

glossolalia (glos-so-lal'ĭ-ă) [" + *lalia*, babble]. Repetition of senseless remarks not related to the subject or situation involved.

glossology (glos-sol'o-jĭ) [" + *logos*, study]. 1. Study of the tongue and its diseases. SYN: *glottology*. 2. Science of nomenclature. SYN: *onomatology*.

glossolysis (glos-sol'is-is) [G. *glōssa*, tongue, + *lysis*, loosening]. Paralysis of tongue. SYN: *glossoplegia*.

glosso″pal'atine. Pertaining to the tongue and the palate.

glossopathy (glos-sop'ă-thĭ) [" + *pathos*, disease]. Disease of the tongue.

glossopharyngeal (glos″o-far-in'je-ăl) [" + *pharygx*, pharynx]. Rel. to tongue and pharynx.

   g. nerve. Ninth cranial n. FUNCT: Special sensory (taste), visceral sensory, motor. ORIG: by several roots from the medulla oblongata. DIST: Pharynx, ear, meninges, tongue, tonsils. BRS: Carotid, tympanic, pharyngeal, lingual, tonsillar, and sinus nerve of Hering.

glossohytia (glŏs-sō-fī'tĭ-ă) SYN: *hyperkeratosis linguae*. Black or hairy tongue, characterized by the appearance on the dorsum of the tongue of a dark furlike patch consisting of hypertrophied filiform papillae, pigment, and shed epithelial cells. Cause unknown.

glossoplasty (glos-so-plas'tĭ) [" + *plassein*, to form]. Reparative surgery of the tongue.

glossoplegia (glŏs-sō-ple'jĭ-ă). SYN: *glossolysis*. Paralysis of tongue, usually unilateral. ETIOL: Cerebral hemorrhage, disease, or injury which involves the hypoglossal nerve.

glossopto'sis [" + *ptōsis*, a dropping]. A dropping of the tongue downward out of normal position.

glosso″pyros'is. A burning sensation of the tongue.

glossorrhaphy (glos-sor'ă-fĭ) [" + *raphē*, suture]. Suture of wound of the tongue.

glossos'copy [" + *skopein*, to examine]. Inspection of the tongue.

glossospasm (glos'so-spazm) [" + *spasmos*, spasm]. Spasmodic contraction of muscles of the tongue.

glossotomy (glos-ot'o-mĭ) [" + *tomē*, incision]. Incision of tongue.

glosso″trich'ia. Hairy tongue, due to greatly elongated filiform papillae which gives the tongue a hairy appearance.

gloss'y [M.E. *glōse*]. Smooth and shining.

   g. skin. Shiny appearance of the skin due to atrophy or injury to nerves.

glot'tic [G. *glōttis*, back of tongue]. Of or pert. to the tongue, or the glottis.

glottis (glŏt'is) [G. *glottis*, back of tongue]. The sound-producing apparatus of the larynx consisting of the two *vocal folds* and the intervening space, the *rima glottidis*. A leaf-shaped lid of fibrocartilage (the epiglottis) protects this opening.

   g., edema. The accumulation of fluid in the tissues lining the larynx. It may result from irritation of the larynx from improper use of the voice, excessive use of tobacco or alcohol, chemical fumes, acute infections, or more serious conditions such as tuberculous or syphilitic laryngitis.

   SYM: Hoarseness, and later complete aphonia, extreme dyspnea at first on inspiration, but later on expiration also. Stridulous respiration, barking cough when epiglottis is involved.

   g. spuria. Space situated bet. the false vocal cords.

glotti'tis [" + -*itis*, inflammation]. Inflammation of the tongue. SYN: *glossitis*.

glottol'ogy [" + *logos*, study]. The study of the tongue and its diseases. SYN: *glossology*.

glucase (glu'kās) [G. *glukus*, sweet]. An old term for a ferment converting starch into glucose.

glucatonia (glu-ka-to'nĭ-ă) [" + *a-*, priv. + *tonos*, tone]. Reduction of blood sugar brought about by insulin therapy. Insulin shock.

glucide (glū'sīd) [G. *glukus*, sweet]. 1. One of a large class of organic compounds including the carbohydrates and glucosides.* 2. USP. White crystalline powder 500 times sweeter than sugar having no food value. USES: Substitute for sugar in diabetes. One-quarter gr. (0.015 Gm.) in the place of an ordinary lump of sugar.

gluciphore (glu'sĭ-fōr) [" + *phorein*, to carry]. An atomic group which, when combined with other tasteless atoms called auxoglucs, forms sweet compounds. SEE: *auxogluc*.

glucohe'mia [" + *aima*, blood]. Sugar in the blood. SYN: *glycosemia*.

gluco″neogenesis [G. *glukus*, sweet, + *neos*, new, + *genesis*, origin]. The formation of glucose from noncarbohydrate sources such as proteins, and possibly fats. It occurs in the liver under such conditions as low carbohydrate intake or starvation.

glu'cose [L. *glucosum* from G. *glukus*, sweet]. 1. A liquid obtained from the incomplete hydrolysis of starch. It is a thick syrupy liquid, sweet in taste, containing d-glucose (dextrose), dextrins and other carbohydrates. It is used for nutritive purposes and in various pharmaceutical and food preparations. 2. Dextrose ($C_6H_{12}O_6$), a crystalline monosaccharide, more specifically dextro- or d-glucose.

Glucose is the most important carbohydrate in body metabolism. It is formed during digestion from the hydrolysis of di- and polysaccharides, esp., starch, and absorbed into the blood of the portal vein. In its passage through the liver excess glucose is converted into glycogen (*glycogenesis*). The concentration of sugar in the blood is approximately 0.1 per cent (100 mg.) the amount being maintained at a fairly constant level (80 to 120 mg.) through the action of insulin produced by the Islets of Langerhans of the pancreas. Failure of the pancreas to produce adequate insulin results in *hyperinsulinism* in which the blood sugar (glucose) level may rise to 200 mg. or higher. When above the renal threshold (about 180 mg.), glucose appears in the urine (glycosuria), a symptom of diabetes. Inadequate production of insulin or injection of insulin as in insulin shock treatment, reduces the blood sugar below normal, a condition known as *hypoglycemia, q.v.*

In the tissue gluecose may be (a) converted into glycogen, (b) converted into fat, or (c) oxidized to carbon dioxide and water. Free glucose is not used in the tissues until phosphorlyated by ATP (adenosinetriphosphate). This occurs through the action of an enzyme, hexokinase, with the resultant production of glucose-6-phosphate. Through a complex series of reactions involving several enzymes, the action of certain hormones, and the formation of several intermediate products including lactic and pyruvic acids, oxidation to carbon and water is brought about. Hormones of and ant., lobe of the hypophysis, the adrenal gland (cortex and medulla), thyroid and the gonads play a role in carbohydrate metabolism.

When the blood sugar is below normal fats are consumed. Incomplete combustion leads to the formation of ketone bodies, also a symptom of diabetes. Blood sugar acts as a protein sparer, *q.v.* Nervous tissue is especially dependent upon glucose as its source of energy, the brain being able to oxidize glucose directly.

g. chemistry findings: The glucose found in the blood stream has a dual origin. First, glucose is present normally in both the whole blood and plasma; secondly, the greater percentage of the normal glucose concentration has an exogenous origin—that is, from the food intake. **A. Normal:** 80 to 120 mgm. per 100 cc. **B. Increased:** (1) Acromegaly, (2) Adrenal tumors, (3) Cortical or medullary, (4) Diabetes mellitus, (5) Hemochromatosism, (6) Hyperthyroidism, (7) Hyperpituitarism, (8) Hyperadrenalism, (9) Intracranial pressure, (10) Severe exercise. **C. Decreased:** (1) Addison's disease, (2) Adenoma or carcinoma of islands of Langerhans, (3) Cretinism, (4) Hyperinsulinism, (5) Hypopituitarism, (6) Hypothyroidism, (7) Insulin shock, (8) Muscular dystrophy, (9) Myxedema.

glucose tolerance test. In suspected cases of hyperinsulinism, the test is prolonged to six hours with samples of blood being drawn hourly and analyzed for sugar content If the blood-sugar level continues to drop after 3 hours, falling below 80 mgs. per 100 cc., hyperinsulinism is indicated although other conditions may produce a deficiency in blood sugar (hypoglycemia).

glucosidase. An enzyme which catalyzes the hydrolysis of a glucoside.

glucoside (glū'kō-sĭd) [G. *glukus*, sweet]. A substance glycoside, which upon hydrolysis, yields a sugar, glucose, and one or two additional products. They are numerous and widely distributed in plants. Many glucosides have medicinal properties, for example digitalin and strophanthin, present in digitalis and strophanthus respectively, which have a specific effect upon the heart. SEE: *glycoside.*

glucosin (glu'ko-sīn) [G. *glukus*, sweet]. Any one of a series of bases derived by action of ammonia on glucose.

glucosu'ria [" + *ouron*, urine]. Abnormal amt. of sugar in the urine. SYN: *glycosuria.*

gluelike tumor. Glioma. Also a colloid degenerative cancer or colloma.

Glu'ge's corpuscles. Granular cells containing fat droplets, usually found in degenerating nervous tissue.

glu'side. Saccharin, said to be 300 times as sweet as cane sugar. SYN: *glusidum.*
  DOSAGE: ½ gr. (0.03 Gm.).

glutam'ic acid. SYN: *Glutamic acid.* An amino acid (COOH(CH₂)₂CHNH₂COOH) formed in the hydrolysis of proteins.

glutaminase. An enzyme which catalyzes the breakdown of glutamine into glutamic acid and ammonia.

glutamine. The mono-amide of aminoglutaric acid. It is present in the juices of many plants and is essential in the metabolism of certain bacteria. It is also present in animal tissues such as the brain, liver and kidney.

glutathione (glū-ta-thī'on) [G. *theion*, sulfur]. A tripeptide of glutamic acid, cystein, and glycine.
  Found in small quantities in active animal tissues; takes up and gives off hydrogen; fundamentally important in cellular respiration.

gluteal (glū'tē-ăl) [G. *gloutos*, buttock]. Pertaining to the buttocks.
  g. fold. Crease between the thigh and the buttocks. SEE: *rump.*
  g. reflex. Contraction of gluteal muscles from stimulation of their skin.

glutelin (glū'tē-lĭn). A simple protein found in grain seeds, soluble in alkalies and dilute acids, but not in neutral solutions. SEE: *protein.*

glu'ten [L. glue]. Vegetable albumin, a protein which can be prepared from wheat, corn, and other grain.

glu'tin [L. glue]. The viscid portion of wheat gluten. SYN: *gliadin.*

glutinous (glū'tĭn-us) [L. *glutinōsus, gluey*]. Adhesive; sticky.

gluti'tis [G. *gloutos*, buttock, + *-itis*, inflammation]. Inflammation of muscles of buttocks.

glu'tolin. An albumoid substance found in small amts. in paraglobulin.

glycase (gli'kās) [G. *glykus*, sweet]. The enzyme that converts maltose into dextrose. SEE: *enzyme, ferment.*

glycemia (gli-se'mĭ-ă) [" + *aima*, blood]. Sugar or glucose in the blood. SYN: *glycosemia.**

glyceride (glĭs'er-ĭd) [G. *glykus*, sweet]. An ester of glycerin compounded with an acid.

glycerine (glĭs'er-ĭn) [G. *glykus*, sweet]. USP. SYN: *glycerol.* A trihydric alcohol, tri-hydroxy-propane (C₃H₅(OH)₂) present in chemical combination in all fats. It is an oil, colorless, liquid soluble in all proportions in water and alcohol. It is made commercially by the hydrolysis of fats esp., during the manufacture of soap.
  USES: Extensively as a solvent, as a preservative, as an emollient in various skin diseases, and in form of suppositories as an evacuant.

glycerite (glĭs'er-ĭt) [G. *glykus*, sweet]. Drug dissolved in glycerin. Four official.

glyceri'tum (pl. *glycerita*) [L *glycerite*]. Medicinal substance mixed or dissolved in glycerin.

glycerol (glĭs'er-ol) [G. *glykus*, sweet]. Clear, colorless, syrupy liquid formed by hydrolysis of fat. SYN: *glycerin, q.v.*

  g. trinitrate. Nitroglycerin, USP. Made by the action of nitric acid on glycerin in presence of sulfuric acid.
  Used internally in form of spirit which is 1% in alcohol, and in form of tablets.
  ACTION AND USES: To dilate blood vessels in some cases of angina pectoris.
  DOSAGE: 1 ℳ (0.6 cc.) Tablets, 1/100 gr. (0.6 mg.).

glyc'eryl. The trivalent radical C_3H_5 of glycerol.

glycine (glī'sēn) [G. *glykus*, sweet]. Aminoacetic acid* derived from gelatin and from many proteins. SYN: *glycocin, glycocoll.*

glyco-. Prefix from G. *glykus*, sweet. Used in chemical compounds to indicate the presence of glycerol or similar substance.

gly'cocin. Glycin, *q.v.*

glycoclas'tic [G. *glykus*, sweet, + *klassein*, to break]. Pert. to the hydrolysis and digestion of sugars.

glycogen (glī'kō-jĕn) [G. *glykus*, sweet, + *gennan*, to produce]. It is a polysaccharide $(C_6H_{10}O_5)x$ and is commonly called "animal starch", a whitish powder which can be prepared from mammalian liver and muscle, and other animal tissues.
  Formation of glycogen from carbohydrate sources is called *glycogenesis*; from noncarbohydrate sources, *glyconeogenesis*. The conversion of glycogen to glucose is called *glycogenolysis*.
  It is the form in which carbohydrate is stored in the animal body for future conversion into sugar, and for subsequent use in performing muscular work or for liberating heat.
  It is formed from sugar and a part of the fat and protein in the blood. It is converted when needed by the tissues into glucose. It is a muscle food, and with the contraction of the muscles it breaks down into lactic acid, causing fatigue. Oxygen is then needed to convert lactic acid back into glycogen, at which time some of the lactic acid is burned, producing carbonic acid and heat. Sugar from the blood takes the place of the lactic acid consumed.
  Oxygen and sugar are necessary to prevent fatigue from muscular exertion long continued. SEE: *azoamyly*.

glycogenase (glī'kō-jen-ās) [" + *gennan*, to produce]. An enzyme in the liver which hydrolyzes glycogen.
  Its end product is dextrose.

glycogenesis (glī-ko-jen'es-ĭs) [" + *genesis*, formation]. The formation of glycogen, as occurs in man after the eating of a carbohydrate meal.

glycogenet'ic [" + *gennan*, to produce]. Pert. to the formation of glycogen.

glycogen'ic [" + *gennan*, to produce]. Rel. to glycogen.

glycogenolysis (glī″ko-jen-ol'ĭs-ĭs) [" + + *lysis*, solution]. Conversion of glycogen into dextrose in the liver.

glycogenolytic (glī-ko-jen-o-lĭt'ĭk) [" + + *lysis*, dissolution]. Pert. to the hydrolysis of glycogen.

glycogenosis (glī-ko-jen-o'sĭs) [" + " + *ōsis*]. Abnormal amt. of glycogen in children resulting in an enlarged liver.

glycogeusia (glī-ko-ju'sĭ-ă) [" + *geusis*, taste]. A sweet taste.

glycohemia (glī-ko-he'mĭ-ă) [" + *aima*, blood]. Abnormal amt. of sugar in the blood. SYN: *glycosemia*.

glycol (glī'kol) [G. *glykus*, sweet]. Any one of the dihydric alcohols related to ethylene glycol, $C_2H_4(OH)_2$. The general formula is $C_2H_2n(OH)_2$.
  The glycols are thick, colorless, water soluble liquids similar to glycerol.

glycolipid(e (glī″ko-lip'ĭd) [" + *lipos*, fat]. Compound of fatty acids with a carbohydrate, containing nitrogen, but no phosphoric acid.
  Found in myelin sheath of nerves. SYN: *cerebroside*.

glycolysis (glī-kol'ĭ-sĭs) [" + *lysis*, dissolution]. Hydrolysis of sugar by a ferment in the body.

glycolyt'ic [" + *lysis*, dissolution]. Pert. to hydrolyzing sugar.
  g. enzyme. An enzyme which catalyzes the hydrolysis of sugars.

glycometabol'ic [" + *metabolē*, change]. Rel. to the metabolism of sugar.

glycometabolism (glī″kō-mĕt-ăb'ō-lĭzm) [" + " + *-ismos*, process]. Utilization of sugar* by the body. SYN: *saccharometabolism*. SEE: *metabolism*.

glyconeogenesis (glī″ko-ne-o-jen'e-sĭs) [" + *neos*, new, + *genesis*, formation]. The formation of carbohydrates from noncarbohydrates, such as fat or protein.

glyconucleopro'tein [" + L. *nucleus*, kernel, + G. *prōtos*, first]. A carbohydrate group unduly developed in a nucleoprotein.

glycopenia (glī-ko-pe'nĭ-ă) [" + *penia*, poverty]. Having a tendency to hypoglycemia.

glycopex'ic [" + *pēxis*, fixation]. Pert. to the fixing or storing of sugar.

glycopex'is [" + *pēxis*, fixation]. The storing of glycogen in the liver.

glycophe'nol [G. *glykus*, sweet]. Saccharin, a very sweet crystalline substance. SYN: *gluside*.

glycophilia (glī-ko-fĭl'ĭ-ă) [" + *philein*, to love]. A condition in which there is a marked tendency to hyperglycemia.

glycopolyuria (glī″ko-pol-ĭ-ū'rĭ-ă) [" + *polys*, much, + *ouron*, urine]. Diabetes mellitus with *polyuria* greater than *glycosuria*.

glycopri'val, glycopri'vous [" + L. *privus*, deprived of]. Lacking in or without carbohydrates.

glycoprotein (glī-ko-pro'te-ĭn) [" + *prōtos*, first]. A compound or conjugated protein such as mucin. SEE: *protein*.

glycoptyalism (glī-ko-tī'al-ĭzm) [" + *ptyalon*, saliva, + *ismos*, state of]. Excretion of glucose in the saliva.

glycoregula'tion [" + L. *regula*, rule]. The dietary and insulin control of sugar metabolism.

glycoreg'ulatory [" + L. *regula*, rule]. Rel. to glycoregulation.

glycorrhachia (glī-ko-rak'ĭ-ă) [" + *rachis*, spine]. Sugar in the cerebrospinal fluid.

glycorrhea (glī-ko-re'ă) [" + *roia*, flow]. Discharge of sugar from the body.

glycosecretory (glī″ko-se-kre'to-rī) [" + L. *secretus*, from *secernere*, to separate]. Pert. to or determining the secretion of glucose.

glycose'mia [" + *aima*, blood]. Abnormal amount of sugar in the blood.

glycosialia (glī-ko-sĭ-al'ĭ-ă) [" + *sialon*, saliva]. Sugar in the saliva.

glycosialorrhea (glī″ko-sĭ-al-or-re'ă) [" + " + *roia*, flow]. Excessive secretion of saliva containing sugar.

gly'coside. A substance derived from plants which upon hydrolysis yields a sugar and one or more additional products. Depending on the sugar formed, glycosides are designated *glucosides*, *galactosides*, etc. SEE: *glucoside*.

glycosom'eter [" + *metron*, measure]. Device for determining proportion of sugar in urine in glycosuria.

glycosuria (gli-ko-su'ri-ă) [" + *ouron*, urine]. The presence of sugar (glucose) in the urine.

Traces of sugar, particularly glucose, may occur in normal urine, but are not detected by ordinary qualitative methods. In routine urinalyses the presence of a reducing substance is suspicious of diabetes mellitus until proven otherwise. Glycosuria is a pronounced symptom of diabetes mellitus when the blood sugar level exceeds the renal threshold (about 170 mg. per cent). Normal conditions should show 0.01% of glucose in the blood. SYN: *glucosuria*.

Glycosuria may result from (a) pancreatic (insulin) insufficiency, (b) disorders of the endocrine glands esp., hypophysis adrenals, thyroid, or ovaries, (c) excessive carbohydrate intake, (d) excessive glycogenolysis, (e) reduction of renal threshold.

g., alimentary. Following ingestion of large amounts of starches or sugars.

g. diabetic. G. resulting from hyposecretion of insulin.

g. emotional. G. resulting from emotional states such as worry, or anxiety.

g. pituitary. G. resulting from dysfunction of the ant. pituitary.

g. phloridzin. G. resulting from the injection of phloridzin which reduces the renal threshold for glucose.

g., renal. When glucose is persistent and not accompanied by hyperglycemia.

glycuresis (gli-ku-re'sis) [" + *ourēsis*, urination]. Presence of sugar (glucose) in the urine. SYN: *glycosuria.*

glycuronuria (gli-ku-ro-nu'ri-ă) [*glycuronic acid* + G. *ouron*, urine]. Glycuronic acid in the urine.

glycylglycine (glis-il-glis'in). The simplest form of a polypeptide.

glycyltryptophan (glis"il-trip'tof-ăn). A dipeptide of glycine and tryptophan.

glycyrrhiza (glis-ĭ-rī'ză). The licorice root. SEE: *licorice*.

glyoxalase. An enzyme which catalyzes the conversion of methylglyoxal to lactic acid by the addition of water.

Gm. Abbr. for *gram*.

gnat. Any of a number of small insects belonging to the order Diptera, suborder Orthorrhapha. Term applied generally to insects smaller than mosquitoes. Includes black flies, midges, and sand flies.

g. buffalo. A small dipterous insect belonging to the family Simuliidae, *q.v.*

gnathalgia (nath-al'ji-ă) [G. *gnathos*, jaw, + *algos*, pain]. Pain in the jaw. SYN: *gnathodynia*.

gnathic (nath'ik) [G. *gnathos*, jaw]. Pert. to an alveolar process or to the jaw.

gnathion (nath'i-on) [G. *gnathos*, jaw]. Lowest point of middle line of lower jaw; a craniometric point.

gnathitis (na-thi'tis) [" + *-itis*, inflammation]. Inflammation of the jaw or adjacent soft parts.

gnatho- (nath'o) [G.]. Prefix. Pert. to jaw or cheek.

gnathocephalus (năth-ō-sĕf'ăl-ŭs). A monster in which the head consists principally of the jaws.

gnathodynia (nath-o-din'i-ă) [G. *gnathos*, jaw, + *odynē*, pain]. Pain in the jaw. SYN: *gnathalgia*.

gnathoplasty (nath'o-plas-ti) [" + *plassein*, to form]. Reparative surgery of jaws or cheek.

gnathoschisis (nath-os'kis-is) [" + *schizein*, to split]. Congenital jaw cleft.

Gnathostoma (nă-thŏs'tō-mă). A genus of Nematode worms which infests the stomach walls of domestic and wild animals. They occasionally accidentally infest man.

gnathostomiasis (năth-ō-stō-mī'ă-sis). Infestation with *Gnathostoma, q.v.*

gnosia (no'si-ă) [G. *gnōsis*, knowledge]. The perceptive faculty of recognizing persons, things and forms.

goat-leap pulse. Term applied to an irregular and bounding pulse. SEE: *pulse*.

goat milk. Milk of a goat. AV. SERVING: 240 Gm. Pro. 9.6, Fat 14.4, Carbo. 12.0. Ca 0.128, Mg 0.013, K 0.145, Na 0.079, P 0.103, Cl 0.014, S 0.037. Vit. A+++. SEE: *buttermilk, milk*.

goblet cell. SYN: *mucous cell*. A type of secretory cell found in the epithelium of the intestinal and respiratory tracts; a unicellular gland which secretes mucus. Mucin droplets accumulate in the distal end of the cell, forming a large ovoid mass which causes the cell to become swollen and distorted in shape. The free surface of the cell finally ruptures liberating the mucus. SEE: *cell, gland, secretion, mucus*.

gog'gle eyed. Having an abnormally protruding eye. SYN: *exophthalmic*.

goiter (goi'ter) [L. *guttur*, throat]. An enlargement of the thyroid gland.

ETIOL: It may be due to lack of iodine in diet, thyroiditis, or inflammation from infection, to tumors, or hyper- or hypofunction of the thyroid gland. SYN: *Derbyshire neck. Struma*.

g., aberrant. Supernumerary thyroid enlargement.

g., acute. G. growing rapidly.

g., adenomatous. Thyroid enlargement due to growth of encapsulated adenomata. Nodular goiter.

g., basedowified. SEE: *toxic g*.

g., colloid. One in which there is a great increase of follicular contents.

g., cystic. A g. in which a cyst or a number of cysts are formed. May result from the degeneration of tissue or liquification within an adenoma.

g., diffuse. G. in which the thyroid tissue is diffuse in contrast to its nodular form as in adenomatous goiter.

g., diver, g., diving. Movable g.

g., endemic. G. development in certain localities, especially those in which iodine is deficient in food and water.

g., exophthalmic. SYN: *Grave's, Parry's* or *Basedow's disease, hyperthyroidism, thyrotoxicosis*. A disease resulting from the excessive secretion of the thyroid hormones.

ETIOL: Unknown. Nervous shock, or strain, worry, and fright, may be precipitating factors. Occurs in constitutionally predisposed individuals. Incidence higher in females.

SYM: Bulging eyeballs generally present. Many eye signs, enlarged thyroid, delayed coagulation time, tremor of fingers and muscles of hands, tachycardia, increased metabolism, vomiting and diarrhea, profuse perspiration, nervous irritability, skin eruptions, emaciation, anemia, hyperglycemia. Goiters are more prevalent in fresh water and lake countries, and less so on the sea coast, probably due to the lack of iodine in fresh water. Iodine and iodinized salt are used as remedies and preventatives.

g., fibrous. G. with hyperplastic capsule and stroma of the thyroid gland.

g., follicular. SEE: *parenchymatous g*.

g., hyperplastic. SYN: *parenchymatous goiter*. Condition in which number of secreting cells esp., those lining the follicles is greatly increased.

g., intrathoracic. G. in which a portion of the thyroid tissue lies within the thoracic cavity.

g., lingual. Hypertrophied mass forming a tumor at post. portion of dorsum of tongue.

g., parenchymatous. G. characterized by multiplication of cells lining the follicles or alveoli. There is usually a reduction in colloid and the follicular cavities assume various sizes and are often obliterated by infoldings of their walls. Fibrous tissue may increase markedly. Iodine content of gland is low. Goiter usually of a diffuse nature.

g., perivascular. G. surrounding a large blood vessel.

g., retrovascular. G. development behind a large blood vessel.

g., simple. Thyroid gland hyperplasia unaccompanied by constitutional symptoms.

g., substernal. Enlargement of lower part of thyroid isthmus.

g., suffocative. G. causing shortness of breath due to pressure.

g., toxic. Exopthalmic goiter or goiter in which there is an excessive production of the thyroid hormone.

g., vascular. G. due to distention of blood vessels.

gold-beaters' skin. A membrane from the cecum of the ox for surgical use.

Gold'berger's diet. One for pellagra. Eggs, lean meat, and brewer's yeast.

Gold'flam's disease. Excessive tiring of voluntary muscles and rapid decrease of contractility. SYN: *myasthenia gravis pseudoparalytica*.

gold seed. Thin capillary glass tube covered with gold containing some form of radium.

Golgi apparatus. The internal reticular apparatus of Golgi. A network of irregular wavy threads present in the cytoplasm, of all nerve cells, and many other cells esp., secretory cells.

Golgi's cells. Multipolar nerve cells in the cerebral cortex and post. horns, of spinal cord. There are two types: Type I, those that possess long axons and Type II, those that possess short axons.

Golgi's corpuscle. A sensory nerve ending or receptor found in tendons, or aponeuroses; an end organ of muscle sense. Also called *organ of Golgi*.

Goll's tract (golz). One in post. white column of spinal cord. SYN: *fasciculus gracilis*.

gomphi'asis [G. *gomphios*, molar tooth]. Loosening of the teeth.

gomphosis (gom-fo'sis) [G. *gomphos*, nail, + *ōsis*]. A conical process fitting into a socket in immovable (synarthrosis*) joint. SEE: *joint*.

gon'ad [G. *gonē*, semen]. A generic term referring to both the female sex glands, or ovaries, and the male sex glands, or testis. The embryonic sex gland before differentiation into definitive testis or ovary.

Each forms the cells necessary for reproduction, spermatozoa from the testes, ova from the ovaries.

INTERNAL SECRETIONS: *Female*: The vesicular follicles of the ovaries secrete estrogen, which maintains the nutrition and mature size of the female generative organs; also the *corpus luteum*, producing the luteal secretion (progesterone) which sensitizes the interior membrane of the uterus to contact with the ovum to assist in the implantation of the fertilized ovum.

Male: The interstitial cells of the testes secrete an internal secretion containing androgens which stimulates metabolism, increases muscular strength, and develops secondary sex characteristics.

Hormones from both sexes have been isolated and standardized, and are used in the treatment of conditions arising from an insufficiency of these hormones. SEE: *ovary, testicle*.

gonadal (gon'ă-dal) [G. *gonē*, seed]. Pert. to a gonad. SYN: *gonadial*.

gonadectomy (gon-ă-dek'to-mĭ) [" + *ektomē*, excision]. Excision of a testis or ovary.

gonad'ial [G. *gonē*, semen]. Pert. to a reproductive gland. SYN: *gonadal*.

gonadogen (gon-ad'ō-jĕn) [" + *gennan*, to produce]. Commercial gonadotropic substance from pregnant mare's serum. Induces ovulation and in male growth of genitalia and secondary sex characteristics.

gonadop'athy [" + *pathos*, disease]. Any disease of the sexual glands.

gonadother'apy [" + *therapeia*, treatment]. Treatment by injection of extracts containing testicular or ovarian hormones.

gonadotrope (gon-ad'o-trōp) [" + *tropē*, turning]. One dominated by the sex instinct.

gonadotrophic (gŏ-năd-ō-trŏf'ĭk) [G. *gonē*, semen]. Relating to stimulation of the gonads.

g. hormones. Gonadotrophins, *q.v.* or gonad-stimulating hormones.

gonadotrophin [G. *gonē*, semen, + *trope*, a turning]. A gonad-stimulating hormone.

g's., ant. pituitary. Those produced by the anterior lobe of the hypophysis. Include (a) follicle-stimulating hormone (FSH), (b) leuteinizing hormone (LH). In the male this is called the interstitial cell stimulating hormone (ICSH), (c) luteotrophic hormone (LTH).

g., chorionic. G's. produced by the chorionic villi of the placenta. They are present in the blood and urine of pregnant women and in the blood of pregnant mares. Their presence in urine is the basis of the Ascheim-Zondeck, Friedman, and other pregnancy tests. Also called ant., pituitary-like hormone, pregnancy hormone.

gonadotropism (go-nad-ot'ro-pizm) [" + " + *ismos*, state of]. Domination by the sex impulse.

gon'aduct [" + L. *ductus*, canal]. The seminal duct or the oviduct.

gonagra (gon-a'gră) [G. *gonu*, knee, + *agra*, seizure]. Gout in the knee.

gonal'gia [" + *algos*, pain]. Pain in the knee.

gonangiectomy (gon-an-jĭ-ek'to-mĭ) [G. *gonē*, seed, + *aggeion*, vessel, + *ektomē*, excision]. Excision of the vas deferens or a part of it. SYN: *vasectomy*.

gonarthritis (gon-ar-thri'tis) [G. *gonu*, knee, + *arthron*, joint, + *-itis*, inflammation]. Inflammation of knee joint.

gonarthrocace (gon-ar-throk'ă-se) [" + *kakē*, evil]. White swelling of knee joint.

gonarthromeningitis (gon-ar″thro-men-in-ji'tis) [" + " + *mēninx*, membrane, + *-itis*, inflammation]. Synovitis of the knee joint.

gonarthrotomy (gon-ar-throt'o-mĭ) [" + " + *tomē*, incision]. Incision of knee joint.

gonatag'ra [" + *agra*, seizure]. Gout in the knee.

gonatocele (gon-at′o-sēl) [" + *kēlē*, swelling]. White swelling; tumor of the knee.

gonecyst, gonecystis (gon′e-sist, gon-e-sis′tis) [G. *gonē*, semen, + *kystis*, a bladder]. A seminal vesicle.

gonecystitis (gon-e-sis-ti′tis) [" + " + -*itis*, inflammation]. Inflammation of seminal vesicles.

gonecystolith (gon-e-sis′to-lith) [" + " + *lithos*, stone]. A concretion or calculus in a seminal vesicle.

gonecystopyosis (gon-e-sist″o-pi-o′sis) [" + " + *pyōsis*, suppuration]. Suppuration in a seminal vesicle or gonecyst.

goneitis (go-ne-i′tis) [G. *gonu*, knee, + -*itis*, inflammation]. Inflammation of the knee.

gonepoiesis (gon-e-poi-e′sis) [G. *gonē*, semen, + *poiein*, to make]. The secretion of the semen.

Gongylonema (gŏn-jō-lō-nē′mă). A genus of nematode worms belonging to the suborder Spirurata. They are parasitic in wall of the esophagus and stomach of domestic animals. Occasionally, they are accidental parasites in man. *G. pulchrum* is the species most frequently involved.

goniometer (gon-ĭ-om′et-er) [G. *gōnia*, angle, + *metron*, measure]. Apparatus to measure joint movements and angles.

gonion (go′nĭ-on) [G. *gōnia*, angle]. Point of angle of the mandible or lower jaw.

gonioscope (go′nĭ-o-skōp) [" + *skopein*, to examine]. An instrument for inspecting angle of ant. chamber of eye and for determining ocular motility and rotation.

gono-, gon- [G.]. Prefix meaning *generation, offspring, semen*.

gonocide (gon′o-sīd) [G. *gonē*, semen, + L. *caedere*, to kill]. Destructive to the gonococcus.

gonococ′cal [" + *kokkos*, berry]. Rel. to or caused by gonococci.

gonococcemia (gon-o-kok-se′mĭ-ă) [" + " + *aima*, blood]. Gonococci in the blood.

gonococcic (gŏn-ō-kŏk′sĭk) [" + *kokkos*, berry]. Pert. to the gonococcus.

g. smears. Gonococci are in pairs and tetrads, never in chains. They are biscuit-shaped with concave adjacent surfaces, Gram negative and intracellular. *Stains*: Gram's method, methylene blue.

gonococcide (gon-o-kok′sīd) [" + " + L. *caedere*, to kill]. Destructive to or that which kills gonococci.

gonococcin (gon-o-kok′sin) [" + *kokkos*, berry]. A glycerin extract of gonococci used in the cutireaction test for gonorrhea.

gonococ′cocide [" + *kokkos*, berry, + L. *caedere*, to kill]. Destructive to or an agent which kills gonococci.

gonococcus (gon-o-kok′us) [" + *kokkos*, berry]. The organism causing gonorrhea. *Neisseria gonorrhoeae*.

It is an intracellular biscuit-shaped diplococcus and tends to occur in pairs. It is classified as a Gram negative bacterium and may be found in or on the genitalia, in the blood, the eye, urine, feces, and in boils.

gon′ocyte [G. *gonos*, seed, + *kytos*, cell]. The primitive reproductive cell.

gonohemia (go-no-he′mĭ-ă) [G. *gonē*, semen, + *aima*, blood]. General gonorrhea infection. SYN: *gonococcemia*.

gonophage (gon′o-fāj) [" + *phagein*, to eat]. The bacteriophage produced by the gonococcus.

gon′ophore [" + *phorein*, to carry]. Any body that stores up or activates sex cells, as the spermatic duct, seminal vesicle, oviduct, or uterus.

gonorrhea (gon-o-re′ă) [" + *roia*, flow]. A specific, contagious, catarrhal inflammation of the genital mucous membrane of either sex.

ETIOL: Infection by the gonococcus, *Neisseria gonorrhoeae*.

The disease also may affect other structures of the body, such as the conjunctiva, the oral mucosa, the rectum, or the joints. In the female the parts involved may be the urethra, vulva, vulvovaginal glands, vagina, endocervix, Skene's glands, Bartholin's glands, or fallopian tubes.

SYM: *Male*: Yellow mucopurulent discharge from the penis. Inception in the urethra. May become deep-seated and affect the prostate. Slow, difficult and painful urination, and sometimes rigidity of the penis with great pain.

Female: The labia may become red, hot, tender, and inflamed. A sticky, serous exudate may cover the surfaces. Labia may become so swollen as to prevent inspection. Two strawberry points may show just beneath the external meatus, the latter being red and tender. The urethral canal is inflamed, painful micturition and frequency of urination may occur. Thick, creamy or greenish mucopurulent discharge develops shortly after invasion. Later it subsides and if the cervix is involved, becomes mucopurulent, and in final stages, whitish. The positive diagnosis is made by finding the organism on smear. Very commonly the disease is subacute or chronic from its inception, in the female.

PROG: It may clear up without serious results, or become chronic (involving deeper tissues and producing urethral stricture), or produce complications (prostatitis, epididymitis, orchitis, cystitis, etc., arthritis and endocarditis). No case of acute gonorrhea should be considered as cured until 3 successive negative smears from the cervix, Bartholin's and Skene's glands are obtained, at least 2 of which should be examined immediately after a menstrual period. Even then the case must be regarded with suspicion.

NP: Every precaution for self-protection. Always wash hands after tending patient. Rubber gloves and a gown should be worn. The latter should not be worn in caring for another patient, and gloves should be sterilized after treatment. All linens should be sterilized after using and dressings immediately disposed of. The danger of an infected eye on part of the nurse is very considerable.

PROPHYLAXIS: Modern methods include the oral administration of either a single tablet of crystalline penicillin G (250,000 units) or 4 Gm. of sulfadiazine within 6 hours of exposure.

TREATMENT: Local measures, including urethral instillations, have largely given way to penicillin therapy. Penicillin is specific, and is regarded as superior to sulfadiazine and other sulfonamides. In the absence of response to adequate administration of penicillin, many venereologists assume that the condition is not gonorrhea but a persistent nonspecific urethritis, requiring local procedures (bladder irrigation, urethral instillation, etc.). Local ther-

gonorrheal G-30 **graft**

apy may be required for eradication of foci of infection in the female, involving such structures as Skene's duct, Bartholin's glands, and the cervix.

DOSAGE: Penicillin is given in one intramuscular injection of 300,000 units. Another injection may be needed a day later. In therapeutic resistance, streptomycin may be injected in one dose of 0.3 Gm.

RS: *antiblennorrhagic, arthritis, blennostrumous, clap, gleet, gonococcus, gonotoxemia, rheumatism.*

gonorrhe'al [G. *gonē*, seed, + *roia*, flow]. Of the nature of or pert. to gonorrhea.

g. arthritis, g. rheumatism. Arthritis, or rheumatism resulting from gonorrheal infection.

gonybatia (gŏn-ĭ-bā'shĭ-ă). Walking on the knees, a symptom of certain pathologic conditions.

gonycamp'sis [G. *gonu*, knee, + *kampsis*, bending]. Abnormal curvature of the knee or ankylosis.

gonycrote'sis [" + *krotēsis*, knocking]. Knock-knee.

gonyectyposis (gŏn"ĭ-ek-tĭ-po'sis) [" + *ektyposis*, displacement]. Bowlegs. SYN: *genu varum.*

gonyocele (gŏn'e-o-sēl) [" + *kēlē*, swelling]. Tuberculous synovitis of the knee. SYN: *white swelling.*

gonyoncus (gŏn"ĭ-on'kus) [" + *ogkos*, tumor]. Tumor of the knee. SYN: *white swelling.*

goose'berries. A fruit. COMP: Contain 93% water; also citric acid. Only contain 4% of sugar. AV. SERVING: 100 Gm. Pro. 0.8, Fat 0.4, Carbo. 10.1, Ca 0.035, Mg. 0.014, K 0.197, Na 0.038, P. 0.031, S. 0.011, Fe 0.005. Vit. B+ to ++, C+.

ACTION: The abundance of seeds and skin may cause irritation of the stomach and intestines. IND: Diabetics may use as there is little sugar. SEE: *fruit.*

goose flesh. SYN: *cutis anserina.* A skin reaction caused by erection of skin papillae from cold or shock due to contraction of the arrector pili muscles.

Gordon's reflex (gord'ŏn). Extension of great toe when sudden pressure is made on deep flexor muscles of calf of leg.

gorget (gor'jet) [Fr. *gorge*, throat, because of shape of instrument]. A grooved instrument to protect soft tissues from injury from point of knife.

gouge (gowj). Instrument for cutting away hard tissue of bone.

Goulard's extract (goo'lars). USP. An aqueous solution of lead subacetate, containing 18% lead.

ACTION AND USES: Diluted from 15 to 39 volumes of distilled water, as an astringent in inflammatory conditions of skin, for sprains and bruises.

INCOMPATIBILITIES: Exposure to air, acacia, albumen.

gout (gowt) [L. *gutta*, drop]. Paroxysmal metabolic disease marked by acute arthritis and inflammation of the great toe and of the joints.

ETIOL: Excessive uric acid in blood and deposits of urates of sodium in and around joints.

SYM: Nocturnally painful with swelling and pain around joints.

NP: The painful joints may be wrapped in cotton. They should be elevated and supported on a pillow. The weight of the bedclothes should be carried on a cradle. Hot fomentations may afford some relief. Massage and radiant energy may be employed. Watch for vomiting and purgation resulting from the use of colchicum. Plentiful liquids should be given and the bowels kept open.

DIET: Milk, diluted fruit juices, and farinaceous foods may be given. The diet, however, should be a light one. Meat should not be given more than once a day. Rich game, kidneys, liver, sweetbreads, and duck are prohibited.

g., abarticular. G. which involves structures other than the joints.

g., chronic. Persistent form of g.

g., latent, g., masked. Lithemia without regular symptoms of gout.

g., misplaced, g., retrocedent. Subsidence of joint symptoms followed by severe constitutional upsets.

g., poor man's. G. due to exposure and privation.

g., tophaceous. G. marked by the development of tophi (deposits of sodium urate) in the joints, the external ear, and about the fingernails.

gout'y [L. *gutta*, drop]. Of the nature of, or rel. to, gout.

g. diathesis. Predisposition to gout.

Gowers' tract (gow'erz). One formed of fibers from post. roots of lateral tract of the spinal cord reaching the cerebellum by way of the sup. peduncle. The anterior spinocerebellar tract, *q.v.*

gr. Abbr. for *grain.*

graaf'ian fol'licle. BNA. A mature, vesicular follicle of the ovary.

Beginning with puberty and continuing until the menopause, except during pregnancy a graafian follicle develops each four weeks. Each follicle contains a nearly mature ovum (an oocyte which upon rupture of the follicle, is discharged from the ovary, a process called *ovulation*. Ovulation occurs usually about the 13th day of the menstrual cycle, dated from the first day of the preceding menstrual period. Within the ruptured graafian follicle, the corpus luteum develops. Both the follicle and the corpus luteum are glands of internal secretion, the former secreting estrogens, the latter, progesterone.

gracile (gras'il) [L. *gracilis*, delicate]. Slender; slight.

g. nucleus. Mass of medullary gray matter terminating the funiculus gracilis.

gracilus. A long slender muscle on the medial aspect of the thigh.

grada'tim [L.]. Gradually or by degrees.

Gradenigo's syndrome (grah-den-e'goz). Suppurative otitis media with abducens paralysis and pain in temporal region.

grad'ient. A slope or grade; an increase or decrease of varying degrees; or the curve which represents such.

g. axial. A gradient of physiological or metabolic activity exhibited by embryos and many adult animals, the principal one of which follows the main axis of the body, being highest at the anterior end and lowest at the posterior end.

graduate (grad'u-āt) [L. *gradus*, a step]. 1. A vessel marked by lines for measuring liquids. 2. One who has been awarded an academic or professional degree from a college or university.

grad'uated. Marked by a series of lines indicating degrees of measurement, weight, or volume.

g. tenotomy. Partial surgical division of tendon of an eye muscle.

Graefe's, von, sign (graf'fes). Failure of the upper lid to follow a downward movement of the eyeball when the patient changes his vision from upward, downward. Seen in Graves' disease.

graft [L. *graphium*, grafting knife]. Skin or other living substance inserted into

graft, autoplastic   G-31   **granular**

Gram Conversion into Ounces

Gm.	Oz.	Gm.	Oz.	Gm.	Oz.	Gm.	Oz.
1	0.03	30	1.06	59	2.08	88	3.10
2	0.07	31	1.09	60	2.11	89	3.14
3	0.11	32	1.13	61	2.15	90	3.17
4	0.14	33	1.16	62	2.18	91	3.21
5	0.18	34	1.20	63	2.22	92	3.24
6	0.21	35	1.23	64	2.26	93	3.28
7	0.25	36	1.27	65	2.29	94	3.31
8	0.28	37	1.30	66	2.33	95	3.35
9	0.32	38	1.34	67	2.36	96	3.38
10	0.35	39	1.37	68	2.40	97	3.42
11	0.39	40	1.41	69	2.43	98	3.46
12	0.42	41	1.44	70	2.47	99	3.49
13	0.45	42	1.48	71	2.50	100	3.53
14	0.49	43	1.51	72	2.54	125	4.41
15	0.53	44	1.55	73	2.57	150	5.30
16	0.56	45	1.59	74	2.61	175	6.18
17	0.60	46	1.62	75	2.64	200	7.05
18	0.63	47	1.65	76	2.68	250	8.82
19	0.67	48	1.69	77	2.71	300	10.58
20	0.70	49	1.73	78	2.75	350	12.34
21	0.74	50	1.75	79	2.79	400	14.11
22	0.77	51	1.80	80	2.82	450	15.87
23	0.81	52	1.83	81	2.85	453.6	16.00
24	0.84	53	1.87	82	2.89	500	17.64
25	0.88	54	1.90	83	2.93	600	21.16
26	0.91	55	1.94	84	2.96	700	24.69
27	0.95	56	1.97	85	3.00	800	28.22
28	0.99	57	2.01	86	3.03	900	30.75
29	1.02	58	2.04	87	3.07	1000	35.33

a similar substance to supply an absence or defect by attachment and growth into an integral part of the original substances.
RS: *autograft, skin grafting, transplantation, zoografting*.

g., autoplastic. One taken from another part of the patient.

g. bone. A piece of bone generally taken from the tibia and inserted elsewhere in the body to replace another osseous structure.

Bones for grafting can be kept in icebox until needed. [other person.

g., heteroplas'tic. One taken from an-
g., ovarian. Implantation of a section of an ovary into the muscles of the abdominal wall.

g., skin. Removal of small sections of skin to a raw, clean surface such as a large superficial burn.

g., sponge. Small piece of sponge placed over an ulcerating part to stimulate epidermal growth.

g., Thiersch's. One in which only epidermis and small amt. of dermis are used.

g., Wolfe's. One in which the whole thickness of the skin is used. [animal.

g., zooplas'tic. One taken from an **grain** [L. *granum*]. 1. The seed or seed-like fruit of many members of the grass family, esp., corn, wheat, oats, and other cereals. 2. A weight; 0.065 of a gram. 3. Direction of fibers or layers.

g. poisoning. Poisoning due to a fungus which develops on grain, as ergot. *Gangrenous*: Tingling, pain, spasmodic muscular contractions, blood stasis and gangrene, fingers, toes, nose or ears.

Convulsive: May be similar to gangrenous form followed by nervous disturbance. Headache, slight fever, spasm and cramps of muscles, delirium, epilepsy, dementia.

TREATMENT: Provoke vomiting; wash out stomach; give a purgative; give an enema; give powdered charcoal freely; give peroxide of hydrogen. Collapse should be fought with external heat; whiskey, strychnine, atropine, etc.

gram. Abbr. Gm., gm., g. A unit of weight (mass) of the metric system. It equals approximately the weight of a cubic centimeter or cubic milliliter of water. It is equal to 15.437 grain (Troy).

gramicidin (grăm-ĭ-sĭd'ĭn). An antibiotic obtained from a spore-forming soil bacillus, *B. brevis*. One which is effective against Gram-positive bacteria. It is toxic to animals inducing hemolysis of the blood, consequently its clinical use is restricted principally to topical application.

gramicidin S. An antibiotic related to gramicidin and more effective than gramicidin against *Staph. aureus* and certain species of Gram-negative bacteria.

gram-meter. A unit of work energy equivalent to that expended in raising a weight of 1 gram vertically a height of 1 meter.

gram mol'ecule. The grams of a substance which equal its molecular weight.

Gram-negative organisms will lose the stain and take the color of the counterstain.

Gram-positive organisms will retain the color of the gentian violet stain.

Gram's method. A method for staining bacteria of importance in the identification of bacteria. 1. Prepare a film on a slide, dry and fix with heat. 2. Stain with aniline gentian violet or ammonium oxalate crystal violet 1 min. 3. Rinse in water, then immerse in Gram's iodine solution for 1 min. 4. Rinse off iodine solution then decolorize in 95% ethyl alcohol or acetone. 5. Counterstain with dilute carbolfuchsin or safranine, 30 sec. 6. Rinse with water, blot dry, and examine.

Gran'cher's disease. Massive pneumonia. SYN: *splenopneumonia*.

G.'s sign. Raised pitch of expiratory murmur in pulmonary consolidation.

grand mal (grahn mal) [Fr. great evil]. The typical epileptic attack with or without coma.

gran'ular [L. *granulum*, little grain]. Of the nature of granules. Roughened by prominences like those of seeds.

granular cast   G-32   **granulocytopoiesis**

g. cast. Coarse or fine granule, short and plump, sometimes yellowish, similar to hyaline cast.
Soluble in acetic acid. Seen in inflammatory and degenerative nephropathies. SEE: *cast.*

granula′tion [L. *granulum*, little grain]. 1. Formation of granules, or state or condition of being granular. 2. Fleshy projections formed on the surface of a gaping wound that is not healing by first intention* or indirect union.

Each granulation represents the outgrowth of new capillaries by budding from the existing capillaries and then joining up into capillary loops supported by cells which will later become fibrous scar tissue. Granulations bring a rich blood supply to the healing surface.

OB: When the umbilical cord separates by wet gangrene there is left a raw area and granulation tissue is formed to heal it. If these granulations are left unchecked they will grow beyond the edge of the navel and form an umbilical polypus which is really an exuberant mass of granulation tissue.

g. arachnoidal. SYN: *Pacchionian bodies, arachnoid villi.* Villus-like projections of the subarachnoid layer of the meninges which project into the superior sagittal sinus and other venous sinuses of the brain. Through them cerebrospinal fluid reenters the blood stream.

g. exuberant. An exuberant mass of granulation-tissue formed in the healing of a wound or ulcer; proud flesh.

gran′ule [L. *granulum*, little grain]. 1. A small, grainlike body. 2. In histology: (a) A minute mass in a cell, which has an outline, but no apparent structure; (b) any minute mass; (c) the crossing points of an intracellular reticulum endwise. 3. In pharmacy, a small globule of sugar and gum tragacanth, combined with a medicinal substance. SEE: *chondroconia, chromomere.*

g., acidophil. One which stains with an acid stain such as eosin. Found in eosinophils of the blood and alpha cells of ant. lobe of hypophysis.

g., agminated. Small round or angular particle of disintegrated red blood corpuscle in the blood.

g., albuminous. Cytoplasmic granule in many normal cells, not affected by ether or chloroform, but disappears from view when acetic acid is added.

g., aleuronoid. Pigment cell g.; colorless, myeloid, and colloidal.

g., alpha. Albuminous g. in leukocytes. Coarse, eosinophil, and highly refractive. SYN: *eosinophil g., oxyphil g.*

g., Altmann's. Mitochondria, *q.v.*

g., amphophil. One which stains with both acid and basic dyes; beta granule *q.v.*

g., azurophil. One which takes a stain with azure dyes easily. Found in lymphocytes; and monocytes; small and red or reddish-purple in color; they are inconstant in number being present in about 30% of the cells.

g., basal. SYN: *blepharoplast, q.v.* A small deeply staining granule found in certain protozoa from which the flagellum arises.

g., beta. An azurophil granule found in beta cells of the hypophysis or Islets of Langerhans of the pancreas.

g., chromophil. A granule of chromiphil substance present in the cytoplasm of neurons; Nissel granules.

g., chromatin. Small masses of deeply staining substance suspended within the meshes of the linin network of the nucleus of a cell.

g's cone. The nuclei of the cones, sensory cells of the retina. They form the outer zone of the outer nuclear layer of the retina.

g., delta. Small granules in the delta cells of the pancreas.

g., eosinophil. Acidophil granules, *q.v.* alpha granules.

g., glycogen. Minute particles of glycogen seen in liver cells following fixation.

g., Grawitz's. Found in lead poisoning basophilia, in the red blood corpuscles.

g., iodophil. Found in polymorphonuclear leukocytes and staining easily with iodine. Seen in various acute infectious diseases.

g., Kölliker's interstitial. Appears in various sizes in muscle fiber sarcoplasm.

g., metachromatic. Found in protoplasm of numerous bacteria. Stains deeply; irregular in size. SYN: *Babes-Ernst body, metachromatic body.*

g., Much's. Rod found in sputum of tuberculosis which stains with Gram stain; considered to be a modified tubercle bacillus.

g., neutrophil. Granules such as those found in neutrophil leucocytes which stain with both basic and acid dyes, assuming a neutral tint.

g., Nissel. Chromophil granules found in the cell bodies of neurons; Nissel bodies.

g., oxyphil. SEE: *alpha g.*

g., pigment. Particle of coloring matter seen esp. in pigment cells.

g., Plehn's. Basophilic and seen in conjugating form of *Plasmodium vivax.*

g., protein. Anabolic and catabolic particles of minute size in various proteins.

g., rod. Nucleus of the rod visual cell found in the external nuclear layer of the retina; connected with the rods.

g., Schüffner's. Polychrome methylene blue-staining g. found in parasitized erythrocytes of tertian malaria; coarse and red.

g., secretory. Zymogen granules, *q.v.*

g., seminal. Minute particles in semen, supposed to derive from disintegrated nuclei in nutritive cells from seminiferous tubules.

g., vitelline. SEE: *yolk g.*

g., yolk. Minute particles of fatty and albuminous nutritive substances present in the yolk (deutoplasm) of ova.

g., zymogen. Granules present in gland cells esp., secretory cells of pancreas, chief cells of the gastric glands, and serous cells of the salivary glands. They are the precursors of the enzymes secreted.

granulitis (gran-u-li′tis) [L. *granulum*, little grain, + G. -*itis*, inflammation]. Acute miliary tuberculosis.

gran′uloblast [L. *granulum*, + G. *blastos*, germ]. Mother cell of a granulocyte. A myeloblast, found in bone marrow.

granulocyte (grăn-ū-lō-sīt) [L. *granulum*, little grain, G. *kytos*, cell]. A granular leukocyte. A polymorphonuclear leucocyte (neutrophil, eosinophil, or basophil).

granulocytopenia (gran″u-lo-si″to-pe′nĭ-ă) [" + " + *penia*, poverty]. Abnormal reduction of granulocytes in the blood. SYN: *granulopenia.*

granulocytopoiesis (gran″u-lo-si″to-poi-e′sis) [" + " + *poiein*, to form]. The formation of granulocytes.

granuloma

granulo'ma [L. *granulum*, + G. *oma*, tumor]. A granular tumor or growth, usually of lymphoid and epithelioid cells. They occur in various diseases such as leprosy, cutaneous leishmaniasis, yaws, and syphilis.

  g., apical. Dental granuloma, *q.v.*
  g., annulare. A condition of the skin characterized by development of reddish nodules arranged in the form of a circle.

granuloma, fungoides

  g., coccidioidal. A chronic, generalized granulomatous disease caused by *Coccidioides immitis*. SEE: *Coccidioidomycosis*.
  g., dental. G. developing at the root of a tooth. May contain epithelial rests or colonies of bacteria.
  g., eosinophilic. G. containing eosinophils and usually accompanied by eosinophilia.
  g., fungoides. Mycosis fungoides, *q.v.*

Spirochaetes—All Species

Genus	Species	Colloquial or Old Names	Disease Caused in Man
Pfeifferella	*Pf. mallei.*	Bacillus mallei, or the glanders bacillus.	Glanders.
Pseudomonas	*Ps. pyocyanea.*	Bacillus pyocyaneus.	Suppuration ("blue pus").
Vibrio	*Vib. cholerae.*	Comma bacillus.	Cholera.
Neisseria	*N. meningitidis.*	Meningococcus.	Cerebrospinal meningitis.
	N. gonorrhoeae.	Gonococcus.	Gonorrhea.
	N. catarrhalis.	Micrococcus catarrhalis.	Nasopharyngeal catarrh.
Proteus	*Pr. vulgaris.*	Bact. proteus vulgaris.	Suppuration.
Escherichia	*E coli.*	Bacillus coli.	Occasionally suppuration, cystitis and pyelitis.
Klebsiella	*K. pneumoniae.*	Pneumobacillus or bacillus mucosus capsulatus.	Occasionally pneumonia. ?Rhinoscleroma.
Eberthella	*E. typhosa*	Typhoid bacillus.	Typhoid fever.
Salmonella	*S. paratyphosum (A&B)*	Bacillus paratyphosus, etc. (Salmonella group.)	Paratyphoid fever, gastroenteritis (food poisoning).
Salmonella	*S. enteritidis*		
Salmonella	*S. aertrycke*		
Shigella	*S. dysenteriae*	The dysentery bacilli.	Bacillary dysentery.
Pasteurella	*Past. pestis.*	Bacillus pestis.	Plague.
Haemophilus	*H. influenzae.*	Pfeiffer's bacillus.	Catarrhal inflammation (?Influenza).
	H. pertussis.	Bordet-Gengou bacillus.	Whooping cough.
Brucella	*Br. melitensis.*	Micrococcus melitensis.	Mediterranean fever.
Spirochaete	*Br. abortus.*	Bacillus abortus of Bang.	Undulant fever.
Spirochaetes	All species.		Syphilis, ictero-hemorrhagic jaundice, etc.

The Chief Gram-positive Bacteria

Genus	Species	Colloquial or Old Names	Disease Caused in Man
Actinomyces	*Actino. bovis.*	Streptothrix actinomyces; ray-fungus.	Actinomycosis.
Mycobacterium	*Myco. tuberculosis.*	Tubercle bacillus.	Tuberculosis.
	Myco. leprae.	Leprosy bacillus.	Leprosy.
Corynebacterium	*C. diphtheriae.*	Diphtheria bacillus.	Diphtheria.
	C. hofmannii, C. xerosis, etc.	Diphtheroid bacilli.	Nonpathogenic.
Streptococcus	*Str. pneumoniae.*	Pneumococcus.	Lobar pneumonia, peritonitis, etc.
	Str. pyogenes.		Suppuration, scarlet fever, septicemia.
	Str. viridans.		Endocarditis.
Staphylococcus	*Staph. aureus, albus,* etc.		Suppuration, pyemia, osteomyelitis.
Micrococcus	*M. tetragenus.*		Rarely suppuration.
Sarcina	*Sarcina lutea.*		Rarely suppuration.
Bacillus	*B. anthracis.*	Anthrax bacillus.	Anthrax.
	B. subtilis.	Hay bacillus.	Nonpathogenic.
Clostridium	*Cl. tetani.*	Tetanus bacillus.	Tetanus.
	Cl. botulinum.	Bacillus botulinus.	Botulism.
	Cl. welchii.	Bact. aerogenes capsulatus.	Gas gangrene.

granuloma, infectious   G-34   **gray matter**

g., infectious. Any infectious disease in which granulomas are formed, such as tuberculosis or syphilis. Granulomas are also formed in mycoses, protozoan infections, and in certain metazoal diseases.

g., inguinale. A granulomatous disease common in the tropics caused by Donovan bodies (*Leishmania donovani*). Characterized by purulent lesions of the skin in region of the groin and often involving external genitalia.

g., iridis. G. which develops on the iris.

g., malignant. Lymphogranulomatosis; Hodgkin's disease.

g., pyogenicum. G. containing pyogenic organisms, which develop at the site of a wound. They may also occur at the tip of the fingers along the sides of the nails or beneath the free edge of the nail. They bleed easily and are usually painful to touch. Also called *septic granuloma*.

g., venereal. Lymphogranuloma venereal, *q.v.*

granulomato'sis [L. *granulum*, little grain, + G. *ōma*, tumor, + *-ōsis*]. The development of multiple granulomas.

g. siderot'ica. Brownish (Gamna) nodules in the enlarged spleen.

granulope'nia [" + G. *penia*, poverty]. Abnormal decrease of granulocytes in the blood. SYN: *granulocytopenia*.

granuloplastic (gran″u-lo-plas'tik) [" + G. *plassein*, to form]. Developing granules.

granulopoiesis (gran″u-lo-poi-e'sis) [" + G. *poiein*, to make]. The formation of granulocytes.

granulopo'tent [" + *potentia*, power]. Potentially capable of forming granules.

granulosa. The membrana granulosa, *q.v.*

gran'ulose [" + G. *ōsis*]. The soluble portion of starch.

It is converted into sugar by hydrolysis.

granulo'sis [" + G. *ōsis*]. A mass of minute granules.

g. ru'bia na'si. Disease of the skin of the nose.

ETIOL: Inflammatory infiltration about nose with slightly elevated papules, and dilated sweat glands.

SYM: Moist erythematous patch on numerous macules.

grape'fruit. A citrus fruit. AV. SERVING: 100 Gm. Pro. 0.5, Fat 0.2, Carbo. 10.0. MINERALS: Ca 0.021, Mg 0.009, K 0.161, Na 0.004, P 0.020, Cl 0.005, S 0.010, Fe 0.0003. Vit. A+, B++, C+++, G++.

g. juice. Av. SERVING: 120 Gm. Pro. 0.6, Fat 0.2, Carbo. 15.2. MINERALS: Ca 0.011, Mg 0.009, K 0.106, Na 0.005, P 0.011, Cl 0.002, S 0.009, Fe 0.0003. Vit. A+, B++, C++, G+. SEE: *fruit*.

grapes [Fr. *grappe*, a cluster]. COMP: Contain acid potassium tartrate. Acidity decreases with the age of the grape and sugar increases. The sugar is nearly all glucose and is more abundant than in any other fruit. Mannite, dulcite, and saccharose also represented. Raisins contain more sugar and less water.

AV. SERVING (Concord): 100 Gm. Pro. 1.4, Fat 1.4, Carbo. 14.9. MINERALS: Ca 0.019, Mg 0.010, K 0.197, Na 0.015, P 0.031, Cl 0.005, S 0.024, Fe 0.0003. Vit. A+, B+ to ++, C+ to ++, G+.

grape sugar. Dextrose.

-graph [G.]. Suffix: Pert. to *a writing* or *treatise*.

graph [G.]. A presentation of statistical, clinical, or experimental data by dots and lines.

graphesthe'sia. The sense by which outlines, numbers, words, or symbols traced or written upon the skin are recognized.

graphite (graf'it) [G. *graphein*, to write]. A soft form of carbon. SYN: *plumbago*.

grapho- [G.]. Prefix: To write.

graphology (graf-ol'o-jī) [G. *graphein*, to write, + *logos*, study]. Examination of handwriting in diseases of the nerves as a means of diagnosis.

graphomotor. Pertaining to movements involved in writing.

graphophobia. Abnormal fear of writing.

graphorrhea (graf-o-re'ă) [" + *roia*, flow]. Writing of many meaningless words and phrases; manifested in dementia precox.

graphospasm (graf'o-spazm) [" + *spasmos*, spasm]. Writer's cramp.

grattage (grat-ahzh') [Fr. a scraping]. Removal of morbid growths by rubbing with a brush or harsh sponge.

grave [L. *gravis*, heavy]. Serious; dangerous; severe.

g. wax. Waxlike matter on flesh caused by exposure to moisture with exclusion of air, as a body in the water or underground. SYN: *adipocere*.

gra'vel [Fr. *gravelle*, coarse sand]. Crystalline dust, or concretions of crystals from the kidneys, distinguished from true calculi by the absence of definite structural arrangement.

Generally made up of phosphates, calcium, oxalate, and uric acid.

graveolent (grav'e-o-lent) [L. *gravis*, heavy, + *olere*, to smell]. Fetid; having an unpleasant, strong odor.

Graves' disease. Exophthalmic goiter. SEE: *Moebius' sign*.

gravid (grav'id) [L. *gravida*, pregnant]. Pregnant; heavy with child.

gravida (grav'id-ă) [L.]. A pregnant woman.

grav'idin [L. *gravida*, pregnant]. A substance on surface of standing urine, once considered a sign of pregnancy in women. SYN: *kyestein*.

grav'idism [" + G. *ismos*, state of]. State of being pregnant.

gravid'ity [L. *gravida*, pregnant]. Pregnancy.

gravidocardiac (grav″id-o-kar'di-ak) [" + G. *kardia*, heart]. Pert. to cardiac disorders resulting from pregnancy.

gravimet'ric [L. *gravis*, weight, + G. *metron*, measure]. Determined by weight.

g. method. Examination of blood by weighing.

gravistatic (grav-is-tat'ik) [" + G. *statikos*, standing]. Resulting from gravitation, as in a form of congestion.

gravita'tion [L. *gravitas*, weight]. Force and movement tending to draw every particle of matter together.

grav'ity [L. *gravitās*, weight]. Property of possessing weight.

g., specific. Weight of a substance compared with that of water, air, or hydrogen.

gravocaine (grav'o-kān). Spinal anesthetic mixture used in obstetrics.

gray [A.S. *graey*]. Black or brown mixed with white.

g. matter. Nervous tissue of a grayish color, in which myelinated nerve fibers *do not* predominate. It contains large numbers of cell-bodies of neurons; also called *substantia grisea*.

The term is generally applied to gray portions of the central nervous system, which include the cerebral cortex, basal ganglia, and nuclei of the brain and the gray columns of the spinal cord which form an H-shaped region surrounded by white matter. Sympathetic ganglia and nerves may also be gray.

gray powder. USP. Mercury with chalk, containing about 38% mercury.
USES: Most frequently as a cathartic for children, sometimes as an alterative.
DOSAGE: As a laxative, 4-10 gr. (0.25-0.65 Gm.). As an alterative, ½-1 gr. (0.03-0.06 Gm.).

green. A color intermediate bet. blue and yellow, afforded by rays of wave length bet. 0.000491 and 0.000535 mm. SEE: "chloro-" words.
g. blindness. *Aglaucopsia;* a type of color-blindness in which green colors cannot be distinguished.
g. sickness. A form of anemia in adolescent girls, perhaps due to faulty diet during puberty. SYN: *chlorosis.*
g. soap. A solution of soft soap in alcohol, molded and dried.
g. soft'ening. Cranial abscess with pus of a greenish hue.
g. vit'riol. Ferrous sulfate. SYN: *copperas.*

green'stick fracture. One involving only part of the thickness of a bone. SEE: *incomplete fracture.*

greffotome (gref'o-tōm) [Fr. *greffe,* graft, + G. *tomē,* incision]. Instrument for making tissue grafts.

grenz rays. Roentgen rays with an average wave length of 2 angstroms. SEE: *ray.*

griffe des orteils (grēf daz or-ta') [Fr.]. Muscular atrophy of foot with contraction. SYN: *clawfoot.*

grinder (grĭn'der) [A.S. *grindan,* to gnash]. A molar tooth. SYN: *dens molaris.*

grind'ers' disease. An asthma due to dust inhalation. SYN: *siderosis.*

grip, grippe (grĭp) [Fr. *gripper,* to seize]. Acute, infectious disease marked by fever, prostration, pains in head and back, and by catarrh of respiratory tract. SYN: *influenza, q.v.*

gripes (grīps) [A.S. *gripan,* to grasp]. Intermittent severe pains in bowels. SYN: *colic; tormina, q.v.*

grippotoxin (grĭp-po-tŏks'ĭn) [Fr. *gripper,* to seize, + G. *toxikon,* poison]. The toxin of the influenza bacillus.

gris'tle [A.S.]. Cartilage.

gro'cers' itch. Eczema or psoriasis of the hands due to irritation from handling flour, sugar, etc.

Groff electrosurgical knife. Device for use of cutting current.

groin [A.S. *grynde,* abyss]. The depression between the thigh and trunk. The inguinal region. SEE: *bubonalgia, venereal bubo.*

groove [Danish *groeve,* to dig]. A furrow or elongated channel. SYN: *sulcus.*
g. bicipital. SYN: *intertubercular groove.* Depression for long tendon of the triceps located on ant. surface of humerus.
g. branchial. In the embryo, a groove lined with ectoderm which lies between two branchial arches. SEE: *branchial groove and branchial arches.*
g., carotid. SYN: *cavernous g.* A broad groove on the inner surface of the sphenoid bone lateral to the body. It lodges the carotid artery and the cavernous sinus.
g., costal. SYN: *subcostal groove.* A groove on the lower internal border of a rib. It lodges the intercostal vessels and nerve.
g., costovertebral. SYN: *vertebral g.* A broad groove extending along each side of the vertebrae. It lodges the sacrospinalis muscle and its subdivisions.
g., infraorbital. A groove on the orbital surface of the maxilla which transmits the infraorbital vessels and nerve.
g., intertubercular. The bicipital groove, *q.v.*
g., labial. A groove which develops in each of the primitive jaws. It gives rise to the vestibule separating the lips from the gums.
g., lacrimal. 1. A groove on post. surface of frontal process of the maxilla. 2. A groove on ant. surface of the post. lacrimal crest of the lacrimal bone. The two grooves serve to lodge the lacrimal sac.
g., laryngo-tracheal. A groove along the ventral surface of the ant. portion of the embryonic gut which gives rise to the respiratory organs.
g., malleolar. G. on ant.. surface of distal end of tibia which lodges tendons of the tibialis posterior and flexor digitorum longus muscles.
g., medullary. Neural groove, *q.v.*
g., musculospiral. The radial groove, *q.v.*
g., mylohyoid. G. on inner surface of the mandible which runs obliquely forward and downward lodging the mylohyoid nerve and artery. In the embryo it lodges Meckel's cartilage.
g., nasolacrimal. In the embryo, a g. extending from inner angle of the eye to the primitive olfactory sac. It separates the maxillary and lateral nasal processes and its epithelial lining gives rise to the nasolacrimal duct.
g., nasopalatine. G. on vomer lodging nasopalatine nerve and vessels.
g., neural. A longitudinal g. on dorsal surface of the embryo lying between the neural folds. Upon closure of the folds to form the neural tube, the groove becoming the cavity of the neural tube eventually giving rise to the ventricles of the brain and the central canal of the spinal cord.
g., obturator. A g. at the sup. and post. angle of the obturator foramen through which pass the obturator vessels and nerve.
g. olfactory. A shallow g. on sup. surface of cribriform plate of the ethmoid on each side of the crista galli. It lodges the olfactory bulb.
g., palatine. One of a number of grooves on the inferior surface of the palatine process of the maxilla. They lodge the palatine vessels and nerves.
g., peroneal. 1. A shallow groove on lateral aspect of the calcaneus. 2. A deep groove on inferior surface of the cuboid bone. Each transmits the tendon of the peroneus longus muscle.
g., pharyngeal. A branchial groove, *q.v.*
g., primitive. In the embryo, a shallow groove in the primitive streak of the blastoderm and bordered by the primitive folds.
g., pterygopalatine. The pterygopalatine sulcus. A groove on the maxillary surface of the perpendicular portion of the palatine bone which, with corresponding grooves on the maxilla and pterygoid process of the sphenoid, transmits the palatine nerve and descending palatine artery.
g., radial. The musculospiral groove; a broad shallow groove running in a spiral direction on post. surface of the humerus. It transmits radial nerve and the profunda brachi artery.
g., rhombic. One of seven transverse grooves in the floor of the developing rhombencephalon. They separate the neuromeres.
g., sagittal. The sagittal sulcus; a shallow groove on inner surface of the parietal bones which lodges the sup. saggital sinus.

groove, sigmond   G-36   **gubernaculum, dentis**

g., sigmond. G. on inner surface of the mastoid portion of temporal bone. It transmits the transverse sinus.
g., subcostal. SEE: *costal groove*.
g., tympanic. A. g. at the bottom of the ext. auditory meatus which receives the inferior portion of the tympanic membrane.
g., urethral. A g. on caudal surface of the genital tubercle or phallus bordered by the urethral folds. The latter close transforming the groove into the cavernous urethra.
g., vertebral. SEE: *costovertebral groove*.
g., visceral. A branchial groove, *q.v.*
gross [L. *grossus*, thick]. Not minute; in mass.
g. anatomy. That of organs and parts seen without the aid of a microscope.
g. lesion. One visible to the eye without the aid of a microscope.
Grotthuss, law of. Light is absorbed when its wave length is in resonance with the atoms on which it falls.
ground. Basic substance or foundation; reduced to a powder; pulverized.
g. bundle. Fasciculus proprius, a bundle of nerve fibers which immediately surrounds the gray matter of the spinal cord. It is divided into three regions, the anterior, lateral, and posterior bundles which lie in the corresponding funiculi. These consist principally of short descending fibers.
g. itch. Ancylostomiasis cutis. Inflammation of the skin resulting from the invasion of the larvae of hookworms (*Ancylostoma* or *Necator*).
g. substance. SYN: *matrix, interstitial substance*. The material, fluid, semifluid, or solid which occupies the intercellular spaces in fibrous connective tissue, cartilage, or bone.
group'ing [It. *gruppo*, bunch]. Classification.
g., blood. Classifying blood of different individuals according to agglutinating and hemolyzing qualities before making a blood transfusion.
Human blood has been divided into 4 groups, and the blood of a patient must be compatible with that of the donor. The blood of one belonging to *Group I* may not be given to any patient not belonging to that group, although a donor belonging to *Group II* may give blood to one belonging to *Groups I* or *II*. One belonging to *Group III* may give to *Group II* or *III*, and one belonging to *Group IV* may give to those belonging to any of the 4 groups. SEE: *blood, transfusion*.
g. serum. A serum used for determining the blood group to which unknown cells belong. The grouping serums commonly used are human serums secured from donors and rabbit antiserums prepared commercially.
grow'ing pains. Pains in the limbs of young persons, probably rheumatic.
growth [A.S. *grōwan*, to grow]. The development or increase in size of a living thing, as cyst, excrescence, tumor, benign or malignant.
Methods of growth. 1. By the synthesis of new protoplasm and multiplication of cells. 2. By the intake of water. 3. By the manufacture and deposition of nonliving substances either within or outside of cells.
There are 4 main types of growth:
1. Organs of the *lymphoid* type, such as the thymus and the lymph nodes, grow fastest early in life, reach their peak of development at the age of about 12, and then regress.
2. The *neural* type of organ, such as the brain, cord, eye, and meninges, grows definitely in childhood, but is close to its adult size by the age of 8 years. This size is maintained without regression.
3. The *general* type of growth is seen in the weight of the body, the height of the body, and lengths of various bones, the total weight of the muscles, and various internal organs. It is a slower and steadier growth than the first two, but has a marked acceleration at the time of puberty.
4. The *genital* type of growth is seen in the testes, ovaries, and other genitourinary structures. Their growth is the slowest of these 4 types in infancy, but at puberty they grow faster than the others and cause the striking changes in appearance noted in the reproductive organs.
Not all of the organs of the body are included in the above 4 types. Some structures, such as the mammary glands, have several cycles of growth and regression in a lifetime, and many other peculiarities of particular organs might be mentioned.
gru'el [L. *grutum*, meal]. Any cereal boiled in water.
gru'mose, gru'mous [L. *grumus*, heap]. 1. BACT: Made up of coarse granular bodies in the center. 2. Lumpy, clotted.
Grunfelder's reflex (grŭn'feld-ĕr). Fanlike spreading of toes with upward flexion of great toe resulting from pressure over post. fontanel.
grutum (gru'tum) [L. meal]. 1. Small pink and white patches most frequently on skin of face and scrotum caused by inspissated sebum beneath the horny epidermis. SYN: *milium*. 2. Oaten grits.
gtt. Abbr. of *guttae*, drops.
guaiacol (gwī'ak-ol). USP. A phenol obtained from wood creosote.
ACTION AND USES: Antiseptic and germicide, intestinal antiseptic and expectorant.
DOSAGE: 8 ℳ (0.5 cc.).
g. carbonate. USP. A white crystalline powder used internally as a tasteless, nonpoisonous substitute for guaiacol.
DOSAGE: 15 gr. (1 Gm.).
INCOMPATIBILITIES: Alkali hydroxides, chloral hydrate.
guanase (gwan'ās). An enzyme in a number of glands; it converts guanine into xanthine.
guanidine (gwan'id-in). A crystalline organic compound, $NH:C(NH_2)_2$, found among the decomposition products of proteins.
guanidinemia (gwan'id-ĕn-e'mĭ-ă) [*guanidine* + G. *aima*, blood]. Guanidine in the blood.
guanine (gwah'nin). An organic compound, $C_5H_5N_5O$, which can be extracted from guano and is related to guanidine and xanthine. It is also found in the liver, pancreas, and muscle.
gua'va. Fruit of the guava tree. Av. SERVING: 15 Gm. Pro. 0.2, Fat 0.1, Carbo. 2.6. MINERALS: Ca 0.014, Mg 0.008, K 0.384, P 0.030, Cl 0.045. No sodium, sulfur, or iron.
gubernaculum (gu-ber-nak'u-lum) [L. helm]. A structure which guides; a cordlike structure uniting two structures.
g., dentis. A connective tissue band which connects the tooth sac of an unerupted tooth with the overlying gum.

gubernaculum, testis G-37 **gynandromorphous**

g., testis. A fibrous cord in the fetus which extends from the caudal end of the testis through the inguinal canal to the scrotal swelling. It plays a role in the descent of the testis into the scrotum.

Gubler's line (goob'lerz). The level of superficial origin of the trigeminus or 5th nerve.

G.'s paralysis. Hemiplegia affecting parts on opposite sides of the body. SYN: *alternate* or *crossed hemiplegia*.

G's tumor. A fusiform swelling on wrist in lead palsy.

Gudden's inferior commissure (good'enz in-fe'ri-or com'mis-sure). Fibers of optic tract. SYN: *arcuate c.*

G.'s law. Lesions of the cerebral cortex are not responsible for lesions of peripheral nerves.

guillotine (gil'o-tēn) [Fr. instrument for beheading]. Instrument for excising tonsils and laryngeal growths.

Guinea worm. *Dracunculus medinensis, q.v.*

gul'let [L. *gula*, throat]. The esophagus, *q.v.*

Gull's disease. Atrophy of the thyroid gland and resulting myxedema.

gum (L. *gummi*). 1. The fleshy substance or tissue covering the alveolar processes of the jaws. 2. SYN: gingiva. A substance which is given out or extracted from certain plants which is sticky when moist but hardens upon drying. Roughly any resinlike substance given out by plants.

DIAG: *Bleeding Easily*: Indicates scurvy, excess of salt in the diet, and lack of vegetable acids, or inflammation, as in trench mouth or pyorrhea, etc.

Bluish Red: Indicates mercurial stomatitis or lead poisoning, if bluish line is at edge of teeth.

Greenish Line: At edge of teeth, may indicate copper poisoning.

Purplish Line or Color: Scurvy.

Red Line: In youth, indicates gingivitis, pyorrhea, scurvy.

Spongy g., and Ulceration: Gingivitis, scurvy, stomatitis, leukemia, tuberculosis, diabetes, and digestive disturbances.

RS: *diagnosis, gingiva, oulorrhagia, ulatropia, ulemorrhagia, uletic, ulitis, uloglossitis, uloncus, ulorrhea.*

gumboil (gum'boyl). Gum abscess.

ETIOL: Subperiosteal infection associated with a carious tooth, irritation or injury by a denture.

SYM: Gum is red, swollen, tender, and very painful. A fluctuating swelling may appear containing pus. It may point and break or require incision.

TREATMENT: Hot mouthwashes and applications over gum or externally. Warn patient not to swallow pus. Frequent mouthwashes after being evacuated. SEE: *gum.*

gumma (gum'mă) [L. *gummi*, gum]. A soft tumor of the tissues characteristic of the tertiary stage of syphilis. It is a granuloma varying in size from a millimeter to a centimeter or more in diameter. They may be single or multiple, and tend to be encapsulated. Each consists of a central necrotic mass surrounded by an inflammatory zone and fibrosis. The necrotic portion may be firm or elastic, gelatinous or hyalinized. Infectious organisms may be present. They occur most frequently in the liver but may occur in other organs such as the brain, testis, heart, bone, and skin.

SYM: Depend upon location. Bursting of a gumma leads to a gummatous ulcer, painless, but slow to heal. The base is formed by a "wash-leather" slough but surrounding tissues are healthy. SEE: *syphilis.*

gummose (gum'ōs). A sugar from animal gum. $C_9H_{12}O_6$.

gum'my [L. *gummi*, gum]. Sticky, swollen, puffy.

gun'shot wound. Penetrating or perforating wound which may contain a foreign body, as a bullet. SEE: *wound.*

gun'stock deform'ity. Deformity in which the long axis of the extended forearm turns outwardly from the arm, caused by fracture at the elbow.

gustation (gus-ta'shun) [L. *gustāre*, to taste]. Sense of taste.

gustatory (gus'tat-o-rī) [L. *gustāre*, to taste]. Pert. to sense of taste.

gustom'etry [" + G. *metron*, measure]. Measurement of the degree of the sense of taste.

gut (A.S.). 1. The bowel or intestine. 2. The primitive gut or embryonic digestive tube which includes the fore-gut, mid-gut, and hind-gut. 3. Short term for catgut.

g., blind. Cecum.

gut'ta [L. a drop]. A drop. The amount in a drop varies with the nature of the liquid, being about a minim of water.

g. rosacea. Chronic inflammation of skin of face and nose. SYN: *acne rosacea.*

g. serena. Blindness. SEE: *amaurosis.*

guttadiophot test (gut-ă-di'ă-fōt) [L. a drop]. A test for detecting pathological conditions of the blood. Consists of examining by transmitted light strips of red, green, and blue absorbent paper upon which two drops of blood have been placed.

gutt'ate [L. *gutta*, drop]. Resembling a drop, said of certain cutaneous lesions.

gutta'tim [L.]. Drop by drop.

gut'tur [L.]. The throat.

guttural (gut'u-ral) [L. *guttur*, throat]. Pert. to the throat.

gutturotet'any [" + G. *tetanos*, tension]. Laryngeal spasm of throat with temporary stutter.

Guyon's sign (gwy-onz'). Ballottement of kidney.

Gwath'mey's meth'od or technic. Adm. of rectal anesthetic of ether and olive oil solution in labor. SEE: *anesthesia.*

gymnas'tics [G. *gymnastikos*, pert. to nakedness]. Systematic bodily exercise, esp. in a gymnasium.

g., ocular. Systematic exercise of the eye muscles to improve muscular coordination and efficiency.

g., Swedish. A system of movements made by a patient against a resistance provided by the attendant.

gymnophobia (jim-no-fo'bĭ-ă) [" + *phobos*, fear]. Abnormal aversion to viewing a naked body.

gynander (jin-an'der) [G. *gynē*, woman, — *anēr, andr*- man]. A gynandromorph, *q.v.* A pseudohermaphrodite; an individual possessing both male and female characteristics.

gynandroid (ji-nan'droyd) [" + " + *eidos*, form]. A female having sufficient hermaphroditic sexual characteristics to be mistaken for a man.

gynandromorph. SYN: *gynander.* An individual in which certain parts of the organism are male and certain parts female; if bilateral, one half of the body shows male characteristics and the other half female. Occurs commonly in insects but is sometimes seen in vertebrates.

gynandromorphous (jin-an-dro-morf'us) [" + " + *morphē*, form]. Having the characteristics of both the male and female.

gynandry (ji-nan'dri) [G. *gynē*, woman, + *anēr*, *andro-* man]. Condition of pseudohermaphroditism.

gynatresia (jin-a-tre'zĭ-ă) [" + *a-*, priv. + *trēsis*, perforation]. Atresia* of the vagina.

gynecic (jin-e'sik) [G. *gynē*, woman]. Pert. to women.

gyneco-, gyno- [G.]. Prefix meaning *woman, female*.

gynecologic, gynecological (jin-e-ko-lo'jik, -ji-kal; gīn-e-) [G. *gynē*, woman, + *logos*, study]. Pert. to gynecology, or study of women's diseases.

gynecologist (jin-e-kol'o-jist; gīn-e-kol'o-jist) [" + *logos*, study]. Physician who specializes in the diseases of women.

gynecology (jin-e-kol'o-jĭ; gīn-e-kol'o-jĭ) [" + *logos*, study]. The study of the diseases of the female, particularly of the genital, urinary or rectal organs.

NP: *Preoperative*: Empty bladder. Local preparation from nipple to anus. *Postoperative*: Count and chart pulse every 15 minutes for first few hours. Report immediately any change in rate or volume. Watch for shock or internal hemorrhage. Keep warm and quiet; no visitors. Fluids when tolerated, tap water being best. Hypodermoclysis or infusions in excessive vomiting instead of fluids by mouth. Harris drip for distention and inability to void.

Patient catheterized every 12 hours after operation, then every 8 hours until able to void. Catheterization after voiding to prevent retention, until less than ½ oz. urine is thus obtained after 2 successive voidings. An 80% solution silver nitrate instilled after each catheterization. Thrombophlebitis with embolism is a dreaded complication.

gynecomania (jin-e-ko-ma'nĭ-ă; gīn-e) [" + *mania*, madness]. Abnormal sex desire in the male. SYN: *satyriasis*, q.v.

gynecomastia, gynecomasty, gynecomazia (ji-ne-ko-mas'tĭ-ă, -tĭ, -ma'zĭ-ă) [" + *mastos, mazos*, breast]. Abnormally large mammary glands in the male; sometimes may secrete milk.

gynecopathy (ji-ne-kop'ă-thĭ) [G. *gynē*, woman, + *pathos*, disease]. Diseases peculiar to women.

gynecophonus (jin-e-kof'on-us) [" + *phōnē*, voice]. Having an effeminate voice.

gynephobia (jin-e-fo'bĭ-ă) [" + *phobos*, fear]. Abnormal aversion to the company of women, or fear of them.

gynergen (ji'ner-jĕn) [" + *ergon*, work]. Known as *ergotamine tartrate*, is a salt of one of the alkaloids of ergot.

USES: As a uterine stimulant and in migraine.

DOSAGE: For oral use, 1/60 gr. (0.001 Gm.). Hypodermically, 1/240 gr. (0.00025 Gm.) with the same caution as with ergot.

gynesic (jĭ-ne'sik) [G. *gynē*, woman]. Pert. to the diseases of women.

gyniatrics (jin-ĭ-at'riks) [" + *iatreia*, treatment]. Treatment of diseases of women.

gynopath'ic [" + *pathos*, disease]. Pert. to disease of women.

gynoplastic [G. *gynē*, woman, + *plassein*, to form]. Pertaining to gynoplasty.

gynoplastics (jin-o-plas'tiks) [" + *plassein*, to form]. Reparative surgery of female genitalia.

gynoplasty (jin"o-plas'tĭ) [" + *plassein*, to form]. Plastic surgery of the female reproductive organs.

gyrate (jī'rāt) [G. *gyros*, circle]. 1. Ring-shaped, convoluted. 2. To revolve.

gyration (ji-ra'shun) [G. *gyros*, circle]. A rotary movement.

gyre (jīr) [G. *gyros*, circle]. Convolution. SYN: *gyrus*.

gyrencephalic (ji-ren-sef-al'ik) [" + *egkephalē*, head]. Having a brain marked by numerous convolutions.

gyri (ji'ri) (sing. *gyrus*) [G. *gyros*, circle]. Convolutions of the brain.

gyro- [G.]. Combining form meaning a *circle, spiral, ring*.

gyrochrome (ji'ro-krōm) [G. *gyros*, circle, + *chrōma*, color]. A nerve cell in which the stainable substance occurs in rings.

gyroma (ji-ro'mă) [" + *ōma*, tumor]. Ovarian tumor consisting of a convoluted mass.

gyromele (ji'ro-mēl) [" + *mēlē*, a probe]. Revolving sound for massage and cleansing of stomach, determining its location, size and condition.

gyrometer (ji-rom'et-er) [" + *metron*, measure]. A device for measuring the cerebral gyri.

gyrosa (ji-ro'să) [" + *ōsis*]. Gastric vertigo causing one to close one's eyes to prevent falling, as everything turns round when standing.

gyrose (ji'rōs) [" + *ōsis*]. BACT: Marked by wavy lines or circles applied to bacterial colonies.

gyrospasm (ji'ro-spasm) [" + *spasmos*, spasm]. Spasmodic rotary head movement.

gyrotrope (ji'ro-trōp) [" + *tropē*, a turning]. Cord connecting an electrode with source of an electric current. SYN: *rheotrope*.

gyrous (ji'rus) [G. *gyros*, circle]. Marked by circular lines. SYN: *gyrose*.

gyrus (ji'rus) (pl. gyri) [G. *gyros*, circle]. A convolution of the cerebral hemisphere of the brain. They are separated by shallow grooves (sulci) or deeper grooves (fissures).

g., angular. G. of the parietal lobe embracing post. and of the superior temporal sulcus.

g., annectant. Any of many short folds of gray matter which are formed as a result of short branches or twigs of sulci extending into adjacent gyri. They are inconstant.

g., ant. central. G. of the frontal lobe extending vertically between precentral and central sulci.

gyri breves insulae. Preinsular g.

g., Broca's. Inf. frontal g.

g., callosal. A large g. on medial surface of cerebral hemisphere which lies directly above the corpus callosum, and arches over its anterior end.

g. cerebelli. Layer of the cerebellum.

g., dentate. A g. marked by indentations which lie on the upper surface of the hippocampal gyrus.

g. fornicatus. G. on medial surface of cerebrum which includes the g. cinguli, the isthmus, the hippocampus, hippocampal gyrus and uncus.

g., frontal, inferior. Convolution on external surface of frontal lobe of cerebrum located bet. the sylvian fissure and the inferior frontal sulcus.

g., frontal, middle. G. bet. the superior and inferior frontal sulci.

g., frontal, superior. Convolution of cerebral frontal lobe situated above the superfrontal fissure.

g., fusiform. G. beneath the collateral fissure joining the occipital and temporal lobes.

g., Heschl's. Transverse temporal g.

g., hippocampal. G. situated bet. the hippocampal and collateral fissures.

g., lingual. G. bet. the calcarine and collateral fissures.

g. longus insulae. Lengthy g. composing the postinsula.
g., marginal. SEE: *frontal superior g.*
g., mediotemporal. G. located bet. the mediotemporal and supertemporal fissures.
g., middle temporal. G. located between middle temporal sulcus and superior temporal sulcus.
g., occipital. Any of the gyri on the lateral surface of the occipital lobe. They are inconstant but grouped roughtly into two groups, the *inferior* or *lateral occipital gyri* and the *superior occipital gyri*.
g., occipitotemporal. SEE: *fusiform g.*
g., orbital. One of four g. (ant., post., lat., and med.), forming inf. surface of the frontal lobe.
g., paracentral. Area on mesial aspect of the cerebrum; the paracentral lobule. Lies above cingulate sulcus.
g., parietal. G. on lateral aspect of parietal lobe. Include post. central gyrus, sup. and inf. parietal gyri.
g., postcentral. G. situated bet. the central and postcentral fissures.

g., primary. Fetal cerebral regions marked by the primary fissures.
g. profundi cerebri. Very deep gyri of the cerebrum.
g., rectus. G. on the orbital aspect of the frontal lobe, located bet. the mesial margin and the olfactory sulcus.
g., Retzii, g., sagittal. The supra- and subcallosal gyri.
g., subcallosal. A narrow band of gray matter on median surface of hemisphere below the rostrum of the corpus callosum.
g., subcollateral. SEE: *fusiform g.*
g., supracallosal. A rudimentary gyrus on the upper surface of the corpus callosum.
g., supracallosus. Gray matter layer covering the corpus callosum.
g., supramarginal. G. in the inferior parietal lobule twisting about the upper terminus of the sylvian fissure.
g., temporal. Three gyri (sup. middle, inf.) on lateral surface of temporal lobe.
g. transitivus. SEE: *annectent g.*
g., uncinate. Ant. hooked portion of the hippocampal g.

H

H. or **h.** Abbr. for *haustus* (a draught), *height*, *henry*, *Holzknecht unit*, *hora* or *hour*, *horizontal*, *hypermetropia*. Symb. for *hydrogen*.

H¹. Symb. for *protium*.

H². Symb. for *deuterium*, an isotope of hydrogen.

H & E. Hematoxylin and eosin, a staining method much used in histology.

Haab's reflex. Contraction of pupils without alteration of accommodation or convergence when gazing at a bright object. A sign of a cortical lesion.

habena (ha-be'nă) [L. rein]. 1. A frenum. 2. Bandage for a wound. 3. Pineal gland peduncle. SYN: *habenula*, 2.

habe'nal, habe'nar [L. *habena*, rein]. Pert. to the habena or habenula.

habenula (hab-en'u-lă) [L. strap]. 1. A frenum. 2. A peduncle of the pineal gland. BNA. 3. A narrow bandlike stricture.
    h. urethra'lis. One of 2 whitish bands between the clitoris and *meatus urethra*.

habenul'ar. Pertaining to the habenula, esp., the stalk of the pineal body.
    h. trigone. A depressed triangular area located on the lateral aspect of the post. portion of the third ventricle. Each contains a *medial* and *lateral habernacular nucleus;* also called *habernacular area*.
    h. commissure. A band of transverse fibers connecting the two habenacular areas.

habit [L. *habitus, habēre,* to hold]. SYN: *habitus,* q.v. 1. A motor pattern executed with facility following constant or frequent repetition; an act at first performed in a typical voluntary manner but which after sufficient repetition is performed as a reflex action. Habits result from the passing of impulses through a particular set of neurons and synapses many times. 2. A particular type of dress or garb. 3. Mental or moral constitution or disposition. 4. Bodily appearance or constitution, esp. as related to a disease or predisposition to a disease, as the *apoplectic habit.* 5. Addiction to the use of drug or beverage as the *opium habit, alcoholic habit.*
    h. chorea. SEE: *h. spasm.*
    h., full. Full bloodedness, as in a disease.
    h. spasm. A spasmodic voluntary movement that has become involuntary. Often due to something irritating; sometimes from mimicry. SYN: *tic.*
    h. training. Schedule for 24 hr., adapted and rigidly enforced to train mental cases in habits of cleanliness and to stimulate mental activity.

habit, words pert. to: acolasia, addict, addiction state, alcoholomania, cacoethes, chloroformism, neuron, perversion, synapse, tic.

habitua'tion [L. *habitus,* habit]. Act of becoming accustomed to anything from frequent use.

hab'itus [L. habit]. Indications in appearance of tendency to disease or abnormal conditions.
    h. apoplecticus. Full bloodedness, as in a disease.
    h. enteropticus. Physical state marking enteroptosis.

    h. phthisicus. Predisposition to pulmonary tuberculosis characterized by poor bone development, pallor, etc.

habromania (hab-ro-ma'nĭ-ă) [G. *abros,* cheerful, + *mania,* madness]. A psychosis accompanied by pleasant delusions.

hachement (hash-mon') [Fr. chopping]. Strokes with edge of hand in massage. SYN: *hacking.*

hack'ing [A.S. *haccian,* to chop]. Strokes with edge of hand in massage. SYN: *hachement.*
    h. cough. A frequent, short cough.

Haemadipsa (hē"mă-dĭp'să). A genus of terrestrial leeches found in Asia which attacks man and animals.
    H. zeylanica and ***H. japonica*** are species found in Ceylon and Japan, respectively.

Haemagogus (hē"mă-gŏg'ŭs). A genus of mosquitoes. Includes the species *H. capricorni* which serves as a vector of yellow fever.

Haemophilus (hem-of'ĭl-us) [G. *aima,* blood, + *philein,* to love]. A genus of Bacteriaceae growing best in hemoglobin.
    H. conjunctivit'idis. The cause of "pink eye." SYN: *h. of Koch-Weeks.*
    H. ducrey'ii. The probable pathogenic agent of chancroid. SYN: *Ducrey's bacillus* and *Bacillus ulceris mollis.*
    H. haemolyt'icus. A nonpathogenic agent in the respiratory tract.
    H. influen'zae. Influenza bacillus or Pfeiffer's b. found in respiratory tract during influenza and other diseases.
    h. of Koch-Weeks. Same as *H. conjunctivitidis.*
    H. lacuna'tus. The cause of mild conjunctivitis.
    H. melaninogen'icus. A Gram-negative organism found on the genitalia and in oral cavities.
    H. pertus'sis. The possible cause of whooping cough. SYN: *Bordet-Gengou bacillus.*

Haemosporidia (hē"mō-spō-rĭd'ē-ă). An order of Sporozoa which live in the blood cells of vertebrates and reproduce sexually in invertebrates; includes four important families, *Babesiidae, Theileriidae, Haemoproteidae,* and *Plasmodiidae,* the last including the genus *Plasmodium,* four species of which cause malaria in man.

Haemphysalis (hē"mă-fĭ'să-lĭs). A genus of ticks belonging to the family Ixodidae. Includes the dog tick and rabbit tick.
    H. leporis-palustris. A species of ticks infesting rabbits. Serves as a vector of tularemia and Rocky Mountain spotted fever.

haf'nium. A rare chemical element of at. wt. 178.6. SYMB: Hf.

Hagedorn needle (hā'ge-dorn). A curved surgical needle with flattened sides.

Haines formula. The number of grains of solid in a fluidounce of urine determined by multiplying the last 2 figures of the sp. gr. of a specimen by 1.1.

hair [A.S. *haer*]. 1. A keratinized, threadlike outgrowth from the skin of mammals. 2. Collectively, the threadlike

outgrowths which form the fur of animals, or which grow on the human head.
A hair is a thin flexible shaft of cornified cells which develops from a cylindrical invagination of the epidermis, the *hair follicle*. Each consists of a free portion or *shaft* (scapus pili) and a *root* (radix pili) imbedded within the follicle. The shaft consists of three

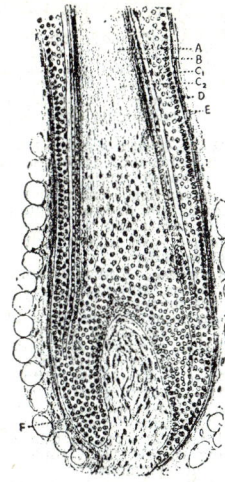

HAIR
Root of hair, longitudinal section.
A. Hair. B. Cuticle of hair. C. Internal root sheath. C₁. Cuticle of root sheath. C₂. Huxley's layer of internal root sheath. D. External root sheath. E. Hair follicle. F. Hair papilla.

layers of cells: the *cuticle* or outermost layer, the *cortex*, forming the main horny portion of the hair, and the *medulla*, the central axis. Hair color is due to pigment in the cortex.
Hairs in each part of the body have a definite period of growth after which they are shed. In man there is a constant gradual loss and replacement of hairs. Hairs of the eyebrows last only three to five months; those of the scalp two to five years. Baldness or *alopacia* results when replacement fails to keep up with hair loss. It may be due to hereditary factors or pathological conditions such as infections or injury from irradiation.
h. bulb *(bulbus pili)*. Lower expanded portion of a hair root. Growth of a hair results from the proliferation of cells of the hair bulb.
h. cell. An epithelial cell possessing fine nonmotile cilia found in the maculae and the organ of Corti of the membranous labyrinth of the inner ear. They are receptors for the senses of position and hearing.
h. dye. May contain silver nitrate or aniline dyes which are often irritating to skin or eyes, causing severe dermatitis or conjunctivitis. Occasionally results in blindness.
F. A. TREATMENT: Wash with sterile salt solution, followed by soap and water, followed by sponging with alcohol; cover with bland ointment, as cold cream or lanolin. The eye should be washed with normal saline and then instil paraffin oil, sweet oil or other bland oil.

h. follicle. An invagination of the epidermis which forms a cylindrical depression, penetrating the corium into the connective tissue which holds the hair root.
Sebaceous glands which secrete an oily fluid, and tiny muscles which cause the hair to stand *(arrectores pili)*, are attached to these follicles.
h., gustatory. A taste-hair. One of several fine hairlike process extending from the ends of gustatory cells in a taste bud. They project through the inner pore of a taste bud.
h. papilla. A projection of the corium which extends into the hair bulb at the bottom of a hair follicle. It contains capillaries through which a hair receives nourishment.
h., pubic. That over the pubes. It assumes the form of a triangle in the female. SYN: *escutcheon*. SEE: *pubic*.
hair′y heart. A heart covered with a rough exudation.
h. tongue. One covered with hairlike papillae.
hala′tion [G. *alōs*, a halo]. Blurring of vision due to light from a wrong direction.
half-life. The time required for a radioactive substance to lose one half of its energy.
half-value layer. SEE: half-value thickness.
h.-v. thickness. The thickness of a substance which, when placed in the path of a given beam of rays, will lower its intensity to ½ of the initial value.
h. ce′rea. Waxy softening of the bones.
halistere′tic [" + *sterēsis*, privation]. Rel. to or affected with halisteresis, *q.v.*
halitosis (hal-i-tos′is) [L. *halitus*, breath, + G. *-ōsis*]. Offensive breath.
halituous (hal-it′u-us) [L. *halitus*, breath]. Covered with moisture. SYN: *vaporous*.
hal′itus [L. breath]. 1. The breath. 2. Warm vapor.
haliver (hal′i-ver) [M.E. *halibut*, holy flounder, halibut, + A.S. *lifer*, liver]. Oil from the halibut's liver. Rich in vitamins A and D.
h. oil. The expressed oil from fresh halibut livers, standardized to contain approximately 100 times the amount of vitamin A, and 10 to 30 times the amount of vitamin D as standard cod liver oil.
USES: In all conditions where cod liver oil is indicated.
DOSAGE: Adults, 10 to 20 ṃ daily; children, 10 drops.
h. o. with viosterol. Haliver oil to which has been added sufficient viosterol to assure a potency of not less than 10,000 vitamin D units per Gm.
USES: Same as for cod liver oil.
DOSAGE: For infants, 8 to 10 drops daily; older children and adults, proportionately increased.
ADM: With a special dropper designed to deliver a certain number of drops to the mouth. [teries in the eye.
Hal′ler's cir′cles. Circles of veins and ar**hal′lex** (pl. *hal'lices*) [L.]. The great toe. SYN: *hallus, hallux*.
hallu′cination [L. *alucinari*, to wander in mind]. PSY: False perception having no relation to reality and not accounted for by any ext. stimuli. May be *visual, auditory, olfactory*, etc.
Commonly, the patient is unable to consider it as not constituting reality, but judgment may at times recognize discrepancies, and even at times deny the hallucination entirely. Usually, then, the patient reacts emotionally and be-

hallucination, extracampine   H-3   **hamulus**

haves as one would to a real situation. An indifferent attitude strongly suggests deterioration. Any sense may be involved, or elaborate combinations may occur. As in dreams, here the patient might be terrified at seeing an approaching assaulter, hear his threats, and feel his blows, and struggle in desperate defense. Emotional tone, delusions, and hallucinations tend to harmonize and this may be ascribed to the last, reflecting rather than determining the others.

Structural disease of the sensory organ and conducting mechanism may favor the formation of hallucinations, e. g., the deafness of an old otitis media often is associated with tinnitus, and at times the paresthesia is associated with phonemes. An irritative lesion of the visual cortex may produce more directly the hallucination, but even here an intact mind probably quickly would recognize the perception as unreal.

Hallucinations must then be considered the product of mental distortion, and the recognition of cause must be based on associated symptoms. It follows that hallucinations with few exceptions are presumptive evidence of a psychosis (insanity). Hypnagogic* hallucinations are notable exceptions.

RS: *acousma, acute hallucinosis, delusion, hallucinosis, illusion.*

h., extracampine. H. of hearing words spoken at a great distance.

h., haptic. One pert. to touching the skin, or to sensations of temperature or pain.

h., hypnogogic. Pre-sleep phenomena having the same practical significance as a dream but experienced while consciousness persists. Includes sense of falling, sinking, or of the ceiling moving.

h., kinetic. Sensation of flying or moving the body or a part of it.

h., microptic. One in which things seem reduced in size.

h., motor. Imaginary perceptions of movement.

h., somatic. Sensation of pain attributed to visceral injury.

h., teleologic. One which advises or guides the subject, such as those of Jeanne d'Arc.

hallucinosis (hăl-lū″sĭn-ō′sĭs) [″ + G. *ōsis*]. The state of having hallucinations more or less persistently. SEE: *hallucination.*

h., acute. PSY: Alcoholic psychosis. SYM: Fear or anxiety and auditory hallucinations.

hal′lus, hal′lux (pl. *hal′luces*) [L.]. The great toe.

h. doloro′sus. Pain in the metatarsophalangeal joint of the great toe due to flat foot.

h. flexus. Hammer toe.

h. valgus. Displacement of great toe toward other toes.

h. varus. Displacement of great toe away from other toes.

halmatogenesis (hal″mă-to-jen′e-sĭs) [G. *alma,* jump, + *genesis,* development]. A sudden deviation of type from one generation to the other one.

ha′lo [G. *alōs,* a halo]. 1. The areola, esp. of the nipple. 2. A ring surrounding the macula lutea in ophthalmoscopic images. 3. A circle of light surrounding a shining body.

h. glaumato′sus. A whitish ring surrounding the optic disk; seen in glaucoma.

h. symptom. Colored circle around lights in glaucoma.

hal′ogen [G. *als,* salt, + *gennan,* to form]. A salt former; one of a group of elements (chlorine, Cl.; bromine, Br.; iodine, I., and fluorine, F.), having very similar properties.

They combine with hydrogen to form acids and with metal to form salts.

haloid (hal′oid) [″ + *eidos,* form]. Resembling salt.

h. salt. A salt made up of a base and a halogen, resembling common salt.

halometer (ha-lom′ē-ter) [G. *alōs,* a halo, + *metron,* measure]. 1. Device for measuring diffraction halo of a red blood cell. 2. Device for measuring the halo around optic disk.

halosteresis (ha-lo-ster-e′sis) [G. *als,* salt, + *sterēsis,* privation]. Deficiency of lime salts in the bones. SYN: *halisteresis.*

Hal′sted's opera′tion. Operation for inguinal hernia and one for amputation of breast with carcinoma.

H.'s suture. An interrupted one for intestinal wounds.

Hal′stern's disease. Endemic syphilis.

ham [A.S. *haum,* haunch]. 1. The popliteal space or region behind the knee. 2. Common name for the thigh, hip, and buttock. 3. The thigh of an animal, esp., the hog, prepared for food.

hamartia (ham-ar′shĭ-ă) [G. *amartia,* defect]. Error in development due to imperfect tissue combination.

hamartoma (ham-ar-to′mă) [″ + *ōma,* tumor]. 1. A tumor due to new growth of blood vessels; opp. to dilatation of preëxisting vessels. 2. A tumor due to failure of development.

hamartomatosis (ham-ar-to-mă-to′sis) [″ + *ōma,* tumor + *-ōsis*]. Existence of multiple hamartomas.

hama′tum [L. *hamatus,* hooked]. The unciform bone, *os hamatum.*

hammer. 1. An instrument with a head attached crosswise to the handle for striking blows. 2. Common name for the malleus, the middle ear bone.

h. percussion. A h. with a rubber head used for tapping surfaces of the body in order to produce sounds for diagnostic purposes. SEE: *plexor.*

h. reflex. A h. used for tapping parts of the body such as a muscle, tendon, or nerve in order to initiate certain reflexes.

ham′mer toe. A toe with dorsal flexion of 1st phalanx and plantar flexion of 2nd and 3rd phalanges.

Hamp′son unit. X-ray unit of measurement.

It is one-fourth of the erythema dose.

hamster. A rodent *Cricetus cricetus* resembling a rat belonging to the family Cricetidae, common in Europe and W. Asia. It is extensively used as a laboratory animal.

ham′string [A.S. *haum,* haunch]. One of the tendons which form the medial and lateral boundaries of the popliteal space.

h's inner. Tendons of the semimembranosus, semitendinosus, and gracilis muscles.

h's outer. The tendon of the biceps femoris.

hamstrings. Three muscles on the posterior aspect of the thigh, the semitendinosus, semimembranosus, and biceps femoris. They flex the leg and adduct and extend the thigh.

ham′ular [L. *hamulus,* a small hook]. Unciform; hook-shaped.

hamulus [L. a small hook]. 1. Any hook-shaped structure. 2. Hooklike process on the hamate bone.

hamulus cochleae   H-4   **haptophoric, haptophorous**

h. cochleae. A hooklike process at the tip of the osseous spiral hamina of the cochlea.
h. lacrimalis. Hooklike process on the lacrimal bone.
h. pterygoideus. Hooklike process at tip of medial pterygoid process of the sphenoid bone.

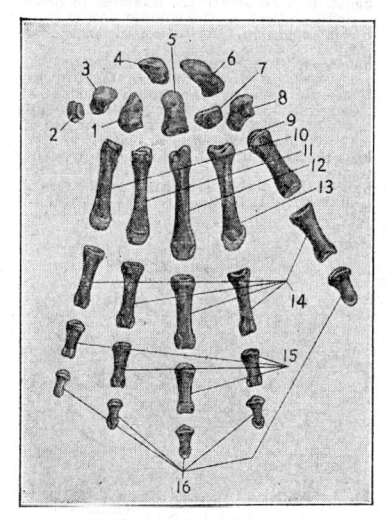

BONES OF THE HAND AND WRIST
1. Hamate. 2. Pisiform. 3. Triquetrum. 4. Lunate. 5. Capitate. 6. Navicular. 7. Lesser multangular. 8. Greater multangular. 9. First metacarpal. 10. Fifth metacarpal. 11. Fourth metacarpal. 12. Third metacarpal. 13. Second metacarpal. 14. First or proximal row of phalanges. 15. Second row of phalanges. 16. Third or distal row of phalanges.

hand [A.S. *hand*]. That part of the body which is distal to but attached to the forearm at the wrist.
It includes the wrist (*ossa carpi*) with its 8 bones, the metacarpus, or body of the hand (*ossa metacarpalia*) having 5 bones, and the phalanges (fingers) with their 14 bones.
hand, words pert. to: "chir-" words, dysgraphia, lumbricalis, macrochira, manus, metacarpus, metacarpus, palmar, skeleton, thenar, trapezium.
hands and skin. Sterilization of hands for surgical operations may be accomplished by preliminary thorough scrubbing (soap and mechanical cleansing alone remove a major part of the organisms), brief immersion in a mild germicidal solution, and finally the wearing of sterilized rubber gloves.
One method commonly used consists of washing the hands thoroughly in hot water and soap, scrubbing energetically with bristle brushes, cleansing nails (80% alcohol for 1 minute), then immersing hands in a 1:1000 mercuric chloride solution for 5 minutes. It is difficult or impossible to disinfect the hands completely, esp. to remove all organisms from around the nails, and hence this partial disinfection is followed by employment of rubber gloves, sterilized by boiling for 20 minutes.

hand'edness. The tendency to use one hand in preference to the other.
h., left. Sinistrality; preferential use of the left hand.
h., right. Dextrality preferential use of the right hand.
hang'ing drop culture. A method of culturing microorganisms by placing a drop of the culture medium containing organisms on a coverslip, then inverting the coverslip over a concavity of a hanging drop slide.
hang'nail [A.S. *hangian* to hang, + *naegel*, nail]. SYN: *agnail*. Partly detached piece of skin at root of a fingernail.
Hanot's disease (han'os). Hypertrophic cirrhosis of liver with jaundice.
Hansen, Gerhard Henrik Armauer. Norwegian physician, 1841-1912.
H's bacillus. *Mycobacterium leprae*, which he discovered in 1871.
H's disease. Leprosy.
Han'son unit. One one-hundredth of the quantity of parathyroid extract solution necessary to elevate by 1 mg. the concentration of calcium in blood serum of a parathyroidectomized dog whose weight is 15 Kg.
hapalonychia (hap-al-o-nik'ĭ-ă) [G. *apalos*, soft, + *onyx, onych-*, nail]. Lack of rigidity of the nails. SYN: *onychomalacia*.
haphalgesia (haf-al-ge'zĭ-ă) [G. *aphē*, touch, + *algēsis*, pain]. A sensation of pain upon touching the skin with an object which is not an irritant.
haphephobia (haf-e-fo'bĭ-ă) [" + *phobos*, fear]. Aversion to being touched by another person.
haplodermatitis (hap'lo-der-mă-ti'tis) [G. *aploos*, simple, + *derma*, skin, + *-itis*, inflammation]. Simple inflammation of the skin. SYN: *haplodermitis*.
hap'lodermi'tis [" + " + *-itis*, inflammation]. Uncomplicated inflammation of the skin.
hap'loid. Possessing half the diploid or normal number of chromosomes found in somatic or body cells. Such is the case of the germ cells, ova or sperms, following the reduction divisions in gametogenesis, the haploid number being 24 in man.
haplop'ia. Single vision; condition in which an object viewed by two eyes appears as a single object in contrast to *diplopia*, in which it appears as two objects.
hap'ten(e [G. *aptein*, to seize]. The portion of an antigen containing the grouping on which the specificity depends.
haptic (hap'tik) [G. *aptein*, to touch]. Pert. to touch. SYN: *tactile*.
hap'tics [G. *aptein*, to touch]. The science of the touch sense.
haptin (hap'tin) [G. *aptein*, to seize]. A cast off receptor.
There are 3 orders of haptin: (a) Antiferment or antitoxin; (b) agglutinin, coagulin, precipitin. (a) and (b) are *uniceptors.* (c) Bacteriolysin, cytolysin, hemolysin. These are *amboceptors.*
haptophile (hap'to-fīl, -fĭl) [" + *philein* to love"]. That portion of a receptor that unites with the haptophore group of a toxin.
haptophore (hap'to-fōr) [" + *pherein*, to bring]. The atom group of an antigen causing a combination with its corresponding antibody. SEE: *Ehrlich's sidechain theory*.
haptophor'ic, haptoph'orous [" + *pherein*, to bring]. Pert. to the action of a haptophore.

har'dening [A.S. heardian, to harden]. 1. Rendering a pathological or histological specimen firm or compact for making thin sections for microscopic study.
2. Increased resistance to changes in temperature of the atmosphere.

If the body is exposed to low temperatures, a contraction of skin vessels takes place, with a corresponding dilatation of the capillaries of the mucous membranes.

Hardening is induced by bathing to cause a prompt skin vascular reaction.

hard'ness [A.S. *heardness*]. 1. Quality of water containing certain substances, esp., soluble salts of calcium and magnesium. These react with soaps forming insoluble compounds which are precipitated out of solution, thus interfering with their cleansing action. 2. That quality of x-rays determining their penetrating power. Hardness lessens as wave lengths become longer.

h. of a gas tube. A term used to qualify the condition of a tube according to the degree of rarefaction of the residual gas.

The higher the vacuum, the harder the tube and the rays emitted, the higher the voltage required to cause a discharge with a cold cathode, and hence the shorter the wave length of the resulting roentgen rays. SEE: *hardness of roentgen, ray*.

hare'lip [A.S. *hara*, hare, + *lippa*, lip]. SYN: *cheiloschisis*. A vertical cleft or clefts in the upper lip. It is congenital resulting from the faulty fusion of the median nasal process and the lateral maxillary processes. It is usually unilateral and on the left side although it may be bilateral. It may involve the lip or the upper jaw alone or both together, and often occurs with cleft palate.

h. suture. A twisted figure-of-eight suture.

harlequin fetus (har'lĕ-kwin). A newly-born infant with *ichthyosis congenita*, SYN: *hyperkeratosis congenitalis*.

Har'rison's groove. Depression on lower edge of the thorax caused by tug of the diaphragm; seen in adenoids and rickets.

Has'ner's valve or fold. SYN: *plica lacrimalis*. A fold of the mucous membrane at the opening of the nasolacrimal duct in the inf. meatus of the nasal cavity.

Has'sall's corpuscles or bodies. SYN: *thymic corpuscle*. Spherical or oval bodies present in the medulla of the thymus. Each consists of central area of degenerated cells surrounded by concentrically arranged flattened or polygonal cells. They are characteristic of the thymus.

Hath'cock's sign. Tenderness just beyond the angle of the jaws when the finger follows on the under surface of the mandible towards the angle. Found in mumps before any swelling can be detected.

haunch (hawnsh) [Fr. *hanche*]. The hips and buttocks.

h. bone. The ilium. SYN: *os coxae*.

Haus'man's stagna'tion test meal. Four tablespoonfuls of boiled rice and a glass of water are given at 9 o'clock at night (a little sugar and milk can be taken on the rice).

If, after fasting until 9 o'clock in the morning, rice residue is not shown microscopically or macroscopically, there is no stagnation (a drop of Lugol's solution stains any starch granules blue so that they are easily seen).

haustra (haws'tra) (sing. *haustrum*) [L. *haurire*, to draw, drink]. The sacculated elevations of the colon.

h. coli. Sacculations of the colon resembling tucks caused by the fact that the gut is longer than the longitudinal bands or taeniae.

haustral (haw'stral) [L. *haurire*, to draw, drink]. Pert. to the colonic haustra.

h. churning. Agitation of the intestinal contents.

haustrum (haw'strum) (pl. *haus'tra*) [L. *haurire*, to draw, drink]. One of the sacculations of the colon caused by longitudinal bands shorter than the gut which causes formation of pouches in the colon. SYN: *haustra coli*.

haus'tus [L. a drink]. A draught of medicine.

haut-mal (o'mahl) [Fr. high evil]. Grand mal when at its height.

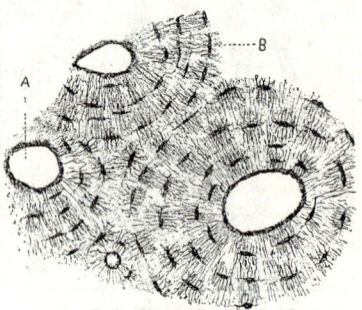

HAVERSIAN SYSTEM OF BONE, MAGNIFIED

Cross section femur, dog. A. Haversian canal. B. Lacunae and canaliculi.

haver'sian canal. Minute vascular canal found in osseous tissue.

h. canaliculi. Delicate canals extending from the lacunae into the matrix of bone. They anastomose with canaliculi of adjacent lacunae forming a network of fine channels which communicate with Haversian and Volkmann's canals. They transmit nutrient materials.

h. gland. A mass of fatty tissue lodged in the acetabular fossa of the innominate bone. Also called *synovial gland*.

h. system. Architectural unit of bone, consisting of a central tube (*h. canal*) with alternate layers of intercellular material (*matrix*) surrounding it in concentric cylinders. Alternating layers of matrix and cells are called *haversian lamellae*. SEE: *bone*.

hay fever. SYN: *allergic coryza, rose cold, vasomotor rhinitis, pollinosis*. An allergic disease of mucous passages of nose and upper air passages induced by external irritation.

SYM: Inflammation, catarrh, watery discharges from the eyes, cold in the head, coryza, headache, asthmatic symptoms.

ETIOL: Air-borne pollens. *Spring type* due to pollens of trees such as oak, elm, hickory, ash; *Summer type* due to pollens of plants such as grasses, plantain, and sorrel; *Fall type* due principally to the pollen of ragweeds. Non-seasonal hay fever may result from (a) inhalation of irritating substances such as the danders of animals, or dust such as hay, straw, or house dust. (b) In-

Hay'garth's deformities 1. Change of climate, sea voyage. 2. Filtration of air by air conditioning, masks, and nasal filters. 3. Drug therapy in which epinephrine, antihistamines, or other drugs are given orally or used as nose drops, or nasal sprays. 4. Prophylactic treatment consisting of injection of pollen extracts made from pollen to which the subject is sensitive.

Hay'garth's deformities, nodes or **nodosities.** Exostoses or bony tumors on joints in arthritis deformans.

ha'zelnut [A.S. *haesel*, hazel, + *hnutu*, nut]. ASH CONST: Ca 0.287, Mg 0.140, K 0.618, Na 0.019, P 0.354, Cl 0.067, S 0.198, Fe 0.0041.

hb. Abbr. for hemoglobin.

h.d. Abbr. for *hora decubitus* (the hour of going to bed).

He. Symb. for helium.

H. D. Abbr. for *hearing distance*.

head [A.S. *heafod*]. 1. Caput. That part of the animal body containing the brain and organs of the sight, hearing, smell, and taste. It includes the facial bones. 2. The proximal end of a bone. 3. The larger extremity of any structure or body.

  h., abnormal fixity of. May be caused by postpharyngeal abscess, occipitocervical myelalgia, arthritis deformans, swollen cervical glands, rheumatism, traumatism of neck, sprains of cervical muscles, congenital spasmodic torticollis, caries of a molar tooth, cicatrices of burns.

  h., abnormal movement of. Habit spasms, such as noddings.

  h., aftercoming. The head of a fetus in a breech presentation.

  h., black. A comedo, *q.v.*

  h. fold. A fold of the blastoderm of a chick which grows caudad under the ant. portion of the neural plate. It brings about the establishment of the head and the foregut.

  h. gut. Part of embryo which develops into stomach, duodenum, and esophagus.

  h., histamine. H. resulting from injection of histamine or excessive histamine in circulating blood. Due to dilatation of branches of the carotid artery.

  h., inability to move the. May be due to caries of cervical vertebrae and diseases of articulation bet. occiput and atlas or paralysis of neck muscles.

  h. kidney. Embryonic kidney.

  h. lock. Interlocking of chins in twin birth.

  h. process. A strand of cells in the embryo extending forward from the primitive knot. Also called *notochordal plate.*

  h., retracted. Seen in acute meningitis, cerebral abscess, tumor, thrombosis of sup. longitudinal sinus, acute encephalitis, laryngeal obstruction, tetanus, hydrophobia, epilepsy, spasmodic torticollis, strychnine poisoning, hysteria, and rachitic conditions. Also in painful neck lesions at the back.

  h., rhythmical nodding of. Seen in aortic regurgitation, chorea, torticollis, *q.v.*

  h. scald. Affection of scalp accompanied by crusts or scales.

head, words pert. to: acromegaly, acromegaly, capitate, caput, "ceph-" words, coryza, face, gyrospasm, macrocephalous, nutation, occipital, sinciput, skeleton, temple, vertex.

head'ache [A.S. *heafod* + *acan*, to ache]. A diffuse pain in different portions of the head and not confined to any nerve distribution area.

It may be *frontal, temporal* or *occipital;* confined to 1 side of head or to region immediately over 1 eye. The character of pain may vary; may be dull ache; acute, almost unbearable pain; intermittent, intense pain; throbbing pain; pressure pain when head feels as if it will burst, or penetrating pain driving through head.

ETIOL: (a) Associated with disorders of alimentary tract, probably due to absorption of toxins, as in indigestion or constipation. (b) Due to toxemia. A constant symptom in nephritis and jaundice; also occurs in septic absorption from foci present in body, as in septic teeth, septic tonsils, infected cranial sinuses. (c) Frequently a symptom at onset of febrile diseases, esp. pneumonia, typhoid fever, scarlet fever, smallpox, erysipelas, tetanus, and influenza. (d) Defective sight and, less commonly, defective hearing are causes. With defective sight, pain may occur over eyes, also at occiput owing to fatigue of visual area, situated in the occipital lobe of the brain. (e) Mental strain, worry, and anxiety will cause headache; this may be associated with eyestrain or be independent of it. (f) Abnormalities in blood pressure give rise to headache. In some cases due to low blood pressure, in which anemia of brain occurs; in other cases blood pressure is high. Sudden changes in blood pressure also cause headache. (g) Changes in intracranial pressure give rise to headache. The acutely painful headache following intrathecal anesthesia is an example, as is the headache associated with meningitis. (h) Diseases of central nervous system are characterized by headache. (i) Any injury resulting in concussion or compression of brain or cord.

Summary:
1. TOXIC FACTORS—
(a) *Of exogenous origin*—Foul air, from poor ventilation, etc.; poisonous gases, including fumes from furnaces or gas fires; drugs (quinine, morphine, etc.); alcohol, tobacco, etc.
(b) *Of endogenous origin* (any absorption of the toxins of bacterial infection or perverted metabolism will cause headache).
Chronic focal infections—Nose and sinuses, teeth, middle ear, pharynx, tonsils, appendix, gallbladder, pelvic viscera.
Fever in general.
Bacteremias—Typhoid fever, malaria, smallpox, tuberculosis, grippe and influenza, puerperal fever, etc.
Systemic diseases—Nephritis with uremia, biliary tract disease (including acute yellow atrophy of the liver), rheumatism, diabetes, anemia, polycythemia, eclampsia, syphilis.
2. GASTROINTESTINAL DISTURBANCES—Dyspepsia, gastric hyper- and hypoacidity, intestinal stasis and constipation.
3. PHYSICO-CHEMICAL DISTURBANCES—Acidosis, alkalosis.
4. CARDIOVASCULAR DISTURBANCES—High blood pressure, low blood pressure, myocardial and valvular insufficiency causing either congestion or anemia.
5. ENDOCRINE DISORDERS — Pituitary, thyroid, suprarenals, ovaries.
6. GYNECOLOGICAL FACTORS (due to functional disturbances of one or more of the above glands)—Puberty, menstruation, pregnancy, menopause.

headache, sick   H-7   **hearing, functional tests for**

7. NEUROLOGICAL FACTORS — Nervous shock; nervous exhaustion; worry, excitement, anger, or nervous tension; migraine; hysteria; epilepsy; psychoneuroses; headache which may be psychic with reflex symptoms to various regions or which may be, itself, a reflex pain secondary to organic disease.

8. DISEASES OF SPECIAL SENSE ORGANS —Iritis, glaucoma, etc.; adenoids, deviated septum, etc.; middle ear affections.

9. ORGANIC DISEASE OF BRAIN—Causing pressure: Tumor, abscess, gumma, cyst, hydrocephaly, intracranial hemorrhage. Intracranial vascular disease; arteriosclerosis; embolism, thrombosis or aneurism; encephalitis.

10. VARIOUS FORMS OF MENINGITIS, including meningismus.

11. FUNCTIONAL CAUSES (almost any disturbance of body function may cause headache)—External pressure and constriction of head; trauma to head; sunstroke; persistent noises; persistent motion (seasickness, train sickness, etc.); irritation of mucous membrane of nose and sinuses by dust, pollen, etc.; fatigue (physical mental); insomnia; eyestrain (uncorrected defects, overwork); spinal puncture usually followed by headache.

TREATMENT: Depends entirely on cause, and there is great danger of headache, which is probably only a symptom, being treated without regard to cause. Provided that due consideration has been given to this, the following points may receive general attention: (a) The diet; (b) adequate rest; (c) the state of the bowels; (d) the amount of urine being passed. Applications of cold to head may relieve, esp. if evaporating lotion is used. A hot bath may help, by stimulating circulation generally. Heat applied to back of neck may relieve by reflex effect. A saline aperient may relieve by producing dehydration, esp. in cases in which blood pressure is high. A stimulant, such as tea, coffee, or sal volatile, may relieve, when headache is due to fatigue or overstrain. Drugs for the relief of headache should be given with care. SYN: *cephalgia.*

h., sick. A nervous headache occurring periodically, usually on 1 side of the head, accompanied by nausea and vomiting.

SEE: *megrim, migraine.*

heal (hēl) [A.S. *hael,* whole]. To cure; to make whole or healthy.

heal′ing [A.S. *hael,* whole]. The restoration to a normal condition, esp. of an inflammation or a wound.

HEALING BY FIRST INTENTION: This process closes the edge of a wound with little or no inflammatory reaction, and in such a manner that no scar is left to reveal the site of the injury. The free bleeding of the cut edges and the intact living cells not affected by the injury make this possible. New cells are formed to take the place of dead ones, and the capillary walls stretch across the wound to join themselves to each other in a smooth surface. New connective tissue may form an almost imperceptible scar which proves temporary.

HEALING BY SECOND INTENTION: This is healing by granulation or indirect union. Granulation tissue is formed to fill the gap between the edges of the wound with a thin layer of fibrinous exudate. It bars out bacteria and aids in checking bleeding by the coagulation of the blood. Connective tissue cells support the new capillaries. This form of healing is slower than that by first intention and its grayish-red surface may become pale and flabby if the healing is too long delayed. If the granulations show above the surface they may have to be removed with caustics. If the granulations first form at the top instead of the bottom of the wound, it may have to be kept open by drainage.

HEALING BY THIRD INTENTION: Of an ulcer, wound, or cavity by filling with granulations. It generally results in the formation of a scar.

COMPLICATIONS IN HEALING: These may result from: (a) The formation of a scar interfering with functioning of the part, and possible deformity; (b) the formation of a *keloid,** the result of overgrowth of connective tissue forming a tumor in the surface of a scar; (c) necrosis of the skin and mucous membrane producing a raw surface that results in an ulcer; (d) a sinus or fistula which may be due to bacteria, or some foreign substance remaining in the wound; (e) proud flesh. This represents excessive granulations, the result of a fungous growth.

health (helth) [A.S. *häelth,* wholeness]. A condition in which all functions of body and mind are normally active.

h., bill of. Public health certificate certifying that passengers on a public conveyance or ship are free of infectious disease.

H., Board of. A public body in charge of the health of a community.

h. certificate. An official statement signed by a physician which attests to the state of health of a particular individual.

H., Department of. Branch of a government (city, county, or nation) for regulation and protection of the people's health.

h., industrial. The health of employees of industrial firms.

h., public. The state of health of the population of a particular community, such as a city, county, state, or nation, as opposed to individual or personal health; community health.

h. nurse, public. One employed by a Board or Dept. of Health to serve the public.

H. Service, Public. A Bureau of the U. S. Treasury Dept.

health′y [A.S. *häelth,* wholeness]. Being in a state of health or enjoying it.

h. pus. Pus of a form without odor, which is less dangerous than the other types.

h. ulcer. Ulcer which heals easily.

hear′ing [A.S. *hēran,* to hear]. The act or power of perceiving sound.

h., after. Perception of sound after the stimulus producing it has ceased to act.

h. aid. An apparatus used by those with impaired hearing for amplifying sound waves.

h. distance. That at which a given sound can be heard. On the prairies a voice may be heard for 2 miles or more.

h., functional tests for. Determination of hearing acuity can be determined by: (1) Determining the distance at which a person can hear a certain sound, such as a watch tick. (2) By the use of *audiometers,* in which electrically produced sounds are conveyed by wires to a receiver applied to the subject's ear. Intensity and pitch of sound can be altered and is indicated on dials. Results are plotted on a graph known as an *audiogram.* (3) By bone conduction tests in which a device such as tuning fork or an apparatus which converts an electrical current into mechanical vibrations is applied to the skull. Such is of value in distinguishing between perceptive and transmission deafness.

h. hallucinations. Subjective sensations of sound such as "hearing voices" when none actually exists.

heart (hart) [A.S. *heorte*]. A hollow, muscular, contractile organ, the center of the circulatory system. Its wall possesses three layers, the outer *epicardium*, a serous layer, the middle ventricles being known as *ventriculus dexter* (right) and *v. sinister* (left).

Contraction of the heart chambers is called *systole;* relaxation with accompanying dilation, *diastole*. The complete series of events which occurs in a single heart beat is known as the *cardiac cycle*. In a normal beating heart, each cycle lasts about 0.85 sec. The heart is divided perpendicularly from base to apex by the *interauricular* and *interventricular septa*, the right side having no communication with the left. The right side receives *deoxygenated* blood from the tissues and pumps it to the lungs; the left side receives oxy-

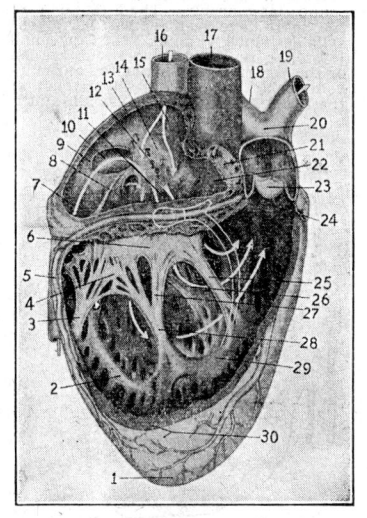

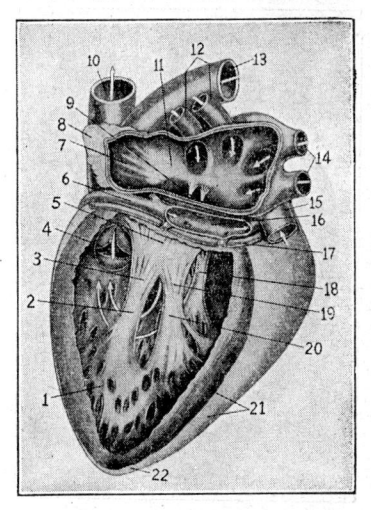

RIGHT AURICLE AND VENTRICLE OF HEART

Both chambers laid open, the anterior wall of each having been removed. The arrows indicate the course of the blood. 1, Apex of heart; 2, columnae carneae; 3, papillary muscles; 4, chordae tendinae; 5, right coronary artery; 6, tricuspid valve; 7, opening of inferior vena cava; 8, eustachian valve; 9, annulus ovale; 10, fossa ovalis; 11, auriculoventricular orifice; 12, foramina thebesii; 13, right auricle; 14, atrium; 15, opening of superior vena cava; 16, superior vena cava; 17, aorta; 18, right branch of pulmonary artery; 19, left branch of pulmonary artery; 20, pulmonary artery; 21, pectinate muscles; 22, auricular appendix; 23, posterior flap of pulmonary valve; 24, infundibulum; 25, papillary muscles; 26, papillary muscles of posterior flap; 27, chordae tendinae; 28, papillary muscles; 29, moderator band; 30, muscular wall.

LEFT AURICLE AND VENTRICLE OF HEART

The arrows indicate the course of the blood. 1. Columnae carneae; 2, papillary muscles; 3, chordae tendinae; 4, orifice of aorta; 5, anterior flap of mitral valve; 6, anterior cardiac vein; 7, pectinate muscles; 8, auricular appendix; 9, auriculoventricular orifice; 10, aorta; 11, cavity of the left auricle; 12, right pulmonary veins; 13, pulmonary artery; 14, left pulmonary veins; 15, vena cava inferior; 16, coronary sinus; 17, transverse branch of the right coronary artery; 18, papillary muscles of the posterior flap; 19, chordae tendinae; 20, papillary muscles; 21, muscular wall; 22, apex.

myocardium, composed of cardiac muscle, and the inner *endocardium,* a layer which lines the chambers of the heart and covers the valves. The heart is enclosed in a fibroserous sac, the *pericardium,* the space between the pericardium and the epicardium forming the *pericardial cavity*.

CHAMBERS: Each lower cavity is the *ventriculum,* or ventricle; each upper one the *atrium,* or auricle. The right auricle is called the *atrium dexter,* and the left one the *atrium sinistrum,* the 2

genated blood from the lungs and pumps it to the tissues.

The atria, serving as receiving chambers, are thin walled; the ventricles, serving as pumping chambers, are thick walled.

Accelerator impulses are conveyed over nerves and ganglia of the sympathetic division. Preganglionic neurons which lie in the thoracic portion of the spinal cord synapse with postganglionic neurons located in the cervical ganglia of sympathetic trunk whose axons pass to the heart. Impulses over these nerves known as *augmentor nerves* increase rate and force of heart beat. Impulses regulating the heart arise in the cardiac center in the medulla oblongata.

Afferent fibers: these pass through the vagus trunks to the medulla. Some

heart   heart, auscultation of

are *depressor* fibers originating in receptors in the base of the aorta. Impulses over these fibers reflexly slow the heart rate. Others are *pressor fibers* originating in receptors in the vena cavae and rt. atrium. These reflexly increase heart beat. Fibers conveying pain impulses are also present.

VALVES: The auriculoventricular orifice bet. each auricle and ventricle. 1. *Valvula tricuspidalis* (tricuspid) guards the opening bet. the *atrium dexter* and the *ventriculus dexter*. 2. *Valvula bicuspidalis* (bicuspid or mitral valve), bet. the *atrium sinistrum* (left auricle)

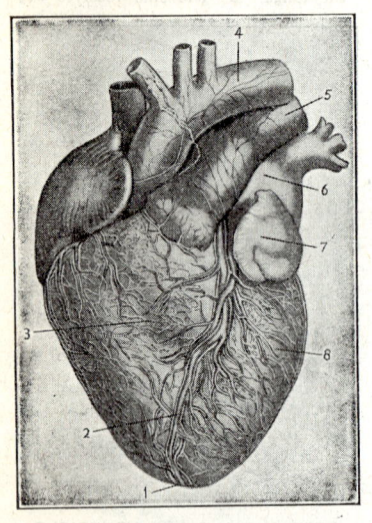

STERNOCOSTAL SURFACE OF HEART

1. Apex. 2. Anterior descending branch of left coronary artery. 3. Right ventricle. 4. Aorta. 5. Pulmonary artery. 6. Left atrium. 7. Left auricle. 8. Left ventricle.

and the *ventriculus sinister* (left ventricle). 3. *Valvulae semilunares* (semilunar valves) guard the orifice bet. the *ventriculus dexter* and the pulmonary artery. 4. *Valvulae semilunares aortae* (aortic valves) guard the orifice bet. the *ventriculus sinister* and the aorta.

NERVE SUPPLY: *Inhibitory*: Vagus or pneumogastric, acceleratory: By way of the sympathetic ganglia of the autonomic system and phrenic nerve. *Afferent*: A depressor nerve running from the heart to a cardio-inhibitory center in the medulla, through the sheath of the vagi nerves, causing reflex inhibition of the heart. Efferent fibers: *Inhibitory impulses* are conveyed by preganglionic fibers of the vagus nerve, which synapse with post-ganglionic neurons located in terminal ganglia in the wall of the heart. They are distributed to the S-A node and other conductile tissue of the heart.

WORK OF HEART. Two to 3 oz. of blood are driven into the arteries by each heartbeat. The power exerted by the heart is said to equal that necessary to lift 80 lb. 1 ft. each minute. The human heart beats 72 times per minute, 104,000 times a day, 38,000,000 times during a year. At every stroke 5 cu. in. of blood are forced out into the body, or 500,000 cu. in. a day. In terms of work this is the equivalent of raising 1 ton to a height of 41 ft. every 24 hr.

h., armoured. Condition characterized by deposit of calcareous matter in the pericardium.

h., athletic. Hypertrophy of the heart as a result of strenuous physical activity. Of little or no significance in the absence of diseased valves.

h., auscultation of. Shows intensity, quality, and rhythm of heart sounds and detects the presence of any adventitious sounds, as murmurs. The 2 sounds over the heart have been represented by the syllables "lubb," "dupp." The first sound (systolic) results from the contraction of the ventricle, tension of the auriculoventricular valves, and the impact of the heart against the chest wall, and is

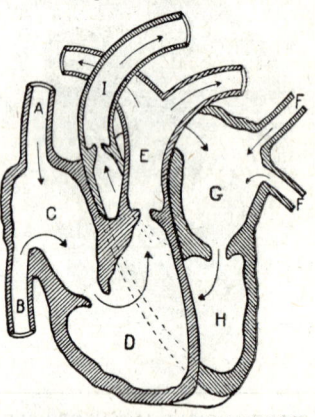

CIRCULATION OF THE BLOOD THROUGH THE HEART

A. Superior vena cava. B. Inferior vena cava. C. Right atrium. D. Right ventricle. E. Pulmonary artery. F. Pulmonary veins. G. Left atrium. H. Left ventricle. I. Aorta.

synchronous with the apex beat and carotid pulse. This sound is prolonged and dull; after the first sound is a short pause, then the second sound (diastolic), which results from the closure of the aortic and pulmonary valves. This sound is short and high pitched. After the second sound a longer pause follows before the first is heard again.

INTENSITY: Both sounds are accentuated in: (1) Excitement of heart from any cause; (2) anemia; (3) cardiac hypertrophy; (4) subjects with thin chest walls; (5) consolidation of the lung, as in phthisis and pneumonia. *Accentuation of the aortic second sound results from*: (a) Hypertrophy of the left ventricle; (b) high arterial tension, as in arteriosclerosis and Bright's disease; (c) aortic aneurysm. *Accentuation of the pulmonary second sound results from*: (a) Pulmonary obstruction, as in emphysema, pneumonia and the congestion of the lungs following mitral disease; (b) hypertrophy of the right ventricle. *Weakness of both sounds is noted in*: (a) General obesity; (b) general debility; (c) degeneration or dilatation of

heart block

the heart; (d) pericardial or pleural effusion; (e) emphysema.

REDUPLICATION — HEART SOUNDS: Probably due to a lack of synchronous action in the valves of the 2 sides of the heart, and results from many conditions, but notably from increased resistance in the systemic or the pulmonary circulation, as in arteriosclerosis of chronic nephritis and in emphysema. Frequently noted in mitral stenosis and pericarditis.

ADVENTITIOUS SOUNDS: *Murmurs*: A murmur is an abnormal sound heard over the heart or blood vessels and may result from: (1) Obstruction or regurgitation at the valves following endocarditis; (2) dilatation of the ventricle or relaxation of its walls rendering the valves relatively insufficient; (3) aneurysm; (4) a change in the blood constituents, as in anemia; (5) roughening of the pericardial surfaces, as in pericarditis; (6) irregular action of the heart.

Murmurs produced within the heart are termed endocardial, those outside exocardial; those produced in aneurysms, bruits; those produced by anemia, hemic murmurs.

Hemic murmurs: They are soft and blowing in character, usually systolic in time, heard best over pulmonary valves. Associated with symptoms of anemia, and disappear with the latter.

Aneurysmal murmur or bruit. Usually loud, booming in character, systolic in time, heard best over the aorta or base of heart and is often associated with an abnormal area of dullness and pulsation, and with symptoms resulting from pressure on neighboring structures.

Pericardial friction sounds. Pericardial murmurs or friction sounds are superficial, rough, and creaking in quality, to and fro in time, not transmitted beyond the precordium and may be modified by pressure of the stethoscope.

PROCEDURE: Patient should be recumbent when beginning examination; then, having elicited all the signs possible, repeat with patient sitting or standing and note any variations from change of position. First listen while patient is breathing naturally, then while holding breath, and finally have patient take 3 or 4 forced inspirations. Explore whole thoracic cavity and endeavor to localize the points at which heart sounds, both normal and abnormal, are heard with the greatest intensity. Proceed from below upward, from left to right.

VALVES: *Location for auscultation*: *Aortic*, 3rd intercostal space; close to left side of sternum. *Pulmonary*, in front of aorta, behind junction of 3rd costal cartilage with sternum, left side. *Tricuspid*, behind middle of sternum about level of 4th of costal cartilage. *Mitral*, behind 3rd intercostal space about 1 in. to the left of sternum.

h. block. Condition in which the conductive tissue of the heart (S-A node and the bundle of His its branches) fails to conduct impulses normally from the auricle to the ventricles. Such results in altered rhythm of heart beat with loss of every other, or of every 3rd beat, the auricular systole not always being followed by the ventricular systole, the bundle of His failing to transmit the regular systolic impulse. The ventricle contracts regularly at a much slower rate than the auricle. The contractions begin at the sino-auricular node, or normal point, but they are interrupted before they reach their destination. The pulse is very slow, usually under 30.

ETIOL: (a) Structural changes as from tumor or degeneration or embryonic maldevelopment. (b) Toxic effects of drugs or the toxins of infections. (c) Nutritional or functional factors.

h. block aborization. B. in which there is interference in terminal fibers of the Purkinje system.

h. block, atrioventricular. B. in which impulses are impeded at the A-V node.

h. block, bundle-branch. B. in which impulses are blocked in one of the branches of the bundle of His, resulting in ventricles beating independently of each other.

h. block, complete. Condition in which there is a complete dissociation between auricular and ventricular systoles. Ventricles may beat at a rate of 30 to 40 per min. while auricles are beating the normal 70 beats per min.

h. block, congenital. H. b. present at birth due to improper development of the impulse-conducting system.

h. block, incomplete. H. b. in which conduction time of impulses is prolonged; usually recognized only by electrocardiograph; partial h.b.

h. block, interventricular. Bundle-branch block, q.v.

h. block, partial. One of 2 or 3 impulses passes to ventricle; pulse is thus 40-50.

h. block, sinoatrial. H. b. in which there is interference in the passage of impulses from the S-A node. May be partial or complete.

h., boatshaped. H. in which l. ventricle is dilated and hypertrophied as a result of aortic regurgitation.

h., dilatation of. Enlargement of heart due to stretching of its walls. VARIETIES: 1. Dilatation with thickening of walls. 2. Dilatation with thinning of walls. SYM: So long as the associated hypertrophy keeps pace with the dilatation no symptoms result, but otherwise dyspnea, cough, dyspepsia, scanty urine, dropsy, feeble pulse. TREATMENT: Rest, light, nutritious diet—improve general condition.

h. disease. Any pathological disorder of the heart.

Intravenous injections of epsom salt are being tried to detect the early stages.

h. failure. 1. Cessation of the beat of the heart. 2. A syndrome or clinical condition resulting from failure of the heart to maintain adequate circulation of blood. May result from failure of the right or left ventricle or both.

ETIOL: Hypertension, infections, valvular insufficiency, coronary disease, congenital malformations, arteriosclerosis, atherosclerosis.

SYM: Dyspnea, cardiac asthma, stasis in systemic or portal circulation, edema, cyanosis, hypertrophy of heart. Symptoms vary depending on which side of the heart is affected.

h. f., backward. H. f. in which venous return to the heart is reduced with resulting venous stasis and congestion. Due principally to failure of the right ventricle.

h. f., congestive. Condition characterized by weakness, breathlessness, abdominal discomfort, edema in lower portions of body resulting from venous stasis and reduced outflow of blood. Also called *myocardial insufficiency*, *cardiac decompensation*.

h. f., forward. H. f. in which forward flow of blood to the tissues is inadequate due to failure of the left ventricle.

h., fatty degeneration of. Cardiac muscle has been metamorphosed into fat. SYM: All signs of heart failure, *viz.*: dyspnea; asthma; cough; weak, irregular pulse; poor digestion; attacks of syncope. PROG: Unfavorable. Death may occur on slight exertion. TREATMENT: Rest of body and mind—light, nutritious diet—medication called for by individual condition.

h., fatty infiltration of. Abnormal amount of fat deposited in and upon heart. SYM: Shortness of breath, increased by exertion. Weak but regular pulse, precordial distress, tendency to pulmonary congestion, with resulting bronchitis and sluggish digestion. PROG: Favorable. TREATMENT: Regulated diet: fats, sugars and starches restricted; exercise; Turkish baths.

h., fibroid. SYM: Same as fatty degeneration, condition dependent upon atheroma or sclerosis of coronary arteries. TREATMENT: Same as in fatty heart.

h., hairy. H. in which pericardium possesses a hairy appearance resulting from deposit of an exudate or shreds of fibrin. Occurs in pericarditis. Also called *cor villosum, shaggy heart.*

h., hypertrophy of. Enlargement due to overgrowth of its muscle. VARIETIES: 1. *Simple h.* Thickened muscle and cavities normal size. 2. *Excentric h.* Thickened muscle and cavities dilated. 3. *Concentric h.* Thickened muscle and cavities diminished in size. Always congenital. SYM: Unless advanced, no symptoms. Extreme hypertrophy, has precordial distress, palpitation. Strong pulse. Sometimes flushed face, ringing in ears, flashes of light, headache, and disturbed sleep. TREATMENT: Graduated exercise, light diet, sedatives.

h., irritable. Neurocirculatory asthenia, or effort syndrome. Syndrome characterized by breathlessness, palpitation, weakness and exhaustion. Also called *soldiers heart.*

h., palpation of. Not only determines position, force, extent, and rhythm of apex beat, but also detects existence of any fremitus or thrill. A thrill is a vibratory sensation likened to that received when the hand is placed on the back of a purring cat. Thrills at base of heart may result from valvular lesions, atheroma of aorta, aneurysm, and from roughened pericardial surfaces, as in pericarditis. A presystolic thrill at apex is almost pathognomonic of mitral stenosis.

h., palpitation of. May result from dyspepsia; excitement, mental or physical; organic heart disease; exophthalmic goiter; overwork, as the "irritable heart" of untrained recruits; anemia; hysteria; or an independent neurosis. Also: *endocarditis, myocarditis, pericarditis* due to infection, to trauma, circulatory disturbances, disorders of metabolism, nutrition, and growth.

h., percussion of. Determines shape and extent of cardiac dullness. The normal area of superficial or absolute percussion—dullness (part uncovered by lung) is detected by light percussion and extends from the 4th left costo-sternal junction to the apex beat; from the apex beat to the juncture of the xiphoid cartilage, with the sternum, and thence up left border of the sternum. The normal area of deep percussion dullness (the heart projected on the chest wall) is detected by firm percussion and extends from 3rd left costosternal articulation to the apex beat; from apex beat to junction of the xiphoid cartilage with the sternum; and hence up right border of sternum to the 3rd rib. The lower level of the cardiac dullness fuses with the liver dullness and can rarely be determined. The area of cardiac dullness is increased in: (1) Hypertrophy and dilation of the heart; (2) pericardial effusion. It is apparently increased in shrinking of the lungs, as in phthisis. The area of cardiac dullness is diminished in: (1) Emphysema; (2) pneumothorax; (3) pneumocardium (rare); (4) gaseous distention of stomach.

h. reflex. A cardiac reflex; any reflex in which the stimulation of a sensory nerve brings about an increase or decrease in heart rate. Ex.: Bainbridge's reflex in which stimulation of sensory receptors in rt. atrium by increased venous return results in increase of heart rate.

h. sounds. SEE: *h., auscultation of.*

h. test. Master has determined the efficiency of the heart by the number of steps a normal individual can ascend in a given time without increasing the heart rate more than 10 beats per minute and without increasing the blood pressure. The following rates were established:

	Age	Weight	Ascent or Steps
Man	20-24	130-139 lbs.	25
"	45-	150-159	21
"	45-	190-	19
Woman	40-	130-	20
"	53-	156	17

heart'burn. Acid liquid raised from the stomach, causing sensation of burning in the esophagus. SYN: *pyrosis.* SEE: *ardor ventriculi.*

heat [G. *heito*, fever]. 1. Condition of being hot; warmth. 2. High temperature. 3. A form of energy manifested to the senses, as in the effects of fire, sun's rays, etc. 4. Sexual excitement in lower mammals; period of such excitement. SYN: *estrus.* 5. To make hot. 6. To become warm.

Heat is constantly being produced within the body as a result of exothermic chemical processes occurring in metabolic activities. Ultimately all heat produced in the body results from oxidative processes. Body temperature (normally 98.6° F. or 37° C.) is the result of a balance between heat produced (*thermogenesis*) and heat loss (*thermolysis*).

The temperature of the body is not uniform. Oral temperatures range from 96.6° F. to 100° F. (ave. 98.6° F.). Axillary temperature averages 0.5° F. lower; rectal temperature averages 0.6° higher.

Reducing the temperature of the skin reflexly brings about a constriction of the blood vessels, thus reducing heat loss and conserving heat within the body. The application of heat reflexly induces the dilation of blood vessels thus increasing blood flow to the skin with consequent increase in heat loss.

The application of heat to the skin reflexly produces effects in the deeper portions of the body. In general, internal organs are reflexly related to the region of the skin lying directly over them, and the effects are the same as those produced in the cutaneous area stimulated. Heat application induces muscle relaxation, increased blood sup-

The mode of elimination of body heat and the per cent of heat lost through each of the following is:

Radiation	55%	
Convection and Conduction	15%	94%
Evaporation through skin and lungs	24%	
Warming inspired air	2%	
Elimination of CO_2 from lungs	3%	6%
Warming ingested food and water and loss through feces and urine	1%	

Figures are approximate and vary with physiological activity of the body.

---

ply and stimulates metabolic activity. Physiological effects resulting are hyperemia, sedation of sensory or motor activity, and attenuation of bacteria. Application of cold tends to produce the opposite effects. Heat, by stimulating circulation and dilating blood vessels, has a tendency to spread infection, and for this reason is no longer used in suspected appendicitis.

Relaxation of muscular tissue results in relief of pain, which may be due to rigidity and tension in tissues. Local hot applications may have some reflex effect on deep organs, as in cases of lobar pneumonia, when the lung is known to be in a state of congestion; local heat is applied in order to relieve, probably, the congestion of the lung by inducing a superficial hyperemia.

H., APPLICATION OF, GENERAL. May be dry, as in the form of electric and radiant heat and hot air baths, or moist, when water or water vapor is used. The *effect* is first to produce a slight contraction of vessels in skin, thus increasing blood pressure and driving blood into the internal organs; this makes patient feel that his head is full and bursting. This effect is, however, only of very short duration, and discomfort can be avoided by application of cold compress or ice bag to head.

The true effect follows immediately, when blood vessels in skin are dilated, due to relaxation of involuntary muscle contained in their walls; the skin is reddened, increased blood supply to the sweat glands causes them to act freely, and waste products are better eliminated and heat is lost to the body. For this reason applications of heat are most often used to increase sweating and so relieve work of kidneys in cases of renal disease.

During a general application of heat it is necessary to watch the patient carefully, noting any apparent discomfort caused, also state of pulse and respiration and color.

H., APPLICATION OF LOCAL. May be dry or moist. Dry applications include hot absorbent wool, rubber hot-water bottles, bags of hot salt or bran previously heated in an oven, radiant heat, electric pads, and diathermy.

H., APPLICATION OF, MOIST. Considered more penetrating than dry heat, thus more readily relaxing muscular spasm and relieving pain due to this. Hot compresses of hypertonic saline will relieve edema and tension in tissues which may be causing great pain.

Ex: Fomentations or stupes, either simple or medicated; poultices such as bread, linseed, linseed and mustard, linseed and charcoal, and antiphlogistine. A starch poultice may also be applied hot.

h., atomic. That amount which will raise an atom from 0° to 1° C.

h., body, loss of. The skin is supposed to lose 87.5 cal., the lungs 10.7 cal., and through excreta, 1.8 cal. In a healthy adult man weighing 154.28 lb., loss in elimination has been estimated in the table above.

h., conductive. A term applied to heat transferred by conduction from poultices, bags, etc.

h., convective. That supplied from heated particles of gases or liquids, such as superheated air, melted paraffin, incandescent light apparatus, or the whirlpool bath.

h., conversive. A term used to designate heat generated in the tissues by a current of electricity or by some form of radiant energy.

h. cramps. Severe, intermittent, spasmodic cramping of muscles in abdomen and extremities.

ETIOL: Profuse sweating due to deficiency of salt in the tissues. Often found in individuals who have been drinking large volumes of water and perspire profusely for long period of time; not fatal.

SYM: Hypochloremia. In addition to free sweating, cramps are felt in the legs and in other regions accompanied by fever, rapid pulse, pains, increased blood pressure, and loss of weight.

F. A. TREATMENT: Adm. ¼ teaspoonful of ordinary table salt (sodium chloride) in glass of water. Repeat at 5- to 30-minute intervals until cramping ceases. May be prevented by adding salt to drinking water on hot days, particularly to hard working individuals.

As a *preventive*, 100–300 gr. of salt per day is necessary to compensate for each 2 quarts of sweat excreted. The salt aids in holding the water in the tissues. If the supply of salt is lowered, thirst calls for more water, but the intake of water is dependent upon the increase of the salt. Local applications of heat to reduce pain and salt solution by mouth or injection. SEE: *cramps, salt.*

h., diathermy. Electrical energy is converted into heat by the use of diathermy and short wave.

h., dry. May be adm. in form of hot, dry pack; hot water bottle; electric light bath; heliotherapy; hot bricks; resistance coil; electric pad or blanket; hot air bath, or therapeutic lamp.

h. exhaustion. Must not be mistaken for heatstroke, *q.v.* Usually affects adults, esp. the debilitated and fatigued.

SYM: Dizziness, nausea, faintness, weakness. Unconsciousness often follows. Skin pale, cool, moist; pulse rapid; respiration shallow and hurried.

heat, initial   H-13   **hebephrenia**

Prog: Favorable under proper treatment.
F. A. Treatment: Lower head and shoulders; elevate lower extremities. Stimulate with aromatic spirits of ammonia to nostrils. Hot, black coffee or tea. External heat and massage. No cold drinks.

h., initial. Muscular heat produced (a) during contraction when tension is increasing, (b) during maintenance of tension, and (c) during relaxation when tension is diminishing.

h., latent. The heat which is required to convert a solid into a liquid or a liquid into a gas at the same temperature.

h., latent, of fusion. That which is required to convert 1 Gm. of a solid into liquid at the same temperature, e. g., when 1 Gm. of ice at 0° C. is converted into water at 0° C.; this process requires 80 calories, and until it is completed there will be no rise of temperature.

h., latent, of vaporization. That required to change 1 Gm. of a liquid at its boiling point to vapor at the same temperature. The latent heat of steam is 540 calories; therefore, when steam cools to liquid, each Gm. gives out 540 calories. This explains why it is that a scald from steam is much more severe than one caused by boiling water.

h., luminous. That derived from light. This may be borne better than other forms of radiation. Light may be converted into heat. Short infrared rays penetrate subcutaneous tissues to a greater extent than long, invisible rays.

h., mechanical equivalent of. The value of heat units in terms of work units. One calorie equals 426.5 grammeters or 3.085 foot-pounds.

h., moist. May be applied as hot bath pack, hot wet pack, hot foot bath, fomentations, poultices or vapor bath. Warnings: Watch for chill, fainting, dizziness, headache, collapse, faintness, increased pulse, weakness. Cold applications to head should be used during and after treatment. Opinion regarding therapeutic use of heat or cold differs.

h., molecular. Result of multiplying a substance's molecular weight by its specific heat.

h., prickly. Vesicles due to obstruction or acute inflammation of sweat glands. Syn: *miliaria*.

h., radiant. Heat given off from a heated body and which passes through the air in form of waves.

h. rays. Visible rays from 4000-7000 A. U. and infrared rays from 6000-14,000 A. U.

h. recovery. Muscular heat produced after relaxation is complete.

h., sensible. Heat producing a temperature rise when absorbed by a body.

h., specific. The heat or number of calories needed to raise the temperature of 1 gram of a substance 1° C.

h. therapy. Use of heat in treatment of the body.

h. therapy, wet. Application of heat by hot water, steam and mud baths, and the hot pack, etc.

h. unit. A calorie, q.v.

heat'stroke. Result of direct exposure to high temperatures or to sun, usually in adults; esp. those who have been taking alcoholic beverages or who are debilitated or fatigued.

Sym: Early symptoms are dizziness, weakness, nausea, spots before the eyes and ringing in the ears. Bright red, dry skin; rapid, strong pulse, later becoming weak. Unconsciousness usually follows. Temperature may reach 108°; occasionally 112°. Latter patients usually do not recover.

F. A. Treatment: Patient should be cooled off in any conceivable manner. Remove clothing. Apply cold cloths, or pour cold water over person. Gently massage to help circulate blood. Cold water irrigations of the bowel are of value. Do not give stimulants of any sort. Heatstroke is a grave emergency, and must be treated promptly.

hebeosteotomy (he″be-os-te-ot′o-mĭ) [G. *ĕbĕ*, pubes, + *osteon*, bone, + *tomē*, incision]. Section of the pubic bone in order to enlarge the pelvic opening for facilitation of delivery. Syn: *pubiotomy*.

hebephrenia (hē-bĕ-frē′nĭ-ă) [G. *ĕbĕ*, puberty, + *phrēn*, mind]. A type of schizophrenic reaction characterized by infantile behavior, regression and deterioration, shallow emotional responses, illogical and senseless thought processes and actions, delusions and hallucinations. Patient may laugh often without cause, talk incoherently and excessively, undergo rapid mood change. Occurs often at age of or following puberty.

Heatstroke versus Heat Exhaustion

Heat or Sunstroke. *Definition:* A condition or derangement of the heat-control centers due to exposure to the rays of the sun or very high temperatures	**Heat Exhaustion.** *Definition:* A state of very definite weakness produced by the loss of the normal fluids and sodium chloride of the body
History: Exposure to sun's rays	*History:* Exposure to heat, usually indoors
Differential Symptoms:	**Differential Symptoms:**
Face: Red, dry, and hot	*Face:* Pale, cool, and moist
Skin: Hot, dry, and no diaphoresis	*Skin:* Cool, clammy, with profuse diaphoresis
Temperature: High, 108° to 110° F.	*Temperature:* Slight elevation to subnormal
Pulse: Full, strong, bounding	*Pulse:* Weak, thready, and rapid
Respirations: Dyspneic and sonorous	*Respirations:* Shallow and quiet
Muscles: Tense and possible convulsions	*Muscles:* Tense and contracted
Eyes: Pupils are dilated but equal	*Eyes:* Pupils are normal
Treatment: Absolute rest with head elevated. Cold packs to prolong radiation of body heat	**Treatment:** Keep patient quiet; head should be lowered. Keep body warm to prevent shock symptoms
Drugs: Allow no stimulants; give infusions of normal saline (to force fluids)	*Drugs:* Aromatic spirits of ammonia. Salt tablets and fruit juices in abundant amounts

hebephrenic (he-be-fren'ĭk) [" + *phrēn*, mind]. Pert. to hebephrenia.

Heb'erden's asthma. Paroxysms of severe pain about heart and down left arm, with sense of oppression. SYN: *angina pectoris, q.v.*

   H.'s disease. Arthritis deformans.

   H.'s nodes. Hard nodules or enlargements of tubercles at the distal phalanges of fingers; seen in osteoarthritis.

hebetic (he-bet'ĭk) [G. *ēbē*, puberty]. Pert. to or occurring at the time of puberty.

hebet'omy [G. *ēbē*, pubes, + *tomē*, incision]. Section through pelvis to aid obstructed delivery. SYN: *pubiotomy*.

hebetude (heb'e-tūd) [L. *hebetūdō; hebere*, to be dull]. Mental dullness, as seen in exhaustive conditions.

   There may be latent conditions suddenly manifesting themselves during the course of a disease not concerned with such a condition but aggravated by the sickness, such as a sudden appearance of hysteria, or the development of a phobia, hallucinations, or delusions.

hebosteotomy (he-bos-te-ot'o-mĭ) [G. *ēbē*, pubes, + *osteon*, bone, + *tomē*, incision]. Enlargement of pelvic diameter by section of the pelvis to aid delivery. SYN: *hebotomy, pubiotomy*.

hebot'omy [" + *tomē*, incision]. Section through the pubis to facilitate labor. SYN: *hebeosteotomy, pubiotomy*.

hecateromeric (hek-a″ter-om-er'ĭk) [G. *ekateros*, each of two, + *meros*, part]. Having processes on a spinal neuron, one supplying each side of the spinal cord.

hecatomeric (hek-at-o-mer'ĭk) [G. *ekateros*, each of two, + *meros*, part]. Having a process which divides into two parts, as that of a spinal sensory neuron, one passing to each side of the spinal cord.

hectic (hek'tĭk) [G. *ektikos*, habitual]. Habitual or constitutional.

   h. fever. A form of fever that occurs in connection with some organic disease, that is attended by some continuous and exhausting drain upon the system, as in pulmonary consumption or abscess of liver or kidney.

   h. flush. The bright pink-red spot that appears on the cheek during a paroxysm of hectic fever.

hec'togram [G. *ekaton*, hundred, + *gramma*, weight]. One hundred grams, or 1543.7 grains.

hec'toliter [" + *litra*, a pound]. One hundred liters.

hec'tometer [" + *metron*, measure]. One hundred meters.

hedge'hog crys'tals. Globular crystals of ammonium urate with spines found in urine.

hedonia. Excessive cheerfulness; amenomania.

hedonism (he'don-izm) [G. *ēdonē*, pleasure, + *ismos*, state]. A theory or standard of conduct in which the principal object of life is pleasure.

hedrocele (hed'ro-sēl) [G. *edra*, anus, + *kēlē*, hernia]. Hernia; prolapse through the anus. SYN: *proctocele*.

heel [A.S. *huela*, heel]. Post. extremity of foot. SYN: *calx*.

   h. bone. Bone at back of tarsus. SYN: *os calcis; calcaneum, calcaneus*.

   RS: *calcaneum, calcaneodynia, calcigrade, calx; os calcis*.

Hegar's sign (hay'garz). Sign present during 2nd and 3rd month of pregnancy, due to: (1) Softening of lower segments of uterus; (2) at this stage, the ovum does not fill the uterine cavity, so there is an empty space in its lower part. On bimanual examination the lower part of uterus is easily compressed bet. fingers in the vagina and those of the other hand.

Heidenhain's demilunes (hi'den-hinz). Crescent-shaped groups of serous cells at the base of or along the sides of the mucous alveoli of the salivary glands, esp., sublingual and submaxillary; also called *crescents of Gianuzzi*.

height (hīt) [A.S. *hiehthu*]. Distance to which anything rises above that surface on which it rests.

Heine-Medin disease (hi'ne-ma'dĭn). Acute infectious disease accompanied by motor paralysis and muscular atrophy, frequently with permanent deformity. SYN: *acute anterior poliomyelitis.**

Heister, spiral valve of. A spiral fold of the mucous membrane lining the cystic duct. It serves to keep the lumen open.

helcoid (hel'koid) [G. *elkos*, ulcer, + *eidos*, form]. Resembling an ulcer.

helcology (hel-kol'o-jĭ) [" + *logos*, study]. The study of ulcers.

helcoplasty (hel-ko-plas-tĭ) [" + *plassein*, to form]. Grafting healthy skin on ulcers. SEE: *dermatoplasty*.

helco'sis [" + *ōsis*]. The development of an ulcer. SYN: *ulceration*.

helicine (hel'is-in) [G. *elix*, coil]. Pert. to a helix or coil; spiral.

   h. arteries. Term applied to tortuous arteries in cavernous tissue of the penis and clitoris, and in the uterus.

helicoid (hel'ĭ-koyd) [" + *eidos*, resemblance]. Resembling a helix or spiral.

helicopodia (hel'ĭ-ko-po'dĭ-ă) [G. *elix*, coil, + *pous, pod-*, foot]. A peculiar movement in which the foot, when brought forward, drags and describes a partial arc. Results in a gait such as seen in spastic hemiplegia.

helicotrema (hĕl-ĭ-kō-tre'mă [G. *elix*, coil, + *trema*, a hole]. The opening at the tip of the cochlear canal where the scala tympani and scala vestibuli unite.

heliencephalitis (he″lĭ-en-sef-al-i'tis) [G. *elios*, sun, + *egkephalos*, brain, + *-itis*, inflammation]. Inflammation of the brain as the result of sunstroke.

heliopho'bia [" + *phobos*, fear]. Abnormal fear of the sun's rays esp. by one who has suffered a sunstroke.

helio'sis [" + *-ōsis*]. Sunstroke.

heliotherapy (he-lĭ-o-ther'ă-pĭ) [" + *therapeia*, treatment]. The therapeutic application of radiation from the sun which includes infrared, ultraviolet and visible radiation. SEE: *solarium*.

heliotropism (he-lĭ-ot'rō-pĭzm) [" + *trepein*, to turn, + *ismos*, state of]. Chemotropism induced by the action of sunlight; the tendency of an organism to turn toward or grow toward sunlight.

he'lium [G. *elios*, sun]. A gaseous element (He). It is given off by radium and other radioactive elements as charged helium ions known as alpha rays.

   Because of its low density, it being next to the lightest element known, it is mixed with air or oxygen and used in the treatment of various respiratory disorders. Because of its low solubility, it is mixed with air supplied to workers laboring under high atmospheric pressure, as in caissons. It reduces time required in adjustment to increasing or decreasing air pressure and reduces the danger of "bends".

he'lix [G. *elix*, coil]. Margin of the external ear.

Hel'ler's test. A test for the presence of albumin in urine.

   Pour ½ in. of pure nitric acid into a clean test tube, and carefully overlay it with an equal quantity of urine. The

Height and Weight Table
(Five pounds either way is not considered abnormal)

Men

Ages	21-24	25-29	30-34	35-39	40-44	45-49	50-54	55-60
5' 2"	124	128	131	133	136	138	138	138
5' 3"	127	131	134	136	139	141	141	141
5' 4"	131	135	138	140	143	144	145	145
5' 5"	134	138	141	143	146	147	149	149
5' 6"	138	142	145	147	150	151	153	153
5' 7"	142	147	150	152	155	156	158	158
5' 8"	146	151	154	157	160	161	163	163
5' 9"	150	155	159	162	165	166	167	168
5'10"	154	159	164	167	170	171	172	173
5'11"	159	164	169	173	175	177	177	178
6' 0"	165	170	175	179	180	183	182	183
6' 1"	170	177	181	185	186	189	188	189

Women

Ages	17-19	20-24	25-29	30-34	35-39	40-44	45-49	50-54	55-60
5' 0"	113	114	117	119	122	125	128	130	131
5' 1"	115	116	118	121	124	128	131	133	134
5' 2"	117	118	120	123	127	132	134	137	137
5' 3"	120	122	124	127	131	135	138	141	141
5' 4"	123	125	127	130	134	138	142	145	145
5' 5"	125	128	131	135	139	143	147	149	149
5' 6"	128	132	135	137	143	146	151	153	153
5' 7"	132	135	139	143	147	150	154	157	156
5' 8"	136	140	143	147	151	155	158	161	161
5' 9"	140	144	147	151	155	159	163	166	166
5'10"	144	147	151	155	159	163	167	170	170

Infants

	Height in.	Weight lb.		Height in.	Weight lb.
At birth	19½	7½	7 months	24½	17
1 month	20½	8½	8 "	25	18½
2 months	21	10½	9 "	25½	20
3 "	22	12	10 "	26	20½
4 "	23	13¾	11 "	26½	21
5 "	23½	15	12 "	27	22½
6 "	24	16			

presence of albumin is indicated by the appearance of an opaque ring at the junction of the fluids; also known as the "cold" test. RS: *albumin, urine.*

Hel'lin's law. Occurrence of twins once in 80 pregnancies, triplets once in 6400 pregnancies, quadruplets once in 512,000 pregnancies.

hel'minth [G. *elmins, elminth-,* worm]. 1. A worm-like animal. 2. More specifically any parasitic, either free-living or parasitic, belonging to the phyla Platyhelminthes (flat-worms), Acanthocephala (spiney-headed worms), nenathelminthes (thread or round worms) or Annelida (segmented worms).

helminthagogue (hel-minth'ag-og) [" + *agōgos,* leading]. A remedy that expels worms. SYN: *vermifuge.*

helminthemesis (hel-min-them e-sis) [" + *emesis* vomiting]. The vomiting of intestinal worms.

helminthiasis (hel-min-thi'a-sis) [G. *elmins, elminth-,* worm]. Having intestinal parasites or worms.

helmin'thic [G. *elmins, elminth-,* worm]. 1. Pertaining to worms. 2. Pert. to that which expels worms. SYN: *anthelmintic; vermifugal.*

helminthicide (hĕl-mĭn'thĭ-sīd) [" + L. *caedere,* to kill]. A worm-expelling drug. SYN: *vermicide.*

helminthoid. Wormlike or resembling a worm.

helminthol'ogy [" + *logos,* study]. The study of intestinal vermiform parasites.

helmintho'ma [" + *ōma,* tumor]. A parasitic worm tumor.

helminthophobia (hel-min-tho-fo'bĭ-ă) [" + *phobos,* fear]. Morbid dread of worms or delusion of being infested by them.

helmitol (hel'mi-tol). A methenamine compound, claimed to be well tolerated, and suitable for prolonged use.
USES: In cystitis, and other conditions where methenamine is indicated.
DOSAGE: From 10-15 gr. (0.6-10 Gm.) dissolved in water.

heloma (he-lo'mă) [G. *ēlos,* nail, + *ōma,* tumor]. A callosity or corn. SYN: *clavus.*

helosis (he-lo'sis) [" + *-ōsis*]. The state of having corns.

helotomeia (he-lo-to-mi'ă) [" + *tomē,* incision]. Corn surgery.

helot'omon [" + *tomē,* incision]. Surgical knife for cutting corns.

helotomy (he-lot'o-mĭ) [" + *tomē,* incision]. Surgical treatment of corns.

Helweg's bundle. SYN: *Helweg's tract, Bechterew's bundle.* A tract in cervical region of spinal cord. Fibers arise from cell bodies in olive of the medulla and upper region of cord.

hemabarometer (hem"ab-ar-om'et-er) [G. *aima,* blood, + *baros,* weight, + *metron,* measure]. Device for determining sp. gr. of blood.

hemachrome (hem'a-krōm) [" + *chrōma,* color]. The red coloring substance of blood. SEE: *hemoglobin.*

hemachro'sis [" + *chrōsis,* coloring]. Abnormal redness of blood.

hemacytom'eter [" + *kytos,* cell, + *metron,* measure]. Apparatus for counting blood corpuscles.

hemacytozoon (hem-a-sī-to-zo'on) [" + *zōon,* animal]. A protozoan parasite infesting red blood corpuscles.

hemad (he'mad) [A.S. *hem,* border, + L. *ad,* toward]. Toward the ventral or hemal aspect of the body. Opp. to neural or dorsal.

hemadostenosis (hem″a-do-sten-o′sis) [G. *aimas, aimad-*, blood stream, + *stenōsis*, narrowing]. Contraction of blood vessels.

hemadromom′eter [G. *aima*, blood, + *dromos*, course, + *metron*, measure]. Device for recording rapidity of flow of blood. SYN: *hemodromometer*.

hemadynamometer (hem″a-dī′na-mom′e-ter) [" + *dynamis*, power, + *metron*, measure]. Device for determining blood pressure.

hemadynamometry (hem″a-di-nă-mom′e-trī) [" + " + *metron*, measure]. Measurement of blood pressure.

hemafa′cient [" + L. *facere*, to make]. A blood producing agent. SYN: *hematopoietic, sanguifacient*.

hemafecia (hem-ă-fe′sĭ-ă) [" + L. *faex, faec-*, dregs]. Feces containing blood.

hemagglutination (hem″ag-glu-tin-a′shun) [" + L. *agglutināre*, to paste to]. The clumping of red blood corpuscles.

hem′agglu′tinin [" + L. *agglutināre*, to paste to]. An antibody that induces clumping of red blood corpuscles.

hemagogue (hem′ag-og) [" + *agōgos*, leading]. An agent that favors the flow of blood or of the menses. SYN: *emmenagogue*.

he′mal [G. *aima*, blood]. 1. Pert. to the blood or blood vessels. 2. Pert. to side of the body in which the heart is located.
  h. arch. The ribs, breastbone, and that part of the vertebrae, which together enclose the heart and viscera.
  h. gland. A hemal or hemolymph node.
  h. node. SYN: *hemal gland, hemolymph gland or node*. A body resembling a lymph node in structure but associated with blood vessels instead of lymph vessels. Present in certain ungulates.

hemanal′ysis [" + *analysis*, a dissolving]. A blood analysis. SEE: *blood*.

hemangiectasis (hem″an-jĭ-ek′ta-sis) [" + *aggeion*, vessel, + *ektasis*, dilatation]. Dilatation of blood vessels.

hemangioblastoma (hem-an″jĭ-o-blas-to′-mă) [" + " + *blastos*, germ, + *ōma*, tumor]. Hemangioma of the brain of a capillary nature.

hemangioendothelioma (hem″an-jĭ-o-en″-do-the-lĭ-o′ma) [" + " + *endon*, within, + *thēlē*, nipple, + *ōma*, tumor]. An overgrowth of the endothelium of the minute capillary vessels frequently on the cerebral meninges.

hemangioma (hem-an-jĭ-o′ma) (pl. *hemangiomata*) [" + " + *ōma*, tumor]. An angioma consisting of blood vessels.

hemangiomatosis (hem″an-jĭ-o-ma-to′sis) [" + " + " + *-ōsis*]. Multiple angiomata of blood vessels.

hemangiosarcoma (hem″an-jĭ-o-sar-ko′mă) [" + " + *sarx*, flesh, + *ōma*, tumor]. A mixed sarcoma and hemangioma. SYN: *angiosarcoma*.

hemaphein (hem-af-e′in) [G. *aima*, blood, + *phaios*, tawny]. Brown coloring matter in the blood; a decomposition product of hematin.

hemapoiesis (hem-ap-oi-e′sis) [" + *poiein*, to form]. Blood formation. SYN: *hematopoiesis*.

hemapoietic (hem-ap-oi-et′ĭk) [" + *poiein*, to form]. Pert. to hemapoiesis. SYN: *hematogenic, hematoplastic*.

hemapophysis (hĕm-ă-pof′is-is) [G. *aima*, blood, + *apo*, from, —*physis*, growth]. Portion of a developing vertebra which forms a rib and costal cartilage.

hemarthros (hem-ar′thros) [" + *arthron*, joint]. Bloody effusion into cavity of a joint. SYN: *hemarthrosis*.

hemarthrosis (hem-ar-thro′sis) [" + " + *-ōsis*]. Effusion of blood in a joint cavity.

hematachometer (hem-at-ak-om′et-er) [" + *tachus*, swift, + *metron*, measure]. Device for determining rapidity of the circulation.

hemataerom′eter [" + *aēr*, air, + *metron*, measure]. Device for measuring gases in the blood.

hematalloscopy (hem-at-al-os′ko-pī) [" + *allos*, other, + *skopein*, to examine]. Examination to distinguish one kind of blood from another.

hematapostema (hem″at-ap-os-te′mă) (pl. *hematapostemata*) [" + *apostēma*, abscess]. Abscess containing extravasated blood.

hemateikon (hem-ăt-ī′kon) [G. *aima*, blood, + *eikon*, image]. A microscopic picture of the blood.

hematemesis (hem-at-em′e-sis) [" + *emesis*, vomiting]. Vomiting of blood.
  SYM: Blood often clotted and mixed with food, acid in reaction. Subsequent stools may be tarry; associated symptoms point to stomach. If of gastric origin, the blood is generally dark and acid. If of pharyngeal origin, it is bright red and alkaline in reaction. In pulmonary tuberculosis, loss of blood may be from a teaspoonful to 2 quarts. It occurs in 60% of patients. Coldness, or followed by a rise in temperature, shock, collapse.
  TREATMENT: Absolute rest, nothing by mouth, nourishment through rectal enemas. No stimulants. May take broth. Have patient lie down; cold applications—ice bag to abdominal region. Keep quiet. Surgery may be necessary. SEE: *hemoptysis, hemorrhage*.

hematencephalon (hem-at-en-sef′a-lŏn) [" + *egkephalos*, brain]. Cerebral hemorrhage.

hematherapy (hem-a-ther′ă-pī) [" + *therapeia*, treatment]. Adm. of fresh blood in treatment of disease.

hemathermal [G. *aima*, blood, + *thermē*, heat]. SYN: *homothermal*. Warm blooded, applied to animals whose blood remains at a fairly constant temperature.

hemather′mous [" + *thermē*, heat]. Warm blooded. SYN: *hemathermal, hematothermal*.

hemathidrosis, hematidrosis (he-mat-hĭ-dro′sis) [" + *idrōs*, sweat, + *-ōsis*]. Condition of sweating blood.

hematic (he-mat′ĭk) [G. *aima*, blood]. 1. Rel. to the blood. 2. A remedy for anemia.

hematim′eter [" + *metron*, measure]. Apparatus for counting blood corpuscles in a cu.mm. of blood. SYN: *hematometer, hemocytometer*.

hem′atin [G. *aima*, blood]. An acid radicle or brown amorphous substance that unites with globin in the formation of hemoglobin.
  It can be prepared from hemoglobin by the action of acids, alkalies, or enzymes. It is the iron-containing pigment of hemoglobin.
  h. hydrochloride. The hydrochloric acid ester of hematin, crystalline in form.
  Crystals dark brown and often seen in groups. SYN: *Teichmann's crystals*.

hematinemia (hem-ă-tin-e′mĭ-ă) [hematin + G. *aima*, blood]. Hematin in the circulating blood.

hematinic (hem-a-tin'ik) [G. *aima*, blood].
SYN: *hematic*. 1. Pert. to blood. 2. An agent which increases the amount of hemoglobin in the blood.

hematinometer (hem-at-in-om'et-er) [" + *metron*, measure]. Device for determining quantity of hemoglobin in blood.

hematinu'ria [" + *ouron*, urine]. Hematin in the urine. SYN: *hemoglobinuria*.

hematischesis (hem-ă-tis'ke-sis) [" + *schesis*, checking]. Arrest of bleeding or hemorrhage.

hemato'bium [" + *bios*, life]. A parasite that lives in the blood. SYN: *hematozoon*.

hematoblast [G. *aima*, blood + *blastos*, germ]. 1. A hemocytoblast, *q.v.* 2. Old term for blood platelet.

hematocele (hem'at-o-sēl) [" + *kēlē*, hernia]. 1. A blood cyst. 2. Effusion of blood into a cavity. 3. Swelling due to effusion of blood into the *tunica vaginalis testis*.

    h., parametric, pelvic, retrouterine. Tumor formed by blood effusion in the *cul-de-sac* of Douglas walled off by adhesions.

    ETIOL: Usually leakage from a fallopian tube, the seat of ectopic gestation.

    TREATMENT: Rest, applications of cold and pressure to limit increase of size. Aspiration may be needed or incision if there are clots.

    h., pudendal. A bloody tumor of the labium.

hematocelia (hem″ă-to-se'lǐ-ă) [" + *koilia*, cavity]. Hemorrhage into the peritoneal cavity.

hematoceph'alus [G. *aima*, blood, + *kephalē*, head]. Fetus born with infusion of blood in the head.

hematochezia (hem″ă-to-ke'zǐ-ă) [" + *chezein*, to go to stool]. Passage of stools containing blood.

hematochromato'sis [" + *chrōma*, color, + *-ōsis*]. A condition showing staining of tissues with blood pigment. SYN: *hemochromatosis*.

hematochyluria (hem″ă-to-ki-lū'rĭ-ă) [" + *chylos*, juice, + *ouron*, urine]. Blood and chyle in the urine in *Filaria* infections.

hematocolpometra (hem″at-o-kol″po-me'-tra) [" + *kolpos*, vagina, + *mētra*, uterus]. Retention of menstrual blood in the vagina and uterus.

hematocolpos (hem-at-o-kol'pos) [" + *kolpos*, vagina]. Retained menstrual blood in the vagina from an imperforate hymen.

hematocrit(e (hem'ă-to-krīt) [" + *krinein*, to separate]. 1. Centrifuge for separating solids from plasma in the blood. 2. The volume of erythrocytes packed by centrifugation in a given volume of blood. The hemocrit is expressed as the percentage of total blood volume which consists of erythrocytes or as the volume in cubic centimeters of erythrocytes packed by centrifugation in 100 cc. of blood. Normal values—45 for males, 41 for females.

hematocryal (hem-at-o-kri'al) [" + *kryos*, cold]. Possessing cold blood.

hematocrystallin (hem-at-o-kris'tal-in) [" + *krystallos*, crystal]. The coloring matter of the blood. SYN: *hemoglobin*.

hematocyst (hem'at-o-sist) [" + *kystis*, a bladder]. A blood cyst.

hematocyte (hem'at-o-sīt) [" G. *aima*, blood, + *kytos*, cell]. A blood corpuscle.

hematocytoblast (hem″ă-to-si'to-blast) [" + " + *blastos*, germ]. A cell in bone marrow.

    Granular leukocytes of myeloid origin are assumed to be derived from it. SYN: *leukoblast, lymphoidocyte, myeloblast*.

hematocytolysis (hem″ă-to-si-tol'is-is) [" + " + *lysis*, dissolution]. Dissolution of blood corpuscles freeing hemoglobin. SYN: *hemolysis*.

hematocytometer (hem-at-o-si-tom'et-er) [" + " + *metron*, measure]. Device for determining number of corpuscles in given quantity of blood.

hematocytozoon (hem″ă-to-si-to-zo'on) [" + " + *zōon*, animal]. A parasite which lives in red blood corpuscles.

hematocyturia (hem″ă-to-si-tū'rĭ-ă) [" + " + *ouron*, urine]. Red blood corpuscles in urine; hematuria* as differentiated from hemoglobinuria.*

hematodyscrasia. A pathological condition of the blood.

hematodystrophy (hem″ă-to-dis'tro-fī) [" + *dys*, bad, + *trophē*, nutrition]. Any disorder of blood, such as anemia.*

hematogenesis (hem″ă-to-jen'es-is) [" + *genesis*, formation]. The development of blood corpuscles. SYN: *hematopoiesis*.

hematogenic, hematogenous (hem-a-to-jen'ik, -ă-toj'en-us) [" + *gennan*, to produce]. Pert. to formation of blood. SYN: *hematopoietic*.

hematoglob'ulin [" + L. *globus*, globe]. Coloring matter of blood. SYN: *hemoglobin, oxyhemoglobin*.

hematohidrosis (hem″ă-to-hī-dro'sis) [" + *idrōs*, sweat, + *-ōsis*]. Excretion of bloody sweat. SYN: *hemathidrosis*.

hematohistioblast (hem″ă-to-his'tĭ-o-blast) [" + *istos*, tissue, + *blastos*, germ]. A polymorphous white blood cell of large size forming connective tissue.

hematoid (he'mă-toid) [G. *aima*, blood, + *eidos*, resemblance]. Resembling blood.

hematoidin (hem-ă-toy'dĭn) [" + *eidos*, resemblance]. An iron-free principle in remains of old blood clots.

hematokolpos (hem-at-o-kol'pos) [" + *kolpos*, vagina]. Collection of blood in the vagina. SYN: *hematocolpos*.

hematokrit (hem'at-o-krīt) [" + *krinein*, to separate]. Device for determining number of corpuscles in the blood. SYN: *hematocrit*.

hem'atolith [" + *lithos*, stone]. Concretion in a blood vessel wall. SYN: *hemolith*.

hematol'ogist. One who specializes in the study of the blood.

hematology (hem-at-ol'o-gĭ) [" + *logos*, science]. The science of the blood.

hematolymphangioma (hem″ă-to-limf-an″-jĭ-o'mă) [" + L. *lympha*, lymph, + G. *aggeion*, vessel, + *ōma*, tumor]. A tumor consisting of dilated blood vessels and lymphatics.

hematolysis (hem-at-ol'is-is) [" + *lysis*, dissolution]. A term applied to (a) diminished coagulability, or (b) to the destruction or disorganization of the blood and its corpuscles. SEE: *hemolysis*.

hematolytic (hem-at-o-lit'ik) [" + *lysis*, dissolution]. Pert. to hematolysis. SYN: *hemolytic*.

hematoma (hem-ă-to'mă) [G. *aima*; blood, + *ōma*, tumor]. A blood tumor.

    h. auris. One beneath perichondrium of ear cartilage.

    h., pelvic. One affecting cellular tissue of pelvis. TREATMENT: Cold applications, rest, compression, massage.

    h., subdural. H. located beneath the dura, usually the result of head injuries.

    h., vulvar. H. occurring on the vulva. SYM: Distention and purplish swelling.

    TREATMENT: Surgical; light pack which is removed in 24 hours at latest.

hematomediastinum (hem″ă-to-me″dĭ-ăs-ti′num) [" + L. *mediastinus*, in the middle]. Blood effusion into the mediastinum.

hematometer (he-mă-tom′et-er) [" + *metron*, measure]. Device for determining the properties of blood.

hematometra (he″mă-to-me′tră) [" + *mētra*, uterus]. 1. Hemorrhage in the uterus. 2. Accumulation of menstrual blood in the womb. SEE: *hematocolpos, hydrometra, pyometra*.

hematom′etry [" + *metron*, measure]. Determination of varieties and number of blood cells and percentage of hemoglobin in the blood.

hematomphalocele (hem″at-om-fal′o-sēl) [" + *omphalos*, navel, + *kēlē*, hernia]. Effusion of blood into an umbilical hernia.

hematomyelia (he-mă-to-mī-e′lĭ-ă) [" + *myelos*, marrow]. Hemorrhage of blood into the spinal cord.

hematomyelitis (hem″ă-to-mi-el-i′tis) [" + " + *-itis*, inflammation]. Inflammation of spinal cord with bloody effusion.

hematomyelopore (hem-at-o-mī′el-o-pōr) [" + " + *poros*, opening]. Porous condition of the spinal cord resulting from hemorrhages.

hematonephrosis (hem-ă-to-nē-fro′sis) [" + *nephros*, kidney, + *ōsis*]. Blood distending the pelvis of the kidney.

hematon′ic [" + *tonos*, tone]. A blood tonic given to raise the percentage of hemoglobin.

hematopathol′ogy [" + *pathos*, disease, + *logos*, study]. The study of morbid conditions of the blood.

hematopericar′dium [" + *peri*, around, + *kardia*, heart]. Bloody effusion into the pericardial sac.

hematoperitone′um [" + *peritonaion*, peritoneum]. Bloody effusion into the peritoneal cavity. SYN: *hemoperitoneum*.

hematopex′in [" + *pēxis*, fixation]. That which coagulates blood. SYN: *hemopexin*.

hematopex′is [" + *pēxis*, fixation]. Coagulation of the blood. SYN: *hemopexia*.

hem′atophage [" + *phagein*, to eat]. A phagocytic cell which destroys red blood corpuscles.

hematophagia (hem-at-o-fa′jĭ-ă) [" + *phagein*, to eat]. 1. Subsistence on blood. 2. Adm. of blood as a treatment.

hematophagous (hem-ă-tof′ag-us) [" + *phagein*, to eat]. Living on blood.

hematophilia (hem-at-o-fil′ĭ-ă) [G. *aima*, blood, + *philein*, to love]. Congenital condition characterized by defective blood coagulation causing copious hemorrhages. SYN: *hemophilia*.

hematophobia (hem″ăt-ō-fō′bĭ-ă) [G. *aima, aimat-*, blood, + *phobos*, fear]. Abnormal aversion to the sight of blood.

hematophthalmia (he-ma-tof-thal′mĭ-ă) [" + *ophthalmos*, eye]. Blood in the vitreous humor.

hematophyte (hem′ă-to-fīt) [" + *phyton*, plant]. Plant organism or bacteria in the blood.

hematopla′nia [" + *planē*, wandering]. Condition of vicarious menstruation.

hematoplas′tic [" + *plassein*, to form]. Pert. to formation of blood. SYN: *hematopoietic*.

hematopneic (hem-ă-to-pne′ĭk) [" + *pnein*, to breathe]. Rel. to oxygenation of the blood.

hematopoiesis (he″mă-to-poi-e′sis) [" + *poiein*, to form]. The formation of red blood corpuscles.

Tissues which can produce red corpuscles are said to be *hematopoietic*, as, for instance, the red bone marrow.

hematopoietic (hem″ă-to-poy-et′ĭk) [" + *poiein*, to make]. Rel. to blood-making processes. SYN: *hematogenic, hematoplastic*.

hematoporphyrin (hem″at-o-por′fĭr-ĭn) [" + *porphyra*, purple]. Iron-free hematin; a decomposition product of hemoglobin in the urine in certain conditions.

hematoporphyrinuria (hem″ă-to-por″fĭ-rĭn-u′rĭ-ă) [" + " + *ouron*, urine]. Hematoporphyrin in urine.

hematoposia (hem″ă-to-po′sĭ-ă) [" + *posis*, a draught]. Drinking of blood. SEE: *hematophagia*.

hematorrhachis (he-mă-tor′ră-kis) [" + *rachis*, spine]. Hemorrhage into the spinal cord.

hematorrhea (he-mă-tor-re′ă) [" + *roia*, flow]. Profuse hemorrhage.

hematosalpinx (he-mă-to-sal′pinks) [" + *salpigx*, tube]. Retained menstrual fluid in the fallopian tube.

hematoscheocele (hem-ă-tos′ke-o-sēl) [" + *oscheon*, scrotum, + *kēlē*, hernia]. Blood accumulated in the scrotum.

hematoscope (he′mat-o-skōp) [" + *skopein*, to examine]. Device for examining the blood.

hematoscopy (hem-at-os′ko-pĭ) [" + *skopein*, to examine]. Examination of the blood.

hematose (hem′at-ōs) [" + *-ōsis*]. Full of blood.

hematosepsis (hem-at-o-sep′sis) [" + *sēpsis*, putrefaction]. Blood toxemia. SYN: *septicemia*.

hematosin (hem-at-o′sin) [G. *aima*, blood]. Decomposition product of hemoglobin. SYN: *hematin*.

hematosis (he-ma-to′sis) [" + *-ōsis*]. 1. The formation of blood and the development of the red blood corpuscles. 2. The oxygenation of blood in the lungs.

hematospec′troscope [" + L. *spectrum*, image, + G. *skopein*, to examine]. Spectroscope for inspecting the blood.

hematospectros′copy [" + " + G. *skopein*, to examine]. Examination of the blood with the hematospectroscope.

hematospermatocele (hem″ă-to-sper-mat′o-sēl) [" + *sperma*, seed, + *kēlē*, tumor]. A blood-filled spermatocele.

hematospermia (he-mă-to-sper′mĭ-ă) [" + *sperma*, seed]. Bloody semen.
 h. spuria. When coming from the prostatic urethra.
 h. vera. When coming from the seminal vessels.

hematostatic (he-mat-o-stat′ik) [G. *aima*, blood, + *stasis*, a standing]. SYN: *hemostatic*. 1. Retaining blood in a part. 2. Pertaining to the arrest of blood flow in a hemorrhage.

hematosteon (hem-ă-tos′te-on) [" + *osteon*, bone]. Bleeding into the medullary cavity of a bone.

hematother′mal [" + *thermē*, heat]. Warm blooded. SYN: *hemathermal; hemathermous*.

hematothorax (hem-at-o-tho′raks) [" + *thōrax*, chest]. Blood in the chest. SYN: *hemothorax*.

hematotox′ic [" + *toxikon*, poison]. Pert. to toxemia.

hematotrachelos (he″mat-o-trak′e-los) [" + *trachēlos*, neck]. Retained menstrual blood in cervix uteri causing distention.

hematotympanum (hem-at-o-tĭm′pan-um) [" + *tympanon*, drum]. Blood in the middle ear.

hematoxylin. A colorless crystalline compound, $C_{16}H_{14}O_6$, obtained by extraction

hematozoon   H-19   **hemicardia**

with ether from logwood. Upon oxidation it is converted into hematein, which stains certain structures a deep blue color. It is an excellent nuclear stain, and widely used in histological work.

hematozoon (he-mat-o-zo′on) [" + *zōon*, animal]. Any living organism in the blood.

hematozymosis (hem-at-o-zi-mo′sis) [" + *zymōsis*, fermentation]. Blood fermentation.

hematuria (he-ma-tu′ri-a) [G. *aima*, blood, + *ouron*, urine]. Blood in the urine.
    SYM: Urine may be slightly smoky, reddish, or very red.
    ETIOL: Lesion of urinary tract, or blood dyscrasia, contamination during menstruation or puerperium, prostatic disease, tumors, poisoning, esp. carbolic acid and cantharides, malaria and toxemias and calculus.
    DIAG: If well mixed with urine, probably from kidneys. If clotted in tubular casts of ureters, from kidneys or ureters. If passed at beginning of urination, from the urethra; if at the end, from bladder.
    h., renal. Urine smoky, sometimes bright red.
    h., urethral. Always bright red. Precedes urination.
    h., vesical. Urine bright red, not uniform.

hemaurochrome (hem″ă-u′ro-krōm) [" + *ouron*, urine, + *chrōma*, color]. A hematin derivative found in the urine in sarcoma and carcinoma, malaria, anemias and other disorders. Supposed to result from dissolution of red blood corpuscles.

heme. $C_{34}H_{32}O_4N_4FeOH$, an iron-containing protoporphyrin derived from hemin when hemin is treated with sodium hydroxide. Heme can combine with a large number of organic nitrogenous substances to form *hemochromogens*. Formerly called *hematin*.

hemeralopia (hem-er-al-o′pi-ă) [G. *ēmera*, day, + *alaos*, blind, + *ōps*, eye]. Day blindness or night blindness, found particularly in macular lesions. Term formerly erroneously applied to nightblindness or *nyctalopia* (inability to see in dim light).
    The latter, *nyctalopia*, indicates inability to see in dim light though otherwise vision is normal.
    In day blindness, the sight is poor in sunlight and in good illumination; it is good at dusk, at twilight, and in poor illumination. This is noted in albinism, retinitis with central scotoma, toxic amblyopia, coloboma of the iris and choroid, opacity of the crystalline lens or cornea, and in conjunctivitis with photophobia.

hemi- [G.]. Prefix meaning *half*.

hemiacephalus. A monster with a markedly defective head. SEE: *anencephalus*.

hemiachromatopsia (he-mī-ak-ro-mat-op′-sī-ă) [G. *ēmi*, half, + *a*-, priv. + *chrōma*, color, + *opsis*, vision]. Color blindness in one-half, or in corresponding halves, of the visual field.

hemialbumin (hem-ĭ-al-bu′min) [" + L. *albumen*, white of egg]. A product resulting from the digestion of albumin. SYN: *antialbumin*.

hemialbumose (hem-ĭ-al′bū-mōs) [" + L. *albumen*, white of egg]. An albumoid product from the digestion of certain proteins. It occurs in bone marrow.

hemialbumosu′ria [" + " + G. *ouron*, urine]. Hemialbumose in the urine.

hemialgia (hem-ĭ-al′jĭ-ă) [" + *algos*, pain]. Pain in one-half of the body.

hemiamaurosis (hem″ĭ-am-aw-ro′sis) [" + *amaurosis*, darkness]. Blindness in one-half the visual field. SYN: *hemianopia*.

hemiamblyopia (hem″ĭ-am-blĭ-o′pĭ-ă) [" + *amblys*, dim, + *ōps*, sight]. Blindness in half the visual field. SYN: *hemianopsia*.

hemiamyosthenia (hem″ĭ-am″ĭ-os-the′nĭ-ă) [" + *a*-, priv. + *mys*, *myo*-, muscle, + *sthenos*, strength]. Absence of normal muscular power on 1 side of the body. SYN: *hemiparesis*.

hemianacusia (hem″ĭ-an-a-kŭ′sĭ-ă) [G. *ēmi*, half, + *an*-, priv. + *akousis*, hearing]. Deafness in 1 ear.

hemianalgesia (hem″ĭ-an-al-ge′sĭ-ă) [" + " + *algos*, pain]. Lack of sensibility to pain (analgesia) on 1 side of the body.

hemianesthesia (hem″ĭ-an-es-the′zĭ-ă) [" + " + *aisthēsis*, sensation]. Anesthesia of one-half of the body.

hemianopia, hemianopsia (hem-ĭ-an-op′ĭ-ă, sĭ-ă) [" + " + *ōps*, eye]. Blindness for one-half field of vision in 1 or both eyes.
    h., altitudinal. Blindness in upper or lower half in each eye.
    h., binasal. Affection of nasal half of visual field in each eye.
    h., bitemporal. Affection of temporal half of visual field in each eye.
    h., complete. H. of half of each eye.
    h., crossed. Bitemporal or binasal hemianopsia.
    h., heteronymous. SEE: *crossed h.*
    h., homonymous. Blindness of nasal half of 1 eye and temporal half of the other or right-sided or left-sided h. of corresponding sides in both eyes.
    h., incomplete. H. of less than half of each eye.
    h., quadrant. Affection of symmetrical quadrant of the field in each eye.
    h., unilateral, uniocular. Hemianopsia affecting only 1 eye.

hemianosmia (hem″ĭ-an-os′mĭ-ă) [G. *ēmi*, half, + *an*-, priv. + *osmē*, smell]. Loss of smell in 1 nostril.

hemiapraxia (hem″ĭ-ă-prak′sĭ-ă) [" + *a*-, priv. + *prassein*, to do]. Incapacity to exercise purposeful movements on 1 side of the body.

hemiarthrosis (hem-ĭ-ar-thro′sis) [" + *arthron*, joint, + *ōsis*]. A false articulation bet. 2 bones. SYN: *synchondrosis*.

hemiasynergia (hem″ĭ-as-in-er′jĭ-ă) [" + *a*-, priv. + *syn*, with, + *ergon*, work]. Lack of coördination of parts affecting 1 side of the body.

hemiataxia (hem-ĭ-ă-taks′ĭ-ă) [" + *ataxia*, lack of order]. Impaired muscular coordination causing awkward movements of the affected side of the body.

hemiathetosis (hem″ĭ-ath-et-o′sis) [" + *athetos*, without fixed position, + *-ōsis*]. Slow change of position; athetosis of 1 side of the body.

hemiatrophy (hem-i-at′ro-fī) [" + *atrophia*, atrophy]. Impaired nutrition resulting in atrophy of 1 side of the face or other part; marked by white or yellow macules on affected side.

hemiballism (hem-ĭ-bal′izm) [" + *ballismos*, jumping]. Jerking and twitching movements of 1 side of the body. SYN: *hemichorea*.

he′mic [G. *aima*, blood]. Pert. to blood. SYN: *hemal*.

hemicanities (hem″ĭ-kan-ish′ĭ-ēz) [G. *ēmi*, half, + L. *canities*, gray hair]. Grayness (*canities*) of hair on 1 side only.

hemicardia (hem-ĭ-kar′dĭ-ă) [" + *kardia*, heart]. Half of a 4-chambered heart.

hemicellulose (hem-ĭ-sel'lu-lōs) [G. *aima*, blood, + L. *cellula*, little cell]. One of a group of polysaccharides which differ from cellulose in that they may be hydrolyzed by dilute mineral acids and from other polysaccharides in that they are not readily digested by amylases. Includes pentosans, galactosans (agar agar), and pectins.

hemicentrum (hem-ĭ-sen'trum) [" + *kentron*, center]. Either lateral half of the centrum of a vertebra.

hemichorea (hem-ĭ-ko-re'ă) [" + *choreia*, a dancing]. Convulsive movements (*chorea*) of but 1 side of the body.

hemichromatopsia (hem"ĭ-kro-mat-op'sĭ-ă) [" + *chrōma*, color, + *opsis*, vision]. Blindness to color in one-half of the visual field. SYN: *hemiachromatopsia*.

hemicrania (hem-ĭ-kra'nĭ-ă) [" + *kranion*, skull]. 1. Unilateral head pain, usually migraine. 2. Monstrosity having only one-half of the skull developed.

hemicraniectomy (hem"ĭ-kra-nĭ-ek'to-mĭ) [" + " + *ektomē*, excision]. Surgical division of cranial vault from before, backward, exposing half of the brain.

hemicraniosis (hem"ĭ-kra-nĭ-o'sis) [" + + *ōsis*]. Enlargement of half of cranium or face.

hemidiaphoresis (hem"ĭ-dĭ-ăf-or-e'sis) [" + *dia*, through, + *pherein*, to carry]. Sweating on 1 side of the body.

hemidi'aphragm [" + " + *phragma*, wall]. Paralysis affecting only one-half of the diaphragm.

hemidro'sis [" + *idrōsis*, sweat]. Bloody sweating. SYN: *hemathidrosis*.

hemidyser'gia [" + *dys*, bad, + *ergon*, work]. Lack of coördination of muscles (*dysergia*) on 1 side of the body.

hemidysesthesia (hem"ĭ-dis-es-the'sĭ-ă) [" + " + *aisthēsis*, sensation]. Impaired sensation (*dysesthesia*) of one-half of the body.

hemidystrophy (hem"ĭ-dis'tro-fĭ) [" + + *trophē*, nourishment]. Inequality in development of the 2 sides of the body.

hemiep'ilepsy [" + *epilēpsia*, seizure]. Epilepsy with convulsions confined to 1 lateral half of the body.

hemifa'cial [G. *ēmi*, half, + L. *faciēs*, face]. Pert. to 1 side of the face.

hemigastrectomy (hem"ĭ-gas-trek'to-mĭ) [" + *gastēr*, belly, + *ektomē*, excision]. Excision of pyloric end of the stomach for hourglass contraction.

hemigeusia (hem-ĭ-gu'sĭ-ă) [" + *geusis*, taste]. Loss of sense of taste on 1 side of the tongue.

hemiglossi'tis [" + *glōssa*, tongue, + *-itis*, inflammation]. Vesicular eruption on one-half of the tongue and inner surface of cheek. Herpetic in character.

hemihidro'sis [" + *idrōsis*, perspiration]. Sweating on only 1 side of the body. SYN: *hemidiaphoresis*.

hemihyperesthesia (hem"ĭ-hĭ-per-es-the'sĭ-ă) [" + *yper*, over, + *aisthēsis*, sensation]. Abnormal tactile and painful sensitiveness of 1 side of the body.

hemihyperidrosis (hem"ĭ-hĭ-per-i-dro'sis) [" + " + *idrōsis*, sweating]. Excessive perspiration confined to 1 side of the body.

hemihyperto'nia [" + " + *tonos*, tone]. Exaggerated tonicity of muscles on 1 lateral half of the body.

hemihyper'trophy [" + " + *trophē*, nourishment]. Muscular overgrowth (*hypertrophy*) of one-half of the body or face.

hemihypesthesia (hem"ĭ-hĭ-pes-the'sĭ-ă) [" + *ypo*, under, + *aisthēsis*, sensation]. Diminished sensibility on 1 side of the body.

hemihypotonia (hem"ĭ-hĭ-po-to'nĭ-ă) [" + " + *tonos*, tone]. Partial loss of tonicity of muscles on 1 side of the body.

hemilat'eral [" + L. *latus*, side]. Rel. to 1 side only.

hemin (he'min) [G. *aima*, blood]. SYN: *heme hydrochloride*. A brownish red crystalline salt of heme formed when hemoglobin is heated with glacial acetic acid and sodium chloride. Used as a test to reveal the presence of blood.

h. crystals. Teichmann's crystals, formed when the above test is made.

heminephrectomy. Excision or removal of a portion of a kidney.

hemineurasthenia (hem"ĭ-nu-răs-the'nĭ-ă) [G. *ēmi*, half, + *neuron*, nerve, + *astheneia*, weakness]. Neurasthenia affecting 1 side of the body only.

hemiopia (hem-ĭ-o'pĭ-ă) [" + *ōps*, eye]. Blindness in half of the visual field. SYN: *hemianopia*.

hemiopic (hem-ĭ-op'ik) [" + *ōps*, eye]. Pert. to hemiopia.

hemiparal'ysis [" + *paralyein*, to loosen from the sides]. Paralysis of 1 side of the body only.

hemiparanesthesia (hem"ĭ-par-an-es-the'sĭ-ă) [" + *para*, beyond, + *an*-, priv. + *aisthēsis*, sensation]. Anesthesia of 1 lower extremity or lower half of 1 side.

hemiparaplegia (hem"ĭ-par-ă-ple'jĭ-ă) [" + " + *plēgē*, stroke]. Paralysis of the lower half of 1 side of or of 1 leg.

hemipar'esis [" + *paresis*, paralysis]. Slight paralysis of 1 side of the body.

hem"iparesthe'sia [" + *para*, beyond, + *aisthēsis*, sensation]. Numbness of 1 side of body.

hemipeptone (hem-ĭ-pep'tōn) [" + *peptein*, to digest]. One of the 2 compounds of peptone in pepsin digestion which later forms leucin, tyrosin, and amino acids.

hemiplegia (hem-i-ple'jĭ-ă) [" + *plēgē*, a stroke]. Paralysis of only one-half of the body.

ETIOL: A brain lesion involving upper motor neurons and resulting in paralysis of the opposite side of the body. May result from cerebral apoplexy, softening or tumors of the cerebrum.

NP: Elevate head and shoulders. Apply cold to head, hot water bottle to feet. See that tongue does not obstruct breathing. Avoid stimulants. Do not move patient until arrival of doctor.

Take a 4-hr. chart for day or two. Turn patient frequently to avoid hypostatic pneumonia. Watch for bedsores, retention of urine, which should be measured and tested for albumin and sugar. Avoid burning with hot water bottles. Do not discuss patient when apparently unconscious.

SEE: *Benedict's syndrome, paralysis, thalamic syndrome*.

h., alternate. Affecting 1 side of face and trunk and opposite of extremities.

h., capsular. H. resulting from a lesion of the internal capsule.

h., cerebral. Due to brain lesion.

h., crossed. Alternate h; cruciate h. q.v.

h. cruciata. Medulla lesion involving the crossed arm and uncrossed leg fibers of the pyramids paralyzing 1 arm and the opposite leg.

h. facial. Paralysis of muscles of one side of face.

h., spastic. H. accompanied by spasms, usually occurring in infants.

h., spinal. H. resulting from a lesion of the spinal cord. SEE: *Brown-Sequard's paralysis*.

hemiplegic (hem-i-ple'jik) [G. *ēmi*, half, + *plēgē*, stroke]. Pert. to hemiplegia.

Hemiptera. The true bugs; an order of insects characterized by piercing and sucking mouth parts; 1st pr. of wings leathery at base and membranous at tip, 2nd pair of wings membranous; incomplete metamorphosis. Includes bedbugs, kissing bugs, and several other species which are pests or transmitters of pathogenic organisms.

hemirachischisis (hēm-ĭ-rā-kĭs'sĭs). Rachischisis in which protrusion of the spinal meninges does not occur; *spina bifida occulta*, q.v.

hemisec'tion [G. *ēmi*, half, + L. *sectio*, a cutting]. SYN: *bisection*. The act of dividing a part or an organ into two halves; bisection.

hemispasm (hem'ĭ-spazm) [" + *spasmos*, spasm]. Spasm of only 1 side of the body or face.

hemisphere (hem'is-fēr) [" + *sphaira*, sphere]. Either half of the cerebrum or cerebellum.

h., dominant. The cerebral hemisphere in which the higher cortical functions, esp. those relating to speech and certain motor activities, are associated; the left one in right-handed individuals. Results in phenomenon known as "cerebral dominance."

Hemis'pora stella'ta. A variety of fungus causing mycosis.

hemispore (hem'ĭ-spōr) [G. *ēmi*, half, + *sporos*, seed]. A spore which reproduces by division of terminal part of a hyphus.*

hemisporosis (hem-ĭ-spo-ro'sis) [" + *sporos*, seed, + *ōsis*]. Infection with a fungus (*Hemispora stellata*) resulting in swellings of bone and other tissue of a gummatous nature. They may later ulcerate.

hemistrumectomy (hem"ĭ-strŭ-mek'to-mĭ) [" + L. *struma*, goiter, + G. *ektomē*, excision]. Excision of about one-half of a goiter.

hemisyndrome (hem-ĭ-sĭn'drōm) [" + *syndromē*, a running with]. One indicating a unilateral lesion of the spinal cord.

hemisystole (hĕm-ĭ-sĭs'tō-le) [G. *ēmi*, half, + *systole*, a contracting]. One pulse beat to every two heart beats. Results from failure of the ventricle to contract every other time.

hem"iterat'a. Individuals possessing congenital malformations but not to such a degree as to be designated a monster.

hemiteric, hemiteratic (hem-ĭ-ter'ĭk, -terat'ik) [" + *teras*, monster]. Congenitally deformed, but not marked as monstrous.

hem'lock [A.S. *hemléac*]. 1. A species of fir tree. 2. Volatile oil extracted from hemlock tree.
  POISONING: SYM: Nausea, vomiting, diarrhea, salivation, pupils dilated.
  TREATMENT: Empty stomach by means of a stomach pump or an emetic. Give a teaspoonful of tannic acid in glass of water. Stimulate.

he'mo. Prefix meaning pertaining to the blood. See also *haemo- haem- hema-* and *hemato*.

hem"oagglutina'tion [G. *aima*, blood, + L. *agglutināre*, to paste to]. The clumping of red blood corpuscles.

hem"oagglu'tinin [" + L. *agglutināre*, to paste to]. An agglutinin which clumps the red blood corpuscles.

hemoalkalim'eter [" + Arab. *alkali*, the kali plant, + G. *metron*, measure]. A device for estimating degree of alkalinity of blood.

hemobilinuria (hem"o-bĭl-ĭn-ū'rĭ-ă) [" + L. *bilis*, bile, + G. *ouron*, urine]. Urobilin in the blood and urine.

hem'oblast [" + *blastos*, germ]. Immature red blood corpuscles; a blood platelet. SYN: *hematoblast*. A *hematocytoblast*.

hemoblastosis (hem-o-blas-to'sis) [" + " + *-ōsis*]. Changes occurring in or increase in amount of the blood forming tissues.

hemocatheresis (hem"o-kath-er-e'sis) [" + *kathairesis*, destruction]. Dissolution of red blood corpuscles as in the spleen.

hemocatheretic (hem"o-kath-er-et'ik) [" + *kathairetikos*, destructive]. Destructive to blood corpuscles.

hemochorial (hēm-ō-kor'ĭ-al). Pertaining to the relationship between blood of the mother and the chorionic ectoderm. SEE: *placenta, hemochorial*.

hemochromatosis (hem"o-krō-mat-ō'sis) [" + *chrōma*, color, + *-ōsis*]. A disease of pigmentation of the skin and viscera, sometimes associated with diabetes and has been called *bronzed diabetes*.

hem'ochrome [" + *chrōma*, color]. The red pigment of the blood.

he'mo-chro'mogen [G. *aima*, blood, + *gennan*, to produce). General term applied to compounds of heme with nitrogen-containing substances such as a protein.

hemochromometer (hem-o-kro-mom'et-er) [G. *aima*, blood, + *chroma*, color, + *metron*, measure). A colorimeter used for estimating the amount of hemoglobin in the blood.

hemocla'sia, hemoc'lasis [" + *klasis*, destruction]. Disintegration of red blood corpuscles. SYN: *hemolysis*.

hemoclas'tic [" + *klasis*, destruction]. Destructive of erythrocytes. SYN: *hemolytic*.

he"moconcentra'tion. SYN: *anhydremia*. An increase in the number of red blood cells resulting from a decrease in the volume of plasma.

hemoco'nia [G. *aima*, blood, + *konis*, dust]. SYN: *hemokonia*. Minute colorless bodies in blood thought to be the products of disintegration of red blood cells. Also called *blood dust*.

hemoconio'sis [" + " + *-ōsis*]. Having an abnormal amt. of hemokonia in the blood. SYN: *hemokoniosis*.

hem'oculture [" + L. *cultura*, development]. A bacteriological blood culture.

hemocyte (hem'o-sīt) [" + *kytos*, cell]. Blood corpuscle.

he'mocy'toblast [G. *aima*, blood, + L. *cultura*, + *blastos*, germ). The common lymphoid stem cell found in bone marrow from which all blood cells are thought to arise.

hemocytoblastoma (hem"o-sī"to-blas-to'-mă) [" + " + " + *ōma*, tumor]. A tumor containing embryonic blood cells.

hemocytocatheresis (hem"o-sī"to-kath-er-e'sis) [" + " + *kathairesis*, destruction]. The dissolution of blood corpuscles.

hem"ocytogen'esis (hem"o-sito-jen'e-sis) [G. *aima*, blood + *kytos*, cell, + *genesis*, development]. SYN: *hematopoiesis*. The formation of blood cells.

hemocytology (he-mo-si-tol'o-jĭ) [" + " + *logos*, study]. The science of blood cells.

hemocytolysis (hem-o-si-tol'is-is) [" + " + *lysis*, dissolution]. Dissolution of the blood corpuscles. SYN: *hematocytolysis, hemolysis*.

hemocytometer (hem-o-si-tom'et-er) [" + " + *metron*, measure]. Device for de-

hemocytopoiesis

termining relative number of corpuscles in the blood.

hemocytopoiesis (hem″o-si″to-poy-e′sis) [" + " + *poiein*, to form]. The development of blood cells.

hemocytotripsis (hem″o-si″to-trip′sis) [" + " + *tripsis*, a crushing]. Fragmentation of the red blood corpuscles.

hemocytozoon (hem″o-si″to-zo′on) [" + " + *zōon*, animal]. An animal microparasite of the blood cells. SYN: *hematobium*.

hemo′dia. Extreme sensitivity of the teeth.

hemodiagno′sis [G. *aima*, blood, + *dia*, through, + *gnōsis*, knowledge]. Examination of the blood for diagnostic purpose.

hemodi′astase [" + *diastasis*, separation]. An amylolytic ferment in the blood.

he″modilu′tion. An increase in the volume of blood plasma resulting in reduced concentration of red blood cells.

hemodromometer (hem″o-dro-mom′et-er) [" + *dromos*, course, + *metron*, measure]. Device for determining the blood's velocity.

hemodynam′ics [" + *dynamis*, power]. The study of circulation of the blood.

hemodynamometer (hem″o-di-na-mom′et-er) [" + " + *metron*, measure]. Device for measuring blood pressure.

hemodystrophy (hem-o-dis′tro-fī) [" + *dys*, bad, + *trophē*, nutrition]. Imperfect nutrition of the blood. SYN: *hematodystrophy*.

he″mo-en″dothe′lial. Pertaining to the relationship between blood of the mother and the endothelium of chorionic vessels. SEE: *placenta, hemoendothelial*.

hemoferrum (hem-o-fer′um) [" + L. *ferrum*, iron]. The iron element of hemoglobin. SYN: *oxyhemoglobin*.

he″moflag′ellate. Any flagellate protozoan parasite of the blood. Includes trypanosomes and leishmanias.

hemofuscin (hem-o-fus′in) [" + L. *fuscus*, brown]. Brown coloring matter derived from hemoglobin.

hemogenesis (hem-o-jen′es-is) [" + *genesis*, formation]. Blood formation. SYN: *hematogenesis*.

hemoge′nia [" + *gennan*, to produce]. A hemorrhagic condition of the blood forming apparatus.

hemogen′ic [" + *gennan*, to produce]. Rel. to the production of blood.

hemoglobin (hem-o-glo′bin) [G. *aima*, blood, + L. *globus*, globe]. A chromoprotein of red color; the coloring substance of the red blood corpuscles.

The amount of hemoglobin in the blood averages 14 to 16 grams per 100 cc. One gram of hemoglobin can combine with 1.34 cc. of oxygen, the resulting compound being oxyhemoglobin.

Hemoglobin is a crystallizable, conjugated protein consisting of an iron-containing pigment called *heme* or *hematin*, and a simple protein, *globin*. In the lungs it combines readily with oxygen to form a loose, unstable compound called *oxyhemoglobin*, a process called *oxygenation*. In the tissues where oxygen tension is low, oxyhemoglobin decomposes and oxygen is liberated. The resulting compound is *reduced hemoglobin*. Hemoglobin is a weak acid and in the red corpuscles is combined with potassium, an alkali, to form potassium hemoglobinate (an alkali), which acts to buffer carbonic acid formed from carbon dioxide entering the blood from the tissues. The buffering action is accomplished by a mechanism known as the *chloride shift*.

H-22

Hemoglobin liberated from disintegrating red blood cells is removed from circulation by the cells of the reticuloendothelial system, esp., those of the liver and spleen. The globin in converted to amino acids and reutilized. Iron from the iron-containing portion is stored in the liver and spleen and reutilized; the noniron containing pigment is converted to *bilirubin* which is excreted as one of the bile pigments.

hemoglobinemia (hem″o-glōb-in-e′mĭ-ă) [" + " + G. *aima*, blood]. Presence of hemoglobin in the blood plasma.

hemoglobinocholia (hem″o-glō″bĭn-o-ko′lĭ-ă) [" + " + G. *cholē*, bile]. Hemoglobin in the bile.

hemoglobinolysis (hem″o-glo-bin-ol′ĭ-sis) [" + " + G. *lysis*, dissolution]. Dissolution of hemoglobin.

hemoglobinometer (hem″o-glo-bin-om′et-er) [" + " + G. *metron*, measure]. Device for determining the hemoglobin in the blood.

hemoglobinopepsia (hem″o-glo″bĭn-o-pep′sĭ-ă) [" + " + G. *pepsis*, digestion]. Destruction of hemoglobin. SYN: *hemoglobinolysis*.

hemoglobinophilic (hem-o-glo-bin-o-fil′ik) [G. *aima*, blood, + L. *globus*, globe, + G. *philein*, to love]. Pert. to organisms which grow better in presence of hemoglobin.

hemoglo′binous [" + L. *globus*, globe]. Pert. to or containing hemoglobin.

hemoglobinuria (hem″o-glo-bin-u′rĭ-ă) [G. *aima*, blood, + L. *globus*, globe, + G. *ouron*, urine]. The presence of hemoglobin in the urine, but free from red blood corpuscles.

Occurs when hemoglobin from disintegrating red blood cells or from rapid hemolysis of red cells exceeds renal threshold.

ETIOL: Scurvy, purpura, or certain drugs, such as arsenic, phosphorus, or typhus fever, or pyemia.

SEE: *Buhl's disease, Winckel's disease*.

h., epidemic. H. of the newborn characterized by jaundice, cyanosis, and fatty degeneration of heart and liver: Winckel's disease.

h., march. H. occurring esp. in young soldiers following strenuous exercise.

h., paroxysmal. Intermittent, recurring attacks of h. following exposure to cold or strenuous exercise. Results from increased fragility of red blood cells, or presence of a thermolabile autohemolysin.

h., toxic. H. resulting from: toxic substances such as muscarine, or snake venom; toxic products of infectious diseases, such as yellow fever, typhoid fever, syphilis and certain forms of hemolytic jaundice; organisms such as *Plasmodium* which destroy red blood cells; foreign proteins in blood as may follow blood transfusion or serum therapy.

hem″oglobinu′ric [" + " + G. *ouron*, urine]. Rel. to or marked by hemoglobinuria.

h. fever. Malarial hemoglobinuria.

hem′ogram [" + *gramma*, a writing]. A graph of the differential blood count. SEE: *Schilling's h*.

hemohistioblast (hĕm″ō-hĭs′tĭ-ō-blăst) [G. *aima*, blood, + *istos*, tissue, + *blastos*, germ]. SYN: *hematohistioblast*. Free macrophages which sometimes appear in the blood in certain diseases, esp., those of a septic nature.

he′moid [" + *eidos*, resemblance]. Having the appearance of blood.

hemoko′nia (pl. *hemokoniae*) [" + *konis*, dust]. Minute, highly refractive body in the blood, said to be disintegrated par-

hemokonia

ticle of blood corpuscle. SYN: *blood dust, blood mote.*

hemokoniosis (hem″o-ko-nĭ-o'sis) [" + " + -*ōsis*]. Abnormal amount of hemokoniae in the blood.

hem'olith [" + *lithos*, stone]. A calculus in the wall of a blood vessel.

hem'olymph [" + L. *lympha*, lymph]. Blood and lymph.

hemol'ysin [" + *lysis*, dissolution]. An agent in a serum destructive of erythrocytes.*

hemolysis (hĕm-ŏl'ĭ-sĭs) [G. *aima*, blood, + *lysis*, dissolution]. The destruction of red blood cells with the liberation of hemoglobin which diffuses into the fluid surrounding them. Also called "laking" of the blood. May occur as a result of the effects of bacterial toxins, snake venoms, immune bodies (hemolysins), and hypotonic saline solutions.

Their stroma is ruptured or dissolved, and the hemoglobin is liberated into the plasma. As a result, the blood, examined grossly, appears to be more transparent and to have a richer, red color; under the microscope the dissolution of the red corpuscles can be observed.

When the hemolysis occurs within the blood vessels, the body is unable to retain the hemoglobin, which is lost through the kidneys and imparts a red color to the urine. A condition called *hemoglobinuria, q.v.*

Injection of a hypotonic saline solution or distilled water into the blood stream induces hemolysis and may result in death. The red blood cells swell, and become globular; their membranes stretch and hemoglobin is liberated. All solutions injected intravenously must be isotonic to the blood. Hemolysis may result from infection by certain disease organisms, e.g. certain streptococci, staphylococci, the tetanus bacillus, and the scarlet fever organism. Hemolysis also occurs in smallpox, diphtheria, and following severe burns. SEE: *fragility test*, *laked.*

hemolytic (hem-o-lĭt'ĭk) [G. *aima*, blood, + *lysis*, dissolution]. Pert. to the breaking down of red blood corpuscles.

h. unit. The amount of inactivated immune serum which causes complete hemolysis of 1 cc. of a 5% emulsion of washed red blood corpuscles, in the presence of complement.

hemolytopoietic (hem-ol-it″o-poi-et'ĭk) [" + " + *poiein*, to form]. Rel. to processes of production and destruction of blood cells.

hem'olyze. To produce hemolysis.

hemomediastinum (hem″o-me-dĭ-as-ti'num) [" + L. *mediastinus*, in the middle]. Effusion of blood into mediastinal spaces. SYN: *hematomediastinum.*

hemometra (he-mo-me'trā) [" + *mētra*, uterus]. Retention of blood within the uterus. SYN: *hematometra.*

hemonephro'sis [" + *nephros*, kidney, + *ōsis*]. Blood in pelvis of the kidney. SYN: *hematonephrosis.*

hemopath'ic [" + *pathos*, blood]. Rel. or due to disease of the blood.

hemopathol'ogy [" + " + *logos*, study]. The science of blood disorders.

hemop'athy [" + *pathos*, disease]. A disease of the blood.

hemoperitone'um [" + *peritonaion*, peritoneum]. Effusion of blood into the peritoneal cavity.

hemopex'in [" + *pēxis*, fixation]. Enzyme which coagulates the blood.

hemopex'is [" + *pēxis*, fixation]. Blood coagulation.

hem'ophage [" + *phagein*, to eat]. A cell destroying red blood corpuscles by phagocytosis.

hemophagocyte (hem-o-fag'o-sīt) [" + *kytos*, cell]. A white blood corpuscle which ingests other blood corpuscles, esp. red.

RS: *anemia, blood, leukocyte.*

hemophilia (hem-o-fĭl'ĭ-ă) [G. *aima*, blood, + *philein*, to love]. An hereditary blood disease characterized by greatly prolonged coagulation-time. The blood fails to clot and abnormal bleeding occurs. It is a sex-linked hereditary trait, being transmitted by normal heterozygous females who carry the recessive gene. It occurs almost exclusively in males.

ETIOL: Failure of the blood to form thrombin. This may be due to failure of platelets to release thromboplastin, failure of prothrombin to react normally to thromboplastin; the presence of a factor inhibiting the formation of thrombin, or absence of a substance present in normal blood plasma which shortens coagulation time.

SYM: Abnormal tendency to bleed. May cause swelling of the joints.

PROG: Unfavorable; one-half of those afflicted die before the 8th year.

TREATMENT: In an emergency, blood transfusions, followed by adm. of ferrous sulfate, 3 gr. (0.2 Gm.), 4 times daily. Adequate fluids and full nourishing diet. Aspirin, codeine or morphine for pain. Injection of placental extracts sometimes reduces clotting time of blood.

Subject should carry notice on person that he or she is a *hemophiliac* so that in case of accident requiring an operation the surgeon may be forewarned and take necessary precautions. SEE: *angiostaxis, blood.*

hemophiliac (hem-o-fĭl'ĭ-ak) [" + *philein*, to love]. One afflicted with hemophilia.

he″mophil'ic. 1. Fond of blood, said of bacteria which grow well in culture media containing hemoglobin. 2. Pertaining to hemophilia or hemophiliacs.

Hemophilus (hē-mŏf'ĭl-us) [G. *aima*, blood, — *philein*, to love]. A genus of bacteria belonging to the family Parvobacteriaceae. Small, pleomorphic, nonmotile, gram-negative, rod-shaped hemophilic organisms.

H. ducreyi. Ducrey's bacillus, the causative organism of chanchroid or soft chancre.

H. duplex. Morax-Axenfeld bacillus, the causative organism of angular conjunctivitis.

H. influenzae. Pfeiffer's bacillus, Koch-Weeks bacillus. An organism found in respiratory infections and formerly thought to be the cause of influenza, but now considered to be a secondary invader. It is the causative organism of influenzal meningitis.

H. pertussis. Bordet-Gengou bacillus, the causative organism of whooping cough.

H. suis. Species which, in conjunction with a filtrable virus, causes swine influenza.

hemophobia (he-mo-fo'bĭ-ă) [" + *phobos*, fear]. Aversion to seeing blood or to bleeding.

hemophor'ic [" + *pherein*, to carry]. Conveying blood.

hemophthal'mia, hemophthal'mus [" + *ophthalmos*, eye]. Effusion of blood into eyeball.

hemoplas'tic [" + *plassein*, to form]. Blood-forming. SYN: *hematoplastic, hematopoietic.*

hemopneumothorax **hemorrhage, carotid artery**

hemopneumothorax (hem″o-nu-mo-tho′-raks) [" + *pneuma*, air, + *thōrax*, chest]. Blood and air in the pleural cavity.

hemopoie′sis [" + *poiein*, to make]. Formation of red blood corpuscles. SYN: *hematopoiesis*.

hemoptysis (hĕm-ŏp′tis-is) [G. *aima*, blood, + *ptyein*, to spit]. Expectoration of blood arising from hemorrhage of the larynx, trachea, bronchi, or lungs.
SYM: Attack sudden. Salty taste. Blood frothy, bright red.
TREATMENT: Cold applications over chest.
NP: Patient must be kept perfectly quiet in bed in a semirecumbent position with bed slightly elevated. No movement or excitement permitted and no visitors. No talking by patient, who should be reassured. No hot drinks. Light diet.
In tuberculosis, in absence of doctor in case of hemorrhage, follow these rules:
1. Support the patient with pillows in a semirecumbent position; if the bleeding side is known, incline him towards that side, and, if any feeling of suffocation, loosen clothing about throat and chest.
2. If there be thirst, give iced water in sips.
3. Open the window.
Keep patient warm. He will probably complain of cold. In that case apply hot water bottle to feet.
4. Keep patient calm and comforted.
5. Do not adm. any drugs until doctor comes, and on no account give stimulants. An injection of morphia may probably be prescribed. Should patient faint hemorrhage will, in all probability, cease. This is often Nature's means of cure.
SEE: *bleeding, hemorrhage, hematemesis*.
The table (p. H-22) gives the more important distinguishing features between hemoptysis and hematemesis, *q.v.*

h., endemic. Paragonimiasis. SEE: *h. parasitic.*

h., parasitic. Spitting of blood resulting from infection of the lungs by *Paragonimus westermani, q.v.* A parasitic fluke.

hemorrhage (hem′o-raj) [G. *aima*, blood, + *rēgnunai*, to burst forth]. Abnormal discharge of blood, either external or internal; venous, arterial, or capillary from blood vessels into tissues, into or from the body.
Venous blood is dark red; flow is continuous. Arterial blood is bright red; flows in jets. Capillary blood is of a reddish color; exudes from tissue.
SYM: When visible, diagnosis is obvious. When internal, diagnosis may be made from the general condition. Patient is in shock; pulse weak, rapid and irregular; face pale; skin cold, moist and flabby.
F. A. TREATMENT: Depends upon location. Remove all dirt with absorbent cotton, using moisture of the blood, not water; apply sterilized sponge; bandage firmly; elevate limb. Patient should recline. Very cold or very hot water contracts vessels. Warm water increases bleeding. Do not use alum, iron solutions, etc., if avoidable. Make pressure on arteries leading to heart. Elevate the part. Tourniquet. A handkerchief or strap tied loosely around the limb, with stick against knot, turning it until part is compressed, will answer all purposes. If an open wound, apply anti-

---

Hemoptysis	Hematemesis
1. Probable previous history of tuberculosis.	1. Probable previous history of gastric or duodenal trouble.
2. Blood is coughed up.	2. Blood is vomited.
3. Blood is frothy, bright red, and alkaline in reaction.	3. Blood is usually (not always) dark, usually not frothy, and acid in reaction. Often clotted.
4. Blood may be mixed with sputum.	4. Blood may be mixed with food.
5. There is some dyspnea, pain, and a tickling sensation in the chest.	5. There is often nausea and pain referred to stomach.

---

septic dressing and a firm bandage. Loosen tourniquet every 12 to 20 minutes. Re-tighten if bleeding has not stopped.

h., accidental. OB. AND GYN: H. caused by premature rupture of the placenta. SEE: *ablatio placentae.*

h., antepartum. Hemorrhage appearing before the onset of labor.

h., armpit. Place sterile gauze sponge into wound; apply pressure over pad and bandage over shoulder and under armpit. Also bandage under opposite armpit over shoulder already bandaged.

h., armpit and elbow (between). Insert sterile gauze sponge into wound and apply pressure over pad; or tourniquet.

h., arterial. In arterial bleeding (red) the blood ordinarily comes through in waves or spurts, unless the torn artery is deep or buried, when the flow may be steady.
F. A. TREATMENT: It is usually necessary: (1) To make pressure along the course of artery, somewhere between heart and bleeding point, by means of fingers (digital pressure) on the pressure points. (2) Then by a tourniquet above the point of injury. (3) Elevate the part. (4) Apply an antiseptic. (5) A sterile dressing. (6) A *firm* bandage. (7) Gradually release tourniquet after 12 to 15 minutes; if bleeding, retighten. *Do not give* stimulants until bleeding is controlled.

h., capillary. Bleeding from minute blood vessels, present in all bleeding; when large vessels are not injured they may be controlled by simple elevation and pressure as with sterile compress.
TREATMENT: Astringents, styptic. Best is simply dry compress applied with pressure.

h., carotid artery. Usually accompanied by bleeding from the jugular veins and may be fatal in a short time.
F. A. TREATMENT: Compression with the thumbs transversely across the neck, both above and below the wound, the fingers directed around the back of the neck to aid in compression. It may be more desirable to pack the wound with sterile gauze and compress it with the

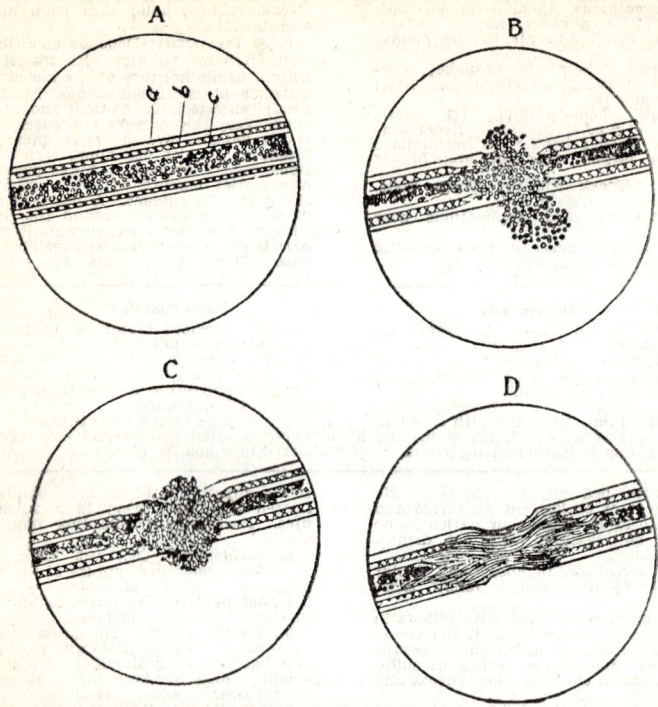

ARREST OF HEMORRHAGE

Temporary and permanent, diagrammatic. A, Normal small artery: a, outer coat, adventitia; b, middle coat, muscular; c, inner coat, intima. B, Artery torn across. Retraction of middle and inner coats; contraction of muscular coat. C, Clotting of blood outside and inside the vessel; temporary arrest. D, Obliteration of the lumen of the vessel with fibrous tissue; permanent arrest.

closed fist. Wounds of the jugular vein are sometimes the cause of air embolism.

h., cerebral. Escape of blood into tissues of brain.

ETIOL: hypertension, arteriosclerosis, or atherosclerosis, infections.

SYM: Unconsciousness, slow pulse, stertorous breathing; hemiplegia, death. May be speech disturbance, incontinence of bladder and rectum, or constipation according to location of damaged brain tissue.

TREATMENT: Ice bag over head and heat at feet.

h., consecutive. Some time after an injury, 20 to 24 hours after an operation.

TREATMENT: Compress applied to main artery and wound. Elevate parts. Reopen and tie bleeding vessels.

h., contact. Hemorrhage from the cervix uteri coming on as a result of exertion, or contact during coitus, douching, or instrumentation.

h., elbow and hand (bet.). Put pad in elbow, apply bandage over it as a tourniquet.

h. of foot. Apply pad and pressure and bandage.

h. of hand. Fill hand with sterile gauze sponge, clasp fingers around it and bandage; apply bandage just above elbow.

h. of knee. At the knee, or below, apply pad as stated with pressure, or put a pad under knee and bandage leg at that place.

h., lung. Blood bright red and frothy, frequently coughed up.

TREATMENT: Rest in cool bed, shoulders and head raised. Small pieces of ice to swallow.

h., pancreas. H. of dark blood in vomitus with slimy mucus, coming from pancreas, usually occurring in inflammation of pancreas. SEE: *hemorrhagic pancreatitis.*

h., peticial. H. in form of small rounded spots of petecia occurring in the skin or mucous membranes.

h., postmenopausal. Bleeding from the vagina after the menopause has been established.

h., postpartum. SEE: *uterine h.*

h., primary. Immediately following any trauma.

h., secondary. H. occurring some time after primary h. It may occur after twenty-four hrs. or at time of separation of ligature, usually between 7th and 10th day. Due to sepsis.

h., stomach. Blood dark, perhaps clotted or mixed with stomach contents, usually vomited.

TREATMENT: Ice to swallow, and ice

cracked and placed in towel over pit of stomach.

h., thigh. Upper part near groin. Insert pad of iodoform gauze into wound and apply pressure or press thumb in center of fold of groin against bone until bleeding stops below groin. Pad as above or tourniquet with pad under.

h., typhoid. It occurs in about 7% of cases. Loss may be 1 quart. It may occur singly or in succession, the latter being more serious than large hemorrhages. They take place at the end of the 2nd week and during the 3rd week of the disease.

h., unavoidable. Ceaseless, painless bleeding. SEE: *placenta previa*.

h., uterine. One into cavity of uterus. ETIOL: Common causes are (1) trauma, (2) congenital abnormalities, (3) pathological processes, such as tumors, (4) infections, esp., of alimentary, respiratory, and genitourinary tracts, (5) generalized vascular disorders such as various purpuras and (6) coagulation defects.

TREATMENT: A wet, sterile packing is used by some but condemned by others. A retained placenta, when present and causing hemorrhage, should be removed with uterine forceps. A relaxed uterus may need a hypodermic injection of pituitrin. The patient may probably need transfusion.

There are 3 varieties:

Essential uterine h. H. occurring in connection with pelvic, uterine, or cervical diseases. SYN: *metropathia haemorrhagica*. SEE: *fibrosis uteri*.

Intrapartum h.: Hemorrhage coming on during labor.

Postpartum h.: Occurring after 3rd stage of labor. Due to inversion, rupture, lacerations, relaxation of the uterus and hematoma. Mortality in cases due to rupture, 60% to 85%.

TREATMENT: Lower head, elevate hips, grasp uterus with hand and make firm compression; follow this with copious injections of hot water (110° to 120° F.).

h., venous. Characterized by steady, profuse bleeding of rather dark blood.

F. A. TREATMENT: Elevate the part, apply an antiseptic about injury, a sterile dressing and make pressure. Elevation and pressure control most venous bleeding. Tourniquets rarely essential. If the bleeding is very severe, may be necessary to compress arteries supplying the part.

GENERAL TREATMENT: Depends upon part affected.

1. Lower blood pressure by keeping patient quiet. Avoid worry and stimulants. Small drinks of cold water if bleeding is not internal.
2. Elevate bleeding part if possible.
3. Apply cold to contract blood vessels.
4. If external, apply pressure in *arterial* bleeding bet. wound and heart (above bleeding point); in *venous* bleeding, pressure over wound in slight cases; below it in more serious ones, and farthest from heart. In capillary bleeding, pressure over part.
5. Have hypodermic of morphia ready for doctor in severe internal bleeding.
6. Watch for shock.

Subsequent treatment designed to maintain low blood pressure.

h., vicarious. H. from a part due to suppression in another part. SEE: *vicarious menstruation*.

hemorrhage, words pert. to: aerteriversion, angiostrophy, anthemorrhagic, atopomenorrhea, autotransfusion, bleeding, bloody weeping, cephalin, chemise, clotting, coagulation, -time, enterorrhagia, hematorrhea, hemophilia, oxalic acid, rhinorrhagia, unavoidable h., Werlhoff's disease, wound.

hemorrhagenic (hem-o-rǎ-jen'ik) [G. *aima*, blood, + *rēgnunai*, to burst forth, + *gennan*, to form]. Producing hemorrhage.

hemorrhagic (hem-or-aj'ik) [" + *rēgnunai*, to burst forth]. Pert. to or marked by hemorrhage.

h. disease of the newborn. Due to inadequate supply of prothrombin received from mother or delay in establishment of bacterial flora of intestine which produces vitamin K. Adm. of vit. K. corrects the condition.

h. fever. Condition peculiar of NE Asia which occurred among United Nations forces from 1951 on. Characterized by prostration, anorexia, vomiting, and petecial hemorrhages. Etiology unknown.

hemorrha'gin [G. *aima*, blood, + *regnunai*, to burst forth]. SYN: *endotheliolysin*. A cytolysin present in venom of snakes and other toxins responsible for hemorrhages and effusion of blood by effecting solvent action upon capillary endothelium.

h. unit. Quantity of venom needed to produce vascular hemorrhage in 3-day-old chick embryos.

hemorrhagiparous (hem-o-rǎ-jip'ǎ-rus) [" + " + L. *parēre*, to produce]. Producing hemorrhage. SYN: *hemorrhagenic*.

hemorrhea (hem-or-e'ǎ) [" + *roia*, flow]. Hemorrhage.

hemorrhoid (hem'o-roid) [G. *aimorrois*, vein liable to discharge blood]. A tumor in form of dilated blood vessels in the anal region. SEE: *hemorrhoidectomy, piles*.

h., external. Cutaneous and thrombotic, outside the sphincter.

TREATMENT: Sitz baths; hot or cold applications; petrolatum; or surgical treatment.

h., internal. Venous, arterial and capillary, within the sphincter but beneath the mucous membrane.

TREATMENT: Local applications of heat or cold. Laxatives. Rest in bed. Operation, ligature, injection, ointment, excision, crushing, clamp, and cautery.

hemorrhoidal (hem-o-roy'dal) [G. *aimorrois*, veins liable to discharge blood]. 1. Rel. to hemorrhoids. 2. Pert. to certain anal arteries, *arteria hemorrhoidalis*.

hemorrhoidectomy (hem-o-roi-dek'to-mī) [" + *ektomē*, excision]. Surgical excision of hemorrhoids.*

DRESSING, etc.: Petrolatum, gauze, sponges, gauze strips 3 and 8 in. wide, cotton and T bandages, 6 towels, leg holders, Thiersch's solution for irrigation, gynecologic suit, Dudley or Kelly's pad.

NP: *Preoperative*: The patient is placed in lithotomy position. A towel, wet with antiseptic solution, is placed over external genitalia. The operating field is thoroughly scrubbed with soap and water and flushed with an iodine solution of 3% strength. The patient is draped with leggings; lithotomy sheet.

Postoperative: Knees tied together until anesthetic is worn off. Head and shoulders elevated on pillows. Keep weight off buttocks. Retard bowel action 3-5 days. Cool fluids; avoid foods stimulating peristalsis. Swab margin of anus with 2% cocaine before stool. Bathe

hemosalpinx   H-27   **hepatic amebiasis**

after with an antiseptic and renew dressing. After a week give daily bath. Inspect dressing carefully. Repack as necessary. Re-dress 2nd day with petrolatum gauze or dry dressing. Watch for retention of urine and possibility of hemorrhage.

hemosal'pinx [G. *aima*, blood, + *salpigx*, tube]. Blood accumulated in an oviduct. SYN: *hematosalpinx*.

he″mosid′erin. An iron-containing pigment derived from hemoglobin from disintegration of red blood cells.

he″mosidero′sis. Condition characterized by the deposition, esp. in liver and spleen, of hemosiderin. Occurs in diseases in which there is marked red cell destruction such as hemolytic anemia and malaria. Hemosiderin may be deposited in pulmonary lymphatics in congenital and rheumatic heart disease.

hemosozic (hem-o-so′zĭk) [" + *sozein*, to save]. 1. Protective of blood corpuscles. 2. Rel. to an antiserum (*antihemolysin*) that prevents hemolysis.

hemospasia (hem-os-pa′zĭ-ă) [" + *spacin*, to draw]. Withdrawal of blood by cupping or leeching.

hemosper′mia [" + *sperma*, seed]. Bloody semen. SYN: *hematospermia*.

hemosta′sia, hemos′tasis [" + *stasis*, a stopping]. 1. Arrest of bleeding or of circulation. 2. Stagnation of blood.

hem′ostat [" + *statikos*, standing]. 1. Device or medicine which arrests the flow of blood. 2. Compressor for controlling hemorrhage of the tonsils.

hemostatic (hem-o-stat′ĭk) [" + *statikos*, standing]. 1. Checking hemorrhage. 2. Any substance which checks bleeding without being directly applied to the bleeding areas. EX: *calcium lactate, ergot, whole blood*.

hemostyp′tic [" + *styptikos*, astringent]. An astringent that stops bleeding; chemically hemostatic.

hemotachometer (hem-o-tak-om′et-er) [" + *tachos*, swiftness, + *metron*, measure]. Device for measuring velocity of the blood.

hemotherapeu′tics [" + *therapeutikē*, medical practice]. The use of blood, by transfusion or otherwise, in treatment of disease.

hemother′apy [" + *therapeia*, treatment]. Blood transfusion or drinking as a therapeutic measure. SYN: *hemotherapeutics*.

hemothorax (hem-o-tho′raks) [" + *thōrax*, chest]. Bloody fluid in the pleural cavity caused by rupture of small blood vessels, due to inflammation of the lungs in pneumonia, or to pulmonary tuberculosis, or to a malignant growth.

hemothy′mia [" + *thymos*, anger]. An irresistible impulse to murder.

hemoto′nia [" + *tonos*, tension]. The tension of the solid elements of the blood.

hemotox′in [" + *toxikon*, poison]. A toxin destructive of red blood cells. SYN: *hemolysin*.

hemotrip′sia [" + *tripsis*, a rubbing]. Hemorrhage in 1 part that induces hemorrhage in another part.

hemotrophic (hĕm-ō-trŏf′ĭk). Pertaining to nutrient substances carried in the blood.

   h. nutrition. Nutrition of the fetus by substances in the maternal blood which pass to the blood of the fetus through vessels within the villi.

hemotropic (hē-mō-trŏf′ĭk). Attracted to or having an affinity for blood or blood cells.

hemotym′panum [" + *tympanon*, drum]. Blood in the middle ear.

hem′ozin. A dark pigment found within malarial organisms (plasmodia). It is derived from the disintegration of hemoglobin.

hem′ozoon. A hematozoon, *q.v.*

henbane (hen′bān). SYN: *Hyoscyamus, q.v.*

Henle's ampul′la. A vas deferens dilatation just above the ejaculatory duct.

   H.'s layer. Outer layer of cells of inner root sheath of hair follicle.

   H.'s loop. A U-shaped portion of a renal tubule lying between the proximal and distal convoluted portions. Consists of a thin descending limb and a thicker ascending limb.

   H.'s membrane. Bruch's layer forming inner boundary of the choroid.

   H.'s sheath. SYN: *endoneurium*. Connective tissue support of individual nerve fibers in a funiculus.

He′noch's angina. Form of angina with gangrenous patches found in mucosa of air passages in scarlet fever and diphtheria. SYN: *necrotic angina*.

   H.'s purpura. Purpura with intestinal disturbances. Infectious disease of children.

   SYM: Erythema, urticaria, purpura, gastroenteric disorders, and perhaps arthritis.   [inductance.

henry (hĕn′rē). Unit designating electrical

Hensen's cells. Tall columnar cells which form the outer border cells of the organ of Corti of the cochlea.

   H.'s disk. Band in center of the A disk of a sarcomere of striated muscle. During contraction it appears lighter than the remaining portion and in its center, a dark stripe, the M stripe, is seen.

   H.'s stripe. A dark band on the under surface of the tectorial membrane.

he′par [G. *ēpar*, liver]. The liver, *q.v.*

heparin (hĕp′ă-rĭn) [G. *ēpar*, liver]. A mucoitin polysulfuric acid which has been isolated from the liver, lung, and other tissues. It is produced by the mast cells of the liver and by basophil leukocytes. It inhibits coagulation by preventing conversion of prothrombin to thrombin by forming an antithrombin, and by preventing liberation of thromboplastin from blood platelets. The action of heparin requires the presence of a co-factor found in serum albumin of the plasma.

   USES: In prevention and treatment of thrombosis and embolism. Sometimes employed concurrently with *dicumarol, q.v.*

   RS: *dicumarol, menadione sodium bisulfite, vitamin K.*

hep′arinize [G. *ēpar*, liver]. To inhibit coagulation of blood with heparin.

hepatalgia (hep-at-al′jĭ-ă) [G. *ēpar, ēpat-*, liver, + *algos*, pain]. Pain in the liver. SYN: *hepatodynia*.

hepatal′gic [" + *algos*, pain]. Pert. to hepatalgia.

hepatatrophia (he-pat-ă-tro′fĭ-ă) [" + *atrophia*, atrophy]. Atrophied condition of the liver.

hepatauxe (hep″at-awk′se) [" + *auxē*, increase]. Enlargement or hypertrophy of the liver.

hepatectomy (hep-ă-tek′to-mĭ) [" + *ektomē*, excision]. Excision of part or all of liver.

hepat′ic [G. *ēpar, ēpat-*, liver]. Pertaining to the liver.

   h. amebiasis. Infection of the liver by *Entameba histolytica* resulting in hepatitis and abscess formation. Usually a sequel to amebic dysentery.

h. duct. The canal that receives bile from the liver. It unites with cystic duct to form the common bile duct.
h. flexure. The right bend of colon under the liver. The junction of the ascending and transverse colon.
h. lobes. Divisions of the liver.
h. veins. The 3 vessels returning blood from the liver and discharging into the inferior vena cava.
h. zones. Venous, arterial, and portal hepatic regions.
hepaticoduodenostomy (he-pat″ĭ-ko-du″-o-de-nos′to-mĭ) [" + L. *duodenum*, duodenum, + G. *stoma*, opening]. Making an artificial opening bet. hepatic duct and duodenum.
hepaticoenterostomy (he-pat″ĭ-ko-en-ter-os′to-mĭ) [" + *enteron*, intestine, + *stoma*, opening]. Operation for artificial opening bet. hepatic duct and intestine.
hepaticogastrostomy (he-pat-ĭ-ko-gas-tros′to-mĭ) [" + *gastēr*, stomach, + *stoma*, opening]. The operation for a passage bet. the hepatic duct and the stomach.
hepaticolithotripsy (he-pat-ĭ-ko-lĭth′o-trĭp-sĭ) [" + *lithos*, stone, + *tripsis*, a crushing]. The crushing of a biliary calculus in the hepatic duct.
hepaticos′tomy [" + *stoma*, opening]. Establishment of permanent fistula into hepatic duct.
hepaticot′omy [" + *tomē*, incision]. Incision into the hepatic duct.
hepatin (hep′at-in) [G. *ēpar*, *ēpat-*, liver]. 1. Carbohydrate formed in the liver, which is changed to dextrose to meet body requirements. SYN: *glycogen*. 2. A hepatic hormone supposed to be useful in reducing high blood pressure. SYN: *hephormone*.
hepatitis (hep-ă-tī′tĭs) [G. *ēpar*, *ēpat*, — liver, + *-itis*, inflammation]. Infectious inflammation of the liver. Children and those under 30 are more apt to have it. Recovery is a matter of two months.
SYM: Enlarged and painful liver, nausea, loss of appetite, raised temperature, perhaps rigors. SEE: *icterus, jaundice, liver.*
ETIOL: Virus A. Incubates 10 to 50 days. Virus B. Causes serum hepatitis. Incubates from 2 to 5 months. TREAT: High caloric diet, bed rest and a great amount of food. No alcohol. Gamma globulin for Type A.
h., acute parenchymatous. Acute yellow atrophy of liver.
h., amebic. Hepatic amebiasis, *q.v.*
h., chronic interstitial. Cirrhosis of liver.
h., epidemic. H. caused by a filtrable virus characterized by parenchymal lesions of the liver. Occurs in epidemic or endemic form. Occurs in two forms (1) *homologous serum hepatitis* caused by parenteral introduction of the virus and (2) *infectious hepatitis* resulting from ingestion of the virus in contaminated food or water. Also called *infective jaundice, epidemic jaundice.*
h. externa. Perihepatitis.
h., homologous serum. Infectious or epidemic hepatitis, *q.v.*; hepatitis resulting from transfusion of blood, serum, or plasma containing the causative virus.
h., infectious. Epidemic hepatis, *q.v.*
h., virus. Epidemic hepatitis, *q.v.*
hepatiza′tion [G. *ēpar*, *ēpat-*, liver]. The 2nd and 3rd stages in consolidation in lobar pneumonia, the tissue changing into a liverlike substance.

FIRST STAGE: *Red h.* exudate tinged with blood.
SECOND STAGE: *Gray, yellowish, or mottled h.* Preceding degeneration of the exudate.
THIRD AND FINAL STAGE: *Yellow h.* Exudate becomes purulent.
hepato- [G.]. Prefix: The liver.
hepatocele (he-pat′o-sēl) [G. *ēpar*, *ēpat-*, liver, + *kēlē*, hernia]. Hernia of the liver.
hepatocholangiocystoduodenostomy (hep″-at-o-ko-lan″jĭ-o-sis″to-du-o-de-nos′to-mĭ) [" + *cholē*, bile, + *aggeion*, vessel, + *kystis*, bladder, + L. *duodenum* + G. *stoma*, opening]. Establishment of drainage of bile ducts into the duodenum through the gallbladder.
hepatocholangioduodenostomy (hep″at-o-ko-lan″jĭ-o-du-o-de-nos′to-mĭ) [" + " + L. *duodenum* + G. *stoma*, opening]. Establishment of drainage of bile ducts into the duodenum.
hepatocholangioenterostomy (hep″at-o-ko-lan″jĭ-o-en-ter-os′to-mĭ) [" + " + " + *enteron*, intestine, + *stoma*, opening]. Establishment of a passage bet. the liver and intestine.
hepatocholangiogastrostomy (hep″at-o-ko-lan″jĭ-o-gas-tros′to-mĭ) [" + " + " + *gastēr*, belly, + *stoma*, opening]. Establishment of drainage of bile ducts into the stomach.
hepatocholangiostomy (hep″at-o-ko-lan-jĭ-os′to-mĭ) [" + " + " + *stoma*, opening]. Establishment of free drainage by opening into the gall duct.
hepatocirrhosis (hep-ă-to-sĭ-ro′sis) [" + *kirros*, tawny, + *ōsis*]. Cirrhosis of liver.
hepatocol′ic [" + *kōlon*, colon]. Rel. to both liver and colon.
hepatocys′tic [" + *kystis*, bladder]. Rel. to the liver and gallbladder, or the gallbladder.
hepatoduodenos′tomy [" + L. *duodenum* + G. *stoma*, opening]. Establishment of an opening from the liver into the duodenum. SYN: *hepaticoduodenostomy.*
hepatodynia (hep-at-o-din′ĭ-ă) [" + *odynē*, pain]. Pain in the liver.
hepatodys′entery [" + *dys*, painful, + *enteron*, intestine]. Inflammation of the liver causing dysentery.
hepatoenter′ic [" + *enteron*, intestine]. Rel. to the liver and intestines.
hepatogas′tric [" + *gastēr*, belly]. Rel. to the liver and stomach.
hepatogenic (hep-ă-to-jen′ĭk) [" + *gennan*, to produce]. Having its origin in the liver.
hepatogenous (hep-a-toj′en-us) [" + *gennan*, to produce]. Originating in the liver.
hepatog′raphy [G. *ēpar*, *ēpat-*, liver, + *graphein*, to write). 1. Treatise on human liver. 2. Roentgenography of the liver.
hepatohemia (hep″ă-to-he′mĭ-ă) [" + *aima*, blood]. Liver congestion.
hep′atoid [G. *ēpar*, *ēpat-*, liver, + *eidos*, form]. Having the structural form of the liver.
hepatolentic′ular [" + L. *lenticula*, lentil, lens]. Rel. to lenticular nucleus and the liver.
h. degeneration. Progressive lenticular degeneration in cirrhosis of the liver. SYN: *Wilson's disease.*
hepatolith (hep′at-o-lĭth) [" + *lithos*, stone]. A biliary concretion in the liver.
hepatolithiasis (hep-a-to-lĭth-ī′a-sis) [" + *lithos*, stone]. Calculi or concretions in the liver.
hepatol′ogist [" + *logos*, study]. A specialist in diseases of the liver.

hepatolysin (hep-ă-tol'ĭ-sin) [" + *lysis*, dissolution]. A cytolysin destructive to hepatic cells.

hepatol'ysis [" + *lysis*, dissolution]. Liver cell destruction.

hepatolyt'ic [" + *lysis*, dissolution]. Destructive to tissues of the liver.

hepatoma (hep-ă-to'mă) [" + *ōma*, tumor]. A tumor of the liver.

hepatomalacia (hep"a-to-mal-a'sĭ-ă) [" + *malakia*, softening]. Softening of the liver.

hepatomegaly (hē-pă-to-meg'ă-lĭ) [" + *megas*, large]. Enlargement of the liver.

hepatomelanosis (hep"ă-to-mel-an-o'sis) [" + *melas*, black, + *-ōsis*]. Pigmented deposits or melanosis in the liver.

hepatonephri'tis [" + *nephros*, kidney, + *-itis*, inflammation]. Inflammation of both liver and kidneys.

hepatonephromegaly (hep"ă-to-nef"ro-meg'ă-lĭ) [" + " + *megas*, large]. Hypertrophy of both liver and kidney or kidneys.

h. glycogenica. Von Gierke's disease, characterized by hypertrophy of liver and excess accumulation of glycogen resulting from failure of glycogenolysis to occur.

hepatopathy (hep-a-top'ă-thĭ) [" + *pathos*, disease]. Disease of the liver.

hepatoperitonitis (hep"ă-to-per"ĭ-to-ni'tis) [" + *peritonaion*, peritoneum, + *-itis*, inflammation]. Inflammation of the peritoneal covering of the liver. Syn: *perihepatitis.*

hep'atopexy [G. *ēpar, ēpat-*, liver, + *pēxis*, fixation]. Fixation of a movable liver to abdominal wall.

hepatophag(e (hep'ă-to-făj) [" + *phagein*, to eat]. A phagocyte that attacks liver cells.

hep"atopto'sia, hepatopto'sis [" + *ptōsis*, a dropping]. Downward displacement of the liver.

hep"atopul'monary [" + L. *pulmō*, lung]. Rel. to both liver and lungs.

hepatore'nal [" + L. *rēn*, kidney]. Pert. to both liver and kidneys.

hepatorrhaphy (hep-a-tor'ă-fĭ) [" + *raphē*, suture]. The suturing of a wound of the liver.

hepatorrhea (hep-at-o-re'ă) [" + *roia*, flow]. 1. Bilious diarrhea. 2. Morbid flow from the liver.

hepatorrhex'is [" + *rēxis*, rupture]. Rupture of the liver.

hepatos'copy [" + *skopein*, to examine]. Inspection of the liver.

heptose. Any sugar containing seven carbon atoms in its molecule.

hepatospleni'tis [" + *splēn*, spleen, + *-itis*, inflammation]. Inflamed condition of both liver and spleen.

hepatosplenomegaly (hep"ă-to-sple"no-meg'ă-lĭ) [" + " + *megas*, large]. Enlargement of both liver and spleen.

hepatostomy (hep-a-tos'to-mĭ) [" + *stoma*, opening]. The making of an artificial fissure into the liver.

hep"atother'apy [" + *therapeia*, treatment]. 1. Treatment of liver disease. 2. The use of liver or liver extract.

hepatotomy (hep-ă-tot'o-mĭ) [" + *tomē*, incision]. Incision into the liver.

hepatotoxemia (hep"ă-to-toks-e'mĭ-ă) [" + *toxikon*, poison, + *aima*, blood]. Autointoxication due to malfunctioning of the liver.

hepatotox'in [" + *toxikon*, poison]. A cytotoxin specific for liver cells.

hephestic (he-fes'tĭk). Pert. to a blacksmith.

h. hemiplegia, h. spasm. A hemiplegia and spasm of blacksmiths of the others, marked by paresis of arm muscles.

heptachromic (hep"tă-kro'mĭk) [G. *epta*, seven, + *chrōma*, color]. Possessing normal color vision.

hep'tad [" + L. *ad*, to]. Any element with a valency of seven.

heptosu'ri-a [G. *epta*, seven, " + " + G. *ouron*, urine]. Heptose in the urine.

herb [L. *herba*, grass]. A plant with a soft stem containing little wood.

herbiv'orous [" + *vorāre*, to eat]. Vegetarian; living on grasses and herbs.

herd [A.S. *heord*]. Any large aggregation of people or animals.

h. instinct. The urge to remain one of the social group and to conform to social patterns and general opinions. An aversion to excessive individualism.

hered'itary [L. *hereditarius*, an heir]. Transmitted from one's ancestry.

h. ataxia. Hereditary spinal ataxia.* Syn: *Friedreich's ataxia.*

heredity (hē-rĕd'ĭ-tĭ) [L. *hereditas*, heir]. Innate capacity of an individual to develop traits and characteristics (body size and form, skin and hair color, intellectual capacity, tendency to certain diseases) possessed by its ancestors. Such is dependent upon the presence of genes (hereditary factors or determiners) in the chromosomes of the fertilized ovum from which the individual develops.

RS: *chromosome, gene, genetics, linkage, sex.*

heredo- [L.]. Prefix: *heredity.*

heredoataxi'a [L. *heres, hered-*, heir, + G. *ataxia*, lack of order]. Hereditary spinal ataxia. Syn: *Friedreich's ataxia.*

Hering-Breuer reflex. Reflex inhibition of inspiration resulting from stimulation of pressoreceptors by inflation of the lungs.

Hering's nerves. Afferent nerve fibers leading from carotid sinus via glossopharyngeal nerve to the brain. They are pressoreceptor nerves responding to changes in blood pressure which reflexly control heart rate. An increase in pressure diminishes heart rate.

Her'ing's theory. A theory of color vision in which it is assumed that the retina possesses three photochemical substances, which depending on their decomposition or resynthesis, to produce different color sensations by their stimulation of different nerve endings.

heritage (her'ĭt-aj) [L. *heres*, heir]. All the characteristics transmitted by parents to their children.

hermaphrodism (her-maf'ro-dizm). Hermaphroditism, *q.v.*

hermaphrodite (her-maf'ro-dĭt) [G. *Hermaphroditos*, son of Hermes and Aphrodite, who was man and woman combined]. One possessing genital and sexual characteristics of both sexes. Syn: *androgyne.*

The clitoris is usually enlarged, resembling the penis of the male.

RS: *gynandroid, gynandromorphous, gynandry.*

hermaph'roditism (G. *Hermaphroditos*, son of Hermes and Aphrodite, who was man and woman combined, + *ismos*, state of). Syn: *hermaphrodism.* Condition in which both ovarian and testicular tissue exist in the same individual. Occurs rarely in humans.

h., complex. Having internal and external organs of both sexes.

h., dimidiate. Lateral h. *q.v.*

h., false. Pseudohermaphroditism; possession of the sex glands of one sex (ovary or testis) but accompanied by secondary sexual characteristics and external genitalia of the opposite sex.

h., lateral. Possession of a testis on one side and an ovary on the other.
h., spurious. False hermaphroditism.
h., transverse. Having the outward organs indicating 1 sex, and the internal ones the other.
h., true. Double sex.
h., unilateral. H. in which an ovary and a testis or an ovotestis are present on one side and either an ovary or testis present on the other side.
hermet'ic [G. *ermēs*, Hermes]. Airtight.
hermetical (her-met'ik-al) [G. *ērmes*, Hermes]. Airtight.

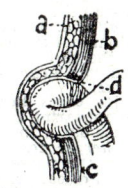

DIAGRAM OF HERNIA

a. Skin and superficial fascia; b. muscular and aponeurotic layer; c, peritoneum; d, neck of the sac.

hernia (hĕr'nĭ-ă). [G. *ernos*, a young shoot]. SYN: *rupture*. The protrusion or projection of an organ or a part of an organ through the wall of the cavity which normally contain it.
ETIOL: Failure of certain normal openings to close during development; weakness resulting from debilitating illness, old age, or injury, prolonged distention as from tumors, pregnancy, or corpulence; increased intraabdominal pressure resulting from lifting heavy loads, or coughing.
TREATMENT: 1. Surgery. 2. Mechanical reduction; taxis. 3. In very large hernias, mechanical devices or trusses may be used.
h., abdominal. H. through the abdominal wall.
h., acquired. H. which develops any time after birth in contrast to one present at birth (congenital hernia). Usually the result of excessive strain on the muscular wall. Frequently occurs following injuries or operations.
h., bladder. Protrusion of the bladder or a part of bladder through normal or abnormal orifice.
h., cerebral. H. of the brain through the cranial wall.
h., Cloquet's. A type of femoral hernia.
h., complete. H. in which sac and its contents have passed through the aperture.
h., concealed. H. that is imperceptible when palpated.
h., congenital. H. existing from birth.
h., crural. SEE: *femoral h.*
h., cystic. Bladder hernia. SYN: *cystocele.*
h. of diaphragm. There are three groups: congenital, acquired or traumatic, and esophageal. In the latter, a portion of the diaphragm is pushed through the esophageal hiatus into the stomach; or h. protruding through the diaphragm.
h. direct. SEE: *inguinal hernia.*
h., diverticular. Protrusion of intestinal congenital diverticulum.
h , encysted. Scrotal protrusion, which, enveloped in its own sac, passes into the tunica vaginalis.

h., epigastric. H. of the intestine through an opening in the midline above the umbilicus.
h., fascial. Protrusion of muscular tissue through its fascial covering.
h., femoral. Descending of intestines besides femoral vessels and through femoral ring.
h., funicular. H. into the umbilical or spermatic cord.
h., hiatus. Protrusion of the stomach upward into the mediastinal cavity through the esophageal hiatus of the diaphragm.
h., Holthouse's. SEE: *inguinocrural h.*
h., incarcerated. H. completely obstructing the bowels.
h., incomplete. H. which has not gone completely through the aperture.
h., indirect. SEE: *inguinal hernia.*
h., inguinal. Protrusion of the hernial sac containing the intestine at the inguinal opening. In *indirect lateral*, or *oblique inguinal hernia,* the sac protrudes through the internal inguinal ring into the inguinal canal often descending into the scrotum; in *direct medial inguinal hernia* the hernial sac protrudes through the abdominal wall in the region of Hesselbach's triangle, a region bounded by the rectus abdominus muscle, inguinal ligament, and inf. epigastric vessels. Inguinal hernia accounts for about 80% of all hernias.
h., inguinocrural. H. which is femoral and inguinal.
h., internal. H. which occurs within the abdominal cavity. May be intraperitoneal or retroperitoneal.
h., interstitial. SYN: *intermuscular hernia.* Form of inguinal hernia in which the hernial sac lies between layers of the abdominal muscles.
h., irreducible. H. which cannot be returned to its original position out of its sac by manual methods.
h., labial. Protrusion of a loop of bowel into the labium majus.
h., lateral. SEE: *inguinal hernia.*
h., lumbar. In lumbar regions or loins.
h., medial. SEE: *inguinal hernia.*
h., mesocolic. H. bet. the layers of the mesocolon.
h., nuckian. H. into canal of Nuck.
h., oblique. SEE: *inguinal hernia.*
h., obturator. H. through the obturator foramen.
h., omental. H. containing a portion of the omentum.
h., ovarian. Presence of an ovary in a hernial sac.
h., phrenic. Projecting through the diaphragm into 1 of the pleural cavities.
h., posterior vaginal. H. of Douglas' sac downward bet. rectum and post. vaginal wall. SYN: *enterocele.* *
h., properitoneal. Protrusion through the peritoneum and into the abdominal wall.
h., reducible. H. which can be replaced by manipulation.
h., retroperitoneal. H. into peritoneal sac extending behind the peritoneum into the iliac fossa.
h., Richter's. H. in which only a portion of wall of intestine protrudes, the main portion of the intestine being excluded from the hernial sac and the lumen remaining open.
h., scrotal. One that descends into the scrotum.
h., strangulated. One so tightly constricted that gangrene results if operation does not relieve. Not reducible by ordinary means.
h., umbilical. Occurring at the navel.

More frequent in women. TREATMENT: Surgical.

h., uterine. Presence of the uterus in the hernial sac.

h., vaginal. Hernial protrusion of the vagina.

h., vaginolabial. Hernia of a viscus into the posterior end of the labium majus.

h., ventral. If stretching and thinning of an abdominal scar occur, pressure from the abdomen may cause protrusion of part of the gut. It is then protected only by a layer of thin scar tissue.

hernia, words pert. to: archocele, Bassini's operation, Beclard's h., bubonocele, cardioclasia, caryorrhexis, cephalocele, ceratocele, cerebroma, herniotomy, liparocele, rupture, strangulated h.

her'nial [G. *ernos*, a young shoot]. Pert. to a hernia.

h. sac. The pouch of peritoneum pushed before a hernia and into which it descends.

her'niated [G. *ernos*, a young shoot]. Having a hernia.

herniation (her-nĭ-a'shun) [G. *ernos*, a young shoot]. Development of a hernia.

her″nioenterot'omy [″ + *enteron*, intestine, + *tomē*, incision]. Herniotomy at same time as enterotomy.

her'nioid [″ + *eidos*, resemblance]. Resembling a hernia.

herniolaparotomy (her″nĭ-o-lap-ă-rot'o-mĭ) [″ + *lapara*, loin, + *tomē*, incision]. Abdominal section for the cure of hernia.

herniol'ogy [″ + *logos*, study]. The science of hernia.

her'nioplasty [″ + *plassein*, to form]. Surgical operation for hernia.

her″niopunc'ture [″ + L. *punctura*, puncture]. Puncture of a hernia with hollow needle for withdrawal of fluid or gas.

herniorrhaphy (her-nĭ-or'ră-fĭ) [″ + *raphē*, for suture]. Surgical operation for hernia.

herniotomy (hēr-nĭ-ŏt'ō-mĭ) [G. *ernos*, a young shoot, + *tomē*, incision]. Cutting for the relief of hernia; an operation for the correction of irreducible hernia, esp. strangulated hernia.

NP: Paint area with iodine, 3½ or 7% as ordered. Place sterile towel over chest and abdomen, place lap ring (small sheet about a yard square, with opening in center) over area of incision. Place regular lap sheet on abdomen and open it. Place 4 towels around area of incision, 2 lengthwise and 2 crosswise.

When the operator is finished with an instrument, discard it into a basin of lysol solution (it may then be removed for resterilization and meanwhile has not contaminated anything). While the skin is being sutured prepare final dressing. The operating nurse washes off her gloves thoroughly before removing them. She then assists in replacing the dressing. In bilateral hernias, each side should be draped and treated as a separate operation.

DRESSING: Borosalicylic acid powder, 4:1, with collodion dressing, sheets, towels, gauze sponges, gauze compresses, safety pins, bandages, cotton, bichloride solution, alcohol, plenty of hot and cold normal saline solution for hands. One pillow under head until otherwise ordered, knee roll under knees, prevent strain on abdominal muscles—assist in turning, etc. The surgeon's requisites vary with the operator.

hero'ic [G. *ērōikos*, pert. to a hero, daring]. Pert. to treatment which, if not successful, increases danger.

heroin (her'o-in). A narcotic derived from morphine, commonly used by addicts.

POISONING: SYM: Resemble those of morphine, but act more markedly on respiration, causing headache, restlessness, cramps, and cyanosis.

TREATMENT: Resembles that of morphine poisoning.

he'roinism [*heroin* + G. *ismos*, condition]. Addiction to habitual use of heroin.

herpangina (her-pan'jĭ-nă) [G. *erpēs*, herpes, + L. *angina*, a choking]. A disease of children marked by fever and small ulcers in the throat.

ETIOL: Thought to be caused by group A Coxsackie viruses.

herpes (her'pez) [G. *erpēs*, herpes]. 1. A form of vesicles appearing in clusters on inflammatory base but with no tendency to rupture; in *herpes zoster* they are distributed along the nerve trunks. 2. Inflammatory skin disease characterized by formation of groups of vesicles. SEE: *tetter, zona.*

h. cincinnatus. Dermatitis herpetiformis, an inflammatory skin disease of a herpetic nature.

h. desquamans. Tinea imbricata, *q.v.*

h. facialis. A form of *h. simplex* which occurs on the face usually about the mouth; commonly called *cold sore.*

h. febrilis. SYN: *h. facialis, q.v.* Fever sores or blisters on the lips.

h. genitalis. Herpetic lesions on the male or female genitalia.

h. iris. Erythema iris; a type of erythema multiforme in which the vesicles occur in concentric rings.

h. labialis. SYN: *h. facialis, q.v.* Fever blister, cold sore, h. of the face.

h. menstrualis. Herpetic lesions seen on the lips at the time of the menstrual period. [genitals.

h. praeputialis. Herpes of the male

h. simplex. So-called fever blisters.

SYM: Occurrence of clusters of vesicles on erythematous edematous base on face or genital regions marked by itching and localized hyperemia, the lesions drying up and shedding yellowish crusts in 10-14 days if unmolested.

ETIOL: A medium-sized virus which is found in early vesicles but usually absent in later pus-filled vesicles. Indigestion, febrile and toxic states, physical fatigue, and emotional disturbances are precipitating factors. The virus apparently lives within the body cells between recurrent manifestations.

h. zoster. SYN: *shingles, zona.* An acute, infectious, inflammatory disease of the skin.

SYM: Usually unilateral.

ETIOL: A large filtrable virus related to that causing chicken pox. Usually, precipitating causes are systemic disease, trauma, exposure to wind or cold, or ingestion or injection of drugs, esp. arsenic.

PATH: The skin vesicles are usually confined to the epidermis accompanied by inflammation of the underlying corium. The nerve, its sensory ganglion and post. horn of the gray matter may show inflammatory reaction.

PROG: Acute course conferring immunity. Hemorrhagic, gangrenous and supraorbital cases are serious.

TREATMENT: Avoidance of temperature changes. Phenacetin, aspirin, sodium salicylate. Antiseptic dusting powder covered with cotton. After crusting, lubricate. Mild galvanic current for neuralgia. Recent successful

herpetic   H-32   **heterograft**

method of treatment has been intramuscular injections of pituitrin. Thiamin chloride (vitamin B₁) has aided materially in helping the lesions clear quickly.

herpet'ic [G. *erpēs*, herpes]. Pert. to herpes. [herpes zoster.
   h. neuralgia. Painful neurosis with
   h. sore throat. Herpetic tonsillitis.

herpet'iform [" + L. *forma*, form]. Resembling herpes.

her'petism [" + *ismos*, state of]. Predisposition to herpetic eruption.

hersage (ār-sazh') [Fr. a harrowing]. Splitting of a nerve trunk into separate fibers.

Herter's infantilism. Celiac disease; a form of infantilism resulting from defective fat and calcium absorption. Resembles sprue in adults.

hertz'ian waves. Electromagnetic vibrations that have wave lengths of a centimeter or longer.

hes'peridin. A derivative of a white glycoside found in ripe and unripe citrus fruits. Decreases capillary fragility and prevents localized hemorrhage.

Hesselbach's hernia (hes'el-bakhs). A lobated hernia which passes through the cribriform fascia.
   H.'s triangle. The triangular space bounded by Poupart's ligament below, ext. border of rectus muscle internally, and epigastric artery ext.

heteradenia (het-er-ad-e'nĭ-ă) [G. *eteros*, other, + *adēn*, gland]. 1. Glandular substance in a part not provided with glands. 2. Abnormal glandular tissue.

heteradenic (het-er-ad-e'nĭk) [" + *adēn*, gland]. Pert. to heteradenia.

heteradenoma (het″er-ad-en-o'mă) (pl. *heteradenomata*) [" + " + *ōma*, tumor]. A heteradenic tissue tumor; any hyaline cylindroma.

heterecious (het-er-e'shus) [" + *oikos*, house]. Living upon different hosts at different stages of development.

heterecism (hĕt″er-ē'sĭzm) [" + *oikos*, house]. Development of different cycles of existence on different hosts, said of certain parasites.

heteresthesia (het-er-es-the'zĭ-ă) [" + *aisthēsis*, sensation]. Variation in degree (plus or minus) of sensory response to cutaneous stimuli.

heteroagglutinin. An agglutinin formed as result of injection of an antigen from an animal of a different species; an agglutinin capable of agglutinating blood cells of other species of animals.

heteroal'bumose [" + L. *albumen*, white of egg]. Albumose insoluble in water but soluble in saline solutions, in acid or alkaline solutions. SYN: *hemialbumose*.

heteroautoplasty (het″er-o-aw'to-plas-tĭ) [" + *autos*, self, + *plassein*, to form]. Grafting skin from 1 person to another.

heteroblas'tic [" + *blastos*, germ]. Having origin in tissue of another kind. Opp. of homoblastic.

heterocel'lular. Composed of different kinds of cells.

heterochiral (hĕt-er-o-kī'răl). Pertaining to the other hand.

het″erochro'matin. A type of chromatin that stains less distinctly than the *euchromatin*, forming clear discs interposed between dark bands on chromosomes. In interphasic nuclei it constitutes the chromocenters. It is thought that it controls certain metabolic activities of cells. SEE: *euchromatin*.

heterochromatosis (het″er-o-kro-ma-to'sis) [" + *chrōma*, color, + *ōsis*]. 1. Pigmentation of skin from foreign substances. 2. Difference in color. SYN: *heterochromia*.

heterochromia (het-er-o-kro'mĭ-ă) [" + *chrōma*, color]. A difference in color.
   h. iridis. Different color of iris in the 2 eyes; the lighter colored iris is atrophic due to previous iridocyclitis, congenital or otherwise.

het″erochrom'osome (hĕt-er-ō-krō'mō-sōm). An allosome; a chromosome which differs from the ordinary chromosomes or autosomes; the X and Y or sex chromosomes. Also called *accessory chromosome*.

heterochromous (het-er-ō-krō'mŭs) [G. *eteros*, other, + *chrōma*, color]. With abnormal difference in coloration.

heterochro'nia [" + *chronos*, time]. Denoting an abnormal time for the occurrence of a phenomenon or production of a structure.

heterochron'ic [" + *chronos*, time]. Occurring at different or at abnormal times.

heterochylia (het-er-o-ki'lĭ-ă) [" + *chylos*, juice]. A change in character of the gastric juice without apparent cause.

heterocinesia (het-er-o-si-ne'sĭ-ă) [" + *kinēsis*, movement]. Movements the reverse of those the patient is instructed to make.

heterocladic. Pertaining to an anastomosis between branches of two different arteries, in contrast to *homocladic*, q.v.

heterocri'sis [" + *krisis*, division]. Irregular crisis with abnormal symptoms.

heterocyclic (het-er-o-si'klĭk) [" + *kyklos*, circle]. Pert. to ring compounds which contain other atoms in addition to carbon atoms as part of the ring.

heteroder'mic [" + *derma*, skin]. Pert. to a method of skin grafting when grafts are taken from another person. SEE: *dermatoheteroplasty*.

het'erodont [" + *odous, odont-*, tooth]. Having teeth of various shapes.

heteroecious (hĕt″er-ē'shŭs) [G. *eteros*, other, + *oikos*, house]. Existing upon different hosts during different phases of development.

heteroecism (hĕt″er-ē'sĭzm) [" + *oikos*, house]. Existence during different phases of development upon different hosts, said of certain parasites.

heteroer'otism [" + *erōs*, love, + *ismos*, state of]. Sexual desire for another person.

het'erogamet'ic. Pertaining to the production of unlike gametes, applied esp. to a male which produces two types of sperm, one containing the X chromosome, the other the Y chromosome.

het″erogam'y. The union of gametes which are dissimilar in size and structure. Occurs in higher plants and animals. SEE: *isogamy*.

heterogeneous (hĕt-er-ō-je'nē-ŭs) [G. *eteros*, other, + *gennos*, type]. Of unlike natures composed of unlike substances. In contrast to homogeneous, q.v.
   h. vaccine. That made from some source other than patient's own organism. Opp. of *autogenous*.

heterogen'esis [G. *eteros*, other, + *genesis*, production]. Alternation of generations; mode of reproduction in which an asexual generation alternates with a sexual generation, or a dioecious generation alternates with a parthenogenetic generation. Occurs in lower forms such as coelenterates and trematodes.

heterogenet'ic [" + *gennan*, to produce]. Rel. to heterogenesis.

het'erograft [" + L. *graphium*, grafting knife]. A graft taken from another individual or an animal of a different

heterography **heterotopy**

species than the one for whom it is intended. SEE: *autograft, isograft.*

heterog'raphy [" + *graphein,* to write]. Writing different words from those the writer intended.

heteroinfec'tion [G. *eteros,* other, + L. *in,* in, + *facere,* to make]. SYN: *exogenous infection.* Infection by virus originating outside of the body.

het'eroinocula'tion [" + " + *oculus,* bud]. Inoculation from other organisms.

heterola'lia [" + *lalia,* babbling]. The use of meaningless words instead of those intended.

heterol'ogous [" + *logos,* relation]. Made up of cell tissue not normal to the part, as certain new growths.

heterol'ogy [G. *eteros,* other, + *logos,* relation]. Difference from the normal in structure or method of growth.

heterolysin (het-er-ol'is-in) [" + *lysis,* solution]. Lysins formed from an antigen from an animal of a different species. SEE: *autolysin, hemolysin.*

heterolysis (het-er-ol'is-is) [" + *lysis,* solution]. Hemolytic action of blood serum of an animal upon corpuscles of another species. SEE: *isolysis.*

heteromeric (het-er-o-mer'ik) [" + *meros,* part]. 1. Pert. to spinal neurons with processes to opposite side of cord. 2. Possessing a different chemical composition.

heterometaplasia (het″er-o-met-ă-pla′zĭ-ă) [" + *meta,* beyond, + *plassein,* to form]. Transformation of tissue to a tissue foreign to the part where produced.

heteromorphous (het-er-o-mor'fus) [" + *morphē,* form]. Deviating from the normal type.

heteronomous (het-er-on'o-mus) [" + *nomos,* law]. Abnormal; differing from type.

heteronymous (het-er-on'ĭ-mus) [" + *onyma,* name]. 1. Expressed in or having different names. 2. On opposite sides.

h. diplopia. Having a false image on same side as the sound eye.

heteroös'teoplasty [" + *osteon,* bone, + *plassein,* to form]. Grafting of bone, esp. with a graft from an animal.

heteropathy (het-er-op'ă-thĭ) [" + *pathos,* disease]. 1. Abnormal reaction to irritation or to stimuli. 2. Creation of a morbid condition to neutralize another disorder.

heterophany (het-er-of'ă-nĭ) [" + *phainein,* to appear]. Having different expressions of the same disorder.

heterophasia (het-er-o-fa'zĭ-ă) [" + *phasis,* speech]. Expression of meaningless words instead of those intended. SYN: *heterolalia, heterophemy.*

heterophe'mia, heteroph'emy [" + *phēmē,* speech]. Expressing 1 thing when another is intended. SYN: *heterolalia, heterophasia.*

heterophil(e (het'er-o-fīl) [" + *philein,* to love]. 1. Pert. to an antibody reacting with other than the specific antigen. 2. Pert. to a tissue or microörganism that takes a stain other than the ordinary one.

heterophonia (het-e-ro-fo'nĭ-ă) [G. *eteros,* other, + *phōnē,* voice]. Change of voice.

heterophoralgia (het-er-o-for-al'jĭ-ă) [" + *phoros,* bearing, + *algos,* pain]. Deviation of 1 eye accompanied by pain.

heteropho'ria [G. *eteros,* other, + *phoros,* bearing]. The tendency of the eyes to deviate from their normal position, esp., when one eye is covered; latent deviation or squint.

ETIOL: Imbalance or insufficiency of ocular muscles.

heterophthalmos (het-er-of-thal'mus) [" + *ophthalmos,* eye]. Difference in appearance of the eyes due to the irides differing in color. SEE: *heterochromia.*

Heterophyes (hĕt-ĕr-ō-fī'ēs). A genus of flukes belonging to the family Heterophyidae, q.v.

H. heterophyes. A species of intestinal fluke commonly infesting man. In heavy infestations may cause diarrhea, nausea, and abdominal discomfort.

heterophyiasis (hĕt-ĕr-ō-fī-ăs'ĭs). Infestation by any fluke belonging to the family *Heterophyidae,* q.v.

Heterophyidae. A family of Trematoda (flukes) which infests the intestines of dogs, cats and other mammals including humans. Infestations are common in Egypt and in the Far East. Includes the genera Heterophyes, Haplorchis, Diorchitrema and Metagonimus. Intermediate hosts are snails, and the cercaria encysting in fishes, esp., mullets, or frogs. The eggs of foreign species may cause serious damage to organs, esp., the heart.

heteroplasia (het-er-o-pla'sĭ-ă) [" + *plassein,* to mold]. Production of a part where it does not belong.

heteroplastic (het-er-o-plas'tĭk) [" + *plassein,* to form]. Rel. to heteroplasia.

het'eroplasty [" + *plassein,* to form]. Grafting with tissue from another person or an animal.

heteroploid. Possessing a chromosome number that is a multiple of the haploid number common for the species.

heteroproteose. An intermediate product formed in the hydrolysis of proteins to peptones.

heteropsia (het-er-op'sĭ-ă) [" + *opsis,* vision]. Inequality of vision in the 2 eyes.

heteroptics. Pervision of vision such as seeing objects that do not exist or misinterpreting what is seen.

heteropyknosis. The property whereby various parts of a chromosome stain with varying degrees of intensity; thought to be due to variations in concentration of nucleic acid.

heteros'copy [" + *skopein,* to examine]. Finding range of vision in strabismus.

heteroserotherapy (het-er-o-se-ro-ther'ă-pĭ) [" + L. *serum,* whey, + G. *therapeia,* treatment]. Treatment by serum from another person.

heterosex'ual [" + L. *sexus,* sex]. Having normal attraction for the opposite sex. SEE: *homosexual.*

het'erosexual'ity [" + L. *sexus,* sex]. The normal state of love for one of the opposite sex.

heterosis. Hybrid vigor; condition in which the offspring of individuals belonging to different races or species possess greater vitality, sturdiness, and resistance to disease, or unfavorable environmental conditions.

heterotax'ia [G. *eteros,* other, + *taxis,* arrangement]. Abnormal position of organs or parts. SEE: *dextrocardia, situs inversum viscerus.*

heteroto'pia [" + *topos,* place]. Displacement of an organ or part.

heterotop'ic [" + *topos,* place]. Misplaced; pert. to heterotopia.

heterotopous (het-er-ot'o-pus) [" + *topos,* place]. Pert. esp. to teratomata consisting of tissues out of normal placement.

heterotopy (het-er-ot'o-pī) [" + *topos,* place]. Displacement of an organ or a portion of the body.

heterotoxin ["+ *toxikon*, poison]. A toxin introduced from without the patient's body.

heterotrans'plant [G. *eteros*, other, + L. *trans*, across, + *plantare*, to plant]. An organ tissue, or structure taken from an animal and grafted into, or on, another animal of a different species. Such transplants usually atrophy.

heterotrichosis (het″er-o-tri-ko'sis) [" + *trichōsis*, growth of hair]. Growth of different kinds or color of hairs on the scalp, or body.

heterotroph (het″er-o-trŏf). An organism which obtains its energy by the oxidation of organic compounds, such as *heterotrophic bacteria*. SEE: *autotrophic*.

heterotro'pia [" + *tropos*, a turn]. Manifest deviation of the eyes due to absence of binocular equilibrium. SEE: *strabismus*.

heterovac'cine [" + L. *vaccinus*, pert. to a cow]. A vaccine from a source other than that of the disease for which it is intended.

heteroxanthine (het″er-o-zan'thin) [" + *xanthos*, yellow]. Methyl xanthine found in the urine.

heterozygosis (hĕt-ēr-ō-zō-gō'sis). Condition in which the two members of a pair of genes in the zygote differ from each other; the result of cross breeding. SEE: *homozygosis*.

heterozygote. An individual in which the members of one or more pairs of genes are unlike.

heterozygous (hĕt-ēr-ō-zī'gŭs). Genetically impure, not breeding true. Having one or many pairs of genes in the phase of heterozygosis resulting from cross-breeding. Having unlike genes. SEE: *homozygons*.

hettocyrtosis (het-o-sir-to'sis) [G. *ēttōn*, less, + *kyrtōsis*, curvature]. A slight curvature of the spine.

Heublein method (hoyb'lĭn). Low voltage doses of x-ray given over the entire body for cancer.

Huebner's disease (hoib'ners). Syphilitic endarteritis of the brain.

heurteloup (hert-loo'). An artificial leech; a cupping apparatus.

hexa- [G.]. Prefix: *Six*.

hexaba'sic [G. *ex*, six, + *basis*, base]. Having 6 replaceable hydrogen atoms.

hexachlorophene (hĕx″ă-klō'rō-fēn). A bacteriocidal and bacteriostatic compound, used in emulsions and soaps for preoperative cleansing of skin and mucous membranes and for hand scrubs. SEE: *phisohex*.

hexachro'mic [" + *chrōma*, color]. Not being able to distinguish more than 6 of the 7 colors of the spectrum or to distinguish violet from indigo.

hexad (heks'ad) [G. *ex*, six]. The atom of an element having a valence of 6.

hexadactylism (hĕks-ă-dăk'tĭl-ĭsm). Possession of six fingers or six toes.

Hexapoda (hek-ă-pŏd'ă). The insects or six-legged arthropods.

hexatomic (hĕks-ă-tŏm'ĭk) [G. *ex*, six, + *atomos*, indivisible]. Pertaining to a compound consisting of six atoms, or a compound having six replacable hydrogen or univalent atoms.

hexavac'cine [" + L. *vaccinus*, pert. to a cow]. A vaccine made from 6 different microörganisms.

hexavalent (hĕks″ă-vă'lĕnt) [G. *ex*, six, + L. *valere*, to have power]. SYN: *sexivalent*. Having a valence of six.

hexokinase. An enzyme present in muscle tissue which catalyzes the phosphorylation of glucose. It has also been isolated from yeast.

hex'one, or **hex'one base** [G. *ex*, six]. One of the amino acids, as histidine, arginine and lysine, so called because they contain chains of 6 carbon atoms.

hexon'ic [G. ex, six]. Rel. to hexone bases.

hexosephosphate (hex-ōs-fŏs'făt) [G. *ex*, six, + *phosphas*, phosphate]. A phosphoric acid ester of glucose. One of several esters (Cori, Robison, *et al.*) formed in the muscles and other tissues in the metabolism of carbohydrates.

hex'oses [G. *ex*, six]. Monosaccharides of the general formula $C_6H_{12}O_6$; the group includes particularly dextrose and levulose, *q.v.*

hexyl-chloro-m-cresol (hĕks″ĭl-klō″rō-mkrĕs'ŏl). New antiseptic effective against staphylococcus and *Streptococcus pyocyaneus*.

Hex'ylresor'cinol solu'tion. S.T. 37. SEE: *caprokol*.

Hey's lig'ament. The semilunar lateral margin (falciform margin) of the fossa ovalis which lies between iliac and pubic portions of the fascia lata.

Hg. SYMB: *mercury (hydrargyrum)*.

HgCl₂. Mercuric chloride; corrosive sublimate.

Hg₂Cl₂. Mercurous chloride; calomel.

HgI₂. Mercuric iodide.

HgO. Mercuric oxide.

HgS. Mercuric sulfide.

HgSO₄. Mercuric sulfate.

hia'tus [L. an opening]. 1. An opening, a foramen. 2. The vulva.

h. aorticus. Opening in diaphragm through which pass the aorta and the thoracic duct.

h. canalis facialis. Opening on superior (ant.) portion of petrous portion of temporal bone. It transmits the great superficial pretrosal nerve and branch of facial and petrosal branch of middle meningeal artery.

h. esophagous. Opening in diaphragm through which passes the esophagus.

h. Fallopii. H. canalis facialis, *q.v.*

h. maxillaris. Opening of maxillary sinus into the nasal cavity, located on nasal surface of maxillary bone.

h. semilunaris. The groove in the external wall of middle meatus of nasal fossa into which the antrum of Highmore, frontal series, and ant. ethmoid cells open.

hiccough, hiccup (hik'up) [probably of imitative origin]. Spasmodic periodic closure of the glottis following spasmodic lowering of the diaphragm, causing a short, sharp, inspiratory cough. SYN: *singultus*.

ETIOL: It may be caused by indigestion, an overloaded stomach, irritation under surface of diaphragm, alcoholism, new growths of the pleura, or certain cerebral lesions, or a hysteria or an influenza. May be due to a disturbance of the phrenic nerve and diaphragm and if prolonged it has serious significance. The time of occurrence and whether accompanied by a burning sensation in the throat, or by an unpleasant sensation, should be noted.

TREATMENT: Warm applications to the diaphragm, protrusion of tongue, holding of breath, drink of water, cold to the spine, are remedies tried successfully in simple cases. Inhibition over the 3rd and 4th cervical vertebrae is sometimes successful. The A.M.A. has reported an almost instantaneous cure by an injection of chlorpromazine.

Hicks' (Braxton) sign. Uterine intermittent contractions at end of 3rd mo. of pregnancy, or in presence of tumor.

hide'bound disease' [A.S. *hyd*, a skin, + *bindan*, to tie up]. Hardening and thickening of the skin with loss of elasticity. SYN: *scleroderma*.

hidradenitis (hi-drad-en-i'tis) [G. *idrōs*, sweat, + *adēn*, gland, + *-itis*, inflammation]. Inflammation of sweat glands by staphylococcus, usually in the axillae.

hidroadenoma (hī-drăd-ē-nō'mă) [G. *idros*, sweat, + *aden*, gland, + *oma*, tumor]. SYN: *syringocystadenoma*. Adenoma of the sweat glands.

hidroa (hi-dro'ă) [G. *idrōs*, sweat]. 1. Vesicles due to retention of sweat. SYN: *sudamina*. 2. Any bullous eruption. SYN: *hydroa*.

hidrocystoma (hi-dro-sis-to'mă) [" + *kystis*, cyst, + *ōma*, tumor]. A cystic tumor of a sweat gland.

hidropoiesis (hī-drō-poy-ē'sĭs) [G. *idros*, sweat, + *poiēsis*, formation]. The formation of sweat.

hidropoiet'ic [" + *poiēsis*, formation]. Pert. to hidropoiesis. SYN: *sudorific*.

hidrorrhea (hi-dro-re'ă) [" + *roia*, flow]. Abnormal sweating.

hidrosadenitis (hi-dros-ad-en-i'tis) [" + *adēn*, gland, + *-itis*, inflammation]. Inflammation of sweat glands. SYN: *hidradenitis*.

hidroschesis (hi-dros'kes-is) [" + *schesis*, a holding]. Retention of perspiration.

hidrosis (hi-dro'sis) [G. *idrōs*, sweat, + *ōsis*]. 1. Formation and excretion of sweat. 2. Excessive sweating.

hidrot'ic. SYN: *diaphoretic, sudorific*. 1. Causing the secretion and excretion of sweat. 2. Any drug or medicine that induces sweating.

hieralgia (hi-er-al'jĭ-ă) [G. *ieron*, sacrum, + *algos*, pain]. Pain in the region of the sacrum.

hierophobia (hī'er-ō-fō-bī'ă). Abnormal fear of sacred things, or persons connected with religion.

high blood pressure. Abnormal pressure in arteries at height of pulse wave.
DIET: Moderate protein d. Fruits, vegetables. Protein allowance for adults, 55-60 Gm. per day. Milk, eggs, no alcohol. Restrict coffee, tea, and tobacco.
TREATMENT: Many drugs and some surgical procedures are used to bring blood pressure to normal.
RS: *blood, blood pressure, hypertension, hypotension, pulse pressure*.

high Calory diet. One that provides maintenance and extra heat and energy. *Indicated:* 1. To prevent loss of weight. 2. In wasting diseases. 3. In high basal metabolism. 4. After long illness. 5. In deficiency caused by anorexia, poverty, poor dietary habits. 6. During lactation when 1000 to 1200 extra Cal. are indicated.
Three meals plus lunch bet. Milk, eggs as under normal conditions, a slight excess of proteins and fats. Fermentable and bulky foods to be avoided.
Breakfast: Three oz. cream, extra butter. *Dinner:* Salad with mayonnaise, extra butter, 3 oz. cream. *Supper:* Same as for dinner. Each in addition to the general diet, with a 10 A. M. and 2:30 P. M. high caloric lunch, and a glass of milk at 8 P. M.

high cellulose diet. The general diet plus the following: *Breakfast:* Bran muffin or a tablespoon of bran added to a cereal, and extra large serving of fruit. 10 A. M.: Fruit juice. *Dinner:* Salad, extra serving of vegetables, fruit. *Supper:* Salad, extra serving of vegetables and fruits.

high frequency treatment. High frequency current passed through the body to produce heat in the tissues. RS: *circuit, current, diathermy*.

High'more, antrum of. The air sinus in the maxillary bone. SEE: *antracele, antrum*.

H.'s body. Fibrous tissue mass, a prolongation of albuginea testis, projecting forward across posterior border of testis. SYN: *mediastinum testis*.

highmori'tis. Inflammation of the maxillary sinus or antrum of Highmore. SYN: *antritis, sinusitis maxillaris*.

hill'ock. A small eminence or projection.
h., anal. One of two small eminences which lie lateral and posterior to the cloacal membrane, and later, the anal fissure in the embryo.
h., axon. SYN: *implantation cone*. A small conical elevation on the cell body of a neuron from which the axon arises. It is devoid of Nissl bodies.
h., seminal. The *colliculus seminalis*, q.v.

Hil'ton's law. The trunk of a nerve which sends branches to a particular muscle; also sends branches to the joint moved by that muscle and to the skin overlying the insertion of the muscle.
H.'s line. A white one at junction of skin of perineum and anal mucosa.
H.'s muscle. The compressor sacculi laryngis muscle.
H.'s sac. Pit along external portion of false vocal cords. SYN: *sacculus laryngis*.

hi'lum, hi'lus [L. a trifle]. 1. Depression or recess at exit or entrance of duct into a gland, or of nerves and vessels into an organ. 2. The root of the lungs at level of 4th and 5th dorsal vertebrae.

himantosis (hi-man-to'sis) [G. *imantōsis*, a long strap]. Abnormal lengthening of the uvula.

hind'brain [A.S. *hindan*, behind, + *bragen*, brain]. The most caudal of the three divisions of the embryonic brain; the *rhombencephalon*. It differentiates into the *metencephalon* which gives rise to the cerebellum and pons and the *myelencephalon*, which gives rise to the medulla oblongata.

hind-gut. The caudal portion of the entodermal tube which develops into the alimentary canal. It gives rise to the ileum, colon, and rectum.

hind kidney. The metanephros, the most caudal of three embronic kidneys. It persists and develops into the permanent kidney. SEE: *metanephros*.

hinge joint. An articulation which permits flexion and extension about a single axis; *ginglymus*.

Hin'ton's test. Agglutination test for syphilis.

hip [A.S. *hype*]. 1. Upper part of thigh, formed by the femur and innominate bones. 2. The region on each side of the pelvis.
h. bone. Os coxa or os innominatum. Its 3 portions are: (a) The ilium (pl. *ilia*); (b) ischium (pl. *ischia*), and (c) pubis (pl. *pubes*).
h., dislocation of. Dislocations of the hip are very often accompanied by a fracture and it is extremely difficult even for a well-trained surgeon to distinguish a pure dislocation from a fracture dislocation without an x-ray.
DIAG: If person has great difficulty in straightening the hip following an accident. It is always accompanied by pain. The knee on the injured side resistantly points inwardly toward the other knee and it is difficult to straighten the leg.
SYM: Pain, rigidity, loss of function, and the dislocation may be obvious by

hip, dislocation of, backward H-36 **hippuric acid**

the abnormal position in which the leg is held, or by seeing or feeling the head of the femur in an abnormal position.
F. A. TREATMENT: Place the patient on a large splint as in a fractured back. In addition, place a large pad, such as a pillow, under the knee of the affected side. Treat for shock.

h., dislocation of, backward. Onto the dorsum ilii or sciatic notch. SYM: 1. Inward rotation of thigh, with flexion, inversion, adduction, shortening. 2. Pain, tenderness. 3. Loss of function and immobility. TREATMENT: (a) Patient anesthetized. (b) Dorsal position, leg flexed on thigh, latter upon abdomen. (c) Adduct thigh, rotate outward; circumduction outwardly across abdomen, back to straight position. (d) Possibly traction, even incision and direct replacement.

h., dislocation of, downward. Rare. TREATMENT: (a) Traction in flexed position. (b) Outward rotation and extension.

h., dislocation of, forward. Through obturator foramen, on pubis, in perineum, or through fractured acetabulum. SYM: 1. Pain, tenderness, and immobility. 2. In pubic and suprapubic forms, shortening; lengthening in obturator and perineal forms. TREATMENT: (a) Hyperextension and direct traction. (b) Flexion, abduction with inward rotations, adduction. SEE: *os coxae*.

hip joint. Articulation bet. femur and innominate bone. A ball and socket (enarthrosis) formed by the head of the femur fitting into a concavity, the acetabulum.

h. j., arthritis of. Usually occurring before age of 14 years. VARIETIES: Arthritic, acetabulum, femoral. SYM: Divided into 3 stages, cardinal symptoms, wasting, spasm, lameness, pain, swelling, deformity. PROG: Influenced by circumstances. Tendency toward recovery. TREATMENT: Tonics, hygiene, mechanical and surgical treatment.

h. j. disease. May be: 1. Tubercular. 2. Pustular (pyogenic). 3. Fracture. 4. Congenital deformities. 5. Dislocation of. 6. Dystrophies of (internal glandular). 7. Perthe-Legge's of. SYM: *General*: 1. Early—pain, limp, muscle spasm. 2. Later—muscle wasting, swelling, deformity. TREATMENT: *General*: Build up patient's general health by: 1. Diets. 2. Fresh air and sunshine. 3. Tonics. *Specific*: Varies with disease. *General to all*: Put on spica plaster cast, surgery or mechanical manipulation.

hip lift (artificial respiration). Following application of the prone-pressure, or Schafer, method, operator leans forward and inserts his clenched fist under one hip, elevating it about 2 inches; then with the other fist under the other hip, it is lifted 4 to 6 inches, producing a rotary motion on the stationary hip. This is alternated with the back-pressure method. This procedure provides more than twice the amount of air in respiration than the prone-pressure method.

hip lift–back pressure (artificial respiration). This method combines alternate lifting of the hips with pressure on the midback (just below the scapulas), with the fingers spread and the thumbs about an inch from the spine. As the operator lifts the hips, he rocks backward; and as he exerts back pressure, he rocks forward. In each phase, he keeps the arms straight, so that the work of lifting and pressing is distributed over the shoulders and back, rather than being imposed primarily on the arms. Active inspiration results from lifting the hips and active expiration from pressure on the midback.

hip roll–back pressure (artificial respiration). This is a modification of the hip lift–back pressure method in which a roll is substituted for the lift in order to increase the ease of performance. The operator kneels astride the prone subject as described for the hip lift; instead of lifting both hips, he uses the knee on which he is kneeling as a fulcrum on which to roll the victim. The operator keeps his arm straight and rolls himself in the same direction in which he rolls the victim. Great care must be exercised to insure that the victim is rolled up onto the operator's knee or thigh so that both hips are raised from the ground.

hippocam'pal [G. *ippokampos*, seahorse]. Pert. to the hippocampus.

h. commissure. SYN: *psalterium* or *lyra*. A thin sheet of fibers passing transversely under post. portion of the corpus callosum. They connect the medial margins of the crura of the fornix.

h. fissure. Fissure above the temporal lobe on mesial surface of cerebrum.

h. formation. Olfactory structures lying along the medial margin of the pallium. It includes the hippocampus, dentate gyrus, supracallosal gyrus, longitudinal striae, subcallosal gyrus, diagonal band of Broca, and hippocampal commissure.

hippocam'pus, ma'jor [G. *ippokampos*, seahorse]. Elevation of floor of inf. horn of lat. ventricle of the brain, occupying nearly all of it.

h., digitations of. Three or four shallow grooves on ant., portion of hippocampus.

h. minor. SYN: *calcaravis*. A small elevation on mesial wall of lat., ventricle formed by end of the calcarine fissure.

Hippocrates (hĭ-pŏk'rā-tēz) [B.C. 460-359 or 377). Greek physician who is referred to as the "father of medicine."

hippocrat'ic fa'cies. The appearance of the face before impending death.
SYM: Dark brown, livid, or lead colored skin; hollow appearance of eyes, collapse of temples, sharpness of nose, lobes of ears contracting and turning outward. SEE: *facial*.

h. oath. Oath exacted of his students by Hippocrates in which they swore to revere him as they would a parent, prescribe for the good of the patient, give no deadly drug, perform no abortions, cut no stones, leaving that work to the stone cutter, act only for the welfare of the patient and keep his secrets, and also to keep themselves from intentional illdoing and seduction.

In part, some of these points are still the accepted standard for the ethical physician today.

hip'pulin(e [G. *ippos*, horse]. An estrogenic substance, obtained from urine of pregnant mares.

hippu'ria [G. *ippos*, horse; + *ouron*, urine]. Large quantities of hippuric acid in the urine.

hippu'ric acid. An acid formed and excreted by the kidneys. It is formed in the human body from the combination of benzoic acid and glycine, the synthesis taking place in the liver and to a limited extent by the kidney. Seven to 15 gr. (0.5 to 1.0 Gm.) is eliminated every 24 hr. It is increased by eating prunes, greengage plums, cranberries, and some vegetables. They increase acidity of the urine, as the hippuric acid remains unburned.

hippur'icase. SYN: *hippurase, histozyme*. An enzyme found in the liver, kidney, and other tissues which catalyzes the synthesis of hippuric acid from benzoic acid and glycine.

hippus (hip'us) [G. *ippos*, horse]. Rhythmical and rapid dilatation and contraction of the pupils. Tremor of iris, spasmodic in character.

    h., respiratory. Dilatation during inspiration, and contraction of pupil during expiration.

Hirschberg's reflex (hĭrsh'bĕrg). Adduction of foot when sole at base of great toe is irritated.

Hirschsprung's disease (hirsh'sprungs). Congenital hypertrophic dilatation of the colon. [Hairy.

hirsute (hĭr-sūt) [L. *hirsutus*, shaggy].

hirsuties (hur-sū'shĭ-ēz) [L. *hirsutus*, shaggy]. Excessive growth of hair.

hirsutism (hur'sūt-ĭsm). Condition characterized by the excessive growth of hair or the presence of hair in unusual places.

hirudicide (hi-ru'dĭs-īd) [L. *hirūdō*, a leech, + *caedere*, to kill]. Any substance that destroys leeches.

hir'udin. A substance present in the secretion of the buccal glands of the leech which prevents coagulation of the blood. It inactivates thrombin.

Hir'udinea. A class of annelida. They are hermaphroditic, lack setae or appendages, and usually possess two suckers. Includes the blood-sucking leeches. A number of species, including *H. medicinalis*, were formerly used extensively for blood-letting.

hir"udini'asis. Infestation by leeches. In *external h.*, leeches attach themselves to the skin and suck blood. After the leeches drop off, bleeding may continue as a result of the action of hirudin. Bites may become infected or ulcerate.

    h. internal. Results from accidental ingestion of leeches in drinking water, which may attach to wall of pharynx, nasal cavity, or larynx.

Hirudo. A genus of leeches belonging to the family Gnathobdellidae.

His, bundle of. The *atrioventricular bundle*, A-V bundle, a group of modified muscle fibers, Purkinje fibers forming a part of the impulse conducting system of the heart. It arises in the atrioventricular node and continues in the interventricular septum as a single bundle, the *crus commune* which divides into two trunks which pass respectively to the right and left ventricles, fine branches passing to all parts of the ventricles. It conducts impulses from the atria to the ventricles which initiate ventricular contraction.

histaffine (his'tă-fēn) [G. *istos*, tissue, + L. *affinis*, having affinity for]. 1. Having affinity for tissues. 2. A hypothetical substance in the blood serum assumed to fix certain constituents of normal and esp. pathological tissues.

histaminase (hĭs-tăm'ĭn-ās). An enzyme widely distributed in the body which inactivates histamine. It is used in the treatment of certain allergies and other conditions resulting from release of excessive quantities of histamine.

histamine (his'ta-mēn). 1. A substance in the body found wherever tissues are damaged. Red flush of a burn is due to the local production of histamine; product of histidine catabolism.

    2. An amine found in almost all animal tissues, and produced by the action of putrefactive bacteria.

Injected under the skin, if the circulation is normal, it produces a wheal surrounded by a flare, suggesting a mosquito bite. Thought to be 1 cause of shock. Given intravenously, causes gastric secretion, flushing of skin, lowered blood pressure, and headache.

    h. cataphoresis. Method of treating rheumatic afflictions in which histamine solution is applied to the skin by the positive pole of the galvanic current.

    h. phosphate. USP. A chemically made product, which may be produced from citric acid by a lengthy process.

USES: Most frequently as a diagnostic agent in determining the acid secreting power of the stomach.

histamine'mia [*histamine* + G. *aima*, blood]. Histamine in the blood.

histamin'ia. Shock induced by histamine in the body.

his'tase [G. *istos*, tissue, + *ase*, enzyme]. An enzyme which digests tissue.

histen'zyme [" + *en*, in, + *zymē*, leaven]. An enzyme in renal tissues which splits up hippuric acid into benzoic acid and glycocol. SYN: *histozyme*.

his'tidase. An enzyme present in the liver which acts on 1-histidine. It splits the imidazole ring with the resultant formation of glutamic and formic acids and ammonia.

histidine (his'tid-ēn). An amino acid, $C_6H_9N_3O_2$, obtained by hydrolysis from tissue proteins and necessary for tissue repair and growth.

his'tiocyte (hĭs'tĭ-ō-sīt) [G. *istos*, web, + *kytos*, cell]. SYN: *macrophage, clasmatocyte, pyrrhol cells, adventitial cells, resting wandering cells*. A cell present in all loose connective tissues. It may exhibit active ameboid movement and show marked phagocytic activity. These cells take up readily substances such as trypan blue, colloidal carbon, and other foreign substances of a particulate nature. Histiocytes belong to the reticuloendothelial system.

histiogenic (his-tĭ-o-jen'ĭk) [" + *gennan*, to form]. Formed by the tissues. SYN: *histogenous*.

his'tioid [" + *eidos*, form]. Resembling or composed of 1 of the body tissues. SYN: *histoid*.

his"tioir'ritative [" + L. *irritāre*, to excite]. Irritative to connective tissue.

histio'ma [" + *ōma*, tumor]. A tissue tumor.

histo- [G.]. Prefix: *Relation to tissue*.

his'toblast [G. *istos*, tissue, + *blastos*, germ]. A tissue cell.

histochromatosis (his"to-kro-mă-to'sis) [" + *chrōma*, color, + *ōsis*]. Name of disorders of reticuloendothelial system.

histoclas'tic [" + *klastos*, breaking]. Decomposing tissue.

histocyte (his'to-sīt) [" + *kytos*, cell]. A tissue cell. SYN: *histoblast*.

histiocytoma. A tumor containing histiocytes.

histocyto'sis [" + " + *ōsis*, intensive]. Histocytes in the blood in unusual numbers.

    h., lipoid. Niemann-Pick disease, *q.v.*

his"todiagno'sis [" + *dia*, through, + *gnōsis*, knowledge]. Diagnosis made from examination of the tissues.

histodial'ysis [" + *dialysis*, a loosening]. Disintegration of tissue. SYN: *histolysis*.

histogenesis (his-to-jen'e-sis) [" + *genesis*, formation]. Development into differentiated tissues of the germ layer; origin and development of tissue.

histogenetic (his-to-jen-et'ik) [" + *genesis*, formation]. Pert. to histogenesis.

histogenous (his-toj'en-us) [" + *gennan*, to form]. Made by the tissues.

histogram (his'to-gram) [" + *gramma*, a writing]. A graph showing frequency distributions.

histog'raphy [" + *graphein*, to write]. A written description of the tissues.

histohem'atin [" + *aima*, blood]. A hemoglobin pigment in various tissues.

histohematogenous (his"to-hem-ă-toj'en-us) [" + " + *gennan*, to form]. Arising from both the tissues and the blood.

histoid (his'toid) [" + *eidos*, form]. 1. Resembling one of the tissues. 2. Developed from a single tissue, as *fibroma*.

histokinesis (his-to-kin-e'sis) [" + *kinēsis*, movement]. Movement through the tissues of the body.

histolog'ical [" + *logos*, knowledge]. Pert. to microscopic tissue anatomy.

histol'ogy [" + *logos*, study]. Study of the microscopic structure of tissue.
 h., normal. Study of healthy tissue.
 h., pathologic. Study of diseased tissue.

histolysis (his-tol'is-is) [" + *lysis*, dissolution]. Disintegration of tissues.

histolyt'ic [" + *lysis*, dissolution]. Pert. to histolysis.

histo'ma [" + *ōma*, tumor]. A tumor composed of tissue. SYN: *histioma*.

his'ton(e [G. *istos*, web]. A class of simple proteins derived from cell nuclei which interferes with coagulation, yielding certain amino acids (the histone or hexone bases) as a result of hydrolysis.
 The thymus histone and globin, or hemoglobin, are the only important ones in foods.

histonec'tomy [G. *istos*, tissue, + *ektomē*, excision]. Periarterial excision of parts of the sympathetic nerve.

histon'omy [" + *nomos*, law]. The law governing development and structure of tissues.

histonu'ria [" + *ouros*, urine]. Excretion of histon in the urine seen in leukemia and certain fevers.

histopathol'ogy [" + *pathos*, disease, + *logos*, study]. Histology of diseased tissues.

histophysiol'ogy [" + *physis*, nature, + *logos*, study]. Study of functions of cells and tissues.

Histoplas'ma. A genus of parasitic fungi.
 H. capsulatim. The causative agent of histoplasmosis, *q.v.*

histoplas'min. An antigen prepared from cultures of *Histoplasma capsulatum* and used as a skin test for the diagnosis of histoplasmosis.

histoplasmo'sis [" + *plasma*, plasma, + *ōsis*]. A disease due to infection by *Histoplasma capsulatum*.
 SYM: Primary infections may be asymptomatic. The respiratory tract is often involved giving rise to pulmonary calcifications which are often mistaken for tubercular calcifications. In severe infections resulting from exposure to massive doses of the fungus such as occurs in closed areas the following symptoms may occur: emaciation, irregular fever, leukopenia and splenomegaly.

historeten'tion [" + L. *rē*, back, + *tenēre*, to hold]. Retention of substances in the tissues.

historrhexis (his-tor-rek'sis) [" + *rēxis*, rupture]. Disintegration of tissue by a noninfectious agent.

histother'apy [" + *therapeia*, treatment]. Administration of animal tissues. SYN: *cytotherapy, organotherapy.*

histothrom'bin [" + *thrombos*, a clot]. A thrombin derived from connective tissue.

histotome (his'to-tōm) [" + *tomē*, incision]. Instrument for cutting tissue for study of its minute structure. SYN: *microtome.*

histotomy (hĭs-tŏt'ō-mī) [G. *ismos*, web, + *tomē*, incision]. SYN: *microtomy.* 1. Dissection of tissue. 2. The cutting of thin sections of tissue for microscopic study.

histotox'ic. Pertaining to a poisonous condition within the cells.
 h. anoxia. Anoxia in which oxidative processes of tissues are depressed or abolished, in cyanide poisoning.

his'totribe [" + *tribein*, to crush]. Instrument for crushing the tissues to stop bleeding.

his'totroph. Nutritive substances other than the mother's blood which the embryo utilizes in early development. These include endometrial tissues which have been destroyed during implantation, extravasated blood, and glandular secretions. SYN: *embryotroph.*

histotrophic (his-to-trof'ik) [" + *trophē*, nourishment]. 1. Pertaining to or favoring the formation of tissue. 2. Pertaining to histotroph, *q.v.*
 h. nutrition. Nutrition of the embryo in which histotroph serves as a source of nourishment. *Cf. hemotrophic nutrition.*

histotrop'ic [" + *tropē*, a turning]. Having attraction for tissue cells, as certain parasites, stains, or chemicals.

histozo'ic. Living within or on tissues, said of certain protozoan parasites.

histozyme (his'to-zīm) [" + *zymē*, leaven]. A renal enzyme which converts hippuric acid into benzoic acid and glycocol, causing fermentation.

histrion'ic [L. *histriō*, an actor]. Theatrical, dramatic.
 h. mania. Dramatic gestures, expressions and speech in certain psychiatric states.
 h. spasm. Facial spasm, tics.

hives [of uncertain origin]. Eruption of very itchy wheals, caused by an allergic substance or food. SYN: *nettle rash, urticaria, q.v.*
 Sudden sharp changes in climate (allergy to heat and cold) may produce hives in some persons.

Hl. Abbr. for *latent hyperopia.*
Hm. Abbr. for *manifest hyperopia.*
HNO$_2$. Symb. for *nitrous acid.*
HNO$_3$. Symb. for *nitric acid.*
HO. Symb. for *holmium.*
H$_2$O. Symb. for *water.*
H$_2$O$_2$. Symb. for *hydrogen peroxide.*

hoarse'ness [A.S. *hās*, harsh]. A rough quality of the voice.
 ETIOL: 1. Simple chronic inflammations, secondary to chronic nasopharyngitis (infected teeth, chemical irritants, tobacco, alcohol, etc.). 2. Specific chronic laryngitis, syphilis, tuberculosis, rhinoscleroma, leprosy. 3. Neoplasms, papilloma, angioma, fibroma, singer's nodes, carcinoma. 4. Paralyses. 5. Prolapse of ventricle of larynx.

hob'nail liv'er. One with irregular surface. ETIOL: Cirrhosis from alcoholism.

Hochsinger's sign (hōk'zing-ers). 1. Indicanuria as a sign of tuberculosis in children. 2. Closure of fist in tetany caused by pressure on inner side of biceps muscle.

Hodara's disease. Trichorrhexis nodosa, *q.v.*

hodegetics (hod″e-jet′iks) [G. *odēgētikos*, suitable for guiding]. Medical ethics and etiquette.

Hodgkin's disease (hoj′kins). A chronic, infectious disease producing enlargement of lymphoid tissue, spleen, and liver, and sometimes kidneys.

SYM: Enlargement of lymph nodes beginning in the cervical region, then the axillary, inguinal, mediastinal and mesenteric. Heart is weak, pressure in various parts, lymphoid infiltration of blood vessels, secondary anemia, presence of eosinophiles, and fibrosis of glands. It may appear in several forms: Acute, localized, latent with relapsing pyrexia, splenomegalic form, lymphogranulomatosis, lymphadenia ossium.

hodoneuromere (hod-o-nu′ro-mēr) [G. *odos*, path, + *neuron*, nerve, + *meros*, part]. Portion of the primitive trunk including neurons and processes.

Hofbauer cell. A large cell found in the connective tissue of chorionic villi. It is thought to be phagocytic.

Hoffman's atrophy. Spinal muscular atrophy, a familial condition which occurs in children.

holarthritis (hol-ar-thri′tis) [″ + *arthron*, joint, + *-itis*, inflammation]. Inflammation of all or many joints. SYN: *polyarthritis*.

Hol′den's line. A wrinkle or indistinct furrow in the groin.

holergasia (hōl′ēr-găs′ĭ-ă) [G. *alos*, whole, + *ergon*, work]. A major psychoses affecting the personality by great excitement, fits of depression, stupor and confusional states.

holergastic (hol′er-gas′tik) [G. *olos*, whole, + *ergon*, work]. Pert. to major psychoses affecting the personality by great excitement, fits of depression, stupor and confusional states.

hol′ism. SYN: *organicism*. Belief or doctrine that the whole is more than the sum of its parts. In biol. the principle may apply to the entire organism, individual organs, or to cells.

holist′ic. Pertaining to holism.

hol′low-back. Ant. post. spinal curvature. SYN: *lordosis*.

Holm′gren's test. Matching colored skeins of yarn for testing color blindness.

holoblas′tic ova [G. *olos*, whole, + *blastos*, germ]. Cleavage with segmentation of the entire yolk. Complete division of the egg as opposed to partial or *meroblastic cleavage*.

holocrine (hol′o-krin) [G. *olos*, whole, + *krinein*, to secrete]. Pert. to a secretory gland or its secretions consisting of altered cells of the same gland. Opp. of *merocrine*, q.v.

holodiastol′ic [″ + *diastellein*, to expand]. Rel. to the entire diastole.

holomastigote (ho-lo-mas′tĭ-gōt) [″ + *mastix, mastig-*, lash]. Having flagella all over the surface.

holorrachischisis (hol-o-ră-kis′ki-sis) [″ + *rachis*, spine, + *schisis*, fissure]. Complete spina bifida.

holosystol′ic [″ + *systellein*, to draw together]. Rel. to the entire systole.

holotetanus (hol-o-tet′an-us) [″ + *tetanos*, tetanus]. General tetanus. SYN: *holotonia*, q.v.

holoto′nia [″ + *tonos*, tension]. Muscular spasm of the entire body. SYN: *holotetanus*.

holoton′ic [″ + *tonos*, tension]. Pert. to or affected by holotonia.

holotrichous (hŏl-ŏt′rĭ-kŭs). Covered entirely with cilia, said of certain protozoa and bacteria.

holozo′ic. Resembling an animal as to its method of nutrition in which organic materials serve as a source of energy.

Holt′house's hernia. Inguinal hernia protruding along folds of the groin.

Holtz static machine. Machine for producing static electricity by induction.

Holzknecht unit (holts′knekt). Abbr. *H*. An x-ray unit of measurement; 1/5 the erythema dose.

homax′ial [G. *omos*, the same, + *axōn*, axis]. Having all axes alike, as a sphere.

homeo- [G.]. Prefix: Likeness or resemblance.

homeomorphous (ho-me-o-mor′fus) [G. *omoios*, like, + *morphē*, form]. Of like shape but not of same composition.

hom″eoös′teoplasty [″ + *osteon*, bone, + *plassein*, to form]. Grafting of a piece of bone like the one upon which it is grafted.

homeopathic (ho-me-o-path′ik) [″ + *pathos*, disease]. Pert. to homeopathy.

homeopathist (ho-me-op′ă-thist) [″ + *pathos*, disease]. One who practices homeopathy.

homeopathy (ho-me-op′ă-thĭ) [″ + *pathos*, disease]. School of medicine founded by Dr. S. C. F. Hahnemann which assumes that such agents cure disease, as in health produce similar symptoms and that the more finely a drug is divided the more potent it becomes.

homeoplasia (ho-me-o-pla′zĭ-ă) [″ + *plassein*, to form]. Formation of new tissue similar to that already existing in a part.

homeoplas′tic [″ + *plassein*, to form]. Rel. to or resembling the structure of adjacent parts.

homeostasis (hō-mē-ōs′tā-sĭs) [G. *omoios*, like, + *stasis*, a standing]. 1. State of equilibrium of the internal environment. 2. The state of relative constancy of the body fluids (blood, lymph, tissue fluid) as to their chemical and physical properties.

homeostat′ic [″ + *statikos*, standing]. Pert. to homeostasis.

homeotherapy (ho″me-o-ther′ă-pī) [″ + *therapeia*, treatment]. Treatment or prevention of disease with a substance similar but not identical with the active causative agent. Ex: *jennerian vaccination*.

homeotransplant (ho″me-o-trans′plant) [″ + L. *trans*, across, + *plantāre*, to plant]. Tissue from one individual transplanted into another.

homeotransplantation (ho″me-o-transplan-ta′shun) [″ + ″ + *plantāre*, to plant]. Tissue transplantation from one to another of the same species.

homergy (hom′er-jĭ) [G. *omos*, same, + *ergon*, work]. Normal metabolism and its results.

homesickness [A.S. *hām*, home, + *seōc*, ill]. Abnormal desire to return home. SYN: *nostalgia*.

Home's lobe (hōm). Median lobe of prostate gland which frequently hypertrophies in older men.

homicide (hom′i-sĭd) [L. *homō*, man, + *caedere*, to cut]. 1. Murder. 2. A murderer.

homiculture (hom′ĭ-kult-chur) [″ + *cultura*, cultivation]. Application of the laws of breeding to the human species. SYN: *eugenics, stirpiculture*.

homo- [G.]. Prefix: Likeness.

homocen′tric [G. *omos*, same, + *kentron*, center]. Having the same center.

  h. rays. Light rays from the same center.

homochronous (hō-mō-krŏn'ŭs). Occurring at the same time, or at the same age in each generation.

homogamet'ic. Producing one kind of gamete as regards the sex chromosome. In humans, the XX female is the homogametic sex as all ova produced contain the X chromosome. SEE: *heterogametic*.

homogeneous (ho-mo-je'ne-us) [" + *genos*, kind]. Uniform in structure, composition or nature.

homogenesis (ho-mo-jen'e-sis) [" + *genesis*, development]. Reproduction of offspring similar to the parents. Opp. of *heterogenesis*.

homogenize (hō-mŏj'en-īz). To make homogeneous; to produce a uniform emulsion or suspension of two substances normally immiscible.

homogentis'ic acid. Alkaptone; an acid in the urine due to incomplete oxidation of tyrosine.

homogeny (ho-moj'en-ĭ) [G. *omos*, same, + *genos*, race]. Reproduction of offspring similar to parents.

homoglandular (ho-mo-glan'du-lar) [" + L *glandula*, a little acorn]. Rel. to the same gland.

homoiopodal (ho-moi-op'o-dal) [G. *omoios*, like, + *pous*, *pod-*, foot]. With only 1 kind of process, as nerve cells.

homolat'eral [G. *omos*, same, + L. *latus*, side]. Pert. to or on the same side. SYN: *ipsilateral.**

homolog, homologue (ho'mo-log) [" + *logos*, relation]. 1. An organ or part common to a number of species. 2. One that corresponds to a part or organ in another structure.

homologous (ho-mŏl'ō-gŭs) [G. *omos*, same, + *logos*, relation]. Similar in fundamental structure and in origin but not necessarily in function: e. g., the arm of man, forelimb of a dog, and the wing of a bird are homologous structures.

 h. organs. Structures which are morphological equivalents as the arm of man and forelimb of quadrupeds; penis of male and clitoris of female. Homologous organs indicate relationship, or descent from a common ancestor.

 h. series. Compounds with a similar chemical structure and properties, arranged in order of their molecular complexity, such as *methane* and *ethane*.

 h. tissues. Those identical in structure.

 h. vaccine. One from the microorganism infecting the patient. SYN: *autogenous vaccine*.

homology (hō-mŏl'ō-jĭ) [G. *omos*, same, + *logos*, relation]). Similarity in structure and in origin.

 h., serial. Anterior-posterior correspondence of parts of an organism which occur in a serial fashion, as the appendage of a crayfish, or the fore- and hind limbs of quadrupeds.

homolysin (hō-mŏl'ĭs-ĭn) [G. *omos*, same, + *lysis*, solution]. SYN: *isolysin*. An agent in a serum destructive of erythrocytes.

homonomous (hō-mŏn'ŏm-ŭs) [G. *omos*, same, + *nomos*, law]. Pertaining to parts arranged in a series which are similar in form and structure as metameres of a segmented animal or the fingers and toes.

homonymous (ho-mon'im-us) [" + *onyma*, name]. Having the same name.

 h. diplopia. D. in which the image seen by the right eye is on the right side and *vice versa*.

homophil (ho'mo-fĭl) [" + *philein*, to love]. Pert. to an antibody reacting only with a specific antigen.

homoplas'tic [" + *plassein*, to form]. Having similar form and structure.

ho'moplasty [" + *plassein*, to form]. Repair by tissue similar to the one replaced.

Homo sapiens. The species to which all races of modern man belong.

homosex'ual [" + L. *sexus*, sex]. 1. An invert, one sexually attracted to another of the same sex. 2. Pert. to attraction to another of same sex.

ho"mosexual'ity [" + L. *sexus*, sex]. A condition in which the libido is directed toward one of the same sex.

homostim'ulant [" + L. *stimulāre*, to arouse]. Stimulating the organ that an extract is derived from.

homotherm'al [G. *omos*, same, + *therma*, heat]. SYN: *warm-blooded*. Condition in which the body temperature is maintained at a fairly constant level regardless of the temperature of the environment.

homotonic (ho-mo-ton'ĭk) [" + *tonos*, tension]. Of uniform tension.

homotype (ho'mo-tīp) [" + *typos*, type]. One organ or part similar in form and function to another, as 1 of 2 paired parts or organs.

homotypic (ho-mo-tip'ĭk) [" + *typos*, type]. Of the same form and type.

homozygote (hō-mō-zī'gŏt). A homozygous individual; an individual developing from like gametes and thus possessing like pairs of genes for any hereditary characteristic.

homozygous (hō-mō-zī'gŭs). 1. Produced by similar gametes. 2. Pure bred. 3. Said of an organism when all germ cells transmit identical genes resulting from inbreeding.

homunculus (hō-mŭn'kŭl-ŭs). A dwarf in which the parts of the body develop in their normal proportions.

hook [A.S. *hōk*, an angle]. A curved instrument.

 h., blunt. One used in extraction of fetus or in embryotomy.

hook-up. Term used in speaking of the method of arranging circuits, appliances and electrodes in the giving of any particular treatment; as, for instance, the hook-up for direct sparks.

hook'worm. A parasitic nematode belonging to the superfamily Strongyloidea, esp., *Ancylostoma duodenale* and *Necator americanus*, q.v.

hook'worm disease. A condition brought about by the presence of the hookworm in the intestinal tract. SYN: *ankylostoma, uncinariasis*.

hoop'ing cough. An acute, infectious disease characterized by a catarrhal stage, followed by a peculiar paroxysmal cough, ending in a prolonged crowing or whooping inspiration. SEE: *pertussis, whooping cough*.

hordeolum (hor-de'o-lum) [L. barleycorn]. Inflammation of a sebaceous gland of the eyelid. SYN: *sty*, q.v.

 h. internum. Suppuration of Zeiss or meibomian glands.

horismascope (hor-ĭz'mă-skŏp) [G. *orizma*, a boundary, + *skopein*, to examine]. A U-shaped tube for an acid test for albumin in the urine.

horizocardia (ho-ri"zo-kar'dĭ-ă) [G. *orizōn*, horizon, + *kardia*, heart]. Horizontal position of the heart on the diaphragm.

horizon'tal posi'tion [G. *orizōn*, horizon]. Lying supine with feet extended. Employed in palpation and auscultation of

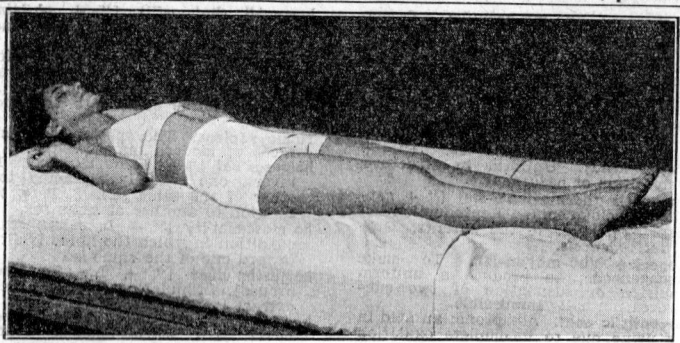

Posed by professional model   *Photo by Whitaker*

HORIZONTAL POSITION

fetal heart beat and in operative procedures.

h. p., abdominal. The patient lies flat on the abdomen with feet extended. Employed in examination of back and spinal column.

hor'mion [G. *ormion*, a little chain]. Junction of post. border of the vomer with the sphenoid bone.

hor'mone [G. *ormanein*, to excite]. 1. A chemical substance originating in an organ, gland, or part, which is conveyed through the blood to another part of the body, stimulating it to increased functional activity, and increased secretion.
Contains amino acids which may be the precursors of hormones.
2. The secretion of the ductless glands, such as insulin, by the pancreas.
They are active in minute quantities and do not supply energy. A hormone that induces an excitatory effect is called an *autocoid*; an inhibitory effect, a *chalone*.

h., adrenocortical. H. secreted by the cortex of the adrenal gland. All are steroids, some twenty eight or more having been isolated from cortical extracts. They fall into three groups (1) *corticoids* which regulate water and salt metabolism, *e. g.*, desoxycortisterone, (2) *cortisteroids* which regulate carbohydrate metabolism (dehydrocorticosterone, cortisterone, 11-hydroxycortisterone, 17-hydroxy-11-dehydrocortisterone, also called Kendall's compound E or cortisone) and (3) *androgenic corticoids*, some of which have a masculinizing effect, others feminizing or progestational effects.

h., adrenocorticotrophic. SYN: *adrenotrophin, corticotrophin, ACTH.* A hormone secreted by the ant., lobe of the hypophysis which stimulates the adrenal cortex.

h., androgenic. SYN: *male sex hormones.* Includes *testosterone, androsterone,* and *dehydroandrosterone.* H. which regulates the development and maintenance of the male secondary sexual characteristics; an androgen, *q.v.* Androgens are secreted by the interstitial tissue of the testis and by the adrenal cortex of both sexes.

h., anterior pituitary. H. secreted by ant. lobe of the hypophysis. Includes the somatotrophic, (SH), thyrotrophic, (TH) gonadotrophic, (folliclestimulating (FSH), interstitial-cell stimulating ICSH, luteotrophic, (LH), lactogenic, and adrenocorticotrophic ACTH hormones.

h., A.P.L. Anterior pituitary-like hormone. A chorionic gonadotrophin secreted by the placenta and found in the urine of pregnant women and serum of pregnant mares. Used in pregnancy tests, *q.v.*

h., chromatophorotropic. Intermedin, *q.v.*

h., corpus luteum. Progestin, *q.v.*

h., corticoadrenal. Adrenocortical hormones, *q.v.*

h., diabetogenic. H. antagonistic to insulin.

h., estrogenic. A hormone which stimulates the development of and maintenance of female sexual characters. As estrogen, *q.v.* Estrogens are secreted by the ovary, the placenta, and the adrenal cortex in both sexes. *Female hormones.* Include estradiol, estrone estriol.

h., follicle, h., follicular. H. secreted by the ovarian follicles; an estrogen.

h., follicle-stimulating. (FSH) . . , H. secreted by the ant., lobe of hypophysis which stimulates development of the ovarian follicles.

h., gastric. Gastrin, *q.v.*

h., gonadotropic. Ant. pituitary h. affecting the gonads. SEE: *folliclestimulating h., interstitial cell-stimulating h., luteinizing h., luteotrophic h.*

h., growth. Ant. pituitary h. promoting normal growth.

h., interstitial cell-stimulating (ICSH). SEE: *luteinizing hormone.*

h., intestinal. A hormone produced by the mucosa of the intestine. SEE: *secretin, cholecystokinin.*

h., lactogenic. SYN: *prolactin, luteotrophin.* Luteotrophic hormone, *q.v.*

h., luteal. SYN: *progesterone, q.v.* H. produced by the corpus luteum.

h., luteinizing. SYN: *interstitial cellstimulating hormone* (ICSH) (LH). H. produced by the ant. lobe of hypophysis which induces ovulation and the formation of the corpus luteum. Also stimulates development of interstitial cells of the testes.

h., luteotrophic. H. produced by ant., lobe of hypophysis which stimulates the secretion of progesterone by the corpus luteum and secretion of milk by the mammary gland.

h., ovarian. A h. produced by the ovary. SEE: *estradiol, estrone, estriol, progesterone.*

h., pancreatic. H. produced by the islets of Langerhans of the pancreas. SEE: *insulin* and *lipocaic.*

h., parathyroid. H. secreted by the parathyroid glands which regulates calcium and phosphorus metabolism. Deficiency results in tetany. SEE: *parathyrin, parathormone*.
h., placental. H. secreted by the placenta. Includes estrogens and chorionic gonadotrophin.
h., post. pituitary. H. secreted by post. lobe of hypophysis. Includes *pitressin*, which produces vasopressor and antidiuretic effects and *ditocin* (oxytocin) which causes contraction of smooth muscles of the uterus.
h.'s, sex, female. Estrogenic hormones, *q.v.*
h.'s, sex, male. Androgenic hormones, *q.v.*
h., testicular. H. produced by the interstitial tissue of the testis, e. g., *testosterone, androsterone*, and *dehydroandrosterone, q.v.*
h., thyroid. H. secreted by the thyroid gland. Among them are three iodine-containing compounds: *thyroglobulin, diiodotyrosine*, and *thyroxin*.
h., thyrotrophic. H. produced by ant. lobe of hypophysis which regulates development and functioning of the thyroid gland.
h., wound. Traumatin.
hormon'ic [G. *ormanein*, to excite]. Rel. to or acting as a hormone. SYN: *hormonal*.
hormonogenesis (hor″mon-o-jen'e-sis) [" + *genesis*, production]. Production of an internal secretion. SYN: *hormonopoiesis*.
hormonogenic (hor″mon-o-jen'ik) [" + *gennan*, to produce]. Producing hormones. SYN: *hormonopoietic*.
hormonol'ogy [" + *logos*, study]. The study of hormones.
hormopoiesis (hor-mo-poi-e'sis) [" + *poiēsis*, formation]. The production of hormones. SYN: *hormonopoiesis*.
hormopoietic (hor-mo-poi-et'ik) [" + *poiēsis*, formation]. Rel. to hormones and their formation. SYN: *hormonopoietic*.
horn. SYN: *cornu*. A cutaneous outgrowth composed chiefly of keratin. A horn-like projection.
h., dorsal. SYN: *posterior column*. Post. projection of gray matter of the spinal cord.
h., ventral. SYN: *anterior column*. Anterior projection of gray matter of the spinal cord.
Hor'ner's syndrome. Anidrosis, enophthalmos, miosis, and ptosis from paralysis of cervical sympathetic nerves.
hor'net sting. Sting by a hornet.
A general urticaria may result from the sting of this insect.
TREATMENT: Remove the stinger; apply tincture of iodine and cold compresses. Weak alkaline solutions are beneficial and subsequent soothing lotions such as zinc oxide or calamine lotion may be used.
hor'ny [A.S. horn]. Resembling or consisting of horn.
h. epithelium. The horny granulations in trachoma of the skin.
h. layer. Horny layer of the skin. SYN: *stratum corneum*.
horopter (hor-op'ter) [G. *oros*, limit, + *optēr*, observer]. Sum of all points in the binocular vision.
horripilation (hor-ĭ-pi-la'shun) [L. *horrēre*, to bristle, + *pilus*, hair]. Goose flesh. SYN: *cutis anserina*.
horse'shoe fis'tula. A fistulous tract in a semicircle in front or behind the anus.
h. kidney. A congenital abnormality. The 2 kidneys are united at their lower poles forming a horseshoe mass generally at a lower level than normal.
hos'pital [L. *hospitalis*, pert. to a guest]. Institution for treatment of the sick and wounded.
h., base. A hospital unit within the lines of an army for reception of wounded and patients from the front, as well as for cases within the line itself.
h., camp. An immobile military unit for care of sick and wounded in camp.
h., cottage. A collection of detached cottages for care of the sick.
h., evacuation. A mobile advance hospital unit to take the place of field hospitals and to supplement base hospitals.
h., field. A portable military hospital beyond the zone of conflict and beyond the dressing stations.
hos'pitalism [L. *hospitalis*, pert. to a guest, + G. *ismos*, state]. 1. Morbid conditions due to lack of ventilation in a hospital. 2. A neurasthenic condition affecting nurses, doctors, and others who spend the greater part of their time in a hospital. 3. Term applied to psychoneurotic condition in which one is a frequent patient of hospitals.
hospitalization. Removal of a patient to and confinement in a hospital.
host [L. *hostis*, a stranger]. 1. The organism from which a parasite obtains its nourishment. 2. In embryology, the larger and relatively normal of conjoined twins. 3. In transplantation of tissue, the individual which receives the graft.
h., accidental. A host other than the usual or normal host.
h., alternate. Intermediate host, *q.v.*
h., definitive. The final host, or host in which the parasite reaches sexual maturity. 2. The vertebrate, when the intermediate host is an invertebrate.
h., final. The definitive host, *q.v.*
h., intermediate. H. in which a parasite passes through its larval or asexual stages of development. The invertebrate host, when final host is a vertebrate.
h., primary. The final host, *q.v.*
h., reservoir. A host other than the usual or normal one in which a parasite is capable of living and serving as a source of infestation.
h., secondary. The intermediate host, *q.v.*
hot. 1. Possessing a high temperature. 2. Actively conducting a current. 3. Contaminated with dangerous radioactive material.
h. flashes. Crises of vasodilation in skin of head, neck, and chest accompanied by sensation of suffocation and sweating. Occurs commonly during menopause.
hot eye. Temporary eye congestion in gout.
Hot'tentot ap'ron. Excessive elongation of the labia minora seen in Hottentot women. SYN: *velamen vulvae*.
H. deformity. Abnormal fatness of the buttocks. SYN: *steatopygia*. [ing.
hot'tentotism. Abnormal form of stutter-
hot water bag. Rubber bag of various shapes and sizes for applying dry heat to circumscribed areas and for keeping moist applications warm.
hourglass contrac'tion. Excessive, irregular contraction of an organ at its center, as the pregnant uterus during 3rd stage of labor.
The placenta is held in upper part of uterus by a tightly constricting band bet. lower and upper uterine segments. SYN: *ectasia*. RS: *labor, stomach*.
h. stomach. Division of stomach (in

house fly   H-43   **humerus**

form of an hourglass) by a muscular constriction; often associated with gastric ulcer.

house fly. *Musca domestica*, a fly belonging to the order Diptera. Serves as a transmitter of organisms of many infectious diseases.

house'maid's knee. A traumatism resulting from kneeling which produces a swelling of the bursa, ant. to the patella.

house physician. The senior interne in a hospital responsible for the orders of the attending physician.

house staff. The internes and externes of a hospital acting under direction of the general staff.

house surgeon. The senior surgical member of the hospital staff who acts for the attending surgeon in his absence.

Houston's muscle (hūs'tonz). The ant. part of the *musculus bulbo-cavernosus*.

    H.'s valves. The folds of mucous membrane or valves formed by them in rectum; supposed to keep feces from entering the anus too rapidly. SYN: *plica transversalis recti*.

Howard's method (artificial respiration) (Benjamin Douglas Howard, American physician, 1840-1900). The patient is placed on his back, with head lower than his abdomen with his hands under his head. Pressure is exerted upon the lower ribs rhythmically every few seconds.

Howell-Jolly bodies. Coarse granules seen in erythrocytes in slides of stained blood. They are thought to be nuclear particles.

Howship's lacunae. Small pits, grooves or depressions found where resorption of bone is occurring. They are usually occupied by osteoclasts, *q.v.*

    H.'s symptom. Paraesthesia, or pain in obturator hernia, on inner side of thigh.

HPO₃. Metaphosphoric acid.
H₃PO₂. Hypophosphorous acid.
H₃PO₃. Orthophosphorous acid.
H₃PO₄. Orthophosphoric acid.
H₄P₂O₆. Hypophosphoric acid.

Hr factors. Structures including *Hr agglutinogens* and *Hr antigens*, on surface of the red blood cells responsible for reactions with *Hr antiserums*. A number of related factors of human blood, so named because of their reciprocal relationship to the Rh factors. Two main factors, Hr' and Hr'' have been identified. The theoretically possible Hr₀ factor has not been found, but instead recently a different factor Hr has been identified. These blood factors are important because sensitization may give rise to dangerous blood transfusion reactions. The baby of a sensitized Hr-negative pregnant woman may develop the blood disease, erythroblastosis fetalis, just as with sensitized Rh-negative mothers.

h.s. Hora somni, bedtime.
H. S. Abbr. for *house surgeon*. [gen.
H₂S. Hydrogen sulfide, sulfureted hydro-
H₂SO₃. Sulfurous acid.
H₂SO₄. Sulfuric acid.

H-substance. A substance similar to or identical with histamine, *q.v.*

Ht. Symb. for *total hyperopia*.

Hub'bard tank. One used for underwater exercises.

Hughes reflex (ūs). Sudden downward movement of penis when the prepuce or gland of a completely relaxed penis is pulled upward.

Húguier's canal (ū-ghe-a'). A canal through which the chorda tympani nerve exits from the cranium.

    H.'s circle. Anastomosis around the isthmus of the uterus.

    H.'s diseases. Lupus of vulva, and uterine fibroma.

    H.'s glands. Two tiny vaginal glands.

Huhner test. One for sterility in the male. SEE: *test*.

hum [of imitative origin]. A soft continuous sound.

    h., venous. Sound from large veins in certain anemias. SYN: *bruit de diable*.

hu'man [L. *humanus*, pert. to man]. Pert. to or characterizing man or mankind.

    h. bite. Wound caused by human teeth.

    SYM: Intense swelling, edema, and foul discharge may develop. The organisms most frequently found in wounds from such bites are a fusiform bacillus, and a spirillum of streptococcus.

    TREATMENT: If lymphangitis, moderate fever, and leukocytosis occur, a wide incision may be necessary with hot wet pack applied to the whole arm or hand that has been injured. Smears should be taken from the drainage. Induration in the palm of the hand may occur. All such victims need the immediate attention of a physician.

humectant. A moistening or diluent agent.

humeral (hu'mer-al) [L. *humerus*, shoulder]. Pert. to the humerus.

humeroradial (hū″mer-o-ra'dĭ-ăl) [" + *radius*, wheel spoke, ray]. Pert. to humerus and radius, esp. in comparison of their length.

humeroulnar (hū″mer-o-ul'năr) [" + *ulna*, forearm]. Pert. to the humerus and ulna, esp. in comparison of their length.

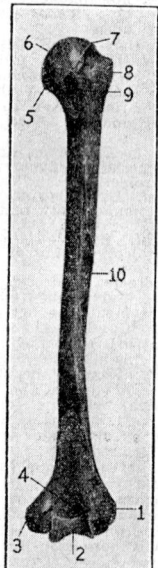

HUMERUS
Anterior view of left humerus. 1. Lateral epicondyle; 2. trochlea; 3. medial epicondyle; 4. coronoid fossa; 5. anatomical neck; 6. head; 7. anatomical neck; 8. greater tubercle; 9. lessor tubercle; 10. body.

hu'merus [L. shoulder]. Upper bone of arm from the elbow (articulating with the ulna and radius) to the shoulder joint, where it articulates with the scapula.

h., fracture of. 1. If the fracture is of the upper end the arm is abducted on a wire splint for about 4 weeks. Movements of the elbow and wrist are started early and movements (active) of shoulder in about a fortnight, or 3 weeks. 2. Fracture of shaft and lower end. The limb is put in plaster in a position midway between pronation and supination with the humerus at right angles to the forearm. Movement of the shoulder, wrist, and finger is allowed at once.
RS: *acromiohumeral, capitellum, cubitus, glenoid cavity.*

hu'mid [L. *humidus*, moist]. Moist, damp.

h. gangrene. G. with serous exudation and rapid decomposition. SEE: *gangrene.*

humidifier (hu-mid'i-fi-er) [L. *humidus*, moist]. Apparatus to increase moisture content of the air in a room.

humid'ity [L. *humiditās*, moisture]. Moisture in the atmosphere.

If air was saturated at a temperature of 70° F., water would condense on all objects if the temperature fell to 68° F.

THE SATURATION OF THE AIR OCCURS AT:
If It Contains
50°   4.2 grains of water per cu. ft.
60°   5.8 grains of water per cu. ft.
70°   7.9 grains of water per cu. ft.
90°   14.3 grains of water per cu. ft.

The air can contain at 90° almost twice as much as at 70° F. The relative humidity at 70° F. would be 50% if the air held 3.88 grains of water per cu. ft. A room with a humidity of from 40-50° F. means the presence of 1½ gal. of water every 24 hours if it represents a content of 10 cu. ft., or 8 or more gal. for a 6-room house. SEE: *relative humidity.*

humor [L. fluid]. 1. Any fluid or semifluid substance in the body. 2. In ancient medicine, the four "juices" or fluids (blood, phlegm, black bile, yellow bile) of which the body was thought to be composed.

h., aqueous. A watery fluid in the anterior and posterior chambers of the eye.

h., crystalline. The fluidlike substance of the crystalline lens of the eye.

h., vitreous. The vitreous body, *q.v.* A semifluid, transparent substance occupying the space between the lens and retina of the eye.

hu'moral [L. *humor*, fluid]. Pertaining to body fluids or substances contained in them.

h. control or **correlation.** The control of various bodily activities by chemical substances, esp., hormones transported by the blood or lymph. In contrast to *nervous control* brought about through nerve impulses.

humpback [origin uncertain]. Curvature of the spine. SYN: *kyphosis.*

hung'er [A.S. *hungur*]. 1. A sensation resulting from lack of food, characterized by dull or acute pain referred to the epigastrium or lower part of chest. Usually accompanied by weakness and an overwhelming desire to eat. Hunger pains coincide with powerful contractions of the stomach. Distinguished from *appetite* in that the latter is a pleasant sensation based on previous experience which causes one to seek food for the purpose of tasting and enjoying. 2. To have a strong desire.
RS: *addephagia, air h., appetite, bulimia, hormone, limosis.*

h., air. Dyspnea, breathlessness.

h. contractions. Those observed, and often felt, in the normal empty stomach. They may be painful. A series of such contractions is followed by a period of rest, after which they may return with greater intensity unless food is taken. Digestion may be activated under such conditions.

h. cure. Restricted diet or fasting for cure of disease. SYN: *nestiatria, nestitherapy.*

h. day. One on which a diabetic is restricted to broth only.

h., hormone. Deficiency of special hormone in an organ.

hungry. Craving food.

hunte'rian chancre. Indurated, syphilitic chancre. SEE: *chancre.*

Hun'ter's canal. *Canalis adductorius.*

H.'s chancre. Hunterian chancre.

Huschke's canal (hoosh'kēz). One formed by juncture of the *annulus tympanicus* tubercules.

H.'s foramen. Perforation found in arrested development near inner extremity of tympanic plate.

H.'s teeth. Tiny, toothlike protuberances at edge of cochlear labium vestibulare.

H.'s valve. Plica lacrimalis.

Hutchinson's patch (hŭtsh'ĭn-sŏn). Salmon-colored area in the cornea seen in syphilitic keratitis. SYN: *salmon patch.*

H's. teeth. A congenital condition; pegged, lateral incisors and notched central incisors along the cutting edge. A sign of congenital syphilis.

Hux'ley's layer. Inner layer of nucleated cells forming the inner root sheath of a hair follicle.

hyalin (hī'a-lĭn) [G. *yalos*, glass]. 1. A substance obtainable from the products of amyloid, colloid, or hyaloid degeneration. 2. Basement substance of hyaline cartilage.

hyaline (hī'al-en, hī'al-ĭn) [G. *yalos*, glass]. Crystalline, glassy, translucent. SEE: *casts, degeneration.*

h. bodies. Homogeneous substance; the result of colloid degeneration and found in degenerated cells.

h. cartilage. The true cartilage. Smooth and pearly. It covers the articular surfaces of bones.

h. casts. The commonest form of cast. They are transparent, pale, and homogeneous with rounded ends, and they indicate nephropathy.

hyalino'sis [" + *ōsis*]. Waxy or hyaline degeneration.

hyalinu'ria [" + *ouron*, urine]. Hyalin present in the urine.

hyalitis (hi-al-i'tis) [" + *-ītis*, inflammation]. Inflammation of the vitreous humor.   [vitreous.

h., asteroid. Spherical bodies in the

h. puncta'ta. A form marked by minute opacities in the vitreous humor.

h. suppurati'va. A purulent inflammation of the vitreous humor.

hyalo- [G.]. Prefix: Transparent.

hyaloenchondroma (hī"a-lo-en-kon-dro'-mä) [G. *yalos*, glass, + *en*, in, + *chondros*, cartilage, + *ōma*, tumor]. A chondroma composed of hyaline cartilage.

hyalogen (hi-al'o-jen) [" + *gennan*, to produce]. A protein substance in cartilage and the vitreous humor.

hyaloid (hī'al-oid) [" + *eidos*, form]. Hyaline, glassy.

h. artery. Present in the fetus. Supplies nutrition to lens. Disappears in later months of gestation.

h. canal. Lymph channel in vitreous extending from optic disc to post. capsule of lens; contains hyaloid artery in fetus. [the vitreous humor.

h. membrane. That which envelops

hyaloiditis (hī"al-oid-i'tis) [" + " + -*itis*, inflammation]. Inflammation of the hyaloid membrane of the vitreous humor. Syn: *hyalitis*.

hyaloma (hī-ăl-ō'mă) [G. *yalos*, glass, + *ōma*, tumor]. Syn: *colloid milium*. A small yellow papule which develops in the corium of the skin as a result of colloid degeneration.

hyalomere (hī'al-o-mēr) [" + *meros*, part]. Homogeneous part of a blood platelet, pale in color, as contrasted with the chromomere.

hyalomu'coid [" + L. *mucus*, mucus, + G. *eidos*, form]. Mucoid in vitreous body.

hyalonyxis (hī"al-o-niks'is) [" + *nyxis*, puncture]. Puncture of vitreous body.

hyalophagia (hī"al-o-fa'jī-ă) [" + *phagein*, to eat]. The eating of glass by the demented.

hyalophagy (hi-al-of'aj-ī) [" + *phagein*, to eat]. Eating of glass by the demented. Syn: *hyalophagia*.

hyalopho'bia [" + *phobos*, fear]. Fear of touching glass.

hyaloplasm (hī'ăl-ō-plăzm) [G. *yalos*, glass, + *plasma*, a thing formed]. Syn: *hyalomitome*. The fluid portion of protoplasm. The basic ground substance; also called basic or fundamental protoplasm.

h., nuclear. Clear substance filling the meshes of the nuclear reticulum. Syn: *karyolymph, nuclear sap.*

hyaloserositis (hī"al-o-se-ro-si'tis) [" + L. *serōsus*, serous, + G. -*itis*, inflammation]. Inflammation of a serous membrane with fibrinous exudate undergoing hyaline transformation.

h., progressive multiple. "Phthisis of serous membranes."

hyalotome (hi-al'o-tōm) [G. *yalos*, glass]. Fluid portion of protoplasm.

hyaluron'ic acid. An acid mucopolysaccharide found in the ground substance of connective tissue which acts as *a* binding and protective agent. Also found in the synovial fluid, vitreous and aqueous humors.

hyaluronidase (hī"ă-lūr-ŏn'ĭ-dās). Syn: *Duran-Reynals spreading factor.* An enzyme found in the testes and other tissues and present in semen. It depolymerizes hyaluronic acid thus increasing the permeability of connective tissues by dissolving the substances that hold body cells together. It acts to disperse the cells of the corona radiata about the newly ovulated ovum.

hybrid. The offspring of unlike parents; a heterozygous individual.

hybridization. The mating of individuals which differ in one or more pairs of genes; cross breeding.

hydan'toin. A colorless base, glycolyl urea, $C_3H_4N_2O_2$, from urea or allantoin.

hydatid (hī'da-tĭd) [G. *ydatis*, a drop of water]. 1. A cyst formed in the tissues, esp. liver, resulting from the development of the larval stage of the dog tapeworm, *Echinococcus granulosus.* The cysts develop slowly forming a hollow bladder from the inner surface of which hollow brood capsules are formed. These are attached by slender stalks or they may fall free into the fluid-filled cavity of the mother cyst. Scolices form on the inner surface of the older brood capsules. In older cysts there is a granular deposit of brood capsules and scoleces called *hydatid sand*. Hydatids may grow for years sometimes attaining an enormous size. See: *Echinococcus granulosus*. 2. A small cystic remnant of an embryonic structure.
Treatment: surgical.

h. fremi'tus. A tremulous sensation felt on palpating a hydatid tumor.

h. mole. Degenerative process in chorionic villi, which gives rise to multiple cysts and rapid growth of uterus with hemorrhage. Diag: Indicated by the latter and expulsion of some of the cysts. Treatment: (a) Packing to con-

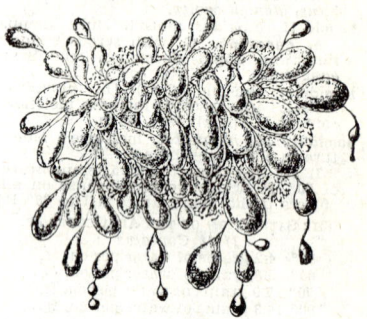

HYDATID MOLE
The entire placenta is transformed into a large number of edematous vesicles which resemble a bunch of grapes. Only a small part of the placenta is represented in this picture.

trol bleeding; (b) curettage week or 2 after expulsion.

h. of Morgagni. Cystlike remnant of the mullerian duct which is attached to the fallopian tube.

h., sessile. Morgagnian h. connected with a testicle.

h., stalked. Morgagnian hydatid connected with a fallopian tube.

hydatidiform (hi-dat-id'if-orm) [" + L. *forma*, shape]. Having the form of a hydatid.

hydatidocele (hi-dat-id'o-sēl) [" + *kēlē*, tumor]. Hydatid cyst of scrotum or testicle.

hydatido'ma [" + *ōma*, tumor]. A tumor consisting of hydatids.

hydatidosis (hi-dat-ĭ-do'sis) [" + *ōsis*]. Condition caused by infestation with hydatids.

hydatidostomy (hi-dat-id-os'to-mi) [" + *stoma*, opening]. Evacuation of a hydatid cyst.

hydat'iform [" + L. *forma*, form]. Having the form of a hydatid.

hy'datism [" + *ismos*, state of]. The sound produced by fluid in a cavity.

hydradenitis (hi-drad-en-i'tis) [G. *idrōs*, sweat, + *adēn*, gland, + -*itis*, inflammation]. Inflammation of a sweat gland.

hydradeno'ma [" + " + *ōma*, tumor]. Tumor of a sweat gland.

hydraeroperitoneum (hi-dra-er-o-per-it-o-ne'um) [G. *ydōr*, water, + *aēr*, air, + *peritonaion*, peritoneum]. Collection of fluid and gas in the peritoneal cavity.

hydragogue (hy'dra-gog) [" + *agōgos*, leading]. Drug promoting watery evacuation of the bowels.

Ex: *magnesium sulfate, sodium phosphate, solution of magnesium citrate.*

hydramnion, hydramnios (hi-dram'nĭ-on, -ōs) [" + *amnion,* a caul on a lamb]. An excess of liquor amnii which leads to overdistention of the uterus and the possibility of malpresentations.
The normal amount is about 1-2 pt. It may increase to 4-6 pt., and in rare cases to very much more.
Liquor amnii is secreted by the fetus, and abnormal amounts are probably due to some abnormality of the fetus. Nearly half the cases occur in twin pregnancies. Hydramnios begins about 5th month of pregnancy and the pressure of the enlarged uterus gives rise to breathlessness, edema, cyanosis, and varicose veins in the mother. The uterus is large for the date given and the fetus may be felt bobbing about in the liquor and the fetal heart is not easily heard.

hydrargyrum (hi-drar'jir-um) [" + *argyros,* silver]. Mercury or quicksilver. See: *mercury.*

hydrarthrosis (hi-drar-thro'sis) [" + *arthron,* joint, + *ōsis*]. Serous effusion in a joint cavity; white swelling.

hydrase. An enzyme which catalyzes the addition of or the withdrawal of water from a compound without hydrolysis occurring.

hydrate (hi'drat) [G. *ydōr,* water]. A crystalline substance formed by water combining with various compounds.

hydrated (hi'dra-ted) [G. *ydōr,* water]. Combined chemically with water.

hydration. The chemical combination of a substance with water.

hydrazine (hi'draz-in). 1. A colorless gas, H₄N₂, with peculiar odor; soluble in water. 2. One of a class derived from hydrazine.

hydre'mia [G. *ydōr,* water, + *aima,* blood]. Excess of watery fluid in the blood.

hydrencephalocele (hi-dren-sef'al-o-sēl) [" + *egkephalos,* brain, + *kēlē,* tumor]. A hernia through a cranial defect of brain substance and meninges, in which fluid occupies the space between the two.

hydrencephalus (hi-dren-sef'al-us) [" + *egkephalos,* brain]. Accumulation of fluid in the cerebral ventricles or outside of the brain. Syn: *hydrocephalus.*

hydrepigastrium (hi-drep-ĭ-gas'trĭ-um) [" + *epi,* upon, + *gastēr,* belly]. Accumulation of fluid bet. the peritoneum and the abdominal muscles.

hydriatics (hi-drī-at'ĭks) [" + *iatikos,* healing]. Application of water in treatment of disease. Syn: *hydrotherapeutics.*

hydriatric (hi-dri-at'rik) [" + *iatrikos,* healing]. Pert. to treatment of disease with water, as hydriatric procedures or hydriatric institutions.

hydriat'rist [" + *iatrikos,* healing]. One who practices hydrotherapy.

hy'drid [G. *ydōr,* water]. Chemical compound containing hydrogen and an element or radical.

hy'drion. The hydrogen ion (H +).

hydro- [G.]. Prefix: Water; also hydrogen.

hydro'a [G. *ydōr,* water]. Chronic inflammatory skin disease.
Sym: Bullae, erythema, itching, papules, pustules, and vesicles.
Syn: *dermatitis herpetiformis, pemphigus pruriginosus.*

hydroappen'dix [" + L. *appendere,* to hang]. Watery fluid distending the vermiform appendix.

hydrobilirubin (hi"dro-bil-ĭ-ru'bĭn) [" + L. *bilis,* bile, + *ruber,* red]. A brownish red bile pigment perhaps identical with stercobilin and urobilin.

hydrobromate (hi-dro-bro'māt) [" + *bromos,* stench]. A salt of hydrobromic acid.

hydrocarbon [G. *ydōr,* water, + L. *carbo,* carbon]. A compound made up only of hydrogen and carbon.
Hydrocarbons may exist as aliphatic chain compounds in which the carbon atoms are arranged in the form of a chain, or as aromatic or cyclic compounds in which the carbon atoms form one or more rings.
h., saturated. H. in which the carbon atoms are linked by a single electron pair and in which all valences are satisfied.
h., unsaturated. H. in which carbon atoms share two or three pairs of electrons.

hydrocele (hi'drō-sēl) [G. *ydōr,* water, + *kēlē,* hernia]. The accumulation of serous fluid in a saclike cavity, esp., the tunica vaginalis testis; serous tumors of the testes or associated parts.
Treatment: aspiration, surgical.
h., acute. Most common, majority of cases bet. 2nd and 5th years. H. occurring suddenly, usually the result of inflammation of the epididymis or testis.
Sym: Convulsions, coma, headache, insomnia, nocturnal deliriums, spasmodic muscular contractions.
h., cervical. H. in the neck resulting from accumulation of serous fluid in persistent cervical duct or cleft.
h., chronic. H. usually seen in men of middle age. May result from filariasis.
h., congenital. That present at birth, resulting from failure of closure of the vaginal process.
Sym: Increased size of head, emaciation of body. Prominent eyes with downward glance, wrinkled face, weakness, inability to walk, feeble voice.
Prog: Generally unfavorable within 5 years.
h., encysted. H. in the vaginal process in which openings to the scrotal and peritoneal cavities are closed.
h. feminae. H. in labium majus or canal of Nuck.
h. muliebris. H. feminae, *q.v.*
h. spinalis. Spina bifida.

hydrocenosis (hi-dro-sen-o'sis) [" + *kenōsis,* an emptying]. Evacuation of a dropsical fluid by tapping or by a hydragogue. Syn: *paracentesis.*

hydrocephal'ic [G. *ydōr,* water, + *kephalē,* head]. Pert. to hydrocephalus.

hydrocephalocele (hi-dro-sef'al-o-sēl) [" + *kēlē,* hernia]. Watery hernia of the brain. Syn: *hydrencephalocele.*

hydroceph'aloid [" + " + *eidos,* resemblance]. Resembling or pert. to hydrocephalus.
h. disease. One of infants similar to hydrocephalus.
Sym: Depressed fontanels, pulse irregular, tendency to vomit.

hydrocephalus (hi-dro-sef'a-lŭs) [G. *ydor,* water, + *kephalē,* head]. The increased accumulation of cerebrospinal fluid within the ventricles of the brain. Results from interference with normal circulation and absorption of the fluid, esp., destruction of the foramina of Magendie and Lushka. This may result from developmental anomalies, infection, injury, or brain tumors.
In children the head is usually globular or pyramidal in shape. Face disproportionately small. Eyes hidden in sockets and turned upward. Sutures separated, with bulging fontanels and thin cranial bones.

In older individuals after skull has formed there are headache, vomiting, choked disks, atrophy of optic nerve, mental disturbances.

h., communicating. H. in which normal communication between fourth ventricle and subarachnoid space is maintained.

h., congenital. Chronic type occurring in infancy. Also called *infantile h.*

h., external. Accumulation of fluid in subdural spaces.

h., internal. Accumulation of fluid within ventricles of the brain.

h., secondary. H. following injury or infections such as meningitis or syphilis.

hydrochlorate (hi-dro-klo′rāt) [" + *chlōros*, green]. Any salt of hydrochloric acid.

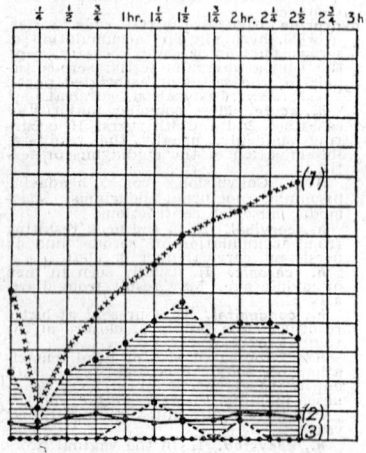

HYDROCHLORIC ACID

The shaded part indicates the normal limits of Hydrochloric Acid.
(1) The upper line (of crosses) is Hyperchlorhydria.
(2) The middle (straight line) is Hypochlorhydria.
(3) The bottom (dotted line) indicates Achlorhydria.

hy″drochlo′ric acid (HCl) [G. *ydōr*, water, + *chlōros*, green]. An aqueous solution of hydrogen chloride, containing 35 to 38% (HCl). Crude commercial hydrochloric acid is known as *muriatic acid*.

It is a normal constituent of gastric juice amounting to 0.4 to 0.5% and is produced by the parietal cells of gastric glands. It serves the following functions: 1. Converts pepsinogen into pepsin and produces an acid medium favorable for the activity of pepsin. 2. Dissolves and disintegrates nucleoproteins and collagen. 3. Hydrolyzes sucrose. 4. Precipitates caseinogen. 5. Inhibits multiplication of bacteria, esp., putrefactive lactic acid fermentation, and certain pathogenic forms. 6. Stimulates secretion of secretin by the duodenum. 7. It inhibits the action of ptyalin and thus stops salivary digestion in the stomach.

Average amount found in the food content of stomach is about 0.2% due to dilution and neutralization by alkaline contents. In pernicious anemia there is an absence of this acid (achlorhydria).

SEE: *achlorhydria, hypochlorhydria,*
hyperchlorhydria, parietal cells.

h.a. dilute. Aqueous solution of 10% HCl.

hydrocholecystis (hi-dro-ko-le-sis′tis) [G. *ydōr*, water, + *cholē*, bile, + *kystis*, bladder]. Dropsy of gallbladder.

hydrocholeresis. Choleresis. Choleresis in which water content of the bile is increased resulting in production of bile with reduced specific gravity, viscosity, and total solid contents.

hydrocirsocele (hi-dro-sir′so-sēl) [" + *kirsos*, varix, + *kēlē*, tumor]. Hydrocele with varicose veins of spermatic cord.

hydrocollidine (hi-dro-kol′id-ēn) [" + *kolla*, glue]. A poisonous ptomaine from putrefying fish or animal flesh.

hydrocolpos (hi-dro-kol′pos) [" + *kolpos*, vagina]. Retention cyst of the vagina containing watery, nonsanguineous fluid, or mucus.

hydroconion (hi-dro-ko′nĭ-on) [" + *konis*, dust]. An atomizer.

hydrocra′nia [" + *kranion*, skull]. Water on the brain. SYN: *hydrocephalus.*

hy′drocyst [" + *kystis*, a bladder]. A cyst containing watery fluid.

hydrocysto′ma [" + " + *ōma*, tumor]. Disease marked by small hydrocysts. Sudamina on the face, esp. in women after middle age. SYN: *hidrocystoma.*

hydrodiascope (hi-dro-di′ă-skōp) [" + *dia*, through, + *skopein*, to examine]. Device to correct astigmatism.

hydrodictiotomy (hi″dro-dik-ti-ot′o-mī) [" + *dictyon*, retina, + *tomē*, incision]. Incision of retina for edema.

hydroelec′tric bath. Administration of an electrically charged bath.

hydroencephalocele (hi″dro-en-sef′al-o-sēl) [G. *ydōr*, water, + *egkephalos*, brain, + *kēlē*, hernia]. Brain substance expanded into a watery sac protruding through a cleft in the cranium. SYN: *hydrencephalocele.*

hy′drogel [" + L. *gelāre*, to congeal]. A colloid containing water that solidifies in gelatinous form.

hy′drogen (H) [G. *ydōr*, water, + *gennan*, to produce]. An element existing as a colorless, odorless, tasteless gas. It has an atomic weight of 1.008 and atomic number of 1. It possesses one valence electron. Three isotopes of hydrogen (*protium, deuterium,* and *tritium*) exist having atomic weight of 1, 2, and 3, respectively.

OCCURRENCE: H. occurs in its free state in natural gases and volcanic eruptions only in minute quantities. It is present in the sun and stars and on the earth it comprises about 1% of all known terrestrial matter. It occurs principally as hydrogen oxide (water, H_2O) and is a constituent of all hydrocarbons. It is present in all acids and in ionic form is responsible for the properties characteristic of acids. It is present in nearly all organic compounds and is a component of all carbohydrates, proteins, and fats.

USES: It is highly inflammable and used in the oxy-hydrogen flame in welding, in hydrogenation of oils for solidifying purposes, as a reducing agent, and in many syntheses.

h. acceptor. In oxidation reduction reactions a substance which receives hydrogen atoms from another substance. SEE: *coenzyme.*

h. donator. In oxidation-reduction reactions a substance which gives up hydrogen atoms to another substance, the acceptor.

hy′drogenate [" + *gennan*, to produce]. To bring about a combination with hydrogen.

hydrogenation (hi-dro-jen-a'shun) [" + *gennan*, to produce]. A process of changing an unsaturated fat to a solid, saturated fat by the addition of hydrogen in the presence of a catalyst, as olein and stearin.

hydrogen dioxide (di-oks'īd) [" + " + *di*, two, + *oxys*, acid]. Hydroden peroxide (H₂O₂) *q.v.* Used in form of 3% aqueous solution. ACTION AND USES: Antiseptic and cleansing agent.

hydrogen ion. A protron, the positively charged nucleus of a hydrogen atom.

 h. ion concentration. The relative proportion of hydrogen ions in a solution, the factor responsible for the acidic properties of a solution.

 h. ion or pH scale. A scale used to express the degree of acidity or alkalinity of a solution. It extends from 0.00 (total acidity) to 14 (total alkalinity), the numbers running in reverse order of H-ion concentration. The pH value is the negative logarithm of the H-ion concentration of a solution, expressed in gram ions (moles) per liter.

 As the hydrogen ion concentration decreases, a change of 1 pH unit means a ten-fold increase in hydrogen-ion concentration or true acidity. Thus a solution with a *p*H of 1.0 is ten times more acid than one with a *p*H of 2.0 and 100 times more acid than one with a *p*H of 3.0. A *p*H of 7.0 indicates neutrality.

 As the hydrogen-ion concentration varies in a definite reciprocal manner with the hydroxyl ion (OH—) concentration, a *p*H reading above 7.0 indicates alkalinity. The blood and body fluids are slightly alkaline having a *p*H of about 7.4.

hydrogen peroxide [G. *ydōr*, water, + *gennan*, to form, + L. *per*, through, + G. *oxys*, acid]. H₂O₂, a colorless, syrupy, liquid with an irritating odor and acrid taste. It decomposes readily, liberating oxygen.

 USES: As a commercial bleaching agent, as an oxidizing and reducing agent. In a 3% solution, as a mild antiseptic, germicide, and cleansing agent.

 h. p., solution of. The action kills bacteria because of its oxidizing power. The most important use is as an antibacterial agent, although its germicidal activity is generally greatly overestimated. In the presence of organic matter (pus, blood, etc.) this compound is so rapidly broken down that it has little efficiency. In contact with tissues its germicidal power is very limited, owing to the fact that organic matter decomposes it. As long as there is effervescence caused by its application to a wound there is no great destruction of bacteria.

 It is of value chiefly as a cleansing agent for suppurating wounds and inflamed mucous membranes. It is esp. useful for this purpose because of the development of gas, which tends to loosen adherent deposits. Its value in cleansing infected wounds and freely suppurating ulcers is probably due more to removal of organic detritus* which forms a breeding place for the microorganisms rather than to its antibacterial action.

 Its styptic action—probably due to activation of the fibrin ferment of the blood and consequent more rapid coagulation—as well as its harmless nature, make it a very popular antiseptic for household use. It is sometimes injected into deep cavities to determine the presence of pus, which will be indicated by effervescence. Because of its lack of toxicity it is a favored disinfectant for application to various mucous membranes, esp. those of the nose and throat. Diluted with equal parts of water used as a gargle in pharyngitis, or mouthwash in stomatitis.

hydroglossa (hi-dro-glos'ă) [" + *glōssa*, tongue]. Cystic tumor beneath the tongue. SYN: *ranula*.

hydrogymna'sium [" + *gymnasion*, exercising]. Pool for underwater exercises.

hydrogymnas'tics [" + *gymnastikos*, pert. to nakedness]. Underwater exercises.

hydrohematonephrosis (hi″dro-hem″at-o-nef-ro′sis) [" + *aima*, blood, + *nephros*, kidney, + *ōsis*]. Blood and urine in pelvis of the kidney.

hydrohepatosis (hī″dro-hep-at-o′sis) [" + *ēpar*, *ēpat-*, liver, + *ōsis*]. Accumulation of fluid in the liver.

hydrohymenitis (hi″dro-hi-men-i′tis) [" + *ymēn*, membrane, + *-ītis*, inflammation]. Any inflammation of a serous membrane.

hydrokinet'ics [G. *ydōr*, water, + *kinēsis*, motion]. Science of fluids in motion.

hydrolase (hi'dro-lās) [" + *ase*, enzyme]. An enzyme that causes hydrolysis. SYN: *hydrolyst*.

hydrology (hī-drŏl′ō-jī) [G. *ydōr*, water, + *logos*, science]. The science of water in all its aspects.

hydrolysis (hi-drol'ĭ-sīs) [G. *ydōr*, water, + *lysis*, solution]. Any reaction in which water is one of the reactants, more specifically the combination of water with a salt to produce an acid and a base, one of which is more dissociated than the other. The reverse of neutralization. A chemical decomposition in which a substance is split into simpler compounds by the addition of and the taking up of the elements of water.

 Reactions of this kind are extremely frequent in life processes. The conversion of starch to maltose, of fat to glycerol and fatty acid, and of protein to amino acids, are examples of hydrolysis, as are more of the other reactions involved in digestion. A simple example is the reaction in which the hydrolysis of ethyl acetate yields acetic acid and ethyl alcohol: $C_2H_5C_2H_3O_2 + H_2O = HC_2H_3O_2 + C_2H_5OH$. Such reactions can be reversed, usually; the reversed reaction is called neutralization, esterification, or condensation. SEE: *assimilation, enzyme*.

hydrolyst (hi'drol-ist) [" + *lysis*, solution]. A ferment that produces hydrolysis.

hydrolyt'ic [" + *lysis*, solution]. Rel. to hydrolysis.

hydrolyze. To cause to undergo hydrolysis.

hydroma (hi-dro'mă) [" + *ōma*, tumor]. A collection of serous fluid in a cyst.

hydromel (hi'dro-mel) [" + *meli*, honey]. Mixture of honey and water.

hydromeningitis (hi-dro-men-in-ji'tis) [" + *mēnigx*, membrane, + *itis*, inflammation]. 1. Inflammation of membranes of brain with serous effusion. 2. Inflammation of Descemet's membrane.

hydromeningocele (hi″dro-men-in′go-sēl) [" + " + *kēlē*, hernia]. Protrusion of meninges or spinal cord in a sac of fluid.

hydrom'eter [" + *metron*, measure]. An instrument which measures the density of a liquid by the depth to which a graduated scale sinks into the liquid.

hydrometra (hi-dro-me′tră) [" + *mētra*, uterus]. Collection of watery fluid or mucus in the uterus.

hydromphalus (hi-drom'fal-us) [" + *omphalos*, navel]. Watery tumor at the umbilicus.

hydromyelia (hi"dro-mi-e'li-ă) [G. *ydōr*, water, + *myelos*, marrow]. Increased fluid in central canal of spinal cord. SYN: *hydrorrhachis*.

hydromyelocele (hi-dro-mi'el-o-sēl) [" + " + *kēlē*, hernia]. Protrusion of sac with cerebrospinal fluid through a spina bifida.

hydromyoma (hi-dro-mi-o'mă) [" + *mys*, *myo-*, muscle, + *ōma*, tumor]. Cystic fibroid, usually uterine, filled with fluid.

hydronephrosis (hi"dro-nef-ro'sis) [" + *nephros*, kidney, + *ōsis*]. Collection of urine in the kidney pelvis owing to obstructed outflow, forming a cyst by production of distention and atrophy of organ.
  DIAG: Large, fluctuating, soft mass in region of kidney, appearing and disappearing as retained urine passes into the ureters and bladder.
  TREATMENT: Aspiration, nephrectomy, or nephrotomy.

hydroparasalpinx (hi"dro-par-ă-sal'pinks) [" + *para*, beside, + *salpigx*, tube]. Accumulation of serous fluid in the accessory tubes of the fallopian tube.

hydroparotitis [" + *para*, near, + *ous*, *ot-*, ear, + *itis*, inflammation]. Accumulation of fluid in the parotid gland.

hydropathic [" + *pathos*, disease]. Rel. to hydropathy.

hydropathy (hi-drop'a-thi) [" + *pathos*, disease]. A term now used to denote the empirical application of water in the treatment of disease. SEE: *hydrotherapy*.

hydropericarditis [" + *peri*, around, + *kardia*, heart, + *itis*, inflammation]. Serous effusion accompanying pericarditis.

hydropericardium (hi"dro-per-ĭ-kar'dĭ-um) [" + " + *kardia*, heart]. Pericardial dropsy. Accumulation of water in pericardial sac without inflammation.
  SYM: Distress in region of heart; dysphagia, disturbed cardiac action and dyspnea. [cause of attack.
  TREATMENT: Paracentesis. Governed by

hydroperinephrosis (hi"dro-per-ĭ-ne-fro'sis) [" + " + *nephros*, kidney, + *ōsis*]. Accumulation of serum of connective tissue surrounding the kidney.

hydroperion (hi-dro-per'ĭ-on) [G. *ydōr*, water, + *peri*, around, + *ōon*, egg]. Fluid supposedly present between decidua capsularis and decidua parietalis.

hydroperitoneum [" + *peritonaion*, peritoneum]. Accumulation of fluid in peritoneal cavity. SYN: *ascites*.

hydrophilism. Tendency of tissues to attract and hold water.

hydrophilous (hi-drof'ĭl-ŭs) [" + *philein*, to love]. Taking up moisture. SYN: *bibulous*.

hydrophobia (hī-drō-fō'bĭ-ă) [G. *ydōr*, water, + *phobos*, fear]. SYN: *lyssa*. 1. Morbid fear of water. 2. Common name for rabies, *q.v.*, resulting from bite of a rabid animal.

hydrophobophobia. Morbid fear of contracting hydrophobia, sometimes resulting in a hysterical condition resembling hydrophobia.

hydrophthalmos (hī-drof-thăl'mŏs) [G. *ydōr*, water, + *ophthalmos*, eye]. SYN: *buphthalmia*, *infantile glaucoma*. Distention of the eyeball due to accumulation of fluid within it.

hydrophysometra (hi"dro-fĭ-so-me'tră) [" + *physa*, gas, + *mētra*, uterus]. Presence of water and gas in the uterus.

hydropic [G. *ydrōpikos*, pert. to dropsy]. Dropsical or pert. to dropsy.

hydropigenous (hi-dro-pij'en-us) [G. *ydrōps*, dropsy, + *gennan*, to produce]. Producing dropsy.

hydropneumatosis (hi"dro-nu-mă-to'sis) [" + *pneuma*, air, + *ōsis*]. Liquid and gas in the tissues producing combined edema and emphysema.

hydropneumogony (hī-dro-nu-mog'ō-nī) [" + " + *gonu*, knee]. Diagnosis of joint effusion by injecting air in joint.

hydropneumopericardium (hī-dro-nu"mo-per-ĭ-kar'dĭ-um) [" + " + *peri*, around, + *kardia*, heart]. Serous effusion with gas in the pericardium.

hydropneumoperitoneum (hi"dro-nu"mo-per-ĭ-to-ne'um) [" + " + *peritonaion*, peritoneum]. Gas and serous fluid in the peritoneal cavity.

hydropneumothorax (hi"dro-nu"mo-tho'-raks) [" + " + *thōrax*, chest]. Gas and serous effusion in pleural cavity. SYN: *pneumohydrothorax*.

hy'drops, hydrop'sy [G. *ydrōps*, dropsy]. Dropsy or edema.
  h. abdominis. Dropsy of the abdominal cavity; ascites.
  h., endolymphatic. H. labyrinthine, *q.v.*
  h. fetalis. Erythroblastosis fetalis, *q.v.*
  h. folliculi. Accumulation of fluid in graffian follicle of ovary.
  h. gravidarum. Edema accompanying pregnancy.
  h., labyrinthine. Dilatation due to an accumulation of fluid in the endolymphatic space of the ear. A characteristic of Meniere's disease, *q.v.*
  h. tubae. Collection of fluid in an oviduct. Hydrosalpinx.
  h. t. profluens. A hydrops of the tube in which the distention becomes so great that the tube is forced to empty itself by the pressure, the emptying taking place via the uterine cavity. SYN: *intermittent hydrosalpinx*.
  h. vesicae fel'leae. Fluid in the gallbladder causing distention.

hydropyonephrosis (hi"dro-pi"o-nef-ro'sis) [G. *ydōr*, water, + *pyon*, pus, + *nephros*, kidney, + *ōsis*]. Dilatation of kidney pelvis with pus and urine.

hydrorheostat (hi-dro-re'o-stat) [" + *reos*, current, + *istanai*, to place]. A rheostat with water resistance.

hydrorrhachis (hi-dro'ră-kis) [" + *rachis*, spine]. Condition of increased cerebrospinal fluid bet. membranes and spinal cord or its central canal or cavities.

hydrorrhachitis (hi-dro-ra-ki'tis) [" + " + *itis*, inflammation]. Serous effusion from the spinal cord or its membranes with inflammation of the cord.

hydrorrhea (hi-dror-re'ă) [" + *roia*, flow].
1. Copious watery discharge from any part.
2. Nasal, watery discharge from the nose.
  h. gravidarum. Discharge of a watery fluid from the vagina during pregnancy, sometimes mistaken for amniotic fluid.

hydrosalpinx (hi-dro-sal'pinks) [" + *salpigx*, tube]. Distention of fallopian tube by clear fluid.
  h., intermittent. A discharge of watery fluid from the oviduct. SYN: *hydrops tubae profluens*.

hydrosarcocele (hi-dro-sar'ko-sēl) [" + *sarx*, flesh, + *kēlē*, hernia]. Hydrocele with chronic swelling of testis.

hydrosol. The fluid state of a colloidal solution; a sol. State of a colloidal solution in which the colloid particles, separated by water in a continuous phase, are free to move about. SEE: *hydrogel*.

hydrosphygmograph (hi-dro-sfĭg'mo-grăf) [" + *sphygmos*, pulse, + *graphein*, to write]. A sphygmograph with indicator consisting of a column of water.

hydro'sis [" + *-ōsis*]. A wrong spelling of hidrosis.

hydrostat'ic [" + *statikos*, standing]. Pert. to the pressure of liquids in equilibrium and that exerted on liquids.
 h. test. Putting lungs of a dead infant in water. If they float, the infant was born alive.

hydrostat'ics [G. *ydōr*, water, + *statikos*, standing]. Science of properties of fluids in equilibrium.

hydrosudotherapy (hi"dro-sū"do-ther'a-pĭ) [" + L. *sudor*, sweat, + G. *therapeia*, treatment]. Treatment of disease by sweating and hydrotherapy.

hydrosyringomyelia (hī"dro-sir-in"go-mi-e'lĭ-ă) [" + *syrigx*, tube, + *myelos*, marrow]. Distention of central canal of spinal cord with effusion of fluid and formation of cavities.

hydrotaxis. The response of an animal toward or away from moisture. SEE: *hydrotropism*.

hydrotherapeu'tics [" + *therapeutikè*, treatment]. Treatment of disease with water. SYN: *hydrotherapy*.

hydrotherapist (hi-dro-ther'ă-pist) [" + *therapeia*, treatment]. One who practices hydrotherapy.

hydrotherapy (hi-dro-ther'ă-pĭ) [" + *therapeia*, treatment]. Scientific application of water in treatment of disease. RS: *bath, cold, compress, douche, pack*.
 The therapeutic effects of hydrotherapy are as follows:
 Brief Hot Tub and Shower Baths: Relieve fatigue but may cause cerebral congestion and wakefulness unless cold compresses are used on the head.
 Cold Baths and Applications: Abstract heat and stimulate reaction, esp. if followed by friction and percussion. They contract the small blood vessels when applied locally.
 Cold and Hot Applications: One followed by the other causes *revulsion*, relieving congestion of internal organs.
 Gradually Elevated Hot Tub and Vapor Baths: Relax all muscles of the body.
 Hot Baths: Relax tissues including capillaries of skin, drawing blood from deeper tissues; also relieve pain.
 Warm and Hot Baths and Applications: They soothe cutaneous nerves, and nerves of internal organs in reflex relation with skin areas to which heat is applied.
 SEE: *Kneipp cure*.

hydrothionammonemia (hi"dro-thī"on-am-o-ne'mĭ-ă) [" + *theion*, sulfur, + L. *ammonia*, ammonium, + G. *aima*, blood]. Ammonium sulfide in the blood.

hydrothionemia (hi"dro-thi-on-e'mĭ-ă) [" + " + *aima*, blood]. Condition caused by hydrogen sulfide in the blood.

hydrothionuria (hi-dro-thi-on-u'rĭ-ă) [" + " + *ouron*, urine]. Condition caused by hydrogen sulfide in the urine.

hydrothorax (hi-dro-tho'raks) [G. *ydōr*, water, + *thōrax*, chest]. Dropsy of the chest, or effused fluid in pleural cavity.
 SYM: Dyspnea, absence of vesicular breath sounds, murmur, flatness over location of fluid.
 TREATMENT: According to cause. Aspiration.

hydro'tis [" + *ous, ot-*, ear]. Serous effusion in the internal ear or tympanum.

hydrotomy (hi-drot'o-mĭ) [" + *tomē*, dissection]. Dissection of tissue by forcible injection of water into the vessels.

hydrotropism. Response of plants toward (positive h.) or away (negative h.) from moisture.

hydrotym'panum [" + *tympanon*, drum]. Dropsy of the middle ear.

hydroure'ter [" + *ourētēr*, ureter]. Dropsy of the ureter.

hydrovarium (hi-dro-va'rĭ-um) [" + L. *ovarium*, ovary]. Dropsy or cyst of the ovary.

hydroxide (hi-droks'īd) [G. *ydōr*, water, + *oxys*, acid]. A compound which contains the hydroxyl (OH) group. Ex: NaOH (sodium hydroxide, or caustic soda).

hydroxy acids (hi-droks'ĭ). Acids containing 1 or more hydroxyl groups in addition to the carboxyl group, as *lactic acid*.

hydroxyethylapocupreine (hĭ-drok"sĭ-ĕth"-ĭl-a"pō-ku'pre-ĭn). Derivative of quinine effective in stopping growth of all types of pneumonia germs.

hydrox'yl. The univalent radical OH which, when combined with a metallic ion or a radical which acts as a metal (*e. g.*, NH₄), forms a hydroxide. Commonly called a base or alkali.

hydrozone (hi'dro-zōn) [G. *ydōr*, water, + *ozein*, to smell]. A bactericide of an aqueous solution of pure hydrogen dioxide.

hydruria (hi-dru'rĭ-ă) [" + *ouron*, urine]. Increase of watery constituents of the urine with diminished solids in proportion. SYN: *polyuria*.

hygiene (hi'jĕn) [G. *ygiēinos*, healthful]. The study of health and observance of health rules.
 h., community. That branch of hygiene which deals with the health of a large group of individuals such as a city, state, or nation, and esp. the control of communicable diseases.
 h., industrial. That branch of hygiene which deals primarily with health of industrial workers, esp., prevention of occupational diseases.
 h., mental. Science of developing and maintaining mental health, preventing neurosis and mental unsoundness.
 h., military. That branch of hygiene that deals with the health of men in military service.
 h., oral. Scientific care of teeth and mouth.
 h., social. The prevention and treatment of venereal disease.

hygienic (hi-jĭ-en'ĭk) [G. *ygiēinos*, healthful]. 1. Pert. to health or its preservation. 2. In a healthy condition.

hygien'ics [G. *ygiēinos*, healthful]. A system for promoting health.

hygienist (hĭ'ji-en-ĭst) [G. *ygiēinos*, healthful]. A specialist in hygiene.
 h., dental. One trained in dental prophylaxis to assist a dentist.

hygienization (hĭ"jĕn-i-za'shun) [G. *ygiēinos*, healthful]. The establishment of sanitary conditions and rules of hygiene.

hy'gric [G. *ygros*, moisture]. Pert. to moisture.

hygro- [G.]. Prefix: Rel. to moisture.

hygroma (hi-gro'mă) (pl. *hygromata*) [" + *ōma*, tumor]. A sac or bursa containing fluid.

hygroscopic (hi-gro-skop'ĭk) [" + *skopein*, to examine]. 1. Pert. to hygroscopy. 2. Absorbing moisture readily. SYN: *bibulous, hydrophilous*.

hygros'copy [" + *skopein*, to examine]. Estimation of the quantity of moisture in the atmosphere.

hygrostomia (hi-gro-sto'mĭ-ă) [" + *stoma*,

mouth]. Excess flow of saliva. SYN: *ptyalism, salivation.*
hyla (hi'lă) [G. *ylē*, matter]. A lateral extension of the *aquaeductus cerebri.* SYN: *paraqueduct.*
hylo'ma [" + *ōma*, tumor]. A tumor composed of or in the hylic tissues, such as *hypohyloma,* and *mesohyloma.*
hymen (hi'men) [G. *ymēn*, membrane]. A membranous fold wholly or partially occluding the vaginal orifice.
Its rupture is no longer considered as a loss of virginity.
RS: *carunculae myrtiformes, defloration, hymenorrhaphy, hymenotomy, imperforate.*
 h. annularis. Hymen with a ring-shaped opening in the center.
 h. biforis. One with 2 parallel openings with a thick septum between.
 h. cribriformis. One with many small perforations.
 h. denticulatis. One with an opening with serrated edges.
 h., fenestrated. Same as cribriform.
 h. imperforatus. A hymen with no opening in it.
 h., lunar. H. shaped like the moon.
 h., ruptured. Hymen that has been torn by coitus, injury or operation.
 h. septus or *h., septate.* Hymen in which the opening is separated by a thin septum.
 h., unruptured. The normal hymen.
hymenal (hi'me-nal) [G. *ymēn*, membrane]. Pert. to the hymen.
hymenectomy (hi-men-ek'to-mǐ) [" + *ektomē*, excision]. 1. Removal of a membrane. 2. Removal of the hymen.
hymenitis (hi-men-i'tis) [" + *-itis*, inflammation]. Inflammation of the hymen or a membrane.
Hymenolepis (hi-men-ol'ep-is) [G. *ymēn,* membrane, + *lepis*, rind]. A genus of tapeworm. Parasitic in birds and mammals.
 H. nana. The dwarf tapeworm, a parasite in the intestine of rats and mice and commonly found in man. It averages about 1 in. in length and differs from other tapeworms in that it is capable of completing its complete life cycle within a single host. It causes severe toxic symptoms, esp. in children.
hymenology (hi-men-ol'o-jǐ) [" + *logos*, science]. Science of the membranes and their diseases.
hymenorrhaphy (hi-men-or'af-ǐ) [" + *raphē*, suture]. Plastic operation on the hymen, occluding the vagina.
hymenotome (hi-men'ō-tōm) [" + *tomē*, incision]. Knife used to divide membranes.
hymenotomy (hi-men-ot'o-mǐ) [" + *tomē*, incision]. 1. Incision of the hymen. 2. Dissection of a membrane.
hyo- [G.]. Prefix: Connection with hyoid bone.
hyobasioglossus (hi″o-ba″sǐ-o-glos'us) [G. *yoeidēs*, shape like letter U, + *basis*, base, + *glōssa*, tongue]. The part of hyoglossal muscle attached to the hyoid bone. SYN: *basioglossus.*
hyoepiglottic (hi″o-ep-ǐ-glot'ik) [" + *epiglōttis*, epiglottis]. Rel. to hyoid bone and epiglottis.
hyoepiglottidean (hi″o-ep-i-glot-id'ē-an) [" + *epiglōttis*, epiglottis]. Rel. to hyoid bone and epiglottis. SYN: *hyoepiglottic.*
hyoglos'sal [" + *glōssa*, tongue]. 1. Pert. to the hyoglossus. 2. Extending to the tongue from the hyoid bone.
hyoglossus. A muscle arising from body and greater cornu of hyoid bone and inserted into dorsum of tongue.
ACTION: Draws down sides and retracts tongue.
hy'oid [G. *yoeidēs*, U-shaped]. Bone at ant. surface of neck at root of the tongue, suspended from styloid processes by the stylohyoid ligament.
It is shaped like the Greek letter U.
 h. arch. Second branchial arch.

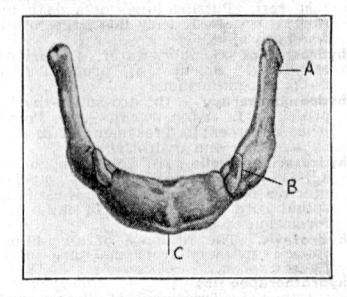

HYOID BONE
A. Greater cornu. B. Lesser cornu. C. Body.

hyopharyngeus (hi-o-far-in'je-us) [" + *pharygx*, gullet]. Middle pharyngeal constrictor.
hyoscine (hi'o-sin) Scopolamine.
Hyoscyamus (hi-o-si'am-us) [G. *ys*, a pig, + *kyamos*, bean]. USP. Dried leaves of the plant *Hyoscyamus niger.* SYN: *henbane.*
ACTION AND USES: Same as belladonna.
DOSAGE: Tincture, 30 ♏ (2 cc.), and of the extract, 3 gr. (0.2 Gm.).
POISONING: Related to atropine, *q.v.* SYN: *henbane.*
hypacousia, hypacusia, hypacusis (hip-ă-koo'sǐ-ă, -kū'sǐ-ă, -sis) [G. *ypo*, under, + *akousis*, hearing]. Impaired hearing.
hypalbuminosis (hip″al-bū-min-o'sis) [" + L. *albumen*, white of egg, + G. *ōsis*]. Deficiency in proportion of albumin in blood.
hypalgesia (hi-pal-je'zǐ-ă) [" + *algēsis*, pain]. Lessened sensitivity to pain. SEE: *hyperalgesia.*
hypalgia (hi-pal'jǐ-ă) [" + *algos*, pain]. Lessened sensitivity to pain. SYN: *hypalgesia.*
hypamnios (hi-pam'nǐ-os) [" + *amnion*, caul of a lamb]. Deficiency in amt. of amniotic fluid.
hypanakinesis (hi-pan-a-kin-e'sis) [" + *anakinēsis*, exercise]. Lowered rate of movement of stomach or intestines.
hypaxial (hi-paks'ǐ-al) [" + *axōn*, axis]. Situated beneath the body axis.
hyper- [G.]. Prefix: Above, excessive, or beyond.
hyperacidaminuria (hi″per-as″id-am-in-ū'-rǐ-ă) [G. *yper*, above, + L. *acidus*, sour, + *amine* + G. *ouron*, urine]. Presence of an excess of amino acids in the urine. SYN: *acidaminuria.*
hyperacid'ity [" + L. *acidus*, sour]. 1. An excess of acid. 2. An excess of acid in the stomach. SEE: *hyperchlorhydria.*
DIET: Three meals and 2 lunches per day. Provide protein to combine with the acid. Moderate amt. of fat to inhibit secretion of acid. Avoid bulky foods, condiments, and extremes of temperature in foods.
hyperacuity (hi-per-a-kū'ǐ-tǐ) [" + L. *acuitās*, sharpness]. Abnormal acuteness, as of vision.

hyperacusis (hi-per-a-ku'sis) [" + *akousis*, hearing]. Abnormal sensitivity to sound. Sometimes found in hysteria.

hyperadenosis (hi"per-ad-en-o'sis) [" + *adēn*, gland, + *ōsis*]. Lymph gland enlargement. SEE: *Hodgkin's disease*.

hyperadiposis, hyperadiposity (hi"per-ad-ĭ-po'sis, -pos'ĭ-tĭ) [" + L. *adeps, adip-*, fat, + *ōsis*]. Excessive fatness.

hyperadrenalemia (hi"per-ad-re"nal-e'mĭ-ă) [" + L. *ad*, toward, + *rēnalis*, pert. to a kidney, + G. *aima*, blood]. Excess of adrenal secretion in the blood.

hyperadre'nalism [" + " + " + G. *ismos*, state of]. Excess of adrenal secretion.

hyperadre'nia [" + " + *rēn*, kidney]. Condition caused by abnormal activity of adrenal glands.

hyperalbuminosis (hi"per-al-bu-min-o'sis) [" + L. *albumen*, white of egg, + G. *ōsis*]. Increased albumin in the blood.

hyperalgesia (hi-per-al-je'zĭ-ă) [" + *algēsis*, pain]. Excessive sensibility to pain; opp. of hypalgesia.

hyperalgia (hi-per-al'jĭ-ă) [" + *algos*, pain]. Excessive sensitivity to pain.

hyperanacinesia, hyperanacinesis (hi"per-an"ă-sin-e'sĭ-ă, -sis) [" + *anakinēsis*, exercise]. Unusual movement, as of the intestines or stomach.

hyperanakine'sis [" + *anakinēsis*, exercise]. Unusual mechanical activity, as of the stomach or intestines.

hyperaphia (hi-per-a'fĭ-ă) [G. *yper*, above, + *aphē*, touch]. Excessive sensitiveness to touch.

hyperaphic (hi-per-af'ĭk) [" + *aphē*, touch]. Marked by extreme sensitiveness to touch.

hyperazoturia (hi-per-az-ot-u'rĭ-ă) [" + *a-*, priv. + *zōē*, life, + *ouron*, urine]. Excessive amt. of nitrogenous matter in the urine.

hyperbilirubinemia (hi"per-bil-ĭ-rū-bĭn-e'mĭ-ă) [" + L. *bilis*, bile, + *ruber*, red, + G. *aima*, blood]. Excessive amt. of bilirubin in the blood.

hyperbrachycephaly (hi"per-brak-ĭ-sef'a-lĭ) [" + *brachys*, short, + *kephalē*, head]. Excessive degree of brachycephaly; having a cephalic index over 85.

hyperbu'lia [" + *boulē*, will]. Morbid wilfulness.

hypercalcemia (hi-per-kal-se'mĭ-ă) [" + L. *calx*, lime, + G. *aima*, blood]. An excessive amt. of calcium in the blood.

hypercalciuria (hi"pĕr-kăl-sĭ-ū'rĭ-ă) [" + " + G. *ouron*, urine]. An excessive quantity of calcium in the urine.

hypercap'nia [" + *kapnos*, smoke]. Undue amt. of carbon dioxide in the blood.

hypercatharsis (hi-per-ka-thar'sis) [" + *katharsis*, purge]. Excessive bowel movement.

hypercementosis (hi"per-se-men-to'sis) [" + L. *cementum*, cement, + G. *ōsis*]. Overgrowth of tooth cement (*cementum*).

hypercenesthesia (hi-per-sen-es-the'sĭ-ă) [" + *koinos*, common, + *aisthēsis*, sensation]. SYN: *euphoria*. Exaggerated feeling of well-being.

hyperchloremia (hi-per-klor-e'mĭ-ă) [" + *chlōros*, green, + *aima*, blood]. Increase in chloride content of the blood.

hyperchlorhydria (hi-per-klor-hid'rĭ-ă) [" + " + *ydōr*, water]. An excess of hydrochloric acid in the gastric secretion.

The amount secreted above what is needed to combine with albumoid and basic substances is known as free HCl.

The normal amount of free hydrochloric acid averages 0.4 to 0.5%. Total acidity is expressed in terms of "clinical units" or the number of c.c. of 0.1 N sodium hydroxide solution required to bring the stomach contents to end point of titration. If stomach contents give values above 60 and after the second hour instead of declining remain high or continue to rise, *hyperchlorhydria* exists. It is common occurring in about 5% of population. If values are below 20 after test meals, hypochlorhydria exists. Excess of HCl causes a burning sensation in the stomach in the absence of ingested food. It also gives rise to gas from this acid's decomposition, and this may cause gastric ulcer. It is more frequent in nervous types, ulcers and chronic gastritis. Two pathological conditions commonly accompanying hyperacidity are duodenal ulcer and pyloric obstruction. SEE: *hydrochloric acid*.

DIET: Small, frequent meals to absorb the HCl. Bland foods and those which will not stimulate the secretion of this acid. Proteins, such as gelatin, eggs, and milk, but little meat or meat broths. Fats, such as cream and butter, permissible as they inhibit the secretion of gastric juice. No sweets, bulky foods, cabbage, onions, or condiments. Cereals; toast; custards; soft, strained, cooked fruits allowable. SYN: *gastrosuccorrhea*. SEE: *gastritis, hypochlorhydria*.

hyperchlorida'tion [G. *yper*, above, + *chlōros*, green]. A dosing with large amounts of sodium chloride.

hypercholestere'mia [" + *cholē*, bile, + *stereos*, stiff, + *aima*, blood]. Excess of cholesterol in the blood. SYN: *hypercholesterinemia*.

hypercholesterine'mia [" + " + *stereos*, solid, + *aima*, blood]. Excess of cholesterol in the blood.

hypercholesterolemia (hi"per-ko-les"ter-ol-e'mĭ-ă) [" + " + " + *aima*, blood]. Excessive amt. of cholesterol in the blood.

hypercholesterolia (hi"per-ko-les"ter-o'lĭ-ă) [" + " + *stereos*, stiff]. Excessive cholesterol in the bile.

hypercholia (hi-per-ko'lĭ-ă) [" + *cholē*, bile]. Abnormal secretion of bile.

hyperchromasia (hi"per-kro-ma'sĭ-ă) [" + *chrōma*, color]. Excessive pigmentation. SYN: *hyperchromatism*.

hyperchromatic (hi"per-kro-mat'ĭk) [" + *chrōma*, color]. Overpigmented.

h. cell. A cell or a part of a cell which contains more than the normal number of chromosomes and hence stains more densely.

hyperchro'matism [" + " + *ismos*, state of]. 1. Excessive pigmentation. 2. Increased staining capacity of any structure. SYN: *hyperchromatosis*.

hyperchromatopsia (hi"per-kro-ma-top'-sĭ-ă) [" + " + *opsis*, vision]. Defect of vision in which all objects appear colored.

hyperchromato'sis [G. *yper*, above, + *chrōma*, color, + *ōsis*]. Excessive pigmentation, esp., of the skin.

hyperchromemia (hi"per-kro-me'mĭ-ă) [" + " + *aima*, blood]. Condition of a high color index of the blood.

hyperchromia (hi-per-kro'mĭ-ă) [" + *chrōma*, color]. Excessive pigmentation. SYN: *hyperchromatism*.

hyperchromic (hĭ-pĕr-krōm'ĭk) [" + *chrōma*, color]. Pert. to excessive pigmentation.

hyperchylia (hi-per-ki'lĭ-ă) [" + *chylos*, juice]. Abnormal secretion of gastric juice.

hypercinesia (hi-per-sin-e'sĭ-ă) [" + *kinēsis*, motion]. Abnormal mobility.

h., professional. Occupational neurosis.

hypercri'nism [" + " + *ismos*, state of]. Condition due to excessive activity of any endocrine gland.

hypercryalgesia (hi-per-kri-al-je'sĭ-ă) [G. *yper*, above, + *kryos*, cold, + *algēsis*, pain]. SYN: *hypercryesthesia*. Excessive sensitivity to cold.

hypercryesthe'sia [" + " + *aisthēsis*, sensation]. Excessive allergy to cold. SYN: *hypercryalgesia*.

hypercyanosis (hi″per-si″an-o'sĭs) [" + *kyanos*, dark blue, + *ōsis*]. Extreme cyanosis.

hypercyanotic (hi-per-si-an-ot'ik) [" + *kyanos*, dark blue]. Denoting extreme cyanosis.

hypercyesis (hi-per-si-e'sĭs) [" + *kyēsis*, gestation]. Presence of more than 1 fetus in a uterus because of fertilization of a second ovum within a short time, at different menstrual periods. SYN: *superfetation*.

hypercythemia (hi-per-si-the'mĭ-ă) [" + *kytos*, cell, + *aima*, blood]. Condition of having an excessive number of red blood corpuscles.

hypercytosis (hi-per-si-to'sĭs) [" + " + *ōsis*]. Abnormal increase in leukocytes in the blood. SYN: *hyperleukocytosis*.

hyperdactyl'ia [G. *yper*, above, + *dactylos*, finger]. State of having supernumerary fingers or toes.

hyperdiastole (hi″per-di-as'to-le) [" + *diastellein*, to draw apart]. Extreme cardiac diastole.

hyperdicrot'ic [" + *dikrotos*, beating double]. Abnormally dicrotic.

hyperdistention (hi″per-dis-ten'shun) [" + L. *distendere*, to stretch out]. Excessive inflation.

hyperdiure'sis [" + *dia*, through, + *ourein*, to urinate]. Excessive urination. SYN: *polyuria*.

hyperdyna'mia [" + *dynamis*, force]. Muscular restlessness or extreme violence.

h. uteri. Abnormal uterine contractions in labor.

hypereccrisia, hypereccrisis (hi-per-ek-kris'ĭ-ă, -ek'kris-is) [" + *ek*, out, + *krisis*, separation]. Abnormal amt. of excretion.

hypereccritic, hyperecritic (hi-per-ek-rit'-ik) [" + *ekkritikos*, excreting]. Pert. to an abnormal amt. of excretion or hypereccrisis.

hyperemesis (hi-per-em'e-sis) [G. *yper*, above, + *emesis*, vomiting]. Excessive vomiting.

h. gravidarum. One of the toxemias of early pregnancy characterized by excessive vomiting.

ETIOL: Occurs most frequently in highly sensitive, neurotic individuals, and although it may begin on a neurotic basis the constant vomiting brings on the definite toxic changes. In the severe cases there is definite pathological evidence of the condition, the liver showing changes of a necrotic nature in the center of the lobules.

SYM: The condition may start as a simple vomiting of early pregnancy, but with combined vomiting of first gastric contents, and later of bile, there is developed a chloride depletion, an acidosis, and, finally, with severe and continued vomiting the pathological changes in the liver take place.

The findings are those of a patient who is pregnant and who vomits constantly, loses weight rapidly, dehydrates, develops a rapid pulse, has rise in temperature, and acetone in the urine. Liver function tests may reveal evidences of impaired function if the condition is allowed to progress.

TREATMENT: In early cases, rest in bed; restrictions of fluids taken by mouth, fluids given per rectum or by hypodermoclysis; saturation of the patient with soporifics. In the average case where nervous irritability is a factor the patient should be kept in a darkened, quiet room free from all visitors.

Any malposition of the uterus, or any cervical pathology should be taken care of immediately. With rigid management of this type, and no relief from symptoms, and if the pulse and temperature rise and there is definite evidence of liver damage (jaundice), therapeutic abortion should be resorted to.

The necessity for emptying the uterus should occur only rarely if the patient is seen early, and the proper treatment instituted at once. When the patient improves and food is again taken by mouth, it should consist of thick gruels and dry toast with very little liquid nourishment.

h. lactentium. Vomiting in nursing infants.

hyperemia (hi-per-e'mĭ-ă) [" + *aima*, blood]. 1. Congestion. An unusual amount of blood in a part. 2. A form of macula; red areas on skin which disappear on pressure. 3. PT: Increase in the quantity of blood flowing through any part of the body; as undue redness of the skin, caused by the application of heat.

h., active, h., arterial. H. caused by increased blood inflow.

h., Bier's, h., constriction. Passive hyperemia* produced by application of an elastic bandage and by suction.

h., leptomeningeal. Pia-arachnoid congestion.

h., passive, h., venous. H. caused by decreased blood outflow.

hyperemization (hi″per-e-mi-za'shun) [G. *yper*, above, + *aima*, blood]. Hyperemia produced artificially for therapeutic purposes.

hyperemotiv'ity [" + L. *ēmotum, ēmovēre*, to move out]. Excessive emotivity or response to stimuli.

hyperendocrin'ia [" + *endon*, within, + *krinein*, to separate]. Pert. to hyperendocrinism.

hyperendocrinism (hi″per-en-dok'rĭ-nizm) [" + " + " + *ismos*, state of]. Abnormal increase of internal secretion.

hyperendocrisia (hi″per-en-do-kris'ĭ-ă) [" + + *krisis*, a separation]. Excessive increase of internal secretions. SYN: *hyperendocrinism*.

hypereosinophilia (hi″per-e″o-sin-o-fĭl'ĭ-ă) [" + *ēōs*, dawn (rose colored), + *philein*, to love]. Excessive leukocytosis with increase of eosinophils.

hyperephidrosis (hi″per-ef-ĭ-dro'sĭs) [" + *epi*, upon, + *idrōs*, sweating]. Abnormal sweating.

hyperepinephria (hi″per-ep″ĭ-nef'rĭ-ă) [" + + *nephros*, kidney]. Excessive adrenal secretion with arterial tension.

hyperepinephrine'mia [" + " + *nephros*, kidney, + *aima*, blood]. Undue proportion of adrenalin in the blood. SYN: *hyperadrenalemia*.

hy″perequilib'rium [" + L. *aequus*, equal, + *libra*, balance]. A tendency to vertigo when turning.

hypererethism (hi-per-er'eth-izm) [" + *erethisma*, stimulation]. Excessive irritability.

hyperergasia (hi-per-er-ga'sĭ-ă) [" + *ergasia*, work]. Unusual functional activity.

hyperergia (hi-per-er'jĭ-ă) [" + *ergon*, work]. Excessive or increased functional activity. SYN: *hyperergasia*.

hy″perergy (hī'per-er-jī) [G. *yper*, above, + *ergon*, energy]. Hypersensitivity or condition in which there is an exaggerated response.

hypererythrocythemia (hi″per-er-ith″ro-si-the'mĭ-ă) [" + *erythros*, red, + *kytos*, cell, + *aima*, blood]. Excess of red corpuscles in the blood.

hyperesophoria (hi″per-es-o-fo'rĭ-ă) [" + *esō*, inward, + *phorein*, to bear]. A tending of visual lines upward and inward. SYN: *heterophoria*.

hyperesthesia (hi″per-es-the'zĭ-ă) [G. *yper*, above, + *aisthēsis*, sensation]. Unusual sensibility to sensory stimuli, such as pain or touch. SYN: *algesia*.

 h., acoustic, h., auditory. Abnormal sensitivity to sound.

 h., cerebral. H. caused by a cerebral lesion.

 h., gustatory. Oversensitivity of taste.

 h., muscular. Muscular sensitivity to pain and tiredness.

 h., optic. Abnormal sensitivity to light.

 h. sexualis. Abnormal increase in the sexual impulse.

 h., tactile. Abnormal sensitivity of touch.

hyperesthet′ic [" + *aisthēsis*, sensation]. Pert. to hyperesthesia.

hyperexophoria (hi″per-eks-o-fo'rĭ-ă) [" + *exō*, outward, + *phorein*, to bear]. A tendency of visual lines upward and outward.

hyperextension (hi″per-eks-ten'shun) [" + L. *extendere*, to stretch out]. Extreme or abnormal extension.

hyperfunction. Excessive activity.

hypergalactia (hi-per-gal-ak'shĭ-ă) [" + *gala*, milk]. Excessive milk secretion.

hypergenesis (hi-per-jen'es-is) [" + *genesis*, development]. Redundancy of organs or parts; overproduction. SYN: *hyperplasia*.

hy″pergen′italism (hi-per-jen'it-al-izm) [G. *yper*, above, + L. *genitalis*, genital, + G. *ismos*, state of]. SYN: *Precocious puberty*. Excessive development of the genital organs.

 ETIOL: Disturbances in endocrine secretions of the adrenal gland, or gonads, or hypothalmic disorders.

hypergeusesthesia, hypergeusia (hi″per-gu-ses-the'sĭ-ă, -gu'sĭ-ă) [" + *geusis*, taste]. Excessive acuteness of sense of taste.

hyperglan′dular [" + L. *glandula*, a little acorn]. Having excessive glandular secretions.

hyperglobu′lia [" + L. *globulus*, globule]. Having an excessive number of red blood corpuscles. SYN: *hypercythemia, polycythemia.*

hyperglobulinemia (hi-per-glob-u-lĭn-e'mĭ-ă) [" + " + G. *aima*, blood]. Excessive globulin in the blood.

hyperglycemia (hi-per-gli-se'mĭ-ă) [" + *glykus*, sweet, + *aima*, blood]. Increase of blood sugar from 0.15 to 0.2 or 0.3% or more, as in diabetes.

 This condition increases susceptibility to infection and it often precedes diabetic coma. SEE: *hypoglycemia*.

hyperglycistia (hi-per-glis-is'tĭ-ă) [G. *yper*, above, + *glykus*, sweet, + *istos*, tissue]. Excess of glucose in the tissues.

hyperglycogenolysis (hi-per-gli-ko-jen-ol'-is-is) [" + " + *gennan*, to form, + *lysis*, dissolution]. Excessive conversion of glycogen into glucose by hydrolysis.

hyperglycoplasmia (hi″per-gli″ko-plas'-mĭ-ă) [" + " + *plasma*, matter formed]. Excessive sugar in the plasma of the blood.

hyperglycorrhachia (hi″per-gli″ko-ra'kĭ-ă) [" + " + *rachis*, spine]. Excess of sugar in the cerebrospinal fluid.

hyperglycosemia (hi-per-gli-ko-se'mĭ-ă) [" + " + *aima*, blood]. Excessive sugar in the blood. SYN: *hyperglycemia*.

hyperglycosuria (hi-per-gli-ko-su'rĭ-ă) [" + " + *ouron*, urine]. Excessive sugar in the urine. SEE: *glycosuria*.

hypergnosis (hi″per-no-sis) [" + *gnōsis*, knowledge]. All that is involved in projection of conflicts with the environment, evidenced in paranoia, q.v.

hypergonadism (hi-per-gon'ad-izm) [" + *gonē*, semen, + *ismos*, state of]. Excessive internal secretion of the sexual glands.

hyperguanidinemia (hi″per-gwan-ĭ-dēn-e'-mĭ-ă) [" + *guanidine* + *aima*, blood]. Abnormal amt. of guanidine in blood.

hyperhedonia, hyperhedonism (hi-per-he-do'nĭ-ă, -he'don-izm) [" + *ēdonē*, pleasure, + *ismos*, state of]. 1. Abnormal pleasure in anything. 2. Abnormal sexual excitement.

hyperhepatia (hi″per-he-pa'shĭ-ă) [" + *epar, epat-*, liver]. Overfunctioning of the liver.

hyperhor′monism [" + *ormanein*, to arouse, + *ismos*, state of]. Excessive activity of the endocrine glands.

hy″perhydro′sis [G. *yper*, above, + *idrōs*, sweat, + *ōsis*]. Excessive sweating.

 ETIOL: Functional disorder of sweat glands, caused by debilitating disease, stimulants, neurasthenia. Increased in rheumatic, malarial, relapsing and septic fever. At night, in pulmonary tuberculosis, and at crisis in pneumonia. In Graves' disease, neuralgia, migraine and following certain drugs and hot drinks. Locally (hands and feet), in hysteria, fright, vagitonia, nervous irritability, and exophthalmic goiter. SEE: *sweat*.

 h. oleosa. Increased and altered sebaceous secretion. SYN: *seborrhea*.

hyperhypocytosis (hi″per-hi″po-si-to'sis) [" + *ypo*, under, + *kytos*, cell, + *ōsis*]. Decrease of white corpuscles (leukopenia), esp. with relative increase of neutrophils.

hyperinose′mia [" + *is, in-*, fiber, + *aima*, blood]. Abnormal coagulability of the blood; excess of fibrinogen in the blood. SYN: *hyperinosis*.

hyperino′sis [G. *yper*, above, + *is, in-*, fiber, + *ōsis*]. Excessive fibrinogen in the blood. SYN: *hyperinosemia*.

hyperinsulinism (hi-per-in'su-lin-izm) [" + L. *insula*, island, + G. *ismos*, state of]. An excessive amount of insulin in the blood.

 ETIOL: Tumor or islets of Langerhans, or excessive sensitivity of the islet tissue to an increase in blood-sugar level. May also occur following injection of an excess of insulin.

 SYM: The hypoglycemic picture: hunger, weakness, sweating, staggering, diplopia—rarely convulsions—coma, and death. Occasionally spontaneous. Symptoms similar to but more chronic than in insulin shock. SEE: *insulin, insulin shock, shock.*

hyperinvolution (hi-per-in-vo-lu′shun) [" + L. *involvere*, to roll in]. 1. Reduction in size of uterus below normal after childbirth. 2. Reduction in size below normal of any organ following hypertrophy. SYN: *superinvolution*.
  h. uteri. Extreme atrophy of the uterus seen following prolonged lactation or severe puerperal sepsis.
hyperisoton′ic [" + " + *tonos*, tension]. Noting 1 of 2 solutions having greater osmotic pressure. SYN: *hypertonic*.
hy″perkalem′ia. Excessive amount of potassium in blood plasm.
hyperkeratomycosis (hi″per-ker″at-o-mi-ko′sis) [" + *keras*, horn, + *mykēs*, fungus, + *ōsis*]. Hypertrophy of horny layer of the epidermis due to a parasitic fungus.
hyperkerato′sis [" + " + *ōsis*]. 1. Overgrowth of cornea. 2. Overgrowth of the horny layer of the epidermis. SYN: *keratodermia, keratosis.*
  h. congenitalis. Hyperkeratosis in the harlequin fetus.
hy″perketonur′ia. Excessive quantity of ketones in urine.
hyperkine′sia, hyperkine′sis [" + *kinēsis*, motion]. Excessive amt. of mobility. SYN: *hypercinesia*.
hyperlacta′tion [" + L. *lactare*, to suckle]. Excessive milk secretion. SYN: *superlactation*.
hyperleukocyto′sis [" + *leukos*, white, + *kytos*, cell, + *ōsis*]. Excessive quantity of leukocytes. SYN: *leukocytosis.*
hy″perlipe′mia (hi-per-lip-e′mĭ-ă) [G. *yper*, above, + *lipos*, fat, + *aima*, blood]. Excessive quantity of fat in the blood.
hyperlipo′sis [" + " + *ōsis*]. 1. Abnormal fat; adiposity. 2. Excessive fatty degeneration.
hyperlithuria (hi-per-lith-u′rĭ-ă) [" + *lithos*, stone, + *ouron*, urine]. Excessive excretion of lithic (uric) acid in the urine.
hypermas′tia [" + *mastos*, breast]. 1. Excessively large mammary gland. 2. Presence of abnormal number of mammary glands. SYN: *polymastia, polymazia*.
hypermature (hi-per-mat-ūr′) [G. *yper*, above, + L. *maturus*, ripe]. Overmature; past maturity.
hypermegasoma (hi″per-meg-ă-sō′mă) [" + *megas*, large, + *sōma*, body]. Excessive bodily development. SYN: *gigantism*.
hypermenorrhea (hi-per-men-o-re′ă) [" + *mēn*, month, + *roia*, flow]. 1. Too frequent menstrual periods. 2. Abnormal menstrual flow.
hypermetaplasia (hi-per-met-ă-pla′sĭ-ă) [" + *metaplasis*, transformation]. Overactivity in tissue replacement or transformation from one type of tissue to another, as cartilage to bone.
hyperme′tria [" + *metron*, measure]. Unusual range of movement.
hypermetrope (hi-per-met′rōp) [" + " + *ōps*, eye]. One who is farsighted. SYN: *hyperope*.
hypermetro′pia [" + " + *ōps*, eye]. Farsightedness. Opp. of *myopia*. SYN: *hyperopia*.
hy″permetrop′ic [" + " + *ōps*, eye]. Pert. to farsightedness.
hypermnesia (hi-perm-ne′zĭ-ă) [" + *mnēsis*, memory]. 1. Great ability to remember names, dates, and details. 2. An exaggeration of memory involving minute details of a past experience. It may occur in mentally unstable individuals after a shock.

hypermorph (hi′per-morf) [" + *morphē*, form]. One whose length of limb and consequent standing height is high in proportion to the sitting height. SEE: *hypomorph, mesomorph*.
hypermotil′ity [" + L. *motiō*, motion]. Unusual motility. SYN: *hyperkinesia*.
hypermyatrophy (hi″per-mi-at′ro-fĭ) [" + *mys, myo*-, muscle, + *atrophia*, atrophy]. Unusual wasting of muscle.
hypermyesthesia (hi″per-mi-es-the′sĭ-ă) [" + " + *aisthēsis*, sensation]. Muscular sensitivity.
hypermyotonia (hi-per-mi-o-to′nĭ-ă) [" + " + *tonos*, tone]. Excessive muscular tonus.
hypermyotrophy (hi-per-mi-ot′rō-fĭ) [" + " + *trophē*, nourishment]. Abnormal muscular development.
hyperneocytosis (hi″per-ne″o-sī-to′sis) [" + *neos*, new, + *kytos*, cell, + *ōsis*]. Abnormal increase of leukocytes in the blood (*leukocytosis*) including immature forms. SYN: *hyperleukocytosis*.
hy″pernephro′ma [G. *yper*, above, + *nephros*, kidney, + *ōma*, tumor]. A tumor of the kidney or other organ which contains adrenal tissue. It can be identified by presence of chromaffin cells.
hyperneurotization (hi-per-nū-rot-i-za′shun) [" + *neuron*, nerve]. Grafting of a motor nerve into a muscle to increase its energy.
hypernitremia (hi-per-nī-tre′mĭ-ă) [" + *nitron*, niter, + *aima*, blood]. Excess of nitrogen in the blood.
hypernoia (hi-per-noy′ă) [" + *nous*, mind]. Excessive mental activity or imagination. SYN: *hyperpsychosis*.
hypernor′mal [G. *yper*, above, + L. *norma*, rule]. Abnormal.
hypernormocytosis (hi″per-nor″mo-sī-to′sis) [" + " + G. *kytos*, cell, + *ōsis*]. An increased proportion of neutrophils in the blood.
hypernutri′tion [" + L. *nutrīre*, to nourish]. Supernutrition; overfeeding.
hyperontomorph (hī-per-ŏn-tō-môrf) [G. *yper*, above, + *ōn*, being, + *morphē*, form]. 1. A person with a long thin body and short intestine. 2. One with a tendency to hyperthyroidism.
hyperonychia (hi-per-o-nik′ĭ-ă) [" + *onyx*, nail]. Overgrowth (hypertrophy) of the nails.
hyperope (hi′per-ōp) [" + *ōps*, eye]. One who is farsighted. SYN: *hypermetrope*.

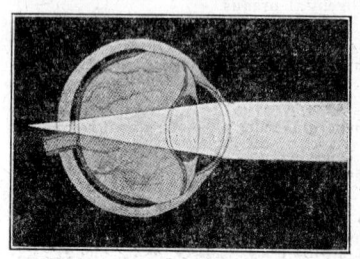

HYPEROPIA
Parallel light rays come to a focus behind the retina. SEE: *ametropia, myopia*.

hypero′pia [" + *ōps*, eye]. Farsightedness.
Parallel rays come to a focus behind the retina due to flattening of the globe

of the eye, or to error in refraction. SYN: *hypermetropia*.
  h., absolute. H. in which the eye cannot accommodate.
  h., axial. H. caused by shortness of the eye's anteroposterior axis.
  h., facultative. H. which can be corrected by accommodation.
  h., latent. H. in which the error of refraction is overcome and disguised by ciliary muscle action.
  h., manifest. Total amount of h. which can be measured by a convex lens.
  h., relative. H. in which vision is clear only when excessive convergence is made.
  h., total. Complete h. combining both latent and manifest types.

hyperorchidism (hi-per-or'kid-izm) [" + *orchis*, testicle, + *ismos*, state of]. Abnormal activity of testicular secretion.

hyperorexia (hi-per-o-reks'ĭ-ă) [" + *orexis*, appetite]. Abnormal hunger.
  Usually satisfied by frequent small meals, as in gastric diseases, diabetes, hysteria, psychosis, hyperthyroidism and brain tumors.
  It is found in helminthiasis, diabetes, hysteria, convalescence from acute diseases, psychosis, hyperthyroidism, brain tumors, diseases of the stomach in which hypermotility and hypersecretion are present. SYN: *bulimia*.

hyperorthocytosis (hi″per-or″tho-si-to'sis) [" + *orthos*, straight, + *kytos*, cell, + *ōsis*]. Increased white blood cells with normal proportion of various forms and without immature forms.

hyperos'mia [G. *yper*, above, + *osmē*, smell]. Abnormal sensitiveness to odors.

hyperosto'sis [" + *osteon*, bone, + *ōsis*]. Abnormal growth of osseous tissue. SYN: *exostosis*.

hyperova'ria [" + L. *ovarium*, ovary]. Precocity of libido in young girls due to excessive ovarian secretion as the result of unusual and premature development of the ovaries.

hyperpancreatism (hi″per-pan'kre-ă-tizm) [" + *pagkreas*, pancreas, + *ismos*, state of]. Abnormal activity of the pancreas with trypsin in excess of other ferments.

hy'perparasit'ism. Condition in which a parasite lives in or upon another parasite.

hyperparathyroidism (hi″per-par-a-thi'roy-dizm) [" + *para*, beside, + *thyreos*, shield, + *eidos*, form, + *ismos*, state of]. Condition due to increase of the parathyroid secretions.

hyperpep'sia [" + *pepsis*, digestion]. 1. Unusually rapid digestion. 2. Indigestion with hyperchlorhydria.

hyperpepsinia (hi″per-pep-sin'ĭ-ă) [" + *pepsis*, digestion]. Excess of pepsin in the gastric secretion.

hyperperistalsis (hi″per-per-ĭ-stal'sis) [" + *peri*, around, + *stalsis*, contraction]. Overactive peristalsis.

hyperphalangism (hi-per-fal'an-jizm) [" + *phalagx*, a line, + *ismos*, state of]. Having an extra phalanx on a finger or toe. SYN: *polyphalangism*.

hyperphasia (hi-per-fa'zĭ-ă) [" + *phasis*, speech]. Loss of control of the organs of speech.

hyperphonesis (hi-per-fō-ne'sis) [" + *phonē*, voice]. Increase in voice or percussion sound in auscultation.

hyperphonia (hi-per-fo'nĭ-ă) [" + *phonē*, voice]. Stuttering or stammering due to excessive innervation of vocal muscles.

hyperphoria (hi-per-fo'rĭ-ă) [" + *phorein*, to bear]. Tendency of 1 eye to turn upward. SEE: *anophoria*.

hyperphosphatemia (hi-per-fos-fă-te'mĭ-ă) [" + L. *phosphās*, phosphate, + G. *aima*, blood]. Abnormal amt. of phosphorus in the blood. SYN: *hyperphospheremia*.

hyperphosphaturia (hi″per-fos-fă-tū'rĭ-ă) [" + " + G. *ouron*, urine]. Increased amt. of phosphates in the urine.

hyperphospheremia (hi″per-fos-fer-e'mĭ-ă) [G. *yper*, above, + L. *phosphās*, phosphate, + G. *aima*, blood]. Abnormal amt. of phosphorous compounds in the blood. SYN: *hyperphosphatemia*.

hyperphragia (hi″per-frăg'ĭ-ă). Excessive mental activity occurring esp. in the manic phase of manic-depressive psychosis.

hyperphragic (hi″per-frăg'ic). Pertaining to hyperphragia, *q.v.*

hyperphrenia (hi-per-fre'nĭ-ă) [" + *phrēn*, mind]. 1. Unusual intellectual activity. 2. Genius.

hyperpiesia, hyperpiesis (hi″per-pi-e'zĭ-ă, -sis) [" + *piesis*, pressure]. Abnormally high blood pressure.

hyperpietic (hi″per-pi-et'ik) [" + *piesis*, pressure]. Rel. to extremely high blood pressure.

hyperpituitarism (hi″per-pit-u'ĭ-tar'ism) [G. *yper*, above, + L. *pituita*, mucus, + G. *ismos*, state of]. Condition resulting from overactivity of the *hypophysis cerebri* or its ant. lobe. SEE: *acromegaly, gigantism*.

hyperplasia (hi-per-plā'zĭ-ă) [G. *yper*, above, + *plassein*, to form]. An increase in size of a tissue or organ resulting from proliferation of cells or the development of additional tissue of which the organ is composed but excluding tumor formation; excessive formation of tissue.
  h., fibrous. Connective tissue cell increase following any inflammation or in chronic visceral fibrosis.
  h., lipoid. Increase in cells containing lipoid.

hyperplas'mia [" + *plasma*, matter formed]. 1. Abnormal increase within certain organs of leukocytes which do not appear in the blood. SYN: *aleukemia*. 2. Increase in size of red blood cells through absorption of fluids.

hyperplastic (hi-per-plas'tik) [" + *plassein*, to form]. Rel. to hyperplasia.

hyperpnea (hi-perp-ne'ă) [" + *pnoē*, breath]. An increased respiratory rate or breathing which is deeper than that seen in resting subjects. A certain degree of hyperpnea is normal after exercise.
  ETIOL: Pain, respiratory disease, febrile or cardiac disease, disease of diaphragm, of blood, of abdominal viscera, or due to certain drugs, hysteria, or atmospheric conditions.

hyperporo'sis [" + *pōros*, callus, + *ōsis*]. Excessive callous formation after a bone fracture.

hyperpragic (hi-per-prā'jĭk) [" + *praxis*, action]. Denoting excessive activity.

hyperprax'ia [G. *yper*, above, + *praxis*, action]. Excessive activity.

hyperprochoresis (hi″per-pro-ko-re'sis) [" + *pro*, forward, + *choreia*, dance]. Unusually rapid passage of food through the alimentary tract due to increased peristalsis. SYN: *hyperperistalsis, hyperanacinesia, tormina nervosa*.

hyperprosexia (hi-per-pro-seks'ĭ-ă) [" + *prosezein*, to heed]. PSY: Fixation of an idea to the exclusion of other ideas, as in compulsion states.

hyperproteinemia (hi″per-pro″te-in-e′-mĭ-ă) [" + *prōtos*, first, + *aima*, blood]. Excess of protein in the blood plasma.

hy″perpro″teinu′ria [" + " + *ouron*, urine]. Excess of protein in the urine.

hyperproteosis (hi″per-pro-te-o′sis) [" + " + *ōsis*]. A condition resulting from an excess of protein in the diet.

hyperpselaphesia (hi″perp-sel-af-e′zĭ-ă) [" + *psēlaphēsis*, touch]. Morbid sensitivity to touch.

hyperpsycho′sis [" + *psychē*, mind, + *ōsis*]. Overfunctioning of the mind.

hyperpyre′mia [" + *pyreia*, fuel, + *aima*, blood]. Excess of heat and energy producing substances in the blood.

hyperpyretic (hi″per-pi-ret′ĭk) [" + *pyrexia*, fever]. Pert. to high body temperature (hyperpyrexia).

hyperpyrexia (hi″per-pi-reks′ĭ-ă) [" + *pyrexia*, fever]. Elevation of systemic temperature, above 106° F.
Produced by following physical agents: Baths, diathermy, radiofrequency current, hot air, radiant heat, electric blankets.

hyperpyrex′ial [" + *pyrexia*, fever]. Denoting high body temperature.

hyperreflex′ia [" + L. *reflexus*, bent back]. Increased action of the reflexes.

hyperres′onance [" + L. *resonāre*, to resound]. Increased resonance caused by percussion.

hy″persaliva′tion. Excessive secretion of saliva.

hypersecretion (hi-per-se-kre′shun) [G. *yper*, above, + L. *secernere*, to secrete]. Abnormal amt. of secretion.

hy″persensibil′ity [" + L. *sensibilitās*, sensibility]. Hypersensitivity of the body to a foreign protein or drug. SYN: *anaphylaxis*, q.v.

hypersensitiveness (hĭ″per-sĕn′sĭ-tĭv-nĕs) [" + L. *sensitivus*, sensitive]. Excessive and abnormal susceptibility to the action of a given agent, as pollen or foreign protein. SEE: *allergy, anaphylaxis, hay fever.*

hy″persensitiv′ity. Abnormal sensitivity to a stimulus of any kind.

hypersensitiza′tion [" + L. *sensitivus*, sensitive]. An abnormally increased susceptibility to infection.

hyperskeocytosis (hi″per-ske″o-si-to′sis) [" + *skaios*, left, + *kytos*, cell, + *ōsis*]. Leukocytosis with many immature forms. SYN: *hyperneocytosis.*

hypersom′nia [" + L. *somnus*, sleep]. A toxic condition conducive to sleeping an excessively long time.

hypersphyxia (hi-per-sfĭks′ĭ-ă) [" + *sphyxis*, pulse]. High blood pressure with increased activity of the circulation.

hypersthe′nia [" + *sthenos*, strength]. Abnormal strength or excessive tension, as in the insane.

hypersthen′ic [" + *sthenos*, strength]. Denoting excessive strength, or tension.

hypersthenuria (hi″per-sthen-u′rĭ-ă) [" + " + *ouron*, urine]. Dilute condition of the urine with elevation of the freezing point.

hy″persuscep′tibil′ity [" + L. *suscipere*, to take, + *habilis*, apt]. Unusual susceptibility to a disease or to physical, esp. pathological, conditions. SEE: *allergic, allergy, anaphylactin, anaphylactogenic, anaphylaxis, anatoxic.*

hypersystole (hi-per-sĭs′to-lē) [" + *systolē*, contraction]. Unusual force or duration of the systole.

hypersystol′ic [" + *systolē*, contraction]. 1. Pert. to hypersystole. 2. Person with undue heart contractions.

hypertarachia (hi-per-tă-rak′ĭ-ă) [" + *tarache*, disorder]. Excessive irritability of the nervous system.

hypertelorism (hi-per-tel′or-izm) [" + *tēlē*, far, + *orizein*, to separate]. Abnormal width between 2 paired organs.

   h., ocular. Abnormal width bet. the eyes.

hy″pertens′in. SYN: *angiotonin*. An active vasoconstrictor (pressor) agent formed in an ischemic kidney. It is a polypeptid formed from the action of renin, an enzyme produced by the renal cortex, on hypertensinogen.

hy″pertens′inase. SYN: *angiotonase*. An enzyme present in normal kidney tissue which inactivates hypertensin. It is also present in other organs and tissues.

hy″pertensin′ogen. A pseudoglobulin present in blood plasma which is the precursor of hypertensin, q.v.

hyperten′sion [G. *yper*, above, + L. *tensiō*, tension]. 1. Tension or tonus above normal. 2. A condition in which patient has a higher blood pressure than normal for his age.
ETIOL: The primary factor in hypertension is an increase in peripheral resistance resulting from vasoconstriction or narrowing of peripheral blood vessels.
One hundred and sixty millimeters systolic pressure constitutes the beginning of high blood pressure which may run well above 200 or even as high as 280. Persistent high blood pressure may eventuate in apoplexy or heart failure.
Recent research has attributed it, in part, to calcium formation on walls of blood vessels. It is treated by redissolving the calcium into the blood by means of electrolysis.

   h., essential. SYN: *hyperpiesia*. H. which develops in the absence of kidney disease. Its cause is unknown. Also called primary or benign hypertension.

   h., benign. H. of slow onset which is usually without symptoms.

   h., Goldblatt. Hypertension which resembles renal hypertension produced in experimental animals.

   h., malignant. Severe form of h. in which occlusion of peripheral vessels occurs resulting from hyperplasia and degenerative changes in intima.

   h., renal. H. resulting from kidney disease. H. produced experimentally by constriction of renal arteries. It is due to a humoral substance *renin*, produced in an ischemic kidney.
RS: *blood pressure, diastolic p., hypotension, pulse, pulse pressure, systolic p.*

hyperten′sive [" + L. *tensiō*, tension]. Marked by a rise in blood pressure.

   h. diseases. Noninfectious ones with increased blood pressure.

hyperthe′lia [" + *thēlē*, nipple]. The presence of more than 2 nipples.

hyperthermalgesia (hi″per-therm-al-je′zhĭ-ă) [" + *thermē*, heat, + *algesia*, pain]. Unusual sensitiveness to heat.

hyperther′mia (hi-per-ther′mĭ-ă) [G. *yper*, above, + *thermē*, heat.] SYN: *hyperpyrexia*. 1. Unusually high fever. 2. Treatment of disease by raising bodily temperature, accomplished by introduction of the malaria organism, injection of foreign proteins, or by physical means.

hyperthermoesthesia (hi-per-therm-o-es-the′sĭ-ă) [" + " + *aisthēsis*, sensation]. Unusual sensitiveness to heat. SYN: *hyperthermalgesia.*

hyperthrombinemia (hi″per-throm-bin-e′mĭ-ă) [" + *thrombos*, clot, + *aima*, blood]. Excess of thrombin in the blood causing coagulation.

hyperthymergastic reaction (hi″per-thi-mer-gas′tik) [" + *thymos*, mind, + *ergasia*, work]. A syndrome of a psychic disorder in which circumscribed attacks exhibit elated excitement, delusions of self-exaltation, euphoria, and other symptoms, including inability to conform to environment, and rebellion against inhibitions.

hyperthymia (hi-per-thi′mĭ-ă) [" + *thymos*, mind]. 1. Morbid sensitiveness. 2. Cruelty or foolhardiness. 3. Moral insanity.

hyperthy′mism, hyperthymiza′tion [" + " + *ismos*, state]. Excess secretion of the thymus gland.

hyperthyrea (hī-per-thi′re-ă) [" + *thyreos*, shield]. Excessive activity of the thyroid.

hyperthyreosis (hi″per-thi-re-o′sis) [" + " + *ōsis*]. Overactivity of the thyroid. SYN: *hyperthyrea, hyperthyroidation*.

hyperthyroidation (hi″per-thi-roy-da′-shun) [" + " + *eidos*, form]. Excessive action of thyroid gland. SYN: *hyperthyrea*.

hyperthyroidism (hi-per-thi′roid-izm) [" + " + " + *ismos*, state of]. A condition caused by excessive secretion of the thyroid glands which overstimulates the basal metabolism, causing an increased demand for food to prevent oxidization of body tissues.

It may take 2 forms: exophthalmic goiter* or Graves' disease and toxic adenoma.

SYM: Autonomic imbalance; exaggeration of all functions, rapid pulse, psychic disturbances, excitement, restlessness, tremors, diarrhea, loss of weight, increased metabolism.

NP: Mental and physical rest with freedom from worry and excitement imperative. A cool, bracing climate away from the seashore desirable. Exercise during hot weather aggravates symptoms. Winter months often bring improvement.

In severe cases confinement in bed, perhaps for several weeks or months. Light, fresh air, and sunshine are needed and sometimes a change of room desirable. Visitors should not be permitted prior to operation or in severe cases, and the nurse should attempt to allay all nervousness on part of patient. Simple diversions help to allay restlessness. Bedclothes during hot weather reduced to a minimum. Encourage patient to drink plenty of water. Bowels should be evacuated daily. Warm baths and frequent rubs are conducive to rest. Patient's position should be changed frequently. Hydrotherapy may be prescribed, and cold applications used to allay palpitation. An accurate record of pulse should be kept and the weight recorded at regular intervals. Regular nursing procedures should be followed for daily care of patient.

DIET: The doctor and the dietition may indicate the needed calories and prescribe the diet. Ordinarily, diet should be light and nourishing, with 2 or 3 pints of milk per day. No coffee or alcohol. Fish, eggs, fat bacon, chicken, custard, bread, vegetables and fruit are permitted. Red meats should be avoided.

RS: *Basedow's disease, cretinism, goiter, myxedema, thyroid*.

hyperthyro′sis [" + " + *ōsis*]. Excess of thyroid secretion in the blood. SYN: *hyperthyroidation*.

hyperto′nia [G. *yper*, above, + *tonos*, tension]. Abnormal tension of arteries or muscles.

hyperton′ic [" + *tonos*, tension]. 1. Having a higher osmotic pressure than blood.
Pert. to a solution of higher osmotic pressure than another.
2. Being in a state of greater than normal tension or of incomplete relaxation. Said of muscles. Opp. of *hypotonic*.*

hypertonic′ity [" + *tonos*, tension]. Excess muscular tonus or intraocular pressure. SYN: *hypertonia*.

hypertonus (hi-per-to′nus) [" + *tonos*, tension]. Increased tension, as muscular tension in spasm.

hypertoxic′ity [" + *toxikon*, poison]. The state of being excessively poisonous.

hypertrichiasis (hi″per-tri-ki′a-sis) [" + *thrix, trich-*, hair]. Abnormal growth of hair.

ETIOL: Congenital or obscure causes. May be due to adrenal or gonad disturbances. Noted in Addison's disease and in patients bedridden with pulmonary tuberculosis. SYN: *hypertrichosis*.

hypertrichophobia (hi″per-trik-o-fo′bĭ-ă) [" + " + *phobos*, fear]. Fear of hair on the body.

hypertrichophrydia (hi″per-trik-of-rid′ĭ-ă) [" + " + *ophrys*, eyebrow]. Undue length of the eyebrows.

hypertrichosis (hi″per-tri-ko′sis) [" + " + *ōsis*]. Abnormal growth of hair. SYN: *hypertrichiasis*.

hypertrophia (hi-per-tro′fĭ-ă) [" + *trophē*, nourishment]. Increased size of an organ, or of the body, due to growth. SYN: *hypertrophy*.

hypertrophic (hi-per-trof′ik) [" + *trophē*, nourishment]. Pert. to hypertrophy.

hypertrophy (hi″per′tro-fi) [G. *yper*, above, + *trophē*, nourishment]. SYN: *hypertrophia*. Increase in size of an organ or structure which does not involve tumor formation. Term is generally restricted to an increase in size or bulk not resulting from an increase in number of cells or tissue elements, as in the hypertrophy of a muscle. Term sometimes used to apply to any increase in size as a result of functional activity. SEE: *hyperplasia*.

h., adaptive. H. in which an organ increases in size to meet increased functional demands, as h. of the heart which accompanies valvular disorders.

h., cardiac. H. of the heart; increase in size of the heart resulting from hypertrophy of muscle tissue but without increase in size of cavities.

h., compensatory. H. resulting from increased function of an organ due to a defect, or due to impaired function of the opposite of a paired organ.

h., concentric. H. in which the walls of an organ become thickened, with no enlargement, but with diminished capacity.

h., eccentric. Hypertrophy of an organ with dilatation.

h., false. H. with degeneration of 1 constituent of an organ and its replacement by another.

h., Marie's. Chronic arthral enlargement subsequent to chronic periostitis.

h., numerical. H. caused by increase in structural elements.

h., physiological. That due to natural rather than pathological factors.

h., pseudomuscular. A disease usually of childhood, characterized by paralysis, depending upon degeneration of the muscles which, however, become enlarged from a deposition of fat and connective tissue.

SYM: Weakness of muscles, child is awkward, stumbles and seeks support in walking. As paralysis increases, the muscles, particularly those of the calf, thigh, buttocks and back, enlarge. Upper extremities less frequently affected. In erect posture feet are wide apart, abdomen protrudes and spinal column shows a marked curvature with convexity forward. Patient rises from recumbent position by grasping the knees or by resting the hands on the floor in front of him, extending the legs and pushing the body backwards. Gait is waddling. In course of few years paralysis becomes so marked patient is unable to leave his bed; atrophy of muscles follows.

PROG: Utterly unfavorable.

TREATMENT: Constitutional; graduated exercises, massage, electricity.

h., simple. H. due to increase in size of structural parts.

h., true. H. caused by increase in size in all the different tissues composing a part.

h., vicarious. H. of an organ when another organ of allied function is disabled or destroyed.

hypertro'pia [G. *yper*, above, + *tropē*, a turning]. Vertical strabismus upward.

hyperuresis (hi-per-ū-re'sis) [" + *ourēsis*, urination]. Excess of urinary secretion. SYN: *enuresis, polyuria.*

hyperuricemia (hi″per-ū-ris-e'mĭ-ă) [" + *ouron*, urine, + *aima*, blood]. Abnormal amt. of uric acid in the blood.

hyperuricu'ria [" + " + *ouron*, urine]. Undue amt. of uric acid in the urine.

hypervas'cular [" + L. *vasculus*, vessel]. Excessively vascular.

hypervenosity (hi″per-ve-nos'ĭ-tĭ) [" + L. *venōsus*, pert. to a vein]. Excessive development of the venous system. SYN: *supervenosity.*

hy″perventila'tion [G. *yper*, above, + L. *ventilatio*, ventilation]. Hyperpnea as occurs in forced respiration; increased inspiration and expiration of air as a result of increase in rate or depth of respiration, or both. Results esp. in carbon dioxide depletion (acapnia) with accompanying symptoms (fall in blood pressure, vasoconstriction, and sometimes syncope).

h. syndrome. A condition common during sleep. Faster and deeper breathing causes a loss of carbon dioxide from the lungs producing numbness of the hands, fingers and of other parts of the body, prickling of skin, trembling feeling, racing of heart, light-headedness, fainting, cramps of muscles, esp. leg cramps, a spastic and painful condition resulting in tetany and possibly death.

hyperviscos'ity [" + L. *viscōsus*, gummy]. Excessive viscosity or exaggeration of adhesive properties. Seen in anemias and inflammatory diseases.

hypervitaminosis (hi″per-vī-tăm-ĭn-o'sĭs) [" + L. *vīta*, life, + *amine* + *ōsis*]. A condition caused by an excessive amount of vitamin.

hypervolemia (hi″per-vol-e'mĭ-ă) [" + L. *volumen*, volume, + G. *aima*, blood]. Plethora of blood. Occurs only in cases of administration of massive doses of vitamins A & D.

hypesthesia (hi-pes-the'zĭ-ă) [G. *ypo*, under, + *aisthēsis*, sensation]. Lessened sensibility to touch.

hypha (hi'fa) [G. *yphē*, web]. A filament of mold, or part of a mold mycelium.

hyphedonia (hĭp-he-dō'nĭ-ă) [G. *ypo*, under, + *ēdonē*, pleasure]. Abnormal diminution in gratification of desires.

hyphemia (hi-fe'mĭ-ă) [" + *aima*, blood]. 1. Blood in the ant. chamber of the eye in front of iris. 2. Oligemia.

hyphex (hi'fĕks). A name for both hexamethonium chloride, and I-hydrazin-ophthalazine, effective in treatment of the hypertensions.

hyphidrosis (hip-hid-ro'sĭs) [" + *idrōs*, sweat]. Diminished secretion of sweat.

Hyphomycetes (hi″fo-mi-se'tēs) [G. *yphē*, web, + *mykes*, fungus]. The *Fungi Imperfecti*. Filamentous fungi with branched or unbranched threads. SYN: *molds.*

hypinosis (hip-in-o'sĭs) [G. *ypo*, under, + *is, in–*, fiber, + *ōsis*]. Deficiency of fibrin in the blood.

hypnagogic (hip-nag-oj'ĭk) [G. *ypnos*, sleep, + *agōgos*, leading]. 1. Inducing sleep or induced by sleep. SYN: *hypnotic.* 2. PSY: Pert. to hallucinations or dreams just before loss of consciousness. SEE: *hypnogenic zones.*

h. state. A transitional state bet. sleeping and awaking and delusions which may result therefrom.

hypnalgia (hip-nal'jĭ-ă) [" + *algos*, pain]. False sense of pain experienced in a dream.

hyp'nic [G. *ypnos*, sleep]. Causing sleep. SYN: *somnifacient, somniferous.*

hyp'nocyst [" + *kystis*, a cyst]. A quiescent cyst or 1 whose activity is in abeyance.

hyp″nogenet'ic [" + *gennan*, to produce]. Producing sleep.

h. spots. Areas which, on being stimulated, produce sleep. SYN: *hypnogenic zones.*

hypnogenic zones (hip-no-jen'ĭk) [" + *gennan*, to produce]. Areas on the body which, when stimulated, produce sleep, esp. a sleep resembling somnambulism.

The area may be the elbow or the popliteal spaces. SEE: *hypnagogic.*

hypnoidal (hip-noy'dal) [" + *eidos*, resemblance]. Pert. to a condition between sleep and waking, resembling sleep.

hypnoidiza'tion [" + *eidos*, form]. Induction of hypnosis.

hypnolepsy (hĭp'no-lep-sĭ) [" + *lēpsis*, seizure]. Irresistible sleepiness. SYN: *narcolepsy.*

hypnology (hip-nol'o-jĭ) [" + *logos*, study]. Scientific study of sleep.

hyp″nophob'ia. Morbid fear of falling asleep.

hypnopompic (hip-no-pom'pĭc) [" + *pompy*, procession]. Dreams persisting after return of consciousness.

hypnosis (hip-no'sĭs) [" + *ōsis*]. A subconscious condition in which the objective manifestations of mind are more or less inactive, accompanied by abnormal sensibility to impressions, the subject responding to these impressions, unrestrained by the reasoning faculties. SEE: *autohypnosis, braidism, hypnotism, sleepwalking, somniloquy.*

hypnosophy (hip-nos'o-fĭ) [" + *sophia*, wisdom]. The study of sleep.

hypnother'apy [" + *therapeia*, treatment]. Treatment by hypnotism, or by inducing prolonged sleep.

hypnot'ic [G. *ypnos*, sleep]. 1. Pert. to sleep or hypnosis. 2. An agent that induces sleep or which dulls the senses. Ex: *chloral hydrate, sulfonethylmethane.*

hypnot'ics [G. *ypnos*, sleep]. Drugs which cause insensibility to pain by inhibiting

afferent impulses, or the cortical centers of the brain receiving sensory impressions, and thus causing partial or complete unconsciousness.
They include: *Sedatives, analgesics, anesthetics,* and *intoxicants, q.v.* They should yield not unpleasant after effects and result in natural sleep.
They are sometimes called *narcotics, somnifacients,* and *soporifics, q.v.,* when used to induce sleep.
NP: They should not be administered without a physician's order.
Ex: *Mild*: Bromides; sodium bromide, dose 5-30 gr.; potassium bromide, dose 5-30 gr.; or ammonium bromide, dose 5-30 gr.
Aspirin, dose 5-15 gr., acts as a mild hypnotic.
Stronger: Trional, 5-10 gr.; veronal, 5-10 gr.; sulfonal, 5-20 gr.—this should be given early in the evening, as it takes several hours to act.
Chloral, 5-20 gr., often used in conjunction with bromide to obtain a more powerful hypnotic effect. Chloral is a heart depressant.
Chloralamide, dose 10-30 gr., is a safer drug to use than chloral, as it is less depressing to the heart.
Narcotics: Opium, morphia and its derivatives are narcotics.

hypnotism (hip'no-tizm) [" + *ismos*, state of]. An induced sleeplike state during which patient is peculiarly susceptible to the suggestions of the hypnotist.
hyp'notist [G. *ypnos*, sleep]. One who practices hypnotism.
hypnotize (hip'no-tīz) [G. *ypnos*, sleep]. To put under hypnotism.
hy'po [G. *ypo*, under]. 1. A hypochondriac. 2. Popular name for hypodermic injection.
hypo- [G.]. Prefix: Less than, below.
hy"poacid'ity [G. *ypo*, under, + L. *acidus*, sour]. A condition caused by lowered hydrochloric secretion.
Secondary to other disorders, such as pernicious anemia.
TREATMENT: Dilute HCl by mouth.
DIET: Fruit juices and meat broths before meals. Nourishing diet.
hypoade'nia [" + *adēn*, gland]. Defective activity of the glands.
hypoadre'nalism, hypoadre'nia [" + L. *ad*, to, + *rēnalis*, pert. to kidney, + G. *ismos*, state of]. Adrenal insufficiency.
hypoalimenta'tion [" + L. *alimentum*, nourishment]. Insufficient nourishment. SYN: *subalimentation.*
hypoalonemia (hi"po-al-o-ne'mĭ-ă) [" + *als*, salt, + *aima*, blood]. Lack of salts in the blood.
hypoazoturia (hi"po-az-ot-ū'rĭ-ă) [" + *a-*, priv. + *zōē*, life, + *ouron*, urine]. Diminished urea in the urine.
hypobaropathy (hi"po-bar-op'ă-thī) [" + *baros*, pressure, + *pathos*, disease]. Symptoms produced by diminished air pressure, mountain sickness, aviator's sickness.
hyp'oblast [G. *ypo*, under, + *blastos*, germ]. The inner cell layer or *endoderm* which develops during gastrulation. The external layer is called epiblast.
hypoblastic (hi-po-blas'tik) [" + *blastos*, germ]. Pert. to the inner layer of the blastoderm.
hypobulia (hi-po-bu'lĭ-ă) [" + *boulē*, will]. Lack of will power.
hypocalcemia (hi"po-kal-se'mĭ-ă) [" + L. *calx*, lime, + G. *aima*, blood]. Abnormally low blood calcium.

hypocalcia (hi-po-kal'sĭ-ă) [" + L. *calx*, lime]. Lack of calcium in the system.
hypocap'nia [" + *kapnos*, smoke]. Lack of carbon dioxide in the blood.
hypochloremia (hi"po-klo-re'mĭ-ă) [" + *chlōros*, green, + *aima*, blood]. Having deficiency of the chloride contents of the blood.
hypochlorhydria (hi-po-klor-hī'drĭ-ă) [" + " + *ydōr*, water]. Diminished secretion of hydrochloric acid.
Less than 25° throughout Ewald test. Small amount and low acid may be indicative of carcinoma or anemia. May be found in subacute and chronic gastritis, peptic ulcers, infections, advanced tuberculosis, early carcinoma, and neuroses. SEE: *achlorhydria, hyperchlorhydria.*
hy"pochloriza'tion [" + *chlōros*, green]. Reduction of sodium chloride in the diet in nephritis and epilepsy.
hypochloruria (hi-po-klo-ru'rĭ-ă) [G. *ypo*, under, + *chlōros*, green, + *ouron*, urine]. Diminution of chlorides in the urine.
hypocholesteremia (hi"po-ko-les-ter-e'mĭ-ă) [" + *cholē*, bile, + *stereos*, solid, + *aima*, blood]. Lowered cholesterin in the blood.
hypochon'dria [" + *chondros*, cartilage]. Abnormal concern about health with false belief of suffering from some disease. SYN: *hypochondriasis.*
hypochon'driac [" + *chondros*, cartilage]. 1. Pert. to the region of the hypochondrium,* or upper lateral region on each side of the body and below the thorax; beneath the ribs.
2. One having a morbid fear of disease.
h. region. Part of abdomen beneath lower ribs on both sides of epigastrium. SYN: *hypochondrium.*
hypochondriacal (hi"po-kon-dri'ă-kal) [" + *chondros*, cartilage]. Affected with a morbid interest in health and disease.
hypochondrial reflex (hi-pō-kon'drĭ-ăl). A sudden inspiratory act resulting from sudden pressure below costal border.
hypochondriasis (hi"po-kon-dri'ă-sĭs) [" + *chondros*, cartilage]. Morbid anxiety about one's health; a frequent symptom of depressed states. SYN: *hypochondria.*
hypochon'drium [" + *chondros*, cartilage]. That part of the abdomen beneath the lower ribs on each side of the epigastrium.
hypochromasia (hi"po-kro-ma'sĭ-ă) [" + *chrōma*, color]. Lack of hemoglobin in the red blood cells.
hypochromatosis (hi"po-kro-mă-to'sĭs) [" + " + *ōsis*]. Disappearance of the chromatin or nucleus in a cell. SYN: *chromatolysis.*
hy"pochrom'ia [G. *ypo*, under, + *chrōma*, color]. Condition of the blood in which the red blood cells have a reduced hemoglobin content.
hypochromic (hī-pō-krōm'ĭk) [" + *chrōma*, color]. Pert. to hypochromia.
hypochro'sis [" + *chrōma*, coloring]. Lack of color in the blood because of low hemoglobin.
hypochylia (hi-po-kī'lĭ-ă) [" + *chylos*, juice]. Lack of normal secretion of gastric juice.
hypocinesia (hi-po-sin-e'sĭ-ă) [" + *kinēsis*, motion]. Diminished power of movement.
hypocolasia (hi-po-ko-la'zĭ-ă) [" + *kolasis*, hindering]. Functional weakness of the inhibiting mechanism.
hypocondylar (hi-po-kon'dĭ-lar) [" + *kondylos*, condyle]. Below a condyle.

hy'pocone. The distolingual cusp of an upper molar tooth.
hy″pocon'id. The distobuccal cusp of a lower molar tooth.
hypocrinism (hi-po-kri'nizm) [" + *krinein*, to separate, + *ismos*, state of]. Deficient secretion of any gland, esp. an endocrine.
hypocyclosis (hi″po-si-klo'sis) [G. *ypo*, under, + *kyklos*, circle]. Deficient accommodation.
  h., ciliary. Weakness of ciliary muscle.
  h., lenticular. Lack of elasticity in crystalline lens.
  Both forms interfere with accommodation.
hypocystotomy (hi-po-sis-tot'o-mī) [" + *kystis*, a bladder, + *tomē*, incision]. Perineal opening of the bladder.
hypocytosis (hi-po-si-to'sis) [" + *kytos*, cell, + *ōsis*]. Lack of normal number of blood corpuscles.
hypodermatomy (hi-po-der-mat'o-mī) [" + *derma*, skin, + *tomē*, incision]. Subcutaneous incision or section, as of a muscle or tendon.
hypoder'mic [" + *derma*, skin]. Under, or inserted under the skin, as a *hypodermic injection*.
  It may be given *subcutaneously, intracutaneously*, or into the skin; *intramuscularly*, or into a muscle; *intraspinally*, or into the spinal canal; or *intravenously*, into a vein.
  It is given to secure prompt action of a drug, when the drug cannot be taken by mouth, when it may not be readily absorbed in the stomach or intestines, when it might be changed by action of the gastric secretions, or to act as an anesthetic about the site of injection.
  h., antitoxin, serum, and vaccine. Subcutaneously in infrascapular region, infraclavicular region, or post. portion of axilla. May also be adm. intramuscularly or intravenously, all by a physician.
  h., intracutaneous. Usually adm. by a physician.
  h., intramuscular. Given in gluteal or in lumbar region. Used when a drug is not easily absorbed or when it is irritating and when large quantity of liquid is to be used.
  h., intravenous. SITE: Median basilic, or median cephalic vein. To be adm. by a physician.
  h., subcutaneous. Given in front of thighs, or outer surface of arms and forearm.
hypodermoclysis, hypodermatoclysis (hi″-po-der-mok'lis-is, -mat-ok'lis-is) [" + *klysis*, injection]. The injection of fluids into the subcutaneous tissues to supply the body with liquids quickly, as after shock or hemorrhage, diarrhea, or when the blood coagulation time is too long; in fact, it may be given in any condition in which it is impossible to give sufficient water by mouth or by rectum.
  When it is necessary to maintain a larger amount of water in the tissues in order to keep up proper metabolism, hypodermoclysis may be ordered. The purpose is about the same as that of intravenous infusions.
  SOLUTIONS USUALLY USED: Physiological salt solution. Normal salt solution is generally used because it is one of the principal constituents of the blood.
  The solution may be made with pre-pared tablets, as is done in many institutions, or 9/10 of 1% may be made very easily by taking 9/10 of 1% common table salt and adding it to each 100 parts of water until the required amount is prepared; this is then boiled. Usually not more than 2 parts are given, or 1 dram for each pound of body weight for each 15 minutes.
  Care must be taken that it does not evaporate, as the content will be hypertonic solution if the steam is not contained.
  There are other solutions given by this method as preferred by the attending physician. If the solution is not of the right percentage, hemolysis* may occur. Other solutions adm. intravenously are not generally given by hypodermoclysis.
  TEMPERATURE OF SOLUTION: It is very essential that solution be of the proper temperature, which should be from 108°-115° F., in the flask, as it cools rapidly while passing through the tubing. It is very necessary also that it be warm enough during the entire course of the flow.
  SITE OF INJECTION: The thighs are not used by some authorities as the needles are not supposed to penetrate near the course of large blood vessels. Here the femoral vein is too close to the site of an injection. (a) In the loose tissues at the base of the breasts; (b) in the thighs or buttocks (care being taken to avoid the large blood vessels); (c) in the axillary line (esp. for men); (d) beneath the skin of the abdomen (half way between the navel and the ant. sup. spine); (e) and intraperitoneally in children.
hypodynamia (hi″po-di-na'mĭ-ă) [G. *ypo*, under, + *dynamis*, energy]. Vital debility. SYN: adynamia.
hypoeccrisia (hi-po-ek-ris'ĭ-ă) [" + *ek*, out, + *krisis*, separation]. Imperfect excretion.
hypoeccritic (hi″po-ek-krit'ik) [" + *ekkritikos*, secreting]. 1. Retarding normal excretion. 2. Pert. to insufficient or defective excretion.
hypoendocrinism (hi″po-en-dok'rĭ-nizm) [" + *endon*, within, + *krinein*, to separate, + *ismos*, state of]. Insufficiency of internal secretion in 1 or more glands.
hypoendocrisia (hi″po-en-do-kriz'ĭ-ă) [" + " + *krisis*, separation]. Insufficiency of endocrine secretion. SYN: *hypoendocrinism*.
hypoeosinophilia (hi″po-e″o-sin-o-fil'ĭ-ă) [" + *eōs*, dawn (rose colored), + *philein*, to love]. Diminished quantity of eosinophil leukocytes of the blood.
hypoepinephria (hi-po-ep-ĭ-nef'rĭ-ă) [" + *epi*, upon, + *nephros*, kidney]. Insufficiency of the adrenal secretion.
hy″poer'gy. Hyposensitiveness, *q.v.*
hypoesophoria (hi″po-es-o-fo'rĭ-ă) [" + *esō*, inward, + *phorein*, to bear]. Downward and inward deviation of the eye.
hypoesthe'sia [" + *aisthēsis*, sensation]. Dulled sensitivity to touch.
hypoexophoria (hi″po-eks-o-fo'rĭ-ă) [" + *exō*, outward, + *phorein*, to bear]. Downward and outward deviation of the eye.
hypogas'tric [" + *gastēr*, belly]. Pert. to lower middle of the abdomen or hypogastrium.
  h. artery. *Arteria iliaca interna.*
  h. plexus. Sympathetic nerve plexus in the pelvis.
  h. region. The hypogastrium. SEE: *abdominal region*.
hypogas'trium [" + *gastēr*, belly]. Region

hypogenesis   H-62   **hypomorph**

below the umbilicus, or navel, between the right and left inguinal regions.

hypogen'esis [" + *genesis*, development]. Cessation of growth or development at an early stage, causing defective structure. SYN: *ateliosis*.

hypogenitalism (hī-pō-jĕn'ĭt-ăl-izm) [G. *ypo*, under, + L. *genitalis*, a genital + G. *ismos*, state of]. Condition in which the genital organs are underdeveloped. Characterized by reduced size of genital organs, failure of testes to descend in some cases, and incomplete development of secondary sex characters. SEE: *hypogonadism*.
     Gonadotropic hormones from urine of pregnant mares aid in causing testicular descent and growth of the genitalia.

hypogeusia (hi-po-gū'sĭ-ă) [" + *geusis*, taste]. Blunting of sense of taste.

hypoglobu'lia [" + L. *globulus*, globule]. Lack of cellular elements of the blood. SYN: *cytopenia, hypocytosis*.

hypoglos'sal [" + *glōssa*, tongue]. Situated under the tongue.
    h. alternating hemiplegia. Medulla lesion paralyzing the tongue by involving the 12 fibers as they course through the uncrossed pyramid. The pathology may extend across the midline or dorsally, involving the medial fillet, causing contralateral anesthesia.
    h. nerve. A mixed nerve. It carries afferent proprioceptive impulses as well as efferent motor impulses.
     ORIG: Medulla oblongata.
     DIST: Extrinsic and intrinsic muscles of tongue.

hypoglot'tis [" + *glōssa*, tongue]. 1. Undersurface of tongue. 2. Cystic tumor of floor of mouth. SYN: *ranula*.

hypoglyce'mia [" + *glykos*, sweet, + *aima*, blood]. Deficiency of sugar in the blood. A condition in which there is less than 80 mg. of sugar per 100 cc. of blood.
     ETIOL: Hyperfunction of the islands of Langerhans may cause it or injection of excessive quantity of insulin. SEE: *coma, hyperglycemia, hyperinsulinism*.
     SYM: acute fatigue, restlessness, malaise, marked irritability and weakness. In severe cases, mental disturbances, delirium, coma, and possibly death.

hypoglycemic (hi-po-gli-se'mik) [" + " + *aima*, blood]. Pert. to or causing hypoglycemia.
    h. shock. Production of shock by artificial production of hypoglycemia by intramuscular adm. of insulin in the treatment of schizophrenia. RS: *insulin, schizophrenia, shock*.

hypoglycogenolysis (hī″pō-glī-kō-jen-ol'-ĭ-sis) [" + " + *gennan*, to produce, + *lysis*, solution]. Defective hydrolysis of glycogen (glycogenolysis).

hypognathous (hī-pog'na-thus) [G. *ypo*, under, + *gnathos*, jaw]. Having a lower jaw longer than the upper one.

hypogonadism (hi-po-go'nad-izm) [" + *gonē*, semen, + *ismos*, state of]. Defective internal secretion of the gonads.

hypohepatia (hī″pō-he-pă'tĭ-ă) [" + *ēpar, ēpat-*, liver]. Deficient liver function.

hypohidrosis (hi-po-hi-dro'sis) [" + *idrōs*, sweat, + *ōsis*]. Diminished perspiration. SYN: *hyphidrosis*.

hy″pohydrochlo'ria diet [" + *ydōr*, water, + *chlōros*, green]. (a) Avoid excessive quantities of fats and salts. (b) Avoid overeating. (c) Avoid much liquid. 1. Potato. 2. Dextrinized cereals. 3. Nuts. 4. Egg yolk. 5. Fruits. 6. Jellies. (d) Small amts. of broth or meat stimulate activity of the stomach.

hypohyloma (hi″po-hi-lo'mă) [" + *ylē*, matter, + *ōma*, tumor]. A tumor formed by embryonic tissue. Derived from hypoblast tissue.

hypohypophysism (hi″po-hi-pof'ĭs-izm) [" + *ypo*, under, + *phyein*, to grow, + *ismos*, state of]. Diminished activity of ant. lobe of the hypophysis. SYN: *hypopituitarism*.

hypoinosemia (hi-po-in-o-se'mĭ-ă) [" + *is, in-*, fiber, + *aima*, blood]. Decreased formation of fibrin in the blood.

hypoin'sulinism [" + L. *insula*, island, + G. *ismos*, state of]. Insufficient secretion of insulin. SYN: *diabetes mellitus*.

hypoisotonic (hi″po-is-o-ton'ĭk) [" + *isos*, equal, + *tonos*, tension]. Denoting a solution having lesser osmotic pressure than another solution.

hypokinesia (hi-po-kin-e'zĭ-ă) [" + *kinesis*, motion]. Decreased motor reaction to stimulus.

hypokinet'ic [" + *kinēsis*, motion]. Pert. to hypokinesia.

hypokolasia (hi″po-kol-a'sĭ-ă) [" + *kolasis*, hindrance]. Imperfect inhibitory power.

hypolem'nal. Situated below a sheath or membrane.

hypolepidoma (hi-po-lep-id-o'mă) [" + *lepis, lepid-*, rind, + *ōma*, tumor]. A hypoblastic tissue tumor.

hypoleukocytosis (hi″po-lū″kō-sī-to'sĭs) [G. *ypo*, under, — *leukos*, white, — *kytos*, cell, — *ōsis*]. SYN: *leukocytopenia*. A lessening of leukocytes in blood.

hypoliposis (hī-pō-lĭp-ō-sĭs) [G. *ypo*, under, + *lipos*, fat, + *ōsis*]. Deficiency of fat in the tissues.

hypologia (hi-po-lo'jĭ-ă) [G. *ypo*, under, + *logos*, word]. A cerebral symptom marked by inadequate speech.

hypolymphemia (hi-po-lim-fe'mĭ-ă) [" + L. *lympha*, lymph, + G. *aima*, blood]. Decreased lymphocytes in the blood with normal number of leukocytes.

hypomania (hi-po-ma'nĭ-ă) [" + *mania*, madness]. Mild mania without much change in behavior, but accompanied by sound associations and distractibility.

hypoma'niac [" + *mania*, madness]. Pert. to maniacal exaltation, or one so affected.

hypomastia, hypomazia (hi-po-mas'tĭ-ă, -ma'zĭ-ă) [" + *mastos, mazos*, breast]. Condition of having abnormally small breasts.

hy″pomelanchol'ia [" + *melas*, black, + *cholē*, bile]. Melancholia without delusions.

hypomenorrhea (hi″po-men-or-re'ă) [" + *mēn*, month, + *roia*, flow]. Deficient menstrual flow.

hypomere (hi'po-mēr) [" + *meros*, part]. That portion of the mesoderm that later forms the pleuroperitoneal walls.

hypometabolism (hi″po-me-tab'o-lizm) [" + *metabolē*, change, + *ismos*, state of]. Lowered metabolism.

hypometria (hi-po-met'rĭ-ă) [" + *metron*, measure]. Shortened range of movement.

hypometropia (hī″pō-mĕ-trŏp'ĭ-ă). Myopia or shortsightedness.

hypomicron (hī″pō-mĭ'krŏn). A submicron; a particle invisible under an ordinary microscope but capable of being recognized under an ultramicroscope.

hypomnesia, hypomnesis (hi-pom-ne'zĭ-ă, -nē'sĭs) [" + *mnēsis*, memory]. Impaired memory.

hypomorph (hi'po-morf) [" + *morphē*, form]. One with short limbs who is short when standing in proportion to

hypomotility when sitting. The opposite of *hypermorph*, *q.v.* SEE: *mesomorph*.
hypomotility (hī-pō-mō-tĭl'ĭ-tĭ). Hypokinesia, *q.v.*
hypomyotonia (hi″po-mi-o-to′nĭ-ă) [" + *mys*, *myo*-, muscle, + *tonos*, tension]. Lacking in muscular tonus.
hypomyxia (hi-po-miks'ĭ-ă) [" + *myxa*, mucus]. Diminished secretion of mucus.
hyponanosoma (hī-pō-năn-ō-sō′mă). Extreme dwarfishness.
hyponatremia (hī-pō-nă-trē′mĭ-ă). Subnormal concentration of sodium in the blood.
hyponeocytosis (hi″pō-ne″o-si-to′sis) [" + *neos*, new, + *kytos*, cell, + *ōsis*]. Decreased number of leukocytes (leukopenia) with immature cells in the blood.
hyponoia (hi-po-noy'ă) [" + *nous*, mind]. Sluggish mental activity or imagination. SYN: *hypopsychosis*.
hyponychium (hi-po-nik′ĭ-ŭm) [G. *ypo*, under, + *onyx*, *onych*-, nail]. The nail bed. SYN: *matrix unguis*.
hypopancreatism (hi″po-pan′kre-ă-tizm) [" + *pagkreas*, pancreas, + *ismos*, state of]. Diminished activity of the pancreas.
hypoparathyreosis (hi″po-par-ă-thī-re-o′sis) [" + *para*, beside, + *thyreos*, shield, + *ōsis*]. A condition due to lessened or absent secretion of the parathyroids. SYN: *hypoparathyroidism*.
hypoparathyroidism (hi″po-păr-ă-thī′royd-izm) [" + " + " + *eidos*, form, + *ismos*, state of]. Insufficient secretion of the parathyroid glands.
hypopep′sia [" + *pepsis*, digestion]. Impaired digestion due to lack of pepsin.
hypopepsinia (hi-po-pep-sin′ĭ-ă) [" + *pepsis*, digestion]. Deficient pepsin in the gastric juice.
hypophar′ynx [G. *ypo*, under, + *pharynx*, pharynx]. The laryngopharynx; the lowermost portion of the pharynx which leads to the larynx and esophagus.
hypophonesis (hi-po-fō-ne′sis) [" + *phōnē*, voice]. A diminished sound in auscultation or in percussion fainter than usual.
hypophonia (hi-po-fo′nĭ-ă) [" + *phōnē*, voice]. Abnormally weak voice due to incoördination of speech muscles.
hypophoria (hi-po-fo′rĭ-ă) [" + *phorein*, to bear]. Tendency of one visual axis to fall below the other one.
hypophosphatemia (hi″po-fos-fă-te′mĭ-ă) [" + L. *phosphas*, phosphate, + G. *aima*, blood]. Phosphates below normal in the blood.
hypophrenia (hi-po-fre′nĭ-ă) [G. *ypo*, under, + *phrēn*, mind]. Subnormal mentality.
hypophren′ic [" + *phrēn*, mind]. 1. Pert. to subnormal mentality. 2. A feebleminded person.
hypophrenosis (hi-po-fre-no′sis) [" + *ōsis*]. Feeblemindedness.
hypophyseal (hi-po-fiz′e-al) [" + *physis*, growth]. Pert. to the hypophysis.
hypophysectomy (hi″po-fĭ-sek′to-mī) [" + " + *ektomē*, excision]. Excision of the hypophysis cerebri.
hypophysis (hi-pof′ĭ-sis) (pl. *hypophyses*) [" + *physis*, growth]. 1. Any undergrowth. 2. BNA. The pituitary body.
  h. cerebri. SYN: *pituitary gland*, *q.v.* A gland of internal secretion lying in the sella turcica of the sphenoid bone. It consists of two portions, the *adenohypophysis* and the *neurohypophysis*. These are differentiated into the anterior and posterior lobes which are attached to the hypothalamus of the brain by the hypophyseal stalk.
hypophysitis (hi-pof-is-i′tis) [" + " + -*itis*, inflammation]. Inflammation of the pituitary body.
hypopiesis (hi-po-pi-e′sis) [" + *piesis*, pressure]. Subnormal arterial pressure.
hypopinealism (hi-po-pin′e-al-izm) [" + L. *pineus*, pert. to pine cone, + G. *ismos*, state of]. Diminished secretion of the pineal body.
hypopituitarism (hi-po-pit-u′ĭ-tă-rizm) [G. *ypo*, under, + L. *pituita*, mucus, + G. *ismos*, state of]. A condition resulting from diminished secretion of pituitary hormones, esp. those of the anterior lobe.
hypoplasia (hi-po-pla′zĭ-ă) [" + *plasis*, formation]. Defective development of tissue. RS: *tissue*.
hypoporosis (hī″pō-pō-rō′sĭs). Deficient development of a callus at site of a bone fracture.
hypoproteinemia (hī″pō-prō-tē-ĭn-ē′mĭ-ă) [" + *prōtos*, first, + *aima*, blood]. Decrease in the normal quantity of protein in the blood.
hypoproteino′sis. Condition resulting from protein deficiency in diet.
hypoprothrombinemia (hī″-pō-prō-thrŏm″-bĭ-nē-mĭ-ă). Deficiency of prothrombin in the blood.
hypopselaphesia (hī-pop-sel-af-e′zĭ-ă) [" + *psēlaphēsis*, touch]. Blunted tactile sense.
hypopsychosis (hī-pŏ-sī-kō′sĭs) [G. *ypo*, under, + *psychē*, mind, + *osis*]. SYN: *hyponoia*. Weakness of the function of thought.
hypoptyalism (hi-po-ti′al-izm) [" + *ptyalon*, saliva, + *ismos*, state of]. Decreased salivary secretion.
hypopyon (hi-po′pĭ-on) [" + *pyon*, pus]. Pus in ant. chamber of the eye in front of iris but behind cornea, seen in corneal ulcer.
hyporeflex′ia [" + L. *reflexus*, bent back]. Diminished function of the reflexes.
hyposalemia (hi-po-sal-e′mĭ-ă) [" + L. *sal*, salt, + G. *aima*, blood]. Decreased amt. of salts in the blood. SYN: *hypochloremia*.
hypo′saliva′tion. Abnormal decrease in flow of saliva.
hyposar′ca [" + *sarx*, flesh]. Extreme dropsy (anasarca) of subcutaneous connective tissue.
hyposecre′tion [" + L. *secrētus*; *secernere*, to separate]. Lowered amt. of secretion.
hypo′′sen′sitive [G. *ypo*, under, + L. *sentīre*, to feel]. Having reduced ability to respond to stimuli.
hy′′posensitiza′tion [" + L. *sentīre*, to feel]. Production of hyposensitiveness.
hyposialadenitis (hi″po-si″al-ad-en-i′tis) [" + *sialon*, saliva, + *adēn*, gland, + -*itis*, inflammation]. Submaxillary salivary gland inflammation.
hyposmia (hi-poz′mĭ-ă) [G. *ypo*, under, + *osmē*, smell]. Defect in sense of smell.
hypospadia, hypospadias (hi-po-spa′dĭ-ă, -as) [" + *span*, to draw]. Congenital opening of the male urethra upon the undersurface of the penis; also an urethral opening into vagina. RS: *penis*, *urethra*.
hyposphresia (hī″pō-sfrē′sĭ-ă). Hyposmia, *q.v.*
hypospyhxia (hi-po-sfik′sĭ-ă) [" + *sphyxis*, pulse]. Sluggish circulation due to abnormally low blood pressure.
hypostasis (hi-pos′tas-is) [" + *stasis*, a halt]. Deposit; sediment. Opposite of *epistasis*.
hypostatic (hi-po-stat′ik) [G. *ypo*, under, + *statikos*, standing). 1. Of or per-

hyposteatolysis

taining to hypostasis. 2. In genetics, hidden or suppressed, said of a gene whose effect is suppressed by the presence of another gene.

hyposteatolysis (hi-po-ste-at-ol′is-is) [" + *stear*, fat, + *lysis*, loosening]. Diminished emulsification of fats during digestion.

hyposthenia (hi-po-sthe′nĭ-ă) [" + *sthenos*, strength]. Subnormal strength; an enfeebled state; weakness.

hypostheniant (hi-pos-the′nĭ-ant) [" + *sthenos*, strength]. Reducing vital forces; debilitant.

hyposthenic (hi-pos-then′ĭk) [" + *sthenos*, strength]. Debilitant.

hyposthenuria (hi-pos-then-u′rĭ-ă) [" + " + *ouron*, urine]. The secretion of urine of low specific gravity, chiefly in chronic nephritis.

  h., tubular. H. resulting from trauma of renal tubule epithelial cells.

hypostypsis (hi-po-stip′sis) [" + *stypsis*, a contracting]. State of being slightly astringent.

hypostyptic (hi-po-stip′tĭk) [" + *stypsis*, a contracting]. Slightly astringent.

hy″posuprare′nalism [" + L. *supra*, above, + *rēn*, kidney, + G. *ismos*, state of]. Suprarenal inactivity.

hyposynergia (hi″po-sin-er′jĭ-ă) [" + *syn*, with, + *ergon*, work]. Poor coordination.

hyposystole (hi-po-sis′to-le) [G. *ypo*, under, + *systolē*, contraction]. A weak or lowered systolic contraction.

hypotaxia (hi-po-taks′ĭ-ă) [G. *ypo*, under, + *taxis*, arrangement]. State of reduced control over voluntary actions such as occurs in early stages of hypnotism.

hypoten′sion [G. *ypo*, under, + L. *tensiō*, tension]. 1. Decrease of systolic and diastolic blood pressure below normal. 2. Deficiency in tonus or tension.

Below 90 systolic and 50 diastolic is pathologic. If hypotension follows hypertension the condition is serious. If the diastolic blood pressure drops in proportion to the systolic pressure and the systolic pressure does not go below 80 points, the patient will respond to the administration of stimulants.

Patients with a systolic pressure of 180 points or over should be kept in bed under observation and for treatment. A patient with a systolic pressure of 90 points or less should also remain in bed for treatment.

It occurs in shock and collapse, in hemorrhages, infections, fevers, cancer, anemia, neurasthenia, Addison's disease and in other debilitating or wasting diseases, and approaching death.

Hypotension causes an accumulation of blood in the veins and slows down the arterial current. Capillary circulation is interfered with as are other functional processes of the body. Thyroid tablets are frequently used for this condition.

  h., orthostatic. H. occurring when a person assumes an erect position.
  h., postural. H. occurring upon suddenly arising from a recumbent position or from standing still.

hypoten′sive [" + L. *tensiō*, tension]. Denoting low blood pressure.

hypotensor (hi-po-ten′sor) [" + L. *tensus*, *tendere*, to stretch]. Agent that lowers blood pressure.

hypothalamus (hi-po-thal′am-us) [G. *ypo*, under, + *thalamos*, chamber]. The portion of the diencephalon comprising the ventral wall of the third ventricle below the hypothalamic sulcus and in-

hypothyroidism

cluding structures forming ventricular floor, including the optic chiasma, tuber cinereum, infundibulum, and mammillary bodies. It lies beneath the thalamus and laterally is continuous with the subthalmic regions. It contains a number of nuclei which are of importance in the control of visceral activities, such as maintenance of water balance, sugar and fat metabolism, regulation of body temperature and secretion of endocrine glands. It is the chief subcortical region for the integration of sympathetic and parasympathetic activities.

hypothenar (hi-poth′en-ar) [" + *thenar*, palm]. The fleshy prominence on inner side of the palm next to the little finger.
  h. eminence. Prominence on palm below little finger.

hypother′mal [" + *thermē*, heat]. 1 Tepid. 2. Subnormal temperature below 98.6° F.

hypother′mia [G. *ypo*, under, + *thermē*, heat]. 1. Having a body temperature below normal. 2. Frozen sleep. Refrigeration treatment for schizophrenia and cancer. 32° F. externally and 75° F. internally for 24 to 72 hours.

hypothesis (hi-pŏth′ĕ-sĭs) [G. *ypo*, under, + *thesis*, a placing]. 1. An assumption not proved by experiment or observation. It is assumed for the sake of testing its soundness or to facilitate investigation of a class of phenomena. 2. A conclusion drawn before all the facts are established and tentatively accepted as a basis for further investigation.

hypothrombinemia (hi″po-throm-bin-e′-mĭ-ă) [" + *thrombos*, clot, + *aima*, blood]. Deficiency of thrombin in the blood, making hemophilia possible.

hypothergasia (hi″po-thi″mer-ga′sĭ-ă) [" + *thymos*, mind, + *ergasia*, energy]. A condition of physical and mental depression.

hypothymergastic reaction (hi″po-thi-mer-gas′tik) [" + " + *ergasia*, energy]. Psychic disorder producing a sense of lonesomeness, sadness, and depression. Opp. of *hyperthymergastic reaction, q.v.*

hypothymia (hi-po-thi′mĭ-ă) [" + *thymos*, mind]. Decreased emotional response to stimuli.

hypothymism (hi-po-thi′mizm) [" + " + *ismos*, state of]. Thymus inactivity.

hypothyrea (hi-po-thi′re-ă) [" + *thyreos*, shield]. Thyroid insufficiency. SYN: *hypothyreosis.*

hypothyreosis (hi″po-thi-re-o′sis) [" + " + *ōsis*]. 1. Thyroid insufficiency. 2. Condition resulting from lack of thyroid secretion. SYN: *myxedema.*

hypothyroid (hi-po-thi′royd) [" + " + *eidos*, form]. Marked by insufficiency of thyroid secretion.

hypothyroida′tion [" + " + *eidos*, form]. Condition causing insufficient thyroid secretion.

hypothyroidea (hi″po-thi-roi′de-ă) [" + " + *eidos*, form]. Diminished thyroid secretion. SYN: *hypothyreosis.*

➤ **hypothyroidism** (hi-po-thi′roid-izm) [" + " + " + *ismos*, state of]. A condition due to deficiency of the thyroid secretion, resulting in a lowered basal metabolism. A lesser degree of cretinism.

SYM: May be obesity; dry skin and hair, both of which become lusterless. Low blood pressure, slow pulse, sluggishness of all functions, depressed muscular activity, goiter.

TREATMENT: Thyroid organotherapy, as adm. of desiccated thyroid* or thyroxin. Increase iodine in diet if iodine is deficient.

hypothyrosis / **hysteresis**

NP: Constipation is a marked feature of this disease, as is slow metabolism, with a subnormal temperature. Guard against chilling, as the patient feels the cold and the pulse is often feeble. Measures for overcoming constipation will be in order. If thyroid extract is ordered, watch for signs of hyperthyroidism. Observe the patient carefully and watch for overexertion during treatment with thyroid extract.

hypothyrosis (hi-po-thi-ro′sis) [G. *ypo*, under, + *thyreos*, shield, + *ōsis*]. Insufficiency of thyroid secretion. SYN: *hypothyreosis*.

hypotonia (hi-po-to′nĭ-ă) [″ + *tonos*, tone]. 1. Reduced tension; relaxation of arteries. 2. Loss of tonicity of the muscles or intraocular pressure.

hypotonic (hi-po-ton′ik) [″ + *tonos*, tone]. 1. Pert. to defective muscular tone or tension. 2. A solution of lower osmotic pressure than another.

hypotoxicity (hi″po-toks-is′ĭ-tī) [″ + *toxikon*, poison]. A reduced toxic quality; only slightly poisonous.

hypotrichosis (hi″po-tri-ko′sis) [″ + *thrix, trich-*, hair, + *ōsis*]. Abnormal deficiency of hair.

hypotrophy (hi-pot′ro-fī) [″ + *trophē*, nourishment]. Progressive degeneration and functional loss of cells and tissues. SYN: *abiotrophy*.

hypotropia (hi-po-tro′pĭ-ă) [″ + *tropē*, a turning]. Ventrical strabismus downward.

hypouresis (hi″po-u-re′sis) [″ + *ourēsis*, urination]. Insufficient urination.

hypouricuria (hi″po-u-rī-ku′rĭ-ă) [″ + *ouron*, urine, + *ouron*, urine]. Deficient uric acid in the urine.

hypourocrin′ia [″ + ″ + *krinein*, to separate]. Deficient urinary secretion.

hypovaria (hi-po-va′rĭ-ă) [″ + L. *ovarium*, ovary]. Deficient internal secretion of the ovary and consequent retardation of puberty in girls.

hypovenosity (hi″po-ven-os′ĭ-tī) [″ + L. *venōsus*, pert. to a vein]. Incomplete development of the venous system in an area, resulting in atrophy, or degeneration.

hy″poventila′tion [″ + L. *ventilātiō*, ventilation]. Subnormal amt. of air in the lungs.

hypovitaminosis (hi″po-vi-tam-in-o′sĭs) [″ + L. *vita*, life, + *amine* + G. *ōsis*]. A condition due to a lack of vitamins in the diet.

hypovolemia (hi″po-vo-le′mĭ-ă) [″ + L. *volumen*, volume]. Diminished blood supply. SYN: *oligemia, oligohemia*.

hypoxanthine (hi″pō-zan′thin) [″ + *xanthos*, yellow]. A leukomaine, $C_5H_4N_4O$, in muscles and tissues in a stage of urea and uric acid formation. It is formed during protein decomposition. In small amts. it is normal in urine.

hypoxemia (hi-poks-e′mĭ-ă) [″ + *oxys*, acid, + *aima*, blood]. Insufficient oxygenation of the blood.

hypoxia (hī″pŏks′ĭ-ă). Anoxia; lack of an adequate amount of oxygen in inspired air such as occurs at high altitudes; reduced oxygen content or tension.

hypsibrachycephalic (hip″se-brak-e-sef-al′ĭk) [G. *ypsi*, high, + *brachys*, broad, + *kephalē*, head]. Having a broad and high skull.

hypsicephalic (hip″si-sef-al′ĭk) [″ + *kephalē*, head]. Having a skull with a cranial index above 75.1°.

hypsicephaly (hip-si-sef′al-ī) [″ + *kephalē*, head]. The condition of having a skull with a cranial index over 75.1°.

hypsiconchous (hip-sĭ-kong′kus) [″ + *kogchē*, shell]. Having an orbital index above 85°.

hypsiloid (hip′sil-oid) [G. *ypsilon*, U or Y, + *eidos*, form]. U- or Y-shaped. SYN: *hyoid*.

  h. **cartilage.** Y-cartilage.
  h. **ligament.** Ligamentum iliofemorale.

hypsistaphylia (hip-sĭ-staf-il′ĭ-ă) [G. *ypsi*, high, + *staphylē*, uvula]. Having a narrow, high palatal arch.

hypsistenocephalic (hip-sist-en-o-sef-al′-ik) [″ + *stenos*, narrow, + *kephalē*, head]. Having a cranial index over 75.1°. SYN: *hypsicephalic*.

hypsoceph′alous [″ + *kephalē*, head]. Having a cranial index over 75.1°. SYN: *hypsicephalic*.

hypsokine′sis [G. *ypsos*, height, + *kinēsis*, motion]. Tendency to fall backward when standing; seen in paralysis agitans.

hypsonosus (hip-son′o-sus) [″ + *nosos*, disease]. Mountain sickness; balloon sickness.
  SYM: Epistaxis, headache, nausea.

hypsophobia (hip-so-fo′bĭ-ă) [″ + *phobos*, fear]. Fear of being at great heights. SYN: *aerophobia*.

hypurgia (hi-pur′jĭ-ă) [G. *ypourgia*, help]. Any minor factors which change the course of a disease, esp. for the better.

hys′tera [G. *ystera*, uterus]. The uterus.

hysteral′gia [″ + *algos*, pain]. Neuralgia of the uterus.

hysterectomy (his-ter-ek′to-mī) [G. *ystera*, uterus, + *ektomē*, excision]. Removal of the uterus. The presence of tumors, both benign and malignant, is a common cause. The uterus may be removed through the abdominal wall or through the vagina.

NP: The patient is placed in dorsal position. The table is ready to be tipped into the Trendelenburg position. As soon as incision is made through the peritoneum, table should be put into Trendelenburg position. This procedure is the same for all abdominal pelvic work.

This position allows the intestines and abdominal organs to fall backwards from pelvis, so that they may be easily packed off with large pads or with a large roll of packing. The procedure following incision is the same as for the appendix.

DRESSING, ETC.: Borosalicylic acid powder, 4:1; 1 yard sterilized gauze; pad of cotton; aseptic adhesive strips; abdominal bandage. Perineal straps and safety pins, towels, gauze compresses, sheets, laparotomy sheet. Watch intake and output closely, prevent bladder distention, turn frequently. SEE: *laparotomy*.

  h., **abdominal.** Removal of the uterus through an abdominal incision.
  h., **chemical.** Destruction of the endometrium by strong caustic substances.
  h., **Porro.** Subtotal hysterectomy following cesarean section.
  h., **subtotal.** Removal of the uterus, leaving the cervix uteri in place.
  h., **supracervical.** Same as subtotal.
  h., **supravaginal.** Same as subtotal.
  h., **total.** Removal of body and cervix.
  h., **vaginal.** Removal of the uterus through the vagina.

hystere′sis [G. *ysterēsis*, a coming too late]. Failure of related phenomena to keep pace with each other.

hystereurynter (his-ter-ū-rin'ter) [G. *ystera*, uterus, + *eurynein*, to stretch]. An instrument for dilating the os uteri.

hysteria (his-te'rĭ-ă) [G. *ystera*, uterus]. A condition presenting somatic symptoms, simulating almost every type of physical disease, and a series of mental manifestations.

The mental attitude is calm; there is a not unfriendly aloofness, but psychotic indifference is quite another matter, and not seen in hysteria. There may be easy laughing and crying—episodes of emotionalism possibly without any apparent explanation, and even occurring in sleep. Episodic states known as fugues (sleeping-walking is a similar affair, occurring in sleep). In these, certain dissociated (repressed) ideas, emotions and goals develop a reality sufficient to constitute a secondary personality which now functions apart from the primary personality.

When the primary consciousness reasserts itself, there is a forgetting (amnesia) of the secondary state. The multiplication or alternation of personalities is quite distinct from schizophrenic splitting in which incongruities and confusion result from the co-existence of each phase of the personality more or less continuously.

An accurate definition is difficult because of extreme diversity of symptoms; a psychoneurosis found in a patient of low vitality, characterized by psychic weakness and undue susceptibility to autosuggestion.

ETIOL: Variable, as in most psychic disturbances. It occurs in both sexes before and after adolescence and at periods of emotional and physical stress, as alternating crying and laughing.

SYM: Emotional instability, various sensory disturbances and a marked craving for sympathy which sometimes leads to fraud.

Paroxysmal convulsive: Preceded by intense pain in ovarian regions and head, and sensations of ball rising in throat (*globus hystericus*). Consciousness may not be lost. No injury is sustained, which aids in differential diagnosis.

Interparoxysmal: Motor, sensory or psychic. May be paralysis, tremor, incoördination, or internal disorders; local hyperesthesia, anesthesia or paresthesia.

TREATMENT: Hygienic, hydropathic, massage, electricity, diet, suggestive therapeutics. Complete isolation from sympathetic individuals. Place patient in a quiet place devoid of spectators. Cold applications to head, face, and neck are helpful. Quiet, firm suggestions are important. Sedatives are to be used under the direction of a physician.

RS: *anthysteric, apsithyria, atremia, cachinnation, deafness, globus hystericus, ox-eyes*.

h. major. Very severe h. accompanied by epileptiform convulsions.

h. minor. Mild form of h. without loss of consciousness.

hyste'riac [G. *ystera*, uterus]. A hysterical person.

hyster'ic, hyster'ical [G. *ystera*, uterus]. Pert. to hysteria.

h. ataxia. Loss of sensation in leg muscles and skin in hysteria.

h. chorea. A form of h. with choreiform movements.

hystericoneuralgic (his-ter-ĭk-o-nū-ral'-jĭk) [" + *neuron*, nerve, + *algos*, pain]. Pert. to pain of hysterical origin, but resembling neuralgia.

hysteritis (his-ter-i'tis) [" + *-itis*, inflammation]. Inflammation of the uterus.

hysterobubonocele (his″ter-o-bu-bon'o-sēl) [" + *boubōn*, groin, + *kēlē*, hernia]. Inguinal hernia surrounding the uterus.

hysterocat'alepsy [" + *kata*, down, + *lēpsis*, seizure]. Major hysteria with cataleptic symptoms.

hysterocele (his'ter-o-sēl) [" + *kēlē*, hernia]. Hernia of the uterus, esp. when gravid.

hysterocervicotomy (his″ter-o-ser-vĭ-kot'-o-mĭ) [" + L. *cervix*, neck, + G. *tomē*, incision]. Cesarean section through the vagina. SYN: *hysterotrachelotomy*.

hysterocleisis (his-ter-o-kli'sis) [" + *kleisis*, closure]. Surgical closure of the os uteri.

hysterocystocleisis (his″ter-o-sis″to-kli'-sis) [" + *kystis*, a bladder, + *kleisis*, a closure]. Operation fastening the cervix uteri in the wall of the bladder.

hysterodynia (his″ter-o-din'ĭ-ă) [G. *ystera*, uterus, + *odynē*, pain]. Uterine pain. SYN: *hysteralgia*.

hysteroepilepsy (his″ter-o-e'pi-lep-sĭ) [" + *epilēpsia*, seizure]. Major hysteria with violent epileptiform convulsions.

In addition to usual symptoms of epilepsy, anger, disgust, joy, surprise and other emotions are dramatically expressed when final stage (delirium) is reached.

hysterofrenic (his″ter-o-fren'ĭk) [" + L. *frenāre*, to restrain]. Arresting an attack of hysteria, noting pressure areas having this effect.

hysterogastrorrhaphy (his″ter-o-gas-tror'-af-ĭ) [" + *gastēr*, belly, + *raphē*, suture]. Fixation of uterus to gastric wall. SYN: *hysteropexy*.

hysterogen'ic [" + *gennan*, to produce]. Causing a hysterical attack.

hysteroid (his'ter-oid) [" + *eidos*, resemblance]. 1. Resembling hysteria. 2. Pert. to hysteria.

hysterokataphraxis (his″ter-o-kat″ă-fraks'-is) [" + *kataphraxis*, a fencing in]. The operation of supporting the uterus by metallic sutures.

hysterolaparotomy (his″ter-o-lap-ă-rot'-o-mĭ) [" + *lapara*, flank, + *tomē*, incision]. Uterine incision through abdominal wall; abdominal hysterectomy.

hysterolith (his'ter-o-lith) [" + *lithos*, stone]. A calculus in the uterus.

hysterology (his-ter-ol'o-jĭ) [" + *logos*, knowledge]. Sum of what is known about the uterus.

hysterolox'ia [" + *loxos*, slanting]. Oblique flexion of the uterus.

hysterolysis (his-ter-ol'ĭ-sis) [" + *lysis*, loosening]. Operation of loosening the uterus from its adhesions.

hysteromalacia (his-ter-o-mal-a'sĭ-ă) [" + *malakia*, softening]. Uterine softening.

hysteroma'nia [" + *mania*, madness]. 1. Hysterical mania. 2. Nymphomania.*

hysterometer (his-ter-om'et-er) [" + *metron*, measure]. Device for measuring the uterus.

hysterom'etry [G. *ystera*, uterus, + *metron*, measure]. Measurement of the size of the uterus.

hysteromyoma (his-ter-o-mi-o'mă) [" + *mys, myos*, muscle, + *ōma*, tumor]. Myoma or fibromyoma of the uterus.

hysteromyomectomy (his″ter-o-mi″o-mek'-to-mĭ) [" + " + *ektomē*, excision]. Excision of a uterine fibroid.

hysteromyotomy (his″ter-o-mī-ot′o-mī) [" + " + *tomē*, incision]. Uterine incision for removal of a solid tumor.

hysteroneurosis (his″ter-o-nū-ro′sis) [" + *neuron*, nerve, + *ōsis*]. A reflex neurosis due to uterine irritation.

hystero-oöphorectomy (his″ter-o-o-o″of-o-rek′to-mī) [" + *ōon*, ovum, + *phoros*, bearing, + *ektomē*, excision]. Removal of the uterus and 1 or both ovaries.

hysteropathy (his-ter-op′ath-ī) [" + *pathos*, disease]. Any uterine disorder.

hysteropexy (his′ter-o-peks″ī) [" + *pēxis*, fixation]. Abdominal fixation of uterus.

hysterophore (his′ter-o-fōr) [" + *phorein*, to carry]. Uterine pessary.

hystero′pia [" + *ōps*, eye]. A hysterical visual defect.

hysteropsychosis (his″ter-o-si-ko′sis) [" + *psychē*, mind, + *ōsis*]. Mental disorder due to uterine disease.

hysteroptosia, hysteroptosis (his-ter-op-to′sī-a, -sis) [" + *ptōsis*, a dropping]. Prolapse of the uterus.

hysterorrhaphy (his-ter-or′ă-fī) [" + *raphē*, sewing]. Suture of womb.

hysterorrhexis (his-ter-o-reks′is) [" + *rēxis*, rupture]. Rupture of the uterus, esp. when pregnant.

hysterosalpingography (his″ter-o-sal-pĭn-gog′ră-fī) [" + *salpigx*, tube, + *graphein*, to write]. X-ray of the uterus and oviducts.

hysterosalpingo-oöphorectomy (his″ter-o-sal″pĭn-go-o″o-for-ek′to-mī) [" + " + *ōon*, ovum, + *phoros*, bearing, + *ektomē*, excision]. Surgical removal of uterus, oviducts, and ovaries.

hysterosalpingostomy (his″ter-o-sal-ping-os′to-mī) [" + " + *stoma*, opening]. Anastomosis of the uterus with the distal end of the fallopian tube after excision of a strictured portion of the tube.

hysteroscope (his′ter-o-skōp) [" + *skopein*, to examine]. Instrument for examining the uterine cavity.

hysteroscopy (his-ter-os′ko-pī) [" + *skopein*, to examine]. Inspection of the uterus by use of mirror.

hys′terospasm [G. *ystera*, uterus, + *spasmos*, a spasm]. Uterine spasm.

hysterostomatocleisis (his″ter-o-sto-mat″-o-klī′sis) [" + *stoma*, opening, + *kleisis*, closure]. Operation for vesicovaginal fistula.

Closure of the cervix uteri, making the vesical and uterine cavities into a common cavity by means of the opening between them.

hysterostomatomy (his″ter-o-sto-mat′o-mī) [" + " + *tomē*, incision]. Surgical enlargement of the os uteri; incision of the os or cervix uteri.

hysterosyph′ilis [" + *syn*, with, + *philein*, to love]. A hysterical manifestation due to syphilis.

hysterosystole (his″ter-o-sis′to-le) [" + *systolē*, contraction]. A delayed contraction of the heart after its normal time; opp. to *extra systole*.

hysterotabetism (his″ter-o-ta′bet-izm) [" + L. *tabes*, a wasting away, + G. *ismos*, state of]. Condition of hysteria and tabes combined.

hysterotokotomy (his″ter-o-to-kot′o-mī) [" + *tokos*, birth, + *tomē*, incision]. Cesarean operation.

hys′terotome [" + *tomē*, incision]. Instrument for incision of the uterus.

hysterotomotokia (his″ter-o-tom″o-to′-kī-ă) [" + " + *tokos*, birth]. Cesarean section.

hysterotomy (his-ter-ot′o-mī) [" + *tomē*, incision]. 1. Incision of the uterus. 2. Cesarean section, *q.v.*

hysterotrachelorrhaphy (his″ter-o-tra-kel-or′ă-fī) [" + *trachēlos*, neck, + *raphē*, sewing]. A plastic operation for a lacerated cervix by paring the edges and suturing them together.

hysterotrachelotomy (his″ter-o-trak-el-ot′o-mī) [" + " + *tomē*, incision]. Surgical incision of neck of uterus.

hysterotraumatic (his″ter-o-traw-mat′ik) [" + *trauma*, wound]. Pert. to traumatic hysteria.

hysterotraumatism (his″ter-o-traw′mă-tizm) [" + " + *ismos*, state of]. Hysteric symptoms due to or following traumatism.

hysterotris′mus [" + *trismos*, a spasm]. Uterine spasm.

hysterovagino-enterocele (his″ter-o-vaj″-in-o-en′ter-o-sēl) [" + L. *vagina*, sheath, + G. *enteron*, intestine, + *kēlē*, hernia]. Hernia surrounding uterus, vagina, and intestines.

hystriciasis, hystricism (his-trĭ-si′a-sis, his′trĭ-sizm) [G. *ystrix*, hedgehog]. 1. Erection of hairs like the spines of a hedgehog. 2. A skin disease.

SYN: Thickened epidermis, warty growths, elongated and hypertrophied papillae. SYN: *ichthyosis hystrix*.

hyther (hī′ther) [G. *ydōr*, water, + *thermē*, heat]. The combined effect of humidity and temperature of atmosphere upon the body.

I

i. Abbr. for *optically inactive*.
I. Chem. symb. for *ampere* and *iodine*.
ianthinopia (ī-ăn-thī-no'pĭ-ă) [G. *ianthinos*, violet colored, + *opsis*, vision]. Violet vision.
-iasis [G.]. Suffix: Same as *-osis*, meaning the state or condition of, as *psoriasis*.
iatraliptics (i-ă-tră-lĭp'tĭks) [G. *iatreia*, cure, + *aleiphein*, to anoint]. Treatment by inunction.
iatric (i-at'rik) [G. *iatros*, physician]. Medical.
iatrochem'istry [" + *chēmeia*, chemistry]. Seventeenth century opinion that chemistry is the basis of all physiological phenomena.
iatrogenic illness (ī-ăt-rŏg'ĕn-ĭk). Condition of anxiety produced in a patient by injudicious statements of a physician.
iatrogeny (ī''ă-trŏg'ĕn-ĭ). Condition induced by a physician.
  i. disorder. Condition involving adverse effects induced by a physician in the care of his patients. Term implies that such effects could have been avoided by proper and judicious care on the part of the physician. The development of anxiety neuroses through thoughtless and ill-considered remarks, development of drug habituation, and the injudicious use of therapeutic measures are examples.
iatrology (i-at-rol'o-jĭ) [" + *logos*, science]. Medical science.
iatrotechnics (i-at-ro-tek'nĭks) [" + *technē*, art]. The art and technic of medicine and surgery.
ice (īs) [A.S. *is*]. Water frozen at temperature below 32° F. (0° C.).
  i. bag, i. cap, i. collar. Devices for holding ice to be applied to a patient to obtain the effect of continuous cold in a circumscribed area.
  The affected part should always be covered with several thicknesses of cloth to prevent freezing.
  i. cravat. Ice pack applied around the neck.
  i., dry. Carbon dioxide in a solid form. Its temperature is —78.5° C. (—110° F). Used as a commercial refrigerant; also used for therapeutic refrigeration in such skin diseases as *lupus erythematosus*.
Iceland moss (īs'land). A lichen. It contains a form of starch; a slightly tonic demulcent. SYN: *Cetraria*.
ichnogram (ĭk'no-gram) [G. *ichnos*, footstep, + *gramma*, a writing]. A footprint, taken standing.
ichor (i'kor) [G. *ichōr*, serum]. Thin, fetid discharge from an ulcer or from a wound.
ichoremia (i-kor-e'mĭ-ă) [" + *aima*, blood]. Septic or toxic blood poisoning due to presence of ichorous matter. SYN: *ichorrhemia*.
ichorous (i'kor-us) [G. *ichōr*, serum]. Resembling ichor or watery pus.
ichorrhea, ichorrhoea (i-ko-re'ă) [" + *roia*, flow]. Profuse discharge of ichorous fluid.
ichorrhemia (i-kor-re'mĭ-ă) [" + *aima*, blood]. Toxic or septic blood poisoning due to presence of ichorous matter. SYN: *ichoremia*.

ichthammol (ĭk'tha-mol). A reddish brown, viscous fluid obtained by the destructive distillation of certain bituminous shale.
  USES: As a mild antiseptic and local stimulant in certain skin diseases.
  DOSAGE: Externally, 5-10% ointment or solution.
  INCOMPATIBILITIES: Mineral acids, alkalies, calomel, resorcin, potassium iodide, etc.
ichthyism (ĭk'thĭ-ĭzm) **icthyismus** (ĭk''thĭ-ĭz'mŭs) [G. *ichthys*, fish, + *ismos*, state of]. Poisoning from eating stale or unfit fish.
ichthyo- [G.]. Combining form meaning *fish*.
ichthyoid (ĭk'thĭ-oyd) [G. *ichthys*, fish, + *eidos*, form]. Fishlike.
ichthyol (ĭk'thĭ-ōl) [" + L. *oleum*, oil]. A brand of ichthammol.
  DOSAGE: 5-10 gr. (0.3-0.6 Gm.).
ichthyophobia (ĭk-thĭ-o-fo'bĭ-ă) [" + *phobos*, fear]. Aversion to fish.
ichthyosis (ĭk-thĭ-o'sĭs) [" + *ōsis*]. Fishskin disease. Congenital abnormality of the skin characterized by dryness, harshness, scaliness.
  ETIOL: Congenital with hereditary tendency probably as a result of persisting embryonic epidermis. Hypothyroidism may play a part in acquired cases, which are rare.
  SYM: As noted, confined to skin, subject to irritation, giving rise to eczema, etc., with formation of spinous, nutmeggrater-like lesions at pilosebaceous orifices.
  PATH: Dermal, affecting horny layer, prickle layer, papillae.
  PROG: Milder, clear up with adolescence. Severe, may be ameliorated.
  TREATMENT: Pilocarpine, thyroid internally. Locally, oils and greases after baths containing bran, borax, or sodium carbonate. SYN: *sauriosis*.
  i. follicularis. I. in which sebaceous and epithelial material accumulate about the hair follicles.
  i. hystrix. A form with warts.
  i. sebacea. Functional disorder of the sebaceous glands. SYN: *seborrhea*.
  i. simplex. I. with cutaneous roughening and dryness. SYN: *xeroderma*.
ichthyotic (ĭk-thĭ-ot'ĭk) [G. *ichthys*, fish]. Rel. to ichthyosis.
I. C. N. Abbr. for *International Council of Nurses*.
iconolagny (ī-kon'o-lag-nĭ) [G. *eikōn*, image, + *lagneia*, lewdness]. Sexual passion stimulated by pictures or statues or objects.
ICSH. Abbr. for *Interstitial-cell-stimulating hormone* secreted by ant. lobe of hypophysis.
icterepatitis (ĭk-ter-ĕ-pă-ti'tis) [G. *ikteros*, jaundice, + *ēpar*, liver, + *itis*, inflammation]. Hepatitis associated with jaundice.
icteric (ĭk-ter'ĭk) [G. *ikteros*, jaundice]. Pert. to jaundice.
  i. fever. Jaundice combined with pernicious malaria.
  i. index. A number obtained by matching blood serum in a colorimeter

against a standard solution of potassium dichromate (1:10,000), which gives a color approximately same as bilirubin.

A test for determining the intensity of the yellow color of blood serum. Since serum color depends upon bile pigment, the index is an indication of the concentration of this pigment in the blood. Valuable in study of jaundice.

The serum is diluted to known strength and then compared; the reading of the standard, divided by the reading of the serum and multiplied by the dilution gives the icteric index. Normal serum gives a value of 5. In patients with visible jaundice values above 15 are obtained.

icteritious (ik-ter-ish'us) [G. *ikteros*, jaundice]. Yellowish; resembling jaundice. SYN: *icteroid*.

icteroane'mia [" + *an-*, priv. + *aima*, blood]. Icterus associated with anemia, hemolysis and splenic enlargement.

icterogenic, icterogenous (ik-ter-o-jen'ĭk, -oj'en-us) [" + *gennan*, to produce]. Causing jaundice.

icterohepatitis (ik″ter-o-hep-ă-ti'tis) [" + *ēpar*, liver, + *itis*, inflammation]. Liver inflammation with jaundice.

icteroid (ik'ter-oyd) [" + *eidos*, form]. Resembling jaundice; yellow-hued.

icterus (ik'te-rus) [G. *ikteros*, jaundice]. Jaundice, *q.v.* Pigmentation of the tissues, membranes and secretions with bile pigments.

   i. castren'sis gravis. Serious camp jaundice. SYN: *Weil's disease.*

   i. castren'sis levis. Mild camp disease of catarrhal form.

   i. cythemoly'tic. A form caused by absorption of bile formed in excess quantities due to hemolysis.

   i. febri'lis. Weil's disease.

   i. gravis. Acute yellow atrophy of liver with cerebral disorders.

   i., hemolytic or *nonobstructive.* Rare chronic form, frequently congenital, with periodic attacks of intense hemolysis.

   SYM: Much the same as in obstructive icterus,* but staining not so intense. Sometimes found in acute yellow atrophy, the anemias and infectious fevers. Enlarged spleen.

   TREATMENT: Rest, liquid diet, treat the cause, splenectomy.

   i. me'las. Black jaundice.

   i. neonatorum. Jaundice of the newborn. A type of hemolytic jaundice. It may be benign or malignant.

   i., obstructive. Jaundice caused by obstruction to the flow of bile in the common or hepatic duct.

   ETIOL: Duodenal catarrh, cholangitis, carcinoma, gumma, gallstones, cirrhosis of liver, cysts, parasites in ducts, pressure by tumors, hepatic abscess.

   SYM: Skin, mucous membrane and secretions stained yellow; first noticed in the conjunctivae. Stool light or claycolored, urine dark, pulse low, temperature slightly subnormal. In extreme cases, delirium, convulsions, coma.

   i. precox. Jaundice of secondary syphilis.

   i., suppression. ETIOL: Caused by toxins in body which destroy the liver cells and red blood cells.

   SYM: Feces may be darker than normal, not clay-colored; no excessive amount of bile pigment in urine.

   PROG: Quick recovery or speedy death.

   i. typhoides. Acute yellow atrophied condition of liver.

ictom'eter [L. *ictus*, stroke, + G. *metron*, measure]. An instrument for estimating the force of apex beat.

ic'tus [L. stroke]. 1. A beat or stroke. 2. An attack.

   i. cordis. A term applied to heartbeat.

   i. epilepticus. Epileptic convulsion.

   i. sanguinis. Apoplexy.

   i. solis. Sunstroke.

id [G. *idios*, own]. 1. BIOL: A biological germ structure carrying the heredity qualities; "an ancestral germ plasm."

   PSY: The unconscious undominated by its ego, but by its own impulsions, which are of an instinctive nature, such as the pleasure urge. 2. A suffix indicating certain secondary skin eruptions which appear some distance from site of primary infection. If etiologic agent of primary infection is known, the secondary lesion is designated by adding "id" as *tuberculid, trichophytid.*

idant (id'ant) [G. *idios*, own]. A chromosome containing all the ids regarded as hereditary factors.

-ide. CHEM: An ending indicating a binary compound, as *sodium chloride.*

ide'a [G. form, from *idein*, to see]. A mental image; a concept.

   i., autochthonous (aw-tok'thon-us). An unaccountable one.

   i., compulsive. A persistent, obsessional impulse or thought.

   i., dom'inant. One controlling all one's actions and thoughts.

   i., fixed. One that completely dominates the mind, as a delusion.

   i. of reference. An impression that the conversation or actions of others have reference to oneself.

idea, flight of. Rapid speech, often disconnected and incoherent, in certain mental diseases.

ideation (i-de-a'shun) [G. *idea, form, from, idein*, to see]. The process of thinking; formation of ideas.

   It is slow in dementias, depressions, and other organic brain diseases, and in narcotic intoxications, but quickened in early stage of intoxications. It is unduly active in manic-depressive insanity.

idée fixe (ē-dā fēks') [Fr.]. An obsession; a fixed idea. SEE: *idea.*

iden'tical [L. *identicus*, the same]. Exactly alike.

   i. twins. Twins developed from 1 fertilized cell. SEE: *Hellin's law, twins.*

identifica'tion [" + *facere*, to make]. 1. A kind of daydream, as when one identifies himself with the hero of a book or play. 2. The process of determining the sameness of a thing or person with that described or known to exist.

   i., anthropometric. The Bertillon system of i., *q.v.*

   i., Bertillon system of. A system based on physical characteristics.

   i., Galton system of. A system based on fingerprints.

   i., palm and sole system of. A system based on prints of the palmar surface of hand and the plantar surface of the foot.

ideo- [G.]. Prefix: Pert. to mental images.

ideogenous (i-de-oj'en-us) [G. *idea*, form, + *gennan*, to produce]. Stimulated by an idea.

ideometabolism. Metabolic changes induced by mental or emotional factors.

ideomo'tion [" + L. *motus*, moving]. Muscular automatic movement activated by a dominant idea.

ideomo'tor [" + L. *motus*, moving]. Pert. to ideomotion.

ideophrenic (id-e-o-fren'ĭk) [" + *phrenitikos*, insane]. Marked by abnormal ideas of a perverted nature.

ideoplastia (ĭd-ē-ō-plăs'tĭ-ă). Condition of the mind of a hypnotized person in which he is capable of receiving and responding to suggestions of the hypnotist.

ideovascular (ĭd″ē-ō-văs′kūl-ar). Pertaining to vascular changes induced by ideas, memories, or emotions.

idio- [G.]. Prefix: Individual, distinct, in compound words.

idioc'rasy [G. *idios*, own, + *krasis*, temperament]. Peculiarity which renders one susceptible to certain habits or drugs.

idiocratic (ĭd″ĭ-o-krăt′ĭk) [" + *krasis*, temperament]. Pert. to idiocrasy.

id'iocy [G. *idiōteia*, uncouthness]. Mental deficiency usually congenital. SEE: *idiot*.

i., amaurotic family. Form of i. seen in infants and small children in which there is increasing failure of vision and eventually death.

i., Aztec. I. combined with microcephalia.

i., complete or profound. I. in which primitive instincts are lacking, even that of self-preservation.

i., cretinoid. Endemic i. accompanied by stunted growth and frequently by goiter.

i., diplegic. I. marked by paralysis of all extremities in infants.

i., epileptic. I. accompanied by epilepsy.

i., genetous. I. of congenital origin.

i., hemiplegic. Hemiplegic manifestations in infants.

i., hydrocephalic. I. accompanied by chronic hydrocephalus.

i., intrasocial. I. in which mentality permits some occupation.

i., microcephalic. SEE: *Aztec i.*

i., Mongolian. Congenital form of i. in which person has Mongolian features, the nose being broad, the eyes slanting and the skull flat.

i., paralytic. I. combined with paralysis.

i., paraplegic. I. combined with paraplegia.

i., sensorial. Mental deficiency caused by loss of 1 of the special senses.

i., traumatic. I. caused by an injury received in infancy or in early childhood.

idiog'amist [G. *idios*, individual, + *gamos*, marriage]. One incapable of the sexual act with more than a few persons because of sexual discrimination.

idiogenesis (ĭd-ĭ-ō-jĕn′-ĕs-ĭs). Of self origin or origin without known cause, esp. with reference to idiopathic disease.

idioglos'sia [" + *glōssa*, tongue]. Inability to articulate properly so that the sounds emitted are like those of an unknown language.

idioisolysin (ĭd″ĭ-o-i-sol′ĭ-sin) [" + *isos*, equal, + *lysis*, solution]. A hemolysin active against the cells of an individual of the same species.

idiolysin (id-i-ol'ĭ-sin) [" + *lysis*, solution]. A lysin in the blood not formed in response to injection of an antigen.

idiometritis (id-ĭ-o-me-tri′tis) [" + *mētra*, uterus, + *itis*, inflammation]. Inflammation of the uterine parenchyma.

idiomus'cular [" + L. *musculus*, a muscle]. Pert. to the muscles independent of nerve control.

i. contraction. Motion produced by degenerated muscles without nerve stimulus.

idioneurosis (id-ĭ-o-nū-ro′sis) [" + *neuron*, nerve, + *ōsis*]. Any functional neurosis arising without stimuli.

idiopathic (id-ĭ-o-path′ĭk) [" + *pathos*, disease]. Pert. to conditions without clear pathogenesis, or disease without recognizable cause, as of spontaneous origin.

idiopathy (id-ĭ-op′ă-thĭ) [" + *pathos*, disease]. A primary disease without apparent external cause. SYN: *autopathy*.

idiophrenic (id-ĭ-o-fren′ĭk) [" + *phrēn*, mind]. Pert. to or originating in the mind alone.

i. psychosis. An organic disease of the brain producing a mental disorder.

idioreflex. A reflex resulting from a stimulus which arises within the organ in which the reflex takes place.

idiosome (id′ĭ-o-sōm) [" + *sōma*, body]. Spermatid's attraction sphere.

idiosyncrasy (ĭd-ĭ-o-sĭn′krā-sĭ) [" + *sygkrasis*, a mixture]. 1. Special characteristics by which persons differ from each other. 2. That which makes one react differently from others. A peculiar or individual reaction to an idea, an action, or some substance, as unusual susceptibility. SYN: *idiocrasy*.

i. to drug. When no effects are produced from large doses of a drug, or unusual effects from small doses or from certain drugs. Ex: *digitalis, hypnotics, mercury, potassium iodide*, and *salicylates*.

i. of effect. When small doses of a drug create a poisonous or opposite effect, an unusual or no effect.

i. to x-ray. Natural or an inherent tendency on the part of the skin to react vigorously to minute doses of x-rays.

idiosyncratic (ĭd″ĭ-o-sĭn-krăt′ĭk) [" + *sygkrasis*, a mixture]. Pert. to an idiosyncrasy. SYN: *idiocratic*.

id'iot [G. *idiōtēs*, an uncouth person]. One with a congenital condition of feeblemindedness, or a serious intelligence defect, a mental age less than 3 years, or an intelligence quotient of less than 20. SEE: *idiocy*.

The idiot must be cared for as a child. Idiocy may be identified by a peculiar expression about the eyes, mouth open, and tongue protruding, with enlargement of the face.

RS: *amaurotic family idiocy, Aztec, cephalone, degenerate, imbecile, moron.*

i., amaurotic. One born apparently normal but who, in a few months after birth, develops symptoms of idiocy, inability to hold the head up, imperfect vision and sometimes the macula shows a cherry-red spot. Failure of vision, paralysis and death follow.

i., Aztec. A microcephalic i.

i., complete or profound. One devoid of all primitive instincts, even that of self-preservation.

i., hydrocephalic. I. with chronic enlargement of head and atrophy of the brain.

i., microcephalic. One with skull too small for proportions of balance of body.

i., Mongolian. One who has a Mongolian cast of countenance, the nose being broad, the eyes slanting, and the skull flat.

idiot'ic [G. *idiōtēs*, an uncouth person]. Like an idiot; said of an idea or action.

idiotrophic (id″ĭ-o-trof′ĭk) [G. *idios*, own, + *trophē*, nourishment]. Capable of securing its own nourishment.

idiotrop′ic [" + *tropē*, a turning]. Turning inward mentally. Individual.
   i. type. An introvert type satisfied by his own emotions, and by inner contemplation and pursuits, who is content to live apart from social contacts.

idiotypic (id-ĭ-o-tĭp′ĭk) [" + *typos*, type]. Rel. to heredity.

idioventricular (id-ĭ-o-ven-trĭk′u-lar) [" + L. *ventriculus*, little belly]. Pert. to the cardiac ventricle alone when dissociated from the auricle.

idrosis (id-ro′sis) [G. *idrōs*, sweat]. Excessive sweating. SYN: *hidrosis*.

ig″niextirpa′tion [L. *ignis*, fire, + *exstirpāre*, to root out]. Cautery excision

ig″nioperation [" + *operari*, to work]. An operation by cautery.

ignipuncture (ig″ni-punk′tur) [" + *punctura*, a piercing]. The use of heated needles in cauterization by puncture.

ignis (ig′nis) [L. fire]. Fire; cautery. SYN: *moxa*.
   i. sa′cer. An inflammatory skin disease. SYN: *herpes zoster*.
   i. Sanc′ti Anto′nii. Acute febrile disease with localized inflammation. SYN: *erysipelas; St. Anthony's fire.*

ileac (il′e-ak) [L. *ileum*, ileum fr. G. *eilein*, to twist]. Pert. to the ileum.

ileëctomy (il-e-ek′to-mĭ) [" + G. *ektomē*, excision]. Excision of the ileum.

ileitis (il-ē-i′tis) [L. *ilium*, flank, + G. *—itis*, inflammation]. Inflammation of the ileum. The membrane becomes inflamed and ulcerates, the affected portion becoming thick, rigid, and edematous and the lumen progressively narrowed. The lymph glands enlarge and the adjacent mesentery becomes thickened. Most often found in the terminal ileum, but it may spread to other parts of the bowel and to the cecum. Adhesions may be formed. Pain is centered around the umbilicus and right lower quadrant with general distention. Diarrhea alternates with constipation. Vomiting may occur. The stools show occult blood, and mucous shreds if bowels are loose.
   i., regional. A nonspecific inflammatory, granulomatous lesion involving the terminal ileum. Age of average subject twenty-seven and a half years. It is nontuberculous. May be acute or chronic. The acute form simulates appendicitis. The chronic form may extend over many years, with diarrhea, abdominal pain, anemia, loss of weight, fistula formation, and eventually obstructive intestinal symptoms. Stools are soft and grayish or brown in color with abundant fecal particles.

ileocecal (il-e-o-se′kăl) [" + *caecus*, blind]. Rel. to the ileum and cecum.
   i. valve. Sphincter muscles which guard the aperture of the ileum at the cecum, where the small intestines open into the ascending colon. It prevents food material from reëntering the small intestines. SEE: *Bauhin's valve.*

ileocecum (il-e-o-se′kum) [" + *caecus*, blind]. The ileum and cecum combined.

ileocol′ic [" + G. *kōlon*, colon]. Pert. to the ileum and colon. SEE: *ileocecal.*
   i. valve. Passage where food is prevented from reëntering small intestines.

ileocolitis (il-e-o-ko-li′tis) [" + " + -*itis*, inflammation]. Inflammation of mucous membrane of the ileum and colon.

ileocolostomy (il-e-o-ko-los′to-mĭ) [" + + *stoma*, opening]. Anastomosis between ileum and colon.

ileocolotomy (il-e-o-ko-lot′o-mĭ) [" + " + *tomē*, incision]. Incision of ileum and colon.

ileoproctostomy (il″e-o-prok-tos′tō-mĭ) [" + G. *prōktos*, rectum, + *stoma*, opening]. Establishment of opening bet. ileum and rectum.

ileorectostomy (il″e-o-rek-tos′tō-mĭ) [" + L. *rectum*, rectum, + G. *stoma*, opening]. Formation of passage bet. ileum and rectum. SYN: *ileoproctostomy.*

ileosigmoidostomy (il″e-o-sig-moid-os′to-mĭ) [" + G. *sigma*, letter S, + *eidos*, form, + *stoma*, opening]. Surgical opening between the ileum and sigmoid flexure.

ileostomy (il-e-os′to-mĭ) [" + G. *stoma*, opening]. Creation of a surgical passage through abdominal wall into ileum.

ileotomy (il-e-ot′o-mĭ) [" + G. *tomē*, incision]. Incision into the ileum. SYN: *ileostomy.*

ileotransversostomy (il″e-o-trans-ver-sos′-to-mĭ) [" + *transversus*, crosswise, + G. *stoma*, opening]. Connection of the ileum with the transverse colon.

iletin (i′le-tĭn). Insulin, q.v.

il′eum (pl. *ilea*) [L. fr. G. *eilein*, to twist]. Lower 3rd portion of small intestines, from the jejunum to the ileocecal valve. It is about 12 ft. long. SEE: Illus. below.

ileus (il′e-us) [G. *eileos*, intestinal colic]. Obstruction of small intestine.
   Originally meant colic due to intestinal obstruction.
   SYM: *Acute obstruction; sudden pain, paroxysmal, then continuous; constipation; persistent fecal vomiting; abdominal distention; collapse.*
   RS: *intussusception, occlusion, congenital strangulation, torsion, volvulus.*
   i., adynamic. That caused by intestinal muscle paralysis.
   i., dynamic, i., hyperdynamic. That caused by intestinal muscle contraction.
   i., mechanical. That produced by an obstruction.
   i., paralyticus. SEE: *adynamic i.*

il′iac [L. *iliacus*, pert. to ilium]. Rel. to the ilium. SEE: *psoas muscle for illustration.*

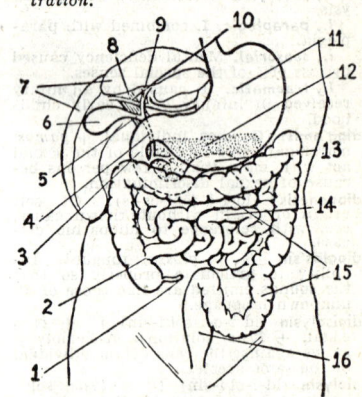

THE ILEUM

1. Appendix. 2. Ileocecal valve. 3. Duodeum. 4. Common bile duct. 5. Cystic duct. 6. Gallbladder. 7. Liver. 8. Portal vein. 9. Hepatic duct. 10. Hepatic artery. 11. Stomach. 12. Pancreas. 13. Jejunum. 14. Ileum. 15. Large intestine. 16. Rectum.

iliac, crest   I-5   **image**

    i. crest. The hip. Upper free margin of the ilium. SYN: crista iliaca.
    i. fascia. Transversalis fascia over ant. surface of the iliopsoas muscle.
    i. fossa. Fossa iliaca, *q.v.*
    i. region. Inguinal region on either side of hypogastrium.
    i. roll. Sausage-shaped mass in left i. fossa. Caused by induration of sigmoidal walls.
    i. spine. Spina iliaca.

iliocolotomy (il-ī-o-kol-ot′o-mĭ) [L. *ilium*, + G. *kōlon*, colon, + *tomē*, incision]. Opening into the colon in the iliac or inguinal region.

iliofemoral (il-i-o-fem′or-al) [" + *femoralis*, pert. to femur]. Pert. to the ilium and femur.

ilioinguinal (il″ī-o-in′gwĭ-nal) [" + *inguinalis*, pert. to groin]. Pert. to the groin and iliac regions.

iliolumbar (il-ĭ-o-lum′bar) [" + *lumbus*, loin]. Rel. to the iliac and lumbar regions.

iliometer (il-ĭ-om′e-ter) [" + G. *metron*, measure]. Device for measuring the iliac spines.

iliopectineal (il″ī-o-pek-tin′e-al) [" + *pecten*, a comb]. Rel. to the ilium and the pubes.

iliopsoas (il-ĭ-o-so′as) [" + G. *psoa*, loin]. The compound iliacus and psoas magnus muscles.
    i. abscess. An abscess in the psoas and iliacus muscles.

iliosacral [" + *sacralis*, pert. to sacrum]. Pert. to the sacrum and ilium.

iliotibial [" + *tibialis*, pert. to tibia]. Pert. to the ilium and tibia.
    i. band. A thick, wide fascial layer from the iliac crest to the knee joint.

il′ium [L. flank]. 1. The haunch bone. The wide upper portion of the innominate bone. 2. The flank. SYN: *os ilium*. SEE: *hip bone, Meckel's diverticulum, sacroiliac*.

ill (ĭl) [Ice. *illr*, sick, evil]. Indisposed; not healthy; diseased.

illaqueation (il″ă-kwe-a′shun) [L. *illaqueāre*, to ensnare]. Turning an inverted eyelash by drawing a loop of thread behind it.

illegal (ĭl-lē′găl) [L. *in*, not, + *lēgalis*, pert. to law]. Contrary to authorized law.

illegitimate (il″le-jĭt′ĭ-mĭt) [" + *legitimus*, according to law]. 1. Not according to law; not authorized. 2. Born out of wedlock.

illness (ĭl′nĕs) [Ice. *illr*, sick, + A.S. *-ness*, state of]. 1. State of being sick. 2. Ailment.

illuminating gas. This is a mixture of various combustile gases, including hydrogen and carbon monoxide.
    Its poisonous effects are largely due to carbon monoxide, *q.v.*
    TREATMENT: Resuscitation, *q.v.*

illumination (il-lu-min-a′shun) [L. *illumināre*, to light up]. 1. The lighting up of a part for examination or an object under a microscope. 2. Amt. of light thrown upon anything.
    i., axial. Light transmitted along the axis of a microscope.
    i., central. Axial illumination, *q.v.*
    i., darkfield. I. of an object under a microscope in which the central or axial light rays are stopped and the object illuminated by light rays coming from the sides, the object then appearing light against a dark background. Used to observe extremely small objects such as spirochetes, colloid particles, etc.
    i., direct. I. of an object under a microscope by directing light rays upon its upper surface.
    i., focal. The concentration of light upon an object by means of a mirror or a system of lenses.
    i., oblique. Illumination of an object from 1 side.
    i. (by) transmitted light. I. in which the light is directed through the object. Light may come directly from a light source or be reflected by a mirror.

illum′inism. Condition in certain psychotic states in which the patient has delusions of talking or communing with supernatural or exalted beings.

illu′sion [L. *illusiō*, fr. *illudere*, to mock]. PSY: Inaccurate perception; misinterpretation of sensory impressions, whereas a hallucination has no source in fact.
    Vague stimuli favor illusions, but essentially it is a disorder of ideation, as in toxic and exhaustive deliria. If an illusion becomes fixed it is said to be a *delusion*.

illu′sional [L. *illusiō*, fr. *illudere*, to mock]. Pert. to, or of the nature of, an illusion.

image (im′ij) [L. *imagō*, likeness]. 1. A mental picture with a likeness of an objective reality. 2. A more or less ac-

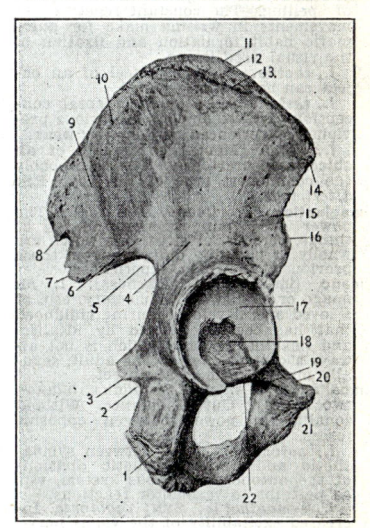

THE ILIUM
1. Tuber ischiadicum. 2. Incisura ischiadica minor. 3. Spina ischiadica. 4. Linea glutaea inferior. 5. Incisura ischiadica major. 6. Linea glutaea anterior. 7. Spina posterior inferior. 8. Spina posterior superior. 9. Linea glutaea posterior. 10. Ala ossis ilium. 11. Labium mediale. 12. Linea intermedia. 13. Labium laterale. (11, 12 and 13 make up the cristae iliacae.) 14. Spina anterior superior. 15. Corpus ossis ilium. 16. Spina anterior inferior. 17. Facies lunata. 18. Fossa acetabuli. 19. Crista obturatoria. 20. Pecten ossis pubis. 21. Tuberculum pubicum. 22. Incisura acetabuli. (From Sabotta-McMurrich: *Atlas of Human Anatomy*, 1930, G. E. Stechert & Co., New York.)

curate likeness of a thing or person. 3. The picture of an object such as that produced by a lens or mirror.

i., after. A retinal impression which persists after the stimulus is removed. A *positive* after-image having the same color as the original; a *negative* after-image possesses complimentary colors.

i., direct, i., erect. Picture from rays not yet focused.

i., double. Condition occurring in strabismus when the visual axes of the eyes are not directed toward the same object. The *false* image is formed in the eye that deviates; *true image* in the other eye. SEE: *diplopia.*

i., false. SEE: *i., double.*

i., inverted. I. that is turned upside down.

i., real. I. formed by convergence of rays of light from an object.

i., true. SEE: *i., double.*

i., virtual. SEE: *direct i.*

imagery (im'a-je-rī) [L. *imagō*, likeness]. Imagination; the calling up of events or mental pictures.

Mental imagery may be of various types, *viz.:*

i., auditory. When sounds can be recalled to mind, as thunder, wind, etc.

i., motor. When movement only is recalled, as the passing of a train. Motor-mindedness is recognized in the mastery of spelling. The constant repetition of movements in writing make for automatic habit formation and fixation of the visual word-image.

i., tactile. When the feel of an object can be readily recalled.

i., taste and **i., smell.** Mental conception of taste or odor sensations previously experienced. Often very weak.

i., visual. Mental conception of an object seen previously. This is probably the commonest type of imagery. RS: *afterimage.*

imagination [L. *imagō*, likeness]. The power of forming mental images of things, persons, or situations which are wholly or partially different from those previously known or experienced.

imago (im-a'gō) [L. likeness]. 1. An image or shadow. 2. A memory, esp. of a loved one, developed during childhood that has become clouded by idealism and imagination, and which is not always a correct one. 3. The adult, sexually mature form of an insect.

imbal'ance [L. *in*, not, + *bilanx*, *bilanc-*, two scales]. Out of balance. Without equality in power between opposing forces.

i., autonomic. An i. between sympathetic and parasympathetic divisions of the autonomic nervous system, esp. as pertains to vasomotor reactions.

i., sympathet'ic. SYN: *vagotonia.* Increased excitability of the vagus nerve.

i., vasomotor. Involving impulses to blood vessels resulting in excessive vasoconstriction or vasodilation.

imbecile (im'be-sil) [L. *imbecillus*, weak, silly]. 1. One with defective mentality, but with intelligence greater than that of an idiot,* and with less than that of a moron. One with a mental age between 3 and 7 years, or a child with an intelligence quotient between 20 and 49, inclusive. RS: *degenerate, idiot, moron, pervert.*

2. Without strength of mind or body; esp. mentally weak. 3. Stupid.

imbecil'ity [L. *imbecillitās*]. A state of mental deficiency intermediate between that of an idiot and a moron. SEE: *imbecile.*

imbed' [L. *im*, in, + A.S. *bedd*, bed]. In histology, to surround with a firm substance, such as paraffin or collodium, preparatory to cuttings sections. SEE: *embed.*

imbibition (im″bi-bish'un) [L. *imbibere*, to drink]. The absorption of fluid by a solid body without a chemical change in either.

imbricate, imbricated (im'bri-kāt) [L. *imbricāre*, to tile]. Overlapping, as tiles; overlapping aponeurotic layers.

imbrication (im-brī-ka'shun) [L. *imbricāre*, to tile]. 1. Overlapping, as tiles. 2. The overlapping of aponeurotic layers in abdominal surgery.

imida′zole or **imina′zole.** An organic compound characterized structurally by the presence of the heterocyclic ring

$$\begin{array}{c} H-C-N-H \\ \| \\ H-C-N=C-H \end{array}$$

which occurs in histidine and histamine.

imide-. Prefix: A compound with the bivalent atom group (NH).

immature (im-ma-tūr′) [L. *in*, not, + *maturus*, ripe]. Not fully developed or ripened.

imme′diate [″ + *mediāre*, to be in middle]. Direct without intervening steps.

i. agglutination. Healing by first intention.

i. auscultation. A. by ear applied to the body. SEE: *auscultation.*

i. cause. A cause directly originating a disease.

i. contagion. Contagion by direct contact.

i. union. Healing by first intention.

immedicable (im-med′i-ka-bl) [″ + *medicabilis*, curable]. Incurable.

immersion (im-er′shun) [″ + *mergere*, to dip]. Placing a body under water, or another fluid.

In microscopy, the act of immersing the objective (then called an i. lens) in water, oil, etc., preventing total reflection of rays falling obliquely upon peripheral portions of the objective.

i., homogeneous. I. in which the stratum of air between objective and cover glass is replaced by a medium which deflects as little as possible the rays of light passing through the cover glass.

i. lens, oil. A special lens used with cedar oil and producing a high magnification; useful in studying bacteria.

immiscible (im-mis′i-bl) [″ + *miscere*, to mix]. Pert. to that which cannot be mixed, as oil and water.

immobiliza′tion [″ + *mobilis*, movable]. The making of a part or limb immovable.

NP: Watch for loosening of splints and extensions and prevent pressure sores.

immune (im-ūn′) [L. *immunis*, safe]. 1. Protected or exempt from a disease. 2. Exempt from a certain disease by vaccination or inoculation.

i. bodies. Substances in those afflicted with an infectious disease formed by the tissues and possessing power to destroy or injure the disease-producing agent, or to neutralize its poisons.

They are found in the serum of coagulated blood, in blood plasma, and in lymph; they are also called antibodies,* and are classified as those of the 1st, 2nd, and 3rd order.

Each is the result of a specific antigen or disease-producing factor which acts only upon the same antigen. They have not been isolated, but are determined by the effect they cause. If the antigen is poisonous it is called a *toxin,* and its antibody is called an *antitoxin.* I. b. of 1st order: The antitoxins. I. b. of the 2nd order: The agglutinins and precipitins. I. b. of the 3rd order: Bacteriolysins and hemolysins.

RS: *anaphylaxis, antibody, ceptor, immunity, immunology, opsonins, precipitin, proteolysis, toxin.*

immunifacient (im-u-nĭ-fa'shent) [" + *facere,* to make]. Making immune.

immun'ity [L. *immunitas,* exemption]. The state of being resistant to injury, particularly by poisons, foreign proteins, and invading parasites.

Such resistance may be due in specific instances to the presence in the blood of antibodies, such as: 1. *Antitoxins,* which counteract bacterial toxins. 2. *Precipitins,* which render a foreign protein insoluble. 3. *Opsonins,* which increase the ability of leukocytes to ingest bacteria. 4. *Agglutinins,* which cause clumping of foreign cells. 5. *Lysins,* which dissolve such cells.

i., acquired. I. resulting from the development of active or passive immunity; opp. of natural or innate immunity.

i., active. I. resulting from the development within the body of substances which renders a person immune. This may result from having the disease or by the injection of the infectious organism, usually attenuated, or products produced by the organism.

i., congenital. I. present at birth. It may be natural or acquired, the latter being dependent upon antibodies received from the blood of the mother.

i., local. I. which is limited to a given area or tissue of the body.

i., natural. A more or less permanent immunity to disease with which an individual is born, the result of natural inherent factors. It may be the heritage of an individual, a race, or a species. It may be due to the natural presence of immune bodies, but other factors such as diet, differences in metabolism or temperature or adaptive features of infective organisms may be involved.

i., passive. Produced by actual injection of sera containing the antibodies into the subject to be protected.

immunity, words pert. to: antianaphylaxis, antivirus, aphylactic, autarcesiology, autarcesis, autarcetic, Ehrlich theory, immune, i. bodies.

immuniza'tion [L. *immunitās,* safety]. Becoming immune or the process of rendering a patient immune. SEE: *autoimmunization, immunity.*

immunizing unit. A unit which expresses an antitoxin's strength. It varies with different antitoxins. SYN: *antitoxic unit.*

immunochemistry (im-mu″no-kem'ĭs-trĭ) [L. *immunis,* safe, + G. *chēmeia,* chemistry]. The chemistry of immunization. The chemistry of antigens, antibodies, and their relations to each other.

immunogenic (im-u-no-jen'ĭk) [" + G. *gennan,* to produce]. Inducing immunity.

immunologic (im-mu-no-loj'ĭk) [" + G *logos,* science]. Pert. to immunology.

i. diseases. These are due to the action of antibodies, as in allergic hypersensitiveness to antigens, or to specific reactivity of the tissues.

The phenomenon of anaphylaxis needs to be understood to gain a knowledge of immunology. SEE: *anaphylaxis, serum sickness.*

immunol'ogy [" + *logos,* study]. The study of immunity to diseases, as: 1. I. to microbic diseases. 2. Serology. 3. Immunologic diseases.

SEE: *serology, serum, toxins, vaccination.*

immunopro'tein [L. *immunis,* safe, + G. *protos,* first]. Any protein immune body or substance that confers immunity.

immunotherapy (im-mu-no-ther'ă-pĭ) [" + G. *therapeia,* treatment]. The production of immunity.

immunotox'in [" + G. *toxikon,* poison]. An antitoxin.

immunotransfusion (im-mu-no-trans-fu'-zhun) [" + *trans,* across, + *fusus,* poured]. Transfusion of blood from one who has been immunized by an autogenous vaccine.

immunpro'tein [" + G. *prōtos,* first]. A bacteriolytic substance formed by the injection of attenuated bacterial cultures.

impac'ted [L. *impactus,* pressed on]. Pressed firmly together so as to be immovable. Term may be applied to a fracture in which ends of bones are wedged together; a tooth so placed in jaw bone that eruption is impossible; a fetus wedged in the birth canal; cerumen; calculi, or accumulation of feces in the rectum.

impaction (im-pak'shun) [L. *impactiō,* a pressing together]. 1. Condition of being tightly wedged into a part; overloading of an organ, as the feces in the bowels.

impal'pable [L. *in,* not, + *palpāre,* to touch]. Felt with difficulty; hardly perceptible to the touch.

impal'udism [L. *in,* into, + *palus,* marsh, + G. *ismos,* state of]. Malaria. SYN: *paludism.*

im'par [L. unequal]. Unpaired. SYN: *azygous.*

imparidigitate (im-par-ĭ-dij'ĭ-tāt) [" + *digitus,* finger. SYN: *perissodactylous.* Having uneven number of fingers or toes.

impe'dance [L. *impedīre,* to hinder]. Resistance due to self induction, as that met by alternating currents in passing through a conductor; virtual as distinguished from ohmic resistance.

The resistance due to the inductive and condenser characteristics of a circuit is called *reactance.*

imper'ative [L. *imperativus,* commanding]. Obligatory; not controlled by the will; involuntary.

i. concept. An idea which dominates one, as a fear or doubt.

impercep'tion [L. *in,* not, + *percipere,* to perceive]. Inability to form a mental picture; lack of perception.

imper'forate [" + *per,* through, + *forus,* a gangway]. Without an opening.

i. hymen. A hymen without an opening. Seldom discovered before puberty. Menstruation is interfered with and incision of hymen becomes necessary. SEE: *hymen.*

imperfora'tion [L. *imperforātus,* not open]. State of being closed or occluded. SYN: *atresia.*

imperious acts. Tics and motions not under control of the will. Urges of compulsion states. SEE: *impulsion.*

imper'meable [L. *in,* not, + *permeāre,* to pass through]. Not allowing passage, as of fluids; impenetrable.

imper'vious [" + *per,* through, + *via,* way]. Unable to be penetrated.

impetiginous (im-pe-tij'ĭn-us) [L. from *impetere,* to attack]. Rel. to impetigo.

impetigo (im-pe-tī′go) [L. from *impetere*, to attack]. Inflammatory skin disease marked by isolated pustules which become crusted and rupture. Occurs principally around mouth and nostrils. SYN: *scrumpox*. [Children esp. afflicted.

i. contagiosa. A contagious form.
SYM: Discrete, thin-walled vesicles and bullae which become pustular and thin crusted, appearing in crops. They may be flat and umbilicated with no tendency to rupture, and they are filled with a straw-colored fluid. They dry up as thin yellow crusts. No itching.
ETIOL: Microbic, streptococci and staphylococcic.
PATH: Papillary layer inflammation involving rete and stratum corneum.
TREATMENT: Soaking off crusts (soapy water containing sodium carbonate), ointment. Painting with bacterial specifics. Penicillin and the broad spectrum antibiotics.

i. herpetiformis. Rare form occurring usually in puerperal women and accompanied by serious systemic disturbance.

i. syphilit′ica. A pustular syphilide.

i. variolo′sa. Pustules in late stage of smallpox. SYN: *melitagra* (2).

im′plant. 1. To transfer a part, to graft, to insert. 2. That which is implanted, such as a piece of tissue, a pellet of medicine, or a tube or needle of radioactive substance.

implantation (im-plan-ta′shun) [L. *in*, into, + *plantare*, to plant]. 1. Grafting. 2. Artificial placing of a substance under the skin into the blood, into the uterine canal, etc. 3. Embedding of the developing blastocyst in the uterine mucosa.

i., hypodermic. Introduction of an implant under the skin.

i., parenchymatous. Introduction of medicinal substance into a neoplasm.

i., teratic. Union of a fetal monster with a nearly normal fetus.

im′plants [L. *in*, into, + *plantare*, to plant]. Capillary tubes of glass, gold, or platinum, containing radioactive substances for insertion into tissue.

impon′derable [L. *in*, not, + *pondus*, weight]. Having no appreciable weight; incapable of being weighed.

im′potence, im′potency [" + *potentia*, power]. Weakness. Inability to copulate. Failure of sexual power.
TREATMENT: Diet, hygiene, aphrodisiac drugs, glandular products, retraining of the mental processes, correction of local infections or congestions, prostatic massage, surgery, and sexual rest.

i., anatomic, i., organic. I. caused by a defect in the genitalia.

i., atonic. I. resulting from paralysis of nervi erigentes which convey impulses bringing about erection.

i., functional. I. not due to an organic or anatomical defect; usually of psychogenic origin.

i., paretic. Failure of impulse.

i., psychic. Due to mental disturbance.

i., symptomatic. Due to poor health, drugs, presence of disease, etc.

impotent (im′pō-tĕnt) [" + *potentia*, power]. 1. Unable to copulate. 2. Sterile; barren. [potence.

impoten′tia [" + L. *potentia*, power]. Im-

i. coeun′di. Inability on part of the male to engage in the sexual act.

i. erigen′di. Loss of power of erection.

impregnate (im-preg′nāt) [L. *impregnare*, to make pregnant]. 1. To render pregnant. To fertilize an ovum. 2. To saturate.

impreg′nated [L. *impregnare*, to make pregnant]. 1. Rendered pregnant. 2. Saturated.

i. carbon. Electrode having a carbon shell with core of various metals or salts of metals for use in a carbon arc lamp.

impregnation (im-preg-na′shun) [L. *impregnare*, to make pregnant]. Fertilization of an ovum; fecundation.

i., artificial. Artificial implantation* of semen in the uterine canal.

impres′sio [L. impression]. A mark, as of 1 part upon another.

i. cardi′aca. Depression on surface of liver for the heart. BNA.

i. col′ica. Depression on under surface of right lobe of liver. BNA.

i. digitata. A depression on the inner cranial surface.

i. duodena′lis. Depression on under surface of liver beside the gallbladder indicating position of duodenum. BNA.

i. gas′trica. Hollow under left lobe of liver indicating position of stomach. BNA.

i. rena′lis. Hollow on under surface of right lobe of liver adjacent to the right kidney. BNA.

impres′sion [L. *impressiō*]. 1. A hollow or depression in a surface. 2. Effect produced upon the mind by external stimuli. 3. Plastic imprint of the jaw and teeth for making a denture.

i., digitate. I. on inner surface of frontal bone for convolutions of the cerebrum.

i., maternal. An effect supposedly produced upon the developing fetus by mental impressions such as strong emotions or shock experienced by the mother during pregnancy. Such is supposed to account for malformations or the marking of the fetus.

impulse (im′puls) [L. *impulsus*, from *impellere*, to drive out]. 1. Act of driving onward with sudden force. 2. An incitement of the mind, prompting an unpremeditated act. 3. PHYS: A change transmitted through certain tissues, esp. nerve fibers and muscles, resulting in physiological activity or inhibition.

i., cardiac. 1. The heart beat felt at the left side of the chest at the 5th intercostal space. 2. I. transmitted over the conductile tissue of the heart which are responsible for the contraction of the chambers of the heart.

i., ectopic. A cardiac impulse arising in some part of the heart other than the sinoatrial node.

i., enteroceptive. Afferent nerve impulses arising from stimuli originating in receptors located in internal organs.

i., excitatory. One which stimulates activity.

i., exteroceptive. Afferent nerve impulses arising from stimuli originating in sense organs located on the body surface.

i., inhibitory. One which lessens activity.

i., morbid. An uncontrollable desire to perform an abnormal act.

i., nervous. A self-propagated excitatory state transmitted along a nerve fiber. It is the result of physicochemical changes occurring in the membrane of the nerve fiber. The impulse on reaching the termination of the fiber may (a) induce an impulse in another nerve cell or (b) induce activity in a tissue such as in muscles (contraction) or in glands (secretion), or (c) give rise to a sensation in the higher nervous centers.

i., proprioceptive. Afferent nerve im-

impulsion   I-9   **incombustible**

pulses arising from stimuli originating in joints, muscles, or tendons, or other sensory endings which respond to pressure or stretch.

impul'sion [L. *impulsus*, from *impellere*, to drive out]. Idea to do something or commit some act or crime suddenly imposed upon the subject which tortures him until the act is accomplished.

Clear consciousness of the proposed act followed by an agonizing struggle, defeat, and sense of relief following the act are characteristics of impulsions, obsessions, and of inhibitions. Impulsions may include: (1) *Folie du doute*, or doubting mania; (2) obsessive fears of contact or delirium of touch; (3) agoraphobia; (4) dipsomania; (5) pyromania; (6) kleptomania; (7) homicidal or suicidal impulsion; (8) onomatomania; (9) arithmomania; (10) exhibitionism. SEE: *cerebrifugal, cerebripetal, imperious acts.*

In. Chem symbol for indium.

in- [L.]. Prefix: *Not, in, inside, within;* also *intensive action.*

inac'tivate [L. *in*, not, + *activus*, acting]. To make inactive.

inactiva'tion [" + *activus*, acting]. Rendering anything inert by using heat or other means.

    i. **of complement.** Loss of activity caused by heating serum to about 55° C. (131° F.) for half an hour.

inadequacy (in-ad'e-kwa-sĭ) [" + *adaequare*, to be equal]. Insufficiency; incompetence.

    i., renal. Inability of kidney to produce normal amt. of urine with proper proportion of solids and of a sp. gr. more than 1.014.

inalimental (in-al-im-en'tal) [" + *alimentum*, food]. Unfit as food; not nutritious.

inan'imate [" + *animatus*, alive]. 1. Not alive; not animate. 2. Dull, lifeless.

inani'tion [L. *inanis*, empty]. A condition due to lack of any food material essential to the body, such as general underfeeding, undernutrition, or caloric insufficiency.

ETIOL: It may be due to other causes than the food supply, such as faulty mastication, stenosis of alimentary canal, etc.

inappetence (in-ap'pe-tens) [L. *in*, not, + *appetere*, to long for]. Lack of craving or desire, esp. for food.

inartic'ulate [" + *articulus*, joined]. 1. Not jointed; without joints. 2. Unable to pronounce distinct syllables or express oneself intelligibly. 3. Not given to expressing oneself verbally.

in artic'ulo mor'tis [L.]. At the time of death.

inassim'ilable [L. *in*, not, + *assimilis*, similar]. Not capable of being utilized by the body for nutrition.

inborn. Innate or inherent, said of characteristics both structural and functional which are inherited or developed during intrauterine development.

in'breeding [L. *in*, into, + A.S. *brēdan*, to cherish]. Producing offspring from those closely related.

incandes'cent [L. *incandescere*, to glow]. Glowing with light; white hot.

incar'cerated [L. *in*, into, + *carcer*, prison]. Imprisoned, confined, constricted, as an irreducible hernia.

incarcera'tion [" + *carcer*, prison]. Legal confinement; imprisonment of a part; constriction.

inca'rial bone. Os incae; interparietal bone.

incep'tion [L. *inceptio*, taking in, beginning]. 1. The beginning of anything. 2. Ingestion. 3. Intussusception.

incest (in'sest) [L. *incestus*, unchastity, incest]. Coitus between those of near relationship, a pathological phenomenon found in acquired or congenital states of mental weakness.

in'cidence [L. *incidere*, to meet with]. The rate of occurrence of any event or condition, as i. of a disease; the falling or impinging upon, touching, or affecting in some way.

in'cident [L. *incidere*, to meet with]. 1. A happening, event, or occurrence. 2. Apt. to happen, esp. in connection with some other event. 3. Falling or striking, as a ray of light.

incineration (in-sin-er-a'shun) [L. *in*, into, + *cinis, ciner-*, ash]. Destruction by fire. SYN: *cremation.*

incipient (in-sip'ĭ-ent) [L. *incipere*, to begin]. Beginning.

incise' [L. *incisus*, from *incidere*, to cut into]. To cut, as with a sharp instrument.

incised (in-sizd') [L. *incisus*, cut into]. Cut with a knife.

    i. **wound.** One clearly cut.

incision (in-sizh'un) [L. *incisiō*, from *incidere*, to cut into]. A cut made with a knife, esp. for surgical purposes.

incisive (in-si'siv) [L. *incisivus*, cutting into]. 1. Cutting; having the power of cutting. 2. Rel. to the incisor teeth.

    i. **bone.** Ant. or medial part of the sup. maxilla.

incisor (in-si'zor) [L. *incisor*, a cutter]. 1. That which cuts. 2. That which applies to the incisor teeth. 3. One of the cutting teeth, 4 in each jaw between the cuspids. SEE: *dentition.*

    i., prostatic. Surgical knife for incision of an enlarged prostate.

incisu'ra (pl. *incisurae*) [L. a cutting into]. An incision or notch.

incisure (ĭn-sīz'ŭr) [L. *incisura*, a cutting into]. A notch or slit.

    i's. **of Schmidt and Lantermann.** Oblique lines on medullated nerve fiber sheaths.

inclina'tion [L. *inclinere*, to slope]. Leaning from the normal, or from the vertical, as a tooth.

inclinometer (in-kli-nom'et-er) [" + G. *metron*, measure]. Device for measuring ocular diameter from vertical and horizontal lines.

inclu'sion [L. *inclusus*, enclosed]. Being enclosed or included.

    i., cell. Lifeless, temporary, constituent of the protoplasm of a cell. SEE: *cell.*

    i., blennorrhea. SYN: *ophthalmia neonatorum.* An inflammatory disease of the conjunctiva of newborn infants.

    i. **bodies.** Bodies present in the nucleus or cytoplasm of certain cells in cases of infection by filtrable viruses. SEE: *Negri bodies.*

    i., fetal. A twin monstrosity in which one, the parasite, is completely enclosed within its host, the *autosite.*

incoercible (in-ko-er'sib-l) [L. *in*, not, + *coercere*, to restrain]. Uncontrollable; not able to be held in check.

    i. **vomiting.** Uncontrollable vomiting.

incoherence (in-ko-her'ens) [" + *cohairens*, adhering]. Inability to express oneself coherently, or to present ideas in a related order; sometimes due to interruption of one's thought processes.

incoherent (in-ko-he'rent) [" + *cohairens*, adhering]. Not coherent or understandable.

incombus'tible [" + *combustus*, burned]. Incapable of being burnt.

incompatibil'ity [" + *compatī*, to suffer with]. State which renders admixture of remedies unsuitable through chemical action, insolubility, formation of poisonous or explosive compounds; difference in solubility, or opposite action.
 The quality of not being mixed without chemical changes, or without antagonizing the action of ingredients in a compound.
 i., physiological. A condition in which 1 or more substances in a mixture have a different physiological action than other substances in the mixture.
incompat'ible [" + *compatī*, to suffer with]. 1. Not capable of uniting in solution. 2. Antagonistic in action, said of some drugs.
 i. transfusion. A transfusion in which the isoagglutinins of the recipient react with the red blood cells of the donor resulting in intravascular agglutination and hemolysis.
incom'petence, incom'petency [" + *competere*, to be suitable]. Inadequate ability to perform the function or action normal to an organ or part.
 i., aortic. Regurgitation of blood through the aortic valves.
 i. of cardiac valves. Condition in which heart valves permit the return of blood beyond them when closed.
 i., ileocecal. Inability of ileocecal valve to stop the return of the material from the colon to the ileum.
 i., mental. Mental inability to retain charge of oneself or possessions.
 i., muscular. Imperfect closure of the cardiac valve due to weak action of papillary muscles.
 i., pyloric. Weakness of pyloric aperture which permits undigested food to leave the stomach and enter the duodenum.
 i., relative. Excessive dilatation of a cardiac cavity which makes perfect closure of opposite cardiac valve impossible.
 i., valvular. Leaky condition of 1 or more cardiac valves.
incom'petent [" + *competere*, to be suitable]. 1. One legally unable to execute a contract, such as a feebleminded or insane person. 2. Incapable.
incompres'sible [L. *in*, not, + *compressus*, pressed together]. Compact; not compressible.
incon'tinence [" + *continere*, to stop]. 1. Inability to retain urine, semen, or feces, through loss of sphincter control, cerebral or spinal lesions. 2. Lack of sexual restraint.
 i., active. Discharge of feces and urine in the normal way at regulated intervals but involuntarily.
 i., intermittent. Loss of control of bladder on sudden pressure or movement, because of interruption of voluntary path above the lumbar center.
 i. of milk. Excessive milk flow. SYN: *galactorrhea.*
 i., overflow. I. caused by pressure of urine retained in the bladder.
 i., paralytic. Constant voiding of small amt. of urine and feces due to relaxation of sphincters from lumbar center destruction.
 i., passive. Urinary i. of a form in which there is a full bladder that doesn't empty normally, but urine drips away upon pressure.
 i. of urine. Inability to control urination. Sphincter muscle always relaxed. SEE: *enuresis, scatacratia.*

incontinen'tia [" + *continere*, to stop]. Incontinence.
 i. alvi. Fecal i.
 i. urinae. Involuntary continual dripping of urine.
incoör'dinate [" + *coordināre*, to arrange]. 1. Not able to make coördinate muscular movements. 2. Unable to adjust one's work harmoniously with others.
incoördination (in-co-or-di-na'shun) [" + *coordināre*, to arrange]. Inability to produce harmonious, rhythmic, muscular action, but not due to weakness.
 ETIOL: The condition may be sensory, due to failure of afferent impulses to be transmitted from muscles, bones, and joints to coördination centers, or motor, due to disturbance in tone or harmony bet. simultaneously acting muscle groups. SYN: *asynergy.*
increment (in'kre-ment) [L. *incrementum*]. 1. Increase or addition. 2. To increase or add to.
incre'tin. A fraction of secretin, a hormone extracted from the duodenal mucosa, which induces hypoglycemia by increasing the output of insulin.
incre'tion [L. *incrētus*, sifted in]. 1. Internal secretion. 2. Functional activity of an endocrine gland.
incretogenous (in-kre-toj'en-us) [" + G, *gennan*, to produce]. Pert. to the internal secretions.
incrusta'tion [L. *in*, on, + *crusta*, crust]. Formation of crusts or scabs.
incubation (in-ku-ba'shun) [L. *incubāre*, to lie on]. 1. The interval between exposure to infection and the appearance of the first symptom. 2. BACT: The period of culture development. 3. The care of a premature infant in an incubator. 4. The development of an impregnated ovum. SYN: *latent period.* SEE: Table I-11.
in'cubator [L. *incubāre*, to lie on]. 1. Apparatus for rearing premature babies in which the temperature may be regulated. 2. Apparatus for cultivating bacteria. 3. An apparatus for artificially hatching eggs.
incubus (in'ku-bus) [L. *incubāre*, to lie upon]. 1. A burden. 2. A nightmare.
in'cudal [L. *incus*, anvil, from *incudere*, to forge]. Rel. to the incus.
incudectomy (in-ku-dek'to-mī) [" + G. *ektomē*, excision]. Surgical removal of the incus.
incudiform (in-ku'dĭ-form) [" + *forma*, shape]. Like an anvil in shape.
In"cudomal'leal [" + *malleus*, a hammer]. Rel. to the incus and malleus and articulation of the anvil and hammer in the tympanum.
incudostapedial (in-kŭ-do-stā-pē'dĭ-ăl) [" + *stapes*, a stirrup]. Pert. to the incus and stapes and articulation bet. anvil and stirrup in the tympanum.
incu'rable [L. *in*, not, + *curāre*, to care for]. SYN: *immedicable.* 1. Not capable of being cured. 2. A person with an incurable disease.
in'cus (pl. *incī*) [L. *anvil*]. The middle of the 3 ossicles in the tympanum; the anvil.
incyclophoria (in-si-klo-fo-ri'a). Median or negative cyclophoria; the turning of the eye inward toward the nose.
incyclotrophia (ĭn-sī-klō'trō'fĭ-ă). Cyclotropia in which the eye turns inward towards the nose.
in d. *In dies;* daily.
indagation (in-da-ga'shun) [L. *indagāre*, to search]. An investigation, esp. examination of the genitalia at termination of puerperium.
indenization (in-den-ĭ-za'shun) [L. *in*, into, + O. Fr. *deinzein*, from L. *de intus*,

Incubation and Isolation Periods in Common Infections

	Incubation Period	Isolation of Patient
Chickenpox.	Two to 3 weeks.	From school and from non-immune friends.
Common cold.	One to 2 days.	In bed for 2 days.
Conjunctivitis of newborn.	Usually 2 days.	Strict until smears are negative.
Diphtheria.	Usually 2 to 5 days.	Sixteen days after onset, or until 2 negative cultures.
Dysentery, amebic.	Two days to 4 weeks.	None.
Dysentery, bacillary	Two to 7 days.	As long as stools remain positive.
Encephalitis.	Four to 21 days.	One week after onset.
German measles.	Two to 3 weeks.	From school and nonimmune friends.
Gonorrhea.	One to 8 days.	No sexual contact until cured.
Influenza.	One to 3 days.	During acute stage.
Malaria.	Usually 2 weeks.	Protected from mosquitoes.
Measles.	Eight to 10 days.	Five days after appearance of rash.
Meningitis.	Usually a week.	Two weeks after onset.
Mumps.	Usually 18 days.	Until the glands recede.
Paratyphoid fevers.	About a week.	Until stools are negative.
Pneumonia, lobar.	One to 3 days.	Until bacteria in the sputum cease to be abundant.
Poliomyelitis.	One to 2 weeks.	Two weeks from onset.
Puerperal infections.	One to 3 days.	Transfer from maternity wards.
Rabies.	Usually 2 to 6 weeks.	Strict; danger to attendants.
Scarlet fever.	Up to a week.	Three weeks after onset.
Septic sore throat.	One to 3 days.	During disease: no handling of milk!
Smallpox.	Eight to 16 days.	Strict: in screened hospital wards.
Syphilis.	About 3 weeks.	Should be enforced until surface lesions are healed in noncoöperative patients.
Tetanus.	Four days to 3 weeks.	None.
Trachoma.	Unknown.	Until lesions disappear.
Tuberculosis.	Variable.	In "open" cases until properly educated.
Tularemia.	About 4 days.	None.
Typhoid fever.	Usually 1 to 3 weeks.	Until cultures of feces and urine are negative.
Typhus fever.	Usually 12 days.	Lice and fleas are dangerous.
Undulant fever.	One to 5 weeks.	None.
Whooping cough.	Usually a week.	For 3 weeks after spasmodic cough.
Vincent's angina.	Variable.	Preferably during the acute stage.

from within]. Arrest and development of cells in a part to which they have been carried by metastasis. SYN: *innidiation*.

indenta′tion [" + *dens, dent-,* tooth]. A depression or hollow.

index (in′deks) (pl. *indices*) [L. an indicator]. 1. The forefinger. 2. The ratio between the measurement of a given substance compared with that of a fixed standard.

i., alveolar. Degree of jaw prominence.
i., cephalic. Skull breadth multiplied by 100 and divided by its length.
i., cerebral. Ratio of greatest transverse to the greatest anteroposterior diameter of the cranium.
i., color. The proportion of hemoglobin to each red blood corpuscle, the normal being regarded as 100. SYN: *blood quotient*.
i., gnathic. Degree of jaw prominence expressed by a number.
i., gonoöpsonic. Opsonic i. in gonococcal infection.
i., hemorenal. Ratio of blood's electrical resistance to urine's.
i., opsonic. The ratio of number of bacteria which are ingested by leukocytes contained in normal serum, compared with the number ingested by leukocytes in the patient's own blood serum.
i., pelvic. Ratio of pelvic conjugate and transverse diameters.
i., phagocytic. Average of bacteria ingested per leukocyte of blood.
i., refractive. Refraction coefficient.
i., thoracic. Ratio of thoracic anteroposterior diameter to transverse diameter.

indican (in′dĭ-kăn). Potassium salt of indoxyl-sulfate, found in sweat and urine, and formed from indol.
When in excess in urine it indicates putrefaction of proteins.

indicanemia (in″dĭ-kan-e′mĭ-ă) [*indican* + G. *aima*, blood]. Indican in the blood.

indicanu′ria [" + G. *ouron*, urine]. Excess of indoxyl-sulfate of potassium, a derivative of indol, in urine.
In normal urine it is found in small quantities.

indica′tion [L. *indicāre*, to point out]. That which indicates the proper treatment.
  i., causal. That shown by a knowledge of the cause of a disease.
  i., morbid. That shown by diagnosis.
  i., symptomatic. That shown by symptoms.

in′dicator [L. *indicāre*, to show]. A substance which can be used to distinguish acid from alkali. (In a more general sense, any substance which can be used to determine the completeness of a chemical reaction, as in volumetric analysis.) The colors of indicators in common use are as in the table below.
  USES: 1. In titration of ammonia and other weak bases. 2. Topfer's reagent, for determining free acid in gastric juice. 3. In titrating weak acids and for determining combined acid in gastric juice.

indif′ferent [L. *in*, not, + *differre*, to differ]. Neutral; tending in no specific direction.

indigenous (in-dij′en-us) [L. *indigenus*, born in]. Native to a country or region.

indigestible (in-dĭ-jes′tĭ-bl) [L. *in*, not, + *digerere*, to separate]. Not digestible.

indiges′tion [L. *in*, not, + *digerere*, to separate]. SYN: *dyspepsia*. Incomplete or imperfect digestion, usually accompanied by one or more of the following symptoms: pain, nausea, and vomiting, heartburn and acid regurgitation, accumulation of gas and belching. It may be due to unimportant functional causes or it may be a symptom of a serious organic or functional disease.

indigitation (in-dĭj-ĭ-ta′shun) [L. *in*, in, + *digitus*, finger]. Displacement of intestines by intussusception.* SYN: *invagination.**

indigouria (ĭn′dĭ-gō-ū′rĭ-ă) [G. *indikon*, Indian dye, + *ouron*, urine]. Indigo in the urine.

indirect′ [L. *indirectus*, not kept straight]. Not direct.
  i. cell division. Amitosis. Single cell division in which a mitotic figure is not formed.
  i. reflexes. 1. Passive flexion of 1 part following flexion of another. 2. Passive flexion of 1 leg causing similar movement of opposite leg.

indisposi′tion [L. *in*, not, + *dispositus*, arranged]. Disorder; any slight or temporary illness.

indol(e. SYN: *ketol*. A solid, crystalline substance, C₈H₇N, found in feces. It is the product of bacterial decomposition of tryptophane and is largely responsible for the odor of feces. In intestinal obstruction it is absorbed and eliminated in the urine in the form of indican, *q.v.*

indolaceturia (in-dol-as-ē-tu′rĭ-ă) [*indol* + L. *acetum*, vinegar, + G. *ouron*, urine]. Excretion of a considable amt. of indolacetic acid in the urine.

in′dolent [L. *in*, not, + *dolere*, to feel pain]. 1. Indisposed to action. 2. Inactive; not developing; sluggish.
  i. ulcer. One that is sluggish but not painful.

indologenous (in-dol-oj′en-us) [*indol* + G. *gennan*, to produce]. Causing the production of indol.

indolu′ria. The presence of indol in urine.

indoxyl (in-dok′sil) [G. *indikon*, indigo, + *oxys*, sharp]. An oily substance, C₈H₇NO, sometimes found in urine of the apparently healthy, formed from the decomposition of tryptophane.

indoxylemia (in-doks-ĭ-le′mĭ-ă) [" + " + *aima*, blood]. Indoxyl in the blood.

indoxyluria (in-doks-il-u′rĭ-ă) [" + " + *ouron*, urine]. Excretion of indoxyl in urine.

induced (in-dūsd′) [L. *inducere*, to lead in]. Produced; caused. [tentionally.
  i. abortion. One brought about in-

induc′tance [L. *inducere*, to lead in]. That property of an electric circuit by virtue of which a varying current induces an electromotive force in that circuit or a neighboring circuit.
It is susceptible of measurement. The unit of inductance, or "self-induction," is the *henry.*

induction (in-duk′shun) [L. *inducere*, to lead in]. 1. The process of causing or producing, as an abortion. 2. The generation of electric current in a body by electricity in another body near it. 3. In Embry. the production of a specific morphogenic effect by a chemical substance from one part of the embryo to another. Also called *evocation.*

inductor′ium. An induction coil, *q.v.*

inductotherm (in-duk′to-therm) [" + G. *therme*, heat]. Device for producing pyrexia by electricity.

inductothermy. Treatment of disease by artificial production of fever by electromagnetic induction.

in′durate [L. *in*, in, + *durus*, hard]. 1. To harden. 2. Hardened.

in′durated [" + *durus*, hard]. Hardened.

indura′tion [" + *durus*, hard]. 1. The act of hardening. 2. An area of hardened tissue.
  SEE: *Chaussier's areola, sclerosis, skin.*
  i., cyanotic. An i. from long continued venous hyperemia, pressure on vessels causing transudation of blood and serum and formation of a dark, hard mass.
In the liver, spleen, etc., it leads to absorption of more or less of the paren-

Colors of Indicators

	Color toward acid	toward alkali	Range of pH
Bromcresol purple	yellow	purple	5.2- 6.8
Bromthymol blue	yellow	blue	6.0- 7.6
Congo red (1)	blue	red	3.0- 5.0
Dimethylaminoazobenzene (2)	red	yellow	2.9- 4.0
Litmus	red	blue	4.5- 8.3
Methyl orange	red	orange	3.1- 4.4
Methyl red	red	yellow	4.2- 6.3
Phenol red	yellow	red	6.8- 8.4
Phenolphthalein (3)	colorless	red	8.3-10.0

induration, fibrous, of the lung **infant feeding**

chyma and to formation of new connective tissue.
   i., fibrous, of the lung. A form of interstitial pneumonia. Hardened pigment forms red points on the lung.
   i., specific. The initial lesion of syphilis.
in'durative [" + *durus,* hard]. Pert. to induration.
indu'sium. 1. A membranous covering. 2. The amnion.
   i. griseum. The supracallosal gyrus, a rudimentary gyrus located on the upper surface of the corpus callosum.
inebriant (in-e'brĭ-ant) [L. *inebrius,* drunken]. 1. Any intoxicant. 2. Making drunk.
ine'briate [L. *inebrius,* drunken]. To make drunk or to become intoxicated.
inebriation (in-e-bri-a'shun). State of intoxication, *q.v.* SYN: *drunkenness, intoxication.*
inelas'tic [L. *in,* not, + G. *elastikos,* elastic]. Not elastic.
inemia (in-e'mĭ-ă) [G. *is, in-,* fiber, + *aima,* blood]. Excess fibrin or presence of inosite (muscle sugar) in the blood. SYN: *inosemia.*
inert' [L. *iners, inert-,* unskilled, idle]. Not active; sluggish.
inertia (in-er'shĭ-ă) [L. inactivity]. 1. Tendency of a body to remain in repose. 2. Sluggishness; lack of activity.
   i., uterine. Absence or weakness of uterine contractions in labor.
in extremis (in-eks-tre'mis) [L.]. At the point of death.
in'fant [L. *infans*]. 1. A babe. 2. A child not over 2 years of age. 3. In law, a minor, or one under legal age.
   i., artificial feeding of. *Precautions*: 1. The feedings must be given *exactly* on time.
   2. Temperature of feeding should be 100° F. Test heat by shaking some of it on the back of the hand. See that bottle is not overheated and that it does not burn infant by coming in contact with it.
   3. Nipples should be kept in a boric acid solution and not fitted to bottle until ready to give. They should not be handled more than necessary, and before touching them one should be assured that the hands are clean. See that the hole in nipple permits a free, but not too rapid, flow of milk. The hole should not be too small. It may be enlarged with a heated needle.
   4. See that infant is changed before bringing in the feeding.
   5. In administering feeding, head and shoulders should be raised higher than the infant's abdomen, but it is better to hold infant while giving the feeding. See that the child is properly protected from drafts or cold. If being fed when in a reclining position the formation of gas may result in belching of the feeding. Change position of bottle as level of the fluid changes.
   6. See that nothing disturbs the child while being fed and that the feeding is not interrupted. Close observation is essential, as the baby must receive all the feeding, which will not be the case if it is regurgitated or lost from belching. Interruptions may cause air-swallowing, which results in gas distention and a feeling of fullness that may cause a rejection of necessary nourishment.
   7. If an accumulation of gas interferes with the feeding, the usual methods of expelling the gas should be employed, such as holding the child over the shoulder and patting it on the back. This should also be done after each feeding in order to expel any air.
   8. Do not rock a baby after it has been fed.
   9. Water should be given bet. feedings to maintain elimination and other body needs.
   9. The habit of finger sucking should not be permitted, as air-swallowing always results therefrom.
   CARE OF NIPPLES AND BOTTLES: Both bottles and nipples should be soaked in cold water. Wash bottles with hot water and soap, using a brush for the purpose, and sterilize them by boiling in hot water. The nipples after being boiled may be kept in a boric acid solution.
   i. development. For 3 days after birth a baby loses weight; in the next 4 days, however, it should regain its loss and weigh as much as it weighed at birth. From 1 year old to 10 years the yearly gain in the child should be 4 or 5 pounds; from 10 to 16 years the yearly growth should be about 8 pounds. Should hold up head by 4th month, sit up before 7th month, walk by 12th to 15th month, talk before 18th month.
   i. feeding. The infant should not go to breast for at least 12 hours after delivery. If this limit is up at night, the next morning will be soon enough for the first nursing. The regular nursing schedule is not necessary until the milk comes in. The 3- or 4-hour nursing interval depends upon the physician, hospital, and the condition of the mother and the baby. The 3-hour interval is advocated by some physicians during the first 2 or 3 weeks. This keeps the breasts emptied, thereby relieving congestion, and increases the amount of the baby's fluid intake in 24 hours. Others prefer the 4-hour interval, especially if the infant is large.
   The early cessation of night feedings is an advantage of the 3-hour schedule rarely attained in the 4-hour régime. The individual breast is stimulated by the 15-minute nursing period. Followed by the 6-hour rest period, this combination provides for maximum functioning.
   COMPLEMENTARY FEEDING: This is an artificial feeding used to round out a breast feeding that is inadequate. It is better given immediately after the breast feeding rather than before it. It abets the utilization of breast milk without interfering with it, while supplying any breast milk deficiency that may exist.
   SUPPLEMENTAL FEEDING: An artificial

Infant Development

Age	Length Inches	Weight Pounds	Girth Inches
At birth	19.5	7	13
1 month	20.5	7.75	..
2 months	21	9.5	..
3 months	22	11	..
4 months	23	12.5	15
5 months	23.5	14	..
6 months	24	15	16
7 months	24.5	16	..
8 months	25	17	..
9 months	25.5	18	..
10 months	26	19	..
11 months	26.5	20	..
12 months	27	21	17

feeding replacing breast feeding, one or several times daily. It is not as generally used as the complementary, since it operates against the stimulation of breast milk production, and so tends to reduce it even further.

COMPOSITION OF ARTIFICIAL FOOD: The basis of artificial infant feedings is cow's milk, which is modified by the addition of water and a carbohydrate. Sometimes lactic acid is added, although lemon juice, orange juice, and even dilute hydrochloric acid may be used. Estimation of the composition of the formula should be based upon the physiologic requirements of the infant. No less than 1½ oz. (45 cc.) of milk per lb. (450 Gm.) of body weight be sufficient for this purpose, and may be increased to 2 oz. (60 cc.) per lb. of body weight within a week or 10 days. Calculation is based upon a 4% fat milk and allows for introducing a weak but sustaining food.

Carbohydrate requirement in 24 hours is 1/10 oz. (3 Gm.) to each lb. (450 Gm.) of body weight, exclusive of the 4% already in the milk. Fluid requirement is 3 oz. (90 cc.) to every lb. of body weight in 24 hours.

Unless an infant is immature or premature, there is no clinical reason for employing concentrated foods, such as evaporated milk, etc.

i., immature. One born near term, but underweight and poorly developed.

i., mature. One born at the end of 270-290 days.

i., premature. One born before term, but viable, having a birth weight of 5½ lb. (2500 Gm.) or less, with a "crown-heel" length of 47 cm. or less; the birth weight being the most important factor. Includes larger number of immature infants. The younger the fetus at birth, the greater are its handicaps in carrying out its required body functions, and thus it needs far greater care than a normal or mature infant.

ARTIFICIAL FEEDING OF: The breast feedings are excessive quantities for artificial feeding. Slower and smaller increases of weight may be expected on artificial feedings.

Small feeding with a low fat content of concentrated mixtures which precipitate with a finely divided curd is desirable.

If fresh sweet milk is used as a basis it should be boiled 5 minutes over a direct flame, but this is not necessary when lactic acid milk is used. Evaporated milk, dried sweet or lactic acid milk, or condensed milk may be used as a safe substitute for sweet milk.

Carbohydrates are first added in 2% quantities and increased to 5% as required. Orange juice may be added by the 3rd week to counteract effect of the boiled milk. Begin with 5 drops daily and increase to 2 tablespoonfuls, twice a day, by the end of the 8th week.

Cod liver oil should be fed before the end of the 3rd week, 2 drops daily, increasing to 60 drops by the 8th week. This is best divided into 2 feedings.

The feeding may be done with a medicine dropper. A nursing bottle also may be used, but the nipple should have a small bulb, or the rubber end of a medicine dropper.

i. pulse. At birth, 120-150 per min.; at the end of 1st year, 120-110; 3rd-4th yr., 100; at puberty, pulse is that of an adult.

i. respiration. At birth, 30-60 per min.; 1st yr., 25-30; 5th yr., 22-25; 14th yr., 20. SEE: *pulse, respiration, temperature.*

i. temperature. Normal (rectal), 98°-99° F. Subnormal more important than in adults.

infanticide (in-fan'tis-īd) [L. *infans*, infant, + *caedere*, to kill]. 1. The killing of an infant. 2. One who takes the life of an infant.

infantile (in'fan-tīl) [L. *infans*, infant]. Pert. to infancy.

i. hernia. Oblique inguinal hernia back of the peritoneal funicular process.

i. liver. Biliary cirrhosis* of children.

i. paralysis. Acute ant. poliomyelitis.*

i. tet'anus. Tetanus which begins with stiffening of jaw muscles. SYN: *trismus nascentium* or *neonatorum*.

infantilism (in-fan'til-izm) [" + G. *ismos*, condition]. A condition in which the mind and body make slow development. Failure to attain adult characteristics, physical or psychic.

i., angioplastic. I. due to defective development of vascular system.

i., Brissaud's. Infantile myxedema.

i., cachectic. I. caused by chronic infection or poisoning.

i., celiac. I. caused by celiac disease.

i., dysthyroidal. I. caused by defective thyroid.

i., hepatic. I. combined with cirrhosis of liver.

i., hypophysial. SYN: *pituitary i., Lorain-Levi dwarfism.* Dwarfism resulting from hyposecretion of growth promoting and gonadotrophic hormones of ant. lobe of the hypophysis.

i., Herter's. I. of the intestines.

i., idiopathic. Variety of arrested physical development, of unknown cause.

i., intestinal. I. associated with chronic intestinal disorder, causing the child to gain no weight nor to grow.

i., Lorain-Levi. Hypophysial i., *q.v.*

i., lymphatic. A form of i. associated with lymphatism.

i., myxedematous. SYN: *cretinism.* SEE: *Brissaud's i.*

i., pancreatic. I. caused by defect in pancreatic function.

i., partial. Arrest in development of a lone tissue or part.

i., pituitary. Hypophysial i., *q.v.*

i., renal. I. caused by defect in renal function.

i., reversive. I. commencing subsequent to completion of bodily growth.

i., sex. Continuation of childish traits, esp. sex characteristics beyond the age of puberty.

i., symptomatic. I. caused by poor tissue development.

i., tardy. SEE: *reversive i.*

i., toxemic. SEE: *intestinal i.*

i., universal. Dwarfed stature, otherwise fairly normal development, except for absence of secondary sexual characteristics.

in'farct [L. *infacire*, to stuff into]. An area of tissue in an organ or part which undergoes necrosis following cessation of blood supply. May result from occlusion or stenosis of supplying artery or more rarely occlusion of vein draining tissue. Usually conical in shape.

i., anemic. I. in which blood pigment is lacking or decoloration had occurred. Also called white or pale infarct.

i., bland. I. in which infection is absent.

i., calcareous. I. in connective tissue in which calcareous salts have been deposited.
i., cicatrized. I. which has been replaced or encapsulated by fibrous tissue.
i., pale. An anemic infarct, *q.v.*
i., red. An i. which is swollen and red as a result of hemorrhage. Also called *hemorrhagic infarct*.
i., uric acid. I. in kidney of a newborn infant due to obstruction of renal tubules by uric acid crystals.
i., white. An anemic infarct, *q.v.*
infarc'tion [L. *infarcire*, to stuff into]. 1. Formation of an infarct. 2. Stoppage of a canal or passage, esp. by engorgement.
i., cardiac. Myocardialial infarction, *q.v.*
i., myocardial. I. in cardiac muscle, usually resulting from coronary thrombosis.
i., pulmonary. I. in lung usually resulting from pulmonary embolism.
infect. To cause pathogenic organisms to be present in or upon, as to *infect* a wound.
infection [L. *inficere*, to taint]. The state or condition in which the body or a part of it is invaded by a pathogenic agent (microörganism or virus) which, under favorable conditions, multiplies and produces effects which are injurious.

Localized infection is usually accompanied by inflammation, but inflammation may occur without infection.

The physician is esp. concerned with 3 conditions: (a) Infections arising without known injury; (b) those arising in wounds of accidental origin, and (c) infections of operative wounds.

ETIOL: The principal causes of infections are agents belonging to the following groups: viruses, bacteria, Rickettsias, fungi, and animal parasites.

Unknown Injury: Inflammations may result from slight abrasions, but most of these infections are now attributed to *focal* infection, such as those of the tonsils and teeth, accessory sinuses, chronic middle ear infection, infection of wounds, or of the gastrointestinal tract.

Known Injury: Many of these are due to wounds. The character of the instrument causing the wound may influence the infection, as in the case of a rusty nail.

Operative Wounds: These infections may occur as the direct result of the operative technic, such as the use of blunt instruments, or too vigorous wiping with sponges, and other surgical causes, and by postoperative exposure to sepsis.

SYM: The symptoms of infection are those of inflammation. The 5 classical symptoms of the earlier medical writers are: *Dolor*, pain; *calor*, heat; *rubor*, redness; *tumor*, swelling, and *functio laesa*, disordered function.

Pain: This is esp. prominent when the infection is confined within retaining cavities. The pain is in proportion to the virulence and extent of the infection.

Redness and Swelling: Not evident when infection is within some rigid tissue or deep within some cavity; more apparent when superficial structures are involved. Discoloration would be a better term than "'redness," as the color is more bluish or purple in advanced infections, while tuberculosis infections have long been called "white swellings."

Heat: Heat may not be evident on the surface, but there may be considerable elevation of body temperature even with small infections.

Disordered Function: This depends upon the part affected as well as upon the virulence. With almost all acute infections there is an increase of white cells and of polymorphonuclear leukocytes, a percentage of over 85% of the latter being of more import than leukocytosis.*

The degree of prostration is out of proportion to the extent of the injury. There have been many deaths from infection following pricks of needles, small splinters of bone, a trifling cut, or an infection from the bristle of a brush, in which streptococcus was the inciting cause. In this type of infection a red streak may be seen running up the extremity from the site of injury, and following the superficial lymphatics. This red line is absent in staphylococcus infections of the lymphatic vessels.

Infection may be *local* or *general*. Local infections may be at the portal of entry, or remote if transferred by the blood or lymph.

SITE OF: Microörganisms may gain entry to the tissues through the *gastrointestinal tract*, as in typhoid fever, or through the *respiratory tract*, as in tuberculosis and common colds, or through *wounds*, as in rabies, or from *contaminated objects*, as in tetanus, or from *bites of insects*, as in malaria and yellow fever.

The Commoner Protozoal Infections of Man

Disease	Primary Site of Infection	Parasite	Mode of Transmission
Malaria: (1) Benign tertian (2) Benign quartan (3) Malignant	Erythrocytes	(1) *Plasmodium vivax* (2) *Plasmodium malariae* (3) *Plasmodium falciparum*	Mosquito (*Anopheles*)
Sleeping sickness	Blood plasma	*Trypsanosoma gambiense*	Tsetse fly (*Glossina palpalis*)
Rhodesian sleeping sickness	Blood plasma	*T. rhodesiense*	Tsetse fly (*Glossina morsitans*)
Kala-azar	Reticuloendothelial cells and plasma	*Leishmania donovani*	The sand fly (*Phlebotomus argentipes*)
Amebic dysentery	Wall of large intestine	*Entamoeba histolytica*	Fecal (cyst) contamination of food and water

infection, acute   **infectious disease**

Lowered vitality and resistance make possible *subinfection* from bacteria whose normal habitat is in the body. All infections of mucous membranes are mixed infections. Foci of infections may be primary or secondary.

METHODS OF: *Air-borne Infection*: Pathogenic organisms in the respiratory tract, discharged from the mouth or nose, may be borne on the air and settle on food, clothing, walls and floors, and if they are of the type which resists drying for a long period they may remain virulent until transmitted to another person. Coughing, sneezing, and expectorating may be responsible for "droplet infection," as bacteria are expelled into the air.

Animal Carriers: Some microorganisms may be carried from an animal to man by *direct contact, indirect transfer, or by intermediary hosts*.

Contact Infection: This is the result of transmission from person to person, as in kissing, coming in contact with those afflicted with communicable diseases, or with utensils handled by one with an infection.

Food-borne Infection: Bacteria may be communicated through food. Root and salad vegetables may carry bacteria from the soil or from manure. Cooking safeguards by destroying microorganisms on food.

Human Carriers: Some parasites may live in or upon the bodies of those who themselves do not suffer from them, but may be carried by them to others. Carriers may be: (a) *Contact* carriers, or those who never show symptoms; (b) *incubationary* carriers, or those in whom the infection is starting but has not completed the incubation period, and (c) *convalescent* carriers, or those who have recovered but who still harbor the organism causing their disease.

Insect Vectors*: An insect may act as a physical carrier, as the housefly, which may transmit the typhoid bacillus, or one that acts as an active intermediate host, such as the Anopheles mosquito, which transmits malaria.

Prenatal Infection: This is the result of the fetus being infected from the mother's blood stream, or from contiguity with the maternal membranes.

Soil-borne Infection: Soil-borne, spore-forming organisms commonly enter the body through wounds, as in tetanus and gas gangrene.

Water-borne Infection: Organisms producing typhoid, dysentery, cholera, and amebic infections may be carried through a water supply, or water in public pools used for bathing. These organisms may pass into the water from the feces of an infected person and be communicated to others.

i., acute. Appears suddenly and runs a short course.

i., a. exacerbation. Recurrence after a period of quiescence.

i., apical. I. located at the tip of root of a tooth.

i., chronic. One having a protracted course.

i., concurrent. Existence of two or more infections at the same time.

i., droplet. Acquired by inhalation.

i., endogenous. I. caused by bacteria, normally nonpathogenic inhabiting the digestive tract.

i., focal. One occurring in a focus or cavity, and acting as a focus for dissemination of infectious material to other parts of the body. Ex: Apical tooth abscess causing infection of heart or joints.

i., food. SEE: *Food infections*.

i., local. I. caused by germs lodging and multiplying at one point in a tissue and remaining there, as a *boil*.

i., low grade. Loosely used term for a subacute or chronic infection with only mild inflammation and without pus formation.

i., metastatic. Local i. caused by germs circulated from a focus of infection.

i., mixed. Caused by 2 or more organisms.

i., pyogenic. I. resulting from pus-forming organisms.

i., secondary. One in which the organisms implant themselves upon an existing primary infection in tissues.

i., simple. Due to a single species of organism.

i., subacute. Intermediate bet. acute and chronic.

i., terminal. One occurring in the late stage of a disease. Generally acute and septic, usually causing death.

infectious (in-fek'shus) [L. *inficere*, to make into]. 1. Capable of being transmitted with or without contact. 2. Pert. to a disease due to a microörganism. 3. Producing infection. SEE: *eruptive*.

i. disease. Any disease caused by growth of pathogenic microörganisms in the body. May or may not be contagious.

Tabulation of Infectious Diseases

CHICKENPOX: *Incubation period*: Four to 27 days. *Eruption appears*: First 4 days. *Begins to fade*: About 4th day. *Quarantine*: About 22 days. *Infection ceases*: When every scab has disappeared.

DIPHTHERIA: *Incubation period*: One to 7 days. *Quarantine*: Nine days after exposure. *Infection ceases*: In 4 weeks if examination of nose and throat is negative and if there are no discharges or albuminuria.

GERMAN MEASLES (Rötheln): *Incubation period*: Seven to 18 days or longer. *Eruption appears*: Second to 4th day. *Begins to fade*: Fourth to 7th day. *Quarantine*: Two days. *Infection ceases*: Not less than 7 days from appearance of rash.

INFLUENZA: *Incubation period*: One to 4 days. *Quarantine period*: Five days. *Infection ceases*: Three days after normal temperature if all discharges have ceased.

MEASLES: *Incubation period*: Eight to 14 days. *Eruption appears*: Fourth day. *Begins to fade*: Fifth to 7th day. *Quarantine*: Sixteen days. *Infection ceases*: Not less than 2 weeks from appearance of rash.

MUMPS: *Incubation period*: Nineteen to 22 days. *Quarantine*: Twenty-four days. *Infection ceases*: Not less than 3 weeks and at least 1 week after subsidence of swelling.

SCARLET FEVER: *Incubation period*: One to 5 days. *Eruption appears*: Second day. *Begins to fade*: Fifth day. *Quarantine*: Seven days. *Infection ceases*: Not less than 4 weeks if no albuminuria and no discharge from nose or ears.

SMALLPOX: *Incubation period*: Twelve to 14 days. *Eruption appears*: Third or 4th day. *Begins to fade*: Ninth or 10th day. *Quarantine*: Sixteen days. *Infection ceases*: When every scab has disappeared.

Fungus Infections

Disease	Causative Organisms	Structures Infected	Microscopic Appearances
Ringworm (tinea, pityriasis, etc.).	*Microsporon* (*audouini*, etc.).	Horny layer of epidermis and hairs, chiefly of scalp.	Fine septate mycelium inside hairs and scales. Spores in rows and mosaic plaques on hair surface.
Ringworm (tinea, pityriasis, etc.).	*Trichophyton* (*tonsurans*, etc.).	Hairs of scalp, beard, and other parts. Also nails.	Mycelium of chained cubical elements and threads in and on hairs. Often pigmented.
Favus.	*Achorion* (*schönleinii*, etc.).	Yellow disks in epidermis round a hair. All parts of body; also nails.	Vertical hyphae and spores in epidermis. Sinuous branching mycelium and chains in hairs.
Epidermophytosis (Dhobie itch, etc.).	*Epidermophyton* (*inguinale*, etc.).	Inflamed patches in inguinal, axillary and interdigital folds. Hairs not affected.	Long, wavy, branched and segmented hyphae and spindle-shaped cells in stratum corneum.
Thrush (and tonsillomycosis).	*Monilia*.	White patches on tongue, mouth, and throat. Some inflammation.	Yeastlike budding cells and oval, thick-walled bodies in epidermis. Some broad hyphae.
Thrush (and tonsillomycosis).	*Oidium* (*albicans*).	White patches on tongue, mouth, and throat. Some inflammation.	Large hyphae and oval bodies, chains of spores at ends of hyphae.
Fungal granuloma (sporotrichosis and blastomycosis).	*Sporotrichon* (*beurmanni*, etc.).	Inflammatory thickening of skin with suppuration.	Oval spores and yeastlike cells in tissues and pus.
Fungal granuloma (sporotrichosis and blastomycosis).	*Cryptococcus*.	Inflammatory thickening of skin with suppuration.	Budding yeastlike cells, short hyphae and large capsulated spheroids in tissues and pus.
Aspergillosis (and bronchomycosis).	*Aspergillus* (*fumigatus*, etc.).	Pustules in external ear. Inflammatory and necrotic foci in lungs.	Branched hyphae and spore-bearing fructifications in pus or sputum.

infecundity   I-18   **inflammation**

TYPHOID FEVER: *Incubation period*: Seven to 21 days. *Eruption appears*: Seventh to 9th day. *Begins to fade*: Twenty-first day. *Quarantine*: Twenty-three days. *Infection ceases*: After 3 consecutive negative reports from bacteriological examination of feces and urine.

TYPHUS FEVER: *Incubation period*: Five to 14 days. Variable. *Eruption appears*: Fourth to 8th day. *Begins to fade*: Fourteenth day. *Quarantine*: Sixteen days. *Infection ceases*: After 4 weeks.

WHOOPING COUGH: *Incubation period*: Seven to 14 days, but whooping may not appear for 3 weeks. *Quarantine*: Sixteen days. *Infection ceases*: Three to 5 weeks.

NOTE: Period of quarantine varies in different states. SEE: *quarantine;* also, *names of infectious diseases.*

infecundity (in-fe-kun′dĭ-tĭ) [L. *infecunditās*, sterility]. Barrenness; sterility in women.

Inferior (in-fē′rĭ-or) [L. *inferus*, below]. Beneath; lower.

inferiority complex. PSY: A repressed state of mind in which one feels himself inferior to others. Such a group of ideas may be manifested by the assumption of superiority, often resulting in over-compensation. OPP: *superiority complex.* RS: *complex.*

infest′ [L. *infestāre*, to attack]. The harboring of parasites.

infesta′tion [L. *infestāre*, to attack]. The harboring of animal parasites, esp. macroscopic forms such as helminthes. *Infestation* is applied to forms which do not multiply within the body in contrast to *infection* which is applied to those which multiply.

infibulation (in-fib-u-la′shun) [L. *in*, in, + *fibula*, clasp]. 1. Fastening the labia of the vagina together, or the prepuce over the glans penis. 2. Joining the lips of wounds by clasps.

Infiltrate (in-fĭl′trāt) [L. *in*, into, + *filtrare*, to strain through]. 1. To pass into or through a substance or a space. 2. The material that has infiltrated.

infiltration (in-fĭl-tra′shun) [L. *in*, into, + *filtrare*, to strain through]. The process of a substance passing into and being deposited within the substance of a cell, tissue, or organ. Ex: I. of a tissue or organ with blood corpuscles, or of a cell by fatty particles.

It must not be confused with degeneration, as in the latter condition the foreign substances are from changes within the cell.

   i., amyloid. I. of tissue or viscera with a glycoprotein.

   i. anesthesia. Injection of a cocaine or similar solution. SEE: *anesthesia.*

   i., calcareous. Deposits of calcium or magnesium salts within a tissue.

   i., cellular. I. of cells, esp. blood cells, into tissues; invasion by cells of malignant tumors into adjacent tissue.

   i., fatty. Deposit of fat in the tissues, or oil or fat globules in the cells.

   i., glycogenic. Glycogen deposit in cells.

   i., pigmentary. Of pigments.

   i., purulent. Pus cells in a tissue.

   i., serous. With diluted lymph.

   i., urinous. With urine.

   i., waxy. Amyloid degeneration.

in′finite distance. 1. A distance without limits. 2. In vision, light rays coming from a point of any distance beyond 20 feet are practically parallel and accommodation is unnecessary.

infirm. Weak or feeble, esp. from old age or disease.

infir′mary (L. *infirmarium*). A hospital; a place for the care of sick or infirm persons.

infirmity. 1. Weakness. 2. A sickness or illness.

inflamma′tion [L. *inflammāre*, to flame within]. Tissue reaction to injury, either direct or referred.

It is a defensive reaction to irritation, *chemical, bacterial, mechanical,* or *toxic.* It produces degeneration of the injured area, and repair ensues by aid of the tissue cells.

Inflammation is a conservative process modified by whatever produces the reaction, but it should not be confused with *infection;* the two are relatively different conditions, although one may arise from the other.

ETIOL: The reaction of tissue to injury of any kind may be the result of: (a) Blows and foreign bodies; (b) chemicals; (c) electricity; (d) heat and cold (thermic causes); (e) microörganisms; (f) surgical operations (traumatic causes).

GENERAL SYMPTOMS: *Dolor*, pain; *calor*, heat; *rubor*, redness; *tumor*, swelling, and *functio laesa*, disordered function. In addition to the symptoms mentioned, the absorption of some of the constituents of inflammatory lymph may cause a slight rise of temperature (99°-101° F.), headache, loss of appetite, and a general feeling of discomfort.

PATHOLOGICAL CHANGES: (a) Vascular dilatation and changes in the blood. (b) Exudation of fluid from blood vessels into tissues with comcomitant swelling; migration of leukocytes into the tissues; gelation of fibrinogen in intercellular spaces. If the injury is not too severe, these processes reach their maximum in six to eight hours, after which reparative processes take place. Blood vessels return to normal size, normal blood flow is re-established. Leukocytes degenerate or re-enter circulation, cellular disintegration or proliferation occurs in which injured cells are replaced; swelling disappears with resorption of tissue fluid and digestion of fibrin.

Each type of cell has a particular rôle to play in the inflammatory process. The *monocytes** and *macrophages** are great scavengers for all kinds of dead tissue. The *polymorphs** are active in autolysis* and the destruction of bacteria, and the *lymphocytes** form a barrier against the spread of irritants and probably form the fundamental tissue from which the healing scar develops. These cells appear in inflammatory conditions at stated intervals, and in a definite order or succession; the macrophage, for instance, antedating the polymorph by a week, and the lymphocyte by several days.

NOMENCLATURE: Most words denoting inflammation end with the suffix *itis*, which in itself pertains to inflammatory conditions. This suffix should *not* be pronounced as "etis." The principal inflammations of the various systems are:

   Ear: Otitis externa, interna and media, mastoiditis.

   The Eye: Conjunctivitis, dacryocystitis, iritis, keratitis, optic neuritis, panophthalmitis, uveitis.

   Gastrointestinal Tract: Appendicitis, colitis, cholangitis, cholecystitis, duodenitis, enteritis, gastritis, hepatitis,

pancreatitis, peritonitis, periproctitis, peridontitis, parotitis, proctitis.
Miscellaneous Organs: Arthritis, carbuncle, dermatitis, furuncle, myositis, osteitis, osteomyelitis, periostitis, phlegmon, cellulitis, tendovaginitis.
Nervous System: Encephalitis, leptomeningitis, myelitis, neuritis, pachymeningitis, polyneuritis.
Respiratory System: Bronchitis, empyema, laryngitis, pharyngitis, pleurisy, pleuritis, pneumonia, rhinitis.
Urinary System: Balanitis, cystitis, cervicitis, epididymitis, endometritis, mastitis, myometritis, nephritis, oöphoritis, pyelitis, prostatitis, perimetritis, parametritis, pyometra, pyosalpinx, orchitis, seminal vesiculitis, salpingitis, salpingo-oöphoritis, urethritis.
Vascular System: Aortitis, endarteritis, endocarditis, epicarditis, lymphangitis, lymphadenitis, myocarditis.
i., acute. I. in which the onset is rapid and the course relatively short.
i., adhesive. One conducive to the healing of wounds.
i., alterative. SYN: *parenchymatous.* I. of an organ in which degeneration of parenchymal cells is accompanied by proliferation of other cells.
i., bacterial. I. induced by the growth of bacteria.
i., catarrhal. I. of a mucous membrane characterized by the excessive secretion of mucus.
i., chronic. I. which progresses slowly, is of long duration, and usually results in the formation of scar tissue.
i., exudative. One in which there is a large accumulation of blood cells and serum.
i., fibrinous. I. in which the exudate is rich in fibrin.
i., hemorrhagic. I. in which red blood cells are conspicuous in the exudate.
i., interstitial. I. involving principally the noncellular or supporting elements of an organ.
i., purulent. I. in which pus is formed.
i., reactive. One about a foreign body or a focus of infection.
i., serous. I. in which the exudate is composed principally of serum.
i., suppurative. Purulent i., *q.v.*
i., toxic. This is one due to toxin or poison.
inflam'matory [L. *inflammāre*, to flame within]. Rel. to or marked by inflammation.
inflation (in-fla'shun) [L. *in*, into, + *flāre*, to blow]. Distention of a part by air, gas, or liquid.
inflection (in-flek'shun) [" + *flectere*, to bend]. 1. An inward bending. 2. Change of tone or pitch of the voice; nuance.
influence machine. A particular type of "static machine." Probably the only type used in physical therapy.
influenza (in-flu-en'za) [It. *influence*]. Grippe, an acute infectious disease characterized by fever, extreme prostration, pain in head and back, and generally by catarrh of respiratory or gastrointestinal tract. SYN: *la grippe.*
ETIOL: The causative agent is a virus, of which two types have been identified, type A and type B. A number of bacteria, esp. Pfeiffer's bacillus (*Hemophilus influenzae*), pneumococci, streptococci, and staphylococci have been found in the lungs in fatal cases, but these are considered to be secondary invaders.
EPIDEMIOLOGY: Usually more prevalent in winter and spring. Young adults, in robust health, appear to be particularly susceptible. This disease is contagious and is spread, in all probability, by immune carriers. It may occur endemically, or epidemically, and pandemics have been witnessed.
INCUBATION: One to 4 days.
SYM: Begins abruptly with lassitude, malaise, chilliness, severe pain in head and back, fever from 101°-103° F. Prostration out of proportion to the fever. Eyes injected, sneezing, hoarseness, and hard paroxysmal cough. In most cases, catarrh of respiratory tract is unusually marked. Less frequently, gastrointestinal symptoms predominate. With latter, there may be diarrhea and abdominal pain.
COURSE: Ordinarily runs from 4 to 5 days, and may terminate by crisis or speedy lysis. Pulse rate usually not increased in proportion to fever; may be 90 to 100. Blood pressure low; nosebleed not uncommon. Examination of blood demonstrates a leukopenia. Urinalysis generally demonstrates presence of albumen and casts.
In some epidemics, a striking symptom is a peculiar cyanosis, which is, in all likelihood, of toxic origin. In addition to the respiratory and gastrointestinal forms referred to, a nervous and fulminating type are sometimes described. In the latter forms, terms used to designate them are suggestive of predominating symptoms encountered.
COMPLICATIONS: Pneumonia, pleurisy, empyema, chronic bronchitis, abscess of lung, sinusitis, otitis media, pericarditis, myocarditis, and very rarely endocarditis; peripheral neuritis, meningitis, and encephalitis are still more rare.
DIFFERENTIAL DIAGNOSIS: Typhoid fever, smallpox in the prodromal stage, cerebrospinal meningitis, and pulmonary tuberculosis.
PROG: As a rule, outcome is favorable in absence of pulmonary complications. In patients with cyanosis, severe nerve disturbances, or bloody expectoration, prognosis must be extremely guarded.
NP: *Prophylactic*: Isolation of patients, disinfection of sputum, and application of aseptic methods in handling sufferers by attendants is of utmost importance; also, sometimes, the wearing of suitable masks. The avoidance of public gatherings and general application of hygienic methods deserve consideration. The use of certain vaccines may play a part in prevention.
Active: Isolation, absolute rest, good ventilation, and a selected diet. No specific treatment; care largely symptomatic. Alcohol and strychnine sometimes recommended as stimulants and codeine may afford relief for cough.
influenzal (in-flu-en'zal) [It. *influence*]. Relating to influenza.
infolding. Process of inclosing within a fold; an operation employed in the treatment of stomach ulcer in which the walls on either side of the lesion are sutured together.
infra- [L.]. Prefix: *Below.*
infraäxillary (in″frå-aks'il-a-rī) [L. *infrā*, beneath, + *axilla*, little axis]. Below the axilla.
in″fraclavic′ular [" + *clavicula*, little key]. Below the clavicle.
infracostal (in-frå-kos'tal) [" + *costa*, rib]. Below a rib.
infraction. An incomplete fracture of a

infraglenoid

bone in which parts do not become displaced.

infraglenoid (in″fră-glē′noyd) [" + G. *glēnē*, cavity, + *eidos*, form]. Beneath the glenoid fossa. SYN: *subglenoid*.

infrahyoid (in-fră-hi′oid) [" + G. *yoeidēs*, U-shaped]. Below the hyoid bone.

inframam′mary [" + *mamma*, breast]. Below the mammary gland.

inframar′ginal [" + *margō*, a margin]. Below any edge or margin.

i. convolution. The sup. temporal one.

inframax′illary [" + *maxilla*, little jaw]. Below the jaw; submaxillary.

infraocclu′sion [" + *occlusio*, a shutting up]. Location of a tooth below the line of occlusion.

infraorbital (in-fră-or′bĭ-tal) [" + *orbita*, track]. Beneath the orbit.

infrapatellar (in″fră-pă-tel′ăr) [" + *patella*, a small plate]. Below the patella.

infrapu′bic [" + *pubes*, hair on genitals]. Below the pubis.

in′frared rays. Invisible heat rays beyond red end of spectrum.

Their wave length ranges from 7,700 to 500,000 Angström units. Long-wave infrared rays (15,000-150,000 A.U.) are emitted by all heated bodies and exclusively by bodies of low temperature such as hot-water bottles and electric-heating pads; short-wave infrared rays (7,200-15,000 A.U.) are those emitted by all incandescent bodies.

SOURCES: The sun, electric arc, incandescent globe, and so-called infrared burners.

USES: Their energy is transformed into heat in a superficial layer of the tissues. They are used therapeutically to stimulate local and general circulation and for relief of pain. They are also used to detect traces of selenium, a deadly poison, in foods, and in alloys and steel. SEE: *radiation, ray*.

infrascap′ular [L. *infrā*, below, + *scapula*, shoulder blade]. Beneath the shoulder blade.

infraspi′nous [" + *spīna*, a thorn]. Beneath the scapular spine.

infraster′nal [" + G. *sternon*, chest]. Beneath the sternum.

infratrochlear (in″fră-trok′le-ăr) [" + *trochlea*, pulley]. Beneath the trochlea.

infric′tion [L. *in*, on, + *frictiō*, rubbing]. Rubbing of ointments into the skin. SYN: *inunction*.

infundibuliform (in-fun-dib′u-lĭ-form) [L. *infundibulum*, funnel, + *forma*, form]. Funnel-shaped.

i. fascia, i. process. The membranous layer investing the spermatic cord.

infundib′ulin [L. *infundibulum*, funnel]. A 20% solution of an extract of the post. lobe of the hypophysis.

infundibulum (in-fun-dib′u-lum) [L. funnel]. 1. Funnel-shaped passage or body. 2. Tube connecting the frontal sinus with the middle nasal meatus. 3. Stalk of the pituitary gland. 4. Any renal pelvis division. 5. Cavity formed by fallopian fimbriae. 6. Terminus of a bronchiole. 7. Terminus at upper end of cochlear canal. 8. Conelike upper ant. angle of right cardiac ventricle, from which the pulmonary artery arises. SYN: *conus arteriosus*.

infu′sible [L. *infusiō*, an infusion]. 1. Not capable of being fused or melted.

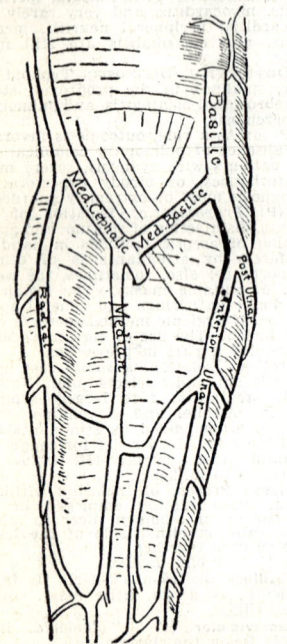

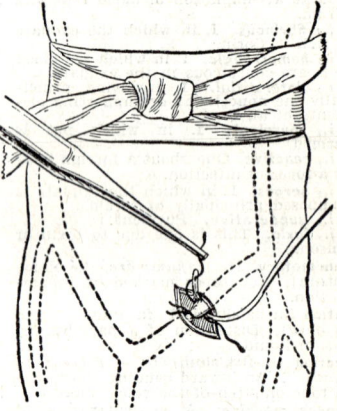

2. Incision method showing the incision made, the distal end of the vein tied, and a second ligature being passed under the proximal end of the vein.

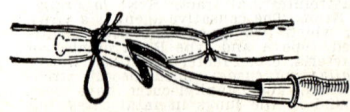

1. The superficial veins of forearm.

3. Incision method, showing cannula tied in place.

INFUSION, INTRAVENOUS SALINE

infusion   I-21   **inheritance, cytoplasmic**

2. Capable of being made into an infusion.

infusion (in-fu'zhun) [L. *infusiō*, from *in*, into, + *fundere*, to pour]. 1. Steeping a substance in cold or hot water below boiling point to obtain its active principles. 2. Product obtained by such a process. SYN: *infusum*. 3. Introduction of a liquid into a vein.
    RS: *apothem, autoinfusion, autoreinfusion, infiltration, intravenous.*
    i., intravenous. Injection of a solution directly into a vein, usually the cephalic or median basilic vein. Normal saline intravenous solutions are usually temporary in effect due to loss of water in tissues. SEE: *Illustration*, I-20.

infusodecoction (in-fu"zo-de-kok'shun) ["+ *dē*, down, + *coquere*, to boil]. 1. Infusion followed by decoction. 2. A medicine made from a crude drug steeped in cold water and then in boiling water.

infusor (in-fu'zor) [L. *infusum*, an infusion]. Instrument for injecting a liquid slowly into a vein.

Infusoria (in-fu-so'rĭ-ă) [L. *infusum*, infusion]. Name formerly applied to a class of *Protozoa*, now called *Ciliata*.

infu'sum [L. infusion]. Liquid preparations made by treating vegetable substances with hot or cold water.
    The drug is not subjected to boiling, as in making decoctions. When the strength and method of preparation are not otherwise specified, they are made by treating 5 parts of the coarsely comminuted drug with boiling water to make 100 parts. None are official.

ingesta (in-jes'tă) [L. *ingestum*, from *ingerere*, to carry in]. Food and drink received into the body through the mouth.

inges'tion [L. *ingestum*, from *ingerere*, to carry in]. The process of taking material (particularly food) into the gastrointestinal tract, or by which a cell takes in foreign particles.

Ingras'sias' apoph'yses. The lesser wings of the sphenoid.

ingravescent (in-grav-es'ent) [L. *in*, upon, + *gravescī*, to grow heavy]. Becoming more severe.

ingredient [L. *ingrediens*, entering]. Any part of a compound or a mixture; a unit of a more complex substance.

in'growing [L. *in*, into, + A.S. *grōwan*, to grow]. Growing inward.
    i. nail. One growing into the flesh. SYN: *onyxia.*

inguen (in'gwen) [L. groin]. The groin.

inguinal (in'gwi-nal) [L. *inguinalis*, pert. to the groin]. Pert. to the region of the groin.
    RS: *bubo, bubononcus, groin, hernia, hysterobubonocele.*
    i. canal. The one carrying the spermatic cord in the male, and the round ligament in the female. It is 1½ in. long; a potential source of weakness and may be the site of a hernia.
    i. glands. Those of the groin.
    i. hernia. Hernia in inguinal region.
    i. ligament. SYN: *Poupart's ligament.* A fibrous band extending from ant., sup., iliac spine to the pubic tubercle.
    i. reflex. One in females resembling cremasteric* reflex in males.
    i. region. The groin. The iliac region on either side of the pubes.
    i. ring. Int. opening of the i. canal (abdominal i. ring), and the end of the i. canal (subcutaneous i. ring).

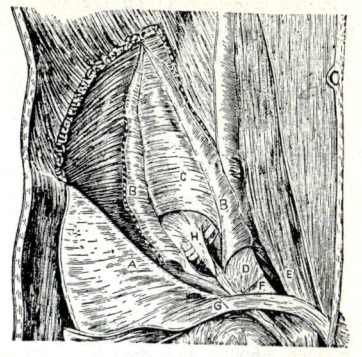

INGUINAL CANAL
A, External oblique muscle; B, internal oblique muscle; C, transversalis muscle; D, conjoined tendon; E, rectus abdominis with sheath opened; F, transversalis fascia; G, cremaster; H, infundibular fascia.

inguinodynia (in"guin-o-din-ĭ-ah). Pain in the groin or inguinal region.

inhal'ant [L. *in*, in + *halāre*, to breathe]. That which may be inhaled.

inhalation (in-ha-la'shun) [" + *halāre*, to breathe]. 1. Act of drawing in of breath, vapor, or gas into the lungs; inspiration. 2. Introduction of dry or moist air or vapor into the lungs for therapeutic purposes, such as *amyl nitrite* to relieve attack of angina pectoris, *aromatic spirits of ammonia* used to overcome fainting.
    SUBSTANCES INHALED: *Calomel:* The fumes from burning calomel are sometimes used for inhalation in syphilis of the throat.
    Oxygen to relieve depressed breathing.
    Steam inhalations are given to overcome spastic conditions of the larynx and bronchi, to soften mucus, to aid in absorption of oxygen, to reduce dryness of mucous membranes and to provide heat and moisture to the membranes of the lungs and appendages; also in croup.
    Stramonium to relieve spasmodic attacks of asthma.
    Stramonium leaves and *belladonna* are used for local effect, the fumes relaxing the involuntary muscles of the bronchial tubes. SEE: *anemopathy, steam tent.*

inhale' [" + *halāre*, to breathe]. To draw in the breath; to inspire.

inhaler (in-ha'ler) [" + *halāre*, to breathe]. Device for inhaling medicinal vapors or steam.

inhe'rent [" + *haerere*, to stick]. Intrinsic; belonging to anything naturally, originally, not as result of circumstances.
    i. cauterization. Deep cauterization.

inheritance. The sum total of all that is inherited; that which is the result of hereditary factors within the egg and sperm.
    i., blending. Type of i. in which characteristics of male and female parents appear to be blended in offspring. May result from lack of dominance or equal contributions of several pairs of multiple factors.
    i., cytoplas'mic. I. of traits due to self-duplicating mutable units present

inherited

in the cytoplasm of an egg such as plastids in plants.

inherited. Received from one's ancestors; not acquired.

inhibition (in-hĭb-ĭsh'ŭn) [L. *inhibitus,* from *inhibere,* to restrain]. 1. Act of repressing or state of being repressed; restraint. 2. PHYS: A stopping of an action or function of an organ. 3. PSY: Restraint of 1 mental process almost simultaneously by another opposed mental process; an inner impediment to free activity.

The best example of this important physiological phenomenon is the slowing or stopping of the heart which can be produced by electrical stimulation of the vagus.

i., psychic. Arrest of an impulse, thought, action, or speech. The term is commonly applied to the denial of the sex instinct. SYN: *suppression.*

inhib'itor [L. *inhibere,* to restrain]. That which inhibits. For example: A chemical substance which stops enzyme activity or a nerve which suppresses activity of an organ innervated by it.

inhibitory (in-hĭb'ĭ-to-ri) [L. *inhibere,* to restrain]. Restraining, preventing.

i. nerve. A nerve which carries impulses which act to slow down or inhibit action in the organ or tissue supplied by its fibers.

inhibitrope (in-hĭb'ĭ-trōp) [" + G. *tropē,* a turning]. One in whom certain stimuli cause partial arrest of function.

iniac, inial (in'ĭ-ak, -ăl) [G. *inion,* nape of neck]. Pert. to the inion.

inion (in'ĭ-on) [G. nape of neck]. 1. Occiput. 2. Back portion of neck. 3. External occipital protuberance.

initial (in-ish'al) [L. *initium,* beginning]. Incipient; rel. to the beginning, or commencing.

initis (in-ī'tĭs) [G. *ĭs, ĭn-,* fiber, + *ĭtis,* inflammation]. 1. Inflammation of fibrous tissue. 2. Inflammation of a tendon. 3. Inflamed condition of a muscle. SYN: *myositis.*

inject' [L. *injectus,* from *injicere,* to throw in]. To introduce fluid into the body or its parts artificially.

injec'ted [L. *injectus,* thrown in]. Filled by injection of fluid; congested.

injection (in-jeck'shun) [L. *injectus,* from *injicere,* to throw in]. 1. Forcing of a fluid into a vessel or cavity or under the skin. 2. Substance introduced in this manner. 3. State of being injected; congestion.

NP: Nurse should wash her hands first. Any substance injected must be sterile. Dosage must be exact. See that the needle is not loose. Cleanse site, after withdrawal of needle, with iodine or alcohol. All air must be expelled from the syringe before using.

RS: *aquapuncture, autoplasmotherapy, Casoni's reaction, cirsenchysis, douche, enema.*

i., air. Spinal i. of air to locate a growth, degree of central atrophy in general paresis, and to find cause of epilepsy.

i., colonic. Into the colon.

i., epidural. Spinal i. given to relieve pain in limbs in tabes dorsalis or tabes paresis and in gastric crisis.

i., hypodermic. A subcutaneous one, generally in front of thighs, or outer part of arms or forearms.

i., intracardial. Into the heart.

i., intracutaneous. Injections into the skin, a method employed in giving of serums and vaccines when a local reaction is desired.

i., intramuscular. Into intramuscular tissue, usually in front of thigh or in 1 of the buttocks.

i., intra''peritoneal. I. into the peritoneal cavity.

i., intravenous.* Into a vein.

i., lipiodol. Spinal i. to locate spinal cord block or tumor.

i., rectal. Into the rectum; an enema.

i., sclerosing. I. into a vessel or into a tissue of a substance which will bring about obliteration of the vessel or hardening of the tissues.

i. spinal. I. into the spinal canal.

i., subcutaneous. I. beneath the skin. SYN: *hypodermic i.*

i., vaginal. A douche.

inject'ors [L. *injicere,* to throw in]. Various instruments for injecting medicinal fluids, making hypodermic injections and for transfusion of blood and intravenous injection.

in'jury [L. *injuria,* a hurt or wrong]. A hurt or damage.

SYM: There may be progressive fall in blood pressure; subnormal temperature; shallow, rapid breathing; cold, clammy, pale skin constituting shock. There is disturbance of blood balance, exhaustion of adrenal glands, blood vessel dilatation and bleeding into capillaries, draining arteries and veins, decreasing return flow to the heart and inducing collapse.

TREATMENT: Avoid rough handling, the loss of fluids, body heat, and exposure of tissue in burns. Cover all wounded surfaces, apply heat and plenty of fluid if conscious, or, if shock is profound, fluids may be administered intravenously. Solutions of glucose are of great value. Blood transfusion may be necessary if there is hemorrhage. One to 2 pints of hot coffee or tea if patient is conscious. Hot water bottle against liver. In case of broken bones and laceration, stop hemorrhage, make comfortable, but do not move patient until physician arrives.

i., egg-white. I. resulting from biotin deficiency. It is produced in experimental animals by feeding raw egg white or its amtibiotin component, avidin.

i., steering wheel. I. following automobile accidents in which driver is thrown forward against steering wheel resulting in contusion of heart.

ink poisoning. Many of the poisonings ascribed to ink are in the form of dermatitis. Several types of materials may be responsible. Ordinary ink may cause irritation, either because of irritating nature, or because of susceptibility of particular skins. Sometimes cleaning materials used in removing ink stains have been found to be causative agents.

SYM: Redness, occasionally small pustules and cracking.

F. A. TREATMENT: Wash with alcohol, soap and water. Rinse carefully, apply a bland dressing, as calomel, cold cream, etc.

in'lay [L. *in,* in, + A.S. *lecgan,* to lie]. A solid filling made to the shape of a cavity of a tooth and cemented into it.

in'let [" + A.S. *lǣtan,* to let go]. Passage leading to a cavity.

i. of the pel'vis. The upper opening into the pelvic cavity.

innate [" + *natus,* born]. Inborn; inherent.

innervate (ĭn-nur'vāt) [" + *nervus,*

innervation (in-er-va'shun) [" + *nervus*, nerve]. 1. Stimulation of a part through the action of nerves. 2. The distribution and function of the nervous system. 3. The nerve supply of a part.

 i., collateral. Supply of nervous force through an adjacent nerve tract to a part of which original nerve supply has been injured or destroyed.

 i., double. I. of an organ with both sympathetic and parasympathetic fibers.

 i., reciprocal. I. of antagonistic muscles of a limb by which impulses of central origin which induce an action such as flexion bring about inhibition of the opposing extensors.

innidiation (in-nid-ī-a'shun) [" + *nidus*, nest]. Multiplication of cells in a part to which they have been carried by metastasis.

innocent (in'o-sent) [L. *in*, not, + *nocere*, to injure]. Benign; not malignant. SYN: *innocuous.*

innoc'uous [L. *innocuus*]. Harmless.

innominate (in-nom'ĭ-nāt) [L. *innominatus*, unnamed]. Nameless.

 i. artery. Right artery arising from the arch of the aorta, dividing into the right subclavian and right common carotid arteries.

 i. bone. *Os innominata.* The hip bone, composed of the *ilium, ischium*, and *pubis*; united to form the pelvis by the sacrum and coccyx.

 i. veins. Right and left vein, each formed by union of internal jugular with subclavian veins.

innoxious (in-ok'shus) [L. *in*, not, + *noxius*, harmful]. Not harmful.

inochondritis (in″o-kon-drī'tis) [" + *chondros*, cartilage, + *itis*, inflammation]. Inflammation of a fibrocartilage.

inochondroma (in″o-kon-dro'mă) [" + " + *ōma*, tumor]. A chondroma or tumor with much fibrous tissue; fibrochondroma.

inoculability (in-ok-u-lă-bil'ĭ-tī) [L. *inoculāre*, to engraft]. Quality of being susceptible to transmission of infection by inoculation.

inoc'ulable [L. *inoculāre*, to engraft]. 1. Transmissible by inoculation. 2. Susceptible to a transmissible disease. 3. Capable of being inoculated.

inoc'ulate [L. *inoculāre*, to engraft, from *in*, on, + *oculus*, bud]. To inject a pathologic microörganism or virus into the body.

inoculation (in-ok-u-la'shun) [L. *inoculāre*, to engraft]. Intentional introduction of a virus into the system as a preventive against the acquisition of certain diseases; it may be antidiphtheritic, antirabic, antitetanic or antityphoid.

 i., animal. The injection of pathogenic organisms into laboratory animals for the purpose of determining their presence, the virulence of the organisms, the action of drugs upon them, or to induce antibody formation.

inoc'ulum [L. *in*, on, + *oculus*, bud]. A substance or virus introduced by inoculation.

inocyst (in'o-sĭst) [G. *is, in-*, fiber, + *kystis*, a bladder]. A fibrous capsule.

inocystoma (in″o-sis-to'mă) [" + " + *ōma*, tumor]. Fibrous tumor undergoing cystic degeneration.

inoepithelioma (in″o-ep-ĭ-the-lĭ-o'mă) [" + *epi*, upon, + *thēlē*, nipple, + *ōma*, tumor]. Epithelioma containing fibrous tissue.

ino'genous [" + *gennan*, to produce]. Forming tissue or produced from it.

inohymenitis (in-o-hī-men-i'tis) [" + *ymēn*, membrane, + *itis*, inflammation]. Inflammation of any fibrous membrane or of an aponeurosis.

inoliomyoma (in″o-lī-o-mī-o'mă) [" + *leios*, smooth, + *mys, myo-*, muscle, + *ōma*, tumor]. A smooth muscle tissue tumor.

in'olith [" + *lithos*, stone]. A concretion formed from fibrous tissue.

inoma (in-o'mă) [" + *ōma*, tumor]. A fibrous tumor. SYN: *fibroma.*

inomyoma (in-o-mi-o'mă) [" + *mys, myo-*, muscle, + *ōma*, tumor]. A fibrous tissue myoma. SYN: *fibromyoma.*

inomyositis (in-o-mi-o-sī'tis) [" + " + *itis*, inflammation]. Chronic muscular inflammation with connective tissue hyperplasia. SYN: *fibromyositis.*

inomyxo'ma [" + *myxa*, mucus, + *ōma*, tumor]. A mixed myxoma and fibroma. SYN: *fibromyxoma.*

inoneuroma (in″o-nu-ro'mă) [" + *neuron*, nerve, + *ōma*, tumor]. A mixed neuroma and inoma. SYN: *fibroneuroma.*

inop'erable [L. *in*, not, + *operārī*, to work]. Unsuitable for being operated upon without danger of death.

inopex'ia [G. *is, in-*, fiber, + *pēxis*, fixation]. Tendency of the blood to spontaneous coagulation in the vessels.

inorgan'ic [L. *in*, not, + G. *organon*, an organ]. 1. In chemistry, occurring in nature independently of living things, substances not containing carbon. 2. Not pert. to living organisms.

 i. acid. An acid composed of inorganic constituents. SYN: *acid, mineral.*

 i. chemistry. C. dealing only with inorganic compounds.

 i. compound. One without carbon.

inosclerosis (in-o-skle-ro'sĭs) [G. *is, in-*, fiber, + *sklērōsis*, hardening]. Increased fibrous tissue density.

inos'copy [" + *skopein*, to examine]. Diagnosis by examining fibrinous deposits in body fluids.

inos'culating [L. *in*, in, + *osculum*, little mouth]. Directly communicating; anastomosing.

inosculation (in-os-ku-la'shun) [" + *osculum*, little mouth]. Union of two vessels; anastomosis.*

inosemia (īn-ō-sē'mĭ-ă) [G. *is, in-*, fiber, + *aima*, blood]. 1. An excessive amount of fibrin in the blood. 2. The presence of inositol in the blood.

inosin'ic acid [G. *is, in-*, fiber, + L. *acidus*, sour]. A mononucleotide present in muscular tissue which upon hydrolysis yields hypoxanthine and d-ribose-5-phosphoric acid.

inosite (in'o-sīt) [G. *is, in-*, muscle]. Inositol, *q.v.*

inositis (in-o-sī'tis) [G. *is, in-*, fiber, + *itis*, inflammation]. Inflammation of fibrous tissue.

inositol (in'o-sī'tol). SYN: *Inosite, Bios, I, mouse antialopecia factor, muscle sugar.* Hexahydroxycyclohexane, a sugar-like crystalline substance $(C_6H_6(OH)_6)$ found in the liver, kidney, skeletal and heart muscle; and also present in the leaves and seeds of most plants. It is a vitamin, deficiency of which in experimental animals results in loss of hair, eye defects, and retardation of growth.

inosituria (in″o-si-tu'rĭ-ă) [" + *ouron*, urine]. Inosite in the urine.

inosteotoma (in″os-te-ō-to'mă) [" + *stear, steat-*, fat, + *oma*, tumor]. Fatty tumor with fibroma.

inosuria (in-o-su'rĭ-ă) [G. *is, in-*, fiber, + *ouron*, urine]. Inosite in the urine. SYN: *inosituria*.

in'quest [L. *in*, into, + *quaerere*, to seek]. 1. A legal medical examination of a corpse to ascertain the cause of death. 2. The act of inquiring.

insaliva'tion [" + *saliva*, spittle]. The process of mixing saliva with food, as in chewing.

insalu'brious [L. *in*, not, + *saluber*, healthful]. Not healthy or contributing to health.

insane (in-sān') [" + *sanus*, sound]. Mentally deranged; pert. to insanity.

insan'itary [" + *sanus*, sound]. Not conducive to health; unhealthful, esp. pert. to filth.

insan'ity [L. *insanitās*]. Legal term for mental derangement; a psychosis. A general term for unsoundness of mind or any mental disorder or psychosis. In legal medicine, the state or mental condition characterized by (1) inability to distinguish between right and wrong; (2) possession of delusions or hallucinations which prevent an individual from looking after his own affairs with ordinary prudence or which render him a menace to others; (3) actions resulting from impulses of such intensity that they cannot be resisted.

The common law recognizes 4 forms: *lunacy, idiocy, accidental loss of understanding,* and *deprivation of understanding*. Only a few states permit divorce for insanity, and then the condition must have continued for a sufficient number of years to indicate incurability.

LUCID INTERVALS: An insane person during lucid intervals, may enter into a legal contract, a marriage, a business, buying and selling, providing at the time he or she is capable of entering into such matters with an understanding of all that is implied. The mental capacity *at the time* determines the validity of such acts and *not the condition before or after*.

RS: *paresis, phobia, psychosis, restraint*.

 i., affective. Affective psychosis, *q.v*.
 i., alcoholic. Alcoholic psychosis, *q.v*.
 i., alternating. Manic-depressive psychosis, *q.v*.
 i., choreic. I. accompanying Huntington's chorea.
 i., circular. Alternating i., *q.v*.
 i., climateric. Mental illness occurring during or near the time of the menopause.
 i., communicated. Folie a deux in which delusions of one person are transmitted to and accepted by a second person.
 i., compulsive. I. in which the actions of a person are the result of obsessions or impulses over which he has no control.
 i., cyclic. Circular or alternating insanity, *q.v*.
 i., delusional. I. in which delusions or hallucinations are characteristic.
 i., emotional. SEE: *psychosis, affective*.
 i., imitative. A form of folie a deux in which the insane actions of one are imitated by another.
 i., imposed. Folie a deux in which delusions and hallucinations of one are imposed on another with whom he is closely associated.
 i., impulsive. I. characterized by the commission of acts, usually of a violent nature, as a result of sudden uncontrollable impulses.
 i., induced. Communicated i., *q.v*.
 i., manic-depressive. Manic-depressive psychosis, *q.v*.
 i., moral. I. characterized by the commission of immoral acts although reasoning and intellectual processes are normal.
 i., senile. I. due to degenerative processes of old age.
 i., toxic. I. resulting from the effects of a poison, such as alcohol, opium, or other drugs.

insatiable (in-sā'shĭ-a-bl) [L. *insatiabilis*]. Incapable of being satisfied or appeased.

inscriptio (in-skrip'shyo) [L. a writing]. Inscription. [ing a muscle. BNA.
 i. tendin'ea. Tendinous band travers-

inscription (in-skrip'shun) [L. *in, upon,* + *scribere*, to write]. Body of a prescription which gives the names of the drugs prescribed and dosage.

in'sect [L. *insectum*]. Common name for any of the class *Insecta*, of the phylum *Arthropoda*. Insects of medical importance are flies, mosquitoes, lice, fleas, and the true bugs.
 i. bites and *stings*. In general, insects when they bite inject an acid substance resembling formic acid, consequently they may be relieved by alkalies, such as ammonia water, baking-soda paste, or even soap rubbed on the wound.
 Bees, wasps, and hornets when they sting inject an unknown organic substance for which there is no specific antidote. If a "stinger" is found in the wound it should be removed.

insect, words pert. to: "acar-" words, bedbug, bee stings, bites, chiggers, foreign bodies, hornet, jiggers, pediculosis, phthiriasis, tularemia, vermin, wasp.

insecta. SYN: *Hexapoda*. A class of the phylum *Arthropoda* characterized by three distinct body divisions (head, thorax, abdomen), three pairs of jointed legs, trachea, and usually two pairs of wings. Insects are of medical significance in that some are parasitic, some serve as carriers or vectors of pathogenic organisms, and some are annoying pests causing injury by their bites or their stings.

insecticide (in-sek'tĭ-sĭd) [L. *insectum*, insect, + *caedere*, to kill]. 1. An agent used to exterminate insects. 2. Destructive to insects.

insemination (in-sem-in-a'shun) [L. *in*, into, + *semen*, seed]. 1. Discharge of semen from the penis into the vagina during coitus. 2. Fertilization of an ovum.
 i., artificial. Artificial injection of semen into the uterine canal. Sometimes resorted to in sterility of the husband. Legal complications as to heritage and inheritance may arise and psychological results may be disastrous to all concerned. SEE: *impregnation*.

insen'sible [L. *in*, not, + *sensibilis*, sensible]. 1. Unconscious; without feeling or consciousness. 2. Not perceptible.

inser'tion [L. *in*, into, + *serere*, to plant]. 1. The manner or place of attachment of a muscle to the bone that it moves. 2. A putting into.
 i., velamentous. Attachment of the umbilical cord to the edge of the placenta.

insheathed. Enclosed, as by a sheath or capsule; encysted.

insidious (in-sĭd'ĭ-us) [L. *insidiōsus*, cunning]. Stealthy, treacherous, hidden; not apparent, as a disease that does not exhibit early symptoms of its advent.

in'sight. PSY: Understanding of oneself or of any nervous or mental difficulties one may have.

insipid. Without taste; lacking in spirit or animation.
in si′tu [L.]. In position.
insolation (in-so-la′shun) [L. *insolāre*, to place in the sun]. 1. Any exposure to the rays of the sun. 2. Heat- or sunstroke.
   EXPOSURE: Not more than twice a day and not more than five minutes at a time to begin with and never more than 90 minutes. Temperature, pulse, blood and urine should be observed after each treatment in those who are sick.
   Dermatitis is always a danger even to the well. The public needs to be warned against undue exposure to the sun's rays which may result as dangerously as any other burn. SEE: *heat, heat exhaustion, heat stroke, heat therapy.*
insoluble (in-sol′u-bl) [L. *in*, not, + *solvere*, to dissolve]. Incapable of solution or of being dissolved.
insomnia (in-som′nĭ-ă) [" + *somnus*, sleep]. Chronic inability to sleep, or sleep prematurely ended or interrupted by periods of wakefulness.
   ETIOL: Heavy late meal; with some coffee and other stimulants, including sugar in any form; overtiredness, mental fatigue, worry, excitement and principally the fear of being unable to sleep.
   NP & TREATMENT: Remove exciting cause. Train the mind in self-control, remove fear of lack of sleep. Do not try to sleep if too wakeful. Sit up and read until tired. Hot foot bath, drink of hot water or milk before retiring. Small amount of plain food before retiring permitted.
   Change of occupation if necessary and possible. Physical exercise during day, and a walk in fresh air at night after dinner. Cold wet cloths about wrists. Constitutional treatment. No mental work after dinner. Those complaining about insomnia generally secure more sleep than they realize. Some require much less sleep than others. Inability to sleep continuously through the night is not a pathological condition. SEE: *agrypnotic, anhypnosis, anthypnotic, sleep, somnambulism, vigil.*
inspect′ [L. *inspectus;* from *inspicere*, to examine]. To examine visually.
inspec′tion [L. *inspectus;* from *inspicere*, to examine]. The ocular examination of the external surface of the body. SEE: *abdominal, chest, and circulatory system.*
inspersion (in-sper′shun) [L. *in*, upon, + *spersus;* fr. *spargere*, to sprinkle]. Sprinkling with powder or a fluid.
inspiration (in-spir-a′shun) [L. *in*, in, + *spirāre*, to breathe]. Inhalation; drawing air into the lungs. Opp. of *expiration, q.v.*
   Inspiration may be costal or abdominal, the latter being deeper. The breaking point reached in from 23-77 seconds, is the limit of ability to hold the breath.
   RATE: 16-18 respirations per minute in an adult. SEE: *respiration.*
   MUSCLES OF: Ext. intercostals, diaphragm, levatores costarum, pectoralis minor, scaleni, serratus post., sup., sternocleidomastoid.
   RS: *air, apnea, asphyxia, breathing, Cheyne-Stokes respiration, dyspnea, hyperpnea, lungs, respiration, ventilation.*
   i., crowing. Peculiar noise in laryngismus stridulus* or spasmodic croup.*
   i., external. Interchange of gases in the lungs.
   i., forcible, difficult, labored. I. in which the muscles of i. are assisted by inspiratory auxiliaries (*i. e.*, muscles attached to chest which by contraction increase the thoracic cavity directly or indirectly by furnishing fixed support whereby other muscles may act more advantageously). If movements become excessively labored, there is brought into coördinate action every muscle in the body which can either directly or indirectly increase the cavity of the thorax.
   i., full. I. in which lungs are filled as completely as possible (voluntarily, as in determining the amount of complemental air, or involuntarily, as in cardiac dyspnea).
   i., internal. Interchange of gases in the tissues.
inspiratory (in-spi′ră-tor-ĭ) [" + *spirāre*, to breathe]. Pert. to inspiration.
inspissate (in-spis′āt) [" + *spissāre*, to thicken]. To thicken by evaporation or absorption of fluid.
inspissated (in′spis-sā-ted) [" + *spissāre*, to thicken]. Thickened by absorption, evaporation or dehydration.
inspissation (in-spis-sa′shun) [" + *spissāre*, to thicken]. 1. Thickening by evaporation or absorption of fluid. 2. Diminished fluidity or increased thickness.
in′step [origin uncertain]. Arch on upper surface of foot in the middle, in front of ankle.
instillation (in-stil-a′shun) [L. *in*, into, + *stillāre*, to drop]. Pouring in a liquid, drop by drop.
in″stillator. An apparatus for introducing, drop by drop, liquids into a cavity.
instinct (in′stinkt) [L. *instinctus*, impulse]. 1. Inherent (racial) patterns of expression normally manifested under suitable conditions, usually heavily loaded with emotional value (libido in its widest sense). Innate urges, principally voluntary, with which one is born and which are necessary for the preservation of life. An innate, complex, coordinated, behavior pattern characteristic of a race or species and usually having an adaptive value. 2. An urge, uncontrolled by reason, to react to stimuli of an emotional nature.
   The term is often misapplied to *intuition*. Some only recognize: 1. *Self-preservation.* 2. *Sex.* 3. *Herd instinct.* Others include: 4. *Flight* or *fear.* 5. *Repulsion.* 6. *Curiosity.* 7. *Pugnacity.* 8. *Self-assertion.* 9. *Self-abasement.* 10. *Parental i.* 11. *Reproduction.* 12. *Acquisitiveness.* 13. *Construction.* Undoubtedly some of these are acquired characteristics. Fisk says the "mother instinct" is only an acquired characteristic.
instinct′ive [L. *instinctus*, impulse]. Determined by instinct.
instrument (in′stru-ment) [L. *instrumentum*, tool]. A tool or piece of apparatus.
instrumental (in-stru-men′tal) [L. *instrumentum*, tool]. 1. Pert. to instruments. 2. Being the cause of anything.
   i. delivery. Delivery of a fetus with forceps.
instrumenta′tion [L. *instrumentum*, tool]. The use of instruments, and their care.
instruments, care and sharpening of. After operation collect, count and unlock instruments. Cleanse by rinsing with warm water to remove blood, and again with hot water and potash soap, place under hot water faucet and allow boiling water to run on them, dry at once with gauze.
   To remove rust use cleanser sparingly, else surface of instrument will be injured in course of time.
   Reliable sterilization of instruments before an operation can always be assured by boiling in a 1% solution of carbonate of soda for 15 minutes. Car-

bonate of soda prevents rusting of the instruments. The dipping of an instrument into alcohol or even pure carbolic acid cannot be relied upon for making it surgically clean.

SHARPENING: *Washita stone* is best for dull instruments as it cuts away the metal faster. Arkansas stone is better for finishing. Glycerin is best lubricant. Entire edge of knife should be covered in one sweep. Hold knife at angle of 30°. All knives should be honed before used. Blunt instruments should be kept highly polished. Rub with fine emery paper and polish with rouge and chamois skin or gauze. Do not use emery paper on saws. Sharpen with three-cornered files. Silver instruments should not come in contact with rubber, or be exposed to atmosphere. Wrap in dry gauze.

insufficiency (in-suf-fish'en-sĭ) [L. *in*, not, + *sufficiens*, sufficient]. The condition of being inadequate for its purpose.
 i., **aortic.** An imperfect closure of the aortic valves.
 i., **cardiac.** Inability of heart to function normally.
 i., **gastric.** Inability of the stomach to empty itself.   [function properly.
 i., **hepatic.** Inability of the liver to
 i., **mitral.** In which the mitral valve inefficiently closes with rhythmic action of the heart.
 i., **muscular.** Condition in which a muscle is unable to exert its normal force and bring about normal movement of the part to which it is attached. Term applied esp. to eye muscles.
 i. **of the ocular muscles.** Absence of dynamic equilibrium of ocular muscles.
 i., **renal.** Inability of the kidney to remove waste products from the blood at the normal rate.
 i., **valvular.** Imperfect cardiac valve closure, permitting leakage of blood.

insuf'flate [L. *insufflāre*, to blow into]. 1. To blow in, as in the lungs of a newborn infant. 2. To blow a medicated powder or medicinal vapor into a cavity.

insuffla'tion [L. *insufflāre*, to blow into]. The act of blowing a vapor or powder into a cavity, as the lungs.

insufflator (in'suf-fla-tor) [L. *insufflāre*, to blow into]. Device for blowing powders into a cavity.

in'sula [L. island]. 1. The central lobe (island of Reil) of the cerebral hemisphere. It is a triangular area of the cerebral cortex lying in the floor of the lateral fissure. 2. Any round cutaneous body or patch.

insular (ins'u-lar) [L. *insula*, island]. Rel. to any insula.

insula'tion [L. *insulāre*, to make into an island]. 1. The protection of a body or substance with a nonconducting medium so as to prevent the transfer of electricity, heat, or sound. 2. The material or substance which insulates.
 The electrical resistance of an insulator is expressed in megohms, a unit representing a million ohms.

in'sulator (L. *insulāre*, to make into an island]. That which insulates; specifically, a substance or body that interrupts the transmission of electricity to surrounding objects by conduction; anything that exerts great resistance to the passage of an electric current by conduction. SEE: *nonconductor*.

in'sulin [L. *insula*, island]. 1. A hormone secreted by the beta cells of the islets of Langerhans of the pancreas. Called the *antidiabetic hormone*. It can be readily crystallized as a zinc salt although nickel, calcium, and cobalt also are effective. It is a protein with a maximum molecular weight of 48,000. Insulin is essential for the proper oxidation and utilization of blood sugar (glucose) and for maintenance of the proper blood sugar level. Inadequate secretion of insulin results in improper metabolism of carbohydrates and fats and brings on diabetes characterized by hyperglycemia and glycosuria. Insulin when injected into a diabetic produces the following effects: normal storage of glycogen in the liver and muscle tissue; reduction in blood sugar level; disappearance of ketosis and hyperlipemia; prevention of excessive breakdown of protein; increase in respiratory quotient; and increase in resistance to infective diseases. The secretion of insulin is primarily dependent upon the concentration of blood glucose, an increase of blood sugar bringing about an increase in the secretion of insulin.
 First discovered and used successfully by Sir F. G. Banting in diabetes. Not a cure, and not necessary in every case. Makes possible a greater metabolism of carbohydrates without evidence of glycosuria. Prepared from animal pancreas.
 DOSAGE: Should always be expressed in units rather than in cubic centimeters or minims. There is no average dose of insulin for diabetics; each case must be studied individually. The dose depends upon the amount of dextrose in such a diet as the patient is unable to metabolize; *i. e.*, the total dextrose minus the dextrose excretion. A convenient formula is:

Average grams of d-glucose excreted
―――――――――――――――――――――――――――――――――― =
                  1.5

sufficient units of insulin to render most patients aglycosuric. In general, it is advisable to keep the volume per injection at from ½–¾ cc., choosing the strength which will give the required number of units in this volume or less.
 ADM: The long-acting (depot) insulins are usually taken in a single dose for the 24 hours before breakfast subcutaneously. The older, short-acting insulins are usually reserved for emergencies (diabetic coma) and for those rare individuals who cannot tolerate the depot type.
 i., **amorphous.** I. to which zinc or other metallic ions have not been added.
 i., **crystalline.** I. which has been precipitated in the presence of zinc or other metallic ions.
 i., **depot.** Insulin that is absorbed slowly from the site of injection.
 i., **globin.** I. combined with globin from blood. It forms a clear solution producing effects longer than those of regular insulin but shorter than those of protamine insulin.
 i., **hexamine.** I. combined with hexamethylene tetramine.
 i. **histone.** Insulin to which has been added the simple protein histone derived from the thymus.
 i. **histone zinc.** Histone insulin to which zinc has been added. The hypoglycemic effect is more prompt, though prolonged, than with protamine zinc insulin. It makes possible a continuously normal blood sugar level and freedom from glycosuria in many.
 i., **NPH.** Abbr. for *neutral-protamine-Hagedorn*, a mixture containing 0.5 mg. of protamine to each 100 units of insulin. Quick-acting, with effects of long duration.

i., protamine. I. combined with protamine, a simple protein derived from the spermatozoa of fishes.

i., protamine zinc. A preparation of insulin, modified by the addition of protamine and a zinc salt.

USES: Same as for unmodified insulin, but has a more prolonged action; its administration is usually but once a day.

i., protamine zinc, clear (soluble). A water-clear preparation with more protamine zinc and glycerin than that present in p. z. insulin.

i. shock. Condition resulting from an overdose of insulin resulting in reduction of blood sugar level below normal (hypoglycemia).

SYM: Excessive hunger, thirst, and nervousness, fear and excitability. Rapid pulse, flushing, pallor and sweating, fainting, convulsions, coma.

TREATMENT: Eating sugar or candy, orange juice, glucose, other carbohydrates and injections of glucose into the blood if patient is unconscious. Adrenalin is of great though transient value.

i. shock therapy. The treatment of schizophrenia and other mental disorders by the injection of insulin. Sufficient insulin is injected to produce unconsciousness, the dosage being carefully regulated during course of treatment. When a deep coma is reached, the patient is brought out of the comatose condition by the administration of glucose followed by a meal rich in carbohydrates.

It is a dangerous procedure with a relatively high mortality and should be employed only by those who are fully equipped, fully qualified, and thoroughly familiar with all aspects of this method. It is essential to have available at all times suitable solutions of dextrose for interrupting the hypoglycemic state which is artificially created.

i. tannate. A combination of insulin with tannic acid.

i. tolerance. The degree to which the body responds to the injection of insulin.

insulinemia (in-su-lin-e'mĭ-ă) [" + G. *aima*, blood]. An undue amt. of insulin in the blood.

insulinogenic (in-su-lin-o-jen'ik) [" + G. *gennan*, to produce]. Caused by hyperinsulinism.

insulinoid (in'su-lin-oid) [" + G. *eidos*, resemblance]. Resembling or having the properties of insulin.

insulogenic (in-su-lo-jen'ik) [" + G. *gennan*, to produce]. Produced by overproduction or overadministration of insulin. SYN: *insulinogenic*.

insulo'ma [" + G. *ōma*, tumor]. A tumor of the island of Reil or of the islands of Langerhans.

insulopath'ic [" + G. *pathos*, disease]. Rel. to or caused by abnormal insulin secretion.

insusceptibility (in"sus-sep"tĭ-bil'ĭ-tĭ) [L. *in*, not, + *susceptus*, undertaken]. Incapability of becoming infected with a germ disease. SYN: *immunity*.

integration (in-te-gra'shun) [L. *integrāre*, to make whole]. 1. Assimilation. 2. A harmonious relationship of the parts constituting the whole of anything.

i., primary. Early recognition of the body and its psyche as apart from one's environment.

i., secondary. The process involved in developing the adult personality, through sublimation of the sex instinct and its components.

integrator (in'te-gra-tor) [L. *integrāre*, to make whole]. Device for measuring body surfaces.

integument (in-teg'u-ment) [L. *integumentum*, a covering]. 1. A covering. 2. The skin, consisting of the *corium* or *dermis*, and *epidermis*.

integumentary (in-teg-ū-men'tă-rĭ) [L. *integumentum*, a covering]. Rel. to the integument. SYN: *cutaneous, dermal*.

in'tellect [L. *intellectus*; from *intelligere*, to understand]. The mind, or understanding; conscious brain function.

intellec'tual [L. *intellectus*; from *intelligere*, to understand]. 1. Pert. to the mind. 2. Possessing intellect.

intel'ligence [L. *intelligere*, to understand]. The capacity to comprehend relationships. The ability to think; the ability to solve problems and to adjust to new situations.

There must be no emotional distortion. If intelligence-testing is to be accurate, a series of graded questions must be asked; the further one can go in answering them correctly, the greater is supposed to be one's intelligence.

i. quotient (IQ). An index of mental age or intelligence determined through the subject's answers to arbitrarily chosen questions, obtained by dividing the mental age by the chronological age and multiplying by 100. After the age of 15, IQ is merely a standard score which places an individual in reference to the scores of others within his age group.

IQ	Classification
Above 140	"Near" genius or genius.
120-140	Very superior intelligence.
110-120	Superior intelligence.
90-110	Normal, or average, intelligence.
80-90	Dullness.
70-80	Very dull, deficiency, dullness.
Below 70	Definite feeblemindedness.

i. test. A test designed to determine the intelligence of an individual. A number of tests have been devised including the Binet t., Babcock-Levy t., Stanford-Binet t., and others. Tests are used as a basis for determining intelligence quotient (IQ), *q.v.*

intem'perance [L. *in*, not, + *temporāre*, to moderate]. Excess in the use of anything; lack of moderation.

inten'sifying [L. *intensus*, intense, + *facere*, to make]. Making intense.

i. screen. A thin sheet of celluloid or other substance coated with a finely divided substance which fluoresces under the influence of roentgen rays and is intended to be used in close contact with the emulsion of a photographic plate or film for the purpose of reinforcing the image. A fluorescent screen.

inten'simeter [" + G. *metron*, measure]. An instrument, often a selenium cell or ionization chamber, designed to measure the intensity of a beam to about 14,000 Angström units.

intensity (in-ten'sĭ-tĭ) [L. *intensus*, tight, intense]. 1. The degree or extent of activity, strength, force, electric current, etc. 2. The state or quality of being intense.

i. of roentgen rays. The attribute of a beam of roentgen rays which determines the rate of ionization of air at a given point, under the conditions stipulated in the definition of roentgen. It is

expressed in roentgens per unit of time. SEE: *rays.*
intensive (in-ten'siv) [L. *intensus,* intense]. Rel. to or marked by intensity.
intention (in-těn'shŭn) [L. *intensiō,* a stretching]. 1. A natural process of healing. 2. Goal or purpose.
  i., first. Healing without granulation or suppuration.
  i., second. Healing by adhesion of two granulated surfaces with suppuration.
  i., third. Healing of an ulcer, wound, or cavity by filling by granulation and followed by cicatrization. SEE: *first i., granulation, resolution, second i., third i.*
  i. tremor. One exhibited or intensified when attempting coördinated movements.
inter- [L.]. Prefix: In the midst, between.
interartic'ular [L. *inter,* between, + *articulus,* joint]. 1. Bet. two joints. 2. Situated bet. two articulating surfaces.
interatrial (ĭn"ter-āt'rĭ-ăl) [" + *atrium,* hall]. Located bet. the atria of the heart. SYN: *interauricular.*
interauricular (ĭn"ter-aw-rĭk'u-lar) [" + *auricula,* auricle]. 1. Situated bet. the auricles or pinnae. 2. Interatrial.
in'terbrain [" + A. S. *braegan,* brain]. The hinder original part of the forebrain including the *thalamus,* pineal body (*epithalamus*) and geniculate bodies (*metathalamus*). SYN: *diencephalon, thalamencephalon.*
intercadence (ĭn-ter-kā'dens) [" + *cadere,* to fall]. A supernumerary pulse wave bet. two regular beats.
intercalary (ĭn-ter'kal-a-rĭ) [" + *calāre,* to call]. 1. Inserted between as something in addition; extraneous. 2. Pert. to an upstroke on a pulse tracing which comes bet. two pulse beats, intercalated.

intercalated (ĭn-ter'kal-at-ed) [L. *inter,* between, + *calāre,* to call]. 1. Inserted between as something in addition; extraneous. 2. Pert. to an upstroke on a pulse tracing which comes between two pulse beats, intercalary.
  i. disks. SEE: *disk, intercalated.*
  i. ducts. Short, narrow ducts which lie between secretory ducts and the terminal alveoli in the parotid and submaxillary glands and the pancreas.
intercarot'ic [" + G. *karoun,* to stupefy]. Bet. the ext. and int. carotid arteries.
in"tercartilag'inous [" + *cartilāgō,* cartilage]. Connecting or bet. cartilages.
intercellular (ĭn-ter-sel'u-lar) [" + *cellula,* little cell]. Bet. the cells of a structure.
interchondral (ĭn-ter-kon'dral) [" + G. *chondros,* cartilage]. Bet. cartilages. SYN: *intercartilaginous.*
intercilium (ĭn-ter-sil'ĭ-um) [" + *cilium,* eyelid]. The space bet. the eyebrows. SYN: *glabella.*
interclavic'ular [" + *clavicula,* little key]. Bet. the clavicles.
intercolumnar (ĭn-ter-kŏ-lum'nar) [" + *columna,* column]. Bet. columns.
  i. fascia. A membrane bet. pillars of the abdominal ring, enclosing the spermatic cord.
  i. fibers. Intercrural fibers.
intercon'dylar, intercon'dyloid, intercon'dylous [" + G. *kondylos,* condyle]. Bet. two condyles (the rounded eminence at the articular end of a bone).
intercos'tal [" + *costa,* rib]. Bet. the ribs.
  i. muscles, external. Outer layer of muscles between the ribs, originating on the lower margin of each rib, being

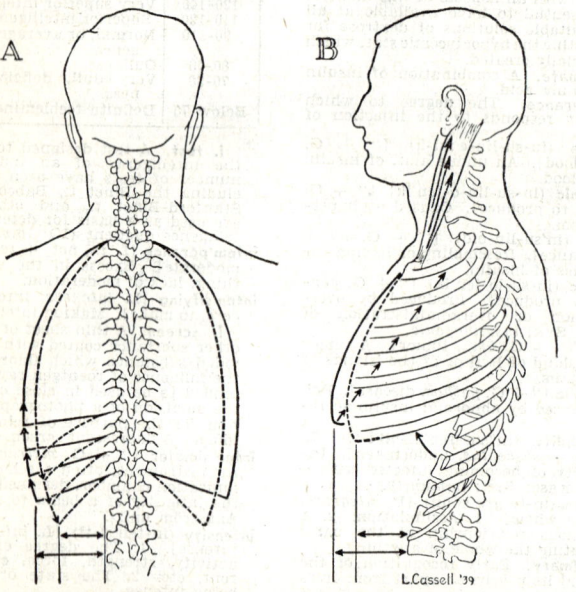

CHANGES IN SIZE OF THORAX DURING INSPIRATION
A. Back view. The contraction of the external intercostal muscles raises the ribs, makes them flare laterally, and so increases the transverse diameter of the thorax.
B. Side view. The contraction of the sternocleidomastoid muscle aids the external intercostals in raising the ribs, and so increases the anteroposterior diameter of the thorax. (Highly schematic.)

intercostal muscles, internal   I-29   **international x-ray unit**

inserted on the upper margin of the next rib. They elevate the ribs, enlarging the thorax thus functioning in inspiration. SEE: Fig. p. I-28.
   i. muscles, internal. Those bet. the ribs lying beneath the external intercostals; function uncertain.

intercos″tohumera′lis [" + " + *humerus*, shoulder]. 1. The post. lateral branch of second intercostal nerve supplying the skin of the arm. 2. Similar branch of the third intercostal nerve.

in′tercourse [" + *cursus*; from *currere*, to run]. 1. Social contacts. 2. The sexual act. SYN: *coition, coitus, copulation.*

intercris′tal [" + *crista*, crest]. Bet. two crests of a bone, organ, or process.

intercrural (in″ter-kru′răl) [L. *inter*, between, + *crus, crur-*, limb]. Bet. two crura.

intercur′rent [" + *currere*, to run]. 1. Intervening. 2. Pert. to a disease attacking a patient with another malady.

intercusp′ing. The fitting together of the surfaces of opposing teeth.

interden′tal [" + *dens, dent-*, tooth]. Bet. the teeth.

interdentium (in-ter-den′shĭ-um) [" + *dens, dent-*, tooth]. The space bet. any two contiguous teeth.

interdigita′tion [" + *digitus*, fingers]. 1. Interlocking of toothed or fingerlike processes. 2. Processes so interlocked.

interfascic′ular (in-ter-fas-ik′u-lar) [" + *fasciculus*, bundle]. Bet. fasciculi.

interfem′oral (in-ter-fem′or-ăl) [" + *femoralis*, pert. to the thigh]. Bet. the thighs.

interference. Clashing or colliding.
   i. of impulses. Condition in which two excitation waves, upon approaching each other and meeting in any part of the heart, are mutually extinguished.

interfib′rillar, interfib′rillary [" + *fibrilla*, a small fiber]. Bet. fibrils.

interfi′lar [" + *filum*, thread]. Bet. the fibrils of a reticulum.

interganglion′ic [" + *gagglion*, a swelling]. Bet. ganglions.

interglob′ular [" + *globulus*, globule]. Bet. [globules.
   i. spaces. Gaps in dentin due to failure of calcification. SYN: *Czermak's spaces.*

interlo′bar [" + *lobus*, lobe]. Bet. lobes.

interlobi′tis [" + " + G. *-itis*, inflammation]. Inflammation of the pleura separating the pulmonary lobes.

interlob′ular [" + *lobulus*, lobule]. Bet. lobules of an organ.   [the lung.
   i. emphysema. Air bet. the lobes of

intermar′riage [" + *maritāre*, to marry]. 1. Marriage bet. persons of two different races or tribes. SYN: *miscegenation.* 2. Marriage bet. blood relations.

intermax′illary [L. *inter*, between, + *maxilla*, jaw]. Between two maxillae.

intermediary (in-ter-me′dĭ-ă-rĭ) [" + *mediāre*, to divide]. 1. Situated bet. two bodies. 2. Occurring bet. two periods of time.
   i. amputation. One performed during the stage of inflammatory fever.
   i. body. An amboceptor; an immune body. SEE: *Ehrlich's side-chain theory.*
   i. metabolism. The series of intermediate compounds formed during digestion before the final excretion or oxidation products are eliminated from the body.

intermedin (in-ter-me′din) [" + *mediāre*, to divide]. A pituitary hormone from pars intermedia of hypophysis. It is of little significance in humans; in lower forms it acts on chromatophores (pigment cells).

intermediolat′eral [" + " + *latus, later-*, side]. Intermediate but not central.
   i. tract of spinal cord. A lateral tract bet. the dorsal and ventral horns.

intermeningeal (in-ter-men-in′je-ăl) [" + *mēnigx*, membrane]. Bet. the meninges.

intermenstrual. Between the menses, or menstrual periods.

intermis′sion [" + *missus*; from *mittere*, to send]. 1. Interval bet. two paroxysms of a disease. 2. Temporary cessation of symptoms.

intermit′tence [" + *mittere*, to send]. 1. Condition marked by intermissions in the course of a disease or of a process. 2. A loss of one or more pulse beats.

intermittent (in-ter-mit′ent) [" + *mittere*, to send]. Ceasing at intervals.
   i. fever. One in which there is complete absence of symptoms bet. paroxysms of the fever. SEE: *malaria, undulant fever, remittent fever for Illus.*
   i. pulse. One in which a beat is dropped at intervals; significant of cardiac exhaustion; serious in pneumonia.
   i. temperature. One that reaches the normal line at intervals during the course of a fever.

intermus′cular [" + *musculus*, muscle]. Bet. muscles.

intern (in′tern) [L. *internus*, within]. An assistant resident physician or surgeon on a hospital staff, usually a recent graduate. Cf. *externe.*

inter′nal [L. *internus*, within]. Within the body. Within or on the inside; enclosed, inward. Opp. of external.
   i. bleeding. Internal hemorrhage, q.v.
   i. capsule. SEE: *capsule, brain (internal of).*
   i. ear. The vestibule, semicircular canals, and cochlea.
   i. injury. Any injury not visible from the outside, as injury to the organs occupying the thoracic, abdominal, or cranial cavities.
   SYM: Vary with structures involved. Ordinarily, profound shock, patient is pale, cold, perspiring freely with an anxious expression; may be semicomatose. Pain usually intense at first, and may continue, or gradually diminish as patient grows worse.
   In severe injuries, pain may not be manifested. The pulse is very feeble, fast, often irregular. Patient may be very restless, breathless, and usually has shallow respiration.
   F. A. TREATMENT: Above all, patient should be kept very quiet and warm. Do not give anything by mouth, and do not give stimulants, as they may exaggerate bleeding. Transportation must be done very cautiously. Patient's head and shoulders should be lowered and extremities elevated at least 45°. This may be done by placing patient on a chair, box, or a folded coat. Massage and a firm bandage of the extremities may be helpful in maintaining circulation. Most of these patients require operation.
   i. medicine. Medicine as opposed to surgery.
   i. secretion. That of the ductless glands which, entering the blood stream, activates other glands and organs. SYN: *hormones*, q.v.
   SEE: *secretion, ductless gland, endocrine.*

international unit. One defined and adopted by the International Conference for Unification of Formulae.

international x-ray unit of intensity. Quantity of x-radiation, which, when secondary electrons are fully utilized and wall

interne   I-30   **interval, presphygmic**

effect of chamber is avoided, produces in 1 cc. of atmospheric air at 0.0° C. and 76 cm. mercury pressure, such a degree of conductivity that one electrostatic unit of charge is measured at saturation current. Designated by r.

interne (in'tern) [L. *internus*, within]. An assistant resident physician or surgeon on a hospital staff, usually a recent graduate. SYN: *intern*. SEE: *externe*.

intern'ist [L. *internus*, within]. One who treats internal diseases; not a surgeon.

in'ternode [L. *inter*, between, + *nodus*, node]. Space bet. adjacent nodes.

internun'cial [" + *nuncius*, messenger]. Acting as a connecting medium.
   i. neuron. One between two other neurons in a neural pathway.

interocep'tive [L. *inter*, within, + *ceptus;* from *capere*, to take]. In nerve physiology, concerned with sensations arising within the body itself, as distinguished from those (as, for instance, sight) arising outside the body.

interoceptor (in"ter-o-sep'tor) [" + *ceptus;* from *capere*, to take]. A receptor activated by stimuli within the body.
   i., general. An end organ carrying sensations of hunger, thirst, visceral pain, nausea, sexual and circulatory sensations.
   i., special. One for smell and taste.

interofec'tive [" + *affectus;* from *afficere*, to influence]. 1. Pert. to that which concerns the interior of an organism. 2. Cannon's term concerning the autonomic nervous system.

in"tero-infe'rior. Pert. to an inward and downward position.

interol'ivary [L. *inter*, between, + *oliva*, olive]. Bet. the olivary bodies.

interor'bital [" + *orbita*, orbit]. Bet. the orbits.

interos'seous [" + *os*, bone]. Situated or occurring bet. bones, as some muscles and ligaments.

interpalpebral (in-ter-pal'pe-bral) [" + *palpebra*, eyelid]. Bet. the eyelids.

interpari'etal [" + *paries, pariet-*, wall]. 1. Bet. walls. 2. Bet. the parietal bones. 3. Bet. the parietal lobes of the cerebrum.
   i. bone. SYN: *inca bone; incarial bone.*
   i. suture. Sagittal suture.

interparoxys'mal [" + G. *paroxysmos*, spasm]. Bet. paroxysms.

interpeduncular (in"ter-pe-dunk'u-lar) [" + *pedunculus*, peduncle]. Bet. peduncles.

interphalangeal (in"ter-fă-lan'jē-ăl) [" + *phalagx*, phalanx]. In a joint bet. two phalanges.

interpolar (in"ter-po'lar) [" + *polus*, pole]. Bet. two poles.
   i. path. Path of galvanic current through tissues bet. poles.

interprox'imal [" + *proximus*, next]. Bet. two adjoining surfaces.
   i. space. Triangular space bet. two adjacent teeth.

interpu'bic [" + *pubes*, pubes]. Bet. the pubic bones.

interpu'pillary [" + *pupula*, pupil]. Bet. the pupils.
   i. distance. Distance between centers of the two pupils of the eyes.

interre'nal [" + *rēn*, kidney]. Bet. the kidneys.

interrupt'er [" + *ruptus*, broken]. A mechanical or electrolytic device for making and breaking (closing and opening alternately) an electrical circuit. Such a device is ordinarily employed in low voltage, direct current circuits.

interscapil'ium [" + *scapula*, shoulder blade]. Area bet. the shoulders or scapulae.

interscap'ular [" + *scapula*, shoulder blade]. Bet. the scapulae.
   i. reflex. Scapular muscular contraction following percussion or stimulus bet. the scapulae.

intersca'pulum [" + *scapula*, shoulder blade]. Section of back bet. shoulder blades. SYN: *interscapilium*.

intersex. An individual having both male and female characteristics; a sex intergrade.

inter'stice [L. *interstitium*, a thing standing bet.]. A space or gap in a tissue or structure of an organ.

interstitial (in-ter-stish'al) [L. *interstitium*, thing standing bet.]. 1. Placed or lying bet.; pert. to interstices or spaces. 2. Occupying space bet. essential parts of an organ which comprises its proper tissue; opp. to *parenchymatous*.
   i. cells of testes. Cells of Leydig, located in groups between the seminiferous tubules. They produce the internal secretion (testosterone) of the testes.

intersystole (in-ter-sis'to-le) [L. *inter*, bet., + G. *systolē*, contraction]. The period bet. the end of the auricular systole and the commencement of the ventricular systole.

intertrigo (in-ter-tri'go) [" + *tritum;* from *terere*, to rub]. A superficial dermatitis in the folds of the skin. SEE: *erythema intertrigo*. SYN: *paratrimma*.

intertrochanteric (in"ter-tro-kăn-ter'ik) [" + G. *trochantēr*, runner]. Bet. the femur's two trochanters.
   i. line. The ridge bet. the greater and lesser trochanters of femur on post. aspect of the bone.

intertubular (in-ter-tu'bu-lar) [" + *tubulus*, tubule]. Bet. or among tubules.

interureteral (in"ter-u-re'ter-al) [" + G. *ourētēr*, ureter]. Bet. the two ureters. SYN: *interureteric*.

interureteric (in"ter-u-re-ter'ik) [" + G. *ourētēr*, ureter]. Bet. the ureters. SYN: *interureteral*.

intervaginal (in-ter-vaj'in-al) [" + *vagina*, sheath]. 1. Bet. sheaths. 2. Within the vagina.

interval (in'ter-val) [" + *vallum*, a breastwork]. 1. The space or time bet. two objects or periods. 2. Break in the course of a disease or bet. paroxysms.
   i., a.-c., i., atriocarotid, i., auriculocarotid. In a venous pulse-tracing, the interval between onset of the presystolic wave (a) and the systolic (c) wave. It indicates the time required for impulses to travel from S-A node to ventricle, normally about 0.2 sec.
   i., a-s-V-s. That bet. beginning of atrial systole and ventricular systole, measured in man from an electrocardiogram.
   i., c.-a., i., cardio-arterial. The time bet. apex beat and radial pulsation.
   i., focal. Distance bet. ant. and post. focal point of the eyes.
   i., isometric. Bet. onset of ventricular systole and opening of the semilunar valves. SYN: *presphygmic, q.v.*
   i., lucid. Brief remission of symptoms in a psychosis.
   i., passive. The rest period of the heart.
   i., postsphygmic. I. bet. closure of semilunar valves and opening of semilunar valves and opening of atrioventricular valves.
   i., presphygmic. Brief period bet. the ventricular systole and opening of the semilunar valves.

intervascular (in-ter-vas′ku-lar) [" + *vasculum*, a vessel]. Situated bet. blood vessels.
interventric′ular [" + *ventriculum*, a small cavity]. Bet. the ventricles.
interver′tebral [" + *vertebra*, joint]. Situated bet. two adjacent vertebrae.
  i. disc. Broad and flattened disc of fibrocartilage bet. the bodies of vertebrae, as in *symphysis*.*
intes′tinal [L. *intestinum*, intestine]. Pert. to the intestines.
  i. digestion. The mixture of food and secretions described under duodenal* digestion moves on rapidly through the jejunum and is then detained for some hours in the lone remaining part of the small intestine, the ileum.
  i. d., chemical. The hydrolysis of starches and sugars to monosaccharides is accomplished by enzymes provided by the pancreatic and intestinal juices. The fats are emulsified by the bile, and then hydrolyzed by the action of the lipase (steapsin) of the pancreatic juice.
  The digestion of proteins, begun in the stomach by the pepsin, is carried on by the trypsin of the pancreatic juice, by the erepsin of the intestinal juice, and by other enzymes. The result is a rather fluid mixture of food and secretions, stained with bile. The products of the chemical action are monosaccharoses, fatty acids, glycerol, and amino acids, and they are actively absorbed.
  i. d., mechanical. Both digestion and absorption are accelerated by a continual mixing and moving of the intestinal

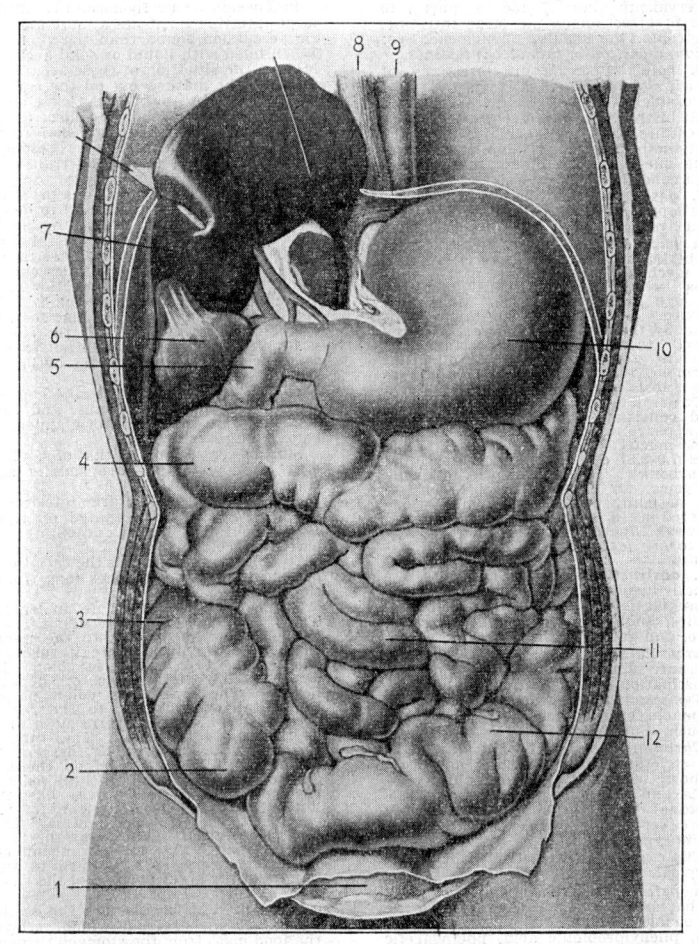

INTESTINAL TRACT
1. Bladder. 2. Cecum. 3. Ascending colon. 4. Transverse colon. 5. Duodenum.
6. Gallbladder. 7. Liver. 8. Esophagus. 9. Aorta. 10. Stomach. 11. Small intestine.
12. Sigmoid flexure.

intestinal flora — intestine, small

contents. A column of chyme may be broken into segments by contractions of the circular intestinal musculature; the segments may reunite and then again divide at the same point or elsewhere (rhythmic segmentation). A column may suddenly move several cm., remain stationary for a time, and then either return or advance.

The area of the absorbing surface is increased by the presence of permanent circular folds in the intestine; the entire surface is studded with fine villi which stud the folds as well as the spaces bet. them. At the end of the ileum the advance of the chyme is halted by the ileocolic sphincter. Peristalsis driving chyme towards it thus results in a churning effect. The sphincter opens at intervals to allow chyme to spurt into the first section of the large intestine, the colon. For ensuing phenomena, SEE: *colon, digestion in the,* also *intestines*.

i. flora. Bacteria in intestines of which *Bacillus acidophilus* is the most favorable.

At birth no bacteria are present in the intestines. Favorable bacteria may protect the body from invasion by unfavorable ones, which cannot thrive in an acid condition.

i. gases. Carbon dioxide, hydrogen, methane, methylmercaptan, and sulfureted hydrogen.

i. juice. A secretion of the crypts of Lieberkühn. The secretion is induced by mechanical stimulation of the mucosa which brings about secretion through local reflexes in Meissmer's plexus. A chemical substance produced by the intestinal mucosa, also induced secretion. This substance is thought to be secretin, a duodenal hormone, and by others to be a different substance called *enterocrinin*.

COMP. I. juice varies in composition and consistency. It is usually cloudy in appearance due to presence of cells and mucus. Its reaction is alkaline (pH 7.0-8.5) due to presence of sodium bicarbonate. It contains the following enzymes: an enzyme complex consisting of many peptidases, formerly considered as a single enzyme (*erepsin*), a weak *lipase, maltase, sucrase* (*invertase*), *lactase*. SEE: *Intestinal digestion*.

i. obstruction. *Acute*: Small intestine usually involved. Due to intussusception, strangulation, volvulus (twists), foreign bodies, knots, adhesions, tumors, stricture, and gallstones in intestines.

SYM: Pain localized and intense. Temperature subnormal or normal, vomiting, constipation and distention of abdomen.

TREATMENT: Irrigation of colon and stomach, cracked ice, but no food by mouth. Surgical.

Chronic: Involves large intestine. Due to stricture, inflammation, abscesses, tumors, fecal matter or chronic peritonitis, and gallstones may obstruct feces. Gradual constipation, pain becoming more severe in few days followed by acute symptoms.

TREATMENT: Diet restricted, enemas, surgical.

i. putrefaction. The chemical changes by bacteria in the intestine, forming the following: indol, skatol, paracresol, phenol, phenylpropionic acid, phenylacetic acid, paraoxyphenylacetic acid, hydroparacumaric acid, fatty acids, carbon dioxide, hydrogen, methane, methylmercaptan, and sulfureted hydrogen.

i. reflex. Intestinal contraction and relaxation above a portion of bowel which is stimulated.

intestine (in-tes′tin) [L. *intestinum*]. The alimentary canal extending from the pylorus to the anus.

It is nearly six times the length of the body, and is divided into the small intestine and the large intestine or colon.

PALPATION OF THE I.: *Fecal accumulations*. Feel like tumor but hard and resistant; but if one finger be pressed steadily upon them for 1 or 2 minutes will at last indent like a large snowball; most frequently collect in descending colon. "There is not the slightest elasticity about them and indentation remains after pressure is removed" (Simpson).

PERCUSSION OF I.: In normal condition large intestine furnishes a more amphoric percussion sound than the stomach. When filled with liquid or solid accumulations, the situation of these accumulations can be marked out on the surface by dullness on percussion. As these accumulations most frequently collect in the descending colon the percussion sound over this portion is usually less resonant than over the ascending or transverse colon.

According to Dr. Bennet, in a practical point of view it is often useful to determine whether a purgative by the mouth or an enema is likely to open bowels most rapidly. If there is dullness in left iliac fossa in the track of descending colon, that portion of the intestine must be full of feces, and an enema is indicated. If the sound in left iliac fossa is tympanitic and in right dull the enema is of little service, as it will not extend to the cecum, and purgatives by mouth are indicated.

i., large. The large intestine extends from the ileum to the anus, and consists of cecum with vermiform appendix, colon, and rectum.

Mucous coat resembles that of small i., *q.v.*, although glands are smaller and there are no villi.

The beginning of the large intestine is the *cecum*, a pouch situated on right side, about 2x3 inches, adjoining the ascending colon.

Attached to the cecum is the *vermiform appendix*, about 3-4 inches long, function unknown.

The colon averages 4-6 ft. in length. The first portion of *ascending colon* extends from the cecum to the under surface of the liver where it turns to the left as the *transverse colon*. Its bend is the right colic or hepatic flexure. The transverse colon passes horizontally to the left to the region of the spleen where it turns downward as the *descending colon*. This turn is the *splenic flexure*. The descending colon continues downward on the left side of the abdomen until it reaches the pelvic brim and curves like the letter **S** and is placed in front of the sacrum to become the *rectum*. This **S**-shaped section is known as the "*sigmoid colon*." The rectum, about 6-8 inches long, passes downward to terminate in the lower opening of the tract, the *anus* or *anal opening*.

i., small. This begins with the *duodenum*, 8-10 inches long, which receives the food mass from the stomach through the pylorus, the bile from the liver and gallbladder, and the pancreatic juice from the pancreas. It connects with the *jejunum*, about 8 ft. long, which is usu-

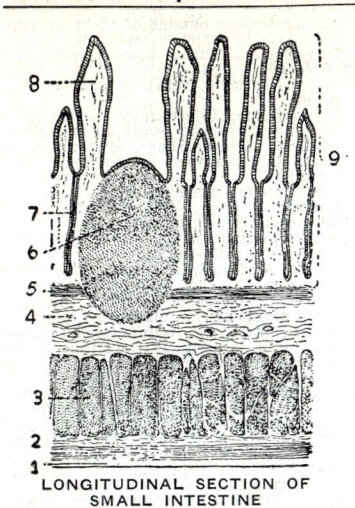

intestine, words pert. to   I-33   **intrafebrile**

LONGITUDINAL SECTION OF SMALL INTESTINE
1. Serous coat. 2. Longitudinal muscular fibers. 3. Circular muscular fibers. 4. Submucosa. 5. Muscularis mucosae. 6. Solitary nodule. 7. Intestinal gland. 8. Villus. 9. Mucosa.

ally empty after death. The jejunum, in turn, joins the *ileum* or twisted intestine, about 12 ft. long, which is attached to the large intestine by the *ileocecal* or *colic valve* that controls passage of food into large i.

In the wall of the small intestine are found Brunner's glands, intestinal glands (crypts of Lieberkühn), blood and lymph vessels (lacteals), and lymphatic tissue in the form of solitary nodules or aggregated nodules (Peyer's patches. SEE: Fig. above).

The inner surface is thrown into folds (circular folds) and lining the entire surface are minute fingerlike *villi* through which the products of digestion (simple sugars, amino acids, and fatty acids and glycerol are absorbed. There are over five million villi providing an absorbing surface of over 100 feet. Villi range from 1.48 to ⅛ of an inch in length.

intestine, words pert. to: abenteric, alvine, alvinolith, angulation, anthrax, antiperistalsis, antistalsis, apenteric, ascaridiasis, atavicosis, Brunner's glands, celiac disease, celiopyosis, Cercomonas intestinalis, Chilomastix mesnili, cholecystenterorrhaphy, choledochoenterostomy, cholera infantum, chyle, chilifaction, circumintestinal, colic, colon, copremia, crepitation, diarrhea, digestion, int., dysentery, "enter- words," flora, ileitis, ileocecal, ileus, "ilio- words," indigitation, intestinal digestion, intestinal flora, intestinal juice, intestinal obstruction, intussusception, invertin, mesentery, obstipation, tormina, valvulae conniventes, villi, villus.

intestinum (ĭn-tĕs-tī'nŭm) [L.]. Intestine.
   i. rectum. BNA. The rectum.

in'tima [L. innermost]. Innermost coat of a structure, as a blood vessel. SYN: *tunica intima.*

intimal (in'tim-al) [L. *intima,* innermost]. Pert. to the inner coat of a blood vessel, the intima.

intimi'tis [" + G. *-itis,* inflammation]. Inflammation of an intima.

intol'erance [L. *in,* not, + *tolerāre,* to bear.] Inability to endure or incapacity for bearing, as pain, or the effects of a drug or other substance.

intoxicant. An agent which produces intoxication.

intoxica'tion [" + G. *toxikon,* poison]. 1. State of being intoxicated, esp. of being poisoned by a drug or toxic substance. 2. Intoxicated from overindulgence in alcoholic beverages. 3. Drunk. SEE: *alcoholism, autointoxication.*

The determination of alcohol content is frequently of value in the diagnosis of intoxication from alcohol, especially in differentiating other disorders. Normally the alcohol content of body tissues and fluids is negligible. Upon ingestion of alcoholic fluids the alcohol rapidly increases in the blood and is excreted in the urine. The urine concentration will generally be slightly less than that of the blood. To be representative the tests must be made immediately. Results are expressed as "milligrams of alcohol per cubic centimeter of blood or urine." One milligram per cubic centimeter represents a condition of *"decent and decorous,"* 2 milligrams *"distinctly drunk,"* 3 milligrams *"drunk and disorderly,"* 4 milligrams *"dead drunk."*
   i., acid. I. resulting from acidosis.
   i., alkaline. I. resulting from alkalosis.
   i., intestinal. Autointoxication.
   i., water. I. resulting from excessive intake or undue retention of water.

intra- [L.]. Prefix meaning *within.*

in"traäbdom'inal [L. *intra,* within, + *abdominalis,* pert. to abdomen]. Within abdomen.
   i. pressure. Pressure within the abdomen.

intraärte'rial [" + G. *artēria,* artery]. Within the atria of the heart.

intraärticular (in-tră-ar-tik'u-lar) [" + *articulus,* joint]. Within a joint.

intracap'sular [" + *capsula,* little box]. Within a capsule.
   i. fracture. One occurring within the capsule of a joint.

intracartilaginous (in"tra-kar-tĭ-laj'in-us) [" + *cartilagō,* gristle]. Within a cartilage or cartilaginous tissue.

intracellular (in-tra-sel'u-lar) [" + *cellula,* cell]. Within cells.

intracra'nial [" + G. *kranion,* skull]. Within the cranium or skull.

intracuta'neous [" + *cutis,* skin]. Within the substance of the skin. SYN: *intradermal.*
   i. reaction. One following injection of tuberculin into the skin.

intracys'tic [" + G. *kystis,* bladder]. Inside a bladder or cyst.

intrad (in'trad) [L. *intra,* within]. Inwardly; toward the inner part.

intrader'mal [" + G. *derma,* skin]. Within the skin. SYN: *intracutaneous.*

intradermoreaction (in"tra-derm"o-re-ak'shun) [" + " L. *rē,* back, + *actus;* from *actere,* to do]. One resulting from the injection of a reagent into substance of the skin.

intraduct (in'tră-dukt) [" + *ductus,* a canal]. Inside a duct.

in"traduode'nal [" + *duodeni,* twelve]. Within the duodenum.

intradu'ral [" + *durus,* hard]. Within or enclosed by the dura mater.

intrafeb'rile [" + *febris,* fever] During the febrile stage.

intrafilar [" + *filum*, thread]. Within a network.
  i. mass. The fluid portion of protoplasm. SYN: *hyaloplasm, paramitome, paraplasm*.
intragem'mal. Within a bud or the expanded ending of a nerve, as a taste bud.
intraligamen'tary [" + *ligamentum*, a binding]. Within the leaves of a ligament.
  Usually used in referring to fibroid tumors or cysts of the ovary that have grown within the broad ligament.
intraligamentous (in″tra-lig-ă-men'tus) [" + *ligamentum*, a binding]. Within a ligament.
intralob'ular [" + *lobulus*, lobule]. Within a lobe.
intraloc'ular [" + *loculus*, a cavity]. Within the cavity of any structure.
intralum'bar [" + *lumbus*, a loin]. Within the lumbar region or portion of the spinal cord.
intraluminal (in-tră-lu'mĭ-nal) [" + *lumen, lumin-*, light]. Within interior of any tubular structure. SYN: *intratubal*.
intramastoiditis (in-tra-mas-toid-i'tis) [" + G. *mastos*, breast, + *eidos*, form, + *-itis*, inflammation]. Inflammation of the antrum and mastoid process. SYN: *endomastoiditis*.
intramu'ral [" + *murus*, a wall]. Within the walls of a hollow organ or cavity.
intramus'cular [" + *musculus*, a muscle]. Within a muscle.
  i. injection. Hypodermic injection of drugs into a muscle.
intranas'al. Within the nasal cavity.
intraoc'ular [" + *oculus*, eye]. Within the eyeball.
intraor'al. Within the mouth.
intraparietal (in-tra-pă-ri'e-tal) [" + *paries, pariet-*, wall]. 1. Within the parietal lobe of the cerebrum. 2. Intramural.
intraperitone'al [" + G. *peritonaion*, peritoneum]. Within the peritoneal cavity.
intrapleu'ral [" + G. *pleura*, rib]. Within the pleural cavity.
intrapon'tine [" + *pons, pont-*, bridge]. Within the *pons Varolii*.
intrapsychic, intrapsychical (ĭn-tra-sī'kĭk, kī-kăl) [L. *intra*, within, + G. *psychē*, mind]. Having a mental origin or basis, such as conflicts and complexes.
intrapul'monary [" + *pulmō, pulmon-*, lung]. Within the lung cavity.
intrapyretic (in-tră-pi-ret'ik) [" + G. *pyretos*, fever]. During the period of fever. SYN: *intrafebrile*.
intraspi'nal [" + *spina*, spine]. 1. Ensheathed, within a sheath. 2. Within the spinal canal. SYN: *intrathecal*.
intrathecal (in-tra-the'kal) [" + G. *thēkē*, sheath]. Intraspinal; within spinal canal.
intrathoracic (in-tră-tho-ras'ĭk) [" + G. *thōrax, thorak-*, chest]. Within the thorax.
intratracheal (in″tră-trak'e-ăl) [" + G. *tracheia*, trachea]. Introduced into, or inside, the trachea.
  i. anesthesia. A. administered through a catheter passed down the trachea.
in″tratu'bal [" + *tuba*, hollow tube]. Within a tube, esp. the fallopian tube.
in′tratympan'ic [" + G. *tympanon*, drum]. Within the tympanic cavity.
intrau'terine [" + *uterus*, womb]. Within the uterus.
  i. douche. D. for washing out interior of the uterus. SEE: *douche*.
intravasation (in-trav-a-sa'shun) [" + *vas*, vessel]. Passage into the blood vessels of matter formed outside of them through traumatic or pathological lesions.
intravas'cular. Within blood vessels.
intravenous (in-tra-ve'nus) [L. *intra*, within, + *vena*, vein]. Within or into a vein.
  i. infusion. Injection into a vein of an isotonic solution to secure an immediate result as in hemorrhage, to stimulate in shock or collapse and to dilute poisons in toxemia.
  SOLUTIONS: Normal saline, Dawson's, Locke's, Fischer's, Ringer's, glucose, 5-10%, sodium bicarbonate, 4%.
  TEMPERATURE: 98.6°; body temperature.
  QUANTITY: 250-500 cc.
  SITE: Median basilic or median cephalic vein.
  Preparation same as for i. injection but a needle or cannula is used, pointing toward heart. The vein must be exposed if cannula is used. Introduction should be very slow, taking at least 15 minutes for 500 cc.
  i. injection. Surface over skin is sterilized, tourniquet or bandage applied to middle of arm, the median cephalic or median basilic vein at front of elbow being used. Hypodermic needle is inserted in the vein, pointing upward. Pressure should be loosed before injection, which should be given very slowly.
  i. medication. The injection of a sterile solution of a drug or an infusion into a vein.
  Neosalvarsan, among other drugs, may be administered best intravenously to prevent pain and tissue reaction. A danger exists which should be minimized by best possible technic.
  i. treatment. This may consist of (*a*) intravenous injection or (*b*) intravenous infusion. The *injection* is usually known as the introduction of a solution into a vein with a hypodermic syringe. The *infusion* is usually known as the introduction of a solution in a larger quantity—250-500 cc. by means of a burette, needle, and rubber tubing.
intraventricular (in-tra-ven-trik'u-lar) [" + *ventriculus*, ventricle]. Within a ventricle.
intravi'tal [" + *vita*, life]. During period of living.
  i. stain. One which when introduced into a living organism is taken up by living cells.
in′tra vi′tam [L.]. During life.
intrin'sic [L. *intrinsicus*, on the inside]. Located entirely within or pertaining exclusively to a part.
  i. muscles. Those which have their origin and insertion entirely within a structure, as the intrinsic muscles of the tongue, larynx, or eye.
intro- [L.]. Prefix meaning *in* or *into*.
introdu'cer [L. *intrō*, into, + *ducere*, to lead]. Device for controlling, directing and placing an intubation tube within the trachea. SYN: *intubator*.
introitus (in-tro'it-us) [" + *ire*, to go]. Any aperture in the body.
  i. canalis sacralis. Terminal opening of spinal canal at end of sacrum.
  i. laryngis. Upper opening of larynx.
  i. vaginae. Ext. orifice of vagina.
introjec'tion [" + *jectus;* from *jacere*, to throw]. PSY: Identification of the self with another, or with some object, the victim assuming the supposed feelings of the other personality.
intromission (in-tro-mish'un) [" + *missus;* from *mittere*, to send]. An insertion or placing of one part into another, as the entry of the penis into the vagina.

intromittent (in-tro-mit′ent) [" + *mittere*, to send]. Conveying or injecting into a cavity or body, as the ejaculation of semen into the vaginal canal.
  i. organ. Penis, which carries seminal fluid into body of the female.
introspec′tion. Looking within, esp. examination of one's mind.
introsusception (in-tro-sus-sep′shun) [" + *suscipere*, to receive]. Invagination. 1. Growth of cells from within by the sythesis of new protoplasm from foodstuffs. 2. The invagination, slipping, or folding of one part of the intestine into an adjoining segment, usually the distal segment. 80% of cases occur in children under two. SYN: *intussusception*.
  PROG: Usually death unless surgery is resorted to.
introversion (in-tro-ver′shun) [" + *versio*, a turning]. 1. Turning inside out of a part or organ. 2. PSY: The condition of an introvert, *q.v.* Invertism: dwelling within one's self and withdrawal from the external environment, as characterized in such pathological states as hypochondriasis,* melancholia,* and schizophrenia.*
in′trovert [" + *vertare*, to turn]. 1. PSY: A personality reaction type characterized by the withdrawal from reality, fantasy formation, and stress on the subjective side of life adjustments, seen pathologically in extreme form in schizophrenia. OPP: *extrovert, q.v.* 2. *v.* To invaginate.
intubate (in′tu-bāt) [L. *in*, into, + *tuba*, a tube]. To insert a tube in a part, esp. the larynx. SYN: *invaginate*.
intubation (in-tu-ba′shun) [" + *tuba*, a tube]. Insertion of a tube into the larynx through the glottis for entrance of air, or to dilate a stricture.
  Tube used is 1½-3 inches long. Usually allowed to remain 5 days. Sometimes for months.
  POSITION: Patient held upright in lap of assistant, head upon assistant's left shoulder, arms secured by wrapping sheet about patient's body or being grasped by elbows. Another assistant stands behind patient with hands firmly grasping the head and holding gag in place. Patient so held that body, neck and head are kept naturally in a straight line.
  NP: Never leave patient alone, do not feed for two or three hours after intubation; nursing infants may go to breast, soft diet to others; keep on back or in sitting position.
in′tubator [" + *tuba*, a tube]. Device used in inserting a tube into the larynx.
intumesce (in-tu-mes′) [L. *intumēscere*, to swell up]. To enlarge or swell.
intumes′cence [L. *intumēscere*, to swell up]. A swelling or the process of enlarging. SYN: *tumefaction*.
intumescent (in-tu-mes′ent) [L. *intumēscere*, to swell up]. Swelling or becoming enlarged.
intussusception (in-tus-sus-sep′shun) [L. *intus*, within, + *suscipere*, to receive]. 1. Growth of cells by deposit of particles bet. those already existing. 2. Invagination.
  The slipping of one part of an intestine into another part just below it. Noted chiefly in children—more common in males—usual seat ileocecal region.
  PROG: Death usually results from gangrene, peritonitis, or collapse. Sometimes a favorable termination from sloughing and adhesion of serous surfaces. SEE: *ileus*.
intussuscep′tum [" + *suscipere*, to receive]. The inner segment of intestine which has been pushed into another segment.
intussuscipiens (in″tus-sus-sip′ĭ-ens) [" + *suscipiens*, receiving]. That portion of intestine which receives the intussusceptum.
inulase (in′u-lās). An enzyme that converts inulin into levulose.
in′ulin. 1. A polysaccharide found in plants yielding levulose. 2. An expectorant.
inunction (in-unk′shun) [L. *in*, into, + *unguere*, to anoint]. Ointment or medicated substance rubbed into the skin, to secure a local or a more general or systemic effect.
  Medicated substances include cocoa butter, cod liver oil and mercurial compounds. If mercury is absorbed there may be danger of salivation or damage to the kidneys. Belladonna may be ordered by a physician.
inus′tion [" + *ustus;* from *urere*, to burn]. Cauterization; burning.
in u′tero [L.]. Within the uterus.
in vac′uo. Within a cavity or a space from which air has been exhausted.
invaginate (in-vaj′ĭn-āt) [L. *in*, into, + *vagina*, sheath]. 1. To ensheath. 2. To insert one part of a structure within a part of the same structure. 3. Intussusception. 4. In Emb., to grow in or from an ingrowth or in pocketing, esp. the ingrowth of the wall of the blastula which results in the formation of the gastrula.
invag′inated [" + *vagina*, sheath]. Enclosed in a sheath; ensheathed.
invagina′tion [" + *vagina*, sheath]. 1. The process of becoming ensheathed. SYN: *intussusception*. SEE: *evagination*.
in′valid [L. *in*, not, + *validus*, strong]. 1. Not well; weak. 2. A sickly person.
invasin. Hyaluronidase, *q.v.*
inva′sion [L. *in*, into, + *vasus;* from *vadere*, to go]. 1. That period of a disease following entrance of of infective organisms and preceding the appearance of symptoms. 2. The entrance of bacteria or other infectious organisms into the body and their distribution to the tissues.
invermina′tion [" + *verminare*, to be wormy]. Infestation by intestinal worms. SYN: *helminthiasis*.
inverse-square law. The intensity of radiation at any distance is inversely proportional to the square of the distance bet. the irradiated surface and a point source.
inversion (in-ver′shun) [L. *in*, into, + *versio*, a turning]. 1. Turning inside out of an organ, *e. g.*, the uterus. 2. In chemistry, the process of converting sucrose (which rotates the plane of polarized light to the right) into a mixture of dextrose and levulose, which mixture rotates the plane to the left.
  The resulting mixture is called invert sugar, and the enzyme which catalyzes this conversion is called invertase. SEE: *enzyme*.
  i., psychic. Lack of harmony bet. the physical and psychic self or sex.
  i., sexual. Deviation from normal sex relationship, diametrically opposite, *i. e.*, sexual interest in one of the same sex. SYN: *homosexuality*.
  i., uterine. A condition in which the fundus of the uterus protrudes through the cervix, and in some cases through the vaginal introitus. May be acute or chronic, the acute type usually occurring immediately postpartum as a result of

invert   I-36   **iodine, radioactive**

too vigorous placental expression or pulling on the placental cord when the placenta is fixed in the uterus. The chronic type is usually due to tumors of the fundus uteri that pull themselves and the uterus through the cervix.

in'vert [" + *vertere*, to turn]. 1. One who, or that which is opposite the normal. SEE: *homosexual.** 2. (in-vert'). To turn inside out or upside down.

   i. sugar. A term usually applied to a mixture of levulose and dextrose, formed by inversion of sucrose by enzyme, invertase. SEE: *carbohydrate, inversion, sugar.*

invertase (in-ver'tās) [" + *vertere*, to turn]. A sugar-splitting ferment or enzyme found in the intestinal juice. It causes the inversion of sugar.

inver'tebrate. Without a backbone; an animal lacking a spinal column.

invertin (in-ver'tin). An intestinal ferment which converts cane sugar into invert sugar. SYN: *invertase.*

invest'ing [L. *in*, in, + *vestire*, to clothe]. Ensheathing, encircling with a sheath or coating, as tissue; surrounding.

invest'ment. A covering or sheath.

invet'erate [" + *vetus, veter-*, old]. Chronic; firmly seated, as a disease or a habit.

in vit'ro [L.]. In a glass, as in a test tube.

in vi'vo [L.]. In the living body.

in'volucre, involu'crum [L. *in*, in, + *volvere*, to wrap]. 1. A sheath or covering. 2. The covering of newly formed bone enveloping sequestrum in infection of bone.

invol'untary [L. *in*, not, + *voluntās*, will]. Independent of or even contrary to volition.

involution (in-vo-lu'shun) [L. *in*, into, + *volvere*, to roll]. 1. A turning or rolling inward. 2. The reduction in size of the uterus following delivery. 3. The retrogressive change in vital processes or in an organ after fulfilling their functions, such as that which follows the menopause. 4. A backward change. 5. Diminishing of an organ in vital power or in size. 6. In Bact., digression from the usual morphological type such as occurs in certain bacteria esp. when grown under unfavorable conditions.

   i. forms. Bacteria possessing abnormal and unusual forms.

   i. of uterus. Return of uterus by absorption to normal size after childbirth.

   i., senile. Shriveling of an organ or part from old age.

   i., sexual. Cessation of menstrual function. SYN: *climacteric, menopause.**

involutional (in-vō-lu'shŭn-ăl) [" + *volvere*, to roll]. Concerning involution or a turning inward.

   i. melancholia. M. associated with senile and presenile types and manic-depressive group.

   Occurs in the climacteric period, somewhat more frequently in women than in men. Stands alone in the classification of the psychoses.

   SYM: 1. No evidence of physical disease. 2. Irregular menstruation or cessation. 3. Anemic. 4. Loss of weight. 5. Foul breath and coated tongue. 6. Expression of being miserable. 7. Temperature usually subnormal. 8. Diminished perspiration. 9. Sleeplessness. 10. Movements slow. 11. Dry and sallow skin. 12. Pulse feeble. 13. Flabby muscles. 14. Decreased urine. 15. Shallow respiration. 16. Constipation. 17. Digestion upset. 18. Large joints more or less rigid. 19. Delusions frequent. 20. May refuse food. 21. *May commit suicide.*

   FORMS OF: *Simple*: 19, absent; 21, possible. *Delusional*: Very marked. *Agitated*: Reverse of No. 10, noisy expressions; 18, smaller joints continually in motion; picking at skin.

iodalbin (ī-ō-dal'bin). A compound of iodine and albumen containing approximately 21.5% iodine.

   USES: Same as the inorganic iodides.

   DOSAGE: Average, 5-10 gr.(0.3-0.6 Gm.).

Iodamoeba (ī-ōd-ă-mēb'ȧ). A genus of nonpathogenic amebas found in the intestinal tract. Their cysts are peculiar in that they are irregular in shape, nucleus usually single, and they possess a vacuole filled with glycogen which stains brown in iodine.

   I. butschlii. SYN: *I. williamsi.* A small, sluggish ameba found in the large intestine of man. Also found in monkeys and pigs. It is nonpathogenic.

iodeikon (ī-ō'de-kon). Brand of soluble iodophthalein.

   USES: For x-ray study of the gallbladder.

iodine (ī'ō-din) [G. *iōdēs*, violet colored]. A nonmetallic element belonging to the halogen group. It is a black, crystalline substance having a density of about five. It melts at 114° C. and boils at a slightly higher temperature, giving off a characteristic violet vapor. SYM: I. Atomic no., 53; atomic weight, 126.92.

   FUNCTIONS: Development and functioning of the thyroid gland, formation of thyroxine and prevention of goiter; regulation of basal metabolic rate. The amount of iodine in the entire body averages 50 mg., of which one-third to one-fifth (10-15 mg.) is found in the thyroid. Iodine content of the blood varies from 5 to 10 micrograms per 100 cc. Daily requirement for iodine is about 100 micrograms. A growing child or a pregnant woman needs several times as much as an adult. Those under emotional strain and the adolescents likewise need more iodine.

   SYM. OF DEFICIENCY: A def. of iodine in the diet leads to simple goiter characterized by thyroid enlargement and hypothyroidism. This may result in retardation of physical, sexual, and mental development in the young, a condition called *cretinism*.

   SOURCES: *Ex*. Broccoli, cod liver oil, iodized salt, fish, esp. halibut and salmon, shell fish. *Good*: Barley, bran, butter, carrots, cherries, corn, green beans, loganberries, oatmeal, spinach, peas, asparagus. The iodine content of vegetables depends upon the locality in which grown.

   POISONING: SYM: Brown stains on mouth and throat, which appear shriveled; burning sensation in throat followed by vomiting and diarrhea. The vomitus is yellow or brown; dizziness.

   F. A. TREATMENT: Empty stomach by means of stomach pump or an emetic. Give starch, flour and water, or barley and water in large quantities. Stimulate if necessary.

   INCOMPATIBILITIES: *alkaloids.*

   USES: Tincture of iodine (a 2 or 3% solution in alcohol) is used as a disinfectant and germicide. It is used as a preventative of simple goiter and, in the form of Lugol's solution, is invaluable in the treatment of exophthalmic goiter. Dosage is 10 to 40 minims daily. It is also used in the treatment of syphilis and tuberculosis.

   i., radioactive. I^{131}, an isotope of I with an atomic weight of 131. Used in diagnosis of thyroid disorders and in the treatment of toxic goiter and thyroid carcinoma.

i., tincture of. A solution of 20 gm. iodine and 24 gm. sodium iodide in 1000 cc. of dilute alcohol.

iod'inin. A purple pigment produced by certain bacteria which inhibits the growth of streptococci, esp. *Streptococcus hemolyticus.* It is effective in very dilute solutions.

iodism (i'o-dizm) [G. *iōdēs,* violet colored]. Condition induced by prolonged use of iodine or its compounds. SEE: *iodine poisoning.*

i'odize [G. *iōdēs,* violet colored]. To administer or impregnate with iodine.

i'odized [G. *iōdēs,* violet colored]. Impregnated with iodine.

i. salt. Salt containing 1 part sodium or potassium iodide to 5000 parts of sodium chloride. SEE: *salt.*

io'doform [G. *iōdēs,* violet colored, + L. *forma,* form]. USP. Yellow powder made by the action of iodine on acetone in the presence of an alkali.

ACTION AND USES: A local analgesic, antiseptic, and stimulant.

DOSAGE: Externally in the form of a dusting powder, or as a surgical dressing in the form of gauze impregnated with the drug.

INCOMPATIBILITIES: Mercuric oxide, calomel, silver nitrate, tannin, balsam of Peru.

io'doformism [" + " + G. *ismos,* state of]. Poisoning caused by iodoform.

iodophilia (i-ō-dō-fil-i-ă). Condition in which certain cells, esp. polymorphonuclear leukocytes show a pronounced affinity for iodine, the cells acquiring a brownish-red color. Seen in pathologic conditions such as acute infections and anemia.

i., intracellular. I. in which color changes occur within the cells.

i., extracellular. I. in which substances in the plasma outside the cells are colored.

iodother'apy [" + *therapeia,* treatment]. Use of iodine medication.

i'odum [L.]. Iodine.

i'on [G. *iōn,* going]. Molecular constituent, *i. e.,* one or more atoms, carrying an electric charge.

A free-wandering particle carrying an electric charge, consisting of an atom or group of atoms into which the molecules of an electrolyte are divided; or one of the electrified particles into which the molecules of a gas are divided by ultraviolet rays, gamma rays, or x-rays, or by other ionizing agents.

Ions occur (1) in gases, esp. at low pressures, under the influence of strong electrical discharges, x-rays, and radium. and (2) in solutions of acids, bases, and salts. Such moving particles render the gas or solution capable of conducting the electric current, and on reaching the electrodes they are discharged.

Ions which carry *positive* charges and which consequently discharge at the negative electrode (cathode) are called cations; examples are the hydrogen in aqueous solutions of acids and the sodium in aqueous solutions of sodium chloride.

Ions which carry *negative* charges will appear at the positive electrode (anode) and are, therefore, called anions; an example is the chlorine in aqueous solutions of hydrochloric acid or of sodium chloride. Thus in the reaction

$HCl \rightarrow H^+ + Cl^-$

is represented the ionization of hydrogen chloride (hydrochloric acid) when dissolved in water; it means that when the electric current is passed through the solution hydrogen gas will appear as bubbles at the cathode, while chlorine will appear at the anode.

ion'ic [G. *iōn,* going]. Pert. to ions.

i. medication. The introduction of chemical ions into the superficial tissues for medicinal purposes by means of a direct current.

The basic rules are: Like forms of electricity repel each other; unlike forms attract each other. Bases, metallic radicals, and alkaloids are electropositive and should be placed at the positive pole. Acids and acid radicals are electronegative and should be placed at the negative pole. Ex: Potassium iodide for the introduction of free iodine should be placed at the negative pole, cocaine hydrochloride for local anesthesia at the positive pole. SYN: *iontophoresis 2, q.v.*

ionization [G. *ion,* going]. The dissociation of compounds (acids, bases salts) into their constituent ions.

ionize [G. *ion,* going]. To separate into ions; ionization, *q.v.*

i"onom'eter [" + *metron,* measure]. An instrument consisting of an ionization chamber, an electroscope and an electric charging current designed to measure the amount of radiation used by roentgen rays or radium and to measure the intensity of the rays themselves. SEE: *roentgenometer.*

ionotherapy (i''on-o-ther'ă-pi) [" + *therapeia,* treatment]. 1. Introduction of ions into the body. 2. [G. *ion,* violet]. Treatment of disease with violet rays. SYN: *iontophoresis, 1.*

iontophoresis (i-on"to-fo-re'sis) [" + *phorein,* to carry]. 1. Process of electrical current traveling through salt solution causing migration of metal ion to negative pole and radical ion to positive pole. 2. Introduction of various ions into tissues through the skin by means of electricity. SYN: *ionic medication.*

iontoquantimeter (i-on''to-kwon-tim'e-ter) [" + L. *quantus,* how much, + G. *metron,* measure]. Instrument used to measure the amount of radiation used by, and the intensity of, roentgen rays. SEE: *roentgenometer.*

iontoradiometer (i-on"to-ra-di-om'e-ter) [" + L. *radius,* ray, + G. *metron,* measure]. Instrument for measuring the amount and intensity of roentgen rays. SEE: *roentgenometer.*

iontotherapy (i-on"to-ther'ă-pī) [" + *therapeia,* treatment]. Treatment by forcing ions into the body electrically.

iophobia (i-o-fo'bĭ-ă) [G. *ios,* poison, rust, + *phobos,* fear]. 1. Fear of being poisoned. SYN: *toxicophobia.* 2. Fear of touching any rusty object.

iotacism (i-o'ta-sizm) [G. *iōta,* letter i]. Defective utterance marked by constant substitution of an ē sound (Greek iota) for other vowels.

ipecac (ip'-e-kak). USP. A dried root of a plant (*ipecacuanha*), grown in Brazil.

ACTION AND USES: Specific against amebic dysentery. Also an expectorant, emetic, and diaphoretic.

DOSAGE: As expectorant, 1 gr. (0.06 Gm.); as emetic, 15 gr. (1.0 Gm.). SEE: *emetine.*

ipral sodium (ip'ral). A proprietary derivative of barbital; a persistent acting hypnotic.

DOSAGE: 2-4 gr. (0.12-0.25 Gm.)

ipsation (ip-sa'shun) [L. *ipse,* self]. Practice of masturbation.

ipsilateral, ipsolateral (ip-si-lat′er-al, ip-so) [L. *ipse*, same, + *latus*, later-, side]. On the same side. Affecting the same side of the body.
Thus, when the right patellar tendon is tapped, a knee-jerk is observed on the same side. Said of findings (paralysis) appearing on same side of body as brain or spinal cord lesion producing them. Opp. of *crossed, contralateral.* SYN: *homolateral.*

IQ. Abbr. for *intelligence quotient.*

Ir. Abbr. for *internal resistance.*

iral′gia [G. *iris*, iris, + *algos*, pain]. Pain felt in the iris. SYN: *iridalgia.*

iridadenosis (ir″ĭ-dăd-e-nō′sis). A glandular affection of the iris.

iridal (ir′ĭd-al) [G. *iris*, *irid-*, iris]. Rel. to the iris.

iridalgia (ir-id-al′jĭ-ă) [" + *algos*, pain]. Pain felt in the iris. SYN: *iralgia.*

iridauxesis (ir″ĭ-dawk-se′sis) [" + *auxēsis*, increase]. Increase in size of the iris. SYN: *iridoncus.*

iridectome (ir-id-ek′tōm) [" + *tomē*, a cutting]. Instrument for cutting the iris.

iridectomesodialysis (ir-ĭ-dek″to-mes″o-dī-al′ĭ-sis) [" + *ektomē*, excision, + *mesos*, middle, + *dialysis*, loosening]. Formation of an artificial pupil, by separating adhesions on inner margin of iris.

iridectomize (ir-id-ek′to-mīz) [" + *ektomē*, excision]. To excise a portion of the iris.

iridec′tomy [" + *ektomē*, excision]. Surgical removal of a portion of iris.
 i., optical. I. done for purpose of making an artificial pupil.

iridectropium (ir-ĭ-dek-tro′pĭ-um) [" + *ektropion*, eversion]. Partial eversion of the iris.

iride′mia [" + *aima*, blood]. Bleeding from the iris.

iridencleisis (ir″id-en-klī′sis) [" + *egklein*, to lock in]. Iris inclusion operation; the iris being incarcerated in the wound, thereby forming a fistula lined with iris tissue. Performed in glaucoma.

iridentropium (ir″ĭ-den-tro′pĭ-um) [" + *entropion*, inversion]. Partial inversion of the iris.

irideremia (ir-id-er-e′mĭ-ă) [" + *erēmia*, lack]. Partial or total absence of the iris. SEE: *aniridia.*

iridesis (i-rid′ē-sis [" + *desis*, a binding]. Formation of an iris artificially, by ligation.

iridic (ir-id′ik) [G. *iris*, *irid-*, iris]. Rel. to the iris. SYN: *iridal.*

ir′ido- [G.]. Combining form, pert. to the iris.

iridoavulsion (ir″ĭ-do-av-ul′shun) [G. *iris, irid-*, iris, + L. *avulsio*, tearing away]. Tearing away (avulsion) of the iris.

iridocapsulitis (ir″id-o-kap-sū-lī′tis) [" + L. *capsula*, little box, + G. *-itis*, inflammation]. Iritis with inflammation of the capsule of the lens.

iridocele (i-rid′o-sēl) [" + *kēlē*, hernia]. Protrusion of a portion of the iris through a defect in the cornea.

iridochorioiditis, iridochoroiditis (ir″ĭ-do-ko″rĭ-oy-dī′tis) (ir″ĭ-do-ko-roy-dī′tis) [" + *chorioeidēs*, skinlike]. Inflamed condition of both iris and choroid.

ir″idocolobo′ma [" + *kolobōma*, mutilation]. Congenital defect or fissure of the iris.

iridocyclectomy (ir″ĭ-do-si-klek′to-mĭ) [" + *kyklos*, circle, + *ektomē*, excision]. Surgical removal of iris and ciliary body.

iridocyclitis (ir″id-o-si-klī′tis) [" + " + *-itis*, inflammation]. Inflammation of iris and ciliary body.

iridocystectomy (ir″ĭ-do-sis-tek′to-mĭ) [" + *kystis*, a bag, + *ektomē*, excision]. Plastic formation of an artificial pupil.

iridodesis (ir-id-od′es-is) [" + *desis*, a binding]. Ligature of part of iris to form an artificial one. SYN: *iridesis.*

ir″idodiagno′sis [" + *dia*, through, + *gnōsis*, knowledge]. Diagnosis of disease by changes in color and form of the iris.

iridodialysis (ir″id-o-dī-al′is-is) [" + *dialysis*, loosening]. The separation of the outer margin of the iris from its ciliary attachment, usually due to trauma, forming an artificial pupil.

iridodila′tor [" + L. *dilatāre*, to dilate]. Substance causing dilatation of the pupil.

iridodonesis (ir″id-o-do-ne′sis) [" + *donēsis*, tremor]. Tremulousness of iris, seen in an aphakik eye or one with subluxated lens. SYN: *hippus.*

iridokinesis (ir″id-o-kĭn-e′sis) [" + *kinēsis*, motion]. The contracting and expanding movements of the iris.

iridoleptynsis. Thinning or atrophy of the iris.

iridology (ir-ĭ-dol′o-jĭ) [" + *logos*, study]. The study of changes in the iris during course of a disease.

iridomalacia (ir″id-o-ma-la′sĭ-ă) [" + *malakia*, softening]. Softening of the iris.

iridomedialysis (ir″id-o-med-ī-al′ĭ-sis) [" + L. *medius*, in middle, + G. *dialysis*, loosening]. Separation of inner marginal adhesions of iris. SYN: *iridomesodialysis.*

iridomesodialysis (ir″id-o-mes″o-dī-al′ĭ-sis) [" + *mesos*, middle, + *dialysis*, loosening]. Separation of adhesions around the inner border of iris.

iridomo′tor [" + L. *motor*, motion]. Rel. to movements of the iris.

iridon′cus [G. *iris*, iris, + *ogkos*, tumor]. Tumefaction of the iris or development of a tumor.

ir″idoparal′ysis [" + *paralysis*, a loosening]. Paralysis of the iris. SYN: *iridoplegia.*

iridoparelkysis (ir″i-do-par-el′kĭ-sis) [" + *parelkysis*, protraction]. Dislocation of pupil due to prolapse of the iris.

iridoperiphacitis, iridoperiphakitis (ir″ĭ-do-per″ĭ-fă-sī′tis, -per″ĭ-fă-kī′tis) [" + *peri*, around, + *phakos*, lens, + *itis*, inflammation]. Inflammation of the iris and ant. portion of capsule of the lens.

iridoplegia (ir″id-o-ple′jĭ-ă) [" + *plēgē*, stroke]. Paralysis of sphincter of iris.
 i., accommodative. Inability of iris to contract when stimulated by accommodation.
 i., complete. I. in which the iris fails to respond to any stimulation.
 i., reflex. Absence of light reflex with retention of accommodation reflex (Argyll-Robertson pupil*).

iridoptosis (ir″id-o-dop-to′sis) [" + *ptōsis*, a dropping]. Prolapse of the iris.

iridorrhexis (ir″id-or-reks′is) [" + *rēxis*, rupture]. Rupture of or a tearing of the iris away from its attachment.

iridosclerotomy (ir″id-o-skle-rot′o-mĭ) [" + *sklēros*, hard, + *tomē*, incision]. Piercing of the sclera and of the border of the iris.

iridosteresis (ir″ĭ-do-stē-re′sis) [" + *sterēsis*, loss]. Removal of the iris or a portion of it.

iridot′asis [" + *tasis*, a stretching]. Stretching the iris for glaucoma.

iridotomy (ir-ĭ-dot′o-mĭ) [" + *tomē*, incision]. Incision of iris without excising a piece, done for the purpose of making a new aperture in the iris when the pupil is closed.
Indicated in eyes that had been operated on for cataract but which have lost

their sight through subsequent iridocyclitis. Also done in seclusio pupillae.
NP: All dressings, sponges, cotton, gauze, compresses, drains, towels, sheets, safety pins, etc., must be sterilized before using.

i'ris [G.]. The colored contractile membrane suspended between the lens and the cornea in the aqueous humor of the eye, separating the ant. and post. chambers of the ball and perforated in the center by the pupil. It regulates by contraction and dilatation the entrance of light.

ANAT: The free inner edge rests on the lens when the pupil is contracted or partially dilated. The iris separates the ant. and post. chambers of the eyeball. The iris contains two muscles, the sphincter pupillae (circular fibers) about one millimeter wide, and the dilator pupillae (meridionally arranged fibers) extending from sphincter pupillae to root of iris. The former is supplied through the oculomotor nerve with parasympathetic fibers derived from the ciliary ganglion; the latter by sympathetic fibers from the sup. cervical ganglion.

The color of the iris depends on the pigment in the stroma cells and in the cells of the retinal layers.

SEE: *aniridia, aquocapsulitis, choroidoiritis, heterochromia iridis, "irid-" words*.

i. bombé. Seen in annular post. synechia (seclusio pupillae). The iris is bulged forward by the pressure of the aqueous humor which cannot reach the ant. chamber.

i., chromatic asymmetry of. Difference in color of the two irides. One may be blue or gray and the other brown. May occur in early iritis or cyclitis. A normal condition except in those of neuropathic tendencies.

i. contraction reflex. Normal contraction on exposure to light.

i., piebald. Dark discoloration in irregularly shaped area. May be in one or both eyes.

I'rish moss. A genus of seaweeds; *chondrus crispus*.

iritic (i-rit′ĭk) [G. *iris*, iris]. Rel. to the iris.

iri′tis [″ + *itis*, inflammation]. Inflammation of the iris.

SYM: Pain, photophobia, lacrimation, diminution of vision; the iris appears swollen, dull, and muddy; the pupil is contracted, irregular and sluggish in reaction.

TREATMENT: *Constitutional* (sweating, catharsis, etc., internal medication for pain, and directed toward etiological factors). *Local* (atropine, dionin, local heat in form of compresses, dark glasses).

i., plastic. I. in which the fibrinous exudate forms new tissue.

i., primary. When the process develops in the iris itself. Seen in general diseases as syphilis, tuberculosis; metastatic in infectious diseases, gonorrhea and focal infections; also occurs in trauma and sympathetic ophthalmia.

i., purulent. One with a purulent exudate.

i., secondary. When the inflammation spreads from neighboring parts as diseases of cornea and sclera.

i., serous. Serum forming the exudate.

iritomy (i-rit′o-mĭ) [″ + *tomē*, incision]. Formation of an artificial pupil. SYN: *iridotomy*.

i'ron [A.S. *iren*] (L. *ferrum*). SYMB: Fe. A metallic element widely distributed in nature. Atomic weight 55.85. Its compounds (oxides, hydroxides, salts) exist in two forms: ferrous, in which iron has a valence of two, and ferric in which it has a valence of three. It is widely used in the treatment of certain forms of anemia. Its compounds have an astringent and styptic action.

Iron is essential for the formation of chlorophyll in plants, although it is not a constituent of chlorophyll. It is an essential constituent of hemoglobin.

FUNCTIONS: Iron is necessary for life, being an essential component of hemoglobin and essential for the formation of red blood corpuscles and also a component of certain respiratory enzymes, esp. the cytochrome system. It plays a role in the nutrition of epithelial tissues. There are approximately 3 Gm. of iron in the adult body, distributed as follows: 65% in hemoglobin, 15% in the reticuloendothelial tissues (liver, spleen, bone marrow) and 20% in remaining tissues. Iron is stored in the tissues principally as *ferritin*. Iron is absorbed from the food in the small intestine; it passes, in the blood, to the bone marrow; here it is used in making red corpuscles. A corpuscle, after circulating in the blood for a few weeks, is destroyed by the liver, and its iron is used over again. About 0.012 Gm. of iron is lost by a woman in the course of each average menstrual period; hence the normal, nonpregnant woman does not need much more iron than does a man.

Copper in the food is necessary for the utilization of iron. It is stored in the body and is reused repeatedly. The infant's food is poor in iron so it draws upon its store to such an extent that its reserve supply may be exhausted before the child is six months old. 10-16 mg. of iron per day are necessary in the diet of the average person. 0.015 Gm. is the normal amt. obtained from daily intake of food, this being equal to the daily loss. 25 mg. are needed in anemia.

Iron also acts as a means of transportation of oxygen. It is needed for tissue respiration, the development of blood cells, hemachromagen synthesis and for the normal complexion. Various forms of iron are used in medicine.

Manganese and cobalt, in addition to copper, are necessary for proper utilization of iron.

Iron, as a component of hemoglobin, is essential in the transportation of oxygen. It is needed for tissue respiration, the development of blood cells, hemachromagen synthesis, and for the normal complexion. Various forms of iron are used in medicine.

DEFICIENCY SYM: Anemia, lowered vitality, pale complexion, retarded development, decreased red blood cells and hemoglobin.

Sometimes a disturbance in iron metabolism occurs in which an iron-containing pigment, *hemosiderin*, and *hemofuscin* are deposited in the tissues. This gives rise to *hemochromatosis*. Excessive deposition of hemosiderin in the tissues such as may occur as a result of excessive breakdown of red cells is called *hemosiderosis*.

SOURCES: *Ex*. Almonds, asparagus, bran, beans, cauliflower, celery, chard, dandelions, Boston brown bread, Graham bread, egg yolk, kidney, lettuce, liver, oatmeal, oysters, soy beans, whole wheat. *Good*: Apricots, beans, greens, beets, beef, cabbage, cucumbers, currants, dates, duck, goose, lamb, molasses, oranges, parsnips, peppers, peas, potatoes, prunes, radishes, raisins, rhubarb, pineapples, tomatoes, peanuts, turnips, cornmeal, mushrooms. There is less iron in carrots and milk than in other foods. Recent investigations show that only 50% of the iron in spinach and some other vegetables is assimilable by the body.

i. arc. One of the commonly employed sources of ultraviolet radiation for therapeutic purposes.

i., high diet. Foods rich in iron and blood building substances are emphasized, *i. e.,* liver, beef heart, kidney, red meats, green leafy vegetables (esp. spinach), apricots, peaches, raisins, apples, prunes, molasses.

irot'omy [G. *iris*, iris, + *tomē*, incision]. Formation of an artificial pupil. SYN: iridotomy, iritomy.

irra'diate [L. *irradiāre*, to illumine]. To administer x-rays or other forms of radiation.

irra'diating [L. *irradiāre*, to illumine]. Diverging or spreading out from a common center.

irradia'tion [L. *irradiāre*, to illumine]. 1. Therapeutic application of roentgen rays, radium rays, ultraviolet rays or other radiation to a patient. 2. Application of form of radiation to an object or substance to give it therapeutic value, or increase that which it already has. 3. Phenomenon in which a bright object on a dark background appears larger than a dark object of the same size on a bright background. 4. The spreading in all directions from a common center for exam. nerve impulses, the sensation of pain.

R.S.: *Grenz ray, heliotherapy, radium, roentgen ray and ultraviolet.*

i., interstitial. Therapeutic irradiation by the insertion into the tissues of capillary tubes containing radon.

i. of reflexes. The spread of a reflex to an increasing number of motor units upon increasing the strength of the stimulus.

irreducible (Ir-re-du'sĭ-bl) [L. *in*, not, + *rē*, back, + *ducere*, to lead]. Not capable of being reduced, or made smaller.

irrel'evance [" + *relevans*, raising]. PSY: Giving an answer not in harmony with question.

irrespirable (ir″rĕ-spī'ra-bl) [" + *re-*, again, + *spirāre*, to breathe]. Unfit for breathing as a gas, or incapable of being breathed.

ir'rigate [L. *in*, into, + *rigāre*, to carry water]. To wash out with a fluid.

ir'riga'tion [" + *rigāre*, to carry water]. The cleansing of a canal by the injection of water or other fluids, as an enema, or the washing of a wound.

From 2-3 pt. of saline or antiseptic solution at 103° F. are used for wounds.

i., bladder. Washing out of bladder for treatment of inflammation.

NP: *Articles Needed*: The same as for a catheterization plus: Sterile funnel about 3 in. diameter. Solution ordered, in sterile pitcher, covered and warmed to 105° F. Bedpan.

If medication is ordered for instillation following irrigation have it ready in medicine glass covered with fold of sterile gauze.

Note: The irrigating can with tubing and a tapered glass connector may be used instead of the pitcher and funnel. A return-flow or double glass catheter may be used. This must have a 6 in. piece of small caliber rubber tubing on its inflow branch to connect with glass connector.

Procedure: 1. The patient may be placed on the bedpan and catheterized or she may be catheterized first and the pan put in place after that. 2. Catheterize but do not remove catheter. 3. Attach funnel to free end of catheter. Do not put your fingers *inside funnel*. 4. Hold funnel up and pour full of solution, allowing almost all of it to run in, then refilling. Do this 3 times and the 4th time fill funnel and turn it down quickly toward bedpan. This will siphon off contents of bladder. 5. Repeat until amount of solution ordered has been used or until solution returns clear. 6. If irrigating can is used, attach small end of connector to catheter and let 4 oz. of solution flow in gently. Detach catheter and allow fluid to run out into bedpan. Repeat. 7. If return-flow catheter is used just keep solution running gently, as it will return by other side of catheter. 8. Run medication ordered through catheter as soon as irrigation is finished. 9. Care for patient and equipment. 10. Record treatment.

BLADDER IRRIGATION: *Time. By whom done. Solution used*: Kind. Amount. Temperature. *Appearance of return flow*: Bloody. Mucus shreds, etc. *Medication instilled. Reaction of patient.*

i., colonic. The flushing of the colon with water. SEE: colonic i., enema.

ir'riga'tor [" + *rigāre*, to carry water]. Device with hose attachment used for purpose of flushing or washing a part or cavity with fluids.

i., Hyam's. Instrument for applying prolonged irrigation to the urethra, cervix, and vagina, with hot solutions at an exact temperature under accurate control.

ir″ritabil'ity [L. *irritāre*, to tease]. 1. Excitability. 2. The ability to respond in a specific way to a change in environment, a property of all living tissue. 3. Condition in which a person, organ, or a part responds excessively to a stimulus. 4. Quick response to annoyance; impatience.

i., muscular. Normal response of muscle to a stimulus.

i., nervous. Response of a nerve to stimulus.

ir'ritable [L. *irritāre*, to tease]. 1. Capable of reacting to a stimulus. 2. Sensitive to stimuli.

i. heart. SYN: *neurocirculatory asthenia,* q.v., *effort syndrome, soldier's heart.* A syndrome characterized by forceful uncomfortable heart beats, tachycardia, auricular flutter and fibrillation, faintness, fatigue and other symptoms.

i. joint. A condition sometimes following a sprain, marked by recurring attacks of acute or subacute inflammation.

ir'ritant [L. *irritāre*, to tease]. An agent which, when used locally, produces more or less local inflammatory reaction. Anything which induces or gives rise to irritation. Ex. *iodine*.

i. poisons. These include a large number of poisons of great variety, not including the corrosive acids or alkalies. They cause pain in the mouth, esophagus, and stomach, nausea, vomiting, and great thirst, abdominal cramping, bloody diarrhea, and diminished urine.

TREATMENT: Varies. SEE: *name of poison.*

irrita'tion [L. *irritāre*, to tease]. 1. Reaction to that which is irritating. 2. Extreme reaction to pain or pathological conditions. 3. Normal response to stimulus of a nerve or muscle.

i., spinal. A neurasthenic condition

characterized by tenderness along the spinal column, numbness and tingling in the limbs, and susceptibility to fatigue.

i., sympathetic. The response of an organ to irritation in another organ.

ir′ritative [L. *irritāre*, to tease]. Pert. to that which causes irritation.

irrumation (ir-ru-ma′shun) [L. *irrumāre*, to give suck]. Form of perversion marked by intromission of the penis into another individual's mouth. SYN: *fellatio*.

Isambert's disease (e-zahm-bairz′). Tuberculosis ulceration of the larynx and pharynx.

ischemia (is-ke′mĭ-ă) [G. *ischein*, to hold back, + *aima*, blood]. Local and temporary anemia due to obstruction of the circulation to a part.

ischesis (is-ke′sis) [G. *ischein*, to hold back]. Suppression of a discharge, esp. a normal one.

ischiac, ischiadic (is′kĭ-ăk, is-kĭ-ad′ik) [G. *ischion*, hip]. SYN: *ischiatic*. Pert. to the hipbone, esp. the ischium.

ischial (is′kĭ-al) [G. *ischion*, hip]. Pert. to the ischium.

ischialgia (is-kĭ-al′jĭ-ă) [" + *algos*, pain]. Neuralgic pain in the hip. SYN: *sciatica*.

ischiatic (is-ki-at′ĭk) [G. *ischion*, hip]. Pert. to the ischium or hipbone. SYN: *sciatic*.

ischiatitis (is-ki-ă-ti′tis) [" + -*itis*, inflammation]. Sciatic nerve inflammation.

ischidrosis (is-kĭ-dro′sis) [G. *ischein*, to hold back, + *idrōsis*, sweat]. Suppression of perspiration.

ischio- [G.]. Prefix: pert. to the *ischium*.

ischiobulbar (is′kĭ-o-bul′bar) [G. *ischion*, hip, + L. *bulbus*, bulb]. Rel. to the ischium and urethral bulb.

ischiocavernosus. 1. A muscle extending from the ischium to the penis or clitoris. It assists in the erection of these structures. 2. Pert. to the ischium and corpora cavernosa of the penis or clitoris.

ischiocele (is′kĭ-o-sēl) [" + *kēlē*, hernia]. Hernia through the sciatic notch.

ischiococcygeus (is′kĭ-o-kok-sĭj′e-us) [" + *kokkyx*, coccyx]. 1. Musculus coccygeus. 2. Post. portion of the levator ani.

ischiofemoral (is′kĭ-o-fem′or-al) [" + L. *femur, femor-*, thigh]. Rel. to the ischium and femur.

ischiofib′ular [" + L. *fibula*, buckle]. Rel. to the ischium and fibula.

ischiohebotomy (is′kĭ-o-he-bot′o-mĭ) [" + *ēbē*, pubes, + *tomē*, a cut]. Division of ascending ramus of the pubes, and of the ischiopubic ramus. SYN: *ischiopubiotomy*.

ischiomenia (is-ki-o-me′nĭ-ă) [G. *ischein*, to check, + *mēnes*, menses]. Suppression of the menses. SYN: *ischemenia*.

ischioneuralgia (is-ki-o-nu-ral′jĭ-ă) (G. *ischion*, hip, + *neuron*, nerve, + *algos*, pain]. Neuralgic pain in the hip. SYN: *sciatica*.

ischiopubic (is-kĭ-o-pu-bĭk) [" + L. *pubes*, the pubes]. Rel. to the ischium and pubes.

ischiopubiotomy (is′kĭ-o-pu-bĭ-ot′o-mĭ) [" + " + G. *tomē*, incision]. Division of the ischiopubic ramus and ascending ramus of the pubes. SYN: *ischiohebotomy*.

is″chiorec′tal [" + L. *rectus*, straight]. Pert. to the ischium and rectum.

i. abscess.* Collection of pus in fatty cavity on either side of rectum.
If it breaks internally into the rectum an anal fistula may result.

ischium (is′kĭ-um) [Pl. *is′chia*] [G. *ischion*, hip]. Post. and inferior parts forming the lower portion of innominate or hipbone.

ischochymia (is-ko-kĭ′mĭ-ă) [G. *ischein*, to check + *chymos*, chyme]. Retention of food in dilatation of the stomach.

ischogalactic (is-ko-gal-ak′tik) [" + *gala, galakt-*, milk]. 1. Causing suppression of breast milk. 2. Agent which checks milk secretion. SYN: *antigalactic, lactifuge*.

ischomenia (is-ko-me′nĭ-ă) [" + *mēnes*, menses]. Menstrual suppression or retention.

ischuretic (is-ku-ret′ik) [" + *ouron*, urine]. 1. Relieving or pert. to ischuria. 2. That which relieves urinary retention or suppression.

ischuria (is-ku′rĭ-ă) (" + *ouron*, urine]. Suppression or retention of the urine.

island (i′land) [A.S. *igland*]. A structure detached from surrounding tissues, or characterized by difference in structure; an islet.

i. of Langerhans. An islet of Langerhans, *q.v.*

i., pancreatic. An islet of Langerhans, *q.v.*

i. of Reil. The *insula*, a lobe of the cerebral cortex comprising a triangular area lying in the floor of the lateral or sylvian fissure. It is overlapped and hidden by the gyri of the fissure which constitute the operculum of the insula.

islet (i′lět) [Fr. *isle*, island]. A tiny isolated mass of 1 kind of tissue within another type.

i's. of Langerhans. Isolated masses of cells located in the pancreas, consisting of three types of cells: alpha or A cells, beta or B cells, and D cells. The islets produce the internal secretions of the pancreas which include *insulin*, the antidiabetogenic hormone, and *glucogon*, a hyperglycemic-glycogenolytic factor (HFC). Destruction or impairment of the functioning of the islets gives rise to diabetes, *q.v.*

-ism [G. *ismos*). Suffix: Condition, or theory of principle or method.

iso- [G.]. Combining form meaning equal.

isoagglutinin (i-so-ag-glū′tin-in) [G. *isos*, equal, + L. *agglutināre*, to glue to]. Antibody in a serum which agglutinates the blood cells of those of the same species from which it is derived.
RS: *agglutinin, blood grouping, isohemagglutinin*.

i″so-ag-glu′tin-o-gen. One of two substances designated A and B which may be present in red blood cells. Cells containing these substances become agglutinated when mixed with serum containing corresponding isoagglutinins (anti-A or anti-B).

isobare (i′so-bār) [" + *baros*, weight]. One of two or more chemical bodies having same atomic weight, and which may have similar or unlike properties.

i'sobody [" + A.S. *bodig*, body]. An antibody acting on animals of the same species, from which it is derived.

isocel′lular [" + L. *cellula*, little cell]. Composed of equal and similar cells.

isochromatic (i-so-kro-mat′ik) [" + *chrōma*, color]. Having the same color.

isochromatophile (i′so-kro-mat′o-fil or fĭl) [" + *philein*, to love]. Having same affinity for a dye.

isochronal (i-so-kro′nal) [" + *chronos*, time]. Acting in uniform time, or taking place at regular intervals.

isochron′ic [" + *chronos*, time]. Performed in uniform time or at regulated intervals. SYN: *isochronal*.

isochronous (i-sok′ro-nus) [" + *chronos*, time]. Performed in equal time. SYN: *isochronal*.

isochroous (i-sok'ro-us) [" + *chroa*, color]. Of uniform color. SYN: *isochromatic*.

isocolloid (i-so-kol'oyd) [" + *kollōdēs*, glutinous]. A colloid having the same composition in every transformation.

isocom'plement [" + L. *complēre*, to complete]. One from the same individual or species which provides the amboceptor.

isocoria (i-so-ko'rĭ-ă) [" + *korē*, pupil]. Equality of diameter of pupils.

i″so-cort'ex. SYN: *homogenetic cortex*. The neopallial cortex consisting of six horizontal layers of nervous tissue.

isocytotoxin (i″so-si″to-tok'sĭn) [" + *kytos*, cell, + *toxikon*, poison]. A cytotoxin destructive to cells of the same species from which it is derived.

isodactylism (i-so-dak'til-izm) [" + *daktylos*, finger, + *ismos*, state]. Condition of having fingers and toes of equal length.

isodiametric (i″so-di-a-met'rik) [" + *aia*, across, + *metron*, measure]. Having equal diameters.

isoelectric (i-so-e-lek'trik) [" + *elektron*, amber]. Having equal electric potentials.

i″soenerget'ic [" + *energeia*, energy]. Showing equal force.

isogam'ete [" + *gametē*, husband or wife]. A cell which, through conjugation or fusion with a similar cell, reproduces.

isogenesis (i-so-jen'es-is) [G. *isos*, equal, + *genesis*, production]. Similarity in morphological development.

i'sograft [" + L. *graphium*, grafting knife.] A graft taken from another individual or animal of the same species. OPP: *autograft*. SEE: *heterograft*.

isohemagglutinin (i″so-hem-ag-glu'tin-in) [" + *aima*, blood, + L. *agglutināre*, to glue to]. Substance normally present in most human blood serum and responsible for the clumping of corpuscles observed when incompatible bloods are mixed.

The clumping is ascribed to the interaction of an agglutinogen in the corpuscles with a specific agglutinin in the foreign serum. In transfusions, the corpuscles of the donor are exposed to an overwhelming quantity of the recipient's plasma; therefore the agglutinogen content of the donor's corpuscles and the agglutinin content of the recipient's serum are the factors which determine compatibility.

Assuming that there are but two possible agglutinogens, red corpuscles from a given donor may contain both, either, or neither. If the agglutinin, *alpha*, can react only with agglutinogen A, one can construct a table from which compatibilities can be deduced (Jansky system). See table.

Literature, particularly rules as to inheritance of blood groups, must be interpreted cautiously because of the wide use of an alternative system of numbering in which groups I and IV of the above system are interchanged. SEE: *blood grouping, table, below*.

i″sohemol'ysin [" + *aima*, blood, + *lysis*, dissolution]. Substance destroying red blood corpuscles of animals of the same species from which it is obtained. SEE: *hemolysin*.

i″sohemol'ysis [G. *isos*, equal, + *aima*, blood, + *lysis*, dissolution]. Action of an isohemolysin.

isohypercytosis (i″so-hi″per-si-to'sis) [" + *yper*, above, + *kytos*, cell, + -*ōsis*]. Increase of leukocytes, the proportion of varieties being unchanged.

isohypocytosis (i″so-hi″po-si-to'sis) [" + *ypo*, under, + *kytos*, cell, + -*ōsis*]. Decrease in number of leukocytes with proportion of varieties unchanged.

isoiconia (i″so-i-ko'nĭ-ă) [" + *eikōn*, image]. Equality in size of two retinal images.

isoiconic (i″so-i-kon'ĭk) [" + *eikōn*, image]. Having equal retinal images.

is″oimmuniza'tion. Immunization of an individual against the blood of an individual of the same species, esp. the development of Rh-agglutinins in an Rh-mother in response to agglutinogens present in transfused Rh + blood or developed in a Rh + fetus.

i'solate [It. *isolare;* from L. *insulāre*, to detach]. 1. To separate or detach from other persons, as during an infectious disease. 2. To free from a chemical combination.

isola'tion [It. *isolare;* from L. *insulāre*, to detach]. Limitation of movement and social contacts of patient suffering from, or a known carrier of communicable disease, in contradistinction to *quarantine*, which limits the movements of exposed or contact persons. SYN: *sequestration* 2. SEE: *quarantine*.

i. ward. Hospital ward where patients suffering from communicable diseases may be kept apart from the rest of the patients.

isoleucine (i-so-lu'sēn). An amino-acid formed during hydrolysis of fibrin and other proteins.

isolophobia (i-so-lo-fo'bĭ-ă) [L. *insulāre*, to detach, + G. *phobos*, fear]. Fear of being alone.

isolysin (i-sol'is-in) [G. *isos*, same, + *lysis*, dissolution]. Substance which dissolves red corpuscles of animals of the same species from which it is obtained. SYN: *isohemolysin*.

isol'ysis [" + *lysis*, dissolution]. Destruction of red blood corpuscles produced by an isolysin. SYN: *isohemolysis*. SEE: *hemolysis*.

isolyt'ic [" + *lysis*, dissolution]. Rel. to isolysins.

isomer (i'so-mer) [" + *meros*, part]. One of a set of chemical substances having an equal number of atoms, but different order of atomic arrangement in the molecule. SEE: *metamer, polymer*.

isomeric (i-sō mer'-ĭk) [G. *isos*, same, + *meros*, part]. Pertaining to isomerism, q.v.

isomerism (i-som'er-izm) [" + *meros*, part, + *ismos*, state of]. State of being composed of compounds of the same number of atoms, but having different atomic arrangement in the molecule. SEE: *metamerism, polymerism*.

isomet'ric [G. *isos*, equal, + *metron*, measure]. Having equal dimensions. OPP: *isotonic*.

i. contraction. C. of a muscle in which shortening is prevented. Tension is developed, but no mechanical work performed, all energy being liberated as heat.

i. contraction phase. The first phase in contraction of the ventricle in which ventricular pressure increases but there is no decrease in volume of contents because semilunar valves are closed.

i. muscle. PHYS: Contraction in which a muscle increases its tension without shortening.

isometro'pia [" + " + *ōps*, eye]. Same refraction of the two eyes.

isomor'phism [" + *morphē*, form, + *ismos*, state of]. Condition marked by possession of the same form.

isomorphous (i-so-mor'fus) [" + *morphē*, form]. Possessing the same shape.

isonormocytosis (i″so-nor″mo-si-to'sis) ["

isopathy I-43 **ivy poisoning**

+ L. *norma*, rule, + G. *kytos*, cell, + *-ōsis*]. State of having leukocytes normal in number and proportion of varieties.

isop′athy [" + *pathos*, disease]. Therapeutic administration of the virus that caused the disease.

isophoria (i-so-fo′rĭ-ă) [" + *phorein*, to carry]. Equal tension of vertical muscles of the eyes with visual lines in same horizontal plane, both hyperphoria* and hypophoria* being absent.

iso″plastic. Term applied to a graft taken from one individual and transplanted to another of the same species.

i″sose″rother′apy [" + L. *serum*, whey, + G. *therapeia*, therapy]. Treatment with serum from one having had the same disease as the patient.

isose′rum [" + L. *serum*, whey]. A serum from one having the disease for which a patient is to receive treatment.

Isospora. A genus of *Sporozoa* belonging to the order *Coccidia*.
 I. hominis. A parasitic protozoan inhabiting the small intestine of man. It is nonpathogenic.

isosthenuria (i-sos-the-nu′rĭ-ă) [" + *sthenos*, strength, + *ouron*, urine]. The decreased variation in specific gravity of nephritic urinary specimens.

isostimula′tion [" + L. *stimulāre*, to excite]. Cell stimulation by injection of the same cell substance.

isother′apy [" + *therapeia*, treatment]. Treatment by active causal agent of a disease. SYN: *isopathy*.

isother′mal [" + *thermē*, heat]. Of an equal degree of heat.

isothermognosis (i″so-ther-mog-no′sis) [" + " + *gnosis*, knowledge]. Abnormal perception in which stimulation by pain, heat, and cold are all felt as heat.

isoto′nia [" + *tonos*, tone, tension]. The maintenance of equal tension in two solutions or substances.

isotonic (G. *isos*, equal, + *tonos*, tension). 1. Having the same tension or tone. 2. Having the same osmotic pressure, *i.e.*, isosmotic. OPP: *isometric*.
 I. muscle contraction. Muscle contraction in which tension developed is less than resistance of load, hence muscle shortens and mechanical work is performed.
 I. solutions. Those having the same osmotic pressure.

isotonicity (i-so-to-nis′ĭ-tĭ) [G. *isos*, equal, + *tonos*, tension]. The state or condition of being isotonic.

isotope (i′so-tōp) [G. *isos*, equal, + *topos*, part]. One of a series of chemical elements which have nearly identical chemical properties but which differ in their atomic weights.

isotropic (i-so-tro′pĭk) [" + *tropos*, a turning]. 1. Possessing similar qualities in every direction. 2. Having equal refraction.

isotyp′ical [" + *typos*, type]. Belonging to the same variety or classification.

issue (is′shu) [O. Fr.; from L. *exire*, to go out]. 1. Offspring. 2. A suppurating sore maintained by a foreign body in the tissue and acting as a counterirritant.
 I. pea. Small round foreign body used in tissues as a counterirritant.

-ist (G. *istēs*). Suffix: One who or an agent that does.

isthmectomy (is-mek′to-mĭ) [G. *isthmos*, narrow passage, + *ektomē*, excision]. Excision of an enlarged isthmus, esp. of the thyroid gland. SYN: *median strumectomy*.

isthmian (is′mĭ-an) [G. *isthmos*, narrow passage]. Rel. to an isthmus.

isthmitis (is-mi′tis) [" + *-itis*, inflammation]. Inflammation of the throat or fauces.

is″thmocholo′sis [" + *cholē*, bile, + *-ōsis*]. Catarrh of fauces accompanied by bilious disturbances.

isthmoparalysis (is″mo-par-al′ĭ-sis) [" + *paralysis*, a loosening]. Paralysis of the muscles of the fauces. SYN: isthmoplegia.

isthmoplegia (is″mo-ple′jĭ-ă) [" + *plēgē*, a stroke]. Faucial paralysis.

isth′mospasm [" + *spasmos*, spasm]. Isthmian spasm, as of the fauces or of the fallopian tubes.

isthmus (is′mus) [G. *isthmos*, narrow passage]. 1. A narrow passage connecting two cavities. 2. A narrow structure connecting two larger parts. 3. A constriction bet. two larger parts of an organ, or anatomical structure.
 i., aortic. Constriction in fetal aorta between ductus arteriosus and left subclavian artery. Sometimes persists in adults.
 i. of eustachian tube. Narrow portion of eustachian tube.
 i. faucium. Path bet. fauces and mouth.
 i., pharyngeal. Opening between naso- and oral pharynx.
 i. of thyroid. Band joining thyroid lobes.
 i. of uterine tube. The narrow portion nearest the uterus.
 i. of uterus. Transverse constriction between cervix and body.

isu′ria [G. *isos*, equal, + *ouron*, urine]. Excretion of urine at a uniform rate, hour by hour.

itch [A. S. *giccan*, to itch]. 1. Irritation of skin, inducing desire to scratch. SYN: *pruritus*. 2. Scabies. SEE: Names in alphabetical order.
 ETIOL: Many diseases, bacteria, molds, animal parasites, allergy, urticaria, and possibly some mental states. Ex: Body louse, chilblains, folliculitis, heat and irritation, jaundice, cancer, and particularly diabetes.
 TREATMENT: Depends upon cause. Calcium used if due to allergy. Rest, soothing lotions, and freedom from mental distress.
 i. mite. Sarcoptes scabiei.

itch′ing. Pruritus; irritation of the skin, causing desire to rub or scratch the part.

-ite [G.]. Suffix denoting *of the nature of*. In chemistry a salt of an acid having the termination *-ous*.

i′ter [L. a way]. Passageway bet. two anatomical parts.

i′teral. Pert. to an iter.

ithycyphosis, ithyokyphosis (ith″ĭ-si-fo′sis, ith″ĭ-o-ki-fō′sis) [G. *ithus*, straight, + *kyphos*, humped]. Kyphosis with backward projection.

ithylordosis (ith″ĭ-lor-do′sis) [" + *lordōsis*, a bending forward]. Lordosis without lateral curvature of the spine.

-itis (ī′tis) [G.]. Suffix: *inflammation of*.

I.U. Abbr. for *immunizing unit. International unit.*

i′vy poisoning. Dermatitis caused by contact with poison ivy.
 The plant is easy to recognize, inasmuch as its leaflets are always in groups of three and rather thick and shiny. The toxic principle is found only in the sap. The sap, fresh or dry, is found in or on practically all parts of the plant.
 IMMUNITY: There is no absolute immunity to ivy poisoning though the susceptibility varies enormously even in the same individual.
 SYM: Always an interval bet. time of contact of poison with skin and first appearance of symptoms, varying from

a few hours to several days, and depending on amount of poisoning, on susceptibility of the patient, and possibly condition of skin. Moderate itching or burning sensation soon followed by small blisters; later manifestations vary. May be swelling, or a flat area (papules); or diffuse swelling, skin becoming red and swollen, swelling being deep and boggy. This may not come on for several days.

As blisters increase some break and skin is covered with constant coating of serum, accompanied by marked discomfort, which feels like a combination of burning, itching, heaviness, and increased sensitiveness, and there is limitation of motion. May have increase in temperature, and prostration. Duration varies from several days to approximately two or three weeks.

F. A. TREATMENT: Locally, most advisable treatment is to wash carefully soon after contact with a yellow soap and water, followed by repeated swabbings of alcohol. After this procedure, do not bathe as there is tendency to spread to unaffected parts. A 5% solution of ferric chloride has long been used, and 10% sodium thiosulfate as a wet dressing is helpful. The antihistaminic drugs, benadryl, pyribenzamine, etc., aid in overcoming the dermatitis and may be given in large dosage at bedtime, since they have a tendency to cause sleepiness. Paraldehyde in a dose of ½ ounce also is useful to give a restful night. Cortisone and ACTH often give dramatic results but should be reserved for the very severe cases.

Ixo'des. A genus of ticks, many of which are parasitic on man and animals. They are of importance as transmitters of disease to domestic animals and man. Among pathogenic organisms transmitted are those causing tick paralysis in domestic animals and tularemia in man.

ixodiasis (iks-o-di'a-sis) [G. *ixōdēs*, like birdlime]. 1. Lesions of the skin caused by tick bites. 2. Any disease caused by ticks, as Rocky Mountain fever.

ixodic (iks-od'ik). Pert. to or caused by ticks.

Ixodidae. A family of ticks belonging to the order *Acarina*, class *Arachnida*. Comprises the hard-bodied ticks including the genera *Ixodes, Amblyomma, Hyalomma, Haemaphysalis, Rhipicephalus, Boöphilus* and *Dermacentor*. All are parasitic and of importance as pests or in the transmission of disease in domestic animals and man. Among diseases transmitted are Rocky Mountain spotted fever, anaplasmosis, tularemia, brucellosis, and several others.

ixomyelitis (iks-ō-mī-e-li'tis) [G. *ixōdēs*, like birdlime, + *myelos*, marrow, + *-itis*, inflammation]. Inflammation of the spinal cord in the lumbar region.

J

J. Symb. for the *joule* and for *Joule's equivalent*.

Jaboulay's button (zhab-oo-lā'). Two cylinders which may be screwed together for lateral intestinal anastomosis.

Jaccoud's sign (zhă-koo'). 1. Movement of chest wall in adherent pericardium, indicating leukemia. 2. Irregular and low pulse with raised temperature in adult tuberculous meningitis.

jack'et [Fr. *jaquette;* from Sp. *jaco,* jacket]. A plaster of Paris or leather bandage applied to the trunk to immobilize spine or correct deformities.

   j., Sayre's. Plaster of Paris jacket used as a support for deformity of the spinal column.

   j., strait. Device for restraining the arms of a violently insane person. SYN: *camisole.*

   j., Willock's respiratory. A type of jacket for strengthening the respiratory movements in emphysema of the lungs.

jack-knife or reclining position. The patient lies on the back with shoulders elevated, thighs flexed on abdomen, legs on thighs, the thighs being at right angles to the abdomen. Employed when passing a urethral sound.

jack'screw. A threaded screw to expand the arch in regulating teeth.

jackson'ian epi'lepsy. A localized form with spasms confined to one part or one group of muscles. SEE: *epilepsy.*

Ja'cob's mem'brane. Retinal layer of rods and cones.

   J.'s ulcer. Epithelioma, usually of the face, which slowly eats away soft tissue and bones. SYN: *rodent ulcer.**

Ja'cobson's car'tilage. One of two narrow longitudinal cartilages lying along ant. portion of inferior border of nasal septum. They are rudimentary in man.

   J.'s nerve. Nervus tympanicus.

   J.'s organ. SYN: *vomeronasal organ.* Rudimentary sac in nasal septum.

   J.'s sulcus. Portion of middle ear containing branches of tympanic plexus.

Jacquemier's sign (zhak-me-āz'). Blue or purplish color of the vaginal mucosa, indicating pregnancy.

jactitation (jak-ti-ta'shun) [L. *jactitāre,* to toss]. Convulsive movements. Restless tossing. Changing from one posture to another, usually characteristic of severe mental and febrile affections.

   j., periodic. Chorea.

Jadelot's lines, furrows, or **traits** (zhad-loz'). Three lines on the face, said to indicate disease in children.

   J.'s labial l. Down from corner of mouth; seen in respiratory diseases.

   J.'s nasal l. From lower border of ala nasi about outer side of orbicularis oris muscle; seen in abdominal disorders.

   J.'s ocular l. From inner canthus toward glenoid fossa; observed in cerebral disease.

Jaeger's test types (ya'gerz). Lines of type of various sizes, printed on a card for testing close visual acuteness.

jail fever. Typhus fever, *q.v.*

Jaksch's anemia or **disease** (yakshs). Infantile anemia with lymphatic enlargement and changes in spleen. SYN: *infantile pseudoleukemia.*

jal'ap, USP. The dried tuberous root of the plant of the same name.

   ACTION AND USES: Purgative, in the form of compound powder.

   DOSAGE: 15 gr. (1.0 Gm.).

James' pow'der. Official antimonial powder.

James'town weed. Antispasmodic and local anodyne. Old name for Jimson weed (stramonium), *q.v.*

   POISONING: F. A. TREATMENT: Same as atropine, *q.v.*

Janet's disease (zhă-nez'). A neurosis characterized by obsessions and phobias.

   SYN: *psychasthenia.*

Japanese method (of resuscitation). Drawing forward the tongue and making rapid passes with paper fans soaked in water and aqua ammonia. The object is to get as much of the vapor of ammonia into the lungs as possible.

jar'gon [O. Fr., a chattering]. Unintelligible speech. SYN: *paraphasia.*

jar"gonapha'sia [" + G. *a-,* priv., + *phasis,* speech]. A form of aphasia* in which words are jumbled so that speech is unintelligible. SYN: *paraphasia.*

Jar'vis' snare. A snare for removing growths.

jaundice (jawn'dis). SYN: *icterus, q.v.* A condition characterized by yellowness of skin, white of eyes, mucous membranes and body fluids, due to deposition of bile pigment resulting from excess bilirubin (hyperbilirubinemia) in the blood. It may result from obstruction of bile passageways, excess destruction of red blood cells, or disturbances in functioning of liver cells.

   j., acatheretic. Form caused by functional hepatic cell disorder.

   j., acholuric. J. without bile pigment in the urine.

   j., black. J. to an extreme degree; icterus melas.

   j., catarrhal. J. resulting from inflammation of the liver. Now considered identical with infectious hepatitis, *q.v.*

   j., congenital. J. occurring at or shortly after birth due to maldevelopment of biliary apparatus.

   j., congenital hemolytic. SYN: *chronic acholuric j., spherocytic anemia.* A familial, hereditary disorder characterized by increased fragility of red blood cells, splenomegaly, and hemolytic anemia.

   j., hematogenous. Hemolytic jaundice, *q.v.*

   j., hemolytic. An inherited, chronic disease marked by increased fragility of red blood cells. Characterized by anemia, increased destruction of red blood cells, absence of bile pigment in urine, and splenomegaly.

   j., hepatocanalicular. J. resulting from changes in the bile canaliculi, the liver cells remaining relatively normal.

   j., hepatocellular. J. resulting from changes in liver cells.

   j., hepatogenous. ETIOL: Due to catarrh of bile duct and duodenum, pressure from tumors or blood vessels, parasites, stricture of gallduct or obstruction by gallstones.

   SYM: Yellow skin and mucous membranes. Light-colored feces, dark urine, nausea, itching anorexia, and mental depression.

j., homologous serum. A form resembling infectious hepatitis. Follows injection of homologous serum containing inducing agent.

j., infectious. Infectious hepatitis, *q.v.*

j., malignant. Acute yellow atrophied condition of the liver.

j. of newborn. J. affecting newborn infants. SYN: *icterus neonatorum.*

j., obstructive. That due to a mechanical impediment to the bile flow.

SYM: 1. Symptoms of gastroduodenal catarrh usually precede, *i. e.*, coated tongue, anorexia, fetid breath, epigastric distress, vomiting, and perhaps diarrhea; yellow skin and conjunctivae, light stools and dark urine. 2. In acute cases slight fever and swelling of the liver, which is tender to touch.

PROG: Favorable; duration, few days to several weeks.

TREATMENT: Rest, liquid diet, constitutional remedies, surgery.

j., parenchymatous. Hepatocellular j., *q.v.*

j., posthepatic. J. resulting from obstruction of flow of bile ducts. May be incomplete or complete.

j., prehepatic. A rare benign form in which there is no demonstrable liver damage. Also called *familial nonhemolytic jaundice.*

j., regurgitation. J. due to bile entering lymph channels of the liver and thence being conveyed to the blood. May result from biliary obstruction or lesions involving bile capillaries.

j., retention. J. resulting from inability of liver cells to remove bile pigment from circulation.

j., spirochetal. SYN: *Weil's disease.* An acute infectious disease due to a spirochete, *Leptospira icterohaemorrhagiae.*

j., toxic. J. resulting from bacterial toxins or poisons such as phosphorus, arsphenamine, carbon tetrachloride, etc.

j., xanthochromic. J. without bile pigment in the urine, but with yellowish discoloration of soles and palms.

jaw [Mid. Eng. *jawe;* from A. S. *cheowen,* to chew]. Either or both the maxillary and mandibular bones, bearing the teeth and forming mouth framework.

j., dislocation of the. Such dislocations are uncomfortable and extremely embarrassing to the patient. They may occur on either side, in which instance the tip of the jaw is pointed away from the dislocation.

On the normal side, just in front of the ear, may be felt a little hollow or depression which is often tender. If both sides of the jaw are dislocated, the jaw is pushed downward and forward. In either event, there is pain and difficulty in speech and the condition is often accompanied by shock. Backward dislocation of the jaw is rare.

CAUSES: Dislocations of the jaw are most often caused by a blow to the face or a fall on the chin, but occasionally they are caused by chewing large chunks of food, by yawning, or by hearty laughing. Individuals who have frequent dislocations of the jaw should be under a doctor's care to prevent recurrence.

REDUCTION OF: These dislocations are reduced by placing well padded thumbs inside of the mouth on the lower molar (back) teeth with the fingers running along the jawbone as a lever. The thumbs should be pressed downward towards the patient's lips and the fingers upward towards the patient's nose. Give a twisting motion to the jaw and at the same time with the wrist and elbows press backward toward the neck. The jaw gliding over the ridge of bone may be felt and just as this occurs the jaw usually snaps into place. When this motion is noted, it is desirable to move the thumbs outwardly towards the cheeks to avoid the thumbs being crushed bet. the molars.

This snapping into place is due to an involuntary spasm of the muscles pulling the jaw as though an overstretched rubber band were attached to it. Following the reduction, an immobilizing bandage or double cravat should be applied.

j. jerk reflex. Clonic movement resulting from percussing or stroking lower jaw.

j., lock. 1. Tonic spasm of jaw muscles preventing opening of mouth. 2. Tetanus, *q.v.*

j., lumpy. SYN: *actinomycosis, q.v.* Fungous disease affecting the jaw, brain, lungs and gastrointestinal tract. Common in cattle and sometimes affecting humans.

j., swelling of. LOWER: May be due to alveolar abscess, a cyst, gumma, sarcoma, or actinomycosis. UPPER: Occurs in alveolar abscess, parotid tumor, parotitis, carcinoma, sarcoma, and necrosis of bone or disease of antrum.

jaw, words pert. to: admaxillary, alveolar, alveolate, alveolus, anisognathous, biomaxillary, brachygnathia, epulis, gnathic, hypognathous, jerk j., mandible, maxilla, maxillary, ramus, submaxillary, tetanus, trismus.

jaw winking. Elevation of the upper eyelid when there is depression of the lower jaw.

jec'orin. A glucopholipin found in the liver, spleen, muscles, and other tissues.

jecorize (jĕk″ŏr-īz). To treat a food substance in such a way that it possesses the therapeutic value of cod liver oil, as the exposure of milk to ultraviolet rays.

jecur (je′kur) [L.]. The liver.

jejunal (je-jŭ′nal) [L. *jejunum,* empty]. Rel. to the jejunum.

jejunectomy (jej-ū-nek′to-mĭ) [″ + G. *ektome,* excision]. Excision of part or all of the jejunum.

jejunitis (jej-ū-ni′tis) [L. *jejunum,* empty, + G. -*itis,* inflammation]. Inflammation of the jejunum.

jejuno- [L.]. Combining form referring to the jejunum.

jeju″nocolos′tomy [L. *jejunum,* empty, + G. *kōlon,* colon, + *stoma,* mouth]. Formation of artificial passage bet. jejunum and colon.

jejunoileitis (jĕ-jun″o-il-e-i′tis) [″ + ″ + -*itis,* inflammation]. Inflamed condition of jejunum and ileum.

jejunoileostomy (je-ju″no-il-e-os′to-mĭ) [″ + G. *ileum,* ileum, + *stoma,* mouth]. Formation of a passage bet. jejunum and ileum.

jejunojejunostomy (je-ju″no-je-ju-nos′to-mĭ) [″ + *jejunum,* empty, + G. *stoma,* mouth]. Formation of a passage bet. two parts of the jejunum.

jejunostomy (jĕ-jū-nos′to-mĭ) [″ + G. *stoma,* mouth]. Surgical creation of a permanent opening into the jejunum.

jejunotomy (je-ju-not′o-mĭ) [″ + G. *tome,* incision]. Surgical incision into the jejunum.

jejunum (je-ju″num) [L. empty]. The second portion of the small intestine

extending from the duodenum to the ileum. It is about 8 feet in length, comprising about two-fifths of the small intestine.
Said to be empty after death.
j., inflammation of. SYM: Absence of diarrhea; colic, distention of abdomen, borborygmus, flocculent or semisolid stools, containing undigested food, unchanged bile, and some mucus. Tenderness over midabdomen relieved by pressure.

jel'ly [L. *gelāre*, to freeze]. A thick semisolid, gelatinous mass.
  j., contraceptive. A jelly introduced into the vagina for the prevention of conception. It may act as an occlusive agent or it may serve as a vehicle for spermacidal substances.
  j., mineral. Petrolatum, petroleum jelly.
  j., petroleum. Petrolatum.
  j., vaginal. A jelly introduced into the vagina for therapeutic or contraceptive purposes.
  j., Wharton's. Soft gelatinous connective tissue that constitutes the matrix of the umbilical cord.

Jen'ner's stain. Eosin methylene blue stain.

jerk (jerk) [Imitative Origin]. 1. A sudden muscular movement. 2. Term applied to certain reflex actions resulting from striking or tapping a muscle or tendon. SEE: *reflex*.
  j., elbow. External stimulation of triceps when stretched, produces involuntary extension of forearm.
  j., jaw. Result of striking lower jaw with mouth open. Indicative of cerebral lesion.
  j., knee. Forward jerk of foot upon striking patellar tendon, when knee is flexed at right angles. Absent in locomotor ataxia, infantile paralysis, meningitis, diabetes, destructive lesions of lower part of cord and certain forms of paralysis. Increased in affections of pyramidal areas, brain tumors, spinal irritability and sclerosis, lateral or cerebrospinal. SYN: *patellar tendon reflex*.
  j., wrist. When hand is held down at arm's length, the hand being in extreme extension, lateral clonic movements of the hand occur; normal phenomenon.

jig'ger (*Dermatophilus penetrans*). SYN: chigoe, nigua. Common name for parasitic fleas belonging to the species *Tunga penetrans, q.v.*

jim'son weed. Stramonium, *q.v.*

Jocasta complex (jo-kas'tă). A term implying a mother and son complex from part taken by Jocasta, mother in the Oedipus complex, who was the wife and mother of Oedipus.

jodum (yo'doom) [G.]. Iodine.

Joffroy's reflex (jof'roy). Twitching of gluteal muscles when pressure is made against buttocks.
  J.'s sign. 1. Absence of facial muscle contraction when eyes turn upward in exophthalmic goiter. 2. Inability to do simple sums in arithmetic. An early sign of general paralysis.

johim'bine. Alkaloid aphrodisiac.*

joint [L. *junctura*, a joining]. An articulation. The point of juncture bet. two bones. SEE: *Table in Appendix*.
A joint is usually formed of fibrous connective tissue and cartilage. It is classified as being immovable (*synarthrosis*), slightly movable (*amphiarthrosis*), and freely movable (*diarthrosis*).
SYNARTHROSIS: Joint in which the 2 bones are separated only by an intervening membrane, as the cranial sutures.

AMPHIARTHROSIS: 1. Joint having a fibrocartilaginous disk bet. the bony surfaces (*symphysis*), as the symphysis pubis. 2. Joint with a ligament uniting the 2 bones (*syndesmosis*), as the tibiofibular articulation.
DIARTHROSIS: Joint in which the adjoining bone ends are covered with a thin cartilaginous sheet and joined by ligament lined by a synovial membrane, which secretes a lubricant.
Grouping is according to motion: Ball and socket (*enarthrosis*), hinge (*ginglymus*), condyloid, pivot (*trochoid*), gliding (*arthrodia*), and saddle joint.
Movements of joints are of 4 kinds: *Gliding*, in which 1 bony surface glides on another without angular or rotatory movement; *angular*, occurring only bet. long bones, increasing or decreasing the angle bet. the bones; *circumduction*, occurring in joints composed of the head of a bone and an articular cavity, the long bone describing a series of circles, the whole forming a cone, and *rotation*, in which a bone moves about a central axis without moving from this axis. In angular movement, if it occurs forward and backwards, it is called *flexion* and *extension*; away from the body, *abduction*, and toward the median plane of the body, *adduction*.
INJURIES: Contusions, sprains, dislocations and penetrating wounds.
  j., amphidiarthrodial. J. both ginglymoid and arthrodial.
  j., arthrodial. SEE: *gliding j.*
  j., ball and socket. J. in which round end of one bone fits into cavity of another bone. SYN: *enarthrosis*.
  j., biaxial. J. possessing two chief movement axes at right angles to each other.
  j., bilocular. J. separated into two sections by interarticular cartilage.
  j., bleeders'. J. hemorrhage in hemophiliacs.
  j., Brodie's. Arthrodial neuralgia due to hysteria.
  j., Budin's. Congenital cartilaginous band bet. squamous and condylar parts of the occipital bone.
  j. capsule. The sacklike structure which encloses the ends of bones in a diarthrodial joint. Consists of an outer *fibrous* and an inner *synovial* layer and contains synovial fluid.
  j. cavity. The articular cavity or space enclosed by the synovial membrane and articular cartilages. It contains synovial fluid.
  j., Charcot's. A disease in advanced syphilis. Wasting away of muscles below the joint.
  j., Chopart's. Union of remainder of tarsal bones with os calcis and astragalus.
  j., cochlear. Hinge j. permitting lateral motion.
  j., compound. J. made up of several bones.
  j., condyloid. J. permitting all forms of angular movements except axial rotation.
  j., Cruveilhier's. Atlanto-odontoid j.
  j., diarthrodial. A joint characterized by the presence of a cavity within the capsule separating the bony elements, thus permitting considerable freedom of movement.
  j., dry. Arthritis of chronic villous type.
  j., ellipsoid. J. having two axes of motion through the same bone.
  j., enarthrodial. SEE: *ball and socket j.*

Joints, Table Comparing Diseases of[1]

	Acute Rheumatism	Rheumatoid Arthritis	Osteoarthritis	Gout
Age	Children and young adults	25 and over	Middle and old age	Middle and old age
Sex	Either	Chiefly women	Either	Chiefly men
Cause	Unknown? allergic reaction to streptococci	Often focal sepsis (streptococci)	Trauma, old age, degenerative changes	Uric acid in blood, due to disordered purin metabolism
Joints	Usually large joints, subsiding in one and commencing in another	Multiple, including small joints of hands and feet	Usually one large joint, e. g., hip, knee, shoulder	Several, e. g., great toe, knee, elbow, hands.
Pyrexia	At onset	In acute stages	Nil	During acute attack
Permanent Deformity	Nil	Spindle-shaped joints. Often gross deformity	Often slight	Deformity mainly from "chalky" deposits
Heart	Often affected	Not affected	Not affected	Often arteriosclerosis

[1]Sears' *Medicine for Nurses*.

j., false. False j. formation subsequent to a fracture.
j., flail. J. which is extremely relaxed, the distal portion of limb being almost beyond the control of the will.
j., ginglymoid. J. having only forward and backward motion, like a hinge.
j., gliding. Diarthrosis permitting a gliding motion.
j., hemophiliac. SEE: *bleeders' j*.
j., hinge. SEE: *ginglymoid j*.
j., immovable. SYN: *synarthrosis*. J. in which a cavity is lacking between the bones.
j's., intercarpal. Articulations which the carpal bones form in relation to one another.
j., irritable. Inflamed spasmodic condition of joint of unknown cause.
j., Lisfranc's. Tarsometatarsal j.
j., midcarpel. J. separating the navicular, lunate, and triangular bones from the distal row of carpal bones.
j., mixed. J. with surfaces joined by fibrocartilaginous disks.
j. mouse. Loose cartilage or other body in a joint.
j., movable. SEE: *diarthrodial j*. SYN: *diarthrosis*.
j., m., slightly. SYN: *amphiarthrosis*.
j., multiaxial. SEE: *ball and socket j*.
j., pivot. SYN: *rotary j., trochoid j*. A joint which permits rotation of a bone, the joint being formed by a pivot-like process which turns within a ring, or by a ringlike structure which turns on a pivot.
j., polyaxial. SEE: *ball and socket j*.
j., receptive or **reciprocal.** Saddle joint, q.v.
j., rotary. A pivot joint, q.v.
j., saddle. A joint in which the opposing surfaces are reciprocally concavoconvex.
j., screw. A cochlear j., q.v.
j., simple. J. composed of two bones.
j., spheroid. Multiaxial j. with spheroid surfaces.
j., spiral. SEE: *cochlear j*.
j., synarthrodial. SEE: *immovable j*.
j., tomato. Pain in the joints wrongly attributed to eating too many tomatoes.

j., trochoid. SEE: *rotary j*.
j., uniaxial. J. moving on a single axis.
j., unilocular. J. with a single cavity.
joint, words pert. to: abarthrosis, abarticular, acampsia, amarthritis, ambo, amphiarthrosis, amphidiarthrosis, ankylosed, ankylosis, aparthrosis, "arthr-words," articular, articulate, articulation, articulus, artus, biarticular, Bouchard's nodules, capsula articularis, capsular ligament, "capsul-" words, carpitis, Charcot's j., Chauffard's syndrome, clasp-knife rigidity, condylarthrosis, coxa, diarthrosis, dysarthria, dysarthrosis, elbow, enarthrosis, ginglymoid, ginglymus, gomphosis, haversian glands, hinge j., hydrarthrosis, junctura, luxation, manipulation, meningosis, metrotherapy, mobilization, nearthrosis, olecranarthritis, olecranon, omarthritis, orthopedics, osteoarthritis, pyarthrosis, schindylesis, socket, suture, symphysis, synarthrodia, synarthrosis, synchondrosis, syndesmosis, synovia, synovial membrane, synovitis, syntaxis, trochoides.
Jolles' test (yŏl'es). Test for biliary pigments in urine.
joule (jool). Work done in one second by current of one ampere against a resistance of one ohm.
Joule's equivalent (jools). Amt. of work which, if converted into heat, will raise temperature of one pound of water 1° F.
J.'s law. 1. Rate of heat production in a part of a circuit is equal to the resistance of that part of the circuit multiplied by the square of the current. 2. In gas expansion, with no change in the amount of heat in a given quantity of gas, and no external work performed, there is no change in temperature.
jugal [L. *jugum*, yoke]. 1. Connected or united as by a yoke. 2. Pertaining to the malar or zygomatic bone.
j. bone. Malar or zygomatic bone.
j. process. Temporal bone process forming zygomatic arch. SYN: *zygomatic process*.
juga'le [L. *jugum*, yoke]. The point at the margin of zygomatic process.
jugate [jū'gāt) [L. *jugatus*, joined]. 1. Coupled, yoked. 2. Having ridges.

ju′gular [L. *jugulum*, throat]. Pert. to the throat.

j. foramen. Opening formed by jugular notches of the occipital and temporal bones.

j. fossa. Depression in the petrosal portion of the temporal bone for the jugular vein.

j. ganglion. Nodes of vagus root and glossopharyngeal nerve in j. foramen.

j. process. Projection from occipital bone toward the temporal bone.

j. veins. *External*, receives the blood from the ext. of the cranium and the deep parts of the face. It lies superficial to the sternocleidomastoid muscle as it passes down the neck to join the subclavian vein. *Internal*, receives blood from the brain and superficial parts of the face and neck. It is directly continuous with the transverse sinus, accompanying the internal carotid as it passes down the neck, and joins with the subclavian vein to form the innominate vein. SEE: *Illustration, below.*

They are more prominent during expiration than during inspiration. Also during cardiac decompensation.

jugulate (jug′u-lāt) [L. *jugulāre*, to cut the throat]. To arrest quickly a process or disease by therapeutic measures.

jugula′tion [L. *jugulāre*, to cut the throat]. Sudden arrest of a disease by therapeutic means.

jug′ulum [L. neck]. Neck or throat.

ju′gum [L. a yoke]. Ridge or furrow connecting two points.

j. penis. Forceps for temporarily compressing the penis.

j. petrosum. Eminence on petrous section of temporal bone showing the position of sup. semicircular canal. SYN: *arcuate eminence.*

juice [L. *jus*, broth]. Liquid that exudes or is expressed from any part of an organism.

j., alimentary. The digestive juices.

j., gastric. Secretions of the stomach, consisting of water, salts, pepsin, and free hydrochloric acid. SEE: *gastric juice.*

j., intestinal. A clear, yellowish, viscid fluid; alkaline in reaction, secreted by Lieberkühn's crypts. SYN: *succus entericus.* SEE: *intestinal juice.*

j., pancreatic. A clear, viscid, alkaline

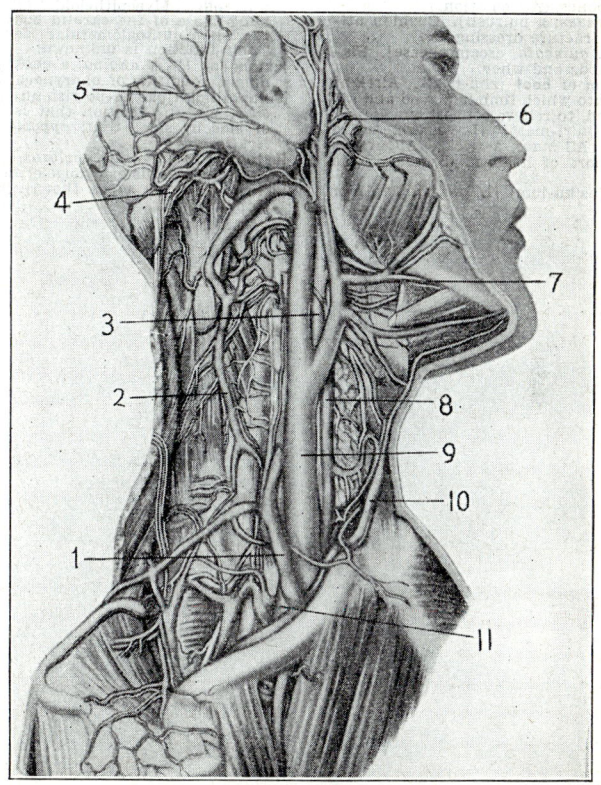

VEINS OF RIGHT SIDE OF NECK
1. External jugular vein. 2. Posterior jugular vein. 3. Carotid artery. 4. Occipital veins. 5. Posterior auricular veins. 6. Temporal veins. 7. Facial vein. 8. Superior thyroid vein. 9. Internal jugular vein. 10. Anterior jugular vein. 11. Subclavian vein.

jujitsu, jiujitsu digestive juice of the pancreas poured into the duodenum. It contains the enzymes *trypsin, amylase,* and *lipase* or *steapsin*.

jujitsu, jiujitsu. A system of physical training for developing the art of self-defense without weapons in which the opponent's weight and strength are used to his disadvantage. Esp. developed in Japan.

jumentous (jū-men′tus) [L. *jumentum*, beast of burden]. Like that of a horse, said of odor of urine.

jum′per. One with nervous disorder who is startled easily or who jumps at sound of a loud noise. SEE: *palmus*.

junction (junk′shun) [L. *junctiō*, a joining]. The place of union or coming together of two parts.

   j., mucocutaneous. A jct. between the skin and a mucous membrane.

   j., myoneural. SYN: *motor end-plate.* Meeting point of a nerve with the muscle to which it is distributed.

   j., sclerocorneal. Meeting point bet. the sclera and the cornea marked on the external surface of the eyeball by the outer scleral sulcus.

junctura (junk-tu′rā) [L. a joining]. Suture of bones. Articulation.

junk [L. *juncus*, a bulrush]. Cushion utilized in fracture dressing.

junk′et [It. *guincata*, cream cheese]. Flavored curds and whey.

Junod's arm or **boot** (zhu-nōz′). Airtight casing into which limb is placed and air exhausted, to relieve congestion.

jurymast (ju′ri-mast) [L. *jurāre*, to be right, + AS *masc*, a stick]. Apparatus for support of head in disease of the spine.

jusculum (jus′ku-lum) [L. broth]. Broth or soup.

Juster's reflex. Finger extension instead of flexion when palm of hand is irritated.

jus′to ma′jor [L. larger than normal]. Bigger than normal, as a *pelvis*.

   j. mi′nor [L. smaller than normal]. Smaller than normal, as a *pelvis*.

Jus′tus' test. A test for syphilis determined by the reaction on hemoglobin of a dose of mercury.

jute (jūt) [Sanskrit *jūta*, matted hair]. Fiber used in dressings.

juvantia (ju-van′shĭ-ā) [L. *juvāre*, to aid]. Adjuvant medicines which intensify action of other drugs or assist them.

juvenile. 1. Pert. to youth or childhood. 2. Young; immature.

   j. cell. A metamyelocyte or white blood cell.

juxta- [L. near to]. Prefix: Close proximity.

jux″taartic′ular [" + *articulus*, joint]. Situated close to a joint.

juxtaglomerular. Near or adjacent to a glomerulus.

   j. apparatus. A structure consisting of myoepitheloid cells forming a cuff surrounding the arteriole leading to a glomerulus of the kidney.

   j. cells. Myoepitheloid cells resembling those of the carotid body present in the juxtaglomerular apparatus. Their function is unknown.

juxtangi′na [" + *angina*, a choking]. Inflamed condition of pharyngeal muscles.

juxtaposition (juks″ta-po-zish′un) [" + *positiō*, place]. Position that is adjacent or side by side. SYN: *apposition, contiguity*.

juxtapylor′ic [" + G. *pylōros*, pylorus]. Near the pylorus or pyloric orifice.

juxtaspi′nal [" + *spina*, thorn]. Near the spinal column.

K

K Chem. symb. for *kalium*, potassium.
Ka. Abbr. for *cathode*.
Ka'der's opera'tion. Surgical formation of a gastric fistula with feeding tube inserted through valvelike flap.
Kaes' feltwork. Nerve fiber network in cerebral cortex.
kaf'fir pox. Modified smallpox with pustules not umbilicated and without a secondary rise in temperature. SYN: *alastrim*.
Kahl'baum's disease. Cyclic dementia with marked muscular tension. SYN: *katatonia, q.v.*
Kahl'er's disease. Destructive bone marrow disease. SYN: *multiple myeloma, q.v.*
Kahn test. 1. A flocculation test for the diagnosis of syphilis.
Positive reaction based upon appearance of a white precipitate when an alcoholic extract of normal heart muscle is added to the blood serum of one afflicted with syphilis.
2. Test for presence of carcinoma.
kaif (kīf) [Arabic *gaif*, quiescence]. A dreamy, tranquil state induced by drugs.
kainophobia (ki-no-fo'bĭ-ă) [G. *kainos*, new, + *phobos*, fear]. Abnormal aversion to new situations and things. SYN: *neophobia*.
kais'erling, Kais'erling's solution. Liquid used in preserving pathological specimens.
kakergasia (kak-er-gas'ĭ-ă) [G. *kakos*, bad, + *ergasia*, work]. 1. Minor psychosis; a term used in place of "neurosis" and "psychoneurosis" when psychodynamic and not primarily nervous. 2. Poor mental functioning. SYN: *merergasia*.
kakergastic (kak-er-gas'tik) [" + *ergasia*, work]. Pert. to minor psychoses.
Applied to those still relatively normal, afflicted with vagaries not of a holergastic* nature. SYN: *merergastic*.
kakesthe'sia [" + *aisthēsis*, sensation]. 1. Any disorder of sensibility. 2. Malaise.
kakidro'sis [" + *idrōsis*, sweat]. Unpleasant odor of the sweat. SYN: *bromidrosis*. [neuritis. SYN: *beriberi*.
kak'ke [Japanese]. Endemic form of poly-
kakosmia (kak-oz'mĭ-ă) [G. *kakos*, bad, + *osmē*, smell]. Perception of bad odors which do not exist. SYN: *cacosmia, parosmia*.
kakotrophy (kak-ot'rof-i) [" + *trophē*, nourishment]. Malnutrition. SYN: *cacotrophy*.
kala azar (kă''la-a'-zar) [Native, "black fever"]. SYN: *Leishmaniasis*. Visceral leishmaniasis, an infectious disease, common in the East. There are several types which differ as to preference for children or adults, incidence in domestic animals, and transmitting agent. The disease is characterized by lesions of the reticuloendothelial system, esp. the liver and spleen. It is often fatal.
ETIOL: *Leishmania donovani*, a flagellated protozoan. The organism is transmitted by sandflies of the genus *Phlebotomus*; however, direct infection through nasal secretions, urine, and feces is possible.
kaliemia (kal-ĭ-e'mĭ-ă) [L. *kali*, potash, + G. *aima*, blood]. Potassium in the blood.
kaligenous (ka-lij'en-us) [" + G. *gennan*, to produce]. Forming potash.

kalimeter (kal-im'e-ter) [" + G. *metron*, measure]. Device for determining degree of alkalinity of a substance. SYN: *alkalimeter*.
ka'lium [L.]. (K) Potassium. A mineral element necessary to the growth of cells, esp. those of the muscles and blood. SEE: *potassium*.
kallikrein (kăl-ĭk're-ĭn). A vasodilator substance obtained from normal urine. Its origin is unknown, although it is present in the pancreas in considerable amounts.
kaolin (kā'o-lin). A yellowish white powder, occurring as a decomposition product of feldspar.
USES: Internally as an absorbent; externally, as a protective by absorbing moisture.
DOSAGE: ½ oz. (15 Gm.).
kaolinosis (kā''o-lin-o'sĭs). Pneumokoniosis caused by inhaling kaolin particles.
kaomagma (kā''ō-mag'mă). A 20% suspension of colloidal kaolin in 2½% aluminum hydroxide.
USES: In intestinal inflammation, dysentery, colitis, etc.
DOSAGE: ½ oz. (15 cc.).
k. with mineral oil. Kaomagma with 20% mineral oil.
Dosage: ½ oz. (15 cc.).
Kapo'si's disease. Diffuse atrophic skin condition. SYN: *xeroderma pigmentosum, q.v.*
Karell cure (ka'rel). Rest in bed, milk sipped in small amounts (not over a quart a day for 5 or 6 days), for treatment of cardiac disease, high blood pressure, and renal insufficiency.
K. diet. A saltless diet constituting a fraction of usual normal diet, given in small quantities at definite intervals, gradually increased by adding other foods; intended to relieve the vital organs. For the first 7 days 200 cc. of milk constitutes diet, given every 4 hours bet. 8 A. M. and 8 P. M., after which soft boiled egg and toast, unsalted butter, cereal, and cream soups are added twice a day, and after 10th day chopped meat, vegetables, and rice boiled in milk, custard, and dextrimaltose are added.
Diet low in calories, vitamins, and iron.
K. d., modified. Found useful when milk is not well tolerated. Food value, water, and salt content only slightly changed.
karyo- [G. *karyon*, nucleus]. Prefix: Referring to a cell's nucleus.
kar''yochromat'ophil [" + *chrōma*, color, + *philein*, to love]. Having nucleus which stains.
karyochrome (kar'ĭ-o-krōm) [" + *chrōma*, color]. The cell of a nerve with an easily staining nucleus.
karyoc'lasis [G. *karyon*, nucleus, + *klasis*, a breaking]. SYN: *karyorrhexis*. The fragmentation of a cell nucleus.
karyogamy (kar-ĭ-og'ă-mĭ) [" + *gamos*, marriage]. Union of nuclei in cell conjugation.
karyogen (kar'ĭ-o-jen) [" + *gennan*, to produce]. A compound of iron in certain cell nuclei.
karyogenesis (kar''ĭ-ō-jĕn'ĕ-sĭs) [G. *karyon*, nucleus, + *genesis*, production].

karyokinesis Formation and development of a cell nucleus.
karyokinesis (kar″ĭ-o-kin-e′sis) [" + *kinēsis*, movement]. 1. Changes taking place in a nucleus during indirect cell division. SYN: *mitosis*. 2. In a narrower sense, nuclear division only.
karyokinetic (ka″rĭ-o-kĭ-net′ĭk) [" + *kinēsis*, movement]. 1. Pert. to karyokinesis. 2. Ameboid.
karyolobism (kar″ĭ-o-lo′bizm) [G. *karyon*, nucleus, + L. *lobus*, lobe, + G. *ismos*, state of]. Condition in which the nucleus of a cell is lobed as in polymorphonuclear leukocytes.
kar′yolymph [" + L. *lympha*, lymph]. Fluid in meshes of the nucleus. SYN: *nuclear sap*.
karyolysis (kar-ĭ-ol′ĭ-sis) [" + *lysis*, dissolution]. The destruction of a nucleus or loss of affinity for basic dyes. SYN: *chromatolysis*.
karyolyt′ic [G. *karyon*, nucleus, + *lysis*, dissolution]. Producing or rel. to karyolysis.
karyomitome (kar-ĭ-om′ĭ-tōm) [" + *mitos*, web]. Network of the cell nucleus.
karyomitosis (kar″ĭ-o-mit-o′sis) [" + "-*osis*]. Nuclear changes in cell division. SYN: *karyokinesis*.
karyomorphism (kar″ĭ-o-mōr′fizm) [" + *morphē*, form, + *ismos*, state of]. The form of a cell nucleus.
karyon (kar′ĭ-on) [G.]. The cell nucleus.
karyophage (kăr′ĭ-ō-fāj) [G. *karyon*, nucleus, + *cleus*, + *phagein*, to eat]. An intracellular protozoan parasite which destroys the nucleus of a cell.
karyorrhexis (kar″ĭ-o-rek′sis) [" + *rēxis*, rupture]. Fragmentation of the chromatin in nuclear disintegration.
karyosome (kar′ĭ-ō-som) [G. *karyon*, nucleus, + *soma*, body]. SYN: *chromatin nucleolus*. 1. Chromatin mass at nodes of nuclear network. 2. A spherical mass of chromatin designated *false nucleolus* to differentiate it from the true nucleolus.
karyotheca (kar″ĭ-o-the′kă) [" + *thēkē*, sheath]. The enveloping membrane of a cell nucleus.
kata- [G.]. Prefix: Down.
katab′olism [G. *kata*, down, + *ballein*, to throw, + *ismos*, stage of]. The breaking down process in metabolism. SYN: *catabolism*.
kataphrax′is [" + *phraxis*, a blocking]. Surgical formation of metallic supports for an organ.
kataplasia (kăt-ă-plā′sĭ-ă). SYN: *cataplasia*. Reversion of a degenerating or atrophied cell to the form of a developing or embryonic cell.
katastalsis (kat-ă-stal′sis) [G. *katastellein*, to check]. SYN: *catastalsis*. Term for gastric downward moving wave of contraction which occurs without a preceding wave of inhibition.
katathermometer (ka″ta-ther-mom′e-ter) [G. *kata*, down, + *thermē*, heat, + *metron*, measure]. A thermometer for measuring the efficiency of ventilation and cooling and drying processes, *i. e.*, the measurement of the cooling power (or, in a very warm atmosphere, of the warming power) of the atmosphere exerted on surface of the thermometer, approximately body temperature (37.0° C. or 98.6° F.) in millicalories (1/1000 Gm. calories) per square centimeter per second and to find air velocities.
The dry kata gives the cooling power by radiation and convection. The wet kata gives the cooling power by radiation, convection, and evaporation.

katatonia (kat-a-tō′ni-a) [" + *tonos*, tension). SEE: *catatonia*.
katelectrotonus (kat″el-ek-trot′o-nus) [" + *electron*, amber, + *tonos*, tension]. Increased excitability in a muscle or nerve in area near cathode during passage of a current. SYN: *catelectrotonus*, *q.v.*
katharom′eter [G. *katharos*, pure, + *metron*, measure]. Electrical device to measure basal metabolic rates.
kathisophobia (kath-ĭ-so-fo′bi-a) [G. *kathizein*, to sit down, + *phobos*, fear]. Fear of sitting down, and subsequent inability to sit still.
kation (kat′ĭ-on) [G. *kation*, descending]. Element appearing at the cathode or negative pole in electrochemical decomposition. SYN: *cation*.
katotro′pia [" + *tropos*, a turning]. Tendency of the eyeball to drop too far downward. SYN: *katophoria*.
KBr. Potassium bromide.
KC₂H₃O₂. Potassium acetate.
KCl. Potassium chloride.
KClO. Potassium hypochlorite.
KClO₃. Potassium chlorate.
K₂CO₃. Potassium carbonate.
kefir, kefyr (ke′fer) [Caucasian]. A preparation of curdled milk.
kelectome (ke′lek-tōm) [G. *kēle*, tumor, + *tomē*, incision]. Instrument for removing specimen of tumor tissue.
kelis (ke′lis) [G. *kēlis*, stain, scar]. 1. Skin disease with pigmented pink and purple patches and lesions leaving scars. SYN: *morphea*. 2. Skin tumor of dense tissue. SYN: *keloid*.
Kel′log's inspiratory lift-exercise. Abdominal exercise for the puerperium.
Kel′ly pad. A drainage pad for the operating table or bed made by wrapping one end of a rubber sheet over a rolled small blanket, forming a bolster; the bolster is twisted round like a horseshoe to form the pad, the free part of the sheet forming the apron. Also commercial inflatable rubber pad of horseshoe shape used in same way.
keloid (ke′loid) [G. *kēlis*, scar, + *eidos*, form]. 1. Scar tissue. 2. A new growth of the skin consisting of dense tissue; most common in the colored race.
k., acne. SYN: *dermatitis papillaris capillitii*. Hypertrophic scars on nape of neck at border of scalp.
ETIOL: Suppurative folliculitis.
k., Addison's. Skin disease with pigmented patches and lesions. SYN: *morphea, q.v.*
k., Alibert's. Growth of fibrous tissue usually at the site of a scar resembling a true keloid.
ETIOL: Predisposition a factor; essential cause unknown.
SYM: Oval, elongated, or irregularly shaped mass, single or lobulated, tender, painful, with burning or pricking sensation. Ranges in size from that of a bean to that of a hand. It sends out clawlike processes as it increases in size.
PROG: Usually permanent if removed, but sometimes returns.
TREATMENT: X-rays, radium, carbon dioxide snow.
k. en plaque. Circumscribed hard plate elevated a little over surface and imbedded in the skin.
keloidosis (ke-loi-do′sis) [" + *-ōsis*]. The formation of keloids.
kelotomy (ke-lot′o-mĭ) [G. *kēle*, hernia, + *tomē*, incision]. Operation for strangulated hernia through tissues of the constricting neck.

Kenny treatment. Treatment originated by Sister Kenny, an Australian nurse, for anterior poliomyelitis. Consists of application of hot, moist packs to affected muscles and early re-education of muscles, first through passive exercise and then by active movements as soon as possible. Rigid fixation of paralyzed limbs is disparaged.

kenogenesis (ken-o-jen'ē-sis) [G. *koinos*, common, + *genesis*, formation]. Deviation from the normal in course of development.

kenophobia (ken-o-fō'bĭ-ă) [G. *kenos*, empty, + *phobos*, fear]. Fear of empty spaces.

kephalin (kef'a-lĭn) [G. *kephalē*, head]. Commercial headache remedy. SYN: *cephalin*.

ker'asin. A cerebroside isolated from brain tissue.

keratalgia (ker-a-tal'jĭ-ă) [G. *keras, kerat-*, horn, + *algos*, pain]. Neuralgia of the cornea.

keratectasia (ker-a-tek-ta'sĭ-ă) [" + *ektasis*, extension]. Conical protrusion of the cornea.

keratectomy (ker-ă-tek'to-mĭ) [" + *ektomē*, excision]. Excision of portion of cornea.

keratiasis (ker-ă-tī'a-sis) [G. *keras, kerat-*, horn]. Horny wart formation.

kerat'ic [G. *keras, kerat-*, horn]. Rel. to horn. SYN: *corneous, horny*.

ker'atin [G. *keras, kerat-*, horn]. A scleroprotein substance in hair, nails, and horny tissue, insoluble in gastric juice. Used for coating pills which should not be dissolved in the stomach.

keratinous (ker-at'in-us) [G. *keras, kerat-*, horn]. Pert. to or composed of keratin.

keratitis (ker-ă-tī'tis) [" + *-itis*, inflammation]. Inflammation of cornea.

k., aspergillar. K. of cornea due to infection from a mold.

k., band shaped. Whitish or grayish band extending across the cornea.

k. bullosa. The formation of large, quite resistant blebs in the cornea of blind trachomatous eyes with increased tension.

k., deep. SEE: *interstitial k.*

k., dendritic. Superficial branching corneal ulcers. [ity in middle of cornea.

k. disciformis. Gray disk-shaped opac-

k., fascicular. Corneal ulcer resulting from phlyctenules which spread from limbus to center of cornea accompanied by fascicle of blood vessels.

k., herpetic. Vesicular keratitis in herpes zoster. [pus in ant. chamber.

k., hypopyon. Serpiginous ulcer with

k., interstitial. Deep form of nonsuppurative k. with vascularization, occurring usually in syphilis and rarely in tuberculosis. Commonly found between 5th and 15th years. [and loss in vision. SYM: Pain, photophobia, lacrimation,

k., lagophthalmic. Desiccation of cornea due to defective closure of lids.

k., mycotic. Produced by mold fungi.

k., neuroparalytic. Dull and slightly cloudy insensitive cornea seen in lesions of fifth nerve.

k., parenchymatous. SEE: *interstitial k.*

k., phlyctenular. Circumscribed inflammation of conjunctiva and cornea accompanied by formation of small projections called phlyctenules which consist of accumulations of lymphoid cells. The phlyctenules soften at the apices, forming ulcers.

k., punctate. Cellular deposits on post. surface of cornea seen in diseases of uveal tract.

k., purulent. K. with formation of pus.

k., sclerosing. Triangular opacity in deeper layers of cornea, associated with scleritis.

k., superficial punctate. Small gray spots in superficial layers of cornea, beneath Bowman's membrane, occurring in young persons.

k., trachomatous. K. with abnormal membrane on cornea. SYN: *pannus*.

k., traumatic. K. caused by wound of the cornea.

k., vasculonebulous. SEE: *trachomatous k.*

k., xerotic. Softening, desiccation and ulceration of cornea. SYN: *keratomalacia*.

TREATMENT: *Local:* Calomel dusted on the eyeball, yellow oxide of mercury ointment 1-2%; hot compresses, atropine, antiseptic solutions. *General:* Proper diet with elimination of sweets and plenty of fresh air, cod liver oil, good general hygiene.

kerato-, kerat- [G.]. Combining form: Rel. to horny substances or to the cornea.

keratocele (ker-ă'to-sēl) [G. *keras, kerat-*, horn, + *kēlē*, hernia, tumor]. Protrusion or herniation of Descemet's membrane through the floor of corneal ulcer.

keratoconjunctivitis (kĕr"a-tō-kŏn-jŭnk-tĭ-vī'tis). Inflammation of the cornea and the conjunctiva.

k., epidemic. An acute, self-limited infection due to a virus.

k., flash. K. resulting from exposure of the eyes to intense ultraviolet irradiation.

k., virus. Epidemic k., *q.v.*

keratoconus (ker-at-o-ko'nus) [" + *kōnos*, cone]. Conical protrusion of center of cornea without inflammation.

keratoderma (ker-ă-tō-dĕr'mă) [G. *keras, kerat-*, horn, + *derma*, skin]. 1. Keratodermia, *q.v.* 2. The cornea.

keratodermatitis (ker"ă-tō-der-mă-tī'tis) [" + " + *-itis*, inflammation]. Inflammation of the horny layer of the skin with proliferation.

ker"atoder'mia [G. *keras, kerat-*, horn, + *derma*, skin]. 1. Hypertrophy of the stratum corneum or horny layer of the epidermis, esp. on the palms of hands and soles of feet producing a horny condition of the skin.

keratogenous (ker-ă-tŏj'en-us) [" + *gennan*, to produce]. Causing horny tissue development.

ker"atoglo'bus [" + L. *globus*, circle]. Globular protrusion and enlargement of cornea seen in congenital glaucoma.

keratohelcosis (ker"a-to-hel-ko'sis) [" + *elkōsis*, ulceration]. Corneal ulceration.

keratohyalin. A substance present in the form of granules in the cytoplasm of cells in the stratum granulosum and thought to be a precursor of keratin.

ker'atoid [" + *eidos*, form]. Horny or resembling horn or corneal tissue.

keratoiditis (ker"ă-toid-ī'tis) [" + " + *-itis*, inflammation]. Inflammation of the cornea.

keratoiritis (ker"a-to-i-rī'tis) [" + *iris*, iris, + *-itis*, inflammation]. Inflammation of the cornea and iris.

keratoleptynsis (ker"ă-to-lep-tin'sis) [" + *leptynein*, to make thin]. Removal of the corneal surface, then covering the area with bulbar conjunctiva.

keratoleukoma (ker"ă-to-lu-ko'mă) [" + *leukos*, white, + *ōma*, tumor]. White corneal opacity.

keratolysis (ker-ă-tŏl'is-is) [" + *lysis*, loosening]. 1. Loosening of horny layer of the skin. 2. Shedding of the skin at regular intervals.

keratolytic   K-4   **ketogenic diet**

keratolyt'ic [" + *lysis*, loosening]. Rel. to or causing keratolysis. SYN: *desquamative*.

kerato'ma [G. *keras, kerat-*, horn, + *ōma*, tumor]. 1. A callosity. 2. A horny growth. SYN: *keratosis*.

keratomalacia (ker″at-o-ma-la′sĭ-ă). SYN: *xerotic keratitis*. Softening of the cornea seen in early childhood due to deficiencies of vitamin A.

keratome (ker′at-ōm) [" + *tomē*, incision]. Knife for incising the cornea.

keratometer (ker-at-om′et-er) [" + *metron*, meter]. An instrument for measuring the curves of the cornea.

keratomycosis (ker″at-o-mĭ-ko′sis) [" + *mykes*, fungus, + *ōsis*]. Fungous growth on the cornea.

ker″atono′sis [" + *nosos*, disease]. Any noninflammatory disease of the horny layer of the skin.

keratonyxis (ker″ă-to-niks′is) [" + *nyssein*, to puncture]. Corneal puncture, esp. surgical puncture.

keratoplasty (ker′ă-to-plas″tĭ) [" + *plassein*, to form]. Plastic operation on the cornea.

ker″atopro′tein [" + *prōtos*, first]. The protein of the hair, nails, epidermis, etc.

keratorrhexis (ker″a-to-rek′sĭs) [" + *rēxis*, rupture]. Corneal rupture.

keratoscleritis (ker″ă-to-skle-ri′tis) [" + *sklēros*, hard, + -*itis*, inflammation]. Inflammation of both cornea and sclera.

keratoscope (ker′at-o-skōp) [" + *skopein*, to examine]. An instrument for examination of the cornea.

keratos′copy [" + *skopein*, to examine]. Examination of the cornea and its reflection of light.

keratose (ker′ă-tōs) [G. *keras, kerat-*, horn]. Horny.

keratosis (ker-a-tō′sĭs) [G. *keras, kerat-* horn, + *osis*]. 1. Horny growth. 2. Any condition of the skin characterized by the formation of horny growths or excessive development of the horny growth.

   k. blennorrhagica. Condition associated with gonorrheal arthritis characterized by development of horny growths, esp. on hands and feet.

   k. climatericum. A skin disease occurring in women during the menopause, characterized by a circumscribed hyperkeratosis of the palms and soles.

   k. follicular. SYN: *Darier's disease, iothyosis follicularis, psorospermosis*.

   k. palmaris et plantaris. Chronic disorder showing thickening of horny layer of palms and soles.

   ETIOL: Congenital, usually hereditary, occurring in several generations.

   PROG: Alleviation but no cure.

   TREATMENT: Keratolytics, x-rays.

   k. pilaris. Inflammatory disorder, chronic in course.

   SYM: Accumulation of horny material at follicular orifices, giving to affected surfaces a nutmeg-graterlike appearance, commonly in those with rough, dry skin. Most pronounced in winter, on lateral aspects of thighs and upper arms, with possible extension to legs, forearms and scalp.

   TREATMENT: Tonics in anemic and debilitated. Locally, green soap, alkaline baths, rosewater ointment or glycerin lotion. In bearded region soothing cream and "once-over" shaving with very keen razor. SYN: *pityriasis pilaris*.

   k. seborrheica. Flat, rough, crusted or scaly keratic lesion.

   ETIOL: Inherent peculiarity of skin—harshness with evidence of long-standing dry seborrhea, with long continued exposure to strong sunlight and sudden temperature changes.

   SYM: Keratoid, nevoid, acanthoid or verrucose types, occurring in elderly and in those with long-standing dry seborrhea, on face, scalp, interscapular or sternal regions and backs of hands, yellowish, grayish, brownish sharply circumscribed lesions covered with a firmly adherent scale, greasy or velvety, on trunk or scalp, but harsh, rough and dry on face or hands. Never disappear spontaneously and are potentially malignant.

   TREATMENT: Earlier keratoid lesions removed by bland grease with subsequent occasional lubrication of site. Avoidance of alkaline soaps and water. For verrucose, nevoid, and advanced keratoid forms, carbon dioxide snow. Those showing malignant change are treated as carcinoma of the skin. SYN: *senile wart, seborrheic wart*.

   k. seni'lis. Dry, harsh skin of the aged.

keratotome (ker′ă-to-tōm) [" + *tomē*, incision]. A knife for incising the cornea. SYN: *keratome*.

keratotomy (ker-at-ot′o-mĭ) [" + *tomē*, incision]. Incision of cornea.

keraunoneurosis (kĕ-raw″no-nū-ro′sis) [G. *keraunos*, lightning, + *neuron*, nerve]. A neurosis from fear of a thunderstorm or from lightning stroke.

keraunophobia (kĕ-raw″no-fo′bĭ-ă) [" + *phobos*, fear]. Dread of thunder and lightning.

kerectomy (ke-rek′to-mĭ) [G. *keras*, cornea, + *ektomē*, excision]. Excision of a portion of the cornea.

kerion (ke′rĭ-on). A form of *tinea tonsurans* with swollen discharging lesions.

   k. celsi. SYN: *tinea kerion*. Inflammation of the hair follicles of the beard and scalp with formation of pustules.

kerither′apy [G. *keros*, wax, + *therapeia*, treatment]. Treatment of burns and denuded surfaces with liquid paraffin.

Kerk′ring's folds or valves. Transverse folds of intestinal mucous membranes. SYN: *plicae circulares, valvulae conniventes*.

kernic′terus. A form of icterus neonatorum occurring in infants in which nuclear masses of the brain and spinal cord undergo pathologic changes accompanied by deposition of bile pigment within them.

Ker′nig's sign. A symptom of meningitis, evidenced by reflex contraction and pain in the hamstring muscles when attempting to extend the leg after flexing the thigh upon the body.

ketogenesis (ke-to-jen′ĕ-sis) [*ketone* + G. *genesis*, production]. Production of ketones or acetone substances.

ketogenic diet (ke-to-jen′ik) [" + G. *gennan*, to produce]. One that produces acetone or ketone bodies, or mild acidosis. Highly beneficial in epilepsy.

   Protein maintenance allowable. Carbohydrates are increased 10 Gm. per month after 3 months. Protein increased and alternated with carbohydrates 6 to 9 months later, and fat reduction 12 months later. Yeast for vitamin B and calcium lactate to insure adequate calcium, recommended by Peterman. Both fats and proteins yield antiketogenic as well as ketogenic derivatives.

   Carbohydrates yield no ketogenic bodies and are 100% antiketogenic. Fats yield 90% ketogenic bodies and are 10% antiketogenic.

   Proteins yield 46% ketogenic bodies and

ketohexose — kidney

are 54% antiketogenic. The ratio usually necessary to produce ketosis is: ketogenic to antiketogenic 2.5 to 1, or 3 to 1.

	For a 10 yr. old child	For a 5 yr. old child
	% cals.	Cals.
Carbohydrates	60	60
Protein	136	72
Fat	1593	1188
Total	1789	1320

Minimum protein, high fat, low carbohydrate. Fatty acid glucose varies with the ease with which ketosis is attained and with the intensity of ketosis desired.

ketohex′ose. A nonsaccharide consisting of a six-carbon chain and containing a ketone group, in addition to alcohol groups. EXAM: *fructose.*

ke′tol. Crystalline substance formed in intestine and pancreas during putrefaction and digestion.

ketol′ysis [" + G. *lysis,* dissolution]. The dissolution of acetone or ketone bodies.

ketolyt′ic [" + *lysis,* dissolution]. Pert. to ketolysis.

ketone (ke′tōn). Oxidation product of a secondary alcohol. Organic chemical substance of the general formula $\begin{smallmatrix}R\\R\end{smallmatrix}\!\!>\!\!CO$.

The simplest example is *acetone.* The ketone acids in the body are the end products of fat metabolism.

   k. bodies. A group of compounds produced during the oxidation of fatty acids, which includes acetoacetic acid, B-hydroxybutyric acid, and acetone. SEE: *ketosis.*

   k. threshold. Ketone level in the blood above which ketone bodies appear in the urine.

ketonemia (ke-to-ne′mĭ-ă) [*ketone* + G. *aima,* blood]. Acetone bodies in the blood. SYN: *acidosis.*

ketonuria (ke-ton-u′rĭ-ă) [" + G. *ouron,* urine]. Acetone bodies in the urine.

ketopla′sia [" + G. *plassein,* to form]. The formation or excretion of ketones.

ketoplas′tic [" + G. *plastikos,* formed]. Pert. to ketoplasia or formation of ketones.

ke′tose. A carbohydrate containing the ketones.

ketosis (kē-tō′sĭs) [*ketone* + G. *-ōsis,* disease]. The accumulation in the body of the ketone bodies: acetone, betahydroxybutyric acid, and aceto-acetic acid.

It is frequently associated with acidosis and is often miscalled acidosis. Ketosis results from the incomplete combustion of fatty acids, generally from carbohydrate deficiency or inadequate utilization, and is commonly observed in starvation, high fat diet, pregnancy, following ether anesthesia, and most significantly in diabetes mellitus. Large quantities of these ketone bodies may be eliminated in the urine (ketonuria). The presence of ketosis is easily determined by testing for the presence of acetone or diacetic acid in the urine, a ketonuria being 1 of the first evidences of beginning acidosis in diabetes. SEE: *acidosis.*

17-ke′tosteroid. One of a group of neutral steroids having a ketone group in position 17. They are produced by the adrenal cortex and gonads and appear normally in the urine. Among them are androsterone, dehydroisoandrosterone, and 11-hydroxyisoandrosterone.

Key-Ret′zius foram′ina. Passages in the pia mater carrying the choroid plexus to the fourth ventricle.

Kg. Abbr. for *kilogram.*
KHCO₃. Potassium bicarbonate.
KHSO₄. Potassium bisulfate.
KI. Potassium iodide.
kibe (kīb) [Welsh *cibi,* chilblain]. Inflamed patch on hands or feet caused by exposure to cold. SYN: *chilblain, q.v.*
kid′ney [A. S. *cwith,* womb, + Ice. *nyra,* kidney]. One of two glandular, bean-shaped bodies, purplish-brown in color, situated at the back of the abdominal cavity, one on each side of the spinal column which excrete waste matter in the form of urine.

The upper level is opp. the 12th thoracic (dorsal) vertebra, the lower level opp. the 3rd lumbar vertebra. The right kidney is slightly lower than the left one. WEIGHT: 120-180 Gm. (4-6 oz.). Size, about 11.5 cm. (4½ in.) long, 5-7.5 cm. (2-3 in.) broad, and 2.5 cm. (1 in.) thick.

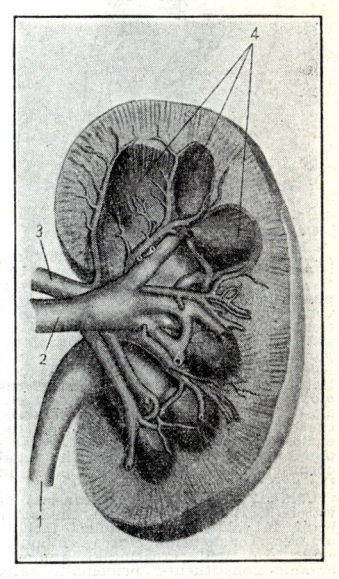

INTERIOR OF KIDNEY
DISTRIBUTION OF VESSELS
1. The ureter. 2. Renal vein. 3. Renal artery. 4. Renal pyramids.

Each kidney is embedded in fatty tissue known as an adipose *capsule,* and surrounded by the renal fascia, a sheath of fibrous tissue, which helps to hold the kidney in place. The concave border of the kidney faces the median line, the center of the concave border opening into a fissure called the *hilum.*

The ureter enters the kidney through the hilum into the *pelvis* of the kidney. The outer portion of the kidney is the *cortex,* a mass of cortical substance; the inner portion (medullary substance) is the *medulla.*

Within the cortical substance are found the arteries, veins, convoluted tubules, and glomerular capsules, while the medulla contains the renal pyramids, conical masses with papillae projecting into the cuplike cavities (calyces) of the pelvis.

Each kidney contains from 8 to 18 pyramids made up of collecting tubules, lymphatics, and blood vessels, the pyramids being penetrated by the cortical substance and supporting them; these extensions are known as the renal columns, or columns of Bertini.

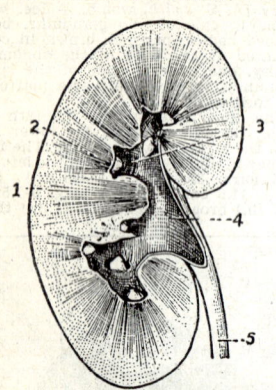

RIGHT KIDNEY, POSTERIOR VIEW OF SECTION
1. Cortex. 2. Renal pyramid. 3. Calyx. 4. Pelvis. 5. Ureter.

The cortical and medullary substance is composed of renal tubules, connective tissue, blood vessels, nerves, and lymphatics. The *renal tubule* or *nephron* constitutes the structural and functional unit of the kidney. Each consists of a *capsule, proximal convoluted portion, loop of Henle* and *distal convoluted portion*, which leads to a collecting duct. The capsule, called the *glomerular* or *Bowman's capsule*, encloses a globular mass of capillaries, the glomerulus. The capsule and the enclosed glomerulus comprise the *malpighian* or *renal corpuscle*. The renal corpuscles are located principally in the cortex.

URINE FORMATION: Urine consists of water (95%) and solids (5%), the latter being in solution. The solids include organic constituents (urea, hippuric acid, uric acid, creatinine) and inorganic constituents, principally salts of sodium and potassium. The kidneys remove these substances from the blood thus acting to maintain homeostasis of the blood and body fluids. Urine is formed by the processes of *filtration* and *reabsorption*. As blood passes through the glomerulus, water and dissolved substances are filtered through the capillary walls and the inner or visceral layer of Bowman's capsule, resulting in formation of the *glomerular filtrate*. Blood cells and colloidal substances such as proteins are retained within the capillaries. The glomerular filtrate passes through the renal tubules to the collecting ducts, during the course of which all of the sugar and some of the salts and other substances are *selectively reabsorbed* into the capillaries surrounding the tubule. There is some evidence that the cells of the tubules may add by the process of secretion some substances such as urea and uric acid to the urine. The final product now known as *urine* passes through straight *collecting ducts* into larger collecting ducts (*papillary ducts*) which open on the tips of the renal papillae. There urine is discharged into the minor calyces of the renal pelvis, and then is conveyed by the ureters to the bladder. Periodically the bladder discharges its contents to the outside through the *urethra* (*micturition*).

Substances which are entirely or almost entirely reabsorbed during passage through the tubule are known as *high threshhold substances*. These include glucose and chlorides of sodium, potassium, calcium, and magnesium. These are important blood constituents and excreted only when their concentrations in the blood are above normal. *Low* or *nonthreshold substances* are those which are reabsorbed only in limited quantities or not at all. These are usually waste products of metabolism such as urea, uric acid, and creatine which appear in considerable quantities in the urine.

The formation of urine is a continuous process, the rate of filtration being dependent primarily upon the blood pressure within the glomeruli. Osmotic pressure exerted by proteins within the blood plasma tends to hold water and dissolved substances within the blood vessels so that the effective filtration pressure (45 mm. Hg) is the difference between capillary blood pressure (70 mm. Hg) and osmotic pressure (25 mm. Hg). General blood pressure and the velocity of blood flow are primary factors in the rate of urine formation.

The volume of urine excreted daily varies from 1000 cc. to 2000 cc. (av. 1500 cc.). The amount varies with water intake, nature of diet, degree of body activity, environmental and body temperature, age, blood pressure, and many other factors. Pathological conditions may affect the volume and nature of the urine excreted.

NERVE SUPPLY: From renal plexuses forming rich networks about renal vessels. Include both sympathetic and parasympathetic (vagal) fibers.

SYMPTOMS OF KIDNEY DISORDER: Lumbar pain, renal colic, disturbances in micturition (anuria, oliguria, or pain on micturition), presence of blood, pus, or abdominal substances in the urine, tenderness or swelling in costovertebral region, enlargement or diminution in size of kidney, edema.

KIDNEY EXAMINATION: By palpation, intravenous pyelography, cystoscopy, panendoscopy.

k., amyloid. K. which is the seat of amyloid degeneration.

k., branny. K. in which spots of fatty degeneration give it the appearance of containing bran.

k., contracted. The small k. of chronic interstitial or diffuse nephritis.

k., cystic. One that has undergone cystic degeneration.

k., embolic contracted. A contracted k. in which embolic infarction of the renal arterioles produces degeneration of renal tissue, and hyperplasia of fibrous tissues produces irregular contraction.

k., fatty. One with fatty infiltration or degeneration of tubular, glomerular, or capsular epithelium, or of vascular connective tissue.

k., floating. One which is displaced and movable.

k., gouty. One with necrosis of renal connective tissue.

k., granular. A slow form of chronic nephritis, in which the size is diminished, and color is red with hard, fibrous, and granular texture.

k., hobnail. Granular k.

k., hogback. Pigback k., *q.v.*

k., horseshoe. Congenital malformation with sup. or inf. extremities united by an isthmus of renal or fibrous tissue, in the form of a horseshoe.

k., lardaceous. Chronic nephritis, often secondary to syphilis, with infiltration with lardaceous matter, of the malpighian bodies, arteries, tubes, and epithelium.

k., large mottled. A type of chronic parenchymatous nephritis.

k., large red. One resembling that of acute parenchymatous nephritis.

k., large white. A chronic parenchymatous nephritis, resulting from an acute inflammation, the organ exceeding 12 oz. in weight.

k., movable. Displaced or loosened. SYM: Dragging, heavy pains in abdomen, worse when erect; melancholia, hysteria, gastrointestinal disturbance; sensitive enlarged or abnormally placed k. TREATMENT: Dietetic. Surgical. SYN: *nephroptosis.*

k., pigback. A congested k. bearing a longitudinal ridge on its vertex. Common in alcoholic subjects.

k., polycystic. K. bearing many cysts.

k., red contracted. Gouty kidney.

k., sacculated. A condition in which the organ has been absorbed and only the distended capsule remains.

k., senile. One with atrophy of the glomeruli and tubules seen in old age.

k., small red granular. Granular k.

k. stones. SYN: renal calculus, q.v. renal lithiasis. Concretions present in the pelvis of the kidney. They are composed principally of oxalates, phosphates, and carbonates and vary in size from small granular masses to an inch in diameter. When level of urinary colloids is high there is an absence of stones. This level is higher in Negroes and in women than in men. Administration of hyaluronidase prevents stone formation and checks increase of size of same. It releases intercellular ground substance of human tissues and a colloid that coats individual salt crystals with a protective jellylike coating. SEE: *colloid, hyaluronidase.*

k., surgical. Suppurative pyelonephritis following operation upon urinary tract.

k., syphilitic. One with fibrous bands running across it, also caseating gummata, due to syphilis.

k., wandering. A floating k.

k., waxy. SEE: *lardaceous k.*

Kienböck unit. Measurement of x-ray dosage; 1/10 of erythema dose.

Kier'nan's spaces. The spaces bet. the lobes of the liver.

Kiesselbach's area (ke'sel-bahks). An area on the ant. inferior portion of the nasal septum. The commonest site for septal bleeding.

Kil'ian's pelvis. Pelvis affected with osteomalacia. SYN: *pelvis spinosa.*

kilo- [G.]. One thousand.

kil'ogram [G. *chilioi,* a thousand, + *gramma,* a weight]. One thousand grams or 2.2 lbs. avoirdupois. ABBR: kg.

kiloliter (kil'o-lē-ter) [Fr. *kilolitre*]. One thousand liters.

kil'ometer [Fr. *kilomètre*]. One thousand meters, or 3281 feet (roughly 0.6 of a mile). ABBR: km.

kilonem. A unit of nutrition equivalent to 667 calories, the energy provided by one liter of milk.

kil'ovolt [G. *chilioi,* a thousand, + *volt*]. One thousand volt unit.

kil'owatt. A unit of electrical energy equal to one thousand watts. ABBR: kv.

kilurane (kil'u-ran). A unit of radioactivity, equivalent to one thousand uranium units.

kinanesthesia (kin″an-es-the'zĭ-ă) [G. *kinein,* to move, + *an-,* priv., + *aisthēsis,* sensation]. Inability to see extent of movement, or direction resulting in ataxia.

kinase (kin'ās) [G. *kinein,* to move]. An organic substance which activates a proenzyme or zymogen.

kinemat'ics [G. *kinein,* to move]. Science of motion.

kineplastic [G. *kinein,* to move, + *plastikos,* formed]. Pert. to kineplasty.

kin'eplasty [" + *plassein,* to form]. A form of amputation so that motion is imparted to an artificial limb.

kinergety (kin-er'jet-ĭ) [" + *ergon,* energy]. The potential capacity for kinetic energy.

kinesalgia (kin-es-al'jĭ-ă) [G. *kinēsis,* movement, + *algos,* pain]. Pain attending muscular movement.

kinesia (kin-e'sĭ-ă) [G. *kinesis,* motion]. SYN: *kinectosis.* Sickness caused by motion, as seasickness, car sickness.

kinesialgia (ki-ne-si-al'jĭ-ă) [" + *algos,* pain]. Pain caused by muscular movements. SYN: *kinesalgia.*

kinesiatrics (ki-ne-sĭ-at'riks) [" + *iatrikos,* curative]. Treatment involving active and passive movements. SYN: *kinesitherapy.*

kinesim'eter. An apparatus for determining the extent of movement of a part.

kinesiodic (ki-ne-sĭ-od'ik) [" + *odos,* path]. Pert. to paths through which motor impulses pass.

kinesiology (kin-es-ĭ-ol'ō-jĭ) [G. *kinesis,* motion, + *logos,* study]. The study of muscles and muscular movement.

kinesioneurosis (ki-ne″sĭ-o-nū-ro'sis) [" + *neuron,* nerve, + *-ōsis*]. Functional disorder marked by tics and spasms.

k., external. K. affecting external muscles.

k., vascular. K. of the vasomotor system.

k., visceral. K. affecting muscles of internal organs.

kinesipathy (ki-ne-sip'a-thĭ). Treatment by movement. SYN: *kinesitherapy.*

kinesis (kin-e'sis) [G.]. Motion.

kinesither'apy [G. *kinēsis,* motion, + *therapeia,* therapy]. Treatment by movements.

kinesod'ic [" + *odos,* path]. Rel. to the conveyance of motor impulses.

kinesthesia (kin-es-the'zĭ-ă) [" + *aisthēsis,* sensation]. 1. Ability to perceive extent or direction, or weight of movement. 2. Illusion of gliding through space.

kinesthesiometer (ki″nes-the-zĭ-om'ĕ-tĕr) [" + " + *metron,* measure]. Instrument for testing the muscular reaction.

kinesthet'ic [" + *aisthēsis,* sensation]. Rel. to kinesthesia.

kinetic (ki-net'ĭk) [G. *kinesis,* motion]. Pert. to or consisting of motion.

kinetosis (ki-ne-to'sis) [" + *-ōsis*]. Any disorder caused by motion, such as seasickness, car sickness, etc. SYN: *kinesia.*

kinetotherapy (kī-net″o-ther'ă-pĭ) [" + *therapeia,* treatment]. Treatment that employs active and passive movements. SYN: *kinesitherapy.*

king's evil. Constitutional condition characterized by glandular swellings in neck and inflammation of joints and mucosa. So called, because it was thought curable by touch of a king. SYN: *scrofula.*

kinom′eter [G. *kinein*, to move, + *metron*, measure]. Instrument which measures displacements of the uterus.

kinomom′eter [" + *metron*, measure]. Device which measures degree of motion of fingers and toes.

ki′otome [G. *kiōn*, column, + *tomē*, incision]. Instrument for amputating the uvula.

kiotomy (ki-ot′o-mĭ) [" + *tomē*, incision]. Use of the kiotome in amputating the uvula.

Kisch's reflex (kĭsh). SYN: *auriculopalpebral reflex*. Closure of an eye resulting from stimulation of heat or some tactile irritant on the ext. auditory meatus or deeper portions of canal up to tympanum.

Kite apparatus. Apparatus for reëducation of weak muscles and for assistance in overcoming contractures of forearm, wrist and fingers.

Klaus′ner's reaction or test. Serum of an assumed syphilitic is covered with distilled water in a test tube. Turbidity at plane of contact will show if syphilis is present.

Klebsiella (kleb-sĭ-el′ă). A genus of bacteria of the family Enterobacteriaceae. They are short, plump, gram-negative bacilli which form capsules. They are nonmotile and do not form spores. Frequently associated with respiratory infections. Commonly called the Friedlander group.

K. capsulatus. Encapsulated rods, singly or in chains in catarrhal inflammations of respiratory tract.

K. ozenae. Species associated with ozena. SEE: *ozena*.

K. pneumoniae. Friedlander's bacillus in certain pneumonias. Also found as a secondary invader in other respiratory infections such as bronchitis or sinusitis.

K. rhinoscleromatis. The cause of rhinoscleroma.

Klebs-Loeffler bacil′lus (klebs-lef′ler). The bacillus of diphtheria. SYN: *corynebacterium diphtheriae*. SEE: *diphtheria*.

Klem′perer's test meal. Milk, 500 cc.; 2 rolls, 70 Gm. This is given on an empty stomach and aspirated 2 hr. later.

kleptolagnia (klep″to-lag′nĭ-ă) [G. *kleptein*, to steal, + *lagneia*, lust]. Sexual gratification derived from stealing.

kleptomania (klep-to-ma′nĭ-ă) [" + *mania*, madness]. Impulsive stealing, the motive not being in the intrinsic value of the article to the patient. There is often deep regret following the act.

kleptoma′niac [" + *mania*, madness]. 1. A psychopathic personality suffering from impulsive stealing. 2. Pert. to kleptomania.

kleptophobia (klep-to-fo′bĭ-ă) [" + *phobos*, fear]. Morbid fear of stealing.

Klieg eye (klēg). Conjunctivitis, lacrimation and photophobia from exposure to the intense lights used in making moving pictures.

Kline test, Kline-Young test. A microscope slide precipitation test for presence of syphilis.

Klon′dike bed. Outdoor sleeping bed that protects patient from draughts.

klotogen (klot′o-jen]. A standardized concentrate of vitamin K in peanut oil.

USES: In obstructive jaundice to prevent hemorrhage due to prolonged coagulation time of the blood.

DOSAGE: *Prophylactic*: 1000 units given with 10 gr. bile salts, during meals, 3 times daily for 4 days. *Therapeutic*: 10,000 units by duodenal tube, followed by sufficient amount of bile salts dissolved in warm water.

Klumpke's paralysis (kloomp′kez). Atrophic paralysis of forearm.

Knapp's forceps. A forceps with blades like rollers for expressing trachomatous granulations on the palpebral conjunctiva.

knead′ing [A. S. *cnedan*, to press a man]. A form of massage, consisting of grasping, wringing, lifting, rolling, or pressing part of a muscle or group of muscles. SYN: *pétrissage*.

knee [A. S. *cneōw*]. The ant. aspect of the leg at the articulation of the femur and tibia; also the articulation itself, covered anteriorly with the patella or kneecap. Formed by the femur, tibia, and patella.

R.S.: *geniculate, geniculum, "genu-" words, "gon-" words, housemaid's k., patella, popliteal*.

k., Brodie's. A chronic, fungoid synovitis of the knee joint in which the affected parts become soft and pulpy.

k. chest position. Resting upon the knees and chest with forearms supporting the head. SEE: *position*.

k., dislocations of the. Displacement of the knee.

Dislocations of the knee in themselves are unusual. The so-called dislocation of the knee is usually due to various injuries of the joint and of the complicating structures of the knee, such as the tearing of the crushed tendons or

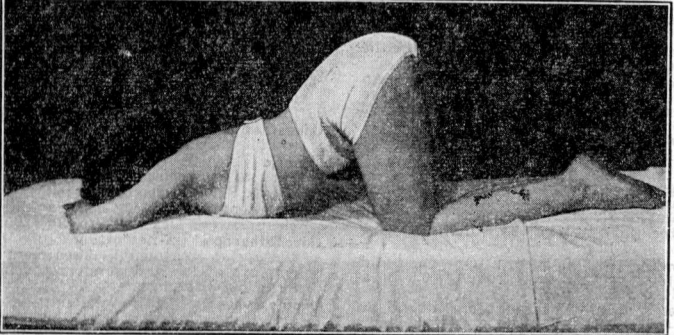

Posed by professional model   *Photo by Whitaker*
KNEE-CHEST OR GENUPECTORAL POSITION.

knee, game   K-9   **kolytic**

ligaments, or slipping of the cartilages, etc., and should be treated either by a straight splint, as in a fracture of the kneecap, or 2 splints, one on either side of the knee, as in a fracture, and the patient should be transported to a hospital as quickly as possible.

k., game. A lay term for internal derangement of knee joint.
PATH: Usually a torn semilunar cartilage, a fracture of the tibial spine, or an injury to the collateral or cruciate ligaments.
SYM: Pain or instability, locking, and weakness.
F. A. TREATMENT: Immobilize with a post. splint plus heat and massage. Surgical exploratory arthrotomy may be necessary.

k., housemaid's. Inflamed condition of the bursa in front of the patella, with accumulation of fluid therein, frequently seen in scrubwomen.

k., in-. The condition in which the knees come together while the ankles are far apart, caused by an outward distortion of the leg throwing knee inside the normal line. SYN: *genu valgum, knock-k.*

k. of the internal capsule. The curve at the meeting place of the ant. and post. limbs of the internal capsule.

k. jerk reflex. The reflex contraction or clonic spasm of the quadriceps muscle, produced by sharply striking the ligamentum patellae when the leg hangs loosely flexed at right angles. It is seen normally in health, but is usually absent in locomotor ataxia, multiple neuritis, lesions of the lower portion of the spinal cord, lesions of the ant. gray horns of the cord, meningitis, infantile paralysis, pseudohypertrophic paralysis, atrophic paralysis, etc., and increased in spinal irritability, lesions of the pyramidal tract, cerebral tumors, sclerosis of the brain and cord, etc. SYN: *patellar reflex.* SEE: *jerk.*

k. joint. The articulation of the femur and tibia.

k., knock-. An outward distortion of the leg, throwing knee inside the normal line. SYN: *genu valgum, in-k.*

k., lawn tennis. A sprain of int. semilunar cartilage of k. joint.

k., locked. Condition in which the leg cannot be extended. Usually due to displacement of semilunar cartilage.

k., out-. Bowleg. SYN: *genu varum.*

knee′cap. The patella.

kneel′ing-squat′ting posi′tion. The patient stoops with knees pressed against the abdomen, and with trunk erect; employed in childbirth in difficult cases.

Kneipp cure (nĭp). Application of water in various forms and degrees of temperature in the cure of disease, esp. wading in cold, dewy grass. SYN: *hydrotherapy.*

kneippism (nĭp′izm). Walking barefoot in dewy grass, bathing in cold water, etc., as a cure of disease.

knife (nīf) [A. S. *cnif*]. A cutting instrument.

k., electric. A knife carrying a high frequency cutting current.

knit′ting [A. S. *cnittan*, to make knots]. The union of pieces of a fractured bone.

KNO₃. Potassium nitrate, niter, saltpeter.

knock-knee. Condition of having the knees turned inward. SYN: *genu valgum, in-knee.*

knockout drops. Colloquial name for chloral hydrate given in alcoholic beverages to produce rapid coma.

knot. 1. An intertwining of a cord or cord-like structure so as to form a lump or knob. 2. In surgery, the intertwining of the ends of a suture, ligature, bandage, or sling so that the ends will not slip or become separated. 3. In anatomy, an enlargement forming a knob-like structure.

k., false. An external bulging of the umbilical cord resulting from the coiling of the umbilical blood vessels.

k., Hensen's. SYN: *Hensen's node.* A knoblike structure at the anterior end of the primitive streak.

k., primitive. Hensen's knot, *q.v.*

k., syncytial. A protuberance formed by many nuclei of the syntrophoblast and found on surface of a chorionic villus.

k., true. A knot formed by the fetus slipping through a loop of the umbilical cord.

Koag′amin. Commercial preparation of blood coagulant.

K. O. C. Abbr. of *cathodal opening contraction.* SYN: *COC.*

Kocher's reflex (kō′kĕr). Contraction of abdominal muscles following moderate compression of testicle.

Koch's bacil′lus (kŏks). SYN: *Mycobacterium tuberculosis.* The bacillus of tuberculosis.

K.'s law or postulates. To prove an organism the cause of a disease or lesion; 1st, microörganism in question must appear in lesion at all times; 2nd, pure cultures must be obtained from it; 3rd, pure cultures when inoculated into susceptible animals must reproduce the disease or pathological condition and, 4th, the organism must be obtained again in pure culture from the inoculated animal.

K.'s lymph. Tuberculin.

K.'s phenomenon. Local inflammatory reaction resulting from injection of tuberculin into the skin of a person who has been previously exposed to the tubercle bacillus.

KOH. Potassium hydroxide.

Kohlrausch's fold or **valve** (kōhl′rowshs). Fold of mucous membrane extending into rectum; rectal valve. SYN: *plica transversales recti.*

koilonychia (koy-lo-nik′ĭ-ă) [G. *koilos,* hollow, + *onyx, onych-,* nail]. Malformation of the fingernails; outer surface is concave.

koinotropic type (koin′o-trop-ĭk) [G. *koinos,* common, + *tropos,* a turning]. Term applied to one who can give and take, as the "good mixer."

ko′la. Cardiac and nerve stimulant derived from *Sterculia acuminata.* Its principal ingredients are caffeine, theobromine, and colatin.

Kol′mer test. 1. A modification of the Wassermann test. 2. Complement fixation test for some infectious diseases.

kolp- [G.]. Prefix: Vagina.

kolpi′tis [G. *kolpos,* vagina, + *-ītis,* inflammation]. Inflammation of vaginal mucous membrane. SYN: *colpitis.*

kolpot′omy [" + *tomē,* incision]. A vaginal operation. SYN: *colpotomy, elytrotomy.*

kol′yone. [G. *kōlyein,* to hinder]. 1. An antacid opposing action of a hormone. 2. An endocrine that diminishes activity of cells. SYN: *chalone, colyone.*

kolypeptic (ko-lĭ-pep′tĭk) [" + *pepsis,* digestion]. Retarding digestion.

kolyphrenia (kol-ĭ-fre′nĭ-ă) [" + *phrēn,* mind]. Exaggerated mental inhibition.

kolyseptic (ko-lĭ-sep′tĭk) [" + *sēpsis,* putrefaction]. Antiseptic.

kolytic (ko-lit′ĭk) [G. *kōlyein,* to hinder].

Hindering or presenting or checking, as a reaction to a stimulus.

Kondoleon's operation (kŏn-dō′lē-ŏn). Surgical removal of layers of subcutaneous tissue to relieve elephantiasis.

koniocortex. The cortex of the sensory areas, so named because of its granular appearance.

koniol′ogy [G. *konis*, dust, + *logos*, study]. Science of dust and its effects. SYN: *coniology*.

koniometer (ko-nĭ-om′ĕ-ter) [" + *metron*, measure]. Device for estimating amt. of dust in the air.

koniosis (ko-nĭ-o′sĭs) [" + *-ōsis*, intensive]. Any morbid condition caused by dust. SYN: *coniosis*.

kopf-tet′anus. Tetanus developing subsequent to head wounds.

kopiopia (ko-pĭ-o′pĭ-ă) [G. *kopos*, fatigue]. Eyestrain. SYN: *copiopia*.

Kop′lik's spots. Small red spots with bluish white centers on the oral mucosa, particularly in the region opposite the line of juncture of the molar teeth.

A diagnostic sign in measles before the rash appears. Not infrequently, the spots disappear as the eruption develops.

kopophobia. Abnormal fear of fatigue or exhaustion.

Kopp's asthma. SYN: *laryngismus stridulus*. Spasm of the glottis in infants not over two years of age. Thought to be due to an enlarged thymus.

koronion (ko-ro′nĭ-on) [G. *korōnē*, crest]. Apex of coronoid process of the mandible.

koroscopy (kor-os′ko-pĭ) [G. *korē*, pupil, + *skopein*, to examine]. Shadow test for refraction of the eye.

Korsakoff's psychosis or syndrome (kor′sak-ofs). One characterized by a psychosis with a polyneuritis, disorientation, muttering delirium, insomnia, illusions and hallucinations, painful extremities, rarely a bilateral wrist drop, more frequently bilateral foot drop with pain or pressure over the long nerves.

Occurs as a sequel to chronic alcoholism. SYN: *polyneuritic psychosis*.

Kott′mann's reaction or test. A blood serum reaction test to indicate whether or not the thyroid gland is functioning.

koumiss (koo′mĭs) [Tartar]. Fermented milk beverage. SYN: *kumyss*.

Kraepelin's classification (kra′pă-linz). A classification of mental disease into 2 groups: the manic-depressive and the schizophrenic.

kraurosis (kraw-rō′sĭs) [G. *krauros*, dry]. Atrophy and dryness of skin and any mucous membrane, esp. of the vulva.

The subcutaneous fat of the mons pubis and labia disappears, clitoris and prepuce atrophy, and stenosis of the vaginal orifice is common. Fissures may develop. Epithelioma are prone to occur most frequently in postmenopausal women or those who have had ovaries removed.

ETIOL: Probably hypoestrinism.

k. penis. SYN: *balanitis xerotica obliterans, Stuhmer's disease*. Condition in which the glans penis atrophies and becomes shriveled.

k. vul′vae. An atrophy of the skin and mucosa, seen in elderly women which pathologically consists of a marked atrophy of the vulvar skin, and which is characterized clinically by severe itching.

The skin has a white marblelike appearance, and frequently shows excoriations as a result of the scratching. A large percentage of these cases, if allowed to go on without operative interference, undergo malignant degeneration. SYN: *leukoplakic vulvitis*.

Krause's end bulb. An encapsulated sensory receptor found widely distributed in connective tissue underlying the skin and mucous membranes. It is the end organ for cold sensations.

K.'s glands. Small mucous acinous glands located beneath the fornix conjunctiva. They are accessory lacrimal glands and open into the fornix.

K.'s membrane. Thin, dark disk transversely crossing through and bisecting clear zone of a striated muscle and bisecting the clear zone (isotropic disk) of a striated muscle fiber. Also called the Z disk. The portion between two Z disks constitutes a sarcomere.

K.'s valve. Mucous membrane fold at juncture where lacrimal sac narrows into nasal duct. SYN: *Béraud's valve*.

kreatine (kre′at-in). Creatine, *q.v.*

kreatinine (kre-at′in-in). Creatinine, *q.v.*

kreotox′in [G. *kreas*, flesh, + *toxikon*, poison]. A poison in flesh due to a microorganism. [Meat poisoning.]

kreotox′ism [" + " + *ismos*, state of].

kresep′tol. A cresol disinfectant more active than the solution cresol compound, USP, made with a specially purified cresol free from objectionable impurities present in ordinary official cresol.

ACTION: Antiseptic, germicidal, disinfectant, and deodorant.

USES: For cleansing and disinfecting wounds and sores, for disinfecting the hands, surgical instruments, towels, bed linen, sickroom utensils, closets, drains, and excreta, such as sputum, urine, or feces.

kresol (kre′sol). USP: Brownish yellow fluid from coal tar, used as a germicide. SYN: *cresol, q.v.*

Krishaber's disease (krēs-ă-bairs′). Neurosis marked by dizziness, sleeplessness, palpitation and syncope.

Kromayer lamp (kro′mĭ-er). Water cooled, mercury quartz lamp for local ultraviolet treatments.

Krompecher's tumor (krŏm′pekh-ers). Rodent ulcer. SYN: *Jacob's ulcer*.

Kronecker's center (krŏn′ek-ers). The inhibitory center of the heart.

Krönig's area or field (kra′nĭg). Resonant region in the thorax over the apices of the lungs.

Kruk′enberg's tumor. A malignant tumor of the ovary, usually bilateral, and secondary to malignancies, esp. of the gastrointestinal tract.

Histologically these tumors consist of myxomatous connective tissue and cells having a signet ring arrangement of their nuclei. The epithelial tissue resembles malignancy of the original site.

kryp′ton [G. *kryptos*, hidden]. A gaseous element found in small amts. in the atmosphere. SYMB: *Kr*.

K$_2$SO$_4$. Potassium sulfate.

kumiss, kumyss (koo′mĭs). 1. Cow's milk with sugar and yeast after fermentation. 2. Fermented mare's milk. SYN: *koumiss*.

Kund′rat's lymphosarco′ma. Lymphosarcoma which affects adjacent glands, but does not invade neighboring organs.

Kussmaul's coma (koos′mawls). Diabetic coma.*

kyestein, kyesthein (ki-es′te-in) [G. *kyēsis*, conception]. A scum which floats on the standing urine of pregnant women.

kyllosis (ki-lo′sĭs) [G. *kyllos*, twisted]. Clubfoot.

ky′matism [G. *kyma*, wave, + *ismos*, state of]. Twitching of isolated segments of muscle. SYN: *myokymia*.

ky'mogram. A tracing or recording made by a kymograph.
kymograph (kī'mō-grăf) [G. *kyma*, wave, + *graphein*, to write]. An apparatus for recording wavelike or cyclic activity. Widely used in physiology to record activities such as blood pressure changes, muscle contractions, respiratory movements, etc. Consists of a drum rotated by a spring or electric motor. Drum is covered by a paper upon which the record is made.
ky'moscope [" + *skopein*, to examine]. Device for measuring variations in blood pressure.
kyogenic (ki-o-jen'ĭk) [G. *kyēsis*, pregnancy, + *gennan*, to produce]. Inducing pregnancy.
kypho- [G.]. Prefix: Humped.
kyphorachitis (kī"fō-rä-kī'tĭs). Rachitic deformity involving thorax and spinal column. Results in development of anteroposterior hump.
kyphoscoliosis (kī"fō-skŏl-ĭ-ō'sĭs). Lateral curvature of the spine accompanying anteroposterior hump.
kyphosis (ki-fo'sis) [G. humpback]. SYN: *humpback, spinal curvature*. Exaggeration or angulation of normal posterior curve of spine. Gives rise to condition commonly known as humpback, hunchback, or Pott's curvature. Also refers to excessive curvature of the spine with convexity backward. The former may be due to congenital anomaly, disease (tuberculosis, syphilis), malignancy, or compression fracture. The latter may result from faulty posture, osteo- or rheumatoid arthritis, rickets, or other conditions.
kyphotic (ki-fot'ik) [G. *kyphōsis*, humpback]. Affected by or pert. to kyphosis.
ky'rin. A protein resisting tryptic digestion, which yields amino acids when treated with an acid.
kyrtorrhachic (kir-to-rak'ik) [G. *kyrtos*, curved, + *rachis*, spine]. Spinal curvature with concavity backward.
kysthitis (kis-thi'tis) [G. *kysthos*, vagina, + *-itis*, inflammation]. Inflammation of the vagina. SYN: *colpitis, vaginitis*.
kysthoptosis (kis-thop-to'sis) [" + *ptōsis*, a falling]. Prolapse of the vagina.
kyto- [G.]. Prefix; denoting cell. SEE: *cyto-*.

L

L. Abbr. for *Latin, Lactobacillus, left, length, lithium, light sense, liter.*

lab, lab ferment [Ger. *lab*, rennet]. Milk-curdling ferment in rennet. SYN: *zymogen.*
  l. zymogen. Preparatory substance from which a ferment or enzyme is formed.

Labarraque's solution (lăb-ar-ăk'). Chlorinated soda solution; a disinfectant.

Labbe's vein (lă-ba'). Vein connecting lateral to sup. longitudinal sinus.

la'bia (sing. *labium*) [L.]. 1. Lips. 2. The lips of the vulva.
  RS: *clitoris, Hottentot's apron, mons veneris, nymphas, nymphoncus, smegma, vagina.*
  l. majora. The 2 folds of cellular adipose tissue extending from the *mons veneris** to the perineum, lying on either side of the vulva, lozenge shaped, and having an outer and an inner surface, the inner surface resembling the mucous membrane of the vagina, and the outer part being skin covered by pubic hair.
  Richly supplied by lymphatics and contain many sebaceous glands. They join each other by their inner surface and completely close the vulva in young girls, or the vulva is closed below and open above. Later, the vulva opens or gaps below, and the labia become more flabby. There are exceptions, as in children, in whom the labia do not project, leaving the vulva open, and in fat women in whom the labia do not become flabby but close over the vulva.
  l. minora. Two mucocutaneous folds of membrane within the labia majora lying on the inner and upper portion of the labia majora, the upper portion ensheathing the clitoris.
  In young children covered by the labia majora but are exposed in adult women. The labia sometimes project from the vulva like an appendage. SYN: *nymphae.*

labial (la'bĭ-al) [L. *labium*, lip]. 1. Pert. to the lips. 2. Letter formed by the lips.
  l. glands. Many racemose glands bet. labial mucosa and orbicularis muscle opening on lip's inner surface.

labialism (la'bĭ-al-izm) [L. *labialis*, pert. to lip, + G. *ismos*, state of]. Defective speech in which labial sounds are stressed.

labidometer (la-bĭ-dom'et-er) [G. *labis*, forceps, + *metron*, measure]. Forceps for measuring fetal head in pelvis.

labile (lab'ĭl) [L. *labī*, to glide]. Not fixed; unsteady; easily disarranged.
  l. elements. Tissue cells which multiply by indirect nuclear division. SEE: *mitosis.*

lability (lab-il'ĭt-ĭ) [G. *labi*, to glide]. State of being unstable or changeable.

labimeter (lab-im'et-er) [G. *labis*, forceps, + *metron*, measure]. Forceps (or attachment to) for measuring fetal head. SYN: *labidometer.*

labioalveolar (lab″ĭ-ō-ăl-ve'ol-ar) [L. *labium*, lip, + *alveolus*, little hollow]. Pert. to lips and tooth sockets.

labiocervical (lab″ĭ-ō-ser'vĭ-kăl) [" + *cervix, cervic-*, neck]. Pert. to lips, and the neck of a tooth.

labioglossolaryngeal (la″bĭ-o-glos″o-lar-in′je-ăl) [" + G. *glōssa*, tongue, + *larynx*, larynx]. Pert. to lips, tongue, and larynx.
  l. paralysis. A neurosis characterized by progressive paralysis of the parts mentioned.

labioglossopharyngeal (la″bĭ-o-glos″o-far-in′je-ăl) [" + " + *pharynx*, throat]. Pert. to the lips, tongue, and pharynx.

labiograph (la′bĭ-o-grăf) [" + G. *graphein*, to write]. Device for registering the lip movements in speaking.

labiology (lā-bĭ-ol′o-jĭ) [" + G. *logos*, study]. Study of the lip movements in speaking or singing.

labiomancy (la′bĭ-o-man″sĭ) [" + G. *manteia*, foretelling]. Interpreting speech by reading lip movements.

labiomental (la-bĭ-ō-men′tal) [" + *mentum*, chin]. Pert. to the lower lip and chin.

labiomycosis (la″bĭ-o-mī-ko′sis) [" + G. *mykēs*, fungus, + -*ōsis*]. Any disease of the lips due to presence of a fungus.

labiopalatine (la″bĭ-ō-pal′ă-tīn) [" + *palatum*, palate]. Relating to the lips and palate.

labioplasty (la′bĭ-o-plas″tĭ) [" + G. *plassein*, to form]. Plastic surgery of the lips. SYN: *cheiloplasty.*

labictenaculum (la″bĭ-o-ten-ak′u-lum) [L. *labium*, lip, + *tenaculum*, a hook]. Instrument for holding lips during an operation.

la′bium (pl. *labia*) [L. lip]. A lip or a structure like one. SEE: *labia.*
  l. cerebri. Margin of the cerebral hemispheres overlapping the corpus callosum.
  l. inferius. Lower lip.
  l. majus (pl. *labia majora**). One of 2 lateral boundaries of the vulva with adipose tissue and hair.
  l. majus pudendi. Fold of integument forming lateral boundary of the vulva.
  l. minus (pl. *labia minora**). One of 2 inner lips of vulva within the labia majora.
  l. minus pudendi. Lesser, inner lip of vulva. SYN: *nympha.*
  l. superius. The upper lip.
  l. tympanicum. Outer edge of organ of Corti.
  l. urethrae. Lateral margin of meatus urinarius externus.
  l. uteri. Thickened margin of the cervix uteri.
  l. vestibulare. Vestibular or inner edge of organ of Corti.

la′bor [L. work]. The physiological process by which the fetus is expelled from the uterus at term.
  Normal appearance 280 days after last menstruation.
  Labor is divided into 3 stages:
  FIRST STAGE: *Dilatation*: Lasting from the onset of uterine contractions until the cervix uteri is dilated completely.
  SECOND STAGE: *Expulsion*: From the time of complete dilatation until the expulsion of the fetus.
  THIRD STAGE: *Placental*: From the time of expulsion of the fetus until the expulsion of the placenta.

labor   L-2   **labor, false**

PREPARATION: Well ventilated, sunny room; temperature 65° during labor, 70° after. Bed with fresh, well-aired linen and a pad previously prepared, of heavy paper covered with cotton wool, the whole covered with cheese-cloth, large enough to cover middle third of bed. This receives the discharge and is easily removed and replaced by a similar fresh one, keeping the bed in good condition.

The patient is given enema if bowels have not moved freely within 12 hours; bladder emptied if nature does not attend to it.

The vulva and mons veneris and thighs rendered thoroughly aseptic (patient will have taken a bath as soon as indications appeared that labor was drawing near); pubic hair about vulva shaved or closely clipped. Long stockings, made of canton flannel or tennis flannel, reaching to the hips, should be drawn on, protecting limbs from exposure. The gown to be worn turned up and smoothly fastened out of the way above the waist, an old sheet or cloth pinned comfortably about the waist next to body.

After the third stage, by removing soiled pad, stockings and old sheet, gown may be brought down and patient is in good condition for rest without being disturbed.

A large number of old soft white cloths should be at hand aseptically clean, in case of hemorrhage. Also a number of vulva pads prepared for receiving the lochia; vessels of boiled water, cooled and kept tightly covered, should be provided and plenty of boiled hot water be at hand. Many obstetricians carry with them a stout strap with stirruplike ends for the hands, which may be thrown about the foot of bed to aid in expulsive movements.

FIRST STAGE: Ascertain amount of dilation and the presentation. In ordinary cases only physician and nurse desired in room; cold water or other cool, refreshing beverage only refreshment required unless protracted.

Ordinarily full dilation is accomplished within 6 hours. Sometimes in a very short time, at others much longer. Patient may walk about or make herself comfortable till second stage. Should then take her position on the pad on left side with breech near edge of bed, thighs flexed at right angles on abdomen and legs on thighs, feet against foot of bed as support during the expulsive efforts. Or the dorsal position (on the back) may be assumed. Pains become stronger and closer together.

SECOND STAGE: During last of first stage or beginning of second, the membranes rupture and a portion of liquor amnii is discharged.

Pains come every 3 minutes or closer; head advances, and fetus is soon expelled; as head appears, attendant should bear his right hand upon the perineum in such a manner as to encircle the labia as much as possible with thumb and fingers, and while drawing down with these upon the labia must press gently forward and upward upon the perineum with the palm of same hand.

Ascertain that cord is not about child's neck. Have at hand a saucer of warm olive oil and as body advances rub it into all the places covered with the vernix which will then easily be removed later. Have at hand a cup of warm, sterilized water; after cleansing hands in the bowl which has been at hand throughout, containing some antiseptic, as creolin or lysol or whatever is preferred, dip bit of absorbent cotton in the sterilized water and thoroughly wash child's eyes and dry with bit of the cotton.

If by this time cord has stopped pulsating (usually in about 5 minutes), tie a ligature about 5 inches from the abdomen, another an inch nearer the placenta and cut between them. After thoroughly cleaning the cord and allowing blood to flow from it toward abdomen, take ends of first ligature and tie cord tightly one-half inch from abdomen (after ascertaining that no part of intestine protrudes into cord); this leaves a loop of umbilical cord which prevents hemorrhage or entrance of infection.

As the child is fully expelled the sheet covering the mother should be dropped between her and the child, who should be wrapped in a warm blanket at hand to receive him. The remaining portion of liquor amnii follows the expulsion and uterus contracts upon itself. This ends second stage.

THIRD STAGE: Return of pain (usually a lull after completion of second stage); this marks expulsion of placenta—may occur within 20 minutes or not for hours. Uterus is found low down, hard, globular and size of fetal head.

Expulsion of placenta without retention of shreds of membrane may be accomplished by twisting movement on cord as placenta appears in vulva, contraction of uterus and avoidance of hemorrhage may be aided by gentle massage of uterus through abdominal wall. After expulsion of placenta examine perineum to see if there is any laceration; if deep, repair at once, tie knees together to prevent pulling apart of wound. If tear is slight, leave for nature to heal and avoid infection. Caution used on changing pad at vulva not to tear out stitches by too hasty removal of pad.

Allow few moments' rest, then quickly remove all soiled bedding and apparel, bring down the pinned up gown, draw down shades and leave patient to rest; on no account have any conversation at this time.

From time to time feel if uterus is contracting as desired and that there is no hemorrhage. If labor is complicated by malpositions different tactics must be pursued in the different stages to suit the individual case.

There is still no ideal anesthetic. The current varyingly successful methods of amnesia, analgesia, and anesthesia are: morphine-scopolamine, sodium amytal, paraldehyde and rectal ether, ether-oil, pentobarbital with or without scopolamine, nitrous oxide and oxygen alone or with ether, ether alone, nitrous oxide and ethylene, evipal, pentothal, pernocton, pantopon, epidural anesthesia and pudendal nerve block. SEE: *pregnancy*.

l., artificial. Labor brought on by the use of ecbolics or hydrostatic bags.

l., complicated. Any complication occurring during the course of labor.

l., dry. Labor after most of the amniotic fluid has been drained away.

l., false. Uterine contractions coming on before the onset of actual labor.

l., induced. Labor brought on by the use of ecbolic hydrostatic bags, or any other method that may be used.

l., instrumental. Labor completed by mechanical means, such as the use of forceps.

l., missed. The patient goes through actual labor but the fetus dies and is not expelled. [fetuses.

l., multiple. Labor with 2 or more

l., precipitate. Rapidly completed labor that occurs without the aid of an accoucheur.

l., premature. Labor coming on between the 7th month of gestation and full term.

l., spontaneous. Labor that is completed without external aid.

labor, words pert. to: abortion; acyesis; "amni-" words; ante partum; aponia; aponic; asynclitism; bag of waters, bag, hydrostatic; ballottement; basilysis; basiotripsy; bipara; biparous; bradytocia; breech presentation; brow presentation; bruit, placental; caput succedaneum; caul; cephalhematoma; cephalic version; cephalotomy; cesarean section; cesarotomy; chorda umbilicalis; cleidotomy; conception; conjugate; Crede's method; cross birth; delivery; disengagement; dystocia; ecbolic; eclampsia; embryectomy; embryo; embryoctony; embryotocia; embryulcia; encyesis; eutocia; fetus; fixity; gestation; Hegar's sign; hourglass contraction; impetigo herpetiformis; maneuver; mimetic; obstetrician; obstetrics; placenta; puerpera; puerperal; puerperium; quintuplets; restitution; Schultze's method; show; synclitism; vagitus; xerotocia.

laboratory (lab'or-a-to-rĭ) [L. *laboratorium*, work place]. A place equipped for analytical or experimental work.

Laborde's method (respiration stimulation). Stimulation of the respiratory center in asphyxiation by a series of rhythmical traction movements upon the tongue.

labrocyte (lab'ro-sīt) [G. *labros*, greedy, + *kytos*, cell]. Large leukocyte containing basophil granules.

Seen in normal blood and in leukemia.
SYN: *mast cell.*

la'brum (pl. *labra*) [L. lip]. Lip.

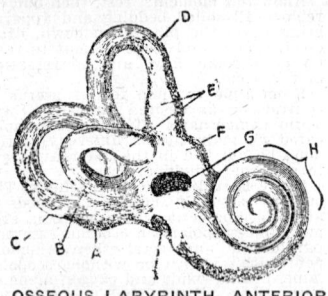

OSSEOUS LABYRINTH, ANTERIOR VIEW
A. Ampulla. B. External semicircular canal. C. Posterior semicircular canal. D. Superior semicircular canal. E. Ampullae. F. Vestibulum. G. Fenestra ovalis. H. Cochlea. I. Fenestra rotunda.

labyrinth (lab'ĭ-rinth) [G. *labyrinthos*, a maze]. 1. Intricate communicating passages. 2. The internal ear consisting of osseous and membranous labyrinths.

l., bony. Osseous labyrinth, *q.v.*

l., ethmoidal. Membranous labyrinth, *q.v.*

l. of kidney cortex. Cortical substance of that part of kidney arranged around the uriniferous tubules of medullary rays in the cortex.

l., Ludwig's. Spaces bet. the cortical arches and Bertin's columns.

l., membranous. Structure in osseous labyrinth consisting of utricle and saccule of vestibule; 3 membranous, semicircular canals, and membranous portion of cochlea.

l., olfactory. The ethmoidal labyrinth, *q.v.*

l., osseous. Consists of vestibule, 3 semicircular canals, and cochlea. Channeled out of substance of petrous bone.

labyrinthectomy (lab-ĭ-rin-thek'tō-mĭ) [" + *ektomē*, excision]. Excision of the labyrinth.

labyrinthine (lab-ĭ-rĭn'thĭn) [G. *labyrinthos*, a maze]. 1. Pert. to a labyrinth. 2. Intricate or involved, as a labyrinth.

labyrinthitis (lab-ĭ-rĭn-thi'tis) [" + *-itis*, inflammation]. Inflammation (acute or chronic) of labyrinth.

ETIOL: Primary infection, complication of influenza, otitis media, or of meningitis.

SYM: Vertigo, vomiting, nystagmus.

TREATMENT: Rest in bed. If pus is present surgery indicated. Limited fluids, saline aperients. Sedatives may be indicated.

RS: *Meniere's disease.*

labyrinthotomy (lab-ĭ-rin-thot'o-mĭ) [" + *tomē*, incision]. Incision of the labyrinth.

lac (lak) [L.]. 1. Milk. 2. Milky medicinal substance.

lacerate (las'er-āt) [L. *lacerāre*, to tear]. To tear, as into irregular segments.

lacerated (las'er-a-ted) [L. *lacerāre*, to tear]. Torn; broken.

lacera'tion [L. *lacerāre*, to tear]. A wound or irregular tear of the flesh.

l. of cervix. Bilateral, stellate, or unilateral tear of the cervix uteri caused by childbirth.

l. of perineum. Injury to perineum caused by childbirth. If extending through sphincter ani muscle it is *complete.*

lacertus (lă-ser'tus) [L.]. 1. Muscular part of the arm. 2. A muscular or fibrous band.

l. cordis. Muscular tissue bands on inner cardiac surface. SYN: *trabecula carneae.*

l. fibro'sus. Aponeurotic band from the biceps tendon to the bicipital or semilunar fascia of forearm.

lacrimal (lak'rim-ăl) [L. *lacrima*, tear]. Pert. to the tears.
RS: *canaliculus,* "*dacry-*" *words, puncta, tear ducts, tears.*

l. bone. One at inner side of the orbital cavity.

l. duct. Duct which conveys the secretion from the glands to the conjunctival sac.

l. gland. The gland which secretes the tears.

l. reflex. Secretion of fluid resulting from irritation of corneal conjunctiva.

l. sac. Upper dilated portion of nasolacrimal duct situated in groove of lacrimal bone. Upper part is behind internal tarsal ligament. Measures 12

lacrimalin   L-4   **lactate**

mm. in vertical and 6 mm. in transverse diameter.

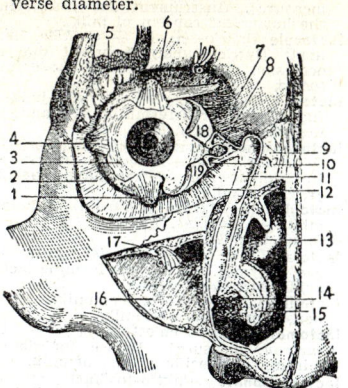

THE LACRIMAL APPARATUS.

1, Inferior rectus muscle; 2, lower eyelid; 3, eyeball; 4, lateral rectus muscle; 5, lacrimal gland; 6, superior rectus muscle; 7, upper lacrimal duct; 8, lacrimal caruncle; 9, medial palpebral ligament; 10, inferior lacrimal duct; 11, lacrimal sac; 12, lower eyelid; 13, middle meatus; 14, opening into inferior meatus; 15, inferior turbinate; 16, maxillary sinus; 17, infraorbital nerve.

lacrimalin (lak-rim′a-lĭn) [L. *lacrima*, tear]. Lacrimal substance supposed to induce a flow of tears.

larcimase (lak′rim-ās). Enzyme from tears.

lacrima′tion [L. *lacrima*, tear]. Secretion and discharge of tears.

lacrimotomy (lak-rim-ot′o-mĭ) [" + G. *tomē*, incision]. Incision of lacrimal duct.

lactac′idase [L. *lac*, milk]. Enzyme in lactic acid bacteria.

lactacidemia (lakt-as-id-e′mĭ-ă) [" + *acidus*, sour + G. *aima*, blood]. Lactic acid in the blood. SYN: *lacticemia*.

lactacidogen (lak-ta-sid′o-jen) [" + " + G. *gennan*, to produce]. The assumed intermediary substance in the transformation of glycogen to lactic acid during muscular contraction.

lactaciduria (lakt-a-sid-ū′rĭ-ă) [" + " + G. *ouron*, urine]. Lactic acid excreted in the urine.

lactagogue (lak′tă-gog) [L. *lac*, milk, + G. *agōgos*, leading]. Agent which induces secretion of milk.

lactalase (lak′tă-lās) [" + *ase*, enzyme]. Ferment converting dextrose into lactic acid.

lactalbu′min [" + *albumen*, coagulated white of egg]. The albumin of milk and cheese; a soluble simple protein.

When milk is heated, the lactalbumin coagulates and appears as a film over the top of the milk.

COMP: Carbon 52.19, hydrogen 7.18, nitrogen 15.77, oxygen 23.13, and sulfur 1.73.

lac′tase [L. *lac*, milk, + *ase*, enzyme]. An intestinal sugar splitting enzyme converting lactose into dextrose and galactose; found in intestinal juice.

SEE: *enzyme, maltase, sucrase, sugar*.

lactate (lak′tāt). [L. *lac*, milk]. A salt derived from lactic acid.

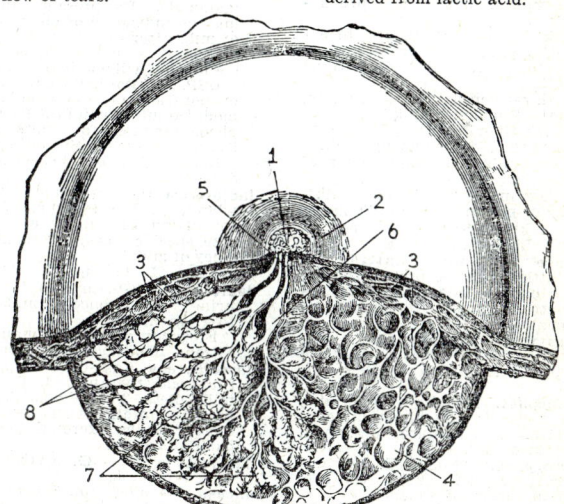

LACTIFEROUS GLAND.

Dissection of the lower half of the female mamma, during the period of lactation. In the left hand side of the dissected part, the glandular lobes are exposed and partially unravelled; and on the right hand side the glandular substance has been removed to show the reticular loculi of the connective tissue in which the glandular lobules are placed: 1. Upper part of the mammilla or nipple. 2. Areola. 3. Subcutaneous masses of fat. 4. Reticular loculi of the connective tissue which support the glandular substance and contain the fatty masses. 5. One of three lactiferous ducts shown passing toward the mammilla where they open. 6. One of the sinus lactei or reservoirs. 7. Some of the glandular lobules which have been unravelled. 8. Others massed together.

lactation (lak-ta'shun) [L. *lactatiō*, a suckling]. 1. The period of suckling in mammals. 2. The function of secreting milk.
  DIET: The mother during this period needs additional calcium to offset its loss in the milk. One qt. of milk, an egg, and meat are needed once a day. Fruits, vegetables, and whole grain cereal should be added.

lacteal (lak'te-al) [L. *lac*, milk]. 1. Pert. to milk. 2. An intestinal lymphatic that takes up chyle and passes it to the lymph circulation, and by way of the thoracic duct to the blood vascular system.
  SEE: *absorption, lymphatic*.

lactescence (lak-tes'ens) [L. *lactescere*, to become milky]. Condition of becoming, or resembling milk.

lac'tic [L. *lac*, milk]. Pert. to milk.
  l. acid. CH$_3$.CH(OH).COOH. An acid formed when milk sours through the action of sugar on certain microörganisms in the air.
  l. fermentation. The fermentation of milk and milk products.
  RS: *enzyme, fatigue, ferment, fermentation*.

lacticemia (lakt-ĭ-se'mĭ-ă) [" + G. *aima*, blood]. Lactic acid in the blood. SYN: *lactacidemia*.

lactiferous (lakt-if'er-us) [" + *ferre*, to bear]. Secreting and conveying milk.
  l. ducts. Ducts of the mammary gland.
  l. glands. 1. The mammary glands. 2. Montgomery's glands consisting of 20 to 24 glands in the areola of the nipples. SEE: *Ill., p. L-5*.

lactification (lak"tĭ-fĭ-ka'shun) [" + *facere*, to make]. Lactic acid production.

lactifuge (lak'tĭ-fuj) [" + *fugāre*, to expel]. 1. Stopping milk secretion. 2. Agent stopping milk secretion. SYN: *ischogalactic*.

lactigenous (lak-tij'en-us) [" + *gennan*, to produce]. Producing milk.

lactigerous (lak-tij'er-us) [" + *gerere*, to carry]. Secreting or conveying milk.

lac'tin [L. *lac*, milk]. Lactose, sugar of milk.

lactinated (lakt'in-āt-ed) [L. *lac*, milk]. Containing or prepared with milk sugar.

lactivorous (lakt-iv'or-us) [" + *vorāre*, to devour]. Living upon milk.

lactobacilline (lakt-o-bas'il-in) [" + *bacillus*, little rod]. A preparation of lactic acid bacilli (1) to counteract intestinal putrefaction, (2) to cause lactic acid fermentation.

Lactobacillus (lakt-o-bă-sil'us) [" + *bacillus*, little rod]. A genus of bacteria producing acid in milk and other substances.
  L. acidophilus. A lactic acid forming organism found in the intestinal contents of infants. It produces lactic acid fermentation of milk.
  L. boasoppleri. Nonmotile Gram-positive rods found in gastric contents especially in cancer of stomach.
  L. bulgaricus. Forms the sour milk known as yoghurt.
  L. caucasicus. Kephir-producing ferment.
  L. helveticus. Type found in Swiss cheese.
  L. odontolyticus. Thought to be a cause of dental caries.
  L. panis. Type occurring in sour dough.

lactobutyrometer (lakt"o-bu-tĭ-rom'et-er) [" + G. *boutyron*, butter, + *metron*, measure]. Instrument for estimating the butter fat content of milk.

lactocele (lakt'o-sēl) [" + G. *kēlē*, hernia]. Cystic tumor of breast due to occlusion of a milk duct. SYN: *galactocele*.

lactocrit (lakt'o-krĭt) [" + *kritēs*, judge]. Instrument for determining the amt. of fatty substance in milk.

lactodensimeter (lakt-o-den-sim'et-er) [" + *densus*, thick, + G. *metron*, measure]. Instrument for determining specific gravity of milk.

lactoglobulin (lak"tō-glob'ū-lĭn) [L. *lac*, milk, + *globulus*, globule]. A protein found in milk.

lactolase (lak'to-lās) [L. *lac*. milk. + *ase*, enzyme]. An enzyme forming lactic acid. SYN: *lactacidase*.

lactolin (lakt'o-lĭn) [L. *lac*, milk]. Condensed or evaporated milk.

lactometer (lak-tom'et-er) [" + G. *metron*, measure]. Device for determining the specific gravity of milk.

lactophosphate (lakt'o-fos"făt) [" + *phosphās*, phosphate]. A salt derived jointly from lactic and phosphoric acid.

lactorrhea (lakt-or-re'ă) [" + G. *roia*, flow]. Discharge of milk between nursings and after weaning of offspring. SYN: *galactorrhea*.

lactoscope (lak'to-skōp) [" + G. *skopein*, to examine]. Device for determining quality of milk.

lac'tose [L. *lac*, milk]. C$_{12}$H$_{22}$O$_{11}$+H$_4$O, A disaccharide which on hydrolysis yields glucose and galactose.
  Bacteria can convert it into lactic and butyric acids, as in the souring of milk. 4-7% are found in the milk of all mammals. Its presence in the urine may be indicative of obstruction to flow of milk after cessation of nursing. Commercially, a fine powdered, white substance that will not dissolve in cold water.
  USP. Crystalline sugar obtained from evaporation of cow's milk. Used as modified milk for infant feeding, or supplementary food for adults, as a diluent. SYN: *milk sugar*. SEE: *disaccharose*.
  DOSAGE: 1-6 oz. (30.0-180.0 Gm.) per day.

lactoserum (lakt-o-sēr'um) [" + *serum*, whey]. 1. Blood serum of an animal inoculated with milk; used to precipitate specific caseins from milk. 2. The whey of milk. [lactose.

lacto'sum [L. *lac*, milk]. USP. term for

lactosuria (lak-to-su'rĭ-ă) [" + G. *ouron*, urine]. Occurrence of milk sugar (lactose) in the urine.
  Frequent during pregnancy and lactation. Identified by osazone crystals.

lactotherapy (lakt-o-ther'ă-pĭ) [" + G. *therapeia*, therapy]. 1. Treatment with milk diet. 2. Medicinal treatment of nursing infant with drugs given to mother to be excreted in milk. SYN: *galactotherapy*.

lac"totox'in [" + G. *toxikon*, poison]. A milk ptomaine.

lacuna (la-ku'na) (pl. *lacunae*) [L. a pit]. 1. A small, hollow space, such as that found in bones, in which lie the osteoblasts. 2. A gap or hiatus.
  l., absorption. Howship's l., *q.v.*
  l., bone. One of the isolated ovoid spaces bet. osseous lamellae, connected by canaliculi, containing a protoplasmic body or bone cell.
  l. cerebri. Cerebral infundibulum.
  l., haversian. One of those bet. the haversian lamellae.

lacuna, Henle's

l., Henle's. One of those separating the muscular fasciculi of the heart.

l., Howship's. 1. An absorption pit next to the periosteum. 2. A recess in bone filled with granulation tissue resulting from caries.

l., intervillous. Sinus of maternal portion of placenta from which are suspended fetal placental villi.

l. magna. Largest of orifices in Littre's glands.

l. Morgagni. Recess in mucous membrane of male urethra.

l. of the cornea. One of those bet. laminae of the cornea.

l. pharyngis. Pit at pharyngeal end of eustachian tube.

l. of the urethra. One of those in mucous membrane of the urethra, esp. along the floor and in the bulb.

l. vasorum. Internal aperture of femoral canal.

lacunar (la-kū'nar) [L. *lacuna*, pit]. Pert. to lacuna.

lacunula (la-kū'nu-lă) [L. little pit]. Small or minute lacuna.

lacus (la'kus) [L. lake]. Collection of fluid in small hollow or cavity.

l. derivitionis. Venous space in tentorium cerebelli.

l. lacrimalis. Space at inner canthus of eye where tears collect.

l. sanguineus. Uteroplacental sinus.

l. seminalis. Vault of vagina after insemination.

Laënnec's cirrhosis (lan-eks'). Atrophic cirrhosis of liver. SYN: *hobnail liver*.

L.'s pearls. Round gelatinous masses in asthmatic sputum.

L.'s râle. Modified subcrepitant râle due to mucus in bronchioles.

L.'s thrombus. Globular thrombus in heart.

lag [Welsh *llag*, slow]. 1. Period of time bet. application of stimulus and resulting reaction. SYN: *lag phase*. 2. Early period following bacterial inoculation into culture medium.

lagena (laj-ē'nă) [L. flask]. Upper extremity of ductus cochlearis.

lageniform (laj-en'ī-form) [" + *forma*, shape]. Flask-shaped.

lagging (lăg'ĭng) [Welsh *llag*, slow]. Retarded movement of chest in pulmonary tuberculosis.

lagophthalmos, lagophthalmus (lag-of-thal'mos, -mus) [G. *lagōs*, hare, + *ophthalmos*, eye]. Incomplete closure of palpebral fissure when lids are shut, resulting in exposure and injury to bulbar conjunctiva and cornea.

ETIOL: Contraction of a scar of eyelid, atony of orbicularis palpebrarum, exophthalmos. Incomplete closure of the lids during sleep is seen in hysteria, in exhausted adults, and often in healthy children. SYN: *hare's eye*.

lag phase [Welsh *llag*, slow, + G. *phasis*, appearance]. The period after a stimulus is administered to the time of its response. SEE: *lag*.

la grippe (la grip') [Fr. the grip]. Acute infectious disease of respiratory or gastrointestinal tract. SYN: *influenza*, q.v.

laity (lā'ĭ-tĭ) [G. *laos*, the people]. Portion of public nonprofessional in field of special professions.

laked [A.S. *lacu*, lake]. Said of the blood in hemolysis* or disintegration of the red blood corpuscles, freeing the hemoglobin into the blood plasma.

lak'ing [A.S. *lacy*, lake]. Freeing of hemoglobin from red blood corpuscles.

laky (lăk'ĭ) [A.S. *lacu*, lake]. Resembling a lake, as (1) postcoital collection in vagina below cervix in normal conditions, (2) color of lake pigment, or (3) red transparency following hemolysis of blood serum.

laliatry (lal-i'a-trĭ) [G. *lallein*, to babble, + *iatria*, therapy]. Study and treatment of speech disorders and defects.

lalla'tion, lal'ling [G. *lallein*, to babble]. A babbling form of stammering. Infantile form of speech. The constant use of "l" instead of "r."

lalognosis (lal-og-no'sis) [" + *gnōsis*, understanding]. Understanding of prattle or speech.

laloneurosis (lal-o-nū-rō'sis) [" + *neuron*, nerve, + *-ōsis*]. Speech impairment of neurotic origin.

lalop'athy [G. *lallein*, to babble, + *pathos*, disease]. Any disorder affecting the speech.

lalophobia (lal-ŏ-fō'bĭ-ă) [" + *phobos*, fear]. Morbid reluctance to speak due to fear of stammering or committing errors.

laloplegia (lal-o-ple'jĭ-ă) [" + *plēgē*, stroke]. A paralysis of speech muscles without affecting action of tongue.

lalorrhea (la-lor-re'ă) [" + *roia*, flow]. Abnormal flow of speech.

lamarckism or **Lamarck's theory** (lam-ark'-ism). Theory that structural changes are due to innate needs, and that these acquired characteristics may be transmitted to descendants.

lamb (lăm) [A.S.]. The young of sheep.

	Av. Serv.	Pro.	Fat	Car.
1. Roasted	115 Gm.	35.2	6.8	..
2. Quarters	75 Gm.	2.9	0.5	6.2

1. Ca 0.058, Mg 0.118, K 1.694, Na 0.421, P 1.078, Cl 0.378, S 1.146, Fe 0.0150.
1. Vit. A— to +, B+, G+.
2. Vit. A+++.

lambda (lam'dă) [G. *lambda*, letter L]. Point or angle of junction of lambdoid and sagittal sutures.

lambdacism (lam'dă-sizm) [G. *lambda*, letter L]. 1. Stammering of *l* sound. 2. Inability to pronounce *l* sound properly.

lambdoid, lambdoidal (lam'doid, lam-doid'-al) [" + *eidos*, form]. Shaped like Greek letter L.

l. ligament. Ligamentum fundiforme pedis.

l. suture. Suture bet. the occipital and 2 parietal bones.

Lamblia intestinalis (lam'blĭ-ă in-test-ĭ-nal'ĭs). Flagellate protozoan parasite found in intestine.

lambliasis (lăm-blī'ă-sĭs). Condition of infection with Lamblia intestinalis, marked frequently by symptoms of dysentery.

lamella (lam-el'ă) (pl. *lamellae*) [L. a little plate, leaf]. 1. A medicated disc of gelatin inserted under lower eyelid and against the eyeball used as a local application to eye. 2. A thin plate or scale.

l., bone. Thin layer of ground substance of osseous tissue.

l., concentric. Plate of bone surrounding a haversian canal.

l., fundamental. A general name for all periosteal, intermediate, and medullary bone lamellae.

l., intermediate. Bone lamella filling irregular spaces bet. concentric lamellae.

l., medullary. The osseous lamella surrounding and forming wall of medullary cavity of tubular bones.

l., periosteal. Bone lamella next to and parallel with the periosteum, forming ext. portion of bone.

l., triangular. Small fibrous lamina

bet. choroid plexuses of 3rd ventricle of the brain.
l., vitreous. Inner boundary of the choroid.
SYN: *Bruck's membrane, lamina basalis.*
lamellar (lam-el'lar). Arranged in thin plates or scales.
lam'ina (pl. *laminae*) [L. a thin plate]. 1. A thin, flat layer or membrane. 2. The flattened part of either side of the arch of a vertebra.
l. basalis. Layer of chorioid touching retinal pigmented layer.
l., Bowman's. Basement membrane beneath epithelium of cornea.
l. cartilaginis cricoideae. Flat, platelike, post. portion of cricoid cartilage.
l. c. thyroideae. One of the alae of the thyroid cartilage.
l. choriocapillaris. BNA. Choroid's middle layer containing close mesh of capillaries. SYN: *membrane, Ruysch's.*
l. choroidea inferior. Choroid plexus of the 4th ventricle.
l. cinerea. Gray substance bet. optic chiasm and callosum.
l. conchae. Surface of lateral mass of ethmoid bones.
l. cribrosa. Cribriform plate of the ethmoid bone.
l. c. ant. inferior. Ant. portion of inferior fossula containing openings for passage of divisions of cochlear branch of auditory nerve.
l. c. sclerae. Innermost lamella of sclera which stretches over the foramen sclerae, forming a diaphragm which is perforated by numerous openings for passageway of optic nerve fibers.
l. lentis. Concentric layer forming the crystalline lens.
l. mastoidea. Basal plate of mastoid process.
l. medullaris. Layer of medullated nerve fibers, the thickened ext. layer of the typical cerebral cortex.
l., medullary, external. Outer of 2 white laminae in nucleus lentiformis.
l., medullary, inner. Internal medullary. Layer of fibers passing from thalamus to the red nucleus.
l. propria of the membrana tympani. Middle fibrous layer of tympanic membrane.
l. quadrigemina. Layer of gray matter forming roof of aqueduct of Sylvius and supporting the corpora quadrigemina.
l. spiralis. One which divides the int. of spiral canal of cochlea into 2 scalae and divides into l. spiralis ossea, and l. spiralis membrana.
l. suprachoroidea. Outermost layer of the choroid.
l. vitreous. Smooth, transparent membrane covering inner surface of choroid.
laminated (lam'in-āt-ed) [L. *lamina*, thin plate]. Arranged in layers or laminae.
lamination (lam-in-ā'shun) [L. *lamina*, thin plate]. 1. Layerlike arrangement. 2. In embryotomy, the slicing of the skull.
laminec'tomy [" + G. *ektomē*, excision]. The excision of a vertebral post. arch.
NP: Keep patient off back in position specified by physician.
laminitis (lă-mĭn-i'tis) [" + G. *-itis*, inflammation]. Inflammation of a lamina.
lamp, therapeutic [G. *lampein*, to give light]. Device for producing and applying light, heat, radiation, and various forms of radioactivity for the treatment of disease.

l., Birch-Hirschfeld. Carbon arc lamp with a filter of uviol glass and a quartz lens system for phototherapy in ophthalmology.
l., carbon arc. A lamp for the passage of electric current through 2 carbon rods, the ends of which are opp. each other but a little distance apart, varying according to kinds of carbons employed. Carbon may be plain or cored with metals or impregnated with metallic salts. Comparatively little energy shorter than 2900 A° is emitted.
USES: To reproduce general physiological effects of sunlight.
l., cold quartz. A low vapor pressure, low amperage, high potential, glow discharge similar to the Geissler tube. Power consumed is small, consequently no great rise in temperature of burner. About 95% of the radiation of wave lengths less than and including 3130 A° is emitted in the resonance line at 2537 A°.
USES: For local bactericidal effect.
l., cold red light. Is emitted by neon glow discharge tube like the neon signs.
l., colored. Colored bulbs absorb some radiation emitted, reduce the efficacy of the lamps for heating, and become hotter for the same output of radiant energy than clear bulbs; are more likely to burst.
l., Cooper Hewitt vapor. Commercial illuminant in long tube of flint glass; is a low vapor pressure glow discharge tube.
l., Duke-Elder. Mercury vapor arc slit lamp apparatus with quartz lens system for ultraviolet radiation therapy in eye conditions.
l., electrodeless high frequency induction. One in which bulb is evacuated and contains a globule of mercury, whose vapor is excited to luminescence through high frequency from 5000 volt secondary of the transformer, passing through the helix surrounding the bulb.
USES: Same as mercury quartz lamp.
l., Finsen. A carbon arc lamp operating at 50 volts and 50 amperes so constructed that radiation is concentrated on an area 1 inch square; a water-cooled quartz system to remove infrared radiation and a compression quartz piece to dehematize the skin.
l., hot quartz. Quartz mercury arc lamp for ultraviolet radiation.
l., induced ultraviolet glow. Glow discharge is produced through an inductive effect. The quartz burner has the form of a sphere and a high frequency coil is wound around this sphere. This coil forms the primary winding of a high frequency transformer and the secondary winding is represented by the mercury vapor arc inside the sphere.
l., Kromayer. A water-cooled mercury quartz lamp, *q.v.*, named after its inventor, Dr. Kromayer.
l., Mazda. A trade name for sun lamps which are known as Mazda S-1 and S-2, differing only in size. The globe is of special size which absorbs radiation of wave lengths shorter than 2800 A°. USES: Home treatment under physician's supervision.
l., mercury glow. A lamp producing suitable ionization by means of electrons emitted from a hot cathode. Only a relatively low voltage is required to excite resonance radiation in the glow discharge through mercury vapor. This type of radiation is in the better ultraviolet glow lamp in a bulb of special

lamp, mercury quartz   L-8   **laparocystidotomy**

glass. It absorbs almost completely all rays shorter than 2800 A°. Operating temperature is low and glow discharge through mercury vapor practically fills the special glass bulb.

l., mercury quartz. Burner containing in quartz tube fluid mercury. One type has 2 columns of mercury representing 2 electrodes, and some burners have a pure tungsten anode and a mercury cathode. Cooling may be by air or water.

l., mercury vapor. Operates at a high vapor pressure, and relatively high temperature and low voltage. SEE: *hot quartz l.*

l., neon glow. One that emits cold red light. Same as neon signs. Little therapeutic effect. SEE: *cold red light lamp.*

l., quartz mercury. SEE: *mercury quartz.*

l., S-1 and S-2 ultraviolet. It consists of a special ultraviolet transmitting glass bulb of same shape as an ordinary light bulb. In this are a tungsten filament, 2 tungsten electrodes, and a drop of mercury. Electric current forms a mercury vapor arc between the highly incandescent tungsten electrodes. A satisfactory source of ultraviolet lamp for home use. A source of ultraviolet radiation.

l., sky light. Radiation from the whole sky in summer has more ultraviolet shorter than 3660 A° than direct sunlight.

l., sun. SEE: *Mazda lamp.*

l., tungsten filament. A gas-filled tungsten lamp is useful as a source of visible and short infrared radiations, but even when enclosed in a bulb that transmits ultraviolet rays from 2800 to 3100 A° it emits but little ultraviolet of these wave lengths, although recognized as effective in preventing rickets.

l., uviol. An electric lamp with a globe of uviol glass. SEE: *Ulilampe.*

l., ultraviolet. SEE: *carbon arc, Duke-Elder, mercury quartz, cold quartz, Finsen, Mazda, mercury glow, neon glow, S-1 and S-2, tungsten filament lamp,* and *uviarc.*

l., violet ray. 1. Helical-shaped carbon filament, incandescent lamp in bulb of blue glass. It has no therapeutic effect, excepting that of heat. 2. A glass tube attached to a spark coil which emits a blue glow when it touches the body. It should not be used as a source of ultraviolet rays.

l., water-cooled carbon arc. A carbon arc of 20-30 amperes with concentration apparatus of quartz lenses and watery solution of cobalt and copper sulfates. USES: In the Finsen method for local treatment of lupus vulgaris.

l., water-cooled quartz mercury vapor arc. A small quartz mercury vapor arc lamp enclosed in a double-walled metal box with a quartz window for generation and application of ultraviolet rays. Water is circulated between the walls to conduct away the intense heat. SYN: *Kromayer lamp.*

lamphonia (lam-pro-fō'nĭ-ă) [G. *lampros*, clear, + *phōnē*, voice]. Marked distinctness or clearness of voice.

lamprophonic (lam-prō-fōn'ik) [" + *phōnē*, voice]. Possessing a clear voice.

lance (lans) [L. *lancea*, spear]. 1. Two-edged surgical knife. 2. To incise with a lancet.

lancet (lan'sĕt) [L. *lancea*, spear]. Pointed surgical knife with 2 edges.

lancinating (lăn'sĭ-nāt-ing) [L. *lancināre*, to tear]. Sharp or cutting, as pain.

Lancisi's nerves (lan-che'zĭ). Striae in corpus callosum. SYN: *striae longitudinales, q.v.*

Landouzy-Dejerine atrophy (lan-dū-ze'da-zhĕ-rēn'). Atrophy of muscles of face and scapulohumeral group.

Landry's paralysis (lăn-drē'). A form of paralysis in which loss of motor power in lower extremities gradually extends to upper extremities and to circulatory and respiratory centers without sensory manifestations, trophic changes, etc. SYN: *acute ascending paralysis.*

land scurvy. Severe variety of purpura with hemorrhage of the mucosa. SYN: *purpura hemorrhagica.*

Lane's disease (lān). Chronic intestinal stasis.

L.'s kinks. Bending or twisting of intestine at various points as result of upright position of body.

L.'s operation. Short circuiting of the colon for chronic constipation, colitis, or obstruction.

Langerhans' islands (lahng'er-hahns). Cellular masses in interstitial tissue of pancreas, from which insulin is secreted. Failure of this secretion is associated with diabetes.*

SEE: *diabetes, insulin, pancreas.*

Lange's test (lăng'ĕ). Diagnosis of cerebrospinal syphilis by degree of gold precipitation in varying concentrations of colloidal gold solution and spinal fluid—4/10% salt solution.

Lang'hans layer. Deep layer of chorionic villi, composed of cells.

lanolin, anhydrous (lan'o-lin), USP. The purified, fatlike substance obtained from the wool of sheep.

USES: As an ointment base, having the property of absorbing water, and the advantage of not becoming rancid.

l., hydrous, USP. Wool fat containing about 25% water.

USES: Same as for l., anhydrous.

lanugo (lan-oo'go) [L. *lana*, wool]. 1. Downy hair covering the body. 2. Fine downy hairs that cover the body of the fetus, esp. when premature.

l. pudendarum. The pubic hair.

laparectomy (lap″ă-rĕk'tō-mĭ) [G. *lapara*, loin, + *ektomē*, excision]. Excision of strips or gores in abdominal wall. SYN: *enterectomy.*

laparo- [G.]. Combining form pert. to the *flank* and to operations *through the abdominal wall.*

laparocholecystotomy (lap″ar-o-kol″e-sis-tot'o-mĭ) [" + *cholē*, bile, + *kystis*, bladder, + *tomē*, incision]. Incision into gallbladder through abdomen.

laparocolostomy (lap″ar-ō-kō-lŏs'tō-mĭ) [" + *kōlon*, colon, + *stoma*, opening]. Formation of permanent opening into colon through abdominal wall.

laparocolotomy (lap″ar-ō-kō-lot'ō-mĭ) [" + " + *tomē*, incision]. Incision of colon through abdominal wall, forming an artificial opening. SYN: *laparocolostomy.*

laparocolpotomy (lap″ar-ō-kol-pot'ō-mĭ) [" + *kolpos*, vagina, + *tomē*, incision]. Incision over Poupart's ligament dissecting peritoneum to vagina which is incised transversely, enabling dilation of cervix and extraction of child through os uteri. SYN: *celioelytrotomy, laparoelytrotomy.*

laparocystectomy (la″pa-ro-sis-tek'to-mĭ) [" + *kystis*, bladder, + *ektomē*, excision]. Removal of an extrauterine fetus or of contents of a cyst through an abdominal incision.

laparocystidotomy (lap″ar-o-sĭst-ĭ-dŏt'ō-mĭ) [G. *lapara*, loin, + *kystis*, bladder,

+ *tomē*, incision]. Bladder incision through the abdominal wall.

laparocystotomy (lap″ar-o-sis-tot′o-mĭ) [" + "*tomē*, incision. Incision of abdomen to remove contents of a cyst or an extrauterine fetus.

laparoelytrotomy (lap″ar-o-el-ĭ-trot′o-mĭ). Abdominal incision to aid in removal of fetus. SEE: *cesarean operation*.

laparoenterostomy (lăp″ă-rō-ĕn-tĕr-ŏs′tō-mĭ) [" + *enteron*, intestine, + *stoma*, opening]. Formation of aperture into intestine through abdominal wall.

laparoenterotomy (lap″ar-o-en-ter-ot′o-mĭ) [" + " + *tomē*, incision]. Opening into intestinal cavity by incision through the loins.

laparogastrostomy (lăp″ăr-ō-găs-trŏs′tō-mĭ) [G. *lapara*, loin, + *gastēr*, belly, + *stoma*, opening]. Formation of permanent gastric fistula through abdominal wall. SYN: *celiogastrostomy*.

laparogastrotomy (lap″a-ro-gas-trot′o-mĭ) [" + " + *tomē*, incision]. Abdominal incision into stomach.

laparohepatotomy (lăp″ăr-ō-hĕp-ă-tŏt′ō-mĭ) [" + *ēpar*, *ēpat-*, liver, + *tomē*, incision]. Incision of the liver through abdominal wall from side.

laparohysterectomy (lap″ar-o-his-ter-ek′to-mĭ) [" + *ystera*, uterus, + *ektomē*, excision]. Abdominal removal of uterus.

laparohystero-oöphorectomy (lap″ar-o-his″ter-o-o″o-for-ek′to-mĭ) [" + " + *ōon*, ovum, + *phoros*, bearer, + *ektomē*, excision]. Removal of uterus and ovaries through an abdominal incision. POSITION: Dorsal.

laparohysteropexy (lap″ar-o-his′ter-o-peks-ĭ) [" + " + *pēxis*, fixation]. Abdominal fixation of the uterus.

laparohysterosalpingo-oöphorectomy (lăp″-ăr-ō-hĭs″tĕr-ō-săl-pĭn″gō-ō″ō-fō-rĕk′tō-mĭ) [G. *lapara*, loin, + *ystera*, uterus, + *salpigx*, tube, + *ōon*, ovum, + *phoros*, bearer, + *ektomē*, excision]. Removal of uterus, fallopian tubes, and ovaries through abdominal incision. SYN: *celiohysterosalpingo-oöthecectomy*.

laparohysterotomy (lap″ar-o-his-ter-ot′o-mĭ) [" + " + *tomē*, incision]. Abdominal incision into uterus. SEE: *cesarean section*.

laparoileotomy (lap″ar-o-il-e-ot′o-mĭ) [" + *eilein*, to twist]. Abdominal incision into ileum.

laparokelyphotomy (lăp″ăr-ō-kĕl-ĭ-fŏt′ō-mĭ) [" + *kelyphos*, eggshell, + *tomē*, incision]. 1. Removal of an extrauterine fetus by laparotomy. 2. Suprapubic cystotomy. SYN: *laparocystotomy*.

laparomyitis (lăp-ăr-ō-mĭ-ī′tĭs) [G. *lapara*, loin, + *mys*, muscle, + *-itis*, inflammation]. Inflammation of muscular portion of abdominal wall.

laparomyomectomy (lap″ar-o-mi-o-mek′to-mĭ) [" + " + *ōma*, tumor, + *ektomē*, excision]. Abdominal excision of a muscular tumor.
Preparation same as for cesarean operation, minus the obstetrical appliances. POSITION: Dorsal.

laparonephrectomy (lap″ar-o-ne-frek′to-mĭ) [" + *nephros*, kidney, + *ektomē*, excision]. Renal excision abdominally.

laparorrhaphy (lăp-ăr-or′ră-fĭ) [" + *raphē*, suture]. Abdominal wall suture. SYN: *celiorrhaphy*.

laparosalpingectomy (lap″ar-o-sal-pin-jek′to-mĭ) [" + *salpigx*, tube, + *ektomē*, excision]. Abdominal excision of a fallopian tube.

laparosalpingo-oöphorectomy (lăp″ăr-ō-săl-pĭn″gō-ō″ŏf-ō-rĕk′tō-mĭ) [" + " + *ōon*, ovum, + *phoros*, bearer, + *ektomē*, excision]. Removal of fallopian tubes and ovaries through abdominal incision. SYN: *celiosalpingo-oöthecectomy*.

laparosalpingotomy (lăp″ăr-ō-săl-pĭn-gŏt′-ō-mĭ) [" + " + *tomē*, incision]. Incision of oviduct through abdominal wall. SYN: *celiosalpingotomy*.

laparoscopy (lăp-ăr-ŏs′kō-pĭ) [" + *skopein*, to examine]. Abdominal exploration employing instruments. SYN: *celioscopy*.

laparosplenectomy (lap″ar-o-splen-ek′to-mĭ) [" + *splēn*, spleen, + *ektomē*, excision]. Abdominal excision of the spleen.

laparosplenotomy (lăp″ăr-ō-splĕn-ŏt′ō-mĭ) [" + " + *tomē*, incision]. Incision of the spleen through abdominal wall.

laparotomy (lap-ar-ot′o-mĭ) [" + *tomē*, incision]. The surgical opening of the abdomen; an abdominal operation.
PREPARATION: *General*: Except in emergency cases, the preparatory treatment should be begun three days before operation, during which time the patient is strictly confined to light, nutritious diet, and receives each day a warm bath, laxative, and, in operations on uterus or vagina, a vaginal douche. Patients having stricture of the esophagus, pylorus, or intestines are not given cathartic, but with physician's permission a high enema. For pyloric or intestinal obstruction wash out the stomach. On evening before operation, previous to shaving abdomen, denude pubes with scissors and apply a potash soap poultice. After an hour remove the poultice; shave entire abdomen, pubes and genitalia, scrub with hot water and potash soap; wrap cotton on the end of probe to clean umbilicus. Wash with sterile water and scrub again, using benzine and soap; rinse with warm water; dry with gauze; sponge with alcohol, then use warm bichloride solution 1:1000 and cover field of operation with a 3-yard compress of sterile gauze, saturated with a warm solution of bichloride, strength 1:3000 or 1:5000, oiled muslin or waxed paper pad of cotton, and enclose all in a snug abdominal bandage, held in place with perineal straps. Iodine followed by alcohol is preferred by some physicians.
Abdominal hysterectomy: The vagina should be disinfected as follows: Wrap gauze around index finger and mop with hot water and soap; then use clear water, give a douche of bichloride 1:4000 and pack cervix with a strip of iodoform gauze. One hour before operation remove gauze and give corrosive sublimate douche and mop vagina thoroughly with alcohol before repacking.
Patient should receive supper and no breakfast. Specimens of urine should be in a sterile bottle for examination. Five hours before operation give a high enema of castile suds followed by a small one of clear water to rinse bowel. Before leaving the room the patient is attired in clean clothing, including a pair of stockings; then the hair, if long, is plaited tightly in two braids.
POSTOPERATIVE NURS: In the treatment after a laparotomy the nurse should carefully observe the condition of the patient, and give timely information of the onset of serious complications, most important of which are shock, secondary hemorrhage, and peritonitis.
Patient is carefully removed from operating room without raising head or chest, to the bed, which has been previously prepared with a rubber and a

draw sheet, and well supplied with hotwater bottles for armpits and lower extremities.

Cover the bottles that they may not burn the insensible patient, as much harm has been done in this way. Patient is placed in the dorsal (recumbent) position with limbs flexed to relax the abdominal muscles, and a pillow placed under the knees to support them. This position is retained for 48 hours during which patient is constantly watched. At termination of this period patient may be turned on either side.

Pulse and temperature should be immediately taken after every operation; temperature should be taken in the rectum (never take aged person's temperature in the axilla). Hypodermic syringe, brandy, strychnine, nitroglycerine, digitalis, flannel bandages and blocks to elevate the foot of bed should be kept in readiness.

No food by mouth should be given during the first 48 hours. In cases of persistent vomiting, stimulants and food are administered by rectum. After a laparotomy, mouth should be frequently sponged and lips moistened. A piece of ice wrapped in gauze and rubbed over the lips is very soothing to the patient, and in cases of extreme thirst very hot water may be given in ½ oz. doses, but as seldom as possible. Small pieces of ice in the form of ice pills are sometimes allowed.

Hot water being a stimulant, is preferred to ice, which is a sedative, another objection being the germs it contains, though it may control the nervous vomiting by rubbing across the lips. In such cases it is best to relieve the thirst by rectal or subcutaneous injections of physiologic solution, thus securing complete rest for the stomach. In absence of bad symptoms toward end of second day patient may have a little peptonized milk, chicken broth or kumiss, varying in amount from ½-4 oz., according to condition of patient, increasing the quantity gradually.

Majority of laparotomy cases require a cathartic as soon as they recover from effects of operation. A teaspoonful of sulfate of magnesia dissolved in hot water and given every hour till bowels move freely is the best course to pursue in relieving the patient and guarding against peritonitis. If patient is vomiting and unable to take a cathartic, and is not relieved by an enema of equal parts (pt. each) of milk and molasses heated to 100° F., give a high enema of magnesium sulfate 2 oz., glycerin 4 oz., pt. of water; use rectal tube. A hot bag applied over bladder often prevents retention of urine.

If obliged to catheterize, which should not be done under 8 hours after operation, use a soft rubber catheter; see that it has been boiled and afterwards kept aseptic. SEE: *ventrotomy*.

laparotrachelotomy (lap″ar-o-tra-kĕl-ot′o-mī) [G. *lapara*, loin, + *trachēlos*, neck, + *tomē*, incision]. Cesarean section with the incision through the lower segment of the uterus.

laparotyphlotomy (lăp″ăr-ō-tī-flŏt′ō-mī) [" + *typhlon*, cecum, + *tomē*, incision]. Incision of cecum through lateral abdominal incision.

laparouterotomy (lăp″ăr-ō-ū-tĕr-ŏt′ō-mī) [" + L. *uterus*, womb, + G. *tomē*, incision]. Incision of uterus through abdominal wall. SYN: *laparohysterotomy*.

lapis (la′pis) [L.]. Stone.

laqueus (lak′we-us) [L. noose]. A noose-shaped band, fillet, or cord.
  l. umbilicalis. The umbilical cord.

lard [L. fat]. Av. SERVING: 15 Gm. Fat 15.0. VITAMINS: A: — to + D: — to +.

lardaceous (lar-dā′shus) [L. *lardum*, fat]. Resembling lard; waxy, fatty.
  l. disease. Amyloid degeneration. The organs affected present a white waxy appearance due to the deposit of a firm translucent substance called *lardacein* or *amyloid* which when treated with iodine produces a dark mahogany-brown color.

larocaine (lar′o-kān). Registered trademark for a medicinal preparation for topical application and for injection.
  USES: As local anesthetic.

larva (lar′vă) [L. ghost, mask]. An immature stage in insect life after it has emerged from the egg and before it assumes adult form.
  l. migrans. An extensive skin eruption due to a parasitic larva which burrows under the epidermis. SYN: *cercaria*.

laryngalgia (lăr-ĭn-găl′jĭ-ă) [G. *larygx*, larynx]. Neuralgia of the larynx.

laryngeal (lar-in′je-al) [G. *larygx*, larynx]. Pert. to the larynx.
  l. reflex. Cough as result of irritation of larynx or fauces.

laryngectomy (lar-in-jek′to-mī) [" + *ektomē*, excision]. Excision of larynx.
  PREPARATION: Similar to tracheotomy, plus additional ligatures, sponge or tampon cannula. Best done in two operations—performing tracheotomy week or two before the main operation.

laryngismal (lar-ĭn-jĭs′măl) [G. *larygx*, larynx]. Concerning or resembling affection with laryngeal spasm.

laryngismus (lar-in-jis′mus) [" + *ismos*, condition of]. Spasm of the larynx.
  SYM: Face pale—later cyanosed; eyes rolled up, body arched; thumbs turned into palm, legs extended, soles turned inward. In a few seconds the spasm relaxes.
  PROG: Favorable. In very young, death may result from suffocation.
  TREATMENT: During paroxysm cold water may be dashed on face and head or few drops of amyl nitrite or chloroform inhaled from handkerchief. In the interval search for cause—gums may need lancing or gastrointestinal tract need attention. Child should be placed under best hygienic conditions; food plain and nutritious, constitutional treatment.
  l., infantile. One occurring in children less than one year old, who are poorly nourished.
  l. stridulus. A paroxysmal neurosis characterized by spasm of the adductors of the larynx and not excited by any local inflammation.
  ETIOL: Early life (within first 2 years), male sex, and the rachitic diathesis are predisposing causes; often accompanies tetany. The discharge of motor force apparently rises in the medulla and may be excited by reflex irritation as in teething and gastrointestinal troubles.
  SYM: Attacks often and sudden; may occur on awakening from sleep — are characterized by a sudden arrest in breathing and tonic muscular swelling; can be detected by finger on throat. Spasm relapses, and air is drawn in through glottis with shrill crowing sound

—may occur several times a day or weeks apart.
PROG: Extremely grave.
TREATMENT: Correct diet, cod-liver oil, and calcium lactate. When symptoms are not urgent, leeches may be applied over larynx and astringent solutions sprayed over the edematous tissues. If symptoms persist, parts may be scarified. If this fails to relieve dyspnea tracheotomy may be performed. SYN: *cantus galli.*

laryngitic (lar-in-jĭt′ĭk) [G. *larygx,* larynx]. 1. Resulting from laryngitis. 2. Rel. to laryngitis.

laryngitis (lar-in-jī′tis) [" + *-itis,* inflammation]. Inflammation of larynx.

l., acute catarrhal. Acute congestive laryngitis; catarrhal inflammation of laryngeal mucosa and the vocal cords.
SYM: Hoarseness and aphonia and occasionally pain on phonation and deglutition.
ETIOL: Improper use of voice, exposure to cold and wet, extension from infections in nose and throat, inhalation of irritating vapors and dust, associated with systemic diseases as whooping cough, measles, etc.
TREATMENT: Complete rest of voice, promotion of elimination by catharsis, diaphoresis, liquid or soft diet, medicated steam inhalations such as compound tincture of benzoin, codeine for cough and pain. SEE: *croup.*

l., atrophic. L. leading to diminished secretion and glandular atrophy of the mucous membrane.
SYM: Tickling sensation in throat, hoarseness, cough, dyspnea when crusts are thick and accumulate on vocal cords so as to narrow the breathing aperture.
TREATMENT: Iodides internally, inhalants and medicated sprays to loosen the crusts; strict attention to associated nose and throat pathology.

l., chronic. A type due to a recurrent irritation, or following the acute form. Often secondary to sinus or nasal pathology, improper use of voice, excessive smoking or drinking.
SYM: Tickling in throat, amblyphonia and huskiness of voice, dysphonia.
TREATMENT: Correction of preëxisting nose and throat pathology, discontinuance of alcohol and tobacco, avoidance of excessive use of voice and proper vocal placement, topical application of 2-5% silver nitrate solution.

l., c. hypertrophic. Hypertrophy of tissues accompanying chronic l.

l., diphtheritic. Invasion of larynx by diphtheria bacilli, usually with formation of membrane.

l., membranous. Characterized by inflammation of larynx with the formation of a false membrane of nondiphtheritic origin.
TREATMENT: Free catharsis, inhalation of medicated vapors to loosen the membrane, administration of ipecacuanha for emesis. SEE: *membranous croup.*

l., phlegmonous. Inflamed larynx with purulent infiltration or abscesses.

l., syphilitic. ETIOL: Due to syphilis.
SYM: Hoarseness, cough, simple catarrh, formation of broad condylomata, follicular hyperplasia, syphiloma, syphilitic perichondritis.
Secondary stage in form of mucous patches or tertiary in form of gumma. Secondary syphilis is a diffuse infection and one sees luetic patches spread over large areas of larynx.
In tertiary syphilis the gummatous lesion can occur in any part of larynx. There is marked redness over the infiltrated area as well as in the surrounding mucous membrane. When there is breaking down, the resultant ulceration is deep with sharp edges. Pain is usually absent and fixation of the cord is late. Cicatrization and deformity follow healing of gumma.
TREATMENT: Antiluetic.

l., tuberculous. Secondary to pulmonary tuberculosis.
SYM: Hoarseness, amblyphonia or aphonia, pain in swallowing, cough. Lesion located in: 1. Interarytenoid area. 2. Vocal cords. 3. Epiglottis. 4. False cords. Lesions are relatively pale; ulceration occurs early.
TREATMENT: Vocal hygiene, absolute rest of voice, orthoform powder sprayed in larynx. Aqueous solutions of lactic acid 20-80% applied to affected areas by applicator, galvanocautery, heliotherapy to affected areas by means of mirrors, alcoholic injection of sup. laryngeal nerve (one or both sides), resection of sup. laryngeal nerve, gastrostomy to keep patient's larynx at rest, since swallowing produces motion of larynx.

l., ulcerative. Chronic l. with ulceration of the mucous membrane.

laryn′go- [G.]. Prefix: Pert. to the *larynx.*

laryngocele (lar-in′go-sēl) [G. *larygx, larygg-,* larynx, + *kēlē,* hernia]. 1. Dilatation of larynx. 2. Protrusion of laryngeal mucosa.

laryngocentesis (lăr-in″gō-sĕn-tē′sĭs) [" + *kentēsis,* puncture]. Incision or puncture of the larynx.

laryngofissure (lar-ing″go-fish′ur) [" + L. *fissura,* a cleft]. The operation of opening the larynx by a median line incision through the thyroid cartilage.

laryngograph (lar-ing′o-grăf) [" + *graphein,* to write]. Device for making a record of laryngeal movements.

laryngography (lăr-in-gŏg′ră-fī) [" + *graphein,* to write]. Description of larynx.

laryngologist (lar-in-gol′o-jĭst) [" + *logos,* study]. Specialist in laryngology.

laryngol′ogy [" + *logos,* study]. The practice of medicine dealing with the treatment of diseases of the larynx.

laryngometry (lăr-in-gŏm′ĕ-trī) [G. *larygx, larygg-,* larynx, + *metron,* measure]. Systematic measurement of larynx.

laryngoparalysis (lăr-in″gō-par-ăl′ĭ-sĭs) [" + *para,* beside, + *lyein,* to loosen]. Paralysis of muscles of larynx.

laryngopathy (lăr-in-gop′ă-thī) [" + *pathos,* disease]. Any disease of the larynx.

laryngophantom (lăr-in-gō-fan′tŏm) [" + *phantasma,* image]. Plastic model of the larynx.

laryngopharyngeal (lar-in″gō-far-in′jē-ăl) [" + *pharygx,* pharynx]. Rel. jointly to larynx and pharynx.

laryngopharyngectomy (lăr-in″gō-făr-in-jek′tō-mī) [" + " + *ektomē,* excision]. Removal of the larynx and pharynx.

laryngopharyngitis (lăr-in″gō-făr-in-jī′tĭs) [" + " + *-itis,* inflammation]. Inflammation of the larynx and pharynx.

laryngopharynx (lăr-in-gō-făr′ĭnks) [" + *pharygx,* pharynx]. Lower portion of the pharynx that extends from the cornua of the hyoid bone or vestibule of the larynx to the lower border of the cricoid cartilage.

laryngophony (lăr-in-gof′ō-nī) [G. *larygx, larygg-,* larynx, + *phōnē,* voice]. Voice sounds heard in auscultating the pharynx.

laryngoplasty (lăr-in-gō-plăs-tī) [" + *plassein,* to form]. Plastic reparative surgery of larynx.

laryngoplegia (la-ring″go-plē′jĭ-ă) [" + *plēgē*, stroke]. Paralysis of laryngeal muscles.

laryngorhinology (lăr-ĭn″gō-rīn-ŏl′ō-jĭ) [" + *ris, rin-*, nose, + *logos*, study]. Science treating with diseases of the larynx and nose.

laryngorrhagia (lăr-ĭn-gor-ră′jĭ-ă) [" + *rēgnunai*, to flow forth]. Laryngeal hemorrhage.

laryngorrhea (lăr-ĭn-gor-rē′ă) [" + *roia*, flow]. Excessive discharge of laryngeal mucus. SYN: *blennorrhea*.

laryngosclerorma (lăr-ĭn-gō-sklē-rō′mă) [" + *sklēros*, hard, + *ōma*, tumor]. Scleroma affecting the larynx.

laryngoscope (lar-ĭn′go-skōp) [" + *skopein*, to examine]. Instrument for examining the larynx.

l., solar. Two mirrors, one reflecting sun rays into mouth, again reflected into larynx by laryngeal mirror. Newer modifications use an alloy of aluminum and magnesium in reflecting mirrors.

laryngoscopic (lar-ĭn-gō-skōp′ĭk) [G. *larygx, larygg-*, + *skopein*, to examine]. Pert. to observation with aid of small long handled mirror for reflecting interior of larynx.

laryngoscopy (lar-ĭn-gos′kō-pĭ) [" + *skopein*, to examine]. Examination of interior of larynx.
NP: Instrument should be warmed. Parts should be cocainized.

l., direct. That done with laryngeal speculum or laryngoscope.
NP: Mouth is held open with a gag.

l., indirect. That done with a mirror.
NP: Nurse should stand behind patient with left hand on head, holding patient's tongue with right hand to steady it.

laryngospasm (lăr-ĭn′gō-spazm) [" + *spasmos*, spasm]. Spasm of laryngeal muscles.

laryngostenosis (lar-ing″go-ste-nō′sis) [" + *stenōsis*, a narrowing]. Stricture of larynx.

l., compression. From causes outside the larynx as result of abscesses, tumors, goiter, etc.

l., occlusion. ETIOL: May be due to congenital bands or membranes, foreign bodies, tumors, cicatricial contraction following ulceration as in diphtheria and tertiary syphilis, penetrating wounds or corrosive fluid.
SYM: Dyspnea, esp. on inspiration and exertion. Loud breathing which becomes a stridulous choking respiration; pulse small and frequent; face anxious and cyanotic.
PROG: Grave.
TREATMENT: Depends on cause. Tracheotomy is often the temporary and almost always the final expedient.

laryngostomy (lăr-ĭn-gos′tō-mĭ) [" + *stoma*, opening]. Establishing permanent opening through neck into larynx.

laryngotracheitis (lăr-ĭn″gō-tra-kē-ī′tĭs). Inflamed condition of the larynx and trachea.

laryngostroboscope (lar-in-go-stro′bo-skōp) [" + *strobos*, whirl, + *skopein*, to view]. Instrument for inspection of vibration of vocal cords.

laryngotomy (lar-in-got′o-mĭ) [" + *tomē*, incision]. Incision of larynx.

laryngotracheotomy (lar-in′go-tra-ke-ot′o-mĭ) [" + *tracheia*, windpipe, + *tomē*, incision]. Incision of larynx with section of upper tracheal rings.

laryngoxerosis (lăr-ĭn″gō-zēr-ō′sĭs) [" + *xērōsis*, dryness]. Abnormal dryness of the larynx.

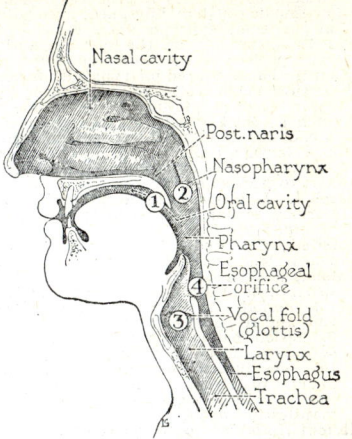

THE LARYNX
Seen in its relation to: 1. The mouth cavity. 2. Nasopharynx. 3. Glottis. 4. Esophagus.

larynx (lar′inks) (*Pl. larynges*) [G. *larygx*]. The organ of voice, the enlarged upper end of trachea; musculocartilaginous structure lined with mucous membrane.
BLOOD SUPPLY: Inf. thyroid, branch of thyroid axis and sup. thyroid, branch of ext. carotid.
CARTILAGES: Thyroid, cricoid, epiglottis, two arytenoids, two cartilages of Santarini articulating with arytenoids, and two cartilages of Wrisberg in aryepiglottic folds.
NERVES: From int. and ext. branches of sup. laryngeal.
NP: *Diseases of*: Patient should stay in bed and, in any event, he should avoid changes of atmosphere which may cause an attack of coughing. Room temperature should be maintained at the proper level, and drafts avoided. Movements may set up coughing, so patient should rest quietly. The voice is generally affected in abnormal conditions of the larynx, so voice also should be rested. To keep silence, however, may cause patient to become depressed. The nurse needs to entertain the patient but she should not ask the patient questions unless they may be answered by a nod of the head. The patient will need encouragement in continuing inhalations ordered.
When possible for the patient to use the voice, instructions should be given to use the diaphragm and abdominal muscles rather than the muscles of the throat. In chronic laryngitis cold water may be applied to the neck morning and night. The nose, throat, and larynx must be kept cleaned by sprays as ordered.
In edema of the larynx sucking ice, or application of ice to the neck may be helpful. Astringent sprays and saline purges may be ordered by the doctor.
RS: *Bouchut's method, cricoarytenoid, epiglottis, glottis, "laryng-" words, prominentia laryngea, vestibule, vocal cord.*

l., foreign bodies in. SYM: When a

lascivia   L-13   **law, Colles'**

foreign body enters it produces violent spasmodic cough and dyspnea; fixed pain at particular spot and loss of voice.

TREATMENT: If on the spot promptly raise patient by the heels and slap him on the back. Search pharynx with finger and extract object. Induce vomiting by inserting finger in throat. Feed foods such as thick gruels, mashed potatoes, bread, etc., to carry object into stomach. Use laryngoscopic mirror and extract substance with forceps—may need to resort to tracheotomy.

lasciv'ia [L. *lascivīre*, to be wanton]. Abnormal sexual desire. SYN: *nymphomania,* satyriasis.**

lassitude (las'ĭ-tūd) [L. *lassitūdō*, weariness]. Weariness; exhaustion.

latency (lā'těn-sĭ) [L. *latēre*, to be hidden]. State of being concealed or hidden.

   l. period. 1. Interval bet. stimulation and response to it. SYN: *lag phase.* 2. Period bet. pregenital or infantile sexuality and onset of puberty or genital sexuality, occurring bet. ages of about 4 to 11 years. 3. Period of incubation in which a disease exists without manifesting itself.

la'tent [L. *latēre*, to be concealed]. 1. Lying hidden. 2. Quiet; not active.

   l. content. PSY: That part of a dream that cannot be brought into the objective consciousness through any effort of will to remember.

   l. heat. Heat that disappears during evaporation or melting.

   l. period. 1. Time bet. a stimulus and its response. SYN: *lag phase.* 2. PSY: Time bet. ages of 4 to about 11 years separating infantile sexuality from onset of puberty or genital sexuality. SYN: *latency period, 2.* 3. Time during which a disease is supposed to be existent without manifesting itself; period of incubation.

laterad (lat'ĕr-ăd) [L. *latus, later-,* side, + *ad,* toward]. Toward a side or lateral aspect.

lateral (lat'er-al) [L. *latus, later-,* side]. Pert. to the side.

   l. sinus. Transverse and sigmoid portion of two cranial venous sinuses. Extends from occipital protuberance to jugular bulb.

latericeous, lateritious (lat-ĕr-ĭ'shŭs) [L. *later,* a brick]. Resembling brick dust.

lateroflexion (lăt"ĕr-ō-flek'shun) [L. *latus, later-,* side, + *flexus;* from *flectere,* to bend]. Bending or curvature toward a side.

lateroprone, laterosemiprone position (lăt"-ĕr-ō-prōn', -sĕm'ĭ-prōn). Patient on left side leaning on chest, right knee and thigh drawn up, left arm back of patient. SYN: *Sims' position, q.v., for illustration.*

lateropulsion (lat-er-o-pul'shun) [" + *pulsus,* driving]. Involuntary tendency in cerebellar and labyrinthine disease to fall to one side.

lateroversion (lăt-ĕr-ō-vĕr'shun) [" + *versiō,* a turning]. Tendency or a turning toward one side.

lathyrism (lath'ĭr-izm) [G. *lathyros,* vetch]. Chick-pea poisoning. SYN: *lupinosis.*

Nervous disorders and tremors with cramps in arms and legs.

TREATMENT: Provoke vomiting, wash out stomach, stimulants.

latrine (la-trēn') [L. *latrina*]. A public privy.

la'tus [L. side]. The flank or side.

laud'able [L. *laudabilis,* praiseworthy]. Healthy; normal; said of *pus.*

laudanum (law'dan-um). Tincture of opium. POISONING: SEE: *morphine.*

laugh (lăf) [M. E. *laughen*, to laugh]. Sound produced by laughing. SYN: *risus.*

   l., sardonic. Spasm of facial muscles producing a grinning effect. SYN: *risus sardonicus.*

laughing gas (laf'ing) [M. E. *laughen*, to laugh]. Nitrous oxide gas.

laughter reflex (lăf'tĕr). Uncontrollable laughter resulting from tickling or pretense of tickling.

lavage (la-vazh') [Fr.; from L. *lavāre*, to wash]. Washing out of a cavity.

   l., gastric. Washing out of the stomach. A stomach tube or catheter is used with solution of sterile water, or normal saline, or 2% boracic acid, or 1-5% sodium bicarbonate.

QUANTITY OF SOLUTION: Not more than 10 oz. at a time repeated until fluid runs clear.

TEMPERATURE AND TIME: 105° F. Preferably before breakfast. POSITION: Semirecumbent or low enough to prevent inhalation of returning fluid. In poisoning, save siphoned fluid for examination. If patient is unconscious use a mouth gag.

PURPOSE: To remove irritants or poisons, to relieve nausea or vomiting, to cleanse the stomach preoperatively or postoperatively. In latter case to prevent nausea. SEE: *bladder irrigation, colonic irrigation.*

law [A. S. *laga,* law]. In the scientific sense, a statement which is found to hold true uniformly for a whole class of natural occurrences.

RS: *Allen's, Camerer's, inverse square, Joule's, Nerst's.*

   l., Ampère's. The directing force of electric currents on mobile magnets causes the latter's austral pole to deviate to the left of current.

   l., Avoga'dro's. If temperature and ext. pressure are the same, all gases contain same number of molecules in equal volumes.

   l., Behring's. Blood and serum of an immunized subject confers immunity when injected into another.

   l., Bell-Magendie's. In spinal nerves the ant. roots contain only motor fibers and post. roots sensory fibers.

   l., Bell's. Ant. spinal nerve roots are motor, and post. roots are sensory.

   l's, Bertholle's. 1. When two salts react because of a solvent, if a new salt can be produced less soluble, this salt will be produced. 2. When dry heat is applied to "two salts, if a new salt can be produced more volatile, this salt will be produced."

   l., Boudin's. There is an antagonism existing bet. malarial and tuberculous disease.

   l., Boyle's. The volume occupied by a fixed quantity of every gas is inversely proportional, and density directly proportional, to pressure applied to the gas.

   l., Brew'ster's. For any substance the polarizing angle is equal to that angle of incidence at which the portion of light that is reflected is at right angles to the portion refracted.

   l's, Bunsen's. Chemical principles governing reactions occurring bet. compound bodies when one of them is present in considerable excess.

   l., Charles'. When pressure is constant, volume of a gas varies as the absolute temperature.

   l., Colles'. A syphilitic father may beget a syphilitic child without apparently infecting the mother, and this mother cannot be infected by nursing the child.

l. of conservation of energy. Energy can be neither created nor destroyed.

l., Coulomb's (koo'looms). 1. Electrified particles attract or repel each other with a force directly proportionate to the quantity of electricity acting, and inversely proportional to the square of the distance between the particles. 2. The force of torsion is proportional to the angle of torsion.

l., Courvoisier's. When the common bile duct is obstructed by a calculus, dilatation of gallbladder is rare; when otherwise obstructed, dilatation is common.

l., Dalton's. 1. The tension of a mixture of several gases or of a gas and a vapor equals the sum of tensions which each would separately possess. 2. The tension and amount of vapor which will saturate a given space at a given temperature are the same whether the space is empty or filled with a gas.

l. of definite proportions. Two or more chemicals when united to form a new substance do so in a constant and fixed proportion by weight.

l., Delboeuf's. If in any species a number of individuals, bearing a ratio not infinitely small to the entire number of births, are in every generation born with a particular variation neither beneficial nor injurious, and if not counteracted by reversion, the proportion of the new variety to the original form will increase till it approaches indefinitely near to equality.

l., Donders'. SEE: *Listing's law*.

l., Du Bois-Reymond's. A nerve through which a galvanic current is passed is stimulated by the making or breaking of the current or by any sudden change in its intensity.

l., Dulong and Petit's. The specific heat of any solid elementary body is in inverse ratio to its atomic weight.

l. of eccentricity of sensation. A sensation is referred to the termination or end organ of the stimulated nerve and not to the nerve center.

l's. of electrolysis, Faraday's. 1. Electrolysis cannot take place unless the electrolyte is a conductor. 2. The electrolytic action is same in all parts of the electrolyte. 3. The same electric current decomposes quantities of the electrolytes directly proportional to their chemical equivalents. 4. The quantity of an electrolyte decomposed is directly proportional to quantity of electricity passing through it.

l., Fechner's. The intensity of sensation is proportional to the logarithm of the strength of the stimulus.

l., Gay-Lussac's. 1. The tension of a gas varies directly with temperature if volume remains the same. 2. When gases or vapors react on each other the volumes both of the factors and of the products of the reaction always bear to each other some very simple numerical ratio. 3. Air and all of less liquefiable gases have a coefficient of expansion of $1/273$.

l., Godélier's. Tuberculous disease of the peritoneum is always accompanied by similar disease of the pleura.

l., Graham's. The rate at which a gas diffuses through a porous membrane is inversely proportional to the square root of the density of the gas.

l., Haeckel's fundamental biological. The ontogeny is a short repetition of the phylogeny of a species.

l., Head's. "When a painful stimulus is applied to a part of low sensibility in close central connection with a part of much greater sensibility, the pain produced is felt in the part of higher sensibility rather than in the part of lower sensibility to which the stimulus was actually applied."

l. of the heart. Other things being equal, the stroke volume of the heart varies as the extent of diastolic filling; or, the energy of contraction is a function of the initial length of the muscle fibers.

l., Henry's. Dalton's law, *q.v.*

l., Hilton's. A nerve trunk supplying any joint supplies the muscles which move the joint and skin over insertion of such muscles.

l., Hooke's. If a body is distorted within limits of perfect elasticity, the force with which it reacts is proportional to amount of distortion.

l. of the intestine. Moderate distention of the intestine at a point causes relaxation below (aborally to the point) and contraction above.

l., Kirchoff's. When a beam of light is passed through a transparent body the latter absorbs those luminous rays which it is capable of emitting when heated to incandescence.

l., Koch's, Koch's postulate. To prove an organism to be the cause of a given disease or lesion: 1st, the microörganism in question must appear in the lesion at all times; 2nd, pure cultures must be obtained from it; 3rd, cultures must reproduce the disease in animals and pure cultures must be again obtained from these lesions.

l., Lambert's cosine. The intensity of radiation received by an absorbing surface varies as the cosine of the angle of incidence for parallel rays.

l., Listing's. If, with normal eyes and parallel visual lines, the visual line passes from the primary position into any other position, the rotatory movement of the eyeball in this secondary position is of such a kind as if it had been turned round a fixed axis, lying perpendicular to the first and second direction of the visual line.

l. of Magendie. Same as l. of Bell.

l., Malaguti's. When solutions of two different salts are mixed, "metathesis occurs and 4 salts result, the proportions of salts to each other being dependent on strength or intensity of force with which the respective basic and acid radicles are united."

l., Mariotte's. Boyle's law, *q.v.*

l. of mass action. In chemical reactions the amount of change taking place is proportional to action mass of the reacting substance.

l., Mendel's. Offspring do not inherit characteristics from parents in equal or intermediate proportions, certain characteristics of 1 parent predominating and being transmitted to offspring in full measure.

These characteristics are termed *dominant*. Those of the other parent are called *recessive*. In second generation ¾ of offspring will inherit dominant characteristics, the remaining ¼ recessive traits.

l., Metchnikoff's. Phagocytes attack and destroy invading bacteria by intracellular digestion.

l., Mikulicz's. Anesthetic is not to be

l. of molecular weights. The weight of a molecule is the sum of the weights of its atoms and the relative molecular weight of a compound is equal to sum of the atomic weights of its components divided by two.

l. of multiple proportions. When two substances unite to form a series of chemical compounds the proportions in which they unite are simple multiples of one another or of one common proportion.

l., Nysten's. Rigor mortis travels progressively from muscles of mastication, through the face, neck, trunk and arms, reaching the legs and feet last.

l., Ohm's. The relations bet. resistances, amount of current and electromotive force as $C = \dfrac{E}{R}$, in which C = current, E = electromotive force, and R = resistance.

l., periodic. The physical and chemical properties of chemical elements are periodic functions of their at. wt. Natural classification of elements according to their at. wt.; when arranged in order of their at. wt. or atomic numbers, elements show regular variations in most of their physical and chemical properties.

l., Pfeiffer's. The blood serum of an animal immunized against bacteria will destroy bacteria used for immunization by bacteriolysis.

l., Pflüger's, of contraction and stimulation. A l. expressing relation of strength and direction of a galvanic current to its stimulating action upon a nerve.

l., Profeta's. The nonsyphilitic child of a syphilitic mother is immune against the acquired disease.

l. of projection. Stimulation of any point on the retina gives a visual sensation, projected outward along secondary axes from point stimulated through the nodal point.

l., psychophysical. To increase the intensity of a sensation in arithmetical progression one must increase the strength of stimulus in geometric progression.

l. of reciprocal proportions. In chemistry, the l. that the proportions in which two elementary bodies unite with a third one are simple multiples or simple fractions of the proportions in which these two bodies unite with each other.

l., Ritter and Valli's. The l. of increased inherent (e. g., electric) excitability in a nerve when separated from its center. The heightened irritability begins at proximal and extends toward distal end, eventually disappearing in same order.

l., Rubner's. 1. *L. of constant energy consumption*: Rapidity of growth is proportional to intensity of the metabolic processes. 2. *L. of constant growth quotient*: The same proportional part, or growth quotient, of total energy is utilized for growth.

l. of sines. Sine of angle of incidence equals the sine of angle of refraction multiplied by a constant quantity.

l., Stokes'. Muscles beneath an inflamed serous or mucous membrane are paralyzed.

l., Van't Hoff's, of temperature coefficient. In chemical reactions the intensity of reaction is doubled for each rise of 10° in temperature.

l., Virchow's. The cell elements of tumors are derived from preëxisting tissue cells.

l. of volumes. SEE: *Gay-Lussac's law*.

l., Waller's, of degeneration. If a spinal nerve is completely divided, the peripheral portion undergoes fatty degeneration, while the proximal part preserves its original character.

l., Weber's. When a stimulus is continually increased the smallest increase of sensation which we can appreciate remains the same, if the proportion of the increase of stimulus to the whole stimulus remains the same.

l., Wolff's. Changes in form and function of bones result in definite changes in their internal structure.

lax (lăks) [L. *laxus*, slack]. Without tension.

laxative (lak'să-tĭv) [L. *laxāre*, to loosen]. A mildly purgative medicine; an aperient or mild cathartic producing one or two evacuations without pain or tenesmus. Ex: *Olive oil, liquid petrolatum, etc.*

l. diet. One promoting free intestinal elimination; fresh fruits, lemonade, stewed raisins, prunes, asparagus, cauliflower, spinach, tomatoes, figs, buttermilk, sweet potatoes, sweet corn, pea and bean puree, carrots, greens, nuts, whole grains, yeasts. Vitamin B essential for good elimination.

layer (lā'ẽr) [M. E. *leyer*]. A sheetlike section.
SYN: *stratum*.

l., ambiguous. Second layer of cerebral cortex.

l., bacilar. Rod and cone layer of retina.

l., claustral. Layer of gray matter bet. external capsule and insula.

l., ganglionic. A layer of angular cells in cerebral cortex.

l., horny. Outer layer of the skin; stratum corneum.

l., osteogenetic. The innermost or bone-forming layer of the periosteum.

lazaret'to [It. *lazzaro*, a leper]. 1. A quarantine station. 2. Hospital for treatment of contagious diseases. SYN: *pesthouse*.

leaching (lēch'ing) [A.S. *leccan*, to wet]. Extraction of a substance from a mixture by washing the mixture with a solvent in which only the desired substance is soluble. SYN: *lixiviation*.

lead (lĕd). SYMB: *Pb*. A metallic element [*plumbum*]. At. wt. 206.9. Its compounds are poisonous.

l. acetate. USP. Sugar of lead.
ACTION AND USES: An astringent, saturated alcoholic solution; is used as a lotion in ivy poisoning. Seldom used internally.
DOSAGE, Av.: Internally, 1 gr. (0.6 Gm.).

l. colic. That due to lead poisoning.

l. encephalopathy. Disease of brain caused by lead poisoning.

l. line. Bluish line on gums in lead poisoning.

l. pipe contraction. Cataleptic condition during which limbs remain in any position in which placed.

l. poisoning, acute. ETIOL: From large overdosage. SYM: Metallic taste in mouth, burns in throat and gullet. Later abdominal cramps and prostration. F. A. TREATMENT: Wash out stomach. Give of magnesium sulfate (epsom salts) or sodium sulfate which precipitates the lead and helps remove the lead by purging.

l. p., chronic. ETIOL: Exceedingly common. Exposure in the industries; from food when lead vessels are used in its preparation; from cosmetics; or in children from nipple shields, chewing lead toys or objects covered with lead paints.

SYM: Anorexia, nausea, vomiting, salivation, anemia, the lead line on the gums, purging, abdominal pains, muscle cramps and pains in the joints. One of the most typical findings is the abdominal pain known as *lead colic*. There may be impairment of any part of the nervous system, often leading to muscle atrophy and the characteristic foot or wrist drop. Various blood changes may be found, especially the "stippling" of the red cells.

TREATMENT: Stop exposure to lead. The use of sodium or magnesium sulfate, the cautious employment of iodides in increasing doses and symptomatic management as indicated. This often requires opiates for the gastrointestinal symptoms, physiotherapy, and other measures of general care. Ketogenic diet is being highly recommended.

lead (lēd) [A.S. *laēdan*, to guide]. An electrocardiograph record.

The 3 common leads are: Lead I, right arm to left arm; lead II, right arm to left leg; lead III, left arm to left leg.

leaf (lēf) [A.S.]. A plant organ usually shooting out from the side of a stem or branch; somewhat flattened and oval in shape, and green in color. Ex: *Belladonna, hyoscyamus, digitalis.*

leaflet (lēflĕt) [A.S. *lēaf*, leaf]. One of the subdivisions of a compound leaf. Ex: *Senna, pilocarpus.*

lean (lēn) [A.S. *hlaēne*, without flesh]. Without flesh, emaciated.

DIET FOR: Diet as for tuberculosis or neurasthenia. Milk, 2 pints with or bet. meals; 2 eggs; meat, 6-8 oz.; bread, 12 oz.; potatoes, 4 oz.; milk puddings, 4 oz.; thick soup, 5 oz.; butter or other fat, 2 oz.; sugar, 4 oz. in any form; plenty of liquids with meals; tea, coffee, cocoa, water, cod-liver oil. SEE: *macies.*

Leber's disease (lā'bĕr). Congenital atrophy of the optic nerve that is inherited.

L.'s plexus. Plexus of venules in rete bet. Schlemm s canal and Fontana's spaces. [the urethra.

Lecat's gulf (lā-kăts'). Bulbous portion of

lechery (letch'er-ĭ) [Fr. *lecher*, to lick]. Lewdness; sensualism.

lechopyra (lek-o-pī'ra) [G. *lechō*, parturient woman, + *pyr*, fever]. Puerperal fever.

lecithin (les'ĭth-ĭn) [G. *lekithos*, egg yolk]. A fatty substance, of the group called phospholipins, found in blood, bile, brain, egg yolk, nerves, and other animal tissues, and yielding stearic acid, glycerol, phosphoric acid, and choline on hydrolysis. They are all derivatives of glycerin.

DOSAGE: 3-8 gr. (0.2-0.5 Gm.).

USES: In cases of poor nutrition, rickets, anemia, diabetes, tuberculosis.

lectual (lekt'ū-ăl) [L. *lectus*, bed]. Pert. to a bed or couch.

l. disease. Bed-confining disease.

Lederer's anemia (lĕd'ĕr-ĕrs). Acute hemolytic anemia.

leech (lētch) [A.S. *laece*]. A bloodsucking water worm.

METHOD OF APPLYING: Apply near a bone. Eyelids and scrotum should never be leeched and only circumjacent tissues of inflamed areas. Wash skin with soap and water. Apply sugar and milk over marked area, arrange the lint. Keep in water 1 hour before applying. Put leech in a test tube tail first. Invert tube over the required spot. If the leech does not bite, the skin may be pricked with a sterile needle.

Leeches must never be covered from the nurse's view. They suck for about 20-30 minutes and then fall off, but must never be pulled off, as teeth may be left in the wound. They can be removed by salt, which causes relaxation. If a leech is applied near an orifice it must be fixed by a thread through its tail.

AFTER REMOVAL: Apply a hot fomentation if bleeding is to be encouraged. If bleeding is to be stopped, apply an ordinary dressing. Sometimes pressure is necessary, and if persistent the wound may have to be cauterized.

To KILL: Place in carbolic, 1 to 20. If required for future use, place first in salt and water, then in clean water.— *Helen M. Gration, S.R.N.*

SEE: *abstraction.*

l., artificial. Cup and exhaust pump or syringe for drawing blood.

leek [A.S. *laec*]. AV. SERVING: 100 Gm. Pro. 1.4, Fat 0.2, Carbo. 2.4. Ca 0.058, Mg 0.014, K 0.199, Na 0.081, P 0.006, Cl 0.024, S 0.072, Fe 0.0006. Vit. B+, C+.

ACTION: Similar to onions but less nutritive and richer in essences.

Lee's ganglion (lē). Cervical ganglion formed from 3rd and 4th sacral nerves and hypogastric and ovarian plexuses.

left'-hand'edness. Condition of being more adept in use of left hand. SYN: *sinistrality.*

left lateral recumbent position. The English or obstetrical position. Patient on left side, right knee and thigh drawn up. Used in rectal operations and obstetrics.

leg (lĕg) [M.E.]. One of the 2 lower extremities, including the femur, tibia, fibula, and patella; spec. the part between the knee and ankle.

RS: *acnemia, acragnosis, anxietas tibiarum, Barbadoes, bayonet, bowleg, Buerger's disease, calf, crural, crus, saphena, sura, systremma, tibia.*

l., Anglesey. A form of jointed artificial leg.

l., badger. Inequality in the length of the legs.

l., baker. Genu valgum, or knockknee.

l., bandy. Same as bowleg.

l., Barbadoes. Elephantiasis of the legs.

l., bayonet. Uncorrected backward displacement of the knee bones, followed by ankylosis at the joint.

l., bird. Reduction in size of the leg from atrophy of the muscles.

l., boomerang. A disease of the leg bones occurring among Australian natives, causing a curvature of the leg resembling a boomerang.

l., bow-. Genu varum; an outward curving of the legs at the knees.

l., lawn tennis. Rupture of plantaris muscle accompanied by excruciating disabling pain in the posterior region of the knee.

l., milk. Phlebitis of the femoral vein occasionally following parturition and typhoid fever. It is characterized by swelling of the leg, usually without redness. Called also white leg. SYN: *phlegmasia alba dolens.*

l., scissor. Cross leg deformity; a result of double hip disease, in which the patient walks with the legs crossed.
l. type. Inherited progressive muscular atrophy.
l., white. See: *milk leg*.
leggings (lĕg'gĭngs) [M.E. *leg*, leg]. Sterile leg coverings used on patient while in operating room.

legitimacy (lē-jĭt'ĭm-ă-sĭ) [L. *legitimus*, lawful]. 1. Condition of being legal. 2. Condition of being born in wedlock.
legume (lĕ'gūm) [L. *legumen*, pulse]. Fruit or pod of beans, peas, lentils, etc.
  COMP: *Nitrogen:* Equal to that in meat. It is called *legumin,* forming with water a paste resembling gluten, but easier to digest.

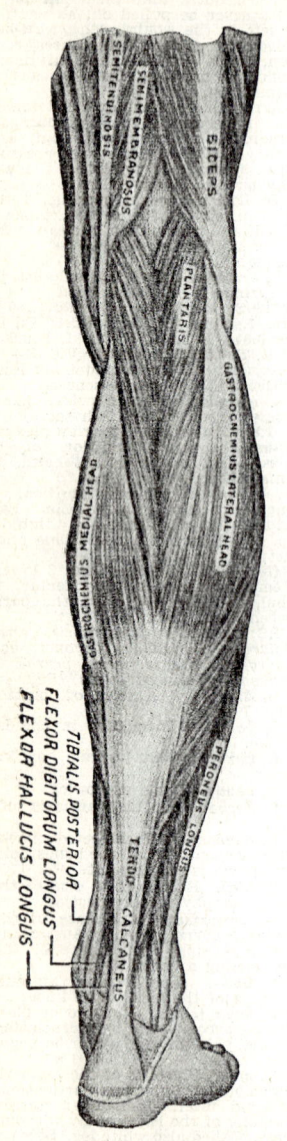

LEG'S POSTERIOR MUSCLES. 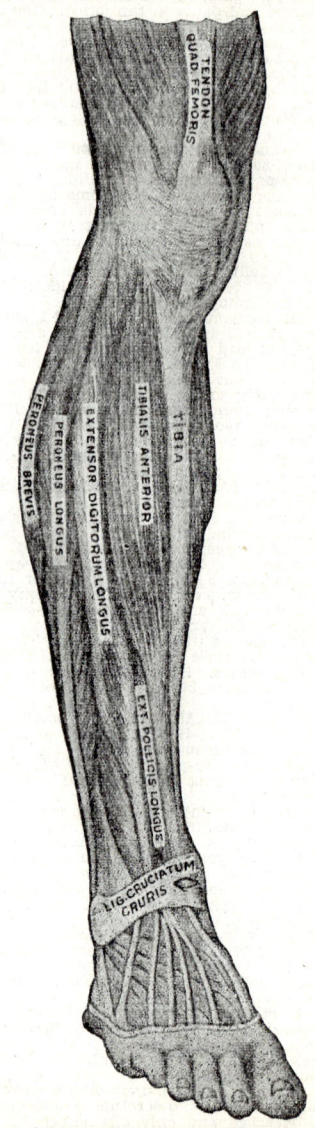   LEG'S ANTERIOR MUSCLES.

VITAMINS (*Sprouted*): A good source of Vit. B and probably Vit. G. Vit. A and C in small amounts.

CARBOHYDRATES: Superior to those in meat. Generally they are in the form of starch in about the same proportion as the cereals, but with more cellulose.

ASH: Twice that of meat or bread. Potash is abundant and soda is present. Alkalinity higher than that of other vegetables. Organic phosphoric acid is high, only exceeded in cheese, oatmeal, and yolk of egg. Iron is found only in the lentils, but lime and magnesium, also nuclein and lecithin, are plentiful in the others as well.

ABSORPTION: They take up large amounts of water. 10.58 oz. of dried peas make 42.38 oz. of puree, while intestinal absorption is lower than that for milk, bread, meat or rice.

EFFECT OF PREPARATION: *Soaking*: The water transforms some of the starch into amylodextrin and modifies the cellulose, assisting in their digestion and absorption.

COOKING: Soft water should be used, as the carbonate of lime in hard water forms an insoluble combination. Add baking soda to hard water. Too much water lowers the nutritive value, wastes the aromatic essences, mineral salts and diminishes digestibility. Cook in small amount of water, over a slow fire in an airtight vessel.

ACTION: About the same as cereals. The great amount of albumin in legumes may overtax gastric action. Too large quantities may overtax the alimentary canal and cause gaseous and acid fermentation. In the intestines, the albumin and starch react at once on the pancreas and the glandular system, while the cellulose reacts on the muscular system. They are heavy in nitrogen and nuclein, and should be considered as less expensive substitute for meat.

IND: *Adolescence and Childhood*: The phosphorus, lime and magnesium in legumes are very valuable in the construction of tissue, as well as in convalescence and tuberculosis. Thick soups may be used when the entire pea or bean would not be tolerated by the stomach.

CONTRA: Dyspepsia, dilatation, gastritis, anemia, neurasthenia, enterocolitis, enteritis, enteroptosis, hyperchlorhydria, gout, gravel, rheumatism, neuralgia, scleroma, Bright's disease, and cardiac affections. *Diabetes*: Slow to digest, and because rich in carbohydrates they should be limited. *Obesity*: There is a tendency to transform them into fatty substances in the liver, therefore they should be avoided. *Gastric troubles*: The hyperacidity arrests the digestion of starch, provoking putrefaction. SEE: *beans, peas, lentils*.

legumelin (leg-u′mel-in) [L. *legumen*, pulse]. An albumin present in many leguminous seeds, as in peas. SEE: *legume, legumlin*.

legu′min [L. *legumen*, pulse]. A protein contained in legumes; vegetable casein. COMP: It is made up of 51.72% carbon, 6.95% hydrogen, 18.04% nitrogen, 22.905% oxygen and 0.385% sulfur.

leiodermia (lī-ō-dēr′mĭ-ă) [G. *leios*, smooth, + *derma*, skin]. Skin disease characterized by abnormal glossiness and atrophy.

leiomyofibroma (lī″ō-mī″ō-fī-brō′mă) [″ + *mys, my-*, muscle, + L. *fibra*, fiber, + G. *ōma*, tumor]. Tumor containing leiomatous, myomatous and fibromatous elements.

leiomyoma (lī″ō-mī-ō′mă) [″ + ″ + *ōma*, tumor]. Myoma of unstriped muscle fibers.

leiomyosarcoma (lī″ō-mī″ō-săr-kō′mă) [″ + ″ + *sarx*, flesh, + *ōma*, tumor]. Combined leiomyoma and sarcoma.

leiphemia (lī-fē′mĭ-ă) [G. *leipein*, to fail, + *aima*, blood]. Thinness, impoverishment, or depravity of the blood.

Leishmania (lēsh-man′ĭ-ă). A genus of organisms, one of which, *L. donovani*, causes kala-azar.

leishmaniasis, leishmaniosis (lēsh-măn-ī′ă-sĭs, -ī-ō′sĭs). Infection with a species of *Leishmania*, affecting the skin, nasal cavities and pharynx, one form causing oriental boil, another kala azar.

lememia (lem-ē′mĭ-ă) [G. *loimos*, plague, + *aima*, blood]. The presence of plague bacilli in the blood.

lemic (lē′mĭk) [G. *loimos*, plague]. Rel. to plague or epidemic disease.

lemmocyte (lem′mō-sīt) [G. *lemma*, husk, + *kytos*, cell]. A cell which becomes a neurilemma cell.

lemniscus (lem-nĭs′kŭs) [G. *lēmniskos*, a fillet]. A bundle of sensory fibers (lateral or ext. and median or int.) in the medulla, and pons. SYN: *fillet, laqueus*. [to contagious diseases.

lemoid (le′moyd) [G. *loimos*, plague]. Pert.

lemol′ogy [″ + *logos*, study]. Study of contagious diseases.

lem′on [Persian *limūn*, lemon]. Contains citric acid. AV. SERVING: 100 Gm. Pro. 1.00, Fat 0.7, Carbo. 7.4. ASH: Ca 0.036, Mg 0.007, K 0.175, Na 0.004, P 0.022, Cl 0.002, S 0.011, Fe 0.0006.

l. juice. AV. SERVING: 15 Gm. Carbo. 1.5. ASH: Ca 0.024, Mg 0.010, K 0.127, Na 0.009, P 0.010, Cl 0.003, S 0.006.

VITAMINS: Same for both. A+, B++, C+++, G++.

A base forming fruit, alkalinity 5 cc. per 100 Gm., 12 cc. per 100 cal.

ACTION: Stimulating and refreshing.

IND: May be used in place of vinegar, spices, and aromatic substances by those who cannot use the latter. Diabetics may use. A fine antiscorbutic; good in Barlow's disease. Six to 8 lemons per day may be used in rheumatism except as stated above.

CONTRA: As they are supposed to increase calcification of arteries and deposit of chalky matter in the tissues, avoid use in pulmonary tuberculosis, and in acute articular rheumatism.

lemoparalysis (le″mo-par-al′ĭs-ĭs) [G. *laimos*, gullet, + *para*, beside, + *lyein*, to loosen]. Paralysis of esophagus.

lemostenosis [″ + *stenōsis*, a narrowing]. Stricture of esophagus.

lenigallol (len-ĭ-gal′ŏl). A derivative of pyrogallic acid (triacetyl pyrogallol).

USES: In eczema, psoriasis, and other skin conditions.

DOSAGE: In 1-6% ointment, usually with zinc oxide.

lenitive (len′ĭ-tĭv) [L. *lenire*, to soothe]. 1. Demulcent, soothing, slightly laxative. 2. A palliative.

lens (lĕnz) (pl. *lentēs*) [L. *lentil*, lens]. A transparent refracting medium; usually made of glass.

RS: *capsitis, capsulociliary, circle of diffusion, posterior chamber, vitreous chamber.*

l., achromatic. One for correction of

aberration of refrangibility, or chromatic aberration.
l., bifocal. Having a double focus.
l., concave spherical. Formed of prisms with their apices together, therefore, thin at the center and thick at the edge. Used in myopia.
l., convex spherical. Formed of prisms with their bases together, therefore, thick at the center and thin at the edge. Used in hyperopia.
l., crystalline. Transparent, colorless structure in eye; biconvex in shape, enclosed in a capsule and held in place just behind the pupil by the suspensory ligament. Consists of cortex and nucleus. Function is to focus rays so they form a perfect image on the retina.
l., cylindrical. Segment of a cylinder parallel to its axis, used in correcting astigmatism.
lenticonus (len-ti-ko'nus) [" + *conus*, cone]. Conical protrusion of ant. or post. surface of lens.
lentic'ular [L. *lenticulāris*, pert. to a lens]. 1. Lens shaped. SYN: *lentiform.* 2. Pert. to a lens.
l. fossa. Depression in ant. surface of vitreous for reception of the crystalline lens.
l. glands. Glands of the gastric mucosa.
lenticulostriate (len-tĭk″ū-lō-strī'āt) [" + *striatus*, streaked]. Rel. to the lenticular nucleus and corpus striatum.
lentiform (lent'ĭ-form) [L. *lens, lent-*, lentil, lens, + *forma*, shape]. Lentil or lens shaped. SYN: *lenticular.*
lentiginous (lĕn-tĭj'ĭn-ŭs) [L. *lentigō*, freckle]. 1. Affected by lentigo. 2. Covered with very small dots.
len'tigo (pl. *lentigines*) [L. freckle]. Small brown macules or yellow-brown pigmented areas on skin sometimes caused by exposure to sun and weather. SYN: *ephelis, freckle.*
len'til [L. *lens, lent-*, lentil]. 1. European, leguminous plant with pods containing edible seeds. 2. The seed of this plant.
AV. SERVING (dried) : 60 Gm. Pro. 15.4, Fat 0.6, Carbo. 32.8.
ASH CONST. (dry) : Ca 0.107, Mg 0.101, K 0.877, Na 0.062, P 0.438, Cl 0.050, S 0.277, Fe 0.0086.
VITAMINS: A+, B++.
ACTION: Antitoxic.
In digestion 40% of the protein is lost and 10% in lentil flour. SEE: *legume.*
lentitis (lĕn-tī'tĭs) [" + G. *-itis*, inflammation]. Inflammation of the optic lens. SYN: *phakitis.*
leontiasis (lē-ŏn-tī'ă-sĭs) [G. *leōn, leont-*, lion]. Lionlike expression about face, accompanying certain diseases.
l. ossea. Enlargement and distortion of facial bones, giving one the appearance of a lion. The condition is rare and not fatal. SYN: *leontiasis.*
leotropic (lē-ō-trop'ĭk) [G. *laios*, left, + *tropos*, a turning]. Running from right to left in a spiral form. OPP: *dexiotropic.*
leper (lĕp'ĕr) [G. *lepros*, scaly]. Person afflicted with leprosy.
lepidic (lep-ĭd'ĭk) [G. *lepis, lepid-*, rind, scale]. Indicating absence of definite stroma between cells, especially in tissue of lining membrane.
l. tissue. Lining membrane tissue.
l. tumor. Rind tumor. SYN: *lepidoma.*
lep'ido- [G.]. Combining form: Referring to scales.
lepidoma (lep-ĭ-dō'mă) [G. *lepis, lepid-*, rind, + *ōma*, tumor]. Neoplasm originating from a lepidic tissue. SYN: *lepidic tumor, rind tumor.*
lepidosis (lĕp-ĭd-ō'sĭs) [" + *-ōsis*, intensive]. Any scaly or desquamating eruption. SYN: *lepra, 2; pityriasis.*
lepocyte (lep'ō-sīt) [G. *lepos*, rind, + *kytos*, cell]. Nucleated cell with cell wall.
lepothrix (lep'o-thriks) [G. *lepos*, scale, + *thrix*, hair]. Condition in which shaft of the hair is incased in hardened, scaly, sebaceous matter.
lepra (lĕp'ră) [G. *lepra*, leprosy]. 1. Leprosy, but commonly used only in conjunction with other words to denote types of leprosy. 2. A dermatosis with desquamation.
l. alba. Skin is anesthetic and white, and different forms of paralysis follow.
l. anesthetica. Leprosy with anesthetic areas on body.
l. Arabum. Tubercular leprosy.
l. maculosa. Form with pigmented cutaneous areas.
l. mutilans. Final stage of true leprosy, or mutilation stage.
leprid(e (lĕp'rĕd) [G. *lepra*, leprosy]. Leprous cutaneous lesion.
leprology (lĕp-rol'ō-jĭ) [" + *logos*, study]. The study of leprosy and methods of treating it.
leproma (lĕp-rō'mă) [" + *ōma*, tumor]. Tubercular lesion of leprosy.
leprosy (lep'ro-sĭ) [G. *lepra*, leprosy]. A chronic, infectious disease in which there may be lesions of skin, membranes, or nerve tissue.
In many respects, this infection resembles tuberculosis, and for many years was regarded as incurable, a conclusion no longer considered true.
Divided into 2 main types, *tubercular* and *anesthetic, q.v.*, below.
ETIOL: Due to *Bacillus leprae*, or Hansen's bacillus. May occur at practically any age. Not easily transmissible, though considered contagious.
INCUBATION: Anywhere from 1 to 30 years.
SYM: Onset very gradual. May be malaise, headache, chilliness, mental depression, and numbness in portions of the body where disease later makes its appearance.
COMPLICATIONS: Mostly surgical amputations and treatment of deformities may be required.
DIFFERENTIAL DIAG: Tuberculosis and esp. syphilis are the 2 diseases most likely to be considered.
PROG: Unfavorable; nevertheless, in recent years many cures have been reported. In other instances, the progress of the disease has been checked for prolonged periods.
TREATMENT: Isolation usually required, though the real danger of infection from ordinary contact is not great. Diamino diphenyl sulfone, usually referred to as DDS, has become the drug of choice and is given by mouth in maximum daily doses of 200 mg., or 300 mg. two or three times a week. Many cases are being cured on this regime. The hygienic surroundings of the patient are an important factor, as well as avoiding secondary infections. SEE: *lepra.*
l., anesthetic. The peripheral nerves are invaded by the leprosy bacillus and discolored spots follow. These may have the appearance of iodine stains, sometimes with a reddish periphery. Skin and appendages atrophy, bones undergo necrosis, and phalanges drop off 1 by 1.

leprosy, Italian   L-20   **lettuce**

l., Italian. SEE: *Lombardy l.*
l., Lombardy. Deficiency disease caused by lack of Vitamin B_2. SYN: *pellegra*, q.v.
l., nodular. L. with granulation of tissues. SYN: *leproma.*
l., trophoneurotic. Anesthetic leprosy.
l., tubercular. Spots of erythema appear on body, become pigmented and hyperanesthetic and develop into tubercles from size of pea to walnut. Face, extremities, and genitals are the parts most commonly affected — occasionally mucous membranes, esp. of nose and throat, are invaded. Hair, eyebrows, and lashes drop out, eyes become inflamed, features distorted, voice husky. Disease may last years. Both the anesthetic and tubercular varieties are frequently seen in same patient.

leprotic (lĕp-rot′ĭk) [G. *lepra*, leper]. 1. Rel. to leprosy. 2. Affected with leprosy. SYN: *leprous.*

leprous (lĕp′rŭs) [G. *lepra*, leper]. 1. Pert. to leprosy. 2. Affected by leprosy. SYN: *leprotic.*

leptodermic (lep-tō-dĕr′mĭk) [G. *leptos*, slender, + *derma*, skin]. Possessing a thin skin.

leptomeninges (lep″tō-men-ĭn′jēs) [″ + *mēnigx*, membrane]. Pia mater and arachnoid as distinct from dura mater, because of their thinner and more delicate structure.

leptomeningitis (lep″tō-men-in-jī′tis) [″ + ″ + -*itis*, inflammation]. Inflammation of the pia and arachnoid membranes.
  ETIOL: Meningococcus or other pathogenic organism.
  SYM: Acute headache, pain in back, rigidity of spine, irritability, drowsiness ending in coma.
  Clinically, it cannot be distinguished from pachymeningitis, q.v.

leptopellic (lep-tō-pel′ĭk) [″ + *pellis*, a bowl (pelvis)]. Having an abnormally narrow pelvis.

leptophonia (lĕp-tō-fō′nĭ-ă) [″ + *phōnē*, voice]. Weakness or feebleness of voice.

leptorhine, leptorrhine (lep′tor-rīn) [″ + *ris*, *rin*-, nose]. Having a very thin or slender nose.

leptosome (lĕp′tō-sōm) [″ + *soma*, body]. Person of thin, slight stature.

Leptospira (lĕp-tō-spī′ră) [G. *leptos*, thin, + *spaira*, coil]. Genus of spirochetes; thin, spiral, and hook-ended.
  L. icterohaemorrha′giae. Species causing acute infectious jaundice.
  L. icteroi′des. Species causing yellow fever.

leptospirosis (lĕp″tō-spī-rō′sĭs) [″ + ″ + -*ōsis*, intensive]. Condition resulting from Leptospira infection.

leptothricosis (lep″tō-thri-kō′sĭs) [″ + *thrix*, hair]. Disease from Leptothrix infection.

Leptothrix (lĕp′tō-thrĭks) [″ + *thrix*, hair]. A genus of bacteria often with long filaments.

Leptotrich′ia bucca′lis. An organism inhabiting the buccal cavity normally.

Leptus autumnalis (lep′tŭs) [G. *leptos*, slender]. Parasitic mite larvae causing itch and sometimes wheals.

les′bian [G. *lesbios*, pert. to island of Lesbos]. 1. Pert. to lesbianism, or perverted sexual desire in women for those of their own sex only. 2. One who practices lesbianism.

les′bianism. Perversion in which sexual desire of women is only for one of their own sex.
  Named from the Island of Lesbos wherein the practice of sapphism was reputed to have been general in ancient days. It may be expressed physically or psychically. SEE: *sapphism, tribadism, urningism.*

lesion (le′zhun) [L. *laesio*, a wound]. 1. Morbid change in tissue formation locally. 2. An injury or wound. 3. Single infected patch in a skin disease.
  Primary lesions include *macules; vesicles; blebs,* or *bullae; pustules; papules; tubercles; wheals,* and *tumors,* q.v. Secondary lesions are the result of primary lesions. They may be *crusts, excoriations, fissures, pigmentations, scales, scars,* and *ulcers,* q.v.
  RS: *abscess, boil, carbuncle, Cazenave's lupus, cerebropsychosis, chancre, chancroids, Chaussier's areola, felon, gumma, moles, pimples, rash, sebaceous cysts, tumefactions, verruca, wound.*

l., degenerative. L. caused by or showing degeneration.
l., diffuse. L. spreading over a large area.
l., discharging. 1. Brain l. discharging nervous impulses. 2. L. discharging an exudate.
l., focal. L. of small definite area.
l., indiscriminate. L. affecting separate systems of the body.
l., initial, of syphilis. Hard chancre.
l., irritative. L. stimulating or exciting activity in part of body where it is situated.
l., local. L. of nervous origin giving rise to local symptoms.
l., peripheral. One of nerve endings.
l., primary. First l. of a disease, esp. used in referring to chancre of syphilis.
l., structural. One causing change in tissue.
l., systematic. One confined to organs of common function.
l., toxic. One resulting from sepsis.
l., vascular. One of a blood vessel.

le′thal [G. *lēthē*, oblivion]. Pert. to or that which causes death.

lethargic (leth-ar′jĭk) [G. *lēthargos*, drowsiness]. 1. Affected with lethargy. 2. Rel. to lethargy. 3. Sluggish.

lethargy (leth′ar-jĭ) [G. *lēthargos*, drowsiness]. 1. A condition of functional torpor or sluggishness; stupor. 2. A state analogous to hypnotism, or the first stage of hypnotism.
  RS: *carus, cataphora, coma vigil, dual and multiple personality, noctambulism, somnambulism, vigilambulism.*

l., African. Sleeping sickness.
l., hysteric. The sleep of hypnotic lethargy, the state in which many cases of apparent death and resurrection are found.
l., lucid. Retention of intellect but loss of will power with a consequent total lack of muscular response. The subject knows what is going on, resents it, perhaps, but is unable to exercise sufficient will to bring about muscular defense.
  ETIOL: Fear, fascination, shock. This unrecognized condition may be responsible for many instances of rape, or of yielding to such an attack.

lethologica (lĕth-ō-loj′ĭk-ă) [G. *lēthē*, forgetfulness, + *logos*, word]. Temporary inability to remember a word or name, or an intended action.

let′tuce [L. *lactuca*, lettuce]. COMP: Contains a small amount of an opium principle. AV. SERVING: 50 Gm. Pro. 0.6, Fat 0.2, Carbo. 0.5. VITAMINS: A++, B++, C+++, D+, E+, G++. The green leaves of lettuce contain 30% more Vit. A than the inner white leaves.

leuc-   **leukocyte**

ASH: Ca 0.043, Mg 0.017, K 0.339, Na 0.027, P 0.042, Cl 0.074, S 0.014, Fe 0.0007. A base forming food; alkalinity 7.4 cc. per 100 Gm., or 38.7 cc. per 100 cal. ACTION: Slightly soporific. A mineralizer and alkalizer.

leuc-. For words beginning thus, see *leuk-* words.

leucine (lū'sēn) [G. *leukos*, white]. Alpha-amino-isobutyl] acetic acid, $CH_3.(CH_2)_3.CH(NH_2).COOH$, an amino acid found among the products of the digestion of proteins.

leucinosis (lū-sin-ō'sĭs) [" + -*ōsis*, intensive]. Excess of leucine in the body.

leucinuria (lū-sin-ū'rĭ-ă) [" + *ouron*, urine]. Presence of leucine in urine.

leucitis (lū-sī'tis) [" + -*itis*, inflammation]. Inflammation of the sclera. SYN: *scleritis*.

leukanemia (lū-kă-ne'mĭ-ă) [" + *a*-, priv. + *aima*, blood]. Leukemia with marked anemia.

leukasmus (lū-kas'mŭs) [G. *leukasmos*, growing white]. Congenital absence of pigment in bands or patches of the skin. SYN: *leukoderma*.

leukemia (lu-ke'mĭ-ă) [" + *aima*, blood]. Disease characterized by a great excess of the white corpuscles with hyperplasia of the spleen or of the lymphatics or changes in the bone marrow.
TREATMENT: Radioactive sodium phosphate. High caloric diet, rest, fresh air, blood transfusions, iron therapy.
NP: Watch for local mouth infections, terminal septicemia, and bronchopneumonia as complications. Myelogenous forms are prone to such infections as boils, erysipelas, grippe, influenza and pneumonia. Good nursing care is very important in all forms of this disease. Hemorrhages from nose and mouth often require packing and hemostatics.
SYN: *leukocythemia*.
SEE: *Auer's bodies, chloroleukemia*.

l., lymphatic. That in which the lymphatic glands are the seat of hyperplasia, with a marked increase in lymphocytes in blood; acute form occurs in children and young adults; spleen is slightly enlarged.

l., myelogenous. That in which the medulla, esp. of the ribs, sternum and vertebrae, is converted into a pulpy material.
SYM: General manifestations of anemia—enlargement of spleen, liver or lymphatic glands. Febrile paroxysms (101°-103° F.), hemorrhage from mucous membranes, digestive disturbances, dimness of vision. There is marked increase in the leukocytes; proportion to red corpuscles may be 1-50 or even 1-10. This leukocytosis results from an increase of the eosinophiles and from the presence of myelocytes.
PROG: Occasional recovery. More fatal in adults than children, death usually resulting in 3-4 years.
TREATMENT: Iron or arsenic in certain forms, x-ray or radium. Removal of spleen gives negative results. Nourishing food. Good hygiene.

l., pseudo-. A disease characterized by hyperplasia of the lymphatic structures, and by progressive anemia, without a marked increase of the white corpuscles.
SYM: General symptoms of anemia—enlargement of lymphatic glands, which usually begins in the neck — spleen somewhat enlarged, febrile paroxysms.

PROG. AND TREATMENT: Same as for leukemia. SYN: *Hodgkin's disease*.

l., splenic. That in which spleen is enlarged from congestion and hyperplasia.

leukemic (lū-kēm'ĭk) [G. *leukos*, white, + *aima*, blood]. 1. Rel. to leukemia. 2. Affected with leukemia.

leukemoid (lū-kē'moid) [" + " + *eidos*, form]. Having symptoms of leukemia.

leu'ko-, leuk- [G.]. Combining forms signifying *deficiency of color*.

leu'koblast [G. *leukos*, white, + *blastos*, germ]. 1. Immature cell in red marrow of bones supposed to develop into erythrocyte. 2. Undeveloped leukocyte. SYN: *myeloblast*.

leukocidin (lū-ko-sid'in) [" + L. *cidus*, from *caedere*, to kill]. An exotoxin that attacks leukocytes. SYN: *leukotoxin, q.v.*

leukocytal (lū-kō-sī'tăl) [" + *kytos*, cell]. Rel. to leukocytes.

leukocyte (lū'ko-sīt) [G. *leukos*, white, + *kytos*, cell]. 1. White blood corpuscle. 2. Any unpigmented ameboid cellular mass in blood, lymph, or pus, or a wandering connective tissue cell.
The principal varieties are *polymorphonuclear neutrophiles* (65%), *large lymphocytes* (10%), *small ones* (20%), *basophiles** (2%), *eosinophiles** (3%).
The leukocytes act as scavengers and resist infection. They have an ameboid power of movement. They are able to penetrate tissue and then return to the blood stream. When invading bacteria overcome them, the dead bodies of the white blood corpuscles collect in the form of pus, causing an abscess if a ready outlet is not found. Different types combat various kinds of infection.
One cu. mm. of blood contains 5000-10,000 colorless corpuscles normally.
FUNCTIONS: (a) Phagocytosis and other defensive activities; (b) aid to other body cells in growth and repair; (c) aid in absorption, varying during the day, and in different parts of the circulatory system, from the intestine; (d) participation in clot formation; (e) special chemical activities (secretion) which maintain the normal composition of the blood plasma.
A greatly diminished number of erythrocytes is found in the anemias, and a greatly increased number of leukocytes (leukocytosis) is indicative of the presence of inflammatory products. A leukocyte count is usually a preoperative routine if infection is suspected, such as in appendicitis. A count may also be taken following an operation to be sure that no infection from a wound is present.
HOW TO RECOGNIZE: White blood cells are round, edges occasionally broken, nucleated, granular, having a grayish color, sometimes clumped, and can be stained as polynuclears from other places.
MICROSCOPIC EXAMINATION: They are usually in pieces of mucus and can be stained by ordinary blood stains.
Two determinations are usually made regarding the leukocytes: their *total number* (total count), and the *percentage of each type* (differential count). Decrease below the normal is called *leukopenia*. Relative increase or decrease of any particular type is denoted by adding the suffix "philia" (denoting increase) or "penia" (denoting decrease), as: neutrophilia, granulocytopenia, neutropenia, eosinophilia, etc.
Sometimes immature white cells are

leukocyte, alpha   L-22   **leukoderma**

Tabular Summary of Leukocytes

Cells	Nucleus	Cytoplasm Color	Cytoplasm Granules	Per Cent
Polymorphonuclear cells or granulocytes.	Polymorphic	None		
Neutrophile.	Polymorphic	None	Fine. Neutral stain.	65
Eosinophile.	Polymorphic	None	Coarse. Stain with acid dye.	4
Basophile.	Polymorphic	None	Coarse. Stain with basic dye.	1
Lymphocytes or agranulocytes.	Circular	None		25
Large.			None.	
Small.			None.	
Monocytes, transitionals, etc.				5
				100

discharged into the blood stream and may be observed in blood smears; myelocytes, myeloblasts, or lymphoblasts. Their presence is always indicative of disease.

In a smear of blood, all of the white cells are not alike; they vary in size, in shape, in appearance, and in color which they assume when stained. Some of the cells contain minute granules, and these cells are called granulocytes, the cytoplasm of others is granular. It is seen that the granules in some cells stain bright red, and the cells are called eosinophiles; in others, deep blue, and these are called basophiles. In most of the cells, however, the granules take a neutral purplish color, and these are called neutrophiles. There are 2 types of nongranular cells, the lymphocytes and the monocytes.

Not all leukocytes are formed in the same place, nor in the same manner. Granulocytes are formed in the bone marrow, arising from large cells called megakaryocytes. Lymphocytes are formed in the lymph nodes; monocytes from the cells lining the capillaries in various organs, perhaps principally in the spleen and bone marrow.

   l., alpha. One of those disintegrating during coagulation of the blood.
   l., beta. One of those which do not disintegrate during coagulation.
   l., endothelial. Large wandering cell with phagocytic properties.
   l., hyaline. Large mononuclear l. SYN: *monocyte.*
   l., polymorphonuclear. L. with irregularly-shaped nucleus and fine granular cell. They predominate in purulent fluids due to pneumo-, strepto-, and staphylococcus, and sometimes in acute tuberculous fluids.

leukocyte, words pert. to: agranulocyte, agranulocytosis, alexocyte, alpha l., anisohypercytosis, anisonormocytosis, antibody, band form, blood, blood count, corpuscle, eosinophil(e, erythrocyte, granulocyte, immunity, macrophage, microcyte, monocyte, neutrophil, phagocyte, thrombocyte, trephone.

leukocythemia (lū-ko-sī-the′mĭ-ă) [G. *leukos,* white, + *kytos,* cell, + *aima,* blood]. Blood disease characterized by excess of white blood corpuscles and enlargement of spleen, lymphatic glands and bone marrow. SYN: *leukemia, q.v.*

leukocytic (lū-kō-sit′ĭk) [" + *kytos,* cell]. Pert. to leukocytes.

leukocytoblast (lū-kō-sīt′ō-blast) [" + " + *blastos,* germ]. Leukocyte mother cell.

leukocytogenesis (lū″kō-sīt″ō-jen′ē-sĭs) [G. *leukos,* white, + *kytos,* cell, + *genesis,* formation]. Leukocyte formation. SYN: *leukopoiesis.*

leukocytoid (lū′kō-sī-toid) [" + " + *eidos,* form]. Resembling a leukocyte.

leukocytol′ogy [" + " + *logos,* study]. The study of leukocytes and their function.

leukocytolysis (lū-kō-sī-tol′ĭ-sĭs) [" + " + *lysis,* dissolution]. Destruction of leukocytes.

leukocytoma (lū-kō-sī-tō′mă) [" + " + *ōma,* tumor]. 1. Tumor composed of cells resembling leukocytes. 2. Tumorlike mass of leukocytes.

leukocytometer (lū″ko-sī-tom′et-er) [" + " + *metron,* measure]. Device for counting white blood corpuscles.

leukocytopenia (lū″kō-sīt″ō-pē′nĭ-ă) [" + " + *penia,* want]. Subnormal number of leukocytes in peripheral blood. SYN: *leukopenia.*

leukocytoplania (lū″kō-sīt″ō-plā′nĭ-ă) [" + " + *planē,* wandering]. Wandering of leukocytes through blood vessel walls. SYN: *leukopedesis.*

leukocytosis (lū″ko-sī-to′sis) [G. *leukos,* white, + *kytos,* cell, + *-ōsis*]. Increase in the number of leukocytes (above 10,000 per cu. mm.) in the blood, generally caused by presence of infection.

Leukemias, however, release immature leukocytes due to abnormal condition of blood forming organs. Leukocytosis is present in all infections excepting influenza, leprosy, malaria, measles, mumps, typhoid, and uncomplicated tuberculosis.

Fifteen thousand to thirty thousand is the usual count in leukocytosis, sometimes 50,000 or 75,000; in leukemias 500,000-1,000,000 per cu. mm. Leukocytosis is early and marked in severe infections when the patient's resistance is good; if infection and resistance are less marked it obtains later and in a lesser degree and disappears more quickly. No leukocytosis may occur in unusually virulent infection, such as diphtheria, pneumonia, sepsis, etc.

leukocytotherapy (lū″kō-sī″tō-thĕr′ă-pī) [" + " + *therapeia,* treatment]. Treatment with leukocytic extracts.

leukocyturia (lū″ko-sī-tu′rĭ-ă) [" + " + *ouron,* urine]. Leukocytes in the urine.

leukoderma (lū-ko-der′mă) [" + *derma.*

leukodiagnosis — L-23 — leukotoxin

skin]. Deficiency of pigmentation of the skin, esp. in patches. SYN: *leukopathia.* Classed as congenital, acquired and syphilitic.

leukodiagnosis (lū-ko-dī-ag-nō'sĭs) [" + *dia,* through, + *gnōsis,* knowledge]. Diagnosis by observance of number, variety, or reaction of leukocytes.

leukokeratosis (lū″kō-kĕr-ă-tō'sĭs) [" + *keras,* horn, + -*ōsis*]. White patch formation on the surface of mucosa of tongue, cheek and gums. SYN: *leukoplakia.*

leukolysin (lū-kol'ĭ-sĭn) [" + *lysis,* dissolution]. Serum constituent destructive to leukocytes.

leukolysis (lū-kol'ĭ-sis) [" + *lysis,* dissolution]. Destruction of leukocytes. SYN: *leukocytolysis.*

leuko'ma [" + -*ōma,* tumor]. A white, opaque corneal opacity.

l. adherens. Corneal scar with incarcerated iris tissue.

leukomaine (lū-kō'ma-ēn, -ma-ĭn) [G. *leukōma,* whiteness]. Nitrogenous alkaloid developed in living tissue as distinguished from one in dead tissue, or one of vegetable origin.
These alkaloids represent 2 groups, the uric acid and the creatinine group. SEE: *anticreatinine.*

leukomainemia (lū-kō-mā-ĭn-ē'mĭ-ă) [" + *aima,* blood]. 1. Excess of leukomaines in blood. 2. Retention of excretory products in the blood.

leukomatous (lū-kōm'ă-tŭs) [" + *ōma,* tumor]. 1. Pert. to leukoma. 2. Suffering from leukoma.

leukomyelitis (lū″ko-mī-ĕ-li'tis) [G. *leukos,* white, + *myelos,* marrow, + -*itis,* inflammation]. Inflammation of spinal cord's marrow or white substance.

leukomyelopathy (lū″kō-mī-ĕl-ŏp'ăth-ĭ) [" + " + *pathos,* disease]. Disease involving white matter of spinal cord or myelon.

leukonecrosis (lū″ko-nĕ-krō'sĭs) [" + *nekrōsis,* deadness]. Dry, light colored or white gangrene.*

leukonychia (lū-kō-nik'ĭ-ă) [" + *onyx, onych-,* nail]. "Gift spots," white spots or streaks on the nails, due probably to air in interstitial corneal spaces, with local trauma as cause of production.

leukopathia (lū-kō-păth'ĭ-ă) [" + *pathos,* disease]. 1. Absence of pigment in skin. SYN: *leukoderma.* 2. Disease involving leukocytes.

leukopedesis (lū-kō-ped-ē'sĭs) [" + *pēdan,* to leap]. Passage of leukocytes through walls of blood vessels. SYN: *leukocytoplania.*

leukopenia (lū-kō-pe'nĭ-ă) [" + *penia,* lack]. Abnormal decrease of white blood corpuscles usually below 5000 per cu. mm.

l., malignant. An acute infection with extreme leukopenia. SYN: *agranulocytosis.*

leukophlegmasia (lū-kō-flĕg-mā'zĭ-ă) [" + *phlegmasia,* inflammation, fever]. Dropsical tendency with general edema and pale, flabby skin.

leukoplakia (lū-kō-plā'kĭ-ă) [G. *leukos,* white, + *plax,* plate]. Formation of white spots or patches on the mucous membrane of the tongue or cheek.
They are smooth, irregular in size and shape, and hard and occasionally fissure. May become malignant. SYN: *leukoma, psoriasis buccalis, smoker's tongue.*

l. buccalis. L. of the mucosa of the cheek.

l. lingualis. L. of the tongue.

leukoplasia (lū-kō-pla'zĭ-ă) [" + *plax,*

plate]. White patch formation on buccal mucosa. SYN: *leukoplakia, q.v.*

leukopoiesis (lū″kō-poi-ē'sĭs) [G. *leukos,* white, + *poiēsis,* formation]. Leukocyte production. SYN: *leukocytogenesis.*

leukopoietic (lū″kō-poi-et'ĭk) [" + *poiein,* to make]. Forming leukocytes.

leukoprotease (lū-ko-pro'te-ās) [" + *prōtos,* first, + *ase,* enzyme]. An enzyme in polynuclear leukocytes that digests protein.

leukorrhagia (lū-ko-ra'jĭ-ă) [" + *rēgnunai,* to flow forth]. Profuse white vaginal discharge. SYN: *leukorrhea, q.v.*

leukorrhea (lū-kōr-e'ă) [" + *roia,* flow]. An abnormal, white or yellowish mucous discharge from the cervical canal or the vagina.
There is frequently a normal physiological leukorrhea which is present just preceding and following menstruation. Leukorrhea may be abnormal because of increase in amount, changes in color, variations in consistency, odors, types of bacterial content, and the appearance of blood.
ETIOL: Pathological states of the endocervix and vagina.
SYM: Usually indications of acute inflammation, pain, heat, redness of parts involved, which may subside as discharge increases. Pain in groins, hypogastrium, sacral regions and small of back. Urethra often implicated, causing painful micturition. Symptoms which may occur in connection with chronic leukorrhea are innumerable. Reaction of discharge is acid, may be any consistency: thin and watery or viscid and tenacious.
TREATMENT: Remove the etiological factor. Constitutional. Improve general health, outdoor exercise, regular habits; plain, nutritious diet. Injections of hot, sterile water (95°-100° F.). Mild antiseptic douches.
SYN: *blennelytria.*

l., uterine. May affect mucous surface of cervix only, or fundus.
SYM: Pain, weight and dragging sensation in back and bearing down pains. Discharge at first serous and bloody, soon becomes thick yellowish or greenish, ropy, fluid or purulent. After drying, leaves yellow or greenish stain on linen and stiffens it. Afterward discharge becomes whiter, milky. May become chronic—discharge is alkaline in reaction.
Examined through speculum, cervix is found swollen, edematous, and red, and from the os pours forth a clear albuminous looking fluid, mucopus or long, tenacious shreds of cervical mucus.
PROG: Favorable in both though cure is often tedious.
TREATMENT: Same as vaginal form. Find and remove any special etiological factor.
SYN: *uterine catarrh.*

leukosarcoma (lū-kō-sar-kō'mă) [G. *leukos,* white, + *sarx,* flesh, + *ōma,* tumor]. An unpigmented sarcoma.

leukosis (lū-ko'sis) [" + -*ōsis,* intensive]. 1. Unnatural pallor. 2. Presence of an abnormal number of leukocytes in blood. 3. Increase in leukocyte forming tissue.

leukothrombin (lū″ko-throm'bin) [" + *thrombos,* a clot]. A fibrin factor derived from leukocytes in the blood which helps to form thrombin.

leukotoxic (lū-ko-toks'ĭk) [" + *toxikon,* poison]. Destroying leukocytes.

leukotoxin (lū-ko-toks'ĭn) [" + *toxikon,* poison]. An exotoxin that attacks white

leukous L-24 Leyden jar

[Diagram: hierarchical levels from Pyramidal Level of Cortex (Polymorphic) → Voluntary Movement; Level of Basal Ganglia (Thalamo-Striate Level) → Instinctive Movement; Level of Midbrain → Posture Movements; Level of Medulla → Vital Movements (of Heart, Lungs, Digestive Organs); Spinal Level → Simple Reflex Movement; Sensory End Organ.]

From Pearn's *Mental Nursing Simplified*, Baillière, Tindall & Cox, London, Eng.

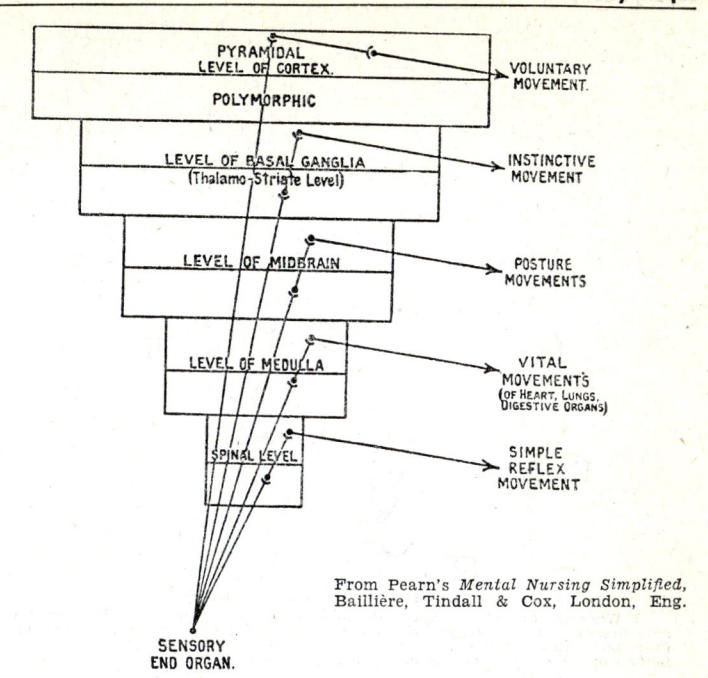

LEVEL OF ACTIVITIES

blood cells. SYN: *leukocidin, leukolysin*. SEE: *erythrotoxin*.

leukous (lū'kŭs) [G. *leukos*, white]. White, esp. rel. to the skin.

leukotrichia (lū-kō-trik'ĭ-ă) [" + *thrix, trich-*, hair]. Whiteness of the hair. SYN: *canities*.

levator (le-vā'tor) [L. lifter]. 1. A muscle that raises a part; opposed to *depressor*. 2. An instrument which lifts depressed portions.

   l. ani. A broad muscle helping to form the floor of the pelvis.

   l. palpebrae superioris. A muscle which elevates the upper eyelid.

level of activities. Connector neurons are grouped into "levels" corresponding to different stages of development: (a) spinal cord level; (b) medullary level; (c) midbrain level; (d) basal ganglial level; (e) cortical level. Each level is responsible for certain activities but yet controlled by the one above it.

le'ver. Rigid bar used to modify direction, force, and motion. SEE: *Ill., p. L-25*.

   l., Davy's. A rigid rod for compressing the common iliac artery.

levocardiogram (lev-ō-kar'dĭ-ō-grăm) [L. *laevus*, left, + G. *kardia*, heart, + *gramma*, a writing]. Part of cardiogram representing effect or action of left ventricle.

levoduction (lev-ō-dŭk'shun) [" + *ducere*, to lead]. Movement or drawing toward the left, esp. of an eye.

levogyrous (lev-ō-jī'rŭs) [" + *gyrāre*, to turn]. Causing to turn toward the left, applied esp. to substances that turn polarized light rays to the left. SYN: *levorotatory*.

levophobia (lev-ō-fō'bĭ-ă) [" + G. *phobos*, fear]. Morbid dread of objects on the left side of the body.

levorotation (lev"ō-rō-tā'shŭn) [" + *rōtāre*, to turn]. Twisting or turning to the left.

levorotatory (lev"ō-rō'tă-tō-rĭ) [" + *rōtāre*, to turn]. Causing to turn toward the left, applied esp. to substances that turn polarized light rays to the left. SYN: *levogyrous*.

levotorsion (lev-ō-tor'shŭn) [L. *laevus*, left, + *torsiō*, a twisting]. A twisting to the left. SYN: *levorotation*.

levoversion (lev-ō-vĕr'shun) [" + *versiō*, a turning]. A turning to the left. SYN: *levotorsion, levorotation*.

lev'ulose [L. *laevus*, left]. Fructose, or fruit sugar, a monosaccharide and a hexose, having the same empirical formula as dextrose, $C_6H_{12}O_6$.

It is an example of the carbohydrates, *q.v.* One of the 3 simple sugars. It is formed in the body by the digestion of sucrose. It is found in plants and fruits, in honey, corn syrup and syrup resulting from the inversion of sucrose.

DOSAGE: 1-2 oz. (30.0-60.0 Gm.).

levulosemia (lev-ŭ-lō-sē'mĭ-ă) [" + G. *aima*, blood]. Presence of levulose in the blood.

levulosuria (lev-ŭ-lō-sū'rĭ-ă) [" + G. *ouron*, urine]. Presence of levulose in the urine, usually in a form of diabetes.

Leyden jar (lī'den). A glass jar coated partially, inside and out, with metal or tinfoil, or coated outside with metal

LEVERS IN THE HUMAN BODY

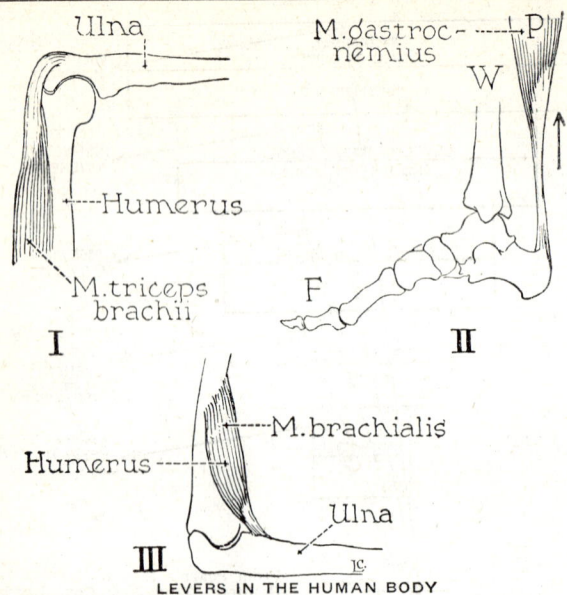

I. When the arm is held above the head, extension of the elbow involves the ulna as a first-class lever. II. Rising on the ball of the foot involves the calcaneus and other bones of the foot as a second-class lever. III. When the arm is held at the side, flexion of the elbow involves the ulna as a third-class lever.

and having salt solution inside; it is used as a capacitor.

Leydig's cells (li'dig). Interstitial tissue cells in the testicles, believed to be responsible for internal secretion of the testicles.

Li. Symbol for *lithium*.

liberomotor (lĭb″ĕr-o-mō'tŏr) [L. *liber*, free, + *motor*, mover]. 1, Pert. to voluntary movement. 2. Free from motor energy.

libidinous (lĭ-bĭd'ĭ-nŭs) [L. *libidinōsus*, pert. to desire]. Characterized by lust or lewdness. SYN: *lascivious, salacious*.

libido (lĭ-bī'dō, -bē'dō) [L. desire]. 1. The sexual drive, conscious or unconscious. 2. The emotional craving activating human behavior.

Repressions are believed to create a psychoneurosis.* SEE: *freudian, object choice*.

lichen (li'ken) [G. *leichen*, lichen]. Any form of papular skin disease; usually noting *l. planus*.

 l. **acuminatus.** A form of *l. ruber* with papulosquamous type of eruption.

 l. **agrius.** Eczema of acute papular type.

 l. **disseminatus.** Form in which the eruption is placed unevenly.

 l. **pilaris.** Form affecting hair follicles. SYN: *keratosis pilaris*.

 l. **planus.** Inflammatory skin disease of many varieties.

 SYM: Begins with pinhead size papules, reddish or violaceous, glistening, then coalescing, forming rough, scaly patches; acute, subacute, or chronic itching situated on extremities. According to type of lesion the disease may be *Lichen planus atrophicus, erythematosus, hypertrophicus, linearis, ruber moniliformis*, etc.

 ETIOL: Unknown. Nervous exhaustion a contributory factor. Probably systemic.

 PROG: Exceedingly chronic but favorable.

 TREATMENT: Hygienic regimen. Mercury, arsenic, and iron internally. Locally, soothing antipruritic ointment.

 l. **ruber.** Form with red, papular lesions and constitutional symptoms. Extremely rare. Most common in poorly nourished, middle aged males.

 SYM: Small, red, glazed, acuminated papules. No tendency to coalesce—associated with itching and failure of general health.

 PROG: Chronic course. May prove fatal through exhaustion.

 l. **scrofulosus.** Form with red papules occurring chiefly in children of strumous diathesis.

 SYM: Small, pale red, or salmon colored, scaly papules, most frequent on trunk. Itching absent.

 PROG: Chronic course.

 TREATMENT: In all forms, good nourishing diet, good hygiene, constitutional remedies in each individual case.

 l. **spinulosus.** Form with spine developing in each follicle. SYN: *keratosis pilaris, q.v.*

 l. **tropicus.** Form with redness and inflammatory reaction of the skin. SYN: *miliaria rubra, prickly heat*.

lichenification (lī-ken″ĭ-fĭ-kā'shun) [G. *leichēn*, lichen]. 1. Cutaneous thickening and hardening from continued irritation. 2. Changing of an eruption into resemblance to lichen.

lichenoid (li′ken-oid) [G. *leichēn*, lichen, + *eidos*, form]. Resembling lichen.

licorice (lik′ō-ris). A dried root of *Glycyrrhiza glabra* and allied species used as demulcent, laxative, and expectorant. SYN: *glycyrrhiza*.

lid reflex. Closure of eyelids resulting from direct corneal irritation.

Lieben's test (lē′ben). A test for acetone in the urine by caustic and iodine.
Yellow phosphate precipitates and iodoform indicates presence of acetone.

Lieberkuhn's crypts (lē′ber-kün, lē′berkün). Tubular glands on the intestinal mucosa surface.
They resemble depressions over the mucous membrane of the small and large intestines, their orifices appearing as minute dots between the villi. They are larger in the colon and increase in size toward the rectum. SYN: *L.'s follicles, L.'s glands*.

Liebig's extract (lē′big). Variety of beef extract.

lie detector. An instrument for determining such minor but definite physical changes under the stress of lying (or any other emotion) as variations in respiratory rhythm and sweating of the hands. Increased perspiration lessens resistance to passage of electrical current.

lien (li′en) [L. spleen]. The spleen.

lienal (li′en-ăl) [L. *lien*, spleen]. Rel. to the spleen. SYN: *splenic*.

lienculus (li-en′kü-lŭs) [L. little spleen]. An accessory spleen.

lienitis (li-en-i′tis) [L. *lien*, spleen, + G. -*itis*, inflammation]. Inflammation of the spleen. SYN: *splenitis*.

lienocele (li-en′ō-sēl) [″ + G. *kēlē*, hernia]. Splenic hernia. SYN: *splenocele*.

lienomalacia (li″en-o-mal-a′sĭ-ă) [″ + G. *malakia*, softening]. Softening of the spleen.

lienomedullary (li″en-ō-med′ŭ-la-rĭ) [″ + *medulla*, marrow]. Rel. to both spleen and bone marrow.

lienomyelogenous (li″en-ō-mī-ĕl-oj′ĕ-nŭs) [″ + G. *myelos*, marrow, + *gennan*, to produce]. Derived from both the spleen and bone marrow.

lienomyelomalacia (li″en-ō-mī″el-o-mă-lā′-sĭ-ă) [″ + ″ + *malakia*, softening]. Softening of the spleen and bone marrow.

lienopancreatic (li″en-ō-păn-krē-at′ĭk) [″ + G. *pagkreas*, pancreas]. Rel. to the spleen and pancreas.

lienopathy (li-en-op′ă-thĭ) [″ + G. *pathos*, a disease]. Any disorder of the spleen. SYN: *splenopathy*.

lienorenal (li″en-ō-rē′nal) [″ + *rēnalis*, pert. to a kidney]. Rel. to the spleen and kidney.

lienotoxin (li″en-ō-toks′ĭn) [″ + G. *toxikon*, poison]. Cytotoxin having specific action on splenic cells. SYN: *splenotoxin*.

lienteric (li-en-ter′ik) [G. *leienteria*, smooth intestine]. 1. Pert. to diarrhea with stools containing undigested food. 2. Affected with lientery.

lientery (li′en-ter-ĭ) [G. *leienteria*, smooth intestine]. Diarrhea with undigested foods in the stools.

lienunculus (li-en-un′kŭ-lŭs) [L. little spleen]. 1. Detached mass of splenic tissue. 2. Detached part of spleen.

life (lif) [A.S.]. 1. State of being alive; quality manifested by metabolism, growth, reproduction, and internal adaptation to environment; state in which the organs of an animal or plant are capable of performing all or any of their functions. 2. Time bet. birth and death.
RS: *anima, antibiosis, antibiotic, apothanasia, archebiosis, "bio-" words, vital, vitality*.

ligament (lĭg′a-ment) [L. *ligamentum*, a band]. A band of flexible connective tissue connecting the articular ends of bones, or supporting viscera, fasciae or muscles.
Ligaments are composed of fibrous material, folds of thickened peritoneum, and remains of fetal structures.
RS: *desmitis, syndesmitis, syndesmosis, vinculum*.

l., accessory. A l. which supplements another one, esp. one on lateral surface of a joint.

l., acromioclavicular. One extending from clavicle to the acromial process of the scapula.

l., adipose. Mucous l. of the knee joint.

l.'s, alar. Two crescentic folds of synovial membrane extending upward on each side of the mucous l. of the knee joint.

l., annular. A circular l.

l., appendiculoövarian. The ligament that runs from the broad l. to the vermiform appendix.

l., arterial. A fibrous cord constituting the remains of the ductus arteriosus of the fetus.

l., atloaxoid. One uniting the atlas and axis.

l.'s, atloöccipital. Those uniting atlas and occipital bone.

l.'s, auricular. The ant., post., and sup. auricular l.'s uniting external ear to side of head.

l., Barkow's. Ant. and post. l.'s of elbow joint.

l., Béraud's. Suspensory ligament of the pericardium.

l., Bertin's. Iliofemoral l.

l., Bigelow's. Iliofemoral ligament. SYN: *Bertin's l*.

l., broad, of the liver. A wide, sickle-shaped fold of peritoneum, attached to lower surface of diaphragm and internal surface of right rectus abdominis muscle, and to the convex surface of liver.

l., broad, of uterus. Folds of peritoneum attached to lateral borders of uterus from insertion of fallopian tube above to the pelvic wall. It consists of 2 leaves between which are found the remnants of the wolffian ducts, cellular tissues, and the major blood vessels of the pelvis.

l., Burn's. Falciform process of fascia lata.

l., calcaneoastragaloid interosseous. A strong bundle of fibers extending from furrow on upper surface of os calcis, bet. its surfaces of articulation with the astragalus.

l., calcaneofibular. A thick, flattened, cylindrical l., bet. the apex of ext. malleolus and outer surface of os calcis.

l., Camper's. Deep perineal fascia.

l.'s, capsular. Heavy fibrous structures, lined with synovial membrane, surrounding articulations.

l., Carcassonne's. Triangular ligament of urethra.

l.'s, carpal. Those uniting carpal bones.

l., caudal. Bundles of fibrous tissue uniting dorsal surfaces of the 2 lower coccygeal vertebrae and superjacent skin.

l., central. Thin distal portion of spl-nal cord. SYN: *filum terminale*.

l., check. One that restrains motion of a joint, esp. the lateral odontoid l.'s.

l., ciliary. One joining iris to corneosclera.

l., conoid. Post. portion of coracoclavicular l.

l., coracoacromial. Broad triangular one attached to the outer edge of coracoid process of the scapula, and to tip of acromion.

l., coracoclavicular. One uniting clavicle and the coracoid process of the scapula.

l., coracohumeral. Broad l. attached to outer margin of coracoid process of the scapula and attached to the clavicle.

l., corniculopharyngeal. Fibrous tissue connecting cartilage of Santorini and cricoid cartilage.

l., coronary, of liver. A fold of peritoneum extending from post. edge of liver to diaphragm.

l.'s, costocentral. Ones uniting head of a rib with bodies of its vertebrae.

l., costocolic. One attaching splenic flexure of colon to diaphragm.

l., costocoracoid. One joining first rib and coracoid process of the scapula.

l.'s, costotransverse. One uniting ribs with transverse processes of vertebrae.

l., costotransverse, middle. One consisting of parallel fibers extending bet. a vertebra and its adjacent rib.

l.'s, costovertebral. Those uniting the ribs and vertebrae.

l., cotyloid. A fibrocartilaginous ring attached to margin of acetabulum.

l.'s, craniovertebral. Those extending bet. cranium and the vertebrae.

l., cricopharyngeal. A ligamentous bundle bet. upper and post. border of cricoid cartilage and ant. wall of pharynx.

l., cricosantorinian. Ligamentous bands uniting cartilages of Santorini with the cricoid cartilage.

l.'s, cricothyroid. Ones uniting cricoid and thyroid cartilages.

l., cricotracheal. The ligamentous structure uniting upper ring of trachea and the cricoid cartilage.

l., crucial. Cruciform l.

l., cruciform. A structure consisting of one l. crossing another.

l. crural. Poupart's l.

l., deltoid. Int. lateral l. of ankle.

l., dentate. Processes of pia mater extending across the subdural space on either side of spinal cord.

l., falciform. SEE: *great sacroischiadic l.*

l., falciform, of the liver. SEE: *broad l. of the liver.*

l., gastrophrenic. SEE: *phrenicogastric l.*

l., gastrosplenic. Fold of peritoneum extending bet. the cul-de-sac of stomach and hilum of spleen. SYN: *gastrosplenic epiploön*.

l., Gimbernat's. Triangular flat expansion of aponeurosis of abdominal ext. oblique muscle.

l., glenohumeral. Fibers of the coracohumeral l. passing into the joint, and inserted into inner and upper part of bicipital groove.

l., glenoid. 1. Fibrocartilaginous ring attached to margin of glenoid fossa of the scapula. 2. One which extends bet. palmar surfaces of phalanges and corresponding metacarpal bone.

l., glenoideobrachial. Thickened area of the shoulder's capsular ligament which is inserted into the lesser tuberosity of the humerus.

l., hepaticoduodenal. A fold of peritoneum from transverse fissure of liver to vicinity of the duodenum and right flexure of colon, forming ant. boundary of foramen of Winslow.

l., Hunter's. Round l. of the uterus.

l., ileopectineal. A portion of the pelvic fascia attached to the ileopectineal line and to capsular l. of hip joint.

l., iliofemoral. Bundle of fibers forming the upper and ant. portion of the capsular l. of the hip joint.

l., iliotrochanteric. Part of capsular ligament of hip joint.

l., infundibulopelvic. The upper free edge of the broad l. in which the ovarian artery is found.

l., inguinal. SEE: *Poupart's l.*

l., interclavicular. Bundle of fibers bet. sternal ends of the clavicles, attached to interclavicular notch of sternum.

l.'s, interspinal, interspinous. Those extending from sup. margin of a spinous process of one vertebra to lower margin of one above.

l.'s, intervertebral. Fibrocartilaginous disks bet. vertebra.

l., lateral. One on side of a joint or on ext. side of a structure.

l.'s, lateral, of the liver. Folds of peritoneum extending from lower surface of diaphragm to adjacent borders of right and left lobes of the liver.

l., lateral occipitoatlantal. A ligament on each side bet. transverse processes of atlas and jugular process of the occipital bone.

l.'s, lateral odontoid. Strong l.'s extending bet. sides of odontoid process of the axis and inner sides of condyles of the occipital bone.

l.'s, lateral patellar. Membranous triangular ones extending on each side from condyle of femur and lateral margin of patella to inf. patellar l. and extensor tendons of the leg.

l., odontoid, middle. One extending bet. apex of odontoid process of the axis and ant. margin of foramen magnum.

l., palpebral. Ligament bet. ext. border of orbit and eyelid tissue and bet. nasal process of sup. maxilla and margins of the tarsi.

l., phrenicogastric. A fold of peritoneum bet. esophageal end of stomach and the diaphragm.

l., posterior crucial. One arising from behind spine of the tibia and ext. semilunar fibrocartilage and connecting with the inner femoral condyle.

l., posterior, of knee joint. A flat thickening of the capsule l. of the knee.

l., Poupart's. The lower portion of the aponeurosis of the ext. oblique muscle of the abdomen. SYN: *crural arch, femoral arch.*

l., pterygomaxillary. Band of fiber extending bet. apex of internal pterygoid plate of sphenoid bone and the post. extremity of internal oblique line of inferior maxilla.

l., pubic. The post. margin of sup. crus of the falciform process of the fascia lata.

l., reticular. One holding a muscle to a bone.

l., rhomboid. A strong structure extending from tuberosity of clavicle to outer surface of the cartilage of the first rib.

l., round. One resembling a round cord.
l., round, of the forearm. A small one bet. the coronoid process of ulna and a point below tuberosity of the radius.
l., round, of uterus. A long, round, fibrous band passing from fundal side of uterus, to be inserted into connective tissue of mons Veneris.
l., sacroischiadic, -ischiatic, or -sciatic, great. Triangular l. attached by its base to sides of sacrum and coccyx and to post. inf. spine of ilium, and by its apex to tuberosity of the ischium.
l., sacroischiadic, lesser; sacrosciatic, lesser. Short l. arising from the lateral margin of lower portion of sacrum and of upper portion of coccyx, in front of and blended with the great sacroischiadic l.
l.'s, stomach. The lesser omentum and the phrenicogastric l.
l., stylohyoid. A thin fibroelastic cord bet. lesser cornu of hyoid bone and apex of styloid process of the temporal bone.
l., stylomaxillary, stylomyloid. A broad fibrous band of tissue extending bet. styloid process of temporal bone and lower part of post. border of ramus of the inferior maxilla.
l., suprascapular. A thin fibrous band of tissue extending from base of coracoid process of scapula to inner margin of suprascapular notch.
l., supraspinal, supraspinous. One uniting apices of spinous processes of vertebrae.
l., suspensory. One suspending an organ.
l.'s, suspensory, of mamma. Fibrous processes of layer of fascia covering ant. surface of the mamma.
l., suspensory, of mesentery. The root of the mesentery.
l., suspensory, of the penis. A triangular bundle of fibrous tissue extending from ant. surface of the symphysis pubis and adjacent structures to dorsum of the penis.
l.'s, suspensory, of the uterus. The broad l.'s, the round ones, and the rectouterine folds of the uterus.
l.'s, sutural. Thin, fibrous layers interposed bet. articulating surfaces of bones united by suture.
l., tarsal. The tarsoörbital fascia.
l., transverse, of atlas. A strong l. passing over odontoid process of the axis.
l., transverse, of hip joint. A ligamentous band extending across cotyloid notch of the acetabulum.
l., transverse, of knee joint. A fibrous band extending from ant. margin of external semilunar fibrocartilage of knee to extremity of the internal semilunar fibrocartilage.
l., trapezoid. Ant. ext. portion of the coracoclavicular l.
l. of Treitz. Fold of peritoneum from duodenojejunal junction to left crus of diaphragm.
l., triangular. Triangular portion of the aponeurosis of ext. oblique muscle.
l., uteroövarian. Attaches the inner surface of the ovary to the uterine horn.
l., uterorectosacral. Arises from the sides of the cervix and passes upwards and backwards, passing around the rectum, to the second sacral vertebra.
l., vaginal, of the testicle. Obliterated portion of the tunica vaginalis.
l., vesicoumbilical. L. connecting bladder and umbilicus. SYN: *urachus*.
l., vesicouterine. The fold of peritoneum that attaches the bladder to the ant. wall of the uterus.
l., Winslow's. Posterior l. of the knee joint.
l., Y-shaped, of Bigelow. Iliofemoral l.
l. of Zinn. Membranous structure forming common tendon of origin for ext., inf., and int. recti muscles of the eye.

ligamentopexis (lĭg-ă-mĕn″tō-peks′ĭs) [L. *ligamentum*, band, + G. *pēxis*, fixation]. Suspension of uterus on the round ligaments.
ligamentous (lig-a-men′tŭs) [L. *ligamentum*, band]. 1. Rel. to a ligament. 2. Like a ligament.
ligamentum (lĭg-a-men′tum) (pl. *ligamenta*) [L. a band]. Ligament.
l. arcuatum. The ligamentous part of the diaphragm, external and internal.
l. arteriosum. A fibrous cord, from pulmonary artery to arch of aorta, the remains of the ductus arteriosus of the fetus.
l. cruciatum atlantis. Cruciform ligament.
l. cruciatum cruris. An X-shaped process of the deep fascia of the leg. SEE: *leg for illustration.*
l. dentatum, denticulatum. A delicate band of connective tissue on each side of the myelon.
l. nuchae. A thin, fibrous membrane connecting the trapezial muscles.
l. palpebrale. Ligamentous band, external and internal, bet. outer margin of the orbit and tissues of eyelids.
l. patellae. A strong, flat band securing the patella to the tibia.
l. pectinatum. The spongy tissue filling up sinus of ant. chamber of eye at junction of cornea and sclera, forming the root of the iris.
l. spirale. A projecting band attached to wall of the cochlea, upon which is inserted the lamina spiralis membranacea.
l. subflavum. Yellow elastic tissue connecting the lamina of the vertebrae from axis downward.
l. suspensorium. Suspensory ligament, *q.v.*
l. teres. 1. A triangular band of fibers arising from the margins of the cotyloid notch at bottom of the acetabulum. 2. Round ligament of the forearm. 3. Middle costotransverse ligament.
ligate (lī′gāt) [L. *ligāre*, to bind]. To apply a ligature.
ligation (lī-gā′shun) [L. *ligāre*, to bind]. The application of a ligature. SYN: *cirsodesis.*
ligature (lĭg′a-tūr) [L. *ligatūra*, a binding]. 1. Process of binding or tying. 2. A band or bandage. 3. A ligament. 4. A thread or wire for tying blood vessels.
The cord or material used in tying or binding, as an artery; catgut, kangaroo gut, silk, either the plaited silk or the Chinese twisted silk. In some cases dentists' floss silk as it does not slip easily. SEE: *catgut.*
light (līt) [A. S. *lĭhtan*, to shine]. The sensation produced by electromagnetic radiation which falls on the retina.
The radiation itself is also called light over the range of wavelengths which produces sensation, and regarding this range it is also called infrared and ultraviolet light. Radiant energy producing a sensation of luminosity on the retina limited to a wavelength of from 4000 to 7000 angstroms.* SEE: *rays.*
l., axial. L. with rays parallel to each other and to optic axis.

l., diffused. Rays broken by refraction.

l., polarized. L. in which waves vibrate in one direction only.

l., red. Cold, red light is emitted by neon glow discharge tube. Intensity of total radiation is low.

l. reflex. Reflection of light from normal eardrum membrane.

l., refracted. Rays bent from original course.

l., sun-. Radiation from the sun.

l. therapy. A limited term used by some physicians to designate the therapeutic application of radiation in the visible spectrum; some include also ultraviolet radiation.

l., transmitted. That which passes through an object.

l. unit. A foot candle. This is the amt. of light measured one foot from a standard candle. The light intensity of the average room is from 3 to 10 foot candles, whereas 25-100 would be better. At noon, on a clear day, the sun gives 10,000 candle ft. of light; under a tree we get 1,000; on a porch, 500; on a fairly cloudy day, 200. The term foot candle takes the place of "candle power."

light, words pert. to: aclastic, "actin-" words, anacamptics, Blondlot rays, catadioptric, circumpolarization, etiolate, "fluor-" words, Fraunhofer's lines, Grotthus' law, half-value thickness, "phot-" words, "radi-" words, ray, reflection, reflector, refraction, spectrum.

light (līt) [A. S. *lēohte*, not heavy]. 1. Not heavy. 2. Pale.

l. diet. All foods allowed in soft diet* plus whole grained cereals, easily digested raw fruits and vegetables. Foods not pureed or ground.

light'ening [A. S. *lēohte*, not heavy]. Uterine descent into pelvis during primary stage of labor.

ligula (lĭg'ū-là) [L. a strap]. Strip of white substance on the margin of the fourth ventricle.

limb (lĭm) [A. S. *lim*]. 1. An arm or leg. 2. Appendage resembling an arm or leg. 3. An extremity.
RS: *acampsia, acroagnosis, anisomelia, appendicular, artificial, cineplastics, extremity, macrocolia, melagra, melitagra, member.*

l., pelvic. A lower extremity.

l., thoracic. An upper extremity.

limbic (lĭm'bĭk) [L. *limbus*, a border]. Pert. to a limbus or border. SYN: *marginal*.

limbus (lĭm'bŭs) [L. border]. The edge or border of a part.

l. conjunctivae. The edge of conjunctiva overlapping the cornea.

lime (līm) [A. S. *līm*, glue]. CaO. A substance obtained from limestone.
It constitutes about 1.5% of the body weight and is found in the blood, tissues, and esp. in the bones and teeth.
In liquid form it stabilizes the nervous system and it is stored throughout the body, the amount even in the bones being unstable. It increases in the aged, making the bones brittle, and a deficiency in the younger children may be responsible for rickets. The amount in the daily diet is not sufficient during pregnancy and an added amount is necessary. It is obtained through the ingestion of calcium foods, such as milk. SEE: *calcium*.

l. water. Solution of lime and distilled water. INCOMPATIBILITIES: Sodium bicarbonate.

lime [Fr. *limo*]. Av. SERVING: 40 Gm. Pro. 0.3, Fat trace, Carbo. 4.9. VITAMINS: A+, B+, C++. Lemons have a much higher antiscorbutic value. ASH CONST: Ca 0.055, Mg 0.014, K 0.350, Na 0.062, P 0.036, Cl 0.039, S 0.010-0.003.

l. juice. Av. SERVING: 15 Gm. Pro. 0.1, Carbo. 1.2. VITAMINS: A+, B+, C++. Fe 0.003.

limen (lī'mĕn) [L. threshold]. Edge, threshold.

liminal (lĭm'ĭ-nàl) [L. *limen, limin-*, threshold]. Hardly perceptible; rel. to the threshold of consciousness.

limitans (lĭm'ĭ-tăns) [L. *limitāre*, to limit]. 1. Used in conjunction with other words to denote limiting. 2. Used synonymously to indicate membrane limitans.

limo'sis [G. *limos*, hunger]. Abnormal hunger; depraved appetite.

limotherapy (lim-ō-ther'ă-pī) [" + *therapeia*, treatment]. Treatment by restriction of diet, or fasting.

lincture (lĭnk'tūr), **linctus** (-tŭs) [L. *linctus*, a licking]. Medicine to be taken by licking.

line (līn) [L. *linea*]. Boundary mark or narrow mark.

l., abdominal. Line indicating abdominal muscle boundaries.

l., adrenal. In defective adrenal activity, white line seen on abdomen following drawing of fingernail across it.

l., alveobasilar. One from nasion to alveolar point.

l., alveolonasal. From alveolar to nasion.

l. of anus, inferior sinuous. Convoluted l. at junction of mucous membrane of rectum with integument at anus.

l., auriculobregmatic. From auricular point to bregma.

l., axillary (ant., post. and mid-). Downward from axilla.

l., base. From infraorbital ridge through middle of external auditory meatus to midline of occiput.

l., basiobregmatic. From basion to bregma.

l., Baudelocque's. Ext. conjugate diameter of pelvis.

l.'s, Beau's. Transverse lines on the fingernails.

l., biauricular. From one auditory meatus over vertex to other.

l., blue. One on gums in chronic lead poisoning.

l., Borsieri's. White l. made by fingernail in early stages of scarlet fever.

l., Burton's. SEE: blue l.

l., Camper's. One from ext. auditory meatus to just below nasal spine.

l., Clapton's. Green line on gums in copper poisoning.

l., Corrigan's. Purplish line on gums in copper poisoning.

l., costoarticular. From sternoclavicular joint to point on 11th rib.

l., costoclavicular. Line midway bet. nipple and sternum border.

l. of demarcation. Division bet. healthy and diseased tissue.

l., Douglas'. Curved lower edge of post. sheath of rectus abdominis muscle just below level of iliac crest.

l. of Douglas, semicircular. Curved lower edge of int. layer of aponeurosis of the obliquus abdominis internus.

l., ectental. Bet. ectoderm and entoderm on embryo.

l., Ellis'. Curved line at upper border of a pleuritic effusion.

l., facial. Straight line touching glabella and point at lower border of face.

l. of femur, internal supracondylar. Inner of 2 ridges into which linea aspera of femur divides.

line of fibula, oblique   L-30   **lingula cerebelli**

l. of fibula, oblique. Prominent ridge on int. surface of shaft of fibula.

l. of fixation. Imaginary l. drawn from subject viewed to the fovea centralis.

l., gingival. 1. Line of junction of cementum and enamel of a tooth. 2. One on neck of tooth where gum is attached.

l., iliopectineal. Bony ridge marking brim of pelvis.

l. of ilium, curved (sup., inf. and mid-). Prominent lines of iliac region.

l. of ilium, intermediate. Ridge upon crest of ilium bet. inner and outer lip.

l. of inferior maxilla, internal oblique. Ridge on int. surface of lower jaw.

l., interauricular. One joining the 2 auricular points.

l.'s, intercellular. The narrow intervals bet. contiguous cells of epithelium or endothelium.

l., intercondylar, intercondylean. Transverse ridge joining condyles of femur above the intercondyloid fossa.

l., interjugal. One joining the jugal points.

l., intermalar. One joining malar points.

l., intertrochanteric. Ridge upon post. surface of femur ext. bet. greater and lesser trochanters.

l., intertuberal. One joining inner borders of ischial tuberosities below small sciatic notch.

l., mammary. From one nipple to other.

l., mammillary. Vertical line through center of nipple.

l., median. One joining any 2 points in the periphery of the median plane of the body, or one of its parts.

l., nasobasilar. Through basion and nasion.

l., nuchal (sup., inf. and mid-). Inf. and sup. curved lines of occiput and ext. occipital protuberance.

l.'s of occipital bone, curved. Two lines on either half of outer surface of occipital bone.

l. of occipital bone, superior curved. Semicircular l. passing outward and forward from ext. occipital protuberance.

l., parasternal. Line midway bet. nipple and sternum border.

l. of parietal bone, superior curved. Ridge upon outer surface of parietal bone.

l., parturient. Axis of the birth canal.

l., pectineal. That portion of iliopectineal l. formed by the os pubis.

l. of radius, oblique. Prominent ridge from lower part of bicipital tuberosity downward and outward to form ant. border of the bone.

l., scapular. Downward from lower angle of scapula.

l., semilunar. Curved tendinous condensation of aponeurosis of obliquus abdominis externus.

l., sight. From center of pupil to viewed object, imaginary.

l., spinoumbilical. Imaginary l. drawn from ant. sup. spine of ilium to umbilicus.

l., sternal. Median line of sternum.

l., sternomastoid. From bet. heads of sternomastoid muscle to mastoid process.

l., supraorbital. Across forehead above root of ext. angular process of frontal bone.

l., temporal. Curved l. on outer surface of parietal bone just below parietal eminence.

l.'s, test. Those for detecting fracture or shortening of neck of femur.

l. of tibia, oblique. Rough ridge crossing post. surface of tibia obliquely downward.

l., umbilicopubic. That portion of median l. extending from umbilicus to symphysis pubis.

l., visual. One that extends from object to macula lutea passing through the nodal point.

linea (lĭn'ē-ä) (pl. *lineae*) [L. line]. An anatomical line.

l. alba. The white line of connective tissue in middle of abdomen from sternum to the pubis.

l. albicans. L. on abdomen in advanced pregnancy, in dropsy or tumor.

l. aspera. A longitudinal ridge on sup. surface of middle third of the femur.

l. costoarticularis. A line bet. the sternoclavicular articulation and point of the 11th rib.

l. cruciatae. The 4 ridges upon inner surface of the occipital bone.

l. directionis pelvis. The axis of pelvic canal.

l. eminens. A ridge on post. surface of the patella.

l. eminens cartilaginis cricoideae. Vertical ridge in middle line of post. half of the cricoid cartilages.

l. eminens transversa ossis hyoidei. Horizontal ridge crossing ant. surface of body of hyoid bone.

l. eminentes. Ridges upon ant. surface of scapula in subscapular fossa.

l. ni'gra. Black line or discoloration of the abdomen seen in pregnant women during latter part of term. It runs from above the umbilicus to the pubes.

l. obliqua cartilaginea. An oblique line extending downward and outward from tubercle of thyroid cartilage.

l. quadrati. An eminence commencing about middle of post. intertrochanteric line, and descending vertically for about 2 inches along post. surface of shaft of femur.

l. sternalis. Median line of the sternum.

l. terminalis. BNA. Bony ridge on inner surface of ilium continued on to pubis which divides true and false pelvis.

l. transversae ossis sacralis. Ridges formed by lines of union of the 4 sacral vertebrae.

linear (lĭn'ē-ar) [L. *linea*, line]. Pert. to, or resembling, a line.

l. measure. Measure of length.

Linear Measure	
12 inches (in.)	=1 foot (ft.)
3 feet	=1 yard (yd.)
16.5 feet	=1 rod (rd.)
320 rods	=1 mile (mi.)
1760 yards	=1 mile
5280 feet	=1 mile

lingism (lĭng'ĭzm). Exercise cure or treatment, esp. without the aid of apparatus. SYN: *kinesitherapy*.

Ling's cure, L.'s system (ling). Treatment by movements.

lingua (lĭng'gwä) [L. tongue]. Tongue, or tonguelike structure.

lingual (lĭn'gwal) [L. *lingua*, tongue]. 1. Pert. to the tongue. 2. Tongue-shaped.

lingula (lĭn'gū-lä) [L. little tongue]. Tongue-shaped process, esp. lingula cerebelli.

l. cerebelli. Tongue of cerebellum

prolonged forward on upper surface of sup. medullary velum.

l. of sphenoid. Ridge between the body and ala magna of the sphenoid.

l. Wrisbergi. Connecting fibers of motor and sensory roots of the trifacial nerve.

lin′iment [L. *linimentum*, smearing substance]. A liquid containing a medicament and oil, alcohol or water for use externally, applied by friction method.

linimentum (lĭn-ĭm-en′tum) [L. smearing substance]. Liquid preparation for external use and usually applied with rubbing. Four are official.

li′nin [L. *linum*, flax]. An achromatic, threadlike substance which forms the nuclear network of a cell; the nucleoplasm is found in its reticulum, in the form of granules.

linitis (lĭn-I′tis) [G. *linon*, web, + *-itis*, inflammation]. Inflamed condition of gastric cellular tissue.

l., plastic. L. with hypertrophy of connective tissue about the stomach.

lin′seed [A.S. *līnsǣd*]. Seeds of the common flax.

l. poultice. One made from crushed linseed which is heated. Test for heat with hand before applying.

l. tea. A soothing demulcent drink for colds. Add 1 tablespoonful of linseed to 1 pint of water. The juice of a lemon may be added and sugar. Some use ¼ oz. of liquorice and ¼ oz. of candy. It is then simmered in a saucepan for half an hour, strained, and served hot.

lint (lĭnt) [L. *linteum*, made of linen]. 1. Linen scraped until soft and woolly for dressing wounds. 2. Cotton fiber.

lintin (lĭn′tĭn) [L. *linteum*, made of flax]. Prepared absorbent cotton; fabric used in dressings.

liomyofibroma (lī-ō-mī-ō-fī-brō′mă) [G. *leios*, smooth, + *mys*, *myo-*, muscle, + L. *fibra*, fiber, + G. *ōma*, tumor]. Tumor in which lioma, myoma, and fibroma are characterized.

lip [A.S. *lippa*]. 1. Soft structure around the oral cavity, externally. 2. One of the lips of the pudendum (*labium majus* or *minus*).

Diagnostic examination incomplete unless lips are everted to expose buccal surfaces. Conditions affecting lip are: *Chancre*: It is not unusual to have the initial lesion of syphilis appear upon the lip as an indurated base, with a thin secretion, accompanied by enlargement of the submaxillary glands. Innocent extragenital syphilitic infection may take place on the lips. *Condyloma latum*: This appears as a mucous patch, flattened, coated with gray exudate, with strictly delimited area, usually at the angle of the mouth. *Eczema*: Dry fissures, often covered with a crust, bleeding easily, and occurring on both lips. *Epithelioma*: May be confused with chancre. Seldom appears before the age of 40, but there are exceptions. It may appear as a common cold sore, a painless fissure or other break of the lower lip. Less than 5% occur on upper lip. A crust or scab covers the lesion, leaving a raw surface if removed. Pain does not appear until well advanced. *Herpes*: Appears on the lips in malaria, pneumonia, typhoid, acute coryza, and other febrile diseases. *Tuberculous ulcer*: At inner portion of lip close to angle of mouth. Pathological examination necessary for verification.

RS: *buccal, cheilitis, "chil-" words, labia, labium, labrum*.

l., bluish or purplish. May appear in the aged, in those exposed to great cold, and in carbon monoxide poisoning.

l., dry. May be seen in fevers, or be caused by drugs such as atropine, by thirst, or exhaustion.

l., fissured. May occur after exposure to cold, in certain forms of indigestion, and in children in congenital syphilis. The dribbling of saliva, and a toothless condition may cause fissures in the corners of the mouth.

l., hare. Slit appearance of upper lip due to developmental failure of continuity.

l., pale. May be seen in anemia and wasting diseases, in prolonged fever, and after a hemorrhage.

l. rashes. These may be manifestations of typhoid fever, meningitis, or pneumonia. In secondary syphilis, chancre, cancer, and epithelioma, mucous patches may appear.

l. reading. Catching meaning of a speaker by watching movements of his lips without hearing his words.

l. reflex. Reflex movement of lips when angle of mouth is suddenly and lightly tapped during sleep.

lipacidemia (lĭp″ă-sĭ-dē″mĭ-ă) [G. *lipos*, fat, + L. *acidus*, acid, + G. *aima*, blood]. Fatty acid in the blood.

lipaciduria (lĭp″ă-sĭ-dū′rĭ-ă) [" + " + G. *ouron*, urine]. Fatty acids in the urine.

liparocele (lĭp′ă-ro-sēl) [" + *kēlē*, hernia]. 1. Scrotal hernia containing fat. 2. A fatty tumor.

liparous (lĭp′ăr-ŭs) [G. *lipos*, fat]. Obese; fat.

liparomphalus (lĭp-ă-rom′fă-lŭs) [" + *omphalos*, navel]. Fatty tumor located at, or involving, the umbilical cord.

lipase (lī′pās, lī′pās) [G. *lipos*, fat, + *ase*, enzyme]. A lipolytic or fat splitting enzyme found in the blood, pancreatic secretion and tissues.

Emulsified fats of cream and egg yolk are changed in the stomach to fatty acids and glycerol by gastric lipase.

lipasuria (lĭp-ăs-u′rĭ-ă) [" + " + G. *ouron*, urine]. Lipase in the urine.

lipectomy (lĭ-pek′to-mĭ) [" + *ektomē*, excision]. Excision of fatty tissues.

lipemia (lĭ-pē′mĭ-ă) [" + *aima*, blood]. Fat in the blood.

l. retinalis. Condition in which retinal vessels appear reddish white, or white; found in cases of lipemia.

lipid(e (lĭp′ĭd, lĭp′īd) [G. *lipos*, fat]. A comprehensive term for fats and soaps. SYN: *lipin, lipoid, q.v.*

lipin (lĭp′ĭn) [G. *lipos*, fat]. Term for fat and fatlike substances.

They may be simple, compound, or derived. SEE: *fat, lipoid*.

lipiodine (lĭp-ī′ō-dīn) [" + *iōdēs*, violet-hued]. Solid form of iodipin.

lipiodol (lĭp-ī′ō-dŏl) [" + " + L. *oleum*, oil]. An iodized oil obtained by fixation of iodine in poppyseed oil.

It contains 40% of pure iodine by weight. It is opaque to x-rays and used for radiological diagnosis. It is introduced into cavities by a catheter, into the trachea for outlining the bronchial tree by x-ray, and spinally to locate tumors. It is eliminated completely and does not cause iodism.

l. injection. May be cisternal, lumbar, or both, depending upon whether the suspected block is near the cisterna magna or below it. Two cubic centimeters are injected into spinal canal. There are 2 forms of lipiodol: *ascending* and *descending*. If tumor is near the cisterna, descending lipiodol is given intraspinously; if position is uncertain or halfway bet. cisterna and lumbar region, both forms are given. If there is a block in the canal, the picture shows a dark mass through which the lipiodol has not passed, and a light streak where the lipiodol is present.

lipo-, lip- [G.]. Combining forms pert. to fat.

lipoarthritis (lip-ō-arth-rī'tĭs) [G. *lipos*, fat, + *arthron*, joint, + *-itis*, inflammation]. Inflammation of fatty tissues of joints.

lipoblast (lĭp'ō-blast) [" + *blastos*, germ]. Immature fat cell.

lipoblastoma (lĭp-ō-blast-ō'mă) [" + " + *-ōma*, tumor]. Tumor of fatty tissue. SYN: *adipoma, lipoma*.

lipocaic (lĭp-ō-kā'ĭk) [G. *lipos*, fat]. Pancreatic hormone controlling hepatic fat supply.
Recently, it has been used successfully to clear up psoriasis.

lipocardiac (lĭp″ō-kar'dĭ-ăk) [" + *kardia*, heart]. 1. Pert. to fatty heart degeneration. 2. Sufferer from fatty degeneration of heart.

lipocele (lĭp'ō-sēl) [" + *kēlē*, hernia]. Presence of fatty tissue in a hernial sac. SYN: *adipocele, liparocele*.

lipocere (lĭp'ō-sēr) [" + L. *cera*, wax]. Waxy substance resulting from exposure of fleshy tissue to moisture with the exclusion of air. SYN: *adipocere*.

lipochondroma (lĭp″ō-kŏn-drō'mă) [G. *lipos*, fat, + *chondros*, cartilage, + *-ōma*, tumor]. Tumor both fatty and cartilaginous.

lipochrome (lĭp'ō-krōm). Colored substance of fatty nature.
Ex: *Carotin*, the fat-soluble yellow pigment found in carrots, sweet potatoes, egg yolk, butter, body fat and corpus luteum. SEE: *carotene*.

lipoclasis (lĭp-ok'lă-sĭs) [" + *klasis*, breaking]. Splitting up of fat. SYN: *lipolysis, lipodieresis*.

lipoclastic (lĭp-ō-klas'tĭk) [" + *klastikos*, broken]. Fat splitting. SYN: *lipolytic*.

lipocyte (lĭp'ō-sīt) [" + *kytos*, cell]. Fat cell.

lipodieresis (lĭp-ō-dī-er'ĕ-sĭs) [" + *dia*, apart, + *airein*, to take]. Splitting or destruction of fat. SYN: *lipoclasis*.

lipodystrophy (lĭp-ō-dĭs'trō-fĭ) [" + *dys*, bad, + *trophē*, nourishment]. Disturbance or defectiveness of fat metabolism.
   l., intestinal. Disease characterized principally by fat deposits in intestinal and mesenteric lymphatic tissue and by fatty diarrhea, loss of weight and strength, and arthritis.

lipoferous (lĭp-ŏf'ĕr-ŭs) [" + *pherein*, to carry]. Causing or carrying fat.

lipofibroma (lĭp″ō-fī-brō'mă) [G. *lipos*, fat, + L. *fibra*, fiber, + G. *-ōma*, tumor]. Tumor indicating lipoma and fibroma.

lipogenesis (lĭp-ō-jĕn'ĕ-sĭs) [" + *genesis*, formation]. Fat formation.

lipogenetic (lĭp-ō-jĕn-ĕt'ĭk) [" + *gennan*, to produce]. Fat producing. SYN: *lipogenic, lipogenous*.

lipogenic (lĭp-ō-jĕn'ĭk) [" + *gennan*, to produce]. Fat producing. SYN: *lipogenetic, lipogenous*.

lipogenous (lĭp-ŏj'ĕn-ŭs) [" + *gennan*, to produce]. Producing fat. SYN: *lipogenetic, lipogenous*.

lipogranuloma (lĭp″ō-gran-ŭ-lo'mă) [" + L. *granulum*, granule, + G. *-ōma*, tumor]. Inflammation of fatty tissue with granulation and development of oily cysts.

lipoid (lĭp'oid) [" + *eidos*, form]. 1. Substance resembling fats in appearance and solubility, but containing other groups than the glycerol and fatty acids which make up the true fats.
Ex: cholesterol, kephalin and lecithin, *q.v.* SYN: *lipid*.
2. Similar to fat.

lipoidemia (lĭp-oi-dē'mĭ-ă) [" + " + *aima*, blood]. Lipoids in the blood.

lipoidosis (lĭp-oi-do'sĭs) [" + " + *-ōsis*, intensive]. Presence of anisotropic lipoids in tissue.

lipoiduria (lĭp-oi-dū'rĭ-ă) [G. *lipos*, fat, + *eidos*, like, + *ouron*, urine]. Lipoids in the urine.

lipolipoidosis (lĭp″ō-lĭp-oi-dō'sĭs) [" + *lipos*, fat, + *eidos*, form, + *-ōsis*]. Infiltration of fats and lipoids into a tissue.

lipolysis (lip-ol'is-is) [" + *lysis*, dissolution]. The decomposition of fat.

lipolytic (lĭp-ō-lĭ'tĭk) [" + *lysis*, dissolution]. Having ability to hydrolyze fats.
   l. digestion. The conversion of neutral fats by hydrolysis into fatty acids and glycerol; fat splitting.
   l. enzyme. Fat splitting ferment. SYN: *lipase*. SEE: *enzymes*.

lipoma (lĭ-po'mă) [" + *-ōma*, tumor]. A fatty tumor. SEE: *chondrolipoma*.
They are frequently multiple, but not metastatic.
   l. arborescens. Excrescence of fatty tissue within a tendon sheath.
   l. colloides. A myxolipoma.
   l., cystic. One containing cysts.
   l., diffuse. One not definitely circumscribed.
   l. diffusum renis. Condition in which fat displaces parenchyma of the kidney.
   l. durum. One in which there is marked hypertrophy of the fibrous stroma and capsule.
   l., hernial. A lipocele.
   l. myxomatodes. A lipomyxoma.
   l., nasal. A fibrous growth of the subcutaneous tissue of the nostrils.
   l., osseous. One in which the connective tissue has undergone calcareous degeneration.
   l. telangiectodes. A rare form containing a large number of blood vessels.

lipomatosis (lĭp-ō-mă-to'sĭs) [G. *lipos*, fat, + *-ōma*, tumor, + *-ōsis*, intensive]. Excessive deposit of fat in the tissues. SYN: *liposis, obesity*.
   l. renis. Fatty infiltration of renal parenchyma. SYN: *lipoma diffusum renis*.

lipomatous (lĭp-ō'mă-tŭs) [" + *-ōma*, tumor]. 1. Of the nature of lipoma. 2. Affected with lipoma.

lipometabolic (lĭp″ō-met-ă-bol'ĭk) [" + *metabolē*, change]. Rel. to metabolism of fat.

lipometabolism (lĭp-ō-mĕ-tab'ol-ĭzm) [" + " + *ismos*, state of]. Fat metabolism.

lipomyxoma (lĭp″ō-miks-ō'mă) [" + *myxa*, mucus, + *-ōma*, tumor]. Tumor indicating lipoma and myxoma.

lipopectic (lĭp-ō-pek'tĭk) [" + *pēxis*, fixation]. Characterized by lipopexia.

lipopexia (lĭp-ō-pek'sĭ-ă) [" + *pēxis*, fixation]. Accumulation of fat in the body. SYN: *adipopexia*.

lipophage (lĭp'o-fāj) [" + *phagein*, to eat]. Cell absorbing fat.

lipophagic (lĭp'o-fā'jĭk) [" + *phagein*, to eat]. Consuming, destroying, or absorbing fat. SYN: *lipolytic*.

lipophil (lĭp'ō-fĭl) [" + *philein*, to love].
1. A fat absorber or solvent. 2. Absorbing fat.
lipophrenia (lĭp-ō-frē'nĭ-ă) [" + *phrēn*, mind]. Mental failure or collapse.
liposarcoma (lĭp-ō-sar-kō'mă) [" + *sarx*, flesh, + *-ōma*, tumor]. Sarcoma with fatty elements.
lipo'sis [" + *-ōsis*, intensive]. Accumulation of fat in a part.
lipothymia (lĭ-po-thī'mĭ-ă) [G. *leipein*, to leave, + *thymos*, mind]. Faintness; syncope.*
lipotropic (lĭp-ō-trŏp'ĭk) [G. *lipos*, fat, + *trope*, a turning]. Said of a basic dye having an affinity for fat.
lipotropy (lĭp-ot'rō-pĭ) [" + *tropos*, a turning]. The affinity of a basic dye for fat.
lipoxeny (lĭp-oks'ē-nĭ) [G. *leipein*, to leave, + *xenos*, host]. Desertion of host by parasitic organism.
Lipschuetz cell (lĭp'shŭtz). Cell with single and double granules in its protoplasm, which are stainable with hematoxylin. SYN: *centrocyte*.
lipuria (lĭ-pu'rĭ-ă) [G. *lipos*, fat, + *ouron*, urine]. Fat in the urine.
liquefacient (lĭk-we-fā'shent) [L. *liquere*, to flow, + *facere*, to make]. 1. Agent which produces a conversion into liquid. 2. Converting into liquid.
liquefaction (lĭk-we-fak'shun) [" + *facere*, to make]. The conversion of a solid into a liquid.
liquescent (lĭk-wes'sent) [L. *liquescere*, to become liquid]. Becoming liquid. SYN: *deliquescent*.
liqueur (lĭ-ker') [Fr.]. Alcoholic spirit. Aromatically flavored, often colored, and sweetened. A cordial.
liquid (lĭk'wĭd) [L. *liquidus*, flowing]. 1. Flowing easily. 2. Substance which flows without being melted. SEE: *emulsion*, *liquefacient*, *liquefaction*.
l. air therapy. Therapeutic application of low temperatures. SEE: *refrigeration*.
l. measure. Measure of liquid capacity.

Liquid Measure	
4 gills (gi.)	= 1 pint (pt.)
2 pints	= 1 quart (qt.)
4 quarts	= 1 gallon (gal.)
63 gallons	= 1 hogshead
2 hogsheads	= 1 pipe
2 pipes	= 1 tun

li'quid di'et. Coffee with hot milk, tea, water, albumin water, milk in all forms, milk and cream mixtures, cocoa, cream soups strained, fruit juices, meat juices, beef tea, clear broths, gruels, meat soups strained, eggnogs. SEE: *fluid diet*.
l. d., full. Restricted liquid diet plus gruels, strained fruit juice, tomato juice, strained cream soups, milk and cream beverages, albumins, plain gelatin, custard, plain ice cream, junket, coffee, tea.
l. d., high caloric. Full liquid diet reinforced with lactose, glucose, dextrimaltose, ice cream, ices, coffee, tea, etc.
l. d., or fluid, without milk. Cereal water, strained fruit and strained vegetable juices, albumins, plain gelatin, water ices, ginger ale, clear fat-free broth, beef juice, coffee, tea, etc.
l. d., restricted. Fat-free broth, tea (no cream), ginger ale, bland fruit juice, such as pear, white cherry, or peach juice.
l. d., surgical. Strained fruit juices,

ginger ale, fat-free broth, strained cream soup, milk and cream beverages, albuminized fruit juices, tea, coffee, gelatin beverage if ordered.
liquor (lĭk'er) [L. a liquid]. 1. Any liquid or fluid. 2. An alcoholic beverage. 3. PHARM: Solution of medicinal substance in water.
l. amnii. The fluid in the amniotic sac in which the fetus floats.
l. folliculi. The fluid contained in the graafian follicle.
l. lymphae. Fluid portion of lymph.
l. puris. Liquid portion of pus.
l. sanguinis. Blood serum or plasma.
l. solutions. Aqueous solutions of nonvolatile substances presenting the greatest variety in strength, character, and method of preparation. They are usually very active medicinal preparations. There are 21 official solutions.
lisping (lĭsp'ĭng) [A.S. *wlisp*, stammering or lisping]. Substitution of sounds due to defect in speech, as of *th* sound for *s* and *z*.
lissotrichy (lĭs-sot'rĭ-kĭ) [G. *lissos*, smooth, + *thrix, trich-*, hair]. Condition of having straight hair.
lis'terism. Theory and practice of antisepsis.
liter (lē'tĕr) [Fr. *litre*, from G. *litra*, a pound]. Metric fluid measure; 1000 cc., 270 fl. drams, 61 cu. in., 33.8 fl. oz., 1.056 qt. SEE: *metric system*.
lithagogue (lĭth'ă-gŏg) [G. *lithos*, stone, + *agōgos*, leading]. 1. Agent which expels calculi. 2. Expelling calculi.
lithectasy (lĭth-ek'ta-sĭ) [" + *ektasis*, dilatation]. Removal of a stone from bladder by dilation of the urethra.
lithemia (lĭth-e'mĭ-ă) [" + .*aima*, blood]. Excess of lithic or uric acid in the blood due to imperfect metabolism of the nitrogenous substances. SYN: *uricemia*. SEE: *oxypathy*.
lithiasis (lĭth-ī'ă-sĭs) [G. *lithos*, stone].
1. Formation of calculi and concretions.
2. Uric acid diathesis.
l. biliaris. Gallstones.
l. nephritica. Stone formation in the kidneys. SYN: *nephrolithiasis*.
l. renalis. Kidney stones.
lithiatry (lĭth-ī'ă-trī) [" + *iatreia*, healing]. Medical treatment of calculus.
lithic acid (lĭth'ĭk) [G. *lithos*, stone]. Acid found in urine. SYN: *uric acid*.
litho-, lith- [G.]. Prefixes: Pert. to *stone* or *calculus*.
lithocenosis (lĭth-ō-sĕn-ō'sĭs) [G. *lithos*, stone, + *kenōsis*, evacuation]. Removal of crushed fragments of calculi. SYN: *litholapaxy, lithotrity*.
lithoclast (lĭth'ō-klăst) [" + *klan*, to crush]. Forceps for breaking up large calculi. SYN: *lithotrite*.
lithoclasty (lĭth'ō-klăs-tĭ) [" + *klan*, to crush]. The crushing of a stone into fragments that it may pass through natural channels.
lithoclysma (lĭth-ō-klĭs'mă) [" + *klysma*, a cluster]. Injection of calculary solvents into urinary bladder.
lithocystotomy (lĭth"ō-sĭs-tot'o-mĭ) [G. *lithos*, stone, + *kystis*, bladder, + *tomē*, incision]. Incision of bladder to remove calculus.
lithodialysis (lĭth"ō-dī-al'ĭ-sĭs) [" + *dialysis*, a breaking up]. Fragmentation or solution of calculi. SYN: *litholysis*.
lithogenesis (lĭth-ō-jen'ĕ-sĭs) [" + *genesis*, formation]. Formation of concretions.
lithokonion (lĭth-ō-kō'nĭ-on) [" + *konian*,

litholapaxy L-34 **litmus paper**

to pulverize]. Instrument for pulverizing vesical calculi.
litholapaxy (lĭth-ol'a-păks-ĭ) [" + *lapaxis*, removal]. The operation of crushing a stone in the bladder followed by immediate washing out of the crushed fragments through a catheter.
lithology (lĭth-ol'ō-jĭ) [" + *logos*, science]. The science dealing with calculi.
litholysis (lĭth-ol'ĭ-sĭs) [" + *lysis*, dissolution]. Dissolving of calculi. SYN: *lithodialysis*.
lithometer (lĭth-om'ĕ-tĕr) [" + *metron*, measure]. Instrument for estimating size of calculi.
lithometra (lĭth-ō-me'tră) [" + *metra*, uterus]. Uterine tissue ossification.
lithomyl (lĭth'ō-mĭl) [G. *lithos*, stone, + *myle*, mill]. Instrument for crushing a vesical stone. SYN: *lithokonion*.
lithonephrotomy (lĭth"o-nĕ-frot'ō-mĭ) [" + *nephros*, kidney, + *tome*, excision]. Incision of kidney for removal of renal calculus.
lithontriptic (lĭth-on-trip'tĭk) [" + *tribein*, to crush]. An agent that tends to dissolve calculi.
Ex: *Lithium citrate, potassium citrate,* and *ammonium benzoate*.
lithopedion (lĭth"ō-pe'dĭ-ŏn) [" + *paidion*, child]. A fetus which has died and become petrified.
lithophone (lĭth'o-fōn) [" + *phōne*, sound]. Instrument for determining by sound the presence of calculi in the bladder.
lithoscope (lĭth'o-skōp) [" + *skopein*, to examine]. Instrument for examining stone in bladder.
lithotome (lĭth'o-tōm) [" + *tome*, incision]. Instrument for performing lithotomy.
lithotomy (lith-ot'o-mĭ) [" + *tome*, incision]. Incision into bladder for removing a stone.
NP: See that retention catheter is kept draining at all times. Watch intake and output of urine.
l., bilateral. Incision across perineum.
l., high. Suprapubic incision.
l., lateral. Front of rectum to one side of raphe.
l., median. In median line in front of anus.
l. position. Upon the back with thighs flexed upon abdomen and legs upon thighs, which are abducted. SYN: *dorsosacral*.
l., rectal. Through the rectum.
l., vaginal. Through vaginal wall.
lithotony (lĭth-ot'ō-nĭ) [" + *toncs*, a stretching]. Removal of a calculus through small incision instrumentally dilated.
lithotresis (lĭth-ō-tre'sĭs) [G. *lithos*, stone, + *trēsis*, boring]. Drilling or boring of holes in a calculus to facilitate crushing.
lithotripsy (lĭth'ō-trĭp-sĭ) [" + *tripsis*, a rubbing]. Crushing of a calculus in bladder or urethra.
lithotriptic (lĭth-o-trip'tĭk) [" + *tripsis*, a rubbing]. 1. An agent that dissolves calculi. 2. Pert. to lithotripsy. SYN: *lithontriptic*.
lithotrite (lĭth'o-trīt) [" + L. *tritus*, a rubbing]. Instrument for crushing stone in the bladder. SEE: *lithotrity*.
lithotrity (lith-ot'rĭ-tĭ) [" + L. *tritus*, a rubbing]. Crushing of a stone to small fragments in the bladder. SEE: *litholapaxy*.
lithous (lĭth'ŭs) [G. *lithos*, stone]. Rel. to a calculus or stone. SYN: *calculous*.
lithoxiduria (lĭth"oks-ĭ-dū'rĭ-ă) [" + *oxide* + G. *ouron*, urine]. Presence of xanthic oxide in the urine.
lithuresis (lith-u-re'sĭs) [" + *ourēsis*, urination]. Passage of calculus through the urethra during urination.
lithureteria (lĭth"ū-re-tē'rĭ-ă) [" + *ourētēr*, ureter]. Disease of the ureter due to presence of calculi.
lithuria (lĭth-u'rĭ-ă) [" + *ouron*, urine]. Excess of uric acid and urates in the urine.
litmus (lĭt'mus) [O.N. *litr*, lichen dye, + *mosi*, moss]. A blue dyestuff made by fermenting certain coarsely powdered lichens.
l. paper. Chemically prepared blue paper which is turned red by acids, and

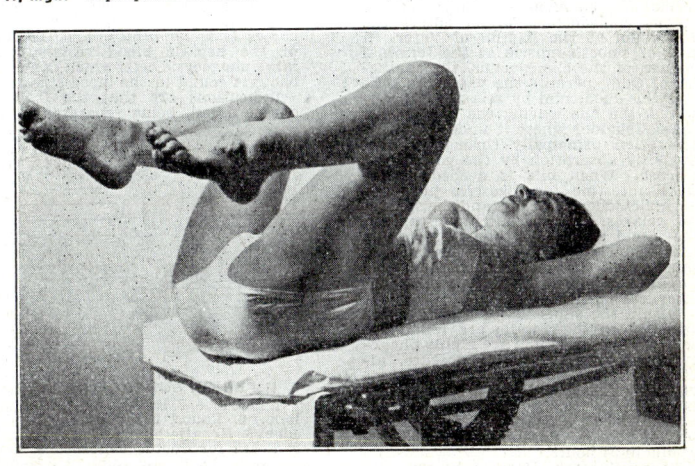

Posed by professional model *Photo by Whitaker*
Courtesy of Mount Vernon Hospital
LITHOTOMY OR DORSOSACRAL POSITION.

remains blue in alkali solutions; used as test for acid in urine. SEE: *indicator*.

litter (lĭt′tēr) [Fr. *litiere*, from *lit*, a bed]. A stretcher for carrying the wounded or the sick.

Little's disease (lĭt′tls). Congenital spastic paralysis on both sides (diplegia), although it may be *paraplegic* or *hemiplegic* in form.

ETIOL: Possible birth injury.

SYM: Child dribbles, is feebleminded, possibly an idiot. Stiff, awkward movements, legs crossed and pressed together, arm adducted, forearm flexed, hand pronated, scissors gait.

PROG: Poor.

TREATMENT: Lumbar puncture or aspiration of hemorrhage, palliative surgery, orthopedic devices.

livedo (lĭv-ē′dō) [L. a dark spot]. Patchy or general dark discoloration of the skin. SYN: *lividity*.

liver (lĭv′er) [A.S. *lifer*]. Large gland in the body, 30x15x8 cm., 1500 to 1800 Gm. in wt., situated on right side beneath the diaphragm; right hypochondriac, epigastric, and part of left hypochondriac regions, level with bottom of sternum, undersurface, concave, covers stomach, duodenum, hepatic flexure of colon, right kidney and suprarenal capsule, secretes bile and aids metabolism.

The liver, the largest organ of the body, is completely covered by a tough fibrous sheath, Glisson's capsule, which is thickest at the transverse fissure. At this point, the capsule carries the blood vessels and hepatic duct which enter the organ at the hilus. Strands of connective tissue originating from the capsule enter the liver parenchyma and form the supporting network of the organ and separate the functional units of the liver, the hepatic lobules.

The many intrahepatic bile passages converge and anastomose, finally leading into the hepatic duct, the excretory channel of the liver. This structure receives the cystic duct on the end of which is situated the gallbladder. The union of the cystic and the hepatic ducts forms the common bile duct or the ductus choledochus, which enters the duodenum at the papilla of Vater. A ring of smooth muscle at the terminal portion of the choledochus, the sphincter of Oddi, permits the passage of bile into the duodenum by relaxing. Briefly stated, the bile leaving the liver enters the gallbladder where it undergoes concentration principally through loss of fluids by absorption by the gallbladder mucosa. When bile is needed in the small intestine for digestive purposes, the gallbladder contracts and the sphincter relaxes, thus permitting escape of the viscid gallbladder bile. Ordinarily, the sphincter of Oddi is contracted, shutting off the duodenal entrance and forcing the bile to enter the gallbladder after leaving the liver.

Within the sinusoids of the liver and attached to their walls are found the cells of Kupffer, which are highly phagocytic. Their function is obscure, although it is established that they are normally concerned with blood destruction.

Has 5 lobes, 5 ligaments, 5 fissures, 5 sets of vessels, secretes 600 to 1200 cc. of bile in 24 hours.

BLOOD SUPPLY: Hepatic artery and portal vein. The liver is sometimes classed as a ductless gland, though no internal secretion has ever been discovered. Great interest has centered about it since it was discovered that liver extract or whole liver by mouth is efficacious in the treatment of pernicious anemia. This property is not known to be due to any internal secretion.

FUNCTIONS: It is concerned with the products of digestion. It is primarily a gland which secretes bile. The bile stimulates other secretions, promotes peristalsis, and checks bacterial action. The bile contains both useful and excrementitious substances; to the former class belong the bile salts, needed in digestion of fats; to the latter belong the bile pigments, which impart the characteristic color to the feces.

In addition to being a gland, however, the liver is an important aggregate of tissues with other complicated functions. It stores fat and glycogen and it prevents poisons from reaching the blood stream and organs of the body.

It is the first organ to receive the blood draining from the mesenteric area and saturated with the products of digestion and decomposition from the intestines. From this blood it removes glucose to synthesize glycogen; it removes ammonia, amino acids, amines, and uric acid to form urea, and removes or detoxifies other substances which would otherwise get into the general blood stream.

It is able to modify fats (by desaturation) absorbed from the intestine. The sugar which has been synthesized to glycogen can either be oxidized for the sake of the heat so liberated, or released into the blood stream as glucose to keep the level of blood sugar constant.

The liver destroys effete red corpuscles, and the bile pigments excreted in the bile are the waste from this destruction. The liver synthesizes the fibrinogen which is necessary for the clotting of blood, and also produces an antithrombin which prevents the clotting within the blood vessels. It is largely responsible for the production of antibodies (SEE: *immunity*) and the linings of the hepatic blood vessels contain large phagocytic cells which can destroy bacteria found in the blood stream.

Indications are that the liver is a double organ, being separated by a di-

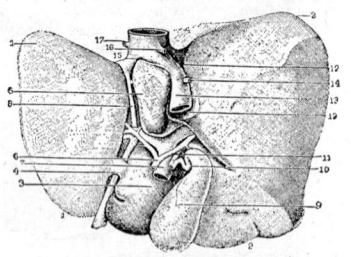

INFERIOR SURFACE OF LIVER
1. Left lobe. 2. Right lobe. 3. Quadrate lobe. 4. Round ligament. 5. Caudate lobe. 6. Hepatic artery. 7. Portal vein. 8. Fossa for ductus venosus. 9. Gallbladder. 10. Cystic duct. 11. Hepatic duct. 12. Fossa for vena cava. 13. **Vena cava**. 14. Right inferior phrenic vein. 15. **Hepatic vein**. 16. **Right renal vein**. 17. **Left renal vein**.

viding membrane, each half having its own circulatory system independent of the other half.

NERVE SUPPLY: Hepatic plexus.

DIFFERENTIAL DIAGNOSIS OF DISEASES OF THE LIVER: *Fecal accumulations* can often be diagnosed only after the trial of remedies, which, acting freely on the bowels, remove the accumulation and cause the disappearance of the supposed hepatic enlargement.

Disease of Stomach: Cancer is only disease likely to be confounded with enlargement of liver; usually can be distinguished from hepatic enlargement by the tympanitic quality of the percussion sound over the cancerous mass, and by mobility of the mass.

Displacements: Downward from extensive pleuritic effusion, and from pneumothorax are recognized by the presence of the signs of these thoracic diseases.

Enlargement of Right Kidney: Sometimes must be diagnosed from tumor of undersurface of right lobe of liver. As patient lies on back the enlargement instead of passing up under ribs dips down so as to allow finger to pass vertically between ribs and tumor. Furthermore, the position of an enlarged kidney is not altered by deep inspiration.

Enlargement of Spleen and Ovarian Tumors: Are distinguished from enlargement of the liver by shape of tumor, and by continuous and increasing flatness of percussion sound as we pass toward the normal position of these organs.

Percussion sound elicited over these tumors is never flat, but has a tympanitic quality, caused by the subjacent intestines. SEE: *ovary* for *differential diagnosis;* also *spleen*.

PALPATION OF THE LIVER:

l., cancer of. Irregular nodules of various sizes are distinctly felt through the abdominal wall projecting from that portion or the enlarged organ which is below the free border of the ribs. These prominences are usually harder than the surrounding hepatic tissue and there is more or less tenderness on pressure over them. May or may not be accompanied by ascites.

l., cirrhosis of. Little nodules will often be felt on undersurface of liver, by making firm pressure with ends of fingers under free border of ribs. Sometimes when there is great dropsical accumulation no information from palpation can be obtained until after performance of paracentesis.

l., congestion of. Space immediately below ribs is occupied by a smooth, hard, resisting enlargement, corresponding to the natural shape of liver. Usually not tender on pressure.

l., fatty. A soft, cushionlike enlargement is readily detected below margin of ribs on right side, and in epigastrium, extending not infrequently as low as the umbilicus, outer surface rounded and not well defined, is never tender on pressure.

l., hydatid tumors of. Sometimes the enlarged portion below the ribs has an elastic or even fluctuating feeling, and if a large cyst be near surface may give sense of fluctuation. Surface over these enlargements is smooth, organ not tender on pressure—growth slow.

l., waxy. Palpation shows that portion of organ below the ribs is dense, firm and resistant; outer surface smooth—lower margin sharp and well defined. Pain and tenderness rarely present. When excessive, almost always accompanied by ascites.

PERCUSSION OF THE LIVER: In healthy state right lobe of liver occupies right hypochondrium, lying completely in hollow formed by the diaphragm, rarely descending below free border of ribs, or extending upward above the 5th intercostal space; left lobe reaches across to left of median line an inch or more, upper boundary is determined by percussing with moderate force from right nipple downward, until flatness of the percussion sound indicates a solid organ has been reached. Indicate this point with aniline pencil. Percuss downward from axilla and from point a little to right of median line in front till a change occurs in percussion sound. Indicate these with pencil. A line drawn through these points marks upper border of liver, generally corresponds to base of ensiform cartilage in front, on median line, to the 5th intercostal space on line of right nipple, to 7th rib in axillary region, and 9th rib in dorsal region. Lower boundary determined by percussing downward from the line of flatness already found, and noting where the tympanitic sounds of the stomach and large intestine occur. Usually found to correspond anteriorly to free border of ribs and to a point 3 inches below ensiform cartilage on median line; laterally, in the axillary region, to the 10th intercostal space, and posteriorly in dorsal region to 12th rib. Flatness of left lobe usually reaches 2 inches to left of median line. Vertical measurements very nearly as follows: On right of median line in front 3 inches; on a line with right nipple 4 inches; in axillary region 4½ inches; in dorsal region 4 inches. Smooth edge of lower margin of liver in health in thin subjects esp. can be distinctly felt behind free border of ribs. The gallbladder is found where lower border of liver passes under ribs on right side just within nipple line. In examination of children it must be remembered that liver is proportionately larger than in adults.

l., atrophy of. Percussion shows rapid diminution in size which is never accompanied by ascites.

l., cancer of. Area of dullness always increased, sometimes extremely so. Organ found to occupy greater portion of epigastrium, extending beyond the median line into left hypochondrium, pushing diaphragm upward, and often descending below ribs to crest of ilium.

l., cirrhosis of. Normal area of hepatic dullness is diminished. Limits determined as follows: If abdominal cavity is distended with dropsical accumulations patient should be placed partly on left side so liquid will gravitate from hepatic region; percussion dullness then, instead of extending to free border of ribs, will often give place to tympanitic resonance an inch or more above their free border, and instead of extending across median line will rarely reach that line. Vertical measurement of hepatic dullness on a line with right nipple often does not exceed 2½ inches.

l., congestion of. A flat sound is elicited an inch or 2 below margin of ribs on right side. Obstruction of the bile ducts will produce an enlargement of liver similar to congestion by preventing outflow of bile; in addition to the slight uniform area of hepatic dullness a globular projection is sometimes found at a point corresponding to the transverse fissure, which has the elastic feel of deep-seated fluid; this tumor is the distended gallbladder.

l., fatty. Flatness over whole surface of abdomen corresponding to enlargement of liver.

Hepatitis, Acute: Physical sign similar to congestion, except that excessive tenderness exists on pressure over that portion of the organ which descends below the ribs.

l., hydatid tumors of. When small cannot be detected by physical examination, but when larger or superficially seated are recognized by abnormal increase in area of hepatic dullness, and by globular form of enlargement on surface of organ. Sometimes these cysts are so large as to cause organ to fill a large portion of abdominal and encroach on right pleural cavity. Sometimes percussion over a large hydatid cyst will give rise to a characteristic vibration, known as hydatid fremitus. This vibration is produced by the impulse of smaller cysts contained in a large one. Hydatid liver encroaching on the thoracic cavity gives rise to flatness on percussion, and absence of respiratory sound from base of chest upward as far as tumor extends; upper boundary of flatness is arched. Distinguished from pleuritic effusion in that change in position of body does not change line of percussion dullness. Enlargement not uniform.

l., waxy. Often becomes so large as to fill whole abdominal cavity; growth slow, often extending over 2 or 3 years. Enlargement uniform, area of hepatic dullness consequently increased on percussion, in every direction; more, however, in front than behind.

DISEASES OF:

l., abscess of. Temperature up in evening, low in morning; sweats and chills; liver enlarged, painful, tender, may be bulging and fluctuation. Pus may be detected by aspirating needle.
PROG: Embolic (multiple) abscesses generally fatal. Traumatic abscesses, or those due to an amebic dysentery may terminate favorably after spontaneous or induced evacuation.

l., acute yellow atrophy of. A rare and grave disease, characterized anatomically by a rapid destruction of the liver tissues, and manifested by jaundice and hemorrhages, a reduction in size of liver and of marked cerebral phenomena. SYM: (1) Malaria, slight fever, coated tongue, nausea, vomiting and jaundice. (2) Nervous symptoms follow, as severe headache, delirium, convulsions and coma; these sometimes precede the jaundice. (3) Urine is scanty, contains albumin, blood, tube casts and crystals of leucine and tyrosine. (4) Hemorrhages are common, the skin may be covered with ecchymoses and bleeding from the mucous membranes may occur. (5) Hepatic dullness diminished; splenic, increased. PROG: Generally fatal. TREATMENT: Constitutional and palliative.
TREATMENT: Constitutional. Hot applications. Single abscesses, invoke surgical aid.

l., amyloid. An enlargement of liver, due to the deposition of an albuminoid substance. SYM: Failure of general health with anemia. Liver is enlarged, smooth, firm and painless. Spleen and kidneys share in the degeneration so the spleen enlarged and urine albuminous. PROG: Unfavorable. TREATMENT: Remedies must be directed to the causal disease, usually prolonged suppuration, syphilis, tuberculosis or chronic malaria. Nutrition or tonics indicated.

l., cancer of. Male sex, heredity and traumatism predisposing factors. SYM: (1) Severe pain and tenderness; (2) cachexia, i. e., loss of flesh and strength with pallor; (3) pressure symptoms, jaundice common, but ascites rare; (4) liver enlarged, surface is nodular and the central depression or umbilications can often be detected; (5) symptoms of the primary growth which is usually in the stomach. Fever generally absent, but secondary perihepatitis or suppuration of cancerous nodules may reduce it. PROG: Fatal; duration from few months to year. TREATMENT: Palliative, constitutional in first stage.

l., cirrhosis of, atrophic. A chronic disease characterized anatomically by a hyperplasia of the connective tissue and destruction of the secreting cells shown chiefly by symptoms of portal obstruction. In advanced stage, liver small, firm, gray color and covered with numerous granulations ("hobnails"). SYM: Coated tongue, anorexia, fullness and distress after eating; vomiting of frothy mucus, flatulence, constipation and dark urine. As obstruction becomes greater, portal blood finds new channels, and the superficial abdominal veins enlarge, notably about the umbilicus, forming the so-called "caput medusae"; hemorrhoids result from the same cause. PROG: Unfavorable except in first stages.

l., c. of, hypertrophic. In which the connective tissue hyperplasia starts from the periphery of the capillary bile ducts instead of from ramifications of portal vein as in atrophic form. SYM: Jaundice marked, liver large, yellow and surface smooth or finely granular, spleen swollen. Disease may last 1 or 2 years, but abrupt termination may occur at any time in convulsions and coma. TREATMENT: Constitutional.

l., fatty. Infiltration of liver with fat. Occurs under 2 opposite conditions. One in which there is general obesity, and fat accumulates in the liver in common with the other parts; the other form in which there is general emaciation and a consequent impairment of the oxygenating power of the blood. TREATMENT: Constitutional for the cause.

l., hobnail. That of atrophic cirrhosis.

l., hydatid cysts of. Formed by embryos of the *Taenia echinococcus*, a small tapeworm inhabiting the intestines of the dog; eggs are accidentally ingested by man and embryos liberated in stomach, and migrate to any part, liver most commonly affected through portal vein. The fixed embryo soon develops into a cyst which is composed of an external laminated layer and an internal breeding layer. The cyst contains a clear, nonalbuminous fluid which has a S. G. of 1.005 to 1.007, and is rich in chlorides; larvae develop from the breeding layer, are provided with 4 suckers and a circle of hooklets.

SYM: Small cysts excite no symptoms, often slow development, irregular enlargement of the liver; if superficial an elastic or fluctuating mass can be felt on palpation. On percussion a peculiar vibratory sensation (hydatid thrill) may be imparted to the hand—aspiration yields a clear fluid, containing hooklets and chlorides. PROG: Guardedly favorable. TREATMENT: When large, aspirate. If fluid collects again open and drain.

l., hyperemia of. Liver enlarged and filled with blood.

l., h. of, active. Commonly due to dietetic indiscretions (biliousness), may result from overindulgence in alcohol—hot climates. SYM: Coated tongue, fetid breath, anorexia, pain and tenderness in epigastric and hypogastric regions, nausea, vomiting, sick headache and sometimes slight jaundice; liver may be enlarged.

l., h. of, passive. SYM: Same, though less marked. Liver often quite large and in extreme cases such as follow tricuspid regurgitation it may pulsate. PROG: In simple active congestion good. In passive depends on cause. TREATMENT: Dietetic; constitutional; hygienic. In passive congestion direct treatment to the cause. In obstinate cases, the concentrated salines may be employed as purgatives.

l., inflammation of. SYM: (1) Symptoms of gastroduodenal catarrh usually precede, *i. e.*, coated tongue, anorexia, fetid breath, epigastric distress, vomiting and perhaps diarrhea; (2) obstructive jaundice indicated by yellow skin and conjunctivae, light stools and dark urine; (3) in acute cases slight fever and swelling of the liver, which is tender to touch. PROG: Favorable; duration, few days to several weeks. TREATMENT: Rest, liquid diet, constitutional remedies. SYN: *hepatitis*.

l., nutmeg. That of amyloid and heart disease, and fatty infiltrations. It has a peculiar mottled appearance and dilatation of capillaries.

l. spots. Yellowish-brown spots on skin following some digestive disturbances.

liver, words pert. to: anhepatia; anhepatogenic; anticholagogue; arginase; azorubin S; bile; -acids; -calculi; -colic; -pigments; "bili-" words; capsule, Glisson's; cardiohepatic; chloasma; choleresis; cirrhosis; facies hepatica; flexure; "glyco-" words; "hepa-" words; jaundice; perihepatitis.

liv'er (as food). CALVES: Contains 1 to 16% glycogen, lecithin and phosphorus, fats and nuclein.

AV. SERVING: 115 Gm. Pro. 27.6, Fat 9.8. VITAMINS: A++ to +++, B++, C++, D+ to ++, G+++.

The liver stores more Vit. A and G than other parts of the animal; 10 times more of Vit. G, and 200 to 400 times more of Vit. A, depending upon the animal's food.

Liver may be assumed to contain about 15 mg. of iron for every 100 Gm. of protein, and 44.1 mg. of copper per kilo of fresh calf liver.

ACTION: Liver supplies some protective substance necessary for the stroma of red cells but not for the formation of hemoglobin. It does not affect gastric secretion.

IND: In anemias (½ lb. or more per day) and diseases of the bone marrow, neurasthenia, and phthisical persons. Recommended for adolescents and convalescents. Easily digested. One hundred and forty degrees Fahrenheit coagulates the albumin and destroys its useful ferments.

l., goose. Av. SERVING: 100 Gm. Pro. 16.66, Fat 15.9, Carbo. 3.7. SYN: *paté de foie gras*.

liv'er ex'tract. A standardized concentrate of the antianemic principles of fresh liver.

DOSAGE: According to the red cell count, from 200 to 500 Gm. of fresh liver equivalent, daily.

livid (lĭv'ĭd) [L. *lividus*, dark in color]. 1. Ashen, cyanotic. 2. Discolored.

lividity (lĭv-ĭd'ĭ-tĭ) [L. *lividus*, dark in color]. 1. Skin discoloration, as from a bruise or venous congestion. 2. State of being livid.

Livierato's reflex (lĭv-yär-ä'tō). Reduction of area of cardiac dullness resulting from manual friction of precordial and epigastric areas.

livor (lī'vor) [L. a dark spot]. 1. Lividity, *q.v.* 2. Cutaneous dark spot on dependent portion of a cadaver.

lixiviation (lĭks"ĭv-ĭ-ā'shŭn) [L. *lixivia*, lye]. Separation of soluble from insoluble substances by washing and filtration.

loa loa (lō'ă lō'ă). An infection of the conjunctiva or of the connective tissues of the body caused by a subgenus of *Filaria*.

lobar (lō'bar) [G. *lobos*, lobe]. Pert. to a lobe.

l. pneumonia. Inflammation of 1 or more lobes of the lungs. SEE: *pneumonia, lobar*.

lobate (lō'bāt) [L. *lobatus*, lobed]. 1. Pert. to a lobe. 2. Having a deeply undulated border. 3. Producing lobes.

lobe (lōb) [G. *lobos*]. A globular part of an organ separated by boundaries.

l., caudate. Elevation of hepatic tissue extending bet. spigelian l. and right l.

l., central. Island of Reil, which forms floor of lateral cerebral fossa.

l.'s of the cerebrum. Ant., middle and post. l.'s of brain.

l., crescentic. One of 2 lobes on upper surface of a cerebellar hemisphere.

l., cuneate. A convolution on int. surface of cerebral hemisphere.

l., digastric. A lobe of the lower surface of cerebellum.

l. of the ear. Lower portion of auricle having no cartilage.

l., floating. A projecting portion of right l. of liver which may extend below crest of the ilium.

l., frontal. That part of a cerebral hemisphere in front of central and sylvian fissures.

l., Home's. Pedunculated median lobe of prostate gland, frequently hypertrophied in old age.

l., insular. SEE: *central l.*

l.'s, lateral, of the prostate. The portions on each side of the urethra.

l.'s, lateral, of thyroid gland. The 2 main portions, 1 on each side of trachea, united below by thyroid isthmus.

l., limbic. Marginal section of cerebral hemisphere on medial aspect. SYN: *gyrus fornicatus*.

l., linguiform. Riedel's lobe.

l.'s of the lung. Small divisions containing terminal ramification of a bronchial tube and pulmonary vessels.

l.'s of the mamma. The glandular tissues of mammary gland divided by fibrous or areolar tissue.

l., marginal. First frontal convolution of the cerebrum.

lobe, median   L-39   **locus niger**

l., median. Sup. vermiform process of the cerebrum.
l. of the nose. A rounded eminence at extremity of dorsum of nose.
l., occipital. Caudal region of either hemicerebrum.
l., olfactory. A series of convolutions below horizontal portion of the intraparietal fissure of cerebrum, containing olfactory bulb.
l.'s, optic. Upper pair of corpora quadrigemina.
l.'s, orbital. The convolutions above the orbit.
l.'s of the pancreas. Roundish aggregations of glandular tissue separated by connective tissue.
l., parietal. Upper and lateral portion of hemisphere of cerebrum.
l.'s of the prostate. The lateral l.'s and the middle l. of the gland.
l., quadrate, of cerebellum. Large l. on upper surface of cerebellum.
l., quadrate, of liver. An oblong elevation on lower surface of liver.
l., Riedel's. Floating l., *q.v.*
l., rolandic. Operculum of the insula.
l., semilunar. Post. l. of upper surface of each hemisphere of the cerebellum.
l., spigelian. Irregular quadrangular portion of liver behind fissure for portal vein and bet. fissure for vena cava and ductus venosus.
lobectomy (lō-bĕk'tō-mǐ) [G. *lobos*, lobe, + *ektomē*, excision]. Surgical removal of a lobe of any organ or gland.
lobengulism (lō-ben'gu-lizm) [" + *ismos*, state of]. Condition marked by increase of subcutaneous fat and decrease or complete abeyance of the sexual function.
lobotomy (lŏb-ŏt'ŏ-mǐ). A bilateral small trephination in the plane of the coronal suture through which the white matter of the brain is sectioned, disconnecting the diencephalon, esp. the hypothalmic area from the prefrontal cortex by section of the white fiber connecting pathways subcortically in a plane that passes adjacent to ant. tip of lateral ventricle and post. margin of sphenoid wing for relief of mental disturbances.
lob'ster. Av. SERVING: 100 Gm. Pro. 17.2, Fat 1.9, Carbo. 0.4. VITAMINS: A— to +, B+, G+.
lob'ular [G. *lobulus*, small lobe]. Composed of small lobes.
lobulate, lobulated (lŏb'ū-lāt, -lāt-ed) [L. *lobulus*, small lobe]. 1. Consisting of lobes or lobules. 2. Pert. to lobes or lobules. 3. Resembling lobes. SYN: *lobular*. [small lobe.
lobule (lŏb'ūl) [L. *lobulus*, small lobe]. A
l., fusiform. Inf. temporoöccipital convolution.
l., paracentral. Sup. convolution of ascending frontal and parietal convolutions forming a union of both. [*lobule*.
lobulus (lŏb'ū-lŭs) [L.]. A lobule. SYN:
l. centralis vermis superior. A small lobe at ant. part of sup. vermiform process.
l. epididymidis. Segments into which the epididymis is divided by transverse septa from its tunica albuginea.
l., parietalis. One of 2 portions of the parietal lobe.
l. testiculi. Conical lobules, from 250 to 400, which make up glandular structure of the testicle.
lobulet, lobulette (lŏb-ū-lĕt') [Fr.]. A very small lobule or a part of one.
lobus (lŏb'ŭs) [L., from G. *lobos*]. Lobe.
l. cerebelli anteriores. The lobes forming ant. and sup. portion of hemisphere of the cerebellum.
l. pulmonales. Lobes of the lung.
l. reniculi. Lobes in fetal kidney, later forming malpighian pyramids.
local (lō'kăl) [L. *locus*, place]. Limited to one place or part.
localization (lō-kăl-ǐ-zā'shun) [L. *locus*, place]. 1. Limitation to a definite area. 2. Determination of the seat of an infection. 3. Relation of a sensation to its point of origin.
l., cerebral. Determination of centers of various faculties in particular parts of the brain. [ited region.
localized (lō'kăl-īzd). Restricted to a lim-
lochia (lō'kǐ-ă) [G. *lochia*, pert. to childbirth]. The discharge from the uterus of blood, mucus and tissue, during the puerperal period.
SYM: The first 6 days it is distinctly blood-tinged and is known as *lochia rubra* or *cruenta;* the following 3 or 4 days the discharge becomes brownish and is known as *lochia serosa;* after this it becomes yellowish, turning to white and is known as *lochia alba.*
It is diminished or suppressed in high fever. If offensive it is result of contamination with saprophytic organisms. Position should favor drainage.
lochial (lō'kǐ-al). Pert. to the lochia.
lochiocolpos (lō"kǐ-ō-kŏl'pŏs) [G. *lochia*, pert. to childbirth, + *kolpos*, vagina]. Retention of lochia in the vagina.
lochiometra (lō"kǐ-ō-mē'tră) [" + *mētra*, uterus]. Retention of lochia in the uterus.
lochiometritis (lō"kǐ-ō-mē-trī'tis) [" + " + *-itis*, inflammation]. Puerperal inflammation of the uterus.
lochiopyra (lō-kǐ-op'ǐr-ă) [" + *pyr*, fever]. Puerperal fever.
lochiorrhagia (lo-kǐ-or-ra'jǐ-ă) [" + *rēgnunai*, to break forth]. Excessive flow of lochia.
lochiorrhea (lō"kǐ-or-rē'ă) [" + *roia*, flow]. Abnormal flow of lochia.
lochioschesis (lō-kǐ-os'kē-sǐs) [" + *schesis*, retention]. Retention or suppression of the lochia.
lochometritis (lō"kŏ-mē-trī'tǐs) [G. *lochos*, childbirth, + *mētra*, uterus, + *-itis*, inflammation]. Puerperal inflammation of uterus. [SEE: *tetanus*, *trismus*.
lock'jaw. Tonic spasm of muscles of jaw.
locomotion (lō-kō-mō'shun) [L. *locus*, place, + *motus*, moving]. Movement of a body from one place to another.
locomotor (lō-kō-mō'tor) [" + *motor*, mover]. Pert. to locomotion.
l. ataxia. A sclerosis affecting the post. columns of the spinal cord. SYN: *tabes dorsalis*. SEE: *ataxia, Charcot's arthropathy*.
locular (lŏk'ū-lăr) [L. *loculus*, a small place]. Divided into small cavities.
loculated (lŏk'ū-lāt-ĕd) [L. *loculus*, a small place]. Containing or divided into loculi. SYN: *locular*.
loc'ulus (pl. *loculi*) [L.]. 1. A cell. 2. A small cavity.
lo'cum ten'ens [L. *locus*, place, + *tenere*, to hold]. A substitute. Physician who substitutes for another temporarily.
lo'cus [L. a place]. A spot or place.
l. caeruleus, l. cinereus, l. ferrugineus. A dark-colored depression in floor of 4th ventricle at its upper part.
l. luteus. The true olfactory area of the nose. It has yellow granules in its epithelium.
l. niger. Gray matter separating the

crusta and tegmentum of the crura cerebri. SYN: *substantia nigra*.
Loeffler's bacillus (lĕf'lĕr). The bacillus of diphtheria.
logaditis (lŏ-gă-dī'tĭs) [G. *logades*, conjunctivae, + *-itis*, inflammation]. Inflammation of the sclerotic coat of the eye. SYN: *scleritis*.
logagnosia (lŏg-ăg-nō'sĭ-ă) [G. *logos*, word, + *a-*, priv. + *gnōsis*, knowledge]. Word blindness. SYN: *aphasia*.
logagraphia (lŏg-ă-grăf'ĭ-ă) [" + " + *graphein*, to write]. Loss of ability to express ideas in writing. SYN: *agraphia*.
logamnesia (lŏg-ăm-nē'zĭ-ă) [" + *amnēsia*, forgetfulness]. Aphasia of a sensory character. Inability to recognize spoken or written words.
logomania (lŏg-ō-mā'nĭ-ă) [" + *mania*, madness]. Repetitious, continuous and excessive flow of speech seen in monomania.
logoneurosis (lŏg"ō-nū-rō'sĭs) [G. *logos*, word, + *neuron*, nerve, + *-ōsis*]. Any neurosis marked by speech disorders.
logopathia (lŏg-ō-păth'ĭ-ă) [" + *pathos*, disorder]. Any disorder of speech.
logopedia (lŏg-ō-pē'dĭ-ă) [" + *pais*, *paid-*, child]. Science dealing with speech defects, and their correction.
logoplegia (lŏg-ō-plē'jĭ-ă) [" + *plēgē*, stroke]. Paralysis of the speech organs.
logorrhea (lŏg-or-ē'ă) [" + *roia*, flow]. Unusual loquacity seen in insanity. SYN: *garrulousness*, *logomania*.
logospasm (lŏg'ō-spazm) [" + *spasmos*, spasm]. Spasmodic word enunciation.
-logy [G.]. Suffix meaning *discourse*, *science* or *study of*.
loimic (loi'mĭk) [G. *loimos*, plague]. Pert. to pestilence or plague.
loimology (loi-mŏl'ō-jĭ) [" + *logos*, science]. Science concerned with contagious diseases, esp. plague.
loin (loyn) [O.Fr. *loigne*, long part]. Lower part of back and sides bet. the ribs and pelvis.
long- [L.]. Prefix meaning *long*.
longevity (lŏn-jĕv'ĭ-tĭ) [L. *longaevus*, aged]. 1. Length of life. 2. Unusual length of life. Age was reckoned by the Romans in six stages: *pueritia*, childhood, to 5 years; *adolescentia*, youth, to 18 years; *juventus*, young man, to 25 years; *majores*, man, 25 to 50 years; *senectus*, old man, 50 to 60 years; *crepita aetas*, decrepit, 60 years to death.
long flame arc lamp. According to distance bet. electrodes, carbon arc lamps are either short or long flame.
longsightedness (lawng-sī'tĕd-nĕs) [L. *longus*, long, + A.S. *gesiht*, sight]. Farsightedness. SYN: *hyperopia*, q.v.
Lophotrichea (lŏ-fō-trĭk'ē-ă) [G. *lophos*, tuft, + *thrix*, *trich-*, hair]. Microorganisms possessing flagella in tufts.
lophotrichous (lŏ-fŏt'rĭk-ŭs) [" + *thrix*, *trich-*, hair]. Having bunches of flagella at one end.
lordoma (lŏr-dō'mă) [G. *lordōma*, a bending]. Forward incurvation of the spine. SYN: *lordosis*.
lordoscoliosis (lŏr"dō-skō-lĭ-ō'sĭs) [G. *lordoun*, to bend, + *skoliōsis*, curvation]. Lordosis and scoliosis combined.
lordosis (lor-dō'sĭs) [G. *lordoun*, to bend]. Abnormal ant. convexity of the spine.
lotion (lō'shun) [L. *lotiō*]. Liquid medicinal preparation for local bathing of a part.
loupe (lūp) [Fr.]. A magnifying lens.
louse (lows) [A.S. *lūs*]. Animal parasite infesting hairy parts. SYN: *pediculus*, *Phthirius*. SEE: *nit*.
   l., body. Pediculus corporis.

   l., crab. Phthirius inguinalis.
   l., head. Pediculus capitis.
lousiness [A.S. *lūs*]. State of being infested with lice.
Loven's reflex (lŏv'en). Vasodilation with corresponding increase in size of organ resulting from stimulation of afferent nerve of organ.
Low'man bal'ance board. Tilted board for walking with feet inverted to restore proper muscle balance and to correct static faults.
low protein diet. Breakfast, 413 calories; lunch, 695; supper, 704. Total daily, 1812. No salt except what is used in cooking, which will equal 3 or 4 Gm. per day.
   Breakfast: Fruit, cereal with cream and sugar or milk (2 oz.), toast, plenty of butter, jelly or jam, cocoa or milk (1 cup), and 1 egg.
   Lunch: Cream soup or 1 cup milk, 1 potato, 1 serving of vegetable, large serving salad with mayonnaise, 1 thin slice bread, liberal amt. butter, custard, gelatin, cake, ice cream or blanc mange, 1 serving. One egg may be substituted for cream soup or milk.
   Supper: One serving cereal or 1 large serving of potatoes, 3 oz. of cream or milk, sugar and butter as desired, large serving salad, fruit and vegetable, 1 cup cocoa, 1 egg or 1 glass milk.
   CONTRA: No meat, fish, chicken, meat gravies, soups or broth. Peas and dried beans only 2 or 3 times per week.
loxarthron (lŏks-ar'thron) [G. *loxos*, slanting, + *arthron*, joint]. Oblique deformity of a joint without dislocation.
loxia (loks'ĭ-ă) [G. *loxia*, slanting]. Wry neck. SYN: *torticollis*.
loxotic (lŏks-ot'ĭk) [G. *loxos*, slanting]. Distorted in an awry manner.
loxotomy (lŏks-ot'ō-mĭ) [" + *tomē*, a cutting]. Amputation by oblique section.
lozenge (lŏz'ĕnj) [Fr. diamond-shaped]. Small, dry, medicinal solid to be held in mouth until it dissolves. SYN: *troche*.
lubb (lŭb) [imitative origin]. Word denoting 1st cardiac sound in auscultation. It is pitched low and slightly longer than the 2nd sound. There is a longer pause after the 2nd sound. SEE: *dupp*; *heart*, *auscultation of*.
lubb-dupp (lŭb-dŭp) [imitative origin]. The 2 sounds heard in auscultation marking a complete cycle of the heart. Pause following the cycle is slightly longer than that bet. the 2 sounds.
lubricant (lū'brĭ-kănt) [L. *lubricans*, making smooth]. 1. Agent which makes smooth. 2. Making smooth.
lub'ricating en'ema. One given to soften feces and lubricate anal canal after hemorrhoidectomy, or to soften fecal impaction. SEE: *enema*.
Lucas-Championniere disease (lū-ka"-shawn-pē-ŏn-yair"). Pseudomembranous affection of the bronchi.
   L.-C. method. Early massage and mobilization in treating fractures.
lucid (lū'sĭd) [L. *lucidus*, clear]. Clear, esp. applied to clarity of the mind.
   l. interval. Period of normal mentality bet. psychiatric attacks.
lucidity (lū-sĭd'ĭ-tĭ) [L. *lucidus*, clear]. Quality of clearness or brightness, most especially with regard to mental conditions. SEE: *lucid*.
lucotherapy (lū-kō-ther'ă-pĭ) [L. *lux*, *luc-*, light, + G. *therapeia*, treatment]. Therapeutic use of light rays. SYN: *phototherapy*.
Ludwig's angi'na (lŭd'wĭg). A suppurative inflammation of subcutaneous con-

nective tissue adjacent to a maxillary gland. SEE: *angina.*

Luer's syringe. One made of glass for intravenous and hypodermic use.

lues (lū'ēz) [L. pestilence]. Any pestilential disease; the plague, esp. syphilis.
   l. **venerea.** Syphilis.

luetic (lū-et'ĭk) [L. *lues,* pestilence]. 1. Pert. to syphilis. 2. Affected with syphilis. SYN: *syphilitic.*

luetin (lū'et-ĭn) [L. *lues,* pestilence]. A killed culture of Treponema pallidum for the Noguchi skin test for syphilis.

Lugol's caustic (lū'gol). Aqueous solution of 25% each of iodine and potassium iodide.
   L.'s solution. Iodine, 5%; potassium iodide, 10%, and water to make 100 cc.
   DOSAGE: 3 ℳ (0.2 cc.).
   INCOMPATIBILITIES: Codeine.

lumbago (lŭm-bā'gō) [L. *lumbus,* loin]. Dull, aching pain across loins due to sudden cooling of overheated lumbar muscles, or turning body or rising from sitting posture causes an exacerbation which is sometimes so severe patient cries out.
   PROG: Favorable.
   TREATMENT: Affected muscles should be put at rest. A large piece of adhesive plaster may be applied from the floating ribs to the iliac crests—acupuncture occasionally gives brilliant results—also the continued current. Internal medication.

lumbar (lŭm'băr) [L. *lumbus,* loin]. Pert. to the loins. SEE: *lumbago.*
   l. **nerves.** Five pairs, corresponding with the lumbar vertebrae.
   l. **puncture.** One made into the subarachnoid space of the spinal cord bet. the 2nd and 5th lumbar vertebrae (or more approximately in the 4th lumbar interspace, the middle of the line connecting the iliac crests).
   PURPOSE: For the removal of spinal fluid for diagnostic or other purposes, and for the injection of an anesthetic solution.
   Fluid is often removed to reduce intracranial pressure. Medication (dissolved in fluid previously removed) or anesthetics for cord blocking, etc., may be cautiously introduced.
   The part is cleansed and painted with iodine. A sterile puncture needle is then readily passed directly in the midline, to and through the dura. On removing the stylet, spinal fluid will escape and can be collected in 2 or 3 tubes for examination.
   NP: Patient should be turned on side near edge of bed with back to operator. Thighs flexed on trunk. Nurse holds patient in this position. Articles needed: Sterilized lumbar puncture needles, gloves for physician, iodine, sterilized gauze and sponge, novocain, 0.5% solution, 5 cc. Two sterile test tubes, collodion, cotton. SEE: *cerebrospinal fluid, cisternal puncture, spinal puncture.*
   l. **reflex.** Irritation of the skin over the erector spinal muscles causing contraction of muscles of the back.
   l. **region.** Each side of umbilical region above the iliac, below the hypochondriac.
   l. **vertebrae.** Five bones of spinal column between sacrum and dorsal vertebrae.

lumbarization (lŭm-băr-ĭ-zā'shŭn) [L. *lumbus,* loin]. Coalescence of the 1st sacral vertebra with the last lumbar vertebra.

lumbo- [L.]. Combining form pert. to the *loins.*

lumbocolostomy (lŭm″bō-kō-los'tō-mĭ) [L. *lumbus,* loin, + G. *kolon,* colon, + *stoma,* opening]. Colostomy by lumbar incision.

lumbocolotomy (lŭm-bō-kō-lot'ō-mĭ) [" + " + *tome,* incision]. Incision into the colon through lumbar region.

lumbocostal (lŭm-bō-kos'tăl) [" + *costa,* rib]. Rel. to the loins and ribs.

lumbodynia (lŭm-bō-dĭn'ĭ-ă) [" + G. *odyne,* pain]. Pain and rigidity in the loins. SYN: *lumbago.*

lumbrical (lŭm'brĭ-kăl) [L. *lumbricus,* earthworm]. Like a worm. SYN: *vermiform.*

lumbrica'lis [L. *lumbricus,* earthworm]. One of the muscles of the hand or foot which are wormlike in form.

lumbricide (lŭm'brĭ-sĭd) [" + *caedere,* to kill]. Destructive to, or an agent which destroys lumbricoid worms.

lumbricoid (lŭm'brĭ-koid) [" + G. *eidos,* resemblance]. 1. Resembling an earthworm. 2. Worm parasitic in the intestines.

lumbricosis (lum-brĭ-kō'sĭs) [" + G. *-ōsis,* intensive]. Condition resulting from being infected with lumbricoids.

lumbri'cus [L.]. An earthworm parasitic in intestines.

lumen (lū'mĕn) (pl. *lumina*) [L. light]. 1. The space within an artery, vein, intestine or tube. 2. Unit of light, the amt. of light emitted in a unit solid angle by a uniform point source of 1 international candle.

luminal (lū'mĭ-năl) [L. *lumen, lumin-,* light]. Rel. to lumen of tubular structure, such as a blood vessel.

luminal (lu'min-al). A brand of phenobarbital.*
   DOSAGE: ½ gr. (0.03 Gm.).
   l. **sodium.** A brand of soluble phenobarbital.*

lunacy (lū'nă-sĭ) [L. *luna,* moon. Insanity was formerly thought to be affected by the moon]. Mental derangement. SYN: *insanity, psychosis.*

lu'nar [L. *luna,* moon]. Pert. to the moon, a month, or silver.
   l. **caustic.** Silver nitrate.

lunaria (lŭn-ar'ĭ-ă) [L. *luna,* moon]. Menstruation.

lunatic (lū'nă-tĭk) [L. *luna,* moon]. 1. An insane person. 2. Insane, mad.

lunet, lunette (lū-nĕt') [Fr. *lunette,* from L. *luna,* moon]. A concavo-convex lens for spectacles.

lung (lŭng) [A.S. *lungen*]. ANAT: One of 2 cone-shaped, spongy organs of respiration.
   Connected with the pharynx through the trachea. The base rests on diaphragm and apex rises to an inch above the collarbone, supported by its attachment to the hilum or root structures.
   Right lung has 3 lobes, left one 2. Weight, 1260 Gm., contains 76,000,000 air cells. Averages 18 respirations per minute in adult. Respiration surface, 870 sq. ft. Capacity, 20 cu. in. of air each respiration, 300 cu. ft. every 24 hours.
   The left lung has an indentation for the normal place of the heart, which is called the *cardiac depression.* Behind this is the *hilum* through which the blood vessels and bronchi enter and leave the lung. Lung tissue is composed of multiple tiny *alveoli* or air sacs, which open into *alveolar ducts,* which, in turn, join together to form into large ducts or *bronchioles.* The bronchioles

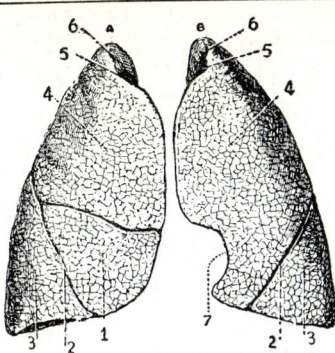

ANTERIOR ASPECT OF LUNGS
A. Right lung. B. Left lung. 1. Middle lobe. 2. Oblique fissure. 3. Lower lobe. 4. Upper lobe. 5. Groove for innominate vein. 6. Groove for subclavian artery. 7. Cardiac notch.

meet to form *bronchi*, which lead into one of the main bronchi and thus into the trachea. The membranous sheath investing the lungs is called the *pleura*.

NERVE SUPPLY: Ant. and post. pulmonary plexus.

BLOOD SUPPLY: Bronchial, pulmonary arteries, and pulmonary veins. Blood passing through lungs gives off carbon dioxide and receives oxygen. The lungs include the lobes, lobules, bronchi, bronchioles, infundibula, and alveoli or air cells. The capacity of the lungs is 230 cu. in.

l. abscess. Circumscribed, suppuration of lung. SYM: High and irregular fever, rigors, sweats and pallor. Dyspnea, cough and purulent expectoration. May be bubbling râles and later cavernous breathing and pectoriloquy.

PROG: Fair, except in embolic abscesses.

TREATMENT: Nutritious food. Remedies called for by general condition. Abscess should be opened and drained.

l., apoplexy of. An effusion of blood into the pulmonary tissues.

SYM: When infarction is large usual symptoms are dyspnea, cough and expectoration of dark blood containing few air bubbles.

TREATMENT: Condition itself not amenable to treatment. Remedies should be directed to the primary disease.

l., cirrhosis of. A chronic disease of the lung, characterized by an overgrowth of fibrous tissue.

SYM: Moderate dyspnea and chronic cough. Expectoration may be slight but is often profuse and fetid from having been retained in bronchiectatic cavities. No fever, and general health may be preserved for many years.

PROG: Incurable—duration from 10-20 years.

TREATMENT: Palliative; consists in good hygiene and use of remedies directed to the bronchiectasis. SYN: *interstitial pneumonia*.

l. collapse. Absence of air from portion of lung. May be congenital and result from deficient respiration.

SYM: When a large area is collapsed in some preëxisting disease, like capillary bronchitis, there is an abrupt increase in the dyspnea and cyanosis without a corresponding rise of temperature.

PROG: Depends upon extent of collapse and gravity of preëxisting disease.

TREATMENT: In congenital form apply alternately hot and cold sponges to spine; keep up external temperature. If these measures fail, gently inflate lung with a catheter. In acquired varieties, direct remedies to the original disease. SEE: *auscultation of lungs, chest; emphysema; tuberculosis*.

l. congestion, active. This results from increased afflux of blood to the lungs.

SYM: Flushed face; dyspnea; short, dry cough, followed by tenacious, blood-streaked expectoration; full, rapid pulse. Slight dullness, crepitant râles and bronchovesicular breathing.

TREATMENT: Rest, liquid diet, and internal remedies as indicated.

l. c., hypostatic. Congestion of dependent portions of the lungs occurring in asthenic diseases which necessitate a protracted recumbent position.

SYM: Dyspnea, cough, scanty expectoration. Slight dullness, subcrepitant râles, and feeble bronchial breathing.

TREATMENT: Development should be prevented by frequent change in position and timely use of cardiac stimulants. Internal remedies.

l. c., passive. Results from obstruction to the flow of blood from the lungs to the heart.

SYM: Dyspnea, hard cough, mucous expectoration containing pigmented cells and râles. Slight dullness, feeble breathing.

TREATMENT: Remedies for underlying cardiac disease as indicated.

l., edema of. Effusion of serous fluid into air vesicles and into interstitial tissue of lungs.

SYM: Extreme dyspnea; rapid, labored breathing; cough with frothy, blood-stained expectoration; cyanosis; cold extremities.

PROG: Grave. Often a final symptom of some pulmonary disease.

TREATMENT: When much cyanosis is present, hot fomentations should be applied to the chest. Hydragogue cathartics indicated. Cardiac stimulants may be given hypodermically.

l., gangrene of. A putrefactive necrosis of lung. Secondary condition to some inflammatory disease of the lung. It is excited by the entrance of bacteria of putrefaction—but unless system is considerably reduced in vitality the tissues, even though diseased, show wonderful resistance and escape putrefaction.

SYM: Are associated with original disease—cough, dyspnea, moderate fever and great prostration generally present. Expectoration is characteristic, is profuse, and has penetrating offensive odor. When allowed to stand in a glass vessel separates into 3 layers. A frothy layer on top, serous in middle, through which hang strings of pus, and at bottom layer of reddish green purulent material.

PROG: Grave.

TREATMENT: Nutritious food. Remedies, inhalations. Surgical interference if strength will permit.

l., hemorrhage from. Hemoptysis.*
l. inflammation. Pneumonia.*
l., iron. Device for inducing respiration artificially.

Patient is placed in airtight compartment except for his head and neck, and then atmospheric pressure inside is raised and lowered by a pulmotor. SEE: *Drinker respirator.*

lung, words pert. to: aeropleura, air vesicle, aluminosis, alveobronchitis, alveolar, alveolus, alveolus pulmoneus, anthracosis, anthrax, anthropotoxin, apicitis, artificial pneumothorax, asbestosis, atelectasis, atmiatrics, atmocausis, atrium, auscultation of, "bronch-" words, byssinosis, byssophthisis, calcicosis, cardiopulmonary, chest, emphysema, hilum, pectoriloquy, "pleur-" words, "pneum-" words, pulmonary, râles, siderosis, silicosis, tuberculosis, vesicular resonance, vomica.

lung motor. Apparatus designed to give artificial respiration. Inferior to prone pressure method.

lunula (lŭ'nu-lă) [L. little moon]. The semilunar white arch or area near the root of the nail.

    l. **lacrimalis.** Small ridge of bone separating antrum of Highmore from the lacrimal groove.

    l. **of valves of heart.** One of 2 narrow portions of flaps of the semilunar and mitral valves.

    l. **scapulae.** Notch behind coracoid process in upper border of the scapula through which passes the suprascapular nerve.

lupiform (lŭ'pĭ-form) [L. *lupus*, wolf, + *forma*, shape]. Resembling lupus.

lupoma (lū-pō'mă) [" + G. *-ōma*, swelling]. Nodule of lupus, esp. a primary one.

lupous (lŭ'pŭs) [L. *lupus*, wolf]. 1. Pert. to lupus. 2. Affected with lupus.

lupus (lŭ'pŭs) [L. wolf]. Tuberculous skin disease, acute or subacute.

    ETIOL: Unknown. Circulatory disorders and trauma predispose.

    SYM: Reddish-brown, soft patches, circumscribed (discoid) or disseminated with raised edges and depressed centers which are white and scarlike when scales drop off. In disseminated type there may be mucous membrane involvement. Sebaceous glands are dilated and often filled with sebum.

    Disease spreads slowly, shows no tendency to ulceration and rarely excites subjective symptoms. Middle life, female sex are predisposing factors.

    PROG: Favorable under prolonged treatment.

    TREATMENT: Hygienic regimen. Locally, soothing lotions, cautiously followed by stimulating agents. Surgical diathermy, curettage, carbon dioxide snow, x-rays, radium.

    l., **disseminated follicular.** L. of face with small and large papules.

    l. **erythematosus.** Superficial inflammation of skin with scaling patches.

    l. **hypertrophicus.** L. with vegetations.

    l. **maculo'sus.** L. with maculae.

    l. **nonex'edens**, L. without ulcerations.

    l. **serpigino'sus.** L. spreading with creeping ulcerations.

    l. **tu'midus.** L. with edematous infiltrations.

    l. **verrucosus.** Lesion consisting of an elevated plaque with indolent inflammatory base and a warty papillary surface.

    l. **vulgaris.** Patches on skin which break down and ulcerate, leaving scars on healing. Most common form of lupus.

Luschka's gland (loosh'kă). The coccygeal gland, a tiny organ near tip of coccyx.

L.'s tonsil. Pharyngeal tonsil bet. nasopharyngeal openings of eustachian tubes. SEE: *adenoids.*

Lust's reflex (lŭst). Dorsal flexion and abduction of foot resulting from percussion of ext. branch of sciatic nerve.

lu'teal [L. *luteus*, yellow]. Pert. to luteum.

    l. **hormone.** A secretion of the corpus luteum. RS: *estrin, gonads.*

lutein (lū'tē-ĭn) [L. *luteus*, yellow]. 1. Yellow pigment derived from corpus luteum, egg yolk, and fat cells or lipochromes. 2. Internal ovarian secretion.
DOSAGE: 2-10 gr. (0.12-0.6 Gm.).

luteinization (lū-tĭn-ĭ-zā'shun). Changes in follicle cells of the graafian follicles which have discharged their ovum, probably induced by the prolan B hormone of the hypophysis.

luteolipoid (lu"tĕ-ō-lĭp'oyd) [" + G. *lipos*, fat, + *eidos*, form]. Substance found in corpus luteum which seems to have hemostatic action during the menstrual period.

luteoma (lū-tē-ō'mă) [" + G. *-ōma*, tumor]. Tumor from the corpus luteum.

luteum (lu'tē-ŭm) [L.]. Yellow.

    l., **corpus.** Yellow cellular mass which forms in position of ruptured graafian follicles in ovary. It persists and enlarges on pregnancy.

lutin (lū'tĭn). Hormone of corpus luteum which aids in preparation of endometrium for fertilized ovum. SYN: *progestin.*

luxation (lŭks-ā'shŭn) [L. *luxāre*, to dislocate]. Displacement of organs or articular surfaces; dislocation of a joint.

lux'us [L. excess]. Excess of anything.

Luy's body. Small ganglion under the optic layer. SYN: *subthalamic nucleus.*

lycanthropy (lĭ-kan'thrō-pĭ) [G. *lykos*, wolf, + *anthrōpos*, man]. Mania in which patient believes himself a wild beast, esp. a wolf. SYN: *lycomania.*

lycomania (lĭ-kō-mā'nĭ-ă) [" + *mania*, madness]. Delusion of being a wild animal, esp. a wolf. SYN: *lycanthropy.*

lye (lī) [A.S. *leáh*]. Liquid from leaching of wood ashes. SEE: *alkalies, NaOH.*

    l. **burns.** Treat with hydrosulfosol,[a] which is safe for use around eyes, nose, and mouth. Spray with h. solution every hr. first 24 hr. [ing in confinement.

ly'ing-in. 1. The puerperal state. 2. Belymph (lĭmf) [L. *lympha*]. The lymph is a body alkaline fluid found in the lymphatic vessels and the cisterna chyli.

It may be transparent and colorless, or milky, or rather yellow, and it clots on standing. It differs from the blood in that it is more diluted and contains no red blood corpuscles. SP. GR.: 1.045.

    CONSTITUENTS: Extractives, fibrin, serum albumin, white blood corpuscles, water, salt. Thoracic duct lymph contains many fat globules and, in addition, cells called lymphocytes and supplied by the lymph glands. Liquid portion is called liquor lymphae.

The lymph is formed in tissue spaces all over the body and is gathered into small vessels which carry it centrally. The lymphatics of the mesentery in particular empty into a large trunk called the cisterna chyli[a] (SEE: *absorption* and *chyle*), carrying the fat which has been absorbed from the intestine. Continuing upwards, it is joined by other lymphatics, and their contents are finally emptied through the thoracic duct into left subclavian vein.

Most of the lymph must pass on its

lymph, animal

way to the blood vessels through the nodes. As the *chyme* washes against the intestinal walls, the digested food is absorbed into the blood and distributed through the mucous membrane. The villi* contain both blood vessels and lacteals, and absorption is carried on through both of them.

The absorption of fatty matter chiefly takes place through the *epithelial cells* of the intestines, and those of the villi. These cells carry it to the lacteals when the particles break up into fat and protein matter.

Absorption is most active in the alimentary canal, the digested material passing into the blood stream through the vessels of the portal circulation and into the lacteals.

l., animal. Vaccine l. from an animal.
l. cell or **corpuscle.** A lymph leukocyte. [lymph structures.
l. channels. Irregular open spaces in
l., inflammatory. Exudate due to inflammation.
l., intercellular. Tissue fluid.
l., intravascular. Chyle; that of the lymph vessels.
l., Koch's. Tuberculin.
l. nodes. Glands scattered along the path of the lymphatics, esp. in the neck, armpits, and at bend of the elbow and knee.

They produce and store white blood corpuscles and act as filters to keep harmful substances out of the system. They also stop cancer cells.

These are small, round or oval bodies not larger than a bean, and many much smaller, situated in the course of the lymphatic vessels, and they look like so many knots in a cord.

l. scrotum. Scrotal lymphatic dilatation.
l. sinuses. Same as l. channels.
l. spaces. Those esp. in connective tissue filled with lymph.

lymphadenectasis (lĭmf″ă-den-ĕkt′ă-sĭs) [L. *lympha*, lymph, + G. *adēn*, gland, + *ektasis*, dilatation]. Dilatation or distention of a lymphatic gland.

lymphade′nia [" + G. *adēn*, gland]. Hyperplasia affecting lymphatic tissue.

l. ossea. Bone marrow hyperplasia accompanied by Bence-Jones protein in urine.

SYM: Neuralgic pains, followed by painful swellings on ribs and skull, and possible occurrence of spontaneous fractures. SYN: *multiple myeloma*.

lymphadenitis (lĭmf″ad-en-i′tis) [" + " + -*itis*, inflammation]. Inflammation of a lymphatic gland.

ETIOL: Drainage of bacteria or toxic matter into lymph nodes.

SYM: Marked increase of tissue; possible suppuration. Swelling, pain, tenderness. Usually accompanies lymphangitis.*

TREATMENT: Hot, moist dressings; incision and drainage if abscesses occur. Similar to other severe infections.

l., tuberculous. ETIOL: Infection.
SYM: Possible loss of weight and strength; gradual onset and enlargement of lymph nodes; may become adherent, necrotic, and discharge pus through skin.

TREATMENT: Elimination of foci; exposure of area to sunlight; deep x-ray in some cases. Surgical removal.

NP: If tuberculosis is cause, same as in that condition. Otherwise, same as in lymphangitis, *q.v.*

lymphadenoma (lĭmf″ă-den-ō′mă) [" + "

lymphatic

+ -*ōma*, tumor]. Hyperplasia of the lymphatic glands. SYN: *lymphoma*.

lymphadenomatosis (lĭmf″ă-den-ō″mă-tō′-sis) [" + " + " + -*ōsis*, intensive]. Condition of general lymphatic engorgement. SYN: *lymphomatosis*.

lymphagogue (lĭmf′ă-gŏg) [L. *lympha*, lymph, + G. *agōgos*, leading]. An agent which stimulates the production or flow of lymph.

lymphangiectasis (lĭmf″ăn-jĭ-ek′tă-sĭs) [" + G. *aggeion*, vessel, + *ektasis*, dilatation]. Dilatation of lymphatic vessels. SYN: *lymphectasia*.

lymphangioendothelioma (lĭmf-ăn″jĭ-ō-en″-dō-thēl-ĭ-ō′mă) [" + " + *endon*, within, + *thēlē*, nipple, + -*ōma*, tumor]. Endothelioma originating from lymph vessels. SYN: *lymphendothelioma*.

lymphangiofibroma (lĭmf-an″jĭ-ō-fī-brō′-mă) [" + " + L. *fiber*, fiber, + G. -*ōma*, tumor]. Fibroma and lymphangioma combined.

lymphangioma (lĭmf″ăn-jĭ-ō′mă) [" + " + -*ōma*, tumor]. Tumor composed of lymphatic vessels.

lymphangiophlebitis (lĭmf-ăn″jĭ-ō-flē-bī′-tis) [" + " + *phleps*, vein, + -*itis*, inflammation]. Inflammation of lymphatic vessels and veins.

lymphangioplasty (lĭmf-an″jĭ-ō-plăs-tĭ) [L. *lympha*, lymph, + G. *aggeion*, vessel, + *plassein*, to form]. Formation of artificial lymphatics.

lymphangiosarcoma (lĭmf-an″jĭ-ō-săr-kō′-mă) [" + " + *sarx*, flesh, + -*ōma*, tumor]. Lymphangioma and sarcoma combined.

lymphangiotomy (lĭmf″an-jĭ-ot′ō-mĭ) [" + " + *tomē*, a cutting]. 1. Dissection of the lymphatics. 2. Anatomy of the lymphatics. SYN: *lymphotomy*.

lymphangitis (limf-an-ji′tis) [" + " + -*itis*, inflammation]. Inflammation of the lymphatics.

ETIOL: Streptococcus infection.

SYM: Onset chill and high fever, moderate swelling and pain. Deep general flush with raised border on affected area if infection is in deep layers of skin.

NP: Applications of heat in the form of baths or fomentations may be ordered. Adm. plenty of fluids. Keep bowels open. Light diet and rest are important. General care given in febrile and painful conditions.

lymphatic (lim-fat′ĭk) [L. *lymphaticus*, pert. to lymph]. Small, transparent vessel that carries lymph.

It conveys toward the heart; contains valves like the veins. The intestinal parts of the lymphatics which take up some of the products of digestion are called *lacteals*.

After the *chyle* enters the lacteals it is known as *lymph*. The lymphatics, or lacteals, carry the food material in the form of lymph, which has not hitherto been taken directly into the blood vessels of the alimentary canal, into the blood stream.

Fluids exuded from the blood vessels into the tissues are gathered up and carried back again to the blood by the lymphatics, so that they serve 2 purposes. They appear like small veins with thin walls, and they are provided with valves. They commence as lymph capillaries, microscopic in size, and empty into 2 trunks which open into the large veins near the heart.

Unlike the blood, the fluid contained in the lymphatics flows only in 1 direction from the small capillaries to the

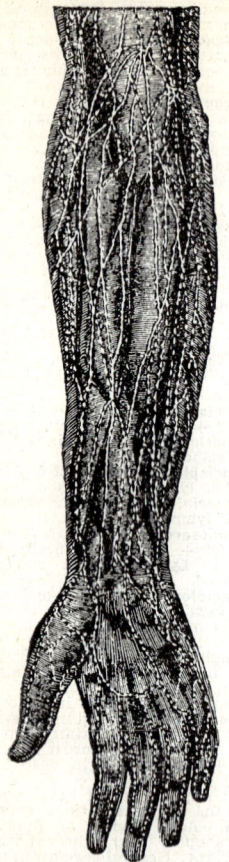

LYMPHATICS

main trunk (the thoracic duct and a smaller duct on the right side) and then to the large veins. When the lymph enters the blood it becomes part of its constituents.

PRINCIPAL GROUPS OF LYMPHATICS: (a) Right internal jugular vein; (b) right subclavian vein; (c) lymphatics of upper extremities; (d) receptaculum chyli; (e) lymphatics of lower extremities; (f) thoracic duct; (g) right subclavian vein; (h) lacteals; (i) lymphatics of lower extremities.

RS: *angioleukasia, angioleukitis, angiolymphitis, angiolymphoma, angiosis, bubo, chylangioma, leukosis, varix,* "*vas-*" *words.*

lymphaticostomy (lĭmf″ăt-ĭ-kos′tō-mĭ) [" + G. *stoma,* opening]. Making of a permanent aperture into a lymphatic duct.

lymphatism (lĭmf′ă-tĭzm) [L. *lympha,* lymph, + G. *ismos,* state of]. 1. The lymphatic temperament. 2. Sluggishness in the vital processes. 3. Excess in lymphoid structures. SYN: *status lymphaticus, q.v.*

lymphatitis (lĭmf-ă-tī′tĭs) [" + G. *-itis,* inflammation]. Inflammation of lymphatic vessel. SYN: *lymphangitis.*

lymphatolysis (lĭmf-ă-tol′ĭ-sĭs) [" + G. *lysis,* dissolution]. Destruction of tissue of lymphatics.

lymphatolytic (lĭm-fat-ō-lĭt′ĭk) [" + G. *lysis,* dissolution]. Destructive to lymphatics.

lymphectasia (lĭmf-ĕk-tā′zĭ-ă) [" + G. *ektasis,* dilatation]. Dilatation of the lymphatics. SYN: *lymphangiectasis.*

lymphedema (lĭmf-ĕ-dē′mă) [" + G. *oidēma,* swelling]. Edema due to obstruction of lymphatics. SYN: *serous edema.*

lympheduct (lĭm′fe-dŭkt) [L. *lympha,* lymph, + *ductus,* a passage]. Duct or vessel for carrying lymph.

lymphemia (lĭmf-ē′mĭ-ă) [" + *aima,* blood]. Hypertrophy of lymphatics with lymphocytes in blood.

lymphendothelioma (lĭmf-ĕn″dō-thēl-ĭ-ō′mă) [" + G. *endon,* within, + *thēlē,* nipple, + *-ōma,* tumor]. Tumor from proliferation and dilatation of lymphatics with overgrowth of myxomatous tissue.

lymphenteritis (lĭmf″ĕn-tĕr-i′tĭs) [" + G. *enteron,* intestine, + *-itis,* inflammation]. Serous infiltration accompanying inflammation of bowels.

lympherythrocyte (lĭmf-ĕr-ĭth′rō-sīt) [L. *lympha,* lymph, + G. *erythros,* red, + *kytos,* cell]. Erythrocyte lacking in hemoglobin.

lymphization (lĭmf-ĭ-zā′shŭn) [L. *lympha,* lymph]. Formation of lymph.

lymphnoditis (lĭmf-nōd-ī′tĭs) [" + *nodus,* knot, + G. *-itis,* inflammation]. Inflamed condition of a lymph node.

lymphoadenoma (lĭmf″ō-ad-en-ō′mă) [" + G. *aden,* gland, + *-ōma,* tumor]. 1. A tumor of lymphoid tissue. 2. Hypertrophied condition of the lymphatics. SYN: *lymphadenoma.*

lymphoblast (lĭmf′ō-blast) [" + G. *blastos,* germ]. A leukocyte of lymphatic origin.

lymphoblastoma (lĭmf-ō-blast-ō′mă) [" + *-ōma,* tumor]. Tumor composed of lymphocytes. SYN: *lymphosarcoma.*

lymphoblasto′sis [" + " + *-ōsis,* intensive]. Excessive number of lymphoblasts in the blood.

lymphocele (lĭmf′ō-sēl) [" + G. *kēlē,* hernia]. Tumor containing lymph. SYN: *lymphocyst.*

lymphocerastism (lĭmf-ō-ser′ăs-tĭzm) [" + G. *kerastos,* mingled, + *ismos,* state of]. Formation of lymph cells.

lymphocyst (lĭmf′ō-sĭst) [" + G. *kystis,* cyst]. Tumor containing lymph. SYN: *lymphocele.*

lymphocyte (lĭmf′ō-sīt) [" + G. *kytos,* cell]. Lymph cell or white blood corpuscle without cytoplasmic granules. They normally number from 25-30% compared with white cells. May increase to 90% in lymphatic leukemia.

l., large. Frequently difficult to classify; characterized by irregular shape, easily indented by any other cell. Protoplasm is larger in amt. than its nucleus which is usually oval and in middle of cell. It stains a faint, even blue. The protoplasm stains palely blue, is very clear, and does not stain for a small area around the nucleus. There may be a few small vacuoles, or eosinophilic granules. SYN: *lymphoblast, macrolymphocyte.*

l., small. Characterized by deeply staining, compact nucleus taking a dark blue. The nucleus occupies all or most

lymphocythemia L-46 **lysis**

of the cell, either in center or at one side. The protoplasm is clear blue. No granules but sometimes a few small vacuoles are seen varying from size of a red cell to twice its size. Form from 15-25% of the white cells of normal blood. Are small lymphocytes. SYN: *microlymphocyte.*
SEE: *blood corpuscles, blood count, lymph.*

lymphocythemia (lĭmf″o-sī-the′mĭ-ă) [" + " + *aima*, blood]. Excess of lymph cells in the blood.

lymphocytopenia (lĭmf″ō-sīt″ō-pē′nĭ-ă) [" + " + *penia*, lack]. Less than normal number of lymphocytes in the blood.

lymphocytopoiesis (lĭmf″ō-sīt″ō-poi-ē′sĭs) [" + " + *poiesis*, production]. Lymphocyte production.

lymphocyto'sis [" + " + *-ōsis*, intensive]. Excess of lymph cells. SYN: *lymphocythemia.*

lymphocytotoxin (lĭmf″o-sīt″ō-toks′ĭn) [" + " + *toxikon*, poison]. A toxin destructive to lymphocytes.

lymphodermia (lĭmf-ō-dĕr′mĭ-ă) [L. *lympha*, lymph, + G. *derma*, skin]. Disease of cutaneous lymphatics.

lymphoduct (lĭmf′ō-dŭkt) [" + *ductus*, duct]. A lymphatic vessel or duct. SYN: *lympheduct.*

lymphogenous (lĭmf-oj′en-ŭs) [" + G. *gennan*, to produce]. Forming lymph.

lymphoglandula (lĭmf″ō-glăn-dū′lă) [" + *glandula*, gland]. A lymph node.

lymphogonia (lĭmf″ō-go′nĭ-ă) [" + G. *gonos*, offspring]. Large lymphocytes with large nuclei appearing in lymphatic leukemia.

lymphogranuloma (lĭmf″ō-grăn-ū-lō′mă) [" + *granulum*, a little granule.. Venereal disease marked by inflammation of lymph glands with enlargement and ulceration. SYN: *l. inguinale.*
l. inguinale, l. venerea. Venereal granuloma of the pudenda with ulcerations. ETIOL: Supposedly Donovan body.

lymphogranulomatosis (lĭmf″ō-grăn-ū-lō″-mă-tō′sĭs) [" + " + *-ōma*, tumor, + *-ōsis*]. 1. Infectious granuloma of the lymphatics. 2. Hodgkin's disease.

lymphoid (lĭmf′oid) [" + G. *eidos*, form]. Resembling lymph. SYN: *adenoid.*

lymphoidectomy (lĭmf-oid-ek′tō-mĭ) [L. *lympha*, lymph, + G. *eidos*, form, + *ektomē*, excision]. Surgical removal of lymphoid tissue.

lymphoidocyte (limf-oid′ō-sīt) [" + " + *kytos*, cell]. Embryonic blood cell bet. a lymphocyte and a lymphoblast.

lymphokinesis (lĭmf″ō-kĭnē′sĭs) [" + G. *kinēsis*, motion]. Endolymphic movement in the semicircular canals.

lympholeukocyte (lĭmf″ō-lū′kō-sīt) [" + G. *leukos*, white, + *kytos*, cell]. One of the type of white corpuscles containing no granules and being mononuclear. It is the larger of the 2 types classed as lymphocytes, being about 3 times the size of a red corpuscle. Approximately 1% of the white corpuscles are lympholeukocytes. SYN: *lymphocyte.*

lymphology (lĭmf-ol′ō-jĭ) [" + G. *logos*, study]. Science of the lymphatics.

lymphoma (lĭmf-o′mă) [" + G. *-ōma*, tumor]. A lymphoid tissue tumor.
l. granulomatosum. Small, white lymphatic nodule in liver in Hodgkin's disease.

lymphomatosis (lĭmf″ō-mă-tō′sĭs) [" + " + *-ōsis*, intensive]. General lymphatic engorgement; general deposition of lymphomata throughout the body.
l. granulomato'sa. Malignant granuloma. SYN: *Hodgkin's disease.*

lymphomatous (lĭmf-ō′mă-tŭs) [" + G. *-ōma*, tumor]. 1. Pert. to a lymphoma 2. Affected with lymphomata.

lymphopath'ia vene'rea [" + *pathos*, disease]. Venereal disease marked by ulceration and enlargement of lymph nodes in inguinal area. SYN: *lymphogranuloma inguinale.*

lymphopathy (lĭmf-op′ă-thĭ) [" + G. *pathos*, disease]. Any lymphatic disease.

lymphopenia (lĭmf-ō-pē′nĭ-ă) [" + G. *penia*, a lack]. Deficiency of lymphocytes in the blood.

lymphoplasm (lĭmf′ō-plăzm) [" + G. *plasma*, a thing formed]. The elastic protoplasmic supporting threads or fibrillar network of cells.

lymphoplasmia (lĭmf-ō-plaz′mĭ-ă) [" + G. *plasma*, a thing formed]. Lack of hemoglobin in red blood corpuscles.

lymphopoiesis (lĭmf-ō-poi-ē′sĭs) [" + G. *poiēsis*, production]. Formation of lymphocytes.

lymphopoietic (lĭmf-ō-poi-et′ĭk) [" + G. *poiein*, to produce]. Forming lymphocytes.

lymphorrhagia (lĭmf-or-rā′jĭ-ă) [L. *lympha*, lymph, + G. *rēgnunai*, to burst forth]. Flow of lymph from ruptured lymph vessels. SYN: *lymphorrhea.*

lymphorrhea (lĭmf-or-rē′ă) [" + G. *roia*, flow]. Internal or external discharge of lymph through a wound. SYN: *lymphorrhagia.*

lymphosarcoma (lĭmf-ō-sar-kō′mă) [" + G. *sarx*, flesh, + *-ōma*, tumor]. Sarcoma of lymph tissue; lymphatic sarcoma.

lymphostasis (lĭmf-os′tă-sĭs) [" + G. *stasis*, a stoppage]. Stoppage of flow of lymph.

lymphotome (lĭmf′o-tōm) [" + G. *tomē*, incision]. Instrument for removing glandular growths from tonsils.

lymphotomy (lĭmf-ot′ō-mĭ) [" + G. *tomē*, incision]. 1. Excision of adenoid growths. 2. Anatomy of lymphatics. SYN: *lymphoidectomy, adenoidectomy.*

lymphotrophy (lĭmf-ot′rō-fĭ) [" + G. *trophē*, nourishment]. Lymph nourishment of cells in regions devoid of blood vessels.

lymphuria (lĭmf-ū′rĭ-ă) [" + G. *ouron*, urine]. Lymph in the urine.

lymphvascular (lĭmf-vas′kū-lar) [" + *vasculus*, a little vessel]. Rel. to the lymphatic vessels.

lyemania (lī-pē-mā′nĭ-ă) [G. *lypē*, sadness, + *mania*, madness]. Dementia with extreme mental depression. SYN: *melancholia.*

lypothymia (lī-pō-thī′mĭ-ă) [" + *thymos*, mind]. Great mental depression or despondency.

lyra (lī′ră) [G. *lyra*, lyre]. Triangular space on ventral surface of corpus callosum bet. post. columns of the fornix.

lysemia (lī-sē′mĭ-ă) [G. *lysis*, solution, + *aima*, blood]. Disintegration of blood.

lysimeter (lī-sĭm′ĕ-ter) [" + *metron*, measure]. Apparatus for determining solubilities.

lysin (lī′sĭn) [G. *lysis*, dissolution]. A specific antibody acting destructively upon cells and tissues.
SEE: *immune body.*

lysine (lī′sēn) [G. *lysis*, dissolution]. An amino acid which is a hydrolytic cleavage product of protein through digestion.
It is essential for growth and repair.

lysis (lī′sĭs) [G. dissolution]. 1. The

lysogenesis gradual decline of a fever or disease. The opp. of *crisis*.* 2. Destruction of blood cells, etc., by a lysin, as when rabbit's red corpuscles are dissolved by dog's serum. SEE: *crisis, hemolysis*.

lysogenesis (lī-sō-jen'ĕ-sĭs) [G. *lysis*, dissolution, + *genesis*, production]. The production of cell-dissolving substance known as lysin.

lysogenic (lī-sō-jen'ĭk) [" + G. *gennan*, to produce]. Producing lysins.

lysol (lī'sŏl). A mixture of cresols made soluble in water by sodium hydroxide. Used as an antiseptic.

POISONING: When swallowed it causes corrosion, edema of the lungs, immobility of pupils, and collapse. Vomiting may occur, death sometimes after symptoms have abated.

TREATMENT: *Prompt use of stomach-pump.*

lysozyme (lī'sō-zīm) [" + *zymē*, leaven]. A bacteria-destructive substance present in tears, and other body secretions, and tissues.

lyssa (lĭs'să) [G. *lyssa*, frenzy]. An acute infectious disease, transferable by inoculation, which particularly attacks the nervous system. SYN: *hydrophobia, rabies*.

lyssin (lĭs'sĭn) [G. *lyssa*, frenzy]. Virus of lyssa. SYN: *hydrophobin*.

lyssodexis (lĭs-sō-deks'ĭs) [" + *dĕxis*, a bite]. Inoculation or infection with lyssin.

lyssoid (lĭs'soid) [" + *eidos*, resemblance]. Resembling lyssa or rabies.

lyssophobia (lĭs-sō-fō'bĭ-ă) [" + *phobos*, fear]. 1. Hysteria resembling rabies. 2. Fear of rabies.

lyterian (lī-tēr'ĭ-an) [G. *lyein*, to dissolve]. Indicative of lysis.

lytic (lĭt'ĭk) [G. *lyein*, to dissolve]. Rel. to lysis or a lysin.

lyze (līz) [G. *lysis*, from *lyein*, to dissolve]. To bring about lysis.

Addendum

lung-heart disease (kôr pŭlmŏnălĕ, *q.v.*). A serious respiratory and heart condition caused by pollution of air by soot, gasoline vapor, sulfur dioxide, or by unburned droplets of such air. It can cause fatal heart failure. It interferes with flow of blood, especially through the right heart which fails. There are more cases than coronary artery disease and hypertension combined. 4000 deaths resulted in England within a five-week period.

M

M. Abbr. for *mille*, a thousand; *misce*, mix.

m. Abbr. for *meter* and *minim;* in chemistry, for *meta-*.

M. A. Abbr. for *meter angle*.

ma. Abbr. for *milliampère*.

M + Am. Abbr. for *compound myopic astigmatism*.

macaro´ni [It.]. Av. SERVING: 75 Gm. Pro. 10.1, Fat 0.7, Carbo. 55.6. ASH: Ca 0.022, Mg 0.037, K 0.130, Na 0.008, P 0.144, Cl 0.073, S 0.172, Fe 0.00012.

Macdowel's frenum (măk-dow´ĕl). Part of post. layer of pectoralis major which extends into muscular substance.

mace (mās) [L. *macis*]. A spice from the nutmeg tree, employed as flavoring similarly to nutmeg.

maceration (măs-ĕr-a´shŭn) [L. *macerāre*, to make soft]. 1. Process of softening a solid by steeping in a fluid. [L. *macer*, lean]. 2. State of emaciation.

Mache unit (mä´kĕ). The unit of measurement of concentration of radium emanation. Abbr. *M. u.*, or German, *M. E.* SEE: *unit*.

machonnement (mash-shŏn-mon´) [Fr.]. Movement of jaws resembling chewing.

macies (mā´shĭ-ēz) [L. wasting]. Atrophy, wasting, emaciation.

MacKenzie exercise apparatus. Mechanical device, devised by Tait MacKenzie for exercise.

macrencephalia, macrencephaly (mak-ren-sē-fa´lĭ-ă, -sef´a-lĭ) [G. *makros*, long, + *egkephalos*, brain]. Abnormal size of brain. SYN: *macrocephalia*.

macro-, macr- [G.]. Combining forms meaning *large, long*.

macrobiosis (măk˝rō-bĭ-ō´sĭs) [G. *makros*, large, + *biōsis*, life]. State of surpassing normal span; longevity.

macroblast (mak´rō-blast) [G. *makros*, large, + *blastos*, germ]. A large, nucleated red blood cell. SYN: *megaloblast*.

macrocephalia (măk-rō-sĕ-fa´lĭ-ă) [" + *kephalē*, brain]. Abnormal largeness of head. SYN: *macrencephalia*.

macrocephalous (măk-ro-sef´ă-lŭs) [" + *kephalē*, brain]. Pert. to or having an excessively large head.
ETIOL: Found in acromegaly, hydrocephalus, rickets, osteitis deformans, leontiasis ossea, myxedema, sporadic cretinism, idiocy, leprosy and hemiatrophy; also in pituitary disturbances.

macrocephaly (măk-rō-sĕf´al-ĭ) [" + *kephalē*, brain]. Abnormal size of head. SYN: *macrocephalia*.

macrocheilia (mak-rō-kī´lĭ-ă) [G. *makros*, large, + *cheilos*, lip]. Abnormal size of lip caused by permanently dilated lymphatic spaces, as in cavernous lymphangioma of the lip. SYN: *macrolabia*.

macrocheiria (mak-rō-kī´rĭ-ă) [" + *cheir*, hand]. Excessive size of the hands. SYN: *macrochiria*.

macrochilia (mak-rō-kī´lĭ-ă) [" + *cheilos*, lip]. Excessive size of the lip, caused by permanently dilated lymphatic spaces. SYN: *macrocheilia*.

macrochiria (mak-rō-kī´rĭ-ă) [" + *cheir*, hand]. Large size of hands.

macrococcus (măk-rō-kok´ŭs) [" + *kokkos*, berry]. A bacterial microörganism, of the largest type recognized. SYN: *megacoccus*.

macrocornea (măk-rō-kor´nē-ă) [" + L. *cornu*, horn]. Abnormal size or projection of the cornea. SYN: *keratoglobus, megalocornea*.

macrocytase (mak-rō-sī´tās) [" + *kytos*, cell, + *ase*, enzyme]. Enzyme in leukocytes capable of digesting organic substance.

mac´rocyte [G. *makros*, large, + *kytos*, cell]. 1. Erythrocyte larger than normal. 2. Large lymphocyte found in pernicious anemia.

macrocythemia (măk˝rō-sī-thē´mĭ-ă) [" + " + *aima*, blood]. Abnormal number of macrocytes in the blood.

macrocytosis (măk˝rō-sī-tō´sĭs) [" + " + *-ōsis*, intensive]. Development of macrocytes, esp. in greater numbers than normal.

macrodactylia (mak˝rō-dak-til´ĭ-ă) [" + *daktylos*, finger]. Excessive size of 1 or more of the digits.

macrodont (mak´rō-dont) [" + *odous, odont-*, tooth]. Having abnormally large teeth. SYN: *megadont*.

macroesthesia (măk˝rō-ĕs-thē´zĭ-ă) [G. *makros*, large, + *aisthēsis*, sensation]. A state in which objects seen or felt appear to be greatly magnified.

macrogenitosomia (mak˝rō-jen˝ĭ-tō-sō´-mĭ-ă) [" + L. *genitālis*, genital, + G. *sōma*, body]. Precocious body development in general, with unusually large genitalia.

macroglia (mak-rog´lĭ-ă) [" + *glia*, glue]. A neuroglia with large multipolar cells. SEE: *glia cell, spider cell*.

macroglos´sia [" + *glōssa*, tongue]. Hypertrophied condition of the tongue.
ETIOL: Usually congenital. May be due to inflammation of the lymphatics, glossitis. Ludwig's angina, acromegaly, myxedema, gumma, carcinoma, trauma, hoof and mouth disease.

macrognathia (mak-rō-nā´thĭ-ă) [" + *gnathos*, jaw]. Abnormal size of jaw.

macrolabia (măk-rō-lā´bĭ-ă) [" + L. *labium*, lip]. Abnormal size of lip. SYN: *macrocheilia*.

macrolymphocyte (mak˝rō-limf´ō-sīt) [" + L. *lympha*, lymph, + G. *kytos*, cell]. A huge lymphocyte.

macromastia (măk-rō-mas´tĭ-ă) [" + *mastos*, breast]. Abnormal size of the breasts.

macromazia (măk-rō-mā´zĭ-ă) [" + *mazos*, breast]. Abnormal development of breasts. SYN: *macromastia*.

macromere (măk´rō-mēr) [" + *meros*, a part]. Blastomere of large size.

mac´ronor´mobiast [" + L. *norma*, rule, + G. *blastos*, germ]. Large, nucleated red blood corpuscle.

mac˝ronor´mocyte [" + " + G. *kytos*, cell]. Huge red blood corpuscle.

mac´ronu´cleus (pl. *macronucleī*) [" + L. *nucleus*, kernel]. Main nucleus of a cell.

macrophage, macrophagus (măk˝rō-fāj, -rof´a-gus) [G. *makros*, large, + *phagein*, to eat]. A large mononuclear leukocyte which ingests other cells.

macrophallus (măk˝rō-făl´ŭs) [" + *phallos*, penis]. Abnormally large penis.

M-1

macropodia (măk-rō-pō'dĭ-ă) [" + *pous,* *pod-,* foot]. Abnormally large feet.
macroprosopia (măk"rō-prō-sō'pĭ-ă) [" + *prosōpon,* face]. Large facial features.
macropsia (mak-rop'sĭ-ă) [" + *opsis,* vision]. Condition in which objects look larger than they really are.
macrorhinia (mak-rō-rĭn'ĭ-ă) [" + *rīs, rin-,* nose]. Excessive size of the nose, either congenital or pathological.
macroscelia (mak-rō-sēl'ĭ-ă) [" + *skelos,* leg]. Abnormal size of the legs.
macroscopic (mak-rō-skop'ĭk) [" + *skopein,* to examine]. Large enough to be seen by the naked eye. OPP: *microscopic.* SYN: *megascopic.*
macroscopy (mak-ros'ko-pĭ) [" + *skopein,* to examine]. Examination of an object with the naked eye.
macrosomatia (mak"rō-sō-mă'shĭ-ă) [" + *sōma,* body]. Abnormally large size of body. SYN: *macrosomia.*
macrosomia (măk-rō-sō'mĭ-ă) [" + *sōma,* body]. Abnormal size of body. SYN: *macrosomatia.*
macrostomia (măk-rō-stō'mĭ-ă) [" + *stoma,* mouth]. Excessively large mouth.
macrotia (mak-ro'shĭ-ă) [G. *makros,* large, + *ous, ot-,* ear]. Abnormal size of ears.
macula (mak'u-lă) (pl. *maculae*) [L. spot]. A blemish, spot, or stain on the skin. SYN: *macule.* SEE: *roseola, vibices.*
  m. acustica. Acoustic nerve termination in both sacculus and utriculus, about 3 mm. in length.
  m. albida. White mark found on liver in some contagious diseases. SYN: *tache blanche.*
  m. atrophica. Glistening white spot on skin following a circumscribed hemorrhage.
  m. caerulea. Steel gray or blue stain of epidermis, without elevation, which does not disappear on pressure, occurring esp. with pediculosis pubis or bites from fleas.
  m., cerebral. Reddened line, becoming deeper and persisting for some time, esp. in tubercular meningitis, by drawing the fingernail across the skin.
  m. corneae. Opaque spot in cornea.
  m., germinal. A nucleolus in an ovular nucleus.
  m. gonorrhoeica. Red spot at orifice of vulvovaginal gland. Seen in gonorrheal vulvitis.
  m. lutea. The yellow spot on the retina, about 1/12 in. (2.08 mm.) to outer side of the optic nerve's exit, the exact center of the retina. Area of acute or central vision. SEE: *choroiditis, areolar and central.*
  m. solaris. A freckle.
macular (măk'ū-lar) [L. *macula,* spot]. 1. Rel. to macules. 2. Having macules.
maculate(d (măk'ū-lāt, -lāt-ĕd) [L. *macula,* spot]. Spotted, as with macules.
maculation (măk-ū-lā'shun) [L. *macula,* spot]. Process of becoming maculate. Development of macules.
macule (mak'ūl) [L. *macula,* spot]. Discolored spot or patch on the skin, neither elevated nor depressed, of various colors, sizes and shapes.
  They consist of *hyperemia, roseola, erythema, telangiectasis, nevi vasculosi, areola, achromia, chloasma, purpura, petechiae, ecchymosis, vibices, albinism, vitiligo, lentigines, nevi pigmentosi, nevi spili, discolorations, q.v.*
  Macules occur in pellagra, pityriasis rosea, pediculosis corporis, rubella, scurvy, serum sickness, peliosis, anemia,
leukemia, cancer, Bright's disease, infectious diseases, poisoning, erysipelas, acne rosacea, nevus pigmentosus, vitiligo, leprosy, morphea, facial hemiatrophy, etc. SYN: *macula, q.v.*
mad. 1. Not rational. 2. Suffering from infection with rabies. SYN: *insane, rabid.*
madarosis (mad-ă-ro'sis) [G. *madaros,* bald]. Loss of cilia or eyelashes and eyebrows.
madescent (mad-es'ent) [L. *madescere,* to become moist]. Slightly moist, or becoming so.
madidans (mad'ĭd-ăns) [L. *madidus,* wet]. Exuding, moist, as in some skin lesions.
ma'dor [L. *madere,* to be wet]. A dripping sweat. [foot. SYN: *mycetoma.*
Madu'ra foot. Fungous disease of the
Magendie's foramen (mă-zhan-de'). The median of 3 openings in the roof of the 4th ventricle which is in front of the cerebellum and behind the *pons varolii,* connecting the ventricle with the subarachnoid space.
  M.'s law. The post. spinal roots are *sensory;* the anterior ones *motor.*
  M.'s solution. Aqueous solution of morphine sulfate, 16 gr. to 1 oz. of water.
  M.'s spaces. Those bet. the arachnoid and pia at level of fissures of brain.
mag'got [origin uncertain]. Larva of an insect.
  m. treatment. A method of treating septic wounds. Meat maggots, introduced into a sloughing septic wound, ingest the necrotic material, leaving the wound with a clean granulating surface. The maggots are then removed and destroyed. SEE: *osteomyelitis.*
magistery (maj'ĭs-tĕr-ĭ) [L. *magister,* master]. 1. Specially compounded remedy. 2. A precipitate.
magistral (măj'ĭs-trăl) [L. *magister,* master]. Concerning medicines prescribed by a physician for a particular case. SEE: *officinal.*
magma (mag'mă) [G. *magma,* from *massein,* to knead]. 1. Mass left after extraction of principle. 2. Salve.
magnesia (măg-nē'zĭ-ă) [G. *magnēs,* a magnet]. Magnesium oxide.
  m., milk of. An aperient composed of magnesium hydroxide and water.
magne'sium [L.]. SYMB: *Mg.* At. wt. 24.32. Sp. gr. 1.74. A white mineral element found in soft tissue, muscles, bones, and to some extent in the body fluids. The entire body contains 0.05% Mg, 70% of which is contained in the bones. The muscles contain less of it than they do calcium. From 0.046 Gm. to 0.52 Gm. have been excreted on the 1st and 31st day of a fast.
  FUNCTIONS: Salts of magnesium and potassium, and other minerals are necessary to maintain osmotic pressure. Magnesium is needed for the ion balance, the activation of enzymes, for muscular activity, nerve stability, and bone structure. It also has a laxative effect.
  DEFICIENCY SYM: Convulsions, nervous conditions, retarded growth, digestive disturbances, spasticity of muscles and nerves, accelerated heart beat, arrhythmia, and vasodilation.
  SOURCES: It is obtained in sufficient quantities in meat, milk, fruits and vegetables to make special dietary planning to include it unnecessary. From 0.14 to 0.67 Gm. have been found in the food for a single day. Indeed, Mg,

magnesium carbonate   M-3   **malaria**

added to a mixed diet, may cause a loss of calcium. Most foods contain almost as much of it as they do of calcium.
   m. car′bonate ($MgCO_3.3H_2O$). USP. A bulky, white, odorless powder.
   ACTION AND USES: Internally, to neutralize acid in stomach, also a laxative.
   DOSAGE: As antacid, 10 gr. (0.6 Gm.); as a laxative, 2 drams (8 Gm.).
   m. citrate solution. USP. A solution containing an amount of magnesium citrate corresponding to approximately 1.6% magnesium oxide.
   ACTION AND USES: Purgative.
   DOSAGE: 12 fl. oz. (350 cc.).
   m. oxide (MgO). USP. Calcined magnesia. *Light* magnesia. A white, very bulky, fine powder.
   ACTION AND USES: Antacid, laxative.
   DOSAGE: As an antacid, 4 gr. (0.25 Gm.); as a laxative, 45 gr. (3 Gm.).
   Heavy. USP. magnesii oxidum ponderosum.
   ACTION AND USES: Same as magnesium, light.
   DOSAGE: Same as magnesium, light.
   m. phosphate tribasic. A white, odorless powder.
   USES: As an antacid and laxative.
   DOSAGE: 15-75 gr. (1.0-5.0 Gm.).
   m. sul′fate (epsom salt) ($Mg-SO_4.7H_2O$). USP. Small, colorless crystals. Saline bitter taste.
   ACTION AND USES: Refrigerant, hydragogue, cathartic, in tetanus and eclamptic conditions.
   DOSAGE: As cathartic, ½ oz. (15 Gm.).
   INCOMPATIBILITIES: Ammonium chloride, soapsuds enema, quinine, ferric chloride, sulfanilamide.

mag′net [G. *magnēs*]. Iron made magnetic by an electric current.
   m., horseshoe. One in shape of a horseshoe.
   m. operation. Removal of metal particles with a magnet.

magnet′ic [G. *magnēs*]. Pert. to a magnet or having magnetism.
   m. field. The space permeated by the magnetic lines of force surrounding a permanent magnet or coil of wire carrying electric current.
   m. induction. The production of magnetic properties in iron or other magnetic metals by the influence of a magnetic field or of a magnet.
   m. lines of force. The lines indicating the direction of the magnetic force in the space surrounding a magnet or constituting a magnetic field.

magnetism (măg′nĕ-tĭzm) [" + *-ismos*, condition]. The property of repulsion and attraction of certain substances.

magnetotherapy (mag″nĕt-ō-ther′ă-pĭ) [" + *therapeia*, treatment]. Application of magnets or magnetism in treating diseases.

magnification (mag-nĭ-fĭ-kā′shun) [L. *magnus*, great, + *facere*, to make]. Process of increasing apparent size of an object, esp. under microscope.

mag′num [L. large]. Largest of the carpal bones.

maidenhead (mād′en-hĕd). Thin, crescentic fold partly closing vaginal opening and once considered a sign of virginity. SYN: *hymen*.

maidism, maidismus (mā′ĭ-dĭzm, -dĭz′mŭs) [L. *mais*, maize]. 1. Another name for pellagra. 2. Poisoning from imperfect maize.

maieusiomania (mī-ū-sī-ō-mā′nĭ-ă) [G. *maieusis*, childbirth, + *mania*, madness]. Insanity following childbirth.

maieusiophobia (mī-ū-sī-ō-fō′bĭ-ă) [" + *phobos*, fear]. Extreme fear of childbirth.

maieutics (mī-u′tĭks) [G. *maieusis*, childbirth]. Obstetrics.

maim (mām) [M.E. *maymen*, to cripple]. 1. To injure seriously; to disable. 2. An injury or hurt.

main or main line (mān) [A.S. *maegen*, power]. P. T. The conductor that delivers the current as it comes in from the street supply or from a motor generator, if one is used.

main (măn) [Fr.]. Hand.
   m. en griffe (ahn-grēf′). Flexion and atrophy of the hand in a claw shape.
   m. succulente (sŭk-kū-lahnt′). Edema of a hand.

Majocchi's disease (mah-yok′ē). Ringform, purplish eruption of lower limbs; *purpura annularis telangiectodes, q.v.*

makro- [G.]. For words beginning thus, see under *macro-*.

mal (mahl) [Fr. from L. *malum*, an evil]. An evil, a sickness or a disorder.
   m. de mer. Seasickness.
   m., grand. A major epileptic attack with convulsions.
   m., petit. A minor attack of epilepsy without convulsions.

mala (ma′lă) [L.]. 1. The cheek. 2. The cheekbone.

malachite green (mal′ă-kīt) [G. *malachē*, a mallow (with green leaves)]. Dye sometimes used in treating trypanosomiasis and as an indicator.

malacia (măl-ā′sĭ-ă) [G. *malakia*, softening]. 1. Softening of tissues of an organ, or of a part of them. 2. A morbid appetite for some specific food, esp. condiments.

malacoma (măl-ă-kō′mă) [G. *malakia*, softening]. Softening of an organ or part of the body. SYN: *malacia, malacosis.*

malacoplakia (mal-ă-kō-plā′kĭ-ă) [" + *plax, plak-*, plaque]. Existence of soft patches in mucous membrane of a hollow organ.
   m., vesical. Soft, funguslike patches on mucosa of the bladder.

malacosarcosis (măl-ă-kō-sar-kō′sĭs) [" + *sarx*, flesh, + *-ōsis*]. Softness of tissue, especially muscular.

malacosis (măl-ă-kō′sĭs) [" + *-ōsis*, intensive]. Softening of an organ or part of the body, abnormally. SYN: *malacia, malacoma.*

malacosteon (mal-ă-kos′tē-ŏn) [G. *malakia*, softening, + *osteon*, bone]. Softening of the bones. SYN: *osteomalacia.*

malacotic (mal-ă-kot′ik) [G. *malakia*, softening]. 1. Soft. 2. Affected with malacia. 3. Rel. to malacia.
   m. teeth. Those of soft texture easily affected by caries.

malacotomy (măl-ă-kot′ō-mĭ) [" + *tomē*, incision]. Incision of soft areas of the body, esp. of the abdominal wall.

malady (mal′ă-dĭ) [Fr. *maladie*, illness, from L. *malum*, an evil]. A condition of ill health. SYN: *disease.*

malaise (mă-lāz′) [Fr.]. Discomfort, uneasiness, indisposition, often indicative of infection.

malar (mā′lar) [L. *mala*, cheek]. Pert. to cheekbones.
   m. bone. A 4-pointed bone on each side of the face, uniting the frontal and sup. maxillary bones with the zygomatic process of the temporal. SYN: *cheekbone.* SEE: *skeleton.*

malaria (ma-lā′rĭ-ă) [It. *malaria*, bad air]. A disease due to circulation and multiplication in the blood of certain parasites (*Plasmodium*).

ETIOL: Result of bites of Anopheles mosquito infested with the etiologic plasmodia. Certain factors tend to perpetuate or facilitate some portion of the cycle necessary in infestation of man. Tropical, subtropical and temperate climates are infested approximately in order named.

SYM: Various derangements of the digestive and nervous systems. Characterized by periodicity, chills, fever and sweats, in the order mentioned, having pathologic manifestations of progressive anemia, splenic enlargement, and deposition in various organs of a melanin, resulting from the biologic activity of the plasmodia.

TREATMENT: Prophylactics. Patients living in malarial districts should avoid the night and early morning air—should sleep in upstairs room. Absolute rest. Light diet. Quinine has long been a popular remedy. Atabrine and plasmochin also used.

RS: *cardiopaludism, hematuria, nonan.*

m., algid. Vomiting and diarrhea, marked prostration, Hippocratic facies, shallow and irregular respiration. Thready, rapid and intermittent pulse. PROG: Death supervenes often in spite of treatment.

m., bilious. Abdominal pain, nausea, vomiting of bile-stained or blood-flecked mucus, feeling of thoracic oppression. PROG: Adequate treatment is usually successful.

m., cephalgic. Unusually severe headache, nausea, vomiting, etc. DIFFERENTIAL DIAG: Meningitis and intracranial lesions.

m., choleriform. Resembles Asiatic cholera. Seizures occur with nausea, vomiting, severe abdominal pain, diarrhea, dehydration. PROG: Treatment is commonly successful.

m., latent. Parasites exist within blood stream, but give rise to no recognizable symptoms. Individuals having this form constitute portion of carriers.

m., masked. Symptoms atypical. Cerebral derangement may be main complaint.

m., pernicious. Onset may be sudden, resembling apoplexy; coma usually comes, however, after obvious, severe, and intense symptoms. Hot skin; petechiae; contracted pupils; Cheyne-Stokes respiration; coated tongue; loss of sphincter control; rapid, irregular, weak pulse; elevated temperature. A remission may occur with profuse perspiration, but other paroxysms follow if treatment is inadequate. ETIOL: *Plasmodium vivax.* PROG: In spite of heroic administrations, death sometimes occurs. Often general collapse, with death in cases where no treatment is instituted.

m., pleuritic and pulmonic. Fever, thoracic pain, cough, dyspnea, sometimes hemoptysis, rales. Periodicity of symptoms may aid diagnosis. Blood findings are conclusive.

m., quartan. Short and less severe paroxysms. Sporulation occurs each 72 hours, causing seizures with that interval.

m., quotidian estivoautumnal. Paroxysms occur with daily periodicity due to 24-hour sporulation. Abrupt rise and fall of temperature.

m., sudoriferous. Sweating is excessive and leads to collapse.

m., syncopal. Characterized by collapse on slightest exertion.

m., tertian. Sporulation each 48 hours. Symptoms more common during the day. Paroxysms divided into chill, fever and sweating stages. Cold stage is usually 10-15 minutes, but may last an hour or more. Febrile stage varies from 4-6 hours.

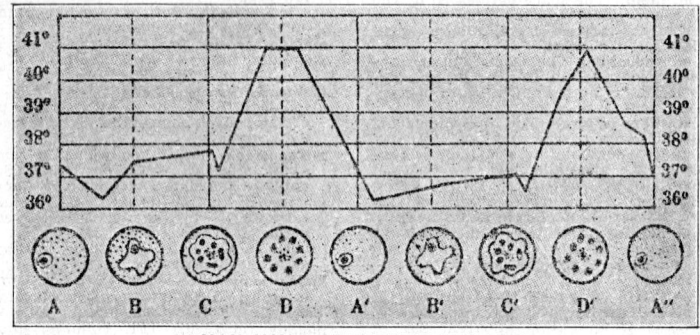

HUMAN CYCLE OF TERTIAN MALARIA.

In the circles A, B, C, D, and A', B', C', and D', which represent red blood corpuscles, malarial parasites are shown growing from the little spore in A and A' to the adult in C and C' and sporulating in D and D'. Above is a temperature curve, the figures on the left indicating the temperature of the patient (given in the Centigrade scale) the vertical lines indicating days. The temperature is highest— i. e., there is a paroxysm—each time the parasite reaches the stage of sporulation, D and D'.

m., delirious. Delusions, hallucinations, maniacal excitement.

m., eclamptic. Chill, fever, severe headache; sometimes nausea and vomiting. Convulsions resembling eclampsia. More common in children.

m., t. estivoautumnal. Indistinct chill, usually only a chilly sensation. Intense headache. profound weakness, marked muscular aching. Marked mental depression. Coated tongue, feeble and accelerated pulse, rapid respira-

malarial M-5 **Malta fever**

tion. Febrile stages may be 36 hours long.

malarial (mă-lar'ĭ-ăl) [It. *malaria*, bad air]. 1. Affected with malaria. 2. Causing malaria. 3. Resembling malaria. 4. Pert. to malaria. SYN: *malarious*.

malarialize (ma-lar'ĭ-al-īz) [It. *malaria*, bad air]. To treat paresis and parasyphilitic conditions by injecting malaria organisms into the body.

malarious (ma-lar'ĭ-ŭs) [It. *malaria*, bad air]. Of the nature of, or afflicted with malaria.

malariology (mă-lar-ĭ-ol'ō-jĭ) [" + G. *logos*, study]. The scientific study of malaria.

malariotherapy (mă-lar-ĭ-ō-ther'ă-pĭ) [" + G. *therapeia*, treatment]. Method of treating paresis and parasyphilitic conditions by injecting malarial organisms into the body.

Malasse'zia. A genus of fungi.
 M. fur'fur. The cause of tinea versicolor.
 M. trop'ica. Cause of tinea flava.

malassimilation (mal"ăs-sĭm-ĭ-lā'shŭn) [L. *malus*, ill, + *assimilāre*, to make like]. Defective, incomplete, or faulty assimilation, esp. of nutritive material.

malaxation (mal-aks-a'shun) [L. *malaxāre*, to soften]. Kneading movement used in massage.

male (māl). 1. Masculine. 2. One of the sex that fertilizes; one potentially capable of producing sperm.
 RS: *female, organs, male generative, virile, virilescence, virilism*.
 m. sex hormone. Hormone found in urine and secreted by the testicles, which regulates development at puberty of male characteristics. SYN: *androsterone.**

malemission (mal-ē-mĭs'shŭn) [L. *malus*, weak, + *ē*, out, + *mittere*, to send]. Failure of semen to be ejaculated from the urethra during coitus.

malformation (măl-for-mā'shŭn) [L. *malus*, bad, + *formatiō*, a shaping]. Deformity; abnormal shape or structure.

malic (mă'lĭk) [L. *malum*, apple]. Pert. to apples.
 m. acid. An acid found in some fruits, such as apples. SEE: *acid*.

malign (mă-līn') [L. *malignus*, of bad kind]. Malignant.

malignancy (mă-lĭg'năn-sĭ) [L. *malignus*, of bad kind]. 1. Opposition to treatment. 2. Severe form of occurrence, tending to grow worse. SYN: *virulence*.

malignant (mă-lĭg'nănt) [L. *malignus*, of bad kind]. Virulent. Growing worse; resisting treatment, said of cancerous growths.

malinger (mă-lĭng'er) [Fr. *malingre*, weak, sickly]. To feign illness, usually to arouse sympathy.

malingerer (mă-lĭng'ger-er) [Fr. *malingré*, sickly, weak]. 1. One who pretends to be ill or to be suffering from a nonexistent disorder to arouse sympathy. 2. One who pretends slow recuperation from a disease once suffered in order to continue to receive benefits of sick insurance.

malis (ma'lĭs) [G. *malis*, distemper]. A cutaneous, parasitic disease.

malleation (măl-lē-ā'shŭn) [L. *malleāre*, to hammer]. Spasmodic action of the hands in which they seem drawn to strike any near object, as spasmodic rapping against thighs, furniture, etc. SEE: *tic*.

malleoincudal (măl"lē-ō-ĭn'kū-dăl) [L. *malleus*, hammer, + *incus*, anvil]. Concerning or pert. to the malleus and incus.

malleolar (măl-lē'ō-lar) [L. *malleolus*, little hammer]. Concerning the malleolus.

malleolus (mă-lē'ō-lus) (pl. *malleolī*) [L. little hammer]. The protuberance on both sides of the ankle joint, the lower extremity of the fibula being known as the *lateral m.*, and the lower end of the tibia as the *medial malleolus*.
 m., ext., lateral, outer. Process on outer edge of fibula at lower end.
 m., int., inner, medial. Round process on inner edge of tibia at lower end.

malleotomy (măl-lē-ot'ō-mĭ) [L. *malleus*, hammer, + G. *tomē*, incision]. 1. Division of the malleus. 2. Division of ligaments to permit separation of the malleoli.

mallet finger (mal'let) [L. *malleus*, hammer]. Loss of power of extension in a finger, causing permanent flexion. SYN: *drop-finger*.
 m. toe. Abnormal flexion or loss of power of extension of a toe. SYN: *hammer toe*.

malleus (mal'ē-ŭs) (pl. *mallei*) [L. hammer]. 1. The largest of the 3 auditory ossicles in the middle ear, attached to the eardrum, and articulating with the incus. 2. Glanders, an acute febrile disease with suppuration and necrosis of cartilage and bone.
 RS: *ear, incus, stapes*.

malnutrition (mal-nū-trĭ'shun) [L. *malus*, bad, + *nutrīre*, to nourish]. Lack of necessary food substances in the body or improper absorption and distribution of them.

maloplasty (mal'ō-plas-tĭ) [L. *mala*, cheek, + G. *plassein*, to form]. Plastic surgery of the cheek.

malpighian (măl-pĭg'ĭ-ăn). Concerning or described by Marcello Malpighi.
 m. bodies. 1. Small, round bodies which commence in the cortex near the uriniferous tubules, forming the m. corpuscle of the kidney and a glomerulus packed into Bowman's capsule. 2. Small glandular patches throughout the spleen.
 SEE: *rete.* [resembling a pouch.
 m. capsule. Envelop. of a m. body
 m. cones. Conical protuberances in the renal medulla, containing the tubules and secreting mechanism.
 m. corpuscle. The capsula glomeruli and capillaries in the kidneys. The water of the urine is secreted therein. SYN: *corpusculum renis*.
 m. glomer'ulus. The blood vessels and coil of capillaries surrounded by the m. corpuscle.
 m. layer. Germinative, mucous and granular layers of the epidermis.
 m. tuft. Capillary inner portion of a m. body.

malposition (măl-pō-zĭ'shŭn) [L. *malus*, bad, + *positus*, from *ponere*, to place]. Faulty or abnormal position or placement, esp. of the body or one of its parts.

malpractice (măl-prak'tĭs) [" + G. *praxis*, an action]. Wrong or injurious treatment, esp. applied to performing illegal abortions.

malpresentation (mal-prē-zen-tā'shun) [" + *praesentatiō*, a presenting]. Abnormal position of fetus rendering natural delivery difficult or impossible.

malt (mawlt) [A.S. *mealt*]. Germinated grain, usually barley, used in fermentation of ale and beer.

Malta fever. An infectious disease caused by *Brucella melitensis*.

Sym: Swelling of the joints and spleen, excessive perspiration, weakness and anemia, and recurrent febrile attacks. **Syn**: *Bruce's septicemia, undulant fever*.

maltase (mawlt'ās) [A.S. *mealt*, grain]. A salivary and pancreatic enzyme which acts on sugar.

It hydrolyzes maltose and dextrin, converting them into dextrose. **See**: *enzyme*.

maltose (mawl'tōs) [A.S. *mealt*, grain]. Malt sugar ($C_{12}H_{22}O_{11}$). A disaccharide converted from starch by hydrolysis, through the action of the intestinal enzyme, *maltase*.

It is found in malt, its products, and in sprouting seeds. **See**: *disaccharose*.

malum (ma'lŭm) [L. an evil]. A disease.

m. perforans pedis. Ulcer of the foot of perforating type. It begins with thickening of the epidermis.

malunion (măl-ūn'yŭn) [L. *malus*, bad, + *unio*, oneness]. Growth of the fragments of a fractured bone in a faulty position, forming an imperfect union.

mamelonation (mam-el-ō-nā'shun) [Fr. *mamelle*, from L. *mamma*, breast]. Nipplelike prominences on a part or organ.

mamma (măm'ă) (pl. *mammae*) [L. breast]. One of 2 glands and structures in the female secreting milk; situated between the 3rd and 6th ribs when not pendulous. **Syn**: *breast*. **See**: *anisomastia, areolitis*.

mammalgia (mam-al'jĭ-ă) [" + G. *algos*, pain]. Pain in the breast. **Syn**: *mastalgia*.

mammary (mam'ă-rĭ) [L. *mamma*, breast]. Pert. to the breast.

m. glands. Two compound glands of the female breast secreting milk. They are made up of lobes and lobules bound together by areolar tissue.

The main ducts are 15 to 20 in number and are known as *lactiferous* ducts, each one discharging through a separate orifice upon the surface of the nipple. The dilatations of the ducts form reservoirs for the milk during lactation.* The pink, or dark colored, skin around the nipple is called the *areola*.* **Syn**: *mammae*.

RS: *breast; b., caked; galactagogue; gynecomastia; mammectomy; mastectomy; mastopathy; nipple*.

mammectomy (măm-mek'to-mĭ) [" + G. *ektome*, excision]. Removal of the breast. **Syn**: *mastectomy*.

mammilla (măm-ĭl'lă) [L. nipple]. 1. Nipple. 2. Any structure resembling a nipple.

mammillary (mam'ĭl-lar-ĭ) [L. *mammilla*, nipple]. Like or concerning a nipple.

mammillated (mam'mĭl-lā-tĕd) [L. *mammilla*, nipple]. Having protuberances like a nipple.

mammillation (măm-ĭl-la'shŭn) [L. *mammilla*, nipple]. 1. Condition of having a granulated appearance or nipplelike projections. 2. A nipplelike protuberance.

mammilliform (mam-mĭl'ĭ-form) [" + *forma*, shape]. Shaped like a nipple.

mammilliplasty (măm-mĭl'ĭ-plăs-tĭ) [" + G. *plassein*, to form]. Plastic operation on a nipple. **Syn**: *thelyplasty*.

mammillitis (măm-mĭl-ī'tĭs) [" + G. *-itis*, inflammation]. Inflammation of a nipple. **Syn**: *thelitis*.

mam'min [L. *mamma*, breast]. Mammary gland hormone causing cessation of the menses.

mammitis (măm-ī'tĭs) [L. *mamma*, breast, + G. *-itis*, inflammation]. Inflamed condition of the breast. **Syn**: *mastitis*.

mammose (mam'ōs) [L. *mamma*, breast]. 1. Having unusually large breasts. 2. Shaped like a breast.

mammotomy (măm-ot'ō-mĭ) [" + G. *tome*, incision]. Surgery of a breast. **Syn**: *mastotomy*.

mammotropin (măm-ŏt'rō-pĭn). Name of lactogenic principle of the ant. pituitary lobe. **Syn**: *prolactin*.

man (măn) [A.S. *mann*]. 1. Member of the human race; a human being. 2. Male member of the species. **See**: "*anthrop-*" words.

mancinism (man'sĭn-ĭzm) [L. *mancus*, crippled]. State of being left-handed.

mandelic acid (man-del'ik). A crystalline compound derived from benzaldehyde.

Uses: In the treatment of urinary infections, esp. pyelitis and cystitis.

Dosage: Usually sodium or ammonium salt, average 12 Gm. per day.

It is necessary that the acidity of the urine be controlled, that the bactericidal effect be received. An additional acidifying agent, as ammonium chloride, is usually required, when the sodium salt is used.

It is advised, because of renal irritation, that the drug be used not longer than 12-14 days.

Incompatibilities: Fluids.

mandible (man'dĭ-bl) [L. *mandibulum*, jaw]. A jawbone, esp. the lower one. The inferior maxilla.

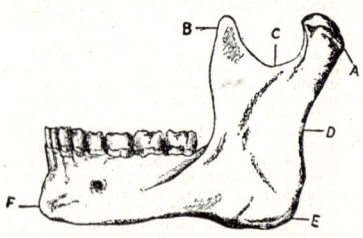

THE MANDIBLE.
A, Condyle; B, Coronoid process; C, Mandibular notch; D, Ramus; E, Angle; F, Mental protuberance.

mandibular (măn-dib'ū-lar) [L. *mandibulum*, jaw]. Rel. to the lower jaw.

m. reflex. Clonic movement resulting from percussing or stroking lower jaw.

m. and m. enema. One given because its ingredients form gases and distend the bowel, thus causing frequent and copious bowel movements. **See**: *enema*.

mandrin (man'drĭn) [Fr.]. A guide for a flexible catheter.

manducation (măn-dū-ka'shŭn) [L. *manducare*, to chew]. The chewing of food. **Syn**: *mastication*.

maneuver (măn-ōō'ver) [Fr. *manoeuvre*, from L. *manu operari*, to work by hand]. **Obs**: Manipulation of the fetus and placenta to aid in delivery. **See**: *labor*.

m., Crede's. Method of expressing the placenta first described by Crede, in which the hand is placed on the fundus of the uterus with the thumb on the ant. wall and the fingers on the post. wall, the placenta being pushed out by pressure in the direction of the birth canal.

m., Leopold's. Method of abdominal palpation for the diagnosis of presentation and position of the fetus in utero.

m., Mauriceau-Smellie-Veit. Method employed to deliver the aftercoming head in breech presentation. Straddling the baby over the right arm, the index finger of that hand is introduced into the mouth of the child and applied over the maxilla; 2 fingers of the other hand are then hooked over the neck, grasping the shoulders. Downward traction is made until the occiput appears under the symphysis pubis. The body of the child is now raised up toward the mother's abdomen and the mouth, nose, brow and occiput are successively brought over the perineum.

m., Muller's. Similar in import and method to that of Munro Kerr.

m., Munro Kerr. A method for determining the presence of disproportion bet. the fetal head and the maternal pelvis. The fetal head is pushed into the pelvis with the right hand on the abdomen, while with 2 fingers of the left hand in the vagina the possibilities of engagement of the head are noted. At the same time the thumb of the left hand feels over the brim of the pelvis to determine the degrees of overlapping.

m., Pinard's. Fingers behind knee and push it toward and past the body, causing flexion of knee. Foot is then grasped and brought down in breech presentation.

m., Prague. A method for the delivery of the aftercoming head in a breech delivery when the occiput is post.

m., Scanzoni. Double application of forceps in post. position of the occiput.

Man'fan's disease. Spastic paraplegia found in children with hereditary syphilis.

manganese (man'gă-nēz) [L. *manganesium*]. SYMB: *Mn.* AT. WT.: 54.93. SP. GR.: 7.2. A metal element found in many foods, and in some plants, and in the tissues of the higher animals.

FUNCTIONS: Its significance in the diet is not clear. It is believed to supplement copper in aiding in the formation of hemoglobin, although some think it has a nutritional function of its own. It seems to aid tissue respiration, and is essential for normal growth. It is a coenzyme necessary for the synthesis of Vitamin C in the body.

DEFICIENCY SYM: Subnormal growth and deficient tissue respiration.

SOURCES: *Ex:* Bananas, bran, beans, beets, blueberries, chard, chocolate, peas. *Good:* Leafy vegetables and whole grains.

POISONING: A rather uncommon industrial poison found usually after prolonged exposure.

SYM: Muscular weakness, peculiar gait, tremors, central nervous system disturbances, salivation.

F. A. TREATMENT: Removal from source of exposure.

mania (mā'nĭ-ă) [G. *mania*, madness]. Mental disease characterized by exaltation or delirium.

m. à pótu. Delirium tremens.
m., Bell's. Periencephalitis in acute form.
m., puerperal. A form of mental derangement occurring occasionally during the puerperium.
m., religious. Mania resulting from excessive religious fervor.
m., transitory. Short attacks of frenzy.
m., unproductive. Behavior characteristic of mania by lack of spontaneity in speech or muteness sometimes seen in manic-depressive psychosis. SEE: *alcoholism.*

mania, words pert. to: aboulomania; acromania; agromania; alcoholomania; amenomania; androphonomania; arithmomania; Bell's disease; bromomania; callomania; camphoromania; chaeromania; choreomania; choromania; dromomania; entheomania; ergasiomania; folie; hypomania; insanity, circular; kleptomania; kleptomaniac; megalomania; micromania; monomania; monomaniac; mythomania; narcomania; necromania; nostomania; nudomania; nymphomania; onomatomania; phaneromania; pharmacomania; potomania; psychosis, manic-depressive; pyromania; theomania; trichotillomania; typhomania; xoanthropy.

maniac (mā'nĭ-ăk) [G. *mania*, madness]. A person with mental disease, usually one disturbed or excited.

maniacal (mă-nī'ăk-ăl) [G. *mania*, madness]. 1. Like a maniac. 2. Affected with mania.

man'ic-depres'sive psychosis. Cyclic or circular affective psychosis in which there are alternating moods of depression and mania. SEE: *psychosis, manic-depressive.*

man'ikin [D. *manneken*, little man]. 1. A model of the human body or its parts. 2. A dwarf.

manipulation (măn-ĭp-ū-la'shŭn) [L. *manipulāre*, to handle]. Any treatment or procedure involving use of the hands.
RS: *massage, osteopathy, spondylotherapy, Swedish movements.*

manipula'tive surgery. Use of manipulation in surgery, bonesetting, etc.

Man'naberg's symptom. Accent of 2nd pulmonic sound in diseases of the abdomen.

man'nerism. Acts which are in keeping with the personality. A peculiar modification of an ordinary movement.

mannite (man'īt). Manna sugar, $C_6H_{14}O_6$, exuded from manna. It is a laxative.

Mann'kopf's sign. Pulse acceleration exhibited on pressing a painful point, seen in neurasthenia.

manometer (măn-om'et-er) [G. *manos*, thin, + *metron*, measure]. Device for determining liquid or gaseous pressure.
m., aural. Instrument for ascertaining mobility of membrane during inflation.

mantle (man'tl) [A.S. *mentel*, a garment]. The cerebral cortex. SYN: *brain mantle, pallium.*

manual (man'ū-al) [L. *manus*, hand]. 1. Pert. to the hands. 2. Performed by or with the hands.

manubrium (man-u'brĭ-um) [L. handle]. 1. The upper bone of the sternum articulating with the clavicle and first pair of costal cartilages. 2. That portion of the malleus* resembling a handle. SEE: *umbo.*
m. sterni. Same as *manubrium, 1.*

manus (ma'nus) [L.]. The hand.

manustupration (man"u-stu-pra'shun) [L. *manustupratiō*, defilement by hand]. Masturbation.

mapharsen (mă-far'sen). A compound containing 29% trivalent arsenic.
USES: As an antiluetic, claiming to have less severe reactions than arsphenamine or neoarsphenamine, and much lower dosage.
DOSAGE: Initially, for women 0.02 Gm. and for men 0.04 Gm. intravenously; second injection, which is usually given from 5-7 days, slightly increased. Maximum dose is regarded as 0.06 Gm. and advised not to be given any patient at the first injection.

marantic (mă-răn'tĭk) [G. *marainein*, to waste]. 1. Pert. to marasmus. 2. Wasting away.

marasmic (mă-raz'mĭk) [G. *marainein*, to waste]. Affected with marasmus; wasting away. SYN: *marantic*.

marasmopyra (mar-az-mo-pi'ră) [G. *marasmos*, wasting, + *pyretos*, fever]. Hectic fever.

marasmus (mar-az'mus) [G. *marasmos*, wasting]. Emaciation, wasting. Infantile atrophy which occurs almost wholly as a sequel to acute diseases, esp. diarrheic diseases of infancy.

Most common from 6-18 months of age. Extreme wasting, child becoming a mere living skeleton.

SYM: May be vomiting and diarrhea, sleep restless, child uncomfortable and in pain, constantly hungry, frets, worries, suffers abdominal pain and headache. Feet edematous, urine scanty, anus and nates chafed and sore from urinal acidity and alkalinity or acidity of evacuations. Prostration becomes extreme, heart weak, abdomen distended, and mesenteric glands enlarged.

PROG: Fair, but recovery is slow.

TREATMENT: Often change of climate or simply from city to country is of great benefit. Keep in fresh air as much as possible. Oil baths.

DIET: Blandest kind of nourishment, as free from starch as possible. Different foods must be tried till one is found to suit the case. Constitutional treatment.

marble bones. Abnormally calcified bones with spotted appearance in a roentgenogram. SYN: *Albers-Schönberg disease, osteosclerosis* fragilis generalisata*.

mareo (mar-a'ō) [Sp. from L. *mare*, sea]. Seasickness. [ness.
  m. de la Cordillera. Mountain sick-

marginal (mar'jĭn-ăl) [L. *margō, margin-*, edge]. Concerning a margin or border.

margination (mar-jĭ-nā'shŭn) [L. *margō, margin-*, edge]. Cleavage of leukocytes to walls of blood vessel in first stages of inflammation.

margin'oplasty [" + G. *plassein*, to form]. Plastic surgery of a border, as of an eyelid.

margo (mar'go) [L.]. A border.

Marienbad (mah-re'ĕn-baht). A spa in Czechoslovakia for cardiovascular disease, urinary disorders, anemia, etc.

Marie's disease (mă-rē'). Chronic condition of enlargement of bones and soft tissues of hands, feet and face. SYN: *acromegaly, hypertrophic pulmonary osteoarthropathy*.
  M.'s sign. Hand tremor seen in exophthalmic goiter.

marihuana (mă-rē-whan'ă). A Mexican name for a poisonous plant. Used in cigarette form, it is a dangerous habit-forming substance. SYN: *Indian hemp; Maria-Juana*.

marine' treat'ment. Routine bathing of the tuberculous patient in sea water; is of tonic value, esp. when combined with heliotherapy.

Mariotte's law (mar-ē-ot'). Boyle's* law.
  M.'s spot. The blind spot of the eye. SYN: *optic papilla*.

maritonucleus (măr"ĭ-tō-nū'klē-ŭs) [L. *maritus*, married, + *nucleus*, kernel]. Nucleus of ovum after being entered by the sperm cell. SYN: *genoblast*.

mark [A.S. *mearc*]. A nevus, bruise, cut or spot on the surface of a body.
  m., birth-. Blemish on the skin at birth.
  m., mother's. Birthmark.

Marmo's method (mar'mōz) (Seratino Marmo, contemporary Italian obstetrician) (artificial respiration). A manner of performing artificial respiration in asphyxiated infants. The accoucheur places his hands in the infant's axillae and thereby raises the subject up in the air and suddenly releases his hands. A sudden drop of a foot or two will cause inspiration to occur, with expiration being effected by pressure of the accoucheur's hands against the chest wall.

marriage (mar'rĭj) [L. *maritāre*, to marry]. State of being united to one of the opposite sex as husband and wife; wedlock. SEE: *misogamy, polyandry, polygamy*.

mar'row [A.S. *mearh*]. The medulla or soft tissues in the hollow of long bones, and medullary cavities, and in the extremities of the long bones.

In adult bone there are red and fat, or yellow, m. The yellow m. is found esp. in medullary cavity of long bones, and the red in spongy bones.

It consists of both fat and red marrow; from 20-80% fat marrow, to 100% red marrow. The marrow may be as high as 5% of body weight in an adult.

The liver seems to have something to do with the production of the red blood cell marrow. These cells may produce many times their volume of mature red blood cells within 2 weeks. The rate of red marrow to fat marrow fluctuates constantly.

FOOD VALUE: Rich in phosphoric fats.

RS: *giant cell, leukomyelitis*.
  m., red. That in cancellous tissue of bone. Concerned with the production, maintenance and disposal of red blood cells and hemoglobin.
  m., spinal. Spinal cord.
  m., yellow. That in the medullary canal of long bones.

marsh fever. Malarial fever.
  m. gas. Methane, *q.v.*

Marsh's test. A test to detect the presence of arsenic.

marsupialization (mar-sū"pĭ-al-ĭ-za'shun) [L. *marsupium*, pouch]. Process of raising the borders of an evacuated tumor sac to the edges of the abdominal wound, and stitching them there to form a pouch.

The interior of the sac suppurates and gradually closes by granulation.

marsupia patellaris (mar-sū'pĭ-ă pă-tel-lā'rĭs) [L.]. The knee joint's alar ligaments.

martial (mar'shal) [L. *mars, mart-*, iron]. Pert. to or containing iron. SYN: *ferruginous*.

Martin's bandage. Rubber bandage for varicose veins, ulcers and other similar conditions.

maschaladenitis (mas-kal-ă-den-ī'tĭs) [G. *maschalē*, armpit, + *adēn*, gland, + *-itis*, inflammation]. Inflammation of axillary glands.

maschaliatry (mas-kal-ĭ-at'rĭ) [" + *iatreia*, healing]. Treatment by axillary inunctions.

masculation (măs-kū-lā'shŭn) [L. *masculus*, a male]. Male sex characteristics formation.

mas'culin [L. *masculus*, a male]. Male sex hormone.

masculine (măs'kū-lĭn) [L. *masculus*, a male]. Having male characteristics.

masculonucleus (mas"kū-lō-nū'klē-ŭs) [" + *nucleus*, kernel]. Male pronucleus. SYN: *arsenoblast*.

mask [Fr. *masque*]. A covering for the

face, as the gauze mask of a surgeon or nurse.
   m., ecchymotic. Traumatic asphyxia.
   m., Fontana's. Fold transversely on a nerve trunk when it has been severed.
   m., Hutchinson's. A feeling of compression over face as though one is wearing a mask. A symptom of tabes dorsalis.
   m., luetic. Blotchy brown pigmentation of cheeks, forehead and temples, seen in tertiary syphilis.
   m., Parkinson's. Immobile facial appearance as a result of encephalitis lethargica. The face is devoid of expression, the skin smooth and without a wrinkle.
   m. of pregnancy. Pigmented spots on the face seen in some pregnant women.
   m., uterine. Mask of pregnancy or uterine disease.

masked (măskd) [Fr. *masque*]. Covered from view.

masochism (mas'o-kĭzm) [named after Sacher-Masoch of Germany]. A psychopathic condition due to weakness and glandular insufficiency, esp. of the gonads and adrenals, which condition demands the stimulation of pain (generally whipping), before the subject is able to react to the sexual stimulus.
   The subject thus expects to dominate indirectly his sexual partner through his own weakness. Masochism demands torture of one's self, or the opp. of sadism, *q.v.* A psychopathic state in males, but also a physiological phenomenon in women, such as an inclination to subordination to man. It is rare in women. SEE: *algolagnia, flagellation.*

masochist (mas'ō-kĭst). A person addicted to masochism.*

mass (măs) [L. *massa*, mass]. Soft, solid preparation for internal use, and of such consistency that it may be molded into pills.
   It is frequently prescribed alone or with other agents, and may be given in pill form or put into capsules. Two masses are official.

mas'sa [L.]. Mass, *q.v.*
   m. innominata. Tubular body on spermatic cord above the epididymis, the remains of post. part of the wolffian body. SYN: *paradidymis.*

massage (mas-săzh') [G. *massein*, to knead]. Manipulation; methodical pressure, friction and kneading of the body. Must always be applied upon the bare skin.
   RS: *anatripsis, effleurage, flagellation, friction, frolement, fustigation, kneading, malaxation, masseur, petrissage, Swedish movements, tapotement, vibration.*
   m., auditory. Massage of the eardrum membrane.
   m., douche. Massage resulting from the application of a douche.
   m., electrovibratory. Massage by means of an electric vibrator.
   m., general. Consists of centripetal stroking in connection with some muscular kneading from the toes upward. Principally used for nervousness, being an important part of the well known "rest cure." Useful in connection with certain baths, duration 30-40 minutes. As soon as a part is massaged, it should be given a few passive rotary movements and afterwards covered up.
   m., hydropneumatic. Massage by means of air forced through a tube at the end of which is a chamber containing water, the water chamber being applied to the part massaged.
   m., introductory. Consists of centripetal strokings around the affected part; as in an affection of the knee joint, where introductory massage should be used on lower part of thigh and somewhat below the knee. Very useful in cases where it is impossible for operator to apply treatment directly to diseased parts.
   m., local. Consists in treatment confined to particular parts.
   m., tremolo. A variety of mechanic massage.
   m., vapor. A treatment of a cavity by a medicated and nebulized vapor under interrupted pressure.
   m., vibratory. Massage by rapidly repeated light percussion with a vibrating hammer or sound.

masseter (mas-sē'tĕr) [G. *masētēr*, chewer]. The muscle which closes the mouth and is the principal muscle in mastication.

masseur (ma-sur') [Fr.]. 1. A man who gives massages. 2. An instrument for massaging.

masseuse (ma-suz') [Fr.]. A woman who gives massages.

massive (măs'ĭv) [Fr. *massif*]. Bulky; consisting of a large mass; huge.
   m. collapse of the lung. Dyspnea and pain in chest, esp. in patients who have suffered severe shock and collapse after abdominal operation or thyroidectomy.
   Patient's condition resembles that of postoperative pneumonia, but the collapsed lung expands in 2-3 days. The condition is a dangerous one.
   TREATMENT: That used for general collapse, Fowler's position, heat to affected side; inhalations of oxygen and carbon dioxide.

massotherapy (măs-ō-ther'ă-pĭ) [G. *massein*, to knead, + *therapeia*, treatment]. Use of massage in treatment of disease.

mastadenitis (măst-ă-den-i'tĭs) [G. *mastos*, breast, + *adēn*, gland, + *-itis*, inflammation]. A mammary gland inflammation.

mastalgia (mast-al'jĭ-ă) [" + *algos*, pain]. Pain in the breast. SYN: *mastodynia.*

mastatrophia (mast-ă-trō'fĭ-ă) [" + *a-*, priv. + *trophē*, nourishment]. Atrophy of breasts. SYN: *mastatrophy.*

mastatrophy (mast-at'rō-fĭ) [" + " + *trophē*, nourishment]. Atrophy of breasts. SYN: *mastatrophia.*

mastauxe (mas-tawk'se) [" + *auxē*, increase]. Excessive size of the breast.

mast cell. A mononuclear leukocyte with basophil granules found in the blood, esp. in leukemia.

mastectomy (mas-tek'to-mĭ) [G. *mastos*, breast, + *ektomē*, excision]. Excision of the breast.
   NP: Patient's gown is removed, care being taken not to chill the patient by exposure. The side arm rest should be attached to table. The patient's arm is extended on the rest. The entire area of operation is then painted with 3½% iodine, extending from wrist to umbilicus and from opposite nipple line, across and around body to middle line of back, with particular attention to axilla. The patient is rolled over on unaffected side, and a sterile sheet slipped underneath painted area and extending over the arm rest. The patient is then rolled back and extended hand is wrapped in a towel. A second towel is wrapped around arm and entire arm covered with sterile sheet. The sterile sheet is

laid over patient from umbilicus to feet. A second sheet extends from neck up over anesthetizing screen. The so-called "thyroid sheet," one which is split part way so as to form 2 "tails" which may be folded under neck and shoulders of patient, is often used. The main part of sheet is brought up over the face. A sheet is placed on unaffected side of patient and extends over midline of body. The sheets should all be clipped into place with towel clips. Four towels are now placed, 2 crosswise and 2 lengthwise, and are clipped into place. The area exposed between towels should extend from midbody line to the axillary line, and from 2 inches above umbilicus to just below clavicle. Thus the axilla and the area of the pectoralis muscles are exposed. Further procedure is routine. Have hot salt water solution ready, as hot wet pads may be needed. A good many ligatures will be used and should be ready. Silkworm gut is used for tension sutures when the skin flaps are approximated. Metal clips (skin clips), silk or interrupted sutures of silkworm gut are used for suture of incision line.

DRAINAGE AND DRESSING: A heavy absorptive dressing is used. The arm is brought across the chest and dressing finished with either a breast bandage or a Velpeau bandage. Strips of iodoform gauze, 3 and 8 inches wide; folded gutta percha tissue for surface drainage; 2 fenestrated tubes, large and medium; borosalicylic acid powder, 4:1; 3 yards gauze; large pad of cotton; 2 aseptic gauze bandages, 7 inches wide, 5 yards long; 6 gauze compresses; gauze sponges; 12 safety pins; 12 towels; 3 sheets; collodion in an aseptic glass, and camel's hair brush. Hot and cold physiologic salt solution. Corrosive sublimate, 1:1000. Support the operated side on a pillow covered with a rubber pillow case. SYN: *mammectomy*.

masthelcosis (măs-thĕl-kō'sĭs) [G. *mastos*, breast, + *elkōsis*, ulceration]. Ulcerated condition of breast.

mastication (măs-tĭ-kā'shŭn) [L. *masticāre*, to chew]. Chewing. The comminution and insalivation of the food in the mouth is the first stage of digestion. Certain muscles close the mouth, raise and lower the mandible, tense the cheeks, and accomplish the highly coordinated movements of the tongue.

The smell and taste of food stimulate sensory nerves, which reflexly elicit both motor and secretory activity in various digestive organs. Thus the salivary glands begin to secrete at once, and both the glands and the musculature of the stomach gradually become active. The saliva dissolves some substances, dilutes materials too concentrated for the stomach, hydrolyzes (due to the salivary enzyme, ptyalin) some of the starch to maltose, and lubricates material to be swallowed.

RS: *absorption, amasesis, enzyme, gastric and salivary digestion.*

masticatory (măs'tĭk-ă-tō-rĭ) [L. *masticāre*, to chew]. 1. Pert. to mastication. 2. Any substance chewed to stimulate secretion of saliva.

mas'tigote [G. *mastix, mastig-*, whip]. A member of the family Mastigophora, or protozoa with flagella.

mastitis (măs-tī'tĭs) [G. *mastos*, breast, + *-itis*, inflammation]. Inflammation of the breast.

Most common in women during lactation, but it may occur at any age.

ETIOL: May be due to entry of disease producing germs through the nipple. In most cases there is a crack or abrasion of the nipple. Infection begins in 1 lobule but may extend.

SYM: The earliest sign is a triangular flush generally underneath the breast. There may be a high temperature and pulse rate, and the patient may become very ill from septic absorption.

TREATMENT: If seen early enough, complete weaning of the baby for 48 hours, support, painting nipple with protargol, 10%, and the whole breast with 10% ichthyol in glycerin will clear up the condition. Otherwise, some authorities advise weaning from the affected breast only, and treatment with antiphlogistine or hot fomentations until inflammation subsides or an abscess forms and is incised. Occasionally the mastitis is secondary to generalized puerperal sepsis.

Testosterone propionate has been giving promising results, but care must be taken not to administer too large a dose.

m., interstitial. Inflammation of glandular substance of the breast.
m., stagnation. Caked breast.
mastocarcinoma (măst"ō-kăr-sĭn-ō'mă) [" + *karkinos*, crab cancer, + *-ōma*, tumor]. Carcinoma of the breast.
mastochondroma (măst"ō-kon-drō'mă) [" + *chondros*, cartilage, + *-ōma*, tumor]. Cartilaginous breast tumor.
mastodynia (măst-ō-dĭn'ĭ-ă) [" + *odynē*, pain]. Neuralgia of the breast.
mastoid (mas'toid) [" + *eidos*, form]. 1. Pert. to mastoid process of the temporal bone. 2. The mastoid process of temporal bone. 3. Formed like a nipple.
m. antrum. Hollow air space in the mastoid process.
m. bone. Mastoid process of temporal bone.
m. cells. Mastoid sinuses.
m. disease. Inflammation of mastoid.
m. operation. Outward drainage of mastoid cells.
m. process. Part of temporal bone; contains antrum, mastoid cells, portion of transverse and sigmoid sinus, facial nerve. SEE: *tegmen*.
mastoidal (măs-toi'dăl) [" + *eidos*, form]. Rel. to mastoid process.
mastoida'le [" + *eidos*, form]. The mastoid process' lowest point.
mastoidalgia (mas-toid-al'jĭ-ă) [" + " + *algos*, pain]. Pain in the mastoid.
mastoidec'tomy [" + " + *ektomē*, excision]. Excision of mastoid cells. Rarely indicated since advent of antibiotics.

NP: Patient in dorsal position with small sand bag under shoulders. The area of operation is painted with iodine (3½%). Two sterile towels placed lengthwise under head and shoulders. One is brought up around head and is kept in place with towel clips. The other covers end of table. A laparotomy sheet is placed over patient, with opening over area of operation.

mastoideocentesis (măs-toid-ē-ō-sen-tē'sĭs) [G. *mastos*, breast, + *eidos*, form, + *kentēsis*, puncture]. Surgical puncture of the mastoid process.
mastoiditis (măs-toid-ī'tĭs) [" + *eidos*, form, + *-itis*, inflammation]. Inflammation of the mastoid process.

COMPLICATIONS: Perisinus abscess, periphlebitis, sinus thrombosis. Involvement is metastatic through blood vessels without erosion of sinus plate or ex-

tension of suppuration directly through sinus plate into the sinus.
SYM: Fever, chills, tenderness over emissary vein, leukocytosis, sepsis.
TREATMENT: Surgical.

m., Bezold's. Abscess underneath insertion of sternocleidomastoid muscle due to pus breaking through the tip cell.

m., zygomatic. Suppuration of cells in root of zygoma with swelling over the zygoma.
TREATMENT: Surgical evacuation of mastoid cells.

mastoidotomy (mas-toid-ot'ō-mǐ) [" + " + tomē, incision]. Incision into mastoid process.

mastology (mast-ol'ō-jǐ) [" + logos, study]. Science or study of the breasts.

mastomenia (mas-to-me'nǐ-ǎ) [" + mēnēs, menses]. Vicarious menstruation from the mammary glands.

mastoncus (mas-ton'kŭs) [" + ogkos, tumor]. Any tumor of the breast.

mastoöccipital (mas"tō-ok-sǐp'ǐ-tǎl) [G. mastos, breast, + L. occipitalis, pert. to occiput]. Rel. to mastoid process and occipital bone.

mastopathy (mǎs-top'ǎ-thǐ) [" + pathos, disease]. A disease of the mammary glands.

mastopexy (mas'tō-pěks-ǐ) [" + pēxis, fixation]. Surgical correction of a pendulous breast by fixation. SYN: mazopexy.

mastoplasia (mǎst-ō-plā'zǐ-ǎ) [" + plassein, to form]. Hyperplasia of mammary gland tissue. SYN: mazoplasia.

mastorrhagia (mǎs-tōr-ā'jǐ-ǎ) [G. mastos, breast, + rēgnunai, to burst forth]. Hemorrhage from the breast.

mastoscirrhus (mǎs-tō-skǐr'ŭs) [" + skirros, hardness]. A hard cancer of breast.

mastotomy (mǎst-ot'ō-mǐ) [" + tomē, incision]. Surgical incision of a breast.

masturbate (mas'těr-bāt) [L. masturbāri, to pollute one's self]. To arouse self-excitement through titillation of the genital organs.

masturbation (mǎs-těr-bā'shŭn) [L. masturbāri, to pollute one's self]. Self-production of an orgasm by titillating the genitals either by hand or some mechanical means.
It is considered morbid or pathological if practiced excessively or as a substitute for normal sexual relations. It is common among the psychopathics. Its harmful effect is due more to a sense of guilt and secrecy than to physical causes and may induce a neurosis or a psychosis.
RS: manustupration, onanism.

m., psychic. When the orgasm ensues through psychic processes such as phantasy and without physical contacts.

match'es. Lucifer matches are usually made of phosphorus, q.v., and potassium chlorate and may be lit by friction.
"Safety" matches contain antimony, sulfide and potassium chlorate and must be lit by striking on the box which is covered with red phosphorus.
POISONING SYM: Gastrointestinal irritation with blood changes.
F. A. TREATMENT: Wash out stomach with water or very dilute potassium permanganate. Repeated catharsis.

maté (mah'ta) [Sp. mate, vessel for preparing leaves]. Paraguay tea made from the leaves of Ilex paraguayensis.
Said to contain caffeine and tannin.
USES: Diaphoretic, diuretic, and for headaches.

materia medica (mǎ-tē'rǐ-ǎ měd'ǐ-kǎ) [L. medical matter]. That branch of science dealing with all drugs used in treatment of diseases, their source, preparation, dosage and use.
RS: active principles, drug action, drug administration, medical preparations, pharmacognosy, pharmacology.

materies morbi (mǎ-tē'rǐ-ēs mor'bǐ) [L. substance of disease]. The matter or substance which is the cause of disease.

mater'nal [L. maternus, pert. to a mother]. 1. Rel. to the mother. 2. From a mother.

maternity (mǎ-ter'nǐ-tǐ) [L. mater, mother]. 1. The condition of motherhood. 2. Lying-in hospital. SEE: accouchée.

maternology (ma-ter-nol'ō-jǐ) [" + G. logos, study]. The scientific study of motherhood.

matrix (mā'trǐks) (pl. matricēs) [L. mother; womb]. 1. The womb. 2. The formative portion of a tooth or nail. 3. The intercellular substance of a tissue. 4. Mold for casting.

m. unguis. Nail bed.

matrixitis (mā-trǐks-ī'tǐs) [" + G. -itis, inflammation]. Inflammation of the bed of a nail. SYN: onychia.

mattoid (mat'oid) [L. mattus, drunken, + G. eidos, form]. Person not in full control of mental faculties, but not to extent of insanity. SYN: paranoiac.

maturate (ma'tūr-āt) [L. maturus, ripe]. 1. To ripen; to mature. 2. To suppurate. SYN: suppurate.

maturation (mǎt-ū-rā'shŭn) [L. maturus, ripe]. 1. Maturing; ripening, as a graafian follicle. 2. Suppuration. 3. Last stage in sex cell formation.

matu'rity [L. maturus, ripe]. State of being mature or fully developed; time when a person becomes capable of reproducing; puberty.

mature (ma-tūr') [L. maturus, ripe]. Fully developed or ripened.

matutinal (ma-tū'tǐ-nǎl) [L. matutinus, morning]. Occurring early in the day, as morning sickness; in the morning.

matzoon (mǎt-zūn') [Armenian]. Milk with a ferment containing lactic acid, bacilli and other organisms.

maxill'a (pl. maxillae) [L. jawbone]. BNA. A jawbone, esp. the upper one; the superior maxilla. SEE: skeleton.

m., inferior. The lower jawbone, or mandible.

m., superior. Upper jawbone.

maxillary (mǎk'sǐ-la-rǐ) [L. maxillaris, pert. to the maxilla]. Pert. to the jaw, esp. the upper.

m. bones. Maxilla sup. and inf., upper and lower jawbones.

m. sinus. The antrum of Highmore; air cavity in sup. maxilla opening into middle meatus of nose.

maxillitis (mǎks"ǐl-ī'tǐs) [L. maxilla, jawbone, + G. -itis, inflammation]. Inflammation of maxilla or maxillary gland.

maximal (maks'ǐ-mal) [L. maximus, greatest]. Greatest possible; highest.

maximum (maks'ǐ-mum) [L. greatest]. 1. The greatest quantity. 2. Height of a disease.

mayidism (mā'ǐd-ǐzm) [L. mais, maize]. Deficiency disease due to lack of Vitamin B. SYN: pellagra, q.v.

Mayo enema. One which causes gas to form in the intestine, inflating the bowel and producing bowel action. SEE: enema.

Mayo-Robson's point. A point just above and to right of the umbilicus, where pressure causes tenderness in pancreatic disease.

"Mazda" lamp. Tungsten filament lamp

enclosed in a bulb of special glass that transmits ultraviolet rays at wave lengths extending from 280-310 millimicrons. Types C X, S-1 and S-2.

mazopexy (mā'zō-pĕks-ĭ) [G. *mazos*, breast, + *pēxis*, fixation]. Correction of a pendulous breast by surgical fixation. SYN: *mastopexy*.

mazoplasia (mā-zō-plā'zĭ-ă) [" + *plasein*, to form]. Hyperplasia of mammary gland tissue. SYN: *mastoplasia*.

McBurney's incision. Abdominal incision employed in appendectomy.

An incision is made parallel to the path of external oblique muscle, about 1-2 inches away from ant. sup. spine of right ilium, cutting through the external oblique to the internal oblique and transversalis, separating their fibers.

McB.'s point. Point of tenderness in acute appendicitis, situated on a line bet. the umbilicus and the right ant. sup. iliac spine, about 1 or 2 inches above the latter.

McCarthy's reflex. Contraction of orbicularis palpebrarum with closure of lids resulting from percussion above supraorbital nerve.

McCormac's reflex. Adduction of 1 leg resulting from percussion of patella tendon of opposite leg.

meal (mēl) [A.S. *mael*, measure, meal]. Portion of food eaten at a particular time to satisfy the appetite. SEE: *test m., Von Leube motor test m., -test m.*

m. deviation. In statistics, a number representing the degree of variation found in a series of observations. The mean is first found; next, by subtraction, the differences bet. the mean and each observation; then the sum of all the differences, treated as positive; then the quotient of this sum by the total number of observations. Thus the mean deviation of the series 5, 6, 7 is $(1+0+1)/3 = 0.67$; the mean deviation for the series 4, 6, 8 is $(2+0+2)/3 = 1.33$.

measles (mē'zls) [Dutch *maselen*]. A highly contagious disease characterized by catarrhal symptoms and the presence of maculopapular eruption.

ETIOL: Believed to be caused by a filtrable virus because of its analogies to other known virus diseases, but the specific virus has not yet been isolated. Measles is the commonest of all so-called contagious diseases. After the age of 4 months, natural immunity may be regarded as practically nonexistent. One attack almost invariably confers immunity, though second occurrences have been recorded.

INCUBATION: Eight to 14 days—rarely longer.

SYM: Onset gradual; coryza, rhinitis, drowsiness, loss of appetite, gradual elevation of temperature for first 2 days, when fever may rise from 101-103° F. Photophobia and cough soon develop, although some recession in the temperature may occur.

About 4th day, fever usually reaches a higher elevation than previously, at times as high as 104-106° F., and with this recurrence the rash appears.

Eruption first appears on face, being seen early as small maculopapular lesions which rapidly increase in size and coalesce in places, often causing a swollen, mottled appearance. The rash ex-

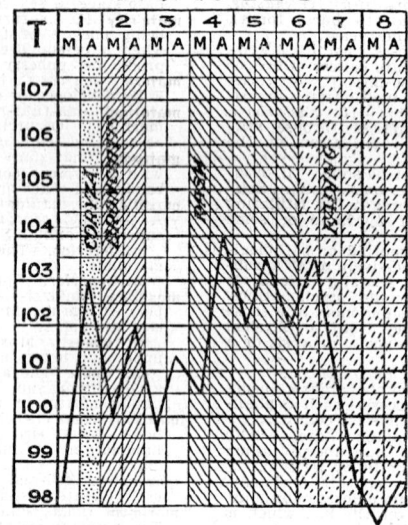

mean (mēn) [L. *medius*, in middle]. In statistics, a number derived from a series of other numbers by a prescribed method of computation. SEE: *median*.

Thus the *arithmetic mean* (commonly called the average) of a series of n numbers is obtained by adding all the numbers and dividing the sum by n. The *geometric mean* is obtained by multiplying all the numbers and taking the nth root of the product.

measles

tends to the body and extremities, and in some areas may assume a deviousness suggestive of scarlet fever.

A cough, present at this time, is due to the bronchitis produced by the inflammatory condition of the mucous membranes that undoubtedly corresponds to the rash seen on the skin. Ordinarily, the rash lasts from 4-5 days and, as it subsides, the temperature declines. Consequently, by the end of 5 days from appearance of rash, temperature should be normal, or approximately normal in uncomplicated cases. Prior to appearance of the eruption, a leukocytosis may be noted. Following presence of rash, a leukopenia may always be expected.

COMPLICATIONS: Bronchopneumonia, the most frequent and most serious complication of measles, and the usual explanation for the fatal case. An otitis* media, followed by a mastoiditis, a brain abscess, or even meningitis, are not rare. Cervical adenitis with marked cellulitis sometimes leads to fatal consequences. Encephalitis is comparatively rare. Tracheitis and laryngeal stenosis, due to edema of glottis, are sometimes seen in the course of measles.

Eye Complications: Frequently feared by parents. Not common in measles, although a marked conjunctivitis may occur.

DIFFERENTIAL DIAG: Scarlet fever, German measles, the prodromal rash of smallpox, or even cases of confluent smallpox may have to be considered. If the measles patient is observed prior to appearance of rash, or sometimes even after rash has developed, a definite decision may be based on the presence of Koplik's spots, *q.v.*

Hemorrhagic spots are also seen on the hard palate and mucous membranes many times before rash is evident on the skin. These spots probably correspond to the typical maculopapular eruption of the disease.

PROG: While usually favorable in the well-nourished child, the seriousness of the possible complications of measles should not be minimized.

TREATMENT AND NP: Patient isolated in a well-ventilated room, since, when a respiratory infection is being dealt with, good ventilation is of utmost importance. Though a room is frequently darkened, this is not a necessary requirement if strong light does not shine in patient's face.

The average measles patient does not care to eat during first few days of illness. Aside from providing plenty of fluids, no unusual effort should be made to force food upon him. Plenty of water, fruit juices and milk, however, are desirable. With fading of rash and reduction of temperature, patient will soon regain his appetite under normal circumstances.

The eyes should receive careful attention, being cleansed with a saturated solution of boric acid, perhaps followed by a few drops of one of the less irritating silver salts.

The cough may be controlled to some extent by any of the drugs ordinarily used for this purpose, or amidopyrine in doses of 1 gr. per year up to 5 years of age may be given 3 to 4 times daily. This remedy appears to lessen cough, and reduce temperature, and to reduce markedly the complications of this disease.

meat

QUARANTINE: It is customary in many states to quarantine until rash has disappeared and temperature has been normal for from 24-48 hours. In the uncomplicated cases, this usually means that the duration of the quarantine will be approximately 10 days from the date of onset. Measles is much more contagious before eruption than it is after eruption has appeared. Consequently, it is not at all likely that the quarantine of measles patients exerts any influence on the control of a measles epidemic. On the other hand, quarantine of susceptible contacts is plainly beneficial in limiting exposures and preventing the spread of infection.

Protection against measles is afforded by intramuscular injections of concentrated ascitic fluid.

SEE: *German m., Koplik's spots, roetheln, rubella, rubeola.*

measure (mē'zhŭr) [Fr. *mesure*, from L. *mensura*, a measuring]. 1. A determined extent or quantity. 2. To determine the extent or amount of an area or substance.

measure, words pert. to: amicron; Angstrom's unit; anthropometry; apothecaries; atmos; atmosphere; atomic weight; avoirdupois; calory; candle, international; c. power; capillus; carbonometry; cardiameter; centesimal; centigram; centiliter; centimeter; centinormal; cephalometry; chloridimetry; chromatoptometry; chromometry; clinical unit; curie; dosage meter; dosimeter; dram; erg; farad; fuel value; gamma; gram; international x-ray unit of intensity; light unit; Mache unit; meter; metric system; microfarad; micron; mil; milliameter; milliampere; millicurie; m. destroyed; millimicron; minimum wave length; molar; ohm; Ohm's law; opsonic index; power; quantimeter; quantum; tension; therm; Troy weight; uncia; unit; velocity; volt; voltage; watt; wattage; watt hour; watt meter; wave length.

meat. Consists of muscle tissue, connective tissue, fat, or the glandular organs. All meats contain proteins and mineral elements and nearly all contain fat. The glandular organs such as liver and kidney contain a considerably higher percentage of certain mineral elements and vitamins than are found in other forms of meat. Muscle tissue (lean meat) is made up of tiny fibers held together by connective tissue (collagen) and desirable juices are held within the walls, and particles of fat are imbedded in the tissue. The tissues and fibers in young animals are tender; as the animal grows older the tissue becomes tougher, in proportion to its food, care and exercise. Little-used muscles of the loin remain more tender; the flesh of poultry raised in a confined area and given a scientifically prepared ration is more tender than that of birds ranging in the open and not specially fed. Fat improves the flavor. It varies little in composition in the different animals and the amount is governed by the food and care of the animal. The best cuts are generously mottled with fat. In beef, pork and poultry some of the fat may be removed before cooking, but in fish it is distributed throughout the fiber.

Nitrogenous extractives, purines and mineral salts give flavor to meat. Lean meat contains about 1% of mineral ash. Clear fat has almost none. The amount of mineral elements in lean meat is

meatal   M-14   **meconium**

proportional to the amount of protein it contains. It is rich in phosphorus, potassium, iron, and it has a good percentage of other minerals, but is deficient in calcium. The ash constituents differ somewhat in the different groups (beef, pork, etc.), and in the same animals at different ages, but in all meats the acid-forming elements are decidedly in excess of the base-forming.

As a source of vitamins, meat is not important except for vitamin G, and in pork, vitamin B. Meat protein is of good quality for tissue building, and it is almost entirely digestible. The less tender cuts of meat are palatable and nutritious when correctly cooked or combined with vegetables, rice and other foods.

Meat has been assailed for several reasons: "It forms acids in the body"; "it is hard on the kidneys"; "it is conducive to 'autointoxication,'" all of which have been proved unwarranted, and objection to purines as precursors of uric acid has been withdrawn. All meat for interstate commerce is subjected to Federal inspection both before and after slaughter; that sold within a state is subject only to state inspection. Meat is preserved by refrigeration, drying, brining, canning, and retail cuts are quick frozen, providing a wide variety.

Meats most commonly used are pork, beef, veal, mutton, lamb and poultry.

DIGESTIBILITY OF MEATS: (1) Mutton quicker than beef. (2) Beef quicker than pork. (3) Pork. (4) Lean meat quicker than fat meat. (5) Fat meat. (6) Young animal quicker than old animal. (7) Old animal. SEE: *flesh, examination of animal; names of meats; purines.*

meatal (mē-ā'tăl) [L. *meatus*, passage]. Pert. to a meatus or passage.

meatometer (mē-ā-tom'ĕt-ĕr) [" + G. *metron*, measure]. Device for measuring a passage or opening.

meat poisoning. Poisoning from eating diseased or putrified animal flesh.

Federal meat inspectors examine over a million head of livestock consigned to the Union Stockyards in Chicago for food purposes every year. Carcasses are condemned for over 40 diseases or conditions rendering them unfit for food. Meat sold within a state is subjected to state regulation only.

SYM: The symptoms depend upon the cause, but (a) cramps, (b) nausea, (c) vomiting, and (d) diarrhea within 24 hours after the ingestion of questionable food are symptoms in common to all forms of food poisoning except *botulism*.* In addition to these symptoms, meat poisoning creates thirst; muscular weakness; pain in the chest or bet. the shoulders; fever; dark, offensive stools; leg and arm cramps; muscular twitching; prickling or numbness of the hands; drowsiness; disturbed vision; yellow skin; hallucinations, and often vertigo and anorexia. Pinched features, blueness of fingers, toes and sunken eyes precede death. SEE: *flesh, examination of animal.*

meatorrhaphy (mē-ăt-or'af-ĭ) [L. *meatus*, passage, + G. *raphē*, a sewing]. Suture of the severed end of a meatus, usually the *meatus urinarius*.

meatoscopy (mē-ăt-os'kō-pĭ) [" + G. *skopein*, to examine]. Instrumental examination of a meatus.

meatotome (mē-at'ō-tōm) [" + G. *tomē*, incision]. Knife with probe or guarded point for enlarging meatus by direct incision.

meatotomy (mē-ā-tot'ō-mĭ) [" + G. *tomē*, incision]. Incision of urinary meatus to enlarge the opening. SYN: *porotomy*.

meatus (mē-ā'tŭs) (pl. *meatūs*) [L. *meatus*, opening]. A passage or opening.

   m. acusticus externus. [BNA.] External auditory canal from tympanum to pinna.

   m. acusticus internus. [BNA.] Canal in the petrous portion of temporal bone, containing facial and auditory nerves and vessels.

   m. audito'rius. Ext. and int. passages of the ear.

   m. nasi communis. Common nasal cavity on either side of septum.

   m. nasi inferior. Space beneath inf. turbinate.

   m. nasi medius. Space beneath middle turbinate.

   m. nasi superior. Space beneath sup. turbinate.

   m. urinarius. External opening of the urethra; usually said of the male.

mechanical rectifier. A device which, by changing contacts at the proper moment in a cycle, changes alternating current into pulsating direct current.

mechanics (mē-kăn'ĭks) [G. *mēchanē*, machine]. Science of force and matter.

mech'anism. PSY: Combination of mental processes by which a result is obtained.

   m., mental. PSY: Method of utilizing energy from instinctive drives with their accompanying emotions to deal with internal and external pressures upon the personality.

mechanology (mĕk-ăn-ŏl'ō-jĭ) [" + *logos*, study]. Study of force and matter.

mechanotherapy (mĕk"an-ō-thĕr'ă-pĭ) [G. *mēchanē*, machine, + *therapeia*, treatment]. Use of various types of mechanical apparatus to perform passive movements and to exercise various parts of the body. Ex: MacKenzie and Zander apparatus.

mecholyl (mĕk'ō-lĭl). Commercial name for acetyl-beta-methylcholine chloride.

   DOSAGE: 3-7½ gr. (0.2-0.5 Gm.).

meckelectomy (mek-el-ek'tō-mĭ) [G. *ektomē*, excision]. Excision of Meckel's ganglion. [pendage of the ileum.

Meck'el's cartilage. A vestigial cecal ap-

   M.'s divertic'ulum. A congenital sac or blind pouch sometimes found in lower portion of the ileum. Strangulation may cause intestinal obstruction. SEE: *diverticulum, diverticulitis.*

   M.'s ganglion. G. located in the sphenomaxillary fossa giving off nerves to eyes, nose and palate. SYN: *sphenopalatine g.* [the gasserian ganglion.

   M.'s space. Area in dura holding

mecometer (mē-kom'ĕt-ĕr) [G. *mēkos*, length, + *metron*, measure]. Device for measuring an infant's length.

meconism (mek'ō-nizm) [G. *mēkōn*, poppy, + *ismos*, condition of]. 1. Opium poisoning. 2. The opium habit.

meconium (me-kō'nĭ-um) [G. *mēkōnion*, poppy juice]. 1. Opium; poppy juice.

2. First feces of a newborn infant, made up of salts, liquor amnii, mucus, bile and epithelial cells; greenish black to light brown, almost odorless and of a tarry consistency.

Evacuated by 3rd or 4th day after birth. Its disappearance should not be hastened, as it is a preventive of early bowel infection. Buttocks should be

medi- greased with petrolatum to prevent meconium from drying on the skin.

medi- [L.]. Prefix: The *middle*.

media (mē'dĭ-ă) [L. middle]. 1. Middle or muscular coat of an artery. SYN: *tunica media.* 2. Plural of *medium.*

me'dial [L. *medius,* middle]. 1. Pert. to middle. 2. Internal.

me'dian [L. *medius,* middle]. 1. Middle; central. 2. In statistics, a number obtained by arranging the given series in order of size and taking the middle number; one then has as many greater as there are less. Thus, in the series 5, 7, 8, 9, 10 the median is 8. SEE: *mean.*

  m. artery. An interosseous branch.

  m. line. The sagittal line, an imaginary line from the top and middle of the head through the sagittal suture to the floor. The parts nearest to it are called mesial, and those farthest from it lateral.

  m. nerve. One of motion and sensation having its origin in the brachial plexus.

mediastinal (mē-dĭ-ăs-tī'năl) [L. *mediastinus,* in middle]. Rel. to the mediastinum.

mediastinitis (mē-dĭ-as-tī-nī'tĭs) [" + G. *-itis,* inflammation]. Inflammation of tissue of the mediastinum.

mediastinopericarditis (mē-dĭ-ăs″tĭ-nō-pĕr″ĭ-kăr-dī'tĭs) [" + G. *peri,* around, + *kardia,* heart, + *-itis,* inflammation]. Inflammatory condition of mediastinum and pericardium.

mediastinum (mē-dĭ-ăs-tī'nŭm) [L. in the middle]. 1. A septum or cavity bet. 2 principal portions of an organ. 2. The folds of the pleura and intervening space bet. right and left lung. The interpleural space. It contains the thoracic viscera. SEE: *chylcmediastinum.*

  m. testis. Partial testicular septum.

mediate (mē'dĭ-āt) [L. *mediatus,* in the middle]. 1. Accomplished by indirect means. 2. Intermediate.

medicable (mĕd'ĭ-kă-bl) [L. *medicārī,* to heal]. Amenable to cure.

medical (mĕd'ĭ-kal) [L. *medicārī,* to heal]. Pert. to medicine.

  m. jurisprudence. Principles of medicine in their application to questions of law.

  m. preparations. SOLID SUBSTANCES: Capsule or *capsula;* cachet, confection or *confectio;* cerate or *ceratum;* extract or *extractum;* lozenge or *trochiscus;* lamella*; ointment or *unguentum;* plaster or *emplastrum;* powder or *pulvis;* pill or *pilula;* paper or *charta;* sterule* or *sterula;* suppository or *suppositorium;* tablet or *tabella;* vescette.*

  FLUIDS: Fluidextract, or *fluidextractum;* tincture or *tinctura;* infusion or *infusum;* decoction or *decoctum;* wine or *vinum;* oleoresin or *oleoresina.*

  SUSPENSIONS: Mixture or *mixtura;* emulsion or *emulsum.*

  SOLUTIONS: Water or *aqua;* mucilage or *mucilago;* solution or *liquor;* elixir or *elixir;* syrup or *syrupus;* spirit or *spiritus;* glycerite or *glyceritum;* vinegar or *acetum.* [or *oleatum.*

  MISC: Liniment or *linimentum;* oleate

RS: alkaloid, active principle, names *of preparations, drugs with two names; antidote; dosage; drug action; drugs and their administration; names of individual drugs in alphabetical order; names of poisons; poison; poisoning; preparations usually given by rectum; prescription writing.* [cine or medicine.

med'icament [L. *medicamentum*]. A medicine

RS: *epispastic, errhine, escharotic, evacuant, medical preparations, rubefacient, saponin, sedative, specific, vesicant, vesicatory.*

medicate (mĕd'ĭ-kāt) [L. *medicārī,* to heal]. 1. To treat a disease with drugs. 2. To impregnate with medicinal substances.

medication (mĕd-ĭ-kā'shŭn) [L. *medicārī,* to heal]. 1. Treatment with remedies. 2. Impregnation with medicine.

  m., hypodermic. Treatment by injection of remedies beneath the skin.

  m., ionic. Introduction of ions of drugs into the body by cataphoresis.

  m., substitutive. Medical therapy to cause a nonspecific inflammation to counteract a specific one.

medication, words pert. to: alterant, amyctic, analeptic, analgetic, antilepsis, antileptic, antimalarial, antiphlogistic, antipruritic, antipyic, antipyretic, antipyrotic, antirheumatic, antiscorbutic, antiseptic, antisialic, antisialogogue, antispasmodic, antisyphilitic, antizymotic, aperient, carminative, catheresis, caustic, cerate, cumulative.

medicinal (mĕ-dĭ'sĭn-ăl) [L. *medicina,* medicine]. Pert. to medicine.

  m. enema. One to which some drug or medication has been added, for retention or absorption, particularly in cases where medication cannot be adm. by mouth. SEE: *enema.*

medicine (mĕd'ĭ-sĭn) [L. *medicina*]. 1. A drug. 2. The art of preventing, caring for, and assisting in the cure of disease, and the care of the injured. 3. Treatment of disease medically as distinguished from surgery.

  m., clinical. Observation and treatment at the bedside.

  m., eclectic. Selection from all systems of medicine.

  m., forensic. Application of medical knowledge to legal affairs.

  m., patent. A medicine for which a patent has been granted. SEE: *patent* medicine.*

  m., preventive. The practice of preventing disease.

  m., proprietary. Medicine in which proprietary interests have been secured by patent, copyright of labels, or secrecy of composition. SEE: *proprietary medicine.*

medicine, rectal administration of. In diseases of the rectum and adjacent parts, medication is often applied by way of the anus, esp. if medication cannot be adm. by mouth, as in persistent nausea or emesis, during unconsciousness or delirium, or on account of the bad taste of the medication.

Almost any drug other than those of a corrosive nature may be adm. through the rectum.

The medication should be given in as small an amount of solution as possible, in order to prevent irritation and expulsion. The preparation should be given in a small, well-greased catheter (with a funnel) into an empty rectum and colon. The colon should be cleansed at least 1 hour previous to giving the enema.

A purgative enema may be used for this purpose. The time elapsing bet. the 2 enemas should be an hour, as there must be no peristaltic action when the medication is introduced. Of course, there must be no fecal content to absorb the medicated solution.

Four points must be kept in mind: (1) The rectum must be free of fecal material.

(2) The medicinal substance must be readily soluble.
(3) The solution must have the consistency of thin starch, with a temperature of 100° F.
(4) The enema must be given slowly and not be too hot but at body temperature so as not to stimulate peristalsis. A wad of cotton should be held against the anal region to aid retention. The patient should lie on the left side while the injection is being given, in order to allow the solution to reach the ascending colon more easily.
A normal salt solution of 4 oz. with 5% of glucose is a common medicated enema. Gelatin or some astringent, such as alum solution, may be given.
SEE: *enema, preparations usually given by rectum.*

medicinerea (měd″ĭ-sĭn-ē′rē-a) [L. *medius*, middle, + *cinerea*, ashen]. Internal gray matter of the claustrum and lenticula of the brain.

medicochirurgical (měd″ĭ-kō-kĭ-rur′jĭ-kăl) [L. *medicus*, medical, + G. *cheir*, hand, + *ergon*, work]. Concerning both medicine and surgery.

medicolegal (měd″ĭ-kō-lē′găl) [" + *legalis*, legal]. Rel. to medical jurisprudence or forensic medicine.

med′icus [L.]. A physician.

medinal (med′ĭ-nal). Soluble barbital, barbital sodium.
USES: Sedative and hypnotic.
DOSAGE: 5-15 gr. (0.3-1.0 Gm.).

medio- [L.]. Prefix meaning *the middle*.

mediopontine (mē″dĭ-ō-pon′tĭn) [L. *medius*, middle, + *pons, pont-*, bridge]. Rel. to center of the pons Varolii.

mediotarsal (mē″dĭ-ō-tar′săl) [" + G. *tarsos*, tarsus]. Rel. to the middle of the tarsus.

medipeduncle (mē″dĭ-pē-dun′kl) [" + *pedunculus*, a stem]. Cerebellar middle peduncle.

medium (mēd′ĭ-ŭm) (pl. *media*) [L. middle]. 1. An agent through which an effect is obtained. 2. Substance used for the cultivation of microörganisms. SYN: *culture medium*. 3. Substance through which impulses are transmitted.

medulla (mē-dul′lă) [L. marrow]. 1. The marrow. 2. Substance in the kidneys below the cortex. 3. Medulla oblongata. 4. Spinal cord. SEE: *accelerating center, cardioinhibitory center.*

m. of kidneys. Renal pyramids.
m. nephrica. Pyramids of kidneys.
m. oblongata. Enlarged portion of spinal cord in cranium after it enters the foramen magnum of the occipital bone; the lower portion of the brain stem.
m. ossium. Marrow in bone.
m. spinalis. Spinal cord.

medullary (med′ŭ-lar-ĭ) [L. *medulāris*, pert. to marrow]. Concerning marrow, or any medulla.

medullated (med′ŭ-lāt-ĕd) [L. *medulla*, marrow]. Covered by or containing marrow or medulla.
m. nerve fiber. A white nerve fiber.

medullispinal (me-dŭl″ĭ-spī′năl) [" + *spina*, thorn]. Rel. to the spinal cord.

medullitis (měd-ū-lī′tĭs) [" + G. *-itis*, inflammation]. Inflammation of marrow. SYN: *myelitis.*

medullization (měd-ŭ-lĭ-zā′shŭn) [L. *medulla*, marrow]. Conversion to marrow abnormally.

medulloarthritis (měd″ŭ-lō-ar-thrī′tĭs) [" + G. *arthron*, joint, + *-itis*, inflammation]. Inflammation of marrow elements of bone ends.

medulloblastoma (měd″ŭ-lō-blas-tō′mă) [L. *medulla*, marrow, + G. *blastos*, germ, + *-ōma*, tumor]. Malignant nerve tissue tumor.

medulloceli (měd-ŭ′lō-sĕl) [" + *cellula*, little box]. Marrow cell. SYN: *myelocyte.*

medulloepithelioma (měd″ŭ-lō-ep″ĭ-thĕl-ĭ-ō′mă) [" + G. *epi*, upon, + *thēlē*, nipple, + *-ōma*, tumor]. Tumor composed of retina epithelium and of neuroepithelium. SYN: *neuroepithelioma, glioma.*

mega-, meg- [G.]. Combining forms meaning *great, large.*

megabacterium (měg″ă-băk-tēr′ĭ-ŭm) [G. *megas*, large, + *baktērion*, little rod]. One of the largest bacterium.

megabladder (měg′ă-blăd-ēr) [" + A.S. *blaedre*]. Permanent abnormal distention of the urinary bladder. SYN: *megalocystis.*

megacephalic (měg-ă-sěf-al′ĭk) [" + *kephalē*, head]. Having an abnormally large head. SYN: *macrocephalous.*

megacoccus (měg-ă-kok′ŭs) [" + *kokkos*, berry]. A large size coccus. SYN: *macrococcus.*

megacolon (meg-ă-ko′lon) [" + *kōlon*, colon]. Extremely dilated colon.
Usually congenital, and occurs also in infancy or childhood. In congenital cases, acetylcholine is used as a diagnostic test. SEE: *Hirschsprung's disease.*

megacoly (měg′ă′kol-ĭ) [" + *kōlon*, colon]. Dilatation of the colon.

megadont (měg′ă-dont) [G. *megas*, large, + *odous, odont-*, tooth]. Possessing very large teeth. SYN: *macrodont.*

megadyne (meg′ă-dīn) [" + *dynamis*, power]. A unit equal to one million dynes.*

megakaryocyte (měg″ă-kar′ĭ-ō-sīt) [" + *karyon*, nucleus, + *kytos*, cell]. Large bone marrow cell with large or multiple nuclei. SYN: *megaloblast, myeloplax.*

megalakria (měg-ă-lak′rĭ-ă) [" + *akros*, extremity]. Trophic disorder marked by progressive enlargement of head, hands, feet, and thorax. SYN: *acromegaly.*

megalgia (měg-al′jĭ-ă) [" + *algos*, pain]. Very severe pain.

megalo- [G.]. Combining form meaning *large, great.*

megaloblast (měg′ă-lō-blăst) [G. *megas*, large, + *blastos*, germ]. A large size nucleated red blood corpuscle, from 11-20 microns in diameter, oval and slightly irregular. SYN: *macroblast.*

megalocardia (měg-ă-lō-kar′dĭ-ă) [" + *kardia*, heart]. Cardiac hypertrophy. SYN: *cardiomegaly.*

megalocephalic (měg-ă-lō-sef-al′ĭk) [" + *kephalē*, head]. Having an abnormally large skull. SYN: *megacephalic, macrocephalic.*

megalocephaly (meg″ă-lō-sef′ă-lĭ) [" + *kephalē*, head]. Abnormal size of the head. SYN: *macrocephaly.*

megalocornea (měg′ă-lō-kor′nē-ă) [G. *megas*, large, + L. *cornū*, horn]. An enlarged cornea.

megalocystis (měg″ă-lō-sĭs′tĭs) [" + *kystis*, bladder]. Abnormal, permanent enlargement of the bladder. SYN: *megabladder.*

megalocyte (měg′ăl-ō-sīt) [" + *kytos*, cell]. Red blood corpuscle larger than average.

megalodactylous (měg″ă-lō-dak′tĭl-ŭs) [" + *daktylos*, finger]. Having very large digits.

megalodontia (měg″ă-lō-don′shĭ-ă) [G.

megaloenteron M-17 **melanocarcinoma**

megas, large, + *odous, odont-*, tooth]. Abnormal size of teeth.
megaloenteron (mĕg″ă-lō-ĕn'tĕr-on) [" + *enteron*, intestine]. Excessive size of the intestine. SYN: *enteromegaly*.
megalogastria (mĕg″ă-lō-gas'trĭ-ă) [" + *gastēr*, belly]. Excessive size of stomach. SYN: *gastromegaly*.
megaloglossia (mĕg″ă-lō-glos'sĭ-ă) [" + *glōssa*, tongue]. Enlargement of the tongue. SYN: *macroglossia*.
megalohepatia (mĕg″ă-lō-hē-pat'ĭ-ă) [" + *ēpar, ēpat-*, liver]. Abnormal enlargement of the liver. SYN: *hepatomegaly*.
megalokaryocyte (meg-ă-lō-kar'ĭ-ō-sīt) [" + *karyon*, nucleus, + *kytos*, cell]. A large bone marrow cell with multiple nuclei. SYN: *megakaryocyte*.
megalomania (meg″a-lo-mā'nĭ-ă) [G. *megas*, large, + *mania*, madness]. A psychosis characterized by ideas of personal exaltation and delusions of grandeur.
megalomelia (mĕg″ă-lō-mēl'ĭ-ă) [" + *melos*, limb]. Abnormally large size of the limbs. SYN: *macromelia*.
megalonychosis (mĕg″ă-lō-nĭ-kō'sĭs) [" + *onyx, onych-*, nail, + *-ōsis*]. Hypertrophy of the nails.
megalopenis (mĕg″ă-lō-pē'nĭs) [" + L. *penis*, penis]. Abnormally large penis. SYN: *macrophallus*.
megalophthalmus (mĕg-ă-lŏf-thal'mus) [" + *ophthalmos*, eye]. Abnormally large eyes.
megalopsia (meg-a-lop'sĭ-ă) [" + *opsis*, vision]. An affection of the eyes in which objects appear enlarged. SYN: *macropsia*.
megaloscope (meg′a-lo-skōp) [" + *skopein*, to examine]. A speculum that magnifies.
megalosplenia (mĕg″ă-lō-splēn'ĭ-ă) [" + *splēn*, spleen]. Hypertrophy of the spleen. SYN: *splenomegaly*.
megalosyndactyly (mĕg″ă-lō-sin-dak'til-ĭ) [" + *syn*, with, + *daktylos*, finger]. A condition of large and webbed digits.
megaloureter (mĕg-ă-lō-ūr'ĕ-tĕr) [G. *megas*, large, + *ourētēr*, ureter]. Increase in diameter of the ureter.
megarectum (mĕg-ă-rek'tŭm) [" + L. *rectum*, straight]. Excessive dilatation of the rectum.
megaseme (mĕg'ă-sēm) [" + *sēma*, sign]. 1. Having an orbital aperture with an index exceeding 89, said of a skull. 2. A megaseme skull.
Megas'toma [" + *stoma*, mouth]. A protozoan.
M. intestinale. A protozoan inhabiting the intestine.
megophthalmus (mĕg-of-thal'mŭs) [" + *ophthalmos*, eye]. Abnormally large eyes. SYN: *buphthalmus, megalophthalmus*.
megrim (mē'grĭm) [O.Fr. migraine]. 1. Sick headache. SYN: *migraine, q.v.* 2. A whim. 3. Vertigo.
meibomian cyst (mī-bō'mĭ-ăn). Small tumor on eyelid, the result of inflammation of a m. gland. SYN: *chalazion*.*
m. gland. One of the sebaceous follicles bet. the tarsi and conjunctiva of eyelids.
Meinicke reaction or **test** (mi'nĭk-e). Tests for syphilis. 1. Flocculur reaction. 2. Turbidity reaction. 3. Clearing reaction.
meiocardia (mī″ō-kar'dĭ-ă) [G. *meiōn*, less, + *kardia*, heart]. Systole; heart contraction.
Meissner's corpuscles (mīs'nĕr). Laminated, ovoid corpuscles attached to nerve fibers; found at tips of fingers and toes, in skin over lips, the mammary glands and genitals.
M.'s plexus. One in submucosa of small intestine. Derived from the myenteric plexus.
mel [L.]. Honey.
melaena (mel-e'na) [G. *melaina*, black, black bile]. 1. Black vomit. 2. Tarry evacuations. SEE: *melena*.
melagra (mĕl-a'gră) [G. *melos*, limb, + *agra*, seizure]. Pain in the limbs. SYN: *melalgia*.
melalgia (mĕl-al'jĭ-ă) [" + *algos*, pain]. Neuralgia of the limbs. SEE: *meralgia*.
melancholia (mĕl-an-kō'lĭ-ă) [G. *melas, melan-*, black, + *cholē*, bile]. Depression of mental condition, with or without delusions or violent mania, characterized by great apathy.
Some classify it as the *depressed* state of mania or the *excited* state of *manic depressive insanity*.
m., affective. Involving or due to the emotions.
m. agita'ta. M. with much motor excitement.
m. attonita. Characterized by mental and physical stupor.
m., climacteric. Occurring at the menopause.
m., convulsive. Occurring in connection with jacksonian epilepsy.
m., involution. Despondency, suicidal tendencies, feelings of unworthiness and mental agitation occurring between 45 and 60 years of age.
m., panphobic. Characterized with dread of everything.
m., paretic. Preceding paresis.
m., puberty. M. with feelings of inferiority.
m., sexual. M. associated with fear of impotence, venereal disease, unsatisfied sexual desires.
m. simplex. Without delusions, a mild form.
m. stuporo'sa. SEE: *m. attonita*.
m., suicidal. Having impulse to commit suicide combined with melancholia.
melanedema (mĕl-an-e-dē'mă) [G. *melas, melan-*, black, + *oidēma*, swelling]. Black deposit in the lungs; melanosis of the lungs. SYN: *anthracosis*.
melanemia (mĕl-an-e'mĭ-ă) [" + *aima*, blood]. Unnaturally dark color of blood, due to presence of melanin or free, dark pigment.
Seen mainly in pernicious anemia.
melanephidrosis (mĕl-ăn-ĕf-ĭ-drō'sĭs) [" + *ephidrōsis*, sweating]. Black sweat. SYN: *melanidrosis*.
mélangeur (mā-lon-jher′) [Fr. mixer]. Apparatus for drawing and diluting blood specimens for microscopic examination.
melanidrosis (mĕl-an-ĭd-rō'sĭs) [G. *melas, melan-*, black, + *idrōsis*, sweat]. Black sweat. SYN: *melanephidrosis*.
melaniferous (mĕl-an-if'ĕr-ŭs) [" + L. *ferre*, to carry]. Containing melanin or some other black pigment.
mel'anin [G. *melas, melan-*, black]. The pigment which gives color to hair, skin and the choroid of the eye, and is present in some cancers, as in *melanoma*.
Melanin can be prepared chemically.
melanism (mĕl'ăn-ĭzm) [" + *ismos*, state of]. Excessively black pigmentation of the organs and tissues. [*darkness*.
melano- [G.]. Prefix meaning *black* or
melanoblastoma (mĕl″ă-nō-blăs-tō'mă) [" + *blastos*, germ, + *-ōma*, tumor]. A tumor containing melanin.
melanocarcinoma (mĕl″ă-nō-kar-sĭn-ō'mă)

melanocyte M-18 **membrana granulosa**

["+ *karkinos*, crab cancer]. A cancer which is darkly pigmented.
melanocyte (mel″an-ō'sīt) ["+ *kytos*, cell]. Pigmented leukocyte.
melanoderma (měl″an-ō-der'mă) ["+ *derma*, skin]. A dark skin discoloration.
melanogenesis (mel″an-ō-jěn'ē-sǐs) ["+ *genesis*, production]. Formation of melanin.
melanoglossia (měl″ăn-ō-glǒs'sǐ-ă) [G. *melas*, *melan-*, black, + *glōssa*, tongue]. Black tongue. SYN: *glossophytia*.
melanoid (měl'ă-noid) ["+ *eidos*, form]. 1. Concerning or resembling melanosis. 2. Melanin which is chemically prepared.
melanoleukoderma (mel″an-ō-lū-kō-der'mă) ["+ *leukos*, white, + *derma*, skin]. Mottled skin.
 m. col′li. Mottled skin of neck sometimes seen in syphilis. SYN: *collar of Venus, venereal collar*.
melano′ma ["+ *-ōma*, tumor]. A pigmented mole or tumor. SYN: *nevus pigmentosus*.
melanomatosis (měl-an-ō-mat-ō'sǐs) ["+ " + *-ōsis*, intensive]. Formation of melanomas on or beneath the skin.
melanonychia (měl-ă-nō-nik'ǐ-ă) [G. *melas*, *melan-*, black, + *onyx*, *onych-*, nail]. Black pigmentation of the nails.
melanopathy (mel-an-op'ă-thǐ) ["+ *pathos*, disease]. 1. Dark pigmentation of skin. 2. Disease with dark pigmentation of the skin. SYN: *melanoderma, melasma*.
melanophore (mel'an-ō-fōr) ["+ *phoros*, a bearer]. Cell carrying dark pigment.
melanoplakia (měl″ă-nō-plā'kǐ-ă) ["+ *plax*, *plak-*, a flat plate]. Condition marked by pigmented patches on the buccal mucosa.
mel′anorrhag′ia [" + *rēgnunai*, to burst forth]. Black feces. SYN: *melanorrhea*.
melanorrhea (měl-an-or-re'ă) ["+ *roia*, flow]. Black stools. SYN: *melena, 2*.
melanosarcoma (měl″ă-nō-sar-kō'mă) [G. *melas*, *melan-*, black, + *sarx*, *sark-*, flesh, + *-ōma*, tumor]. Sarcoma containing melanin.
melanoscirrhus (měl-ă-nō-skir'rŭs) ["+ *skirros*, hard]. Black pigmented cancer. SYN: *melanocarcinoma*.
melanosis (měl-an-ō'sǐs) ["+ *-ōsis*, intensive]. Unusual deposit of black pigments in different parts of body.
 m. lenticularis. Rare skin disease, beginning in early youth, characterized by scattered pigment discolorations, ulcers, atrophy, etc. SYN: *xeroderma pigmentosum*.
melanot′ic [G. *melas*, *melan-*, black]. 1. Blackish in color. 2. Pert. to melanosis.
melanuria (měl-an-u'rǐ-ă) ["+ G. *ouron*, urine]. Dark pigments in urine.
melasma (měl-az'mă) [G. a black spot]. Any discoloration of the skin. SYN: *nigredo cutis*.
 m. gravidarum. Discoloration of the skin during pregnancy.
 m. suprarenale. Hypofunction of the suprarenals with cutaneous pigmentation and severe anemia. SYN: *Addison's disease, q.v.*
melena (měl-ē'nă) [G. *melaina*, black, black bile]. 1. Black vomit. 2. Evacuations resembling tar, due to action of intestinal juices on free blood. Common in the newly born.
melenemesis (mel-e-nem'ē-sǐs) ["+ *emesis*, vomit]. Black vomit caused by blood that has been acted upon by the gastric juice. SYN: *melena, 1*.
melicera, meliceris (měl-ǐ-sēr'ă, -ǐs) [G. *meli*, honey, + *kēros*, wax]. Cyst containing matter of honeylike consistency.

melissopho′bia [G. *melissa*, bee, + *phobos*, fear]. Insane fear of bee or wasp stings.
melitagra (měl-ǐ-tag'ră) [G. *meli*, *melit-*, honey, + *agra*, seizure]. A form of eczema with soft crusts resembling honey.
melitemia (mel-ǐ-te'mǐ-ă) ["+ *aima*, blood]. Sugar in the blood. SYN: *glycemia*.
melitis (měl-ǐ'tǐs) [G. *mēlon*, cheek, + *-itis*, inflammation]. Inflammation of cheek.
melitoptyalism (měl″ǐt-ō-tī'al-ǐzm) [G. *meli*, *melit-*, honey, + *ptyalon*, saliva]. Saliva containing glucose. SYN: *glycoptyalism*.
melituria (mel-ǐ-tu'rǐ-ă) [" + *ouron*, urine]. Diabetes mellitus; excretion of sugar in urine.
mellite (mel'ǐt) [G. *meli*, *melit-*, honey]. Any medicated preparation of honey.
melodiotherapy (mel-ō″dǐ-ō-ther'ă-pǐ) [G. *melōdia*, music, + *therapeia*, treatment]. Treatment by music. SYN: *musicotherapy*.
melomania (mel-ō-mā'nǐ-ă) [G. *melos*, song, + *mania*, madness]. Insane love for music.
meloncus (měl-on'kŭs) [G. *mēlon*, cheek, + *ogkos*, tumor]. Tumor of the cheek.
mel′on [G. *mēlon*, apple]. COMP: Principally water and carbohydrates, the latter nearly all in the form of sugar.
 ACTION: A good cleanser. Often used in semi-fasting; esp. watermelon.
 IND: If fully ripened dyspeptics may use in small quantities. Good in constipation and in clogged conditions of the system.
 CONTRA: The sugar in melons is not sufficient to prohibit for diabetics. In irritable conditions of the digestive system they should be avoided. SEE: *cantaloupe, muskmelon, watermelon*.
meloplasty (mel'ō-plas-tǐ) [G. *mēlon*, cheek, + *melos*, limb, + *plassein*, to form]. Reparative surgery of a cheek or limb.
melosis (mel-ō'sǐs) [G. *mēlōsis*, probing]. 1. Act of probing, as in a wound or ulcer. 2. Act of using a catheter.
melt′ing point. Temperature at which conversion of a solid to a liquid begins.
mem′ber [L. *membrum*]. An organ or part of the body, esp. a limb. [brane.
membrana (mem-brā'na) [L.]. Mem-
 m. adventitia. Any covering membrane not made up of the tissues of organ so covered.
 m. basila′ris. Membrane forming floor of ductus cochlearis.
 m. basilaris of the cochlea. Portion of lamina spiralis membranacea of cochlea into which bases of Corti's and Deiter's cells are inserted. [*cidua*.
 m. caduca vera. SEE: *membrana de-*
 m. capsularis genu. Capsular ligament of knee.
 m. cellulosa. SEE: *membrana decidua*.
 m. chorii. The chorion.
 m. communis. Membrane common to 2 structures.
 m. decidua. BNA. Membrane lining the uterus during pregnancy and cast off in parturition. SYN: *decidua*.
 m. eboris. Layer of odontoblasts bet. tooth pulp and wall of pulp cavity.
 m. elastica laryngis. Layer of yellow elastic tissue subjacent to mucosa of larynx helping to form the true vocal cords.
 m. flaccida. Shrapnell's membrane.
 m. germinativa. The blastoderm.
 m. granulosa. Layer of granular cells forming lining of maturing graafian vesicle.

m. humoris aquei. Membrane of Descemet.
m. intercipientes. Membranes separating one space from another, as the diaphragm.
m. limitans externa retinae. A very delicate membrane in the retina bet. outer granular layer and layer of rods and cones.
m. limitans interna retinae. The hyaloid capsule.
m. pituito'sa. Schneiderian membrane lining the nasal fossa.
m. prolifera. The blastoderm.
m. propria. A thin layer of connective tissue upon which rests the epithelium.
m. pupillaris. Thin, vascular, transparent membrane closing the fetal pupil during the development of the eye.
m. ruyschiana. Middle layer of the choroid, bet. the vitreous lamina and the layer of larger blood vessels.
m. succingens. Visceral layer of the pleura.
m. tectoria. Corti's membrane covering organ of Corti in the ear.
m. tympani. The drum membrane, or tympanic membrane.
m. tympani reflex. Reflection of light from normal eardrum membrane.
m. tympani secundaria. A m. closing the fenestra ovalis.
m. vestibularis Reissneri. Membrane separating cochlear canal from the scala vestibuli.
m. vi'brans. Tenser part of membrane of eardrum.
m. vocalis. Mucous m. covering the vocal bands.
membrane (mem'brān) [L. *membrana*]. A pliable layer of substance lining, separating or enveloping the internal parts of the body.
m., arachnoid. Middle layer of membranes covering brain and spinal cord.
m., basement. Delicate m. underlying epithelium of mucous surfaces, and serving as a support for delicate structures.
m. bone. Bone originating in a membrane.
m., Bowman's. Thin homogeneous m. separating corneal epithelium from proper substance of the cornea.
m., brain and spinal cord. Pia mater, inner m.; dura mater, outer m., and arachnoid, middle m.
m., Bruch's. The lamina basalis constituting the inner layer of the choroid.
m., Corti's. Membrane covering organ of Corti in ear.
m., costocoracoid. Dense fascia bet. the pectoralis minor and subclavius muscles.
m., cricothyroid. M. connecting thyroid and cricoid cartilages of the larynx.
m., croupous. False yellowish-white m. in the larynx during croup.
m., Débove's. Layer bet. epithelium and basement m. of mucosa of the bronchi, trachea and intestinal tract.
m., decidual. M. covering the fetal envelope.
m., Descemet's. Elastic m. forming lining surface of the cornea.
m., diphtheritic. Fibrinous false m. on mucous surfaces in diphtheria.
m., drum. The tympanic membrane.
m., elastic. One formed by elastic tissue fibers, as in the coats of arteries, etc.
m., false. Fibrinous exudate on a mucous surface of a membrane, as in diphtheria.

m., fenestrated. The tunica intima of an artery.
m., fetal. The chorion, amnion, or allantois.
m., germinal. The blastoderm.
m., homogeneous. A fine m. covering villi of the placenta.
m., hyaline. 1. Basement* m. 2. M. bet. outer root sheath of a hair follicle and inner fibrous layer.
m., hyaloid. One investing the vitreous humor of the eye, seen on longitudinal section.
m., Krause's. Dark membranous band limiting the sarcomere in striated muscle.
m., meconic. A m. forming a layer in rectum of the fetus.
m., medullary. Endosteum.*
m., mucous. M. lining cavities and canals communicating with the air and kept moist by secretion of mucus.
m., Nasmyth's. Epithelial m. covering enamel of teeth in the fetus; also for a short time after birth.
m., obturator. Fibrous m. closing the obturator foramen.
m., palatine. One covering buccal roof.
m., periodontal. One covering roots of teeth.
m., pseudoserous. M. resembling serous membrane.
m., pupillary. Transparent m. closing the fetal pupil. If it persists after birth it is known as persistent p. membrane.
m., pyogenic. Granular lining of an abscess or fistula.
m., pyophylactic. Protective lining of an abscess that prevents reabsorption.
m., Reissner's. M. separating the cochlear canal from the scala vestibuli. SYN: *membrana vestibularis Reissneri.*
m., Ruysch's. Choroid's middle layer composed of a close capillary network.
m., schneiderian. Mucosa of the nasal fossae. SYN: *membrana pituitosa.*
m., semipermeable. M. allowing passage of water but not substances in solution.
m., serous. One covered with endothelial cells lining closed cavities and forming inner coat of a blood vessel.
m., Shrapnell's. That portion of the tympanic m. filling the notch of Rivinus.
m., synovial. M. lining a joint and secreting synovia.
m., tectorial. Corti's membrane.
m., Tenon's. Fibroelastic m. surrounding the eyeball. SYN: *Tenon's capsule.*
m., thyrohyoid. One joining the hyoid bone and the thyroid cartilage.
m., tympanic. The drum membrane.
m., virginal. The hymen.
m., vitreous. Descemet's membrane.
m., yolk. Ext. capsule of the ovum.
membrane, words pert. to: arachnopia, basement, basilemma, Cargile, caryomitome, celarium, cephalomeningitis, cerebromeningitis, cerosis, descemetitis, Descemet's, dialysis, encysted, endothelial cell, epithelial, lamella, lamina, leukoplakia, meninges, mucous, obturator, pars flaccida, sarcolemma, sheath, Shrapnell's, synovial, theca, thecal puncture, thecitis, tunica.
membraniform (mem-bran'i-form) [L. *membrana*, membrane, + *forma*, shape]. Resembling or of the nature of a membrane. SYN: *membranoid, membranous.*
membranocartilaginous (měm″brăn-ō-kăr-tĭl-aj′ĭ-nŭs) [" + *cartilāgō, cartilagin-*, cartilage]. 1. Pert. to membrane and

cartilage. 2. Derived from both membrane and cartilage.

membranoid (měm′brȧ-noid) [" + G. *eidos*, resemblance]. Resembling a membrane. SYN: *membraniform, membranous.*

membranous (měm′brȧn-ŭs) [L. *membrana*, membrane]. 1. Rel. to a membrane. 2. Resembling a membrane. SYN: *membraniform, membranoid.*

membrum virile (měm′brŭm vĭr-īl′e) [L. male member]. The penis.

memory [L. *memoria*, memory]. The mental registration of past experience, knowledge, ideas, sensations and thoughts.

Registration of experience is favored by clear comprehension during intense consciousness, but it may occur during catatonic stupor (here stupor refers not to a clouding of consciousness, but to a type of behavior).

Retention of memory differs greatly with individuals, as well as with structural and psychological variations. Memory recall, esp. its intentional recall, means the reproduction of a memory in consciousness. Clear comprehension greatly favors retention. Recall may fail because the memory has been obliterated, or functionally because the stream of ideas is that which one does not wish to remember. Various memory defects occur in many diseases.

Memory is confused or obliterated in *maniacal* states, lively in *paranoia*, abolished in *senile psychosis* and *organic brain disease*, but undisturbed in *depressions*. In dementia from senile causes there is accurate m. for remote events but none for recent occurrences.

RS: *anamnestic, association center, mnemic, mnemonics, retention, r. defect.*

menacme (měn-ăk′mē) [G. *mēn*, month, + *akmē*, top]. The pinnacle (acme) of the menstrual life of a woman.

menadione sodium bisulfite (mē-nȧ′dē-ōn). USP term for synthetic *vitamin K, q.v.*, derived from vitamin K_3.

USES: In prophylaxis, management, or treatment of hypothrombinemia, hemorrhagic disease of newborn, and vitamin K deficiency induced by prolonged antibiotic therapy (reduced intestinal flora), faulty nutrition, intestinal absorption, hepatic disease, or biliary disturbance.

DOSAGE: Oral: 4 mg. daily (capsules). Parenteral: 4 mg. daily. In hypothrombinemia emergency associated with *dicumarol*, 72 mg. intravenously (1 cc. per minute).

RS: *dicumarol, heparin, vitamin K.*

menarche (měn-ȧr′kē) [" + *archē*, beginning]. Beginning of menstruation.

In a group of 100 subjects it was found that the menarche occurred:
In 8 between ages 11 and 11.99 years
In 22 between ages 12 and 12.99 years
In 32 between ages 13 and 13.99 years
In 23 between ages 14 and 14.99 years
In 11 between ages 15 and 15.99 years
In 4 between ages 16 and 16.99 years

Mendel's law. Inherited characters are *dominant* or *recessive*. Dominant ones are recognizable in the individual (as red hair, etc.). Recessive characters are not manifest in the individual, though he transmits them to his progeny, either as dominant or recessive characters. Two persons mating with the same recessive character are virtually certain to have children with that character dominant. [5th toes.

M.'s reflex. Dorsal flexion of 2nd to

menhidrosis (měn-hī-drō′sĭs). Vicarious menstruation through the sweat glands. SYN: *menidrosis.*

menidrosis (měn-ĭ-drō′sĭs) [G. *mēn*, month, + *idrōs*, sweat]. Vicarious menstruation through sweat glands. SYN: *menhidrosis.*

Ménière's disease (mā-nē-ārs′). Disturbance in labyrinth seen in great variety of conditions, as drug poisoning, circulatory disturbances, infectious diseases, as in the exanthemata, and chancre of syphilis, blood dyscrasias, neuritis of vestibular branch of 8th nerve, and tumors of cerebellopontine angle.

SYM: Sudden onset of tinnitus, deafness, nausea, vomiting and dizziness. May last from several days to months.

TREATMENT: Should be directed toward underlying cause. Symptomatic treatment is eliminative, sedative and withholding fluids on the basis of edema of labyrinth as cause of symptoms.

Relief obtained by performing Dandy's operation of severing equilibrium branch of auditory nerve.

meningeal (men-ĭn′jē-ăl) [G. *mēnigx, mēnigg-*, membrane]. Rel. to the meninges.

meningeorrhaphy (mē-nĭn-jē-or′rȧ-fī) [" + *raphē*, a sewing]. Suture of any membranes, esp. those of brain and spinal cord.

meninges (měn-ĭn′jēz) (sing. *meninx*) [G. *mēnigx, mēnigg-*, membrane]. 1. Membranes. 2. The 3 membranes investing the spinal cord and brain: the *dura mater*, external; the *arachnoid*, middle, and *pia mater*, internal.

meningina (me-nĭn-jī′nȧ) [G. *mēnigx*, membrane]. The pia mater and adjacent layer of the arachnoid combined. SYN: *pia-arachnoid.*

meninginitis (me-nĭn-jī-nī′tĭs) [" + *-ītis*, inflammation]. Inflammation of the pia-arachnoid membrane. SYN: *leptomeningitis, piarachnitis.*

meningioma (me-nĭn-jī-ō′mȧ) [" + *-ōma*, tumor]. Tumor of the meninges.

meningism (men-ĭn′jĭzm) [" + *ismos*, state of]. Irritation of the brain and spinal cord with simulation of meningitis, but without actual inflammation.

meningitic (me-nĭn-jĭt′ĭk) [G. *mēnigx*, membrane]. Pert. to meningitis.

meningitis (men-ĭn-jī′tĭs) [" + *-ītis*, inflammation]. Inflammation of the membranes of spinal cord or brain.

SEE: *choriomeningitis, Kernig's sign, leptomeningitis, pachymeningitis.*

m., acute. SYM: Moderate, irregular fever, loss of appetite, constipation, intense headache, intolerance to light and sound, contracted pupils, delirium, retraction of head, convulsions and coma.

PROG: Unfavorable though recovery is not impossible.

NP: The room should be dark and kept quiet. Bowels may be kept open with the aid of aperients. Retention of urine must be guarded against, as distention is apt to occur. The eyes and mouth must be kept cleansed, and pressure points upon the back should be guarded against. The foot of the bed should be raised after each injection. Headache may be relieved by an icebag or cold compresses. Special nursing technic as may be necessary. Isolation and asepsis are indicated. All discharges should be burned. The eyes should be protected from the light, and all noise and everything that might disturb the patient should be avoided.

A bed cradle may be necessary to relieve pressure and friction. Sudden excitement may cause a convulsion, so quiet is absolutely necessary. Change the patient's position frequently but avoid jarring the bed. Hypostatic pneumonia must be guarded against. A cleansing bath with an alcohol rub should be a daily procedure. All body prominences need special attention to prevent pressure sores. Mouth hygiene is also called for morning and night. The intake and output of fluids must be recorded. During the acute stage restraints may be necessary.

DIET: A fluid diet is necessary during the acute stage, but later as much nourishment should be given as possible, as the disease is an exhaustive one. Milk, eggs, beef tea, water, fruit juices and sugar may be given freely. A more solid diet may be given during convalescence. With stuporous patients nasal feeding is necessary. Children and some adults may have to be fed with a spoon, or a medicine dropper.

TREATMENT: Patient should be placed in a darkened, well-ventilated room. Ice bag to head. When robust wet cups or leeches may be applied to neck. Constipation relieved by enemas. Remedies called for in individual case. Sulfanilamide and its derivatives are used successfully now in pneumococcic, meningococcic and beta hemolytic streptococcus meningitis. [brain of the meninges.

m., basilar. Inflammation at base of
m., cerebral. Acute or chronic m. of brain membranes. [cord.
m., cerebrospinal. M. of brain and
m., chronic. ETIOL: Generally results from injury, syphilis, sunstroke, or caries of the bone.
TREATMENT: Same as for acute m.
m., c., epidemic. A specific infectious disease caused by invasion of meningococci, characterized anatomically by inflammation of the cerebrospinal meninges, and clinically by intense pain in head, back and limbs, convulsions, irregular fever and frequently by a petechial eruption.

SYM: Abrupt chill, vomiting and pain as mentioned, muscles of neck and back become rigid and contracted. Opisthotonos may be present; mind soon affected (delirium); nystagmus; strabismus; ptosis; irregular, sluggish pupils; partial deafness or blindness; extreme cutaneous hyperesthesia, so that slightest touch causes pain, may all be present. Temperature ranges generally between 101°-103° F. May be about normal or very high. Pulse full, rapid; urine may contain albumin and sugar. Blotchy, purpuric rash over whole body may be present. Duration, few hours to several weeks. Three forms: Fulminant, abortive, intermittent.

PROG: Guarded. Mortality varies in different epidemics from 20-80%.
TREATMENT: Liquid diet. Ice bags to head and along spinal column. Medication to suit the case. Sponging with cool water or cold pack.
m., influenzal. A form caused by a bacterium which can be seen under a microscope in severe cases. It is in no way related to epidemic influenza. *Hemophilus* is the offending bacterium.
m., otitic. M. as a complication of otitis. [poisoning.
m., septicemic. M. due to septic blood

m., serous. Serous exudation in m. into cerebral ventricles.
m., spinal. M. of spinal cord membranes.
m., tuberculous. An acute inflammation of the cerebral meninges excited by the tubercle bacillus.
SYM: Loss of flesh, gradual wasting of strength, evening rise of temperature, restlessness, irritability, and sleeplessness may exist for some time before acute symptoms come on. These are severe headache, occasional convulsions, delirium, vomiting, fever, optic neuritis.
meningitophobia (me-nin-jit-ō-fō'bī-ă) [G. *mēnigx, mēnigg-,* membrane]. Meningism due to fear of brain disease.
meningoarteritis (me-nĭn-gō-ăr-tĕr-īt'ĭs) [" + *artēria,* artery, + *-itis,* inflammation]. Inflammatory condition of the meningeal arteries.
meningocele (men-ĭn'gō-sēl) [" + *kēlē,* hernia]. Congenital hernia, the meninges protruding through an opening of the skull or spinal column.
meningocerebritis (me-nĭn-gō-ser-e-brī'tĭs) [" + L. *cerebrum,* brain, + G. *-itis,* inflammation]. Inflamed condition of brain and meninges. SYN: *meningo-encephalitis.*
meningococcemia (me-nĭn-gō-kŏk-sē'mī-ă) [" + *kokkos,* berry, + *aima,* blood]. Meningococci in the blood.
meningococcus (men-in-go-kok'us) (pl. *meningococci*) [G. *mēnigx, mēnigg-,* membrane, + *kokkos,* berry]. The microörganism responsible for cerebrospinal meningitis. SEE: *coccus, Neisseria meningitidis.*
meningocortical (me-nin-gō-kor'tĭ-kal) [" + L. *cortex, cortic-,* bark]. Pert. to the meninges and the cortex.
meningoencephalitis (men-ĭn"go-en-sef-al-ī'tĭs) [" + *egkephalos,* brain, + *-itis,* inflammation]. Inflammation of meninges and cerebral cortex of the brain.
meningoencephalocele (me-nĭn"gō-en-sĕf'ăl-ō-sēl) [" + *egkephalos,* brain, + *kēlē,* hernia]. Hernia of brain and meninges.
meningoencephalomyelitis (me-nĭn"gō-en-sĕf"ăl-ō-mī-ĕl-ī'tĭs) [" + " + *myelon,* marrow, + *-itis,* inflammation]. Inflammation of the brain, spinal cord, and their meninges.
meningomalacia (me-nĭn-gō-mă-lā'sī-ă) [" + *malakia,* softening]. Softening of any membrane.
meningomyelitis (men-ĭn"gō-mī-ĕl-ī'tĭs) [G. *mēnigx, mēnigg-,* membrane, + *myelon,* marrow, + *-itis,* inflammation]. Inflammation of spinal cord and its membranes; less commonly of the dura mater, also.
meningomyelocele (me-nĭn"gō-mī'ĕl-ō-sēl) [" + " + *kēlē,* hernia]. Hernia of spinal cord and membranes.
meningopathy (me-nĭn-gop'ă-thī) [" + *pathos,* disease]. Any pathological condition of the meninges.
meningorhachidian (me-nĭn"gor-ră-kid'ĭ-an) [" + *rachis,* spine]. Concerning the spinal cord and meninges.
meningorrhagia (me-nĭn"gor-ra'jī-ă) [" + *rēgnunai,* to burst forth]. Meningeal hemorrhage. SYN: *meningorrhea.*
meningorrhea (me-nĭn-go-rē'ă) [" + *roia,* flow]. Meningeal hemorrhage. SYN: *meningorrhagia.*
meningosis (men-ĭn-gō'sĭs) [" + *-ōsis,* intensive]. Membranous joining of bones, as in the infant.
meningotyphoid (me-nĭn"gō-tī'foid) [G. *mēnigx, mēnigg-,* membrane, + *typhos,*

meninguria stupor, + *eidos*, form]. Typhoid fever with symptoms of meningitis.

meninguria (me-nĭn-gū'rĭ-ă) [" + *ouron*, urine]. Presence of membraniform shreds in urine.

meninx (me'nĭnks) (pl. *meninges*) [G. *mēnigx*, membrane]. Any membrane, but esp. one of the coverings of the brain or spinal cord.

meniscitis (men-ĭs-kī'tĭs) [G. *mēniskos*, crescent, + *-ītis*, inflammation]. Inflamed condition of an interarticular cartilage.

meniscocyte (men-ĭs'kŏ-sīt) [" + *kytos*, cell]. A crescent-shaped red blood cell.

meniscocytosis (men-is"ko-sĭt-ō'sĭs) [" + " + *-ōsis*, intensive]. Crescent cells in the blood; sickle cell anemia.

meniscus (men-ĭs'kus) [G. *mēniskos*, crescent]. 1. Concavo-convex lens. 2. Interarticular fibrocartilage of crescent shape, found in certain joints. SYN: *meniscus articularis*.
m. articularis. [BNA.] SEE: *meniscus*, 2.

menocelis (men-ō-sē'lĭs) [G. *mēn*, month, + *kēlis*, spot]. Spotted cutaneous condition sometimes seen in women failing to menstruate.

menofor'mōn [" + *ormanein*, to excite]. A commercial ovarian hormone.

menolipsis (men-ō-lĭp'sĭs) [" + *leipsis*, a failing]. Temporary absence or retention of menses.

menolysin (měn-ol'ĭs-ĭn) [" + *lysis*, a destruction]. Commercial preparation for treating amenorrhea and dysmenorrhea.

menometrorrhagia (měn"ō-mět-ror-rā'-jĭ-ă) [G. *mēn*, month, + *mētra*, uterus, + *rēgnunai*, to burst forth]. Abnormal hemorrhagic condition of uterus, esp. bet. menstrual periods.

Cure of this condition has been effected by correcting body weight and basal metabolic rate, and by using blood from lactating amenorrheic women.

menopause (měn'ō-pawz) [G. *mēn*, month, + *pausis*, cessation]. That period which marks the permanent cessation of menstrual activity.

Ceases bet. 45 to 50 years of life. The menses may stop suddenly or there may be a decreased flow each month until there is a final cessation, or the interval bet. periods may be lengthened until complete cessation is accomplished.

Average Age of Women at Menopause

Per Cent	Age
12	36-40
26	41-45
41	46-50
15	51-55

Six per cent had their menopause before 35 or after 55.

SYM: The menopause is usually accompanied by elevation of blood pressure, hot and cold flashes, feeling of weakness, and, in some cases, marked mental derangements.

In women of *plethoric* type symptoms are those of congestion—flushes of heat, rush of blood to face and head, uterine and other hemorrhages, leukorrhea, and even diarrhea. In *chlorotic* subjects, sallow complexion, semichlorotic skin, weak pulse and various other indications of debility. In *nervous* subjects, the overanxious look, the terror-stricken expression as if apprehensive of seeing some frightful object, the face bedewed with perspiration, and remarkable tendency to hysteria are symptoms often met.

The unusual development of hair on chin and lip generally coincides with final cessation of menses; so does an unusual power of generating heat, indicated by throwing off clothing and opening doors and windows. There is often rheumatism of shoulder or thigh or swelling of joints. Often nymphomania is present. May be ulcers and polypi of uterus and carcinoma of this organ and of the breasts.

Anatomically there is marked atrophy of the external pudendi, and atrophy of the uterus, tubes and ovaries; the vagina becomes conical in shape, and the mucous membrane becomes smooth and atrophic.

NP & TREATMENT: Constitutional as indicated by special symptoms of the case. An utter change of surroundings where possible. As many restful vacations as possible. Great care in diet, exercise, clothing, etc. Plain, simple food, consisting for most part of vegetables, fruits, fresh beef and mutton. All stimulating food and beverages should be avoided. Daily exercise in open air, riding or walking; clothing warm, comfortable and adapted to the season. Frequent bathing and friction of skin; absence of worry.

Estrogen in large doses, estradiol dipropionate, thyroid extract and sedatives have been used effectively in this condition. Large doses of female sex hormone may loosen painful or stiff shoulders and thighs. Ovarian therapy and the use of bromides. SYN: *change of life, climacteric*.

RS: *involution, menses, menstruation, sexual involution*.

menophania (men-ō-fa'nĭ-ă) [G. *mēn*, month, + *phainein*, to show]. First appearance of the menses at puberty.

menoplania (men-ō-plā'nĭ-ă) [" + *planē*, a wandering]. Vicarious menstruation; menstruation through other than the normal outlet, as through the nose.

menorrhagia (men-ō-ra'jĭ-ă) [" + *rēgnunai*, to burst forth]. Excessive bleeding at the time of a menstrual period, either in number of days or amount of blood or both.

ETIOL: *Endocrine Disturbances*: Pituitary gland, thyroid and ovary. *General Systemic Diseases*: Hypertension, diabetes mellitus, blood dyscrasias, chronic nephritis. *Malpositions of the Uterus*: Retroversion and retroflexion. *New Growths of the Uterus*: Particularly fibroids of the intramural and submucous types, adenomyosis of the uterus, fibrosis of the uterus with hyperplastic changes of the endometrium. *Conditions of the Cervix Uteri*: Erosions, polypi. *Inflammations in the Pelvis*: Acute salpingitis, acute metritis, acute endometritis, chronic metritis and endometritis.

NP & TREATMENT: The specific treatment of this condition depends upon the direct etiological factor. In urgent cases place patient on hard mattress in cool room and elevate the hips. If this does not diminish the flow, apply piece of ice to mouth of uterus. This failing, bandage extremities as described under hemorrhage (postpartum) or plug vagina.

During attack all food and drink should be taken moderately cold. Avoid stimulating food and beverages. Careful constitutional treatment should be given to remove cause of the disorder. Menorrhagia can be curtailed temporarily by the use of ecbolics (fluid extract of ergot and hydrastis). In cases in which the bleeding occurs near the

menorrhalgia   M-23   **menstruation**

time of the menopause, the use of radium or the removal of the uterus by either abdominal or vaginal hysterectomy.

menorrhalgia (men-or-ral'jĭ-ă) [G. *mēn*, month, + *roia*, flow, + *algos*, pain]. Painful menstruation. SYN: *dysmenorrhea*.

menorrhea (měn-or-ē'ă) [" + *roia*, flow]. 1. Normal menstruation. 2. Free or profuse menstruation. SYN: *menorrhagia*.

menoschesis (men-os'kĕ-sis) [G. *mēn*, month, + *schesis*, retention]. Suppression of menses.

menosepsis (men-o-sep'sĭs) [" + *sēpsis*, putrefaction]. Septic poisoning from retained menstrual discharge.

menostasis (men-os'tă-sĭs) [" + *stasis*, a halting]. Suppression of menses. SYN: *amenorrhea.**

menostaxis (men-ō-stak'sĭs) [" + *staxis*, dripping]. Prolonged menstruation.

menotox'in [" + *toxikon*, poison]. A toxin which develops in women during menstruation.

menoxenia (men-ok-se'nĭ-ă) [" + *xenos*, strange]. Abnormal menstruation.

menses (men'sēz) [L. pl. of *mensis*, month]. Monthly flow of bloody fluid from the uterus; catamenial flow.

menstrua (men'strŭ-ă) (pl. of *menstruum*) [L.]. The menses.

menstrual (men'strŭ-ăl) [L. *menstruāre*, to discharge the menses]. Pert. to menstruation. SYN: *catamenial*.

   m. cycle. Interval, averaging about 28 days, from 1 menstrual period to another in which uterus undergoes changes.

   It is divided into 4 periods: 1. Postmenstrual or period of recuperation, 4-5 days. 2. Proliferative or estrogen phase, 14 days. 3. Premenstrual, secretory or progestin phase, 5 days. 4. Menstrual or period of dismantling, 4 days.

menstruant (men'strŭ-ănt) [L. *menstruāre*, to discharge the menses]. 1. In the condition of menstruating. 2. One who menstruates.

menstruate (men'strŭ-āt) [L. *menstruāre*]. To discharge menses.

menstruation (měn-strŭ-ā'shŭn) [L. *menstruāre*, to discharge the menses]. Periodic flow of blood from the uterus, containing disintegrated structural elements of the endometrium at more or less regular intervals throughout the active sexual life of women.

Menstruation is brought about by hormones originating in the ant. pituitary body, graafian follicle and corpus luteum. It has its onset at puberty (11-15 years of age), having a definite *habitus*, occurring most often at 28-, 30-, 26- and 21-day intervals and lasting anywhere from 3 to 7 days.

The blood originates in the endometrium, where definite cyclic changes can be noted, so that the endometrium can be divided into 4 histological stages.

POSTMENSTRUAL STAGE OR PERIOD OF REPAIR AND REGENERATION: About 5 days during which the mucous membrane returns to its normal state.

PROLIFERATIVE OR ESTROGEN PHASE: Period of about 14 days in which estrogen is secreted by corpus luteum and follicle matures and ovulation occurs. There is proliferation and differentiation of cells of membrana granulosa.

PREMENSTRUAL STAGE: About 5 days before menstruation, when the mucous membrane becomes congested with blood and thickens.

MENSTRUATION OR PERIOD OF DEGENERATION: A period of about 4 days during which capillary hemorrhage takes place and epithelium of the mucous membrane is expelled. During menstruation, from one-half to two-thirds of the endometrium is extruded.

Normal menstruation should not be accompanied by any pain, but there is usually menstrual molimen, consisting of feeling of fullness in the pelvis, bearing down sensation, fullness in the breasts, slight nausea and headache, and occasionally herpes menstrualis or other skin eruptions. When the pain is severe enough to require the use of analgesic drugs there is dysmenorrhea. As a rule, the menstrual blood does not coagulate, though there may be very small clots.

The total amount of blood lost in a

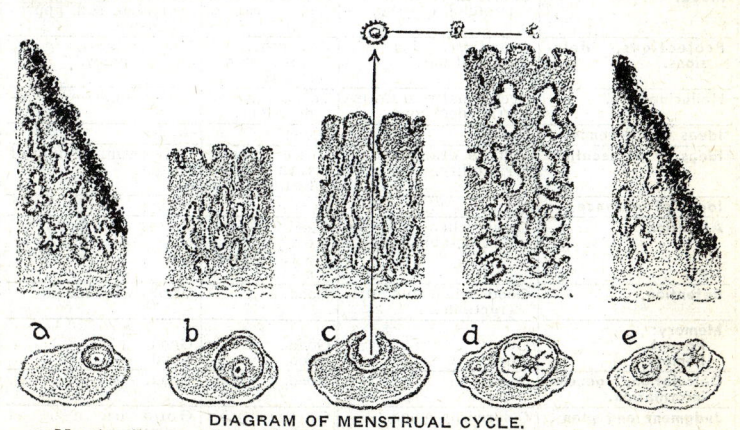

DIAGRAM OF MENSTRUAL CYCLE.
a. Menstruation graafian follicle beginning to develop. b. Endometrium growing and follicle ripening. c. Endometrium in rest stage. Follicle ruptures and sets ovum free about fourteenth day (ovulation). d. Endometrium in premenstrual or pregravid stage. Corpus luteum developing. Ovum degenerating. e. Corpus luteum degenerating. Menstruation recurs.

normal period is about 2 oz. In terms of pads used during a normal period, 20 is the maximum number. Beyond that number the condition is menorrhagic.

Safe period judged to be period bet. 18th day after menstruation up to the next period and first 9 days following it, including the flow, in a 28-day cycle. Not considered altogether safe.

m., anovulatory. Menstruation with no pregravid endometrium, or corpus luteum. Occurs in a small number of women, esp. sterile ones. The bleeding arises from a proliferative type of endometrium instead of a pregravid or secretory type.

m., climacteric. First menstruation.

m., ovular. A true menstruation resulting from the action of ovarian hormones, estrogen, or progesterone upon the endometrium.

m., vicarious. Menstruation from other than the uterine passage. SEE: *atopomenorrhea.*

menstruous (men'strŭ-ŭs) [L. *menstruāre*, to discharge the menses]. Rel. to menstruation.

menstruum (men'strŭ-um) [L. menstrual fluid; it was believed that this fluid had solvent qualities]. A solvent; a medium. SEE: *vehicle.*

mensuration (men-sŭ-rā'shŭn) [L. *mensurātiō*, a measuring]. The process of measuring. SEE: *chest, measure.*

mentagra (men-tag'ra) [L. *mentum*, chin, + G. *agra*, seizure]. Inflammation of the hair follicles, esp. of the beard, with pustular eruptions. SYN: *sycosis.*

mentagrophyton (men-tag-rof'ĭ-ton) [" + " + *phyton*, a plant]. The fungus which is the cause of sycosis.

men'tal [L. *mens, ment-,* mind; *mentum,* chin]. 1. Rel. to the mind. 2. Rel. to the chin.

RS: *acatalepsy, cataleptic, cataphrenia, cenopsychic, cerebrasthenia, cerebropsychosis.*

m. age. Age of a person mentally, determined by a group of mental tests. SEE: *age, mental; Binet.*

m. apparatus. A term that includes the ego, the id, and the super ego.

m. deficiency. May be due to following causes: Postinfectional, posttraumatic (natal and postnatal), epilepsy, endocrine disorders, growths, prenatal influences, undiagnosed causes.

m. fog. Clouding of consciousness.

m. hygiene. Science of maintaining healthy mental and emotional responses and preventing development of insanity and neurosis.

m. status. A chart of various mental

Mental Status Chart

Mental Status	Manic	Depressive	Agitated-Depression
General attitude and behavior.	Overactive, overproductive, prankish, playful, frequently abusive and destructive, sometimes assaultive.	Slow—retarded and feels depressed.	Agitated, restless, appears depressed, hair pulling, picking at the body.
Talk.	Excess of talk, rhyming, punning, flight of ideas, clang association.	Slow, retarded slowness of thinking.	Agitated, complaining —tendency to harp.
Orientation.	Correct, misidentification.	Correct.	Correct.
Mood.	Cheerful, elated, irritable if crossed.	Depressed, sad, downhearted, blue.	Anxious, gloomy, depressed, sad, apprehensive.
Projections, delusions.	Grandiose, boastful, pretentious.	Unworthiness, guilt, inadequacy.	Unworthiness, guilt, inadequacy.
Hallucinations.	Occasionally to dramatize delusions.	To dramatize delusions.	To dramatize delusions.
Ideas of reference.	None.	None.	None.
Ideas of persecution.	Mild to dramatize irritability.	None except with guilty feeling.	Only with a feeling of guilt.
Ideas of influence.	None.	None.	None.
Attention.	Good when not too distractable.	Good when not occupied with depression.	Varies with mood.
Retention.	Good when not distractable.	Good.	Varies with mood.
Memory: Recent. Remote.	Good. Good.	Good. Good.	Good. Good.
Calculation, general information.	Good.	Good.	Good.
Judgment and plans.	Colored by mood.	Colored by mood.	Good on neutral topics.
Insight, recognition, understanding.	Good. May be good.	Good. May be good.	Good. May be good.
Prognosis.	Good.	Good.	Good.

Mental Status Chart (*Continued*)

Mental Status	Schizophrenia	Paranoid	Organic	Delirium
General attitude and behavior.	Indifferent, apathetic, negativistic, cataleptic, bizarre, impulsive, stereotyped activity, unexplained smiling, outbursts of laughter.	Superior, intellectually, personality remains intact, alert, sensitive, suspicious.	General slump in deportment and personal appearance.	Restless, picking at bedclothes.
Talk.	Mute, blocking, high flown, grandiloquent word salad.	Intelligent, clever, alert, aggressive, defends delusions.	May or may not change.	Drift.
Orientation.	Actually correct, double orientation.	Correct.	Disorientated.	Cloudy, disorientated.
Mood.	No dominant change, episodically irritable, morose, silly.	Suspicious, alert.	Mild, euphoric.	Variable, fear, jocose, euphoria depressed.
Projections, delusions.	Persecution, bodily changes, passivity feeling.	Delusions of persecution are prominent. Organized, systematized.	Grandeur.	May be present, not fixed.
Hallucinations.	Prominent.	To dramatize delusions.	None.	Variable.
Ideas of reference.	Prominent.	Prominent.	None.	Absent.
Ideas of persecution.	Attitude of suspicion.	See delusions.	None.	None.
Ideas of influence.	External, occult forces, hypnotism.	None.	Some.	None.
Attention.	Diverted by dreaminess.	Good.	Unusually good.	Poor, momentary.
Retention.	Good.	Good.	Somewhat impaired.	Poor.
Memory: Recent. Remote.	Good. Good.	Good. Good.	Poor. Good.	Poor. Good.
Calculation, general information.	Good.	Good.	Apt to be reduced.	Temporarily disturbed.
Judgment and plans.	Good except in ambitions.	Affected by delusional content.	Impaired.	Good if examinable.
Insight, recognition, understanding.	Good except in ambitions.	Lacking.	Lacking.	Usually present.
Prognosis.	Poor.	Poor.	Remission with treatment.	Always good.

states appears on pages M-24 and M-25.

men′tha [L.]. Mint.
   m. piperita. Peppermint.
   m. pulegium. Pennyroyal.
   m. viridis. Spearmint.

men′thol. USP. Colorless crystals obtained from oil of peppermint or other mint oils.
   ACTION AND USES: Counterirritant, as an antiseptic and as a stimulant for inflamed mucous membranes, esp. for nose and throat.
   DOSAGE: 1 gr. (0.06 Gm.).

mentim′eter [L. *mens, ment-*, mind, + G. *metron*, measure]. Measurement of mental capacity.

ment′ism [" + G. *ismos*, state of]. Involuntary creation of mental images.

mentula (men′tŭ-lă) [L.]. The penis.

mentulagra (men-tŭ-lag′ră) [L. *mentula*,

mentulate M-26 **mercury salicylate**

penis, + G. *agra*, seizure]. Painful involuntary erection of the penis, sometimes curved. SYN: *chordee, priapism*.
mentulate (men'tū-lāt) [L. *mentula*, penis]. Possessing a large penis.
mentulomania (měn″tū-lō-mā'nĭ-ă) [" + G. *mania*, madness]. Mental state characterized by addiction to masturbation.
men'tum [L.]. The chin. SYN: *genion*.
mephit'ic [L. *mephitis*, foul exhalation]. Noxious, foul, as a poisonous odor.
 m. air or gas. Carbon dioxide.
meralgia (mer-al'jĭ-ă) [G. *měros*, thigh, + *algos*, pain]. Neuralgia of the thigh. SEE: *sciatica*.
 m. paresthet'ica. Affection of nerves of the thigh causing itching, tingling, pain, burning, and sometimes numbness.
merbaphen (měr'băf-ěn). USP. A compound of mercury of about 33% mercury.
 USES: As a diuretic.
 DOSAGE: From 1-2 cc. of a 10% solution, intramuscularly, or intravenously. Give first a tolerance test of ½ cc.
 INCOMPATIBILITIES: Acids and ferric chloride.
Mercier's bar or barrier (mer-se-ā'). A curved fold at neck of bladder, forming post. margin of trigonum vesicae.
mercupurin (měr-kū″pū-rĭn) [L. *mercurius*, mercury, + *purum*, pure, + *uricum*, uric acid]. A proprietary diuretic.
mercurial (mer-kū'rĭ-al) [L. *mercurialis*, pert. to mercury]. 1. Pert. to mercury. 2. A substance containing mercury.
 m. palsy. Paralysis induced by mercurial poisoning.
 m. rash. Rash caused by application of mercurial preparations locally.
mercurialism (mer-kū″rĭ-al-ĭzm) [" + G. *ismos*, state of]. Chronic poisoning by mercury seen as a result of continuous administration of mercury.
 Also occurs in workmen who labor on the metal, or inhale its vapors.
 SYM: Soreness of gums and loosening of teeth; increased salivation; fetor of breath; griping, and diarrhea.
mercurialization (mer-kū″rĭ-al-ĭ-zā'shŭn) [L. *mercurius*, mercury]. Condition of influencing with mercury.
mercurialized (měr-kū'rĭ-a-līzd) [L. *mercurius*, mercury]. 1. Impregnated with mercury. 2. Influenced by or treated with mercury.
mercuric (mer-ku'rik) [L. *mercurius*, mercury]. Rel. to bivalent mercury.
 m. chloride (HgCl$_2$). A common compound of mercury formerly used in the household as an antiseptic, as a douche, and to destroy household pests.
 One part to 1000 of water is used to free the hands or skin from bacteria. This solution used in strength of 1:2000 or 1:4000 may be used for wound irrigation. It should be remembered that this disinfectant coagulates albumen, that it corrodes metal instruments, and causes local dermatitis. No metallic instrument should ever be placed in contact with mercuric chloride. Since it has been put up in blue coffin-shaped tablets in a notched bottle, poisoning has been less common.
 POISONING: SYM: *Acute*: Those of any severe gastrointestinal irritation, with pain, cramping, constriction of the throat, vomiting, and a metallic taste in the mouth. Stronger solution causes a white coating due to coagulation. Abdominal pain may be so severe as to cause fainting, bloody diarrhea, bloody vomitus, scanty urine, prostration, convulsions and unconsciousness.
 SYM: *Chronic*: Bad breath, loosening of teeth, fever, urinary difficulties, nausea, diarrhea, sore tongue, paralyses, weakness and death.
 F. A. TREATMENT: Evacuate stomach, wash out with milk. Administration of sodium formaldehyde sulfoxylate given by mouth and intravenously reduces mercuric salts to insoluble salts of low toxicity. This process also takes place in the tissues. Given intravenously, its effects last for several hours. SEE: *nephrosis*.
 m. oxide (HgO). A powder, usually yellow in color. Used in ointments. When red, it is used to dress sores in syphilis.
mercurin (mer'ku-rĭn). The sodium salt of an organic mercurial compound, containing about 40% mercury.
 USES: As a powerful diuretic, contraindicated in chronic nephritis and renal disease.
 DOSAGE: In the form of cocoa butter suppository, containing 0.5 Gm.
mercurochrome (mer-kū″ro-krōm) [L. *mercurius*, mercury, + G. *chrōma*, color]. A compound containing about 23% mercury, used as a germicide in 1 to 4% solution.
mer'curol [L. *mercurius*, mercury]. A mercuric acid compound used in infections of the genitourinary tract and the conjunctiva.
 DOSAGE: ½-2 gr. (0.03-0.12 Gm.).
mercurous (mer-kū'rus, mer'ku-rus) [L. *mercurius*]. Rel. to monovalent mercury.
 m. chloride (HgCl) (Calomel). USP. This is a heavy white powder used in small doses in medicine as a laxative.
 It is used in powder form as an application in ulcers and skin rashes.
 DOSAGE: Mild, as laxative, in fractional doses, 2½ gr. (0.15 Gm.).
 POISONING: SYM: Salivation, abdominal discomfort, and diarrhea.
 F. A. TREATMENT: SEE: *mercuric chloride*.
 INCOMPATIBILITIES: Iodoform, soluble iodides, soluble hydroxides.
mercury (mer'ku-rĭ) (quicksilver) [L. *mercurius*]. SYMB: Hg. A silvery liquid element most commonly used in thermometers, barometers, dentistry and medicine. When heated, gives off poisonous fumes.
 POISONING: SYM: In large doses, increased salivation, abdominal cramps, interference with kidney function, etc.
 TREATMENT: SEE: *mercuric chloride*.
 m., ammoniated. USP. White precipitate.
 USES: Externally, as an antiseptic in certain skin conditions, as acne, psoriasis, etc.
 DOSAGE: Externally, 5 to 10% ointment.
 m. bichloride. USP. Corrosive sublimate.
 USES: Germicide.
 INCOMPATIBILITIES: Albumen, alkalies, borax, etc.
 SEE: *mercuric chloride, nephrosis*.
 m. iodide, red. USP. Mercury biniodide.
 USES: Alterative, germicide.
 DOSAGE: Average, 1/15 gr. (0.004 Gm.).
 m. iodide, yellow. USP. Protiodide of mercury.
 USES: Same as for mercury iodide, red.
 DOSAGE: Average, 1/6 gr. (0.01 Gm.).
 INCOMPATIBILITIES: Soluble iodides.
 m. mass. USP. Blue mass.
 USES: Cathartic.
 DOSAGE: 5 gr. (0.3 Gm.).
 m. salicylate. USP.

mercury succinimide   M-27   **mesenteritis**

USES: Antiluetic, antiseptic.
DOSAGE: Average, 1 gr. (0.06 Gm.), intramuscularly.
m. succinimide.
USES: Same as for m. salicylate.
DOSAGE: Subcutaneously, mainly, 1/6 gr. (0.01 Gm.).
m. vapor arc. An electric discharge through mercury vapor.
mere (mēr) [G. *meros*, part]. One of the sections into which a zygote splits.
meridrosis (mer-id-rō′sĭs) [G. *meros*, part, + *idrōsis*, perspiration]. Local perspiration.
merinthophobia (mĕr-ĭn-thō-fō′bĭ-ă) [G. *mērinthos*, a cord, + *phobos*, fear]. Morbid fear of being tied.
Merismopedia (mer-is-mō-pē′dĭ-ă) [G. *merisma*, division, + *pedion*, plane]. A genus of bacteria including all micrococci which divide into 2 planes.
merispore (mer′ĭ-spōr) [G. *meros*, a part, + *sporos*, a seed]. A secondary spore resulting from the division of another spore.
mero- [G.]. Combining form meaning *the thigh*.
meroblastic (mer-ō-blast′ĭk) [G. *meros*, a part, + *blastos*, germ]. Pert. to a yolk in an ovum which contains nutritive material as well as the germinal protoplasm with cleavage taking place only in the protoplasm. OPP: *holoblastic*.
merocele (mer′ō-sēl) [G. *mēros*, thigh, + *kēlē*, hernia]. Hernia of the thigh.
merocoxalgia (mer′′ō-koks-al′jĭ-ă) [" + L. *coxa*, hip, + G. *algos*, pain]. Painful condition of the thigh and hip.
merocrine (mer′o-krīn) [G. *meros*, a part, + *krinein*, to secrete]. Pert. to a secretory gland, part of whose cells produce secretions without injury to the balance of the cells. OPP: *holocrine*, *q.v.*
meroergasia (mĕr′′ō-ĕr-gă′zĭ-ă) [" + *ergasia*, work]. Partial mental disorder with symptoms of emotional instability. SEE: *holergastic*.
merogenesis (mĕr′′ō-jen′ĕ-sĭs) [" + *genesis*, production]. Multiplication or reproduction by segmentation.
merology (mer-ol′ō-jĭ) [" + *logos*, study of]. Anatomy of the elementary tissues.
meromicrosomia (mĕr′′ō-mī′′krō-sō′mĭ-ă) [" + *mikros*, small, + *sōma*, body]. Abnormal smallness of some part or structure of the body.
meronecrosis (mer′′ō-nĕk-rō′sĭs) [" + *nekros*, dead]. Necrosis of cells.
meroparesthesia (mer′′ō-păr-ĕs-thē′sĭ-ă) [G. *mēros*, limb, + *para*, beside, + *aisthēsis*, sensation]. Change in the extremities' tactile reactions.
meropia (mer-o′pĭ-ă) [G. *meros*, part, + *ōps*, vision]. Partial blindness.
merorrhachischisis (mĕr-or-ră-kis′kĭ-sis) [" + *rachis*, spine, + *schisis*, fissure]. Fissure of a portion of the spinal cord.
meroscope (me′rō-skōp) [G. *meros*, part, + *skopein*, to examine]. Device used in performing meroscopy.
meroscopy (mĕr-os′kō-pĭ) [" + *skopein*, to examine]. Auscultation of the separate parts of the cardiac cycle.
merosmia (mĕr-os′mĭ-ă) [" + *osmē*, odor]. Inability to detect certain odors.
merosystolic (mĕr-ō-sĭs-tol′ĭk) [" + *systolē*, a contraction]. Rel. to a portion of the systole.
merotomy (mer-ot′o-mē) [" + *tomē*, incision]. Division into sections or segments.
merozoite (mer-ō-zō′ĭt) [" + *zōon*, animal]. A spore formed in schizogenous reproduction of protozoa.

mersalyl (mer′sal-ĭl). A complex mercurial preparation in the form of a white crystalline powder, containing 39.6% mercury.
USES: Chiefly as a diuretic.
DOSAGE: 8 ℳ (0.5 cc.) of a 10% solution, intravenously, or intramuscularly (never subcutaneously), at intervals of 3-5 days, as may be required. Initial dose should be 0.5 cc. as a tolerance test.
merthiolate (mer-thī′ō-lāt). An organic combination containing about 50% mercury, and less toxic than bichloride, used as a disinfectant in solutions of 1:5000 to 1:1000, aqueous, or in the form of a tincture, as an ointment, 1:2000. *For ophthalmic use*, 1:5000 ointment, or 1:10,000 aqueous.
Méry's glands (ma-rē′). Two bulbourethral glands. SYN: *Cowper's glands*.
mesad (mes′ăd) [G. *mesos*, middle, + L. *ad*, toward]. Toward a median point.
mesal (mes′ăl) [G. *mesos*, middle]. In a middle line or plane.
mesameboid (mes-ă-mē′boid) [" + *amoibē*, change, + *eidos*, shape]. A wandering cell of the mesoderm.
mesaortitis (mĕs-ā-or-tī′tĭs) [" + *aortē*, aorta, + *-itis*, inflammation]. Inflammation of the middle aortic coat.
mesaraic, mesareic (mes-ar-ā′ĭk, -e′ĭk) [" + *araia*, belly]. Rel. to the mesentery. SYN: *mesenteric*.
mesarteritis (mĕs-ar-tĕr-ī′tĭs) [" + *artēria*, artery, + *-itis*, inflammation]. Inflammation of the tunica media or middle coat of an artery.
mesaticephalic (mĕs-ăt′′ĭ-sef-al′ĭk) [G. *mesatos*, medium, + *kephalē*, head]. Having a skull with a length-breadth index of 75-80 degrees, or of medium length.
mesatipellic, mesatipelvic (mĕs-ăt′′ĭ-pĕl′-lĭk, -pel′vĭk) [" + *pellis*, pelvis]. Having a pelvis with an index bet. 90 and 95 degrees.
mesectic (mĕs-ek′tĭk) [G. *mesos*, middle, + *echein*, to have]. Using up a normal amount of oxygen. SEE: *mionectic*, *pleonectic*.
mesencephal (mĕs-ĕn′sĕf-ăl) [G. *mesos*, middle, + *egkephalos*, brain]. Middle area of brain. SYN: *mesencephalon*, *midbrain*.
mesencephalon (mes-en-sef′al-on) [G. *mesos*, middle, + *egkephalos*, brain]. The midbrain consisting of the corpora quadrigemina, the crura cerebri, and the aqueduct of Sylvius.
mesenchyma (mes-en′kim-ă) [" + *egchyma*, infusion]. Portion of embryonic mesoderm that produces connective tissue.
mesenter′ic [" + *enteron*, intestine]. Pert. to the mesentery.
mesenteriolum (mes-en-ter-ĭ-ō′lum) [L. *mesenteriŏlum*, little mesentery]. A small mesentery, as that of a diverticulum of the intestine.
mesenteriopexy (mes-en-ter′ĭ-ō-peks-ĭ) [G. *mesos*, middle, + *enteron*, intestine, + *pēxis*, fixation]. Fixation of a torn mesentery.
mesenteriorrhaphy (mes′′en-ter-ĭ-or′ra-fĭ) [" + " + *raphē*, a sewing]. Suturing of the mesentery.
mesenteriplication (mĕs′′ĕn-tĕr-ĭ-plĭ-kā′-shun) [" + " + L. *plicāre*, to fold]. Taking tucks in the mesentery surgically.
mesenteritis (mes′′ĕn-tĕr-ī′tĭs) [" + " + *-itis*, inflammation]. Inflamed condition of the mesentery.

mesenteron (mes-en′ter-on) [G. *mesos*, middle, + *enteron*, intestine]. Middle portion of the embryonic digestive tract.

mesentery (mes′en-ter-ĭ) [" + *enteron*, intestine]. A peritoneal fold, connecting the intestine with the post. abdominal wall.

m., proper. That of the small intestine.

Mesocolon is the name given to that of the colon; *mesocecum*, that of the cecum, and *mesorectum*, that of the rectum.

mesiad (mes′ĭ-ad) [" + L. *ad*, toward]. Toward the middle line. SYN: *mesad*.

mesial (me′sĭ-ăl) [G. *mesos*, middle]. Toward the middle line, esp. of the dental arch. SEE: *median line*.

mesion (mes′ĭ-on) [G. *mesos*, middle]. The imaginary plane dividing the body into right and left symmetric halves. SYN: *meson*.

mesiris (mes-ī′ris) [" + *iris*, iris]. Middle portion of the iris.

mesmeric (mes-mer′ĭk). Rel. to or induced by hypnotism; fascinating.

mesmerism (mes′mer-izm). Originally the theory of Mesmer, it now means therapeutics employing hypnotism or hypnotic suggestion.

mesoaortitis (mes″o-ā-or-tī′tis) [G. *mesos*, middle, + *aortē*, artery, + -*itis*, inflammation]. Inflamed condition of aortic middle coat. SYN: *mesaortitis*.

mesoappendicitis (mes-ō-ap-pen-dĭ-sī′tis) [" + L. *appendix*, an appendage, + G. -*itis*, inflammation]. Inflamed condition of the mesoappendix.

mesoappendix (mes″ō-ap-pen′dĭks) [" + L. *appendix*, an appendage]. Mesentery of the vermiform appendix.

mesoblast (mes′o-blast) [" + *blastos*, germ]. Embryonic middle layer of the blastoderm, bet. the hypoblast and epiblast from which arise the bone, skin, connective tissue, muscles, internal genitalia and excretory organs. SYN: *mesoderm*. SEE: *acroblast*.

mesobronchitis (mes″ō-bron-kī′tis) [G. *mesos*, middle, + *brogchos*, windpipe, + -*itis*, inflammation]. Inflammation of the middle layer of the bronchi.

mesocardia (mes-ō-kar′dĭ-ă) [" + *kardia*, heart]. Location of the heart in the middle line of the thorax, being a normal position in fetal stage, but a malposition in life.

mesocardium (mes-ō-kar′dĭ-um) [" + *kardia*, heart]. 1. Portion of mediastinal pleura attached to pericardium. 2. Embryonic membrane connecting the heart with the body wall and the intestine.

mesocecum (mes-ō-se′kŭm) [G. *mesos*, middle, + L. *caecum*, blind gut]. Mesentery attaching the cecum.

mesocele (mes′ō-sēl) [" + *koilia*, hollow]. Sylvian aqueduct in the brain.

mesocephalic (mes-ō-sef-al′ĭk) [" + *kephalē*, head]. 1. Pert. to the midbrain. 2. Having a medium sized head.

mesocephalon (mĕs-ō-sef′ă-lon) [" + *kephalē*, head]. The midbrain.

mesocolic (mes-ō-kol′ĭk) [" + *kōlon*, colon]. Concerning the mesocolon.

mesocolon (mĕs-ō-kō′lon) [" + *kōlon*, colon]. Mesentery connecting colon with post. abdominal wall.

mesocolopexy (mĕs″ō-kŏ′lō-peks-ĭ) [G. *mesos*, middle, + *kōlon*, colon, + *pēxis*, fixation]. The taking of tucks in the mesocolon and then suturing it to make it shorter. SYN: *mesocoloplication*.

mesocoloplication (mĕs″ō-kō″lō-plĭ-kā′shun) [" + " + L. *plicāre*, to fold]. The operation of shortening the mesocolon by taking a tuck in it.

mes′ocord [" + *chordē*, cord]. A portion of umbilical cord attached to placenta.

mesoderm (mĕs′ō-derm) [" + *derma*, skin]. The middle layer of cells in the germinal membrane of an embryo. SYN: *mesoblast*, q.v. SEE: *ectoderm*, *entoderm*.

mesodmitis (mĕs-od-mī′tis) [G. *mesodmē*, partition, + -*itis*, inflammation]. Inflamed condition of the mediastinum. SYN: *mediastinitis*.

mesoduodenum (mĕs″ō-dū-ō-dē′nŭm) [" + L. *duodeni*, twelve]. Mesentery connecting duodenum to abdominal wall.

mesogastric (mĕs-ō-gas′trĭk) [" + *gastēr*, belly]. 1. Pert. to umbilical region. 2. Pert. to the mesogastrium.

mesogastrium (mĕs″ō-gas′trĭ-ŭm) [G. *mesos*, middle, + *gastēr*, belly]. 1. The umbilical region. The part of the mesentery of the embryo attached to the primitive stomach.

mesoglia (mĕs-og′lĭ-ă) [" + *glia*, glue]. Neuroglia tissue cell of moderate size. SYN: *oligodendroglia*.

mesognathic (mĕs-og-nā′thĭk) [" + *gnathos*, jaw]. Having a gnathic index bet. 98 and 103.

mesognathion (mĕs-og-nā′thĭ-on) [" + *gnathos*, jaw]. The intermaxillary or premaxillary bone.

mesohyloma (mes-ō-hī-lō′mă) [" + *ylē*, matter, + -*ōma*, tumor]. Tumor derived from the mesothelium.

mesoileum (mes-ō-il′ē-ŭm) [" + L. *ileum*, from G. *eilein*, to twist]. Mesentery of the ileum.

mesojejunum (mes-ō-jĕ-jū′nŭm) [" + L. *jejunum*, empty]. Mesentery of the jejunum.

mesol′obus [" + L. *lobos*, lobe]. Corpus callosum.

mesometritis (mes-o-me-trī′tis) [G. *mesos*, middle, + *mētra*, uterus, + -*itis*, inflammation]. Inflammation of the uterine musculature. SYN: *myometritis*.

mesometrium (mes-o-me′trĭ-um) [" + *mētra*, uterus]. 1. The uterine musculature. 2. BNA. The broad ligament below the mesovarium.

mesomorph (mes′ō-morf) [" + *morphē*, form]. A well-proportioned person of medium height. SEE: *hypermorph*, *hypomorph*.

mesom′ula [" + *sōma*, body]. An early embryonic stage when there is a mass of mesenchyma enclosed in mesoderm and entoderm.

meson (mes′on) [G. *mesos*, middle]. Imaginary plane dividing body into symmetric halves. SYN: *mesion*.

mesonephric (mes-ō-nef′rĭk) [" + *nephros*, kidney]. Rel. to the mesonephron.

m. duct. Embryonic duct which becomes *vas deferens* in the male and rudimentary in the female. SYN: *wolffian duct*.

mesonephron, mesonephros (mes-ō-nef′ron, -ros) [" + *nephros*, kidney]. Embryonic excretory organ. SYN: *wolffian body*.

mesoneuritis (me-sō-nū-rī′tis) [" + *neuron*, nerve, + -*itis*, inflammation]. Inflammation of the substance of a nerve or of its lymphatics.

mesoömentum (mes″ō-ō-men′tŭm) [" + L. *omentum*]. Mesentery of the omentum.

mesopexy (mes′ō-peks-ĭ) [" + *pēxis*, fixation]. Operation of shortening the mesentery by taking a tuck in it.

mesophilic (mes-ō-fĭl′ĭk) [G. *mesos*, middle, + *philein*, to love]. Preferring moderate temperature, as some bacteria which develop best at body temperature.

mesophryon (mes-of'rĭ-on) [" + *ophrys*, eyebrow]. Midpoint in smooth space bet. the eyebrows. SEE: *glabella*.

mesopneumon (mes-ō-nū'mŏn) [" + *pneumōn*, lung]. Meeting point of 2 pleural layers at hilus of the lung.

mesorchium (mes-or'kĭ-um) [" + *orchis*, testicle]. Peritoneal fold which holds fetal testes in place.

mesorectum (měs-ō-rěk'tŭm) [" + L. *rectus*, straight]. Mesentery of the rectum.

mes″oret′ina [" + L. *retina*, from *rētē*, a net]. Middle or mosaic layer of retina.

mesoropter (mes-ō-rop'ter) [G. *mesos*, middle, + *oros*, boundary, + *optēr*, observer]. Normal eye position with muscles at rest.

mesorrhachischisis (měs″or-ră-kĭs'kĭ-sĭs) [" + *rachis*, spine, + *schisis*, cleft]. Fissure of a portion of the spinal cord. SYN: *merorrhachischisis*.

mesorrhaphy (mes-or'ră-fĭ) [" + *raphē*, a sewing]. Suture of the mesentery. SYN: *mesenteriorrhaphy*.

mesorrhine (mes'or-rīn) [" + *ris*, rin-, nose]. With a nasal index variously quoted to range anywhere bet. 47 and 53.

mesosalpinx (měs″ō-sal'pĭnks) [G. *mesos*, middle, + *salpigx*, tube]. BNA. The free margin of the upper division of the broad ligament, within which lies the oviduct.

mesoseme (mes'ō-sēm) [" + *sēma*, sign]. Possessing an orbital index bet. 83 and 90.

mesosigmoid (měs-ō-sĭg'moid) [" + *sigma*, letter S, + *eidos*, form]. Mesentery of the sigmoid flexure.

mesosternum (mes″ō-ster'nŭm) [" + *sternon*, chest]. The middle or second section of the sternum. SYN: *gladiolus*.

mesothelium (měs-ō-thē'lĭ-ŭm) [" + *thēlē*, nipple]. The layer of cells, derived from the mesoderm lining the primitive body cavity; in the adult it becomes the epithelium covering the serous membranes.

mesothenar (mes-ō-thē'nar) [" + *thenar*, palm]. The adductor pollicis muscle.

mesotropic (mes-ō-trŏp'ĭk) [" + *tropē*, a turning]. Situated in or turned toward the median plane of a body, member or organ.

mesoturbinate (měs-ō-tur'bĭ-nāt) [" + L. *turbō*, a top]. Middle turbinate bone.

mesovarium (měs-ō-va'rĭ-ŭm) [" + L. *ovarium*, ovary]. BNA. The portion of the peritoneal fold that connects the ant. border of the ovary to the post. layer of the broad ligament.

meta-, met- [G.]. Combining forms meaning *after, between, with*.

metabasis (mĕt-ab'ă-sĭs) [G. *meta*, beyond, + *basis*, a going]. Change of any kind in the progress of a disease.

metabiosis (mĕt-ă-bī-ō'sĭs) [" + *biōsis*, way of life]. Dependence of an organism for its existence upon another and giving no recompense.

metabolic (met-a-bol'ĭk) [G. *metabolē*, change]. Rel. to metabolism.

metabolimeter (mē-tab″ō-lim'e-tĕr) [" + *metron*, measure]. Device for measuring rate of basal metabolism.

metabolin (mē-tab'ō-lin) [G. *metabolē*, change]. Any metabolism product.

metab′olism [" + *ismos*, state of]. The sum of the tissue changes, physical and chemical, whereby the bodily mechanisms function, plus the mechanisms by which energy and needed substances are made available to the bodily tissues. SEE: *Table, p. M-30*.

Thus, a complete account of the metabolism of a fat would describe the chemical form in which it is transported by the blood and lymph, its storage and mobilization, the changes necessary to make it part of the body structures, and its final excretion from the body as carbon dioxide, water, or abnormal products such as acetone. Similarly, one can speak of carbohydrate metabolism, mineral metabolism, etc. Its processes consist of catabolism* and anabolism.*

END PRODUCTS: In the muscles, glycogen is decomposed whenever work is done. In each of these decompositions, many intermediate reactions occur which have proved very difficult to unravel; the *ultimate* fate of carbohydrate, however, is represented by the following reaction:

$$C_6H_{12}O_6 + 6 O_2 \rightarrow 6 CO_2 + 6 H_2O$$

This means that, given enough oxygen (6 molecules for each molecule of glucose), carbohydrates can be converted completely into carbon dioxide and water with no other residue. It also tells the chemist that for every 6 molecules of oxygen so used, 6 molecules of carbon dioxide are produced, or (since equal volumes of gases contain equal numbers of molecules) that for every liter of oxygen used up, a liter of carbon dioxide is produced. That is, when the body is oxidizing carbohydrates,

$$\frac{\text{liters of } CO_2 \text{ exhaled in 1 hour}}{\text{liters of } O_2 \text{ absorbed in 1 hour}} = 1.00$$

This equation is interesting because it shows the comparatively simple relationship that exists among the 4 substances concerned. It also enters into the considerations on which determinations of the basal metabolic rate (BMR) are based.

PHYSIOLOGICAL EXAMPLES: When benzoic acid unites with amino glycine, they form hippuric acid represented by the following equation:

$$C_6H_5COOH + H_2N(CH_2)COOH \rightarrow C_6H_5-(CO)(NH)(CH_2)COOH$$

This reaction occurs whenever the benzoic acid, which is somewhat poisonous, is taken into the body. This illustrates one way in which the body protects itself against poisons. Glycine is always available for this purpose, as it is the product of protein digestion, and is always found in circulating blood after a meal. This process represents the formation of a complex substance from a simpler one.

THE RESPIRATORY QUOTIENT: This is the numerical relationship between carbon dioxide exhaled and the oxygen absorbed in metabolism of foods, as shown in the second equation under "end products." The fraction which is the first member of the equation is called the respiratory quotient. The statement can be abbreviated by saying that "The R. Q. of carbohydrates is one."

RS: *acetone, a. bodies, amino acids, amylolopsin, amylolopsis, amylolytic, amylose, anabolism, basal, biostatics, cacochymia, catabolism, degeneration, fatty d., glutathion, waste*.

m., basal. The number of calories per 24 hours per square meter of body surface liberated by a person in muscular relaxation (but not sleep) and in the postabsorptive state. It is usually cal-

DIAGRAM OF NORMAL METABOLIC FOOD CHANGES

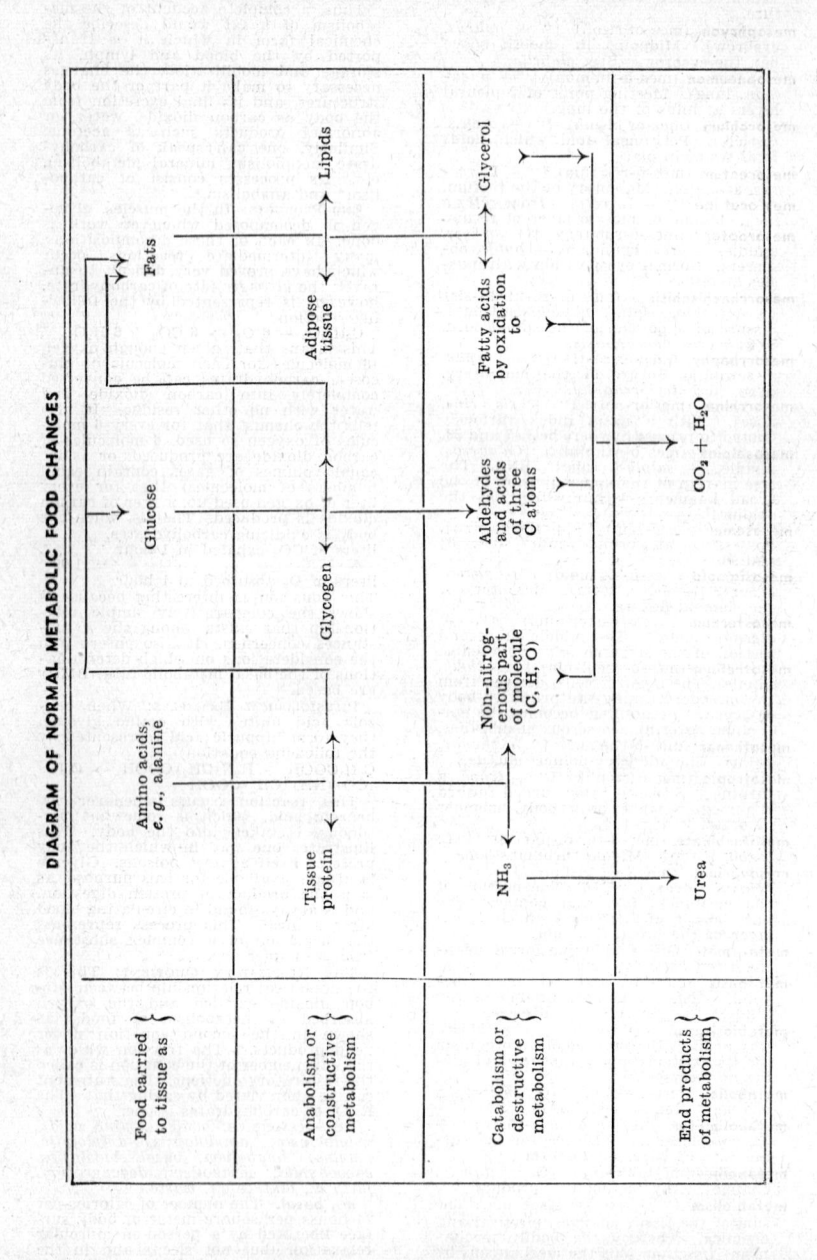

Food carried to tissue as	Amino acids, *e.g.*, alanine	Glucose		Fats
Anabolism or constructive metabolism	Tissue protein	Glycogen	Adipose tissue	Lipids
Catabolism or destructive metabolism	NH$_3$ • Non-nitrogenous part of molecule (C, H, O)	Aldehydes and acids of three C atoms	Fatty acids by oxidation to	Glycerol
End products of metabolism	Urea		$CO_2 + H_2O$	

culated from the rate of oxygen consumption, since the utilization of 1 liter of oxygen under the above conditions by normal persons on a mixed diet is accompanied by the release of 4.825 cal. of heat. Also called basal metabolism rate.

m., constructive. Transformation of matter into protoplasm. SYN: *anabolism, q.v.*

m., destructive. Decomposition of protoplasm into waste products. SYN: *catabolism, q.v.*

m. energy. M. expressed in terms of energy.

metabolite (mē-tab'ō-līt) [G. *metabolē*, change]. Any product of metabolism.

metacar'pal [G. *meta*, beyond, + *karpos*, wrist]. Pert. to the bones of the metacarpus, or bones of the hand. SEE: *skeleton.*

metacarpus (met-ă-kar'pus) [" + *karpos*, wrist]. The 5 metacarpal bones of the palm of the hand. SEE: *carpometacarpal.*

metacele (met'ă-sēl) [" + *koilia*, hollow]. Caudal portion of 4th ventricle of brain.

metachromasia, metachromatism (mĕt-ă-krō-mā'zī-ă, -krom'ă-tĭzm) [G. *meta*, change, + *chrōma*, color]. Change of color, esp. one produced by staining.

metachromatic (met"ă-krō-mat'ĭk) [" + *chrōma*, color]. Pert. to metachromatism.

m. bodies or **granules.** Granules in protoplasm which stain deeply and differently from the surrounding ones; seen in various bacteria.

metachromatin (met-ă-krōm'ă-tin) [" + *chrōma*, color]. Basophil portion of chromatin.

metachromophil (met-a-krōm'ō-fĭl) [" + " + *philein*, to love]. Not reacting normally to staining.

metachrosis (met-ă-krō'sĭs) [" + *chrōa*, color]. Change of color in animal life.

metachysis (me-tak'ĭs-ĭs) [G. *meta*, beyond, + *chysis*, effusion]. 1. Blood transfusion. 2. The introduction of any substance directly into the blood stream by mechanical means.

metacoele (met'a-sēl) [" + *koelia*, hollow]. Post. part of 4th ventricle of brain.

metacyesis (met-ă-sī-ē'sĭs) [" + *kyesis*, pregnancy]. Extrauterine gestation.

metagaster (met-ă-gas'ter) [" + *gastēr*, belly]. Permanent embryonic intestinal canal derived from the protogaster.

metagen'esis [" + *genesis*, formation]. Alternation of generation.

metagglutinin (met-ag-glū'tĭn-ĭn) [" + L. *agglutināre*, to glue]. An agglutinin in an antigen which acts on closely related organisms of the antigen.

metagrippal (met-ă-grip'al) [G. *meta*, beyond, + Fr. *grippe*, attack]. Occurring as a consequence of influenza.

metaicteric (met"ă-ik-ter'ĭk) [" + *ikteros*, jaundice]. Occurring as a consequence of jaundice.

metainfective (mĕt-ă-ĭn-fek'tĭv) [" + L. *infectiō*, an infection]. Occurring as a consequence of an infection.

metakinesis (mĕt"ă-kĭn-ē'sĭs) [" + *kinēsis*, motion]. 1. Separation of new cells in cell division. 2. Stage in cell reproduction when chromatic loop divides into 2. SYN: *metaphase, q.v.*

metal fume fever (or braziers' chills). This results from absorbing the fumes in special occupations such as welding, metal founding, torch metal cutting, and galvanizing. Zinc commonest cause of these disturbances.

SYM: Come on late. Chills, weakness, lassitude, profound thirst, followed after some hours by sweating and anorexia; occasionally there is mild inflammation of the eyes and respiratory tract.

F. A. TREATMENT: Fresh air and symptomatic treatment.

metallesthesia (mĕt"al-ĕs-thē'sĭ-ă) [G. *metallon*, metal, + *aisthēsis*, sensation]. Recognition of metals by touching them.

metallic (mē-tal'ĭk) [G. *metallon*, metal]. 1. Pert. to metal. 2. Composed of or resembling a metal.

m. tinkling. A peculiar ringing or bell-like auscultatory sound in pneumothorax over large pulmonary cavities.

metallophobia (mē"tal-ō-fō'bĭ-ă) [" + *phobos*, fear]. Psychiatric fear of metals and metallic objects and of touching them.

metalloscopy (mē-tăl-os'kō-pĭ) [" + *skopein*, to examine]. Determination of the effects of applying metals to the body, and its sensitivity to them.

metallotherapy (mē-tal-ō-ther'ă-pī) [" + *therapeia*, treatment]. Treatment by applying metals to the affected part.

metallur'gy [" + *ergon*, work]. Study and methods of using metals.

metameric (mĕt-ă-mĕr'ĭk) [G. *meta*, across, + *meros*, part]. Rel. to metamerism. SYN: *isomeric.*

metamerid (met-am'er-id) [" + *meros*, part, + *idios*, own]. A substance that is metameric.

metamerism (met-am'er-izm) [" + " + *ismos*, state of]. Isomerism when the component elements are identical and in the same ratio, but their structural arrangement in the molecule is not the same.

metamorphopsia (mĕt"ă-mor-fop'sĭ-ă) [" + *morphē*, form, + *opsis*, vision]. OPHTH: Visual distortion of objects; found in refractive errors, esp. astigmatism, retinal disease, choroiditis, detachment of retina, and tumors of retina and choroid.

metamorphosis (met-ă-mor'fō-sĭs) [G. *meta*, across, + *morphē*, form, + *-ōsis*, intensive]. A structural change during the life of an organism.

m., fatty. Fatty degeneration.

m., viscous. Collection of blood plates in thrombosis.

metanephron, metanephros (met-ă-nĕf'ron, -nef'ros) [" + *nephros*, kidney]. The post. segmental body or primitive embryonic kidney from which the kidney is developed.

metaneutrophil (met-ă-nū'trō-fĭl) [" + L. *neuter*, neither, + G. *philein*, to love]. Not reacting normally with neutral stains.

metanucleus (met-ă-nū'klē-us) [" + L. *nucleus*, kernel]. The egg nucleus after expanding beyond the germinal vesicle.

metaphase (met'ă-fāz) [G. *meta*, beyond, + *phasis*, a shining out]. The stage in cell division during which the chromatic loop divides in two. Chromosomes arrange themselves along an equatorial plate.

metaphen (met'ă-fĕn). A yellow, odorless powder containing about 56% mercury in organic combination.

USES: As a germicide, claimed to be more powerful than bichloride.

DOSAGE: As a tincture for skin sterilization, 1:200. For irrigations for delicate membranes, from 1:2500 to 1:10,000 aqueous solution.

metaphrenia (mĕt-a-frē'nĭ-ă) [G. *meta*, between, + *phrēn*, mind]. A condition in which the libido is withdrawn from its natural associations and directed to the more practical activities of life, such as gainful occupation.

metaphyllin (met"ă-fĭl'ĭn). Theophylline with ethylene diamine.
USES: As a vasodilator and diuretic.
DOSAGE: 1½ gr. (0.1 Gm.).

metaphysis (mē-tăf'ĭ-sĭs) [G. *meta*, after, + *physis*, nature]. End of a long bone's diaphysis or shaft where it meets the epiphysis.

metaplasia (met-ă-plā'zĭ-ă) [" + *plasis*, a molding]. Conversion of 1 kind of tissue into another.

metaplasm (mĕt'ă-plăzm) [" + *plasma*, a thing formed]. Reserve material present in protoplasm, esp. stored nutritive substance.

metaplastic (met-ă-plăs'tik) [" + *plastikos*, formed]. Pert. to or formed by metaplasia.

metaplexus (met-ă-plĕks'ŭs) [" + L. *plexus*, braid]. Choroid plexus of the brain's 4th ventricle.

metapneumonic (met-ă-nū-mŏn'ĭk) [G. *meta*, beyond, + *pneumonia*, lung infection]. Succeeding or as a consequence of pneumonia.

metapophysis (met-ă-pŏf'ĭ-sĭs) [" + *apo*, from, + *physis*, growth]. Mammillary process on the superior articular processes of a vertebra.

metapore (mĕt'ă-pōr) [" + *poros*, a passage]. The aperture of Magendie.

metapro'tein [" + *prōtos*, first]. Derived protein resulting from the action of acids or alkalies, in which the molecule is changed to form protein insoluble in neutral solvents but soluble in alkalies and weak acids.
Group includes the acid and alkali proteins and albumins, syntonin and albuminates. SEE: *protein*.

metapyretic (mĕt"ă-pī-rĕt'ĭk) [" + *pyretos*, fever]. Performed or occurring during fever.

metastable (met"ă-stā'bl) [G. *meta*, change, + L. *stabilis*, stable]. Changing from one condition to another; unstable.
m. solutions. Those of supersaturation in relation to amt. of dissolved substance.

metastasis (mē-tăs'tă-sĭs) [" + *stasis*, a standing]. 1. Movement of bacteria from one part of the body to another. 2. Change in location of a disease or of its manifestations or transfer from one organ or part to another.
The usual application is to the manifestation of a malignancy in a secondary growth arising from the primary growth in a new location. Spread is by the lymphatics or blood stream.

metastasize (me-tas'tă-sīz) [" + *stasis*, a standing]. To invade by metastasis.

metastatic (met-ă-stat'ik) [" + *statikos*, standing]. Pert. to metastasis.

metasternum (met-ă-ster'num) [G. *meta*, after, + *sternon*, sternum]. Last bone of sternum; the ensiform process.

metasyphilis (met-ă-sĭf'ĭ-lĭs) [" + *syn*, with, + *philein*, to love]. 1. Congenital syphilis with no local lesions but presenting general degeneration. 2. Condition due to syphilis. SYN: *parasyphilis*.

metatarsalgia (met-ă-tar-săl'jĭ-ă) [G. *meta*, beyond, + *tarsos*, tarsus]. Neuralgia of the metatarsus. SYN: *Morton's disease*.

metatarsectomy (met"ă-tar-sek'tō-mĭ) [" + " + *ektomē*, excision]. Removal of the metatarsus.

metatarsophalangeal (met"ă-tar"sō-fā-lan'jē-ăl) [" + " + *phalagx, phalagg-*, a phalanx]. Concerning the metatarsus and phalanges.

metatarsus (mĕt-ă-tar'sŭs) [" + *tarsos*, tarsus]. The 5 bones bet. the instep and the phalanges. SEE: *skeleton*.

metathalamus (met-ă-thal'ă-mus) [" + *thalamos*, a chamber]. BNA. The post. part of the thalamus including the 2 geniculate bodies.

metathesis (mē-tath'ĕ-sĭs) [G. *meta*, over, + *thesis*, a placing]. 1. A changing of places. 2. Forcible transference of a disease process from one part to another where it will be more accessible for treatment. 3. Double decomposition chemically.

metatrophia (met-ă-tro'fĭ-ă) [" + *trophē*, nourishment]. A condition due to disorder of nutrition.

metatro'phic [" + *trophē*, nourishment]. 1. Pert. to metatrophia. 2. Requiring lifeless organic matter for food. SYN: *saprophytic*.

metatropism (mĕt-ăt'rō-pĭzm) [G. *meta*, change, + *tropē*, a turning, + *ismos*, state of]. Masculine behavior in women and feminine behavior in men.
Metatropic women favor younger men whom they may dominate. They are usually dictatorial and often found among business and professional women. The metatropic men usually select a woman older than themselves, either very intellectual or very low in the social scale.

metatuberculosis (mĕt"ă-tū-ber-kū-lō'sĭs) [" + L. *tuberculum*, a small nodule]. A condition of tuberculous reactions with nontuberculous lesions.

metaxeny (mē-taks'ĕ-nĭ) [" + *xenos*, host]. Adoption of another host by a parasite when conditions are unfavorable to it with normal host. SYN: *metoxeny*.

Metchnikoff's theory. Microörganisms are ingested by living cells, as by leukocytes and other phagocytes. SYN: *phagocytosis*.

metencephalon (met"ĕn-sĕf'ă-lon) [G. *meta*, after, + *egkephalos*, brain]. BNA. 1. Most caudal portion of the brain or primitive cerebral vesicle from which are developed the cerebellum, pons and pontine portion of 4th ventricle. 2. The cerebellum and pons considered together. SYN: *afterbrain, hindbrain*.

metensomatosis (met"en-sō-mat-ō'sĭs) [" + *en*, in, + *sōma*, body]. Incorporation with, or change into, another body.

meteorism (mē'tē-or-izm) [G. *meteōrizein*, to raise up]. Distention by gas in the abdomen. SYN: *tympanites*.

me'ter [G. *metron*, a measure]. A linear standard of measurement, 39.371 inches.
m. angle. A. of visual axis 1 meter distant.
m. atom. An Angstrom* unit or 1.094 yd. SEE: *metric system*.

methane (CH_4). A combination of carbon with hydrogen; the same as the so-called "fire damp" in mines.
It is colorless, odorless and inflammable. It is one of the waste products of intestinal digestion, being produced in the colon through putrefactive and fermentative processes. SYN: *marsh gas*. [SYN: *wood alcohol*.

methanol (meth'an-ol). Methyl alcohol.

methemoglobin (met"hĕm-ō-glō'bĭn) [G. *meta*, across, + *aima*, blood, + L. *globus*, globe]. A compound closely related to oxyhemoglobin found in the

blood following poisoning by certain substances.
It gives blood a chocolate-brown color and is useless as a carrier of oxygen.

methemoglobinemia (met″hem″ō-glōb″ĭ-nē′mĭ-ă) [" + " + " + G. *aima*, blood]. Presence of methemoglobin in the blood.

methemoglobinuria (met″hem-ō-glōb″ĭ-nū′-rĭ-ă) [" + " + " + G. *ouron*, urine]. Presence of methemoglobin in the urine.

methenamine (mĕth″ĕn-a′mĕn). USP. Formin, hexamethylene, urotropin. Colorless crystals, with sweetish taste.
ACTION AND USES: Urinary antiseptic.
DOSAGE: 5 gr. (0.3 Gm.). Best results obtained by giving alternate doses of an equal amount of sodium acid phosphate.
INCOMPATIBILITIES: Ammonium salts, alkalies, ferric salts.

methionine (meth-ī′ō-nĭn). A sulfur-bearing compound; an essential amino acid.

methomania (meth-ō-mā′nĭ-ă) [G. *methē*, drunkenness, + *mania*, mania]. Psychiatric craving for intoxicating drinks. SYN: *dipsomania*.

methyl (meth′ĭl) [G. *methy*, wine, + *ylē*, substance]. In organic chemistry, the radical CH_3, seen, for instance, in the formula for methyl alcohol, CH_3OH.

  m. alcohol. A colorless liquid with a peculiar alcoholic odor largely used as a solvent for paints, varnishes, etc.
  POISONING: SYM: Different from those of ordinary alcoholism. Depression, weakness, nausea, headache, abdominal cramping, difficult breathing, cold sweats, coma. Well-known blindness which often follows may appear in several hours or not for several days. Sometimes the vision remains blurred, or may become totally blind.
  TREATMENT: Give stimulants often in form of black coffee. Sedatives may be necessary. Saline cathartic.

  m. chloride. Gas obtained by distilling methyl alcohol.
  It has a narcotic action and no distinctive warning features.
  POISONING: SYM: Drowsiness, mental confusion, coma, nausea, vomiting and perhaps convulsions. Anuria occurs and there is an increase in temperature, pulse and respiration.
  TREATMENT: Inhalations of oxygen and 5-7% carbon dioxide; bromides for convulsions. Oxygen and alkalinization and hospitalization.

  m. ether. An anesthetic gas without color.

  m. oxide. SEE: *m. ether*.

  m. parafynol. SEE: *dormison*.

  m. salicylate (sal-is′il-āt). USP. Oil of wintergreen, oil of gaultheria. Produced from distillation of leaves of sweet birch.
  ACTION AND USES: Antiseptic. Internally, same as salicylic acid.
  DOSAGE: Internally, 12 ℔ (0.75 cc.).

  m. violet. Stain employed in histology and bacteriology. SYN: *pyoktanin*.

methylene blue (meth′ĭ-lēn). USP. Methylthionine chloride. A dark green crystalline powder, producing a distinct blue stain.
USES: As a urinary antiseptic, as a test for kidney function, and as an antidote for carbon monoxide and cyanide poisoning.
DOSAGE: Average, 2½ gr. (0.15 Gm.). As an antidote, 50 cc. of a 1% solution, intravenously.

metopantralgia (met″ō-pan-tral′jĭ-ă) [G. *metōpon*, forehead, + *antron*, cavity, + *algos*, pain]. Pain in frontal sinuses.

metopantritis (met-ō-pan-trī′tis) [" + " + *-itis*, inflammation]. Inflamed condition of frontal sinuses.

metopic (met-op′ĭk) [G. *metōpon*, forehead]. Rel. to the forehead.

metopion (met-ō′pĭ-on) [G. *metōpon*, forehead]. Craniometric point in forehead midway bet. frontal eminences.

metopism (met′ō-pĭzm) [" + *ismos*, condition of]. Persistence of the metopic suture in an adult.

metopodynia (met-ō-pō-din′ĭ-ă) [" + *odynē*, pain]. Headache in frontal area of head.

meto′pon [G. forehead]. Cranial ant. lobule.

metoposcopy (met-ō-pos′kō-pĭ) [" + *skopein*, to examine]. The study of physiognomy.

metoxenous (mĕ-toks′ĕn-ŭs) [G. *meta*, across, + *xenos*, host]. Denoting a parasite spending each of its 2 cycles on a different host. SYN: *heterecious*.

metoxeny (mĕ-toks′ĕ-nĭ). Adoption of a new host in each cycle by a parasite having 2 cycles of existence. SYN: *heterecism*.

metra (mē′tra) [G. *mētra*]. The uterus.

metralgia (me-tral′jĭ-ă) [G. *mētra*, uterus, + *algos*, pain]. Pain in the uterus.

metranemia (met-ră-ne′mĭ-ă) [" + *a-*, priv. + *aima*, blood]. Local uterine anemia.

metranoikter (met-ră-nō-ĭk′ter) [" + *anoigein*, to open]. Instrument for dilating cervix uteri by means of 2 or 4 spring blades when a wide, prolonged dilation is necessary.

metrapectic (met-ră-pek′tĭk) [" + *apechein*, to avoid]. Denoting a disease that is transmitted by the mother, who herself is unaffected by it.

metratome (met′ră-tōm) [" + *tomē*, incision]. Instrument for incising the uterus.

metratomy (mĕt-răt′ō-mĭ) [" + *tomē*, a cutting]. Surgical incision of the uterus. SYN: *metrotomy*.

metratonia (mē-tra-to′nĭ-ă) [G. *mētra*, uterus, + *a-*, priv. + *tonos*, tone]. Uterine atony occurring after childbirth.

metratrophia (met-ra-tro′fĭ-ă) [" + *atrophia*, atrophy]. Atrophy of the uterus.

metrauxe (me-trawk′se) [" + *auxē*, increase]. Hypertrophy of the uterus.

metrazol (met′ră-zōl). Pentamethylene tetrazol, cardiazol. A white powder, chemically neutral substance.
USES: As a circulatory and respiratory stimulant, regarded as valuable in shock, in pneumonia, and in other infectious diseases, and in schizophrenia in combination with insulin and curare.
DOSAGE: 1½-4½ gr. (0.1-0.28 Gm.) orally or subcutaneously.

metre (mē′ter) [G. *metron*, measure]. Meter, q.v.

metrechoscopy (mĕt-rĕk-os′kō-pĭ) [" + *ēchō*, sound, + *skopein*, to examine]. Mensuration and auscultation combined with inspection.

metrectasia (mĕt-rĕk-tā′zĭ-ă) [G. *mētra*, uterus, + *ektasis*, dilatation]. Uterine dilatation.

metrectomy (mē-trek′to-mĭ) [" + *ektomē*, excision]. Surgical removal of the uterus. SYN: *hysterectomy*.

metrectopia (met-rek-to′pĭ-ă) [" + *ek*, out, + *topos*, place]. Displacement of the uterus.

metrelcosis (mĕt-rĕl-kō'sĭs) [" + *elkōsis*, ulceration]. Uterine ulceration.

metreurynter (met-rū-rĭn'ter) [" + *eurynein*, to stretch]. An inflatable bag which is inserted in the os uteri and distended to dilate the cervix.

metreurysis (me-trū'rĭ-sĭs) [" + *eurynein*, to stretch]. Dilatation of cervix uteri with the metreurynter.

met'ric sys'tem. One based upon the meter (39.371 inches) as the unit of measurement; the gram (15.432 gr.) the unit of weight; the liter (1.056 qt. liquid, or 0.908 qt. dry measure) as the unit of volume.

CONVERSION RULES: To change grams to grains multiply by 15, or divide by 0.064. To change grains to grams divide by 15, or multiply by 0.064. To change grams to ounces divide by 30. To change ounces to grams or cc. multiply by 30. SEE: *avoirdupois, household measures, table in Appendix, Troy weight.*

metritis (me-trī'tĭs) [G. *mētra*, uterus, + -*ītis*, inflammation]. Inflammation of the uterine musculature accompanied by an extensive increase in fibrous tissue.

metro- [G.]. 1. Combining form (*metron*) meaning rel. to measure or measurements. 2. From *metra*, the *uterus*, meaning rel. to the uterus.

metrocarcinoma (mĕt″rō-kăr-sĭ-nō'mă) [G. *mētra*, uterus, + *karkinos*, crab cancer, + -*ōma*, tumor]. Uterine carcinoma.

metrocele (met'rō-sēl) [" + *kēlē*, hernia]. Uterine hernia.

metroclyst (met'rō-klĭst) [" + *klystēr*, an injection]. Device for douching the uterus.

metrocolpocele (met″rō-kol'pō-sēl) [" + *kolpos*, vagina, + *kēlē*, hernia]. Protrusion of uterus into the vagina which pushes the vaginal wall downward.

metrocystosis (met″rō-sĭs-tō'sĭs) [" + *kystis*, cyst, + -*ōsis*, intensive]. Formation of uterine cysts.

metrocyte (me'trō-sīt) [G. *mētēr*, mother, + *kytos*, cell]. A mother cell.

metrodynia (met-rō-dĭn'ĭ-ă) [G. *mētra*, uterus, + *odynē*, pain]. Uterine pain.

metrofibroma (me-trō-fī-brō'mă) [" + L. *fibra*, fiber, + G. -*ōma*, tumor]. Uterine fibroma.

metromalacosis (me″trō-mal-ă-kō'sĭs) [" + *malakia*, softening, + -*ōsis*, intensive]. Malacia or softening of uterine tissues.

metroma'nia. 1. [G. *mētra*, uterus, + *mania*, madness]. Nymphomania. Insanity caused by uterine disease. 2. [G. *metron*, measure, + *mania*, madness]. Insanity characterized by continuous writing of verses.

metroneuria (me-trō-nū'rĭ-ă) [G. *mētra*, uterus, + *neuron*, nerve]. A uterine nervous affection.

metronome (met'rō-nōm) [G. *metron*, measure, + *nomos*, law]. Apparatus for recording intervals or periods of time.

metroparalysis (met″rō-pă-ral'ĭ-sĭs) [G. *mētra*, uterus, + *paralysis*, a loosening from the side]. Uterine paralysis.

metropath'ia haemorrhag'ica [" + *pathos*, disease, + *aima*, blood, + *rēgnunai*, to burst forth]. Condition of the uterus characterized by hemorrhage, usually accompanied by hypertrophy of the uterine mucous membranes and ovarian cystic disease. SEE: *fibrosis uteri.*

metropathic (me-tro-path'ĭk) [" + *pathos*, disease]. Pert. to or caused by uterine disorders.

metropathy (me-trop'ă-thĭ) [" + *pathos*, disease]. Any uterine disease.

metroperitonitis (me″trō-per-ĭ-tō-nī'tĭs) [" + *peritonaion*, peritoneum, + -*ītis*, inflammation]. Inflamed condition of uterus and peritoneum.

metrophlebitis (me″trō-flē-bī'tĭs) [G. *metra*, uterus, + *phleps, phleb-*, vein, + -*ītis*, inflammation]. Inflamed condition of uterine veins.

metroptosis (met-rop-tō'sĭs) [" + *ptōsis*, a dropping]. Dropping of the uterus.

metrorrhagia (met-ror-ra'jĭ-ă) [" + *rēgnunai*, to burst forth]. Bleeding from the uterus, esp. at any time other than during the menstrual period.

This is most often caused by lesions of the cervix uteri, and its occurrence should always lead one to suspect and search for a malignancy in the genital tract.

metrorrhea (met-ror-rē'ă) [" + *roia*, flow]. Any morbid discharge from the uterus.

metrorrhexis (met-ror-reks'ĭs) [" + *rēxis*, a rupture]. A uterine rupture.

metrorthosis (me-tror-thō'sĭs) [" + *orthōsis*, a straightening]. Correction of uterine displacement.

metrosalpingitis (met-rō-săl-pĭn-jī'tĭs) [G. *mētra*, uterus, + *salpigx, salpigg-*, tube, + -*ītis*, inflammation]. Inflamed condition of uterus and oviducts.

metroscope (met'ro-skōp) [" + *skopein*, to examine]. Instrument for examining the uterus.

metrostaxis (me-tro-stak'sĭs) [" + *staxis*, a dripping]. Persistent but slight hemorrhage from the uterus.

metrostenosis (me-trō-stĕn-ō'sĭs) [" + *stēnōsis*, a narrowing]. Contraction of the uterine cavity.

metrosteresis (me-trō-ster-ē'sĭs) [" + *sterēsis*, loss]. Removal of the uterus. SYN: *hysterectomy, metrectomy.*

metrother'apy [G. *metron*, measure, + *therapeia*, treatment]. Treatment of a condition by measurement, as in restoration of joint function following injury, measuring the angle of joint motion and recording the progress, has a psychologic effect on patient.

metrotome (mē'trō-tōm) [G. *mētra*, uterus, + *tomē*, a cutting]. Instrument used in incising the uterus.

metrotomy (me-trot'ō-mĭ) [G. *mētra*, uterus, + *tomē*, incision]. Incision of the uterus. SYN: *hysterotomy.*

metrourethrotome (met-ro-u-re'thrō-tōm) [G. *metron*, measure, + *ourēthra*, urethra, + *tomē*, incision]. Device for incising the urethra and measuring depth to be incised.

metrypercinesis (met″rĭ-per-sĭn-ē'sĭs) [G. *mētra*, uterus, + *yper*, over, + *kinēsis*, movement]. Excessive contraction of the uterus causing abnormal labor pains.

metycaine (met'ĭ-ka'ĭn). A white crystalline substance formerly known as neothesin.

USES: As a local anesthetic, prompt in action as topical application, or subcutaneous injection.

DOSAGE: As an application to the eye, 2% solution recommended; for infiltration, use ½-1%.

Meynert's commis'sure (mī'nerts). Fibrous tract extending from subthalamic body to base of 3rd ventricle.

M. F. D. Abbr. for *minimum fatal dose.*
Mg. Symb. for *magnesium.*
mg. Symb. for *milligram.*
miasm, miasma (mī'azm, mī-az'mă) [G.

miasma, stain]. A foul emanation or odor.
miasmatic (mī-az-mat′ĭk) [G. *miasma*, stain]. Pert. to miasm.
mication (mi-ka′shun) [L. *micāre*, to glitter]. 1. Rapid winking that is involuntary. 2. A quick motion.
micella (mī-sĕl′ă) [L. a little crumb]. One of the ultramicroscopic units of organized bodies. SYN: *bioblast, tagma*.
mick′ey finn. Slang term for an alcoholic drink which is tampered with voluntarily, in order to produce ill effects in the drinker, as acute nausea or diarrhea. SEE: *knockout drops*.
micrencephalon (mĭk-rĕn-sef′ă-lon) [" + *egkephalos*, brain]. 1. Cerebellum. 2. Smallness of brain; cretinism.
micrencephalous (mi-kren-sef′al-ŭs) [" + *egkephalos*, brain]. Possessing a small brain.
micro-, micr- [G.]. Combining forms denoting *small size* or *extent*.
microaerophilic (mī″krō-a-er-ō-fil′ĭk) [G. *mikros*, small, + *aēr*, air, + *philein*, to love]. Growing at low oxygen tension.
mi′croanal′ysis [" + *analysis*, a loosening apart]. Analytical examination of tiny granules.
microbe (mī′krōb) [G. *mikros*, small, + *bios*, life]. 1. A minute one-celled form of life not distinguishable as to its vegetable or animal nature. 2. Bacteria, germs producing fermentation, putrefaction and disease; microörganism.
microbemia (mī-krō-bē′mĭ-ă) [" + " + *aima*, blood]. Diseased condition caused by presence of microörganisms in the blood]. SYN: *microbiohemia*.
microbian (mī-krō′bĭ-an) [" + *bios*, life]. Rel. to a microbe. SYN: *microbic*.
microbic (mī-krōb′ĭk) [" + *bios*, life]. Concerning microbes. SYN: *microbian*.
microbicidal (mī-krōb-ĭs-ī′dal) [" + " + L. *cidus*, from *caedere*, to kill]. Destructive to microbes.
microbicide (mī-krōb′is-īd) [" + " + L. *cidus*, from *caedere*, to kill]. An agent which is destructive to microbes.
microbiohemia (mī″krōb-ī-ō-hē′mĭ-ă) [G. *mikros*, small, + *bios*, life, + *aima*, blood]. A condition resulting from microbes in the blood. SYN: *microbemia*.
microbiology (mī″krō-bī-ol′ō-jī) [" + " + *logos*, study]. Scientific study of microbes.
microbiophobia (mī″krō-bī-ō-fō′bĭ-ă) [" + " + *phobos*, fear]. An abnormal fear of microbes. SYN: *microphobia*.
microbism (mī′krōb-ĭzm) [" + " + *ismos*, state of]. Infection with microbes.
microbioscope (mī-krō-bī′ō-skōp) [" + " + *skopein*, to examine]. Form of microscope for studying changes in living tissue.
microbiotic (mī-krō-bī-ot′ĭk) [" + *bios*, life]. Of microbic life, or origin.
microblast (mī′krō-blăst) [G. *mikros*, small, + *blastos*, germ]. Minute red blood corpuscle. SYN: *microcyte*.
microblepharism, microblephary (mī-krō-blef′ar-izm, -ar-ī) [" + *blepharon*, eyelid]. Condition of having abnormally small eyelids.
microcalory (mī″krō-kal′ō-rī) [" + L. *calor*, heat]. A unit of heat, the amount required to raise the temperature of 1 cc. of distilled water from 0° to 1° C.
microcardia (mī-krō-kar′dĭ-ă) [" + *kardia*, heart]. Unusually small heart.
microcaulia (mī″krō-kaw′lī-ă) [" + *kaulos*, penis]. Unusually small size of penis.
microcentrum (mī-krō-sĕn′trum) [" + *kentron*, center]. 1. A small nucleus.

SYN: *micronucleus*. 2. Motor or dynamic center of a cell.
microcepha′lia [" + *kephalē*, head]. Abnormal smallness of the head.
microcephalic (mī-krō-sef-al′ĭk) [" + *kephalē*, head]. Having or pert. to a small head; one below 1350 cc. capacity.
microcephalous (mī-kro-sef′al-us) [" + *kephalē*, head]. Having an abnormally small head.
microcephalus (mik-rō-sef′a-lŭs) [G. *mikros*, small, + *kephalē*, head]. 1. Person with an exceptionally small head, esp. an idiot. 2. Fetus with a very small head.
microcephaly, microcephalism (mī-krō-sef′ă-lĭ, -lĭzm) [" + *kephalē*, head]. Abnormal smallness of head often seen in idiocy; it is congenital.
microchemistry (mī-krō-kem′is-trī) [" + *chēmeia*, chemistry]. Chemical work in which the aid of the microscope is required.
Micrococcus (mī″krō-kŏk′ŭs) [" + *kokkos*, berry]. 1. A small coccus. 2. A genus of the Schizomycetes, of the family Coccaceae.
Some are aerobic. They occur singly; or in pairs as *diplococci;* in chains as *streptococci;* in clusters or groups as *staphylococci*.
Micrococci are divided into 3 forms—*chromogenic, pathogenic, zymogenic*.
M. a′cidi lactici. M. in milk; cause of lactic acid fermentation.
M. ascofor′mans. M. occurring in bothriomycosis.
M. bucca′lis. Nonpathogenic organism found in the mouth.
M. capillo′rum. One of the scalp affecting color of hair.
M. catarrha′lis. Neisseria catarrhalis.
M. cereus. A species sometimes seen in pus; nonpathogenic.
M. cit′reus. M. found in osteomyelitis and in water.
M. endocardi′tidis ruga′tus. Form seen in ulcerative endocarditis.
M. fla′vus conjuncti′vae. Form found in the conjunctiva.
M. foetidus. Form found in caries and fetid cases of pharyngitis.
M. gelatino′sus. Form found in milk.
M. gingi′vae pyogenes. Nonmotile M. in alveolar abscess.
M. gonorrhoeae. Neisseria gonorrhoeae.
M. intracellularis meningitidis. Diplococcus intracellularis.
M. lanceolatus. Diplococcus pneumoniae.
M. liquefa′ciens conjuncti′vae. Seen in normal human conjunctiva.
M. loewenber′gii. Seen in nose in ozena.
M. melitensis. Cause of Malta fever.
M. mucilaginosus. Cause of slimy milk.
M. nasa′lis. Found in nasopharynx.
M. neofor′mans. Found in various tumors.
M. of osteomyelitis. Pathogenic in osteomyelitis.
M. pasteu′rii. Found in saliva.
m., pathogenic. Any m. producing disease.
M. pyo′genes ten′uis. Found in large abscesses.
M. restit′uens. Converts peptone into albumin.
M. rosenbach′ii. Derived from pus of abscesses.
M. ro′seus. Found in sputum of influenza.

M. saliva′rius sep′ticus. Found in sputum of puerperal septicemia.
M. tetragenus. A species in sputum and walls of cavities in the lung.
M. urea. A m. decomposing urea into ammonia.
M. urinal′bus. Found in urine in cystitis and pyelonephritis.
M. vir′idis flaves′cens. Seen in lymph of varicella.
M. xanthogen′icus. Seen in yellow fever.
m., zymogenic, zymogenous. Any m. causing fermentation.
microcor′nea [" + L. *cornū*, horn]. Abnormally small cornea.
microcoulomb (mī-krō-kū′lŏm) [G. *mikros*, small, + *coulomb*]. One-millionth part of a coulomb.
microcrith (mī′kro-krith) [G. *mikros*, small, + *krithē*, a barleycorn]. Unit of weight equal to 1 atom of hydrogen.
microcrystalline (mī-krō-kris′tal-īn) [" + *krystallos*, ice]. Composed of microscopic crystals.
microcyst (mī′krō-sīst) [" + *kystis*, a cyst]. A very small cyst.
microcytase (mī-krō-sī′tās) [" + *kytos*, cell, + *ase*, enzyme]. Cytase acting on bacteria and formed by leukocytes.
mi′crocyte [" + *kytos*, cell]. 1. A small multinuclear leukocyte from 3½-6 microns in diameter. 2. Degenerating, small, nonnucleated, red blood corpuscle.
microcythemia (mī′kro-sī-the′mī-ă) [" + " + *aima*, blood]. Abnormally small erythrocytes in the blood.
microdactylia (mī′′krō-dak-til′ī-ă) [G. *mikros*, small, + *daktylos*, digit]. Abnormal smallness of the digits.
microdissection (mī′′krō-dĭ-sek′shŭn) [" + L. *dissectiō*, a cutting apart]. Dissection with aid of the microscope.
microdont (mī′krō-dont) [" + *odous*, *odont-*, tooth]. Possessing very small teeth.
microdontism (mī-krō-don′tizm) [" + " + *ismos*, state of]. Unusual smallness of the teeth.
microfarad (mī-krō-far′ăd) [" + *farad*]. One-millionth of a farad which is the capacity of a condenser which, when charged with 1 coulomb, gives a difference of potential of 1 volt.
microgamete (mī-krō-gam′ēt) [" + *gametēs*, spouse]. Male element in conjugation of protozoa.
microgametocyte (mī-krō-gam-ē′tō-sīt) [" + " + *kytos*, cell]. Mother cell of the microgamete.
microgastria (mī-krō-gas′trī-ă) [G. *mikros*, little, + *gastēr*, belly]. Unusual smallness of the stomach.
microgenitalism (mī′′krō-jĕn′ĭt-ăl-ĭzm) [" + L. *genitalia*, genitals, + G. *ismos*, state of]. Abnormal smallness of the external genitals.
microglia (mī-krog′lī-ă) [" + *glia*, glue]. Neuroglia tissue probably derived from the mesoderm, forming a portion of the adventitial structure of the central nervous system.
microgliacyte (mī′′krō-glī′ă-sīt) [" + " + *kytos*, cell]. Embryonic cell of a neuroglia.
microglos′sia [" + *glōssa*, tongue]. Small size of the tongue.
Etiol: Occurs in anemia, convalescence from typhoid fever, the result of hemorrhage, gumma.
Prog: A local condition which is temporary.
micrognathia (mī-krog-nā′thī-ă) [G. *mikros*, small, + *gnathos*, jaw]. Abnormal smallness of jaws.

microgram (mī′krō-gram) [" + *gramma*, a small weight]. One-millionth part of a gram.
micrograph (mī′krō-graf) [" + *graphein*, to write]. Apparatus for magnifying and recording minute movements.
micrography (mī-krog′ră-fī) [" + *graphein*, to write]. 1. Study of physical appearance and characteristics of microbes. 2. Very minute writing, engraving, etc.
microgyria (mī-krō-jir′ī-ă) [" + *gyros*, circle]. Smallness of cerebral convolutions.
microhepatia (mī-krō-hĕ-pat′ī-ă) [" + *ēpar*, *ēpat-*, liver]. Abnormally small size of the liver.
microhistology (mī-krō-his-tol′ō-jī) [G. *mikros*, small, + *istos*, web, + *logos*, study]. Histology with aid of a microscope.
microhm (mī′krōm) [" + *ohm*]. One-millionth of an ohm.
mi′′croleuk′oblast [" + *leukos*, white, + *blastos*, germ]. A nongranular bone marrow cell. Syn: *myeloblast*.
microliter (mī′′krō-lē-ter) [" + Fr. *litre*, from G. *litra*, a pound]. One-millionth part of a liter.
microlith (mī′krō-lith) [" + *lithos*, stone]. A very tiny calculus.
microlithiasis (mī′′krō-lī-thī′ă-sīs) [" + *lithos*, stone]. The development of very minute calculi.
micrology (mī-krol′o-jī) [G. *mikros*, small, + *logos*, study]. Science of microscopic investigations.
microlymphoidocyte (mī′′krō-lĭm-foid′ō-sīt) [" + L. *lympha*, lymph, + G. *eidos*, form, + *kytos*, cell]. An immature, tiny lymphoidocyte.
micromania (mī-krō-mā′nī-ă) [" + *mania*, madness]. A delusion that one has become small or infantile or insignificant.
micromazia (mī-krō-mā′zī-ă) [" + *mazos*, breast]. Abnormally small size of the breasts.
micrometer (mī-krom′et-er) [" + *metron*, measure]. Device for making microscopic measurements.
micromillimeter (mī-krō-mil′ī-mē-ter) [" + L. *mille*, a thousand, + G. *metron*, measure]. One-millionth part of a millimeter. Syn: *micron*.
micromyces (mī-krom′ī-sēs) (pl. *micromycetes*) [" + *mykēs*, fungus]. Minute fungus.
micromyelia (mī-krō-mī-ē′lī-ă) [" + *myelon*, marrow]. Abnormally small size of spinal cord.
micromyeloblast (mī-krō-mī′el-ō-blast) [" + *blastos*, germ]. A nongranular bone marrow cell. Syn: *myeloblast*.
micron (mī′krŏn) [G. *mikros*, small]. Symb: μ. The millionth part of a meter; the thousandth part of a millimeter; about 1/25,000 part of an inch.
microne (mī′krōn) [G. *mikros*, small]. A colloid particle that is distinguishable with the microscope.
micronucleus (mī-krō-nū′klē-us) (pl. *micronucleī*) [" + L. *nucleus*, kernel]. 1. A small nucleus. 2. The smaller of the 2 nuclei of infusoria considered as containing the inheritable germ substance.
microörganism (mi-kro-or′gan-izm) [" + *organon*, organ, + *ismos*, condition]. Minute living body not perceptible to the naked eye, esp. a bacterium or protozoon.

Microörganisms may be carried from 1 host to another as follows:

micropathology   M-37   **micturition**

Animal carriers: Some organisms are pathogenic for animals as well as man, and may be communicated to man through direct, indirect or intermediary hosts.

By air: Pathogenic microörganisms in the respiratory tract may be discharged from the mouth or nose and settle on food, dishes, clothing and other places. They may carry infection if they resist drying.

Contact infections: These are the result of direct transmission of bacteria from one to another, as in venereal diseases.

Food-borne: Bacteria may reach the body by food affected by the handling of one infected, or by other means.

Human carriers: Persons who have recovered from an infectious disease remain carriers of the organism causing the infection, and may transfer the organism to another host.

Insects: They may be the physical carrier, as the housefly or *Anopheles* mosquito.

Soil-borne: Spore forming organisms in the soil may enter the body through a cut or wound. Vegetables and fruits, esp. roots, need thorough cleansing before being eaten raw.

RS: *bacteria, cataxia, Hyphomycetes, mold, Schizomycetes, virus,* etc.

micropathology (mĭ″krō-path-ol′ō-jĭ) [G. *mikros*, small, + *pathos*, disease, + *logos*, study]. Study of microörganismal diseases and their cell and tissue changes.

microphage, microphagus (mi′kro-fāj, -krof′ag-us) [" + *phagein*, to eat]. A small phagocyte; polymorphonuclear leukocyte; most active in attacking bacteria.

RS: *bacteria, bacteriolysin, leukocyte, opsonin, phagocyte, trephone*.

microphakia (mĭ″krō-fā′kĭ-ă) [" + *phakos*, lens]. Abnormally small lens.

microphallus (mĭ-krō-fal′us) [" + *phallos*, penis]. Abnormally small size of penis. SYN: *microcaulia*.

microphobia (mĭ-krō-fō′bĭ-ă) [" + *phobos*, fear]. Psychopathic fear of microbes. SYN: *microbiophobia*.

microphone (mi′kro-fōn) [" + *phōnē*, sound]. Device for augmenting sound.

microphonia (mĭ-krō-fō′nĭ-ă) [G. *mikros*, small, + *phōnē*, voice]. Weakness of voice.

microphonoscope (mĭ-krō-fō′nō-skōp) [" + " + *skopein*, to examine]. Form of biaural stethoscope for augmenting the sound.

microphotograph (mĭ″krō-fō′tō-graf) [" + *phōs, phot-*, light, + *graphein*, to write]. A photograph of microscopic substance, or substance viewed under a microscope. SYN: *photomicrograph*.

microphthalmia (mi-krof-thal′mĭ-ă) [" + *ophthalmos*, eye]. Abnormally small size of eyes.

microphthalmus (mĭ-krŏf-thal′mus) [" + *ophthalmos*, eye]. 1. Person with unusually small eyes. 2. Condition characterized by abnormally small eyes.

microphysics (mĭ-krō-fĭz′ĭks) [G. *mikros*, small, + *physis*, nature]. The branch of science dealing with the forces controlling ultimate structure of matter.

microphyte (mĭ′krō-fīt) [" + *phyton*, plant]. Any microscopic plant, esp. if parasitic.

micropia (mi-kro′pĭ-ă) [" + *opsis*, vision]. A condition in which objects seem diminished in size. SYN: *micropsia*.

micropodia (mĭ-krō-pō′dĭ-ă) [" + *pous, pod-*, feet]. Unusually small size of the feet.

micropsia (mi-krop′sĭ-ă) [G. *mikros*, small, + *opsis*, vision]. Condition in which objects seem smaller than they usually are.

Seen in paralysis of accommodation, retinitis and choroiditis. SYN: *micropia*.

micropus (mĭ-krō′pus) [" + *pous*, feet]. One with unusually small feet.

micropyle (mi′kro-pīl) [" + *pylē*, gate]. The opening in the ovum for entrance of the spermatozoon.

microscope (mi′krō-skōp) [" + *skopein*, to examine]. Instrument which greatly magnifies very minute objects.

   m., binocular. Microscope for both eyes.

   m., compound. One with 2 or more lenses or lens systems for use in observing the minutest bodies.

   m., simple. One with a simple or single lens.

microscopic, microscopical (mī-krō-skop′-ik, -ĭ-kal) [G. *mikros*, small, + *skopein*, to examine]. 1. Pert. to the microscope. 2. Visible only by using the microscope.

microscopy (mĭ-krŏs′kōp-ĭ) [" + *skopein*, to examine]. Inspection with the microscope.

microseme (mi′krō-sēm) [" + *sēma*, sign]. Possessing an orbital index less than 83.

microsoma (mi-kro-so′mă) [". + *sōma*, body]. 1. Chromatin granule of the cell nucleus. 2. Unusually small stature.

microsome (mi′krō-sōm) [" + *sōma*, body]. 1. Very minute granule in protoplasm. 2. Corpuscle.

microsomia (mi-kro-so′mĭ-ă) [G. *mikros*, small, + *soma*, body]. Abnormally small size of body.

microspectroscope (mi-kro-spek′trō-skōp) [" + L. *spectrum*, image, + *skopein*, to examine]. A combined spectroscope and microscope.

microsphygmia, microsphyxia (mi-kro-sfig′-mĭ-ă, -sfiks′ĭ-ă) [" + *sphygmos*, pulse, — + *sphyxis*, pulse]. Smallness of the pulse.

microsplenia (mi-krō-splē′nĭ-ă) [G. *mikros*, little, + *splēn*, spleen]. Abnormal smallness of the spleen.

Microsporon (mĭk-ros′por-on) [" + *sporos*, seed]. A minute genus of fungi that may cause disease of the skin, hair or nails.

   M. audouini. Species that causes head ringworm or *tinea tonsurans*.

microstat (mĭk′rō-stăt) [" + *istanai*, to stand]. The microscope's stage and finder.

microstomia (mĭ-krō-stō′mĭ-ă) [" + *stoma*, mouth]. Unusual smallness of the mouth.

microtia (mi-kro′shĭ-ă) [" + *ous, ot-*, ear]. Unusually small size of the auricle or external ear.

microtome (mi′kro-tōm) [G. *mikros*, small, + *tomē*, incision]. Instrument for preparing thin sections for microscope.

microtomy (mi-krot′o-mi) [" + *tomē*, incision]. The process of cutting into sections.

microvolt (mi′krō-volt) [" + *volt*]. One-millionth part of a volt.

microzyme (mi′krō-zīm) [" + *zymē*, ferment]. A microörganism causing fermentation.

micturate (mĭk′tū-rāt) [L. *micturire*, to urinate]. To pass the urine. SYN: *urinate*.

micturition (mĭk-tū-rĭ′shŭn) [L. *mic-*

turīre, to urinate]. The voiding of urine. SYN: *urination*.

mid'brain [A.S. *mid*, middle, + *braegen*, brain]. The corpora quadrigemina, the crura cerebri and aqueduct of Sylvius which connect the pons and cerebellum with the hemispheres of the cerebrum. SYN: *mesencephalon, q.v.*

midgut (mid'gut) [" + *gut*, intestine]. Embryonic source of liver, duodenum, pancreas, jejunum and ileum.

midriff (mid'rif) [" + *hrif*, belly]. The diaphragm.

mid'wife [" + *wif*, wife]. A female who practices the art of aiding in the delivery of children.

midwifery (mid-wīf'er-ĭ) [" + *wif*, wife]. The art of assisting at childbirth. SYN: *obstetrics*.

migraine (mī'grān) [Fr. from G. *ēmikrania*, half skull]. Periodic pain in 1 side of the head, principally along the course of the 5th cranial nerve, accompanied by disordered vision, nausea, languor and chill.

ETIOL: Unknown. Frequently hereditary. It may be precipitated by unsuitable food, allergic hypersensitivity, worry or menstrual flow, and it is often considered anaphylactic or endocrine in origin.

SYM: As stated. It is also associated with zigzags of light and vomiting, and at times with diplopia, unilateral sweating and focal symptoms. Sharp, stabbing pains frequently in temperofrontal region. Susceptible to light and sound. Face frequently flushed.

PROG: It must be distinguished from other types of headache, but the history, the course of the disorder, and the peculiar combination of symptoms rarely permit of much uncertainty. Migraine often disappears entirely after 30 years of age.

TREATMENT: Rest in quiet, darkened room during attack. Good ventilation. Feet in mustard bath with cold compress to head. Ergotamine tartrate proves efficacious in most cases, with calcium gluconate and vitamin D bet. attacks. Avoid overwork, alcohol, tea and coffee. Systematic exercise bet. attacks with frequent bathing, then friction.

Recently, oxygen inhalation has seemed successful in overcoming and preventing attacks.

SYN: *browache, hemicrania, megrim*.

migration (mī-grā'shun) [L. *migrāre*, to move from place to place]. Passage of cells, etc., from 1 position to another; *physiological*, as the migration of an ovum from the ovary into the fallopian tube, or *pathological*, as migration of leukocytes through the wall of a blood vessel into surrounding tissues.

m., external, of the ovum. The entrance of an ovum into the oviduct of the opposite ovary.

m., e., of the semen. Passage of semen from 1 oviduct to the opposite ovary.

m., internal, of the ovum. Passage of an ovum (after going through the uterine horn on same side as its ovary) into the opp. horn of a *uterus bilocularis*.

m. of the testicle. Descent of testicle into the scrotum. SYN: *descensus testis*.

m. of white blood corpuscles. Passage of white blood corpuscles through walls of capillaries during acute inflammation.

migratory (mī'grā-tō-rĭ) [L. *migrāre*, to wander from place to place]. 1. Pert. to migrate. 2. Changing or capable of changing positions.

mikro-. For words commencing thus, see *micro-*.

Mikulicz's disease (mik'ū-lits). Chronic hypertrophic enlargement of lacrimal and salivary glands.

M. drain. A method for draining the abdominal cavity after operating.

M.'s law. Patients with hemoglobin below 30% must not be given a general anesthetic.

M.'s mask. Gauze-covered frame worn over nose and mouth during performance of operation.

M.'s pad. Folded gauze pad for packing off the viscera in abdominal operations and used as a sponge in general.

M.'s syndrome. Characteristics of M.'s disease appearing as a complication of another disease.

mil [L. *mille*, a thousand]. One-thousandth part of an inch or liter; equivalent to a cubic centimeter.

mil'dew [A.S. *mildeāw*]. A parasitic fungus, and plant disease produced by it.

Miles' operation. One for carcinoma of the rectum.

miliaria (mil-ĭ-a'rĭ-ă) [L *milium*, millet]. A form of vesicles due to obstruction of the sweat glands. Acute inflammation of the sweat glands.

ETIOL: Exposure to excessive heat, infancy, obesity, debility, overclothing and tendency to hyperhidrosis.*

SYM: Sudden appearance of red patches of small papules. Vesicles are discrete and accompanied by red areolae. They usually appear on the trunk and are accompanied by itching and burning; fever of short duration. They occur in hot weather, in tropical countries, in individuals sweating profusely, and the papules may become eczematous if irritated.

TREATMENT: Mild astringent lotions with bland dusting powder. SYN: *prickly heat, sudamina*.

m. crystallina. Form with vesicles opaque and white.

m. rubra. Same as m. crystallina with the addition of inflammation, lesions being on a slightly inflamed base. SYN: *lichen tropicus, prickly heat*.

miliary (mil'ĭ-ă-rĭ) [L. *miliaris*, like a millet seed]. Resembling millet seed.

m. fever. An infectious disease accompanied by fever.

SYM: Fever, profuse sweating, eruption of minute red and white pimples.

m. tubercles. Small gray nodules in first stage of tuberculosis.

m. tuberculosis. Acute, generalized tuberculosis with minute tubercles in the affected part or organ.

milieu (mēl-yew') [Fr.]. Environment.

milium (mil'ĭ-ŭm) [L. *milium*, millet seed]. Small pink and white nodule below the epidermis, caused by clogged sebaceous glands.

TREATMENT: Mechanical keratolytics (pumice stone, soap or sapolio), salicylic acid and sulfur ointment, electrolysis, or incision and expression of contents.

m., colloid. Tiny papule formed beneath the epidermis due to colloid degeneration.

milk [A.S. *meolc*, milc]. A secretion of the mammary glands, density about 1.032, for feeding the young.

COMP: According to Gautier, there are 2 kinds of bodies held in suspension in the plasm of milk, *viz*: 1. Globules of butter which seem to contain an in-

	Mother's Milk	Cow's Milk
Water	88.3%	87.3%
Mineral salts	0.2%	0.7%
Protein	1.5%	3.5%
Fat	4.0%	4.0%
Sugar (carbohydrate)	6.0%	4.5%
Reaction	Alkaline	Acid

A comparison of mother's milk and cow's milk by Gladys B. Caster, B.S., follows:

Mother's Milk	Cow's Milk
Clean, practically free from bacteria, correct temperature. Cheap.	May be dirty, contains bacteria causing diseases, such as tuberculosis, scarlet fever, typhoid, enteritis, diphtheria. Must be heated for use and is difficult to keep fresh. Clean milk very expensive.
Sucking of the milk provides exercise to the baby's jaw and the pleasure of nestling in to the mother, also delight to the mother. It probably assists involution of the uterus and is the proper physiological sequel to childbirth.	These pleasures are absent. Use of proper teats and correct technic of bottle feeding may replace to some extent jaw exercise.
Protects from infection by virtue of immune bodies in the mother's milk.	Bottle-fed babies have to acquire their immunity unaided, and succumb much more readily to disease.
Composition of the milk:	
Mother's milk undergoes changes during the first few weeks, which adapt it to the needs of the baby.	These modifications cannot be imitated even by "humanizing" the milk.
Protein:	
About two-thirds of the protein is soluble lactalbumen, one-third insoluble caseinogen. Curd flocculent and easy to digest.	About one-quarter is lactalbumen. About three-quarters is caseinogen. Curd tough and dense and difficult of digestion.
Fat:	
Fine emulsion, small globules, small proportion of volatile fatty acids which cause indigestion.	Coarse emulsion, large globules. Large proportion of these acids.
Sugar:	
Lactose similar in quality in both milks, but greater in quantity in human milk.	
Mineral salts:	
Lesser quantity of salts but of a type better adapted to infants' growth and metabolism.	Fewer organic compounds of salts, especially of phosphorus.

finitesimally small amount of fatty substance encapsulated in a very thin, elastic envelope composed of proteid matter. There are about 1,500,000 of these little balloons in the cubic millimeter.

2. Fine granulations of phosphates which are united in a special albuminoid nuclein substance. The albumins of the plasm are casein and lacto-albumins. Milk is curdled by acid or rennet, and is then known as casein. Its protein is coagulated by heat when it assumes the form of albumen. The butyric globules contain butter fat, and the purpose of churning is to break the albumin envelope so each globule of fat may unite in a solid mass of butter, which is the principal constituent of milk.

Carbohydrates: These consist of lactose, or milk sugar.

Mineral substances: These are lime and phosphorus. In infants ¾ of these phosphates of lime in cow's milk are rejected. Phosphorus envelops the casein as nuclein; also present in the form of lecithin. Phosphocarnic acid, or nucleon, is also present. Magnesium is rare; sodium chloride and iron are present. It also contains a number of diastatic ferments of which little is known. Milk is not the best mineralizing or phosphorating food. It sours through the action of germs acting on the lactose in the milk, changing it to lactic acid, which in turn affects the casein, precipitating it and producing curd or whey.

NUTRITIVES: "A glass of milk adds as much to the nutritive value of a meal as a quarter of a loaf of bread or a good slice of beef. A quart of average milk contains the same amount of nutritive ingredients as 0.75 lb. of beef or 6 oz. of bread, or about one-eighth of the whole weight of the milk, one-third of the beef, and two-thirds of the bread consist of actually nutritive ingredients. The other seven-eighths of the milk and one-third of the bread are water, while the two-thirds of the meat which are not actual nutriment are mainly water. As compared with the animal foods, milk contains more carbohydrates and has no refuse. In these two respects it

milk, acidophilus   M-40   **milligram**

resembles more nearly many of the vegetables foods such as flour, oatmeal and the like. The amount of mineral matter is much the same as in the other fresh substances given. There is a larger proportion of water in milk than in most other food material except very succulent fruits and vegetables, so that a given weight contains less dry matter or nutrients than most foods."—*U. S. Dept. Agr.*

Av. SERVING: 240 Gm. *Skimmed*: Pro. 8.9, Fat 0.5, Carbo. 12.0. *Whole*: Pro. 7.9, Fat 9.6, Carbo. 12.0.

VITAMINS: A+++ — +, B++, C+, G+++.

ASH (whole and skimmed): Ca 0.120-0.122, Mg 0.012-0.015, K 0.143-0.149, Na 0.051-0.052, P 0.093-0.096, Cl 0.106-0.110, S 0.034-0.035, Fe 0.00024-0.00025.

ACTION: Milk makes the smallest demands upon the digestive glands of any food unless it be eggs or meat, and decreases the urinary nitrogen. The absence of stimulation is its principal characteristic. A milk diet may cause a feeling of faintness, but this is not due to the lack of nutriment but to the lack of stimulant in the milk. It is a sedative, quieting the liver, heart and blood vessels, suppresses the toxins, neutralizes vascular constriction and defective tension, and relieves the heart action. It is poor in salt, rich in lactose, and it is antitoxic, easy on the kidneys. It is a good diuretic, increasing the output of urine. *Hot milk* produces sleep. *Boiled milk* is constipating. Fat is predominant, carbohydrates are present only in minute quantities. Boiling or skimming reduces the fat; the addition of sugar will supply the carbohydrate, and crackers or bread will reduce the liquid quantity. Milk should be taken slowly and in small amounts, as otherwise it is liable to ferment. Gastric hyperacidity will coagulate the casein, but a little bicarbonate of soda and lime water will modify this tendency. Best digested with a mixed diet. Sterilization lowers its digestibility. Most germs in milk are killed at 168° F. It is pasteurized at 145° F.

m., acidophilus. Milk or soy bean oil inoculated with *B. acidophilus*.

m., bacillary. M. fermented by a *Lactobacillus*.

m., blue. M. altered by the *B. cyanogenes*.

m., butter-. That left after removal of butter following churning.

m., casein. M. prepared with a large quantity of casein and fat, but little sugar and salts.

m., certified. That certified by a Board of Health as pure.

m., condensed. Partly evaporated and sweetened milk.

m., diabetic. M. with small amt. of lactose.

m. ferment. A diastatic ferment found in milk.

m., homog'enized. M. with fats combined with the body of the milk.

m., lactobacillary. M. with cultures of lactic acid bacteria.

m. leg. Acute edema of the leg. SYN: *phlegmasia alba dolens, q.v.*

m. of magnesia. Magnesium hydroxide in permanent suspension.

m., modified. Water and lactose mixed with cream of cow's milk.

m., mother's. That from the mammary glands of a woman. The protein, fat, carbohydrate and mineral salts are exactly balanced to promote growth of the infant. Average composition of mother's milk and cow's milk is shown on p. M-39.

m., pasteurized. M. heated for 30 minutes at 140 or 158°F. (60 or 70° C.) to kill the living bacteria. SEE: *pasteurization*.

m., peptonized. M. partly digested with pepsin and hydrochloric acid, or pancreatic extract and sodium bicarbonate.

m. poisoning. SYM: Headache, vertigo, thirst, vomiting, indigestion, diarrhea, frequently skin eruptions, and possible collapse are the usual symptoms.

TREATMENT: Purgatives, emetics and stimulants are administered.

m., protein. M. with high protein and low carbohydrate and fat content.

m., ropy. That which has become viscid.

m. sickness. Disease of cattle and sheep transmitted to man through milk and butter, characterized by vomiting, pain, constipation, and muscular tremors. SYN: *slows, trembles*.

m., skimmed. M. after removal of cream.

m., sour. M. with lactic acid caused by lactic acid bacteria.

m., sterilized. M. boiled to kill bacteria.

m., sugar of. Lactose.

m. teeth. First or deciduous teeth.

m. tumor. Retention of milk in mammary gland.

m., uterine. White, milklike substance in the gravid uterus bet. villi of the placenta.

m., uviol. M. sterilized by ultraviolet rays.

m., vegetable. The latex of plants.

m., witch's. 1. Colostrumlike fluid in mammary gland of a newborn child due to slight inflammations. 2. M. secreted by the human male at birth and puberty.

milk, words pert. to: ablactation, acidophilus, agalactia, agalorrhea, androgalactozemia, antigalactagogue, aolan, bacillac, beestings, breast, butyrometer, casein, caseinogen, caseous, colostrum, curd, flash-method, "galac-" words, kumiss, lac, "lact-" words, mamma, mammary, matzoon, milk sugar, mother's, pasteurization, peptonized, tyrosis, whey, yoghurt.

milk'pox. Modified form of smallpox prevalent in South Africa. Called *alastrim** in America. SEE: *amaas*.

milli- [L.]. Prefix meaning *a thousandth part*.

milliam'meter [L. *mille*, thousand, + *ampere* + G. *metron*, measure]. Ammeter registering in milliamperes. SEE: *ammeter*.

milliampere (mĭl″-e-ahm-pair′) [" + *ampere*]. P.T. One one-thousandth of an ampere.

m. minute. An electrical unit of quantity, equivalent to that delivered by 1 milliampere in 1 minute.

millicurie (mĭl″ĭ-ku′rē) [" + *curie*]. P.T. One-thousandth of a curie.

m.'s destroyed. A unit of the quantity of radiation furnished by a tube of radon. One millicurie in decaying gives 133.3 millicurie hours of radiation.

m. hour. A practical unit of dosage for radon. One millicurie of radon applied for 1 hour. The biologic effect depends on time, filtration, distance.

milligram (mĭl′ĭ-gram) [L. *mille*, a thousand, + G. *gramma*, a weight]. One-thousandth of a gram.

milliliter (mĭl'ĭ-le-ter) [" + Fr. *litre*, from G. *litra*, a pound]. One-thousandth of a liter. SYN: *1 cc*.

millimeter (mĭl'ĭ-mēt-er) [" + G. *metron*, measure]. One-thousandth of a meter.

millimicron (mĭl-i-mī'kron). One-thousandth of a micron; one-millionth of a millimeter. SYMB: mμ·

mime'sis [G. *mimēsis*, imitation]. Simulation of an organic disease, esp. of one that simulates another; most appropriately said of hysteria.

mimetic, mimic (mi-met'ĭk, mĭm'ĭk) [G. *mimétikos*, pert. to imitation]. Imitative.

 m. convulsion. Facial convulsion.
 m. labor. False labor.
 m. spasm. Spasm of facial muscles.

min. Abbr. for *minim*.

mind (mīnd) [A.S. *gemynd*]. Integration of functions of the brain resulting in intelligence.

No conclusive scientific definition of mind has yet been given.

 m. blindness. A condition in which one does not recognize what is seen due to a brain lesion. A form of aphasia.
 m. deafness. Inability to comprehend what is heard. A form of aphasia.

mind, words pert. to: ablepsia, 2; acalculia; age, mental; agonia; akatamathesia; allophasis; amnestic; anacroasia; anagnosasthenia; anamnesis; ananabasia; anosognosia; anxietas; aphelotic; aphelxia; aphose; aphrasia; apperception; apsychosis; association center; asynesia; ataraxia; audile; autosuggestibility; autosuggestion; barythmia; bradyesthesia; cacothymia; cathexis; conation; concept; delirium; ergasia; eunoia; eupraxia; hallucination; hebetude; hypermnesia; hyperphrenia; hypobulia; hypophrenia; ideation; imagery; intelligence; i. classification; lucid; lypothymia; misologia; misopedia; obfuscation, 2; onomatomania; onomatopoiesis; orthophrenia; paratypic; perception; perseveration; phrenitis; phrenasthenia; pseudocyesis; psychology; psychopathology; recapitulation theory; retention defect; sublimation; unconscious.

mineral (mĭn'er-ăl) [L.L. *minerale*]. 1. A chemical element or compound occurring in nature as a product of inorganic processes. 2. One of the 3 classifications of matter, the others being animal and vegetable.

 m. elements. The human body is composed of the following chemical elements: Oxygen, 65%; carbon, 18%; hydrogen, 10%; nitrogen, 3.0%; calcium, 1.5%; phosphorus, 1.0%; potassium, 0.35%; sulfur, 0.15%; chlorine, 0.15%; magnesium, 0.05%; iron, 0.04%; iodine, 0.00004%, with traces of copper, manganese, zinc, fluorine, silicon, cobalt, aluminum, arsenic and nickel. In the body they are found in the bones, teeth, nails, hair, tissues, fluids and some of the body organs.

As there is a daily loss of these elements from the body they must be resupplied in the food intake, some of them in both organic and inorganic forms.

They help maintain osmosis and influence the elasticity of muscles and nerves, maintaining the solvent power of body fluids and their neutrality. They also supply what is needed for the acidity or alkalinity of the body secretions. Twenty to 30 Gm. of mineral salts are excreted daily by an adult man under normal conditions. SEE: *acid-base balance, body, names of elements*.

 m. oil. Petroleum.
 m. water. W. charged with inorganic salts.

minim (mĭn'ĭm) [L. *minimum*, least]. One-sixtieth part of a fluidram. SYN: *drop*.

minimal (mĭn'ĭ-mal) [L. *minimum*, least]. Least.

 m. dose. Smallest dose producing an effect.

minimum (mĭn'ĭ-mum) [L. least]. Least quantity or lowest limit. SEE: *threshold*.

 m. lethal dose. Smallest quantity of a substance producing death.
 m. wave length. The shortest wave length in a roentgen ray or gamma ray spectrum. It is definitely related to the maximum voltage applied to the roentgen ray tube in accordance with the Planck-Einstein quantum equation.

Minin light (mĭn'ĭn). A lamp for the administration of violet and ultraviolet light, producing local anesthesia.

minor (mī'nor) [L. less]. Less important.

Minot-Murphy diet (mī'nŏt). Diet for pernicious anemia containing large quantities of liver.

minuthesis (mĭn"ū-thē'sĭs) [G. *minythēsis*, a decrease]. 1. Decrease in specific sensitivity resulting from continual stimulation to a sense organ; sense organ fatigue. 2. Decrease in symptoms of a disease. SYN: *miosis*.

miocardia (mī-ō-kar'dĭ-ă) [G. *meiōn*, less, + *kardia*, heart]. Systolic lessening of heart's volume. SYN: *systole*.

mionectic (mī-ō-nek'tĭk) [G. *mionektikos*, taking less]. Pert. to having or using a subnormal amount of oxygen, esp. blood. SEE: *mesectic, pleonectic*.

mioplas'mia [G. *meiōn*, less, + *plasma*, a thing formed]. Abnormal lessening of the amount of blood plasma.

miopragia (mī-ō-prā'jĭ-ă) [" + *prassein*, to perform]. Decrease of functional power.

miosis (mī-ō'sĭs) [G. *meiōsis*, a lessening]. 1. Abnormal contraction of pupils. 2. Period of diminishing symptoms in a disease. 3. Reduction phase in chromosome development.

miot'ic [G. *meiōn*, less]. 1. An agent that causes the pupil to contract, such as eserine and pilocarpine. 2. Pert. to or causing contraction of the pupil. 3. Diminishing. 4. Pert. to chromosome reduction.

mire (mīr) [L. *mirāre*, to look at]. OPHTH: An object used as a test, the images of which denote the amount of astigmatism.

mirror drill. Exercises before a mirror practicing control of convulsive tics.

Patient sitting in front of mirror tries to control movements. When he does, physician begins to distract his attention from his reflection by having patient do calisthenics.

 m. speech. That which reverses the order of words in a sentence or pronounces words backward. SEE: *lalopathy*.
 m. writing. Writing in which the words are reversed, as seen in a mirror.

mis- [A.S. *mis*, wrong]. Prefix implying *not, bad, wrong, improper*, etc.

miscar'riage [A.S. *mis*, wrong, + L. *carrus*, cart]. A term used synonymously with *abortion*, and referring to the interruption of pregnancy prior to the 7th month.

Usually refers to expulsion of fetus, specifically in period bet. 4th month and viability.

misce (mĭs'e) [L. mix]. Abbr. M. Mix. A direction to the pharmacist placed upon a prescription for mixing the preparation.

miscegenation (mis″ej-en-a'shun) [L. *miscere*, to mix, + *genus*, race]. Sex relations or marriage bet. those of different races.

miscible (mĭs'ĭ-bl) [L. *miscere*, to mix]. Capable of being mixed.

misemission (mĭs″ē-mĭs'shun) [A.S. *mis*, bad, + L. *emittere*, to send out]. Failure of seminal emission in coitus.

misocainia (mis-o-kī'nĭ-ă) [G. *misein*, to hate, + *kainos*, new]. An aversion to new ideas. SYN: *misoneism*.

misog'amy [" + *gamos*, marriage]. Abnormal aversion to marriage.

misogyny (mĭs-ŏj'ĭn-ĭ) [" + *gyne*, woman]. Abnormal hatred of women.

misologia (mĭs-o-lo'jĭ-ă) [" + *logos*, word]. Aversion to mental work.

misoneism (mĭ-sō-nē'ĭzm) [" + *neos*, new]. Aversion to new things or new ideas; conservatism.

misopedia (mĭ-sō-pe'dĭ-ă) [" + *pais*, *paid-*, child]. Abnormal dislike for children or the young.

misophobia (mis-ō-fō'bĭ-ă) [A.S. *mis*, bad, + G. *phobos*, fear]. Morbid fear or dread of contamination or filth.

Mist, mist. Abbr. for *mistura*, *q.v.*

mistura [L. mixture]. Preparation intended for internal use, and containing suspended insoluble substances which do not unite chemically.
Should always be shaken before using. There are 2 official mixtures.

mite (mīt) [A.S.]. A minute arachnid, a member of the order Acarina.

mithridatism (mĭth'rĭ-dāt″ĭzm) [Mithridates, a king of Pontus, B. C., supposed to have acquired immunity in this fashion]. Immunity to a poison acquired by taking it in doses of increasing size.

mitigated (mĭt'ĭ-gāt-ed) [L. *mitigāre*, to soften]. Diminished in severity. SYN: *allayed, moderated*.

mitochondria (mĭt″ō-kon'drĭ-ă) (sing. *mitochondrion*) [G. *mitos*, thread, + *chondros*, cartilage]. Granular and filamentous structures in cell cytoplasm.

mito'ma, mi'tome [G. *mitos*, thread]. A fine network support or framework of protoplasm in a cell.

mitosin (mĭt'ō-sĭn) [G. *mitos*, thread]. A hormone aiding in mitosis or maturation of follicles.

mito'sis (pl. *mitoses*) [G. *mitos*, thread, + *-ōsis*]. Indirect nuclear division; the usual process of cell reproduction.
There are 4 phases in mitosis: 1. *Prophase*: The nuclear chromatin granules first form a continuous thread, the skein, and then divide into definite segments forming chromosomes. At the same time the centriole divides and each resulting centriole moves toward opposite poles of the nucleus. The centrioles, surrounded by attraction spheres, appear to be connected by a spindle of delicate fibers, the achromatic spindle. The nuclear membrane and nucleolus fade gradually from sight. 2. *Metaphase*: In this stage each chromosome divides longitudinally, forming 2 daughter chromosomes. The number of the chromosomes is now doubled. 3. *Anaphase*: The daughter chromosomes travel in opposite directions along the achromatic spindle towards the centrosome. Gradually the chromosomes lose their individuality, form a skein of chromosome material and resume their former appearance of being chromosome granules suspended in the linin network. The nuclear membrane and nucleolus reappear. 4. *Telephase*: This stage is primarily concerned with the division of the cytoplasm. A constriction appears in the cytoplasm midway bet. the 2 centrosomes. This constriction deepens until 2 distinct cells form with a nucleus and centriole.

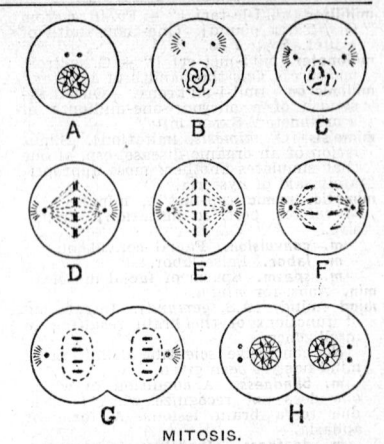

MITOSIS.
Diagram illustrating the four phases of mitotic division in a cell having four chromosomes: A, B, and C illustrate the changes in the centrosome and nucleus during the prophase; D represents the metaphase; E and F, the anaphase; and G and H, the telephase.

mitosome (mĭ'tō-sōm) [" + *soma*, body]. 1. A body giving rise to the middle piece of the spermatozoon. 2. Chromatin mass in a cellular nucleus.

mitotic (mĭ-tot'ĭk) [G. *mitos*, thread]. Pert. to mitosis.

mitral (mĭ'tral) [L. *mitra*, a miter]. Pert. to the bicuspid or mitral valve. SEE: *facies, mitral*. [SEE: *heart*.
  m. disease. That of the mitral valve.
  m. murmur. One produced at the mitral valve. [aperture.
  m. orifice. Left auriculoventricular
  m. regurgitation. Due to failure of valve to close completely, allowing blood to flow back into the auricle.
  m. stenosis. Narrowing orifice of the valve obstructing free flow from auricle to ventricle.
  m. valve. Valve bet. left auricle and left ventricle. SYN: *bicuspidalis, valvula*.

mittelschmerz (mĭt'el-shmärts) [German]. Pain bet. menstrual periods.

mit'tor [L. *mitere*, to rend]. A neuron terminal which transmits impulses to ceptors of the adjoining neuron.

mixed (mikst) [L. *mixtus*, from *miscere*, to mingle]. Consisting of 2 or more interminglings substances.
  m. diet. One consisting of all the food elements in proper proportion. There is no scientific validity to the theory that carbohydrates and proteins should not be eaten together. Over 6000 determinations have been made which proved that the acid response to carbohydrates, to proteins, and to both taken together, is the same and that a mixed

diet does not interfere with gastric secretions or with any of the digestive functions. The presence of protein seems to prolong carbohydrate assimilation.

m. nerves. The spinal nerves containing sensory or afferent, and motor or efferent fibers.

mixture (mĭks'tŭr) [L. *mistura*]. A combination of 2 or more substances without chemical union. SEE: *mistura*.

mm. Abbr. for *millimeter*.

mmm. Abbr. for *micromillimeter*.

Mn. Symb. for *manganese*.

mnemic (nē'mĭk) [G. *mnēmē*, memory]. Relating to memory.

m. hypothesis or **theory.** Stimuli leave engrams (definite traces) on protoplasm, which when frequently repeated set up a habit which persists after the stimuli cease; these engrams possibly may be transmitted to descendants. SYN: *mnemism*. [Mnemic hypothesis, q.v.

mnemism (nē'mĭzm) [G. *mnēmē*, memory].

mnemonics (nē-mŏn'ĭks) [G. *mnēmonikos*, pertaining to memory]. The art of memory culture.

mobile (mō'bĭl) [L. *mobilis*, movable]. Movable.

m. spasm. Tonic spasm with irregular, slow movements of limbs following hemiplegia.

mobility (mō-bĭl'ĭ-tĭ) [L. *mobilitas*]. State or quality of being mobile; facility of movement.

mobilization (mo″bĭl-ĭ-zā'shŭn) [L. *mobilis*, movable]. 1. The making of a fixed or ankylosed part movable. 2. Restoration of motion to a joint.

In fractures Lucas-Championnière advocated the regular administration of a definite dose of movement followed by a period of rest. This he called mobilization.

mobilize (mō'bĭl-īz) [L. *mobilis*, movable]. 1. To incite to physiological action. 2. To render movable; to put in movement.

modal (mōd'al) [L. *modus*, mode]. Pert. to form without reference to substance.

modal'ity [L. *modus*, mode]. 1. Quality of being modal. 2. A method of application or the employment of any therapeutic agent; limited usually to physical agents. The word is avoided by scholarly writers. 3. Any state that modifies the action of a drug. 4. PSY: Whole character of stimuli or sensations determined by the class to which they belong.

mode (mōd) [L. *modus*]. Any class occurring most frequently; a series of variables. SEE: *mean, median*.

modiolus (mō-dī'ō-lŭs) [L. a small measure]. BNA. Central pillar or axial part of cochlea extending from the base to the apex.

modulus (mŏd'ū-lŭs) [L. a small measure]. A unit of physical effects, as a *calorific unit*.

modus (mō'dŭs) [L. method]. A method or a mode.

m. operandi. Method of performing an act.

Moebius' sign (mā'bĭ-ŭs). A symptom in Graves' disease in which one eye converges and the other diverges when looking at the tip of one's nose.

mogigraphia (mŏ-jĭ-grăf'ĭ-ă) [G. *mogis*, with difficulty, + *graphein*, to write]. Writers' cramp.

mogilalia (mŏj-ĭ-la'lĭ-ă) [" + *lalia*, chatter]. Any speech defect, as *stuttering*.

mogiphonia (mŏj-ĭ-fō'nĭ-ă) [" + *phōnē*, voice]. Difficulty in emitting vocal sounds due to strain.

mogitocia (mŏj-ĭ-tō'sĭ-ă) [" + *tokos*, birth]. Difficult birth or parturition.

Mohrenheim's space (mor'en-hīm). Space bet. pectoralis major and deltoid just beneath the clavicle.

moist (moyst) [L. *musteus*, musty]. Damp, wet.

m. chamber. A vessel for keeping microscopic objects moist.

mol(e (mōl). A gram-molecule, a quantity of a chemical compound whose weight in grams equals its molecular weight. Thus 18.016 Gm. of water would be 1 mol.

mo'lar 1. [L. *molēs*, a mass]. Pert. to a mass; not molecular. 2. Pert. to a mole. 3. [L. *molaris*, grinding]. A grinding or back tooth, one of three on each side of the jaws.

The first permanent one erupts at the 6th year; the second one about the 12th year. SEE: *dentition*. 4. Gram-molecule. SYN: *mol, q.v.*

m. solution. One in which there is 1 *mole* of the solute dissolved in each liter of the solution.

molas'ses [L. *mellaceus*, honeylike] (Cane). AV. SERVING: 190 Gm. Pro., 4.6; Carbo., 131.2. VITAMINS: B+. ASH: Ca 0.211, Mg 0.068, K 1.349, Na 0.019, P 0.044, Cl 0.317, S 0.129, Fe 0.0073. SEE: *carbohydrate, sugar*.

mold (mōld) [Icelandic *mugga*, mist]. 1. A fuzzy coating of a fungous nature, on the surface of decaying vegetable matter. 2. A parasitic fungus causing mold. 3. [L. *modulus*, a small measure]. A receptacle into which liquid plastic material is poured to shape it as it dries. 4. To shape a mass, as a *pill.** 5. To shape the fetal head, adapting it to the pelvic inlet.

mold'ing [L. *modulus*, a small measure]. 1. Shaping of the fetal head, adapting itself to pelvic inlet. 2. Manual shaping of infant's features following delivery. 3. A protective border, used in plastic surgery. 4. Casting of a reproduction.

mole (mōl) [AS. *māl*]. 1. A congenital discolored spot elevated above the surface of the skin. SYN: *nevus*.

ETIOL: Not clear. May arise from local or static condition of circulation in a small area. Harmless unless irritated, in which case cancer may appear.

TREATMENT: Protect against irritation. Do not tie a thread about a mole. Electrosurgery.

SEE: *acephalocyst, racemose, melanoma*.

2. [L. *mola*, moistened meal]. A uterine mass arising from a poorly developed or degenerating ovum.

m., blood. A mass made up of blood clots, membranes, and placenta, retained following abortion.

m., Breus'. Malformation of the ovum, a decidual tuberous subchorional hematoma.

m., carneous. Blood mole which has assumed a fleshlike appearance, when retained in uterus for some time.

m., false. One formed from a tumor or polypus.

m., fleshy. SEE: *carneous mole*.

m., hydatid, hydatidiform. A polycystic mass in which the chorionic villi have undergone cystic degeneration.

m., stone. Calcareous degeneration in the uterus.

m., true. Mole representing the degenerated ovum itself.

m., vesicular. SEE: *hydatidiform mole*.

molecular (mō-lek'ū-lar) [L. *molecula*, little mass]. Pert. to a molecule.
　m. layer. 1. Cortical l. of cerebellar or cerebral substance. 2. (Inner). Inner retinal plexiform layer. 3. (Outer). Outer retinal plexiform layer.
　m. lesion. One not even visible through a microscope.
　m. weight. Relative weight attained by totalling the weight of its constituent atoms, using the atomic weight of oxygen, 16, as a unit. SEE: *atomic weight.*
molecule (mŏl'ĕ-kūl) [L. *molecula*, little mass]. 1. The smallest quantity into which a substance may be divided without loss of its characteristics. 2. Any small portions of a substance. 3. A chemical combination of two or more atoms which form a specific chemical compound; the chemical elements are formed by the combination of atoms.
　Combinations of dissimilar atoms form chemical compounds. In normal molecules the positive and negative electric charges exactly balance. Excess or deficiency of either positive or negative charge by the loss or acquisition of electrons results in the formation of an ion.
　The molecule is designated by the number of atoms it contains, as: *monatomic,* (one atom); *diatomic,* (two); *triatomic,* (three); *tetratomic,* (four); *pentatomic,* (five); *hexatomic,* (six), etc. SEE: *cleavage.*
moli'men (Pl. *molimina*) [L. effort]. Effort to establish any normal function, esp. the monthly effort to establish the menses and disturbances experienced at the time.
　m. climacterium virile. A neurasthenia in men bet. 45-55 resulting from change of the testicular secretion.
　m., men'strual. SEE: *molimen.*
Möllgaard treatment (mŭl'gahrd). Treatment of tuberculosis with sanocrysin and sometimes with serum.
mollities (mol-ĭsh'ĭ-ēz) [L.]. Abnormal softening of a part.
　m. ossium. Softening of the bones. SYN: *osteomalacia.*
Moll's glands. Modified sweat glands at border of eyelids. SYN: *ciliary glands.*
molluscous (mol-lŭs'kŭs) [L. *molluscus*, soft]. Concerning molluscum.
molluscum (mol-us'kum) [L. soft]. A mildly infective skin disease characterized by tumor formations on the skin.
　m. contagiosum. The usual mildly contagious form of molluscum.
　SYM: Characterized by small waxy globular epithelial tumors containing semifluid caseous matter or solid masses, healing without scarring though they may suppurate and break down, commonly on face, eyelids, breasts, genitalia and inner surface of thigh. On pressure a substance resembling sebum is expressed.
　ETIOL: Still indefinite. Infection contracted in Turkish baths, bathing pools, and interchangeable bathing suits, etc.
　TREATMENT: Incision, expression of contents, followed by iodine.
　m. fibrosum. A form showing masses of fibrocellular tissue.
　m. simplex. SEE: *m. fibrosum.*
momentum (mō-měn'tŭm) [L. equilibrium, motion]. 1. Quantity of motion. 2. Force of motion acquired by a moving object as a result of continuance of its motion; impetus.
mon'ad [G. *monas*, a unit]. 1. A univalent element. 2. A unicellular organism.
monarthritis (mŏn-ar-thrī'tĭs) [G. *monas*, single, + *arthron*, joint, + *-ītis*, inflammation]. Arthritis affecting a single joint.
monarticular (mŏn-ar-tĭk'ū-lăr) [" + L. *articulus*, joint]. Concerning or affecting one joint.
monaster (mŏn-as'ter) [" + *astēr*, star]. Single starlike figure formed in mitosis.
monathetosis (mŏn"ăth-e-tō'sĭs) [" + *athētos*, not fixed, + *-ōsis*]. Athetosis affecting a single part of the body.
Mondonesi's reflex (mon-dō-na'zĭ). Contraction of facial muscles following pressure on eyeball.
monesthetic (mŏn-ĕs-thet'ĭk) [G. *monas*, single, + *aisthēsis*, sensation]. Affecting only one of the senses.
Mongo'lian id'iocy. Congenital form with resemblance to an Asiatic. SEE: *idiocy.*
Monil'ia [L. *monilis*, necklace]. A genus of parasitic fungi or molds.
monilethrix (mŏn-ĭl'ē-thrĭks) [" + G. *thrix*, hair]. Disease in which the hair becomes brittle and nodulated so that it has a beaded appearance.
moniliform (mŏn-ĭl'ĭ-form) [" + *forma*, shape]. Resembling a necklace or string of beads.
moniliosis (mŏn-ĭl-ī-ō'sĭs) [" + G. *-ōsis*, intensive]. Infection with any species of Monilia.
mono, mon- [G.]. Prefixes: *One, single.*
monoanesthesia (mŏn-ō-ăn-ĕs-thē'sĭ-ă) [G. *monos* + *an-*, priv., + *aisthēsis*, sensation]. Anesthesia of a single member or organ.
monobasic (mŏn-ō-bā'sĭk) [" + *basis*, a base]. Having but one atom of hydrogen replaceable by a base.
monoblepsia (mŏn-ō-blĕp'sĭ-ă) [" + *blepsis*, sight]. 1. OPHTH: Condition marked by a tendency to shut one eye to see clearly.
　Found in anisometropia and in motor anomalies causing diplopia.
　2. Color blindness in which only one color can be seen.
monobrachius (mŏn"ō-brā'kĭ-us) [" + *brachiōn*, arm]. 1. State of having only one arm. 2. Fetus with only one arm.
monobromated (mŏn"ō-brō'māt-ĕd) [G. *monos*, single, + *brōmos*, stench]. Pert. to chemical compound with only one atom of bromine in each molecule.
monocalcic (mŏn-ō-kal'sĭk) [" + L. *calx, calc-*, lime]. Pert. to a chemical compound containing only one atom of calcium in the molecule.
monocelled (mŏn'ō-sĕld) [" + L. *cella*, a chamber]. Composed of a single cell.
monochord (mŏn'ō-kord) [" + *chordē*, cord]. An instrument for testing upper tone audition by means of friction.
monochorea (mŏn"ō-kor-ē'ă) [" + *choreia*, dance]. Chorea which affects but a single part.
monochromatic (mŏn"ō-krō-măt'ĭk) [" + *chrōma*, color]. 1. Having but one color. 2. A color-blind person to whom all colors appear to be of one hue.
monochromator (mŏn-ō-krō'ma-tor) [" + *chrōma*, color]. Instrument for selective transmission of homogeneous radiant energy.
monococcus (mŏn-ō-kŏk'ŭs) [" + *kokkos*, berry]. A form of coccus existing singly instead of as part of the usual group or chain.
monocular (mŏn-ok'ū-lar) [G. *monos*, single, + L. *oculus*, eye]. Concerning or affecting but one eye.
monoculus (mŏn-ok'ū-lŭs) [" + L. *oculus*, eye]. 1. A bandage for shielding one eye. 2. A fetus with only one eye.
monocyesis (mō-nō-sī-ē'sĭs) [" + *kyēsis*,

pregnancy]. Average pregnancy with a single fetus.

monocyte (mŏn′ō-sīt) [" + *kytos*, cell]. A large mononuclear leukocyte.

monocytic (mŏn-ō-sĭt′ĭk) [" + *kytos*, cell]. Concerning or resembling monocytes.

monocytopenia (mŏn″ō-sīt″ō-pē′nĭ-ă) [" + " + *penia*, lack]. Diminished number of monocytes in the blood.

monodactylism (mŏn-ō-dăk′tĭl-ĭzm) [" + *daktylos*, digit]. Condition, usually congenital, of having one digit on a hand or foot.

monodal (mŏ-nod′ăl) [G. *monos*, single, + *odos*, way]. Connected with one terminal of a resonator so that the patient acts as a capacitor for entrance and exit of high frequency currents.

monodiplopia (mŏn″ō-dĭ-plō′pĭ-ă) [" + *diploos*, double, + *ōps*, eye]. Double vision in one eye only.

monogenesis (mŏn-ō-jĕn′ĕ-sĭs) [" + *genesis*, production]. 1. Asexual reproduction. SYN: *parthenogenesis*. 2. Direct development of offspring resembling parent. 3. Theory that all living things develop from a single cell. OPP: *polygenesis*.

monogenous (mŏn-ŏj′en-us) [" + *gennan*, to produce]. Produced or reproducing asexually.

monogerminal (mŏn-ō-jĕrm′ĭn-ăl) [" + L. *germen, germin-*, bud]. Rel. to or developed from a single germ, as *twins*.

monograph (mŏn′ō-grăf) [" + *graphein*, to write]. A treatise dealing with a single subject.

monohemerous (mŏn-ō-hĕm′ĕr-ŭs) [" + *ēmera*, day]. Continuing for only one day.

monohydrated (mŏn-ō-hī′drāt-ed) [G. *monos*, single, + *ydor*, water]. United with only one molecule of water.

monoideaism, monoideism (mŏn-ō-ī-dē′ă-ĭzm, -dē′ĭzm) [" + *idea*, idea]. Domination by only one idea.

monolocular (mŏn″ō-lok′ū-lar) [" + L. *loculus*, a small chamber]. Having only 1 cell or cavity. SYN: *unilocular*.

monoma (mŏn-ō′mă) [" + G. *ōma*, tumor]. Single tumor of uterus.
 SYM: Pain and severe hemorrhage.
 PROG: Fatal ending.

monomania (mŏn-ō-mā′nĭ-ă) [" + *mania*, madness]. Insanity on one subject only, a term found in legal phraseology.

monoma′niac [" + *mania*, madness]. One afflicted with monomania.

monomastigote (mŏn-ō-măs′tĭ-gōt) [" + *mastix, mastig-*, whip]. Possessing only one flagellum.

monomelic (mŏn-ō-mel′ĭk) [G. *monos*, single, + *melos*, limb]. Affecting a single limb.

monomeric (mŏn-ō-mĕr′ĭk) [" + *meros*, part]. Consisting of, or affecting a single piece or segment of a body.

monomicrobic (mŏn″ō-mī-krō′bĭk) [" + *mikros*, small, + *bios*, life]. Caused by one species of microbe.

monomorphic (mŏn-ō-mor′fĭk) [" + *morphē*, form]. Unchangeable in form.

monomyople′gia [" + *mys, myo-*, muscle, + *plēgē*, stroke]. Paralysis of only one muscle.

monomyositis (mŏn″ō-mī-ō-sī′tĭs) [" + + -*itis*, inflammation]. Inflamed condition of only one muscle.

mononeural (mŏn-ō-nū′răl) [G. *monos*, single, + *neuron*, nerve]. Supplied by or concerning a single nerve.

mononeuritis (mŏn″ō-nū-rī′tĭs) [" + " + -*itis*, inflammation]. Inflamed condition of a single nerve.

mononuclear (mŏn-ō-nū′klē-ăr) [" + L. *nucleus*, kernel]. Having one nucleus. SYN: *uninuclear*.

mononucleosis (mŏn-o-nū-klē-ō′sĭs) [" + L. *nucleus*, kernel]. Presence of more than normal number of mononuclear leukocytes in the blood.
 m. infections. Glandular fever with great increase of mononuclear leukocytes in the blood.

monoparesis (mŏn-ō-păr′es-ĭs) [" + *paresis*, weakness]. Paralysis of a single part of body.

monoparesthesia (mŏn″ō-păr-es-thē′sĭ-ă) [" + *para*, beside, + *aisthēsis*, sensation]. Paresthesia of only one region of limb.

monopathy (mŏn-op′ăth-ĭ) [G. *monos*, single, + *pathos*, disease]. 1. A disease attacking only one part of the body. 2. Mental suffering due to solitude or lack of sympathy.

monophagia (mŏn-ō-fā′jĭ-ă) (" + *phagein*, to eat]. 1. Appetite for only one kind of food. 2. The habit of eating of just one meal a day.

monophasia (mŏn-ō-fā′zĭ-ă) [" + *phasis*, speech]. Inability to utter anything but one word or phrase repeatedly.

monophobia (mŏn-ō-fō′bĭ-ă) [" + *phobos*, fear]. Abnormal fear of being alone.

monophyletic (mŏn″ō-fīl-ĕt′ĭk) [" + *phylē*, tribe]. Originating from a single source.

monoplasmatic (mŏn″ō-plăz-măt′ĭk) [" + *plasma*, a thing formed]. Composed of but one tissue or substance.

monoplast (mŏn″ō-plăst) [G. *monos*, single, + *plastos*, formed]. An organism that is unicellular and which keeps the same form throughout its life.

monoplegia (mŏn-ō-plē′jĭ-ă) [" + *plēgē*, stroke]. Paralysis of a single limb, or of one side of the face or body.

monopolar (mŏn-ō-pō′lăr) [" + L. *polus*, pole]. Using 1 terminal only, the ground acting as the 2nd terminal. SEE: *monoterminal*.

monorchid (mŏn-or′kĭd) [" + *orchis*, testicle]. Person having only 1 testicle.

monorchidism, monorchism (mŏn-ōr′kĭd-ĭzm, mŏn′or-kĭzm) [" + *orchis*, testicle]. Condition in which there is only 1 descended testicle.

monorchis (mŏn-or′kis) [" + *orchis*, testicle]. A male having only 1 testicle or but 1 descended testicle.

monosaccharide (mŏn-ō-săk′ăr-id) [G. *monos*, single, + *sakcharon*, sugar]. A sugar which cannot be decomposed into simpler sugars. Ex: *fructose, galactose, glucose*.
 The m. group consist of glucose, fructose, galactose, *q.v*. These sugars are absorbed directly without chemical changes unaffected by enzymes, if not attacked by bacteria. They are soluble, crystallized with difficulty, and fermented by yeast. They maintain the glucose content of the blood and provide for the production of glycogen. SYN: *monosaccharose*.

monosaccharoses (mŏn-ō-săk′ă-rōs-ĕs) [" + *sakcharon*, sugar]. A group name for *monosaccharides, q.v.* Simple sugars which cannot be split into sugars of lower molecular weight.
 They are unaffected by enzymes and enter the blood unchanged, except for the possible action of bacteria. All carbohydrates must be reduced by digestion to monosaccharoses before they may be absorbed by the body, where they are utilized for the production of glycogen. These sugars are very soluble. They ferment without the aid of yeast, and

they are not easily crystallized. SEE: *disaccharoses, polysaccharoses*.

monosome (mŏn'ō-sōm) [" + *sōma*, body]. An accessory chromosome which, without dividing, goes into only 1 of the daughter cells.

monospasm (mŏn'ō-spazm) [" + *spasmos*]. Spasm affecting a single part or organ.

monosymptomatic (mŏn″ō-sĭmp-tō-mat'ĭk) [" + *symptōma*]. Having only 1 dominant symptom.

monosyphilide (mŏn-ō-sĭf'ĭl-ĭd) [" + Fr. *syphilide*]. Characterized by only a single syphilitic lesion.

monoter′minal [" + *terma*, a limit]. Using 1 terminal only in the giving of treatments, the ground acting as the 2nd terminal for the completion of the electrical circuit.

monothermia (mŏn-ō-therm'ĭ-ă) [G. *monos*, single, + *thermē*, heat]. Condition in which bodily temperature is stable.

Monotricha (mŏn-ot'rĭk-ă) [" + *thrix, trich-*, hair]. Bacteria having a single flagellum at 1 pole.

monotrichous (mon-ot'rĭ-kus). Pert. to or having a single flagellum.

monovalent (mon-o-va'lent) [" + L. *valēre*, to have power]. Having the combining power of a single hydrogen atom. SYN: *univalent*.

monoxide (mŏn-ŏk'sīd) [" + *oxys*, sour]. An oxide having only 1 atom of oxygen.

Monro's foramen (mŏn-rō'). Point of communication bet. 3rd and lateral ventricles of the brain.
  M.'s sulcus. Sulcus on 3rd ventricle's lateral wall from the foramen interventriculare to the aditus ad aquaeductum cerebri. SYN: *aulix*.

mons (mŏns) (pl. *montēs*) [L. an elevation]. An anatomical eminence above the surface of the body.
  m. pubis. BNA. Pubic eminence. SYN: *m. Veneris*.
  m. veneris [L. mount of Venus]. A pad of fatty tissue and coarse skin overlying the symphysis pubis in the woman. After puberty covered with short, curly hair called the *escutcheon*. Typically triangular in shape. SEE: *pubes*.

mon′ster [L. *monstrum*]. A malformed fetus. SYN: *teras, teratism*.

monsuparity [" + *parēre*, to give birth to]. The act of bearing a monster.

monstros′ity [L. *monstrositās*]. 1. Monster. 2. Congenital malformation.

Montgom'ery's glands. Small prominences around the nipple of the breast which enlarge during pregnancy and lactation. SEE: *areola, mamma*.

monthlies (mŭnth'lēs). The menses.

monticulus (mon-tĭk'u-lus) [L. little mountain]. A protuberance.
  m. cerebelli. BNA. Protuberance of the superior vermis whose ant. portion is called the *culmen*, the post. portion the *declive*.

mood (mōōd) [A.S. *mōd*, mind, feeling]. Temporary state of mind in regard to or as result of emotion.

moogrol (moo'grŏl). Ethyl chaulmoograte. An oily liquid of faint odor.
  USES: In treatment of leprosy.
  DOSAGE: Intramuscularly, 1 cc. weekly.

morament (mŏr-am'ent) [G. *mōros*, stupid, + *a-*, priv. + L. *mens, ment-*, mind]. A moron of low grade. A person who is mentally defective and without moral sense.

moramentia (mŏr-ă-mĕn′shĭ-ă) [" + " + L. *mens, ment-*, mind]. State of being without moral sense.

Morand's disease (mor-an′). Paresis affecting the lower extremities.

morbid (mor'bĭd) [L. *morbidus*, sick]. 1. Diseased. 2. Pert. to disease.

morbid'ity [L. *morbidus*, sick]. 1. State of being diseased. 2. Prevalence of disease in proportion to the population of a given area.

morbific (mor-bĭf'ĭk) [" + *jacere*, to make]. Causing or producing disease.

morbilli (mor-bĭl'ī) [L. *morbillus*, little disease]. Measles.

mor′bus [L. disease]. Disease.
  m. caducus. Epilepsy.
  m. caeruleus. Cyanosis which is congenital.
  m. coxa'rius. Hip joint disease.
  m. miseriae. Condition due to neglect and want.

morcellation, morcellement (mor-sel-ā'-shŭn, -mon') [Fr. *morceller*, to subdivide]. Method of removing a tumor or organ in pieces.

mordant (mor'dănt) [L. *mordere*, to bite]. A substance which fixes a stain or dye, as *alum* and *phenol*.

mordication (mor″dĭ-kā'shŭn) [L. *mordicāre*, to bite]. Gradual disintegration by chemical process. SYN: *corrosion*.

morgagnian (mor-gan'yē-ăn). Pert. to or described by Morgagni.

Morgagni's caruncle (mor-gan'yē). The middle prostatic lobe.
  M.'s cataract. One that is hypermature with a softened cortex and a hard nucleus. SEE: *cataract*.
  M.'s hy′datid. Remains of müllerian duct attached to testicle or oviduct.
  M.'s liquor. Fluid bet. lens of eye and capsule.
  M.'s ventricle. Ventriculus laryngis. SEE: *ventricle*.

morgue (morg) [Fr.]. A public mortuary; a place for holding dead bodies before disposing of them.

moria (mo'rĭ-ă) [G. *mōria*, folly]. 1. Simple dementia. 2. Foolishness.

moribund (mor'ĭ-bŭnd) [L. *moribundus*, dying]. In a dying condition; dying.

morioplasty (mo′rĭ-ō-plas-tĭ) [G. *morion*, piece, + *plassein*, to form]. Plastic surgery to restore portions of the body which have been lost through accident or disease.

morning or "A. M." care. AIM: Comfort and cleanliness.
  ARTICLES NECESSARY: Basin with warm water. Washcloth and face towel. Toothbrush, mouthwash, and water for mouth hygiene. Emesis basin. Comb and brush. Fresh linen as needed. Bath blanket. Rubbing alcohol and talcum powder.
  PROCEDURE: If in ward screen bed or draw curtains. Offer bedpan before beginning procedure, and supply fresh perineal pad if necessary. Cover patient with bath blanket and fold top bedding to foot of bed. If very disordered, remove to chair. Remove all but 1 pillow. Assist patient with care of mouth, or care for it if patient is not able to. Wash face and hands. Turn patient on side and rub back with alcohol and powder. Patients whose skin is tender should have back washed before the rubbing. If patient is to have bath later the linen need not be changed until that is given. Loosen bottom sheet and draw sheet and pull them tight again, brushing out any crumbs that may be on them. Smooth patient's hair. Fluff and rearrange pillows. Rearrange upper bedding neatly. If patient has a hot water bottle or an ice cap refill them.

Leave fresh water within patient's reach. Leave fresh washcloth and towel.

morn'ing sickness. The nausea and vomiting that affect pregnant women during first few months of pregnancy, particularly in the morning.

Without these symptoms, headache, dizziness and exhaustion may be experienced. It may clear up after the 3rd month and may occur at other times of the day also. It occurs in about 50% of pregnancies.

NP & TREATMENT: Crackers or vanilla wafers on arising. Three to 5 *small* meals per day. Tea helps, some outdoor activities. Psychic causes aggravate, so mental hygiene is desirable. Eat what is craved. Good ventilation during sleep, effervescent drinks. Amytal, 1-2 gr. (0.065-0.13 Gm.).

mo'ron [G. *mōros*, stupid]. A feebleminded person, not beyond the Binet age of 12, having the mentality ordinarily attained between 8 and 12; some authorities state 8 to 11 years. Of greater intelligence than an imbecile. The term implies no moral defect. SEE: *idiot, imbecile.*

moronic (mōr-on'ĭk) [G. *mōros*, stupid]. Feebleminded.

moronity (mōr-on'ĭ-tĭ) [G. *mōros*, stupid]. Feeblemindedness.

Moro's reaction or test. Test to determine the presence of tuberculosis, by application of an ointment of 5 cc. of old tuberculin and 5 Gm. of anhydrous wool fat to the thorax for 1 minute. An eruption of red papules on the skin appears in 24-48 hours in tuberculosis.

M.'s reflex. A defensive reflex, a response consisting of the drawing of the infant's arms across its chest in an embracing manner, in response to stimuli produced by striking the surface on which the infant rests.

morosis (mo-rō'sĭs) [G. *mōros*, stupid, + *-ōsis*]. The mental state of a moron. Feeblemindedness. SYN: *moronity.*

morphea (mor-fē'ă) [G. *morphē*, form]. Skin disease characterized by discrete, circumscribed, grayish or yellowish patches, firm but not hard, bordered by pinkish or purplish areolae on breasts, head, face, lower extremities, with telangiectases on the lesions.

Plaques disappear spontaneously but may leave cicatrixlike marks. Probably a trophoneurosis. SYN: *Addison's keloid, circumscribed scleroderma.*

mor'phia. Morphine, *q.v.*

morphi'na [L.]. Morphine, *q.v.*

morphine (mor'fēn) [L. *morphina*, from *Morpheus*, god of sleep]. Main alkaloid found in opium, occurring in bitter, colorless crystals.

Widely used as analgesic and sedative. Very satisfactory in combination with scopolamine in obstetrics.

POISONING: *Preliminary Symptoms:* Brief mental exhilaration; languor; followed by weariness, sleepiness, pinpoint pupils; rapid, forcible pulse which becomes slow and feeble. Respiration slow and shallow. Unconsciousness, from which patient may be aroused with difficulty. Muscles become relaxed; reflexes diminished; temperature low; skin pale, cold and moist; pupils dilated; coma and death follow.

F. A. TREATMENT: Gastric lavage may be administered and ½% potassium permanganate or 1% tannic acid or powdered charcoal. Large doses of atropine. Hot coffee or tea by mouth and rectum should be administered. Other stimulants injected hypodermically. The reflexes may be stimulated by walking, slapping, or alternate with cold and hot applications, and external heat. Inhalation of oxygen and artificial respiration may be necessary.

m. sul'fate. USP. The sulfate of an alkaloid obtained from opium and occurring as white, feathery crystals, incompatible with alkalies, tannic acid and iodides. [gesic.

ACTION AND USES: Hypnotic and analDOSAGE: 1/8 gr. (0.008 Gm.).

morphinism (mor'fĭn-ĭzm) [L. *morphina*]. Morbid condition due to habitual or excessive use of morphine. Morphine habit.

morphinomania, morphiomania (mor"fĭn-ō-mā'nĭ-ă, fe-ō-mā'nĭ-ă) [" + G. *mania*, madness]. 1. Morbid desire for morphine. 2. Insanity resulting from use of morphine.

morphogenesis (mor"fō-jĕn'ĕ-sĭs) [G. *morphē*, form, + *genesis*, development]. Stimulation of growth and development of form.

morphogenetic (mor"fō-jĕn-et'ĭk) [" + *gennan*, to produce]. Stimulating growth and development of form.

morphology (mor-fol'ō-jĭ) [" + *logos*, study]. Science of external structure and form without regard to function.

morphometry (mor-fom'e-trĭ) [" + *metron*, measure]. The measurement of external portions of forms and organisms.

morphon (mor'fon) [G. *morphoun*, to form]. An individual elemental structure of an organism or person.

morphosis (mor-fō'sĭs) [G. *morphoun*, to form]. Formative process of an organ or part.

morphotic (mor-fot'ĭk) [G. *morphoun*, to form]. Pertaining to or concerning morphosis.

morpio, morpion (mor'pĭ-ō, -pĭ-on) [L.]. The crab louse infesting the pubic area.

mors [L.]. Death.

mor'sus diab'oli [L. "devil's bite"]. Fimbriae of a fallopian tube.

mor'tal [L. *mors, mort-*, death]. 1. Causing death. 2. Subject to death. 3. Human.

mortality (mor-tal'ĭ-tĭ) [L. *mors, mort-*, death]. 1. State of being mortal. 2. The death rate.

mortar (mor'tar) [L. *mortarium*]. Vessel, with a smooth interior, used for powdering or pulverizing drugs with a pestle.

mortification (mor"tĭ-fĭ-kā'shŭn) [L. *mors, mort-*, death, + *facere*, to make]. Death or failure of a tissue, organ or part. SYN: *gangrene, necrosis.*

mortinatality (mor"tĭ-nā-tal'ĭ-tĭ) [" + *natus*, birth]. Ratio of stillbirths to normal births.

mort'ise joint. Ankle joint.

Mor'ton's disease. Neuralgia of the metatarsus.

mortuary (mor'tu-a-rĭ) [L. *mortuarium*, a tomb]. 1. Temporary place for keeping dead bodies before burial. SYN: *morgue.* 2. Rel. to the dead or to death.

morula (mor'ū-lă) [L. *morus*, mulberry]. Solid mass of cells, resembling a mulberry, resulting from segmentation of vitellus of an ovum.

moruloid (mor'u-loid) [" + G. *eidos*, form]. 1. BACT: A colony made up of a mass resembling a mulberry. 2. Resembling a mulberry.

mosquito (mŏs-kē'tō) [Sp. little fly]. 1. A blood-sucking insect of several genera, as *Anopheles, Stegomyia, Culex, Aedes.*

They are the main transmitting agents of various diseases, as *malaria.*
2. Laboratory device for withdrawing blood from a blood vessel.
mossy cell (maws'ĭ). A large neuroglia cell with multiple short processes. SEE: *neuroglia cell.*
moth'er [A.S. *mōdor*]. 1. Female parent. 2. A structure which gives rise to others.
  m. cell. A cell which, by fission or budding, gives rise to similar cells.
  m. cyst. An echinococcus cyst enveloping smaller ones.
  m. liquor. That left after removal of crystals from a solution.
  m.'s mark. A birthmark. SEE: *mark.*
  m.'s star. Single starlike figure in mitosis. SYN: *monaster.*
motile (mō'tĭl) [L. *motilis*, moving]. Able to move spontaneously.
motiline (mo'tĭl-ĭn) [L. *motilis*, moving]. A hormone stimulating contraction.
motility (mō-tĭl'ĭt-ĭ) [L. *motilis*, moving]. Capability of moving spontaneously.
motion (mō'shun) [L. *motio*, movement]. 1. A change of place or position; movement. 2. Evacuation of the bowels. 3. *(Pl.)* Matter evacuated. SEE: *"cine-" words, efferent, "kine-" words, circus movements.*
  m., active. Movements caused by the patient's own intention.
  m., passive. Movements due to an attendant causing the part to be moved.
motor (mō'tor) [L. *motus*, moving]. 1. Causing motion. 2. A part or that which induces movements, as *nerves* or *muscles.*
  m. aphasia. A condition in which the patient understands but cannot express himself in words, or read aloud.
  m. area. Post. part. of frontal lobe ant. to the central sulcus.
  m., electric. Apparatus for the conversion of electric energy into mechanical energy. The reverse of the dynamo.
  m. end plate. Flat expansion ending a motor nerve fiber where it connects with a muscle fiber.
  m. generator. A transforming device consisting of a motor mechanically connected to a generator.
  Such machines are designed to generate direct current when alternating alone is available, or *vice versa.*
  m. nerves. Those causing a muscle or part to move.
  m. oculi. Third cranial nerve.
  m. points. Points where the motor nerve enters the muscle, and where visible contraction can be elicited with a minimal amount of stimulation.
  m. reflex. Any reflex of motor origin; opposite of sensory reflex.
  m., universal. Motor activated by both types of current.
  m. zone. Area affected by stimulation of a motor nerve.
motorial (mō-tor'ĭ-ăl) [L. *motus*, moving]. Concerning motion or a motor center.
motoricity (mō-tor-ĭs'ĭt-ĭ) [L. *motus*, moving]. Capability of movement.
motorium (mō-tōr'ĭ-ŭm) [L. power of motion]. Motor center of a body or organism.
motorius (mō-tōr'ĭ-ŭs) [L. power of motion]. Any motor nerve.
  m. oculi communis. Third cranial nerve. SYN: *motor oculi.*
motorpathy (mō-tōr'păth-ĭ) [L. *motus*, moving, + G. *pathos*, disease]. Treatment of a condition by prescribed movements. SYN: *kinesitherapy, kinetotherapy.*
mottling (mŏt'lĭng) [O.E. *motteley*, many colored]. A condition which is marked by discolored areas.
moulage (moo-lahzh') [Fr.]. 1. A wax model or reproduction, as of a skin condition. 2. Molding of a wax model.
mould (mōld). SEE: *mold.*
moulding (mōld'ĭng). SEE: *molding.*
mounding [origin uncertain]. Lumping, as the mounding of a wasting muscle when struck a quick, firm blow.
mountain fever (mown'těn). 1. A short, remittent fever occurring in mountain regions. 2. SEE: *m. sickness.* 3. Rocky Mountain spotted fever; tick fever; undulant fever.
  m. sickness. Condition characterized by nausea, headache, increased pulse, etc., suffered by those unable to adjust themselves to high altitudes or rare atmosphere. SYN: *mareo de la Cordillera.*
mounting (mownt'ĭng) [L. *mons, mont-,* mountain]. The arrangement of specimens on slides, frames, chart boards, display boards or any background for study.
mouse unit (mows). Least amount of estrus-producing hormone which induces, in a spayed mouse, a characteristic desquamation of the vaginal epithelium.
mouth (mowth) [A.S. *mūth*]. 1. The opening of any cavity. 2. The cavity within the cheeks, containing the tongue and teeth, and communicating with the pharynx.
  Metallic tastes, excess salivation and sore tongue may be due to reverse peristalsis, pernicious anemia, pellagra and sleeping with open mouth. It has been found that dentures, fillings and crowns containing 2 different metals set up galvanic action or low grade electricity, injuring the tissues and through absorption in the body causing organic disorders.
  Excess of saliva or dryness of mouth and throat, erosions of teeth or plates, ulcers, patches, leukoplakia and other symptoms mentioned may also be caused in this way.
  NP: *Aim:* To keep mouth clean and in good condition. *Articles Necessary:* Small tray with glass of fresh water, glass or cup of mouthwash, applicators, tongue depressors, gauze bandage about 2 in. wide, emesis basin, towel, paper bag, liquid albolene or special ointment. *Procedure:* 1. Have all equipment ready on bedside table. 2. Place towel under patient's chin, across chest. 3. Turn patient's head to side and arrange emesis basin close to corner of mouth. 4. Dip applicators in mouthwash and clean teeth, tongue, gums, and roof of mouth. 5. Discard used applicators into paper bag. Do not dip into mouthwash after using. 6. If teeth are difficult to clean make a larger swab by winding several turns of bandage around tongue depressor. 7. Allow patient to rinse mouth with mouthwash, followed by fresh water. Caution him not to expectorate the fluids forcibly, but to let them run gently out at the corner of his mouth. Keep corner wiped clean. 8. If lips are dry or cracked apply liquid albolene or special ointment. 9. If the patient has a high temperature clean the mouth before each feeding. 10. If he is unconscious hold the mouth open with a tongue depressor padded with gauze. 11. Be gentle and thorough.
  RS: *agranulocytosis, Ludwig's; antitrismus; astomatous; bucca; buccal; b. glands; cancrum oris; chalinoplasty; chin jerk; fauces; ora; palate; oral; ori-*

fice; os; stoma; stomatitis; tongue; xerostomia.

m., digestion in. SEE: *salivary digestion*.

m., examination of. Consider size, color, moisture of lips, rashes, abrasions, cysts, fissures, crusts, discoloration, odor of breath, etc. SEE: *mastication*.

movement (moōv'mĕnt) [L. *movēre*, to move]. 1. Act of passing from place to place or changing position of body or its parts. 2. Evacuation of feces.

m., ameboid. Movements resembling that of the ameba by rapid projection or withdrawal from any part of the surface of a process, or change in position and form by flowing of all the protoplasm into 1 of the processes.

m., autonomic. A spontaneous, involuntary m., independent of ext. stimulation.

m., brownian. A peculiar rapid whirling and oscillating m. of minute particles seen under the microscope, as of the granular particles within the salivary corpuscles.

m., ciliary. That of the cilia of a ciliated cell or epithelium.

m., circus. A phenomenon in an animal after injury to 1 corpus striatum, optic thalamus, or crus cerebri, causing it to move about in a circle.

m., disorders of. May be due to injury or disease of (a) muscle, (b) nerve ending, (c) motor nerve, (d) spinal cord, or (e) of the brain.
TYPES OF: Hemiplegia, ataxia, monoplegia, tremors, rigors, choreic, athetosis, convulsions, spasm (clonic or tonic), reflex (hysterical, habit spasm, tics), and spastic paralysis.

m.'s, fetal. Muscular m.'s performed by the fetus in utero.

m., molecular. SEE: *brownian m.*

m., pendular. Swaying movements of the intestine when exposed, due to rhythmic contractions of the circular layer of muscle.

m.'s, respiratory. All the m.'s caused by respiration. SEE: *inspiration, expiration, respiration*.

m. of restitution. A partial rotation of the fetal head, in cases of head presentation.

m., vermicular. Peristalsis.

m. vibratile. Ciliary m.

movement, words pert. to: abduction; abductor; abenteric; aberrant; aberration; acinesia; acroataxia; acrocinesia; acrocinesis; acrocinetic; adduction; adiadochokinesis; akinesia; allocinesia; allokinesis; allokinetic; ambidextrous; ambulant; ambulatory; amyostasia; anapeiratic; anatripsis; anatriptic; apraxia; associated m.; astasia; a. abasia; astrict; athetosis; attollens; autocinesia; autokinesis; autokinetic; bradycinesia; bradykinesia; cardiataxia; cardiocinetic; cardiokinetic; cardioinhibitory; cardiomotility; cardiopaludism; caryocinesis; caryomitosis; cellulifugal; cellulipetal; center, association; centrocinesia; centrostaltic; cephalomotor; cerebellifugal; cerebellipetal; cerebripetal; chemotaxis; chemotropism; chirokinesthesia; cholecystokinin; choreal; choreomania; cinclisis; circumduction; cycle; c., cardiac; dysergia; dysmetria; mobile; motile; motion; motor; palsy; pendulum; relaxed; retroflexion; Swedish; syncinesis.

moxa (mŏk'sa) [Japanese]. Inflammable substance used as a cautery for the skin, or as a counterirritant.

moxibustion (mŏks-ĭ-bŭst'shŭn) [Japanese *moxa*, + L. *combustus*, burned]. Cauterization by means of a cylinder or cone of cotton wool, called a moxa, placed on the skin and fired at the top.

moxosophyra (moks-ō-sof-i'rā) [Japanese *moxa* + G. *sphyra*, hammer]. A hammer heated and used as a cautery.

mu (mū) [Greek letter m]. A micron, 1/1000 of a millimeter or 1/25,000 of an inch.

M. u. Abbr. for Maché unit and mouse unit.

mucedin (mū'se-dĭn) [L. *mucedō*, mucus]. A substance obtained from gluten.

Much-Holzmann reaction (mook-holts'-mahn). Inhibition of hemolysis of erythrocytes by cobra venom in manic-depressive insanity and dementia precox. SYN: *psychoreaction*.

muciferous (mū-sĭf'ĕr-ŭs) [L. *mucus*, mucus, + *ferre*, to carry]. Secreting or producing mucus.

muciform (mū'sĭ-form) [" + *forma*, shape]. Appearing similar to mucus.

mucigen (mū'sĭ-jĕn) [" + G. *gennan*, to produce]. A substance in the mucous membranes that may be converted into mucin.

mucigenous (mū-sĭj'ĕn-ŭs). Producing mucus. SYN: *muciferous*.

mucilage (mū'sĭ-lăj). Vegetable preparation used in pharmaceuticals. SEE: *mucilagō*.

mucilaginous (mū-sĭl-aj'ĭn-ŭs) [L. *mucilāgō*, moldy juice]. Resembling mucilage; slimy; sticky.

mucila'go [L. moldy juice]. Thick, viscid, adhesive liquid, containing gum or mucilaginous principles dissolved in water, usually employed to hold insoluble substances in suspension in aqueous liquids or as a demulcent. There are 2 official mucilages.

mucin (mū'sĭn) [L. *mucus*]. 1. An albuminoid found in mucus and connective tissue, and various secretions such as saliva, bile and the synovial fluid, formed from mucigen, and yielding a slimy solution in water.
2. A commercial preparation made from the gastric mucosa of the hog, used in the treatment of ulcers of the digestive tract.
On decomposition the mucins give dextrose, sulfur and nitrogen among other products. Increase of mucin in the urine indicates irritation and inflammation of the mucous membrane of the urinary tract or vagina.
It forms a protective coating over the ulcer or erosion which prevents irritation from the passing of bile and acid secretions in the duodenum, and from acid conditions irritating peptic ulcer of the stomach.
DOSAGE: Daily, 80-100 Gm. (100 Gm.- 1½ qt., ½ milk and cream, flavored to taste, and divided into 12 hourly doses.)

mucinemia (mū-sĭn-ē'mĭ-ă) [" + G. *aima*, blood]. Mucin in the blood.

mucinogen (mū-sĭn'ō-jĕn) [" + G. *gennan*, to produce]. A glycoprotein which forms mucin.

mucinoid (mū'sĭn-oid) [" + G. *eidos*, resemblance]. Appearing similar to mucin.

mucinuria (mū-sĭn-ū'rĭ-ă) [" + G. *ouron*, urine]. Presence of mucin in the urine.

muciparous (mū-sĭp'ăr-ŭs) [L. *mucus*, mucus, + *parēre*, to bring forth]. Producing or secreting mucus. SYN: *muciferous, mucigenous*.

mucitis (mū-sī'tĭs) [" + G. *-itis*, inflammation]. Inflammation of any mucosa.

muco- [L.]. Combining form, *having relation to mucus*.

mucocele (mū'kō-sēl) [L. *mucus*, mucus, + G. *kēlē*, swelling]. 1. Enlargement of the lacrimal sac. 2. A mucous cyst. 3. A mucous polypus.

mucocutaneous (mū"kō-kū-tā'nē-ŭs) [" + *cutis*, skin]. Concerning a mucous membrane and the skin.

mucodermal (mū-kō-dĕr'măl) [" + G. *derma*, skin]. Pert. to a mucous membrane and the skin. SYN: *mucocutaneous*.

mucoenteritis (mū"kō-ĕn-tĕr-ī'tĭs) [" + G. *enteron*, intestine, + *-itis*, inflammation]. Inflammation of intestinal mucosa.

mucofibrous (mū-kō-fī'brŭs) [" + *fibra*, fiber]. Made up of mucous and fibrous tissues.

mucoglobulin (mū"kō-glŏb'ū-lĭn) [" + *globulus*, globule]. Any protein group to which plastin belongs.

mucoid (mū'koyd) [" + G. *eidos*, resemblance]. 1. Glycoprotein similar to mucin. 2. Muciform similar to mucus.

mucomembranous (mū"kō-mem'brăn-ŭs) [L. *mucus*, mucus, + *membrana*, membrane]. Composed of or rel. to mucosa. SYN: *mucosal*.

mucopurulent (mū-kō-pur'ū-lĕnt) [" + *purulentus*, made up of pus]. Consisting of mucus and pus.

mucopus (mū'kō-pŭs) [" + *pus*, pus]. Mucus combined with or resembling pus.

mucor (mū'kor) [L. mold]. 1. Animal mucus. 2. Mold. 3. (M-). A genus of mold fungi seen on dead and decaying matter.

mucoriferous (mū-kor-ĭf'ĕr-ŭs) [" + *ferre*, to carry]. Covered with mold or a moldlike substance.

mucorin (mū'kor-ĭn) [L. *mucor*, mold]. An albuminoid substance derived from molds.

mucormycosis (mū-kor-mī-kō'sĭs) [" + G. *mykēs*, fungus, + *-osis*]. A fungous disease due to Mucor.

mucosa (mū-kō'să) (pl. *mucosae*) [L. *mucous*]. Mucous membrane.

mucosal (mū-kō'săl) [L. *mucōsa*, mucous]. Concerning any mucous membrane.

mucosanguineous (mū"kō-san-gwĭn'ē-ŭs) [L. *mucus*, mucus, + *sanguineus*, bloody]. Containing mucus and blood.

mucosedative (mū"kō-sĕd'ă-tĭv) [" + *sedativus*, allaying]. Soothing to mucosae of the body. SYN: *demulcent*.

mucoserous (mū"kō-sēr'ŭs) [" + *serum*, whey]. Composed of mucus and serum.

mucosin (mū'kō-sĭn) [L. *mucus*, mucus]. Mucin found in thick, sticky mucus.

mucous (mū'kŭs) [L. *mucus*, mucus]. Having the nature of or resembling mucus.
RS: *mucitis, mucocele, mucopurulent, mucosa, mucus, "myx-" words*.

m. colitis. Inflammation of the mucosa of the colon. SEE: *colitis*.

m. membrane. That lining passages and cavities communicating with the air, and which secretes mucus.

EXAMINATION OF: Examination should reveal degree of moisture, cyanosis, pallor, hyperemia, pigmentation, lesions, or their absence, and hemorrhage.

PALLOR: Seen in all anemias. If temporary, may indicate shock, vasomotor spasm, or may occur in severe hemorrhages.

BLANCHING AND FLUSHING ALTERNATELY: Accompanies aortic regurgitation.

CYANOSIS: SEE: *skin*.

HYPEREMIA OR EXCESSIVE REDNESS: Buccal *mucous membrane*: Due to decayed teeth, traumatism, stomatitis.

Nasal mucosa: Ulceration of nose, rhinitis, inflammation.

Eyes (local irritation): Foreign body, ulcer, inflammation. SEE: *jaundice*.

EXCESSIVE MOISTURE OF MOUTH: Seen in stomatitis, irritation of pneumogastric nerve, ingestion of irritating drugs or foods, nervous disorders, teething, seeing appetizing foods, smelling pleasant odors, and during sexual intercourse.

DRYNESS: Seen in fevers, chronic gastritis, some liver disturbances, excitement, shock, prostration, fatigue, thirst and certain drugs.

m. polypus. Small growth from mucous lining of the cervix or uterus.

m. rashes in mouth. Stomatitis, measles, scarlet fever. ON LIPS: Typhoid fever, meningitis, pneumonia. In secondary syphilis, chancre, cancer and epithelioma mucous patches appear. RS: *baptorrhea, canker, catarrh*.

mucus (mū'kŭs) [L.]. A viscid fluid secreted by mucous membranes and glands, consisting of mucin, leukocytes, inorganic salts, water and epithelial cells.

A good example is the almost ropy secretion from the sublingual and submaxillary glands. Mucus in feces indicates irritation of mucous lining of the intestines and inflammation. It gives a slimy appearance to the stool. If the inflammation is in the small intestines the mucus will be mixed with the stool; if in the colon it will be on surface.

RS: *amyxorrhea, "blenn-" words, expectorant, expectoration, glairy, goblet cell, "muc-" words*.

mulatto (mū-lăt'tō) [Spanish *mulato*, of mixed breed, from L. *mulus*, mule]. First generation born of pure negro and white parentage; popularly anyone of white and negro blood mixed.

Müller's ducts. Embryonic tubes from which the oviducts, uterus and vagina develop in the female; in the male they become atrophied.

M.'s dust bodies. Blood fragments or dust. SEE: *hemokonia*.

M.'s fibers. Finely striated circular fibers of the retina.

M.'s fluid. Solution of 1 part sodium sulfate, 2 parts potassium bichromate in 100 parts of distilled water; used for hardening objects for microscopic examination.

M.'s ganglion. Jugular ganglion.

M.'s muscle. 1. Ciliary circular fibers. 2. Inf. and sup. palpebral muscles. 3. Muscular covering over sphenomaxillary fissure.

M.'s reaction. A sphincterlike muscular r. at the point where the canal of the cervix uteri joins the cavity of the body of the uterus at an advanced stage of pregnancy.

M.'s ring. Muscular ring at junction of cervical canal and the gravid uterus.

M.'s trigone. Portion of *tuber cinereum* folding over the optic chiasm.

mult-, multi- [L.]. Prefixes meaning *many, much*.

multiarticular (mŭl"tĭ-ar-tĭk'ū-lar) [L. *multus*, many, + *articulus*, joint]. Concerning, having, or affecting many joints.

multicapsular (mŭl"tĭ-kap'sŭ-lar) [" + *capsula*, a little box]. Composed of many capsules.

multicellular (mŭl"tĭ-sĕl'ū-lar) [" + *cellula*, small chamber]. Consisting of many cells.

multicuspid, multicuspidate (mul-tĭ-kŭs'-pĭd, -pĭ-dāt) [" + *cuspis*, point]. Having several cusps.

multifid (mŭl'tĭf-ĭd) [" + *fidus*, from *findere*, to split]. Divided into many sections.

multiform (mŭl'tĭ-form) [" + *forma*, shape]. Having many forms or shapes. SYN: *polymorphous*.

multiglandular (mŭl″tĭ-glănd'ū-lar) [" + *glandula*, a little acorn]. Concerning several glands.

multigrav′ida [L. *multus*, many, + *gravida*, pregnant]. A woman who has borne children 2 or more times. SYN: *multipara*.

multiinfection (mŭl″tĭ-ĭn-fĕk'shŭn) [" + *infectio*, an infection]. A mixed infection with several organisms developing at the same time.

multilobular (mŭl″tĭ-lŏb'ū-lar) [" + *lobulus*, a small lobe]. Formed of, or possessing many lobules.

multilocular (mŭl″tĭ-lŏk'ū-lar) [" + *loculus*, a cell]. Having many cells or compartments. SYN: *multicellular*.

multimammae (mul″tĭ-mam'mē) [" + *mamma*, a breast]. Condition of possessing more than the normal number of breasts. SYN: *polymastia*.

multinodal (mul-tĭ-nō'dăl) [" + *nodus*, node]. Having many nodes or knots.

multinodular (mŭl-tĭ-nŏd'ū-lar) [" + *nodulus*, little knot]. Possessing many nodules or small knots.

multinuclear, multinucleate (mul-tĭ-nū'klē-ar, -āt) [L. *multus*, many, + *nucleus*, kernel]. Possessing several nuclei.

multipara (mŭl-tĭp'ă-ră) [" + *parēre*, to bear]. A woman who has borne more than 1 child.

multiparity (mul-tĭ-par'ĭ-tĭ) [" + *parēre*, to bear]. 1. Condition of having borne more than 1 child. 2. Production of more than 1 child at birth.

multiparous (mul-tĭp'ăr-ŭs) [" + *parēre*, to bear]. 1. Having borne more than 1 child. 2. Producing more than 1 child at birth.

multiple (mul'tĭ-pl) [L. *multiplex*, many folded]. 1. Consisting of, or containing more than 1; manifold. 2. Occurring simultaneously in various parts of the body.

   m. personality. Condition in which the subject may develop more than 2 personalities. SEE: *dual personality, vigilambulism*.

multipolar (mul-tĭ-pōl'ar) [L. *multus*, many, + *polus*, a pole]. Possessing more than 2 poles.

multiter′minal [" + G. *terma*, a limit]. Providing several sets of terminals, making possible the use of several electrodes.

multivalent (mul-tĭ-vā'lent) [" + *valēre*, to have power]. Having ability to combine with more than 2 atoms of a univalent element or radical.

mummification (mum″mĭ-fĭ-kā'shun) [Arabian *mūmiyaa*, mummy, + L. *facere*, to make]. 1. Mortification producing a hard, dry mass. SYN: *dry gangrene*. 2. Drying and shriveling of a body, as a dead *fetus*.

mumps (mŭmps) [Dutch *mompen*, to mumble]. An acute, contagious, febrile disease characterized by inflammation of the parotid gland and other salivary glands.

   ETIOL: Causative organism unknown. Probably a filtrable virus.

   SYM: Onset gradual. There may be chilliness, malaise, headache, pain below ears, moderate fever (101-102° F.), sometimes higher, followed by swelling of parotid glands, the enlargement of 1 usually becoming evident a day or 2 before the other. Swelling is below and in front of the ear. It is pyriform in shape, and has a doughy feeling.

   The lobe of the ear is sometimes pushed forward, surrounding tissues are edematous, the features may be greatly distorted. Movements of the jaw are painful and restricted. Saliva may be increased or diminished. Sometimes only 1 parotid is involved. Occasionally, the parotid glands seem to escape, and swelling is confined to the submaxillary gland. Swelling usually lasts from 5 to 7 days.

   COMPLICATIONS: When complications set in, they usually develop about the time the swelling in the parotids subsides. The most common complication in the adult male is orchitis; in the female ovaritis, mastitis and vulvitis. Rarely permanent dullness of hearing follows an attack of mumps.

   DIFFERENTIAL DIAGNOSIS: Cases of symptomatic parotitis must be excluded. Instances of trauma, infections about teeth and mouth, or a blocking of Stensen's duct may be suggestive of mumps.

   PROG: Favorable, although the possibility of sterility may have to be considered in extremely rare instances of double orchitis or double ovaritis.

   TREATMENT: Rest in bed, liquid diet; avoid acids, promote elimination; cold, local applications may control swelling to some extent. SYN: *branks, epidemic parotitis*.

mural (mū'ral) [L. *murus*, a wall]. Pert. to a wall of an organ or part.

muriate (mūr'ĭ-āt) [L. *muria*, brine]. 1. An old synonym for *chloride*. 2. To charge with chlorine or certain chlorine compounds.

muriated (mūr'ĭ-āt-ĕd) [L. *muria*, brine]. Charged with or containing chlorine or certain chlorine compounds.

muriat′ic acid [L. *muria*, brine]. Commercial hydrochloridic acid, *q.v.*

mur′mur [L. *murmur*]. Sound heard in auscultation* due to the more or less forcible closure of the heart's valves.

   Two of the valves give forth a "lubb"* sound and the other 2 a "dupp"* sound, known as the 1st and 2nd heart sounds. A blowing sound is heard if the valve does not close tightly, indicating a leaky valve.

   A slight sound given off first does not necessarily indicate an organic trouble, and heart disease may not result in any murmur; this may also be true in angina pectoris and coronary disorders. Air in the lungs may simulate sounds similar to heart murmurs.

   RS: *auscultation, circulation of blood, heart, hum, venous*.

   m., aneurysmal. Whizzing systolic sound heard over an aneurysm.

   m., aortic obstructive. Harsh systolic one heard with and after the 1st heart sound. Loudest at the base.

   m., a. regurgitant. Blowing, hissing following 2nd heart sound.

   m., apex. Inorganic m. over apex of heart.

   m., arterial. Soft flowing one, synchronous with pulse.

   m., bronchial. M. heard over large bronchi, resembling respiratory laryngeal m.

   m., cardiac pulmonary. M. caused by movement of heart against lungs.

m., diastolic. M. during dilation of heart.

m., direct. M. caused by obstruction of blood in normal course.

m., dynamic. M. due to irregular action.

m., friction. M. caused by rubbing of 2 inflamed mucous surfaces.

m., functional. May be due to changes in the blood and the type of contraction of the heart muscle. They do not indicate organic disease of the heart. They may disappear upon a return to health. They must not be mistaken for true pathological murmurs.

m., hemic. Sound heard on auscultation of anemic persons without a valvular lesion. ETIOL: Abnormal, usually anemic, blood condition.

m., indirect. M. heard when blood flows in abnormal directions.

m., inorganic. M. not due to structural changes.

m., organic. M. due to structural changes.

m., regurgitant. M. due to backward flow of blood current.

m., systolic. M. heard during contraction of heart, due to obstruction.

m., tricuspid. One caused by disease of t. valves.

m., vesicular. One heard in normal breathing.

Murphy's button. Mechanical device used to connect visceral ends of a divided intestine in anastomosis.

M.'s drip or **treatment.** Continuous slow passage of normal saline solution into the rectum; usually used in treating peritonitis.

muscae volitantes (mus'sē vol-ĭ-tan'tēz) [L. flitting flies]. Black specks seen floating in the vitreous humor of the eye and visible to the patient; often seen in myopia.

muscle (mus'el) [L. *musculus*]. Organ composed of contractile tissue which effects the movement of any organ or part of the body.

The outstanding characteristic of muscular tissue is its elasticity. The cellular arrangement varies with each type of muscle tissue, which has little intercellular material and the cells are very close together. The human body has 3 types of muscular tissue:

SMOOTH, NONSTRIATED, ORGANIC: Does not have distinctive cross markings on it which are seen in the other types of muscle tissue. Called *involuntary* because it is not controlled by conscious effort, but works without control of the will. Its cells are elongated with a central nucleus, and are gathered into bundles held together by connective tissue sheaths. Found in blood vessels, skin, ducts of glands and digestive tract.

STRIATED, STRIPED, SKELETAL: Has striped markings. Called *voluntary* because it is controlled by conscious effort. Muscle cells are long and cylindrical, with multiple nuclei arranged about the periphery of the fiber. The cytoplasm (sarcoplasm) contains numerous coarse myofibrils. Cytoplasmic membrane of cell is called the sarcolemma sheath. Muscle fibers grouped into bundles called fascicles. Found in walls of hollow viscera.

CARDIAC: Although striated like the skeletal muscle, it is *involuntary*. Found only in the heart. Fibers contain abundant sarcoplasm and multiple nuclei. Myofibrils run throughout the sarcoplasm. Cell ends untie to form a meshwork. At various intervals, prominent bands, or intercalated disks, cross the fibers.

BLOOD SUPPLY: Obtained from small blood vessels which enter the muscular tissue and subdivide into capillaries which permeate throughout.

NERVE SUPPLY: *Voluntary*: From branches of the peripheral cerebrospinal nervous system. It is because of this that the skeletal muscles are under conscious control. *Involuntary*: Smooth and cardiac receive their nerve supply from autonomic nervous system and function involuntarily without conscious control.

FUNCTION: To bring about changes in position.

SHAPE: Voluntary muscle spindle-shaped, attached to bones by *tendons*, or broad and flat, attached by broad fibrous tissue sheets called *aponeuroses*. Fixed point of attachment is the *origin* of a muscle, the *point of insertion* of a muscle being the more movable point of attachment.

FUNCTIONAL NEEDS: Sufficient blood supply, impulses from nervous system, glucose, oxygen.

CHEMICAL CONSTITUENTS: Proteins, creatine, hypoxanthine, carnine, inosite, phosphocarnic acid, glycogen, sarcolactic acid, fat and mineral salts.

m., abductor. M. which draws away from the midline.

m., adductor. M. which draws toward the midline.

m., antagonistic. M. which neutralizes the function of another.

m.'s, antigravity. M.'s which pull against the force of gravity to maintain posture.

m., appendicular. One of the skeletal muscles of the limbs.

m., articular. A joint muscle.

m., axial. A skeletal m. of the head or trunk.

m., bipennate. M. in which the fibers converge toward a central tendon on both sides.

m. bound. Condition caused by overuse in which muscles are less elastic and bulkier.

m., constrictor. A m. which compresses a part.

m., corrugator. M. drawing the skin up and causing it to wrinkle.

m. curve. A tracing of muscular contraction.

m., digastric. M. with a fibrous insertion bet. 2 fleshy bellies. [part.

m., extensor. M. which straightens a

m., extrinsic. Any m. of different developmental origin from the part on which it acts.

m. fatigue. Contraction of a muscle represents *latency, contraction* and *relaxation*. During contraction the muscle is shortened. The contraction is more or less modified by fatigue, the height of contraction is lowered, the relaxation delayed, lengthening the period of latency. Stimuli occurring in too rapid succession may prevent relaxation. Overexertion spreads the body's lactic acid to muscles not being used which, with a deficiency of oxygen intake, brings about fatigue.

m.'s, fixation. Accessory m.'s which aid in steadying a part.

m., flexor. M. which bends a part.

m., fusiform. A m. resembling a spindle.

Tabular Comparison of the Properties of Three Types of Muscle

	Smooth	Cardiac	Striped
Synonyms	Involuntary Visceral Plain	Myocardium	Voluntary Skeletal Striated
Fibers: Length in micra Thickness Shape Marking	75. 5. Spindles No striation	Blocks Striation	25,000. 75. Cylinders Marked striation
Nuclei	Single	Single	Multiple
Speed of contraction	Very slow	Moderate	Very quick
Effects of cutting related nerve	Slight	Slight	Complete paralysis

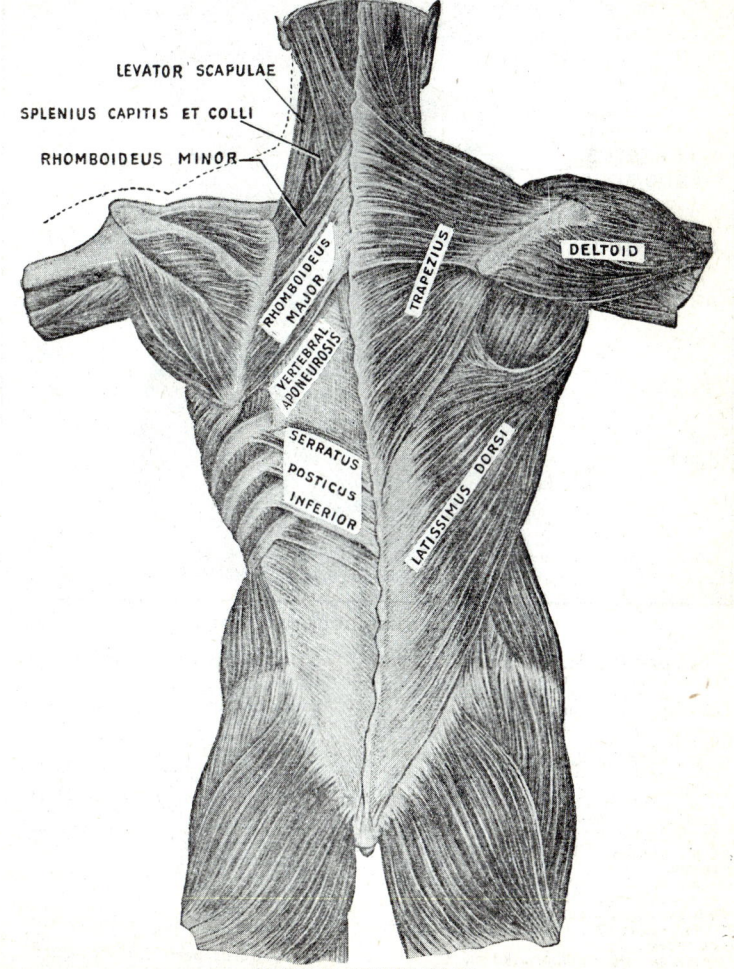

MUSCLES OF THE BACK.

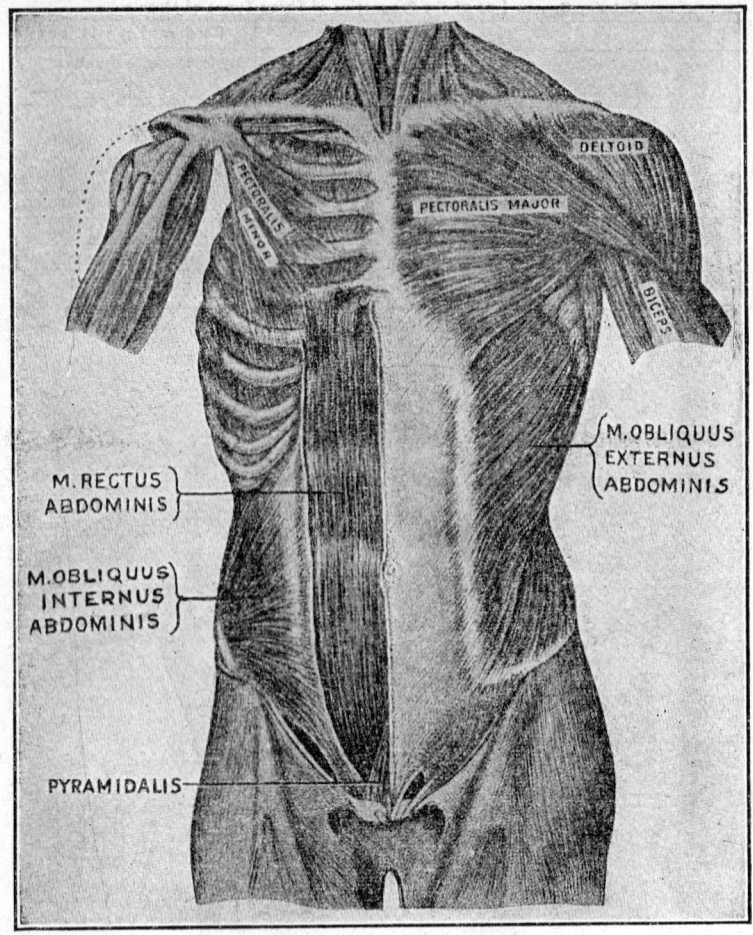

MUSCLES OF THE ABDOMINAL WALL.

m., intrinsic. M. with origin and insertion on the same limb.
m., involuntary. M. not controlled by the will; mainly smooth.
m., joint. M. which produces motion in a joint.
m., nonstriated, m., organic. M. without markings on its fibers; mainly involuntary.
m., pennate. M. with central or lateral tendon toward which fibers converge on 1 or both sides.
m. plasma. Fluid found in muscular tissue.
m. serum. M. plasma without myosin.
m., skeletal. M. which is connected with a bone; mainly striated.
m., skew. M. which pulls a part obliquely.
m., smooth. Nonstriated m.
m., somatic. Skeletal m.
m., sphincter. M. controlling an opening.
m., striated, m., striped. M. with bands dividing its fibers; mainly voluntary.
m. sugar. Sugar found in muscular tissue. SYN: *inosite*.
m.'s, synergistic. M.'s aiding one another in function.
m., unipennate. M. whose fibers converge on only 1 side of a tendon.
m., unstriated, m., unstriped. M. without markings; mainly involuntary.
m., visceral. 1. Any m. not originated in somite of embryo. 2. Any m. of the visceral part of the skull.
m., voluntary. M. whose action is controlled by will; excepting the cardiac m.; all striated m.'s are voluntary.
muscle, words pert. to: accommodation; achalasia; agraphia; algiomotor; algio-

muscular; amphicreatine; "amyo-" words; anisosthenic; anodal closure contraction; aphthongia; astasia; asynergia; asynergy; atactic; ataxia; a., locomotor; ataxiadynamia; ataxy; athermosystaltic; biventer; biventral; cardiomyotomy; carneous column; cavalry bone; celiomyalgia; celiomyositis; charley horse; cheek; cinesalgia; contracture; coördination; diastasis recti; dystrophy; fasciculus; fasciola; flaccid; flexion; flexure; hemiataxia; hypertonia; hypertonic; hypertonus; incoördination; isometric; isotonic; kinesalgia; kinesiology; kinetic; ligament; muscular contraction; muscularis; musculature; "my-" words; origin; peroneal; relaxation, complete; rigor; sprain; staircase-effect; strain; Thomsen's disease; trophoneurosis; unstriated; venter; volley; voluntary; writer's cramp.

mus'cular [L. *musculus*, muscle]. 1. Pert. to muscles. 2. Possessing well developed muscles.

m. **contractions, graduated.** Accomplished by gradually sheathing the core of specially designed faradic coil with operator's right hand which slowly increases the current, while the operator's left hand applies small, active electrode to muscles under treatment.

m. **reflex.** Muscle contraction, either or both isotonic and isometric.

m. **rheumatism.** That affecting the muscles.

muscularis (mŭs-kū-la'rĭs) [L. muscular]. Muscular coat of a hollow organ or tubule.

m. **mucosae.** Unstriated muscular tissue layer of mucous membrane.

musculation (mŭs-kū-lā'shŭn) [L. *musculus*, muscle]. 1. Muscular arrangement in the body. 2. Muscular action. SYN: *musculature.*

mus'culature [L. *musculus*, muscle]. The arrangement of muscles in the body or its parts.

mus'culin [L. *musculus*, muscle]. Muscle tissue globulin or protein.

musculo- [L.]. Combining form *pert. to a muscle.*

musculocutaneous (mŭs"kū-lō-kū-tān'ē-ŭs) [L. *musculus*, muscle, + *cutis*, skin]. 1. Pert. to the muscles and skin. 2. Supplying or affecting the muscles and skin.

musculomembranous (mŭs"kū-lō-mĕm'brăn-ŭs) [" + *membrana*, membrane]. Pert. to or consisting of muscle and membrane.

mus'culus (pl. *musculī*) [L.]. Muscle, *q.v.*

mush'room [Fr. *moucheron*, from L. *muscus*, moss]. Umbrella-shaped fungus which grows on decaying vegetable matter; common in woods and damp places. The poisonous varieties are commonly called toadstools, *q.v.*

COMP: Low in carbohydrates and fats; high in protein but of little alimentary value. Xanthic bodies and toxic elements are present. Their relationship and similarity to poisonous fungi are so close that only those who are thoroughly posted should attempt to gather or purchase them.

AV. SERVING (fresh) : 50 Gm. Fat 0.2. VITAMINS: B+, G+ to ++. ASH CONST: Ca 0.017, Mg 0.016, K 0.384, Na 0.027. P 0.108, Cl 0.021, S 0.051. A base-forming food; alkalinity, 4 cc. per 100 Gm.; 9 cc. per 100 cal.

ACTION: As a seasoning they stimulate gastric secretions.

m. **and toadstool poisoning.** Poisoning from eating wrong species.

TREATMENT: These require an abundance of hot drinks, preferably containing a small amount of table salt; heat to the abdomen; strong tea, and above all atropine or belladonna and morphine, which are physiologic antidotes. Patients are always in shock and need adequate treatment. Diarrhea and emesis are marked and ordinarily need to be allayed rather than stimulated.

mu"sicoma'nia [G. *mousikē*, music, + *mania*, madness]. Insane love of music.

mu"sicother'apy [" + *therapeia*, treatment]. Treatment of mental diseases with music.

musk (mŭsk) [G. *moskos*, from Sanskrit *muska*, testicle]. Dried secretion of the preputial follicles of male musk deer. Used as a stimulant and sedative.

DOSAGE: 1-10 gr. (0.06-0.6 Gm.).

musk'melon [" + G. *mēlon*, apple]. Av. SERVING: 200 Gm. Pro. 1.2, Fat 0.2, Carbo. 11.8. VITAMINS: A++, B++, C++ to +++. ASH: Ca 0.017, Mg 0.012, K 0.235, Na 0.061, P 0.015, Cl 0.041, S 0.014, Fe 0.0003. SEE: *cantaloupe, melon.*

mus'sel [L. *musculus*, little mouse]. Principles and action about the same as those of the oyster, although less liable to cause infection.

mussitation (mŭs-sĭ-tā'shŭn) [L. *mussitāre*, to mutter]. The muttering of delirium or the moving of the lips without sound.

must [L. *mustus*, young, fresh]. Unfermented grape juice.

mus'tard [Fr. *moustarde*]. Yellow powder of mustard seed used as a counterirritant, rubefacient, emetic and stimulant. SEE: *plaster.*

As a condiment: Av. SERVING (prepared): 10 Gm. Pro. 0.4, Fat 0.3, Carbo. 0.7. ASH: Ca 0.402, Mg 0.260, K 0.761, Na 0.056, P 0.755, Cl 0.016, S 1.230. No iron. SEE: *condiments.*

m. **greens.** Av. SERVING: 50 Gm. Pro. 1.2, Fat 0.2, Carbo. 2.00. VITAMINS: A+++, B+, G+++.

mutacism (mū'tă-sĭzm) [G. *mytakīsmos*, fondness for letter m]. Excessive or improper pronunciation and use of letter m or its sound. SYN: *mytacism.*

mutant (mū'tănt) [L. *mutāre*, to change]. In heredity, a sport or variation which breeds true.

mutase (mū'tās) [" + *ase*, enzyme]. 1. Enzyme which accelerates oxidation reduction reactions through activation of oxygen and hydrogen. 2. A food preparation made from leguminous plants high in protein content.

mutation (mū-tā'shŭn) [L. *mutāre*, to change]. 1. Change; transformation; instance of such change. 2. Sudden, permanent variation with offspring differing from parents in a marked characteristic as differentiated from gradual variation through many generations, so called by De Vries. Also person showing such change.

mute (mūt) [L. *mutus*, dumb]. 1. One who is unable to speak. 2. Dumb; without ability to speak.

m., **deaf.** Individual who is unable to hear or to speak.

mutism (mū'tĭzm) [L.]. 1. Condition of being unable to speak. 2. PSY: Persistent inhibition to speech; seen in *dementia precox.*

mut'ton [Fr. *mouton*, from L. *multo* (*n*), sheep]. COMP: NUTRIENTS, E. P. (fore and hind quarters, leg and side). Pro. 15.6-16.7-19.8-16.2%, Fat 30.9-28.1-12.4-29.8%. VITAMINS: Vit A present. A good source of Vit. B. C and G lacking.

Contains more fat and mineral matter than beef but less albumin. Its nutritive value is lower and it is not so easily digested.

mutualism (mū'tū-ăl-ĭzm) [L. *mutuus*, exchanged]. Relationship of 2 organisms living together, both benefiting. SYN: *symbiosis, 2.*

myalgia (mī-al'jĭ-ă) [G. *mys, my-,* muscle. + *algos,* pain]. Tenderness or pain in the muscles; muscular rheumatism.

myameba (mī-ăm-ē'bă) [" + *amoebē,* change]. A muscle cell considered as an organism.

myanesin (mī-ăn'ĕ-sĭn). A synthetic compound injected into a vein for relaxation of muscle tension. It gives relief in poliomyelitis and some types of arthritis.

myasis (mī-ā'sĭs) [G. *myia,* a fly]. Condition which arises from larvae of flies or maggots in the body or upon mucous membranes. SYN: *myiasis.*

myasthenia (mī-ăs-thē'nĭ-ă) [G. *mys, my-,* muscle, + *astheneia,* weakness]. Muscular weakness.

m., angiosclerotic. Vascular changes producing excessive muscular fatigue.

m. gastrica. Loss of muscular tone in coats of the stomach.

m. gravis. Great muscular weakness without atrophy.

Motor impulses flow freely through nerves until they reach end fibers which fail to carry on impulses to motion. May present myasthenic face, inability to swallow, difficult breathing, difficulty in raising the feet, and general prostration.

PROG: Grave.

NP: Adequate rest is imperative, according to severity of the condition. It is best to insist upon complete rest, both physical and mental. Diet is a very important problem. A soft, easily masticated diet (highly nutritious), will aid the difficulty in chewing and swallowing. The patient should chew and swallow slowly with time between each movement, thus allowing the muscles to regain lost power by repeated activity. A nasal tube may be necessary with some patients. All forms of exercise, physical therapy, and electrical treatment are contraindicated. The nurse should not discount the seriousness of these cases.

TREATMENT: Ingestion daily of ephedrine. Guanidine hydrochloride given orally or intravenously is being used with success. A 2% solution in physiological solution of sodium chloride is used for the intravenous administration. Gelatin capsules are used for oral administration. Dosage to suit the case, 10 mg. per kilogram of body weight. Prostigmine bromide is often given with it. SEE: *myasthenic face, myopathy.*

m. pseudoparalytica. Muscular weakness simulating paralysis due to myasthenia.

myasthe'nic [" + *astheneia,* weakness]. Marked by muscular weakness.

m. face. A type of myasthenia, in which 1 side of the face will have a normal smile, and the other side a sneer, when attempting to smile.

Another type exhibits the upper lids apparently closed and the mouth partly open, with evidence of fatigue or exhaustion.

myatonia (mī-ă-tō'nĭ-ă) [" + *tonos,* tone]. Deficiency or loss of muscular power.

m. congenita. M. of early childhood; it is not hereditary. SYN: *Oppenheim's disease.*

myatrophy (mī-at'rō-fī) [" + *atrophia,* atrophy]. Muscular wasting away.

mycelioid (my-se'lĭ-oid) [" + " + *eidos,* form]. Appearing like molds and yeast colonies having filaments radiating from the center.

mycelium (mī-se'lĭ-ŭm) [G. *mykēs,* fungus, + *ēlos,* nail]. Mass of vegetative portion of fungus consisting of hyphae forming molds.

mycethemia (mī-se-thē'mĭ-ă) [" + *aima,* blood]. Fungi in the blood. SYN: *mycohemia.*

mycetism, mycetismus (mī'se-tĭzm, -tĭz'-mŭs) [" + *ismos,* condition]. Poisoning from eating mushrooms.

mycetogenetic, mycetogenic, mycetogenous (mī-sē″tō-jĕn-ĕt'ĭk, -jĕn'ĭk, -toj'-ĕn-ŭs) [G. *mykēs,* fungus, + *gennan,* to produce]. Induced by fungi.

mycetoma (mī-se-tō'mă) [" + *ōma,* tumor]. A disease induced by fungi, seen in India, which attacks the foot. SYN: *Madura foot.*

Myco. Abbr. for *Mycobacterium.*

Mycobacte'rium [G. *mykēs,* fungus, + *baktērion,* little rod]. A genus of bacillary organisms, including those of leprosy and tuberculosis.

mycocyte (mī'kō-sīt) [G. *mykēs,* mucus, + *kytos,* cell]. A cell found in mucous tissue.

Mycoderma (mī-kō-der'mă) [G. *mykēs,* fungus, + *derma,* skin]. Genus of fungi forming membranes in fermenting liquids.

M. ace'ti. Mother of vinegar.

mycoder'ma [G. *mykēs,* mucus, + *derma,* skin]. Mucous membrane.

mycodermatitis (mī″kō-der-mă-tī'tĭs) [" + " + *-itis,* inflammation]. Inflamed condition of a mucous membrane. SYN: *catarrh.*

mycogastritis (mī-kō-gas-trī'tĭs) [" + *gastēr,* belly, + *-itis,* inflammation]. Inflamed condition of mucosa of stomach.

mycohemia (mī-kō-hē'mĭ-ă) [" + *aima,* blood]. Fungi present in the blood.

mycoid (mī'koyd) [G. *mykēs,* fungus, + *eidos,* form]. Funguslike.

m. degeneration. Excessive formation of mucus in catarrhal conditions, or in tumors.

mycology (mī-kol'ō-jī) [" + *logos,* study]. Science of fungi.

mycomyringitis (mī″kō-mī-rin-jī'tĭs) [" + *myrigx,* membrane, + *-itis,* inflammation]. Fungous inflammation of membrana tympani.

mycophylaxin (mī″kō-fĭl-ăks'ĭn) [G. *mykēs,* fungus, + *phylax,* guard]. A phylaxin which destroys microörganisms.

mycosis (mī-kō'sĭs) [" + *-ōsis,* intensive]. Any disease induced by a fungus.

m. favosa. Formation of honeycomblike crusts over hair follicles with itching and unpleasant odor. SYN: *favus, q.v.*

m. fungoides. A rare chronic inflammatory malignant disease probably of septic origin that affects the superficial and deep layers of the skin, and occasionally the mucous membrane.

SYM: Urticarial, erythematous or eczematous patches of irregular shape and size, with well-defined margins usually upon scalp and skin of trunk. Itching intense, and frequently the patches become hypertrophic and firm. Hard nodules varying from size of pea to apple, either sessile or pedunculated, develop on them. These eventually break down and form ulcers that contain sensitive, fungating granulation tissue, and

discharge thin pus and serum. Death results from progressive cachexia.
TREATMENT: Constitutional. Good, nourishing food. Hygienic living. Ulcers may be treated surgically. Cleanliness.

m. leptothrica. Disease caused by *Leptothrix buccalis*, consisting of gray or black deposits on tongue and buccal mucosa usually with constitutional symptoms.

m. tonsillaris benigna. A name applied by Frankel to a peculiar form of pharyngeal disease induced by undue accumulations of Leptothrix upon pharyngeal tissue.

mycosozin (mī-kō-sō'zĭn) [" + *sōzein*, to save]. A sozin that destroys microörganisms.

mycotic (mī-kŏt'ĭk) [G. *mykēs*, fungus]. Caused by or affected with microörganisms.

mydaleine (mīd-ā'le-ēn) [G. *mydaleos*, putrid]. A poisonous ptomaine from putrefied visceral organs, acting mainly on the heart.

mydriasis (mid-rī'ăs-ĭs) [G. *mydriasis*]. Abnormal dilation of the pupil.
ETIOL: Fright, sudden emotion, anemia, 1st and 3rd stages of anesthesia, drugs, coma, hysteria, botulism, irritation of cervical sympathetic nerve.

mydriatic (mid-rī-at'ĭk) [G. *midriasis*. dilatation]. 1. Causing pupillary dilatation. 2. Any drug which dilates the pupil.
EX: *atropine, cocaine, ephedrine, euphthalmine, homatropine*.

myectopia (mī-ĕk-tō'pĭ-ă) [G. *mys, my-*, muscle, + *ek*, out, + *lopos*, place]. Muscle dislocation.

myelalgia (mī-el-al'jĭ-ă) [G. *myelos*, marrow, + *algos*, pain]. Pain of the spinal cord or its membranes.

myelanalosis (mī"el-ă-nal-ō'sĭs) [" + *analōsis*, wasting]. Gradual wasting of spinal cord. SYN: *tabes dorsalis*.

myelapoplexy (mī-el-ap'ō-plĕks-ĭ) [" + *apoplexia*, stroke]. Hemorrhagic effusion into the spinal cord.

myelasthenia (mī-ĕl-ăs-thē'nĭ-ă) [G. *myelos*, marrow, + *astheneia*, weakness]. Spinal exhaustion; neurasthenia arising from spinal causes.

myelateleia (mī-el-ă-tē'lĭ-ă) [" + *ateleia*, imperfection]. Defective development of spinal cord.

myelatrophy (mī-el-at'rof-ĭ) [" + *atrophia*, atrophy]. Wasting of the spinal cord.

myelauxe (mī-el-awks'ē) [" + *auxē*, increase]. Abnormal enlargement of spinal cord and marrow.

myelemia (mī-ĕl-ē'mī-ă) [" + *aima*, blood]. Abnormal number of marrow cells in the blood. SYN: *myelocytosis*.

myelencephalon (mī"ĕl-ĕn-sef'ă-lon) [" + *egkephalos*, brain]. 1. The cerebrospinal axis, composed of the spinal cord and brain. 2. Afterbrain; portion of embryo from which arise the medulla oblongata and the bulbar area of the 4th ventricle.

my'elin [G. *myelos*, marrow]. 1. Fatlike white material composing sheath of a medullated nerve fiber. SYN: *white substance of Schwann*. 2. A lipoid substance seen in animal tissues, as the brain.

myelination (mī-ĕl-ĭn-ā'shŭn) [G. *myelos*, marrow]. Process of acquiring a myelin sheath. SYN: *myelinization*.

myelinic (mī-ĕl-ĭn'ĭk) [G. *myelos*, marrow]. Concerning or composed of myelin.

myelinization (mī"ĕl-ĭn-ĭ-zā'shŭn) [G. *myelos*, marrow]. Acquirement of myelin sheath for nerve fibers. SYN: *myelination*.

myelinogenetic (mī"ĕl-ĭn-ō-jĕn-et'ĭk) [" + *gennan*, to produce]. Producing myelin or a myelin sheath.

myelinosis (mī"ĕl-ĭn-ō'sĭs) [" + -*ōsis*, intensive]. Fatty degeneration during which myelin is produced.

myelitic (mī-el-it'ĭk) [G. *myelos*, marrow]. Concerning myelitis.

myelitis (mi-el-i'tis) [" + -*ītis*, inflammation]. 1. Inflammation of the spinal cord. 2. Inflammation of bone marrow.
SYM: Moderate fever (101°-103° F.), loss of appetite, coated tongue and constipation, followed by pain in back radiating into the limbs. Various forms of paresthesia, as numbness, tingling, burning, etc. Frequently a sense of painful constriction, "girdle pain" at level of the disease. Paralysis soon develops, and may become more or less complete; at first may be retention, later frequently incontinence of feces, anesthesia, more or less complete. Bedsores soon develop. Death may result in few days from extension upward, and involvement of respiratory muscles. In rare cases a spontaneous arrest of inflammation and slow recovery follows, attended with partial paralysis.
SEE: *axophage, osteomyelitis, poliomyelitis*.

m., acute. Simple acute form which develops following injury.

m., bulbar. M. involving the oblongata.

m., central. M. in which the gray matter is esp. involved.

m., c., acute. Resembles acute transverse m., but the trophic disturbances are more marked and duration shorter. Usually fatal in 1 to 2 weeks.
PROG: Always extremely grave.
TREATMENT: If possible place patient on water bed. Both in retention and incontinence of urine catheter should be used twice daily. In incontinence of urine and feces the discharges should be received on cotton, wool or oakum, which should be frequently renewed and parts thoroughly cleansed. In the beginning ice bags or wet cups may be applied to the spine. Frequent baths should be given, milk, eggs, rice, toast, farina, fruit and blanc mange may be given in early stages of disease. Later, more nutritious diet.

m., chronic. Form progressing slowly but steadily.
SYM: Begin with numbness, tingling or burning in lower extremities, followed by loss of power and sensation. Reflexes generally exaggerated. Sphincters soon become involved. Girdle pain at level of disease. Progress slow, 6 months to 10 years.
TREATMENT: Patient should be put at rest. Frequent tepid baths; plenty of sleep; good, nourishing food; moderate exercise that stops short of fatigue. Freedom from mental worry. Constitutional treatment, antisyphilitics where indicated.

m., compression. M. caused by pressure on the cord, as by a hemorrhage.

m., cornual. M. affecting the spinal cord's horns of gray matter.

m., descending. M. affecting successively lower areas of the spinal cord.

m., diffuse. M. involving large sections of the cord.

myelitis, disseminated   M-58   **myelopathy**

m., disseminated. M. with several separated foci on the cord.
m., hemorrhagic. M. with hemorrhage.
m., parenchymatous. M. of nerve substance.
m., sclerosing. M. with hardening of cord, and interstitial tissue growth.
m., systemic. M. affecting only certain tracts of the cord.
m., transverse. M. involving the whole thickness of the cord.
m., t., acute. Acute form of m. involving entire thickness of cord, developing subsequent injury to spinal cord.
m., traumatic. M. due to cord injury.
myelo- [G.]. Prefix denoting *the spinal cord,* or *bone marrow.*
myeloblast (mī'el-ō-blăst) [G. *myelos,* marrow, + *blastos,* germ]. Bone marrow cell which develops into a myelocyte.
myeloblastemia (mī″ĕl-ō-blăst-ē'mĭ-ă) [" + " + *aima,* blood]. Occurrence of myeloblasts in the blood.
myeloblastoma (mī″ĕl-ō-blăst-ō'mă) [" + " + *-ōma,* tumor]. 1. Tumor containing myeloblasts. 2. Myelogenic form of leukemia.
myelobrachium (mī″ĕl-ō-brā'kĭ-ŭm) [" + *brachiōn,* arm]. The restiform body.
myelocele (mī'ĕl-ō-sēl) [" + *kēlē,* hernia]. 1. A form of spina bifida with spinal cord protrusion. 2. [" + *koilos,* hollow]. Central canal of spinal cord.
myelocyst (mī'ĕl-ō-sĭst) [G. *myelon,* marrow, + *kystis,* bladder]. Cyst arising from the spinal cord.
myelocystocele (mī″ĕl-ō-sĭst'ō-sēl) [" + " + *kēlē,* hernia]. Cystic tumor of spinal cord.
myelocystomeningocele (mī″ĕl-ō-sĭst″ō-men-ĭn'gō-sēl) [" + " + *mēnigx,* membrane, + *kēlē,* hernia]. Combined myelocystocele and meningocele.
myelocyte (mī'ĕl-ō-sīt) [G. *myelos,* marrow, + *kytos,* cell]. 1. A large cell in red bone marrow, from which leukocytes are derived. 2. Any gray matter nerve cell.
myelocythemia (mī″ĕl-ō-sī-thē'mĭ-ă) [" + *aima,* blood]. Presence of an excess number of myelocytes in the blood. SYN: *myelocytosis.*
myelocytic (mī″ĕl-ō-sĭt'ĭk) [" + *kytos,* cell]. Characterized by presence of, or pert. to, myelocytes.
myelocytoma (mī″ĕl-ō-sīt-ō'mă) [" + " + *-ōma,* tumor]. Leukemia with leukocytes arising from both myeloid and lymphoid substance. SYN: *chronic myelogenous leukemia.*
myelocytosis (mī″ĕl-ō-sī-tō'sĭs) [" + " + *-ōsis,* intensive]. Myelocytes in large quantities in the blood. SYN: *myelocythemia.*
myelodiastasis (mī″ĕl-ō-dī-as'tă-sĭs) [G. *myelos,* marrow, + *diastasis,* separation]. Destruction and disintegration of spinal cord.
myelodysplasia (mī″ĕl-ō-dĭs-plā'zĭ-ă) [" + *dys,* bad, + *plassein,* to form]. Defective formation of the spinal cord.
myeloencephalic (mī″ĕl-ō-ĕn-sĕf-al'ĭk) [" + *egkephalos,* brain]. Concerning the spinal cord and brain.
myeloencephalitis (mī″ĕl-ō-ĕn-sĕf-ă-lī'tĭs) [" + " + *-ītis,* inflammation]. Inflamed condition of spinal cord and brain.
myelogangliitis (mī″ĕl-ō-găng-lĭ-ī'tĭs) [G. *myelos,* marrow, + *gagglion,* knot, + *-ītis,* inflammation]. Severe choleraic condition due to gangliitis of solar and hepatic plexus.
myelogenesis (mī″ĕl-ō-jĕn'ĕ-sĭs) [" + *genesis,* development]. 1. The development of brain and spinal cord. 2. Development of myelin.
myelogenic, myelogenous (mī-ĕ-lŏ-jen'ĭk, -lŏj'ĕn-ŭs) [" + *gennan,* to produce]. Producing or originating in marrow, or in the spinal column.
myelogeny (mī-ĕl-oj'ĕn-ĭ) [G. *myelos,* marrow, + *gennan,* to produce]. Production of myelin sheaths by bone marrow.
myelogone, myelogonium (mī'ĕl-ō-gōn, mī″-ĕl-ō-gōn'ĭ-ŭm) [" + *gonē,* seed]. 1. Myeloblast. 2. Myeloid white blood cell with a deeply stained nucleolus and a reticulate nucleus stained with eosin.
myelography (mī-ĕl-og'ră-fĭ) [" + *graphein,* to write]. Roentgenographical inspection of the spinal cord.
myeloid (mī'el-oid) [" + *eidos,* form]. 1. Medullary; like marrow. 2. Pert. to the spinal cord. 3. Resembling a myelocyte, but not necessarily originating from bone marrow.
myeloidosis (mī″ĕl-oid-ō'sĭs) [" + " + *-ōsis,* intensive]. Formation of myeloid tissue, esp. abnormal tissue formation.
myelolymphocyte (mī″ĕl-ō-lĭmf'ō-sīt) [" + L. *lympha,* lymph, + G. *kytos,* cell]. Tiny lymphocyte formed abnormally in bone marrow.
myeloma (mī-ĕl-ō'mă) [G. *myelos,* marrow, + *-ōma,* tumor]. 1. Soft growth from medullary cavity of ends of long bones.
   The bone expands and thins out. On light pressure there is an eggshell crackling sound beneath the fingers. It does not give rise to metastases or recur after removal.
   2. Encephaloid tumor. 3. Giant cell sarcoma.
m., multiple. Diffuse hyperplasia of bone marrow with painful swellings on ribs and skull. SYN: *Kahler's disease, lymphadenia ossea.*
myelomalacia (mī″ĕl-ō-mă-lā'sĭ-ă) [" + *malakia,* softening]. Abnormal softening of spinal cord.
myelomatosis (mī″ĕl-ō-mă-tō'sĭs) [" + *-ōma,* tumor, + *-ōsis*]. Disease marked by multiple tumors of the bone marrow, pernicious anemia, and albumosuria. SYN: *multiple myeloma.*
myelomenia (mī-ĕl-ō-mē'nĭ-ă) [" + *mēn,* month]. Vicarious menstrual discharge in the spinal cord.
myelomeningitis (mī″ĕl-ō-men-ĭn-jī'tĭs) [G. *myelos,* marrow, + *mēnigx, mēnigg-,* membrane, + *-ītis,* inflammation]. Inflamed spinal cord and membranes; spinal meningitis.
myelomeningocele (mī″ĕl-ō-men-ĭn'gō-sēl) [" + " + *kēlē,* hernia]. Spina bifida with portion of cord and membranes protruding.
myelomyces (mī-el-ō-mī'sēs) [" + *mykēs,* fungus]. Malignant growth resembling brain substance. SYN: *encephaloma.*
myelon (mī'el-on) [G. *myelos,* marrow]. The spinal cord.
myeloneuritis (mī″ĕl-ō-nū-rī'tĭs) [" + *neuron,* nerve, + *-ītis,* inflammation]. Multiple neuritis and myelitis combined.
myelonic (mī-ĕl-on'ĭk) [G. *myelos,* marrow]. Pert. to the spinal cord.
myeloparalysis (mī″ĕl-ō-pă-ral'ĭ-sĭs) [" + *para,* beside, + *lyein,* to loosen]. Paralysis of the spine.
myelopathy (mī-ĕl-op'ă-thĭ) [" + *pathos,*

myelopetal (mī-ĕl-op′et-ăl) [" + L. *petere*, to seek for]. Proceeding toward the spinal cord.

myelophage (mī′ĕl-ō-fāj) [" + *phagein*, to eat]. A myelin ingesting macrophage.

myelophthisis (mī-ĕl-of′thĭ-sĭs) [" + *phthisis*, a wasting]. Atrophy of the spinal cord. Syn: *myelanalosis.*

my′eloplast [G. *myelos*, marrow, + *plastos*, formed]. A bone marrow cell similar to a leukocyte.

my′eloplax [" + *plax*, plate]. Large, multinuclear, bone marrow cell.

myeloplaxoma (mī″ĕl-ō-plăks-ō′mă) [G. *myelos*, marrow, + *plax*, plate, + *-ōma*, tumor]. Tumor composed of myeloplaxes.

myeloplegia (mī″ĕl-ō-plē′jĭ-ă) [" + *plēgē*, stroke]. Paralysis of spinal origin.

myelopoiesis (mī″ĕl-ō-poy-ē′sĭs) [" + *poiein*, to form]. The development of marrow or myelocytes.

myelorrhagia (mī-ĕl-ōr-rā′jĭ-ă) [" + *rēgnunai*, to burst forth]. Hemorrhage into myelon.

myelorrhaphy (mī-ĕl-or′ra-fī) [" + *raphē*, a sewing]. Suture of a cut or wound of the spinal cord.

myelosarcoma (mī″ĕl-ō-săr-kō′mă) [" + *sarx*, flesh, + *-ōma*, tumor]. Sarcoma of bone marrow cells and tissue. Syn: *osteosarcoma.*

myelosclerosis (mī″ĕl-ō-sklĕr-ō′sĭs) [G. *myelos*, marrow, + *sklērōsis*, hardening]. Sclerosis of the spinal cord.

myelosis (mī-ĕl-ō′sĭs) [" + *-ōsis*, intensive]. Formation of a myeloma or medullary tumor.

myelospongium (mī″ĕl-ō-spon′jĭ-ŭm) [" + *spoggos*, sponge]. Embryonic network from which the neuroglia arises.

my″elother′apy [" + *therapeia*, treatment]. Treatment of disease with extract of spinal cord or bone marrow.

myelotome (mī′ĕl-ō-tōm) [" + *tomē*, incision]. Instrument used to dissect the spinal cord.

myelotomy (mī-ĕl-ot′ō-mĭ) [" + *tomē*, incision]. Dissection of the spinal cord.

myelotoxic (mī-ĕl-ō-toks′ĭk) [" + *toxikon*, poison]. 1. Destroying bone marrow. 2. Pert. to or arising from diseased bone marrow.

myelotoxin (mī″ĕl-ō-toks′ĭn) [" + *toxikon*, poison]. Toxin which destroys marrow cells.

myenergia (mī-ĕn-er′jĭ-ă) [G. *mys*, *my-*, muscle, + *ergon*, work]. Muscular energy.

myenteric (mī-ĕn-ter′ĭk) [" + *enteron*, intestine]. Concerning the myenteron.
 m. **reflex.** Intestinal contraction and relaxation above a portion of bowel which is stimulated.

myenteron (mī-ĕn′tĕr-ŏn) [" + *enteron*, intestine]. Muscular layer of the intestine.

myesthesia (mī-ĕs-thē′zĭ-ă) [" + *aisthēsis*, sensation]. Muscle sensitivity.

myiasis (mī-ī′ă-sis) [G. *myia*, fly]. A disease caused by infestation with the larger pestiferous organisms, such as the larvae of maggots, flies, etc.

myiodesopsia (mī″i-ō-dĕs-op′sĭ-ă) [G. *myiōdēs*, flylike, + *opsis*, vision]. Condition in which spots are seen before the eyes. See: *muscae volitantes.*

myitis (mī-i′tĭs) [G. *mys*, *my-*, muscle, + *-ītis*, inflammation]. Inflamed condition of a muscle. Syn: *myositis.*

mylohyoid (mī″lō-hī′oid) [G. *mylē*, mill, + *yoeidēs*, U-shaped]. Pert. to the hyoid bone and the molar teeth.

myo- [G.]. Combining form pert. to *muscle.*

myoalbumin (mī″ō-al-bū′mĭn) [G. *mys*, *myo-*, muscle, + L. *albumen*, white of egg]. Albumin found in muscular tissue.

myoalbumose (mī-ō-al′bŭ-mōs) [" + L. *albus*, white]. A protein derived from muscle plasma.

myoarchitectonic (mī″ō-ar″kĭ-tĕk-ton′ĭk) [" + *architektōn*, master workman]. Pert. to or resembling structural arrangement of muscle or of fibers.

myoatrophy (mī-ō-ăt′rō-fī) [" + *atrophia*, atrophy]. Muscular wasting.

myoblast (mī′ō-blast) [G. *mys*, *myo-*, muscle, + *blastos*, germ]. An embryonic cell which develops into muscle fiber cell.

myobra′dia [" + *bradus*, slow]. Slow muscular reaction to stimulation.

myocardia (mī-ō-kar′dĭ-ă) [" + *kardia*, heart]. Noninflammatory cardiac failure.

myocardiac, myocardial (mī-ō-kar′dĭ-ăk, -ăl) [" + *kardia*, heart]. Concerning the myocardium.

myocardiograph (mī″ō-kar′dĭ-ō-grăf) [G. *mys*, *myo-*, muscle, + *kardia*, heart, + *graphein*, to write]. Instrument for recording heart movements.

myocardiosis (mī-ō-kăr-dĭ-ō′sĭs) [" + *-ōsis*, intensive]. Noninflammatory cardiac disorder. Syn: *myocardia.*

myocard′ism [" + " + *ismos*, condition]. Tendency toward development of myocardial disorders.

myocarditis (mī-ō-kar-dī′tĭs) [" + " + *-itis*, inflammation]. Inflammation of the cardiac muscular tissue.
 Etiol: Unknown. Perhaps focal infection.
 Physical Signs: Apex beat extremely weak and rapid; pulse irregular and weak; tenderness over precordium, percussion negative, auscultation reveals 1st sound of heart resembling 2nd heart sound, high pitched and wanting in muscular quality.
 NP: In acute myocarditis absolute rest is essential. Years may be added in chronic myocarditis if moderation in all things is observed. Plenty of rest and sleep, light diet, and avoidance of all worry, hurry, and physical strains are very important. High altitudes must be avoided, and climbing stairs should be reduced to a minimum, and haste avoided. The bowels should be kept regular. In some instances graduated exercises may be ordered.
 m., **acute, primary.** Acute interstitial inflammation of the myocardium.
 m., a., **secondary.** Acute inflammation of the heart muscle.
 Etiol: Secondary to acute inflammation of pericardium or endocardium, or may occur during some infectious disease.
 Sym: Marked by primary disease; great weakness; cardiac palpitation with irregularity; small, feeble pulse, and dyspnea; precordial pain and distress.
 m., a., **septic.** Localized, suppurative inflammation of the heart muscle.
 Etiol: Distant infection, suppurating pericardium or endocardium.
 m., **chronic.** Characterized by round cell infiltration of interstitial tissue, followed by parenchymatous changes of muscle fibers.
 Etiol: Nephritis, syphilis, grave anemias, diabetes, rheumatic fever, malaria, toxic substance, or excessive use of al-

cohol and tobacco. Certain wasting diseases, disease of coronary arteries, joint affections, or extension from endocardium and pericardium.
SYM: Cardiac insufficiency. Rapid heart which does not immediately recover from exercise. On first exertion the heart and blood pressure rise quickly but become slower with prolonged exertion.
PHYSICAL SIGNS: Face appears cyanosed, esp. about the lips and ears; also about the fingertips. Apex beat of heart not displaced unless the heart was previously hypertrophied, in which case apex beat will be displaced downward and to the left, or downward if dilatation exists. Pulse weak, blood pressure either low or high. Auscultation reveals a short, feeble 1st sound, lacking in muscular quality with reduplication of that sound. Second sound, esp. the aortic, is accentuated. Systolic murmur at apex over a small area if dilatation exists.
m., Fiedler's. Myocardial progressive failure without infection.
m., fragmentation. F. of the myocardium.
m., indurative. Chronic m. causing hardening of muscular walls of the heart.
m. scarlatinosa. M. associated with scarlet fever.
myocardium (mī-ō-kar'dĭ-ŭm) [" + kardia, heart]. Muscular mass of the heart made up of striated muscular tissue. SEE: Aschoff's bodies.
myocardosis (mī″ō-kăr-dō'sĭs) [G. mys, myo-, muscle, + kardia, heart, + -ōsis, intensive]. 1. Cardiac disorder without known pathological lesion. 2. Any degenerative condition (except myofibrosis) of the heart muscle.
myocele (mī'ō-sēl) [" + kēlē, hernia]. 1. Muscular protrusion through a muscle sheath. 2. [" + koilos, hollow]. Cavity in a muscular segment.
myocelialgia (mī″ō-sē-lĭ-al'jĭ-ă) [" + koilia, belly, + algos, pain]. Abdominal muscle pain.
myocelitis (mī-ō-sē-lī'tĭs) [" + " + -itis, inflammation]. Inflamed condition of abdominal muscles.
myocellulitis (mī″ō-sĕl-ū-lī'tĭs) [G. mys, myo-, muscle, + L. cellula, little chamber, + G. -itis, inflammation]. Myositis combined with cellulitis.
myocerosis (mī″ō-sē-ro'sĭs) [" + kēros, wax]. Waxy degeneration of a muscle.
myochorditis (mī″ō-kor-dī'tĭs) [" + chordē, cord, + -itis, inflammation]. Inflammation of the muscles of the larynx.
myochrome (mī'ō-krōm) [" + chrōma, color]. Reddish pigment derived from hemoglobin and found in muscle. SYN: myohematin.
myochronoscope (mī″ō-krō'nō-skōp) [" + chronos, time, + skopein, to examine] Device for determining time for producing a muscular contraction.
myoclonia (mī-ō-klō'nĭ-ă) [" + klonos, tumult]. Condition of intermittent, clonic spasm or twitching of a muscle or muscles.
myoclonus (mī-ŏk'lō-nŭs) [G. mys, myo-, muscle, + klonos, tumult]. Twitching or clonic spasm of a muscle or group of muscles. SYN: paramyoclonus.
m. multiplex. Condition marked by persistent and continuous muscular spasms.
myocoele (mī'o-sēl) [" + koilos, hollow]. The hollow portion of a myotome; muscle chamber.

myocolpitis (mī″ō-kol-pī'tĭs) [" + kolpos, vagina, + -itis, inflammation]. Muscular tissue inflammation of the vagina.
myocomma (mī-ō-kŏm'mă) [" + komma, cut]. 1. A segment of embryonic muscle along neural tube. SYN: myotome. 2. Septum dividing the myotomes.
myocrismus (mī-ō-kris'mŭs) [" + krizein, to squeak]. A peculiar crackling sound sometimes heard in auscultation resulting from contraction of a muscle.
myocyte (mī'ō-sīt) [" + kytos, cell]. A muscular tissue cell.
myocytoma (mī″ō-sī-tō'mă) [G. mys, myo-, muscle, + kytos, cell, + -ōma, tumor]. Tumor containing muscle cells.
myodemia (mī-ō-de'mĭ-ă) [" + dēmos, fat]. Fatty degeneration of muscular tissue.
Muscular fiber cells become filled with fat granules and are ultimately destroyed.
myodesopsia (mī″ō-des-op'sĭ-ă) [G. myiōdēs, flylike, + opsis, vision]. Vision of muscae volitantes or specks before the eyes. SYN: myiodesopsia.
myodiastasis (mī″ō-di-as'tă-sĭs) [G. mys, myo-, muscle, + diastasis, separation]. Division or rupture of a muscle.
myodynamia (mī″ō-dī-nam'ĭ-ă) [" + dynamis, force]. Muscular force or strength.
myodynamometer (mī″ō-dī-nă-mom'ĕt-ĕr) [" + " + metron, measure]. Device for measurement of muscular strength.
myodynia (mī-ō-dĭn'ĭ-ă) [" + odynē, pain]. Any muscle pain. SYN: myalgia.*
myoedema (mī″ō-ĕ-dē'mă) [G. mys, myo-, muscle, + oidēma, swelling]. 1. Lumping in a wasting muscle when struck. SYN: mounding. 2. Muscular edema.
myoelectric (mī″ō-ĕ-lĕk'trĭk) [" + ēlektron, amber]. Pert. to muscular electrical properties.
myoendocarditis (mī″ō-ĕn″dō-kar-dī'tĭs) [" + endon, within, + kardia, heart, + -itis, inflammation]. Inflammation of the cardiac muscular wall and membranous lining.
myoepithelial (mī″ō-ĕp-ĭ-thē'lĭ-ăl) [" + epi, upon, + thēlē, nipple]. Containing muscular and epithelial cells.
myoepithelium (mī″ō-ĕp-ĭ-thē'lĭ-ŭm) [" + thēlē, nipple]. Epithelium combined with muscular cells; muscle epithelium.
myofascitis (mī″ō-făs-ī'tĭs) [" + L. fascia, band, + G. -itis, inflammation]. Inflamed condition of a muscle and its fascia.
myofibril, myofibrilla (mī-ō-fī'brĭl, -fī-brĭl'lă) (pl. myofibrillae) [G. mys, myo-, muscle, + L. fibrilla, a small fiber]. A tiny fibril found in muscular tissue, running parallel to the cellular long axis, from 1 cell to another.
May be the contractile element.
myofibroma (mī″ō-fī-brō'mă) [" + L. fibra, fiber, + G. -ōma, tumor]. Tumor containing muscular and fibrous tissue.
myofibrosis (mī″ō-fī-brō'sĭs) [" + " + G. -ōsis, intensive]. Increase of connective or fibrous tissue with degeneration of muscular tissue.
myogelosis (mī-ō-jel-ō'sĭs) [" + L. gelāre, to congeal]. Hardening of a portion of muscle.
myogen (mī'ō-jĕn) [" + gennan, to produce]. A protein found in muscle plasma, which is spontaneously coagulable.
myogenesis (mī-ō-jĕn'ĕ-sĭs) [" + genesis, development]. Formation of muscular tissue.
myogenetic (mī″ō-jĕn-et'ĭk) [G. mys,

myo-, muscle, + *gennan*, to produce]. Having origin in muscle. SYN: *myogenic*.
myogen'ic, myog'enous [" + *gennan*, to form]. Arising from muscle.
  m. theory. The cardiac movements start in the heart muscle itself and not in nerve centers in or near the heart; opposed to the neurogenic* theory.
myoglia (mī-og'lĭ-ă) [" + *glia*, glue]. A fibrous network in muscular tissue resembling neuroglia in appearance.
myoglobulin (mī"ō-glob'ū-lĭn) [" + L. *globulus*, globule]. A coagulable globulin seen in muscular tissue.
my'ogram [" + *gramma*, a marking]. A tracing made by the myograph of muscular contractions.
myograph (mī'ō-grăf) [G. *mys*, *myo-*, muscle, + *graphein*, to write]. Instrument for tracing movements caused by muscular contractions.
myographic (mī-ō-graf'ĭk) [" + *graphein*, to write]. Pert. to a myograph, or the tracings made by it.
  m. tracing. A myogram or muscular tracing.
myography (mī-og'ră-fī) [" + *graphein*, to write]. 1. Recording of muscular contractions by a myograph. 2. Description of the muscles and their action.
myohematin (mī"ō-hem'ăt-ĭn) [" + *aima*, blood]. Red pigment from hemoglobin found in muscles. SYN: *histohematin*.
myohysterectomy (mī"ō-hĭs-tĕr-ek'tō-mĭ) [" + *ystera*, uterus, + *ektomē*, excision]. Excision of the body of the uterus, leaving the cervix in place. SYN: *subtotal hysterectomy*.
my'oid [" + *eidos*, resemblance]. Resembling muscle.
myoidema (mī-oi-dē'mă) [" + *oidēma*, swelling]. 1. The mounding of a muscle. 2. Muscular edema. SYN: *myoedema*.
myoideum (mī-oid'ē-ŭm) [G. *mys*, *myo-*, muscle, + *eidos*, resemblance]. Muscle tissue.
my'oidism [" + " + *ismos*, condition]. Muscular contraction responding to a direct stimulus without nervous control.
myoischemia (mī"ō-ĭs-kē'mĭ-ă) [" + *ischein*, to hold back, + *aima*, blood]. Local anemia in a muscle.
myokerosis (mī"ō-kĕ-rō'sĭs) [G. *mys*, *myo-*, muscle, + *kēros*, wax, + *-ōsis*]. Waxy degeneration of muscle or muscular tissue.
myokinesis (mī"ō-kĭn-ē'sĭs) [" + *kinēsis*, motion]. 1. Muscular activity. 2. Surgical displacement of muscular fibers.
myokinetic (mī"ō-kĭn-et'ĭk) [" + *kinēsis*, motion]. Pert. to motile muscular element as contrasted with the myotonic* element.
myokymia (mī-ō-kĭm'ĭ-ă) [" + *kyma*, wave]. Twitching of fibers of a muscle. It may be functional and is also seen in organic affections and general paresis.
myolemma (mī-ō-lĕm'ă) [G. *mys*, *myo-*, muscle, + *lemma*, rind]. Sheath investing a muscle fiber. SYN: *sarcolemma*.
myolin (mī'ō-lĭn) [G. *mys*, *myo-*, muscle]. Substance supposedly found in muscular fibrils.
myolipoma (mī"ō-lĭ-pō'mă) [" + *lipos*, fat, + *-ōma*, tumor]. Muscle tissue tumor containing fatty elements.
myology (mī-ol'o-jī) [" + *logos*, study]. The science or study of the muscles and their parts.
myolysis (mī-ol'ĭ-sĭs) [G. *mys*, *myo-*, muscle, + *lysis*, destruction]. Fatty degeneration and infiltration with destruction of muscular tissue accompanied by separation and disappearance of muscle cells.
myoma (mī-ō'mă) [" + *-ōma*, tumor]. A tumor containing muscle tissue. SEE: *chondromyoma*.
  m. cysticum. A sarcoma containing groups of muscular tissue.
  m., eccentric. M. in muscular wall of a hollow organ projecting externally.
  m. lymphangiectodes. M. containing dilated lymphatic vessels.
  m., nonstriated. A tumor of unmarked muscle tissue. SYN: *leiomyoma*.
  m. striocellulare. Fibroma with striated muscular fibers. SYN: *rhabdomyoma*.
  m. telangiectodes. Coiled blood vessel tumor in muscular fibers.
myomalacia (mī"ō-mă-lā'sĭ-ă) [" + *malakia*, softening]. Softening of muscular tissue. [muscle.
  m. cordis. Softening of the heart
myomatosis (mī-ō-mă-tō'sĭs) [" + *-ōma*, tumor, + *-ōsis*]. The development of myomas.
myomatous (mī-ō'mă-tŭs) [" + *-ōma*, tumor]. Pert. to or resembling a myoma.
myomectomy (mī-ō-mek'tō-mĭ) [" + " + *ektomē*, excision]. 1. Removal of a portion of muscle or muscular tissue. 2. Removal of a myomatous tumor, generally uterine, usually by abdominal section, leaving the uterus in place.
  NP: Same as for cesarean section. Position, dorsal, possibly followed by Trendelenburg's.
myomelanosis (mī"ō-mĕl-ă-nō'sĭs) [G. *mys*, *myo-*, muscle, + *melanosis*, blackening]. Darkening of muscle tissue.
myomere (mī'ō-mēr) [" + *meros*, part]. Embryonic muscular segment along the neural tube. SYN: *myocomma*, *myotome*.
myometer (mī-om'ĕt-ĕr) [" + *metron*, measure]. Device for measurement of muscular contractions.
myometritis (mī"ō-me-trī'tĭs) [" + *mētra*, uterus, + *-itis*, inflammation]. Inflamed condition of the muscular part of the uterus.
myometrium (mī"ō-me'trĭ-ŭm) [" + *mētra*, uterus]. Muscular structure of the uterus.
myomohysterectomy (mī-ō"mō-hĭs-tĕr-ĕk'tō-mĭ) [G. *mys*, *myo-*, muscle, + *-ōma*, tumor, + *ystera*, uterus, + *ektomē*, excision]. Hysterectomy performed to remove a myomatous uterus.
myomotomy (mī-ō-mot'ō-mĭ) [" + " + *tomē*, excision]. Excision of a myoma, usually uterine. SYN: *myomectomy*.
my'on [G. *mys*, *myo-*, muscle]. A muscle.
myonarcosis (mī"ō-năr-kō'sĭs) [" + *narkosis*, a numbing]. Muscular numbness.
myonephropexy (mī"ō-nef'rō-pĕk"sĭ) [" + *nephros*, kidney, + *pēxis*, fixation]. Fixation of a movable kidney by attaching it to a portion of muscular tissue with sutures.
myoneuralgia (mī"ō-nū-răl'jĭ-ă) [" + *neuron*, nerve, + *algos*, pain]. Neuralgia in a muscle.
myoneurasthenia (mī"ō-nūr-ăs-thē'nĭ-ă) [" + " + *astheneia*, weakness]. Neurasthenic muscular relaxation.
myoneure (mī'ō-nūr) [" + *neuron*, nerve]. A nerve cell which aids muscular action.
myoneuroma (mī"ō-nū-rō'mă) [" + " + *-ōma*, tumor]. A neuroma partially composed of muscular elements.
myoneuro'sis [" + " + *-ōsis*, disease]. Any muscular neurosis.
myonicity (mī-ō-nĭs'ĭt-ĭ) [G. *mys*, *myo-*, muscle]. Contraction and relaxation of living muscular tissue.

myonosus (mī-on'o-sŭs) [" + *nosos*, disease]. A disease of muscular tissue. SYN: *myopathy*.

myopachynsis (mī″ō-păk-in'sĭs) [" + *pachynsis*, thickening]. Abnormal thickening of muscle tissue.

myopalmus (mī-o-pal'mŭs) [" + *palmos*, a twitching]. Twitching of muscles.

myoparalysis (mī″ō-pă-ral'ĭ-sĭs) [" + *para*, beside, + *lysis*, loosening]. Paralysis in a muscle.

myopathic (mī-ō-path'ĭk) [" + *pathos*, disease]. 1. Pert. to muscular disease. 2. One suffering from a muscular disease.

  m. facies. Facial expression caused by relaxation of facial muscles.

myopathy (mī-op'ă-thĭ) [G. *mys, myo-*, muscle, + *pathos*, disease]. Any diseased condition of a muscle.

  m., facial. Atrophy of facial muscles.
  SYM: Lips pouted, "twisted" smile. Sometimes ptosis of upper eyelids; inability to whistle or to blow out the cheeks, depending upon the muscles affected.

  m., pseudohypertrophic. A progressive disease occurring bet. the ages of 5 to 10 in which development of muscles becomes deranged.
  SYM: Waddling gait, overdeveloped calves and buttocks. After stooping, inability to stand erect without help. Deformity of spine, contracture of muscle groups. Patient becomes bedridden.

  m., spinal. M. caused by disease or injury of the spinal cord.

myope (mī'ōp) [G. *myein*, to shut, + *ōps*, eye]. One afflicted with myopia or nearsightedness.

myopericarditis (mī″ō-per-ĭ-kar-dī'tĭs) [G. *mys, myo-*, muscle, + *peri*, around, + *kardia*, heart, + *-itis*, inflammation]. Inflammation of the pericardium and cardiac muscular wall.

myoperitonitis (mī″ō-pĕr-ĭ-tō-nī'tĭs) [" + *peritonaion*, peritoneum]. Inflammation of muscular peritoneal tissue.

myophage (mī'ō-fāj) [" + *phagein*, to eat]. A phagocyte that devours muscle tissue.

myophone (mī'ō-fōn) [" + *phōnē*, voice]. Device for conveying sound of muscular contractions.

myo'pia [G. *myein*, to shut, + *ōps*, eye]. Defect in vision so that objects can only be seen distinctly when very close to the eyes; nearsightedness.
  Light rays come to a focus in front of the retina.

  m., axial. M. due to elongation of the axis of the eye.

  m., chromic. Color blindness when viewing distant objects.

  m. of curvature. M. due to curvature of the eye's refracting surfaces.

  m., index. M. resulting from abnormal refractivity of the media.

  m., malignant. Pernicious myopia.

  m., pernicious. M. with progressive disease of the choroid, terminating in blindness.

  m., prodromal. M. in which reading is possible without glasses; seen in incipient cataract.

  m., progressive. M. that increases steadily during adult life.

  m., stationary. Myopia that comes to a stop after adult growth is attained.

  m., transient. M. seen in spasm of accommodation, as in acute iritis or iridocyclitis.

myopic (mī-op'ĭk) [" + *ōps*, eye]. Pert. to or affected with myopia.

  m. crescent. Post. crescentic protrusion seen in myopia.

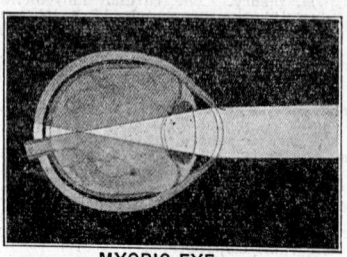

MYOPIC EYE.
Parallel rays of light reaching a focus in front of retina. See: emmetropia, hyperopia.

myoplasm (mī'ō-plazm) [G. *mys, myo-*, muscle, + *plasma*, a thing formed]. The contractile part of the muscle cell, as differentiated from the sarcoplasm.

myoplastic (mī-ō-plăst'ĭk) [" + *plassein*, to form]. Pert. to plastic use of muscle tissue or plastic surgery on muscles.

myoplasty (mī″ō-plas-tĭ) [" + *plassein*, to form]. Plastic surgery of muscle tissue.

myoplegia (mī″ō-plē'jĭ-ă) [" + *plēgē*, stroke]. Muscular paralysis.

myoprotein (mī″ō-prō'tē-ĭn) [" + *prōtos*, first]. A protein found in muscle tissue.

myoproteose (mī″ō-pro'te-ōs) [" + *prōtos*, first]. A protein found in muscle plasma. SYN: *myoalbumose*.

myop'sin [" + *psiein*, to chew up]. A proteolytic ferment in the pancreatic juice.
  Its action is similar to trypsin, which is also present in the pancreatic juice.

myopsychosis (mī″ō-sī-kō'sĭs) [G. *mys, myo-*, muscle, + *psychē*, mind, + *-ōsis*]. A muscular affection connected with a mental disorder.

myorrhaphy (mī-or'ă-fĭ) [" + *raphē*, a sewing]. Suture of a muscle wound.

myorrhexis (mī-or-eks'ĭs) [" + *rēxis*, a rupture]. Rupture of a muscle.

myosalgia (mī-ō-sal'jĭ-ă) [" + *algos*, pain]. Pain in a muscle. SYN: *myalgia*.

myosalpingitis (mī″ō-săl-pĭn-jī'tĭs) [" + *salpigx, salpigg-*, tube, + *-itis*, inflammation]. Inflamed condition of muscular tissue of a fallopian tube.

myosarcoma (mī″ō-sar-kō'mă) [" + *sarx, sark-*, flesh, + *-ōma*, tumor]. Tumor containing both muscular tissue and connective tissue cells.

myosclerosis (mī″ō-sklĕr-ō'sĭs) [" + *sklērōsis*, hardening]. Hardening of muscle.

myoseism (mī'ō-sīzm) [G. *mys, myo-*, muscle, + *seismos*, an earthquake]. Muscular contraction of a jerky nature.

my'osin [G. *mys, myo-*, muscle]. A protein derivative of myosinogen found in the muscle plasma, the coagulation of which produces rigor mortis.
  It is made up of 52.82% carbon, 7.11% hydrogen, 16.67% nitrogen, 22.03% oxygen and 1.27% sulfur.

  m. ferment. A coagulating enzyme in muscle plasma. It converts myosinogen into myosin.

myosinogen (mī″ō-sĭn'ō-jĕn) [" + *gennan*, to produce]. One of 2 main (globulin) proteins in muscular tissue.
  Myosin, a derivative, is formed during rigor mortis. SYN: *myogen*.

myosinose (mī-os'ĭn-ōs) [G. *mys*, *myo*-, muscle]. A proteose resulting from the hydrolysis of myosin.

myosinuria (mī"ō-sĭn-ū'rĭ-ă) [" + *ouron*, urine]. Myosin in the urine.

myo'sis [G. *myein*, to close]. Contraction of the pupil.
ETIOL: Irritation of oculomotor system, paralysis of dilators. Occurs in certain fevers, congestion of iris, in typhus and in early stages of meningitis; also from drug poisoning. Seen in brain lesions, sunstroke and pulmonary congestion. SYN: *miosis, 1.*

myositis (mī-ō-sī'tĭs) [G. *mys, myo*-, muscle, + *-itis,* inflammation]. Inflammation of muscle tissue, generally due to traumatism, to contiguous inflammation, diathetic states, or to parasites. SEE: *fibrositis*.
NP: In suppurative myositis a cold pack and free purgation at the onset may be ordered. After active inflammation has subsided, local heat, massage, and passive motion may help in preventing contractures. If they occur, orthopedic treatment will be necessary. In traumatic myositis fomentations may be applied to the part. Counterirritants may be ordered for acute pain. Rest is essential.

m. a frigore. Muscular rheumatism affecting muscles of back, chest, or neck attributed to sudden chilling of part.

m. fibrosa. SEE: *interstitial m.*

m., interstitial. M. with hyperplasia of connective tissue.

m. ossificans. M. marked by ossification of muscles.

m., parenchymatous. M. of substance of a muscle.

m. purulenta. Suppurative myositis.

m., rheumatic. A common form which may affect muscle tissue, fascia, or connective tissue.

m., traumatic. May be simple, with pain and swelling, or suppurative.

m. trichinosa, m., trichinous. M. due to infestation with trichinae.

myospasm (mī'ō-spăzm) [" + *spasmos*, spasm]. Spasmodic contraction of a muscle.

myosteo'ma [" + *osteon*, bone, + *-ōma*, tumor]. A bony growth found in muscle tissue.

myostroma (mī-ō-strō'mă) [" + *strōma*, a covering]. Framework or basement substance of muscle tissue.

myostromin (mī-ō-strō'mĭn) [" + *strōma*, a covering]. Protein found in muscle framework.

myostypsis (mī"ō-stĭp'sĭs) [" + *stypsis*, a contracting]. 1. A contraction of muscles. 2. Obstruction of any functional movement.

myosuria (mī-ō-sū'rĭ-ă) [" + *ouron*, urine]. Presence of myosin in the urine. SYN: *myosinuria*.

myosuture (mī"ō-sū'chŭr) [" + L. *sutura*, a stitch]. Stitching of a muscle.

myosynizesis (mī-ō-sĭn-ĭ-zē'sĭs) [G. *mys, myo*-, muscle, + *synizēsis*, sitting together]. Adhesion of muscular layers of tissue.

myotactic (mī"ō-tăk'tĭk) [" + L. *tactus*, touch]. Pert. to the muscular sensitivity.

myotasis (mī-ot'ă-sĭs) [" + *tasis*, a stretching]. Stretching of a muscle.

myotat'ic [" + *tasis*, stretching]. Pert. to the stretching of muscles.

myotenontoplasty (mī"ō-ten-on'tō-plast-ĭ) [" + *tenōn, tenont*-, tendon, + *plassein*, to form]. Plastic operation involving muscles and tendons. SYN: *tenontomyoplasty*.

myotenositis (mī"ō-tĕn-ō-sī'tĭs) [" + " + *-itis*, inflammation]. Inflamed condition of a muscle and its tendon.

myotenotomy (mī"ō-tĕn-ot'ō-mĭ) [" + " + *tomē*, incision]. Division of the tendon of a muscle.

myotherapy (mī"ō-ther'ă-pī) [" + *therapeia*, treatment]. Treatment by administration of muscular tissue extract.

myothermic (mī"ō-therm'ĭk) [" + *thermē*, heat]. Pert. to rise in muscle temperature due to its activity.

myot'ic [G. *myein*, to close]. 1. An agent that will contract the pupil of the eye. Ex: *physostigmine, pilocarpine*. 2. Producing contraction of a pupil.

myotility (mī-ō-til'ĭ-tĭ) [G. *mys, myo*-, muscle]. Contractility of a muscle.

myotome (mī'ō-tōm) [" + *tomē*, incision]. 1. Knife for cutting muscles. 2. Muscular portion of primitive segment of the body. SYN: *myocomma, somite*.

myotomy (mī-ot'ō-mĭ) [" + *tomē*, incision]. Division or anatomical dissection of muscles.

myotonia (mī-ō-tō'nĭ-ă) [" + *tonos*, tension]. Tonic spasm of a muscle, or temporary rigidity.
SYN: *Thomsen's disease*.

m. congenita. A disease characterized by tonic spasms of the muscles induced by voluntary movements; usually congenital and transmitted from 1 generation to another.
SYM: Disease appears in early childhood, is manifested by a tonic spasm of the muscles every time they are put in use. In few minutes the rigidity wears away and the movements become free from repeated contractions, the muscles becoming firm and extremely well developed; under electrical treatment the muscles contract and relax slowly.
PROG: Incurable.
TREATMENT: Physical exercise causes improvement.

myoton'ic [" + *tonos*, tension]. 1. Pert. to tonic muscular spasm. 2. Pert. to the tonic muscular element as compared with the myokinetic* or motile element of a muscle.

myotonometer (mī"ō-tō-nom'ĕt-ĕr) [" + *metron*, measure]. Instrument used to measure muscular tonus.

myot'onus [" + *tonos*, tension]. A tonic muscle spasm with temporary rigidity.

myot'rophy [" + *trophē*, nourishment]. Nutrition of the tissues of muscle.

myovas'cular [" + L. *vasculus*, a little vessel]. Pert. to blood vessels and cardiac muscle.

Myriapoda (mĭr-ĭ-ap'ō-dă) [G. *myrios*, numberless, + *pous, pod-*, foot]. Group of arthropods including millepedes and centipedes.

myriapodiasis (mir"ĭ-ăp-ō-dī'ă-sĭs) [" + *pous, pod-*, foot]. Infestation with 1 of the Myriapoda.

myringa (mĭr-ĭn'gă) [L. drum membrane]. The tympanic membrane or eardrum.

myringectomy (mĭr-ĭn-jĕk'tō-mĭ) [" + G. *ektomē*, excision]. Excision of the myringa or eardrum. SYN: *myringodectomy*.

myringitis (mĭr-ĭn-jī'tĭs) [" + G. *-itis*, inflammation]. Inflammation of the tympanum or eardrum.

m. bullosa. M. with blebs or vesicular inflammation of the outer layer.

myringodectomy (mĭ-rĭn-gō-děk'tō-mĭ) [" + G. *ektomē*, excision]. Excision of the tympanum. SYN: *myringectomy*.

myringodermatitis (mĭr-ĭn′gō-dĕr-mă-tī′- tĭs) [" + G. *derma*, skin, + *-itis*, inflammation]. Inflamed condition of outer layer of the membrana tympani.

myringomycosis (mĭr-ĭn″gō-mī-kō′sĭs) [L. *myringa*, drum membrane, + G. *mykēs*, fungus, + *-ōsis*]. Disease of eardrum due to parasitic fungi.

myringoplasty (mĭr-ĭn′gō-plăst-ĭ) [" + G. *plassein*, to form]. Plastic operation on membrana tympani.

myringoscope (mĭr-ĭn′gō-skōp) [" + G. *skopein*, to examine]. Instrument used for examination of the eardrum.

myringotome (mĭ-rĭn′gō-tōm) [" + G. *tome*, incision]. Knife for incising the tympanic membrane.

myringotomy (mĭr-ĭn-got′ō-mĭ) [" + G. *tome*, incision]. Incision of tympanic membrane.

myrrh (mur) [G. *myrra*]. USP. A gum resinous substance of great antiquity, cherished as a constituent of incense and perfume; most important use today is as an aromatic, astringent mouthwash.

mysophobia (mī-sō-fō′bĭ-ă) [G. *mysos*, filth, + *phobos*, fear]. Abnormal aversion to dirt or contamination.

mytacism (mī′tă-sĭzm) [G. *mytakismos*, fondness for letter m]. Excessive or incorrect use of the letter *m* or the *m* sound. SEE: *metacism, mutacism*.

mythomania (mĭth-ō-mā′nĭ-ă) [G. *mythos*, myth, + *mania*, madness]. Abnormal tendency to lie and exaggerate.

mythophobia (mĭth-ō-fō′bĭ-ă) [" + *phobos*, fear]. Abnormal dread of making a false or incorrect statement.

myurous (mī-u′rŭs) [G. *mys, my-*, mouse, + *oura*, tail]. Gradually diminishing or tapering; said of certain symptoms, as the heart beat which, under certain conditions, grows feebler and then stronger.

myxadenitis (mĭks-ad-en-ī′tĭs) [G. *myxa*, mucus, + *adēn*, gland, + *-itis*, inflammation]. Inflamed condition of mucous glands.

myxadenoma (miks-ad-en-ō′mă) [" + " + *-ōma*, tumor]. 1. A tumor with the structure of a mucous gland. 2. A tumor of glandular structure containing mucous elements. SYN: *myxoadenoma*.

myxangitis (miks-an-jī′tĭs) [" + *aggeion*, vessel, + *-itis*, inflammation]. Inflammation of mucous gland ducts.

   m. fibrosa. M. accompanied by hyperplasia.

   m. hyalinosa. M. with hyaline degeneration about the ducts.

myxangoitis (miks″an-gō-ī′tĭs) [" + *aggeion*, vessel, + *-itis*, inflammation]. Inflammation of vessels with mucous discharge.

myxasthenia (mĭks-ăs-thē′nĭ-ă) [" + *astheneia*, weakness]. Imperfect or insufficient secretion of mucus.

myxedema (mĭks-ĕ-dē′mă) [" + *oidēma*, swelling]. A trophic disease due to hypofunction of thyroid gland.

ETIOL: Due to lack of thyroid secretion.

SYM: Characterized by hard edema of subcutaneous tissues, loss and dryness of hair, dullness, lethargy.

   m., congenital. Cretinism.

   The face is "moon-shaped," features coarse, nostrils thick, with thick lips and large mouth.

myxedematoid (miks-ĕ-dēm′ă-toid) [" + *eidos*, resemblance]. Resembling myxedema.

myxedematous (miks-ĕ-dēm′ă-tŭs) [" + *oidēma*, swelling]. Marked by or concerning myxedema.

myxemia (miks-ē′mĭ-ă) [G. *myxa*, mucus, + *aima*, blood]. Accumulation of mucin in the blood. SYN: *mucinemia*.

myxidiotic (miks-ĭd-ĭ-ot′ĭk) [" + *idiōtēs*, private]. Myxedema with few physical symptoms, but marked mental defects.

myxiosis (miks-ĭ-ō′sĭs) [G. *myxa*, mucus]. A mucous discharge or secretion.

myxo-, myx- [G.]. Combining form meaning *of*, or pert. *to mucus*.

myxoadenoma (miks″ō-ăd-en-ō′mă) [G. *myxa*, mucus, + *adēn*, gland, + *-ōma*, tumor]. 1. Glandular tumor containing mucus. 2. Tumor of structure of a mucous gland. SYN: *myxadenoma*.

myxocystoma (mĭks″ō-sĭs-tō′mă) [" + *kystis*, cyst, + *-ōma*, tumor]. 1. A cystic tumor containing mucus. 2. Ovarian cyst with lining structure resembling mucous membrane.

myxocyte (mĭks′ō-sīt) [" + *kytos*, cell]. A typical mucous tissue cell, usually polyhedral or stellate.

myxodermia (mĭks″ō-der′mĭ-ă) [" + *derma*, skin]. 1. Edematous softening of the skin. 2. Disease marked by cutaneous discoloration and softening and muscular contraction.

myxoedema (mĭks-ĕ-dē′mă) [" + *oidēma*, swelling]. Condition due to deficiency of thyroid secretion or removal of the gland. Not congenital.

SYM: Dry skin, hair thin. Susceptible to cold. Slow speech and walking.

myxoenchondroma (mĭks″ō-ĕn-kŏn-drō′mă) [" + *en*, in, + *chondros*, cartilage, + *-ōma*, tumor]. A cartilaginous tissue tumor which has undergone partial mucous degeneration.

myxofibroma (mĭks″ō-fī-brō′mă) [" + L. *fibra*, fiber, + G. *-ōma*, tumor]. Tumor composed of myxomatous and fibrous elements.

myxoglioma (mĭks″ō-glĭ-ō′mă) [G. *myxa*, mucus, + *glia*, glue, + *-ōma*, tumor]. Tumor composed of myxomatous and gliomatous elements.

myxoid (mĭks′oid) [" + *eidos*, resemblance]. Similar to or resembling mucus.

myxoidedema (miks-oid-e-de′mă) [" + " + *oidēma*, swelling]. Severe form of influenza.

myxoinoma (mĭks″ō-ĭn-ō′mă) [" + *is, in-*, fiber, + *-ōma*, tumor]. Tumor composed of mucous and fibrous elements.

myxolipoma (mĭks″ō-lĭ-pō′mă) [" + *lipos*, fat, + *-ōma*, tumor]. Mucous tumor with fatty tissue elements in it.

myxoma (mĭks-ō′mă) [" + *-ōma*, tumor]. A benign mucous tumor. SEE: *chondromyxoma*.

   m., cartilaginous. M. with a firmer consistence than usual or with cells like those of cartilage.

   m., cystic, cystoid. One with parts fluid enough to resemble cysts.

   m., enchondromatous. One with nodules of hyaline cartilage.

   m., erectile. SEE: *telangiectatic m.*

   m., fibrous. A m. composed mainly of fibrous tissues.

   m., intracanalicular, of the mamma. One developing in the interstitial connective tissue of the mamma.

   m. lipomatodes. SEE: *lipomatous m.*

   m., lipomatous. One containing much fat.

   m., telangiectatic, vascular. One of highly vascular structure.

myxomatosis (mĭks″ō-mă-tō′sĭs) [G. *myxa*,

mucus, + -ōma, tumor, + -ōsis]. 1. Formation of multiple myxomas. 2. Degeneration of myxomatous type.

myxomycetes (mĭks″ō-mī-sē′tēs) [" + mykēs, fungus]. Certain species of fungoid organisms; slime molds.

myxomyoma (mĭks-ō-mī-ō′mă) [" + mys, myo-, muscle, + -ōma, tumor]. Muscle tissue tumor that has undergone mucous degeneration.

myxoneuroma (mĭks″ō-nū-rō′mă) [" + neuron, nerve, + -ōma, tumor]. Tumor composed of mucous and nerve tissue elements.

myxoneurosis (mĭks-ō-nū-ro′sĭs) [" + " + -ōsis, intensive]. Neurosis of mucous membranes.
SYM: Excessive secretion, esp. from respiratory or intestinal membrane without active inflammation.

myxopapilloma (mĭks″ō-păp-ĭl-ō′mă) [" + L. papilla, nipple, + ōma, tumor]. Combination myxomatous and papillomatous tumor or tumors.

myxopod (mĭks′ō-pod) [G. myxa, mucus, + pous, pod-, foot]. The earliest form of malarial parasite. SYN: schizont.

myxopoiesis (mĭks″ō-poy-ē′sĭs) [" + poiēsis, formation]. The production of mucus.

myxorrhea (mĭks-or-rē′ă) [" + roia, flow]. Free discharge from mucous surfaces. SYN: blennorrhea.
  m. gastrica. Excessive mucous secretion in the stomach.
  m. intestinalis. Secretion of mucus from the bowel in neurotic persons in times of mental stress.

myxosarcoma (mĭks″ō-săr-kō′mă) [" + sarx, sark-, flesh, + -ōma, tumor]. Mixed tumor, partly myxomatous and partly sarcomatous, having undergone partial degeneration.

myxosarcomatous (mĭks″ō-săr-kō′măt-ŭs) [" + " + -ōma, tumor]. Pert. to or of the nature of myxosarcoma.

myxospore (mĭks′ō-spor) [G. myxa, mucus, + sporos, seed]. Spore embedded in a gelatinous mass, seen in some fungi and protozoa.

Myxosporidia (mĭks-ō-spor-ĭd′ĭ-ă) [" + sporos, seed]. Parasitic sporozoans, most commonly found in epithelial cells of lower vertebrates.

myzesis (mī-zē′sĭs) [G. myzein, to suck]. Sucking.

N

N. Symb. for *nitrogen*.
n. Chemical symb. for *normal*.
Na. Symb. for *sodium*.
nabothian cysts (na-bō'thĭ-ăn). Retention cysts formed by the n. follicles at neck of uterus. SEE: *cyst*.
 n. follicles, n. glands. Mucous follicles of the external os uteri. They contain a glairy fluid.
 ETIOL: Due to closing of mouths of glands by new epithelium of a healed erosion. They always denote an erosion has been present.
 n. menorrhagia. Accumulated mucus in the pregnant uterus, the result of excessive secretion of the uterine glands.
NaBr. Sodium bromide.
N. A. C. G. N. National Association of Colored Graduate Nurses.
NaCl. Sodium chloride.
NaClO. Sodium hypochlorite.
Na₂CO₃. Sodium carbonate.
nacreous (na'kre-us) [Arabian, *nagir*, hollowed out]. Having an iridescent, pearl-like luster, as bacterial colonies.
N. A. D. Abbr. for *no appreciable disease*.
Naegele's obliquity (na'ge-le). Inclination of fetal head, laterally in a flat pelvis.
 N.'s pelvis. An obliquely contracted pelvis, caused by disease in infancy.
NaHCO₃. Sodium bicarbonate.
nail (nāl) [A.S. *naegel*]. A horny cell structure of the epidermis forming flat plates upon the dorsal surface of the terminal phalanges. SYN: *unguis*.
 The *matrix* is the bed, or underlying corium.* Soft cells of the stratum mucosa at the root are responsible for the growth and extension of the nails.
 It takes about 4 months for the nails to grow ½ in.
 Changes in the nails, such as ridges, may occur in defective nutrition or after a serious illness. In achlorhydria, hypochromic anemia, excessive spoon-shaped nails with center depression may occur. In chronic pulmonary conditions and congenital heart disease excessive curving of the nails may be associated with clubbed fingers.
 ATROPHY: May occur as a result of hereditary or congenital tendencies. Permanent atrophy may follow injuries, scars from disease, frostbite, nerve injuries and hyperthyroidism. Sulfur administration sometimes stops this process. Nail shedding is due to the same causes.
 Nails that are fragile or split often may be congenital or due to prolonged contact with chemicals or to too frequent manicuring.
 DISCOLORATIONS: *Black*: In diabetes and other forms of gangrene. *Blueblack*: Common condition, usually due to hemorrhage, bleeding diseases such as hemophilia, and trauma. May be painful and can be relieved by drilling holes in the nails. *Brown*: May be due to arsenical poisoning. *Brownish-black*: This discoloration often indicates chronic mercurial poisoning, due to formation of sulfide of mercury in the tissues. *Cyanosis*: Usually indicates anemia, poor circulation, or venous stasis. *Slate*: This is an early manifestation of argyria and administration of silver should be stopped at once. *White spots*: Striate lesions may be due to trauma and are more frequent in women. Transverse white bands in all nails may be a sign of acute or chronic arsenical poisoning, or rarely of thallium acetate poisoning. SYN: *leukonychia*.
 DRY, MALFORMED: May result from trophic changes resulting from injury to nerve or finger, neuritis, Raynaud's disease, pulmonary osteoarthropathy, syphilis, onychia, scleroderma, acrodermatitis and granuloma fungoides of the fingers.
 STRIATIONS, LONGITUDINAL: Often found in those past middle life; frequently associated with onychorrhexis, splitting at the free margins. Note in association with a focus of infection in the mouth or at root of a tooth. Vitamin deficiency may be a cause. Microscopic examination of nail clippings should be made for ringworm. When hard and brittle, gouty conditions are indicated.
 Transverse lines (Beau's lines): May result from previous interference of nail matrix growth. May be caused by local or systemic conditions. Approximate date of lesion may be determined, as it takes 4-6 months for the nail to grow.
 ULCERS AND ECCHYMOSIS: At base of nails noted in chloral addicts, syphilis and scrofula if not due to trauma. Chancre may be suspected if a small, indolent ulcer appears near the nail, esp. if indurated and associated with enlarged lymph glands above the inner condyle.
 QUINCKE'S CAPILLARY PULSATION: Rhythmic flushing and blanching most frequent in aortic regurgitation and often in anemia.
 n. bed. The end of a finger or toe covered by the nail. SYN: *nail matrix*.
 n. culture. Test tube culture in which the culture grows in the shape of a nail.
 n., eggshell. Nail plate is soft, semitransparent, bends easily, and splits at end. Associated with arthritis, peripheral neuritis, leprosy and hemiplegia. May be the only visible sign of late syphilis.
 n. fold. Groove in the cutaneous tissue surrounding the margins and proximal edges of the nail.
 n., hang. Broken epidermis at edge of the nail. SYN: *agnail*, (1).
 n., ingrowing. Nail with tissue overgrowing its edges.
 n. matrix. The nail bed.
 n., reedy. One marked by longitudinal fissures.
 n. skin. The quick of the nail.
 n. wall. Epidermis covering edges of the nail. SYN: *vallum unguis*.
nail, words pert. to: acronyx, agnail, caconychia, eponychium, leukonychia, lunula, matrix, onychonosus, onychophosis, onychoptosis, onychorrhexis, onyxis, phaneromania, unguis.
naked (nā'kĕd) [A.S. *naced*, nude]. Uncovered, exposed to view, nude, bare.
nanism (na'nizm) [G. *nanos*, dwarf]. Condition of being dwarflike in build.
 n., symptomatic. N. with deficient

dentition, sexual development and ossification.

nanocephalism (nan-ō-sef'ăl-ĭzm) [" + *kephalē*, head]. Condition of having an abnormally small head.

nanocephalous (nan-ō-sef'ă-lŭs) [" + *kephalē*, head]. Having an abnormally small head.

nanocormia (na-nō-kor'mĭ-ă) [" + *kormos*, trunk]. Abnormally dwarfed thorax or body.

nanoid (na'noid) [" + *eidos*, like]. Dwarflike.

nanosomia (na-nō-so'mĭ-ă) [" + *soma*, body]. State of being a dwarf. SEE: *nanism*.

nanous (nan'ŭs) [G. *nanos*, dwarf]. Dwarfed or stunted.

na'nus [G. *nanos*]. 1. A dwarf. 2. Stunted; dwarflike.

NaOH. Sodium hydroxide.

nap (năp) [A.S. *hnappian*, nap]. 1. To slumber. 2. A short sleep; a doze.

nape (năp; năp) [origin uncertain]. Upper back part of neck.

napex (na'peks) [origin uncertain]. Scalp beneath the occipital protuberance.

naphtha (naf'thă) [G. *naphtha*]. 1. A volatile inflammable liquid distilled from carbonaceous substances. 2. Petroleum, esp. more volatile varieties.

naphthalene (naf'thă-lēn) [G. *naphtha*]. A hydrocarbon, one of principal constituents of coal tar.
USES: As a disinfectant, in moth balls, and in manufacture of dyes and explosives.
DOSAGE: 2-10 gr. (0.12-0.6 Gm.).

naphthol (năf'thŏl). Coal tar substance used as an antiseptic and in certain dyes. Also prepared from naphthalene.

napiform (na'pĭ-form) [L. *napus*, turnip, + *forma*, shape]. BACT: Formed like a turnip, as gelatin liquefaction.

naprapathy (nap-răp'ăth-ĭ) [Czech *naprava*, correction, + G. *pathos*, disease]. Method of manipulation practiced by a certain school in the treatment of disease which is based upon the assumption that disease is due to faulty functioning of ligaments.

narcism, narcissism (nar'sĭzm, nar-sĭs'-ĭzm) [G. from *Narkissos*, a mythical character who fell in love with his own image]. 1. Self-love or self-admiration. 2. Voluptuous pleasure derived from observing one's own naked body.

narcissistic (nar-sĭs-sĭst'ĭk). Pert. to narcissism.
n. object choice. Selection of another like one's own self as the object of love, friendship or liking.

narco- [G.]. Prefix: *numbness, stupor.*

narcoanesthesia (nar″kō-ăn-ĕs-thē'zĭ-ă) [G. *narkē*, stupor, + *an-*, priv. + *aisthesis*, sensation]. Anesthesia produced by a narcotic, as scopolamine and morphine.

narcohypnia (nar″kō-hĭp'nĭ-ă) [" + *hypnos*, sleep]. Numbness following sleep.

narcolepsy (nar″ko-lep-sĭ) [" + *lēpsis*, seizure]. Overwhelming attacks of sleep which the victim cannot inhibit. SYN: *sleep epilepsy; sleep, paroxysmal.*

narcoleptic (nar-kō-lĕp'tĭk) [" + *lēpsis*, seizure]. Pert. to or marked by an overwhelming desire to sleep.

narcoma (nar-kō'mă) [" + *kōma*, coma]. Coma or stupor from use of a narcotic.

narcomania (nar-kō-mā'nĭ-ă) [" + *mania*, madness]. 1. Abnormal craving for alcohol or narcotics. 2. Insanity due to use of alcohol or narcotics.

narcomaniac (nar-kō-mā'nĭ-ăk) [" + *mania*, madness]. 1. Pert. to narcomania. 2. One affected by narcomania.

narcomatous (nar-kō-mă'tŭs) [" + *kōma*, coma]. Pert. to a state of stupor from use of narcotics.

nar'cose [G. *narkē*, stupor]. In a stuporous state.

narco'sis [G. *narkē*, stupor, + *-osis*]. Unconscious state due to narcotics.
n., basal. N. produced prior to administration of ether or any general anesthetic.
n., insufflation. General anesthesia produced by administering the anesthetic through a tube passed bet. the vocal cords into the trachea.
n., medullary. General anesthesia induced by a local anesthetic injected in the sheath of the spinal cord in lumbar region. SYN: *spinal anesthesia.*
n. paralysis. P. induced by pressure on a nerve during surgical anesthesia.

narcosomania (nar-kō″sō-mā'nĭ-ă) [" + *mania*, madness]. Morbid craving for, or insanity produced by narcotics. SYN: *narcomania.*

narcot'ic [G. *narkōtikos*, benumbing]. 1. Producing stupor or sleep. 2. Drug producing stupor, complete unconsciousness, and allaying pain.
Narcotics are more powerful than hypnotics. Ex: *chloral hydrate, sulfonal, trional, veronal.*
RS: *anesthetic, depressant, hypnotic, morphine, opiate, opium, pantopon.*

narcotism (nar'kŏt-ĭzm) [G. *narkē*, stupor, + *ismos*, condition]. 1. State of stupor induced by a narcotic. SYN: *narcosis.* 2. An addiction to the use of narcotics.
Addiction may be said to exist when discontinuance causes abstinence symptoms relieved speedily by a dose of the drug. It is this addition to the original purpose in taking the drug that so readily aggravates the need.
TREATMENT: Can ordinarily be successful only under sanitarium conditions positively preventing the use of the drug, and then it consists mostly of substituted sedatives to minimize distress of withdrawal. Relapses are frequent and the building up of a new philosophy of life is sometimes of prime importance.
POISONING: Narcotic or sleep producing poisons as opium and its derivatives, chloral combinations, barbital and its myriad subvarieties, etc.
SYM: Depression, slowing of heart and respiration, sleep, followed by coma.
F. A. TREATMENT: Remove poison by vomiting, purging, dilution of blood, diuretics, intravenous hypertonic glucose. Administer stimulants by all routes.

nar'cotize [G. *narkōtikos*, benumbing]. To render unconscious through the use of a narcotic.

naris (na'rĭs) (pl. *nares*) [L. nostril]. The nostril.
n., anterior. BNA. External nostril.
n., posterior. BNA. Either internal opening into pharynx.
RS: *anosmia, epistaxis, hyperosmia, nose, parosmia, septum, smell.*

nasal (nā'zl) [L. *nasus*, nose]. 1. Pert. to the nose. 2. Uttered through the nose. 3. A nasal bone.
n. bones. The 2 small bones forming the arch of the nose.
n. douche. Injection of fluid into 1 nostril, with fluid passing into the other nostril, escaping by way of the nasopharynx out of the mouth.

Patient should keep mouth open to prevent fluid from entering the throat. Force must not be great. Atomized spray is safer. Container should not be suspended over 6 inches above patient, who should not blow the nose during treatment.

n. feeding. N. gavage, q.v.

n. fossae. Post. nasal and nasopharyngeal cavities.

n. gavage. Feeding through a tube in the nasal passage.

This is resorted to when all other methods fail, and quite often only 1 nasal feeding is necessary to make the patient realize that it is much easier to eat.

NP: Throughout a course of tube feedings in mental cases, the nurse should frequently experiment to see if the patient will eat. Try him with a fully prepared tray. Also offer the tube feeding in a glass that he may drink it. Again, it should be remembered that suggestion is a very powerful factor in the care of the mental patient, so the nurse may see the reflection of her own attitude in the patient's behavior.

ARTICLES NECESSARY: (a) Tray with feeding (consisting usually of milk, eggs, sugar and malted milk, or concentrated broths and purées with milk and cream) heated to 98° F. (b) Pitcher of water (about 100 cc.). (c) Pitcher of orange juice (200 cc.). (d) Basin with ice and nasal tube and funnel. (e) Medicine glass with glycerine. (f) Gown for doctor. (g) Rubber and draw sheet to protect patient. (h) Face towel. (i) Bowl of water to invert funnel in. (j) Any medication ordered.

PROCEDURE: (a) Have patient in bed or in chair, according to the doctor's wishes, usually in a chair, however. (b) Restrain, if a mental patient, with a blanket or sheet or put him in a dry pack if in bed. (c) Protect patient with rubber and draw sheet. (d) Pour water into funnel and clamp tube so no air will enter. (e) Dip end of funnel in glycerine. (f) After tube is inserted, note color of face, invert funnel in water and if air bubbles appear, obstruction is in the trachea and tube should be removed immediately. (g) Fill funnel with feeding and hold slightly above patient's head to allow flow by gravity. (h) Give orange juice and any medication, also water. (i) Hold towel over patient's mouth and keep head raised slightly as patient is more apt to retain the feeding. (j) Remove tube quickly and keep patient quiet for a few minutes, until desire for regurgitation has passed. (k) Entire amount of fluid given at 1 feeding should not exceed 1000 cc.

n. height. Distance bet. lower border of nasal aperture and the nasion.

n. index. The greatest width of the nasal aperture in relation to a line from the lower edge of the n. aperture to the nasion.

n. line. L. from lower edge of the ala nasi curving to outer side of the orbicularis oris muscle, seen in abdominal disorders. SYN: *Jadelot's furrow or line.*

n. obstruction. Commonest causes: (a) Irregular septum; (b) enlarged turbinates; (c) nasal polypi. Many complications result. TREATMENT: Nasal douches, inhalations and operative care: (a) Resection of septum; (b) turbinectomy; (c) removal of polypi; (d) opening and draining sinuses.

n. reflex. Contraction of facial muscles due to irritation of nasal mucosa.

n. width. Maximum width of nasal aperture.

nascent (năs'ĕnt; nā'sĕnt) [L. *nascens*, born]. 1. Just born; incipient or beginning. 2. Pert. to a substance being set free from a compound.

nasion (nā'zĭ-ŏn) [L. *nasus*, nose]. The point where the nasofrontal suture is cut across by the median anteroposterior plane.

nasitis (nā-zī'tĭs) [" + G. *-itis*, inflammation]. Inflammation of the nose.

Nasmyth's membrane (nāz'mĭth). Epithelial m. enveloping enamel of a tooth for short period after birth.

naso- [L.]. Combining form, *rel. to the nose.*

nasoantritis (nā″zō-ăn-trī'tĭs) [L. *nasus*, nose, + G. *antron*, cavity, + *-itis*, inflammation]. Inflammation of nose and antrum of Highmore with rhinitis.

nas″ofron'tal [" + *frons, front-*, forehead]. Pert. to nasal and frontal bones.

nas″ola'bial [" + *labium*, lip]. Connected with or rel. to the nose and lip.

nasolacrimal (nā″zō-lăk'rĭm-ăl) [" + *lacrima*, tear]. Pert. to nose and lacrimal mechanism.

nasology (nā-zŏl'ō-jĭ) [" + G. *logos*, study]. Study of the nose and its diseases.

nasomental (nā″zō-mĕn'tăl) [" + *mentum*, chin]. Pert. to the nose and chin.

n. reflex. Contraction of mentalis muscle with elevation of lower lip and wrinkling of skin of chin resulting from percussion of side of nose.

nasopalatine (nā″zō-păl'ăt-īn) [L. *nasus*, + *palatum*, palate]. Pert. to both nose and palate.

nasopharyngeal (nā″zō-făr-ĭn'jē-ăl) [" + G. *pharygx*, pharynx]. Pert. to the pharynx and nose.

nasopharyngitis (nā″zō-făr-ĭn-jī'tĭs) [" + " + *-itis*, inflammation]. Inflamed condition of the nasopharynx. SYN: *rhinopharyngitis.*

nasopharynx (nā″zō-far'ĭnks) [" + G. *pharygx*, pharynx]. Part of pharynx situated above the soft palate (postnasal space). SYN: *rhinopharynx.*

nasoscope (nā'zō-skōp) [" + G. *skopein*, to examine]. Electrical device for examination of the nasal cavity.

nasoseptitis (nā″zō-sĕp-tī'tĭs) [" + *saeptum*, partition]. Inflamed condition of the nasal septum.

nasosinuitis, nasosinusitis (nā″zō-sīn-ū-ī'tĭs, -sī-nū-sī'tĭs) [" + *sinus*, cavity]. Inflammation of the nasal accessory sinuses and cavities.

nas'tin [G. *nastos*, solid]. Oily substance from streptothrix of leprosy which, combined with benzoyl chloride, is said to produce active immunity against leprosy.

nasus (nā'sŭs) [L.]. The nose.

nasute (nā'sūt) [L. *nasus*, nose]. Having a large or long nose.

natal (nā'tăl) [L. *natus*, birth; *nasci*, to be born]. 1. Pert. to birth or the day of birth. 2. [L. *nates*, buttocks]. Pert. to the nates or buttocks.

natal'ity [L. *natus*, birth; *nasci*, to be born]. The birth rate.

natant (nā'tănt) [L. *natāre*, to swim]. Floating; swimming.

nates (nā'tēz) [L. pl. buttocks]. 1. Gluteal region; fleshy prominences formed by the gluteal muscles and covering of fat and skin. SYN: *buttocks.* 2. The ant., sup. or upper 2 corpora quadrigemina.* SEE: *testes.*

natimortality (nā"tĭ-mor-tăl'ĭ-tĭ) [L. *natus*, one born, + *mortalitās*]. Rate of stillbirths in proportion to birth rate.

native (nā'tĭv) [L. *nativus*, born in]. 1. Born with; inherent. 2. Natural, normal. SYN: *indigenous*. 3. Belonging to, as place of one's birth.
  n. albumin. A protein group found in tissues. SEE: *albumin*.

nativistic theory (nā-tĭv-ĭs'tĭk). The mind forms ideas and possesses an inherent knowledge not derived from sensations or experience.

natremia (na-trē'mĭ-ă) [L. *natrium*, sodium, + G. *aima*, blood]. Sodium in the blood.

natrium (na'trĭ-um) [L. sodium]. SYMB: Na. Sodium.
  This is found abundantly in plants, animal fluids and minerals, as common salt. It is the base of all the salts of soda. It seems necessary to animal life in order to keep proteins in solution and to make the secretions of a proper composition.

na'tron. Sodium carbonate. [sodium.
na'trum. Homeopathic name for soda or
natuary (nă'tū-ar-ĭ) [L. *natus*, birth]. A lying-in ward.

nat'ural [L. *natura*, nature]. Not abnormal or artificial.

na'turopath [" + G. *pathos*, suffering]. One who practices naturopathy.

naturopathy (nā-tūr-op'ă-thĭ). "A therapeutic system embracing a complete physianthropy employing Nature's agencies, forces, processes, and products, except major surgery." *Amer. Naturopathic Ass'n.*

naupathia (naw-path'ĭ-ă) [G. *naus*, ship, + *pathos*, disease]. Seasickness.

nausea (naw'shē-ă; naw'sē-ă) [G. *nausia*, seasickness]. Inclination to vomit; usually preceding emesis if of gastric origin.
  It is present in seasickness, early pregnancy, diseases of the central nervous system, neurasthenia, hysteria, and sometimes in astigmatism. It may be due to the sight or odor of obnoxious matter or conditions, or to mental images of same. It may be present, without vomiting, in certain gallbladder disturbances and in carsickness.
  NP: Report the nature of vomitus, if it occurs, *frequency and time, effect of food and gases, bilious, fecal, profuse, purulent, watery, mucous* and *hematemesis.* SEE: *vomitus*.
  n. gravidarum. Morning sickness of pregnancy.
  n. navalis. Seasickness. SYN: *mal de mer, naupathia.*

nauseant (naw'shē-ănt; naw'sē-ănt) [G. *nausia*, seasickness]. 1. Causing nausea. 2. That which causes nausea.

nauseate (naw'shē-āt; naw'sē-āt) [G. *nausia*, seasickness]. To cause or affect with nausea.

nauseous (naw'shus; naw'shē-ŭs) [G. *nausia*, seasickness]. Producing nausea, disgust or loathing.

navel (nā'věl) [A.S. *nafela*]. The depression or scar in center of abdomen, where the umbilical cord of fetus is attached. SYN: *umbilicus, q.v.*
  RS: *cirsomphalos, umbilical cord, umbilicate.*
  n. string. Umbilical cord.

navicula (nă-vĭk'ū-lă) [L. *navicula*, boat]. Fossa navicularis.*

navicular (nă-vĭk'ū-lar) [L. *navicula*, boat]. 1. Shaped like a boat. 2. Scaphoid bones in the carpus and in the tarsus. SEE: *skeleton.*

N. D. A. National Dental Association.

near point. Closest point of distinct vision, with maximum accommodation.
  It recedes with age, varying from 3 in. in 2 yr. to 40 in. at 60 yr.
  n. p., absolute. For either eye.
  n. p., relative. For both eyes taken together.

nearsight (nēr'sĭt). Ability to see clearly only a short distance. SYN: *myopia.*

near'sight"ed. Able to see clearly only a short distance. SYN: *myopia.*

nearsight'edness. Ability to see distinctly only a short distance. SYN: *myopia.*

nearthrosis (nē-ar-thrō'sĭs) [G. *neos*, new, + *arthron*, joint]. A false joint or abnormal articulation.

nebula (něb'ū-lă) [L. mist, cloud]. 1. Slight haziness. 2. Clouds in urine. 3. Group of oily substances.
  n. corneae. Grayish opacity of the cornea.

nebuliza'tion [L. *nebula*, vapor]. 1. Treatment with spray method. 2. Conversion into a vapor. SYN: *vaporization.*

nebulizer (něb'ū-lī-zěr) [L. *nebula*, mist]. An atomizer or sprayer.

Neca'tor america'nus. The hookworm. SYN: *Ankylostoma americanum.*

neck (něk) [A.S. *hnecca*, nape]. 1. Part of body bet. head and shoulders. 2. The constricted portion of an organ, or that resembling a neck.
  DISLOCATIONS: These are rather common, and it is difficult to distinguish them from a fracture of the neck; therefore, treatment should be the same as for fracture of the neck or spine.
  RS: "cervico-" words, *cervix, collum, nape, nucha, torticollis, trachelos, wry neck.*
  n., anatomical. Constriction just below the head of the humerus. SYN: *collum anatomicum.*
  n., back of. Nape of the neck. SYN: *nucha, scruff.*
  n., Madelung's. Diffuse lipoma of the neck.
  n., Nithsdale. Goiter.
  n., surgical. Narrow part of humerus below the tuberosity. Fracture here is common.
  n. of womb. The cervix uteri.
  n., wry. Torsion of the neck caused by contracted muscles. SYN: *torticollis.*

necrectomy (ně-krěk'to-mĭ) [G. *nekros*, dead, + *ektomē*, excision]. Surgical removal of necrosed tissue.

necremia (něk-rē'mĭ-ă) [" + *aima*, blood]. Death of most of the erythrocytes in the blood; decomposition of the blood.

necro- [G.]. Combining form meaning *pertaining to death.*

necrobiosis (něk-rō-bĭ-ō'sĭs) [G. *nekros*, dead, + *biosis*, life]. Gradual degeneration and death of tissue. SEE: *necrosis.*

necrobiotic (ně"krō-bĭ-ŏt'ĭk) [" + *biosis*, life]. Pert. to or affected by necrosis. SYN: *necrotic.*

necrocytosis (ně"krō-sī-tō'sĭs) [" + *kytos*, cell, + *-ōsis*]. Cellular death or decomposition.

necrogenic, necrogenous (ně-krō-jěn'ĭk, -kroj'ěn-ŭs) [" + *gennan*, to produce]. Caused by, pert. to, or originating in dead matter.

necrology (něk-rol'o-jĭ) [" + *logos*, study]. The study of mortality statistics.

necrologist (něk-rol'ō-jĭst) [" + *logos*, study]. A student of mortality statistics.

necromania (něk-rō-mā'nĭ-ă) [G. *nekros*, dead, + *mania*, madness]. 1. Abnormal interest in dead bodies or in death. 2. Mania with desire for death.

necrometer (něk-rom'ět-ěr) [" + *metron*,

measure]. Device for measurement of dead organs.

necronarcema (ně-krō-nar-sē'mă) [" + *narkē*, stupor]. Rigidity of a dead body. SYN: *rigor mortis*.

necronectomy (něk-rŏn-ěk'tō-mǐ) [" + *ektomē*, excision]. Excision of a necrotic part, esp. of necrotic ossicles.

necroparasite (něk-rō-par'ă-sīt) [" + *parasitos*, food near]. A vegetable organism which lives in dead organic matter. SYN: *saprophyte*.

necrophagous (ně-krŏf'ă-gŭs) [" + *phagein*, to eat]. Feeding or existing on dead bodies or matter.

necrophile (něk'rō-fīl) [" + *philein*, to love]. One who has a morbid interest in or violates dead bodies.

necrophilia (něk-rō-fǐl'ǐ-ă) [" + *philein*, to love]. 1. Sexual perversion with desire for, or coitus with, dead bodies. 2. Strong desire for death. SYN: *necrophilism*.

necrophilism (ně-krŏf'ǐl-ǐzm) [" + *philein*, to love, + *ismos*, condition]. 1. Sexual perversion in which there is insane love for, or violation of, the dead. 2. Strong desire for death.

necrophilous (ně-krŏf'ǐl-ŭs) [" + *philein*, to love]. 1. Having a morbid fondness for, or feeding on, dead tissue. 2. Pert. to or affected with necrophilism.

necrophobia (něk-rō-fō'bǐ-ă) [G. *nekros*, dead, + *phobos*, fear]. 1. Abnormal aversion to dead bodies. 2. Insane dread of death. SYN: *thanatophobia*.

necropneumonia (něk″rō-nŭ-mō'nǐ-ă) [" + *pneumon*, lung]. Pulmonary gangrene.

necropsy (něk'rŏp-sǐ) [" + *opsis*, view]. The scientific examination of a dead body to determine cause of death or pathological conditions. SYN: *autopsy, necroscopy, postmortem*.

necropyoculture (něk″rō-pī-ō-kŭl'tshŭr) [" + *pyon*, pus, + L. *cultura*, culture]. A culture from pus in which the leukocytes are dead.

necrosadism (něk″rō-sā'dǐzm) [" + *sadism*]. Sexual gratification derived from the mutilation of dead bodies.

necroscopy (ně-krŏs'kō-pǐ) [" + *skopein*, to examine]. Scientific inspection of a dead body to find cause of death or pathological condition. SYN: *autopsy, necropsy*.

necrose (něk-rōs') [G. *nekros*, dead]. To cause or to undergo necrosis.

necrosis (něk-rō'sǐs) [G. *nekrōsis*, a killing]. Death of areas of tissue or bone surrounded by healthy parts; death in mass as distinguished from *necrobiosis*, a gradual degeneration. SYN: *gangrene, mortification*.

The dead part in bone is called *sequestrum*; in soft tissue, a *slough* or *sphacelus*. Term is usually applied to bone destruction or small areas of tissue, while gangrene is generally applied to destruction of specific parts or larger areas. RS: *anthraconecrosis, cardionecrosis, sequestrum, sphacelus*.

   n., anemic. N. caused by disturbed circulation in a part.

   n., Balser's fatty. Pancreatitis with gangrenous areas in the fatty tissues.

   n., caseous. SEE: *cheesy n.*

   n., central. N. which affects only the center of a part.

   n., cheesy. N. of tuberculous type with cheeselike formation.

   n., coagulative. N. due to embolic infection or exuding inflammations.

   n., colliquative. N. caused by liquefaction of tissue due to autolysis or bacterial putrefaction.

   n., dry. N. with dryness of the sequestrum.

   n., embolic. N. resulting from an embolus which causes anemic n.

   n., fat. N. in small scattered areas in the fatty tissue.

   n., fibrinous. SEE: *coagulative n.*

   n., focal. Coagulative n. in small scattered areas.

   n., moist. N. with softening and moist condition of the dead bone.

   n., putrefactive. N. caused by bacterial decomposition.

   n., superficial. N. affecting only the bone surface.

   n., thrombotic. N. due to thrombus formation.

   n., total. N. affecting an entire part.

   n. ustilaginea. Dry n. due to ergot poisoning.

necrot'ic [G. *nekrōsis*, a killing]. Rel. to death of a portion of tissue.

necrotomy (něk-rŏt'ō-mǐ) [G. *nekros*, dead, + *tomē*, a cutting]. 1. Dissection of a cadaver. 2. Excision of a sequestrum or other necrotic tissue.

nectarine (něk″ter-ēn'). AV. SERVING: 125 Gm. Pro. 0.8, Carbo. 19.9. VITAMINS: A+, C+.

needle (nēd'l) [A.S. *naedl*]. A pointed instrument for stitching, ligaturing or puncturing.

They may be *straight, half curved, full curved, semicircular,* or *double curved*, sometimes called *"S"* or *sigmoid*-shaped. There are 2 classifications: cutting edge and round point. Cutting edge type is used in skin and dense tissue work, while round point needles are used for more delicate operations. All curved needles are used with a holder, straight usually without a holder.

CARE OF: Wash off, scrub with mild cleanser, benzine and ether, sharpen, oil, and then sterilize.

   n., abdominal. Straight type with sharp point. SYN: *Keith's n.*

   n., aneurysm. N. with handle and hooked, curved point.

   n., aspirating. Long, hollow n. used in extracting fluids from cavities.

   n., Ferguson's. Full, curved, fine n. for intestinal operations.

   n., fistula. N. with shorter curve than ordinary full curved needles, used also in suturing dense tissue.

   n., Hagedorn. 1. Straight, flat n. with round eye. 2. Curved, flat n. bent on edge instead of on the flat, with round eye.

   n. holder. Device similar to a scissors used to hold surgical needles.

   n., hypodermic. N. of different lengths and bores of a hollow type, used in injecting or withdrawing fluid under the skin.

   n., Keith's. SEE: *abdominal n.*

   n. spray. Spray bath through tiny horizontal jets of approximately needle size.

   n., staphylorrhaphy. N. with handle and curved point.

need'ling [A.S. *naedl*]. Treatment by puncturing with a needle. SYN: *discission*.

Used in treatment of a cataract to allow entrance of aqueous humor and bring about absorption of the lens, and of an aneurysm in an effort to thicken and strengthen walls of the sac. Several fine needles are introduced into sac and left to be played upon by the blood

neencephalon (nē-ĕn-sĕf'ă-lŏn) [G. *neos*, new, + *egkephalos*, brain]. The higher nerve centers comprising the cerebral cortex and fibers of pyramidal tracts.

negative (neg'ă-tiv) [L. *negāre*, to deny]. 1. Without positive statement. 2. Lacking results. 3. PSY: Marked by resistance or retreat, as to a suggestion. 4. Directed away from a source of stimulation. 5. Not affirming presence of an organism, as a negative diagnosis.

  n. culture. One not revealing the suspected organism.

  n. electricity. Static e. in which elementary unit is the electron, and which is produced by friction.

  n. electrode. The chemically active pole by which currents leave. SYN: *cathode, negative pole*.

  n. glow. The luminous glow that is adjacent to the cathode in a vacuum tube through which an electrical discharge is passing.

  n. reaction. Absence of a positive indication of disease, as a negative Wassermann reaction for syphilis.

  n. sensation. One caused by stimulus not perceived in consciousness.

  n. sign. Minus sign (—) used in subtraction and to indicate a lack.

negativism (nĕg'ă-tĭv-ĭzm) [L. *negāre*, to deny, + G. *ismos*, state]. Behavior peculiarity marked by not performing suggested actions (*passive negativism*) or in doing the opposite (*active negativism*), as seen in dementia precox.

A patient may refuse to respond to suggestions because of *sluggish mental reflexes*, or from *fear*. Retardation may be slow, or sudden and intense, as in manic depressive insanity. Opposition from fear must be considered apart from dementia precox, in which the patient performs acts directly contrary to those suggested.

Ne'gri bodies. Very minute bodies formed in nerve cells of the brain of one affected by rabies.

Neisseria (nī'sĕ-rī-ă) A genus of Coccaceae, diplococci with flattened spherical shapes.

They are arranged in pairs, nonmotile, gram-negative and parasitic.

  N. catarrhalis. Species found in inflammation of the mucosa. [catarrhs.

  N. flava. Species seen in respiratory

  N. gonorrhoeae. Species causing gonorrhea. SYN: *gonococcus*.

  N. intracellularis. Intracellular organism causing cerebrospinal meningitis. SYN: *meningococcus*.

  N. meningitidis. SEE: *N. intracellularis*.

Nelaton's cath'eter. A flexible, soft rubber catheter.

  N.'s line. One from ant. sup. spine of the ilium to tuberosity of the ischium.

nem. A food value unit, the value in calories of 1 Gm. of mother's milk, equalling about 2/3 calory.

Nemathel'minthes [G. *nēmat-*, thread, + *elminth-*, worm]. A roundworm. SEE: *Platyhelminthes*.

nematoblast (nĕm'ă-tō-blast) [" + *blastos*, germ). Rudimentary spermatozoon from division of the spermatocyte. SYN: *spermatoblast*.

nematocide (nĕm'ă-tō-sīd) [" + *caedere*, to kill]. An agent that kills nematode worms.

Nematoda, Nematodes (nĕm-ăt-ō'dă, -dez) [" + *eidos*, like]. An order of threadlike worms, mostly parasitic.

nematode, nematoid (nĕm'ă-tōd, -ăt-oyd) [" + *eidos*, like]. 1. Filamentous; threadlike. 2. A species of the Nematoda.

nematodiasis (nĕm″ăt-ō-dī'ă-sīs) [" + " + *iasis*, infection]. Infestation by a parasite belonging to the order Nematoda.

nembutal (nĕm'bū-tăl). Pentobarbital sodium. One of the newer barbiturates, believed to have a short hypnotic action, and pronounced sedative effect.

  USES: As a preanesthetic, sedative and hypnotic.

  DOSAGE: As a hypnotic, 1½ gr. (0.1 Gm.).

  SEE: *pentobarbital sodium*.

neo- [G.]. Combining form meaning *new* or *recent*.

neoarsphenamine (nē″ō-ars-fĕn-am'ēn) [G. *neos*, new, + *arsphenamine*]. An arsenic compound containing about 20% arsenic.

Because it is so prone to deterioration, even in ampules, it should never be used unless of a lemon yellow color, should be preserved in a dark, cool place or icebox, and recommended not to be used after 6 months.

  USES: As for arsphenamine; probably less toxic.

  DOSAGE: Average for man, 10 gr. (0.6 Gm.). For women of average weight, 5 gr. (0.3 Gm.) to 7 gr. (0.45 Gm.) maximum. Intravenous injections preferable.

neoarthrosis (nē″ō-ar-thrō'zĭs) [" + *arthron*, joint, + *-ōsis*, increase, invasion]. A false joint. SYN: *nearthrosis*.

ne'oblast [" + *blastos*, germ]. Part of a mesoblastic element from which the vascular and connective structures originate. SYN: *parablast*.

neoblas'tic [" + *blastos*, germ]. Pert. to, or constituting, a new growth of tissue.

neocerebellum (nē″ō-sĕr-ē-bĕl'ŭm) [" + L. *cerebellum*, little brain]. Lateral lobes of the cerebellum, the more recently developed part.

neocinchophen (nē-ō-sĭn'kō-fĕn) [" + *cincophen*]. USP. A tasteless preparation of cinchophen and less likely to cause gastric irritation.

  DOSAGE: 8 gr. (0.5 Gm.).

neocinetic (nē-ō-sĭn-et'ĭk) [" + *kinēsis*, motion]. Pert. to a division of the motor system of peripheral nerves. SYN: *neokinetic*.

neocyte (nē'ō-sīt) [" + *kytos*, cell]. An immature white blood corpuscle.

neocytosis (nē″ō-sī-tō'sĭs) [" + " + *-ōsis*, invasion]. Presence of immature leukocytes in the blood. SYN: *skeocytosis*.

neoencephalon (nē″ō-ĕn-sĕf'ă-lŏn) [" + *egkephalos*, brain]. The higher nerve centers. SYN: *neënchephalon*.

neofetus (nē-ō-fē'tŭs) [" + L. *foetus*, offspring]. Embryo during 8th and 9th week of intrauterine existence.

neoformation (nē″ō-for-mā'shŭn) [" + L. *formātiō*, a shaping]. 1. Regeneration. 2. A neoplasm or new growth.

neogala (nē-og'ăl-ă) [" + *gala*, milk]. The first milk following childbirth. SEE: *colostrum*.

neogenesis (nē-ō-jĕn'ē-sĭs) [" + *genesis*, formation]. Regeneration or re-formation, as of tissue.

neogenetic (nē″ō-jĕn-ĕt'ĭk) [" + *genesis*, formation]. Newly formed; relating to new formations.

neohymen (nē-ō-hī'mĕn) [" + *ymēn*, membrane]. A false or new membrane. SYN: *pseudomembrane*.

neokinetic (nē″ō-kĭn-et'ĭk) [". + *kinēsis*, motion]. Pert. to a division of the motor mechanism of peripheral nerves.

neologism (nē-ol′ō-jĭzm) [" + *logos*, study, + *ismos*, state]. 1. A new word or phrase, or a new meaning attached to an old word or phrase. 2. Psy: A mental condition in which the patient coins new words which are meaningless, or words to which he gives *special* significance without being aware of their normal significance. See: *lalopathy*.

neomembrane (nē-ō-mĕm′brăn) [" + L. *membrana*, membrane]. A false or a new membrane. Syn: *neohymen*.

neomorph (nē′ō-mŏrf) [" + *morphē*, form]. Biol: A new formation or development which is not inherited from a similar structure in an ancestor.

neomycin (nē″ō-mī′sĭn) [" + *mykes*, fungus]. An antibiotic from a species of *Streptomyces*, isolated from soil. Active against gram-positive and gram-negative bacteria, as well as streptomycin-resistant strains of *Mycobacterium tuberculosis*. Toxic to kidneys and eighth nerve, and affects hearing.

neon (nē′ŏn) [G. *neos*, new]. Symb: Ne. An inert, gaseous element in the air derived from liquid argon. At. wt. 20.2.

neonal (nē′ō-năl). A compound of barbituric acid, considered more active.
Uses: Similar in sedative effects to barbital, regarded as useful in neuroses, but like all barbiturates, which may be habit forming, should be used with caution over long periods of time, always at the recommendation of the physician.
Dosage: 1½ gr. (0.1 Gm.).

neonatal (nē″ō-nā′tăl) [G. *neos*, new, + L. *natāre*, to be born]. Concerning the newborn. See: *period*.

neopallium (nē″ō-pal′ĭ-ŭm) [" + L. *pallium*, cloak]. That portion of cerebral hemisphere not belonging to the rhinencephalon or corpus callosum, comprising most of the convoluted cortex and its associated white fibers.
Phylogenetically, it is the new part of the pallium.

neopathy (nē-ŏp′ă-thĭ) [" + *pathos*, disease]. 1. A newly found disease. 2. A new complication or new condition of a disease.

neopenil (nē″ō-pĕn′ĭl) [" + *pen*, penicillin]. A mixture of penicillin and iodine that penetrates scar tissue in the lung, combating infection not affected by other agents. May prove effective in certain brain and kidney conditions.

neophilism (nē-ŏf′ĭl-ĭzm) [" + *philein*, to love, + *ismos*, state]. Morbid love of novelty and new persons and scenes.

neophobia (nē″ō-fō′bĭ-ă) [" + *phobos*, fear]. Fear of new scenes or novelties; aversion to all that is unknown or not understood. Syn: *cainotophobia*.

neophrenia (nē″ō-frē′nĭ-ă) [" + *phrēn*, mind]. Mental deterioration or primary psychical failure in early youth.

neoplasia (nē″ō-plā′zĭ-ă) [" + *plassein*, to form]. The development of new tissues or neoplasms.

neoplasm (nē′ō-plăzm) [" + *plasma*, a thing formed]. A new formation of tissue, abnormally, as a tumor or growth. It serves no useful function, but grows at the expense of the healthy organism.
n., benign. A growth not spreading by metastases or infiltration of tissue.
n., histoid. A n. in which structure resembles the tissues and elements which surround it.
n., malignant. A growth, such as cancer, that infiltrates tissue, metastasizes, and often recurs after removal.
n., mixed. A n. composed of tissues from 2 of the germinal layers.
n., multicentric. A growth arising from a number of distinct groups of cells.
n., organoid. A n. in which the structure is similar to some organ of the body.
n., unicentric. A growth having origin in 1 group of cells.

neoplastic (nē″ō-plăs′tĭk) [G. *neos*, new, + *plastikos*, formed]. Pert. to, or of the nature of, new, abnormal tissue formation.

neoplasty (nē″ō-plăs-tĭ) [" + *plassein*, to form]. Surgical formation or restoration of parts.

neoprontosil (nē″ō-pron′tō-sĭl). A sulfonamide and proprietary preparation of prontosil for parenteral injection, depending for efficacy on liberation of sulfanilamide through reduction in the body. The prontosil preparations have been largely replaced by other sulfonamides. Syn: *azosulfamide*.
Uses: As an antibacterial, especially in hemolytic streptococci, gonococci, and perhaps other infections. Cures gonorrhea of pregnancy.
Dosage: Orally, from 5 to 15 gr. at the discrimination of the physician, proportioned according to body weight of the patient and the condition. In pregnancy, 40 gr. daily in 5-day courses. Subcutaneously or intramuscularly, 15-20 cc. of a 2.5% solution are recommended in severe cases.

neosalvarsan (nē″ō-săl′var-săn). A compound of arsenic. See: *neoarsphenamine*.
Dosage: Intraven., 10 gr. (0.6 Gm.).

neosil′ver arsphenamine (ars″fĕn-ăm′ĕn). A silver derivative of arsphenamine, containing about 20% arsenic and 6% silver. [of neurosyphilis.
Uses: Recommended in the treatment
Dosage: For adults, 0.3-0.4 Gm. intravenously, at intervals of 5-7 days. Course of treatment recommended: 10 or 12 injections, with the same caution observed as in the use of neoarsphenamine.

neo-sil′vol. Colloidal silver iodide compound containing 18-22% silver iodide.
Action and Uses: Antiseptic, useful in infection of mucous membranes.
Dosage: In solutions of 5-40% strength.

neostigmine (nē-ō-stĭg′mĭn). Prostigmine.

neostomy (nē-os′tō-mĭ) [G. *neos*, new, + *stoma*, opening]. Formation of opening into an organ or bet. 2 organs.

neostriatum (nē″ō-strī-ā′tŭm) [" + L. *striatum*, grooved]. The caudate nucleus and outer, darker part of the lenticular nucleus of the brain.
It is the phylogenetically new part of the corpus striatum.

neo-synephrin hydrochloride (nē″ō-sĭn-ef′rĭn). A synthetic alkaloid, with therapeutic effects similar to, but more lasting than, those of ephedrine and adrenalin.
Uses: Chiefly as a vasoconstrictor.
Dosage: ¼-1 cc. of a 1% solution.

neothalamus (nē″ō-thal′am-ŭs) [G. *neos*, new, + *thalamos*, chamber]. The cortical part of the optic thalamus.

neothesin (nē-ō-thes′ĭn). Local anesthetic, one of the cocaine group, used in 1-20% solution.

neothe′sol. A mixture of procaine, refined French almond oil and 2 other chemicals, said to produce local anesthesia lasting for 14 days.
The oil holds and releases the anes-

thetic gradually into the tissues. One injection is sufficient for this period.

nephelometer (něf-ěl-om'ět-ěr) [G. *nephelē*, mist, + *metron*, measure]. Apparatus for measuring the turbidity of a fluid for the number of bacteria in a suspension.

nephelometry (něf-ěl-ŏm'ět-rǐ) [" + *metron*, measure]. The employment of the nephelometer.

nephelopia (něf-el-ō'pǐ-ă) [" + *ōps*, eye]. Dim or cloudy vision from lessened transparency of the ocular media.

nephradenoma (něf-răd-ěn-ō'mă) [G. *nephros*, kidney, + *adēn*, gland, + *-ōma*, tumor]. Renal adenoma.

nephralgia (něf-ral'jǐ-ă) [" + *algos*, pain]. Renal pain.
In absence of other symptoms, may alone be symptomatic of an obstructive renal process, but commonly presents a problem in differential diagnosis.

nephralgic (něf-răl'jǐk) [" + *algos*, pain]. Pert. to renal pain.
n. crises. Ureteral paroxysmal pain in locomotor ataxia.

nephrapostasis (něf-ră-pos'tă-sǐs) [" + *apostasis*, suppuration]. Renal abscess or purulent inflammation of the kidney.

nephrasthenia (ně-frăs-thē'nǐ-ă) [" + *a-*, priv. + *sthenos*, strength]. A slight nephrosis without actual disease of the renal tubules.

nephratony (něf-rat'ō-nǐ) [" + *a-*, priv. + *tonos*, tone]. Lack of normal renal tone.

nephrauxe (něf-rawks'ē) [" + *auxē*, increase]. Renal hypertrophy.

nephrectasia, nephrectasis, nephrectasy (něf-rěk-ta'zǐ-ă, -rěk'tă-sǐs, -tă-sǐ) [G. *nephros*, kidney, + *ektasis*, dilatation]. Renal distention.

nephrectomy (něf-rek'tō-mǐ) [" + *ektomē*, excision]. Removal of a kidney.
ONP: Patient lies on the good side. Lower thigh is flexed to a right angle at hip and the knee is drawn up to same extent. Other lower limb goes straight down the table. Upper extremity in contact with the table is flexed at the elbow, while the arm lies a little on front at side of body. A kidney bridge or sandbag is placed under the loin. The procedure is routine.
The wound should be redraped after kidney is removed and instruments used in its removal discarded. Plenty of heavy drainage tubing, both of plain and cigarette types, should be ready.
NP: Patient should be kept on back without a pillow. Urine should be measured each day. Bland diet throughout illness. Dressing watched for signs of bleeding and changed often. Drainage tube left in for a few days, removed, and dressings changed. Stitches removed in from 10-12 days.
COMPLICATIONS: Suppression of urine and secondary hemorrhage.

nephrelcosis (něf-rěl-kō'sǐs) [" + *elkōsis*, ulceration]. Ulceration of the mucosa of the kidney.

nephrelcus (něf-rěl'kŭs) [" + *elkos*, ulcer]. Renal ulcer.

nephremia (něf-rē'mǐ-ă) [" + *aima*, blood]. Congested state of kidney. SYN: *nephrohemia.*

nephremphraxis (něf"rem-fraks'is) [" + *emphraxis*, obstruction]. Obstruction in the renal vessels.

nephric (něf'rǐk) [G. *nephros*, kidney]. Pert. to the kidney or kidneys. SYN: *renal.*

nephridium (něf-rǐd'ǐ-ŭm) [G. *nephridios*, of a kidney]. An embryonic segment from which are developed part of the ovary or testis, and the excretory portion of the kidney.

nephrin (nef'rin) [G. *nephros*, kidney]. An amino acid derived from protein digestion. SYN: *cystine.*

nephrism (něf'rǐzm) [" + *ismos*, condition]. Aggregate of symptoms produced by chronic kidney disease.

nephritic (něf-rǐt'ǐk) [G. *nephros*, kidney]. 1. Rel. to the kidney. 2. Pert. to nephritis. 3. An agent used in nephritis.

nephritis (ně-frī'tǐs or něf-rī'tǐs) (pl. *nephritides*) [" + *-itis*, inflammation]. Inflammation of the kidney.
ETIOL: Bacteria or their toxins, scarlet fever, diphtheria, septicemia, or toxic drugs, such as mercury, arsenic, alcohol. Malnutrition, exposure to cold and wet. Streptococcus infection of throat, etc.
The glomeruli may be affected, or the tubules. It may be either acute or chronic.
RS: *arteriosclerosis, Bright's disease, glomerulonephritis, kidney, nephrosis.*
n., acute. An inflammatory form involving the glomeruli, the tubules, or the entire kidney. It is of various types, depending on the portion of the kidney involved, degenerative, diffuse, suppurative, hemorrhagic, interstitial and parenchymatous.
n., arteriosclerotic. SEE: *chronic interstitial n.*
n., catarrhal. Acute n. with stoppage of the tubules.
n., cheesy. A chronic form with caseous degeneration and suppuration.
n., chronic. Progressive form in which entire structure of kidney may be affected, or affection may be confined to the glomerular or tubular processes. One variety of nephritis may merge with another, causing a diffuse nephritis. Symptoms depend upon the tissues involved.
n., desquamative. SEE: *acute n.*
n., diffuse, acute. An inflammatory process involving more or less the entire kidney.
SYM: Acute onset; moderate fever; dull lumbar pain; marked edema and anasarca; hypertension; rapid pulse; vomiting; delirium; scanty, highly colored urine, containing large quantities of albumin and blood; bloody, hyaline and granular casts; uremic symptoms may develop.
PROG: Guardedly favorable. May become chronic or death through exhaustive uremia or dropsy.
TREATMENT: Absolute rest in bed until albumin has disappeared. Hot fomentations to loins. Severe cases in pregnancy may require therapeutic abortion or induction of premature labor.
DIET: Milk, buttermilk, citrus fruit juices; later, cereals, fruits, vegetables. Cream and sugar allowable. Limit proteins, salt and fluids.
n., d., chronic. SEE: *interstitial n., chronic.*
n. dolorosa. A form with hypertrophy of the capsule and pain in the kidney.
n., exudative. Form with blood serum exudation.
n., focal. N. with foci of inflammation distributed throughout the kidney.
n., glomerular. A form involving the renal glomeruli. It may be acute or chronic. SEE: *glomerulonephritis.*

n., g., acute. Acute form in which the pulse is rapid, and hypertension, edema and urine containing albumin, blood and casts are present. There is retention of urea and salt.

n., g., chronic. Form almost always following acute glomerular n. It is marked by hyalinization of the glomeruli, arteriosclerosis, hypertension, albuminuria, edema, and later uremic symptoms. Usually fatal. SEE: *glomerulonephritis, chronic.*

n., g., focal, embolic. N. in which emboli lodge in the capillary loops of the glomeruli, occluding them.
ETIOL: Subacute bacterial endocarditis due to *Streptococcus viridans*.
Glomerulus becomes hyalinized and there is blood in the lumen of tubules. Marked by blood, albumen, and hyaline and granular casts in urine. There is no edema or hypertension. TREATMENT: That of endocarditis.

n., g., f., nonembolic. N. in which not all of the glomeruli are affected and those affected are not equally so.
ETIOL: Streptococcus infections.
Marked by blood, albumin, erythrocytes, leukocytes, and granular and hyaline casts in the urine. Lumbar pain and slightly painful urination. Edema and hypertension absent. TREATMENT: Removal of the etiologic disease.

n., hemorrhagic. Acute n. with tubular hemorrhage and subsequent hematuria.

n., idiopathic. N. of unknown etiology.

n., indurative. Chronic n. marked by atrophy of the renal secreting structure and enlargement of the connective tissue stroma.

n., interstitial, acute. Rare form of acute n. in which there occur areas of cellular infiltration irregularly distributed bet. the tubules and around the glomeruli. SEE: *n., glomerular, focal, nonembolic*, for symptoms and treatment.

n., i., chronic. Glomeruli and interstitial tissue involved.
ETIOL: May follow parenchymatous n., alcoholism, lead poisoning, irritating toxins, bacterial infection, syphilis.
SYM: Headache, weakness, digestive disturbances, retinal hemorrhages and eye disturbances, dry skin. Vasomotor disturbances, such as tingling in fingers, with blanching. Hypertension marked. Low sp. gr. of urine, the quantity of which is considerable; as much by night as by day. Trace of albumin, few narrow hyaline casts, and sometimes granular casts. Retention of urea, uric acid, creatinine and protein waste products in blood.
NP: Rest and general hygienic care. Observe diet strictly, care for skin, be particular in collection of urine specimens, avoid stimulation of kidneys, increase elimination of skin and bowels. Treat symptoms as they arise.

n., lipomatous. Fatty infiltration of the renal parenchyma. SYN: *lipomatosis renis*.

n., parenchymatous, acute. Acute form affecting the parenchyma.
SYM: Marked anasarca; scanty urine; much albumin and blood; many granular, hyaline and bloody casts in urine. Great salt retention and moderate retention of nitrogenous products in the blood.

n., p., chronic. Progressive form with loss of strength and flesh.
ETIOL: Infections, fevers, alcoholism, septicemia or consequence of acute nephritis.
SYM: Marked anemia, indigestion, pallor, edema, first of lower eyelids, then general. Gastrointestinal disturbances, increased arterial tension, some hypertrophy of left ventricle, uremic symptoms—vertigo, headache, nausea, sleeplessness, stupor, convulsions, coma. Urine diminished, color and appearance often normal; highly albuminous, with sediment, hyaline, fatty and granular casts, and fatty epithelial cells. Sodium chloride retention in blood. Nitrogen retention if glomeruli are affected.
PROG: Unfavorable.
TREATMENT: Largely dietetic and hygienic. Rest; dry, warm, equable climate. Woolen or silk underclothing.

n., productive. N. with blood serum exudation and dilatation of the connective tissue stroma.

n., saturnine. N. from lead poisoning.

n., suppurative. Purulent form of n.

n., s., acute. Purulent form with abscess formation.

n., s., chronic. Cheesy and tubercular form of n.

n., tubal, n., tubular. N. affecting the renal tubules.

n., tuberculous. N. due to presence of tubercle bacilli.

nephro- [G.]. Prefix: Pert. to the kidney.

nephroabdominal (něf″rō-ăb-dom′ĭ-năl) [G. *nephros*, kidney, + L. *abdominalis*, pert. to abdomen]. Concerning the kidney and abdomen.

nephrocapsectomy (něf″rō-kăp-sek′tō-mǐ) [″ + L. *capsula*, capsule, + G. *ektomē*, excision]. Renal decapsulation for relief of chronic nephritis.

nephrocardiac (něf″rō-kar′dǐ-ăk) [″ + *kardia*, heart]. Concerning the heart and kidney.

nephrocele (něf′rō-sēl) [″ + *kēlē*, hernia]. Renal hernia.

nephrocolic (něf″rō-kŏl′ǐk) [″ + *kōlikos*, pert. to colon]. 1. Severe, colicky pain in ureter due to passage of stone. 2. Concerning the colon and kidney.

neph″rocol′ica [″ + *kōlikos*, pert. to colon]. Colicky cramp in ureter from passage of stone.

nephrocolopexy (něf″rō-kŏl′ō-pěks″ǐ) [″ + *kōlon*, colon, + *pēxis*, fixation]. Surgical suspension of kidney and colon using the nephrocolic ligament.

nephrocoloptosis (něf″rō-kō-lŏp-tō′sǐs) [″ + ″ + *ptōsis*, a dropping]. Condition in which the kidney and colon are displaced downward.

nephrocystanastomosis (něf″rō-sǐst-ăn-ăs″-to-mō′sǐs) [″ + *kystis*, bladder, + *anastomōsis*, outlet]. Surgical formation of a connection bet. kidney and the bladder, in permanent ureteral obstruction.

nephrocystitis (něf″rō-sǐs-tī′tǐs) [G. *nephros*, kidney, + *kystis*, a bladder, + *-itis*, inflammation]. Inflamed condition of kidneys and bladder.

nephrocystosis (něf″rō-sǐs-tō′sǐs) [″ + ″ + *-ōsis*, condition]. Formation of cysts in the kidneys.

n., bacterial. N. having a bacterial etiology.

n., capsular. N. affecting Bowman's capsule.

n., catarrhal. N. with the epithelium desquamated from the tubules.

n., desquamative. SEE: *catarrhal n.*

n., diffuse. A form, acute or chronic, affecting both the parenchyma and the stroma.

n., fibrous. N. affecting the stroma.

n., glomerular. Nephrocytosis especially affecting the glomeruli.
nephrogenetic, nephrogenic, nephrogenous (něf″rō-jĕn-ĕt′ĭk, -jĕn′ĭk, -rŏj′ĕn-ŭs) [" + *gennan*, to develop]. Arising in or from the renal organs.
nephrohemia (něf″rō-hē′mĭ-ă) [" + *aima*, blood]. Renal congestion. SYN: *nephremia*.
nephrohydrosis (něf″rō-hī-drō′sĭs) [" + *ydōr*, water, + -*ōsis*]. Accumulation of renal fluid due to obstruction.
nephrohypertrophy (něf″rō-hī-pĕr′trō-fĭ) [" + *yper*, over, + *trophē*, nourishment]. Overgrowth or dilatation of the kidneys.
nephroid (něf′roid) [" + *eidos*, resembling]. Resembling a kidney; kidney-shaped. SYN: *reniform*.
nephrolith (něf′rō-lĭth) [" + *lithos*, stone]. Stone in the kidney.
nephrolithiasis (něf″rō-lĭth-ī′ă-sĭs) [G. *nephros*, kidney, + *lithos*, stone]. The formation of renal stones. SYN: *lithiasis nephritica, lithiasis renalis*. SEE: *calculus, renal*.
nephrolithotomy (něf″rō-lĭth-ot′ō-mĭ) [" + " + *tomē*, incision]. Renal incision for removal of calculus.
nephrology (něf-rŏl′ō-jĭ) [" + *logos*, study]. Science of the structure and function of the kidney.
nephrolysin (něf-rol′ĭs-ĭn) [" + *lysis*, dissolution]. A toxic principle from animal serum that dissolves kidney cells. SYN: *nephrotoxin*.
nephrolysis (něf-rol′ĭs-ĭs) [" + *lysis*, loosening]. 1. Surgical detachment of an inflamed kidney from adhesions. 2. Destruction of kidney tissue by action of a nephrotoxin.
nephroma (něf-rō′mă) [" + -*ōma*, tumor]. Renal tumor or 1 of renal tissue.
nephromalacia (něf″rō-mă-lā′sĭ-ă) [" + *malakia*, softening]. Abnormal renal softness or softening.
nephromegaly (něf″rō-měg′ă-lĭ) [" + *megas, megal-*, large]. Extreme enlargement of 1 or both kidneys.
nephromere (něf′rō-mēr) [" + *meros*, part]. Segment in embryo from which kidney develops. SYN: *nephrotome*.

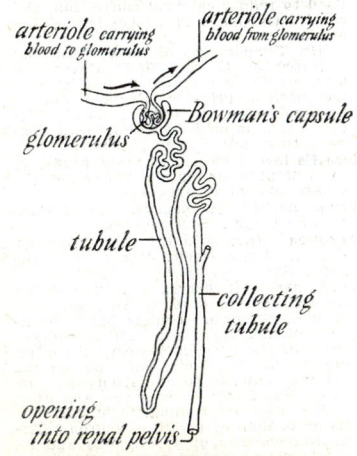

NEPHRON.
Copyright 1939, R. N.—*A Journal for Nurses*.

nephron (něf′ron) [G. *nephros*, kidney]. A unit in the kidney (said to be a million of them in each kidney) representing the excretory function of the organ.
It consists of a malpighian body and a uriniferous tubule, extending from the m. body to the collecting tubule. Most of it is within the cortex of the kidney.
nephroncus (něf-rŏn′kŭs) [" + *ogkos*, tumor]. A renal tumor.
nephroparalysis (něf″rō-păr-ăl′ĭ-sis) [" + *paralysis*, a loosening]. Paralyzed renal function.
nephropathy (něf-rop′ă-thĭ) [" + *pathos*, disease]. Disease of the kidney.
This term includes inflammatory (nephritis), degenerative (nephrosis), and sclerotic (arteriosclerotic) lesions of the kidney.
nephropexy (něf′rō-pěks-ĭ) [" + *pexis*, fixation]. Surgical attachment of a floating kidney.
nephrophthisis (něf-rŏf′thĭs-ĭs) [" + *phthisis*, a wasting]. 1. Tuberculosis of the kidney, with caseous degeneration. 2. Suppurative nephritis with wasting of the kidney substance.
nephroptosis (něf-rŏp-tō′sĭs) [" + *ptōsis*, a dropping]. Prolapse or downward kidney displacement.
ETIOL: Shape of lumbar recess, pregnancy, emaciation, enteroptosis are predisposing factors, with trauma the exciting cause.
SYM: (1) None. (2) Symptoms not referable to kidney (nervous and digestive disorders or pain). (3) Painful paroxysms simulating renal colic; kidney found anywhere in abdomen; albuminuria; painful, scanty and frequent micturition.
TREATMENT: Bed rest, truss, surgery. SEE: *nephrectomy, nephropexy*.
nephropyelitis (něf″rō-pī-ĕl-ī′tĭs) [G. *nephros*, kidney, + *pyelos*, pelvis, + -*itis*, inflammation]. Inflammation of the renal pelvis and substance. SYN: *pyelonephritis*.
nephropyosis (něf″rō-pī-o′sĭs) [" + *piōsis*, suppuration]. Purulence of a kidney.
nephrorrhagia (něf-ror-ā′jĭ-ă) [" + *rēgnunai*, to burst forth]. Renal hemorrhage into pelvis and tubules.
nephrorrhaphy (něf-ror′ă-fĭ) [" + *raphe*, a stitch]. Suture of a floating kidney to the post. wall of the abdomen.
nephrosclerosis (něf″rō-sklĕ-ro′sĭs) [" + *sklērōsis*, a hardening]. Renal sclerosis or hardening. SEE: *nephritis, chronic interstitial*.
nephrosis (něf-rō′sĭs) [G. *nephros*, kidney]. Condition in which there are degenerative changes in the kidneys without the occurrence of inflammation.
Besides the true or lipoid n., there are 3 general forms: amyloid, necrotic, and that of pregnancy.
n., amyloid. N. due to deposition of amyloid within the walls of the renal blood vessels and at the base of the cells of the tubules. Marked degeneration of kidney tissue results.
SYM: Albumin, hyaline, granular and waxy casts in urine. Polyuria present when there is no edema, and oliguria in presence of edema, with high specific gravity. Kidney function is normal. Increased globulin and cholesterol in blood and lipids in the urine.
ETIOL: Chronic suppuration in the body, tuberculosis, syphilis, Hodgkin's disease, chronic dysentery, chronic malaria, chronic gonorrhea, and in malignant tumors. Occasionally unknown.

nephrosis, dehydration

TREATMENT: Etiologic disease.

n., dehydration. Condition arising in the absence of sufficient fluids in the body. These may be lost in vomiting, severe diarrheas, or the intake may be inadequate.

SYM: Marked oliguria with albumin and casts in urine. Uremia may occur. Severe degenerative changes take place in the kidney.

n., Epstein's. A chronic metabolic form occurring with endocrine disturbances.

n., febrile. Condition in which mild changes take place in the kidneys of patients with acute infectious diseases, manifested by traces of albumin in urine.

n., larval. SEE: *febrile n.*

n., lipoid. A chronic disease of unknown etiology in which large amounts of albumin are lost in urine, resulting in depletion of the plasma protein and development of nephrotic edema. It is probably due to disordered metabolism. Occurs mainly in children and young adults.

SYM: Gradual development of edema, which reaches a high degree. Oliguria, albumin, casts of hyaline and granular type and lipids in urine. Blood serum proteins markedly reduced, but nitrogenous constituents remain normal. Blood cholesterol and globulin elevated. Hypertension absent. Anemia occurs.

PROG: Few weeks to several months.

TREATMENT: Etiologic disease, if known, high protein diet, and thyroid extract, salt and fluid restriction.

n., necrotic or necrotizing. Condition in which there is extensive death of the kidney tubules.

ETIOL: Metal poisoning, usually bichloride of mercury, and severe dehydration following intestinal or pyloric obstruction.

PATH: Lesions not confined to kidney. In kidney diffuse extensive necrosis of tubular epithelium with tubules filled with casts.

SYM: If absorption has taken place, oliguria followed by anuria; sore throat and mouth, salivation, some vomiting, weakness. Uremia and anuria set in with increasing weakness and drowsiness, ending in death. Few elements present in the tubules owing to the blocked tubules. Blood urea, nitrogen and nonprotein nitrogen high.

PROG: Depends on amount absorbed.

TREATMENT: Immediate, if possible, to prevent absorption (induced vomiting; stomach lavage, with 1:1000 calcium sulfide solution, followed by 300-400 cc. acacia mucilage; same colonically if necessary). Counteracting acidosis by washing out secreted mercury and treatment of kidney itself. If anuria persists for more than 3 days decapsulation is to be considered.

n. of pregnancy. Degenerative change in the kidney during pregnancy.

ETIOL: Generalized arterial constriction with increase in blood pressure and other symptoms follow hypertension.

SYM: A trace or large amounts of albumin in urine, with hyaline or fatty casts and a few erythrocytes present. Edema, oliguria, hypertension. Later, eclamptic symptoms, headache, vertigo, nausea, vomiting and convulsions.

TREATMENT: Rest in bed, limitation of food and fluid intake, sedatives. SEE: *eclampsia, toxemia of pregnancy.*

n., true. SEE: *lipoid n.*

N-11

nerve

nephrostoma, nephrostome (nē-fros'tō-mă, něf'ros-tōm) [G. *nephros*, kidney, + *stoma*, mouth]. The internal orifice of a Wolffian tubule, connected with the celom in the human embryo.

nephrostomy (něf-ros'to-mǐ) [" + *stoma*, mouth]. Formation of an artificial fistula into the renal pelvis.

nephrotic (něf-rot'ǐk) [G. *nephros*, kidney]. Rel. to, or caused by, nephrosis.

nephrotome (něf'rō-tōm) [" + *tomē*, a section]. Embryonic bridge of cells, connecting primitive segments along neural tube to the somatopleure and splanchnopleure, from which arises the urogenital system.

nephrotomy (něf-rot'ō-mǐ) [" + *tomē*, incision]. Incision (not exploratory) of the kidney.

NP: Accurate recording of intake and output of fluid; watch orders for collecting of specimens; watch drainage from catheter if used.

nephrotoxin (něf'rō-tōks'ǐn) [" + *toxikon*, poison]. A specific toxin which destroys renal cells.

nephrotresis (něf-rō-trē'sǐs) [" + *trēsis*, piercing]. Formation of a permanent excretory opening in the kidney through the loin.

nephrotyphus (něf-rō-tī'fŭs) [" + *typhos*, stupor]. Typhus fever complicated by hemorrhage of the kidney.

nephroureterectomy (nef'rō-ū-rē"těr-ěk'-tō-mǐ) [" + *ourētēr*, ureter, + *ektomē*, excision]. Surgical excision of kidney with the ureter or part of it.

nephrozymosis (něf"rō-zī-mō'sǐs) [" + *zymē*, ferment, + *-ōsis*]. Condition in which there is an infectious, fermentative disease of the kidney. SEE: *zymosis.*

nephrydrosis (něf-rǐ-drō'sǐs) [" + *ydōr*, water, + *-ōsis*]. Water collected in the renal pelvis due to obstruction. SYN: *hydronephrosis, nephrohydrosis.*

nepiology (nē-pǐ-ol'ō-jǐ) [G. *nēpios*, infant, + *logos*, study]. Pediatrics concerned with young infants.

Nep'tune gir'dle. Compress of linen covered by flannel which encircles the trunk from lower end of sternum to the pubes. Used in applying wet packs, esp. cold. Used to reduce cerebral congestion, visceral irritation and congestion of int. organs.

NP: Temperature of linen wrung out of water bet. 42° and 50° F. Cover with blanket. Patient should first be given a foot bath of 104°-110° F. for 5 minutes with cold compress over forehead. Girdle to remain on 1-6 hr. Forehead compress to remain during treatment.

Nernst's law (něrnst). Current necessary to stimulate a muscle varies as the square root of its frequency.

nerval (ner'văl) [L. *nervus*, sinew]. Concerning nerves. SYN: *neural.*

nervation (ner-vā'shŭn) [L. *nervus*, sinew]. Arrangement of nerves in the body. SYN: *neuration.*

nerve (nerv) [L. *nervus*, sinew; probably from G. *neuron*, sinew]. An association of filamentous or cordlike bands or fibers of nervous tissue which connect parts of the nervous system with other organs of the body, and conducting nervous impulses to and from these organs. SEE: *Table of nerves in Appendix.*

The essential component of nervous tissue is the nerve cell or *neuron.** The neuron consists of a *cell body* and its *processes,* whose number determines the shape of the cell body. The cell body contains a spherical, large, central nucleus and 1 or more nucleoli, containing only a small quantity of chromatin. The cytoplasm contains 2 characteristic structures, *neurofibrillae* and *Nissl bodies*. Neurofibrillae are fine fibers running throughout the cytoplasm and continuing on into the cell processes. Nissl bodies are chromophilic granules.

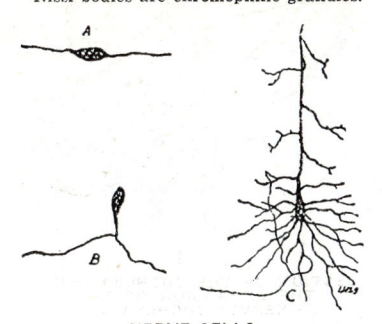

NERVE CELLS.

A. Unipolar cell; B, bipolar cell; C, multipolar cell.

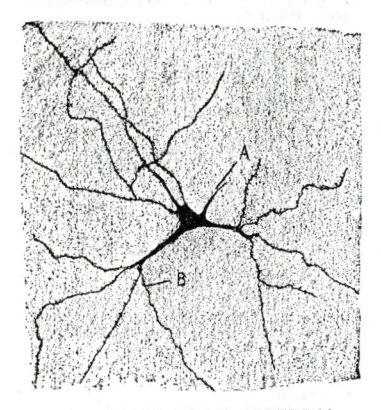

NERVE CELL FROM CEREBRAL CORTEX.

A. Axis cylinder, directed towards periphery. B. Dendrites.

Nerve processes leading from the cell body are of 2 types: the short and bushy protoplasmic process or *dendron*, and the *axon*, which branches infrequently and is longer. The dendron is also called a *dendrite* and normally carries impulses toward the cell body, while the axon normally carries impulses away from the cell body. The axon is also referred to as a *neurite*. As a rule, each nerve cell has a single axon and numerous dendrites. The processes of the nerve cells seem to be interlaced. The point at which the axon of 1 neuron and the dendrite of another *seem* to meet is known as the *synapse*. At this junction the nerve impulse jumps a tiny gap from the axon to the dendrite.

The processes derive nourishment from the cell body. Their essential function is to conduct impulses.

The neuron's function is to receive impulses and convey them to other cells. Each neuron has a distinct polarity. The *unipolar* cells are those having a single process, and are found in the spinal ganglia. *Bipolar* cells are those having processes extending from either end of the cell, and are found in the sympathetic ganglia. The *multipolar* cells are pyramidal in shape, with many processes leaving at various places, and are found in the brain and spinal cord. The other main element of nervous tissue is the *neuroglia*, which is similar to connective tissue in function, for it supports the nerve cells.

The *nerve fiber* is composed of axons and their associated structures. The axon or core of the nerve fiber is also known as the *axis cylinder* or *neuraxon*. The axis cylinder is covered by a fatty *myelin sheath*, and this, in turn, is surrounded by a nucleated layer of tissue, the *neurilemma*. At regular intervals, there are interruptions, the *nodes of Ranvier*, which divide the fiber into segments. This type of fiber is known as a *medullated* or *myelinated* fiber and is white. There is another type of fiber which does not have a myelin sheath and this is known as the *unmyelinated* or *nonmedullated fiber*, and is gray or yellow in color.

Neurons carrying impulses to the center are known as *receptor, sensory*, or *afferent*. Those which carry impulses from the center to the periphery are known as *effector, motor*, or *efferent*. Another group of neurons carries impulses from afferent to efferent neurons and is known as *connecting, central, association*, or *internuncial*. When an impulse causes secretion, the nerve is known as *secretory*. The fibers are also designated by the same names, afferent, efferent, etc. Nerves composed of motor fibers are called *motor nerves*. Those composed of sensory fibers only are *sensory nerves*, while those having both types of fibers are *mixed nerves*.

Bundles of nerve fibers are gathered together by a connective tissue sheath, the *endoneurium*, to form *fasciculi*, also known as *nerve tracts, fillets*, or *funiculi*. These, in turn, are held together by a connective tissue, the *perineurium*, and surrounded by a sheath called the *epineurium*. The fasciculi contained in the epineurium form a *nerve trunk*. Thus, nerves are branches of nerve trunks. The nerve trunk at intervals has visible bulges composed of masses of cell bodies, which are named according to their location. The *ganglion* is the name of the mass lying outside the brain and spinal cord. *Nucleus* is the mass found inside the substance of the brain or spinal cord.

The nerve terminates in a specialized part known as an *end organ, end capsule, end plate, end bulb, nerve ending*, or *arborization*. Endings of efferent nerves are known as *effector* or *motor*. Afferent nerve endings are *receptor* or *sensory*. Nerve endings in various parts of the body have special names, as touch or tactile corpuscles in skin.

There is evidence to show that nerve centers and sense organs are affected by fatigue, but not nerve fibers. A nerve cell will give off carbon dioxide when stimulated, showing that metabolic processes are involved in the activity of nerve impulse. The neuron may function as a reservoir of energy which may be depleted to such an extent as to cause physical and mental exhaustion.

n., afferent. One which transmits impulses from the periphery to a nerve center.

n. block. The prevention of stimuli from reaching consciousness by infiltrating the nerve supply of the field with novocain or other regional anesthetic, or by pressure, as in surgical operations.

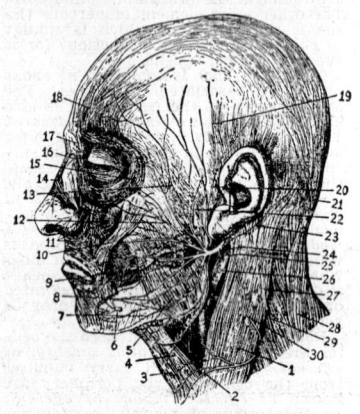

n. f., medullated. N. f. with myelin sheath bet. the axis cylinder and the neurilemma.

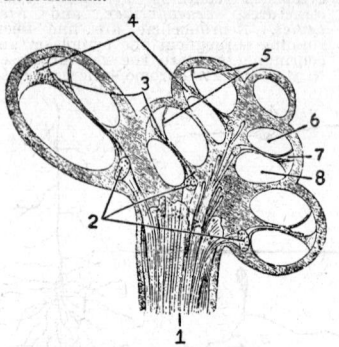

SECTION OF THE COCHLEA, WITH THE EXPANSION OF THE NERVUS COCHLEAE.

1. N. cochleae. 2. Ganglia. 3. Organon spirale. 4. Ligamentum spirale. 5. Membrana vestibularis Reissneri. 6. Scala vestibuli. 7. Scala media. 8. Scala tympani.

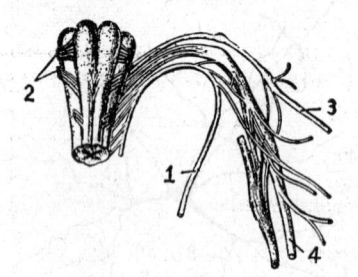

THE FACIAL PORTION OF THE FACIAL NERVE.

1. Musculus sternocleidomastoideus. 2. Nervus subcutaneus colli medius. 3. M. sternohyoideus. 4. M. omohyoideus. 5. M. masseter. 6. N. mentalis. 7. N. maxillaris inferior. 8. N. subcutaneus. 9. Stensen's duct. 10. M. zygomaticus. 11. N. infraorbitalis. 12. N. zygomaticus. 13. N. temporofrontalis. 14. N. nasociliaris. 15. M. orbicularis orbitae. 16. N. infratrochlearis. 17. N. supratrochlearis. 18. N. frontalis. 19. N. auriculotemporalis. 20. N. auriculotemporalis. 21. N. occipitalis major. 22. N. anastomaticus. 23. N. auricularis posterior profundus. 24. N. stylohyoideus. 25. N. digastricus posterior. 26. M. digastricus. 27. N. occipitalis minimus. 28. M. cucullarius. 29. M. splenius. 30. N. auricularis magnus.

DIAGRAM OF THE ORIGIN OF THE 9TH, 10TH, 11TH, AND 12TH PAIRS OF CRANIAL NERVES.

1. Nervus recurrens. 2. N. hypoglossus. 3. N. glossopharyngeus. 4. N. vagus.

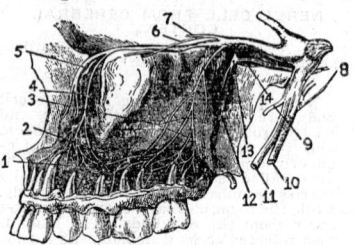

n., calorific. N. increasing heat in a part upon stimulation.

n. cell. The essential component of nervous tissue, consisting of a cell body and processes. Syn: *neuron.* See: *nerve.*

n. center. A group of cells concerned with those impulses controlling or regulating a bodily function.

n., centrifugal. See: *efferent n.*

n., centripetal. See: *afferent n.*

n., compound. See: *mixed n.*

n., depressor. An afferent n., which, when stimulated, depresses the vasomotor centers.

n., efferent. One transmitting impulses from a nerve center to the periphery.

n. ending. Terminal point of a nerve.

n., excitatory. N. transmitting impulses which stimulate function.

n. fiber. A unit of a nerve trunk composed of an axis cylinder, a myelin sheath and a neurilemma. See: *nerve.*

THE SECOND DIVISION OF THE TRIGEMINAL NERVE.

1. Plexus dentalis. 2. Ansa supramaxillaris. 3. N. dentalis posterior. 4. N. dentalis anterior. 5. N. infraorbitalis. 6. N. malaris. 7. N. temporalis. 8. Chorda tympani. 9. N. buccinatorius. 10. N. mandibularis. 11. N. lingualis. 12. N. alveolaris superior. 13. Sphenopalatine ganglion. 14. N. sphenopalatinus.

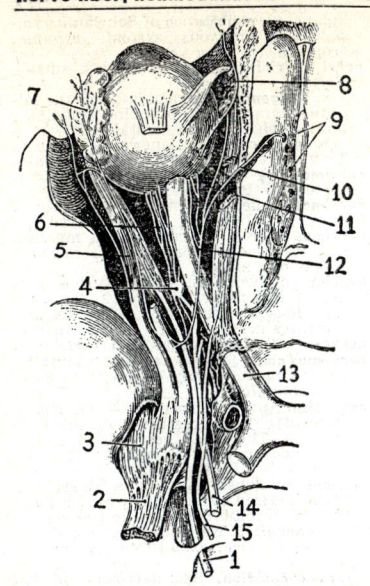

OCULOMOTOR, TROCHLEAR, AND ABDUCENT NERVES.

1. Nervus abducens. 2. N. trigeminus. 3. Gasserian ganglion. 4. Ciliary ganglion. 5. N. lacrimalis. 6. N. ciliaris. 7. Lacrimal gland. 8. N. supratrochlearis. 9. Lamina cribrosa. 10. N. ethmoidalis. 11. N. infratrochlearis. 12. N. nasociliaris. 13. N. opticus. 14. N. oculomotorius. 15. N. trochlearis.

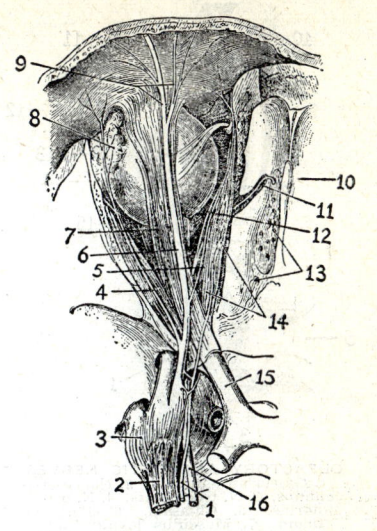

THE FIRST DIVISION OF THE TRIGEMINAL NERVE.

1. Nervus trochlearis. 2. N. trigeminus. 3. Gasserian ganglion. 4. N. lacrimalis. 5. N. infratrochlearis. 6. N. frontalis. 7. Musculus levator palpebrae superioris. 8. Lacrimal gland. 9. N. supraorbitalis. 10. Crista galli. 11. N. ethmoidalis. 12. N. supratrochlearis. 13. Lamina cribrosa. 14. M. obliquus superior. 15. N. opticus. 16. N. oculomotorius.

n. f., nonmedullated. One consisting of only an axis cylinder and a neurilemma.

n. fibril. A fine fiber in the cytoplasm and cell processes of a neuron. SYN: *neurofibrilla*.

n., frigorific. A sympathetic n. causing a lowering in temperature on stimulation.

n. grafting. Insertion of a piece of healthy nerve, usually from an animal, to replace a degenerated portion in the human. SYN: *neuroplasty*.

n. hillock. Small bulge where a nerve fiber enters a muscle.

n. impulse. Name for the excitatory process which travels along a nerve fiber when stimulated.

n., inhibitory. One which, upon stimulation, lessens activity in a part.

n., mixed. One containing both afferent (sensory) and efferent (motor) fibers.

n., motor. One containing motor fibers and conveying motor impulses. SYN: *efferent n.*

n. plexus. A group of nerves intertwined like a braid.

n., pressor. An afferent n., which, when stimulated, excites vasomotor activity, increasing its function.

n., secretory. N. whose stimulation excites secretion in a part.

n., sensory. N. which conducts impulses from a sensory organ to a nerve center.

n., somatic. A sensory or motor n.

n. storm. Sudden attack of nervousness or nervous disorder.

n. stretching. Stretching of a nerve or nerve trunk to relieve pain.

n., sympathetic. N. of the sympathetic system which supplies the internal viscera and coats of blood vessels.

n. tract. Group of nerve fibers connected by a sheath. SYN: *fasciculus*. SEE: *nerve*.

n., trophic. N. aiding in nutritional regulation of a part.

n. trunk. An aggregation of nerve fiber bundles or fasciculi, bound together by a sheath, the epineurium. SEE: *nerve*.

n., vasoconstrictor. One which contracts a blood vessel upon stimulation.

n., vasodilator. One which dilates blood vessels upon stimulation.

n., vasomotor. N. which controls the caliber of a blood vessel.

nerve, words pert. to: abducens; accelerans; accessorius; acoustic; acusticus; afferent; alemmal; anastomose; Andersch's; aneuria; aneurosis; archeokinetic; Arnold's; Auerbach's plexus; axis cylinder process; axolysis; axon; axone; axoneuron; beneceptor; block; cardiasthenia; cardioneurosis; casserian ganglion; catastaltic; cavity pulp; cell, pyramidal; celluloneuritis; center; centric; centrotherapy; cerebrifugal; cerebrin; cerebripetal; chiropractic; chiropractor; chronaxy; cranial; dendrite; dendron; effector; efferent; end organ; excitation; fasciculis; fasciola; fiber; fi-

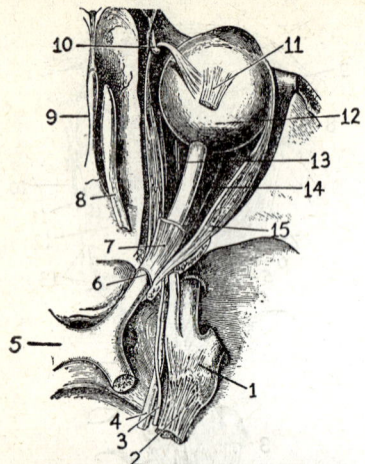

OLFACTORY AND OPTIC NERVES.
1. Gasserian ganglion. 2. Nervus trigeminus. 3. N. trochlearis. 4. N. oculomotorius. 5. Chiasma. 6. Foramen opticum. 7. Musculus levator palpebrae superioris. 8. N. olfactorius. 9. Crista galli. 10. Trochlea. 11. M. rectus superior. 12. Bulbus. 13. M. rectus interior. 14. M. rectus inferior. 15. M. rectus exterior.

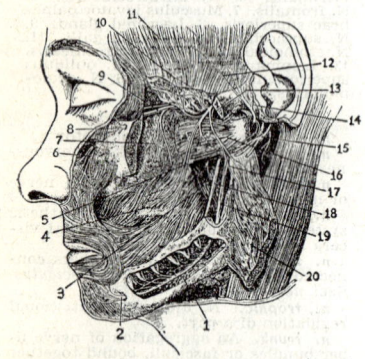

THIRD DIVISION OF THE TRIGEMINAL NERVE.
1. Nervus alveolaris inferior. 2. N. mentalis. 3. Musculus pterygoideus internus. 4. M. buccinator. 5. N. buccinator. 6. N. infraorbitalis. 7. N. alveolaris superior. 8. N. zygomaticus. 9. N. supramaxillaris trigeminus. 10. N. temporalis profundus. 11. M. temporalis. 12. Temporalis superficialis. 13. N. pterygoideus interior. 14. N. membranae tympani. 15. N. facialis. 16. M. pterygoideus externus. 17. N. massetericus. 18. N. lingualis. 19. N. mandibularis. 20. M. masseter.

bril; fibrillation; ganglion; ganglion, Arnold's; impulse; incident; innervation; mesoneuritis; mixed; motor; myelin; name of each; nervous; nervus; "neur-" words; organule; origin; plexus; polarity; radix; receptor; reflex; reinforcement; sciatica; sclerosis; sensory; splanchnic; substance of Schwann; sympathetic; -nervous system; synapse; trophic.

nervi (nĕr'vĭ) [L. pl. of *nervus*, sinew]. Nerves.
  n. erigentes [L. raising nerves]. Minute sacral nerve branches supplying rectum, bladder and genitalia.
  n. nervorum [L. sinews of sinews]. Tiny nerves distributed to nerve trunks.
nervimotil'ity [L. *nervus*, sinew, + *motor*, a mover]. Power of nerve motion.
nervimotor (nĕr-vim-ō'tor) [" + *motor*, a mover]. Concerning a motor nerve.
nervimus'cular [" + *musculus*, a muscle]. Rel. to nerves and muscles, or to nerve supply of a muscle.
nervine (nĕr'vēn) [L. *nervus*, a sinew]. 1. Acting as a nerve sedative. 2. An agent that lessens irritability of nerves and increases nerve energy. [*nerve*.
nervo- [L.]. Combining form *pert. to a*
nervomus'cular [" + *musculus*, a muscle]. Rel. to nerve supply of muscles. SYN: *nervimuscular*.
nervosism (nĕr'vō-sĭzm) [" + G. *ismos*, state of]. 1. Neurasthenia or nervousness. 2. The idea that morbid conditions depend upon alterations of nerve force.
nervous (nĕr'vus) [L. *nervus*, sinew]. 1. Characterized by instability of nerve action; excitability. 2. Pert. to the nerves.
  n. debility. Nervous fatigue with resultant physical exhaustion. SYN: *neurasthenia*.
  n. exhaustion. SEE: *nervous debility*.
  n. impulse. The excitatory process set up in nerve fibers by stimuli.
  It is probably in the nature of a wave of electrochemical disturbance traveling at the comparatively slow rate (even in fastest conducting mammalian nerves) of 50-80 meters per second. The velocity varies in different fibers according to the diameter.
  n. prostration. SEE: *nervous debility*.
  n. system. A system of extremely delicate nerve cells, elaborately interlaced with each other, collectively consisting of the brain, cranial nerves, spinal cord, spinal nerves, autonomic ganglia, ganglionated trunks and nerves, maintaining the vital function of reception and response to stimuli.
  With this system belong the sense organs, which are the eye, ear, apparatus for taste and smell, and the skin.
  Gray's Anatomy divides it into three parts: 1. *The Central Nervous s.* including the brain and spinal cord. 2. *The Peripheral Nervous s.* including the cranial and spinal nerves, which directs the function of those parts of the brain concerned with skeletal muscular activity, consciousness, and mental activity, as well as the end organs of all sensory nerves. 3. *The Autonomic Nervous s.* This controls, involuntarily, the function of smooth muscle tissue, the heart, and the glands. It is divided into the *sympathetic* and the parasympathetic branches. SEE: *autonomic n.s.* also: *central nervous s., sympathetic n.s.*, and *parasympathetic s.*
nervousness (nĕr'vŭs-nĕs) [L. *nervus*, sinew]. Morbid excitability of the nervous system associated with unrest.
nervule (nĕr'vŭl) [L. *nervulus*, a little sinew]. A small nerve.
nestiatria (nĕs-tĭ-ă-trī'ă) [G. *nēstis*, hunger, + *iatreia*, therapy]. Therapeutic use of hunger cure. SYN: *nestotherapy*.
nestiostomy (nĕs-tĭ-os'tō-mĭ) [G. *nēstis*,

jejunum, + *stoma,* mouth]. The surgical formation of a permanent jejunal fistula through the abdominal wall.

nes'tis [G. *nēstis,* fasting]. 1. Jejunum. 2. Fasting.

nestither'apy [G. *nēstis,* hunger, + *therapeia,* treatment]. Use of hunger cure therapeutically.

nestother'apy [G. *nēstis,* hunger, + *therapeia,* treatment]. Therapeutic use of fasting or reduced diet.

net knot. Chromatin mass in a cell nucleolus forming a nucleolus. SYN: *karyosome.*

net′tle rash. Skin rash with intense itching, resembling condition produced by stinging with nettles. SYN: *hives, urticaria.*

net'work [A.S. *net,* net, + *wyrcan,* to work]. Fiber arrangement in a structure resembling a net. SYN: *rete, reticulum.*

neu (nū) [G. *neuron,* sinew]. A nerve fiber sheath. SYN: *neurilemma.*

Neumann's disease (noi'mănz). Malignant form of pemphigus with growths. SYN: *pemphigus vegetans, q.v.*

neura (nū'ră) (sing. *neuron*) [G. *neuron,* sinew]. Nerves.

neurad (nū'răd) [G. *neuron,* sinew, + L. *ad,* to]. Toward the neural axis or aspect.

neuradynamia (nū-ră-dĭ-nā'mĭ-ă) [" + *a-,* priv. + *dynamis,* power]. Nervous disorder with extreme fatigue. SYN: *neurasthenia.*

neuragmia (nū-rag'mĭ-ă) [" + *agmos,* break]. The bruising or ripping of a nerve trunk above or below a ganglion.

neural (nū'răl) [G. *neuron,* sinew]. Pert. to nerves or connected with the nervous system.

n. **spine.** Spinous vertebral process.

neuralgia (nū-ral'jĭ-ă) [" + *algos,* pain]. Severe, lancinating pain along the course of a nerve.

ETIOL: Pressure on nerve trunks, faulty nerve nutrition, changes in root ganglia, toxins, neuritis.

SYM: According to the part affected. SEE: *geniculate, sciatica.*

n., **cardiac.** Angina pectoris.

n., **degenerative.** N. caused by degenerative changes in the nerves or nerve cells.

n., **epileptiform.** Spasmodic facial n. SYN: *tic douloureux.*

n., **facialis vera.** Geniculate n.

n., **Fothergill's.** Trigeminal n.

n., **geniculate.** N. with paroxysmal lancinating pain in the ear.

n., **hallucinatory.** Impression of local pain without actual peripheral pain.

n., **Hunt's.** Geniculate n.

n., **idiopathic.** N. without structural lesion or pressure from a lesion.

n., **intercostal.** Pain follows course of intercostal nerves; frequently associated with eruption of herpes zoster; spots of tenderness near vertebral column, in middle of nerve, and near sternum. May be dependent upon spinal caries, or thoracic aneurysm.

n., **mammary.** N. of the breast. SYN: *mastodynia.*

n., **Morton's.** N. of joint of 3rd and 4th toes.

n., **nasociliary.** N. of eyes, brows and root of nose.

n., **occipital.** Involves upper cervical nerves. A spot of tenderness found bet. mastoid process and upper cervical vertebrae. May be due to spinal caries.

n., **otic.** Geniculate n.

n., **reminiscent.** Continued mental impression of pain after n. has ceased.

n. **(of) sphenopalatine ganglion.** SYN: *Sluder's n.* SYM: Pain on one side of face, radiating to eyeballs, ear, occipital and mastoid areas of skull; sometimes to nose, upper teeth and shoulder of same side. PROG: good.

n., **stump.** Pressure on nerves in stump after amputation, causing pain.

n., **symptomatic.** N. not primarily involving the nerve structure.

n., **trifacial.** N. involving 1 or more branches of the trifacial nerve.

SYM: Tender points correspond to supraorbital, infraorbital, and mental foramina. Often violent spasm of muscles. In long standing cases hair on affected side sometimes becomes coarse and bleached.

ETIOL: Frequently a reflex from caries of teeth, nasal disease, or some distant center of infection.

PROG: For attack, good; permanent cure, guarded.

TREATMENT: Quiet, cool, well-ventilated room, cold applications, hot fomentations, or hot salt bags. Trace course of nerve with oil of peppermint or oil of cloves. Bet. attacks, improve nutrition, give constitutional remedies. Surgical interference, nerve stretching, section, or removal of a portion of the nerve.

SYN: *tic douloureux, prosopalgia.*

neuralgic (nū-ral'jĭk) [G. *neuron,* sinew, + *algos,* pain]. Of, or concerning, neuralgia.

neuramebimeter (nu″răm-ē-bĭm'ĕt-ĕr) [" + *amoibē,* response, + *metron,* a measure]. Device for determining time of response of a nerve to a stimulus.

neuranagenesis (nu″ran-a-jen'ē-sĭs) [" + *ana,* up, + *genesis,* formation]. Regeneration or reformation of nerve tissue.

neurangio′sis [" + *aggeion,* vessel, + *-ōsis,* condition]. A vascular neurosis.

neurapophysis (nū-ră-pof'ĭ-sĭs) [" + *apo,* from, + *physis,* growth]. 1. Either side of the neural arch in a vertebra. 2. Spinous process of a vertebrae.

neurarthropathy (nū-rar-throp'ă-thĭ) [" + *arthron,* joint, + *pathos,* disease]. Disease of the joints and nerves.

neurasthenia (nū-răs-thē'nĭ-ă) [G. *neuron,* sinew, + *astheneia,* weakness]. An ill-defined disease commonly following depressed states characterized by a sense of weakness or exhaustion, or by the symptoms of various types of organic disease without the existence of organic disease in a degree sufficient to justify the subjective complaints of the patient.

SYM: Fatigue; weakness; headache; sweating; polyuria; tinnitus and vertigo; photophobia; fear; easy exhaustion on the slightest effort; inability to concentrate; irritability and complaint of poor memory; poor sleep; numerous, constantly varying aches and pains; vasomotor disturbances.

The neurasthenic is often physically asthenic with a long, narrow thorax, small muscles and undernourished. The face is thin, alert, and often suggests chronic suffering. Much of this is the result of the neurasthenia, but it suggests also a physical type, inherently predisposed to develop the disease.

Freud believes the disease is probably a frustration (esp. sexual) which possibly complicates the symptoms by an element of renunciation as well.

PROG: Favorable, if cause can be removed.
TREATMENT: Largely hygienic and dietetic. Where there has been great inactivity give regular physical exercise. Weak and anemic require rest. Frequent bathing with salt water followed by friction massage. Tobacco and alcohol interdicted, tea and coffee used sparingly. Constitutional remedies. SEE: *apokamnosis.*

n., sexual. Disorder arising from excessive fear due to statements of quacks, associates, etc., concerning early masturbation as a cause of imbecility or insanity.

n., traumatic. Either the expression of actual brain change, too slight to be objectively demonstrable, or a true, latent neurasthenic reaction brought to light by injury or the hope of compensation for injury.

neurastheniac, neurasthenic (nū-răs-thē′-nĭ-ăk, -nĭk) [G. *neuron,* sinew, + *astheneia,* weakness]. 1. Suffering from or concerning neurasthenia. 2. Individual suffering from neurasthenia.

neurataxia, neurataxy (nū-ră-tăk′sĭ-ă, nū′-ră-tăk-sĭ) [″ + *ataxia,* lack of order]. Functional nervous disorder. SYN: *neurasthenia, q.v.*

neuration (nū-rā′shŭn) [G. *neuron,* sinew]. Arrangement or distribution of nerves. SYN: *nervation.*

neuratrophia, neuratrophy (nū-ă-trō′fĭ-ă, -răt′rō-fĭ) [″ + *atrophia,* a wasting]. Atrophy of the nervous tissue or deficient nutrition of the nervous system.

neuraxial (nū-răks′ĭ-ăl) [″ + *axon,* axis]. Concerning a neuraxis.

neuraxis (nū-răks′ĭs) [″ + *axon,* axis]. 1. An axis cylinder of a nerve cell. 2. The cerebrospinal axis.

neuraxitis (nū-răks-ī′tĭs) [″ + ″ + *-itis,* inflammation]. 1. Inflamed condition of a neuraxis. 2. Encephalitis.

n., epidemic. Epidemic encephalitis.

neuraxon(e (nū-răks′ŏn) [″ + *axon,* axis]. The axis cylinder process of a nerve cell. SYN: *axon.* SEE: *nerve.*

neure (nūr) [G. *neuron,* sinew]. A nerve cell. SYN: *neuron.*

neurectasy, neurectasia, neurectasis (nū-rĕk′ta-sī, -rĕk-tā′zĭ-ă, -rĕk′ta-sĭs) [″ + *ektasis,* a stretching]. Surgical nerve stretching.

neurectomy (nū-rĕk′tō-mĭ) [″ + *ektomē,* excision]. Partial or total excision or resection of a nerve.

neurectopia, neurectopy (nū-rĕk-tō′pĭ-ă, nūr-ĕk′tō-pĭ) [″ + *ek,* out, + *topos,* place]. Displacement or abnormal position of a nerve.

neurenergen (nū-rĕn′ĕr-jĕn) [″ + *ergon,* work, + *gennan,* to produce]. Substance said to supply energy to the neurons.

neurenteric (nū-rĕn-tĕr′ĭk) [″ + *enteron,* intestine]. Rel. to the neural canal and intestinal tube of the embryo.

n. canal. Temporary canal of the embryo bet. the medullary and intestinal tubes.

neurepithelium (nūr″ĕp-ĭ-thē′lĭ-ŭm) [″ + *epi,* upon, + *thēlē,* nipple]. 1. Epithelial structures forming the terminations of nerves of special sense. 2. Embryonic layer from which arises the cerebrospinal axis. SYN: *neuroepithelium.*

neurergic (nū-rĕr′jĭk) [G. *neuron,* sinew, + *ergon,* work]. Concerning the activity of a nerve.

neurexairesis (nū-rĕks-ī-rē′sĭs) [″ + *exairein,* to draw out]. Ripping or tearing out of a nerve to relieve neuralgia.

neuriatry (nū-rī′a-trī) [″ + *iatreia,* treatment]. Study and treatment of diseases of nervous system. SYN: *neurology.*

neurilemma (nū″rĭ-lĕm′ă) [″ + *lemma,* rind]. An elastic nerve fiber sheath. SEE: *nerve, substance of Schwann.*

neurilemmitis (nū″rĭ-lĕm-mī′tĭs) [″ + ″ + *-itis,* inflammation]. Inflamed condition of a neurilemma.

neurility nū-rĭl′ĭ-tĭ) [G. *neuron,* sinew]. Ability of nerve fibers to conduct stimuli.

neurimotility (nū-rĭ-mō-tĭl′ĭ-tĭ) [″ + L. *motilis,* able to move]. Power of neural motion. SYN: *nervimotility.*

neurimo′tor [″ L. *motor,* a mover]. Concerning a motor nerve.

neurine (nū′rĕn) [G. *neuron,* sinew]. 1. An albuminous substance in nerve tissue. 2. Poisonous ptomaine found in decomposition of protagon, fungi and fish. 3. An extract of nerve tissue used therapeutically. 4. A name for nerve energy.

neurinoma (nū-rĭn-ō′mă) [″ + *-ōma,* swelling]. A tumor derived from connective tissue in a nerve fiber. SYN: *neurofibroma.*

neurinomatosis (nū″rĭn-ō-mă-tō′sĭs). Condition of having multiple neurinomas on nerve fibers. SYN: *neurofibromatosis.*

neurite (nū′rīt) [G. *neuron,* sinew]. The axis cylinder process of a neuron. SYN: *axon, neuraxon.*

neuritic (nū-rĭt′ĭk) [G. *neuron,* sinew]. Concerning, or suffering from, neuritis.

neuritis (nū-rī′tĭs) [G. *neuron,* sinew, + *-itis,* inflammation]. Inflammation of a nerve or nerves, usually associated with a degenerative process.

ETIOL: Colds; traumatism, poisons, infections, esp. from diphtheria; scarlet fever, typhoid fever, measles, malaria, pneumonia, pertussis, beriberi; drugs, such as alcohol, arsenic, lead, mercury, etc.

SYM: Neuralgia in part affected; hyperesthesia, paresthesia, dysesthesia, hypesthesia, or anesthesia; muscular atrophy of part supplied by affected nerve; paralysis; lack of reflexes.

NP: Rest in bed, water or air bed. Uniformity of pressure on body. Temperature of water in water bath must be maintained by frequent replacement of cooling water with warm water. Hot water bags or electric heating pads under covers but not next to skin, as lack of sensibility to heat on part of patient may lead to burns. Cradles may be necessary. Padded splints with little bandage compression to affected parts. No sudden change of position. Place limb in suspended towel to move it. No rubbing. Later diathermy under direction of physician, also massage, using mildest of manipulations. Avoid all strain on patient. SEE: *polyneuritis.*

n., adventitial. Inflammation of nerve sheath.

n., ascending. N. along a nerve trunk away from periphery.

n., axial. Parenchymatous n.

n., degenerative. N. with rapid degeneration of nerve.

n., descending. N. along nerve trunk toward the periphery.

n., diphtheritic. N. following diphtheria.

n., disseminated. Segmental n.

n., endemic. Beriberi or multiple n.

n., interstitial. N. of connective tissue of a nerve.

n., intraocular. N. of retinal region of optic nerve.

SYM: Disturbed vision, contracted field, enlarged blind spot, fundus find-

neuritis, migrans N-18 **neurocladism**

ings such as exudates, hemorrhages and abnormal condition of blood vessels.
TREATMENT: Depends on etiology such as brain tumors, meningitis, syphilis, nephritis, diabetes, etc.
  n., migrans, n., migrating. A roving n.
  n., multiple. Inflammation of many spinal nerves at the same time.
  SYM: *Acute*: Chill; fever, 102-103° F.; headache; pain in back; malaise; coated tongue; loss of appetite; constipation; loss of power, esp. in legs and extensor muscles; abolition of reflexes; atrophy of muscles; more or less anesthesia; tenderness over nerve trunks. *Chronic*: Pains in limbs, hyperesthesia, paresthesia, irregular areas of anesthesia, loss of power, abolition of deep reflexes, tenderness over nerve trunks, wasting of muscles, impaired electrical contractility; edema of hands and feet.
  PROG: Guardedly favorable. Acute form may prove fatal from involvement of respiratory muscles.
  TREATMENT: Acute cases, absolute rest, limb in splint later, and in chronic cases, massage, electricity, general treatment.
  SYN: *polyneuritis*. SEE: *beriberi*.
  n. nodosa. N. with formation of nodes on nerves.
  n., optic. N. of optic nerve.
  n., parenchymatous. N. of nerve fiber substance.
  n., peripheral. N. of terminal nerves or of end organs.
  n., retrobulbar. N. of optic nerve behind eyeball.
  SYM: Loss of vision in affected eye. (a) *Acute*: Seen in sinus disease; orbital cellulitis; poisons, as lead and alcohol; multiple sclerosis. (b) *Chronic*, or *toxic amblyopia*: Seen in excessive tobacco and alcohol users. SYM: Central scotoma.
  n., rheumatic. N. with symptoms of rheumatism.
  n., segmental. N. affecting segments of a nerve interspersed with healthy segments.
  n., senile. N. in feet and legs of the elderly.
  n., simple. Inflammation of single nerve trunk.
  SYM: Severe pain along course of nerve which is tender to touch, burning, numbness, tingling. At first hyperesthetic, later, anesthetic. Muscular power impaired, fibrillar tremors, reflexes diminished, or lost. Sometimes eruption of herpes follows affected nerves. Skin may become glossy; nails brittle, lusterless. Advanced cases, wasting and impaired electrocontractility; occasionally effusion into joints. In some cases febrile symptoms. Symptoms of chronic form are similar.
  PROG: Guardedly favorable in acute case. Chronic, after trophic changes, grave.
  TREATMENT: Rest part in splint, elevated; hot or cold applications; electricity, general treatment.
  n., sympathetic. N. of opposite nerve without attacking nerve center.
  n., tabetic. N. in locomotor ataxia.
  n., toxic. N. from alcohol.
  n., traumatic. N. following an injury.
neuro- [G. *neuron*, sinew, nerve]. Combining form *rel. to a nerve*.
neuroamebiasis (nū-rō-ă-mē-bī'ă-sĭs) [G. *neuron*, sinew, + *amoibē*, change, + *iasis*, infection]. Neuritis occurring as a sequela to amebic dysentery.

neuroanatomy [" + *ana*, up, + *tomē*, a cutting]. Study of structure of the nervous system.
neuroarthritis (nū"rō-ar-thrīt'-ĭzm) [" + *arthron*, joint, + *ismos*, condition]. Tendency toward contraction of nervous and gouty disorders.
neuroarthropathy (nū"rō-ar-throp'ăth-ī) [" + " + *pathos*, disease]. Disease of a joint combined with disease of the central nervous system.
neurobiology (nū"rō-bī-ol'ō-jī) [" + *bios*, life, + *logos*, study]. Biological approach in studying the nervous system.
neurobion (nū-rō-bī'on) [" + *bios*, life]. A hypothetical particle connected with renewal of nerve tissue.
neurobiotaxis (nū"rō-bī"ō-tak'sĭs) [" + " + *taxis*, order]. Migration of nerve cells during development toward source of nutrition and stimulation.
neuroblast (nū'rō-blăst) [" + *blastos*, germ]. 1. An embryonic cell giving rise to a neuron. 2. Immature neuron.
neuroblastoma (nū"rō-blăs-tō'mă) [G. *neuron*, sinew, + *blastos*, germ, + *-ōma*, tumor]. A tumor composed of immature or embryonic neurons.
neurocanal (nū"rō-kă-năl') [" + L. *canalis*, passage]. The central canal of the spinal cord.
neurocardiac (nū"rō-kar'dĭ-ăk) [" + *kardia*, heart]. 1. Pert. to the nerves supplying the heart or nervous system and the heart. 2. Concerning a cardiac neurosis.
neurocele (nū'rō-sēl) [" + *koilia*, cavity]. Ventricles and cavities in the cerebrospinal axis.
neurocentral (nū"rō-sĕn'trăl) [" + *kentron*, center]. Pert. to the centrum of a vertebra and the neural arch.
neurocentrum (nū"rō-sĕn'trŭm) [" + *kentron*, center]. A vertebral element which unites with another on opposite side to form a neural arch, from which vertebral spine develops.
neuroceptor (nū"rō-sep'tor) [" + L. *ceptor*, a receiver]. A dendritic terminus which receives a stimulus from an adjoining nerve process.
neurochemistry (nū"rō-kĕm'ĭs-trī) [" + *chēmeia*, chemistry]. Physiological chemistry dealing with nervous tissue.
neurochitin (nū-rō-kī'tĭn) [G. *neuron* + *chitōn*, tissue]. The substance supporting nerve fibers in nervous tissue.
neurochondrite (nū"rō-kon'drĭt) [" + *chondros*, cartilage]. One of the primordial cartilaginous elements from which arises the neural arch of a vertebra.
neurochorioretinitis (nū"rō-kō"rī-ō-rĕt-ĭn-ī'tĭs) [" + *chorion*, skin, + L. *rētē*, a net, + G. *-itis*, inflammation]. Inflammation of choroid and retina combined with optic neuritis.
neurochoroiditis (nū"rō-kō-roi-dī'tĭs) [" + *chorion*, skin, + *eidos*, like, + *-itis*, inflammation]. Inflamed condition of the choroid coat and optic nerve.
neurocirculatory (nū"rō-sur'kū-lă-tō"rī) [" + L. *circulatiō*, circulation]. Pert. to circulation and the nervous system.
  n. asthenia. A combination of nervous and circulatory disturbances with fatigue and precordial pain, usually seen in soldiers. SYN: *irritable heart, soldier's heart*. SEE: *asthenia*.
neurocity (nū-ros'ĭt-ī) [G. *neuron*, sinew]. Nerve force.
neurocladism (nū-rok'lăd-ĭzm) [" + *klados*, branch, + *ismos*, state]. Reunion of ends of a divided nerve by attraction

of processes of nerve cells. SYN: *odogenesis.*

neuroclonic (nū″rō-klon'ĭk) [" + *klonos,* spasm]. Marked by spasms of nervous origin.

neurocoele (nū″rō-sēl) [" + *koilia,* cavity]. System of cavities in cerebrospinal axis. SYN: *neurocele.*

neurocranium (nū″rō-krā'nĭ-ŭm) [" + *kranion,* skull]. The part of the skull enclosing the brain.

neurocrine (nū′rō-krīn) [" + *krinein,* to secrete]. Concerning an endocrine influence on the nervous system.

neurocrinia (nū-rō-krĭn'ĭ-ă) [" + *krinein,* to secrete]. Endocrine stimulus of nervous system.

neurocutaneous (nū″rō-kū-tā'nē-ŭs) [" + L. *cutis,* skin]. Pert. to the nervous system and skin.

neurocyte (nū′rō-sīt) [G. *neuron,* sinew, + *kytos,* cell]. A nerve cell. SYN: *neuron.*

neurocytoma (nū″rō-sī-tō'mă) [" + " + *-ōma,* tumor]. A tumor formed of cells, usually ganglionic, of nervous origin. SYN: *neuroma, 2.*

neurodealgia (nū″rō-dē-al'jĭ-ă) [G. *neurōdēs,* retina, + *algos,* pain]. Pain in the retina.

neurodendrite, neurodendron (nū″rō-děn'drīt, -dron) [G. *neuron,* sinew, + *dendron,* tree]. Protoplasmic branched process of a nerve cell. SYN: *dendrite, dendron.*

neurodermatitis (nū″rō-děr-mă-tī'tĭs) [" + *derma,* skin, + *-itis,* inflammation]. Cutaneous inflammation of neural origin, or accompanied by nervous disorder, marked by itching.

neurodermatosis (nū″rō-děr-mă-tō'sĭs) [" + " + *-ōsis,* condition]. Any skin disease of neural origin.

neurodiagnosis (nū″rō-dī-ăg-nō'sĭs) [" + *dia,* through, + *gnōsis,* knowledge]. Diagnosis of nervous disorders.

neurodocitis (nū″rō-dō-sī'tĭs) [" + *-itis,* inflammation]. Lesion of nerve roots due to pressure.

neurodynamia (nū″rō-dī-nam'ĭ-ă) [" + *dynamis,* power]. Nervous energy or force.

neurodynamic (nū″rō-dī-nam'ĭk) [" + *dynamis,* power]. Concerning nervous force or energy.

neurodynia (nū″rō-dĭn'ĭ-ă) [G. *neuron,* nerve, + *odynē,* pain]. Pain in a nerve or nerves. SYN: *neuralgia.*

neuroelectricity (nū″rō-ē-lěk-trĭs'ĭ-tĭ) [" + *ēlektron,* amber]. Electricity generated by the nervous system.

neuroelectrotherapeutics (nū″rō-ē-lěk″trō-ther-ă-pū'tĭks) [" + " + *therapeutikē,* treatment]. Electricity in treatment of neural diseases.

neuroenteric (nū″rō-ěn-ter'ĭk) [" + *enteron,* intestine]. Pert. to the embryonic intestinal tube and neural canal. SYN: *neurenteric.*

neuroepidermal (nū″rō-ěp-ĭ-dŭr'măl) [" + *epi,* upon, + *derma,* skin]. Pert. to or giving rise to nervous system and epidermis.

    n. layer. Ext. or outermost layer of the blastoderm which gives rise to epidermis and nervous system. SYN: *ectoderm, epiblast.*

neuroepithelioma (nū″rō-ěp″ĭ-thē-lĭ-ō'mă) [" + " + *thēlē,* nipple, + *-ōma,* tumor]. A tumor of neuroepithelium in a nerve of special sense.

neuroepithelium (nū″rō-ěp″ĭ-thē'lĭ-ŭm) [" + " + *thēlē,* nipple]. 1. A specialized epithelial structure forming the termination of a nerve of special sense. 2. Embryonic layer of the epiblast from which the cerebrospinal axis is developed.

neuroequilibrium (nū″rō-ē″kwĭ-lĭb'rĭ-ŭm) [G. *neuron,* sinew, + L. *aequus,* equal]. Balance of neural tension.

neurofibril, neurofibrilla (nū-rō-fī'brĭl, -fī-brĭl'ă) (pl. *neurofibrils, neurofibrillae*) [" + L. *fibrilla,* a small fiber]. A tiny fiber in the cytoplasm of a neuron which continues on into the nerve processes. SEE: *nerve.*

neurofibroma (nū″rō-fī-brō'mă) (pl. *neurofibromata* or *-mas*) [" + L. *fibra,* fiber, + G. *-ōma,* tumor]. A tumor of connective tissue of a nerve including medullated layer of a nerve fiber. SYN: *neuroma, false; pseudoneuroma.*

neurofibromatosis (nū″rō-fī-brō″mă-tō'sĭs) [" + " + " + *-ōsis,* increase]. Condition in which there are tumors of various sizes on peripheral nerves.

    They may be neuromas or fibromas.

neurofibrositis (nū″rō-fī″brō-sī'tĭs) [" + " + G. *-itis,* inflammation]. Inflammation of nerve fibers and sensory nerve fibers in muscular tissue.

neurofil (nū′rō-fĭl) [" + L. *filum,* a thread]. A mass of fibers arising at the beginning of the axis cylinder and enveloping the neuron.

neurogangliitis (nū″rō-gan-glĭ-ī'tĭs) [G. *neuron,* sinew, + *gagglion,* knot, + *-itis,* inflammation]. Inflamed condition of a neuroganglion.

neurogang'lion [" + *gagglion,* knot]. A mass of neurons on a nerve trunk acting as a nerve center. SEE: *nerve.*

neurogen (nū′rō-jen) [" + *gennan,* to produce]. A substance which supposedly liberates nervous force at the synapse.

neurogenesis (nū″rō-jěn'ē-sĭs) [" + *genesis,* production]. 1. Growth or development of nerves. 2. Development from nervous tissue.

neurogenetic (nūr″ō-jěn-et'ĭk) [" + *genesis,* production]. 1. Pert. to nerve formation. 2. Pert. to origin in nerves.

neurogenic, neurogenous (nū-rō-jěn'ĭk, -rŏj′ěn-ŭs) [" + *gennan,* to produce]. Originating in nerve cells.

    n. theory. Cardiac muscle fibers move only in response to neural stimuli. OPP: *myogenic theory.*

    n. tonus. Tonic muscular contraction due to stimuli from nerve centers.

neurogeny (nū-rŏj'ěn-ĭ) [" + *gennan,* to produce]. 1. Nerve development or growth. 2. Formation from nervous tissue.

neuroglia (nū-rŏg'lĭ-ă) [G. *neuron,* sinew, + *glia,* glue]. Connective tissue forming the supporting substance of the nerve cells of the cerebrospinal axis.

    It, unlike other connective tissue, is derived from the ectoderm.*

    RS: *astroglia, bindweb, macroglia, mesoglia, microglia, oligodendroglia.*

    n. cell. Spider and mossy cell in the neuroglia. SYN: *glia cell.*

neurogliac (nū-rŏg'lĭ-ăk) [" + *glia,* glue]. Pert. to the supporting tissue of nerve cells.

neurogliacyte (nū-rŏg'lĭ-ă-sīt) [" + " + *kytos,* cell]. Any one of the cells found in neuroglial tissue.

neurogliar, neuroglic (nū-rŏg'lĭ-ăr, -lĭk) [" + *glia,* glue]. Pert. to or resembling the supporting tissue of nerve cells.

neuroglioma (nū″rō-glĭ-ō'mă) [" + " + *-ōma,* tumor]. Tumor of neurogliar tissue. SYN: *glioma.*

neuroglioma, ganglionar

n., ganglionar, n., ganglionare. Glioma with ganglion cells.

neurogliosis (nū″rō-glī-ō′sĭs) [" + " + *-ōsis,* increase]. Development of numerous neurogliomas.

neurogram (nū′rō-grăm) [" + *gramma,* a mark]. The impression left upon the physical brain following any cerebral experience which is retained as unconscious memory. SEE: *engram.*

neurography (nū-rog′ră-fĭ) [G. *neuron,* sinew, + *graphein,* to write]. 1. A study or description of the nervous system. 2. Formation of neurograms in the brain.

neurohematology (nū″rō-hem″at-ol′ō-jĭ) [" + *aima,* blood, + *logos,* study]. The study of hemic changes in neural diseases.

neurohistology (nū″rō-hĭs-tol′ō-jĭ) [" + *istos,* tissue, + *logos,* study]. The study of nervous tissue.

neurohypophysis (nū″rō-hī-pof′ĭs-ĭs) [" + *ypo,* under, + *physis,* growth]. Post. portion of the pituitary gland.

neuroid (nū′roid) [" + *eidos,* resemblance]. 1. Resembling nervous substance or nerves. 2. Neurapophysis, *q.v.*

neuroinduction (nū″rō-ĭn-dŭk′shŭn) [" + L. *in,* into, + *ductus,* leading]. Suggestion.

neuroinidia (nū″rō-ĭn-id′ĭ-ă) [" + L. *in,* not, + *nidus,* nest]. Insufficient nutrition of nerve cells.

neuroinoma (nū″rō-ĭn-ō′mă) [" + *is, in-,* fiber, + *-ōma,* tumor]. A connective tissue tumor arising from a nerve fiber. SYN: *neurofibroma.*

neuroinomato′sis [" + " + " + *-ōsis,* increase]. Multiple tumors of the peripheral nerves, either fibromas or neuromas. SYN: *neurofibromatosis.*

neurokeratin (nū″rō-ker′ă-tĭn) [G. *neuron,* sinew, + *keras, kerat-,* horn]. The variety of keratin found in myelinated nerve fibers.

neurokinet (nū-rō-kin′ĕt) [" + *kinein,* to move]. An apparatus for neural stimulation by mechanical percussion.

neurokyme (nū′rō-kīm) [" + *kyma,* wave]. Energy of the nerve impulse and of all nervous activity.

neurolabyrinthitis (nū″rō-lăb-ĭr-ĭn-thī′tĭs) [" + *labyrinthos,* a maze, + *-itis,* inflammation]. Inflammation of the nerves of the labyrinth.

neurolemma (nū″rō-lem′ă) [" + *lemma,* a rind]. 1. Sheath of a nerve fiber. 2. Rarely used name for retina.

neurologic, neurological (nū-rō-loj′ĭk, -ĭ-kal) [" + *logos,* study]. Pert. to the study of nervous diseases.

neurologist (nū-rol′ō-jĭst) [" + *logos,* study]. A specialist in diseases of nervous system.

neurology (nū-rol′ō-jĭ) [G. *neuron,* sinew, + *logos,* study]. The branch of medicine that deals with the nervous system and its diseases.

neurolymph (nū′rō-lĭmf) [" + L. *lympha,* fluid]. The cerebrospinal fluid.

neurolysin (nū-rol′ĭs-ĭn) [" + *lysis,* destruction]. A substance which destroys nerve cells.

neurolysis (nū-rol′ĭs-ĭs) [" + *lysis,* a loosening; a degeneration]. 1. Exhaustion of a nerve or nerves from prolonged stimulation. 2. Stretching of a nerve to relieve tension. 3. Loosening of adhesions surrounding a nerve. 4. Disintegration of nerve tissue.

neurolytic (nū-rō-lit′ĭk) [" + *lysis,* destruction]. Concerning neurolysis.

neuroma (nū-rō′mă) [G. *neuron,* sinew, + *-ōma,* tumor]. 1. A tumor of a nerve fiber. 2. A tumor composed of ganglion cells, or cells of nervous origin.

n., amputation. N. occurring on a stump after amputation.

n., amyelinic. N. of a nerve fiber that has no myelin sheath.

n. cutis. N. of the derma.

n., cystic. N. with cystic formations.

n., false. Tumor arising from connective tissue of nerves, including the myelin sheath. SYN: *neurofibroma, pseudoneuroma.*

n., ganglionated. N. composed of nerve cells.

n., multiple. Condition in which many neuromas develop in the body. SYN: *neuromatosis.*

n., myelinic. N. composed of medullated nerve fibers.

n., plexiform. Congenital n. involving all branches of a nerve. Usually found around head and are painless.

n. telangiectodes. N. with an abundance of blood vessels contained within it.

n., traumatic. N. occurring in wounds or on an amputation stump.

n., true. Tumor of nerve fibers or cells of nervous origin. SYN: *neuroma.* SEE: *ganglioneuroma.*

neuromalacia (nū″rō-mal-a′sĭ-ă) [" + *malakia,* softening]. Pathological softening of neural tissue.

neuromast (nū′rō-măst) [" + *mastos,* hill]. A clump of neuroepithelium composing a sense organ. SYN: *nerve hillock.*

neuromatosis (nū-rō″mă-tō′sĭs) [" + *-ōma,* tumor, + *ōsis,* increase]. Multiple neuromas occurring in the body.

neuromatous (nū-rō′mă-tŭs) [" + *-ōma,* tumor]. Rel. to a neuroma.

neuromechanism (nū″rō-měk′ăn-ĭzm) [" + *mēchanē,* machine]. The neural structure controlling organic and systemic function.

neuromelitococcosis (nū″rō-mel″ĭ-tō-kok-kō′sĭs) [" + *meli, melit-,* honey, + *kokkos,* berry, + *-ōsis,* increase]. Undulant fever with pronounced neural disturbances.

neuromere (nū′rō-mēr) [G. *neuron,* sinew, + *meros,* part]. 1. Embryonic segment from which a portion of the nervous system arises. 2. A segment of the cerebrospinal nervous system.

neuromimesis (nū-rō-mĭm-ē′sĭs) [" + *mimēsis,* imitation]. Resemblance of hysteria to organic disease.

neuromittor (nū-rō-mit′or) [" + L. *mittor,* one who sends]. Nerve terminus which sends a stimulus to the neuroceptor of an adjacent nerve.

neuromotor (nū-rō-mō′tor) [" + L. *motor,* a mover]. Pert. to efferent nerve impulses.

neuromuscular (nū″rō-mus′kū-lăr) [" + L. *musculus,* a muscle]. Concerning both nerves and muscles.

neuromyelitis (nū″rō-mī-ĕl-ī′tĭs) [" + *myelos,* marrow, + *-itis,* inflammation]. Inflamed condition of spinal neural and medullary substance.

neuromyon (nū-rō-mī′ŏn) [" + *mys, myo,-* muscle]. The nerve elements of a muscle.

neuromyositis (nū″rō-mī″ō-sī′tĭs) [" + " + *-itis,* inflammation]. Inflammation of both nerves and muscles of a part.

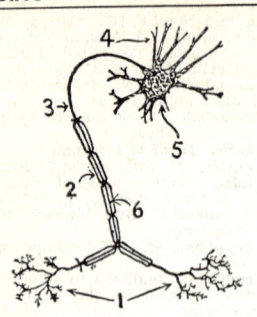

NEURON.
1. Terminal branches. 2. Neurilemma.
3. Axon. 4. Dendrites. 5. Cell body.
6. Myelin sheath.

neuron(e (nū'rŏn) [G. *neuron*, sinew]. Basic unit of nervous tissue, nerve cell and its processes, the dendrite and the axon. SYN: *nerve cell*.
RS: *amphicyte, nerve, receptor, synapse*.

n., central. Connecting or internuncial neuron interposed between other neurons.

neuronatrophy (nū-rŏn-at′rō-fī) [" + *atrophia*, a wasting]. Any nervous disease caused by sclerosing of the neurons.

neuronephric (nū″rō-něf′rĭk) [" + *nephros*, kidney]. Concerning the neural and renal systems.

neuroneuronitis (nū″rō-nū″rŏn-ī′tĭs) [" + *neuron*, sinew, + *-itis*, inflammation]. Inflammation of both nerve cells and roots of the spinal cord. SYN: *neuronitis*.

neuron′ic [G. *neuron*, sinew]. Concerning a nerve cell.

neuronitis (nū-rŏn-ī′tĭs) [" + *-itis*, inflammation]. Inflammation, or degenerative inflammation of nerve cells.

neuronophage (nū-ron′ō-fāj) [" + *phagein*, to eat]. A phagocyte which eats neurons.

neuronophagia, neuronophagy (nū-ron-ō-fā′jĭ-ă, -of′ă-jĭ) [" + " + *phagein*, to eat]. Destruction of nerve cells by phagocytes.

neuronosis (nū″rō-nō′sĭs) [" + *nosos*, disease]. Any disease of neural origin.

neuronyxis (nū-rō-nĭks′ĭs) [" + *nyxis*, a piercing]. Neural puncture.

neuroparalysis (nū″rō-pă-ral′ĭs-ĭs) [" + *para*, beside, + *lyein*, to loosen]. Paralysis due to a nervous disorder.

neuropath (nū′rō-păth) [G. *neuron*, nerve, + *pathos*, disease]. One predisposed to neural disorders.

neuropathic (nū-rō-păth′ĭk) [" + *pathos*, disease]. Rel. to neural disorders.

neuropathogenesis (nū″rō-păth″ō-jĕn′ĕ-sĭs) [" + " + *genesis*, production]. Development of a neural disease.

neuropathology (nū″rō-pă-thol′ō-jĭ) [" + " + *logos*, study]. The study of the diseases of the nervous system and the structural and functional changes occurring in them.

The diseases are divided into congenital defects in development, those in which an inherent tendency to degeneracy reveals itself only after a period of time, and finally those in which destructive influences act upon a brain initially normal. The latter group are mainly inflammatory, toxic, traumatic, mechanical and neoplastic in type. Circulatory impairment, disuse and overactivity also contribute to the development of nervous diseases.

neuropathy (nū-rop′ă-thĭ) [" + *pathos*, disease]. Any disease of the nerves.

neurophage (nū′rō-fāj) [" + *phagein*, to eat]. A phagocyte that absorbs cells. SYN: *neuronophage*.

neurophonia (nū″rō-fō′nĭ-ă) [" + *phōnē*, voice]. A tic or spasm of muscles of speech resulting in an involuntary cry or sound.

neurophthisis (nū-rof′thĭ-sĭs) [" + *phthisis*, wasting]. Atrophy of nerve tissue.

neurophysiology (nū″rō-fĭz-ĭ-ol′ō-jĭ) [" + *physis*, growth, + *logos*, study]. Physiology of the nervous structure of the body.

neuropil, neuropile, neuropilem (nū′rō-pĭl, -pīl, nū″rō-pī′lěm) [G. *neuron*, sinew, + *pilos*, felt]. 1. Network of unmyelinated fibrils into which nerve processes of central nervous system divide. 2. Terminus of a nerve fiber.

neuroplasm (nū′rō-plăzm) [" + *plasmos*, a thing formed]. Protoplasmic content of a neuron.

neuroplasmic (nū″rō-plaz′mĭk) [" + *plasmos*, a thing formed]. Concerning the protoplasm of a neuron.

neuroplasty (nū″rō-plăs-tĭ) [" + *plassein*, to form]. Reparative surgery of the nerves.

neuroplexus (nū″rō-plěks′ŭs) [" + L. *plexus*, a braid]. An intertwined bundle of nerves.

neuropodium (nū″rō-pō′dĭ-ŭm) [" + *pous, pod-*, foot]. The delicate terminal fibril of an axis cylinder process.

neuropore (nū′rō-pōr) [" + *poros*, an opening]. Embryonic opening from neural canal to exterior.

neuropsychiatry (nū″rō-sī-kī′ă-trī) [" + *psychē*, mind, + *iatreia*, healing]. Study and treatment of nervous and mental diseases.

neuropsychic (nū″rō-sī′kĭk) [" + *psychē*, mind]. Pert. to neural phenomena from a psychic point of view.

neuropsychology (nū″rō-sī-kol′ō-jĭ) [G. *neuron*, sinew, + *psychē*, mind, + *logos*, study]. The science of connection of neurological and psychological facts.

neuropsychopathy (nū″rō-sī-kop′ăth-ĭ) [" + " + *pathos*, disease]. A neurosis in combination with a mental disease.

neuropsychosis (nū-rō-sī-kō′sĭs) [" + " + *-ōsis*, condition]. Neurosis complicated by mental symptoms.

neuropyra (nū-rō-pī′ră) [" + *pyr*, fire]. Fever induced or accompanied by nervousness.

neuropyretic (nū″rō-pī-ret′ĭk) [" + *pyretos*, fever]. Rel. to nervous fever.

neurorecidive (nū″rō-rěs′ĭ-dĭv) [" + L. *recidere*, to fall back]. Nervous symptoms in syphilis following a salvarsan injection. SYN: *neurorelapse*.

neurorecurrence (nū″rō-rē-kŭr′ănz) [" + L. *rē*, back, + *currere*, to run]. Nervous manifestation as a sequel to salvarsan injection. SYN: *neurorelapse*.

neurorelapse (nū″rō-rē-lăps′) [G. *neuron*, sinew, + L. *relapsus*, fallen back]. Nervous symptoms in syphilis subsequent to an injection of salvarsan. SYN: *neurorecidive, neurorecurrence*.

neuroretinitis (nū″rō-rět″ĭn-ī′tĭs) [" + L. *rētē*, net, + G. *-itis*, inflammation]. Inflamed condition of optic nerve and retina.

neurorrhaphy (nū-ror′ă-fī) [" + *raphē*, a sewing]. Suturing of ends of a severed nerve.

Neurorrhyctes hydrophobiae (nū″rō-rĭk′-tēs hī-drō-fō′bĭ-ē) [" + *oryktēs*, a digger, + *ydōr*, water, + *phobos*, fear]. Supposed microörganisms of rabies. SYN: *Negri bodies*.

neurosarcokleisis (nū″rō-săr″kō-klī′sĭs) [" + *sarx, sark-,* flesh, + *kleisis,* closure]. Operation for relief of neuralgia by resection of a wall of the osseous canal carrying a nerve and transplanting the nerve to soft tissues.

neurosarcoma (nū″rō-săr-kō′mă) [" + " + *-ōma,* tumor]. A sarcoma containing neuromatous components.

neurosclerosis (nū″rō-sklĕ-rō′sĭs) [" + *sklērōsis,* a hardening]. Hardening of nervous tissue.

neurosensory (nū″rō-sĕn′sō-rī) [" + L. *sensōrius,* pert. to a sensation]. Concerning a sensory nerve.

neurosis (nū-rō′sĭs) [G. *neuron,* sinew, + *-ōsis,* disease]. Functional disorder of the nervous system without demonstrable physical lesion.

Included among the neuroses are neurasthenia, psychasthenia, anxiety neurosis and hysteria, *q.v.* In general, they manifest themselves as bodily disturbances, without structural abnormality, or as mental disturbances quite distinct from the psychoses. The personality as such is not essentially changed; it mirrors, and reacts to reality as does the normal individual. Conduct may be inefficient and inadequate but it is not antisocial. Emotional reaction may be intensified or dulled but not sufficiently to change the individual basically. Feelings, ideas, failings are not projected or explained by external forces. Language is not distorted though enunciatory difficulties are rather frequent and aphonia is not uncommon.

The neurotic does not violate his ethical standards in the presence of clear consciousness, though during a period of hysterical amnesia he may not escape from a situation that conscious duty would avoid. He has good insight but may falsely consider his symptoms the onset or evidence of insanity. SEE: *pruritus, psychoneurosis, psychosis.*

n., accident. A nervous disorder caused by injury or an accident.

n., anxiety. N. in which fear or apprehension is the essential symptom. SEE: *anxiety n.*

n., association. N. in which association of ideas causes mental repetition of an experience.

n., compensation. N. developing after an accident in people who think they can obtain compensation by being ill.

n., compulsion. N. marked by overpowering impulse to perform acts against the will.

n., expectation. Condition in which anticipation of an occurrence produces nervous symptoms.

n., fatigue. Neurasthenia, *q.v.*

n., obsessional. Uncontrollable obsessions dominating the victim's behavior; a psychoneurosis.

n., occupational, n., professional. N. in a group of muscles caused by constant repetition of an act, as in playing the piano.

n., sexual. Disorder of sex function, as impotence.

n., traumatic. SEE: *accident n.*

n., war. Disorder with or without physical cause brought on by conditions of war. SYN: *shellshock.*

neuroskeleton (nū″rō-skĕl′ĕt-ŏn) [G. *neuron,* sinew, + *skeleton,* skeleton]. The true skeleton or internal bony framework which aids in protection of parts of central nervous system. SYN: *endoskeleton.*

neurosome (nū′rō-sōm) [" + *sōma,* body]. 1. The cell body of a neuron. 2. One of the tiny fragments in the ground substance of the nerve cell protoplasm.

neurospasm (nū′rō-spăzm) [" + *spasmos,* spasm]. Spasmodic muscular twitching due to a nervous disorder.

neurosplanchnic (nū-rō-splănk′nĭk) [" + *splagchna,* viscera]. Concerning the cerebrospinal and sympathetic nervous systems.

neurospongioma (nū″rō-spŭn-jĭ-ō′mă) [" + *spoggos,* sponge, + *-ōma,* tumor]. A tumor composed of neurogliar tissue. SYN: *neuroglioma.*

neurospongium (nū″rō-spŭn′jĭ-ŭm) [" + *spoggos,* sponge]. 1. A meshwork of nerve fibrils in the cytoplasm of a neuron. 2. The reticular layer of the retina.

neurosthenia (nū″rō-sthē′nĭ-ă) [" + *sthenos,* strength]. Abnormal response of nerves to stimuli.

neurosurgery (nū″rō-sur′jĕ-rĭ) [G. *neuron,* sinew, + L. *chirurgia,* from G. *cheir,* hand, + *ergon,* work]. Surgery of the nerves and nerve structure.

neurosuture (nū″rō-sū′chŭr) [" + L. *sutura,* a stitch]. Stitching of ends of a cut nerve. SYN: *neurorrhaphy.*

neurosyphilis (nū″rō-sĭf′ĭ-lĭs) [" + *syphilis*]. Syphilis affecting the nervous structures. SEE: *dementia paralytica.*

neurotabes (nū″rō-ta′bēz) [" + L. *tabescere,* to waste]. Multiple neuritis complicated by ataxic symptoms.

neurotagma (nū-rō-tag′mă) [" + *tagma,* arrangement]. Linear arrangement of the neuron's structural elements.

neurotension (nū″rō-tĕn′shŭn) [" + L. *tensiō,* a stretching]. Operative stretching of a nerve. SYN: *neurectasis.*

neurothecitis (nū″rō-the-sī′tĭs) [" + *thēkē,* sheath, + *-ītis,* inflammation]. Inflamed condition of a nerve sheath.

neurotherapeutics (nū″rō-thĕr-ă-pū′tĭks) [" + *therapeutikē,* treatment]. Treatment of disorders of the nervous system. SYN: *neurotherapy.*

neurotherapy (nū-rō-ther′ă-pĭ) [" + *therapeia,* treatment]. Treatment of neural disorders. SEE: *psychotherapy.*

neurothlipsis (nū″rō-thlĭp′sĭs) [" + *thlipsis,* pressure]. Irritation or pressure on a nerve.

neurotic (nū-rot′ĭk) [G. *neuron,* sinew]. 1. One suffering from instability of the nervous system. 2. Nervous or pert. to a neurosis. 3. A nervine or sedative.

neuroticism (nū-rŏt′ĭ-sĭzm) [" + *ismos,* state of]. A condition or trait of neurosis.

neurotization (nū-rot-ĭ-zā′shŭn) [G. *neuron,* sinew]. 1. Acquisition of nervous substance. 2. Renewal of a nerve after division. 3. Surgical introduction of a nerve into a paralyzed muscle.

neurotology (nū″rō-tol′ō-jĭ) [" + *ous, ot-,* ear, + *logos,* study]. The study of ear lesions in combination with neural complications.

neurotome (nū′rō-tōm) [" + *tomē,* a slice]. 1. Fine knife used in the division of a nerve. 2. An embryonic segment from which arises a part of the nervous system.

neurotomy (nū-rot′ō-mĭ) [" + *tomē,* an incision]. Division or dissection of a nerve.

neurotonia (nū″rō-tō′nĭ-ă) [″ + *tonos*, tone]. Nerve stretching.

neurotonic (nū″rō-ton′ĭk) [″ + *tonos*, tension]. 1. Concerning neural stretching. 2. Stimulating a disordered nervous system.

neurotony (nū-rot′ō-nĭ) [G. *neuron*, sinew, + *tonos*, a stretching]. Nerve stretching.

neurotoxic (nū″rō-toks′ĭk) [″ + *toxikon*, poison]. Poisonous to the nerve cells.

neurotoxin (nū″rō-toks′ĭn) [″ + *toxikon*, poison]. A toxin that attacks nerve cells. SYN: *neurolysin*.

neurotrauma (nū-rō-traw′mă) [″ + *trauma*, wound]. Nerve lesion. SYN: *neurotrosis*.

neurotripsy (nū′rō-trip-sĭ) [″ + *tripsis*, a rubbing]. Surgical crushing of a nerve.

neurotrophasthenia (nū″rō-trof-ăs-thē′nĭ-ă) [″ + *trophē*, nourishment, + *astheneia*, weakness]. Malnutrition of the nervous system.

neurotrophy (nū-rot′rō-fĭ) [″ + *trophē*, nourishment]. Nutrition of the nerves.

neurotropic (nū″rō-trop′ĭk) [″ + *tropos*, a turning]. 1. Pert. to, or having a chemical affinity for nervous tissue. 2. Pert. to neurotropism.

neurotropism (nū-rot′rō-pĭzm) [″ + ″ + *ismos*, condition]. Attraction which nutritive elements, basic dyes, and microörganisms have for nervous tissue.

neurotrosis (nū″rō-trō′sĭs) [″ + *trōsis*, a wound]. A lesion of a nerve. SYN: *neurotrauma*.

neurovaccine (nū″rō-văk′sēn) [″ + L. *vaccinus*, pert. to a cow]. A standardized vaccine virus of specific strength secured by cultivation in a rabbit's brain.

neurovaricosis (nū″rō-văr-ĭ-kō′sĭs) [″ + L. *varicōsus*, pert. to a swollen vein]. Multiple swellings along the pathway of a nerve.

neurovascular (nū″rō-văs′kū-lăr) [″ + L. *vasculus*, a small vessel]. Concerning both the nervous and vascular systems.

neurovegetative (nū″rō-věj′ē-tā-tĭv) [″ + L. *vegetāre*, to arouse]. Noting the vegetative nervous system.

neutral (nū′trăl) [L. *neuter*, neither]. 1. Neither alkaline nor acid. 2. Indifferent; having no positive properties.

n. diet. One in which total basic ash is equal to or exceeded by the total acid ash. A slight excess of acids is usually planned. Protein allowance, 0.65-1 Gm. per Kg. ideal body weight. All food prepared and served without salt.

n. principle. A proximate principle of neutral reaction, not otherwise classified. Ex: *aloin, elaterin*.

neutralization (nū-tral-ĭ-zā′shŭn) [L. *neuter*, from *ne*, not, + *uter*, either, one of two]. 1. The opposing of one force or condition with an opposite force or condition to such degree as to cause counteraction that permits neither to dominate. 2. The reaction in which the hydrogen ion of an acid and the hydroxyl ion of a base unite to form water, the other producing a salt.

neutralize (nū′tral-īz) [L. *neuter*, from *ne*, not, + *uter*, either, one of two]. 1. To counteract. 2. CHEM: To destroy peculiar properties of or effect of; to make inert.

neutroclusion (nū″trō-klū′zhŭn) [″ + *occlusiō*, a closing before]. State in which the anteroposterior occlusal positions of the teeth or the mesiodistal positions are normal, but malocclusion of the other positions exists.

neutron (nū′trŏn) [L. *neuter*, neither]. Elementary particle with approximately the mass of a hydrogen atom, but without any electric charge. [nucleus.
It is a constituent of the atomic

neutropenia (nū-trō-pē′nĭ-ă) [″ + G. *penia*, lack]. Abnormally small number of neutrophil cells in the peripheral blood stream.

neutrophil(e (nū′trō-fĭl, -fīl) [″ + G. *philein*, to love]. 1. Staining easily with neutral dyes. 2. A leukocyte which stains easily with neutral dyes. SEE: *polymorphonuclear leukocyte*.

neutrophilia (nū″trō-fĭl′ĭ-ă) [″ + G. *philein*, to love]. Increase in the number of neutrophile leukocytes.

neutrophilic, neutrophilous (nū-trō-fĭl′ĭk, -trof′ĭ-lŭs) [″ + G. *philein*, to love]. Staining readily with neutral dyes. SYN: *neutrophil*.

neutrotaxis (nū″trō-taks′ĭs) [″ + G. *taxis*, arrangement]. The attracting or repelling power of neutrophil leukocytes.

nevoid (nē′voyd) [L. *naevus*, birthmark, + G. *eidos*, form]. Resembling a nevus.

n. elephantiasis. Enlarged scrotum due to distention of lymphatics and hyperplasia of tissues. SYN: *lymph scrotum*.

nevolipoma (nē-vō-lip-ō′mă) [″ + G. *lipos*, fat, + *-ōma*, tumor]. Rare lipoma containing numerous blood vessels, probably a degenerated nevus.

nevose (nē′vōs) [L. *naevus*, birthmark]. Spotted or marked with nevi. SEE: *nevus*.

nevus (nē′vŭs) [L. *naevus*, birthmark]. 1. A congenital discoloration of a circumscribed area of the skin due to pigmentation. SYN: *birthmark, mole*. 2. Circumscribed vascular tumor of the skin, usually congenital, due to hyperplasia of the blood vessels. SEE: *angioma*.

n. angiectodes. SEE: *n. vascularis*.

n. angiomatodes. Extensive diffuse angiomatous condition of the subcutaneous tissues.

n. araneus. Acquired or congenital dilatation of the capillaries, marked by red lines radiating from a central red dot. SYN: *spider n*.

n., capillary. N. of dilated capillary vessels, elevated above the skin. TREATMENT: Ligature, excision.

n., cutaneous. N. formation on the skin.

n. flammeus. Reddish discoloration of the face or neck, usually not elevated above the skin. A serious deformity due to large size and color. TREATMENT: Freezing, cautery, escharotics.

n. lipomatodes. Fatty connective tissue tumor, probably a degenerated nevus, containing numerous blood vessels. TREATMENT: Excision, caustics, electrolysis. SYN: *nevolipoma*.

n. maternus. A birthmark.

n. pigmentosus. Congenital pigment spot varying in color from light yellow to blackish. SYM: Color as stated, variable in size, single or multiple, with many names according to cutaneous changes. PROG: Potentially malignant. TREATMENT: Small ones destroyed by electrolysis or carbon dioxide snow. Excision in presence of inflammation. X-rays, radium and electrodesiccation.

n. pilosus. A n. covered with hair.

n., spider. SEE: *n. araneus*.

n. spilus. Pigmented n. with smooth surface.

n., strawberry. SEE: *n. vascularis*.

n., telangiectatic. N. containing dilated capillaries.

n. vascularis, n. vasculosus. N. in which superficial blood vessels are enlarged.

They are usually congenital and of variable size and shape, slightly elevated, reddish or purplish, on face, head, neck and arms, though no region is exempt; permanent, or disappearing spontaneously, leaving white or pigmented atrophic scars.

TREATMENT: Puncture followed by collodion, electrolysis (superficial growths), surgery for deep-seated, x-rays cautiously employed.

SYN: *strawberry n.*

n. venosus, n. venous. N. formed of dilated venules.

n. verrucosus. N. with a raised wart-like surface.

new growth. Any morbid new formation, as a tumor. SYN: *neoplasm.*

nexus (neks'us) [L. *nectere,* to bind]. A connection or link; a binding together.

N. F. Abbr. for *National Formulary.*

NH₃. Ammonia.

NH₄Cl. Ammonium chloride.

Ni. Symb. for nickel. [*acid.*

niacin (nī'ă-sĭn). A synonym for *nicotinic*

n. amide. A synonym for *nicotinamide.*

niccolum (nĭk'ō-lŭm) [L.]. Nickel, *q.v.*

nickel (nĭk'el) [L. *niccolum*]. SYMB: Ni. Metallic element with an at. wt. of 58.6, salts of which are used medicinally.

n. arc. One that emits strongly at 230 and esp. at 350 millimicrons.

Nicolaier's bacillus (nĭk-ō-lī'er). The *Bacillus tetani.*

Nicolas-Favre disease (nē″kō-lă făvr'). Venereal disease marked by involvement of inguinal lymph glands with an exuding lesion. SYN: *Frei's disease, lymphogranuloma venerea.* [found in the blood.

Nicol'lia. A genus of parasitic protozoa

nicotinamide (nĭk″ō-tĭn'ă-mīd). Member of vitamin-B complex, used in management or prevention of pellagra. The peripheral flush that often accompanies therapy with nicotinic acid, *q.v.,* is avoided with nicotinamide. SYN: *niacinamide.*

nicotine (nĭk'ō-tēn, -tĭn). A poisonous alkaloid found in all parts of the tobacco plant, but esp. in the leaves.

When pure, it is a colorless oily fluid with little odor but a sharp, burning taste. On standing or in crude materials, it becomes deep brown with a characteristic smell.

POISONING: SYM: Hot, burning sensation in mouth, extending to stomach, followed by nausea, increased salivation, vomiting, diarrhea, restlessness, confusion and weakness. Convulsions may appear either locally or generally. Respiration and pulse very rapid.

F. A. TREATMENT: Wash out stomach and administer finely divided charcoal to absorb nicotine. Stimulants, massage, artificial respiration and inhalation of oxygen important adjuncts.

nicotinic acid (nĭk″ō-tĭn'ĭk). The antipellagra principle of vitamin-B complex.

USES: In pellagra, in cutaneous circulatory deficiency (frostbite, acne vulgaris), in trigeminal neuralgia, in multiple sclerosis, in certain cases of deafness, and in Ménière's syndrome.

DOSAGE: 50-500 mg. daily, in divided doses.

SYN: *niacin.*

nicotinism (nĭk'ō-tēn-ĭzm, -tĭn-ĭzm). Poisoning from excessive use of tobacco or nicotine.

nictitate (nĭk'tĭ-tāt) [L. *nictitāre,* to wink]. To wink.

nictitating (nĭk'tĭ-tāt-ĭng) [L. *nictitāre,* to wink]. Winking or blinking.

n. spasm. Clonic spasm of eyelid with continuous winking.

nictation, nictitation (nĭk-tā'shŭn, nĭk-tĭ-tā'shŭn) [L. *nictitāre,* to wink]. The act of involuntary winking due to a nervous disorder.

nidal (nī'dal) [L. *nidus,* nest]. Pert. to a nucleus or an implanted fertilized ovum.

nidation (nī-da'shŭn) [L. *nidus,* nest]. 1. Periodic intramenstrual preparation of endometrial epithelium. 2. Implantation of fertilized ovum in the uterine endometrium. 3. Formation of a colony or nest.

nidulus (nĭd'ū-lŭs) [L. *nidulus,* small nest]. Point of origin of a nerve.

nidus (nī'dŭs) [L. nest]. 1. A cluster; nest-like structure. 2. Focus of infection. 3. A nucleus or origin of a nerve.

n. avis. SEE: *n. hirundinis.*

n. hirundinis. Depression on each side of inf. surface of cerebellum in which is lodged the tonsil.

night blindness (nīt blĭnd'nĕs) [A.S. *neaht,* night, + *blind,* without sight]. Absence of or defective vision in the dark. SYN: *nyctalopia, nyctotyphlosis.*

Nightingale, Florence (nīt'ĭn-gāl). Originator of modern nursing.

N. oath or pledge. "I solemnly pledge myself before God and in the presence of this assembly to pass my life in purity and to practice my profession faithfully. I will abstain from whatever is deleterious and mischievous, and will not take or knowingly administer any harmful drug. I will do all in my power to elevate the standard of my profession, and I will hold in confidence all personal matters committed to my keeping, and all family affairs coming to my knowledge in the practice of my calling. With loyalty will I endeavor to aid the physician in his work and devote myself to the welfare of those committed to my care."

nightmare (nīt'măr) [" + *mara,* incubus]. A bad dream accompanied by great fear and a feeling of suffocation, once believed to be caused by a female monster or spirit that sat upon the dreamer. SYN: *oneirodynia.* SEE: *antephialtic.*

nightshade (nīt'shăd) [A.S. *nihtscada*]. Any of the species of *Solanum.* SEE: *atropine, belladonna.*

night sweat (nīt swĕt) [A.S. *neaht,* night, + *swat,* sweat]. Profuse sweating during sleep at night.

Often an early sign of disease with intermittent temperature. In children, it occurs in rickets, in debilitated states and in those with a tendency toward tuberculosis. Patient should be rubbed down, sponged, and changed into dry clothing.

night terrors (nīt tĕr'ĕrs) [" + L. *terror,* state of fear]. Form of nightmare in children causing them to awaken in terror, screaming.

Fear continues for a period after the return to consciousness. SYN: *pavor nocturnus.*

nightwalking (nīt'wauk'ĭng) [" + *wealcan,* to revolve]. State in which individual walks about habitually while sleeping. SYN: *somnambulism.*

nigra (nī'gră) [L. black]. Mass of gray matter bet. the dorsal and pedal parts of the crus cerebri. SYN: *substantia nigra.*

nigral (nī'grăl) [L. *niger,* black]. Rel. to the substantia nigra.

nigredo (nī-grē'dō) [L. blackness]. Blackness.
  n. cutis. N. of the skin. SYN: *melasma*.
  n. nativa. Natural dark dermal pigmentation.
nigrescence (nī-gres'ĕns) [" + *nigrescere*, to grow black]. The process of becoming black or the blackness produced.
nigricans (nī'grĭ-kăns) [L.]. Blackened.
nigri-, nigro- [L.]. Combining forms meaning *pert. to blackness*.
nigrismus (nī-grĭz'mŭs) [L.]. Black pigmentation. SYN: *melasma, nigredo*.
nigrities (nī-grĭsh'ĭ-ēz) [L. blackness]. Blackness; black pigmentation.
  n. linguae. A black pigmentation of the tongue. SYN: *glossophytia*.
nihilism (nī'ĭ-lĭzm) [L. *nihil*, nothing, + G. *ismos*, state of]. 1. Disbelief in beneficial properties of medicine. 2. PSY: A delusion that everything is unreal.
nikethamide (nī-keth'ă-mīd). The diethyl amide of nicotinic acid, *q.v.*
Nikolsky's sign (nī-kol'skĭ). Condition of the external layer of the skin in which it can be rubbed off by slight friction or injury.
ninth cranial nerve. Glossopharyngeal nerve. SEE: *Appendix, cranial nerves.*
  n.-day erythema. A nontoxic e. which sometimes appears on the 9th day in a course of medication.
niphablepsia (nĭf"ă-blĕp'sĭ-ă) [G. *nipha*, snow, + *ablepsia*, blindness]. Blindness caused by light glare on snow.
niphotyphlosis (nĭf"ō-tĭf-lō'sĭs) [" + *typhlosis*, blindness]. Snow blindness. SYN: *niphablepsia*.

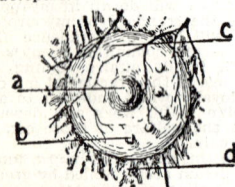

NIPPLE.
a. Nipple; b. Montgomery's follicles; c. primary areola; d. secondary areola.

nipple (nĭp'l) [earlier *neble, nible*, possibly diminutive from A.S. *neb*, a little protuberance]. 1. The protuberance in each breast from which, in the female, the lactiferous ducts discharge. SYN: *mammilla, papilla, teat.* 2. Artificial substitute for female n. to be used on a nursing bottle.
  The nipple contains erectile tissue and is surrounded by a pink or brownish area called the areola. It is supplied with a row of small sebaceous glands around its base called Montgomery's follicles, which secrete an oily substance to keep it supple.
  NP: During pregnancy, they should be washed well with soap and water and dried with a rough towel. Excessively dry nipples may be massaged with cold cream or lanolin. Cracked and sore nipples result from misuse of the nipple due to the baby's chewing.
  Retracted nipples are caused by deficiency of muscle tissue or flattening of the erectile tissue, and are lower than the surrounding area.
  RS: *acromastitis, halo, mammary, mammillation, Paget's disease of n., thelalgia, thelitis.*

  n. shield. Mechanical device to protect the nipple during lactation period.
nirvanin (nĭr-van'en). Colorless, soluble, crystalline local anesthetic, less toxic than cocaine.
Nissl's bodies or **granules** (nĭs'el). Granular bodies scattered throughout the cell body of a neuron or nerve cell, which stain with cytoplasm of the basic dyes and are supposed to represent a store of nervous energy.
  They appear as microscopic dots and they shift their location when the nerve cell has become fatigued. They are present in all stages of vital activity. When the arrangement of these bodies is altered, disease, senility and death ensue. The key to the preservation of life may be found in these granules.
  SYN: *chromophilic* or *tigroid bodies*.
  N.'s degeneration. Slow d. of a neuron following division of nerve fiber supplying it.
nisus (nī'sŭs) (pl. *nisŭs*) [L. effort]. 1. An effort or struggle. 2. The desire for coitus on the part of certain animals in the spring. 3. Contraction of the muscles of the abdomen and diaphragm in the expulsion of the feces or urine.
  n. formativus. The effort of fertilized ovum to take on the characteristics of the species from which it is derived.
nit (nĭt) [A.S. *hnitu*]. The egg of a louse or any other parasitic insect. SEE: *pediculosis*.
niter (nī'ter) [G. *nitron*, soda]. 1. Saltpeter, potassium nitrate. 2. A salt or ester of nitric acid.
  n., sweet spirit of. Spirit of nitrous ether; *spiritus aetheris nitrosi, U.S.P.*
niton (nī'tŏn). Inert gas in radium emanation. SYMB: Nt. AT. WT.: 222.4. SYM: *radon*.
nitrate (nī'trāt) [G. *nitron*, soda]. A salt of nitric acid.
ni'trated [G. *nitron*, soda]. Combined with nitric acid or a nitrate.
nitra'tion [G. *nitron*, soda]. Combination with nitric acid or a nitrate.
nitrato (nī-trā'tō). Combining form denoting presence of nitrate group; NO_3.
nitre (nī'tĕr) [G. *nitron*, soda]. 1. A salt or ester of nitric acid. 2. Potassium nitrate. SYN: *niter*.
nitremia (nī-trē'mĭ-ă) [G. *nitron*, soda, + *aima*, blood]. Abnormal quantity of nitrogen in the blood.
ni'tric acid. HNO_3. A colorless, corrosive, poisonous liquid in concentrated form, employed as a caustic and disinfectant in treatment of venereal ulcers, poisoned wounds, and esp. the bites of rabid animals. It is widely used in industries and in chemical laboratories.
  POISONING: SYM: Are essentially same as those produced by sulfuric acid. Pain, burning, vomiting, thirst and shock, except that stains become intensely yellow.
  TREATMENT: Dilute with large volumes of water. Neutralize with weak alkalies, as magnesia, soapsuds, baking soda and chalk. Follow by soothing drinks. SYN: *aqua fortis*.
  n. a., fuming. Combination of nitric acid which emits fumes of a choking nature. SEE: *fumes*.
nitrification (nī"trĭ-fĭ-ka'shun) [G. *nitron*, soda, + L. *facere*, to make]. Process brought about by bacteria, in which nitric acid and nitrates are liberated in the soil by oxidation of nitrogen in ammonium salts.
nitrifying (nī'trĭ-fī'ĭng) [" + L. *facere*, to make]. Liberating nitrous and nitric

pertension of 180 or above, hypotension of 80 or below, decompensated heart lesions, obesity, diabetes, dyspnea, alcoholism, or in advanced pulmonary tuberculosis.
HYPERANESTHESIA FROM: The patient should be given oxygen under pressure, the rectum should be dilated and respiratory stimulation administered. Carbon dioxide may also be given.
In labor it is given alone or with ether or ethylene.
SYN: *laughing gas.*
niveau diagno'sis (nē-vo') [Fr. level diagnosis]. Determination of the exact level of a lesion.
N. L. N. E. Abbr. *National League of Nursing Education.*
N. N. R. Abbr. for *New and Nonofficial Remedies*, the title of a book published by the American Medical Association, listing and describing the articles that stand accepted by the Council on Pharmacy and Chemistry of the A. M. A.
These include simple nonproprietary and nonofficial substances sufficiently important for inclusion, and simple pharmaceutical preparations which are believed to be useful to physicians.
No. Abbr. L. *numero*, to the number of.
N₂O. Nitrous oxide.
N₂O₃. Nitrogen trioxide.
N₂O₅. Nitrogen pentoxide.
noble cells. Those of the organs, muscles and nerves as differentiated from wandering and connective tissue cells.
Noble's enema. One dram of turpentine mixed well with glycerin, 2 ounces; mix 3 ounces of magnesium sulfate with 4 ounces of water, and pour the 2 mixtures together.
nociassociation (nō"sĭ-ă-sō'sĭ-ā'shŭn) [L. *nocere*, to hurt, + *association*]. Discharge of nervous energy as exhibited in form of shock, exhaustion, etc., following stimuli of the nature of trauma and operations.
nociceptive (nō"sĭ-sept'ĭv) [" + *ceptus*, receiving]. Having the ability to receive painful stimuli.
nociceptor (nō"sĭ-sĕp'tōr) [" + *ceptor*, a receiver]. A peripheral mechanism for reception of stimuli of pain.
nociinfluence (nō"sĭ-ĭn'flōō-ĕns) [" + *influens*, a flowing in]. Harmful or injurious influence.
nociperception (nō"sĭ-pĕr-sĕp'shŭn) [" + *perceptio*, apprehension]. The perception by the nerve centers of injurious influences or painful stimuli.
Noct. [L.]. Abbr. for *night.*
noctalbuminuria (nŏk"tăl-bū-mĭn-ū'rĭ-ă) [L. *nox, noct-*, night, + *albumen*, white of egg, + G. *ouron*, urine]. Excess of albumin voided in urine at night. SYN: *nyctalbuminuria.*
noctambulism (nŏk-tăm'bū-lĭzm) [" + *ambulāre*, to walk, + G. *ismos*, state of]. Sleep walking. SYN: *somnambulism.*
noctiphobia (nŏk"tĭ-fō'bĭ-ă) [" + G. *phobos*, fear]. Fear of the night and darkness. SYN: *nyctophobia.*
nocturia (nŏk-tū'rĭ-ă) [" + G. *ouron*, urine]. Urination, esp. excessive, during the night. SYN: *nycturia.* SEE: *enuresis.*
noctur'nal [L. *nocturnus*, at night]. Pert. to or occurring in the night. OPP: *diurnal.* SEE: *"nyct-" words.*
n. enuresis.* Urinary incontinence during sleep at night. SYN: *bedwetting.*
nocuity (nŏk-ū'ĭt-ĭ) [L. *nocere*, to harm]. Injuriousness; harmfulness.

nodal (nō'dăl) [L. *nodus*, knot]. Pert. to a protuberance.
n. points. One of 2 points situated on axis of a lens that any incident ray sent through 1 will produce a parallel emergent ray sent through the other.
n. rhythm. Cardiac rhythm with origin at auriculoventricular node.
nodding (nŏd'ĭng) [origin uncertain]. Quick inclination of the head downward. SYN: *nutation.*
n. spasm. Nodding of the head due to spasm of the sternomastoid muscles. SYN: *salaam convulsion.*
node (nōd) [L. *nodus*, knot]. A knot, knob, protuberance or swelling.
n., auriculoventricular. Commencement of bundle of His in right auricle of heart.
n's., Bouchard's. N's. on 2nd joints of the fingers in gastric dilatation.
n's., Féréol's. N's that are subcutaneous and seen in acute rheumatism.
n's., gouty. N's. seen in gout.
n's., Haygarth's. Swelling of joints in arthritis deformans.
n's., Heberden's. N. on fingers seen in hypertrophic arthritis.
n's., Hensen's. Cell proliferation in the impregnated ovum, the beginning of the primitive streak. [node.
n., Keith and Flack's. Sinoauricular
n., lymph. Mass of lymphoid tissue along the course of lymphatic vessels.
n's., Meynet's. Those in capsules of joints and tendons in rheumatism.
n's., Parrot's. Osteophytes around ant. fontanel seen in hereditary syphilis.
n. piedric. Node on the hair shaft seen in piedra.*
n's. of Ranvier. Round constrictions of the myelinated nerve fibers.
n's., Schmidt's. The medullated interannular segments of a nerve fiber.
n., singer's. Trachoma of vocal cords.
n., sinoauricular. One at entrance of sup. vena cava into right auricle where cardiac rhythm originates. SYN: *pacemaker.*
n's., solitary lymph. Small lymph nodes over entire mucous membrane of the intestines.
n., syphilitic. Circumscribed swelling at end of long bones due to congenital syphilis. Sensitive and painful during inflammation, esp. at night. SEE: *Parrot's n.*
nodose (nō'dōs) [L. *nodōsus*, knotted]. Swollen or knotlike at intervals; marked by nodes or projections.
nodosity (nō-dŏs'ĭ-tĭ) [L. *nodositās*, a knot]. 1. A protuberance or knot. 2. Condition of having nodes.
nodular (nŏd'ū-lăr) [L. *nodulus*, a little knot]. Containing or resembling nodules.
nodule (nŏd'ūl) [L. *nodulus*, a small knot]. 1. A small node. 2. Tiny protuberance on inferior cerebellar vermiform process at its ant. extremity. SEE: *chalarosis, cladosporiosis.*
n., Albini's. N's. on free edges of auriculoventricular valves in infants.
n's., apple jelly. Elevations on leprous ulcers. They are of reddish color.
n's., Arantius'. Central fibrous tubercles in segments of semilunar valves. SYN: *corpora Arantii.*
n's., Aschoff's. Those in myocardium, seen in rheumatism.
n's., Bianchi's. SEE: *Arantius' n's.*
n's., Bouchard's. N's. on finger joints in gastric dilatation.
n's., endolymphangeal. Small ones

acid from ammonium salts; said of bacteria.

n. bacteria. Those which liberate nitric and nitrous acids from free nitrogen and ammonia.

nitrile (nī'trĭl, nī'trĭl). An organic compound in which the nitrogen of ammonia exists with all 3 of the hydrogen atoms displaced.

nitrogenization (nī"trō-jen-ĭz-ā'shŭn) [" + gennan, to produce]. The act of combining a substance with nitrogen or 1 of its compounds.

nitrogenous (nī-troj'ĕn-ŭs) [G. nitron, soda, + gennan, to produce]. Pert. to or containing nitrogen.

Foods which contain nitrogen are the proteins; those which do not contain

Nonprotein Nitrogenous Constituents of Whole Blood

Total nonprotein nitrogen	25-30 mg. per 100 cc.
Urea nitrogen	12-15 mg. per 100 cc.
Uric acid	2- 4 mg. per 100 cc.
Creatinine	1- 2 mg. per 100 cc.

nitrite (nī'trīt) [G. nitron, salt]. A salt of nitrous acid.

nitritoid (nī'trĭ-toyd) [" + eidos, resemblance]. Resembling a nitrite.

n. crisis. A syndrome resembling symptoms produced by the use of a nitrite, usually occurring after arsphenamine injection.

nitrituria (nī-trī-tū'rĭ-ă) [" + ouron, urine]. Nitrites or nitrates present in the urine.

nitro- [G.]. Combining form denoting (a) presence of niter in some form, (b) presence of the group NO_2.

nitrobacteria (nī"trō-băk-tē'rĭ-ă) [G. nitron, soda, + bakterion, little rod]. Bacteria in the soil which convert ammonium salts into nitric acid and nitrates by oxidation. SEE: nitrogen cycle.

nitrofurazone (nī-trō-fu'ră-zōn). A synthetic antibiotic for topical application in some skin diseases and in preparation for skin grafting. SYN: furacin.

nitrogen (nīt'rō-jen) [" + gennan, to produce]. SYMB: N. A colorless, odorless, tasteless, gaseous element occurring free in the atmosphere, forming 4/5 of its volume. Atomic weight, 14,008.

One of the important elements in all proteins, essential to plant and animal life for tissue building. Nitrogen is generally found in organic nature only in the form of compounds, as ammonia, nitrites, and nitrates which are transformed by plants into proteins, and, being consumed by animals, are converted into animal proteins of the blood and tissues, leaving the body in form of urea, creatinine and ammonia.

RS: azotation, azote, azotification, azotized.

n. cycle. The return of nitrogen from animal life to the soil, from which plants derive their supply, and in turn its return to animal life through plants taken as food.

n. equilibrium. Condition during which nitrogen excreted in the urine equals amt. taken in by the body in the food.

n. lag. Time required after a given protein is ingested until an equal amt. of nitrogen is excreted in the urine as that ingested.

n. mustard. A term embracing certain therapeutic mustard compounds. Three are in use: HN2, R48, and TEM (triethylene melamine). Used in Hodgkin's disease, lymphosarcoma, giant follicular lymphoblastoma, chronic lymphoid and myeloid leukemia, rheumatoid arthritis, and nephritis.

n., nonprotein. A nitrogenous component of the blood that is not a protein.

n. partition. Percentage of nitrogen in the urine shown by each nitrogenous constituent.

nitrogen are the fats and carbohydrates. The retention of nitrogenous products in the blood is marked in kidney diseases.

nitroglycerin (nī"trō-glĭs'ẽr-ĭn) [" + glycerin]. Any nitrate of glycerol, specifically the trinitrate, a heavy, oily, explosive, colorless liquid obtained by treating glycerol with nitric and sulfuric acids.

USES: Explosive constituent of dynamite and in medicine it has the action of nitrites and is a vasodilator.

nitromuriatic acid (nī"trō-mū-rĭ-at'ĭk) [" + L. muriaticus, briny]. A mixture of 1 part nitric and 3 parts hydrochloric acid used in commercial industries because it dissolves all the metals including platinum and gold.

POISONING: SYM: Same as those of nitric acid poisoning. TREATMENT: Same. SYN: aqua regia.

nitron (nī'tron) [G. soda]. Molecular weight of a radium emanation.

nitrous (nī'trŭs) [G. nitron, soda]. Containing nitrogen in its lowest valency.

n. oxide. N_2O. Colorless, sweet-tasting gas with pleasing smell causing temporary general anesthesia when inhaled.

It is usually used in dentistry and minor surgery and before ether or chloroform.

It is not toxic or inflammable. It is given in a mixture of 90% nitrous oxide gas and 10% oxygen. If used with ether it may be inflammable. The patient may easily be asphyxiated if it is not administered properly.

SIGNS: Deep signs of nitrous oxide anesthesia are a slight increase in respirations, some dyspnea, cyanosis becomes deeper, eyeballs are fixed, either upward or downward. There is muscular rigidity, cyanosis increases to a grayish pallor, pupils become fixed in a dilated form, and respirations become paralyzed.

ACTION: Slightly stimulating to cardiac and respiratory systems; lowers body temperature, raises blood pressure, and has no irritating effects on the glands or kidneys. It has very little effect on body chemistry. Nitrous oxide is a favorable anesthetic when complete relaxation is not required. Gas anesthesia is never induced for brain surgery. Nitrous oxide and oxygen are always safe when properly used in a mixture, but nitrous oxide is dangerous when used without oxygen. Should never be given with less than 1/6 part of oxygen or not over 1/15 of oxygen to produce an even anesthesia.

CONTRAINDICATIONS: Not to be given in advanced conditions of anemia, in hy-

within lymphatic vessels formed by adenoid tissue.
   n's., epicardial. Those over epicardial vessels.
   n's., Gamna. Yellowish-brown ones in the spleen in certain enlargements. SYN: *tabac n's.*
   n's., Leishman's. Pinkish ones seen in certain types of Oriental sore.
   n's., lymph. L. glands found throughout the lymphatics.
   n's., lymphatic, lymphoid. Adenoid tissue localized in masses of nucleated corpuscles.
   n's., Morgagni. SEE: *n's. of Arantius.*
   n's., tabac. SEE: *Gamna n's.*
nodulus (nod′ū-lŭs) (pl. *noduli*) [L.]. Nodule.
   n. lymphatici aggregati. BNA. Lymphoid tissue nodules on mucosa of small intestines. SYN: *Peyer's patches.*
nodus (nō′dŭs) [L.]. Node.
noematachograph (nō-ē″mă-tak′ō-grăf) [G. *noēma*, understanding, + *tachus*, swift, + *graphein*, to write]. Device for recording time taken in mental activity.
noematachometer (nō-ē″mă-tak-om′ĕt-ēr) [″ + ″ + *metron*, measure]. Device for measurement of the time taken in a simple perception. SYN: *noematachograph.*
Noguchi's test (no-goo′tshe). 1. Skin test for syphilis. A few drops of luetin are injected beneath the skin. A positive result appears within 1 day, increases in size, and lasts several days. This test is more constant in tertiary syphilis and in latent forms than the Wassermann reaction.
   2. A modified Wassermann test for syphilis. Extracts of animal heart muscle, as antigen, human corpuscles, complement serum from guinea pigs and hemolytic amboceptor from rabbits are materials used in it. Results are based on amt. of inhibition of hemolysis.
   3. A test for general paresis as shown by the globulin content of spinal fluid when mixed with butyric acid and normal sodium hydroxide solution.
noise (noyz) [O.Fr. *noise*, strife, brawl; possibly derived from G. *nausea*, seasickness]. Sound of any sort, usually a loud, harsh one. SEE: *odynacusis.*
noli-me-tangere (nō′lĭ-mē-tan′jĕ-rē) [L. touch me not]. Cancerous ulcer, generally of the face, which eats away bone and soft tissue.
noma (nō′mă) [G. *nomē*, a spreading]. A gangrenous progressive condition, generally found in children, spreading from the mucous membrane of the cheek or gum to the cutaneous surface. SYN: *cancrum oris, stomatitis, gangrenous.*
   n. pudendi, n. vulvae. A similar condition affecting the labia majora.
no′madism [G. *nomas*, roaming about]. PSY: Impulse to wander.
nomenclature (nō″mĕn-klā″chur) [L. *nomenclatura*, a name calling]. System of technical or scientific names. SYN: *terminology.*
nomogram (nŏm′ō-gram) [G. *nomos*, law, + *gramma*, a mark]. Representation by graphs, diagrams or charts of the relationship bet. numerical variables.
nomography (nō-mog′ră-fĭ) [G. *nomographia*, a writing of laws]. A graphic representation of the relation bet. numerical variables.
nomotopic (nŏm-ō-tŏp′ĭk) [G. *nomos*, law, + *topos*, place]. Occurring at the normal site.

non- [L.]. Prefix denoting *not, negation.*
nona-, non-, [L.]. Prefix meaning *ninth.*
nona (nō′nă) [L. *nonus*, ninth]. Acute or chronic infectious disease of central nervous system. SYN: *encephalitis lethargica, sleeping sickness.*
nonan (nō′năn) [L. *nonus*, ninth]. Having increased symptoms or reappearing every 9th day, as the paroxysms of malaria.
non compos mentis (nŏn kŏm″pŏs měn′tĭs) [L.]. Not of sound mind.
nonconductor (nŏn″kŏn-dŭk′tōr) [L. *non*, not, + *con*, with, + *ductor*, a leader]. A substance that does not conduct or conducts with difficulty heat, sound, or electricity.
   Strictly speaking, there is no perfect nonconductor. On the application of a sufficiently high voltage, current may be caused to flow through materials usually spoken of as nonconductors. SYN: *insulator.*
nonelectrolyte (nŏn″e-lek′tro-līt) [″ + *ēlectron*, amber, + *lytos*, dissolved]. A nonconducting solution.
nonipara (nō-nĭp′ăr-ă) [L. *nonus*, ninth, + *parēre*, to bring forth]. A woman who has given birth 9 times.
nonlax′ative diet. Low residue diet* with boiled milk and toasted crackers. No strained oatmeal, vegetable juice, or fruit juice given. Fats and concentrated sweets are restricted.
nonpolar (nŏn-pō′lĕr) [L. *non*, not + *polus*, a pole]. Not having separate poles; sharing electrons.
   n. compound. One formed by the sharing of electrons.
nonpro′tein [L. *non*, not + G. *prōtos*, first]. Any substance not a protein.
   n. nitrogen. 1. A nitrogenous constituent of blood that is not a protein. 2. Sum of all nonprotein nitrogen in the blood. SEE: *nitrogen.*
non repetat [L.]. Do not repeat.
nonrestraint (nŏn″rē-strănt′) [L. *non*, not, + *rē*, back, + *stringere*, to bind back]. Treatment of the insane without using mechanical restraint.
nonseptate (nŏn-sĕp′tăt) [″ + *saeptum*, a partition]. Having no dividing walls.
nonsexual (nŏn-sĕk′shū-ăl) [″ + *sexus*, sex]. Without sex. SYN: *asexual.*
nontoxic (nŏn-tŏks′ĭk) [″ + G. *toxikon*, poison]. Not poisonous or productive of poison.
nonunion (nŏn-ūn′yŭn) [L. *non*, not, + *uniō*, oneness]. Failure of bone fragments to knit together.
no′nus [L.]. 1. Ninth. 2. Hypoglossal or *ninth* cranial nerve.
nonviable (nŏn-vī′ă-bl) [″ + *via*, life]. Incapable of life or of living.
nookleptia (nō-ō-klep′tĭ-ă) [G. *nous*, mind, + *kleptein*, to steal]. An obsession that one's thoughts are being stolen by others.
noöpsyche (no′o-sī-ke) [″ + *psychē*, soul]. Reasoning or intellectual processes.
N. O. P. H. N. Abbr. *National Organization for Public Health Nursing.*
norm (norm) [L. *norma*, rule]. A type or standard pattern.
nor′ma [L. rule]. A line used to define the various aspects of the cranium.
   n. frontalis. Cranial outline viewed from the front.
   n. inferior. Cranial outline of inferior aspect.
normal (nor′măl) [L. *norma*, rule]. 1. Standard; performing proper functions; natural; regular. 2. BIOL: Not affected

by experimental treatment; occurring naturally and not because of a disease or experimentation. 3. PSY: (a) Free from mental disorder; (b) of average development or intelligence. 4. CHEM: A term used to describe a solution so made that 1 liter contains 1 gram equivalent of the solute.

In the case of acids and bases formed by univalent radicals, a normal solution is the same as *molar*, as in the case of HCl. In the case of H_2SO_4, however, the normal solution would be half as strong as the molar, and in the case of H_3PO_4 it would be one-third.

n. body temperature. 98.6° F.

n. formula of response. PT: A condensed statement of the results of stimulating motor nerves with direct current. A large flat electrode (indifferent) is placed over a convenient surface (*e. g.*, the back of the neck) while a more pointed electrode (different) is held over the motor nerve to be studied.

In the formula CCC (cathodal closing contraction) means the height of the contraction seen in the muscle concerned with the different electrode is the cathode and when the circuit is closed; AOC (anodal opening contraction) means the height of the contraction when the different electrode is the anode and the circuit is opened. The formula for normal nerves is CCC ACC AOC COC. In degenerating nerves this order is changed.

n. pulse. 72-80 beats per minute.
n. respiration. 18-24 per minute.
n. salt. An ionic compound containing no replaceable hydrogen or hydroxyl ions.
n. solution. Solution containing 1 Gm., molecular weight, of dissolved substance divided by the hydrogen equivalent of the substance per liter of solution.

normalization (nŏr-măl-ĭ-zā'shŭn) [L. *norma*, rule]. Modification or reduction to normal.

normergic (norm'ẽr'jĭk). Reacting or pertaining to that which reacts in a normal manner.

normoblast (nor"mō-blăst) [L. *norma*, rule, + G. *blastos*, germ]. A nucleated red blood corpuscle similar in size to an ordinary erythrocyte.

normochromasia (nŏr"mō-krō-mā'zĭ-ă) [" + G. *chrōma*, color]. Average staining capacity in a cell or tissue.

normocyte (nor'mō-sīt) [" + G. *kytos*, cell]. An average-sized red blood corpuscle. SYN: *erythrocyte*.

normocytosis (nor"mō-sī-tō'sīs) [" + " + -*ōsis*, condition]. A normal state of the corpuscular elements of the blood.

normoglycemia (nor"mō-glī-sē'mĭ-ă) [" + G. *glykus*, sweet, + *aima*, blood]. Normal state of sugar content of the blood.

normoglycemic (nor"mō-glī-se'mĭk) [" + " + *aima*, blood]. Having a normal amount of sugar in the blood.

normoörthocytosis (nor"mō-or"thō-sī-tō'-sīs) [L. *norma*, rule, + G. *orthos*, correct, + *kytos*, cell, + -*ōsis*, increase]. Increase in the blood of the number of leukocytes, but with normal proportion of the different varieties.

normoplasia (nor"mō-pla'zĭ-ă) [" + *plasis*, a formation]. A specific variation in the character of a cell within normal limits.

normoskeocytosis (nor"mō-skē"ō-sī-tō'sīs) [" + *skaios*, left, + *kytos*, cell, + -*ōsis*, condition]. Normal number of the leukocytes of the blood with deviation* to the left, *i. e.*, with immature forms present.

normosthenuria (nor"mō-sthĕn-ū'rĭ-ă) [" + G. *sthenos*, strength, + *ouron*, urine]. Urination of normal amount and specific gravity.

normotonic (nor"mō-ton'ĭk) [" + G. *tonos*, tension]. 1. Having normal muscular tonus. 2. One who has normal muscle tonus.

normotopia (nor"mō-tō'pĭ-ă) [" + G. *topos*, place]. Situation in the regular place.

normotopic (nor"mō-top'ĭk) [" + *topos*, place]. In the right location; pert. to the normal situation.

normovolemia (nor"mō-vō-lē'mĭ-ă) [" + *volūmen*, volume, + G. *aima*, blood]. Normal state of blood volume.

Norris' corpuscles. Colorless red blood corpuscles not visible in the blood plasma.

Norwe'gian itch. Severe form of scabies marked by pustules and crusts, seen usually in leprosy.

nose (nōz) [A.S. *nosw*]. Projection in center of face; the organ of olfaction and the entrance which warms, moistens and filters the air for the respiratory tract. SYN: *nasus, organon olfactus*.

ANAT: The external portion of the nose is a triangle of cartilage and bone covered with skin and lined with mucous membrane. Internally, a septum divides nose into 2 chambers. Each chamber contains 3 *meatuses* which are found underneath the corresponding turbinates. Orifices of frontal, ant. ethmoid and maxillary sinuses are in middle meatus. Orifices of post. ethmoids and sphenoids are in sup. meatus.

Sinuses, Communicating: Ethmoidal, frontal, maxillary, sphenoidal.

Nerves: Facial, olfactory, ophthalmic and maxillary.

Blood Supply: Ext. and int. maxillary arteries from the ext. carotid and ethmoidal artery from the int. carotid.

EXAMINATION OF: Note shape, size, color, state of the alae nasi, discharge, interference with respiration, evidences of injury, deflected or perforated septum, enlarged turbinates, and tenderness over frontal and maxillary sinuses.

DIAG: COLOR: *Chronic red n*: Dilated capillaries the result of alcoholism, lupus erythematosus, acne rosacea, pustules, boils and digestive disorders. ULCERATION, SUPERFICIAL: Tuberculous ulcer, epithelioma, syphilis. SIZE AND SHAPE: *Broad and Coarse*: Cretinism, myxedema, acromegaly. *Sunken*: Syphilis or injury. *Pinched with Small Nares*: Hypertrophied adenoid tissue or chronic obstructions; also tumors. DISCHARGES: *Inoffensive watery discharge*: Present in nasal catarrh, early stages of measles, hay fever, acute irritation of lining membranes. *Offensive discharges*: Nasopharyngeal diphtheria, lupus, local infection, impacted foreign bodies, caries, rhinitis, glanders, syphilitic infection.

FOREIGN BODY IN THE NOSE: SYM: Irritation of nose resulting in coughing or watery or purulent discharge. Occasionally pain and obstruction of nose. If not recognized immediately it often causes a foul discharge on the affected side of the nose. There may be obstruction to breathing in 1 nostril. If the foreign body is very small, symptoms may be absent.

NOSE.

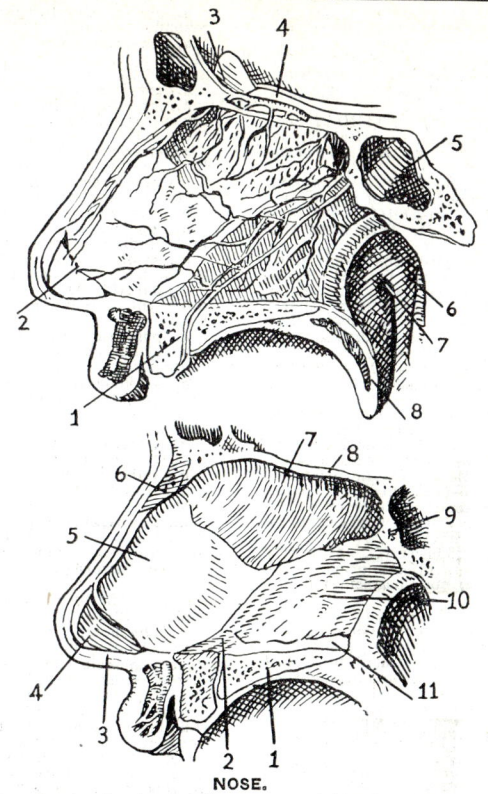

Nasal septum, showing its structural arrangement, blood, and nerve supply. *Above:*
1. Incisor canal. 2. Little Kisselbach triangle. 3. Crista galli. 4. Olfactory bulb.
5. Sphenoid sinus. 6. Rosenmueller's fossa. 7. Pharyngeal orifice of eustachian tube.
8. Soft palate. *Below:* 1. Hard palate. 2. Septal or medial crest of maxillary bone.
3. Columella. 4. Medial crus of major alar cartilage. 5. Quadrangular cartilage.
6. Nasal process. 7. Perpendicular plate of ethmoid. 8. Cribriform plate of ethmoid.
9. Rostrum of sphenoid. 10. Vomer. 11. Septal or medial crest of palatine bone.

TREATMENT: Vigorous blowing of the nose is dangerous as it may spread infection to the various cavities and sinuses about the nose or to the ear. Do not attempt to fish the body out with a hairpin or other object, as this often results in pushing the body into the throat and it may drop into the larynx or trachea. Attempts to dislodge may cause it to slip further in the nose or down the throat, from where it occasionally drops into the windpipe. Foreign bodies in the nose rarely need emergency measures. Instill a drop or 2 of oil (such as mineral oil) into the affected nostrils and take the patient to a physician.

n., saddle. Nose with depressed bridge seen in tertiary syphilis due to gummatous destruction of septal supporting structure, and following operations which are complicated by suppuration and destruction of supporting framework.

nose, words pert. to: agger nasi; ala nasi; alinasal; anosmia; aporrhinosis; apostaxis; bulb, olfactory; bulla ethmoidalis; choana narium; columella nasi; epistaxis; hyperosmia; naris; "nas-" words; nostril; parosmia; rhinalgia; rhinitis; "rhino-" words; septum; sinus, accessory; sinusitis; smell; vestibule; vibrissae; vomer; xeromycteria.

nosebleed (nōz'blēd) [A.S. *nosu*, nose, + *blēdan*, to bleed]. Hemorrhage from nose. SYN: *epistaxis*.

nosema (no-sē'mă) [G. *nosēma*, disease]. 1. Ailment (nosema) or disease. 2. A genus of Microsporidia.

noso- [G.]. Combining form meaning *pert. to disease*.

nosochthonography (nos″ok-thon-og'ră-fī) [G. *nosos*, disease, + *chthōn*, earth, + *graphein*, to write]. Study of geography of diseases; medical geography. SYN: *nosogeography*.

nosocomium (nŏs″ō-kō'mĭ-ŭm) [" + *komein*, to care for]. A hospital or infirmary.

nosode (nos'ōd) [" + *eidos*, appearance].

A bacterial vaccine used in treatment of the disease of which it is the causative agent.

nosogenesis, nosogeny (nos″ō-jĕn′ĕ-sĭs, nos-oj′en-ĭ) [" + *gennan*, to produce]. The development and progress of a disease.

nosogeography (nos″ō-jē-og′ră-fĭ) [" + *gē*, earth, + *graphein*, to write]. Study of medical geography. SYN: *nosochthonography*.

nosography (no-sog′ră-fĭ) [" + *graphein*, to write]. The description of a disease.

nosohemia (nŏs-ō-hē′mĭ-ă) [G. *nosos*, disease, + *aima*, blood]. Disease of the blood.

nosointoxication (nos″ō-ĭn-tok″sĭ-kā′shŭn) [" + *in*, into, + *toxikon*, poison]. Pathological interference with metabolic processes resulting in autointoxication.

nosology (no-sol′o-jĭ) [" + *logos*, disease]. The science of description, or the classification of diseases.

nosomania (nos″ō-mā′nĭ-ă) [" + *mania*, madness]. 1. The delusion that one is diseased. 2. Morbid fear of disease.

nosomycosis (nos″ō-mī-kō′sĭs) [" + *mykēs*, fungus, + *-ōsis*]. Any disease caused by a parasitic fungus or Schizomycete.

nosonomy (nos-on′ō-mĭ) [" + *nomos*, law]. The science of disease classification.

nosoparasite (nos″ō-par′ă-sīt) [" + *para*, beside, + *sitos*, food]. A microörganism associated with a disease which it modifies but does not cause.

nosophobia (nō″sō-fō′bĭ-ă) [G. *nosos*, disease, + *phobos*, fear]. Abnormal aversion to illness, or to a particular affection.

nosopoietic (nō″sō-poy-ĕt′ĭk) [" + *poiein*, to form]. Producing or causing disease.

nosotherapy (nos″ō-ther′ă-pĭ) [" + *therapeia*, treatment]. Treatment of 1 disease by voluntarily introducing another microörganism into the body.

nosotoxicosis (nos″ō-tok″sĭ-kō′sĭs) [" + *toxikon*, poison, + *-ōsis*]. Disorder caused by toxic products of another disease.

nosotoxin (nos″ō-tok′sĭn) [" + *toxikon*, poison]. Any toxin productive of or associated with disease.

nosotrophy (nos-ot′rō-fĭ) [" + *trophē*, nourishment]. Nursing care and feeding of the sick.

nostalgia (nos-tal′jĭ-ă) [G. *nostos*, a return home, + *algos*, pain]. Homesickness. SEE: *cainotophobia*.

nostology (nŏs-tol′ō-jĭ) [" + *logos*, study]. The study of physiological stages of senility.

nostomania (nos″tō-ma′nĭ-ă) [" + *mania*, madness]. Nostalgia* verging on insanity.

nos′tril [A.S. *nosu*, nose, + *thyrl*, a hole]. Apertures of the nose. SYN: *naris*. SEE: *nose*.

n. reflex. Reduction of opening of naris on affected side in lung disease in proportion to lessened alveolar air capacity on affected side.

nostrum (nŏs′trŭm) [L. our]. A patent or a quack remedy.

notal (nō′tăl) [G. *nōton*, back]. Concerning the back. SYN: *dorsal*.

notalgia (nō-tal′jĭ-ă) [" + *algos*, pain]. Painful condition of the back. SYN: *dorsalgia*.

notch (nŏtsh) [A.S. *nocke*]. A rather deep indentation or narrow gap in the edge of a part. SYN: *incisura*.

n., acetabular. Notch in the margin of the acetabulum opp. the obturator foramen.

n., aortic. One in sphygmogram from rebound at aortic valve closure.

n., clavicular. One at the upper angle of the sternum with which the clavicle articulates.

n., cotyloid. SEE: *acetabular n.*

n., interclavicular. A rounded one at top of manubrium of sternum, bet. surfaces articulating with the clavicles.

n., interlobar. One in ant. margin of liver, separating left and right lobes.

n's., intervertebral. The ones constituting the intervertebral foramina.

n., ischiatic. Sacrosciatic, q.v.

n., jugular. One which forms the post. and middle portions of jugular foramen.

n., nasal. A deep gap at inner margin of facial surface of maxilla.

n., parotid. One bet. ramus of mandible and mastoid process of temporal bone.

n., popliteal. A shallow depression separating tuberosities of head of tibia posteriorly.

n. of Rivinus. The one in the upper and ant. portion of osseous ring attached to which is the tympanic membrane.

n's., sacrosciatic. Two n's. on post. border of innominate bone.

n., sigmoid. One bet. the condyle and the coronoid process of ramus of mandible.

n., suprascapular. One sometimes converted into a foramen by a ligament or bony process, in upper border of scapula.

n., suprasternal. SEE: *interclavicular n.*

note (nōt) [L. *nota*, a mark]. A sound of definite pitch.

n. blindness. Inability to recognize musical notes, due to a central lesion.

notencephalocele (no″tĕn-sef′al-ō-sēl) [G. *nōton*, back, + *egkephalos*, brain, + *kēlē*, hernia]. Protrusion of brain substance at the back of the head.

notifi′able diseases. The laws of the various states require that certain diseases when existing shall be reported to the local health authorities, such as a Board of Health. A fine may be levied for not doing so. Among the diseases generally required to be reported are: All communicable or contagious diseases, such as smallpox, scarlet fever, relapsing fever; diphtheria or membranous croup; enteric fevers, such as typhoid fever; erysipelas; puerperal pyrexia and sepsis; cholera; typhus; cerebrospinal fever; acute anterior poliomyelitis; polioencephalitis; encephalitis lethargica; tuberculosis; dysentery; pneumonia; epidemic diarrhea; chickenpox; gonorrhea; syphilis. SEE: *quarantine, reportable diseases*.

notochord (nō′tō-kord) [G. *nōton*, back + *chordē*, cord]. The embryonic spinal cord.

notomyelitis (nō″tō-mī-ĕ-lī′tĭs) [" + *myelos*, marrow, + *-itis*, inflammation]. Inflamed condition of the spinal cord.

noumenal (nŭ′mē-năl) [G. *nooumenon*, a thing perceived]. Pert. to rational intuition opposed to sensual perception.

noumenon (nŭ′mē-nŏn) [G. *nooumenon*, a thing perceived]. An object of rational apprehension as opposed to perception.

nourishment (nur′ĭsh-mĕnt) [L. *nutrire*, to nurse]. 1. Act of nourishing or of being nourished. 2. Sustenance; nutriment. SEE: *trophic, trophic center*.

novaspirin (nō-văs′pĭr-ĭn). A crystalline substance of the aspirin type, representing about 62% salicylic acid. Per-

nucleus (nū'klē-ŭs) (pl. *nuclei*) [L. little kernel]. 1. A central point about which matter is gathered, as in a calculus. SYN: *core*.
2. The vital body in the protoplasm of a cell, the essential agent in growth, metabolism, reproduction and transmission of characteristics of a cell.
3. A group of nerve cells or mass of gray matter in the central nervous system, esp. the brain.
4. CHEM: Heavy central atomic particle in which most of the mass and total positive electric charge are concentrated.

The nucleus of a cell usually is a round or oval mass of protoplasm sheathed in a *membrane* and containing a hyaline ground substance which is formed of a network and 1 or more *nucleoli*. *Chromatin* granules are found in the network. The network is called *linin*.
RS: *circumnuclear, "karyo-" words.*

n., abducent. A gray n., the origin of abducens nerve, on floor of 4th ventricle, behind trigeminal n.

n., accessory auditory. A ganglionic mass at the convergence of the 2 roots or divisions of the auditory nerve.

n. ambiguus. BNA. N. of the glossopharyngeal and vagus nerves in oblongata.

n. amygdaloid. A mass of gray matter forming the ant. extremity of descending cornu of lateral ventricle.

n., angular. SEE: *Bechterew's n.*

n., arcuate. The largest of the masses of cinerea in the arciform fibers of the pyramids on the ventral side.

n., auditory. Nest of nerve cells where auditory nerves arise.

n., Bechterew's. N. giving origin to roots of auditory nerve.

n., Burdach's. Upper part of cuneate fasciculus in oblongata.

n., caudate. Portion of striated body projecting into lateral ventricle.

n., chromatic. Principal nucleus of a cell.

n. cinereum. Gray matter of the restiform bodies.

n., cuneate. SEE: *Burdach's n.*

n., daughter. N. produced by the division of mother nucleus.

n., Deiter's. Main terminal n. of the vestibular nerve in oblongata.

n., dentate. Indented layer of gray matter in center of white substance of cerebellum. SYN: *corpus dentatum*.

n., ectoblastic. One in cells of the epiblast.

n., emboliform. A small mass of gray matter in central white substance of the cerebellum.

n. fasti'gii. BNA. Small mass of gray matter in white substance of vermis of the cerebellum.

n. funiculi gracilis. BNA. Elongated mass of gray matter in dorsal pyramid of medulla oblongata.

n., germinal. N. resulting from union of male and female pronuclei.

n., gonad. Reproductive n. of a cell.

n., gray. Gray substance of spinal cord.

n., hypoglossal. Large multipolar nerve cells in inf. triangle of 4th ventricle.

n. hypothalamicus. BNA. A lenslike mass of gray matter in the subthalamic region of the hypothalamus.

n., intraventricular. SEE: *caudate n.*

n., lenticular. In corpus striatum, gray matter of its extraventricular portion.

n. lentis. N. of crystalline lens.

n., mother. One that divides into 2 or more parts called *daughter nuclei*.

n., motor. A ganglionic mass in the central nervous system giving origin to motor nerve fibers.

n., oculomotor. N. of the oculomotor nerve.

n., olivary. One of 2 bands of gray matter, 1 in the medulla below the olive, the other on inner side of facial n. in the pons.

n. pulposus. Gelatinous mass in center of intervertebral disks.

n., pyramidal. Band of gray matter near olivary n. in the medulla.

n. quintus. Trigeminal nerve nucleus.

n. ruber. BNA. Mass of red colored gray matter in crus cerebri close to optic thalamus.

n., subthalamic. SEE: *n. hypothalamicus.*

n., vesicular. N. having deeply staining membranes and pale center.

n. vestibularis. SEE: *Bechterew's n.*

n., vitelline. One formed by union of male and female pronuclei within the vitellus.

n., white. Central white substance of corpus dentatum of olive.

nude (nūd) [L. *nudāre*, to strip]. 1. Bare; naked; unclothed. 2. An unclothed body.

nudi- [L.]. Combining form denoting *uncovered, naked.*

nudomania (nū-dō-ma'nĭ-ă) [L. *nudāre*, to strip, + G. *mania*, madness]. Abnormal desire to be nude.

nudophobia (nū-dō-fō'bĭ-ă) [" + G. *phobos*, fear]. Abnormal fear of being unclothed. SEE: *gymnophobia.*

Nuel's space (nū'ĕl). Space bet. outer rods of Corti and Deiter's cells and hair cells in organs of Corti.

Nuhn's gland (noon). Mucous gland on each side of frenulum of the tongue. SYN: *Blandin's gland.*

nullipara (nŭl-ĭp'ă-ră) [L. *nullus*, none, + *parēre*, to bear]. A woman who has borne no children.

nulliparity (nŭl-ĭ-par'ĭ-tĭ) [" + *parēre*, to bear]. Condition of not having given birth to a child.

nulliparous (nŭl-lĭp'ăr-ŭs) [" + *parēre*, to bear]. Never having borne a child.

numb (nŭm) [A.S. *numen*, taken]. 1. Insensible; lacking in sensation of power and motion, esp. from cold. 2. To render senseless or inert.

number (nŭm'bĕr) [L. *numerus*, number]. 1. A total of units. 2. A symbol graphically representing an arithmetical sum.
RS: *mean, median, modality, mode, numeral.*

numbness (nŭm'nĕs) [A.S. *numen*, taken]. Lack of sensation in a part, esp. from cold. SEE: *narcohypnia.*

numeral (nū'mĕr-ăl) [L. *numerus*, number]. 1. Denoting or pert. to a number. 2. A word or figure expressing a number.

num'miform, num'mular [L. *nummus*, a coin, + *forma*, shape]. 1. Coin-shaped, said of some mucous sputum. 2. Arranged like a stack of coins.

nummulation [L. *nummus*, a coin]. The formation of a coin-shaped mass.

nunnation (nŭn-ā'shŭn) [Arabic *nun*, letter N]. Frequent and abnormal use of the n sound.

nupercaine (nu'per-kān). A white powder or crystals manufactured from cinchoninic acid.
USES: As a local anesthetic of prolonged action. More toxic than cocaine.

nuptiality (nŭp″shĭ-ăl'ĭ-tĭ) [L. *nuptiae*, wedding]. 1. The number of marriages

novasurol   **nucleotoxin**

haps less powerful than aspirin, but believed to be tolerated better.
USES: Same as aspirin.
DOSAGE: 10-15 gr. (0.65-1 Gm.). [acids.
INCOMPATIBILITIES: Iron compounds,
novasurol (nō-vǎs'ū-rōl). SEE: *merbaphen*.
novatropine (nov-at'rō-pēn). The methyl bromide of the alkaloid homatropine, less active and less toxic than atropine.
USES: Chiefly in gastrointestinal spasm.
DOSAGE: 1/24 gr. (2.5 mg).
novocain (nō'vō-kǎn). A commercial brand of procaine hydrochloride, USP.
The noxious principle in novocain is supposed to have been eliminated in procain.
DANGERS OF NOVOCAIN: Lowers blood pressure, produces convulsions accompanied by complete dilatation of the pupils, hallucinations, delusions and death. For all cocaine preparations, the barbituric preparations act as an antidote, causing a relaxation of the muscles and lowering brain tension. They act as a buffer for novocain poisoning and should always be given preoperatively before giving novocain.
DOSAGE: *Infilt.*, 4 gr. (0.25 Gm.); *instill.*, 1½ gr. (0.1 Gm.).
noxa (noks'ǎ) (pl. *noxae*) [L. injury]. Anything harmful to health.
noxious (nok'shus) [L. *noxius*, injurious]. Harmful; not wholesome.
NPH insulin. Abbr. for *neutral-protamine-Hagedorn insulin*. SEE: *insulin, NPH*.
NPN. Abbr. for *nonprotein nitrogen*.
n-rays. Rays discovered by Blondlot in 1903 making certain bodies luminous.
nubecula (nū-bek'ū-la) [L. little cloud]. Cloudiness of the cornea or the urine.
nubile (nū'bǐl) [L. *nubere*, to marry]. Pert. to a girl who has attained puberty and who is thus able to marry.
nubility (nū-bǐl'ǐ-tǐ) [L. *nubere*, to marry]. Marriageableness, said of female at puberty, the final state of sex development.
nucha (nū'kǎ) [L.]. Nape of neck.
nuchal (nū'kal) [L. *nucha*, back of neck]. Pert. to the neck or *nucha*.
Nuck's canal or diverticulum (nook). Peritoneal pouch descending along round ligament of uterus.
nuclear (nū'klē-ǎr) [L. *nucleus*, a kernel]. Resembling or concerning a nucleus.
   n. cell division. Changes occurring in a nucleus in indirect cell division. SYN: *karyokinesis*. [cell nucleus.
   n. fibril. Tiny f. of chromatin in a
   n. sap. Liquid of a cell nucleus found within the meshwork.
nuclease (nū'klē-ās) [L. *nucleus*, kernel, + *ase*, enzyme]. Any enzymes in animals and plants which facilitate hydrolysis of nuclein and nucleic acids.
nucleate (nū'klē-āt) [L. *nucleatus*, having a kernel]. 1. Having a nucleus. 2. To form a nucleus. 3. A salt or ester of nucleic acid.
nucleation (nū"klē-ā'shŭn) [L. *nucleus*, kernel]. Nucleus formation.
nuclei (nū'klē-ī) [L.]. Pl. of nucleus.
nucle'ic acid, nuclein'ic acid. Acid which, combined with proteins, forms nuclein.
DOSAGE: 1-5 gr. (0.06-0.3 Gm.).
nuclein (nū'klē-ǐn) [L. *nucleus*, a kernel]. A normal chemical constituent of a cell nucleus, a colorless, shapeless substance obtained by hydrolysis of nucleoproteins or cells containing nucleic acid and proteins rich in phosphorus.
Said to increase number of white blood cells and therefore increase resistance to infection. N. derived from glands is given therapeutically.
DOSAGE: *Hypoderm.* of 0.5% solut., 8 ℳ (0.5 cc.).
   n. bases. Adenine, guanine, xanthine, hypoxanthine. SYN: *xanthine bases*.
nucleo- [L.]. Pertaining to a *nucleus*.
nucleoalbumin (nū"klē-ō-ǎl-bū'mǐn) [L. *nucleus*, kernel, + *albus*, white]. A protein compound composed of protein and an undefined phosphorus. Former name for phosphoprotein, *q.v.*
nucleoalbuminuria (nū"klē-ō-al-bu"mǐ-nū'rǐ-ǎ) [" + " + G. *ouron*, urine]. Nucleoalbumin found in urine.
nucleoalbumose (nū"klē-ō-ǎl'bū-mōs) [" + *albus*, white]. Partly hydrated nucleoalbumin found in the urine of patients with osteomalacia.
nucleochylema (nū"klē-ō-kī-lē'mǎ) [" + G. *chylos*, juice]. The chylema of the cell nucleus differentiated from that of the cytoplasm.
nucleofugal (nū-klē-of'ū-gǎl) [" + *fugere*, to flee]. Moving from a nucleus in the cell.
nucleohiston(e (nū"klē-ō-hǐs'ton, -tōn) [" + *istos*, tissue]. A substance in leukocytes, lymph and thymus glands, composed of nuclein and histone.
nucleoid (nū'klē-oyd) [" + G. *eidos*, resemblance]. Resembling a nucleus.
nucleolar (nū-klē'ō-lǎr) [L. *nucleolus*, a little kernel]. Pert. to a nucleolus.
nucleoliform (nū-klē'ō-lǐ-form) [" + *forma*, shape]. Like a nucleolus.
nucleolin (nū-klē'ō-lǐn) [L. *nucleolus*, little kernel]. The substance composing the nucleolus. SYN: *plastin*.
nucleolus (nū-klē'ō-lŭs) (pl. *nucleoli*) [L. little kernel]. A spherical body within the cell nucleus. SYN: *karyosome, plasmosome*.
nucleomicrosome (nū"klē-ō-mī"krō-sōm) [L. *nucleus*, kernel, + G. *mikros*, tiny, + *sōma*, body]. Any 1 of the minute granules making up a nucleoplasmic fiber.
nucleon (nū'klē-ōn) [L. *nucleus*, kernel]. Acid substance found in muscle, blood, milk which is related to the nucleins and yields peptone.
nucleopetal (nū-klē-op'ět-ǎl) [" + *petere*, to seek]. Seeking or moving toward the nucleus.
   n. movement. The attraction of a male pronucleus toward the female pronucleus.
nucleoplasm (nū'klē-ō-plǎzm) [" + *plasma*, a thing formed]. 1. Protoplasm of a nucleus. SYN: *karyoplasm*. 2. Reticular substance of a nucleus. 3. Ground substance of a nucleus.
nucleoprotein (nū"klē-ō-prō'tē-ǐn) [" + G. *prōtos*, first]. The combination of 1 of the proteins with nucleic acid to form a conjugated protein found in cell nuclei.
nucleoreticulum (nū"klē-ō-rē-tǐk'ū-lŭm) [" + *reticulum*, network]. Any mesh framework in a nucleus.
nucleospindle (nū"klē-ō-spǐn'dl) [" + A.S. *spinel*]. Spindle-shaped body occurring in karyokinesis.*
nucleotherapy (nū"klē-ō-thěr'ǎ-pī) [" + G. *therapeia*, treatment]. The use of nuclein in therapy.
nucleotide (nū'klē-ō-tīd) [L. *nucleus*, kernel]. Compound of nucleic acid and a base, formed by hydrolysis of nucleic acid.
nu"cleotox'in [" + G. *toxikon*, poison]. A toxin acting upon or produced by cell nuclei.

in proportion to the population. 2. Wedding. 3. Conjugal character.
nurse (ners) [L. *nutrix*, a nurse]. One who cares for the sick or wounded, esp. a registered nurse. SEE: *nutrix*.

n., charge. One in charge of a single hospital ward.

n., community; n., district. A visiting nurse.

n., dry. An infant's nurse who does not suckle the child.

n., general duty. One not specializing.

n., graduate. One who is a graduate of an accredited school of nursing.

n., head. A supervisor at the head of a hospital nursing staff.

n., health. A community nurse.

n., practical. One with experience in nursing but who is not a graduate of a school of nursing.

n., private. A nurse in charge of a single patient.

n., private duty. One not a member of a hospital staff who is called in to care for an individual patient in the hospital.

n., probationer. One under observation in a nursing school before being admitted as a student.

n., public health. A graduate nurse employed by a Board of Health.

n., registered. A graduate nurse who has been registered and legally licensed to practice by state authority.

n., school. A registered nurse whose duties are to supplement the work of the physician in medical inspection of pupils.

n., trained. A registered nurse.

n., visiting. A registered nurse, employed by an association to care for the sick poor in their homes.

n., wet. A woman who gives suck to infants of others.

nurse (ners) [L. *nutrix*, a nurse]. 1. To feed an infant at the breast. 2. To care for an invalid. 3. To care for a young child. 4. To suckle.

nur'ses' contracture. Tetany sometimes seen in nurses.

nur'sing [L. *nutrix*, nurse]. 1. Scientific care of the sick by a graduate, registered nurse. 2. Loosely applied to any care of the sick. 3. Suckling at the female breast, as an infant. 4. Lactation.

nutation (nū-tā'shŭn) [L. *nutātiō*, a nodding]. Nodding, as of the head.

n. of sacrum. Partial rotation of the sacrum on its transverse axis to give greater space for passage of the fetus.

nutriceptor (nū″trĭ-sĕp'tor) [L. *nutriens*, feeding, + *ceptōr*, a receiver]. One which reacts with nutritive matter to nourish a cell.

nutrient (nū'trĭ-ĕnt). 1. Food that supplies the body with its necessary elements. 2. Nourishing.

Those containing carbon are *organic* food nutrients. Organic food nutrients may or may not contain nitrogen. Nutrients used for body fuel are fat, proteins and carbohydrates. Energy is obtained by the oxidation of certain food nutrients.

RS: *calory, carbohydrate, fat, food, mineral, nitrogen, pabulum, protein.*

nutriment (nū'trĭ-mĕnt) [L. *nutrimentum*, nourishment]. That which nourishes; nutritious substance.

nutriology (nū″trĭ-ol'ō-jĭ) [L. *nutrīre*, to nourish, + G. *logos*, study]. The science of use of foods in diet and therapy.

nutrition (nū-trĭ'shŭn) [L. *nutritiō*, a feeding]. 1. Absorption of food elements and transformation into living tissue, the processes of which include *ingestion, digestion, absorption, assimilation* and *excretion, q.v.* 2. Nourishing substance.

Nutrients are stored by the body in various forms, and drawn upon when the food intake is not sufficient in the following order: usable gases; water as needed; body carbohydrates, such as sugar or glycogen; lactic acid and then the fats are utilized; large globules of neutral fat, and the fats that bear a relation to other fats, as glycogen does to sugar.

These are not easily utilized and harm results, or a too large consumption of fats may induce acidosis. The albumins and proteins are then consumed, and if this continues death ensues.

nutrition, words pert. to: angiotrophic, athrepsia, athreptic, atrophy, bathmism, cachexia, cacotrophy, cardiotrophotherapy, hemiatrophy, inanition, paratrophic, vasotrophic, vivification, waste products.

nutritional (nū-trĭsh'ŭn-ăl) [L. *nutritiō*, a feeding]. Rel. to nutrition.

nutritious (nū-trĭsh'ŭs) [L. *nutritius*, feeding]. Affording nutriment. SYN: *nutritive*.

nutritive (nū'trĭ-tĭv) [L. *nutritius*]. Pert. to the process of assimilating food; having the property of nourishing.

n. enema. One of predigested foods to give sustenance to a patient unable to take nourishment in the usual way. SEE: *enema.*

nutritorium (nū-trĭt-o'rĭ-ŭm) [L. *nutritorius*, nutritive]. The entire body mechanism directly concerned with nutrition.

nutritory (nū'trĭ-tō″rĭ) [L. *nutritorius*, nutritive]. Nutritive, nourishing.

nutrix (nū'trĭks) [L.]. A woman nurse.

nux vomica (nŭks vom'ĭ-ka). A poisonous seed from an East Indian tree, containing several alkaloids, the principal ones being brucine and strychnine, *q.v.* USP.
DOSAGE: 1½ ℳ (0.1 cc.).

nyctalbuminuria (nĭk″tăl-bū″min-ū'rĭ-ă) [G. *nyx, nykt-*, night, + L. *albus*, white, + G. *ouron*, urine]. A cyclic albuminuria occurring at night. SYN: *noctalbuminuria.*

nyctalgia (nĭk-tal'jĭ-ă) [″ + *algos*, pain]. Pain during the night.

nyctalopia (nĭk-tă-lō'pĭ-ă) [″ + *alaos*, blind, + *ōps*, eye]. 1. A condition in which person cannot see well in a faint light or at night. Seen in retinitis pigmentosa and in the Laurence-Biedl syndrome, and also as a result of secondary atrophy of the optic nerve. SYN: *night blindness.* 2. Incorrectly, having better sight at night or in semi-darkness than by day; night vision. SEE: *hemeralopia.*

nyctamblyopia (nĭk″tam-blĭ-ō'pĭ-ă) [″ + *amblyōpia*, poor sight]. Poor vision at night without visible eye changes.

nyctaphonia (nĭk-tă-fō'nĭ-ă) [″ + *a-*, priv. + *phōnē*, voice]. Hysterical loss of voice during the night.

nycthemerus (nĭk-them'ĕ-rŭs) [G. *nychthemeros*]. 1. Space of a day and a night. 2. Pert. to a night and day. SYN: *ephemeral.*

nycterine (nĭk'tĕr-ĭn) [G. *nyx, nykt-,* night]. 1. Taking place at night. 2. Obscure.

nyctohemeral (nĭk″to-hē'mer-al) [″ + *ēmeraa*, day]. Rel. to both day and night.

nyctophilia (nĭk″to-fĭl'ĭ-ă) [″ + *philein*, to love]. A predilection for darkness or for night. SYN: *scotophilia.*

nyctophobia (nĭk″tō-fō′bĭ-ă) [" + *phobos*, fear]. Abnormal dread of the night, or of darkness.

nyctophonia (nĭk″tō-fō′nĭ-ă) [" + *phōnē*, voice]. Hysterical loss of voice only during the day.

nyctotyphlosis (nĭk″tō-tĭf-lō′sĭs) [" + *typhlōsis*, blindness]. Poor vision at night. SYN: *night blindness, nyctalopia*.

nycturia (nĭk-tū′rĭ-ă) [" + *ouron*, urine]. Urination, esp. excessive, during the night. SYN: *nocturia*. SEE: *enuresis*.

nygma (nĭg′mă) [G. *nygma*, a puncture]. A puncture wound.

nym′pha (pl. *nymphae*) [G. *nymphē*, a maiden]. One of the labia minora,* the small folds of mucous membrane forming the inner lips of the vulva.
So called from the nymphs, or goddesses of the fountain. SYN: *labium minus pudendi*.
 n. pendulae. Stretched pendulous nymphae.

nymphectomy (nĭm-fĕk′tō-mĭ) [" + *ektomē*, excision]. Excision of hypertrophied nymphae.

nymphitis (nĭm-fī′tĭs) [" + *-itis*, inflammation]. Inflamed condition of the nymphae.

nymphocaruncular sul′cus (nĭm″fō-kăr-ŭn′kŭ-lăr) [" + L. *caruncula*, little mass of flesh]. The depression bet. the hymen and the labium minus, on either side.

nymphohymenal sul′cus (nĭm″fō-hī′mĕn-ăl) [" + *ymēn*, membrane]. Trench bet. labium minus and the hymen on either side.

nympholepsy (nĭm′fō-lĕp-sĭ) [" + *lēpsia*, a seizure]. 1. Frenzied ecstasy usually erotic in nature. 2. Operative removal of the nymphae.

nymphomania (nĭm″fō-mā′nĭ-ă) [" + *mania*, madness]. Abnormally excessive sexual desire in the female. SYN: *furor femininus, furor uterinus*. SEE: *satyriasis*.

nymphomaniac (nĭm″fō-ma′nĭ-ăk) [G. *nymphē*, maiden, + *mania*, madness]. 1. Woman who is afflicted with excessive sexual desire. 2. Marked by excessive sexual desire.

nymphoncus (nĭm-fon′kŭs) [" + *ogkos*, a swelling]. Swelling or tumor of the nymphae.

nymphotomy (nĭm-fot′ō-mĭ) [" + *tomē*, a cutting]. 1. Removal of the nymphae. SYN: *nymphectomy*. 2. Incision into a nympha. 3. Removal of the clitoris.

nystagmic (nĭs-tag′mĭk) [G. *nystazein*, to nod]. Rel. to or suffering from condition of involuntary eyeball movements.

nystagmiform (nĭs-tag′mĭ-form) [" + L. *forma*, shape]. Pert. to or suffering from involuntary eyeball motion.

nystagmograph (nĭs-tag′mō-grăf) [" + *graphein*, to write]. Apparatus for recording the oscillations of the eyeball in nystagmus.

nystagmoid (nĭs-tag′moyd) [" + *eidos*, resemblance]. Similar to, or resembling nystagmus.

nystagmus (nĭs-tag′mŭs) [G. *nystazein*, to nod]. Constant involuntary movement of the eyeball.
 ETIOL: (1) Congenital, seen in bilateral amblyopia. (2) Occupational, as in miners and train dispatchers. (3) Labyrinthine irritability. (4) Nervous diseases.
 n., aural. N. due to disorder in the labyrinth of the ear.
 n., Cheyne's. N. with rhythmical movements of the eye.
 n., lateral. Horizontal movement of eyes from side to side.
 n., palatal. Spasm of levator palati muscle.
 n., rotatory. Rotation of the eyes about the visual axis.
 n., vertical. Up and down ocular movements.
 n., vestibular. That due to ear disturbances.

Nysten's law (nĭ′stĕn). Rigor mortis begins with muscles of mastication and progresses down the body affecting legs and feet last. SEE: *rigor mortis*.

nyxis (niks′ĭs) [G. *nyxis*, a pricking]. Puncture or piercing. SYN: *paracentesis*.

O

O. Symb. of *oxygen* and abbr. for various terms, as: *oculus*, eye; *octarius*, pint.
o-. Abbr. for *ortho-*, most commonly used in chemical terminology.
O_2. Symb. for the *two eyes*.
O_3. Symb. for *ozone*.
oakum (ō′kŭm) [A.S. *ācumba*, tow]. Loose fiber obtained by unravelling old hemp ropes, used occasionally as a surgical dressing.
oarialgia (ō″ăr-ĭ-ăl′jĭ-ă) [G. *ōarion*, little egg, + *algos*, pain]. Ovarian pain. SYN: *ovarialgia*.
oaric (ō-ă′rĭk) [G. *ōarion*, little egg]. Pert. to an ovary. SYN: *ovarian*.
oario-, oari- [G.]. Prefix pert. to the ovary.
oariopathy (ō″ăr-ĭ-op′ăth-ĭ) [G. *ōarion*, little egg, + *pathos*, disease]. Any disease of the ovary.
oariotomy (ō″ă-rĭ-ot′ō-mĭ) [" + *tomē*, incision]. Incision into an ovary or surgical removal of a tumor or the ovary itself. SYN: *ovariotomy*.
oaritis (ō-ă-rī′tĭs) [" + *-itis*, inflammation]. Inflamed condition of an ovary. SYN: *ovaritis*.
oarium (ō-ā′rĭ-um) (pl. *oaria*) [L., from G. *ōarion*, little egg]. An ovary. SYN: *ovarium*.
oasis (ō-ā′sĭs) (pl. *ōāsēs*) [G. *oasis*, a dry spot]. Area of healthy tissue surrounded by a diseased portion.
oat (ōt) [A.S. *āte*, oat]. Grain or seed of a cereal grass used as an article of diet.
oatmeal (ōt′mēl) [" + *melu*, meal]. COMP: Cellulose heavy. Rich in fats and lecithins.
  AVERAGE SERVING: 20 Gm. Pro. 3.2, Fat 1.4, Carbo. 13.5.
  VITAMINS: A— to +, B++, E+.
  ASH CONST: Ca 0.069, Mg 0.110, K 0.344, Na 0.062, P 0.392, Cl 0.069, S 0.202, Fe 0.0038.
  An acid forming food. Potential acidity, 12 cc. per 100 Gm., or 3 cc. per 100 calories.
  ACTION: Stimulating, laxative, fattening and nutritive.
ob- [L.]. Combining form meaning *towards, against, in the way of*.
O. B. Abbr. for *obstetrics*.
obcordate (ŏb-kor′dāt) [L. *ob*, against, + *cor*, cord-, heart]. Inversely heart-shaped.
obdormition (ŏb-dor-mĭsh′ŭn) [" + *dormire*, to sleep]. Numbness followed by tingling in a limb produced by pressure of the nerve trunk supplying it.
  Limb is commonly referred to as being asleep.
obduction (ŏb-duk′shŭn) [" + *ducere*, to lead]. Scientific inspection of a dead body to learn pathological conditions and cause of death. SYN: *autopsy, necropsy*.
obelion (ō-bē′lĭ-ŏn) [G. *obelos*, spit]. A craniometric point on the sagittal suture bet. the 2 parietal foramina.
obese (ō-bēs′) [L. *obesus*, fat]. Extremely fat. SYN: *corpulent*.
obesity (ō-bē′sĭ-tĭ) [L. *obesitās*, corpulence]. Abnormal amount of fat on the body. SYN: *adiposity, corpulence, polysarcia*.
  Term usually not employed unless individual is from 20-30% over average weight for his age, sex and height. There are 2 general classifications, *exogenous*, that caused by excessive food intake, and *endogenous*, that caused by some abnormality within the body, endocrine, nervous, or due to faulty salt and water metabolism.
  ENDOCRINE CAUSES: (1) Hypothyroidism, producing a decreased metabolic rate and insufficient energy output to balance the caloric intake; not a very frequent cause; (2) adrenal hyperfunction, apparently causing exaggerated metabolism; (3) pituitary dysfunction, in which there is lack of regulation of fat metabolism, and (4) testicular and ovarian hypofunction, the most important of the endocrine factors causing obesity.
  The second of the endogenous factors, nervous abnormality, has been determined by recent investigations which point to a central nervous lesion as being responsible for adiposity. The question of how it affects weight regulation is still problematical. The third endogenous cause is defective salt and water metabolism, which leads to retention of fluid in the tissues. This is associated with overweight, but is not a true obesity. It probably results from an early excess production of prolan, resulting in early puberty and excess of pitressin, causing water retention.
  ETIOL: Sex, obesity being more frequent in the female; race; climate; heredity, and occupation.
  TREATMENT: (1) Prophylaxis, in children of families with a tendency to obesity, in the form of moderate dieting and exercise; (2) dieting; (3) organotherapy, consisting of the administration of thyroid, pituitary or ovarian extracts; (4) dinitrophenol, a very dangerous and toxic metabolic stimulant causing cataracts and in some cases death, and (5) benzedrine sulfate in combination with a relatively low calory diet. Benzedrine stimulates nervous energy, produces a sense of well being, and reduces the desire for food. When used in cases of obesity with hypertension, it has caused a lowering of the blood pressure.
  Diet should be below maintenance requirements so far as energy units are concerned and must be provided with all other essential nutrients. Maintenance requirements are based on what the average weight should be. 1000-1200 calories per day is a slow reduction regimen; 600-800 calories is more rapid, but examination should be made in the 600-800 calory diet for the presence of acetone, and all essential nutrients must be included. Acidosis may result, as body fat may overbalance necessary glucose for the oxidation of fat.
  DIET: The average basic diet is 1000 calories a day, consisting of 90 Gm. of carbohydrate, 75 Gm. of protein, and 38 Gm. of fat. Vegetables and fruits low in carbohydrates, skimmed milk, cottage cheese twice a week in place of meat, eggs, lean meat and vitamin concen-

obesity, endogenous   O-2   **obstruction, intestinal**

trates, if extended for any length of time. Avoid concentrated carbohydrates, fats, whole grain cereals only sparingly.
RS: *carbohydrate, emaciation, fat, height, protein, starch, sugar, vitamin, weight.*

o., endogenous. O. caused by some abnormality within the body, endocrine, nervous, or due to faulty salt and water metabolism.

o., exogenous. O. due to excessive intake of food.

o., hyperplasmic. O. caused by increased quantity of body protoplasm.

o., hypoplasmic. O. due to lowering of body protoplasm and increase in fat and water content.

obex (ō'běks) [L. a band]. BNA. A thin, triangular band of nervous substance over the calamus scriptorius in roof of cranial 4th ventricle.

obfuscation (ŏb-fŭs-kā'shŭn) [L. *obfuscāre*, to darken]. 1. Clouding or dimming, as of the cornea. 2. Mental confusion.

ob'ject [L. *objectum*, a thing thrown before]. That which is visible or tangible to the senses.

o. blindness. Affection in which brain fails to recognize things seen correctly by eyes. SEE: *apraxia.*

o. choice. Selection of love object decided by a fixation developed in pregenital stage.

o. glass, o. lens. Microscope lens closest to the object.

o. libido. Love or interest expressed external to oneself upon persons, objects, causes. SEE: *anaclitic choice.*

o. symbolism. A concept formed, or an emotion incited by seeing an object, as in ideas like *heart* of stone, the *brow* of a hill, the *lap* or *bosom* of *nature*, etc.

objective (ob-jek'tiv) [L. *objectivus*, pert. to something thrown before]. 1. Perceptible to other persons, said of symptoms. 2. Directed toward external things. 3. The lens of a microscope which is closest to the object.

o. symptoms. Those apparent to physical means of diagnosis.

obligate (ŏb'lĭ-gāt) [L. *obligāre*, to bind to]. 1. To make necessary or to require. 2. Compulsory, bound.

o., aerobic. A microbe that must have oxygen in order to live.

o., anaerobic. A microörganism that lives only without oxygen.

o. parasite. One that can exist only at the expense of another plant or organism.

oblique (ŏb-lēk') [L. *obliquus*, slanting]. Slanting; diagonal.

o. muscles. Two muscles of the eye; also 2 in the abdomen and 2 muscles of the atlas.

obliquimeter (ŏb-lĭk-wĭm'ĕt-ĕr) [" + G. *metron*, measure]. Apparatus for indicating the angle of the pelvic brim with the upright body.

obliquity (ŏb-lĭk'wĭ-tĭ) [L. *obliquus*, slanting]. The state of being oblique.

o., Litzmann's. Inclining of the fetal head until the post. parietal bone presents to the uterine canal.

o., Nägele's. Presentation of the fetal head with ant. parietal bone toward the uterine canal with oblique biparietal diameter in relation to the pelvic brim.

o., Roederer's. Presentation of fetal head with occiput at pelvic brim.

obliquus (ŏb-lĭk'wŭs) [L. slanting]. A name applied to several muscles. SEE: *Table of Muscles in Appendix.*

o. reflex. Contraction of ext. obliquus muscle in toto on application of stimulus to skin of thigh below Poupart's ligament.

obliteration (ŏb-lĭt"ĕr-ā'shŭn) [L. *obliterāre*, to deface]. Extinction or complete occlusion of a part by means of surgery, degeneration or disease.

oblongata (ŏb"lŏn-ga'tă) [L. *ob*, before, + *longus*, long]. The medulla oblongata; the cylindrical extension of the spinal cord as it enters the brain, about an inch long, reaching to the pons, and forming part of base of 4th ventricle.
RS: *erection center, oliva, olivary body.*

oblongatal (ŏb"lŏn-gă'tal) [" + *longus*, long]. Rel. to the medulla oblongata.

obmutescence (ŏb-mū-tĕs'ĕns) [L. *obmutescere*, to become dumb]. Loss of vocal power. SYN: *aphonia.*

obnubilation (ŏb-nū-bĭl-ā'shŭn) [L. *obnubilāre*, to befog or darken]. An impaired or confused state of mind.

obscure (ŏb-skūr') [L. *obscurus*, dark]. Hidden, indistinct, as the cause of a condition.

observerscope (ob-ser'ver-skōp). Type of endoscope having 2 branches, so that 2 persons can inspect the same place simultaneously.

obses'sion. An uncontrollable desire to dwell on an idea or an emotion, or to perform a specific act.
It is not uncommon among normal persons, but if not banished may become all compelling and developing into a "compulsion neurosis." A dominating condition in certain psychoses.

o's., impulsive. Those accompanied by action. They sometimes become manias.

o's., inhibitory. O's. accompanied by impediments to action. They represent the phobias, q.v.

o's., intellectual. Recurring and persistent o's. unaccompanied by action. Typical of the habitual worriers.

obses'sional neuro'sis. A psychoneurosis marked by obsessions controlling the behavior of the individual. SYN: *compulsion neurosis.*

obsolete (ŏb'sō-lĕt) [L. *obsoletus*, fallen into disuse]. Indistinct or absent; noting an organ or characteristic having a functional counterpart in an earlier stage.

obstetric, obstetrical (ŏb-stĕt'rĭk, -rī-kăl) [L. *obstetrix*, a midwife, from *obstāre*, to stand before]. Pert. to obstetrics or midwifery.

o. forceps. Instrument used to facilitate delivery of the fetus.

obstetrician (ŏb-stĕt-rĭsh'ăn) [L. *obstetrix*, -ic-, a midwife]. A physician or one who treats women during pregnancy and parturition.

obstetrics (ob-stet'riks) [L. *obstetrix*, a midwife]. Scientific management of women during pregnancy, childbirth and the puerperium.
RS: *childbirth, labor, maieutics, maneuver, midwife, parturition, pregnancy.*

obstipation (ŏb-stĭp-ā'shŭn) [L. *obstipāre*, to stop up]. 1. The act or condition of obstructing. 2. Obstinate or extreme constipation due to an obstruction.

obstruction (ŏb-strŭk'shŭn) [L. *obstructus*, built up before]. 1. Blocking of a structure that prevents it from functioning normally. 2. A thing that impedes; an obstacle.

o., intestinal. Blockage of the lumen of the intestine. SEE: *intestinal o.*

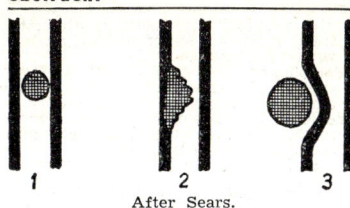

After Sears.
DIAGRAM ILLUSTRATING OBSTRUCTION.
1. Foreign body in the lumen. 2. Disease of the duct wall. 3. Pressure from outside.

obstruent (ŏb'strū-ĕnt) [L. *obstruens*, blocking]. 1. Blocking up. 2. That which closes a normal passage in the body; an astringent.

obtund (ŏb-tŭnd') [L. *obtundere*, to beat against]. To dull or blunt, as sensitivity or pain.

obtundent (ŏb-tŭn'dĕnt) [L. *obtundere*, to beat against]. 1. Deadening sensibility of a part, or reducing irritability, soothing. 2. A soothing remedy.

obturation (ŏb-tū-rā'shŭn) [L. *obturāre*, to stop up]. Closure of a passage or opening.
  o. of teeth. Filling of a cavity.

obturator (ŏb'tū-rā"tor) [L. *obturāre*, to stop up]. 1. Anything that obstructs or closes a cavity or opening. 2. Rel. to the o. membrane. 3. Bridge for spanning the gap in the cleft palate.
  o. foramen. The one in the anterior part of the os innominatum bet. pubis and ischium.
  o. membrane. The sturdy one occluding the o. foramen.
  o. muscles. Two muscles on each side in the pelvic region which rotate the thighs outward. SEE: *Table of Muscles in Appendix, psoas for illustration.*

obtuse (ŏb-tūs') [L. *obtusus*, blunted]. 1. Not pointed or acute; dull or blunt. 2. Stupid; dull mentally.

obtusion (ŏb-tū'zhŭn) [L. *obtusio*, from *obtundere*, to beat against]. Blunting or weakening of normal sensation, as in certain diseases.

occipital (ŏk-sĭp'ĭ-tăl) [L. *occiput*, back of head]. Concerning the back part of the head.
  o. bone. Bone in lower back part of skull bet. the parietal and temporal bones.
  o. lobe. Post. lobe of the cerebral hemisphere which is shaped like a 3-sided pyramid.

occipitalis (ŏk-sĭp"ĭ-tā'lĭs) [L. pert. to back of head]. The posterior portion of the occipitofrontalis muscle at back of the head.

occipito- [L.]. Combining form showing relationship bet. the occiput and another part.

occiput (ŏk'sĭ-pŭt) [L.]. The back part of the skull.

occlude (ō-klŭd') [L. *occludere*, to shut up]. To close up, obstruct or join together, as the masticatory surfaces of the teeth.

occlusio pupillae [L. a closing up of the pupil]. Condition in which the pupil is closed by a membrane.

occlusion (ō-klū'zhŭn) [L. *occlusio*, a closing up]. 1. The closure, or state of being closed, of a passage. SYN: *imperforation*.
  May be acquired or congenital.
  2. Adsorption of gas by a substance which doesn't thereby lose its characteristic property.
  3. Relation of the teeth when the jaws are closed.

oc'cult [L. *occultus*, hidden]. Obscure; hidden, as a hemorrhage.
  o. blood. Blood in such minute quantity that it can only be recognized by microscopic or chemical means.

occupa'tion neuro'sis. A functional disorder of a part, caused by certain occupations, as writer's cramp.

occupa'tional ther'apy. Use of any activity or occupation for purposes of treatment.

ochlesis (ŏk-lē'sĭs) [G. *ochlēsis*, a crowding]. Any disease caused by conditions of overcrowding.

ochlophobia (ŏk-lō-fō'bĭ-ă) [G. *ochlos*, crowd, + *phobos*, fear]. Abnormal dread of crowds or populated places.

ochrodermia (ō"krō-der'mĭ-ă) [G. *ōchros*, pale yellow, + *derma*, skin]. A yellow state of the skin.

ochrometer (ō-krom'ĕt-ĕr) [G. *ōchros*, pallor, + *metron*, measure]. Device for estimating the capillary blood pressure by compression of a finger until its skin becomes blanched.

ochronosis, ochronosus (ō-krō-nō'sĭs, -sŭs) [G. *ōchros*, yellow, + *nosos*, disease]. A rare condition marked by dark pigmentation of the ligaments, cartilage, fibrous tissues, skin and urine.

octa-, octo- [G.]. Combining forms meaning *eight*.

octan (ŏk'tăn) [G. *oktō*, eight]. Reappearing on every 8th day, as a fever.

octane (ŏk'tān) [G. *oktō*, eight]. A hydrocarbon of the paraffin series. CH_3-$(CH_2)_6CH_3$.

octarius (ŏk-ta'rĭ-ŭs) [L.]. Pint.

octavalent (ŏk"tă-vā'lĕnt) [G. *oktō*, eight, + L. *valere*, to have power]. Having a valence of 8.

octipara (ŏk-tĭp'ă-ră) [" + L. *parere*, to bear]. A woman who has given birth to 8 children.

octoroon (ŏk-tō-roon') [G. *oktō*, eight]. One who has one-eighth negro blood and seven-eighths white blood; progeny of a white person and a quadroon.

ocular (ŏk'ū-lăr) [L. *oculus*, eye]. 1. Concerning the eye or vision. 2. Eyepiece of a microscope.

oculist (ŏk'ū-lĭst) [L. *oculus*, eye]. A specialist in diseases of the eye.

oculocephalogyric re'flex (ŏk"ū-lō-sĕf"ă-lo-gī'rĭk). Associated movements of eye, head and body in focalizing vision upon an object.

oculogyration (ŏk"ū-lō-jī-rā'shŭn) [L. *oculus*, eye, + G. *gyros*, circle]. Motions of the eyeball.

oculogyric (ŏk"ū-lō-jī'rĭk) [" + G. *gyros*, circle]. Producing or concerning movements of the eye.

oculomotor (ŏk"ū-lō-mō'tor) [" + *motor*, mover]. Rel. to eye movements. SYN: *oculogyric*.
  o. nerve. The 3rd cranial nerve.

oculomotorius (ŏk"ū-lō-mō-tor'ĭ-ŭs) [L.]. The oculomotor or 3rd cranial nerve.
  The *motor oculi* of the eye.
  FUNCT: Motor. Supplies 5 of the 7 eye muscles.
  ORIGIN: Floor, aquaeductus cerebri.
  DIST: All eye muscles except ext. rectus and sup. oblique. SEE: *cranial nerves.*

oculomycosis (ŏk"ū-lō-mī-kō'sĭs) [L. *oculus*, eye, + G. *mykēs*, fungus, + *-ōsis*]. Any disease of the eye or its parts caused by a fungus.

oculonasal (ŏk"ū-lō-nā'sal) [" + *nasus*,

nose]. Concerning both the eye and the nose.

oculoreaction (ok″ū-lō-rē-ak′shŭn) [" + rē, back, + actus, acting]. A reaction in the eye, upon the instillation of toxins of tuberculosis and typhoid.
More severe in persons suffering from the disease.

oculozygomatic (ok″ū-lō-zī-gō-mat′ĭk) [" + G. zygon, yoke]. Pert. to the eye and zygoma.

o. line. Line bet. inner canthus of eye and cheek supposedly indicating neural disorders.

oculus (ok′ū-lŭs) [L.]. Eye.

O. D. Abbr. for oculus dexter, right eye.

od (ŏd) [G. odos, way]. The supposed magnetic force which acts upon the nervous system to produce hypnotism.
An obsolete theory.

odaxesmus (o-daks-ĕz′mŭs) [G. odaxēsmos, a biting]. 1. The biting of the tongue, lip or cheek during an epileptic attack. 2. Itching or biting sensation, a paresthesia.

odaxetic (o-dăks-ĕt′ĭk) [G. odaxēsmos, a biting]. Producing a stinging or itching sensation.

Oddi's sphincter (ŏd′dī). A contraction at the opening of the common bile duct at the ampulla of Vater.

odogenesis (ō-dō-jĕn′ĕ-sĭs) [G. odos, path, + genesis, formation]. The re-establishment of connections bet. the divided ends of a nerve by nerve process attraction. SYN: neurocladism.

odontagra (ō-dŏn-tăg′ră) [G. odous, odont-, tooth, + agra, seizure]. Toothache, esp. when originating from gout.

odontalgia (o-don-tal′jĭ-ă) [" + algos, pain]. Toothache. SYN: odontodynia.
o., phantom. Pain felt in the area from which a tooth has been pulled.

odontatrophy (ō″dŏn-tăt′rō-fī) [" + atrophia, atrophy]. 1. Decay of the teeth. 2. Imperfect development of the teeth.

odontectomy (ō-dŏn-tek′tō-mĭ) [" + ektomē, excision]. Surgical removal of a tooth.

odonterism (ō-don′tĕr-ĭzm) [" + erismos, quarrel]. Chattering of the teeth.

odontia (ō-dŏn′shĭ-ă) [G. odous, odont-, tooth]. 1. Pain in a tooth. SYN: odontalgia. 2. Condition or abnormality of the teeth.

odontiasis (ō″dŏn-tī′ăs-ĭs) [" + iasis, disease]. 1. Cutting of the teeth. SYN: dentition, teething. 2. Disease caused by teething.

odontitis (ō-dŏn-tī′tĭs) [" + -ītis, inflammation]. Inflammation of the pulp of a tooth.

odonto-, odont- [G.]. Combining form meaning tooth.

odontoblast (ō-don′tō-blăst) [G. odous, odont-, tooth, + blastos, germ]. One of the cells which fill the pulp chamber of the teeth.
They produce the dentine and deposit it in layers on inside of the teeth for years after they have erupted.

odontobothrion (ō-don′tō-both′rĭ-ŏn) [" + bothrion, pit]. Socket of a tooth.

odontodynia (ō-dŏn′tō-dĭn′ĭ-ă) [" + odynē, pain]. Toothache. SYN: odontalgia.

odontogen (ō-don′tō-jĕn) [" + gennan, to produce]. The substance from which dentine arises.

odontogenesis, odontogeny (ō-don″tō-jĕn′ĕ-sĭs, -toj′ĕn-ĭ) [" + genesis, production]. The origin and formation of the teeth.

odontoid (ō-don′toyd) [" + eidos, resemblance]. Toothlike.

o. process. The toothlike projection from upper surface of the body of the 2nd cervical vertebrae.

odontology (ō-dŏn-tol′ō-jĭ) [" + logos, study]. The science of dealing with the teeth and their care. SYN: dentistry.

odontoma (ō-dŏn-tō′mă) [G. odous, odont-, tooth, + -ōma, tumor]. Tumor of a tooth or of the dental tissue.
o., coronary. Bony tumor at crown of a tooth.
o., follicular. Bony shell in gums below tooth margin, usually after 2nd dentition.
ETIOL: Excessive number of dental follicles.
SYM: Crepitating to pressure. They often contain 1 or more teeth. SYN: cyst, dentigerous.
o., radicular. Bony tumor at root of a tooth.

odontonecrosis (ō-don″tō-nĕ-krō′sĭs) [" + nekros, dead, + -ōsis, intensive]. Decay or gangrene of a tooth.

odontopathy (ō-don-top′ăth-ī) [" + pathos, disease]. Any disease of the teeth.

odontophobia (ō-don″tō-fō′bĭ-ă) [" + phobos, fear]. 1. Abnormal aversion to the sight of teeth. 2. Abnormal fear of dental surgery.

odontoplerosis (ō-don″tō-plē-rō′sĭs) [G. odous, odont-, tooth, + plērōsis, filling]. The filling of a dental cavity.

odontoprisis (ō-don″tō-prī′sĭs) [" + prisis, sawing]. Grinding of the teeth.

odontorrhagia (ō-don″tō-rā′jĭ-ă) [" + rēgnunai, to burst forth]. Hemorrhage from a tooth socket following extraction.

odontorthosis (ō-don-tŏr-thō′sĭs) [" + orthos, straight]. Operation of straightening irregular teeth.

odontosis (ō-don-tō′sĭs) [" + -ōsis, intensive]. 1. Development of teeth. 2. Eruption of teeth.

odontotherapy (ō-don′tō-ther′ă-pī) [" + therapeia, treatment]. Care of diseased teeth.

odontotripsis (ō-don″tō-trĭp′sĭs) [" + tripsis, a rubbing]. Natural abrasion of the teeth.

odontotrypy (ō-dŏn-tot′rĭ-pī) [" + trypan, to bore]. 1. Drilling of a tooth. 2. Perforation of a tooth to draw off pus from an inner abscess.
Different locations of abscess call for different treatment.

odor (ō′der) [L. smell]. 1. That quality of a substance which renders it perceptible to sense of smell. 2. Any smell, esp. a sweet scent. 3. Any sensation of sense of smell.
Each odoriferous substance causes its own sensation. Odors have been classed as (a) pure odors, (b) those mixed with sensations from the mucous membrane, (c) those mixed with the sensation of taste.
PURE ODORS: These are aromatic, burning, fragrant, fetid, or nauseating, and repulsive odors.
Another classification is spicy, flowery, fruity, resinous, foul, scorched.
RS: antibromic, "brom-" words, capric, deodorant, effluvium osmolagnia, osphresiolagnia, pungent, smell.

odoriferous (ō″der-ĭf′ĕ-rŭs) [" + ferre, to bear]. Bearing scent, having an odor; fragrant; perfumed.

odorous (ō′der-us) [L. odor, smell]. Having an odor, scent or fragrance.

odynacusis (ō-dĭn-ă-kū′sĭs) [G. odynē, pain, + akusis, hearing]. A condition in which noises cause pain in the ear.

odynometer (ō-dĭn-om′ĕt-ĕr) [" + metron, measure]. Device for measuring pain.

odynophagia (ō-dĭn-ō-fā'jĭ-ă) [" + *phagein*, to eat]. Pain upon swallowing.

odynophobia (ō"dĭn-ō-fō'bĭ-ă) [" + *phobos*, fear]. Abnormal dread of pain.

odynopoeia (ō"dĭn-ō-pē'ă) [" + *poiein*, to make]. Induction of labor pains.

Oedipus com′plex (ē'dĭ-pŭs). Abnormally intense love of the child for parent of the opposite sex retained in adulthood.
Usually involves jealous dislike of the other parent. Most commonly love of a boy for his mother. SEE: *complex*.

Oertel's terrain cure (er'tel). Graduated exercise, mountain climbing, diet, and reduction of fluids for heart cases, obesity, circulatory diseases, etc.

offi′cial. Said of medicines authorized as standard in the U. S. Pharmacopeia, and in the National Formulary.

officinal (of-ĭs'in-al) [L. *officina*, shop]. Regularly kept in a druggist's stock. SEE: *magistral*.

Ogata's method (ō-gah'tă) (M. Ogata, Japanese physician) (respiratory stimulation). 1. Resuscitation in asphyxia by stroking the chest. 2. A manner of stimulating respiration by shaking the body in conjunction with artificial respiration.

-OH. Hydroxyl group.

ohm (ōm). Practical unit of resistance, the resistance through which a difference of potential of 1 volt will produce a current of 1 ampere.
The international or legal ohm is the resistance offered by a column of mercury 106.3 cm. long, 14.45 Gm. in mass, and of constant cross section at 0° C.

O.'s law. The law determined experimentally by the physicist Ohm, which states that the strength of an electric current in a direct current circuit varies directly as the applied electromotive force, and inversely as the resistance of the circuit; or, the current *i* expressed in amperes equals the electromotive force E in volts, divided by the resistance R in ohms:

$$i = \frac{E}{R}$$

-oid [G.]. Suffix meaning *having the form of, or likeness of*, as *ovoid*.

oidiomycetes (ō-ĭd"ĭ-ō-mī-sē'tēs) [*Oidium* + G. *mykēs*, fungus]. A group of fungi including the Oidium.

oidiomycosis (ō-ĭd"ĭ-ō-mī-kō'sĭs) [*Oidium* + G. *mykēs*, fungus, + *-ōsis*]. Disease due to infection by an Oidium.

Oidium (ō-ĭd'ĭ-ŭm) [G. *ōion*, egg]. 1. A genus of fungi of the family *Moniliaceae*. 2. (oidium) A fungus of this genus.
O. albicans. A microscopic fungus that causes thrush.
O. lactis. White mold on bread and sour milk.
O. Schoenlein′ii. Fungus of favus. SYN: *Achorion Schoenleinii*.
O. tonsurans. Fungus of ringworm. *Trichophyton tonsurans*.

oikomania (oy-kō-mā'nĭ-ă) [G. *oikos*, house, + *mania*, madness]. Nervous disorder induced by unhappy home surroundings.

oikophobia (oy"kō-fo'bĭ-ă). Morbid dislike of the home. SYN: *ecomania*.

oil (oyl) [L. *oleum*]. A greasy liquid not miscible with water, usually obtained from a mineral, vegetable or animal source.
According to character, oils are subdivided principally as *fixed* or *fatty*, and *volatile* or *essential*.

Ex: Fixed—*Castor oil, olive oil, cod-liver oil.* Volatile—*Oils of mustard, peppermint, rose.*
RS: *oleaginous, oleate, oleic, olein, oleum, unctuous.*

ointment (oynt'mĕnt) [Fr. *oignement*]. A fatty, soft substance having antiseptic or healing properties.
Its base is usually vaseline, lard or lanolin to which the medicament is added. Applied on linen. It should be spread from the center outwards, so that edges are completely covered. SYN: *salve, unguent.*

okra (ō'kra). AVERAGE SERVING: 50 Gm. Pro. 0.8, Fat 0.1, Carbo. 2.00. VITAMINS: A++, B++, C+. ASH CONST: Ca 0.071, Mg 0.010, K 0.035, Na 0.043, P 0.019, Fe 0.006. No calcium or sulfur.

ol. Abbr. for *oleum*, oil.

O. L. A. Abbr. for L. *occipito laevo anterior*, fetal presentation with the occiput toward the maternal left acetabulum.

old age. Human life after 70 years.
DISEASES COMMON TO: *Aortic, apoplexy, bronchopneumonia, chronic bronchitis, cancer, cerebral disorders, emphysema, myocarditis, prostatic, senile dementia.*
o. sight. Defective changes in vision due to advancing old age.

olea (ō'lē-a) [L. oils, olive]. 1. L. for *olive*. 2. Pl. of *oleum, oils*.

oleaginous (ō-lē-ăj'ĭ-nŭs) [L. *oleaginus*, oily]. Greasy; oily; unctuous.

oleate (ō'lē-āt) [L. *oleatum*]. 1. Any salt of oleic acid. 2. Salt of oleic acid dissolved in an excess of the acid.

oleatum (ō-lē-at'ŭm) [L.]. Preparation made by dissolving metallic salts or alkaloids in oleic acid. SYN: *oleate*, 2.

olecranal (ō-lĕk'răn-ăl) [G. *ōlekranon*, elbow]. Concerning the olecranon.

olecranarthritis (ō-lĕk"răn-ar-thrī'tĭs) [G. *ōlekranon*, elbow, + *arthron*, joint, + *-itis*, inflammation]. Inflamed condition of the elbow joint.

olecranarthrocace (ō-lĕk"răn-ar-throk'ă-sē) [" + " + *kakē*, badness]. Tuberculous ulceration of the elbow joint.

olecranarthropathy (ō-lĕk"răn-ar-throp'ăth-ĭ) [" + " + *pathos*, disease]. Any disease of the elbow joint.

olecranoid (ō-lĕk'răn-oyd) [" + *eidos*, resemblance]. Similar to the olecranon.

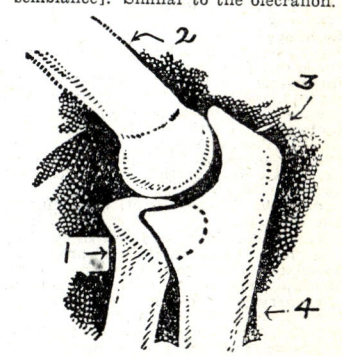

OLECRANON.
1. Radius. 2. Humerus. 3. Olecranon. 4. Ulna.

olecranon (ō-lĕk'răn-ŏn, ō"lē-krā'nŏn) [G. elbow]. BNA. A large process of the ulna projecting behind the elbow joint

oleic   O-6   **oligophosphaturia**

and forming the bony prominence of the elbow.
FRACTURE OF: Prevent spasm of triceps muscle to avoid separation of fragments. Latter may have to be wired.
TREATMENT: Similar to that for fracture of patella, q.v. SEE: *skeleton*.

oleic (ō-lē'ĭk) [L. *oleum*, oil]. Derived from or pert. to oil.
  o. acid. A colorless, oily liquid prepared from fats, the salts of which are *oleates*.

olein (ō'lē-ĭn) [L. *oleum*, oil]. An oleate of glyceryl found in nearly all fixed oils and fats; an important part of oils. SYN: *triolein*.

oleo- [L.]. Combining form meaning *oil*.

oleoarthrosis (ō″lē-ō-ar-thrō'sĭs) [L. *oleum*, oil, + G. *arthron*, joint, + *-ōsis*]. Therapeutic introduction of oil into a joint.

oleoinfusion (ō″lē-ō-ĭn-fū'zhŭn) [" + *in*, into, + *fusus*, poured]. Combination of a drug and oil.

oleomargarine (ō″lē-ō-mar'jă-rēn) [" + *margarine*]. Artificial butter from fats of beef, soy bean, cottonseed, etc.

oleoresin (o″le-o-rez'in) [" + *resina*, resin]. Extract of plant containing resinous substance and oil, prepared by dissolving the crude drug in ether, acetone or alcohol.

oleosaccharum (ō-lē-ō-sak'ăr-ŭm) [" + G. *sakcharon*, sugar]. A substance compounded of sugar and volatile oil.

oleotherapy (ō″lē-ō-ther'ă-pĭ) [" + G. *therapeia*, treatment]. Therapeutic injection of oil. SYN: *eleotherapy*.

oleothorax (ō-lē-ō-thō'răks) [" + G. *thōrax*, chest]. Therapeutic injection of oil into the pleural cavity.

oleum (ō'lē-ŭm) [L.]. Oil.
  o. morrhuae. Cod-liver oil.
  o. percomorphum. Mixture of oils from livers of various members of order Percomorphi. More potent than cod-liver oil in Vitamins A and D.
  o. ricini. Castor oil.

olfactie (ŏl-făk'tĭ) [L. *olfacere*, to smell]. Unit of smell; the threshold of stimulation for an odor.

olfaction (ŏl-fak'shŭn) [L. *olfacere*, to smell]. The sense of smell. Smelling.

olfactive (ŏl-fak'tĭv) [L. *olfacere*, to smell]. Pert. to the sense of smell. SYN: *olfactory*.

olfactology (ŏl-făk-tol'ō-jĭ) [" + G. *logos*, study]. Scientific investigation of sense of smell.

olfactometer (ŏl″fak-tom'et-ĕr) [" + G. *metron*, measure]. Apparatus for testing the power of the sense of smell.

olfactory (ŏl-făk'tō-rĭ) [L. *olfacere*, to smell]. Pert. to smell.
  o. area. A. in the hippocampal convolution. Ant. portion of the callosal gyrus and the uncus.
  o. bulb. Enlarged ant. extremity of the o. nerve. [nix.
  o. bundle. Mass of fibers in the for-
  o. lobe. A cranial lobe projecting from ant. lower part of each cerebral hemisphere.   [nasal organ.
  o. nerves. The nerves supplying the First pair of cranial nerves.
Differs from other nerves in being composed exclusively of nonmedullated fibers. FUNCT: Special sense of smell. ORIG: Olfactory bulb. DIST: Nasal mucous membrane. BRS: It has 20 brs.
  o. organ. The nose.

oligemia (ol-ig-e'mĭ-ă) [G. *oligos*, little, + *aima*, blood]. Deficient amount of blood in the body. SYN: *oligohemia*.

oligergasia (ol-ĭ-gĕr-ga'sĭ-ă) [" + *ergasia*, work]. Psychic disorder from deficiency due to imperfect development.

olighydria (ol-ĭ-gĭd'rĭ-ă) [" + *ydōr*, water]. Deficient perspiration.

oligo-, olig- [G.]. Combining form meaning *small* or, in the plural sense, *few*.

oligocholia (ol-ĭg-ō-kō'lĭ-ă) [G. *oligos*, little, + *cholē*, bile]. Lack of bile.

oligochromemia (ol″ĭg-ō-krō-mē'mĭ-ă) [" + *chrōma*, color, + *aima*, blood]. Lack of sufficient hemoglobin in the blood.

oligochylia (ol-ĭ-gō-ki'lĭ-ă) [" + *chylos*, juice]. Deficiency of chyle.

oligochymia (ol-ĭg-ō-ki'mĭ-ă) [" + *chymos*, juice]. Deficiency of chyme.

oligocystic (ol-ĭ-gō-sĭst'ĭk) [" + *kystis*, a bladder]. Having just a few cysts, as a tumor.

oligocythemia (ol″ĭ-gō-sī-thē'mĭ-ă) [" + *kytos*, cell, + *aima*, blood]. Deficiency in number of red blood corpuscles.

oligocytosis (ol″ĭ-gō-sī-tō'sĭs) [" + " + *-ōsis*, intensive]. Deficiency of red blood corpuscles. SYN: *oligocythemia*.

oligodactylia (ol-ĭ-gō-dăk-tĭl'ĭ-ă) [" + *daktyllos*, digit]. Subnormal number of fingers or toes.

oligodendroglia (ol″ĭ-gō-den-drog'lĭ-ă) [" + *dendron*, a tree, + *glia*, glue]. Adventitial cells found in central nervous system, with characteristic vinelike processes. SYN: *mesoglia*.

oligodipsia (ol-ĭ-gō-dĭp'sĭ-ă) [G. *oligos*, few, + *dipsa*, thirst]. Abnormal lack of desire for fluids.

oligodynamic (ŏl″ĭ-gō-dī-năm'ĭk) [" + *dynamis*, power]. Effective in a small quantity.

oligoerythrocythemia (ol″ĭ-gō-er″ĭth-rō-sī-thē'mĭ-ă) [" + *erythros*, red, + *kytos*, cell, + *aima*, blood]. Deficiency of hemoglobin or red blood corpuscles.

oligogalactia (ol″ĭ-gō-gă-lak'tĭ-ă) [" + *gala, galakt-*, milk]. Deficient milk secretion.

oligogenics (ol-ĭ-gō-jĕn'ĭks) [" + *gennan*, to produce]. Limitation of the number of offspring by artificial mediums such as contraceptives. SYN: *birth control*.

oligoglobulia (ol″ĭ-gō-glŏb-ū'lĭ-ă) [" + L. *globulus*, globule]. Deficiency of red blood corpuscles. SYN: *oligocythemia*.

oligohemia (ol″ĭ-gō-hē'mĭ-ă) [" + *aima*, blood]. Insufficiency of blood in the body. SYN: *oligemia*.

oligohydramnios (ol″ĭg-ō-hī-dram'nĭ-ŏs) [" + *ydōr*, water, + *amnion*, amnion]. Abnormally small amount of amniotic fluid.

oligohydruria (ol″ĭ-gō-hī-drū'rĭ-ă) [G. *oligos*, few, + *ydōr*, water, + *ouron*, urine]. Highly concentrated urine.

oligoleukocythemia (ol″ĭ-gō-lū″kō-sī-thē'-mĭ-ă) [" + *leukos*, white, + *kytos*, cell, + *aima*, blood]. Reduction in leukocytic content of blood. SYN: *leukopenia*.

oligoleukocytosis (ol″ĭ-gō-lū″kō-sī-tō'sĭs) [" + " +]. Decreased number of leukocytes in the blood. SYN: *leukopenia, oligoleukocythemia*.

oligomania (ol-ĭ-gō-mā'nĭ-ă) [" + *mania*, madness]. Insanity involving only a few mental faculties.

oligomastigate (ol-ĭ-gō-mas'tĭ-gāt) [" + *mastix, mastig-*, whip]. Characterized by 2 flagella.

oligomenorrhea (ol″ĭg-ō-mĕn-ō-rē'ă) [" + *mēn*, month, + *roia*, flow]. Scanty or infrequent menstrual flow.

oligopepsia (ol-ĭ-gō-pĕp'sĭ-ă) [" + *pepsis*, digestion]. Insufficient digestive tone.

oligophosphaturia (ol″ĭ-gō-fŏs-făt-ū'rĭ-ă) [" + *phosphas*, phosphate, + *ouron*,

oligophrenia   O-7   **omentum**

urine]. Scanty amount of phosphates in the urine.

oligophrenia (ol″ĭg-ō-frē′nĭ-ă) [G. *oligos*, few, + *phrēn*, mind]. Mental deficiency due to faulty development. SYN: *imbecility*.

oligoplasmia (ŏl″ĭg-ō-plăz′mĭ-ă) [" + *plasmos*, a thing formed]. Insufficient amt. of blood plasma.

oligopnea (ol-ĭg-op′nē-ă) [" + *pnoia*, breath]. Infrequent respiration. SYN: *hypopnea*.

Respiration shallow or abnormally deep; rate as slow as 6-10 per minute. Usually accompanied by slow pulse, although high in some conditions.

ETIOL: Cerebral compression, meningeal or pontine hemorrhage, cerebral or cerebellar tumors, abscess, gumma of meninges, osteoma of cranium, some forms of meningitis, trauma of brain, drug poisoning, shock, constitutional diseases, etc.

oligoposia (ol-ĭ-gō-pō′sĭ-ă) [" + *posis*, drink]. Inadequate use of liquids in diet. SYN: *oligoposy*.

oligoposy (ol-ĭ-gop′ō-sĭ) [" + *posis*, drink]. Insufficient use of liquids in the diet. SYN: *oligoposia*.

oligoptyalism (ol-ĭ-gō-tī′ă-lĭzm) [" + *ptyalon*, saliva]. Insufficient secretion of saliva. SYN: *oligosialia*.

oligoria (ol-ĭ-gō′rĭ-ă) [G. *oligoria*, apathy]. A form of melancholia in which there is apathy toward things and people.

oligosialia (ol″ĭ-gō-sĭ-a′lĭ-ă) [G. *oligos*, few, + *sialon*, saliva]. Scanty salivary secretion. SYN: *oligoptyalism*.

oligospermia (ŏl″ĭ-gō-spĕr′mĭ-ă) [" + *sperma*, seed]. Paucity of spermatozoa in seminal fluid.

It may be temporary or permanent. SEE: *aspermatism*.

oligotrophia (ŏl″ĭ-gō-trof′ĭ-ă) [" + *trophē*, nourishment]. Insufficient nourishment.

oligotrophy (ol-ĭ-gō′trō-fĭ) [" + *trophē*, nourishment]. Inadequate nutrition.

oliguresis (ol-ĭg-ū-rē′sĭs) [" + *ourēsis*, urination]. Scantiness of urine; infrequent urination.

oliguria (ol-ĭg-ū′rĭ-ă) [" + *ouron*, urine]. Diminished amt. and frequency of urination.

ETIOL: Seen after profuse perspiration, bleeding, and diarrhea. Also in retention of urine due to brain disease, drug poisoning, deep coma.

oliva (ō-lī′vă) [L. olive]. BNA. An olive-shaped gray body behind the ant. pyramid of the medulla oblongata. SEE: *olivary body*.

ol′ivary [L. *oliva*, olive]. Shaped like an olive; oval.

   o. body. One of 2 oval prominences on each side of the ant. surface of the medulla oblongata just below the pons.

olive. AVERAGE SERVING (green): 25 Gm. Pro. 0.3, Fat 6.9, Carbo. 2.9. AVERAGE SERVING (ripe) : 20 Gm. Pro. 0.3, Fat 5.0, Carbo. 0.8. ASH (green): Ca 0.122, Mg 0.002, K 1.526, Na 0.128, P 0.014, Cl 0.004, S 0.027, Fe 0.0029. VITAMINS (green): A++. A base-forming food. Alkalinity, 45 cc. per 100 Gm.

   o. oil enema. Mix 4 oz. of olive oil with 1 dr. of turpentine, beating the mixture well so as to break the oil globules.

This will cause sufficient peristalsis to move the bowels.

olive (ŏl′ĭv) [L. *oliva*, olive]. Oliva, BNA.

   o., inferior. Olivary body.

   o., superior. Layer of gray matter with a core in the cerebellar hemispheres. SYN: *nucleus dentatus*.

-ology [G.]. Suffix meaning *science of, knowledge, study of*.

olophonia (ol-ō-fōn′ĭ-ă) [G. *oloos*, destroyed, + *phōnē*, voice]. Malformation of vocal organs with resulting unnatural speech.

Olshausen's sign (ŏls′how-zĕn). If a tumor ant. to uterus is found in an unmarried woman it will probably be a dermoid* cyst.

-oma [G.]. Suffix denoting *a tumor*.

omagra (ō-mag′ră) [G. *ōmos*, shoulder, + *agra*, seizure]. Attack of gout in the shoulder.

omalgia (ō-mal′jĭ-ă) [" + *algos*, pain]. Neuralgia of shoulder.

omarthritis (ō-mar-thrī′tĭs) [" + *arthron*, joint, + *-itis*, inflammation]. Inflamed condition of the shoulder joint.

Ombrédanne's mask (ŏm-brā-dăhn′). Mask for ether administration in exact dosage.

ombrophobia (ŏm-brō-fō′bĭ-ă) [G. *ombros*, rain, + *phobos*, fear]. Fear and anxiety induced by storms, threatening clouds, or rain.

ombrophore (om′brō-for) [" + *phoros*, a carrier]. Portable apparatus for administering shower baths.

omental (ō-měn′tăl) [L. *omentum*, covering]. Pert. to the omentum, the peritoneal fold supporting the viscera.

omentectomy (ō-měn-těk′tō-mĭ) [" + G. *ektomē*, excision]. Surgical removal of a portion of the omentum.

omentitis (ō-měn-tī′tĭs) [" + G. *-itis*, inflammation]. Inflamed condition of omentum.

omentopexy (ō-měn′tō-pěks″ĭ) [" + *pēxis*, fixation]. Fixation of the omentum to the abdominal wall.

omentorrhaphy (ō-měn-tor′ră-fĭ) [" + G. *raphē*, a sewing]. Suture of the omentum.

omentosplenopexy (ō-men″tō-splē′nō-pěks-ĭ) [" + G. *splēn*, spleen, + *pēxis*, fixation]. Fixation of the spleen and omentum. Omentopexy and splenopexy.

omentotomy (ō-měn-tot′ō-mĭ) [" + G. *tomē*, incision]. Surgery of the omentum.

omentum (ō-měn′tŭm) (pl. *omenta*) [L. a covering]. A fold of peritoneal layers connecting and supporting the viscera.

The omenta are the *great o.*, or *gastrocolic*; the *gastrosplenic o.*, and the *lesser*, or *gastrohepatic o*.

PALPATION OF: Cancerous and tubercular enlargements are distinguished by

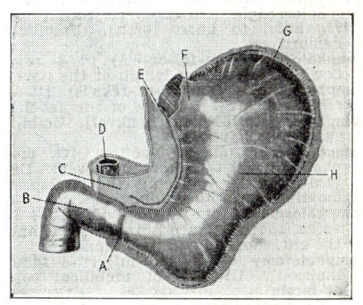

STOMACH AND LESSER OMENTUM.
A. Pylorus. B. Duodenum. C. Lesser omentum. D. Portal vein. E. Left gastric artery. F. Cardiac part. G. Fundus. H. Body.

omentum, great   O-8   **one-two-three enema**

the fact that they extend across the abdomen; and cannot be traced backward; they do not ascend behind the ribs; are rough, hard, and uneven.
RS: *abdomen, caul, epiploon, kidney, ovary, spleen.*
o., great. It is suspended from the greater curvature of the stomach. It contains fat and aids in keeping the intestines warm, and preventing friction. SYN: *epiploon majus.*
o., lesser. It passes from the lesser curvature of stomach to transverse fissure of the liver. SYN: *epiploon minus.*
omitis (ō-mī'tĭs) [G. *ōmos*, shoulder, + *-itis*, inflammation]. Inflamed condition of the shoulder.
omni- (om'nĭ) [L.]. Prefix meaning *all.*
omnip'otence of thought. PSY: Infantile concept of reality whereby one expects his wishes to be instantly accomplished, as a child that gains its objectives through crying, comes to believe in his own omnipotence because of a parent's surrender to his demands.
omnivorous (ŏm-nĭv'ō-rŭs) [L. *omnis*, all, + *vorāre*, to eat greedily]. Living on all kinds of food.
omo- [G.]. Combining form meaning *shoulder* or *pert. to the shoulder.*
omodynia (ō-mō-dĭn'ĭ-ă) [G. *ōmos*, shoulder, + *odynē*, pain]. Pain of the shoulder.
omohyoid (ō-mō-hī'oyd) [" + *yoeidēs*, y-shaped]. 1. Concerning the scapula and the hyoid bone. 2. Muscle attached to the hyoid bone and the scapula.
omophagia (ō-mō-fā'jĭ-ă) [G. *ōmos*, raw, + *phagein*, to eat]. The custom of eating foods raw, esp. flesh.
omphal-, omphalo [G.]. Combining form *relating to the navel.*
omphalectomy (ŏm-făl-ek'tō-mĭ) [G. *omphalos*, navel, + *ektomē*, excision]. Surgical removal of the umbilicus.
omphalic (om-fal'ĭk) [G. *omphalikos*, pert. to the navel]. Concerning the umbilicus.
omphalitis (ŏm-făl-ī'tĭs) [G. *omphalos*, navel, + *itis*, inflammation]. Inflamed condition of the navel.
omphalocele (ŏm-făl'ō-sēl) [G. *omphalos*, navel, + *kēlē*, hernia]. Hernia of the navel. SEE: *hernia.*
omphalomesenteric (om"fal-ō-měs-ěn-ter'-ĭk) [" + *mesenterion*, mesentery]. Concerning the umbilicus and mesentery.
omphaloncus (om-fal-on'kŭs) [" + *ogkos*, tumor]. Umbilical tumor or swelling.
omphalophlebitis (ŏm"făl-ō-flē-bī'tĭs) [" + *phleps*, vein, + *-itis*, inflammation]. Inflamed condition of umbilical veins.
omphalorrhagia (ŏm"făl-ŏr-rā'jĭ-ă) [" + *rēgnunai*, to burst forth]. Umbilical hemorrhage.
omphalorrhea (om-fal-or-ē'ă) [" + *roia*, flow]. Discharge of lymph at the navel.
omphalorrhexis (om-fal-or-rĕks'ĭs) [" + *rēxis*, rupture]. Rupture of the navel.
omphalos (om'făl-ŏs) [G. navel]. Umbilicus. SYN: *navel.*
omphalosotor (om-fal-ō-sō'tor) [G. *omphalos*, navel, + *sōtēr*, preserver]. Device used in replacing the prolapsed umbilical cord at childbirth.
omphalospinous (om-fal-ō-spī'nŭs) [" + L. *spina*, thorn]. Concerning the navel and the ant. sup. spine of the ilium.
omphalotomy (om-făl-ot'ō-mĭ) [" + *tomē*, incision]. Division of umbilical cord at birth.
DRESSING: Cotton gauze, borated calendula powder.
omphalotripsy (om'făl-ō-trĭp'sĭ) [" + *tripsis*, a rubbing]. Severing of the umbilical cord by a crushing method.

onanism (ō'năn-ĭzm). Coitus interruptus,* so named because it was practiced by the Biblical character Onan, but the term is used also, erroneously, to designate masturbation, *q.v.*
onanist (ō'năn-ĭst). One who practices coitus interruptus or, erroneously, masturbation.
Onanoff's reflex (ŏn-ăh-nŏf'). Contraction of bulbocavernous muscle resulting from compression of glans penis.
onchocerca (ŏng-kŏ-ser'kă) [G. *ogkos*, hook, + *kerkos*, tail]. A genus of filarial worms.
onchocerciasis (ŏng-kŏ-ser-kī'ăs-ĭs) [" + " + *iasis*, infestation]. Condition produced by infestation with 1 of the species of Onchocerca. SYN: *onchocercosis.*
oncogenesis (ong"kō-jĕn'ĕ-sĭs) [G. *ogkos*, mass]. Tumor formation and development.
oncogenous (ong-koj'ĕ-nŭs) [" + *gennan*, to produce]. Forming or producing tumors.
oncograph (ŏng'kō-grăf) [" + *graphein*, to write]. Device attached to oncometer for making record of the internal organs' size.
oncology (ŏng-kŏl'ō-jĭ) [" + *logos*, study]. The branch of medicine dealing with tumors.
oncolysis (ŏng-kol'ĭ-sĭs) [" + *lysis*, dissolution]. The absorption or dissolution of tumor cells.
oncolytic (ong-kō-lĭt'ĭk) [" + *lysis*, dissolution]. Destructive to tumor cells.
oncoma (ong-kō'mă) [G. *ogkōma*, a swelling]. A tumor or swelling.
Term is no longer commonly used.
oncometer (ŏng-kom'ĕt-ĕr) [G. *ogkos*, mass, + *metron*, measure]. Apparatus for measurement of variations in size of the internal organs. SEE: *plethysmograph.*
oncosis (ŏng-kō'sĭs) [" + *-ōsis*, intensive]. 1. A condition characterized by the development of tumors. 2. A swelling or tumor.
oncosphere (ong"kō-sfēr) [G. *ogkos*, hook, + *sphaira*, sphere]. Embryonic stage of a tapeworm in which it has hooks.
oncothlipsis (ŏng-kō-thlĭp'sĭs) [G. *ogkos*, tumor, + *thlipsis*, pressure]. Pressure due to presence of a tumor.
oncotic (ŏng-kŏt-ĭk) [G. *ogkos*, tumor]. Concerning, caused, or marked by swelling.
oncotomy (ŏng-kot'ō-mĭ) [" + *tomē*, incision]. The operation of cutting into a tumor, abscess, or boil.
oncotropic (ong-kō-trop'ĭk) [" + *tropos*, a turning]. Possessing special attraction for tumor cells. SYN: *tumoraffin.*
oneiric (ō-nī'rĭk) [G. *oneiros*, dream]. Resembling, rel. to, or accompanied by dreams.
oneirism (ō-nī'rĭzm) [" + *ismos*, state of]. A condition of cerebral automatism resembling the prolongation of a dream after waking.
oneirodynia (ō-nī-rō-dĭn'ĭ-ă) [" + *odynē*, pain]. Painful dreaming; nightmare.*
o. activa. Walking while sleeping. SYN: *somnambulism.*
o. gravans. A bad dream. SYN: *nightmare.*
oneirology (ō-nī-rol'ō-jĭ) [" + *logos*, study of]. The scientific aspect of dreams.
oneiroscopy (o-nī-ros'kō-pĭ) [" + *skopein*, to examine]. Analysis of dreams in the diagnosis of the individual's mental state.
one-two-three enema. One consisting of

oniomania

one oz. magnesium sulfate, *two* oz. glycerin, and *three* oz. water. SEE: *enema.*

oniomania (ō-nĭ-ō-mā'nĭ-ă) [G. *ōnios,* for sale, + *mania,* madness]. A psychoneurotic symbolism evidenced by an abnormal urge to spend money.

onion (ŭn'yŭn) [L. *uniō,* onion]. AVERAGE SERVING (white): 50 Gm. Pro. 0.8, Fat 0.2, Carbo. 4.0. VITAMINS: A— to +, B+, C++, G+. ASH CONST: Ca 0.034, Mg 0.016, K 0.178, Na 0.016, P 0.045, Cl 0.021, S 0.070, Fe 0.0006. A base forming food; alkalinity, 1.5 cc. per 100 Gm., or 3.1 cc. per 100 cal. ACTION: Appetizer and stimulant to gastric tract. Onions cause flatulence and irritability, although boiling reduces this tendency.

oniric (ō-nī'rĭk) [G. *oneiros,* dream]. Concerning a dream. SYN: *oneiric.*

onirism (ō-nī'rĭzm) [" + *ismos,* state]. Dreamlike hallucination in a waking state. SYN: *oneirism.*

onkinocele (ŏng-kĭn'ō-sēl) [G. *ogkos,* mass, + *is, in-,* fiber, + *kēlē,* swelling]. Inflammation, with swelling, of a tendon sheath.

onomatology (ŏn-o-mă-tol'ō-jĭ) [G. *onoma,* name, + *logos,* study]. Science of names. SYN: *nomenclature, terminology.*

onomatomania (ŏn-ō-mă-tō-mā'nĭ-ă) [" + *mania,* madness]. An abnormal or morbid impulse to dwell upon and repeat certain words, their imagined hidden meanings and significance, or to try to recall frantically a particular word.

onomatophobia (ŏn-ō-mă-tō-fō'bĭ-ă) [" + *phobos,* fear]. Condition in which there is abnormal fear of hearing a certain name or word, because of an imaginary dreadful meaning attached to it.

onomatopoiesis (ŏn-ō-mă-tō-poy-ē'sĭs) [" + *poiein,* to make]. Imitation of natural sounds by the use of created, usually meaningless, imitative words and sounds.

onto- [G.]. Combining form, *being.*

ontogenesis (ŏn″tō-jĕn'ĕ-sĭs) [G. *ōn, ont-,* being, + *genesis,* formation]. Origin and development of the individual. SYN: *ontogeny.*

ontogeny (ŏn-toj'ĕn-ĭ) [" + *gennan,* to produce]. 1. The history of the development of an individual. 2. The belief that the human species was an act of special creation. SYN: *ontogenesis.* SEE: *phylogeny.*

onychatrophia (ŏn″ĭ-kă-trō'fĭ-ă) [G. *onyx, onych-,* nail, + *a-,* priv. + *trophē,* nourishment]. Wasting away of the nails.

onychauxis (ŏn″ĭ-kawk'sĭs) [" + *auxein,* to increase]. Hypertrophy of the nails.

onychia (on-ĭk'ĭ-ă) [G. *onyx, onych-,* nail]. Inflammation of the nail bed with suppuration and, frequently, loss of the nail. SYN: *onychitis.* SEE: *paronychia.*

  o. lateralis. Suppuration of tissues in the area lateral to fingernail.

  o. maligna. Type in debilitated persons in which there is fetid ulceration and loss of the nail.

  o. parasitica. Any parasitic disease of the nails.

onychitis (on-ĭk-ī'tĭs) [" + *-itis,* inflammation]. Inflammation of the nail bed. SYN: *onychia.*

onychocryptosis (ŏn″ĭ-kō-krĭp-tō'sĭs) [" + *kryptein,* to conceal]. Ingrowing of the toenail.

onychograph (ŏn-ĭk'ō-grăf) [" + *graphein,* to write]. Device for making record of capillary blood pressure under the fingernails.

onychogryposis (ŏn″ĭ-kō-grĭ-pō'sĭs) [" + *gryposis,* a curving]. Abnormal growth of the nails with inward curvature.

onychoid (on'ĭ-koyd) [" + *eidos,* resemblance]. Similar to a nail, esp. a fingernail.

onycholysis (ŏn-ĭ-kol'ĭ-sĭs) [" + *lysis,* destruction]. Loosening or detachment of the nail from the nail bed.

onychoma (on-ĭ-kō'mă) [G. *onyx, onych-,* nail, + *-ōma,* tumor]. Tumor of the nail or the nail bed.

onychomalacia (ŏn″ĭ-kō-mă-lā'sĭ-ă) [" + *malakia,* softening]. Unnatural softening of the nails. SEE: *hapalonychia.*

onychomycosis (ŏn″ĭ-kō-mī-kō'sĭs) [" + *mykēs,* fungus, + *-ōsis*]. Disease of the nails due to a parasitic fungus.

onychonosus (ŏn-ĭ-kon'ō-sŭs) [" + *nosos,* disease]. Any disease of the nails.

onychopathy (ŏn-ĭ-kop'ăth-ĭ) [" + *pathos,* disease]. Any disease of the nails. SYN: *onychonosus.*

onychophagy (ŏn-ĭ-kof'ă-jĭ) [" + *phagein,* to eat]. The practice of nail biting.

onychophosis (ŏn-ĭk-ō-fō'sĭs) [" + *yphē,* web]. Accumulation of horny layers of epidermis under the toenail.

onychophyma (ŏn″ĭ-kō-fī'mă) [G. *onyx, onycho,* nail, + *phyma,* a growth]. Painful degeneration of the nail with hypertrophy.

onychoptosis (ŏn-ĭk-ŏp-tō'sĭs) [" + *ptōsis,* a falling]. Dropping off of the nails.

onychorrhexis (ŏn″ĭ-kō-rĕk'sĭs) [" + *rēxis,* a rupture]. Nail splitting.

onychosis (ŏn-ĭ-kō'sĭs) [" + *-ōsis,* disease]. Any diseased condition of the nails. SYN: *onychopathy.*

onychotomy (ŏn-ĭ-kot'ō-mĭ) [" + *tomē,* incision]. Surgical incision of a fingernail or toenail.

onychotrophy (ŏn-ĭ-kŏt'rō-fĭ) [" + *trophē,* nourishment]. Nourishment of the nails.

onyx (on'ĭks) [G. *onyx,* nail]. 1. A fingeror toenail. 2. Pus collection bet. the corneal layers of the eye.

onyxis (ŏn-ĭk'sĭs) [G. *onyx,* nail]. Ingrowing of the nails.

onyxitis (ŏn-ĭk-sī'tĭs) [" + *-itis,* inflammation]. Inflamed condition of matrix of a nail, with suppuration and loss of the nail. SYN: *onychia.*

oö- [G.]. Combining form denoting an *egg,* or the *primordial cell* that develops into an ovule.

oöblast (ō'ō-blăst) [G. *ōon,* egg, + *blastos,* germ]. A cell derived from the germinal epithelium which gives rise to an ovum.

oöcyesis (ō″ō-sī-ē'sĭs) [" + *kyēsis,* pregnancy]. Ectopic pregnancy in the ovary.

oöcyst (ō'ō-sĭst) [" + *kystis,* bladder]. 1. An encased oöspore, before or after cell division. 2. The membrane enclosing the oöspore.

oöcyte (ō'ō-sīt) [" + *kytos,* cell]. The early or primitive ovum before it has developed completely.

oögenesis (ō″ō-jĕn'ĕ-sĭs) [" + *genesis,* formation]. Formation and development of the ovum.

oögonium (ō″ō-gō'nĭ-ŭm) (pl. *oögonia*) [" + *gonē,* generation]. 1. The primordial cell from which an oöcyte originates. 2. Descendant of primordial cell from which the oöcyte arises. 3. Female element of a fungus, which forms the oöspore when fertilized.

oökinesis (ō″ō-kĭn-ē'sĭs) [" + *kinēsis,* movement]. The movements of division taking place in an ovum during maturation, fertilization, and segmentation, esp. active changes of the vitellus.

oöphor- [G.]. Form indicating *ovary*.

oöphoralgia (ō″ŏf-ō-ral′jĭ-ă) [G. *ōon*, egg, + *phoros*, bearing, + *algos*, pain]. Neuralgic pain in an ovary.

oöphorauxe (ō″ŏf-ō-rawks′ē) [" + " + *auxein*, to increase]. Ovarian enlargement.

oöphorectomy (ō″ŏf-ō-rĕk′tō-mĭ) [" + + *ektomē*, excision]. Excision of an ovary. SYN: *ovariectomy*.
POSITION: Dorsal, followed perhaps by Trendelenburg.

oöphorin (ō-ŏf′ō-rĭn) [" + *phoros*, bearing]. A commercial hormone preparation made from cow and swine ovaries.

oöphoritis (ō″ŏf-o-rī′tis) [" + " + -*itis*, inflammation]. Inflamed condition of the ovary. SYN: *ovaritis, q.v.*
o., follicular. Inflammation of the graafian follicles.

oöphorocystosis (ō-ŏf″ō-rō-sĭs-tō′sĭs) [" + " + *kystis*, cyst, + -*ōsis*]. Development of an ovarian cyst.

oöphoroepilepsy (ō-of″ō-rō-ĕp′ĭ-lĕp-sĭ) [G. *ōon*, egg, + *phoros*, bearing, + *epilēpsia*, seizure]. Epilepsy caused by irritation or disease of the ovary.

oöphorohysterectomy (ō-ŏf″ō-rō-hĭs-tĕr-ĕk′tō-mĭ) [" + " + *ystera*, uterus, + *ektomē*, excision]. Surgical removal of the uterus and ovaries. SYN: *oöthecohysterectomy*.

oöphoroma (ō-ŏf-ō-rō′mă) [" + " + -*ōma*, tumor]. Malignant ovarian tumor.

oöphoromania (ō-ŏf″ō-rō-mā′nĭ-ă) [" + " + *mania*, madness]. Insanity arising from an ovarian disease.

oöphoron (ō-ŏf′ō-rŏn) [" + *phoros*, bearing]. An ovary. SYN: *oötheca.*

oöphoropeliopexy (ō-ŏf″ō-rō-pe′lĭ-ō-pĕk-sĭ) [" + " + *pēlios*, pelvis, + *pēxis*, fixation]. Suture of a displaced ovary to the pelvic wall.

oöphoropexy (ō-ŏf′ō-rō-pĕk″sĭ) [G. *ōon* + *phoros*, bearing, + *pēxis*, fixation]. Fixation of a displaced ovary. SYN: *oöphoropeliopexy*.

oöphorosalpingectomy (ō-ŏf″ō-rō-săl-pĭn-jĕk′tō-mĭ) [" + " + *salpigx*, tube, + *ektomē*, excision]. Excision of an oviduct and ovary. POSITION: Dorsal.

oöphorostomy (ō-ŏf-ō-rŏs′tō-mĭ) [" + " + *stoma*, opening]. Creation of artificial opening into ovarian cyst for drainage.

oöphorrhagia (ō″ŏf-ōr-ra′jĭ-ă) [" + " + *rēgnunai*, to burst forth]. Hemorrhage from an ovulatory site severe enough to cause clinical symptoms or signs.

oöphorrhaphy (ō-ŏf-or′ă-fĭ) [" + " + *raphē*, a sewing]. Suture of a displaced ovary to the pelvic wall.

oösperm (ō′ō-spĕrm) [" + *sperma*, seed]. The cell formed by union of the spermatozoon with the ovum; the fertilized ovum.

oötheca (ō-o-thē′kă) [G. *oothēkē*, ovary]. An ovary.

oöthecohysterectomy (ō-o-thē″kō-hĭs-tĕr-ĕk′tō-mĭ) [" + *ystera*, uterus, + *ektomē*, excision]. Excision of the uterus and ovaries.

oötherapy (ō″o-ther′ă-pĭ) [G. *ōon*, egg, + *therapeia*, treatment]. Treatment with ovarian substance.

opacity (o-păs′ĭ-tĭ) [L. *opacitās*, darkness]. 1. Darkness; shading from light. 2. Lack of transparency. 3. Mental dullness.

opaque (ō-pāk′) [L. *opacus*, dark]. 1. Dark. 2. Not transparent. 3. Stupid.

open (ō′pĕn) [A.S.]. 1. Not shut. 2. Uncovered, exposed, as to air. 3. To make an aperture in, as to open a boil. 4. Interrupted, said of an electric circuit, when current cannot pass.

operable (ŏp′ĕr-ă-bl) [L. *operārī*, to work]. 1. Practicable. 2. Admitting of treatment by operation with reasonable expectation of cure.

operate (ŏp′ĕr-āt) [L. *operatus*, worked]. 1. To perform an excision or incision or to make a suture on the body or any of its organs or parts to restore health. 2. To produce an effect, as a drug.

operation (ŏp-ĕr-ā′shŭn) [L. *operatiō*, a working]. 1. The act of operating. 2. A surgical procedure to restore health. 3. Action of a drug.
PREPARATION FOR:
Abdominal: Shave entire abdomen and pubic hair. Cleanse umbilicus.
Anal and perineal: Shave genital area.
Arm: Shave axilla, and from shoulder to below elbow.
Breast: Shave axilla and well around the breast. If radical operation, also chest from sternum to spine, and from costal margin to clavicle.
Cerebellar: In males and children, shave the whole head and back of neck to scapulae; in females, back of head from above ears down to scapulae.
Cerebral: Shave entire head unless otherwise ordered.
Chest: Shave from median line to median line, including back.
Elbow: Shave from middle of upper arm, to fingers; also axilla.
Forearm: Shave from hand to shoulder.
Hernia: Shave genital area and lower abdomen to umbilicus; also down front of thighs to middle of thighs.
Knee: Shave from thigh to foot.
Kidney: Shave from scapula to sacrum, and spine to ant. median line.
Leg: Shave from thigh to ankle.
Neck, lateral: Shave 2 inches behind ear on side indicated; cheek in males.
Rectal: SEE: *abdominal*.
Spine: Shave entire back if necessary.
Thigh: Shave from groin to foot; also genital area.
Thyroid: Shave lower neck in front if necessary.
SEE: *Name of operation, in alphabetical order.*

o., home. PREPARATION FOR: In private houses a room should be selected that is least frequented. Often kitchen is best for the purpose. Carpets, curtains, and all unnecessary furniture should be removed.
If time permits, the disinfection of the empty room should be commenced by fumigating with sulfur dioxide for 12 hours. Burn 3 pounds of sulfur for every 1000 cubic feet of air space in the room. The sulfur must be burned in an iron kettle placed in a wash tub partly filled with water, and doors and windows should be tightly closed to prevent escape.
After the expiration of 12 hours, or if time does not permit fumigation, ceilings, doors, floors, windows, etc., and all objects in the room must be scrubbed with hot soda solution to be followed by scrubbing with a solution of corrosive sublimate, 1:1000, or carbolic acid, 5%. Color the solutions to prevent accidents.
The microbes floating in the air should be precipitated by moisture in form of steam or spray; by so doing the air is purified and the microbes become attached to the moist floor, which should

be kept moist till operation is finished. For cleaning the wallpaper Von Esmarch has recommended rubbing with soft bread.

When possible, room should be prepared the day before the operation, and doors and windows closed. The kitchen table can be converted into an operating table that will answer every purpose by placing upon it a blanket properly folded and covering the same with a clean sheet. The kitchen stove does excellent service in sterilizing everything that can be sterilized by heat, wash basins, pans, water, instruments, etc.

Napkins and towels that are to be used during operation should be boiled for 5 minutes in soda solution. Sterile water, hot and cold, and saline solution must be kept in readiness, as well as sterile vessels for use during operation.

For major operations temperature of room should be kept at not less than 75° F., and warm blankets, bottles filled with hot water, or warm bricks must be kept in readiness. A hypodermic syringe, strychnine tablets, capsules of nitrite of amyl, alcoholic stimulants, ether and chloroform must be kept within easy reach of the anesthetizer. Brushes for hand and surface disinfection must be rendered sterile by exposing them to live steam for 30 minutes, or boiling in soda solution for from 5 to 10 minutes.

Should gowns not be on hand, night shirts are excellent substitutes, and in absence of these, clean sheets wrapped about body, with towels for the arms secured with safety pins, answer admirably.

Nurse should wear cotton dress and over it an aseptic gown. Hair and beard of operator and assistants may be covered with aseptic gauze. Antiseptic solution should be within easy reach, if hands become bloody or contaminated. SEE: *laparotomy.*

   o., major. One involving danger to life.

   o., minor. O. not serious or risking life.

   o., radical. O. performed to effect complete cure.

   o., subtotal. One in which not quite all of the organ is removed, as subtotal removal of thyroid gland.

operative (op′ĕr-ă-tĭv) [L. *operativus,* working]. 1. Effective, active. 2. Pert. to or brought about by an operation. 3. A drug that is acting.

   o. procedure. A surgical operation.

opercular (ō-pur′kū-lăr) [L. *operculum,* a cover]. Concerning a covering.

operculum (ō-pur′kū-lŭm) (pl. *opercula*) [L. a covering]. 1. Any covering. 2. Plug of mucus which fills up the opening of the cervix upon impregnation. 3. BNA. Convolutions covering the island of Reil.

ophiasis (ō-fī′ăs-ĭs) [G. *ophis,* snake]. Baldness occurring in windy streaks upon the head.

ophidiophobia (ō-fĭd″ĭ-ō-fō′bĭ-ă) [G. *ophidion,* snake, + *phobos,* fear]. Abnormal fear of snakes.

ophidism (ō′fĭd-ĭzm) [G. *ophis,* snake, + *ismos,* condition]. Poisoning from snake bite.

ophiotoxemia (ō″fĭ-ō-tŏk-sē′mĭ-ă) [" + *toxikon,* poison, + *aima,* blood]. Poisoning due to venom injected by a snake.

ophiotoxin (ō-fĭ-ō-tŏk′sĭn) [" + *toxikon,* poison]. A poison in cobra venom.

ophritis, ophryitis (ŏf-rī′tĭs, -rē-ī′tĭs) [G.

ophrys, eyebrow, + *-itis,* inflammation]. Inflammation of the eyebrow.

ophryon (ŏf′rē-ŏn) [G. *ophrys,* eyebrow]. Meeting point of the facial median line with a transverse line across the forehead's narrowest portion.

ophthalmagra (ŏf-thăl-măg′ră) [G. *ophthalmos,* eye, + *agra,* seizure]. Gouty or rheumatic inflammation of the eye, with pain.

ophthalmalgia (ŏf-thăl-măl′jĭ-ă) [" + *algos,* pain]. Pain in the eye.

ophthalmatrophy (ŏf-thăl-măt′rō-fĭ) [" + *atrophia,* a wasting]. Atrophy of eyeball.

ophthalmectomy (ŏf-thăl-mĕk′tō-mĭ) [" + *ektome,* excision]. Excision of an eye.

   DRESSING: Antiseptic gauze, iodoform, rubber drainage tube, bichloride solution, 1:5000.

   POSITION: Dorsal.

ophthalmia (ŏf-thăl′mĭ-ă) [G. *ophthalmos,* eye]. Severe inflammation of the eye, usually including the conjunctiva.

   o., catarrhal. Conjunctivitis of a severe, frequently purulent, form.

   o., Egyptian. Granular conjunctivitis. SYN: *trachoma.*

   o., gonorrheal. Severe, purulent form due to infection with gonococcus.

   o., granular. Severe purulent conjunctivitis with formation of granules on the eyelids. SYN: *trachoma.*

   o., metastatic. Sympathetic inflammation of the choroid due to pyemia or metastasis.

   o., migratory. SEE: *sympathetic o.*

   o. neonatorum. Severe purulent conjunctivitis in the newborn.

   ETIOL: Infection with gonococcus responsible for great majority of cases. Condition causes about 25% of all blindness in children.

   PROPHYLAXIS: Introduction of a few drops of a silver salt into each eye at birth.

   o., neuroparalytic. Corneal inflammation due to a nerve lesion.

   o., phlyctenular. Vesicular formations on epithelium of conjunctiva or cornea.

   o., purulent. Purulent inflammation of eye, usually due to gonococcus.

   o., scrofulous. SEE: *phlyctenular o.*

   o., spring. Conjunctivitis in the spring of the year.

   o., sympathetic. Plastic or serous uveitis in one eye caused by some disorder in the other eye.

   SYM: Photophobia, lacrimation, pain, deposits on post. surface of cornea. Exudate appears in pupillary area with post. synechia, seclusio pupillae, secondary atrophy with blindness.

   TREATMENT: Removal of exciting eye early in the disease. Atropine, heat, salicylates, potassium iodide.

   o., varicose. O. seen in varicose veins of the conjunctiva.

ophthalmiatrics (ŏf-thăl-mĭ-at′rĭks) [G. *ophthalmos,* eye, + *iatreia,* treatment]. The treatment of eye diseases.

ophthalmic (ŏf-thăl′mĭk) [G. *ophthalmos,* eye]. Pert. to the eye.

   o. nerve. A branch of the trigeminal or trifacial nerve (5th cranial n.). It is sensory and its branches are the *lacrimal, frontal,* and *nasociliary,* etc.

ophthalmitis (ŏf-thăl-mī′tĭs) [" + *-itis,* inflammation]. Inflamed condition of the eye.

ophthalmo- [G.]. Combining form *pert. to the eye.*

ophthalmoblennorrhea (ŏf-thăl″mō-blĕn-ŏr-rē′ă) [G. *ophthalmos,* eye, + *blenna,*

ophthalmocele O-12 **opiate**

mucus, + *roia*, flow]. Purulent inflammation of the eye or conjunctiva, usually due to the gonococcus.
ophthalmocele (ŏf-thăl'mō-sēl) [" + *kēlē*, swelling]. Abnormal protrusion of the eyeballs. SYN: *exophthalmos*.
ophthalmocopia (ŏf-thăl-mō-kō'pĭ-ă) [" + *kopos*, fatigue]. Ocular fatigue; eyestrain. SYN: *asthenopia, q.v.*
ophthalmodesmitis (ŏf-thăl"mō-dĕs-mī'tĭs) [" + *desmos*, ligament, + *-itis*, inflammation]. Inflammation of tendons of the eye.
ophthalmodiagnosis (ŏf-thăl"mō-dī-ăg-nō'sĭs) [" + *dia*, through, + *gnōsis*, knowledge]. Diagnosis of eye conditions by means of the ophthalmoreaction.*
ophthalmodynia (ŏf-thăl-mō-dĭn'ĭ-ă) [" + *odynē*, pain]. Pain in the eye. SYN: *ophthalmalgia*.
ophthalmofundoscope (ŏf-thăl"mō-fŭnd'ō-skōp) [G. *ophthalmos*, eye, + L. *fundus*, base, + G. *skopein*, to examine]. Apparatus used in examining the fundus of the eye.
ophthalmography (ŏf-thăl-mŏg'răf-ĭ) [" + *graphein*, to write]. Description of the eye, and its disorders.
ophthalmogyric (ŏf-thăl-mō-jī'rĭk) [" + *gyros*, circle]. Causing or concerning ocular movements. SYN: *oculogyric*.
ophthalmolith (ŏf-thăl'mō-lĭth) [" + *lithos*, stone]. A calculus of the lacrimal duct.
ophthalmologist (ŏf-thăl-mol'ō-jĭst) [" + *logos*, study]. One who treats the eye and its disorders.
ophthalmology (ŏf-thăl-mol'ō-jĭ) [" + *logos*, study]. The science dealing with the eye and its diseases.
ophthalmomalacia (ŏf-thăl"mō-măl-a'sĭ-ă) [" + *malakia*, softening]. Shrinkage or softness of eye.
ophthalmometer (ŏf-thăl"mŏm'ĕt-ĕr) [G. *ophthalmos*, eye, + *metron*, measure]. Instrument for making measurements of corneal astigmatism.
ophthalmometry (ŏf-thăl-mom'ĕt-rĭ) [" + *metron*, measure]. Measurement of the ocular defects and refractive powers.
ophthalmomycosis (ŏf-thăl"mō-mĭ-kō'sĭs) [" + *mykēs*, fungus, + *-ōsis*]. Any fungous disease of the eye.
ophthalmomyitis (ŏf-thăl"mō-mī-ī'tĭs) [" + *mys, my-*, muscle, + *-itis*, inflammation]. Inflammation of the ocular muscles.
ophthalmomyositis (ŏf-thăl"mō-mī-ō-sī'tĭs) [" + " + *-itis*, inflammation]. Inflamed condition of the eye muscles. SYN: *ophthalmomyitis*.
ophthalmomyotomy (ŏf-thăl"mō-mī-ot'ō-mĭ) [" + " + *tomē*, incision]. Surgical section of the muscles of the eyes.
ophthalmoneuritis (ŏf-thăl"mō-nū-rī'tĭs) [" + *neuron*, sinew, + *-itis*, inflammation]. Inflamed condition of the optic nerve.
ophthalmopathy (ŏf-thăl-mop'ă-thĭ) [G. *ophthalmos*, eye, + *pathos*, disease]. Any eye disease.
ophthalmophlebotomy (ŏf-thăl"mō-flē-bŏt'ō-mĭ) [" + *phleps, phleb-*, vein, + *tomē*, incision]. Incision of the eye to overcome congestion of conjunctival veins.
ophthalmophthisis (ŏf-thăl-mŏf'thĭs-ĭs) [" + *phthisis*, a wasting]. Softening or shrinking of the eyeball. SYN: *phthisis bulbi*.
ophthalmoplasty (ŏf-thăl'mō-plăs"tĭ) [" + *plassein*, to form]. Ocular plastic surgery.

ophthalmoplegia (ŏf-thăl"mō-plē'jĭ-ă) [" + *plēgē*, stroke]. Paralysis of ocular muscles.
  o. externa. Paralysis of extraocular muscles.
  o. interna. Paralysis of intraocular muscles.
  o., nuclear. O. due to lesion of nuclei of origin of the ocular motor nerves.
  o. partialis. Paralysis of not all of ocular muscles.
  o. progressiva. Form in which all muscles become involved slowly.
  o. totalis. Paralysis of both internal and external ocular muscles.
ophthalmoptosis (ŏf-thăl-mŏp-tō'sĭs) [" + *ptōsis*, a dropping]. Protrusion of the eyeball. SYN: *exophthalmos*.
ophthalmoreaction (ŏf-thăl"mō-rē-ăk'-shŭn) [" + L. *rē*, back, + *actus*, acted]. Reaction of the conjunctiva resulting on instillation of a drop of tuberculin or typhoid fever toxin into the eye of persons suffering from the diseases.
ophthalmorrhagia (ŏf-thăl-mō-rā'jĭ-ă) [G. *ophthalmos*, eye, + *rēgnunai*, to break forth]. Ocular hemorrhage.
ophthalmorrhea (ŏf-thăl-mō-rē'ă) [" + *roia*, flow]. Flow of blood from eye.
ophthalmorrhexis (ŏf-thăl-mō-rĕks'ĭs) [" + *rēxis*, rupture]. Rupture of an eyeball.
ophthalmoscope (ŏf-thăl'mō-skōp) [" + *skopein*, to examine]. Instrument for examining interior of the eye.
ophthalmoscopy (ŏf-thăl-mŏs'kō-pĭ) [" + *skopein*, to examine]. The examination of the interior of the eye.
  o., direct. Examination in which image in interior of eye is upright.
  o., indirect. Examination in which image in interior of eye is inverted.
ophthalmostat (ŏf-thăl'mō-stăt) [" + *statos*, standing]. Instrument used to hold the eye still during an operation.
ophthalmostatometer (ŏf-thăl"mō-stăt-om'ĕt-ĕr) [" + " + *metron*, measure]. Instrument for ascertaining position of eyes.
ophthalmothermometer (ŏf-thăl"mō-thĕr-mom'ĕt-ĕr) [G. *ophthalmos*, eye, + *thermē*, heat, + *metron*, measure]. Instrument for determining local temperature in eye diseases.
ophthalmotonometer (ŏf-thăl"mō-tō-nŏm'-ĕt-ĕr) [" + *tonos*, tension, + *metron*, measure]. Instrument for determining tension within globe of eye.
ophthalmotoxin (ŏf-thăl"mō-toks'ĭn) [" + *toxikon*, poison]. Cytotoxin derived on injection of emulsions of the ciliary body.
ophthalmotrope (ŏf-thăl'mō-trōp) [" + *tropē*, a turning]. Instrument for showing the movements of the ocular muscles.
ophthalmotropometer (ŏf-thăl"mō-trō-pom'ĕt-ĕr) [" + " + *metron*, measure]. Instrument for measuring the eye movements.
opiate (ō'pĭ-āt) [G. *opion*, poppy juice]. 1. A drug derived from opium. 2. A drug inducing sleep. 3. To deaden, to put to sleep.
  They include the bromides. The principal opiates are opium and its derivatives, such as morphine. They are all habit-forming.
  NP: Given only under a doctor's orders. When possible patient should not know the nature of the drug given. Otherwise, warn patient of its dangers unless given by a physician.
  Opiates should be kept separate from other drugs and guarded from patient.

opiomania O-13 **opium**

Physician prescribing narcotics must have his own registry number, and place it on every narcotic prescription. A prescription for an opiate cannot be refilled. A new one must be written by the physician

SEE: *depressant, narcotic, sedative, etc.*
opiomania (ō"pĭ-ō-mā'nĭ-ă) [" + *mania*, madness]. Morbid addiction to use of opium or its derivatives.
opiophagism (ō-pĭ-ŏf'ă-jĭzm) [" + *phagein*, to eat, + *ismos*, condition]. Addiction to the use of opium, esp. the eating of it.
opisthenar (ō-pĭs'the-năr) [G. *opisthen*, behind, + *thenar*, palm]. Back of the hand.
opisthion (ō-pĭs'thĭ-ŏn) [G. *opisthion*, rear]. Craniometric point at middle of lower border of foramen magnum.
opistho-, opisth- [G.]. Combining form meaning *backward, behind*.
opisthognathism (ō"ĭs-thŏg'nă-thĭzm) [G. *opisthen*, behind, + *gnathos*, jaw, + *ismos*, state of]. Skull abnormality marked by a retreating lower jaw.
opisthoporeia (ō-pĭs"thō-pō-rī'ă) [G. *opisthen*, behind, + *poreia*, a walking]. Involuntary walking backward due to loss of motor control.
Opisthorchis (ō-pĭs-thor'kĭs) [" + *orchis*, testicle]. A genus of parasitic fluke worms with testicles near the post. end of the body.
  O. sinensis. Common form causing the liver fluke disease of Asia.
opisthotic (ŏp"ĭs-thŏt'ĭk) [" + *ous, ot-*, ear]. 1. Located behind the ear or in the int. ear. 2. An opisthotic element or bone.
  o. center. Petrous bone's ossification center.

because it is a respiratory depressant. (3) Also a heart depressant, but is administered in some heart cases to produce sleep and so improve condition of heart by relieving fatigue. It slows the pulse. (4) Sedative to the nervous system; promotes rest and sleep by relieving excitability and fear. It relieves pain. (5) Applied locally will relieve pain; therefore used in liniments and plasters; and as a preparation of gall and opium ointment in treatment of painful hemorrhoids. Inhibits all secretions of the body except perspiration, which it increases. It also contracts the pupils, even in small doses.

DOSAGE: Opium: 1 gr. (0.06 Gm.). Tr. opium (laudanum): 10 ♏ (0.6 cc.). Tr. opium camphorated (paregoric): Adult, 1 dram (4 cc.).

POISONING: SYM: Excitement that may pass unnoticed as characteristic symptoms develop. Drowsiness, limpness and flaccidity of muscles; sleep, passing on to stupor and coma. Pupils contracted to pinpoint size. Reflexes abolished. Pulse slow and weak at first; later irregular and sometimes quick and running. Respirations depressed, sometimes as slow as 8 or 10 a minute, and with coma become stertorous. Temperature is subnormal, skin cold and covered with sweat. The face becomes livid and, unless treated successfully, patient will die of asphyxia.

TREATMENT: First, send for a doctor; in the meantime, administer *emetics*, such as mustard and water, or better, wash out the stomach with a solution of potassium permanganate (1:3000). A pint should be left in the stomach. *Caf-*

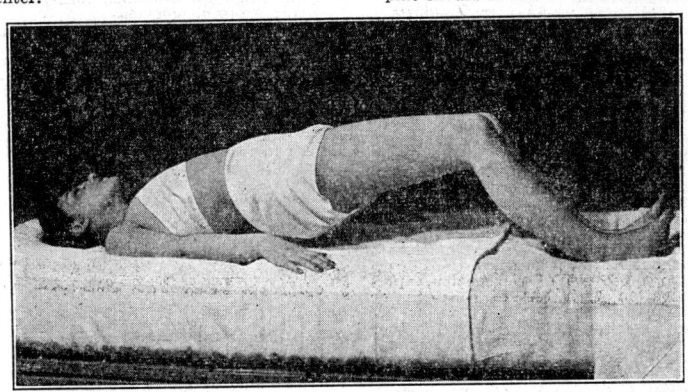

Posed by professional model   OPISTHOTONOS   *Photo by Whitaker*

opisthotonos (ŏp"ĭs-thŏt'ō-nŏs) [" + *tonos*, tension]. An arched position of the body with feet and head on the floor caused by a tetanic spasm.
  Seen in severe cases of meningitis and tetanus. SEE: *emprosthotonos, pleurothotonus, posture.*
opium (ō'pĭ-ŭm) [G. *opion*, poppy juice]. USP. The dried juice obtained from the unripe capsule of the poppy.
  ACTION: Resembles that of morphine.
  USES: (1) As a sedative in forms of indigestion and diarrhea. (2) It diminishes the secretions of bronchial tubes and relieves spasm; given to suppress ineffective coughing. Caution indicated

feine is probably the best physiological antidote, and may be given as such, or in the form of coffee, by mouth or rectum. Other measures to keep person awake are the use of *ammonia* by mouth and inhalation; *atropine, strychnine*, or *camphor* by needle; *cold water* to the head and face; *exercise; artificial respiration, etc. Apomorphine hydrochloride*, being a powerful hypnotic, should not be used as the emetic for opium poisoning except in cases of extreme urgency that are seen early. In emptying the stomach, it is best to use a stomach tube as emetics may be much delayed in their action due to the depressing effect on the vomiting center by the absorbed narcotic. Inhalations of oxygen are of unquestionable benefit in many cases. *Strychnine* by hypodermic has been highly recommended. Note breathing and, if very slow, promote by intermittent artificial respiration; keep covered with blankets and apply hot water bottles; keep skin dry by continually wiping the deposit of perspiration from it.

opiumism (ō'pĭ-ŭm-ĭzm) [G. *opion*, poppy juice, + *ismos*, state of]. 1. Addiction to use of opium. 2. Physical condition resulting from overuse of opium.

opo- [G.]. Prefix meaning *derived from juice*.

opohypophysin (ō"pō-hī-pof'ĭ-sĭn) [G. *opos*, juice, + *ypo*, under, + *physis*, growth]. Commercial preparation used in treating acromegaly.

opomam'min [" + *mamma*, breast]. Commercial animal udder extract used in diseases of the uterus.

opoövariin (ō"pō-ō-va'rē-ĭn) [" + L. *ovarium*, ovary]. Commercial preparation of animal ovaries used in hysteria and diseases of the ovary.

opopros'tatin [" + *prostatēs*, prostate]. Commercial preparation of animal prostate glands used in hypertrophied prostate.

opotherapy (ō-pō-thĕr'ă-pĭ) [" + *therapeia*, treatment]. 1. Treatment of disease by using animal organs or extracts from them. SYN: *organotherapy*. 2. Use of juice in treatment of disease.

Oppenheim's disease (ŏp'ĕn-hīm). A rare congenital disorder marked by atony of entire bodily musculature. SYN: *amyotonia congenita*.

oppilation (ŏp"pĭ-lā'shŭn) [L. *oppilātiō*, a closure]. 1. An obstruction. 2. Act or state of being obstructed. 3. Constipation.

oppilative (ŏp'pĭ-lā-tĭv) [L. *oppilāre*, to stop up]. 1. Closing the pores. 2. Constipating. 3. Obstructive. 4. A constipating agent.

opponens (op-pō'nĕns) [L. placed against]. Opposing, a term applied to muscles of hand or foot by which 1 of the lateral digits may be opposed to 1 of the other digits. SEE: *Table of Muscles in Appendix*.

opposition (ŏp-pō-sĭ'shŭn) [L. *oppositio*, a placing against]. Refusal of certain psychopaths to accept suggestions or directions because of retardation,* preoccupation with bizarre concepts, or from fear of the results.
In dementia precox not only do they oppose suggestions, but perform acts directly opposite to those suggested. SEE: *negativism*.

opsialgia (ŏp-sĭ-al'jĭ-ă) [G. *ōps*, face, + *algos*, pain]. Neuralgic pain of the face.

opsinogen (ŏp-sĭn'ō-jĕn) [G. *opsōnein*, to prepare food for, + *gennan*, to produce]. A substance which stimulates formation of opsonins.

opsinogenous (ŏp-sĭn-oj'ĕn-ŭs) [" + *gennan*, to produce]. Capable of forming opsonins.

opsiometer (ŏp-sĭ-ŏm'ĕt-ĕr) [G. *opsis*, vision, + *metron*, measure]. Apparatus for the measurement of vision. SYN: *optometer*.

opsiuria (ŏp-sĭ-ū'rĭ-ă) [G. *opson*, food, + *ouron*, urine]. Condition in which excretion of urine is more rapid during fasting than after a meal.

opsogen (ŏp'sō-jĕn) [G. *opsōnein*, to prepare food for, + *gennan*, to produce]. Substance stimulating the formation of opsonins. SYN: *opsinogen*.

opsomania (ŏp-sō-mā'nĭ-ă) [G. *opson*, a dainty, + *mania*, madness]. Morbid desire for some special article of food.

opsone (ŏp'sōn) [G. *opsōnein*, to prepare food for]. Substance in blood serum whose function is to render cell and microörganisms attractive to phagocytes. SYN: *opsonin*.

opsonic (ŏp-son'ĭk) [G. *opsōnein*, to prepare food for]. Pert. to opsonins or their use in therapy.
o. index. A measure of the resistance of a patient to bacterial invasion.
Determined by the ratio bet. the number of bacteria destroyed and ingested by the leukocytes in normal blood serum, as compared with the number ingested by leukocytes under the influence of the patient's own serum.
A special technic is followed. The white corpuscles are fixed, stained, and examined under the microscope. The number of germs in 100 leukocytes are counted. The total is then divided by 100, showing the patient's phagocytic index. This is divided by average from normal blood serum and result is the opsonic index.

opsoniferous (op-so-nif'er-us) [" + L. *ferre*, to carry]. Carrying or producing opsonin.

opsonification (ŏp-sŏn"ĭ-fĭ-kā'shŭn) [" + L. *facere*, to make]. Effect of opsonins in rendering cells or bacteria phagocytized more readily.

opsonin (ŏp'sō-nĭn) [G. *opsōnein*, to prepare food for]. Substance in blood serum which acts upon microörganisms and other cells, making them more attractive to phagocytes.
Some opsonins are formed as the result of special stimuli as specifics for certain species of bacteria. They do not make any appreciable change in bacteria or kill them, but unite with them. They are also formed for other elements, such as the red blood corpuscles.
The amt. of opsonin in the blood can be increased by immunization.

opsonization (ŏp-sŏn-ĭ-zā'shŭn) [G. *opsōnein*, to prepare food for]. Action of opsonins in making cells or bacteria more attractive to phagocytes. SYN: *opsonification*.

opsonize (ŏp'son-īz) [G. *opsōnein*, to prepare food for]. To render more attractive to phagocytes.

opsonocytophagic (ŏp"sŏn-o-sī-tō-fā'jĭk) [" + *kytos*, cell, + *phagein*, to eat]. Pert. to phagocytic action of blood when serum opsonins are present.

opsonogen (ŏp-spn'ō-jĕn) [" + *gennan*, to produce]. A stimulant to opsonin formation.

opsonology (ŏp-sō-nol'ō-jĭ) [" + *logos*, study]. Study of opsonins and their function and action.

opsonometry (ŏp-sō-nŏm'ĕt-rĭ) [" + G. *metron*, measure]. Estimation of amt. of opsonins in the blood serum. SEE: *opsonic index*.

opsonophilia (ŏp-sŏn-ō-fĭl'ĭ-ă) [" + *philein*, to love]. Attraction for opsonins.

opsonophil'ic [" + *philein*, to love]. Attractive to opsonins.

opsonotherapy (ŏp-sŏn-ō-thĕr'ă-pĭ) [" + *therapeia*, treatment]. Treatment by stimulation of a specific opsonin with bacterial vaccines. SYN: *vaccine therapy*.

optesthesia (ŏp-tĕs-thē'zĭ-ă) [G. *optikos*, pert. to the eye, + *aisthēsis*, sensation]. Visual sensibility; perception of visual stimuli.

optic (op'tĭk) [G. *optikos*, pert. to the eye]. Pert. to the eye or the sight.
  o. chiasm, o. commissure. The crossing of the optic nerve fibers in the brain.
  o. disk. Area in retina for entrance of optic nerve; the blind spot.
  o. foramen. Groove for optic nerve and ophthalmic artery at the orbit's apex.
  o. lobes. Upper pair of corpora quadrigemina of the brain.
  o. nerve. Second cranial n. FUNCT: Special sense of sight. ORIG: Occipital lobe, cortical center. DIST: Retina.
  o. papilla. SEE: optic disk.
  o. thalamus. Mass of gray substance at base of brain which connects with fibers of optic tract. SEE: *thalamic syndrome*. [chiasm and visual center.
  o. tract. Fibers running bet. optic
optical (ŏp'tĭ-kăl) [G. *optikos*, pert. to the eye]. Pert. to vision or the eye.
  o. activity. CHEM: The property of rotating the plane of polarized light. Measurement of this property is called polarimetry, and is useful in the determination of optically active substances like dextrose. Particularly the sugars are classified according to this criterion. Optical activity in a substance can be detected by placing it bet. polarizing and analyzing prisms.
optician (ŏp-tĭsh'ăn) [G. *optikos*, pert. to the eye]. One who makes optical apparatus.
optico- [G.]. Combining form meaning relating to the eye or vision.
opticociliary (ŏp"tĭ-kō-sĭl'ĭ-ăr-ĭ) [G. *optikos*, pert. to the eye, + L. *ciliaris*, pert. to eyelash]. Concerning the optic and ciliary nerves.
opticopupillary (ŏp"tĭ-kō-pū'pĭl-ĕr-ĭ) [" + L. *pupilla*, pupil]. Concerning optic nerve and the pupil.
optics (ŏp'tĭks) [L. *optikos*, pert. to vision]. The science dealing with light and its relation to vision.
optimum (ŏp'tĭm-ŭm) (pl. *optima*) [L. *optimus*, best]. The condition which is most conducive to favorable activity.
  o. temperature. That t. which is most suitable for development of bacterial cultures. [*sion or eye*.
opto- [G.]. Combining form meaning *vi-*
optogram (ŏp'tō-grăm) [G. *optos*, seen, + *gramma*, mark]. Image of ext. object fixed on the retina by photochemical bleaching action of light on the visual purple.
optometer (ŏp-tŏm'ĕt-ĕr) [" + *metron*, measure]. Instrument for measurement of the eye's refractive power.
optometrist (ŏp-tŏm'ĕt-rĭst) [" + *metron*, measure]. Person who measures the eye's refractive powers and fits glasses to correct ocular defects.
optometry (ŏp-tŏm'ĕt-rĭ) [" + *metron*, measure]. Measurement of the visual refractive power and correction of visual defects with eyeglasses.
optomyometer (ŏp"tō-mī-ŏm'ĕt-ĕr) [" + *mys, my-*, muscle, + *metron*, a measure]. Instrument for determining strength of the muscles of the eye.
optophone (ŏp'tō-fōn) [" + *phōnē*, voice]. Instrument converting light energy into sound energy. Used by the blind.
optostriate (ŏp-tō-strī'āt) [" + L. *striatus*, grooved]. Concerning the optic thalamus and the corpus striatum.
ora (ō'ra) [L.]. Plural of os, mouth.
ora (ō'ră) [L.]. A border or margin.
  o. serrata retinae. BNA. Notched ant. edge of retina.
orad (ō'răd) [L. *os, or-,* mouth, + *ad*, toward]. Toward the mouth or oral region.
oral (ō'răl) [L. *os, or-,* mouth]. Concerning the mouth.
oralogy (ō-răl'ō-jĭ) [" + G. *logos*, study of]. 1. The science of oral hygiene. 2. Study of diseases of the mouth.
orange (ŏr'ĕnj) [Persian *nārang*, orange]. Contains citric acid, sugar and considerable cellulose. AVERAGE SERVING: 100 Gm. Pro. 0.8, Fat 0.2, Carbo. 11.6. VITAMINS: A— to ++, B+, C+++, G++.
  ASH CONST: Ca 0.045, Mg 0.012, K 0.177, Na 0.012, P 0.021, Cl 0.006, S 0.011, Fe 0.0002.
  o. juice. AVERAGE SERVING: 120 Gm. Pro. 0.7, Carbo. 15.7. VITAMINS: A+ to ++, B+, C+++. ASH CONST: Ca 0.029, Mg 0.011, K 0.182, Na 0.008, P 0.016, Cl 0.003, S 0.008, Fe 0.0002.
  ACTION: Similar to that of lemons, *q.v.* Somewhat laxative although claimed to be constipating in some forms of intestinal disorders. A good mineralizer. SEE: *fruit, lemon, lime.*
orbicular (ŏr-bĭk'ū-lăr) [L. *orbiculus*, a small circle]. Circular.
  o. bone. Ossicle frequently becoming attached to the incus. SYN: *os orbiculare.*
  o. ligament. Circular l. about the neck of the radius. SYN: *ligamentum orbiculare.*
  o. muscle. Muscle about an opening.
  o. process. End of long process of the incus. SYN: *lenticular process.*
orbicularis (ŏr"bĭk-ū-la'rĭs) [L. *orbiculus*, little circle]. Muscle surrounding an orifice; a sphincter muscle.
  o. oculi. Muscle encircling the opening of orbit of the eye.
  o. oris. Circular muscle surrounding the mouth.
  o. palpebrarum. SEE: *o. oculi.*
orbit (ŏr'bĭt) [L. *orbita*, track]. The bony, pyramid-shaped cavity of the skull which holds the eyeball. It is formed by the frontal, malar, ethmoid, maxillary, lacrimal, sphenoid, and palatine bones. It is pierced posteriorly by the optic foramen to receive the optic nerve and ophthalmic artery.
orbita (ŏr'bĭ-tă) (pl. *orbitae*) [L. wheel track]. BNA. Latin term for orbit.
orbital (ŏr'bĭ-tăl) [L. *orbita*, track]. Concerning the orbit.
orbitale (or-bĭ-tā'lē) [L. *orbita*, track]. Lowest point on lower orbital margin.
orbitotomy (or-bĭt-ŏt'ō-mĭ) [" + G. *tomē*, incision]. Surgical incision into the orbit.
orchectomy (ŏr-kĕk'tō-mĭ) [G. *orchis*, testicle, + *ektomē*, excision]. Surgical removal of a testicle.
  DRESSINGS, ETC: Small drainage tube, sterilized gauze, borosalicylic acid powder, 4:1. SYN: *orchidectomy.*
orcheoplasty (ŏr'kē-ō-plăs-tĭ) [" + *plassein*, to form]. Plastic repair work of the scrotum.
orchialgia (or-kĭ-ăl'jĭ-ă) [" + *algos*, pain]. Pain in the testes. SYN: *orchiodynia.*
orchic (ŏr'kĭk) [G. *orchis*, testicle]. Concerning the testicle.
orchichorea (or"kĭ-kō-rē'ă) [" + *choreia*, a dance]. Involuntary jerking movements of the testicles.
orchidalgia (or-kĭ-dăl'jĭ-ă) [G. *orchis, orchid-*, testicle, + *algos*, pain]. Neuralgia in the testicles. SYN: *orchialgia.*
orchidectomy (ŏr"kĭd-ĕk'tō-mĭ) [" + *ektomē*, excision]. Removal of a testicle surgically. SYN: *orchectomy.*
orchidin (ŏr'kĭd-ĭn) [G. *orchis, orchid-*,

testicle]. Proprietary preparation of testicular extract.

orchido- [G.]. Combining form, meaning *testicle*.

orchidocele (or'kĭ-dō-sēl) [G. *orchis, orchid-*, testicle, + *kēlē*, hernia]. Scrotal hernia.

orchidocelioplasty (or″kĭd-ō-sēl′ĭ-ō-plăs″-tĭ) [" + *koilia*, belly, + *plassein*, to form]. Surgical transfer of an undescended testicle to the abdominal cavity.

orchidoncus (ŏr-kĭ-dong′kŭs) [" + *ogkos*, mass]. A neoplasm of the testicle.

orchidopexy (or'kĭd-ō-pĕks″ĭ) [" + *pēxis*, fixation]. Surgical transfer of an imperfectly descended testicle into the scrotum and suturing it there.

orchidoplasty (ŏr′kĭd-ō-plăs″tĭ) [" + *plassein*, to form]. Operative transfer of an undescended testicle to the scrotum.

orchidoptosis (ŏr″kĭd-ŏp-tō′sĭs) [" + *ptōsis*, a falling]. Dropping of the testicle.

orchidotomy (ŏr-kĭ-dŏt′ō-mĭ) [G. *orchis, orchid-*, testicle, + *tomē*, incision]. Incision into the testes.

orchiectomy (ŏr-kĭ-ĕk′tō-mĭ) [" + *ektomē*, excision]. Surgical excision of a testicle. SEE: *castration*.

orchiencephaloma (or″kĭ-ĕn-sef-ă-lō′mă) [" + *egkephalos*, brain, + *-ōma*, tumor]. Tumor of brainlike substance in the testicle. SEE: *orchiomyeloma*.

orchiepididymitis (or″kĭ-ep″ĭ-dĭd-ĭ-mī′tĭs) [" + *epi*, upon, + *didymos*, testis, + *-itis*, inflammation]. Inflamed condition of a testicle and epididymis.

orchiocele (or'kĭ-ō-sēl) [" + *kēlē*, mass]. 1. Scrotal hernia. SYN: *orchidocele*. 2. A tumor of the testicle.

orchiodynia (ŏr-kĭ-ō-dĭn′ĭ-ă) [" + *odynē*, pain]. Testicular pain. SYN: *orchialgia, orchidalgia*.

orchiomyeloma (or″kĭ-ō-mī-ĕ-lō′mă) [G. *orchis*, testicle, + *myelos*, marrow, + *-ōma*, tumor]. Tumor of the testicle composed of marrowlike cells.

orchioncus (ŏr-kĭ-ong′kŭs) [" + *ogkos*, tumor]. Neoplasm of the testicle. SYN: *orchidoncus*.

orchioneuralgia (or″kĭ-ō-nū-răl′jĭ-ă) [" + *neuron*, sinew, + *algos*, pain]. Neuralgia of the testicles. SYN: *orchialgia*.

orchiopathy (or″kĭ-ō-op′ăth-ĭ) [" + *pathos*, disease]. Any diseased condition of the testes.

orchiopexy (or'kĭ-ō-peks″ĭ) [" + *pēxis*, fixation]. The suturing of an undescended testicle in the scrotum. SYN: *orchidopexy, orchiorrhaphy*.

orchioplasty (or'kĭ-ō-plas″tĭ) [" + *plassein*, to form]. Plastic repair of the testicle.

orchiorrhaphy (ŏr-kĭ-or′ră-fĭ) [" + *raphē*, a sewing]. The suturing of an undescended testicle to surrounding tissue in the scrotum. SYN: *orchidopexy, orchiopexy*.

orchiosceocele (or-kĭ-os′kĕ-ō-sēl) [" + *oschē*, scrotum, + *kēlē*, hernia]. Scrotal hernia with enlargement or tumor of testicle.

orchioscirrhus (or-kĭ-ō-skĕr′rŭs) [G. *orchis*, testicle, + *skirros*, hard]. Testicular hardening due to tumor formation.

orchis (or′kĭs) [G.]. A testicle.

orchitic (or-kit′ĭk) [G. *orchis*, testicle, + *-itis*, inflammation]. Concerning or caused by orchitis.

orchitis (ŏr-kī′tĭs) [" + *-itis*, inflammation]. Inflammation of a testis due to trauma, metastasis, mumps, or infection elsewhere in the body.

SYM: Swelling, severe pain, possibly gangrene, chills, fever, vomiting, hiccough, delirium. May end in atrophy of organ.

TREATMENT: In mumps, prevention by confining patient to bed first 8 days; locally by immobilization of organ and ice cap.

For acute pain, relief of tension by incision of tunica albuginea, after exposure of organ through scrotal incision, to prevent gangrene. Orchidectomy in suppurative forms, referably to kidney, evidenced by pain increased by exercise, tenderness, frequent urination.

Palliative treatment is orthopedic training in proper posture, etc., improvement in general vitality, combating psychasthenia by overfeeding, massage, hygiene, etc., abdominal support.

o., gonorrheal. O. due to gonococcus.

o., metastatic. O. due to infection from organisms in blood stream.

o., syphilitic. SYM: Begins painlessly in body of gland as a rule, apt to be bilateral; causes dense, irregular, knotty induration, but not much increase in size.

TREATMENT: Antisyphilitics.

o., tuberculous. Form generally arising in the epididymis. It may be accompanied by formation of chronic sinuses, and destruction of tissues.

SYM: Little or no pain. Begins as hard, irregular enlargement at lower and post. aspect of gland, gradually increasing, sometimes extends along vas deferens. Later whole gland undergoes caseous degeneration.

TREATMENT: If unilateral, castration; if bilateral, palliative and symptomatic treatment until evidence of complete destruction. Sinuses and abscesses curetted and treated antiseptically, general health improved.

orchitolytic (or″kĭt-ō-lĭt′ĭk) [G. *orchis*, testicle, + *lysis*, destruction]. Destructive to testicular tissue.

orchotomy (ŏr-kŏt′ō-mĭ) [" + *tomē*, incision]. 1. Incision into a testicle. 2. Erroneously, excision of the testes. SYN: *orchectomy*.

orcin, orcinol (or'sĭn, -ol). Antiseptic derived from lichens, used in skin disorders.

orderly (or'dĕr-lĭ) [L. *ordō*, order]. Male attendant in a hospital, other than doctors or interns, responsible for care or preparation of male patients.

They shave male patients preparatory to operation, catheterize them, and assist nurses in lifting.

orexigenic (ō-rĕk-sĭ-jĕn′ĭk) [G. *orexis*, appetite, + *gennan*, to produce]. Stimulating the appetite.

oreximania (ō-rĕk-sĭ-mā′nĭ-ă) [" + *mania*, madness]. Abnormal desire for food.

organ (or′găn) [G. *organon*, organ]. A part of the body having a special function.

Most organs are in pairs. Any 1 organ may be extirpated and the remaining 1 will perform all necessary functions peculiar to it. Even the right half of the brain may be removed without being fatal. From one-third to two-fifths of some organs may be removed without interference with their functions.

RS: *carreau, name of each in alphabetical order, viscus*.

o., accessory. One having a subordinate function.

o., acoustic. SEE: *o. of Corti*.

Average Size, Weight and Capacity of Various Organs and Parts of the Body

Name	Size	Weight	Capacity
Bladder	5 x 3 x 5 in.		½ to 1 pt.
Esophagus	8 to 9 in.		
Fallopian tubes	4 in. long, 1/16 in. diameter.		
Gallbladder	3 to 4 in. long, 1 in. wide.		8 to 10 dr.
Heart	5 x 3½ x 2½ in.	8 to 12 oz.	4-6 oz. in each ventricle.
Intestines—Duodenum	8 to 10 in. long.		
Intestines—Jejunum	8 ft. long.		
Intestines—Ileum	12 ft. long.		
Intestines—Cecum	2 x 3 in. pouch.		
Intestines—Vermiform appendix	3 to 6 in. long.		
Intestines—Colon	4 to 6 ft. long.		1 gal.
Intestines—Rectum	6 to 8 in. long.		
Kidney	4 x 2½ x 1½ in.	4 to 6 oz.	
Lung—Three right lobes		22 oz.	
Lung—Two left lobes		20 oz.	
Liver	12 x 6 x 3 in.	3 to 5 lb.	
Ovaries	1½ x ¾ x ⅓ in.	½ oz. each.	
Prostate Gland	1 x 1½ x ¾ in.	¾ oz.	
Pharynx	4½ in. long.		
Pancreas	7 x 2 x 1 in.	2 to 4 oz.	
Spleen	5 x 3 x 2 in.	6 to 10 oz.	
Stomach	12 x 4 in.	4 to 5 oz.	3 pt.
Spinal cord	17 to 18 in. long.	1 to 1½ oz.	
Suprarenal Capsule	1½ to 2 in. long.	1 to 2 dr.	
Thoracic duct	18 to 20 in. long.		
Trachea	4 to 5 in. long, ¾-in. diameter.		
Thyroid gland	3 in. long.	1 to 2 oz.	
Thymus gland	2 x 1½ in. long.	½ oz.	
Testes	1-in. diameter, 1½ in. long.	6 to 8 dr. each.	
Uterus	3 x 2 x 1 in.	1 to 3 oz.	
Ureter	12 to 16 in.		
Urethra—Male	8 to 9 in. long.		
Urethra—Female	1½ in. long.		

o., appendicular. The limbs.
o., cell. Basic part of a cell, as a nucleus.
o. of Corti. Terminal acoustic apparatus in the cochlea. SEE: *Claudius' cell, ear.*
o., end. A termination of a nerve, usually bulbous, and of sensory or motor function.
o., endocrine. An organ yielding internal secretions. SEE: *endocrine.*
o., excretory. One secreting waste products of the body.
o's. of generation. The reproductive organs, external and internal. SEE: *genitalia, male and female.*
o. of Giraldes. A small body on the spermatic cord, above the epididymis. SYN: *paradidymis.*
o's., Golgi's. Spindle-shaped structure in muscles.
o., Jacobson's. Rudimentary canal opening in the nasal septum.
o., Meyer's. Area on both sides of post. portion of the tongue.
o. of Rosenmüller. Residual sexual portion of the wolffian body in the broad ligament. SYN: *epoöphoron, parovarium.*
o. of Ruffini. End organ of the fingertips.
o., sense. One consisting of a nerve and its terminus, which convert a stimulus into a sensation.
o., vomeronasal. SEE: *Jacobson's o.*
o., Weber's. Residual prostatic pouch in the male, the remains of the müllerian ducts.
organic (or-găn'ĭk) [G. *organon*, organ].
1. Pert. to an organ or organs. 2. Structural. 3. Pert. to or derived from animal or vegetable forms of life.
o. acid. Any acid containing or derived from the carboxyl group.
o. chemistry. Branch dealing with carbon compounds.
o. disease. One indicating that the structures of an organ are affected.
o. food nutrients. Those nutrients containing carbon.
o. reaction types. PSY: A general term applied to those psychoses induced by structural brain changes.
In general, a character change is manifested in behavior and disposition. The patient is less stable than before, emotional instability, irritability and anger outbursts being frequent. His attention fluctuates widely; gradually he deteriorates; early or later, memory, comprehension, ideation, and orientation become defective.
ETIOL: Alcohol, narcotics, trauma, syphilis, drugs, poisons, chronic infections, encephalitis, brain tumors among many others.
o. sensation. One which arises from the organs of the body.
Muscles, joints, and tendons give us a sense of *position and movement*, without touching anything. This sense is also given by the internal ear. A sense of *hunger* and *thirst* may arise from the alimentary system. The circulatory, urinary, respiratory, and sexual systems also stimulate sensations.

organism (or'găn-ĭzm) [G. " + ismos, condition]. Any correlated living thing.
organization (or"găn-ĭ-zā'shŭn) [G. organon, organ]. 1. Process of correlating. 2. Systematic arrangement. 3. That which is organized; an organism.
organize (or'găn-īz) [G. organon, organ]. 1. To correlate or systematize. 2. To furnish with organs.
organogenesis, organogeny (or-găn-ō-jen'-ĕ-sĭs, -oj'ĕn-ĭ) [" + gennan, to produce]. The formation and development of body organs from embryonic tissues.
organography (or-găn-og'ră-fĭ) [" + graphein, to write]. The description of the body organs.
organoleptic (or-găn-ō-lep'tĭk) [" + lēpsis, a seizure]. 1. Affecting an organ, esp. the organs of special sense. 2. Susceptible to sensory impressions.
organology (or-găn-ol'ō-jĭ) [" + logos, study]. The science dealing with the body organs.
organoma (or-găn-ō'mă) [" + -ōma, tumor]. A tumor composed of definite organs or parts of organs and so arranged as to be a part of the organ or organs concerned.
organon (or'găn-ŏn) [G. & L. organ]. An organ.
 o. auditus. BNA. Organ of hearing.
 o. gustus. BNA. Organ of taste.
 o. olfactus. BNA. Organ of smell.
 o. spirale. BNA. Spiral organ in the cochlea. SYN: *organ of Corti*.
 o. visus. BNA. The organ of sight.
 o. vomeronasale. BNA. Canal opening into nasal septum. SYN: *Jacobson's organ*.
organopexia (or"găn-ō-pĕk'sĭ-ă) [G. organon, organ, + pēxis, fixation]. Surgical fixation of an organ that is detached from its proper position.
organoscopy (or-găn-os'kŏ-pĭ) [" + skopein, to examine]. Examination of the internal organs of the body.
organotherapy (or"găn-ō-thĕr'ă-pĭ) [" + therapeia, treatment]. The treatment of disease by preparations of the endocrine glands of animals, or by extracts made from the same.
organotrope, organotropic (or-găn'ō-trōp, -trŏp'ĭk) [" + tropos, a turning]. Having affinity for tissues, noting substances acting on the organs of the body.
organule (or'găn-ūl) [G. organon, organ]. 1. An essential element of a cell or organ. 2. End organ of sensory receptors for the reception of specially complex sensations, such as the *taste bud* of the tongue, the retinal *rods* and *cones* of the eye, and the *organ of Corti* in the internal ear.
orgasm (or'găzm) [G. organ, to swell, to lust]. 1. Paroxysmal emotional excitement. 2. An instance of it, specifically, the climax of sexual passion.
oridine (or'ĭ-dēn). The calcium salt of iodized fatty acids containing 23-25% organic iodine. [iodine.
 USES: A more easily tolerated form of
 DOSAGE: 1/6 gr. (10 mg.) iodine.
Orien'tal sore. An ulcerating, chronic, nodular skin lesion prevalent in the Orient and the tropics, due to parasites of the genus Leishmania.
orientation (or"ĭ-ĕn-tā'shŭn) [L. oriens, the east]. Ability to comprehend and to adjust one's self in an environment with regard to time, location, and identity of persons. [psychoses.
 Partially or completely absent in some
orifice (or'ĭ-fĭs) [L. orificium]. Mouth, entrance or outlet to any aperture.
 o., anal. The anus.
 o., auriculoventricular. Opening in front and lower part of left and right ventricles of the heart, oval in form, connecting with the auricle.
 o., cardiac. Opening of esophagus into stomach.
 o., pyloric. Opening from stomach into the duodenum. SEE: *pylorus*.
orificial (or-ĭ-fĭ'shĭ-ăl) [L. orificium, outlet]. Pert. to or forming an orifice.
orificialist (or-ĭ-fĭsh'ăl-ĭst) [L. orificium, outlet]. One who practices orificial surgery in the treatment of diseases.
origin (or'ĭ-jĭn) [L. origo, beginning]. 1. The source of anything; a starting point. 2. The beginning of a nerve. 3. The more fixed attachment of a muscle.
ornithosis (or-nĭ-tho'sĭs). A virus disease of birds, communicated to man. The causative agent closely resembles the virus of psittacosis.
orodiagnosis (or"ō-dī-ăg-nō'sĭs) [G. oros, serum, + dia, through, + gnōsis, knowledge]. Diagnosis by using serums or serum reactions.
oroimmunity (o"rō-ĭm-mū-nĭ-tĭ) [" + L. immunitās, safety]. Immunity acquired by injection of serum from a person or animal who has active immunity against the disease in question.
orolingual (ō"rō-lĭn'gwăl) [L. os, or-, mouth, + lingua, tongue]. Concerning the mouth and tongue.
oronasal (ō"rō-nā'zăl) [" + nasus, nose]. Concerning the mouth and nose.
oropharynx (ō"rō-far'ĭnks) [" + G. pharygx, pharynx]. Portion of pharynx between the soft palate and hyoid bone.
orotherapy (ō"rō-thĕr-ă-pĭ) [" + G. therapeia, treatment]. 1. Treatment of disease with serums. SYN: *serotherapy*. 2. Use of whey in treatment.
Oro'ya fever. An acute endemic Chilian disease caused by *Bartonella bacilliformis*.
 SYM: Intermittent fever, pernicious anemia, pains in joints, long bones, and head.
orrhoimmunity (or"rō-ĭm-mū'nĭ-tĭ) [G. orros, serum, + L. immunitās, safety]. Immunity acquired by serum injections from an animal or individual who is actively immunized against the disease in question. SYN: *passive immunity*.
orrhology (or-rol'ō-jĭ) [" + logos, study]. The study of serums and their reactions. SYN: *serology*.
orrhomeningitis (or"rō-men-ĭn-jī'tĭs) [" + mēnigx, membrane, + -itis, inflammation]. Inflammation of a serous membrane.
orrhoreaction (or"rō-rē-ăk'shŭn) [" + L. rē, back, + actus, acted]. A reaction from injection of serum.
orrhorrhea (or"rō-rē'ă) [" + roia, flow]. 1. A flow of serum. 2. A watery discharge. SYN: *seriflux*.
orrhosis (or-rō'sĭs) [" + -ōsis, intensive]. Formation of serum.
orrhotherapy (or"rō-thĕr'ă-pĭ) [" + therapeia, treatment]. 1. Serum therapy. 2. Whey cure.
or'tal-so'dium. A barbituric acid derivative similar to, but more active than barbital.
 USES: As a hypnotic.
 DOSAGE: 3-6 gr. (0.2-0.4 Gm.).
ortho- [G.]. Combining form meaning *straight, right*.
orthoarteriotony (or"tho-ăr-tē-rĭ-ot'ō-nĭ) [G. orthos, straight, + artēria, artery, + tonos, tension]. Normal arterial blood pressure.
orthobiosis (or"thō-bĭ-ō'sĭs) [" + bios, life, + ōsis, increase]. Hygienic living.
orthocephalic (or"thō-sē-făl'ĭk) [" +

kephalē, head]. Noting a head with a height-length index bet. 70 and 75.
orthochorea (or″thō-kō-rē′ă) [″ + *choreia*, dance]. Movements of chorea in erect posture.
orthochromatic (or″thō-krō-mat′ĭk) [″ + *chrōma*, color]. Having normal color.
orthochromophil (or″thō-krō′mō-fĭl) [″ + ″ + *philein*, to love]. Staining normally with neutral dyes.
orthocrasia (or″thō-krā′sĭ-ă) [″ + *krasis*, temperament]. Condition in which the body reacts normally to drugs, proteins, and treatment in general.
orthocytosis (or″thō-sī-tō′sĭs) [G. *orthos*, straight, + *kytos*, cell, + *-ōsis*, condition]. The presence in the blood of mature cells only.
orthodiagraph (or″thō-dī′ă-grăf) [″ + *dia*, through, + *graphein*, to write]. An instrument for accurately recording the outlines and positions of organs or foreign bodies as seen by radiographic apparatus.
orthodontia (or″thō-don′shĭ-ă) [″ + *odous, odont-*, tooth]. Division of dentistry dealing with prevention and correction of irregularities of the teeth.
orthoform (or′thō-form). Colorless, crystalline powder used as an anesthetic.
  DOSAGE: 8-15 gr. (0.5-1.0 Gm.).
orthogenesis (or″thō-jĕn′ĕ′sĭs) [G. *orthos*, straight, + *genesis*, development]. A biological principle that variations in an animal species begin to assume a definite direction, resulting in evolution of a new type, irrespective of ext. factors. SEE: *kinetic system*.
orthogenics (or″thō-jĕn′ĭks) [″ + *genikos*, relating to reproduction]. The science dealing with defects, mental and physical, that hinder normal development. SYN: *eugenics*.
orthoglycemic (or″thō-glī-sē′mĭk) [″ + *glykus*, sweet]. Having an average amount of sugar in the blood.
orthognathous (or-thog′nă-thŭs) [″ + *gnathos*, jaw]. Having straight jaws.
orthograde (or′thō-grād) [″ + L. *gradus*, a step]. Walking with the body vertical or upright.
ortholiposis (or″thō-lĭ-pō′sĭs) [″ + *lipos*, fat, + *-ōsis*]. 1. Normal amount of liposin in blood serum. 2. Condition of normal proportion of weight to height.
orthometer (or-thom′ĕt-ĕr) [″ + *metron*, measure]. Device for determining the degree of protrusion of the eyes.
orthomorphia (or-thō-mor′fĭ-ă) [G. *orthos*, straight, + *morphē*, form]. Correction of a deformity.
orthoneutrophil(e (or″thō-nū′trō-fĭl, -fīl) [″ + L. *neuter*, neither, + G. *philein*, to love]. Staining normally with neutral dyes.
orthopedia (or″thō-pē′dĭ-ă) [″ + *pais, paid-*, child]. Prevention or correction of deformities. SYN: *orthopedics*.
orthopedic (or″thō-pē′dĭk) [″ + *pais, paid-*, child]. Concerning orthopedics; prevention or correction of deformities.
  o. surgery. Surgical prevention and correction of deformities. SYN: *orthopedics*.
orthopedics (or″thō-pē′dĭks) [″ + *pais, paid-*, child]. The treatment of chronic affections of the spine and joints and the prevention and correction of deformities.
orthopedist (or″thō-pē′dĭst) [″ + *pais, paid-*, child]. One who corrects deformities and treats diseases of the joints and spine.
orthopercussion (or″thō-pĕr-kŭsh′ŏn) [″ + L. *percussio*, a striking through]. Percussion with the distal phalanx of the percussing finger held perpendicularly to the surface percussed.
orthophoria (or″thō-fō′rĭ-ă) [G. *orthos*, straight, + *pherein*, to bear]. Parallelism of visual axes, the normal muscle balance.
orthophrenia (or″thō-frē′nĭ-ă) [″ + *phrēn*, mind]. The normal mental state of one who shares his emotional life with the family or a group.
orthopnea (or-thŏp-nē′ă) [″ + *pnein*, to breathe]. Respiratory condition in which breathing is possible only when person sits or stands in erect position.
  ETIOL: Seen in grave cardiac diseases, bronchial and cardiac asthma, edema of lungs, severe emphysema, pneumonia, angina pectoris, spasmodic croup, aneurysm or tumor pressing down on pneumogastric nerve.
  SYM: Respiratory rate, slow or rapid; sitting or standing posture necessary, muscles of respiration forcibly used; patient feels necessity of bracing himself in order to breathe. Anxious expression, face cyanosed. Struggle to inhale and exhale.
  RS: *dyspnea, hyperpnea, hypopnea, oligopnea, posture, respiration*.
orthopraxy (or′thō-prăk-sī) [″ + *prassein*, to make]. Correction and prevention of deformities by mechanical means. SYN: *orthopedics*.
orthopsychiatry (or″thō-sī-kī′ă-trī) [″ + *psychē*, soul, + *iatreia*, treatment]. The study and treatment of conduct disorders, esp. in the young.
orthoptic (or-thŏp′tĭk) [″ + *optikos*, pert. to vision]. Concerning the correction of a deviating eye.
  o. training. Eye muscle exercises for educating the fusion faculty; used in the treatment of squint.
orthoroentgenography (or″thō-rĕnt-gĕn-og′ră-fī) [″ + roentgen, + G. *graphein*, to write]. Measurement of size and position of internal organs accurately, using radiographic apparatus. SEE: *orthodiagraph*.
orthoscope (or″thō-skōp) [G. *orthos*, straight, + *skopein*, to examine]. Instrument for examining the eyes through a layer of water.
orthoscopic (or″thō-skŏp′ĭk) [″ + *skopein*, to examine]. 1. Having correct vision. 2. Seen without distortion. 3. Made to correct optical distortion.
orthoscopy (or-thŏs′kō-pī) [″ + *skopein*, to examine]. Ocular examination with an orthoscope.
orthostatic (or′thō-stăt-ĭk) [″ + *statos*, standing]. Concerning an erect position.
orthostatism (or′thō-stăt-ĭzm) [″ + ″ + *ismos*, condition]. An upright standing position of the body.
orthotast (or′thō-tăst) [″ + *tassein*, to arrange]. Instrument for straightening bone curvatures.
orthotherapy (or″thō-ther′ă-pī) [G. *orthos*, straight, + *therapeia*, treatment]. Correction of posture as a means of treatment.
orthotonos, orthotonus (or-thŏt′ō-nos, -nŭs) [″ + *tonos*, tension]. Tetanic spasm marked by rigidity of the body in a straight line. SEE: *Illus. O-20*.
orthuria (orth-ū′rĭ-ă) [″ + *ouron*, urine]. Average frequency of urination.
oryzenin (ō-rī′zĕn-ĭn) [G. *oryza*, rice]. Concentrated antineuritic vitamin obtained from rice bran. SYN: *Vitamin B₁ or F*.
O. S., o. s. Abbr. for L. *oculus sinister*, left eye.

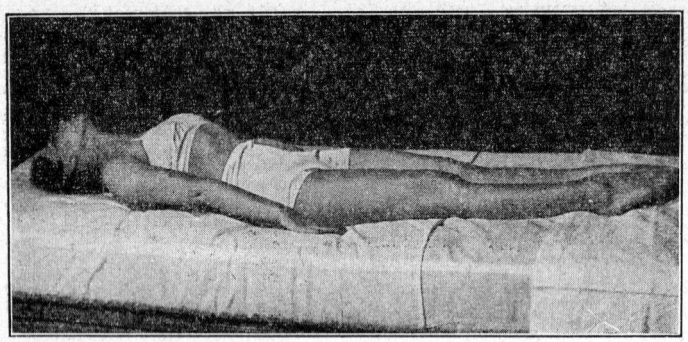

Posed by professional model ORTHOTONOS *Photo by Whitaker*

os (ŏs) (pl. ō*ra*) [L.]. Mouth, opening. BNA.
   o. externum. Portion of the cervix uteri opening into the vaginal canal.
   o. internum. Portion of the cervix uteri opening into the uterus.
   o. uteri. Mouth of the uterus.

os (ŏs) (pl. *ossa*) [L.]. Bone.

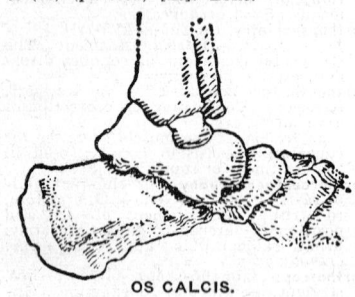

OS CALCIS.

   o. calcis. Heel bone. SYN: *calcaneum*.
   o. coxae. Hipbone.
   o. hamatum. Hooked bone in second row of carpus. SYN: *unciform bone*.
   o. hyoideum. U-shaped bone at the base of the tongue.
   o. ilium. Haunch bone.
   o. innominatum. SEE: *o. coxae*.
   o. interparietale. A bone, occasionally separate, found bet. the frontal, parietal, and sup. occipital bones.
   o. magnum. A carpal bone, the third in the second distal row.
   o. orbiculare. Tiny bone in the ear which usually becomes attached to the incus.
   o. peroneum. Bone occasionally found in tendon of peroneus longus muscle.
   o. planum. 1. Flat bone. 2. Orbital plate of ethmoid bone.
   o. pubis. The pubic bone.
   o. unguis. Lacrimal bone.

osazone (ō'să-zōn, ō″să-zōn'). Any of a series of compounds resulting from heating sugars with acetic acid and phenylhydrazine.

oscedo (os-sē'dō) [L. yawning]. 1. Yawning. 2. White spots on the mucosa of the mouth. SYN: *aphthae*.

oscheal (os'kē-ăl) [G. *oscheon*, scrotum]. Concerning the scrotum.

oscheio-, oscheo- [G.]. Combining forms meaning the *scrotum*.

oscheitis (ŏs-kē-ī'tĭs) [G. *oscheon*, scrotum, + *-itis*, inflammation]. Inflamed condition of the scrotum.

oscheocele (os'kē-ō-sēl) [" + *kēlē*, swelling]. 1. A scrotal swelling or tumor. 2. Scrotal hernia. SYN: *oscheoma*.

oscheohydrocele (os″kē-ō-hī'drō-sēl) [" + *ydōr*, water, + *kēlē*, hernia]. Collection of fluid in the sac of a scrotal hernia.

oscheolith (os'kē-ō-lĭth) [" + *lithos*, stone]. A concretion in the scrotal sebaceous glands.

oscheoma (ŏs-kē-ō'mă) [" + *-ōma*, tumor]. Scrotal tumor. SYN: *oscheoncus*.

oscheoncus (ŏs-kē-on'kŭs) [" + *ogkos*, tumor]. A tumor of the scrotum.

oscheoplasty (os'kē-ō-plăs-tĭ) [" + *plassein*, to form]. Plastic surgical repair of the scrotum.

oschitis (os-kī'tĭs) [G. *oscheon*, scrotum, + *-itis*, inflammation]. Inflamed condition of the scrotum. SYN: *oscheitis*.

oscillation (ŏs″sĭl-ā'shŭn) [L. *oscillāre*, to swing]. A swinging, pendulumlike movement; a vibration.

oscillogram (ŏs'ĭl-ō-grăm) [" + G. *gramma*, a mark]. Record made by the oscillograph.

oscillograph (ŏs'ĭl-ō-grăf) [" + G. *graphein*, to write]. Machine for recording electric vibrations, as of the heart or blood pressure.

oscillometer (ŏs-ĭl-om'ĕt-ĕr) [" + G. *metron*, measure]. Machine to measure oscillations.

oscillometry (ŏs-ĭl-om'ĕ-trĭ) [" + G. *metron*, measure]. The measurement of oscillations with a machine.

oscilloscope (ŏs-ĭl'ō-skōp) [" + G. *skopein*, to examine]. An instrument for making visible the presence or the nature and form of oscillations or irregularities of an electric current.

oscitation (ŏs-ĭ-tā'shŭn) [L. *oscitāre*, to yawn]. Yawning, gaping.

oscodal (os'kō-dăl). A cod liver oil concentrate containing vitamins A and D.
   ACTION AND USES: Same as cod-liver oil.
   DOSAGE: In tablet form, 1-2 tablets t. i. d.

osculum (os'kŭ-lŭm) [L. a little mouth]. Any tiny aperture or pore.

-ose. Chemical suffix indicating (a) the presence of carbohydrates, as *glucose*; (b) primary alteration product of a protein, as *proteose*.

-osis [G.]. Suffix denoting *caused by, state of, disease, intensive*.

Osler's disease (ŏs'lĕr). Rare disease of

the blood in which the red cells are increased in number, the spleen becomes enlarged and cyanosis of the mucosa and skin. SYN: *erythremia, polycythemia.*

osmatic (ŏz-măt'ĭk) [G. *osmaein*, to smell]. Having a keen sense of smell.

osmatism (ŏz'mă-tĭzm) [G. *osme*, odor, + *ismos*, condition]. A well-developed sense of smell.

osme (ŏz'mē) [G.]. 1. An odor. 2. The sense of smell.

osmesis (ŏz-mē'sĭs) [G. *osmēsis*, smelling]. The sense of smell; act of smelling.

osmesthesia (ŏz-mĕs-thē'zĭ-ă) [G. *osmē*, smell, + *aisthēsis*, sensation]. Olfactory sensibility; power of perceiving and distinguishing odors.

osmic acid (ŏz'mĭk) [G. *osmē*, smell]. 1. Volatile, colorless compound formed by heating osmium in air. 2. Compound of osmium trioxide and water (H_2OsO_4).

osmicate (ŏz'mĭ-kāt) [G. *osmē*, smell]. To impregnate or stain with osmic acid.

osmics (ŏz'mĭks) [G. *osmē*, smell]. The science of odors.

osmidrosis (ŏz-mĭd-rō'sĭs) [" + *idrōsis*, perspiration]. Condition in which perspiration has a very strong odor. SYN: *bromidrosis.*

osmium (ŏz'mĭ-ŭm) [G. *osmē*, smell]. A metallic element; symb. Os.

osmo- [G.]. Combining form. 1. (osme) *odor* or *smell*, and 2. (osmos) *threat* or *push.*

osmodysphoria (ŏz-mō-dĭs-fō'rĭ-ă) [" + *dys*, bad, + *pherein*, to bear]. Abnormal dislike of certain odors.

osmogen (ŏz'mō-jĕn) [G. *ōsmos*, impulse, + *gennan*, to produce]. Substance from which an enzyme or ferment is derived.

osmolagnia (ŏz-mō-lăg'nĭ-ă) [G. *osmē*, a smell, + *lagneia*, lust]. Erotic satisfaction derived from odors, usually of the body.

osmology (ŏz-mŏl'ō-jĭ) [" + *logos*, study]. 1. The study of odors. SYN: *osphresiology.* 2. [G. *ōsmos*, a thrusting]. Study of osmosis.

osmometer (oz-mŏm'ĕt-ĕr) [G. *osmē*, smell, + *metron*, measure]. 1. Device for measuring acuity of sense of smell. 2. [G. *ōsmos*, a pushing]. Device for measuring velocity of fluids diffused through membranes.

osmonosology (ŏz"mō-no-sŏl'ō-jĭ) [G. *osmē*, smell, + *nosos*, disease, + *logos*, study]. Branch of medicine dealing with diseases of the organs of smell.

os'mophilic [G. *ōsmos*, a thrusting, + *philein*, to love]. Readily diffused through a membrane.

osmose (ŏz'mōs) [G. *ōsmos*, a thrusting]. 1. To subject to osmosis. 2. To undergo osmosis.

osmosis (ŏz-mō'sĭs) [" + -*ōsis*, intensive]. The passage of solvent through a partition separating solutions of different concentrations.

Pressure varies with amt. of substance in solution and with temperature variations, being greater when the temperature is higher.

Liquid of low pressure always passes through membrane to liquid of higher pressure until both are equal.

The two kinds are *endomosis*, which is the passage into a vessel, and the reverse of this is called *exosmosis*, or the passage of a substance from within outward.

RS: *absorption, dialysis, diffusion, diosmosis, hypotonic, isotonic.*

osmotherapy (os-mō-ther'ă-pĭ) [G. *ōsmos*, a thrusting, + *therapeia*, treatment].

Treatment by changing the osmotic pressure of blood and tissues, as by injection of hypertonic solutions into the blood.

osmotic (ŏz-mŏt'ĭk) [G. *ōsmos*, a thrusting]. Pert. to osmosis, the passage of solutions of different concentration through a membrane.

o. pressure. Unbalanced pressure causing phenomena of osmosis and diffusion.

Closely related to gas pressure. The cells of the body are accustomed to an osmotic pressure of about 7 atmospheres. Of this, more than 6 atmospheres are contributed by sodium chloride and other minerals dissolved in the body fluids.

osphresiolagnia (ŏs-frē"zĭ-ō-lag'nĭ-ă) [G. *osphrēsis*, smell, + *lagneia*, lust]. Excitement of an erotic nature aroused by odors.

osphresiology (ŏs-frē-zĭ-ŏl'ō-jĭ) [" + *logos*, study]. Science of odors and the sense of smell. SYN: *osmology.*

osphresiometer (ŏs-frē-zĭ-ŏm'ĕt-ĕr) [" + *metron*, measure]. Apparatus for measuring the acuteness of the sense of smell. SYN: *osmometer, 1.*

osphresis (ŏs-frē'sĭs) [G. *osphrēsis*, smell]. The sense of smell. SYN: *olfaction.*

osphretic (ŏs-fret'ĭk) [G. *osphrēsis*, smell]. Concerning the sense of smell. SYN: *olfactory.*

osphus (ŏs'fŭs) [G. *osphys*, loin]. Loin.

osphyalgia (ŏs-fĭ-al'jĭ-ă) [" + *algos*, pain]. Pain of the loins or hips. SEE: *lumbago, sciatica.*

osphyitis (ŏs-fĭ-ī'tĭs) [" + -*itis*, inflammation]. Inflammation in the lumbar region.

osphyomyelitis (ŏs"fī-ō-mī-ĕl-ī'tĭs) [" + *myelos*, marrow, + -*itis*, inflammation]. Inflamed condition of the lumbar region of the spinal cord.

os pubis (ŏs pū'bĭs) [L. *os*, bone, + *pubis*, pubes]. A bone that in adult life unites with the ilium and ischium to form the pelvis. Irregular shape, divided into a horizontal, ascending, and descending ramus. The outer extremity constitutes approximately one-fifth of the acetabulum. The inner unites in middle line with corresponding part of the bone of opp. side, forming the symphysis pubis.

ossa (ŏs'ă) (sing. *os*). Bones.
  o. innominata. The hipbones.
  o. triquetra. Tiny bones in cranial sutures. SYN: *wormian bones.*

ossagen (ŏs'ă-jĕn) [L. *ossa*, bones, + G. *gennan*, to produce]. Proprietary powder made from red bone marrow, containing calcium salts.

ossein (ŏs'ē-ĭn) [L. *ossa*, bones]. The organic substance of bones. SYN: *ostein.*

osseous (ŏs'ē-ŭs) [L. *osseus*, bony]. Bonelike; concerning bones. SYN: *bony.*

ossicle (ŏs'ĭ-kl) [L. *ossiculum*, little bone]. Any small bone, as 1 of the 3 bones of the ear, the *malleus, incus,* or *stapes.*

ossicula (ŏs-ĭk'ū-lă) [L. pl.]. Little bones.

ossiculectomy (ŏs"ĭk-ū-lĕk'tō-mĭ) [L. *ossiculum*, little bone, + G. *ektomē*, excision]. Excision of an ossicle, especially one of the ear.

ossiculotomy (ŏs"ĭk-ū-lŏt'ō-mĭ) [" + G. *tomē*, incision]. Surgical incision of 1 or more of the ossicles of the ear.

ossiculum (ŏs-ĭk'ū-lŭm) [L.]. Tiny bone, esp. 1 of the 3 in the middle ear.

ossiferous (ŏs-ĭf'ĕr-ŭs) [L. *os*, bone, + *ferre*, to bear]. Composed of, or forming bone or bony tissue.

ossific (ŏs-ĭf'ĭk) [" + *facere*, to make]. Producing or becoming bone.

ossification (ŏs″ĭ-fĭ-kā′shŭn) [" + *facere*, to make]. 1. Formation of bone substance. 2. Conversion into bone. SEE: *center, epiotic, centrosclerosis.*

ossify (ŏs′ĭ-fī) [" + *facere*, to make]. To turn into bone.

ostalgia (ŏs-tăl′jĭ-ă) [G. *osteon,* bone, + *algos,* pain]. Pain in a bone. SYN: *osteodynia.*

osteanabrosis (ŏs″tē-ăn-ă-brō′sĭs) [" + *anabrōsis,* eating up]. Wasting away of bone.

osteanagenesis (ŏs″tē-ăn-ă-jĕn′ĕ-sĭs) [" + *anagenesis,* reproduction]. Regeneration or re-formation of bone.

ostearthritis (ŏs″tē-ăr-thrī′tĭs) [" + *arthron,* joint, + *-itis,* inflammation]. Inflamed condition of bones and joints.

ostearthrotomy (ŏs″tē-ăr-thrŏt′ō-mĭ) [" + " + *tomē,* incision]. Surgical excision of the articular end of a bone.

ostectomy, osteëctomy (ŏs-tĕk′tō-mĭ, -tē-ĕk′tō-mĭ) [" + *ektomē,* excision]. Surgical excision of a bone or a portion of one.

osteëctopia (ŏs″tē-ĕk-tō′pĭ-ă) [" + *ek,* out, + *topos,* place]. Dislocation of a bone.

ostein (ŏs′tē-ĭn) [G. *osteon,* bone]. Organic matter of bone. SYN: *ossein.*

osteitis (ŏs-tē-ī′tĭs) [" + *-itis,* inflammation]. Inflammation of a bone.

 o., condensing. A form in which the marrow changes into bone. SYN: *osteopsathyrosis, q.v.*

 o. deformans. Chronic form with thickening and hypertrophy of the long bones and deformity of the flat bones.
 SYM: Slow and insidious in onset. Pain in lower limbs, esp. the tibia. Frequent fractures. Waddling gait. Skull becomes enlarged, so that the face appears small and triangular in shape with the head pushed forward. Stature shortens. Occurs only in adults.
 TREATMENT: Constitutional and palliative. SYN: *Paget's disease.* SEE: *Pott's disease.*

 o. fibrosa. O. in which fibrous tissue replaces bony tissue. SYN: *Recklinghausen's disease.*

 o. f. cystica. O. fibrosa with cyst formation on bones.

 o., gummatous. Chronic o. associated with syphilis.

 o., rarefying. Form in which the bone tissue becomes cancellated.

 o., sclerosing. SEE: *condensing o.*

ostemia (ŏs-tē′mĭ-ă) [G. *osteon,* bone, + *aima,* blood]. Congestion of blood in a bone.

ostempyesis (ŏs-tĕm-pī-ē′sĭs) [" + *empyēsis,* suppuration]. Purulent inflammation within a bone.

osteo- [G.]. Combining form meaning *bone.*

osteoaneurysm (ŏs″tē-ō-an′ū-rĭzm) [G. *osteon,* bone, + *aneurysma,* a widening]. Aneurysm, or dilatation of a blood vessel filled with clotted blood, occurring within a bone.

osteoarthritis (ŏs″tē-ō-ăr-thrī′tĭs) [" + *arthron,* joint, + *-itis,* inflammation]. Primarily a disease of the bones with joint involvement and formation of bony excrescences.
 Degenerative form of arthritis* with tendency to fixation.

osteoarthropathy (ŏs″tē-ō-ar-thrŏp′ăth-ĭ) [" + " + *pathos,* disease]. Any involvement of bones and joints, esp. when associated with disease of the central nervous system, the pleura, and lungs.

 o., hypertrophic pulmonary. An affection characterized by enlargement and curving of the nails of fingers or toes and enlargement of wrist and interphalangeal joints.
 Distal ends of tibia and fibula may be affected or enlargement of lower jaw.
 ETIOL: Found in pulmonary tuberculosis, chronic bronchitis, bronchiectasis, congenital heart disease, and chronic cardiac affections.

osteoarthrotomy (ŏs″tē-ō-ar-thrŏt′ō-mĭ) [" + " + *tomē,* incision]. Excision of joint end of a bone. SYN: *ostearthrotomy.*

osteoblast (ŏs-tē-ō-blăst) [G. *osteon,* bone, + *blastos,* germ]. Small germinal cell from which bone grows.

osteocampsia (ŏs″tē-ō-kămp′sĭ-ă) [" + *kampein,* to bend]. Curvature of a bone, as in osteomalacia.

osteocarcinoma (ŏs″tē-ō-kăr-sĭn-ō′mă) [" + *karkinos,* crab cancer, + *-ōma,* tumor]. 1. Osteoma and carcinoma combined. 2. Carcinoma of a bone.

osteocele (ŏs′tē-ō-sēl) [" + *kēlē,* swelling]. 1. Hardening or bony tumor of testis or scrotum. 2. Bony matter forming in hernial sac.

osteocephaloma (ŏs″tē-ō-sĕf-ă-lō′mă) [" + *kephalē,* head, + *-ōma,* tumor]. Encephaloma, a malignant neoplasm of brainlike texture in a bone.

osteochondritis (ŏs″tē-ō-kŏn-drī′tĭs) [" + *chondros,* cartilage, + *-itis,* inflammation]. 1. Inflammation of bone and cartilage. 2. Inflammatory condition in which calcification is defective, with a layer of soft, yellowish-white tissue forming bet. the cartilaginous and calcified parts of a rib.

 o. deformans juvenilis. Chronic inflammation of head of femur in childhood resulting in atrophy and shortening of neck of femur and wide, flat head.

osteochondroma (ŏs″tē-ō-kŏn-drō′mă) [" + " + *-ōma,* tumor]. Tumor composed of both cartilaginous and bony substance.

osteochondrophyte (ŏs″tē-ō-kŏn′drō-fīt) [" + " + *phyton,* growth]. A tumor composed of cartilage and bone.

osteoclasia, osteoclasis (ŏs″tē-ō-klā′zĭ-ă, -ŏk′lă-sĭs) [G. *osteon,* bone, + *klasis,* a breaking]. 1. Fracture of a bone, surgically, to remedy a deformity. 2. Bony tissue destruction.

osteoclast (ŏs′tē-ō-klăst) [" + *klan,* to break]. 1. Device for fracturing bones for therapeutic purposes. 2. Giant, multinuclear cell* found in depressions on the surface of a bone causing entire resorption of bone substance.
 These depressions are called *Howship's lacunae.* The bone appears eroded or as if gnawed.

osteocope (ŏs′tē-ō-kōp) [" + *kopos,* pain]. Severe pain of the bone, esp. at night, usually symptomatic of syphilis.

osteocopic (ŏs″tē-ō-kŏp′ĭk) [" + *kopos,* pain]. Concerning pain in the bone.

osteocranium (ŏs″tē-ō-krā′nĭ-ŭm) [" + *kranion,* skull]. The bony fetal cranium, as differentiated from the cartilaginous cranium.

osteocystoma (ŏs″tē-ō-sĭs-tō′mă) [" + *kystis,* a bladder, + *-ōma,* tumor]. Cystic tumor of a bone.

osteodermia (ŏs″tē-ō-dĕr′mĭ-ă) [" + *derma,* skin]. Bony portions forming in the skin.

osteodynia (ŏs″tē-ō-dĭn′ĭ-ă) [G. *osteon,* bone, + *odynē,* pain]. Persistent pain in a bone. SYN: *ostealgia.*

osteodystrophia (ŏs″tē-ō-dĭs-trō′fĭ-ă) [" + *dys,* ill, + *trophē,* nourishment]. Defective bone development.

o. juvenilis. Defective bone formation in children, in which bone substance is replaced by fibrous tissue. SEE: *osteitis fibrosa.*

osteoencephaloma (ŏs″tē-ō-ĕn″sĕf-ă-lō′mă) [" + *egkephalos,* brain, + *-ōma,* tumor]. Malignant bone tumor, of brainlike texture.

osteoepiphysis (ŏs″tē-ō-ĕp-ĭf′ĭs-ĭs) [" + *epi,* upon, + *physis,* growth]. A small piece of bone which later becomes attached to the larger one.

osteofibroma (ŏs″tē-ō-fī-brō′mă) [" + L. *fibra,* fiber, + G. *-ōma,* tumor]. Tumor of bony and fibrous tissues. SYN: *fibroosteoma.*

osteogen (ŏs′tē-ō-jĕn) [" + *gennan,* to produce]. Substance of the inner periosteal layer from which bone is formed.

osteogenesis, osteogeny (ŏs″tē-ō-jĕn′ē-sĭs, -ŏj′ē-nĭ) [" + *gennan,* to produce]. Formation and development of bone taking place in connective tissue or in cartilage.

o. imperfecta. A congenital bone disease causing the bones to fracture easily.

osteography (ŏs-tē-og′raf-ĭ) [G. *osteon,* bone, + *graphein,* to write]. Descriptive treatise on the bones.

osteohalisteresis (ŏs″tē-ō-hăl-ĭs-tĕr-ē′sĭs) [" + *als,* salt, + *sterein,* to deprive]. Deficiency of the mineral constituents in bone causing softening.

osteoid (ŏs′tē-oyd) [" + *eidos,* resemblance]. 1. Resembling bone. 2. A bone tumor.

o. sarcoma. A rapidly forming sarcoma with bone tissue in it. SYN: *osteosarcoma.*

osteology (ŏs-tē-ol′ō′jĭ) [" + *logos,* study]. The science of structure and function of bones.

osteolysis (ŏs-tē-ol′ĭs-ĭs) [" + *lysis,* dissolution]. Softening and destruction of bone, as in caries.

osteoma (ŏs-tē-ō′mă) (pl. *osteomata*) [" + *-ōma,* tumor]. A bony tumor; a hard tumor of bonelike structure developing on a bone, and sometimes on other structures.

o., cancellous. One that is soft and spongy. Its thin and delicate trabeculae enclose large medullary spaces similar to cancellous bone.

o., cavalryman's. Bony outgrowth of femur at the insertion of the adductor femoris longus.

o. dentale. A hard, bony outgrowth from the jawbone.

o. durum. A tumor composed of hard bony tissue.

o., heteroplastic. An o. in an organ or tissue in which bone does not normally occur.

o. medullare. An osteoma containing medullary spaces.

o. spongiosum. Soft, spongy tumor in bone.

osteomalacia (ŏs″tē-ō-măl-ā′sĭ-ă) [" + *malakia,* softening]. Softening of the bones. SYN: *malacosteon, mollities ossium.*

A disease marked by increasing softness of the bones, so that they become flexible and brittle and cause deformities. It is attended with rheumatic pains. The limbs, spine, thorax, and pelvis esp. are affected; anemia and signs of deficiency disease present; the patient becomes weak, and finally dies from exhaustion. It occurs chiefly in adults.

o. apsathyros. A form in which bones become flexible like wax.

o. carcinomatosa. Diffuse cancerous infiltration of medullary tissue of bones with softening.

o. fracturosa, o. fragilis, o. psathyra. O. in which the bones become brittle.

osteomalacic (ŏs″tē-ō-măl-ā′sĭk) [G. *osteon,* bone, + *malakia,* softening]. Concerning or characterized by softening of the bone.

osteomalacosis (ŏs″tē-ō-măl-ă-kō′sĭs) [" + " + *-ōsis,* intensive]. Softening of the bone. SYN: *osteomalacia.*

osteomatoid (ŏs-tē-ō′mă-toyd) [" + *-ōma,* tumor, + *eidos,* resemblance]. Resembling a tumor of bone tissue.

osteomere (ŏs′tē-ō-mēr) [" + *meros,* part]. One of a series of similar bone segments, such as any of the vertebrae.

osteometry (ŏs-tē-om′et-rĭ) [" + *metron,* measure]. The study of the measurement of bones.

osteomiosis (ŏs″tē-ō-mĭ-ō′sĭs) [" + *meiōsis,* a lessening]. Bone disintegration.

osteomyelitis (ŏs″tē-ō-mī-ĕl-ī′tĭs) [G. *osteon,* bone, + *myelos,* marrow, + *-itis,* inflammation]. Inflammation of bone marrow, or of the bone and marrow.

SYM: Pain over affected part, fever, sweats, leukocytosis, overlying muscles usually rigid, skin inflamed, pain on pressure over affected part. Suppuration may occur.

TREATMENT: Prompt and adequate doses of antibiotics. Sedation for pain and anxiety. Aspiration of abscess. Blood transfusions and saline infusions. Immobilization of affected extremity. Foods and liquids by mouth. Surgery if abscess persists.

o. fibrosa. Fibroid change in bone in osteitis deformans.

o., hemorrhagic. Bone marrow inflammation with cyst formation.

o., hunger. O. in those not properly nourished, displaying early symptoms of osteomalacia.

o., malignant. Malignant bone marrow tumor.

o. variolosa. O. as a complication of smallpox.

osteoncus (ŏs-tē-on′kŭs) [" + *ogkos,* tumor]. A bone tumor. SYN: *exostosis, osteoma.*

osteonecrosis (ŏs″tē-ō-nē-krō′sĭs) [" + *nekrōsis,* death]. Death of bone.

osteoneuralgia (ŏs″tē-ō-nū-ral′jĭ-ă) [" + *neuron,* nerve, + *algos,* pain]. Pain of a bone.

osteonosus (ŏs-tē-on′ō-sus) [" + *nosos,* disease]. Any disease of bone.

osteopath (os′tē-ō-păth) [" + *pathos,* disease]. A practitioner of osteopathy, *q.v.*

osteopathic (ŏs″tē-ō-păth′ĭk) [" + *pathos,* disease]. Concerning therapeutic bone manipulation.

osteopathology (os-tē-ō-path-ol′ō-jĭ) [G. *osteon,* bone, + *pathos,* disease, + *logos,* study]. Any bone disease.

osteopathy (ŏs-tē-op′ăth-ĭ) [" + *pathos,* disease]. 1. Any bone disease.

2. "A school of medicine based upon the theory that the body is a vital mechanical organism whose structural and functional integrity are coördinate and that the perversion of either is disease, while its therapeutic procedure is chiefly manipulative correction, its name indicating the fact that the bony framework of the body largely determines the structural relation of its tissues." *Committee on Osteopathic Terminology.*

osteopecilia (ŏs″tē-ō-pē-sĭl′ĭ-ă) [" + *poikilia*, spottedness]. Disease marked by spontaneous fractures and spotted marble appearance of bones following abnormal skeletal calcification. SYN: *Albers-Schönberg disease*.

osteopedion (ŏs″tē-ō-pe′dĭ-ŏn) [" + *paidion*, child]. A calcified or hardened fetus. SYN: *lithopedion*.

osteoperiosteal (ŏs″tē-ō-per-ĭ-os′tē-ăl) [" + *peri*, around, + *osteon*, bone]. Concerning bone and its periosteum, the protective membrane.

osteoperiostitis (ŏs″tē-ō-per-ĭ-ŏs-tī′tĭs) [" + " + *-itis*, inflammation]. Combined inflammation of a bone and its protective membrane, the periosteum.

osteopetrosis (ŏs″tē-ō-pĕt-rō′sĭs) [" + L. *petra*, stone, + G. *-ōsis*, disease]. Excessive calcification of bones causing spontaneous fractures and marblelike appearance. SYN: *osteosclerosis fragilis generalisata*.

osteophage (ŏs″tē-ō-fāj) [G. *osteon*, bone, + *phagein*, to eat]. Large multinuclear cell which causes absorption of bone. SYN: *osteoclast, 2*.

osteophlebitis (ŏs″tē-ō-flē-bī′tĭs) [" + *phleps, phleb-*, vein, + *-itis*, inflammation]. Inflammation of veins of a bone.

osteophone (ŏs′tē-ō-fōn) [" + *phōnē*, voice]. Device used by the deaf for conducting sound through facial bones.

osteophyma (ŏs″tē-ō-fī′mă) [" + *phyma*, growth]. A swelling or growth of bone.

osteophyte (ŏs′tē-ō-fīt) [" + *phyton*, plant]. A bony excrescence or outgrowth, usually branched in shape.

osteoplastic (ŏs″tē-ō-plăs′tĭk) [" + *plastikos*, formed]. 1. Pert. to bone repair. 2. Concerning bone formation.

osteoplastica (ŏs″tē-ō-plăs′tĭ-kă) [" + *plastikos*, formed]. An inflammatory disease of the bone with fibrous degeneration and formation of cysts, the femur, humerus and tibia esp. being affected. SYN: *osteitis fibrosa cystica*.

osteoplasty (ŏs″tē-ō-plăs″tī) [G. *osteon*, bone, + *plassein*, to form]. Plastic repair of the bones.

osteopoikilosis (ŏs″tē-ō-poy-kĭ-lō′sĭs) [" + *poikilos*, spotted]. Disease of bones marked by excessive calcification in spots, causing spontaneous fractures and spotted marble appearance. SYN: *Albers-Schönberg disease*.

osteoporosis (ŏs″tē-ō-por-ō′sĭs) [" + *poros*, a passage]. Increased porosity of bone.
SYM: Softening of bone, widening of haversian canals, absorption of calcareous matter. SEE: *osteomalacia*.

o., parachitic. O. with tendency to develop into rickets. Congenital.

osteoporotic (ŏs″tē-ō-pō-rot′ĭk) [" + *poros*, passage]. Concerning enlarged bone spaces.

osteopsathyrosis (ŏs″tē-op-sath″ĭ-rō′sĭs) [" + *psathyros*, fragile]. Fragility or brittleness of bones.
Congenital condition of unknown etiology, in which the long bones appear normal in appearance and chemical composition, but are extremely brittle.
SYM: Breaks may occur upon bathing infant or turning him over, following minor injuries, chewing, bending the knee, etc. Breaks almost painless with slight swelling and only evidence is unwillingness of the child to use his injured limb.
PROG: Condition tends to improve and usually disappears by the 21st year.
TREATMENT: Good hygiene, nourishing diet, supports to prevent breaks. Bones knit quickly with normal amount of callus. SYN: *fragilitas ossium*.

osteorrhagia (ŏs″tē-ō-rā′jĭ-ă) [" + *rēgnunai*, to burst forth]. Hemorrhagic flow of blood from a bone.

osteorrhaphy (ŏs″tē-or′ăf-ĭ) [" + *raphē*, a sewing]. Suture of bone or the wiring of bone fragments.

osteosarcoma (ŏs″tē-ō-sar-kō′mă) [G. *osteon*, bone, + *sarx, sark-*, flesh, + *-ōma*, tumor]. A malignant sarcoma of the bone. SYN: *myelosarcoma*.

osteosarcomatous (ŏs″tē-ō-sar-kō′măt-ŭs) [" + " + *-ōma*, tumor]. Concerning or like an osteosarcoma.

osteosarcosis (ŏs″tē-ō-sar-kō′sĭs) [" + " + *-ōsis*, intensive]. Conversion of bone into a fleshy mass.

osteosclerosis (ŏs″tē-ō-sklē-rō′sĭs) [" + *sklēros*, hard, + *-ōsis*, intensive]. Hardening of bone with increased heaviness.

o. congenita. Defective development of cartilage at epiphyses of long bones resulting in dwarfism. SYN: *achondroplasia*.

o. fragilis generalisata. Abnormal calcification of the bones, causing spontaneous fractures and spotted marblelike appearance in a roentgenogram. SYN: *Albers-Schönberg disease; marble bones; osteitis, condensing; osteopetrosis; osteopoikilosis*.

osteoscope (ŏs″tē-ō-skōp) [" + *skopein*, to examine]. Appliance used to test x-ray machines by observing certain bones of the forearm which are considered as a standard.

osteoseptum (ŏs″tē-ō-sĕp′tŭm) [" + L. *saeptum*, a dividing]. The bony area of the nasal septum.

osteosis (ŏs″tē-ō′sĭs) [G. *osteon*, bone, + *-ōsis*, condition]. Formation of bony tissue. SYN: *osteogenesis*.

o. cutis. Diffuse thickening of skin and subcutaneous tissue. Rare.

osteospongioma (ŏs″tē-ō-spon-jĭ-ō′mă) [" + *spoggos*, sponge, + *-ōma*, tumor]. A spongy neoplasm of the bone. SYN: *osteoma spongiosum*.

osteosteatoma (ŏs″tē-ō-stē-ăt-ō′mă) [" + *stear, steat-*, fat, + *-ōma*, tumor]. A fatty tumor with bony elements.

osteostixis (ŏs″tē-ō-stiks′ĭs) [" + *stixis*, a puncture]. Therapeutic puncture of a bone.

osteosuture (ŏs″tē-ō-sūt′chūr) [" + L. *sutura*, a stitch]. Suture or wiring of bone fragments. SYN: *osteorrhaphy*.

osteosynovitis (ŏs″tē-ō-sin-ō-vī′tĭs) [" + *syn*, with, + *ōon*, egg, + *-itis*, inflammation]. Inflammation of a synovial membrane and the surrounding bones.

osteosynthesis (ŏs″tē-ō-sĭn′the-sĭs) [" + *synthēsis*, a joining]. Surgical fastening of the ends of a fractured bone mechanically.

osteotabes (ŏs″tē-ō-tā′bēz) [G. *osteon*, bone, + *tabes*, a wasting]. Atrophy of the bone in infants, beginning with wasting of the marrow and gradually the rest of the bone.

osteotelangiectasia (ŏs″tē-ō-tĕl-ăn″jĭ-ĕk-tā′zĭ-ă) [" + *telos*, end, + *aggeion*, vessel, + *ektasis*, a stretching]. 1. Dilatation of a bone's small blood vessels. 2. Sarcomatous tumor of the bone containing dilated blood vessels.

osteothrombosis (ŏs″tē-ō-thrŏm-bō′sĭs) [" + *thrombōsis*, a clotting]. Clot formation in the veins of a bone.

osteotome (ŏs′tē-ō-tōm) [" + *tomē*, a cutting]. A chisel bevelled on both sides for cutting through bones.

osteotomy (ŏs″tē-ot′ō-mĭ) [" + *tomē*, in-

cision]. The surgical section of a bone.
  o., cuneiform. The excision of a wedge of a bone.
  o., linear. Lengthwise division of a bone.
  o., MacEwen's. Supracondylar section of the femur for correction of knock-knee.
  o., subtrochanteric. Gant's operation, division of shaft of femur below lesser trochanter to correct ankylosis of hip joint.
  o., transtrochanteric. Section of the femur through the lesser trochanter for deformity about the hip joint.
osteotrite (ŏs'tē-ō-trīt) [" + *tribein*, to crush]. Instrument used to scrape away diseased bone.
osthexia (ŏs-thĕks'ĭ-ă) [G. *osteon*, bone, + *exis*, condition]. Excessive ossification, esp. in abnormal places.
ostial (ŏs'tĭ-ăl) [L. *ostium*, a little opening]. Concerning an orifice.
ostitis (ŏs-tī'tĭs) [G. *osteon*, bone, + *-itis*, inflammation]. Inflammation of a bone. SYN: *osteitis*, q.v.
ostium (ŏs'tĭ-ŭm) (pl. *ostia*) [L. a small opening]. Any small opening.
  o. abdominale. Fimbriated extremity of a fallopian tube.
  o. arteriosum. BNA. Arterial orifice, of ventricle of the heart into the aorta, or pulmonary artery.
  o. internum. Uterine end of a fallopian tube. SYN: *o. uterinum tubae.*
  o. pharyngeum. Pharyngeal opening of the auditory tube.
  o. tympanicum. Tympanic opening of the auditory tube.
  o. uterinum tubae. BNA. Uterine opening of an oviduct.
  o. vaginae. Ext. opening of the vagina.
ostraco-, ostrac- [G.]. Combining form meaning *hard shell.*
ostreotoxismus (ŏs″trē-ō-tŏks-ĭz'mŭs) [G. *ostreon*, oyster, + *toxikon*, poison]. Poisoning from eating diseased oysters.
Ostrow'ski manumo'bilizer. Apparatus to mobilize finger by stretching contractures and loosening adhesions.
otacoustic (ō″tă-koos'tĭk) [G. *ōtakoustein*, to listen]. 1. Aiding or concerning the hearing. 2. Device to aid hearing.
otalgia (ō-tăl'jĭ-ă) [G. *ous*, *ōt-*, ear, + *algos*, pain]. Pain of the ear.
  TREATMENT: *Local:* Heat in the form of compresses or hot water bottle, warm glycerin dropped in ear. Incision of drum if bulging is present. *General:* Active elimination, sedatives. SYN: *earache.*
otaphone (ō'tă-fōn) [" + *phōnē*, voice]. A device used to aid in hearing.
otectomy (ō-tĕk'tō-mĭ) [" + *ektomē*, excision]. Surgical excision of the contents of the tympanum.
othelcosis (ō-thĕl-kō'sĭs) [" + *elkōsis*, ulceration]. Ulceration or suppuration of the ear.
othematoma (ō″thĕm-ă-tō'mă) [" + *aima*, blood, + *-ōma*, tumor]. Effusion of blood between perichondrium and cartilage of pinna.
  Common in fighters or wrestlers or in the insane.
othemorrhea (ō-thĕm-or-rē'ă) [" + " + *roia*, flow]. Bleeding from the ear.
othygroma (ō-thī-grō'mă) [G. *ous*, *ōt-*, ear, + *ygros*, moist, + *-ōma*, tumor]. Edema of ear lobe.
otiatrics (ō-tĭ-ăt'rĭks) [" + *iatrikos*, healing]. Treatment of ear diseases.
otic (ō'tĭk) [G. *ous*, *ōt-*, ear]. Concerning the ear.

oticodinia (ō″tĭk-ō-dĭn'ĭ-ă) [" + *dinē*, a whirl]. Vertigo due to ear disease.
otitic (ō-tĭ'tĭk) [" + *-itis*, inflammation]. Concerning inflammation of the ear.
otitis (ō-tī'tĭs) [G. *ous*, *ōt-*, ear, + *-itis*, inflammation]. Inflamed condition of the ear.
  It is differentiated as *externa, media,* and *interna,* depending upon the portion of the ear which is inflamed.
  TREATMENT: Depends on type of otitis. (1) External otitis, such as furunculosis and eczema, treated conservatively. (2) Exudative catarrh treated by inflation. (3) Acute catarrhal otitis media, use local heat, and resort to active elimination and sedatives. (4) Acute suppurative otitis media, liberal incision in drum membrane. (5) Chronic suppurative otitis media, dry treatment. Clean canal thoroughly, then follow with iodine, dusting powder in ear, and dry strips of gauze for drainage. (6) Circumscribed otitis interna and diffuse serous otitis interna, treated conservatively with absolute rest in bed. (7) Diffuse purulent suppurative otitis interna, treated surgically.
  o., furuncular. Furuncle formation in ext. meatus.
  o. labyrinthica. Inflammation of the labyrinth.
  o. mastoidea. Inflamed condition of the mastoid spaces.
  o. mycotica. Fungous inflammation.
  o. parasitica. Inflammation caused by a parasitic fungus.
  o. sclerotica. Inflammation of inner ear accompanied by hardening of the aural structures.
oto-, ot- [G.]. Combining form meaning *ear.*
otoantritis (ō″tō-ăn-trī'tĭs) [G. *ous*, *ōt-*, ear, + *antron*, cavity, + *-itis*, inflammation]. Inflamed condition of mastoid antrum.
otobiosis (ō″tō-bĭ-ō'sĭs) [" + *bios*, life, + *-ōsis*, condition]. Disease of the ear caused by presence of *Otobius.*
Otobius (ō-tō'bĭ-ŭs) [" + *bios*, life]. Genus of ticks probably transmitting relapsing fever.
  Certain species bite the ear.
otoblennorrhea (ō″to-blĕn-or-rē'ă) [" + *blenna*, mucus, + *roia*, flow]. Mucous discharge from ear.
otocatarrh (ō″tō-kă-tar') [" + *katarrein*, to flow down]. Catarrhal discharge of the ear.
otocerebritis (ō″tō-sĕr-ē-brī'tĭs) [" + L. *cerebrum*, brain, + G. *-itis*, inflammation]. Cerebral inflammation resulting from disease of the middle ear.
otocleisis (ō-tō-klī'sĭs) [" + *kleisis*, a closure]. Occlusion of ear.
otoconia, otoconite, otoconium (ō″tō-kō'nĭ-ă, -tok'ō-nīt, -tō-kō'nĭ-ŭm) [G. *ous*, *ōt-*, ear, + *konis*, dust]. Concretion of calcium carbonate on the membranous labyrinth of the ear. SYN: *ear dust, otolith.*
otocrane (ō'tō-krān) [" + *kranion*, skull]. The cavity in the petrous bone wherein lodges the internal ear.
otocyst (ō'tō-sĭst) [" + *kystis*, bladder]. Primordial chamber from which arises the membranous labyrinth. SYN: *auditory vesicle.*
otodynia (ō″tō-dĭn'ĭ-ă) [" + *odynē*, pain]. Pain in the ear. SYN: *otalgia.*
otoencephalitis (ō″tō-ĕn-sĕf-ăl-ī'tĭs) [" + *egkephalos*, brain, + *-itis*, inflammation]. Inflammation of brain resulting

otoganglion   O-26   **ounce**

from disease of the middle ear. SYN: *otocerebritis.*

otoganglion (ō″tō-găng′lĭ-on) [" + *ganglion*, knot]. Ganglion located below foramen ovale distributing to the tensor tympani and the tensor palati. SYN: *ganglion, otic.*

otography (ō-tog′ră-fĭ) [" + *graphein*, to write]. Anatomical description of the ear.

otolith (o′to-lith) [G. *ous, ōt-*, ear, + *lithos*, stone]. One of the calcareous deposits resting on sensory nerve fibers within the utricle and saccule; part of the static apparatus. SEE: *otoconia.*

otological (ō″tō-lŏj′ĭ-kl) [" + *logos*, study]. Rel. to study of diseases of the ear.

otologist (ō-tŏl-ō-jĭst) [" + *logos*, study]. One versed in diseases of the ear. SYN: *aurist.*

otology (ō-tol′ō-jĭ) [" + *logos*, study]. The science of the ear, its function, and diseases.

otomassage (ō″tō-mă-säj′) [" + *massein*, to knead]. Application of massage to tympanic membrane and auditory ossicles.

otomyasthenia (ō″tō-mĭ-ăs-thē′nĭ-ă) [" + *mys, my-*, muscle, + *astheneia*, weakness]. 1. Weakened condition of the ear muscles. 2. Defective hearing caused by paresis of the tensor tympani and stapedius muscles.

Otomyces (ō″tō-mĭ′sēz) [" + *mykēs*, fungus]. Fungus infesting the ear.
   O. hageni. Form with green conidia, affecting ext. canal.
   O. purpureus. A dark red variety.

otomycosis (ō″tō-mĭ-kō′sĭs) [" + " + *-ōsis*, condition]. Fungous infection of ext. auditory meatus of the ear. SYN: *otitis mycotica.*

otoncus (ō-tŏng′kŭs) [" + *ogkos*, tumor]. An aural tumor.

otonecrectomy, otonecronectomy (ō″tō-něk-rěk′tō-mĭ, -rō-něk′tō-mĭ) [G. *ous, ōt-*, ear, + *nekros*, dead, + *ektomē*, excision]. Excision of necrosed areas from the ear.

otoneuralgia (ō″tō-nū-răl′jĭ-ă) [" + *neuron*, sinew, + *algos*, pain]. Pain in the ear. SYN: *otalgia.*

otoneurasthenia (ō″tō-nū-răs-thē′nĭ-ă) [" + " + *astheneia*, weakness]. Neurasthenia caused by ear disease.

otoneurology (ō″tō-nū-rŏl′ō-jĭ) [" + " + *logos*, study]. Study of ear conditions in conjunction with neural complications. SYN: *neurotology.*

otopathy (o-top′ăth-ĭ) [" + *pathos*, disease]. Any diseased condition of the ear.

otopharyngeal (ō″tō-far-ĭn′jē-ăl) [" + *pharygx*, pharynx]. Concerning the ear and pharynx.
   o. tube. Passage bet. tympanic cavity and the pharynx. SYN: *eustachian tube.*

otophone (o′tō-fōn) [G. *ous, ōt-*, ear, + *phōnē*, voice]. Device for assisting deaf to hear.

otopiesis (ō″tō-pĭ-ē′sĭs) [" + *piesis*, a pressing]. 1. Sinking in or depression of the membrana tympani. 2. Pressure on the labyrinth causing deafness.

otoplasty (ō′tō-plăs-tĭ) [" + *plassein*, to form]. Plastic surgery of the ear to correct defects.

otopolypus (ō″tō-pol′ĭp-ŭs) [" + *polus*, many, + *pous*, foot]. Smooth growth occurring in the ear.

otopyorrhea (ō″tō-pī-ō-re′ă) [" + *pyon*, pus, + *roia*, a flow]. Purulent ear discharge.

otopyosis (ō″tō-pī-ō′sĭs) [" + " + *-ōsis*, infection]. Ear disease marked by discharge of pus.

otorhinolaryngology (ō″tō-rī-nō-lăr-ĭn-gōl′ō-jĭ) [" + *ris, rin-*, nose, + *larygx*, larynx, + *logos*, study]. The science of ear, nose, and larynx and their functions and diseases.

otorhinology (ō″tō-rī-nŏl′ō-jĭ) [" + " + *logos*, study]. Branch of medicine dealing with ear and nose diseases.

otorrhagia (ō-tō-rā′jĭ-ă) [G. *ous, ōt-*, ear, + *rēgnunai*, to flow]. Discharge of blood from ear.

otorrhea (ō-tō-rē′ă) [" + *roia*, flow]. Inflammation of ear with purulent discharge.
   SYM: Membrana tympani may be partially or completely destroyed; deafness, tinnitus, no pain, repeated attacks of nasopharyngitis.
   TREATMENT: Frequent dry cleansing, iodine dusting powder, tubal inflation. SEE: *otitis.*

otosalpinx (ō″tō-săl′pĭnks) [" + *salpigx*, tube]. Passage connecting pharynx and tympanic cavity. SYN: *eustachian tube.*

otoscleronectomy (ō″tō-sklē-rō-něk′tō-mĭ) [" + *sklēros*, hard, + *ektomē*, excision]. Surgical excision of sclerosed and ankylosed ear ossicles.

otosclerosis (ō″tō-sklē-rō′sĭs) [" + *sklērōsis*, a hardening]. Disease of the ear characterized by a patent eustachian tube, normal drum membrane, conversion into sponge of the bony capsule of the labyrinth and fixation of the stapes due to ankylosis in the oval window. Possibly hereditary. The disease results in chronic progressive deafness.

otoscope (ō′tō-skōp) [" + *skopein*, to examine]. Device for examination of the ear.

otosis (ō-tō′sĭs) [" + *-ōsis*, intensive]. Mishearing of spoken sounds.

otosteal (ō-tos′tē-ăl) [G. *ous, ōt-*, ear, + *osteon*, bone]. Concerning the bones or ossicles of the ear.

ototomy (ō-tŏt′ō-mĭ) [" + *tomē*, incision]. Incision into or dissection of the ear.

oturia (ō-tū′rī-ă) [" + *ouron*, urine]. Delusion of urinous discharge from the ear due to metastasis. [eye.
O. U. Abbr. for L. *oculus uterque*, for each
ouabain (wăh-băh′ĭn). A glucoside prepared from *Strophanthus gratus*, but more active. USP. Syn. for *G. strophanthin.*
   USES: Same as for digitalis, but less tendency to cumulative action.
   DOSAGE: 1/120 gr. (0.0005 Gm.), intravenously.

Oudin current (oo-dan′). A high frequency oscillating current of higher voltage than the current used ordinarily, employed in therapeutic treatment.
   O. resonator. A coil of wire with an adjustable number of turns, designed to be connected to a source of high frequency current, such as a spark gap and induction coil, for the purpose of applying a convective discharge of high voltage current to a patient.

oulitis (oo-lī′tĭs) [G. *oulon*, gum, + *-ītis*, inflammation]. Inflamed condition of the gums. SYN: *ulitis.*

oulorrhagia (oo-lō-rā′jĭ-ă) [" + *rēgnunai*, to burst forth]. Hemorrhage from the gums. SYN: *ulorrhagia.*

ounce (ouns) [L. *uncia*, a twelfth]. A measure of weight.
   In *apothecaries* or *troy* weight, 1/12

ounce, fluid lb. [480 gr. (31.103 Gm.)]. Symb. ℥.
In *avoirdupois* measure, 1/16 lb. [437.5 gr. (28.349 Gm.)]. Abbr. oz.
  o., fluid. For liquid medicines, 8 fluid drams [1/16 pint (29.6 cc.)].
out'patient. One receiving treatment at a hospital without being an inmate.
ova (ō'vă) (pl. of *ovum*) [L., from G. *ōon*, egg]. Reproductive cells of the female. 2. Eggs. SEE: *ovary, ovum.*
oval (ō'văl) [L. *ovum*, egg]. 1. Like or concerning an ovum, the reproductive cell of the female. 2. Shaped like an egg.
  o. window. Oval-shaped aperture in the middle ear.
ovalbumin (ō-văl-bū'mĭn) [" + *albumen*, white of egg]. Albumin in egg whites.
ovalocyte (o'văl-ō-sīt) [" + G. *kytos*, cell]. Egg-shaped red blood corpuscle.
ovalocytosis (ō-văl″ō-sī-tō'sĭs) [" + " + *-ōsis*, intensive]. Oval red blood corpuscles in the blood.
ovaraden (ō-văr-ā'dĕn) [L. *ovarium*, ovary]. A powdered extract from animal ovaries used as a sedative, nerve tonic, and in disorders of the female genitalia.
ovaralgia, ovarialgia (o-var-al'jĭ-ă, -ĭ-al'-jĭ-ă) [L. *ovarium*, ovary, + G. *algos*, pain]. Ovarian pain. SYN: *oarialgia.*
ovarian (ō-vā'rĭ-ăn) [L. *ovarium*, ovary]. Concerning or resembling the ovary.
  o. cyst. A sac containing fluid which develops in the ovary proper.
    It consists of 1 or more chambers containing fluid. These *loculi*, or chambers, may contain an enormous amt. of fluid. Not malignant but may prove fatal if not removed, because of twisting of the pedicle which causes gangrene, or because of pressure. Dermoid cyst contains a cheesy substance composed of fat, hair, sebaceous matter, bone, or teeth. Solid tumors, if benign, are usually fibroid.
ovariectomy (ō-vā-rĭ-ĕk'tō-mĭ) [" + G. *ektomē*, excision]. Excision of an ovary or a portion of it. SYN: *oöphorectomy.*
ovario- [G.]. Combining form meaning *ovary.*
ovariocele (ō-va'rĭ-ō-sēl) [L. *ovarium*, ovary, + G. *kēlē*, mass]. Ovarian tumor or hernia.
ovariocentesis (ō-vā-rĭ-ō-sĕn-tē'sĭs) [" + G. *kentēsis*, a piercing]. Puncture and drainage of an ovarian cyst.
ovariocyesis (ō-vā-rĭ-ō-sī-ē'sĭs) [" + G. *kyēsis*, pregnancy]. Pregnancy in the ovary, instead of in the uterus.
ovariodysneuria (ō-vā″rĭ-ō-dĭs-nū'rĭ-ă) [" + G. *dys*, ill, + *neuron*, sinew]. Neuralgia in an ovary.
ovariohysterectomy (ō-vā″rĭ-ō-hĭs-tĕr-ĕk'tō-mĭ) [" + G. *ystera*, uterus, + *ektomē*, excision]. Excision of the ovaries and uterus. SYN: *oöphorohysterectomy.*
ovariorrhexis (ō-vā'rĭ-ō-rĕks'ĭs) [" + G. *rēxis*, a rupture]. Rupture of an ovary.
ovariosalpingectomy (ō-vā″rĭ-ō-săl-pĭn-jĕk'tō-mĭ) [" + G. *salpigx*, tube, + *ektomē*, excision]. Removal of an ovary and oviduct. SYN: *oöphorosalpingectomy.*
ovariosteresis (ō-va″rĭ-ō-ster-ē'sĭs) [L. *ovarium*, ovary, + G. *sterēsis*, loss]. Complete eradication of an ovary.
ovariostomy (ō-vā-rĭ-ŏs'tō-mĭ) [" + G. *stoma*, opening]. Creation of an opening in an ovarian cyst for drainage.
ovariotomist (ō-va″rĭ-ot'ō-mĭst) [" + G. *tomē*, incision]. A surgeon who performs operations on the ovary.
ovariotomy (ō-va″rĭ-ŏt'ō-mĭ) [" + G. *tomē*, incision]. Incision into or removal of an ovary, or of an ovarian tumor.
ovariotubal (ō-va″rĭ-ō-tū'băl) [" + *tuba*, a narrow duct]. Concerning the ovary and the oviducts.
ovariprival (ō-vā″rĭ-prī'văl) [" + *privāre*, to remove]. Resulting from loss of the ovaries.
ovaritis (ō-va-rī'tĭs) [L. *ovarium*, ovary, + G. *-itis*, inflammation]. Inflamed condition of an ovary.
  Usually involved secondarily in inflammation of the oviducts or pelvic peritoneum. May involve the substance of the organ (*oöphoritis*) or its surface (*perioöphoritis*), and may be acute or chronic.
  o., acute. Acute, severe inflammation of the ovary.
  ETIOL: Postabortal or postpartum infection, gonorrheal infection of the oviducts or pelvic peritoneum, tuberculous infection of same area, or may be due to streptococcus, staphylococcus, or colon bacillus. Occasionally, from cervicitis or in course of acute infectious diseases.
  SYM: Ovary swollen and edematous. Interstitial substance infiltrated with round cells and leukocytes. May become suppurative or abscess may form. Sometimes a tuboövarian cyst develops.
  DIAG: Usually determined at operation.
  TREATMENT: Rest in bed, heat to abdomen, hot douches and bland nourishing diet. Avoid purgation.
  o., chronic. Inflammation of ovary over a long period of time.
  SYM: Marked production of fibrous tissue in interstitial portion as well as about surface of organ. Surface studded by small, cystlike bodies which develop into larger cysts, causing cystic degeneration. Inflammatory exudate forms upon surface of ovaries. Severe pain may be felt, which is aggravated by any excitation. Leukorrhea present and sometimes amenorrhea.
  TREATMENT: Usually complete extirpation of the organ necessary.
ovarium (ō-va'rĭ-ŭm) (pl. *ovaria*) [L.]. Ovary.
ovary (ō'va-rĭ) [L. *ovarium*, ovary, egg holder]. One of 2 glands in the female, producing the reproductive cell, the ovum, and 2 known hormones.
  They are 2 almond-shaped bodies, lying in the fossa ovarica on either side of the pelvic cavity, attached to the uterus by the uteroövarian ligament and lying close to the fimbria ovarica of the fallopian tube. About 4 cm. long, 2 cm. wide, and 1½ cm. thick. Each ovary is supported by 3 ligaments, *ligamentum ovarii proprii, infundibulopelvic ligament* and the *broad ligament* or *mesovarium.*
  The ovary is divided into 2 parts, the *cortex* and the *medulla.* In the cortex are the primary oöcytes and the developing graafian follicles. The medullary portion consists mainly of the vascular supply of the organ. The outer covering of the ovary is known as the *tunica albuginea ovarii.* The surface of the ovary in early life is smooth and in later life is markedly pitted as an end result of the atrophy of the corpus luteum.
  BLOOD SUPPLY: Mainly derived from the ovarian artery which reaches it through the infundibulopelvic ligament.
  FUNCTION: The production of a sex hormone, corpus luteum hormone, and the preparation and production of ova.

Hyperfunction produces early dentition, rapid growth of hair, early menstruation, and appearance of pubic and axillary hair; enlarged sexual organs, unusual mental development, early adolescence. Hypofunction causes obesity, poor development of breasts and secondary sex characteristics, absence of sexual desire, amenorrhea, irregular menstruation, low basal metabolism, tall skeleton.

DISEASES: The ovary, being in close proximity to the fallopian tube, which has contact with the outside air, is frequently subjected to acute inflammation. It is also frequently subjected to cyst formation, both proliferating and nonproliferating cysts. Among the common nonproliferating cysts are those that follow atresia of graafian follicles. The most common proliferating cysts are the papillary adenocystoma and the pseudomucinous cyst. The malignant tumors of the ovary are papillary adenocarcinoma, Krukenberg tumor, sarcoma and the rare teratoma.

PALPATION FOR OVARIAN TUMORS: When small, have an elastic feel; when large, soft and fluctuating. In some cases, detected by passing hand lightly over abdomen; in others, deep pressure required.

PERCUSSION OF OVARIES: Sound is flat over that portion of the abdomen which comes in contact with inner surface of abdominal wall, while at sides and above where intestines have been pushed aside and upward by the tumor, percussion sound will be tympanitic; by this change in percussion sound boundaries of tumor are known.

DIFFERENTIAL DIAG: Ovarian tumor may be confounded with uterine enlargements, as pregnancy, fibroid tumors of uterus, ascites, hydatids of the omentum, fecal accumulations in intestines, and enlargements of liver, spleen, and kidneys.

They are distinguished from uterine tumors by their consistency, outline, difference in connection and relative position to uterus, and by fact that in uterine tumors the cavity of uterus as determined by uterine sound is always elongated.

Diagnosis bet. ovarian and abdominal dropsy is made: *first*, by observing the shape of abdomen when patient lies on back. Ovarian tumors project forward in the center, while in ascites the abdominal enlargement is uniform. *Second*, in ovarian tumors the percussion sound is dull as high as tumor extends, while at same time there will be tympanitic resonance in most dependent portion of abdominal cavity; in ascites the depending portion of abdomen is always flat, the percussion resonance being confined to the epigastric and umbilical regions. *Third*, in ovarian tumor, the relative line of flatness and resonance is not altered by change in posture of patient as it is in ascites. Hydatids of omentum cannot be distinguished from ovarian tumors by physical signs, but the fact that omental enlargements are first noticed above the umbilicus and gradually enlarge downward, while ovarian tumors are first noticed low down in abdomen and enlarge upward, will in most cases be sufficient for diagnosis.

DOSAGE: 5 gr. (0.3 Gm.).

ovary, words pert. to: adnexitis; agenitalism; albuginea; castrate; cell, interstitial; conception; corpus albicans; dysovarism; facies ovarica; fimbria ovarica; fimbriate; fimbriation; folliculoma; graafian follicle; hyperovaria; Krukenberg's tumor; menstruation; mesosalpinx; mesovarium; oarialgia; oaric; oaritis; "oöphor-" words; "ov-" words; pyoövarium; spay; spermatozoon; stroma; teratoma; tunica albuginea.

ovate (ō'vāt) [L. *ovum*, egg]. BACT: Having the outline of an egg.

overdetermination (ō″vĕr-dē-tĕr-mĭ-nā′-shŭn) [A.S. *ofer*, above, + L. *determinãre*, to limit]. PSY: The idea that every symptom and dream may have several meanings, being determined by more than a single association.

overproduction (ō″vĕr-prō-dŭk′shŭn) [" + L. *producere*, to beget]. Destruction of an organic element is followed by overproduction of the element during the reparative process, as excessive callus development after a bone fracture. SYN: *Weigert's law*.

overri′ding [" + *rīdan*, to ride]. The slipping of 1 end of a fractured bone past the other part.

ov′ertone [" + G. *tonos*, a stretching]. A harmonic.

o., psychic. A dimly perceived associated impression about a mental image.

overwork (ō'vĕr-wŭrk) [" + *worc*, work]. Excessive work causing exhaustion. SEE: *ergasthenia*.

ovestrin (o-ves′trĭn) [L. *ovarium*, ovary]. Hormone from the ovary stimulating the gonads.

ovi- [L.]. Combining form meaning *egg*.

ovi al′bumin (ō'vĭ ăl-bū′mĭn) [L.]. White of egg.

o. vitellum. Egg yolk.

ovicapsule (ō″vĭ-kăp′sŭl) [L. *ovum*, egg, + *capsula*, a little box]. The sac enclosing the ovum; outer layer of a graafian follicle. SYN: *ovisac*.

oviduct (ō'vĭ-dŭkt) [" + *ductus*, a path]. One of 2 muscular tubes on either side of the uterus, about 4 in. long, forming the path conveying the ovum from the ovary to the uterus.

They are lined with mucous membrane and sheathed by ciliated epithelium.

One end is attached to the uterus. The other, or abdominal end, is composed of fringed parts or *fimbriae,* one of which, the *fimbria ovarica*, reaches close to the ovary, *q.v.* SYN: *fallopian tube*.

oviferous (ō-vĭf′ĕr-ŭs) [" + *ferre*, to bear]. Containing or producing ova.

ovification (ō-vĭ-fĭ-kā′shŭn) [" + *facere*, to make]. The production of ova. SYN: *ovulation*.

oviform (ō'vĭ-form) [" + *forma*, shape]. 1. Having the shape of an egg. 2. Resembling an ovum.

ovigerm (ō'vĭ-jĕrm) [" + *germen*, germ]. The cell which produces or develops into an ovum.

ovigerous (ō-vĭj'ĕr-ŭs) [" + *gerere*, to bear]. Producing or carrying ova. SYN: *oviferous*.

ovination (ō-vĭn-ā′shŭn) [L. *ovinus*, pert. to a sheep]. Inoculation with sheep pox virus.

Ovipara (ō-vĭp′ăr-ă) [L. *ovum*, egg, + *parēre*, to bear]. Animals which deposit the ova outside of their bodies. Opp. of *Vivipara*.

oviparous (ō-vĭp′ăr-ŭs) [" + *parēre*, to produce]. Producing eggs hatched outside the body.

ovisac (ō'vĭ-săk) [" + G. *sakkos*, a bag].

ovi vitellus

Outer layer of graafian follicle. SYN: *ovicapsule*.
ovi vitellus (o'vĭ vī-tĕl'ŭs) [L.]. Egg yolk; pharmaceutical term when used in preparation of emulsions.
ovo- [L.]. Combining form meaning egg.
ovoferrin (ō″vō-fĕr'rĭn) [L. *ovum*, egg, + *ferrum*, iron]. Commercial name for an albuminate of iron used in anemia.
ovogenesis (ō″vō-jĕn'ĕ-sĭs) [" + G. *genesis*, production]. Production of ova. SYN: *oögenesis*.
ovoglobulin (ō″vō-glŏb'ū-lĭn) [" + *globulus*, globule]. The globulin found in egg white. SEE: *albumen, protein*.
ovoid (ō'voyd) [" + G. *eidos*, form]. Egg shaped. SYN: *oviform*.
  o., fetal. The egg-shaped mass into which the uterine contractions mold the fetus.
ovolemma (ō″vō-lĕm'ă) [" + G. *lemma*, husk]. Membrane enclosing the vitellus of the ovum.
ovomucoid (ō″vō-mū'koyd) [" + *mucus*, mucus, + G. *eidos*, form]. A glycoprotein principle from egg white.
ovoventer (ō″vō-vĕn'tĕr) [" + *venter*, belly]. The impregnated ovum's centrosome, q.v.
ovovitellin (ō″vō-vī-tĕl'lĭn) [" + *vitellus*, yolk]. Protein found in an egg yolk.
ovoviviparous (ō″vō-vi-vip'ă-rŭs) [" + *vivus*, alive, + *parēre*, to bear]. Reproducing by hatching the eggs within the body.
ovula (ō'vū-lă) (sing. *ovulum*) [L.]. Little eggs.
  o., Nabothi. Distended mucous follicles in tissues of the cervix uteri.
ovular (ō'vū-lăr) [L. *ovulum*, little egg]. Concerning an ovule or ovum.
ovulation (ō-vū-lā'shŭn) [L. *ovulum*, little egg]. The lunar monthly ripening and rupture of the mature graafian follicle and the discharge of the ovum from the cortex of the ovary, normally occurring 13 times a year.
"As the follicle increases in size, it comes to the surface of the ovary and bursts. The ovum may enter the fallopian tube. It may meet a spermatozoon and be fertilized, or it may escape into the abdominal cavity and die.
"Rupture of a ripe follicle takes place bet. the 12th and 16th day after beginning of menstruation. The empty follicle then fills up with blood clot and new cellular tissue formed from the lining of *membrana granulosa* and is called the *corpus luteum*.
"This continues to grow for 3 days and the tissue is thrown into folds. If fertilization does not take place the corpus luteum then turns yellow (lutein = yellow) and begins to degenerate, atrophies, and remains as a small white scar on the surface of the ovary—the corpus albicans (albicans = white). After fertilization occurs no more follicles ripen, and the corpus luteum persists, and goes on developing until the 3rd month of pregnancy, when it is large enough to be felt as a small swelling on surface of the ovary. It then degenerates and finally disappears."—*Faber's Encyclopedia*.
RS: *anovular, conception, menstruation, ovary, ovum, safe period, spermatozoon*.
ovulatory (ō'vū-lă-tō-rĭ) [L. *ovulum*, a little egg]. Concerning ovulation.
ovule (ō'vūl) [L. *ovulus*, a little egg]. 1. The unimpregnated ovum before leaving graafian follicle. 2. Any egglike structure.
  o., Nabothi's. Distended mucous follicles in the cervix uteri. SYN: *ovula Nabothi*.
  o., primitive. A rudimentary ovum inside the ovary.
ovulin (ō'vū-lĭn) [L. *ovulum*, little egg]. An internal secretion of the ovary, supposed to be 1 of the elements in the hormone oöphorin.
ovulum (ō'vū-lŭm) [L.]. The ovum contained within the graafian follicle.

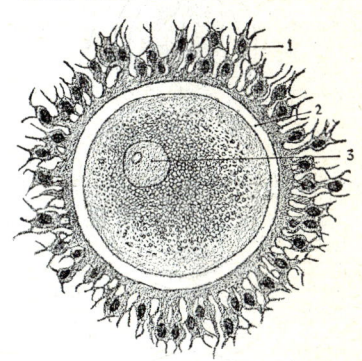

OVUM AND SPERM.
Ovum and sperm (Waldeyer), showing comparative size ovum, diameter 1/125 inch, sperm length 1/450 inch.

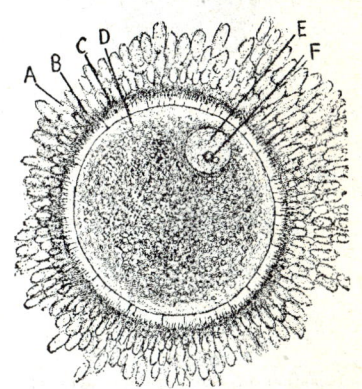

MATURE OVUM.
A. Cells of zona radiata. B. Epithelium of follicle. C. Vitelline membrane. D. Yolk with yolk granules. E. Germinal vesicle (nucleus). F. Germinal spot (nucleolus).

ovum (o'vum) (pl. *ova*) [L. egg]. 1. The fully developed globular cell, about 1/125 of an inch in diameter, which is capable, upon fertilization, of developing into an organism similar to the parent; female sexual cell or egg. 2. An egg.
The various parts of the ovum have been named as follows: The protoplasm is known as the *vitellus* or *yolk*; the outer layer is referred to as the *ectoplasm* or *zona pellucida* or *zona radiata*;

ovum   O-30   **oxaluria**

the inner layer, the cell membrane, is the *vitelline membrane;* the nucleus is called the *germinal vesicle,* and the nucleolus, the *germinal spot.*

The cellular layers proliferate, becoming cuboid in shape, and in the center a clear albuminous fluid, the *liquor folliculi,* forms. The follicular cells surrounding the fluid-filled cavity are known as the *membrana granulosa.* The layer surrounding the egg cell, or *oöcyte,* is known as the *discus proligerus.*

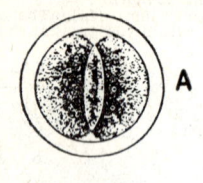

As the follicular layer enlarges to form the *graafian follicle,* the term for the developed ovum, containing the above, before it leaves the ovary, there is a slight protrusion of the ovarian surface when the follicle has matured. Its rupture through the ovarian surface frees the ovum, which then proceeds ordinarily into the fallopian tube and into the uterus, which process is known as *ovulation,* and occurs bet. the 12th and 16th day following the onset of menstruation. It usually takes the ovum from 5 to 7 days to go from the ovary to the uterus. SEE: *menstruation.*

Normally, only 1 graafian follicle matures each month, coming alternately from the 2 ovaries.

o., alecithal. One in which there is little or no food yolk.

o., apoplectic. One having an extravasation of blood.

o., blighted. One with arrested development after impregnation.

o., centrolecithal. One having a large central food yolk.

o., holoblastic. One having a largely formative yolk.

o., meroblastic. One having a large yolk.

o., permanent. One ready for fertilization.

o., primitive. Cell from which ovule arises.

ovum, words pert. to: amphicytula, amphigastrula, amphimorula, archeocyte, archiblast, archiblastic, archiblastoma, archigaster, archistome, arsenoblast, binovular, blastid, calyx ovum, conception, corpus hemorrhagicum, corpus luteum, cytula, denidation, fertilization, genotype, germ, germinal, germination, germ plasm, graafian follicle, impregnate, impregnation, incubation, menstruation, micropyle, oöblast, oöcyte, "ov-" words, spermatozoon, vitelline, vitellus, viviparous.

oxacid (ŏk′să-sĭd) [G. *oxys,* sour, + L. *acidum,* acid]. An acid of which oxygen is a constituent.

oxal-, oxalo-. CHEM: Combining forms indicating derivation from *oxalic acid.*

oxalate (ŏk′să-lāt) [G. *oxalis,* sorrel]. A salt of oxalic acid.

About 5-20 mg. of the oxalates are excreted in urine per day.

oxalemia (ŏk″să-lē′mĭ-ă) [" + *aima,* blood]. An abnormal amount of oxalates in the blood.

oxalic acid (ŏk′săl′ĭk) [G. *oxalis,* sorrel]. A white crystalline powder often used about the home as a stain remover or bleach, resembling epsom salts in appearance.

Recent research has revealed that oxalic acid has the effect of marked and rapid reduction of blood coagulation time, with indication of its value in treating hemorrhage, jaundice, etc.

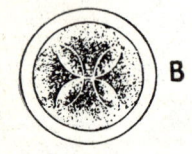

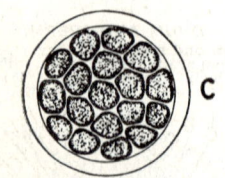

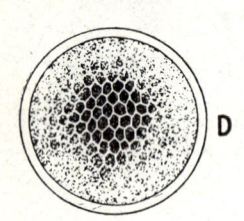

SOURCES: Cranberries, chard, rhubarb, gooseberries, spinach, beet leaves. When eating these should be accompanied by liberal portions of calcium foods, such as eggs, beans, and milk.

POISONING: SYM: Erosive action on swallowing; sour taste; burning in mouth, throat and stomach; great thirst; bloody vomitus; collapse; sometimes convulsions and coma.

TREATMENT: Soapsuds are of no value against oxalic acid since they form poisonous oxalates which may be absorbed and do further damage. Use powdered chalk, calcium carbonate or magnesium carbonate. Dilute the poison and cause vomiting. SEE: *acid, poisoning.*

o. a. diathesis. Chronic state of oxalemia.

oxalism (ŏk′săl-ĭzm) [" + *ismos,* state of]. Poisoning from oxalic acid or an oxalate.

oxaluria (ok-sa-lŭ′rĭ-ă) [" + *ouron,* urine]. The abnormal excretion of oxalates in the urine, esp. calcium oxalate.

Presence of oxalates does not always indicate oxaluria when found in standing urine, because of their insolubility. May be due to ingestion of certain vege-

OVUM.
Diagram of the various stages of cleavage of the yolk.

oxalylurea

tables (tomatoes) or the imperfect oxidation of carbohydrates.
ETIOL: When not due to foods, may be due to oxaluria diathesis, dyspepsia, gout, debility, lithemia, skin disease, constipation, neurasthenia, hemophilia, overeating and lack of exercise.

oxalylurea (ok″sa-lĭl-ū-rē′ă). An oxidation product of uric acid.

oxidase (ŏk′sĭ-dās) [G. *oxys*, sour]. 1. A ferment whose action causes the oxidation process. 2. The inherent substance of the living cell nucleus possessing the power of freeing active oxygen.

oxidation (ŏk″sĭ-dā′shŭn) [G. *oxys*, sour]. The process by which a substance combines with oxygen, generally involving a change from a lower to a high positive valence. In the human body the rate of oxidation depends upon cell activity, not the intake of oxygen or food. SEE: *carbonemia*.

oxide (ŏk′sīd) [G. *oxys*, sharp]. Any chemical compound in which oxygen is the negative radical.

oxidize (ŏk′sĭ-dīz) [G. *oxys*, sour]. 1. To combine with oxygen. 2. To increase the ratio of the negative to the positive radical within a chemical compound, or to form a compound with the principle in question being the positive radical by combining with it any substance that will become the negative radical. SYN: *oxygenize, q.v.*

oxidosis (ŏk″sĭ-dō′sĭs) [″ + -*osis*, condition]. Decrease in normal alkaline content of blood. SYN: *acidosis*.

oxonemia (ŏk″sō-nē′mĭ-ă) [L. *oxone*, acetone, + G. *aima*, blood]. Excess of acetone bodies found in the blood. SYN: *acetonemia*.

oxonuria (ŏk″sō-nū′rĭ-ă) [″ + G. *ouron*, urine]. Abnormal number of acetone bodies in urine. SYN: *acetonuria*.

oxos (ŏk′sŏs) [G.]. Vinegar.

oxy- [G.]. Combining form meaning sharp, keen, acute, acid, pungent.

oxyacoia, oxyakoia (ŏk″sĭ-ă-koy′ă) [G. *oxys*, keen, + *akoē*, hearing]. Abnormal sensitiveness to noises, as in facial paralysis, esp. if the stapedius muscle is involved.

oxyacusis (ŏk″sĭ-ă-kū′sĭs) [″ + *akousis*, hearing]. Abnormally acute hearing. SYN: *hyperacusis*.

oxyblepsia (ŏk″sĭ-blĕp′sĭ-ă) [″ + *bleps*, vision]. Extraordinary acuteness of vision.

oxyburserasin (ŏk″sĭ-bŭr-sĕr-ā′zĭn). An extract of resin of myrrh used to aid in healing internal lesions.

oxybutyria (ŏk″sĭ-bū-tĭr′ĭ-ă) [G. *oxys*, sharp, + *boutyron*, butter]. Oxybutyric acid in the blood or in the urine.

oxycephalia (ŏk″sĭ-sĕf-ā′lĭ-ă) [″ + *kephalē*, head]. State of having a high and pointed skull.

oxycephalous (ŏk-sĭ-sĕf′ă-lŭs) [″ + *kephalē*, head]. Denoting a head that is pointed and conelike.

oxychinolin (ŏk″sĭ-kĭn′ō-lĭn) [″ + *chinosol*]. A quinoline derivative used in disinfecting wounds.

oxychloride (ŏk″sĭ-klō′rīd) [″ + *chlōros*, green]. A compound of oxygen and a metal chloride.

oxychlorine (ŏk″sĭ-klō′rēn) [″ + *chlōros*, green]. Commercial dressing for wounds.

oxychromatic (ŏk″sĭ-krō-măt′ĭk) [G. *oxys*, sour, + *chrōma*, color]. Staining readily with acid dyes.

oxychromatin (ŏk″sĭ-krō′mă-tĭn) [″ + *chrōma*, color]. That part of chromatin which stains readily with acid dyes.

oxygen

oxycinesia (ŏks″ĭ-sĭn-ē′zĭ-ă) [G. *oxys*, keen, + *kinēsis*, movement]. Pain experienced on moving.

oxydase (ŏk′sĭ-dās) [″ + *ase*, enzyme]. A ferment causing oxidation. SYN: *oxidase*.

oxydasis (ŏk-sĭ-dā′sĭs) [G. *oxys*, sour]. The process of oxidation produced by an oxydase.

oxydesis (ŏk-sĭ-dē′sĭs) [″ + *desis*, a binding]. Acid fixing capacity, esp. as evidenced in the blood by buffer salts.*

oxydetik (ŏk-sĭ-dē′tĭk) [″ + *desis*, binding]. Concerning the acid fixation capacity.

oxyecoia (ok″sĭ-ē-koy′a) [G. *oxys*, sharp, + *akoē*, hearing]. Abnormal sensitivity to noises. SYN: *oxyacoia, q.v.*

oxyesthesia (ŏk″sĭ-ĕs-thē′zĭ-ă) [″ + *aisthēsis*, sensation]. Abnormal acuteness of sensation. SYN: *hyperesthesia*.

oxygen (ŏk′sĭ-jĕn) [G. *oxys*, sharp, since oxygen was formerly considered an essential element of acids, + *gennan*, to produce]. SYMB: O. 1. A nonmetallic element occurring free in the atmosphere as a colorless, odorless, tasteless gas; at. wt., 16. 2. Chlorine used for bleaching purposes.

It is a constituent of animal, vegetable and mineral substances comprising by weight 3/4 of the animal, 4/5 of the vegetable, and 1/2 of the mineral world, and by volume, 1/5 of the atmosphere, and by weight 8/9 of water.

It is essential to respiration of most forms of animal and plant life, and is the most important and abundant element discovered, composing about 21% of the atmosphere's total volume. When O combines with another substance, the process is called *oxidation*. When combination takes place rapidly enough to produce light and heat, the process is called burning or *combustion*. O combines readily with other elements to form oxides.

It is the only element that enters the animal organism in a free state. It is absorbed by plants in the form of water and carbon dioxide being converted by them into organic substances utilized for the food of man, and in turn is returned to the atmosphere by man in form of waste products of water and carbon dioxide, thus maintaining the balance of oxygen and carbon dioxide in the atmosphere.

It represents 65% of the elements in the body; 12% in venous, and 20% in arterial blood.

USES: O is employed largely in the treatment of anemia; pulmonary tuberculosis; pneumonia; poisoning by illuminating gas; or by narcotics, as opium and the barbiturates; heart disease, etc.

In the treatment of pneumonia, there is considerable difference of opinion as to the use of oxygen at all or, if used, as to when to begin, how much to employ, and how to administer. Many begin administration when the diagnosis of pneumonia is made; others only when signs of anoxemia appear. Another large group do not use it at all in the treatment of this disease.

Among the most common methods in use are the open cone, nasal catheter, the oxygen tent, and the oxygen chamber. The modern tent is the most uniformly satisfactory. O is also used subcutaneously.

Oxygen is employed frequently with ether or other agents used for the induction of general anesthesia. Follow-

ing extensive surgery it reduces reactions to anesthetic. Also employed in septicemia, gas gangrene, peritonitis, and intestinal obstruction.
RS: anoxemia, anoxia, anoxic, anoxybiosis, asthenoxia, autointoxication, cyanosis, element, hydrogen, ozone, ozonize.
o. therapy. Treatment by inhalation of oxygen, as in pneumonia.

oxygenase (ŏk"sĭ-jĕn-ās) [G. *oxys*, sharp, + *genan*, to produce, + *ase*, enzyme]. A substance in the tissues which takes up oxygen to form an organic peroxide.*

oxygenation (ŏk"sĭ-jĕn-ā'shŭn) [" + *gennan*, to produce]. Impregnation or combination with oxygen, as the aeration of the blood in the lungs.

oxygenic (ŏk"sĭ-jĕn'ĭk) [" + *gennan*, to produce]. Concerning, resembling, containing, or consisting of oxygen.

oxygenium (ŏk"sĭ-jē'nĭ-ŭm) [L.]. Oxygen.

oxygenize (ŏk"sĭ-jĕn-īz) [" + *gennan*, to produce]. To impart oxygen to a substance either by causing chemical union of the substances or by causing absorption or solution of the oxygen by the substance. SYN: *oxidize*.

oxygeusia (ŏk"sĭ-gū'sĭ-ă) [" + *geusis*, taste]. Abnormally keen sense of taste.

oxyhemoglobin (ŏk"sĭ-hem-ō-glō'bĭn) [" + *aima*, blood, + L. *globus*, a sphere]. The combined form of hemoglobin and oxygen.
Hemoglobin with oxygen is found in arterial blood and is the oxygen carrier to the body tissues. SYN: *hematoglobulin*. SEE: respiration.

oxyhemoglobinograph (ŏk"sĭ-hem-ō-glō-bĭn'ō-grăf). Device for recording amount of oxygen in the blood; a photoelectric cell is attached to the ear lobe, which is blue if the blood is short of oxygen and red if oxygen is sufficient. The result is recorded on a tape.

oxyhemoglobinometer (ŏk"sĭ-hem-ō-glo"-bĭn-ŏm'ĕt-ĕr) [" + " + G. *metron*, a measure]. Apparatus for measurement of oxygen in the blood.

oxyhydrocephalus (ŏk"sĭ-hī-drō-sĕf'ăl-ŭs) [G. *oxys*, sharp, + *ydōr*, water, + *kephalē*, brain]. Pointed head shape type of hydrocephalus.

oxyiodide (ŏk"sĭ-ī'ō-dīd) [" + *iōdēs*, violet colored]. Compound of iodine and oxygen with an element or radical.

oxylalia (ŏk"sĭ-lā'lĭ-ă) [G. *oxys*, swift, + *lalein*, to speak]. Abnormal rapidity of speech.

oxyntic (ŏk-sĭn'tĭk) [G. *oxynein*, to make acid]. Producing or secreting acid. SEE: *cell*.
o. gland. Gland of tubular form found in the body and fundus of the stomach secreting acid of gastric juice.

oxyopia (ŏk"sĭ-ō'pĭ-ă) [G. *oxys*, sharp, + *ōps*, sight]. Unusual acuteness of vision.

oxyopter (ŏk"sĭ-ŏp'tĕr) [" + *opsis*, vision]. A unit of visual acuity, being the reciprocal of the visual angle, in degrees.

oxyosis (ŏk"sĭ-ō'sĭs) [G. *oxys*, sharp, + *-ōsis*, condition]. Decrease in normal alkalinity of the blood. SYN: *acidosis, q.v.*

oxyosmia (ŏk"sĭ-oz'mĭ-ă) [" + *osmē*, odor]. Unusual acuity of sense of smell. SYN: *oxyosphresia*.

oxyosphresia (ok"sĭ-ŏs-frē'zĭ-ă) [" + *osphrēsis*, smell]. Abnormal acuity of the sense of smell.

oxyparaplastin (ok"sĭ-păr-ă-plăs'tĭn) [" + *para*, beside, + *plassein*, to form]. Part of paraplastin staining readily with acid dyes.

oxypathia, oxypathy (ok"sĭ-păth'ĭ-ă, -sĭp'- ăth-ĭ) [G. *oxys*, sharp, + *pathos*, feeling]. 1. Unusual acuity of sensation. 2. An acute condition. 3. Condition of inability to eliminate unoxidizable acids which combine with fixed alkalies of the tissues and harm the organism. SEE: *arthritism, lithemia*.

oxyperitoneum (ŏk"sĭ-pĕr-ĭ-tō-nē'ŭm) [" + *peritonaion*, peritoneum]. Introduction of oxygen into the peritoneal cavity.

oxyphil(e (ok"sĭ-fĭl, -fīl) [" + *philein*, to love]. 1. Staining readily with acid dyes. 2. A cell which stains readily with acid dyes.

oxyphilous (ŏk-sĭf'ĭl-ŭs) [" + *philein*, to love]. Having an affinity for acid dyes. SYN: *oxyphil, 1*.

oxyphonia (ok"sĭ-fō'nĭ-ă) [" + *phōnē*, voice]. An abnormally sharp or shrill voice.

oxyplasm (ŏk"sĭ-plăzm) [" + *plasmos*, a thing formed]. The part of the cytoplasm staining readily with acid dyes.

oxyproline (ŏk"sĭ-prō'lēn) [G. *oxys*, sharp]. An amino acid, a decomposition product of proteins.

oxypurine (ŏk"sĭ-pu'rēn) [G. *oxys*, sharp, + L. *purus*, pure, + *urina*, urine]. An oxidation product of purine.
Group includes hypoxanthine, xanthine, uric acid.

oxyrhine (ŏk"sĭ-rīn) [" + *ris*, nose]. 1. Having a sharp pointed nose. 2. Possessing an acute sense of smell.

oxyrygmia (ok"sĭ-rĭg'mĭ-ă) [" + *erygmos*, eructation]. Belching up of acid. SEE: *eructation*.

oxysalt (ŏk"sĭ-sawlt) [" + L. *sal*, salt]. A salt of an acid of which oxygen is a component.

oxysepsin (ŏk"sĭ-sep'sĭn) [" + *sēpsis*, putrefaction]. An oxidized toxin prepared from cultures of bacilli of tuberculosis in advanced stages.

oxysepsis (ok"sĭ-sĕp'sĭs) [" + *sēpsis*, putrefaction]. 1. Decay with development of acidity. 2. Putrefaction developing soon after death.

oxysparteine (ok"sĭ-spăr'te-ēn) [" + L. *spartium*, broom]. White crystalline oxidation product of sparteine, used as a cardiac stimulant.

oxytocia (ok"sĭ-tō'shĭ-ă) [G. *oxys*, swift, + *tokos*, childbirth]. Unusual rapidity of childbirth.

oxytocic (ok"sĭ-tō'sĭk) [" + *tokos*, birth]. 1. Agent which stimulates uterine contractions. 2. Accelerating childbirth.

oxytocin injection (ŏk"sĭ-to'sĭn) [" + *tokos*, birth]. USP term for an aqueous solution containing the oxytocic fraction of the post. pituitary gland.
USE: To stimulate uterine contraction after delivery of placenta, thus avoiding postpartum hemorrhage.
DOSAGE: From 3 to 15 ℳ (0.2–1 cc.) intramuscularly (from 2 to 10 USP oxytocic units).
SYN: *pitocin*.

oxytoxin (ok"sĭ-tŏk'sĭn) [G. *oxys*, sharp, + *toxikon*, poison]. An oxidation product of a toxin.

oxytropism (ok"sĭt'rō-pīzm) [" + *tropē*, a turning, + *ismos*, condition]. The tendency of living cells to be attracted by or respond to the stimulus of oxygen.

oxytuberculin (ŏk"sĭ-tū-bĕr'kū-lĭn) [" + L. *tuberculum*, a swelling]. An oxidized tuberculin.

oxyuriasis (ŏk"sĭ-ŭ-rī'ăs-ĭs) [G. *oxys*, sharp, + *oura*, tail, + *iasis*, infection]. Infestation with pinworms of genus Oxyuris.

oxyuricide (ŏk"sĭ-ŭ'rĭ-sīd) [" + " + L.

oxyurid

caedere, to kill]. Destructive to, or an agent that destroys pinworms.
oxyurid (ŏk″sĭ-u′rĭd) [" + *oura*, tail]. Pinworm.
oxyurifuge (ŏk″sĭ-ŭ′rĭ-fŭj) [" + " + L. *fugere*, to flee]. An agent killing pinworms.
Oxyuris (ŏk″sĭ-ŭ′rĭs) [" + *oura*, tail]. Genus of nematode worms, the pinworms.
　O. vermicularis. Common pinworm infesting the intestines and causing intense nocturnal itching of the anus.
oxyvaselin (ŏk″sĭ-vas′ĕ-lēn) [G. *oxys*, sharp, + Ger. *wasser*, water, + G. *elaion*, olive oil]. Commercial ointment base containing oxygen. SYN: *vasogen*.
oyster (oi′ster) [G. *ostreon*]. Shellfish eaten raw or cooked.
　AVERAGE SERVING: 120 Gm. PRO. 6.8, Fat 1.3, Carbo. 4.0. VITAMINS: A+, B++, C+, G++.
　ASH CONST: Ca 0.052, Mg 0.037, K 0.091, Na 0.459, P 0.155, Cl 0.590, S 0.187, Fe 0.0045.
　An acid forming food with potential acidity of 15 cc. per 100 Gm., or 30 cc. per 100 cal.
　ACTION: Changes in the liquor of oysters may give rise to toxicity with rising temperature, headaches, eruptions, gastrointestinal troubles, infection or food poisoning.
Oz., oz. Abbr. for *ounce*.
ozena (ō-zē′nă) [G. *ozein*, to smell]. Disease of the nose characterized by atrophy of the turbinates and mucous membrane accompanied by considerable crusting and discharge and a very offensive odor.
　It is present in various forms of rhinitis.

ozostomia

ozocerite (ō″zō-sē′rĭt) [" + *kēros*, wax]. Mineral wax used as an ointment base. SEE: *ceresin*.
ozochrotia (ō″zō-krō′shĭ-ă) [" + *chrōs*, skin]. Strong odor given off by the skin. SYN: *bromidrosis*.
ozokerite (ō″zō-kē′rĭt) [" + *kēros*, wax]. Mineral wax which is employed as an ointment base. SYN: *ozocerite*.
ozonator (ō′zō-nā-tor) [G. *ozein*, to smell]. Device for generating ozone.
ozone (ō′zōn) [G. *ozein*, to smell]. A form of oxygen in which 3 atoms of the element combine to form the molecule, O_3.
　It gives an odor of chlorine or sulfurous acid gas when mixed with air. Used as a disinfectant and antiseptic.
ozon′ic e′ther. A mixture of hydrogen peroxide, ether, and alcohol, used in a test for blood in the urine, and in treating diabetes and whooping cough.
ozonization (ō-zō-nĭ-zā′shŭn) [G. *ozein*, to smell]. The act of converting to, or impregnating with ozone.
ozonize (ō′zō-nīz) [G. *ozein*, to smell]. 1. To convert oxygen to ozone, *i. e.*, 3 atoms to the molecule of free oxygen. 2. To impregnate the air of a substance with ozone.
ozonometer (ō″zō-nom′ĕt-ĕr) [" + *metron*, a measure]. An apparatus for estimating the quantity of ozone in the atmosphere.
ozonophore (ō-zō′nō-fōr) [" + *pherein*, to carry]. 1. A red blood corpuscle. 2. A protoplasmic granule of a cell.
ozonoscope (ō-zō′nō-skōp) [" + *skopein*, to examine]. A device for showing the presence or amount of ozone.
ozostomia (ō″zō-stō′mĭ-ă) [G. *ozē*, stench, + *stoma*, mouth]. Fetid breath.

P

P. Symb. of *phosphorus*.
P., p. Abbr. for *para, pupil, pulse, position*; also for *postpartum*.
P₂. Abbr. for *pulmonic second sound*.
PABA. Abbr. for *paraaminobenzoic acid*, *q.v.*
pabular (pab'ū-lar) [L. *pabulum*, food]. Pert. to nourishment.
pabulin (păb'ū-lĭn) [L. *pabulum*, food]. Albuminous and fatty product found in the blood following digestion.
pabulum (păb'ū-lŭm) [L.]. Food; nourishment.
pacchionian bodies (păk-ē-ō'nĭ-ăn). Enlarged villi, small pedunculated or rounded growths of fibrous tissue along longitudinal fissure of the cerebrum growing on arachnoid membrane.
   p. corpuscle. Small granulation on surface of the dura mater along longitudinal fissure.
   p. depressions. Small pits produced on inner surface of skull by protuberance of p. bodies.
   p. fossae. Depressions upon inner surface of the skull in which are lodged the p. bodies. SYN: *p. depressions*.
   p. glands. SEE: *p. bodies*.
pacemaker (pās'māk-ēr) [L. *passus*, a step, + A.S. *macian*, to make]. The sinuauricular node, so named because cardiac rhythm commences here, taking place near the spot where the large veins empty into the auricle.
pachemia (păk-ē'mĭ-ă) [G. *pachys*, thick, + *aima*, blood]. Abnormal thickening of the blood. SYN: *pachyemia*.
pachismus (păk-ĭz'mŭs) [" + *ismos*, condition]. Condensation or thickening of an organ or part.
pachometer (păk-ŏm'ĕt-ēr) [" + *metron*, measure]. Device for determining a body's thickness. SYN: *pachymeter*.
pachy-, pach- [G.]. Combining form meaning *thick, large, heavy, massive*.
pachyacria, pachyakria (păk-ĭ-ăk'rĭ-ă) [G. *pachys*, thick, + *akron*, end]. 1. Hypertrophy of soft portions of the extremities. 2. Chronic disease due to overfunction of hypophysis, in which there is enlargement of the face and extremities. SYN: *acromegaly*.
pachyblepharon (păk"ĭ-blĕf'ăr-ŏn) [G. *pachys*, thick, + *blepharon*, eyelid]. A thickening of border of eyelid.
pachycephalic (păk"ĭ-sĕf-al'ĭk) [" + *kephalē*, brain]. Possessing a thick skull. SYN: *pachycephalous*.
pachycephalous (păk"ĭ-sĕf'ăl-ŭs) [" + *kephalē*, brain]. Thick skulled. SYN: *pachycephalic*.
pachycephaly (păk"ĭ-sĕf'ăl-ĭ) [" + *kephalē*, brain]. Unusual thickness of the walls of the skull.
pachychilia (păk"ĭ-kī'lĭ-ă) [" + *cheilos*, lip]. Unusual thickness of the lips.
pachycholia (păk"ĭ-kō'lĭ-ă) [" + *cholē*, bile]. Thickening or inspissation of the bile.
pachychromatic (păk"ĭ-krō-măt'ĭk) [" + *chroma*, color]. Possessing a coarse chromatin network.
pachycolpismus (păk-ĭ-kŏl-pĭz'mŭs) [G. *pachys*, thick, + *kolpos*, vagina, + *ismos*, condition]. Chronic inflammation of vagina with thickened vaginal walls. SYN: *pachyvaginitis*.
pachydactylia, pachydactyly (păk"ĭ-dăk-tĭl'ĭ-ă, -dăk'tĭ-lĭ) [" + *daktylos*, digit]. Condition marked by unusually large fingers and toes.
pachyderma (păk-ĭ-der'mă) [" + *derma*, skin]. Unusual thickness of the skin.
pachydermatocele (păk"ĭ-der-măt'ō-sēl) [" + " + *kēlē*, swelling]. A pendulous state of the skin with thickening. SYN: *dermatolysis*.
pachydermatosis (păk"ĭ-der-măt-ō'sĭs) [" + " + *-ōsis*, condition]. Chronic hypertrophy of the skin. SYN: *pachydermia*.
pachydermatous (păk-ĭ-der'mă-tŭs) [" + *derma*, skin]. Possessing a thick skin.
pachydermia (păk-ĭ-der'mĭ-ă) [G. *pachys*, thick, + *derma*, skin]. Progressive hypertrophy of skin and subcutaneous tissues, usually associated with lymphangitis and edema.
   ETIOL: Results from obstruction of lymphatics; most common cause, presence of a parasite, *Filaria bancrofti* and *Filaria sanguinis hominis*.
   SYM: Recurring attacks of erysipelatoid inflammation. Part is red, swollen, painful; lymphatics may be traced as branching red lines; fever. After each attack part becomes a little more enlarged, till finally it is enormously swollen, skin thickened and roughened; papillae unusually prominent. Legs and genitals usually affected. In p. of scrotum mass may weigh 50 to 100 pounds.
   PROG: In early stages may be arrested, otherwise incurable.
   TREATMENT: Acute attacks, rest; firm bandaging; sometimes amputation in p. of scrotum. In p. of leg, ligation of main artery. Constitutional treatment.
   SYN: *Barbados leg, elephantiasis*.
   p. laryngis. Irregular thickening and hypertrophy of mucous membrane in the larynx seen in chronic laryngitis.
   p. vesica. Condition in which there is a thickened mucous membrane in the urinary bladder.
pachyemia (păk-ĭ-ē'mĭ-ă) [G. *pachys*, thick, + *aima*, blood]. Thickness or coagulation of the blood.
pachyglossia (păk"ĭ-glŏs'sĭ-ă) [" + *glōssa*, tongue]. Unusual thickness of the tongue.
pachygnathous (păk-ĭg'năth-ŭs) [" + *gnathus*, jaw]. Having a thick or large jaw.
pachygyria (păk-ĭ-jī'rĭ-ă) [" + *gyros*, a circle]. Flat, broad formation of the cerebral convolutions.
pachyhematous (păk-ĭ-hĕm'ăt-ŭs) [" + *aima*, blood]. Having thickened blood.
pachyhemia (păk-ĭ-hē'mĭ-ă) [" + *aima*, blood]. A thickened state of the blood.
pachyleptomeningitis (păk-ĭ-lĕp-tō-mĕn-ĭn-jī'tĭs) [G. *pachys*, thick, + *leptos*, thin, + *mēnigx*, membrane, + *-itis*, inflammation]. Inflammation of pia and dura of the brain and spinal cord.
pachylosis (păk-ĭ-lō'sĭs) [G. *pachylos*, thick]. A rough, dry, thickened, chronic condition of skin. SYN: *xerosis*.
pachymeningitis (păk-ĭ-mĕn-ĭn-jī'tĭs) [G. *pachys*, thick, + *mēnigx*, *mēnigg-*, mem-

pachymeningitis externa

brane, + -*itis*, inflammation]. Inflamed condition of the dura mater.
Inflammation of the pia, dura, and arachnoid membranes is sure to extend to either or both of the others, and the consequence in any form is suppuration, abscess, effusion into the ventricles and softening of cerebral tissue if brain is involved.
ETIOL: Possible spread of infection from cranial wounds, inflammation of mastoid bone secondary to otitis media, or of frontal sinus or by means of blood stream.
SYM: Headache, malaise, moderate fever. Extradural abscess of pus forms with intracranial pressure preceded by vomiting.
SEE: *leptomeningitis, meningitis.*
p. externa. Inflammation of outer layer of dura mater.
p., hemorrhagic. Circumscribed effusion of blood on inner surface of dura with inflammation.
Secondary to chronic cardiac disease, renal disease, the infectious fevers, chronic alcoholism or insanity.
SYM: Often obscure. Where marked, there is headache, failure of memory, impairment of intellect, stupor, contracted pupils, local convulsions, or palsies.
PROG: Unfavorable.
TREATMENT: Grave cases should be treated as apoplexy.
p. interna. Inflammation of inner layer of dura mater.
pachymeninx (păk-ĭ-mē'nĭnks) [G. *pachys,* thick, + *meninx,* membrane]. Membrane known as the dura mater.
pachymeter (păk-ĭm'ĕt-ĕr) [" + *metron,* measure]. Instrument for measuring thickness. SYN: *pachometer.*
pachynsis (păk-ĭn'sĭs) [G. *pachynsis,* a thickening]. Thickening of a substance or part, usually abnormal.
pachyntic (păk-ĭn'tĭk) [G. *pachynsis,* a thickening]. Thickening, abnormally thickened.
pachyonychia (păk″ĭ-ō-nĭk'ĭ-ă) [G. *pachys,* thick, + *onyx, onych-,* nail]. Thickening of finger or toe nails.
pachyostosis (păk″ĭ-ŏs-tō'sĭs) [" + *osteon,* bone, + -*osis,* disease]. Thickening of the bones.
pachyotia (păk-ĭ-ō'shĭ-ă) [" + *ous, ōt-,* ear]. Abnormal thickness of the ears.
pachypelviperitonitis (păk″ĭ-pĕl″vĭ-pĕr-ĭt-ō-nī'tĭs) [" + L. *pelvis,* basin, + G. *peritonaion,* peritoneum, + -*itis,* inflammation]. Inflammation of the pelvic and peritoneal membranes with hypertrophy and thickening of their surfaces.
pachyperitonitis (păk-ĭ-pĕr-ĭt-ō-nī'tĭs) [" + *peritonaion,* peritoneum, + -*itis,* inflammation]. Inflammation of the peritoneum with thickening of the membrane.
pachypleuritis (păk-ĭ-plū-rī'tĭs) [" + *pleura,* a side, + -*itis,* inflammation]. Inflamed condition of the pleura with thickening of the membrane.
pachypodous (pak-ĭp'ō-dŭs) [" + *pous, pod-,* foot]. Having massive feet.
pachysalpingitis (păk-ĭ-săl-pĭn-jī'tĭs) [G. *pachys,* thick, + *salpigx,* tube, + -*itis,* inflammation]. Chronic inflammation of an oviduct with thickening of the muscular coat.
pachysalpingoövaritis (păk″ĭ-săl-pĭn″gō-ō-văr-ī'tĭs) [" + " + L. *ovarium,* ovary, + G. -*itis,* inflammation]. Chronic inflamed condition of an ovary and oviduct with thickening of the membranes.

pachysomia (păk-ĭ-sō'mĭ-ă) [" + *sōma,* body]. Pathological thickening of the soft parts of the body, as in acromegaly.
pachyvaginalitis (păk″ĭ-văj-ĭn-ăl-ī'tĭs) [" + L. *vagina,* sheath, + G. -*itis,* inflammation]. Inflamed condition of the tunica vaginalis with thickening of the membrane.
pachyvaginitis (păk″ĭ-văj-ĭn-ī'tĭs) [" + " + -*itis,* inflammation]. Chronic inflammation of the vagina with thickening of the membranes. SYN: *pachycolpismus.*
pacinian corpuscles (pă-sĭn'ĭ-ăn). Oval bodies which are end organs of sensory nerve fibers of the skin.
p. fluid. Solution used in making a count of erythrocytes.
pacinitis (pă-sĭn-ī'tĭs) [G. -*itis,* inflammation]. Inflammation of the end organs of the skin, the pacinian corpuscles.
pack (păk) [Gaelic, *pakke*]. 1. A dry or moist, hot or cold blanket or sheet wrapped around a patient. 2. To fill up a cavity.
p., cold wet sheet. This pack is a physiologic sedative and hypnotic employed for relief of restlessness, insomnia, and used extensively in psychiatric conditions. Effects are similar to those of any cold application except they are more intense as greater area is covered by the pack. Cooling of the skin ensues, contraction of the muscles with, perhaps, shivering, *cutis anserina* (gooseflesh), and pallor, with checked and then quickened respiration and perhaps gasping, and checked insensible perspiration. The internal temperature is raised and circulatory reaction begins instantly; thermic reaction being established in from 5 to 20 minutes, with a return to normal physiological functioning. As blood is withdrawn from the brain, sleep is induced. Action takes place and reaction begins during the *cool stage* of the pack; the *neutral stage* is reached when the surface of the body, the sheets, and the moist air within the pack have reached the normal skin temperature, 92° to 94° F. *A superheated stage* may ensue but it must be prevented if sedation* and not elimination is desired.
NP: No definite length of time for this treatment can be prescribed but it should continue while the patient is quiet. The first sign of undue redness or warmth is a signal for instant removal of the pack, or if the patient becomes restless and does not become quiet within 40 minutes the treatment should be discontinued. A second pack usually proves effectual. The period of sedation is from ½ to 3 hours.
The patient is enveloped in from 1 to 3 cotton sheets wrung out of cold water. The smooth moist fabric is held snugly against the skin by a large woolen blanket, and an additional blanket may be used to prevent the loss of heat, or cooling from without. The exact temperature of the water used depends upon the patient as indicated.
Robust, flushed and excited patient, 48° F.; average vitality, restless or sleepless patient, 60° to 70° F.; frail patients, 92° to 106° F.
The room must be warm, well ventilated, and quiet, with a subdued light. The bowels should be emptied before the treatment and the urine voided. Water is given if the patient is thirsty and demands it, *but not otherwise.*
p., dry. Procedure used in combination with hot bath. When patient leaves

hot bath he is placed in dry, warm sheet and wrapped in several warm blankets.
p., full. SEE: *pack, wet sheet.*
p., half. Wet sheet pack but in this type the moist fabric and dry blanket extend from the axilla to below the knees.
p., hot bath. SEE: *pack, dry.*
p., hot blanket. The envelopment of a patient in moist blanket wrung from very hot water (150° to 160° F.). Given to relax contracted muscles, relieve convulsions, or induce profuse perspiration.
p., ice. If ice bag is not available, a local cold application may be made by folding a soft towel so it will fit the area and filling it with crushed ice.
p., neutral wet sheet. SEE: *pack, wet sheet.*
p., one sheet. Same as wet sheet pack except only 1 large sheet, 84 x 96 in., is used.
p., partial. SEE: *half and three-quarter packs.*
p., three-quarter. Pack using same temperatures as wet sheet pack but the body is enveloped from below upward as far as the armpits.
p., wet sheet. The envelopment of patient in 1, 2 or 3 linen or soft cotton sheets that have been wrung out of water which is hot, cold or lukewarm, depending on the purpose. These are held against the body by large woolen blankets.
Temperature of the water used for the sheets varies.
packer (păk'ẽr) [Gaelic *pakke*, a pack]. Device for packing a cavity, as the uterus or rectum with gauze, etc.
packing (păk'ĭng) [Gaelic *pakke*, a pack]. 1. The process of filling a cavity or wound with gauze sponges, etc. 2. Material used to fill a cavity or wound.
pad (păd) [origin uncertain]. Soft cushion or bag to relieve or give pressure, support an organ or part, etc.
Usually cotton, oakum, jute or wood wool. Surgical cotton is not suitable for open wounds or broken surfaces. Oakum or marine lint is too irritating to place in direct contact with skin.
p., abdominal. Pad for absorbing fluids from surgical wounds, etc., of abdomen. Stock sizes 6 x 7 and 8 x 9 in.
p., dinner. Pad placed on stomach prior to application of a plaster cast.
Pad is then removed, leaving space for abdominal distention after meals.
p., kidney. Air or water pad fixed on abdominal belt for compression over a movable kidney.
p.'s, knuckle. Nodules on dorsal sides of the fingers.
p., Malgaigne's. Mass of fat in knee joint on either side of the patella's upper end.
p., Mikulicz's. One of folded gauze used in surgery.
p., sucking. Mass of fat on inner cheek assumed to aid in sucking.
p., surgical. Soft rubber pad with apron and inflatable rim for drainage of escaping fluids, used in operations and obstetrics.
Pagenstecher's ointment (păhg'ĕn-stĕk-ĕr). Ophthalmic ointment composed of a base of yellow oxide of mercury.
P.'s thread. Suture thread made of linen dipped in celluloid.
Paget's disease (păj'ĕt). 1. Chronic inflammation of bones with thickening and distortion. SYN: *osteitis deformans.*
2. A cancerous dermatosis of nipple area in women, though extramammary cases have been reported.
ETIOL: Exciting cause unknown. Whether it is primary or secondary with reference to malignancy has not yet been settled.
Serum phosphatase used for diagnosis and prognosis.
SYM: Insidious beginning as sharply circumscribed eczematous inflammatory area on areola with itching. Later, crusting from sticky, viscid exudation. Never heals spontaneously, nor does it respond to antieczematous treatment. Extends peripherally with retraction and fissuring of nipple. After 1 or 2 years a superficial ulcerating or deep nodular carcinoma develops.
PROG: Good in early cases under proper treatment. If advanced and extensive, prognosis is same as in breast cancer.
TREATMENT: X-rays, radium, and amputation. Early radical excision is best. SEE: *mastectomy.*
pain (pān) [G. *poinē*, penalty]. 1. A protective mechanism of the body; an unpleasant reaction to massive stimulation of the sensory nerves, calling attention to derangement of function, disease or injury of a part. 2. In the plural refers to contractions of uterus in childbirth.
Marked by a desire to avoid or escape it. It is present in diseases such as neuritis, neuralgia, and in diseases of the central nervous system, or disorders affecting it. It may be observed by its nature, its cause or origin, its duration, its severity, or the disease or disorder as well as the region in which it occurs. Varieties of pain include the nature of pain, or its character.
FACTS TO NOTE IN OBSERVING PAIN: *Nature*: Severe. Sharp. Dull. Lancinating. Throbbing. *Time*: Exact time. Duration of: Sudden. Slow in developing. Remittent. *Food*: Increased by taking food? How soon after? Decreased by taking food? How soon after? Induced by sight or thought of food? By what foods is pain affected? *Location*: Exact region or area, or relation to an organ. *Cause*: Any that might be responsible. *Mental Condition*: Any producing pain. *Miscellaneous*: Any other factors that may cause pain.
p., abdominal. Increased with respiration; experienced in broken ribs, intercostal neuralgia, wounds, herpes zoster, pleurisy, pleurodynia, myalgia, periostitis, acute peritonitis, colic; hepatic, gastric, or renal ulcer; gallbladder disorders; carcinoma in late stages, and gummata of this region.
p., absence of. In disorders in which pain should be expected may indicate pressure on the brain. The sudden abatement of pain, when other symptoms continue to be bad, is not a good sign.
p., after-. That following labor, caused by contraction and retraction of uterine muscles during involution.
p., angina pectoris. Paroxysmal, severe pain radiating from the heart to shoulder, thence down the arm, or rarely from the heart to the abdomen. Lasts from a few seconds to several minutes.
p., appendicitis. If acute, abdominal pain, usually severe, generally throughout the abdomen, followed by localization of pain in right lower quadrant of abdomen with tenderness over right rectus muscle with rigidity.
p., bearing-down. Straining and tenesmus with uterine contractions.

p., boring. P. of a severe, piercing type.
p., cardiac. SEE: *epigastric pain.*
p., cardialgic. SEE: *epigastric pain.*
p., causalgic. A spontaneous pain, esp. burning in character, when associated with anesthesia, or hyperesthesia in a given nerve. SEE: *causalgia.*
p., cephalgic. Head pain, *q.v.*
p., continuous. May indicate persistent obstruction; also a tendency to suppuration.
p., cramplike. Muscular spasm such as epigastric pain. Significance depends upon location of pain.
p., dull. Continuous mild throbbing which attends inflammation of mucous membranes.
p., ear. May indicate inflammation of the ext. auditory canal, except in young children. It also may indicate a furuncle in the meatus, or middle ear disease. SYN: *otodynia.*
p., epigastric. Severe pain occurring in paroxysms in gastric disorders.

If to the left of the spine, with epigastric tenderness occurring soon after a meal, gastric ulcer is indicated. If it occurs several hours after eating and is then relieved by food, duodenal ulcer is indicated. If the pain is constant and not relieved by food or by alkalies, carcinoma may be suspected.

Heartburn indicates acute gastritis. Epigastric pain and tenderness occurring in paroxysms, with pain in the right shoulder, indicate gallbladder disease. Epigastric pain with slow pulse, occurring in paroxysms, acute and sharp, with tenderness over the umbilicus, indicates pancreatic disease.

In general, may accompany any gastric or intestinal disorder, as well as pleural and some cardiac affections. SEE: *cardialgia.*

p., false. One mistaken for a true labor pain.
p., fixed. Indicates derangement at some special point; the sharper the pain, the deeper seated the trouble.
p., fulgurant. Sudden shooting p., esp. experienced in locomotor ataxia.
p., gallbladder. In upper right abdominal quadrant, dull pain just below the last rib in infection, or sharp pain in same area radiating to the back and up under right shoulder, esp. if calculi are present. SEE: *epigastric pain.*
p., gastralgic. Severe pain occurring in paroxysms in gastric disorders. If pain is constant and not relieved by food or by alkalies, carcinoma may be suspected. Heartburn indicates acute gastritis. Epigastric pain and tenderness occurring in paroxysms, with pain in the right shoulder, indicate gallbladder disease. Epigastric pain with slow pulse, occurring in paroxysms, acute and sharp, with tenderness over the umbilicus, indicates pancreatic disease. In general, epigastric pain may accompany any gastric or intestinal disorder, as well as pleural and some cardiac affections. SEE: *epigastric pain.*
p., girdle. One resembling sensation of a constricting cord around the waist, often associated with syphilis.
p., gnawing. May denote disease of the spinal column, gastric disturbance, and aneurysms.
p., growing. That felt in the joints of growing children.
p., head. It may be due to mental exertion or sympathetic irritation, or intestinal or liver derangements unless it results from catarrh.

(a) If around the eyes and nose it indicates trouble with the eyes, nose, or stomach.
(b) If in the center of the forehead above the nose, it may denote constipation, decayed teeth, or errors of refraction.
(c) Ache in the center of the forehead may result from nasal or intestinal trouble.
(d) Ache over each eye indicates stomach trouble.
(e) A tight, bandlike sensation all around the head above the eyes indicates anemia or similar condition.
(f) Ache in the upper center of the forehead denotes nasal trouble.
(g) Ache over the entire top of head may result from uterine trouble, debility, anemia, stomach or bladder disorders.
(h) Side of the head over the ear denotes anemia or bad blood conditions.
(i) If the pain is near the center of the back head level with the top of the ear, it indicates eye trouble.
(j) An ache just below the center of the back of head indicates constipation from colon difficulties.
(k) If the pain is just back of the ear it may indicate mastoid complications.
(l) If the ache is back of the neck at the base of the brain, it indicates a nervous condition or spinal irritation.
(m) A pain a little to 1 side and below the base of the brain may denote derangement of the stomach and irritation of the spine. SYN: *cephalalgia.*

p., hunger. Pain due to need for food.
p., ideogenous. Self-induced pain of mental origin.
p., inflammatory. Pain in presence of inflammation which is increased by pressure.
p., lancinating. A short, sharp, cutting pain.
p., lingual. Pain in tongue which may be due to local lesions, glossitis, fissures, pernicious anemia and malignancies.
p., lung. SEE: *pulmonary pain.*
p., mental. One of psychic origin; mental distress or grief. May, if persistent, cause true physical pathological states.
p., migraine. Headache accompanied by nausea and vomiting. It may arise from a number of causes, esp. those of neurological origin. SEE: *migraine, sick headache.*
p., mind. Pain occurring subsequent to a mental operation or of mental origin. SYN: *psychalgia.*
p., neuralgic. Pain, frequently paroxysmal, occurring along the branches of a nerve. Temporarily relieved by heat or pressure. May be of rheumatic origin, a tic or inflammation of nerves or nerve trauma.
p., noise. Pain of ear caused by a noise. SEE: *odynacusis.*
p., osteocopic. Pain in bones. SEE: *osteocope.*
p., paresthesic. Stinging or tingling sensation manifested in central and peripheral nerve lesions. SEE: *paresthesia.*
p., pseudomyelic. False sensation of movement in a paralyzed limb, or 1 of no movement in a moving limb. Not a true pain. SEE: *pseudomyelia paresthetica.*
p., pulmonary. Sharp pain in the region of the lungs. Indicates that the

pain, referred, reflex   P-5   **palatoplasty**

pleurae are involved. There is no pain when lung substance is involved.

p., referred, p., reflex. Pain seeming to arise in an area or point other than at its origin, as pain from appendicitis which often seems to occur in areas other than that of the appendix. SYN: *synalgia.*

p., regional. Pain in a specific area and its significance.

p., remittent. P. which subsides temporarily. Characteristic of neuralgia and colic.

p., shifting. Present in rheumatism, hysteria and locomotor ataxia.

p., shooting. SEE: *fulgurant p.*

p., soul. SEE: *mind pain.*

p., sympathetic. SEE: *referred p.*

p., tenesmic. P. accompanying urination or defecation. SEE: *tenesmus.*

p., thermalgesic. Pain caused by heat. SEE: *thermalgesia.*

p., thoracic. A sharp pain over the sternum, often running down the arm to the elbow.

Indicative of angina pectoris, although it must not be confused with pain from gastric pressure in the region of the heart, caused by an accumulation of gas.

It is increased with respiration, experienced in broken ribs; intercostal neuralgia; wounds, herpes zoster; pleurisy; pleurodynia; myalgia; periostitis; acute peritonitis; colic; hepatic, gastric, or renal ulcer; gallbladder disorders; carcinoma in late stages, and gumma of this region. SEE: *abdominal pain.*

p., ulcer *(gastric or duodenal)* : Sharp, lancinating, or dull and gnawing in precordium, radiating to left of spine posteriorly, on a level with the 10th rib. Burning sensation may be felt in epigastrium. Pain may occur from 10 to 15 minutes after eating, as soon as an excess of hydrochloric acid is secreted. If ulcer is near cardia, pain ensues soon after eating; if near pylorus, pain may not ensue for 2 or 3 hours after eating.

p., urethral. Pain at end of the urethra, without soreness, which may denote presence of gravel or stone in the urinary bladder.

pain, words pert. to: "alg-" words, amphicrania, analgesia, analgia, angor, anodyne, anodynia, aortalgia, aponia, cardiodynia, carotidynia, causalgia, celialgia, celiomyalgia, cephalalgia, cephalodynia, chiropodalgia, chondralgia, chondrodynia, cinesalgia, clavus, colalgia, colpalgia, colpodynia, cryalgesia, cryesthesia, dolor, dysthymia, fulgurant, fulminant, haphalgesia, hemialgia, hemicrania, hypalgesia, hypalgia, hyperalgesia, hypnalgia, kinesalgia, lancinating, mastalgia, megalgia, myalgia, neuralgia, notalgia, nyctalgia, oarialgia, odynacusis, omalgia, oöphoralgia, orchialgia, orchidalgia, ostalgia, otalgia, oxycinesia, photalgia, rachialgia, rectalgia, rhinalgia, stitch, synalgia, thelalgia, thermalgesia, thermalgia, thermohyperalgesia, vaginodynia, visceralgia, xiphodynia.

painters' colic (pān'tērs). Colic accompanying lead* poisoning.

SYM: Vomiting, abdominal pains, marked prostration, paralysis, profound collapse, if not averted.

TREATMENT: Remove patient from source of trouble, as from a newly-painted room; hot applications to abdomen; stimulants, and warmth in bed. SEE: *lead poisoning.*

palatable (pǎl'ǎt-ǎ-bl) [L. *palatum*, palate]. Pleasing to the palate or taste, as food.

palatal (pǎl'ǎt-ǎl) [L. *palatum*, palate]. Pert. to the roof of the mouth, the palate.

p., paralysis of. May occur in diphtheria, or complications of it, and in severe septic sore throat and quinsy.

SYM: Slight cough on drinking, or regurgitation of fluid intake. Difficulty in pronouncing words containing the letter "m."

NP: Absolute rest. Jellied fluids. No ordinary fluid while there is tendency to regurgitation.

p. reflex. Swallowing induced by stimulation of soft palate.

palate (pǎl'ǎt) [L. *palatum*, palate]. 1. The horizontal structure separating the mouth and the nasal cavity; the roof of the mouth. 2. Mental taste.

DISORDERS: *Koplik's Spots*: A rash frequently seen upon the palate in measles.

Secondary Syphilis: Indicated by mucous patches on the palate.

Herpes of the Throat: Shown by vesicles in circles upon the pharyngeal walls and soft palate.

Swelling of Uvula: Noted in inflammations of pharynx and tonsil, in nephritis, severe anemia, angioneurotic edema, and general debility. In diphtheria and Vincent's angina, a membranous exudate appears. In purpura hemorrhagica and some hemorrhagic diatheses, bloody extravasation appears.

Paralysis: May result from diphtheria, bulbar paralysis, neuritis, basal meningitis, tumor at base of brain and vertebral caries.

Anesthesia: Seen in involvement of 2nd division of the 5th nerve.

RS: *Avellis' syndrome, Bednar's aphthae, cheilognathopalatoschisis, cleft, "palat-" words, "staphyl-" words, "uran-" words, "uvul-" words.*

p., artificial. Hard substance molded to fill a cleft in the palate.

p. bones. Bones forming post. part of hard palate and lateral nasal wall bet. the int. pterygoid plate of sphenoid bone and sup. maxilla.

p., cleft. One with congenital opening bet. 2 parts of palate.

p., falling. Abnormally long uvula.

p., hard. Ant. part supported by the maxillary and palatine bones.

p., soft. Post. muscular, membranous fold partly separating the mouth and pharynx. SYN: *velum*. SEE: *Illus., p. P-6.*

palatine (pǎl'ǎ-tīn) [L. *palatum*, palate]. 1. Concerning the palate. 2. The palate bones, *q.v.*

p. arches. Archlike folds or double pillars of mucous membrane formed by descent of the soft palate as it descends toward the pharynx.

p. artery. One of 2 arteries in the face.

p. bone. Palate bones, *q.v.*

palatitis (pǎl-ǎt-ī'tĭs) [" + G. *-itis*, inflammation]. Inflamed condition of the palate.

palatoglossus (pǎl"ǎt-ō-glŏs'ŭs) [" + G. *glōssa*, tongue]. Muscle forming under surface of soft palate, which lifts rear of tongue and narrows the fauces. SEE: *Table of Muscles in Appendix.*

palatognathous (pǎl-ǎt-ǒg'nǎ-thŭs) [" + G. *gnathos*, jaw]. Having a congenital fissure in the palate.

palatopharyngeus (pǎl"ǎt-ō-fǎr"ĭn-jē'ŭs) [" + G. *pharygx, pharygg-*, pharynx]. Muscle arising from soft palate which narrows the fauces. SEE: *Table of Muscles in Appendix.*

palatoplasty (pǎl'ǎt-ō-plǎs"tǐ) [" + G.

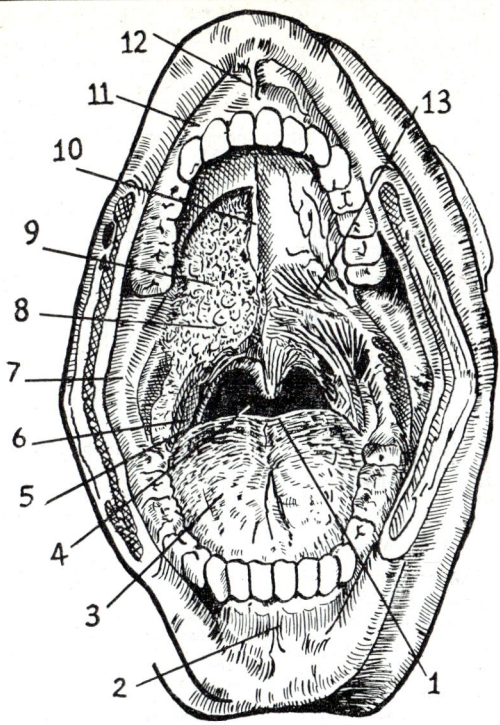

THE HARD AND SOFT PALATE.

The dissection to the left shows the large mass of glandular tissue extending the full length of the palate; to the right the musculature of the soft palate and faucial pillars. 1. Isthmus of faucies. 2. Inferior lip frenulum. 3. Tongue surface (dorsum linguae). 4. Oropharyngeal cavity (nasopharynx). 5. Uvula. 6. Palatine tonsil. 7. Buccal cavity. 8. Soft palate. 9. Palatine glands. 10. Hard palate. 11. Gum (gingiva). 12. Superior lip frenulum. 13. Tensor.

plassein, to form]. Plastic surgery of the palate, usually to correct a cleft. SYN: *staphylorrhaphy, uranoplasty*.
palatoplegia (păl″ăt-ō-plē′jĭ-ă) [" + G. *plēgē*, stroke]. Paralysis of muscles of the soft palate. SEE: *palate*.
palatorrhaphy (păl-ă-tor′ă-fĭ) [" + G. *raphē*, a sewing]. Operation for uniting of a cleft palate. SYN: *staphylorrhaphy*.
palatoschisis (păl-ă-tŏs′kĭs-ĭs) [L. *palatum*, palate, + *schisis*, a fissure]. Palate with cleft in it. SYN: *uranoschisis*.
palatostaphylinus (păl″ăt-ō-stă-fĭl-ī′nŭs) [" + G. *staphylē*, uvula]. Group of muscular fibers going from post. nasal spine of palate bone to uvula, helping to raise it.
paleëncephalon, paleoencephalon (pā″lē-ĕn-sĕf′ă-lŏn, -ō-ĕn-sĕf′ă-lŏn) [G. *palaios*, old, + *egkephalos*, brain]. Phylogenetically older portion of the brain which includes all of it except the cerebral cortex and its allied structures.
paleogenesis (pā″lē-ō-jĕn′ĕ-sĭs) [" + *genesis*, production]. Reproduction of ancestral characteristics without change, in a later generation, esp. abnormalities.
paleogenetic (pā″lē-ō-jĕn-ĕt′ĭk) [" +

genesis, production]. Having origin in a previous generation.
paleokinetic (pā″lē-ō-kĭn-ĕt′ĭk) [" + G. *kinēsis*, motion]. Noting a peripheral motor nervous system controlling automatic associated movements and phylogenetically older than system controlling voluntary movement. SEE: *neokinetic*.
paleontology (pā″lē-ŏn-tŏl′ō-jĭ) [G. *palaios*, old, + *onta*, existing things, + *logos*, study]. Branch of biology dealing with ancient plant and animal life of the earth. SEE: *phylogeny*.
paleopathology (pā″lē-ō-păth-ŏl′ō-jĭ) [" + *pathos*, disease, + *logos*, study]. The study of diseases in remains of bodies and fossils of ancient times.
paleostriatal (pā″lē-ō-strī-ā′tăl) [" + L. *striatus*, ridged]. Concerning the primitive portion of the corpus striatum.
paleostriatum (pā″lē-ō-strī-ā′tŭm) [" + L. *striatus*, ridged]. Primitive portion of corpus striatum, the globus pallidus. SEE: *neostriatum*.
paleothalamus (pā″lē-ō-thăl′ă-mŭs) [" + *thalamos*, chamber]. Medial portion of thalamus, the medullary, or noncortical

palikinesia   P-7   **palsy**

part which is phylogenetically older. SEE: *thalamus*.

palikinesia (păl″ĭ-kĭn-ē′zĭ-ă) [G. *palin*, again, + *kinēsis*, motion]. Continued, involuntary, repetitious movements.

palilalia (păl-ĭ-lā′lĭ-ă) [" + *lalein*, to speak]. Pathologic repetitious use of words and phrases.

palinal (păl′ĭn-ăl) [G. *palin*, backward]. Moved or moving backward.

palindromia (păl-ĭn-drō′mĭ-ă) [" + *dromos*, a running]. The recurrence of symptoms of a disease or its turn for the worse. SYN: *relapse*.

palindromic (păl-ĭn-drŏm′ĭk) [" + *dromos*, a running]. Recurring, as the symptoms of a disease. SYN: *relapsing*.

palinesthesia (păl″ĭn-ĕs-thē′zĭ-ă) [" + *aisthēsis*, sensation]. Return of power of sensation, as after recovery from anesthesia or coma.

palingenesis (păl″ĭn-jĕn′ĕ-sĭs) [" + *genesis*, formation]. 1. Regeneration or restoration of an organism or part of one. 2. Reappearance of ancestral characteristics, esp. abnormal ones. SYN: *atavism, paleogenesis*.

palingraphia (păl″ĭn-grăf′ĭ-ă) [" + *graphein*, to write]. Pathologic repetition of words or phrases in writing.

palinphrasia, paliphrasia (păl-ĭn-frā′zĭ-ă, -ĭ-frā′zĭ-ă) [" + *phrasis*, speech]. Pathological condition in which there is coherent speech but certain words or phrases are frequently repeated. SYN: *palilalia*.

pallanesthesia (păl″ăn-ĕs-thē′zĭ-ă) [G. *pallein*, to shake, + *anaisthēsia*, anesthesia]. Loss of vibration sensation of skin and bones. SYN: *apallesthesia*. SEE: *pallesthesia*.

pallescence (pă-lĕs′ĕns) [L. *pallescere*, to grow pale]. Diminution of body color; a pale appearance. SYN: *pallor*.

pallesthesia (păl-ĕs-thē′zĭ-ă) [G. *pallein*, to shake, + *aisthēsis*, sensation]. The sensation of vibration felt in skin or bones, as that produced by a tuning fork when held against the body.

palliate (păl′ĭ-āt) [L. *pallium*, a cloak]. To ease or reduce in violence, to allay temporarily, as pain, without curing.

palliative (păl′ĭ-a-tĭv) [L. *pallium*, a cloak]. 1. Serving to relieve or alleviate, without curing. 2. An agent which alleviates or eases. [color, pale, wan.

pallid (păl′ĭd) [L. *pallidus*, pale]. Lacking

pallidal (păl′ĭ-dăl) [L. *pallidus*, pale]. Concerning the pallidum of the brain.

pal′lidin [L. *pallidus*, pale]. A preparation made from the lung substance of congenital syphilitics, which is used in the skin test for syphilis.

pallidum (păl′ĭd-ŭm) [L. pale]. The globus pallidus of the lenticular nucleus in the corpus striatum.

pallium (păl′ĭ-ŭm) [L. cloak]. The cerebral cortex with its adjacent white substance, considered as a cover for rest of the brain. SYN: *brain mantle*.

pallor (păl′or) [L. *pallere*, to be pale]. Lack of color; paleness. SEE: *skin*.

palm (pahm) [L. *palma*, hand]. Ant. or flexor surface of the hand from wrist to fingers. SYN: *vola manus*. SEE: *antithenar, thenar*.

palmar (păl′mar) [L. *palma*, hand]. Concerning the palm of the hand.

p. **or Darwinian reflex.** A grasping reflex in infants, more highly developed in some than in others. It gradually disappears and is absent after 4 or 5 months. It persisted in 100 infants up to the age of 4 months.

palmaris (păl-mā′rĭs) [L. *palma*, hand]. One of 2 muscles, *p. brevis* and *p. longus*. SEE: *Table of Muscles in Appendix*.

palm-chin reflex. Contraction of chin muscles resulting when thenar eminence of hand is strongly irritated by a sharp object.

palmiacol (pal-mī′ăk-ōl). Proprietary creosote derivative used in lung diseases.

palmic (pal′mĭk) [G. *palmos*, a beat]. 1. Concerning palpitation or pulse. 2. Concerning palmus, q.v.

palmitic acid (pal-mĭt′ĭk). $CH_3(CH_2)_{14}$-COOH. A fatty acid found in solid fats, animal, and vegetable, palm oil, some waxes and many fatty oils.

palmitin (pal′mĭt-ĭn). An ester of glycerol and palmitic acid, derived from fat of both animal and vegetable origin.

palmomen′tal reflex. Contraction of chin muscles when thenar eminence of hand is strongly irritated by a sharp object.

palmus (păl′mŭs) [G. *palmos*, a throb]. 1. Palpitation; a throb. 2. Jerking; a disease with convulsive nervous twitching of the leg muscles, similar to jumping. 3. Heartbeat.

palpable (păl′pă-bl) [L. *palpāre*, to stroke]. Perceptible, esp. by touch.

palpate (păl′pāt) [L. *palpāre*, to touch]. To examine by touch; to feel.

palpation (păl-pā′shŭn) [L. *palpatiō*, a feeling]. Process of examining by application of the hands to the external surface of the body to detect evidence of disease in the various organs.

RS: *abdomen, bladder, chest, heart, intestines, kidney, liver, omentum, ovary, peritoneum, spleen, uterus*.

palpatometer (păl-pă-tom′ĕt-ĕr) [L. *palpāre*, to feel, + G. *metron*, a measure]. Device for determining arterial tension.

palpebra (pl. *palpebrae*) (păl′pe-bră, păl-pē′bră) [L. eyelid]. An eyelid.
p. **inferior.** The lower eyelid.
p. **superior.** The upper eyelid.

palpebral (păl′pe-brăl) [L. *palpebra*, eyelid]. Concerning an eyelid.
p. **cartilages.** Thin plates of condensed tissue forming the framework of the eyelid. SYN: *tarsal cartilages*.
p. **fissure.** The opening bet. the eyelids.
p. **follicles.** Sebaceous follicles in eyelids whose secretion prevents their sticking together. SYN: *meibomian glands*.
p. **muscle.** The orbicularis palpebrarum which closes the eyelid.

palpebrate (păl′pē-brāt) [L. *palpebra*, eyelid]. 1. To wink. 2. Possessing eyelids.

palpitant (păl′pĭ-tănt) [L. *palpitāre*, to quiver]. Throbbing; trembling.

palpitate (păl′pĭ-tāt) [L. *palpitāre*, to quiver]. 1. To cause to throb. 2. To throb or beat intensely or rapidly, usually said of the heart.

palpitation (păl-pĭ-tā′shŭn) [L. *palpitāre*, to quiver]. Rapid, violent or throbbing pulsation, as an abnormally rapid throbbing, or fluttering of the heart.
ETIOL: It may be reflex from the stomach, coronary arteries, or uterus; in chronic heart affection, overwork, or it may be the result of a psychic condition. SEE: *heart*.
p., arterial. That felt in course of an artery.

palsy (pawl′zĭ) [M.E. *palesie*, from G. *paralysis*, a disabling at the side]. 1. Temporary or permanent loss of sensation, or of ability to move, or to control

palsy, Bell's   P-8   **pancreas**

movement. 2. A person disabled by palsy. SYN: *paralysis*.

p., Bell's. P. of the facial nerve at its periphery.

p., birth. P. arising from an injury received at birth.

p., crutch. P. resulting from pressure on axilla from use of a crutch.

p., Erb's. A paralysis of the deltoid, biceps, long supinator, and brachialis anticus muscles due to lesion and degenerative changes in spinal cord. Other muscles may sometimes become affected.

p., lead. P. of the forearm as a result of lead poisoning.

p., night. Form of paresthesia in which numbness is a symptom, esp. at night.

p., shaking. Progressive muscular weakness and tremor with impaired voluntary motion. SYN: *paralysis agitans, Parkinson's disease*.

p., wasting. Chronic condition in which there is atrophy and paralysis of muscles which grow progressively worse. SYN: *progressive muscular atrophy*.

paludal (păl'ū-dăl) [L. *palus*, a marsh]. Concerning, or originating in, marshes. SYN: *malarial*.

paludism (păl'ū-dĭzm) [" + G. *ismos*, condition]. Swamp fever. SYN: *malaria, q.v.*

pampiniform (păm-pĭn'ĭ-form) [L. *pampinus*, a tendril, + *forma*, shape]. Convoluted like a tendril.

p. plexus. 1. A mesh of spermatic or ovarian veins. 2. Network of nerves supplying the testicles.

pampinocele (păm-pĭn'ō-sēl) [" + G. *kēlē*, swelling]. A swollen, painful condition of the veins of the spermatic cord. SYN: *varicocele*.

pan-, pant- [G.]. Combining form meaning *all*.

panacea (păn-ă-sē'ă) [G. *pas, pan-*, all, + *akeisthai*, to heal]. A remedy for all ills.

panagglutinin (păn-ăg-lū'tĭn-ĭn) [" + L. *agglutināre*, to glue to]. Substance capable of agglutinizing corpuscles of every blood group.

Panama fever (păn-ă-mă'). Severe, pernicious, malarial fever peculiar to Panama.

panaris (pă-nā'rĭs, pa'nă-rĭs) [L. *panaricium*, whitlow]. Inflammation and infection of part of digit around the nail. SYN: *felon, paronychia, whitlow*.

panarthritis (păn-ar-thrī'tĭs) [G. *pas, pan-*, all, + *arthron*, joint, + *-itis*, inflammation]. 1. Inflammation of all parts of a joint. 2. Inflamed condition of all the joints in the body.

panasthenia (păn-ăs-thē'nĭ-ă) [" + *astheneia*, weakness]. Generalized weakness or exhaustion without evidence of organic disease. SYN: *neurasthenia, q.v.*

panatrophy (păn-ăt'rō-fĭ) [" + *a-*, priv. + *trophē*, nourishment]. 1. Wasting away of an entire structure. 2. Generalized wasting away of the body.

pancarditis (păn-kăr-dī'tĭs) [" + *kardia*, heart, + *-itis*, inflammation]. Inflamed condition involving all the structures of the heart.

panchreston (păn-krē'stŏn) [" + *chrestos*, useful]. A remedy for every disease. SYN: *panacea*.

panchromia (păn-krō'mĭ-ă) [" + *chroma*, color]. Power of staining with numerous dyes.

pancreas (păn'krē-ăs) [G. *pas, pan-*, all, + *kreas*, flesh]. A racemose compound gland, situated behind the stomach in front of the 1st and 2nd lumbar vertebrae, in a horizontal position, its head firmly attached to the duodenum and its tail reaching to the spleen.

The gland is composed of lobules which form lobes connected by strands of tissue, with ducts which lead from the lobules into a main one, the *pancreatic duct*, or duct of Wirsung, which in turn is connected with the duodenum.

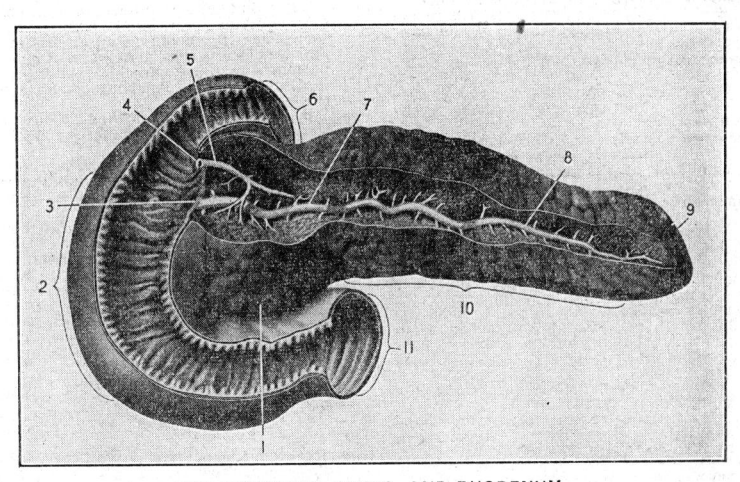

THE PANCREAS, DUCTS, AND DUODENUM.

1. Uncinate portion of duodenum. 2. Descending portion of duodenum. 3. Orifice of greater pancreatic duct. 4. Duodenal papilla. 5. Lesser pancreatic duct. 6. Superior portion of duodenum. 7. Greater pancreatic duct. 8. Greater pancreatic duct. 9. Tail of pancreas. 10. Body of pancreas. 11. Inferior portion of duodenum.

Scattered throughout the substance are differentiated masses of cells which are the *islands of Langerhans.**

FUNCTION: Production of internal and external secretion. *Pancreatic* juice, an external secretion, is produced by the lobules and passes into the duodenum during digestion, which it aids. The internal secretion, called *insulin*, is elaborated by the islands of Langerhans. The function of insulin is the control of carbohydrates, but it is supposed that other endocrines coöperate with the islands of Langerhans to control carbohydrate metabolism.

Disease of these islands causes hypofunction, and a lack of insulin resulting therefrom is the immediate cause of *diabetes mellitus.** Diabetes mellitus is characterized by the inability of the body to properly utilize carbohydrates and fats. The blood sugar rises to an abnormal height and when it reaches a high level the kidneys allow it to pass through into the urine.

Hyperfunction of the islands of Langerhans causes *hypoglycemia*.

Pancreatic affections upset the digestion of proteins, fats, and perhaps nuclear substances.

RS: *achylia pancreatica, Balser's fatty necrosis, Cammidge's reaction, duodenal digestion, enzyme, insula, island of Langerhans, islet, "pancr-" words, Wirsung's duct.*

p., accessory. Small mass of tissue close to the pancreas, apparently detached from it.

p., little. Semidetached lobular part of post. surface of head of the p., sometimes having a separate duct opening into the principal one.

p., Willis'. SEE: *little pancreas.*

pancreatalgia (păn″krē-ăt-ăl′jĭ-ă) [G. *pas, pan-*, all, + *kreas*, flesh, + *algos*, pain]. Painful condition of the pancreas.

pancreatectomy (păn″krē-ăt-ĕk′tō-mĭ) [" + " + *ektomē*, excision]. Operation for removal of part or all of the pancreas.

pancreatemphraxis (păn″krē-ăt-ĕm-frăk′sĭs) [" + " + *emphraxis*, stoppage]. Congestion of pancreas due to obstruction of pancreatic duct causing swelling of the gland.

pancreathelcosis (păn″krē-ăth-ĕl-kō′sĭs) [" + " + *elkōsis*, ulceration]. Ulcerated condition of the pancreas or its suppurative inflammation.

pancreatic (păn-krē-ăt′ĭk) [G. *pas, pan-*, all, + *kreas*, flesh]. Concerning the pancreas.

p. juice. An external secretion of the pancreas which acts on food following action of gastric juice in the stomach.

It is activated by the hormone secretin which reaches that organ through the blood. The p. juice begins to flow when the acid contents of the stomach pass through the pylorus.* Bile also aids this process.

The p. juice is a clear, viscid, alkaline fluid. Sp. gr., 1.0008.

It contains *trypsin, amylopsin, steapsin* (lipase), the proenzyme trypsinogen, and alkali.

From 500 to 800 cc. are secreted every 24 hr. It is discharged into the duodenum through the duct of Wirsung.

Amylopsin hydrolyzes starch to maltose; steapsin hydrolyzes fats to fatty acids and glycerol; trypsinogen, by the action of enterokinase in the duodenum, is converted into the active form trypsin which hydrolyzes proteins to amino acids. The alkali neutralizes the acidity of the chyme entering the duodenum from the stomach.

RS: *duodenal digestion, enzyme, pancreas, secretion.*

pancreaticocholecystostomy (păn″krē-ăt′-ĭ-kō-kō″le-sĭs-tos′tō-mĭ) [G. *pas, pan-*, all, + *kreas*, flesh, + *cholē*, bile, + *kystis*, bladder, + *stoma*, opening]. Surgical creation of passage bet. the gallbladder and a fistulous pancreas.

pancreaticoduodenal (păn″krē-ăt′′ĭ-kō-dū-ō-dē′năl) [" + " + L. *duodeni*, twelve]. Concerning the duodenum and a fistulous pancreas.

pancreaticoduodenostomy (păn″krē-ăt′′ĭ-kō-dū′′ō-dē-nŏs′tō-mĭ) [" + " + " + G. *stoma*, opening]. Surgical creation of a passage bet. a fistulous pancreas and duodenum.

pancreaticogastrostomy (păn″krē-ăt′′ĭ-kō-găs-trŏs′tō-mĭ) [" + " + *gastēr*, belly, + *stoma*, opening]. Surgical creation of a passage bet. a fistulous pancreas and the stomach.

pancreatin (păn′krē-ăt-ĭn) [" + *kreas*, flesh]. 1. One of the active ferments of the pancreas. 2. USP. A mixture of enzymes obtained from pancreas of ox or hog.

ACTION AND USES: Chiefly as a digestant. Inactive in presence of acid, should be adm. in combination with an alkali, as sodium bicarbonate.

DOSAGE: 8 gr. (0.5 Gm.)

pancreatism (păn′krē-ăt-ĭzm) [" + " + *ismos*, state of]. Normal activity and functioning of the pancreas.

pancreatitis (păn″krē-ă-tī′tĭs) [G. *pas, pan-*, all, + *kreas*, flesh, + *-ītis*, inflammation]. Inflamed condition of the pancreas.

p., acute. Form characterized by necrosis, suppuration, gangrene, and hemorrhage.

SYM: Sudden and intense pain in epigastric region, vomiting, belching of gas, sometimes hiccough, collapse. Rigidity and tenderness over umbilicus. Constipation, slow pulse, possible jaundice.

p., centrilobar. P. about divisions of the pancreatic duct.

p., chronic. Form marked by formation of scar tissue in pancreas associated with malfunction.

Pain mild or severe. Pain has tendency to radiate to left side. Jaundice, weakness, emaciation, diarrhea. SEE: *pancreas*.

p., hemorrhagic. Form with hemorrhage into pancreatic tissue.

SYM: Paroxysms of deep seated pain in epigastrium, nausea, retching, constipation. Slight rise in temperature, blood and mucus in vomitus, dyspnea, feeble pulse, delirium, tympanites, jaundice, hiccough, cyanosis, collapse.

p., perilobar. Fibrosis of the pancreas bet. acinous groups.

p., purulent. P. with suppuration.

p., suppurative. Form marked by development of many small abscesses.

SYM: May be those of acute or chronic form.

pancreatoduodenectomy (păn″krē-ă-tō-dū′′ō-dē-něk′tō-mĭ) [G. *pas, pan-*, all, + *kreas*, flesh, + L. *duodeni*, twelve, + G. *ektomē*, excision]. Excision of the head of the pancreas and the adjacent portion of the duodenum.

pancreatogenic, pancreatogenous (păn″-krē-ă-tō-jĕn′ĭk, -tŏj′ĕ-nŭs) [" + " +

pancreatolith P-10 **panophthalmia purulenta**

gennan, to produce]. Produced in or by the pancreas; having origin in the pancreas.

pancreatolith (păn-krē-ăt'ō-lĭth) [" + " + *lithos*, stone]. A calculus of the pancreas.

pancreatolithectomy (păn″krē-ăt-ō-lĭth-ĕk'tō-mĭ) [" + " + " + *ektomē*, excision]. Removal of a concretion from the pancreas. SYN: *pancreatolithotomy*.

pancreatolithotomy (păn″krē-ăt-ō-lĭth-ot'-ō-mĭ) [" + " + " + *tomē*, an incision]. Removal of a concretion from the pancreas. SYN: *pancreatolithectomy*.

pancreatolysis (păn″krē-ăt-ŏl'ĭ-sĭs) [" + " + *lysis*, dissolution]. Destruction of the pancreatic substance.

pancreatolytic (păn″krē-ăt-ō-lĭt'ĭk) [" + " + *lysis*, dissolution]. Destructive to the pancreatic tissues. SYN: *pancreolytic*.

pancreatomy (păn-krē-at'ō-mĭ) [G. *pas, pan-*, all, + *kreas*, flesh, + *tomē*, incision]. Operation into the pancreas. SYN: *pancreatotomy*.

pancreatoncus (păn-krē-ăt-ong'kŭs) [" + " + *ogkos*, tumor]. A pancreatic tumor.

pancreatopathy (păn″krē-ăt-op'ă-thĭ) [" + " + *pathos*, disease]. Any pancreatic disease.

pancreatotomy (păn-krē-ă-tŏt'ō-mĭ) [" + " + *tomē*, incision]. Surgical incision into the pancreas. SYN: *pancreatomy*.

pancreëctomy (păn-krē-ĕk'tō-mĭ) [" + " + *ektomē*, excision]. Partial or total excision of the pancreas. SEE: *preparation for hysteropexy*.

pancreolithotomy (păn″krē-ō-lĭth-ŏt'ō-mĭ) [" + " + " + *lithos*, stone, + *tomē*, incision]. Surgical removal of a pancreatic concretion.

pancreolytic (păn-krē-ō-lĭt'ĭk) [" + " + *lysis*, dissolution]. Destructive to the pancreas.

pancreon(e (păn'krē-ōn) [G. *pas, pan-*, all, + *kreas*, flesh]. A commercial digestive powder obtained from pancreatin.

pancreopathy (păn-krē-ŏp'ăth-ĭ) [" + " + *pathos*, disease]. Any diseased condition of the pancreas. SYN: *pancreatopathy*.

pandemia (păn-dē'mĭ-ă) [G. *pas, pan-*, all, + *dēmos*, the people]. Epidemic affecting the major portion of the population of a district.

pandemic (păn-dĕm'ĭk) [" + *dēmos*, the people]. 1. Affecting the majority of the population; said of a disease. 2. A disease affecting the majority of the population of a large region, or which is epidemic at the same time in many different parts of the world.

Pander's layers (păn'dĕr). The mesoblastic layer in which the blood vessels are first formed in the embryo.

pandiculation (păn-dĭk-ū-lā'shŭn) [L. *pandiculārī*, to stretch oneself]. Stretching of the limbs and yawning, as on awakening from normal sleep.

pang (păng) [M.E. *prange*]. 1. A paroxysm of extreme agony. 2. A sudden attack of any emotion.

pangenesis (păn-jĕn'ĕs-ĭs) [G. *pas, pan-*, all, + *genesis*, production]. Darwin's theory of reproduction in which each cell of the parent is represented by a particle in the reproductive cell, and thus each part of the organism reproduces itself in the progeny.

The chromosome theory has been employed both to substantiate and refute this.

panhidrosis (păn-hĭd-rō'sĭs) [" + *idrōsis*, perspiration]. Perspiration over the entire surface of the body. SYN: *panidrosis*.

panhydrometer (păn″hī-drŏm'ĕt-ĕr) [" + *ydōr*, water, + *metron*, measure]. Apparatus for obtaining specific gravity of any fluid.

panhysterectomy (păn-hĭs-tĕr-ĕk'tō-mĭ) [" + *ystera*, uterus, + *ektomē*, excision]. Excision of entire uterus including the cervix uteri.

NP: Preparation same as for ovariohysterectomy. SEE: *hysterectomy*.

panhysterokolpectomy (păn-hĭs″tĕr-ō-kŏl-pĕk'tō-mĭ) [" + " + *kolpos*, vagina, + *ektomē*, excision]. Total excision of the uterus and vagina.

panidrosis (păn-ĭd-rō'sĭs) [" + *idrōsis*, perspiration]. General perspiration over the body's entire surface.

panighao (păn-ĭ-gä'ō). Eruption due to presence of larva of uncinaria under the skin. SYN: *ground itch*.

panis (păn'ĭs) [L.]. Bread.

p., mica. Bread crumb.

panmyelophthisis (păn″mī-ĕl-of'thĭ-sĭs) [G. *pas, pan-*, all, + *myelos*, marrow, + *phthisis*, a wasting]. General wasting away of the bone marrow.

panmyelosis (păn″mī-ĕl-ō'sĭs) [" + " + *-ōsis*, intensive]. Increase in all the constituents of the bone marrow.

panneuritis (păn″ū-rī'tĭs) [" + *neuron*, sinew, + *-itis*, inflammation]. Generalized neuritis.

p. endemica, p. epidemica. Deficiency disease in which there is lack of vitamin B₁. SYN: *beriberi*.

panniculitis (pan-ĭk-ū-lī'tĭs) [L. *panniculus*, a small piece of cloth, + G. *-itis*, inflammation]. Inflamed condition of a layer of fatty connective tissue in the abdomen.

SYM: Pain and tenderness and hypertrophy of tissue in parts where fat is the thickest.

TREATMENT: Massage. Improvement of circulation in affected parts.

panniculus (păn-ĭk'ū-lŭs) [L. a small piece of cloth]. A layer or sheet of tissue.

p. adiposus. The superficial fascia with fat in its areolar substance.

p. carnosus. Thin layer of muscular tissue in superficial fascia.

pannus (păn'ŭs) [L. cloth]. Newly formed vascular tissue involving the upper half of the front of the cornea.

The area is cloudy, and its surface is uneven as it is covered with a film of new capillary blood vessels. May cover entire cornea. Seen in trachoma, acne rosacea, eczema, and as a result of irritation in granular conjunctivitis.

panopeptone (păn-ō-pep'tōn) [L. *panis*, bread, + G. *peptein*, to digest]. Commercial invalid food composed of bread and peptonized beef.

panophobia (păn-ō-fō'bĭ-ă) [G. *pas, pan-*, all, + *phobos*, fear]. Morbid fear of some unknown evil or of everything in general; general apprehension. SYN: *pantophobia*.

panophthalmia, panophthalmitis (păn-ŏf-thăl'mĭ-ă, -mī'tĭs) [G. *pas, pan-*, all, + *ophthalmos*, eye, + *-itis*, inflammation]. Inflammation of entire eye.

p. purulenta. Severe form with suppuration.

SYM: Fever, pain, headache, vomiting, loss of sight, ant. chamber and vitreous filled with pus.

PROG: Unfavorable.

TREATMENT: Hot, moist compresses; incision, and evisceration.

panoptic (păn-ŏp′tĭk) [" + *opsis*, sight]. Making every part visible; completely visible.
 p. stain. Stain which causes every part of the tissue to be differentiated.
panoptosis (păn-ŏp-tō′sĭs) [" + *ptōsis*, a dropping]. General prolapse of the abdominal organs.
panosteitis (păn″ŏs-tē-ī′tĭs) [" + *osteon*, bone, + *-itis*, inflammation]. Inflammation of every structure of a bone.
panotitis (păn-ō-tī′tĭs) [" + *ous*, *ōt-*, ear, + *-itis*, inflammation]. Inflammation involving all the parts of the ear.
panparnit (păn-par′nĭt). Trade name for synthetic antispasmodic used in paralysis agitans (Parkinsonism). Diminishes muscular rigidity and relieves tremor.
panphobia (păn-fō′bĭ-ă) [" + *phobos*, fear]. Groundless fear of everything.
panspermia (păn-spĕr′mĭ-ă) [" + *sperma*, seed]. The theory that distribution of disease germs is widespread, accounting for apparent cases of spontaneous generation. SEE: *biogenesis*.
pansphygmograph (păn-sfĭg′mō-grăf) [G. *pas*, *pan-*, all, + *sphygmos*, pulse, + *graphein*, to write]. Apparatus for registering cardiac movements, the pulse wave, and chest movements at one time.
pansporoblast (păn-spō′rō-blăst) [" + *sporos*, seed, + *blastos*, germ]. Reproductive area in the myxosporidia having both germinal and vegetative nuclei.
pant (pănt) [O.Fr. *pantaisier*, to be breathless]. 1. To breathe hard; to gasp for breath. 2. A short or labored breath.
 ETIOL: Produced by overexertion physically, as in running, or from fear.
pantachromatic (păn″tă-krō-măt′ĭk) [G. *pas*, *pan-*, all, + *a-*, priv. + *chrōma*, color]. Entirely colorless.
pantalgia (păn-tăl′jĭ-ă) [" + *algos*, pain]. Pain felt over the entire body.
pantatrophia, **pantatrophy** (păn-tăt-rō′fĭ-ă, -tat′rō-fĭ). Complete lack of nourishment to a part with resultant wasting.
panthodic (păn-thŏd′ĭk) [" + *odos*, way]. Radiating to all parts of the body, esp. applied to nervous impulses.
panting (pănt′ĭng) [O.Fr. *pantaisier*, to be breathless]. 1. Breathing hard; gasping for breath. 2. Labored breathing.
pantophobia (păn-tō-fō′bĭ-ă) [" + *phobos*, fear]. Morbid, groundless fear of everything in general. SYN: *panophobia*.
pantopon (păn′tō-pŏn) [" + *opion*, poppy juice]. Registered trade-mark for a brand of purified opium alkaloids. Oral and parenteral administration.
 USES: In all disorders where the analgesic, sedative-hypnotic or narcotic effect of an opiate is needed.
 DOSAGE: From 1/24 to 1/3 gr. (0.0025-0.02 Gm.).
pantoscopic (păn″tō-skŏp′ĭk) [G. *pas*, *pan-*, all, + *skopein*, to examine]. Viewing everything; adjusted to both close and far objects.
 p. glasses. Glasses with 2 segments of different focal lengths for near and far objects. SYN: *bifocal spectacles*.
pantothenic acid (păn-tō-then′ĭk) [G. *pas*, *pant-*, all, + *tithēnai*, to be]. Newly synthesized vitamin found in yeast, molasses, rice hulls, and liver.
 Belief that this acid is necessary to humans is based on several discoveries: (1) It appears to be an essential part in all living things; (2) baby chicks deprived of it develop serious skin disorders; (3) when hens lack this vitamin their eggs almost all fail to hatch; (4) it is powerful stimulant of growth.
pantothermia (păn″tō-thĕr′mĭ-ă) [" + *thermē*, heat]. Condition in which there is variation in bodily temperature without apparent reason.
panturbinate (păn-tur′bĭ-năt) [" + L. *turbinatus*, shaped like a top]. All of the turbinate structure.
pap (păp) [L. *papa*, infant's cry for food]. 1. Any soft, semiliquid food. 2. [M.E. *pappe*, nipple]. The nipple.
papain (pa-pā′ĭn, pa′pă-ĭn). A digestive ferment obtained from the papaw fruit.
 USES: As a digestant.
 DOSAGE: 2-4 gr. (0.12-0.25 Gm.).
papaverine hydrochloride (pă-păv′ĕr-ēn) [L. *papaver*, poppy]. The salt of an alkaloid obtained from opium.
 USES: Antispasmodic, especially in gastric and intestinal distress, and recommended in bronchial spasm.
 AVERAGE DOSE: ½ gr. (0.03 Gm.).
paper (pā′pĕr) [G. *papyros*, a paper]. 1. A substance mechanically woven into thin sheets or strips, with many uses, as for filtering. 2. A piece of paper specially prepared, as by having a medicinal preparation spread out on it.
papilla (pă-pĭl′ă) (pl. *papillae*) [L. nipple]. 1. The nipple of the breast; any nipplelike protuberance. 2. A small, soft, sensitive eminence in the skin possessing a tactile function.
 p., acoustic. Organ of Corti.
 p., circumvallate. One of the large papillae near the base on the dorsal aspect of the tongue, arranged in a V-shape.
 p., duodenal. The slight eminence in duodenum indicating opening of ductus choledochus communis.
 p., filiform. One of the very slender papillae at tip of the tongue.
 p., fungiform. One of the broad, flat papillae resembling a fungus, chiefly found on dorsal central area of tongue.
 p., gustatory. Taste papilla of tongue; one of those possessing a taste bud.
 p., hair. A conical process of the corium in which a hair is nourished.
 p., lacrimal. An elevation in edge of eyelid for the lacrimal puncta.
 p., lingual. Tiny eminence covering ant. two-thirds of tongue, including circumvallate, filiform, fungiform, and conical papillae.
 p., nerve. P. of skin containing tactile corpuscles. SEE: *tactile corpuscles*.
 p., optic. Terminus of optic nerve where it enters the eyeball.
 p., primary. A p. arising directly from the corium.
 p., renal. Apex of a malpighian pyramid in the kidney.
 p., secondary. P. arising from a primary p.
 p., simple. An undivided p. arising directly from the corium.
 p., tactile. SEE: *nerve p.*
 p., taste. SEE: *gustatory p.*
 p., vascular. P. of skin to the tips of which extend 1 or more capillary loops.
 p. of Vater. SEE: *duodenal p.*
papillary (păp′ĭ-lar-ĭ) [L. *papilla*, nipple]. 1. Concerning a nipple or papilla. 2. Resembling or composed of papillae.
 p. body. Papillary layer of the corium. SYN: *pars papillaris*.
 p. muscles. Muscular eminences in ventricles of the heart.
 p. tumor. Neoplasm composed of or resembling enlarged papillae. SEE: *papilloma*.

papillate (păp'ĭl-āt) [L. *papilla*, nipple].
BACT: Having nipplelike growths on the surface, as a culture.

papillectomy (păp-ĭl-ĕk'tō-mĭ) [" + G. *ektome*, excision]. Excision of any papilla or papillae.

papilledema (păp-ĭl-e-dē'mă) [" + *oidēma*, swelling]. Edema and inflammation of the optic nerve at its point of entrance into the eyeball.
ETIOL: Intracranial pressure, often caused by tumor of the brain pressing on optic nerve.
PROG: Unless relieved, blindness may result very rapidly. SYN: *choked disk, optic neuritis.*

papilliferous (păp-ĭl-ĭf'ĕr-ŭs) [" + *ferre*, to carry]. Having or containing papillae.

papilliform (pă-pĭl'ĭ-form) [" + *forma*, shape]. 1. Having the characteristics or appearance of papillae. 2. BACT: Denoting a shallow saucerlike form.

papillitis (păp-ĭl-ī'tĭs) [" + G. *-itis*, inflammation]. Inflammation of optic disk with edema. SYN: *choked disk, optic neuritis.*

papilloadenocystoma (păp"ĭl-ō-ăd"ē-nō-sĭs-tō'mă) [" + G. *adēn*, gland, + *kystis*, a cyst, + *-ōma*, tumor]. A tumor composed of elements of papilloma, adenoma and cystoma.

papillocarcinoma (păp"ĭl-ō-kăr-sĭn-ō'mă) [" + G. *karkinos*, crab cancer, + *-ōma*, tumor]. 1. A malignant tumor of hypertrophied papillae. 2. Carcinoma with papillary growths.

papilloma (pl. *papillomata*) (păp-ĭ-lō'mă) [" + G. *-ōma*, tumor]. 1. Any benign epithelial tumor. 2. Epithelial tumor of skin or mucous membrane consisting of hypertrophied papillae covered by a layer of epithelium.
Included in this group are *warts, condylomas*, and *polypi.* SEE: *acanthoma.*

p. durum. A hardened p., as a wart.
p., hard. P. which develops from squamous epithelium.
p. molle. A p. with only a thin, horny layer covering it.
p., soft. P. formed from columnar epithelium.
p., urethral. A painful urethral caruncle or fibrocellular tumor arising from the urethra.

papillomatosis (păp"ĭl-ō-mă-tō'sĭs) [" + " + *-ōsis*, disease]. 1. Widespread formation of papillomata. 2. Condition of being afflicted with many papillomata.

papilloretinitis (păp"ĭl-ō-rĕt-ĭn-ī'tĭs) [" + *rētē*, net, + G. *-itis*, inflammation]. Inflamed condition of the papilla and retina extending to the optic disk.

papoid (pa'poyd). Commercial powder given to stimulate digestion.

paprika (păp'rĭ-ka, păp-rē'kă) [G. *peperi*, pepper]. ASH CONST: Ca 0.229, Mg 0.164, K 2.075, Na 0.178, P 0.341, Cl 0.155. No iron or sulfur. VITAMINS: C+++. SEE: *condiment, pepper.*

papula (păp'ū-lă) [L.]. A pimple. SYN: *papule.*

papular (păp'ū-ler) [L. *papula*, pimple]. Of the nature of or concerning pimples.
p. fever. Mild fever with maculopapular eruptions and rheumatoid pains.

papulation (păp-ū-lā'shŭn) [L. *papula*, pimple]. 1. The development of papules. 2. The stage of pimple formation in a disease.

papule (păp'ūl) [L. *papula*, pimple]. Red elevated area on the skin, solid and circumscribed, varying from the size of a pinhead to that of a pea.
P.'s often precede vesicular or pustular formation and may appear in erythema multiforme, eczema papulosum, prurigo, syphilis, measles, smallpox, and they may develop after the use of bromides, iodides, coal tar preparations, etc.
In *measles* they are small and run together, forming crescent-shaped patches; in *smallpox* they are hard and feel like shot, terminating in umbilicated vesicles and exciting itching. In *prurigo* they are small, pale, deep seated, and accompanied by intense itching; in *syphilis* they are dark colored and widely distributed, especially on the trunk and surfaces of the extremities. They do not cause itching. In *eczema* they are small, often associated with pustules and vesicles, and are closely aggregated; there is intense itching and the skin is thickened. In *erythema multiforme* they are found with macules and tubercles, and are bright red or purple and flat, appearing especially on the extremities. They do not suppurate or cause itching, but are accompanied by rheumatic pains and prostration. SEE: *Casoni's reaction.*

p., dry. Hard one that is primary lesion of syphilis.
p., moist; p., mucous. A syphilitic eruption of papules with flat tops. SYN: *condyloma lata.*

papuliferous (păp"ū-lĭf'ĕr-ŭs) [L. *papula*, pimple, + *ferre*, to bear]. Having papules or pimples.

papulo- [L.]. Combining form meaning *a pimple, a papule.*

papyraceous (păp-ĭ-rā'shŭs) [L. *papyraceus*, made of papyrus, from G. *papyros*, parchment]. Parchmentlike.
OB: Denoting a fetus retained in the uterus beyond natural term that has assumed a mummified appearance.

Paquelin's cautery (păk-lăn'). A hollow, platinum pointed cautery apparatus kept at a constant temperature by means of benzene vapor.

par [L. pair]. A pair, esp. a pair of cranial nerves.
p. vagum. The vagus or 10th pair of cranial nerves.

para-, par- [G.]. Combining forms meaning *alongside of, by, past, beyond, the opposite, abnormal, irregular.*

paraaminobenzoic acid (păr"ă-ăm-ĭ-nō-bĕn-zō'ĭk). Commonly abbrev. PABA. A member of the vitamin B complex. Used in arthritis, rheumatic fever, fibrositis, gout, scleroderma, dermatomyositis. Inhibits bacteriostatic action of sulfonamides; hence contraindicated during sulfonamide therapy.

paraaminosalicylic acid (păr"ă-ăm-ĭ-nō-săl-ĭ-sĭl'ĭk). Commonly abbrev. PAS. An adjuvant to streptomycin or dihydrostreptomycin in treatment of tuberculosis. Valuable both for inhibitory effect on tubercle bacillus and for ability to delay development of streptomycin-resistant organisms.

paraänesthesia (păr"ă-ăn-ĕs-thē'zhĭ-a) [G. *para*, beside, + *an-*, negative, + *aisthēsis*, sensation]. Anesthesia of two corresponding sides, esp. of lower half of body.

paraäppendicitis (păr"ă-ăp-ĕnd-ĭ-sī'tĭs) [" + L. *appendix*, + G. *-itis*, inflammation]. Inflammation involving the connective tissue adjacent to the appendix. SYN: *perityphlitis.*

parabiosis (păr"ă-bī-ō'sĭs) [" + *biōsis*, living]. 1. Temporary suppression of

parabiotik   P-13   **paraffin**

excitability and conductivity of a nerve. 2. Anatomical and physiological joining of 2 separate organisms, naturally or artificially formed. SEE: *Siamese twins.*
parabiotik (păr"ă-bī-ŏt'ĭk) [" + *biōsis*, living]. Concerning parabiosis.
parablast (păr'ă-blăst) [" + *blastos*, germ]. Part of the embryonic mesoblast from which arise the vascular and connective tissue structures.
parablastic (păr"ă-blăst'ĭk) [" + *blastos*, germ]. Pert. to the embryonic layer giving rise to the vascular and connective tissue structures.
parablastoma (păr"ă-blăst-ō'mă) [" + " + -*ōma*, tumor]. A tumor composed of parablastic tissue.
parablepsia, parablepsis (păr"ă-blĕp'sĭ-ă, -sĭs) [G. *para*, irregular, + *blepsis*, vision]. Abnormality of the visual sensations.
parabulia (păr-ă-bū'lĭ-ă) [" + *boulē*, will]. Perversion or abnormality of will power.
paracentesis (păr-ă-sĕn-tē'sĭs) [G. *para*, beside, + *kentēsis*, a puncture]. Puncture of a cavity with evacuation of fluid by tapping, as in dropsy.
NP: Watch pulse and respirations for signs of collapse during procedure and following.
   p., abdominal. Tapping of the abdomen.
   p. capitis. P. of the cranium.
   p. cordis. Surgical puncture of the heart.
   p. pericardii. P. of the pericardial sac.
   p. pulmonis. Removal of fluid from a lung.
   p. thoracis. Drainage of fluid from the cavity of the chest. SEE: *aspiration.*
   p. tunicae vaginalis. P. of the tunica vaginalis.
   p. tympani. Drainage or irrigation through incision of the tympanic membrane.
   p. vesicae. Puncture of the wall of the urinary bladder.
paracentetic (păr"ă-sĕn-tĕt'ĭk) [G. *para*, beside, + *kentēsis*, a piercing]. Concerning paracentesis.
paracentral (păr"ă-sĕn'trăl) [" + *kentron*, center]. Located near the center.
   p. lobule. Cerebral convolution on mesial surface joining the upper terminations of the ascending parietal and frontal convolutions.
parachlorphenol (păr"ă-klor-fē'nol). Strong antiseptic and disinfectant used in lupus and erysipelas.
paracholia (păr"ă-kō'lĭ-ă) [G. *para*, abnormal, + *cholē*, bile]. Condition of disturbed bile secretion.
parachordal (păr-ă-kor'dăl) [G. *para*, beside, + *chordē*, a cord]. 1. Noting the 2 plates of cartilage, 1 on either side of the ant. portion of the notochord.* 2. A parachordal cartilage.
parachroma (păr-ă-krō'mă) [" + *chrōma*, color]. Discoloration, as that of the skin.
parachromatin (păr"ă-krō'mă-tĭn) [" + *chrōma*, color]. The portion of the nucleoplasm that forms the spindle threads in karyokinesis.
parachromatopsia (păr"ă-krō-mă-tŏp'sĭ-ă) [" + " + *opsis*, vision]. Color blindness.
parachromatosis (păr"ă-krō-mă-tō'sĭs) [" + " + -*ōsis*, disease]. Any 1 of the diseases in which the skin is pigmented.
parachromophoric (păr"ă-krō'mō-for'ĭk) [" + " + *phoros*, a carrier]. Excreting pigment, but retaining it within the organism.

parachymosin (păr"ă-kī-mō'sĭn) [" + *chymos*, juice]. The ferment found in the stomach of both pig and human being.
paracinesia, paracinesis (păr"ă-sĭn-ē'zĭ-ă, -sĭs) [G. *para*, abnormal, + *kinēsis*, motion]. Condition in which there is perversion of motor powers; motor abnormality.
paracmastic (păr-ăk-măs'tĭk) [" + *akmē*, point]. Denoting the period of decrease of symptoms. RS: *acmastic, epacmastic.*
paracolpitis (păr"ă-kŏl-pī'tĭs) [" + *kolpos*, vagina, + -*itis*, inflammation]. Inflammation of tissues adjoining the vagina.
paracolpium (păr"ă-kol'pĭ-ŭm) [" + *kolpos*, vagina]. The vascular and connective tissue alongside the vagina.
paracrisis (păr-ăk'rĭ-sĭs, păr"ă-krī'sĭs) [" + *krisis*, a separation]. Any abnormality of the secretions.
paracusis (păr-ă-kū'sĭs) [" + *akousis*, a hearing]. Any abnormality or disorder of the sense of hearing.
   p. acris. Excessively acute hearing.
   p. duplicata. The hearing of 1 sound as 2. SYN: *diplacusis.*
   p. loci. Difficulty in estimating the direction of sound.
   p. willisiana. An apparent ability to hear better in a noisy place, found in deafness due to stapes fixation and adhesive processes.
paracyesis (păr-ă-sī-ē'sĭs) [G. *para*, beside, + *kyēsis*, pregnancy]. Extrauterine pregnancy.
paracystitis (păr"ă-sĭs-tī'tĭs) [" + *kystis*, bladder, + -*itis*, inflammation]. Inflamed condition of connective tissues and other structures around the urinary bladder.
paracystium (păr-ă-sĭs'tĭ-ŭm) [" + *kystis*, bladder]. The connective tissue surrounding the urinary bladder.
paradenitis (păr"ăd-en-ī'tĭs) [" + *adēn*, gland, + -*itis*, inflammation]. Inflammation of areolar tissues close to a gland.
paradidymis (păr-ă-dĭd'ĭ-mĭs) [" + *didymos*, testicle]. BNA. The atrophic remnants of the tubules of the wolffian body, situated on the spermatic cord above the epididymis. SYN: *massa innominata, organ of Giraldès, parepididymis.*
paradoxic, paradoxical (păr"ă-dŏk'sĭk, -sĭ-kal) [G. *paradoxos*, contrary to opinion]. Seemingly contradictory, but demonstrably true.
   p. contraction. Contraction of a muscle when its origin and insertion are suddenly relaxed or its length shortened, suddenly.
   p. flexor reflex. Extension of great toe when sudden pressure is made on deep flexor muscles of calf of leg.
   p. movement. When diaphragm is paralyzed, it is forced upward during inspiration, and downward during expiration—the reverse of normal.
   p. respiration. A lung is breathing paradoxically when it expands during expiration and contracts during inspiration.
paraffin (păr'ă-fĭn) [L. *parum*, too little, + *affinis*, allied]. 1. A waxy, white, tasteless, odorless mixture of solid hydrocarbons obtained from petroleum. 2. A saturated hydrocarbon of the methane series.
ACTION AND USES: Medically, chiefly as a protective covering for burns and to give stiffness to ointments.

p., hard. Solid p. with a melting point bet. 45° C. and 60° C.
p., liquid. Liquid hydrocarbon. SYN: *liquid petrolatum.*
p., soft. A semisolid p. SEE: *petrolatum.*
paraffinoma (păr″ă-fĭn-ō′mă) [" + " + G. *-ōma,* tumor]. A tumor which arises at site of injection of paraffin.
paraffinum (păr-ă-fe′nŭm) [L.]. Paraffin, *q.v.*
paraformaldehyde (par″ă-fōr-măl′dĕ-hīd). A white, powdered antiseptic and disinfectant, a polymer of formaldehyde.
paragammacism (păr″ă-găm′mă-sĭzm) [G. *para,* beside, + *gamma,* Greek letter G, + *ismos,* condition]. Inability to pronounce "g" and "k" sounds, with substitution of other consonants for them.
paraganglin (păr″ă-găng′lĭn). Commercial intestinal tonic prepared from the medulla of the suprarenal glands of oxen.
paraganglioma (păr″ă-găng-lĭ-ō′mă) [G. *para,* beside, + *gagglion,* knot, + *-ōma,* tumor]. 1. Tumor composed of cells resembling medullary tissue of the adrenals. 2. Tumor of the adrenal medulla.
paraganglion (pl. *paraganglia*) (păr″ă-găng′lĭ-ŏn) [G. *para,* beside, + *gagglion,* knot]. 1. Any structure supplementing, or in the neighborhood of, a ganglion. 2. A mass of cells in the medullary portion of the adrenal bodies. 3. Chromaffin mass found along the branches of the sympathetic nervous system. SEE: *chromaffinoma.*
parageusia, parageusis (păr-ă-gū′sĭ-ă, -sĭs) [" + *geusis,* taste]. Disorder or abnormality of the sense of taste.
May follow the use of certain drugs, such as the bromides, tartar emetic, or potassium iodide. May be present in gastrointestinal catarrh, jaundice, and conditions producing a furred tongue, as a "bad taste." Functional nerve derangements, hysteria, and the hallucinations of the insane often present perversion of taste. An unpleasant, sour, sticky, or bitter taste experienced upon awakening in the morning, which may be more or less persistent, is associated with gastrointestinal conditions. SEE: *taste.*
paraglobulin (păr″ă-glŏb′ŭ-lĭn) [" + L. *globulus,* a small sphere]. A globulin found in blood plasma, lymph, and other body fluids, associated with coagulation.
paraglobulinuria (păr″ă-glŏb-ū-lĭn-ū′rĭ-ă) [" + " + G. *ouron,* urine]. Excretion of paraglobulin in the urine.
paraglossa (păr-ă-glŏs′să) [" + *glōssa,* tongue]. 1. Enlargement of the tongue. 2. Congenital hypertrophy of the tongue.
Paragonimus (păr″ă-gŏn′ĭm-ŭs). Genus of trematode worms.
P. westermanii. Lung fluke.
paragraphia (păr-ă-grăf′ĭ-ă) [G. *para,* besides, + *graphein,* to write]. The writing of letters or words other than those intended, due to partial lesion of the visual word center in the brain.
parahepatitis (păr″ă-hĕp-ă-tī′tĭs) [" + *ēpar, ēpat-,* liver, + *-ītis,* inflammation]. Inflamed condition of parts immediately adjacent to the liver.
parainfection (păr″ă-ĭn-fĕk′shŭn) [" + L. *in,* into, + *facere,* to make]. The symptomatology of an infectious disease without evidence of the presence of the microörganism causing the disease.
parakeratosis (păr″ă-kĕr-ă-tō′sĭs) [" + *keras, kerat-,* horn, + *-ōsis,* infection]. Any disorder affecting the horny layer of the epidermis.

p. psoriasiformis. Scab formation resembling that of psoriasis.
p. scutularis. Scalp disease with hairs encircled by epidermic crust formation.
paralalia (păr-ă-lā′lĭ-ă) [" + *lalein,* to babble]. Any speech defect, characterized by sound distortion.
p. literalis. Stammering, *q.v.*
paralambdacism (păr″ă-lăm′dă-sĭzm) [G. *para,* beside, + *lambda,* Greek letter L, + *ismos,* condition]. Inability to sound the letter "l" correctly, substituting some other letter for it.
paralbumin (păr-ăl-bū′mĭn) [" + L. *albumen,* white of egg]. An albumin found in fluid content in ovarian cysts and in ascites.
paraldehyde (păr-ăl′dĕ-hīd). USP. $C_6H_{12}O_3$. A liquid polymer of aldehyde which is colorless, with characteristic unpleasant odor and taste.
Made by action of hydrochloric acid on acetic aldehyde.
ACTION AND USES: Hypnotic, having low toxicity and prompt action as a sedative. Recently has been used as an analgesic in obstetrics, esp. in combination with rectal ether.
DOSAGE: 30 minims (2 cc.) in sweetened water or lemonade.
POISONING: SYM: Resemble those of chloral hydrate, cardiac and respiratory depression, dizziness, collapse with partial or complete anesthesia. Odor on the breath is a constant distinct sign.
F. A. TREATMENT: Same as for chloral hydrate, *q.v.*
paraldehydism (păr-ăl′dĕ-hīd-ĭzm). Poisoning from an overdose of paraldehyde, *q.v.*
paralepsy (par′ă-lĕp″sĭ) [G. *para,* besides, + *lēpsis,* seizure]. Temporary attack of mental inertia and hopelessness, or sudden alteration in mood or mental tension. SYN: *psycholepsy.*
paralexia (păr-ă-lĕk′sĭ-ă) [" + *lexis,* speech]. Inability to comprehend printed words or sentences with substitution of meaningless combinations of words.
paralgesia (păr-ăl-jē′zĭ-ă) [" + *algēsis,* pain]. Any unusual sensation which is painful.
paralgia (păr-al′jĭ-ă) [" + *algos,* pain]. Sensation both abnormal and painful.
parallagma (păr-ăl-ăg′mă) [G. *parallagma,* alternation]. Overlapping or displacement of the fragments of a fractured bone.
parallax (păr′ă-lăks) [G. *parallax,* in turn]. Apparent displacement of a part due to change in observer's position.
paralogia (păr-ă-lō′jĭ-ă) [G. *para,* beside, + *logos,* understanding]. A disorder of the reasoning; a psychosis.
paralysin (păr-ăl′ĭs-ĭn) [" + *lysis,* solution]. An antibody causing clumping of cells or bacteria. SYN: *agglutinin.*
paralysis (pă-ral′ĭ-sĭs) [G. *paralyein,* to disable at the side]. Temporary suspension or permanent loss of function in a living part, esp. loss of sensation or voluntary motion.
Any voluntary movement depends on the integrity of 2 motor neurons; 1 arising in the motor cortex, coursing across the brain stem and ending in the ant. gray horn of the spinal cord, and the lower neurons arising in the ant. horn cell and passing to the muscle. If the latter are destroyed, the muscle loses tone, atrophies (withers away) and shows reaction of degeneration (R. D.).

The flaccidity and absent muscular reflexes reveal the loss of tonus. If the upper neuron is paralyzed, the patient is equally unable to move the affected part, but the intact lower neuron may permit other motor centers to act on the muscle. In addition, tone is increased, there is no R. D. and no atrophy save that of disease. So-called pathological reflexes may appear in addition to the increase of normal deep reflexes.

Paralyses are divided into 2 groups, *spastic*, when due to lesion of upper motor neuron, and *flaccid*, when due to lesion of lower motor neuron.

Psychic inhibition of motor function occurs most characteristically in hysteria, but the evidence of organic disease is always lacking in these hysterical paralyses.

RS: *anesthecinesia; ballism; Bell's phenomenon; celluloneuritis; diplegia, acute, anterior; Duchenne's disease; Gradenigo's syndrome; hemiplegia; monoparesis; monoplegia; nerve; oxyacoia; palsy; paraparesis; paraplegia; paresis; quadriplegia; Volkmann's p.*

p. of accommodation. Inability of the eye to adjust itself to various distances due to paralysis.

p., acoustic. Nervous deafness.

p., acute ascending. Rapidly progressing form of paralysis which begins in the feet and slowly ascends. Fatal. SYN: *Landry's p.*

p., acute atrophic. SEE: *infantile p.*

p., acute infectious. SEE: *infantile p.*

p. agitans. A basal ganglion disease of late life producing a picture of rigid tremulousness progressive in its course, and marked by weakness, delay of voluntary motion, a peculiar festinating gait, and muscular contraction, causing peculiar and characteristic positions of the limbs and head. The disease is attended with excessive sweating and feelings of heat and cold. While movement is slow, there is no true paralysis. The face appears expressionless, there is general flexion attitude, the balance tends to be lost (in a forward direction). Many of these cases follow encephalitis lethargica; others are essentially senile. SEE: *Parkinson's disease.*

p., alcoholic. P. due to habitual drunkenness.

p., anesthesia. P. which develops following administration of anesthesia.

p., anterior spinal. Inflamed condition of the ant. horns of the spinal cord's gray matter. [from arsenic.

p., arsenical. P. following poisoning

p., ascending. P. beginning with the lower limbs and progressing upward.

p., association. SEE: *bulbar p.*

p., Bell's. Facial paralysis.

ETIOL: Lesion of the facial nerve or of its nucleus; a neuritis of this nerve. Pressure on nerve as it reaches the face through its bony canal near the ear.

SYM: One side of entire face may be affected, or corner of mouth may drop, eyelid may droop or be unable to close, may be unable to close lips or to speak, or loss of control of eye.

TREATMENT: Fly blister behind the ear on affected side until blister appears, or better, infrared lamp or heat sufficient to keep skin red for several days to lessen swelling of nerve. Adhesive strips to hold up sagging tissues. Salicylates and iodides may be indicated.

p., Bernhardt's. Pain and hyperesthesia on the outer femoral surface from lesion or disease of the external cutaneous nerve of the thigh.

p., birth. P. caused by injury received at birth.

p., brachial. Paralysis of 1 or both arms.

p., brachiofacial. P. of the face and an arm.

p., Brown-Sequard's. P. of motion on 1 side and of sensation on the other.

p., bulbar. P. caused by changes in the motor centers of the oblongata.

p., central. Any paralysis from a lesion of the brain or spinal cord.

p., cerebral. P. due to lesion of some portion of the cerebrum.

p., complete. P. in which there is total loss of function.

p., compression. P. due to pressure on a nerve, as by a crutch or during sleep.

p., crossed. P. of the face on 1 side of the body and the limbs on the opposite side.

p., crutch. P. due to pressure in the armpit.

p., decubitus. P. due to pressure on a nerve from lying in 1 position for a long time.

p., diver's. P. due to increase in atmospheric pressure, evidenced on return to normal atmosphere. SYN: *caisson disease.*

p., Erb's. 1. SEE: *birth p.* 2. Partial p. of the brachial plexus.

p., exhaustion. P. due to prolonged voluntary movements involving exhaustion of the nerve centers.

p., facial. SEE: *Bell's p.*

p., general. Progressive loss of power and the mental faculties resulting eventually in dementia and death. SYN: *paresis.*

p., ginger. P. of the limbs after drinking Jamaica ginger.

p., glossolabial. SEE: *bulbar p.*

p., histrionic. Paralysis of certain facial muscles, producing a facial expression of some emotion.

p., hysteric. One that may simulate any form of paralysis; it appears to have no adequate causative lesion.

p., incomplete. Partial paralysis of the body or a part.

p., infantile. Motor paralysis with atrophy of a group of muscles following an acute infectious disease in children which is transmitted by a filtrable virus. SEE: *acute anterior poliomyelitis.*

p., jake. SEE: *ginger p.*

p., Klumpke's. Wasting p. of the arms and hands.

p., Kussmaul's; p., Landry's. SEE: *acute ascending p.*

p., lead. P. following poisoning by lead.

p., local. P. of a single muscle or 1 group of muscles.

p., nuclear. P. caused by lesion of a nucleus.

p., obstetrical. SEE: *birth p.*

p., periodic. P. which recurs and abates temporarily.

p., progressive bulbar. SEE: *bulbar p.*

p., pseudobulbar. P. caused by cerebral center lesions, which simulates the bulbar types of paralysis.

p., reflex. P. caused by irritation of a periphery. In some cases, secondary changes occur in the spinal cord, and the paralysis ceases to be truly reflex.

p., spastic spinal. Congenital sclerosis of spinal cord's lateral columns with

muscular rigidity and exaggerated reflexes. SYN: *Little's disease.*
p., spinal. SEE: *p., anterior spinal.*
p., wasting. Progressive wasting away of the muscles. SEE: *progressive muscular atrophy.*
paralytic (păr-ă-lĭt'ĭk) [G. *para*, beside, + *lyein*, to loosen]. 1. Concerning paralysis. 2. One afflicted with paralysis.
p. dementia. Progressive paralysis with mental deterioration. SYN: *paresis.*
p. ileus. P. of intestinal wall with distention and symptoms of acute obstruction and prostration.
ETIOL: It may occur after any abdominal operation.
paralyzant (păr"ă-līz'ănt) [" + *lyein*, to loosen]. 1. Causing paralysis. 2. A drug or other agent that induces paralysis.
paralyze (păr'ă-līz) [" + *lyein*, to loosen]. 1. To cause temporary or permanent loss of muscular power or sensation. 2. To render ineffective.
paramastigote (păr"a-măs'tĭ-gōt) [" + *mastix, mastigg-*, a whip]. Possessing an accessory flagellum adjacent to a larger one.
paramastitis (păr-ă-măs-tī'tĭs) [" + *mastos*, breast, + *-itis*, inflammation]. Inflammation around the mamma.
paramecium (par-ă-mē'cĭ-um) [G. *paramēkēs*, rather long]. Genus of infusorians, rather long in shape and sometimes seen by the naked eye.
paramenia (păr-ă-mē'nĭ-ă) [" + *mēniaia*, menses]. Irregular, abnormal or difficult menstruation.
parametric (păr-ă-mĕt'rĭk) [" + *mētra*, uterus]. 1. Concerning the area near the uterus. 2. Rel. to the parametrium, the tissue surrounding the uterus.
parametrismus (păr-ă-mē-trĭz'mŭs) [G. *para*, beside, + *mētra*, uterus, + *trismos*, a spasm]. Muscular spasm in the broad ligament accompanied by pain.
parametritis (păr"ă-mē-trī'tĭs) [" + " + *-itis*, inflammation]. Inflamed condition of parametrium, the cellular tissue adjacent to uterus. SYN: *cellulitis, pelvic.*
parametrium (păr-ă-mē'trĭ-ŭm) [" + *mētra*, uterus]. Fat and connective tissue around the uterus.
paramimia (păr-ă-mĭm'ĭ-ă) [G. *para*, beside, + *mimeisthai*, to imitate]. PSY: Disturbance of association tracts bet. motor and sensory centers resulting in misuse of gestures.
paramitome (păr-ă-mī'tōm) [" + *mitos*, a thread]. Fluid portion of protoplasm of cells. SYN: *hyaloplasm, paraplasm.*
paramnesia (păr"-ăm-nē'zĭ-ă) [" + *a-*, priv. + *mnēsis*, memory]. 1. The use of words without meaning. 2. Inability to distinguish imaginary or suggested experiences from those which have actually occurred.
paramorphia (păr-ă-mor'fĭ-ă) [" + *morphē*, form]. Abnormality of shape.
paramusia (păr"ă-mū'zĭ-ă) [" + *amousia*, want of harmony]. Loss of ability to render music accurately.
paramyoclonus (păr"ă-mī-ō-klō'nŭs) [" + *mys, my-*, muscle, + *klonos*, tumult]. Clonic spasm of symmetrical groups of muscles.
paramyosinogen (păr"ă-mī"ō-sĭn'ō-jĕn) [" + *mys, my-*, muscle, + *gennan*, to produce]. Protein derived from muscle plasm.
paramyotonia (păr"ă-mī"ō-tō'nĭ-ă) [" + " + *tonos*, tone]. A disorder marked by muscular spasms and abnormal muscular tonicity.
p. ataxia. Tonic muscular spasm when making any movement, with slight ataxia or paresis.
p. congenita. Congenital condition of tonic muscular spasms when body is exposed to cold. SYN: *Thomsen's disease.*
p., symptomatic. Temporary muscular rigidity when first trying to walk, as in paralysis agitans.
paranephrine (păr"ă-nĕf'rĭn) [" + *nephros*, kidney]. Commercial preparation of extract of the adrenal glands which controls hemorrhage and raises blood pressure.
paranephritis (păr"ă-ne-frī'tĭs) [G. *para*, beside, + *nephros*, kidney, + *-itis*, inflammation]. 1. Inflamed condition of the suprarenal capsules. 2. Inflammation of connective tissue about kidney. SYN: *perinephritis.*
paranephros (păr-ă-nĕf'rŏs) [" + *nephros*, kidney]. A suprarenal or adrenal capsule.
paranesthesia (păr"ăn-ĕs-thē'zĭ-ă) [" + *an-*, negative, + *aisthēsis*, sensation]. Anesthesia of the lower portion of the body.
paranoia (păr-ă-noy'ă) [" + *nous*, mind]. A chronic, psychotic entity characterized by fixed but ever-expanding systematized delusions of persecution.
General characteristics are sensitive, suspicious, jealous, brooding nature; excessive self-consciousness; fixed ideas, developed into well-systematized, logical delusions, megalomania, rare hallucinations, repressed homosexuality, inability to make concessions.
The 3 chief stages are: (1) Self-analytical, introverted, hypochondriacal period; (2) persecution period; (3) delusion period.
Paranoid personality is sometimes applied to borderline cases in which the attitude is not sufficiently controlling to prevent contact with reality. The individual may finally become expanded and attempt to explain his delusions in terms flattering to himself.
Delusions are fixed in type, systematized and always directed toward same individual or group. They are coherent. Delusions never are bizarre. There is no evidence of derangement of personality. Patient cannot be trusted and may be dangerous. SEE: *paranoid reaction type.*
p., alcoholic. This condition simulates true paranoia. Delusions of suspicion, conspiracy, and of superiority are present.
paranoiac (păr-ă-noy'ăk) [" + *nous*, mind]. 1. One suffering from paranoia. 2. Concerning or afflicted with paranoia.
paranoid (păr'ă-noyd) [G. *para*, beside, + *nous*, mind, + *eidos*, like]. 1. Resembling paranoia. 2. A person afflicted with paranoia.
p. reaction type. Individual who has fixed, systematized delusions, is suspicious, has a persecution complex and is resentful, bitter, and a megalomaniac.
Many states approach true paranoia and resemble it, but lack 1 or more of its distinguishing features. Some of these are: (a) Transitory p. states due to toxic conditions; (b) p. type of schizophrenia; (c) p. states due to alcoholism.
In the paranoid-reaction types, the delusions tend to scatter and shift from individual to individual, or group to group, and tend also to be more bizarre. Types are: (a) Delusions of persecution; (b) delusions of jealousy; infidelity on the part of someone loved by the in-

paranoid violence   **paraplegic**

dividual; (c) delusions of erotomania; of being loved by someone who *does not* love him; (d) delusions of megalomania; the delusions of greatness which are invariably present.
The type of individual that develops a paranoid reaction is ambitious, aggressive, suspicious, and one who has a feeling that someone is imposing on him. Many of these individuals have been inventive geniuses. Severe physical handicaps or failures are often basis for delusions and feelings of mistreatment. Always a tendency to make the other person responsible for the discrepancy bet. desires and satisfactions.

p. violence. NP: In dealing with all types of paranoids:
Do not handle without an assistant. Shout, call, or signal for aid. Don't back away or have back to patient. Don't use more force than necessary. Don't force patient over hard edges of furniture. Don't exert force over patient's chest. Keep pressure off of ribs. Avoid patient's knee or fist in the abdomen. If patient is prone, hold down by shoulders and just above knees or control limbs at wrists and ankles. Remove patient's shoes when under control. Keep close to patient; bend his wrists forward. Have a layer of cloth, sheet, blanket, patient's clothes, anything between patient's skin and yours when holding him, to prevent bruising.

paranomia (păr″ă-nō′mĭ-ă) [G. *para*, beside, + *onoma*, name]. Form of aphasia in which there is inability to remember correct name of objects shortly after seeing or using them.

paranuclein (păr″ă-nū′klē-ĭn) [" + L. *nucleus*, a kernel]. A protein which does not yield nitrogenous bases when decomposed. SYN: *nucleoalbumin*.

paranucleus (păr″ă-nū′klē-ŭs) [" + L. *nucleus*, a kernel]. A small body lying close to a cell nucleus.

paraomphalic (păr″ă-ŏm-făl′ĭk) [" + *omphalos*, navel]. Adjacent to the navel. SYN: *paraumbilical*.

paraoperative (păr″ă-ŏp′ĕr-ă-tĭv) [" + L. *opus*, *oper-*, work]. Concerning all the details and the accessories of operation and preparation of the patient.

paraosteoarthropathy (păr″ă-ŏs″tē-ō-ăr-thrŏp′ăth-ĭ) [" + *osteon*, bone, + *arthron*, joint, + *pathos*, disease]. Paralysis of lower portion of the body in addition to bone and joint disease.

paraparesis (păr″ă-păr-ē′sĭs, -păr′ē-sĭs) [" + *paresis*, paralysis]. Partial paralysis affecting the lower limbs.

parapathia (păr-ă-păth′ĭ-ă) [G. *para*, beside, + *pathos*, disease]. Emotional aspects of a disorder.

parapedesis (păr″ă-pĕd-ē′sĭs) [G. *para*, beside, + *pedēsis*, a bending]. Secretion through other than normal channels.

parapeptone (păr″ă-pĕp′tōn) [" + *peptein*, to digest]. Intermediate digestion product of albumin. SEE: *peptone*.

paraphasia (păr-ă-fā′zĭ-ă) [" + *a-*, priv. + *phasis*, speech]. The misuse of words or word combinations spoken; a form of aphasia.

paraphemia (păr″ă-fē′mĭ-ă) [" + *phēmē*, speech]. A disorder marked by consistent use of the wrong words, or mispronunciation of words.

paraphia (păr-ā′fĭ-ă) [" + *aphē*, touch]. Irregularity of the sense of touch.

paraphimosis (păr″ă-fĭ-mō′sĭs) [" + *phimoein*, to muzzle]. 1. Strangulation of glans penis due to retraction of foreskin. 2. Retraction of eyelid in back of eyeball.

paraphobia (păr-ă-fō′bĭ-ă) [" + *phobos*, fear]. A mild form of phobia.

paraphonia (păr″ă-fō′nĭ-ă) [" + *phōnē*, voice]. Partial loss or weakness or abnormal change of the voice.

paraphora (păr-ăf′ō-ră) [G. a wandering]. 1. A mental disorder of minor degree. 2. The unsteadiness due to drunkenness.

paraphrasia (păr-ă-frā′zĭ-ă) [G. *para*, beside, + *phrasis*, speech]. Disorder characterized by incoherent speech. SYN: *paraphasia*.

paraphrenia (păr-ă-frē′nĭ-ă) [" + *phrēn*, mind]. 1. Dementia precox according to Freud. 2. Paranoid dementia precox according to Kraepelin, behavior disorders and personality defects not being marked.

p. confabulans. P. marked by memory distortions.
p. expansiva. P. with delusions of grandeur, exaltation and moderate excitement.
p., phantastica. P. with unsystematized delusions.
p. systematica. P. with progressive delusions of persecution, followed by delusions of grandeur, but personality shows no deterioration.

paraphrenitis (păr″ă-frē-nī′tĭs) [G. *para*, beside, + *phrēn*, mind, diaphragm, + *-itis*, inflammation]. 1. Inflammation of the tissues around the diaphragm. 2. Mental delirium or derangement.

paraphronia (păr″ă-frō′nĭ-ă) [" + *phrēn*, mind]. A psychosis with change of the patient's disposition and character.

paraplasm (păr′ă-plăzm) [" + *plasma*, a thing formed]. 1. Any abnormal new formation or malformation. 2. The fluid portion of protoplasm. SYN: *hyaloplasm*.

Paraplasma flavigenum (păr-ă-plăz′mă flă-vĭj′ĕn-ŭm). A parasitic organism in the red blood cells in yellow fever, assumed to be the cause of it. SYN: *Seidelin bodies*.

paraplastic (păr-ă-plăs′tĭk) [G. *para*, beside, + *plastikos*, formed]. 1. Pert. to fluid portion of protoplasm. 2. Misshapen; deformed.

paraplastin (păr-ă-plăs′tĭn) [" + *plassein*, to form]. A substance found in a cell's nucleus and cytoplasm which resembles parachromatin.

paraplectic (păr-ă-plĕk′tĭk) [G. *paraplēktikos*, striking at the side]. Afflicted with paralysis of lower extremities. SYN: *paraplegic*.

paraplegia (păr-ă-plē′jĭ-ă) [G. *para*, beside, + *plēgē*, a stroke]. Paralysis of lower portion of the body and of both legs due to injury to spinal cord. SEE: *paralysis*.

p., alcoholic. P. of spinal origin due to use of alcohol.
p., ataxic. Lateral and post. sclerosis of spinal cord, combined, and resulting symptoms.
p., cerebral. P. from bilateral cerebral lesion.
p., cervical. P. of both arms.
p. dolorosa. P. due to pressure of a neoplasm on post. minor roots. Very painful.
p., ideal. Reflex p. due to excitement.
p., peripheral. P. from neoplastic pressure on nerves with severe pain.
p., spastic. P. from primary lateral sclerosis of spinal cord.
p., s., primary. P. from degeneration in pyramidal tracts.

paraplegic (păr-ă-plē′jĭk) [G. *para*, be-

side, + *plēgē*, a stroke]. Concerning, or affected with, paraplegia. SYN: *paraplectic*.
parapleuritis (păr″ă-plū-rī′tĭs) [" + *pleura*, a side, + *-itis*, inflammation]. 1. Inflammation in the thoracic wall. 2. Mild inflammation of the pleura. 3. Pain in the pleura. SYN: *pleurodynia*.
paraplexus (păr″ă-plĕk′sŭs) [" + L. *plexus*, a braid]. The choroid plexus of the lateral ventricle of the brain.
parapophysis (păr″ă-pŏf′ĭ-sĭs) [" + *apo*, beneath, + *physis*, a growth]. Elevation on side of a vertebra on which head of a rib fits.
parapoplexy (păr-ăp′ō-plĕk-sĭ) [" + *apoplēxia*, a striking down]. A mild or slight apoplexy with partial stupor; a stupor resembling apoplexy. SYN: *pseudoapoplexy*.
parapraxia, parapraxis (păr-ă-prak′sĭ-ă, -sĭs) [" + *praxis*, a doing]. Disturbed mental processes producing inaccuracy and forgetfulness and tendency to misplace things and make slips of speech or pen.
paraproctitis (păr″ă-prŏk-tī′tĭs) [" + *prōktos*, anus, + *-itis*, inflammation]. Inflamed condition of tissues near the rectum.
parapsia, parapsis (păr-ăp′sĭ-ă, -sĭs) [G. *para*, beside, + *apsis*, touch]. Any disorder of touch. SYN: *paraphia*.
parapsoriasis (păr″ă-sō-rī′ă-sĭs) [" + *psōriasis*, itching]. A chronic disorder of the skin marked by scaly red lesions.
parapyknomorphous (păr″ă-pĭk-nō-mor′fŭs) [" + *pyknos*, thick, + *morphē*, form]. Having cell particles placed so as to stain only moderately well.
paraqueduct (păr-ăk′wē-dŭkt) [" + L. *aequeductus*, a water passage]. A lateral protuberance of the aqueduct of the cerebrum.
parareflexia (păr″ă-rē-flĕk′sĭ-ă) [" + L. *reflectere*, to turn back]. Irregularity or disorder of the reflexes.
pararenal (păr″ă-rē′năl) [" + L. *rēn*, kidney]. Near the kidneys.
pararhotacism (păr″ă-rō′tă-sĭzm) [" + *rho*, letter R, + *ismos*, condition]. Constant erroneous use of letter r or the placing of undue emphasis on letter r.
pararrhythmia (păr-ăr-ĭth′mĭ-ă) [" + *a-*, negative, + *rhythmos*, rhythm]. Disturbed or disordered cardiac rhythm.
pararthria (păr-ărth′rĭ-ă) [" + *arthron*, articulation]. Disordered articulation of speech.
parasalpingitis (păr″ă-săl-pĭn-jī′tĭs) [G. *para*, beside, + *salpigx, salpigg-*, tube, + *-itis*, inflammation]. Inflamed condition of tissues around an oviduct or a eustachian tube.
parasigmatism (păr″ă-sĭg′mă-tĭzm) [" + *sigma*, letter S, + *ismos*, condition]. Imperfect pronunciation of the letter S. SYN: *lisping*.
parasite (păr′ă-sīt) [" + *sitos*, food]. An organism that lives within, upon, or at expense of another organism known as the host.
RS: *cenosite, chromophytosis, host, saprophyte*.
 p., external. One which lives on the outer surface of its host, bugs, fleas, and lice.
 p., facultative. P. capable of living independently of its host at certain times.
 p., internal. One living within its host, as worms and flukes.
 p., obligate. P. completely dependent on its host.

parasitic (păr-ă-sĭt′ĭk) [" + *sitos*, food]. Like, caused by, or concerning, a parasite.
parasiticide (păr″ă-sĭt′ĭ-sīd) [" + " + L. *caedere*, to kill]. 1. Killing parasites. 2. An agent that will kill parasites. Ex: sulfur, iodine, mercurial ointment.
parasitifer (păr-ă-sit′ĭ-fĕr) [" + " + L *ferre*, to carry]. Organism which acts as the host of a parasite.
parasitism (păr″ă-sīt-ĭzm) [" + " + *ismos*, condition]. 1. The parasitic condition or state. 2. Disease caused by infestation with parasites.
parasitogenic (păr″ă-sī″tō-jĕn′ĭk) [G. *para*, beside, + *sitos*, food, + *gennan*, to produce]. 1. Caused by parasites. 2. Favoring parasite development.
parasitology (păr″ă-sī-tŏl′ō-jĭ) [" + *sitos*, food, + *logos*, study]. The study of parasites, their effect on the human system, and their elimination.
parasitophobia (păr″ă-sī″tō-fō′bĭ-ă) [" + " + *phobos*, fear]. Unusual fear of parasites.
parasitotropic (păr″ă-sī″tō-trŏp′ĭk) [" + " + *tropos*, a turning]. Having attraction for parasites.
paraspadia (păr-ă-spā′dĭ-ă) [G. *paraspaein*, to draw aside]. Condition in which the urethra has an opening into 1 side of the penis.
paraspasm (păr′ă-spazm) [G. *para*, beside, + *spasmos*, a spasm]. 1. Muscular spasm of the lower extremities. 2. Spastic paralysis of the lower extremities.
parasteatosis (păr″ă-stē-ă-tō′sĭs) [" + *stear, steat-*, tallow, + *-ōsis*, disease]. Any disordered condition of the sebaceous secretions.
parasternal (păr″ă-stern′ăl) [" + *sternon*, chest]. Along the side of the sternum.
 p. line. Imaginary vertical line running midway bet. sternal margin and line passing through the nipple.
 p. region. Area bet. sternal margin and parasternal line.
parasthenia (păr″ăs-thē′nĭ-ă) [" + *sthenos*, strength]. Condition characterized by abnormal functioning of organic tissue at odd intervals.
parastruma (păr-ă-strū′mă) [" + L. *struma*, goiter]. Goiterlike tumor due to hypertrophy of a parathyroid gland.
parasympathetic (păr″ă-sĭm-pă-thet′ĭk) [" + *sympathētikos*, suffering with]. Term applied to the division of the autonomic* nervous system whose fibers arise from the midbrain, the medulla oblongata and sacral portion of the spinal cord.
 The parasympathetic division causes constricting of the pupil, of the arterioles and bronchioles, contraction of the smooth muscle of the stomach and intestines, slowing up of the heart, and stimulates secretion of most glands in the body. SEE: *sympathetic nervous system*.
 p. bodies. Coccygeal gland and the intercoracoid body.
parasynovitis (păr-ă-sĭn-ō-vī′tĭs) [G. *para*, beside, + *syn*, with, + *ōon*, egg, + *-itis*, inflammation]. Inflamed condition of tissues about a synovial sac.
parasyphilitic (păr″ă-sĭf-ĭl-ĭt′ĭk) [" + *syn*, with, + *philos*, love]. Marking diseases assumed to be indirectly due to syphilis, but with none of the usual lesions of that disease.
parasystole (păr-ă-sĭs′tō-lē) [" + *systolē*, contraction]. Abnormally prolonged interval of rest following the cardiac systole.
paratarsium (păr-ă-tar′sĭ-ŭm) [" + *tar-*

paratenon P-19 **parencephalous**

sos, tarsus]. The covering and connective tissues of the tarsus of the feet.
paratenon (păr"ă-těn'ŏn) [" + *tenōn*, tendon]. Fatty tissue surrounding a tendon.
paratereseomania (păr"ă-te-rē"sē-ō-mā'-nĭ-ă) [G. *paratērēsis*, observation, + *mania*, madness]. Insane desire to investigate new scenes and subjects.
paratherapeutic (păr"ă-thĕr-ă-pū'tĭk) [G. *para*, beside, + *therapeutikē*, treatment]. Caused by the treatment used for another disease.
parathesin (păr"ăth'e-sĭn). Proprietary analgesic and local anesthetic.
parathormone (păr-ă-thor'mōn) [G. *para*, beside, + *thyroid* + *ormanein*, to excite]. 1. The substance secreted by the parathyroid glands. 2. Commercial name for this substance.
parathymia (păr"ă-thī'mĭ-ă) [" + *thymos*, mind]. Disordered state of the emotions.
parathyrin(e (păr-ă-thī'rĭn, -rēn) [" + *thyroid*]. The active constituent of the parathyroid glands.
parathyroid (păr"ă-thī'royd) [G. *para*, beside, + *thyreos*, shield, + *eidos*, form]. 1. Located close to the thyroid gland. 2. One of 4 small epithelial bodies about the size of a pea on the back of and at lower edge of the thyroid gland.
  They control the calcium-phosphorus balance of the body. The loss of the calcium promotes excitability, muscular contractions and a condition simulating epilepsy. They also are concerned with the neutralization of certain toxic wastes generated in the gastrointestinal tract as a result of the action of proteolytic bacteria. Their removal or severe injury leads to tetany.
  Tumors of these glands or hyperfunction of them is associated with decalcification of the bones, weakness and loss of muscle tone. Osteitis fibrosa cystica is probably due to hypersecretion of the parathyroids.
  DOSAGE: Sol. *subcut.* or *intramusc.*, 3-6 gr. (0.2-0.4 Gm.).
  Parathormone is the substance excreted by these glands, and a commercial preparation of it is used in deficiency of secretion. Secretion with Vitamin D may promote metabolism of calcium and phosphorus.
parathyroidectomy (păr"ă-thī-royd-ĕk'tō-mĭ) [G. *para*, beside, + *thyreos*, shield, + *eidos*, form, + *ektomē*, excision]. Excision of one or more of the parathyroid glands.
parathyroprivia (păr"ă-thī"rō-prĭv'ĭ-ă) [" + " + L. *privus*, deprived of]. Condition which supervenes when the parathyroids are removed.
parathyroprivic, parathyroprivous (păr-ă-thī-rō-prĭv'ĭk, -us) [" + " + L. *privus*, deprived of]. Resulting from loss of function of, or removal of, parathyroid glands.
paratoloid (păr-ăt'ō-loyd). Substance containing extract from the tubercle bacillus. SYN: *tuberculin*.
paratoxin (păr-ă-tŏk'sĭn) [G. *para*, beside, + *toxikon*, poison]. Product composed of bile, without its pigment, and cholesterol which is used in treating tuberculosis.
paratrichosis (păr"ă-trĭ-kō'sĭs) [" + *thrix, trich-*, hair, + *-ōsis*, disease]. Any disorder of hair growth, as growth in abnormal places.
paratrimma (păr-ă-trĭm'mă) [" + *tribein*, to rub]. Chafing; irritation of the skin. SYN: *intertrigo*.
paratrophic (păr-ă-trō'fĭk) [G. *para*, beside, + *trophē*, nourishment]. 1. Requiring living substances for food; parasitic. 2. Pert. to abnormal nutrition. 3. Pert. to adiposis dolorosa.
paratrophy (păr-ăt'rō-fī) [" + *trophē*, nourishment]. 1. Localized fatty swellings and nerve lesions in various regions of the body. SYN: *Dercum's disease, adiposis dolorosa.* 2. Defective nutrition. SYN: *dystrophy.*
paratuberculosis (păr"ă-tū-bĕr"kū-lō'sĭs) [" + L. *tuberculus*, a tubercle, + G. *-ōsis*, disease]. Disease resembling tuberculosis, but in which the tubercle bacillus cannot be demonstrated.
paratyphlitis (păr"ă-tĭf-lī'tĭs) [" + *typhlos*, blind, + *-ītis*, inflammation]. Inflammation of the connective tissue close to the cecum.
paratyphoid (păr-ă-tī'foyd) [G. *para*, near, + *typhos*, fever, + *eidos*, like]. Similar to typhoid.
  p. fever. An infectious fever resembling typhoid.
  ETIOL: The *paratyphoid bacillus* of 2 varieties not identical with the *B. typhosus* of Eberth.
  SYM: Fever rises more quickly than in typhoid, more diarrhea, less cause for hemorrhages and perforation, recovery quicker and disease milder than typhoid. The ulcers are in lower end of small intestine in typhoid but more are in the upper end of the large intestine in paratyphoid. Widal* test is negative.
  TREATMENT: Triple vaccine, quarantine, disinfectants, screening against flies, cleanliness, pasteurization of milk, no raw foods, protection of other foods.
paratypic (păr-ă-tĭp'ĭk) [G. *para*, beside, + *typos*, type]. Relating to differences due to the influences of environment; diverging from a type.
paraumbilical (păr"ă-ŭm-bĭl'ĭk-ăl) [" + L. *umbilicus*, navel]. Close to the navel.
paraurethral (păr"ă-ū-rē'thrăl) [" + *ourēthra*, urethra]. Located close to the urethra.
parauterine (păr"ă-ū'tĕr-ĭn) [" + L. *uterus*, womb]. Around the uterus.
paravaginal (păr"ă-văj'ĭn-ăl) [" + L. *vagina*, sheath]. Around the vagina.
paravaginitis (păr"ă-văj-ĭn-ī'tĭs) [" + " + G. *-itis*, inflammation]. Inflammation of the cellular tissue surrounding the vagina.
paraxanthine (păr-ăk-săn'thĭn) [G. *para*, beside, + *xanthos*, yellow]. A poisonous leukomaine occurring in healthy urine and in excess in gout.
paraxial (păr-ăk'sĭ-ăl) [" + L. *axis*, axis]. On either side of the axis of the body, or 1 of its parts.
paraxin (păr-ăk'sĭn). Commercial diuretic.
paraxon (păr-ăks'ŏn) [G. *para*, beside, + *axon*, axis]. A collateral branch of a nerve cell's axis cylinder process.
parched (parchd) [M.E. *parchen*]. Dried to extremity.
paregoric (păr-e-gŏr'ĭk) [G. *parēgoros*, soothing]. 1. Soothing. 2. Camphorated tincture of opium, a narcotic containing drug which in large doses is poisonous.
  TREATMENT FOR POISONING: Same as for morphine, *q.v.*
parencephalia (păr"ĕn-sĕf-ă-lī'ă) [G. *para*, beside, + *egkephalos*, brain]. Congenital malformation of the cerebrum.
parencephalitis (păr"ĕn-sĕf-ă-lī'tĭs) [" + " + *-itis*, inflammation]. Inflamed condition of the cerebellum.
parencephalous (păr-ĕn-sĕf'ă-lŭs) [" + *egkephalos*, brain]. 1. Having a con-

parenchyma

genital cerebral deformity. 2. Concerning the cerebellum.

parenchyma (păr-ĕn'kĭ-mă) [" + *en*, in, + *chein*, to pour]. The essential parts of an organ which are concerned with its function in contradistinction to its framework.

The uriniferous tubules of the kidneys are the parenchymatous tissue.

p. disease. Disease affecting the principal tissue of an organ.

parenchymatitis (păr-ĕn-kī-mă-tī'tĭs) [" + " + " + -*itis*, inflammation]. Inflamed condition of parenchyma, or substance of a gland.

parenchymatous (păr-ĕn-kĭm'ăt-ŭs) [" + " + *chein*, to pour]. Concerning the essential substances of an organ.

p. neuritis. Neuritis of the axis cylinder and its myelin sheath.

p. pain. Pain arising at peripheral end of a nerve.

parent (păr'ent) [L. *parēre*, to bring forth]. A father or a mother; one who begets offspring.

RS: *brood cell, daughter cell, mother cell*.

p. fixation. Continuation of the child-parent affiliation into the adult state, so that the person so afflicted is unable to become interested in a person of the opposite sex.

parenteral (păr-ĕn'tĕr-ăl) [G. *para*, beside, + *enteron*, intestine]. Situated or occurring outside of the intestines, as by a subcutaneous method.

p. digestion. Digestion of foreign substances by body cells as opposed to *enteral digestion*, which occurs in the alimentary canal.

p. therapy. Introduction of a substance, esp. nutritive material, into the body by means other than the intestinal tract.

parepididymis (par"ep-ĭ-dĭd'ĭ-mĭs) [" + *epi*, on, + *didymos*, testis]. A small body to front of the spermatic cord above the epididymis. SYN: *paradidymis*.

parergastic reactions (păr-ĕr-găst'ĭk) [" + *ergon*, work]. A general term used by A. Meyer for the essentials involved in schizoid types but without relation to prognosis.

paresis (păr'e-sĭs, pă-rē'sĭs) [G. weakness]. 1. Partial or incomplete paralysis. 2. An organic mental disease with somatic, irritative and paralytic focal symptoms and signs running a slow, chronic, progressive course and tending to a fatal termination.

Comprises 10-20% of total admissions to mental hospitals.

ETIOL: Diffuse and focal involvement of brain and spinal cord due to syphilis, usually occurring from 5 to 15 years after primary infection and frequently precipitated by trauma of the head.

PATH: A diffuse meningoencephalitis with degenerative changes dependent upon vascular and toxic factors.

SYM: May simulate any psychoneuroses or psychoses. Pupillary changes, facial tremors, tremors of the lips and tongue, speech disturbances. Usually Argyll-Robertson pupil, impaired vision, headache, speech slurred with letters and syllables often omitted. Epileptic convulsions. Unequal exaggeration of the reflexes. Always a positive Wassermann reaction of spinal fluid, with increase of protein and lymphocytes. Colloidal gold curve changes, reading often being 5555544431. Memory defective, expansive delusions, depression, dementia.

TREATMENT: Fever therapy, esp. inoculation with malaria or diathermy. SYN: *dementia paralytica, general paralysis of insane.* SEE: *Bayle's disease, malaria, syphilis.*

p., juvenile. General p. due to hereditary syphilis, seen in children.

paresq-analgesia (păr"ĕs-ō-ăn-ăl-jē'zĭ-ă) [G. *paresis*, weakness, + *an-*, negative, + *algēsis*, pain]. Painlessness with paralysis of the arms.

paressine (păr'ĕs-ēn). Commercial preparation of paraffin, gum and wax, used as a covering in burns and frostbites.

paresthesia (păr-ĕs-thē'zĭ-ă) [G. *para*, beside, + *aisthēsis*, sensation]. Abnormal sensation without objective cause, such as numbness, pricking, etc.; heightened sensitivity.

Experienced in central and peripheral nerve lesions and in locomotor ataxia.

paretic (pă-rĕt'ĭk, pă-rē'tĭk) [G. *paresis*, weakness]. Affected with or concerning paresis.

pareunia (păr-ū'nĭ-ă) [G. *pareunos*, lying beside]. Sexual intercourse. SYN: *coition, coitus, copulation*.

parhormone (păr-hor'mōn) [G. *para*, beside, + *ormanein*, to secrete]. A waste product having a hormonelike function. SEE: *hormone*.

paridrosis (păr-ĭ-drō'sĭs) [" + *idrōsis*, perspiration]. Any disordered secretion of perspiration.

paries (pā'rĭ-ēs) (pl. *parietes*) [L. a wall]. The enveloping wall of any structure; applied especially to hollow organs.

parietal (pă-rī'ĕ-tăl) [L. *pariēs, pariet-*, wall]. Pert. to, or forming, the wall of a cavity. SEE: *suture, sagittal*.

p. bone. A bone on each side of the cranium or skull.

p. cells. Large cells on margin of the peptic glands of stomach which supposedly secrete hydrochloric acid. SYN: *border cells*.

p. lobe. A central portion of the cerebrum bet. the parieto-occipital and rolandic fissures above the horizontal branch of the fissure of Sylvius.

parietes (pă-rī'ĕ-tēs) [L.]. Plural of paries; walls of an organ or hollow part.

Paris green (păr'ĭs grēn). A compound of copper and arsenic, *q.v.*; acetoarsenite of copper.

Parkinson's disease (par'kĭn-sŭn). A chronic nervous disease characterized by a fine, slowly spreading tremor, muscular weakness and rigidity and a peculiar gait.

SYM: Onset may be abrupt; generally insidious. First symptom is a fine tremor beginning in hand or foot which may spread till it involves all the members. At first paroxysmal but becomes almost continuous.

Face becomes expressionless. Speech slow and measured, later muscular rigidity. Head bowed, body bent forward, arms flexed, thumbs turned into palms, knees slightly bent. Gait characteristic by this time; steps grow faster and faster, body inclines more and more forward until patient falls, seeks some support; this is termed festination.

Occasionally a tendency to fall backwards, retropulsion replaces festination; numbness, tingling, sensation of heat.

PROG: Recovery rarely if ever occurs. Duration indefinite.

TREATMENT: Regulated diet; rest of mind and body; frequent bathing followed by friction, massage, electricity, constitutional remedies. SYN: *palsy*, *shaking, paralysis agitans.* SEE: *paralysis.*

P.'s mask. Expressionless appearance of the face. Eyebrows are raised, wrinkles are smoothed out, and there is immobility of the facial muscles.
A typical symptom seen in P.'s disease and in postencephalitic states.

P.'s syndrome. Symptoms of P.'s disease.

paroccipital (pă̆r-ŏk-sĭp'ĭt-ăl) [G. *para*, near, + L. *occiput*, occiput]. 1. Close to the occipital bone. 2. The paramastoid process.

parodontitis (păr″ō-don-tī'tĭs) [" + *odous*, *odont-*, tooth, + *-itis*, inflammation]. Inflamed condition of tissues around a tooth.

parodynia (păr-ō-dĭn'ĭ-ă) [L. *parere*, to bring forth, + G. *odynē*, pain]. 1. Labor pains. 2. Difficult or abnormal labor or birth. SYN: *dystocia.*

p. perversa. Presentation with fetus lying transversely across the uterus. SYN: *cross birth.*

parogen (păr'ō-jĕn). An ointment and liniment base containing liquid petrolatum, oleic acid and ammoniated alcohol.

paroidin (păr-oy'dĭn). Commercial preparation of parathyroid extract used in treatment of tetany.

parolivary (păr-ŏl'ĭ-va-rī) [G. *para*, near, + L. *oliva*, olive]. Situated close to the olivary body.

p. bodies. Nuclei in medulla oblongata, lying close to the olivary bodies.

paromphalocele (păr-om'fă-lō-sēl″) [" + *omphalos*, navel, + *kēlē*, hernia]. Hernia or tumor close to the umbilicus.

paroniria (păr-ō-nī'rĭ-ă) [" + *oneiros*, dream]. Abnormal dreaming of a terrifying nature.

p. ambulans. Sleepwalking.

p. salax. Restlessness in sleep with lascivious dreams and nocturnal emissions.

paronychia (păr-ō-nĭk'ĭ-ă) [" + *onyx*, *onych-*, nail]. Acute or chronic infection of marginal structures about the nail.

ETIOL: Trauma, infection, systemic disease (syphilis, tuberculosis, leprosy).

SYM: Redness, swelling and suppuration around nail edge.

TREATMENT: Specific, in specific disease. Hot soaks (1% lysol), painting beneath nail fold (chrysarobin in chloroform, salicylic acid ointment). Surgery in severe cases.

SYN: *felon, onychia, runaround, whitlow.*

p. tendinosa. Inflammation of sheath of a digital tendon. ETIOL: Sepsis.

paroöphoron (păr-ō-ŏf'ō-rŏn) [G. *para*, near, + *ōon*, egg, + *phoros*, bearer]. Remnant in the broad ligament of the urinary portion of the wolffian body corresponding to the paradidymis in the male.

parophthalmia (păr-ŏf-thăl'mĭ-ă) [" + *ophthalmos*, eye]. Inflamed condition of tissue around the eye.

paropsis (păr-op'sĭs) [" + *opsis*, vision]. Any disorder of sense of sight.

parorchidium (păr-ŏr-kĭd'ĭ-ŭm) [" + *orchis*, orchid-, + testicle]. Abnormal position or nondescent of a testicle. SYN: *ectopia testis.*

parorexia (păr-ō-rĕk'sĭ-ă) [" + *orexis*, appetite]. An abnormal or perverted craving for special or strange foods. SEE: *appetite, taste.*

parosmia (păr-ŏz'mĭ-ă) [" + *osmē*, odor]. Any disorder or perversion of the sense of smell; a false sense of odors or perception of those which do not exist.
Agreeable ones are considered offensive and disagreeable odors are accepted as pleasant. SEE: *kakosmia*. SYN: *parosphresia.*

parosphresia, parosphresis (păr″ŏs-frē'-zĭ-ă, -sĭs) [" + *osphrēsis*, a smelling]. Disordered sense of smell. SYN: *parosmia, q.v.*

parosteitis, parostitis (păr-ŏs-tē-ī'tĭs, -tī'-tĭs) [G. *para*, beside, + *osteon*, bone, + *-itis*, inflammation]. Inflammation of tissues next to the bone.

parosteosis, parostosis (păr-ŏs-tē-ō'sĭs, -tō'sĭs) [" + " + *-ōsis*, disease]. 1. Bone formation outside of the periosteum. 2. Bone development in an unusual location.

parotid (pă-rŏt'ĭd) [" + *ous*, *ot-*, ear]. 1. Located near the ear. 2. Parotid gland.

p. duct. One 2 in. long from ant. border of the parotid gland crossing the masseter and piercing the buccinator, and buccal mucous membrane.
It opens in the mouth opposite 2nd upper molar. The transverse facial artery is above the duct and buccal branch of 7th nerve below. SYN: *Stenson's duct*. SEE: *saliva.*

p. gland. Largest of the salivary glands situated on side of the face below and in front of the ear.

DOSAGE: 5 gr. (0.3 Gm.).

parotidectomy (pă-rŏt-ĭd-ĕk'tō-mĭ) [" + " + *ektomē*, excision]. Excision of parotid gland. [adenectomy.
NP: Modification of preparation for

parotiditis (pă-rŏt-ĭ-dī'tĭs) [" + " + *-itis*, inflammation]. Inflamed condition of the parotid gland. SYN: *mumps,* parotitis.*

p., epidemic. Acute, infectious, contagious inflammation and swelling of parotid gland; mumps.

parotidoscirrhus (pă-rŏt″ĭd-ō-skĭr'ŭs) [" + " + *skirros*, hardness]. 1. Hardening of the parotid gland. 2. A scirrhous cancer of the parotid area.

parotitis (pă-rō-tī'tĭs) [G. *para*, near, + *ous*, *ot-*, ear, + *-itis*, inflammation]. Inflammation of the parotid gland, either simple or epidemic (mumps).
ETIOL: Mumps is caused by a filtrable virus found in the saliva. It is only mildly contagious.
Complications of parotitis are ovaritis in the female and orchitis in the male, and occasionally nephritis and meningoencephalitis. SYN: *mumps, q.v.; parotiditis.*

parous (pa'rus) [L. *parēre*, to bring forth]. Parturient; fruitful; having borne at least 1 child.

parovarian (par-ō-vār'ĭ-ăn) [G. *para*, near, + L. *ovarium*, ovary]. 1. Situated near or beside the ovary. 2. Pert. to the parovarium, a residual structure in the broad ligament.

parovariotomy (păr-ō-vă-rĭ-ŏt'ō-mĭ) [" + " + G. *tomē*, a cutting]. Removal of a parovarian cyst.

parovarium (păr″ō-vār'ĭ-ŭm) [" + L. *ovarium*, ovary]. Vestigial remnant of the wolffian body found in broad ligament representing the sexual portion. SYN: *epoöphoron.*

paroxyl (păr-ŏk'sĭl). Commercial amebicide. SEE: *acetarsone.*

paroxyntic (păr-ŏk-sĭn'tĭk) [G. *paroxynein*, to excite]. Like a convulsion; paroxysmal.

paroxysm (păr'ŏk-sĭzm) [G. *para*, beside, + *oxynein*, to sharpen]. 1. A sudden, periodic attack or recurrence of symptoms of a disease; an exacerbation of the symptoms of a disease. 2. A fit or convulsion of any kind. 3. Sudden emotional state, as of fear, grief, or joy.
paroxysmal (păr-ŏk-sĭz'măl) [" + *oxynein*, to sharpen]. 1. Occurring in or concerning paroxysms. 2. Of the nature of a paroxysm.
parresine (păr'ĕs-ēn). A commercial paraffin mixture used as a protective covering for wounds and burns.
par'rot fever. Contagious disease transmitted by parrots and characterized by high fever and disorder of the lungs. SYN: *psittacosis*, *q.v.*
Parrot's disease (păr-ō'). The pseudoparalysis of the extremities in infants caused by syphilis.
 P.'s nodes. Bony nodules on skull of infants with syphilis.
 P.'s sign. 1. In meningitis, pupils dilate upon pinching the skin of neck. 2. SEE: *P.'s nodes*.
 P.'s ulcer. Lesions of thrush or stomatitis.
Parry's disease (păr'ē). Swelling of the thyroid gland with increased rate of basal metabolism in hypersecretion of the thyroid gland. SYN: *goiter*, *exophthalmic*; *hyperthyroidism*, *q.v.*
pars (parz) [L. *pars*, *part-*, a part]. A part.
 p. basilaris. Basilar process of the occipital bone.
 p. caeca oculi. The blind spot of the eye.
 p. carnea diaphragmatis. Muscular portion of diaphragm.
 p. carnosa urethrae. Membranous portion of urethra.
 p. cartilaginea tubae Eustachii. Cartilaginous portion of eustachian tube.
 p. cavernosa. Cavernous portion of urethra.
 p. cephalica nervi sympathici. Plexuses, ganglia, and nerves derived from sympathetic nerve.
 p. cervicalis nervi sympathici. Ganglia, plexuses, and branches of sympathetic nerve in neck.
 p. ciliaris retinae. Portion of retina situated in front of ora serrata.
 p. flaccida. A portion of membrane which fills the notch of the eardrum above the notch of Rivinus. SYN: *Shrapnell's membrane*.
 p. frontalis ossis frontis. Upper, larger portion of frontal bone, excluding orbits and nasal process.
 p. genitales. The genitals.
 p. intestinalis choledochi. Portion of ductus choledochus communis that pierces duodenum.
 p. nervosa. Post. lobe of the pituitary gland.
 p. olfactoria. Part of ant. cerebral commissure of brain the fibers of which, in the shape of a horseshoe, turn toward basal mass of head of corpus striatum.
 p. papillaris. Papillary cutaneous layer.
 p. scleralis corneae. Corneal substance proper.
 p. tendinea diaphragmatis. Tendinous portion of diaphragm.
 p. urethrae cavernosa. Cavernous portion of urethra.
 p. urethrae membranacea. Membranous portion of urethra.
pars'ley [M.E. *persely*, parsley]. Av. SERVING: 1 Gm. Pro. trace. Fat trace. Carbo. 0.1. VITAMINS: A+++, B++, C+++.

pars'nips [M.E. *pasnepe*, parsnip]. Av. SERVING: 120 Gm. Pro. 1.3, Fat 0.6, Carbo. 13.2. VITAMINS: A+, B++. ASH CONST: Ca 0.059, Mg 0.034, K 0.518, Na 0.004, P 0.076, Cl 0.030, S 0.036, Fe 0.0006. A base-forming food; alkalinity 12 cc. per 100 Gm., 18 cc. per 100 cal. ACTION: Easy to digest. Antiflatulent.
parthenogenesis (păr'thĕn-ō-jĕn'ē-sĭs) [G. *parthenos*, virgin, + *genesis*, production]. 1. Reproduction without fertilization of egg by a male. 2. Reproduction by fission or division. SYN: *asexual reproduction*.
 p., synthetic. Introduction of chemical stimulus into an egg with its subsequent development, in place of natural fertilization by the male.
parturient (păr-tū'rĭ-ĕnt) [L. *parturiens*, desiring to bring forth]. 1. Concerning childbirth or parturition.* 2. Bringing forth; giving birth. 3. A woman giving birth.
 p. canal. Path from uterine cavity to vulva.
 p. woman. One in labor.
parturifacient (păr-tū-rĭ-fā'shĕnt) [" + *facere*, to make]. 1. Inducing or accelerating labor. 2. Drug used to cause delivery of the fetus.
parturiometer (păr-tū-rĭ-ŏm'ĕt-ĕr) [" + G. *metron*, measure]. Instrument for determining the expulsive force of the uterus.
parturition (păr-tū-rĭsh'ŭn) [L. *parturitio*, childbirth]. Act of giving birth to young. SYN: *childbirth*; *delivery*.
parturition, words pert. to: accouchement, accoucheur, accoucheuse, afterbirth, afterpains, axis traction, bradytocia, Braune's canal, childbirth, dystocia, labor, mogitocia, multipara, nullipara, obstetrics, oxytocia, parturient, parturifacient, postpartum, sextipara, unipara.
partus (păr'tŭs) [L. *partus*, from *parere*, to bring forth]. Labor; parturition.
 p. agrippinus. Breech presentation in delivery.
 p. caesareus. Delivery by cesarean method.
 p. difficilis. Difficult labor. SYN: *dystocia*.
 p. immaturus. Premature labor.
 p. maturus. Labor at term.
 p. serotinus. Prolonged or delayed labor.
 p. siccus. Dry labor with little amniotic fluid.
parulis (păr-ŭ'lĭs) [G. *para*, near, + *oulon*, gum]. Abscess in a gum. SYN: *gumboil*.
parumbilical (păr-ŭm-bĭl'ĭ-kăl) [" + L. *umbilicus*, navel]. Close to the navel.
paruria (păr-ū'rĭ-ă) [" + *ouron*, urine]. Any abnormality in discharge of urine.
parvicellular (păr-vĭ-sĕl'ū-lăr) [L. *parvus*, small, + *cellula*, a little box]. Concerning, or composed of, tiny cells.
parvule (păr'vūl) [L. *parvulus*, very small]. A small pill, pellet, or granule.
PAS. Abbrev. for *paraäminosalicylic acid*, *q.v.*
Paschen bodies (pă'shĕn). Particles supposed to be the pathogenic virus of vaccinia and variola found in great numbers in skin exanthemas.
passage (păs'aj) [L. *passus*, a step]. 1. A communication bet. cavities and body structures or with the ext. surface of an organ. 2. Act of passing. 3. An evacuation of the bowels. 4. Introduction of a probe or catheter, etc.
 p's., alveolar. Sacculated communications into which the bronchioles are transformed and into which infundibula open.

p., lacrimal. Lacrimal and nasal ducts.
passion (păsh'ŭn) [L. *passiō*, suffering].
1. Suffering. 2. Great emotion, esp. sexual excitement.
p., ileac. Intestinal colic due to obstruction. SEE: *ileus*.
passional (păsh'ŭn-ăl) [L. *passiō*, suffering]. Exciting or concerning any passion. SEE: *emotional*.
p. attitudes. The stages of hysteria, as an attitude indicating any great emotion.
passive (păs'ĭv) [L. *passivus*, enduring].
1. Submissive. 2. Acted upon. 3. Not active.
p. congestion. Congestion due to obstruction in a part.
p. exercise. Muscular exercise without any effort on part of patient.
p. hyperemia. Blood in a part due to decreased outflow.
p. motion. Same as p. exercise. SEE: *exercise, p.*
p. movement. SEE: *p. exercise*.
passivism (păs'ĭ-vĭzm) [" + G. *ismos*, condition]. Sexual perversion with subjugation of the will by that of another, usually of the male by the female.
paste (pāst) [G. *pastē*, barley broth]. 1. To cause to adhere. 2. Any ointment whose base is a nonfatty material. 3. A mixture of flour and water, used as an adhesive. 4. A moist, doughy, plastic substance.
Pasteurella (păs-tĕr-ĕl'ă). Genus of family Bacteriaceae, characterized by bipolar staining.
P. pestis. Organism causing bubonic plague.
P. tularensis. Organism causing tularemia.
pasteurellosis (păs-ter-ĕl-ō'sĭs) [G. *-ōsis*, disease]. Disease caused by infection with bacteria of the *Pasteurella* group inducing hemorrhagic septicemia.
pasteurization (păs-tĕr-ī-zā'shŭn). Partial sterilization and the arrest of fermentation in a fluid by heating it for 30 minutes at 60°-70° C., without destroying its chemical composition.
In p. of milk, bacilli are destroyed at 167° F. in 10 minutes, 158° F. in 15 minutes, 155° F. in 30 minutes. It decreases the content of Vitamin C and Vitamin B. The curd in most cases is softer, in some tougher, while other cases are not affected.
Pasteurized milk being variable in this respect, boiled milk has some advantages as a soft curd results in the stomach. Use of fruit juice remedies any possible harm from lack of vitamins lost in pasteurization. SEE: *milk*.
Pasteur treatment (păs-tĕr'). Inoculation with increasingly virulent doses of dead organism causing rabies prepared from spinal cords of infected rabbits, for prevention of hydrophobia.
pastille (păs-tēl') [L. *pastillus*, a little roll]. 1. A small cone used to fumigate or scent the air of a room. 2. A medicated disk used for local action on the mucosa of the throat and mouth. SYN: *lozenge, troche*. 3. PT: Small disk of paper coated with barium platinocyanide or other substances, used to estimate the amount of x-rays administered, also for testing the intensity of ultraviolet radiations.
The green color changes to brown when exposed to roentgen rays.
p. radiometer. An instrument consisting of a color index by means of which the color changes in the pastilles, before and after exposure to roentgen rays, may be gauged. At one time it was used frequently to estimate the quantity of roentgen rays but is now practically obsolete.
patch (pătsh) [M.E. *pacche*]. A blotch distinct from surrounding surface in character and appearance.
p., herald. Oval patch of efflorescence showing before the general eruption of pityriasis rosea; often several days before.
p., Hutchinson's. Salmon-yellow area seen on cornea in syphilitic keratitis.
p., mucous. A syphilitic eruption having an eroded, moist surface; generally on mucous membrane of mouth or ext. genitals or on surface subject to moisture and heat. SYN: *condyloma latum*.
p., opaline. Whitish patch in mouth, sometimes observed in syphilis.
p's, Peyer's. Masses of lymphoid follicles found on mucous membrane of small intestine. SYN: *noduli lymphatici aggregati*.
p., salmon. Salmon-colored area of cornea in ocular syphilis.
p. test. One to detect hypersensitiveness to food, pollen or other substances by applying suspected substance to an area on the skin.
A small square of clean linen cloth should be covered with substance suspected. Cloth is laid on skin of chest or upper arm and another piece of cloth laid over it and fastened with adhesive. Remove at end of 24 hr. If irritation is present, the substance may be suspected and the individual is probably sensitive to it.
Substances with which the patient comes in contact may be used for the test. SEE: *allergy, eczema*.
patella (pă-tĕl'ă) [L. a small pan; kneepan]. The kneecap, or kneepan; a lens-shaped sesamoid bone situated in front of the knee, in the tendon of the quadriceps extensor.
RS: *acromyle, beat knee, housemaid's knee, knee, rotula*.
p., floating. A patella which floats up from the condyles due to a large effusion in the knee.
p., fracture of. TREATMENT: Suture of bone fragments. A plaster is then put on, reaching from the toes to the groin, remaining on for 6-8 weeks. Then gradual exercise and weight upon the leg for a few weeks, after which patient may walk.
p., rider's painful. Tenderness and pain in the patella due to horseback riding.
patellapexy (pă-tĕl'ă-pĕk"sĭ) [L. *patella*, kneepan, + G. *pēxis*, fixation]. Fixation of the patella to the lower end of the femur to stabilize the joint.
patellar (pă-tĕl'ăr) [L. *patella*, kneepan] Concerning the patella.
p. paradoxic reflex. Contraction of ant. muscles when leg is forcibly flexed and immediately released.
p. reflex. Involuntary jerk of leg due to sudden spasm of quadriceps following percussion of patellar ligament. SYN: *knee jerk reflex*.
patelliform (pă-tĕl'ĭ-form) [" + *forma*, shape]. Of the shape of the patella.
patellofemoral (pă-tĕl"ō-fĕm'or-ăl) [" + *femur, femor-*, thigh]. Concerning the patella and the femur.
patency (pā'tĕn-sē) [L. *patens*, from *patere*, to be open]. The state of being freely open.
patent (păt'ĕnt, pā'tĕnt) [L. *patens*, from *patere*, to be open]. 1. Wide open; evi-

patent medicine — **pathophobia**

dent; accessible. 2. Protected by a trade mark, as a patent medicine. 3. Secured by law for exclusive manufacture. SYN: *patulous*.

pat'ent med'icine. Packaged remedy for public use which is protected by letters patent and sold without a physician's prescription.
The law requires that it be labeled with names of active ingredients, the quantity or proportion of the contents, directions for its use, and that it may not have misleading statements as to curative effects on the label. SEE: *prescription*.

pathema (pă-thē'mă) [G. *pathēma*, a suffering]. Disease.

pathergasia (păth-ĕr-gā'zĭ-ă) [G. *pathos*, disease, + *ergon*, work]. Any form of malfunctioning, constitutional or structural, which inhibits self-adjustment.

pathetic (pă-thĕt'ĭk) [G. *pathētikos*, suffering]. 1. Arousing the tender emotions, as sorrow. 2. Denoting the sup. oblique muscle or its nerve.
  p. muscle. Sup. oblique muscle of the eye.
  p. nerve. One of 4th cranial pair of nerves supplying the sup. oblique muscle of the eye.

patheticus (pă-thĕt'ĭk-ŭs) [G. *pathētikos*, suffering]. 1. Fourth cranial, or trochlear, nerve which supplies sup. oblique muscle of the eye. 2. Superior oblique muscle of the eye.

pathetism (path'ĕt-ĭzm) [G. *pathein*, to suffer, + *ismos*, condition]. State of overcoming another's will by suggestion. SYN: *hypnotism, mesmerism*.

pathfinder (păth'fīnd-ĕr) [A.S. *paeth*, road, + *findan*, to locate]. Instrument for locating stricture of the urethra.

pathic (păth'ĭk) [G. *pathos*, disease]. 1. Concerning disease. 2. Suffering. 3. [G. *pathikos*, passive]. One whose sexual perversion causes his submission to unnatural relations.

pathoanatomy (păth″ō-ăn-ăt'ō-mĭ) [G. *pathos*, disease, + *ana*, apart, + *tomē*, a cutting]. Dissection and study of diseased organs.

pathobiology (păth″ō-bī-ŏl'ō-jĭ) [" + *bios*, life, + *logos*, study]. The study of disease. SYN: *pathology*.

pathobolism (păth-ŏb'ō-lĭzm) [" + (*meta*)-*bolism*, *metabolē*, change, + *ismos*, condition]. A condition of abnormal or perverted metabolism; seen in diabetes.

pathocrine (păth'ō-krīn, -krēn, -krĭn) [" + *krinein*, to secrete]. Concerning an endocrine disorder.

pathocrinia (păth-ō-krĭn'ĭ-ă) [" + *krinein*, to secrete]. Abnormal or disordered endocrine function.

pathodixia (păth-ō-dĭk'sĭ-ă) [" + L. *dicere*, to say, from G. *deiknunai*, to show]. Exhibitionism in reference to an injury or to disease.

pathodontia (păth'ō-dŏn'shĭ-ă) [" + *odous, odont*-, tooth]. Branch of dentistry dealing with diseases of the teeth.

pathoformic (păth-ō-for'mĭk) [G. *pathos*, disease, + L. *forma*, shape]. Concerning the beginning symptoms of a condition, as a mental disease.

pathogen (păth'ō-jĕn) [" + *gennan*, to produce]. A microörganism or substance capable of producing a disease.

pathogenesis (păth-ō-jĕn'ĕ-sĭs) [" + *genesis*, development]. Origination and development of a disease.
  p., drug. 1. Morbid symptoms of disease produced by a drug. 2. Observation of all symptoms which may be produced by a drug.

pathogenetic, pathogenic (păth″ō-jĕn-ĕt'ĭk, -jĕn'ĭk) [" + *gennan*, to produce]. Productive of disease. SYN: *morbific*.
  p. organism. One that produces disease in the body.

pathogeny (păth-ŏj'ĕn-ĭ) [" + *gennan*, to produce]. The origin or growth of a disease. SYN: *pathogenesis*.

pathognomonic (păth-ŏg-nō-mŏn'ĭk) [" + *gnōmonikos*, showing]. Indicative of a disease, esp. of 1 or more of its characteristic symptoms.

pathologic, pathological (păth-ō-lŏj'ĭk, -ĭkăl) [" + *logos*, study]. 1. Concerning pathology. 2. Diseased; due to a disease. SYN: *morbid*.
  p. histology. Histology of diseased tissues.
  p. reflex. One resulting in diseased states.

pathologist (pă-thŏl'ō-jĭst) [G. *pathos*, disease, + *logos*, study]. A specialist in diagnosing the morbid changes in tissues removed at operations and postmortem examinations.

pathology (pă-thŏl'ō-jĭ) [" + *logos*, study]. 1. Study of the nature and cause of disease which involves changes in structure and function. 2. Condition produced by disease.
  p., cellular. That which is based upon microscopic changes in body cells during disease.
  p., comparative. The observation of pathological conditions, spontaneous or artificial, in the lower animals or in vegetable organisms as compared to those of human body.
  p., experimental. Study of diseases induced intentionally, esp. in animals.
  p., general. The general facts of p. derived from a comparison of particular diseases with each other.
  p., geographical. P. in its relations to geographical conditions.
  p., medical. The p. of disorders, the treatment of which does not call for operative interference.
  p., special. The p. of particular diseases.
  p., surgical. The p. of surgical diseases.

patholysis (pă-thŏl'ĭ-sĭs) [G. *pathos*, disease, + *lysis*, destruction]. 1. Dissolution or destruction of disease. 2. Dissolution of diseased tissue.

pathomania (păth-ō-mā'nĭ-ă) [" + *mania*, madness]. Moral insanity; irresistible tendency toward forbidden conduct with retention of reasoning power.

pathometabolism (păth″ō-me-tăb'ō-lĭzm) [" + *metabolē*, change]. 1. Metabolism in disease. 2. Disordered metabolism.

pathometry (păth-ŏm'ĕt-rĭ) [" + *metron*, measure]. The estimate of the incidence of a disease.

pathomimesis (păth″ō-mĭm-e'sĭs) [" + *mimēsis*, imitation]. Intentional or unconscious as well as conscious imitation of a disease.

pathomorphism (păth-ō-mor'fĭzm) [" + *morphē*, form, + *ismos*, condition]. Study of abnormal form and structure of organisms.

pathonomy (păth-ŏn'ō-mĭ) [" + *nomos*, law]. Science of the laws of diseased conditions.

pathophilia (păth-ō-fĭl'ĭ-ă) [G. *pathos*, disease, + *philein*, to love]. Adjustment of habits to conditions made mandatory by some chronic disease.

pathophobia (păth-ō-fō'bĭ-ă) [" + *phobos*, fear]. Morbid apprehension of disease.

pathophoresis (păth″ō-for-ē′sĭs) [" + *phoros*, carrying]. The transmission of disease-producing organisms.

pathophoric (păth-ō-for′ĭk) [" + *phoros*, carrying]. Carrying or transmitting disease, as certain insects.

pathopleiosis (păth″ō-plī-ō′sĭs) [" + *pleion*, greater]. The tendency to magnify the gravity of one's disease.

pathopoiesis (păth″ō-poy-ē′sĭs) [" + *poiein*, to make]. The method of disease production.

pathopsychology (păth″ō-sī-kŏl′ō-jĭ) [" + *psyche*, soul, + *logos*, study]. The branch of psychology dealing with mental processes during disease.

patient (pā′shĕnt) [L. *patiens*, *patient*-, suffering]. 1. Enduring pain or injury. 2. A person who is receiving treatment for disease.

patulous (păt′ū-lŭs) [L. *patulus*, open]. Open; exposed. SYN: *patent*.

paulocardia (pawl″ō-kar′dĭ-ă) [G. *paula*, pause, + *kardia*, heart]. 1. Sensation of momentary stoppage of heartbeat. 2. Undue prolongation of the rest period in the cardiac cycle.

pavement (păv′mĕnt) [L. *pavire*, to pave]. Any structure resembling a tiled floor, or pavement.

p. epithelium. Flattened, single layer of epithelial cells resembling a tiled floor.

pavilion (păv-ĭl′yŭn) [O.Fr. *paveillon*]. 1. A flaring expansion at the extremity of a canal or tube. 2. A tent-shaped structure.

p. of the pelvis. The flare of the ilia, the expanded part of the pelvis.

pavor (pā′vor) [L.]. Anxiety, dread.

p. nocturnus. Night terror during sleep in children and the aged.

Pavy's disease (pā′vē). Albuminuria which recurs at periodic intervals.

Pb. SYMB: *plumbum*, lead.

p.c. Abbr. L. *post cibos*, after meals.

pea (pē) [G. *pison*]. COMP: Richer in proteins than other vegetables except lentils, but poorer in carbohydrates. Av. SERVING (fresh and dried): 75-100 Gm. Pro. 5.3-24.6, Fat 0.4-1.00, Carbo. 11.14-57.5. VITAMINS: A++ to +++ — +, B++ — ++, C+++ — 0, G++ — +. Ca 0.028-0.084, Mg 0.038-0.149, K 0.285-0.903, Na 0.013-0.104, P 0.127-0.400, Cl 0.024-0.035, S 0.063-0.0219, Fe 0.0017-0.0057.

peach (pētsh) [L. *persicum*, peach]. Av. SERVING (fresh): 150 Gm. Pro. 0.8, Fat 0.2, Carbo. 13.2. Av. SERVING (dried): 50 Gm. Pro. 2.0, Fat 0.4, Carbo. 36.1. VITAMINS (fresh): A+ to ++, B+, C++. VITAMINS (dried): A—, B+, C+. ASH CONST. (fresh and dried): Ca 0.016-0.034, Mg 0.010-0.056, K 0.214-0.830, Na 0.022-0.082, P 0.024-0.146, Cl 0.004, S 0.009-0.212, Fe 0.00033-0.0012. A base forming food; alkalinity 5 cc. per 100 Gm., 12.2 cc. per 100 cal.

p. stones. SEE: *cyanide poisoning*.

peanut (pē′nŭt). Av. SERVING: 60 Gm. Pro. 15.5, Fat 23.3, Carbo. 14.6. VITAMINS: A+, B++, G+. ASH CONST: Ca 0.071, Na 0.180, K 0.654, Na 0.050, P 0.399, Cl 0.056, S 0.224, Fe 0.0020.

p. butter. Av. SERVING: 15 Gm. Pro. 3.8, Fat 7.5, Carbo. 1.7. VITAMINS: A+, B++, G+.

pear (păr) [L. *pirum*]. Av. SERVING (fresh): 150 Gm. Pro. 0.6, Fat 0.6, Carbo. 12.5. VITAMINS: A+, B++, C+, E+, G++. ASH CONST: Ca 0.015, Mg 0.011, K 0.132, Na 0.016, P 0.026, Cl 0.011, S 0.010, Fe 0.0003.

ACTION: Heavy in the stomach unless cooked. Dried pears are highly nutritive and contain malic acid.

pearl (pĕrl) [O.Fr. *perle*]. 1. Small, tough mass in sputum in asthma. 2. Small, hollow glass capsule containing a fluid for inhalation, as amyl nitrite.

p., epithelial. Concentric squamous epithelial cells in carcinoma.

p., gouty. Sodium urate concretion on cartilage of the ear seen in people with gout.

pecan (pē-kăn′) [Algonquin *paccan*]. Av. SERVING: 25 Gm. Pro. 2.4, Fat 17.60, Carbo. 3.8. VITAMINS: A+ to ++, B++. ASH CONST: Ca 0.089, Mg 0.152, K 0.332, P 0.335, Cl 0.050, S 0.113, Fe 0.0026.

peccant (pek′ant) [L. *peccāre*, to sin]. Corrupt; producing disease. SYN: *pathogenic*, *unhealthy*, *morbid*.

peccatiphobia (pĕk-ăt-ĭ-fō′bĭ-ă) [" + G. *phobos*, fear]. Abnormal dread of sinning.

peciloblast (pē-sĭl′ō-blăst) [G. *poikilos*, variable, + *blastos*, germ]. Large, malformed, red blood cell. SYN: *poikiloblast*, *poikilocyte*.

pecilocyte (pē-sĭl′ō-sīt) [" + *kytos*, cell]. Large red blood cell of irregular shape. SYN: *peciloblast*, *poikiloblast*, *poikilocyte*.

pecilocythemia (pē-sĭl″ō-sī-thē′mĭ-ă) [" + " + *aima*, blood]. Pecilocytes in the blood. SYN: *pecilocytosis*.

pecilocytosis (pē-sĭl″ō-sī-tō′sĭs) [" + " + -*ōsis*, disease]. Pecilocytes in the blood stream. SYN: *pecilocythemia*.

pecilothermal (pē-sĭl″ō-ther′măl) [" + *therme*, heat]. 1. Not constant in temperature, denoting cold blooded animals. 2. Capable of developing in varying degrees of temperature.

Pecquet's cistern (pē-ka′). A reservoir for chyle at lower end of the thoracic duct. SEE: *chylocyst*, *receptaculum chyli*.

P.'s duct. Passage from the cisterna chyli to the joining point of the left subclavian and int. jugular veins, acting as a lymph channel.

P.'s reservoir. SEE: *P.'s cistern*.

pectase (pĕk′tās) [G. *pektos*, congealed, + *ase*, enzyme]. Enzyme facilitating the conversion of pectin into pectic acid.

pecten (pĕk′tĕn) [L. comb]. 1. The pubic bone. 2. A comblike organ. 3. Middle portion of anal canal.

p. band. Fiberlike induration of the iliopectineal line.

p. commissurae anterioris. Transverse fibrous bundles of the ant. cerebral commissure.

p. pubis. Ridge on horizontal ramus of the os pubis from its spine, continuous with the *linea arcuata* of the ilium.

p. sclerae. Opening on sclera for passage of the optic nerve.

pectenitis (pĕk-tĕn-ī′tĭs) [" + G. -*itis*, inflammation]. Inflamed condition of the sphincter ani.

pectenosis (pĕk′tĕn-ō′sĭs) [" + G. -*ōsis*, disease]. Fibrosis of the pecten which produces the p. band.

pectic acid (pĕk′tĭk) [G. *pektos*, congealed]. An acid derived from pectin by hydrolyzing the methyl ester group which is found in many fruits.

pectin (pĕk′tĭn) [G. *pēktos*, congealed]. A white, amorphous, plant carbohydrate that forms a gelatinous mass in the cooking of fruits and vegetables, causing them to "jell." SEE: *pectose*.

pectinate (pĕk′tĭn-āt) [L. *pecten*, comb]. Having teeth like a comb.

pectineal (pĕk′tĭn′ē-ăl) [L. *pecten*, comb]. Relating to the os pubis or the pectineus muscle.

pectineal line

p. line. The line or ridge on the os pubis separating the true from the false pelvis. SYN: *iliopectineal line, linea terminalis.*

p. muscle. Muscle on upper inner portion of thigh aiding in adduction and flexion.

pectineus (pek-tĭn-ē′-us) [L. *pecten, pectin-*, comb]. A flat, quadrangular muscle at upper and inner part of thigh arising from iliopectineal line and inserted bet. lesser trochanter and linea aspera of the femur, which flexes and adducts the outward thigh. SEE: *Table of Muscles in Appendix.*

pectiniform (pĕk-tĭn′ĭ-form) [" + *forma,* shape]. Toothed like a comb. SYN: *pectinate.*

pectization (pĕk-tĭ-zā′shŭn) [G. *pēktos,* congealed]. In colloidal chemistry, coagulation.

pectoral (pĕk′tō-răl) [L. *pectus, pector-*, breast]. 1. Concerning the chest. 2. Efficacious in relieving chest conditions, as a cough.

pectoralgia (pĕk-tō-ral′jĭ-ă) [" + G. *algos,* pain]. Neuralgic pain in the breast.

pectoralis (pĕk-tō-rā′lĭs) [L.]. One of 4 muscles of the breast.

p. major. A large triangular muscle extending to the humerus which draws the arm forward and downward and aids in chest expansion. SEE: *muscles, abdominal wall, for illustration.*

p. minor. Muscle beneath p. major, extending to scapula, which lowers the scapula and depresses the shoulder point. SEE: *muscles, abdominal wall, for illustration.*

pectoriloquy (pĕk-tō-rĭl′ō-kwĭ) [L. *pectus, pector-*, breast, + *loqui,* to speak]. The distinct transmission of vocal sounds to the ear through the chest wall in auscultation.*

The words seem to emanate from the spot which is auscultated. Heard over cavities which communicate with a bronchus; areas of consolidation near a large bronchus; over pneumothorax when the opening in the lung is patulous; over some pleural effusions. SEE: *chest.*

p., aphonic. In auscultation, whispered sound heard over a lung with a cavity or pleural effusion.

p., whispering. Sound over a lung with a cavity of limited extent when patient whispers, in auscultation of the chest.

pectorophony (pĕk-tō-rof′ō-nĭ) [" + G. *phōnē,* voice]. Exaggeration of vocal sounds heard on auscultation of the chest. SYN: *pectoriloquy.*

pectose (pĕk′tōs) [G. *pēktos,* congealed]. A substance found in some fruits and vegetables that yields pectin when it is boiled.

pectunculus (pĕk-tun′kŭ-lŭs) [L. little comb]. One of the tiny longitudinal ridges on the sylvian aqueduct.

pectus (pĕk′tŭs) [L.]. The chest; breast; thorax.

p. carinatum. Abnormal prominence of the sternum. SYN: *chicken* or *pigeon breast.*

pedal (pĕd′ăl, pē′dăl) [L. *pēs, ped-*, foot]. Concerning the foot.

pederast (pĕd′ĕr-ăst) [G. *pais, paid-*, youth, + *erastēs,* lover, from *eran,* to love]. One who indulges in the unnatural, illegal habit of sexual intercourse with men, esp. young boys, through the anus.

pederasty (pĕd′ĕr-ăs-tĭ) [" + *erastēs,* lover, from *eran,* to love]. Illicit coitus by the anus with males, esp. with young boys. SYN: *sodomy.*

pedialgia (pĕd-ĭ-al′jĭ-ă, pē-dĭ-) [G *pedion,* foot, + *algos,* pain]. Pain of the foot.

pediatric (pē-dĭ-ăt′rĭk) [G. *pais, paid-*, child, + *iatreia,* treatment]. Concerning the treatment of children.

pediatrician (pē-dĭ-ă-trĭsh′an) [G. *pais, paid-*, child, + *iatrikos,* healing]. A specialist in treatment of children's diseases. SYN: *pediatrist.*

pediatrics (pē-dĭ-ăt′rĭks) [" + *iatreia,* treatment]. Medical science relating to hygienic care of children and treatment of diseases peculiar to them. SYN: *pediatry.*

pediatrist (pē″dĭ-ăt′rĭst) [" + *iatrikos,* healing]. Physician who specializes in treatment of children's diseases.

pediatry (pĕd′ĭ-ăt-rĭ, pē-dĭ′ăt-rĭ). The treatment of children's diseases. SYN: *pediatrics.*

pedicellation (pĕd″ĭ-sĕl-ā′shŭn) [L. *pediculus,* a little foot; stalk]. Formation and development of a pedicle.

pedicle (pĕd′ĭ-kl) [L. *pediculus,* a little foot]. 1. The stem which attaches a new growth. 2. The bony process projecting backward which connects the lamina of a vertebra on either side.

pedicular (pē-dĭk′ū-lar) [L. *pediculus,* a louse]. 1. Infested with or concerning lice. 2. [L. *pediculus,* a little foot]. Concerning a stalk or stem.

pediculate (pē-dĭk′ū-lāt) [L. *pediculus,* a little foot]. Having a pedicle or stem. SYN: *pedunculate.*

pediculation (pē-dĭk-ū-lā′shŭn) [L. *pediculus,* a louse; a little foot]. 1. Infestation with lice. 2. Development of a pedicle.

pediculicide (pē-dĭk′ū-lĭ-sīd) [L. *pediculus,* a louse, + *caedere,* to kill]. Destroying or that which destroys lice.

pediculophobia (pē-dĭk″ū-lō-fō′bĭ-ă) [" + G. *phobos,* fear]. Abnormal dread of lice. SYN: *phthiriophobia.*

pediculosis (pē-dĭk-ū-lō′sĭs) [" + G. *-ōsis,* infestation]. Lousiness; infestation with lice. SEE: *pediculus,* 2.

pediculus (pē-dĭk′ū-lŭs) [L. stem, louse]. 1. A pedicle. 2. [capitalized] Genus of parasitic insects; lice.

P. capitis. A form affecting the scalp.
ETIOL: Contracted by close contact, common brush and comb, and interchanging headgear.
SYM: Itching, and in long standing, neglected cases, matted hair with disgusting odor, and possibly impetigo or eczematous dermatitis resulting from inflammation, scratching, infection.
TREATMENT: Petroleum cap; soaking scalp in petroleum and wearing close fitting cap for 12 to 24 hours, guarding against open flame, then scrubbing with soap and water. Emollient ointment in presence of inflammation.
Larkspur cap may be applied in same manner.
Long hair should be rolled to the head and covered well, or it may be advisable with the consent of the patient to cut off the hair, in which case it should be burned at once. When removing the head covering, the bed and the surrounding area should be well covered with newspapers or towels. The hair should then be brushed and combed with a fine-tooth comb, and all dead insects must be burned at once.
To loosen nits or eggs, moisten the hair in hot vinegar and comb out with

Pediculus corporis — a fine-tooth comb. Kerosene will kill both nits and pediculi, but it is disagreeable and irritating to the scalp. It may be diluted one-half with olive oil. No injury will be done to the hair from this treatment.

P. corporis. The body louse which causes red or purple eruptions on skin as the result of its bite.

They are small in size, and confined to covered parts of the body, esp. the trunk, the insect living in the clothing, in the interscapular, shoulder, and waist region. From scratching, secondary eczema may develop.

TREATMENT: Sterilization of clothing. Pressing of seams with hot iron. Thorough scrubbing of body with soap and water.

P. pubis. The crab louse affecting the genital, abdominal and presternal regions, often the result of body contacts. SYN: *morpio*.

TREATMENT: Thorough cleansing with soap and water, followed by bichloride of mercury, dilution (1:1000), tincture Cocculus indicus (1:3).

P. vestimenti. SEE: *P. corporis*.

pedicure (pĕd'ĭ-kŭr) [L. *pĕs, ped-*, foot, + *cura*, care]. 1. Care of the feet. 2. A chiropodist or one who cares for the feet. 3. The care, painting, and polishing of the toenails.

pediluvium (pĕd-ĭ-lū'vĭ-ŭm) [" + *luere*, to wash]. A foot bath.

pedionalgia (pĕd-ĭ-ō-nal'jĭ-ă) [G. *pedion*, foot, + *algos*, pain]. Neuralgic pain in the sole of the foot. SYN: *metatarsalgia*.

pediophobia (pē-dĭ-ō-fō'bĭ-ă) [G. *pais, paid-*, child, + *phobos*, fear]. Unnatural dread of young children or of dolls.

pedobaromacrometer (pē″dō-băr″ō-măk-rŏm'ĕt-ĕr) [" + *baros*, weight, + *makros*, long, + *metron*, measure]. Apparatus for determining measurement and weight of infants.

pedobarometer (pē″dō-băr-om'ĕt-ĕr) [" + " + *metron*, measure]. Apparatus for weighing infants.

pedodontia, pedodontics (pē″dō-don'shĭ-ă, -tĭks) [" + *odous, odont-*, tooth]. Phase of dentistry dealing with care of children's teeth.

pedodontist (pē″dō-dŏn'tĭst) [" + *odous, odont-*, tooth]. Dentist who specializes in care of children's teeth.

pedograph (pĕd′ō-grăf) [L. *pĕs, ped-*, foot, + G. *graphein*, to write]. Imprint of the foot on paper.

pedologist (pē-dŏl'ō-jĭst) [G. *pais, paid-*, child, + *logos*, study]. One who has made a study of children and their development.

pedology (pē-dŏl'ō-jĭ) [" + *logos*, study] The study of children and their development.

pedometer (pē-dom'ĕt-ĕr) [G. *pais, paid-*, child, + *metron*, measure]. 1. Device for measurement of infants. 2. (pĕd-ŏm'ĕt-ĕr) [L. *pĕs, ped-*, foot, + G. *metron*, measurement]. Watch which indicates number of steps taken in walking.

pedomorphism (pē″dō-mor'fĭzm) [G. *pais, paid-*, child, + *morphē*, form, + *ismos*, condition]. Retention of juvenile characteristics in the adult.

pedonosology (pē″dō-nŏs-ŏl'ō-jĭ) [" + *nosos*, disease, + *logos*, study]. The study of children's diseases. SYN: *pediatrics*.

pedophilia (pē″dō-fĭl'ĭ-ă) [" + *philein*, to love]. 1. Fondness for children. 2. PSY: Unnatural desire for sexual relations with children.

peduncle (pē-dung'kl) [L. *pedunculus*, a little foot]. 1. A stem or stalk. SYN: pedicle. 2. A brachium of the brain; a band connecting parts of the brain. SYN: *pedunculus*. SEE: *cimbia, crus, sessile*.

p., callosal. Fibrous band from sylvian fissure to area under the callosum.

p., cerebral. White bundle from upper part of the pons to the cerebrum. SYN: *crus cerebri*.

p., pineal. A band from either side of the pineal gland to the ant. pillars of the fornix.

peduncular (pē-dŭn'kū-lar) [L. *pedunculus*, a little foot]. Concerning a peduncle.

pedunculate, pedunculated (pē-dŭn'kū-lāt, -ĕd) [L. *pedunculus*, a little foot]. Possessing a stalk or peduncle. SYN: *pediculate*.

pedunculus (pē-dŭn'kū-lŭs) [L. a little foot]. A stalk or peduncle, *q.v.*

p. ant. callosi. Ant. extremity of the *corpus callosum*.

p. flocci. Constricted part of a cerebellar lamina.

p. pulmonum. Root of the lung.

p. trigoni cerebralis ant. Ant. pillar of the fornix.

peinotherapy (pī-nō-thĕr'ă-pĭ) [G. *peina*, hunger, + *therapeia*, treatment]. Hunger cure for disease. SYN: *pinotherapy*.

pelada, pelade (pē-la'dă, -lăd) [Fr., from L. *peler*, to strip of hair]. 1. Loss of hair on circumscribed areas of the scalp. SYN: *alopecia areata*. 2. Disease resembling pellagra, caused by infected maize.

pelage (pē-lahj') [Fr.]. The hair of the body collectively.

pelicology (pĕl-ĭk-ŏl'ō-jĭ) [G. *pelika*, pelvis, + *logos*, treatise]. The science of the pelvis and its relation to other structures in the body.

pelidisi (pĕl-ĭd-ē'sē) [coined term]. Pirquet's unit index for the nutritive development of children.

It is obtained by division of cube root of 10 times the weight (grams) by sitting height (centimeters). Quotient of less than 95 indicates undernutrition.

pelioma (pĕl-ĭ-ō'mă) [G. *peliōma*, a livid spot]. A livid cutaneous patch. SYN: *ecchymosis*.

peliosis (pĕl-ĭ-ō'sĭs) [G. *peliōsis*, a livid spot]. A disease marked by purple patches on the mucous membranes and skin. SYN: *purpura*.

p. rheumatica. An acute affection characterized by inflammation of the joints.

A form of rheumatism. SYM: Sore throat, urticaria, moderate fever, purpuric spots over extremities or trunk. Tenderness, swelling, and pain in joints. SYN: *purpura rheumatica,, Schonlein's disease*.

pellagra (pĕl-ā'gră, pĕ-lăg'ră) [L. *pellis*, skin, + G. *agra*, seizure]. An endemic deficiency disease affecting chiefly cerebrospinal and digestive systems resulting from improper diet.

ETIOL: Due to absence of vitamin B in diet. Begins in spring or autumn as a rule. Frequently found in alcoholics.

SYM: May be a mixture of symptoms from 3 different deficiencies, nicotinic acid, riboflavin and thiamin chloride or may occur alone. Lesion appears on parts of body exposed to air and light; face, neck, back of hands and feet. Intense, rapidly extending erythema; bright red or brown swelling, itching, burning. Spreading edge of patches much elevated and darker than central

pellagra sine pellagra   P-28   **pelvis**

portion. Gastrointestinal and nervous disturbances. SEE: *Italian leprosy, Lombardy leprosy, rosa asturica*.

TREATMENT: Nicotinic* acid with vitamin B$_6$ and G for the neuritis that accompanies this disease. Recently pyrazine -2, 3-dicarboxylic acid and pyrazine monocarboxylic acid have been used successfully in treating pellagra.

DIET: Brewer's yeast; abundance of milk, eggs, lean meat and perhaps calves' liver.

p. sine pellagra. Former name for condition due to riboflavin deficiency.

TREATMENT: Constitutional and administration of riboflavin. Dusting with cooling powder to relieve itching. SEE: *ariboflavinosis*.

pellagracein (pĕl-ă-gra′sē-ĭn). Poisonous substance in decomposed cornmeal. SYN: *pellagrazein*.

pellagragenic (pĕ-lā-gră-jĕn′ĭk) [L. *pellis*, skin, + G. *agra*, seizure, + *gennan*, to produce]. Producing pellagra.

pellagrazein (pĕl-ă-grā′zē-ĭn). Poisonous substance in cornmeal that has decomposed. SYN: *pellagracein*.

pellagrin (pĕ-lā′grĭn, -lăg′rĭn) [L. *pellis*, skin, + G. *agra*, seizure]. A person afflicted with pellagra.

pellagrous (pĕ-lā′grŭs, -lăg′rŭs) [" + G. *agra*, seizure]. Concerning or affected with pellagra.

pellet (pĕl′ĕt) [L. *pila*, a ball]. A tiny pill or small ball of medicine or food.

pelletierine tan′nate (pĕl″ē-tēr′ēn). USP. A mixture of the tannates of alkaloids obtained from the pomegranate.

ACTION AND USES: Anthelmintic and teniafuge.

DOSAGE: 4 gr. (0.25 Gm.) in capsule, after adm. of a mild purgative, previous fasting, followed by a purgative.

pellicle (pĕl′ĭ-kl) [L. *pellicula*, a little skin]. 1. A thin piece of cuticle or skin. 2. Film or surface on a liquid. SYN: *scum*.

pellotine (pĕl′ō-tēn). A white, crystalline alkaloid used as a hypnotic.

pellucid (pĕ-lū′sĭd) [L. *pellucidus*, shining through]. Translucent; transparent.

p. zone. Clear layer covering the oöcyte. SYN: *zona pellucida*.

pelveoperitonitis (pĕl″vē-ō-pĕr-ĭ-tō-nī′tĭs) [L. *pelvis*, basin, + G. *peritonaion*, peritoneum, + *-itis*, inflammation]. Inflammation of the peritoneum situated in the pelvic region. SYN: *pelviperitonitis*.

pelvic (pĕl′vĭk) [L. *pelvis*, basin]. Pert. to the bony basin of trunk formed by innominate bones, sacrum, and coccyx.

p. girdle. Arch made by the innominate bones.

p. inlet. Upper pelvic entrance, the brim of the pelvis forming its boundary.

p. outlet. Lower pelvic opening.

pelvilithotomy (pĕl″vī-lĭ-thŏt′ō-mī) [" + G. *lithos*, stone, + *tomē*, a cutting]. Removal of a stone from the renal pelvis. SYN: *nephrolithotomy, pelviolithotomy, pyelolithotomy*.

pelvimeter (pĕl-vĭm′ĕt-ĕr) [" + G. *metron*, measure]. Device for measuring the pelvis.

pelvimetry (pĕl-vĭm′ĕt-rī) [" + G. *metron*, measure]. Measurement of the pelvic dimensions or proportions. SEE: *pelvis, Illus., pp. P-33 and P-34*.

pelviolithotomy (pĕl″vī-ō-lĭ-thŏt′ō-mī) [" + G. *lithos*, stone, + *tomē*, a cutting]. Incision of the renal pelvis to remove a calculus.

pelvioperitonitis (pĕl″vī-ō-pĕr-ĭ-tō-nī′tĭs) [" + G. *peritonaion*, peritoneum, + *-itis*, inflammation]. Inflammation of the peritoneum lining the pelvic region.

pelvioplasty (pĕl′vī-ō-plăs″tī) [" + G. *plassein*, to form]. Enlargement of the outlet of the pelvis. SYN: *hebotomy, symphyseotomy*.

pelvioscopy (pĕl″vī-ŏs′kō-pī) [L. *pelvis*, basin, + G. *skopein*, to examine]. Inspection of the pelvis.

pelviotomy (pĕl-vī-ŏt′ō-mī) [" + G. *tomē*, a cutting]. 1. Incision of pelvic bones, esp. in case of difficult labor. 2. Incision into the renal pelvis.

pelviperitonitis (pĕl″vī-pĕr-ĭ-tō-nī′tĭs) [" + G. *peritonaion*, peritoneum, + *-itis*, inflammation].

pelvis (pĕl′vĭs) (pl. *pelves*) [L. basin]. 1. Any basin-shaped structure or cavity. 2. The bony structure formed by the innominate bones, the sacrum, the coccyx and the ligaments uniting them, which serves as a support for the post. portion of the limbs. 3. The area included within these bones.

It is separated into a *false*, or superior pelvis, and a *true*, or inferior one, by the iliopectineal line, and the upper margin of the symphysis pubis, the circumference of this area constituting the *inlet* of the true pelvis. Lower border of true pelvis is formed by the coccyx, the protuberances of the ischia, the ascending rami of the ischia, the descending rami of the ossa pubis and the sacrosciatic ligaments, and is termed the *outlet*.

The floor of the pelvis is formed by the perineal fascia, levator ani and the coccygeus.

DIAMETERS: All diameters are larger in the female than in the male.

EXTERNAL: *Interspinous*: Distance bet. outer edges of the ant. sup. iliac spines, diameter normally measuring 26 cm. (10 in). *Intercristal*: Distance bet. outer edges of the most prominent portion of the iliac crests, diameter normally being 28 cm. (11 in.). *Intertrochanteric*: Distance bet. most prominent points of the femoral trochanters, 32 cm. (12½ in.). *Oblique* (right and left): Distance from 1 post. sup. iliac spine to the opposite ant. sup. iliac spine, 22 cm. (8½ in.), right being slightly greater than the left. *External conjugate*: Distance from the undersurface of the spinous process of last lumbar vertebra to the upper margin of ant. surface of the symphysis pubis, 20 cm. (7¾ in.). SYN: *Baudelocque's diameter*.

INTERNAL: *True conjugate*: Anteroposterior diameter of the pelvic inlet, 11 cm. (4¼ in.), the most important single diameter of the pelvis. *Diagonal conjugate*: Distance bet. the promontory of the sacrum to undersurface of symphysis pubis, 13 cm. (5 in.), 2 cm. being deducted for the height and inclination of symphysis to obtain diameter of conjugate. *Transverse*: Distance bet. ischial tuberosities, 11 cm. (4¼ in.). *Anteroposterior* (of outlet): Distance bet. the lower border of symphysis and tip of sacrum, 11 cm. (4¼ in.). *Anterior sagittal*: Distance from undersurface of symphysis to center of line bet. the ischial tuberosities, 7 cm. (2¾ in.). *Posterior sagittal*: Distance from the center of line bet. ischial tuberosities to the tip of the sacrum, 10 cm. (4 in.).

RS: *acanthopelvis, brim, Claudius' fossa, diameter, endopelvic, pelvic cavity, pelvimetry, pelviotomy.*

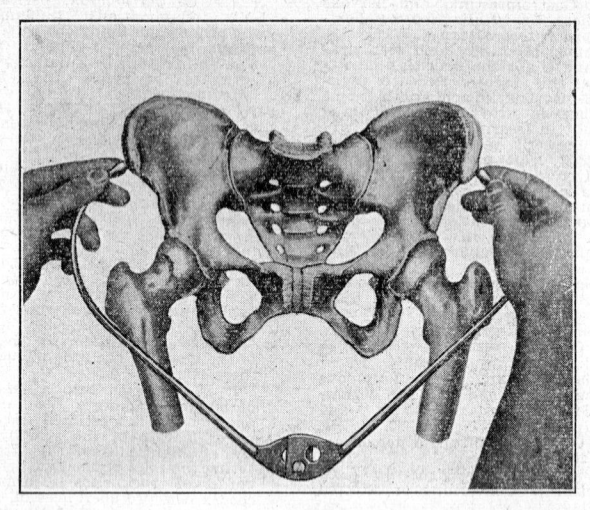

Measuring the intraspinous diameter of the pelvis.

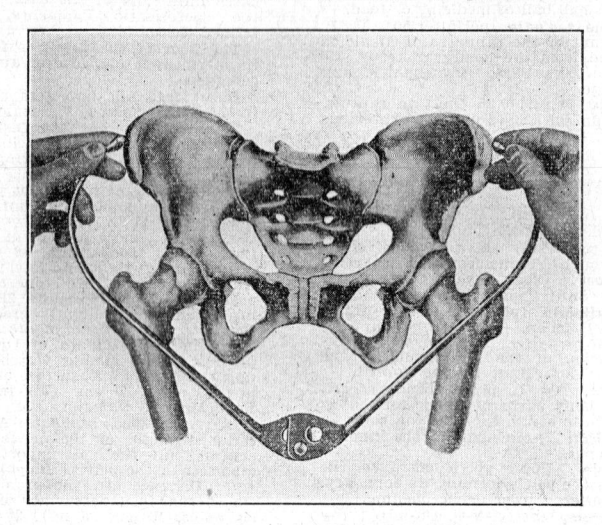

Measuring the intracrestal diameter.
EXTERNAL PELVIMETRY.

p. aequabiliter justo major. One symmetrically above standard in all its dimensions.
p. aequabiliter justo minor. One with all equally below standard.
p., beaked. One with the pelvic bones laterally compressed and pushed forward so that outlet is narrow and long.
p., brim of. SEE: *inlet of pelvis.*
p., caoutchouc. Same as India rubber pelvis.

p., Capuron's cardinal points of. Four points within the pelvic inlet, the 2 sacroiliac articulations and the 2 iliopectineal eminences.
p., cordate. P. which has a heart shape.
p., coxalgic. One deformed subsequent to hip joint disease.
p., dwarf. An aequabiliter justo minor pelvis.

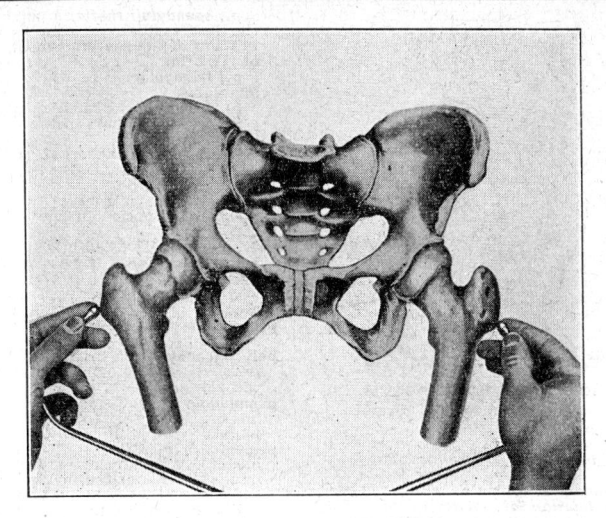

Measuring the bitrochanteric diameter.

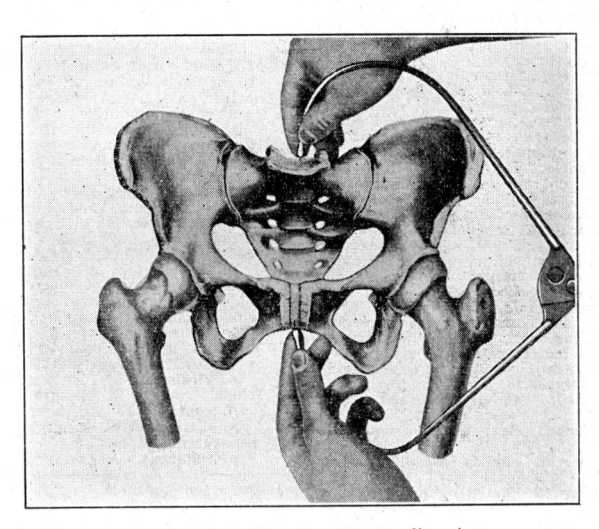

Measuring the external conjugate diameter.

EXTERNAL PELVIMETRY (*Continued*)

p., dynamic. The pelvis as related to force, as in labor.
p., elastic. An osteomalacic pelvis.
p., false. Portion above the iliopectineal line.
p., fissured. A rachitic pelvis with ilia pushed forward so as to be almost parallel.
p., fracture of. Bed rest most important. A firm binder is applied round the pelvis and, if the displacement is severe, the legs are placed in Braun's splints with extension. Movements of all joints are allowed. If the fracture is severe the bladder or intestines may be injured; a catheter is usually passed as soon as possible after the accident to see if the urethra or bladder has been injured. The patient must be carefully watched and the urine measured and tested.

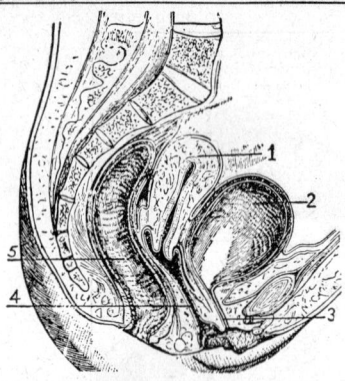

SECTION OF FEMALE PELVIS.
1. Uterus. 2. Bladder. 3. Urethra. 4. Vagina. 5. Rectum.

p., giant. SEE: *p. aequabiliter justo major.*
p., Hauder's. Same as *pelvis spinosa.*
p., inclination of, obliquity of. The angle between the axis of the pelvis and that of the body.
p., India rubber. A pelvis, the bones of which may be stretched out of normal position in osteomalacia. SYN: *caoutchouc p.*
p., inverted. SEE: *split pelvis.*
p., Kilian's. SEE: *osteomalacic pelvis.*
p., kyphotic. Deformed p. characterized by increase of the conjugate diameter at the brim with reduction of the transverse diameter at the outlet.
p., lordotic. Deformed p. in which the spinal column has an ant. curvature in the lumbar region.
p., malacosteon. SEE: *rachitic p.*
p., masculine. A woman's pelvis that is funnel-shaped like that of a man.
p., Nägele's. Oblique pelvis. Distorted p. in which the conjugate diameter takes an oblique direction.
p., osteomalacic. P. distorted as a consequence of osteomalacia.
p., Prague. SEE: *spondylolisthetic p.*
p., pseudoösteomalacic. A rickety pelvis similar to that of a person affected with osteomalacia.
p., rachitic. One deformed from rickets.
p., reduced. SEE: *aequabiliter justo minor.*
p., reniform. Pelvis shaped like a kidney.
p., Robert's. One with an embryonic sacrum and narrowing of the transverse and oblique diameters.
p., Rokitansky's. SEE: *spondylolisthetic p.*
p., rostrate. SEE: *beaked p.*
p., rotunda. A tympanic depression in the inner wall, at the bottom of which is the fenestra rotunda.
p., round. One with a circular inlet.
p., rubber. An osteomalacic p.
p., scoliotic. Deformed p. due to spinal curvature.
p., simple flat. One whose deformity is a shortened anteroposterior diameter.
p. spinosa. A rachitic pelvis with a pointed crest of the pubis.
p., split. One with a congenital division at the symphysis pubis.
p., spondylolisthetic. A pelvis in which the last lumbar vertebra is dislocated in front of the sacrum causing occlusion of the brim.
p., triangular. One whose inlet is triangular.
p., triradiate. SEE: *beaked p.*
p., true. The part of the p. below the iliopectineal line.
pelvitherm (pĕl'vĭ-thurm) [L. *pelvis*, basin, + G. *thermē*, heat]. Device for heating the pelvis.
pelvitomy (pĕl-vĭt'ō-mĭ) [" + G. *tomē*, incision]. Incision of the pelvis to aid delivery.
pelvoscopy (pĕl-vŏs'kō-pĭ) [" + G. *skopein* to examine]. Inspection of a pelvis.
pelycalgia (pĕl-ĭ-kăl'jĭ-ă) [G. *pelyx*, pelvis, + *algos*, pain]. Pain in the pelvic area.
pelycogram (pĕl'ĭ-kō-grăm) [" + *gramma*, a writing]. An x-ray of the pelvis.
pelycography (pĕl-ĭ-kŏg'ră-fĭ) [" + *graphein*, to write]. Treatise describing the pelvis.
pemphigoid (pĕm'fĭ-goyd) [G. *pemphix*, blister, + *eidos*, like]. Similar to pemphigus.
pemphigus (pĕm'fĭ-gŭs) [G. *pemphix*, a blister]. An acute or chronic disease of adults characterized by occurrence of successive crops of bullae appearing suddenly on apparently normal skin, and which disappear leaving pigmented spots. It may be attended by itching and burning and constitutional disturbance.

ETIOL.: Unknown.

TREATMENT: Care of general health. In severe and extensive cases patient to be kept on air or water mattress; continuous bath therapy, tonics, arsenic, arsphenamine, carron oil bath, ultraviolet irradiation. In *p. foliaceous* and *p. vegetans*, autogenous serum. Locally, large quantities of powder, soothing lotions.

p. acutus. Butcher's p. Constitutional symptoms severe and outcome often fatal. Bullae 1-10 cm. in diameter often containing blood and serum. If coalescing, denuded areas are formed.
p. benignus. A mild form of p.
p. chronicus, p. vulgaris. Uncomplicated form in which replacement of epidermis follows. Lesions round or oval, thin walled, tense, translucent, contents bilateral in distribution, developing suddenly, without scarring resulting.
p. circinatus. P. with circular eruptions. [the groin and axilla.
p. contagiosa. An infective type of
p. disseminatus. P. marked by widely separated bullae.
p. foliaceus. Rare type. Large flaccid bullae developing rapidly, rupture soon, leaving moist, raw surface covered with seropurulent fluid. Bullous contents are purulent from beginning with sickening odor. Chronic course.
p. neonatorum. P. soon after birth, generally due to septic infection but sometimes leutic. [tinuous itching.
p. pruriginosus. P. with severe, con-
p. syphiliticus. A form due to syphilis.
p. vegetans. Resembles *p. vulgaris* in beginning, but instead of drying up, the lesions persist, resulting in papillary excrescences with no tendency to heal, secreting foul-smelling seropurulent fluid and sodden decomposing masses of epidermis.
penatin (pĕn'ă-tĭn). A derivative of penicillin more powerful than the latter, affecting germs nonresistant to penicil-

lin, and in dilutions of from one to ten to four hundred million parts.

pendular (pĕn'dū-lẽr) [L. *pendulus*, from *pendere*, to hang]. Hanging so as to swing by an attached part; oscillating like a pendulum.

pendulous (pĕn'dū-lŭs) [L. *pendulus*, from *pendere*, to hang]. Swinging freely like a pendulum; hanging.

pendulum (pĕn'dū-lŭm) [L. *pendulus*, swinging]. Body suspended from a fixed point and free to swing to and fro.

  p. movements. To and fro movement which churns the contents of intestine during digestion, mixing them with ferments without peristaltic action.

  p. rhythm. Disordered cardiac rhythm; the diastolic sound resembles the systolic sound so that the completed cardiac cycle sounds like the ticking of a clock.

penetrate (pĕn'e-trāt) [L. *penetrāte*, to go within]. To enter into the interior of.

penetrating (pĕn'e-trāt-ĭng) [L. *penetrāre*, to go within]. Entering beyond the exterior.   [lens.

  p. power. Penetrating capacity of a

  p. wound. Wound affecting the interior of an organ or cavity.

penetration (pĕn"e-trā'shŭn) [L. *penetrāre*, to go within]. 1. Process of entering within a part. 2. Capacity to enter within a part. 3. Power of a lens to give a clear focus at varying depths.

penetrometer (pĕn-y-trŏm'ĕt-ĕr) [" + G. *metron*, measure]. FT: An instrument that compares roughly the comparative absorption of roentgen rays in various metals, esp. silver, lead and aluminum; hence, it gives a rough estimation of hardness of roentgen rays.

Best known are those of Benoist, Walter, and Wehnelt.

penicillin (pen-ĭ-sĭl'ĭn, pen-ĭ-sĭl'ĭn). A substance from a family of molds known as Penicillium. Effective in gram-positive coccal, bacillary, clostridial, and some actinomycotic infections. Effective also in spirochetal disease and in gonococcal and meningococcal infections.

It is not a normal body-substance. It may be allergic and should not be given if the patient has ever experienced allergy, rash, or swollen joints from its use. Skin tests should be made before giving. Many sudden deaths following administration have been reported.

penicilliosis (pen"ĭs-ĭl-ĭ-ō'sĭs) [L. *penicillum*, pencil]. Infection with the fungi of the genus Penicillium.

Penicillium (pen-ĭs-ĭl'ĭ-ŭm) [L. *penicillum*, pencil, brush]. A genus of molds seen on fruit, bread, cheese, etc., which affects the skin and mucosa of man.

penile (pē'nĭl, -nīl) [L. *penis*, penis]. Pert. to the penis. SYN: penile.

  p. reflex. 1. Sudden downward movement of penis when the prepuce or gland of a completely relaxed penis is pulled upward. 2. Contraction of bulbocavernous muscle on percussing dorsum of penis. 3. Contraction of bulbocavernous muscle resulting from compression of glans penis.   [male organ.

penis (pē'nĭs) (pl. *penes*) [L.]. Generative

It is a cylindrical, pendulous organ suspended from the front and sides of the pubic arch. It is composed of 3 columns of cavernous tissue, the whole being covered with skin, the 2 lateral columns being known as the *corpora cavernosa penis.* The 3rd or median column contains the urethra, known as the *corpus cavernosum urethrae.*

The head of the penis is known as the *glans penis* in which the urethral orifice is situated, and it is covered with a movable hood known as the *foreskin* or *prepuce,** under which is secreted a lubricating substance called *smegma.**

Hyperemia of the genitals fills the corpora cavernosa with blood as the result of libido, thus causing an *erection.**

The hyperemia is lowered following ejaculation of the seminal fluid and the organ returns to its normal condition.

Normally the penis is about 4 or more inches long when distended.

  p. cerebri. The pineal gland.

  p., clubbed. A condition when the penis is curved during erection.

  p. lunatus. Painful curved erection in gonorrhea. SYN: *chordee, q.v.*

  p. muliebr!s. Clitoris,* the erectile organ of the female.

  p. palmatus. One enclosed by the scrotum.

  p. webbed. Same as *p. palmatus.*

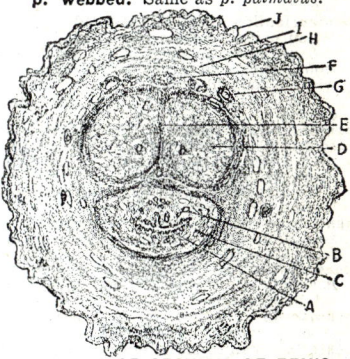

TRANSVERSE SECTION OF PENIS.
A. Lumen of urethra. B. Mucosa urethrae. C. Corpus cavernosum urethrae. D. Corpus cavernosum penis. E. Arteria profunda penis. F. Arteria dorsalis penis. G. Vena dorsalis penis. H. Nervus dorsalis penis with pacinian corpuscles. I. Musculus ischiocavernosus. J. Musculus bulbocavernosus.

penis, words pert. to: anaspadias, apellous, "balan-" words, cavernitis, chordée, circumcision, condyloma, cord, corpora cavernosa, Cowper's gland, erectile, erection, erector, foreskin, frenulum, hypospadias, mentulagra, mentulate, mentulomania, nervi erigentes, peotomy, "phall-" words, prepuce, prostate, scrotum, seminal vesicles, testes, urethra, vas deferens.

penischisis (pen-ĭs'kĭs'-ĭs). Epispadias, hypospadias, paraspadias, or any fissured condition of the penis.

penitis (pē-nī'tĭs) [L. *penis*, penis, + G. *itis*, inflammation]. Inflammation of the penis.

penniform (pĕn'ĭ-form) [L. *penna*, feather, + *forma*, shape]. Feather-shaped.

pennyroyal (pĕn'ĭ-roi'ăl). Name for various plants, esp. Hedeoma and Mentha, which yield commercial oil used as emmenagogue, carminative, and stimulant.

pennyweight (pĕn'ĭ-wāt). Troy weight containing 24 gr. or 1/20 of an ounce.

pension neurosis (pĕn'shan nū-rō'sĭs). A condition which develops subsequent to an injury in the belief that compensation can be obtained by being ill. SEE: *neurosis, compensation.*

penta-, pent- [G.] Combining form meaning *five.*

pentad (pĕn'tăd) [G. *pente,* five]. 1. A radical or element with a valence of 5. 2. Group of 5.

pental (pĕn'tăl) [G. *pente,* five]. C_5H_{10}. Trimethylethylene, a hydrocarbon, used as an anesthetic in minor surgery.

pentamethylendiamine (pĕn″tă-mĕth″ĭl-ĕn-dī'ăm-ēn) [G. *pente,* five]. A pathogenic ptomaine occurring in tissue decomposition. SYN: *cadaverine, q.v.*

pentane (pĕn'tān) [G. *pente,* five]. C_5H_{12}. One of the hydrocarbons of the methane series used as an anesthetic.

pentavalent (pĕn″tă-vā'lĕnt, -tăv'ă-lent) [G. *pente,* five, + L. *valens,* having power]. Having a valence of 5. SYN: *quinquivalent.*

pentene (pĕn'tēn) [G. *pente,* five]. A liquid hydrocarbon used as an anesthetic.

pentnucleotide (pĕpt-nū'klē-ō-tīd). A solution prepared from yeast nucleic acid.
USES: Recommended in certain infectious conditions, accompanied by a low white blood cell count.
DOSAGE: From 10 to 20 cc. intramuscularly.

pentobarbital sodium (pĕn″tō-bar'bĭ-tăl sō'dĭ-ŭm). A barbituric acid derivative used as an analgesic, sedative, and hypnotic, prior to anesthesia.
Used in labor with or without scopolamine. SYN: *nembutal.*

pentosazon (pĕn″tō-sa'zŏn). Abnormal substance in urine which is incapable of fermentation.

pentose (pĕn'tōs) [G. *pente,* five]. $C_5H_{10}O_5$. A simple sugar with 5 atoms of oxygen in the molecule.

pentosemia (pĕn″tō-sē'mĭ-ă) [*pentose* + G. *aima,* blood]. Pentose in the blood.

pentoside (pĕn'tō-sīd). Pentose combined with some other substance.

pentosuria (pĕn″tō-sū'rĭ-ă) [*pentose* + G. *ouron,* urine]. A condition in which pentose is found in the urine.

pentothal sodium (pĕn'tō-thăl so'dĭ-ŭm). Commercial barbituric acid derivative used as an anesthetic and hypnotic.
CONTRAINDICATIONS: In arteriosclerosis.

peonin (pē'ō-nĭn). A dye used as a hydrogen ion concentration test.

peotillomania (pe″ō-til-ō-mā'nĭ-ă) [G. *peos,* penis, + *tillein,* to pull, + *mania,* madness]. A tic resulting in constant pulling at the penis. SYN: *pseudomasturbation.*

peotomy (pē-ŏt'ō-mĭ) [″ + *tomē,* incision]. Amputation of the penis.

pepo (pē'pō) [G. *pepōn,* ripe]. USP. Pumpkin seed which is used as an agent to remove tapeworms.
DOSAGE: 1 oz. (30 cc.).

pepper (pĕp'ĕr) [G. *peperi,* pepper]. A spice which is used as a condiment, stimulant, carminative, counterirritant and antiperiodic.
ASH CONST. (black and white, dry): Ca 0.440-0.425, Mg 0.156-0.113, K 1.140-none in white pepper, Na 0.131-none in white pepper, P 0.188-0.233, Cl 0.312-0.029, no sulfur or iron in either.
(Green, fresh): AV. SERVING: 25 Gm. Pro. 0.2, Fat trace, Carbo. 1.00. VITAMINS: A++, B++, C+++. Ca 0.006, Mg 0.010, K 0.139, P 0.026, Cl 0.013, S 0.014.

peppermint (pĕp'ĕr-mĭnt). USP. The top and leaves of the plant Mentha piperita from which oil of peppermint is derived. USES: Aromatic stimulant, carminative, and flavoring agent.

pepsic (pĕp'sĭk) [G. *peptein,* to digest]. 1. Concerning digestion. 2. Concerning pepsin. SYN: *peptic.*

pepsin (pĕp'sĭn) [G. *pepsis,* digestion]. The chief enzyme of gastric juice which converts proteins into proteoses and peptones.
It is formed in the pyloric glands. It may be obtained as a powder, and with the help of hydrochloric acid, it will digest proteins in the test tube.
USP: An enzyme obtained from the glandular layer of the fresh stomach of the hog. Assayed to digest 3000 times its weight of freshly coagulated egg albumen.
ACTION AND USES: Acts only in acid medium. Useful to aid digestion of protein food in the stomach; sometimes combined with hydrochloric acid in cases of acute dyspepsia.
DOSAGE: 8 gr. (0.5 Gm.).

p. unit. Standard amount for measurement of ratio of pepsin to gastric juice.

pepsinia (pĕp-sĭn'ĭ-ă) [G. *pepsis,* digestion]. Secretion of pepsin in gastric juice. SEE: *apepsinia, hyperpepsinia, hypopepsinia.*

pepsinogen (pĕp-sĭn'ō-jĕn) [″ + *gennan,* to produce]. A gastric ferment that is converted into pepsin in the stomach during digestion.

pepsinum (pĕp-sī'nŭm) [L. digestion]. A ferment in the gastric juice which hydrolyzes protein into proteoses and peptones in presence of an acid. SYN: *pepsin, q.v.*

peptarnis (pĕp-tar'nĭs) [G. *peptein,* to digest]. Preparation of beef peptones.

peptenzyme (pĕpt-ĕn'zīm) [″ + *en,* in, + *zymē,* leaven]. Commercial digestive stimulant made of gastric glands.

peptic (pĕp'tĭk) [G. *peptein,* to digest]. 1. Concerning digestion. 2. Concerning pepsin.

p. cells. Those of the gastric glands secreting pepsin.

p. ulcer. A gastric or duodenal ulcer.
ETIOL: Arises without obvious exciting cause, but is probably due to the digestive action of highly acid gastric juice on a part of the stomach, whose nutrition has been impaired by some local disturbance of the circulation; anemia; trauma; focal infection. Has been found in many cases of brain lesions, and worry is not only a predisposing cause but a retarding influence upon recovery from digestive erosions. There seems to be a decided correlation between this condition and the nervous system. Emotional strain and overwork are important factors to be considered. The worriers, the excitable and emotional types are prone to digestive ulcers.
Ulcer is round or oval, usually at pylorus or duodenum, on post. wall, near lesser curvature; has punched out appearance.
SYM: General symptoms of dyspepsia; loss of flesh and strength. Severe pain increased by eating; may radiate to back; may be paroxysmal; may be worse in certain positions. Local tenderness. Persistent vomiting after partaking of food; gastric juice unnaturally acid. Hemorrhage is common; varies from trace to quart or more. In some cases only symptoms of dyspepsia present. In others all symptoms may be absent and hemorrhage or perforation first indication.

peptide   P-34   **percolation**

PROG: Guardedly favorable. Hemorrhage or perforation may occur without warning and relapses from new ulcers not uncommon.

NP: Alkalinization. Banthine or probanthine. Bed rest, at first, in calm, quiet atmosphere. Daily bath and oral hygiene. Watch for complications of hemorrhage and perforation. Examine vomitus and stools for blood. In hemorrhage, ice cap over epigastric area, no food or fluid by mouth, no movement. Report pain immediately as it is first sign of perforation.

TREATMENT: Absolute rest in bed, alkaline Sippy treatment. Mucin therapy, metaphen and iron therapy in presence of hemorrhage. Lavage contraindicated. Stomach cleansed by sipping hot water before breakfast. Hemorrhage requires absolute rest, ice bag to stomach; pellets of ice by mouth. Remedies as indicated.

DIET: Frequent feedings; bland, smooth, liquid or semi-liquid foods; high protein feedings to keep the acid in combination; high fat to inhibit acid secretion and increase energy value of food; alkaline powders at intervals bet. feedings to combine with HCl to keep stomach neutral. In acute ulcer, Sippy diet recommended, q.v. With normal progress, after 1 week at the most, soft, bland foods; purée of vegetable and fruit; custards, and toast may be added. Number of feedings is decreased if increased amount is given at each feeding and intervals of feeding extended to 6 small meals a day, each to consist of from 10 to 12 oz. Diet should be low in cellulose. SYN: *gastric ulcer.*

peptide (pĕp′tĭd) [G. *peptein*, to digest]. Compound formed by hydrolytic cleavage of peptones and which contains 2 or more amino acids.

A class of substances prepared by synthesis from amino acids and intermediate in molecular weight and chemical properties bet. the amino acids, which may be made artificially, and the proteins, which may not.

RS: *dipeptide, polypeptide, tripeptide.*

peptidolytic (pĕp″tĭd-ō-lĭt′ĭk) [″ + *lysis*, dissolution]. Causing the splitting up or digestion of peptides.

peptinotoxin (pĕp-tĭn-ō-tŏk′sĭn) [″ + *toxikon*, poison]. Poisonous ptomaine found in the body as a result of disordered or defective digestion.

peptization (pĕp-tĭ-zā′shŭn) [G. *peptein*, to digest]. In the chemistry of colloids, the process of making a colloidal solution more stable; conversion of a gel to a sol.

peptize (pĕp′tīz) [G. *peptein*, to digest]. To disperse an insoluble material to a colloidal solution.

peptogenic, peptogenous (pĕp-tō-jĕn′ĭk, -tŏj′ĕn-ŭs) [″ + *gennan*, to produce]. 1. Producing peptones. 2. Promoting digestion.

peptoid (pĕp′toyd) [″ + *eidos*, resemblance]. A product of protein digestion which does not give the biuret reaction.

peptolysis (pĕp-tŏl′ĭ-sĭs) [G. *peptein*, to digest, + *lysis*, dissolution]. The splitting up or hydrolysis of peptones.

peptolytic (pĕp-tō-lĭt′ĭk) [″ + *lysis*, dissolution]. Pert. to the splitting up of peptone.

peptone (pĕp′tōn) [G. *peptōn*, digesting]. Secondary protein formed through the action of gastric (pepsin) and pancreatic (trypsin) juices on albumins.

They are nitrogenous compounds soluble in water and are not coagulated by boiling.

RS: *amphopeptone, hemipeptone, peptide, protein, proteose.*

peptonemia (pĕp-tō-nē′mĭ-ă) [″ + *aima*, blood]. Peptones in the blood.

peptonization (pĕp″tō-nĭ-zā′shŭn) [G. *peptōn*, digesting]. Process of changing protein substance into peptones by action of proteolytic enzymes.

peptonized milk (pĕp′tō-nīzd) [G. *peptōn*, digesting]. This is milk that has been predigested by the addition of pancreatic extract and sodium bicarbonate, before feeding, to prevent formation of tough curds in stomach.

To make peptonized milk, take 250 cc. of milk and add contents of a Fairchild's peptonizing tube. Stir the mixture thoroughly and set aside in a warm place for 20 minutes. The mixture should not be boiled, but should be set in a pan of very hot water to heat when ready to use.

1. Another formula is the following: Dissolve 1 Fairchild peptonizing powder in 4 oz. of cold water to which 12 oz. of fresh milk should be added. This should be placed in a water bath at 105° F. for 15 minutes and then placed on ice for use.

2. Another combination is peptonized milk. 3 ounces, with 1 egg stirred into it. The egg should be cut with a spoon or scissors, but never beaten. It may be added with salt to the milk.

peptonoid (pĕp′tō-noyd) [G. *peptein*, to digest]. A substance similar to a peptone.

peptonuria (pĕp-tō-nū′rĭ-ă) [″ + *ouron*, urine]. Excretion of peptones in the urine.

peptotoxin (pĕp″tō-tŏks′ĭn) [″ + *toxikon*, poison]. A poisonous product found in an early stage of protein decomposition.

per- [L.]. Prefix meaning *through, by, by means of.* In chemistry, the *maximum of an element in a combination.*

peracidity (pŭr-ăs-ĭd′ĭt-ĭ) [L. *per*, throughout, + *acidus*, sour]. Abnormal acidity.

peracute (pŭr-ăk-ūt′) [″ + *acutus*, keen]. Very acute or violent.

per anum (pŭr ā′nŭm) [L.]. Through or by way of the anus.

percaine (pŭr′kā-ĭn). A quinoline derivative used as a local anesthetic, which is powerful and toxic.

perception (pŭr-sĕp′shŭn) [L. *perceptiō*, a seeing through]. 1. Process of being aware of objects; consciousness. 2. The process of receiving sensory impressions. 3. The elaboration of a sensory impression; the ideational association modifying, defining, and usually completing the primary impression or stimulus.

Vague or inadequate association occurs in confused and depressed persons.

RS: *aphose, bradyesthesia, chirokinesthesia, phose, word center.*

perceptivity (pŭr-sĕp-tĭv′ĭ-tĭ) [L. *perceptus*, from *percipere*, to see through]. Power to receive sense impressions.

percolate (pŭr′kō-lāt) [L. *percolāre*, to strain through]. 1. To seep through a powdered substance. 2. Any fluid that has been filtered or percolated. 3. To strain a fluid through powdered substances in order to impregnate it with soluble principles of such substances.

percolation (pŭr″kō-lā′shŭn) [L. *percolāre*, to strain through]. 1. Filtration. 2. Process of exhausting virtues of a drug of powdered composition by filtering a liquid solvent through it.

percolator (pŭr'kō-lā″tŭr) [L. *percolāre*, to strain through]. Apparatus used for extraction of a drug with a liquid solvent.

per contiguum (pŭr kŏn-tĭg'ū-ŭm) [L.]. Touching, as in the spread of an inflammation from 1 part to a contiguous structure.

per continuum (pŭr kŏn-tĭn'ū-ŭm) [L.]. Continuous, as the spread of an inflammation from part to part.

percuss (pŭr-kŭs') [L. *percussus*, from *percutere*, to strike through]. To tap parts of the body to aid diagnosis by sound emitted.

percussion (pŭr-kŭsh'ŭn) [L. *percussiō*, a striking through]. Tapping the body lightly but sharply to determine position, size and consistency of an underlying structure, the presence of fluid or pus in a cavity and resonance, pitch and resistance by the sound emitted.

Immediate percussion is performed by striking the surface directly with the fingers. Not often employed except over the clavicles where bones themselves act as pleximeters.

Mediate p. is performed by using fingers of one hand as a plexor, and those of the opposite hand as a pleximeter, or using a piece of glass, ivory, or hard rubber as a pleximeter and small hammer as plexor. Use of fingers preferable, as only in this way can resistance be determined.

RS: *abdomen, bladder, boxnote, chest, heart, intestines, kidney, liver, ovary, palpation, spleen, uterus.*

p., auscultatory. Percussion combined with auscultation.

p., finger. Striking of the finger resting upon the body with a finger of the other hand.

percussor (pŭr-kŭs'or) [L. striker]. Device used for diagnosis by percussion, consisting of hammer with rubber or metal head. SEE: *emballometer*.

percutaneous (pŭr″kū-tā'nē-ŭs) [L. *per*, through, + *cutis*, skin]. Effected through the skin, as in inunction and friction.

pereirine (pĕ-rā'rēn). An alkaloid obtained from pereira bark which is used as a tonic, antiperiodic, and antipyretic.

perflation (pŭr-flā'shŭn) [L. *perflāre*, to blow through]. The process of blowing air into a cavity to expand its walls or to force out secretions or other matter.

perforans (pŭr'fō'rāns) [L. boring through]. Perforating or penetrating, as a nerve or muscle.

perforate (pŭr'fō-rāt) [L. *perforāre*, to pierce through]. 1. To puncture or to make holes. 2. Pierced with holes.

perforation (pŭr″fō-rā'shŭn) [L. *perforāre*, to pierce through]. 1. The act or process of making a hole, such as that caused by ulceration. 2. Hole made through substance or part.

p. of stomach or intestine. SYM: Abdominal crisis due to escape of contents of the perforated viscus into the peritoneal cavity. Peritonitis certain unless operated upon in time. Onset is accompanied by acute pain over perforated area spreading all over the abdomen which is rigid. Face is anxious with beads of perspiration on it. Nausea and vomiting will occur. Pulse rapid and feeble, respiration rapid and shallow. Temperature drops, but rises as peritonitis sets in, when pulse becomes fuller.

TREATMENT: Surgical. Pending operation give no fluids. Complete rest. No talking. Apply warmth. SEE: *peritonitis*.

perforator (pŭr'fō-rā-tor) [L. a piercing device]. Instrument for piercing the skull and other bones.

p., tympanum. Instrument for perforating the tympanum.

perfrication (pŭr-frĭ-kā'shŭn) [L. *perfricāre*, to rub]. Thorough rubbing with an ointment or embrocation. SYN: *inunction*.

perfusion (pŭr-fū'zhŭn) [L. *perfundere*, to pour through]. Passing of a fluid through spaces.

peri- [G.]. Prefix meaning *around, about*.

periacinal, periacinous (pĕr″ĭ-ăs'ĭ-năl, -ŭs) [G. *peri*, around, + L. *acinus*, grape]. Placed around an acinus.

periadenitis (pĕr-ĭ-ă-dē-nī'tĭs) [" + *adēn*, gland, + *-itis*, inflammation]. Inflamed condition of tissues surrounding a gland.

perialienitis (pĕr″ĭ-ā″lĭ-ĕn-ī'tĭs) [" + L. *alienus*, foreign, + G. *-itis*, inflammation]. Noninfectious inflammation around a foreign body. SYN: *perixenitis*.

periamygdalitis (pĕr″ĭ-ăm-ĭg″dăl-ī'tĭs) [" + *amygdalē*, tonsil, + *-itis*, inflammation]. Inflammation of connective tissue around the tonsil. SYN: *peritonsillitis*.

periangiocholitis (pĕr″ĭ-ăn″jĭ-ō-kō-lī'tĭs) [" + *aggeion*, vessel, + *cholē*, bile, + *-itis*, inflammation]. Inflamed condition of tissues around the bile ducts.

periangitis (pĕr″ĭ-ăn-jī'tĭs) [" + " + *-itis*, inflammation]. Inflamed condition of tissue around a blood or lymphatic vessel.

periaortitis (pĕr″ĭ-ā-or-tī'tĭs) [" + *aorte*, aorta, + *-itis*, inflammation]. Inflamed condition of adventitia and tissues around the aorta.

periapical (pĕr″ĭ-ăp'ĭ-kăl) [G. *peri*, around, + L. *apex*, tip]. Around the apex of the root of a tooth.

periappendicitis (pĕr″ĭ-ă-pĕn-dĭ-sī'tĭs) [" + L. *appendix*, that which hangs, + G. *-itis*, inflammation]. Inflamed condition of appendix with its surrounding tissues. SYN: *perityphlitis*.

p. decidualis. Decidual cells in the peritoneum of the appendix vermiformis in cases of tubal pregnancy due to adhesions bet. fallopian tubes and the appendix.

periarterial (pĕr″ĭ-ar-tē'rĭ-ăl) [" + *artēria*, artery]. Placed around an artery.

periarteritis (pĕr″ĭ-ar-tĕr-ī'tĭs) [" + " + *-itis*, inflammation]. Inflammation of ext. coat of an artery.

p. gummosa. Gummas in the blood vessels in syphilis.

p. nodosa. A multiple, circumscribed inflammation of an outer arterial coat resulting in the formation of nodules along its course.

periarthric (per″ĭ-ar'thrĭk) [" + *arthron*, joint]. Surrounding a joint. SYN: *circumarticular*.

periarthritis (pĕr″ĭ-ar-thrī'tĭs) [" + *arthron*, joint, + *-itis*, inflammation]. Inflammation of area around a joint.

periarticular (pĕr″ĭ-ar-tĭk'ū-lăr) [" + L. *articulus*, a joint]. Surrounding a joint. SYN: *circumarticular*.

periaxial (pĕr-ĭ-ăks'ĭ-ăl) [" + *axēn*, axis]. Located around an axis.

periaxillary (pĕr″ĭ-ăk'sĭl-ĕ-rī) [G. *peri*, around, + L. *axilla*, armpit]. About the axilla.

periblast (pĕr'ĭ-blăst) [" + *blastos*, germ].

peribronchiolitis

Protoplasm around a cell nucleus. SYN: *periplast*.
peribronchiolitis (pĕr″ĭ-brŏng″kĭ-ō-lī′tĭs) [" + L. *bronchiolus*, bronchiole, + *-itis*, inflammation]. Inflammation of area around the bronchioles.
peribronchitis (pĕr″ĭ-brŏng-kī′tĭs) [" + *brogchos*, windpipe, + *-itis*, inflammation]. Inflammation of all tissues surrounding the bronchi or bronchial tubes.
pericardiac, pericardial (pĕr-ĭ-kar′dĭ-ăk, -ăl) [" + *kardia*, heart]. Concerning the pericardium.
pericardicentesis (pĕr″ĭ-kar″dĭ-sĕn-tē′sĭs) [" + *kardia*, heart, + *kentēsis*, puncture]. Surgical piercing of the pericardium.
pericardiectomy (pĕr″ĭ-kar-dĭ-ĕk′tō-mĭ) [" + " + *ektomē*, excision]. Excision of part or all of the pericardium.
pericardiocentesis (pĕr″ĭ-kar″dĭ-ō-sĕn-tē′sĭs) [G. *peri*, around, + *kardia*, heart, + *kentēsis*, puncture]. Surgical perforation of the pericardium. SYN: *pericardicentesis*.
pericardiolysis (pĕr″ĭ-kar″dĭ-ŏl′ĭ-sĭs) [" + " + *lysis*, dissolution]. Separation of adhesions bet. the visceral and parietal pericardium.
pericardiomediastinitis (pĕr″ĭ-kar″dĭ-ō-mē-dĭ-ăs″tĭ-nī′tĭs) [" + " + L. *mediastinum* + G. *-itis*, inflammation]. Inflamed condition of the pericardium and mediastinum.
pericardiophrenic (pĕr-ĭ-kar″dĭ-ō-fren′ĭk) [" + " + *phrēn*, diaphragm]. Concerning the pericardium and diaphragm.
pericardiopleural (pĕr″ĭ-kar″dĭ-ō-plū′răl) [" + " + *pleura*, rib]. Concerning the pericardium and pleura.
pericardiorrhaphy (pĕr″ĭ-kar″dĭ-or′ă-fī) [" + " + *raphē*, a sewing]. Suture of a wound in the pericardium.
pericardiostomy (pĕr″ĭ-kar″dĭ-ŏs′tō-mĭ) [G. *peri*, around, + *kardia*, heart, + *stoma*, opening]. Formation of an opening into the pericardium for drainage.
pericardiosymphysis (pĕr″ĭ-kar″dĭ-ō-sĭm′fĭ-sĭs) [" + " + *symphysis*, a joining]. Adhesion bet. the layers of the pericardium.
pericardiotomy (pĕr″ĭ-kar-dĭ-ŏt′ō-mĭ) [" + " + *tomē*, a cutting]. Incision of membranous sac around heart.
pericarditic (pĕr-ĭ-kar-dĭt′ĭk) [" + *kardia*, heart]. Concerning the pericardium.
pericarditis (pĕr-ĭ-kar-dī′tĭs) [G. *peri*, around, + *kardia*, heart, + *-itis*, inflammation]. Inflammation of pericardium.

SYM: Moderate fever, precordial pain and tenderness, dry cough, dyspnea and palpitation. Pulse, first rapid, forcible, then weak and irregular.

First stage: Auscultation reveals to and fro friction sound heart over 4th left intercostal space near sternum. Inspection and palpation sometimes reveal a diffuse apex beat. Friction rub may sometimes be palpated.

Second stage: Serofibrinous effusion. Bulging of precordium. Increased area of dullness, triangular in shape, base down. Heart sounds muffled, distant, feeble. Purulent effusion yields similar signs, but in addition high, irregular fever; sweats; chills, and progressive pallor; sometimes edema over the precordium. In doubtful cases the aspirating needle reveals pus.

PROG: Fair in early stages. In purulent and fibrinous, extremely grave.

TREATMENT: In severe cases, apply leeches, ice bag poultice; absolute rest; light diet; internal remedies; aspiration of fluid when present in large quantity.
p. adhesiva. Form in which the layers of pericardium adhere.
p. callosa. A chronic form with signs of obstructed return flow of venous blood to the heart, but with no other symptoms.
p. externa. Inflammation of exterior surface of the pericardium.
p., fibrinous. Membrane is covered with butterlike exudate which organizes and unites the pericardial surfaces.

SYM: Precordial bulging, a weak apex beat with loud sounds, a systolic retraction at apex and over large part of precordium, peculiar diastolic collapse of jugular veins, feeble apex beat with a forcible impulse over body of heart. Signs of heart failure, as dyspnea, dropsy, cyanosis.
p. obliterans. Pericardial inflammation causing adhesions and obliteration of the pericardial cavity.
pericardium (pĕr″ĭ-kar′dĭ-ŭm) [G. *peri*, around, + *kardia*, heart]. The double, membranous, cone-shaped, fibroserous sac enclosing the heart and the roots of the great blood vessels.

It is composed of a serous inner layer and a fibrinous outer layer.

Its base is attached to the diaphragm, its apex extending upward as far as the first subdivision of the great blood vessels. It is attached in front to the sternum, laterally to the mediastinal pleura and posteriorly to the esophagus, trachea, and principal bronchi.

Normally, p. contains a thin serous fluid.

RS: *Broadbent's sign, camera cordis, cardiopericarditis, cardiosymphysis, chylopericarditis, hydropericardium,* "*pericard-*" words.
p. externum. The outer fibrous layer of the pericardium.
p. internum. Serous inner layer of the pericardium.
pericardosis (pĕr″ĭ-kar-dō′sĭs) [" + " + *-ōsis*, disease]. Bacterial infection of the pericardium.
pericecal (pĕr-ĭ-sē′kăl) [" + L. *caecum*, blind]. Situated around the cecum.
pericecitis (pĕr-ĭ-sē-sī′tĭs) [" + " + G. *-itis*, inflammation]. Inflamed condition of area around the cecum. SYN: *perityphlitis*.
pericementitis (pĕr″ĭ-sĕm-ĕn-tī′tĭs) [" + L. *caementum*, cement, + G. *-itis*, inflammation]. Progressive necrosis of the alveoli of the teeth. SYN: *periodontitis*.
pericementoclasia (pĕr″ĭ-sĕm-ĕn-tō-klā′zĭ-ă) [" + " + G. *klasis*, a breaking]. Dissolution of the pericementum with alveolar absorption. SYN: *pyorrhea alveolaris*.
pericementum (pĕr″ĭ-sĕm-ĕn′tŭm) [" + L. *caementum*, cement]. Fibrous tissue covering the root of a tooth.
pericholangitis (pĕr″ĭ-kō-lăn-jī′tĭs) [G. *peri*, around, + *cholē*, bile, + *aggeion*, vessel, + *-itis*, inflammation]. Inflammation of tissues surrounding a bile duct. SYN: *periangiocholitis*.
pericholecystitis (pĕr″ĭ-kō-lē-sĭs-tī′tĭs) [" + " + *kystis*, a sac, + *-itis*, inflammation]. Inflammation of tissues situated around the gallbladder.
perichondral, perichondrial (pĕr-ĭ-kon′drăl, -drī′ăl) [" + *chondros*, cartilage]. Concerning the membrane covering cartilage.
perichondritis (pĕr″ĭ-kŏn-drī′tĭs) [" + "

perichondrium   P-37   **perilymphangitis**

+ -*itis*, inflammation]. Inflamed condition of perichondrium.
perichondrium (pĕr-ĭ-kŏn'drĭ-ŭm) [" + *chondros*, cartilage]. Membrane of fibrous connective tissue around surface of cartilage.
perichondroma (pĕr"ĭ-kŏn-drō'mă) [" + " + -*ōma*, tumor]. A tumor arising from fibrous tissue which covers cartilage.
perichordal (pĕr-ĭ-kor'dăl) [" + *chordē*, cord]. Placed around the notochord.
perichorioidal, perichoroidal (pĕr"ĭ-kō-rĭ-oy'dăl, -roy'dăl) [G. *peri*, around, + *chorioeidēs*, skinlike]. Situated around the choroid coat.
perichrome (pĕr'ĭ-krōm) [" + *chrōma*, color]. A nerve cell in which the tigroid mass is arranged in rows through the protoplasm.
pericolic (pĕr-ĭ-ko'lĭk) [" + *kōlon*, colon]. Around or encircling the colon.
pericolitis (pĕr"ĭ-kō-lī'tĭs) [" + " + -*ītis*, inflammation]. Inflammation of area around the colon.
pericolonitis (pĕr"ĭ-kō-lŏn-ī'tĭs) [" + " + -*ītis*, inflammation]. Inflamed condition of region around the colon.
pericolpitis (pĕr"ĭ-kŏl-pī'tĭs) [" + *kolpos*, vagina, + -*ītis*, inflammation]. Inflammation of connective tissues surrounding the vagina.
periconchal (pĕr-ĭ-kŏng'kăl) [" + *cogchē*, concha]. Around the concha of the ear.
    p. sulcus. Groove on post. surface of the auricle.
periconchitis (pĕr"ĭ-kŏng-kī'tĭs) [" + " + -*ītis*, inflammation]. Inflamed condition of the lining of the orbit.
pericorneal (pĕr"ĭ-kor'nē-ăl) [G. *peri*, around, + L. *cornu*, horn]. Placed around the cornea.
pericranitis (pĕr"ĭ-krā-nī'tĭs) [" + *kranion*, skull, + -*ītis*, inflammation]. Inflamed condition of pericranium.
pericranium (pĕr"ĭ-krā'nĭ-ŭm) [" + *kranion*, skull]. Fibrous membrane surrounding the skull bone; periosteum of the skull.
    p. internum. Lining surface of the skull. Syn: *endocranium*.
pericystitis (pĕr"ĭ-sĭs-tī'tĭs) [" + *kystis*, a bladder, + -*ītis*, inflammation]. Inflamed condition of tissues about the bladder.
pericytial (pĕr-ĭ-sĭsh'ăl) [" + *kytos*, cell]. Placed around a cell.
peridectomy (pĕr-ĭ-dĕk'tō-mĭ) [" + *ektomē*, excision]. 1. Operation for relief of pannus. 2. Circumcision. Syn: *peritomy*.
peridendric (pĕr-ĭ-dĕn'drĭk) [" + *dendron*, a tree]. Surrounding a dendrite of a nerve cell.
peridental (pĕr-ĭ-dĕn'tăl) [G. *peri*, around, + L. *dens*, *dent*-, tooth]. Surrounding a tooth or part of one. Syn: *periodontal*.
peridentoclasia (pĕr"ĭ-dĕn-tō-klā'zĭ-ă) [" + " + G. *klasis*, a breaking]. Breaking down of tissues about the teeth.
peridesmitis (pĕr"ĭ-dĕz-mī'tĭs) [" + *desmos*, band, + -*ītis*, inflammation]. Inflammation of the areolar tissue around a ligament.
peridesmium (pĕr"ĭ-dĕz'mĭ-ŭm) [" + *desmos*, band]. The connective tissue membrane sheathing a ligament.
peridiastole (pĕr-ĭ-dī-ăs'tō-lē) [" + *diastolē*, a setting apart]. Interval before onset of the diastole following the systole.
perididymis (pĕr-ĭ-dĭd'ĭ-mĭs) [" + *didymos*, testicle]. The tunica albuginea of testicles.
perididymitis (pĕr"ĭ-dĭd"ĭ-mī'tĭs) [" + "

+ -*ītis*, inflammation]. Inflammation of tunica albuginea of the testicles.
peridiverticulitis (pĕr"ĭ-dī-vĕr-tĭk"ū-lī'tĭs) [G. *peri*, around, + L. *diverticulāre*, to turn aside, + G. -*ītis*, inflammation]. Inflammation of tissues situated around an intestinal diverticulum.
periductal (pĕr-ĭ-duk'tăl) [" + L. *ductus*, a passage]. Situated about a duct.
periduodenitis (pĕr"ĭ-dŭ"o-dē-nī'tĭs) [" + L. *duodeni*, twelve, + -*ītis*, inflammation]. Inflammation around the duodenum due to adhesions attaching it to the peritoneum.
periencephalitis (pĕr"ĭ-ĕn-sĕf-ă-lī'tĭs) [" + *egkephalos*, brain, + -*ītis*, inflammation]. Inflamed condition of the surface of the brain.
periencephalomeningitis (pĕr"ĭ-ĕn-sĕf-ă-lō-mĕn-ĭn-jī'tĭs) [" + " + *mēnigx*, membrane, + -*ītis*, inflammation]. Inflamed condition of cerebral cortex and the meninges.
periendothelioma (pĕr"ĭ-ĕn"dō-thē-lĭ-ō'mă) [" + *endon*, within, + *thēlē*, nipple, + -*ōma*, tumor]. A tumor arising from the endothelium of the lymphatics and the perithelium of blood vessels.
perienteritis (pĕr"ĭ-ĕn-tĕr-ī'tĭs) [G. *peri*, around, + *enteron*, intestines, + -*ītis*, inflammation]. Inflamed condition of peritoneal lining of intestines.
periepithelioma (pĕr"ĭ-ĕp"ĭ-thē"lĭ-ō'mă) [" + *epi*, upon, + *thēlē*, nipple, + -*ōma*, tumor]. A tumor arising in the endothelial lining of blood vessels or lymphatics, as that of the suprarenal body.
periesophagitis (pĕr"ĭ-ē-sŏf-ă-jī'tĭs) [" + *oisophagos*, esophagus, + -*ītis*, inflammation]. Inflamed condition of tissues around the esophagus.
perifistular (pĕr-ĭ-fĭs'tū-ler) [" + L. *fistula*, pipe]. Located around a fistula.
perifolliculitis (pĕr"ĭ-fō-lĭk"ū-lī'tĭs) [" + L. *folliculus*, a little sac, + -*ītis*, inflammation]. Inflamed condition of area around the hair follicles.
perigangliitis (pĕr"ĭ-găng-lĭ-ī'tĭs) [" + *gagglion*, knot, + -*ītis*, inflammation]. Inflamed condition of region around a ganglion.
perigastritis (pĕr"ĭ-găs-trī'tĭs) [" + *gastēr*, belly, + -*ītis*, inflammation]. Inflammation of peritoneal lining of stomach.
periglottis (pĕr-ĭ-glŏt'tĭs) [G. *peri*, around, + *glōtta*, tongue]. The mucosa covering of the tongue.
perihepatitis (pĕr"ĭ-hĕp-ă-tī'tĭs) [" + *ēpar*, *ēpat*-, liver, + -*ītis*, inflammation]. Inflammation of peritoneal covering of the liver, usually occurring in circumscribed areas.
perijejunitis (pĕr"ĭ-jĕj-ū-nī'tĭs) [" + L. *jejunum*, empty, + G. -*ītis*, inflammation]. Inflamed condition of tissues around the jejunum.
perikaryon (pĕr"ĭ-kăr'ĭ-ŏn) [" + *karyon*, nucleus]. Nerve cell exclusive of the nucleus.
perilabyrinthitis (pĕr"ĭ-lăb-ĭr-ĭn-thī'tĭs) [" + *labyrinthos*, a maze, + -*ītis*, inflammation]. Inflammation of tissues and parts about the labyrinth.
perilaryngitis (pĕr"ĭ-lăr-ĭn-jī'tĭs) [" + *larygx*, larynx, + -*ītis*, inflammation]. Inflamed condition of tissues around the larynx.
perilymph (pĕr-ĭ-lĭmf) [" + L. *lympha*, serum]. The pale, limpid fluid contained in the space bet. the membranous and bony labyrinth of the internal ear.
perilymphangitis (pĕr"ĭ-lĭmf-ăn-jī'tĭs) [G. *peri*, around, + L. *lympha*, serum, +

perimeningitis   P-38   **perineurial**

aggeion, vessel, + *-itis*, inflammation]. Inflammation of tissues around a lymphatic vessel.

perimeningitis (pĕr″ĭ-mĕn-ĭn-jī′tĭs) [" + *meningx*, membrane, + *-itis*, inflammation]. Inflamed condition of the dura mater. SYN: *pachymeningitis*.

perimeter (pĕr-ĭm′ĕt-ēr) [" + *metron*, measure]. 1. The outer edge or periphery of a body or measure of the same. 2. Device for determining the extent of the field of vision.

perimetric (pĕr-ĭ-mĕt′rĭk) [" + *metron*, measure]. Concerning the outer surface of a body.

perimetritis (pĕr″ĭ-me-trī′tĭs) [" + *metra*, uterus, + *-itis*, inflammation]. Inflammation of the peritoneal covering of the uterus.

May be associated with parametritis.

perimetrium (pĕr-ĭ-mē′trĭ-ŭm) [" + *metra*, uterus]. Peritoneum covering uterus.

perimetry (pĕr-ĭm′ĕ-trĭ) [" + *metron*, measure]. 1. Circumference, edge, border of a body. 2. Measurement of the scope of the field of vision with a perimeter.

perimyelitis (pĕr″ĭ-mī-ē-lī′tĭs) [" + *myelos*, marrow, + *-itis*, inflammation]. 1. Inflammation of the pia mater and arachnoid of the brain or spinal cord. SYN: *leptomeningitis*. 2. Inflammation of the endosteum, or membrane around medullary cavity of a bone.

perimyelography (pĕr″ĭ-mī-ē-lŏg′ră-fĭ) [" + " + *graphein*, to write]. X-ray examination around the spinal cord.

perimyoendocarditis (pĕr″ĭ-mī″ō-ĕn″dō-kar-dī′tĭs) [" + *mys*, *my-*, muscle, + *endon*, within, + *kardia*, heart, + *-itis*, inflammation]. Inflammation of the muscular wall of the heart, its epithelial lining and the membrane surrounding it.

perimysial (pĕr-ĭ-mĭs′ĭ-ăl) [G. *peri*, around, + *mys*, muscle]. Concerning, or of the nature of, perimysium; sheathing a muscle.

perimysiitis (pĕr-ĭ-mĭs-ĭ-ī′tĭs) [" + " + *-itis*, inflammation]. Inflamed condition of the perimysium, the sheath surrounding a muscle.

perimysium (pĕr-ĭ-mĭs′ĭ-ŭm) [" + *mys*, muscle]. The connective tissue sheath that envelops each primary bundle of muscle fiber.

perineal (pĕr-ĭ-nē′ăl) [G. *perinaion*, perineum]. Concerning or situated on the perineum.

   p. body. Mass of tissue composed of skin, muscle, and fascia bet. vagina and rectum in the female, and the urethra and rectum in the male. [of perineum.
   p. fascia. Three layers bet. muscles
   p. hernia. Hernia perforating the perineum. SYN: *perineocele*.
   p. section. Surgical incision through perineum. SYN: *perineotomy*.

perineo- [G.]. Combining form for *region bet. the anus and the scrotum, or the vulva.*

perineocele (pĕr-ĭ-nē′ō-sēl) [G. *perinaion*, perineum, + *kēlē*, hernia]. Hernia in the region of the perineum.

perineocolporectomyomectomy (pĕr-ĭ-nē″ō-kŏl″pō-rĕk″tō-mī-ō-mĕk′tō-mĭ) [" + *kolpos*, vagina, + L. *rectus*, straight, + G. *mys*, *myo-*, muscle, + *-oma*, tumor, + *ektomē*, excision]. Excision of a myoma by incising the perineum, vagina, and rectum.

perineoplasty (pĕr-ĭ-nē′ō-plăs″tĭ) [" + *plassein*, to form]. Reparative surgery on the perineum.

perineorrhaphy (pĕr″ĭ-nē-ŏr′ă-fĭ) [" + *raphē*, a sewing]. Suture of the perineum usually following labor.

NP: After operation a towel should be pinned around the limbs to hold them in position until anesthetic wears away. Give external irrigation to perineum following each use of bedpan as sepsis must be avoided. Keep stitches dry, sterile dressing secured with a T-bandage which may be removed for urination. Swab with antiseptic, dry and put on fresh dressing. Warm glycerin packs are sometimes ordered to relieve pain and reduce edema.

It is difficult for patient to assume a comfortable position in which to lie. Prop up first on one and then the other side. The patient cannot sit upright. Keep bowels from acting during first 5 days. Fluid diet and light jellies. After 5th day a mild aperient. 4-5 oz. of warm olive oil per rectum before aperient acts. Warn against straining. Stitches removed about 12th day.

   p., anterior. Rectifying cystocele.*
   p., colpo-. Removal of part of post. vaginal wall and suturing torn perineal body.
   p., posterior. Removal of rectocele.

perineosynthesis (pĕr-ĭ-nē″ō-sĭn′the-sĭs) [" + *synthesis*, a placing together]. Plastic operation for repair of a lacerated perineum; performed by grafting vaginal mucosa over area.

perineotomy (pĕr″ĭ-nē-ŏt′ō-mĭ) [" + *tomē*, a cutting]. Operation of incising the perineum.

perineovaginal (pĕr-ĭ-nē″ō-văj′ĭn-ăl) [" + L. *vagina*, sheath]. Concerning the perineum and vagina.

perinephric (pĕr-ĭ-nĕf′rĭk) [G. *peri*, around, + *nephros*, kidney]. Located or occurring around the kidney.
   p. abscess. Abscess formation in peritoneal membrane surrounding the kidney.

perinephritis (pĕr″ĭ-ne-frī′tĭs) [" + " + *-itis*, inflammation]. Inflammation of peritoneal tissues around the kidney. SYN: *paranephritis*.

perinephrium (pĕr-ĭ-nĕf′rĭ-ŭm) [" + *nephros*, kidney]. The connective and fatty tissue surrounding the kidney.

perineum (pĕr-ĭ-nē′ŭm) [G. *perinaion*, perineum]. The space lying bet. the vulva and the anus in the female; bet. scrotum and the anus in male. Structures comprising the pelvic floor occupying the outlet of the pelvis.

It is made up of skin, muscle and fasciae. The muscles of the perineum are the ant. portion of the intact levator ani muscle, the transverse perineal muscle and the sphincter muscles of the vagina. RS: *bodies, perineal, "perine-" words.*

   p., tears of the. There are 3 degrees of severity, being caused by overstretching of vagina and perineum in delivery, malposition increasing the tears.

COMPLICATIONS: Hemorrhage, infection, cystocele, rectocele, descent of uterus, perhaps loss of bowel control.

TREATMENT: Surgery.

NP: Spray wound after each urination and bowel movement with mild antiseptic solution. Compound licorice at night, enema every morning in 3rd degree tears. Anal stitches removed the 12th day. Dressing of balsam of Peru in castor oil.

   p., watering-pot. One riddled with fistulas from urethral stricture.

perineurial (pĕr″ĭ-nu-rī′ăl) [G. *peri*, around, + *neuron*, sinew]. Concerning

perineuritis

the perineurium, the sheath around a bundle of nerve fibers.

perineuritis (pĕr″ĭ-nū-rī'tĭs) [" + " + -itis, inflammation]. Inflammation of the sheath enveloping nerve fibers.

perineurium (pĕr-ĭ-nū'rĭ-ŭm) [" + neuron, sinew]. Connective tissue sheath investing a nerve fiber funiculus or bundle.

periocular (pĕr-ĭ-ŏk'ŭ-ler) [" + L. oculus, eye]. Located around the eye. SYN: circumocular.

period (pēr'ĭ-ŏd) [" + odos, a way]. 1. The time during which anything or at which anything takes place, which is limited by a recurring event. 2. The menses. 3. Time occupied by a disease in running its course, or by a division of the total, as an incubation period.

p., childbearing. The p. in the female during which she is capable of procreation; puberty to the menopause.

p., incubation. Time from moment of infection until appearance of first symptom.

p., latent. 1. The time bet. stimulation and the resulting response. 2. Time bet. 4 and 11 years separating infantile sexuality from onset of puberty, the genital sexuality.

p., menstrual. Time for an individual act of menstruation.

p., neonatal. The first 30 days of infant life.

At this time the mortality of all infants under 1 yr. is greatest (67%); usual causes are prematurity, birth injuries, and sepsis.

p., puerperal. The p. bet. delivery and first menstruation thereafter; or bet. delivery and normal involution.

periodic (pēr-ĭ-ŏd'ĭk) [G. peri, around, + odos, way]. Recurring after definite intervals.

p. law. That which states that the chemical and physical properties of the chemical elements are periodic junctions of their atomic weights.

periodicity (pĕr″ĭ-ō-dĭs'ĭ-tĭ) [" + odos, way]. 1. State of being regularly recurrent. 2. PT: The rate of rise and fall or interruption of a unidirectional current. 3. Recurrence of the menses.

periodontal (pĕr″ĭ-ō-dŏn'tăl) [" + odous, odont-, tooth]. Located about a tooth.

periodontitis (pĕr″ĭ-ō-dŏn-tī'tĭs) [" + " + -itis, inflammation]. Inflammation of the tissues sheathing a tooth.

periodontium (pĕr-ĭ-ō-dŏn'shĭ-ŭm). The dental periosteum; pericementum.

periodontoclasia (pĕr″ĭ-ō-dŏn″tō-klā'zĭ-ă) [" + " + klasis, a breaking]. Dissolution of membrane around a tooth.

periodontology (pĕr″ĭ-ō-dŏn-tŏl'ō-jĭ) [" + " + logos, disease]. Phase of dentistry dealing with treatment of diseases of the tissues around the teeth.

periodoscope (pĕr″ĭ-ŏd'ō-skōp) [G. peri, around, + odos, way, + skopein, to examine]. Table or dial for calculation of expected date of confinement.

periomphalic (pĕr″ĭ-ŏm-făl'ĭk) [" + omphalos, eye]. Located around umbilicus.

perionychium (pĕr″ĭ-ō-nĭk'ĭ-ŭm) [" + onyx, onych-, nail]. The epidermis surrounding a nail.

perionyxis (pĕr″ĭ-ō-nĭk'sĭs) [" + onyx, nail]. Inflammation of epidermis surrounding a nail.

perioöphoritis (pĕr″ĭ-ō-ŏf″ō-rī'tĭs) [" + oophoron, ovary, + -itis, inflammation]. Inflammation of the surface membrane of the ovary. SYN: perioöthecitis.

perioöphorosalpingitis (pĕr″ĭ-ō-ŏf″ō-rō-săl″pĭn-jī'tĭs) [" + " + salpigx, tube, + -itis, inflammation]. Inflamed condition of tissues around an ovary and oviduct.

perioöthecitis (pĕr″ĭ-ō″o-the-sī'tĭs) [" + ōon, egg, + thēcē, box, + -itis, inflammation]. Inflammation of the peritoneal tissues around the ovary. SYN: perioöphoritis.

perioöthecosalpingitis (pĕr″ĭ-ō″o-the″kō-săl-pĭn-jī'tĭs) [G. peri, around, + thēcē, box, + salpigx, tube, + -itis, inflammation]. Inflammation of peritoneal membrane around the ovary and oviduct. SYN: perioöphorosalpingitis, perisalpingoövaritis.

perioptometry (pĕr″ĭ-op-tŏm'ĕt-rĭ) [" + optos, visible, + metron, a measure]. Measurement of the visual field.

periorbita (pĕr″ĭ-or'bĭ-tă) [" + L. orbita, orbit]. Periosteum of the socket of the eye.

periorbital (pĕr″ĭ-or'bĭ-tăl) [" + L. orbita, orbit]. Surrounding the socket of the eye. SYN: circumorbital.

periorbititis (pĕr″ĭ-or-bĭ-tī'tĭs) [" + " + G. -itis, inflammation]. Inflamed condition of the periorbita.

periorchitis (pĕr″ĭ-or-kī'tĭs) [" + orchis, testicle, + -itis, inflammation]. Inflamed condition of the tissues investing a testicle.

p. hemorrhagica. Chronic hematocele of the tunica vaginalis coat of the testis.

periosteal (pĕr″ĭ-ŏs'tē-ăl) [" + osteon, bone]. Concerning the periosteum.

periosteitis (pĕr″ĭ-ŏs-tē-ī'tĭs) [G. peri, around, + osteon, bone, + -itis, inflammation]. Inflammation of membrane investing a bone, the periosteum. SYN: periostitis.

periosteoedema (pĕr″ĭ-os″tē-ō-ĕ-dē'mă) [" + " + oidema, swelling]. Edema of the periosteum, the membrane surrounding a bone.

periosteoma (pĕr″ĭ-ŏs-tē-ō'mă) [" + " + -ōma, tumor]. 1. An abnormal growth surrounding a bone. 2. Tumor of the periosteum, the tissue surrounding a bone.

periosteomedullitis (pĕr″ĭ-os″tē-ō-mĕd-ŭ-lī'tĭs) [" + " + L. medulla, marrow, + G. -itis, inflammation]. Inflamed condition of the periosteum and of bone marrow. SYN: periosteomyelitis.

periosteomyelitis (pĕr″ĭ-ŏs″tē-ō-mī′ĕ-lī'tĭs) [" + " + myelos, marrow, + -itis, inflammation]. Inflamed condition of the marrow and investing sheath of a bone.

periosteophyte (pĕr″ĭ-ŏs'tē-ō-fīt) [" + " + phyton, growth]. Abnormal bony growth on periosteum, or arising from it.

periosteorrhaphy (pĕr″ĭ-ŏs-tē-or'ă-fĭ) [" + " + raphē, a sewing]. Joining by suture the margins of a severed periosteum.

periosteotome (pĕr″ĭ-ŏs′tē-ō-tōm) [G. peri, around, + osteon, bone, + tomē, a cutting]. Instrument for cutting the periosteum or removing it from the bone.

periosteotomy (pĕr″ĭ-ŏs-tē-ŏt'ō-mĭ) [" + " + tomē, an incision]. Incision into the periosteum.

periosteous (pĕr″ĭ-ŏs'tē-ŭs) [" + osteon, bone]. Concerning, or of the nature of, periosteum. SYN: periosteal.

periosteum (pĕr″ĭ-ŏs′tē-ŭm) [" + osteon, bone]. The fibrovascular membrane that invests and nourishes the bone.

It extends over the whole surface except at the cartilaginous articulations.

p. externum. P. covering ext. surfaces of bones.

p. internum. Int. p. lining the medullary canal of a bone.

periostitis (pĕr-ĭ-ŏs-tī'tĭs) [" + " + -itis,

periostitis, albuminous   P-40   **perisinusitis**

inflammation]. Inflamed condition of membrane investing a bone, the periosteum.
ETIOL: Infectious diseases may be responsible.
SYM: Pain over part, esp. under pressure, fever, sweats, leukocytosis, skin inflamed, rigidity of overlying muscles.

p., albuminous. P. with albuminous serous fluid exudate beneath the membrane affected.

p., alveolar. Inflammation of the peridental membrane. SYN: *periodontitis*.

p., dental. P. of a tooth sheath.

p., diffuse. P. of the long bones.

p., hemorrhagic. P. with extravasation of blood under the periosteum.

periostoma (pĕr″ĭ-ŏs-tō′mä) [G. *peri*, around, + *osteon*, bone, + -*ōma*, tumor]. A bony neoplasm around a bone or arising from its membranous sheath.

periostomedullitis (pĕr″ĭ-ŏs″tō-mĕd-ū-lī′tĭs) [" + " + L. *medulla*, marrow, + G. -*itis*, inflammation]. Inflammation of the marrow or sheath of a bone. SYN: *periosteomedullitis, periosteomyelitis*.

periostosis (pĕr″ĭ-ŏs-tō′sĭs) [" + " + -*ōsis*, disease]. A bony neoplasm around a bone or arising from it.

periostotomy (pĕr″ĭ-ŏs-tŏt′ō-mī) [" + " + *tomē*, incision]. Incision of the periosteum, the sheath covering a bone. SYN: *periosteotomy*.

periotic (pĕr-ĭ-ōt′ĭk) [" + *ous, ōt-*, ear]. Situated around the internal ear.

p. bone. The mastoid and petrous portions of the temporal bone.

peripachymeningitis (pĕr″ĭ-pak″ĭ-mĕn-ĭn-jī′tĭs) [" + *pachys*, thick, + *mēninx*, membrane, + -*itis*, inflammation]. Inflamed condition of connective tissue bet. the dura mater and the bone.

peripancreatitis (pĕr-ĭ-păn-krē-ă-tī′tĭs) [G. *peri*, around, + *pagkreas*, pancreas, + -*itis*, inflammation]. Inflammation of the peritoneal tissues covering the pancreas.

peripatetic (pĕr-ĭ-pă-tĕt′ĭk) [" + *patein*, to walk]. Moving from place to place, as in walking typhoid.

periphacitis (pĕr-ĭ-fă-sī′tĭs) [" + *phakos*, lens, + -*itis*, inflammation]. Inflamed condition of the capsule of the crystalline lens of the eye.

peripherad (pĕr-ĭf′ĕr-ăd) [" + *pherein*, to bear, + L. *ad*, to]. In the direction of the periphery.

peripheral (pĕr-ĭf′ĕr-ăl) [" + *pherein*, to bear]. Located at or pert. to the periphery.

periphery (pĕr-ĭf′ĕ-rĭ) [" + *pherein*, to bear]. Outer layer or a surface of a body; part away from the center.

periphlebitis (pĕr″ĭ-flē-bī′tĭs) [G. *peri*, around, + *phleps*, vein, + -*itis*, inflammation]. Inflamed condition of external coat of a vein or tissues around it.

periphoria (pĕr-ĭ-fō′rĭ-ă) [" + *phoros*, a bearer]. Tendency for the cornea to deviate from its normal axis. SYN: *cyclophoria*.

periphrastic (pĕr-ĭ-frăs′tĭk) [" + *phrazein*, to speak]. Relating to the use of superfluous words in expressing a thought.

periphrenitis (pĕr″ĭ-frĕn-ī′tĭs) [" + *phrēn*, diaphragm, + -*itis*, inflammation]. Inflamed condition of the structures around the diaphragm.

periplast (pĕr′ĭ-plăst) [" + *plassein*, to form]. 1. Peripheral protoplasm of a cell exclusive of the nucleus. 2. Matrix of a part or organ. 3. A cell wall. SYN: *periblast*.

peripleural (pĕr″ĭ-plū′răl) [" + *pleura*, rib]. Encircling the pleura.

peripleuritis (pĕr-ĭ-plū-rī′tĭs) [" + " + -*itis*, inflammation]. Inflamed condition of the connective tissues bet. the pleura and wall of the chest.

periplocin (pĕr-ĭp′lō-sĭn). $C_{30}H_{48}O_{12}$. Glucoside of *Periploca graeca*, used in treating diseases of the heart.

peripneumonia (pĕr″ĭp-nū-mō′nĭ-ă) [G. *peri*, around, + *pneumōn*, lung]. Inflammation of the lungs alone or in combination with pleurisy.

p. notha. Congestion of the lungs; term used by older writers.

periproctitis (pĕr″ĭ-prŏk-tī′tĭs) [" + *prōktos*, anus, + -*itis*, inflammation]. Inflammation of areolar tissues in region of the rectum and anus. SYN: *perirectitis*.

periprostatic (pĕr″ĭ-prŏs-tăt′ĭk) [" + *prostatēs*, prostate]. Surrounding or occurring about the prostate.

periprostatitis (pĕr″ĭ-prŏs-tă-tī′tĭs) [" + " + -*itis*, inflammation]. Inflamed condition of tissues surrounding the prostate.

peripylephlebitis (pĕr″ĭ-pī″le-flē-bī′tĭs) [" + *pylē*, gate, + *phleps, phleb-*, vein, + -*itis*, inflammation]. Inflamed condition of tissues about the portal vein.

peripylic (pĕr″ĭ-pī′lĭk) [" + *pylē*, gate]. Situated around the portal vein.

peripyloric (pĕr″ĭ-pī-lor′ĭk) [G. *peri*, around, + *pylōros*, pylorus]. Extending around the pylorus.

perirectal (pĕr″ĭ-rĕk′tăl) [" + L. *rectus*, straight]. Extending around the rectum.

perirectitis (pĕr″ĭ-rĕk-tī′tĭs) [" + " + G. -*itis*, inflammation]. Inflamed condition of tissues about rectum and anus. SYN: *periproctitis*.

perirenal (pĕr″ĭ-rē′năl) [" + L. *rēn*, kidney]. Extending around the kidney. SYN: *circumrenal, perinephric*.

perirhinal (pĕr″ĭ-rī′năl) [" + *ris, rin-*, nose]. Located about the nose or nasal fossae.

perirhizoclasia (pĕr″ĭ-rī″zō-klā′zĭ-ă) [" + *riza*, root, + *klasis*, a breaking]. Inflammation and destruction of tissues extending around the roots of a tooth.

perisalpingitis (pĕr″ĭ-săl-pĭn-jī′tĭs) [" + *salpigx, salpigg-*, tube, + -*itis*, inflammation]. Inflamed condition of peritoneal coat about the oviduct.

perisalpingoövaritis (pĕr″ĭ-săl-pĭn″gō-ō-văr-ī′tĭs) [" + " + L. *ovarium*, ovary, + G. -*itis*, inflammation]. Inflammation of peritoneal tissues surrounding the fallopian tubes and ovaries. SYN: *perioöphorosalpingitis, perioöthecosalpingitis*.

periscle′rium [G. *peri*, around, + *sklēros*, hard]. Fibrous tissue encircling ossifying cartilage.

periscopic (pĕr″ĭ-skop′ĭk) [" + *skopein*, to examine]. Viewing on all sides.

perish (pĕr′ĭsh) [L. *perīre*, to come to nothing]. To disintegrate or die, esp. by other than natural causes.

perisigmoiditis (pĕr″ĭ-sĭg-moi-dī′tĭs) [G. *peri*, around, + *sigma*, Greek letter S, + *eidos*, like, + -*itis*, inflammation]. Inflamed condition of peritoneal tissues around sigmoid flexure of the colon.

perisinuitis (pĕr″ĭ-sĭ-nū-ī′tĭs) [G. *peri*, around, + L. *sinus*, cavity, + G. -*itis*, inflammation]. Inflamed condition of tissue about a sinus, esp. a cerebral one. SYN: *perisinusitis*.

perisinusitis (pĕr″ĭ-sī-nū-sī′tĭs) [" + " + G. -*itis*, inflammation]. Inflammation of membranes about a sinus, esp. a cerebral sinus. SYN: *perisinuitis.*

perispermatitis (pĕr″ĭ-spĕr-mă-tī′tĭs) [" + *sperma*, seed, + *-itis*, inflammation]. Inflamed condition of tissues about spermatic cord.

p. serosa. Hydrocele of spermatic cord.

perisplanchnic (pĕr″ĭ-splănk′nĭk) [" + *splagchnon*, viscus]. Extending around a viscus or the viscera.

perisplanchnitis (pĕr″ĭ-splănk-nī′tĭs) [" + " + *-itis*, inflammation]. Inflamed condition of the tissues around the viscera. SYN: *perivisceritis.*

perisplenitis (pĕr″ĭ-splē-nī′tĭs) [" + *splēn*, spleen, + *-itis*, inflammation]. Inflammation of peritoneal coat of the spleen, the splenic capsule.

perispondylitis (pĕr″ĭ-spŏn-dĭl-ī′tĭs) [" + *spondylos*, vertebra, + *-itis*, inflammation]. Inflamed condition of the parts around a vertebra.

perissad (pĕr-ĭs′ăd, per′ĭs-ad) [G. *perissos*, odd]. 1. Radical or element of odd valence. 2. Having odd valence.

perissodactylous (pĕr-ĭs″ō-dăk′tĭ-lŭs) [" + *daktylos*, digit]. Having an odd number of toes.

peristalsis (pĕr-ĭs-tăl′sĭs) [" + *stalsis*, contraction]. Peculiar, contractile, muscular, vermicular, involuntary movements of any hollow tube of the body, esp. of the alimentary canal.

It consists of contractions of successive portions of the circular muscles followed by relaxation, and propels the food content onward. In the stomach, muscular contraction begins in the middle part and moves toward the pylorus, but there is no peristalsis in the cardiac part of the stomach. A peristaltic wave may, in the intestine, move in either direction and may or may not be preceded by a wave of bulging (relaxation).

RS: *bradystalsis, digestion, intestinal, intestine.*

p., mass. Forced peristaltic movements of short duration moving contents from 1 section of the colon to another, occurring 3 or 4 times daily.

p., reverse. Backward movement of the intestines, a pathological condition often seen in intestinal and pyloric obstruction, and in the presence of diverticula and diverticulitis.

TREATMENT: Atropine.

peristaltic (pĕr″ĭ-stăl′tĭk) [G. *peri*, around, + *stalsis*, contraction]. Concerning, or of the nature of, peristalsis.

p. unrest. Increased peristalsis or abnormal motility of the intestinal tract.

peristaphyline (pĕr″ĭ-stăf′ĭ-lĭn) [" + *staphylē*, uvula]. About the uvula.

peristole (pĕr-ĭs′tō-lē) [" + *stellein*, to place]. The tonic power of the stomach to contract around its contents.

peristome (pĕr′ĭs-tōm) [" + *stoma*, mouth]. Channel leading from the mouth in protozoa.

peristrumitis (pĕr″ĭ-strŭ-mī′tĭs) [" + L. *struma*, goiter]. Inflamed condition of tissues around a goiter. SYN: *perithyroiditis.*

perisynovial (pĕr″ĭ-sĭn-ō′vĭ-ăl) [" + *syn*, with, + *ōon*, egg]. Extending around a synovial structure.

perisystole (pĕr″ĭ-sĭs′tō-lē) [" + *systolē*, contraction]. The period preceding the systole in the cardiac rhythm.

peritectomy (pĕr″ĭ-tĕk′tō-mĭ) [G. *peri*, around, + *ektomē*, excision]. Surgical removal of a ring of conjunctiva around the cornea.

peritendineum (pĕr″ĭ-tĕn-dĭn′ē-ŭm) [" + L. *tendō*, tendon]. The sheath of tissues investing a tendon.

peritendinitis (pĕr″ĭ-tĕn-dĭn-ī′tĭs) [" + " + G. *-itis*, inflammation]. Inflamed condition of the sheath of a tendon. SYN: *peritenonitis.*

peritenonitis (pĕr″ĭ-tĕn-on-ī′tĭs) [" + *tenōn*, tendon, + *-itis*, inflammation]. Inflammation of sheath investing a tendon. SYN: *peritendinitis.*

perithelioma (pĕr″ĭ-thē-lĭ-ō′mă) [" + *thēlē*, nipple, + *-ōma*, tumor]. A tumor derived from the perithelial layer of the blood vessels.

perithelium (pĕr-ĭ-thē′lĭ-ŭm) [" + *thēlē*, nipple]. Fibrous outer layer of the blood vessels and capillaries.

perithyroiditis (pĕr″ĭ-thī-roy-dī′tĭs) [" + *thyreos*, shield, + *eidos*, form, + *-itis*, inflammation]. Inflammation of capsule or tissues sheathing the thyroid gland. SYN: *peristrumitis.*

peritomy (pĕr-ĭt′ō-mĭ) [G. *peri*, around, + *tomē*, incision]. 1. Excision of narrow strip of conjunctiva around the cornea in treatment of pannus. 2. Circumcision.

Operation also consists in dividing the conjunctival vessels running over the limbus.

peritoneal (pĕr″ĭ-tō-nē′ăl) [G. *peritonaion*, peritoneum]. Concerning the peritoneum.

p. cavity. Region bordered by parietal layer of the peritoneum containing all the abdominal organs exclusive of the kidney. SEE: *cholascos.*

peritonealgia (pĕr″ĭ-tō-nē-al′jĭ-ă) [" + *algos*, pain]. Pain of the peritoneum.

peritoneocentesis (pĕr″ĭ-tō-nē″ō-sĕn-tē′sĭs) [" + *kentēsis*, a puncture]. Piercing of the peritoneal cavity to obtain fluid. SEE: *paracentesis.*

peritoneoclysis (pĕr″ĭ-tō-nē″ō-klī′sĭs) [" + *klysis*, a washing out]. Introduction of fluid into the peritoneal cavity.

peritoneopathy (pĕr″ĭ-tō-nē-op′ăth-ĭ) [" + *pathos*, disease]. Any disordered condition of the peritoneum.

peritoneopexy (pĕr″ĭ-tō-nē′ō-pĕks″ĭ) [" + *pēxis*, fixation]. Fixation of the uterus by way of the vagina.

peritoneoplasty (pĕr″ĭ-tō-nē′ō-plăs″tĭ) [" + *plassein*, to form]. Reparative surgery to prevent re-formation of loosened adhesions.

peritoneoscope (pĕr″ĭ-tō-nē′ō-skōp) [G. *peritonaion*, peritoneum, + *skopein*, to examine]. Long, slender telescope with a tiny electric light on the end as well as a forceps for grasping a small metal fragment or for clamping a bleeding artery in the peritoneum.

peritoneoscopy (pĕr″ĭ-tō-nē-ŏs′kō-pĭ) [" + *skopein*, to examine]. Examination of peritoneal cavity with the peritoneoscope.

peritoneotomy (pĕr″ĭ-tō-nē-ŏt′ō-mĭ) [" + *tomē*, a cutting]. Process of incising the peritoneum.

peritoneum (pĕr-ĭ-tō-nē′ŭm) [G. *peritonaion*]. The serous membrane reflected over the viscera, and lining the abdominal cavity.

PALPATION: If palmar surface of hand be applied to side of abdomen at level of the liquid in ascites, and light percussion be performed on the opposite side, a sense of fluctuation will be communicated to the hand.

RS: *abdominal cavity, chyloperito-*

neum, Douglas' cul-de-sac, mesenteric, mesenteritis, mesentery, perihepatitis.
  p., abdominal. That part of the p. lining inner surfaces of the abdominal parietes.
  p., genitourinary. Retrovesical folds.
  p., parietal. P. lining abdominal and pelvic walls and undersurface of diaphragm.
  p., subduodenal. Peritoneal folds and ligaments below the duodenum.
  p., supraduodenal. Peritoneal folds and ligaments above the duodenum.
  p., visceral. The p. that invests the abdominal organs except the kidneys.
peritonism (pĕr'ĭ-tō-nĭzm) [G. *peritonaion*, peritoneum, + *ismos*, condition]. A false peritonitis with symptoms of peritonitis and abdominal rigidity and tenderness, but with no inflammation of the peritoneum.
peritonitic (pĕr-ĭ-tō-nĭt'ĭk) [" + *-itis*, inflammation]. Affected with or concerning peritonitis.
peritonitis (pĕr"ĭ-tō-nī'tĭs) [G. *peritonaion*, peritoneum, + *-itis*, inflammation]. Inflammation of the peritoneum, the membranous coat lining the abdominal cavity and investing the viscera.
  RS: *celiopyosis, celitis, endoperitonitis, pachypelviperitonitis.*
  p., acute diffuse. Generalized p. of a large area.
  ETIOL: Rupture of an intraäbdominal viscus, as the appendix or stomach. Infection may take place directly from an adjacent organ which is inflamed, or from the blood stream in patients with septicemia.
  SYM: Chill; fever, 102°-103° F.; rapid, wiry pulse; abdominal pain and tenderness so intense abdominal respiration and bodily movement inhibited; patient on back, thighs flexed; features pinched, and anxious; teeth showing by raised lips; vomiting persistent; bowels usually constipated; hiccough; abdominal distention.
  PROG: Guarded.
  TREATMENT: Surgical intervention. Absolute bed rest; sips of water by mouth; saline or glucose solution parenterally; heat to abdomen; repeated gastric lavage; sedatives; foot of bed raised. Recent additions to treatment have been the inhalation of concentrated oxygen, and in cases complicating appendicitis, the administration of sulfanilamide.
  p., adhesive. P. in which the visceral and parietal layers stick together by means of adhesions.
  p., chronic. Usually tuberculous, cancerous or syphilitic; occurs in chronic alcoholism.
  SYM: Fever slight or absent. Pain not severe; paroxysms; usually diffuse tenderness; anemia and emaciation may be marked.
  PROG: Guarded.
  TREATMENT: Rest; light diet; constitutional treatment, when effusion is great; paracentesis. Laparotomy.
  DIET: Milk diet, meat juices, raw eggs, no vegetables or fruit. Avoid causes of distention.
  p. deformans. Chronic p. with thickened membrane and adhesions contracting and causing retraction of the intestines.
  p., diffuse. P. which is not found in only a circumscribed area.
  p., local. P. confined to 1 limited area of the peritoneum.
  p., pelvic. Infection of the peritoneal lining of the pelvic cavity.
  p., plastic. A form binding the bowels together with adhesions.
  p., puerperal. P. which develops following childbirth.
  p., septic. P. caused by a pyogenic bacterium.
  p., serous. P. in which there is liquid exudation.
  p., traumatic. P. due to injury or wound infection.
  p., tuberculous. P. caused by numerous tubercle bacilli on the peritoneum.
peritonsillar (pĕr"ĭ-ton'sĭl-ăr) [G. *peri*, around, + L. *tonsilla*, tonsil]. Extending around a tonsil.
peritonsillitis (pĕr-ĭ-tŏn-sĭl-ī'tĭs) [" + " + G. *-itis*, inflammation]. Inflamed condition of tissues around the tonsils. SYN: *periamygdalitis.*
peritrichous (pĕr-ĭt'rĭk-ŭs) [" + *thrix, trich-*, hair]. BACT: Having cilia or flagella covering the entire surface.
perityphlitis (pĕr"ĭ-tĭf-lī'tĭs) [" + *typhlos*, blind, + *-itis*, inflammation]. Inflamed condition of tissues around the cecum and appendix. SYN: *appendicitis.*
periureteritis (pĕr"ĭ-ū-rē"tĕr-ī'tĭs) [" + *ourētēr*, ureter, + *-itis*, inflammation]. Inflamed condition of parts about the ureter.
periurethral (pĕr"ĭ-ū-rē'thrăl) [" + *ourēthra*, urethra]. Located about the urethra.
periuterine (pĕr"ĭ-ū'tĕr-ĭn) [" + L. *uterus*, womb]. Located about the uterus. SYN: *perimetric.*
perivaginitis (pĕr"ĭ-văj-ĭn-ī'tĭs) [G. *peri*, around, + L. *vagina*, sheath, + G. *-itis*, inflammation]. Inflammation of region around the vagina. SYN: *pericolpitis.*
perivascular (pĕr"ĭ-văs'kū-ler) [" + L. *vasculus*, a little vessel]. Located around a vessel, esp. a blood vessel.
perivasculitis (pĕr"ĭ-văs-kū-lī'tĭs) [" + " + G. *-itis*, inflammation]. Inflamed condition of tissues surrounding a blood vessel. SYN: *periangitis.*
perivisceritis (pĕr"ĭ-vĭs"ĕr-ī'tĭs) [" + L. *viscus, viscer-*, internal organ, + G. *-itis*, inflammation]. Inflamed condition of the tissues surrounding the viscera.
perixenitis (pĕr"ĭ-zĕn-ī'tĭs) [" + *xenos*, strange, + *-itis*, inflammation]. Inflammation of the region around a foreign body.
perlèche (pĕr-lăsh') [Fr.]. Contagious disorder marked by fissures and epithelial desquamation at corners of the mouth, esp. seen in children.
permanent (pŭr'măn-ĕnt) [L. *per*, through, + *manere*, to remain]. Enduring; without change.
  p. teeth. Teeth developing at the 2nd dentition. SEE: *dens permanens.*
permanganate (pĕr-man'găn-āt). Any one of the salts of permanganic acid.
permeable (pŭr'mē-ă-bl) [L. *per*, through, + *meare*, to pass]. Capable of or allowing the passage of fluids into or through. SEE: *pervious, porous.*
pernicious (pĕr-nĭsh'ŭs) [L. *perniciōsus*, destructive]. Destructive; fatal; harmful.
  p. anemia. Severe, often fatal, form of blood disease, marked by progressive decrease in red blood corpuscles, muscular weakness, and gastrointestinal and neural disturbances. SEE: *anemia, pernicious.*
  p. trend. PSY: An abnormal departure from conventional ideas and

social interests. Pregenital interests are manifested.

pernio (pŭr′nĭ-ō) [L. chilblain]. Congestion and swelling of the skin, due to cold.

SYM: Attended with severe burning or itching; ulceration may result from vesicles and bullae which sometimes form. SYN: *chilblain.*

perniosis (pŭr-nĭ-ō′sĭs) [L. *perniō*, chilblain, + G. *-ōsis*, disease]. A skin disorder due to cold. SEE: *chilblain, pernio.*

pernocton (pŭr-nŏk′tŏn). Barbituric acid derivative used as an anesthetic and hypnotic, as in labor.

pero (pē′rō) [L. boot]. The soft outer layer of the olfactory lobe of the brain from which the olfactory nerves arise.

perogen (per′ō-jĕn). A preparation composed of 2 separate mixtures which are united in making an oxygen bath.

peronaeus (pĕr-ō-nē′ŭs) [G. *peronē*, pin]. A group of leg muscles controlling motion of the foot.

peroneal (pĕr-ō-nē′ăl) [G. *peronē*, pin]. Concerning the fibula.

peroneo- [G.]. Combining form, *pert. to the fibula.*

peroneum (pĕr-ō-nē′ŭm) [G. *peronē*, pin]. The fibula. SYN: *os peroneum.*

peroneus (pĕr-ō-nē′ŭs) [L., from G. *peronē*, pin]. One of several muscles of the leg causing motion in the foot.

peronin (pĕr′ō-nĭn). Proprietary powder, benzylmorphine hydrochloride, used in treating coughs.

DOSAGE: ⅓ gr. (0.02 Gm.).

Peronospora (pĕr-ō-nŏs′pō-rä) [G. *peronē*, point, + *sporos*, seed]. Genus of fungi causing mildew formation.

peroral (pĕr-or′ăl) [L. *per*, through, + *os, or-*, mouth]. Via the mouth.

per os [L.]. By mouth.

peroxidase (pĕr-ŏks′ĭ-dăs) [L. *per*, through, + *oxys*, acid, + *ase*, enzyme]. An enzyme which hastens the decomposition of peroxides, esp. of hydrogen peroxide.

The presence of this enzyme in the tissues is the cause of the bubbling seen when peroxide is poured over a cut in the skin. SEE: *catalase.*

peroxide (pŭr-ŏk′sĭd) [" + G. *oxys*, acid]. In chemistry, a compound containing more oxygen than do the other oxides of the element in question.

Examples are the peroxides of hydrogen, H_2O_2; sodium, Na_2O_2; magnesium, MgO_2, and nitrogen, NO_2.

perplication (per-plĭ-kā′shŭn) [" + *plicāre*, to fold]. Inserting the cut end of an artery through an incision in its own wall to arrest bleeding.

per primam, per primam intentionem (per prē′măm ĭn-tĕn-tĭ-ō′nĕm) [L.]. By first intention. SEE: *first intention, healing.*

per rectum (per rĕk′tŭm) [L.]. By the rectum; through the rectum.

persalt (pursawlt). CHEM: A salt containing largest possible amount of an acid radical.

per secundam (per se-kun′dăm) [L.]. By second intention. SEE: *healing, second intention.*

perseveration (pŭr-sĕv-ĕr-ā′shŭn) [L. *perseverāre*, to persist]. Continued repetition of a meaningless word or phrase, or repetition of answers which are not related to successive questions asked.

persimmon (pur-sĭm′ŭn) [Algonquin]. Av. SERVING (American): 50 Gm. Pro. 0.4, Fat 0.4, Carbo. 14.9. VITAMINS: A+, C+. ASH CONST: Ca 0.002, Mg 0.009, K 0.292, Na 0.011, P 0.021, Cl 0.002, S 0.005.

personal (pŭr′sō-năl) [L. *persona*, a person]. Characteristic of an individual.

p. equation. In scientific observation, factors depending on personal qualities of individual observers.

personality (pŭr-sō-năl′ĭ-tĭ) [L. *persona*, person]. That which constitutes the distinction of person. PSY: Totality of an individual's characteristics; the integrated group of emotional trends, interests and behavior tendencies of an individual. SEE: *idiosyncrasy.*

p., double. SEE: *dual p.*

p., dual. Mental dissociation in which 1 individual shows in alternation 2 very different personalities. SEE: *dual personality.*

p., multiple. State in which 3 or more personalities alternate in the same individual. SEE: *multiple personality.*

p., psychopathic. One who, while possessing normal intelligence, by reason of heredity or congenital conditions, becomes constitutionally lacking in moral sensibilities, emotional control and inhibitions of the will.

Constitutional imbalance in the pattern of the mind, but not a disorder of function such as is observed in actual neuroses and psychoses. In other words, such a personality represents a borderline state. The inferiority of the psychopath is *emotional and not intellectual.*

p., split. Dissociation of ideas not amenable to conscious control, as in schizophrenia.

RS: *consciousness, disassociation, dual p., multiple p., somnambulism, vigilambulism.*

perspiration (pŭr-spĭr-ā′shŭn) [L. *per*, through, + *spirāre*, to breathe]. 1. Sweat. 2. Secretion and exudation of fluid by sweat glands of the skin, about 700 cc. per day.

Perspiration is increased by: (a) Temperature and humidity of the atmosphere; (b) diluted blood; (c) exercises; (d) pain; (e) nausea; (f) nervousness; (g) mental excitement; (h) dyspnea; (i) diaphoretics.

It is decreased by: (a) Colds; (b) diarrhea; (c) voiding large quantities of urine; by using certain drugs.

p., sensible. P. which occurs so as to form drops.

p., insensible. P. which evaporates as fast as formed, leaving no moisture on the skin.

perspiration, words pert. to: adiaphoresis, adiapneustia, anhidrosis, anhidrotic, anidros, bromohyperhidrosis, bromidrosis, chlorophidrosis, chromidrosis, diaphoresis, meridrosis, panidrosis, polyidrosis, secretion, sudor, sudorific, sweat, -center, sweating, transpiration, uridrosis.

perspire (pŭr-spĭr′) [L. *per*, through, + *spirāre*, to breathe]. To excrete fluid through the skin. SYN: *sweat.*

perstriction (pĕr-strĭk′shŭn) [L. *per*, through, + *strictus*, from *stringere*, to tighten]. Ligation of a bleeding vessel for the arrest of hemorrhage.

persulfate (pŭr-sŭl′făt). One of a series of sulfates containing more sulfuric acid than the others in same series.

per tertiam intentionem (per tĕr′tĭ-ăm ĭn-tĕn-tĭ-ō′nĕm) [L.]. By third intention. SEE: *healing, third intention.*

Perthes' disease (păr′tăs). One in which changes take place in bone at head of femur with deformity resulting.

SYM: Similar to tuberculous hip joint

per tubam

disease. SYN: *osteochondritis deformans juvenilis*.

per tubam (pĕr tū'băm) [L.]. Through a tube.

pertussin (pĕr-tŭs'ĭn) [L. *per*, through, + *tussis*, cough]. Proprietary cough remedy.

pertussis (pĕr-tŭs'ĭs) [" + *tussis*, cough]. An acute, infectious disease characterized by a catarrhal stage, followed by a peculiar paroxysmal cough, ending in a whooping inspiration.

ETIOL: Due to the *Bordet-Gengou bacillus*. Usually prevalent in spring and early summer, though endemic at all seasons. Most common in infants and young children, though may occur in adults. Most contagious, early. Danger of contagion rapidly diminishes after the catarrhal stage.

INCUBATION: Seven to 10 days.

SYM: A blood count shows a marked lymphocytosis which may vary from 20,000 to 10,000. Often divided into 3 stages; first, *catarrhal*. At this time the symptoms chiefly suggestive of the common cold—slight elevation of fever, sneezing, rhinitis, and dry cough. Irritability and loss of appetite.

After from 7 to 10 days, the second, or *paroxysmal stage*, sets in. The cough is more violent, and consists of a series of several short coughs, followed by long drawn inspiration, during which the typical whoop is heard, this being occasioned by the spasmodic contraction of the glottis.

With the beginning of each paroxysm, patient often assumes a worried expression, sometimes even one of terror. The face becomes cyanosed, eyes injected, veins distended. With conclusion of the paroxysm, vomiting is common. At this time also, there may be epistaxis, subconjunctival hemorrhages, or hemorrhages in other portions of body.

Number of paroxysms in 24 hours may vary from 3 to 4 up to 40 or 50. Following an indefinite period of several weeks, the stage of *decline* begins, the paroxysms grow less frequent and less violent. Nutrition of child improves, and after a period which may be prolonged for several months, the cough finally ceases.

COMPLICATIONS: Pneumonia is one of the fatal consequences of whooping cough. Various types of hemorrhages, occasionally a subdural hemorrhage after a hemiplegia in a case of whooping cough. Permanent heart defects may also develop from overengorgement of heart as result of strain at time of paroxysms. Various types of hernias are sometimes produced and patient seems more disposed to tuberculosis than prior to attack. Loss of weight and malnutrition also may be regarded as complications of this serious infection.

DIFFERENTIAL DIAG: Early, either a common cold or measles may be suspected, or sometimes simple bronchitis.

During recent years, unusual efforts have been made to develop a reliable method for early diagnosis. For this purpose, the use of chocolate agar plates has been urged, with the idea of determining whether or not the Bordet-Gengou bacillus is present on culture media which is inoculated by the cough of a patient before the paroxysmal stage had developed. A marked leukocytosis, ordinarily evident during catarrhal stage, is also suggestive of whooping cough. This is particularly true in view of the mildness of the constitutional symptoms at this time.

PROG: The disease is exceptionally fatal in the very young and in negroes, and is one of the comparatively few infectious diseases that may occur during the first few weeks of life. In children over 5 years, complications are not usually so severe nor are the sequelae so serious.

TREATMENT: Vaccine made from the Bordet-Gengou bacillus often appears to be of value in preventing onset of whooping cough. In the actual treatment of the sufferer, hygienic conditions are of great importance.

A patient should have an abundance of fresh air and sunlight, and the sleeping room should be well ventilated. The child should be disturbed as little as possible, since mere handling may be sufficient to bring on a paroxysm. Feeding should be in small amounts at frequent intervals, rather than in the 3 customary meals a day. In this manner, there is greater opportunity for patient to retain and digest the small quantities of nourishment between paroxysms.

Constipation should be avoided, and sedatives may be of value. It is esp. important that patient be isolated during catarrhal stage.

A quarantine period of from 2 to 3 weeks is probably sufficient for protection of susceptibles, even though paroxysms of coughing may continue for a period of months. This statement is made on the basis of practical experience and owing to the fact that it is scarcely ever possible to isolate the causative organism after the paroxysmal stage has developed.

DIET: Ordinary diet. Carbonate of soda in milk reduces tenacity and vicidity of mucus, and assists in its expulsions. Lime water and milk for vomiting; white of egg and lemon water.

In pertussis complicated by pneumonia, sulfapyridine with sodium bicarbonate, adm. rectally if necessary, when vomiting is present. Dosage is 1½ gr. per lb. of body wt. for first 24 hr. Thereafter, 1 gr. per lb. continued for 5 to 7 days after temperature subsides. Limit fluids.

SYN: *whooping cough*.

pertussoid (pĕr-tŭs'oyd) [L. *per*, through, + *tussis*, cough, + G. *eidos*, resemblance]. 1. Of the nature of whooping cough. 2. A cough generally similar to that of whooping cough.

peruol (pĕr'ū-ŏl). Oil derived from balsam of Peru used in scabies.

perversion (pŭr-vŭr'zhŭn) [L. *per*, through, + *versio*, a turning]. Deviation from the normal path, as in function.

p., sexual. Maladjustment of sexual life in which satisfaction is sought in ways deviating from the accepted normal.

Substitution of sadism, peeping, or touching the object of one's libido, or gloating upon some possession of that object rather than the normal expression through heterosexual coition; it may take many forms of expression, such as homosexuality.

pervert (pŭr-vŭrt') [L. *per*, through, + *vertere*, to turn]. 1. v. To turn from the normal. 2. (pŭr'vŭrt). n. One who has turned from the normal or right path, esp. sexually.

p., sexual. One whose sex conduct is not normal.

Many of them suffer from mental diseases, such as dementia, senility, epilepsy, and from general paralysis.
Most of them are mental degenerates suffering from psychic or physical defects. Heredity plays a part in some instances. Diseases of the nervous system, alcoholism, and infections also may be responsible in part. Stigmata or malformations are often present.

pervigilium (pĕr-vĭ-jĭl'ĭ-ŭm) [L. *per*, through, + *vigil*, awake]. Inability to sleep. SYN: *insomnia, wakefulness*.

pervious (pŭr'vĭ-ŭs) [L. *per*, through, + *via*, way]. 1. Capable of being penetrated. 2. Penetrating. SYN: *permeable*.

pes (pl. *pĕ'dēz*) (pēz) [L. *pēs, ped*, foot]. The foot or a footlike structure.

  p. accessorius. A white projection in the brain at the juncture of descending and post. cornua of lateral ventricle.

  p. anserinus. Three primary branches of the facial nerve after leaving the stylomastoid foramen.

  p. cavus. Abnormal hollowness of the sole of the foot.

  p. corvinus. Wrinkles at outer ocular canthus. SYN: *crow's foot*.

  p. equinus. Deformity marked by walking without touching heel to the ground. SYN: *talipes equinus, q.v.*

  p. hippocampi. Lower portion of the hippocampus major.

  p., infraorbital. Terminal radiating branches of the infraorbital nerve after exit from the infraorbital canal.

  p. planus. Flatfoot.

  p. valgus. Clubfoot in which sole turns outward. SYN: *talipes valgus*.

  p. varus. Clubfoot in which sole turns inward. SYN: *talipes varus*.

pessary (pĕs'ăr-ĭ) [G. *pessos*, oval pebble]. 1. A device to insert into the vagina to hold the uterus in position. 2. A vaginal suppository.

  p., cup. One which has a cup-shaped hollow that fits over the os uteri.

  p., diaphragm. Cup-shaped rubber p. used as a contraceptive device.

  p., Gariel's. Inflatable hollow rubber p.

  p., Hodge's. P. used to correct retrodeviations of the uterus.

  p., lever. P. designed according to the principles of a lever.

  p., ring. Round pessary.

  p., stem. P. with stem which fits into the uterine canal.

pessima (pĕs'ĭ-mă) [L.]. A skin affection characterized by pustular lesions, hard and yellowish, surrounded by areola of inflammation appearing over surface of body causing a checkerboard appearance.
TREATMENT: Constitutional.

pest (pĕst) [L. *pestis*, plague]. 1. Fatal epidemic disease, esp. the plague. 2. A destructive insect.

  p.-house. Hospital for those infected with a pestilential or communicable disease.

pestiferous (pĕst-ĭf'ĕr-ŭs) [" + *ferre*, to carry]. Producing a pestilence; carrying infection. SYN: *pestilential*.

pestilence (pĕst'ĭl-ĕns) [L. *pestilentia*, a widespread epidemic]. 1. An epidemic contagious disease, specifically bubonic plague. 2. An epidemic caused by such a disease.

pestilential (pĕst-ĭ-lĕn'shăl) [L. *pestilentia*, a widespread disease]. Concerning or causing a pestilence. SYN: *pestiferous*.

pestis (pĕs'tĭs) [L. plague]. The plague.

pestle (pĕs'l) [L. *pistillum*, pestle]. Device for macerating drugs in a mortar.

petechiae (pe-tē'kĭ-ē) [Italian *peteche*, a flea bite]. 1. Small, purplish, hemorrhagic spots on the skin which appear in certain severe fevers and are indicative of great prostration, as in typhus. 2. Red spots from bite of a flea.

petechial (pe-tē'kĭ-ăl) [Italian *peteche*, a flea bite]. Marked by presence of petechiae.

petit mal (pĕt'ē măhl) [F. little illness]. Mild form of epileptic attack.
Consciousness may be lost, but there is an absence of convulsions. SEE: *epilepsy, pyknolepsy*.

Petit's canal. Canal encircling the lenticular periphery.

  P.'s sinuses. Hollows in aortic and pulmonary arteries behind semilunar valves. [nal muscular wall.

  P.'s triangle. One on lateral abdomi-

petrifaction (pĕt-rĭ-făk'shŭn) [L. *petra*, stone, + *facere*, to make]. Process of changing into stone or hard substance.

petrified (pĕt'rĭ-fīd) [L. *petra*, stone]. Changed into stone; rigid.

petrify (pĕt'rĭ-fī) [L. *petra*, stone]. Convert into stone; make rigid.

pétrissage (pā-trē-sazh') [Fr.]. A kneading movement in massage.
Performed generally by: (a) The tips of the thumbs; (b) with index finger and thumb; (c) with palm of hand.
It is used principally on the extremities. The operator picks up a special muscle or tendon and, placing 1 finger on each side of the part, proceeds in centripetal motion with a firm pressure. SYN: *kneading*.

petro- [L.]. Combining form meaning *stone*. Pert. to petrous portion of temporal bone.

petrolatoma (pĕt″rō-lă-tō'mă) [L. *petra*, stone, + *oleum*, oil, + G. *-ōma*, tumor]. Tumor or swelling caused by introduction of liquid petrolatum under the skin.

petrolatum (pĕt-rō-lă'tŭm) [" + *oleum*, oil]. USP. A purified semi-solid mixture of hydrocarbons obtained from petroleum.
ACTION AND USES: As a base for ointments and as a lubricant.

  p. liquid. USP. A mixture of liquid hydrocarbons obtained from petroleum.
ACTION AND USES: A vehicle for medicinal substances for local applications. Light p. employed as a spray. Heavy p. given internally in treatment of constipation.
DOSAGE: 4 drams (15 cc.). SEE: *mineral oil, paraffin, liquid*.

petroleum (pĕt-rō'lē-ŭm) [L. *petra*, stone, + *oleum*, oil]. An oily inflammable liquid found in the upper strata of the earth, a hydrocarbon mixture.

petrolization (pĕt-rŏl-ĭ-zā'shŭn) [G. *petra*, stone, + L. *oleum*, oil]. The application of kerosene to pools of water for the extermination of mosquito larvae.

petromastoid (pĕt″rō-măs'toyd) [L. *petrōsus*, stony, + G. *mastos*, breast, + *eidos*, form]. Concerning petrous and mastoid portions of the temporal bone.

petrosa (pĕt-rō'să) [L. stony]. The petrous part of the temporal bone.

petrosal (pĕt-rō'săl) [L. *petrōsus*, stony]. Of, pert. to, or situated near, the petrous portion of the temporal bone.

petrosalpingostaphylinus (pĕt″rō-săl-pĭn′-gō-stăf-ĭl-ī'nŭs) [G. *petra*, stone, + *salpigx*, tube, + *staphylē*, uvula]. The levator palati muscle which elevates the soft palate.

petrositis (pĕt″rō-sī'tĭs) [" + *-itis*, inflam-

phantom P-48 **pharyngoparalysis**

one would escape through revelling in imaginative possibilities.
RS: *delirium, delusion, hallucination, hysteria, illusion, phobia.*

phantom (făn'tŭm) [G. *phantasma*, an appearance]. 1. An apparition. 2. A model of the body or of 1 of its parts.
  p. corpuscle. A colorless erythrocyte.
  p. tumor. An apparent tumor due to muscular contractions or flatus seen in hysterics. SEE: *pseudocyesis.*

pharmacal (făr'măk-ăl) [G. *pharmakon*, drug]. Concerning pharmacy.

pharmaceutical (făr-mă-sū'tĭk-ăl) [G. *pharmakeutikos*, pert. to a drug]. Concerning drugs or pharmacy.

pharmaceutics (făr-mă-sū'tĭks) [G. *pharmakon*, drug]. Science of dispensing medicines. SYN: *pharmacy.*

pharmacist (făr'mă-sĭst) [G. *pharmakon*, drug]. A druggist; one licensed to prepare and dispense drugs. SYN: *apothecary.*

pharmaco- [G.]. Combining form meaning *drug, medicine, poison.*

pharmacodiagnosis (făr"mă-kō-dī-ăg-nō'sĭs) [G. *pharmakon*, drug, + *dia*, through, + *gnosis*, knowledge]. Use of drugs in making a diagnosis.

pharmacodynamics (făr"mă-kō-dī-năm'ĭks) [" + *dynamis*, power]. Study of drugs and their reactions.

pharmacognosy (făr"mă-kog'nō-sī) [" + *gnosis*, knowledge]. The science of crude drugs, their physical, botanical and chemical properties.

pharmacography (făr"mă-kog'ră-fī) [" + *graphein*, to write]. Treatise on the properties of drugs.

pharmacology (făr-mă-kŏl'ō-jī) [" + *logos*, a study]. The study of the effects of drugs upon the physical organism. SYN: *pharmacodynamics.*

pharmacomania (făr"mă-kō-mā'nĭ-ă) [" + *mania*, madness]. Abnormal desire for giving or taking medicines.

pharmacopedia (făr"mă-kō-pē'dĭ-ă) [" + *paideia*, education]. Information concerning drugs and their preparation.

pharmacopeia (făr"mă-kō-pē'ă) [G. *pharmakon*, drug, + *poiein*, to make]. Authorized treatise on drugs and their preparation, esp. a book containing formulas and information concerning drugs which is a standard for their preparation and dispensation.

The United States Pharmacopeia was adopted as standard in 1906.

pharmacophobia (făr"mă-kō-fō'bĭ-ă) [" + *phobos*, fear]. Abnormal fear of taking medicines.

pharmacopsychosis (făr"mă-kō-sī-kō'sĭs) [" + *psyche*, soul, + *-osis*, disease]. Addiction to drugs.

pharmacotherapy (făr"mă-kō-thĕr'ă-pī) [" + *therapeia*, treatment]. Use of medicine in treatment of disease.

pharmacy (făr'mă-sī) [G. *pharmakon*, drug]. 1. The practice of compounding and dispensing medicinal preparations. 2. A drugstore. 3. A medicinal preparation.

pharyngalgia (făr-ĭn-găl'jĭ-ă) [G. *pharynx*, pharynx, + *algos*, pain]. Pain in the pharynx. SYN: *pharyngodynia.*

pharyngeal (far-ĭn'jē-ăl) [G. *pharynx*, pharynx]. Concerning the pharynx.
  p. arches. Cartilaginous embryonic framework forming various structures in neck. SYN: *visceral arches.*
  p. reflex. Attempt to swallow following any application of stimulus to pharynx.
  p. spine. Small elevation on inf. surface of basilar process of occipital bone for attachment of pharynx.
  p. tonsil. Lymphoid tissue on post. sup. wall of the pharynx.
  p. tubercle. SEE: *p. spine.*

pharyngectomy (făr-ĭn-jĕk'tō-mī) [" + *ektome*, excision]. Partial excision of the pharynx to remove growths, abscesses, etc.

pharyngemphraxis (făr-ĭn-jĕm-frăks'ĭs) [" + *emphraxis*, stoppage]. Pharyngeal obstruction.

pharyngismus (făr-ĭn-jĭz'mŭs) [" + *ismos*, condition]. Spasm of the muscles in the pharynx. SYN: *pharyngospasm.*

pharyngitis (făr-ĭn-jī'tĭs) [" + *-itis*, inflammation]. Inflammation of pharynx, usually associated with rhinitis.
  p., acute. SYM: Malaise, slight rise in temperature, dysphagia, pain in throat, postnasal secretion.
  TREATMENT: *Local:* Intranasal medication, gargles, lozenges, topical application to oral pharynx. *General:* Catharsis, salicylates, fluids.
  p., atrophic. Chronic form with some atrophy of mucous glands and abnormal secretion. SYN: *p. sicca.*
  p., chronic. Associated with pathology in nose and sinuses, mouth breathing, excessive smoking and chronic tonsilitis.
  SYM: Dryness and irritation of throat, cough.
  TREATMENT: Intranasal medication and removal of sinus pathology, tonsillectomy, cauterization of hypertrophic lymph follicles if present on post. pharyngeal wall.
  p., croupous. P. with the false membrane of croup.
  p., diphtheritic. Sore throat with general symptoms of diphtheria.
  p., follicular. SEE: *granular p.*
  p., gangrenous. G. inflammation of mucous membrane of pharynx. SYN: *angina maligna, cynanche maligna.*
  p., granular. P. with granulations seen on the pharynx. SYN: *clergyman's sore throat.*
  p. hypertrophica. A chronic form with thickened, red mucous membrane on each side with a glazed central portion.
  p. sicca. SEE: *atrophic p.*
  p. ulcerosa. P. with fever, pain and the formation of ulcerations.

pharyngo- [G.]. Combining form pertaining to the pharynx.

pharyngoamygdalitis (făr-ĭn"gō-ăm-ĭg-dăl-ī'tĭs) [G. *pharynx*, pharynx, + *amygdalon*, tonsil, + *-itis*, inflammation]. Inflamed condition of the pharynx and tonsil.

pharyngocele (făr-ĭn'gō-sēl) [" + *kele*, hernia]. Hernia through pharyngeal wall.

pharyngodynia (făr-ĭn"gō-dĭn'ĭ-ă) [" + *odyne*, pain]. Pain in the pharynx. SYN: *pharyngalgia.*

pharyngolaryngitis (făr-ĭn"gō-lăr-ĭn-jī'tĭs) [" + *larygx*, larynx, + *-itis*, inflammation]. Inflamed condition of pharynx and larynx.

pharyngolith (făr-ĭn'gō-lĭth) [" + *lithos*, stone]. Concretion in pharyngeal walls.

pharyngology (făr-ĭn-gŏl'ō-jī) [" + *logos*, a study]. Branch of medicine dealing with the pharynx.

pharyngomycosis (făr-ĭn"gō-mī-kō'sĭs) [" + *myke*, fungus, + *-osis*, disease]. Disease of pharynx due to fungi.

pharyngoparalysis (făr-ĭn"gō-păr-ăl'ĭ-sĭs) [G. *pharynx*, pharynx, + *paralysis*, a loosening at the side]. Paralysis of the muscles of the pharynx. SYN: *pharyngoplegia.*

pharyngopathy (făr-ĭn-gŏp'ăth-ĭ) [" + *pathos*, disease]. Any disorder of the pharynx.

pharyngoperistole (făr-ĭn″gō-pĕr-ĭs'tō-lē) [" + *peristolē*, a drawing out]. Narrowing or stricture of the lumen of the pharynx.

pharyngoplasty (făr-in'gō-plăs″tĭ) [" + *plassein*, to form]. Reparative surgery of the pharynx.

pharyngoplegia (făr-ĭn″gō-plē'jĭ-ă) [" + *plēgē*, a stroke]. Paralysis of muscles of pharynx. SYN: *pharyngoparalysis*.

pharyngorhinitis (făr-ĭn″gō-rī-nī'tĭs) [" + *ris, rin*, nose, + *-itis*, inflammation]. Inflamed condition of the nasopharynx.

pharyngorhinoscopy (făr-ĭn″gō-rī-nŏs'kō-pĭ) [" + " + *skopein*, to examine]. Inspection of the nasopharynx and posterior nares.

pharyngoscope (făr-ĭn'gō-skōp) [G. *pharygx*, pharynx, + *skopein*, to examine]. Instrument for examination of the pharynx.

pharyngoscopy (făr-ĭn-gos'kō-pĭ) [" + *skopein*, to examine]. Examination of the pharynx.
NP: Watch for difficult breathing and cyanosis from edema. Steam inhalations are sometimes ordered.

pharyngospasm (făr-ĭn'gō-spăzm) [" + *spasmos*, a spasm]. Spasmodic contraction of muscles of the pharynx. SYN: *pharyngismus*.

pharyngotherapy (făr-ĭn″gō-thĕr'ă-pĭ) [" + *therapeia*, treatment]. Treatment of pharyngeal disturbances or diseases.

pharyngotome (făr-ĭn'gō-tōm) [" + *tomē*, an incision]. Instrument for incision of the pharynx.

pharyngotomy (făr-ĭn-gŏt'ō-mĭ) [" + *tomē*, a cutting]. Incision of the pharynx.

pharynx (pl. *pharynges*) (făr'ĭnks) [G. *pharygx*, pharynx]. A musculomembranous tube from oral cavity to esophagus.
Communicates with post. nares, eustachian tube, mouth, esophagus and larynx. *Nasopharynx* part above the palate, *oropharynx* bet. palate and hyoid bone, and *laryngopharynx* part below *the hyoid bone*.
NERVES: Autonomic, vagus, glossopharyngeal.
BLOOD VESSELS: Branches from the ext. carotid artery.
FUNCTION: Passage for air, and food to the stomach; also a resonating cavity.
RS: *clergyman's sore throat, epipharynx, nasopharynx, oropharynx, pharyngitis, pharyngoscopy, Rosenmuller's cavity, -fossa*.

phase (fāz) [G. *phasis*, a showing]. 1. A stage of development. 2. A transitory appearance.

phas'ic re'flex. Normal response to stimulation indicated by coördinated movement.

phasin (fā'sĭn). A plant substance which causes erythrocyte agglutination.

phatne (făt'nē) [G. *phatnē*, socket]. Socket for a tooth.

phatnoma (făt-nō'mă) [" + *-ōma*, tumor]. Tumor of a tooth socket.

phatnorrhagia (făt″nō-rā'jĭ-ă) [" + *rēgnunai*, to burst forth]. Hemorrhage from the socket of a tooth.

phatnorrhea (făt-nō-rē'ă) [" + *roia*, flow]. Purulent disintegration of dental periosteum. SYN: *pyorrhea alveolaris*.

phediuretin (fĕd-ū-rē'tĭn). A phenol derivative used as an anodyne and diuretic.

phenacaine (fē'nă-kān, fĕn'ă-kān). A local anesthetic resembling cocaine, but more rapid in effect.

phenacetin (fē-năs'e-tĭn). White crystalline compound commercially prepared as an antipyretic.
DOSAGE: 5 gr. (0.3 Gm.).

phenalgin (fē-năl'jĭn). A commercial analgesic and antipyretic.

phenate (fē'nāt). A salt of phenic acid.

phenazone (fĕn'ă-zōn). SEE: *antipyrine*.

phenegol (fē'nē-gŏl). Antiseptic and emetic formed from mercuric potassium salt of nitroparaphenolsulfonic acid.

phenetidin(e (fĕn-ĕt'ĭ-dēn). A basic amino derivative used in manufacture of medicine.

phenetidinuria (fĕn-ĕt″ĭd-ĭn-ū'rĭ-ă). Phenetidin in the urine.

phenetsal (fĕn-ĕt'săl). A phenetidin derivative, with effects resembling salol.
USES: Intestinal antiseptic, antirheumatic, and antipyretic.
DOSAGE: 5 to 15 gr. (0.3 to 1 Gm.).
INCOMPATIBILITIES: Ferric chloride.

phengophobia (fĕn-gō-fō'bĭ-ă) [G. *pheggos*, light, + *phobos*, fear]. Abnormal dread of light. SYN: *photophobia*.

phenic acid (fē'nĭk). Carbolic acid, *q.v.*

phenobarbital (fē″nō-bar'bĭ-tăl). A derivative of veronal.
ACTION AND USES: A hypnotic sedative and antispasmodic.
DOSAGE: ¼ to 2 gr. (0.015–0.12 Gm.).

phenobarbital sodium (soluble phenobarbital). More rapidly absorbed than phenobarbital.
USES: Same as p., but adapted for subcutaneous and rectal use.
DOSAGE: From ½ to 5 gr. (0.03-0.3 Gm.). [monia salts.
INCOMPATIBILITIES: Chloral, acids, am-

phenocoll (fē'nō-kŏl). A white crystalline base from coal tar compounds which are used as analgesics and antipyretics.

phenol (fē'nŏl). C_6H_5OH, USP. 1. A crystalline, colorless or light pink, solid melting at 43° C., obtained from the distillation of coal tar, having a characteristic odor, and dangerous because of its rapid corrosive action on tissues. SYN: *carbolic acid*.* 2. Any of the aromatic hydroxyl derivatives of benzene of which phenol is the type.
Lister began antiseptic surgery in 1867 with the use of phenol sprays.
ACTION AND USES: Antiseptic and germicide. Liquified phenol contains 87% of pure phenol, mixed with water. A protoplasmic poison which precipitates proteins but penetrates deeply. One-half to 5 per cent solutions most generally used as antiseptics. Stronger solutions used for cauterization. Phenol in concentrations of ½ to 1 per cent is used to stop itching.
DOSAGE: 1 gr. (0.06 Gm.).
POISONING: SYM: Strong solutions cause burning, pain and later anesthesia. The skin and mucous membrane first become pale, then grayish white, opalescent and finally brown to black. Even a 5 per cent solution may cause local gangrene. It is absorbed from intact skin wounds and mucous membrane to cause general effects, including collapse and coma. When taken by mouth, it causes whitish discoloration of mucous membranes, intense burning, nausea and vomiting, followed shortly by faintness, weakness and collapse. Pulse slow and weak. Perspiration is increased, and it causes renal damage.
F. A. TREATMENT: It is not advisable to depend upon emetics as ipecac or

mustard, as the anesthetic effect of the phenol may prevent their action. A well-lubricated small stomach tube should be employed with due caution. It should be remembered that alcohol is an antidote for the local action of the drug, but does not prevent the absorption and systemic effects, so that alcohol should not be administered only, but should be removed (with the phenol) from the stomach. Following this, demulcents such as olive oil, cream, or mucilage of tragacanth should be given. Lime water is frequently used as a chemical antidote, also the sulfates, sodium sulfate being the salt of choice. About an ounce of the latter preparation may be introduced through the tube after the stomach has been emptied. Large amounts of liquid petrolatum have been recommended as an antidote. Shock should be combated. A guarded prognosis should always be given, for should the patient improve at first, damage to the mucous membrane and absorption of phenol may lead to serious complications later. Skin burns with phenol should be first cleansed with a solution of alcohol and then treated as burns from any other cause.

p. coefficient. The germicidal efficiency of phenol as a standard in testing disinfectants in comparison of their potency. SEE: *carbolic acid, phenol.*

p. red. An indicator used in determining hydrogen ion concentration.

phenolin (fĕn'ō-lĭn). Antiseptic prepared from cresol.

phenolization (fē"nō-lĭ-zā'shŭn). Treatment with phenol.

phenology (fē-nŏl'ō-jĭ) [G. *phainein*, to shine out, + *logos*, a study]. Branch of biology dealing with the development of animal and plant life as affected by climate.

phenolphthalein (fē"nŏl-thăl'ē-ĭn, fē"nŏl-thăl'ēn). USP. A white, yellowish, crystallized powder, produced by the interaction of phenol and phthalic anhydride.
ACTION AND USES: As a laxative.
DOSAGE: 1 gr. (0.06 Gm.). SEE: *indicator.*

phenolsulfonphthalein (fē"'nŏl-sul''fŏn-thăl'ēn). Phenol compound used to test renal function and as an indicator. SYN: *phenol red.*

phenoltetrachlorphthalein (fē"nŏl-tĕt"rä-klōr-thăl'ēn). A phenol compound used to test function of the liver and as a purgative.

phenoluria (fē"nŏl-ū'rĭ-ă) [*phenol* + G. *ouron,* urine]. Elimination of phenols in the urine.

phenomenon (fē-nŏm'ē-nŏn) [G. *phainomenon,* appearing]. A change perceivable by the senses that occurs in an organ or vital function; a symptom.

p., Bell's. Rolling of the eyeballs upward and outward when an attempt is made to close the eye affected in peripheral facial paralysis.

phenopyrine (fē"nō-pī'rēn). Antiseptic composed of equal parts of antipyrine and phenol.

phenoresorcin (fē"nō-rē-sor'sĭn). Compound of resorcin and phenol.

phenosalyl (fē"nō-săl'ĭl). An external antiseptic compound of phenol, salicylic acid, menthol and lactic acid.

phenyl (fĕn'ĭl). In chemistry, the univalent radical of phenol, C_6H_5.

phenyl salicylate (săl-ĭs'ĭl-āt). USP. Compound of salicylic acid and phenol.
ACTION AND USES: Intestinal antiseptic.
DOSAGE: 5 gr. (0.3 Gm.).

phenylhydrazine (fĕn"ĭl-hī'drā-zēn). Oily nitrogenous base used as a test for presence of sugar.

pheochrome (fē'ō-krōm) [G. *phaios,* dark, + *chrōma,* color]. Staining readily with chromium salts. SYN: *chromaffin.*

pheochromoblast (fē"ō-krō'mō-blăst) [" + " + *blastos,* germ]. A primitive cell which develops into a cell that stains readily with chromium salts, as in adrenal body.

pheochromocyte (fē"ō-krō'mō-sīt) [" + " + *kytos,* cell]. A cell staining readily with chromium salts.

pheochromocytoma (fē"ō-krō-mō-sī-tō'mă) [" + " + " + -*ōma,* tumor]. A tumor in the adrenal medulla arising from overgrowth of pheochromocytes.

phesin (fē'sĭn). A commercial antipyretic and antineuralgic.

phial (fī'ăl) [G. *phialē,* a bowl]. A small vessel for medicine; a vial.

phimosis (fī-mō'sĭs) [G. a muzzling]. Stenosis or narrowness of preputial orifice so that the foreskin cannot be pushed back over the glans penis.
TREATMENT: Circumcision. SEE: *capistration.*

p. vaginalis. Narrowness or closure of the vaginal orifice.

phisoderm (fī'sō-derm). Trade name for sudsing, emollient, detergent cream, about 40 per cent more active than soap, used for cleansing skin, hair, scalp, and genital mucosa. Active in cold, hot, soft, hard, or sea water.

phisohex (fī'sō-hĕks). Trade name for phisoderm combined with hexachlorophene, used for 2-minute preoperative scrub or wash and preparation of patient. Renders skin virtually sterile, with prolonged antisepsis.

phlebalgia (flĕb-ăl'jĭ-ă) [G. *phleps, phleb-,* vein, + *algos,* pain]. Pain in varices or venules within or around a nerve.

phlebangioma (flĕb-ăn-jĭ-ō'mă) [" + *ageion,* vessel, + -*ōma,* tumor]. An aneurysm occurring in a vein.

phlebarteriectasia (flĕb"ăr-tē"rĭ-ĕk-tā'-zĭ-ă) [" + *artēria,* artery, + *ektasis,* dilatation]. Varicose aneurysms; dilatation of blood vessels.

phlebarteriodialysis (flĕb"ăr-tē"rĭ-ō-dī-ăl'-ĭs-ĭs) [" + " + *dialysis,* separation]. Arteriovenous aneurysm.

phlebectasia, phlebectasis (flĕb-ĕk-tā'zĭ-ă, -ĕk'tă-sĭs) [" + *ektasis,* dilatation]. Venous dilatation. SYN: *varicosity.*

phlebectomy (flĕb-ĕk'tō-mĭ) [" + *ektomē,* excision]. Surgical removal of a vein.

phlebectopia (flĕb-ĕk-tō'pĭ-ă) [" + *ek,* out, + *topos,* place]. Abnormal position of a vein.

phlebemphraxis (flĕb-ĕm-frăk'sĭs) [G. *phleps, phleb-,* vein, + *emphraxis,* a stopping]. Artificial obstruction of a vein.

phlebhepatitis (flĕb-hĕp-ă-tī'tĭs) [" + *ēpar, ēpat-,* liver, + -*itis,* inflammation]. Inflammation of the hepatic vein.

phlebin (flĕb'ĭn) [G. *phleps, phleb-,* vein]. A pigment assumed to be present in venous blood.

phlebismus (flĕb-ĭz'mŭs) [G. *phleps, phleb-,* vein, + *ismos,* condition]. Venous congestion and dilatation.

phlebitis (flē-bī'tĭs) [" + -*itis,* inflammation]. Inflammation of a vein.
ETIOL: Infectious traumatism; typhoid fever; varicose veins.
SYM: Pain and tenderness along course of vein; discoloration of skin; inflammatory swelling, and acute edema

phlebitis nodularis necrotisans   P-51   **phlogogenic, phlogogenous**

below obstruction; rapid pulse; rigors; elevation of temperature; dry, brown tongue; pain in joints, if pyemia has developed.
TREATMENT: Keep patient perfectly still, limb elevated. Fomentations may give relief. Abscesses should be opened. Nourishing food; constitutional treatment. Do not forget possibility of a thrombus or embolism.
  p. nodularis necrotisans. Circumscribed inflammation of cutaneous veins resulting in nodules which ulcerate.
  p., puerperal. Venous inflammation following childbirth.
  p., sinus. Inflammation of a sinus of the cerebrum.
phlebocholosis (flĕb″ō-kō-lō′sĭs) [G. *phleps, phleb-*, vein, + *cholos*, maimed]. Diseased condition of a vein.
phleboclysis (flĕb-ŏk′lĭ-sĭs) [" + *klysis*, injection]. The introduction of an isotonic solution of dextrose or other substances into a vein.
  p., drip. Injection, intravenously, drip by drip. SEE: *Murphy drip procedure*.
phlebogram (flĕb′ō-grăm) [" + *gramma*, a mark]. A tracing of venous movement.
phlebolite, phlebolith (flĕb′ō-līt, -lĭth) [" + *lithos*, a stone]. A venous concretion, caused by calcification of a thrombus.
phlebology (flĕb-ŏl′ō-jĭ) [" + *logos*, study]. The science of veins and their diseases.
phlebometritis (flĕb″ō-mē-trī′tĭs) [" + *metra*, uterus, + *-itis*, inflammation]. Inflammation of uterine veins.
phlebomyomatosis (flĕb″ō-mī″ō-mă-tō′sĭs) [" + *mys, my-*, muscle, + *-oma*, tumor, + *-osis*, disease]. Thickening of the tissue of a vein from overgrowth of muscular fibers.
phlebopexy (flĕb′ō-pĕks″ĭ) [G. *phleps, phleb-*, vein, + *pēksis*, fixation]. Extraserous transplantation of the testes for varicocele, with preservation of venous network.
phleboplasty (flĕb′ō-plăs″tĭ) [" + *plassein*, to form]. Plastic repair of a wounded vein.
phleborrhaphy (flĕb-or′ăf-ĭ) [" + *raphē*, a sewing]. Suture of a vein.
phleborrhexis (flĕb-or-rĕks′ĭs) [" + *rēxis*, a rupture]. Rupture of a vein.
phlebosclerosis (flĕb″o-sklē-rō′sĭs) [" + *sklērōsis*, a hardening]. Fibrous hardening of a vein's walls.
phlebostasia, phlebostasis (flĕb-ō-stā′zĭ-ă, -ŏs′tă-sĭs) [" + *stasis*, a standing]. Compression of veins temporarily removing an amount of blood from the general circulation. SYN: *phlebotomy, bloodless.*
phlebothrombosis (flĕb″ō-thrŏm-bō′sĭs) [" + *thrombos*, a clot]. Clotting in a vein; phlebitis with secondary thrombosis.
phlebotome (flĕb′ō-tōm) [G. *phleps, phleb-*, vein, + *tomē*, a cutting]. Lancet used in cutting a vein.
phlebotomist (flĕb-ŏt′ō-mĭst) [" + *tomē*, an incision]. One who advocates and practices blood letting.
phlebotomy (flĕb-ŏt′ō-mĭ) [" + *tomē*, an incision]. Opening a vein. SYN: *venesection, q.v.*
  p., bloodless. Compression of veins of the extremities, cutting off some of the blood from the general circulation. SYN: *phlebostasia.*
phlegm (flĕm) [G. *phlegma*, inflammation]. 1. Thick mucus, esp. that from the respiratory passages. 2. One of the 4 "humors" of early physiology.
phlegmasia (flĕg-mā′zĭ-ă) [G. *phlegmasia*, inflammation]. Inflammation.
  p. alba dolens. Acute edema, esp. of leg from venous obstruction, usually thrombosis.
Formerly regarded as peculiar to the lying-in state but occurs at other times, even attacks men and is not confined to the lower extremities, as the arms are occasionally seat of the disease.
SYM: Usually begins, esp. in lying-in women, with slight rigors, and febrile phenomena, pain in lower part of abdomen follows, extends to hips and back, passes under Poupart's ligament and thence down the thigh into calf of leg. Sometimes proceeds from calf upwards. Whole extremity becomes excessively swollen, hot and painful, but not red, hence the name. The lochia and milk may or may not be suppressed. Constitutional disturbance and fever become greatly increased.
Tenderness on pressure most marked along course of femoral vein and veins of the affected region together with associated lymphatics may be felt to be hard and cordlike. Sometimes marked by faint red line. Progress rapid, which frequently doubles size of limb in 24 hours or less; parts within pelvis become irritable; often difficulty in evacuating bladder and rectum; glands in groin sometimes swell and suppurate, and abscesses may form in different parts of limb.
TREATMENT: Elevate limb and apply warm fomentations. Where suppuration is inevitable, poultices of linseed meal beneficial. Constitutional remedies. During inflammatory stage diet should be very simple. Later, milk, broths, soft boiled eggs, fruits, vegetables, etc. Strict cleanliness and ventilation.
NP: Complete rest, immobilization of the limb. There is danger of a piece of thrombus* becoming detached to form an *embolus.** No excitement. Six weeks in bed. SYN: *milk leg, white leg.*
  p., cellulitic. Septic inflammation of connective tissue of the leg following childbirth.
  p. malabarica. Inflammation with hypertrophy and induration of the skin. SYN: *elephantiasis.*
  p., thrombotic. SEE: *p. alba dolens.*
phlegmatic (flĕg-măt′ĭk) [G. *phlegmatikos*, inflamed]. Of sluggish or calm temperament. SYN: *apathetic.*
phlegmon (flĕg′mŏn) [G. *phlegmonē*, inflammation]. Acute suppurative inflammation of subcutaneous connective tissue.
  p., bronze. Gaseous p. after a renal operation causing bronze spots near incision.
  p., diffuse. D. inflammation of subcutaneous tissues with sepsis.
  p., gas. P. with extensive emphysema.
phlegmonous (flĕg′mŏn-ŭs) [G. *phlegmonē*, inflammation]. Pert. to inflammation of subcutaneous tissues.
phlogistic (flō-jĭs′tĭk) [G. *phlogistos*, burnt]. Pert. to or inducing inflammation.
phlogocyte (flō′gō-sīt) [G. *phlogōsis*, inflammation, + *kytos*, cell]. A typical cell in tissue during inflammation. SYN: *irritation cell, plasma cell, stimulation cell.*
phlogocytosis (flō″gō-sī-tō′sĭs) [" + " + *-osis*, disease]. Presence of many phlogocytes in the peripheral circulation.
phlogogenic, phlogogenous (flō-gō-jĕn′ĭk,

phlogosin P-52 **phoresis**

-goj'ĕn-ŭs) [" + *gennan*, to produce]. Producing or exciting inflammation.
phlogosin (flō-gō'sĭn) [G. *phlogōsis*, inflammation]. Substance, isolated from cultures of *Staphylococcus aureus*, producing suppuration.
phlogosis (flō-gō'sĭs) [G. inflammation]. 1. Inflammation. 2. Erysipelas.
phloretin (flor'e-tĭn). Product derived from phlorizin used as a febrifuge.
phlorizin (flor'ĭz-ĭn). A bitter, white, crystalline glucoside used as an antiperiodic and tonic.
phlyctena (flĭk-tē'nă) [G. *phlyktaina*, a blister]. A thin ichor or lymph containing vesicle, esp. one of many after a first degree burn.
phlyctenoid (flĭk-tē'noyd) [" + *eidos*, resemblance]. Resembling a blister or pustule.
phlyctenosis (flĭk-tē-nō'sĭs) [" + -*ōsis*, disease]. Appearance of blisters or pustules.
phlyctenula (flĭk-tĕn'ū-lă) [G. *phlyktaina*, a blister]. A tiny vesicle or pustule, esp. that seen on the cornea.
phlyctenular (flĭk-tĕn'ū-lăr) [G. *phlyktaina*, a blister]. Resembling or pert. to vesicles or pustules.
phlyctenule (flĭk-tĕn'ūl) [G. *phlyktaina*, a blister]. A small vesicle or blister, as on cornea or conjunctiva.
phlyctenulosis (flĭk-tĕn-ū-lō'sĭs) [" + -*ōsis*, intensive]. The formation of many phlyctenules.
phlyzacium (flĭ-za'sĭ-um) [G. *phlyzakion*, inflammation]. 1. A minute pustule. 2. Inflammatory disease of the skin with large, superficial pustules. SYN: *ecthyma*.
-phobia [G.]. Suffix meaning *dread, horror, fear*.
phobia (fō'bĭ-ă) [G. *phobos*, fear]. Any abnormal fear.
RS: Words beginning with the following forms: *acaro-, acro-, aero-, agora-, aichmo-, ailuro-, algo-, amaxo-, amycho-, andro-, anemo-, anthropo-, aphe-, api-, astra-, astro-, ataxo-, auto-, automyso-, bacillo-, ballisto-, basi-, batho-, bato-, belone-, bromidrosi-, cainoto-, carcinomato-, cardio-, carno-, catoptro-, ceno-, chero-, cholero-, claustro-, copro-, dora-, eremo-, ereuto-, ergasio-, ergo-, erythro-, gato-, gephyro-, gymno-, gyne-, haphe-, hemo-, klepto-, lysso-, maieusio-, mono-, myso-, mytho-, necro-, neo-, noso-, nudo-, nycto-, ochlo-, odonto-, ombro-, ophidio-, pan-, pharmaco-, photo-, poly-, pono-, psychro-, pyro-, rhabdo-, rhypo-, scoto-, sito-, symbolo-, syphilo-, thanato-, topo-, toxico-, tricho-, trichopatho-, xeno-, zoo-*.
phobic (fō'bĭk) [G. *phobos*, fear]. Concerning a phobia.
phobophobia (fō"bō-fō'bĭ-ă) [" + *phobos*, fear]. Morbid fear of acquiring a phobia.
phonacoscope (fō-năk'ō-skōp) [G. *phōnē*, voice, + *skopein*, to examine]. A device for increasing the percussion note or voice sounds.
phonacoscopy (fō-năk-ŏs'kō-pĭ) [" + *skopein*, to examine]. Inspection of the chest with the phonacoscope.
phonal (fō'năl) [G. *phōnē*, voice]. Concerning the voice.
phonasthenia (fō"năs-thē'nĭ-ă) [" + *astheneia*, weakness]. Abnormal voice sounds due to functional fatigue.
phonation (fō-nā'shŭn) [G. *phōnē*, voice]. Process of uttering vocal sounds.
phonatory (fō'nă-tō-rĭ) [G. *phōnē*, voice]. Concerning utterance of vocal sounds.
p. bands. Vocal cords.
phonautograph (fōn-aw'tō-grăf) [" + *autos*, self, + *graphein*, to write]. Device for registering the voice's vibrations.
phoneme (fō'nēm) [G. *phōnēma*, sound]. Auditory hallucination of voices and spoken words.
May include neologisms. They may repeat a thought or the part of a sentence just read.
phonendoscope (fō-nĕn'dō-skōp) [G. *phōnē*, voice, + *endon*, within, + *skopein*, to examine]. A stethoscope magnifying sounds.
phonendoskiascope (fō-nen"dō-skī'ăs-kōp) [" + " + *skia*, shadow, + *skopein*, to examine]. Device for observing the cardiac movements and for hearing heart sounds.
phonetics (fō-nĕt'ĭks) [G. *phōnētikos*, spoken]. Science of speech and pronunciation. SYN: *phonology*.
phonic (fō'nĭk) [G. *phōnē*, voice]. Concerning the voice or sound.
phonism (fō'nĭzm) [" + -*ismos*, condition]. An auditory sensation occurring when another sense is stimulated. SEE: *synesthesia*.
phono- [G.]. Combining form meaning *sound, voice*.
phonocardiography (fō"nō-kar-dĭ-ŏg-ră-fī) [" + *kardia*, heart, + *graphein*, to write]. Mechanical registration of heart sounds.
phonogram (fō'nō-grăm) [" + *gramma*, a mark]. A graphic curve indicating intensity and duration of a sound.
phonograph (fō'nō-grăf) [" + *graphein*, to write]. Appliance used for reproduction of sounds.
phonology (fō-nŏl'ō-jĭ) [" + *logos*, a study]. Science of vocal sounds. SYN: *phonetics*.
phonomassage (fō"nō-măs-sazh') [" + *massein*, to knead]. Exciting movements of the ossicles of the ear by means of noise directed through the ext. auditory meatus.
phonometer (fō-nŏm'ĕt-ĕr) [" + *metron*, measure]. Device for determining intensity of vocal sounds.
phonomyoclonus (fō"nō-mī-ok'lō-nŭs) [G. *phōnē*, voice, + *mys, myo-*, muscle, + *klonos*, a contraction]. Invisible fibrillary muscular contractions revealed by auscultation.
phonomyogram (fō"nō-mī'ō-grăm) [" + " + *gramma*, a writing]. A recording of sound produced by action of a muscle.
phonomyography (fō"nō-mī-ŏg'ră-fĭ) [" + " + *graphein*, to write]. The recording of sounds made by contracting muscular tissue.
phonopathy (fō-nŏp'ăth-ĭ) [" + *pathos*, disease]. Any disease of organs affecting speech.
phonophore (fō'nō-fōr) [" + *phoros*, carrying]. 1. An ossicle of the ear. 2. A form of binaural stethoscope.
phonopneumomassage (fō"nō-nu"mō-măs-săzh') [" + *pneuma*, air, + *massein*, to knead]. Massage of the middle ear, and by forcing air into the ext. auditory meatus.
phonopsia (fō-nŏp'sĭ-ă) [" + *opsis*, vision]. Perception of certain sounds which cause a subjective color sensation.
phonoscope (fō'nō-skōp) [G. *phōnē*, voice, + *skopein*, to examine]. Device for recording photographs of heart sounds.
phoresis (fō-rē'sĭs) [G. *phorēsis*, from *phorein*, to bear]. PT: The migration of ions through a membrane by the action of an electric current.
The direction of migration is some-

times distinguished by the use of the terms "cataphoresis" and "anaphoresis" for migrations toward cathode and anode, respectively.

phorology (fō-rol'ō-jī) [G. *phorein*, to carry, + *logos*, study]. Science dealing with disease carriers.

phorometer (fō-rŏm'ĕt-ēr) [" + *metron*, measure]. Device for examination of the extrinsic ocular muscles.

phorotone (fō'rō-tōn) [" + *tonos*, tension]. Device for exercising eye muscles.

phose (fōz) [G. *phōs*, light]. A subjective sensation of light or color. SEE: *centraphose*, *centrophose*, *chromophose*, *peripheraphose*, *peripherophose*.

phosphatase (fŏs'fāt-ās). An enzyme which splits phosphoric acid esters.

phosphate (fŏs'fāt) [G. *phōs*, light, + *pherein*, to carry]. A salt of phosphoric acid.

They are present in the blood in small amounts and help to form buffers which are of small value in the blood, but more important in their effects in the excretion of acid products by the kidneys.

Two to 3 Gm. of phosphoric acid are excreted in 24 hours.

Decreased p. excretion seen in nephritic acidosis.

Increased p. in urine occur in convalescence from acute fevers, in diabetes, leukemia, disease of the bones, following violent exercise, worry, mental strain, hot baths, and often the use of some drugs.

p., test for in urine. To half an inch of urine add a few drops of uranium nitrate and a few drops of sodium acetate solution. The presence of phosphates is indicated by a greenish precipitate.

phosphatemia (fŏs-fă-tē'mĭ-ă) [" + " + *aima*, blood]. Phosphates in the blood.

phosphatide (fŏs'fă-tīd) [" + *pherein*, to carry]. One of a group of fatty substances containing phosphoric acid.
An example is lecithin. SYN: *phospholipide*, *phospholipin*.

phosphatine (fŏs'fă-tĭn). One of a class of phosphorous compounds found in brain tissue.

phosphatometer (fŏs-fă-tŏm'ĕt-ēr) [G. *phōs*, light, + *pherein*, to carry, + *metron*, a measure]. Device for measuring the amount of phosphates in the urine.

phosphatoptosis (fŏs-fă-tŏp-tō'sis) [" + + *ptōsis*, a dropping]. Spontaneous precipitation of phosphates in urine.

phosphaturia (fŏs-fă-tū'rĭ-ă) [" + " + *ouron*, urine]. Phosphates in the urine.
They often cause renal calculi. May be associated with mental strain, anxiety or neurasthenia. SYN: *phosphoruria*, *phosphuria*.

SYM: Cloudy urine, opaque and pale. Reaction alkaline. Pearly- or pinkish-white deposits of phosphates in standing urine.

phosphene (fŏs'fēn) [" + *phainein*, to show]. A subjective sensation of light caused by pressure upon the eyeball.

phosphide (fŏs'fīd) [G. *phōs*, light, + *pherein*, to carry]. Binary compound of phosphorus with an element or radical.

phosphite (fŏs'fīt) [" + *pherein*, to carry]. A salt of phosphoric acid.

phosphocreatine (fŏs"fō-krē'ă-tēn). A compound found in muscle of equal parts of phosphoric acid and creatine.

phospholipid (fŏs"fō-lĭp'ĭd) [G. *phōs*, light, + *pherein*, to carry, + *lipos*, fat]. A lipoid substance containing phosphorus, fatty acids and nitrogenous base, as lecithin. SYN: *phosphatide*.

phospholipin (fŏs"fō-lĭp'ĭn) [" + " + *lipos*, fat]. A lipoid compound containing phosphorus. SYN: *phosphatide*.

phosphonecrosis (fŏs"fō-nē-krō'sĭs) [G. *phōs*, light, + *pherein*, to carry, + *nekros*, dead, + *-ōsis*, disease]. Necrosis of the alveolar process in those working with phosphorus.

phosphopenia (fŏs"fō-pē'nĭ-ă) [" + " + *penia*, lack]. Lack of phosphorus in the body.

phosphoprotein (fŏs"fō-prō'tē-ĭn) [" + " + *prōtos*, first]. One of a group of proteins in which the protein is combined with phosphorus other than lecithin or nucleic acid.
Formerly called nucleoalbumin.

phosphorated (fŏs'fō-rā-tĕd) [" + *phorein*, to carry]. Impregnated with phosphorus.

phosphorenesis (fŏs"fō-rĕn'ĕ-sĭs) [" + *phorein*, to carry]. Any condition of the body due to excess of calcium phosphate.

phosphorescence (fŏs-fō-rĕs'ĕns) [" + *phorein*, to carry]. PT: The induced luminescence that persists after cessation of the irradiation that caused it.

phosphoretted (fŏs"fō-rĕt-ĕd) [" + *phorein*, to carry]. Impregnated with, or charged with phosphorus.

phosphorhidrosis (fŏs"for-hĭd-rō'sĭs) [G. *phōs*, light, + *phorein*, to carry, + *idrōsis*, sweating]. Secretion of phosphorescent perspiration. SYN: *phosphoridrosis*.

phosphoric acid (fŏs-for'ĭk) [" + *phorein*, to carry]. One of 3 oxygen acids of phosphorus. SEE: *acid*.

phosphoridrosis (fŏs"for-ĭd-rō'sĭs) [" + " + *idrōsis*, perspiration]. Secretion of perspiration that is luminous. SYN: *phosphorhidrosis*.

phosphorism (fŏs'for-ĭzm) [G. *phōs*, light, + *phoros*, carrying, + *ismos*, condition]. Chronic poisoning from P.

phosphorous acid (fŏs-fō'rŭs) [" + *phoros*, carrying]. Crystalline acid formed when phosphorus is oxidized in moist air. SEE: *acid*.

phosphoruria (fŏs"for-ū'rĭ-ă) [" + " + *ouron*, urine]. Phosphorus in the urine in excess of normal. SYN: *phosphaturia*, *phosphuria*.

phosphorus (fŏs'fĕr-ŭs) [G. *phōs*, light, + *phoros*, carrying]. SYMB: P. At. wt. 31.04. A nonmetallic element not found in a free state but in combination with alkalies.

It occurs in 2 forms: the yellow, crystalline, waxy, poisonous form, and the allotropic, reddish-brown, nonpoisonous powder which is toxic only because it often contains 0.4 to 0.6% yellow phosphorus. Calcium phosphate is in all fertile soils, and it is essential to the growth of plant life. This is the only form in which it can be absorbed by plants, and through vegetable life it enters into the food of men and animals.

The element phosphorus is taken into the body at the rate of about 1 Gm. per day in the form of various foods like milk, in which one finds a phosphoprotein, casein, plus other phosphorus-containing substances. In the blood, phosphorus can be found in the form of phosphates and phospholipins both in the corpuscles and, either dissolved or suspended, in the plasma; it is also found as calcium phosphate in the bones and teeth. At any given time the body

phosphotal P-54 **photoncia**

of an adult is likely to contain about 70 Gm. of phosphorus in various forms. What is not needed by the body is excreted as phosphate in the urine, and the amount so excreted by an adult will be roughly equal, in 24 hours, to the amount taken in.

FUNCTIONS: It constitutes an important part of bone, nerves and brain, and aids in building bone and teeth. In bone, it exists as phosphate of calcium and other alkaline earths, forming 60% of the bones. In the cells, it consists of nuclein, various phosphorized fats, such as lecithin, cerebrin, and cholesterin.

It activates enzymes, is essential in the metabolism of fats and carbohydrates, and exerts buffer effects in blood and muscles. It is necessary to maintenance of the neutral condition of the blood which it brings about as a soluble salt in conjunction with the carbonates and protein. About 0.38 Gm. per day is necessary, although the gross quantity should be 1.32 Gm. to allow for loss. It leaves the body in the same organic condition in which it enters the vegetable kingdom.

DOSAGE: 1/100 gr. (0.0006 Gm.).

DEFICIENCY SYM: Perverted appetite, retarded growth, loss of weight, weakness, rickets, imperfect bone and teeth development.

It is found in the protein of food. Ex: Almonds, beans, barley, bran, cheese, cocoa, chocolate, eggs, lentils, liver, milk, oatmeal, peanuts, peas, walnuts, whole wheat, and rye. *Good*: Asparagus, beef, cabbage, carrots, celery, cauliflower, chards, chicken, clams, corn, cream, cucumbers, egg plant, fish, figs, prunes, pineapples, pumpkin, raisins, string beans; also in meats.

POISONING: SYM: Acute irritation of gastrointestinal tract, followed by symptoms resembling acute yellow atrophy of liver, and marked blood changes. Bloody vomitus, garlic odor of breath, cramps, headache, liver and kidney damage. Profound weakness, hemorrhage, heart failure. Occasionally nervous symptoms predominate. Metabolism changes.

F. A. TREATMENT: Prolonged gastric lavage, part of which should contain a small amount of copper sulfate or potassium permanganate which may aid in oxidizing the phophorus. This should, of course, be washed out. Oils, creams and fats should be avoided. Sodium bicarbonate tends to reduce acidosis. Otherwise treat symptomatically. Blood transfusion is helpful.

phosphotal (fŏs'fō-tăl). Commercial phosphorus and creosote compound.
phosphuria (fŏs-fū'rĭ-ă) [G. *phōs*, light, + *phoros*, a bearer, + *ouron*, urine]. Excess of phosphorus in the urine. SYN: *phosphaturia, phosphoruria.*
photalgia (fō-tăl'jĭ-ă) [G. *phōs, phot-*, light, + *algos*, pain]. Pain produced by light. SYN: *photodynia.*
photaugiophobia (fō-tăw-jĭ-ō-fō'bĭ-ă) [" + *augē*, glare, + *phobos*, fear]. Intolerance of bright light.
phote (fōt) [G. *phōs, phot-*, light]. The unit of photochemical energy, 1 lumen per square centimeter, employed in determination of color solidity in comparison with average noonday solar light.
photesthesis (fō-tĕs-thē'sĭs) [" + *aisthesis*, sensation]. Sensitivity to light.
photic (fō'tĭk) [G. *phōs, phot-*, light]. Concerning light.
photism (fō'tĭzm) [" + *ismos*, condition]. A subjective sensation of color or light produced by a stimulus of another sense, such as smell, hearing, taste, or touch. SEE: *synesthesia.*
photo- [G.]. Combining form meaning *light*.
photobiotic (fō"tō-bī-ŏt'ĭk) [G. *phōs, phot-*, light, + *bios*, life]. Capable of living only in the light.
photocauterization (fō"tō-kaw-tĕr-ĭz-ā'shŭn) [" + *kautērion*, a branding iron]. Cauterization using radioactive means, as x-rays.
photoceptor (fō"tō-sĕp'tor) [" + L. *ceptor*, a receiver]. A nerve ceptor receiving light ray sensations.
photochemistry (fō"tō-kĕm'ĭs-trĭ) [" + *chemeia*, chemistry]. Phase of science dealing with chemical changes produced by light rays.
photodynamic (fō"tō-dī-năm'ĭk) [" + *dynamis*, force]. Pert. to the effect of light on organisms.
photodynia (fō"tō-dĭn'ĭ-ă) [" + *odynē*, pain]. Pain produced by rays of light. SYN: *photalgia.*
photodysphoria (fō"tō-dĭs-fō'rĭ-ă) [" + *dys*, bad, + *phorein*, to carry]. Extreme intolerance of light. SYN: *photophobia, phengophobia.*
photoelectricity (fō"tō-ē-lĕk-trĭ'sĭ-tĭ) [G. *phōs, phot-*, light, + *ēlektron*, amber]. Electricity formed by action of light.
photogene (fō'tō-jĕn) [" + *gennan*, to produce]. Prolonged retinal image. SYN: *after-image.*
photogenic, photogenous (fō"tō-jĕn'ĭk, -tŏj'ĕn-ŭs) [" + *gennan*, to produce]. Induced by or inducing light.
photograph'ic radiom'eter. PT: An instrument containing a half-tone color index for strips of photographic paper after exposure to roentgen rays and after development, used to estimate the quantity of roentgen rays.
photohemotachometer (fō"tō-hem"ō-tăk-ŏm'ĕt-ĕr) [G. *phōs, phot-*, light, + *aima*, blood, + *tachus*, swift, + *metron* measure]. Device for photographing velocity of blood current.
photoinactivation (fō"tō-ĭn-ăk-tĭ-vā'shŭn) [" + L. *in*, not, + *activus*, acting]. Inactivation of complement by use of light rays.
photokinetic (fō"tō-kĭn-ĕt'ĭk) [" + *kinēsis*, motion]. Reacting with motion to stimulus of light.
photoluminescence (fō"tō-lū-mĭn-ĕs'ĕns) [" + L. *lumen*, light]. PT: The power of an object to become luminescent when acted on by light.
photolysis (fō-tŏl'ĭs-ĭs) [" + *lysis*, dissolution]. Dissolution or disintegration under stimulus of light rays.
photolytic (fō"tō-lĭt'ĭk). Dissolved by stimulus of light rays.
photomania (fō"tō-mā'nĭ-ă) [" + *mania*, madness]. 1. A psychosis produced by prolonged exposure to intense light. 2. A psychotic desire for light.
photometer (fō-tŏm'ĕt-ĕr) [G. *phōs, phot-*, light, + *metron*, measure]. PT: A device for measuring the intensity of light.
photometry (fō-tom'ĕt-rĭ) [" + *metron*, measure]. Measurement of light rays.
photomicrograph (fō"tō-mī'krō-grăf) [" + *mikros*, small, + *graphein*, to write]. Enlarged photograph of an object under the microscope.
photon (fō'tŏn) [G. *phōs, phot-*, light]. A light particle comparable to an electron.
photoncia (fō-tŏn'sĭ-ă) [" + *ogkos*, tumor]. Swelling caused by the action of light.

photonosus (fō-ton'ō-sŭs) [" + *nosos*, disease]. Disease due to prolonged exposure to intense light.

photoperceptive (fō″tō-pĕr-cĕp'tĭv) [" + *percipere*, to receive]. Capable of perceiving light.

photophilic (fō-tō-fĭl'ĭk) [" + *philein*, to love]. Seeking or fond of light.

photophobia (fō″tō-fō'bĭ-ă) [" + *phobos*, fear]. Unusual intolerance of light.
 Occurs in measles and rubella, meningitis, and inflammations of the eyes. SYN: *phengophobia, photodysphoria*.

photophone (fō'tō-fōn) [" + *phōnē*, voice]. Device for production of sound by action of light.

photophore (fō'tō-fōr) [G. *phōs, phot-*, light, + *phoros*, a bearer]. Apparatus for examining cavities by electricity.

photopia (fō-tō'pĭ-ă) [" + *ōps*, eye]. Adjustment of eye muscles to light.

photopsia, photopsy (fō-tŏp'sĭ-ă, fō'tŏp-sĭ) [" + *opsis*, vision]. Subjective sensation of sparks or flashes of light in retinal, optic, or brain diseases.

photoptarmosis (fō″tō-tar-mō'sĭs) [" + *ptarmōsis*, sneezing]. Sneezing caused by the action of light.

photoptometer (fō-tŏp-tŏm'ĕt-ĕr) [" + *opsis*, vision, + *metron*, measure]. Device for determining acuteness of vision.

photoreceptive (fō″tō-rē-sĕp'tĭv) [" + *receptor*, a receiver]. Capable of perceiving light rays.

photoreceptor (fō″tō-rē-sep'tor) [" + *receptor*, a receiver]. Nerve ceptor sensitive to light stimuli.

photoscope (fō'tō-skōp) [G. *phōs, phot-*, light, + *skopein*, to examine]. A variety of fluoroscope used to observe light.

photoscopy (fō-tŏs'kō-pī) [" + *skopein*, to examine]. Examination with a fluorescent screen. SYN: *fluoroscopy, skiascopy*.

photosensitization (fō″tō-sĕn-sĭ-tĭ-zā'shŭn) [" + *sensitivus*, feeling]. Process by which phenomena are produced in living system by substances not normally present in these systems which sensitize them to light.

photosensitizer (fō″tō-sĕn-sĭ-tĭ'zĕr) [" + *sensitivus*, feeling]. Sensitizing substance used in light therapy to produce photosensitization, such as fluorescein dyes.

photosynthesis (fō″tō-sĭn'the-sĭs) [" + *synthesis*, a placing together]. The process by which plants are able to manufacture carbohydrates from the air in the presence of light.
 Only plants containing chlorophyll are capable of thus producing sugars. The red and blue waves of the spectrum are absorbed by the chlorophyll, but all other rays are rejected. CO_2 and H_2O are also necessary factors.
 When grape sugar is formed, the plant splits up CO_2, uses the carbon by photosynthesis, and liberates the oxygen. The sources of energy for this disruption are the blue and red rays which are absorbed by the plant. To make 1 Gm. of synthetic sugar the plant uses 750 cu. ft. of CO_2.

phototaxis (fō″tō-tăks'ĭs) [" + *taxis*, arrangement]. PT: The reaction and movement of cells and microörganisms under the stimulus of light.

phototherapy (fō″tō-thĕr'ă-pī) [" + *therapeia*, treatment]. Light therapy, the use of light in treating disease.
 By custom the term denotes also the application of the invisible, infrared or heat and ultraviolet, or actinic rays. SEE: *actinotherapy*.

photothermal (fō″tō-thĕr'măl) [G. *phōs, phot-*, light, + *thermē*, heat]. Concerning heat produced by light.

 p. radiation. Radiation of heat by a source of light, as that from an electric bulb.

phototoxis (fō″tō-toks'ĭs) [" + *toxikon*, poison]. Disorder produced by effects of overexposure to light or radiation.

photuria (fō-tū'rĭ-ă) [" + *ouron*, urine]. Excretion of phosphorescent urine.

phren (frĕn) [G. *phrēn*, mind, diaphragm]. 1. The mind. 2. The diaphragm.

phrenalgia (frĕ-năl'jĭ-ă) [" + *algos*, pain]. 1. Pain of mental origin or caused by a mental process. SYN: *psychalgia*. 2. Pain in the diaphragm.

phrenasthenia (fren-ăs-thē'nĭ-ă) [" + *astheneia*, weakness]. Mental deficiency.

phrenetic (fren-ĕt'ĭk) [G. *phrēn*, mind]. 1. Maniacal; frenzied. 2. A maniac.

phrenic (frĕn'ĭk) [G. *phrēn*, mind, diaphragm]. 1. Concerning the diaphragm; as the p. nerve. 2. Concerning the mind.

 p. avulsion. Elevation of a side of the diaphragm and semi-collapse of corresponding lung by means of excision of part of the phrenic nerve.

 p. nerve. One arising in the cervical plexus before entering the thorax and passing to the diaphragm.
 A motor nerve to the diaphragm with sensory fibers to the pericardium. SYN: *nervus phrenicus*.

phrenicectomy (fren-ĭs-ĕk'tō-mĭ) [" + *ektomē*, excision]. Resection of a part of the phrenic nerve.
 Used to collapse the lung on 1 side by paralyzing the diaphragm.

phrenicoexairesis (fren″ĭ-kō-ĕks-ī-rē'sĭs) [" + *ek*, out, + *airein*, to take]. Excision of part of the phrenic nerve.

phrenicotomy (fren-ĭk-ŏt'ō-mĭ) [" + *tomē*, a cutting]. Cutting of the phrenic nerve to produce immobilization of a lung by inducing a paralysis of 1 side.
 This causes the diaphragm to rise, it compresses the lung, and diminishes respiratory movement, thus resting the viscus.

phrenitis (frĕ-nī'tĭs) [" + *-itis*, inflammation]. 1. Acute delirium or frenzy. 2. Inflammation of the brain. SYN: *encephalitis*. 3. Inflammation of the diaphragm.

phreno- [G.]. Combining form meaning *mind, midriff*.

phrenocardia (frē″nō-kar'dĭ-ă) [" + *kardia*, heart]. Cardiovascular neurasthenia.
 SYM: Cardiac arrhythmia, dyspnea with psychic disturbances, and submammary pain.

phrenocolopexy (frē″nō-kō'lō-pĕks″ĭ) [" + *kōlon*, colon, + *pēxis*, fixation]. Suture of the transverse colon to the diaphragm.

phrenodynia (frē″nō-dĭn'ĭ-ă [" + *odynē*, pain]. Pain in the diaphragm.

phrenograph (fren'ō-grăf) [G. *phrēn*, diaphragm, mind, + *graphein*, to write]. Device for registering movements of diaphragm.

phrenology (frē-nol'ō-jī) [" + *logos*, study]. Study of the shape of the skull as indicative of characteristics and mental faculties.

phrenopathy (frē-nŏp'ăth-ĭ) [" + *pathos*, disease]. Any mental disorder.

phrenopericarditis (frē″nō-pĕr-ĭ-kar-dī'-tĭs) [" + *peri*, around, + *kardia*, heart,

-itis, inflammation]. Attachment of the heart by adhesions to the diaphragm.
phrenoplegia (frē-nō-plē'jĭ-ă) [" + *plēgē*, a stroke]. 1. A sudden psychopathic attack. 2. Paralysis of the diaphragm.
phrenosin (fren'ō-sĭn) [G. *phrēn*, mind, diaphragm]. A nitrogenous principle obtained from brain substance.
phrictopathic (frĭk-tō-păth'ĭk) [G. *phriktos*, shuddering, + *pathos*, disease]. Pert. to or having a shuddering sensation; applied to a shuddering sensation due to irritating a hysterical anesthetic area.
phthiocol (thĭ'ō-kōl). Oily yellow pigment found in tubercle bacilli.
phthiriasis (thĭr-ī'ăs-ĭs) [G. *phtheir*, louse]. Condition of being infested with lice. SYN: *pediculosis*.
 p. palpebrarum. Presence of lice on the eyelashes.
phthiriophobia (thĭr″ĭ-ō-fō'bĭ-ă) [" + *phobos*, fear]. Abnormal dread of lice.
Phthirius (thĭr'ĭ-ŭs) [G. *phtheir*, louse]. Genus of crab louse.
phthisic (tĭz'ĭk) [G. *phthisis*, a wasting]. 1. Affected with pulmonary consumption. 2. Asthma. 3. One afflicted with phthisis or asthma.
phthisical (tĭz'ĭk-ăl) [G. *phthisis*, a wasting]. Concerning, or afflicted with, phthisis.
phthisicky (tĭz'ĭ-kĭ) [G. *phthisis*, a wasting]. Suffering from asthma or phthisis.
phthisis (tĭ'sĭs) [G. a wasting]. 1. Pulmonary consumption. SEE: *tuberculosis*. 2. Any wasting or atrophic disease.
 p., abdominal. Intestinal tuberculosis.
 p., black. Lung disease from inhaled coal dust. SYN: *anthracosis*.
 p. bulbi. Atrophy of eyeball following intraocular inflammation.
 p., fibroid. 1. Interstitial pneumonia. 2. Pulmonary tuberculosis with dense layers of fibrous tissues surrounding a cavity.
 p. mesenterica. Tuberculosis of the mesentery glands.
 p., miner's. SEE: *black p*.
 p., pulmonary. Tuberculosis of the lungs.
 p., stonecutter's. A wasting form of bronchopneumonia due to inhalation of stone dust with consequent irritation. SYN: *chalicosis*.
phygogalactic (fī″gō-găl-ăk'tĭk) [G. *pheugein*, to avoid, + *gala*, milk]. Checking or that which checks or arrests milk secretion. SYN: *galactophygous, ischogalactic, lactifuge.*
phylacogen (fī-lăk'ō-jĕn) [G. *phylax*, guard, + *gennan*, to produce]. Commercial bacterial culture filtrate which stimulates defensive protein formation in the body.
phylacogogic (fī-lăk-ō-gŏj'ĭk) [" + *agōgos*, leading]. Stimulating the formation of protective antibodies.
phylactic (fī-lăk'tĭk) [G. *phylaxis*, protection]. Concerning or producing phylaxis.
 p. agent. One with protective power.
 p. power. That of an organism to ward off infection.
phylaxin (fī-lăks'ĭn) [G. *phylaxis*, protection]. Substance warding off infection. SEE: *mycophylaxin, toxophylaxin.*
phylaxis (fī-lăks'ĭs) [G. protection]. The active defense of the body against infection.
phyllo- [G.]. Combining form meaning *leaf*.
phylogenesis (fī-lō-jĕn'ĕ-sĭs) [G. *phylon*, tribe, + *genesis*, generation]. The growth of a group, race or species.
phylogenetical (fī″lō-jĕn-ĕt'ĭk-ăl) [" + *genesis*, generation]. Concerning the development of a race or group.
phylogeny (fī-lŏj'ĕ-nĭ) [" + *gennan*, to produce]. Development and growth of a group or race.
phylum (fī'lŭm) [G. *phylon*, tribe]. One of the primary divisions of the animal or plant kingdom.
phyma (fī'mă) (pl. *phymata*) [G. *phyma*, growth]. A small, rounded skin tumor.
phymatoid (fī'măt-oyd) [" + *eidos*, resemblance]. Like a tumor.
phymatosis (fī-mă-tō'sĭs) [" + *-ōsis*, disease]. A disease marked by the presence of phymata or small nodules in the skin.
phyon(e (fī'ŏn) [G. *phyos*, growth]. 1. The growth factor of the ant. pituitary body. 2. Commercial preparation of growth factor of ant. pituitary body.
physaliform, physalliform (fĭs-al'ĭ-form) [G. *physallis*, bubble, + L. *forma*, shape]. Resembling a bleb or bubble.
physaliphore (fĭs-ăl'ĭf-or) [" + *phoros*, carrying]. A round cavity in a cancer cell.
physalis (fĭs'ăl-ĭs) [G. *physallis*, bubble]. Huge brood cell from a cancer or sarcoma.
physic (fĭz'ĭk) [G. *physikos*, natural]. 1. The art of medicine and healing. 2. A medicine, esp. a cathartic. 3. Drugs in general.
physical (fĭz'ĭk-ăl) [G. *physikos*, natural]. Concerning the body.
 p. examination. Examination of the body by auscultation, palpation, percussion and inspection.
 p. signs. Disease symptoms revealed by physical examination.
 p. therapist. PT: A medical graduate skilled in physical therapy.
 p. therapy. The therapeutic use of physical agents other than drugs.
It comprises the use of physical, chemical and other properties of heat, light, water, electricity, massage, exercise, and radiation. SEE: *breeze, static*.
 p. t. technician or aide. A lay assistant or a nurse trained to apply the physical measures of treatment which have been prescribed by a physician.
 p. unit. Coulomb, erg, dyne, etc. SEE: *unit*.
physician (fĭ-zĭsh'ăn) [O. Fr. *physicien*, from G. *physikos*, natural]. A person authorized by law to treat diseases with medicines.
physicist (fĭz'ĭs-ĭst) [G. *physikos*, natural]. One who is versed in the science of physics.
physico- [G.]. Combining form meaning *physical, natural*.
physics (fĭz'ĭks) [G. *physis*, nature]. The study of forces and properties of matter, and of natural phenomena.
physinosis (fĭz-ĭn-ō'sĭs) [" + *nosos*, disease]. A disease caused by physical agents.
physio- [G.]. Combining form meaning *nature*.
physiognomy (fĭz-ĭ-ŏg'nō-mĭ) [G. *physis*, nature, + *gnōmōn*, a judge]. 1. The countenance. 2. Assumed ability to see the mental or moral character and qualities by the face.
physiognosis (fĭz-ĭ-ŏg-nō'sĭs) [" + *gnosis*, knowledge]. Diagnosis determined from one's facial expression and appearance of the eyes.
physiological (fĭz″ĭ-ō-lŏj'ĭk-ăl) [G. *physis*,

physiological chemistry   P-57   **pigment, urinary**

nature, + *logos,* study]. 1. Normal; not diseased. 2. Concerning body function.
   p. chemistry. Chemistry of living organisms. SEE: *biochemistry.*
   p. salt solution. One teaspoonful of salt to a pint of water is a normal salt solution. It may be abbreviated as N. S. Sol.
   p. s. s. enema. The distention made by this enema excites peristalsis and evacuation. Often ordered when there is dehydration. SEE: *enema.*
physiology (fĭz-ĭ-ŏl′ō-jĭ) [G. *physis,* nature, + *logos,* study]. The science of the functions of cells, tissues, and organs of the living organism. SEE: *cerebrophysiology, chemophysiology.*
physiotherapy (fĭz-ĭ-ō-thĕr′ă-pĭ) [" + *therapeia,* treatment]. Treatment with physical and mechanical means, as massage, electricity, etc.
   The term "physical therapy" has supplanted it in medical usage.
physo- [G.]. Combining form meaning *bladder, bellows, bubble.*
physocele (fĭ′sō-sēl) [G. *physa,* air, + *kēlē,* tumor]. 1. A tumor filled with gas or circumscribed swelling due to gas. 2. A gas-distended hernial sac.
physohematometra (fĭ″sō-hem-ăt-ō-mē′tră) [" + *aima,* blood, + *mētra,* uterus]. Gas and blood distending the uterus.
physohydrometra (fĭ″sō-hī-drō-mē′tră) [" + *ydōr,* water, + *mētra,* uterus]. Air or gas and serum in the uterus.
physometra (fĭ-sō-mē′tră) [" + *mētra,* uterus]. Air or gas in the uterine cavity.
physopyosalpinx (fĭ″sō-pī″ō-săl′pĭnks) [" + *pyon,* pus, + *salpigx,* tube]. Pus and gas in the fallopian tube.
physostigmine salicylate (fĭ-sō-stĭg′mĕn săl-ĭs′ĭl-āt). USP. The salicylate of an alkaloid obtained from the dried Calabar bean.
   ACTION AND USES: To increase intestinal peristalsis and produce contraction of pupil by local action.
   DOSAGE: In eye, solutions 1%. Internally 1/30 gr. (0.002 Gm.).
phytalbumin (fī-tăl-bū′mĭn) [G. *phyton,* plant, + L. *albumen,* white of egg]. An albumin from plants and vegetables.
phytalbumose (fī-tăl′bū-mōs) [" + L. *albumen,* white of egg]. An albumose found in plants and vegetables.
phytase (fī′tās) [" + *ase,* enzyme]. A liver and blood ferment which splits phytin.
   DOSAGE: 4-15 gr. (0.25-1.0 Gm.).
phyto-, phyt- [G.]. Combining forms meaning a *plant,* or *that which grows.*
phytobezoar (fī″tō-bē′zōr) [" + Persian *bād-zahr,* antidote]. A stone composed of vegetable matter found in the stomach. SYN: *food ball.*
phytosis (fī-tō′sĭs) [" + *-ōsis,* disease]. Any disease of vegetable parasitic origin.
pia (pī′ă) [L. tender]. Innermost cerebrospinal membrane.
   p. arachnoid (ă-răk′noyd). The pia mater and arachnoid membranes, when regarded as 1 structure.
   p., cerebral. The pia of the brain, containing in its meshes ramifications of cerebral vessels. [brain.
   p., external. Pia covering ext. of the
   p., internal. Pia within the ventricles of the brain.
   p. mater. Innermost vascular membrane covering the spinal cord, nerves, and brain.

   p., spinal. SEE: *pia mater.*
pia-arachnitis (pī-ă-ăr-ăk-nī′tĭs) [L. *pia,* tender, + G. *arachnē,* spider, + *-itis,* inflammation]. Inflammation of the arachnoid and pia mater. SYN: *leptomeningitis.*
pial (pī′al). Concerning the pia mater.
pialyn (pī′al-ĭn) [G. *piar,* fat, + *lyein,* to loosen]. A fat-splitting enzyme. SYN: *lipase, steapsin.*
pian (pī-ăn′) [Fr.]. Contagious skin disease of the tropics. SYN: *frambesia, yaws.*
pianists' cramp (pē′ăn-ĭsts). Spasm or professional neurosis of muscles of fingers and forearms from piano playing.
piarachnitis (pi-ăr-ăk-nī′tĭs) [L. *pia,* tender, + G. *arachnē,* spider, + *-itis,* inflammation]. Inflamed condition of the arachnoid and pia mater.
piarachnoid (pī-ăr-ăk′noyd) [" + " + *eidos,* like]. The pia and arachnoid considered as one.
piarrhemia (pī-ar-ē′mĭ-ă) [G. *piar,* fat, + *aima,* blood]. Fat or lipids in the blood. SYN: *lipemia.*
pica (pī′kă) [L. magpie]. A perversion of appetite, with craving for substance not fit for food.
   Condition seen in pregnancy, chlorosis, hysteria, helminthiasis and in certain psychoses. SEE: *appetite, taste.*
piceous (pĭ′sē-ŭs). Like pitch.
Pick's syndrome (pĭk). 1. Effusions in the serous cavities with cardiac decompensation and ascites. 2. Progressive dementia.
picrate (pĭk′rāt). A salt of picric acid.
picric ac id (pĭk′rĭk) [G. *pikros,* bitter]. Bitter yellow crystalline substance formed by action of nitric acid on phenol or allied compounds.
   Used as a dye, an antiseptic and in treating burns.
picro-, picr- [G.]. Combining forms meaning *bitter.*
picrocarmine (pĭk-rō-kar′mĭn). A stain used in microscopy.
picroformal (pĭk-rō-for′mal). Solution of picric acid, formaldehyde and water used as a fixing agent.
picrol (pĭk′rōl). Antiseptic powder used as a dressing.
piebald skin (pī′bawld). Skin with spots or pigmentation or patches with loss of pigment. SEE: *leukoderma, vitiligo.*
piedra (pĭ-ā′dră) [Spanish, stone]. Disease in which hard nodules form on the hair shafts.
   Composed of fungous masses of *Trichosporon giganteum.*
   p. nostras. P. affecting the beard.
piesesthesia (pī-es-ĕs-thē′zĭ-ă) [G. *piesis,* pressure, + *aisthēsis,* sensation]. Sensibility to pressure. SYN: *pressure sense.*
piesimeter, piesometer (pī-ē-sĭm′ĕt-ĕr, -sōm′ĕt-ĕr). Device for measurement of skin's sensitiveness to pressure.
pigment (pĭg′mĕnt) [L. *pigmentum,* paint]. Any coloring matter. SEE: *albino, "chrom-" words.*
   p., biliary. Bilirubin, biliverdin, *q.v.*
   p., blood. Hematin, hemoglobin, oxyhemoglobin, *q.v.*
   p., endogenous. A pigment produced within the body, as melanin.
   p., exogenous. A pigment produced outside the human body.
   p., hematogenous. P. from hemoglobin of erythrocytes.
   p., hepatogenous. P. from hemoglobin destruction in the liver. SYN: *bile pigment.*
   p., urinary. Urobilin, *q.v.*

pigment, uveal

p., uveal. That in cells on inner or post. surface of the iris, choroid, and ciliary processes.

pigmentary (pĭg'mĕn-tĕr-ĭ) [L. *pigmentum*, paint]. Concerning, or like, a pigment.

pigmentation (pĭg-mĕn-tā'shŭn) [L. *pigmentum*, paint]. Localized coloration due to deposition of pigments.
RS: *albinism, carotenosis, "chrom-" words*.

p., lymphatic. Arrest of granules of pigment by lymph nodules in tattooing.

pigmentolysin (pĭg″mĕn-tŏl'ĭ-sĭn) [" + G. *lysis*, dissolution]. An antibody that destroys pigment.

pigmentolysis (pĭg″mĕn-tŏl'ĭ-sĭs) [" + G. *lysis*, dissolution]. Disintegration of pigment.

pigmentophage (pĭg-mĕn'tō-fāj) [" + G. *phagein*, to eat]. Cell which absorbs pigment.

pigritis (pĭ-grī'tĭs) [L. *piger*, slow, + G. *-itis*, inflammation]. Stuporous condition due to alcoholism.

piitis (pī-ī'tĭs) [L. *pia*, tender, + G. *-itis*, inflammation]. Inflamed condition of the pia mater.

Pil. Abbr. of L. *pilula*, pill, or pl. *pilulae*, pills.

pilar, pilary (pī'lar, pĭl'ă-rĭ) [L. *pilaris*, pert. to the hair]. Concerning, or covered with, hair.

pilaster (pī-lăs'tĕr) [L. *pila*, pillar]. A prominent bone on the femur.

pile (pH) [L. *pila*, a ball, a pillar]. 1. A single hemorrhoid. See: *piles*. 2. The hair. 3. A battery for production of electricity.

pileous (pī'lē-ŭs) [L. *pilus*, hair]. Hairy; hirsute.

piles (pīls) [L. *pila*, a mass]. Dilated blood vessels in the rectal mucosa forming a vascular tumor. Syn: *hemorrhoids, q.v.*

pileus (pī'lē-ŭs) [L. a cap]. A nipple shield.

p. ventriculi. The upper part of the duodenum. Syn: *duodenal bulb*.

piliation (pĭl-ĭ-ā'shŭn) [L. *pilus*, hair]. Formation and development of hair.

piliform (pĭl'ĭ-form) [" + *forma*, shape]. Hairlike.

pill (pĭl) [L. *pilula*, from *pila*, a ball]. Medicine in the form of a tiny rounded mass to be taken whole.

pillar (pĭl'ĕr) [L. *pila*, a column]. An upright support; column, or structure resembling a column.

p. of the abdominal ring. One of the columns on either side of abdominal ring.

p's., ant., of fornix. Two diverging columns extending downward from ant. extremity of body of the fornix.

p's. of Corti. Two layers resting on membrana basilaris in the ear. Syn: *rods of Corti*.

p's. of diaphragm. Bundles of tendinous fibers arising on right side from ant. surfaces of 1st, 2nd, and 3rd lumbar vertebrae and the intervertebral fibrocartilages, and on the left side from the ant. surfaces of 2nd and 3rd lumbar vertebrae, passing upward and outward, to form an arch over the aorta.

p., ext., of abdominal ring. Outer aponeurotic margin of ext. abdominal ring, formed by portion of Poupart's ligament.

p's. of the fauces. Folds of mucous membrane, one on each side of the fauces, *q.v.*, and bet. which is situated the tonsil.

p., int., of abdominal ring. Inner aponeurotic margin of ext. abdominal ring.

p's., posterior, of fornix. Two bands forming prolongation of fornix posteriorly.

p's., Uskow's. Two folds of embryo fastened to dorsolateral body wall.

pilleus, pilleum (pĭl'ē-ŭs, -ŭm) [L. a cap; caul]. A membrane sometimes covering a baby's head at birth. Syn: *caul*.

p. ventriculi. The 1st portion of the duodenum. Syn: *pyloric cap*.

pillion (pĭl'yŭn) [L. *pellis*, skin]. Artificial leg, esp. in form of a stump.

pilo- [L.]. Combining form meaning *hair*.

pilocarpine hydrochlor'ide (pī″lō-kar'pĕn). Hydrochloride of an alkaloid obtained from leaves of the plant.
Action and Uses: Increases secretion of salivary mucus and sweat glands. Used internally as a diaphoretic, esp. in nephritis.
Dosage: 1/12 gr. (0.005 Gm.).

p. ni'trate. USP. Nitrate of the alkaloid obtained from pilocarpus.
Action, Uses, and Dosage: Same as pilocarpine hydrochloride.

pilocystic (pī-lō-sĭs'tĭk) [L. *pilus*, hair, + G. *kystis*, a bladder]. Encysted and containing hair, said of a dermoid cyst.

pilomotor (pī-lō-mō'tor) [" + *motor*, a mover]. Causing the movements of hairs, as the *arrectores pilarum*.

p. reflex. Gooseflesh formation when skin is stroked.

pilonidal (pī-lō-nī'dăl) [" + *nidus*, nest]. Containing hairs in a cyst in nest formation.

p. fistula. F. near the rectum resulting from a growth of subcutaneous hair.

p. sinus. A p. fistula.

pilose (pī'lōs) [L. *pilus*, hair]. Hairy, downy.

pilosebaceous (pī″lō-sē-bā'shŭs) [" + *sebaceus*, fatty]. Concerning the hair and sebaceous glands.

pilosis (pī-lō'sĭs) [L. *pilus*, hair, + G. *-osis*, intensive]. Excessive formation of hair.

pilosity (pī-lŏs'ĭ-tĭ) [L. *pilus*, hair]. Hairiness.

pilous (pī'lŭs) [L. *pilus*, hair]. Covered with hair; hirsute.

Piltz's reflex (pĭltz). Change in size of pupil on sudden fixation of attention.

pilula (pĭl'ū-lă) (pl. *pilulae*) [L. pill]. A small, solid body of medicine of a globular, ovoid or lenticular shape, intended to be swallowed whole and produce medicinal action.
May be ordered to be made extemporaneously by the druggist, or ready-prepared pills may be used. The latter usually are coated with sugar, gelatin, chocolate, etc. The gelatin-coated pills are the most desirable, as a rule, for many reasons. Pills are not prescribed as often as formerly. Five different pills are official.

pilular (pĭl'ū-lar) [L. *pilula*, pill]. Pert. to, or of the nature of, pills.

pilus (pī'lŭs) (pl. *pili*) [L. hair]. A hair.

pimel- [G.]. Combining form or prefix meaning *fat* or *associated with fat*.

pimelitis (pĭm-ĕl-ī'tĭs) [G. *pimelē*, fat, + *-itis*, inflammation]. Inflammation of adipose and of connective tissue in general.

pimeloma (pĭm-ĕl-ō'mă) [" + *-ōma*, tumor]. A fatty tumor. Syn: *lipoma*.

pimelorrhea (pĭm-ĕl-or-ē'ă) [" + *roia*, flow]. Discharge of fat in loose stools.

pimelosis (pĭm-ĕl-ō'sĭs) [" + -ōsis, intensive]. 1. A conversion into fat. 2. Fatty degeneration of any tissue. 3. Corpulence; obesity.

pimeluria (pĭm-ĕl-ū'rĭ-ă) [" + ouron, urine]. Excretion of fat or oil in urine. SYN: lipuria.

pimple (pĭm'pl) [A.S. pimpel]. A tiny, sharp-pointed protuberance of the skin, sometimes going on to suppuration. SYN: papule, pustule.
Often seen on the skin of the adolescent. They have little diagnostic value, but are supposed to result from faulty nutrition or interference with capillary circulation. Patients should be warned, when necessary, not to pick at pimples, as infection may take place and blood poisoning result.

pincement (pans-mong') [Fr. pinching]. Pinching or nipping of the flesh in massage.

pineal (pī'nē-ăl, pĭn'ē-ăl) [L. pineus, pine cone]. 1. Shaped like a pine cone. 2. The small red gland attached to post. part of 3rd ventricle of brain.
Included with endocrine system although no known hormone is produced. The physiology of this gland is entirely obscure. Because pineal extracts tend to retard the growth and development of experimental animals, some observers believe that the pineal hormone is an antagonist of that of the thymus, and that normal growth depends upon a proper balance bet. the two; perhaps pituitary hormones regulate the rate at which these 2 glands discharge their antagonistic hormones.
FUNCTION: Unknown. Such knowledge as we have is derived from observation of cases of teratoma. These are sometimes associated with marked sexual and somatic overgrowth leading to the condition known as pubertas praecox or macrogenitosomia praecox. Whether this is due to a lack of pineal secretion or to a hyperfunction of the gland is not known. SYN: epiphysis.
RS: acervulus, apinealism, apophysis, endocrine, glands.

pinealectomy (pī"nē-ăl-ĕk'tō-mĭ) [L. pineus, pine cone, + G. ektomē, excision]. Removal of the pineal body.

pinealism (pī'nē-ăl-ĭzm) [" + G. ismos, condition]. Disorder caused by abnormality of the secretion of the pineal body.

pinealoma (pī-nē-ăl-ō'mă) [" + G. ōma, tumor]. A tumor of the pineal body.

pinealopathy (pī"nē-ăl-op'ăth-ĭ) [" + G. pathos, disease]. Any disorder of the pineal gland.

pineapple (pīn'ăp-l) [A.S. pīn, pine, + aeppel, apple]. COMP: Very rich in cane sugar. Contains tartaric acid.
AV. SERVING (fresh and juice): 150-120 Gm. Pro. 0.6-0.4, Fat 0.5-0.4, Carbo. 13.9-15.4. VITAMINS: A++ — + to ++, B++ — ++, C++ — + to ++, G+ — +. ASH CONST. (fresh only): Ca 0.018, Mg 0.011, K 0.321, Na 0.016, P 0.028, Cl 0.051, S 0.009, Fe 0.0005.
ACTION: Easy to digest. Juice very valuable.
IND: Sore throat. SEE: fruit.

pine tar (pīn). USP. A product obtained from the distillation of pine wood.
ACTION AND USES: Externally, a stimulant in dermatitis; internally, a stimulant to bronchial mucous membrane.
DOSAGE: 8 gr. (0.5 Gm.) Externally, 50% ointment in petrolatum. SYN: pix liquida.

pinguecula (pĭn-gwĕk'ū-lă) [L. pinguis, fat]. BNA. Yellowish thickening of bulbar conjunctiva, triangular in shape, on inner and outer margins of the cornea.
Base of triangle is toward the limbus. Yellowish color is due to increase in the elastic fibers.

pinhole (pĭn'hōl) [A.S. pinn, a pin, + hol, hole]. Small perforation made by, or size of that made by, a pin. [women.
p. os. A very small os uteri in young
p. pupil. Extreme contraction of the iris.
It is seen in locomotor ataxia, after use of miotics, in some brain diseases, and in opium poisoning.

piniform (pĭn'ĭ-form) [L. pineus, pine cone, + forma, shape]. Shaped like a pine cone.

pink disease (pĭnk). Rare disease of children marked by swelling and redness of feet and hands, sweating, itching and polyarthritis. SYN: acrodynia,* erythredema.
p. eye. Epidemic form of acute conjunctivitis* from Koch-Weeks bacillus.

pinna (pĭn'ă) (pl. pinnae) [L. wing]. The auricle or projecting part of the ext. ear.
It collects and directs sound waves upon the eardrum.
p. nasi. Protruding cartilaginous extension on each nostril. SYN: ala nasi.

pinocytosis (pī"nō-sī-tō'sĭs) [G. pinein, to drink, + kytos, cell]. Term for the absorption of liquids by phagocytic cells.

pinotherapy (pī-nō-thĕr'ă-pī) [G. penia, hunger, + therapeia, treatment]. Hunger cure. SYN: nestotherapy, peinotherapy.

pint (pĭnt) [O.Fr. pinte]. Measure of capacity equal to one-half a quart; 16 fluid ounces; 28.875 cu. in. SEE: Table of weights and measures in Appendix.

pin'ta. An endemic So. Amer. disease of the skin.

pinworm (pĭn'wurm). Parasitic worm found in the intestines and rectum. SYN: ascaris, oxyuris.

pioepithelium (pī"ō-ĕp-ĭ-thē'lĭ-ŭm) [G. pion, fat, + epi, upon, + thēlē, nipple]. Epithelium that has undergone fatty degeneration, or which contains fat globules.

pionemia (pī-ō-nē'mĭ-ă) [" + aima, blood]. Fat in the blood. SYN: lipemia.

pioscope (pī'ō-skōp) [" + skopein, to examine]. Device for estimating the fat content of milk.

piper (pī'pĕr) [L.]. Pepper.

pipet, pipette (pī-pĕt') [Fr. pipette, a tiny pipe]. Narrow glass tube with both ends open for transferring and measuring liquids, using suction principle.

Pirogoff's amputation (pĭr'ō-gŏf). Foot amputation, removing part of the os calcis.

Piroplasma (pī"rō-plăz'mă) [L. pirum, pear, + G. plasma, a thing formed]. A genus of Sporozoa, some of which are parasitic to man and beast.
p. hominis. A parasite assumed to cause Rocky Mountain spotted fever.

piroplasmosis (pī"rō-plăz-mō'sĭs) [" + " + -ōsis, condition]. An infection caused by Piroplasma.

Pirquet's test (pēr-kā'). Test for tuberculosis by means of a skin reaction.

pisiform (pī'sĭ-form) [L. pisum, pea, + forma, shape]. 1. Name of small, pealike sesamoid bone of the wrist. 2. Peashaped.

pit (pĭt) [A.S. pytt, hole]. 1. A tiny hollow or pocket. SYN: depression, fossa. 2. To be or become marked with a shallow depression; to cause a depression on pressure in edema.

p's., nasal; p's., olfactory. Two small depressions on ant. cerebral vesicle, from which the nasal fossae develop.
p. of the stomach. 1. Depression at end of the ensiform process. 2. The center of the abdominal region above the navel.
p's., stomach. Openings of gastric tubules in the mucous surface of the stomach. SYN: *stomach cells, stomach ducts.*
p., tear. The lacrimal sinus.
pithecoid (pĭth'ē-koyd) [G. *pithēkos*, ape, + *eidos*, like]. Apelike; resembling an ape.
pithiatism (pĭth-ī'ăt-ĭzm) [G. *peithein*, to persuade, + *iatos*, curable]. 1. Hysteria induced by suggestion. 2. Mental disorder cured by suggestion.
pithiatric (pĭth-ĭ-at'rĭk) [" + *iatrikos*, healing]. Capable of being soothed or relieved by persuasion or by suggestion.
pithing (pĭth'ĭng). Destruction of the central nervous system by the piercing of brain or spinal cord, as in vivisection, etc. SYN: *decerebration.*
pitocin (pĭt-ō'sĭn). Brand name for an aqueous solution containing the oxytocic fraction of the post. pituitary gland. SEE: *oxytocin injection.*
Pitres's sections (pē-trē'). Series of 6 coronal vertical brain sections for study of this organ.
pitressin (pĭt-rĕs'ĭn). A product obtained from the post. lobe of the pituitary gland.
USES: For increasing blood pressure, the muscular contraction of the intestinal tract, and diminishing urinary output.
DOSAGE: From 5 to 15 ℞ (0.3-1 cc.) intramuscularly. SEE: *vasopressin.*
pitting (pĭt'ĭng) [A.S. *pytt*, hole]. The formation of pits or depressions or scars, as in smallpox.
pituglandol (pĭt-ū-glăn'dōl). Commercial extract of infundibular area of pituitary body.
pituita (pĭt-ū'ĭ-tă) [L. phlegm]. A glairy or viscid mucus, as a thick nasal secretion.
pituitarism (pĭt-ū'ĭ-tă-rĭzm) [" + G. *ismos*, condition]. Any disorder of the pituitary gland.
pituitary (pĭt-ū'ĭ-tăr-ĭ) [L. *pituita*, phlegm]. 1. Concerning phlegm. 2. The pituitary body.
DOSAGE: Anterior, 5 gr. (0.3 Gm.); posterior, sol. subcut., intramusc., or intranasally, 15 gr. (1.0 Gm.).
p. body, p. gland. Small, reddish body; weight 5 to 10 grains; situated in sella turcica or pituitary fossa of sphenoid bone, just back of root of nose.
It is composed of the ant. lobe and the post. lobe. The *anterior lobe* is derived embryologically from the upper part of the pharynx, Rathke's pouch. The *posterior lobe* comes down from the floor of the midbrain and is known as the pars nervosa. These lobes are differently functionally.
FUNCTIONS: The ant. lobe elaborates at least 2 groups of hormones. The growth hormone has to do with the growth and development of the bones and of the voluntary muscle system and probably with the viscera.
Overabundance of the growth hormone during the early years of life leads to a condition of gigantism. If this overfunction or *hyperpituitarism* occurs in later life, acromegaly results. The basophilic cells of the ant. lobe sometimes indulge in hypersecretion. This condition is called pituitary basophilism. A peculiar painful obesity develops about the face, neck and trunk.
Hypertension frequently occurs. There are various pains about the head, eyes and trunk, purplish striae on the abdomen and an excess growth of hair about the face and trunk. Frequently there is loss of calcium from the bones.
The sex hormones have to do with the growth, development and function of the genital apparatus, particularly with menstruation. For this reason, the p. body is sometimes called the motor of the ovary. The ant. lobe is believed to elaborate 2 sex hormones. One known as Prolan A or Rho I stimulates the follicles; the other Prolan B or Rho II, also called the luteinizing hormone, hastens the production of the corpora lutea.
The Germans claim to have isolated a metabolism hormone from this lobe which has to do particularly with obesity.
The post. lobe or pars nervosa elaborates a product which presides over or is concerned with the metabolism of carbohydrates, water and to a less degree fat metabolism. It is concerned with sleep, the maintenance of blood pressure and the regulation of body temperature.
There is a 3rd portion of this gland known as the pars intermedia, smaller and less important than the 2 lobes just mentioned, which possibly has something to do with the pigment metabolism of the body.
p. extract. Extract of the internal secretions of the pituitary gland.
p. membrane. Schneiderian membrane of nose.
pituitotrope (pĭt-ū'ĭt-ō-trōp) [L. *pituita*, phlegm, + G. *tropos*, a turning]. A person exhibiting tendencies to being overinfluenced by the pituitary gland.
pituitotropic (pĭt-ū'ĭt-ō-trōp'ĭk) [" + G. *tropos*, a turning]. Concerning or marked by pituitotropism.
pituitotropism (pĭt-ū'ĭt-ō-trō'pĭzm) [" + " + *ismos*, condition]. Bodily constitution in which the pituitary influence dominates.
pituitrin (pĭt-ū'ĭt-rĭn). A solution of the dried powdered post. lobe of the pituitary body of cattle.
ACTION AND USES: Used to stimulate contraction of blood vessels, peristalsis in intestines, and uterine contractions in labor.
DOSAGE: 15-30 ℞ (1-2 cc.). 1:1000 solut. intramusc.
pituitrism (pĭt-ū'ĭt-rĭzm) [L. *pituita*, phlegm, + G. *ismos*, condition]. Any disorder of the pituitary gland.
pityriasis (pĭt-ĭr-ī'ăs-ĭs) [G. *pityron*, bran, + *iasis*, disease]. A skin disease characterized by branny scales.
p. alba atrophicans. Cutaneous disorder with scaling and atrophy. SYN: *atrophoderma albidum.*
p. capitis. Dandruff. SYN: *dermatitis seborrhoica.*
p. lichenodes seborrhoica chronica. Maculopapular erythrodermia.
p. linguae. Transitory benign plaques of the tongue. [*rosea.*
p. maculata et circinata. SEE: *p.*
p. nigra. The dark brown or black patches in p. versicolor in warm climates.
p. pilaris. SEE: *p. rubra.*
p. rosea. A skin disease characterized by development of distributed patches which are circinate in outline,

pityriasis rubra

slightly scaly, a faint red color. SYN: *p. maculata et circinata*.

Acute inflammatory disease marked by a macular eruption on the trunk, obliquely to the ribs. Rose red and somewhat scaly with a clearing in the center, or reddish ring-shaped patches symmetrically distributed over the limbs.

ETIOL: Unknown.

SYM: Macular or circinate lesions; yellowish, salmon or red; rounded, oval or irregular; thinly covered with fine branny scales, increasing in size; when centers clear up, giving rise to slightly elevated reddish rings with fawn-colored centers, coalescence of rings resulting in segmental or gyrate lesions of various sizes. Spontaneous disappearance.

TREATMENT: Salicin internally. Locally: antipruritics.

p. rubra. Persistent general exfoliative dermatitis.

p. rubra pilaris. A chronic disease with formation of subacute inflammatory papules around the hair follicles. These coalesce and form infiltrated plaques of scaling dermatitis.

p. versicolor. Contagious skin disease marked by yellow patches, scales and itching.

pityroid (pĭt'ĭr-oyd) [G. *pityron*, bran, + *eidos*, like]. Branny; resembling bran.

pix (pĭks) [L.]. Pitch.

p. liquida. Tar.

placebo (plă-sē'bō) [L. I shall please]. Inactive substance given to satisfy patient's demand for medicine, such as a bread pill.

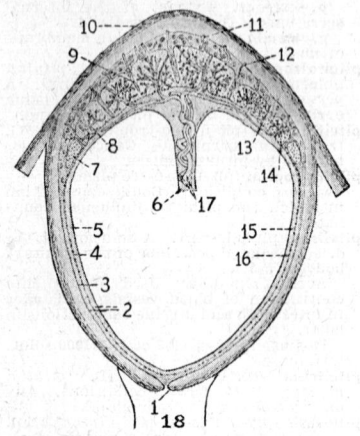

PLACENTA AND ITS RELATION TO THE UTERUS. (Diagrammatic.)

The fetus is not represented. 1. Cervix. 2. Chorion leve. 3. Decidua vera and reflexa. 4. Remains of trophoblast. 5. Amnion. 6. Umbilical cord. 7. Marginal sinus. 8. Villus, floating. 9. Septum. 10. Uterine wall. 11. Maternal vein. 12. Artery. 13. Spongy layer. 14. Intervillous space. 15. Mesoderm. 16. Ectoderm. 17. Umbilical vessels. 18. Vagina.

placenta (plă-sĕn'ta) (pl. *placentae*) [L. a flat cake, from G. *plakous*]. The oval or discoid spongy structure in the uterus through which the fetus derives its nourishment.

ANAT: The placenta is made up of a number of cotyledons. It presents 2 surfaces, *maternal* and *fetal*. To the placenta are attached the membranes (amnion and chorion) and the umbilical cord which is situated somewhere near the center of the fetal surface.

The cord is approximately 50 cm. long at full term. In the cord are found the umbilical artery and veins surrounded by Wharton's jelly.

The maternal surface of the placenta is rough because of irregular separation from the uterus. Its weight is approximately one-fifth the weight of the child.

PHYS: It aerates the blood of the fetus by directing the interchange of gases bet. the fetal and maternal blood.

The placenta either elaborates or is the storehouse for 3 substances that are apparently hormones. One is the *elin*, or the ovarian hormone; the 2nd is *emmenin*, which is effective in the treatment of dysmenorrhea, and the 3rd is an anterior pituitarylike substance which is said to be valuable in the treatment of menorrhagia.

RS: *ablatio placentae, abruptio placentae, childbirth, delivery obstetrics, placentation, placentoma, retroplacental, secundines*.

p. accreta. A placenta in which the cotyledons have invaded the uterine musculature and, as a result of this, separation of the placenta is very difficult or even impossible.

p., adherent. One that remains adherent to the uterine wall after normal period following childbirth.

p., annular. A p. that extends like a belt around the interior of the uterus.

p., basal; p., basilar. A free central p., 1 in which the ovules are borne on a column rising free from the bottom of the ovary.

p., battledore. A form of insertion of the umbilical cord into margin of the p. in which it spreads out to resemble a battledore.

p., bell-shaped. Domelike p.

p. bipartitia. One that is divided into 2 separate parts.

p., circinate. One that is cup-shaped.

p., cirsoides. P. with appearance of varicose veins.

p., cordiform. A p. having a marginal indentation giving it a heart shape.

p., deciduate. A p. of which the maternal part escapes with delivery.

p., diffused. A villous* p.

p., discoid. P. which constitutes practically 1 mass, circumscribed and circular in form.

p., disseminated. SEE: *villous p.*

p., domelike. One in which the chorionic villi persist at the upper pole of chorion, disappearing from lower pole.

p., double. A placental mass of the 2 placentae of a twin gestation.

p. duplex. Same as *p. bipartitia*.

p. fenestratum. One so formed that at some point not involving the periphery, its substance is lacking, the chorion being free from villi at that point and transparent like a window.

p., fetal. That part of the p. formed by aggregation of chorionic villi in which the umbilical vein and arteries ramify.

p., free central. Same as *basal p.*

p., fundal. One attached to the uterine wall within the fundal zone.

p., horseshoe. A formation in which the 2 placentae of a twin gestation are united.

p., incarcerated. One retained in the uterus by irregular uterine contractions after delivery.
p., lateral. One attached to lateral wall of uterus.
p., marginate. One with a large amount of tissue elevated on the edge.
p., maternal. That part of the p. originally consisting of the superficial part of the decidua serotina, and forming a thin, translucent, whitish gray layer attached to uterine surface of the fetal p. so as to be separable only in small pieces.
p., membranous. A thinning of the p. from atrophy.
p., nondeciduate. One that does not shed the maternal portion.
p. previa. Placenta which is implanted in the lower uterine segment. There are 3 types: *Centralis, lateralis,* and *marginalis. P. p. centralis* is the condition where the placenta has been implanted in the lower uterine segment and has grown to completely cover the cervical os. *P. p. lateralis* is the condition when the placenta lies just within the lower uterine segment. *P. p. marginalis* is the condition where the placenta partially covers internal 'cervical os.
SYM: Slight hemorrhage, recurrent with greater severity; appears 7th or 8th month; gradual anemia, pallor, rapid weak pulse, air hunger, low blood pressure.
DIAG: Painless bleeding during last 3 months; placenta in lower portion of uterus.
PROG: Depends upon control of hemorrhage and asepsis.
TREATMENT: Conserve blood supply during delivery and before; prevent and control postpartum hemorrhage; combat anemia before and after labor; prevention of sepsis.
p. reniformis. A kidney-shaped half of a *p. dimidiata*.
p., retained. One not expelled for 2 hours after 2nd stage of labor.
p. sanguinis. A blood clot.
p. spuria. An outlying portion of p. which has not maintained its vascular connection with the decidua vera.
p. succenturiata. An accessory p.
p. tripartita. A 3-lobed p.
p., triple. A placental mass of 3 placentae of a triple gestation.
p., uterine. Same as *maternal p*.
p., velamentous. A p. having the umbilical cord attached at 1 end.
p., villous. A placental formation with cotyledons scattered and having the form of chorionic villi.
p., zonary. Same as *annular p*.
placental (plă-sĕn'tăl) [L. *placenta*, a flat cake]. Relating to the placenta.
p. bruit, p. souffle. Sound heard in auscultation over the placenta in pregnancy due to circulation of the blood.
placentation (plă-sĕn-tā'shŭn) [L. *placenta*, a flat cake]. The process of formation and attachment of the placenta.
placentin (plă-sĕn'tĭn) [L. *placenta*, a flat cake]. Extract of placenta used for cutaneous reaction in testing for pregnancy.
placentitis (plă-sĕn-tī'tĭs) [" + G. *-itis*, inflammation]. Inflamed condition of placenta.
placentography (plă-sĕn-tŏg'ră-fī) [" + G. *graphein*, to write]. Examination of the placenta by x-ray.

placentoid (plăs-ĕn'toyd) [" + G. *eidos*, like]. Like the placenta.
placentolysin (plă-sĕn-tŏl'ĭs-ĭn) [" + G. *lysis*, dissolution]. A lysin obtained by injecting placental tissue into an animal, the serum thus obtained being destructive to placental cells of the species of animal from which the placenta was taken.
placentoma (plă-sĕn-tō'mă) [" + G. *-ōma*, tumor]. A new growth derived from retained placental tissue.
placentotherapy (plă-sĕn"tō-thĕr'ă-pĭ) [" + G. *therapeia*, treatment]. Therapeutic use of placental extract.
Placido's disk (pla-sē'dō). A disk marked with black and white circles used in determining amt. and character of corneal astigmatism.
placuntitis (plă-kŭn-tī'tĭs) [G. *plakous*, a flat cake]. Inflamed condition of the placenta. SYN: *placentitis*.
pladarosis (plad-ar-ō'sĭs) [G. *pladaros*, soft, + *-ōsis*, disease]. A soft growth like a wart on the eyelid.
plagiocephalia (plă-gĭ-ō-sĕf-ā'lĭ-ă) [G. *plagios*, oblique, + *kephale*, head]. Inequality of development of the two sides of the skull.
plagiocephalic (plă-jĭ-ō-sĕf-ăl'ĭk) [G. *plagios*, oblique, + *kephalē*, head]. Marked by or relating to plagiocephaly.*
plagiocephalism, plagiocephaly (plă"jĭ-ŏ-sĕf'ăl-ĭzm, plă"jĭ-ō-sĕf'ă-lĭ) [" + " + *ismos*, condition]. Condition of malformation of the skull, it being developed more ant. than post.
plague (plāg) [G. *plēgē*, a stroke]. 1. Any widespread contagious disease of great mortality. 2. An acute infection caused by *Pasteurella pestis*. Has a pneumonic or a septicemic form. Streptomycin has reduced mortality to 5-10%. SYN: *black death, bubonic p*.
p., ambulatory. Mild but often fatal. Patient does not take to his bed.
plane (plān) [L. *planus*, flat]. 1. A level surface. 2. An ideal p. as a standard of reference by which positions of parts of a body are indicated.
p's., Addison's. Planes used as landmarks in thoracoabdominal topography.
p., Aeby's. One perpendicular to the median plane of the cranium through the *basion* and *nasion*.
p., alveolocondylar. One tangent to the alveolar point and most prominent points on lower aspects of condyles of the occipital bone.
p., Baer's. One through upper border of the zygomatic arches.
p., coccygeal. The 4th parallel one of the pelvis.
p., coronal. Vertical p. at right angles to a sagittal p. dividing the body into ant. and post. portions.
p., datum. An assumed horizontal plane from which craniometric measurements are taken.
p., Daubenton's. One passing through the opisthion and inferior borders of the orbits.
p's., focal. Two p's. through ant. and post. principal foci of a dioptric system and perpendicular to the line connecting the two.
p., glabello-occipital. The vertical p. of maximum anteroposterior diameter of the skull.
p., Hodge's. One parallel to the plane of the pelvic inlet and passing through the 2nd sacral vertebra and upper border of the os pubis.

p's., inclined, of the pelvis. According to Lusk, "The sciatic spines divide the pelvic cavity into 2 unequal sections. In the larger, anterior section, the lateral walls slope toward the symphysis and arch of the pubes, while posteriorly the walls slope in the direction of the sacrum and coccyx. The declivities in front of the spines are termed the anterior inclined p's. of the pelvis, over which rotation of the occiput takes place in the mechanism of normal labor. Behind the spines the lateral slopes are known as the posterior inclined p's."

p., Listing's. A transverse vertical plane perpendicular to anteroposterior axis of eye, containing center of motion of the eyes; in it also lie the transverse and vertical axes of voluntary ocular rotation.

p., Meckel's. One through the auricular and alveolar points.

p., medial; p., median; p., mesial. One usually anteroposterior dividing a body or organ into 2 equal and symmetrical parts. The median p. of the body is known as the *meson*.

p., Morton's. One passing through the most projecting points of the parietal and occipital protuberances.

p., nuchal. Outer surface of occipital bone between the foramen magnum and the sup. curved line.

p., occipital. Outer surface of occipital bone above the sup. curved line.

p., orbital. 1. Orbital surface of the maxilla. 2. One passing through the visual axis of the eye.

p's., parallel, of the pelvis. Those intersecting at right angles the axis of the pelvic canal. The 1st is the p. of the superior strait; the 2nd the p. extending from middle of the sacral vertebra to level of the subpubic ligament; the 3rd the p. at level of spines of the ischia; the 4th at the outlet.

p's. of the pelvis. Imaginary ones touching the same parts of the pelvic canal on both sides.

p., popliteal. The popliteal space.

p. of refraction. One passing through a refracted ray of light and drawn perpendicular to the surface at which refraction takes place.

p. of regard. One through the fovea of the eye and fixation point.

p., sagittal. The median anteroposterior p. of the body.

p., sternal. Ant. surface of sternum.

p., temporal. Depressed area on side of skull below the inf. temporal line.

p., visual. One passing the visual axis of the eye.

planocellular (plă″nō-sĕl'ū-lăr) [L. *planus*, flat, + *cellula*, a little box]. Composed of or concerning flat cells.

planoconcave (plă″nō-kŏn'kăv) [" + *concavus*, hollow]. Flat on 1 side and concave on the other.

planoconvex (plă″nō-kŏn'vĕks) [" + L. *convexus*, arched]. Flat on 1 side and on the other convex.

planocyte (plă″nō-sīt) [G. *plane*, a wandering, + *kytos*, cell]. A meandering cell. SYN: *ameboid cell*.

plant (plănt) [L. *planta*, a sprout]. Organized being of vegetable life that is nonsentient and lacks voluntary motor power. SEE: *chloroplast*.

p. acids. Acids containing carbon; organic acids found in many fruits.

planta (plan'tă) [L. sole]. BNA. The sole of the foot.

plantar (plăn'tăr) [L. *planta*, sole]. Concerning the sole of foot.

p. arch. Vascular arch in sole of foot. The union of the plantar and dorsalis pedis arteries in the sole. SYN: *arcus plantaris*.

p. reflex. Contraction of toes upon irritation of the sole.

plantaris (plăn-tăr'ĭs) [L.]. An extensor muscle found in the calf of the leg.

planuria (plăn-ū'rĭ-ă) [G. *plane*, a wandering, + *ouron*, urine]. The voiding of urine from an abnormal passage of the body.

plaque (plăk) [Fr. a spot]. 1. A patch on the skin or on a mucous surface. 2. A blood platelet.*

plasma (plăz'mă) [G. *plasma*, a thing formed]. 1. The liquid part of the lymph and of the blood. 2. Protoplasm, cell substance outside the nucleus. 3. An ointment base of glycerol and starch.

In the blood, the corpuscles and platelets float in it. It consists of serum and protein substances in solution.

The blood plasma consists of water in which numerous chemical compounds, both solids and gases, are dissolved. Among the important constituents may be mentioned the following: Water, electrolytes, sugar, proteins, nonprotein nitrogenous compounds, fats and lipoids, bile pigment or bilirubin, gases.

In general, plasma is a medium for circulation of blood cells, carries nutritive substances to various structures, and removes from them waste products of metabolism. It makes possible chemical communication bet. different portions of the body carrying minerals, hormones, vitamins and antibodies.

Different constituents of the plasma have specific functions within the blood. The proteins, bicarbonates, carbon dioxide, chlorides, phosphates, and ammonia serve to keep the acid base equilibrium of the blood constant, when acid or base substances are added to it. The proteins, esp. albumin, by virtue of their osmotic pressure, tend to prevent undue leakage of fluids out of the capillaries, and to maintain a proper exchange of fluid bet. capillaries and tissues.

Plasma, if normal, is thin and colorless when free from corpuscles, or it has a faint yellow tinge when seen in thick layers.

After clotting of the blood, the liquid squeezed out by the clot is called blood serum. If whole blood is prevented from clotting either by chilling it or by adding anticoagulants, such as sodium citrate, it can be centrifuged. The clear fluid which then occupies the upper half of the centrifuge tube is called plasma. SEE: *blood, coagulation, serum*.

p., blood. Fluid in which float the corpuscles.

p., germ. Protoplasm of the germinal cell.

p., histogenetic. Protoplasm controlling tissue development.

p., lymph. Lymph without its corpuscles.

p., muscle. Muscle juice that forms myosin on coagulation.

p., somatic. That of body cells other than the germ cells.

plasmacule (plăz'mă-kūl) [L. *plasmacula*, little plasm]. One of the minute particles said to be found in the blood plasma giving it its vital power. SYN: *hemokonia*.

plasmacyte (plăz'mă-sīt) [G. *plasma*, a

plasmacytosis P-64 **plaster cast**

thing formed, + *kytos*, cell]. A plasma cell, 1 of those found in connective tissue with an eccentrically placed round nucleus and filled with a chromatin mass that stains deeply.

plasmacytosis (plăz-mă-sĭ-tō'sĭs) [" + " + *-ōsis*, intensive]. Plasma cells in the blood.

plasmameba (plăz-mă-mē'bă) [" + *amoibē*, a change]. An amebic, parasitic organism in blood during dengue, possibly causing that disease.

plasmapheresis (plăz-mă-fĕr'ē-sĭs) [" + *aphairesis*, a taking away]. The removal of fluid portion of blood from the body by venesection, centrifugalization, and replacement of the corpuscles into the blood stream.

plasmase (plăz'mās) [" + *ase*, enzyme]. Substance in serum which combines with fibrinogen to form fibrin. SYN: *fibrin ferment*.

plasmasome (plăz'măs-ōm) [" + *sōma*, body]. A leukocyte granule; nucleolar substance (nonchromatin staining) in the cytoplasm.

plasmatic (plăz-măt'ĭk) [G. *plasma*, a thing formed]. 1. Relating to plasma. 2. Formative or plastic.
 p. layer. Blood plasma adjacent to the capillary walls. SYN: *plasmic*.

plasmatorrhexis (plăz″măt-ō-rĕks'ĭs) [" + *rēxis*, a rupture]. Rupture of a cell with loss of its plasma from internal pressure due to swelling.

plasmic (plăz'mĭk) [G. *plasma*, a thing formed]. Concerning plasma. SYN: *plasmatic*.

plasmochin (plăz'mō-kĭn). An oxyquinoline derivative, in the form of a tasteless salt.
 USES: In malaria.
 DOSAGE: Adult, 1/3 gr. (0.02 Gm.).

plasmocyte (plăz'mō-sīt) [G. *plasma*, a thing formed, + *kytos*, cell]. 1. Any cell except blood corpuscles free in blood plasma. 2. A parasite in the blood plasma.

plasmodium (plăz-mō'dĭ-ŭm) (pl. *plasmodia*) [" + *eidos*, form]. Protoplasm formed by 2 or more amebiform bodies fusing with each other.

Plasmodium (plăz-mō'dĭ-ŭm) [" + *eidos*, form]. Genus of malarial parasites. The causative agent of malaria.
 P. falciparum. The parasite of pernicious anemia.
 P. malariae. A protozoan parasite found in the blood of those with malaria.

plasmogen (plăz'mō-jĕn) [" + *gennan*, to produce]. Essential part of protoplasm.

plasmology (plăz-mŏl'ō-jĭ) [" + *logos*, a study]. The study of the cells and plasma. SYN: *histology*.

plasmolysis (plăz-mŏl'ĭs-ĭs) [" + *lysis*, dissolution]. Shrinking of cytoplasm in a living cell due to loss of water by osmosis.

plasmorrhexis (plăz-mor-ĕks'ĭs) [" + *rēxis*, rupture]. Rupture of a cell with loss of plasma. SYN: *erythrocytorrhexis, erythrorrhexis, plasmatorrhexis*.

plasmoschisis (plăz-mos'kĭs-ĭs) [G. *plasma*, a thing formed, + *schisis*, a splitting]. The splitting of a cell.

plasmosome (plăz-mō-sōm) [" + *sōma*, body]. 1. The nucleolus of a cell. 2. A granular structural element of a cell.

plasmotomy (plăz-mŏt'ō-mĭ) [" + *tomē*, incision]. Mitosis in which the cytoplasm divides into 2 or more masses.

plasmotropism (plăz-mŏt'rō-pĭzm) [" + *tropein*, to turn, + *ismos*, condition]. The action of spleen, liver and bone marrow, causing the destruction of red blood cells.

plasmozyme (plăz'mo-zīm) [" + *zymē*, a leaven]. A substance in blood plasma which probably becomes thrombin when activated by thrombokinase. SYN: *thrombogen*.

plasome (plăz'ōm) [G. *plassein*, to form, + *sōma*, a body]. Smallest hypothetical unit of protoplasm capable of life.

plasson (plăs'ŏn) [G. *plassōn*, forming]. Primitive protoplasm in the cytode or non-nucleated stage.

plastein (plăs'tē-ĭn) [G. *plassein*, to form]. One of several proteinlike substances produced by the action of proteolytic enzymes, as pepsin, on digestion products of protein.

plaster (plăs'tŭr) [G. emplastron]. Medicinal preparation, to be used externally, in which the constituents are formed into a tenacious mass of substance harder than an ointment and spread upon muslin, linen, skin or paper.
 It may be *mustard, belladonna,* to check secretions or to allay pain; *capsicum*, as a counterirritant; *cantharides*, or Spanish fly, as a vesicant* used in arthritis with synovitis, and in pleural effusions. Cantharides is readily absorbed if used in large quantities and it is eliminated through the kidneys and may induce nephritis. The urine should be watched for 24 hours after application.
 p., adhesive. Plaster made of resin, wax and olive oil used to immobilize a part, to relieve pressure upon sutures, to protect wounds, to secure traction in fractures, to exert pressure, to hold dressings in place, etc.
 Hair on the area should first be removed before applying any plaster. It should never be applied to abraded or raw surfaces. In re-applying, dead scarf skin should be removed. Surface should be dry and clean. Removal should be made by stripping from both ends up to the wound, first moistening with benzine or ether.
 p. bandage. Bandage stiffened with plaster of Paris.
 p., blistering. P. made of cantharides.
 p., court-. P. made of isinglass on silk, used for superficial wounds.
 p. jacket. P. for the trunk made of plaster of Paris.
 p., mustard. P. made of powdered mustard paste spread on cloth, used as a rubefacient.
 p. of Paris. Calcined gypsum mixed with water to form a paste which sets rapidly, used to make casts and stiff bandages.
 p., porous. Perforated p.
 p., resin; p., rosin. P. containing resin, wax and lead plaster, used as a soothing agent, esp. for children.
 p., rubber. SEE: *adhesive p*.
 p., warming. P. of cantharides and pitch employed as a counterirritant.

plas′ter cast. Rigid dressing made of gauze impregnated with plaster of Paris, used to immobilize an injured part, esp. in bone fractures.
 NP: Patient's position is indicated by fracture. A fracture table should be used when possible and various parts should be in readiness. Place a plaster bandage end up in tepid water. When about saturated water is gently squeezed by pressing both ends (otherwise the plaster will be forced out through the ends of bandage). As 1 bandage is passed to doctor, another is placed in

water. There should be extra plaster of Paris in perforated cans so it can be shaken on in smoothing the cast.
plastic (plăs'tĭk) [G. *plastikos*, formed]. 1. Capable of being molded. 2. Contributing to building tissues.
   p. bronchitis. Bronchitis with fibrin exudate adhering in the form of a cast to the bronchial tubes.
   p. force. The impetus that builds tissues; generative force.
   p. linitis. Cirrhosis of the stomach.
   p. lymph. The exudate covering inflamed serous surfaces, as in wounds.
   p. surgery. The restoration and repair of external physical defects by use of grafts of bone or tissues. SEE: *chalinoplasty*.
plasticity (plăs-tĭs'ĭ-tĭ) [G. *plastikos*, formed]. The ability to be molded.
plastid (plăs'tĭd) [G. *plastidēs*, molded]. Area having special chemical activity in the cells for the production of special substances, such as the starch grains in plant cells; a cytode or elementary organism.
plastidule (plăs'tĭd-ūl) [G. *plastidēs*, molded]. Smallest unit of protoplasm capable of life.
plastin (plăs'tĭn) [G. *plassein*, to form]. 1. The principal proteid of protoplasm. 2. Chromatin granules in a cell nucleus. SYN: *linin*.
plastocyte (plăs'tō-sīt) [G. *plastos*, formed, + *kytos*, cell]. A blood platelet.
plastocytopenia (plăs"tō-sī"tō-pē'nĭ-ă) [" + " + *penia*, lack]. Lack of the normal number of blood platelets.
plastocytosis (plăs"tō-sī-tō'sĭs) [" + " + -*ōsis*, intensive]. Abnormal increase in the quantity of blood platelets.
plate (plāt) [G. *platys*, flat]. A flattened process, chiefly of bone. SYN: *lamina, lamella*.
   p., approximation. A disk of decalcified bone used in intestinal surgery.
   p., auditory. Bony roof of the ext. auditory meatus.
   p., axial. The primitive streak of the embryo.
   p., blood. Platelet.
   p., bone. Flat, round or oval decalcified bone metal or hard rubber disk, employed in pairs, used in approximation.
   p., culture. Bacterial culture in agar or gelatin on a plate.
   p., dorsal. One of 2 prominences of the notochord in the embryo.
   p., end-. Termination expanded of a nerve fibril in muscular tissue.
   p., foot. Flat portion of stapes. BNA. *basis stapedis*.
   p., medullary or **neural.** Central portion of the ectoderm developing into neural canal.
   p., palate. Part of the palate bone forming a lateral half of roof of mouth.
   p., tympanic. Bony plate between ant. wall of the ext. auditory meatus and the tympanum.
platelet (plāt'lĕt) [G. *platys*, flat]. A round or oval disk, 1/3 to 1/2 the size of an erythrocyte found in the blood.
   Platelets number from 200,000 to 800,-000 per cm. They contain no hemoglobin. SEE: *blood*.
platiculture (plă"tĭ-kŭl'chur) [G. *platys*, flat, + L. *cultura*, cultivation]. Cultivation of bacterial plates. SYN: *plate culture*.
platinum (plăt'ĭn-ŭm) [Spanish *plata*, silver]. Heavy silver-white metal. SYMB: Pt. At. wt. 195.2. Sp. gr. 21.5.
platy- [G.]. Combining form meaning *broad*.

platycelous (plăt-ĭ-sē'lŭs) [G. *platys*, broad, + *koilos*, hollow]. Concave ventrally and convex dorsally, said of vertebrae.
platycephalic, platycephalous (plăt"ĭ-sē-făl'ĭk, -sĕf'ă-lŭs) [" + *kephalē*, head]. Having a wide skull with vertical index less than 70.
platycnemia, platycnemism (plat-ĭk-nē'mĭ-ă, -mĭzm) [" + *knēmē*, knee, + *ismos*, condition]. 1. Having an unusually broad tibia. 2. Broadlegged.
platycnemic (plăt-ĭk-nē'mĭk) [" + *knēmē*, knee]. Having unusually broad tibiae.
platycyte (plăt'ĭs-īt) [" + *kytos*, cell]. A form of cell found in tubercle nodules.
   It is bet. a leukocyte and a giant cell in size.
Platyhelminthes (plăt"ĭ-hĕl-mĭn'thēz) [" + *elmins, elminth-*, worm]. A phylum of flatworms. SEE: *Cestoda, Trematoda*.
platyhieric (plat-e-hi-er'ĭk). Having a broad sacrum with a sacral index over 100.
platymeric (plăt-ĭ-mē'rĭk) [G. *platys*, broad, + *mēros*, thigh]. Having an unusually broad femur.
platyopia (plăt-ĭ-ō'pĭ-ă) [" + *ōps*, visage]. Having a very broad face, the nasomalar index being less than 107½°.
platypellic, platypelvic (plăt"ĭ-pĕl'ĭk, -vĭk) [" + *pella*, a basin]. Having a broad pelvis.
platypodia (plăt-ĭ-pō'dĭ-ă) [" + *pous, pod-*, foot]. Condition of being flatfooted.
platyrrhine (plăt'ĭr-ĭn) [" + *ris, rin*, nose]. 1. Having a very wide nose in proportion to length. 2. Pert. to a skull with a nasal index bet. 51.1 and 58.
platysma myoides (plăt-ĭz'mă mī-oy'dēz) [G. *platysma*, plate, + *mys, my-*, muscle, + *eidos*, form]. Broad, thin muscular layer on either side of the neck under the superficial fascia.
platysmal reflex. Dilation of pupil resulting from sharp pinching of platysma myoides.
platyspondylisis (plăt"ĭ-spŏn-dĭl'ĭs-ĭs) [G. *platys*, flat, + *spondylos*, vertebra]. Flatness of the vertebral bodies.
platytrope (plăt'ĭ-trōp) [" + *tropē*, a turning]. One of a pair of bilateral symmetrical parts of the body on either side.
Plaut's angina (plawt's ăn-jī'nă). Ulceromembranous form of contagious disease of the oral mucosa, with inflammation of the tonsil. SYN: *trench mouth, Vincent's angina*.
pleasure principle. PSY: The avoidance of pain and the seeking of pleasure, indicative of the early stages of man's development. SYN: *hedonism*.
pledget (plĕj'ĕt) [origin uncertain]. Small, flat, lint compress, used to apply or absorb fluid, as a protector, to exclude air, etc.
plegaphonia (pleg-af-ō'nĭ-ă) [G. *plēgē*, stroke, + *a-*, neg. + *phōnē*, voice]. A sound produced in percussion of the larynx when the glottis is open during auscultation of the chest.
pleio-, pleo-, plio- [G.]. Combining forms meaning *more*.
pleochroic, pleochromatic (plē-ō-krō'ĭk, -măt'ĭk) [G. *pleōn*, more, + *chroa*, color]. Pert. to property of crystals and some other bodies of showing various colors when seen from different axes.
pleocytosis (plē"ō-sī-tō'sĭs) [" + *kytos*, cell, + -*ōsis*, intensive]. Increased number of lymphocytes in the cerebrospinal fluid.
pleomastia, pleomazia (plē"ō-măs'tĭ-ă,

-mā'zĭ-ă) [" + *mastos, mazos*, breast].
The state of having more than 2 mammae. SYN: *polymastia*.
pleomorphic (plē-ō-mor'fĭk) [" + *morphē*, form]. Having many shapes.
pleomorphism (plē-ō-mor'fĭzm) [" + " + *ismos*, condition]. 1. Property of crystallizing into 2 or more different forms. 2. Occurrence of more than 1 form in a life cycle.
pleomorphous (plē-ō-mor'fŭs) [" + *morphē*, form]. Having many shapes or crystallizing into several forms.
pleonasm (plē'ō-năzm) [G. *pleonasmos*, exaggeration]. State of having more than normal number of organs or parts.
pleonectic (plē-ō-něk'tĭk) [G. *pleonexia*, greediness]. 1. Being saturated with more than the normal amount of oxygen, said of blood. 2. Relating to excessive urge to possess; greedy. SEE: *mesectic, mionectic*.
pleonexia (plē"ō-něk'sĭ-ă) [G. greediness]. Having morbid desire for possession.
plesiomorphous (plē-sĭ-ō-mor'fŭs) [G. *plesios*, close, + *morfē*, form]. Of like or nearly the same in form.
plessesthesia (plĕs-ĕs-thē'zĭ-ă) [G. *plēssein*, to strike, + *aisthēsis*, sensation]. Palpatory percussion with left middle finger pressed against body and the index finger of right hand percussing in contact with left finger.
plessimeter (plĕs-ĭm'ĕt-er) [" + *metron*, a measure]. A disk held over the body which is struck in mediate percussion. SYN: *pleximeter*.
plessor (plĕ'sor) [G. *plēssein*, to strike]. A hammer for performing percussion. SYN: *plexor*.
plethora (plĕth'ō-ră) [G. *plēthōrē*, fullness]. 1. Overfullness of blood vessels or of the total quantity of blood or other fluid in the body. 2. Congestion causing distention of blood vessels. SEE: *sanguine*.
plethoric (plĕth-or'ĭk) [G. *plēthōrē*, fullness]. Pert. to or characterized by plethora; overfull.
plethysmograph (plē-thĭz'mō-grăf) [G. *plēthysmos*, increase, + *graphein*, to write]. Device for finding variations in size of a part, due to vascular changes.
pleura (pl. *pleurae*) (plū'ră) [G. *pleura*, a side]. Serous membrane that enfolds lungs and is reflected upon the walls of the thorax and diaphragm. SEE: *mediastinum, thorax*.
p., costal or **parietal layer.** Extends from roots of the lungs covering the sides of the pericardium to chest wall and backward to the spine. The visceral and costal pleural layers are separated only by a lubricating secretion. These layers may become adherent or separated by fluid or air in diseased conditions.
p. diaphragmatica. That covering upper surface of diaphragm.
p. pericardiaca. That covering the pericardium.
p. phrenica. SEE: *p. diaphragmatica*.
p. pulmonalis. BNA. The pleura investing the lungs and fissures bet. the lobes.
p., visceral. Invests the lungs and enters into and lines the interlobar fissures. It is loose at the base and at sternal and vertebral borders to allow for lung expansion.
pleural (plū'răl) [G. *pleura*, a side]. Concerning the pleura.
p. cavity. Space bet. the parietal and visceral layers of the pleura. SEE: *chylothorax*.

pleuralgia (plū-răl'jĭ-ă) [" + *algos*, pain]. Pain in the pleura, or in the side. SYN: *neuralgia, intercostal*.
pleurapophysis (plū-ră-pop'ĭs-ĭs) [" + *apo*, from, + *physis*, a growth]. A rib or a vertebral lateral process.
pleurectomy (plū-rĕk'tō-mĭ) [" + *ektomē*, excision]. Excision of part of the pleura.
pleurisy (plū'rĭs-ĭ) [G. *pleura*, a side]. Inflammation of pleura—may be primary or secondary; unilateral, bilateral or local; acute or chronic; fibrinous, serofibrinous or purulent. SEE: *Andral's decubitus*.
NP: In simple pleurisy, absolute rest is essential with plenty of sunlight and fresh air if there is no rise in temperature. Routine nursing is in order, but the patient should not be permitted to exert himself and he should be kept cheerful. Assistance should be given in moving the patient. Fluids should be given to eliminate body poisons. Five meals per day of a high caloric character may be given. The doctor may strap the affected side to help immobilize the chest. Counterirritants such as an icebag may be indicated.
p., acute. Chilliness, stabbing pain or stitch in affected side, intensified by coughing or deep breathing. Fever, 101°-103°; cough short, dry, partially suppressed; face pale, anxious; patient usually lies on affected side. An effusion of any kind remaining unabsorbed constitutes a chronic p.
p., diaphragmatic. Inflammation of diaphragmatic pleura.
SYM: Intense pain under margin of ribs, sometimes referred into abdomen, with tenderness on pressure; thoracic breathing; tenderness over phrenic nerve referred to supraclavicular region in neck or same side; hiccough; extreme dyspnea.
p., dry. Condition in which the pleural membrane is covered with a fibrinous exudate.
It clings together, causing pain during respiration. There is slight pain when apical pleura is inflamed, but acute stabbing pain in costal or diaphragmatic pleural inflammation.
p., embolic. P. resulting from a pulmonary embolus.
p., encysted. P. with effusion limited by adhesions.
p., fibrinous. Pain severe and continuous. Aspiration gives negative results, later much retraction of affected side.
p., hemorrhagic. P. with hemorrhage.
p., interlobar. P. in interlobar spaces.
p., purulent. High, irregular fever; sweats; chills; anemia; sometimes pitting from edema of surface; purulent effusion found on aspiration.
p., secondary. Infectious p. resulting from some specific inflammation.
p., serofibrinous. P. with fibrinous exudate and serous effusion.
p., suppurative. SEE: *purulent p*.
p., tuberculous. Most common cause of pleurisy that is apparently primary is tuberculosis. May be secondary to pulmonary phthisis. Effusion apt to be bloody, but presents same symptoms as ordinary serofibrinous pleurisy.
PROG: Depends largely on character and amount of effusion. Favorable as a rule.
TREATMENT: Absolute rest, light diet. Aconite often removes entire trouble. Other remedies as required. Locally, hot fomentations, hot water bags, or strapping of chest.

pleuritic P-67 **plexus**

DIET: (a) Acute: As in pneumonia. (b) With effusion: Dry diet, salt-free diet.
pleuritic (plū-rĭt'ĭk) [G. *pleura*, a side]. Relating to, or like, pleurisy.
pleuritis (plū-rī'tĭs) [" + -*itis*, inflammation]. Inflammation of the pleura. SYN: *pleurisy.*
pleurocele (plū'rō-sēl) [" + *kēlē*, a swelling]. 1. Hernia of lungs or of pleura. 2. A serous pleural effusion.
pleurocentesis (plū″rō-sĕn-tē'sĭs) [" + *kentēsis*, a piercing]. Surgical puncture of the pleural cavity. SYN: *thoracentesis.*
pleurocentrum (pl. *pleurocentra*) (plū-rō-sĕn'trŭm) [" + *kentron*, center]. The lateral element of the centrum or vertebral column.
pleurocholecystitis (plū″rō-kō-lē-sĭst-ī'tĭs) [" + *cholē*, bile, + *kystis*, bladder, + -*itis*, inflammation]. Inflamed condition of the pleura and gallbladder.
pleuroclysis (plū-rŏk'lĭs-ĭs) [" + *klysis*, an injection]. Injection of fluid into the pleural cavity.
pleurodynia (plū″rō-dĭn'ĭ-ă) [" + *odynē*, pain]. Pain in intercostal muscles of sharp intensity, due to chronic inflammatory changes in chest fasciae; pain of the pleural nerves.
p., epidemic diaphragmatic. Epidemic disease with sudden attack of pain in the chest, fever, and a tendency to recrudescence on the 3rd day. SYN: *devil's grip.*
pleurogenic (plū-rō-jĕn'ĭk) [G. *pleura*, a side, + *gennan*, to produce]. Arising in the pleura. SYN: *pleurogenous.*
pleurogenous (plū-rŏj'ĕn-ŭs) [" + *gennan*, to produce]. Having origin in the pleura. SYN: *pleurogenic.*
pleurography (plū-rŏg'ră-fī) [" + *graphein*, to write]. X-ray examination of the lungs and pleura.
pleurohepatitis (plū″rō-hĕp-ă-tī'tĭs) [" + *ēpar*, *ēpat-*, liver, + -*itis*, inflammation]. Inflammation of pleura and the liver.
pleurolith (plū'rō-lĭth) [" + *lithos*, stone]. A calculus in the pleura.
pleurolysis (plū-rŏl'ĭ-sĭs) [" + *lysis*, a loosening]. Loosening of pleura that has become thickened from intrathoracic fascia, to relieve contraction of the lungs. SYN: *pneumolysis.*
pleuroparietopexy (plū″rō-păr-ī'ĕt-ō-pĕk″-sī) [" + L. *pariēs*, *pariet-*, wall, + G. *pēxis*, fixation]. Fastening the lung to the wall of the chest by binding the visceral pleura to the wall of its cavity.

pleuropericarditis (plū″rō-pĕr″ĭ-kar-dī'tĭs) [G. *pleura*, side, + *peri*, around, + *kardia*, heart, + -*itis*, inflammation]. Pleuritis accompanied by pericarditis.
pleuroperitoneal (plū″rō-pĕr-ĭ-tō-nē'ăl) [" + *peritonaion*, peritoneum]. Relating to the pleura and peritoneum.
p. cavity. The body cavity. SYN: *celom.*
pleuropneumonia (plū″rō-nū-mō'nĭ-ă) [" + *pneumōn*, lung]. Pleurisy accompanied by pneumonia.
pleuropneumonolysis (plū″rō-nū-mōn-ŏl'ĭ-sĭs) [" + " + *lysis*, a loosening]. Resection of 1 or more ribs from 1 side to collapse the lung in unilateral pulmonary tuberculosis.
pleurorrhea (plū″rō-rē'ă) [" + *roia*, a flow]. Effusion of fluid into the pleura.
pleuroscopy (plū-rŏs'kō-pī) [" + *skopein*, to examine]. Inspection of the pleural cavity through an incision into the thorax.

Posed by professional model
PLEUROTHOTONOS.
Photo by Whitaker

pleurothotonos (plū-rō-thŏt'ō-nos) [G. *pleurothen*, from the side, + *tonos*, tension]. Tetanic spasm in which the body position is arched to 1 side.
ETIOL: Spinal affection or acute pleural involvement.
RS: *emprosthotonos, opisthotonos, orthotonos, position, posture.*
pleurotomy (plū-rŏt'ō-mī) [G. *pleura*, a side, + *tomē*, incision]. Incision of the pleura.
pleurotyphoid (plū-rō-tī'foyd) [" + *typhos*, fever, + *eidos*, form]. Typhoid fever with pleural involvement.
pleurovisceral (plū″rō-vĭs'ĕr-ăl) [" + L. *viscus*, *viscer-*, viscera]. Concerning the pleura and the viscera.
plexal (plĕks'ăl) [L. *plexus*, a braid]. Pertaining to, or of the nature of, a plexus.
plexalgia (plĕks-ăl'jĭ-ă) [" + G. *algos*, pain]. General fatigue, multiple pains, excitability, paresthesia and insomnia seen in soldiers after long exposure to cold and wet; a symptom complex.
plexiform (plĕk'sĭ-form) [" + *forma*, shape]. Resembling a network or plexus.
pleximeter (plĕks-ĭm'ĕt-ĕr) [" + G. *metron*, measure]. Device made of many kinds of material, for receiving the blow of the percussion hammer.
plexor (plĕks'or) [G. *plēxis*, a stroke]. Hammer or other device for striking upon the pleximeter in percussion.
plexus (plĕk'sus) (pl. *plexūs* or *plexuses*) [L. a braid]. A network of nerves or

blood vessels. SEE: *rete, table of plexuses* in Appendix.
pliability (plī-ă-bĭl'ĭ-tĭ) [Fr. *plier*, to bend]. Capacity of being bent or twisted easily.
plica (plī'kă) (pl. *plicae*) [L. a fold]. A fold.
  p. circularis. One of the transverse folds in the intestinal mucosa.
  p. epiglottica. One of 3 folds of mucosa bet. the tongue and the epiglottis.
  p. lacrimalis. Mucosal fold at the lower orifice of the nasolacrimal duct.
  p. neuropathica. Curly hair due to a nervous disorder.
  p. palmatae. Radiating fold in the uterine mucosa.
  p. polonica. Tangled matted hair in which crusts and vermin are embedded.
  p. semilunaris. Mucosal fold at the inner canthus of the eye.
  p. transversalis recti. One of the mucosal folds in the rectum.
plicate (plī'kăt) [L. *plica*, fold]. Braided or folded.
plication (plī-kā'shŭn) [L. *plicāre*, to fold]. Stitching folds in an organ's walls to reduce its size.
plicotomy (plī-kŏt'ō-mĭ) [" + G. *tomē*, a cutting]. Section of the post. fold of the tympanic membrane.
plombage (plŭm-bazh') [Fr. *plomber*, to plug]. A method of collapsing the apex of lung by stripping the parietal pleura from the chest wall at the site of desired collapse and packing the space bet. the lung and chest wall with a foreign substance, such as adipose tissue, muslin, gauze, or paraffin wax.
plough (plow) (*nasal*). Triangular gouge used with Woake's forceps for excision of nasal tissue.
plug (plŭg) [M.D. *plugge*, plug]. A mass obstructing or for closing a hole.
  p., cervical. One forming in cervix after conception for duration of pregnancy.
  p., laryngeal. Bulb-shaped laryngeal dilator.
  p., suprapubic urethral. A stem mounted upon a disk used to maintain the patency of an artificial suprapubic urethra and to prevent dribbling of urine.
  p., vaginal. Closed tube for maintaining patency of vagina following operation for fistula.
plumbago (plŭm-bā'gō) [L. lead ore]. Graphite; a native carbon.
plumbic (plŭm'bĭk) [L. *plumbicus*, leaden]. Pertaining to, or containing, lead.
plumbism (plŭm'bĭzm) [L. *plumbum*, lead, + G. *ismos*, condition]. Poisoning from lead, *q.v.*
plumbotherapy (plŭm"bō-ther'ă-pĭ) [" + G. *therapeia*, treatment]. Treatment of disease with lead.
plumbum (plŭm'bŭm) [L. lead]. Lead; a bluish-white metal. SYMB: Pb. At. wt. 207.10. Sp. gr. 11.38. SYN: *lead*.
plumose (plū'mōs) [L. *pluma*, feather]. Having a delicate, feathery growth.
plumper (plŭm'pĕr). Pad for filling out sunken cheeks, sometimes in form of extended artificial dentures.
pluri- [L.]. Combining form meaning several.
pluriceptor (plū-rĭ-sĕp'tor) [L. *plus, plur-*, more, + *ceptor*, a receiver]. A receptor which has more than 2 groups uniting with the complement.
pluridyscrinia (plū"rĭ-dĭs-krĭn'ĭ-ă) [" + G. *dys*, bad, + *krinein*, to secrete]. Disorder of several endocrine organs at the same time.
pluriglandular (plū"rĭ-glăn'dū-ler) [" + *glans*, a kernel]. Concerning more than 2 glands.
  p. syndrome. Term concerned with any group of endocrinologic symptoms.
plurigravida (plū-rĭ-grăv'ĭd-ă) [" + *gravida*, pregnant]. A woman who has had 2 or more children.
plurilocular (plū-rĭl-ŏk'ū-lar) [" + *loculus*, a cell]. Composed of many cells. SYN: *multilocular*.
plurimenorrhea (plū-rĭ-mĕn-ō-rē'ă) [" + *mēn*, month, + *roia*, flow]. Abnormal frequency of menstrual periods.
pluripara (plū-rĭp'ă-ră) [" + *parēre*, to bring forth]. A woman who has given birth to 3 or more children.
pluripar'ity [L. *plus, plur-*, more, + *parēre*, to bring forth]. Condition of having borne 3 or more children.
plutomania (plū"tō-mā'nĭ-ă) [G. *ploutos*, wealth, + *mania*, madness]. Delusion that one is very rich.
pnein (nē'ĭn) [G. *pneia*, breath]. A substance assumed to be present in the tissues which hastens their oxidizing activities.
pneocardiac reflex (nē-ō-kar'dĭ-ăk) [G. *pnein*, to breathe, + *kardia*, heart]. Change in rate and rhythm of heart and circulatory changes as blanching, flushing or sweating, when an irritant vapor enters air passages.
pneodynamics (nē"ō-dī-năm'ĭks) [" + *dynamis*, force]. Branch of science which treats of respiration. SYN: *pneumodynamics*.
pneograph (nē'ō-grăf) [" + *graphein*, to write]. Apparatus for registering respiratory movements.
pneometer (nē-ŏm'ĕt-ĕr) [" + *metron*, a measure]. Instrument for measuring lung respiration. SYN: *spirometer, q.v.*
pneophore (nē'ō-for) [" + *phoros*, bearing]. Device to aid artificial respiration.
pneopneic reflex (nē-ŏp-nē'ĭk) [" + *pnein*, to breathe]. Change in respiratory depth and rate, coughing, suffocation and pulmonary edema, when an irritant vapor enters air passages.
pneoscope (nē'ō-skōp) [" + *skopein*, to examine]. Device for measuring movements of respiration.
pneumarthrosis (nū-mar-thrō'sĭs) [G. *pneuma*, air, + *arthron*, joint, + *-ōsis*, intensive]. Accumulation of gas or air in a joint.
pneumascope (nū'mă-skōp) [" + *skopein*, to examine]. 1. Device for estimating gas in expired air. 2. Instrument for internal auscultation of the thorax. 3. Device for discovering foreign bodies in mastoid sinuses. 4. Apparatus for measurement of the movements of respiration. SYN: *pneumatoscope*.
pneumathemia (nū-mă-thē'mĭ-ă) [" + *aima*, blood]. Accumulation of air or gas in blood vessels.
pneumatic (nū-măt'ĭk) [G. *pneumatikos*, pert. to air]. 1. Concerning gas or air. 2. Relating to respiration. 3. Relating to rarefied or compressed air.
  p. cabinet. Cabinet for treatment of a part with rarefied or compressed air.
pneumatinuria (nū"măt-ĭn-ū'rĭ-ă) [G. *pneuma*, air, + *ouron*, urine]. Excretion of urine containing free gas. SYN: *pneumaturia*.
pneumatocardia (nū"-măt-ō-kar'dĭ-ă) [" + *kardia*, heart]. Air or gas in the heart chambers.
pneumatocele (nū-măt'ō-sēl) (" + *kēlē*,

pneumatodyspnea   P-69   **pneumodynamics**

hernia]. 1. Hernial protuberance of lung tissue. 2. A swelling containing a gas or air, esp. of the scrotum. SYN: *pneumonocele.*

pneumatodyspnea (nŭ″măt-ō-dĭsp-nē′ă) [" + *dys*, bad, + *pneia*, breath]. Dyspnea caused by pulmonary emphysema.

pneumatogram (nū-măt′ō-grăm) [" + *gramma*, a mark]. A tracing or record made by a pneumatograph.

pneumatograph (nū-măt′ō-grăf) [" + *graphein*, to write]. Device for registering respiratory movements. SYN: *pneograph.*

pneumatology (nū-mă-tŏl′ō-jĭ) [" + *logos*, a study]. Science of gases and air, their chemical properties and use in treatment.

pneumatometer (ʀū-măt-ŏm′ĕt-ĕr) [G. *pneuma*, air, + *metron*, a measure]. Device for measuring quantity of air involved in inspiration and expiration. SYN: *spirometer.*

pneumatometry (nū-măt-ŏm′ĕt-rĭ) [" + *metron*, measure]. Measurement of respiratory force as a means of diagnosis.

pneumatorachis (nū-măt-or′ă-kĭs) [" + *rachis*, spine]. Air in the spinal canal.

pneumatoscope (nū-măt′ō-skōp) [" + *skopein*, to inspect]. 1. Device for ascertaining presence of foreign bodies in mastoid sinuses. 2. Apparatus used to measure the gas in expired air. 3. Apparatus for internal thoracic auscultation. 4. Instrument used to measure the respiratory movements. SYN: *pneumascope.*

pneumatosis (nū-mă-tō′sĭs) [" + *-ōsis*, intensive]. Accumulation in any part of the body of gas, esp. in the intestinal tract.

ETIOL: Air swallowing, simultaneous spasm of cardia and pylorus.

pneumatotherapy (nū″măt-ō-thĕr′ă-pĭ) [" + *therapeia*, treatment]. Treatment by means of rarefied or compressed air.

pneumatothorax (nū″măt-ō-thō′răks) [" + *thōrax*, chest]. Air or gas accumulation in the pleural cavities. SYN: *pneumothorax.**

pneumaturia (nū-măt-u′rĭ-ă) [G. *pneuma*, air, + *ouron*, urine]. Excretion of urine containing free gas.

pneumatype (nŭ″mă-tīp) [" + *typos*, type]. Deposit of moisture on glass from the breath exhaled through the nostrils with the mouth closed for purpose of diagnosis.

pneumectomy (nū-mĕk′tō-mĭ) [G. *pneumōn*, lung, + *ektomē*, excision]. Excision of all or part of a lung.

pneumo-, pneumono- [G.]. Combining forms meaning *air; lung.*

pneumobacillus (nū″mō-bă-sĭl′ŭs) [" + L. *bacillus*, a little rod]. The bacillus causing pneumonia. SYN: *B. pneumoniae.*

pneumocele (nŭ″mō-sēl) [" + *kēlē*, hernia]. 1. A swelling containing air or gas, esp. of the scrotum. 2. Hernia of lung tissue through chest wall. SYN: *pneumatocele.*

pneumocentesis (nŭ″mō-sĕn-tē′sĭs) [" + *kentēsis*, a piercing]. Paracentesis* or surgical puncture of a lung to evacuate a cavity.

pneumocephalus (nŭ″mō-sĕf′ă-lŭs) [" + *kephalē*, head]. Gas or air in the cavity of the cranium.

pneumocholin (nŭ″mō-kō′lĭn) [" + *cholē*, bile]. Commercial preparation of pneumococci in sodium taurocholate used as prophylactic agent in Type I.

pneumochysis (nū-mŏk′ĭs-ĭs) [" + *chysis*, a pouring]. Edema of the lung.

pneumococcal (nū-mō-kŏk′ăl) [G. *pneumōn*, lung, + *kokkos*, berry]. Concerning or caused by pneumococci.

pneumococcemia (nū″mō-kŏk-sē′mĭ-ă), Presence of pneumococci circulating in the blood.

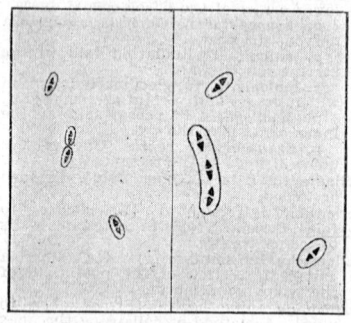

pneumococcolysis (nū″mō-kŏk-ŏl′ĭ-sĭs) [" + " + *lysis*, destruction]. Destruction or lysis of pneumococci.

PNEUMOCOCCUS TYPING
(Schematized.)

The sputum is mixed with typing sera. Left, negative reaction; the capsule is thin, the flame shaped cocci are close together; right, positive reaction; the capsules are much swollen, pushing the cocci apart.

pneumococcus (nū-mō-kŏk′ŭs) [" + *kokkos*, berry]. The pathogenic microorganism causing pneumonia of which there are 33 known strains or types.

Types I, II, III, V, VII, VIII and XIV cause over 80% of all cases, with I and II causing 60 to 70%. SEE: *Illus., above.*

Antipneumococcic serum may be had for all of the types including the newly discovered 33rd.

Temperature of solution: 100° F. Desensitizing treatment may be necessary before injection if patient is sensitive to horse serum. SEE: *pneumonia.*

p. antibody solution. A colorless, clear, aqueous solution containing antibodies from antipneumococcic serum in normal saline, combining Types I-II-III. It is free from serum proteins, is miscible with body fluids and quickly absorbed.

ADMINISTRATION: *Adults:* Intravenously. *Children:* Intramuscularly.

p., how to recognize in sputum. Detected by paired arrangements and slightly curved, long, thin appearance. Commonly seen in clumps, in short chains of 4 to 6. It takes a gram-positive stain.

pneumoconiosis (nū″mō-kō-nĭ-ō′sĭs) [G. *pneumōn*, lung, + *konis*, dust, + *-ōsis*, disease]. A condition of the respiratory tract due to inhalation of dust particles.

An occupational disorder such as that caused by mining or stonecutting.

RS: *anthracosis, chalicosis, monoconiosis, siderosis, silicosis.*

pneumoderma (nū-mō-dĕr′mă) [" + *derma*, skin]. Emphysema under the skin.

pneumodynamics (nū″mō-dī-năm′ĭks) [" + *dynamis*, force]. Branch of science

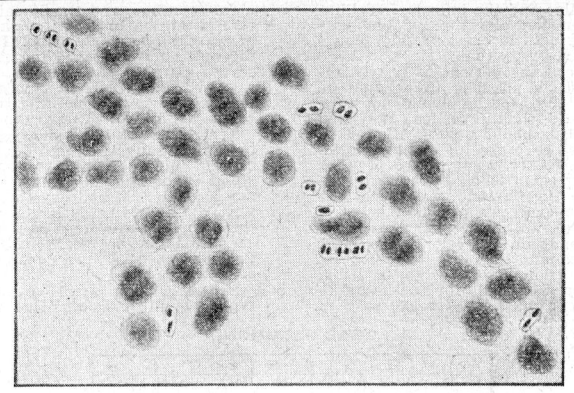

PNEUMOCOCCI IN PUS.
Empyema, diplococci, varying in shape and size, surrounded by capsules are distributed among the pus cells.

treating with force employed in respiration.
pneumoempyema (nū″mō-ĕm-pī-ē′mă) [" + *en*, in, + *pyon*, pus]. Empyema accompanied by an accumulation of gas.
pneumoenteritis (nū″mō-ĕn-tēr-ī′tĭs) [" + *enteron*, intestine, + -*itis*, inflammation]. Pneumonia and enteritis combined.
pneumogalactocele (nū″mō-găl-ăk′tō-sēl) [" + *gala*, *galakt*, milk, + *kēlē*, hernia]. A breast tumor containing milk and gas.
pneumogastric (nū″mō-găs′trĭk) [G. *pneumōn*, lung, + *gastēr*, stomach]. Concerning the lungs and stomach.
 p. nerve. The 10th cranial nerve.
 FUNCT: Motor and sensation.
 ORIG: Medulla oblongata.
 DIST: Lungs, larynx, heart, esophagus, stomach and much of the abdominal viscera. SYN: *vagus nerve*. SEE: *cranial nerves*.
pneumogram (nū′mō-grăm) [" + *gramma*, a mark]. Device for recording respiratory movements. SYN: *pneumatogram*.
pneumograph (nū′mō-grăf) [" + *graphein*, to write]. Device for measuring and recording movements of respiration.
pneumography (nū-mŏg′ră-fĭ) [" + *graphein*, to write]. 1. A descriptive treatise on the lungs. 2. A tracing of the respiratory movements.
pneumohemopericardium (nū″mō-hem″ō-pĕr-ĭ-kar′dĭ-ŭm) [" + *aima*, blood, + *peri*, around, + *kardia*, heart]. The accumulation of air and blood in the pericardium.
pneumohemorrhagia (nū″mō-hem-or-hā′-jĭ-ă) [" + " + *rēgnunai*, to burst forth]. Hemorrhage into pulmonary air cells; apoplexy of the lungs.
pneumohemothorax (nū″mō-hem″ō-thō′-răks) [" + " + *thōrax*, chest]. Gas or air and blood collected in the pleural cavity.
pneumohydropericardium (nū″mō-hī″drō-pĕr-ĭ-kar′dĭ-ŭm) [G. *pneumōn*, lung, + *ydōr*, water, + *peri*, around, + *kardia*, heart]. Air and fluid accumulated in the pericardium.
pneumohydrothorax (nū″mō-hī-drō-thō′-răks) [" + " + *thōrax*, chest]. Gas or air and fluid in the pleural cavity.
pneumohypoderma (nū″mō-hī-pō-dĕr′mă)

[" + *ypo*, under, + *derma*, skin]. Air in the tissues under the skin.
pneumokidney (nū″mō-kĭd′nĭ) [" + M.E. *kydney*, kidney]. X-ray of the kidney following introduction of oxygen into renal pelvis. SYN: *pneumopyelography*.
pneumolith (nū′mō-lĭth) [" + *lithos*, stone]. A pulmonary calculus.
pneumolithiasis (nū″mō-lĭth-ī′ăs-ĭs) [" + *lithos*, stone]. Formation of concretions in the lungs.
pneumology (nū-mŏl′ō-jĭ) [" + *logos*, a study]. The scientific study of diseases of the lungs and air passages.
pneumolysis (nū-mŏl′ĭs-ĭs) [G. *pneumōn*, lung, + *lysis*, a loosening]. Separation of an adherent lung from costal pleura.
pneumomalacia (nū″mō-mă-lā′sĭ-ă) [" + *malakia*, a softening]. Abnormal softening of the lung.
pneumomassage (nū″mō-măs-sazh′) [" + *massein*, to knead]. Massage of the tympanum with air to cause movement of the ossicles.
pneumomelanosis (nū″mō-mĕl-ăn-ō′sĭs) [" + *melas*, *melan*-, black, + -*ōsis*, disease]. Pigmentation of lung seen in pneumoconiosis.
pneumometer (nū-mŏm′ĕt-ēr) [" + *metron*, measure]. Instrument for measuring amt. of air inspired and expired in respiration. SYN: *spirometer*, *q.v.*
pneumomycosis (nū″mō-mī-kō′sĭs) [" + *mykēs*, fungus, + -*ōsis*, disease]. A fungous pulmonary disease. SYN: *pneumonomycosis*.
pneumomyelography (nū″mō-mī-ĕl-ŏg′ră-fĭ) [" + *myelos*, marrow, + *graphein*, to write]. X-ray inspection of the spinal canal.
pneumonectasia, pneumonectasis (nū-mŏn-ĕk-tā′zĭ-ă, ĕk′tă-sĭs) [G. *pneumōn*, lung, + *ektasis*, dilatation]. Distention of lungs with air.
pneumonectomy (nū-mŏn-ĕk′tō-mĭ) [" + *ektomē*, excision]. Removal of a lung. SYN: *pulmonectomy*, *pneumectomy*.
pneumonemia (nū-mō-nē′mĭ-ă) [" + *aima*, blood]. Congestion of the lungs.
pneumonia (nū-mō′nĭ-ă) [G. *pneumōn*, lung]. Inflammation of the lungs with exudation into the lung tissue and high temperature.
 ETIOL: Pneumococcus, streptococcus hemolyticus, staphylococcus, Friedlan-

pneumonia   P-71   pneumonia, chronic interstitial

der's bacillus and the influenza bacillus.

Sym: Sudden elevation of temperature, chill, pain in chest or side, blood-tinged or rusty sputum.

NP: Afford the patient as nearly absolute rest as possible. He should be turned in the bed; he should not turn himself. He should be fed, not feed himself. He should not be allowed to talk except to make his wants known. If he is restless or in pain, drugs or other therapeutic agents should be used as prescribed by the physician. All measures to promote comfort should be taken.

A careful watch over the patient's general condition: his color, his general appearance, and his pulse, temperature, and respiration. Cyanosis, or a rising respiratory rate, calls for the administration of oxygen, or for increase in the amount of oxygen if it is already being given. The nurse must understand how to regulate the flow of oxygen and to adjust the temperature of the oxygen tent. High fever demands tepid sponges or the use of antipyretics. Any marked change in the patient's general condition should be reported to the doctor at once.

Measures to prevent and combat abdominal distention. The bowels must act daily; to accomplish this an enema or flush may be given, or the physician may prescribe a laxative. If distention appears, a rectal tube is inserted, pituitrin, or prostigmine may be given by hypodermic, and turpentine stupes may be used.

If specific serum is given, the nurse must watch carefully for manifestations of serum reactions—shortness of breath, sneezing, lacrimation, urticaria, signs of shock, or rising temperature. If any reaction occurs, the doctor should be notified at once. Adrenalin should always be at hand when serum is to be administered.

If sulfapyridine is being given, the nurse must be on the lookout for toxic manifestations, and should call the doctor's attention to them: to skin rashes, or jaundice, or bloody urine. The nurse's ingenuity may be taxed in getting nauseated patients to take or to retain sulfapyridine. Often it is best to have the patient take something to eat just before his dose of sulfapyridine is due.

Treatment: Antipneumococcus serum, oxygen, sulfapyridine and a new derivative of quinine which is effective in stopping the growth of all types of pneumococcus germs, hydroxyethylapocupreine. Sulfapyridine is given with fruit juices or milk or water and taken with a small amount of bicarbonate of soda. Promises to be a very effective method of treatment.

Serum is now available for the 33 types of pneumococcus causing pneumonia. A unit is the amount of serum which will protect a mouse against 1,000,-000 lethal doses of pneumococci.

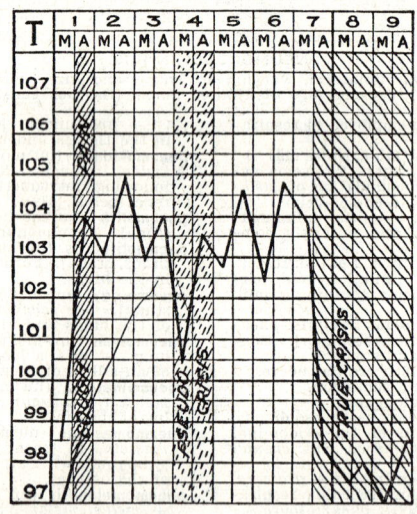

p., acute lobar. Pneumonia of one or more lobes of the lungs.

p., broncho-. See: *catarrhal p.*

p., catarrhal. Inflammation of terminal bronchioles and air vesicles, with scattered areas of consolidation, usually secondary to bronchitis.

Sym: Onset gradual; prostration, cough, fever moderately high, 101-104° F., and very irregular. Dyspnea marked; respirations, 50 to 80 per minute; pulse, 120 to 180; cough painful, with muco-purulent expectoration. Face pale, anxious, lips blue.

Prog: Always guarded. Most fatal in extremes.

Treatment: No draft; temperature, uniformly 70°. Moist atmosphere. Liquid or semi-liquid diet. Remedies conforming to special phase of disease.

p., chronic interstitial. Chronic disease of lung with overgrowth of fibrous tissue.

Sym: Moderate dyspnea and chronic cough, expectoration, slight or profuse, fetid, from being retained in bronchi-

ectatic cavities. No fever. May live years.
PROG: Incurable. Duration, 10 to 20 years.
TREATMENT: Palliative. Good hygienic regulations, remedies directed to bronchiectasis.
p., croupous. SEE: *lobar p.*
p., double. That affecting both lungs or both lobes of 1 lung.
p., hypostatic. Pneumonia caused by constantly remaining in same position. Gravity causes blood to become congested in 1 part of the lung. Infection aids development of true pneumonia.
NP: Change position of patient frequently and whenever patient is uncomfortable. Have patient breathe deeply several times each hour for full aeration of lungs. Short, shallow breaths predispose to pulmonary complications. Deep respirations after an upper abdominal incision cause pain.
DIET: No routine diet; adjust to patient. Nutrition increased preoperatively by rectum, and postoperatively by hypodermoclysis. *First Day*: Hot fluids; no milk or orange juice until ordered. *Second Day*: Tea, broth, ginger ale, etc. *Third Day*: Soapsuds enema and cathartic, then diet of milk, custards, milk-toast, cereals, soft eggs, stewed fruits. *Fourth and Fifth Days*: Regular diet if tolerated. *This is also a general postoperative diet.*
p., lobar. An acute specific disease characterized by inflammation of lungs, followed by a rapid infiltration of their alveoli.
SYM: Decided chill, sharp pain in side, rapid rise of temperature; latter often reaches its maximum in 24 hr. (104°-105° F.), and generally continues high with slight diurnal remissions till 9th day, when it falls by crisis or occasionally by lysis. SEE: *Illus., p. P-71.*
Dyspnea—respirations 40 to 80 per minute. Cough, at first short, dry; later rusty, translucent, tenacious sputum. Face flushed, lips cyanosed, often with herpetic eruption, tongue heavily furred, bowels constipated. Urine scanty, high colored, deficient in chlorides, often albuminous. In severe cases delirium.
PROG: Guarded. Average mortality, 20%.
TREATMENT: Absolute rest—liquid or semi-liquid diet. Delirium with high fever, cold pack or tepid bath. Remedies to suit individual case.
NP: SEE: *pneumonia above.*
p., typhoid. Pneumonia associated with typhoid symptoms; headache; muttering delirium; stupor; dry, brown tongue, etc.
TREATMENT: Similar to above. Brandy or whisky or other alcoholic stimulants are questionable. Watch pulse and tongue.
p. virus. P. caused by a virus. SYN: *pneumonitis.*
SYM: High fever, severe cough, slow pulse. Little or no expectoration. White cells sometimes decreased in number. Mild form runs 5 to 10 days. More severe form produces fever during 2nd week, lasting 15-18 days, or even 25 days.
TREATMENT: Oxygen. Sulfa drugs only aid in preventing infection with pneumococcus and streptococcus.
pneumonic (nū-mon'ĭk) [G. *pneumōn*, lung]. Concerning the lungs or pneumonia.

p. phthisis. Tuberculosis of an entire pulmonary lobe.
pneumonitis (nū-mō-nī'tĭs) [" + *-itis*, inflammation]. 1. Inflammation of the lung. SYN: *pneumonia.* 2. A virus form of pneumonia. SYN: *Virus pneumonia.**
pneumono- (nū-mon-ō) [G.]. Prefix: *pert. to the lungs.*
pneumonocele (nū-mō'nō-sēl) [G. *pneumōn*, lung, + *kēlē*, hernia]. A pulmonary hernia. SYN: *pneumocele.*
pneumonocirrhosis (nū"mō-nō-sĭr-ō'sĭs) [" + *kirros*, orange]. Interstitial pneumonia; cirrhosis of the lung.
pneumonoconiosis (nū"mō-nō-kō-nī-ō'sĭs) [" + *konis*, dust, + *-osis*, disease]. Fibrous inflammation or chronic induration of the lungs resulting from inhalation of dust. SEE: *anthracosis, chalicosis, siderosis.*
pneumonograph (nū-mō'nō-grăf) [" + *graphein*, to write]. Roentgen ray picture of the lungs.
pneumonography (nū-mō-nŏg'ră-fī) [" + *graphein*, to write]. The taking and developing of x-ray pictures of the lungs.
pneumonolysis (nū-mō-nŏl'ĭs-ĭs) [" + *lysis*, loosening]. Loosening of an adherent lung from the pleura. SYN: *pneumolysis.*
pneumonomelanosis (nū"mō-nō-měl-ăn-ō'sĭs) [" + *melas, melan-*, black, + *-osis*, disease]. Pigmentation and disease of the lung due to inhalation of dust.
pneumonometer (nū-mō-nŏm'ĕt-ēr) [G. *pneumōn*, lung, + *metron*, measure]. Device to measure amt. of inspired and expired air during respiration. SYN: *spirometer.*
pneumonomoniliasis (nū"mō-no-mō"nĭl-ī'ăs-ĭs) [" + L. *monile*, necklace]. Infestation of lungs and bronchi by Monilia.
pneumonomycosis (nū-mō-nō-mī-kō'sĭs) [" + *mykēs*, fungus, + *-osis*, disease]. Disease of the lungs caused by schizomycetes. SYN: *pneumomycosis.*
pneumonopathy (nū-mō-nŏp'ăth-ī) [" + *pathos*, disease]. Any diseased condition of the lung.
pneumonoperitonitis (nū"mō-nō-pěr"ĭ-tō-nī'tĭs) [" + *peritonaion*, peritoneum, + *-itis*, inflammation]. Peritonitis with gas in the peritoneal cavity.
pneumonopexy (nū-mō'nō-pěk'sī) [" + *pēxis*, fixation]. Surgical attachment of the lung to the chest wall. SYN: *pneumopexy.*
pneumonophthisis (nū"mō-nŏf'thĭs-ĭs) [" + *phthisis*, a wasting]. Tuberculosis of the lungs.
pneumonorrhaphy (nū-mō-nor'ă-fī) [" + *raphē*, a sewing]. Suture of a lung.
pneumonosis (nū-mō-nō'sĭs) [G. *pneumōn*, lung, + *-osis*, disease]. Any pulmonary disease.
pneumonotomy (nū-mō-nŏt'ō-mī) [" + *tomē*, incision]. Incision into the lung. SYN: *pneumotomy.*
pneumopaludism (nū"mō-păl'ū-dĭzm) [" + L. *palus*, swamp, + G. *-ismos*, condition]. Malarial symptom complex of the lungs.
SYM: Bronchophony without râles, expectoration, or friction; bronchial respiratory murmurs; percussion resonance at 1 apex; coughing in paroxysms.
pneumoparesis (nū"mō-păr-ē'sĭs) [" + *paresis*, paralysis]. Progressive congestion of the lungs.
ETIOL: Vasomotor deficiency, imperfect innervation, respiratory failure.
pneumopericardium (nū"mō-pěr-ĭ-kar'dĭ-ŭm) [" + *peri*, around, + *kardia*,

pneumoperitoneum P-73 **pneumotyphus**

heart]. Air or gas in the pericardial sac.
ETIOL: Traumatism or communication bet. the esophagus, stomach, or lungs and the pericardium.
SYM: Unusual metallic heart sounds, tympany over precordial area.

pneumoperitoneum (nū″mō-pĕr-ĭ-tō-nē′ŭm) [G. *pneumōn*, lung, + *peritonaion*, peritoneum]. Condition in which air or gas is collected in the peritoneal cavity.
May be artificially injected to treat tuberculous peritonitis or where pneumothorax is impossible.
INDICATIONS: Tuberculous peritonitis with or without fluid; tuberculous enterocolitis; tuberculosis of the mesentery; persistent vomiting in tuberculous patient (adhesions or after left phrenic operation); tuberculosis of the lungs in any case where pneumothorax is indicated but impossible or ineffective on account of irremovable pleural adhesions; advanced cases of bilateral pulmonary tuberculosis in which all functioning lung is needed. Unlike pneumothorax, pneumoperitoneum never increases dyspnea.

pneumoperitonitis (nū″mō-pĕr-ĭ-tō-nī′tĭs) [G. *pneumōn*, lung, + *peritonaion*, peritoneum, + *-itis*, inflammation]. Peritonitis with gas accumulation.

pneumopexy (nū″mō-pĕks″ĭ) [" + *pēxis*, fixation]. Surgical attachment of a lung to the thoracic wall.

pneumopleuritis (nū″mō-plū-rī′tĭs) [" + *pleura*, a side, + *-itis*, inflammation]. Inflamed condition of lungs and pleura.

pneumopleuroparietopexy (nū″mō-plū″rō-pă-rī′ĕt-ō-pĕk″sĭ) [" + " L. *pariēs*, wall, + G. *pēxis*, fixation]. The operation of attaching the lung with its parietal pleura to the border of a thoracic wound.

pneumopyelography (nū″mō-pī-ĕ-lŏg′ră-fĭ) [" + *pyelos*, pelvis, + *graphein*, to write]. Making of a skiagram of the renal pelvis and ureters after they are injected with oxygen.

pneumopyopericardium (nū″mō-pī″ō-pĕr-ĭ-kar′dĭ-ŭm) [" + *pyon*, pus, + *peri*, around, + *kardia*, heart]. Air, gas and pus collected in the pericardial sac.

pneumopyothorax (nū″mō-pī″ō-thō′rāks) [" + " + *thōrax*, chest]. Air and pus collected in the pleural cavity.

pneumoradiography (nū″mō-rā-dĭ-ŏg′ră-fĭ) [" + L. *radius*, a ray, + G. *graphein*, to write]. Injection of air into a part for taking an x-ray picture.

pneumorrachis (nū-mor-rā′kĭs) [G. *pneumōn*, lung, + *rachis*, spine]. Gas accumulation in the spinal canal.

pneumorrhagia (nū-mor-ā′jĭ-ă) [" + *rēgnunai*, to burst forth]. Pulmonary hemorrhage. SYN: *hemoptysis*.

pneumosan (nū″mō-san) [G. *pneumōn*, lung]. Commercial remedy for pulmonary tuberculosis.

pneumoscope (nū′mō-skōp) [" + *skopein*, to examine]. Device for estimating the respiratory force.

pneumoserosa (nū″mō-sē-rō′să) [" + L. *serum*, whey]. Introduction of air into a joint cavity.

pneumoserothorax (nū″mō-sē-rō-thō′rāks) [" + " + G. *thōrax*, chest]. Air or gas and serum collected in the pleural cavity.

pneumosilicosis (nū″mō-sĭl-ĭ-kō′sĭs) [" + L. *silex*, *silic-*, flint, + G. *-ōsis*, disease]. Silica particles in the lungs.

pneumotachograph (nū″mō-tăk′ō-grăf) [G. *pneuma*, air, + *tachus*, swift, + *graphein*, to write]. Device for registering velocity of inspiration and expiration of air.

pneumotherapy (nū-mō-ther′ă-pĭ) [G. *pneumōn*, lung, + *therapeia*, treatment]. 1. Treatment of diseases of the lungs. 2. Use of compressed air in treatment. SYN: *pneumatotherapy*.

pneumothermomassage (nū″mō-ther″mō-măs-azh′) [G. *pneuma*, air, + *thermē*, heat, + *massein*, to knead]. Application to the body of air of varying temperature and pressure.

pneumothorax (nū-mō-thō′rāks) [" + *thōrax*, chest]. A collection of air or gas in the pleural cavity.
The gas enters as the result of a perforation through the chest wall or the pleura covering the lung (visceral pleura). This perforation may be the result of an injury or the rupture of an emphysematous bleb or superficial lung abscess; the most common latter condition being a tuberculous abscess in the presence of pulmonary tuberculosis.
SYM: The onset is sudden, usually with a severe sticking pain in the side and marked dyspnea. Fluid very frequently is found, developing within 48 hours (hydropneumothorax). The physical signs are those of a distended unilateral chest, tympanitic resonance, absence of breath sounds, and with fluid, a splash or succussion on shaking patient.

p., artificial. Pneumothorax induced intentionally by artificial means employed in the treatment of pulmonary tuberculosis or pneumonia.
Pneumothorax gives the diseased lung temporary rest. The lung collapses when the air enters the pleural space which is not possible if there are adhesions. Twenty per cent of cases have no free pleural space.
Scattered adhesions may afford only a partial collapse. Forty per cent is the estimated number of indicated cases. Effusion may occur in about one-third of the cases. Hazards are small.
NP: Explain to patient. Instruct not to cough or to warn doctor when so impelled. Patient lies on affected side, arm overhead, and held by nurse. Observe color of face, respiration, and pulse. Record intrapleural pressure. Watch for pleural shock and effusion. Pain in side, weak pulse, dyspnea, sweating are instances. Doctor gives hypodermics or inhalation of oxygen. Complications may be: (a) Air embolism from puncture of a vein; (b) puncture of lung; (c) surgical emphysema.
Postoperative care: Rest for an hour after. Four hour record of temperature for 48 hours. Report dyspnea, as it is serious.

p., spontaneous. Spontaneous entrance of air into the pleural cavity.
The pressure may collapse the lung and displace the heart.
SYM: Pain, dyspnea, cyanosis, prostration, collapse, death, perhaps in a few minutes.

p., valvular. That which is characterized by an opening through the pleura which has a slit with a valvelike action allowing the air to pass in but not out.

pneumotomy (nū-mŏt′ō-mĭ) [G. *pneumōn*, lung, + *tomē*, a cutting]. Incision of the lung.

pneumotoxin (nū″mō-tŏks′ĭn) [" + *toxikon*, poison]. A toxin produced by the pneumococcus.

pneumotyphus (nū″mō-tī′fŭs) [" + *typhos*, fever]. 1. Typhoid fever with pneumonia

pneumouria

at onset. 2. Development of pneumonia during typhoid fever.

pneumouria (nū″mō-ū'rĭ-ă) [G. *pneuma*, air, + *ouron*, urine]. Excretion of urine with free gas. SYN: *pneumaturia*.

pneumoventricle (nū″mō-vĕn'trĭ-kl) [″ + L. *ventriculus*, little belly]. Air accumulation in the cerebral ventricles.

pneumoventriculography (nū″mō-vĕn-trĭk″ū-lŏg'ră-fĭ) [″ + ″ + G. *graphein*, to write]. Radiography of the lateral ventricles of the brain, after removal of fluid content and injection with air. SYN: *ventriculography*.

pneusimeter, pneusometer (nū-sĭm'ĕt-ĕr, -sŏm'ĕt-ĕr) [G. *pneusis*, a breathing, + *metron*, a measure]. Device used as a spirometer to measure vital capacity of the chest in respiration.

pnigophobia (nĭ-gō-fō'bĭ-ă) [G. *pnigos*, choking, + *phobos*, fear]. Morbid fear of choking; sometimes experienced in angina pectoris.

pock (pŏk) [A.S. *poc*, pustule, pouch]. A pustule of an eruptive fever, esp. of smallpox.
  p.-marked. Pitted or marked with cicatrices of smallpox pustules.

pocket (pŏk'ĕt) [Fr. *pochet*, little pouch]. A saclike cavity.

pocketing (pŏk'ĕt-ĭng) [Fr. *pochet*, little pouch]. Method of treating the pedicle in ovariotomy by enclosing it within the edges of the wound.

podagra (pŏd-ăg'ră) [G. *pous*, *pod*-, foot, + *agra*, seizure]. Gout, esp. of the foot's joints or of the great toe.

podalgia (pod-ăl'jĭ-ă) [″ + *algos*, pain]. Pain in the feet.

podalic (pŏd-ăl'ĭk) [G. *pous*, *pod*-, foot]. Pert. to the feet.
  p. version. Shifting position of a fetus to bring the feet to the outlet in labor.

podarthritis (pŏd-ar-thrī'tĭs) [″ + *arthron*, joint, + *itis*, inflammation]. Inflammation of joints of the feet. SYN: *podagra*.

podiatrist (pŏd-ī'ăt-rĭst) [G. *pous*, *pod*-, foot, + *iatreia*, treatment]. Specialist in foot diseases. SYN: *chiropodist*.

podiatry (pŏd-ī'ăt-rĭ) [″ + *iatreia*, healing]. Treatment of foot disorders. SYN: *chiropody*.

podo-, pod- [G.]. Combining forms meaning *foot*.

podobromidrosis (pŏd″ō-brō-mĭ-drō'sĭs) [″ + *bromos*, stench, + *idrōsis*, perspiration]. Offensive perspiration of the feet.

pododynamometer (pŏd″ō-dī-năm-ŏm'ĕt-ĕr) [″ + *dynamis*, force, + *metron*, measure]. A device for testing strength of the leg and foot muscles.

pododynia (pŏd-ō-dĭn'ĭ-ă) [″ + *odynē*, pain]. Pain in the feet, esp. a neuralgic pain in the heel with swelling and redness.

podogram (pŏd'ō-grăm) [″ + *gramma*, a mark]. An imprint of the sole of the foot.

podology (pŏd-ŏl'ō-jĭ) [″ + *logos*, a study]. The study of the anatomy and physiology of the foot.

podophyllum (pŏd-ō-fĭl'ŭm) [G. *pous*, *pod*-, foot, + *phyllon*, leaf]. USP. Mandrake; May apple. An herb grown extensively in eastern U. S. and parts of the South.
  p., resin of.
    ACTION AND USES: Cathartic.
    DOSAGE: 1/6 gr. (0.01 Gm.).

pogoniasis (pō-gō-nī'ăs-ĭs) [G. *pōgōn*, beard, + *iasis*, disorder]. 1. Excessive growth of the beard. 2. Growth of a beard in a woman.

pogonion (pō-go'nĭ-ŏn) [G. *pōgōn*, beard]. The most anterior projecting midpoint of the chin.

-poietic (poy-ĕt'ĭk) [G.]. Suffix meaning making or producing.

poikilocyte (poy'kĭl-ō-sīt) [G. *poikilos*, spotted, + *kytos*, cell]. A large, irregular, malformed blood corpuscle.

poikilocytosis (poy″kĭl-ō-sī-tō'sĭs) [″ + ″ + -*ōsis*, intensive]. Variation in shape of red blood corpuscles; a condition characterized by poikilocytes in the blood.

poikiloplastocyte (poy″kĭl-ō-plăs'tō-sīt) [″ + *plastos*, formed, + *kytos*, cell]. A blood platelet of irregular form.

poikilothermal (poy″kĭl-ō-thĕr'măl) [″ + *thermē*, heat]. Varying in temperature according to environment.

point (poynt) [O.Fr. *point*, a prick, a dot]. 1. The sharp end of any object. 2. Point at which an abscess is about to rupture on a surface. SEE: *fixation*. 3. A minute spot. 4. Position in space, time, or degree.
  p., absolute near. The nearest p. at which normal vision is retained.
  p., anterior focal. Same as focal p.
  p., anterior nodal. SEE: *nodal p's*.
  p., apophysial. Tender spot over a vertebral spinous process, beneath which neuralgic nerves exit.
  p., auricular. Center of external orifice of auditory canal.
  p., Boas'. Tender spot in gastric ulcer left of 12th thoracic vertebra.
  p., boiling. The temperature at which a liquid vaporizes.
  p., Brewer's. Costovertebral triangle which in kidney infection is tender.
  p., Broca's. Center of the ext. auditory meatus; the *auricular point*.
  p's., Capuron's. Four fixed points in pelvic inlet, the iliopectineal eminences and the sacroiliac joints.
  p's., cardinal. Six p's. determining direction of light rays emerging from and entering the eye and of 4 points of the pelvic inlet toward 1 of which the head of the fetus is presented. SEE: *principal p's*, *focal p's*, *nodal p's*.
  p., craniometric. One of the fixed points of the skull used in craniometry.
  p., critical, of gases. Temperature at or above which a gas can no longer be liquefied by pressure.
  p., critical, of liquids. Temperature above which no pressure may retain a body in a liquid form.
  p's., deaf, of the ear. Point at lower end of tragus and 1 where helix intersects line of motion when vibrating tuning fork held in front of ear cannot be heard when started from the lower edge of the zygoma and moved backward toward the occiput.
  p., dew. The temperature at which moisture begins to be deposited as dew.
  p., disparate. Points on the retinae unequally paired.
  p., external orbital. The prominent 1 at outer edge of orbit above the frontomalar suture.
  p., far. The point (20 ft. or more) at which distinct vision is possible without aid of the muscles of accommodation. It is nearer than 20 ft. according to degree of myopia. There is no far point in the hypermetropic eye.
  p., fixation. That at which the 2 visual axes converge.
  p., freezing. Temperature at which liquids become solid.

p's., hysterogenic. Circumscribed areas of the body which produce symptoms of a hysterical aura, and eventually a hysterical attack when rubbed or pressed.
p's., identical retinal. P's. in the 2 retinae upon which the images are seen as one.
p., jugal. Posterior border of frontal process of the malar bone where cut by a line tangent to upper border of zygoma.
p., lacrimal. Outlet of lacrimal canaliculus. SYN: *puncta lacrimalia.*
p., Lanz's. One on line bet. 2 ant. sup. iliac spines, 1/3 distant from right spine, indicating origin of the vermiform appendix.
p., Lian's. One at junction of outer and middle thirds of a line from the umbilicus to ant. sup. spine of ilium where trocar may be introduced safely for paracentesis.
p., malar. The most prominent p. on ext. tubercle of the malar bone.
p., Mayo-Robson's. 1. One just above and right of the umbilicus, pressure over which causes tenderness in the pancreas. 2. One on 1/3 of distance from umbilicus to right nipple showing greatest tenderness in gallbladder inflammation.
p., McBurney's. One bet. 1½ and 2 in. above ant. sup. spine of ilium, on line bet. the ilium and umbilicus, where pressure shows tenderness in acute appendicitis.
p., Morris'. Point of tenderness on pressure on line bet. umbilicus (1½ in. from it) and right ant. sup. spine of ilium. Present in irritation near the vermiform appendix.
p., motor. The p. at which a motor nerve enters a muscle, where an electrode may produce the maximum electrical contraction of that muscle.
p., Munro's. One halfway bet. left ant. iliac spine and the umbilicus.
p's., nasal genital. Point at ant. end of lower turbinated bone, and 1 at the tuberculum septi, irritation of which, when in a hyperesthetic state, produces pain in the hypogastrium and in sacral region.
p., near. Nearest one at which the eye can accommodate for distinct vision.
p's., nodal. An ant. and post. cardinal p. on the surface of lens of the eye so related that every ray directed toward the ant. p. is represented after refraction by a ray emanating from the post. p.
p's., painful. Points over which a neuralgic nerve is tender on pressure.
p's., pressure. The p's. of emergence of the infraorbital and supraorbital, and sometimes branches of facial nerve, in vicinity of margins of the orbit, pressure upon which may arrest blepharospasm.
p's., principal. Two p's. so situated that the optical axis is cut by the 2 principal planes.
p., Robson's. SEE: *Mayo-Robson's point.*
p's., Valleix's. Tender spots upon pressure over the course of a nerve in neuralgia.
pointillage (pwăhn-tĭ-yahzh') [Fr.]. Massage with the finger tips.
points douloureux (pwăhnt doo-loo-rōō'). Painful points in peripheral neuralgia when the nerves pass through bony canals or openings in fascia. SYN: *Valleix's points.*

Poiseuille's law (pwă-sŭ-ēz'). The rapidity of the capillary current is in proportion to the square of the diameter of their capillary tubes.
P.'s layer or **space.** The inert capillary current in which leukocytes move slowly, the erythrocytes moving more rapidly in the middle current.
poison (poy'zn) [L. *potiō*, a poisonous draft]. Any substance which, taken into the system, will produce an injurious or deadly effect.
poison ivy. SEE: *ivy poison.*
poison, words pert. to: *alkaloid, active principles, names of preparations, drugs with 2 names; antidote; convulsant; corrosive; dosage; drug action; drugs and their administration; irritant; medical preparations; names of individual drugs in alphabetical order (over 500 in*

Classification of Poisons

CORROSIVES:
 Strong mineral acids:
  Sulfuric.
  Nitric.
  Hydrochloric.
 Vegetable acids:
  Oxalic.
 Organic derivatives:
  Carbolic acid.
 Alkalies:
  Strong alkalies.
  Alkaline carbonates.
SPECIFIC IRRITANTS:
 The above diluted.
 Lime.
 Zinc.
 Silver, etc.
SIMPLE IRRITANTS:
 Arsenic.
 Mercury.
 Antimony.
 Phosphorus.
 Iodine, etc.
NEURAL IRRITANTS:
 Opium.
 Prussic acid.
 Chloroform.
 Belladonna.
 Aconite.
 Strychnine.
 Conium.
 Tobacco.
 Phenol.

all); names of poisons; poisoning; preparations usually given by rectum; prescription writing; virulent; virus.
poisoning (poy'zn-ĭng) [L. *potiō*, a poisonous draft]. 1. The state produced by introduction of a poison into the system. 2. Administration of a poison.
 GENERAL: SYM: Somewhat slow in onset. Include gastrointestinal irritation with nausea, cramping and vomiting, systemic effects on brain, heart, kidneys, liver, etc. They also cause local irritation, as preparations of arsenic, antimony, copper, mercury, and silver.
 FIRST AID: Avoid becoming excited. Send for a physician immediately. Notify him of the character of emergency.
 Recognition of poison if possible; by looking at bottle, or by observing burns, stains, odor, or symptoms. SEE: *name of specific poison.*
 Dilute at once with large doses milk or water. Soap water may be useful, but should be avoided if alkalies are present. Diluting the poison delays absorption.
 Removal from alimentary tract by emesis, lavage, and catharsis as indi-

Some Common Poisons and Treatment

Poison	Lavage or Emetic	Antidote	Other Treatment
Aconite.	Lavage or emetic.	Tr. digitalis or liq. atropinae, ♏ii.	Keep flat with head low. Stimulants. Treat for shock. Unceasing artificial respiration.
Alcohol.	Lavage or emetic.		Strychnine, gr. 1/20. Cold douche, etc. Leave coffee in stomach after lavage.
Ammonia.	None.	Weak acetic acid or vinegar.	Olive oil and demulcents. Treat shock. Morphine. (Tracheotomy may be necessary.)
Antimony (*tartar emetic*).	Not usually required.	Tannin.	Alcohol. Strong tea or coffee. Warmth. Treat shock. Keep prone. Give demulcents.
Arsenic.	Lavage or emetic.	Dialyzed iron, ʒi every 2 hours for some hours.	Large dose of castor oil to clear out intestines. Demulcent drinks.
Belladonna and atropine.	Lavage or emetic.	Tannin or tea, morphine, gr. ½.	Free stimulation. Artificial respiration.
Camphor.	Lavage or emetic.		Stimulants. Alternate hot and cold douches. Oils.
Carbolic, lysol, etc.	Lavage with very soft tube.	Mag. sulf.	Albumen water, oil, milk. Treat shock.
Caustic potash. Caustic soda.	Neither.	Dilute vinegar or lemon juice.	Treat shock. Oils and butter. Demulcents.
Chloral hydrate.	Lavage or emetic.	Strychnine, gr. 1/20, or atropine, gr. 1/25.	Stimulants. Artificial respiration. External warmth. Rouse patient.
Cocaine.	Lavage or emetic.	Strychnine, gr. 1/20.	Stimulants. Artificial respiration. External warmth. Rouse patient.
Corrosive sublimate. Digitalis.	SEE: Mercury. Emetic and lavage (*zinc sulfate, gr. 1/2*).	Opium and tannin.	Keep in horizontal position. Free stimulation. Alcohol.
Fungi.	Emetic or lavage.	Atropine or morphine.	Free stimulation and friction.
Hydrochloric acid (*spirits of salt*).	Same as for sulfuric acid.		
Hydrocyanic acid (*prussic acid*).	Lavage or rapid emetic.	Ammonia inhalation. Ferrisulf.	Alternate hot and cold douches. Artificial respiration. Treat for shock.

Some Common Poisons and Treatment *(Continued)*

Poison	Lavage or Emetic	Antidote	Other Treatment
Iodine.	Emetic or lavage (*used continuously*).	Starch in water.	Demulcent drinks. Bread, arrowroot, flour.
Laudanum (*opium*).	SEE: Morphine.		
Lead salts.	Lavage or emetic.	Sulfate of zinc.	Demulcents. Epsom salts. White of egg.
Mercury.	Emetic or lavage.		Demulcents. Treat for shock. White of egg.
Morphine.	Lavage with pot. permanganate or emetic (*apomorphine, gr.* 1/10).	Pot. permanganate. Atropine.	Stimulation. Prevent sleep. Artificial respiration if necessary.
Nitric acid.	Neither.	Alkalies.	Demulcents. Magnesia, lime water, or albumen water.
Nux vomica.	SEE: Strychnine.		
Opium.	SEE: Morphine.		
Oxalic acid.	Lavage or emetics.	Lime water and chalk.	Castor oil. Free stimulation. Demulcents. Treat shock.
Phosphorus.	Lavage or emetics. ($CuSO_4$.)	Permanganate of potash, gr. 5, in 1 oz. of water. Also $CuSO_4$, gr. 5.	Avoid oils but give French oil of turpentine. Purgatives. Demulcents.
Ptomaines.	Lavage with Condy's fluid.		Purgation and colonic lavage. Salines. Strychnine. Treat for shock.
Silver nitrate (*lunar caustic*).	Lavage and emetics.	Large doses of common salt.	White of egg, milk, and water.
Soda, caustic.	SEE: Caustic soda.		
Strychnine.	Lavage before spasms appear. Emetic (*apomorphine, gr.* 1/10).	Tannin or charcoal. Chloral, pot. bromide.	Chloroform inhalation. Morphine. Artificial respiration.
Sulfuric acid (*oil of vitriol*).	Neither.	Dilute alkalies, *e. g.*, lime, soap, chalk, magnesia, etc.	Wall plaster in warm water. Oils. Demulcents.
Tobacco.	Emetics.	Tannin.	Free stimulation. Strychnine. Recumbent position.
Turpentine.	Emetics.	Mag. sulf.	Albumen water or milk.
Veronal.	Lavage.	Strychnine.	Artificial respiration. Keep warm.
Zinc chloride.	Cautious lavage, emetic (*apomorphine, gr.* 1/10).		Tannin. Egg albumen. Oils. Give demulcents freely.

Faber's Pocket Encyclopedia.

cated. SEE: *emetics;* may be dangerous in corrosive poisoning.

The administration of antidotes. SEE: *antidote.*

Elimination of poison from system.

Counteract the effects of the poison. SEE: *name of specific poisoning.*

Treat collapse. Avoid strong stimulants, without specific instructions.

LOCAL IRRITANTS: Represented by acids, alkalies, and caustics.

SYM: Burning, color changes of skin and mucous membrane, gastrointestinal irritation with nausea, vomiting and cramping.

F. A. TREATMENT: Dilute with large volumes of water, following by diluted antidote, then soothing substances as oils, egg whites, cream, etc.

LOCAL EFFECTS OF: *Corrosives*: Chemical decomposition, as seen in the effects of strong mineral acids and alkalies; *irritation or inflammation*: Varies from simple redness to ulceration and gangrene; *local specific effects*: Produced on sentient extremities of nerves as felt on local application of prussic acid.

NP: Keep any receptacle containing poison taken, as well as specimens of vomitus, sputum, urine, or feces. Make note of all said by the patient, and do not repeat any of it to anyone but the physician or court officials.

Never administer any drug without first looking at label on bottle. Do not take any medicine from a bottle when the light is so dim the label may not be read easily. Keep poisonous drugs separate from other medicines and out of the reach of children. The law requires that all poisonous drugs bear a label printed *in red.* Odd-shaped bottles for poisons is another precaution.

The nurse may not legally administer an overdose of any poisonous drug, even though prescribed by a physician. His attention must be called to the assumed mistake, and even then she is within her rights in refusing to administer the prescription.

DISEASES SIMULATING POISONS: *Acute indigestion, intestinal obstruction, appendicitis, cholera and c. morbus, hepatic colic, gastritis, gastroenteritis, renal colic, peritonitis, peptic ulcer,* may give symptoms similar to *irritant poisons. Cerebral hemorrhage, epilepsy, hysteria, organic heart disease, meningitis, thrombosis,* and *uremia* may offer symptoms similar to those of *narcotic poisons.*

p., acid. SEE: *acid p.*
p., alkali. SEE: *alkali p.*
p., atropine. SEE: *atropine p.*
p., belladonna. SEE: *belladonna p.*
p., blood. SEE: *bacteremia, pyemia, septicemia, toxemia.*
p., convulsive. SEE: *convulsive p.*
p., corrosive. SEE: *corrosive p.*
p., fish. Treat as for *black widow spider.*
p., ivy. SEE: *ivy p.*
p., mushroom. SEE: *mushroom p.*
p., narcotic. SEE: *name of.*
p., sedative. SEE: *sedative p.*
p., toadstool. SEE: *toadstool p.*
p., unknown. In case no information is available about the character of the poison taken, and the symptoms and signs are not characteristic, it is evident that the exact antidote cannot be administered.

In such instances it is often helpful to be able to administer antidotes which in themselves are harmless and may prove efficacious.

Many combinations of this character have been described. One of the best is the following: Pulverized charcoal, 2 parts; magnesium oxide (magnesia), 1 part; tannic acid, 1 part; Fuller's earth, kaolin or hydrous magnesium silicate, 1 part. This mixture may be administered in doses of 1 heaping teaspoonful mixed in water. It may be repeated several times, as none of the ingredients are harmful and they may be very advantageous.

The charcoal and Fuller's earth act physically by absorption of the drugs, thus retarding their absorption. The tannic acid acts chemically by precipitating many drugs, and physiologically, by coating the lining of the stomach with a coagulum which delays absorption, and the magnesia neutralizes acids and is a good antidote for arsenic, and acts mechanically by incorporating the undissolved poison in the stomach and thus delays its absorption.

poisoning, words pert. to: acid; alkali; alkaloid; allantiasis; antidote; artificial respiration; atriplicism; atropinism; brass-founder's disease; bromatoxism; bromoderma; carbolism; carboxyhemoglobin; cellulotoxic; chalcosis; cinchonism; Clapton's lines; daturine; duboisine; emetic; first aid; food; grain; hemlock; heroin; ink; lavage, gastric; matches; meat; milk; nicotine; oxalic acid; oxygen; plumbism; ptomaine; rough-on-rats; saturnism; Scheele's green; sedative; sodium hydroxide; strychnine; sulfur dioxide; tellurium; tin; toadstool; tobacco; "tox-" words; "venen-" words, verdigris.

poisonous plants. *Do not eat:* castor bean, chinaberry, European bittersweet, wild or black cherry, horsenut, poisonous hemlock, laurel, mushroom or death cup, black nightshade or deadly nightshade, Jimson weed. *Do not touch:* poison ivy, poison oak, snow-on-the-mountain, showy lady-slipper, poison sumac.

poitrinaire (pwah-trē-nār′) [Fr.]. One with chronic disease of the chest or with pulmonary tuberculosis.

polar [L. *polus,* pole, from G. *polos,* axis]. Concerning a pole.

p. compounds. Those formed by an exchange of electrons.

polarimeter (pō-lar-ĭm′ĕt-ẽr) [" + G. *metron,* a measure]. Instrument for measuring amount of polarization of light, or rotation of polarized light.

polarimetry (pō-lar-ĭm′ĕt-rĭ) [" + G. *metron,* a measure]. Measurement of the amount and rotation of polarized light.

polariscope (pō-lar′ĭ-skōp) [" + G. *skopein,* to examine]. Apparatus used in measurement of polarized light.

polarity (pō-lar′ĭ-tĭ) [L. *polus,* pole]. P.T. 1. The quality of having poles. 2. The exhibition of opposite effects at the 2 extremities.

polarization (pō-lăr-ĭ-zā′shŭn) [L. *polus,* pole]. 1. Condition in a ray of light in which vibrations occur in only 1 plane or in curves. 2. In a galvanic battery, collection of hydrogen bubbles on negative plate and oxygen on the positive plate, whereby generation of current is impeded.

pole (pōl) [L. *polus,* a pole, from G. *polos,* axis]. 1. The extremity of any axis about which forces acting on it are symmetrically disposed. 2. One of 2 points in a magnet, cell, or battery having opposite physical qualities.

p., animal. One opposite the yolk in

an ovum near which is the protoplasm of the germinal vesicle.
p., antigerminal. That of an ovum opp. the germinal p. where is situated the food yolk.
p., cephalic. End of the ovoid formed by the fetus at which the head is formed.
p's. of the chorion. The upper and lower extremities of the chorion, analogous to the fundus and os uteri.
p's. of the eye. The ant. and post. extremities of the optic axis.
p., frontal. Most projecting part of the ant. extremity of both cerebral hemispheres.
p., germinal. The p. of an ovum at which the development begins.
p's. of the kidney. The kidney's upper and lower extremities.
p., negative. That electrode or cathode portion of a battery connected with its electropositive element.
p., nutritive. Antigerminal* p.
p., occipital. The post. extremity of the occipital lobe.
p., pelvic. Breech of a fetus.
p., placental, of the chorion. Spot at which the domelike placenta is situated.
p., positive. That electrode (anode) or other portion of the apparatus of a battery connected with its electronegative element.
p's. of the testicle. The upper and lower extremities of a testicle.
p., vegetative. Part of the egg containing the food yolk.
p., vitelline. Antigerminal* pole.
policlinic (pŏl-ĭ-klĭn'ĭk) [G. *polis*, city, + *klinē*, bed]. A city hospital or clinic for outpatients. SYN: *polyclinic.*
polioclastic (pŏl″ĭ-ō-klăs'tĭk) [G. *polios*, gray, + *klastos*, breaking]. Destructive of the gray matter of the nervous system.
polioencephalitis (pŏl″ĭ-ō-ĕn-sĕf″ăl-ī'tĭs) [G. *polios*, gray, + *egkephalos*, brain, + *-itis*, inflammation]. An infectious inflammatory disease of the gray matter of the brain.
SYM: Fever, vomiting, convulsions.
p. acuta. Acute inflammation of the cerebral cortex giving rise to infantile cerebral palsy in children.
p., anterior superior. P. of the 3rd ventricle and ant. portion of the 4th of the brain.
p., infective. Encephalitis lethargica.
p., inferior. Bulbar paralysis.
polioencephalomeningomyelitis (pŏl″ĭ-ō-ĕn-sĕf″ăl-ō-men-ĭng-ō-mī-ĕl-ī'tĭs) [" + *egkephalos*, brain, + *mēnigx*, membrane, + *myelos*, marrow, + *-itis*, inflammation]. Inflammation of the gray matter of the brain and spinal cord and their meninges.
polioencephalomyelitis (pŏl″ĭ-ō-ĕn-sĕf″ăl-ō-mī-ĕl-ī'tĭs) [" + " + *myelos*, marrow, + *-itis*, inflammation]. Inflamed condition of the gray matter of the brain and spinal cord. SYN: *Heine-Medin disease.*
polioencephalopathy (pŏl″ĭ-ō-ĕn-sĕf″ăl-ŏp'-ăth-ĭ) [" + " + *pathos*, disease]. Diseased condition of the gray matter of the brain.
poliomyelencephalitis (pŏl″ĭ-ō-mī-ĕl-ĕn″-sĕf-ăl-ī'tĭs) [" + *myelos*, marrow, + *egkephalos*, brain, + *-itis*, inflammation]. Poliomyelitis with polioencephalitis.
poliomyeliticidal (pŏl″ĭ-ō-mī-ĕl-ĭt-ĭs-ī'dăl). Having power to destroy or neutralize poliomyelitis virus.
poliomyelitis (pŏl″ĭ-ō-mī-ĕl-ī'tĭs) [G. *polios*, gray, + *myelos*, marrow, + *-itis*, inflammation]. Inflammation of the gray matter of the spinal cord.
p., acute anterior. An acute infectious inflammation of ant. horns of the spinal cord.
While commonly referred to as infantile paralysis, this designation is not accurate because the infection is not confined to infants, nor is paralysis present in every instance.
According to modern conception, this is an acute, infectious, systemic disease in which paralysis may, or may not, occur. Some believe that it is the lymphatic system which is primarily involved. When paralysis develops, the ganglion in the ant. gray horns of the cord shows distinctive changes and marked atrophy of muscles, and contractions may be late manifestations of the disease.
ETIOL: The actual cause was thought to be a filtrable virus, although a minute coccus has been described by several investigators. Susceptibility is greatest among children under 5 years of age. Epidemics, when they occur, usually reach their peak during the warmest seasons of the year, esp. July and August.
INCUBATION: Probably varies from 2 to 7 days in most instances.
SYM: Onset is often abrupt, though the ordinary manifestations of a severe cold, or some gastrointestinal disturbances may come on gradually, accompanied by slight elevation of temperature, frequently enduring for not more than 3 days. At the end of this period, paralysis may, or may not, develop. The extent of any paralysis necessarily depends upon degree of nerve involvement. Consequently, paralysis may be confined either to 1 small group of muscles, or affect 1 or all extremities. In some instances, the respiratory muscles are also involved, and it is in these cases that death is so likely to ensue. In the average paralytic case it is the extensor muscles in particular that are concerned.
COMPLICATIONS: Any paralysis occurring in this disease may be regarded as a complication. Atrophy of muscles, and ultimate deformities may likewise be classed in a similar way. Aside from bronchopneumonia, which may develop in very severe cases, other complications are surprisingly few.
DIFFERENTIAL DIAG: Among the diseases confused with this infection are the various types of meningitis, rheumatism, traumatic conditions, tuberculosis involving bones or joints, and occasionally scurvy or rickets in infants.
PROG: Ordinarily, the outcome as to life is good. It is only the bulbar and respiratory cases in which death is likely to occur. In fact, these 2 types constitute nearly all of the fatal cases. Even in those cases where paralysis is present, complete restoration of the parts may finally be brought about. In the more severe types, however, some deformity is very likely to remain.
TREATMENT: Salk vaccine as preventive. Rest in bed when acute. Keep paralyzed parts warm with woolen stockings or flannel, and promote elimination. Support any affected limb with padded wire splints or sandbags. Use a cradle in order that bedclothing does not press on toes if the foot is paralyzed. No massage, electricity, or mechanical manipulations of any description prior to 3 weeks from onset of the paralysis.

poliomyelitis, anterior

SPECIFIC TREATMENT: Convalescent human serum is the only remedy that offers any real hope from a curative standpoint. This is used by means of intramuscular, intravenous, or intraspinal injection. Sometimes all 3 are resorted to. It should be given before the development of paralysis when there is any possibility of administration at such a time. After 4 weeks, in many cases, plaster casts or mechanical appliances will be needed to prevent the development of impending deformities. At this time, too, massage and muscle training may be used.
Electricity is employed on a much smaller scale than some years ago. There is not loss of sensation in this disease, but early in its course the patient may be hyperesthetic; consequently, with the adoption of any treatment, the production of pain must receive consideration. While the quarantine period varies in different states, 3 weeks of isolation is probably sufficient.
Recent method of treatment has been intravenous injections of glucose for muscular pain and muscle transplantation in paralysis.

p., anterior. Inflamed state of spinal cord's ant. horns.

p., chronic, anterior. Progressive wasting of the muscles.

poliomyelopathy (pŏl″ĭ-ō-mī-ĕl-ŏp′ăth-ĭ) [G. *polios*, gray, + *myelos*, marrow, + *pathos*, disease]. Any diseased condition of the gray matter of the spinal cord.

polioplasm (pĕl″ĭ-ō-plăzm) [″ + *plasma*, a thing formed]. Granular protoplasm.

poliosis (pŏl-ĭ-ō′sĭs) [″ + *-osis*, condition]. Absence of pigment in the hair. SYN: *calvities; grayness*.

Po'lish plait. Matted hair due to disease of the scalp and want of cleanliness. SYN: *plica polonica*.

politzerization (pō-lĭt-zĕr-ĭ-zā′shŭn). The inflation of the middle ear using a Politzer bag.

Politzer's bag (pŏl′ĭts-ĕr). Soft rubber bag with rubber tip for inflating the middle ear.

pollaccine (pŏl-ăk′sĭn). A pollen preparation used in testing for sensitivity and in treatment of asthma and hay fever.

pollakiuria (pŏl-ăk-ĭ-ū′rĭ-ă) [G. *pollakis*, often, + *ouron*, urine]. Abnormally frequent passage of urine.

pollen (pŏl′ĕn) [L. powder]. The male element in flowering plants.

pollenogenic (pŏl″ĕn-ō-jen′ĭk) [″ + G. *gennan*, to produce]. Due to the pollen of plants or producing plant pollen.

pollenosis (pŏl-ĕn-ō′sĭs) [″ + G. *-osis*, disease]. Hay fever; disease due to pollen.

pollex (pŏl′ĕks) [L. thumb]. The thumb.

p. flexus. Permanent flexion of the thumb.

p. pedis. The great toe. SYN: *hallux*.

pollinosis (pŏl-ĭn-ō′sĭs) [L. *pollen*, powder, + G. *-osis*, disease]. Nasal congestion of mucous membranes due to contact with pollen. SYN: *hay fever*.

pollution (pol-ū′shun). 1. State of making impure or defiling. 2. Emission of semen at other times than in coition.

polonium (pō-lo′nĭ-ŭm). Radioactive metal isolated from pitchblende. SYN: *radium F*.

polus (pō′lŭs) [L.]. Pole.

poly- [G.]. Prefix meaning *many* or *much*.

poly. (pŏl′ĭ). Abbr. for *polymorphonuclear leukocyte*.

polyadenia (pŏl″ĭ-ăd-ē′nĭ-ă) [G. *polys*, many, + *adēn*, gland]. Enlargement of the lymph glands. SYN: *pseudoleukemia*.

polyadenomatosis (pŏl″ĭ-ăd-ē-nō-mă-tō′sĭs) [″ + ″ + *-oma*, tumor, + *-osis*, disease]. Adenomas in many glands.

polyadenous (pŏl-ĭ-ad′ē-nŭs) [″ + *adēn*, gland]. Involving or relating to many glands.

polyalgesia (pŏl″ĭ-ăl-je′zĭ-ă) [″ + *algēsis*, sensation]. A single stimulus of a part, producing sensation in many parts.

polyandry (pŏl″ĭ-an′drĭ) [″ + *aner, andr-*, man]. The practice of having more than 1 husband at the same time. SEE: *polygamy*.

polyarteritis (pŏl″ĭ-ar-ter-ĭ′tĭs) [″ + *artēria*, artery, + *-itis*, inflammation]. Inflammation of more than 1 or 2 arteries at the same time.

p. nodosa. P. with nodules on smaller arterial branches.

polyarthric (pŏl″ĭ-ar′thrĭk) [″ + *arthron*, joint]. Affecting or pert. to several joints.

polyarthritis (pol-ĭ-ar-thrī′tis) [G. *polys*, many, + *arthron*, joint, + *-itis*, inflammation]. Inflammation of a number of joints.

p. rheumatica acuta. Acute articular rheumatism.

p., vertebral. Intervertebral inflammation of the disks without vertebral caries.

polyarticular (pŏl″ĭ-ar-tĭk′ū-lar) [″ + L. *articulus*, a joint]. Affecting many joints. SYN: *multiarticular*.

polyatomic (pŏl″ĭ-ă-tom′ĭk) [″ + *atomon*, atom]. Having several atoms or more than 2 replaceable hydrogen atoms.

polyaxon (pol-ĭ-ak′son) [″ + *axōn*, axis]. Neuron with more than 2 axons.

polyblast (pŏl′ĭ-blăst) [″ + *blastos*, a germ]. Large mononuclear phagocyte present in inflammation derived from an embryonic wandering cell.

polyblennia (pŏl-ĭ-blĕn′nĭ-ă) [″ + *blennos*, mucus]. Secretion of more mucus than normal.

polyceptor (pŏl-ĭ-sep′tor) [G. *polys*, many, + L. *ceptor*, a receiver]. An amboceptor having several complementophile groups.

polycholia (pŏl-ĭ-kō′lĭ-ă) [″ + *cholē*, bile]. Abnormal secretion of bile.

polychrest (pol′ĭ-krĕst) [″ + *chrēstos*, useful]. A medicine useful in many diseases.

polychromasia (pŏl″ĭ-krō-mā′zĭ-ă) [″ + *chrōma*, color]. Quality of having many colors.

polychromatic (pŏl″ĭ-krō-măt′ĭk) [″ + *chrōma*, color]. Multicolored.

polychromatophil(e (pŏl″ĭ-krō-măt′ō-fĭl) [″ + ″ + *philein*, to love]. Stainable with more than 1 kind of stain.

polychromatophilia (pŏl″ĭ-krō-măt-ō-fĭl′ĭ-ă) [″ + ″ + *philein*, to love]. 1. The quality of being stainable with more than 1 stain. 2. Polychromatophil cells in the blood to excess.

polychromemia (pŏl-ĭ-krō-mē′mĭ-ă) [G. *polys*, many, + *chrōma*, color, + *aima*, blood]. Increase in the blood's coloring matter.

polychromia (pŏl″ĭ-krō′mĭ-ă) [″ + *chrōma*, color]. Increased or excessive pigmentation.

polychylia (pŏl″ĭ-kī′lĭ-ă) [″ + *chylos*, juice]. Excessive secretion of chyle.

polyclinic (pŏl-ĭ-klĭn′ĭk) [″ + *klinē*, bed]. Hospital or clinic treating many diseases; a general hospital.

polyclonia (pŏl″ĭ-klō′nĭ-ă) [″ + *klonos*, tumult]. A disease characterized by many clonic spasms but distinct from chorea or tic.

polycoria (pŏl-ĭ-kō′rĭ-ă) [″ + *korē*, pu-

polycrotic P-81 **polymeria**

pil]. The state of having more than 1 pupil in 1 eye.
polycrotic (pŏl-ĭ-krŏt'ĭk) [" + *krotos*, a beat]. Having several pulse waves for each cardiac systole.
polycrotism (pŏl-ĭk'rŏt-ĭzm) [" + " + *ismos*, a beat]. Condition of having several pulse waves for each cardiac systole.
polycyesia, polycyesis (pŏl-ĭ-sī-ē'zĭ-ă, -sĭs) [G. *polys*, many, + *kyēsis*, pregnancy]. 1. Pregnancy with more than 1 fetus in the uterus. 2. Frequent pregnancy.
polycystic (pŏl-ĭ-sĭs'tĭk) [" + *kystis*, a bladder]. Composed of many cysts.
polycythemia (pŏl'ĭ-sī-thē'mĭ-ă) [" + *kytos*, cell, + *aima*, blood]. An excess of red blood cells. SEE: *erythrocytosis*.
 p. megalosplenica, p., myelopathic, p. rubra, p., splenomegalic, p. vera. A slowly progressive disease characterized by an increased number of red blood cells and increase in total blood volume.
 SYM: Weakness, fatigue, vertigo, tinnitus, irritability, enlarged spleen, skin and mucosa have a red cyanosis. Basal metabolism increased and bone marrow shows increased cellularity.
 ETIOL: Unknown.
 TREATMENT: Permanent cure cannot be achieved today, but remissions of many months can be produced. Venesection, phenylhydrazine derivatives, roentgen-ray therapy and Fowler's solution, in combination or singly. SYN: *erythremia*, *Osler's disease*, *Vaquez's disease*.
polycytosis (pŏl'ĭ-sī-tō'sĭs) [G. *polys*, many, + *kytos*, cell, + *-ōsis*, disease]. Increased number of red and white blood corpuscles in the blood.
polydactylism (pŏl'ĭ-dăk'tĭ-lĭzm) [" + *daktylos*, digit, + *-ismos*, condition]. State of having supernumerary fingers or toes.
polydipsia (pŏl-ĭ-dĭp'sĭ-ă) [" + *dipsa*, thirst]. Excessive thirst.
polyemia (pol-ĭ-ē'mĭ-ă) [" + *aima*, blood]. Abnormal amount of blood in the system. SYN: *polycythemia*.
 p. aquosa. Physiological excess of water in the blood after drinking much fluid.
 p. hyperalbuminosa. Excessive amt. of albumin in the blood plasma.
 p. polycythaemica. An increase of red corpuscles.
 p. serosa. Increase of blood serum.
polyesthesia (pŏl'ĭ-ĕs-thē'zĭ-ă) [" + *aisthēsis*, sensation]. Disturbed sensation of touch in which an external stimulus or touch is felt as several.
polyesthetic (pŏl'ĭ-ĕs-thĕt'ĭk) [" + *aisthēsis*, sensation]. Exciting sensation in several different points when only 1 is stimulated.
polygalactia (pŏl'ĭ-găl-ăk'shĭ-ă) [" + *gala, galakt-*, milk]. Excessive secretion or flow of milk.
polygamy (pō-lĭg'ă-mĭ) [G. *polys*, many, + *gamos*, marriage]. Practice of having several wives or husbands at the same time, esp. wives.
polygen (pŏl'ĭ-jĕn) [" + *gennan*, to produce]. 1. Serum derived from more than 1 antigen. 2. Element capable of combining in several proportions.
polygenesis (pŏl'ĭ-jĕn'ĕ-sĭs) [" + *genesis*, development]. Theory that 2 or more branches of the human race evolved independent of each other.
polyglandular (pŏl'ĭ-glăn'dū-lar) [" + L. *glandula*, a little kernel]. Pert. to or affecting many glands. SYN: *pluriglandular*.

polyglobulia, polyglobulism (pŏl'ĭ-glō-bū'-lĭ-ă, -glŏb'ū-lĭzm) [" + L. *globulus*, globule, + G. *-ismos*, condition]. Increase in number of red corpuscles in the blood. SYN: *polycythemia*.
polygram (pŏl'ĭ-grăm) [" + *gramma*, a mark]. Sphygmographic record made by polygraph of pulse beats simultaneously.
polygraph (pŏl'ĭ-grăf) [" + *graphein*, to write]. A device which records simultaneously tracings of several different pulsations, as arterial and venous pulse waves, apex beat of heart, and other pulsations. SYN: *sphygmograph*.
polygroma (pŏl-ĭ-grō'mă) [G. *polys*, many, + *ygros*, moist, + *-ōma*, tumor]. A large sac distended with fluid. SYN: *hygroma*.
polygyria (pŏl-ĭ-jī'rĭ-ă) [" + *gyros*, circle]. Excess of the number of convolutions in the brain.
polyhedral (pŏl-ĭ-hē'drăl) [" + *edra*, base]. Having many surfaces.
polyhemia (pŏl'ĭ-hē'mĭ-ă) [" + *aima*, blood]. Abnormal increase in amount of the blood. SYN: *polyemia*.
polyhidrosis (pŏl-ĭ-hī-drō'sĭs) [" + *idrōsis*, perspiration]. Excessive perspiration.*
polyhydramnios (pŏl-ĭ-hī-drăm'nĭ-ŏs) [" + *ydōr*, water, + *amnion*, amnion]. An excess of amniotic fluid in the bag-of-waters in pregnancy. SEE: *amnion*.
polyhydruria (pŏl'ĭ-hī-drū'rĭ-ă) [" + *ouron*, urine]. Excessive amt. of water in urine.
polyhypermenorrhea (pŏl'ĭ-hī-pĕr-mĕn-ō-rē'ă) [G. *polys*, many, + *yper*, over, + *mēn*, month, + *roia*, flow]. Frequent menstruation with excessive discharge.
polyhypomenorrhea (pŏl-ĭ-hī-pō-mĕn-ō-rē'ă) [" + *ypo*, under, + *mēn*, month, + *roia*, flow]. Frequent menstruation with scanty discharge.
polyinfection (pŏl'ĭ-ĭn-fĕk'shŭn) [" + L. *infectio*, a making in]. Infection with 2 or more microörganisms. SYN: *multiinfection*.
polykaryocyte (pŏl-ĭ-kar'ĭ-ō-sīt) [" + *karyon*, nucleus, + *kytos*, cell]. A cell possessing several nuclei.
polyleptic (pŏl'ĭ-lĕp'tĭk) [" + *lēpsis*, a seizure, from *lambanein*, to seize]. Characterized by numerous remissions and exacerbations, as malaria.
polymastia, polymazia (pŏl-ĭ-măs'tĭ-ă, -mă'zĭ-ă) [" + *mastos, mazos*, breast]. Condition of having more than 2 mammae.
polymastigote (pŏl-ĭ-măs'tĭ-gōt) [" + *mastix, mastig-*, whip]. Possessing several flagella.
polymenia (pŏl-ĭ-mē'nĭ-ă) [G. *polys*, many, + *mēn*, month]. Excessive and frequent menstrual flow. SYN: *menorrhagia*, *polymenorrhea*.
polymenorrhea (pŏl'ĭ-mĕn-or-rē'ă) [" + " + *roia*, a flow]. Excessive menstrual flow occurring too frequently. SYN: *menorrhagia, polymenia*.
polymer (pŏl'ĭ-mer) [" + *meros*, a part]. One of 2 or more compounds of same elements in same proportion by weight, but differing in molecular weight, formed by polymerization, as paraformaldehyde from formaldehyde.
 A substance A is said to be a polymer of the substance B if A contains the same elements in the same proportions as B but its molecular weight is a multiple of B's. Thus, acetic acid, $C_2H_4O_2$, is a polymer of formaldehyde, CH_2O.
polymeria (pŏl-ĭ-mē'rĭ-ă) [" + *meros*, a part]. 1. Condition of having super-

numerary parts of the body. 2. A chain of atoms.

polymeric (pŏl-ĭ-mĕr'ĭk) [" + *meros*, a part]. 1. Consisting of the same elements in same proportions by weight, but differing in molecular weight. 2. Said of muscles derived from more than 1 myotome.

polymerism (pŏl'ĭ-mĕr-ĭzm, pō-lĭm'ĕr-ĭzm) [" + *meros*, part, + *ismos*, condition]. 1. Condition of having more than normal number of parts. 2. Isomerism in which the molecular weights of the polymers are multiples of each other.

polymerization (pŏl"ĭ-mĕr-ĭ-zā'shŭn) [" + *meros*, part]. Process of changing into another compound having same elements in same proportions, but a higher molecular weight.

polymitus (po-lĭm'ĭ-tŭs) [G. *polys*, many, + *mitos*, thread]. Stage in reproduction of microörganisms with threads of protoplasm which, being detached, constitute the microgamete.

polymorphic (pŏl-ĭ-mor'fĭk) [" + *morphē*, form]. Occurring in more than 1 form.

polymorphism (pŏl-ĭ-mor'fĭzm) [" + " + -*ismos*, condition]. 1. Capacity for appearing in many forms. 2. Existence of several types in the same group or species. SYN: *pleomorphism*.

polymorphocellular (pŏl"ĭ-mor-fō-sĕl'ū-lar) [" + " + L. *cellula*, a small chamber]. Composed of cells of many forms.

polymorphonuclear (pŏl"ĭ-mor-fō-nū'klē-ar) [" + " + L. *nucleus*, a kernel]. Having nuclei of varied forms, esp. a common variety of leukocytes.

The cell nucleus is blue, lobated and variable in shape. About twice the size of a red blood cell. The protoplasm is pinkish in color with a few granules of a lilac tint. They make up about 70% of the leukocytes.

p. leukocyte, p. neutrophil leukocyte. Finely granular cell with an affinity for acid and neutral dyes with an irregularly formed nucleus. SEE: *leukocyte*.

polymorphous (pŏl-ĭ-mor'fŭs) [" + *morphē*, form]. Appearing in many forms. SYN: *polymorphic*.

p. perverse. PSY: Term for pregenital expressions of sex activities natural in babies, but which become abnormal when expressed in adult life. Ex: *cruelty, exhibitionism*.

polymyoclonus (pŏl-ĭ-mī-ŏk'lō-nŭs) [G. *polys*, many, + *mys, myo-*, muscle, + *klonos*, tumult]. A shocklike muscular contraction, occurring in various parts at the same time. SYN: *myoclonus multiplex, paramyoclonus*.

polymyositis (pŏl-ĭ-mī-ō-sī'tĭs) [" + " + -*itis*, inflammation]. Simultaneous inflammation of many muscles.

polymyxin (pŏl-ĭ-mĭks'ĭn). An antibiotic isolated in 1947 from *Bacillus polymyxa*. Most effective against gram-negative bacteria *(Pyocyaneus)* and useful against streptomycin-resistant organisms but not *Proteus*. Dangerously toxic when injected. An intestinal antiseptic when given by mouth.

polynesic (pŏl-ĭ-nē'sĭk) [" + *nēsos*, an island]. Appearing in many separate locations or foci.

polyneural (pŏl-ĭ-nū'răl) [" + *neuron*, sinew]. Pert. to, innervated, or supplied by, many nerves.

polyneuralgia (pŏl"ĭ-nū-ral'jĭ-ă) [" + " + *algos*, pain]. Neuralgia in several nerves.

polyneuritic (pŏl"ĭ-nū-rĭt'ĭk) [" + " + -*itis*, inflammation]. Suffering from inflammation of several nerves at once.

p. psychosis. P. seen in chronic alcoholism with disturbed orientation, polyneuritis, hallucinations, falsification of memory, etc.

polyneuritis (pŏl-ĭ-nū-rī'tĭs) [" + " + -*itis*, inflammation]. A neuritis involving 2 or more nerves; usually a large number.

ETIOL: Alcoholism, beriberi, metallic poisoning, certain infectious diseases.

TREATMENT: Thiamin chloride, vitamin B₁, has been used successfully.

RS: *beriberi*; celluloneuritis; neuritis, multiple; vitamin*.

polynuclear (pŏl"ĭ-nū'klē-ar) [G. *polys*, many, + L. *nucleus*, a kernel]. Possessing more than 1 nucleus.

polynucleosis (pŏl"ĭ-nū-klē-ō'sĭs) [" + " + G. -*ōsis*, disease]. Many polynuclear cells in the blood or in a pathologic exudate. SYN: *leukocytosis, polymorphonuclear*.

polyodontia (pŏl"ĭ-ō-dŏn'shĭ-ă) [" + *odous, odont-*, tooth]. State of having supernumerary teeth.

polyopia, polyopsia (pŏl-ĭ-ō'pĭ-ă, -ŏp'sĭ-ă) [" + *opsis*, vision]. Multiple vision; perception of more than 1 image of the same object.

polyorchidism (pŏl"ĭ-or'kĭd-ĭzm) [" + *orchis*, testicle, + -*ismos*, condition]. Condition marked by having more than 2 testicles.

polyorchis (pŏl"ĭ-or'kĭs) [" + *orchis*, testicle]. One with more than 2 testicles.

polyorrhomenitis (pŏl"ĭ-or"rō-mĕn-ī'tĭs) [" + *orros*, serum, + *ymēn*, membrane, + -*itis*, inflammation]. Malignant inflammation and wasting of serous membranes. SYN: *Concato's disease*.

polyotia (pŏl-ĭ-ō'shĭ-ă) [G. *polys*, many, + *ous, ot-*, ear]. State of having more than 2 ears.

polyp (pŏl'ĭp) [" + *pous*, foot]. A tumor with a pedicle, esp. on mucous membranes of *nose, bladder, rectum, uterus*. SYN: *polypus*.

polyparesis (pŏl"ĭ-par'ĕs-ĭs) [" + *paresis*, relaxation]. General progressive paralysis of paralytic dementia.

polypathia (pŏl-ĭ-păth'ĭ-ă) [" + *pathos*, disease]. The presence of several diseases at 1 time, or their frequent recurrence.

polypeptide (pŏl-ĭ-pĕp'tĭd) [" + *peptein*, to digest]. A union of 3 or more amino acids. SEE: *peptide*.

polypeptidemia (pŏl"ĭ-pĕp-tĭd-ē'mĭ-ă) [" + " + *aima*, blood]. Polypeptides present in the blood.

polypeptidorrhachia (pŏl"ĭ-pĕp-tĭd-ō-rā'kĭ-ă) [" + " + *rachis*, spine]. Polypeptides in the cerebrospinal fluid.

polyphagia (pŏl-ĭ-fā'jĭ-ă) [G. *polys*, many, + *phagein*, to eat]. Eating abnormally large amounts of food at a meal.

RS: *anorexia, acoria, bulimia, parorexia, taste*.

polyphalangism (pŏl"ĭ-făl-ăn'jĭzm) [" + *phalanx*, phalanx, + *ismos*, condition]. An extra number of phalanges on a finger or toe.

polypharmacy (pŏl-ĭ-far'mă-sĭ) [" + *pharmakon*, drug]. 1. Excessive use of drugs or overdose of a drug. 2. Prescription of many drugs given at 1 time.

polyphobia (pŏl-ĭ-fō'bĭ-ă) [" + *phobos*, fear]. Excessive or abnormal fear of a number of things.

polyphrasia (pŏl-ĭ-frā'zĭ-ă) [" + *phrasis*, speech]. Excessive talkativeness, a manifestation of insanity. SYN: *verbigeration*.

polyplast (pŏl'ĭ-plăst) [" + *plastos*, formed]. 1. Composed of many different substances. 2. Experiencing many structural modifications during development.

polyplastic (pŏl-ĭ-plăs'tĭk) [G. *polys*, many, + *plastos*, formed]. 1. Having had many evolutionary modifications. 2. Having many substances in cellular composition.

polyplastocytosis (pŏl″ĭ-plăs-tō-sī-tō'sĭs) [" + " + *kytos*, cell, + *-ōsis*, intensive]. Increase of blood platelets formation.

polyplegia (pŏl-ĭ-plē'jĭ-ă) [" + *plēgē*, a stroke]. Paralysis affecting several muscles.

polypnea (pŏl-ĭp-nī'ă) [" + *pnoia*, breath]. Very rapid breathing. SYN: *panting*.

polypodia (pŏl″ĭ-pō'dĭ-ă) [" + *pous*, *pod-*, foot]. Possession of more than normal number of feet.

polypoid (pŏl'ĭ-poyd) [" + *pous*, foot, + *eidos*, like]. Like a polyp.

polyposis (pŏl-ĭ-pō'sĭs) [" + " + *-ōsis*, intensive]. The presence of numerous polypi.

p. ventriculi. Warty condition of the gastric mucosa accompanied by catarrh and hypertrophy.

polypotome (pol-ĭp'o-tōm) [G. *polys*, many, + *pous*, foot, + *tomē*, a cutting]. Instrument for excision of a polypus.

polypus (pŏl'ĭ-pŭs) (pl. *polypi*) [" + *pous*, foot]. A pedunculate tumor growing from a mucous membrane.

Commonly found in vascular organs such as the nose, uterus and rectum. They bleed easily and should be removed surgically. SYN: *polyp*.

p., bleeding. Angioma of nasal mucous membrane.

p., cellular. Mucous polypus.

p., cervical. A polyp, either fibrous or mucous, on the cervical mucosa.

p., fibrous. A pedunculated fibroid tumor within the uterine or cervical cavities.

p., fleshy. A submucous myoma in the uterus.

p., placental. A polyp composed of retained placental tissue.

polyrrhea, polyrrhoea (pol-ĭr-rē'ă) [G. *polys*, many, + *roia*, flow]. Excessive secretion of fluid.

polysaccharid (pŏl″ĭ-săk′kă-rĭd) [" + *sakcharon*, sugar] ($C_6H_{10}O_5$) n. One of a carbohydrate group which on hydrolysis yields 2 or more molecules of simple sugars. Ex: Starch, which on hydrolysis yields maltose.

polysaccharose (pŏl″ĭ-săk'ă-rōs) [" + *sakcharon*, sugar]. The name for 1 of a *group* of carbohydrates which yields simple sugar.

They include the following: Starch, dextrin, pectose, cellulose, gums, glycogen and insulin. SYN: *polysaccharide*. SEE: *disaccharose*.

polysarcia (pŏl″ĭ-sar′shĭ-ă) [" + *sarx*, *sark-*, flesh]. Fleshiness; obesity.

polysarcous (pŏl″ĭ-sar′kŭs) [" + *sarx*, *sark-*, flesh]. Very fleshy; fat.

polyscelia (pŏl″ĭ-sē′lĭ-ă) [" + *skelos*, leg]. Condition of having more than the normal number of legs.

polyscope (pŏl'ĭ-skōp) [" + *skopein*, to examine]. Instrument for illumination and examination of cavities.

polyserositis (pŏl″ĭ-sē-rō-sī'tĭs) [G. *polys*, many, + L. *serum*, whey, + *-ītis*, inflammation]. General progressive inflammation of all the serous membranes.

polysinuitis, polysinusitis (pŏl″ĭ-sĭn-ū-ī'tĭs, -sī″nŭs-ī'tĭs) [" + L. *sinus*, a hollow, + G. *-ītis*, inflammation]. Inflammation of several sinuses simultaneously.

polyspermia, polyspermism (pŏl″ĭ-sper′mĭ-ă, -mĭzm) [" + *sperma*, seed]. 1. Excessive secretion of seminal fluid. 2. Entrance of several spermatozoa into 1 ovum.

polystichia (pŏl-ĭ-stĭk'ĭ-ă) [" + *stichos*, a row]. Condition in which there are more than 2 rows of eyelashes.

polysyphilide (pŏl″ĭ-sĭf'ĭl-ĭd) [" + *syn*, with, + *philos*, love]. Having numerous syphilitic lesions.

polythelia, polythelism (pŏl-ĭ-thē'lĭ-ă, -lĭzm) [" + *thēlē*, nipple, + *-ismos*, condition]. Presence of more than 1 nipple on a mamma.

polytocous (pŏl-ĭt'ō-kŭs) [" + *tokos*, birth]. Producing several offspring at 1 time.

polytrichia, polytrichosis (pŏl-ĭ-trĭk'ĭ-ă, -ō'sĭs) [G. *polys*, many, + *thrix*, *trich-*, hair, + *-ōsis*, intensive]. Excessive growth of hair. SYN: *hypertrichiasis*.

polytrophia, polytrophy (pŏl-ĭ-trō'fĭ-ă, -ĭt'-rō-fĭ) [" + *trophē*, nourishment]. Excessive or abundant nutrition.

polyuria (pŏl-ĭ-ū'rĭ-ă) [" + *ouron*, urine]. Excessive secretion and discharge of urine.

The urine does not, as a rule, contain abnormal constituents. Several hundred ounces a day may be voided. It is pale in color. Sp. gr. 1.000 to 1.002 and higher in diabetes.

ETIOL: Seen in diabetes insipidus, convalescence of typhoid fever, hysteria, nervous persons, renal congestion, and when taking large quantities of liquid.

polyvalent (pŏl-ĭ-vă'lĕnt, pō-lĭv'a-lent) [" + L. *valēre*, to be strong]. 1. Multivalent; having a combining power of more than 2 atoms of hydrogen.

p. serum. One with antibodies produced by injecting several strains of microörganisms of the same species or by injecting different species.

p. vaccine. One produced from cultures of a number of strains of the same species.

pomade (po'măd) [Fr., from L. *pomum*, apple]. A perfumed ointment, esp. 1 for the hair. SYN: *pomatum*.

pomatum (pō-mā'tŭm) [L. *pomum*, apple]. A perfumed unguent, esp. 1 used on the hair. SYN: *pomade*.

pompholyx (pŏm′fō-lĭks) [G. *pompholyx*, bubble]. Acute inflammatory affection characterized by bullae limited to hands and feet.

ETIOL: Not known. Occurs in 2nd to 4th decade, in coffee and tobacco users, and in those with lowered vitality.

SYM: Symmetrical eruptions of crops of deeply seated vesicles and bullae with itching, hyperemia, lasting 4-6 weeks. Secondary infection may occur.

TREATMENT: Hygienic regimen, mercurial purge followed by saline, alkaline diuretics, tonics. Locally, soothing stringents. SYN: *chiropompholyx*.

pomphus (pŏm'fŭs) (pl. *pomphi*) [G. *pomphos*, a blister]. A blister or a circumscribed elevation on the skin; a wheal.

pomum (pō'mŭm) [L.]. An apple.

p. Adami. Prominence in middle line of throat, caused by junction of 2 lateral wings of the thyroid cartilage.

p. oculi. The pupil.

ponogen (pŏn'ō-jĕn) [G. *ponos*, pain, + *gennan*, to produce]. Any waste matter of tissues derived from the nervous system. SYN: *fatigue poison*.

ponograph (pŏn'ō-grăf) [" + *graphein*, to write]. Device for measuring and registering sensitiveness to pain or fatigue.

ponopalmosis (pŏn″ō-păl-mō'sĭs) [" +

palmos, palpitation, + *-ōsis,* intensive]. Palpitation of the heart produced by slight exertion. SYN: *neurocirculatory asthenia.*

ponophobia (pŏn-ō-fō'bĭ-ă) [" + *phobos,* fear]. 1. Abnormal distaste for exerting one's self. 2. Dread of pain.

pons (pl. *pontes*) [L. bridge]. 1. A process of tissue connecting 2 or more parts. 2. Pons Varolii, *q.v.*

  p. **hepatis.** Part of liver extending sometimes from quadrate lobe to left lobe across the umbilical fissure.

  p. **Varolii.** The eminence caused by a convex mass of white nerve tissue connecting cerebrum, medulla oblongata and cerebellum.

  Named for Costanzo Varolio, anatomist of Bologna, 1544-75.

  RS: *cerebellopontile, cerebellopontine, cerebropontile.*

pontic (pŏn'tĭk) [L. *pons, pont-,* bridge]. 1. An artificial tooth set in a bridge. 2. Concerning the pons.

ponticular (pŏn-tĭk'ū-lar) [L. *pons, pont-,* bridge]. Relating to the ponticulus or ridge bet. the pyramids of the pons and oblongata.

ponticulus (pŏn-tĭk'ū-lŭs) [L. a little bridge]. The transverse ridge bet. the pyramids of the pons and oblongata. SYN: *propons.*

pontile, pontine (pŏn'tīl, -tēn) [L. *pons, pont-,* bridge]. Pert. to the pons Varolii.

  p. **hemiplegia.** One due to lesion of the pons. The arm and leg on 1 side and face on the other are affected.

  p. **nuclei.** The gray matter in the pons.

pontocaine hydrochlo'ride (pŏn'tō-kān). A white crystalline powder, the base of which belongs to the procaine type.

  USES: As a local anesthetic, useful for surface anesthesia in the eye, ear, nose and throat.

  DOSAGE: ½% strength recommended for the eye, 2% for nose and throat.

popliteal (pŏp-lĭt-ē'ăl, -lĭt-ē'ăl) [L. *poples, poplit-,* the ham]. Concerning the post. surface of the knee.

popliteus (pŏp-lĭt'ē-ŭs, -lĭt-ē'ŭs). Muscle located in hind part of the knee joint which flexes the leg and aids it in rotating. SEE: *Table of Muscles in Appendix.*

poradenitis (pŏr-ăd-ē-nī'tĭs) [G. *pōros,* pore, + *adēn,* gland, + *-itis,* inflammation]. Formation of small abscesses in the iliac glands.

porcellaneous, porcellanous (pŏr-sĕ-lā'nē-ŭs, -sel'ăn-ŭs) [Italian *porcellana,* the porcelain shell]. Translucent or white like porcelain, as the skin.

porcupine disease (por'kŭ-pīn) [L. *porcus,* swine]. A chronic skin disease with scaly epidermal plates. SYN: *ichthyosis.*

pore (pōr) [G. *póros,* a pore]. A small orifice in membrane or tissue, the mouth of a duct, for absorption or excretion; as orifices of sweat glands of skin.

  Pores open on the surface of the skin, and are controlled by papillary muscles, contracting in cold and dilating in heat.

  RS: *absorb, absorption, skin, stoma.*

porencephalia, porencephalus (pōr-ĕn-sĕf-ā'lĭ-ă, -sĕf'ă-lŭs) [" + *egkephalos,* brain]. Condition in which cavities exist in substance of the cerebrum, communicating usually with ventricles.

porencephalitis (pōr-ĕn-sĕf-ăl-ī'tĭs) [" + " + *-itis,* inflammation]. Inflammation of the brain with development of depressions on its surface.

porencephalous (por-ĕn-sĕf'ăl-ŭs) [" + *egkephalos,* brain]. Affected with depressions on the brain surface.

pork (pōrk) [L. *porcus,* swine]. COMP: NUTRIENTS: Nutritive value greater than that of beef. Av. SERVING: 230 Gm.

	Prot.	Fat
1. Chops, E. P.	38.2	69.2
2. Ribs, E. P.	17.3	31.1
3. Sausage, A. P.	13.0	44.2
4. Side, E. P.	9.1	55.3
5. Tenderloin, A. P.	18.9	13.0

	Carbo.	Fuel Value	Cal.
1.		100 Gm. =	333
2.		100 Gm. =	345
3.	1.1	100 Gm. =	769
4.		100 Gm. =	454
5.		100 Gm. =	526

ASH CONST: Ca 0.006, Mg 0.012, K 0.169, Na 0.042, P 0.108, Cl 0.038, S 0.115, Fe 0.0015.

VITAMINS: A— to +, B++, G++.

pornography (pōr-nŏg'ră-fī) [G. *pornē,* prostitute, + *graphein,* to write]. 1. Obscene writing or painting. 2. Description of prostitutes or prostitution.

porocele (pō'rō-sēl) [G. *pōros,* callus, + *kēlē,* hernia]. Scrotal hernia with indurated and thickened coverings.

porocephaliasis, porocephalosis (pō"rō-sĕf-ăl-ī'ă-sĭs, -ō'sĭs) [G. *pōros,* pore, + *kephalē,* head]. Infection with a species of Porocephalus.

Porocephalus (pō"rō-sĕf'ă-lŭs) [" + *kephalē,* head]. A genus of parasites for their larvae which infest animals and man.

porokeratosis (pō"rō-kĕr-ăt-ō'sĭs) [G. *pōros,* callus, + *keras,* a horn, + *-ōsis,* disease]. Skin disease marked by thickening of stratum corneum in linear arrangement, followed by its atrophy.

  It appears on smooth areas. It is irregular in form and size, with circumscribed outline and affects hands and feet, forearms and legs, the face, neck and scalp.

poroma (pō-rō'mă) [" + *-ōma,* tumor]. Inflammatory hardening or callosity.

porosis (pō-rō'sĭs) [" + *-ōsis,* disease]. 1. A callus formed about the ends of a fractured bone. 2. A thickened induration. 3. A condition marked by pore formation.

porosity (pō-rŏs'ĭ-tĭ) [G. *pōros,* pore]. 1. The state of being porous. 2. Pore.

porotomy (pō-rŏt'ō-mĭ) [" + *tomē,* a cutting]. Incision of urethral meatus to enlarge it.

porous (pō'rŭs) [G. *pōros,* a pore]. Full of pores; able to admit passage of a liquid.

porphyria (por-fī'rĭ-ă) [G. *porphyra,* purple]. Porphyrin in the blood.

porphyrin (por'fī-rĭn) [G. *porphyra,* purple]. One of a group forming basis of animal and plant respiratory pigments, obtained from hemoglobin and chlorophyll.

porphyrinuria (por"fī-rĭn-ū'rĭ-ă) [" + *ouron,* urine]. The excretion of porphyrin in the urine.

porphyrization (por"fĭr-ĭ-zā'shŭn) [G. *porphyra,* purple]. Process of pulverizing.

porphyruria (por-fĭr-ū'rĭ-ă) [" + *ouron,* urine]. Excretion of porphyrin in urine.

porrigo (pō-rī'gō) [L. dandruff]. Any disease of scalp involving scaling or loss of hair.

  p. **decalvans.** Baldness in patches. SYN: *alopecia areata.*

  p. **favosa.** Tiny, contiguous ulcer and crust formation. SYN: *favus.**

  p. **furfurans.** Ringworm of the scalp. SYN: *tinea* tonsurans.*

p. larvalis. Eczema of the scalp with impetigo.

Porro's operation (por'ōz). Removal of a pregnant uterus, the ovaries and tubes through an incision in the abdominal wall.

porta (por'tăh) [L. gate]. 1. The point of entry of nerves and vessels into an organ or part. 2. Passage bet. the 3rd and lateral ventricles of the brain. SEE: *hilum*.
   p. hepatis. The fissure of the liver where the portal vein enters.
   p. lienis. Hilus of the spleen where vessels enter.
   p. pulmonis. Pulmonary hilus for entry and exit of the bronchi, nerves, and vessels.
   p. renis. Hilus of the kidney for entry of the vessels.

portal (por'tăl) [L. *porta*, a gate]. Concerning a porta or entrance to an organ, esp. that through which the blood is carried to liver.
   p. circulation. That of blood brought by the portal vein into the liver and out by the hepatic vein.
   p. system. Branches of portal vein by which blood is taken up from abdominal viscera and carried through portal capillaries of liver, finally entering inf. vena cava.
   p. vein. One formed by the veins of the splanchnic area conveying its blood into the liver.
   It is made of the combined sup. and inf. mesenteric, splenic, gastric, and cystic veins.

port-caustic (pōrt'kaws'tĭk) [Fr.]. Contrivance for handling a caustic.

porte-, port- (pōrt) [Fr. *porter*, to carry, from L. *portāre*, to carry]. To carry.

porte-caustic (pōrt″kŏs-tēk′) [Fr. *porter*, to carry, + *caustique*, caustic]. Device for handling a caustic.

porte-fillet (pōrt″fĭl′ĕt) [" + *fillet*, a thread]. Appliance for passing a cord around a fetus, employed in breech presentation.

portenoeud (pōrt-ned′) [" + *noeud*, a knot]. Instrument for applying a ligature around an artery or the pedicle of a tumor.

portio (pŏr′shĭ-ō) [L. a part]. A part.
   p. dura. The 7th cranial or facial nerve.
   p. intermedia. A small nerve bet. the facial and acoustic nerves, the sensory root of the facial n. SYN: *pars intermedia of Wrisberg*.
   p. major. BNA. The larger sensory part of the trigeminal nerve.
   p. minor. BNA. The smaller motor part of the trigeminal nerve.
   p. mollis. The 8th cranial or acoustic nerve.
   p. vaginalis. The part of the cervix within the vagina.

port-wine mark or **stain.** A purplish-red, superficial birthmark. SYN: *nevus.**

porus (pō′rūs) [L., from G. *poros*, a passage]. A meatus or foramen; a tiny aperture in a structure; a pore.
   p. acusticus externus. Ext. acoustic or auditory meatus.
   p. acusticus internus. Int. acoustic or auditory foramen.
   p. opticus. Aperture containing the optic disk, the point where the optic nerve pierces the sclera.

posiomania (pŏs″ĭ-ō-mā′nĭ-ă) [G. *posis*, a drink, + *mania*, madness]. Addiction to alcoholic drinks. SYN: *dipsomania*.

position (pō-zĭsh′ŭn) [L. *positiō*, a placing, from *ponere*, to place]. 1. Place in which a thing is put. 2. Manner in which a body is arranged, as by the nurse or physician for examination. 3. OB: The relation of some arbitrarily chosen portion of the child in the pelvis to the right or left side of the mother, the occiput, chin, and sacrum being the points used. SEE: *posture*.
   p., dorsal. P. in which patient is on his back.
   p., d. elevated. On back, head and shoulders elevated at angle of 30° or more. Employed in digital examination of genitalia and in bimanual examination.
   p., d. recumbent. On back, extremities moderately flexed and rotated outward. Employed in application of obstetrical forceps, repair of lesions following parturition, vaginal examination, bimanual palpation. SEE: *dorsal recumbent p. for illustration*.
   p., dorsosacral. Same as *lithotomy p.*
   p., Edebohl's. Same as *Simon's p.*
   p., Elliott's. P. in which supports are placed under small of back so that patient resembles a double inclined plane.
   p., English. SEE: *left lateral recumbent p.*
   p., erect. Occiput and heels on line, also nose, groins, and great toes in same vertical plane. Employed in practice of ballottement, differentiation of tumors, cystic and solid hernia.
   p., Fowler's. Position when the head of the patient's bed is raised above the level about 1½ ft. SEE: *Fowler's p. for illustration*.
   p., genucubital. Patient on knees, thighs upright, body resting on elbows, head down on hands. Employed when not possible to use the classic knee-chest position.
   p., genupectoral. Patient on knees, thighs upright, head and upper part of chest resting on table, arms crossed above head. Employed in displacement of prolapsed fundus, dislodgment of impacted head, management of transverse presentation, replacement of retroverted uterus or displaced ovary, flushing of intestinal canal.
   p., horizontal. Lying supine, feet extended. Employed in palpation, in auscultation of fetal heart and in operative procedures. SEE: *horizontal p. for illustration*.
   p., h. abdominal. Patient flat on abdomen, feet extended. Employed in examination of back and spinal column.
   p., jackknife. Patient on back, shoulders elevated, legs flexed on thighs, thighs at right angles to abdomen. Employed when passing urethral sound.
   p., knee-chest. SYN: *genupectoral p.* SEE: *knee-chest p. for illustration*.
   p., knee-elbow. SEE: *genucubital p.*
   p., kneeling-squatting. Patient stooping, knees pressed on abdomen, trunk erect. Employed in childbirth in difficult cases and in uncivilized nations.
   p., lateroprone. Same as *Sims' p.*
   p., laterosemiprone. Same as *Sims' p.*
   p., left lateral recumbent. Patient on left side, right knee and thigh drawn up. Employed in childbirth.
   p., lithotomy. Patient on back, thighs flexed on abdomen, legs on thighs, thighs abducted. Employed in operation on genital tract, in vaginal hysterectomy, diagnosis and treatment of diseases of urethra and bladder.

position, obstetrical

p., obstetrical. SEE: *left lateral recumbent p.*

p., prone. P. in which patient is lying face downward.

p., reclining. SEE: *jackknife p.*

p., side, semiprone. Same as *Sims' p.*

p., Simon's. Exaggerated lithotomy position. Patient flat on back, legs flexed on thighs, thighs on abdomen, hips somewhat elevated, thighs strongly abducted. Employed in operations on vagina.

p., Sims'. Patient on left side, right knee and thigh drawn well up above left, left arm back of patient and hanging over edge of table, chest inclined forward so that patient rests upon it. Employed in curettement of uterus, intrauterine irrigation after labor, tamponade of vagina, rectal exploration, operations on cervix. SEE: *Sims' position for illustration.*

p., Trendelenburg. Dorsal position, body elevated at angle of about 45°, feet and legs hanging over end of table, head down. Employed in abdominal surgery to favor gravitation upward of abdominal viscera.

p., Walcher. The patient with hips on the edge of the table and the lower extremities hanging down.

position, words pert. to: aboral, acathisia, accubation, adduct, adduction, adductor, adoral, anaclisis, anteflexion, antelocation, anteposition, anterior, "antero-" words, anteversion, anticheirotonus, anticlinal, anticus, apex, aspect, atropic, attitude, dorsal, dorsosacral, Edebohl's, emprosthotonos, erect, Fowler's, genupectoral, horizontal, in situ, jackknife, jactitation, kneeling squatting, lateroprone, left lateral recumbent, lithotomy, opisthotonos, orthotonos, posture, pronation, prone, recumbent, sedentary, side, Simon's, Sims', supination, supine, Trendelenburg's, vertical, Walcher's.

positive (pŏz'ĭt-ĭv) [L. *positivus*, ruling]. 1. Definite; affirmative; opposed to negative. 2. Indicating the reaction in laboratory work. 3. Indicating an abnormal condition in examination and diagnosis. 4. Indicates pathological change in postmortem examination. 5. Noting a quantity greater than zero.
Indicated by the plus (+) sign.

p. pole. The electrode of a battery which is connected with the negative plate. SEE: *anode.*

posological (pŏs"ō-lŏj'ĭ-kăl) [G. *posos*, how much, + *logos*, a study]. Concerning dosage.

posology (pō-sŏl'ō-jĭ) [" + *logos*, a study]. Branch of scientific study dealing with dosage.

possession (pō-zĕsh'ŭn) [L. *possessio*, a sitting before]. State of being dominated by an idea, a passion or a mental obsession.

p., demoniacal. Belief of being under the influence of an evil spirit or demon.

post- [L.]. A prefix meaning *behind* or *after.*

postabortal (pŏst"ăb-or'tăl) [L. *post*, after, + *abortius*, abortion]. Happening subsequent to abortion.

postaxial (pŏst-ăks'ĭ-ăl) [" + G. *axōn*, axis]. Situated or happening behind an axis.

postcava (pŏst-kā'vă) [" + *cavus*, a hollow]. The ascending or inf. vena cava.

postcaval (pŏst-kā'văl) [" + *cavus*, hollow]. Concerning the postcava.

postcentral (pŏst-sĕn'trăl) [" + G. *kentron*, center]. 1. Situated or happening

P-86

postgeniculatum, postgeniculum

behind a center. 2. Located behind the fissure of Rolando.

postcibal (pŏst-sī'băl) [" + *cibum*, food]. Occurring after meals.

postclavicular (pŏst"klă-vĭk'ū-lăr) [" + *clavicula*, a little key]. Located or occurring behind the clavicle.

postclimacteric (pŏst-klī"mă-k-tĕr'ĭk, -mak'tĕr-ĭk) [L. *post*, after, + G. *klimaktēr*, round of a ladder]. Occurring after the menopause.

postcoital (pŏst-kō'ĭt-ăl) [" + *coitiō*, a coming together]. Subsequent to sexual intercourse.

postcommissure (pŏst-kŏm'ĭs-ūr) [" + *commissura*, a joining together]. The post. commissure of the brain.

postconnubial (pŏst-kŏn-ū'bĭ-ăl) [" + *connubium*, marriage]. Occurring after marriage.

postconvulsive (pŏst-kŏn-vŭl'sĭv) [" + *convulsiō*, a pulling together]. Occurring after a convulsion.

postcornu (pŏst-kor'nū) [" + *cornū*, a horn]. The post. horn of the lateral ventricle of the brain.

postdiastolic (pŏst-dī-ăs-tŏl'ĭk) [" + *diastolē*, a sending apart]. Occurring after the cardiac diastole.

postdicrotic (pŏst-dī-krŏt'ĭk) [L. *post*, after, + G. *dikrotos*, beating double]. Occurring after the dicrotic pulse wave.

p. wave. A recoil or second wave (not always present) in a sphygmographic tracing.

postencephalitis (pŏst"ĕn-sĕf-ăl-ī'tĭs) [" + *egkephalos*, brain, + *-itis*, inflammation]. The condition sometimes remaining after convalescence from epidemic encephalitis.

postepileptic (pŏst"ĕp-ĭ-lĕp'tĭk) [" + G. *epi*, upon, + *lēpsis*, a seizure]. Following an epileptic seizure.

posterior (pŏs-tē'rĭ-or) [L. after]. 1. Toward the dorsal or back aspect; opposed to anterior. 2. Situated behind; coming after. [*situated back.*

postero- [L.]. Prefix meaning *hinder,*

posteroexternal (pŏs"tĕr-ō-ĕks-tŭr'năl) [L. *posterus*, behind, + *externus*, outer]. On the outer side of a back aspect, as the p. column of the spinal cord.

posterointernal (pŏs"tĕr-ō-ĭn-tŭr'năl) [" + *internus*, inner]. On the inner side of a back part.

posterolateral (pŏs"tĕr-ō-lăt'ĕr-ăl) [" + *latus*, *later-*, a side]. Located behind and at the side of a part.

posteromedian (pŏs-tĕr-ō-mē'dĭ-ăn) [" + *medius*, middle]. Located at the middle of a posterior aspect.

posterosuperior (pŏs-tĕr-ō-sū-pē'rĭ-or) [" + *superior*, upper]. Located behind and above a part.

posterula (pŏs-tĕr'oo-lă) [L. *posterus*, after]. Portion of nasopharynx bet. the salpingopalatal fold and the post. nares, a small space between the turbinal bones and the posterior nares.

postesophageal (pŏst"ē-sō-făj'ē-ăl) [L. *post*, after, + G. *oisophagos*, gullet]. Located behind the esophagus.

postethmoid (pŏst-ĕth'moyd) [" + G. *ethmos*, sieve, + *eidos*, form]. Located behind the ethmoid bone.

postfebrile (pŏst-fē'brĭl) [" + *febris*, fever]. Occurring after a fever.

postgeminum (pŏst-jĕm'ĭn-ŭm) [" + *geminus*, twin]. The post. pair of corpora quadrigemina.

postgeniculatum, postgeniculum (pŏst"jē-nĭk-ū-lā'tŭm, -nĭk'ū-lŭm) [" + *geniculum*, a little knee]. The inner elevation on optic thalamus, the internal geniculate body of the brain.

posthetomy (pŏs-thĕt′ō-mĭ) [G. *posthē*, prepuce, + *tomē*, a cutting]. Surgical removal of all or part of the foreskin. SYN: *circumcision*.

posthioplasty (pŏs′thĭ-ō-plas″tĭ) [" + *plastos*, formed]. Plastic surgery of the prepuce or foreskin.

posthitis (pŏs-thī′tĭs) [" + *-itis*, inflammation]. Inflamed condition of the foreskin.

posthumous (pŏs′tū-mŭs) [L. *postumus*, last]. Born after the father's death.
Sometimes refers to a child taken from dead body of mother.

posthypnotic (pŏst″hĭp-nŏt′ĭk) [L. *post*, after, + G. *ypnos*, sleep]. Occurring or performed subsequent to the hypnotic state.
   p. suggestion. One offered during the hypnotic state influencing a later action when individual returns to normal state.

posticus (pŏs-tī′kŭs) [L.]. Posterior.

postmedian (pŏst″mē′dĭ-ăn) [L. *post*, after, + *medius*, middle]. Behind the middle transverse line of the body.

post-mortem (pŏst-mor′tĕm) [L.]. After death.
   p. examination. Dissection of a dead body to ascertain cause of death and the changes wrought by disease. SYN: *autopsy*.

postnatal (pŏst-nā′tăl) [L. *post*, after, + *natus*, birth]. Happening after birth.

postoblongata (pōst-ŏb-long-gah′tă) [" + *ob*, toward, + *longus*, long]. Caudal portion of the oblongata below the pons.

postocular (pōst-ŏk′ū-lar) [" + *oculus*, eye]. Behind the eye.
   p. neuritis. Inflammation of the optic nerve behind the eyeball.

postolivary (pōst-ŏl′ĭv-a-rĭ) [" + *oliva*, olive]. Behind the olivary body; back of the ant. pyramid of the medulla.

postoperative (pōst-ŏp′ĕr-ā-tĭv) [" + *operatus*, from *operāri*, to work]. After or following a surgical operation.
   POSTOPERATIVE CARE: 1. When you are called to the operating room to get a patient, take a towel and emesis basin with you. 2. See that ether bed is ready and furniture moved so stretcher can be gotten close to it. 3. Be careful when handling unconscious patient. Remember that it will be a difficult task because he is a dead weight and not able to help himself. Get assistance. 4. See that there are no drafts, but plenty of fresh air. Do not let direct light shine on patient's face. 5. When he vomits keep head turned to one side so vomitus will not be swallowed or inhaled. 6. Change gown when wet or soiled, rubbing patient dry with bath towel under the bedclothes. 7. Watch him carefully when consciousness begins to return, for it is at this time he becomes restless. 8. Note pulse, respiration and other symptoms at intervals as required by the routine of your hospital.

postoperculum (pōst-ō-per′kū-lŭm) [" + *operculum*, a cover]. The fold covering the insula that is formed of part of the supertemporal gyrus. SYN: *operculum temporal*.

postoral (pōst-ō′răl) [" + *os, or-*, mouth]. Behind or in the posterior part of the mouth.

postpallium (pōst-păl′ĭ-ŭm) [L. *post*, after, + *pallium*, cloak]. That part of the cerebral cortex behind the fissure of Rolando.

postpaludal (post-pal′ū-dăl) [" + *palus, palud-*, swamp]. After a malarial attack.

postparalytic (pōst-par-ă-lĭt′ĭk) [" + *para*, beside, + *lyein*, to loosen]. Subsequent to an attack of paralysis.

postpartum (pōst-par′tŭm) [L. *post*, after, + *partus*, birth]. After parturition.
   p. hemorrhage. Hemorrhage which occurs after childbirth.
   NP: If hemorrhage occurs, regardless of the use of safe and preventive measures, drastic ones for its control must be employed.
   Extra hypodermics of oxytocic drugs may be used. An icebag placed on fundus is used as early routine postpartum measure by some physicians. Massage of uterus with a piece of ice on the abdomen is frequently used when bleeding persists. Packing the lower segment of uterus and vagina is an excellent method of controlling hemorrhage. The large tubular packer is preferred here to a dressing forceps to avoid contamination of the packing by contact with the vulva and vaginal tract. Packing the vagina may be done by the nurse, if absolutely necessary, when a physician is not available. A hot intrauterine douche may be used by the doctor in place of the packing. The temperature of the solution should always be 120° F. This is sufficiently hot to stimulate the uterus to contract. Cooler douches simply wash out the clots, causing more bleeding, and fail to stimulate contractions.
   If the above procedures fail to halt the hemorrhage, the physician may insert 1 hand into the fundus and at the same time massage the uterus with the other hand on the abdomen. A sterile pair of long gloves should be ready in this case. Keep the patient warm during this time. Elevate the lower extremities as soon as possible. Oxytocic drugs may be ordered intravenously by some physicians. Note the pulse and general condition frequently. Stimulants are given as necessary.
   Blood transfusions are generally given to maintain and increase the patient's resistance. Massage the uterus. The fingertips may be kept lightly on the fundus to discover any relaxation. Give massage only when relaxation occurs. Hypodermoclysis and intravenous injections are used if patient is unable to take and retain fluids. Force fluids as soon as patient's condition warrants, but do not take a chance on making the patient vomit, as retching may start another hemorrhage.
   When tolerated, the patient may be given a limited number of mouth preparations of ergot, preferably the ones that are not nauseating. These keep the uterus contracted and lessen the chance of infection to which the patient has been predisposed by the loss of blood, lowered resistance, and much manipulation. Perfect asepsis must be maintained at all times. Remember that since this patient is predisposed to sepsis, her general resistance must be built up and maintained by plenty of fluids, nourishing foods and, above all, rest.

postpontile (pōst-pŏn′tĭl) [L. *post*, after, + *pons, pont-*, bridge]. Situated behind the pons Varolii.
   p. recess. The foramen caecum.

postpyramid (post-pir′am-id) [L. *post*, after, + G. *pyramis*, pyramid]. 1. The posterior pyramid of the cerebellum. 2. The gracile funicle.

postpyramidal (post-pĭ-răm′ĭd-al). Referring to a postpyramid.

p. nucleus. Mass of gray matter in post. column of the medulla. SYN: *nucleus funiculi gracilis.*
postural (pos′tū-răl) [L. *postura*, position]. Pert. to or effected by posture.
p. drainage. Drainage of secretions from the bronchi or a cavity in the lung by placing the patient's head lower than the area to be drained.
Used in bronchiectasis and before operation for lobectomy.* The position aggravates coughing, resulting in expectoration of much sputum, 5-10 oz. in bad cases. 5-10 minutes morning and evening is recommended. High protein diet to replace protein lost.

port. Seen in spasmodic asthma, emphysema, dyspnea, abdominal dropsy, effusions into the pleural and pericardial cavities, and in late stages of diseases of the heart.
p., orthotonos. Neck and trunk extended rigidly in straight line, in tetanus, strychnine poisoning, rabies or meningitis.
p., pleurothotonos. Lateral position with body arched in acute pleural involvement or spinal affection.
p., prone. Posture assumed after abdominal colic or because of tuberculosis of spine, eroded vertebrae, abdominal pain or gastric ulcer.

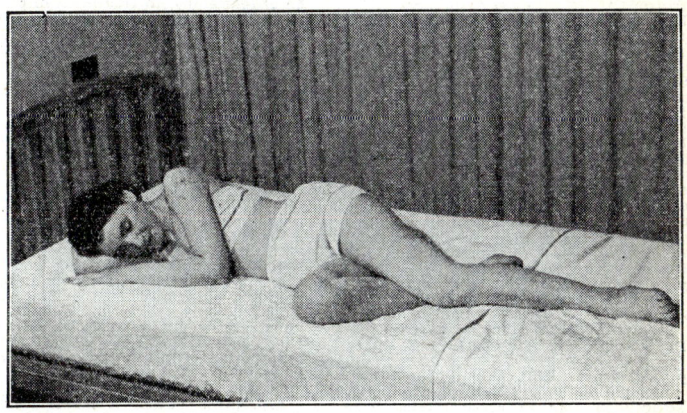

Posed by professional model   *Photo by Whitaker*
UNILATERAL POSTURE FOR COMFORT.

posture (pŏs′tūr) [L. *postura*, position]. 1. The adaptation of the body to the laws of gravity. SYN: *body mechanics.* 2. Attitude or position of the body.
p., coiled. Body on 1 side with legs drawn up to meet the trunk. Noted in cerebral diseases, hepatic, intestinal or renal colic.
p., dorsal inertia. Patient on back, with tendency to slip down in bed or to either side. Seen in great weakness, in acute infectious diseases such as typhoid, in mental apathy or muscular weakness.
p., dorsal, rigid. P. on back with both legs drawn up. Seen in peritonitis, meningitis, ascites, tympanites. In appendicitis the right leg is drawn up. Also occurs in pelvic inflammation or peritonitis of right side, renal calculus in right ureter, and in psoas abscess.
p., emprosthotonos. The body is incurved and rests upon the forehead and feet with face downward. It is rarely seen in tetanus and strychnia poisoning.
p., opisthotonos. An uncommon dorsal position in which the body rests upon the head and heels, with the trunk arched upward. It is seen in strychnia poisoning, tetanus, hysteria, epilepsy, the convulsions of rabies, and to a slight extent in meningitis. In the latter case, the neck is rigid and the head retracted, seeming to press into the pillow. SEE: *opisthotonos.*
p., orthopnea. Patient sitting upright, hands or elbows resting upon some sup-

p., semireclining. Used in diseases of heart and interference with respiration in asthma and pleural effusions.
p., unilateral. Patient on right side in acute pleurisy, lobar pneumonia of right side and in a greatly enlarged liver, or left side in lobar pneumonia, or pleurisy on that side, and in large pericardial effusions.
postuterine (pōst-ū′tĕr-ĭn) [L. *post*, after, + *uterus*, womb]. Situated behind the uterus.
postvermis (pōst-vĕr′mĭs) [" + *vermis*, worm]. The inferior vermiform process of the cerebellum.
potable (pō′tȧ-bl) [L. *potabilis*, from *potāre*, to drink]. Suitable for drinking.
Potain's apparatus (po-tan′). A form of aspirator.
P.'s disease. Pleural and pulmonary edema.
P.'s sign. Dullness on percussion of the aorta in dilatation, extending from the *manubrium sterni* toward the third costal cartilage on the right, the base of the sternum in segment of a circle to the right marking the upper limit.
potamophobia (pŏt″ȧm-ō-fō′bĭ-ȧ) [G. *potamos*, river, + *phobos*, fear]. A morbid fear of large bodies of water.
potash (pŏt′ȧsh). SEE: *potassium carbonate* or *potassium hydroxide, q.v.*
potassa sulfurata (pō-tăs′ȧ sŭl-fū-rā′ta). USP. (Liver of sulfur.) Greenish yellow pieces containing 12.8% sulfur in the combination as a sulfide. [diseases.
USES: Externally, in parasitic skin

DOSAGE: For application in 5% solution.
INCOMPATIBILITIES: Acids, alcohol, acid salts.

potassemia (pō-tăs-sē'mĭ-ă) [L. *potassa*, + G. *aima*, blood]. Presence of excessive quantity of potassium in the blood.

potassic (pō-tăs'ĭk) [L. *potassa*, potash]. Composed of or containing potash.

potassium (pō-tăs'ĭ-ŭm) [L. *potassa*, potash]. SYMB: K. At. wt. 39.10. Sp. gr. 0.865. An alkaline mineral element found in combination with other elements in the body.

FUNCTIONS: Salts of magnesium and potassium maintain osmotic pressure and the ion balance. Potassium has a buffer action and is necessary to normal growth.

DEFICIENCY: SYM: Disorders of the nervous system, loss of weight, poor digestion, irregular heart action, and poor muscular control.

SOURCES: Found in most foods. *Ex*: Bran, beans, olives, molasses, spinach, raisins, parsnips, potatoes. *Good*: Apricots, asparagus, bananas, beets, beef, cabbage, cantaloupe, carrots, cherries, celery, coconut, chocolate, turnips, dates, figs, grapes, nuts, lettuce, milk, peaches, peas, pineapples, prunes, squash, tomatoes. SYN: *kalium*.

p. acetate. USP. A white powder or crystalline flakes.
ACTION AND USES: Alkaline diuretic.
DOSAGE: 15 gr. (1 Gm.).

p. bicarbonate. USP. White crystals or powder.
ACTION AND USES: To neutralize acid of stomach and lessen acidity of urine.
DOSAGE: 15 gr. (1 Gm.). SEE: p. chromate.

p. bitartrate. USP. Cream of tartar. A white powder or crystalline salt.
ACTION AND USES: Diuretic, cathartic and refrigerant.
DOSAGE: 30 gr. (2 Gm.).

p. bromide. USP. White cubical crystals of powder.
ACTION AND USES: Nerve sedative.
DOSAGE: 15 gr. (1 Gm.).

p. chlorate. USP. An explosive, white crystalline salt, used in diseases of mouth and throat.
In large doses causes destruction of red blood corpuscles. Used in manufacture of fireworks, explosives, flashlight powder, toothpastes, mouthwashes, etc.
DOSAGE: Tablet, 5 gr. (0.3 Gm.).
POISONING: SYM: Large doses cause abdominal discomfort, vomiting, diarrhea, hematuria with nephritis and disturbances of the blood.
F. A. TREATMENT: Stomach should be washed out. Otherwise treatment must be symptomatic.

p. chromate. Used as dye, furniture stain, in manufacture of batteries, in photography and in medicine for cauterization.
SYM: May be inhaled or contact the nose from fingers, causing deep, indolent ulcers. When taken by mouth has a disagreeable taste, causes cramping, pain, vomiting, diarrhea, slow respiration; may affect liver and kidneys.
F. A. TREATMENT: Treat as an acid, dilute and give weak alkalies as chalk, baking soda, magnesia, etc., followed by soothing mucilaginous drinks. Treat symptomatically.

p. citrate. USP. Transparent prismatic crystals. [sium acetate.
ACTION AND USES: Similar to potas-
DOSAGE: 15 gr. (1 Gm.). [benzoate.
INCOMPATIBILITIES: Caffeine sodium

p. cyanide. SEE: *cyanide*.
p. hydroxide. Grayish-white compound used in various shops, and in preparation of soap.
POISONING: SYM: Nausea; soapy taste; burning pain in mouth which causes bloody, slimy vomitus; abdominal cramping; bloody purging and prostration.
TREATMENT: Dilute with weak, acidulated water such as vinegar, lemon juice, orange juice, grape juice. Household oils likewise reduce the free alkali, but more slowly. Follow with olive oil, sweet melted butter or lard.

p. iodide. USP. Colorless or white crystals having a faint odor of iodine.
ACTION AND USES: To increase bronchial secretions; in treatment of certain metallic poisons, and syphilis.
DOSAGE: 5 gr. (0.3 Gm.).

p. permanganate. USP. Dark purple prisms, odorless, with sweet taste.
ACTION AND USES: Deodorant, germicide and astringent. Internally, an antidote in phosphorous poisoning and snake bite. Used for disinfectant and deodorant action as an application in gangrenous ulcers, cancerous sores, diphtheria and gonorrhea. In diluted solutions it may be used as a gargle or mouthwash (¼%), to disinfect the hands (1%), and for other purposes.
Concentrated solutions irritate and even corrode the skin, and when swallowed induce gastroenteritis. The solutions have considerable power as disinfectants, owing to their oxidizing power which destroys bacteria. They fail to penetrate deeply in an active form and this renders them of less value than many other disinfectants, except for use in very superficial infections.
DOSAGE: 1 gr. (0.06 Gm.).

p. sulfate. USP. A laxative and a purgative, but because of its irritant qualities not to be recommended.
DOSAGE: 15 gr. (1 Gm.).

p. sulfite. $K_2SO_3 + H_2O$. A white, crystalline antiseptic salt.
USES: To check fermentation, both internally and externally.
DOSAGE: 3-10 gr. (0.2-0.666 Gm.).

potato (pō-tā'tō). COMP: Deficient in protein and fat; also in salt (sodium chloride) and water is in excess. This lowers the nutritive value. Young potatoes contain more juice and protein and less starch. They should be supplemented with milk, butter and eggs, and always used with salt. Potash and soda make them higher in alkalinity than fresh vegetables.
They contain 0.003 purine. Nitrogen is low, half of it being in the form of glutaric acid (asparagin, leucine, tyrosine). The ash has only a small amount of phosphoric acid and magnesium and a still smaller amount of lime, but it contains as much as 60% of potassium. This makes the use of salt with potatoes necessary, as potassium splits the sodium chloride (common salt) in the blood and forms a chloride of potassium, which, if in excess, is eliminated through the urine, and this loss of sodium chloride must be made up by the use of salt.
The potassium in the potato is in part combined with organic acids and partly with phosphoric acid, making the ash strongly alkaline. The carbohydrates are the only nutritive elements the potato has. Heat changes its starch to sugar and in sprouting potatoes this

change is absolute. Cold, if long continued, reverses this process. They are antiscorbutic.

The sprouting potato contains *solanin*, from 0.04 to 0.60 Gm. per kilogram and should never be used, as this is a dangerous poison. If used, cut out the sprouts and their roots.

NUTRIENTS (white): Av. SERVING: 100 Gm. Pro. 2.2, Fat 0.1, Carbo. 18.

NUTRIENTS (sweet): Av. SERVING: 150 Gm. Pro. 2.7, Fat 1.1, Carbo. 39.2.

VITAMINS (white): A+, B++, C++, G++. (Sweet): A++ to +++, B++, C++.

ASH CONST. (white and sweet): Ca 0.014-0.018, Mg 0.028, K 0.429-0.347, Na 0.021-0.039, P 0.058-0.045, Cl 0.038-0.094, S 0.030-0.024, Fe 0.00013-0.0005.

A base-forming food; alkaline potentiality 7 cc. units per 100 Gm., 8.6 cc. per 100 cal.

ACTION: The intestinal absorption is imperfect which lessens the food value. The method of cooking changes the nutritive value and ease of digestion.

COOKING: *Boiled:* The weight is not appreciably diminished by boiling, but part of the essential salts is lost. By adding common salt, or by boiling with the jackets on, much of this loss is compensated. Steaming also helps. *Baked:* Baked, they lose ¼ of their weight of water. The addition of milk and butter and salt adds to their nutritive value. Esp. good for dyspeptics. *Fried:* The addition of fat and the elimination of water doubles their food value, but this process adds to their difficulty of digestion. This also applies to potato salad. Following is the order of ease in digestion:

EASE OF DIGESTION: PROTEIN: 23% is lost in digestion. STARCH: 5% is lost in digestion. 1st. Mealy potatoes. 2nd. Mashed potatoes. 3rd. Unmashed potatoes. 4th. Waxy potatoes. *Stomach:* Potatoes are said to be the easiest of all vegetables on the stomach. The cellulose is tender and small, and the starch is fine. *Intestines:* The carbohydrates stimulate pancreatic secretion and the cellulose stimulates peristalsis. Putrefaction is not frequent. They improve the tone of the entire digestive system and their alkalinity aids oxidation and the combustion of waste material.

CONTRA: Avoid in obesity. Soggy potatoes and fried potatoes cause indigestion.

potency (pō'těn-sĭ) [L. *potentia*, power]. 1. Strength of a medicine. 2. Ability of male to perform coitus. 3. Strength; force; power.

potent (pō'těnt) [L. *potens, potent-*, powerful]. 1. Powerful. 2. Highly effective medicinally. 3. Having power of procreation.

potentia coeundi (pō-těn'shĭ-ă kō-ĕ-ŭn'dē). Complete ability to perform sexual intercourse in a normal manner.

potential (pō-těn'shăl) [L. *potentia*, power]. 1. Latent; existing in possibility. 2. PT: The condition of electrical tension in a body, manifested by the production of electrical effects in other bodies of different potential, or in a different state of electrical tension.

When 2 bodies of different potential are brought together, a current passes from the high to the low potential which is capable of doing work.

potion (pō'shŭn) [L. *potiō*, draft]. A drink or draught; a dose of poison or liquid medicine.

potomania (pō-tō-mā'nĭ-ă) [G. *potos*, a drinking, + *mania*, madness]. Delirium tremens, *q.v.*

Pott's disease (pŏts). Caries or osteitis of the vertebrae, usually of tuberculous origin; tubercular inflammation of bodies of the vertebrae.

A disease usually found in children between ages of 3 and 10 years, of poor parents, and esp. those of tubercular families. No age or class exempt, however. SYN: *spondylitis*.

SYM: Child will complain of pain in region supplied by the nerves arising from affected segment of the cord. If disease is lumbar, pains are abdominal and apt to be associated with vesical irritability; if dorsal, pains are epigastric or intercostal, and respiration sometimes irregular and hurried from failure of respiratory muscles to take the full share in the work; if cervical, neuralgic pain or numbness in hands, a tickling cough and difficult deglutition. Pains apt to be symmetrical.

Increase of pain on jumping or flexing or rotating spine is extremely significant. If child can jump painlessly from chair to floor it is almost certain no inflammation of the body of a vertebra exists. If vertebra be crowded together by pressure on head or shoulders while patient sits or stands, or while he lies face downward across knees of surgeon, pain much increased.

If stretched, so spine is elongated, relief follows. Involuntary immobilization of spine, as a result of pain on movement, is very characteristic military attitude. If child is asked to look at something behind him he turns whole trunk. If requested to pick up something from floor, he stoops by bending the thighs upon the trunk and knees upon thighs; never by flexing spinal column in usual way.

In *walking* moves as if on ice, sliding or shuffling along so as to avoid jar of successive steps. In *standing* he fixes upper portion of column by aid of trapezii and other scapular muscles, action of which at same time raises shoulders and throws arms out from sides. In *standing* or *sitting* there is an involuntary transfer of the weight of head and shoulders and parts above diseased area to the pelvis, by means of the upper extremities. Hands placed upon the hips and arm muscles are tense. In walking about room lays hold of furniture for aid. Spinal abscess occurs later, position varies with seat of caries. Paralysis may occur, always motor at first, not affecting sensation at all.

TREATMENT: 1. Endeavor to secure resolution of the tuberculous ostitis. 2. Limit destruction of tissue and resulting deformity. 3. Promote ankylosis. 4. Evacuate pus. 5. Remove a sequestrum or the focus of carious bone. 6. Relieve cord from pressure by pus, bone, or most commonly, by products of an ext. pachymeningitis. Rest in bed in recumbent position. Gentle massage, friction, alcohol baths. Cod-liver oil inunctions. Food nutritious and abundant. Extension — plaster or other jackets — jury masts, etc. Tuberculosis in any part must be dealt with accordingly. Good nourishing food, fresh air, sunshine, and constitutional remedies plus surgical aid, when feasible. SEE: *gibbosity*.

P.'s fracture. Fracture of lower end of fibula with dislocation of foot outwards and backwards.

After reduction, foot and leg are put in plaster in which a walking iron is incorporated. The patient is able to walk, and plaster is removed in about 6 weeks.

pouch (powch) [Fr. *poche*, pocket]. Any pocket or sac. SYN: *sacculation*.

p., Broca's. A sac in tissues of the labia majora.

p., laryngeal. Blind pouch of mucosa entering the ventral portion of the ventricle of the larynx.

p., pressure. An esophageal bulge due to weakness of the wall.

p., rectouterine. Pouch bet. ant. rectal wall and post. uterine wall. SYN: *Douglas' cul-de-sac*.

poultice (pōl'tĭs) [L. *puls, pult-*, porridge]. A hot, moist mass of linseed, bread, mustard, or soap and oil bet. 2 pieces of muslin applied to the skin to relieve congestion or pain, to stimulate absorption of inflammatory products, and to hasten suppuration. SYN: *cataplasm*. SEE: *plaster, sinapism*.

p., bread. The crumb of bread is moistened by pouring boiling water over it; the water is then pressed out, and the bread mash spread between old linen and applied.

p., charcoal. Used for foul septic wounds. It can either be made in the same way as a mustard poultice in the proportion of 1 to 3, or an ordinary linseed poultice can be made and the charcoal powdered over the top; the former method is the more usual.

p., flaxseed. AIM: To apply moist heat for the relief of congestion and the promotion of suppuration.

ARTICLES NECESSARY: Tray. Old muslin twice the size the finished plaster is to be. Flaxseed meal. Tablespoon, teaspoon. Saucepan, 1 to 2 qt. size. Boiling water. Sodium bicarbonate. Vaseline, or mineral oil in medicine glass. Applicators. Oiled muslin a little larger than the finished plaster. Bandage or binder if needed. Towel. Emesis basin or paper bag.

PROCEDURE: 1. Assemble equipment. 2. Put water in saucepan and bring to rapid boil. 3. Spread muslin on tray. 4. Sprinkle flaxseed meal into boiling water, stirring constantly until it is about the consistency of "breakfast cereal," or until it will drop off the spoon in lumps. 5. Take from fire and beat well. 6. Add ½ to 1 teaspoonful of sodium bicarbonate, stir in well but do not beat hard. 7. Spread on one-half the muslin, leaving a 2 in. margin around plaster. 8. Turn edges of muslin up and fold other half over. 9. Lay on tray, cover with towel, add oiled muslin, oil and swabs, and carry to bedside. 10. Cover area to be poulticed (unless poultice is to be put over dressings) with oil or vaseline. Apply poultice, raising it frequently to accustom the patient's skin to the heat. 11. When patient can bear heat without discomfort, cover poultice with oiled muslin and then with towel. Fasten with bandage or binder if needed. 12. Change poultices each ½ hour or as ordered. Do not let them get cold. 13. Make fresh poultice each time. The old one cannot be reheated. 14. Renew oil as necessary. 15. When treatment is completed wipe excess oil from skin and cover area with old flannel or a towel.

p., jacket. One made both for the chest and back; used in acute lobar pneumonia.

p., linseed. Have everything heated before commencing. Pour 1 teacupful of boiling water into hot bowl and add heated linseed (about 3 cupfuls) handful by handful, stirring all the time. Should be a stiff paste which does not stick to the sides of the bowl.

On the flannel spread the paste ¼ to ½ in. thick with the hot moist spatula, fold over the edges of the flannel. The poultice is then rolled on itself, carried bet. 2 hot plates to the bedside. Apply to the part, cover with wool and bandage. The fresh poultice is rolled on as the old one is removed. The skin must not be exposed.

p., mustard. Dry mustard is added to the dry linseed in proportions of 1 to 8 for adults, but 1 to 12 to 1 to 16 for children; the poultice is then made as for an ordinary linseed poultice.

p., starch. Used in eczema and other skin affections.

A thick paste of 3ii of starch is made, to which is added 1 dram of boracic acid to water, 1 pint; the mixture is boiled to burst the starch granules, and is then spread on old linen and applied to the part; it is renewed 4-hourly.

pound (pownd) [L. *pondus*, a weight; pound]. SYMB: lb. A measure of weight, commonly 12 or 16 ounces.

p., avoirdupois. Sixteen ounces, 7000 grains. [pound 1 foot high.

p., foot-. Power necessary to raise 1

p., troy. Twelve ounces, 5760 grains.

Poupart's ligament (pōō-parz'). The ligament which is the lower border of aponeurosis of external oblique muscle bet. ant. sup. spine of the ilium and spine of the pubis. SYN: *inguinal ligament*.

powder (pow'dĕr) [Fr. *poudre*, powder]. 1. Aggregation of particles. 2. Fine particles of 1 or more substances that may be passed through fine meshes. 3. A dose of such a powder, contained in a paper.

power (pow'er) [M.E. *pouer*, from L. *posse*, to be able]. 1. PT: Rate at which work is done. 2. Capacity for action.

The electrical unit of power is the watt, *q.v.*

pox (pŏks) [M.E. *pokkes*, pits]. 1. An eruptive, contagious disease. 2. A papular eruption that becomes pustular.

SEE: *chickenpox, smallpox, etc*.

P. P. D. Abbr. *purified protein derivative*, substance used in intradermal test for tuberculosis.

P. P. F. Abbr. meaning the *pellagra preventive factor* in vitamin B.

PPLO. Pleuro-pneumonia-like microörganisms found in the throat, saliva, sputum, bladder, and urine, growing in masses. They may be an underlying cause of some infectious diseases.

Ppt. Abbr. for *precipitate*.

Pr. Abbr. for *presbyopia*.

P. r. [L.]. Abbr. of *punctum remotum* meaning *far point*.

practice (prăk'tĭs) [G. *praktikē*, business]. Phase of medicine dealing with professional diagnosis and treatment of disease.

practitioner (prăk-tĭsh'ŭn-ĕr) [G. *praktikē*, business]. One who practices the profession of medicine.

prae-. For words beginning thus, see *pre-*.

pragmatagnosia (prăg″măt-ăg-nō′zĭ-ă) [G. *pragma*, object, + *agnōsia*, lack of recognition]. Inability to recognize objects once familiar.

pragmatamnesia (prăg″măt-ăm-nē′zĭ-ă) [" + *amnēsia*, forgetfulness]. Inability to

recall the appearance of an object.
  p., visual. Name for the mental condition making possible pragmatamnesia.
pragmatic (prăg-măt'ĭk) [G. *pragma*, a thing done]. Pert. to, or concerned with, the practical side of anything.
pragmatism (prăg'mă-tĭzm) [" + *ismos*, condition]. A belief that the practical application of a principle should be the determining factor.
pragmatist (prăg'mă-tĭst) [G. *pragma*, a thing done]. One who believes that practical application should be the determining factor of a principle.
prasoid (prā'soyd) [G. *prason*, leek, + *eidos*, form]. 1. Leek green. 2. Commercial mixture of globularin and globularetin used in treatment of rheumatism and gout.
praxinoscope (prăk-sĭn'ō-skōp) [G. *praxis*, action, + *skopein*, to examine]. Contrivance for studying the larynx.
pre- [L.]. Prefix meaning *before*, or *in front of*.
preagonal (prē-ăg'ō-năl) [L. *prae*, before, + G. *agōnia*, agony]. Pert. to condition immediately before death agony.
prealbuminuric (prē"ăl-bū"mĭn-ū'rĭk) [" + *albumen*, white of egg]. Before the appearance of albuminuria.
preanal (prē-ā'năl) [" + *anus*, anus]. In front of the anus.
preanesthetic (prē"ăn-ĕs-thĕt'ĭk) [" + G. *anaisthēsia*, lack of sensation]. Preliminary drug given to facilitate induction of general anesthesia.
preantiseptic (prē"ăn"tĭ-sĕp'tĭk) [" + G. *anti*, against, + *sēpsis*, decay]. Before the adoption of antisepsis in surgery.
preaortic (prē-ā-or'tĭk) [" + G. *aortē*, aorta]. Located in front of the aorta.
preataxic (prē-ăt-ăk'sĭk) [" + G. *ataxia*, disorder]. Before the onset of ataxia.
preaxial (prē-ăk'sĭ-ăl) [" + G. *axōn*, axis]. In front of the axis of a limb or of the body.
precancerous (prē-kăn'sĕr-ŭs) [" + *cancer*, crab]. Taking place before the development of a carcinoma.
precava (prē-kā'vă) [" + *cavus*, hollow]. The descending or superior vena cava.
precentral (prē-sĕn'trăl) [" + G. *kentron*, center]. In front of a center, as the central fissure of the brain.
  p. convolution. The ascending frontal convolution.
prechordal (prē-kor'dăl) [" + G. *chordē*, cord]. In front of the primitive backbone or notochord.
precipitant (prē-sĭp'ĭ-ănt) [L. *praecipitāre*, to cast down]. A substance bringing about precipitation.
precipitate (prē-sĭp'ĭ-āt). 1. A deposit separated from a suspension or solution by precipitation, the reaction of a reagent, which causes the deposit to fall to the bottom or float near the top. 2. To separate as a precipitate. 3. Hasty.
precipitation (prē-sĭp"ĭ-tā'shŭn). Process of a substance being separated from a solution by action of a reagent.
  p. test. One in which positive reaction is indicated by formation of a precipitate in the solution being tested.
precipitin (prē-sĭp'ĭt-ĭn). Substance, formed in blood serum, producing precipitation of solubles utilized for biological identification of unknown proteins, for determining types of pneumococcus, for diagnosis of echinococcus, etc., and to discriminate bet. human and animal blood.
  The injected protein is called the *antigen* and the antibody produced is the *precipitin.* SEE: autoprecipitin, precipitinogen.
precipitinogen (prē-sĭp"ĭt-ĭn'ō-jĕn) [" + G. *gennan*, to produce]. Any protein which, acting as an antigen, stimulates the production of a specific precipitin.
precipitoid (prē-sĭp'ĭt-oyd) [" + G. *eidos*, form]. Precipitin which can no longer cause precipitation due to subjection to heat.
precipitophore (prē-sĭp'ĭt-ō-fōr) [" + G. *phoros*, a bearer]. Group in a precipitin which produces precipitation. OPP: haptophore precipitum.
preclinical (prē-klĭn'ĭ-kăl) [L. *prae*, before, + G. *klinikos*, pert. to a bed]. Before the development or onset of disease.
  p. medicine. Practice of health examinations at stated intervals in order to detect presence of disease.
preclival (prē-klī'văl) [" + *clivus*, slope]. In front of the cerebellar clivus.
precoital (prē-kō'ĭt-ăl) [" + *coitiō*, a going together]. Prior to sexual intercourse.
precommissure (prē-kŏm'ĭs-ūr) [" + *commissura*, a joining together]. The ant. commissure of the brain.
preconscious (prē-kŏn'shŭs) [" + *conscius*, aware]. Not present in consciousness but able to be recalled as desired.
preconvulsive (prē-kŏn-vŭl'sĭv) [" + *convulsiō*, a pulling together]. Before a convulsion.
precordia (prē-kor'dĭ-ă) [" + *cor*, *cord-*, heart]. The epigastric region including ant. part of lower thorax. SYN: epigastrium, precordium.
precordial (prē-kor'dĭ-ăl) [L. *prae*, before, + *cor*, *cord-*, heart]. Pert. to the precordia or epigastrium.
precordialgia (prē"kor-dĭ-ăl'jĭ-ă) [" + " + G. *algos*, pain]. Pain in the chest or precordial area.
precordium (prē-kor'dĭ-ŭm) [" + *cor*, *cord-*, heart]. A rectangular space over the heart, its blood vessels and the pericardium.
  Above it is the 2nd rib, below the 6th rib, the left boundary is the left midclavicular line, the right boundary is the right parasternal line. It includes the thoracic organs in front of the heart. SYN: precordia.
precornu (prē-kor'nū) [" + *cornu*, horn]. Anterior horn of lateral ventricle of the brain.
precuneus (prē-kū'nē-ŭs) [" + *cuneus*, wedge]. 1. The division of the mesial surface of a cerebral hemisphere bet. the cuneus and the paracentral lobule. 2. The quadrate lobule of the cerebellum.
prediastolic (prē-dī-ăs-tŏl'ĭk) [" + G. *diastolē*, a sending apart]. Before the diastole, or interval in the cardiac cycle that precedes it.
predicrotic (prē-dī-krŏt'ĭk) [" + G. *dikrotos*, beating double]. Preceding the dicrotic wave of the sphygmographic tracing.
predigestion (prē-dĭ-jĕs'chŭn) [L. *prae*, before, + *digestiō*, a carrying apart]. Artificial proteolysis or digestion of proteins and amylolysis of starches before ingestion for use in illness.
predisposing (prē-dĭs-pōz'ĭng) [" + *disponere*, to dispose]. Conferring a tendency to or susceptibility to disease.
predisposition (prē"dĭs-pō-zĭ'shŭn) [" + *disponere*, to dispose]. A tendency to develop a certain disease, either acquired or hereditary, such as nervous disorders, malformations, etc.

p., acquired. Principally subject to diseases made possible by lowered resistance. This class includes such factors as age, sex, climate, racial differences, environment and occupation.

preëclampsia (prē″ĕk-lămp′sĭ-ă) [" + G. *ek*, out, + *lampein*, to flash]. A toxemia of pregnancy characterized by hypertension which increases, headaches, albuminuria, and edema of the lower extremities.

If this condition is neglected or not treated properly, the patient may develop true eclampsia.

Recent method of determining preeclamptic state in 88% of the cases has been by findings of high levels of A. P. L. in the blood serum and low levels of estrogen during 5th, 6th or 7th month. SEE: *eclampsia*.

preflagellate (prē-flăj′ĕl-āt) [" + *flagella*, whip]. Before the flagellate stage; noted in protozoa.

prefrontal (prē-fron′tăl) [" + *frons, front-*, front]. 1. The middle portion of the ethmoid bone. 2. In ant. part of the frontal lobe of the brain.

pregeniculatum, pregeniculum (prē″jē-nĭk″ū-lā′tŭm, -nĭk′ū-lŭm) [" + *geniculum*, a little knee]. The external geniculate body; 1 of 2 flattened bodies on the post. inf. part of the optic thalamus.

pregenital (prē-jĕn′ĭt-ăl) [L. *prae*, before, + *genitalia*, genitals]. PSY: Relating to that period when erotic interest is not yet organized about the reproductive organs and functions.

preglobulin (prē-glŏb′ū-lĭn) [" + *globulus*, a small sphere]. A proteid in cell protoplasm derived from cytoglobulin.

pregnancy (prĕg′năn-sĭ) [L. *praegnans*, with child]. The condition of being with child.

SYM: Amenorrhea, nausea and vomiting, inordinate appetite, pigmentation of the areola of the breasts, the development of Montgomery's tubercles around the nipple, changes in the uterus (softening and progressive enlargement), vaginal discoloration and frequent urination.

The positive signs are: Aschheim-Zondek test positive, hearing of the fetal heart tones, and finding of the fetus on x-ray. The term of pregnancy is 280 days. SEE: *Table, p. P-95*.

PHYSICAL CHANGES DURING: *The Uterus*: (a) Changes shape, size and consistency. (b) Lining undergoes changes. (c) Peritoneal covering enlarges. (d) Muscles increase enormously. (e) Blood vessels penetrate through uterine muscle. (f) Cervix, vagina, and vulva become softer.

The Vaginal Canal: (a) Elongation caused by rising of uterus in pelvis. (b) Mucosa thickens. (c) Secretion increased. (d) Increased vascularity, and more elastic.

Abdominal Changes: (a) Growing distention and flattened navel. (b) Striae gravidarum.

The Breasts: (a) Enlarged and painful. (b) Skin thin and sensitive. (c) Nipples erectile and enlarged, and darker. (d) Escape of colostrum. (e) Primary and secondary areola. (f) Tingling sensation.

Endocrine Glands: (a) Thyroid increases in size and activity. (b) Parathyroids enlarge, secretion increases. (c) Pituitary increases its activity. One of its hormones contracts blood vessels. One contracts uterus. Some affect follicles and corpus luteum. (d) Placenta gives forth hormones, affecting ovaries and corpus luteum.

Circulatory System: (a) Increased activity. (b) Increased blood supply, with increased white corpuscles. (c) Blood pressure should be normal. (d) Varicose veins common.

Skeletal Changes: (a) Pelvic joints soften. (b) Pelvic joints more movable. (c) Bones and teeth affected.

Respiratory Changes: (a) Lungs impeded in late pregnancy. (b) Breathing deeper and more frequent.

Digestive Tract: (a) Nausea and vomiting in early pregnancy. (b) Appetite affected. (c) Loss of weight in early pregnancy with slight anemia. (d) Basal metabolism raised in later pregnancy. (e) Constipation frequent.

The Liver: Enlarged and displaced in late pregnancy.

Skin: (a) Sudoriparous and sebaceous glands very active. (b) Deposit of brown pigment (mask of pregnancy). (c) Linea nigra.

The Weight: (a) Loss during first months. (b) Increased later.

Posture: (a) Changes, as enlargement of abdomen advances. (b) Sacroiliac joints and symphysis pubis more movable. (c) Painful locomotion and backache; waddling gait.

The Urinary Tract: (a) Increased kidney activity. (b) Failure of kidneys produces nephritic toxemia. (c) Ureters, especially right one, dilated. (d) Pressure on bladder with increased circulation. (e) Frequent urination. (f) Bladder lifted into abdomen and pressure diminished. (g) Bladder later pressed upon by presenting part. (h) Urinary output varies. (i) Presence of albumen abnormal. (j) Sugar found in later part of pregnancy. May be diabetes or glycosuria. (k) No blood sugar change.

DISORDERS OF: *Nausea and Vomiting*: (a) May be marked when stomach is empty. (b) May occur at any time. (c) Food may help on arising. (d) Four or 5 small meals per day. (e) Psychic causes may be responsible.

Constipation and Flatulence: (a) Pressure of uterus on intestines may be a cause. (b) Laxative diet and exercise may aid. (c) Intestinal stasis may cause flatulence. (d) Gas-forming foods should be avoided.

Muscular Cramps: (a) Retention of waste products a cause. (b) Poor circulation may cause (a). (c) Pressure on foot, extension of leg helps. (d) Rest between periods of standing needed. (e) Tetany may ensue because of deficient calcium supply. (f) Calcium and vitamin D indicated.

Pressure Edema: (a) May occur during last weeks. (b) Better in morning; worse at night. (c) Frequent rest and elevation of limbs indicated. (d) May be due to calcium deficiency. (e) Toxemia must be ruled out by frequent blood pressure and urinalysis.

Headache: (a) Intestinal intoxication and constipation causes. (b) Eyestrain may be suspected. (c) Temporary hypertrophy of pituitary common. (d) Sinusitis most common cause. (e) May be due to toxemia. (f) Blood pressure and urinalysis checked.

Neuralgic Pains: (a) Pressure of fetal head upon sciatic nerve suspected. (b) Rest periods and abdominal support indicated. (c) Knee-chest position after retiring.

pregnancy, abdominal

Toothache: (a) May be due to caries induced by deficient calcium. (b) Acid condition of gums may be a cause. (c) Magnesia as a mouthwash indicated in (b). (d) Frequent dental examinations desirable.

Backache: (a) Abnormal balance caused by protruding abdomen. (b) Proper shoes indicated for (a). (c) Intraabdominal pressure may be a cause. (d) Flatulence aggravates (c); enemas may help it. (e) Knee-chest position at night may help. (f) Gastric hyperacidity may induce high backaches. (g) Alkalies may temporarily help (f).

Dyspnea: (a) Pressure of uterus upward on transverse colon and stomach. (b) Aggravated by flatulence, especially when lying down. (c) Alkalies may help. (d) Pillows under head and shoulder indicated. (e) Reëxamination of heart indicated.

Vaginal Discharge: (a) Increased blood supply to glands of cervix. (b) Cleanliness but no douches indicated. (c) Foul or blood-tinged or profuse discharge should be reported.

Pruritus or Itching: (a) Breasts, abdomen, and vulva may be affected. (b) Stretching of skin of abdomen a cause in that area. (c) If general, a toxic or nervous origin may be cause. (d) Acid-forming organism may cause vulvar itching. (e) Alkaline solutions, bland ointment, talcum for (e). (f) Sugar in urine may cause pruritus of vulva.

Heartburn: (a) Hyperacidity may be responsible, due to oversecretion of hydrochloric acid; also nervous tension. (b) Sedation, frequent small meals, no highly seasoned foods. (c) Organic acids from fermentative changes may be responsible. (d) Alkalies must not be taken too close to a meal. (e) Discomfort may be felt in the back. (f) Hydrochloric acid administered by the doctor.

Salivation: (a) May be associated with extreme nausea and vomiting. (b) Usually an expression of neurosis. (c) Mild astringents may be employed. (d) If due to a toxemia, refer to the physician.

Varicose Veins: (a) Congenitally acquired; aggravated by pregnancy. (b) May occur in pelvis, vulva, and legs; marked on right side. (c) Round garters, tight clothing, standing to be avoided. (d) Rest and supporting bandage indicated. (e) Elevation of lower limbs while sleeping. (f) Sims position, pillow under hips to shift uterus.

Hemorrhoids: (a) Avoid constipation. (b) Ointments, wet compresses, suppositories on doctor's orders. (c) Carbolized or mentholated vaseline in absence of (b). (d) Incision by surgeon.

p., abdominal. Implantation of the ovum in the abdominal cavity.

p., bigeminal. Pregnancy with twins *in utero.*

p., cervical. Implantation of the ovum in the cervical canal.

p., cornual. Pregnancy in 1 of the horns of a bicornuate uterus.

p., ectopic. SEE: *extrauterine p.*

p., extrauterine. Pregnancy outside the uterine cavity.

p., heterotropic. Combined intrauterine and extrauterine pregnancies.

p., interstitial. P. occurring in the uterine wall which forms part of the oviduct.

p., mask of. Area of brown pigmentation sometimes appearing on the face during pregnancy.

p., multiple. State of having more than 1 fetus in the uterus at the same time.

p., ovarian. Implantation of the fertilized ovum in the substance of the ovary.

p., phantom. Enlargement of the abdomen simulating pregnancy. SEE: *pseudocyesis.*

p. table. SEE: Table for calculation of expected date of delivery from the first day of the last menstrual period.

pregnancy, words pert. to: Aaron's sign; Abderhalden's reaction; abortion; acromphalus; acyesis; Ahlfeld's sign; alochia; amnion; amniorrhexis; amniorrhea; amnios; amniotic; amniotitis; Aschheim-Zondek test; Beccaria's sign; Bercovitz's test; Brouha's test; celiocolpotomy; childbirth; chloasma gravidarum; conception; congenital; cyesiognosis; cyesiology; cyesis; decidua; deciduoma; deciduomatosis; ectopic; eclampsia; embryo; enceinte; encyopyelitis; fertility; fetal; fetation; feticide; fetus; Friedman test; gestation; gravid; gravida; gravidity; hyperemesis gravidarum; hypercyesis; interstitial; labor; linea nigra; maieusiophobia; maieutics; menstruation; miscarriage; monocyesis; multigravida; multipara; multiparity; nabothian menorrhagia; nullipara; obstetrics; paracyesis; parturition; placenta; plurigravida; pseudocyesis; quadripara; quickening; quintipara; Rubin test; sterility; stria gravidarum; striae; superfetation; toxemia; unigravida; unipara; uterogestation; vomiting, pernicious, of.

pregnant (prĕg'nănt) [L. *praegnans,* with child.] Having conceived; with child. SYN: *gravid.*

pregnenolone (prĕg-nĕn'ō-lōn). A relatively nontoxic steroid hormone, with a formula closely related to that of cortisone. Used in rheumatoid arthritis, fibrositis, dermatomyositis.

pregniotin (prĕg-nī'ŏt-ĭn). Preparation, no longer available commercially, of antigen from human placenta which was supposed to determine pregnancy when injected intradermally.

pregravidic (prē-grăv-ĭd'ĭk) [L. *prae,* before, + *gravida,* pregnant]. Before pregnancy.

prehallux (prē-hăl'ŭks) [" + *hallux,* the great toe]. A supernumerary bone or accessory *naviculare pedis* or sometimes a prolongation inward of it on the foot.

prehemiplegic (prē-hĕm-ĭ-plē'jĭk) [" + G. *emi,* half, + *plēgē,* a stroke]. Occurring before an attack of hemiplegia.

prehensile (prē-hĕn'sĭl) [L. *prehendere,* to seize]. Capable of grasping.

prehension (prē-hĕn'shŭn) [L. *prehensio,* from *prehendere,* to seize]. The act of grasping or seizing.

prehyoid (prē-hī'oyd) [L. *prae,* before, + G. *yoeidēs,* U-shaped]. Before the hyoid bone.

prehypophysis (prē"hī-pof'ĭs-ĭs) [" + G. *ypo,* under, + *physis,* growth]. The anterior and larger part of the hypophysis or pituitary gland.

preimmunization (prē-ĭm"ū-nĭ-zā'shŭn) [" + *immunis,* safe]. Immunization produced artificially in very young infants.

preinsula (prē-ĭn'sū-lă) [" + *insula,* island]. The cephalic area of the island of Reil, the insula, a group of several small convolutions at bottom of the fissure of Sylvius.

Preiser's disease (prī'zĕr). A porous condition of bone, osteoporosis, caused by

PREGNANCY TABLE

Find the date of the first day of the last menstrual period in the top line and the date below this will be the expected day of delivery.

	1	2	3	4	5	6	7	8	9	10	11	12	13	14	15	16	17	18	19	20	21	22	23	24	25	26	27	28	29	30	31
Jan.	1	2	3	4	5	6	7	8	9	10	11	12	13	14	15	16	17	18	19	20	21	22	23	24	25	26	27	28	29	30	31
Oct.	8	9	10	11	12	13	14	15	16	17	18	19	20	21	22	23	24	25	26	27	28	29	30	31	(1	2	3	4	5	6	7 Nov.
Feb.	1	2	3	4	5	6	7	8	9	10	11	12	13	14	15	16	17	18	19	20	21	22	23	24	25	26	27	28			
Nov.	8	9	10	11	12	13	14	15	16	17	18	19	20	21	22	23	24	25	26	27	28	29	30	(1	2	3	4	5			Dec.
Mar.	1	2	3	4	5	6	7	8	9	10	11	12	13	14	15	16	17	18	19	20	21	22	23	24	25	26	27	28	29	30	31
Dec.	6	7	8	9	10	11	12	13	14	15	16	17	18	19	20	21	22	23	24	25	26	27	28	29	30	31	(1	2	3	4	5 Jan.
Apr.	1	2	3	4	5	6	7	8	9	10	11	12	13	14	15	16	17	18	19	20	21	22	23	24	25	26	27	28	29	30	
Jan.	6	7	8	9	10	11	12	13	14	15	16	17	18	19	20	21	22	23	24	25	26	27	28	29	30	31	(1	2	3	4	Feb.
May	1	2	3	4	5	6	7	8	9	10	11	12	13	14	15	16	17	18	19	20	21	22	23	24	25	26	27	28	29	30	31
Feb.	5	6	7	8	9	10	11	12	13	14	15	16	17	18	19	20	21	22	23	24	25	26	27	28	(1	2	3	4	5	6	7 Mar.
June	1	2	3	4	5	6	7	8	9	10	11	12	13	14	15	16	17	18	19	20	21	22	23	24	25	26	27	28	29	30	
Mar.	8	9	10	11	12	13	14	15	16	17	18	19	20	21	22	23	24	25	26	27	28	29	30	31	(1	2	3	4	5	6	7 April
July	1	2	3	4	5	6	7	8	9	10	11	12	13	14	15	16	17	18	19	20	21	22	23	24	25	26	27	28	29	30	31
April	7	8	9	10	11	12	13	14	15	16	17	18	19	20	21	22	23	24	25	26	27	28	29	30	(1	2	3	4	5	6	7 May
Aug.	1	2	3	4	5	6	7	8	9	10	11	12	13	14	15	16	17	18	19	20	21	22	23	24	25	26	27	28	29	30	31
May	8	9	10	11	12	13	14	15	16	17	18	19	20	21	22	23	24	25	26	27	28	29	30	31	(1	2	3	4	5	6	7 June
Sept.	1	2	3	4	5	6	7	8	9	10	11	12	13	14	15	16	17	18	19	20	21	22	23	24	25	26	27	28	29	30	
June	8	9	10	11	12	13	14	15	16	17	18	19	20	21	22	23	24	25	26	27	28	29	30	(1	2	3	4	5	6	7	July
Oct.	1	2	3	4	5	6	7	8	9	10	11	12	13	14	15	16	17	18	19	20	21	22	23	24	25	26	27	28	29	30	31
July	8	9	10	11	12	13	14	15	16	17	18	19	20	21	22	23	24	25	26	27	28	29	30	31	(1	2	3	4	5	6	7 Aug.
Nov.	1	2	3	4	5	6	7	8	9	10	11	12	13	14	15	16	17	18	19	20	21	22	23	24	25	26	27	28	29	30	
Aug.	8	9	10	11	12	13	14	15	16	17	18	19	20	21	22	23	24	25	26	27	28	29	30	31	(1	2	3	4	5	6	7 Sept.
Dec.	1	2	3	4	5	6	7	8	9	10	11	12	13	14	15	16	17	18	19	20	21	22	23	24	25	26	27	28	29	30	31
Sept.	7	8	9	10	11	12	13	14	15	16	17	18	19	20	21	22	23	24	25	26	27	28	29	30	(1	2	3	4	5	6	7 Oct.

trauma and affecting the carpal scaphoid bone of the wrist.
prelimbic (prē-lĭm'bĭk) [L. *prae*, before, + *limbus*, border]. Situated before a margin.
 p. fissure. Ant. part of the fissure of the corpus callosum and marginal gyri of the brain.
prelipoid (prē-lĭp'oyd) [" + G. *lipos*, fat, + *eidos*, form]. Before conversion into the lipoid state.
 p. substance. Nerve tissue broken down, but not yet converted into fat.
prelum (prē'lŭm) [L.]. A press.
 p. abdominale. Squeezing of abdominal viscera in defecation, urination, and parturition, bet. the diaphragm and abdominal wall.
premature (prē-mă-tūr'). Not mature; before term or full development.
 p. beat. A cardiac contraction occurring before the normal one. SYN: *extrasystole.*
 p. infant. One born before term. ETIOL: Uterine disease, shock, accident, toxemia of pregnancy, syphilis or any serious organic disease.
 p. labor. Onset of labor before full term.
premaxilla (prē"măks-ĭl'ă) [" + *maxilla*, upper jaw]. The intermaxillary bone forming median ant. part of sup. maxillary bones.
premaxillary (prē-măk'sĭ-lĕr-ĭ) [" + *maxillaris*, pert. to the upper jaw]. Located before the maxilla.
 p. bone. The intermaxillary bone. SYN: *incisive bone.*
premedication (prē-mĕd-ĭ-kā'shŭn) [" + *medicari*, to heal]. Induction of unconsciousness by internal drugs prior to administration of inhalation anesthesia.
premenstrual (prē-mĕn'strū-ăl) [L. *prae*, before, + *menstruāre*, to menstruate]. Before menstruation.
premenstruum (prē-mĕn'strū-ŭm) [" + *menstruum*, monthly fluid]. The period prior to menstruation.
premolar (prē-mō'lĕr) [" + *moles*, a mass]. 1. A bicuspid tooth. 2. Before a molar tooth.
premonition (prē-mŏ-nĭsh'ŭn) [" + *monēre*, to warn]. A feeling of an impending event.
premonitory (prē-mŏn'ĭ-tō-rĭ) [L. *praemonitorius*, warning before]. Giving a warning; foreboding or forewarning.
premonocyte (prē-mŏn'ō-sīt) [L. *prae*, before, + G. *monos*, alone, + *kytos*, cell]. An embryonic cell transitional in development prior to a monocyte.
premunition (prē-mū-nĭsh'ŭn) [" + *munitiō*, a fortification]. Immunity conferred by preventive vaccination.
premunitive (prē-mū'nĭ-tĭv) [" + *munitiō*, a fortification]. Pert. to, or resulting from, preventive vaccination.
premyelocyte (prē-mī'ĕl-ō-sīt) [" + G. *myelos*, marrow, + *kytos*, cell]. An embryonic myeloblast.
prenarcosis (prē-nar-kō'sĭs) [" + G. *narkōsis*, stuporous condition]. Induction of unconsciousness by int. drugs before general inhalation anesthesia. SYN: *premedication.*
prenatal (prē-nā'tl) [" + *natalis*, pert. to birth]. Before birth.
 p. care. The care of the pregnant woman during the period of gestation. This care consists of periodic examinations for the determination of the blood pressure, weight, urinalysis, changes in the size of the uterus, and condition of the fetus as determined by the heart tones and position. By such examinations, changes in the condition of the patient can be noted and toxemias prevented by the institution of treatment as soon as any abnormal signs are present.
preoperative preparation. 1. Prepare area indicated according to technic of your hospital. 2. Be sure the water and liquid soap you use for shaving and cleansing the skin are warmed; cold liquids on the abdomen give the patient a disagreeable shock. 3. See that patient is attended by his clergyman if this has not already been done before he came to the hospital. This is *absolutely essential* in the case of Catholic patients. 4. Try to have the patient get as much sleep as possible. If he is wakeful and you do not wish to give sedative early, try to find some reading matter for him. 5. Give the enemas ordered for the morning as late as you can if he is asleep so as to give him as much rest as possible. 6. Get order for catheterization if you think it will be needed. 7. *Never* send a patient to the operating table with a full bladder. 8. Give preanesthetic medication, or basal anesthetic, at *exactly* the time specified. 9. See that dentures are removed and placed in a glass of water which is marked with the patient's name and room number. 10. See that women do not have make-up on face or nails and that they are not wearing hair pins or "bobbie" pins. 11. Tie the wedding ring in place. 12. Do not use straight pins in patient's gown or operating cap. 13. Wrap blankets well around neck when he is placed on stretcher to keep drafts out. 14. Do not forget chart when taking him to surgery. 15. Do not chatter with other nurses you meet on the way or while waiting with the patient before he is anesthetized. 16. Do not forget to reassure anxious relatives who may not like to disturb you with many questions and who do not understand all that is going on as well as you do.
preoperculum (prē"ō-pĕr'kū-lŭm) [L. *prae*, before, + *operculum*, a cover]. The frontal part of the convolutions covering the island of Reil, the operculum.
preoptic (prē-ŏp'tĭk) [" + G. *optikos*, pert. to vision]. In front of the optic lobes.
preoral (prē-ō'răl) [" + *os, or-*, mouth]. In front part of the mouth.
prepallium (prē-păl'ī-ŭm) [" + *pallium*, a cloak]. The part of the brain cortex ant. to the fissure of Rolando.
preparalytic (prē"-păr-ă-lĭt'ĭk) [" + G. *para*, at the side, + *lyein*, to loosen]. Before the appearance of paralysis.
preparations usually given by rectum. These are the following:
 Asafetida: Two drams of asafetida in 4 to 6 oz. of water. Another mixture is 1 oz. of milk of asafetida and 1 pt. of warm water, or to 12 oz. of warm water add 4 oz. of asafetida emulsion prepared by agitating ½ dram. of asafetida powder in 4 oz. of hot water.
 Chloral hydrate: Ten to 30 gr. dissolved in 3 oz. of olive oil, warmed; or 3 oz. of very warm milk, or 3 oz. of thin, boiled cornstarch water. This makes a good preparation or a base in which to hold the medicine in suspension. The patient's pulse should be taken 5 minutes before and 5 minutes after the administration to determine the heart action. If untoward effects are noticed, action may be taken to prevent further absorption.

Glycerin: This is added, 1 oz. to a pt. of solution of plain water. It will cause a good evacuation. One ounce of glycerin to 1 oz. of water will cause irritation of the lower bowel and precipitate an evacuation. This may be given with a bulb syringe.

Alum: The alum enema consists of 1 qt. of warm water and 1 oz. of powdered alum. This enema has a tendency to dry up intestinal fermentations.

Paraldehyde: Dosage, 1 to 4 cc. may be mixed with water in the proportion of 1 to 8 and in this ratio it may be mixed with thin starch water for rectal medication. There should be about 3 oz. of starch water.

Sodium bicarbonate: One tablespoonful or 4 Gm. to 500 cc. or 1 pt. of water aids in the expulsion of the bowel content. The neutralizing action of the acidity of the bowel content brought about by the sodium bicarbonate solution leaves the bowel soothed and with a bland reaction.

Sodium bromide: Ten to 60 gr. dissolved in plain water water, 2 to 4 oz.

RS: *alkaloids, active principles, drugs with 2 names, names of preparations; antidotes; dosage; drug action; drugs and their administration; medical preparations; names of individual drugs in alphabetical order; names of poisons; poison; poisoning; prescription writing.*

prepatellar (prē-pă-těl′ar) [L. *prae*, before, + *patella*, pan]. In front of the patella.

p. bursitis. Inflammation of the bursa in front of patella. SYN: *housemaid's knee*. SEE: *bursitis*.

prephthisis (prē-tī′sĭs) [″ + G. *phthisis*, a wasting]. 1. The pretuberculous stages of pulmonary phthisis. 2. Predisposition to tuberculosis.

prephyson (prē-fī′son) [″ + G. *physis*, growth]. Hormone elaborated by the ant. pituitary lobe which aids in metabolic regulation.

prepuce (prē′pūs) [L. *praeputium*, prepuce]. The foreskin or fold of skin over the glans penis in the male.

Excision constitutes *circumcision*, a practice becoming more widely adopted among Gentiles for inhibitory and prophylactic purposes. A sebaceous secretion under the prepuce is called *smegma*.* It acts as a lubricant.

RS: *acrobystiolith, acrobystitis, acroposthitis, aposthia, frenulum, penis, phimosis, smegma, urethra* (of male).

p. of the clitoris. Fold of the labia minora which covers the clitoris. SEE: *clitoris*.

preputial (prē-pū′shăl) [L. *praeputium*, prepuce]. Concerning the prepuce.

p. glands. Small sebaceous glands of the corona of the penis which secrete an odoriferous discharge. SYN: *Tyson's glands*.

preputium (prē-pū′shĭ-ŭm) (pl. *preputia*) [L. *praeputium*, prepuce]. The fold of skin which covers the glans penis. SYN: *prepuce, q.v.*

p. clitoridis. Prepuce of the clitoris, the 2 layers of the labia pudendi minora which split at their junction anteriorly.

presbyacusia, presbyacousia (prĕz″bĭ-ă-kū′sĭ-ă) [G. *presbys*, old, + *akousis*, hearing]. Hearing less acutely, due to old age. SYN: *presbycusis*.

presbyatrics, presbyatry (prĕz-bĭ-ăt′rĭks, prĕz′bĭ-ăt-rī) [″ + *iatrikos*, healing]. That branch of medicine dealing with the diseases of old age.

presbycusis, presbykousis (prĕz-bĭ-kū′sĭs) [″ + *akousis*, hearing]. Impairment of acute hearing in old age. SYN: *presbyacusia*.

presbyophrenia (prĕz-bĭ-ō-frē′nĭ-ă) [″ + *phrēn*, mind]. Senile psychotic syndrome involving confabulation and disorientation with preservation of mobility, loquacity, and good spirits. SYN: *Wernicke's syndrome*.

presbyopia (prĕz-bĭ-ō′pĭ-ă) [″ + *ōps*, eye]. Defect of vision in advancing age involving loss of accommodation or recession of near point.

Usually occurs between 40 and 45 years of age. SEE: *farsightedness*.

presbytiatrics (prĕz-bĭt-ī-ăt′rĭks) [″ + *iatrikos*, healing]. Science of old age and its treatment. SYN: *geriatrics, presbyatrics, presbyatry*.

prescription (prē-skrĭp′shŭn) [L. *praescriptio*, a writing before, an order]. A written order for dispensing drugs signed by a physician. [parts:

A prescription consists of 4 main SUPERSCRIPTION: Represented by the symbol ℞ which signifies *Recipe*, from the Latin *recipere*, meaning to take.

INSCRIPTION: Containing the ingredients. This again is generally constructed of 4 parts: (a) The *basis* or principal drug; (b) the *adjuvant*, which assists the action of the basis; (c) the *corrective*, which diminishes unpleasant taste or pain or griping, etc.; (d) the *vehicle* to hold the drugs either in solution or suspension.

SUBSCRIPTION: Directions to the dispenser as to the manner of preparation of the drugs.

SIGNATURE: Directions to the patient with regard to the manner of taking, dosage, etc.; finally, the physician's signature and the date must be added.

p. carbons. PT: Carbons impregnated with various substances for use in treatment of specific conditions.

prescription writing. LATIN USAGE IN PRESCRIPTIONS: An official Latin name is in the nominative case. *Drugs*: Written in the genitive case, as the prescription is an order, meaning "take thou." Word "*of*": This is not written in Latin but is indicated by the ending of a word: *Quinina*, of course, means "quinine," but changing the termination to "ae" we have "*quininae*," meaning of *quinine*.

ALKALOIDS: Written the same as in English, except that the final "e" is changed to "a" to form the nominative case, as *quinina*, for the English quinine. To form the genitive case, the final "e" is changed to "ae," as *quininae*.

ACTIVE PRINCIPLES: These, such as glucosides, resinoids and others, add "um" to the nominative, and "i" to the genitive, as Strophanthin becomes *strophanthinum* to form the Latin nominative, and *strophanthini*, to form the Latin genitive.

ACIDS: The names of these are formed in the same way as those of alkaloids, except that the adjective is formed in the same way and follows the nominative, as *Acidum Hydrochloricum*, or the genitive, *Acidi Hydrochlorici*.

METALS: Latin names of metals, except those of a few known to the ancients, are the same as English forms ending in "um," as in *Sodium*, forming the Latin nominative, but ending in "i" to form the genitive, *Sodii*.

SALTS: Written first with the name of the *base* in its genitive form, next the *acid radical* in the nominative, followed

Terms Used in Prescription Writing

Abbreviation	Word or Phrase	English Equivalent
āā or a	ana	of each
abs. feb.	absente febre	fever being absent
ad	ad	to, up to
add.	adde	add
ad. feb.	adstante febre	fever being present
adhib.	adhibendus	to be administered
ad. lib.	ad libitum	at pleasure
admov.	admove	apply
ante cib. or A. C.	ante cibum	before food
aq. bull.	aqua bulliens	boiling water
aq. dest.	aqua destillata	distilled water
aq. font.	aqua fontis	spring water
aq. pur.	aqua pura	pure water
bene	bene	well
b. i. d.	bis in die	twice daily
bull.	bulliat	let (it) boil
c̄	cum	with
cap.	capsula	a capsule
chart. or cht.	chartula	a small medicated paper
coch. mag.	cochleare magnum	a tablespoonful
coch. med.	cochleare medium	a dessertspoonful
coch. parv.	cochleare parvum	a teaspoonful
collyr.	collyrium	an eyewash
comp.	compositus	compounded of
cong.	congius	a gallon
cont. rem.	continuantur remedia	continue the medicine
cras mane sum.	cras mane sumendus	take tomorrow morning
cuj. lib.	cujus libet	of any you please
d., det.	da, detur	give, let be given
d. d. in d.	de die in diem	from day to day
dent. tal. dos.	dentur tales doses	give of such doses
dieb. alt.	diebus alternis	every other day
dieb. tert.	diebus tertiis	every 3rd day
dil.	dilue, dilutus	dilute, diluted
dim.	dimidius	one-half
div.	divide	divide
div. in p. aeq.	dividatur in partes aequales	let it be divided into equal parts
donec alv. sol. ft.	donec alvus soluta fuerit	until bowels are open
dos.	dosis	dose
dur. dolor.	durante dolore	while pain lasts
emp.	emplastrum	plaster
emuls.	emulsio	an emulsion
ft.	fiat	let be made
garg.	gargarisma	a gargle
grad.	gradatim	by degrees
gr.	granum	a grain
gtt.	gutta, guttae	a drop, drops
guttat.	guttatim	by drops
haust.	haustus	a draught
hor. decub.	hora decubitus	bed hour
hor. som. or h. s.	hora somni	bed time
hor. 1 spat.	horae unius spatio	one hour's time
ind.	indies	daily
inf.	infusum	let it infuse
int.	intime	thoroughly
lin.	linimentum	a liniment
lot.	lotio	a lotion
M.	misce	mix
mac.	macera	macerate
man. prim.	mane primo	first thing in the morning
mas.	massa	mass
med.	medicamentum	a medicine
m. et n.	mane et nocte	morning and night
mitt.	mitte	send
mitt. x tal.	mitte decem tales	send 10 like this
mod.	modicus	moderate sized
mod. praesc.	modo praescripto	in the manner written
moll.	mollis	soft
mor. dict.	more dicto	in the manner directed
mor. sol.	more solito	as accustomed
ne tr. s. num.	ne tradas sine nummo	deliver not without the money
no.	numerus	number
noct. maneq.	nocte maneque	night and morning

Abbreviation	Word or Phrase	English Equivalent
non. rep., n. r.	non repetatur	let it not be repeated
o.	octarius	a pint
omn. bih.	omni bihoris	every 2nd hour
omn. hor.	omni hora	every hour
om. ¼ h.	omni quadrantae horae	every 15 minutes
om. mane vel. noc.	omni mane vel nocte	every morning or night
p. c.	post cibum	after meals
pil.	pilula	a pill
p. p. a.	phiala prius agitata	the bottle being first shaken
p. r. n.	pro re nata	as occasion arises
pro. rat. aet.	pro ratione aetatis	according to patient's age
pulv.	pulvis	powder
q. h.	quaque hora	every hour
q. l.	quantum libet	as much as pleases
q. s.	quantum sufficiat	as much as suffices
quotid.	quotidie	daily
red. in pulv.	redactus in pulverem	reduced to powder
repetat., rep.	repetatur	to be repeated
sec. a., or s. a.	secundum artem	according to art
semih.	semihora	half an hour
sig.	signa	write
sing.	singulorum	of each
sol.	solutio	solution
s. o. s.	si opus sit	if need exists
solv.	solve	dissolve
ss.	semi or semisse	a half
stat.	statim	immediately
st.	stet or stent	let it (or them) stand
subind.	subinde	frequently
sum.	sume	take
sum. tal.	sumat talem	take 1 such
suppos.	suppositoria	a suppository
tab.	tabella	a tablet
tere	tere	rub
tere bene	tere bene	rub well
t. i. d.	ter in die	thrice daily
trit.	tritura	triturate or grind
ult. praes.	ultimus praescriptus	the last ordered
ut dict.	ut dictum	as directed
vitel.	vitellus	yolk of an egg

Weights and Measures.

- ℳ Minimum, -i, n., minim, of a fluidram.
- Gtt. Gutta, -ae, f., a drop.
- gr. Granum, -i, n., a grain.
- ℈ Scrupulus, -i, m., a scruple, 20 grains.
- ℨ Drachma, -ae, f., a dram, 60 grains.
- f ℨ Fluidrachma, -ae, f., a fluidram, 60 minims.
- ℥ Uncia, -ae, f., a troy ounce, 480 grains.
- f ℥ Fluiduncia, -ae, f., a fluidounce, 8 fluidrams.
- lb. Libra, -ae, f., a pound (troy), 5760 grains.
- O. Octarius, -i, m., a pint, 16 fluidounces.
- C. Congius, -i, m., a gallon, 8 pints.
- ss. Semis, indecl., a half.

Quantities are designated by Roman numerals following the symbol for denomination.
SEE: charting.

by the *qualitative adjective*, also in the nominative, as *Ferri Sulfas Exsiccatus*, exsiccated sulfate of iron.

NAMES OF PREPARATIONS: Show the *class* to which it belongs first, the name of the *ingredient* next, and the *qualifying* adjective last, as *Syrupus Scillae Compositus* (Compound Syrup of Squills). First and last words are in nominative case and middle one in genitive.

DRUGS WITH TWO NAMES: Both should be in the genitive, as *Liquor Potassi Arsenitis*. *-ate endings*: The Latin nominative ends in "as," as *sulfas*, for sulfate, and the genitive in "atis," as *sulfatis*. *-ite endings*: If the English word ends in "ite," as *"sulfite,"* the Latin nominative ends in "is," as *sulfis*, and the genitive in "itis," as *sulfitis*. *-ide endings*: If an English word has this ending, as "Bromide," the Latin nominative ends in "um," dropping the final "e" in the English form, as *Bromidum*; the genitive dropping the "um" to add "i," as *Bromidi*.

-a, -us, -um endings: English words with these endings are the same in the Latin nominative, but the genitive is formed by changing "a" to "ae," or the "us" or "um" to "i." *-in endings*: An English word having this ending adds "um" (usually) to form the Latin nominative as Benzoin and *Benzoinum*, the genitive being formed by merely adding "i," as *Benzoini*. *-ol endings*: The Latin nominative is the same as the English, as in "Phenol," but "is" is added to form the genitive, as *Phenolis*. *-al endings*: To form the Latin nominative, "um" is added, as Chloral and *Chlo-*

ralum. To form the genitive, "i" is added to the English form, as *Chlorali*.

There are, of course, exceptions to the foregoing. Many Latin words have the same form as in English. Fortunately, perhaps, most drugs are indicated in prescription by abbreviations which may not discriminate bet. the Latin nominative and genitive.

RS: *alkaloids, active principles, drugs with 2 names, names of preparations; antidotes; dosage; drug action; drugs and their administration; medical preparations; names of individual drugs in alphabetical order (500+ in all); names of poisons; poison; poisoning; preparations usually given by rectum.*

presentation (prē-zĕn-tā′shŭn) [L. *praesentatio*, a placing before]. OB: Term applied to the manner of the fetus presenting itself to the examining finger at the mouth of the uterus.

Thus longitudinal (normal) and transverse (pathological) presentation.

p., breech. When pelvic extremity presents.

Breech presentation is divided into 3 types: *Complete breech*, when the thighs are flexed on the abdomen and the legs flexed upon the thighs; *frank breech*, when the legs are extended over the ant. surface of the body, and *footling*, when a foot or feet present; footling can be single, double, or if the leg remains flexed, knee presentation.

p., brow. When the brow presents.

p., cephalic. Presentation of the head in any position.

p., face. When the head is sharply extended so that the face presents.

p., footling. Presenting feet first.

p., placental. Presentation of the placenta first. SYN: *placenta previa*.

p., sinciput. When the large fontanel presents.

p., transverse. With fetus lying crosswise.

p. vertex. P. of the upper and back part of the head.

presphenoid (prē-sfē′noyd) [L. *prae*, before, + G. *sphēn*, wedge, + *eidos*, form]. Ant. region of the body of the sphenoid bone.

presphygmic (prē-sfĭg′mĭk) [" + G. *sphygmos*, pulse]. Pert. to period preceding the pulse wave.

prespinal (prē-spī′năl) [" + *spina*, thorn]. Before the spine, or ventral to it.

prespondylolisthesis (prē-spŏn″dĭl-ō-lĭs-thē′sĭs) [" + G. *spondylos*, vertebra, + *olisthanein*, to slip]. A congenital defect of a lumbar vertebra without displacement, which predisposes to spondylolisthesis.

pressinervoscopy (prĕs″ĭ-nĕr-vŏs′kō-pĭ) [L. *pressus*, from *premere*, to press, + *nervus*, a nerve, + G. *skopein*, to examine]. Diagnosis by pressing upon the pneumogastric and sympathetic nerves.

pressor (prĕs′ōr) [L. *pressor*, from *premere*, to press]. 1. Stimulating, increasing the activity of a function, especially of vasomotor activity, as a nerve. 2. A substance in the pituitary body capable of raising blood pressure.

p. base or **substance.** One of several products of intestinal putrefaction found in normal urine which, when injected, raises blood pressure in animals.

p. nerves. Those nerves which under stimulation cause reaction of the vasomotor centers.

p. reflex. Any reflex in which the response to stimulation is increased activity of a motor center.

p. X. An animal extract which raises blood pressure and decreases kidney function.

pressure (prĕsh′ūr) [L. *pressura*, a squeezing]. 1. A compression. 2. Stress or force exerted on a body, as by tension, weight, pulling, etc. 3. PSY: Quality of sensation aroused by moderate compression of the skin. 4. In physics, the quotient obtained by dividing a force by the area of the surface on which it acts.

RS: *atmosphere, blood, hypertonic, isotonic.*

p., after-. A feeling of p. which remains for a few seconds after removal of a weight or other pressure.

p., arterial. P. of blood in the arteries.

p., atmospheric. P. of weight of atmosphere; at sea level it averages about 760 mm. of mercury.

p., blood. P. exerted by blood against the walls of blood vessels.

For young men the systolic general arterial blood pressure is about 120 mm. of mercury and the systolic, about 70. There is a wide range of normal variation, due to constitutional, physical, and psychic factors. For women the figures are lower; for older people they are higher. There is little difference in the b. p. of the 2 arms.

p., diastolic. Arterial pressure during dilatation of the heart cavities; diastole.

p., intracranial. P. of the cerebrospinal fluid, which in a recumbent position is from 60 to 120 mm.

p., intraocular. Normal tension within the eyeball, equal to 25 mm. of mercury.

p., intrathoracic. P. within the thorax but outside of the lungs. In quiet expiration it is about — 4.5 mm., and in forced inspiration, as high as — 30 mm., but in quiet inspiration, — 7.5 mm.

p., intraventricular. P. within the ventricles of the heart during different phases of diastole and systole.

p., osmotic. The force with which the solvent passes through a semipermeable septum bet. solutions, which is measured by determining the hydrostatic (mechanical) pressure which must be opposed to the osmotic force to bring the passage to a standstill. The osmotic p. of blood serum and of solutions isotonic* with it is 6.7 atmospheres.

p. palsy. Temporary paralysis due to pressure on a nerve trunk.

p. paralysis. Paralysis due to pressure on the spinal cord.

ETIOL: Injury, tumor, gummata.

p. points. Areas for exerting pressure to control bleeding.

For control of hemorrhage, pressure above bleeding point when an artery passes over a bone may be sufficient. The principal p. points are:

(a) Two inches above clavicle, over common *carotid artery*, backwards, against spine. (b) At side of face in front of ear, over *temporal artery*. (c) Behind mastoid process, over *occipital artery*. (d) Behind clavicle, pressing *subclavian artery* down on to 1st rib. (e) The *axillary artery* by compression in axilla. (f) The *brachial artery* compressed by pressure at inner edge of biceps muscle halfway down arm, and also above bend of elbow, before artery divides into *radial* and *ulnar arteries*. (g) On thumb side of wrist against radius, to compress the radial. (h) On little finger side of wrist against ulna, to compress ulnar. (i) In palm, opp. root of abducted thumb, over deep palmar arch. (j) *Abdominal artery* may be compressed against lumbar vertebrae, to left of middle line, when patient lies on his back. (k) By abduction and ext. rotation of thigh, head of femur is brought forward into groin and *femoral artery* may be compressed against it, in this position. (l) In popliteal space over *popliteal artery*. (m) At front of bend of ankle over *ant. tibial artery*. (n) Behind int. malleolus, over *post. tibial artery*, as it passes into foot.

p., pulse. The difference between systolic and diastolic pressures; normally about 120, —70 equalling 50 mm.

p. sore. A bed* sore, one caused by pressure on a certain area or by a splint. SYN: *decubitus.*

p., systolic. Arterial pressure at time of the contraction of the ventricles; the cardiac systole.

presternum (prē-stẽr'nŭm) [L. *prae*, before, + G. *sternon*, chest]. The upper part of the sternum. SYN: *manubrium, sterni.*

presuppurative (prē-sŭp'ū-rā-tĭv) [" + *sub*, under, + *puris*, pus]. Relating to period of inflammation before suppuration.

presylvian fissure (pre-sĭl'vĭ-ăn) [L. *prae*, before]. The anterior division of the sylvian fissure.

presystole (prē-sĭs'tō-lē) [" + G. *systolē*, contraction]. The period in the heart's cycle just before the systole.

presystolic (prē-sĭs-tol'ĭk) [" + *systolē*, contraction]. Before the systole of the heart.

pretarsal (prē-tar'săl) [" + G. *tarsos*, tarsus]. In front of the tarsus.

pretibial (prē-tĭb'ĭ-ăl) [" + *tibia*, shin]. In front of the tibia.

preurethritis (prē″ū-re-thrī'tĭs) [" + G. *ourēthra*, urethra, + *-itis*, inflammation]. Inflammation around the urethral orifice of the vaginal vestibule.

preventive (prē-věn'tĭv) [L. *praevenīre*, to come before]. Warding off. SYN: *prophylactic.*

p. medicine. That branch of medicine concerned with the prevention of disease.

preventorium (prē-věn-to-rī'ŭm) [L. *praevenīre*, to come before]. An institution for those threatened with tuberculosis.

prevertebral (prē-vẽr'te-brăl) [L. *prae*, before, + *vertebra*, vertebra]. In front of a vertebra.

prevertiginous (prē-ver-tĭj'ĭn-ŭs) [" + *vertigō*, dizziness]. Having a tendency to fall forward. SYN: *dizzy.*

prezymogen (prē-zī'mō-jĕn) [" + G. *zymē*, leaven, + *gennan*, to produce]. A granular substance in the cell nucleus which changes into zymogen when discharged into the cytoplasm. SYN: *prozymogen.*

priapism (prī'ăp-ĭzm) [G. *Priapos*, god of procreation, + *-ismos*, condition]. Abnormal, painful and continued erection of the penis due to disease, usually without sexual desire.

ETIOL: May be due to lesions of the cord above the lumbar region, or turgescence of corpora cavernosa without erection may exist. It may be reflex from peripheral sensory irritants, from organic irritation of nerve tracts or nerve centers when libido may be lacking or from psychical irritation with libido present in satyriasis.

RS: *erection, gonorrhea, satyriasis.*

priapitis (prī-ăp-ī'tĭs) [" + *-itis*, inflammation]. Inflammation of the penis.

prickle cell (prĭk'l). A cell with rod-shaped processes connecting with similar adjoining cells.

p. layer. Outer layer of the epidermal stratum mucosum. SYN: *stratum spinosum.*

prickly heat (prĭk'lĭ hēt). Noncontagious, cutaneous eruption of red pimples, with itching and tingling of the affected parts, seen usually in hot weather.

ETIOL: Inflammation of skin around sweat ducts. SYN: *lichen tropicus, miliaria.*

Priessnitz compress (prēs'nĭtz). A wet cold compress. SEE: *Neptune girdle.*

primae viae (prī'mē vī'ē) [L. first passages]. The alimentary canal; the secondary ones consisting of the lacteals.

primary (prī'mă-rĭ) [L. *primus*, first]. First in time or order. SYN: *principal.*

p. amputation. One before inflammation has set in.

p. bubo. An adenitis, of simple character, of an inguinal gland. SYN: *bubon d'emblée.*

p. cell. PT: A device consisting of a container, 2 solid conducting elements and an electrolyte, for the production of electric current by chemical energy.

p. dementia. A psychosis of youth. SYM: Extreme apathy, listlessness, without perception of environment.

p. hemorrhage. Bleeding at time of an injury.

p. lesion. 1. An original one from which a 2nd one originates. 2. Lesion of syphilis, a chancre.*

p. sore. The initial s. or hard chancre of syphilis.

primate (prī'māt) [L. *primus*, first]. Highest order of Primates, mammals, including man and the apes, monkeys, lemurs and marmosets.

prime (prīm) [L. *primus*, first]. Period of greatest health and strength.

primigravida (prī-mĭ-grăv'ĭ-dă) [" + *gravida*, pregnant]. A woman during her 1st pregnancy.

primipara (prī-mĭp'ă-ră) [" + *parēre*, to bear offspring]. A woman who has had or who is giving birth to her 1st child.

primiparity (prī-mĭp-ăr'ĭt-ĭ) [" + *parēre*, to bear offspring]. Condition of having given birth to only 1 child.

primiparous (prī-mĭp'ă-rŭs) [" + *parēre*, to bear offspring]. Pert. to a primipara, woman giving birth to, or having had, 1st child.

primitiae (prī-mĭsh'ĭ-ē) [L. *primus*, first]. Liquor amnii appearing before the fetus at birth. SEE: *amnion, bag of waters, liquor amnii, labor.*

primitive (prĭm'ĭ-tĭv) [L. *primitivus*, from *primus*, first]. Original; early in point of time; embryonic.

p. groove. The longitudinal depression in the dorsum of the embryonic area opposite the p. streak.

p. streak. The dark line near the posterior extremity of the embryo indicating the first growth of the secondary mesoderm.

primordial (prī-mor'dĭ-ăl) [L. *primordium*, the beginning]. Existing first.

princeps (prĭn'sĕps) [L. *princeps*, chief]. 1. Original; first. 2. A principal artery.

principal (prĭn'sĭ-păl) [L. *princeps, princip-*, chief]. 1. Chief. 2. Outstanding.

principle (prĭn'sĭ-pl) [L. *principium*, foundation]. A constituent of a compound representing its essential properties.

p., proximate. A substance that may be extracted from its complex form

without destroying or altering its chemical properties.
p., ultimate. Any element within a compound body.

priscol (pris'kŏl). A drug used for quick relief of pain, spasm, cramps and tenderness in early stages of poliomyelitis. It promotes rest and quiet sleep at night, and makes possible straightening of arms and legs.

prism (prĭzm) [G. *prisma*]. A solid with sides which are parallelograms whose bases are similar plane figures.

prismoptometer (prĭz-mŏp-tŏm'ĕt-ẽr) [" + *opsis*, vision, + *metron*, measure]. Device for estimating abnormal refraction of the eye by using prisms.

privates (prī'vĕts) [L. *privatus*, peculiar to an individual]. The ext. genitalia of the male or female.

p. r. n. [L. *pro re nata*]. As circumstance may require.

pro- [L. & G.]. Prefix meaning *for, in front of, before, from, in behalf of, on account of*, etc.

proamnion (prō-ăm'nĭ-ŏn) [G. *pro*, before, + *amnion*, amnion]. The primitive amnion, at the cephalic extremity which at first is without the mesoderm.

proband (prō'bănd). One selected as the basis for a genetic or hereditary study as the original one having a physical or mental disorder.

probang (prō'băng). Rod and sponge used in treatment of larynx.
p., foreign body. Web catheterlike tube with circle of bristles or sponge tip for removal of foreign bodies from the esophagus.

probationary (prō-bā'shŭn-ar-ĭ) [L. *probatio*, a trial]. One who is on trial. Waiting, as for admission or for a test.
p. ward. One for the temporary detention of patients suspected of having a communicable disease.

probationer (prō-bā'shŭn-ẽr) [L. *probatio*, a trial]. A person on trial for a time, as a newly admitted student nurse.

probe (prōb) [L. *probāre*, to test]. Slender, flexible rod for exploring suppurative tracts, cavities, or for locating foreign bodies.
VARIETIES: Bullet, bullet-electric, ear, nasal, rectal, urethral, uterine.

procaine hydrochlor'ide (prō'kān). USP. White, colorless, crystalline compound.
ACTION AND USES: A safe local anesthetic said to be less noxious than cocaine. Used like cocaine.
DOSAGE: Subcutaneously (having no effect when applied on the surface), from ½ to 1%. SYN: *novocain*, q.v.

procatarctic (prō"kăt-ark'tĭk) [G. *pro*, before, + *katarchein*, to begin]. Predisposing or inciting, as the cause of a disease.

procatarxis (prō"kăt-ark'sĭs) [" + *katarchein*, to begin]. Inception of a disease through a predisposing cause.

procelous (prō-sē'lŭs) [" + *koilos*, hollow]. Concave anteriorly.

procephalic (prō-sē-făl'ĭk) [" + *kephalē*, a head]. Of or relating to the ant. part of the head.

process (prŏs'ĕs) [L. *processus*, a going before]. 1. A method of action. 2. State of progress of a disease. 3. A projection, as of the extremity of a bone.
p., acromion. Summit of the acromion.
p., alveolar. Thick curved border of either maxilla containing the alveoli.
p., basilar. Narrow part of the base of occipital bone, in front of foramen magnum, articulating with the sphenoid bone. SYN: *pars basilaris*.

p., ensiform. The xiphoid cartilage of the sternum.
p., ethmoidal. A small projection on the upper surface of the inferior turbinated bone which articulates with the uncinate p. of the ethmoid bone.
p., lenticular. A knob on the malleus in the ear which articulates with the stapes.
p., mastoid. Projection of mastoid process of the temporal bone.
p., orbicular. SEE: *p., lenticular*.

processus (prō-sĕs'ŭs) (pl. *processūs*) [L.]. Process or processes.
p. brevis. Short process of the malleus; also, short process of the incus.
p. clavatus. A thickening on posterior pyramid of medulla, near apex of 4th ventricle.
p. cochleariformis. Bony plate bet. the canal for eustachian tube from that of tensor tympani.
p. e cerebello ad medullam. Inf. peduncle of the cerebellum.
p. e cerebello ad pontem. The center peduncles of cerebellum.
p. e cerebello ad testes. Superior cerebellar peduncles.
p. gracilis. The long process below neck of the malleus.
p. hamatus. SEE: *p., uncinnatus processus*.
p. lenticularis. Knob at tip of incus articulating with the stapes.
p. longus. 1. Long process of incus. 2. Long process of malleus.
p. uncinatus. Sickle-shaped 1 on inner surface of the ethmoidal labyrinth.

Prochownick's diet (pro-kŏv'nĭk). A restricted one for women with a narrow pelvis who are pregnant. Carbohydrates and liquids are reduced.

Prochownick's method (artificial respiration). A manner of administering artificial respiration in asphyxia of the newborn by compression of the infant's chest while the head hangs backward.

procidentia (prō-sĭ-dĕn'shĭ-ă) [L. a falling forward]. A complete prolapse, esp. of the uterus which lies outside of the vulva, with inverted vaginal walls.
ETIOL: Generally due to injury of pelvic floor. SEE: *decensus uteri*.

procreate (prō'krē-āt) [L. *prō*, forward, + *creāre*, to create]. To beget; to bring forth young.

procreation (prō"krē-ā'shŭn) [" + *creāre*, to create]. The act or state of bringing forth young. SYN: *reproduction*.

proctagra (prŏk-tag'ră) [G. *prōktos*, anus, + *agra*, seizure]. Sudden rectal pain.

proctalgia (prŏk-tăl'jĭ-ă) [" + *algos*, pain]. Pain in or about the anus and rectum.

proctatresia (prŏk-tăt-rē'zĭ-ă) [" + *a-*, priv. + *trēsis*, perforation]. Imperforate condition of the anus.

proctectomy (prŏk-těk'tō-mĭ) [" + *ektomē*, excision]. Excision of the rectum or anus.
NP: Keep wound clean by irrigating with solution ordered.

proctenclisis (prŏk-těn-klī'sĭs) [" + *egkleiein*, to shut in]. Stricture of the anus or rectum.

procteurynter (prŏk-tū-rĭn'tĕr) [" + *eurynein*, to widen]. Instrument for dilation of the anus or rectum.

proctitis (prŏk-tī'tĭs) [" + *-itis*, inflammation]. Inflammation of rectum and anus. SYN: *bicho, rectitis*.
p., catarrhal, acute and chronic. SYM: Mucus in each stool and some blood, finally dysenteric stool.

p., diphtheritic. Diphtheritic membrane forms over surface of mucous membrane, forms sort of albuminous membrane. Headache, roaring in ears. Constipation, gas, neurasthenia, bloating.

p., dysenteric. May result from ordinary diarrhea, affects upper part the most. May have ulcers, afterwards cicatricial scars.

p., gonorrheal. Gonorrheal infection.

p., traumatic. SYM: Pain, pressure as if bowels were going to move; irritable; mucous membrane red, eroded. Surface tissues sensitive to touch. Chronic constipation.

procto-, proct- [G.]. Combining forms meaning the *anus* and *rectum*.

proctocele (prŏk'tō-sēl) [G. *prōktos*, anus, + *kēlē*, hernia]. A protrusion of the rectal mucosa.

p., vaginal. Prolapsus of the vaginal mucosa.

proctoclysis (prŏk-tŏk'lĭ-sĭs) [" + *klysis*, a washing out]. A continuous injection into the rectum and colon in which the solution is introduced drop by drop.

THERAPEUTIC PURPOSES: (a) To supply fluid in postoperative cases when fluids cannot be taken otherwise. (b) In suppression of kidney functioning, to flush the kidneys and stimulate elimination. (c) To supply the body with fluid as in hemorrhage, vomiting, or in diarrhea. (d) To stimulate the body when in shock, by raising the blood pressure. (e) To relieve thirst as in persistent vomiting. (f) To dilute toxic substance as in septicemia. (g) To promote elimination in infectious conditions. (h) To help prevent or overcome acidosis.

SOLUTIONS USED: The solution usually consists of a normal saline solution, a sodium bicarbonate solution, or plain tap water at body temperature. Normal salt solution half strength is frequently used. This need not be a sterile solution unless so ordered. Sodium bicarbonate of 2% to 5% strength. A glucose solution of 5% to 15% strength may be ordered for its nutritive value. A combination of these may also be ordered: as a normal saline with glucose and sodium bicarbonate, 5% and 2%, respectively, or other combinations may be given as an order.

METHOD: 15-30 drops per minute continuously for 36 hr. SEE: *enteroclysis*.

TEMPERATURE: This should be not less than 105° F. to begin with, although some advocate 118° to 120° F. SYN: *Murphy drip*.

proctococcypexia, proctococcypexy (prŏk"tō-kŏk-sĭ-pĕk'sĭ-ă, -kŏk'sĭ-pĕk"sĭ) [" + *kokkyx*, coccyx, + *pexis*, fixation]. Suture of rectum to the coccyx.

proctocolitis (prŏk"tō-kō-lī'tĭs) [" + *kolon*, colon, + *-itis*, inflammation]. Inflamed condition of colon and rectum.

proctocolonoscopy (prŏk"tō-kō"lŏn-ŏs'kō-pī) [" + *kolon*, colon, + *skopein*, to examine]. Examination of interior of rectum and lower colon.

proctocystotomy (prŏk"tō-sĭs-tŏt'ō-mĭ) [G. *prōktos*, anus, + *kystis*, bladder, + *tomē*, a cutting]. Incision into the bladder through the rectum.

proctodeum (prŏk-tō-dē'ŭm) [" + *daiein*, to divide]. The primitive fold which becomes the anus.

proctodynia (prŏk-tō-dĭn'ĭ-ă) [" + *odynē*, pain]. Pain in the rectum or about the anus.

proctologist (prŏk-tŏl'ō-jĭst) [" + *logos*, a study]. One who specializes in diseases of the rectum and anus.

proctology (prŏk-tŏl'ō-jĭ) [" + *logos*, a study]. Phase of medicine dealing with treatment of diseases of rectum and anus.

proctoparalysis (prŏk-tō-păr-ăl'ĭs-ĭs) [" + *para*, at the side, + *lyein*, to loosen]. Paralysis of the anal sphincter muscle.

proctopexia, proctopexy (prŏk-tō-pĕks'ĭ-ă, prŏk'tō-pĕks"ĭ) [" + *pexis*, fixation]. Suture of the rectum to some other part.

proctophobia (prŏk"tō-fō'bĭ-ă) [G. *prōktos*, anus, + *phobos*, fear]. Abnormal apprehension in those suffering from rectal disease.

proctoplasty (prŏk'tō-plăs-tĭ) [" + *plastos*, formed]. Plastic surgery of the anus or rectum.

proctoplegia (prŏk"tō-plē'jĭ-ă) [" + *plēgē*, a stroke]. Paralysis of the anal sphincter. SYN: *proctoparalysis*.

proctoptosis (prŏk-tŏp-tō'sĭs) [" + *ptōsis*, a dropping]. Prolapse of the rectum. SEE: *procidentia*.

proctorrhaphy (prŏk-tŏr'ă-fī) [" + *raphē*, a sewing]. Suturing of rectum or anus.

proctorrhea (prŏk-tŏr-ē'ă) [" + *roia*, a flow]. Mucous discharge from the anus.

proctoscope (prŏk'tō-skōp) [" + *skopein*, to examine]. Instrument for inspection of the rectum.

proctoscopy (prŏk-tŏs'kō-pĭ) [G. *prōktos*, anus, + *skopein*, to examine]. Instrumental inspection of the rectum.

proctosigmoiditis (prŏk"tō-sĭg-moyd-ī'tĭs) [" + *sigma*, letter S, + *eidos*, form, + *-itis*, inflammation]. Inflamed condition of the rectum and sigmoid.

proctospasm (prŏk'tō-spăzm) [" + *spasmos*, a contracting]. Rectal spasm.

proctostenosis (prŏk"tō-stĕn-ō'sĭs) [" + *stēnōsis*, a narrowing]. Stricture of the anus or rectum.

proctostomy (prŏk-tŏs'tō-mĭ) [" + *stoma*, a mouth]. Creation of a permanent opening into the rectum.

proctotome (prŏk'tō-tōm) [" + *tomē*, a cutting]. Knife for incision into rectum.

proctotomy (prŏk-tŏt'ō-mĭ) [" + *tomē*, a cutting]. Incision of the rectum or anus.

POSITION: Simon's.

DRESSING: Iodoform gauze, T-bandage.

proctotoreusis (prŏk-tō-tō-rū'sĭs) [" + *toreusis*, boring]. The making of an opening in an imperforate anus.

proctovalvotomy (prŏk-tō-văl-vŏt'ō-mĭ) [" + L. *valva*, valve, + G. *tomē*, a cutting]. Incision of the rectal valves.

procumbent (prō-kŭm'bĕnt) [L. *procumbere*, to lean forward]. Lying face down.

procursive (prō-kŭr'sĭv) [L. *procursivus*, running forward]. Having an involuntary tendency to run forward, as in p. epilepsy.

prodromal (prŏd'rō-măl) [G. *prōdromos*, running before]. Pert. to the initial stage of a disease; the interval bet. the earliest symptoms and the appearance of the rash or fever.

p. rash. One that precedes the true rash of an infectious disease.

prodrome (prō'drŏm) [G. *prōdromos*, running before]. A symptom indicative of an approaching disease.

product (prŏd'ŭkt) [L. *producere*, to beget]. Anything which is made naturally or artificially. SEE: *catabolin, catabolite*.

production (prō-dŭk'shŭn) [L. *productiō*, a begetting, a formation]. Development or formation of a substance. SEE: *chromoparic*.

productive (prō-dŭk'tĭv) [L. *producere*, to beget]. Forming, as new tissue.

p. inflammation. Inflammation pro-

proenzyme

ducing new tissue with or without an exudate.

proenzyme (prō-ĕn'zīm) [G. *prō*, before, + *en*, in, + *zymē*, a leaven]. 1. Substance from which an enzyme is derived. 2. Microörganism causing fermentation. SYN: *zymogen*.

proferment (prō-fer'měnt) [" + L. *fermentum*, leaven]. 1. Substance which develops into an enzyme. 2. Microörganism causing fermentation.

professional (prō-fĕsh'ŭn-ăl) [L. *professio*, from *profiteri*, to profess]. 1. Pert. to a profession. 2. Caused by the practice of a profession, as *writer's cramp*.

proflavine powder (prō-flā'vĭn). A powder used for dusting wounds, apparently overcoming infection where sulfanilamide fails.

profondometer (prō-fŏn-dŏm'ĕt-ēr) [L. *profundus*, deep, + G. *metron*, a measure]. Device for locating a foreign body with the fluoroscope.

progeny (prŏj'ĕn-ĭ) [L. *progeniēs*, offspring]. Offspring.

progeria (prō-jē'rĭ-ă) [G. *pro*, before, + *gēras*, old age]. Premature senility supervening upon infantilism. Rare.
ETIOL: Unknown.
SYM: Skin becomes loosened and wrinkled, baldness is common, and arteries become hardened.

progesterone (prō-jĕs'tĕr-ōn). The hormone found in corpora lutea which prepares the endometrium for nidation of the embryo.
It has been used successfully in treatment of spasmodic rhinorrhea to reduce congestion and discharge.

progestin (prō-jĕs'tĭn). A corpus luteum hormone which prepares the endometrium for the fertilized ovum. SYN: *progesterone*.

proglossis (prō-glŏs'ĭs) [G. *pro*, before, + *glōssa*, tongue]. The tip of the tongue.

prognathism (prŏg'nă-thĭzm) [" + *gnathos*, jaw, + *ismos*, condition]. Projection of jaws beyond upper face.

prognathous (prŏg'năth-ŭs) [" + *gnathos*, jaw]. Having jaws projecting forward beyond rest of the face.

prognosis (prŏg-nō'sĭs) [G. *prognōsis*, foreknowledge]. Prediction of course and end of disease, and outlook based on it.
p. anceps. Doubtful prognosis.
p. fausta. Favorable prognosis.
p. infausta. Unfavorable prognosis.

prognostic (prŏg-nŏs'tĭk) [G. *prognōsis*, foreknowledge]. Affording an indication as to outcome of a disease.

prognosticate (prŏg-nŏs'tĭ-kāt) [G. *prognōstikon*, knowing before]. To make a statement on the probable outcome of an illness.

progonasyl (prō-gō-nă'zĭl) [Gr. *pro*, before, + *gōnē*, sexual]. A medicinal vegetable and mineral oil containing an emulsifier and iodine, used to spread over vaginal tissues as a preventive against venereal disease for both sexes.

progressive (prō-grĕs'ĭv) [L. *progressus*, stepping forward]. Advancing.
p. muscular atrophy. Gradual advancing atrophy of groups of muscles due to spinal cord degeneration. SEE: *atrophy*.
p. ossifying myositis. Tendency to bony deposits in the muscles with chronic inflammation.

progynon (prō'jĭn-ŏn). Commercial preparation of female sex hormone extracted from the placenta.

proiosystole (prō-ĭ-ō-sĭs'tō-lē) [G. *prōi*, early, + *systolē*, contraction]. A cardiac contraction occurring before its normal time.

proiosystolia (prō-ĭ-ō-sĭs-tō'lĭ-ă) [" + *systolē*, contraction]. A condition marked by occurrence of systoles before the normal time.

proiotia (prō-ĭ-ō'shĭ-ă) [G. *prōi*, early]. Genital precocity.

projectile vomiting. Vomiting not preceded by nausea in which the stomach contents are forcibly ejected.
Seen in some cerebral diseases and in pyloric obstruction.

projection (prō-jĕk'shŭn) [L. *pro*, forward, + *jacere*, to throw]. 1. The act of throwing forward. 2. A part extending beyond the level of its surroundings. 3. PSY: Distortion of a perception as a result of its repression, resulting in such a phenomenon as hating without cause one who has been dearly loved, seen in paranoiac delusions of persecution.
p., erroneous. Inability to correctly judge the position of an object due to weak ocular muscles.

prolabium (prō-lā'bĭ-ŭm) [L. *pro*, forward, + *labium*, lip]. The exposed ext. red border of the lip.

prolactin (prō-lăk'tĭn) [" + *lac*, milk]. Hormone, derived from the ant. pituitary lobe, which stimulates lactation. SYN: *galactin, mammotropin*.

prolamin(e (prō-lăm'ĭn, prō'lă-mĭn). Any one of a class of proteins found in seeds, soluble in alcohol, and insoluble in water and absolute alcohol. SYN: *gliadin*.

prolan (prō'lan). A hormone from the ant. pituitary body. It consists of:
p. A. Which stimulates the ovary to formation of ripe graafian follicles and the secretion of estrin, and
p. B. Which acts on the ovary to stimulate the formation of progestin by the corpora lutea. SEE: *hormone, prolactin*.

prolapse (prō-lăps') [L. *pro*, before, + *lapsus*, from *labi*, to fall]. 1. A dropping of an int. part of the body, as of the uterus or rectum. 2. To drop down, noted of an organ. SYN: *ptosis*.
p. of the cord. Expulsion of umbilical cord prematurely. SEE: *labor*.
p. of rectum. Seen in children under 3 years of age. Sometimes in old people.
ETIOL: Probably poor development of muscles of the pelvic floor and ext. sphincter. May be associated with constipation, phimosis, rectal polypus, or threadworms.
SYM: Lining of rectum stretches on straining at stool and is separated from its muscular coat. When sphincter grows weaker condition becomes permanent. Blood and mucus pass, control is lost; continual irritation causes soreness.

prolapsus (prō-lăp'sŭs) [L. a dropping]. A falling or downward displacement of some part of the body, as the uterus.
p. ani. Dropping down of the anus.
p. uteri. Dropping down of the uterus. SYN: *descensus uteri*.

prolepsis (prō-lĕp'sĭs) [G. *pro*, before, + *lēpsis*, a seizure]. Return of paroxysmal attacks at successively shorter intervals.

proleptic (prō-lĕp'tĭk) [" + *lēpsis*, a seizure]. Recurring before the time expected, said of paroxysms.

proleukemia (prō-lū-kē'mĭ-ă) [" + *leukos*, white, + *an-*, negative, + *aima*, blood]. A condition marked by both leukemia and pernicious anemia. SYN: *leukanemia*.

proleukocyte (prō-lū'kō-sīt) [" + " + *kytos*, cell]. An undeveloped leukocyte. SYN: *leukoblast*.

proliferate (prō-lĭf'ĕr-āt) [L. *proles*, offspring, + *ferre*, to bear]. To increase by reproduction of similar forms.
proliferation (prō-lĭf"ĕr-ā'shŭn) [" + *ferre*, to bear]. 1. Reproduction rapidly and repeatedly of new parts, as by cell division. 2. Process or result of rapid reproduction. SEE: *auxesis*.
proliferous (prō-lĭf'ĕr-ŭs) [" + *ferre*, to bear]. 1. Multiplying, as by formation of new tissue cells. 2. Bearing offspring.
  p. cyst. One with epithelial lining, proliferating and projecting from inner surface of the cyst.
prolific (prō-lĭf'ĭk) [" + *facere*, to make]. Fruitful; reproductive. SYN: *fertile*.
proligerous (prō-lĭj'ĕr-ŭs) [" + *gerere*, to bear]. Producing offspring. SYN: *germinating*.
  p. disk. Collection of cells of the graafian vesicle surrounding the ovum. SYN: *discus proligerous*.
prolin(e (prō'lēn, -lĭn). An important amino acid, formed by protein decomposition, having the formula: $C_4H_9N.$-$COOH$.
promegaloblast (prō"mĕg'ăl-ō-blăst) [G. *pro*, before, + *megas, megal-*, large, + *blastos*, germ]. A cell intervening bet. a megaloblast and a lymphoidocyte.
promin (prō'mĭn). Commercial preparation of follicular sex hormone.
prominentia (prŏm-ĭn-ĕn'shĭ-ă) [L.]. A projection.
  p. laryngea. BNA. The laryngeal prominence; Adam's apple. SYN: *pomum adami*.
promontory (prŏm'ŭn-tō-rĭ) [L. *promontorium*, a projection]. A projecting process or part.
  p. of the sacrum. P. between upper extremity of the sacrum and 5th lumbar vertebra.
promyelocyte (prō"mī'ĕl-ō-sīt) [G. *pro*, before, + *myelos*, marrow, + *kytos*, cell]. 1. A large mononuclear myeloid cell seen in the blood in leukemia. 2. Cell development bet. myeloblast and a myelocyte, resembling a myeloblast.
pronation (prō-nā'shŭn) [L. *pronāre*, to bend forward]. The act of lying with face downward, or having the palms face downward. The opp. of *supine*.
pronaus (prō'nă-ŭs) [G. *pro*, before, + *naos*, temple]. The vestibule of the vagina.
prone (prōn) [L. *pronāre*, to bend forward]. Lying horizontal, with face downward; of the hand, with the palms turned downward. OPP: *supine*.
pronephron, pronephros (prō-nĕf'rŏn, -rŏs) [G. *pro*, before, + *nephros*, kidney]. The primitive kidney. SEE: *wolffian duct*.
pronograde (prō'nō-grād) [L. *pronāre*, to bend forward, + *gradus*, a step]. Walking on hands and feet or resting with the body in a horizontal position. OPP: *orthograde*.
pronometer (prō-nŏm'ĕt-ĕr) [" + G. *metron*, a measure]. Device for showing amount of pronation or supination of forearm. [fanilamide derivative.
prontosil (prŏn'tō-sĭl). A less toxic sulUSES: Same as sulfanilamide, *q.v.*
prontylin (prŏn'tĭl-ĭn). A commercial brand of sulfanilamide, *q.v.*
pronucleus (prō-nū'klē-ŭs) [L. *pro*, before, + *nucleus*, nut]. Nucleus of the ovum, the female p., or of the spermatozoon, the male p., after the fertilization of the ovum.
proötic (prō-ŏt'ĭk, -ō'tĭk) [G. *pro*, before, + *ous, ot-*, ear]. In front of the ear.
propagation (prŏp-ă-gā'shŭn) [L. *propagāre*, to fasten forward]. Act of reproducing or giving birth. SYN: *generation*, *reproduction*.
propagative (prŏp'ă-gā-tĭv) [L. *propagāre*, to fasten forward]. Pert. to or taking part in reproduction.
propalinal (prō-păl'ĭn-ăl) [G. *pro*, before, + *palin*, back]. Applied to a backward and forward movement, as of the jaws.
prop cells (prŏp). 1. Nerve cells bet. the granular and molecular layers of the cerebellar cortex. SYN: *Purkinje's cells*. 2. Columnar or fusiform cells bet. rods and hair cells of the organ of Corti. SYN: *Deiter's cells*.
propeptone (prō-pĕp'tōn) [G. *pro*, before, + *peptein*, to digest]. An intermediate product in the digestive conversion of protein into peptone. SYN: *hemialbumose*.
propeptonuria (prō"pĕp-tō-nū'rĭ-ă) [" + *ouron*, urine]. Excretion of propeptone in the urine. SYN: *hemialbumosuria*.
properdin. SEE: p. P-132.
prophase (prō'fāz) [G. *pro*, before, + *phasis*, an appearance]. First stage of indirect cell division.
  SEE: *centriole*, "*meta-*" words, *mitosis*, "*tele-*" words.
prophylactic (prō-fĭl-ăk'tĭk) [G. *prophylaktikos*, guarding]. 1. Warding off dis-

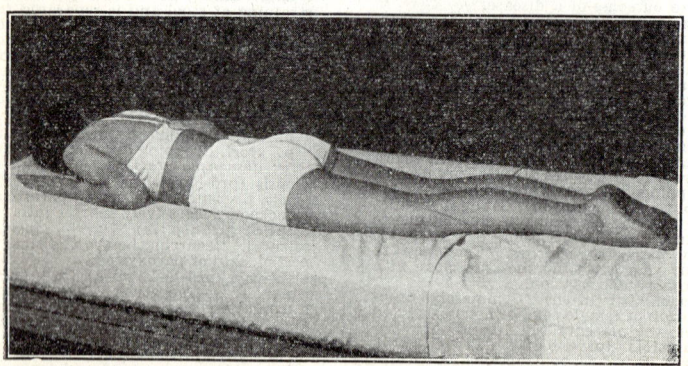

Posed by professional model   PRONE POSITION.   *Photo by Whitaker*

ease. 2. Agent which wards off disease.

prophylaxis (prō-fĭl-ăks'ĭs) [G. *prophylassein*, to guard against]. 1. Observance of rules necessary to prevent disease. 2. In dentistry, cleansing of the teeth's surface.

proplex, proplexus (prō'plĕks, prō-plĕk'sŭs) [L. *pro*, before, + *plexus*, a braid, a network]. The choroid plexus of the lateral ventricles of the cerebrum.

propons (prō'pŏnz) [" + *pons*, bridge]. White fibers passing transversely across the ant. margin of the pyramid and just below the pons Varolii. SYN: *ponticulus*.

proposote (prō'pō-sōt). A condensation product containing 50% creosote.
ACTION AND USES: Same as creosote.
DOSAGE: 5-10 ♏ (0.3-0.6 cc.).

proprietary medicine (prō-prī'ĕ-tar'ĭ) [L. *proprietarius*, pert. to property]. "Any chemical, drug or similar preparation used in the treatment of diseases, if such article is protected against free competition, as to name, product, composition or process of manufacture, by secrecy, patent or copyright, or by another means." *American Medical Association*. SEE: *patent medicine*.

proprioceptive (prō"prī-ō-sĕp'tĭv) [L. *proprius*, one's own, + *ceptus*, from *capere*, to take]. Noting impulses from afferent nerves in an organism stimulated by its own tissues.

proprioceptor (prō"prī-ō-sep'tor) [" + *ceptor*, a receiver, from *capere*, to take]. A receptor stimulated by action of the organism itself. SEE: *receptor*.

proptometer (prŏp-tŏm'ĕt-ĕr) [G. *proptōsis*, protrusion, + *metron*, a measure]. An instrument for measuring extent of exophthalmos.

proptosis (prŏp-tō'sĭs) [G. *proptōsis*, protrusion]. A downward displacement, as of the uterus or of the eyeball in exophthalmic goiter, or in inflammatory conditions of the orbit.

propulsion (prō-pŭl'shŭn) [L. *propulsus*, from *propellere*, to force forward]. 1. A tendency to push or fall forward in walking. 2. A condition seen in paralysis agitans. SEE: *festination*.

propylthiouracil (prō"pĭl-thī-ō-ū'ră-sĭl). Antithyroid drug used in treatment of hyperthyroidism, thyroiditis, and thyrotoxicosis. Also employed for preoperative therapy and in cases where surgery is contraindicated.
DOSAGE: *Severe hyperthyroidism*, 50 mg. every 8 hours. *Milder hyperthyroidism*, 50 mg. twice daily.

pro re nata (prō rā nah'tă) [L.]. According to the circumstances.

prorennin (prō-rĕn'ĭn) [L. *pro*, before, + *rennin*]. The preliminary material which is converted into rennin. SYN: *mother substance, renninogen, zymogen*.

prorsad (pror'săd) [L. *prorsum*, forward]. Toward the anterior or front.

prosecretin (prō"sē-kre'tĭn) [L. *pro*, before, + *secretiō*, a secretion]. Preliminary substance which develops into secretin.
It is secreted by the mucosa of small intestines and stimulates the digestive glands and activates their secretions. Prosecretin is converted into active secretin by the hydrochloric acid of the chyme.

prosector (prō-sĕk'tor) [" + *sector*, from *secāre*, to cut]. One who prepares cadavers for dissection or dissects for demonstration.

prosencephalon (prŏs-ĕn-sef'ăl-ŏn) [G. *pros*, before, + *egkephalos*, brain]. Part of embryonic brain from which arise the cerebral hemispheres, corpora striata, corpus callosum, olfactory lobes and the fornix. SYN: *forebrain*.

prosodemic (prŏs-ō-dĕm'ĭk) [G. *prosō*, forward, + *dēmos*, people]. Spread by individual contact; said of a disease.

prosogaster (prŏs-ō-găs'tĕr) [" + *gastēr*, belly]. Embryonic forerunner of the digestive tract. SYN: *foregut*.

prosopalgia (prŏs-ō-păl'jĭ-ă) [G. *prosōpon*, face, + *algos*, pain]. Neuralgic pain in the trigeminal nerve and its branches. SYN: *prosopodynia*.

prosopantritis (prŏs-ō-păn-trī'tĭs) [" + *antron*, a hollow, + -*itis*, inflammation]. Inflamed condition of the frontal sinuses.

prosopectasia (prŏs"ō-pĕk-tā'zĭ-ă) [" + *ektasis*, dilatation]. Abnormal size of the face.

prosoplasia (prŏs"ō-plā'zĭ-ă) [G. *prosō*, forward, + *plassein*, to form]. 1. Progressive cellular changes toward a more complex state. 2. Unusual cell differentiation beyond the normal.

prosopodiplegia (prŏs"ō-pō-dī-plē'jĭ-ă) [G. *prosōpon*, face, + *dis*, double, + *plēgē*, a stroke]. Paralysis of 1 lower extremity and the face.

prosopodynia (prŏs"ō-pō-dĭn'ĭ-ă) [" + *odynē*, pain]. Pain in the face. SYN: *tic douloureux*.

prosoponeuralgia (prŏs"ō-pō-nū-răl'jĭ-ă) [" + *neuron*, sinew, + *algos*, pain]. Facial neuralgia. SYN: *prosopalgia*.

prosopoplegia (prŏs"ō-pō-plē'jĭ-ă) [" + *plēgē*, stroke]. Paralysis of the face.

prosopoplegic (prŏs"ō-pō-plē'jĭk) [" + *plēgē*, a stroke]. Relating to, or afflicted with, facial paralysis.

prosoposchisis (prŏs-ō-pŏs'kĭ-sĭs) [" + *schisis*, a cleft]. Congenital cleft of the face.

prosopospasm (prŏs"ō-pō-spazm) [" + *spasmos*, a spasm]. Facial spasm.

prosopotocia (prŏs"ō-pō-tō'shĭ-ă) [" + *tokos*, birth]. Presentation of the face in parturition.

prostatalgia (prŏs-tă-tal'jĭ-ă) [G. *prostatēs*, prostate, + *algos*, pain]. Pain of the prostate gland.

prostatauxe (pros-tat-awks'e). Enlargement of the prostate gland.

prostate (prŏs'tāt) [G. *prostatēs*]. A male body, partly glandular, partly muscular, surrounding proximal portion of the male urethra and the neck of the bladder, consisting of a median lobe and 2 lateral lobes, the glandular matter emptying through ducts into the post. urethra, and the muscular fibers encircling the urethra.

FUNCTION: The secretion of the prostatic fluid, 1 of the seminal fluids. It is about the size of a horse chestnut, weighing about 25 Gm. Often affected by gonorrhea, and frequently enlarges after middle age, closing down upon the urethra and causing slow urination. It may impede it altogether.
Retention may cause urine to back up and seriously affect the kidneys. About 40-50% of all men over 60 have prostatic trouble.

TREATMENT: Enlarged prostate frequently treated through the rectum with finger massage. Electrosurgery is also employed, through the urethra. Extirpation sometimes resorted to.
Injection of artificially prepared chemicals and the use of some by inunction have had some favorable results. In prostatic obstruction, transurethral

prostatic resection has been utilized favorably.

RS: *endocrine, generation, organs of male, gland, "prostat-" words, semen.*

prostatectomy (prŏs-tă-tĕk'tō-mĭ) [G. *prostatēs*, prostate, + *ektomē*, excision]. Excision of part or all of the prostate gland.

The operation procedure is same as that for the cystotomy. In this operation some operators control hemorrhage with packs 4 in. wide and 2 yd. long. These pads are dipped in a small sterile dish filled with thromboplastin.

NP: It is very essential that these packs be made with edges turned in and sewed together, otherwise a thread of gauze may be left behind. Raw edged gauze should never be used in the bladder, nor in fact at any time by the operating surgeon.

COMPLICATIONS: Retention of urine, hematuria, cystitis, infection of kidney, pyelitis, infective nephritis, renal failure.

prostatic (prŏs-tăt'ĭk) [G. *prostatēs*, prostate]. Concerning the prostate gland.

p. calculus. A stone in the prostate.

p. plexus. 1. Veins around the base and neck of the bladder and prostate gland. 2. Nerves from the pelvic plexus to the prostate gland, erectile tissue of the penis, and to the seminal vesicles.

p. urethra. Part of the urethra surrounded by the prostate gland.

prostatism (prŏs'tă-tĭzm) [G. *prostatēs*, prostate, + *-ismos*, condition]. Condition induced by chronic prostatic disease.

Usually due to a hormone hyperplasia or a sclerotic condition of the prostate causing obstruction to the outflow of urine through the urethra and attended by a morbid state of mind.

prostatitis (prŏs-tă-tī'tĭs) [" + *-itis*, inflammation]. Inflamed condition of the prostate gland.

May be a complication of gonorrheal infection.

p., acute. Discomfort and pain in perineal area. Frequent urination; later, retention of urine. If severe, marked malaise, rise of temperature, constipation, thirst, furred tongue, rigors and vomiting.

p., chronic. Dull, aching pain in perineal region. Discharge from the penis.

prostatocystitis (prŏs″tăt-ō-sĭs-tī'tĭs) [G. *prostatēs*, prostate, + *kystis*, bladder, + *-itis*, inflammation]. Inflammation of the prostatic urethra involving the bladder.

prostatocystotomy (prŏs″tăt-ō-sĭs-tŏt'ō-mĭ) [" + " + *tomē*, a cutting]. Surgical incision of the prostate and the bladder.

prostatodynia (prŏs″tăt-ō-dĭn'ĭ-ă) [" + *odynē*, pain]. Pain in the prostate gland. SYN: *prostatalgia*.

prostatomegaly (prŏs″tăt-ō-mĕg'ăl-ĭ) [" + *megas, megal-*, large]. Enlargement of the prostate gland.

prostatometer (prŏs-tăt-ŏm'ĕt-ĕr) [" + *metron*, a measure]. Device for measuring enlargement of the prostate.

prostatomyomectomy (prŏs″tăt-ō-mī-ō-mĕk-tō-mĭ) [" + *mys, my-*, muscle, + *ektomē*, excision]. Surgical excision of a prostatic myoma.

prostatomy (prŏs-tăt'ō-mĭ) [" + *tomē*, a cutting]. Incision into the prostate.

prostatorrhea (prŏs-tăt-or-rē'ă) [G. *prostatēs*, prostate, + *roia*, flow]. Abnormal discharge from the prostate gland.

prostatotomy (prŏs-tă-tŏt'ō-mĭ) [" + *tomē*, a cutting]. Incision into prostate gland.

prostatovesiculectomy (prŏs″tăt-ō-vĕs-ĭk″-ū-lĕk'tō-mĭ) [" + L. *vesiculus*, a little sac, + G. *ektomē*, excision]. Removal of the prostate gland and seminal vesicles.

prostatovesiculitis (prŏs″tăt-ō-vĕs-ĭk-ū-lī'tĭs) [" + " + G. *-itis*, inflammation]. Inflammation of the seminal vesicles and prostate gland.

prosternation (prō-stĕr-nā'shŭn) [G. *pro*, before, + *sternon*, chest]. Habitual flexion of the trunk forward. SYN: *camptocormia*.

prostheon (prŏs'thē-ŏn) [G. *prosthios*, foremost]. The alveolar point; midpoint of lower border of upper alveolar arch.

prosthesis (prŏs'thē-sĭs) [G. *pros*, to, + *thesis*, a placing]. 1. Replacement of a missing part by an artificial substitute. 2. An artificial organ or part.

p., dental. Mechanical dentistry.

p., maxillofacial. Repair and artificial replacements of face and jaw.

p., paraffin. Subcutaneous injection of paraffin to restore the natural contour of a part or to replace cartilaginous part of the nasal septum.

prosthetics (prŏs-thĕt'ĭks) [" + *thesis*, a placing]. The making and application of an artificial part to remedy a want or defect of the body, as a wooden leg.

prosthetist (prŏs'thē-tĭst) [" + *thesis*, a placing]. 1. Specialist in artificial dentures. 2. Maker of artificial limbs.

prosthodontist (prŏs-thō-dŏn'tĭst) [" + " + *odous, odont-*, tooth]. A dentist who specializes in the mechanics of making and fitting artificial teeth.

prostigmin (prō-stĭg'mĕn). Registd. trademark for a brand of neostigmine; a synthetic parasympathetic stimulant for oral and parenteral use.

Recently used in cases of simple glaucoma and in acute and chronic deafness, and in trigeminal neuralgia.

p. bromide. USES: Orally, for the treatment of myasthenia gravis. USP. Syn: *neostigmine b*.

DOSAGE: 0.015 Gm.

p. methylsulfate. USES: For prevention and treatment of postoperative distention. USP. Syn: *neostigmine methylsulfate*.

DOSAGE: For prophylactic, 1 cc. 1-4000; for treatment, 1 cc. 1-2000 solution.

prostitution (prŏs-tĭ-tū'shŭn) [L. *prostituere*, to prostitute]. Profession practiced, esp. by women, in which sexual gratification is exchanged for hire.

Said to be the oldest profession. Although not engaged in it as a profession, the woman who, without affection, accepts money, gifts, or maintenance in exchange for sexual gratification prostitutes her body.

It is a neurosis found esp. in the hypothyroid, hypoadrenal female, generally of low intelligence and without culture. The prostitute, however, may be of either sex, the male prostitute being inf. to the female. Many female prostitutes have a father fixation complex. SEE: *parent-fixation*.

prostration (prŏs-trā'shŭn) [L. *prostratus*, spreading before]. Absolute exhaustion.

p., nervous. General physical and nervous exhaustion. SYN: *neurasthenia*.

protagon (prō'tăg-ŏn) [G. *prōtos*, first, + *agein*, to lead]. White, crystalline mixture of lipids obtained from the brain.

protamine (prō'tă-mĕn) [" + *amine*]. One

of a class of simple proteins which are strongly basic, noncoagulable in heat and yield diamino acids when hydrolyzed.
Found in fish sperm and named from the fish from which it is derived. SEE: *clupeine, salmine, sturine.*

p. insulin, p. zinc insulin. Preparations of insulin which are more slowly dissolved and absorbed by body tissues than ordinary insulin. Act longer and keep the blood sugar normal for 20 to 24 hr. One injection is sufficient for this period.

protan (prō'tăn). A chemical combination of casein and tannic acid, containing 50% tannic acid.
USES: Intestinal astringent, in diarrhea.
DOSAGE: For children, 5 to 10 gr. (0.3-0.6 Gm.).

protanopia (prō-tăn-ō'pĭ-ă) [G. *prōtos*, first, + *an-*, negative, + *opsis*, vision]. Defect in color vision in which there is condition of red blindness.

protargol (prō-tar'gŏl). A compound of silver albumose containing approximately 8% silver.
USES: Antiseptic, for use in local infections.
DOSAGE: For application to mucous membrane from 0.5% to 2%.
INCOMPATIBILITIES: Alcohol, ferric chloride, mercuric chloride.

protean (prō'tē-ăn) [G. *Prōteus*, a god who changed shapes at will]. Having the ability to change form, as the ameba. 2. [G. *prōtos*, first]. One of the primary derivatives of protein resulting from action of water, enzymes or dilute acids.

protease (prō'tē-as) [G. *prōtos*, first, + *ase*, enzyme]. A protein-splitting enzyme.*

protectin (prō-tĕk'tĭn) [L. *protectus*, shielding]. A substance in blood serum protecting corpuscles against a hemolytic action.

protective (prō-tĕk'tĭv) [L. *protectus*, shielding]. 1. Covering or guarding. 2. An agent that will mechanically protect the part to which applied. Ex: *collodion, plaster.* SYN: *dressing.*

proteid (prō'tē-ĭd) [G. *prōtos*, first]. One of a class of constituents essential to all living organisms. SYN: *protein, q.v.*

proteidin (prō'tē-ĭd-ĭn) [G. *prōtos*, first]. A bacteriolytic substance formed in the body.

proteidogenous (prō'tē-ĭd-ŏj'ĕn-ŭs) [" + *gennan*, to produce]. Producing proteins.

protein (prō'tē-ĭn, prō'tēn) [G. *prōtos*, first]. One of a class of nitrogenous compounds which occur naturally, give amino acids when hydrolyzed, and are essential to all living organisms.
The following classification suggests the nature of the substances in this group:

p., conjugated. Those containing the protein molecule with some other molecule or molecules. *Chromoproteins*: Ex: hemoglobin. *Glycoproteins*: Ex: mucin. *Lecithoproteins*: Compounds of lecithins or similar substances with the protein molecule. *Nucleoproteins. Phosphoproteins*: Ex: casein.

p., derived. The product of hydrolytic changes of the protein molecule with only slight alteration. Primary derivatives include: (a) *Proteans;* (b) *metaproteins;* (c) *coagulated proteins*, and secondary derivatives representing further cleavage include: *proteoses, peptones* and *peptides.*

COMPOSITION: Proteins are composed of carbon, hydrogen, oxygen, nitrogen, phosphorus, sulfur, and iron which make up the greater part of plant and animal tissue. Amino acids represent the elements in proteins, 22 of which may be combined to form various proteins. Different protein foods contain a different number and kind of amino acids and more than 1 kind of nitrogen. Complete proteins are those containing all the amino acids necessary to the body.

Proteins consist of the following: (1) *Albumins* (1% of the body). Ex: (a) Albumen (white of egg); (b) serum albumin (in blood); (c) lactalbumin (in milk). Soluble in cold water, but coagulated on heating; then no longer dissolved by hot or cold water. Coagulated albumins are rendered soluble in the stomach by peptase, being changed at the same time into albumoses and peptones. (2) *Globulins*: Ex: (a) Serum globulin (in blood); (b) myosin (in muscle); (c) crystallin (in the eye); (d) ovoglobulin (in egg yolk). These are not soluble in water alone, but in weak solutions of salt. (3) *Albumoses* and *peptones*: Products of the digestive secretions acting upon albumins and other proteins. Soluble in water. (4) *Coagulated proteins*: Ex: fibrin (in blood). Fibrin is derived from fibrinogen and clots the blood when it is exposed to the air.

FUNCTIONS: Proteins furnish heat and energy to the body; they repair worn out or waste tissue, and build new tissue.
They are oxidized in the body, thus liberating heat. One Gm. supplies 4 calories of heat. It is said that 0.65 Gm. of protein will care for the wear of 1 kilogram of body tissue or body weight. That amount is the minimum requirement as a basal protein level.

Children require from 2 to 3 Gm. per kilogram of body weight. Weight should always be calculated at the normal level. Age also is a factor in determining protein requirements, the amount decreasing with the age. Physical work demands increased protein requirement, as is the case during menstruation, lactation, and convalescence. Excess protein in the diet means an elimination of nitrogen through the urine.

SOURCES: Milk, eggs, cheese, and meat are the best sources. Proteins are found in both vegetable and animal forms. The principal animal proteins are ovalbumin in eggs, lactoalbumin in milk, serumalbumin in serum, myogen or myosinogen in striated muscle tissue, crystallins found in the lens of the eye, fibrinogen in blood clots, ovoglobulin in eggs, lactoglobulin in milk, serumglobulin in serum, myosin in striated muscle tissue, thyreoglobulin in thyroid, globin in blood, thymus histones in thymus, collagen and gelatin in connective tissue, elastin and keratin. Nucleoprotein is found in the thymus, pancreas, liver, animal cells and glands; chondroprotein is found in tendons and cartilage; mucin and mucoids are found in various secreting glands and animal mucilaginous substances; caseinogen in milk; vitellin in egg yolk; hemoglobin in blood, and lecithoprotein in blood, brain and bile.

Blood proteins are determined on blood plasma. Normal value for total protein, about 7.5%; albumin, 4.5%; globulin,

2.5%; fibrinogen, 0.5%. The amount of albumin in proportion to the amount of globulin is referred to as the *albuminglobulin* ratio. Decrease of the plasma proteins is called *hypoproteinemia*. Increase above the normal is unimportant.
p. high diet. 1.5-2 Gm. pro. per kg. ideal body weight.
p. low diet. 0.65 Gm. pro. per kg. ideal body weight. Supplied by means of pro. of good biological value.
p. sensitization. Condition in which patient is hypersensitive to foreign proteins, so that severe reaction occurs upon their administration.
p. shock therapy. Introduction into the body of a nonspecific protein substance, such as milk, egg albumin, or whole blood in treatment of disease. Sometimes used in rheumatoid arthritis, disseminated sclerosis, gonorrhea and syphilis.
p., simple. Those which produce alpha amino acids on hydrolysis. *Albumins*: Soluble in water and coagulated by heat. Ex: egg albumen. *Globulins*: Insoluble in water, soluble in salt solutions, coagulated by heat. Ex: edestin, from hemp seed. *Glutelins. Prolamines* (alcoholsoluble proteins): Ex: gliadin, from wheat. *Albuminoids*: Ex: keratin, from corn. *Histones. Protamines*: Ex: salmon, from the ripe sperm of salmon.
protein, words pert. to: albuminate, albuminolysis, albuminose, albuminous, albumose, aleuron, amino acid, archon, chondrin, chondroprotein, chromoprotein, coagulated, dipeptide, gelatin, gliadin, globulin, gluten, glycoprotein, histone, metaprotein, myosin, myosinogen, myosinose, nucleoprotein, protamine, protean, protease, proteid, scleroprotein, syntonin.
proteinase (prō'tē-in-ās) [G. *prōtos*, first, + *ase*, enzyme]. A colloid enzyme which splits protein.
proteinemia (prō-tē-ĭn-ē'mĭ-ă) [" + *aima*, blood]. Excessive amount of protein in the blood.
proteinic (prō-tē-ĭn'ĭk) [G. *prōtos*, first]. Relating to protein.
proteinivorus (prō-tē-ĭn-ĭv'ō-rŭs) [" + L. *vorāre*, to devour]. Living on protein.
proteinogenous (prō-tē-ĭn-ŏj'ĕn-ŭs) [" + *gennan*, to produce]. Developing from a protein.
proteinophobia (prō"tē-ĭn-ō-fō'bĭ-ă) [" + *phobos*, fear]. Aversion to foods containing protein.
proteinotherapy (prō"tē-ĭn-ō-thĕr'ă-pī) [" + *therapeia*, treatment]. Treatment by the injection of proteins not normally present in the body.
proteinuria (prō-tē-ĭn-ū'rĭ-ă) [" + *ouron*, urine]. Protein or albumin in the urine.
proteoclastic (prō"tē-ō-klăs'tĭk) [" + *klastos*, broken]. Having the ability to split up proteins.
proteogens (prō'tē-ō-jĕns) [G. *prōtos*, first, + *gennan*, to produce]. Preparations of plant proteins for injection hypodermically.
proteolysin (prō-tē-ŏl'ĭs-ĭn) [" + *lysis*, dissolution]. A specific substance causing decomposition of proteins.
proteolysis (prō-tē-ŏl'ĭs-ĭs) [" + *lysis*, dissolution]. 1. The conversion of proteins by ferments into peptones. 2. The process of disintegrating dissolved antigens by immune sera, lysin being the antibody.
proteolytic (prō-tē-ō-lĭt'ĭk) [" + *lysis*, dissolution]. In the chemistry of enzymes, hastening the hydrolysis of proteins.

proteometabolism (prō"tē-ō-mē-tăb'ō-lĭzm) [" + *metabolē*, change, + *ismos*, condition]. Digestion, absorption, and assimilation of proteins.
proteopeptic (prō"tē-ō-pĕp'tĭk) [" + *peptein*, to digest]. Pert. to the digestion of protein.
proteopexic (prō-tē-ō-pĕks'ĭk) [" + *pēxis*, fixation]. Pert. to fixation of proteins within the organism.
proteopexy (prō"tē-ō-pĕks'ĭ) [G. *prōtos*, first, + *pēxis*, fixation]. The fixation of proteins within the body.
proteose (prō'tē-ōs) [G. *prōtos*, first]. One of the class of intermediate products of proteolysis bet. protein and peptone.
p., primary. First formed products during proteolysis of proteins.
p., secondary. P. resulting from further hydrolysis of primary proteoses.
proteosotherapy (prō"tē-ōs-ō-thĕr'ă-pī) [" + *therapeia*, treatment]. Treatment by introduction of foreign proteose intravenously, or subcutaneously. SYN: *protein therapy.*
proteosuria (prō"tē-ōs-ū'rĭ-ă) [" + *ouron*, urine]. Proteose in urine. SYN: *albumosuria.*
proteotherapy (prō"tē-ō-thĕr'ă-pī) [" + *therapeia*, treatment]. Introduction of proteins parenterally in treating disease. SYN: *proteinotherapy.*
proteotoxin (prō"tē-ō-tŏk'sĭn) [" + *toxikon*, poison]. Product from reaction bet. serum of a host and a foreign protein. SYN: *anaphylatoxin, endotoxin.*
proteuria (prō-tē-ū'rĭ-ă) [" + *ouron*, urine]. Proteins in the urine. SYN: *proteinuria.*
Proteus (prō'tē-ŭs) [G. *Prōteus*, a god of many forms]. A genus of family Bacteriaceae found in intestines and decaying material, which cause protein decomposition.
prothesis (prŏth'ĕs-ĭs) [G. *pro*, before, + *thesis*, a placing]. Replacement by an artificial part. SYN: *prosthesis.*
prothrombase (prō-thrŏm'bās) [" + *thrombos*, a clot]. A substance which becomes a fibrin ferment when activated by thrombokinase. SYN: *prothrombin, thrombogen.*
prothrombin (prō-thrŏm'bĭn) [" + *thrombos*, a clot]. A chemical substance existing in circulating blood, and which, through the medium of *thrombokinase*, interacts with calcium salts to produce thrombin. SYN: *thrombogen.*
protistologist (prō-tĭs-tŏl'ō-jĭst) [G. *prōtista*, the very first, + *logos*, study]. One who studies the Protista, the unicellular organisms.
protistology (prō-tĭs-tŏl'ō-jĭ) [" + *logos*, study]. The science of Protista or animal unicellular plant and microörganisms. SYN: *microbiology.*
proto- [G.]. 1. A prefix signifying *first*. 2. The lowest of a series of compounds having the same elements.
protobe (prō'tōb) [G. *prōtos*, first, + *bios*, life]. d'Herelle's term for the bacteriophage. SYN: *protobios.*
protobiology (prō"tō-bī-ŏl'ō-jī) [" + *bios*, life, + *logos*, study]. The phase of science dealing with the forms more minute than bacteria, as the ultraviruses and bacteriophages.
protobios (prō-tō-bī'ōs) [" + *bios*, life]. A term suggested by d'Herelle for the minute forms parasitic to other organisms. SYN: *bacteriophage.*
protoblast (prō'tō-blăst) [" + *blastos*, a germ]. 1. A naked cell with no cell wall yet formed. 2. Blastomere of segment-

protoblastic   P-110   **prototrophic**

ing ovum which is parent cell of a part or organ.

protoblastic (prō″tō-blăs′tĭk) [" + *blastos*, germ]. Pert. to a protoblast.

protocol (prō′tō-kŏl) [" + *kolla*, glue (first notes glued)]. 1. A clinical report from first notes taken. 2. Minutes of a meeting. 3. Description of steps taken in an experiment.

protoerythrocyte (prō″tō-ĕr˝th′rō-sīt) [G. *prōtos*, first, + *erythros*, red, + *kytos*, cell]. An embryonic erythroblast with deeply staining nucleus.

protogala (prō-tŏg′ăl-ă) [" + *gala*, milk]. A mother's first milk after birth of a child. SYN: *colostrum*.

protogaster (prō″tō-găs′tẽr) [" + *gastēr*, belly]. Embryonic part from which stomach arises. SYN: *foregut*.

protogen (prō′tō-jĕn) [" + *gennan*, to produce]. 1. Any albuminoid substance which, when heated, does not coagulate. 2. Dietary preparation formed by action of formaldehyde on egg albumin.

protoglobulose (prō″tō-glŏb′ū-lōs) [" + L. *globulus*, a small sphere]. A primary product in the digestion of protein.

protoleukocyte (prō″tō-lū′kō-sīt) [" + *leukos*, white, + *kytos*, cell]. A minute lymphoid cell in red bone marrow and in the spleen.

protomyosinose (prō″tō-mī-ō′sĭn-ōs) [" + *mys*, *my-*, muscle]. An albumose formed in the primary digestion of protein.

proton (prō′tŏn) [G. *prōtos*, first]. 1. Embryonic trace which is forerunner of a part. 2. PT: The nucleus of the hydrogen atom.

It is assumed to be the unit of positive charge of electricity. SEE: *atom, atomic theory, electron*.

proton(e (prō′tŏn) [G. *prōtos*, first]. Any 1 of the peptonelike substances formed as primary decomposition products of the protamines.

protonephron, protonephros (prō″tō-nĕf′-ron, prō-tō-nĕf′rŏs) [" + *nephros*, kidney]. The primitive kidney of the embryo. SYN: *pronephros, wolffian body*.

protoneuron (prō″tō-nū′rŏn) [" + *neuron*, sinew]. A bipolar neuron connecting a sense organ with the central nervous system.

protoplasm (prō′tō-plăzm) [" + *plasma*, a thing formed]. 1. A vaguely used word for the essential, living material in an organism. 2. The primitive organic cell matter.

It contains not less than 12, and sometimes more, elements, such as carbon, calcium, chlorine, hydrogen, iron, magnesium, nitrogen, oxygen, phosphorus, potassium, sulfur, and sodium.

It is a thick, viscous, colorless material with large amt. of water, and is the seat of active chemical changes in the body. SYN: *cytoplasm*.

RS: *blastema, blastid, caryenchyma, cell, chromidiosis, chromplastid*.

protoplasmic (prō″tō-plăz′mĭk) [G. *prōtos*, first, + *plasma*, a thing formed]. Pert. to protoplasm or composed of it.
p. process. A dendrite. SEE: *nerve*.

protoplast (prō′tō-plăst) [" + *plassein*, to form]. 1. First hypothetical specimen of a race. 2. A primitive cell. 3. A unicellular organism. 4. Vital substance of an organism. SYN: *protoplasm*.

protospasm (prō′tō-spăzm) [" + *spasmos*, a spasm]. One which begins in 1 area and which extends to other parts.

prototoxin (prō″tō-tŏks′ĭn) [" + *toxikon*, poison]. Dissociation product of a toxin, having greatest affinity for the antitoxin.

prototrophic (prō″tō-trō′fĭk) [" + *trophē*,

Classification of Pathogenic Protozoa
Kingdom: Animals   Phylum: Protozoa

Class	Genus	Species
Sarcodina (locomotion by pseudopodia).	Endamoeba	E. histolytica E. coli E. gingivalis
	Dientamoeba	D. fragilis
	Endolimax	E. nana
	Iodamoeba	I. williamsi
Flagellata (locomotion by flagella).	Borellia	B. recurrentis B. vincenti B. refrigens B. bronchiale
	Leptospira	L. icterohaemorrhagiae L. icteroides
	Treponema	T. pallidum T. microdentium T. pertenue
	Trypanosoma	T. gambiense T. cruzi T. lewisi
	Leishmania	L. donovani L. tropica L. infantum
	Trichomonas	T. hominis T. vaginalis T. buccalis
	Chilomastix	C. mesnili
	Giardia	G. lamblia
Sporozoa (no organs of locomotion. Propagate by spores).	Isospora	I. hominis
	Plasmodium	P. malariae P. vivax P. falciparum
Infusoria (supplied with cilia).	Balantidium	B. coli B. minutum

nourishment]. Requiring simple inorganic elements as food.
protovertebra (prō″tō-vĕr′te-bră) [" + L. *vertebra*, vertebra]. Primitive vertebra in the notochord. SYN: *metamere, somite*.
protoxoid (prō-tŏks′oyd) [" + *toxikon*, poison]. Hypothetical nonpoisonous substance from prototoxin which has stronger affinity for the antitoxin than the toxin has. SEE: *toxoid*.
protozoa (prō-tō-zō′ă) (sing. *protozoon*) [G. *prōtos*, first, + *zōon*, animal]. The division of animal kingdom characterized by being unicellular and reproducing by fission.
protozoacide (prō-tō-zō′ă-sīd) [" + " + L. *cidus*, from *caedere*, to kill]. Destructive to, or that which kills, protozoa.
protozoal (prō″tō-zō′ăl) [" + *zōon*, animal]. Pert. to protozoa, unicellular organisms.
  p. diseases. Those produced by single-celled organisms, such as amebic dysentery, malaria and syphilis.
protozoan (prō-tō-zō′ăn) [" + *zōon*, animal]. 1. One organism of the protozoa. 2. Pert. to protozoa. SEE: *Cercomonas intestinalis*.
protozoology (prō″tō-zō-ŏl′ō-jī) [" + " + *logos*, study]. Phase of science dealing with study of protozoa.
protozoon (prō″tō-zō′ŏn) (pl. *protozoa*) [" + *zōon*, animal]. Unicellular organism. SEE: *protozoa*.
protozoophag(e (prō″tō-zō′ō-făg, -făj) [" + " + *phagein*, to eat]. A phagocyte which ingests protozoa.
protozootherapy (prō″tō-zō-o-thĕr′ă-pī) [" + " + *therapeia*, treatment]. Treatment of conditions due to protozoa.
protractor (prō-trăk′tōr) [L. *pro*, forward, + *tractōr*, that which draws]. 1. Instrument for removing foreign bodies from wounds. 2. A muscle that draws a part forward. OPP: *retractor*.
protuberance (prō-tū′bĕr-ăns) [" + *tuberare*, to bulge]. 1. A part that is prominent beyond a surface, like a knob. 2. Quality of projecting.
proud flesh (prowd). A mass of excessive granulation, formed when a wound shows no other sign of healing or tendency to cicatrization.
provertebra (prō-vĕr′tĕ-bră) [L. *pro*, before, + *vertebra*, vertebra]. A mesoblastic segment on the notochord of the embryo from which vertebra arises. SYN: *protovertebra, somite*.
proviron (prō-vī′rŏn). A hormone producing secondary male characteristics.
provisional (prō-vĭzh′ŭn-ăl) [L. *provisiō*, a providing before]. Serving a temporary use.
provitamin (prō-vī′tăm-ĭn) [L. *pro*, before, + *vita*, life, + *amine*]. A substance which may be inactive, but which can be transformed in the body to the corresponding active vitamin. They can function as vitamins.
Prowazekia (prō-wă-zē′kĭ-ă). A genus of flagellate protozoans.
prowazekiasis (prō-wă-zē-kī′ăs-ĭs). Infestation with Prowazekia.
proximad (prŏk′sĭm-ăd) [L. *proximus*, next, + *ad*, toward]. Toward the proximal or central point.
proximal (prŏks′ĭm-ăl) [L. *proximus*, nearest]. Nearest the point of attachment.
proximate (prŏks′ĭm-ăt) [L. *proximus*, nearest]. 1. Next to; immediate. 2. In chemistry, elemental, the opposite of ultimate.

Thus, a proximate analysis of a substance may be designed to determine the presence or amount of carbonate or oxalate as distinguished from total carbon.
In a material of vegetable or animal origin, the effects of administration may be determined either by the elements (*e. g.*, iodine) or the proximate principles (*e. g.*, alkaloids) it contains.
  p. principles. Organic constituents which with other elements make up living tissue, such as the albuminoids, carbohydrates, fats, and proteins.
proximoataxia (prŏk-sĭ-mō-at-ăk′sĭ-ă) [" + G. *ataxia*, lack of order]. Lack of coordination in muscles of the proximal area of an extremity, as the arm, forearm, thigh, or leg.
prozymogen (prō-zī′mō-jĕn) [G. *pro*, before, + *zymē*, leaven, + *gennan*, to produce]. An intranuclear substance that becomes zymogen. SYN: *prezymogen*.
prune (prōōn) [L. *pruna*]. COMP: Contains malic acid and sugar.
  AV. SERVING (fresh and dried) : 50-100 Gm. Pro. 0.5-2.1, Fat 0.1-0.0, Carbo. 6.7-73.0.
  VITAMINS (both) : A++, B+ and ++, C— + and none, G++ dried only.
  ASH CONST. (dried only): Ca 0.054, Mg 0.055, K 1.030, Na 0.069, P 0.105, Cl 0.017, S 0.037, Fe 0.003. A good source of iron and ranks with raisins.
pruriginous (prū-rĭj′ĭn-ŭs) [L. *prurigō*, itch, from *prurire*, to itch]. Pert. to, or of the nature of, prurigo.
prurigo (prū-rī′gō) [L. itch, from *prurire*, to itch]. A chronic skin disease marked by constantly recurring, discrete, pale, deep-seated, intensely itchy papules on extensor surfaces of limbs.
Superimposed exanthematous manifestations may mask the true nature.
ETIOL: Exciting cause unknown. Hygienic factors are supplementary.
PROG: Guarded. It begins in childhood and may last a lifetime.
TREATMENT: Constitutional and local. Hygienic regimen. Locally, antipruritics.
  p. aestivalis. P. recurring every summer and continuing during hot weather.
  p. agria. Very severe p. with great itching.   [eruption of milk teeth.
  p. infantilis. P. in children during
  p. nodularis. Eruption in skin of hard nodules with great itching.
  p. simplex. Simple form of p. with recurring tendency.
pruritus (prū-rī′tūs) [L. itching, from *prurire*, to itch]. Severe itching.
May be symptomatic, or occur idiopathically as a neurosis without structural change.
ETIOL: Predisposing factor is cutaneous hyperesthesia. Localized causes are present in p. ani, p. vulvae, focal infection, mycotic infection, bath itch, etc.
TREATMENT: Exciting or contributory cause to be located and removed. Hygienic regimen. Pilocarpine, phenacetin, bromide. Colon vaccine for protein shock. In anal and vulvar pruritus, examination by competent gynecologist or proctologist before cutaneous therapy is instituted. In bath avoid too sudden changes of temperature. For dry skins, avoid frequent soap and water bathing. Soft, nonirritating underclothing, soothing lotions, oil rubs, antipruritics.
  p. aestivalis. P. with prickly heat occurring in hot weather. SYN: *summer itch*.
  p. ani. Itching about the anus. May

be due to threadworms, fistula in ani, hemorrhoids, or irritation. [lesion.
p., essential. P. without apparent skin
p. hiemalis. Winter itch, occurring in cold weather. [tive skin changes.
p. senilis. P. in aged with degenera-
p., symptomatic. P. as a symptom of some other disorder.
p. vulvae. Disorder marked by severe itching of ext. female genitalia. Often an early sign of diabetes mellitus.
Prussak's space (proos'ăk). Tiny space in middle ear bet. Shrapnell's membrane laterally and neck of malleus medially.
prussic acid (prŭs'ĭk, proō'sĭk). A violent and rapid poison. SYN: *acid, hydrocyanic, q.v.*
psalis (sā'lĭs) [G. *psalis*, arch]. The cerebral fornix, a fibrous arch connecting cerebral hemispheres.
psalterium (săhl-tē'rĭ-ŭm) [G. *psalterion*, harp]. Longitudinal fibers on floor of the aqueduct of Silvius, the post. portion of cerebral fornix. SYN: *lyra.*
psammoma (săm-ō'mă) [G. *psammos*, sand, + *-oma*, tumor]. A small tumor of the brain, the choroid plexus and other areas, containing calcareous particles.
psammosarcoma (săm″ō-sar-kō'mă) [" + *sarx*, flesh, + *-oma*, tumor]. A sarcoma composed of spots of calcareous degeneration.
psammotherapy (săm″ō-thĕr'ă-pĭ) [" + *therapeia*, treatment]. The application of sand baths in treatment.
pselaphesia, pselaphesis (sĕl-ă-fē'zhĭ-ă, -sĭs) [G. *psēlaphēsis*, touch]. 1. Active sense of touch, including muscle sense. 2. Plucking at bedclothes with the fingers, a sign observed in low delirium. SYN: *carphology.*
psellism, psellismus (sĕl'ĭzm, sĕl-ĭz'mŭs) [G. *psellizein*, to stammer]. Defective pronunciation, stuttering or stammering.
p. mercurialis. Jerking, hurried, unintelligible speech in mercurial tremor.
pseudacousma (sū″dă-kŭz'mă) [G. *pseudēs*, false, + *akousma*, a thing heard]. Condition in which all sounds are heard falsely, seeming to be altered in quality of pitch, or imaginary sounds are heard.
pseudacusis (sū″dă-kū'sĭs) [" + *akousis*, hearing]. State in which sounds are heard falsely or imagined. SYN: *pseudacousma.*
pseudaphia (sū-dăf'ĭ-ă) [" + *aphē*, touch]. A false or defective perception of touch. SEE: *paraphia, pseudesthesia.*
pseudarthritis (sū″dar-thrī'tĭs) [" + *arthron*, joint, + *-itis*, inflammation]. Hysterical disease of the joints.
pseudarthrosis (sū-dar-thrō'sĭs) [" + " + *-osis*, disease]. A false joint developing after a fracture that has not united.
pseudesthesia (sū-dĕs-thē'zĭ-ă) [" + *aisthēsis*, sensation]. 1. An imaginary or false sensation, as that after amputation felt in the lost part. 2. Sense of feeling not caused by ext. stimulation. SEE: *paraphia, pseudaphia.*
pseudo- (sū'dō) [G. *pseudēs*, false]. A prefix meaning *false.*
pseudoanemia (sū″dō-ăn-ē'mĭ-ă) [G. *pseudēs*, false, + *an-*, negative, + *aima*, blood]. Pallor of mucous membranes and skin without other signs of true anemia.
pseudoangina (sū″dō-ăn-jī'nă) [" + L. *angina*, a choking]. False symptoms resembling angina pectoris of nervous origin.
SYM: Functional attacks in cardiac region but not associated with any disease of the heart or its vessels.

pseudoapoplexy (sū″dō-ăp'ō-plĕk-sĭ). Condition simulating apoplexy but not accompanied by cerebral hemorrhage.
pseudoataxia (sū″dō-ă-tăks'ĭ-ă) [" + *ataxia*, lack of order]. Condition resembling ataxia not due to *tabes dorsalis.*
pseudobacterium (sū″dō-băk-tē'rĭ-ŭm) [" + *baktērion*, a little rod]. Any microscopic cell similar to a bacterium.
pseudoblepsia, pseudoblepsis (sū″dō-blĕp'-sĭ-ă, -sĭs) [" + *blepsis*, sight]. False or imaginary vision. SYN: *parablepsia, pseudopsia.*
pseudobulbar paralysis (sū″dō-bŭl'ber) [" + *bolbos*, a swollen end]. Paralysis resembling bulbar paralysis, but due to lesion of cortical centers.
pseudocartilaginous (sū″dō-kar-tĭ-lăj'ĭn-ŭs) [G. *pseudēs*, false, + L. *cartilāgō*, gristle]. Pert. to, or formed of, a substance resembling cartilage.
pseudocast (sū'dō-kăst) [" + M.E. *casten*, a throwing off]. A sediment in urine resembling a true cast.
pseudocele (sū'dō-sēl) [" + *koilos*, hollow]. The 5th ventricle of the brain. SYN: *cavum septi pellucidi.*
pseudochorea (sū″dō-kō-rē'ă) [" + *choreia*, a dance]. Hysterical state resembling chorea. SYN: *spurious chorea.*
pseudochromesthesia (sū″dō-krō-mĕs-thē'zĭ-ă) [" + *chrōma*, color, + *aisthēsis*, sensation]. A condition in which sounds, esp. of the vowels, seem to induce a sensation of a distinct visual color. SEE: *phonism, photism.*
pseudocirrhosis (sū″dō-sĭr-ō'sĭs) [" + *kirros*, orange yellow, + *-osis*, disease]. A condition with symptoms of cirrhosis of liver, due usually to pericarditis.
SYM: Cyanosis, ascites, dyspnea.
pseudocoele (sū'dō-sēl) [G. *pseudēs*, false, + *koilos*, hollow]. The 5th ventricle of brain. SYN: *pseudocele.*
pseudocoloboma (sū″dō-kŏl-ō-bō'mă) [" + *koloboma*, imperfection]. A scarcely noticeable scar on the iris from an embryonic fissure.
pseudocrisis (sū-dō-krī'sĭs) [" + *krisis*, a separation]. A temporary fall of body temperature which may be followed by a rise.
pseudocroup (sū'dō-kroop) [" + A.S. *kropan*, to shout aloud]. False croup. SYN: *laryngismus stridulus.*
pseudocyesis (sū″dō-sī-ē'sĭs) [" + *kyēsis*, pregnancy]. A condition in which the abdomen enlarges and the menses cease when the patient thinks that she is pregnant but is not.
Usually seen in woman very desirous of having children, due to an abnormal mental state in which the woman sometimes imagines she has had sexual intercourse with a man she would like to have as lover or husband. Men have been accused of being the father of an unborn child or guilty of fornication or adultery because of this.
Under anesthesia the enlargement of the abdomen disappears. SYN: *phantom pregnancy.*
pseudocyst (sū'dō-sĭst) [G. *pseudēs*, false, + *kystis*, bladder]. A dilatation resembling a cyst.
pseudodementia (sū″dō-dē-mĕn'shĭ-ă) [" + L. *de-*, negative, + *mens, ment-*, mind]. Exaggerated indifference to environment without impairment of mind.
pseudodiphtheria (sū″dō-dĭf-thē'rĭ-ă) [" + *diphthera*, membrane]. A condition resembling diphtheria but not due to Klebs-Löffler bacillus.
p. bacillus. A nonpathogenic one resembling the true diphtheria bacillus.

pseudoedema (sū"dō-ē-dē'mä) [" + *oidēma*, a swelling]. A puffy condition of the skin simulating edema.

pseudoemphysema (sū"dō-ĕm-fĭz-ē'mä) [" + *emphysēma*, an inflation]. A bronchial condition with blocking simulating emphysema.

pseudoencephalitis (sū"dō-ĕn-sĕf-ă-lī'tĭs) [" + *egkephalos*, brain, + *-itis*, inflammation]. A false encephalitis, due to profuse diarrhea.

pseudoerysipelas (sū"dō-ĕr-ĭ-sĭp'ĕl-ăs) [" + *erythros*, red, + *pella*, skin]. An inflammation of subcutaneous cellular tissue simulating erysipelas.

pseudoesthesia (sū"dō-ĕs-thē'zĭ-ă) [G. *pseudēs*, false, + *aisthēsis*, sensation]. An imaginary sensation or a false one. SYN: *pseudesthesia*.

pseudoganglion (sū"dō-găn'glĭ-ŏn) [" + *gagglion*, knot]. A slight thickening of a nerve resembling a ganglion.

pseudogeusesthesia (sū"dō-gū-sĕs-thē'zĭ-ă) [" + *geusis*, taste, + *aisthēsis*, sensation]. A sense of color accompanying sensations of taste.

pseudogeusia (sū"dō-gū'sĭ-ă) [" + *geusis*, taste]. A subjective sensation of taste not produced by external stimulus.

pseudoglioma (sū"dō-glī'ō-mă) [" + *glia*, glue, + *-ōma*, tumor]. Exudate in the vitreous giving a yellowish reflex as seen in glioma of retina.

pseudoglobulin (sū"dō-glŏb'ū-lĭn) [" + L. *globulus*, little globe]. One of 2 globulins comprising paraglobulin, *q.v.*

pseudoglottis (sū"dō-glŏt'ĭs) [" + *glōttis*, glottis]. Area bet. false vocal cords.

pseudohemoptysis (sū"dō-hē-mŏp'tĭs-ĭs) [" + *aima*, blood, + *ptyein*, to spit]. Spitting of blood which does not arise from the bronchi or the lungs.

pseudohermaphroditism (sū"dō-hĕr-măf'rō-dīt"ĭzm) [G. *pseudēs*, false, + *Hermaphroditos*, mythical two-sexed god]. A congenital abnormality of the ext. genitalia and of the body in which one resembles the other sex; not a true hermaphroditism. SEE: *hermaphroditism*.

p. femininus. One with a large clitoris resembling the penis and with hypertrophied labia majora resembling the scrotum, thus resembling a male.

p. masculinus. A male with a small penis and perineal hypospadias, and scrotum without testes, the condition resembling the vulva.

pseudohernia (sū-dō-hĕr'nĭ-ă) [G. *pseudēs*, false, + L. *hernia*, rupture]. An empty hernial sac simulating a strangulated, inflamed hernia.

pseudohydrophobia (sū"dō-hī-drō-fō'bĭ-ă) [" + *ydor*, *ydr-*, water, + *phobos*, fear]. Disorder simulating hydrophobia in its symptoms. SYN: *lyssophobia*.

pseudohypertrophic (sū"dō-hī-pĕr-trō'fĭk) [" + *yper*, above, + *trophē*, nourishment]. Pert. to a false hypertrophy.

p. paralysis. Paralysis with enlargement and loss of motion of muscles.

pseudohypertrophy (sū"dō-hī-pĕr'trō-fĭ) [" + " + *trophē*, nourishment]. Increase of size of an organ or part with diminution of function.

pseudoleukemia (sū"dō-lū-kē'mĭ-ă) [" + *leukos*, white, + *aima*, blood]. Progressive anemia with lymphomata, generally fatal. SYN: *Hodgkin's disease*.

p., infantile. Anemia in children caused by rachitic tendencies.

pseudoleukocythemia (sū"dō-lū"kō-sī-thē'mĭ-ă) [" + " + *kytos*, cell, + *aima*, blood]. Progressive anemia with lymphomata, characteristic of several conditions. SYN: *pseudoleukemia*.

pseudologia (sū-dō-lo'jĭ-ă) [" + *logos*, a study]. Falsification in writing or in speech, a form of pathological lying.

p. fantastica. Pathological lying; one of the forms of the psychopathic state. A moral deficiency exists and punishment therefore is useless.

pseudomania (sū"dō-mā'nĭ-ă) [G. *pseudēs*, false, + *mania*, madness]. 1. A psychosis in which the patient falsely accuses himself of crimes which he thinks he has committed. 2. Pathological lying.

pseudomasturbation (sū"dō-măs-tur-bā'shŭn) [" + L. *manus*, hand, + *stuprāre*, to rape]. A nervous habit of pulling at the penis. SYN: *peotillomania*.

pseudomelanosis (sū"dō-mĕl-ăn-ō'sĭs) [" + *melas*, *melan-*, black, + *-ōsis*, disease]. Discoloration of tissues after death.

pseudomembrane (sū"dō-mĕm'brăn) [" + L. *membrana*, membrane]. A false membrane, as in diphtheria.

pseudomembranous (sū"dō-mĕm'brā-nŭs) [" + L. *membrana*, membrane]. Pert. to or marked by false membranes.

pseudomeningitis (sū"dō-mĕn-ĭn-jī'tĭs) [" + *mēnigx*, membrane, + *-itis*, inflammation]. A condition resembling symptoms of meningitis without lesions of meningeal inflammation.

pseudomnesia (sū"dŏm-nē'zĭ-ă) [" + *mnēsis*, memory]. A memory perversion in which patient remembers that which never occurred.

Pseudomonas (sū-dō-mō'năs) [" + *monas*, single]. A genus of saprophytic bacteria found in soil and water which produces blue-green pigment.

pseudomucin (sū-dō-mū'sĭn) [G. *pseudēs*, false, + L. *mucus*, mucus]. A variety of mucin found in proliferative ovarian cysts.

pseudomyelia paresthetica (sū"dō-mī-ē'lĭ-ă păr-ĕs-thĕt'ĭk-ă). False sense of motion in paralyzed limb or of no motion in a moving limb. SEE: *pain*.

pseudoneuroma (sū"dō-nū-rō'mă) [" + *neuron*, sinew, + *-ōma*, tumor]. A growth of connective tissue of a nerve including medullary layer of nerve fiber. SYN: *neurofibroma*.

pseudonuclein (sū"dō-nū'klē-ĭn) [" + L. *nucleus*, a nut]. A combination of albumin with metaphosphoric acid. SYN: *paranuclein*.

pseudoparalysis (sū"dō-pă-răl'ĭ-sĭs) [" + *para*, at the side, + *lyein*, to loosen]. A loss of muscular power not due to lesion of the nervous system.

pseudoparaplegia (sū"dō-păr-ă-plē'jĭ-ă) [" + " + *plēgē*, a stroke]. Seeming paralysis of the lower extremities without impairment of the reflexes.

pseudoparasite (sū"dō-păr'ă-sīt) [" + " + *sitos*, food]. 1. Anything resembling a parasite. 2. Organism which can live as a parasite, although it is normally not one. SYN: *commensal*. SEE: *facultative parasite*.

pseudoparesis (sū"dō-păr-e'sĭs, -păr'e-sĭs) [" + *paresis*, relaxation]. A condition simulating paresis but unlike the ordinary forms and due to hysteria.

pseudopepsin (sū"dō-pĕp'sĭn) [G. *pseudēs*, false, + *pepsis*, digestion]. A proteolytic ferment secreted by some of the gastric glands.

pseudopeptone (sū"dō-pĕp'tōn) [" + *peptein*, to digest]. A mucoid substance derived from egg white.

pseudophthisis (sū-dōf-thī'sĭs, -dō-tī'sĭs) [" + *phthisis*, a wasting]. Progressive emaciation not due to pulmonary tuberculosis.

pseudoplegia (sū″dō-plē′jĭ-ă) [" + *plēgē*, a stroke]. Paralysis of hysterical origin. SYN: *pseudoparalysis*.

pseudopod (sū′dō-pŏd) [" + *pous, pod-*, foot]. Protruding protoplasmic process of a temporary nature in protozoa for taking up food and aiding in locomotion. SYN: *pseudopodium*.

pseudopodium (sū″dō-pō′dĭ-ŭm) (pl. *pseudopodia*) [" + *pous, pod-*, foot]. A temporary protruding process of a protozoan aiding in locomotion and prehension of food. SYN: *pseudopod*.

pseudopsia (sū-dŏp′sĭ-ă) [" + *opsis*, vision]. Visual hallucinations or false perceptions. SYN: *pseudoblepsis*.

pseudorabies (sū″dō-rā′bēz, -rā′bĭ-ēz) [G. *pseudēs*, false, + L. *rabere*, to rage]. condition with rash resembling scar- of the disease. SYN: *lyssophobia, pseudohydrophobia*.

pseudoscarlatina (sū″dō-skar-lă-tē′nă) [" + L. *scarlatina*, scarlet]. A septic febrile condition with rash resembling scarlatina.

ETIOL: Gonorrhea, puerperal infection, food or blood poisoning.

pseudosclerosis (sū″dō-sklē-rō′sĭs) [" + *sklērōsis*, a hardening]. A condition with the symptoms, but without the lesions, of multiple sclerosis of the nervous system.

pseudosmia (sū-dŏz′mĭ-ă) [" + *osmē*, smell]. An olfactory hallucination or perversion of the sense of smell.

pseudostoma (sū-dŏs′tō-mă) [" + *stoma*, a mouth]. An apparent aperture bet. endothelial cells that have been stained.

pseudosyphilis (sū″dō-sĭf′ĭ-lĭs) [" + *syn*, with love, + *philos*, love]. A nonspecific condition resembling syphilis.

pseudotabes (sū″dō-tā′bēz) [" + L. *tabēs*, a wasting]. A neural disease simulating tabes dorsalis.

pseudotetanus (sū″dō-tĕt′ăn-ŭs) [G. *pseudēs*, false, + *tetanos*, tension]. Persistent muscular contractions resembling tetanus.

pseudotuberculosis (sū″dō-tū-ber″kŭ-lō′sĭs) [" + L. *tuberculus*, tubercle, + G. -*ōsis*, disease]. Disease like tuberculosis not caused by the tubercle bacillus.

pseudotympany (sū″dō-tĭm′pă-nĭ). Flattening of arch of diaphragm, swelling of abdomen with increased respiration.
It disappears under anesthesia and is of purely nervous origin. SYN: *accordion abdomen*.

pseudotyphoid (sū″dō-tī′foyd) [" + *typhos*, fever, + *eidos*, resemblance]. Condition resembling typhoid fever, not caused by the typhoid bacillus.

pseudoxanthoma (sū″dō-zăn-thō′mă) [" + *xanthos*, yellow, + -*ōma*, tumor]. Chronic degenerative cutaneous disease marked by yellow patches and stretching of the skin; resembles xanthoma.

psilosis (sī-lō′sĭs) [G. *psilōsis*, a stripping]. 1. Falling out or removal of hair.
2. Tropical diarrhea of severe, often fatal form. SYN: *sprue*.
ETIOL: Disease of pancreas, invasion by bacteria, mold; or fat deficiency.
SYM: Diarrhea, large, lightly-colored, acid stools containing fat. No pain or tenesmus. Inflamed, eroded and cracked tongue and mouth, angina.

psittacosis (sĭt-ă-kō′sĭs) [G. *psittakos*, parrot, + -*ōsis*, disease]. A fatal, infectious disease of parrots and other birds that may be transmitted to man.
SYM. (in man): Headache, epistaxis, nausea, chill followed by fever, constipation, sometimes pulmonary disorders.

psoas (sō′ăs) [G. *psoa*, loins]. One of 2 muscles of the loins. SEE: *Table of Muscles in Appendix, Illus., below*.
p. abscess. A cold a. in sheath of the psoas major muscle.
It follows the sheath of this muscle until it reaches the surface and points. It generally occurs above Poupart's ligament in the iliac fossa or near the attachment of the psoas muscle to the femur.

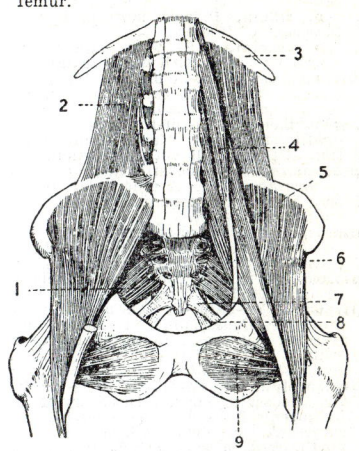

PSOAS, ILIACUS AND OBTURATOR EXTERNUS.
1. Pyriformis; 2. Quadratus lumborum; 3. Twelfth rib; 4. Psoas minor; 5. Psoas major; 6. Iliacus; 7. Sacrospinous ligament; 8. Sacrotuberous ligament.

ETIOL: Usually tuberculous disease of vertebrae accompanied by pus.

psoitis (sō-ī′tĭs) [" + -*ītis*, inflammation]. Inflammation of the psoas muscles or of the area of the loins.

psora (sō′ră) [G. *psōra*, itch]. 1. An itching disease of the skin; scabies. 2. Psoriasis, an erythematous, scaling, cutaneous eruption. 3. Hahnemann's name for the theory that chronic diseases are a manifestation of a suppressed itch or an itch dyscrasia.

psorelcosis (sō-rĕl-kō′sĭs) [" + *elkōsis*, ulceration]. Ulceration occurring as a result of scabies.

psoriasis (sō-rī′ăs-ĭs) [G. *psōriasis*, an itching]. Chronic inflammatory skin disease of many varieties characterized by formation of scaly red patches on extensor surfaces of body.
ETIOL: Unknown.
SYM: Begins in adult life as flat-topped papule covered with thin, grayish-white scale spreading peripherally; lesions coalescing; centers regressing, forming circinate lesions. Under the dry scales are red bleeding points (papillae).
TREATMENT: Hygienic regimen, tonics, arsenicals internally. Recently, pancreatic hormone, lipocaic, given orally, has successfully cleared up psoriasis. Locally, salicylic acid, mineral or wood tar, ammoniated mercury, betanaphthol, pyrogallol. Ointments to be rubbed in thoroughly.
DIET: Low protein because of positive nitrogen metabolism in this disease. 4.5 Gm. nitrogen with calories made up of

psoriasis buccalis   P-115   **psychiatry, words pert. to**

fats and carbohydrates. Sugar, candy, oysters, and ice cream may be used. Fruits and vegetables may be substituted. SEE: *Bazin's disease*.
p. buccalis. Variety with white patches on tongue and cheek. SYN: *leukoplakia buccalis*.
p. circinata. Form with ring-shaped lesions with healing beginning in the center.
p. diffusa. P. with more or less coalescence of lesions.
p. punctata. P. with papular red eruptions tipped with white scales.
psorocomium (sō-rō-kō'mĭ-ŭm) [G. *psōra*, itch, + *komein*, to care for]. Hospital for patients with the itch.
psorophthalmia (sō-rŏf-thăl'mĭ-ă) [" + *ophthalmos*, eye]. Marginal inflammation of the eyelids with ulceration.
psorosperm (sō'rō-sperm) [G. *psōra*, itch, + *sperma*, seed]. A unicellular, protozoan, parasitic organism. SYN: *coccidium, sporozoon*.
psorospermosis (sō"rō-sperm-ō'sĭs) [" + " + *-ōsis*, condition]. Morbid condition caused by presence of psorosperms.
psorous (sō'rŭs) [G. *psōra*, itch]. Related to or affected with itch.
psychalgia (sī-kăl'jĭ-ă) [G. *psychē*, soul, mind, + *algos*, pain]. 1. Mental distress or pain, esp. in melancholia. 2. Pain of hysterical origin. SYN: *mind* or *soul pain, phrenalgia*.
psychanalysis (sī-kăn-ăl'ĭ-sĭs) [" + *analysis*, a loosening apart]. Discovery of the pathogenic links bet. the objective and subjective consciousness by a system of recall. SYN: *psychoanalysis, q.v.*
psychanopsia (sī-kăn-ŏp'sĭ-ă) [" + *an-*, negative, + *opsis*, vision]. Sight with failure to recognize anything seen, due to brain lesion. SYN: *psychic blindness*.
psychasthenia (sī-kăs-thē'nĭ-ă) [" + *astheneia*, weakness]. A neurotic condition marked by sense of inadequacy, unreality, anxiety and doubt.

A neurosis characterized by obsessions, phobias, tics, and compulsions. Obsessions are intrusive ideas which the patient cannot dismiss from consciousness and yet clearly recognizes as pathologic. (Delusions are false ideas not recognized as abnormal.)

There may be associated restlessness, palpitation, fatigue, or irritability. A definite sense of dread or fear is associated with phobias. The anxiety is rationalized, as a fear of syphilis (syphilophobia), or cancer (carcinomatophobia), or insanity (psychopathophobia), or contamination (mysophobia), among many others.

Obsessions and phobias may occur at the onset or during the course of other diseases, notably schizophrenia. Frequently, obsessive impulses dominate behavior. These may be peculiar (touching lampposts, avoiding lines on sidewalk), or distinctly antisocial. In the latter event, it is indicative of a condition more serious than a neurosis. SYN: *anxiety neurosis, q.v.; Janet's disease*.
psychataxia (sī"kă-tăk'sĭ-ă) [G. *psychē*, soul, + *ataxia*, lack of order]. Disordered power of concentration.
psyche (sī'kē) [G. *psychē*, soul, mind]. All that constitutes the mind and its processes. SYN: *soul*.
psycheclampsia (sī-kĕk-lămp'sĭ-ă) [" + *eklampsis*, a flashing out]. Acute mania or mental convulsions.
psychiatric (sī-kĭ-ăt'rĭk) [" + *iatrikos*, healing]. 1. Pert. to psychiatry, the science dealing with mental ailments. 2. One who has a psychosis or tendency toward one.
p. habits. *The Confused*: May not realize the incongruity of an act as related to the environment.
The Deluded: May have phobias or specific fears which control some of their habits.
The Depressed: May ignore everything because of their misery, which engages all of their attention.
The Excited: May be unable to concentrate.
The Feeble: May be unable to control themselves because of weakness.
The Hallucinated: Habits may be affected by "voices," etc.
psychiatrist (sī-kī'ă-trĭst) [G. *psychē*, soul, + *iatreia*, healing]. A physician who specializes in study and treatment of mental disorders.
psychiatry (sī-kī'ă-trĭ) [" + *iatreia*, healing]. That branch of medicine which treats of mental and neurotic disorders and the pathologic, or psychopathologic changes associated with them.
psychiatry, words pert. to: abalienation; abalienatio mentis; aberration; abnormality; abreaction; abulia; acatalepsy; acatamathesia; acataphasia; acousma; acousmatagnosis; acousmatamnesia acrasia; Adler's organ inferiority; affect; agnosia; agraphia; agrypnia; ahypnia; akathisia; akinesia; alcoholism; alexia; algesia; algolagnia; algopsychalia; alienation; alienism; alienist; alliteration; allophasis; allopsychic; allotropic; alogia; Alzheimer's disease; ambitendency; ambivalence; amentia; amimia; amnesia; amnestic; amok; amoralia; amusia; anaclitic choice; anacroasia; anal erotic; ananabasia; ananastasia; anandria; anergastic; anhedonia; anoesia; anoia; anomia; anorexia; apandria; apanthropia; apastia; apathy; aphasia; aphemesthesia; aphemia; aphonia; aphrasia; aphrenia; aphronesia; aphthenxia; apodemialgia; apraxia; aprosexia; apsithyria; apsychosis; asemasia; asemia; asitia; association; assonance; asterognosis; asyllabia; asymbolia; asynesia; atactilia; atavism; ataxaphasia; ataxia, intrapsychic; ataxophemia; ateliosis; athymia; atrabiliary; attitude; autism; autistic thinking; autoanalysis; automatism; autoecholalia; autophagy; autophilia; autophobia; autoplastic; autopsychosis; autosuggestion; autosynoia; avulsion; behaviorism; blocking; bradylalia; bradylexis; brain storm; catatonia; catharsis; cenesthesia; censor; chorea; claustrophilia; claustrophobia; complex; compulsion; conation; condensation; confabulation; conflict; constellation; coprolagnia; coprolalia; coprophilia; cretinism; cryptesthesia; cycloid; cyclothymia; deafness; delire de toucher; delirium; delusion; dementia; depersonalization; depression; dereistic; determinism; disassociation; disorientation; displacement; distractibility; divagation; dysbulia; dyschiria; dyscinesia; dysmnesia; dysphremia; dysthymia; echolalia; echomania; echomimia; ego; egocentric; ekphorize; electra complex; emotion; emotivity; empathy; eremophobia; erethism; ergasiomania; ergasiophobia; erotism; erotomania; erythrophobia; eschrolalia; eviration; exhibitionism; extrovert; fabrication; fastidium; fear; feeblemindedness; fixation; folie; free association; fuge; furor amatorius; Ganser's syndrome; geophagia; graphorrhea; hallucination;; hallucinosis; haphalgesia; hebephrenia; heterolalia; holergastic; hy-

perhedonia; hyperognosis; hyperprosexia; hypersthenia; hyperthymia; hypnagogic; hypnoidal; hypnosis; hypnotic; hypnotism; hypochondria; hypochondriac; hypochondriasis; hypophrenia; hysteria; idea; idiocy; idiophrenic psychosis; idiot; idiotropic type; illusion; image; imago; imbecile; imperious act; impulsion; incoherency; incompetent; infantilism; inhibition; insanity; instinct; integration; intelligence; intraphysical; introjection; introversion; introvert; kakergastic reaction; katatonia; kinesthesia; Korsakoff's psychosis; latent content; lethargy; lethologica; logamnesia; logopathia; logorrhea; malingerer; masochism; melancholia; mesmerism; mestatropism; metaphrenia; mind; misocainea; misologiamisopedia; moramentia; moria; moron; morosis; narcissism; narcotism; necrophilia; negativism; neologism; neurosis; noctambulism; non compos mentis; nooklepsia; nunnation; object choice; obsession; oligergasia; oligopnea; omnipotence of thought; oneiric; oneirism; oneirodynia; organic reaction type; orthopsychiatry; overdeterminism; overtone; paragraphia; paralexia; paralogia; paramimia; paramnesia; paranoia; paranomia; parapathia; paraphasia; paraphonia; parapraxis; parent-fixation; parergastic reaction; paresis; pathergasia; pavor nocturnus; pedophilia; periphrastic; perseveration; personality; phantasia; phantasm; phantasmatomoria; phantasy; phantom; phoneme; pica; pithiatism; pleasure principle; pragmatism; pragmatagnosia; preconscious; pseudoalgia; psychasthenia; psychiatrist; psyche; psychic; psychoanalysis; psychobiological; psychobiology; psychogenesis; psychogenic; psycholepsy; psychology; psychologist; psychoneurosis; psychopath; psychopathology; psychosis; psychotherapy; rationalization; reaction; reality principle; recapitulation theory; repression; resistance; restraint; retardation; rut formation; safety symbolism; satyriasis; schizoid; schizophrenia; scotomization; sexual bondage; shell shock; sterotypy; stupor; subconscious; subjective; sublimation; subliminal; suggestion; surrogate; sycophancy; symbiosis; symbol; symbolism; syntonic; threshold of consciousness; transfer; transference; transvestism; trend; twilight state; tyrannism; unconscious; vervigeration; vesania; vigil; vigilambulism; vision; voice; word blindness; word salad; zeloptypia.

psychic (sī'kĭk) [G. *psychē*, soul, mind]. 1. Concerning the mind, or soul. 2. One said to be endowed with semisupernatural powers, such as the ability to read the mind of others, or to foresee coming events; one apparently sensitive to nonphysical forces.

p. blindness. Sight without recognition of that which is seen.

p. contagion. Communication of another's nervous disorder by imitation, as a tic.

p. deafness. Inability to recognize sounds heard.

p. determinism. The theory that mental processes are determined by conscious or unconscious motives, and are never irrelevant.

p. force. One generated apart from physical energy.

p. infection. Mental condition due to an influence upon the mind.

psychical (sī'kĭ-kăl) [G. *psychē*, soul]. Pert. to mind or soul. SYN: *psychic*.

psychinosis (sī-kĭn-ō'sĭs) [" + *nosos*, disease]. Any functional disease affecting the mind.

psychoanalysis (sī″kō-ăn-ăl'ĭ-sĭs) [" + *analysis*, a loosening apart]. Method of obtaining a detailed account of past and present mental and emotional experiences and repressions, in order to determine the source and eliminate the pathologic mental or physical state produced by these mechanisms.

Largely a system that is the creation of 1 man, Sigmund Freud, and originally, the outgrowth of his observations of neurotics. Frequently, the term often is used synonymously with freudianism, but more commonly for a rather more extensive system of psychologic fact and theory applying both to normal and abnormal groups.

The process is based upon the theory that such abnormal phenomena are due to repression of painful or undesirable past experiences, which, although totally forgotten, later manifest themselves in various abnormal ways. Psychoanalysis, therefore, makes an effort to bring up such forgotten memories into the conscious mind. The patient is thus enabled to view the occurrence in its true perspective, and so loses its harmful effect. There are 2 main methods: (1) Dream analysis; (2) the method of free association.

Includes a study of the ego in relation to reality, and more particularly the herd, and the conflicting goals so created. This conflict is "solved" by repressing 1 component. This repressed or censored emotion-laden complex of ideas exists in the so-called "subconscious," manifesting itself in the hidden content of dreams, in neuroses and tension states.

Quite unaware of the influence of the subconscious, anger outbursts, rationalization of unfair attitudes, slips of the tongue, etc., occur. Repressed material is largely sexual and the peculiar conditioning of the patient is chiefly determined by the emotional experiences of the earlier years. Reactions of inferiority may result in a compensatory reaction of goodness, ambition, etc. Sublimation is the escape of creative interest on levels not socially taboo. This, however, is not accepted by all psychologists.

psychobiological formula (sī″kō-bī-ō-lŏj'ĭ-kăl). A series of questions, used in studying a psychobiological problem, as to what constitutes the facts of mental phenomena, the factors and their grouping, and the conditions and results involving such facts and how they may be tested or modified.

psychobiology (sī″kō-bī-ŏl'ō-jī) [G. *psychē*, soul, + *bios*, life, + *logos*, a study]. Study of mental life and behavior in its interrelationship with other biological processes.

A concept dealing with objective and determinable factors pertaining to behavior and the condition in which they are manifested and influences modifying them, with their effects.

psychocardiac reflex (sī″kō-kar'dĭ-ăk). Change in circulatory rate and consciousness of heart thumping resulting from memory of, or subconscious dream state recollection of, an emotional impression or experience.

psychochrome (sī'kō-krōm) [G. *psychē*, soul, + *chrōma*, color]. Color impression resulting from sensory stimulation of a part other than the visual organ. SEE: *psychochromesthesia*.

psychochromesthesia (sī″kō-krŏm-ĕs-thē′-zĭ-ă) [" + " + *aisthēsis*, sensation]. Color sensation produced by the stimulus of sense organ other than that of vision.

psychocoma (sī-kō-kō′mă) [" + *kōma*, stupor]. Condition of mental stupor.

psychocortical (sī″kō-kor′tĭ-kăl) [" + L. *cortex*, rind]. Pert. to the cerebral cortex as the seat of sensory, motor, and psychic functions.

p. center. The cerebral center supposed to be the seat of motor, sensory, and psychic activity.

psychodometry (sī″kō-dŏm′ĕ-trĭ) [" + *odos*, way, + *metron*, measure]. Measurement of rate of mental activity.

psychodynamics (sī″kō-dī-năm′ĭks) [" + *dynamis*, power]. The scientific study of mental action or force.

psychogenesis (sī″kō-jĕn′ĕs-ĭs) [G. *psychē*, soul, + *genesis*, formation]. The origin and development of mind; the formation of mental traits.

psychogenetic (sī″kō-jĕn-ĕt′ĭk) [" + *genesis*, to produce]. 1. Originating in the mind, as a disease. 2. Concerning formation of mental traits.

psychogenia (sī″kō-jē′nĭ-ă) [" + *gennan*, to produce]. Disease resulting from disturbed psychic activity.

psychogenic (sī-kō-jĕn′ĭk) [" + *gennan*, to produce]. 1. Of mental origin. 2. Concerning the development of the mind. SYN: *psychogenetic*.

psychogram (sī′kō-grăm) [" + *gramma*, a writing]. A subjective visualization of a mental concept.

psychokinesia (sī″kō-kĭn-ē′zĭ-ă) [" + *kinēsis*, motion]. Explosive or impulsive maniacal action due to defective inhibition. SYN; *psycheclampsia*.

psycholepsy (sī′kō-lĕp′sĭ) [" + *lēpsis*, a seizure]. Sudden alteration of moods in which mental inertia and hopelessness are manifested.

psycholeptic (sī′kō-lĕp′tĭk) [" + *lēpsis*, a seizure]. Concerning sudden shifting of moods, particularly to 1 marked by hopelessness and mental inertia.

psychological (sī″kō-lŏj′ĭ-kal) [G. *psychē*, soul, mind, + *logos*, a study]. Pert. to study of the mind in all of its relationships, normal and abnormal.

psychologist (sī-kŏl′ō-jĭst) [" + *logos*, study]. One who specializes in the mental phenomena of consciousness and behavior or mental activity.

psychology (sī-kŏl′ō-jĭ) [" + *logos*, a study]. The science which deals with the mental processes, both normal and abnormal and their effects upon behavior. There are 2 main approaches to the study: (1) Introspective, *i. e.*, looking inwards, or self-examination of one's own mental processes. (2) Objective, *i. e.*, studying the minds of others. In this latter there are 4 chief lines of attack: (a) The experimental method; (b) the comparative method; (c) the genetic method; (d) the pathological method. SEE: *esthetic morality, "psych-" words*.

p., abnormal. The study of irregular or pathological mental phenomena.

p., experimental. Study of mental acts by tests and experiments.

p., genetic. Study of the evolution of mind in the individual and the race.

psychometry (sī-kŏm′ĕt-rĭ) [G. *psychē*, soul, mind, + *metron*, a measure]. Measurement of work accomplished, time consumed, and precision of mental operations; intelligence testing.

psychomotor (sī-kō-mō′tor) [" + L. *motor*, a mover]. Concerning, or causing, voluntary movement.

psychoneurosis (sī″kō-nū-rō′sĭs) [" + *neuron*, sinew, + *-ōsis*, disease]. A functional disease or disorder of mental origin without demonstrable lesion. Value of reality remains unchanged, but the individual uses reality to excess or to a minimum.

Includes hysteria, psychasthenia and neurasthenia. [*sis*.

SEE: *neurosis, psychoanalysis, psycho-*

p., defense. Condition due to attempt to dismiss from the mind ideas and sensations that are painful. This results in buried subconscious memories producing psychoneurosis.

psychoneurotic (sī″kō-nū-rŏt′ĭk) [G. *psychē*, soul, mind, + *neuron*, sinew]. Pert. to a functional disorder of mental origin.

psychonomy (sī-kŏn′ō-mĭ) [" + *nomos*, law]. The science of the laws of the mind and its functions.

psychonosis (sī″kō-nō′sĭs) [" + *nosos*, disease]. Any mental disorder.

psychoparesis (sī″kō-păr-ē′sĭs, -par′ĕ-sĭs) [" + *paresis*, relaxation]. Weakness or enfeeblement of the mind.

psychopath (sī′kō-păth) [" + *pathos*, disease]. One with a constitutional lack of moral sensibility, although possessing normal intelligence. SYN: *psychopathic personality*.

psychopathic (sī″kō-păth′ĭk) [" + *pathos*, disease]. 1. Concerning or characterized by a mental disorder. 2. Concerning treatment of mental disorders.

p. personality. "One who, though possessing normal intelligence, is or becomes, by reason of heredity or congenital conditions, constitutionally lacking in moral sensibility, emotional control, and the inhibition of will."—Dr. C. H. Patten.

A constitutional imbalance in the pattern of the mind, but not a disorder of function, such as is observed in the actual neuroses and psychoses. Psychopathics are attractive but cannot be depended upon. Judgment is poor; they are easily pleased or displeased, and are above the average in intelligence. Usually antisocial.

p., transportation of. 1. Be sure you have necessary legal papers.

2. Learn all you can about patient before starting.

3. Ascertain, if suicidal, epileptic, destructive, or dangerous.

4. If so (No. 3), do not travel with patient without assistance.

5. See that patient has nothing that may be used for violence or self-destruction.

6. If on train or boat, use a compartment.

7. If patient is dangerous, notify the transportation company in advance.

8. Do not hesitate to call upon local police or trainmen if necessary.

9. Be sure you have enough money for the journey and your own return.

10. Ascertain names of physicians who may be called en route if needed.

11. Secure copy of inventory of patient's effects from hospital, with statement as to any bruises or injuries suffered by patient.

psychopathology (sī″kō-păth-ŏl′ō-jĭ) [G. *psychē*, soul, mind, + *pathos*, disease,

+ *logos*, a study]. Cause and nature of diseased mental processes.

psychopathosis (sī″kō-păth-ō′sĭs) [″ + ″ + *-ōsis*, disease]. Any disease of the mind in the psychopathic group.

psychopathy (sī-kŏp′ăth-ĭ) [″ + *pathos*, disease]. Any mental disease, esp. 1 characterized by defective character or personality.

p., bisexual. Disorder including those who find sexual gratification from either sex.

p., sexual. A term for the group of disorders in which exist perversions of sex.

psychophysical (sī″kō-fĭz′ĭ-kăl) [″ + *physikos*, natural]. Concerning the relation of the physical and the mental.

p. law. Intensity of sensation increases as the logarithms of the stimuli.

psychophysics (sī″kō-fĭz′ĭks) [″ + *physikos*, natural]. 1. The study of mental processes in relation to physical processes. 2. The study of stimuli in relation to the effects they produce.

psychophysiology (sī″kō-fĭz-ĭ-ŏl′ō-jĭ) [″ + *physis*, nature, + *logos*, study]. Physiology of the mind; science of the correlation of body and mind.

psychoplegic (sī-kō-plē′jĭk) [G. *psychē*, mind, soul, + *plēgē*, a stroke]. An agent reducing excitability of the cerebrum.

psychoreaction (sī″kō-rē-ăk′shŭn) [″ + L. *re*, back, + *agere*, to lead]. Ability of serum from one having dementia precox or manic-depressive psychosis to inhibit hemolysis caused by cobra venom. SYN: *Much-Holzmann reaction.*

psychorhythmia (sī″kō-rĭth′mĭ-ă) [″ + *rythmos*, rhythm]. Involuntary repetition by the mind of its former actions.

psychorrhea (sī-kor-ē′ă) [″ + *roia*, a flow]. A disorder manifested by an incoherent stream of thought.

psychosensory (sī″kō-sĕn′sor-ĭ) [″ + L. *sensorius*, pert. to sensation]. 1. Understanding and interpreting sensory stimuli. 2. Concerning perceptions not arising in sensory organs, as hallucinations.

psychosexual (sī″kō-sĕks′ū-ăl)[″ + L. *sexus*, sex]. Concerning the emotional components of sexual instinct.

p. development. Evolution of personality through infantile and pregenital periods to sexual maturity.

psychosin (sī-kō′sĭn) [G. *psychē*, mind, soul]. A cerebroside occurring in brain tissue.

psychosis (sī-kō′sĭs) (pl. *psychoses*) [G. *psychē*, mind, soul]. Any mental derangement. SEE: *neurosis, psychoneurosis, psychotherapy.*

A condition manifested in the behavior, emotional reaction and ideation of the patient. He fails to mirror reality as it is, reacts erroneously to it, builds up false concepts regarding it, and his behavior responses are peculiar, abnormal, inefficient, or definitely antisocial.

All this does not include amentia, because defective intelligence merely lessens comprehension of reality but does not distort it, or the psychopathic personality, as here the patient reacts badly because of intrinsic emotional differences playing upon an undistorted world of reality.

Delusions or hallucinations strongly suggest a psychosis, as does marked indifference, depression and excitement. Antisocial behavior occurs with psychopathic personalities and mental defectiveness. When epileptic, it suggests the occurrence of an episodic psychosis known as an equivalent.

CLASSIFICATION: Divided into 3 main groups according to etiology: *Organic*, including all those in which brain damage can be demonstrated neuropathologically, such as senile dementia, meningoencephalitic lues (general paresis), and others. *Toxic*, which include all cases in which mental phenomena could be supposed to be caused by a toxic agent, such as psychoses from alcohol, drugs, etc. *Functional*, including all those cases in which an organic or toxic factor has not yet been ascertained, such as dementia precox, manic-depressive group, and so forth.

Below are listed some of the diseases or conditions in connection with which psychoses develop and the form that they take:

Psychoses with syphilitic meningoencephalitis (general paresis), or *with other forms of syphilis of the central nervous system*: (1) Meningovascular type (cerebral syphilis). (2) With intracranial gumma.

Psychoses with or following infectious diseases; infective-exhaustive psychosis: (1) With tuberculous meningitis.* (2) With meningitis (unspecified). (3) With acute chorea.* (4) With typhoid, influenza, pneumonia, scarlet fever, diphtheria, malaria, encephalitis, prolonged parturition. (5) Postinfectious psychoses, schizophrenia or manic-depressive type.

Psychoses due to drugs or other exogenous poisons: (1) Due to metals. (2) Due to gases. (3) Due to opium and derivatives. (4) Due to other drugs.

Alcoholic psychoses: (1) Pathological intoxication. (2) Delirium tremens. (3) Korsakoff's* psychosis. (4) Acute alcoholic hallucinosis.* (5) Chronic alcoholism of various types.

Senile psychoses: (1) Simple deterioration. (2) Presbyophrenic type. (3) Delirious and confused types. (4) Depressed and agitated types. (5) Paranoid type. (6) Presenile or Alzheimer's disease. (7) Other types.

Paranoia and paranoid conditions: (1) Paranoia.* (2) Paranoid conditions.

Psychoses with psychopathic personality: (a) With pathological sexuality. (b) With emotional instability. (c) With asocial or amoral trends. (d) Mixed types.

Undiagnosed psychoses.

Manic - depressive psychoses*: (1) Manic type. (2) Depressive type. (3) Circular type. (4) Mixed type. (5) Atypical type.

*Dementia precox** (schizophrenia*): (1) Simple type. (2) Hebephrenic* type. (3) Catatonic* type. (4) Paranoid type.

Traumatic psychoses: (1) Traumatic delirium. (2) Posttraumatic personality disorders. (3) Posttraumatic mental deterioration. (4) Rare condition following head injury.

*Psychoses with cerebral arteriosclerosis.**

Psychoses with disturbances of circulation: (1) With cerebral embolism.* (2) With cardiorenal disease. (3) Other types (to be specified).

Psychoses with convulsive disorders (epilepsy*): (1) Epileptic deterioration. (2) Epileptic clouded states. (3) Equivalent types.

Involutional psychoses: Melancholia.*

Psychoses due to brain tumors.

Psychoses associated with organic

changes of the nervous system: (1) With multiple sclerosis.* (2) With paralysis agitans.* (3) With Huntington's chorea.* (4) With other brain or nervous diseases.
Psychoses with endocrine dysfunction: (1) Dementia precox. (2) Epilepsy. (3) Feeblemindedness. (4) Organic psychoses. (5) Toxic psychoses. (6) Manic-depressive psychosis. (7) Paranoia. (8) Involutional melancholia.
Methods of treatment include psychotherapy,* shock therapy* (insulin, metrazol, electric), hydrotherapy,* and psychosurgery.*
Management requires meticulous care and great patience. Above all, do not appear alarmed or become excited. Be firm and composed. Patients frequently have hallucinations and often attempt suicide.
F. A. TREATMENT: Cold applications applied to head or neck may be soothing; prolonged warm baths are frequently helpful. Sedatives or drugs when given under a doctor's direction are invaluable. Spectators, excitement, and worried relatives should be banished. If necessary to restrain, this may be done by tying wrists together diagonally, and tying feet together with a double figure-of-eight bandage. Knees and shoulders should be fastened to the bed by broad cravats or similar strips. Such patients must be watched continuously.

p., affective. P. marked by moods of exaltation and depression, with flight or retardation of ideas, and nervous manifestations, hallucinations and delusions. SYN: *manic-depressive p*.

p., alcoholic-delusional. A degenerative process marked by delusions.

p., anxiety. Functional disturbance of mind marked by anxiety, depression and restlessness.

p., barbed wire. A psychosis involving irritability and loss of memory; seen in prisoners of war.

p., circular. Returning in cycles.

p., climacteric. Occurring at the menopause.

p., concurrent. Caused by disease.

p., confusional. Temporary, due to nervous shock.

p., congenital. From birth.

p., depressive. Melancholia.

p., deuteropathic. Secondary to some other disease.

p., diathetic. Inherited.

p., exhaustion. Confusional psychosis following an operation, tragic event, infection or shock.

p., homicidal. Desire to kill.

p., involutional. P. following the menopause, or in senility.

p., manic-depressive. Ordinarily a series of periods of psychotic depression or excessive well-being, appearing in any sequence and alternating with longer periods of relative normalcy.
Though intensity may vary greatly, the manic shows an elated though unstable mood, a flight of ideas, and great physical activity. The case of primary depression finds all exertion exhausting; there is difficulty in thinking or acting and victim is very unhappy.

p., organic. The result of a pathological condition of the central nervous system, such as paresis.

p., paroxysmal. Temporary attacks.

p., perceptional. Illusions and hallucinations.

p., polyneuritic. Korsakoff's p., seen in chronic alcoholism, with hallucinations, falsification of memory, wrist drop and disturbed orientation.

p., recurrent. Occurring at intervals.

p., senile. Due to old age.

p., situation. Transitory p. caused by an unpleasant situation. [agents.

p., toxic. One resulting from toxic

p., traumatic. One resulting from head injuries and belonging to the organic group.

psychosomatic. Pert. to interrelationship between the mind and body.

psychosurgery (sī″kō-sur′jer-ĭ) [G. *psyche*, soul, + G. *cheirourgia*, handwork]. Brain surgery for mental illness. The term includes such procedures as lobotomy,* topectomy,* and thalamotomy.*

psychotechnics (sī″kō-tĕk′nĭks) [G. *psyche*, soul, + *techne*, art]. Application of psychological methods in the study of economic and social problems.

psychotherapy (sī-kō-thĕr′ă-pĭ) [" + *therapeia*, treatment]. Any mental method of treating disease, esp. nervous disorders, by means such as suggestion, hypnotism, psychoanalytic therapy, etc.

psychroalgia (sī-krō-ăl′jĭ-ă) [G. *psychros*, cold, + *algos*, pain]. Painful sensation of cold.

psychroesthesia (sī″krō-ĕs-thē′zĭ-ă) [" + *aisthesis*, sensation]. 1. A sensation of cold in a part of the body, although it is warm. 2. The sensation that perceives cold.

psychrometer (sī-krŏm′ĕ-tĕr) [" + *metron*, a measure]. Device for measuring relative humidity of the atmosphere.

psychrophilic (sī-krō-fīl′ĭk) [" + *philein*, to love]. Preferring cold, as bacteria which thrive best at low temperature.

psychrophobia (sī-krō-fō′bĭ-ă) [" + *phobos*, fear]. Abnormal aversion or sensitiveness to cold.

psychrophore (sī′krō-fōr) [" + *phorein*, to carry]. Apparatus for applying cold to the urethra, or other canal.

psychrotherapy (sī″krō-thĕr′ă-pĭ) [" + *therapeia*, treatment]. Treatment of disease by administration of cold.

psyllium seed (sĭl′ĭ-ŭm). The dried, ripe seed of a plant grown in France, Spain, and India.
USES: As a mild laxative.
DOSAGE: 2 drams (8 Gm.) in orange or prune juice.

ptarmic (tar′mĭk) [G. *ptarmos*, a sneezing]. 1. Causing sneezing. SYN: *sternutatory*. 2. That which causes sneezing.

pterion (tē′rĭ-ŏn) [G. *pteron*, wing]. Point of suture of frontal, parietal, temporal, and sphenoid bones.

pteroylglutamic acid. SEE: *folic acid*.

pterygium (tĕr-ĭj′ĭ-ŭm) [G. *pterygion*, wing]. OPHTH: Triangular thickening of bulbar conjunctiva on the cornea with apex toward pupil.

p., progressive. Stage in which the growth extends toward center of cornea.

p., stationary. Stage in which the head of pterygium remains permanently attached to same point on the cornea.
TREATMENT: Surgical.

pterygoid (tĕr′ĭ-goyd) [" + *eidos*, appearance]. Wing-shaped. SYN: *alate*.

p. fossa. 1. The depression bet. the pterygoid plates of the sphenoid for the origin of the internal pterygoid muscle. 2. The condyloid fossa of the mandible.

p. processes. Two big processes which are part of the sphenoid bone.

pterygomaxillary (tĕr″ĭ-gō-măks′ĭl-ā-rĭ) [" + L. *maxillaris*, pert. to upper jaw]. Concerning the pterygoid process and the upper jaw.

pterygopalatine (tĕr″ĭ-gō-păl′ă-tīn) [" + L. *palatinus*, pert. to the palate]. Relating to the pterygoid process and the palate bone.

ptilosis (tĭl-ō′sĭs) [G. *ptilon*, feather, + *-ōsis*, disease]. Loss of eyelashes.

ptomaine (tō′mān) [G. *ptōma*, dead body]. One of a class of nitrogenous organic bases formed in the action of putrefactive bacteria on proteins and amino acids. Ex: Cadaverine, $NH_2(CH_2)_5NH_2$. SEE: *aporrhegma*.

They are poisonous substances resembling alkaloids resulting from decomposition of proteins. Many are very toxic. Ptomaines are poisonous bodies due to the action of microörganisms.

They are chemical compounds of definite composition and are elaborated by microörganisms breaking down the complex ingredients of animal tissues, just as alcohol is due to the action of yeast breaking down sugar, or as acetic acid is formed from the alcohol of cider or wine by the yeastlike plant which produces vinegar, and which we call "mother" when we find it collected in masses.

The formation of ptomaines quite generally, although not always, accompanies putrefaction (being greatest, it is said, in its early stages).

p. poisoning. An unsatisfactory term for food poisoning which has been dropped from good medical usage.

Ptomaines only occur in the later stages of food decomposition. For many years it was assumed that food poisoning was due to ptomaines. Such, however, is not the case, as many food poisonings are due to bacteria or their products. Food that has developed ptomaines from decomposition would be so offensive to sight and smell that it would cause its immediate rejection by the purchaser. SEE: *food poisoning*.

ptomainemia (tō″mān-ē′mĭ-ă) [G. *ptōma*, corpse, + *aima*, blood]. Conditions caused by ptomaines in the circulating blood.

ptosis (tō′sĭs) [G. *ptosis*, a dropping]. Dropping or drooping of an organ or part, as the upper eyelid from paralysis, or the visceral organs from weakness of the abdominal muscles.

RS: *cataptosis, phalangosis, visceroptosis.*

p., abdominal. Sagging of transverse colon; sometimes almost to the pelvic floor.

ETIOL: Obesity or lack of abdominal muscle tone.

TREATMENT: A properly adjusted abdominal belt may help.

CONTRA: Dependence upon belt rather than on exercising and developing abdominal muscles.

ptyalagogue (tĭ-ăl′ă-gŏg) [G. *ptyalon*, saliva, + *agōgos*, leading]. Causing or that which causes a flow of saliva. SYN: *sialogogue*.

ptyalin (tī′ă-lĭn) [G. *ptyalon*, saliva]. A salivary amylolytic enzyme converting starch into maltose and dextrin. SEE: *enzyme, ptyalinogen, ptyalism, saliva*.

ptyalinogen (tī-ăl-ĭn′ō-jĕn) [" + *gennan*, to produce]. A hypothetical substance in the salivary glands from which ptyalin is formed.

ptyalism (tī′ăl-ĭzm) [" + *-ismos*, condition]. Excessive secretion of saliva.

ETIOL: May be due to pregnancy, stomatitis, rabies, exophthalmic goiter, menstruation and other disorders, including epilepsy, hysteria, nervous conditions and gastrointestinal troubles. May be induced by mercury, iodides, pilocarpine and other drugs. SYN: *salivation*. SEE: *xerostomia*.

ptyalith (tī′ă-lĭth) [" + *lithos*, stone]. A calculus in a salivary gland.

ptyalocele (tī-ăl′ō-sēl) [" + *kēlē*, hernia]. A salivary cystic tumor or cystic dilatation of a salivary duct.

ptyalogenic (tī″ăl-ō-jĕn′ĭk) [" + *gennan*, to produce]. Of salivary origin.

ptyalogogue (tī-ăl′ō-gŏg) [" + *agōgos*, leading]. That which produces saliva. SYN: *sialogogue*.

ptyalogram (tī-ăl′ō-grăm) [G. *ptyalon*, saliva, + *gramma*, a writing]. An x-ray film of the salivary glands.

ptyalography (tī-ăl-ŏg′ră-fī) [" + *graphein*, to write]. X-ray inspection of the salivary glands and ducts. SYN: *sialography*.

ptyalolith (tī′ă-lō-lĭth) [" + *lithos*, stone]. A salivary concretion.

ptyalolithotomy (tī″ăl-ō-lĭth-ŏt′ō-mĭ) [" + " + *tomē*, a cutting]. Surgical removal of a concretion from a salivary duct or gland.

ptyalorrhea (tī″ă-lō-rē′ă) [" + *roia*, flow]. An excessive flow of saliva.

ptyocrine, ptyocrinous (tī′ō-krĕn, tī-ŏk′rĭn-ŭs) [" + *krinein*, to secrete]. Secreting part of the protoplasm, said of a gland cell. OPP: *diacrinous, exocrine*.

puber (pū′bŭr) [L.]. One at onset of puberty.

puberal (pū′bĕr-ăl) [L. *pubertās*, puberty]. Concerning puberty.

puberty (pū′bĕr-tĭ) [L. *pubertās*, puberty]. Period in life at which 1 of either sex becomes functionally capable of reproduction.

A period of rapid change in boys and girls. It occurs in temperate climates bet. the ages of 13 and 16 in boys, and from 12 to 15 in girls, and ends in the attainment of sexual maturity.

In the boy it is marked by appearance of hair on the face and chest, under the axilla, and on the pubes, change of voice, definite enlargement of the penis, and the appearance of erections and erotic dreams with ejaculation. Other physical and psychic disturbances are normal at this period, and end in the appearance of functional spermatozoa in the semen.

In the girl menstruation begins, the breasts enlarge, and hair appears in axilla and on the pubes.

RS: *hebephrenia, hebetic, interstitial, latency period, menacme, nubility*.

pubes (pū′bēz) (sing. *pubis*) [L. pubic hair]. 1. Ant. part of innominate bone; *os pubis*. 2. The pubic region. 3. Hair of the pubic region.

It is a sexual fetish, inspiring passion in the opposite sex.

pubescence (pū-bĕs′sĕns) [L. *pubescĕre*, to become hairy]. 1. Puberty or its approach. 2. Covering of fine, soft hairs on the body. SYN: *lanugo*.

pubescent (pū-bĕs′ĕnt) [L. *pubescĕre*, to become hairy]. 1. Reaching puberty. 2. Covered with downy hair.

pubetrotomy (pū″bē-trŏt′ō-mĭ) [L. *pubes*, pubic hair, + G. *ētron*, belly, + *tomē*, a cutting]. Section through the pubes.

pubic (pū′bĭk) [L. *pubes*, pubic hair]. Concerning the pubes.

p. bone. The lower ant. part of the innominate bone. SYN: *os pubis*.

p. hair. Hair over the pubes which appears at onset of sexual maturity. It is usually lighter in color than hair on the head. It protects vital organs under the pubes. It is a fetish* to some of the opposite sex, exciting the libido, and its abundance is claimed by some to be a mark of sexual vigor. SEE: *escutcheon, fetish, libido*.

pubio-, pubo- [L.]. Combining forms meaning the *pubic hair, pubic bone* or *region*.

pubiotomy (pū″bĭ-ŏt′ō-mĭ) [L. *pubes*, pubic hair, + *tome*, a cutting]. Incision across the pubis in order to enlarge the pelvic passage, facilitating the delivery of the fetus when pelvis is malformed.

pubis (pū′bĭs) [L. pubic hair]. 1. Pubic bone. 2. BNA. Hair over pubic bone. RS: *hebeosteotomy, mens, os pubis*.

pubofemoral (pū″bō-fĕm′or-ăl) [L. *pubis*, pubic hair, + *femur, femor-*, thigh bone]. Pert. to the os pubis and the femur.

puboprostatic (pū″bō-prŏs-tăt′ĭk) [" + G. *prostates*, prostate]. Relating to the os pubis and prostate gland.

pubovesical (pū″bō-vĕs′ĭ-kl) [" + *vesiculus*, a little sac]. Pert. to the os pubis and bladder.

pudenda (pū-dĕn′dă) (sing. *pudendum**) [L. *pudendum*, from *pudere*, to be ashamed]. The ext. genitalia, esp. of the female. SYN: *vulva*.

pudendagra (pū″den-dăg′ră) [" + G. *agra*, seizure]. Pain in the ext. genitals.

p. pruriens. Intense itching of ext. female genitals. SYN: *pruritus vulvae*.

pudendal (pū-dĕn′dăl) [L. *pudendum*, from *pudere*, to be ashamed]. Relating to the ext. genitals of female.

pudendum (pū-dĕn′dŭm) (pl. *pudenda*) [L.]. The ext. genitals, esp. those of the female; the vulva.

p. muliebre. BNA. Ext. genitals of the female.

pudic (pū′dĭk) [L. *pudicus*, modest]. Concerning ext. female genitalia. SYN: *pudendal*.

puericulture (pū-er′ĭ-kŭl″chūr) [L. *puer*, child, + *cultura*, a cultivating]. Science concerned with prenatal care of unborn children and the art of raising and training children.

puerile (pū′ĕ-rĭl) [L. *puer*, boy]. Concerning a child; childlike.

p. respiration. That heard in auscultation of healthy children.

puerilism (pū′ĕr-ĭl-ĭzm) [" + G. -*ismos*, condition]. Childishness.

puerpera (pū-er′pĕr-ă) [L. *puer*, boy, + *parere*, to bear]. Woman during the period following the 3rd stage of labor, lasting until there is complete involution of the pelvic viscera.

puerperal (pū-er′pur-ăl) [L. *puer*, boy, + *parere*, to bear]. Concerning puerperium.

p. eclampsia. Convulsions during puerperium.

p. fever. Septicemia following childbirth. SYN: *childbed fever*.

p. insanity. A psychosis during the puerperium.

p. period. Period immediately following after childbirth.

p. sepsis. A toxemia of puerperium accompanied by a rise in temperature during the first 21 days.

CHARACTERISTICS: (a) Greatest single cause of death due to childbirth. (b) Lowered resistance a danger. (c) Toxemia, anemia, exhaustion in labor, abrasions and lacerations, loss of blood predisposing factors. (d) May be autogenous or heterogeneous. (e) Other foci aside from genitals may be responsible for invasion. (f) Infection may remain localized or it may spread. (g) Infected thrombi from veins of placental site may enter blood stream. (h) Metastatic areas of infection may be caused by (g). (i) Spreading along mucous membranes the infection may reach the tubes, ovaries and peritoneum. (j) Thrombophlebitis in pelvic veins may lead to thrombophlebitis in veins of the leg. (k) Localized infections indicated by fever, rapid pulse, pain and pelvic tenderness. (l) Fever in (k) about 3rd day, 103° F. to 104° F. (m) In endometritis, tenderness confined to uterus, lochia may be scant without odor. (n) Lochia profuse and foul if any membranes are retained. (o) Parametritis in more severe infections. (p) In (o) swelling due to inflammatory exudate, giving place to suppuration after a few days, accompanied by chill and rise in temperature. (q) Peritonitis possible, especially if gonococcus is present. (r) Every spread of disease indicated by rise in temperature, and perhaps chills. (s) Drainage may be necessary. (t) Permanent sterility possible.

PREVENTION: 1. Aseptic technic in all obstetric cases. 2. Masking of those who come in contact with patient. 3. Complete bacteriological survey following any infection to determine possible source. 4. Exclusion of all positive carriers from attendance upon maternity cases. 5. Better intrapartum care of case long in labor, use of least traumatizing type of delivery, avoidance of blood loss and wider use of blood transfusions.

TREATMENT: Active surgical intervention during infection seldom indicated. Good nursing care, high caloric and vitamin diet, restriction of visitors and sources of irritation. All manipulative procedures kept at a minimum. Excellent results have been obtained from use of sulfonamides and antibiotics.

puerperalism (pū-er′pŭr-ăl-ĭzm) [L. *puer*, boy, + *parere*, to bear, + G. *ismos*, condition]. Pathological conditions of the puerperal state.

p., infantile. Any pathogenic condition of the newly born.

p., infectious. Puerperal disease caused by infection.

puerperant (pū-er′pŭr-ănt) [" + *parere*, to bear]. A woman in labor or one who recently has been delivered.

puerperium (pū-er-pē′rĭ-ŭm). Period following the 3rd stage of labor, lasting until involution of pelvic organs takes place; usually 3 to 6 weeks.

RS: *childbed; Kellogg's inspiratory lift exercise; sepsis, puerperal*.

puerperous (pū-ŭr′pŭr-ŭs) [L. *puer*, boy, + *parere*, to bear]. In the period following childbirth. SYN: *puerperal*.

pulmo- [L.]. Combining form meaning *lung*.

pulmoaortic (pŭl″mō-ā-or′tĭk) [L. *pulmo*, lung, + G. *aorte*, aorta]. 1. Concerning the lungs and the aorta. 2. Relating to the pulmonary artery and aorta.

pulmometer (pŭl-mŏm′ĕt-ēr) [" + G. *metron*, a measure]. Device for measuring the lung capacity. SYN: *spirometer*.

pulmometry (pŭl-mŏm′ĕt-rĭ) [" + G. *metron*, a measure]. Determination of capacity of the lungs.

pulmonary (pŭl′mō-na-rĭ) [L. *pulmo, pulmon-*, lung]. Concerning or affected by the lungs. SEE: *caverniloquy*.

p. circulation. Passage of blood from heart to lungs and back again for purification.

The blood flows from the right cardiac ventricle through the lungs, there to be

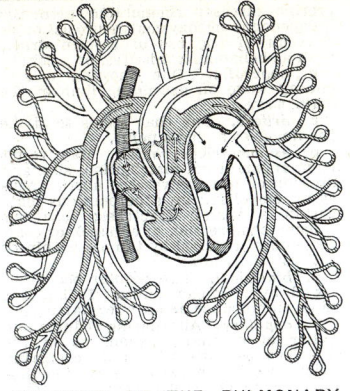

pulmonary incompetence   P-122   **pulse**

DIAGRAM OF THE PULMONARY CIRCULATION.
The shaded areas represent the course of the venous blood; the unshaded, the arterial blood.

oxygenated; then back to the left cardiac auricle.
   p. incompetence, p. insufficiency. Failure of the pulmonary valve to close properly.
   p. reflex. Contraction of lung induced by sudden stimulation of thoracic wall.
   p. stenosis. Narrowing of opening into the pulmonary artery from right cardiac ventricle.
pulmonectomy (pŭl-mō-nĕk'tō-mĭ) [L. *pulmō, pulmon-*, lung, + G. *ektomē*, excision]. Removal of part or all of a lung's tissue. SYN: *pneumonectomy*.
pulmonic (pŭl-mŏn'ĭk) [L. *pulmō, pulmon-*, lung]. 1. Relating to or affecting the lungs. SYN: *pulmonary*. 2. Relating to the pulmonary artery. 3. Having origin at or by the pulmonic valve, as a *murmur*.
   p. circulation. Flow of blood from right cardiac ventricle to the lungs, returning to the left ventricle.
   p. fever. Lobar pneumonia.
pulmonitis (pŭl-mō-nī'tĭs) [" + G. *-itis*, inflammation]. Inflamed condition of the lung. SYN: *pneumonia*.
pulmotor (pŭl-mō'tor) [" + *motor*, a mover]. Apparatus for inducing artificial respiration by forcing oxygen into the lungs, or for expelling gas in case of asphyxiation.
pulp (pŭlp) [L. *pulpa*, flesh]. 1. The soft part of fruit. 2. The soft part of an organ. 3. Chyme.
   p. cavity. Hollow space within a tooth containing dental pulp.
   p. cells. Those in the pulp cavity of any organ.
   p., dental. The soft tissue filling the cavity of a tooth.
   p., digital. Elastic, soft prominence on the palmar or plantar surface of the last phalanx of a finger or toe.
pulpal (pŭl'păl) [L. *pulpa*, flesh]. Relating to pulp.
pulpefaction (pŭl-pĭ-făk'shŭn) [" + *facere*, to make]. Conversion into pulpy substance.
pulpy (pŭl'pĭ) [L. *pulpa*, flesh]. Resembling pulp; flabby. SYN: *pultaceous*.
pulsate (pŭl'sāt) [L. *pulsāre*, to beat]. To throb or beat in rhythm.

pulsatile (pŭl'să-tĭl). Pulsating; characterized by a rhythmic beat. SYN: *throbbing*.
pulsation (pŭl-sā'shŭn) [L. *pulsatiō*, a beating]. The rhythmic beat, as of the heart and blood vessels; a throbbing. SEE: *pulse*.
   ABNORMAL CENTERS OF PULSATION: *Epigastric p.*: May result from: 1. Excited action of heart from any cause. 2. Enlargement of right ventricle. 3. A pulsating aorta noted in certain nervous and anemic patients. 4. Aortic aneurysm. 5. Tumors of left lobe of liver resting on the aorta. *P. in left axillary region*: May result from: 1. Enlargement of heart. 2. A tense purulent effusion in left pleural sac (pulsating empyema). 3. Aneurysm. 4. Chronic disease of left lung and pleura, associated with retraction.
   Unnatural p. in carotids: May result from: 1. Excitement of heart from any cause. 2. Exophthalmic goiter. 3. Anemia. 4. Valvular disease, especially aortic regurgitation. 5. Aneurysm or dilatation of the vessels. 6. Unnatural elasticity of the vessels, noted in certain nervous and anemic patients. *Jugular p.*: The jugular vein often becomes distended in forced expiration and coughing. Sometimes distention noted in adherent pericardium. A true rhythmical venous pulsation usually results from tricuspid regurgitation. A pulsation may be transmitted to the jugular vein from the underlying carotid, but this false pulsation will continue when light pressure is made on root of neck, while the true venous pulse will cease.

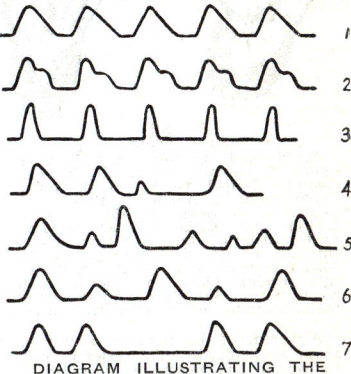

DIAGRAM ILLUSTRATING THE COMMON TYPES OF PULSE.
After Sears.

1. Normal Pulse. Showing fairly sharp onset with more gradual falling away of the beat. 2. Dicrotic Pulse. Showing secondary wave as the beat falls away. 3. Waterhammer Pulse. Showing abrupt onset and sharp falling away of the beat. 4. Pulse with Extra Systole. A small premature wave followed by a pause before the next normal beat. 5. Pulse in Auricular Fibrillation, with irregularity in rhythm and volume of all the beats. 6. Pulsus Alternans. Large and small beats alternate regularly with each other. 7. Pulsus Bigeminus. A coupling of two beats, followed by a pause.

pulse (pŭls) [L. *pulsus*, from *pulsāre*, to beat]. 1. Edible leguminous seeds, as peas, beans. 2. Rhythmical throbbing.

3. Throbbing caused by the regular contraction and alternate expansion of an artery; the periodic thrust felt over arteries in time with the heartbeat.

Normal pulse rate of adult is 70 to 75 and is usually observed in radial artery of the wrist.

POINTS TO BE OBSERVED: Hour, frequency, pressure, regularity, force. Temperature and respiration are of clinical importance to the physician. Right and left radial arteries are usually tested, and differences, if any or absent, should be noted. Pressure should not be too great on artery and thumb should not be used. Count half a minute at a time per minute.

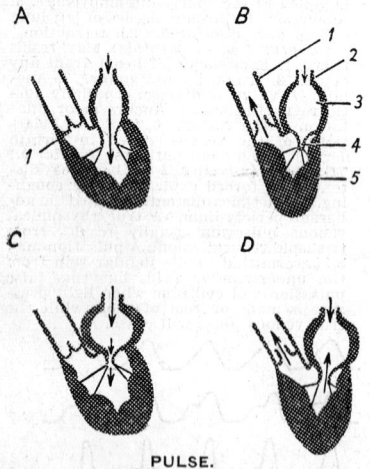

PULSE.
After Sears.

A. Normal diastole. Mitral valve open. 1. Aortic valve. B. Normal systole. Mitral valve closed, aortic valve open. 1. Aorta. 2. Pulmonary veins. 3. Auricle. 4. Mitral valve. 5. Ventricle. C. Mitral stenosis. Hypertrophied left auricle forcing blood through narrowed mitral valve. D. Mitral regurgitation. Ventricular systole forcing blood into aorta, with regurgitation into left auricle owing to inadequate closure of mitral valve.

A tracing of this is called a sphygmogram and consists of a series of waves in which the upstroke is called the *anacrotic* limb, and the downstroke (on which is normally seen the dicrotic notch), the *catacrotic*.

p., accelerated. A common symptom in all fevers. The pulse of the adult rarely exceeds 150 beats per minute even in acute inflammatory infections; when it runs above 170 it *may* portend a fatal issue.

A pulse of 170 is known as *tachycardia*, and in some diseases it is a common symptom. If such an acceleration does not diminish within a short time it is especially unfavorable. A rate of 150 is not necessarily fatal. When quick and bounding it indicates acute fever or inflammation, or may result from a toxic goiter; organic heart disease; pressure at the base of the brain sufficient to paralyze the pneumogastric nerve, as in clot, tumor, and advanced meningitis; shock; reflex irritation, as in ovarian or uterine disease; rheumatoid arthritis; independent paroxysmal neurosis, or be a result of the use of certain drugs, such as belladonna, nitrites, or alcohol.

p., anacrotic. One showing a secondary wave on ascending limb of the main wave.

p., ardent. One that seems to strike the finger at a single point.

p., asymmetrical radial. May result from anomalies of distribution, size, and division of 1 of the vessels; aortic aneurysm; embolism; an atheromatous plate within a vessel; fractures; luxations causing compression of a vessel, or compression of a vessel by tumors within or without the thorax.

p., bigeminal. Two regular beats followed by a longer pause. It has the same significance as an irregular pulse.

p., capillary. Alternating redness and pallor of capillary region, as in the matrices beneath the nails, occurring chiefly where an excessive cardiac impulse coincides with general arterial narrowing.

p., caprizant. An irregular, peculiar, weak pulsation succeeded by a stronger one.

p., catacrotic. One showing 1 or more secondary waves on descending limb of the main wave.

p., changeable. Denotes nervous derangement and sometimes organic heart disease.

p., collapsing. One feebly striking the finger, then subsiding abruptly and completely.

p., Corrigan's. One of aortic insufficiency. SEE: *waterhammer pulse*.

p., dicrotic. A double beat, 1 heartbeat for 2 arterial pulsations, or a seeming weak wave bet. the usual heartbeats. This weak wave should not be counted as a regular beat. It is indicative of low arterial tension, and is noted in fevers, in low states of the nervous system, and sometimes in typhoid fever.

p., febrile. A full, bounding pulse at onset of fever, becoming feeble and weak when fever subsides or on prostration.

p., female. More frequent than male p. by 10 or 15 beats. There is an important correlation bet. the pulse, respiration and temperature which must be considered in most disease states.

p., fine, scarcely perceptible. Denotes great exhaustion and approaching death. May be caused by wasting disease or by hemorrhage.

p. frequency. Depends upon sex, age, exertion, position of body and health. It is higher in children and increases with very old age. It is slower in tall persons than it is in short ones. It is 10 to 12 beats more frequent in standing than sitting. Muscular exertion, as dancing, will raise it from 75 to 125 or higher. Eating and drinking likewise increase heart action. It is less frequent when sleeping or lying down.

p., full. A distended one giving a tense feeling; observed in sthenic inflammation.

p., gaseous. SEE: *hemorrhagic pulse*.
p., goat-leap. SEE: *caprizant p.*
p., hard. One with sensation of hardness due to changes in the arterial wall or to vascular distention.

p., hemorrhagic. A soft, full, and readily compressible 1 marking a distended artery that has lost its tone.

p., hepatic. One due to expansion of

veins of the liver at each ventricular contraction.

p., high-tension. One in which force of beat is relatively increased and which may be roughly estimated by noting the amount of pressure of the fingers that is required to arrest the beat. It is observed in many conditions, notably: cardiac diseases, such as hypertrophy; chronic nephritis; cerebral affections; irritation of the vasomotor center, as in apoplexy, tumors, and beginning meningitis; also after the use of certain drugs, such as digitalis, ergot, and alcoholic stimulants; and in chills, angina pectoris, epileptic and hysterical seizures, lithemia, gout, and uremia.

p., incident. One with 2nd beat weaker than 1st, the 3rd weaker than the 4th, followed by a stroke as strong as the 1st.

p., infrequent. Observed in organic heart disease, especially fatty degeneration, and fibroid induration; jaundice; pressure at base of brain sufficient to irritate the vagus, as in beginning meningitis; and at the close of febrile diseases, as in typhoid fever, and pneumonia. May follow the use of certain drugs, such as digitalis, aconite, and opium. Physiological slowness is noted in repose, during fasting, in the puerperium, and old age; it is habitual in certain people (40 to 60 beats per minute).

p., intermittent. One in which occasional beats are skipped.

Caused by an apparent drop of a heartbeat. It is not inconsistent with health; yet it is commonly an indication of disease, frequently from gastric, hepatic, uterine, and renal causes. It is common in lithemia and fatty degeneration of the heart and is habitual in certain people after exercise, eating, excitement, or after the use of tobacco, tea, coffee, or other stimulants.

p., irregular. One when there is a variation in "force" and "frequency." Has same significance as intermittent pulse. Common in myocarditis and valvular diseases, esp. in mitral regurgitation. Heart trouble may be noted by long continued irregular pulse. Excess of tea, coffee, tobacco, or exercise may cause an irregular pulse.

p., jerking. That of aortic regurgitation, because from a state of emptiness the artery is suddenly filled with blood.

p., jugular. Venous pulse, *q.v.*

p., long. One in which duration of the systolic wave is comparatively long.

p., low-tension. One with sudden onset, short duration and rapid decline; esp. noted in degeneration of the heart, collapse, in debility, fevers, and low states of the nervous system.

p., male. From 70-75 beats per minute, but not an invariable rule, as some are healthy with a pulse rate of 50 or even 90.

p., monocrotous. One with a sphygmogram showing a simple ascending and descending, uninterrupted line and no dicrotism, indicative of a grave condition of the circulation and of impending death.

p., myurous. One with gradually weaker beats of diminishing amplitude.

p., paradoxical. One which is more or less suppressed at close of each full inspiration. Thought to be due to compression of the great vessels by inflammatory adhesions; the latter being stretched during act of inspiration. Frequently noted in adherent pericardium.

p., plateau. One slowly rising but which is maintained.

p. pressure. The difference bet. the systolic and the diastolic pressure.

This is really expressive of the tone of the arterial walls. Ex:

120 is systolic pressure.
100 is diastolic pressure.
───
20 is the pulse pressure.

130 is the systolic pressure.
90 is the diastolic pressure.
───
40 is the pulse pressure.

Normal pulse pressure: The systolic pressure must be about 40 points over the diastolic pressure in comparison. *Abnormal pulse pressure*: A pulse pressure over 50 points and under 30 points is considered abnormal.

p., quick, full, bounding. Indicates inflammation or fever of acute inflammatory character.

p., quick, hard. Characteristic of diphtheria and scarlatina. It also indicates inflammation or fever of acute inflammatory nature.

p., rapid. SEE: *accelerated p.*

p. rate.

Average Normal Expansile

P. of embryo, average per minute	150
At birth	140-130
During 1st year	130-115
During 2nd year	115-100
During 3rd year	100- 90
About 7th year	90- 85
About 14th year	85- 80
In middle life	75- 70
Old age	65- 50

p., regular. When the "force" and "frequency" are the same, that is, when the length of beat and number of beats per minute and the strength are the same.

p., renal. A hard and full one in coma from kidney disease.

p., respiratory. Alternate dilatation and contraction of the large veins of the neck occurring simultaneously with inspiration and expiration following rapid exercise.

p., senile. That of the aged. The sphygmogram shows a high position of the secondary waves in descent with great size of the 1st secondary wave as compared with the 2nd.

p., short. One with a short, quick systolic wave.

p., shuttle. One that feels as though it is floating something solid as well as fluid.

p., slow. A very slow pulse, fully accentuated, often found among the aged, and it is a habitual rate among those inclined to be slow and easy in their actions. Such a pulse rate ranges bet. 40 and 60 beats per minute.

p., sluggish, full. Evinces want of nervous energy. Usual slowness, chiefly met with in chronic softening and tuberculous affections of brain. Also common in diseases attended with coma resulting from concussion or compression of brain.

p., small and rapid. Seen in great prostration from wasting diseases or hemorrhage.

p., soft. One which may be stopped by digital compression.

p., steel hammer. It is abrupt and energetic, as the rebound of a smith's hammer. One observed in arteries near a joint in rheumatism.

p., systolic. The period of the contraction of the heart causing the greatest arterial pressure, which normally is 100. Two or 3 beats followed by a longer pause. It has the same significance as the irregular pulse.

p., thready. A scarcely appreciable one observed in syncope.

p., tremulous. One in which a series of oscillations is felt with each beat.

p., trigeminal. Three regular beats followed by a pause. SEE: *irregular p.*

p., undulating. One that seems to have several successive waves.

p., unequal. One that varies in strength of its beats.

p., vaginal. Arterial p. perceptible in the vagina in inflammatory disease or in pregnancy.

p., venous. Pulsation noted in jugular vein, often noted in tricuspid regurgitation. A venous pulse on dorsum of hand may be due to forcible propulsion of blood through the capillaries, as in aortic regurgitation, with great hypertrophy of left ventricle, or to extreme relaxation of arterioles and capillaries, permitting the transmission of the pulse wave, as in grave cachexia and anemia.

p., vermicular. A small, frequent one with a wormlike feeling.

p., jerking. A jerking p., *q.v.*

p., water-hammer. Characterized by a short, powerful, jerky beat which suddenly collapses. The peculiar pulsation may be distinctly visible, not only in the carotids, but throughout the brachial artery. It is diagnostic of aortic regurgitation during the period of compensation, and its force is due to excessive ventricular hypertrophy and to the large amount of blood expelled with each systole; its sudden recession is due to the incompetent valves failing to support the column of blood. SYN: *Corrigan's p.*

p., wiry. A tense one that feels like a wire or firm cord.

pulse, words pert. to: acrotic, acrotism, Adams-Stokes syndrome, anacrotic, anadicrotic, anadicrotism, anatricrotic, arrhythmia, artery, asphyctic, auricular, bisferious, bradycrotic, bradydiastole, bradysphygmia, cacosphyxia, capricant, cardiopuncture, catacrotism, catadicrotic, catadicrotism, centesis, Corrigan's, diastasis, diastole, diastolic pressure, dicrotic, heart, -block, hemisystole, infant, intercadence, intercalary, phlebogram, pulsate, pulsation, pulsus, respiration, spinal, sphygmoid, sphygmogram, sphygmomanometer, systaltic, systole, systolic pressure, systolic temperature, thermometry, vein.

pulsimeter (pŭl-sĭm'ĕt-ĕr) [L. *pulsus*, a beat, + G. *metron*, measure]. Contrivance for measuring frequency and force of the pulse. SYN: *sphygmometer.*

pul'sion [L. *pulsus*]. A veering of the individual from one side to another.

pulsus (pŭl'sŭs) [L.]. Pulse.

p. alternans. A succession of strong and weak beats alternating.

p. bigeminus. Paired beats.

p. celer. Fast pulse, particularly that associated with high pulse pressure in aortic regurgitation.

p. paradoxus. One in which p. becomes weaker during inspiration.

p. tardus. Slow pulse, particularly seen in aortic stenosis.

pultaceous (pŭl-tā'shŭs) [L. *puls, pult-, pap*]. Resembling a poultice. SYN: *pulpy.*

pulv. [L.]. Abbr. *pulvis*, powder.

pulverization (pŭl-vĕr-ĭ-zā'shŭn) [L. *pulvis*, powder]. The crushing of any substance to powder or tiny particles.

pulverulent (pŭl-vĕr'ū-lĕnt) [L. *pulvis, pulver-*, powder]. Of the nature of, or resembling, powder. SYN: *powdery.*

pulvinar (pŭl-vī'nĕr) [L. cushioned seat]. The post. prominence of the optic thalamus.

pulvinate (pŭl'vĭn-āt) [L. *pulvinus*, cushion]. Very convex; shaped like a cushion.

pulvis (pŭl'vĭs) [L.]. Powder.

The 6 official powders are mixtures of powdered medicinal substances.

pump (pŭmp) [M.E. *pumpe*]. 1. Apparatus that transfers fluids or gases by pressure or suction. 2. To force air or fluid into a cavity, as heart pumps blood.

p., air. Device for forcing air in or out of a chamber.

p., breast. Apparatus for removing milk from the breasts.

p., dental. Apparatus for removing saliva during operation on teeth or jaws.

p., stomach. Apparatus for removing contents of stomach.

pumpkin (pŭmp'kĭn) [G. *pepōn*, ripe]. Av. SERVING: 120 Gm. Pro. 1.2, Fat 0.1, Carbo. 4.8. VITAMINS: A++, B+, C+ to ++. ASH CONST: Ca 0.023, Mg 0.008, K 0.320, Na 0.065, P 0.059, S 0.021, Fe 0.0008. A base forming food; alkaline potentiality, 1.5 cc. per 100 Gm., 5.7 cc. per 100 Cal.

puncta (pŭnk'tă) (sing. *punctum*) [L. *punctum*, point]. Points.

p. dolorosa. Painful points in course of or at exit of nerves affected by neuralgia.

p. lacrimalia. Orifices of lacrimal canaliculi about 6 mm. from inner canthus in the eyelids.

p. vasculosa. Minute red areas which mark the cut surface of white central substance of the brain, from blood escaping from divided blood vessels.

punctate (pŭnk'tāt) [L. *punctum*, point]. Having pinpoint punctures or depressions on the surface; marked with dots.

p. rash. One with minute red points.

punctiform (pŭnk'tĭ-form) [" + *forma*, shape]. 1. Formed like a point. 2. BACT: Referring to pinpoint colonies of less than 1 mm. in diameter.

punctograph (pŭnk'tō-grăf) [" + G. *graphein*, to write]. Device employing radiography for localization of foreign bodies in the tissues.

punctum (pŭnk'tŭm) (pl. *puncta*) [L.]. Point.

p. caecum. Spot in fundus of the eyeball where the optic nerve enters. SYN: *blind spot.* [naliculus.

p. lacrimale. Outlet of lacrimal ca-

p. nasale inferius. Lower portion of suture joining the nasal bones. SYN: *rhinion.*

p. proximum. Point nearest the eye at which an object may be seen clearly. SYN: *near point.*

p. remotum. Farthest spot at which there is clear vision. SYN: *far point.*

p. saliens. First trace of the embryonic heart.

puncture (pŭnk'chūr) [L. *punctura*, a point]. 1. A hole or wound made by a sharp pointed instrument. 2. To make a hole with such an instrument.

p., exploratory. Removal of fluid or pus from a cavity or cyst for examination by piercing it.

p., lumbar. Puncture of the lumbar spinal membranes to relieve dropsy or for examination of spinal fluid. SEE:

puncture, spinal   P-126   **Purkinje's cells**

cisternal p., lumbar p., spinal fluid, spinal puncture.
  p., spinal. See: *lumbar p.*
  p. wound. A wound made by piercing with a sharp instrument.
pungency (pŭn'jĕn-sĭ) [L. *pungere*, to prick]. Quality of being sharp, strong or bitter, as an odor or taste.
pungent (pŭn'jĕnt) [L. *pungere*, to prick]. Acrid, sharp, as applied to an odor or to taste.
P. U. O. Abbr. for *pyrexia of unknown origin*, or for *trench fever.*
pupil (pū'pĭl) [L. *pupilla*, pupil]. The contractile opening at the center of the iris for the transmission of light.
  It contracts when exposed to strong light, and when the focus is on a near object. It dilates in the dark, and when the focus is on a distant object. Average diameter is 4 to 5 mm. Both pupils should be equal.
  Contraction of: May occur in tabes and in nervous diseases.
  Dilatation of: May occur in atrophy of optic nerve, sympathetic irritation and oculomotor nerve weakness.
  May be induced by belladonna (atropine), cocaine, hyoscyamus, gelsemium, muscarine, nicotine, pilocarpine, physostigma, scopola, stramonium.
  RS: *accommodation, adaptation, anissocoria, cat's eye pupil, ciliospinal center, corectasis, corencleisis, eye, hippus, iridoplegia, isocorial, miosis, miotic, mydriasis, mydriatic, myosis, myotic, occlusio pupillae, reflex, seclusio pupillae.*
  p., Argyll* - Robertson. Symptom of locomotor ataxia in which there is accommodation but light reflex is lost.
  p., bounding. Rapid dilatation of pupil alternating with contraction.
  p., occlusion of. One with opaque membrane shutting off the pupillary area.
pupillary (pū'pĭ-lĕr″ĭ) [L. *pupilla*, a pupil]. Concerning the pupil.
  p. contraction reflex. Pupillary contraction resulting from endeavoring forcibly to close eyelids which are held apart.
  p. reflexes. Those concerning passage of light through or dilation or contraction of pupil.
pupillometer (pū-pĭl-ŏm'ĕt-ẽr) [L. *pupilla*, a pupil, + G. *metron*, a measure]. Device for measurement of pupil's diameter.
pupilloscopy (pū-pĭl-os'kō-pĭ) [" + G. *skopein*, to examine]. 1. Measurement of eye refraction by effect of light and shadow on the retina. Syn: *skiascopy.* 2. Examination of the pupil.
pupillostatometer (pū″pĭl-ō-stăt-ŏm′ĕt-ẽr) [" + G. *statos*, placed, + *metron*, a measure]. Device for measuring distance between centers of the pupils.
purgation (pŭr-gā'shŭn) [L. *purgatio*, from *purgare*, to cleanse]. 1. Evacuation of the bowels caused by action of a purgative medicine. Syn: *catharsis.* 2. Cleansing.
purgative (pŭr'gă-tĭv) [L. *purgare*, to cleanse]. 1. Purgation. 2. An agent that will cause watery evacuation of the intestinal contents. Ex: *calomel, castor oil, magnesium sulfate.* See: *catharsis, cathartic.*
  Simple: Produces free discharge from bowels with some griping. *Drastic*: Produces violent action of bowels with cramps and griping. *Saline*: Produces copious watery discharges. *Cholagogue*: Stimulates flow of bile, producing green stools.

  p. enema. A strong, high one that produces evacuation when other enemas fail. See: *enema.*
purge (pŭrj) [L. *purgare*, to cleanse]. 1. To evacuate the bowels by means of a cathartic. 2. A drug that causes evacuation of the bowels.
puriform (pū'rĭ-form) [L. *pus, pur-*, pus, + *forma*, shape]. Resembling pus.

Purines in Food

	Grains per lb.	Per Cent
Vegetables—		
Asparagus	4.16	.021
Beans—Haricot	1.50	.063
Oatmeal	3.45	.053
Onions	.06	.009
Peameal	2.54	.039
Potatoes	.14	.002
Meats—		
Beef Ribs	7.96	.113
Beef Steak	14.45	.206
Beef Sirloin	9.13	.130
Liver	19.26	.275
Ham (fat)	8.08	.115
Ham (neck)	3.97	.056
Mutton	6.75	.096
Sweetbreads	70.43	1.006
Tripe	4.00	.057
Veal (loin)	8.14	.116
Fowls—		
Chickens	9.06	.129
Turkey	8.82	.126
Fish—		
Cod	4.07	.058
Halibut	7.14	.102
Plaice	5.56	.079
Salmon	8.15	.116
Coffee	....	.2

purin(e (pū'rēn, -rĭn) [L. *purum*, pure, + *uricum*, uric acid]. Parent of a group of heterocyclic nitrogen compounds including purine itself, $C_5H_4N_4$, and caffeine, theobromine, theophylline, xanthine, prepared from uric acid.
  They are end products of nucleated protein digestion, but otherwise foreign to the body. They are divided into the following groups: Xanthine, hypoxanthine, and uric acid, belonging to the *oxypurines;* guanine and adenine, belonging to the *aminopurines;* and theophylline, theobromine, and caffeine, belonging to the *methylpurines.* Purines break down to form uric acid. Cereals without the germ are purine-free. See: *meat.*
  p. body, base. Purine or any base derived from it.
  Those mentioned in the foregoing plus paraxanthine and heteroxanthine.
  p. free diet. Any fruit excepting cranberries and prunes. Milk, butter, cream, cheese, rice, flour, tapioca, cabbage, cauliflower, sugar, macaroni, white bread.
  p. low diet. Excludes meat, fish, fowl, spinach, lentils, mushrooms, peas, asparagus, coffee, tea, cocoa, spices, etc.
purinemia (pū-rĭn-ē'mĭ-ă) [*purine* + G. *aima*, blood]. Purine bodies in the blood.
purinom'eter [" + G. *metron*, measure]. Instrument to estimate amt. of purin bodies in urine.
Purkinje's cells (poor-kĭn'yĕ). Large ganglionated cells of middle layer of the cerebellar cortex.

P's. corpuscles. SEE: *P's. cells.*

P's. figures. Dark lines produced by the vessels of the retina.

P's. network. Fibrous network of large muscle cells found in cardiac muscle beneath the endocardium.

P. vesicle. The nuclear portion of an ovum. SYN: *germinal vesicle.*

Purkinje-Sanson's images (poor-kĭn'yĕ-sähn-son'). Three images of 1 object seen in the pupil of the eye.

purohepatitis (pū″rō-hep-ă-tī′tĭs) [L. *pus, pur-,* pus, + G. *ēpar, ēpat-,* liver, + *-itis,* inflammation]. Purulent inflammation of the liver.

puromucous (pū″rō-mū′kŭs) [″ + *mucus,* phlegm]. Both purulent and mucus.

purpura (pŭr′pū-ră) [L. purple] An affection with various manifestations and obscure etiology, characterized by hemorrhages into the skin, mucous membranes, internal organs, and other tissues.

Hemorrhage into the skin shows red, darkening into purple, then brownish-yellow and finally disappearing in from 2 to 3 weeks. They do not disappear under pressure. A primary lesion and a type of macule; may be arthritic or visceral as well as hemorrhagic and chronic.

p. annularis telangiectodes. Eruption of ring-shaped spots on lower limbs with pronounced telangiectasia.

p. haemorrhagica. Severe systemic disease with eruption progressing from legs over entire body. SYN: *land scurvy.*

p., malignant. Cerebrospinal fever.

p., rheumatica. P. with fever, swelling and severe rheumatic pains.

p. senilis. In debilitated and aged persons, ecchymoses and petechiae on legs.

purpuric (pŭr-pū′rĭk) [L. *purpura,* purple]. Pert. to, resembling, or suffering from, purpura.

purpurin (pŭr′pū-rĭn) [L. *purpura,* purple]. An acid dye used to stain nuclei.

purpurinuria (pŭr″pū-rĭn-ū′rĭ-ă) [″ + G. *ouron,* urine]. Purpurin in urine. SYN: *porphyrinuria.*

purring thrill (pŭr′ĭng). Thrill or vibration like a cat's purring, due to mitral stenosis, aneurysm, or valvular erosion of the heart felt by palpation over the precordium.

purulence, purulency (pŭr″ū-lĕns, pŭr″ū-lĕn-sĭ) [L. *purulentia,* a pussy condition]. The state of containing pus. SYN: *suppuration.*

purulent (pŭr′ū-lĕnt) [L. *purulentia,* a pussy condition]. Suppurative; forming or containing pus, *q.v.* SEE: *sputum.*

puruloid (pŭr′ū-loyd) [L. *pus, pur-,* pus, + G. *eidos,* form]. Like pus. SYN: *puriform.*

pus (pŭs) [L.]. Liquid product of inflammation composed of albuminous substances, a thin fluid, and leukocytes or their remains, generally yellow in color.

If *red* it suggests rupture of small vessels. If *blue* or *green* it indicates presence of *B. pyocyaneus.*

ETIOL: *Streptococci, staphylococci, gonococci,* and *pneumococci.*

p., cheesy. Very thick pus.

p., concrete. Fibropurulent coagula seen in infective endocarditis.

p., healthy. Same as laudable pus.

p., ichorous. P. that is thin with shreds of sloughing tissue. It may have a fetid odor.

p., laudable. Obsolete term referring to typical pus considered as essential in healing wounds.

p., sanious. Pus colored by blood.

p., serous. Pus mostly of thin serum containing flakes.

p. in urine. Condition when there are more than the normal number of pus or white blood cells in the urine. It may be due to cystitis, pyelitis, urethritis, tuberculosis of the kidney, or any infection of the genitourinary tract. May also be caused by trauma. SYN: *pyuria.*

TEST FOR PRESENCE OF: Fill a test tube half-full with urine and add some liquor potassae. Slowly pour urine from 1 test tube into another; repeat 2 or 3 times. The mixture will become thick and ropy if pus is present.

The presence of small amounts of pus is best detected by microscopic examination of the centrifuged deposit.

pus, words pert. to: apogenous, apyetous, apyous, archepyon, biocytoculture, burrowing, cell, clap threads, empyema, empyesis, pyemia, "pyo-" words, resorption, saprogenic, suppurate, suppuration.

pustulant (pŭs′tū-lănt) [L. *pustulāre,* to blister]. 1. Causing pustules. 2. Agent which produces the formation of pustules, such as Croton oil and antimony; seldom used any more.

pustular (pŭs′tū-lĕr) [L. *pustulāre,* to blister]. Pert. to, or characterized by, pustules.

pustulation (pŭs-tū-lā′shŭn) [L. *pustulāre,* to blister]. The development of pustules.

pustule (pŭs′tūl) [L. *pustulāre,* to blister]. Small elevation of skin filled with lymph or pus.

Pustules may be circumscribed, flat, rounded or umbilicated. They occur in eczema pustulosum, acne vulgaris, dermatitis herpetiformis, impetigo simplex, ecthyma, varicella, syphilis, or in smallpox.

RS: *achor, Chaussier's areola, pus, pustulant.*

p., malignant. Severe infectious disease with formation of hard pustule and symptoms of collapse. SYN: *anthrax.*

pustulocrustaceous (pŭs″tū-lō-krŭs-tā′-shŭs) [L. *pustulāre,* to blister, + *crusta,* a shell]. Characterized by formation of pustules and crusts.

pustulosis (pŭs-tū-lō′sĭs) [″ + G. *-osis,* disease]. A generalized eruption of pustules.

putamen (pū-tā′mĕn) [L. shell]. BNA. The darker, outer layer of the lenticular nucleus.

putrefaction (pū″trē-făk′shŭn) [L. *putrefacere,* to putrefy]. Decomposition of animal matter, esp. protein, associated with malodorous and poisonous products, such as the ptomaines, mercaptans, and hydrogen sulfide, caused by certain kinds of bacteria and fungi.

Decomposition occurring spontaneously in sterile tissue after death is called autolysis. SEE: *intestinal putrefaction, sepsis.*

putrefactive (pū-trē-făk′tĭv) [L. *putrefacēre,* to putrefy]. 1. Causing, or pert. to, putrefaction. 2. Agent promoting putrefaction.

p. alkaloid. A ptomaine, a base formed by action of bacteria on an amino acid.

putrefy (pū′trē-fī) [L. *putrefacere,* to putrefy]. To cause to decompose offensively.

putrescence (pū-trĕs′ĕns) [L. *putrescere,* to grow rotten]. Decay; rottenness.

putrid (pū'trĭd) [L. *putridus*, rotting]. Decayed; rotten; foul.

putrilage (pū'trĭl-ăj) [L. *putrilāgō*, putrefaction]. Product of putrefaction.

pyarthrosis (pī-ar-thrō'sĭs) [G. *pyon*, pus, + *arthron*, joint]. Pus in the cavity of a joint.

pycnemia (pĭk-nē'mĭ-ă) [G. *pyknos*, thick, + *aima*, blood]. Thickening of the blood. SYN: *pyknemia*.

pycno- (pĭk'no) [G.]. Combining form meaning *dense, thick*.

pycnosis (pĭk-nō'sĭs) [G. *pyknos*, thick, + *-ōsis*, intensive]. 1. Thickening. SYN: *inspissation*. 2. A degenerative cellular change with shrinking of the cell. SYN: *pyknosis*.

pyecchysis (pī-ĕk'ĭs-ĭs) [G. *pyon*, pus, + *ek*, out, + *chein*, to pour]. An effusion of pus.

pyelectasia, pyelectasis (pī-ĕl-ĕk-tā'zĭ-ă, -ĕk'tăs-ĭs) [G. *pyelos*, pelvis, + *ektasis*, dilatation]. Dilatation of the renal pelvis.

pyelitic (pī-ĕ-lĭt'ĭk) [" + *-itis*, inflammation]. Relating to or affected with pyelitis.

pyelitis (pī-ĕl-ī'tĭs) [" + *-itis*, inflammation]. Inflammation of the kidney pelvis and its calices.

ETIOL: Bacterial, metastatic, urogenous (ascending from bladder), or by penetrating wounds.

SYM: Pain in the loins, vesical irritability, swelling, constitutional symptoms, urine cloudy and decreased in amount with increased frequency in acute p., increased in amount in chronic p. and pyelonephritis; albumin and sediment with pus cells, bacteria, and fatty or hyaline casts, and sometimes red blood corpuscles.

PROG: Depends upon character and virulence of infection, accessory etiological factors, drainage of kidney, presence or absence of complications, and general physical condition.

TREATMENT: Recognition and removal of cause (focal infection, etc.), measures to increase resistance of patient, bed rest, milk or buttermilk diet, avoidance of drugs irritating to kidney, condiments of alcohol. Hot water bag, antipyretic drugs, urinary antisepsis. Surgery if necessary (nephrotomy, nephrectomy, pyelotomy). If both kidney and pelvis are affected, urine generally is acid, and pus in form of slugs or balls pass in the urine.

pyelo- [G.]. Combining form meaning the *pelvis*.

pyelocystitis (pī"ĕl-ō-sĭs-tī'tĭs) [G. *pyelos*, pelvis, + *kystis*, bladder, + *-itis*, inflammation]. Inflamed condition of the kidney, pelvis and bladder.

pyelocystostomosis (pī"ĕl-ō-sĭs"tō-sto-mō'sĭs) [" + " + *stoma*, mouth, + *-ōsis*]. Establishment of surgical communication bet. the kidney and the bladder.

pyelogram, pyelograph (pī'ĕl-ō-grăm, -grăf) [" + *gramma*, a mark]. A roentgen picture of the ureter and renal pelvis.

pyelography (pī-ĕ-lŏg'ră-fī) [" + *graphein*, to write]. Radiography of a renal pelvis and ureter.

pyelolithotomy (pī"ĕl-ō-lĭth-ŏt'ō-mĭ) [" + *lithos*, stone, + *tomē*, incision]. Removal of calculus from the pelvis of a kidney through an incision.

pyelometer (pī-ĕl-ŏm'ĕt-ĕr) [" + *metron*, a measure]. Device to measure the pelvic diameters. SYN: *pelvimeter*.

pyelometry (pī-ĕl-ŏm'ĕ-trī) [" + *metron*, a measure]. 1. Measurement of the kidney's pelvis. 2. Measurement of the diameters of the pelvis. SYN: *pelvimetry*.

pyelonephritis (pī"ĕl-ō-nef-rī'tĭs) [G. *pyelos*, pelvis, + *nephros*, kidney, + *-itis*, inflammation]. Inflammation of kidney substance and pelvis.

pyelonephrosis (pī"ĕl-ō-nef-rō'sĭs) [" + " + *-ōsis*, disease]. Disease of the pelvis of the kidney.

pyelopathy (pī-ĕl-ŏp'ăth-ĭ) [" + *pathos*, disease]. Any disease of the pelvis of the kidney. SYN: *pyelonephrosis*.

pyeloplasty (pī'ĕl-ō-plăs"tĭ) [" + *plastos*, formed]. Reparative operation on the kidney pelvis.

pyeloplication (pī"ĕl-ō-plĭ-kā'shŭn) [" + L. *plicāre*, to fold]. Shortening of the wall of a dilated renal pelvis by taking tucks in it.

pyeloscopy (pī-ĕl-ŏs'kō-pĭ) [" + *skopein*, to examine]. Examination of the pelvis of the kidney using an x-ray.

pyelostomy (pī-ĕl-ŏs'tō-mĭ) [" + *stoma*, mouth]. Creation of an opening into the renal pelvis.

pyelotomy (pī-ĕl-ŏt'ō-mĭ) [G. *pyelos*, pelvis, + *tomē*, incision]. Incision of renal pelvis.

NP: Keep patient dry, watch skin for decubitus. If retention catheter present, keep draining at all times. Accurate record of intake and output of urine.

pyelovenous backflow (pī-ĕl-ō-vē'nŭs) [" + L. *vena*, vein]. Drainage from the renal pelvis into the venous system because of back pressure.

pyemesis (pī-ĕm'ĭs-ĭs) [G. *pyon*, pus, + *emesis*, vomiting]. The vomiting of pus.

pyemia (pī-ē'mĭ-ă) [" + *aima*, blood]. Blood poisoning caused by pus absorption; a form of septicemia. Usually occurs in 2nd week of healing process when suppuration is fully established.

SYM: High intermittent temperature with chills — repeated following day — repetition of chills metastatic absc mittent type, wh tion; sweetish odor processes in various parts esp. in lungs. Septic pneumonia, pyema. May result fatally.

TREATMENT: Prophylactic treatment consists in prevention of suppuration. When possible all metastatic abscesses or suppurating joints should be laid open and thoroughly disinfected. Internal remedies. Easily digested food given unsparingly. Ventilation free — patient may be placed in a tent in certain cases.

p., cryptogenic. P., the focus of which is hidden in the deeper tissues.

p., metastatic. Multiple abscess resulting from infected pyemic thrombi.

p., portal. Suppurative inflammation of portal vein.

pyemic (pī-ē'mĭk) [G. *pyon*, pus, + *aima*, blood]. Relating to or affected with blood poisoning.

pyemid (pī-ē'mĭd) [" + *aima*, blood]. A cutaneous eruption in pyemia from metastasis.

pyencephalus (pī-en-sef'al-us) [" + *egkephalos*, brain]. A brain abscess with suppuration within the cranium. SYN: *pyocephalus*.

pyesis (pī-ē'sĭs) [G. *pyon*, pus]. The formation of pus. SYN: *suppuration*.

pygal (pī'găl) [G. *pygē*, rump]. Concerning the buttocks.

pygalgia (pī-găl'jĭ-ă) [" + *algos*, pain]. Pain in the rump or buttocks.

pygo- [G.]. Combining form meaning the *rump*.

pyin (pī'ĭn) [G. *pyon*, pus]. A substance of albuminous nature sometimes present in pus.
pyknemia (pĭk-nē'mĭ-ă) [G. *pyknos*, thick, + *aima*, blood]. Thickening of the blood.
pyknic type (pĭk'nĭk) [G. *pyknos*, thick]. One with broad head, thick shoulders, large chest, short neck and stocky body.
They are often happy, carefree persons whose emotional reactions are obvious. They are interested in others apart from themselves. They are extroverts.* SEE: *asthenic body type*.
pyknocardia (pĭk-nō-kar'dĭ-ă) [" + *kardia*, heart]. Rapid pulse. SYN: *tachycardia*.
pyknohemia (pĭk-nō-hē'mĭ-ă) [" + *aima*, blood]. Thickening of the blood. SYN: *pyknemia*.
pyknolepsy (pĭk-nō-lĕp'sĭ) [" + *lēpsis*, seizure]. Attacks similar to petit mal or minor epileptic seizures, usually occurring in childhood.
pyknometer (pĭk-nŏm'ĕt-ĕr) [" + *metron*, measure]. 1. Device for determining specific gravity of anything. 2. Device for measurement of the thickness of a substance.
pyknomorphous (pĭk"nō-morf'ŭs) [" + *morphē*, form]. Characterized by compact arrangement of the stainable portions, said esp. of certain nerve cells.
pyknophrasia (pĭk"nō-frā'zĭ-ă) [" + *phrasis*, speech]. Thickness of words uttered in speech.
pyknosis (pĭk-nō'sĭs) [" + *-ōsis*, intensive]. Inspissation; thickness, esp. shrinking of cells through degeneration.
pyla (pī'lă) [G. *pylē*, gate]. Opening connecting the 3rd ventricle to the sylvian aqueduct.
pyle- [G.]. Combining form meaning *orifice*, esp. that of the portal vein.
pylemphraxis (pī-lĕm-frăk'sĭs) [G. *pylē*, gate, + *emphraxis*, stoppage]. Occlusion ——— ——al vein.
——————phlebectasis (pī-le——————is) [" + *phleps*, ——, dilatation]. Dis——— ———rtal vein.
——————— (pī-le-flē-bī'tĭs) [" + " + ——*itis*, inflammation]. Inflamed condition of the portal vein, generally suppurative.
p., adhesive. Thrombosis of the portal vein.
p. obturans. P. with obstructed flow in the portal vein.
pylethrombosis (pī-le-thrŏm-bō'sĭs) [" + *thrombos*, a clot, + *-ōsis*, intensive]. Occlusion of portal vein by a thrombus.
pylometer (pī-lŏm'ĕt-ĕr) [" + *metron*, a measure]. Device for measuring obstructions at vesical opening.
pyloralgia (pī"lō-răl'jĭ-ă) [G. *pylōros*, gatekeeper, + *algos*, pain]. Pain around the pylorus.
pylorectomy (pī-lō-rĕk'tō-mĭ) [" + *ektomē*, excision]. Surgical removal of the pylorus.
pyloric (pī-lor'ĭk) [G. *pylōros*, gatekeeper]. Pert. to the opening bet. the stomach and duodenum.
p. cap. Portion of duodenum next to pylorus.
p. gland. A gland of the stomach near the pylorus secreting pepsin.
p. orifice. Opening or passage bet. the stomach and duodenum.
p. stenosis. Narrowing of the pyloric orifice.
Often due to contraction following healing of a peptic ulcer.
pyloristenosis (pī"lō-rī-stĕn-ō'sĭs) [" + *stenōsis*, a narrowing]. Constriction of the pylorus.

pyloritis (pī-lō-rī'tĭs) [" + *-ītis*, inflammation]. Inflamed condition of the pylorus.
pyloro- [G.]. Combining form meaning *gatekeeper*; applied to the *pylorus*.
pyloroduodenitis (pī"lor-ō-dū"ō-dē-nī'tĭs) [G. *pylōros*, gatekeeper, + L. *duodeni*, twelve, + G. *-ītis*, inflammation]. Inflammation of the mucosa of the pylorus and duodenum.
pylorogastrectomy (pī-lō"rō-găs-trĕk'tō-mĭ) [" + *gastēr*, belly, + *ektomē*, excision]. Excision of pyloric portion of the stomach.
pyloromyotomy (pī-lō"rō-mī-ŏt'ō-mĭ) [" + *mys*, *my-*, muscle, + *tomē*, a cutting]. Incision and suture of the pyloric sphincter.
pyloroplasty (pī-lor'ō-plăs"tĭ) [" + *plassein*, to form]. Operation to repair the pylorus, esp. 1 to increase the caliber of the pyloric opening by stretching.
pyloroptosia, pyloroptosis (pī-lo"rŏp-tō'sĭ-ă, -rŏp'tō-sĭs) [" + *ptōsis*, a dropping]. Displacement downward of the pyloric end of the stomach.
pyloroscopy (pī-lō-rŏs'kō-pī) [" + *skopein*, to examine]. Fluoroscopic examination of the pylorus.
pylorospasm (pī-lō'rō-spăzm) [" + *spasmos*, a spasm]. Spasmodic contraction of the pyloric orifice.
pylorostenosis (pī-lō"rō-stĕn-ō'sĭs) [" + *stenōsis*, narrowing]. Contraction of the pylorus.
pylorostomy (pī-lor-ŏs'tō-mĭ) [G. *pylōros*, gatekeeper, + *stoma*, opening]. Formation of an opening through the abdominal wall into the pylorus.
pylorotomy (pī-lor-ŏt'ō-mĭ) [" + *tomē*, a cutting]. Incision of the pyloric submucosa to relieve hypertrophic stenosis.
pylorus (pī-lōr'ŭs) [G. *pylōros*, gatekeeper]. The lower orifice of the stomach opening into the duodenum.
It opens at intervals, the food mass (chyme) passing into the duodenum. The intervals are less as digestion advances but sufficient to permit of the escape of undigested particles.
RS: *cardiopyloric, janitor, stomach*.
p., glands of. Those in the stomach near the pylorus secreting pepsin.
p., spasm of. Usually secondary to hyperperistalsis, hyperacidity, or the ingestion of irritating foods.
pyo-, py- [G.]. Combining forms meaning *pus*.
pyocele (pī'ō-sēl) [G. *pyon*, pus, + *kēlē*, hernia]. A hernia or distended cavity containing pus.
pyocelia (pī-ō-sē'lĭ-ă) [" + *koilia*, cavity]. Pus formation in the abdominal cavity.
pyocephalus (pī"ō-sĕf'ă-lŭs) [" + *kephalē*, head]. Effusion of purulent nature within the cranium.
p., circumscribed. Abscess of the brain.
p., external. Suppuration of the meninges.
p., interval. Pus in the cerebrospinal fluid.
pyochezia (pī"ō-kē'zĭ-ă) [" + *chezein*, to defecate]. Pus in the feces.
pyococcus (pī"ō-kŏk'ŭs) [" + *kokkos*, berry]. A micrococcus which causes suppuration, as the *Streptococcus pyogenes*.
pyocolpocele (pī-ō-kŏl'pō-sēl) [" + *kolpos*, vagina, + *kēlē*, mass]. A vaginal tumor containing pus. SEE: *pyocolpos*.
pyocol'pos [" + *kolpos*, vagina]. Accumulation of pus in the vagina.
pyoculture (pī'ō-kŭl-chŭr) [G. *pyon*, pus, + L. *cultura*, growth]. Comparative

pyocyst P-130 **pyosepticemia**

tests for cultivation of pus from a wound, a portion being left in the collecting tube and a portion being cultivated on bouillon.
If the test is positive, it indicates a struggle bet. the bacteria and the body forces which need therapeutic assistance.
pyocyst (pī′ō-sĭst) [" + *kystis*, sac]. A cyst holding pus.
pyocyte (pī′ō-sīt) [" + *kytos*, cell]. A pus corpuscle, considered a leukocyte. SYN: *pus cell.*
pyodermatitis (pī″ō-dŭr-mă-tī′tĭs) [" + *derma*, skin, + *-itis*, inflammation]. Pyogenic infection of the skin causing a dermatitis.
pyodermatosis (pī″ō-dĕr-mă-tō′sĭs) [" + " + *-osis*, condition]. Any skin condition of pyogenic origin. SYN: *pyodermia.*
pyodermia (pī″ō-der′mĭ-ă) [" + *derma*, skin]. Any suppurative skin disease.
pyofecia (pī″ō-fē′sĭ-ă) [" + L. *faeces*, feces]. Pus in the stools.
pyogenesis (pī″ō-jĕn′ĕs-ĭs) [G. *pyon*, pus, + *genesis*, formation]. The development of pus.
pyogenic (pī-ō-jĕn′ĭk) [" + *gennan*, to produce]. Producing pus.
  p. microörganisms. M. forming pus.
pyohemia (pī″ō-hē′mĭ-ă) [" + *aima*, blood]. Blood poisoning with multiple abscess formation. SYN: *pyemia.*
pyohemothorax (pī″ō-hĕm-ō-thō′răks) [" + " + *thōrax*, chest]. Pus and blood in the pleural cavity. [bling pus.
pyoid (pī′oyd) [" + *eidos*, like]. Resem-
pyoktanin (pī-ŏk′tăn-ĭn) [" + *kteinein*, to kill]. Commercial preparation of methyl violet; a germicide used in cystitis, gonorrhea, and infections of the eyes, ears, nose, and throat.
pyolabyrinthitis (pī″ō-lăb-ĭ-rĭn-thī′tĭs) [" + *labyrinthos*, a maze, + *-itis*, inflammation]. Inflammation with suppuration of the labyrinth of the ear.
pyometra (pī-ō-mē′tră) [G. *pyon*, pus, + *mētra*, uterus]. Retained pus accumulation in the uterine cavity.
pyometritis (pī″ō-mē-trī′tĭs) [" + " + *-itis*, inflammation]. Purulent inflammation of the uterus.
pyonephritis (pī″ō-nef-rī′tĭs) [" + *nephros*, kidney, + *-itis*, inflammation]. Inflammation of the kidney, suppurative in character.
pyonephrolithiasis (pī″ō-nef-rō-lĭth-ī′ăs-ĭs) [" + " + *lithos*, stone]. Pus and calculi formation in the kidney.
pyonephrosis (pī″ō-nef-rō′sĭs) [" + " + *-osis*, condition]. Pus accumulation in the pelvis of kidney.
  ETIOL: Pyelitis, hydronephrosis when infected by pus-producing organisms.
  SYM: Gradual onset. Toxemia, wasting, sallow skin, intermittent temperature or acute onset with rigors, headache, high temperature, thirst, foul tongue, general pains. Albumin and pus in urine. Uremia threatens if both kidneys are affected.
  TREATMENT: Rest, urinary antiseptics, large amounts of water. Sometimes nephrectomy, or nephrotomy.
pyoövarium (pī″ō-ō-vā′rĭ-ŭm) [G. *pyon*, pus, + L. *ovarium*, ovary]. Abscess formation in an ovary.
pyopericarditis (pī″ō-pĕr-ĭ-kar-dī′tĭs) [" + *peri*, around, + *kardia*, heart, + *-itis*, inflammation]. Pericarditis with suppuration.
pyopericardium (pī″ō-pĕr-ĭ-kar′dĭ-ŭm) [" + " + " *kardia*, heart]. Pus formation in the pericardium.
pyoperitoneum (pī″ō-pĕr-ĭ-tō-nē′ŭm) [" + *peritonaion*, peritoneum]. Pus formation in the peritoneal cavity.
pyoperitonitis (pī″ō-pĕr-ĭ-tō-nī′tĭs) [" + " + *-itis*, inflammation]. Purulent inflammation of the lining of peritoneum.
pyophagia (pī″ō-fā′jĭ-ă) [" + *phagein*, to eat]. Swallowing of purulent substance.
pyophthalmia, pyophthalmitis (pī″ōf-thăl′-mĭ-ă, -thăl-mī′tĭs) [" + *ophthalmos*, eye, + *-itis*, inflammation]. Suppurative inflamed condition of the eye.
pyophylactic (pī″ō-fī-lăk′tĭk) [G. *pyon*, pus, + *phylaxis*, protection]. Guarding against formation of pus.
  p. membrane. Lining membrane of an abscess cavity separating it from healthy tissue.
pyophysometra (pī″ō-fī-sō-mē′tră) [" + *physa*, air, + *mētra*, uterus]. Pus and gas accumulation in the uterus.
pyoplania (pī″ō-plā′nĭ-ă) [" + *planos*, wandering]. Spreading of pus by infiltration into tissue.
pyopneumocholecystitis (pī″ō-nū″mō-kō-lē-sĭs-tī′tĭs) [" + *pneuma*, air, + *cholē*, bile, + *kystis*, sac, + *-itis*, inflammation]. Dilatation of the gallbladder with air and pus.
pyopneumocyst (pī″ō-nū″mō-sĭst) [" + " + *kystis*, a bladder]. A cyst enclosing pus and gas.
pyopneumopericardium (pī″ō-nū″mō-pĕr-ĭ-kar′dĭ-ŭm) [" + " + *peri*, around, + *kardia*, heart]. Pus and air or gas in pericardium.
pyopneumoperitonitis (pī″ō-nū″mō-pĕr-ĭ-tō-nī′tĭs) [" + " + *peritonaion*, peritoneum]. Pus and air in the peritoneal cavity complicating peritonitis.
pyopneumothorax (pī″ō-nū″mō-thō′răks) [" + " + *thōrax*, chest]. Pus and gas or air accumulated in the pleural cavity.
  p., subphrenic. Pus and air accumulated below the diaphragm.
pyopoiesis (pī″ō-poy-ē′sĭs) [G. *pyon*, pus, + *poiein*, to make]. Development of pus. SYN: *pyogenesis, suppuration.*
pyopoietic (pī″ō-poy-ĕt′ĭk) [" + *poiein*, to make]. Secreting or forming pus. SYN: *suppurative.*
pyoptysis (pī-ŏp′tĭs-ĭs) [" + *ptyein*, to spit]. Spitting of pus.
pyorrhagia (pī-or-ā′jĭ-ă) [" + *rēgnunai*, to burst forth]. Profuse flow of pus, as when an abscess ruptures.
pyorrhea (pī-ō-rē′ă) [" + *roia*, a flow]. A discharge of purulent matter.
  p. alveolaris. Inflammation of periosteum of the tooth socket.
  SYM: Gums shrink; teeth loosen; infection and constitutional disturbances.
  SYN: *Riggs' disease.*
  p. salivaris. Flow of pus from a salivary duct.
pyosalpingitis (pī″ō-săl-pĭn-jī′tĭs) [G. *pyon*, pus, + *salpigx*, tube, + *-itis*, inflammation]. Retained pus in the oviduct with inflammation.
pyosalpingoöophoritis (pī″ō-săl-pĭn″gō-ō-ŏf-ō-rī′tĭs) [" + " + *ōon*, ovum, + *phoros*, a bearer, + *-itis*, inflammation]. Inflammation of ovary and oviduct with suppuration.
pyosalpinx (pī″ō-săl′pĭnks) [" + *salpigx*, tube]. Pus in the fallopian tube. SEE: *pyosalpingitis.*
pyosapremia (pī″ō-săp-rē′mĭ-ă) [" + *sapros*, rotten, + *aima*, blood]. Purulent infection of the blood; blood poisoning. SYN: *pyemia.*
pyoscheocele (pī-ŏs′kē-ō-sēl) [" + *oscheon*, scrotum, + *kēlē*, tumor]. Swelling and suppuration of the scrotum.
pyosepticemia (pī″ō-sĕp-tĭ-sē′mĭ-ă) [" +

pyosin   P-131   **3-pyridinecarboxylic acid**

sēptikos, putrid, + *aima*, blood]. Condition in which pyogenic and pathogenic bacteria are in the blood; blood poisoning with suppuration. SYN: *septicopyemia*.

pyosin (pī'ō-sĭn) [G. *pyon*, pus]. A substance found in plasma of pus cells.

pyosis (pī-ō'sĭs) [" + -*ōsis*, intensive]. Formation of pus. SYN: *suppuration*.

pyospermia (pī"ō-spĕr'mĭ-ă) [" + *sperma*, seed]. Pus in the semen.

pyostatic (pī"ō-stăt'ĭk) [" + *statikos*, standing]. 1. Agent checking the development of pus. 2. Preventing pus formation.

pyotherapy (pī"ō-thĕr'ă-pī) [" + *therapeia*, treatment]. Treatment of disease with pus.

pyothorax (pī"ō-thō'răks) [" + *thōrax*, chest]. Pus in the pleural cavity. SYN: *empyema*.

   p. subphrenic. An abscess below the diaphragm.

pyotorrhea (pī"ō-tor-ē'ă) [" + *ous, ot-*, ear, + *roia*, flow]. Purulent discharge from the ear.

pyotoxinemia (pī"ō-tŏk-sĭ-nē'mĭ-ă) [G. *pyon*, pus, + *toxikon*, poison, + *aima*, blood]. Infection from toxic products of pus organisms in the blood.

pyoturia (pī"ō-tū'rĭ-ă) [" + *ouron*, urine]. Pus cells in the urine. SYN: *pyuria*.

pyourachus (pī"ō-ū'ră-kŭs) [" + *ourachos*, fetal urinary canal]. Accumulation of pus in the urachus.

pyoureter (pī"ō-ūr'ĕt-ĕr, -ū-rē'tĕr) [" + *ourēter*, ureter]. Pus collection in a ureter.

pyovesiculosis (pī"ō-vĕs-ĭk-ū-lō'sĭs) [" + L. *vesiculus*, a small vessel, + G. -*ōsis*, condition]. Pus collection in the seminal vesicles.

pyramid (pĭr'ăm-ĭd) [G. *pyramis*, a pyramid]. 1. A solid on a base with 3 or more sides, the triangular planes of which meet at an apex. 2. Any part of the body resembling a pyramid. 3. A compact bundle of nerve fibers in the medulla oblongata. 4. Petrous portion of temporal bone.

   p. of cerebellum. A conical projection near the center of the inf. vermiform process.

   p., Ferrein's. Any one of the renal medullary rays.

   p., Lalouette's. Pyramid of the thyroid.

   p., malpighian. Any 1 of the pyramidal masses of the renal cortex made up of glomeruli, blood vessels, and convoluted tubules. SYN: *cones of Malpighi*.

   p. of the medulla. (Ant.) A pair of oblong bodies on ant. surface of the medulla. (Post.) The 2 expanded portions of the funiculus gracilis at lower angle of the 4th ventricle.

   p., renal. Same as *malpighian pyramid*.

   p. of the thyroid. A conical process sometimes arising from the t. gland up to the hyoid bone, the median lobe.

   p. of the tympanum. A hollow projection on inner wall of the tympanum through which passes the stapedius muscle.

pyramidal (pī-răm'ĭd-ăl) [G. *pyramis*, *pyramid*-, pyramid]. In the shape of a pyramid.

   p. bone. The cuneiform bone of the carpus.

   p. cell. Pyramid-shaped cell of cerebral cortex.

   p. tract. A large bundle of medullated nerve fibers in the medulla oblongata carrying motor nerves downward to the spinal cord.

pyramidalis (pī-răm-id-al'ĭs) [G. *pyramis*, pyramid). The muscle which arises from the crest of the pubis and is inserted into the linea alba upward about half way to the navel.

pyramidon (pī-răm'ĭd-ŏn). Proprietary preparation of amidopyrine; a yellowish-white powder.

   USES: As an antipyretic.
   DOSAGE: 5 gr. (0.3 Gm.) every 2 hours.

pyrazine -2, 3- dicarboxylic acid (pīr'ă-zēn dī"kar-bŏk-sĭl'ĭk). Compound used successfully in treating pellagra, *q.v.*

   p. monocarboxylic acid. Compound used successfully in treatment of pellagra.

pyrectic (pī-rĕk'tĭk) [G. *pyrektikos*]. Feverish. SYN: *pyretic*.

pyrenemia (pī-rē-nē'mĭ-ă) [G. *pyrēn*, fruit stone, *aima*, blood]. Condition in which there are nucleated red cells in the blood.

pyrenin (pī-rē'nĭn) [G. *pyrēn*, fruit stone]. The oxyphilic substance found in a nucleolus.

pyrenoid (pī're-noyd) [" + *eidos*, like]. A colorless, highly refractive body in certain protozoan chromatophores.

pyretherapy (pī-rē-thĕr'ă-pī) [G. *pyr*, fever, + *therapeia*, treatment]. 1. Artificial fever treatment. 2. Treatment of febrile conditions. SYN: *pyretotherapy*.

pyretic (pī-rĕt'ĭk) [G. *pyretos*, fever]. 1. Concerning fever. 2. Remedy for fever.

   p. therapy. Treatment of disease by artificial induction of fever, either by physical agents or the inoculation of malarial organisms.

pyreticosis (pī-rĕt-ĭ-kō'sĭs) [" + -*ōsis*, intensive]. Feverishness.

pyreto- [G.]. Prefix meaning *fever*.

pyretogen (pī-rĕt'ō-jĕn) [G. *pyretos*, fever, + *gennan*, to produce]. A substance producing fever.

pyretogenesia, pyretogenesis (pī"rĕt-ō-jĕn-ē'zĭ-ă, -jĕn'ĕs-ĭs) [" + *genesis*, production]. Origin and production of fever.

pyretogenic, pyretogenous (pī"rĕt-ō-jĕn'ĭk, -ŏj'ĕn-ŭs) [" + *gennan*, to produce]. Producing or causing fever.

   p. bacteria. Pathogenic bacteria causing fever.

   p. stage. Period in a fever when it is rising slowly.

pyretography (pī-rĕt-ŏg'ră-fī) [" + *graphein*, to write]. A treatise on fever.

pyretology (pī-rĕt-ŏl'ō-jī) [" + *logos*, a study]. Science of fevers and their characteristics.

pyretolysis (pī-rĕt-ŏl'ĭs-ĭs) [" + *lysis*, a disintegration]. 1. Reduction of fever. 2. Hastening of lysis by elevation of temperature.

pyretotherapy (pī"rē-tō-thĕr'ă-pī) [" + *therapeia*, treatment]. 1. Treatment by artificially raising the patient's temperature. 2. Treatment of fever.

pyretotyphosis (pī"rĕt-ō-tī-fō'sĭs) [" + *typhōsis*, delirium]. The delirious or stuporous symptom of fever.

pyrexia (pī-rĕk'sĭ-ă) [G. *pyressein*, to be feverish]. Condition in which the temperature is above normal. SYN: *fever*.
   Some classify it as:
   Low .... 99°—101° F.
   Moderate .... 101°—103° F.
   High .... 103°—105° F.
   p., local. Acute inflammation of a part.

pyrexial (pī-rĕks'ĭ-ăl) [G. *pyressein*, to be feverish]. Concerning fever.

3-pyridinecarboxylic acid (pīr'ĭd-ēn-kar"-

R

R. Abbr. for *Réaumur, roentgen, respiration, right.* ℞. Symb. for L. *recipe,* to take.

Ra. Chemical symb. for *radium.*

rabbetting (răb'ĕt-ĭng) [Fr. *raboter,* to plane]. Interlocking of the jagged edges of a fractured bone.

rabiate (rā'bĭ-āt) [L. *rabere,* to rage]. Suffering from rabies. SYN: *rabid.*

rabiator (rā'bĭ-ā-tor) [L. *rabere,* to rage]. One affected with rabies.

rabic (răb'ĭk) [L. *rabere,* to rage]. Concerning rabies.

rabicidal (răb-ĭ-sī'dăl) [" + *cidus,* from *caedere,* to kill]. Destructive to causative agent of rabies (*Bacillus lyssae*).

rabid (răb'ĭd) [L. *rabidus,* raving]. Pert. to or affected with rabies. SYN: *rabiate.*

rabies (rā'bēz) [L. *rabies,* from *rabere,* to rave]. An extremely fatal infectious disease communicated to man by bite of a rabid animal, usually a dog. SYN: *hydrophobia, lyssa.* SEE: *dog bite.*

PERIOD OF INCUBATION: Six days to 1 year.

ETIOL: May be a filtrable virus or possibly the protozoon, so-called negri body in nerve cells and their processes.

SYM: Difficult swallowing, malaise, clonic spasms of respiratory muscles, anxiety, depression, increased irritability, pulse and temperature, delirium, paralysis, coma, death.

PROG: Generally fatal.

TREATMENT: If hysteria ensues, increase of temperature, respiration and pulse do not occur. Suspicious bites should be thoroughly disinfected, cups applied, cauterized by hot iron or nitric acid. Patient given inoculation after method of Pasteur.

Attack: *Palliative.* For the convulsions morphine may be employed hypodermically and chloroform by inhalation. Strength sustained by rectal alimentation. Preserve dog alive if possible for examination by health authorities.

race (rās) [Italian *razza*]. 1. A class of individuals with common interests, characteristics, appearance, habits, etc., as if derived from a common ancestor. 2. State of being 1 of a special group. 3. Division of mankind with traits sufficient to mark it as a distinct human type.

racemose (răs'ē-mōs) [L. *racemōsus,* full of clusters]. Resembling a clustered bunch of grapes, as a gland, divided and subdivided, ending in a bunch of follicles.

rachi-, rachio- [G.]. Combining forms meaning *rib of a leaf, ridge, spine.*

rachialbuminimeter (rā″kĭ-ăl-bū-mĭn-ĭm'ĕt-ĕr) [G. *rhachis,* spine, + L. *albumen,* white of egg, + G. *metron,* measure]. Device for estimating amt. of albumin in the cerebrospinal fluid.

rachialbuminimetry (rā″kĭ-ăl-bū-mĭn-ĭm'ĕt-rī) [" + " + G. *metron,* measure]. The estimation of amt. of albumin in the cerebrospinal fluid.

rachianalgesia (rā″kĭ-ăn-ăl-jē'zĭ-ă) [" + *analgesia,* lack of pain]. Spinal anesthesia. SYN: *rachianesthesia.*

rachialgia (ră-kĭ-ăl'jĭ-ă) [" + *algos,* pain]. Pain in the spine.

rachianesthesia (rā″kĭ-ăn-ĕs-thē'zĭ-ă) [" + *an-,* negative, + *aisthēsis,* sensation]. Spinal anesthesia.

rachicentesis (rā″kĭ-sĕn-tē'sĭs) [" + *kentēsis,* a piercing]. Puncture into the spinal canal.

rachidian (ra-kĭd'ĭ-ăn) [G. *rhachis, rachid-,* spine]. Relating to the spinal column.

rachigraph (rā'kĭ-grăf) [" + *graphein,* to write]. Device for outlining the curves of the spine.

rachilysis (ră-kĭl'ĭs-ĭs) [" + *lysis,* a loosening]. Mechanical treatment of lateral curvature of the spine.

rachiocampsis (rā-kĭ-ō-kămp'sĭs) [" + *kampsis,* a bending]. Curvature of spine.

rachiochysis (rā-kĭ-ok'ĭs-ĭs) [" + *chysis,* a pouring]. Accumulation of fluid within the spinal canal.

rachiodynia (rā-kĭ-ō-dĭn'ĭ-ă) [" + *odynē,* pain]. Painful condition of spinal column. SYN: *rachialgia.*

rachiometer (rā-kĭ-ŏm'ĕt-ĕr) [" + *metron,* measure]. Instrument for measuring a curvature of the spine.

rachiomyelitis (rā″kĭ-ō-mī-ĕ-lī'tĭs) [G. *rhachis,* spine, + *myelos,* marrow, + *-itis,* inflammation]. Inflamed condition of spinal cord. SYN: *myelitis.*

rachioplegia (rā'kĭ-ō-plē'jĭ-ă) [" + *plēgē,* a stroke]. Paralysis of spine.

rachiotome (rā'kĭ-ō-tōm) [" + *tomē,* a cutting]. Instrument for dividing the vertebrae.

rachiotomy (rā-kĭ-ŏt'ō-mĭ) [" + *tomē,* a cutting]. Surgical cutting of the vertebral column.

rachis (rā'kĭs) (pl. *rachises*) [G. spine]. The spinal column.

rachischisis (ră-kĭs'kĭs-ĭs) [G. *rhachis,* spine, + *schisis,* cleft]. Spinal column fissure; congenital.

rachistovainization (rā-kĭs-tō-vă-nī-zā'shŭn) [G. *rhachis,* spine]. Spinal injection of stovaine to produce anesthesia.

rachitic (ră-kĭt'ĭk) [G. *rhachis,* spine]. Pert. to or affected with rickets.

r. flat pelvis. Pelvic deformity due to having had rickets in childhood.

r. rosary. Beadlike prominences at junction of the ribs with their cartilages.

rachitis (ra-kī'tĭs) [G. *rhachis,* spine, + *-itis,* inflammatory]. Inflammation of the spine, commonly rickets, *q.v.* SEE: *rachitic beads.*

r. fetalis annularis. Enlargement of epiphyses of long bones; congenital.

r. fetalis micromelica. Congenital shortness of the bones.

rachitome (rā'kĭ-tōm) [" + *tomē,* a cutting]. Instrument employed for opening spinal canal.

radiability (rā-dĭ-ă-bĭl'ĭ-tĭ) [L. *radius,* ray]. Capability of being penetrated readily by the x-ray.

radiad (rā'dĭ-ăd) [L. *radius,* spoke, + *ad,* toward]. In direction of the radial side.

radial (rā'dĭ-ăl) [L. *radius,* spoke]. 1. Radiating out from a given center. 2. Pert. to the radius.

r. reflex. Flexion of forearm resulting when lower end of radius is percussed.

radiant (rā'dĭ-ănt) [L. *radiāre,* to emit

R-1

radiate

rays]. 1. Emitting beams of light. 2. Transmitted by radiation. 3. Emanating from a common center.
RS: *energy, flux, heat, heater.*

radiate (rā′dĭ-āt) [L. *radius*, spoke]. 1. Spreading from a common center. 2. To spread from a common center.

radiation (rā-dĭ-ā′shŭn) [L. *radiāre*, to emit rays]. 1. Process by which energy is propagated through space or matter not affected by it. 2. Emission of rays in all directions from a common center. 3. Treatment with a radioactive substance.

A general term for any form of radiant energy emission or divergence, as of energy in all directions from luminous bodies, roentgen ray tubes, radioactive elements and fluorescent substances.

r., infrared. Near or short infrared extends from 7200 A. U. to 14,000 A. U. Far or long infrared from 15,000 to 150,000 A. U.

r., far ultraviolet. Ultraviolet radiation of short wave length; farthest away from the visible spectrum.

r., photochemical. From a therapeutic standpoint the electromagnetic spectrum divided into photothermal and photochemical radiations. Photochemical r's, penetrate only to fractions of millimeters, are absorbed by protoplasm, and cause physical and biological changes which manifest themselves after several hours from exposure.

r., photothermal. Photothermal radiations penetrate subcutaneous tissues, heat the blood, accelerate vital reactions and act instantaneously. SEE: *photochemical radiation.*

r., solar. Radiations of the sun, 60% in infrared region and 40% visible and ultraviolet, shortest wave length is 2900 A. U.

r., ultraviolet. Radiant energy extending from 3900 to 1800 A. U. Divided into "near ultraviolet," extending from 3900 to 2900 A. U., and "far ultraviolet," from 2900 to 1800 A. U.

r. unit. SEE: *angstrom unit, maché unit.*

r., visible. Visible spectrum may be broken up into different wave lengths representing different colors:

Violet .... 4000-4500 A. U.
Blue .... 4500-4900 " "
Green .... 4900-5500 " "
Yellow .... 5500-5900 " "
Orange .... 5900-6300 " "
Red .... 6300-7800 " "

SEE: *spectrum.*
RS: *heliotherapy, heliotropis, helium.*

radiator (rā′dĭ-ā-tor) [L. *radiator*]. Device for radiating heat or light.

r., infrared. Device for transmitting infrared rays. SEE: *heater, radiant.*

radical (răd′ĭ-kal) [L. *radix, radic-,* a root]. 1. A group of elements acting as a single element, passing without change from 1 compound to another one, but not able to exist in a free state. 2. Anything that reaches the root or origin; original. 3. A foundation or principle.

r. treatment. A treatment that seeks an absolute cure, as r. surgery; not palliative.

radicle (răd′ĭ-kl) [L. *radix, radic-,* root]. 1. A structure resembling a rootlet, as a r. of a nerve or vein. 2. Group of elements unaffected by chemical change, unable to exist in the free state.

radicotomy (răd-ĭ-kŏt′ō-mĭ) [" + G. *tomē*, a cutting]. Section of a nerve, esp. post.

radioepithelitis

spinal nerve roots. SYN: *rhizotomy.* SEE: *radiculectomy.*

radiculalgia (răd-ĭ-kū-lăl′jĭ-ă) [" + G. *algos*, pain]. Neuralgia of roots of nerves.

radicular (răd-ĭk′ū-lar) [L. *radix, radic-,* root]. Concerning a root or radicle.

r. arteries. Those accessory to spinal nerve roots.

r. fibers. Those associated with spinal nerve roots.

r. syndrome. Symptoms due to interference with intradural part of spinal nerve roots.

r. vessels. Those supplying spinal nerves and their roots.

radiculectomy (răd-ĭk-ū-lĕk′tō-mĭ) [" + G. *ektomē*, excision]. 1. Excision of a spinal nerve root. 2. Resection of post. spinal nerve root. SEE: *radicotomy.*

radiculitis (răd-ĭk-ū-lī′tĭs) [" + G. *-itis*, inflammation]. Inflammation of spinal nerve roots, accompanied by pain and hyperesthesia.

radiculomeningomyelitis (răd-ĭk″ū-lō-mē-nĭn″gō-mī-ĕl-ī′tĭs) [" + G. *mēninx*, membrane, + *myelos*, marrow, + *-itis*, inflammation]. Inflamed condition of nerve roots, meninges, and spinal cord. SYN: *rhizomeningomyelitis.*

radioactive (rā″dĭ-ō-ăk′tĭv) [L. *radius*, ray, + *activus*, acting]. Exhibiting radioactivity.

r. constant. That part of the whole amt. of radioactive substance which, in a given unit of time, will disintegrate. SYMB.: λ

radioactivity (rā″dĭ-ō-ăk-tĭv′ĭ-tĭ) [" + *activus*, acting]. The ability to emit rays or particles of matter, which can penetrate various substances, as radium.

r., induced. Temporary r. of a substance which has been within the sphere of influence of a radioactive element.

radioanaphylaxis (rā″dĭ-ō-ăn-ă-fĭ-lăks′ĭs) [" + G. *ana*, against, + *phylaxis*, protection]. Sensitization to radioactive energy.

radiocarpal (rā″dĭ-ō-kar′păl) [L. *radius*, spoke, + G. *karpos*, wrist]. Concerning the radius and carpus.

radiochemistry (rā″dĭ-ō-kĕm′ĭs-trĭ) [" + G. *chemeia*, chemistry]. The phase of chemistry dealing with radioactive phenomena.

radiochroism (rā″dĭ-ō-krō′ĭzm) [" + G. *chroa*, color]. The ability of a substance to absorb radioactive rays.

radiochrometer (rā″dĭ-ō-krŏm′ĕt-ĕr) [" + G. *chrōma*, color, + *metron*, measure]. Device for testing penetrating powers of x-rays and the character of roentgen tubes. SEE: *penetrometer.*

radiode (rā′dĭ-ōd) [L. *radius*, ray]. Metal container for radium, used in therapeutic application.

radiodermatitis (rā″dĭ-ō-der″mă-tī′tĭs) [" + G. *derma*, skin, + *-ōsis*, condition]. Inflammation of the skin caused by roentgen rays or radiation from radioactive elements. SYN: *actinodermatitis, q.v.*

radiodiagnosis (rā″dĭ-ō-dī-ăg-nō′sĭs) [" + G. *dia*, through, + *gnōsis*, knowledge]. Diagnosis by means of x-ray.

radioelement (rā″dĭ-ō-ĕl′e-mĕnt) [" + *elementum*]. An element possessing power of radioactivity.

radioepidermitis (rā″dĭ-ō-ĕp-ĭ-der-mī′tĭs) [" + G. *epi*, upon, + *derma*, skin, + *-itis*, inflammation]. Irritation of the skin caused by radioactive rays.

radioepithelitis (rā″dĭ-ō-ĕp-ĭ-thē-lī′tĭs) [" + " + *thēlē*, nipple, + *-itis*, inflamma-

radiogen   R-3   **radish**

tion]. Disintegration of epithelium due to exposure to irradiation.

radiogen (rā'dĭ-ō-jĕn) [" + G. *gennan*, to produce]. Any substance containing radioactive elements. SYN: *actinogen*.

radiogenic (rā"dĭ-ō-jĕn'ĭk) [L. *radius*, ray, + G. *gennan*, to produce]. 1. Due to irradiation. 2. Producing rays. SYN: *actinogenic*.

radiogenol (rā"dĭ-ō-jĕn'ōl) [L. *radius*, ray, spoke]. A commercial emulsion of radioactive substances for injection into tumors.

radiogram (rā'dĭ-ō-grăm) [" + G. *gramma*, a writing]. X-ray picture, esp. of internal organs. SYN: *actinogram*.

radiograph (rā'dĭ-ō-grăf) [" + G. *graphein*, to write]. A record produced on a photographic plate, film, or paper by the action of roentgen rays or radium; specifically an x-ray photograph.
Roentgenogram and curiegram fully cover the 2 senses which are included in this definition. SYN: *skiagraph*.

radiographer (rā"dĭ-ŏg'ră-fer) [" + G. *graphein*, to write]. A person skilled in making roentgenograms, or radiographs.
Usually, but at the present time not necessarily, applied to physicians who practice diagnostic roentgenology.

radiography (rā-dĭ-ŏg'ră-fĭ) [" + G. *graphein*, to write]. The making of x-ray pictures. SYN: *roentgenography, skiagraphy*.

radiohumeral (rā"dĭ-ō-hū'mĕr-ăl) [" + *humerus*]. Concerning the radius and humerus.

radiologist (rā-dĭ-ŏl'ō-jĭst) [" + G. *logos*, a study]. One who practices diagnosis and treatment by radiant energy.

radiology (rā-dĭ-ŏl'ō-jĭ) [L. *radius*, ray, spoke, + G. *logos*, study]. The branch of science which deals with roentgen rays, radium rays, and other radiations, and their curative properties.

radiolucency (rā"dĭ-ō-lū'sĕn-sĭ) [" + *lucere*, to shine]. Property of being partly or wholly permeable to radiant energy.

radiolus (rā-dĭ'ō-lŭs) [L. *radiolus*, a little spoke]. A sound; a probe.

radiometallography (rā"dĭ-ō-mĕt"ăl-ŏg'ră-fĭ) [L. *radius*, ray, spoke, + G. *metallon*, metal, + *graphein*, to write]. The study of metals by means of x-rays.

radiometer (rā-dĭ-ŏm'ĕt-ĕr) [" + G. *metron*, a measure]. 1. An instrument used to estimate the quantity of roentgen rays, usually with pastilles or pieces of photographic paper.
2. An instrument in which radiant heat and light may be directly converted into mechanical energy as devised by Sir William Crookes.
3. An instrument for measuring intensity of radiant energy.

radion (rā'dĭ-ŏn) [" + G. *ōn*, being]. One of the particles of the alpha, beta rays, or cathode rays, given off by radioactive matter.

radionecrosis (rā"dĭ-ō-nĕ-krō'sĭs) [" + G. *nekrōsis*, death]. Disintegration of tissue by exposure to radiant energy.

radionetics (rā-dĭ-ō-nĕt'ĭks). The application of electronics to the human body.

radioneuritis (rā"dĭ-ō-nū-rī'tĭs) [" + G. *neuron*, sinew, + *-itis*, inflammation]. Neuritis caused by exposure to radioactive substance.

radiopaque (rā-dĭ-ō-pāk') [" + *opacus*, dark]. Impenetrable to the x-ray or other forms of radiation.

radioparent (rā"dĭ-ō-par'ĕnt) [" + *parere*, to appear]. Penetrable by the x-ray or other rays.

radiopelvimetry (rā"dĭ-ō-pĕl-vĭm'ĕt-rĭ) [L. *radius*, ray, spoke, + *pelvis*, basin, + G. *metron*, measure]. Measurement of the pelvis by the x-ray.

radiopraxis (rā"dĭ-ō-prăks'ĭs) [" + G. *praxis*, practice]. Diagnosis or use in treatment of some radioactive substance, as x-ray or ultraviolet ray. SYN: *actinopraxis*.

radioreceptor (rā"dĭ-ō-rē-sĕp'tor) [" + *receptor*, one who receives]. Receptor responding to stimuli of radioactive elements, as to light and temperature. SEE: *receptor*.

radiosclerometer (rā"dĭ-ō-sklē-rŏm'ĕt-ĕr) [" + G. *sklēros*, hard, + *metron*, a measure]. An instrument that records penetration and intensity of the x-ray. SYN: *penetrometer, q.v.*

radioscopy (rā-dĭ-ŏs'kō-pĭ) [" + G. *skopein*, to examine]. Inspection and examination of the inner structures of the body by means of roentgen rays. SYN: *actinoscopy*.

radiosensibility (rā"dĭ-ō-sĕn"sĭ-bĭl'ĭ-tĭ) [" + *sensibilitās*]. Quality of sensitivity to radioactive substances.

radiosensitive (rā"dĭ-ō-sĕn'sĭ-tĭv) [" + *sensitivus*, feeling]. Capable of being destroyed by radiation, as a tumor by x-rays.

radiosurgery (rā"dĭ-ō-sur'jer-ĭ) [L. *radius*, ray, + G. *cheirurgia*, handwork]. The use of radium in surgery.

radiotherapist (rā"dĭ-ō-ther'ă-pĭst) [" + G. *therapeia*, treatment]. One trained in use of radiant energy for therapeutic purposes.

radiotherapy (rā"dĭ-ō-ther'ă-pĭ) [" + G. *therapeia*, treatment]. The treatment of disease by application of roentgen rays, radium, ultraviolet and other radiations.

radiothermitis (rā"dĭ-ō-ther-mī'tĭs) [" + G. *thermē*, heat, + *-itis*, inflammation]. Dermatitis caused by exposure to x-rays or other radiant substances.

radiothermy (rā"dĭ-ō-ther'mĭ) [" + G. *thermē*, heat]. Use of heat, in treatment, obtained from radioactive substances by specially built short wave apparatus.

radiotoxemia (rā"dĭ-ō-tŏks-ē'mĭ-ă) [" + G. *toxikon*, poison, + *aima*, blood]. Toxemia produced by exposure to radioactive substance. SYN: *actinotoxemia*.

radiotransparent (rā"dĭ-ō-trăns-par'ĕnt) [" + *trans*, across, + *parere*, to appear]. Penetrable by x-ray or other forms of radiation.

radiotropic (rā"dĭ-ō-trŏp'ĭk) [L. *radius*, ray, spoke, + G. *tropos*, a turning]. Affected by radiation.

radioulnar (rā"dĭ-ō-ŭl'nar) [" + *ulna*, arm]. Concerning the radius and ulna.

radio wave (rā'dĭ-ō wāv) [L. *radius*, ray, + A.S. *wawe*]. Electric wave produced by or employing radiant energy.* SEE: *radiothermy*.

radish (răd'ĭsh) [L. *radix*, an edible root]. COMP: Contain sulfocyanate of allyl, the active principle of mustard and arsenic. High in oxalic acid; little food value, but desirable for its minerals.
AV. SERVING: 50 Gm. Pro. 0.7, Fat 0.1, Carbo. 1.7.
VITAMINS: A— to +, B++, C+++.
ASH CONST: Ca 0.021, Mg 0.012, K 0.218, Na 0.069, P 0.029, Cl 0.054, S 0.041, Fe 0.0006.
A base-forming food; alkaline potentiality, 2.9 cc. per 100 Gm, 9.8 cc. per 100 cal.
ACTION: An acid stimulant. An appetizer, stimulates saliva, and antiseptic to intestinal tract.

radium (rā'dĭ-ŭm) [L. *radius*, rays]. SYMB: Ra. A metallic element found in very small quantities in pitchblende. At. wt. 226.4. SEE: "*actin-*" *words*.

It does not seem to exist in a free state. It is radioactive and fluorescent, becoming darker on exposure to light.

Radiation is of 3 kinds: (1) The *alpha rays;* (2) *beta rays;* (3) *gamma rays,* which are analogous to the x-rays.

Radium is an unstable substance, and is therefore used mainly in the form of the sulfate. These salts are inserted into fine glass capillary tubes, which for safety are then put into silver or lead containers. Fine needles containing radium salts are also used. Radium emanation is used in the form of tiny tubes or seeds of *radon.* Medically, radium is used extensively in the treatment of cancer and skin conditions.

r. intratumoral application. Implanting radium into tumors for therapeutic purposes.

r. needles. Radium needles contain from 2 to 12½ milligrams of radium element. The usual material employed for needle containers is a steel alloy. The wall thickness is from 0.2 to 0.4 millimeters.

r. emanation. Heavy, colorless, gaseous element given off in disintegration of radium. SYN: *radon.*

Its concentration is measured in terms of the maché unit, abbr. *m. u.*

radiumization (rā"dĭ-ŭm-ĭ-za'shŭn) [L. *radius,* ray]. Exposure to action of radium rays.

radiumologist (rā"dĭ-ŭm-ŏl'ō-jĭst) [" + G. *logos,* a study]. One who specializes in radium therapy.

radiumology (rā"dĭ-ŭm-ŏl'ō-jĭ) [" + G. *logos,* a study]. The science of radium therapy.

radium therapy (rā'dĭ-ŭm ther'ă-pĭ) [" + G. *therapeia,* treatment]. The treatment of disease by means of radium, radon, its emanation, or its active deposit.

radius (rā'dĭ-ŭs) [L. *radius,* a spoke, ray]. 1. The outer and shorter bone of the arm which revolves partially about the ulna. 2. A line extending from a circle's center point to its circumference.

Its head articulates with the *capitulum* of the humerus. Its lower extremity articulates by the ulnar notch with the ulna, and by another articulation with the navicular and lunate bones of the wrist. SEE: *radial, skeleton.*

r., fracture of. *Colles' Fracture*: A fracture and dislocation of lower end of radius, generally caused by falling on the outstretched hand.

May be treated in an unpadded plaster cast applied to the hand and arm from heads of the metacarpals to elbow. The wrist is dorsiflexed, the cast being bandaged or strapped in position. Fingers, elbows and shoulders are used almost at once.

Fracture of Shaft of Radius and Ulna: Two wires may be necessary, both wires being incorporated in the plaster, which extends from hand to about middle of upper arm.

radix (ra'dĭks) (pl. *radices*) [L. root]. 1. The root portion of a cranial or spinal nerve. 2. The root of a plant.

radon (rā'dŏn) [L. *radio,* ray]. A heavy radioactive gas given off in the disintegration of radium. SYN: *niton, radium emanation.*

ragsorters' disease (răg'sort'ers). A febrile pulmonary disease arising in persons who sort paper and rags due to inhalation of bacillus causing anthrax, *q.v.*

railway spine (rāl'wā). A traumatic neurasthenia due to injuries in railway accidents.

raised (rāzd) [M.E. *reisen,* to rise]. BACT: Having a thick, terraced elevated growth with terraced edges.

raisin. AV. SERVING: 60 Gm. Pro. 1.6, Fat 0.1, Carbo. 48.5.
VITAMINS: B+.
ASH CONST: Ca 0.064, Mg 0.083, K 0.820, Na 0.133, P 0.132, Cl 0.082, S 0.051, Fe 0.0021.

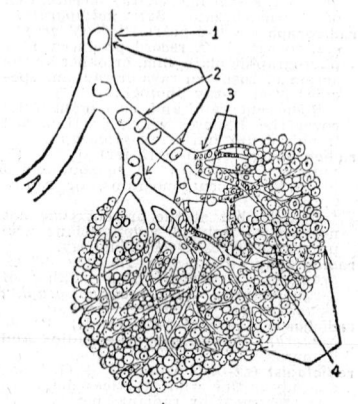

RÂLES.
1. Death rattle. 2. Large moist râles. 3. Small moist râles. 4. Subcrepitant râles.

râle (rahl) [Fr. rattle]. Bubbling sound heard in bronchi in inspiration and expiration in disease.

ETIOL: Produced by movement of air in a tense, walled cavity containing air and communicating with a bronchus; character, large musical and tinkling; condition in which heard, tuberculosis, pneumonia, bronchitis, and abscess cavities. Classified as dry or moist.

RS: *bronchorrhoncus, crepitation, rhoncus, sibilant.*

r., bronchiectatic. Heard over bronchiectatic cavities filled with accumulated secretion. Disappears with expectoration.

r., bubbling medium. Heard in inspiration and expiration; produced by passage of air through mucus in the larger tubes; character, larger than the small bubbling moist r.; heard in capillary bronchitis, esp. in children.

r., cavernous. Heard in inspiration and expiration; produced by passage of air through a small cavity with flaccid walls that collapse with expiration; character, hollow and metallic; heard in the 3rd stage of pulmonary tuberculosis.

r., clicking. Heard in inspiration only; produced by passage of air through softening material in smaller bronchi; character, small, sticky; heard in pulmonary tuberculosis, early stage.

r., coarse. Originates in the larger bronchi.

r., crackling, medium. Heard chiefly in inspiration; produced by fluid in the finer bronchi; character, larger than the small, crackling, dry; heard in softening of the tubercular deposit, or pneumonic exudation.

r., crepitant. Heard at end of inspiration; produced by passage of air into collapsed vesicles containing fibrinous exudation, usually at base of lungs; character, small, like rubbing hair bet. the fingers; heard in pneumonia, in early stage edema of lungs, hypostatic pneumonia. It is localized in pulmonary tuberculosis.

r., dry. Heard in inspiration and expiration; produced by narrowing of the bronchial tubes from thickening of their mucous lining, from spasmodic contraction of the muscular coat, viscid mucus within or pressure from without; character, large and sonorous, small, hissing or whistling; heard in bronchitis, asthma, and localized in beginning pulmonary tuberculosis.

r., friction. Heard in inspiration and expiration, most distinct at end of respiration produced by the rubbing together of serous surfaces roughened by inflammation or deprived of their natural secretions; character, grazing, rubbing, grating, creaking, or crackling; heard in pleurisy and pericarditis.

r., gurgling. Heard in inspiration and expiration; produced by passage of air through fluid in cavities of large bubbles; heard in pulmonary tuberculosis after formation of cavities.

r., moist. Produced by passage of air through bronchi containing fluid.

r., mucous (of Laennec). Heard in inspiration and expiration; produced by viscid bubbles bursting in the bronchial tubes; character, modification of the subcrepitant; heard in pulmonary emphysema.

r. redux, r. de retour. Heard in inspiration and expiration; produced by passage of air through fluid in bronchial tubes; character, crackling, unequal; heard in pneumonia, in the stage of resolution.

r., sibilant. High pitched, whistling, and frequent at end of inspiration.

r., sonorous. Low snoring, greater in volume, continuing during inspiration.

r., subcrepitant. Heard in inspiration and expiration; produced by passage of air through mucus in the capillary bronchial tubes; character, small, moist; heard in capillary bronchitis.

r., submucous. Higher pitched and more numerous than large mucous râle. Heard in interscapular and supramammary regions and indicating involvement of many tubes of small caliber.

rami (rā'mī) (L. *ramus*, a branch. Plural of *ramus*.

ramification (răm-ĭ-fĭ-kā'shŭn) [L. *ramus*, branch, + *ficāre*, to make]. 1. Process of branching. 2. A branch. 3. Arrangement in branches.

ramify (răm'ĭ-fī) [L. *ramificāre*, to make in branches]. To branch; to spread out in different directions.

ramisection (răm″ĭ-sĕk″shŭn, răm″ĭ-sĕk′-shŭn) [L. *ramus*, branch, + *sectĭō*, a cutting]. Section of nerve fibrils bet. the spinal and sympathetic systems.

ramisectomy (răm-ĭs-ĕk′tō-mī) [" + G. *ektomē*, excision]. Excision of a ramus, specifically r. communicans. SEE: *ramisection*.

ramitis (răm-ī′tĭs) [" + G. *-ītis*, inflammation]. A nerve root inflammation.

ramollissement (rah″mo-lēs-mon′) [Fr. *ramollir*, to soften]. Morbid softening of some organ or tissue, esp. of brain.

ramus (rā′mŭs) (pl. *rami*) [L. *ramus*, a branch]. 1. A branch of 1 of the divisions of a forked structure. 2. Post. portion of lower jawbone. 3. BNA. Primary division of a blood vessel or nerve.

r. communicans. Small nerve fiber passing bet. fibers from ant. roots of the spinal cord and a sympathetic ganglion. SEE: *sympathetic nervous system*.

rancid (răn′sĭd) [L. *rancere*, to be rancid]. Offensive; having a sour smell or taste from partial decomposition, as a *fat*.

range of accommodation. Difference bet. least and greatest distance of distinct vision. SEE: *accommodation*.

ranine (rā′nīn) [L. *rana*, a frog]. 1. Pert. to a ranula or to the region beneath the tip of the tongue. 2. Branch of the lingual artery supplying that area.

Ranvier's nodes (ron-vē-ās′). Constrictions in the medullary substance of a nerve fiber at more or less regular intervals. SEE: *nerve*.

ranula (răn′ū-lă) [L. *ranula*, little frog]. A large cystic tumor seen on underside of tongue on either side of the frenum. The swelling may be small or as large as an egg.

SYM: Semitranslucent; soft, large, dilated veins coursing over it. Fullness and discomfort. Usually no pain. Contains clear, glairy fluid, due to dilatation of ducts of salivary glands and to obstruction of those of sublingual mucous glands.

TREATMENT: Empty sac as it refills. Necessary to destroy lining membrane of cyst by caustic, after having excised part of cyst wall.

r., pancreatica. Cystic disease of pancreas due to obstruction of its ducts.

rape (rāp) [L. *rapere*, to snatch]. 1. Coitus with a female without her consent or when she is too young or without sufficient intelligence to give legal consent. SYN: *stupration*.

It is a crime punishable by death in some states. It is very difficult legally to prove rape. Rape of a vigorous girl by an unassisted male is considered almost impossible if the victim is conscious and free to defend herself.

Rape during sleep, under anesthesia, or hypnosis is considered questionable, although there are cases on record of those who claim to have been raped under such conditions. [*tercourse, virginity*.

RS: *age of consent, coitus, sexual in-*

raphania (răf-ā′nĭ-ă) [G. *rhaphanos*, radish]. A spasmodic disease caused by eating seeds of the wild radish; allied to ergotism, *q.v.* SYN: *rhaphania*.

raphe (rā′fē) [G. *rhaphē*, a seam]. 1. A crease or ridge or seam noting union of the halves of a part, as the division of the 2 lateral halves of the scrotum. 2. A suture.

rapport′ [Fr. *rapporter*, to bring back]. PSY: A relationship of sympathy and confidence.

rarefaction (rar″ē-făk′shŭn) [L. *rarefacere*, to make thin]. Process of decreasing density and weight, as of *air*.

The farther from the surface of the earth, the less dense the atmosphere becomes.

r. of bone. The process of making bone more porous because of absorption of lime salts.

ETIOL: General changes in metabolism, caries or rarefying osteitis. SEE: *sclerosis*.

rar′efy″ing os″tei′tis. Chronic bone inflammation marked by development of granulation tissue in marrow spaces with absorption of surrounding hard bone. SEE: *osteitis*.

rash (răsh) [O.Fr. *rasche*, eruption]. Temporary eruption on skin, with little or no elevation. SYN: *exanthema*. SEE: *lesion, roseola*.

r., drug. One caused by use of certain drugs, such as *bromide* or *iodine*. SEE: *idiosyncrasy*.

r., enema. One caused by too much soap in an enema; resembles measles.

r., gum. A red, papular eruption of the mouth, a form of miliaria, seen esp. in infants, due to intestinal disturbances. SYN: *strophulus*.

r., mulberry. R. seen in typhus fever; dusky in color.

r., nettle. Smooth, elevated, itchy, white patches. SYN: *hives, urticaria*.

r., red. SEE: *gum rash*.

r., rose. Any rose-colored rash. SYN: *roseola*.

r., tooth. SEE: *gum rash*.

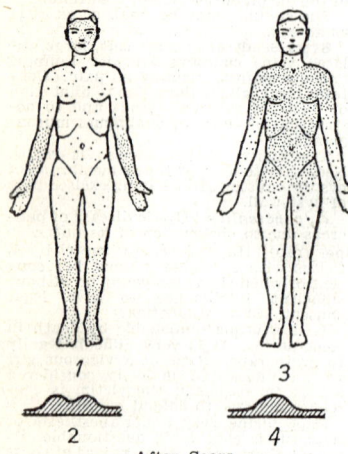

After Sears.
RASH.

1. Smallpox. 2. Vesicle of smallpox with umbilication. 3. Chickenpox. 4. Vesicle of chickenpox, no umbilication.

raspatory (răs′pă-tō″rĭ) [L. *raspatorium*]. File used in surgery, esp. for trimming surfaces of bone.

raspberry (răz′bĕr-ĭ) (red). COMP: Contains 3 times as much cellulose and less ash than strawberry.

AV. SERVING: 75 Gm. Pro. 0.8, Fat 0.4, Carbo. 7.3.

VITAMINS: A++, B+, C+++.

ASH CONST: Ca 0.049, Mg 0.024, K 0.173, Na none, P 0.052, Cl none, S 0.017, Fe 0.0006.

r. juice. AV. SERVING: 120 Gm. Pro. 0.5, Carbo. 10.0.

ASH CONST: Ca 0.021, Mg 0.016, K 0.134, Na 0.005, P 0.012, S 0.009, no Fe or Cl.

rasura, rasure (ră-sū′ră, ră′zhur) [L. *rasura*, a scraping]. 1. Process of scraping or shaving. 2. Scrapings or filings.

rat (răt) [A.S. *raet*]. A rodent found in and around human habitations.

Transmits disease to man, esp. bubonic plague. Its bite causes ratbite fever. White species used for testing purposes in laboratories.

r. unit. Greatest dilution of an estrus-producing hormone which will cause desquamation and cornification of vaginal epithelium during 1st day, if given to a mature spayed rat in 3 injections, 1 every 4 hours.

ratbite fever. An infectious disease transmitted by bite of a rat, caused by infection with *Spirillum minus*.

SYM: Chill followed by febrile attacks at irregular intervals, reddish-blue rash, severe muscular pain.

rate (răt) [L. *rata*, a fixed amount]. 1. Valuation based on comparison with a standard. 2. Measure of a thing.

Rathke's columns (raht′keh). Two cartilages elongated at ant. extremity of chorda dorsalis.

R's. diverticulum, R's. pouch. A pouch in bucco-pharyngeal embryonic membrane from which is developed the ant. lobe of the hypophysis cerebri.

ratio (rā′shĭ-ō) [L.]. Proportion.

ration (rā′shŭn) [L. *ratio*, proportion]. Fixed allowance of food and drink for a certain period.

rational (răsh′ŭn-ăl) [L. *rationalis*, reasoning]. 1. Of sound mind. SYN: *sane*. 2. Reasonable or logical. 3. Employing treatments based on reasoning or general principles, opposed to empiric.

r. formula. A chemical one, written in symbols showing the constituents of a molecule and the atomic arrangement and relationship in it.

r. symptom. One discovered by questioning instead of by physical examination.

rationalization (răsh-ŭn-ăl-ĭ-zā′shŭn) [L. *rationalitās*, reasoning]. PSY: Rational or plausible explanation of behavior or belief activated by unknown motives.

rattle (răt′l) [M.E. *ratelen*, probably of imitative origin]. A sound or râle heard on auscultation.

r., death. A gurgling sound or subcrepitant râle heard in the trachea of the dying.

Rau's process (rowz). Slender, long process of the malleus. SYN: *processus gracilis mallei*.

Rauber's layer (row′ber). The external layer of cells partially composing the ectoderm of the primitive embryo.

raucous (raw′kŭs) [L. *racus*, hoarse]. Hoarse, strident, as the sound of a voice.

rave (rāv) [O.Fr. *raver*, to rave]. To talk irrationally, as in delirium.

raving (rāv′ing) [O.Fr. *raver*, to rave]. 1. Irrational utterance. 2. Talking irrationally.

ravish (răv′ĭsh) [Fr. *ravir*, to seize]. 1. To commit rape upon a girl or woman. 2. To remove or carry away by force.

ray (rā) [L. *radius*, a rod, spoke]. 1. One of a number of lines diverging from a common center. 2. Line of propagation of any form of radiant energy, esp. light or heat; loosely, any narrow beam of light.

RS: *energy; e., radiant; fluorescence; heat; radiation; "roentgen-" words; spectrum; x-ray*.

r., actinic. A solar ray of the spectrum capable of producing chemical changes.

r., alpha. Ray composed of positively charged particles of helium derived from atomic disintegration of radioactive elements.

Velocity from 1/10 to 1/3 that of light. They are completely absorbed by a thin sheet of paper, and possess powerful fluorescent, photographic and ionizing properties. They are less penetrative than the beta rays.

r., antirachitic. Ultraviolet ray from 2700 to 3020 A. U.

r., bactericidal. Ray bet. 1850 and 2600 A. U. which is strongly bactericidal.

r's., Becquerel's. Those from radium, uranium, and other radioactive substances.

r's., beta. Negatively charged electrons expelled from atoms of disintegrating radioactive elements.

They possess strong photographic, fluorescent and ionizing properties. They are identical in character with the cathode rays produced by an electrical discharge in a vacuum tube. Their velocity is approximately that of light. Beta rays are more penetrating than alpha rays; half of the shorter rays from radium are absorbed by about 1 mm. of lead. Silver will absorb about 0.9% of the shortest beta rays.

r's., Blondlot's. SEE: *n. rays*.

r's., border, r's., borderline, r's., Bucky. SEE: *Grenz rays*.

r's., canal. Positive rays in a vacuum tube going from anode toward cathode. Old name for positive ray.

r's., cathode. Negatively charged electrons discharged by the cathode through a vacuum, moving in a straight line, and upon hitting solid matter produce roentgen rays.

r., characteristic. Secondary roentgen rays, the wave lengths of which are determined by the chemical constitution of the object that emits, transmits, or scatters them.

r., chemical. SEE: *actinic ray*.

r., cosmic. SEE: *Millikan's rays*.

r's., delta. Highly penetrative ether waves given off by radioactive substances.

r's., dynamic. Rays which are physically or therapeutically active.

r. fungus. Genus of parasitic fungi with radiating formation.

r., erythema-producing. Ray bet. 1800 and 4000 A. U., which produces erythema; those around 2540 and bet. 2050 and 3100 A. U. being most effective.

r., Finsen (or light). Ultraviolet radiation from the Finsen lamp.

r's., fluorescent roentgen. Secondary rays whose wave lengths are characteristic of the substance which emits them.

r., gamma. Heterogeneous vibrations caused by electronic disturbance in atoms of radioactive elements during their disintegration and appear identical with roentgen rays except that the wave lengths range from about 1.4 to 0.01 angstroms. They have high velocity and penetrative power. They lie bet. ultraviolet and roentgen rays.

r., Grenz. Soft roentgen ray with an average wave length of 2 angstroms (range from 1 to 3 angstroms); obtained with peak voltage of less than 10 kilovolts.

r's., hard. X-rays of short wave length and great penetration.

r's., heat. Visible rays from 4000 to 7000 A. U. and infrared rays from 6000 to 14,000 A. U. The heating effect of visible rays on deeper tissue is proportionately stronger than that of infrared rays, on account of greater penetrating power. SEE: *heat*.

r's., Hertzian. Electromagnetic waves of great wave length. Used in radio communication.

r's., infrared. Radiations just beyond the red end of the spectrum. Their wave lengths range bet. 7700 and 500,000 angstroms. The therapeutic range extends from about 7700 to about 14,000 angstroms.

r's., Lenard's. Cathode rays that have passed outside the discharge tube. SEE: *cathode ray*.

r., luminous. Visible ray.

r., medullary. Cortical protuberance from a bundle of tubules in a renal pyramid.

r's., Millikan. Electromagnetic waves coming from unknown sources, resembling the gamma rays, but their penetration is greater and their wave length shorter.

r's., monochromatic. Rays characterized by a definite wave length, as secondary rays.

r's., n. Radiant energy emitted by active nerves and muscles, affecting a fluorescent screen similarly to x-rays; discovered by Blondlot.

r's., pigment-producing. Rays at 2500 and 3000 A. U. are most effective in causing pigmentation, a local response to irritation of cutaneous prickle-cells.

r., primary. Ray discharged directly from a radioactive substance, as the alpha, beta, and gamma rays.

r., positive. Ray of positively charged ions which, in a discharge tube, go from the anode toward the cathode.

r., roentgen. X-rays discovered by Wilhelm Konrad Roentgen. They have a penetrative power through opaque substances; used for photographing internal organs and parts, and for diagnostic and therapeutic purposes. Hardness of roentgen rays is a descriptive term used to characterize the penetrating power of the roentgen rays. Depending on wave length, the shorter the wave length is, the harder the rays and the greater their penetrating ability. SEE: *intensity, international x-ray unit, roentgen ray, x-ray*.

r's., scattered. Roentgen rays or gamma rays which, in their passage through a substance, have deviated in direction and also may have been changed by an increase in wave length.

r's., Schumann. Rays in the region bounded bet. 1220 and 1850 angstroms.

r's., secondary. Roentgen rays emitted in all directions by any matter irradiated with roentgen rays.

r's., ultraviolet. Invisible rays of the spectrum which are beyond the violet rays, and of varying wave lengths. Of luminous ether which may be refracted, reflected, and polarized, but which will not traverse many substances impervious to the rays of the visible spectrum. They do not affect the retina, but rapidly destroy the vitality of bacteria. They produce photochemical and photographic effects.

r's., x-. SEE: *roentgen rays*.

Raynaud's disease (rā-nōz'). Severe, paroxysmal, vascular disorder causing disturbances of the circulation in the extremities.

Venous stasis follows in 3 stages: Local syncope, asphyxia, and gangrene. A vasomotor neurosis, characterized by local anemia, congestion or gangrene.

SYM: In 1 form, the part, usually a finger or toe, becomes pale, cold, anesthetic. After a time these phenomena disappear and are followed by redness, heat and tingling. Attacks may be excited by cold and come and go without damaging the part. In another form, affected part becomes swollen, dark, red, painful; if attack persists bullae may appear and gangrene develop. Gangrenous areas often symmetrical, involving a finger on each hand, toe on each foot, or both ears. Hemoglobinuria may occur in, or replace an attack.

PROG: Attacks persist, but life not endangered. In rare instances extensive gangrene develops and death follows. Gangrene may be absent in mild forms.

TREATMENT: Patients liable to attacks should be well protected from cold. Frequent bathing and friction. Raynaud advises use of a continuous current, 1 pole over spine, other over affected area. Nitroglycerin.

Rb. Symb. for *rubidium*.
R. C. P. Royal College of Physicians.
R. C. S. Royal College of Surgeons.
R. D. A. Right dorsoanterior presentation position of the fetus.
R. D. P. Right dorsoposterior presentation position of the fetus.
R. E. Abbr. for *radium emanation* and for *right eye*.
re- [L.]. Prefix meaning *back* or *again*.
reaction (rē-ăk'shŭn) [L. *rē*, back, + *actus*, acting]. 1. Mutual action of chemical agents upon each other. 2. Response of a muscle or nerve to stimulation, including its rebound or opp. movement. 3. Emotional and mental state created by a situation.

Response to tests may be (a) *positive*, when definite reactionary changes take place; (b) *negative*, when no changes take place, and (c) *neutral*, when change is only due to agent used.

r., cutaneous deep. PSY: Diminution or abolition of pressure, musculoarticular, or osseous sensibility occurs with conservation of thermic, tactile and pain sensibility.

FORMS OF REACTIONS: *Anesthesia Dolorosa*: Pain associated with anesthesia of a part, as in thalmic lesions.

Dysthesia: Retardation and fusion of sensations or prolonged sensation due to successive stimuli; addition of sensations, errors of location, perception only of the 1st of a series of sensations, disappearance of sensation during prolonged stimulation, polyesthesia when stimulus is single, pain far from point stimulated, perception at symmetrical points (allochiria*), false interpretation of a sensation.

Subjective Sensations: These may include causalgia, paresthesia, pseudomyelia paresthetica, a false sensation, as of movement in a paralyzed limb or part, or sensation of lack of movement in a moving limb.

r. of degeneration. The change in muscle reactivity to electricity, seen in lower motor neuron paralysis.

Response to faradism disappears, while that to galvanism increases. In addition, the anodal closing contraction now equals or exceeds the cathodal closing contraction. In partial r. d. an anodal change alone may be present. The muscle contracts tardily and tends to persist longer than in health.

r. formation. The checking of infantile impulses and tendencies which might become those of an antisocial nature later, or which might hold the individual upon an infantile level and the attributes developed from such partial repressions, such as modesty, shame, or disgust.

r., miostagmin. Diagnostic test for syphilis, malignant tumors and typhoid involving determination of surface tension of blood serum.

r., ophthalmic. Ocular reaction to introduction of toxins of tuberculosis and typhoid fever; more severe in those having the diseases.

r. period. SEE: *reaction time*.

r's. of sensibility. Tests to determine forms of sensibility by pressure, tactile means, heat, pain, etc.

r. time. Time elapsing bet. giving a stimulus word and the response to it.

reactive depression (rē-ăk'tĭv dē-prĕsh'ŭn). PSY: A psychosis resulting from bereavement, sadness or a situation causing such emotions, lasting longer and more marked than the normal reaction.

reagent (rē-ā'jĕnt) [L. *rē*, again, + *agere*, to act]. 1. A substance which may be added to a solution to detect the presence or absence of a certain substance, or to produce a chemical reaction. 2. PSY: Subject of a psychological experiment, esp. one reacting to a stimulus.

reality principle (rē-ăl'ĭ-tĭ) [Fr. *réalité*]. The effect of necessity or external consideration, acting to control self-gratification, or of the ego's self-protective influences.

reapers' keratitis (rēp'ĕrs kĕr-ă-tī'tĭs). Keratitis caused by dust from grain.

Réaumur's thermometer (rā'o-mur). A thermometric scale having 0° for the freezing point, and 80° for the boiling point of water.

Readings changed to Centigrade by multiplying by 5/4, to Fahrenheit by multiplying by 9/4 and adding 32.

rebreathing (rē-brĕth'ĭng) [L. *rē*, again, + A.S. *braeth*, breath]. Administration of oxygen to a patient under a general anesthetic for speedy elimination of the anesthetic.

recall (rē-kawl') [" + A.S. *ceallian*, to call]. PSY: Act of bringing back to mind that which has been previously learned or experienced; reproduction.

recapitulation theory (rē"kă-pĭt-ū-lā'shŭn) [L. *rē*, again, + *capitulum*, a section]. The idea that man's development from the ovum to maturity repeats and represents all the stages of evolution through which he is supposed to have developed.

receiver (rē-sēv'er) [L. *rē*, back, + *capere*, to take]. Container for holding a gas or a distillate.

receptaculum (rē-sĕp-tăk'ū-lŭm) [L. a container]. A vessel or cavity in which a fluid is contained.

r. chyli. Inferior, pear-shaped, expanded portion of the lower end of the thoracic duct, near 1st and 2nd lumbar vertebrae, into which certain lymphatics discharge.

r. seminis. Post. *cul-de-sac* of the vagina, so named because it was once assumed to be a receptacle for the semen during sexual intercourse.

receptor (rē-sĕp'tor) [L. a receiver]. 1. Molecular group in cells which have a special affinity for toxins, amboceptors, etc. SEE: *Ehrlich's side chain theory*. 2. Group of cells functioning in reception of stimuli; a sense organ; endings of afferent (sensory) nerves.

Classified as: (a) *Exterceptors*, those responding to sources external to the body; (b) *interoceptors*, those affected by substances or conditions within the digestive cavities; (c) *proprioceptors*, those affected by that which occurs within the body.

Receptors may also be classified by the nature of the stimuli to which they respond: (a) *Chemo-r.*, responding to the sense of smell or taste; (b) *mechanico-r.*, those responding to the sensation of sound and pressure, and (c) *radio-r.*, those responding to heat, cold, and light. There are other receptors which are not within the foregoing classifications.

r. neuron (sensory). One carrying impulses from the periphery to the center.

recessus (rē-sĕs'ŭs) [L. cavity]. A small hollow or recess.

r. cochlearis. Hollow or inner wall of the labyrinthine vestibule, perforated for passing of nerves supplying the ductus cochlearis.

r. opticus. BNA. Optic recess above the optic chiasm.

r. parotideus. Deep recess in front of the mastoid in which is lodged the parotid gland.

r. pharyngeus. Fossa in nasopharynx on either side of the eustachian tubes.

recipe (rĕs'ĭ-pē) [L. *recipere*, to receive]. 1. [L.]. Take, indicated by the sign ℞. 2. A prescription or formula for a medicine.

recipient (rē-sĭp'ĭ-ĕnt) [L. *recipiens*, receiving]. One who receives anything, esp. the blood in transfusion. SEE: *donor*.

reciprocal (rē-sĭp'rō-kăl) [L. *reciprocus*, turning backward and forward]. Interchangeable in character.

r. reception. Articulation with convex surface in 1 direction and concave surface in another.

Recklinghausen's canals (rĕk'lĭng-howzĕn). Tiny channels conveying lymph in connective tissue which are continuations of the lymphatics, being their roots.

R's. disease. 1. A condition characterized by pigmentation of the skin and multiple neurofibromata of trunk and scalp. SYN: *Von Recklinghausen's disease*. 2. Generalized fibrocystic bone disease. 3. Arthritis with deformity and neoplastic formations.

reclination (rĕk-lĭ-nā'shŭn) [L. *reclināre*, to lean back]. The turning of the eye lens covered with a cataract over into the vitreous to remove it from line of vision.

recline (rē-klīn') [L. *reclināre*, to lean back]. To be in recumbent position; to lie down.

Reclus' disease (rĕ-klū'). Multiple, benign, cystic growths in the mammary gland.

R's. method. The use of cocaine to produce local anesthesia.

R's. operation. Creation of an artificial anus in cancer of the rectum.

reconstituent (rē″kŏn-stĭt'ū-ĕnt) [L. *re*, again, + *constituens*, constituting]. An agent that improves or strengthens 1 or more parts or functions of the body by replacing lost material. Ex: calcium, iron, phosphorus. SYN: *tonic*.

recrement (rĕk'rē-mĕnt) [L. *recrementum*, that which is separated back]. Secretion which, after having performed its function as the saliva or part of the bile, is reabsorbed into the blood.

recrementitious (rĕk″rē-mĕn-tĭsh'ŭs) [L. *recrementum*, that which is separated back]. Of the nature of a secretion which, having performed its function, is reabsorbed into the blood.

recrudescence (rē-krū-dĕs'ĕns) [L. *recrudescere*, to become raw again]. Return of symptoms. SYN: *relapse*.

recrudescent (rē-krū-dĕs'ĕnt) [L. *recru-*

descere, to become raw again]. Assuming renewed activity.

rectal (rĕkt'ăl) [L. *rectus*, straight]. Pert. to the rectum.

r. alimentation. Rectal feeding, q.v.

r. anesthesia. Introduction of anesthetic into rectum for local desensitization, used esp. in labor. SEE: *anesthesia, labor*.

r. crisis. Tenesmus and rectal pain in locomotor ataxia.

r. feeding. The introduction of nutrients in fluid form into the colon through the rectum. SYN: *nutrient enema*, q.v.

r. reflex. The normal desire to evacuate feces present in rectum.

rectalgia (rĕk-tăl'jĭ-ă) [L. *rectus*, straight, + G. *algos*, pain]. Pain in rectum.

rectectomy (rĕk-tĕk'tō-mĭ) [" + G. *ektomē*, excision]. Excision of the rectum or anus. SYN: *proctectomy*.

rectification (rĕk″tĭ-fĭ-kā'shŭn) [" + *-ficāre*, to make]. 1. The process of refining or purifying a substance. 2. Act of straightening or correcting.

rectified (rĕk'tĭ-fīd) [" + *-ficāre*, to make]. Made pure or straight. Set right.

r. spirit. One resulting from fractional or repeated distillation of alcohol, as whisky.

rectifier (rĕk'tĭ-fī'ĕr) [" + *-ficāre*, to make]. A device for obtaining a unidirectional current from an alternating current.

rectitis (rĕk-tī'tĭs) [" + G. *-ītis*, inflammation]. Inflamed condition of the rectum. SYN: *proctitis*.

recto- [L.]. Combining form meaning *straight, the rectum*.

rectocele (rĕk'tō-sēl) [L. *rectus*, straight, + G. *kēlē*, hernia]. Protrusion of posterior vaginal wall with ant. wall of rectum through the vagina.

rectoclysis (rĕk-tŏk'lĭs-ĭs) [" + G. *klysis*, a washing out]. Slow introduction of fluid into rectum. SYN: *Murphy drip, proctoclysis*.

rectococcypexia (rĕk″tō-kŏk-sĭ-pĕks'sĭ-ă) [" + G. *kokkyx*, coccyx, + *pēxis*, fixation]. Fixation of rectum by suturing it to coccyx.

rectocolitis (rĕk″tō-kō-lī'tĭs) [" + G. *kōlon*, colon, + *-ītis*, inflammation]. Inflamed condition of rectum and colon. SYN: *proctocolitis*.

rectocystotomy (rĕk″tō-sĭs-tŏt'ō-mĭ) [" + G. *kystis*, bladder, + *tomē*, a cutting]. Incision of the bladder through rectum, usually to remove a calculus.

rectopexy (rĕk'tō-pĕks-ĭ) [" + G. *pēxis*, fixation]. Fixation of rectum by suturing to another part. SYN: *proctopexy*.

rectophobia (rĕk″tō-fō'bĭ-ă) [" + G. *phobos*, fear]. Morbid fear in those patients with rectal disease.

rectoplasty (rĕk'tō-plăs″tĭ) [L. *rectus*, straight, + G. *plassein*, to form]. Plastic operation on the anus and rectum. SYN: *proctoplasty*.

rectorrhaphy (rĕk-tor'ră-fĭ) [" + G. *raphē*, a sewing]. Suture of rectum and anus. SYN: *proctorrhaphy*.

rectoscope (rĕk'tō-skōp) [" + G. *skopein*, to examine]. A speculum to examine the rectum.

rectosigmoid (rĕk″tō-sĭg'moyd) [" + G. *sigma*, letter S, + *eidos*, form]. Upper part of rectum and adjoining portion of the sigmoid colon.

rectostenosis (rĕk″tō-stĕn-ō'sĭs) [" + G. *stenōsis*, a narrowing]. Stricture of the rectum.

rectostomy (rĕk-tŏs'tō-mĭ) [" + G. *stoma*, a mouth]. Creation of an artificial open-

rectotomy   R-10   **reduction diet, modified**

ing into the rectum to relieve stricture. SYN: *proctostomy, q.v.*

rectotomy (rĕk-tŏt'ō-mĭ) [" + G. *tomē*, an incision]. Incision for stricture of the rectum or other purposes. SYN: *proctotomy, q.v.*

rectourethral (rĕk"tō-ū-rē'thrăl) [L. *rectus*, straight, + G. *ourēthra*, urethra]. Concerning the rectum and urethra.

rectouterine (rĕk"tō-ū'ter-ĭn) [" + *uterus*, womb]. Concerning the rectum and uterus.

rectovaginal (rĕk"tō-văj'ĭn-ăl) [" + *vagina*, sheath]. Concerning the rectum and vagina.

rectovesical (rĕk"tō-vĕs'ĭk-ăl) [" + *vesica*, a small vessel]. Concerning the rectum and bladder.

rectum (rĕk'tŭm) [L. straight]. Lower part of large intestine, about 5 in. (12 cm.) long, bet. sigmoid flexure and the anus.

The centers of the anorectal mechanism are in the 3rd and 4th sacral segments. SYN: *intestinum rectum*.

PREPARATIONS SOMETIMES GIVEN BY RECTUM: (1) *Sodium Bromide*: Ten to 60 gr. dissolved in 2 to 4 oz. of plain warm water.

(2) *Chloral Hydrate*: Ten to 30 gr. dissolved in 3 oz. of warm olive oil, 3 oz. of very warm milk, or 3 oz. of thin, boiled cornstarch water. This makes a good preparation or base in which to hold the medicine in suspension. The patient's pulse should be taken 5 minutes before and at 5-minute intervals for one-half hour after the administration, to observe the heart action. If untoward effects are noticed, action should be taken to prevent further absorption.

(3) *Paraldehyde*: Dosage, 1 to 4 cc., may be mixed with water in the proportion of 1 to 8, and in this ratio it may be mixed with thin starch water for rectal medication. There should be about 3 oz. of starch water.

(4) *Sodium Bicarbonate*: One teaspoonful, or 4 Gm. to 500 cc., or 1 pint, of water aids in the expulsion of the bowel content. The neutralizing action on the acidity of the bowel content brought about by the sodium bicarbonate solution leaves the bowel soothed and with a bland reaction.

(5) *Glycerine*: One oz. is added to a pint of plain water. It will cause a good evacuation. One oz. of glycerine to 1 oz. of water will cause irritation of the lower bowel and precipitate an evacuation. This may be given with a bulb syringe.

(6) *Alum*: The alum enema consists of 1 quart of warm water and 1 oz. of powdered alum. This enema has a tendency to dry up intestinal flora and check fermentation.

(7) *Asafetida*: Two dr. of asafetida in 4 to 6 oz. of water. Another mixture is 1 oz. of milk of asafetida and 1 pint of warm water, or, to 12 oz. of warm water add 4 oz. of asafetida emulsion prepared by agitating ½ dr. of asafetida powder in 4 oz. of hot water. SEE: *enema*.

RS: *anorectal, anus, archocele, archoptosis, archoptima, archorrhagia, archostenosis, caribi, cloaca, colon, feeding, hemorrhoid, "proct-" words, "rect-" words, sigmoid.*

rectus (rĕk'tŭs) [L. straight]. 1. Straight; not crooked. 2. Any straight muscle.

   r. muscles. 1. Two ext. abdominal muscles, 1 on each side, from pubic bone to the ensiform cartilage and 5th, 6th, and 7th ribs. 2. Four short muscles of the eye, *ext., int., sup.,* and *inf.*

recumbent (rē-kŭm'bĕnt) [L. *recumbere*, to lean back]. 1. Lying down. SEE: *left lateral recumbent position, prone.* 2. One who is lying down.

recuperation (rē-kū"per-ā'shŭn) [L. *recuperāre*, to recover]. Restoration to normal health.

recurrence (rē-kŭr'ĕns) [L. *rē*, again, + *currere*, to run]. Return of symptoms after a period of quiescence, as in recurrent fever and in yellow fever. SYN: *relapse.*

recurrent (rē-kur'ĕnt) [" + *currere*, to run]. Returning at intervals, as a fever.

recurrentotherapy (rē-kur"rĕnt-ō-ther'ă-pĭ) [" + " + G. *therapeia*, treatment]. Therapeutic inoculation with organisms of a recurrent fever.

recurve (rē-kurv') [" + *curvus*, curved]. Bend backward.

red (rĕd) [A.S. *rēad*]. A primary color of the spectrum.

   r. blindness. Inability to see red hues. The most frequent color blindness.

   r. blood cell. Blood corpuscle containing hemoglobin. SYN: *erythrocyte, q.v.*

   r. lead. Lead tetroxide, Pb_3O_4; minium.

   r. nucleus. Gray matter in the tegmentum. SYN: *nucleus ruber.*

   r. precipitate. Red mercuric oxide. POISONING: SYM: Similar to mercuric chloride.

   r. softening. Hemorrhagic softening of the brain and cord.

   r. streak. One lasting more than 14 seconds when the skin is stroked with a pressure of about 10 oz. by a hard object followed by a white line in a few seconds which lasts a minute or 2; a reflex vasodilatation.

redintegration (rĕd-ĭn-tē-grā'shŭn) [L. *rē*, again, + *integrāre*, to make whole]. 1. Restitution of a part. 2. Restoration to health. 3. Recall by mental association.

redressment (rē-drĕs'mĕnt) [Fr. *redressement*]. 1. Correction of a deformity. 2. Dressing of a wound more than once.

reduce (rē-dūs') [L. *rē*, back, + *ducere*, to lead]. 1. To restore to usual relationship, as the ends of a fractured bone. 2. To weaken, as a solution. 3. To diminish, as in bulk or weight.

reducible (rē-dūs'ĭ-bl) [" + *ducere*, to lead]. Capable of being replaced in a normal position, as a dislocated bone, a hernia, etc.

reductase (rē-dŭk'tās) [" + " + *ase*, enzyme]. An enzyme accelerating process of reduction of chemical compounds.

reduction (rē-dŭk'shŭn) [L. *reductio*, a leading back]. 1. Restoration to normal position, as a hernia. 2. CHEM: A type of reaction in which hydrogen is taken up by the given compound, or oxygen is removed, or the valence of the metallic element is lowered. *Cf. oxidation.*

   r. diet. One that eliminates fat-producing foods.

Normal metabolism must be preserved. Bulk, mineral, protein, vitamin, and water requirements must be maintained. Energy value should be 600 to 1500 calories below maintenance requirements. Not over 10 to 20 Gm. of fat per day. Carbo., 52 Gm.; Pro., 60 Gm.; Fat, 45 Gm.; Cal., 850.

   r. d., modified, Evans-Strang. 970 Cal. diet: Carbo., 50 Gm.; Pro., 80 Gm.; Fat, 50 Gm. 1500 Cal. diet: Carbo., 115 Gm.;

Pro., 80 Gm.; Fat, 80 Gm. 1800 Cal. diet: Carbo., 180 Gm.; Pro., 85 Gm. Emphasis placed on avoidance of food poor in vitamins and minerals and high in calories. SEE: *obesity diet.*
reduplicated (rē-dū″plĭ-kā″tĕd) [L. *rē*, back, + *duplicāre*, to double]. 1. Doubled. 2. Bent backward upon itself, as a fold.
reduplication (rē-dū″plĭ-kā′shŭn) [" + *duplicāre*, to double]. 1. A doubling, as of the heart sounds in some morbid conditions. 2. A fold.
re-education (rē″ĕd-ū-kā′shŭn) [L. *rē*, again, + *educāre*, to educate]. 1. Training of a disabled or mentally disordered individual to restore to him at least partial competence. 2. Physical means for restoring muscular tone and activity.
referred pain (rē-fĕrd′ pān). Pain felt in a part removed from its point of origin. SYN: *synalgia.*
refine (rē-fīn′) [L. *rē*, back, + M.E. *fine*, finished]. To purify or render free from foreign material.
reflection (rē-flĕk′shŭn) [" + *flectere*, to bend]. 1. Process or condition of bending back. 2. The throwing back of a ray of radiant energy from a surface not penetrated. 3. Mental consideration of some subject matter.
reflector (rē-flĕk′tor) [" + *flectere*, to bend]. Device or surface which reflects waves of radiant energy or sound.
In ultraviolet lamps the reflector absorbs more of the short wave length ultraviolet than of the visible and infrared rays, esp. when the surface is composed of a powdered metal, as aluminum, which has been applied with a lacquer. The total amount of ultraviolet radiation in proportion to the visible and infrared rays is relatively lower in the reflected rays than those direct from the source.
reflex (rē′flĕks) [L. *reflexus*, bent back]. 1. Turned backward. 2. Pert. to a reflex action. 3. An involuntary act in response to a nervous impulse transmitted inward by afferent fibers to a nerve center and outward by efferent fibers to an effector, as a muscle or gland; the process culminating in such an act, called reflex action.
CLASSIFICATION: *Simple*: Reflex involving 1 muscle. *Coördinated*: Reflex involving a group of muscles. *Convulsive*: Reflex in which there is no muscular coordination, the resultant motions being disordered, as in a spasm. *Conditioned*: Reflex which is developed by training and association. Also classified as *superficial*, *deep*, and *organic*.
RS: *Achilles jerk, areflexia, chemoreflex, chin jerk, conditioned, consensual, individual name, intestinal, jerk, reaction, reinforcement, Setschenow's center.*
r. action. The transmission of an impulse from a sensory to a motor nerve. SEE: *reflex,* 3.
r. arc. The structures which are concerned with reflex action, *i. e.*, receptor and effector nerves and a nerve center.
r. center. Spot in spinal cord or brain where a sensory impression is converted into a motor impulse.
r., conditioned. A reflex which arises as a response to some particular situation, the reflex being aroused and modified by association with some past experience. The majority of the bodily acts are reflex in type, *e. g.*, sneezing, blinking, coughing, etc.

r., deep. One caused by stimulation of parts beneath skin, like tendons or bones, as the jaw, elbow, wrist, triceps, knee and ankle jerk reflexes.
r., delayed. One not taking place until some seconds after application of stimulus.
r., elbow jerk, r., biceps. Normal reflex caused by tapping of tendon on the biceps.
r., excitomotor. Organic, as in defecation, urination, respiration.
r., knee jerk. This is illustrative of a series of so-called deep muscular reflexes. If one strikes the patellar tendon, the quadriceps femoris contracts, extending the leg.
The reflex is diminished or destroyed if the motor nerve to the muscles be destroyed as in infantile paralysis, or if the sensory part of the arc be interfered with as in tabes. If, however, the upper motor neuron is destroyed, muscle tone and the motor response are greatly increased. So-called pathologic reflexes under these conditions may appear (see Babinski's sign). Reflexes are also modified by higher centers—*e. g.*, emotional tension increases the knee jerk (and muscle tension generally).
r., myenteric. Contraction above the stimulation point of intestines and relaxation below it.
r., organic. One of natural phenomena as those of defecation and urination.
r., patellar. SEE: *knee jerk.*
r., pathologic. Abnormal reflex due to disease and seen as one of its symptoms.
r., pupillary. A beam of light striking the retina normally causes the pupil to contract (protective against excessive stimulation). The same effect results with accommodation to near objects.
r., superficial (cutaneous). R. caused by irritation of the skin or areas depending upon the spinal cord as a motor center, such as the *scapular, epigastric, abdominal, cremasteric, gluteal,* and *plantar reflexes,* or upon *centers in the medulla,* as *conjunctival, pupillary* and *palatal reflexes.*
r., tendon. Deep r. obtained by tapping skin over tendon of a muscle sharply.
It is exaggerated in disease of an upper neuron, and diminished or lost in disease of lower neuron.
reflexogenic (rē-flĕks″ō-jĕn′ĭk) [L. *reflexus*, bent back, + G. *gennan*, to produce]. Causing a reflex action.
reflexograph (rē-flĕks′ō-grăf) [" + G. *graphein*, to write]. Device for charting a reflex.
reflexometer (rē-flĕks-ŏm′ĕt-ĕr) [" + G. *metron*, a measure]. Instrument for measuring force of the tap required to excite a reflex.
reflexophil (rē-flĕks′ō-fĭl) [" + G. *philein*, to love]. Characterized by activity of, or exaggerated, reflexes.
reflexotherapy (rē-flĕks-ō-ther′ă-pī) [" + G. *therapeia,* treatment]. Treatment by manipulation, anesthetizing, or cauterizing an area distant from seat of the disorder. SEE: *spondylotherapy, zone therapy.*
reflux (rē′flŭks) [L. *rē*, back, + *fluxus*, flow]. A return or backward flow. SYN: *regurgitation,* 2.
refract (rē-frăkt′) [L. *refractus*, from *refringere,* to break back]. 1. To turn back. 2. To deflect a light ray. 3. To detect errors of refraction in the eyes and to correct them.
refracta dosi (rē-frak′tă dō′sĭ) [L.]. In

refraction

divided doses, denoting a definite amt. of a drug taken within a given time in a number of fractional equal parts.

refraction (rē-frăk'shŭn) [L. *refractio*, from *refringere*, to break back]. 1. Deflection from a straight path, as of light rays as they pass through media of different densities; the change of direction of a ray when it passes from one medium to another of a different density. 2. Determination of amount of ocular refractive errors and their correction. SEE: *catadioptric.*

VISUAL DEFECTS: In errors of refraction light rays do not focus directly on the retina, preventing a clear image. This must be corrected by glasses.

RS: *ametropia, anisometropia, astigmatism, emmetropia, hypermetropia, myopia, presbyopia.*

refractionist (rē-frăk'shŭn-ĭst) [L. *refractio*, from *refringere*, to break back]. One skilled in determining and correcting ocular refractive errors by means of glasses.

refractive (rē-frăkt'ĭv) [L. *refractus*, from *refringere*, to break back]. Concerning refraction.

refractometer (rē-frăk-tŏm'ĕt-ĕr) [" + G. *metron*, a measure]. Device for measuring the refractive power, as of the eye.

refractory (rē-frăk'tō-rĭ) [L. *refractus*, from *refringere*, to break back]. Not responsive to ordinary treatment.

r. period. A short period in muscle and nerve functioning after activity when stimuli will not excite tissue.

Thus, the heart muscle ignores stimulation during its period of systole, and will execute premature contractions only if stimulated during diastole.

refractoscope (rē-frăk'tō-skōp) [" + G. *skopein*, to examine]. Device for auscultation of heart sounds.

refracture (rē-frăk'chūr) [L. *rē*, again, + *frangere*, to break]. 1. To break again, as a bone set wrongly. 2. Rebreaking of a fracture previously united in the wrong position.

refrangible (rē-frăn'jĭ-bl) [" + *frangere*, to break]. Capable of refraction.

refresh (rē-frĕsh') [O.Fr. *refreschir*, to renew, from L. *rē*, again, + *friscus*, new]. 1. To restore strength; to relieve from fatigue; to renew; to revive. 2. To scrape epithelial covering from 2 opposing surfaces of a wound to cause them to unite.

refrigerant (rē-frĭj'ĕr-ănt) [L. *rē*, again, + *frigerāre*, to make cold]. 1. Allaying heat or fever; cooling. 2. Medicine or agent which relieves thirst and is cooling or reduces a fever. SEE: *algefacient.*

r. gases. A number of these gases are used in ordinary household mechanical refrigerators; poisoning due to leaks, faulty connections or breakage, and gas dissipated into atmosphere may occur.

Among these gases are methyl chloride, ammonia, sulfur dioxide and more than 20 other gases. Most of these are toxic. Warning agents mixed with these gases are not a guarantee of protection to infants, children, hospital patients, firemen and refrigerator workers.

Methyl chloride is responsible for more poisoning than other refrigerant gases. It has a narcotic action and no distinctive warning features.

SYM: Drowsiness, mental confusion, coma, nausea, vomiting, and perhaps convulsions. Anuria occurs and there is an increase in temperature, pulse and respiration.

TREATMENT: Inhalations of oxygen and 5 to 7% carbon dioxide; bromides for convulsions. Oxygen and alkalinization in hospitalization.

Sulfur Dioxide: As this is a respiratory irritant it is easily detected, so serious poisoning is not likely to occur.

refrigeration (rē-frĭj"ĕr-ā'shŭn) [L. *rē*, back, + *frigerāre*, to make cool]. In physical therapy the therapeutic application of low temperatures, as with solid carbon dioxide.

refusion (rē-fū'zhŭn) [" + *fusio*, a pouring]. 1. Process of melting again. 2. The return of blood to the circulation after being temporarily cut off by a ligature.

regeneration (rē-jĕn"ĕr-ā'shŭn) [" + *generāre*, to beget]. Repair, regrowth, or restoration of a part, as tissues. Opp. of *degeneration*, q.v.

r., pathological. Renewal of injured tissues by pathological rather than by physiological processes.

regimen (rĕj'ĭ-mĕn) [L. guidance, from *regere*, to rule]. 1. Regulation of diet, sleep, exercise, and manner of living to improve or maintain health. 2. Hygiene.

region (rē'jŭn) [L. *regio*, a boundary line]. A portion of the body with natural or arbitrary boundaries. SEE: *abdomen.*

RS: *epigastrium, inguinal, Kiesselbach's area, temple.*

regional (rē'jŭn-ăl) [L. *regio*, a boundary line]. Concerning a region.

registrant (rĕj'ĭs-trănt) [L. *registrans*, registering]. A nurse who is named on the books of a registry as being "on call" for duty.

registrar (rĕj'ĭs-trar) [L. *registrans*, registering]. The official manager of a registry.

registry (rĕj'ĭs-trĭ) [Fr. *registrer*, from L. *registrum*]. An office or book where a list of nurses ready for duty is kept; a placement bureau for nurses.

regression (rē-grĕsh'ŭn) [L. *regressio*, a going back]. 1. Abatement or return of symptoms. 2. Degeneration. 3. PSY: The turning back of the libido, upon encountering difficulties, to an early fixation, from a higher to a lower level. 4. BIOL: Reversion of offspring from the mean of parental traits to normal type.

regressive (rē-grĕs'sĭv) [L. *regressio*, a going back]. Concerning or marked by regression.

regular (rĕg'ū-lar) [L. *regula*, a rule]. 1. Conforming to rule or custom. 2. Methodical, steady in course, as pulse. SYN: *normal, typical.*

r. practitioner. A physician of the regular school of medicine.

r. school. That system of medicine to which the greatest number of physicians belong; erroneously called the *allopathic school;* founded on scientific facts and the knowledge gained by experience.

regurgitant (rē-gŭr'jĭt-ănt) [L. *rē*, back, + *gurgitāre*, to flood]. Throwing or flowing back.

regurgitation (rē-gŭr-jĭ-tā'shŭn) [" + *gurgitāre*, to flood]. 1. Return of solids or fluids to the mouth from the stomach. 2. Reflux of blood from the ventricles into the auricles when the heart valves are defective.

It may be a complication of diphtheria and it occurs in paralysis of the soft palate, and in some digestive disorders. SEE: *taste.*

r., cardiac. Backward flow of blood

rehabilitation   R-13   **remission**

through the *aortic, mitral,* and *tricuspid* valves due to incomplete closure.

rehabilitation (rē″hă-bĭl″ĭ-tā′shŭn) [L. *rehabilitāre*]. Process of restoring, or of undergoing restoration, to health or efficiency, as a person physically handicapped.

rehalation (rē-ha-lā′shŭn) [L. *rē*, again, + *halāre*, to breathe]. Rebreathing process occasionally employed in anesthesia.

Reichart's cartilage (rī′kerts). The hyoid cartilaginous arch of the embryo which becomes the styloid process, stylohyoid ligaments, and lesser cornua of the hyoid bone.

Reichmann's disease (rīk′mahnz). Excessive gastric secretion without intermission. SYN: *gastrochronorrhea, gastrorrhea, gastrosuccorrhea.*

Reid's base line (rēds). One extending from lower edge of the orbit to center of aperture of ext. auditory canal backward to center of occipital bone.

Reil's island (rīlz). Three or more small convolutions at bottom of fissure of Sylvius. SYN: *the insula, island of Reil, q.v.*

reimplantation (rē″ĭm-plăn-tā′shŭn) [L. *rē*, again, + *in*, into, + *plantāre*, to set]. Replacement of a part from where it has been taken out, as a tooth.

reinfection (rē″ĭn-fĕk′shŭn) [″ + *inficere*, to make into]. Infection after recovery or during convalescence from the original disease.

reinforcement (rē″ĭn-fors′mĕnt) [″ + O.Fr. *enforcier*, to strengthen]. Strengthening of the response to one stimulus by concurrent action of another; the exaggeration of a reflex by nervous activity elsewhere.

Thus, during the raising of a heavy weight the knee jerk is stronger.

reinnervation (rē″ĭn-ner-vā′shŭn) [L. *rē*, again, + *in*, into, + *nervus*, nerve]. Anastomosis of a paralyzed part with a living nerve.

reinoculation (rē″ĭn-nŏk-ū-lā′shŭn) [″ + ″ + *oculus*, bud]. A second inoculation with the same virus following a previous one. SEE: *reinfection.*

Reinsch's test (rīnsh′ez). One for presence of arsenic.

reinversion (rē″ĭn-ver′shŭn) [L. *rē*, again, + *in*, into, + *versiō*, a turning]. Correction of an inverted organ, as of an inverted uterus, by pressure on the fundus.

Reissner's canal (rīs′nerz). A canal in the cochlea following convolutions of the lamina spiralis. SYN: *cochlear canal.*

   R's. corpuscles. Epithelial cells covering Reissner's membrane.

   R.'s membrane. Delicate membrane separating the cochlear canal from scala vestibuli. SYN: *membrana vestibularis.*

rejuvenation (rē-jū-ve-nā′shŭn) [L. *rē*, again, + *juvenis*, young]. A return to youthful conditions or to the normal.

   r. operation. One to restore virility or for renewing youth by ligating the vas deferens of the male. SYN: *Steinach's operation.* SEE: *Voronoff's method.*

The x-ray has been used over the ovaries with some success in females.

rejuvenescence (rē-jū-ve-nĕs′ĕns) [″ + *juvenis*, young]. The renewal of youth or return to earlier stage of existence.

relapse (re-lăps′) [L. *relapsus*, slipping back]. Recurrence of grave symptoms during convalescence.

relapsing (rē-lăps′ĭng) [L. *relapsus*, slipping back]. Recurring after beginning of convalescence.

   r. fever. A contagious disease marked by intermittent attacks of high fever.

ETIOL: Species of Borrelia family.

SYM: High temperature, 104° to 105° F., pain in limbs and joints, headache, sometimes rigors and vomiting, malaise and prostration. Fever declines by crisis in about a week followed by another period of fever in 4-6 days. This is repeated until intervals become prolonged and fever ceases.

TREATMENT: Intravenous administration of a preparation of arsenic. Regulate temperature by sponging. SYN: *typhinia.*

relative (rĕl′ă-tĭv) [L. *relativus*, related]. Existing in connection with another object or person.

   r. field. That area in the cerebral cortex in which a lesion may or may not cause a spasm or paralysis.

   r. humid′ity. Ratio of amt. of moisture in the atmosphere to amt. present if air is saturated at the same temperature. SEE: *humidity.*

   r. near point. Nearest point at which clear vision is possible. SEE: *near point.*

relaxant (rē-lăks′ănt) [L. *rē*, back, + *laxāre*, to loosen]. 1. Loosening; laxative. 2. An agent diminishing tension, or loosening the bowels.

relaxation (rē-lăks-ā′shŭn) [″ + *laxāre*, to loosen]. A lessening of tension or activity in a part.

   r., complete. Relaxation, whether general or local, is complete if it proceeds to the zero point of contraction for the part or parts involved.

   r., differential. Absence of an undue degree of contraction in the muscles employed during an act, while other muscles not so needed remain flaccid.

   r., general. R. which includes practically the entire body lying down.

   r., local. R. limited to a particular muscle group or to a part.

relaxed move′ment (rē-lăksd′). Form of bodily movement which the operator carries through without the assistance or resistance of the patient. SYN: *passive exercise.*

relaxin (rē-lăks′ĭn). Extract of corpora lutea which relaxes the pelvic ligaments, as in pregnancy.

relief (rē-lēf′) [O.Fr. *relief*]. Alleviation or removal of a distressing or painful symptom.

   r. incision. One made to relieve tension.

Remak's axis cylinder (ra′mahk). The conducting part of a nerve.

   R's. fibers. The nonmedullated nerve fibers.

   R's. ganglion. A ganglion of nerve cells near the sup. vena cava.

   R's. sign. A double sensation after pricking with a needle, the 2nd one being painful. Seen in *tabes dorsalis.*

   R's. symptom. Delayed appearance of pain.

   R's. type of palsy. Paralysis of muscles of the arm.

remedial (rē-mē′dĭ-ăl) [L. *remedialis*, pert. to a remedy]. 1. Curative; intended for a remedy. 2. Something used as a remedy.

remedy (rĕm′ĕd-ĭ) [L. *remedium*]. 1. Anything that relieves or cures a disease. 2. To cure or relieve a disease. SEE: *catholicon.*

   r., local. Agent to relieve a local condition, as a sore.

   r., systemic. Agent to relieve or cure a disease affecting the entire organism.

remission (rē-mĭsh′ŭn) [L. *remissiō*, a

remittent   R-14   repercussion

sending back]. Lessening of severity, or abatement of symptoms.

remittent (rē-mĭt'ĕnt) [L. *rē*, back, + *mittere*, to send]. Alternately abating and returning at certain intervals.

   r. fever. A malarial* fever with alternate periods of high and low temperature, but not below normal.

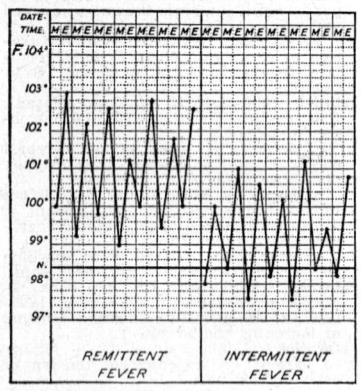

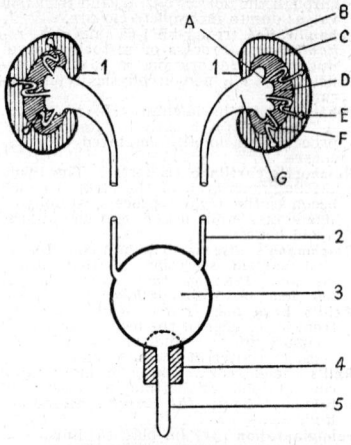

After Sears.

SYM: Malaise, moderate chilliness followed by a fever which daily remits. Maximum temperature ranges from 103° to 106°; while this lasts face is flushed, eyes injected, pulse full and rapid, urine scanty—pain in head and limbs. Delirium sometimes noted; vomiting often occurs—jaundice may develop from destruction of red blood corpuscles. Spleen enlarged. Sometimes resembles typhoid, then termed typhomalaria.

PROG: Favorable—duration, 1-2 weeks.

TREATMENT: Absolute rest. Light diet. Quinine popular remedy. Remedies called for by special symptoms. SEE: *malaria*.

SEE: *Illus., above*.

   r. temperature. One that varies 2 or more degrees but which does not reach the normal.

ren (pl. *renes*) [L.]. The kidney.

   r. amyloides. Amyloid degeneration of the kidneys.

   r. mobilis. Movable kidney.

   r. unguiformis. Horseshoe kidney.

renal (rē'năl) [L. *rēnalis*, pert. to kidney]. 1. Pert. to the kidney. 2. Shaped like a kidney.

renifleur (rä-nĭ-flŭr') [Fr.]. One stimulated sexually by certain odors, esp. by the urine of others.

reniform (rĕn'ĭ-form) [L. *rĕn*, kidney, + *forma*, shape]. Shaped like a kidney.

ren'in. A vasoconstrictor substance formed in an ischemic kidney which produces hypertensive effects.

reniportal (rĕn-ĭ-por'tăl) [" + *porta*, gate]. 1. Concerning the portal system of the kidney. 2. Pert. to the kidney's venous capillary circulation.

renipuncture (rĕn″ĭ-pŭnk'chŭr) [" + *punctūra*, a piercing]. Surgical puncture of capsule of kidney to relieve albuminuria.

rennet (rĕn'nĕt) [M.E. *rennen*, to run]. 1. An infusion of inner coat of calf's stomach. 2. A fluid containing rennin,* a coagulating enzyme, used for making junket.

rennin (rĕn'ĭn) [M.E. *rennen*, to run]. A coagulating enzyme found in the stomach of ruminants, which curdles milk. It is the active principle of rennet. It acts on caseinogen in the presence of calcium ions converting it to insoluble casein. Rennin has been considered to be present in the gastric juice of man but recent experimental evidence indicates that rennin is not produced by the adult human stomach. Coagulation of milk in the stomach is brought about by pepsin.

renninogen, rennogen (rĕn-ĭn'ō-jĕn, rĕn'ō-jĕn) [A.S. *rennen*, to run, + G. *gennan*, to produce]. Antecedent or zymogen glands from which rennin is formed. The inactive form of rennin.

renogastric (rĕn-ō-găs'trĭk) [L. *rĕn*, kidney, + G. *gaster*, belly]. Concerning the kidney and stomach.

renography (rĕ-nŏg'ră-fĭ) [" + G. *graphein*, to write]. Study of the kidney by means of an x-ray picture.

renointestinal (rĕn″ō-ĭn-tĕs'tĭn-ăl) [" + *intestinum*, intestine]. Concerning the kidney and the intestine.

renopathy (rĕn-ŏp'ăth-ĭ) [" + G. *pathos*, disease]. Any pathological condition of the kidneys.

repair (rē-pār') [L. *reparāre*, to prepare again]. To remedy, replace or heal, as a wound or a lost part.

repellent (rē-pĕl'ĕnt) [L. *repellere*, to drive back]. 1. Reducing a swelling. 2. That which lessens a swelling. 3. That which repels as insects.

repercolation (rē″per-kō-lā'shŭn) [L. *re*, again, + *percolāre*, to filter]. Repeated percolation using same materials.

repercussion (rē-per-kŭsh'ŭn) [" + *percussiō*, a striking]. 1. Reciprocal action. 2. Action involved in causing subsidence of a swelling, tumor or eruption. 3. OB: Diagnosis of pregnancy by insertion of a finger into the vagina to push the

repletion R-15 **residue, high, diet**

uterus, causing embryo to rise and fall. SYN: *ballottement*.

repletion (rē-plē'shŭn) [L. *repletio*, a filling up]. 1. Condition of being full or satisfied. 2. Fullness of blood. SYN: *plethora*.

report'able diseases. Diseases which must be reported by the physician to the health authorities.

List of Reportable Diseases
1. Actinomycosis.
2. Acute infectious conjunctivitis (ophthalmia neonatorum).
3. Ankylostomiasis (hookworm).
4. Anthrax.
5. Botulism and other forms of food poisoning.
6. Chancroid.
7. Chickenpox.
8. Cholera (Asiatic).
9. Dengue.
10. Diphtheria.
11. Dog bites.
12. Dysentery (amebic).
13. Dysentery (bacillary and other infectious types).
14. Epidemic (lethargic) encephalitis.
15. Erysipelas.
16. Favus.
17. German measles.
18. Glanders.
19. Gonorrhea.
20. Granuloma inguinale.
21. Impetigo contagiosa (in institutions).
22. Influenza, epidemic.
23. Leprosy.
24. Malaria.
25. Measles.
26. Meningitis, epidemic (cerebrospinal fever, meningococcus meningitis).
27. Mumps.
28. Pellagra.
29. Paratyphoid fever.
30. Plague.
31. Pneumonias, the primary and the pneumonias complicating influenza, measles and whooping cough.
32. Poisonings, heavy metals, drugs, occupational and other poisonings.
33. Poliomyelitis, acute anterior (infantile paralysis).
34. Psittacosis.
35. Puerperal septicemia.
36. Rabies.
37. Rocky Mountain spotted or tick fever.
38. Scarlet fever.
39. Septic sore throat.
40. Smallpox.
41. Syphilis.
42. Tetanus.
43. Trachoma.
44. Trichinosis.
45. Tuberculosis (pulmonary).
46. Tuberculosis (other than pulmonary).
47. Tularemia.
48. Typhoid fever.
49. Typhus.
50. Undulant fever and Malta fever (brucellosis).
51. Vincent's angina and other anginas.
52. Whooping cough.
53. Yellow fever.

reposition (rē-pō-zĭsh'ŭn) [L. *repositio*, a replacing]. Act of replacing a part.

repositor (rē-pŏz'ĭt-or) [L. *repositio*, a replacing]. Instrument for replacing a part.

   r., inversion. Instrument for replacement of an inverted uterus.

   r., uterine. A lever to replace the uterus when out of normal position.

repression (rē-prĕsh'ŭn) [L. *repressus*, from *reprimere*, to check]. PSY: Refusal to entertain distressing or painful ideas, thus submerging them in the unconscious where they continue to exert their influence upon the individual. Psychoanalysis seeks to discover and to release these repressions.

reproduction (rē-prō-dŭk'shŭn) [L. *re-* again, + *productio*, production]. 1. Conscious repetition of recognized sensations. SYN: *recall*. 2. Process by which plants and animals give rise to offspring. 3. Process of regeneration, as of tissue.

   RS: *fertilization, gamete, genetopathy*.

   r., asexual. R. without sexual contact, intercourse, or seminal implantation.

reproductive (rē-prō-dŭk'tĭv) [L. *re*, again, + *producere*, to produce]. Concerning, or employed in, reproduction.

repulsion (rē-pŭl'shŭn) [L. *repulsio*, a thrusting back]. 1. Act of driving back. 2. The force exerted by one body on another to cause separation.

   r., capillary. R. from forces causing movements of liquid in small vessels.

   r., electric. Like charges of electricity repel each other.

resection (rē-sĕk'shŭn) [L. *resectio*, a cutting off]. Partial excision of a bone or other structure.

   r. of a rib for empyema. DRESSING, ETC.: Borosalicylic acid powder, 4:1; strips of iodoform gauze, 3 and 8 in. wide; gauze sponges; 3 yd. gauze; large pad of cotton; 2 gauze roller bandages; safety pins; 6 towels; 3 sheets; 2 large rubber tubular drains.

   NP. (rib): Watch patient closely for signs of shock and hemorrhage. Support but do not remove or interfere with clamps to drains from wound.

resectoscope (rē-sĕk'tō-skōp) [L. *resectus*, cutting back, + G. *skopein*, to examine]. An instrument for resection of prostate gland through the urethra.

resectoscopy (rē-sĕk-tŏs'kō-pĭ) [" + G. *skopein*, to examine]. Resection of the prostate through the urethra.

reserpine. SEE: p. R-33.

reserve (rē-zerv') [L. *reservāre*, to keep back]. 1. That which is held back for future use. 2. Self control of one's feelings and thoughts.

   r. air. Additional amount of air that can be expelled from the lungs over the normal quantity, 1200-1600 cc.

   r., alkali. Alkali content of body available for neutralization of acid. SEE: *alkaline reserve*.

reservoir of Pecquet (rĕz'ĕr-vwor pĕ-kā') [Fr.]. Expansion beginning at the thoracic duct opp. 12th dorsal vertebra. SYN: *receptaculum chyli*.

residual (rē-zĭd'ū-ăl) [L. *residuum*, that is left behind]. 1. Relating to that which is left as a residue. 2. PSY: Any internal aftereffect of experience influencing later behavior.

   r. air. That remaining in the lungs after normal expiration.

   r. urine. That left in bladder after urination; occurring in cases of enlarged prostate.

residue (rĕz'ĭd-ū) [L. *residuum*, that which remains]. That which remains after a part is removed. [roughage.

   r. free diet. One without cellulose or Purées and semisolids and bland foods are included.

   r., high, diet. A diet with increased amounts of cellulose (fiber), water, min-

eral salts, and vitamins (esp. vitamin B).
r., low, diet (solid). An inadequate diet including solid food in which residue is reduced to a minimum. SEE: *non-laxative diet*.
residuum (rē-zĭd'ū-ŭm) [L.]. Residue; the remainder.
resilience (rē-zĭl'ĭ-ĕns) [L. *resiliens*, leaping back]. The quality of coming back to normal after straining, as a stretched rubber band when released. SYN: *elasticity*.
resilient (rē-zĭl'ĭ-ĕnt) [L. *resiliens*, leaping back]. Elastic.
resin (rĕz'ĭn) [L. *resina*]. An amorphous, nonvolatile solid or soft solid substance, a natural exudation from plants; it is practically insoluble in water, but soluble in alcohol. Ex: *Guaiac, rosin*.
resin-P.M.S. SEE: p. R-33.
resinous (rĕz'ĭn-ŭs) [L. *resina*]. Of the nature of or pert. to resin.
resistance (rē-zĭs'tăns) [L. *resistens*, standing back]. 1. Opposition to or the ability to oppose anything, as the power of a fluid to retard that which is passing through it, as the resistance of the air, or opposition of the body to passage of an electric current. Incorrectly used in reference to immunity; or ability of the body to resist infection or disease. 2. The force exerted to penetrate the Unconscious, or to submerge memories in the Unconscious.
r., unit of. Expressed in ohms; 1 ohm of resistance will permit the flow of a current of 1 ampere as the result of a pressure of 1 volt.
resolution (rĕz-ō-lū'shŭn) [L. *resolūtio*]. 1. Decomposition; absorption or breaking down of the products of inflammation. 2. Cessation of inflammation without suppuration. The return to normal.
RS: *exudate, first intention, healing, inflammation, pus, second intention, third intention*.
resolvent (rē-zŏl'vĕnt) [L. *resolvens*, dissolving]. 1. Promoting disappearance of inflammation. 2. That which causes dispersion of inflammation.
resonance (rĕz'ō-năns) [L. *resonantia*, an echo]. 1. A sound heard on percussing or on auscultating a part, esp. the lungs. 2. PT: Resonance of an electric circuit is similar to the resonance of a mechanically vibrating body, such as a tuning fork.
In a diathermy apparatus the frequency is determined by the capacity of the condensers and the inductance of the current, and the frequency is the natural frequency to which the combination of coil and condenser resonates.
r., amphoric. Sound, as that when blowing across the mouth of an empty bottle.
r., bell-metal. Sound heard in pneumothorax in auscultation when chest is percussed with 2 coins.
r., skodaic. Increased percussion sound over upper lung when there is pleural effusion in lower part.
r., tympanic. Hollow percussion sound over large air-filled cavities.
r., vesicular. Normal pulmonary resonance.
r., vocal. The vibrations of the voice transmitted to the ear, normally more marked over the right apex.
Abnormally increased in: (1) Pneumonic consolidation; (2) phthisical infiltration; (3) cavities which freely communicate with a bronchus.
Vocal r. is diminished or absent in: (1) Pleural effusion — air, pus, serum, lymph or blood; (2) emphysema; (3) pulmonary collapse; (4) pulmonary edema; (5) egophony, a modified bronchophony, characterized by a trembling, bleating sound usually heard above the upper border of dullness of pleural effusions; occasionally heard in beginning pneumonia; (6) bronchophony; extreme exaggeration of vocal resonance, the sounds, but not words, are transmitted. Esp. noted over marked consolidations and over certain cavities.
r., whispering. Auscultation sound heard when patient whispers.
resonator (rĕz'ō-nā''tor) [L. *resonare*, to resound]. Apparatus for exhibiting effects of resonance on an electrical circuit in which oscillations of a certain frequency are set up by oscillations of the same frequency in another circuit. When this occurs, the circuits are said to be in syntony.
resorbent (rē-sor'bĕnt) [L. *resorbens*, sucking in]. An agent that promotes the absorption of abnormal matter, as exudates or blood clots. Ex: *Potassium iodide, ammonium chloride*.
resorcin, resorcinol (re-zor'sĭn, -ōl). USP. Nearly colorless, needle-shaped crystals with a sweetish taste.
ACTION AND USES: Antiseptic, most important use is in treatment of certain skin diseases. Sometimes used to check fermentation in the stomach.
DOSAGE: 2 gr. (0.12 Gm.). Externally, 1 to 4% solution or ointment.
INCOMPATIBILITIES: Camphor, chloral, iron, alkalies.
resorption (rē-sorp'shŭn) [L. *resorbere*, to drink in]. 1. Act of removing by absorption of an exudate or pus. 2. Loss by lysis. 3. Absorption not dependent upon mechanical laws of diffusion, as *intestinal absorption*.
respirable (rē-spīr'ă-bl, rĕs'pĭr-ă-bl) [L. *respirāre*, to respire]. Fit or adapted for respiration.
respiration (rĕs-pĭr-ā'shŭn) [L. *respiratio*, breathing]. The act of breathing.
r., abdominal. R. where the diaphragm chiefly exerts itself, while walls of chest are nearly at rest, as in acute pleurisy, pericarditis, fracture of rib.
r., accelerated. Considered accelerated when more than 25 per minute, after 15 years of age.
Frequently occurs in disease. In disease it may be preternaturally frequent, or slow, rising to 60 or 80, or falling to 8 to 10 per minute. Increased frequency may, in health, result from exercise or physical exertion or from mental disturbances. It is present in many disorders of the *lungs*, as in pneumonias, bronchiectasis, advanced pulmonary tuberculosis, consolidation or compression of a lobe or of 1 entire lung, congestion, asthma, emphysema, tumors, aneurysms, diseases of the thorax, hernia, abscess of the diaphragm, and partial obstruction to the entrance of air into the lungs. It may be seen in diseases of the *blood*, such as the anemias; in *kidney* troubles; *febrile disease*; diseases of the *heart*, and as a result of drugs or nervous conditions.
r., artificial. Artificial methods to restore respiration in cases of suspended breathing. SEE: *artificial respiration*.
r., Cheyne-Stokes. Respirations gradually increase in rapidity, and volume, until they reach climax, then gradually subside and cease entirely for from 5 to 50 seconds, when they begin again.

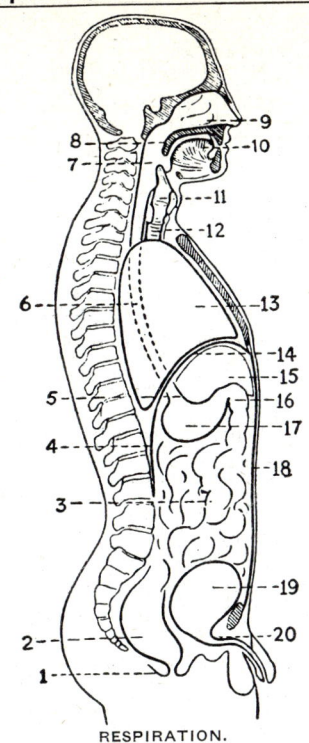

RESPIRATION.
1. Sphincter ani. 2. Rectum. 3. Intestines. 4. Diaphragm. 5. Cardiac sphincter. 6. Esophagus. 7. Pharynx. 8. Soft palate. 9. Nose. 10. Tongue. 11. Rima glottidis. 12. Trachea. 13. Lungs. 14. Diaphragm. 15. Liver. 16. Pylorus. 17. Stomach. 18. Abdominal muscles. 19. Bladder. 20. Sphincters of the bladder.

Due to some disturbance of respiratory center, exact nature of which is as yet undetermined. Usually forerunner of death but may last several months, or few days, and disappear. Ratio between respirations and pulse beats is 1 to 4 or 4.5.

r., decreased. It obtains in uremia, diabetic coma, affections of the brain, in shock, hysteria, stenosis of the larynx, in chronic fibroid phthisis, on approaching death, and in poisoning with opium or its derivatives.

r., edematous. Breathing moist, rattling sounds, due to air passing through fluid from the blood infiltrated into air cells.

r., external. The mechanical process, involving contractions of muscles and movements of ribs and sternum, whereby air is aspirated (inspiration) into the lungs and then released (expiration), liberating carbon dioxide.

The chemical changes in the air thus taken into the lungs are given under *air*; the volumes of air involved in respiratory movements are given under *spirometry*. If the aspiration of air is accomplished chiefly by contraction of the diaphragm, the abdomen will bulge with each inspiration, for the diaphragm, forming at once the floor of the thorax and the roof of the abdominal cavity, is dome-shaped, with its concavity downward; in contracting, it pushes the abdominal viscera down. This type of respiration is called diaphragmatic or abdominal. Its opposite is the costal type, in which the ribs and sternum must be raised and which is seen when the abdomen is confined by tight clothing.

r., forms of. Jerking, spasmodic, stertorous, stridulous, whistling, wavy, lack of evenness, abdominal, or thoracic.

r., frequent. Common in all febrile and inflammatory diseases, esp. in children. As a rule, rapid breathing is a sign of thoracic disease. In hysteria patient often breathes 60 to 70 times per minute. It may occur in acute respiratory affections, lesions of medulla, or it may be induced by atropine, carbon dioxide, cocaine.

r., internal. The carriage of oxygen and carbon dioxide by the blood, the passage of oxygen into the cells, its utilization there and the reverse processes with carbon dioxide.

Oxygen is carried in combination with hemoglobin; oxyhemoglobin gives arterial blood its red color, reduced hemoglobin gives venous blood its blue color. Carbon dioxide is carried in combination with metallic elements in the blood as bicarbonates and also as carbonic acid.

The following table gives the number of cc. of each gas contained in 100 cc. of blood. The higher of the 2 figures for carbon dioxide represents conditions during exercise:

Blood	Oxygen cc.	Carbon dioxide cc.
Arterial blood	18.5	52
Mixed venous blood	15.	55-65

r., method of counting. With the hand in the same position as when taking the pulse, watch the patient's chest, without his knowledge if possible, as breathing is controlled by both the voluntary and involuntary muscles. Count each inspiration and expiration as 1 breath for 1 full minute by watching rise and fall of chest or upper abdomen. When the movements are scarcely perceptible, place the hand gently but firmly on the chest or back and count in this manner. *Note* hour, frequency, any abnormal condition such as pain associated with breathing.

NORMAL EXPANSION: 2 in. in male, 2½ in. in female.

CAPACITY: Normal male 22 years of age, 5.8 feet, 230 to 240 cu. in., 3.5 cu. in. for each in. in height. Female, 19 years, 5.25 feet, 145 to 150 cu. in., 2.3 cu. in. for each in. in height.

r., rate of. It may be preternaturally frequent, or slow, rising to 60 or 80, or falling to 8 or 10 per minute.

In newly born	30-60	per m.
1st year, about	25-30	" "
2nd year, about	20-26	" "
15th year, about	20	" "
21st year:		
Men	16-18	per m.
Women	18-20	" "
50th year	16	" "
70th year	14-16	" "
Usual ratio to pulse	1- 4	" "

Another comparative tabulation is the following:

	Tempera-ture	Ab-normal	Pulse	Ab-normal	Respira-tion	Ab-normal	Age
Rectal	99.6°	99°	140-130	90	44	20	at birth
Rectal	99.6°	100°	130-115	100	35	22	at 1st year
Rectal	99.6°	101°	115-100	110	25	24	at 2nd year
Mouth	98.6°	102°	85- 80	120	20	26	at 15th year
Mouth	98.6°	103°	85- 75	130	18	28	at 25 years
Mouth	98.2°	104°	75- 70	140	16	30	at 50 years
Mouth	98°	105°	65- 50	150	14-16	36	at 70 years

More frequent during exercise, digestion, standing, during emotion, and faster in the spring.

Respiration, Pulse and Temperature Ratio

Respiration	Pulsations	Temperature
18	80	99° F.
19 (plus)	88	100
21	96	101
23	104	102
25 (minus)	112	103
27	120	104
28	128	105
30	136	106

r., slow. Generally result of some structural or functional derangement of the nervous system.

Observed in apoplexy, in effusion of serum within cranium, softening of the brain and in most of the circumstances that occasion coma. It may occur in brain compressions and hemorrhage, and in uremia or be induced by carbon monoxide and opium or its derivatives.

r., thoracic. R. when abdomen does not move, being performed entirely by expansion of the chest. Observed when peritoneum, diaphragm or its pleural cavity is inflamed.

respiration, words pert. to: air, complementary; a., minimal; a., reserve; a., residual; a., supplemental; a., tidal; anapnea; apnea; asphyxia; Biot's breathing; blowing; Buchut's; chest, auscultation of; Cheyne - Stokes; diaphragm; dyspnea; eupnea; hay fever; hyperpnea; hypopnea; infant; inspiration; oligopnea; orthopnea; polypnea; respirator; respiratory; stridor; stridulus; tachypnea; thermometry.

respirator (rĕs′pĭ-rā″tor) [L. *respirāre*, to breathe]. 1. A device by which inspired air is purified, warmed, or medicated when passing through it. 2. A machine for prolonged artificial respiration. SEE: Drinker's respirator.

respiratory (rē-spīr′ă-tō-rĭ, rĕs″pĭ-ră-tōrĭ) [L. *respirāre*, to breathe]. Pertaining to respiration.

r. center. A region in the medulla oblongata which regulates movements of respiration.

r. system. The lungs, pleura, bronchi, pharynx, larynx, tonsils, and the nose.

respirometer (rĕs″pĭr-ŏm′ĕt-ĕr) [" + G. *metron*, a measure]. Instrument to ascertain character of respirations.

rest (rĕst) [A.S. *raestan*, to rest]. 1. Repose of body due to sleep. 2. Freedom from activity, as of mind or body. 3. To lie down; to cease from motion.

r. cure. Method of treatment of nervous diseases described by S. Weir Mitchell, consisting of isolation, rest in bed, forced feeding, massage, and hydrotherapy.

restibrachium (rĕs″tĭ-brā′kĭ-ŭm) [L. *restis*, rope, + G. *brachiōn*, arm]. Bundle of nerve fibers on both sides of the medulla, inferior peduncles of cerebellum. SYN: *corpus restiforme, myelobrachium*.

restiform (rĕs′tĭ-form) [" + *forma*, shape]. Ropelike; rope-shaped.

r. body. Inferior peduncle of the cerebellum. SYN: *corpus restiforme, restibrachium*.

restis (rĕs′tĭs) [L. rope]. The restiform body, the inf. cerebellar peduncle.

restitution (rĕs-tĭt-ū′shŭn) [L. *restitutio*]. 1. A return to a former status. 2. The act of making amends. 3. The turning of the fetal head to the right or left after it has completely emerged through the vulva.

restorative (rē-stōr′ă-tĭv) [L. *restaurāre*, to fix]. An agent that restores lost tone or function. Ex: *Preparations of iron, arsenic, mercury, etc.*

restraint (rē-strānt′) [O.Fr. *restraindre*]. 1. Process of hindering from any action, mental or physical. 2. State of being hindered. 3. That which hinders or restricts; device or method used to keep a patient from injuring himself. SEE: knot.

r. in bed. Move bed against wall, place straight backed chairs along open side of bed. Tie them into place by interlacing with rope and then tying to foot and head of bed, or place a wide board the length of bed on either side and fasten through 3 or 4 holes bored near ends of the boards. Place a folded sheet across chest under each armpit with ends of sheet tied to end of bed. Bring patient's arms along sides and place them in a wide pillow slip under back with the open end of the slip pulled to armpits and closed end tucked under buttocks. The weight of body holds pillow slip in place.

r. of the lower extremities. Tie a sheet across knees and tie feet together with a figure-of-eight bandage. (Start loop under ankles, cross between feet and bring ends around feet and tie on top.)

resuscitation (rē-sŭs-ĭ-tā′shŭn) [L. *resuscitātio*]. Act of bringing one back to full consciousness.

RS: *anabiosis, anastasis, artificial respiration, revivification*.

resuscitator (rē-sŭs′ĭ-tā″tor). An automatic breathing machine that forces oxygen into the lungs under pressure of 4 ounces per square inch when back pressure of 3 ounces trips the machine for exhalation. May be used for several patients at the same time.

retardation (rē-tar-dā′shŭn) [L. *retardāre*, to delay]. 1. A holding back or slowing down; delay. 2. Delayed mental or physical response due to pathological conditions, and seen in manic-depressive psychosis.

retard′ed depres′sion. The depressed state of manic-depressive psychosis.

retch (rĕtch) [A.S. *hrǣcan*, to clear the throat]. To make an involuntary attempt to vomit, *q.v.*

retching (rĕtch′ĭng) [A.S. *hrǣcan*, to clear the throat]. An involuntary attempt to vomit.

rete (rē'tē) (pl. *retia*). A network. A plexus of nerves or blood vessels.
  r. Malpighii. Same as *r. mucosum*.
  r. mirabile. BNA. A plexus formed by sudden division of a vessel into small twigs, which unite again to form 1 vessel, as in the vessel tufts of the kidneys.
  r. mucosum. Three lower layers of the epidermis.

retention (rē-tĕn'shŭn) [L. *retentio*, a holding back]. Retaining in the body that which does not belong there, or which should be excreted, as urine, feces, or perspiration. SEE: *chloruremia*.
  r. cyst. One caused by retention of a secretion in a gland.
    ETIOL: Closure of the gland's duct.
  r. defect. Inability to recall a name, number, or fact shortly after the subject was requested to remember it.
  r. enema. Enema to be retained to provide nourishment, medicate the mucosa or for anesthesia. SEE: *enema, retention*.
  r. memory. It is affected in senile psychoses, paresis, arteriosclerosis, alcoholic hallucinosis and in Altheimer's disease. Memory of long-past events is affected in senile dementia, dementia precox, paresis, epilepsy, and arteriosclerosis.
  r. of urine. This is failure to expel the urine in the bladder.
    This may be due to a number of causes, such as (a) loss of muscle tone of the bladder from anemia, old age, exposure to cold, prolonged operation, or a greatly distended bladder without voiding for a considerable length of time; (b) failure of nerve ending in the bladder to respond to stimulus; (c) failure of nerve centers in the cord to respond; (d) contraction of the urethra from nervousness.
    It is a well-known fact that some are unable to void the urine in the presence of another. Elimination and brain action are closely related. One will affect the other. The sound of running water, will sometimes start the flow of urine.
    INDICATIONS: Disease of spinal cord if not induced by obstruction such as that from calculi, enlarged prostate, or from nervousness.
  r. with overflow. Spasm of sphincter, causing failure to empty the bladder at one voiding, only overflow dribbling away, due to above causes.

reticular (rē-tĭk'ū-lăr) [L. *reticula*, net]. Meshed, as a network, or distributed as the fibers of a leaf.
  r. tissue. Connective tissue formed of a fibrous network containing lymphoid cells. SEE: *tissue*.

reticulated (rē-tĭk'ū-lā-tĕd) [L. *reticula*, network]. Netlike; pert. to a reticulum. SYN: *reticular*.

reticulation (rē-tĭk-ū-lā'shŭn) [L. *reticula*, a net]. The formation of a network mass.

reticulin (rē-tĭk'ū-lĭn) [L. *reticula*, net]. An albuminoid or scleroprotein substance in the connective tissue framework of lymphatic tissues.

reticulocyte (re-tĭk'ū-lō-sīt) [" + G. *kytos*, cell]. A reticulated red blood cell in process of active blood regeneration.

reticulocytopenia (re-tĭk"ū-lō-sī"tō-pē'nĭ-ă) [" + " + *penia*, lack]. Lowering of the number of the reticulocytes of the blood.

reticulocytosis (re-tĭk"ū-lō-sī-tō'sĭs) [" + " + *-osis*, intensive]. Presence of numerous reticulocytes during active blood regeneration. SYN: *reticulosis*.

reticuloendothelial system (re-tĭk'ū-lō-ĕn"-dō-thē'lĭ-ăl). A cell group having the same behavior toward dyes, and with endothelial and reticular qualities. They are found in the bone marrow, liver, spleen, and hemolymph nodes. They are assumed to aid in making new blood cells and in disintegrating old ones.

reticuloendothelioma (re-tĭk"ū-lō-ĕn"dō-thē-lĭ-ō'mă) [L. *reticula*, network, + G. *endon*, within, + *thēlē*, nipple, + *-oma*, tumor]. Reticuloendothelial tissue tumor.

reticuloendotheliosis (re-tĭk"ū-lō-ĕn"dō-thē-lĭ-ō'sĭs) [" + " + *-osis*, intensive]. Hyperplasia of reticuloendothelium.

reticuloendothelium (re-tĭk"ū-lō-ĕn"dō-thē'lĭ-ŭm) [" + " + *thēlē*, nipple]. Tissue of the reticuloendothelial system.

reticuloma (re-tĭk-ū-lō'mă) [" + G. *-oma*, tumor]. Reticuloendothelial cell tumor.

reticulosis (re-tĭk-ū-lō'sĭs) [" + G. *-ōsis*, intensive]. Presence of more than the normal percentage of reticulocytes in the peripheral blood during active blood regeneration.

reticulum (re-tĭk'ū-lŭm) [L. *reticulum*, a little net]. A network in cells.
  r. cell. A parent stem cell which in fetal life is responsible for the formation of the blood elements, the erythrocytes,* leukocytes,* monocytes,* lymphocytes,* and the thrombocytes.*
    It is found in bone marrow, lymph nodes, and elsewhere, but it is not engaged in the formation of blood in normal life unless pathological conditions affect blood metabolism. SEE: *blood*.

retiform (rĕt'ĭ-form) [L. *rēte*, net, + *forma*, shape]. Resembling a network. SYN: *reticular*.

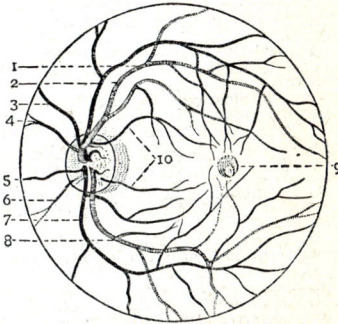

RETINAL VESSELS, DIAGRAM OF
1. Superior temporal artery. 2. Superior temporal vein. 3. Superior nasal vein. 4. Superior nasal artery. 5. Inferior nasal vein. 6. Inferior nasal artery. 7. Inferior temporal vein. 8. Inferior temporal artery. 9. Macula lutea. 10. Macular veins.

retina (rĕt'ĭ-nă) (pl. *retinae*) [L. *rēte*, a net]. Innermost or 3rd tunic of the eye which receives image formed by the lens and is immediate instrument of vision.
  It is the perceptive structure upon which light rays focus, and is formed by the expansion of the optic nerve. Extends from the ora serrata to the optic disk and consists of 10 layers which from without inwards are:
  (1) Layer of pigment epithelium; (2) layer of rods and cones; (3) external limiting membrane; (4) external nuclear layer; (5) external plexiform layer; (6)

internal nuclear layer; (7) internal plexiform layer; (8) layer of ganglion cells; (9) layer of nerve fibers; (10) internal limiting membrane.
COLOR: Normally a purplish red tint, varying with complexion. It is colorless in severe anemia or in ischemia. It is reddened in hyperemia.
RS: *albedo retinae, amphiblestritis, anaxon, angiomatosis retinae, anisoconia, blind spot, chorioretinitis, choroidoretinitis, chlorophane, chromophane, diabetes, disk, eye, glioma, lipemia retinalis, macula lutea, mesoretina, retinitis, yellow spot, Young-Helmholtz theory.*

retinaculum (rĕt-ĭn-ăk'ū-lŭm) [L. halter]. A band or membrane holding any organ or part in its place.
 r. costae ultimatae. Lumbocostal ligament.
 r. ligamenti arcuati. Short, external, lateral ligament of the knee joint.
 r. morgagni of the ileocecal valve. Ridge formed by the coming together of valve segments at each end of opening bet. the ileum and cecum.
 r. peroneorum inferius. Fibrous band over peroneal tendons on outer side of calcaneum.
 r. peroneorum superius. External annular ligament of ankle joint.
 r. tendinum. Annular ligament of the ankle or wrist.

retinal (rĕt'ĭn-ăl) [L. *rētē*, net]. Concerning the retina.

retinitis (rĕt-ĭn-ī'tĭs) [" + G. *-itis*, inflammation]. Inflamed condition of the retina.
SYM: Diminished vision, contractions of fields or scotomata, alteration in size of objects, photophobia.
TREATMENT: Absolute rest of eyes, protection from light, treat underlying cause.
 r., actinic. R. due to exposure to intense light or other forms of radiant energy.
 r. albuminurica. R. associated with chronic kidney disease.
Shows not only general signs of retinitis but is distinguished by white patches in the fundus, esp. surrounding the papilla and in the macular region.
 r., diabetic. R. seen in diabetes. Picture may resemble albuminuric retinitis.
 r. pigmentosa. Chronic progressive degeneration of retina consisting of atrophy of retina with characteristic deposit of pigment.
 r., proliferating. Vascularized masses of connective tissue which project from retina into the vitreous. End result of recurrent hemorrhage from retina into the vitreous. Found in tuberculosis.
 r., syphilitic. R. generally associated with choroiditis.

retinochoroiditis (rĕt″ĭn-ō-kō-royd-ī'tĭs) [L. *rētē*, net, + G. *chorioeidēs*, skinlike, + *-itis*, inflammation]. Inflamed condition of retina and choroid.

retinocystoma (rĕt″ĭn-ō-sĭs-tō-mă) [" + G. *kystis*, sac, + *-ōma*, tumor]. Glioma of the retina.

retinoid (rĕt'ĭn-oyd) [" + *eidos*, resemblance]. Like the retina.

retinopapillitis (rĕt″ĭ-nō-pă-pĭl-ī'tĭs) [" + *papilla*, nipple, + G. *-itis*, inflammation]. Inflamed condition of retina and optic papilla. SYN: *papilloretinitis.*

retinoscope (rĕt″ĭn-ō-skōp) [" + G. *skopein*, to see]. An instrument used in performing retinoscopy.

retinoscopy (rĕt-ĭn-ŏs-kō'pĭ) [" + G. *sko-*

pein, to examine]. Shadow test or refraction of eyes by effect of lights and shadows. SYN: *skiascopy.*
Objective method of refracting the eye by illuminating the eye with a plane or concave mirror and observing the direction of movement of the retinal shadows when the mirror is rotated. Examination is usually done in a dark room with the pupils dilated.

retinosis (rĕt-ĭn-ō'sĭs) [" + G. *-ōsis*, condition]. A degeneration of the retina.

retisolution (rĕt″ĭ-sō-lū'shŭn) [L. *rētē*, net, + *solutio*, dissolution]. Dissolution of the Golgi structures.

retispersion (rĕt″ĭ-spĕr'zhŭn) [" + *spersio*, a scattering]. Transference of Golgi structures to periphery of the cell.

retort (rē-tort') [L. *retortus*, bent back]. A flasklike, long-necked vessel used for distilling.

retothelioma (rē″tō-thē-lĭ-ō'mă) [L. *rētē*, net, + G. *thēlē*, nipple, + *-ōma*, tumor]. A tumor of the retothelium.

retothelium (rē″tō-thē'lĭ-ŭm) [" + G. *thēlē*, nipple]. Cellular layers covering reticular tissue. SYN: *reticuloendothelium, reticulothelium.*

retractile (rē-trăkt'ĭl) [L. *retractilis*, able to be drawn back]. Capable of being drawn back or in.

retraction (rē-trăk'shŭn) [L. *retractio*, from *retrahere*, to draw back]. A shortening. The act of drawing backward or state of being drawn back.
 r. ring. A ridge sometimes felt on uterus above the pubes, marking line of separation bet. upper contractile and lower dilatable segments of the uterus. Seen in prolonged or obstructed labor. SYN: *Bandl's ring.*
 r., uterine. The process by which muscular fibers of the uterus remain permanently shortened to a small degree following each contraction or labor pain.

retractor (rē-trăk'tor) [L. from *retrahere*, to draw back]. 1. Instrument for holding back the margins of a wound. 2. Muscle which draws in any organ or part.

retro- [L.]. Prefix meaning *backward.*

retroauricular (rē″trō-aw-rĭk'ū-lar) [L. *rētrō*, backward, + *auricula*, ear]. Behind the auricle or ear.

retrobuccal (rē″trō-bŭk'ăl) [L. *rētrō*, backward, + *bucca*, cheek]. Concerning the back part of the mouth or area behind the mouth.

retrobulbar (rē″trō-bŭl'bar) [" + G. *bolbos*, a bulb]. 1. Behind the eyeball. 2. Post. to the medulla oblongata.

retrocedent (rē″trō-sē'dĕnt) [" + *cedere*, to go]. Going backward.
 r. gout. G. in which inflammation of the joint disappears with appearance of an internal affection.

retrocervical (rē″trō-sĕr'vĭ-kăl) [" + *cervix*, neck]. Back of the cervix uteri.

retrocession (rē″trō-sĕsh'ŭn) [" + *cessio*, from *cedere*, to go]. 1. A going back; a relapse. 2. Metastasis of a condition from the surface to an internal organ. 3. Indication of an abnormal (further back) position of the uterus.

retroclusion (rē″trō-klū'zhŭn) [" + *clusio*, a shutting]. Passing a pin over and under a vessel in compression of a bleeding artery.

retrocolic (rē″trō-kŏl'ĭk) [" + G. *kōlon*, colon]. Back of the colon.

retrocollic (rē″trō-kŏl'ĭk) [" + *collum*, neck]. Concerning the back of the neck.
 r. spasm. Wryneck with spasms affecting post. muscles of neck.

retrocollis (re″tro-kŏl′ĭs) [L. *retro*, backward, + *collum*, neck]. Spasm of post. muscles of the neck with torsion. SYN: *torticollis*.

retrocursive (re″tro-kŭr′sĭv) [" + *cursio*, from *currere*, to run]. Stepping or turning backward.

retrodeviation (re″tro-de″vĭ-a′shŭn) [" + *deviare*, to turn aside]. Backward displacement, as of an organ.

retrodisplacement (re″tro-dĭs-plas′mĕnt) [" + Fr. *déplacer*, to displace]. Displacement backwards of a part.

retroesophageal (re″tro-e-sŏf-a′je-ăl) [" + G. *oisophagos*, gullet]. Located behind the esophagus.

retroflexed (re″tro-flĕkst) [" + *flexus*, bent, from *flectere*, to turn]. Bent backward.

retroflexion (re″tro-flĕk′shŭn) [L. *retro*, backward, + *flexio*, a bending]. A bending or flexing backward.

  r. of uterus. A condition of the womb in which its body is bent backward at an angle with the cervix whose position usually remains unchanged.

  SYM: Irritability of rectum with retention of stool. Neuralgia of uterus and as consequence of the natural congestion and nervous compression; so-called uterine colic may result from retention of the secretion of the intrauterine mucous membrane. If retroflexion is great enough to occlude uterine canal, dysmenorrhea and sterility result.

  TREATMENT: Constitutional treatment to give strength and tone to tissues of the region. Postural treatment, the knee-chest position so that force of gravity may assist in throwing organ into proper position. Use of uterine elevator. Tampons.

retrogasserian (re″tro-găs-se′rĭ-ăn) [L. *retro*, backward, + *gasserian*]. Referring to the post. root of the gasserian ganglion.

retrograde (rĕt′ro-grād, re′tro-grād) [" + *gradi*, to step]. Moving backward; degenerating from better to worse state.

  r. amnesia.* Loss of memory for events and situations just preceding time of patient's illness.

retrography (re-trŏg′ră-fĭ) [" + G. *graphein*, to write]. Mirror writing, a symptom of certain brain diseases.

retrogression (rĕt″ro-grĕsh′ŭn, re″tro-grĕsh′ŭn) [" + *gressus*, stepping]. 1. Atrophy or degeneration, esp. of tissue. 2. Transition of tissue from a higher to a lower type of structure. SEE: *catagenesis*.

retrogressive changes (re″tro-grĕs′ĭv) [" + *gressus*, stepping]. Changes to lower type of organization, such as in atrophy, degeneration, necrosis, hypertrophy, etc.

retroinfection (re″tro-ĭn-fĕk′shŭn) [" + *infectio*, infection]. Infection communicated by the fetus *in utero* to the mother.

retroinsular (re″tro-ĭn′su-lar) [" + *insula*, island]. Situated behind the island of Reil.

retrolabyrinthine (re″tro-lăb-ĭ-rĭn′thĭn) [L. *retro*, backward, + G. *labyrinthos*, a maze]. Situated behind the labyrinth of the ear.

retrolingual (re″tro-lĭng′gwal) [" + *lingua*, tongue]. Behind the tongue.

retromammary (re″tro-măm′ma-rĭ) [" + *mamma*, breast]. Located behind the mammary gland.

retromandibular (re″tro-măn-dĭb′u-lar) [" + *mandibulum*, jaw]. Located behind the lower jaw.

retromastoid (re″tro-măs′toyd) [" + G. *mastos*, breast, + *eidos*, like]. Situated behind the mastoid process.

retromorphosis (re″tro-mor′fo-sĭs) [" + G. *morphē*, form, + -*ōsis*, intensive]. Change in shape accompanying a transition from a higher to a lower type of structure. SEE: *catabolism*.

retronasal (re″tro-na′zăl) [" + *nasus*, nose]. Relating to or situated at the back part of the nose.

retroöcular (re″tro-ŏk′u-lar) [L. *retro*, backward, + *oculus*, eye]. Located behind the eye.

retroperitoneal (re″tro-pĕr-ĭ-to-ne′ăl) [" + G. *peritonaion*, peritoneum]. Located behind the peritoneum.

retroperitoneum (re″tro-pĕr-ĭ-to-ne′ŭm) [" + G. *peritonaion*, peritoneum]. The space behind the peritoneum.

retroperitonitis (re″tro-pĕr-ĭ-to-ni′tĭs) [" + " + -*itis*, inflammation]. Inflammation behind the peritoneum.

retropharyngeal (re″tro-făr-ĭn′je-ăl) [" + G. *pharygx*, pharynx]. Behind the pharynx.

  r. abscess. Acute or chronic abscess
  Acute: Due to direct infection through injury to post. wall of pharynx or indirectly from inflammation of tonsils.

  SYM: Pain, swelling, difficulty in swallowing, possible edema of glottis, malaise, rise in temperature, fear of suffocation causing anxiety and lack of sleep.

  TREATMENT: Incision of abscess, pus swabbed away.

  Chronic: Often associated with tuberculosis of cervical vertebrae.

  SYM: Stiff neck, rigidity in head movements, little pain on swallowing.

retropharyngitis (re″tro-făr-ĭn-ji′tĭs) [L. *retro*, backward, +G. *pharygx*, pharynx, + -*itis*, inflammation]. Inflammation of the retropharyngeal tissue.

retroplacental (re″tro-plă-sĕn′tăl) [" + *placenta*, a flat cake]. Behind the placenta, or behind both the placenta and the uterine wall.

retroplasia (re″tro-plă′zĭ-ă) [" + G. *plassein*, to form]. Degenerative change of a cell or tissue into a more primary form.

retroposed (re-tro-pōsd′) [" + *posus*, from *ponere*, to place]. Displaced backward.

retropulsion (re″tro-pŭl′shŭn) [L. *retro*, backward, + *pulsio*, a thrusting]. 1. Pushing back of any part, as of the fetal head in labor. 2. A walking or running backward, involuntarily, seen in some nervous disorders.

retrosternal (re″tro-ster′nal) [" + G. *sternon*, chest]. Behind the sternum.

  r. pulse. Venous pulse felt over suprasternal notch.

retrotarsal (re-tro-tar′săl) [" + G. *tarsos*, edge of eyelid]. Located behind the tarsus of the eye.

retrouterine (re″tro-u′tĕr-ĭn) [" + *uterus*, womb]. Located behind the uterus.

retroversion (rĕt″ro-ver′shŭn, re″tro-ver′shŭn) [" + *versio*, a turning]. A turning or state of being turned back.

  r. of uterus. Displacement of the uterus backward with cervix pointing forward toward symphysis pubis.

  Normally, the cervix points toward the lower end of the sacrum with the fundus toward the suprapubic region. Retroversion may be met with in early months of pregnancy and serious complications may result if not corrected.

Retzius, lines of (ret′ze-ŭs). Brownish, concentric lines in the enamel of a tooth.

  R., space of. Triangular s. bet. peritoneum and ant. abdominal wall filled with connective tissue.

R., veins of. Veins forming communications bet. the mesenteric veins and inf. vena cava.

Reuss' test (rois'ez). Test for atropine employing sulfuric acid and an oxidizing agent.

revellent (rĕ-vel'ent) [L. *rĕ*, back, + *vellere*, to draw]. 1. Producing revulsion, the diversion of disease or blood from one part of the body to another. 2. Agent producing revulsion.

revivification (rē-vĭv″ĭ-fī-kā'shŭn) [" + *vivere*, to live, + *-ficāre*, to do]. 1. Attempt to restore life to those apparently dead; restoration to life or consciousness. Also restoring life in local parts, as a limb after freezing. 2. Paring of surfaces to facilitate healing, as in a wound.

revulsant (rĕ-vŭl'sănt) [" + *vulsio*, a pulling]. 1. Causing transfer of disease or blood from one part of the body to another. 2. Drug which draws blood to an inflamed part.

revulsion (rĕ-vŭl'shŭn) [L. *revulsio*, a pulling back]. 1. Act of driving backward, as diverting disease from one part to another by a quick withdrawal of the blood from that part. 2. PT: Circulatory changes obtained by sudden and intense reactions to heat and cold.

The Scotch douche is a powerful revulsive measure. SEE: *counterirritation*.

revulsive (rĕ-vŭl'sĭv) [L. *revulsio*, a pulling back]. 1. Causing revulsion. 2. A counterirritant.

Rh blood factor. An antigenic substance in human blood similar to the A and B factors which determine blood groups; apparently present only in red blood cells. There are no normal agglutinins against it. Positive in 85% of the population.

Rhabditis (răb-dī'tĭs) [G. *rhabdos*, rod]. A genus of small nematode worms, some of which are parasitic.

rhabdo- [G. *rhabdos*, rod]. Combining form meaning *rod*.

rhabdomyoma (răb″dō-mī-ō'mă) [" + *mys*, *my-*, muscle, + *-ōma*, tumor]. A striated muscular tissue tumor.

Rhabdonema (răb″dō-nē'mă) [" + *nēma*, thread]. A genus of minute nematode worms, some of which are parasitic.

rhabdophobia (răb-dō-fō'bĭ-ă) [" + *phobos*, fear]. Abnormal fear of being chastised, or of anything that might be used for such a purpose, as a rod.

rhachialgia (rā″kĭ-ăl'jĭ-ă) [G. *rhachis*, spine, + *algos*, pain]. Pain in the spine.

rhachiocampsis (rā″kĭ-ō-kămp'sĭs) [" + *kampsis*, a bending]. Curvature of spine.

rhachioplegia (rā″kĭ-ō-plē'jĭ-ă) [" + *plēgē*, a stroke]. Spinal paralysis.

rhachioscoliosis (rā″kĭ-ō-skō-lĭ-ō'sĭs) [" + *skoliōsis*, a bending]. Curvature of the spine laterally.

rhachis (rā'kĭs) [G.]. Spinal column.

rhachischisis (rā-kĭs'kĭs-ĭs) [G. *rhachis*, spine, + *schisis*, fissure]. A congenital cleft in the spinal column.

rhachitis (ră-kī'tĭs) [" + *-itis*, inflammation]. Constitutional disease of infancy marked by faulty nutrition and bone deformity. SYN: *rachitis, rickets, q.v.*

rhacoma (ră-kō'mă) [G. *rhakoein*, to rend]. 1. Ragged, irregular abrasion, usually of the skin. 2. Relaxation of integument of scrotum.

rhagades (răg'ăd-ēz) [G. *rhagadēs*, tears]. Linear fissures appearing in skin, esp. at the corner of the mouth or anus, causing pain.

If due to syphilis, they form a radiating scar on healing.

rhagadiform (răg-ăd'ĭ-form) [" + L. *forma*, shape]. Fissured; having cracks.

-rhagia [G.]. Suffix meaning *bleeding*.

rhaphania (răf-ă'nĭ-ă) [G. *rhaphanos*, radish]. Spasmodic disease caused by eating the wild radish. SYN: *raphania*.

rhaphe (rā'fē) [G. *rhaphē*, a seam]. A seam or ridge. SYN: *raphe*.

rhegma (rĕg'mă) [G. *rhēgma*, a tear]. Rupture, fracture or rent, as of vessel walls, a bone, or of an abscess.

rheo- [G.]. Combining form meaning *current, stream*.

rheobase (rē'ō-bās) [G. *rheos*, current, + *basis*, step]. In unipolar testing with the galvanic current using negative as active pole, the minimal voltage required for a response when the make of the current is determined.

This is the rheobase, or threshold of excitation. SEE: *chronaxie*.

rheochord (rē'ō-kord) [" + *chordē*, cord]. Type of rheostat used for measuring resistance of an electric current. SEE: *rheostat*.

rheometer (rē-ŏm'ĕt-ĕr) [" + *metron*, a measure]. 1. Instrument for qualitative determination of presence of an electric current. SYN: *galvanometer*. 2. Device for measuring rapidity of the blood current.

rheonome (rē'ō-nōm) [" + *nemein*, to distribute]. Device for ascertaining the effect of irritation on a nerve.

rheophore (rē'ō-fōr) [" + *phoros*, a carrier]. A cord conducting an electrical current, as one bet. patient and electrical apparatus. SYN: *electrode*.

rheoscope (rē'ō-skōp) [" + *skopein*, to examine]. Device indicating the existence of an electrical current. SYN: *galvanoscope*.

rheostat (rē'ō-stăt) [" + *statos*, standing]. A device maintaining fixed or variable resistance for controlling the amount of current entering a circuit.

rheostosis (rē-ŏs-tō'sĭs) [G. *rheos*, current, + *osteon*, bone]. A hypertrophying and condensing osteitis in streaks, involving long bones.

rheotachygraphy (rē-ō-tă-kĭg'ră-fī) [" + *tachys*, swift, + *graphein*, to write]. Graphic recording of variation of electromotive force in a muscle.

rheotaxis (rē″ō-tăks'ĭs) [" + *taxis*, arrangement]. Reaction to a current of fluid causing the part acted upon to move against the current.

rheotome (rē'ō-tōm) [" + *tomē*, a cutting]. An interrupter with an adjustable speed control.

rheotrope (rē'ō-trōp) [" + *tropos*, a turning]. An instrument for automatically reversing a current of electricity.

rhestocythemia (rĕs″tō-sī-thē'mĭ-ă) [G. *rhaistos*, destroyed, + *kytos*, cell, + *aima*, blood]. Condition of degenerated red blood cells in the peripheral circulation.

rheum, rheuma (rūm, rūm'ă) [G. *rheuma*, a flowing]. Any catarrhal or watery discharge.

r., salt. Moist tetter and similar skin eruptions; chronic eczema.

rheumarthrosis (rū-mar-thrō'sĭs) [" + *arthron*, joint, + *-ōsis*, condition]. Chronic rheumatic pain in the joints; articular rheumatism.

rheumatalgia (rū″mă-tăl'jĭ-ă) [" + *algos*, pain]. Rheumatic pain.

rheumatic (rū-măt'ĭk) [G. *rheuma*, a flowing]. Pert. to rheumatism.

r. fever. Acute articular rheumatism.

rheumaticosis

ETIOL: Supposed to result from a midget microbe, smaller than bacteria but a little larger than an invisible virus, about 1/50,000 in. in diameter. Isolated by the Rockefeller Institute in 1939. It has been called a "pleuropneumonialike organism."
SYM: Fever, sweating, painful and swollen joints. Inflammation frequently spreads to heart.

rheumaticosis (rū″măt-ĭ-kō′sĭs) [" + -*ōsis*, condition]. General condition caused by rheumatism in children.

rheumatid (rū′mă-tĭd) [G. *rheuma*, a flowing]. A skin lesion sometimes seen in rheumatic conditions.

rheumatism (rū′măt-ĭzm) [G. *rheuma*, a flowing, + -*ismos*, condition]. A disease with fever, pain, inflammation and swelling of the joints. SEE: *arthritis*.

r., acute articular, r., inflammatory. Acute general disease, characterized by irregular fever, acid sweat, inflammation of joints and marked tendency to involve the heart.
ETIOL: Possibly a filtrable pleuropneumonialike microörganism.
SYM: Generally begins abruptly or sometimes follows such prodromes as malaise, chilliness and sore throat. The large joints usually affected; are slightly reddened, swollen, intensely painful and tender to touch. Marked tendency not only to spread from joint to joint but to disappear abruptly in one, while it attacks another. Knees, ankles, elbows and wrists most commonly involved, but no joint exempt. In severe cases intensely painful, tender and sometimes rigid.
Fever rises to 102° or 103° F., indefinite in its duration, irregular in course. Perspiration often copious; peculiar sour smell, acid reaction, urine scanty, high colored. On standing, throws down an abundant sediment of urates and uric acid. Tongue heavily coated; appetite lost; bowels constipated; face at first flushed, later becomes anemic.
PROG: Guarded. Most cases end in recovery; some in chronic rheumatism. Small number die of exhaustion; lasts from few days to several weeks.
TREATMENT: Absolute rest in a room well ventilated but free from draft; patient should lie between blankets. Diet consists mainly of milk and vegetables. Meat interdicted. Free use of lemonade or mineral waters. Joints wrapped in cotton wool. Remedies to suit special features of case. Diathermy; shortwave. Remove focus of infection. Large doses of vitamins.
RS: *arthritis, celiomyalgia, dorsodynia, rheumarthrosis, rheumatic fever.*

r., chronic. Usually begins as chronic infection.
SYM: Pain, stiffness, deformity, creaking of joints. Aggravation on approach of stormy weather, joints become swollen and tender.
PROG: Generally unfavorable. Much relief may follow persistent and judicious treatment, but perfect cure rarely attainable.
TREATMENT: Special care in diet, bathing, clothing, exercise, and occupation. Change to dry, warm climate may effect cure. Build up system. Mineral waters.
SYN: *rheumatoid arthritis.*

r., gonorrheal. Joint affections associated with gonorrhea.
May be only more or less severe intermittent arthralgia which soon passes, or may be a chronic inflammation with abundant effusion into joint cavity, chiefly of knee, an acute seroplastic arthritis or a suppurative inflammation. May occur at any period in the course of urethritis, but more often in 3rd or 4th week than later.
SYM: In acute form. Suffering is intense, persistent, worse at night and increased by even slight movements. Parts swollen and hot, skin red. Atrophy of structure above and below quickly produced. Elevation of temperature, acceleration of pulse and loss of strength and weight.
PROG: Terminates in resolution, ankylosis or destruction of the joint; most frequently in ankylosis (fibrous), either partial or complete. Serous accumulation in the joints often remains unchanged for weeks or months.
TREATMENT: Rest, as long as any inflammation present, joint kept immobilized. Most good from quietude and equable compression secured by plaster-of-Paris bandage followed by passive motion soon as feasible. An existing hydrarthrosis may be aspirated and carbolic acid injections used. If suppuration occurs aspiration and thorough antiseptic irrigation may be employed—joint then immobilized with fair prospect of success. If not quick relief, open cavity and drain as when due to other causes. Massage, baths, douches, continued after removal of immobilizing dressings. If ankylosis is present, break up or excise joint.

r., muscular. An affection of the voluntary muscles characterized by pain, tenderness and rigidity.
SYM: Pain generally worse with use of muscles and associated with tenderness, which is esp. marked at tendinous origins and insertion of muscles. Muscles sometimes contracted and rigid.
FORMS: *Cephalodynia*: Characterized by superficial head pain, increased by moving the scalp and with tenderness on pressure. *Lumbago*: Dull, aching pain across loins. *Pleurodynia*: Pain in side increased by deep breathing, coughing, or twisting the body. Respirations are restricted on affected side—diffuse tenderness to touch. *Torticollis*: Head fixed and inclined to one side. Every effort to turn attended with sharp pain.
PROG: Favorable.
TREATMENT: Affected muscles put at rest. In pleurodynia, by strapping affected side as in fracture of ribs. In lumbago, large piece of adhesive plaster from floating ribs to iliac crests. In mild cases plasters and liniments are favorite prescriptions. Internal remedies to suit case. Continued current. Acupuncture.
DIET: *Acute*: Milk, 4 or 5 pints daily, in small quantities, diluted with equal amount of barley, soda, or potash; white of eggs; thin oatmeal gruel; bread and milk. As fever subsides add clear soup flavored with vegetables, milk pudding, scraped meat, pounded chicken, bread and butter, blanc mange, jelly, custard, stewed fruit, grapes, strawberries; then light fish, etc.
Chronic: Light, moderate diet. (a) Tender meat, poultry, or game; fish; green vegetables, onions, celery, lettuce, watercress; milk puddings, junket, custard, jelly; butter, cream, milk; bread; 1 potato; little sugar. Avoid all causes of fermentation. (b) Lactovegetarian diet; sour milk.

r., palindromic. Recurring attacks of acute arthritis and periarthritis at irregularly spaced intervals.

rheumatism (rū-mă-tĭz'măl) [G. *rheuma*, a flow, + *-ismos*, condition]. Of the nature of rheumatism.

r. edema. Rheumatism accompanied by painful subcutaneous swellings.

rheumatoid (rū'mă-toyd) [" + *eidos*, like]. Of the nature of rheumatism.

r. arthritis. Form with inflammation of the joints, stiffness, swelling, cartilaginous hypertrophy, and pain. SEE: *arthritis*.

rheumatopyra (rū″măt-ō-pī′ră, rū-mă-top′-ĭ-ră) [" + *pyr*, fire]. Febrile infectious disease with pain and swelling of the joints and cardiac involvement. SYN: *rheumatic fever*.

rheumatosis (rū-mă-tō'sĭs) [" + *-ōsis*, condition]. Any disorder believed to be of rheumatic origin, as *erythema nodosum*.

rheumic (rū'mĭk) [G. *rheuma*, a flowing]. Concerning a rheum or flux.

r. diathesis. Predisposition to rheumatismal conditions.

rhexis (rĕks'ĭs) [G. *rhēxis*, a rupture]. The rupture of any organ, blood vessel, or tissue.

rhinal (rī'năl) [G. *rhis, rhin-*, nose]. Concerning the nose. SYN: *nasal*.

rhinalgia (rī-năl'jĭ-ă) [" + *algos*, pain]. Pain in nose; nasal neuralgia.

rhinencephalon (rī-nĕn-sĕf'ăl-ŏn) [" + *egkephalos*, brain]. BNA. The olfactory portion of the brain; consisting of the olfactory lobe, the ant. perforated substance, the subcallosal gyrus, and the parolfactory area.

rhinesthesia (rī-nĕs-thē'zĭ-ă) [" + *aisthēsis*, sensation]. The sense of smell.

rhineurynter (rī-nū-rĭn'tĕr) [" + *eurynein*, to dilate]. Elastic bag used for dilating the nostrils.

rhinion (rĭn'ĭ-on) [G. *rhinion*, nostril]. Lower end of the suture bet. nasal bones. A craniometric point. SYN: *punctum nasale inferius*.

rhinitis (rī-nī'tĭs) [G. *rhis, rhin-*, nose, + *-itis*, inflammation]. Inflammation of the nasal mucosa. SEE: *endorrhinitis, ozena*.

r., acute catarrhal. Acute congested condition of nose with increased secretion of mucus. SYN: *common head cold, coryza*.

SYM: Malaise, nasal blockage, discharge, and sneezing.

TREATMENT: Nasal shrinkage and antiseptics such as argyrol, free catharsis, force fluids, rest.

r., atrophic. Chronic inflammation with marked atrophy of mucous membrane with considerable dry crusting and disturbance in the sense of smell.

Usually accompanied by ozena. The throat is dry and, as a rule, contains crusts. A husky voice or hoarseness is often a common accompaniment.

SYM: Fetid odor from nose and throat, with considerable crusting.

TREATMENT: Irrigation and cleansing of the nose with various solutions, narrowing of the nose with various types of intranasal submucous transplants such as bone or ivory, surgical treatment of sinus pathology, diet rich in vitamins and general hygienic measures.

r., chronic hyperplastic. Chronic inflammation of mucous membrane accompanied by polypoid formation and underlying sinus pathology. SEE: *sinus*.

r., chronic hypertrophic. Inflammation of the mucous membrane of the nose characterized by hypertrophy of the mucous membrane of the turbinates and the septum.

SYM: Those of nasal obstruction, postnasal discharge and recurrent head colds.

TREATMENT: Consists in surgical removal of hypertrophic and mulberry ends of inf. turbinates and cauterization of mucosa of inf. turbinates and septum.

r., hyperesthetic. Nonseasonal symptom complex depending on a conditioning predisposition of eyes and respiratory tract.

ETIOL: Hyperplastic sinus disease, allergy, neuromotor instability, etc.

SYM: Nasal blockage, watery discharge from nose, sneezing.

TREATMENT: Exenteration of hyperplastic sinuses, skin tests for irritating substances with immunization, internal medication such as calcium, sedatives, etc. SYN: *vasomotor rhinitis*. SEE: *allergy, hay fever*.

r., intumescent. Chronic rhinitis with unilateral, bilateral or alternating swelling of the inf. turbinates.

ETIOL: Low grade ethmoiditis, irritating dusts, fumes, neuromotor instability.

TREATMENT: Remove underlying cause, cauterize inf. turbinates with chemicals such as trichloracetic acid, silver nitrate and chromic acid, or with electrocautery.

r., specific. Tuberculosis or syphilis with ulceration or gumma in respiratory tract.

r., suppurative. Seen in suppurative sinus disease such as complication of severe rhinitis.

TREATMENT: Shrinkage with ample drainage of sinuses, and along same lines as that of acute rhinosinusitis.

r., vasomotor. SEE: *hyperesthetic r*.

rhino- [G.]. Combining form meaning *the nose*.

rhinoantritis (rī″nō-ăn-trī'tĭs) [G. *rhis, rhin-*, nose, + *antron*, cavity, + *-itis*, inflammation]. Inflamed condition of the nasal cavities and one or both maxillary antra.

rhinobyon (rī-nō-bī'ŏn) [" + *byein*, to plug]. A tampon or plug for the nose.

rhinocanthectomy (rī″nō-kăn-thĕk'tō-mĭ) [" + *kanthos*, corner of the eye, + *ektomē*, excision]. Excision of inner canthus of the eye. SYN: *rhinommectomy*.

rhinocele (rī'nō-sēl) [" + *koilos*, hollow]. The ventricle or hollow of the olfactory lobe or *rhinoencephalon*.

rhinochiloplasty (rī″nō-kī'lō-plăs-tī) [" + *cheilos*, lip, + *plastos*, formed]. Plastic surgery of the nose and upper lip.

rhinocleisis (rī-nō-klī'sĭs) [" + *kleisis*, closure]. Nasal obstruction.

rhinodacryolith (rī″nō-dăk'rĭ-ō-lĭth) [" + *dakryon*, tear, + *lithos*, stone]. A nasal calculus.

rhinodynia (rī-nō-dĭn'ĭ-ă) [G. *rhis, rhin-*, nose, + *odynē*, pain]. Nasal pain. SYN: *rhinalgia*.

rhinogenous (rī-nŏj'ĕn-ŭs) [" + *gennan*, to produce]. Originating in the nose.

rhinolalia (rī-nō-lā'lĭ-ă) [" + *lalia*, speech]. Nasal quality of voice.

r. aperta. R. caused by undue patency of posterior nares.

r. clausa. R. caused by closure of nasal passages.

rhinolaryngitis (rī″nō-lăr-ĭn-jī'tĭs) [" + *larynx*, tube, + *-itis*, inflammation]. Inflammation of mucosa of nose and larynx at the same time.

rhinolite (rī'nō-līt) [" + *lithos*, a stone]. A nasal calculus; stone in the nose.

rhinolith (rī'nō-lĭth) [" + *lithos*, stone]. Nasal concretion.

rhinolithiasis (rī"nō-lĭth-ī'ă-sĭs) [" + " + *-iasis*, condition]. The formation of nasal calculi.

rhinologist (rī-nŏl'ō-jĭst) [G. *rhis, rhin-*, nose, + *logos*, study]. A specialist in diseases of the nose.

rhinology (rī-nŏl'ō-jĭ) [" + *logos*, study]. Science of the nose and its diseases.

rhinomanometer (rī"nō-măn-ŏm'ĕt-ĕr) [" + *manos*, thin, + *metron*, a measure]. A device for measuring the amount of nasal obstruction.

rhinometer (rī-nŏm'ĕt-ĕr) [" + *metron*, a measure]. Device for measurement of the nose.

rhinomiosis (rī-nō-mī-ō'sĭs) [" + *meiōsis*, a lessening]. Surgical reduction in size of the nose.

rhinommectomy (rī-nŏm-mĕk'tō-mĭ) [" + *omma*, eye, + *ektomē*, excision]. Surgical excision of the inner canthus.

rhinomycosis (rī"nō-mī-kō'sĭs) [" + *mykēs*, fungus, + *-ōsis*, condition]. Fungi in mucous membranes and secretions of the nose.

rhinonecrosis (rī"nō-nē-krō'sĭs) [G. *rhis, rhin-*, nose, + *nekrōsis*, death]. Necrosis of the nasal bones.

rhinopathy (rī-nŏp'ă-thĭ) [" + *pathos*, disease]. Any nasal diseases.

rhinopharyngitis (rī"nō-făr-ĭn-jī'tĭs) [" + *pharynx, pharygg-*, pharynx, + *-itis*, inflammation]. Inflamed condition of the nasopharynx.

rhinopharyngocele (rī"nō-făr-ĭn'gō-sēl) [" + " + *kēlē*, a mass]. A nasopharyngeal tumor.

rhinopharyngolith (rī"nō-făr-ĭn'gō-lĭth) [" + " + *lithos*, stone]. Concretion in the nasal pharynx.

rhinopharynx (rī"nō-făr'ĭnks) [" + *pharynx*, pharynx]. Upper portion of pharynx continuous with the nasal passages.

rhinophonia (rī"nō-fō'nĭ-ă) [" + *phōnē*, voice]. A nasal tone in speaking.

rhinophyma (rī-nō-fī'mă) [G. *rhis, rhin-*, nose, + *phyma*, growth]. Lobular hypertrophy of nose, with red coloration, congestion and retention of sebum. SYN: *acne rosacea*.

rhinoplasty (rī'nō-plăs-tĭ) [" + *plastos*, formed]. Plastic surgery of the nose.

rhinopolypus (rī-nō-pŏl'ĭp-ŭs) [" + *polys*, many, + *pous*, foot]. Polypus of the nose.

rhinoreaction (rī"nō-rē-ăk'shŭn) [" + L. *rē*, back, + *actio*, an acting]. Moeller's test for tuberculosis, a nasal tuberculin reaction.

rhinorrhagia (rī-nō-rā'jĭ-ă) [" + *rhēgnūnai*, to burst forth]. Profuse hemorrhage from nose. SYN: *epistaxis, nosebleed*.

rhinorrhea (rī-nō-rē'ă) [" + *rhoia*, a flow]. Thin, watery discharge from nose. Progesterone reduces discharge and congestion.

r., cerebrospinal. Discharge of spinal fluid from nose due to defect in cribriform plate.

rhinosalpingitis (rī"nō-săl"pĭn-jī'tĭs) [" + *salpigx, salpigg-*, tube, + *-itis*, inflammation]. Inflammation of the mucosa of the nose and eustachian tube.

rhinoscleroma (rī-nō-skle-rō'mă) [G. *rhis, rhin-*, nose, + *sklēros*, hard, + *-ōma*, tumor]. Nodular enlargement of nose and other portions of upper air passages.
Pathology usually begins on nasal septum, trachea or larynx. The infection is probably due to *B. rhinoscleromatis*.

SYM: The disease presents a hard, nodular growth, which usually begins at ant. end of nose and spreads to the lower respiratory tract. There is usually no pain and no tendency to ulceration.

TREATMENT: Variable. Surgery is of little value. Tracheotomy may be necessary. Roentgen rays and radium have been used with some success.

rhinoscope (rī'nō-skōp) [" + *skopein*, to examine]. Instrument for examination of the nose.

rhinoscopy (rī-nŏs'kō-pĭ) [" + *skopein*, to examine]. Examination of nasal passages.

r., anterior. E. through anterior nares.

r., posterior. E. through posterior nares usually with small mirror in nasopharynx.

rhinostenosis (rī"nō-sten-ō'sĭs) [" + *stenōsis*, a narrowing]. Obstruction of the nasal passages. SYN: *rhinocleisis*.

rhinotomy (rī-nŏt'ō-mĭ) [" + *tomē*, incision]. Incision of the nose.

rhinovaccination (rī"nō-văk-sĭn-ā'shŭn) [" + L. *vaccinus*, pert. to a cow]. Vaccine applied to the mucosa of the nose.

rhitidectomy (rī-tĭ-dĕk'tō-mĭ) [G. *rhytis*, wrinkle, + *ektomē*, excision]. Removal of wrinkles by operation. SYN: *rhytidectomy*.

rhitidosis (rī-tĭ-dō'sĭs) [" + *-ōsis*, condition]. 1. Wrinkling of face without corresponding signs of age. 2. Wrinkling of the cornea, indicating its disintegration. SYN: *rhytidosis*.

rhizo- [G.]. Combining form meaning *root*.

rhizodontropy (rī-zō-dŏn'trō-pĭ) [G. *rhiza*, root, + *odous, odont-*, tooth, + *tropē*, a turning]. Process of pivoting an artificial crown upon the root of a tooth.

rhizodontrypy (rī-zō-dŏn'trĭ-pĭ) [" + " + *trypē*, a hole]. Puncture of root of a tooth.

rhizoid (rī'zoyd) [" + *eidos*, form]. BACT: 1. Having branched growth as *B. mycoides*; rootlike. 2. A rootlike plant filament.

rhizome (rī'zōm) [G. *rhizōma*, a mass of roots]. A more or less underground and horizontal root stem of a plant. Ex: *hydrastis, valerian, ginger*.

rhizomelic (rī-zō-mĕl'ĭk) [G. *rhiza*, root, + *melos*, limb]. Concerning the hips and shoulders, in man the roots of the extremities.

rhizomeningomyelitis (rī"zō-me-nĭng"gō-mī-ĕl-ī'tĭs) [" + *mēnigx, mēnigg-*, membrane, + *myelos*, marrow, + *-itis*, inflammation]. Inflammation of roots of a nerve, the meninges, and spinal cord. SYN: *radiculomeningomyelitis*.

rhizoneure (rī'zō-nūr) [" + *neuron*, nerve]. A nerve cell having a fiber contributing to formation of a nerve root.

Rhizopoda (rī-zop'ō-dă) [" + *pous, pod-*, foot]. A class of Sarcodina without axial filaments, as the amebas.

rhizotomy (rī-zŏt'ō-mĭ) [" + *tomē*, a cutting]. Section of post. roots of the spinal nerves for pain or spastic paralysis. SYN: *Dana's operation*.

rhodocyte (rō'dō-sīt) [G. *rhodon*, rose, + *kytos*, cell]. A red blood cell.

rhodogenesis (rō"dō-jĕn'ĕs-ĭs) [" + *genesis*, formation]. Regeneration of visual purple bleached by light.

rhodophane (rō'dō-fān) [" + *phainein*, to show]. A red pigment found in retinal cones.

rhodophylaxis (rō-dō-fī-lăks'ĭs) [" + *phylaxis*, protection]. Ability of the retinal epithelium to regenerate visual purple which has been bleached by light.

rhodopsin (rō-dŏp'sĭn) [" + *opsis*, vision]. Visual purple, a pigment in outer segment of retinal rods.

rhombencephalon (rŏm-bĕn-sĕf'ă-lon) [G. *rhombos*, rhomb, + *egkephalos*, brain]. The hind brain (metencephalon) with the after brain (myelencephalon).

rhombocele (rŏm'bō-sēl) [" + *koilos*, a hollow]. Dilatation in the sacral region of the cavity of the spinal cord.

rhomboid (rŏm'boyd) [" + *eidos*, shape]. Shaped like a rhomb.
  r. **fossa**, r. **sinus**. The 4th ventricle of the brain.

rhomboideus (rŏm-boi'dē-ŭs) [L.]. One of 2 muscles beneath the trapezius muscle. SEE: *Muscles, Table of, in Appendix; muscles, back, for illustration*.

rhoncal, rhonchial (rong'kal, rŏng'kĭ-ăl) [G. *rhogchos*, a snore]. Pert. to or produced by a rhonchus, or rattle in the throat.

rhonchus (rŏn'kŭs) [G. *rhogchos*, a snore]. A râle or rattling in the throat, esp. when it resembles snoring.

rhotacism (rō'tăs'ĭzm) [G. *rhōtakeizein*, to overuse letter r]. Overuse or improper utterance of *r* sounds, with too much emphasis upon this letter.

rhubarb (rū'barb) [L. *rhabarbarum*, wild rhubarb]. USP. Extract made from roots of the plant.
  ACTION AND USES: A cathartic and acid stimulant.
  DOSAGE: 15 gr. (1.0 Gm.).
  COMP: High in oxalic acid. Of little food value but desirable for its mineral content.
  AV. SERVING: 90 Gm. Pro. 0.5, Fat 0.6, Carbo. 2.3.
  VITAMINS: C++ to +++.
  ASH CONST: Ca 0.044, Mg 0.017, K 0.325, Na 0.025, P 0.031, Cl 0.036, S 0.013, Fe 0.0010.

rhyostomaturia (rī"ō-sto-mă-tū'rĭ-ă) [G. *rhyas*, fluid, + *stoma*, mouth, + *ouron*, urine]. The elimination of urinary elements by the salivary glands.

rhyparia (rī-pa'rĭ-ă) [G. *rhyparia*, filth]. 1. Foul substance in mouth in low fevers. SYN: *sordes*. 2. Filth.

rhypophagy (rī-pŏf'ă-jĭ) [G. *rhypos*, filth, + *phagein*, to eat]. The eating of filth. SYN: *scatophagy*.

rhypophobia (rī-pō-fō'bĭ-ă) [" + *phobos*, fear]. Abnormal disgust at the act of defecation, feces, or filth.

rhythm (rĭth'ŭm) [G. *rhythmos*, measured motion]. 1. A measured time or movement; regularity of occurrence. 2. Marking the intermenstrual periods of fertility and sterility in the female. SEE: *cacorhythmic*.
  r., **cantering**. Abnormal heart rhythm comparable to the cantering of a horse.
  r., **coupled**. One in which every other heartbeat produces no pulse at the wrist.
  r., **gallop**. Same as *cantering r*.
  r., **idioventricular**. An automatic rhythm in complete heart block.
  r., **nodal**. R. caused by contraction starting from the atrioventricular instead of sinoauricular node.
  r., **pendulum**. R. with the 2 heart sounds alike, with the sound of a ticking clock.
  r., **respiratory**. Successive and measured movements in breathing.
  r., **sinus**. The normal cardiac rhythm proceeding from the sinoauricular node.
  r., **ventricular**. Very slow ventricular contractions in heart block.

rhythmotherapy (rĭth"mō-ther'ă-pĭ) [G. *rhythmos*, measured motion, + *therapeia*, treatment]. Application of different forms of rhythm in treatment of disease.

rhytidectomy (rĭt-ĭd-ĕk'tō-mĭ) [G. *rhytis*, wrinkle, + *ektomē*, excision]. Excision of wrinkles by plastic surgery.

rhytidosis (rĭt-ĭd-ō'sĭs) [" + *-ōsis*, condition]. 1. Wrinkling of the skin. 2. Wrinkling of cornea.
  Occurs in cases of great diminution in tension of eyeball, particularly after the escape of aqueous or vitreous, usually near death. SYN: *rhitidosis*.

rib (rĭb) [A.S. *ribb*]. One of the 24 bones enclosing the chest.
  FRACTURE OF: There is generally pain on breathing deeply or on coughing. The lower part of the chest is strapped after expiration, the strapping being carried around the thorax (novocain may be necessary while this is being done); the strapping is left on for about a month.
  Paravertebral injections of procaine and alcohol at site of involved thoracic nerves facilitate healing and lessen pain.
  RS: *costa, chondrocostal, floating, false, intercostal, true, vertebra*.
  r's., **false**. Five ribs on each side not directly attached to the sternum.
  r's., **floating**. Two lower ribs not attached to the sternum.
  r's., **true**. The upper 7 ribs on each side which join the sternum by separate cartilages.

Ribes' ganglion (rēbz). Small g. of the sympathetic nervous system situated on the ant. communicating artery of brain.

riboflavin (rĭb"ō-flăv-ĭn). This is vitamin B₂ complex and was formerly called bactoflavin.
  USES: Not fully established as yet.
  DOSAGE: Experimentally, 2 to 3 mg., higher in lactation and pregnancy.
  RS: *ariboflavinosis, cheilosis, vitamin*.

rice (rīs) [G. *oryza*]. COMP: Poor in nitrogen and fats; high in carbohydrates. Lowest of all cereals in albumin. Shelled rice contains half as much phosphorus and lime as white bread, while magnesium is lower and iron a little higher. Potassium much higher than in other cereals. Cellulose is higher in bread and residue greater.
  AV. SERVING (brown and white): 20 Gm. Pro. 1.3, Fat 0.5-0.1, Carbo. 15.3-16.2.
  VITAMINS (brown): A+, B++, G+; (white): C+.
  ASH CONST. (brown): P 0.207, Fe 0.0020.
  ASH CONST. (white): Ca 0.009, Mg 0.033, K 0.070, Na 0.025, P 0.096, Cl 0.054, S 0.117, Fe 0.0009. An acid-forming food.
  POTENTIAL ACIDITY: 9 cc. per 100 Gm., 2.6 cc. per 100 cal.
  ACTION: Easier to digest than bread, but large quantities tax the digestive system. In cooking, the starch is partly converted into dextrin. It is highly nutritive and strengthening.
  r. **water stools**. Those of cholera which resemble water in which rice has been boiled.

Richter's hernia (rĭk'terz). Strangulated hernia with only a part of the gut constricted.

rickets (rĭk'ĕts) [origin uncertain]. A disease of metabolism affecting children, characterized by defective nutrition and often resulting in deformities.
  SYM: Restlessness and slight fever at night (101-102° F.), free perspiration about head, diffuse soreness and tenderness of body, pallor, slight diarrhea,

rickets, fetal — enlargement of liver and spleen, delayed dentition and eruption of badly formed teeth, head large and more or less square in outline, craniotabes or skull bones often so thin they crackle like parchment.

Sides of thorax flattened; sternum prominent; nodules can be felt at sternal ends of ribs, forming "rachitic rosary." Deformity may be kyphosis, lordosis or scoliosis. Liver and spleen may be considerably enlarged, long bones are curved and prominent at their extremities. Bowels constipated, abdomen distended.

PROG: Serum phosphatase studies are helpful in making diagnosis and prognosis. Usually favorable. Deformity disappears in 90% of cases.

TREATMENT: Careful regulation of diet, fresh milk, properly diluted for infants; meat juice or raw beef for older children. Fresh air and sunshine. Vitamin D in small regular dose or preferably in 1 large injection of 600,000 international units, and an abundance of calcium and phosphorus in the food. Sunlight or ultraviolet rays. Fresh air and sunshine. Sea bathing, irradiated cod-liver oil, liver, egg yolks, lactophosphate of lime, good hygiene. Surgical treatment for deformities of bones.

RS: *carpopedal spasm, child crowing, rachitis, spasmophilia.*

r., fetal. Defective cartilage formation at epiphyses of long bones in fetus producing a dwarfed body.

r., renal. A disturbance in epiphyseal growth during childhood due to severe chronic renal insufficiency.

Dwarfism and failure of gonadal development result.

PROG: Poor.

TREATMENT: Diet low in meat, milk, cheese and egg yolk and adm. of calcium lactate or calcium gluconate in large doses.

rickettsia (rĭk-ĕt'sĭ-ă). Minute organisms which cause typhus fever, trench fever, Rocky Mountain spotted fever, Q fever, rickettsialpox, and others.

rickety (rĭk'ĕt-ĭ) [origin uncertain]. Affected with or resembling rickets. SYN: *rachitic.*

Riddock's mass reflex. Flexion of 1 or both lower extremities with involuntary emptying of bladder and sweating in lower regions when stimulation is applied below level of a spinal cord injury.

riders' bone (rī'derz). Bony formation in adductor muscle of leg from pressure on the saddle. SYN: *cavalry bone.*

r. leg, r. sprain. Sprain of adductor muscles of the thigh.

ridge (rĭj) [M.E. *rigge*, from A.S. *hrycg*, back of an animal]. Narrow, elongated or elevated border.

r., epicondylic. One of 2 ridges for muscular attachments on the humerus.

r., gastrocnemial. A ridge on post. femoral surface for attachment of gastrocnemius muscles.

r., gluteal. A ridge extending obliquely downward from great trochanter of femur to the attachment of the gluteus maximus muscle.

r., interosseous. A ridge on the fibula for attachment of the interosseous membrane.

r., pronator. Oblique ridge on the ant. surface of ulna, giving attachment to the pronator quadratus.

r., pterygoid. One at angle of junction of temporal and infratemporal surface of great wing of the sphenoid bone.

r., superciliary, r., supraorbital. Curved ridge of the frontal bone over supraorbital arch.

r., supracondylar. Epicondylic r.

r., tentorial. One on upper inner surface of the cranium to which is attached the tentorium.

r., trapezoid. An oblique ridge on the upper surface of the clavicle giving attachment to the trapezoid ligament.

r., wolffian. Ridge in the embryo from which the wolffian body develops.

ridgel, ridgil, ridgling (rĭj'ĕl, -ĭl, -lĭng) [origin uncertain]. One with 1 testicle removed.

Riedel's lobe (rē'dĕl). A tongue-shaped process of liver, frequently found protruding over gallbladder in cases of chronic cholecystitis.

Riegel's test meal (rē'gĕl). Mutton broth, 200 cc.; beefsteak, 200 Gm.; mashed potato, 50 Gm.; bread or rolls, 50 Gm.; water, 200 cc. The stomach contents are expressed in 6 hours.

Riga's disease (rē'gă). Ulceration of frenum of the tongue with membrane formation.

Rigg's disease (rĭg). Formation of pus in teeth sockets with inflammation of the gums. SYN: *pyorrhea alveolaris, q.v.*

rigidity (rĭj-ĭd'ĭ-tĭ) [L. *rigidus*, stiff]. Tenseness; immovability; stiffness; inability to bend or be bent.

rigor (rī'gŏr, rĭg'or) [L. *rigor*, stiffness]. 1. A sudden, paroxysmal chill with high temperature, called the *cold stage*, followed by a sense of heat and profuse perspiration, called the *hot stage.* 2. A state of hardness and stiffness, as in a muscle. Rigor chills may be coarse, fine, diffuse, trembling.

r. mortis. The stiffness seen in corpses.

The rigidity of death which begins after 8, 10 or 20 hr. and may last 9 days. SEE: *dead, care of the; Nysten's law.*

rima (rī'ma) (pl. *rimae*) [L. *rima*, a slit]. A slit, fissure, or crack.

r. cornealis. Groove in the sclera holding edge of the cornea. SYN: *corneal cleft.*

r. glottidis. Interval bet. the true vocal cords. SYN: *glottis vera.*

r. oris. Aperture of the mouth.

r. palpebrarum. Slit bet. the eyelids.

r. pudendi. Space bet. the labia majora. SYN: *pudendal slit, vulvar slit, urogenital cleft.*

r. respiratoria. Space behind the arytenoid cartilages.

r. vestibuli. BNA. Space bet. the false vocal cords. SYN: *glottis spuria.*

r. vocalis. SEE: *r. glottidis.*

rimmose, rimose (rĭm'ōs, rī'mōs) [L. *rimōsus*, full of cracks]. Fissured or marked by cracks.

rimous (rī'mŭs) [L. *rimōsus*, full of cracks]. Filled with cracks or fissures. SYN: *rimmose.*

rimula (rĭm'ū-lă) [L. *rimula*, a little crack]. A minute fissure or slit, esp. of the spinal cord or brain.

rind (rīnd) [A.S. bark]. The skin or cortex of an organ or person.

r. tumor. Neoplasm arising from lining membrane tissue of the embryo. SYN: *lepidoma.*

ring (rĭng) [A.S. *hring*]. 1. Any round organ or band around a circular opening. 2. ANAT: A circular structure. SYN: *annulus.* 3. BACT: A growth like a ring around upper margin of a liquid culture, adhering to the glass more or less closely.

Ringer's solution (rĭng′ẽr). An aqueous solution containing 0.7% sodium chloride, 0.03% potassium chloride, and 0.025% calcium chloride.
USES: In forms of dehydration, and for improving circulation.
DOSAGE: From 500 to 1000 cc., all parenteral routes, chiefly subcutaneously.

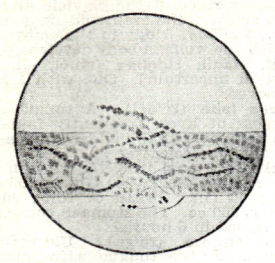

RINGWORM OF HAIR.
Granular threads of the parasite invade and destroy the hair shaft.

ringworm (rĭng′wŭrm). Contagious skin disease due to a species of *Trichophyton*, a fungous parasite.
When attacking the scalp it is called *Tinea* tonsurans*; when on the body it is known as *Tinea circinata*.
SYM: Red ringed patch of vesicles, itching, pain, scaling.
TREATMENT: Paint affected parts with iodine 3 times a day. Expose affected patches to the x-ray. Also powder composed of salicylic acid, 5 Gm.; menthol, 2 Gm.; camphor, 8 Gm.; boric acid, 50 Gm.; starch, 35 Gm., applied 3 times daily for ringworm of the feet. SEE: *athlete's foot*.
r., crusted. Contagious skin affection caused by parasitic fungus with formation of honeycomblike crusts over hair follicles, itching, and moldy odor. SYN: *favus*.
r., honeycomb. SEE: *crusted r.*
Rinne test (rĭn′nĕh). A test to ascertain condition of various parts of the ear with a vibrating tuning fork held over the mastoid process. SEE: *test*.
Riolan's arch (rē-ō-lahn′). Arch of transverse mesocolon.
R's. bouquet. Two ligaments and 3 muscles attached to styloid process of temporal bone.
R's. muscle. Ciliary portion of orbicularis palpebrarum. SYN: *musculus ciliaris*.
ripa (rī′pă) [L. *ripa*, bank]. Any line of reflection of the endyma of the brain from a ventricular surface.
Ripault's sign (rē-pōz′). Change in shape of pupil produced by unilateral pressure upon eyeball, transitory phase during life, but permanent after death.
risorius (rī-sō′rĭ-ŭs) [L.]. Muscular fibrous band arising over masseter muscle and inserted into tissues at the corner of the mouth. SEE: *Muscles, Table of, in Appendix*.
risus (rī′sŭs) [L.]. Laughter; a laugh.
r. sardonicus. A peculiar grin, as seen in tetanus, caused by acute spasm of facial muscles.
Ritter's disease (rĭt′ẽr). 1. Severe inflammation of skin with scaling, seen in infants. SYN: *dermatitis exfoliativa infantum*. 2. Fatal disease of infants, marked by hemorrhage, jaundice and cyanosis.
Ritter-Valli law (rĭt″ẽr-văl′ĭ). Increased irritability from center outward if a nerve is cut off from its center or if the latter is destroyed.
Irritability is soon lost.
ri′valry strife. Alternate sensations of color and shape when the fields of vision of the 2 eyes cannot combine in 1 visual image.
Rivalta's disease (rē-val′tă). Chronic inflammation with lumpy formations and suppuration about the jaws. SYN: *actinomycosis, lumpy jaw*.
Rivinus' canals or ducts (re-ve′nŭs). Ducts of sublingual gland.
R's. glands. Sublingual glands.
R's. ligament. Small portion of the drum membrane in notch of Rivinus. SYN: *Shrapnell's membrane*.
R's. notch. Cleft in upper part of long tympanic ring, filled by Shrapnell's membrane.
riziform (rĭz′ĭ-form) [Fr. *riz*, rice, + *forma*, form]. Resembling rice grains.
RLS person. One who stammers and usually mispronounces these letters.
R. M. A. Abbr. of *right mentoanterior presentation of the fetal face*.
R. M. P. Abbr. of *right mentoposterior presentation of the fetal face*.
R. N. Abbr. for *Registered Nurse*.
Robertson's pupil. Pupil in which there is no light reflex, but power of contraction during accommodation remains unchanged. Same as *Argyll-Robertson pupil*.
roborant (rŏb′ō-rănt) [L. *roborans*, strengthening]. 1. A tonic. 2. Strengthening.
Rochelle salt (rō-shĕll′). USP. Potassium and sodium tartrate, a colorless, transparent powder, having a cooling and saline taste.
ACTION AND USES: Saline cathartic.
DOSAGE: From 1 to 4 drams (4-15 Gm.).
Rocky Mountain spotted fever. An infectious disease caused by a parasite and transmitted by a wood tick; marked by fever, pains in bones and muscles, and profuse reddish eruption.
In the Rocky Mountains and on the Pacific Coast the mortality is 90%. SEE: *spotted fever, tick fever*.
rod (rŏd) [A.S. *rodd*, club]. 1. Slender, straight bar. 2. One of the slender, long sensory bodies in retina responding to faint light. 3. Bacterium shaped like a rod.
r's. and cones. Sensory ending of the retina composing the 2nd layer.
rodent ulcer (rō′dĕnt) [L. *rodere*, to gnaw]. A slow growing, gnawing cancer which steadily eats into tissues, causing great destruction.
The most usual sites are on outer angle of the eye, near side and on tip of nose, and edges of the scalp. SEE: *ulcer, rodent*.
rodonalgia (rō-dŏn-ăl′jĭ-ă) [G. *rhodon*, rose, + *algos*, pain]. Vasomotor condition marked by redness and neuralgic pain of the extremities and swelling, and fever. SYN: *erythromelalgia*.
roentgen (rĕnt′gĕn). The international unit of quantity of roentgen rays adopted by the Second International Congress of Radiology at Stockholm in 1928.
It is the quantity of radiation which, when the secondary electrons are fully utilized and the wall effect of the chamber is avoided, produces in 1 cc. of atmospheric air at 0° C. and 760 mm. of mercury pressure such a degree of

conductivity that 1 electrostatic unit of charge is measured at saturation.

r. rays. Radiation associated with the sudden change in velocity of free electrons (general radiation) or the transfer from higher to lower energy levels of electrons bound in atoms (characteristic radiation).

As in the case of visible light, the properties of roentgen rays fall into 2 groups. With regard to 1 group (diffraction and refraction) these rays act like very short electromagnetic waves, while in the photoelectric effect and in Compton scattering they behave as discrete particles of energy (quanta) traveling in straight lines with the velocity of light. "Roentgen rays" is preferred by medical authorities, but "x-rays" is more generally used by physicists. The wave lengths concerned are usually between 0.005 and 1 millimicron or 0.05 to 10 angstroms or 50 to 10,000 x units.

r. r. crystallography. The study of the arrangement of the atoms in a crystal by the deflection of roentgen rays by the atoms of the crystal.

r. r. photograph. A photograph taken with roentgen rays. SYN: *roentgenogram.*

r. r., quality of. Hardness, that quality of roentgen rays which determines their penetrating power, the hardness increasing as wave length shortens.

r. r., quantity of. The product of intensity and time. Quantity is used here in a sense different from that customary in other fields, such as radiant energy in general. It is not proportional to energy, but rather to the product of energy density and a coefficient expressing the ability to cause ionization.

r. r. spectrometer. An instrument used for determining the wave length of roentgen rays.

r. r. spectrum. The spectrum of a heterogeneous beam of roentgen rays produced by a suitable grating, generally a crystal.

r. r. tube. A glass vacuum bulb containing 2 electrodes. Electrons are obtained either from gas in the tube or from a heated cathode. When suitable potential is applied, electrons travel at high velocity from cathode to anode, where they are suddenly arrested, giving rise to roentgen rays.

roentgenism (rĕnt'gĕn-ĭzm) [*roentgen* + G. *-ismos*, condition]. Disease produced by the use of roentgen rays.

roentgenization (rĕnt-gĕn-ĭ-zā'shŭn). The act of subjecting a patient, animal or other object to the action of roentgen rays.

roentgenocinematography (rĕnt″gĕn-ō-sĭ″-ne-măt-ŏg′ră-fĭ) [*roentgen* + *kinema*, motion, + *graphein*, to write]. Photography with roentgen rays of the internal organs' movements.

roentgenogram (rĕnt′gĕn-ō-grăm) [*roentgen* + G. *gramma*, a mark]. A photographic record made with roentgen rays of the relative transparency of the various parts of an object to roentgen rays.

roentgenographer (rĕnt-gĕn-ŏg′ră-fer) [*roentgen* + G. *graphein*, to write]. A physician skilled in roentgen diagnosis.

Applies specifically to the making of photographic records as distinguished from roentgenoscopy.

roentgenography (rĕnt-gĕn-ŏg′ră-fĭ) [*roentgen* + G. *graphein*, to write]. The art of producing roentgenograms or photography with roentgen rays.

roentgenologist (rĕnt-gĕn-ŏl′ō-jĭst) [*roentgen* + G. *logos*, study]. A physician skilled in roentgen diagnosis, roentgen therapy, or both.

roentgenology (rĕnt-gĕn-ŏl′ō-jĭ) [*roentgen* + G. *logos*, study]. The science of applying roentgen rays for diagnostic and therapeutic purposes.

roentgenometer (rĕnt-gĕn-ŏm′ĕ-tĕr) [*roentgen* + G. *metron*, a measure]. An instrument for measuring the quantity, dosage, or intensity of roentgen rays.

roentgenometry (rĕnt-gĕn-ŏm′ĕ-trĭ) [*roentgen* + G. *metron*, a measure]. Measurement of penetrating capacity of the x-ray and of therapeutic doses of the same.

roentgenoscope (rĕnt′gĕn-ō-skōp) [*roentgen* + G. *skopein*, to examine]. Device for holding the fluorescent screen in roentgen ray examinations. SYN: *fluoroscope.*

roentgenoscopy (rĕnt-gĕn-ŏs′kō-pĭ) [*roentgen* + G. *skopein*, to examine]. The examination of a patient or object by direct visualization of shadows cast on a roentgenoscope, fluoroscope or fluorescent screen by a beam of roentgen rays.

roentgenotherapy, roentgentherapy (rĕnt-gĕn-ō-ther′ăp-ĭ, rĕnt-gĕn-ther′ă-pĭ) [*roentgen* + G. *therapeia*, treatment]. The treatment of disease by exposure of the patient to roentgen rays.

r., radicular. The application of roentgen rays to the roots of nerves where they emerge from the spinal cord.

roentography (rĕn-tŏg′ră-fĭ) [*roentgen* + G. *graphein*, to write]. The making of x-ray pictures. SYN: *roentgenography, skiagraphy.*

roeteln, roetheln (rĕt'ĕln). German measles, *q.v.* SYN: *rubella.*

Rokitansky's disease (rō-kĭt-ăn′skĭ). Acute yellow atrophy of the liver.

Rolan'do's area. Motor area in the cerebral cortex.

R. fissure. Fissure bet. parietal and frontal lobes. SYN: *sulcus centralis.*

roller (rōl′er) [L. *rotula*, a little wheel]. 1. Strip of muslin or other cloth rolled up in cylinder form for surgeon's use. 2. A roller bandage. SEE: *bandage.*

Rollier technic (rōl′ē-ā). Method of using heliotherapy in which the body is gradually exposed to the sun's rays.

romaine (rō-mān') [Fr. *romaine*, Roman]. AV. SERVING: 50 Gm. Pro. 0.5, Carbo. 1.5. VITAMINS: A++, B++.
ASH CONST: Ca 0.045, Mg 0.032, K 0.306, Na 0.016, P 0.053, Cl 0.073, S 0.019, Fe none.

Roman numerals. Those used by the Romans in contradistinction to the Arabic numerals which we now use.

In Roman notations values are increased either by adding 1 or more symbols to the initial symbol, as III for 3, or by subtracting a symbol from 1 or more to the right of it, as IV for 4, IX for 9, etc., as shown in the following table:

Arabic	Roman	Arabic	Roman
1	I	10	X
2	II	11	XI
3	III	12	XII
4	IV	13	XIII
5	V	14	XIV
6	VI	15	XV
7	VII	16	XVI
8	VIII	17	XVII
9	IX	18	XVIII

Arabic	Roman	Arabic	Roman
19	XIX	90	XC
20	XX	100	C
30	XXX	500	D
40	XL	900	CM
50	L	1,000	M
60	LX	1,900	MCM
70	LXX	1,000,000	M̄
80	LXXX		

A line placed over a letter increases its value 1000 times, as M̄ is equal to 1000 times 1000 for which the M stands.

romanopexy (rō-man'ō-pĕks″ĭ) [L. *romanum*, the sigmoid, + G. *pēxis*, fixation]. Fixation of the sigmoid flexure for prolapse of the rectum. SYN: *sigmoidopexy.*

romanoscope (rō-măn'ō-skōp) [" + G. *skopein*, to examine]. Instrument for examining the sigmoid flexure.

Romberg's sign (rŏm'bĕrg). Inability to maintain the body balance when the eyes are shut and the feet close together; seen in tabes dorsalis, severe alcoholic neuritis, etc.

rongeur (ron-zhūr') [Fr. *ronger*, to gnaw]. A gouge forceps, an instrument for removing tiny fragments of bone.

roof nucleus (rūf nū'klē-ŭs). Small mass of gray matter in white substance of vermis of the cerebellum. SYN: *nucleus fastigii.*

root (rūt) [A.S. *rōt*]. 1. The underground part of a plant. Ex: *Stillingia, Glycyrrhiza, Belladonna.* 2. Proximal end of a nerve. 3. Portion of an organ implanted in tissues.
  r. arteries. A. accompanying nerve roots into the spinal cord. SYN: *radicular vessels.*
  r. canal. Pulp cavity of root of tooth.
  r. sheath. Epithelium covering the hair follicle.
  r. zone. Burdach's column of the spinal cord. Outer tract of post. funiculus or white column of the cord. SYN: *fasciculus cuneatus.*

R. O. P. Abbr. for *right occipitoposterior presentation*, *i. e.*, the occiput of fetus being in relation to the right sacroiliac joint of the mother.

rosa (rō'ză) [L.]. Rose.
  r. asturica. Deficiency disease due to lack of vitamin B₂. SYN: *pellagra.*

rosacea (rō-zā'sē-ă) [L. *rosaceus*, rosy]. Chronic hyperemic disease of the skin, esp. of the nose. SYN: *acne° rosacea.*

rose cold or **rose fever.** Summer or June cold; hay fever of early summer attributed to inhaling rose pollen. SEE: *hay fever.*

Rosenbach's sign (rō'zĕn-băhk). One of 4 signs: absence of abdominal reflex in intestinal inflammation.

Rosenheim's enema (rō'zĕn-hīm). A nutrient enema containing cod liver oil, sugar and peptone in a 3% soda solution. SEE: *enema.*

Rosenmüller's body (rō'zĕn-mŭ-ler). Rudimentary tubule in the mesosalpinx bet. the fallopian tube and ovary. SYN: *epoöphoron, parovarium.*

R's. cavity, R's. fossa. Slitlike depression in the pharyngeal wall behind opening of the eustachian tube.

roseo- [L.]. 1. Combining form meaning rose-colored. 2. A prefix in chemical terms.

roseola (rō-zē'ō-lă) [L. *roseus*, rosy]. 1. Skin condition marked by maculae or red spots of varying sizes on the skin; a rose-colored rash. 2. Measles or German measles. SEE: *roseolous, rose rash.*
  r. idiopathica. Macular eruptions not associated with any well-defined symptoms.
  r. symptomatica. Macular eruption occurring in well-defined diseases.

roseolous (rō-zē'ō-lŭs) [L. *roseus*, rosy]. Resembling or pert. to roseola.

rose rash (rōz răsh). Any red colored eruption. SYN: *roseola.*

Roser's position (rō'zer). Head downward for operations on the air passages.

R's. sign. No pulsation of dura mater after trephining, indicative of a subjacent lesion.

rose water (rōz wau'ter). Saturated aqueous solution of the oil of rose.
  ACTION AND USES: To impart agreeable odor to lotions, etc.

rosin (rŏz'ĭn) [L. *resina*]. Substance distilled from oil of turpentine and used as adhesive and stimulant on plasters.

Rossbach's disease (rŏs'băhks). Excessive secretion of gastric juice. SYN: *gastroxynsis, hyperchlorhydria.*

Rossolimo's reflex (rŏs-ō-lē'mō). Extension or abduction of great toe resulting from light percussion or stroking of its plantar surface.

Ross' bodies (rŏs). Bodies sometimes found in tissue fluids in syphilis.
  They are copper-colored, round and dark granules sometimes exhibiting ameboid movements.

rostellum (rŏs-tĕl'lŭm) [L. *rostellum*, little beak]. The ant. part of the head of worms equipped with a row of hooks.

rostral (rŏs'trăl) [L. *rostrum*, beak]. 1. Resembling a beak. 2. Toward the front or cephalic end of the body.

rostrate (rŏs'trāt) [L. *rostrum*, beak]. Having a beak or hook formation.

rostrum (rŏs'trŭm) [L. beak]. Any hooked or beaked structure.

rosulate (rŏs'ū-lāt) [L. *rosulatus*, like a rose]. Shaped like a rosette.

rotate (rō'tāt) [L. *rotāre*, to turn]. To twist or revolve.

rotation (rō-tā'shŭn) [L. *rotatio*, a turning]. Process of turning on an axis.
  r., fetal. Twisting of the fetal head as it follows the curves of the birth canal, downward.

rotator (rō-tā'tor) (pl. *rotatores*) [L. that which turns]. A muscle revolving a part on its axis.
  r., uterine. An elevator or replacer used to push or rotate the uterus when it is out of its natural position.

röteln, rötheln (re'teln) [Ger. *rot*, red]. German measles. SYN: *rubella.*

Rothera's test (rŏth'ĕ-ră). Method for finding acetone bodies in urine. SEE: *acetone.*

rotula (rŏt'ū-lă) [L. *rotula*, little wheel]. 1. The kneecap. SYN: *patella.* 2. A medicated disk. SYN: *lozenge, troche.*

rotular (rŏt'ū-lar) [L. *rotula*, little wheel]. Concerning the patella or kneecap.

rouge (rūzh) [Fr. from L. *rubeus*, red]. A powder prepared by calcining ferrous sulfate used in polishing metal and glass instruments.

roughage (rŭf'ĭj) [M.E. *rough*, from A.S. *rūh*]. Indigestible fiber of fruits, vegetables, and cereals which acts as a stimulant to aid intestinal peristalsis.
  Plenty of water should be added to consumption of roughage. Should not be used in colitis or in intestinal irritation. SEE: *cellulose.*
  r. diet. Diet with large amounts of cellulose, water, mineral salts and vitamins. SYN: *high residue diet.*

rough on rats. A proprietary rat poison.
POISONING: SYM: Pain and burning in stomach. Vomiting and diarrhea which cause great thirst; shock. Extremities are cold; cold sweats; pulse weak and rapid; exhaustion.
F. A. TREATMENT: Empty stomach with stomach pump, or give emetic. Wash stomach out with large quantities of soapy water. SEE: *arsenic, barium.*

rouleau (roo-lō') (pl. *rouleaux*) [Fr. roll]. A group of red blood corpuscles arranged like a roll of coins.

round (rownd) [L. *rotundus*, round]. Circular in shape.
   r. ligament. 1. Curved fibrous cord attached to center of articular surface of head of femur. 2. Two round cordlike structures passing from front of the body of the uterus in ant. wall of broad ligament, below the fallopian tubes, outward through the inguinal canals to soft tissues of the labia majora. 3. Fibrous cord which is the remnant of umbilical vein.
   r.-worm. Common intestinal parasite, esp. in children. SYN: *Ascaris lumbricoides.*

roust (rowst). Delivery room nurse who carries out unsterile tasks.

R. Q. Abbr. for *respiratory quotient.*

-rrhagia (rā'jĭ-ă) [G. *-rrhagia*, from *rhēgnunai*, to burst forth]. Combining form indicating *abnormal discharge, hemorrhage.*

rubber dam. Thin rubber tissue used by dentists, and as covering for dry dressings.
   r. goods, care of. AIM: To preserve the life of the article. To have the article clean and ready for use at any time. To prevent carrying contamination from 1 patient to another.
   TO CLEAN ARTICLES: 1. Wash off with cold water immediately after use. 2. Wash with soap and tepid water, and rinse well. Dry outside. 3. Before storing articles that have been used, wash well with 5% Lysol solution and rinse well with clear water. 4. If boiling, wrap in 1 layer gauze and boil 3 minutes only. 5. Inflate bags and air cushions before storing to prevent adherence.
   THINGS TO REMEMBER: 1. Never stick pins into rubber or into anything near it. 2. Rubber goods are very expensive. 3. Oil ruins rubber. Cover oily dressings well with waxed paper before applying any rubber. 4. Oil softens rubber and partially dissolves it. 5. Never allow contact of acids with rubber. 6. Heat destroys rubber. Never place on or near a radiator to dry. 7. Never pour boiling water on rubber. 8. Do not fold rubber. It cracks. Rubber sheeting should be rolled or hung over a rod. 9. Soak unused rubber sheeting in cold water, occasionally, to prevent its cracking. 10. Do not mix caps and covers on bags and bottles. Have them marked alike. Keep washers on covers. 11. If hard rubber must be boiled, cool quickly and do not *destroy the shape.* 12. Never leave the clamp closed on rubber tubing. 13. Do not bend the tubing at right angles; hang it up loosely to dry, after draining it thoroughly.
   r. tissue. Gutta percha sheets used for protecting dry dressings.

rubedo (rū-bē'dō) [L.]. Temporary redness of the skin. SYN: *blushing.*

rubefacient (rū″be-fā'shĕnt) [L. *rubefaciens*, making red]. 1. Causing redness, as of the skin. 2. Agent which reddens the skin, producing a local congestion, the vessels becoming dilated and the supply of blood increased.
The effect is immediate, but of short duration, as it rapidly disappears when the irritant is removed. When the application is prolonged, it causes a severe inflammation of the skin, which may result in vesication or ulceration.
For this reason, rubefacients need to be applied with some care on children, and others whose skin is thin and sensitive, as the irritation may be unnecessarily severe. The same caution is necessary when applied to the skin of the unconscious, or of patients in whom the sense of pain is impaired. If weak preparation is used for a short time, only a redness is produced.
FRICTION WITH RUBEFACIENT DRUGS: Rubbing a small amount on desired part for a period of from 3 to 10 minutes and then cover with cotton or flannel cloth. This may be repeated 2 or 3 times daily. Those most commonly used are: (a) Camphorated oil. (b) Oil of turpentine (an excellent mixture is camphorated oil, oil of turpentine, and olive oil in equal quantities). (c) Alcohol. (d) Chloroform liniment. (e) Menthol plus camphor mixed with chloral hydrate becomes a liquid and is of value as a rubefacient. (f) Methyl salicylate liniment (oil of wintergreen).
APPLICATION OF MORE POTENT RUBEFACIENTS: (a) *Tincture of iodine:* Painted on lightly (if color is too deep, remove some with alcohol). (b) *Unguentum ichthyolis:* 10 or 20 per cent applied on gauze dressing. (c) *Burow's solution:* Sol. aluminum acetate: Applied as a wet dressing.
SEE: *mustard stupes.*
If the rubefacient action is prolonged, or a stronger strength of preparation is used, a vesicant or epispastic action results. The latter are agents which cause blister formation. The rubefacients include: (a) *Mustard;* (b) *turpentine;* (c) *capsicum;* (d) *flaxseed;* (e) *arnica,* and (f) *liniments.*

rubella (rū-bĕl'lă) [L. *rubellus*, reddish]. Acute infectious disease, resembling both scarlet fever and measles, but differing from these in its short course, slight fever and freedom from sequelae. SYN: *German measles, röteln.*
   INCUBATION: 5-21 days. It produces a maculopapular rash which vanishes by slight desquamation in from 2 to 3 days.
   SYM: Prodromes, slight or altogether absent. Drowsiness, slight fever, sore throat. Eruption 1st or 2nd day. In some cases, rash composed of pale red, scarcely elevated papules, more or less discrete rubella morbilliforme; in others, rash is bright red and diffuse like that of scarlet fever, rubella scarlatiniforme.
   Begins on face, spreads rapidly over whole body, but fades so rapidly that face may be clear before extremities are affected. Slight desquamation frequently present, though not always. Superficial cervical and posterior auricular glands more swollen than in measles. Duration, 3 to 5 days.
   PROG: Good.
   TREATMENT: Rest. Liquid diet. Refrigerants. Sponging with tepid water.
   r. scarlatinosa. A mild, exanthematous, contagious disease similar to scarlatina, measles, and rubella.

rubeola (rū-bē'ō-lă) [L. *rubeus*, reddish]. 1. Acute, contagious disease, marked by fever, catarrhal symptoms and a typical cutaneous eruption. SYN: *measles*. 2. Term occasionally applied to acute infectious disease with mild symptoms and rose-colored macular eruption. SYN: *German measles, rubella*.

rubescent (rū-bĕs'ĕnt) [L. *rubescere*, to grow red]. Growing red; flushing.

rubidium (rū-bĭd'ĭ-ŭm) [L. *rubidus*, red]. A metallic, silvery white metal used for same purpose as sodium salts or potassium. SYMB: Rb. At. wt. 85.44.

rubiginous (rū-bĭj'ĭn-ŭs). Rusty or rust-colored. [mildew].

rubigo (rū-bī'gō) [L. rust, mildew]. Rust;

Rubin's test (rū'bĭn). Transurine insufflation with carbon dioxide to test the patency of the fallopian tubes. SEE: *sterility*.

rubor (rōō'bor) [L. redness]. Discoloration or redness due to inflammation. One of the classical symptoms of inflammation. RS: *calor, dolor, tumor*.

rubrospinal (rū″brō-spī'năl) [L. *ruber*, red, + *spina*, thorn]. Concerning the red nucleus and the spinal cord.

rubrum (ru'brŭm) [L. red]. Reddish nucleus of gray matter in crus cerebri near optic thalamus.

r. scarlatinum. N.F. Scarlet red, a substance used as a healing agent and stain.

ructus (rŭk'tŭs) [L.]. Belching of wind from stomach.

rude respiration (rūd). R. having both bronchial and normal vesicular qualities.

rudiment (rū'dĭm-ĕnt) [L. *rudimentum*, a wild thing]. 1. That which is undeveloped. 2. BIOL: A part just beginning to develop. 3. An organ arrested in an early stage of development. 4. Remains of a part functional only at an earlier stage of an individual or in his ancestors.

rudimentary (rū-dĭm-ĕn'tă-rĭ) [L. *rudimentum*, a wild thing]. 1. Elementary. 2. Undeveloped; not fully formed; remaining from an earlier stage. SYN: *vestigial*.

rufous (rū'fŭs) [L. *rufus*, red]. Ruddy; having a ruddy complexion and reddish hair.

ruga (rū'gă) (pl. *rugae*) [L.]. A fold or crease.

r. vaginae. Transverse ridges of ant. and post. walls of the vagina.

Ruggeri's reflex. Increase in pulse rate when eyes are strongly converged on a near object.

rugose, rugous (rū'gōs, -gŭs) [L. *rugōsus*, wrinkled]. Wrinkled and rough in short, irregular folds. SYN: *corrugated*.

rugosity (rū-gos'ĭ-tĭ) [L. *rugōsitas*, wrinkled condition]. 1. Condition of being folded or wrinkled. 2. A ridge or wrinkle.

Ruhmkorff coil (rōōm'korf). An induction coil with an immovable secondary coil fixed at point of maximum intensity.

rumination (rū-mĭn-ā'shŭn) [L. *ruminăre*, to chew the cud]. Regurgitation, esp. with rechewing, of previously swallowed food.

rump (rŭmp) [M.E. *rumpe*]. Post. end of the back; the gluteal region or buttocks.

Rumpf's symptom (rŭmpf). 1. In neurasthenia, the pulse is quickened to 20 beats per minute if pressure is exerted over a painful spot. 2. Twitching, after strong faradization, in traumatic neuroses.

run (rŭn) [A.S. *rinnan*, to flow]. To exude pus or mucus.

run-around, runround (rŭn'ă-rownd, -rownd). Superficial infection encircling the fingernail. SYN: *felon, paronychia, whitlow*.

rupia (rū'pĭ-ă) [G. *rhypos*, filth]. A cutaneous eruption, usually of tertiary syphilis, which manifests itself at first by large elevations of the epidermis, filled with a clear or bloodstained serum, soon becoming turbid and purulent.

The bulla bursts, allows some fluid to escape and as it desiccates is covered with a crust, which drys, accumulates new layers and becomes covered with greenish-brown scales, sometimes to depth of ½ in. Thickest of all syphilides and presents most extensive ulcerations.

TREATMENT: Constitutional, antisyphilitics.

rupophobia (rū″pō-fō'bĭ-ă) [″ + *phobos*, fear]. Abnormal dislike for dirt or filth. SYN: *rhypophobia*.

rupture (rŭp'tūr) [L. *ruptūra*, a breaking]. A breaking apart, as of an organ. SYN: *hernia*, q.v.

r. of membranes. R. of amniotic sac as normal result of dilatation of the cervix uteri in labor.

r. of perineum. Rupture of p. in labor, a condition the obstetrician seeks to avoid; more frequent in *primiparae*.

r. of tubes. Rupture of a fallopian tube; a serious event in extrauterine pregnancy which may occur without the woman's knowledge of her pregnancy.

r. of uterus. Rare and due to unrelieved obstructed labor.

Russell's bodies (rŭs'ĕl). Hyaline, small, spherical bodies in cancerous and simple inflammatory growths.

Russian bath. Hot vapor bath followed by friction and plunge in cold water.

Rust's disease (rŭst). Tuberculosis of 2 upper cervical vertebrae and their articulations.

rusty (rŭst'ĭ) [A.S. *rustig*]. Reddish in color. Resembling or containing rust. SYN: *rubiginous*.

r. sputum. Reddish sputum expectorated in pneumonia.

rutabaga (rū″tă-bā'gă) [Swedish *rotabagge*]. Av. SERVING: 120 Gm. Pro. 1.3, Fat 0.1, Carbo. 8.7.

VITAMINS: A— to +, B++, C+++. ASH CONST: Ca 0.074, Mg 0.018, K 0.399, Na 0.083, P 0.056, Cl 0.058, S 0.083, Fe trace.

A base forming food, alkaline potentiality 8.5 cc. per 100 Gm., 29.8 cc. per 100 cal.

rut-formation. Loss of interest in environment, fixation upon a single object, and concentration of emotional or other interests in a groove or rut.

ruthenium (rū-thē'nĭ-ŭm). A hard, brittle, metallic element of platinum group. SYMB: Ru. At. wt. 101.7.

rutidosus (rūt-ĭ-dō'sŭs) [G. *rhytis*, wrinkle]. Contraction or puckering of cornea just before death.

rutilizm (rū'tĭl-ĭzm) [L. *rutilis*, red, + G. *-ismos*, condition]. Red-headedness.

rutin. A crystalline glucoside of quercetin, closely related to hesperidin. Derived from buckwheat; said to be a constituent of thirty-eight specific plants.

USES: To restore increased capillary fragility to normal, preventing vascular accidents in patients with hypertension; in various hemorrhagic conditions in which permeability, or capillary fragility is involved.

DOSAGE: 1 tablet (20 mg.) three times daily; more in refractory cases (40 mg. or more).

ruyschian membrane, r. tunic (rīsh'ĭ-an). Middle layer of the choroid. SYN: *lamina choriocapillaris, entochoroidea*.
  r. muscle. Muscular tissue of the fundus uteri.
Rx. Symbol for "take," "recipe." Simple method for writing Rx in metric system: Write for 15 capsules or powders, or for 2 ounces of liquid (60 cc.). Then the dose in grains or minims equals the amount of the drug in the entire Rx.
  EXAMPLE: Sodium salicylate is to be given in doses of 10 grains Morphine sulfate in doses of ¼ grain.

  Rx
Sodii salicylas	10	
Morphinae sulphas		25
Elixir lactopep. qsad	60	

  M. Sig. A teaspoonful (4 cc.) every four hours.
  If the Rx is to be for 4 ounces or 6 ounces, multiply the dose in grains by 2 or 3 respectively for the total amount of grams in the Rx.

rye (rī) [A.S. *ryge*]. COMP: Contains cellulose and sometimes ergot.
  Av. SERVING: 30 Gm. Pro. 3.2, Fat 0.5, Carbo. 21.2.
  VITAMINS: A+, B++, G+.
  ASH CONST. (whole grain): Ca 0.055, Mg 0.150, K 0.453, Na 0.035, P 0.385, Cl 0.025, S 0.170, Fe 0.0039.
  ACTION: Hard to digest. Cellulose may be desirable in constipation.
rytidosis (rĭt-ĭ-dō'sĭs) [G. *rhytis*, a wrinkle, + *-ōsis*, condition]. Wrinkling or contraction of cornea preceding death. SYN: *rutidosis*.
ryzamin-B (rī'ză-mĭn). A proprietary preparation of concentrated vitamin B_1 obtained from rice polishings, and having a potency of 50 I. U. per Gm.
  USES: Neuritis, to stimulate appetite, increase tone of the intestinal tract.
  DOSAGE: As indicated, ½ Gm. being equivalent in B_1 potency to 3 cakes of yeast.

Addenda

Recklinghausen's canals. Rootlets of the lymphatics, minute spaces in connective tissue.
  R's. disease, and syndrome. Pigmentation of skin, multiple small fibrous tumors on same with tenderness along nerves, pain in joints, sluggishness, multiple neurofibromatosis. 2. *Osteitis fibroma cystica*.
  R's. tumor. An adenoliomyo-fibroma on wall of the fallopian tube, or posterior uterine wall.
rejuvenation. The process of aging has been checked in many women by Dr. Wm. H. Masters of the Washington Univ., Medical School of Medicine, by twice weekly injections of half a teaspoon of mixed hormones in oil: one part estrogen to 20 parts androgen, evidently a replacement of substances naturally produced in younger women. Its continual use may be necessary as is insulin in diabetes.
reserpine (rē-serp'ĭn). A chemically pure derivative of *rauwolfia serpentina*. An old snake root remedy used in India for centuries for snake bite, mental illness, anxiety states. It lowers blood pressure. It acts upon the hypothalamus, the seat of emotional behavior, having a tranquilizing action, beginning a reorganizing of the personality.
Resin-P.M.S. A combination of an antibiotic and an iron-exchange resin put out by the Nat'l. Drug Co., Phil. The pure-irons in the resin knock out and replace the harmful ones in the intestines. For relief in summer complaints, ulcerative colitis, irritable colon, and in after effects of certain antibiotics.

S

S. Abbr. for *signa*, mark, term used in prescription writing; *sinister*, left; *semis*, half; *spherical* or *spherical lens*.

S. Symb. of *sulfur;* also L. *sine*, without.

Sabatier's suture (sab-ă-tē-āz'). Method using oiled cardboard inserted into the intestine for closing of wounds.

saber shin. Ant. border of the tibia marked with sharp convexity found in hereditary syphilis.

sabulous (săb'ū-lŭs) [L. *sabulum*, sand]. Gritty; sandy.

saburra (să-bŭr'ră) [L. *saburra*, sand]. Foulness of stomach or mouth; vitiated matter accumulated in stomach from indigestion. SYN: *sordes*.

saburral (să-bŭr'ăl) [L. *saburra*, sand]. 1. Pert. to foulness of mouth or stomach due to accumulation of undigested material. 2. Pert. to sand, as in application of a hot sand bath for relief from pain, as in muscular rheumatism.

sac (săk) [G. *sakkos*, a bag]. A baglike part of an organ; a cavity or pouch, sometimes containing fluid. SEE: *cyst*.
  s., air. An air cell in the lung.
  s., allantoid. Embryonic organ forming part of the umbilical cord, its expanded extremity uniting with the chorion to form the placenta.
  s., amniotic. A thin membrane, containing a serous fluid, enclosing the embryo. SYN: *amnion*.
  s., aneurysmal. Dilatation of a blood vessel forming wall of an aneurysm.
  s., embryonic. The embryo at an early period when it resembles a sac.
  s., fetal. Sac containing the fetus in extrauterine pregnancy.
  s., hernial. Covering of a hernia from a pouch of peritoneum.
  s., lacrimal. Upper dilated portion of the lacrimal duct.
  s., vitelline. Umbilical vessel surrounding the yolk in the embryo.
  s., yolk. Part of vitelline sac which is outside the embryonic body connected to it by umbilical duct. SYN: *umbilical vesicle*.

saccate (săk'āt) [L. *saccatus*, baglike]. 1. Pert. to, like, or enclosed in a sac. SYN: *encysted*. 2. BACT: Marking a sac-shaped form, as in a type of liquefaction.

saccharephidrosis (săk″ă-rĕf-ĭ-drō'sĭs) [G. *sakcharon*, sugar, + *ephidrōsis*, sweating]. Sugar in the perspiration, giving it a sweet odor.

saccharide (săk'ă-rīd) [G. *sakcharon*, sugar]. One of the carbohydrate group containing sugar, made up of mono-saccharoses, disaccharoses, and poly-saccharoses, *q.v.*

sacchariferous (săk-ă-rĭf'ĕr-ŭs) [″ + L. *ferre*, to carry]. Producing or containing sugar.

saccharification (săk″ă-rĭ-fĭ-kā'shŭn) [″ + *-ficāre*, to make]. Process of changing into sugar.

saccharimeter (săk-ă-rĭm'ĕ-tĕr) [″ + *metron*, measure]. Device for determining amount of sugar in a solution. SYN: *saccharometer*. SEE: *hydrometer, polarimeter*.

saccharin (săk'ă-rĭn) [G. *sakcharon*, sugar]. USP. (C₇H₄SO₂-NHCO.) A sweet, white, powdered, synthetic product derived from coal tar, 300 to 500 times as sweet as sugar.
  USES: In diabetes as sugar substitute.
  DOSAGE: ½ gr. (0.03 Gm.) in place of 1 lump of sugar; 2 ½ gr. tablets will sweeten 4 oz. of fluid. SYN: *gluside*, 2.

saccharine (săk'ă-rĭn, -rīn) [G. *sakcharon*, sugar]. Of the nature of, or having the quality of, sugar. SYN: *sweet*.

saccharo- [G.]. Combining form meaning sugar.

saccharogalactorrhea (săk″ă-rō-găl-ăk-tō-rē'ă) [G. *sakcharon*, sugar, + *gala, galakt-*, milk, + *rhoia*, flow]. Excessive lactose secreted in milk.

saccharolytic (săk″ă-rō-lĭt'ĭk) [″ + *lysis*, dissolution]. Able to split up sugar.

saccharometabolic (săk″ă-rō-mĕt-ă-bŏl'ĭk) [″ + *metabolē*, change]. Concerning the metabolism of sugar.

saccharometabolism (săk″ă-rō-mĕ-tăb'ō-lĭzm) [″ + ″ + *-ismos*, process]. The chemical changes involved in utilization of sugar by the body. SYN: *glycometabolism*.

saccharometer (săk-ă-rŏm'ĕt-ĕr) [″ + *metron*, a measure]. Device for determining amount of sugar in a solution. Used in testing urine. SYN: *saccharimeter*.

Saccharomyces (săk″ă-rō-mī'sēz) (pl. *saccharomycetes*) [″ + *mykēs*, fungus]. A genus of fungi, reproducing by budding. SYN: *yeasts*.

saccharomycetolysis (săk″ă-rō-mī-sēt-ŏl'ĭ-sĭs) [″ + ″ + *lysis*, destruction]. Splitting up of sugar by a yeast fungus.

saccharomycosis (săk″ă-rō-mī-kō'sĭs) [″ + ″ + *-ōsis*, condition]. Disease due to yeast fungi. SYN: *blastomycosis*.
  s. hominis. Pyemia induced by a pathogenic yeast.

saccharorrhea (săk-ă-rō-rē'ă) [G. *sakcharon*, sugar, + *rhoia*, flow]. Secretion of sugar in the body fluids, as in urine or perspiration. SEE: *diabetes mellitus, glycosuria*.

saccharose (săk'ăr-ōs) [G. *sakcharon*, sugar]. 1. Sucrose; cane, beet, or maple sugar. 2. One of the group of carbohydrates having the same chemical formula, $C_{12}H_{22}O_{11}$.

saccharosuria (săk″ă-rō-sū'rĭ-ă) [″ + *ouron*, urine]. Saccharose in the urine.

saccharum (săk'ăr-ŭm) [L. sugar]. Sugar, the term being used in the pharmacopeia.
  s. album. Pure or white crystallized sugar.
  s. canadense. Maple sugar.
  s. candidum. Rock candy.
  s. lactis. Sugar of milk. SYN: *lactose*.
  s. purificatum. Pure white sugar.

saccharuria (săk-ă-rū'rĭ-ă) [G. *sakcharon*, sugar, + *ouron*, urine]. Sugar in the urine.

sacciform (săk'sĭ-form) [G. *sakkos*, bag, + L. *forma*, shape]. Bag-shaped or like a sac. SYN: *saccate*.

sacculated (săk'ū-lăt-ĕd) [L. *sacculātus*, baglike]. Consisting of small sacs or saccules.

sacculation (săk″ū-lā'shŭn) [L. *sacculus*, a little bag]. 1. Formation into a sac or sacs. 2. Group of sacs, collectively.

saccule (săk'ūl) [L. *sacculus*, a little bag].
1. A small sac. 2. One of the sacs of the vestibular membrane of the ear, the other being the utricle.
 s., vestibular. SEE: *saccule, 2.*
sacculocochlear (săk″ū-lō-kŏk'lē-ar) [" + *cochlea*, a snail]. Concerning the saccule of the vestibule, and the cochlea.
sacculus (săk'ū-lŭs) (pl. *sacculi* [L. a small bag]. A saccule or little sac.
 s. alveolaris. An air cell of the lung.
 s. chylifer. The receptaculum* chyli.
 s. cordis. Sac surrounding the heart. SYN: *pericardium*.
 s., Horner's. Saccular fold of the rectal mucosa forming anal pocket.
 s. lacrimalis. Expanded portion of nasolacrimal duct.
 s. laryngis. Pouch bet. sup. vocal bands and inner surface of the thyroid cartilage.
saccus (săk'ŭs) [L. a bag). A sac or pouch.
 s. endolymphaticus. BNA. Dilated, blind end of the *ductus endolymphaticus*.
 s. lacrimalis. BNA. The lacrimal sac, into which empty the 2 lacrimal ducts.
sacrad (sā'krăd) [L. *sacrum*, sacred, + *ad*, toward]. In the direction of the sacrum.
sacral (sā'krăl) [L. *sacrum*, sacred]. Relating to the sacrum.
 s. bone. A triangular bone made up of 5 vertebrae just above the coccyx.
 s. canal. Continuation of the vertebral canal in the sacrum.
 s. flexure. Rectal curve in front of the sacrum.
 s. index. Sacral breadth multiplied by 100 and divided by sacral length.
 s. nerves. Two spinal nerves of motion and sensation which emerge from the sacral foramina.
 s. vertebra. Fused segments forming the sacrum.
sacralgia (sā-krăl'jĭ-ă) [" + G. *algos*, pain]. Pain in the sacrum. SYN: *hieralgia*.
sacralization (sā-krăl-ĭ-zā'shŭn) [L. *sacrum*, sacred]. Union of the sacrum and the 5th lumbar vertebra.
sacra media (sā'krā mē'dĭ-ă) [L.]. Middle sacral artery.
sacrectomy (sā-krĕk'tō-mĭ) [" + G. *ektome*, excision]. Excision of part of sacrum.
sacrificial operation. One in which some organ is removed from the patient's good.
sacro- (sā'krō) [L.]. Prefix denoting the *sacrum*.
sacroanterior (sā″krō-ăn-tē'rĭ-or) [L. *sacrum*, sacred, + *anterior*, comparative of *ante*, before]. Denoting a fetus having the sacrum directed forward.
sacrococainization (sā″krō-kō-kăn-ĭ-zā'shŭn) [" + *cocaine*]. Injection of cocaine through the sacrolumbar space into the spinal cord.
sacrococcygeal (sā″krō-kŏk-sĭj'ē-ăl) [" + G. *kokkyx*, coccyx]. Concerning the sacrum and coccyx.
sacrocoxalgia (sā″krō-kŏks-ăl'jĭ-ă) [" + *coxa*, hip, + G. *algos*, pain]. Pain in sacroiliac joint, usually due to inflammation. SEE: *sacrocoxitis*.
sacrocoxitis (sā″krō-kŏks-ī'tĭs) [" + " + G. *-itis*, inflammation]. Inflammation of the sacroiliac joint, frequently tuberculous.
sacrodynia (sā-krō-dĭn'ĭ-ă) [" + *odyne*, pain]. Pain in the region of the sacrum. Sometimes referred in neurasthenia or hysteria.
sacroiliac (sā″krō-ĭl'ĭ-ăk) [L. *sacrum*, sacred, + *iliacus*, pert. to the hipbone].
Of, or pert. to the sacrum and ilium.
 s. disease. Tuberculous disease of the sacroiliac joint.
 s. joint. The articulation bet. the hipbone and sacrum.
 There is no movement normally in this joint in men, but in the pregnant woman it becomes movable, allowing the pelvis to tip slightly during labor.
 s. synchondrosis. Meeting point of the sacrum and ilium.
sacrolumbar (sā″krō-lŭm'bar) [L. *sacrum*, sacred, + *lumbus*, loin]. Of, or concerning the sacrum and loins.
 s. angle. Angle formed by articulation of the last lumbar vertebra and the sacrum.
sacroposterior (sā″krō-pŏs-tē'rĭ-or) [" + *posterior*, comparative of *posterus*, coming after]. Having the fetal sacrum directed backward.
sacrosciatic (sā″krō-sī-ăt'ĭk) [" + *sciaticus*, pert. to hip joint]. Concerning the sacrum and ischium.
sacrospinal (sā″krō-spī'năl) [" + *spina*, thorn]. Relating to the sacrum and spine.
sacrotomy (sā-krŏt'ō-mĭ) [" + G. *tome*, a cutting]. Surgical excision of the lower part of the sacrum.
sacrouterine (sā″krō-ū'tĕr-ĭn) [" + *uterus*, womb]. Concerning the sacrum and uterus.
sacrovertebral (sā″krō-ver-tē-brăl) [" + *vertebra*, vertebra]. Concerning the sacrum and the vertebrae.
 s. angle. Promontory of the sacrum.
sacrum (sā'krŭm) [L. *sacrum*, sacred]. The triangular bone situated dorsal and caudal from the 2 ilia bet. the 5th lumbar vertebra and the coccyx.
 It is formed of 5 united vertebrae wedged in bet. the 2 innominate bones forming the sacroiliac joints, above the coccyx and forming the keystone of the pelvic arch.
 s., assimilation. A sacrum with a lumbar vertebra fused to the sacrum, or 1 with the 1st sacral vertebra free, resembling a lumbar vertebra. SEE: *pelvic, sacroiliac*.
sacto- [G.]. Combining form meaning *stuffed*, as sactosalpinx, an overfilled tube.
sactosalpinx (săk″tō-săl'pĭnks) [G. *saktos*, stuffed, + *salpigx*, tube]. Dilated fallopian tube due to retention of secretions, as in pyosalpinx or hydrosalpinx.
saddle joint (săd'l). Joint with articulating surfaces convex in 1 direction and concave in the other.
 s. nose. A nose with a depressed bridge.
sadism (sā'dĭzm, săd'ĭzm) [Fr. *sadisme*]. A morbid phenomenon named after the Marquis de Sade, a French pervert of the 18th century, in which gratification is obtained by hurting a loved person.
 Sadism is a part of the make-up of a neurotic, a short cut whereby an inferior person acquires a brief superiority over his sexual partner. The suffering of the sadist's victim produced by physical violence, supplies an artificial stimulation which normal sex desire produces in the normal male.
 Sadism is not confined to sex expression; it is a mob characteristic, and one found in slave-driving bosses. SEE: *masochism, algolagnia*.
Saemisch's ulcer (sā'mĭsh). Serpiginous, infectious ulcer of the cornea.
safety symbolism. Engagements to marry, the engagement ring, the wedding, the

wedding ring, marriage, itself, the public announcement of wedding anniversaries, the advent of children, are all symbols which announce to the world that a man or a woman is the possession of one or the other; a warning, as it were, to protect the other partner from the attentions of one of the opposite sex.

sagittal (săj'ĭ-tăl) [L. *sagitta*, arrow]. Arrowlike; in an anteroposterior direction.

   s. line. An anteroposterior line.

   s. plane. A bilateral symmetrical plane representing an imaginary line from the tip of the nose, tip of chin, and the occipital protuberance, dividing the head and the rest of the body medially.

   s. sinus. The sup. longitudinal sinus.

   s. sulcus. Groove on int. surface of skull.

   s. suture. Suture bet. the 2 parietal bones.

sago (sā'gō) [Malay *sagu*]. COMP: A substance prepared from the vegetable cells of various palms. A carbohydrate food made up entirely of starch.
ACTION: Easy to digest. Fattening. Leaves little residue.
IND: Convalescence, emaciated conditions and when little residue is desired.
SEE: *starch, carbohydrate.*

   s. spleen. The spleen in state of amyloid degeneration resembling sago.

Sahli's motor and secretory test meal (sah'lĭ). Test for both motor and secretory functions.
The meal consists of 25 Gm. of flour and 15 Gm. of butter, cooked until brown, to which 350 cc. of water are added, and enough salt to season the mixture.
The mass is boiled for 1 or 2 minutes. The patient's stomach is washed out and then 300 cc. of *soup* mixture are served. The remainder is kept as a standard. At the end of an hour the stomach contents are withdrawn and the quantity noted. 300 cc. of water are now introduced through the tube and the stomach massaged. The diluted meal is then withdrawn and its quantity noted.

Saint Anthony's fire. Any of certain inflammations or gangrenous skin conditions, esp. erysipelas, hospital gangrene, and ergotism, *q.v.*

   Saint Gotthard's disease. Condition due to presence of hookworms in intestinal tract. SYN: *ankylostomiasis.*

   Saint Vitus' dance. Nervous disease with involuntary, jerking motions. SYN: *chorea.*

sajodin (săj'ō-dĭn) USP. A brand of calcium iodobehenate. A preparation from calcium and iodine, containing 17% iodine.
USES: As a substitute for the inorganic iodides.
DOSAGE: 8 gr. (0.5 Gm.).

sal (săl) [L. salt]. Salt.

   s. ammoniac. Chloride of ammonia.

salaam convulsion (sa-lahm') [Arabic *salām*, peace]. Clonic muscular spasm of the trunk resulting in a bowing movement. SYN: *nodding spasm.*

salacious (sa-lā'shŭs) [L. *salax, salac-*, lustful]. Lustful or inciting to lust.

salethyl carbonate. A proprietary salicylic acid derivative.
USES: As an analgesic and antipyretic.
DOSAGE: 5-15 gr. (0.3-1 Gm.).

salicylate (săl'ĭ-sĭl"āt, săl-ĭs'ĭl-āt). Any salt of salicylic acid.

   s., methyl. The principal constituent of oil of wintergreen. It is applied externally for acute rheumatism.

   s., sodium. White crystalline substance with disagreeable taste, in some cases even nauseating.
USES: To reduce pain and temperature.
DOSAGE: 15-30 gr. (1-2 Gm.).

salicylated (săl-ĭs'ĭl-āt-ĕd). Impregnated with salicylic acid.

salicylism (săl'ĭs-ĭl-ĭzm) [*salicylic acid* + G. *-ismos*, condition]. Toxic condition caused by salicylic acid or its derivatives

salicyl-sulfonic acid test. Test for albumen in urine. SEE: *albumen.*

salicyluric acid (săl-ĭs-ĭl-ū'rĭk). Acid in urine after taking salicylic acid or its derivatives.

salifiable (săl-ĭf-ī'ă-bl) [L. *sal*, salt, + *fieri*, to be made]. Capable of forming a salt by combining with an acid.

salihexin (săl-ĭ-hĕks'ĭn). Proprietary salicylic acid derivative combining effects of the salicylates and methenamine.
USES: As an antipyretic, analgesic, and urinary antiseptic.
DOSAGE: 5-10 gr. (0.3-0.6 Gm.).

salimiter (săl-ĭm'ĭt-er) [L. *sal*, salt, + G. *metron*, a measure]. Device for testing strength of saline solutions.

saline (sā'lĭn) [L. *salinus*; of salt]. 1. Containing or pert. to salt; salty. 2. A mineral salt that produces evacuation of the intestinal contents. Ex: *magnesium sulfate, sodium sulfate, potassium citrate,* and *potassium tartrate.*

   s. enema. E. used to excite peristalsis and evacuation.
Magnesium sulfate, 1 oz. in 2 oz. of very warm water (115° F.), given with a small bore tube. SEE: *normal salt solution enema.*

   s. purgative. Any salt producing evacuation, as Epsom salts.

   s. solution. A solution of sodium chloride and distilled water; in biological laboratory parlance, a 0.9% solution of sodium chloride. An isotonic solution.
A normal saline s. consists of 0.85% salt solution, which is necessary to maintain osmotic pressure and the stimulation and regulation of muscular motion. SYN: *physiological salt solution*, *q.v.*

Salisbury treatment (sawlz'bĕr-ĭ). Treatment of obesity with meat and hot water diet.

saliva (să-lī'vă) [L. saliva]. The 1st digestive secretion emitted from the salivary glands into the mouth. SYN: *spittle.*

CHARACTER: It is tasteless, clear, odorless, viscid, and weakly alkaline, being neutralized after being acted upon by the gastric juice in the stomach. Sp. gr. 1.002-1.006. Amount secreted in 24 hr., 45 oz.

CONSTITUENTS: The secretion of the salivary glands has a highly variable composition, that from the parotid glands being the most serous and that from the sublinguals most mucous. The reaction to indicators is also normally variable, and is more frequently acid than alkaline.

FUNCTION: (a) To moisten the food, assist in mastication and deglutition, (b) lubricating the food with mucin, (c) dissolving solid or dry food, (e) secreting ptyalin to act upon starch.

It contains 2 enzymes: (1) *Ptyalin* salivary amylase), a diastatic enzyme changing starch into dextrin, and then

saliva, chorda

into maltose. It can only act in an alkaline solution. (2) *Maltase,* which splits maltose into dextrose.

The saliva also contains (a) mucin, which causes its viscosity and which acts as a lubricant; (b) carbon dioxide, a trace; (c) thiocyanic acid, a trace, an antiseptic and antitoxic; (d) about 99.5% water.

CAUSE OF EXCITATION: Reflex action through the special senses of: (a) Sight, exciting the optic nerve; (b) smell, exciting the olfactory nerve; (c) taste, exciting the glossopharyngeal nerve, supplying the submaxillary, sublingual, and parotid glands.

RS: *angiosialitis, aptyalia, aptyalism, asialia, glycosialia, insalivation, parotid, ptyalin, ptyalinogen, ptyalism, salivary digestion, s. glands, sialagogue.*

s., chorda. S. from the submaxillary gland obtained by irritation of the chorda tympani.

s. sympathetic. S. produced by stimulus to sympathetic nerve fibers supplying the glands; more scanty, but thicker than that of the chorda saliva.

salivant (săl'ĭv-ănt) [L. *saliva,* saliva]. Stimulating or that which stimulates the secretion of saliva.

salivary (săl'ĭv-ĕr-ĭ) [L. *saliva,* saliva]. Pert. to, producing, or formed from, saliva.

s. calculus. Concretion in a salivary duct.

s. corpuscles. Nucleated, spherical bodies in saliva.

s. diastase. Enzyme in saliva acting on starch. SYN: *ptyalin.*

s. digestion. The 1st digestive process taking place in the mouth.

I. PHYSICAL OR MECHANICAL ACTION: (a) Assists in mastication; (b) deglutition; (c) acts as a solvent, by (aa) moistening; (bb) by dissolving, esp. starch into soluble sugar. Temperature of 100° F. facilitates action; 32° F. temporarily stops action; 140° F. destroys action. Acids and strong alkalies stop salivary action.

II. CHEMICAL ACTION: (1) Sets up amylolysis, through the action of the diastatic enzyme, ptyalin, which by hydrolysis converts in the following order: *Sugar* into: (a) Erythrodextrin, a polysaccharide; (b) achroodextrin, a polysaccharide; (c) isomaltose, a disaccharide; (d) maltose, a monosaccharide. *Starch:* Perhaps 1% into dextrose.

(2) PROCESSES (Mouth): 1. *Mechanical:* (a) Mastication; (b) liquification; (c) deglutition (passing of food from the mouth through the pharynx into the esophagus, through the cardiac orifice into the stomach. 2. *Chemical:* Insalivation.

The primary purpose of salivary digestion is to convert starches into sugar, or to break down complex carbohydrates into simpler form. This process is barely started in the mouth, esp. if mastication is not thorough. As the enzyme, ptyalin, acts only in an alkaline solution, it was supposed that salivary digestion soon stopped in the stomach because of the acidity of the gastric juice, but it has been determined that food remains for some time in the pyloric region and that it is more than 20 to 30 minutes after eating before the fundus of the stomach receives and mixes the food mass with gastric juice. The carbohydrates are acted upon when they reach the duodenum, where carbohydrate digestion is completed. Sugars, like other foods, must be chemically acted upon and reduced from complex to simpler forms before absorption becomes possible. Therefore, disaccharides must be reduced to monosaccharides.

III. POSTSALIVARY DIGESTION (stomach and duodenum): After deglutition, the action of ptyalin may continue in the stomach for half an hour or more, or until the accumulation of hydrochloric acid in the fundus of stomach neutralizes and stops its action. Amylolysis, as stated, is completed in the duodenum. Food taken in the later part of the meal may not be acted upon sufficiently by ptyalin because of the presence of hydrochloric acid already secreted in the stomach. The soft palate, and root of tongue secrete mucin and mucinogen.

SEE: *digestion.*

s. glands. Three pairs of glands including the: (1) *Parotid* glands, 1 on each side of the face below the ear; secrete *ptyalin;* (2) *submaxillary* glands, principally in the floor of mouth; secrete *ptyalin* and *mucin;* (3) *sublingual* glands, principally in floor of mouth; secrete *mucin* and *mucinogen;* (4) *buccal* glands, scattered beneath the mucous membrane of lips and cheeks. They form a secretion that is mixed with the saliva.

NERVES: Facial and glossopharyngeal, also the autonomic system.

BLOOD SUPPLY: Branches from the ext. carotid artery. SEE: *saliva, salivary digestion.*

salivation (săl-ĭ-vā'shŭn) [L. *salivātio,* a secreting of saliva]. 1. The secretion of saliva. 2. Excessive secretion of saliva. SYN: *ptyalism.*

salivatory (săl'ĭ-vā'tō-rĭ) [L. *salivātio,* a secreting of saliva]. Producing secretion of saliva. SYN: *salivant.*

salivin (săl'ĭv-ĭn) [L. *saliva,* saliva]. Enzyme in saliva acting on starch. SYN: *ptyalin.*

sallow (săl'ō) [A.S. *salu*]. Of a pale, yellowish color, usually said of complexion or skin.

sallowness (săl'ō-nĕs) [A.S. *salu*]. Brownish-yellow tint combined with pallor of skin; normal to brunettes. SEE: *skin, face, facies.*

salmin(e (săl'mēn, -mĭn). $C_{30}H_{57}N_{14}O_{8}$. A protamine obtained from spermatozoa of salmon. SEE: *protamine, protein.*

sal mirabile (săl mĭ-răb'ĭ-lē) [L.]. A purgative salt. SYN: *Glauber's salt, sodium sulfate, q.v.*

salmon (săm'ŭn) (pl. *salmon*) [M.E. *salmon* from L. *salmo, salmon-,* salmon]. Av. SERVING (canned): 230 Gm. Pro. 50.6, Fat 29.4.

VITAMINS: A+, B+, D+++, G+++.
ASH CONST: Ca 0.109, Mg 0.133, K 1.671, Na 0.373, P 1.148, Cl 0.528, S 1.119, Fe 0.0055.

salmon patch (săm'ŭn). Salmon-colored area of the cornea in syphilitic keratitis. SYN: *Hutchinson's patch.*

Salmonella (săl-mō-nĕl'ă) [L.]. A genus of Gram-negative bacteria, some of them being intestinal pathogens.

S. aertrycke (ā-ĕr'trĭk-ĕ). A medium-sized, motile, Gram-negative rod present in meat poisoning and in paratyphoid fevers.

S. enteritidis. Gärtner's bacillus, a species causing meat poisoning.

S. hirschfeldii. A species found in paratyphoid fever, Type C.

S. paratyphi. A species causing paratyphoid fever, Type A.

S. psittacosis. A species found on parrots.
S. schottmülleri. Species causing paratyphoid fever, Type B.
salmonellosis (săl-mō-nĕ-lō'sĭs) [L. *salmonella* + G. *-ōsis*, condition]. Infestation with bacteria of genus *Salmonella*.
Salmon's operation (să'mŭn). Incision along an anal fistula; back-cut of Salmon.
salpingectomy (săl-pĭn-jĕk'tō-mĭ) [G. *salpigx*, *salpigg-*, tube, + *ektomē*, excision]. Excision of an oviduct.
salpingemphraxis (săl″pĭn-jĕm-frăks'ĭs) [" + *emphraxis*, a stoppage]. Obstruction of the eustachian tube causing deafness, or of a fallopian tube.
salpingian (săl-pĭn'jĭ-ăn) [G. *salpigx*, *salpigg-*, tube]. Concerning an oviduct, or the eustachian tube.
salpingion (săl-pĭn'jĭ-ŏn) [G. *salpigx*, *salpigg-*, tube]. A point at inf. surface of the apex of the petrous portion of temporal bone.
salpingitis (săl-pĭn-jī'tĭs) [G. *salpigx*, *salpigg-*, tube, + *-ītis*, inflammation]. Inflammation of the fallopian tube, or, less commonly, of the eustachian tube.
ETIOL: The condition may be acute, subacute, or chronic. The organisms most often associated with salpingitis are the gonococcus, staphylococcus, streptococcus, colon bacillus, and tubercle bacillus. The latter is the etiological factor in about 8% of the cases, while the gonococcus is responsible for about 75%.
PATH: In *acute* cases, the tube is swollen, particularly the inner coats, and the edema of the peritoneal coat causes an inclusion of the infundibular end and in this manner the tube is closed. There is a plastic exudate on the peritoneal coat, and associated with this there is always a local and sometimes a general peritonitis. The tube lumen is filled with purulent material.
In the *subacute* cases, the characteristic sausage-shaped tumor is present and with it more or less involvement of the ovary, producing either salpingo-oöphoritis or a tuboövarian abscess.
In *chronic* cases any 1 of the following pathologic conditions may be found: Chronic catarrhal salpingitis with thickened tubes, the mucous membrane folds of which are adherent and occasionally form pseudofollicles (pseudofollicular salpingitis); *salpingitis isthmica nodosum*, which is usually bilateral and in which there is a swelling at the cornual end of the tube varying in size from that of a pea to hazelnut. In these nodes there are miliary abscesses lined by normal tubal mucosa.
Hydrosalpinx, in which the tubal ostium is closed, the entire wall is greatly thinned out, the inner lining of the tube is greatly atrophied and the tube is distended by serous fluid; *pyosalpinx*, in which there is a greatly distended tube with a closed ostium, thick walls, and the lumen filled with a sterile purulent material; *tuberculous salpingitis*, in which there is either an acute miliary tuberculosis with the peritoneal coat of the tube studded with small tubercles or nodular tuberculosis simulating s. isthmica nodosum or tuberculous pyosalpinx, the pus in these cases being of a caseous nature.
PATHOGENESIS: Salpingitis may arise by: (a) Ascending infection by way of the mucous membrane of the uterus from the cervix; (b) puerperal or postabortal infection; (c) by way of the blood stream, or (d) by direct contact with the digestive tract.
SYM: The symptoms of acute salpingitis are those of acute pelvic peritonitis, pain in one or both sides of the lower abdomen, chill, nausea, fever, backache, loss of appetite, pain on urination and defecation, feeling of heat in the pelvis, and leukorrhea.
In the subacute stages the symptoms are similar to those present in the acute condition except that they are less intense.
In the chronic cases there are menstrual changes (*dysmenorrhea, menorrhagia*), and sterility is common. When fever persists over a period of 10 to 14 days a complication has usually arisen. The two most frequent complications are pelvic abscess or tuboövarian abscess.
DIAG: The diagnosis is usually made from the history, symptoms, and bimanual examination of the pelvis. On examination there is found an unusual amount of heat in the vagina, with bilateral tender swellings in the region of the adnexa. The white blood count in the acute cases is usually from 15,000 to 20,000, and the sedimentation time of the red blood cells is markedly reduced.
TREATMENT: The treatment of the acute case consists of absolute rest in bed, ice bag to the abdomen, coal tar analgesics for the control of pain. Push fluids. Antibiotics and/or sulfonamides by mouth in adequate dosage. Hot, antiseptic vaginal douches. Elimination should be encouraged without the use of enemas or drastic cathartics. Surgery should not be attempted in the acute case.
In the subacute type if there are frequent attacks and where the patient, for economic reasons, cannot be kept at rest, surgery is indicated. Nonspecific protein therapy has been used in these cases with doubtful efficacy.
In chronic cases where pain and bleeding are important factors radical surgery is indicated. In complicated acute cases with pelvic abscess or tuboövarian abscess drainage through the vagina is necessary.
s. profluens. S. with sudden discharge of secretions gathered in the fallopian tube.
salpingo- [G.]. Combining form meaning *trumpet* or *tube*.
salpingocatheterism (săl-pĭng″gō-kăth'ĕt-ēr-ĭzm) [G. *salpigx*, *salpigg-*, tube, + *katheter*, catheter, + *-ismos*, process]. Application of a catheter to the eustachian tube.
salpingocele (săl-pĭn'gō-sēl) [" + *kēlē*, hernia]. Hernial protrusion of an oviduct.
salpingocyesis (săl-pĭng″ō-sī-ē'sĭs) [" + *kyēsis*, pregnancy]. Pregnancy where fetus begins to develop in an oviduct; tubal pregnancy.
salpingo-oöphorectomy (săl-pĭng″gō-ō″o-for-ĕk'tō-mĭ) [" + *ōŏn*, ovum, + *phoros*, a bearer, + *ektomē*, excision]. Excision of an oviduct and ovary.
OPER. NP: The needle layout, sutures and operating procedure identical with those for hysterectomy. In the operation for a ruptured ectopic pregnancy it is well to have 3 times the usual number of laparotomy pads and packs ready, as well as an extra amount of very warm

salpingo-oöphoritis   S-6   **salt**

saline solution for flushing out the abdominal cavity. This is because there may be a great quantity of both fresh and clotted blood to be removed. POSITION: Horizontal.

salpingo-oöphoritis (săl-pĭng″ōo″o-for-ī′-tĭs) [" + " + " + -*itis*, inflammation]. Inflammation of the tube and ovary. SYN: *salpingo-oöthecitis*.

salpingo-oöphorocele (săl-pĭng″gō-ō-of′or-ō-sēl) [" + " + " + *kēlē*, hernia]. Hernia enclosing the ovary and fallopian tube.

salpingo-oöthecitis (săl-pĭng″gō-ō″ō-thē-sī′tĭs) [G. *salpigx*, *salpigg*-, tube, + *ōon*, ovum, + *thēkē*, box, + -*itis*, inflammation]. Inflammation of a fallopian tube and ovary. SYN: *salpingo-oöphoritis*.

salpingo-oöthecocele (săl-pĭng″gō-ō″o-thē′-kō-sēl) [" + " + " + *kēlē*, hernia]. Hernia of both ovary and fallopian tube.

salpingo-ovariectomy (săl-pĭng″gō-o″var-ĭ-ĕk′tō-mĭ) [" + L. *ovarium*, ovary, + G. *ektomē*, excision]. Surgical removal of an oviduct and ovary. SYN: *salpingo-oöphorectomy*.

salpingopexy (săl-pĭng′ō-pĕks″ĭ) [" + *pēxis*, fixation]. Fixation of a fallopian tube.

salpingopharyngeus (săl-pĭng″ō-făr-ĭn′jē-ŭs) [" + *pharygx*, *pharygg*-, pharynx]. The muscle arising in cartilage of the eustachian tube which raises soft palate.

salpingorrhaphy (săl-pĭng-or′ă-fĭ) [" + *rhaphē*, a seam]. Suture of an oviduct.

salpingosalpingostomy (săl-pĭng″gō-săl-pĭng-gŏs′tō-mĭ) [" + *salpigx*, tube, + *stoma*, a mouth]. The operation of attaching 1 fallopian tube to the other.

salpingoscope (săl-pĭng′gō-skōp) [G. *salpigx*, *salpigg*-, tube, + *skopein*, to see]. Device for examining the nasopharynx and eustachian tube.

salpingostaphylinus (săl-pĭng″gō-stăf-ĭl-ī′-nŭs) [" + *staphylē*, uvula]. The muscle which tightens soft palate. SEE: *Table of Muscles in Appendix*.

salpingostomatomy (săl-pĭng″gō-stō-măt′ō-mĭ) [" + *stoma*, a mouth, + *tomē*, a cutting]. Creation of an artificial opening in a fallopian tube after it has been occluded by inflammation.

salpingostomy (săl-pĭng-ŏs′tō-mĭ) [" + *stoma*, a mouth]. Surgical opening of a fallopian tube which has been occluded, or for drainage.

salpingotomy (săl-pĭng-ŏt′ō-mĭ) [" + *tomē*, a cutting]. Section of a fallopian tube.

salpingo-ureterostomy (săl-pĭng″ō-ūr-ēt″-ĕr-ŏs′tō-mĭ) [" + *ourēter*, ureter, + *stoma*, opening]. Surgical connection of the ureter and the fallopian tube.

salpingysterocyesis (săl-pĭn-jĭs″tĕr-ō-sī-ē′-sĭs) [" + *hystera*, uterus, + *kyēsis*, pregnancy]. Pregnancy partly in a fallopian tube and partly in the uterus.

salpinx (săl′pĭnks) (pl. *salpinges*) [G. *salpigx*]. The fallopian or eustachian tube.

salsify (săl′sĭ-fĭ) [Italian *sassefrica*, goat's beard]. COMP: Contains a compound of inulin. It is a fibrous food, heavier in carbohydrates, protein and fat than carrots, turnips, beets or celery, but it contains less ash than any of them.
Av. SERVING: 100 Gm. Pro. 3.5, Fat 1.0, Carbo. 15.5.
ACTION: Laxative.

salt (sawlt) [A.S. *sealt*]. SYMB: NaCl. 1. White crystalline compound occurring in nature, known chemically as sodium chloride. 2. Containing, tasting of, or treated with salt. 3. To treat with salt. 4. *plural*. Any mineral salt or saline mixture used as an aperient or cathartic, esp. Epsom salts or Glauber's salt. 5. CHEM: A compound consisting of a positive ion other than hydrogen, and a negative ion other than hydroxyl. 6. A chemical compound, usually crystalline, resulting from the interaction of an acid and a base.
RS: *chlorite, normal, rheum, sal, saline, salt-free diet, salt glow, secretion, "sial-"* words.

Natural or common table salt contains sodium chloride (NaCl) with potassium, calcium, and magnesium combinations, and is a necessary ingredient of food. In the preparation of commercial salts, only the sodium chloride remains, with the result that prolonged use in some disturbs the cation* relation which impoverishes the body's potassium, calcium, and magnesium supply, resulting in alteration of the colloid structure of the cells, and disturbing their conduction of, and response to, stimuli. This may set up sympathetic disturbances, such as skin stigmata and allergic diseases.

An equilibrated mixture possessing the same cation relationship as that of blood serum has been used with marked beneficial effect in various forms of dermatitis and in cutaneous tuberculosis. This mixture consists of: Sodium, 32.51%; calcium, 1.42%; magnesium, 0.86%; potassium, 2.7%; chloride, 52.63%; lactate, 3.79%, and citrate, 0.50%.

SOURCES: The sodium chloride of common salt is combined with the chlorine found in foods and with that in the blood and other body fluids, which have a content of 0.85% of these elements or 0.15% of sodium and 0.15% chlorine. They are found in meat, fruits, vegetables, and eggs esp.

Salt also contains impurities that are valuable, such as fluorine, arsenic, bromide and iodide. The process of refining makes some slight changes in salt. Fine salt has less arsenic and iron and iodine than coarse salt and is less valuable for hygienic reasons.

The system is deficient in sodium chloride, so that 2 Gm. per day of common salt seem necessary to maintain the balance required, but it is estimated that 4 to 10 times the necessary amount is consumed by the average person.

ACTION (Physiological): Hydrochloric acid in the stomach is not derived from the sodium chloride in the blood but from the salt in foods. In the intestines it brings about isotonia,* or the maintenance of an equal blood tension, the various salts maintaining normal osmotic pressure in the tissues. It oxidates the unassimilated food substances and moderates the movement of nitrogenous disassimilation. According to Gourund, it may have something to do with the fermentation of hemoglobin and red blood corpuscles.

An excess of salt of potassium is found in foods, esp. vegetables, and this splits sodium chloride into potassium chloride and sodium phosphate which are eliminated from the body as foreign substances, thus creating a loss in sodium chloride which already is deficient in the body. Without salt, less vegetables containing potassium, such as potatoes, would be eaten. Sodium chloride aids the kidneys in eliminating urea, the amines, and leukomaines and glucose in diabetes. An excess of salt causes an infiltration of the tissues and serous cavities, and in some cases causes car-

salt, buffer   S-7   **Salzer's double test meal**

diac fatigue, sluggish pulse, hypertension and nephritis. A decrease in use of salt may decrease the water in the tissues and overstimulate the digestive tract. Salt also increases protein catabolism.

IND: Teaspoonful in a glass of water for colds. May be increased in tuberculosis, dyspepsia from insufficiency, hyperchlorhydria, Addison's disease, lymphangitis and scrofula. In gout it acts as a solvent of uric acid. It is used internally in treatment of severe burns, in prolonged vomiting after abdominal operation, in diabetic acidosis and in strangulation of the bowels, and in cramps, *q.v.*

CONTRA: Discard in nephritis or use very little. Reduce its use in scarlatina to avoid renal complications; also in dropsy, cardiac and hepatic affections with ascites, and in arterial hypertension, infectious phlebitis, hyperchlorhydria and obesity, its use should be curtailed. Prohibit in epilepsy.

   s., buffer. A salt found in the blood which fixes excess amounts of acid or alkali, without a change in hydrogen-ion concentration.

   s., Epsom. Magnesium sulfate.

   s., Glauber's. Sodium sulfate.

   s., iodized. Salt containing 1 part sodium or potassium iodide to 5000 parts of sodium chloride.

   s., Rochelle. Sodium and potassium tartrate.

   s., rock. Native sodium chloride.

   s. solution, normal. SEE: *physiological salt solution.*

   s. s., physiological. Solution containing 0.9% of salt, which resembles in density the proportion in the blood. SYN: *saline solution.*

A stimulant to heart and vasomotor centers and increases bulk of fluid in blood vessels. It increases all secretions of the body. Its action on kidneys is important, as it is a powerful nonirritant diuretic.

Made by adding 1 teaspoonful of salt to a pint of water. This has approximately the same salt tension as the blood plasma, *i. e.*, 0.9%. May be administered by bowel, subcutaneously, or intravenously. Used in the treatment of shock and where hemorrhage has occurred, as it increases the volume of the plasma.

When cold baths are not tolerated well, to reduce high temperatures, enemas of salt solution and ice are sometimes effectual. When there is suppression of urine, and dropsy is not present, it often has a good effect, administered hot, in uremic conditions.

NP: When salt solution is given intravenously or hypodermically, rigid aseptic precautions must be observed. Usually injected in front of thighs or under breasts, as loose tissue is found in these areas. The temperature of the solution is about 100° F., so that when the blood is reached solution will be at body temperature. If the disadvantage of slowness is not very important, injection by rectum is the least risky, as it is not painful and there is no risk of infection. The patient placed on left side, hips are elevated by a pillow, and the solution, by means of a rectal tube, is injected into the rectum. The solution is allowed to run in at the rate of about 1 quart per hour.

saltation (săl-tā'shŭn) [L. *saltātio*, a leaping]. 1. Act of leaping or dancing, as in chorea. 2. Abrupt variation in character of a species. SYN: *mutation.* 3. A spurting forth of arterial blood.

saltatory (săl'ta-tō-rĭ) [L. *saltātio*, a leaping]. Marked by dancing or leaping.

   s. spasm. Tic of muscles of lower extremity, causing convulsive leaping upon attempt to stand. SEE: *palmus.*

salt-free diet. One with no more than 2 Gm. of salt allowed, as in *edema.*

Bread and butter must also be salt-free. No salt added to food eaten. Permissible foods: 1. Milk. 2. Eggs. 3. Custards. 4. Bread. 5. Omelettes. 6. Gelatin and jellies. 7. Meat jelly. 8. Butter (salt-free). 9. Fat meat. 10. Cheese. 11. Sugar. 12. Vegetables. 13. Buttermilk. 14. Whey. 15. Fruit jellies. 16. Chocolate or cocoa. 17. Flavors and spices.

NOTE: The stage of fever in which the heavier of these foods may be taken depends upon the physician's orders.

RS: *salt, sodium chloride.*

salt glow. Name given to a rub of the entire body with moist salt for stimulation.

salt, low diet. No salt allowed on patient's tray. No salty food served.

   s. poor diet. All food prepared and served without the addition of salt, including salt-free bread and butter. Milk intake is limited. Protein caloric fluid level governed by orders of physician.

saltpeter (sawlt"pē'ter) [O.Fr. *salpetre*, from L. *sal*, salt, + *petra*, rock]. A common name for potassium nitrate.

   s., chile. A common name for sodium nitrate. NaNO₃. Crystalline powder, saline in taste and soluble in water.

USES: In diarrhea.

DOSAGE: 1-2 drams (4-8 Gm.).

salt rheum (sawlt room). Any one of a variety of skin affections of the eczematous type. SEE: *eczema.*

salts. Plural of salt. SEE: *salt*, 4.

salubrious (săl-ū'brĭ-ŭs) [L. *salubris*, healthy]. Promoting or favorable to health. SYN: *wholesome.*

salutary (săl'ū-ta-rĭ) [L. *salutaris*, healthy]. Healthful; promoting health; curative.

salvarsan (săl'var-săn) [L. *salvus*, saved, + G. *arsen*, arsenic]. An arsenical, yellowish powder preparation (606) given intramuscularly or intravenously for syphilis.

RS: *arsphenamine, autoserosalvarsan, neoarsphenamine.*

salvatella (săl-văt-ĕl'ă) [L.]. A small vein on the dorsum of the little finger and hand. SYN: *vena salvatella.*

salve (săv) [A.S. *sealf*]. 1. An ointment applied to wounds. 2. PHARM: Any ointment or cerate made with a base of a fat, oil, petrolatum, resin, etc.

salyrgan (săl-ĭr'găn). A synthetic mercurial compound containing about 40% mercury.

ACTION AND USES: Chiefly a diuretic.

DOSAGE: 10% solution intravenously or intramuscularly, 8 ℳ (0.5 cc.) increased to 1 cc. or a maximum of 2 cc., if required. Injections are made at intervals of 3-5 days. SYN: *mersalyl.*

   s. suppositories. Each suppository contains 0.4 Gm. salyrgan.

USES: Same as salyrgan intramuscularly, but given rectally.

DOSAGE: 1 suppository.

Salzer's double test meal (sahlz'er). Beef, 40 Gm., scraped and broiled; milk, 250 cc.; boiled rice, 50 Gm.; 1 soft cooked egg. Four hours later give Ewald-Boas test meal and express 1 hour later.

sanative (săn'ă-tĭv) [L. *sanāre*, to heal]. Of a healing nature. SYN: *curative*.

sanatorium (săn-ă-tō'rĭ-ŭm) (pl. *sanatoriums* or *-ria*) [L. *sanatōrius*, healing]. An establishment for preservation of health or the treatment of the chronically sick; esp. a private one. SYN: *sanitarium*.

sanatory (săn'ă-tō-rĭ) [L. *sanatōrius*, healing]. Curative; conducive to health.

sand (sănd) [A.S.]. Fine grains of disintegrated rock.
  s., auditory. Calcareous concretion in labyrinth of the ear. SYN: *otolith*.
  s. bath. Therapeutic covering of the body with hot sand.
  s., brain. Concretion of matter near base of the pineal gland. SYN: *acervulus cerebri*.
  s. tumor. One in membrane of the brain, choroid plexus, and other areas made up of calcareous particles. SYN: *psammoma*.

Sand'with's bald tongue. Abnormally clean tongue seen in late stages of pellagra.

sane (sān) [L. *sanus*, sane, healthy]. Sound of mind; mentally normal.

Sänger's operation (seng'er). A form of cesarean section by which the uterus is taken out before the fetus.

sanguicolous (săng-gwĭk'ō-lŭs) [L. *sanguis*, blood, + *colere*, to dwell]. Inhabiting the blood, as a parasite.

sanguifacient (săng-gwĭf-ā'shĕnt) [" + *facere*, to make]. Making blood.

sanguiferous (săng-gwĭf'ĕr-ŭs) [" + *ferre*, to carry]. Conducting blood, as the circulatory organs.

sanguification (săng-gwĭf-ĭk-ā'shŭn) [" + *facere*, to make]. Conversion into, or formation of, blood. SYN: *hematopoiesis*.

sanguimotor, sanguimotory (săng'gwĭ-mō'tor, -tō-rĭ) [" + *motor*, a mover]. Pert. to the blood circulation.

sanguinal (săng'gwĭn-ăl) [L. *sanguis*, blood]. A blood preparation used in chlorosis and anemia.
  Evaporated blood and hemoglobin in liquid form consisting of 46 parts of natural blood salts, oxyhemoglobin, 10 parts, and 44 parts of peptonized muscle albumni.

sanguine (săng'gwĭn) [L. *sanguineus*, bloody]. 1. Hopeful. 2. Plethoric, bloody; marked by abundance and active blood circulation. 3. Pert. to or consisting of blood.

sanguineous (săng-gwĭn'ē-ŭs) [L. *sanguineus*, bloody]. 1. Bloody; relating to blood. 2. Having an abundance of blood. SYN: *plethoric*.

sanguinolent (săng-gwĭn'ō-lĕnt) [L. *sanguinolentus*, from *sanguis*, blood]. Containing, or tinged with, blood.

sanguinopoietic (săng"gwĭn-ō-poy-ĕt'ĭk) [L. *sanguis*, blood, + *poiein*, to form]. Generating blood. SYN: *hematopoietic, sanguifacient*.

sanguirenal (săng"gwĭ-rē'năl) [" + *rēn*, kidney]. Pert. to the blood supply of the kidneys.

sanguis (săng'gwĭs) [L.]. Blood.

sanguisuga (săng-gwĭs-ū'gă) [L. *sanguis*, blood, + *sugere*, to suck]. A leech or bloodsucker. SEE: *Hirudo*.

sanies (sā'nĭ-ēz) [L.]. diseased blood]. A thin, fetid, greenish discharge from a wound or ulcer, presenting appearance of pus tinged with blood.

saniopurulent (sā"nĭ-ō-pū'rū-lĕnt) [L. *sanies*, diseased blood, + *purulentus*, full of pus]. Having characteristics of sanies and pus; pert. to a fetid, serous, blood-tinged discharge containing pus.

sanioserous (sā"nĭ-ō-sē'rŭs) [" + *serum*, whey]. Composed of sanies* and serum.

sanious (sā'nĭ-ŭs) [L. *sanies*, diseased blood]. Of the nature of fetid, purulent fluid from an ulcer; sanies.

sanitarium (săn-ĭ-tā'rĭ-ŭm) (pl. *sanitariums* or *-ria*) [L. *sanatōrius*, giving health]. Institution for treatment and recuperation of persons having physical or mental disorders; occasionally limited to place where conditions are prophylactic rather than therapeutic. SYN: *sanatorium*.

sanitary (săn'ĭ-tar-ĭ) [L. *sanitas*, health]. Promoting, or pert. to conditions improving health.

sanitation (săn"ĭ-tā'shŭn) [L. *sanitas*, health]. The use of measure to promote and establish conditions favorable to health, esp. public health. SEE: *assanation, hygiene*.

sanity (săn'ĭt-ĭ) [L. *sanitas*, health, from *sanus*, sound]. Soundness of health or mind; normal mentality. SEE: *sane*.

santal oil (săn'tăl) [L. *santalum*, sandalwood]. USP. Sandalwood oil. A volatile oil distilled from the wood of the plant.
  ACTION AND USES: Expectorant, local and genitourinary irritant with possible antiseptic properties.
  DOSAGE: 8 ℳ (0.5 cc.) in capsules.
  INCOMPATIBILITIES: Alkalies.

santonin (săn'tō-nĭn) [L. *santoninum*]. USP. A colorless crystalline substance obtained from the dried flower heads of the plant *santonica*.
  ACTION AND USES: A vermifuge against the roundworm.
  DOSAGE: 1 gr. (0.06 Gm.).

Santorini's canal (săn-tō-rē'nē). Same as *S's. duct*.
  S's. cartilage. Nodules of cartilage on tips of the arytenoid cartilages.
  S's. duct. An accessory duct of the pancreas.
  S's. fissures. A fissure in cartilage of the ext. auditory meatus and one in the tragus.
  S's. muscle. The risorius muscle, which compresses the cheek and draws angle of mouth out. SEE: *Table of Muscles in Appendix*.
  S's. veins. Veins from scalp passing to the cerebral sinus.

sap (săp) [A.S. *saep*]. 1. Any fluid essential to life and vitality of a living structure. 2. To cause gradual exhaustion of, as the strength.
  s., nuclear. Liquid portion of a cell nucleus. SYN: *karyolymph*.

saphena (să-fē'nă) (pl. *saphenae*) [G. *saphēnēs*, manifest]. Name given to two large veins of the leg.

saphenous (saf-ē'nŭs) [G. *saphēnēs*, visible]. Pert. to or associated with a saphenous vein or nerve in the leg.
  s. nerves. Two nerves accompanying each saphenous vein.
  s. opening. An aperture in the fascia, oval in shape, in inner and upper part of thigh transmitting the saphenous vein below Poupart's ligament. SYN: *fossa ovalis*.
  s. veins. Two veins, long and short, passing up the leg, the long from the foot to the saphenous opening, the short one behind outer malleolus up back of leg joining the popliteal. SEE: *vein*.

sapid (săp'ĭd) [L. *sapidus*, tasty]. Savory; tasty; opp. of insipid.

sapo (sā'pō) [L.]. USP. Soap prepared from pure olive oil and sodium hydroxide.

sapocrinin (săp″ō-krĭn′ĭn) [L. *sapo*, soap, + G. *krinein*, to separate]. The secretion of the intestinal mucous membrane after a soap enema or rub.

saponaceous (săp-ō-nā′shŭs) [L. *saponaceus*, soapy]. Soapy; resembling soap in feel or quality.

saponatus. (să-pō-na′tus). Mixed with soap.

saponification (sa-pŏn″ĭ-fĭ-kā′shŭn) [Fr. *saponifier*, from L. *sapo*, *sapōn-*, soap, + *-ficāre*, to make]. 1. Conversion into soap; chemically, the hydrolysis or the splitting of fat by an alkali yielding glycerol and 3 molecules of alkali salt of the fatty acid, the soap. 2. CHEM: Hydrolysis of an ester into corresponding alcohol and acid (free or in form of a salt).

s. number. In analysis of fats, the number of milligrams of potassium hydroxide needed to neutralize the fatty acids in 1 Gm. of oil or fat.

saponify (sa-pŏn′ĭ-fī) [L. *sapo*, *sapōn-*, soap, + *-ficāre*, to make]. To convert into a soap, as when fats are treated with an alkali to produce a free alcohol plus the salt of the fatty acid.

Thus, stearin, saponified with sodium hydroxide, yields the alcohol glycerol plus the soap sodium stearate.

saponin(e (săp′ō-nĭn, -nēn) [L. *sapo*, *sapōn-*, soap]. Unabsorbable glucoside contained in the roots of some plants forming a lather in an aqueous solution.

They are irritating and produce vomiting and diarrhea if taken internally.

saporific (săp″ō-rĭf′ĭk) [L. *saporificus*, producing taste]. Imparting a taste or flavor.

sapphism (săf′ĭzm) [G. *Sapphō*, Greek poetess]. Sexual desire of women for their own sex.

From Sappho, the reputed instigator of lesbianism.

RS: *amor lesbicus*, *homosexual*, *tribadism*, *urningism*.*

sapremia (săp-rē′mĭ-ă) [G. *sapros*, rotten, + *aima*, blood]. A toxic condition caused by the absorption into the blood of toxins or poisons produced by saprophytes or putrefactive bacteria. SEE: *septicemia*.

sapro- [G.]. Combining form meaning *putrid*.

saprodontia (săp-rō-dŏn′shĭ-ă) [G. *sapros*, rotten, + *odous*, *odont-*, tooth]. Caries of the teeth; tooth decay.

saprogen (săp′rō-jĕn) [" + *gennan*, to produce]. Any microörganism causing or produced by putrefaction.

saprogenic (săp″rō-jĕn′ĭk) [" + *gennan*, to produce]. Causing decay or resulting from it.

saprophilous (săp-rŏf′ĭl-ŭs) [" + *philein*, to love]. Living on decaying or dead substances, as a microörganism. SYN: *saprophytic*.

saprophyte (săp′rō-fīt) [G. *sapros*, rotten, + *phyton*, plant]. Any organism living on decaying or dead organic matter.

Most of the higher fungi are saprophytes. SEE: *parasite*.

saprophytic (săp-rō-fĭt′ĭk) [" + *phyton*, growth]. Living or growing in decaying or dead matter; characteristic of a saprophyte.

sapropyra (săp-rō-pī′ră) [" + *pyr*, fever, fire]. 1. Typhus fever. 2. Any fever caused by putrid infection. SYN: *saprotyphus*.

saprotyphus (săp″rō-tī′fŭs) [" + *typhos*, stupor]. 1. Putrid or typhus fever. 2. Fever due to putrid infection.

saprozoic (săp-rō-zō′ĭk) [" + *zōon*, animal]. Living on decaying or dead organic matter.

sarcin (sar′sĭn) [G. *sarx*, *sark-*, flesh]. A leukomaine found during decomposition of proteins in muscles and other tissues. SYN: *hypoxanthine*.

Sarcina (sar′sĭ-nă) [L. *sarcina*, bundle]. A genus of nonflagellated bacteria of the family *Coccaceae* which has cells dividing in 3 directions.

Majority are harmless and produce pigments.

S. ventriculi. S. found in the stomach of man.

sarcitis (sar-sī′tĭs) [G. *sarx*, flesh, + *-ītis*, inflammation]. Inflammation of muscle tissue. SYN: *myositis*.

sarco- [G.]. Combining form meaning *flesh*.

sarcoadenoma (sar″kō-ăd″en-ō′mă) [G. *sarx*, *sark-*, flesh, + *adēn*, gland, + *-ōma*, tumor]. A fleshy tumor of a gland. SYN: *adenosarcoma*.

sarcoblast (sar′kŏ-blăst) [" + *blastos*, a germ]. 1. A protoplasmic germinal mass. 2. Embryonic cell which develops into a muscle cell.

sarcocarcinoma (sar″kō-kar-sĭn-ō′mă) [" + *karkinos*, crab cancer, + *-ōma*, tumor]. A tumor of malignant growth of sarcomatous and carcinomatous types.

sarcocele (sar′kŏ-sēl) [" + *kēlē*, a mass]. A fleshy tumor of the testicle.

Sarcocystis (sar″kō-sĭs′tĭs) [" + *kystis*, bladder]. A genus of parasitic microörganisms found in the muscles of swine and other animals.

S. miescheriana. A parasite found in pork and beef.

sarcode (sar′kŏd) [G. *sarx*, *sark-*, flesh, + *eidos*, form]. Protoplasm of body of a unicellular animal.

Sarcodina (sar-kō-dī′nă) [" + *eidos*, form]. The lowest class of protozoa including the Amoebae.

sarcoenchondroma (sar″kō-ĕn-kŏn-drō′mă) [" + *en*, in, + *chondros*, cartilage, + *-ōma*, tumor]. Tumor composed of cartilaginous and fleshy elements. SEE: *enchondroma*, *sarcoma*.

sarcogenic (sar″kō-jĕn′ĭk) [" + *gennan*, to produce]. Producing flesh.

sarcoglia (sar-kŏg′lĭ-ă) [" + *glia*, glue]. Protoplasmic matter containing granules and nuclei composing the eminences of Doyen or point of entrance of a motor nerve into a muscular fiber.

sarcoid (sar′koyd) [" + *eidos*, form]. 1. A sarcomalike tumor. 2. Resembling flesh. 3. A nodule or plaque of the skin which leaves atrophic scars.

sarcolemma (sar″kō-lĕm′ă) [" + *lemma*, a rind]. A delicate membrane surrounding each striated muscle fiber. SEE: *muscle*.

sarcology (sar-kŏl′ō-jĭ) [G. *sarx*, *sark-*, flesh, + *logos*, a study]. Branch of medicine dealing with study of the soft tissues of the body.

sarcolysis (sar-kŏl′ĭ-sĭs) [" + *lysis*, a dissolution]. Decomposition of the soft tissues or flesh.

sarcolyte (sar′kŏ-līt) [" + *lyein*, to dissolve]. A multinucleated cell concerned in the decomposition of the soft tissues.

sarcolytic (sar′kō-lĭt′ĭk) [" + *lyein*, to dissolve]. Decomposing flesh.

sarcoma (sar-kō′mă) (pl. *sarcomas*, *-mata*) [G. *sarx*, *sark-*, flesh, + *-ōma*, tumor]. A tumor of nonepithelial, modi-

sarcoma, alveolar   **satyriasis**

fied, embryonic, connective tissue, esp. a malignant one.
  Sarcoma may affect the bones, bladder, kidneys, liver, lungs, parotids, and spleen.
  RS: *chloroma, sarcoid, words ending in "-sarcoma."*

  s., alveolar. S. principally in bone, skin, and muscle with largely developed stroma and alveoli.

  s., angiolithic. Small tumor containing granular calcareous concretions in the cerebral meninges.

  s., chondro-. One composed of masses of cartilage.

  s., fibro-. A malignant tumor with fibrous tissue and many spindle cells and dilated vessels.

  s., giant-celled. S. from cancellous bone tissue with large cells with many nuclei.

  s., lymphangio-. S. arising from endothelium of lymph vessels in a lymph gland.

  s., melanotic. S. containing melanin.

  s., myeloid. Same as giant-celled sarcoma.

  s., myxo-. A tumor of loose connective tissue containing a viscid fluid, mucin.

  s., osteo-. One composed of osseous tissue or bone containing variously shaped cells.

  s., round-cell. One containing small and large closely packed round cells resembling leukocytes.

  s., spindle-cell. One consisting of small and large spindle-shaped cells.

sarcomatoid (sar″kō′mă-toyd) [G. *sarx, sark-*, flesh, + *-ōma*, tumor, + *eidos*, form]. Resembling a sarcoma.

sarcomatosis (sar-kō-mă-tō′sĭs) [" + " + *-ōsis*, condition]. Condition marked by presence and spread of a sarcoma; sarcomatous degeneration.

sarcomatous (sar-kō′măt-ŭs) [" + *-ōma*, tumor]. Of the nature of, or like, a sarcoma.

sarcomere (sar′kō-mēr) [" + *meros*, a part]. A segment into which a muscle fibril is divided by transverse septa.

sarcomphalocele (sar-kŏm-făl′ō-sēl) [" + *omphalon*, umbilicus, + *kēlē*, mass]. Fleshy tumor at the umbilicus.

sarcophagy (sar-kŏf′ă-jī) [" + *phagein*, to eat]. Practice of eating flesh.

sarcoplasm (sar′kō-plăzm) [" + *plasma*, a thing formed]. Hyaline, semifluid, interfibrillary substance of striated muscle fibers.

sarcoplast (sar′kō-plăst) [G. *sarx, sark-*, flesh, + *plassein*, to form]. A cell bet. muscular fibrils developing into muscular fiber.

sarcopoietic (sar″kō-poy-ĕt′ĭk) [" + *poiein*, to form]. Forming muscle or flesh.

Sarcoptes (sar-kŏp′tēz) [" + *koptein*, to cut]. A genus of mites.

  S. scabiei. A species that produces the itch or scabies, *q.v.*

sarcosis (sar-kō′sĭs) [" + *-ōsis*, condition]. 1. The development of multiple fleshy tumors. 2. Abnormal formation of flesh.

sarcosome (sar′kō-sōm) [" + *sōma*, body]. Contractile part of a muscle fibril.

Sarcosporidia (sar″kō-spō-rĭd′ĭ-ă) [" + *sporos*, a seed]. An order of protozoans parasitic in muscle fiber.

sarcosporidiosis (sar″kō-spō-rĭd-ĭ-ō′sĭs) [" + " + *-ōsis*, condition]. Infestation with Sarcosporidia or condition produced by them.

sarcostosis (sar-kŏs-tō′sĭs) [" + *osteon*, bone, + *-ōsis*, condition]. Ossification of fleshy or muscular tissue.

sarcostyle (sar′kō-stīl) [G. *sarx, sark-*, flesh, + *stylos*, a column]. Any one of the fine longitudinal fibrillae of a striated muscle fiber.

sarcotherapeutics (sar″kō-ther-ă-pū′tĭks) [" + *therapeutikē*, art of healing]. Treatment of disease with animal extracts or glands. SYN: *organotherapy*.

sarcotherapy (sar″kō-ther′ă-pī) [" + *therapeia*, treatment]. Use of animal extracts and glands in treatment. SYN: *organotherapy, sarcotherapeutics.*

sarcotic (sar-kŏt′ĭk) [G. *sarx, sark-*, flesh]. 1. Producing or pert. to flesh formation. 2. Agent producing growth of flesh.

sarcous (sar′kŭs) [G. *sarx, sark-*, flesh]. Concerning flesh or muscle.

  s. element. One of the dark prisms of ultimate fibrils of striated muscle fibers.

  s. substance. Substance of a sarcous element.

sardine (sar-dēn′) [L. *sardina*]. AV. SERVING: 50 Gm. Pro. 9.6, Fat 12.8. VITAMINS: B+.

sardon′ic laugh. Old term for a spasmodic affection of facial muscles, giving an appearance of laughter. SYN: *risus sardonicus.*

sartorius (sar-tō′rĭ-ŭs) [L. *sartor*, tailor]. A long, ribbon-shaped muscle of the thigh.
  It aids in flexing the knee; longest muscle in the body. So-called from its use in crossing the legs, as tailors do. SEE: *Table of Muscles in Appendix.*

satellite (săt′ĕl-īt) [L. *satelles*, companion]. 1. ANAT: Structure associated with another, esp. vein accompanying an artery. 2. A tiny lesion near a big one.

satellitosis (săt-ĕl-ī-tō′sĭs) [" + *-ōsis*, condition]. Accumulation of free cell nuclei around the ganglion cells of the cortex of the brain, seen in paralysis and other affections.

satiety (sa-tī′ĕt-ĭ) [Fr. *satiété*, from L. *satis*, enough]. Fullness or gratification beyond desire.

saturated (săt′ū-rā-tĕd) [L. *saturāre*, to saturate]. Holding all of a substance that can be combined.

  s. compounds. Those incapable of additional products, as any in the methane series. SEE: *unsaturated compounds.*

  s. solution. One containing as much of the solid drug as it can dissolve.

saturation (săt″ū-rā′shŭn) [L. *saturatio*]. 1. The holding in solution of all of a solid that can be dissolved therein. 2. Administration of an erythema dose of radiant energy, followed by smaller doses for a period of time.

  s., high frequency. Rarely employed modification of a monoterminal high frequency treatment.

saturnine (săt′ŭr-nīn) [L. *saturnus*, lead]. Concerning or produced by lead.

  s. breath. Sweet breath produced by lead* poisoning.

saturnism (săt′ŭrn-ĭzm) [" + G. *ismos*, condition]. Lead poisoning, *q.v.*

satyriasis (sat-ĭ-rī′ă-sĭs) [G. *satyriasis*]. Great mental excitement with abnormal sex desire in the male.
  It is an acute abnormal psychosexual state, aggravated by psychical or peripheral irritation, neurasthenia, masturbation* and morbid ideas.
  Same as nymphomania* in the female. The symptoms are a partial expression of a general psychosis. The imagination calls forth sensual associations. Satyri-

asis is less frequent than nymphomania. Priapism* is frequently manifested.

satyromania (săt″ĭr-ō-mā′nĭ-ă) [G. *satyros*, satyr, + *mania*, madness]. Excessive sexual desire in the male. SYN: *satyriasis*.

Sauerbruch's cabinet (sow′ĕr-brook). An airtight cabinet for operation on the chest under negative pressure.

The patient's head is outside the cabinet and his body and the surgeon's are within it.

sauerkraut (sow′ĕr-krowt) [Ger. *sauer*, sour, + *kraut*, cabbage]. Av. SERVING: 100 Gm. Pro. 1.5, Fat 0.4, Carbo. 3.5.
VITAMINS: A+, B+, C+ to ++. Ca 0.040, P 0.010, Fe 0.0032.

sauriasis (saw-rī′ăs-ĭs) [G. *sauros*, a lizard, + *-iasis*, infection]. Ichthyosis* with marked thickness of the skin.

sauriderma (saw-rĭ-der′mă) [" + *derma*, skin]. Skin disease with thick, elevated scale formation. SYN: *ichthyosis hystrix*.

sauriosis (saw-rĭ-ō′sĭs) [" + *-osis*, condition]. Cutaneous disorder in which there is cornification of epithelial layers. SYN: *ichthyosis*.

sausage (saw′saj) (pork) [M.E. *sausige*]. Av. SERVING: 35 Gm. Pro. 4.6, Fat 15.5, Carbo. 0.4.
VITAMINS: A— to +, B++.

Savill's disease (sā′vĭl). An epidemic skin disease with papular rash, followed by branny desquamation. May be fatal. SYN: *dermatitis exfoliativa epidemica, epidemic eczema*.

Saviotti's canals (sah-vē-ŏt′ĭ). Artificially formed passages bet. secreting cells of pancreas.

savory (sā′vō-rĭ) [O.Fr. *savouré*, tasty]. Having a pleasant or appetizing taste or odor.

saw (saw) [A.S. *sagu*]. Instrument for cutting, esp. bone, its cutting edge being toothed.

saxifragant (săks-ĭf′răg-ănt) [L. *saxum*, rock, + *frangere*, to break]. Dissolving or breaking calculi, esp. in the bladder.

Sayre's jacket (sārz). A jacket of plaster-of-Paris worn to support the spine in vertebral diseases.

Sb. Symb. for *antimony*.

SbCl₃. Antimony trichloride.

Sb₂O₅. Antimonic oxide; antimony pentoxide.

Sb₄O₆. Antimonious oxide.

scab (skăb) [M.E. *scabbe*]. 1. Crust of a cutaneous sore, wound, ulcer or pustule formed by drying up of the discharge. 2. To become covered with a crust.

scabies (skā′bĭ-ēs) [L. *scabere*, to scratch]. 1. A skin disease caused by an animal parasite, the Acarus scabei. SYN: *itch*. 2. A form of vesicles associated with pustules.

SYM: Papules, vesicles, pustules, burrows and intense itching resulting in eczema. The burrows are discolored, dotted, slightly elevated lines, ranging from ¼ line to ½ line in length, produced by female Acarus and the deposition of her eggs along the passage.

Parts most commonly affected are hands, bet. the fingers, the wrists, axillae, genitalia, beneath the mammae and inner aspect of the thighs. Face and scalp never involved.

PROG: Favorable.

TREATMENT: Take a small strip of white flannel, roll tightly, tie in center, dip end in oil of lavender, rub thoroughly on all parts occupied by the parasite for about 5 minutes night and morning. In 4 to 8 days not a living parasite will be found.

Then give general internal treatment if required, or rub patient thoroughly with soft soap for ½ hr., then give warm bath and when dry rub all over with a solution of 2 parts liquid storax and 1 part glycerine.

Two or 3 repetitions will suffice for a cure in most cases. Externally, parasiticides followed by soothing applications to dermatitis. Remedies to be selected with care to prevent injury to host.

scabrities (skă-brĭsh′ĭ-ēz) [L.]. 1. Scaly, roughened condition of the skin. 2. A morbid roughness of inner surface of eyelids, causing sensation as if sand were in eyes.

s. unguium. Morbid degeneration of the nails, making them rough, thick, distorted and separated from the flesh at the root. Symptomatic of syphilis and leprosy.

scala (skā′lă) [L. ladder]. Any one of the 3 spiral passages of the cochlea. SEE: *ear*.

s. media. It contains the organ of Corti.

s. tympani. BNA. The part of the spiral canal of the cochlea which is situated below the lamina spiralis.

s. vestibuli. BNA. The part of the spiral canal above the lamina spiralis.

scald (skawld) [M.E. *scalden*, from L. *ex*, out, + *calidus*, hot]. 1. Burn to skin or flesh caused by moist heat and hot vapors, as steam. 2. To cause a burn with hot liquid or steam. 3. Cutaneous disease marked by scab formation on the head.

It is deeper than dry heat, and should be treated as a burn, *q.v.* Healing is slower and scar formation greater. SEE: *burn*.

scald head (skawld′ hĕd). Any one of several contagious affections of the scalp excited by Achorion Schönleinii.

SYM: Disease is characterized by 1 or more rounded, yellow, cup-shaped crusts through which project dry, brittle, lusterless hairs. Scaling. Underlying tissue is more or less atrophied and scarred. Associated with some itching, and a peculiar, musty odor. Specially observed in poor, ill-nourished children.

PROG: Favorable. When not treated early it may be followed by permanent baldness.

TREATMENT: Crusts should be removed by oil, or soap and water; affected hairs removed; parasiticides, as mercury, sulfur, are generally used. Child should be cared for hygienically and general health looked after; nourishing food; head kept cool. SEE: *favus*.

scale (skāl) [A.S. *sceale*, scale]. 1. A small, thin, dry exfoliation shed from upper layers of skin. 2. Film of tartar incrusting the teeth. 3. To form a scale on. 4. To shed scales.

5. [M.E. *scole*, balance]. An instrument for weighing.

6. [L. *scala*, ladder]. A graduated or proportioned measure, series of tests, or instrument for measuring quantities or for rating, as individual intelligence. SEE: *Binet*.

Shedding of scales from skin in small amounts is normal. It is also seen in cutaneous disorders such as squamous eczema, seborrhea sicca, psoriasis, ichthyosis, syphilis, lupus erythematosus, pityriasis rosea, and tinea tonsurans. SEE: *macule, rash*.

s., absolute. A scale used for indicating low temperatures based on absolute zero. SEE: *absolute temperature, a. zero*.

s., centigrade. Thermometric scale running from 0°, the melting point of ice, and 100°, the boiling point of water. SEE: *centigrade, thermometer*.

s., Fahrenheit. One in which the freezing point of water is 32° and the boiling point is 212°. SEE: *Fahrenheit, thermometer*.

s., Réamur. Scale which runs bet. freezing point of water at 0° and the boiling point at 80°. SEE: *Réamur, thermometer*.

scalene (skā-lēn') [G. *skalēnos*, uneven]. 1. Having unequal sides and angles, said of a triangle. 2. Designating a scalenus muscle.

s. tubercle. One on upper surface of 1st rib, the insertion of the scalenus anticus muscle. SYN: *Lisfranc's tubercle*.

scaleniotomy (skā-lēn"ĭ-ŏt'ō-mĭ) [" + *tomē*, a cutting]. Incision of scalenus muscles near their insertion to check expansive movements in tuberculosis of the apex of the lung.

scalenus (skā-lē'nŭs) [L. from G. *skalēnos*, uneven]. One of 3 deeply situated muscles on each side of the neck, extending from the transverse processes of 2 or more cervical vertebrae to the 1st or 2nd rib; known as scalenus anterior, medius, posterior. SEE: *Table of Muscles in Appendix*.

s. anticus syndrome, s. syndrome. A symptom complex characterized by brachial neuritis with or without vascular or vasomotor disturbance in the upper extremities.

The pathological condition is due to mechanical irritation or pressure on the brachial plexus and subclavian artery. Diagnosis is made primarily in the presence of clinical symptoms in the upper extremities which are influenced by posture.

SYM: Not clearly defined, but pain, tingling and numbness may occur anywhere from shoulder to fingers. Atrophy of small muscles of the hand or even the deltoid or other muscles of arm. Circulatory changes are less frequently observed than neurological symptoms.

TREATMENT: Since posture, stature, and muscular fatigue affect severity of symptoms, conservative treatment. Correction of posture, avoidance of fatigue and sometimes immobilization of arm and shoulder. When relief is not obtained, operative interference may be considered.

scall (skawl) [O. Norse *skalli*, a bald head]. A crusty eruption of the skin or scalp. SYN: *favus, impetigo, eczema, psoriasis*.

scalp (skălp) [M.E.]. The hairy integument of the head.

In anat. includes skin, dense subcutaneous tissue, occipitofrontalis muscle with the galea aponeurotica, loose subaponeurotic tissue and the cranial periosteum.

RS: *cranium, dandruff, folliculitis, hair, head, porrigo, scald head*.

scalpel (skăl'pĕl) [L. *scalpellum*, little knife]. A straight, small surgical knife with a convex edge and thin, keen blade.

scalpriform (skăl'prĭ-form) [L. *scalprum*, chisel, + *forma*, shape]. In the shape of a chisel.

scalprum (skăl'prŭm) (pl. *scalpra*) [L. *scalprum*, knife]. 1. A toothed instrument for removal of carious bone or for trephining. 2. A large scalpel. 3. Cutting edge of an incisor tooth.

scaly (skā'lĭ) [A.S. *sceale*, scale]. Resembling or characterized by scales.

scan'ning speech. Pronunciation of words in syllables, or slowly and hesitatingly; a symptom of disseminated sclerosis.* SEE: *speech*.

scanty (skăn'tĭ) [M.E. *skant*, short]. Not abundant; insufficient, as a secretion.

scapha (skā'fă) [L. from G. *skaphē*, boat]. BNA. Elongated depression of the ear bet. the helix and antehelix.

scapho- [G.]. Combining form meaning boat.

scaphocephalic, scaphocephalous (skăf"ō-sĕf-ăl'ĭk, -sĕf'ăl-ŭs) [G. *skaphē*, boat, + *kephalē*, head]. Having a deformed head, projecting like a boat's keel.

scaphocephalism (skăf"ō-sĕf'ăl-ĭzm) [" + " + *-ismos*, condition]. Condition of having a deformed head, projecting like the keel of a boat.

scaphoid (skăf'oyd) [" + *eidos*, resemblance]. 1. A proximal, boat-shaped bone of the carpus on radial side. SYN: *os scaphoides*. 2. A boat-shaped bone on inner side of the tarsus between the astragalus and 3 cuneiform bones. 3. Boat-shaped, navicular, hollowed.

s. abdomen. One with hollowed anterior wall.

s. bone. SEE: *scaphoid, 1 and 2*.

scaphoiditis (skăf-oyd-ī'tĭs) [G. *skaphē*, boat, + *eidos*, form, + *-itis*, inflammation]. Inflamed condition of the scaphoid bone.

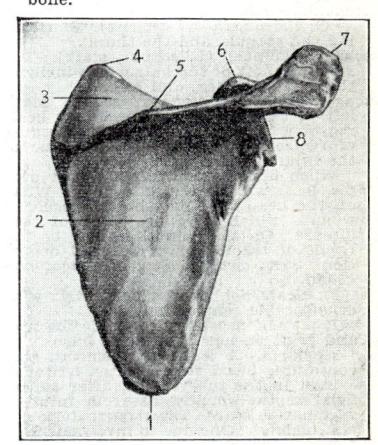

SCAPULA.
1. Inferior angle. 2. Infraspinatous fossa. 3. Supraspinatous fossa. 4. Superior angle. 5. Spine. 6. Coracoid process. 7. Acromion process. 8. Anterior angle.

scapula (skăp'ū-lă) (pl. *scapulae, -as*) [L. shoulder blade]. The large, flat, triangular bone of the shoulder.

It articulates with the clavicle and the humerus. SYN: *shoulder blade*. SEE: *triceps for illustration*.

RS: *acromial, a. angle, acromioclavicular, acromiocoracoid, acromion, angel's wing, glenoid cavity*.

scapula alata

s. alata. Winglike appearance of the scapula in thin and weak muscled persons.

scapulalgia (skăp-ū-lăl'jĭ-ă) [L. *scapula,* + G. *algos,* pain]. Pain in the region of the shoulder blade.

scapular (skăp'ū-lar) [L. *scapula,* shoulder blade]. Of or pert. to the shoulder blade.

s. reflex. Scapular muscular contraction following percussion or stimulus bet. the scapulas.

scapulary (skăp'ū-la-rĭ) [L. *scapula,* shoulder blade]. A shoulder bandage bifurcated with the 2 ends over the shoulders, the single end passing down the back, the 3 fastened to a body bandage.

scapulectomy (skăp-ū-lĕk'tō-mĭ) [" + G. *ektomē,* excision]. Surgical excision of the scapula.

scapulo- [L.]. Combining form meaning *shoulder.*

scapuloclavicular (skăp″ū-lō-klă-vĭk'ū-lar) [L. *scapula,* shoulder blade, + *clavicula,* a little key]. Concerning the scapula and the clavicle.

scapulodynia (skăp″ū-lō-dĭn'ĭ-ă) [" + *odynē,* pain]. Inflammation and pain in the shoulder muscles.

scapulohumeral (skăp″ū-lō-hū'mer-ăl) [" + *humerus,* shoulder]. Concerning the scapula and the humerus.

s. reflex. When inner margin of scapula is percussed upper arm is adducted and rotated outwards.

scapulopexy (skăp″ū-lō-pĕks'ĭ) [" + G. *pexis,* fixation]. Fixation of the scapula to the ribs.

scapulothoracic (skăp″ū-lō-thō-răs'ĭk) [" + G. *thōrax, thōrak-,* chest]. Concerning the scapula and the thorax.

scapus (skā'pŭs) [L. *scapus,* stalk]. The stem or shaft of the hair which includes the *cuticle, cortex,* and *medulla.*

scar (skar) [G. *eschara,* scab]. Mark left in skin or internal organ by healing of a wound, sore or injury because of replacement by connective tissue of the injured tissue.

When first developed it is red or purple, later whitish and glistening. When on the head they may be the result of wounds which have healed or of skin disease. On the skin they may be the result of trauma or of surgical operation. SYN: *cicatrix.* SEE: *cicatricotomy, keloid.*

s., cicatricial. A scar or cicatrix with considerable contraction.

It may be necessary to divide the scar and graft on new skin, as in burns.

s., keloid. A red, raised, smooth scar containing blood vessels, often irritable.

Seen in the tuberculous, after superficial septic wounds, as from infected vaccination scars. TREATMENT: Removal.

s., painful. One due to involvement of a nerve during healing.

The end of the nerve may become bulbous. TREATMENT: Dissection of scar or excision of nerve.

scarfskin (skarf'skĭn) [Fr. *écharpe,* scarf, + O. Norse *skinn*]. Epidermis* or outermost layer of the skin.

scarification (skăr-ĭ-fĭ-kā'shŭn) [L. *scarificatio,* from G. *skariphasthai,* to scratch]. Making of numerous slight incisions in the skin, over a part.

scarificator (skăr'ĭf-ĭk-ā-tor) [L. from G. *skariphasthai,* to scratch]. Instrument for making small incisions in the skin.

scarifier (skăr'ĭ-fĭ-er) [L. *scarificator*]. Instrument used for withdrawal of blood by incision with circular cutting edge and blades operated by springs.

scarlatina (skar-lă-tē'nă) [L. *scarlatina,* from *scarlatum,* red]. An acute, contagious disease characterized by sore throat, fever, punctiform scarlet rash, and rapid pulse. SYN: *scarlet fever.*

ETIOL: Streptococcus, hemolyticus scarlatinae, a hemolytic streptococcus described by the Dicks. Susceptibility may be determined with fair degree of accuracy by means of the Dick test. This is a skin test, the technic of which is practically the same as that of the Schick test. The material for the Dick test consists of a toxic filtrate obtained from the specific scarlet fever hemolytic streptococci. This is diluted 1:1000 and 1/10 cc. is injected intracutaneously. If the individual is susceptible, an area of erythema at least 5/10 cm. in diameter should be present at the point of injection 24 hr. after the test. The absence of such a reaction signifies that the patient is immune.

INCUBATION: Probably never less than 24 hr. May be from 1 to 10 days, with average time of from 2 to 4 days.

SYM: Onset sudden, rarely with a chill, but sometimes with a convulsion in very young children. As a rule, begins with sore throat, temperature from 103° to 104° F., frequent vomiting, followed within 12 to 36 hr. by a rash, first on neck and chest, rapidly extends over body, lastly involving the extremities. Face flushed and may be characterized by the well-known circumoral pallor, the punctiform rash on the remainder of the body, seldom seen on face.

With first eruption, throat is markedly injected, tonsils are swollen, tongue heavily coated, and the papillae are enlarged, projecting through it; the tongue properly described as a "strawberry" tongue. In mild or average case duration of rash is from 2 to 3 days. By the end of 3rd day, the coating has disappeared from tongue, though the papillae are still enlarged, the remainder of tongue presenting a deep red appearance. In this stage, the tongue may be referred to as the "raspberry" tongue.

With disappearance of rash in an uncomplicated case, the temperature closely approaches normal and recovery is uneventful. Extremely mild cases occur in which the rash is very faint and of very short duration, possibly not exceeding 24 hr. Scarlet fever may actually occur without any rash whatsoever. In any form, a leukocytosis is to be expected in the average case. Number of leukocytes may range from 14,000 to 16,000.

MALIGNANT TYPES: *Anginose*: In this form, attention is focused primarily on severity of throat symptoms, the entire mucosa of which may be markedly edematous due to the inflammatory condition. The tissues of the neck are markedly swollen, resulting in a cellulitis, with a brawny cervical induration. Swelling may be so intense that respiratory embarrassment is marked, and a severe degree of toxemia present. Temperature may range from 104° F. upward. Lips sometimes cyanotic and delirium may exist. Membranous patches or sloughs on tonsils or in the pharynx, and profuse nasal discharge may develop. Unusual rapidity of pulse often forecasts the inevitable outcome common in cases of this kind.

Septic: Under this classification are those cases of s. f. in which suppurative processes seem to exist almost from the beginning. Mastoiditis, cervical adenitis, and sometimes suppurative arthritis, which is usually rare in scarlet fever, are seen early in the disease. Sinusitis is also frequent, and though the patient's condition appears desperate from the very onset, chances of final recovery are frequently fairly good after a tedious struggle for existence, which may be prolonged for many weeks.

Toxic: Although this term is frequently applied to various forms of s. f. it should designate that type in which the toxemia is so overwhelming that death often ensues before any rash appears. Diagnosis of this form may be largely dependent on the history of exposure, the unusually high fever, which may rise from 106° to 107° F., and the throat symptoms, as well as early delirium or coma.

COMPLICATIONS: While albuminuria is an ordinary accompaniment of s. f., nephritis, which has always been so closely associated with this disease, is undoubtedly far less frequent than it was many years ago. When nephritis develops, it is most likely to occur during the 2nd or 3rd week of the disease, though at times it comes on long after all acute symptoms have subsided. When there is renal involvement, it is usually a hemorrhagic nephritis. Although a favorable conclusion may be expected, the possibility of uremia must be considered.

Much more frequent complications are otitis media, cervical adenitis, mastoiditis, sinusitis, arthritis; less often, endocarditis, pneumonia, peritonsillar abscess; rarely, a sinus thrombosis, brain abscess, and cancrum oris. May affect any of the personality glands later in life.

DIFFERENTIAL DIAG: Measles, German measles, diphtheria, drug and serum rashes, urticarias of various types, as well as toxic erythemas, may cause confusion. Acute pharyngitis and streptococcic sore throat sometimes present delicate problems in diagnosis.

PROG: Depends chiefly on severity of infection, although severe complications sometimes follow types of the disease that are apparently mild. The fatality rate in any epidemic will be dependent upon type of infection that predominates. In the United States and the European countries, the fatality rate in recent years has ranged very close to 3%, which is about 60% lower than some 30 years ago.

TREATMENT: Active immunization against s. f. may now be accomplished by means of the toxin preparation introduced by the Dicks. Five subcutaneous injections are given at weekly intervals and immunity, which is generally established soon after the final dose, is said to endure for a number of years.

SERUM THERAPY: In the active case, consideration must be given to use of s. f. antitoxin. In the mild case, this form of therapy is not required. The value of s. f. antitoxin in severe cases, while received very enthusiastically by some, is not at this time universally accepted, although it frequently appears to be markedly beneficial in the toxic type of s. f. Convalescent s. f. serum (not available for the general practitioner) is unquestionably of great value in the treatment of s. f. In the use of either serum, it is of the utmost advantage to administer it at the earliest possible time, preferably not later than the 3rd day of the rash. Either of these serums when used are injected intramuscularly.

Gamma globulin and the broad spectrum antibiotics have all been used with good effect.

GENERAL TREATMENT: Isolation, rest, and diet are of utmost importance. *Rest*: Keep the uncomplicated case in bed for a minimum of 2 weeks. The course of attack will determine whether this period of rest should be prolonged. While antiseptic mouthwashes often have a place for cleansing purposes, and serve to refresh the patient to some extent, gargles are not advisable. Occasionally, when itching of the skin is troublesome, olive oil or cocoa butter may be applied. Except in the case of nephritics, hot packs or cold sponging for purpose of lowering temperature should not be used. Laxatives or cathartics must not be neglected when indicated. Routine use of sodium citrate in 10- to 15-gr. doses 3 times daily throughout the course of the disease is beneficial. This may be augmented by addition of an equal amount of sodium bicarbonate. Complications will necessarily be treated as they arise in accordance with their requirements. No surgical interference that would be required in a noncontagious case should be avoided because of the presence of s. f.

DIET: During first few days when throat is highly inflamed, have patient on liquid diet of fruit juices, clear soups without beef stock, milk, orangeade or lemonade, and plenty of water. When temperature reaches normal level, or approximately so, which is usually by the close of a week in the uncomplicated case, a vegetable diet with the continuation of fruit juices and plenty of water, may be ordered. As a rule, exclude red meats until after the 4th week, although not an absolute necessity in all cases. Frequent examinations of urine. Results of these will determine, to some extent, the diet to be provided. *During temperature*: Milk, water, plus fruit syrup or juice, white of egg, and lemon water. *After temperature is normal*: If able to swallow, oatmeal gruel, farinaceous foods, arrowroot, blancmange, jelly, custard, isinglass, raw eggs, beef tea or soup. *Convalescence*: About 3rd or 4th week: Fish, chicken, rabbit, potatoes, cooked fruit, oranges, grapes.

QUARANTINE: Regulated by different states, and it is difficult to set any arbitrary time as suitable for all patients. Evidence of the desquamative process at end of 4 weeks carries no significance in relation to the contagiousness of the disease. It is not the desquamating patient ordinarily who is a menace to the public, but the patient who has a discharging ear or nose who is very likely to transmit infection to susceptibles when coming in contact with them, even though his convalescence has been prolonged over a period of months. From the standpoint of absolute safety, it would be proper to determine that the s. f. patient is free of hemolytic streptococci before being released from quarantine. This can be done to a fair degree by obtaining cultures from the nose, throat, discharging ears, or glands on blood agar plates to determine whether

or not such patient continues to harbor hemolytic streptococci.
  s. anginosa. S. with throat symptoms. SEE: *scarlatina.*
  s. haemorrhagica. S. with blood extravasated into mucous membranes and the skin.
  s. latens. S. without rash, but complicated by nephritis.
  s. maligna. S. with great prostration and severe symptoms. SEE: *scarlatina.*
  s. rheumatica. S. with severe pain. SYN: *dengue.*
scarlatinal (skar-lă-tē'năl) [L. *scarlatum*, red]. Concerning or due to scarlatina.
scarlatinella (skar-lă-tĭn-el'lă) [L.]. A mild disease resembling measles and scarlet fever. SYN: *fourth disease, rubella scarlatinosa.*
scarlatiniform, scarlatinoid (skar-lă-tĭn'ĭ-form, -lăt'ĭ-noyd) [L. *scarlatina + forma*, shape, + G. *eidos*, form]. Resembling scarlatina or its rash.
scarlet (skar'lĕt) [L. *scarlatum*, red]. A bright red color, as that of a rash.
  s. fever. Acute, contagious, febrile disease marked by sore throat, and a scarlet rash. SYN: *scarlatina, q.v.*
  RS: *Amato bodies, Borsieri's line, Dick's method.*

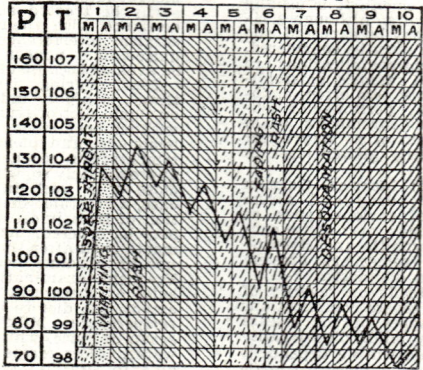

  s. rash. A rose-colored rash, specifically that of German* measles.
scar'let red. An azo dye, of the color its name suggests.
  USES: To stimulate healing of indolent ulcers, burns, wounds, etc.
  DOSAGE: 4 to 8% ointment. SYN: *rubrum scarlatinum.*
Scarpa's fascia (skar'pa). Deep layer of superficial abdominal fascia around edge of the subcutaneous inguinal ring.
  S's. fluid. Fluid in membranous labyrinth of the ear. SYN: *endolymph.*
  S's. foramina. Bony passages opening into the incisor canal for passage of the nasopalatine nerves.
  S's. liquor. SEE: *S's. fluid.*
  S's. membrane. Membrane that closes the fenestra rotunda of the tympanic cavity.
  S's. triangle. Triangular space bounded laterally by inner edge of sartorius, above by Poupart's ligament, and medially by the adductor longus.
scatacratia (skăt-ă-krā'shĭ-ă) [G. *skōr, skat-,* dung, + *akratia,* lack of control]. Fecal incontinence.

scatemia (skăt-ē'mĭ-ă) [" + *aima*, blood]. Intestinal toxemia from retained fecal matter.
scatology (skăt-ŏl'ō-jĭ) [" + *logos*, a study]. 1. Scientific study and analysis of the feces. SYN: *coprology.* 2. Interest in obscene things, esp. literature.
scatoma (skă-tō'mă) [" + *-ōma,* tumor]. Mass of inspissated feces in colon or rectum resembling an abdominal tumor. SYN: *coproma, fecaloma, stercoroma.*
scatophagy (skă-tŏf'ăj-ĭ) [" + *phagein,* to eat]. The eating of excrement. SYN: *coprophagy.*
scatoscopy (skă-tŏs'kō-pĭ) [" + *skopein,* to examine]. Examination of excreta for diagnostic purposes.
scavenger cells (skăv'ĕn-jer) [O.Fr. *escauwage,* inspection]. Wandering phagocytic cells, common in the nervous system, that aid in removing disintegrated tissue.
scelalgia (skē-lăl'jĭ-ă, sē-lăl'jĭ-ă) [G. *skelis,* leg, + *algos,* pain]. Pain in a leg.
  s. puerperarum. Painful swelling of the leg due to septic infection in the puerperium. SYN: *phlegmasia alba dolens.*
Schacher's ganglion (shah'ker). The ophthalmic ganglion.

SCARLET FEVER

Schachowa's spiral tube (shah-ko'vah). Part of a uriniferous tubule bet. a looped tubule and a convoluted one.
Schafer's method of artificial respiration (shā'fer).
  THE POSITION OF PATIENT: Lying prone on abdomen, both arms stretched over head, with one arm flexed at elbow with hand resting under cheek and mouth; mouth directed toward finger tips (downhill), thus allowing the nose and mouth to be free for breathing and prevent aspiration of dirt. Constricting clothing about neck, chest and waist should be loosened. Foreign bodies in mouth *should be removed.* These may be done between strokes. *Do not waste time.*
  THE POSITION OF THE OPERATOR: Kneel on both knees astride one or preferably both thighs as near patient's knees as the respective size of the operator and patient permits.
  METHOD OF PROCEDURE: Operator almost sits on his heels, places palms of his hands just above patient's lowest ribs with fingers and thumbs loosely directed toward armpits. Operator's wrists from

two to six inches apart depending on conformation of patient. Arms and elbows straight. Gradually commence making pressure while rising to a vertical position. Operator's shoulders should never go beyond the wrists in the vertical position, as this would compress abdominal viscera alone. Maximum pressure varies somewhere between 30 to 70 lbs., but this should never be exceeded. This should require two or three seconds. Begin to resume sitting position, and release hands with a quick, sudden, snappy jerk, rest for one to two seconds, then repeat. Entire cycle should occupy about five seconds or 12 to 16 strokes per minute.
INTERPRETATION OF PROCEDURE: Expiration is made efficient (1) by compressing chest in anteroposterior diameter, (2) because curvature of ribs makes the chest narrower during compression, (3) the abdominal viscera, especially the liver, are pushed up in the chest as a piston. This three-fold action expresses a maximum of "bad air." The quick, snappy, sudden release allows these structures to spring back into place, causing a maximum inspiration which is distinctly greater than that induced by a slow release.

Schäffer's reflex (shā'fer). Dorsal flexion of toes and flexion of foot resulting when middle portion of tendo Achillis is pinched.

Schede's method (shā'dĕ). Treatment of caries of bone by scraping away dead tissue and allowing cavity to fill with a blood clot.

S's. operation. A radical thoracoplasty.

Scheele's green (shā'lēz, shēlz). Copper arsenite.
POISONING: TREATMENT: Same as for arsenic, q.v.

schematic (skē-măt'ĭk) [L. schematicus, planned]. Pert. to a diagram or model; showing part for part in a diagram.

s. eye. A diagram or model showing proportions of a typical eye.

Scheurlen's bacillus (shor'lĕnz). A bacillus once thought to cause carcinoma.

Schick's method (shĭk). Injection of a mixture or toxin and antitoxin to cause immunity to diphtheria.

S. test. Injection beneath skin of 1/50 of dose of diphtheria toxin which would be fatal to a guinea pig, as a test of susceptibility to this disease.
Proved within 48 hours by appearance of red spot at point of injection which fades in about 4 days. Otherwise natural immunity is indicated.
As a control, a similar test is given in the other arm but the serum is heated to 75° C. for 10 minutes to destroy the toxin but not the protein. If test is positive, the red spots appear in both arms, thus obviating a possible pseudoreaction from the protein of the toxin. SEE: Dick method, test.

Schiller's test (shĭl'er). One for superficial cancer, esp. of the cervix uteri.
Paint with solution of iodine. Cancer cells not containing glycogen fail to stain, thus revealing their presence.

Schilling's hem'ogram (shĭl'ĭng). Method of taking a differential blood count by separating the polymorphonuclear neutrophils into 4 categories according to number and arrangement of the nuclei in the cells.

schindylesis (skĭn-dĭ-lē'sĭs) [G. schindylēsis, a splintering]. A form of synarthrosis* in which the receptor of a plate of one bone fits into a fissure of another one. SEE: gomphosis, synchondrosis.

schistasis (skĭs'tăs-ĭs) [G. schistos, split]. A splitting; specifically, a congenital fissure of the body.

schistocelia (skĭs-tō-sē'lĭ-ă) [" + koilia, belly]. Congenital abdominal fissure.

schistocyte (skĭs'tō-sīt) [" + kytos, a cell]. 1. A blood cell in process of segmentation. 2. A very tiny red blood corpuscle.

schistocytosis (skĭs"tō-sī-tō'sĭs) [" + " + -ōsis, condition]. 1. Schistocytes in the blood. 2. Segmentation process of blood corpuscles.

schistoglossia (skĭs"tō-glos'ĭ-ă) [" + glōssa, tongue]. A cleft tongue.

schistoprosopia (skĭs"tō-prō-sō'pĭ-ă) [" + prosōpon, face]. Congenital fissure of the face.

schistorrhachis (skĭs"tor'ă-kĭs) [" + rhachis, spine]. Protrusion of membranes through a congenital cleft in lower vertebral column. SYN: spina bifida.

Schistosoma (skĭs"tō-sō'mă) [G. schistos, a cleft, + sōma, body]. A genus of trematode parasitic worms. SYN: flukes.

schistosomiasis (skĭs"tō-sō-mī'ă-sĭs) [" + " + -iasis, infection]. Infestation with Schistosoma.

schistothorax (skĭs"tō-thō'răks) [" + thōrax, chest]. Fissure of the thorax.

schizaxon (skĭs-ăks'ŏn). A neuraxon that divides in 2 equal or nearly equal branches.

schizo- [G.]. Combining form meaning to split.

schizocyte (skĭs'ō-sīt) [G. schizein, to split, + kytos, cell]. 1. A blood cell in process of segmentation. 2. A tiny red blood cell. SYN: schistocyte.

schizocytosis (skĭs"ō-sī-tō'sĭs) [" + " + -ōsis, condition]. Schistocytes in the blood. SYN: schistocytosis.

schizogenesis (skĭz"ō-jĕn'ĕs-ĭs) [" + genesis, production]. BIOL: Reproduction by fission.*

schizogyria (skĭz-ō-jī'rĭ-ă) [" + gyros, a circle]. A break or cleft in the cerebral convolutions.

schizoid (skĭz'oyd) [" + eidos, resemblance]. Similar to schizophrenia, name applied to one unduly given to introspection and the inner rather than the outer life.
It is seen in an exaggerated form in schizophrenia.

Schizomycetes (skĭz"ō-mī-sē'tēz) [" + mykēs, fungus]. Class of plant microorganisms or fungi which multiply by fission.

schizomycosis (skĭz"ō-mī-kō'sĭs) [" + " + -ōsis, condition]. Disease caused by Schizomycetes.

schizont (skĭz'ont) [G. schizein, to split]. A form of protozoa showing alternation* of generation.

schizonychia (skĭz"ō-nĭk'ĭ-ă) [G. schizein, to split, + onyx, onych-, nail]. Split condition of the nails.

schizophasia (skĭz-ō-fā'zĭ-ă) [" + phasis, speech]. Muttered and incomprehensible speech of the schizophrenic.

schizophrenia (skĭz-ō-frē'nĭ-ă) [G. schizein, to split, + phrēn, mind]. One of the most important of the psychoses, characterized by loss of contact with the environment and by disintegration of personality.
This term includes all cases of dementia precox of the older writers. Possibly, it may also apply to numerous borderline cases which would not have been included in dementia precox.

Though presented in a variety of forms, the entity is fairly clear-cut; the *hebephrenic, catatonic,* and *paranoid* types — a very mild symptomatology. Sometimes, in addition, is called "simple." The paranoid type develops extensive delusions of persecution; the catatonic may show stereotyped excitement or simulate a stupor, though lucid and clearly recalling the episode if recovery occurs. A vague sense of being 2 personalities and "changed" occurs in all types. The hebephrenic shows mannerisms, speech anomalies, hysteroid symptoms, delusions, hallucinations, and often a dreamy, ineffectual reaction. The disease tends to develop in certain types and the recognition of these types may offer something in the way of prevention.

+ -*ōsis*, condition]. Any of the types of schizophrenia.
schizothemia (skĭz-ō-thē'mĭ-ă) [" + *thema*, a theme]. PSY: Hysterical resort to reminiscences during a conversation.
schizotrichia (skĭz″ō-trĭk′ĭ-ă) [" + *thrix, trich-*, hair]. Splitting of the hair.
Schlemm's canal (shlĕm). Irregular space or spaces in the sclerocorneal region of the eye.
 S's. ligament. One of 2 ligaments of the shoulder joint. SYN: *glenoideobrachial ligament.*
Schmidt's intestinal test (shmĭt). Test diet given for indigestion.
 For breakfast the following may be served: Milk, ½ liter, or an equal quantity of cocoa made with milk; 1 cooked or raw egg; zwieback or roll, 50 Gm.; butter, 10 Gm.

Schizophrenia (Symptoms)

1. Occurs in young men and women.
2. Poor general health.
3. Memory better than it seems.
4. Hallucinations common, especially of hearing.
5. Loss of emotion or, if shown, it is out of place.
6. Affection absent.
7. May revert to stereotype.
8. Impulsive destructive acts.
9. Negativism.
10. May be catatonic.
11. May be hebephrenic.
12. May recover sufficiently to be discharged.
13. Pulse feeble.
14. Cold, blue, and edematous extremities.
15. Muddy complexion.
16. Conscious, but takes little cognizance of what is going on about them.
17. Delusions frequent but absurd, often of grandeur and persecution.
18. May have attacks of tears or laughter.
19. Facial grin while describing tortures.
20. May have excited activity.
21. May remain in stupor.
22. Grimaces and mannerisms frequent.
23. May pay no attention to calls of nature if disease is advanced.
24. May be paranoid.
25. Disease sometimes changes its form.
26. Complete recovery rare.

Principal Signs: Moodiness, solitary habits, stupor and excitement, delusions and hallucinations.

ETIOL: Unknown. Pituitary and adrenal hormones always deficient.
PROG: Always guarded.
NP: Expert and careful nursing care is required during the administration of shock treatment, as patient's blood sugar is at a low level in insulin therapy and delay may have serious consequences. Constant watching is required while patient is unconscious because of the violent twitchings during convulsions.
TREATMENT: Simplification of the environment, occupational therapy, the building of more healthful approach to one's emotional problems may offer something.
 Recent forms of treatment which are proving successful are: 1. Insulin shock therapy, in which the patient is given sufficient insulin in daily doses to go into a state of shock and convulsions. 2. Administration of metrazol, which produces convulsions and unconsciousness, given 3 or 4 times a week for 12 to 15 treatments. Curare, when given with metrazol, lessens the contractions. 3. Best method to date is a combination of metrazol and insulin. 4. Inhalation of nitrogen 3 times a week for 5 minutes, which deprives the brain of oxygen temporarily; method produces no convulsions and is safer to give than insulin or metrazol. SYN: *dementia precox.*
SEE: *hypoglycemic shock, shock.*
schizophrenic (skĭz″ō-frĕn′ĭk) [G. *schizein*, to split, + *phrēn*, mind]. Afflicted with or person afflicted with schizophrenia.
schizophrenosis (skĭz″ō-frē-nō′sĭs) [" + "

 The midmorning meal consists of ½ liter of oatmeal gruel, made from oatmeal, 40 Gm.; water, 200 cc., and milk, 300 cc.
 Dinner consists of chopped beef, 125 Gm., lightly broiled in butter and raw inside; strained potato purée made from mashed potato, 190 Gm.; milk, 100 cc., and butter, 10 Gm.
 The midafternoon meal is the same as the breakfast, and supper is the same as the midmorning meal.
 This diet is usually maintained for about 3 days. All the food used must be weighed or measured *accurately*. Should the patient not eat the entire amount the portion not eaten must be weighed or measured. All the urine and feces passed are measured and sent to the laboratory for examination. It is also sometimes required that the foods used must first be analyzed.
Schmidt-Strassburger motor test meal. An intestinal motility test meal.
 With the meal, 2 capsules, each containing 5/10 of a gram of charcoal, are given to mark the meal, then the following: Finely chopped meat, 80 Gm.; mashed potato, 200 Gm.; 2 eggs; butter, 49 Gm.; oatmeal gruel made with milk, 1500 cc.; clear soup, 250 cc.; very dry toast or zwieback, 100 Gm.
 In health, it is said this should pass through the intestines in 15 to 25 hr.; in diarrhea due to colitis, in 10 to 15 hr.; in enterocolitis with diarrhea, in 3 to 5 hr.
schneiderian membrane (shnī-dē′rĭ-ăn)

schneiderian reflex   S-18   **scillaren**

The nasal mucosa. SYN: *pituitary membrane*.
   s. reflex. Contraction of facial muscles due to irritation of nasal mucosa.

Schönlein's disease (shen'lin). An acute disease characterized by purpuric spots, urticaria, sore throat, and inflammation of the joints resembling rheumatism. SYN: *peliosis, purpura rheumatica*.
   SYM: Fever, arthritic pains of knees and ankles. In few days petechial to ecchymotic, light red to dark purplish maculations appear upon extremities, trunk or entire body; fadeless under pressure. Subjective symptoms trivial. In fortnight eruption may subside; relapses common. Purpuric spots sometimes make their appearance regularly in afternoon and evening, daily or on days between; pain and stiffness.
   TREATMENT: Constitutional.

Schott method (shŏt). Resisting exercises and special baths in the treatment of heart disease.

Schroeder's method (shrōd'er) (resuscitation). A manner of resuscitating asphyxiated infants by placing the patient in a bath and then bending the body over the abdomen. This movement compresses the thorax and produces a forceful expiration.

Schueller's method (shil'er) (Karl Heinrich Anton Max Schueller, Berlin surgeon, 1843-1907) (artificial respiration). A manner of performing artificial respiration by a series of rhythmic raisings of the thorax by the operator hooking his fingers under the lower ribs.

Schüller's ducts (shil'er). Those of Skene's glands.
   S's. glands. The glands of the urethra.
   S's. phenomenon. Turning to the sound side in walking, in functional hemiplegia, but to the affected side in cases of organic lesion.

Schultze's bundle. Longitudinal mass of descending fibers shaped like a comma, in the fasciculus cuneatus of spinal cord.
   S's. cells. Olfactory cells.
   S's. granule masses. Fine, granular masses formed by breaking up of plaques in the blood.
   S's. method. A method of resuscitating an asphyxiated infant at birth.
   The 1st and 2nd fingers are placed in child's axillae, with thumbs over shoulders. The child is held firmly, and swung at arm's length above head of nurse, which brings the legs of the infant on to the abdomen, thereby compressing the chest. On swinging child down again, the chest becomes expanded, and so inspiration takes place.

Schwabach test (shvah'bahkh). A test for hearing by use of 5 tuning forks, each of a different tone. SEE: *test*.

Schwann's primitive bundle (shvan). A muscular fiber.
   S's. sheath. The neurilemma of a nerve fiber. SYN: *neurilemma*.
   S's. white substance. Myelin of a medullated nerve fiber.

schwannoma (shvan-nō'mă) [Schwann + G. *-ōma*, tumor]. A tumor having its origin in Schwann's sheath.

sciage (se-ahzh') [Fr. a sawing]. A movement in massage resembling that in sawing.

sciatic (sī-ăt'ĭk) [G. *ischiadikos*, pert. to the ischium]. 1. Pert. to the hip or ischium. 2. Pert. to, due to, or afflicted with, sciatica.
   s. nerve. Largest nerve in the body arising from sacral plexus on either side, passing from pelvis to greater sciatic foramen, down back of thigh, where it divides into tibial and peroneal nerves. SEE: *Table of Nerves in Appendix*.
   s. n., great. Has 2 divisions—external and internal popliteal.
   Lesions cause paralysis of flexion and of adduction of toes, abduction and adduction of toes, rotation inward and adduction of foot; of plantar flexion and lowering of ball of foot; anesthesia in cutaneous distribution (ext. popliteal nerve); paralysis of dorsal flexion and adduction of foot; of rotation of ball of foot outward and of raising external border of foot and of extension of toes; also anesthesia in cutaneous distribution.
   s. n., small. Ischiatic nerve; a cutaneous n. supplying skin of buttocks, perineum, popliteal region, and back of thigh.
   Lesions of: Result in flaccidity of affected buttock, difficult extension of thigh.

sciatica (sī-ăt'ĭ-kă) [L. from G. *ischiadikos*, pert. to the ischium]. Inflammation and pain along the sciatic nerve felt at back of thigh running down the inside of the leg. SEE: *meralgia; sciatic, lesions of*.
   ETIOL: Male sex, middle life, gout, rheumatism and syphilis are predisposing causes. Exposure to cold and wet is common exciting cause. Very largely sciatica is a secondary condition resulting from the presence of an intrapelvic growth, or from caries of bone in joint disease. Also impingement on nerve or having one leg a trifle shorter than the other.
   SYM: May begin abruptly or gradually and is characterized by a sharp, shooting pain running down back of thigh. Movement of limb generally intensifies the suffering. Pain may be uniformly distributed along the limb, but not infrequently there are certain spots where it is more intense; numbness, tingling; nerve may be extremely sensitive to touch. Symptoms grow worse at night and on approach of stormy weather. Duration of attack varies from few days to several months. In long standing cases, muscles grow atrophied and rigid.
   PROG: Recovery follows in majority of cases when treatment is instituted early, and is persistently carried out.
   TREATMENT: In acute stage, rest is essential. Hot fomentations. Deep injections of morphine or cocaine may be required to relieve the pain. In rheumatic cases full doses of salicylate of sodium are useful. In chronic case prolonged rest. Deep injections along course of nerve of morphine and atropine, cocaine or plain water; electricity. Improve general health; good, nourishing diet; bags of hot salt; covering part with flannel and running hot iron over it often relieves. Some cases relieved by cold. Nerve stretching by pulling affected leg. Lift in shoe of affected limb.

science (sī'ĕns) [L. *scientia*, knowledge]. 1. Any branch of systematized knowledge considered as a distinct field of investigation or object of study. 2. Knowledge accumulated and classified and made available for work.

scieropia (sī-ĕr-ō'pĭ-ă) [G. *skieros*, shadow, + *opsis*, vision]. Abnormal vision in which things appear to be in shadow.

scillaren (sĭl'lă-rēn) [G. *skilla*, squill]. A mixture of glucosides obtained from squill.

scintillascope

USES: As a heart stimulant, similar in action to digitalis.
DOSAGE: 1/40 gr. (1.6 mg.).

scintillascope (sĭn-tĭl'ă-skōp) [L. *scintilla*, spark, + G. *skopein*, to examine]. Device for estimating physical properties of radium. SYN: *spinthariscope*.

scintillation (sĭn-tĭl-lā'shŭn) [L. *scintilla*, spark]. Sparkling; a subjective sensation, as of seeing sparks.

scirrho- [G.]. Combining form meaning *hard*, as *scirrhus*, a hard tumor.

scirrhoid (skĭr'oyd) [G. *skirrhos*, hard, + *eidos*, form]. Pert. to or like a hard carcinoma or scirrhus.

scirrhoma (skĭr-ō'mă) [" + *-ōma*, tumor]. A hard carcinoma or scirrhus.

scirrhosarca (skĭr-ō-sar'kă) [" + *sarx*, *sark-*, flesh]. Hardening of the flesh, esp. of the newly born. SYN: *sclerema neonatorum*, *scleroderma*.

scirrhous (skĭr'rŭs) [G. *skirrhos*, hard]. Hard, like a scirrhus.

scirrhus (skĭr'ŭs) [G. *skirrhos*, hard]. A hard, cancerous tumor due to overgrowth of fibrous tissue. A hard form of cancer.
Seats of predilection are alimentary tract, esp. pyloric end of stomach and in a few instances glands of the skin. Average duration of life about 30 months.
TREATMENT: Palliative, relieving pain, and making patient comfortable as possible or radical treatment. Prompt extirpation of all diseased tissue.

s., atrophic. Tumor resulting from the fatty degeneration and absorption of the epithelial cells. Perhaps induced by unusually abundant development of the fibrous stroma, contracting so as to diminish the blood supply to the cells. Leaves little more than a mass of fibrous tissue, with here and there a few cells surrounded by débris. Although tumor is slower in its growth and rather diminishes than increases in size its malignancy is not lost, the ultimate result being same. SYN: *witherings*.

s. of breast. SYM: Scirrhus forms an irregular, nodulated, somewhat rounded, stony, hard, heavy mass, inseparable from the glandular tissue, possessing no defined outline, but gradually merging into the healthy mammary tissue, with which it freely moves. Soon it adheres to the skin which becomes dimpled, and later to the pectoral muscle, thus at first being partially, then immovably, fixed to chest wall; grows slowly, nipple gradually becomes retracted, but growth never attains large size.
As a rule, upper axillary segment is attacked, but may originate close to nipple or to inner side of breast. Retraction of nipple due to scirrhus growths differs from that seen in benign growths, in that nipple is actually drawn in, not buried by projection of the tumor mass.
Pain is absent in the early stages; only prominent when tumor is of some size. Sometimes slight stinging pains attract attention to the growth, but generally it is accidentally discovered. Is not tender. When fixed to chest wall and axillary nerves are compressed by secondary lymphatic glandular tumors, pain is severe and almost ceaseless; lancinating, darting or cutting. Cachexia is present when ulceration has taken place and when mental anxiety, prolonged pain or profuse discharge have exhausted the patient; but in nearly every case patient is in robust health when first attacked.
If removed when in first stage and with it pain, worry and discharge cease, patient promptly regains color and flesh. Generally appears between 40th and 50th years. Scirrhus left to itself will involve whole mamma, converting it, with overlying skin and subjacent muscular parietes of chest, into one nodular, stony hard mass with retracted, buried nipple. When this involves a large portion of chest wall, it is called cancer en cuirasse.

s. of testicle. Presents no features peculiar to the locality; is very rare.

s. ventriculi. 1. Induration and diffuse thickening of wall of stomach, esp. of the pylorus. 2. A form of chronic gastritis.

scissor leg (sĭz'or lĕg). Abnormal crossing of both legs, the result of adduction at both hips. SYN: *x-leg*.

s. l. gait. Crossing the legs in walking. SEE: *gait*.

scissors (sĭz'ors) [L. *cisorium* from *caedere*, to cut]. A cutting instrument composed of 2 opposed cutting blades with handles, held together by a central pin. Often used as substitute for knife. Straight, angular, curved on the flat, with sharp, blunt, rounded and probe points.

sclera (sklē'ră) (pl. *sclerae*) [G. *sklēros*, hard]. BNA. The white or sclerotic outer coat of the eye.
It extends from optic nerve to cornea. SYN: *sclerotica*.

scleradenitis (sklē-rad-ĕn-ī'tĭs) [" + *adēn*, gland, + *-itis*, inflammation]. Inflammation and induration of a gland.

scleral (sklē'răl) [G. *sklēros*, hard]. Concerning the sclera.

sclerectasia (sklēr-ĕk-tā'zĭ-ă) [" + *ektasis*, dilatation]. Protrusion of the sclera.

sclerectoiridectomy (sklēr-ĕk″tō-ĭr-ĭ-dĕk′tō-mĭ) [" + *iris*, *irid-*, iris, + *ektomē*, excision]. Formation of a filtering cicatrix in glaucoma by combined sclerectomy and iridectomy.

sclerectoiridodialysis (sklēr-ĕk″tō-ĭr-ĭd-ō-dī-ăl'ĭ-sĭs) [" + " + *dialysis*, a loosening]. Sclerectomy and iridodialysis for relief of glaucoma.

sclerectomy (sklē-rĕk'tō-mĭ) [" + *ektomē*, excision]. 1. Excision of a portion of the sclera. 2. Removal of adhesions in chronic otitis media.

sclerema (sklē-rē'mă) [G. *sklēros*, hard]. Hardening of the skin. SYN: *scleroderma*.

s. neonatorum. Progressive hardening of the skin in the newly born; usually fatal.

scleriasis (sklē-rī'ăs-ĭs) [" + *-iasis*, disease]. Progressive hardening of the skin. SYN: *scleroderma*.

scleriritomy (sklēr-ĭ-rĭt'ō-mĭ) [" + *iris*, iris, + *tomē*, a cutting]. Incision of iris and sclera.

scleritis (sklē-rī'tĭs) [" + *-itis*, inflammation]. Inflammation of the sclera; superficial and deep. SEE: *episcleritis*.

scleroblastema (sklē″rō-blăs-tē'mă) [" + *blastēma*, a sprout]. The embryonic tissue from which formation of bone takes place.

scleroblastemic (sklē″rō-blăs-tĕm'ĭk) [" + *blastēma*, a sprout]. Relating to or derived from scleroblastema.

sclerocataracta (sklē″rō-kăt-ă-răkt-ă) [" + *katarraktēs*, a pouring down]. A hard cataract.

sclerochoroiditis (sklē″rō-kō-roy-dī'tĭs) [G. *sklēros*, hard, + *chorioeidēs*, skinlike, + *-itis*, inflammation]. Inflammation of the sclera and choroid coat of the eye.

s., posterior. Myopic chorioiditis, posterior staphyloma.

scleroconjunctival   S-20   **scleroticotomy**

scleroconjunc′tival. Pertaining to the sclera and conjunctiva.

sclerocornea (sklē″rō-kor′nē-ă) [" + L. *cornu*, a horn]. The sclera and cornea together considered as one coat.

sclerodactylia (sklē″rō-dăk-tĭl′ĭ-ă) [" + *daktylos*, digit]. Induration of the skin of the fingers and toes.

scleroderma (sklē-rō-der′mă) [" + *derma*, skin]. Hard, thickened, rigid disease of the skin resulting in a hidebound condition.

ETIOL: Unknown, but thought to be a trophoneurosis depending upon central nervous system changes.

SYM: Diffuse symmetrical form, occurring in adults, following exposure to cold or wet. Smooth, waxy, edematous skin; later becomes hard, yellowish, and adherent to underlying tissue, causing masklike expression (face) or clawlike appearance of hands (sclerodactylia). When chest is involved respiration may be interfered with.

PROG: Better in circumscribed form than in extensive s.

TREATMENT: Tonics; warm, moist, equable climate; endocrine medication in some. Locally, mildly stimulating ointments (salicylic acid, mercurials), chloroform, liniment.

   s., circumscribed. Skin disease with pink, firm patches which atrophy, leaving scars. SYN: *morphea*.

   s. neonatorum. Hardness and tightness of the skin in early infancy. SYN: *sclerema*.

sclerodermitis (sklē″rō-der-mă-tī′tĭs) [G. *skleros*, hard, + *derma*, skin, + -*itis*, inflammation]. Induration and inflammation of the skin.

sclerogenous (sklē-rŏj′ĕn-ŭs) [" + *gennan*, to produce]. Causing sclerosis or hardening of tissue.

scleroiritis (sklē″rō-ī-rī′tĭs) [" + *iris*, iris, + -*itis*, inflammation]. Inflammation of both sclera and iris.

sclerokeratitis (sklē″rō-ker-ă-tī′tĭs) [" + *keras*, *kerat-*, horn, + -*itis*, inflammation]. Cellular infiltration with inflammation of the sclera and cornea.

sclerokeratoiritis (sklē″rō-ker″ă-tō-ī-rī′tĭs) [" + " + *iris*, iris, + -*itis*, inflammation]. Inflamed condition of the sclera, cornea, and iris.

scleroma (sklē-rō′mă) [" + -*ōma*, tumor]. Indurated, circumscribed area of granulation tissue in mucous membrane or skin. SEE: *sclerosis*.

scleromere (sklē′rō-mēr) [" + *meros*, a part]. Any homologous segment of the skeleton.

scleronyxis (sklē-rō-nĭks′ĭs) [G. *skleros*, hard, + *nyxis*, a piercing]. Puncture of the sclera.

sclerooöphoritis (sklē″rō-ō″ŏf-or-ī′tĭs) [" + *oon*, egg, + *phoros*, a bearer, + -*itis*, inflammation]. Induration and inflammation of the ovary.

sclerophthalmia (sklēr-ŏf-thăl′mĭ-ă) [" + *ophthalmos*, eye]. Congenital condition in which opacity of the sclera advances over the cornea.

scleroprotein (sklē″rō-prō′tē-ĭn) [" + *prōtos*, first]. One of group of simple proteins* forming the skeletal structure of animals marked by their insolubility. They are not suitable for food. Elastin and keratin are examples. SYN: *albuminoid*.

sclerosarcoma (sklē″rō-sar-kō′mă) [" + *sarx*, *sark-*, flesh, + *ōma*, tumor]. A fleshy, fibrous tumor of the gums. SEE: *epulis*.

sclerosed (sklē-rōsd′, sklē″rōsd) [G. *skleros*, hard]. Having sclerosis; hardened. SYN: *indurated*.

sclerosing (sklē-rō′sĭng) [G. *skleros*, hard]. Causing or suffering from sclerosis.

sclerosis (sklē-rō′sĭs) [G. *sklērosis*, a hardening]. An induration of inflammatory nature, esp. of the nervous system; also a chronic thickening of the arteries' coats due to inflammation.

RS: *cerebrosclerosis, Charcot's disease, scleritis*.

   s., Alzheimer's. Hyaline degeneration affecting the small blood vessels of brain.

   s., amyotrophic lateral. Progressive muscular atrophy affecting lateral columns of the spinal cord and ending in bulbar paralysis.

   s., arterial. Hardening of the coats of the arteries. SYN: *arteriosclerosis*.

   s., diffuse. S. affecting large areas of the brain and spinal cord.

   s., disseminated. Condition characterized by inflammatory patches which become sclerosed, freely scattered through the brain and spinal cord.

   s., insular. Multiple sclerosis, q.v.

   s., lateral. S. of a lateral column of the spinal cord.

   s., multiple. Chronic induration in patches scattered over the nervous system.

   s., neural. S. with chronic inflammation of a nerve trunk with branches.

   s., vascular. Same as arterial sclerosis, q.v.

scleroskeleton (sklē″rō-skĕl′ĕ-tŏn) [G. *skleros*, hard, + *skeleton*, skeleton]. Skeletal parts resulting from ossification of fibrous structures, such as ligaments, fasciae, and tendons.

sclerostenosis (sklē″rō-sten-ō′sĭs) [" + *stenōsis*, a narrowing]. Contraction and induration of tissues.

   s. cutanea. Induration of the skin. SYN: *scleroderma*.

sclerostomy (sklē-rŏs′tō-mī) [" + *stoma*, an opening]. Formation of an opening in the sclera.

sclerothrix (sklē′rō-thrĭks) [" + *thrix*, hair]. Brittleness of the hair.

sclerotic (sklē-rŏt′ĭk) [L. *scleroticus*, from G. *skleros*, hard]. 1. Pert. to or affected with sclerosis. 2. Hard.

   s. acid. An amorphous, brown powder from ergot. A hemostatic and oxytocic.

   s. coat. The membrane forming the ext. coat of the eye. SYN: *sclera, sclerotica*.

   s. teeth. Hard, yellowish ones almost immune to caries.

sclerotica (sklē-rŏt′ĭ-kă) [L. from G. *skleros*, hard]. The ext. white coat of the eye. SYN: *sclera, sclerotic coat*.

scleroticectomy (sklē-rŏt-ĭ-sĕk′tō-mī) [L. *scleroticus*, sclerotic, + G. *ektomē*, excision]. Excision of a part of the sclera. SYN: *sclerectomy*.

scleroticochoroiditis (sklē-rŏt″ĭ-kō-kō″roy-dī′tĭs) [" + G. *chorioeidēs*, skinlike, + -*itis*, inflammation]. Inflammation of sclerotic and choroid coats of the eye. SYN: *sclerochoroiditis*.

scleroticonyxis (sklē-rŏt-ĭk-ō-nĭks′ĭs) [" + G. *nyxis*, a piercing]. Puncture of the sclera. SYN: *scleronyxis*.

scleroticopuncture (sklē-rŏt″ĭk-ō-pŭnk′tūr) [" + *punctūra*, a piercing]. Surgical puncture of the sclera. SYN: *scleronyxis, scleroticonyxis*.

scleroticotomy (sklē-rŏt-ĭk-ŏt′ō-mī) [" + G. *tomē*, a cutting]. Incision of the sclerotic coat of the eye. SYN: *sclerotomy*.

sclerotitis (sklē-rō-tī'tĭs) [G. *skleros,* hard, + *-itis,* inflammation]. Inflammation of the sclera. SYN: *scleritis.*

sclerotium (sklē-rō'shĭ-ŭm) [L. from G. *skleros,* hard]. Hardened mass formed of mycelium and food débris, the resting stage of certain fungi.

sclerotome (sklē'rō-tōm) [G. *skleros,* hard, + *tome,* a cutting]. 1. Knife used in incision of the sclera. 2. Embryonic mass of tissue from which part of the skeleton arises.

sclerotomy (sklē-rŏt'ō-mĭ) [" + *tome,* a cutting]. Simple division of sclera.
 s., anterior. Incision at angle of anterior chamber in glaucoma.
 s., posterior. Opening through sclera into the vitreous for detached retina, removal of foreign body, etc.

scolecology (skō"lē-kŏl'ō-jĭ) [G. *skolex,* worm, + *logos,* a study]. The study of parasitic worms. SYN: *helminthology.*

scolectomy (skō-lĕk'tō-mĭ) [" + *ektome,* excision]. Operation for removal of the vermiform appendix. SYN: *appendectomy.*

scoledocostomy (skō-lĕd-ō-kŏs'tō-mĭ) [" + *stoma,* an opening]. Creation of an opening into the vermiform appendix. SYN: *appendicostomy.*

scoliometer (skō-lĭ-ŏm'ĕt-ĕr) [G. *skolios,* crooked, + *metron,* measure]. Device for measuring curves, esp. lateral ones of the spine.

scoliosiometry (skō"lĭ-ō-sĭ-ŏm'ĕ-trĭ) [" + *rachis,* spine]. Pert. to or afflicted with spinal curvature from rickets.

scoliosiometry (skō"lĭ-ō-sĭ-ŏm'ĕ-trĭ) [" + *metron,* a measure]. Measurement of degree of spinal curvature.

scoliosis (skō-lĭ-ō'sĭs) [G. *skoliosis,* curvature]. Lateral curvature of the spine.
 Usually consists of 2 curves, the original one and a compensatory curve in the opp. direction.
 s., cicatricial. S. due to cicatricial contraction resulting from necrosis.
 s., coxitic. S. in the lumbar spine due to tilting of the pelvis in hip disease.
 s., empyematic. S. following empyema and retraction of one side of the chest.
 s., habit. S. due to habitually assumed improper position.
 s., inflammatory. S. due to disease of the vertebrae.
 s., ischiatic. S. due to hip disease.
 s., myopathic. Weakening of spinal muscles causing a lateral curvature.
 s., ocular, s., ophthalmic. S. from tilting of the head in astigmatism.
 s., osteopathic. Same as s. myopathic, *q.v.*
 s., paralytic. Lateral curvature of the spine due to paralysis of the muscles.
 s., rachitic. S. due to rickets.
 s., rheumatic. S. due to rheumatism of dorsal muscles.
 s., sciatic. Lateral curvature in sciatica.
 s., static. That due to difference in length of legs.

scoliosometry (skō"lĭ-ō-sŏm'ĕt-rĭ) [G. *skoliosis,* curvature]. Determination of degree of spinal curvature. SYN: *scoliosiometry.*

scoliotic (skō-lĭ-ŏt'ĭk) [G. *skoliosis,* curvature]. Suffering from or related to scoliosis.

scoliotone (skō'lĭ-ō-tōn) [G. *skolios,* curved, + *tones,* a stretching]. An apparatus for correcting the curve in scoliosis by stretching the spine.

scolopsia (skō-lŏp'sĭ-ă) [G. *skolops,* a pointed thing]. A suture bet. 2 bones which permits reciprocal motion.

scoop (skoop) [M.E. *scope,* a ladle]. Surgical spoon-shaped instrument.
 s., bone. Instrument for scraping or removing necrosed bone or contents of suppurative tracts. Volkmann's, Schede's, Von Brun's, Hebras, Treves.
 s., bullet. Instrument for dislodging bullets.
 s., cataract. Instrument for removing fluids, foreign growths, for exerting pressure or center pressure.
 s., ear. Instrument for removing middle ear granulations.
 s., lithotomy. Instrument for dislodging encysted calculi, removing stones, débris, etc.
 s., mastoid. Instrument used in mastoid operations.
 s., renal. Instrument to dislodge or remove small stones from pelvis of kidney.

scopograph (skŏp'ō-grăf) [G. *skopein,* to examine, + *graphein,* to write]. A fluoroscope and radiographic unit combined in one device.

scopolamine hydrobromide (sko-pol'ă-mēn hī"drō-brō'mĭd) [G. *skopolamin*]. USP. The hydrobromide of alkaloids obtained from plants of the nightshade family.
 ACTION AND USES: As a cerebral sedative and locally as a mydriatic, and with morphine and pentobarbital in labor to produce twilight sleep. SYN: *hyoscine hydrobromide.*
 DOSAGE: 1/120 gr. (0.5 mg.).

scopophobia (skŏp"pō-fō'bĭ-ă) [G. *skopos,* a watcher, + *phobos,* fear]. Abnormal fear of being seen.

scopophobiac (skŏp"pō-fō'bĭ-ăk) [" + *phobos,* fear]. One who is afraid of being seen.

scoptolagniac (skŏp-tō-lăg'nĭ-ăk) [G. *skopein,* to see, + *lagneia,* lust]. One who derives sexual gratification from observing objects or situations. SYN: *voyeur, q.v.* SEE: *scoptophilia.*

scoptophilia (skŏp-tō-fĭl'ĭ-ă) [" + *philein,* to love]. Sexual pleasure derived from visual sources, such as nudity, obscene pictures, etc.

scoptophobia (skŏp-tō-fō'bĭ-ă) [" + *phobos,* fear]. Aversion to being seen.

scoptophobiac (skŏp"tō-fō'bĭ-ăk) [" + *phobos,* fear]. One who dreads being seen.

-scopy [G.]. Combining form meaning *examination.*

scoracratia (skŏr-ăk-ră'shĭ-ă) [G. *skōr,* dung, + *akratia,* lack of control]. Inability to retain the feces. SYN: *scatacratia.*

scorbutic (skor-bū'tĭk) [L. *scorbutus,* scurvy]. Concerning or affected with scurvy.

scorbutus (skor-bū'tŭs) [L. scurvy]. A deficiency disease due to lack of vitamin C in fresh vegetables and fruits. SYN: *scurvy, q.v.* SEE: *deficiency diseases, vitamin.*

scordinema (skor-dĭn-ē'mă) [G. yawning]. Yawning and stretching with heaviness of the head, a prodrome of an infectious disease.

scoretemia (skor-ĕ-tē'mĭ-ă) [G. *skōr,* dung, + *aima,* blood]. Autointoxication resulting from absorption of feces in the intestine. SYN: *scatemia.*

scorpion bite (skor'pĭ-ŏn) [G. *skorpios*]. The symptoms are similar to those from a spider bite.
 Vomiting and mental symptoms often

scotodinia

present. Apply a tourniquet and treat as for the black widow spider* bite.

scotodinia (skō-tō-dĭn'ĭ-ă) [G. *skotos*, darkness, + *dinos*, a whirl]. Vertigo with black spots before the eyes and faintness.

scotogram, scotograph (skŏt'ō-grăm, -grăf) [" + *gramma*, a mark, + *graphein*, to write]. A print from an x-ray plate. SYN: *skiagram*.

scotography (skō-tŏg'ră-fĭ) [" + *graphein*, to write]. Making of x-ray photographs. SYN: *skiagraphy*.

scotoma (skō-tō'mă) (pl. *scotomata*) [G. *skotōma*, darkness]. Islandlike blind gap in the visual field.

　s., absolute. An area in the visual field in which there is absolute blindness.

　s., annular. A scotomatous zone which encircles the point of fixation like a ring, not always completely closed, but leaves the fixation point intact.

　s., central. One which involves the point of fixation, seen in lesions of the macula.

　s., color. Color blindness in the involved area.

　s., flittering. Same as scintillating scotoma.

　s., negative. One not perceptible by the patient.

　s., physiological. Blind spot where optic nerve enters the retina.

　s., positive. One which patient perceives in his visual field as a dark spot.

　s., relative. One in which perception of the object is impaired but not completely lost.

　s., scintillating. An irregular outline around a luminous patch in the visual field following mental or physical labor or eyestrain or in migraine.

scotomagraph (skō-tō'mă-grăf) [G. *skotōma*, darkness, + *graphein*, to write]. Instrument for automatically recording the shape and size of a scotoma.

scotomameter (skō"tō-măm'ĕ-ter) [" + *metron*, a measure]. Instrument for measuring the size of a scotoma.

scotomata (skō-tō'mă-tă) [G.]. Plural of *scotoma*.

scotomatous (skō-tom'ă-tŭs) [G. *skotōma*, darkness]. Relating to, of the nature of, or afflicted with, scotoma.

scotometer (skō-tŏm'ĕt-ĕr) [" + *metron*, a measure]. Device for detecting and measuring a dark spot in visual field.

scotometry (skō-tom'ĕ-trĭ) [" + *metron*, a measure]. The locating and measurement of scotomata.

scotomization (skō-tō-mĭz-ā'shŭn) [G. *skotōma*, darkness]. PSY: A sadistic expression seen in compulsion neuroses and schizophrenia by which the victim indulges in self-punishment as an expression of hatred for another.

scotophilia (skō-tō-fĭl'ĭ-ă) [G. *skotos*, darkness, + *philein*, to love]. Preference for darkness or for the night. SYN: *nyctophilia*.

scotophobia (skō-tō-fō'bĭ-ă) [" + *phobos*, fear]. Abnormal dread of darkness.

scotopia (skō-tō'pĭ-ă) [" + *ōps*, eye]. The adjustment of vision for darkness.

scotoscopy (skō-tŏs'kō-pĭ) [" + *skopein*, to examine]. Examination of internal organs by use of the fluoroscope. SYN: *skiascopy*.

scototherapy (skō"tō-ther'ă-pĭ) [" + *therapeia*, treatment]. Treatment of disease by keeping patient in a dark room and by exclusion of light, as in malaria.

scratch (skrătsh) [M.E. *cracchen*]. A mark

or superficial injury produced by scraping with the nails or a rough surface.

screatus (skre-ā'tŭs) [L. *screātus*, a hawking]. A neurosis characterized by paroxysmal fits of hawking.

scriveners' palsy (skrīv'ner). Occupational neurosis caused by excessive use of the hand in writing. SYN: *writers' cramp*.

scrobiculate (skrō-bĭk'ū-lāt) [L. *scrobiculus*, a little pit]. Having shallow depressions; pitted.

scrobiculus (skrō-bĭk'ū-lŭs) [L. a little pit]. A small groove or pit.

　s. cordis. Pit of the stomach; precordial or epigastric depression.

scrofula (skrŏf'ū-lă) [L. *scrofula*, a breeding sow]. A constitutional, tuberculous condition characterized by glandular swelling in the neck and inflammations of joints and mucous membranes followed by cheesy degeneration; tuberculosis of the glands, joints, bones.

A term formerly applied to all tuberculous affections except those of lungs. Most common in childhood. Two types of the affection.

RS: *king's evil, struma*.

　s., erethistic. Less tendency to glandular enlargement. Individuals are dark colored, nervous temperament subject to catarrhal affections.

　s., torpid. Most characteristic. Such children have light or reddish hair, a sallow or pasty complexion, puff cheeks, protruding lips. Eyelids and conjunctivae often seat of a chronic inflammation. Catarrhal affections of nose and ear often exist; skin is eczematous and cervical glands enlarged.

TREATMENT: Such children should be placed under most hygienic conditions and exposures and fatigues of all kinds should be avoided. Should not be subjected to too rigorous a school discipline. Adults should seek most favorable climate. Deep acting constitutional remedies, as proper diet, heliotherapy.

scrofulide (skrof'ū-līd) [L. *scrofula*, a breeding sow]. Any scrofulous skin disease. SYN: *scrofuloderm, scrofuloderma*.

scrofuloderm, scrofuloderma (skrŏf'ū-lō-derm, -der'mă) [" + G. *derma*, skin]. Any tuberculous skin disease. SYN: *scrofulide*.

scrofulosis (skrŏf-ū-lō'sĭs) [" + G. *-ōsis*, condition]. Predisposition to scrofula.

scrofulous (skrŏf'ū-lŭs) [L. *scrofula*, a breeding sow]. Of the nature of, or afflicted with, scrofula.

scrotal (skrō'tăl) [L. *scrotum*, a bag]. Concerning the scrotum.

　s. reflex. Slow vermicular contraction of scrotal muscle when perineum is stroked or cold applied.

　s. tongue. A furrowed tongue.

scrotectomy (skrō-tĕk'tō-mĭ) [" + G. *ektomē*, excision]. Excision of part of the scrotum.

scrotitis (skrō-tī'tĭs) [" + G. *-ītis*, inflammation]. Inflamed condition of the scrotum.

scrotocele (skrō'tō-sēl) [" + G. *kēlē*, hernia]. Hernia in the scrotum.

scrotum (skrō'tŭm) (pl. *scrota*) [L. *scrotum*, bag]. The double pouch containing the testicles and part of the spermatic cord.

RS: *chimney-sweep's cancer, chyloderma, dartos, oscheal, oscheitis, oscheoncus, rhacoma, urocele*.

　s., lymph. Dilatation of scrotal lymphatics. SYN: *elephantiasis of scrotum*.

scrub'bing. Term applied to sterilization

scrub nurse of the hands for surgical operations.
  METHOD: Scrubbing with soap and water and a nail brush, immersion in a mild germicidal solution and the wearing of sterilized rubber gloves. SEE: *sterilization.*

scrub nurse. Term applied to operating room nurse who hands instruments to the surgeon, and who has previously sterilized her hands and wears sterile rubber gloves.

scruple (skrü'pl) [L. *scrupulus,* a small stone]. Twenty grains apothecaries' weight; 1/3 dram. SYMB: ℈.

Scultetus bandage (skŭl-tē'tŭs). A many-tailed bandage used in compound fractures.
  S. position. One with head low and the body on an inclined plane.

scum (skum) [M.E. *scume*]. BACT: Slimy floating islands of bacteria or impurities on the surface of a culture; an interrupted pellicle of bacterial growth.

scurf (skurf) [A.S. *scurf,* a gnawing]. A branny desquamation of the epidermis, esp. on the scalp. SEE: *dandruff.*

scurvy (skur'vĭ) [origin uncertain]. A disease due to lack of fresh fruits and vegetables and of vitamin C in diet.
  SYM: Preceded by period of ill-health; sallow; loss of energy; pains in legs, limbs and joints. Anemic; great weakness; spongy, bleeding gums; fetor of breath, and loosening of teeth; subcutaneous hemorrhages and hemorrhages from mucous membranes; painful, brawny indurations of muscles.
  PROG: Favorable in early stages.
  TREATMENT: Fresh vegetables and free use of lemon juice. Good hygienic surroundings. In infantile scurvy good results follow use of fresh milk, beef juice and orange juice. Minimum amt. of vitamin C required daily as a preventive of scurvy is 1 oz. of orange, lemon, or grapefruit juice, or a pint of milk, or 1 lb. of cooked potato or cabbage.
  s., infantile. A form of scurvy which sometimes follows the prolonged use of condensed milk, sterilized milk or proprietary foods. SYN: *Barlow's disease.*
  SYM: Anemia, immobility of legs, pseudoparalysis, extreme tenderness, swelling without pitting, thickening of bones from subperiosteal hemorrhage, ecchymoses and tendency to epiphyseal fractures at epiphyses of bones.
  s., land. Disease characterized by hemorrhage of the mucosa, ecchymoses and prostration. SYN: *purpura haemorrhagica.*

scute (skūt) [L. *scutum,* shield]. A plate or thin lamina forming outer wall of the attic separating it from the tympanum.
  s., tympanic. A crescentic plate.

scutiform (skū'tĭ-form) [" + *forma,* a shield]. Shield-shaped.

scutulum (skū'tū-lŭm) (pl. *scutula*) [L. a little shield]. 1. Any of the thin crusts of favus. 2. The shoulder blade. SYN: *scapula.*

scutum (skū'tŭm) [L. shield]. 1. Plate of bone resembling a shield. 2. The thyroid cartilage. 3. The kneecap. SYN: *patella.*
  s. cordis. The sternum.
  s. genu. The patella.
  s. pectoris. The thorax.
  s. thoracis. The sternum.

scybalous (sĭb'ăl-ŭs) [G. *skybalon,* dung]. Of the nature of hard fecal matter.

scybalum (sĭb'ăl-ŭm) (pl. *scybala*). A hard, rounded mass of fecal matter.

scypho- [G.]. Combining form meaning cup.

scyphoid (sī'foyd) [G. *skyphos,* cup, + *eidos,* like]. Cup-shaped.

scythian disease (sĭth'ĭ-ăn). Atrophy of male ext. genitalia with corresponding tendency to perversion and feminine manners.

scytitis (sī-tī'tĭs) [G. *skytos,* skin, + -*itis,* inflammation]. Inflammation of the skin. SYN: *dermatitis.*

scytoblastema (sī″tō-blăs-tē'mă) [" + *blastēma,* a sprout]. Skin in embryonic stage of its development.

scytoblastesis (sī″tō-blăs-tē'sĭs) [" + *blastēma,* a sprout]. The condition and progressive development of the embryonic skin.

séance (sā'ans) [Fr. from *seoir,* to sit]. A treatment, as by electricity or massage.

searcher (serch'er) [M.E. *serchen,* from L. *circāre,* to go about]. Instrument for locating opening of ureter previous to inserting catheter, exploring sinuses, and esp. for detecting stones in the bladder. SYN: *sound.*

seasickness (sē'sĭk-nĕs) [A.S. *sae,* sea, + *sēocness,* illness]. Disorder due to motion of a vessel at sea, or riding in cars, trains, and elevators. A similar condition affects some air travelers.
  ETIOL: Unknown. Supposed to be due to temporary disorder of middle ear mechanism affecting one's equilibrium.
  SYM: Giddiness, vomiting, headache, nausea, and often extreme drowsiness, retching, prostration.
  TREATMENT: Inhalation of oxygen has been quite successful. Following prescription also has been helpful to many:
  Soda bromide, ℥ij; ammon. bromide, ℥ij; aqua menth. pip. fl., ℥iiiss. Sig.—A teaspoonful before meals and at bedtime. Begin 3 days before going on board.
  RS: *mal de mer, naupathia, nausea.*

seat worm (sēt' worm). A genus of nematode worms, *Oxyuris vermicularis,* found in the sigmoid colon and the rectum.

sebaceous (sē-bā'shŭs) [L. *sebaceus,* fatty]. Containing or pert. to sebum, or an oily, fatty matter secreted by the sebaceous glands.
  s. cyst. A cyst filled with sebaceous material from a distended sebaceous gland.
  These are sometimes known as *wens.* They frequently form on the scalp, and consist of a small sac containing sebaceous matter, which may grow to a large size. They may result from impairment of localized circulation and closure of sebaceous glands or ducts. Drainage does not remove them permanently, as they will recur unless entirely extirpated,* which should be done with an electric current or cutting knife. One should never attempt to drain such a cyst without taking every precaution against infection.
  s. gland. Oil-secreting gland of the skin.
  The secretion of these glands keeps the hair from becoming dry and brittle, maintains the moisture of the skin, and forms a covering on surfaces of the skin to prevent undue absorption and evaporation. (SEE: *Illus. p. S-24.*)
  SEE: *seborrhea, sebum, steatoma, steatorrhea.*

sebastomania (sē-băs-tō-mā'nĭ-ă) [G. *sebastos,* reverend, + *mania,* madness]. Religious insanity.

sebiagogic (seb-ĭ-ă-goj'ĭk) [L. *sebum,* tal-

sebiferous   S-24   **sebum**

low, + G. *agōgos*, leading]. Forming fat or sebaceous matter. SYN: *sebiferous, sebiparous*.
sebiferous (sē-bĭf′ĕr-ŭs) [" + *ferre*, to carry]. Producing fatty or sebaceous matter. SYN: *sebiagogic, sebiparous*.
sebip′arous [" + *parēre*, to produce]. Producing sebum or sebaceous matter. SYN: *sebiagogic, sebiferous*.
sebolite, sebolith (sĕb′ō-līt, -lĭth) [" + G. *lithos*, a stone]. Concretion in a sebaceous gland.
seborrhagia (sĕb-ō-rā′jĭ-ă) [" + G. *rhēgnūnai*, to burst forth]. Excessive secretion of sebaceous glands. SYN: *seborrhea*.

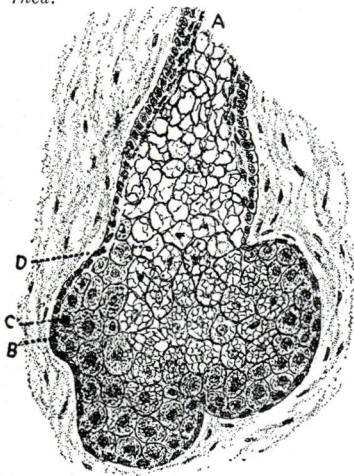

SEBACEOUS GLAND.
(*Meatus auditorium* in man)
A. Epidermis of hair follicle. B. Germinating layer. C. Sebaceous cells in stage of beginning fatty metamorphosis. D. Particles of sebaceous material.

seborrhea (sĕb-or-ē′ă) [L. *sebum*, tallow, + G. *rhoia*, a flow]. Functional disease of the sebaceous glands marked by increase in the amount and often alteration of the quality of the sebaceous secretion.
ETIOL: Reflex venous congestion of skin predisposes, therefore, indigestion, constipation, etc., are contributory.
PROG: Favorable, under prolonged and judicious treatment.
TREATMENT: Constitutional. Keep up general health, avoid constipation. The gastrointestinal tract often requires especial attention. Crusts should be removed by applications of oil, followed by shampooing with alcohol and green soap. Cleanliness, and a thorough rinsing off of the soap used, will effect a great deal. Underlying factor to be remedied or removed. Skin cleansed with soap and water, benzine or carbon tetrachloride. X-rays, sulfur, resorcin.
RS: *dermatitis seborrhoeica, sebaceous, sebum*.
   s. capillitii. Scalp seborrhea.
   s. congestiva. Facial form with elevated patches with red borders and covered with crusts and scars. SYN: *lupus erythematosus*.
   s. corporis. S. of the trunk.
   s. faciei. S. of the face.
   s. nigra, s. nigricans. Dark-colored crusts in seborrhea.
   s. oleosa. S. in which fat elements predominate. Shows shiny skin with widely dilated follicular orifices, many of which contain comedones.
   s. sicca. S. with grayish-brown or yellow scale and crust formation in addition to abnormal oiliness.
Differentiation from seborrheic dermatitis is difficult. This form most frequently observed on scalp and consti-

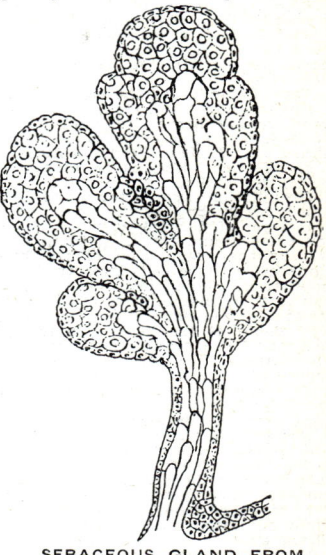

SEBACEOUS GLAND FROM HUMAN SKIN.

tutes what is popularly called dandruff.
Examination reveals an incrustation composed of thin, yellowish-gray scales. In uncomplicated cases the skin is pale, but often from irritation may become hyperemic or inflamed. When allowed to continue, nutrition of hair is interfered with, and baldness results. On the body s. sicca appears as yellowish-gray, slightly elevated patches covered with greasy scales. Outlets of follicles are often dilated. There is generally more or less redness of the skin from hyperemia (seborrheal eczema).
seborrheic (sĕb-or-rē′ĭk) [L. *sebum*, tallow, + G. *rhoia*, flow]. Afflicted with or like seborrhea.
seborrheid (sĕb-ō-rē′ĭd) [" + G. *rhoia*, a flow]. A seborrheic eruption.
seborrhoea (sĕb-or-ē′ă) [" + G. *rhoia*, a flow]. Disease of the sebaceous glands marked by increased discharge and altered quality of the secretion. SYN: *seborrhea, q.v.*
seborrhoic (sĕb-or-ō′ĭk) [" + G. *rhoia*, a flow]. Suffering from or like seborrhea.* SYN: *seborrheic*.
sebum (sē′bŭm) [L. *sebum*, tallow]. A

fatty secretion of the sebaceous glands of the skin.
It varies in different parts of the body; that from the ears is called *cerumen,* that from the foreskin is called *smegma praeputii,* and that which covers the body of the newborn is called *vernix caseosa.*
RS: *sebaceous, seborrhea, smegma.*

secernent (sē-ser'nĕnt) [L. *secerneus,* secreting]. 1. Secreting. 2. A secreting organ.

seclusio pupillae [L.]. Shutting off of the pupil due to adherence of iris to the lenticular capsule. SYN: *synechia, annular posterior.*
  s. p. siderosis bulbi. Deposit of iron pigment within the eyeball.
  Seen in cases of retained iron foreign body in the eye.

seconal (sē'kŏn-ăl). A barbituric acid derivative.
USES: Same as for the barbiturates.
DOSAGE: 1.5 gr. (0.1 Gm.).

second cranial nerve (sĕk'und) [L. *secunda*]. The optic nerve which controls sight. SEE: *Table of Nerves in Appendix.*
  s. intention. Healing by granulation or indirect union.
  Granulation tissue is formed to fill the gap bet. the edges of the wound with a thin layer of fibrinous exudate. It bars out bacteria and aids in checking bleeding by the coagulation of the blood. Connective tissue cells support the new capillaries. This form of healing is slower than that by first intention and its grayish-red surface may become pale and flabby if the healing is too long delayed. If the granulations show above the surface they may have to be removed with caustics. If the granulations first form at the top instead of the bottom of the wound, it may have to be kept open with drainage.
RS: *healing, intention, resolution.*
  s. sight. Alteration in refractive powers of the lens so that reading again is possible without glasses in incipient cataract. SYN: *gerontopia.*
  s. stage of labor. Period bet. complete dilatation of cervix and delivery of the child.
  During this stage pains become severe. It lasts normally 2-4 hr. in primiparae and up to 1 hr. in multiparae.

secondary (sek'ŭn-dar-ĭ) [L. *secondarius,* second]. 1. Next to or following; second in order. 2. Produced by a primary cause. SYN: *subordinate.*
  s. areola. Pigmentation around the nipples during pregnancy. SEE: *areola.*
  s. disease. One following a previous disease.
  s. hemorrhage. 1. One after an injury or operation coming on more than 24 hr. afterward and which is due to sepsis and septic ulceration into a blood vessel. 2. Uterine bleeding due to septic infection or from infant's umbilicus due to same cause. SEE: *hemorrhage.*

secreta (sē-krē'tă) [L.]. The products of secretion.

secretagogue (sē-krē'tă-gog) [L. *secretum,* secretion, + G. *agogos,* leading]. 1. Causing secretion. 2. That which stimulates secreting organs, as "substances present in food or produced by the digestion or decomposition of food which excite the secretion of digestive juice either by acting locally or by being absorbed into the blood or lymph or by causing a hormone to be formed." (A. C. Ivy.)

secrete (sē-krēt') [L. *secretus,* separated].
To separate a constituent from the blood, elaborate and discharge it; said of a gland.

secretin (sē-krē'tĭn) [L. *secretio,* a separation]. 1. A hormone formed in the mucous membrane of the duodenum through the influence of acid contents from the stomach whose function is to stimulate the flow of pancreatic juice. 2. A substance of unknown chemical composition, prepared by extraction from the mucous membrane of the duodenum and causing, when injected intravenously, an increased secretion of pancreatic juice.
Probably formed from a precursor, prosecretin.*
SEE: *duodenal and intestinal digestion, gastrin.*

secretion (sē-krē'shŭn) [L. *secretio,* a separation]. 1. A process in physiology whereby certain materials are separated, by the activity of a gland, from the blood, and made into something useful to the body. 2. Substance secreted. Fluids of the body.
If the useful material flows out through a duct (e. g., saliva) it is called an *external secretion;* if it is returned to the blood or lymph (e. g., insulin) it is called an *internal secretion* or autacoid.*

SECRETIONS OF BODY
(With amount for 24 hours)
BLOOD: Is composed of 14 elements, 79% water, 21% solids, 500 to 600 red corpuscles to 1 white.
BILE: Emulsifies fats and precipitates soluble peptones, 20 to 24 oz. Sp. gr. 1.026-1.032. Reaction alkaline.
CHYLE: Absorbed by lacteals, resembles lymph. Begins to be formed in duodenum, 4-5 lb. Sp. gr. 1.015. Alkaline.
CHYME: Food that has undergone gastric digestion only.
GASTRIC JUICE: An antiseptic juice that converts proteids into peptones. Six to 8 lb. Sp. gr. 1.010. Reaction acid.
INTESTINAL JUICE: Has combined action of saliva, gastric and pancreatic juices. Converts cane into grape sugar and maltose into glucose. Also contains a milk curdling ferment, 10 oz. Sp. gr. 1.011. Reaction alkaline.
LYMPH: Clear, transparent, yellowish fluid devoid of smell with saline taste. Four to 5 lb. Sp. gr. 1.012 to 1.022, alkaline.
MENSTRUAL: Menstrual blood. Two to 4 oz. in entire period.
PANCREATIC JUICE: Emulsifies fats and converts proteids into peptones, 20 oz. Sp. gr. 1.010 to 1.015. Alkaline.
PERSPIRATION: The secretion of sweat glands of skin. About 2 lb. Sp. gr. 1.005. Acid.
SALIVA: Converts starch into sugar. Secreted by salivary glands, 30-40 oz. Sp. gr. 1.002-1.006. Alkaline.
URINE: Forty to 50 oz. Sp. gr. 1.015-2. Acid. Contains 1½ oz. solids, 30-50 gr. urea, 1 gr. uric acid to 33 gr. urea. SEE: *urine.*
  s., antilytic. Watery saliva excreted continuously by submaxillary gland with intact nerves after division of the chorda tympani of the other side.
  s., external. S. discharged from the body.
  s., internal. S. imparted to the blood instead of being eliminated by a duct.
  s., nervous. S. that depends upon activity of secretory nerves.
  s., paralytic. Abundant watery secre-

tion continuously from a gland after section of its secretory nerves.

secretion, words pert. to: acrinia, amyxia, anorrhorrhea, apolepsis, asteatosis, athyrea, athyria, athyroidism, cerumen, ceruminal, ceruminosis, ceruminous, choleresis, chromocrinia, crinogenic, diacrisis, errhine, exsiccant, hormone, interstitial, saliva, sebum, secretagogue, secrete, secretin, semen, smegma, succorrhea.

secretodermatosis (sē-krē″tō-der-mă-tō′sĭs) [L. *secretio*, a separation, + G. *derma*, skin, + *-osis*, condition]. Condition resulting from disorder of the secretory function of the skin.

secretogogue (sē-krē′tō-gŏg) [″ + G. *agogos*, leading]. 1. Causing secretion. 2. That which stimulates secretion.

secretoinhibitory (sē-krē″tō-ĭn-hĭb′ĭ-tō-rĭ) [″ + *inhibere*, to restrain]. Checking secretion.

secretomotor, secretomotory (sē-krē′tō-mō′tor, -ĭ) [″ + *motor*, a mover]. Stimulating or promoting secretion.

secretory (sē-krē′tō-rĭ, sē′krē-tō-rĭ) [L. *secretio*, a separation]. Pert. to or promoting secretion; secreting.
  s. capillaries. Very small canaliculi receiving secretion discharged from gland cells.
  s. fibers. Centrifugal nerve fibers which excite secretion.

sectarian (sĕk-tār′ĭ-ăn) [L. *sectum*, from *secāre*, to cut]. A medical man who "follows a dogma, tenet, or principle based on the authority of its promulgator to the exclusion of demonstration and practice" (Judicial Council A. M. A.).

sectile (sĕk′tĭl) [L. *sectilis*, able to be cut]. Capable of being cut.

section (sĕk′shŭn) [L. *sectio*, from *secāre*, to cut]. 1. Process of cutting. 2. A division or segment of a part. 3. A surface made by cutting.
  s., abdominal. Any abdominal operation. SYN: *laparotomy, q.v.*
  s., cesarean. Incision of uterus for delivery of a fetus through abdominal wall or through the vagina. SEE: *cesarean section*.
  s., frontal. One dividing the body into 2 parts, *dorsal* and *ventral*.
  s., occipital. Transverse s. through middle of the occipital lobe.
  s., parietal. Transverse vertical s. through ascending parietal convolution.
  s., perineal. External incision into urethra to relieve stricture.
  s., sagittal. One parallel with the sagittal suture.
  s., serial. Microscopic sections made and arranged in consecutive order.
  s., sigaultian. Resection of the symphysis pubis. SYN: *symphysiotomy*.
  s., vaginal. Incision into the abdominal cavity through the vagina.

sectioning (sĕk-shŭn′ĭng) [L. *sectio*, a cutting]. The slicing of thin sections of tissue for examination under the microscope.

sector (sĕk′tor) [L. *sector*, a cutter]. The area of a circle included bet. 2 radii and an arc.

sectorial (sĕk-tō′rĭ-ăl) [L. *sector*, a cutter]. Cutting, as teeth.

secundae viae (sē-kŭn′de vī′e) [L. second way]. Secondary passage in the body for nutrients, the lacteals and blood vessels. SEE: *via*.

secundigravida (sē-kŭn″dĭ-grăv′ĭd-ă) [L. *secundus*, second, + *gravida*, a pregnant woman]. A woman in her 2nd pregnancy.

secundinae (sĕk″ŭn-dē′nē) [L. things following]. The membranes discharged after birth of the child. SYN: *afterbirth*.

secundines (sĕk′ŭn-dīns) [L. *secundinae*, things following]. The placenta and fetal membranes expelled during the 3rd stage of labor. SYN: *afterbirth*.

secundipara (sē″kŭn-dĭp′ă-ră) [L. *secundus*, second, + *parēre*, to give birth]. A woman who has borne 2 children at separate labors.

secundum artem (sē-kun′dŭm ar′tĕm) [L.]. In an approved manner; according to rule or science.

S. E. D. Abbr. for *skin erythema dose*.

Sed. [L.]. Abbr. of *sedes*, stool.

sedation (sē-dā′shŭn) [L. *sedatio*, from *sedāre*, to calm]. 1. Process of allaying nervous excitement. 2. State of being calmed.
  Usually effected by means of a drug.

sedative (sĕd′a-tĭv) [L. *sedativus*, calming]. 1. An agent allaying irritability or nerve action. 2. Quieting.
  They may be *general, local, nervous*, or *vascular*.
  TYPES AND EX: *Cardiac*: Bromides, chloral, pilocarpine. *Respiratory*: Chloral, opium. *Gastric*: Bismuth, belladonna. *Nervous*: Antipyrine. *Cerebral*: Bromides and all hypnotics. *Intestinal*: Bismuth, opium. *General*: Opium and all hypnotics.
  s., cardiac. One that decreases the heart's force.
  s. enema. Retention enema given for its soothing action and to allay irritability. SEE: *enema, sedative*.
  s., nervous. S. affecting nervous system.
  s. poisons. TREATMENT: Administer large amounts of fluids and induce vomiting.
  Tea made by boiling to extract the tannic acid should be given repeatedly; a solution of tannic acid, a teaspoonful to a pint may be used, if available. Strong coffee, caffeine, citrate, aromatic spirits of ammonia or other available stimulants should be used. Induce diaphoresis, diuresis and catharsis. Oxygen and artificial respiration may be necessary. The patient should be kept in the Trendelenburg position. External heat, flagellation, massage, talking and other methods of keeping the patient awake are temporarily useful. There is always associated shock.

sedentary (sĕd′ĕn-ta-rĭ) [L. *sedentarius*, from *sedere*, to sit]. 1. Sitting. 2. Pert. to an indoor occupation in which physical exercise is impossible.

sediment (sĕd′ĭ-mĕnt) [L. *sedimentum*, a settling]. The substance settling at bottom of a liquid. SYN: *hypostasis*. SEE: *precipitate*.

sedimentation (sĕd″ĭ-mĕn-tā′shŭn) [L. *sedimentum*, a settling]. Formation or depositing of sediment.
  s. rate. Speed at which erythrocytes settle when an anticoagulant is added to blood. SYN: *suspension stability*.
  In this test, blood to which an anticoagulant has been added is placed in a long, narrow tube, and the speed at which the red cells settle is observed. Various methods of determining the rate have been devised. Some pathologists determine the time required for the cells to settle a certain distance (sedimentation time), while others determine the distance the cells settle in a given time (sedimentation rate), both normally about 5 min. per millimeter. The speed at which the cells settle depends upon the size of the clumps into which the red cells aggregate, and the size of the

clumps appears to depend upon the amount of fibrinogen in the blood. The speed of settling is increased in a variety of infections, in cancer, and in pregnancy, and may be decreased in liver disease.
sedimentator (sĕd-ĭ-mĕn-tā'tor) [L. *sedimentum*, a settling]. A centrifuge for separating urinary sediment.
seed (sēd) [A.S. *saed*, seed]. 1. The part of the fruit containing the germ. Ex: *nux vomica, mustard, colchicum seed*. 2. Sperm; semen. 3. Capsule containing radon, radium, etc., for use in treatment of cancer. 4. Offspring. 5. To introduce microörganisms into a culture medium.
segment (sĕg'mĕnt) [L. *segmentum*, a portion]. 1. A part or section, esp. a natural one, of an organ or body. 2. One of the serial divisions of an animal. SYN: *metamere*.
segmental (sĕg-mĕn'tăl) [L. *segmentum*, a portion]. Relating to or forming a segment.
segmentation (sĕg″mĕn-tā'shŭn) [L. *segmentum*, a portion]. 1. Division into similar parts. SEE: *merogenesis*. 2. Formation of many cells from a single cell. SYN: *cleavage*.
   s. cavity. Central space in blastula stage of segmentation of an ovum.
   s. nucleus. N. developing from union of the male and female pronuclei.
   s., rhythmic. Division of chyme into segments by intestinal contractions. SEE: *intestinal digestion*.
   s. sphere. Cells of an ovum during early stages of segmentation when nucleus is dividing.
segregator (sĕg're-gā-tor) [L. *segregāre*, to separate]. Instrument composed of 2 catheters for securing urine from each kidney separately.
Séguin's signal symptom (sa-ganz'). Contraction of muscles constituting a forerunner of an epileptic attack.
Seidelin bodies (sī'de-lĭn). Parasitic organisms in the erythrocytes in yellow fever, the probable cause of the disease.
Seidlitz powder (sĕd'lĭts, sĭd'lĭtz). Effervescent cathartic composed of tartaric acid, sodium bicarbonate, and sodium and potassium tartrate.
seisesthesia (sī-zĕs-thē'zĭ-ă) [G. *seisis*, concussion, + *aisthēsis*, sensation]. The perception of a concussion.
seismesthesia (sīz-mĕs-thē'zĭ-ă) [G. *seismos*, earthquake, + *aisthēsis*, sensation]. Perception of vibrations.
seismotherapy (sīz-mō-thĕr'ă-pĭ) [" + *therapeia*, treatment]. Treatment of disease by vibratory massage. SYN: *sismotherapy*.
seizure (sē'zhŭr) [M.E. *seizen*, to take possession of]. A sudden attack of pain or of a disease, or of certain symptoms.
   s., psychic. Appearance of morbid sensations, such as palpitation, with temporary disturbance of consciousness.
self-abuse'. Unnatural method of bringing about the venereal orgasm by mechanical friction, in either sex. SYN: *masturbation*.
self-diges'tion. Destruction or disintegration of a cell or tissue by its own juice, as that of the walls of the stomach by the gastric juice occurring in certain diseases of that organ. SYN: *autodigestion*.
self-induc'tance. Tendency in a conductor to oppose changes in current by formation of a counter electromotive force. SEE: *inductance*.
self-lim'ited disease. Disease that, without treatment, runs a definite course within a limited time.
self-pollu'tion. Sexual self-abuse. SYN: *masturbation*.
self-suspen'sion. Suspension of the body for extension by stretching of the vertebral column.
sella turcica (sĕl'a tur'sĭ-ka) [L. Turkish saddle]. Pituitary fossa of middle of the sphenoid bone enclosing the pituitary body.
sellar (sĕl'ar) [L. *sella turcica*, Turkish saddle]. Pert. to the sella turcica, depression for pituitary body in sphenoid bone.
Selters water, Seltzer water (sĕl'ters, sĕlt'ser). Effervescent mineral water containing carbonates of sodium, calcium, chloride of sodium, and magnesium.
semeiology (sē″mĭ-ŏl'ō-jĭ) [G. *semeion*, sign, + *logos*, study]. The branch of medicine dealing with the study of symptoms. SYN: *symptomatology*.
semeiosis (sē-mĭ-ō'sĭs) [" + *-ōsis*, intensive]. Study of disease by symptoms.
semeiotic (sē″mĭ-ot'ĭk) [G. *sēmeiōtikos*, pert. to a sign]. Of or pert. to symptoms. SYN: *symptomatic*.
semeiotics (sē″mĭ-ŏt'ĭks) [G. *sēmeiōtikos*, pert. to a sign]. 1. Phase of medical science treating of symptoms. 2. Symptoms of a disease in a particular case considered as a whole. SYN: *semiotics, symptomatology*.
semel (sĕm'ĕl) [L.]. Once. SEE: *charting, prescription writing*.
semelincident (sĕm-ĕl-ĭn'sĭd-ĕnt) [L. *semel*, once, + *incidens*, falling upon]. Occurring only once in the same person.
semen (sē'mĕn) (pl. *semina*) [L. *sēmen*, seed]. A thick, opalescent, viscid secretion discharged from the urethra of the male at the climax of sexual excitement (orgasm) which fertilizes the female ovum.
   It is the mixed product of various glands (prostate and bulbourethral) plus the spermatozoa which, having been produced in the testicles, are stored in the seminal vesicles.
   RS: *aspermatic; aspermatism; aspermos; azoöspermia; bradyspermatism; coition; coitus; coitus interruptus; copulation; ejaculation; emissio seminis; emission; erection; excitation; fertilization; insemination; libido; orgasm; penis; prostate; sexual intercourse; sperm; sperma; spermatemphraxis; spermatic; spermatorrhea; spermatozoön; vesicle, seminal*.
semenuria (sē″mĕn-ū'rĭ-ă) [L. *sēmen*, seed, + G. *ouron*, urine]. Excretion of semen in the urine. SYN: *seminuria, spermaturia*.
semi- [L.]. Prefix meaning *half*.
semicanal (sĕm″ĭ-kăn-ăl') [L. *semis*, half, + *canalis*, passage]. A duct open on one side.
semicircular (sĕm″ĭ-sĭr'kŭ-lar) [" + *circulus*, a ring]. In the form of a half circle.
   s. canals. Sup. post., and inf. passages forming back part of ear, *q.v.*
semicoma (sĕm″ĭ-kō'mă) [" + G. *kōma*, lethargy]. Mild degree of coma from which it is possible to arouse the patient.
semicomatose (sĕm″ĭ-kō'măt-ōs) [" + G. *kōma*, lethargy]. In a condition of unconsciousness from which patient may be aroused.
semiflexion (sĕm″ĭ-flĕk'shŭn) [" + *flexio*, from *flectere*, to bend]. Position of a segment of a limb midway bet. flexion and extension.

semilunar (sĕm″ĭ-lū′nar) [" + *luna*, moon]. Crescentic in shape.
 s. bone. Halfmoon-shaped bone of carpus.
 s. cartilages. Two crescentic cartilages (int. and ext.) in the knee joint bet. the femur and tibia.
 s. ganglions. Two small nervous ganglions of the abdominal cavity, supplying solar plexus.
 s. lobe. One on upper surface of the cerebellum.
 s. notch. Notch in scapula for passage of the suprascapular nerve.
 s. valves. Valves of aorta and pulmonary artery. SEE: *Arantius' body*.
semimembranosus (sĕm″ĭ-mĕm-brăn-ō′sŭs) [L.]. Large muscle of inner and back part of thigh. SEE: *Table of Muscles in Appendix*.
seminal (sĕm′ĭn-ăl) [L. *sēmen, semin-*, seed]. Concerning the semen.
 s. emission. Involuntary loss of seminal fluid, usually during sleep, esp. in the adolescent male.
 s. filament. Male seed. SYN: *spermatozoon*.
 s. fluid. Semen, male fertilizing fluid.
 s. vesicle. Sac, on either side, in male connected with seminal duct and serving to store semen temporarily. SYN: *vesicula seminalis*.
semination (sĕm-ĭn-ā′shŭn) [L. *seminatio*, a begetting]. Introduction of semen into the uterus during sexual intercourse or artificially. SYN: *insemination*.
 s., artificial. Introduction of prepared semen into the uterus. SYN: *artificial insemination*.
seminiferous (sĕm-ĭn-ĭf′ĕr-ŭs) [L. *sēmen, semin-*, seed, + *ferre*, to produce]. Producing or conducting semen, as the tubules of the testes.
seminoma (sĕm-ĭ-nō′mă) [" + G. *-ōma*, tumor]. A tumor of the testis.
seminormal (sĕm″ĭ-nor′măl) [L. *semis*, half, + *norma*, rule]. One-half the normal standard.
 s. solution. One having half the quantity of the substance in the normal solution.
seminuria (sē″mĭn-ū′rĭ-ă) [L. *sēmen*, seed, + G. *ouron*, urine]. Seminal discharge present in the urine. SYN: *semenuria, spermaturia*.
semiology (sē″mĭ-ŏl′ō-jĭ) [G. *sēmeion*, sign, + *logos*, a study]. Phase of medicine dealing with study of symptoms. SYN: *semeiology, symptomatology*.
semiotic (sē-mĭ-ŏt′ĭk) [G. *sēmeiōtikos*, pert. to a sign]. Like or pert. to symptoms of disease. SYN: *semeiotic, symptomatic*.
semiotics (sē″mĭ-ŏt′ĭks) [G. *sēmeiōtikos*, pert. to a sign]. Scientific study of symptoms as a whole or in one particular case. SYN: *semiology, symptomatology*.
semiparasite (sĕm″ĭ-par′ă-sīt) [L. *semis*, half, + G. *parasitos*, living beside]. 1. Organism usually a parasite, but capable of living as a saprophyte. 2. An organism with mild infectiousness for living tissue.
semipermeable (sĕm″ĭ-per′mē-ă-bl) [" + *per*, through, + *meāre*, to pass]. Half permeable; said of a membrane which will allow fluids but not the dissolved substance to pass through it. SEE: *membrane, osmosis*.
semiprone (sĕm-ĭ-prōn′) [" + *pronus*, prone]. In a position on left side and chest, with both thighs flexed on abdomen, the right higher than the left, and left arm back. SYN: *Sims' position, q.v., for illustration*.

semirecumbent (sĕm″ĭ-rē-kŭm′bĕnt) [" + *recumbere*, to lie down]. Reclining, but not fully recumbent.
semis (sē′mĭs) [L. *semis*, half]. Half. Abbreviated to *ss* after sign indicating the measure in prescriptions.
semisideratio, semisideration (sĕm″ĭ-sĭd-ĕr-ā′shĭ-ō, -ā′shŭn) [" + *sideratio*, a blight]. Paralysis on one side of the body. SYN: *hemiplegia*.
semisopor (sĕm-ĭ-sō′por) [" + *sopor*, deep sleep]. Light coma from which patient can be roused. SYN: *semicoma*.
semispinalis (sĕm″ĭ-spī-na′lĭs) [L.]. Deep layer of muscle of back on either side of spinal column, divided into 3 parts. SEE: *Table of Muscles in Appendix*.
semisulcus (sĕm″ĭ-sŭl′kŭs) [L. *semis*, half, + *sulcus*, a groove]. A slight depression or groove which forms a sulcus by uniting with a similar groove on the adjoining structure.
semisupination (sĕm″ĭ-sŭ-pĭn-ā′shŭn) [" + *supinus*, bent back]. A position halfway bet. supination and pronation.
semitendinosus (sĕm″ĭ-tĕn-dĭn-ō′sŭs) [L.]. Fusiform muscle of post. and inner part of thigh. SEE: *Table of Muscles in Appendix*.
semper- [L.]. Combining form meaning *always*.
senescence (sĕn-es′ĕns) [L. *senescere*, to grow old]. The process of growing old, or the period of old age.
senile (sē′nīl, -nĭl) [L. *senilis*, old]. Pert. to growing old or to the aged.
 Absence of vitamin G in diet has hastened premature senility. Vitamins A, C, and G with liberal amounts of calcium help to insure nutritional conditions through the life cycle.
senilism (sē′nĭl-ĭzm, -nĭl-ĭzm) [" + G. *-ismos*, condition]. Old age, particularly when premature. SEE: *progeria*.
senility (sē-nĭl′ĭ-tĭ) [L. *senilis*, old]. 1. The state of being old. 2. Weakness of old age, mental or physical.
 s., premature. Onset of characteristics before the normal time.
 May be due to dissipation, privation, or congenital structural defects.
 s., psychosis of. Mental disorder in old age.
 SYM: General impairment of all special senses. Many imagined pains. Skin is undernourished and inelastic and wrinkled. Memory and comprehension fail, as well as judgment and mental ability. Marked motor restlessness and often delusions of persecution. Delirium may occur.
 SEE: *caducity, canities, progeria*.
senium (sē′nĭ-ŭm) [L.]. Old age, esp. its debility.
 s. precox. PSY: Mental disorder resembling senile dementia occurring before 60, usually showing incoherent delusions.
senna (sĕn′a) [Arabic *sana*]. USP. The dried leaves of the plant *Cassia acutifolia* and *C. angustifolia*.
 ACTION AND USES: As a purgative acting on the large intestine.
 DOSAGE: 30 gr. (2 Gm.).
Senn's bone plates (sĕn). Plates of decalcified bone used for intestinal anastomoses.
senopia (sĕn-ō′pĭ-ă) [L. *senilis*, old, + G. *ōps*, eye]. Improvement in visual power of old people usually due to incipient cataract. SYN: *gerontopia*.
sensation (sĕn-sā′shŭn) [L. *sensatio*, a feeling]. 1. State resulting when a stimulus is conveyed to the brain by the ac-

tion of an afferent nerve and projected *externally* in the form of sight, smell, taste, hearing, heat, cold, or pressure, or *internally* as in hunger, pain, thirst, fatigue, sexual desire, etc. SEE: *receptor*. 2. Power or act of responding to stimulation.

The "mirroring" of the world of reality within the central nervous system of the individual is a prerequisite to favorable reactions and behavior. This information is obtained in many ways: *Vision* and *hearing* are distant receptors, as (in a modified sense) is smell. *Taste* requires contact with the *taste buds* chiefly located on the tongue. *Touch* is a composite sense appreciating not only contact (such as a strand of cotton) but hot, cold, pain and movement of a part.

A synthesis of all sense modalities in the cortex of the brain results in the keenest possible understanding of the situation and so favors the "best" response.

Sensation may be lost, diminished, or increased. In the realm of touch, one speaks of *anesthesia, hypesthesia,* or *hyperesthesia.* Analgesia indicates an absence of pain sense. Hallucinations are sensory falsifications.

Sense impressions do not register well in imbecility, senility, paresis, epilepsy, arteriosclerosis, or Korsakoff's psychosis.

s., articular. S. caused by moving of joint surfaces.

s., common. The sum total of all bodily sensations.

s., cutaneous. S. through medium of the skin.

s., delayed. S. not experienced immediately following a stimulus.

s., epigastric. A sinking feeling in the stomach.

s., external. Effect upon the mind of any stimuli from peripheral nerves.

s., general. One of the body as a whole and not referred to any particular external object. SEE: *subjective s.*

s., girdle. A painful s., as a bandage tightened about a limb or the trunk as in spinal disease. SYN: *zonesthesia.*

s., gnostic. Nerve sensations, as those of touch and vibration.

s., internal. A subjective one.

s., palmesthetic. S. felt in the skin from vibration.

s., referred. Same as reflex sensation.

s., reflex. S. felt elsewhere than at point of stimulus.

s., subjective. S. not resulting from any external stimulus and perceptible only by the subject.

s., tactile. S. produced through the sense of touch.

s., transferred. Same as a reflex sensation.

sensation, words pert. to: abarognosis, acanthesthesia, achiria, acragnosis, acroagnosis, acroanesthesia, acroesthesia, acroparesthesia, algesia, algesic, algesthesia, algetic, algor, algos, allachesthesia, allesthesia, allochesthesia, allochiria, anakatesthesia, analgesia, anesthesia, anoci-association, anodyne, anodynia, aponia, apselaphesia, ardanesthesia, asphalgesia, baragnosis, baresthesia, barognosis, bathesthesia, bathyanesthesia, bathyhyperesthesia, besoin de respirer, bradyesthesia, cacesthesia, calefacient, eardianesthesia, caumesthesia, cenesthesia, centraphose, ceptor, chaude-pisse, chromophose, cincture s., cinesthesia, cryanesthesia, cryesthesia, dyschiria, dysesthesia, epicritic, esthesia, formication, girdle s., haphonosus, haptodysphoria, hypalgesia, hypalgia, hyperesthesia, hyperthymia, hypesthesia, hypothymia, kinesthesia, mordication, nerve, obdormition, obtusion, odaxesmus, organule, oxyesthesia. palsy, paralysis, paresthesia, polyesthesia, proprioception, sensitization, sensorium, sensory, supersensitiveness, synesthesia, tactile, thermesthesia, threshold stimulus, topesthesia, zonesthesia.

sense (sĕns) [L. *sensus*, a feeling]. 1. To perceive through a sense organ. 2. The general faculty by which conditions outside or inside the body are perceived. 3. Any special faculty of sensation connected with a particular organ. 4. Normal power of understanding.

The most important of the senses are: (1) Sight; (2) hearing; (3) smell; (4) taste; (5) touch and pressure; (6) temperature; (7) weight, resistance, and tension (muscle sense); (8) pain; (9) visceral and sexual sensations; (10) equilibrium; (11) hunger and thirst.

s., acid. Ability of the stomach to regulate as needed the secretion of hydrochloric acid.

s. body. The peripheral termination of nerve of special sensation.

s. capsule. Hollow, cuplike receptacle of a peripheral sense organ.

s., color. The perception of various colors.

s., concomitant. A secondary sensation along with a primary one.

s., cutaneous. Sensation felt through the skin.

s., dermal. A sensation felt through the skin.

s. epithelium. A tract of epithelium having a specialized function of sensation.

s., genesic. The sexual instinct.

s., kinesthetic. SEE: *muscular s.*

s., light. Perception of degree of light.

s., muscle, muscular. Consciousness of muscular movement required in a given act.

s's., nutritive. S's. of smell and taste.

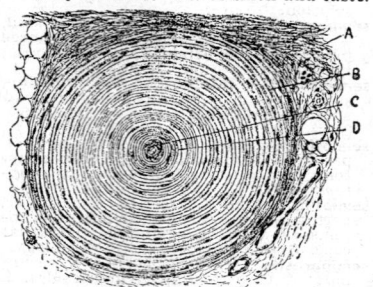

SENSE ORGAN, CUTANEOUS
Transverse section of pacinian corpuscle. Sole of foot of man. A. Connective tissue. B. Outer lamellose sheath. C. Central core. D. Axis cylinder.

s. organ. The organ which gives rise to a nerve impulse which reaching the brain registers in consciousness as a particular sensation.

s., posture. Ability through muscle sense to differentiate positions of the body or its structures.

s., pressure. Faculty of feeling various degrees of pressure on the body surface.

s., seventh. Subjective sensations of internal organs.
s. shock. Condition in hysterics at moment of awakening, the sensation rising from feet or hands and disappearing in the sense of having been struck a blow in the head.
s., sixth. General feeling of normal functioning of the bodily organs. SYN: *cenesthesia.*
s., space. That sense by which we recognize objects in space, their relationship and dimensions.
s's., special. Sight, hearing, smell, touch, and taste.
s., stereognostic. Ability to judge consistency and shape of objects held in the fingers.
s., temperature. Ability to detect differences of temperature.
s., time. Ability to detect differences in time intervals, as in sound.
s., tone. Ability to distinguish bet. different tones.
s., visceral. Perception of the sensations of the internal organs. SYN: *seventh sense.*
sensibilatrice (son-se-be-lăt-rēs) [Fr.]. An immune body. SYN: *amboceptor, q.v.*
sensibilin (sĕn'sĭ-bĭl-ĭn) [L. *sensibilis*, feeling]. A specific antibody formed at first injection of a foreign protein, derived from sensibilisinogen.
sensibilisin (sĕn-sĭ-bĭl'ĭ-sĭn) [L. *sensibilis*, feeling]. A specific antibody produced by introduction of a foreign protein and arising from a substance in it. SYN: *anaphylactin.*
sensibilisinogen (sĕn-sĭ-bĭl-ĭs-ĭn'ō-jĕn). A substance in an antigen that, when injected, produces a specific antibody, *sensibilisin.* SEE: *allergen.*
sensibility (sĕn-sĭ-bĭl'ĭ-tĭ) [L. *sensibilitās*]. Capacity to receive and respond to stimuli.
s., bone. Sensation like that received from the vibration of a tuning fork. SYN: *pallesthesia.*
s., deep. 1. The sensibility existing after an area is made anesthetic. 2. Sensation by which the position of a limb and estimation of difference in weight and tension is apparent.
s., epicritic. The sensibility which makes fine discriminations of touch and temperature.
s., mesoblastic. SEE: *deep s.*
s., palmesthetic. SEE: *bone s.*
s., protopathic. The sensibility to strong stimulations of pain and temperature, which exists in the skin and in the viscera.
s., recurrent. Sensibility in the ant. root of a spinal nerve when distal portion is stimulated after section.
s., somesthetic. Sensory consciousness of bodily movements.
s., splanchnesthetic. Consciousness or sensibility from splanchnic receptors.
sensibilization (sĕn-sĭ-bĭl-ĭz-ā'shŭn) [L. *sensibilitās*, feeling]. 1. The process of making sensitive. 2. Production of hypersusceptibility to a foreign substance by injecting it into the body. SYN: *anaphylaxis, sensitization.*
sensibilizer (sĕn'sĭ-bĭl-ī-zer) [L. *sensibilitās*, feeling]. Substance in blood serum normally or after inoculation which is active in cytolysis. SYN: *amboceptor, immune body, sensitizer.*
sensible (sĕn'sĭ-bl) [L. *sensibilis*, feeling]. 1. Capable of being perceived by the senses; perceptible. 2. Capable of receiving sensations. SYN: *sensitive.* 3. Having reason. SYN: *intelligent.* 4. Conscious, as opposed to insensible.
sensiferous (sĕn-sĭf'ĕr-ŭs) [L. *sensus*, a feeling, + *ferre*, to bear]. Conducting or transmitting sensations.
sensigenous (sĕn-sĭj'ĕn-ŭs) [" + G. *gennan*, to produce]. Producing sensation.
sensimeter (sĕn-sĭm'ĕ-ter) [" + G. *metron*, a measure]. Machine for recording the degree of sensitiveness of various areas of the body.
sensitinogen (sĕn-sĭ-tĭn'ō-jen) [L. *sensus*, feeling, + G. *gennan*, to produce]. The antigens collectively which sensitize the body.
sensitive (sĕn'sĭ-tĭv) [L. *sensitivus*, feeling]. 1. Capable of transmitting a sensation. 2. Able to respond to a stimulus. 3. Subject to destructive action of a complement. 4. Susceptible to suggestions, as a hypnotic. 5. Abnormally susceptible to a substance, as a drug or foreign protein.
sensitization (sĕn"sĭ-tĭ-zā'shŭn) [L. *sentire*, to feel]. 1. A condition of being made sensitive to specific stimulus. 2. Rendering of a cell sensitive to the action of a complement by uniting it with a specific amboceptor. 3. Process of making a person susceptible to a substance by repeated injections of it, as a serum. SYN: *anaphylaxis.*
sensitized (sĕn'sĭ-tīzd). Made susceptible to a specific substance.
s. vaccine. A live culture which has been mixed with its antiserum before introduction.
sensitizer (sĕn'sĭ-tī''zer) [L. *sensitivus*, feeling]. An antibody producing susceptibility to cytolysis. SYN: *amboceptor.*
sensitometer (sĕn-sĭ-tŏm'ĕt-ĕr) [L. *sensitivus*, perceiving, + G. *metron*, a measure]. Device for determining the penetrating power of light.
sensomobile (sĕn-sō-mō'bĭl) [L. *sensus*, sensation, + *mobilis*, able to move]. Capable of responding to a stimulus.
sensomotor (sĕn''sō-mō'tor) [" + *motor*, motion]. Both sensory and motor, esp. a nerve with both afferent and efferent fibers. SYN: *sensorimotor.*
sensoparalysis (sĕn''sō-păr-ăl'ĭ-sĭs) [" + G. *paralyein*, to disable at the side]. Paralysis of a sensory nerve.
sensorial (sĕn-sō'rĭ-ăl) [L. *sensus*, a sensation]. Pert. to the sensorium, the seat of sensation.
sensorimotor (sĕn-sō-rĭ-mō'tor) [" + *motor*, motion]. Both sensory and motor. SYN: *sensomotor.*
sensorium (sĕn-sō'rĭ-ŭm) (pl. *sensoriums, -ria*) [L. *sensōrium*, from *sentīre*, to perceive]. 1. Brain center of a nerve and its special sense organ. 2. The sensory apparatus of the body taken as a whole.
s., clear. Normal correct memory and orientation.
sensory (sĕn'sō-rĭ) [L. *sensorius*]. 1. Conveying impulses from sense organs to the reflex or higher centers. SYN: *afferent.* 2. Pert. to sensation.
s. amusia. Inability to produce or understand musical sounds.
s. aphasia. Loss of memory for words. SEE: *aphasia.*
s. crossway. Part of the internal capsule behind lenticular nucleus at place where afferent fibers send forth sensory impulses to the opposite side.
s. decussation. The sup. pyramidal decussation.
s. epilepsy. Disturbances of sensation that replace epileptic convulsions.
s. nerve. An afferent nerve convey-

sensual   **septicemia**

ing sensory impressions to the sensorium, or one composed of sensory fibers.

sensual (sĕn'shû-ăl) [L. *sensus*, sense]. Concerning or consisting in the gratification of the senses.

sensuous (sĕn'shū-ŭs) [L. *sensus*, sense]. Pert. to or affecting the senses; susceptible to influence through the senses.

sentient (sĕn'shĭ-ĕnt) [L. *sentire*, to perceive]. Capable of sensation. SYN: *sensitive*.

separator (sĕp'ar-ā-tor) [L. *separator*, a separator]. 1. Anything which prevents 2 substances from mingling. 2. Device to prevent mingling in the bladder of urine from the 2 ureters.

separatorium (sĕp-ar-ā-tō'rĭ-ŭm) [L. *separatorium*, from *separāre*, to separate]. Instrument for separating pericranium from skull.

separatory (sĕp'ar-ā-tō"rĭ) [L. *separāre*, to separate]. Device for keeping objects or substances apart. SYN: *separator*.

sepedogenesis (sē"pĕd-ō-jĕn'ĕ-sĭs) [G. *sēpein*, to be rotten, + *genesis*, production]. Development of putrefaction.

sepsis (sĕp'sĭs) [G. *sēpsis*, putrefaction]. Poisoned state due to absorption of pathogenic bacteria and their products into the blood stream. SYN: *putrefaction*, *septicemia*, q.v.

s., gas. S. due to the gas bacillus, *Bacillus aerogenes capsulatus*.

s., intestinal. Poisoning due to ingestion of decaying food.

s. lenta. A more or less localized and slowly developing infection from *Streptococcus viridans*.

s., puerperal. Infection of the genital tract following childbirth.

The infection may be brought about by exogenous or endogenous means. The organisms most commonly associated with this type of infection are *streptococcus*, *staphylococcus*, *gonococcus*, *bacillus coli*, *diphtheria bacillus*, and a putrefactive group of *saprophytic organisms*. The infection may be localized in the uterine cavity, lymphatics, veins and mucous membrane of the vaginal tract.

PATH: In the minor cases of ulceration in the vaginal tract covered by a dirty membrane. In streptococci infection the endometrium is smooth, and the lymphatics are congested with the invading organism. As a rule, the uterine cavity is filled with very little lochia. There is very little or no leukocytic barrier. The saprophytic type shows an endometrial cavity filled with greenish, purulent, foul-smelling shreds. Microscopically, there is a thick layer of leukocytes under the necrotic layer. The uterus shows poor involution. In the event that the infection extends further than the uterus, the parametrium or cellular tissues show edema, serum and in the saprophytic cases, purulent infiltration. Extension of the process to the veins produces infectious thrombi which in turn produce localized abscesses in other parts of the body.

SYM: On the 3rd to the 7th day the patient begins to have general malaise, headache, chilly sensations or true rigors and rise in temperature. The uterus is tender, there is some abdominal distention, and the lochia in the saprophytic type is profuse and foul-smelling, while in the streptococcic type it is decreased in amount and of a serous character. Occasionally there is swelling of the lower limb accompanied by high fever, rapid pulse rate and chills. Upon palpation the femoral vein is found to be tender and cordlike. This is an infectious thrombosis of the femoral vein, and the condition is known as phlegmasia alba dolens.

COURSE: In most instances, after 7 to 10 days, the symptoms subside and the patient's condition is greatly improved, although involution is delayed. In a very severe septicemic case with rapid onset, the prognosis is bad and frequently convalescence is delayed for months. In cases where multiple abscesses develop, the prognosis is very favorable once the abscesses are drained.

TREATMENT: The treatment consists of rest in bed, icebag to the lower abdomen, push fluids, good nutritious diet, and the use of ecbolics in order to keep the uterus involuted. If localized abscesses are formed they should be evacuated. Vaccines have been developed for use in the streptococcic type of infection with questionable efficacy. Sulfanilamide is effective in reducing the toxemia rapidly. In patients who have a low hemoglobin content, transfusion of whole blood is of value in helping the patient to withstand the infection.

The most important part of the treatment is prophylaxis. Precise aseptic technic during examination, labor, and delivery are very important factors. The substitution of rectal for vaginal examination during labor is very desirous. If vaginal examination is found to be necessary it is done under the most strict asepsis. The avoidance of trauma in delivery, and the performance of only the necessary obstetric operations decrease the number of lacerations and thus open less avenues for the entrance of infection. No one in attendance during labor or the puerperium can have any infections that might be transmitted. SEE: *puerperal sepsis*.

sepsometer (sĕp-sŏm'ĕ-ter) [G. *sēpsis*, putrefaction, + *metron*, a measure]. Device for detecting organic impurities in the air. SYN: *septometer*, 2.

septal (sĕp'tăl) [L. *saeptum*, a dividing wall]. Concerning a septum.

septan (sĕp'tăn) [L. *septem*, seven]. Recurring every 7th day, as the paroxysms of malarial fever.

septate (sĕp'tāt) [L. *saeptum*, a partition]. Having a dividing wall.

septectomy (sĕp-tĕk'tō-mĭ) [" + G. *ektomē*, excision]. Excision of a septum, esp. the nasal septum or a part of it.

septemia (sĕp-tē'mĭ-ă) [G. *sēptos*, putrid, + *aima*, blood]. Invasion of the blood by pathogenic bacteria or their toxins. SYN: *septicemia*.

septic (sĕp'tĭk) [G. *sēptos*, putrid]. Caused by or relating to putrefaction.

s. fever, s. infection. Fever or infection due to presence of pathogenic organisms or their products in the blood. SYN: *septicemia*.

s. sore throat. Streptococcic inflammation of throat with fever and marked prostration.

septicemia (sĕp-tĭ-sē'mĭ-ă) [G. *sēptikos*, putrid, + *aima*, blood]. Morbid condition from absorption of septic products into blood and tissues or of pathogenic bacteria which may rapidly multiply there.

Experiments on animals show there are 2 varieties of this form of blood poisoning:

Sapremia, toxemia, or septic intoxication, in which symptoms supervene immediately upon the inoculation. Frequently seen in obstetrical cases in which putrefaction of retained clots or placenta has taken place within uterus.

Poison may be absorbed through mucous membrane of vagina or uterus or through open wounds in these regions or the uterine sinuses. SEE: *sepsis*. Conditions favorable for such a type of poisoning are rare in general surgery, although a large, ill-drained wound or decomposition occurring in the contents of a psoas, or other abscess, is a common cause. May be found in abdominal wounds where extensive injury of peritoneum has favored oozing and accumulation of blood clot in peritoneal cavity.

Septic infection: The symptoms come on less rapidly and death is caused by presence of bacilli or micrococci in the blood.

Since the existence of ptomaines as a product of decomposition has been understood it is generally recognized that the poisons elaborated by bacteria play a prominent part in production of disease. The method is through the diffusion and multiplication of the bacteria from an infected wound even of a trivial character.

The development of the disease is more gradual in this form. Fever curve is of the continuous type, as in sapremia, and as fatal end approaches will range higher. In some cases, as seen occasionally in strangulated hernia, or in gunshot wounds of abdomen, is abnormal.

SYM: Temperature, 105° F. or more. Fever intermittent, some chills, pulse weak and rapid, freedom from pain unless localized. Delirium common and diarrhea not infrequent. Great prostration, headache, anorexia, and a typhoid condition supervene. May be accompanied by vomiting. Tendency to enlargement of lymphatic glands throughout body and more particularly of spleen. Skin pale; dusky, scarlet eruption may occur. Skin hot, dry; later bathed in perspiration; finally becomes cold and clammy. Senses dulled, countenance listless; tongue covered with brownish fur; diarrhea increases; urine concentrated and scanty. Delirium followed by coma, patient becomes moribund.

PROG: Grave.

TREATMENT: Prophylactic treatment consists in application of rules of antiseptic and aseptic surgery. When disease appears, carry out thorough disinfection of entire wound surface. Stitches should be removed and sinuses carefully exposed; all collections of blood clot or decomposing fluids should be washed out with corrosive sublimate, 1:1000, and subsequently the tissues should be disinfected with strong solutions of carbolic acid (1:20 or pure crystals), or chloride of zinc (1:10); wound can then be packed with gauze containing large amount of iodoform powder; or antiseptic poultices can be applied to favor free discharge.

When the wound has deep recesses or pockets, irrigation with boiled water or boric acid (4%) may be used. In abdominal wounds hot water douching of peritoneal cavity followed by drainage. In puerperal fever the antiseptic washing of uterus is valuable. Constitutional treatment to suit special phases. Nutritious diet in such form as not to impede digestion, and to favor rapid assimilation. Inhalations of concentrated oxygen are remarkably beneficial.

RS: *autosepticemia, sapremia, sepsis, toxemia*.

s., bronchopulmonary. S. following operation on the larynx resulting in infected secretions from the wound entering the bronchial tubes.

s., Bruce's. Same as melitensis septicemia.

s., cryptogenic. S. in which cannot be found any primary focus of infection.

s., melitensis. Infectious disease marked by remittent fever, weakness, perspiration, neuralgia, and swelling in the joints. SYN: *Malta fever, undulant fever*.

s., puerperal. S. occurring following childbirth from a lesion in the genital tract. SEE: *puerperal sepsis*.

septicemic (sĕp-tĭ-sē'mĭk) [G. *sēptikos*, putrid, + *aima*, blood]. Relating to, resulting from, or of the nature of, septicemia.

septicophlebitis (sĕp″tĭ-kō-flē-bī'tĭs) [" + *phleps*, vein, + *-itis*, inflammation]. Septic inflammation of a vein.

septicopyemia (sĕp″tĭ-kō-pī-ē'mĭ-ă) [" + *pyon*, pus, + *aima*, blood]. Septicemia and pyemia together.

septiferous (sĕp-tĭf'ĕr-ŭs) [" + L. *ferre*, to bear]. Carrying or transmitting septic poisoning.

septile (sĕp'tĭl) [L. *saeptum*, a partition]. Relating to a septum. SYN: *septal*.

septimetritis (sĕp″tĭ-mē-trī'tĭs) [G. *sēptos*, putrid, + *mētra*, uterus, + *-itis*, inflammation]. Inflammation of uterus due to sepsis.

septipara (sĕp-tĭp'ă-ră) [L. *septem*, seven, + *parēre*, to bring forth]. A woman who has borne 7 children separately or is pregnant for the 7th time.

septivalent (sĕp-tĭ-vā'lĕnt, -tĭv'ă-lĕnt) [" + *valēre*, to be strong]. Having a valency of 7 or combining with or replacing 7 hydrogen atoms.

septometer (sĕp-tŏm'ĕt-ĕr) 1. [L. *saeptum*, a partition]. Calipers for measuring nasal septum. 2. [G. *sēptos*, putrid, + *metron*, a measure]. Device for determining atmospheric impurity.

septopyemia (sĕp″tō-pī-ē-mĭ-ă) [G. *sēptos*, putrid, + *pyon*, pus, + *aima*, blood]. Pyemia and septicemia together. SYN: *septicopyemia*.

septotome (sĕp'tō-tōm) [L. *saeptum*, a partition, + G. *tomē*, a cutting]. An instrument for cutting or removing a section of the nasal septum.

septotomy (sĕp-tŏt'ō-mĭ) [" + G. *tomē*, a cutting]. Incision of a septum, esp. the nasal septum.

septum (sĕp'tŭm) (pl. *septa*) [L. *saeptum*, a partition]. A membranous wall dividing two cavities.

s. atriorum, BNA, **s. auricularum.** A wall bet. the atria of the heart.

s., crural. A mass of fat obstructing the femoral ring.

s. lucidum. 1. A translucent s., the int. boundary of lateral ventricles of the brain. 2. The stratum corneum layer of the epidermis.

s., nasal. The partition which divides the 2 nasal cavities.

Bony portions (perpendicular plate of ethmoid, vomer, maxillary crest and palatine crest). Cartilaginous portion anteriorly. Deviations, abscess, hematoma, ridges—spurs.

s. pectiniforme. Comblike partition that separates the corpora cavernosa.

s., rectovaginal. Partition bet. the rectum and the vagina.

s. scroti. BNA. Partition dividing the 2 chambers of the scrotum.
s. ventriculorum. BNA. Partition bet. the ventricles of the heart.
septuplet (sĕp'tŭp-lĕt) [L. *septuplum*, a group of seven]. One of 7 children born from the same gestation.
séquardin (sā-kwar'dĭn). Commercial sterilized testicular extract.
sequela (sē-kwē'lă) (pl. *sequelae*) [L. a following]. A condition following and resulting from a disease.
sequester (sē-kwĕs'tēr) [L. *sequestrāre*, to separate]. 1. To isolate. 2. A piece of necrosed bone separated from surrounding tissue. SYN: *sequestrum*.
sequestration (sē-kwĕs-tra'shŭn) [L. *sequestrātio*, a separation]. 1. The formation of sequestrum. 2. Isolation of a patient for treatment or quarantine. 3. Reduction of hemorrhage of head or trunk by temporarily stopping circulation with bands on the thighs and arms.
sequestrectomy (sē-kwĕs-trĕk'tō-mĭ) [" + G. *ektomē*, excision]. Excision of a necrosed piece of bone.
sequestrotomy (sē-kwĕs-trŏt'ō-mĭ) [" + G. *tomē*, a cutting]. Operation for removal of a sequestrum, a fragment of necrosed bone. SYN: *sequestrectomy*.
sequestrum (sē-kwĕs'trŭm) [L. *sequestrum*, from *sequestrāre*, to separate]. Fragment of a necrosed bone that has become separated from surrounding tissue.
sera (sē'ră) [L.]. Plural of *serum*.
seralbumin (sĕr-ăl-bū'mĭn) [L. *serum*, whey, + *albumen*, white of egg]. Albumin of the blood.
serial (sē'rĭ-ăl) [L. *series*, a succession]. In numerical order, in continuity or sequence, as in a series.
sericeps (sĕr'ĭ-sĕps) [L. *sericus*, silken, + *caput*, head]. Silk sac used in making traction on fetal head.
series (sēr'ēz) [L. *series*, a succession]. 1. Arrangement of objects in succession or in order. 2. ELECT: A mode of arranging the parts of a circuit by connecting them successively end to end to form a single path for the current. The parts so arranged are said to be "in series."
seriflux (sē'rĭf-lŭks) [L. *serum*, whey, + *fluxus*, a flow]. A profuse, serous, or watery discharge. SYN: *orrhorrhea*.
seriscission (sĕr-ĭ-sĭsh'ŭn) [L. *sericum*, silk, + *scindere*, to cut]. Division of soft tissues, as a pedicle, by tying a silk ligature around it.
sero- [L.]. Combining form *pertaining to serum*.
seroalbuminuria (sē"rō-ăl-bū-mĭn-ū'rĭ-ă) [L. *serum*, whey, + *albumen*, white of egg, + G. *ouron*, urine]. Serum albumin in the urine.
serobacterin (sē"rō-băk'tēr-ĭn) [" + G. *bakterion*, a small rod]. Bacterial vaccine sensitized with serum from an animal partially immunized against the same microörganism. See: *vaccine*.
serochrome (sē"rō-krōm) [" + G. *chrōma*, color]. The pigment which colors the normal serum. SYN: *lipochrome, lutein*.
serocolitis (sē"rō-kō-lī'tĭs) [" + G. *kōlon*, colon, + *-ītis*, inflammation]. Inflammation of serous coat of the colon. SYN: *pericolitis*.
seroculture (sē"rō-kŭl-chŭr) [" + *cultura*, cultivation]. A bacterial culture on blood serum.
serocystic (sē"rō-sĭs'tĭk) [" + G. *kystis*, a cyst]. Composed of cysts containing serous fluid.
serodermatosis (sē"rō-der-mă-tō'sĭs) [" + G. *derma*, skin, + *-ōsis*, condition].

Skin disease with serous effusion into tissues of the epidermis.
serodiagnosis (sē"rō-dī-ăg-nō'sĭs) [L. *serum*, whey, + G. *dia*, through, + *gnōsis*, knowledge]. Diagnosis by observing the reactions of blood serum.
seroenteritis (sē"rō-ĕn-ter-ī'tĭs) [" + G. *enteron*, intestine, + *-ītis*, inflammation]. Inflammation of serous covering of the intestine.
seroenzyme (sē"rō-ĕn'zīm) [" + G. *en*, in, + *zymē*, leaven]. Any enzyme in the blood serum.
serofibrinous (sē"rō-fīb'rĭn-ŭs) [" + *fibra*, fiber]. 1. Composed of both serum and fibrin. 2. Denoting a serofibrinous exudate.
seroglobulin (sē"rō-glŏb'ū-lĭn) [" + *globulus*, a little sphere]. The globulin contained in the blood serum.
serohemorrhagic (sē"rō-hem-or-răj'ĭk) [" + G. *haima*, blood, + *-rrhagia*, from *rhēgnŭnai*, to burst forth]. Consisting of both serum and blood.
serohepatitis (sē"rō-hĕp-ă-tī'tĭs) [" + G. *hēpar, hepat-*, liver, + *-ītis*, inflammation]. Inflammation of the peritoneal covering of the liver.
seroimmunity (sē"rō-ĭm-mū'nĭ-tĭ) [" + *immūnis*, safe]. Immunity conferred by antitoxins or vaccines. SYN: *passive immunity*.
serolactescent (sē"rō-lăk-tĕs'ĕnt) [L. *serum*, whey, + *lac, lact-*, milk]. Resembling serum and milk, as the secretion of Montgomery's glands.
serolemma (sē"rō-lĕm'ă) [" + G. *lemma*, rind]. External layer of the embryonic false amnion.
serolin (sē"rō-lĭn) [" + *oleum*, oil]. A neutral fatty constituent of blood containing cholesterol, the nature of which is unknown.
serolipase (sē"rō-lĭp'ās) [" + G. *lipos*, fat, + *ase*, enzyme]. Lipase found in blood serum.
serologic, serological (sē-rō-lŏj'ĭk, -ăl) [" + G. *logos*, a study]. Pert. to or the study of sera.
serologist (sē-rŏl'ō-jĭst) [" + G. *logos*, a study]. One versed in serology.
serology (sē-rŏl'ō-jĭ) [L. *serum*, whey, + G. *logos*, a study]. The science of serum reactions, diagnosis and treatment.
It treats of the relation of antibodies and antigens, an antigen being a substance which, inoculated into the body, is capable of causing the creation of antibodies.
serolysin (sē-rŏl'ĭs-ĭn) [" + G. *lysis*, dissolution]. A bactericidal substance or lysin found in the blood serum.
seromembranous (sē"rō-mĕm'brăn-ŭs) [" + *membrana*, membrane]. Both serous and membranous; relating to a serous membrane.
seromucoid (sē"rō-mū'koyd) [" + *mucus*, mucus, + G. *eidos*, like]. A substance resembling serum and mucus sometimes found in urine.
seromucous (sē"rō-mū'kŭs) [" + *mucus*, mucus]. Composed of serum and mucus.
seromuscular (sē"rō-mŭs'kū-lar) [" + *musculus*, a muscle]. Referring to the serous and muscular intestinal coats.
seroperitoneum (sē"rō-pĕr-ĭ-tō-nē'ŭm) [" + G. *peritonaion*, peritoneum]. Fluid in the peritoneum. SYN: *ascites, hydroperitoneum*.
serophysiology (sē"rō-fīz-ĭ-ŏl'ō-jĭ) [L. *serum*, whey, + G. *physis*, nature, + *logos*, a study]. The study of the physiology of serum action.
serophyte (sē-rō-fīt) [" + G. *phyton*,

seroplastic   **serrenoeud**

plant]. A microörganism which can grow readily in the body fluids.
seroplastic (sē″rō-plăs′tĭk) [" + G. *plastikos*, formed]. Containing serum and fibrin. SYN: *serofibrinous*.
seropneumothorax (sē″rō-nū-mō-thō′răks) [" + G. *pneuma*, air, + *thōrax*, chest]. Effusion of serum and air in the pleural cavity.
seroprevention (sē″rō-prē-věn′shŭn) [" + *praeventum*, coming before]. Prevention by the injection of serum.
seroprognosis (sē″rō-prŏg-nō′sĭs) [" + G. *pro*, before, + *gnōsis*, knowledge]. Prognosis of disease determined by sero-reactions.
seroprophylaxis (sē″rō-prō-fĭ-lăks′ĭs) [" + G. *pro*, before, + *phylaxis*, protection]. Prevention of a disease by injection of serum. SYN: *seroprevention*.
seropurulent (sē″rō-pū-rū-lĕnt) [L. *serum*, whey, + *purulentus*, full of pus]. Composed of serum and pus, as an exudate.
seropus (sē′rō-pus) [" + *pus*, pus]. A fluid consisting of serum and pus.
seroreaction (sē″rō-rē-ăk′shŭn) [" + *re*, back, + *actio*, action]. 1. Any reaction taking place in serum. SEE: *deviation of complement, fixation of complement*. 2. Reaction to an injection of serum marked by rash, fever, pain, etc. SYN: *serum sickness*.
serosa (sē-rō′să) [L. from *serum*, whey]. A serous membrane.
serosamucin (sē-rō″să-mū′sĭn) [L. *serosus*, serous, + *mucus*, mucus]. Mucoid in serous fluids.
serosanguineous (sē″rō-săn-gwĭn′ē-ŭs) [L. *serum*, whey, + *sanguineus*, bloody]. Containing or of the nature of serum and blood.
seroscopy (sē-rŏs′kō-pĭ) [" + G. *skopein*, to examine]. Examination of serum for diagnostic purposes.
seroserous (sē″rō-sē′rŭs) [" + *serum*, whey]. Pert. to 2 serous surfaces.
serositis (sē″rō-sī′tĭs) [" + G. *-itis*, inflammation]. Inflamed condition of a serous membrane.
serosity (sē-rŏs′ĭ-tĭ) [Fr. *sérosité*, from L. *serum*, whey]. 1. The quality of being serous. 2. A thin, watery, serous fluid, not the real secretion of serous membranes.
serosynovitis (sē″rō-sĭn-ō-vī′tĭs) [L. *serum*, whey, + G. *syn*, with, + *ōon*, egg, + *-itis*, inflammation]. Synovitis with increase of synovial fluid.
serotaxis (sē″rō-tăks′ĭs) [" + G. *taxis*, arrangement]. The drawing of blood serum to the skin surface by application of a solution of caustic potash for diagnostic or therapeutic purposes.
serotherapy (sē″rō-thĕr′ă-pĭ) [" + G. *therapeia*, treatment]. Injection of a specific serum or antitoxin in the treatment of an infectious disease.
   Concerned with producing artificial immunity in a person by injecting the blood serum of an animal which has acquired active immunity* to the disease in question. The degree of protection is not great, usually being limited to days or weeks.
serothorax (sē″rō-thō′răks) [L. *serum*, whey, + G. *thōrax*, chest]. Fluid in the pleural cavity. SYN: *hydrothorax*.
serotina (sĕr-ō-tī′nă) [L. *serotinus*, late]. Part of decidua that becomes maternal portion of the placenta. SYN: *decidua serotina*.
serotoxin (sē-rō-tŏks′ĭn) [L. *serum*, whey, + G. *toxikon*, poison]. A toxin in the blood serum.

serous (sē′rŭs) [L. *serum*, whey]. Having the nature of serum.
   s. cavity. A large lymph space.
   s. effusion. One of serum.
   s. exudate. One consisting mostly of serum.
   s. fluids. Liquids of the body, similar to blood serum, which are in part secreted by serous membranes.
   s. glands. Certain glands secreting a watery fluid, as those found in the digestive tract.
   s. inflammation. One with a serous exudate or inflammation of a serous membrane.
   s. membrane. One with 2 layers of flat endothelial cells lining closed cavities.
serovaccination (sē″rō-văk-sĭn-ā′shŭn) [L. *serum*, whey, + *vaccinus*, pert. to a cow]. Injection of a vaccine to secure passive immunity and also to secure active immunization.
serozyme (sē″rō-zīm) [" + G. *zymē*, leaven]. Substance in the blood which is converted into thrombin. SYN: *thrombogen*.
serpiginous (ser-pĭj′ĭn-ŭs) [L. *serpere*, to creep]. Creeping from one part to another.
   s. ulcer. One extending in one direction, while healing in another direction.
serpigo (ser-pī′gō) [L. *serpere*, to creep]. A creeping eruption, esp. ringworm. SYN: *herpes, ringworm*.
serrate (sĕr′rāt) [L. *serratus*, toothed]. Notched; toothed. SYN: *dentate*.
serration (ser-ā′shŭn) [L. *serratio*, a notching]. 1. Formation with sharp projections like the teeth of a saw. 2. Notch resembling one bet. teeth of a saw.

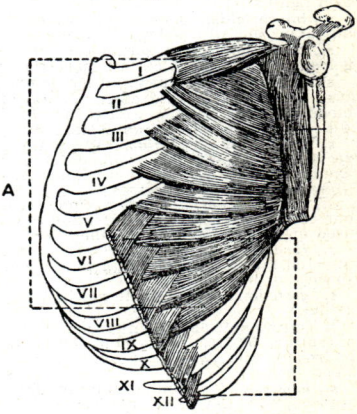

SERRATUS ANTERIOR.
A. Serratus anterior.

serratus muscle (sĕr-ā′tŭs) [L. *serratus*, toothed]. Any of several muscles arising from the ribs or vertebrae by separate slips. SEE: *Table of Muscles in Appendix*.
serrefine (sār-fēn′) [Fr.]. A small, spring wire forceps for compressing bleeding vessels.
serrenoeud (sār-nōōd) [Fr. *serrer*, to squeeze, + *noeud*, knot]. Device employed for constricting uterus near *os internum* with strong steel wire, used for ligating.

serrulate (ser'ū-lāt) [L. *serrulatus*, notched]. Minutely notched.

Sertoli's cells (sĕr-tō'lē). Supporting, elongated, striated cells of seminiferous tubules which nourish spermatids.

S's. column. Elongated cell in a seminiferous tubule giving support to spermatogenic cells.

serum (sē'rum) (pl. *serums, sera*) [L. *serum,* whey]. 1. Any serous fluid, esp. the fluid which moistens the surfaces of serous membranes. 2. The watery portion of the blood after coagulation; a fluid found when clotted blood is left standing long enough for the clot to shrink. 3. Serum from an animal rendered immune against a pathogenic organism, to be injected into a patient with the disease resulting from the same organism. SEE: *plasma, blood.* 4. Whey of milk.

s. albumin. A protein found in blood serum. For properties, see *proteins;* for amount, see *blood.*

s., anticrotalus. S. to overcome the effect of rattlesnake poison.

s., antidiphtheritic. One used to overcome the effects of diphtheria.

s., antimeningococcus. S. antagonistic to meningococcus infection.

s., antiophidic. S. antagonistic to snake poisons.

s., antipneumococcus. S. for pneumococcus infection.

s., antitetanic. S. given to overcome tetanus toxin.

s., antitoxic. One containing the antitoxin of the microörganism against which it is supposed to be protective.

s., antityphoid. A sterilized culture of typhoid bacilli administered by vaccination against typhoid fever.

s., bactericidal. One having no effect on toxins but which destroys bacteria.

s., bacteriolytic. A serum containing a lysin that destroys certain bacteria.

s., Behring's. An antidiphtheritic one.

s., blood. The liquid clear portion of blood without its fibrin and corpuscles.

s., cerebrospinal. Cerebrospinal fluid.

s. coagulation reaction. Weltmann's reaction for differential diagnosis bet. exudative, necrotic processes and proliferative, fibrotic processes.

s., convalescent. Blood serum from one convalescent from an infection to be used on others having the same disease.

s., foreign. Serum from one animal injected into another animal of another species, or into man.

s. globulin. A protein found in blood serum.

It contains 15.85% of nitrogen, 1.11% of sulfur, 52.71% of carbon, 7.01% of hydrogen, and 23.32% of oxygen. SEE: *blood, protein.*

s., immune. A serum containing many amboceptors having a special affinity for a given bacterium. SYN: *specific serum.*

s., inorganic. A solution of various salts in same proportion as in the human blood.

s. lutein. Yellow pigment from serum.

s., Maragliano's. A serum that is antitubercular.

s., Marmorek's. The antitoxin of *Streptococcus pyogenes* and the tubercle bacillus.

s. pains. Joint pains accompanying serum reaction.

s., pooled. Blood s. from several persons, which has been mixed.

s., pregnancy. Blood serum from pregnant women given to premature infants in food.

s. protein. Any protein in blood serum.

Serum p. forms weak acids mixed with alkali salts and this increases the buffer effects of the blood but to a lesser extent than cell protein.

s., Quéry's. An antisyphilitic serum from inoculated monkeys.

s. rash. One first seen at site of an injection of serum.

It remains thickest there but it may invade other parts of the body. It resembles a combination of *urticarial, morbilliform* and *scarlatiniform rashes.*

SYM: Severe irritation; marked swelling of skin, esp. of the face; malaise, and constitutional symptoms.

s. reaction. SEE: *serum sickness.*

s., salvarsanized. One used in cerebrospinal syphilis, taken from a patient half an hour after an intravenous injection of salvarsan.

s., serous (*acute*). Associated with edema of brain. May occur with pneumonia, measles, or other infections, from alcoholism or head injury. SYM: Mild headache, some nuchal rigidity, vomiting, subfebrile or normal temperature. Slow pulse, optic neuritis or choked disks. Spinal fluid clear, moderate increase in cellular content but under pressure. Normal chemistry.

s. sickness. An eruption of purpuric spots, with pain in limbs and joints, following administration of serum, such as streptococcic s.

SYM: Supposed to be anaphylactic. Symptoms appear 5 to 12 days after the injection. Slight fever, skin eruptions, swelling and pain in joints may develop. Hay fever and asthma victims are hypersensitive to serum injections. Adrenalin is used to combat such reactions. Histaminase is a prophylactic and also relieves the condition, as does epinephrine in oil. SYN: *serum reaction.*

s., specific. SEE: *immune s.*

s. test for typhoid fever. SEE: *Widal's serum test.*

s. therapy. Therapeutic use of animal serums. SYN: *serotherapy, q.v.*

s., Trunecek's. Same as *inorganic serum.*

s., Widal's, test. One for typhoid fever. SEE: *Widal.*

serum, words pert. to: agglutinin, agglutinogen, aggressin, antigen, antitropin, antivenin, autoserodiagnosis, autoserotherapy, autoserous, autoserum, chromodiagnosis, complement, icteric index, isohemagglutinin, "lymph-" words, opsonic index, opsonin, orrhorrhea, serology, serous.

serumal (sē-rū'măl) [L. *serum,* whey]. Relating to serum.

s. calculus. One formed about the teeth from serous exudate.

serumuria (sē-rŭm-ū'rĭ-ă) [" + G. *ouron,* urine]. Albumen in the urine. SYN: *albuminuria.*

sesamoid (ses'am-oyd) [G. *sēsamon,* sesame, + *eidos,* form]. Resembling in size or shape a grain of sesame.

s. bone. An oval nodule of bone or fibrocartilage in a tendon playing over a bony surface.

The patella is the largest one.

s. cartilages. Small ones in the side of the wing of the nose.

sesqui- [L.]. Prefix meaning *one and a half.*

sessile (sĕs'ĭl) [L. *sessilis,* low]. Having

setaceous — sheath, nerve

setaceous no peduncle but attached directly by a broad base.
setaceous (sē-tā'shŭs) [L. *setaceus*, bristly]. Resembling a bristle; bristly, hairy.
Setchenoff or **Sechenoff**. SEE: *Setschenow's inhibitory centers.*
seton (sē'tŏn) [L. *seto, seton-*, a thread]. A thread or threads drawn through a fold of skin to act as a counterirritant, or a fistulous tract so produced.
setose (sē'tōs) [L. *seta*, bristle]. Having bristlelike appendages.
Setschenow's inhibitory centers (sĕtsh'ĕn-ŏf). Centers in the spinal cord and oblongata for inhibiting reflex movement.
sev'enth cra'nial nerve. Facial nerve*; *nervus facialis.*
   s. sense. Perception of normal functioning of internal organs. SEE: *visceral sense.*
sevum (sē'vŭm) [L. suet]. Tallow or suet.
sewer gas. Foul air of a sewer. SEE: *carbon monoxide gas.*
sex (sĕks) [L. *sexus*, sex]. 1. The distinctive quality which differentiates bet. male and female. 2. Males or females, collectively.
   s. chromosomes. Chromosomes in a cell determining sex.
sexdigital (sĕks-ĭ-dĭj'ĭ-tăl) [L. *sex*, six, + *digitus*, digit]. Having 6 fingers or toes.
sexivalent (sĕks-ĭ-vā'lĕnt, -ĭv'ăl-ĕnt) [" + *valere*, to be strong]. Capable of combining with 6 atoms of hydrogen.
sexoesthetic inversion (sĕks"o-ĕs-thĕt'ĭk). Inclination to dress as one of the opp. sex. SYN: *eonism, transvestism.*
sextan (sĕks'tăn) [L. *sextanus*, of the sixth]. Occurring every 6th day.
sextigravida (sĕks-tĭ-grăv'ĭd-ă) [L. *sextus*, six, + *gravida*, a pregnant woman]. A woman pregnant for the 6th time.
sextipara (sĕks-tĭp'ă-ră) [" + *parere*, to bear a child]. A woman who has borne 6 children at different pregnancies.
sextuplet (sĕks-tū-plĕt) [L. *sextus*, six]. One of 6 children born of a single gestation.
sexual (sĕks'ū-ăl) [L. *sexualis*, pert. to sex]. 1. Pert. to sex. 2. Having sex.
   s. bondage. An abnormal phenomenon (not perverse) of dependence of one person upon another of the opposite sex, one dominating the other.
   The motives are purely normal except that egoism is the motive of the dominating one. Henpecked husbands, old men who have married young wives and those who have to surrender their rights to secure the love or favor of a woman— these are examples of sexual bondage. Masochism* may develop from such a condition.
   s. intercourse. Sexual congress bet. a male and a female. SYN: *coition, coitus, concubitus, copulation.*
   RS: *clitoris, coitus interruptus, dyspareunia, ejaculation, emission, excitation, penis, semen, telegony, vagina.*
   s. inversion. A perversion in which an abnormal affection for one of the same sex is experienced.
   s. involution. The menopause.
   s. metamorphosis. A perversion in which one adopts the habits and dress of the opposite sex.
   s. psychopathy. A term for the group in which exist perversions of sex, such as *bestiality,* coprolagnism,* exhibitionism,* fetishism,* frottage,* homosexualism,* lesbianism,* masochism,* masturbation,* onanism,* pedophilia,* renifleurs,* sadism,* sodomy,* transvestism,* voyeur.**

   s. reflex. Erection and ejaculation resulting from genital stimulation or indirectly from emotion whether asleep or awake.
sexuality (sĕks-ū-ăl'ĭ-tĭ) [L. *sexus*, sex]. 1. State of having sex; the collective characteristics which mark the differences bet. the male and the female. 2. Undue concern with what is sexual. 3. Constitution and life of individual as related to sex; all the dispositions related to the love life whether associated with the sex organs or not.
shad (shăd) [A.S. *sceadd*]. COMP: E. P. Pro. 18.8%, Fat 9.5%. FUEL VALUE: 100 Gm. equal 164 Cal.
shadowgram, shadowgraph (shăd'ō-grăm, -grăf) [M.E. *shadowe*, darkness, + G. *graphein*, to write]. A print on a photographic plate exposed to x-rays. SYN: *skiagraph.*
shakes (shāks) [A.S. *scacan*, to shake]. Shivering caused by a chill, esp. in an intermittent fever.
shaking (shāk'ĭng) [A.S. *scacan*, to shake]. A passive movement in Swedish massage.
   s. cure. Vibratory movements for treatment of paralysis agitans.
   s. palsy. A basal ganglion disease with progressive rigid tremulousness, peculiar gait, muscular contraction and weakness. SYN: *paralysis agitans.*
shampoo (shăm-poo') [Hindu *champna*, to press]. 1. A thorough cleansing of the entire body or hair and scalp with thick soap lather applied with friction and followed by an affusion with clear water. 2. To thoroughly wash the hair or body.
shank (shăngk) [A.S. *sceanca*]. The tibia or leg from knee to ankle. SYN: *shin.*
shape (shāp) [A.S. *sceapan*, to shape]. 1. To mold to a particular form. 2. Outward form; contour.
   RS: *aliform, arcate, arciform, arcuation, arenoid, asbestiform, asteroid, bacciform, belemnoid, bilateralism, bosselated, bosseation, bulbiform, calculus, caniniform, capreolary, capreolate, carinated, caudate, circle, circumvallate.*
Sharpey's intercrossing fibers (shar'pē). Fibers forming the lamellae constituting the walls of the haversian canals in bone.
   S. perforating fibers. Those which connect the lamellae in walls of the haversian canals.
sheath (shēth) [A.S. *scēath*]. A covering structure of connective tissue, usually of an elongated part, such as the membrane covering a muscle, etc.
   s., arachnoid or **arachnoidean.** Delicate partition bet. pial sheath and dural one of the optic nerve.
   s., crural. The femoral sheath.
   s., dentinal. One lining the dental canals.
   s., dural. A fibrous membrane or ext. investment of the optic nerve.
   s., femoral. The fascial covering of femoral vessels.
   s. of Henle. An extension of perineurium investing fibers composing nerve trunk funiculi.
   s., lamellar. Connective tissue sheath covering bundle of nerve fibers. SYN: *perineurium.*
   s., medullary. Myelin s. surrounding the axis cylinder.
   s., myelin. A fatty, semifluid covering of a nerve fiber; also called the *medulla.* It may insulate the nerve fiber and prevent the escape of the nerve impulse.
   s., nerve. SEE: *lamellar s.*

s., perivascular. Lymphatic tube around the smallest blood vessels.

s., pial. Extension of the pia, closely investing surface of the optic nerve.

s. of Schwann. Membranous covering of myelin sheath of a nerve fiber. SYN: *neurilemma.*

s., synovial. S. membrane lining cavity of a bone through which a tendon glides.

sheet (shēt) [A.S. *sciete,* piece of cloth]. Linen or cotton bedcovering next to the sleeper.

s., draw. One folded under patient so it may be withdrawn without lifting the patient.

shell shock. PSY: Any one of the disorders of motor, sensory and special sense centers; a form of psychoneurosis which occurs during military service and in training camps, but not as a result of exploding shells. SYN: *war neurosis.*

shield (shēld) [A.S. *scild,* shield]. 1. Any protecting device. 2. BIOL: A protective plate.

s. bone. The scapula.

s., Buller's. A watch glass to be worn over the eye to protect it from gonorrheal or ophthalmic infection.

s., embryonic. An area of proliferating cells in the ovum in which the primitive streak appears.

s., nipple. A protective covering to protect sore nipples.

s., phallic. An antiseptic covering for the male genitals during operations.

Shiga's bacillus (shē'gă). The bacillus causing a form of dysentery.

Shigella (shĭ-jel'lă, -gĕl'ă). A genus of the family *Bacteriaceae* containing the dysentery organisms.

shin (shĭn) [A.S. *scinu,* shin]. Anterior edge of tibia. Also, leg bet. the ankle and knee. SYN: *shank.*

shingles (shĭng'lz) [L. *cingulus,* a girdle]. Eruption of acute, inflammatory, herpetic vesicles on the trunk of the body along a peripheral nerve; occasionally elsewhere. SYN: *herpes zoster, q.v.*

ship fever. A fever due to unhygienic conditions aboard ship, usually typhus fever or yellow fever occasionally.

shiver (shĭv'ĕr) [M.E. *chiveren*]. 1. A slight tremor of the skin, as from cold, or from fear. 2. To tremble or shake, as from fear or cold.

shock (shŏk) [M.E. *schokke*]. A depression or cessation of the influences of the nervous system over various important body functions, principally the circulation and respiration.

It may be immediate or delayed, slight or severe, even fatal. Other form resembling faintness, but may be restless and excited. The result of an injury, bleeding, pain, fear, fright, anesthesia, the result of an operation and many other causes.

Every injury is accompanied by some degree of shock and so should be treated promptly. Syncope is caused by an anemia of the brain in certain persons and resembles shock in symptoms and treatment.

RS: *anaphylactic, catalepsy, cataleptic, insulin, nociassociation.*

SYM: Five "P's" denote the outstanding symptoms of shock: Prostration, pallor, perspiration, pulselessness, pulmonary deficiency. They vary in intensity, depending upon patient and injury.

The most outstanding symptoms are: (a) Marked paleness of the skin; (b) a bluish or grayish discoloration (cyanosis) of the lips, nails, tips of the fingers and lobes of the ears; (c) the face is pinched and without expression; (d) there may be a staring of the eyes which often lose their characteristic luster; and (e) the pupils are dilated; (f) the pulse is weak, rapid and irregular; (g) the breathing is increased in rate and it is shallow; and (h) the blood pressure is instantly lowered; (i) there may be urinary retention and incontinence of feces; (j) occasionally there is an unusual restlessness or excitement, and (k) very often the patient expresses an extreme thirst. If conscious the patient seems quite disinterested in the surroundings and complains little of pain even though he may be groaning.

TREATMENT: Keep patient lying down with head lower than body. The lower extremities can be slightly elevated by placing the patient on a box, stool or a folded blanket.

External heat should be applied in the form of hot water bottles, hot bricks, hot plates, etc. A simple means of applying heat is by placing ordinary electric light bulbs within a foot or two of the patient. Avoid disturbing by any noise, questions, or transportation. Do not move patient unnecessarily.

If able to swallow, should be given hot drinks. If bleeding is present it should be controlled. If internal hemorrhage is suspected, or presence of head injuries, no stimulants are permissible. In any other instance they may be given hot, black coffee; hot, strong tea, or other warm drinks. A half teaspoonful of aromatic spirits of ammonia in a glass of warm water may likewise be given by mouth. If the patient cannot swallow, spirits of ammonia may be held to the nostrils intermittently for a few breaths.

A physician should be called promptly. The use of hypodermics and intramuscular and intravenous injections, such as epinephrine, ephedrine, caffeine, etc., or hot enemata, may be recommended by the doctor.

Oxygen may be necessary. Blood transfusion or even artificial respiration may be required, depending on the seriousness of the condition.

Relieve pain by splints, posture, supporting bandages and drugs. Morphine is valuable and when injection is impossible may be placed under tongue for prompt absorption. Alcoholic stimulants are occasionally helpful. Maintain circulation by posture, have patient flat. Lower head and shoulders, elevate all extremities and, if possible, apply snug bandages of all extremities beginning with the lower ones—this forces blood into the general circulation and prevents further peripheral stagnation. Administer fluids by all routes, by mouth, by rectum and intravenously (saline with dextrose is best). Blood transfusion when possible (6% gum acacia in saline when compatible blood is not available).

Respiration may be aided by administration of oxygen preferably mixed with 4 to 10% carbon dioxide as a respiratory stimulant. Constant, kindly, tactful encouragement and extreme gentleness in all procedures are of importance. Atropine sulfate is used in doses of 1/150 to 1/50 gr. to diminish perspiration.

F. A. TREATMENT: Depends on accuracy of diagnosis. In general, treat specific etiologic factor, maintain body heat by hot blankets, water bottles, bricks, etc. If permissible, a hot bath, hot enemas and hot drinks, and massage (do not expose patient unduly). Stimulants used generously except in presence of suspected bleeding or head injury. Strong, hot, black coffee with sugar or strong, hot tea by mouth and by rectum are esp. recommended.

s., aerial. Condition in soldiers from exposure to bursting shells.

s., anaphylactic. Reaction from injection of protein substance to which patient is sensitized.

s., anesthesia. This is not surgical shock, but is due to an overdosage of anesthetic and calls for the immediate cessation of anesthesia.

Artificial respiration and various stimulants should be given at once. The condition is manifested by a weak, rapid pulse; a fall or drop in blood pressure; by cold, clammy skin, and by shallow respirations.

s., apoplectic. Sudden attack of paralysis and coma with hemorrhage into brain and spinal cord. SYN: *apoplexy*.

s., barium. One caused by intravenous injection of barium causing destruction of red blood corpuscles.

s., cardiac. S. caused by overexertion.

s., colloid. One causing symptoms of anaphylaxis when colloids are injected.

s., deferred or delayed. Late manifestation following injury or burns.

May appear in 3 to 30 hours and may be due to transportation, emotional stress, hemorrhage, dehydration, acidosis, or toxemia.

s., electric. The result of passage of electric current.

s., epigastric. Result of a blow or other trauma (surgery) in upper abdomen.

s., erethismic. Excitement, toxic or traumatic delirium following shock.

s., faradic. The result of faradization.

s., heart. Heart failure due to overexertion.

s., hemoclastic. S. resulting from destruction of blood cells.

s., hypoglycemic. SEE: *insulin shock*.

s., injection. S. resulting from injection of various medicaments or foreign proteins.

s., insulin. Condition resulting from overdosages of insulin.

F. A. TREATMENT: Give orange juice, glucose, candy, lump of sugar, etc. If unconscious, inject glucose intravenously. SEE: *insulin*.

s., mental. SEE: *psychic s.* Due to emotional stress or seeing injury, accidents, etc.

s., metabolodispersion. The result of change in colloidal dispersion in the body.

s., peptone or **protein.** Reaction resulting from parenteral administration of a protein.

s., phenolic. S. caused by intravenous injection of phenol.

s., pleural. S. sometimes following thoracentesis.

s., pneumothorax acute. Acute s. resulting upon entrance of air into pleural cavity by perforation from disease or trauma.

s., psychic. S. due to excessive fear, joy, anger, grief.

s., railway. One caused by a railroad accident.

s., secondary. Same as *deferred shock*.

s., sense. A mild nightmare.

s., serum. One occurring as part of reaction to injection of serum.

s., sexual. Prostration or heart failure following coition or rape.

s., shell. An indefinite nervous condition found in soldiers.

s., surgical. Following operations and including traumatic shock, *q.v.*

s., testicular. Result of blow to or torsion of testicles.

s. therapy. Form of treatment in mental illness. Three types are widely used: 1. *Electric shock therapy*, in which convulsions are induced by passage of electricity through the brain; used chiefly in manic depressive psychoses, anxiety states, depression, involutional melancholia, and certain types of schizophrenia. 2. *Insulin shock therapy*, in which hypoglycemia and coma are induced by injection of insulin; used chiefly in schizophrenia. 3. *Metrazol shock therapy*, in which convulsions are induced by injection of metrazol; used chiefly in schizophrenia.

s., traumatic (broad interpretation). Shock due to injury or surgery.

May occur as result of *abdominal injury* from any cause. Shock is proportional to extent of injury. Esp. severe in upper abdomen and more marked when viscera are damaged.

If prolonged, indicates hemorrhage or peritonitis or both.

Cerebral injury: Concussion of brain or skull fracture. May come on immediately or later from edema or intracranial hemorrhage.

Chemical injury: Esp. corrosives, due to pain and effect of chemical and absorption of altered tissue.

Crushing injuries: The nearer the body the greater the shock.

Fracture: Esp. in compound fracture. Often extensive blood loss into tissues and hence body is not able to maintain circulation.

Heart damage: As in angina pectoris, coronary occlusion, or acute dilatation.

Inflammation: As acute general peritonitis or fulminating sepsis anywhere in the body.

Intestinal obstruction: Shock is present when obstruction is acute.

Nerve injury: Contusion of highly sensitive parts, as testicle, solar plexus, eye, urethra, etc.

Operations: May occur even after minor operations, as paracentesis, catheterization, etc.

Perforation or rupture of viscera, as: Acute pneumothorax, ruptured aneurysm, perforated peptic ulcer, perforation in appendicitis, ectopic pregnancy.

Strangulation: As in hernia, intussusception, volvulus.

Thermal injury: As burns, frostbite, heat exhaustion.

Torsion of viscera: As of an ovary, testicle.

s., wound. Same as *traumatic shock*.

shod'dy fever. A condition caused by the inhalation of dust among workers in shoddy factories.

SYM: Feverishness, headache, dryness of mouth, nausea, cough, dyspnea, expectoration.

shoe'makers' cramp or **spasm.** Spasm of muscles of hand and arm occurring in shoemakers.

shortsightedness (short-sīt'ĕd-nĕs). A condition of not being able to see very far. Due to light rays coming to a focus in front of the retina. SYN: *myopia, nearsightedness.*

shot'gun prescrip'tion. One containing many drugs given with hope that one of them may prove effective.

shoulder (shōl'dẽr) [A.S. *sculdor*]. The junction of the clavicle and scapula where the arm meets the trunk.
RS: *omalgia, omarthritis, omitis, scapula*.

  s. blade. The scapula.
  s., dislocation of. Displacement of shoulder joint.
  Very frequently accompanied by a fracture. It is believed by all surgeons that it is wiser to have an x-ray examination of the affected bones because fractures are so often present and attempts to reduce fractured dislocations without knowing of fractures present are very dangerous, sometimes resulting in serious paralysis of the entire upper extremity, or of grave damage to the large blood vessels in the armpit.
  CAUSES: The causes of a dislocation of a shoulder are usually those of falling on an outstretched arm, or a blow to the arm in some unusual position. It is very common among athletes, esp. among football and basketball players. A patient with a dislocated shoulder usually has a deformity with a hollow in place of the normal bulge of the shoulder. There seems to be a slight depression at the outer end of the clavicle, and the patient cannot place his hand at his opposite shoulder and still place his elbow onto his chest. Always compare both sides.
  TREATMENT: Send for a doctor as soon as possible. Lay the patient on the back, with a pillow bet. the shoulders (or folded pad). Place a large, soft pad under the elbow on the affected side and then bind the forearm horizontally across the chest, using an open sling which is reinforced by a broad cravat; bandage, and then apply cold applications to the affected shoulder. Treat for shock.
  s. girdle. The 2 scapulae and 2 clavicles attaching the bones of the upper extremities to the axial skeleton.
  s. joint. Formed by humerus and glenoid cavity of scapula.

show (shō) [A.S. *scēawian*, to look]. The sanguinoserous discharge from the vagina during the first stage of labor or just preceding menstruation.

Shrapnell's membrane (shrăp'nĕl). A small, triangular area of membrane of the eardrum fitting in the notch of Rivinus.

shred'ded wheat. Av. SERVING: 100 Gm. Pro. 10.5, Fat 1.4, Carbo. 77.9. ASH CONST: Ca 0.041, Mg 0.144, K none, Na none, P 0.324, Cl none, S none, Fe 0.0045.

shrimp (shrĭmp) [M.E. *shrimppe*]. Av. SERVING: 65 Gm. Pro. 14.1, Fat 0.5. VITAMINS: A+, ASH CONST: Ca 0.096.

shunt (shŭnt) [M.E. *shunten*, to avoid]. 1. Conductor connecting 2 points in a circuit to form a parallel or derived circuit through which a portion of the current may pass. 2. Conductor providing a low-resistance path for the flow of current.
  When 2 or more electrical devices or resistances are so connected that the current is divided between them, the current through each device or resistance being inversely proportional to the resistance, they are said to be connected "in shunt" parallel or multiple, with one another.

Si. Symb. of *silicon*.

siagonantritis (sī″ăg-ŏn-ăn-trī′tĭs) [G. *si-agōn*, jawbone, + *antron*, cavity, + *-itis*, inflammation]. Inflammation within the antrum of Highmore.

sialaden (sī-ăl′ăd-ĕn) [G. *sialon*, saliva, + *adēn*, gland]. A salivary gland.

sialadenitis (sī-ăl-ăd-ĕn-ī′tĭs) [" + " + *-itis*, inflammation]. Inflamed condition of a salivary gland.

sialadenoncus (sī-ăl-ăd-ĕn-ŏng′kŭs) [" + " + *ogkos*, tumor]. Tumor of salivary gland.

sialagogue (sī-ăl′ă-gŏg) [" + *agōgos*, leading]. Agent increasing flow of saliva. Ex: *pilocarpine, potassium iodide, citric acid*.

sialaporia (sī″al-ap-ō′rĭ-ă) [" + *aporia*, lack]. Deficiency in secretion of saliva.

sialemesis (sī″ăl-ĕm′ĕs-ĭs) [" + *emesis*, vomiting]. Vomiting of saliva or vomiting caused by an excessive secretion of it.

sialine (sī′ăl-ĭn) [G. *sialon*, saliva]. Concerning the saliva.

sialism, sialismus (sī′ăl-ĭzm, sī-ăl-ĭz′mŭs) [" + *-ismos*, condition]. An excessive secretion of saliva. SYN: *ptyalism, salivation*.

sialoadenitis (sī″ăl-ō-ăd-ĕn-ī′tĭs) [" + *adēn*, gland, + *-itis*, inflammation]. Inflammation of a salivary gland. SYN: *sialadenitis*.

sialoaerophagy (sī″ăl-ō-ā-ĕr-ŏf′ă-jī) [" + *aēr*, air, + *phagein*, to eat]. Constant swallowing, thus taking saliva and air into the stomach.

sialoangitis (sī″ăl-ō-ăn-jī′tĭs) [" + *aggeion*, vessel, + *-itis*, inflammation]. Inflamed condition of the salivary ducts.

sialodochitis (sī″ăl-ō-dō-kī′tĭs) [" + *dochē*, receptacle, + *-itis*, inflammation]. Inflamed condition of salivary ducts.

  s. fibrinosa. S. with duct obstructed by a fibrinous exudate.

sialoductitis (sī″ăl-ō-dŭk-tī′tĭs) [" + L. *ductus*, duct, + G. *-itis*, inflammation]. Inflamed condition of Stensen's duct.

sialogenous (si-al-oj′en-us) [G. *sialon*, saliva, + *gennan*, to produce]. Forming saliva.

sialogogic, sialogogue (sī-ăl-ō-gŏj′ĭk, -ăl′-ō-gŏg) [" + *agōgos*, leading]. Producing or promoting a secretion of saliva; or that which stimulates its secretion.

sialography (sī-ăl-ŏg′ră-fī) [" + *graphein*, to write]. Examination of salivary ducts and glands with x-rays. SYN: *ptyalography*.

sialolith (sī-ăl′ō-lĭth) [" + *lithos*, a stone]. A salivary concretion or calculus.

sialolithiasis (sī-ăl-ō-lĭth-ī′ăs-ĭs) [" + *-iasis*, condition]. Presence of salivary calculi.

sialolithotomy (sī″ăl-ō-lĭth-ŏt′ō-mī) [" + " + *tomē*, a cutting]. Removal of a calculus from a salivary gland or duct.

sialoncus (sī-ăl-ŏng′kŭs) [" + *ogkos*, tumor]. A tumor under the tongue caused by obstruction of a salivary gland or duct.

sialoporia (sī″ăl-ō-pō′rĭ-ă) [G. *sialon*, saliva, + *aporia*, lack]. Deficient secretion of saliva.

sialorrhea (sī-ăl-or-ē′ă) [" + *rhoia*, a flow.] Excessive flow of saliva. SYN: *sialism*.

sialoschesis (sī-ăl-ŏs′kĕs-ĭs) [" + *schesis*, suppression]. Suppression or retention of saliva.

sialosemeiology (sī″ăl-ō-sē-mī-ŏl′ō-jī) [" + *semeion*, sign, + *logos*, a study]. Diagnosis based upon examination of the saliva.

sialosis (sī-ăl-ō'sĭs) [" + -ōsis, condition]. The flow of saliva.
sialostenosis (sī"ăl-ō-stĕn-ō'sĭs) [" + stenōsis, a narrowing]. Closure of a salivary duct.
sialosyrinx (sī"ăl-ō-sī'rĭnks) [" + syrigx, a pipe]. 1. Fistula into the salivary gland. 2. A syringe for washing out salivary ducts. 3. Drainage tube for a salivary duct.
sialotic (sī-ăl-ŏt'ĭk) [G. sialon, saliva]. Concerning the flow of saliva.
sialozemia (sī"ăl-ō-zē'mĭ-ă) [" + zēmia, loss]. Involuntary loss of saliva. SYN: salivation.
Siamese twins (sī-ă-mēz'). Congenitally united twins, usually at the hips or buttocks, the members being capable of activity.
sibilant (sĭb'ĭl-ănt) [L. sibilans, hissing]. Hissing or whistling, as a sound heard in a certain râle, q.v.
sibilus (sĭb'ĭl-ŭs) [L. a hissing]. A hissing râle.
sibling (sĭb'lĭng) [A.S. sibb, kin, + -ling, having the quality of]. One of 2 or more children of same parents.
siccant (sĭk'ănt) [L. siccus, dry]. Drying.
siccative (sĭk'ă-tĭv) [L. siccativus, drying]. Drying or that which dries. SYN: siccant.
siccus (sĭk'ŭs) [L. dry]. Not moist; dry.
sick (sĭk) [A.S. seóc, ill]. 1. Not well. SYN: ill. 2. Nauseated or "sick at the stomach." 3. Menstruating.
  s. headache. One with nausea, vomiting, anorexia, etc. SYN: migraine, q.v.
  s. at the stomach. Inclined to vomit. SYN: nauseated.
sick'le cell. Abnormal red blood corpuscle of crescent shape.
  s. c. anemia. A form of anemia in which are present abnormal sickle or crescent-shaped erythrocytes. SEE: anemia.
sicklemia (sĭk-lē'mĭ-ă) [A.S. sicol, sickle, + G. aima, blood]. Sickle cells in the blood.
sick'ness [A.S. seóc, ill]. State of being unwell. SYN: illness.
  s., bleeding. Abnormal tendency to bleed. SYN: hemophilia.
  s., car. Nausea and malaise from riding in street cars, on elevated railroads and railroads.
  s., falling. Epilepsy.
  s., green. Form of anemia with greenish pallor. SYN: chlorosis.
  s., monthly. Menstruation.
  s., morning. Nausea of early pregnancy.
  s., mountain. Nausea and dyspnea caused by being on great elevations.
  s., sea. S. caused by motion of a vessel while at sea.
  s., serum. S. following injection of serum.
  s., sleeping. 1. Infection with genus of Trypanosomes with involvement of central nervous system and ultimately continuous sleeping. SYN: trypanosomiasis. 2. Acute infectious disease with increasing lethargy. SYN: lethargic encephalitis.
Siddall test (sĭd'al). A hormone test for pregnancy in early or late stage.
  One cc. of serum from patient is injected into an immature, virgin, white mouse daily for 4-5 days. It is then killed. If its weight is divided by the weight of its uterus and ovaries and the ratio is less than 400, the test is positive.
side (sīd) [A.S. side]. 1. Left or right part of wall of trunk of body. 2. An outer portion considered as facing in a particular direction.
  s.-chain theory. Theory concerning cell dissolution and immunity; complex molecules react with one another through their side chains when they have definite correspondence in structure. SEE: Ehrlich's theory.
  s. position. Lying on one side, thighs flexed, with underarm behind back. SYN: Sims' position, q.v.
sideration (sĭd-ĕr-ā'shŭn) [L. siderāri, to be struck by a planet]. 1. Therapeutic application of electric sparks. 2. A sudden stroke of disease, as in apoplexy. 3. Lightning stroke.
siderism, sidermus (sĭd'ĕr-ĭzm, -ĭz'mŭs) [G. sidēros, iron, + -ismos, condition]. Therapeutic application of metals to the skin. SYN: metallotherapy.
sidero- [G.]. Combining form meaning iron or steel, as siderosis.
sideroderma (sĭd"ĕr-ō-der'mă) [G. sidēros, iron, + derma, skin]. Bronzed coloration of the skin from disordered hemoglobin disintegration.
siderodromophobia (sĭd"ĕr-ō-drŏ"mō-fō'bĭ-ă) [" + dromos, a way, + phobos, fear]. Morbid fear of railway travel.
siderofibrosis (sĭd"ĕr-ō-fī-brō'sĭs) [" + L. fibra, fiber, + G. -ōsis, condition]. Fibrosis associated with deposits of iron.
siderogenous (sĭd-ĕr-ŏj'ĕn-ŭs) [" + gennan, to produce]. Producing or forming iron.
siderophilous (sĭd-ĕr-of'ĭl-ŭs) [" + philein, to love]. Having a tendency to absorb iron, as the red blood corpuscles.
sideroscope (sĭd"ĕr-ō-skōp) [" + skopein, to examine]. Instrument for finding metal particles in the eye.
siderosis (sĭd-ĕr-ō'sĭs) [" + -ōsis, condition]. 1. Disease of lungs caused by inhalation of metallic dust. SYN: pneumonoconiosis. 2. Deposit of iron pigments in a tissue or in the blood.
  s. bulbi. Iron pigment deposits in the eyeball.
  s., hepatic. Condition in which there is an abnormal amt. of iron in the liver.
Sigault's operation (sē-gō'). Division of the symphysis pubis to aid delivery. SYN: symphyseotomy.
sight (sīt) [A.S. sihth]. 1. Power or faculty of seeing. SYN: vision. 2. Range of sight. 3. A thing or view seen.
  s., day. Night blindness. SYN: nyctalopia.
  s., far-. Rays of light focusing behind the retina. SYN: hyperopia.
  s. meter. Device for measuring intensity of light in foot candles.
  s., near-. Rays of light focusing before the retina. SYN: myopia.
  s., night. Day blindness. SYN: hemeralopia.
  s., old. Loss of accommodation of near point. SYN: presbyopia.
  s., second. Improvement of vision in the aged usually due to incipient cataract.
sight, words pert. to: achromatopsia, afterimage, alexia, amaurosis, amblyopia, ametropia, aniseikonia, anisocoria, anisoiconia, anisometropia, anorthopia, aprosexia, asthenopia, astigmatism, blindness, brachymetropia, Burns' amaurosis, hemeralopia, hypermetropia, hyperopia, myopia, nyctalopia, photophobia, presbyopia, squint.
sigmatism (sĭg'mă-tĭzm) [G. sigma, letter S, + -ismos, condition]. Excessive or defective use of s sounds in speech.
sigmoid (sĭg'moyd) [G. sigma, letter S, +

eidos, form]. Shaped like the Greek letter *sigma, s*.
s. flexure. The lower part of descending colon bet. iliac crest and the rectum, shaped like the letter S.
RS: *cecosigmoidostomy, colon, "sigmoido-"* words.
sigmoidectomy (sĭg-moy-dĕk′tō-mĭ) [" + " + *ektomē*, excision]. Removal of all or part of the sigmoid flexure.
sigmoiditis (sĭg-moy-dī′tĭs) [" + " + *-ītis*, inflammation]. Inflammation of the sigmoid flexure of the colon.
sigmoidopexy (sĭg-moyd′ō-pĕks″ĭ) [" + " + *pēxis*, fixation]. Fixation of the sigmoid to an abdominal incision for prolapse of the rectum.
sigmoidoproctostomy (sĭg-moyd″ō-prŏk-tos′tō-mĭ) [" + " + *prōktos*, rectum, + *stoma*, passage]. Establishment of artificial passage by anastomosis of the sigmoid flexure with the rectum.
sigmoidorectostomy (sĭg-moyd″ō-rĕk-tŏs′-tō-mĭ) [" + " + L. *rectus*, straight, + G. *stoma*, passage]. Anastomosis of sigmoid flexure with the rectum to establish an artificial passage. SYN: *sigmoidoproctostomy*.
sigmoidoscope (sĭg-moy′dō-skōp) [" + " + *skopein*, to examine]. Tubular speculum for examination of sigmoid flexure.
sigmoidostomy (sĭg-moyd-ŏs′tō-mĭ) [G. *sigma*, letter S, + *eidos*, form, + *stoma*, passage]. Creation of an artificial anus in the sigmoid flexure.
sign (sīn) [L. *signum*, mark]. 1. Symbol or abbreviation, esp. one used in pharmacy. 2. Any objective evidence of an abnormal nature in the body or its organs. They are more or less definitive and obvious, and apart from the patient's impressions. Symptoms* are subjective.
s., objective. One recognized by an observer. SYN: *physical s*.
s., physical. One revealed by auscultation, percussion, inspection, etc.
signa (sĭg′nă) [L. *signa*, mark]. A term used in writing prescriptions,* meaning mark. Usually designated S or sig.
signature (sĭg′nă-tūr) [L. *signatura*]. The part of a prescription giving instructions to the patient.
sig′natures, doctrine of. Obsolete belief that medicinal uses of plants can be determined from peculiar visible characters.
silica (sĭl′ĭ-kă) [L. *silex*, flint]. Silicon dioxide, SiO₂.
silicate (sĭl′ĭ-kāt) [L. *silicus*, flintlike]. A salt of silicic acid.
silicic (sĭl-ĭs′ĭk) [L. *silex*, flint]. Pert. to silica or silicon.
s. acid. One of a number of colloid acids.
silicon (sĭl′ĭ-kon) [L. *silex*, flint]. SYMB: Si. A nonmetallic element found in the soil. At. wt. 28.06. Sp. gr. 2.48.
When combined with oxygen, it is absorbed by plants, esp. in the grains, in the form of silicates.
In animal life it seems necessary in the growth of hair, teeth, and nails. The most abundant element, excepting oxygen. Only a trace of silicon is found in the body and that in the skeletal structures. Its function is unknown but its physiological effects are unfavorable. Sherman suggests its presence with fluorine in the bones may be "a mode of disposal rather than a utilization."
silicosis (sĭl-ĭ-kō′sĭs) [L. *silex, silic-*, flint, + G. *-ōsis*, condition]. A condition caused by the inhalation of small particles of stone or stone dust.

SYM: Similar to those of emphysema.
TREATMENT: Insufflation of aluminum powder is said to be successful. SEE: *pneumonoconiosia, -is*.
silicotic (sĭl-ĭ-kŏt′ĭk) [L. *silex, silic-*, flint]. 1. Relating to silicosis. 2. One affected with silicosis.
silicotuberculosis (sĭl″ĭ-kō-tū-bĕr-kū-lō′sĭs) [" + *tuberculus*, a tubercle, + G. *-ōsis*, condition]. Silicosis associated with pulmonary tuberculosis.
siliqua olivae (sĭl′ĭk-wă ō-lī′vē) [L. olive husk]. Nerve fibers encircling the inf. olive of the brain.
siliquose (sĭl′ĭ-kwōs) [L. *siliqua*, pod]. Resembling a 2-valve capsule.
s. cataract. Cataract with a dry, wrinkled capsule.
s. desquamation. Shedding of dried vesicles from the skin.
silver (sĭl′ver) [A.S. *siolfor*]. SYMB: Ag. A white metal widely used in medicine.
s. arsphenamine. A brownish black arsphenamine derivative, containing 19% arsenic and 14% silver.
USES: Same as those of arsphenamine.
DOSAGE (adult): From 0.1 Gm. to 0.3 Gm. given with caution.
s. nitrate. USP. A toxic preparation made from silver. Most of its former uses have passed out of vogue, but it remains important as a germicide and local astringent.
DOSAGE: As an antiseptic in the eyes of newly born, 1/6 ℳ (0.01 cc.); topically as an astringent to the mucous membrane of the throat, from 5 to 10%.
INCOMPATIBILITIES: Aspirin, sodium chloride.
POISONING: When taken by mouth, causes a grayish discoloration of mucous membranes.
SYM: Burning in throat and stomach; rather prompt vomiting. When small amounts of silver are taken over a long period, as in nose or eye drops, patient develops argyria, a peculiar bluish discoloration of all the exposed tissues of body.
F. A. TREATMENT: Large volumes of ordinary table salt in water precipitate the silver as a slightly soluble chloride; follow with egg whites, oils, and other demulcents.
s. picrate. A compound of silver and picric acid, containing 30% silver. Useful as an antiseptic, similar to other preparations of silver.
DOSAGE: Dilutions from 1 to 2%.
s. protein. USP. A combination of silver and protein, containing from 7 to 19% silver. Two strengths are official, the strong and mild.
sil′ver-fork deformity or **fracture.** Deformity in Colles' fracture of wrist and hand resembling curve on back of a fork.
Silves′ter's method. A method of artificial respiration consisting of constant movements of the patient's arms.
Useless in asphyxia neonatorum.
silvol (sĭl′vol). USP. A commercial brand of mild silver protein.
simesthesia (sĭm-ĕs-thē′zĭ-ă) [G. *aisthēsis*, sensation]. Sensibility felt in a bone.
similia similibus curantur (sĭm-ĭl′ĭ-ă sĭm-ĭl′-ĭ-bŭs kū-rahn′tūr) [L. likes are cured by likes]. The homeopathic doctrine that a drug producing pathological symptoms in those who are well will cure such symptoms in disease states.
Simmonds' disease or **syndrome** (sĭm′-mond). Condition in which complete atrophy of the pituitary body causes pre-

Simon's position S-42 **sinistrosis**

mature senility and psychic symptoms. SYN: *pituitary cachexia, q.v.*
Simon's position (zē'mŏn). An exaggerated lithotomy position in which the hips are somewhat elevated with thighs strongly abducted. Employed in operations on the vagina.
simple (sĭm'pl) [L. *simplex,* simple]. 1. Not complex; not compound. 2. Deficient in intellect. 3. A medicinal plant.
 s. *fracture*. Fracture without rupture of ligaments and skin.
 s. *inflammation*. Inflammation without pus or other inflammatory exudates.
 s. *mixed enema*. A soapsuds enema to which is added 1 dram of salt and ½ oz. of molasses.
 s. *reflex*. One acting upon a single muscle.
simples (sĭm'plz) [L. *simplex,* simple]. Medicinal plants.

Infant: 10-12 parts wheat flour to 1 of mustard flour.
sinapized (sĭn'ăp-īzd) [G. *sinapi,* mustard]. Containing mustard.
sincipital (sĭn-sĭp'ĭ-tăl) [L. *sinciput,* half a head]. Concerning the sinciput.
sinciput (sĭn'sĭp-ŭt) [L. *sinciput,* half a head]. 1. Fore and upper part of the cranium. 2. Upper half of the skull. SYN: *calvaria.*
sinew (sĭn'ū) [A.S. *sinu*]. 1. A tendon. 2. Chiefly in the plural, strength; nervous energy; muscular power.
sing. [L.]. Abbr. of *singulorum*, meaning *of each.*
singer's node or **nodule** (sĭn'gerz nōd, nŏd'ūl). A swelling bet. the arytenoid cartilages of singers. SYN: *chorditis nodosa.*
singultus (sĭng-gŭl'tŭs) [L. *singultus,* hiccup]. Hiccups, *q.v.*
sinistrad (sĭn'ĭs-trăd) [L. *sinister, sinistr-,*

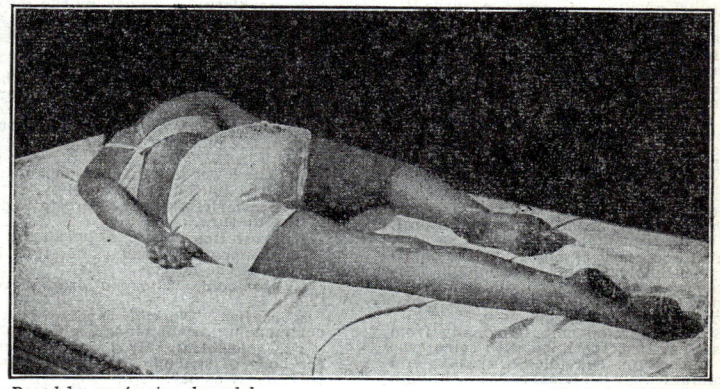

Posed by professional model SIMS' POSITION. *Photo by Whitaker*

Sims' position (sĭmz). A semiprone position; the patient lies on the left side, and the right knee and thigh are drawn up well above the left lower limb. The patient may present an anterior or posterior view. The left arm is placed back of the patient or projecting over the side of the table or bed. The chest is inclined forward so that the patient rests upon it.
 It is assumed in various treatments or operations on the genital crease, or in childbirth, if so ordered by the doctor. SEE: *position, posture.*
simul. (sī'mŭl) [L.]. At once or at the same time.
simulation (sĭm-ū-lā'shŭn) [L. *simulātio,* imitation]. Pretense of having a disease; feigning of illness. Imitation of symptoms of 1 disease by another. SEE: *malingering.*
Sinapis (sĭn-ā'pĭs) [G. *sinapi,* mustard]. Mustard.
sinapiscopy (sĭn-ăp-ĭs'kō-pĭ) [" + *skopein,* to examine]. Use of mustard in testing for sensory disturbance.
sinapism (sĭn'ăp-ĭzm) [" + *-ismos,* process]. A mustard plaster.
 Used to relieve congestion or pain, headache, neuralgia, flatulence, nausea, etc.
 PROPORTIONS: *Adult:* 3-4 parts wheat flour to 1 of mustard flour. *Child:* 8-10 parts wheat flour to 1 of mustard flour.

left, + *ad,* toward]. Toward the left.
sinistral (sĭn'ĭs-trăl) [L. *sinister, sinistr-,* left]. 1. Pert. to or showing preference for the left hand, eye, or foot in certain actions. 2. On the left side.
sinistrality (sĭn'ĭs-trăl'ĭ-tĭ) [L. *sinister, sinistr-,* left]. Left-handedness.
sinistraural (sĭn-ĭs-traw'răl) [" + *auris,* ear]. Having better hearing with the left ear.
sinistro- (sĭn'ĭs-trō) [L.]. Prefix meaning *left.*
sinistrocardia (sĭn-ĭs-trō-kar'dĭ-ă) [L. *sinister, sinistr-,* left, + G. *kardia,* heart]. Displacement of the heart to left of the medial line; opp. of *dextrocardia.*
sinistrocerebral (sĭn-ĭs-trō-ser'ē-brăl) [" + *cerebrum,* brain]. Located in the left cerebral hemisphere.
sinistrocular (sĭn-ĭs-trok'ū-lar) [" + *oculus,* eye]. Having stronger vision in the left eye.
sinistrocularity (sĭn-ĭs-trŏk-ū-lăr'ĭ-tĭ) [" + *oculus,* eye]. Condition of having better vision in the left eye.
sinistrogyration (sĭn-ĭs-trō-jī-rā'shŭn) [" + G. *gyros,* a circle]. Inclination to the left.
sinistromanual (sĭn-ĭs-trō-măn'ū-ăl) [" + *manus,* hand]. Left-handed.
sinistropedal (sĭn-ĭs-trŏp'ĕd-ăl) [" + *pes, ped-,* foot]. Left-footed.
sinistrosis (sĭn-ĭs-trō'sĭs) [L. *sinister,*

sinistr-, left, unlucky, + G. *-ōsis*, condition]. Shell shock.

sinistrotorsion (sĭn-ĭs-trō-tor'shŭn) [" + *torsio*, a turning]. A twisting or turning toward the left.

sinoauricular (sī″nō-aw-rĭk'ū-lar) [L. *sinus*, a curve, + *auricula*, a little chamber]. Pert. to the right cardiac auricle and the sinus venosus.

    s. node. One at entrance of the sup. vena cava into right auricle, regarded as starting point of the heartbeat. SYN: *sinuauricular node*.

sinuauricular (sĭn″ū-aw-rĭk'ū-lar) [" + *auricula*, a little chamber]. Concerning the sinus venosus and the right cardiac auricle.

    s. node. Node at junction of sup. vena cava with right cardiac auricle, regarded as starting point of the heartbeat.

sinuitis (sĭ-nū-ī'tĭs) [L. *sinus*, a curve, + G. *-itis*, inflammation]. Inflammation of a sinus. SYN: *sinusitis*.

sinuotomy (sĭn-ū-ŏt'ō-mĭ) [" + G. *tomē*, a cutting]. Surgical incision into a sinus.

sinuous (sĭn'ū-ŭs) [L. *sinōsus*, winding]. Winding; wavy; tortuous.

sinus (sī'nŭs) (pl. *sinuses, sinūs*) [L. *sinus*, a curve]. 1. A canal or passage leading to an abscess. 2. A cavity within a bone. 3. Dilated channel for venous blood. 4. Any cavity having a relatively narrow opening.
    RS: *antritis, antronasal, antrotympanic, antrum, cephalematocele, lateral, sinusitis, transillumination.*

    s's., accessory nasal. Frontal, maxillary, ethmoidal, and sphenoidal. *Anterior group*: Frontal, maxillary and anterior ethmoids. *Posterior group*: Posterior ethmoids and sphenoid.

    Sinuses develop embryologically from nasal cavities, are lined with same type of epithelium, are filled with air, and communicate with nasal cavities through their various ostia.

    Function of sinuses not definitely known. Various theories give them the same function as nasal cavities, viz. (warming, moistening and filtering the air); aid in resonance and make the skull lighter.

    s., aortic. Saclike dilatation of the aorta.

    s. arrhythmia. Irregularity of heartbeat due to interference with impulses from the sinoauricular node.

    s., basilar. SEE: *transverse s.*

    s., cavernous. A large s. from sphenoidal fissure to apex of petrous portion of temporal bone.

    s., circular. A venous s. around the pituitary body, communicating on each side with the cavernous s.

    s's., circular, of the placenta. A plexus of veins in the maternal portion of placenta.

    s., clinoid. SEE: *circular s.*

    s., coronary, of the heart. A vein in transverse groove bet. left cardiac auricle and ventricle.

    s's., cranial. Venous canals bet. folds of the dura.

    s's., ethmoidal. Air cavities in the ethmoid bone.

    s., frontal. An irregular cavity in frontal bone on each side of midline above the nasal bridge. One may be larger than the other. A duct carries secretions to upper part of nostrils.

    s., genital. The cleft of the vulva.

    s., genitourinary. SEE: *urogenital s.*

    s., great, of the aorta. A dilatation on right side of ascending portion of the aorta.

    s., inferior longitudinal. A venous s. along post. half of lower border of the falx cerebri.

    s., inferior petrosal. A large venous s. from cavernous s., running along lower margin of the petrous portion of the temporal bone.

    s's., intercavernous. The ant. and post. halves of the circular s.

    s., lateral. One of 2 large venous s's. in inner side of skull passing near the mastoid antrum, emptying into the jugular vein.

    s's., lymph. Small spaces throughout the parenchyma of a lymphatic gland.

    s's., mastoid. Cells within mastoid portion of the temporal bone.

    s., maxillary. A cavity in the maxillary bone opening at upper part of antrum into the nose. SYN: *antrum* or *antrum of Highmore*.

    s., occipital. A small venous s. in attached margin of the falx cerebelli extending to margin of the foramen magnum.

    s., placental. A venous passage around edge of the placenta.

    s's., pleural. Spaces in pleural sac along the lower and inf. portions of lung which the lung does not occupy.

    s. pocularis. Lacuna in prostatic part of the urethra.

    s. prostaticus. SEE: *s. pocularis.*

    s. pulmonalis. Atrium of the left auricle of the heart.

    s., rhomboid. The 4th cranial ventricle.

    s. rhythm. Normal cardiac rhythm commencing at the sinoauricular node.

    s's., sphenoidal. Air s's. which occupy the body of sphenoid bone and connect with nasal cavity.

    s., sphenoparietal. 1. A vein uniting the cavernous s. and a meningeal vein. 2. The portion of the cavernous s. below the ensiform process.

    s., straight. One which is continuous with the inf. longitudinal s. and running along junction of the falx cerebri and tentorium.

    s., superior longitudinal. A triangular one along upper edge of the falx cerebri.

    s., superior petrosal. A venous canal running in a groove in the petrous portion of the temporal bone.

    s. tachycardia. Uncomplicated rapid heartbeat.

    s., terminal. A vein encircling the vascular area of the blastoderm.

    s., transverse. 1. S. that unites the 2 inf. petrosal sinuses. 2. Venous network in the dura over basilar process of occipital bone.

    s., urinogenital or **urogenital.** 1. Duct into which, in the embryo, the wolffian ducts and bladder empty and which opens into the cloaca. 2. The common receptacle of genital and urinary ducts.

    s's., uteroplacental. Slanting venous channels from the placenta serving to convey the maternal blood from the intervillous lacunae back into the uterine veins.

    s. of Valsalva. A dilatation of the aorta or pulmonary artery opp. segment of the semilunar valve. SYN: *aortic s.*

    s., venous. One conveying venous blood.

s's., vertebral. Veins within the vertebrae.

sinusitis (sĭ-nŭ-sī'tĭs) [L. *sinus*, a curve, a hollow, + G. *-itis*, inflammation]. Inflammation of a sinus, esp. the accessory nasal ones.
  ETIOL: Possibly deficiency of vitamin A. Seems responsible for increased sinus affections as well as ophthalmia.
  s., acute catarrhal. Inflammation accompanying a similar process in the nose.
  s., acute suppurative. Purulent inflammation with symptoms of pain over the sinus, fever, chills, headache, etc.
  TREATMENT: Conservative, shrinkage in the nose for ventilation, and drainage of the sinus, aeration, constitutional treatment, capillary suction. Rest in bed, catharsis, force fluids, anodynes for pain.
  s., chronic hyperplastic. Polypi present in sinuses and nose and underlying osteitis of sinus walls.
  TREATMENT: *Surgical*: Conservative; removal of polypi and intranasal opening into sinuses for adequate ventilation and drainage. *Radical*: Complete removal of sinus mucosa either through external or intranasal route.
  s., chronic hypertrophic. Inflammation found in conjunction with chronic hypertrophic rhinitis.
  Ideal treatment in these cases is change of climate where the temperature fluctuations are not extreme.

sinusoid (sī'nŭs-oyd) [L. *sinus*, a hollow, a curve, + G. *eidos*, like]. 1. Resembling a sinus. 2. A minute terminal, endothelium-lined space, or passage for blood in tissues of an organ, as the liver.

sinusoidal (sī-nŭs-oyd'ăl) [" + G. *eidos*, like]. Pert. to a sinusoid.
  s. current. Alternating induced electric current, the 2 strokes of which are equal.

sinusoidalization (sī-nŭs-oyd-al-ĭ-zā'shŭn) [" + G. *eidos*, like]. Use of a sinusoidal current.

sinusotomy (sī-nŭ-sŏt'ō-mĭ) [" + G. *tomē*, a cutting]. The operation of incising a sinus.

SiO₂. Silicon dioxide.

siphon (sī'fŏn) [G. *siphōn*, tube]. A tube bent at an angle to form 2 unequal lengths for removing liquids by atmospheric pressure.

siphonoma (sī-fon-ō'mă) [" + *-ōma*, tumor]. A tumor made up of fine tubes.

Sippy diet (sĭp'ē). Treatment of gastric ulcer by diet checking acidity of gastric juice.
  Small amounts of milk and cream every hour and alkaline powders every ½ hr.
  Average mixture: 1½ oz. each of cream and milk given from 7 A.M. to 7 P.M., 13 *feedings*, for 3 to 4 days when an egg is given for breakfast. Next day, 3 oz. soft cereal added to afternoon feeding; another egg the next day, and finally 3 servings of cereal and 3 eggs per day added to the milk and cream. Purée, custards, toast added the next week. Decreased feedings as amt. of each feeding is increased until 6 feedings are given per day.

siriasis (sĭ-rī'ă-sĭs) [G. *seirian*, to be hot]. Sunstroke, *q.v.*

sismotherapy (sĭs-mō-ther'ă-pĭ) [G. *seismos*, a shake, + *therapeia*, treatment]. Therapeutic employment of vibration. SYN: *seismotherapy, vibrotherapeutics*.

sissorexia (sĭs-ō-rĕk'sĭ-ă). Accumulation of blood corpuscles in the spleen.

sistomensin (sĭs-tō-mĕn'sĭn). Commercial preparation containing the luteolipoid of the corpus luteum and used to check excessive menstrual flow.

sitieirgia (sĭt-ĭ-ĭr'jĭ-ă) [G. *sition*, food, + *eirgein*, to bar out]. Hysterical refusal to take food.

sitio-, sito- [G.]. Combining forms meaning *bread*, or *made from grain; food*, as *sitomania*.

sitiology (sĭt-ĭ-ŏl'ō-jĭ) [G. *sition*, food, + *logos*, a study]. Science of nutrition. SYN: *sitology*.

sitiomania (sĭt-ĭ-ō-mā'nĭ-ă) [" + *mania*, madness]. Periodic abnormal appetite or craving for food. SYN: *sitomania*.

sitology (sī-tŏl'ō-jĭ) [G. *sitos*, food, + *logos*, a study]. Science of nutrition and food. SYN: *sitiology*.

sitomania (sī'tō-mā'nĭ-ă) [" + *mania*, madness]. 1. Periodic abnormal craving for food. SYN: *sitiomania*. 2. Periodic abnormality of appetite.

sitophobia (sī'tō-fō'bĭ-ă) [" + *phobos*, fear]. Psychoneurotic abhorrence of food, or morbid dread of, or repugnance to food, whether generally or only to specific dishes.

sitotherapy (sī'tō-ther'ă-pĭ) [" + *therapeia*, treatment]. The therapeutic use of food.

sitotoxism (sī'tō-tŏks'ĭzm) [" + *toxikon*, poison, + *ismos*, condition]. Poisoning by vegetable foods infested with molds or bacteria.

sitotropism (sī-tŏt'rō-pĭzm) [" + *tropos*, a turning, + *-ismos*, condition]. Response of cells to the attraction or repulsion of food elements.

situs (sī'tŭs) [L. position]. A position.
  s. inversus viscerum. Displacement of viscera abnormally to opposite side of the body.
  s. perversus. Malposition of any visceral structure.

sitz bath (sĭtz bath). Bath to sit in with water above and covering the hips. SYN: *hip bath, q.v.* SEE: *bath*.

sixth cranial nerve (siksth). Abducens nerve which supplies the external rectus of the eye. SEE: *cranial nerves*.

skatol(e (skăt'ōl) [G. *skōr, skat-*, dung]. Beta-methyl indole, C₉H₉N, a malodorous, solid, heterocyclic nitrogen compound found in feces, formed by protein decomposition in the intestines and giving them their odor.

skein (skān) [M.E. *skeyne*]. Coiled thread of chromatin seen in the earlier stages of mitosis. SYN: *spireme*.

skelalgia (skē-lăl'jĭ-ă) [G. *skelis*, leg, + *algos*, pain]. Pain in the leg.

skeletal (skĕl'ĕ-tăl) [G. *skeleton*, skeleton]. Pert. to the skeleton.
  s. muscle. One attached to, or one moving some structure.
  s. tissue. Bony, cartilaginous, fibrous, or ligamentous tissues forming the framework of the body.

skeletization (skĕl-ĕt-ĭ-zā'shŭn) [G. *skeleton*, skeleton]. 1. Excessive emaciation. 2. Removal of soft parts of the body leaving only the skeleton.

skeleto- [G.]. Prefix meaning *skeleton*.

skeletogenous (skĕl-ĕt-ŏj'ĕn-ŭs) [G. *skeleton*, skeleton, + *gennan*, to produce]. Forming skeletal structures or tissues.

skeletology (skĕl-ĕ-tŏl'ō-jĭ) [" + *logos*, study]. The study of the skeleton.

skeleton (skĕl'ĕt-ōn) [G. *skeleton*]. The bony framework of the body, consisting of 206 bones, as follows:

    AXIAL GROUP (80 Bones)
  8 cerebral cranials.
 14 visceral cranials.
  1 os hyoideum (hyoid).
  6 ossicula auditus (ossicles, ear bones).
26 columna vertebralis (vertebrae).
24 costae (ribs).
 1 sternum (chest).
80 Total

    APPENDICULAR GROUP (126 Bones)
64 extremitas sup. (32 in each upper extremity).
62 extremitas inf. (31 in each lower extremity).
126 Total

    TRUNK (51 Bones)
Columna vertebralis (vertebrae), 26 Bones
 7 cervicales (cervicals).
12 thoraces (dorsals).
 5 lumbales (lumbar).
 1 os sacrum.
 1 os coccygis.
26 Total

    Ribs (24 Bones)
14 costae verae (true ribs).
 6 costae spuriae (false ribs).
 4 costae vertebrales (floating ribs).
24 Total
1 sternum (chest bone).

    HEAD (29 Bones)
    Cerebral cranials (8 Bones)
1 os frontale (frontal).
2 ossa parietalia (parietals).
1 ossa occipitale (occipital).
2 ossa temporales (temporal).
1 os sphenoidale (sphenoid).
1 os ethmoidale (ethmoid).
8 Total

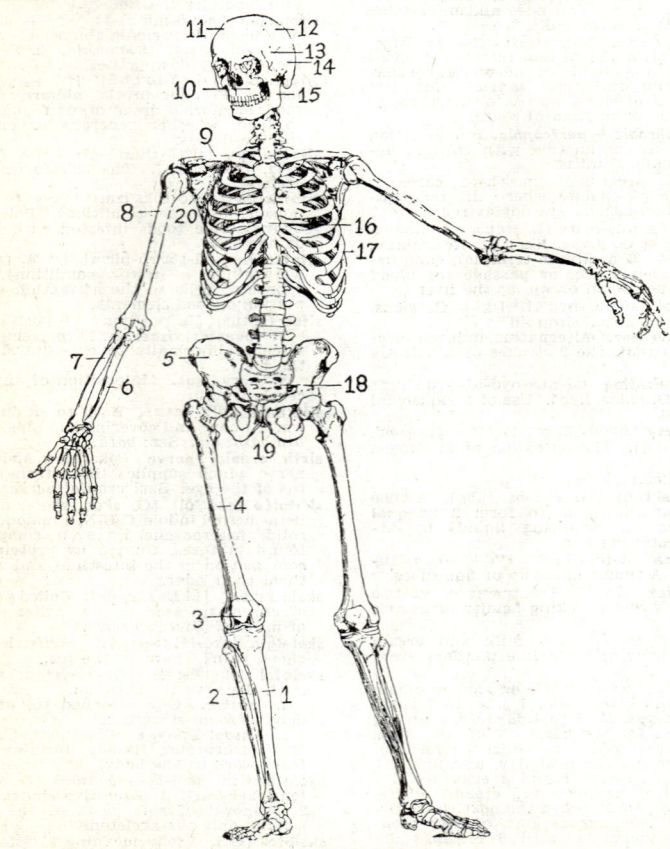

THE SKELETON.

1. Tibia. 2. Fibula. 3. Patella. 4. Femur. 5. Innominate. 6. Ulna. 7. Radius. 8. Humerus. 9. Clavicle. 10. Superior maxillary. 11. Os Frontale. 12. Parietal Bone. 13. Temporal Bone. 14. Occipital Bone. 15. Inferior Maxillary. 16. Sternum. 17. Costae. 18. Sacrum. 19. Coccyx. 20. Scapula.

skeleton S-46 **skin**

Visceral cranials (facial) (14 Bones)
2 ossa maxillae (sup. maxillary).
1 os mandibula (inf. maxillary).
2 ossa zygomatica (malar).
2 ossa lacrimales (lacrimal).
2 ossa nasalia (nasal).
2 conchae nasales inferiores (turbinates).
1 os vomer.
2 ossa palatina (palate).
—
14 Total
1 os hyoideum (hyoid).
EAR: *Ossicula auditus* (ossicles of the tympanum).
2 malleus.
2 incus.
2 stapes.
—
6 Total
EXTREMITAS SUPERIOR (upper extremities) (64 Bones)
(Arm, 5 bones, 10 in both arms)
2 claviculae (clavicle).
2 scapulae (shoulder blade).
2 humeri (arm bone).
2 radii (forearm).
2 ulnae (elbow bone).
—
10 Total
Ossa carpi (wrist bones, 16)
2 ossa naviculare manus (scaphoid).
2 ossa lunatum (semilunar).
2 ossa triquetrum (cuneiform).
2 ossa pisiforme (pisiform).
2 ossa multangulum majus (trapezium).
2 ossa multangulum minus (trapezoid—like a trapezium).
2 ossa capitatum (os magnum).
2 os hamatum (unciform).
16 Total
Hands (38 Bones)
10 metacarpalia (metacarpus).
28 phalanges digitorum manus.
—
38 Total
10 both arms.
16 ossi carpi.
—
64 Total
EXTREMITAS INFERIOR (lower extremities) (62 Bones)
(Leg, 5 bones each, or total of 10)
2 os coxae (hipbone).
2 femur.
2 tibia.
2 fibula.
2 patella (kneepan).
—
10 Total
Ossa tarsi (ankle, 7 bones each, total 14)
2 talus (astragalus).
2 calcaneus (os calis, heel bone).
2 os naviculare pedis (scaphoid).
2 os cuboideum (cuboid).
2 os cuneiforme primus (int. cuneiform).
2 os cuneiforme secundum (middle cuneiforme).
2 os cuneiforme tertium (ext. cuneiform).
—
14 Total
14 ossa tarsi (as above).
10 ossa metatarsalia (metatarsal).
28 phalanges digitorum pedis.
10 leg and hip.
—
62 Total
SUMMARY
28 Head.
1 Hyoid.
51 Trunk.
64 Extremitas superior.
62 Extremitas inferior.
—
206 Total bones in skeleton.

s., appendicular. The bones of the limbs.
s., axial. Bones of the head and trunk.
s., cartilaginous. Structure from which the bones have been formed through ossification.
s., visceral. That part of the skeleton that protects the viscera.
Skene's glands (skēn). Glands lying just inside of and on the post. floor of the urethra, in the female.
If the margins of the urethra are drawn apart and the mucous membrane gently averted, the 2 small openings of Skene's tubules or glands, 1 on each side of the floor of the urethra, become visible. Trauma frequently causes a gaping of the urethra and ectropion of the mucous membrane. In acute gonorrhea these glands are almost always infected.
skenitis (skē-nī'tĭs) [G. -*itis*, inflammation]. Inflamed condition of Skene's glands.
skeocytosis (skē-ō-sī-tō'sĭs) [G. *skaios*, left, + *kytos*, cell, + -*osis*, condition]. Immature white corpuscles in the peripheral blood. SYN: *neocytosis*.
skiagram (skī'ă-grăm) [G. *skia*, shadow, + *gramma*, a mark]. An x-ray picture. SEE: *roentgenogram*.
skiagraph (skī'ă-grăf) [" + *graphein*, to write]. An x-ray picture. SYN: *roentgenograph*.
skiagraphy (skī-ăg'ră-fĭ) [" + *graphein*, to write]. Process of taking pictures with roentgen rays. SYN: *radiography*, *roentgenography*.
skiameter (skī-ăm'ĕt-ĕr) [" + *metron*, a measure]. Device for determining differences in density and penetration of x-rays.
skiascope (skī'ă-skōp) [" + *skopein*, to examine]. 1. Device for examination by the fluoroscope. 2. Examination of the eye employing movement of shadow and light.
skiascopy (skī-ăs'kō-pĭ) [" + *skopein*, to examine]. 1. Retinoscopy or shadow test used in determining the refractive error of an eye. 2. Fluoroscopic inspection of the body.
skin (skĭn) [Old Norse *skinn*]. The integument or external covering of the body.
The skin consists essentially of 2 layers, the *epidermis* and the *corium*. The epidermis (cuticle, scarf skin) is composed of 4 main layers of stratified epithelium. The outermost, the *stratum corneum*, is formed of several layers of flattened cells which have become horny and lost their nuclei and which contains keratin.* They form a protective covering for the body surfaces. Underneath this layer is the *stratum lucidum*, which is formed of translucent flattened cells. The 3rd layer, the *stratum granulosum*, is formed of cells which contain nuclei and are not so flat. The last layer of the epidermis is the *stratum mucosum*, which contains pigment granules. This is sometimes called *prickle cell layer*. The upper portions of this layer are composed of cuboidal cells, the cells nearest the corium being columnar. This columnar layer is sometimes called *stratum germinativum*.
The corium (cutis, dermis, derma, true skin) is formed of connective tissue containing lymphatics, nerves and nerve endings, blood vessels, sebaceous and sweat glands, and elastic fibers. It is divided into 2 layers, a *superficial papillary layer* and a *deep reticular layer*. The papillary layer contains conical **pro-**

tuberances, the papillae, which fit into corresponding depressions in the epidermis. Within each papilla is a capillary loop which furnishes the epidermis with a blood supply. The reticular layer is made up in the main of white fibrous

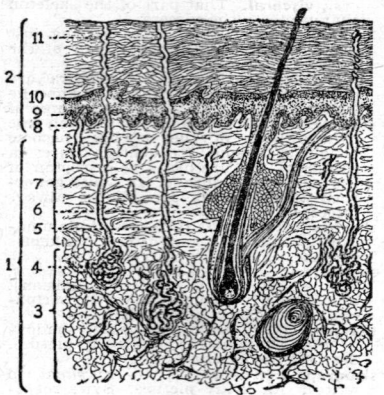

LAYERS OF SKIN.
1. Dermis. 2. Epidermis. 3. Stratum reticulare. 4. Sweat gland. 5. Hair follicle. 6. Sebaceous gland. 7. Stratum papillare. 8. Papilla. 9. Stratum germinativum. 10. Stratum granulosum. 11. Stratum corneum.

tissue supporting the blood vessels and other structures in it. It rests on the subcutaneous connective tissue.

Appendages of the skin are the hair* and nails.*

FUNCTION: 1. Protection against injuries and parasitic invasion. 2. Regulation of body temperature. 3. Aids in elimination.

DIAGNOSIS: *Ashy*: Malignant diseases, cancer, scrofula, chronic interstitial nephritis.

Bronzing: Addison's disease, dyes or metals, early stages of pellagra.

Brownish-yellow Spots (liver spots): Noted in pregnancy (chloasma uterinum), in exophthalmic goiter, and uterine and liver malignancies; also freckles, sunburn, cosmetics, mustard, turpentine, and other irritants.

Cold Sweats: Indicate great prostration, fear or depression of spirits.

Cyanosis: May be congenital; if acquired may be due to asthma, pulmonary tuberculosis, whooping cough, advanced emphysema, croup, tracheal obstruction, aneurysm, foreign body, tumor, dilated heart, goiter, flushing (hyperemia), emotion, febrile disorders, pulmonary tuberculosis, during convulsions, large ovarian tumor, plethora.

Cyanosis Alternating with Pallor: Cerebrospinal diseases, typhoid, vasomotor disturbances, menopause, Gray's argyria, silver salts. May be noted in lips, mucous membranes, fingertips and external ear. If extreme, entire body shows dusky, leaden tint. Indicates lack of oxygen and excess of carbon dioxide in blood. May be due to inflammation of pharynx and larynx, abscess of same, angina Ludovici, croup and disorders affecting respiration. Also to overdose of drugs and asphyxiation by gas.

Discolorations: Seen in icterus, chlorosis, leprosy, resulting from administration of silver nitrate, malignant diseases, and asphyxia from gas.

Edema: Due to imbalance of fluids from capillaries and absorption by lymphatics. Seen in anemia, hydremia, obstruction, inflammation, cardiac, circulatory and renal decompensation. If local, may be due to obstruction of return circulation, heart failure, in which case it will be evident in ankles and often legs, esp. at night. May also be due to renal diseases.

Emphysema: Due to air or gas in cellular tissue.

Hot and Dry: Indicates fever, mental excitement, or excessive use of salted provisions.

Moisture: Lack of noted in ichthyosis. Increased perspiration (hyperhidrosis) may be due to malarial fever; rheumatic, relapsing and septic fever; pneumonic

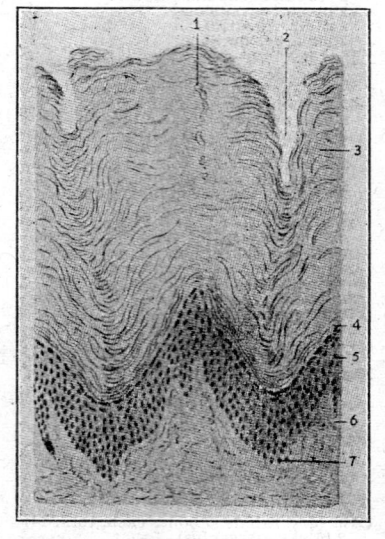

VERTICAL SECTION OF THE SKIN OF THE SOLE. (Diagrammatic)
1. "Fine furrow" corresponding in position to an interpapillary process. 2. Sweat pore. 3. Stratum corneum. 4. Granular layer. 5. Malpighian layer. 6. Basal layer. 7. Interpapillary process.

crisis; pulmonary tuberculosis; Graves' disease; neuralgia; migraine; drugs; hot drinks.

Paleness: Nervous prostration, dropsy, paralysis, malnutrition.

Pallor: Obtains in those living an indoor life, esp. in prisoners and night workers. May be due to lowered circulation, decrease of red blood corpuscles, nonfilling capillaries. Obtains in all anemias. Temporary pallor occurs in syncope, heart weakness, chills, shock, rigors and some vasomotor spasms. If sudden and persistent may be sign of int. hemorrhage. Also seen in lead poisoning, toxic febrile affections. If it gradually becomes permanent may indi-

skin, alligator   S-48   **skull, fractured**

cate chronic febrile disease, chronic gastrointestinal disease, cancer, arsenical poisoning, chronic suppuration, chronic mercurial poisoning, hemorrhages, leukemia, cachexia, nephrosis, nephritis, syphilis, parasitic diseases, tuberculosis, malaria.

Purplish: Interference of circulation common in asthma and typhus.

Rashes: SEE: *rash*.

Temperature: Usually corresponds with internal temperature, unless raised by local applications of heat. If generally cold may be due to poor circulation or obstruction of same, vasomotor spasms, venous or arterial thrombosis, exposure to cold. General abnormal heat seen in febrile disorders, although some of them present a cold and clammy skin.

Redness: Red spots upon pale cheeks, tubercular involvement, worms. Local redness seen in inflammation, skin diseases, chronic alcoholism, vasomotor disturbances, pyrexia and chlorosis. One side of face, lobar pneumonia. Local redness with pain indicates inflammation.

Sallowness: Cachexia, syphilis, chronic gallbladder disease, arthritis deformans, constipation, some anemias, gastric, pancreatic, enteric, or hepatic disorders.

Yellow: Absorption of bile, jaundice, liver derangements. If jaundiced, plethoric, hyperemic, or pigmented, it should be noted in any examination. Rashes, scars, and their cause are also diagnostic. Texture and temperature of skin are important signs. Undue moisture, cold or hot spots on body, dryness of skin are other points to look for in diagnosis. SEE: *face*.

s., alligator. Severe scaling of the skin with formation of thick plates resembling hide of an alligator.

s., deciduous. Shedding of the epidermis. SYN: *heratolysis*.

s., elastic. Skin which has property of great elasticity.

s., glossy. Shining atrophy of the skin.

s. grafting. Grafting of skin from another part of body to repair a defect or trauma. SEE: *Thiersch's graft*.

ONP: Position of patient indicated by location of graft. The area to receive graft requires little or no preparation, the area from which graft is to be taken is washed thoroughly with alcohol (70%). Patient is draped with sterile sheets and towels so that both areas are exposed. A continual saline drip is used while skin is being removed. A wet dressing is applied to area from which the skin is removed and is covered with rubber dam. The area receiving skin is covered with a paraffin-coated mesh.

s., loose. Hypertrophy of the skin.

s., parchment. Atrophy of the skin with stretching.

s., scarf, s., scurf. Cuticle, epidermis, the outer layer of the skin.

s., true. Corium or inner layer of the skin, *q.v.*, above.

skin, words pert. to: abrasion, acanthoma, acanthosis, acarodermatitis, achor, achroma, achromasia, achromodermia, acladiosis, acme, acne, acneform, acrodermatitis, acrodynia, acroscleroderma, actinocutitis, actinodermatitis, adermia, adermogenesis, albaras, allergy, allochromasia, alphus, anetodermia, angiodermatitis, apellous, areatus, areola, arevareva, argyria, argyrosis, arrectores pilorum, asteatosis, atrophoderma, atrophodermatosis, attrition, autodermic, autographism, biotripsis, bronzed, bruise, callosity, cellulocutaneous, ceratum, cheloid, chiropompholyx, chloasma, chromatopathy, chromodermatosis, comedo, contusion, corium, corn, cutaneous, cuticle, cutis, cyanosis cyesedema, "derm-" words, desquamation, eczema, elephantiasis, endermatic, ephelis, epidermis, epidermolysis, epispastics, epithelial, epithelioma, epithelium, erubescence, eruption, erysipelas, erythema, erythemogenic, erythrasma, erythristic, erythromelalgia, escharotic, exanthem, excoriation, excrescence, exfoliation, faveolus, fissure, fistula, flush, follicle, freckle, furfuraceous, geroderma, gerodermia, graft, herpes, heteroautoplasty, hyperemia, ichthyosis, icterus, impetigo, induration, integument, itch, keratoderma, keratodermatitis, keratosis, leprosy, leukoderma, lichen, lupus, macula, macule, melanoderma, melasma, mentum, molluscum, mycosis, nevus, pachydermia, pallor, papilla, papillate, papilloma, papule, pessima, petechiae, pityriasis, pore, prickle, prurigo, pruritus, psoriasis, purpura, pustule, racemose, radiodermatitis, rash, rhacoma, rhagades, rimmose, roseola, rubedo, rubefacient, rubescent, rubiginous, rubor, ruga, sallowness, saltrheum, scabies, scale, scarification, scarf skin, scleroderma, sebaceous, seborrhea, sebum, skin grafting, stigma, stria, suffusion, tache, tegument, telangiectasis, tubercle, xanthochromia, xanthoderma, xanthoma, xeroderma, xeronosus, xerosis, yava skin.

skleriasis (sklē-rī′ăs-ĭs) [G. *sklēros*, hard, + *-iasis*, condition]. Progressive hardening of the skin in patches. SYN: *scleroderma*.

sklero- [G.]. See words beginning with *sclero-*.

Skoda's râles (skō′dă). Bronchial ones heard through consolidated tissue of the lungs in pneumonia.

S's. resonance, S's. tympany. Tympanic resonance above the line of fluid in pleuritic effusion, or above consolidation in pneumonia.

S's. sign. Same as *Skoda's resonance*.

skotogram, skotograph (skō′tō-grăm, -grăf) [G. *skotos*, darkness, + *gramma*, mark, + *graphein*, to write]. A roentgen ray picture. SYN: *skiagram*.

skotography (skō-tŏg′ră-fĭ) [" + *graphein*, to write]. Photography by x-rays. SYN: *skiagraphy*.

skull (skŭl) [M.E. *skulle*, bowl]. The bony framework of the head, composed of 8 cranial bones and the 14 bones of the face. SYN: *calvaria, cranium*. SEE: *skeleton*.

s. cap. Upper round portion of skull covering the brain.

s., fractured. Fractures of the skull can be classified according to whether the fracture is in the vault or the base, but from the point of view of treatment a more useful classification is as follows:

(1) *Simple Uncomplicated Fractures*: Not common.

(2) *Compound Fractures*: If in vault of skull, the bone is depressed and driven inwards with possible damage to brain. Treatment is operative.

Hair should be cut as short as possible for at least 2 in. all around wound and a dressing applied. If fracture of base of skull is compound, it shows by the escape of blood and perhaps cerebrospinal fluid (which is clear) through the ear, nose, or back of mouth, according to location of fracture. Any such escape of blood must at first be assumed to be

skull, fractured S-49 **skull, fractured**

due to a compound fracture of skull. Infection spreading inwards and leading to meningitis unless care is taken is a serious possibility. The ears and nose should be mopped out gently with swabs soaked in weak carbolic—*never syringed*—and a small piece of sterile cotton wool should be left in cavity.

Any fracture of skull may be associated with concussion or other damage to brain, which is of greater importance than the fracture. Unless fracture is compound, treatment depends more on amount of injury brain has sustained than on actual damage to skull. The patient should be kept very quiet in a darkened room. A cold compress or ice bag applied to head, which is kept low. A calomel purge is usually given, or if there is deep unconsciousness 1 ℞ of croton oil may be ordered. Any discharge of blood or fluid should be reported and particular note taken if returning consciousness is followed by a

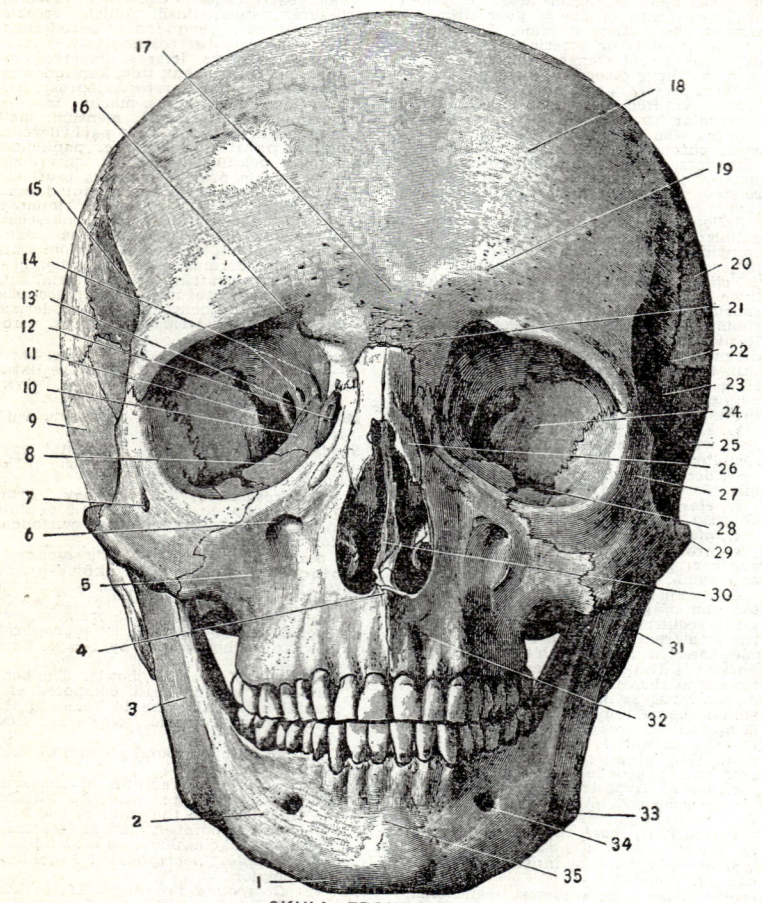

SKULL, FRONT VIEW.

1, Mental tubercle; 2, body of mandible; 3, ramus of mandible; 4, anterior nasal spine; 5, canine fossa; 6, infraorbital foramen; 7, zygomaticofacial foramen; 8, orbital surface of maxilla; 9, squamous temporal; 10, lateral surface of ethmoid; 11, superior orbital fissure; 12, lacrimal bone and groove; 13, optic foramen; 14, ethmoidal foramina; 15, temporal line; 16, supraorbital notch; 17, glabella; 18, frontal eminence; 19, superciliary arch; 20, parietal bone; 21, nasofrontal suture; 22, pterion; 23, great wing of sphenoid; 24, orbital surface of great wing; 25, squamous part of temporal; 26, left nasal bone; 27, zygomatic bone; 28, inferior orbital fissure; 29, zygomatic arch; 30, apertura piriformis; 31, mastoid process; 32, incisive fossa; 33, angle of mandible; 34, mental foramen; 35, symphysis menti. (Robinson, Editor: *Cunningham's Textbook of Anatomy*, 6th Ed., Oxford University Press, New York City, 1931.)

sleep relapse into unconsciousness, as this denotes continued cerebral hemorrhage and is a very grave sign.

sleep (slēp) [A.S. *slāep*, sleep]. A normal (more or less periodic) loss of consciousness, apparently favoring recuperation following the exhaustion entailed in conscious activity.

It is easily differentiated from the lessened consciousness of stupor, in that normal awareness can completely reassert itself when danger threatens and ordinarily continue until sleep can again safely reassert itself.

Metabolism falls to less than 0.25 calories per minute, about that of a dying person. Half as much air is taken in, muscles relax, perspiration increases, blood pressure falls sharply, and output of urine in the bladder decreases. Temperature drops sharply; lowest about the middle hours of sleep.

Emotionalism (*e. g.*, fear) is the great enemy of sleep, and the most common cause of insomnia. Hypersomnia may be a symptom of hypopituitarism.

s., crescendo. Normal sleep with increased movement during the night.

s. drunkenness. The stupor of sleep in drunkenness. SYN: *somnolentia*.

s. epilepsy. Uncontrollable desire to sleep at periodic intervals. SYN: *narcolepsy*. [suggestion.

s., hypnotic. S. induced by hypnotic

s. paralysis. Temporary p. of a part due to pressure during sleep.

s., paroxysmal. SEE: *sleep epilepsy*.

s., pathologic. A term used in encephalitis lethargica (sleeping sickness); here sleep reasserts itself excessively and under conditions not to the best interests of the patient.

s., phy. standards Pg. S-121.

s., twilight. A procedure of spinal injection of scopolamine and morphine to abolish the subsequent memory of pain felt during childbirth, but it does not abolish pain at the time. The patient is delivered in deliriumlike state.

s. walking. Walking in one's sleep. SYN: *somnambulism*.

sleep, words pert. to: agrypnia, ahypnia, antilethargic, anypnia, carotic, carus, hallucination, hypnagogic, hypnogenic, hypnoidal, hypnosis, hypnotic, hypnotism, incubus, insomnia, narcohypnia, narcolepsy, noctambulism, oneirodynia, somnambulism, somnifacient, somniloquy, somnolence, somnolent, sopor, soporific, twilight sleep.

sleeping pills. SEE: p. S-121.

sleep'ing sick'ness. 1. Acute, infectious disease marked by increasing lethargy, drowsiness, muscular weakness and cerebral symptoms. SYN: *encephalitis lethargica, q.v.* 2. African trypanosomiasis caused by a protozoan introduced into the blood and cerebrospinal fluid by the bite of a tsetse fly; characterized by fever, protracted lethargy, weakness, tremors, and wasting.

slimy (slĭm'ĭ) [A.S. *slim*, smooth]. Resembling slime or a viscid substance; of a growth, adhering to needle so it can be drawn out as a long thread.

sling (slĭng) [A.S. *slingan*, sling]. A support for an injured upper extremity.

s., clove hitch. Make clove hitch in center of roller bandage. Fit to hand and carry ends over shoulder. Tie beside neck with square knot, making longer ends. They may be carried over the shoulder, brought under each axilla and tied over chest.

s., cravat. The center of cravat is placed under wrist or forearm and ends tied around neck.

s., folded cravat (lesser arm sling). Place broad fold in position on chest with one end over affected shoulder and other hanging down in front of chest. Flex arm as desired across sling. Bring lower end up over sound shoulder. Knot with other end on affected shoulder.

s., open. The point of the triangle is placed at tip of elbow. The ends brought around at back of neck and tied. The point should be brought forward and pinned or tied in a single knot, forming a cup to prevent elbow from slipping out.

s., simple figure-of-eight roller arm. Flex arm on chest in desired position, then fix bandage with single turn toward uninjured side around arm and chest, crossing elbow just above external epicondyle of humerus. Make 2nd turn overlapping 2/3 of 1st and bring bandage forward under tip of elbow, then upwards, along flexed forearm to root of neck of sound side. Then bring downward over scapula and cross chest and arm horizontally, overlapping, turn above and continue as in progressive figure-of-eight.

s., St. John's. Apply triangle with point downwards under elbow, upper end over sound shoulder. Flex arm acutely on chest. Bring lower end under affected arm and around back to knot with upper end on sound shoulder. Bring point up over elbow and fasten to base. Support is wholly for injured shoulder.

s., swathe arm or cravat. (Use wide cravat or folded muslin band.) Place center under acutely flexed elbow, carry front and upwards across the forearm and over affected shoulder. Proceed obliquely across back to sound axilla. Bring other end around front of arm and across body to sound axilla, where it is pinned to other end, continuing around back to part of sling surrounding affected elbow and pinned again.

s., triangular. With suspension from uninjured side (brachioscapular sling). Place triangle on chest with one end over sound shoulder, the point under affected extremity, fold the base. Flex injured arm outside of triangle. Carry lower end upward under axilla of injured side, back of shoulder and tie with upper end behind back. Bring point of triangle anteriorly and medially around back of elbow and fasten to body of bandage. (This bandage changes point of carrying and also relieves clavicle of injured side of a load.)

s., triangular, reversed (reversed brachiocervical sling). Apply with one end over injured shoulder, point toward the sound side, base vertical under injured elbow. Flex arm acutely over triangle. Lower end is brought upwards over front of arm and over sound shoulder. Pull ends taut and tie over sound shoulder. The point is pulled taut over forearm and fixed to anterior and posterior layers between forearm and arm. (Holds elbow more acutely flexed—the weight is supported by the elbow.)

slough (slŭf) [M.E. *slughe*, a skin]. 1. Dead matter or necrosed tissue separated from living tissue or an ulceration. 2. To separate in the form of dead or necrosed parts from living tissue. 3. To cast off, as dead tissue. SEE: *eschar*.

sloughing (slŭf'ĭng) [M.E. *slughe*, a skin].

The formation of a slough; separation of dead tissue from living tissue.
  s. phagedena. Hospital gangrene.
slow (slō) [A.S. *slāw*, dull]. 1. Mentally dull. 2. Exhibiting retarded speed, as the pulse. 3. Of a morbid condition or fever, not acute. SEE: *"brady-" words*.
slows (slōz). An infectious disease of cattle transmitted to man through milk or butter, marked by severe neural symptoms, constipation, vomiting; frequently fatal. SYN: *milk sickness, trembles*.
sludge (slujh). The semisolid matter deposited in sewage.
  s., activated. Sludge from well-aerated sewage, exposed to oxidizing bacteria, supplying oxidizing organisms sufficient to activate another supply of sewage.
  s., dewatered. Sludge that has been dried.
slugged blood. That found in alcoholics. Individual clumps of cell masses move at a slower rate than normal, making gaps between clumps which sometimes block the blood vessels. It may occur in serious sickness from other causes.
smallpox (smawl'pŏks) [A.S. *smael*, tiny, + *poc*, pustule]. An acute, contagious, febrile disease, the constitutional symptoms of which are followed by successive stages of eruptions. SYN: *variola, q.v.*
  RS: *alastrim, alices, amaas, variolate, varioloid.*
smear, smear culture (smēr) [A.S. *smerian*, to anoint]. 1. BACT: Material spread on a surface, as a microscopic slide or a culture medium. 2. One obtained from infected matter spread over a solidified medium.
Smee's battery or **cell** (smē). A form of electric battery.
smegma (smĕg'mă) [G. *smēgma*, soap]. Secretion of sebaceous glands, specifically, the thick, cheesy, ill-smelling secretion found under the labia minora about the glans clitoridis and under the male prepuce from Tyson's glands. SYN: *sebum*.
  s. clitoridis. BNA. Odoriferous secretion of the glands of the clitoris.
  s. praeputii. BNA. Cheesy odoriferous substance collecting under prepuce in the male, secreted by Tyson's glands.
smegmatic (smĕg-măt'ĭk) [G. *smēgma*, soap]. Pert. to or made up of smegma.
smegmolith (smĕg'mō-lĭth) [" + *lithos*, a stone]. Calcareous mass in the smegma.
smell (smĕl) [M.E. *smellen*, to reek]. 1. To perceive by stimulation of the olfactory nerves. 2. To emit an odor, pleasant or offensive. 3. A chemical sense dependent upon end organs on the surface of the upper part of the nasal septum and the superior nasal conch. 4. Property of a thing affecting the olfactory organs, pleasant or unpleasant. SYN: *odor, scent, stench*.

The sense of smell may be affected by

Differential Diagnosis Between Smallpox and Chickenpox[1]

	Smallpox	Chickenpox
General symptoms	May be severe, with pyrexia, backache, etc., for 3 days before appearance of eruption.	Mild. Appear at same time as rash.
Eruption Type	Third day of illness. Papules before vesicles. Deep, often "shotty." Umbilication of vesicles.	Vesicles from start. Superficial. First day. No umbilication.
Shape	Circular.	May be oval.
Appearance	All spots at same stage of development. Pustules appear on the 8th day.	Successive crops, therefore, all stages present at the same time. Pustules on 2nd day.
Distribution	Maximum on distal parts, not in axillae or groins.	Maximum on trunk, present in axillae.

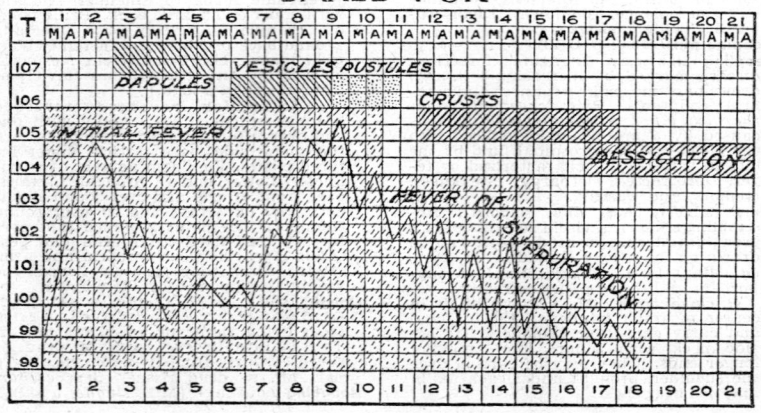

[1]Sears.

many conditions, some of which are the following:
Anosmia*: A loss of the sense of smell. It may be a local and a temporary condition resulting from acute and chronic rhinitis, mouth breathing, nasal polypi, dryness of the nasal mucous membrane, pollens, or very offensive odors. It may also result from the following causes: Disease or injury of the olfactory tract, bone disease near the olfactory nerve, disease of the nasal accessory sinuses, basal meningitis, or tumors or gumma affecting the olfactory nerve. It is sometimes found in locomotor ataxia, and frequently in hysteria and neurasthenia. Disease of 1 cranial hemisphere or of 1 nasal chamber may account for anosmia, and it may be the result of scarlet fever.
Hyperosmia: An increased sensitivity to odors. It occurs among the hypersensitive type and among those susceptible to certain odors.
Kakosmia*: The perception of bad odors where none exist and it may be due to head injuries or occur in hallucinations in certain psychoses.
Parosmia*: A perverted sense of smell. Odors that are considered agreeable are assumed to be offensive and disagreeable odors may be found pleasant to those suffering from certain functional derangements and in some catarrhs.
smell, words pert. to: anodmia, anosmatic, anosmia, anosphresia, aroma, aromatic, cacosmia, dysosmia, hyperosmia, jumentous, kakosmia, odor, odoriferous, olfaction, olfactory, osmesthesia, osphresis, oxyosphresia, parosmia.
smiths' spasm. An occupational neurosis in form of a spasm of the arm and hand in blacksmiths.
smok′er's can′cer or tongue. Cancer of the lip or throat due to irritation from a pipe stem or excessive smoking.
Sn. [L. *stannum*]. Symb. of tin.
snake bite (snāk bīt). All snakes should be considered poisonous, although there are only a few that secrete an amount of venom sufficient to inoculate poison deeply into the tissues.
F. A. TREATMENT: Apply tourniquet, incise and induce bleeding. If swelling persists, incise again. This may be necessary repeatedly. Inject antivenin. If the type of snake cannot be determined, use mixed antivenin. Release tourniquet cautiously at 15- to 20-minute intervals and observe effect.
A tourniquet should not be applied too tightly or remain on too long. Alcoholic stimulants must not be taken and nothing should be done to increase circulation. Do not cauterize with strong acids or depend upon home remedies.
The Antivenin Institute of America, Glenolden, Pa., prepares antivenin for the North American rattler, the copperhead, and the moccasin.
RS: *antivenene, antivenom, antivenomous, ophidiophobia, ophidism, ophiotoxemia, venenation, venene, veneniferous, venom.*
snap′ping hip. Slipping of the hip joint with a snap due to displacement over the great trochanter of a tendinous band.
snare (snār) [A.S. *sneare*, noose]. Device for excision of polypi, tumors, etc., by tightening wire loops around them.
sneeze (snēz) [M.E. *snesen*, from A.S. *fnēosan*, to pant]. 1. To expel air forcibly through the nose and mouth by spasmodic contraction of muscles of expiration due to irritation of nasal mucosa. 2. The act of sneezing.
RS: *sternutation, sternutator, sternutatory.*
Snellen's reflex (snĕl′ĕn). Congestion of ear on same side resulting when distal end of the divided auriculocervical nerve is stimulated.
snore (snōr) [A.S. *snora*, snoring]. 1. To breathe noisily during sleep, due to vibration of the uvula and soft palate. 2. Noisy breathing in sleep or coma. SYN: *rhonchus, stertor.*
snoring râle (snŏr′ing rahl). A sonorous râle, low in pitch, resembling a snore.
snow blind′ness. Irritation of the conjunctiva caused by reflection of the sun on the snow.
SYM: Photophobia, blepharospasm, burning pain in the eyes, hyperemia or temporary blindness. SYN: *chionablepsia, niphablepsia, niphotyphlosis.*
snuffles (snŭf′ls) [Middle Dutch *snuffen*, to snuff]. Obstructed nasal breathing with discharge from the nasal mucosa, esp. in infants, chiefly in congenital syphilis.
soap (sōp) [A.S. *sāpe*, soap]. A cleansing chemical compound formed by an alkali acting on a fatty acid; example: sodium stearate, $NaC_{18}H_{35}O_2$. SEE: *saponification.*
Castile soap is made by saponifying olive oil with sodium hydroxide, and contains mainly sodium oleate, $NaC_{18}H_{33}O_2$.
s. liniment. USP. Liquid opodeldoc. A solution of soap and camphor in alcohol and water. [facient.
ACTION AND USES: Stimulant and rube**s. suds enema.** One given so that the irritating action of the soap will start bowel motion. SEE: *enema.*
sobisminol (so-bĭs′mĭn-ōl). An antisyphilitic for intramuscular injection on solution, and orally in mass.
socia parotidis (sō′shē-ă pă-rŏt′ĭd-ĭs) [L. companion of the parotid]. An accessory parotid gland sometimes detached at beginning of Stenson's duct.
sociology (sō-sĭ-ŏl′ō-jĭ) [L. *socius*, companion, + G. *logos*, a study]. Science of the forms, institutions and functions of human groups.
socket (sŏk′ĕt) [M.E. *soket*, a spearhead]. A hollow in a joint or part for another corresponding organ, as a bone socket or an eye socket. SEE: *ambon.*
soda (sō′dă) [Middle Latin *soda*, headache]. 1. Term loosely applied to various salts of sodium, esp. to caustic soda (sodium hydroxide) and baking soda (sodium bicarbonate). SEE: *sodium.* 2. Short for soda water, which is water charged with carbon dioxide.
sodic (sō′dĭk) [Middle Latin *soda*, headache]. Relating to or containing soda or sodium. [taining sodium.
sodio-. Prefix denoting a *compound con-*
sodium (sō′dĭ-ŭm) [Middle Latin *soda*, headache]. SYMB.: Na. At. wt. 23.00. Sp. gr. 0.97. Melting point 97.5. A metallic element of the alkali group.
It represents 0.15% of the elements of the body. From 0.053 to 2.090 Gm. have been excreted per day during a 31-day fast. The sodium of salt is of more importance than the chlorine.
FUNCTIONS: Sodium salts are found in the fluids of the body, serum, blood, and lymph, and in the tissues, the concentration being lower in the tissues. They are necessary to preserve a balance bet. calcium and potassium to maintain normal heart action and the equilibrium of the body. They regulate osmotic pres-

sure in the cells and fluids, act as an ion balance in tissues, produce a buffer action in the blood, and guard against an excessive loss of water from the tissues.
DEFICIENCY SYM: Weakness, nerve disorders, loss of weight, "salt hunger," miner's cramps, disturbed digestion.
SOURCES: SEE: *names of foods.*

s. acetate. USP. Colorless, odorless, translucent crystals, saline in taste and soluble in water.
ACTION AND USES: Diuretic and laxative.
DOSAGE: 25 gr. (1.5 Gm.).

s. aleurate. The monosodium salt of allyl isopropyl barbituric acid.
ACTION AND USES: Oral or rectal adm. as preanesthesia medication.
DOSAGE: 1 gr. for each 15 lb. of body weight (10 mg. per Kg.).

s. amytal. The monosodium salt of isoamylethylbarbituric acid.
ACTION AND USES: Sedative and hypnotic in control of insomnia; preliminary to surgical anesthesia and in labor.
DOSAGE: 3 gr. (0.2 Gm.) as sedative or hypnotic. 3-9 gr. (0.2-0.6 Gm.) as preliminary anesthetic, depending upon many factors.

s. barbital. SEE: *barbital.*

s. benzoate. USP. A white, odorless powder with sweet taste.
ACTION AND USES: Internally in treatment of rheumatism and as a food preservative.
DOSAGE: Internally, 15 gr. (1 Gm.).

s. bicarbonate. USP. White, odorless powder with saline taste.
ACTION AND USES: In hyperacidity and for acidosis. Externally, mild alkaline wash.
DOSAGE: 15 gr. (1 Gm.).
INCOMPATIBILITIES: Acids, acid salts, ammonium chloride, lime water, ephedrine, hydrochloride, iron chloride.

s. biphosphate. USP. Sodium acid phosphate.
ACTION AND USES: To render urine acid, thereby assisting the action of urotropin.
DOSAGE: 10 gr. (0.6 Gm.).

s. bisulfite. Granular or crystalline powder, sulfurous taste and odor, soluble in water.
ACTION AND USES: Gastric and intestinal fermentation.
DOSAGE: 10-20 gr. (0.6-1/3 Gm.).

s. borate. USP. Borax.
ACTION AND USES: Antiseptic and astringent.
DOSAGE: 1 to 2% solution used as an eyewash.

s. bromide. USP. NaBr. White crystalline powder with saline taste.
ACTION AND USES: Nerve sedative and cerebral depressant.
DOSAGE: 15 gr. (1 Gm.).
INCOMPATIBILITIES: Tincture ferric chloride.

s. cacodylate. USP. The sodium salt of cacodylic acid.
ACTION AND USES: Similar to arsenic.
DOSAGE: Hypodermically, 1 gr. (0.06 Gm.).

s. carbonate. USP. Na_2CO_3. White crystalline powder (washing soda).
ACTION AND USES: An alkali employed chiefly in alkaline baths.
DOSAGE: 5-20 gr. (0.33-1.333 Gm.).

s. chloride. USP. NaCl. Common salt.
ACTION AND USES: In preparation of normal saline solution, emetic and in metabolism.
DOSAGE: 10-60 gr. (0.666-4 Gm.).
INCOMPATIBILITIES: Silver nitrate.

s. citrate. White granular powder, saline in taste and soluble in water.
ACTION AND USES: Diuretic and antilithic.
DOSAGE: 15 gr. (1.0 Gm.).

s. fluoride. White crystalline powder saline in taste, soluble in 25 parts of water.
ACTION AND USES: Epilepsy, tuberculosis, and malaria. Commercially, in etching glassware, for eradication of rats, insects, ants, and other pests, or as a food preservative.
DOSAGE: 1/12-1/6 gr. (0.005-0.01 Gm.).
POISONING: SYM: Optical: conjunctivitis; oral: retching, vomiting, nausea, later cardiac weakness, kidney disturbances, and interference with coagulation of blood.
F. A. TREATMENT: In addition to washing affected areas, precipitate by addition of soluble calcium salts, as lime water, calcium gluconate, calcium lactate. Give emetics and soothing drinks, as milk, cream, egg whites, etc.

s. hexametaphosphate. A salt of metaphosphoric acid.
ACTION AND USES: Water softener, antiperspirant, and in dermatoses due to oil or soap irritation.
DOSAGE: 1-2% solution.

s. hydroxide. A whitish solid; soluble in water, making a clear solution.
USES: Antacid and caustic. In the laundry and in commercial compounds, in cleaning sink traps, toilets, etc., and in the preparation of soap.
ACTION: Use great care in handling it as it rapidly destroys organic tissues.
POISONING: SEE: *potassium hydroxide.*
DOSAGE: 15 ♏ (1 cc.).

s. hyposulfite. Same as s. thiosulfate.

s. iodide. USP. NaI. A salt resembling in appearance and action potassium iodide.
DOSAGE: 5 gr. (0.3 Gm.).

s. morrhuate. The sodium salt of the fatty acids, found in cod-liver oil.
USES: For the obliteration of varicose veins.
DOSAGE: 0.5-1 cc. of 5% solution.

s. nitrate. SEE: *Chile saltpeter.*

s. nitrite. USP. $NaNO_3$. White crystalline powder, characteristic properties of nitroglycerine; effects more lasting.
DOSAGE: 1 gr. (0.06 Gm.).

s. oleate. A white, soft mass; sodium salt of oleic acid.
USES: As a cholagogue.
DOSAGE: 2-10 gr. (0.12-0.6 Gm.).

s. pentothal. SEE: *pentothal s.*

s. phosphate. USP. $Na_2HPO_4.12H_2O$. White crystalline powder.
ACTION AND USES: Similar to magnesium sulfate, but with less disagreeable taste.
DOSAGE: 1 dram (4 Gm.).

s. phosphate effervescent. USP. A mixture of sodium phosphate, sodium bicarbonate, and tartaric acid.
DOSAGE: 2½ drams (10 Gm.).

s. salicylate. USP. White powder or scales with sweet saline taste.
ACTION AND USES: As an analgesic and antipyretic.
DOSAGE: 15 gr. (1 Gm.).
INCOMPATIBILITIES: Caffeine citrate, caffeine sodium benzoate.

s. sulfate (Glauber's salt). USP. Resembles magnesium sulfate in appearance and action.
DOSAGE: 4 drams (15 Gm.).

s. tartrate. $Na_2C_4H_4O_6$—2 H_2O. White soluble crystals.
USES: Diuretic and laxative.

sodium taurocholate   S-54   **solubility**

DOSAGE: 15-60 gr. (1-4 Gm).; 4-8 drams (15-30 Gm.).
   s. taurocholate. Extract of bile from carnivora; a yellowish gray powder soluble in water.
   USES: Cholagogue.
   DOSAGE: 2-6 gr. (0.12-0.4 Gm.).
   s. thiocyanate. NaSCN. A sodium salt.
   USES: Reducing high blood pressure, relieving insomnia due to hypertension, in narcotic addiction, and in crises of tabes dorsalis.
   DOSAGE: 5 gr. (0.3 Gm.).
   s. thiosulfate. USP. White crystalline substance, having a cooling taste.
   ACTION AND USES: Externally, for ringworm, in dermatitis, to remove stains of iodine. Intravenously, as an antidote for metallic poisons.
   DOSAGE: 15 gr. (1 Gm.).
   s. valerianate. White crystalline powder with faint odor and taste of valerian. Soluble in water and of unctuous feel.
   USES: Nervine tonic.
   DOSAGE: 2-5 gr. (0.13-0.3 Gm.).
sodokosis (sŏd-ō-kō′sĭs) [Japanese, rat poison]. Infectious febrile disease caused by infection from bite of a rat. SYN: *rat-bite fever, sodoku.*
sodoku (sō-dō′koo) [Japanese, rat poison]. Infectious febrile disease due to rat bite. SYN: *rat-bite fever, sodokosis.*
sodomy (sŏd′ō-mĭ) [O.Fr. *Sodome*, Sodom]. Anal coitus, usually bet. males; bestiality (*concubitus cum bestia*), and pederasty,* (*concubitus cum persona ejusdem sexus*).
   Not always a psychopathological phenomenon or confined to either sex, although most of those who practice such vices are weak minded.
Soemmering's foramen (sĕm′ĕr-ĭng). Marginal process of the malar bone. SYN: *fovea centralis.*
S's. spot. The macula lutea of the retina.
S's. yellow spot. Same as *S's. spot.*
soft or **convalescent diet.** Fish, egg and cheese dishes, chicken, cereals, bread, toast, butter, nothing not soft, semisolid or liquid. No red meats, vegetables or fruits having seeds or thick skins. No cellulose, raw fruits, or salads.
   s. diet, cold. Suitable for tonsillectomies. All forms of milk and cream, iced cocoa, coffee and tea iced, gelatin, junket, custard, strained cereals and fruits if not seeded, such as berries. No fruit juices unless ordered.
   s. d., light. Medical liquids; cream soups, strained; toast; cream; poached or coddled eggs; mashed potatoes; carrots, peas, and spinach purées; gelatins; junkets; custards; stewed fruits; souffles; jellies; gruels; cereals if strained; ice cream; sherbets.
   s. d., l., surgical. Fluids plus thick water gruels, toast, stewed fruits if strained but no seeded fruits.
   s. d., modified. Small meals, frequent feedings, gradual additions to full liquid diet—crackers, baked potato, soft cooked egg, cream of wheat, farina, strained oatmeal, applesauce, puréed pears, jelly, simple desserts; later, cottage cheese, puréed vegetables, minced tender meat.
soft (sŏft) [A.S. *sōfte*]. Not hard, firm or solid.
   s. palate. The soft post. part of the palate. SYN: *palatum molle, velum pendulum palati.*
   s. sore. A venereal sore, not due to syphilis, caused by Ducrey's bacillus. SYN: *chancroid.*
softening (sŏf′en-ĭng) [A.S. *sōfte*, soft]. Process of becoming soft. SYN: *malacia, mollities.* RS: *words ending in malacia.*
   s., anemic. White softening of the brain from lack of blood.
   s. of the brain. Paresis with progressive dementia. SYN: *encephalomalacia.*
   s., gray. S. of the brain with absorption of fat following yellow s.
   s., hemorrhagic. Red softening, q.v.
   s., mucoid. Myxomatous degeneration.
   s., red. S. of the brain with bleeding into necrosed portions.
   s., white. Same as anemic s.
   s., yellow. S. of brain in a late stage with deposit of changing pigment and fatty degeneration of cells.
sol (sŏl, sōl) [G. *sole*, salt water]. In the chemistry of colloids, a fluid mixture of a colloid and a liquid.
   Thus, a 0.5% solution of gelatin when warm is a sol, being perfectly liquid; after standing in the cold it sets to a gel, q.v.
solanine (sō′lăn-ĭn). A poisonous narcotic alkaloid obtained from potatoes.
solar (sō′lar) [L. *sol*, sun]. Pert. to the sun or its rays.
   s. fever. An infectious febrile disease. SYN: *dengue*, q.v.
   s. ganglion. Ganglion on 5th cranial nerve. SYN: *gasserian ganglion.*
   s. plexus. The celiac plexus behind the stomach and bet. the suprarenal glands, and consisting of 2 large ganglia.
   s. therapy. Treatment with the sun's rays. SYN: *heliotherapy.*
solargentum (sol-ar-jĕn′tŭm). A brand of mild silver protein, containing 19-23% colloidal silver.
solarium (sō-lā′rĭ-ŭm) [L. from *sol*, sun]. A room designed for heliotherapy or for the application of artificial light.
solation (sō-lā′shŭn) [L. *sol*, sun]. In colloidal chemistry, the transformation of a gel into a sol.
solbisminol (sŏl-bĭz′mĭn-ōl). An antisyphilitic drug which can be taken by mouth.
sole (sōl) [A.S. *sole*, from L. *solum*, ground]. Underpart of the foot. SYN: *planta, plantar surface.* SEE: *antithenar, thenar.*
   s. plate. Flattened nucleated mass in which motor nerve endings rest.
   s. reflex. Contraction of muscles when tickling the sole.
solenoid (sō′le-noyd) [G. *sōlēn*, pipe, + *eidos*, like]. Tubular coil used in producing a magnetic field.
   A coil or series of turns of wire spaced equally bet. turns. Usually designates a coil whose length is greater than its diameter. When an electric current flows through a solenoid, it acts in general like a magnet.
solepism (sō′le-pizm) [L. *solus*, alone, + G. *-ismos*, condition]. The theory that nothing may be known objectively, because only may one's own mental processes be known.
soleus (sō′le-ŭs) [L. *solea*, sole of foot]. A flat, broad muscle of calf of leg. SEE: *Table of Muscles in Appendix.*
solid (sŏl′ĭd) [L. *solidus*, a solid]. 1. Not gaseous, hollow, or liquid. 2. A substance not gaseous, liquid, or hollow.
   s. carbon dioxide therapy. Therapeutic application of solid carbon dioxide. SEE: *refrigeration.*
solitary glands or **follicles** (sol′i-tar-ĭ) [L. *solitarius*, from *solus*, alone]. Lymphatic glands in mucous membrane of small intestines not included in Peyer's* patches.
solubility (sŏl′ū-bĭl′ĭ-tĭ) [L. *solubilis*, from *solvere*, to dissolve]. Capability of being dissolved.

soluble (sŏl'ū-bl) [L. *solubilis*, from *solvere*, to dissolve]. Able to be dissolved.

solute (sŏl'ūt) [L. *solutus*, dissolved]. The substance that is dissolved in a solution.

solution (sō-lū'shŭn) [L. *solutio*, a dissolving]. 1. Liquid containing dissolved substance. 2. Process by which a solid is homogeneously mixed with a fluid, or a solid or gas, so that the dissolved substances cannot be distinguished from the resultant fluid. 3. Mixture so formed. 4. Termination of a disease.

The liquid in which the substances are dissolved is called the *solvent** and the substance dissolved, the *solute.** The strength represents the amt. of substance dissolved, represented by ratio, percentage, or grains to the ounce.

s., colloidal. That in which the solute is suspended and not dissolved, such as gelatin, albumin.

s., dilute. One containing a small amount of a dissolved material in proportion to the amount that could be dissolved.

s., inorganic. Watery solution of substances such as alkalies and acids and their salts having such properties as ionization and osmosis.

s., saline, s., salt. Sodium chloride (0.6 to 0.75%) in distilled water. It may be *isotonic*, having the same salt concentration as the blood and the same osmotic power, or *hypotonic*, having a lesser concentration of salt than the blood, thus affecting the integrity of the cells or tissues.

RS: *attraxin, diffusion, dialysis, hydrolysis, osmosis, reaction, saturation, solute, solvent.*

s., saturated. A solution that contains all the solute it can dissolve. This limit is called the *saturation* point.

s., supersaturation. S. in which the saturation point is reached, but when heated it is possible to dissolve more of the solute.

solv. [L.]. Abbr. of *solve*, meaning *dissolve.*

solvent (sŏl'vĕnt) [L. *solvens*, from *solvere*, to dissolve]. 1. Producing a solution; dissolving. 2. A liquid holding another substance in solution.

soma (sō'mă) [G. *sōma*, body]. 1. Body tissues distinguished from germinal or reproductive ones. 2. The body without its appendages. 3. PSY: The body as differentiated from the psyche.

somacule (sō'măk-ūl) [G. *sōma*, body]. A physiological unit; the smallest possible division of protoplasm.

somal (sō'măl) [G. *sōma*, body]. Concerning the body. SEE: *soma.*

somasthenia (sō-măs-thē'nĭ-ă) [" + *astheneia*, weakness]. A condition of chronic bodily weakness. SYN: *somatasthenia.*

somatalgia (sō-măt-ăl'jĭ-ă) [" + *algos*, pain]. Bodily pain.

somatasthenia (sō-măt-ăs-thē'nĭ-ă) [" + *astheneia*, weakness]. Chronic bodily weakness usually with low blood pressure, but *not* neurasthenia. SYN: *somasthenia.*

somatesthesia (sō-măt-ĕs-thē'zĭ-ă) [" + *aisthēsis*, sensation]. The consciousness of the body; bodily sensation.

somatic (sō-măt'ĭk) [G. *sōma*, body]. Concerning the body as distinguished from the viscera or mind; physical.

s. death. Death of the entire body.

s. tissue. All tissue other than the reproductive tissue. SEE: *soma.*

somatoblast (sō-mat'ō-blăst) [" + *blastos*,

a germ]. Any plastidule from which cell material is developed.

somatochrome (sō-mat'ō-krōm) [" + *chrōma*, color]. A nerve cell or group which stains readily.

somatogenetic (sō-mat"ō-jĕn-ĕt'ĭk) [" + *gennan*, to produce]. Facilitating the reproduction of the body.

somatology (sō-măt-ŏl'ō-jĭ) [" + *logos*, a study]. Comparative study of structure, functions and development of the human body.

somatopathic (sō-măt-ō-păth'ĭk) [" + *pathos*, disease]. Organically ill, as distinguished from neuropathic or psychopathic diseases.

somatoplasm (sō-măt'ō-plăzm) [" + *plasma*, a thing formed]. The protoplasmic substance of the body.

somatopleure (sō-mat'ō-plŭr) [G. *sōma*, body, + *pleura*, a side]. The embryonic outer layer together with the epiblast after the mesoderm splits into 2 layers.

somatopsychic (sō-măt-ō-sī'kĭk) [" + *psychē*, mind]. Pert. to both body and mind.

somatopsychosis (sō"mă-tō-sī-kō'sĭs) [" + "+ -ōsis. condition]. Any mental disorder which is a symptom of a bodily disease.

somatoschisis (sō-măt-ŏs'kĭs-ĭs) [" + *schisis*, a cleavage]. Splitting of the vertebral bodies.

somatoscopy (sō-măt-ŏs'kō-pĭ) [" + *skopein*, to examine]. Physical examination of the body.

somatotomy (sō-mă-tŏt'ō-mĭ) [" + *tomē*, a cutting]. Anatomy of the human body.

somatotropic (sō"măt-ō-trŏp'ĭk) [" + *tropos*, a turning]. 1. Having selective attraction for, or influencing body cells. 2. Stimulating growth.

somatropin (sō-măt'rō-pĭn) [" + *tropos*, a turning]. The anterior pituitary lobe's growth-stimulating principle.

somesthesia (som-es-thē'sĭ-ă) [G. *sōma*, body, + *aisthēsis*, sensation]. Awareness of bodily sensations. SYN: *somatesthesia.*

somesthetic (sō-mĕs-thĕt'ĭk) [" + *aisthēsis*, sensation]. Pert. to sensations and sensory structures of the body.

s. area. The region in the cortex in which lie the terminations of the axons of general sensory conduction-paths.

s. path. General sensory conduction-path leading to the cortex.

somite (sō'mīt) [G. *sōma*, body]. 1. Embryonic blocklike segment formed on either side of the neural tube and its underlying notochord. 2. Any one of the embryonic segments.

Each pair of somites forms a vertebra, a pair of muscle segments, and a pair of spinal nerves. SYN: *myocomma, myotome.*

somnambulism (sŏm-năm'bū-lĭzm) [L. *somnus*, sleep, + *ambulāre*, to walk]. 1. A form of hysteria in which behavior and purposeful actions are not subsequently remembered. 2. Sleepwalking, an affection that prompts the sleeping person to perform, unconsciously, acts that naturally belong to the waking state. SYN: *noctambulism, q.v.*

The term has a more comprehensive meaning in psychiatry than that of noctambulism.

somnarium (sŏm-nā'rĭ-ŭm) [L. *somnus*, sleep]. A sanitarium in which sleep therapy is employed in the treatment of neuroses.

somnifacient (sŏm-nĭ-fā'shĕnt) [" + *facere*, to make]. 1. Producing sleep. SYN:

somniferous   S-56   **sound, words pert. to**

hypnotic. 2. A medicine producing sleep. SYN: *soporific, q.v.*
somniferous (sŏm-nĭf'ĕr-ŭs) [" + *ferre*, to bear]. Sleep-producing; pert. to that which promotes sleep.
somnific (sŏm-nĭf'ĭk) [" + *facere*, to make]. Producing sleep.
somniloquy (sŏm-nĭl'ō-kwĭ) [" + *loqui*, to speak]. Act of talking during sleep or in a hypnotic condition.
somnipathy (sŏm-nĭp'ă-thĭ) [" + G. *pathos*, disease]. 1. Any disorder of sleep. 2. Hypnotism.
somnocinematograph (sŏm-nō-sĭn-ē-măt'ō-grăf) [" + G. *kinema*, motion, + *graphein*, to write]. Device for recording motions of those who are asleep.
somnolence (sŏm'nō-lĕns) [L. *somnolentia*, sleepiness]. Prolonged drowsiness or a condition resembling trance which may continue for a number of days; sleepiness.
somnolent (sŏm'nō-lĕnt) [L. *somnolentus*, sleepy]. Sleepy; drowsy.
somnolentia (sŏm-nō-lĕn'shĭ-ă) [L. *somnolentia*, sleepiness]. 1. Drowsiness. 2. The sleep of drunkenness in which the faculties are only partially in repose.
somopsychosis (sŏm"ō-sī-kō'sĭs) [G. *sōma*, body, + *psychē*, mind, + *-ōsis*, condition]. A psychosis in which symptoms are mostly of a bodily nature.
sonic boom (sŏn'ĭk) [L. *sonus*, sound]. Noise caused by shock waves from nose of a plane flying faster than sound. When they hit the ground they may break windows and affect the hearing. They occur when the plane dives. They are imperceptible at 30,000 ft. At 5000 ft. the noise drops to 78 decibels, *q.v.*
sonitus (sŏn'ĭ-tŭs) [L. *sonitus*, sound]. Subjective noises in the ear. SYN: *tinnitus aurium, q.v.*
sonometer (sō-nŏm'ĕt-ĕr) [L. *sonus*, sound, + G. *metron*, a measure]. Device for testing the hearing.
sonorous (sō-nō'rŭs) [L. *sonor*, sound]. Giving forth a loud and rounded sound.
   s., **râle**. A dry or low pitched râle often caused by vibration of mucous secretion in a bronchus.
soot cancer, soot wart (sŏŏt) [A.S. *sōt*, dust]. Epithelioma of the scrotum found in chimney sweepers.
sophistication (sō-fĭs-tĭ-kā'shŭn) [G. *sophistikos*, deceitful]. Adulteration of any substances.
sopor (sō'por) [L. *sopor*, deep sleep]. Deep, lethargic sleep. SYN: *stupor*.
soporific (sō-por-ĭf'ĭk) [" + *facere*, to make]. 1. Inducing sleep. 2. Narcotic; a drug producing sleep.
soporose, soporous (sō'por-ōs, -ŭs) [L. *sopor*, deep sleep]. Marked by or resembling sound sleep or coma.
sorbefacient (sor"bē-fā'shĕnt) [L. *sorbere*, to suck, + *facere*, to make]. Causing or that which causes or promotes absorption.
sordes (sor'dēz) [L. *sordere*, to be dirty]. 1. Foul, brown crusts or accumulations on the teeth and about the lips from foul stomach or secretions of the mouth in low forms of fever. 2. Filth.
   NP: Wash carefully with soft linen moistened with glycerin and borax. Burn the linen after using.
sore (sōr) [A.S. *sār*, sore]. 1. Causing physical pain. 2. A tender or painful ulcer or lesion of the skin.
   s., **bed**. Gangrene of skin due to pressure. SYN: *decubitus, q.v., pressure sore.*
   s., **cold**. Blister on the lips. SYN: *herpes* facialis.* [croid.
   s., **fungating**. A granulating chan-

   s., **hard**. Syphilitic chancre,* primary lesion of syphilis.
   s., **pressure**. A bedsore, *q.v.*
   s., **soft venereal**. Soft, nonsyphilitic, venereal sore occurring on the genitalia. SYN: *chancroid.**
   s. **throat**. Any inflammation of the tonsils, pharynx or larynx.
   s. t., **clergyman's**. Granular pharyngitis with dysphonia. [tis.
   s. t., **diphtheritic**. Croupous tonsilli-
   s. t., **hospital**. Superficial septic inflammation of fauces and pharynx.
   s. t., **septic**. Severe, epidemic, pseudomembranous inflammation of fauces and tonsils caused by the hemolytic streptococcus.
   s. t., **spotted**. Follicular tonsillitis.
   s. t., **ulcerated**. Pharyngitis with formation of gangrenous patches.
   s., **venereal**. SEE: *soft venereal sore.*
sororiation (so-ror-ĭ-ā'shŭn) [L. *sororiāre*, to increase together]. Growth of the breasts at puberty. [required.
s.o.s. Abbr. for *si opus sit*, if necessary or
soterocyte (sō'ter-ō-sīt) [G. *sōtēr*, savior, + *kytos*, cell]. A blood platelet.
souffle (soof'fl) [Fr. *souffle*, a puff]. A soft blowing sound heard in auscultation; a bruit; an auscultatory murmur.
   s., **cardiac**. Heart murmur.
   s., **fetal**. The soft blowing sound heard over the location of the umbilical cord of the fetus *in utero* and synchronous with the fetal heartbeat during late pregnancy.
   s., **funic**, *s.*, **funicular**, *s.*, **umbilical**. Same as fetal souffle. [in malaria.
   s., **splenic**. Sound heard over spleen
   s., **uterine**. Sound caused by blood entering dilated arteries of uterus in last months of pregnancy; synchronous with maternal pulse. It is more frequent than the fetal souffle and is heard as a loud blowing murmur along left side of uterus, and frequently all over it. An enlarged uterus may cause it. That of pregnancy is variable, whereas other forms are constant.
sound (sownd) [L. *sonus*, sound]. 1. Auditory sensations produced by vibrations; noise. It is measured in decibels, *q.v.* and advances geometrically; thus 20 d. represents not twice 10 d, but ten times as much. Conversation represents 90 d's. Exposure to 130 d. for ten minutes in any 24 hrs. should call for a weekly hearing test. A 90 d., noise over an extended period may permanently injure one's hearing. SEE: *decible, noise, sonic boom*. 2. Healthy, not diseased. 3. Heart sounds. 4. [Fr. *sonder*, to probe.] Instrument for introduction into a cavity or canal for diagnosis or treatment. SEE: *diastole, systole, sonic boom.*
   s., **blowing**. Organic murmur as of air from an aperture expelled with moderate force.
   s., **bottle**. Noise as of fluid in a bottle. SYN: *amphoric* murmur.*
   s., **cracked-pot**. A tympanic resonance heard over pulmonary cavities.
   s., **fetal heart**. One made by the fetal heart.
   s., **friction**. One produced by rubbing together of 2 inflamed mucous surfaces.
   s's., **heart**. The "lub" "dub" sounds of the heart.
   s., **to and fro**. Rasping friction sounds of pericarditis.
sound, words pert. to: amphoric, anacamptic, aphthongia, aspirate, auscultation, bell-metal resonance, bourdonnement, capotement, caverniloquy, clang,

clapotage, clapotement, heart, hyperacusis, murmur, râle, resonance, souffle, stridulous, succussion, uterus.
soybean (soi'bēn) [Japanese *shōyu*] (dried, flour, milk in this order): Av. Serving: 100 Gm. each. Pro. 30.2, 45.0, 3.5; Fat 15.3, 11.0, 2.4; Carbo. 33.1, 8.0, 0.6.
Vitamins: B++, ++, none; G++, none, none. (Milk): Ca 0.034, P 0.040.
sozalbumin (sō-zăl-bū'mĭn) [G. *sōzein*, to save, + L. *albumen*, white of egg]. A defensive proteid normally in the body. Syn: *mycosozin, toxosozin*.
sozin (sō'zĭn) [G. *sōzein*, to save]. A protein in the body which destroys microörganisms (a mycosozin) or which counteracts bacterial poisons (toxosozin).
space (spās) [L. *spatium*, space]. An area, region, or segment.
RS: *chondroporosis, circumscribed.*
s., arachnoid. Space beneath the arachnoid membrane.
s., axillary. The axilla or space beneath the arm.
s., epidural. S. bet. the dura mater and vertebral periosteum, or bet. the bones of the cranium and the dura mater, assumed to be lymph spaces.
s's. of Fontana. Spaces bet. the processes of the *ligamentum pectinatum*.
s. nerves. Auditory nerve fibers carrying impulses to the semicircular canals.
s., Nuel's. Space bet. outer hair cells and rods in the organ of Corti.
s., perforated. S. pierced by blood vessels at base of brain. Syn: *substantia perforata*.
s., plantar. S. (1 of 4) bet. fascial layers of the foot. When the foot is infected, pus may be found here.
s., popliteal. S. back of knee joint containing the popliteal artery and vein, and small sciatic and popliteal nerves.
s., Prussak's. S. in tympanum behind Shrapnell's membrane.
s., subarachnoid. S. bet. the pia mater and arachnoid containing the spinal fluid.
s., Tenon's. Lymph s. bet. the sclera and Tenon's capsule.
spaghetti (spă-gĕt'ĭ) [Italian *spaghetto*, little cord]. Av. Serving: 100 Gm. Pro. 12.1, Fat 0.4, Carbo. 75.9. Ca. 0.004, P. 0.025.
spanemia (spăn-ē'mĭ-ă) [G. *spanos*, scarce, + *aima*, blood]. Poverty of blood — diminution of supply of red blood corpuscles. Syn: *anemia*.
Spanish fly (spăn'ĭsh flī). A strong rubefacient and blistering agent, diuretic stimulant to reproductive and urinary organs. Syn: *cantharides*.
spanogyny (spăn-ŏj'ĭ-nĭ) [G. *spanos*, scarce, + *gynē*, a woman]. More males than females; decrease in female births.
spanomenorrhea (spăn"ō-mĕn-ō-rē'ă) [" + *mēn*, month, + *rhoia*, a flow]. Scanty menstruation.
spanopnea (spăn-ŏp-nē'ă) [" + *pnoia*, breath]. Infrequent respiratory functioning; slow and shallow respiration.
sparadrap (spăr'ă-drăp) [L. *sparadrapum*]. A medicated adhesive plaster.
sparer (spăr'er) [A.S. *sparian*, to refrain]. A substance destroyed by catabolism, but which, nevertheless, lessens catabolic action upon other substances.
sparganosis (spar-gă-nō'sĭs). Infestation with a variety of *Sparganum*.
spargosis (spar-gō'sĭs) [G. *spargōsis*, swelling]. 1. Distention of the female breasts with milk. 2. Swelling or thickening of the skin. Syn: *elephantiasis*.
spark coil. Coil consisting of primary and secondary coils with an interrupted current passing through them. Syn: *induction coil*.
s. gaps. Arrangement of opposed points or surfaces, between which an electric spark may jump.
An adjustable gap between needle points or between spheres is used to measure high potentials. For spark-over voltages see American Institute of Electrical Engineers Standardization Rules.
s. g., quenched. A multiple spark gap with numerous electrodes about 0.3 mm. apart and equipped with a copper air-cooling device.
sparteine sulfate (spar'tēn) [L. *spartium*, broom]. The salt of an alkaloid obtained from Scoparius.
Uses: Once regarded as of value in cardiac diseases, and as a diuretic.
Dosage: ½ gr. (0.03 Gm.).
spasm (spăzm) [G. *spasmos*, a convulsion]. An involuntary, sudden movement or convulsive muscular contraction.
The effect depends upon the part affected. *Asthma* is assumed to be due to spasm of muscular coats of smaller bronchi; *renal colic* to spasm of muscular coat of the ureter.
Treatment: In all forms, dietetic, hygienic and psychologic. Electricity — constitutional. Remove underlying cause. See: *tic*.
s., Bell's. Convulsive tic of the face.
s. center. Point in the oblongata where it meets the pons.
s., choreiform. Spasmodic movements resembling chorea.
s., clonic. Intermittent contractions and relaxation of muscles.
s. of esophagus. Paroxysmal dysphagia (inability to swallow), often associated with a sense of constriction in the chest. Little or no loss of flesh.
Prog: For life, good, but indefinite as regards duration.
Treatment: Search for exciting cause and remove. Treatment largely dietetic, hygienic and psychologic. Systematic passage of a bougie may be of great value. A mild electrical current may be applied through the bougie.
s. of glottis. Spasm of laryngeal adductors.
Characterized by intense dyspnea and occurs in spasmodic croup, true croup, ulceration of larynx, laryngismus stridulus, whooping cough, tetany, hysteria, hydrophobia, laryngeal crises of locomotor ataxia, when foreign bodies have lodged in larynx, when aneurysms or mediastinal tumors press on recurrent laryngeal nerve and irritate it.
s., habit. Spasms due to habit.
s., nodding. A psychogenic condition in adults, causing nodding of the head from clonic spasms of the sternomastoid muscles. A similar nodding in babies with head turning from side to side.
s., saltatory. Term employed to designate a condition allied to hysteria, in which a violent spasm seizes the muscles of the leg as soon as the feet touch the ground and as a result patient is thrown violently in the air.
s., tetanic. S. in which contractions continue for a time without interruption.
s., tonic. Continued involuntary contractions.

spasm, toxic

s., toxic. S. due to poison.
spasm, words pert. to: campospasm, carpopedal, child crowing, chirospasm, Chvostek's sign, clonic, clonospasm, clonus, facial, habit, hypertonus, mobile, Raynaud's disease, spasticity, tetanus, tetany, tic douloureux, tonic spasm, trismus.
spasmatic, spasmodic (spăz-măt′ĭk, -mŏd′-ĭk) [G. *spasmos*, a convulsion]. Pert. to, like, or marked by, spasm. SEE: *cholepathia spastica*.
  s. asthma. A. caused by spasm of the bronchioles.
  s. croup. Laryngismus stridulus.
  s. stricture. Temporary narrowing of any canal, as the urethra, due to localized spasmodic muscular contraction of its coat.
spasmodermia (spăz-mō-der′mĭ-ă) [G. *spasmos*, a convulsion, + *derma*, skin]. A spasmodic skin disorder.
spasmodism (spăz′mō-dĭzm) [" + *-ismos*, condition]. Medullary excitation causing various intermittent nervous conditions.
spasmology (spăz-mŏl′ō-jĭ) [" + *logos*, a study]. The study of spasms, their nature and cause.
spasmolygmus (spăz-mō-lĭg′mŭs) [" + *lygmos*, a sob]. 1. Spasmodic hiccup. 2. Spasmodic sobbing.
spasmolysis (spăz-mŏl′ĭs-ĭs) [" + *lysis*, dissolution]. The arrest of a spasm or convulsion.
spasmolytic (spăz-mō-lĭt′ĭk) [" + *lysis*, dissolution]. Checking or that which checks spasms.
spasmomyxorrhea (spăz″mō-mĭks-or-re′ă) [" + *myxa*, mucus, + *rhoia*, flow]. Excessive secretion of intestinal mucus. SYN: *myxorrhea intestinalis*.
spasmophemia (spăz-mō-fē′mĭ-ă) [G. *spasmos*, convulsion, + *phēmē*, speech]. A spasmodic disorder of speech. SYN: *stuttering*.
spasmophilia (spăz-mō-fĭl′ĭ-ă) [" + *philein*, to love]. A tendency to tetany and convulsions; almost always associated with rickets.
spasmotin (spăz′mō-tĭn) [G. *spasmos*, a spasm]. Poisonous ecbolic principle obtained from ergot.
spasmous (spăz′mŭs) [G. *spasmos*, convulsion]. Of the nature of a spasm.
spasmus (spăz′mŭs) [L. from G. *spasmos*, convulsion]. A spasm.
  s. agitans. Paralysis agitans, *q.v.*
  s. bronchialis. Bronchial asthma.
  s. caninus. Spasm of face causing a constant grin. SYN: *risus sardonicus*.
  s. coordinatus. Imitative or compulsive movements, as mimic tics or festination.
  s. cynicus. Spasmodic contraction of muscles on both sides of the mouth.
  s. Dubini. Rhythmic contractions, in rapid succession, of a group or groups of muscles, starting at an extremity or half of the face, and covering a large part or all of the body. PROG: Usually fatal. SYN: *electric chorea*.
  s. glottidis. Spasm of larynx. SYN: *laryngismus stridulus*.
  s. intestinorum. Pain in intestines. SYN: *enteralgia*.
  s. nictitans. A winking movement of the eyelid.
  s. nutans. Nodding spasm.
spastic (spăs′tĭk) [G. *spastikos*, convulsive]. Resembling or of the nature of spasms or convulsions.
  s. gait. A stiff movement with toes seeming to catch together and to drag.

specimen

  s. hemiplegia. Partial hemiplegia with spasmodic muscular contractions.
  s. paralysis. Muscular rigidity accompanying partial paralysis.
  s. paraplegia. P. due to transverse lesions of the cord or sclerosis.
spasticity (spăs-tĭs′ĭ-tĭ) [G. *spastikos*, convulsive]. Hypertension of muscles causing stiff and awkward movements; the result of upper motor neuron lesion.
spatula (spăt′ū-lă) [L. *spatula*, a little sword]. Instrument for spreading or mixing semisolids.
  It is usually flat, thin, somewhat flexible and shaped like a knife.
  s., eye. Blades for separating lips of corneal wounds, arresting hemorrhage or for making pressure; sheet metal or rubber.
  s., nasal. Device for holding mucous flaps in place or to guard against burning from cautery.
spay (spā) [Gael. *spoth*, castrate]. Surgical removal of ovaries, usually said of animals. SEE: *castration*.
specialist (spĕsh′ăl-ĭst) [L. *specialis*, special]. A physician who treats a special type of diseases.
species (spē′shēz) [L. *species*, a kind]. BIOL: Category of classification, a subdivision between a genus and a variety in which all the individuals are almost identical.
specific (spē-sĭf′ĭk) [L. *specificus*, pert. to a kind]. 1. A remedy having a curative effect on a particular disease or symptom. 2. Pert. to a species. 3. A disease always caused by the same organism.
  s. gravity. Weight of a substance compared with an equal volume of water. Water is represented by 1.000.
specificity (spē-sĭ-fĭs′ĭ-tĭ) [L. *specificus*, pert. to a kind]. State of being specific; having a relation to a definite result, or to a particular cause.
specillum (spē-sĭl′lŭm) [L. *specillum*]. 1. Lens. 2. Button-shaped silver probe.
specimen (spĕs′ĭ-mĕn) [L. from *specere*, to look]. A part of a thing intended to show kind and quality of the whole, as a specimen of urine.
  TECHNIC OF COLLECTION: AIM: To get specimen to laboratory in proper condition for examination.
  ARTICLES NECESSARY: Container of the correct type. Labels. Laboratory request slips. Tongue depressors. Sterile swabs.
  PROCEDURES: *Feces*: Have a bedpan warm. Transfer stool with tongue depressor. Do not contaminate container. Keep specimen warm after it is taken.
  For Bacteriological Examination: Have bedpan and tongue depressor sterile (it is presumed that the container, obtained from the laboratory, is sterile).
  Sputum: Collect specimen first thing in the morning before patient uses mouthwash, or eats. Do not contaminate container.
  Gastric Contents: Receive in container. If not possible to send to laboratory at once, keep on ice to prevent deterioration.
  Nasal and Throat Cultures: Use specially prepared culture tubes. Label carefully, "Nasal" and "Throat." Take throat culture from throat, not tongue. If cotton slips off swab into nose, call the doctor. Do not try to remove it yourself.
  Smears: Have 2 clean slides. Take material on sterile swab. Place on slide by rolling, not rubbing, swab along its surface. Cover slide with the other, keeping apart with rubber bands at ends.

specimens nurse may collect

Urine: Routine specimen: Use sterilized bedpan. Wash vulva of woman patient with soap and water before she voids. Send at least 4 oz.

Catheterized specimen: Catheterize directly into specimen bottle. Cover with fold of sterile gauze before putting on paper cap.

Twenty-four hour specimen: Tie a tag bearing patient's name, room number, and the date to a sterile gallon bottle with a cork and place this in a cool spot in the utility or bathroom. Have patient void at 6 A. M. Discard this first urine after measuring. Measure and keep in bottle all urine voided for the next 24 hr., including that at 6 A. M. the next morning. Send all to laboratory if ordered or mix well and send 8 oz. If it is necessary to use a second large bottle, mark in same and indicate bottle No. 1 and No. 2.

IN GENERAL: Have right type of container. Label correctly. Make out laboratory request correctly. Collect specimen as taught. Avoid contamination of: Specimen, outside of container, your own hands. Send to laboratory as promptly as possible.

Specimens the nurse may have a part in collecting for examination and diagnosis. *Amebiasis and amebic dysentery:* If possible, the patient should go to the laboratory for the evacuation in order that the specimen be as fresh and as warm as possible. If the patient is not able to do this, the specimen must be collected in a sterile container free from urine or any other material. No preservatives must ever be used. The warm specimen must be taken to the laboratory at once. As much as can be obtained should be taken so that some part of it containing the parasite may not be omitted.

Anthrax: Material from the abrasion should be collected on a swab, placed in a sterile test tube and sealed. A slide may be prepared and sealed with another slide over it, to be sent at once to the laboratory for examination.

Chancroid: Slides may be prepared for the open lesion and sealed with another slide and taken to the laboratory, properly labeled. The patient may go to the laboratory and the fresh material obtained from the lesion for immediate examination. If blood sample is taken for a blood Wassermann or Kahn test and this should prove negative, then a second specimen should be taken sometime between the 6th and 8th week after the lesion has appeared; the nurse may call the doctor's attention to the fact that this time has elapsed.

Cholera: Specimens of bowel evacuations freshly collected and delivered to the laboratory for immediate examination should never contain any other material.

Diphtheria: The nurse collects swabbings from the nose and throat and deposits these swabs with the material on them in a sterile test tube.

Dysentery (bacillary): The nurse prepares the patient for the withdrawal of blood (5 to 10 cc.), after the patient has reached about the 2nd week of the attack.

Encephalitis (epidemic): The doctor will take specimens of spinal fluid, usually in 2 or 3 test tubes for the laboratory to examine.

Food poisoning: Specimens of the vomitus or of the bowel contents are taken to the laboratory immediately after the specimen is secured. The laboratory technician may be called to take a specimen of the patient's blood, or the doctor may procure a specimen of it. He may also request portions of the suspected food which have not been eaten, or the container in which the food was purchased or in which it was prepared for the table.

Gonorrhea: Slides may be made by swabbing the urethral, vaginal or cervical discharge, spreading a film over the glass and covering it with another slide for protection until given over to the laboratory - technician. Such smears should be spread evenly, allowed to dry in the air, then taken to the laboratory. The doctor may also order 5 to 10 cc. blood to be taken.

Intestinal parasites: The fresh specimen of feces must go to the laboratory at once for immediate examination. It is well to have the container warmed in which to place the specimen for delivery.

Malaria: Slides are prepared with a specimen of the blood just before the expected chill, or from 6 to 8 hr. after the periodic chill. Considerable blood should be smeared on the slides which should be 3 in number.

Meningitis: The doctor does a spinal puncture and collects specimens of this fluid in 3 sterile test tubes. These are to be examined immediately.

Nasopharyngeal swabbings: These should be made in pure, warm blood-agar which is transported immediately to the laboratory for examination. The new thermal containers are of much help in keeping specimens warm until they may be examined. The nurse must see that they are used properly.

Ophthalmia neonatorum: The doctor or the nurse will make a smear from each eye involved, and cover each with a sterile slide for protection while being taken to the laboratory for examination.

Paratyphoid or typhoid fever: The doctor orders a Widal test for blood culture and agglutination tests. Five to 10 cc. of blood are taken. The doctor may order that 2 or 3 drops of blood be collected on a slide or on parchment paper and allowed to dry. If the first tests are negative then other periods are selected for taking more specimens. Usually the 2nd and 3rd week are the best for positive reaction. Besides the blood (Widal) test, specimens of stool and urine must be procured, although the specimen of feces, if only a very small bit, must be submitted. Special containers are on hand for this purpose and the collection of a portion of either is very essential, as this may be the determining factor in releasing the patient or finding the carrier.

Plague: The doctor may order from 5 to 10 cc. of blood for laboratory examination; some discharge from the bubo may be collected or in the case of a pneumonic type a specimen of the sputum may be collected.

Pneumonia: Specimens of sputa may be examined and typed for pneumococci. The sputum must not be mixed with any preservative. Blood culture, spinal fluid, or pleural fluid may be examined for the germs.

Poliomyelitis: Five to 10 cc. of spinal fluid are collected; the first fluid in one tube marked No. 1. The next dripping of fluid may be clearer, and it may not

spectacles S-60 **speech abnormalities**

contain blood due to the puncture made, and so the second tube must contain part of the specimen. The specimen must be examined immediately for cell count, for if the specimen stands it is worthless for the determination of cell content.

Rocky Mountain spotted fever: Five to 10 cc. of blood are taken from a vein for the Weil-Felix (agglutination) test.

Scarlet fever: There is no laboratory test that definitely may diagnose this disease. However, sometimes the doctor may order an examination for hemolytic streptococci.

Septic sore throat: Swabbing the throat and transferring the swabbings to a slide should be made from all violent sore throats to determine the cause.

Syphilis: The patient should go to the laboratory directly from the bedside. Microscopic examinations for *Treponema pallidum* will be made directly from the lesion. Smears of the exudate may be made. Five to 10 cc. of blood are taken for the blood Wassermann or Kahn tests. Spinal fluid may be taken to determine positive reaction. Three tests should be made at intervals of at least 8 weeks after the suspected lesion appears.

Trichiniasis: A section of muscle in 50% glycerol is used for detection of the germ. Ten cubic centimeters of blood are obtained by laking and adding 25 cc. of 2% acetic acid. A portion of the meat suspected of being the source of the infection should also be obtained.

Tuberculosis (pulmonary): A specimen should be obtained early in the morning on awakening, when the patient first coughs after a night of sleep. This coughing may bring out material from the deeper tissues of the respiratory tract.

Tularemia: Five to 10 cc. of blood are taken for the agglutination test. If the patient should have any lesion that is discharging, a film of the discharge should be prepared on a glass slide.

Typhus fever: Five to 10 cc. of blood are taken from the vein for the Weil-Felix (agglutination) test.

Undulant fever: Five to 10 cc. of blood are taken from the vein for agglutination test.

Vincent's angina: A swabbing of the exudate from the mouth and one from the throat are transferred to glass slides.

Whooping cough: Some of the coughed-up material is applied to culture media from which growths may be developed in the incubator.

spectacles (spĕk'tăk-lz) [L. *spectāre*, to see]. Two lenses supported by a nose bridge and side pieces passing over the ears, to aid vision or protect the eyes.

spectro- [L.]. Combining form meaning *appearance, image, form, spectrum*.

spectrocolorimeter (spĕk-trō-kŭl-or-ĭm'ĕt-ēr) [L. *spectrum*, image, + *color*, color, + G. *metron*, measure]. Device for detecting color blindness by isolating a single spectral color.

spectrograph (spĕk'trō-grăf) [" + G. *graphein*, to write]. An instrument designed to photograph spectra on a sensitive photographic plate.

spectrometer (spĕk-trŏm'ĕt-ēr) [" + G. *metron*, a measure]. A spectroscope so constructed that angular deviation of a ray of light produced by a prism or by a diffraction grating thus indicates the wave length.

spectrophotometer (spĕk"trō-fō-tŏm'ĕt-ēr) [" + G. *photos*, light, + *metron*, a measure]. Device for measuring amt. of color in a solution by comparison with the spectrum.

spectrophotometry (spĕk"trō-fō-tŏm'ĕt-rĭ) [" + " + *metron*, a measure]. Estimation of coloring matter in a solution by use of the spectroscope, or spectrophotometer.

spectropyrheliometer (spĕk"trō-pĭr-hē-lĭ-ŏm'ē-tēr) [" + G. *pyr*, fire, + *helios*, sun, + *metron*, a measure]. Instrument to measure solar radiation.

spectroscope (spĕk'tro-skōp) [" + *skopein*, to examine]. An instrument for separating radiant energy into its component frequencies or wave lengths by means of a prism or grating to form a correct spectrum for inspection.

spectroscopy (spĕk-trŏs'kō-pĭ) [" + G. *skopein*, to examine]. The branch of physical science that treats of the phenomena observed with the spectroscope, or those principles on which its action is based; also, the art of using the spectroscope.

spectrum (spĕk'trŭm) [L. image]. Charted band of wave lengths of electromagnetic vibrations obtained by refraction and diffraction of ray of white light.

The visible spectrum consists of the colors from red to violet. The invisible spectrum is composed of hertzian rays, infrared rays, ultraviolet rays and roentgen rays (x-rays), gamma rays and cosmic rays. The rainbow of colors seen when light passes through a prism, the colors being in series and grouped according to their wave lengths.

The 7 colors of the spectrum comprise *white* light. When projected through a prism colors occur as follows: *violet, indigo, blue, green, yellow, orange,* and *red*.

s., invisible. Spectral portion either below the red (infrared) or above the violet (ultraviolet), which is invisible to the eye, the waves being too long or too short to affect the retina.

s., visible. Seven colors from red to violet.

speculum (spĕk'ū-lŭm) (pl. *specula*) [L. *speculum*, a mirror]. 1. Instrument for examination of canals. 2. Membrane separating ant. cornua of lateral ventricles of brain. SYN: *septum pellucidum*.

s., ear. Short, funnel-shaped tubes, tubular or bivalve; former preferable.

s., eye. Device for separating eyelids. Plated steel wire, plain, Von Graefe's, Steven's or Luer's most common.

speech. Verbal expression of one's thought.

s. abnormalities. These are numerous as would be expected from so highly complicated a series of mechanisms underlying language. Primitively, certain crude sounds served as warnings or threats in much the same way as did facial and bodily expressions. As sounds became highly differentiated, each became associated, and gradually identified with a certain idea.

These word-symbols are a most valuable tool in ideation and thinking is very largely dependent on this internal speech. Further identifications have made possible visual symbols (written language); though primitive written language was entirely unrelated—a series of pictures and crude representations.

External speech requires the coördination of larynx, mouth, lips, chest, and abdominal muscles. These have no special enervation for speech but the upper neurons respond to complex motor pattern fields which convert the idea into suitable motor stimuli. Failure here results in pure *motor aphasia* (subcortical aphasia). The patient is able to write and comprehend.

In cortical motor aphasia, writing is disturbed (*agraphia**) and internal speech at least somewhat impaired. *Labialism* is the excessive use of labial sounds.

Absent speech or hoarseness may be part of a hysteria; in epilepsy one finds a monotonous "woody" sound. Aphasias are also described as sensory.

When a word is heard, but the patient has no idea of its meaning, we speak of word-deafness. Similarly, word-blindness means that the written symbol might as well be a foreign word. This is sometimes called *alexia*.* *Aphasia** in right-handed patients is classically referable to left-handed brain lesions, but the concept of centers for internal speech esp. is rather misleading. It is probably a diffuse cortical activity and countless minor distortions occur in addition to those mentioned. Chief of those not enumerated is the slurring speech of *paresis**; here letters and syllables are omitted without recognition of defect, and this further identifies the abnormality. *Dysarthria** describes any defect of articulation; muscular tone disturbances as seen in cerebellar disease, chorea, paralysis agitans, lenticular degeneration, multiple sclerosis producing jerky, monotonous or scanning speech.

Paralysis due to bilateral medullary pathology results in indistinct enunciation (mouthful speech) often entirely unintelligible. *Pseudobulbar palsy* (as in cases of double hemiplegia) adds a slow spastic characteristic. Peripheral nerve lesions, cleft palate, adenoids, myasthenia gravis, merely suggest the many possible modifications.

Stammering and stuttering are probably psychogenic.

Emotional values may be added to speech qualities; tremulousness and tension may render the voice high-pitched, irritating, or unsustained and broken. Emotional flattening may occur in the neuroses and psychoses. In the latter, diagnostic changes may occur in the stream of talk.

Slowing is common in all depressed states. When complete (mutism) it suggests the negativism esp. likely to occur in schizophrenia. Aphoniclike aphasia patients will find some means of communication.

Excessive talk flow is seen in mania and excited states generally. When merely voluble but relevant, it constitutes circumstantiality. If the goal ideal is lost, irrelevancy is associated with a "flight of ideas"—in extreme form a "word salad." The manner of speech often mirrors the mood.

Neologisms are words created by the patient, often of no apparent significance.

Stereotyped speech is constant repetition of a word or phrase. It should be distinguished from *perseveration* in which the repetition is against the intention or wishes of the patient.

Amentia* invariably delays speech appearance and its faulty development is of diagnostic value. Its delayed or non-appearance may be referable to deafness (deaf-mutism). Childish indistinctness (*e. g.*, r's replaced by w's) may persist in feebleminded adults (*lalling-smudging*).

s. center. The 3rd frontal convolution of the brain which controls speech.

s., clipped. Same as scamping speech.

s., echo. Parrotlike repetition of words spoken by others. SYN: *echolalia*.

s., mirror. Reversing the order of syllables of a word.

s., scamping. Omission of consonants or syllables when unable to pronounce them.

s., scanning. A staccatolike speech with pauses bet. syllables.

s., slurring. Slovenly articulation of letters difficult to pronounce.

s., staccato. Slow and laborious speech with each syllable pronounced separately, as in multiple sclerosis.

speech, words pert. to: acataphasia, alliteration, allolalia, alogia, anarthria literalis, anchone, angophrasia, aphasia, aphemia, aphonia, aphrasia, aphthenxia, aphthongia, articulation, asaphia, ataxophemia, baryglossia, barylalia, baryphonia, betacism, bradyarthria, bradylalia, bradyphrasia, bradyphremia, bredouillement, cataphasia, deaf mute, divagation, dyslalia, dysphasia, dysphemia, dysphonia, egophony, hyperplasia, labialism, lalling, lalopathy, laloplegia, monophasia, mute, mutism, nyctophonia, onomatomania, onomatopoiesis, oxylalia, palinphrasia, perseveration, scanning speech, speech center, stammering, stutter, tachyphasia, Wernicke's center.

spend (spĕnd) [L. *dispendere*, to expend]. To ejaculate semen in coitus or masturbate, or during sleep.

sperm (sperm) [G. *sperma*, seed]. 1. The male germ cell. 2. Male fertilizing secretion. SYN: *semen*.

s. cell. A spermatozoon or spermatid.

s. center. The spermatozoon's centrosome during fertilization.

s. nucleus. That of a spermatozoon.

sperma (sper'mă) [G. *sperma*, seed]. 1. Testicular secretion containing the male reproductive cells. SYN: *semen*. 2. Individual male germ cell.

spermacrasia (spĕr″măk-rā′zĭ-ă) [″ + *akrasia*, bad mixture]. Lack of spermatozoa in the semen.

spermatemphraxis (sper-măt-ĕm-frăks′ĭs) [″ + *emphraxis*, stoppage]. An obstruction to emission of semen.

spermatic (sper-măt'ĭk) [G. *sperma*, semen]. Pert. to semen or sperm.

s. arteries. Two long, slender vessels, branches of the abdominal aorta, following each spermatic cord to the testes.

s. cord. The cord suspending the testis composed of *veins*, *arteries*, *lymphatics*, *nerves*, and the *vas deferens*. SEE: *cord*, *infundibuloform*, *varicocele*.

s. duct. Canal for passage of semen.

spermatid (sper'mă-tĭd) [G. *sperma*, seed]. A cell arising by division of the secondary spermatocyte to become a spermatozoon.

spermatin (sperm'ă-tĭn) [G. *sperma*, seed]. A mucilaginous substance in the semen.

spermatism (sper'mă-tĭzm) [G. *sperma*, seed, + *-ismos*, condition]. Ejaculation of semen, voluntarily or otherwise.

spermatitis (sper-mă-tī′tĭs) [″ + *-itis*, inflammation]. Inflammation of the spermatic cord or of the vas deferens. SYN: *deferentitis*, *funiculitis*.

spermato- [G.]. Combining form meaning *sperm, to sow seed*.

spermatoblast (sper-măt'ō-blăst) [G. *sperma, spermato-*, seed, + *blastos*, germ]. The rudimentary spermatozoon. SYN: *spermatid*.

spermatocele (sper-măt'ō-sēl) [" + *kēlē*, mass]. A cystic tumor of the epididymis containing spermatozoa.

spermatocidal (sper"mă-tō-sī'dăl) [" + L. *cidus*, from *caedere*, to kill]. Destroying spermatozoa.

spermatocyst (sper-măt'ō-sĭst) [" + *kystis*, a sac]. 1. A seminal vesicle. 2. Tumor of epididymis containing semen. SYN: *spermatocele*.

spermatocystectomy (sper"măt-ō-sĭs-tĕk'tō-mĭ) [" + " + *ektomē*, excision]. Removal of the seminal vesicles.

spermatocystitis (sper"măt-ō-sĭs-tī'tĭs) [" + " + *-itis*, inflammation]. Inflammation of a seminal vesicle. SYN: *seminal vesiculitis*.

spermatocystotomy (sper"măt-ō-sĭs-tŏt'ō-mĭ) [" + " + *tomē*, a cutting]. Incision into a seminal vesicle for drainage.

spermatocyte (sper-măt'ō-sīt) [G. *sperma*, seed, + *kytos*, cell]. A cell originating from a spermatogonium, and which forms by division the spermatids which give rise to spermatozoa.

spermatogenesis, spermatogeny (sper-măt-ō-jĕn'ē-sĭs, -ŏj'ē-nĭ) [" + *genesis*, produce, + *gennan*, to produce]. The formation of spermatozoa.

spermatogonium (sper-măt-ō-gō'nĭ-ŭm) (pl. *spermatogonia*) [" + *gonē*, generation]. A seminal cell in its formative state; a mass of spermatoblasts.

spermatoid (sper'măt-oyd) [" + *eidos*, form]. 1. Resembling semen. 2. A male germ cell. SYN: *spermatozoid, spermatozoon*.

spermatology (sper-mă-tŏl'ō-jĭ) [" + *logos*, a study]. The study of the seminal fluid.

spermatolysin (sper-măt-ŏl'ĭ-sĭn) [" + *lysis*, dissolution]. A lysin destroying spermatozoa.

spermatolysis (sper-măt-ŏl'ĭ-sĭs) [G. *sperma*, seed, + *lysis*, dissolution]. Dissolution or destruction of spermatozoa.

spermatolytic (sper-măt-ō-lĭt'ĭk) [" + *lysis*, dissolution]. Destroying spermatozoa.

spermatomere, spermatomerite (sper'mă-tō-mēr, sper"mă-tō-mē'rĭt) [" + *meros*, a part]. One of the particles of the nucleus of the spermatozoon into which it divides after fertilization of the ovum.

spermatopathia, spermatopathy (sper"mă-tō-păth'ĭ-ă, sper-măt-ŏp'ă-thĭ) [" + *pathos*, disease]. Disease of sperm cells or their secreting glands or ducts.

spermatophobia (sper-măt-ō-fō'bĭ-ă) [" + *phobos*, fear]. Abnormal fear of being afflicted with spermatorrhea, involuntary loss of semen.

spermatophore (sper-măt'ō-fōr) [" + *phoros*, a bearer]. 1. A capsule surrounding a mass of spermatozoa. 2. Rudimentary undifferentiated male germ cell. SYN: *spermatogonium*.

spermatoplania (sper"măt-ō-plā'nĭ-ă) [" + *planē*, a wandering]. An assumed metastasis of semen.

spermatopoietic (sper-măt-ō-poy-ĕt'ĭk) [G. *sperma*, seed, + *poiein*, to make]. Promoting the formation and secretion of semen.

spermatorrhea (sper-măt-or-ē'ă) [" + *rhoia*, a flow]. Abnormally frequent, involuntary loss of semen without orgasm.

spermatoschesis (sper-măt-ŏs'kĕ-sĭs) [" + *schesis*, a checking]. Suppression of the seminal fluid.

spermatospore (sper-mat'ō-spōr) [" + *sporos*, a seed]. A primitive cell from which spermatozoa arise. SYN: *spermatogonium*.

spermatotoxin (sper-măt-ō-tŏks'ĭn) [" + *toxikon*, poison]. A toxin which destroys spermatozoa. SYN: *spermatoxin*.

spermatovum (sper-măt-ō'vŭm) [" + L. *ovum*, egg]. A fecundated or impregnated ovum.

spermatoxin (sper-mă-tŏks'ĭn) [" + *toxikon*, poison]. A toxin which causes destruction of spermatozoa. It is formed by injecting spermatozoa from animal of another species.

spermatozoa (sper"măt-o-zō'ă) (sing. *spermatozoon*) [" + *zōon*, life]. Male germ cells.

spermatozoid (sper'măt-ō-zoyd) [" + " + *eidos*, like]. 1. Like semen. 2. Male germ cell. SYN: *spermatoid*.

spermatozoon (sper"măt-ō-zō-ŏn) (pl. *spermatozoa*) [G. *sperma*, seed, + *zōon*, life]. The basic or fecundating nature element of the semen.

The spermatozoon has a broad, oval, flattened head with a nucleus and a protoplasmic neck or middle piece and tail. It is about 1/500 in. in length and resembles a tadpole.

It has the power of self-propulsion by means of a flagellum. Developed after puberty from the *spermatids* in the testes in enormous quantities. The head pierces the envelope of the ovum and loses its tail when fusion of the 2 cells takes place.

RS: *acrosome, fertilization, gamete, ovum, semen, sperm, zoosperm, zygote*.

spermaturia (sper-măt-ū'rĭ-ă) [G. *sperma*, seed, + *ouron*, urine]. Semen discharged with the urine.

spermectomy (sper-mĕk'tō-mĭ) [" + *ektomē*, excision]. Resection of a portion of the spermatic cord and duct.

spermic (sper'mĭk)]G. *sperma*, seed]. Concerning sperm, male reproductive cells.

spermicidal (sper"mĭ-sī'dăl) [" + L. *cidus*, from *caedere*, to kill]. Killing spermatozoa.

spermicide (sper'mĭ-sīd) [" + L. *cidus*, from *caedere*, to kill]. An agent which kills spermatozoa.

spermiduct (sper'mĭ-dŭkt) [" + L. *ductus*, a duct]. The ejaculatory duct and vas deferens considered as one.

spermoblast (sper'mō-blăst) [" + *blastos*, a germ]. A cell developing into a spermatozoo. SYN: *spermatoblast* or *spermatid*.

spermolith (sper'mō-lĭth) [" + *lithos*, stone]. A calculus in the seminal vesicle or spermatic duct.

spermolytic (sper-mō-lĭt'ĭk) [" + *lysis*, dissolution]. Causing the destruction of spermatozoa.

spermoneuralgia (sper"mō-nū-răl'jĭ-ă) [G. *sperma*, seed, + *neuron*, nerve, + *algos*, pain]. Neuralgic pain in the testicles and spermatic cord.

spermophlebectasia (sper"mō-flē-bĕk-tā'zĭ-ă) [" + *phleps, phleb-*, vein, + *ektasis*, dilatation]. Varicosity of the spermatic veins.

spermoplasm (sper'mō-plăzm) [" + *plasma*, a thing formed]. The protoplasm of a male germ cell.

spermosphere (sper'mō-sfēr) [" + *sphaira*, a circle]. Mass of spermatoblasts derived from spermatogonia.

spermospore (sper'mō-spōr) [" + *sporos*, seed]. A primitive cell from which spermatozoa originate. SYN: *spermatogonium, spermatospore*.

sp. gr. Abbr. for *specific gravity*.

spes phthisica (spēz' tĭz'ĭk-ă) [L. *spēs*, hope, + *phthisis*, consumption]. A sense of well-being, happiness, and hopefulness in patients ill with tuberculosis.
The cause may be an underlying fear from which the patient tries to escape, and accomplishes it by repression, which manifests itself by characteristic behavior of the opposite extreme.

sphacelate (sfăs'ĕl-āt) [G. *sphakelos*, gangrene]. 1. To affect with gangrene. 2. Gangrenous. SYN: *mortified, necrosed*.

sphacelation (sfăs-ĕl-ā'shŭn) [G. *sphakelos*, gangrene]. Mortification; formation of a mass of gangrenous tissue. SYN: *gangrene, necrosis*.

sphacelism (sfăs'ĕl-ĭzm) [" + *-ismos*, condition]. Condition of being affected with sphacelus, or gangrene. SYN: *necrosis*.

sphaceloderma (sfăs"ĕl-ō-der'mă) [" + *derma*, skin]. Gangrene of the skin, esp. when symmetrical. SEE: *Raynaud's disease*.

sphacelotoxin (sfăs"ĕl-ō-tŏks'ĭn) [" + *toxikon*, poison]. Poisonous principle obtained from ergot used as an ecbolic. SYN: *spasmotin*.

sphacelous (sfăs'ĕl-ŭs) [G. *sphakelos*, gangrene]. Pert. to a slough or patch of gangrene. SYN: *gangrenous, necrosed, necrotic*.

sphacelus (sfăs'ĕl-ŭs) [G. *sphakelos*, gangrene]. 1. A necrosed mass of tissue. SYN: *slough*. 2. Process of becoming gangrenous. SYN: *gangrene, mortification, necrosis*.

sphenion (sfē'nĭ-ŏn) [G. *sphēn*, wedge]. Point at apex of the sphenoidal angle of the parietal bone.

spheno- [G.]. Combining form meaning a *wedge*, the *sphenoid bone*.

sphenoethmoid (sfē"nō-ĕth'moyd) [" + *ēthmos*, sieve, + *eidos*, form]. Pert. to the sphenoid and the ethmoid bones.
s. recess. Groove back and above the sup. concha, or turbinate bone.

sphenoid (sfē'noyd) [G. *sphēn*, wedge, + *eidos*, form]. Cuneiform, or wedge-shaped.
s. bone. Large bone at base of skull bet. *occipital* and *ethmoid* in front, and the *parietals* and *temporal* bones at the side.
s. fissure. Fissure in sphenoid and frontal bones for nerves and blood vessels.

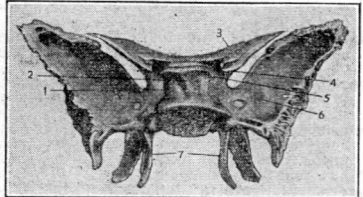

SPHENOID BONE.
(front side)
1. Sella turcica. 2. Dorsum sellae. 3. Small wing. 4. Anterior clinoid process. 5. Posterior clinoid process. 6. Great wing. 7. Pterygoid process.

sphenoiditis (sfē-noy-dī'tĭs) [G. *sphēn*, wedge, + *eidos*, form, + *-itis*, inflammation]. 1. Inflammation of the sphenoidal sinus. 2. Necrosis of the sphenoid bone.

sphenomaxillary (sfē"nō-măks'ĭl-lā-rī) [" + L. *maxilla*, jaw]. Concerning the sphenoid and the maxilla.

sphenopalatine (sfē"nō-păl'ăt-ēn) [" + L. *palatum*, palate]. Concerning the sphenoid and palatine bones.

sphenotresia (sfē-nō-trē'zĭ-ă) [" + *trēsis*, a boring]. Perforating of the basal part of the fetal skull in craniotomy.

sphenotribe (sfē'nō-trīb) [" + *tribein*, to crush]. Instrument for breaking up basal part of fetal cranium.

sphere (sfēr) [G. *sphaira*, a globe]. 1. A ball or globelike structure. 2. The limited space of one's action, esp. that in which one is most capable.
s., hearing. Portions of temporal cranial lobes supposed to be seats of sense of hearing.
s., motor. Region ant. to fissure of Rolando that originates movements when stimulated.
s., segmentation. 1. Cellular mass developed by segmentation of ovum's nucleus. SYN: *morula*. 2. A cell formed by segmentation of nucleus of an ovum.
s., sensory. Region of the central nervous system that perceives sensory impressions. It is post. to the fissure of Rolando.
s., vitelline. SEE: *segmentation sphere, 1*.

spheresthesia (sfē-rĕs-thē'zĭ-ă) [G. *sphaira*, a globe, + *aisthēsis*, sensation]. A morbid sensation, as of swallowing a globe in the throat.

spherical (sfĕr'ĭ-kăl) [G. *sphaira*, a globe]. Having the form of, or pert. to, a sphere. SYN: *globular*.

spherobacteria (sfē"rō-băk-tē'rĭ-ă) [" + *baktērion*, little rod]. A class of organisms to which the micrococci belong.

spheroid (sfē'royd) [" + *eidos*, form]. 1. A body shaped like a sphere. 2. Sphere-shaped.

spherolith (sfē'rō-lĭth) [" + *lithos*, a stone]. A minute concretion in the kidney of the newly born.

spheroma (sfē-ro'mă) [" + *-ōma*, tumor]. A tumor of spherical form.

spherometer (sfē-rŏm'ĕt-ĕr) [" + *metron*, a measure]. Device to ascertain curvature of a surface.

spherospermia (sfē"rō-sper'mĭ-ă) [" + *sperma*, seed]. Round spermatozoa without tails.

spherule (sfĕr'ŭl) [L. *sphaerula*, a little globe]. A very small sphere.

sphincter (sfĭngk'tĕr) [G. *sphigktēr*, a binder]. Circular muscle constricting an orifice. SEE: *tenesmus*.
s. ani. S. that closes the anus, the *external* one being of striated muscle, the *internal* one, of plain muscle.
s., bladder. Plain muscle about opening of bladder into the urethra.
s., cardiac. Plain muscle about the esophagus at cardiac opening into the stomach.
s., ileocecal. Plain muscle about the ileum at its opening into the cecum.
s. of Oddi. Contracted region in common bile duct at ampulla of Vater.
s., pyloric. A thickening of the muscular wall around the pyloric orifice.

sphincteralgia (sfĭngk-tĕr-ăl'jĭ-ă) [G. *sphigktēr*, a binder, + *algos*, pain]. Pain in the sphincter ani muscles.

sphincterectomy (sfĭngk-tĕr-ĕk'tō-mĭ) [" + *ektomē*, excision]. 1. Dissection of any sphincter muscle. 2. Excision of part of the iris' pupillary border; oblique blepharotomy.

sphincterismus (sfĭngk-tĕr-ĭz'mŭs) [" +

ismos, condition]. Spasm of sphincter ani muscles.

sphincteritis (sfĭngk-tĕr-ī'tĭs) [" + *-itis*, inflammation]. Inflammation of any sphincter muscle.

sphincterolysis (sfĭngk-tĕr-ŏl'ĭ-sĭs) [" + *lysis*, dissolution]. Freeing of the iris from the cornea in anterior synechia affecting only the pupillary border.

sphincteroplasty (sfĭngk'tĕr-ō-plăs"tĭ) [" + *plassein*, to form]. Plastic operation upon any sphincter muscle.

sphincteroscope (sfĭngk'tĕr-o-skōp) [" + *skopein*, to examine]. Instrument for inspection of a sphincter.

sphincteroscopy (sfĭngk-tĕr-ŏs'kō-pĭ) [G. *sphigktēr*, a binder, + *skopein*, to examine]. Inspection of the internal anal sphincter.

sphincterotomy (sfĭngk-tĕr-ŏt'ō-mĭ) [" + *tomē*, a cutting]. Cutting of a sphincter muscle.

sphygmic (sfĭg'mĭk) [G. *sphygmos*, pulse]. Relating to the pulse.

sphygmo- [G.]. Combining form meaning the *pulse*.

sphygmobolometer (sfĭg"mō-bō-lŏm'ĕ-tĕr) [G. *sphygmos*, pulse, + *bōlos*, mass, + *metron*, a measure]. Device to measure force of the pulse rather than the blood pressure.

sphygmocardiogram (sfĭg"mō-kar'dĭ-ō-grăm) [" + *kardia*, heart, + *gramma*, a mark]. A tracing made by a sphygmocardiograph of the heartbeat and radial pulse.

sphygmocardiograph (sfĭg"mō-kar'dĭ-ō-grăf) [" + " + *graphein*, to write]. Device for recording the radial pulse and the heartbeat.

sphygmocardioscope (sfĭg"mō-kar'dĭ-ō-skōp) [" + " + *skopein*, to examine]. Device for recording the action of the pulse and heart. SYN: *sphygmocardiograph*.

sphygmochronograph (sfĭg"mō-krō'nō-grăf) [" + *chronos*, time, + *graphein*, to write]. A sphygmograph recording graphically time bet. the heartbeat and the pulse.

sphygmogenin (sfĭg-mŏj'ĕn-ĭn) [" + *gennan*, to produce]. Active principle derived from the suprarenal capsule. SYN: *epinephrine*.

sphygmogram (sfĭg'mō-grăm) [" + *gramma*, a mark]. A tracing of the pulse made by using the sphygmograph.

sphygmograph (sfĭg'mō-grăf) [G. *sphygmos*, pulse, + *graphein*, to write]. Instrument for recording differences of pulse beat in disease and health.

sphygmoid (sfĭg'moyd) [" + *eidos*, form]. Resembling the pulse.

sphygmology (sfĭg-mŏl'ō-jĭ) [" + *logos*, a study]. The study of the pulse.

sphygmomanometer (sfĭg"mō-măn-ŏm'ĕt-ĕr) [" + *manos*, thin, + *metron*, a measure]. Instrument for determining arterial pressure.

sphygmometer (sfĭg-mŏm'ĕt-ĕr) [" + *metron*, a measure]. Instrument for measuring the pulse. SYN: *sphygmograph*.

sphygmometroscope (sfĭg"mō-mĕt'rō-skōp) [" + *metron*, a measure, + *skopein*, to examine]. Instrument for auscultating the pulse by reading diastolic blood pressure.

sphygmophone (sfĭg'mō-fōn) [" + *phōnē*, a voice]. Instrument for hearing the pulse beat.

sphygmoplethysmograph (sfĭg"mō-plĕth-ĭz'-mō-grăf) [G. *sphygmos*, pulse, + *plēthysmos*, increase, + *graphein*, to write]. Device which traces the pulse with its curve of fluctuation in volume.

sphygmoscope (sfĭg'mō-skōp) [" + *skopein*, to examine]. Instrument for showing the heart's movements or pulsations of arteries and veins.

sphygmosystole (sfĭg"mō-sĭs'tō-lē) [" + *systolē*, contraction]. The segment of the pulse wave that corresponds to the heart's systole.

sphygmotonograph (sfĭg"mō-tō'nō-grăf) [" + *tonos*, tone, + *graphein*, to write]. An instrument for recording both blood pressure and pulse pressure.

sphygmotonometer (sfĭg"mō-tō-nŏm'ĕt-ĕr) [" + " + *metron*, a measure]. Instrument for ascertaining elasticity of walls of an artery.

sphyrectomy (sfī-rĕk'tō-mĭ) [G. *sphyra*, malleus, + *ektomē*, excision]. Surgical excision of the malleus.

sphyrotomy (sfī-rŏt'ō-mĭ) [" + *tomē*, a cutting]. Partial excision of the malleus.

spica (spī'kă) [L. *spica*, ear of grain]. A reverse spiral bandage, the turn of which crosses like letter V. SEE: *bandage*.

spicular (spĭk'ū-lar) [L. *spiculum*, a dart]. Pert. to, or resembling, a spicule; dartlike.

spicule (spĭk'ūl) [L. *spiculum*, a dart]. A small, needle-shaped body.

  s., bony. A needle-shaped fragment of bone.

spiculum (spĭk'ū-lŭm) (pl. *spicula*) [L. *spiculum*, a dart]. A sharp, small spike. SYN: *spicule*.

spider bites or **poisoning** (spī'der) [A.S. *spinnan*, to spin]. All spider bites are not dangerous.

  SYM: In general, the victim is often bitten about the genitalia. Local symptoms are slight burning followed in about half an hour by severe radiating pains, often extending long distances from puncture. Sloughing at site and along lymphatics may occur. Collapse, unconsciousness, convulsions, and death sometimes follow.

  s., black widow. It is coal black with a brilliant red or yellow spot on the abdomen. The body is about ½ in. long and the legs extend over 2 in. It is found under rocks, in dark attics, basements, barns, and in outdoor privies. Bite causes excruciating pain. It is very poisonous and its bite may prove fatal.

  SYM: Initially, the sensation resembles the prick of a pin. From a few minutes to several hours later, severe pain radiates from the wound, becoming general and resulting in paroxysmal cramps, often accompanied by nausea, cold sweats, urinary retention and perhaps delirium. The symptoms may last for hours or for 2 or 3 days.

  Avoid all stimulants. Suction is of little value as the toxin is rapidly absorbed. Calcium gluconate intravenously often gives relief from pain. Large doses of morphine, repeated when necessary, given slowly by vein, also controls pain. Heat, a hot tub, and forcing fluids also recommended. Serum treatment is not satisfactory. SEE: *bites*.

  s. cancer. SEE: *spider nevus*.

  s. cells. Branching cells in neuroglia. SEE: *Deiter's cell*, *neuroglia cell*.

  s. fingers. Abnormally long phalanges of the fingers. SYN: *arachnodactyly*.

  s. nevus. A branched growth on the skin of dilated capillaries, resembling a spider. SYN: *nevus araneus*.

Spies' diet. One for pellagra. Brewer's yeast, milk, eggs, lean meat and perhaps calves' liver, all in greater abundance than in Goldberger's* diet.

spigelian line (spī-jē'lĭ-ăn, spē-gā'lĭ-ăn). One marking musculotendinous junction of transversus abdominis muscle.

   s. lobe. A small lobe behind right lobe of liver. SYN: *lobus caudatus of liver*.

spill (spĭl) [A.S. *spillan*, to squander]. An overflow.

   s., cellular. Dissemination of cells through lymph or the blood resulting in metastasis.

spiloma, spilus (spī-lō'mă, spī'lŭs) [G. *spilōma*, spot]. A birthmark. SYN: *nevus*.

spiloplaxia (spī″lō-plăks'ĭ-ă) [G. *spilos*, spot, + *plax*, plate]. A red spot appearing in leprosy.

spina (spī'nă) (pl. *spinae*) [L. *spina*, thorn]. 1. Any spinelike protuberance. 2. The spine.

   s. bifida. Congenital defect in walls of spinal canal caused by lack of union bet. the laminae of the vertebrae.

Lumbar portion is part chiefly affected, 50% of all cases occurring in this region, 12% in lumbosacral, and 27% sacral.

SYM: As result of this deficiency the membranes of the cord are pushed through the opening, forming a tumor known as spina bifida, on account of condition of spine giving rise to the deformity, and as hydrorrhachis on account of the fluid contained in the tumor.

Latter varies in size from that of a walnut or closed fist to that of a child's head. Sometimes covered with skin of normal color and appearance, but oftener skin is thin and translucent, or may be entirely absent, in which case tumor has raw, florid look. The true sac consists of the membranes of the cord blended together and enclosing a liquid, which is ordinarily the cerebrospinal fluid; usually communicates directly with brain, as in the normal condition through the opening in the pia mater at lower border of 4th ventricle.

Pressure on tumor of this variety will, therefore, sometimes cause stupor through pressure upon the brain. When protrusion consists of membranes, the fluid is called a spinal meningocele; when it contains a portion of cord also, a meningomyelocele; when central canal of spinal cord is dilated, forming a cavity of the sac, the tumor is called a syringomyelocele or syringomyelia.

DIAG: Made by following points: 1. Tumor is congenital. 2. It occupies a central position, a peculiarity which characterizes most tumors of intraspinal origin. 3. It may probably be reduced by gentle pressure, or at least greatly diminished in size, the diminution being attested by increased tension of the fontanel and sometimes with stupor, convulsions and other nervous symptoms. 4. Bony margin of the gap in spine can be felt at base of tumor. 5. Tumor becomes more tense where child cries or coughs. 6. It is often translucent and when so, an opaque band or bands, consisting of the spinal cords and nerves, may sometimes be seen upon inner surface of its walls. 7. Apt to be associated with other deformities, such as hydrocephalus, or talipes, or with paraplegia, vesical or rectal paralysis, etc. 8. Cutaneous covering of tumor is often absent. 9. Profuse outgrowth of hair over site of defective arches.

PROG: Usual course of such cases tends towards death which commonly occurs within 6 or 8 months. Spontaneous cure happens very rarely, the vertebral arches growing and developing, and neck and sac correspondingly contracting and finally being shut off from communication with the canal. Oftener the integuments and membranes over tumor ulcerate, contents of sac escape and frequently child dies in convulsions or will perish soon after from a septic meningitis, following infection through ulcerated tract.

TREATMENT: If tumor is small, covered with sound skin, and not growing rapidly, should be enveloped in raw cotton and supported by a loosely fitting elastic bandage, or a layer of cotton brushed over with collodion may be applied to surface. Tumor may shrink and disappear. Tapping, drainage, excision of sac; injection of sac with iodoglycerin solution gives, at present, best hopes of success.

   s. ventosa. Absorption of bone bordering the medulla, appearing to be inflated with air. Seen in cancer or tuberculosis of bone.

spinach (spĭn'ach) [Spanish *espinaca*]. COMP: Oxalates prevail. AV. SERVING: 75 Gm. Pro. 1.6, Fat 0.2, Carbo. 0.8.

VITAMINS: A+++, B++, C+++, G++.

ASH CONST: Ca 0.067, Mg 0.037, K 0.774, Na 0.125, P 0.068, Cl 0.074, S 0.038, Fe 0.0036.

ACTION: Laxative, antitoxic and valuable for its mineral content. SEE: *atriplicism*.

spinal (spī'năl) [L. *spina*, a thorn]. Pert. to the spine or spinal cord.

   s. anesthesia. An anesthetic injected into the spinal canal.

RS: *anesthesia, cisternal puncture, lumbar puncture, spinal puncture*.

   s. canal. Canal of the vertebral column. RS: *intrathecal, spina bifida, spinal puncture*.

   s. column. The vertebral column enclosing spinal cord. Thirty-three bones in all, 7 cervical, 12 dorsal or thoracic, 5 lumbar, 5 sacral vertebrae forming 1 bone and 4 coccygeal vertebrae which, with the sacrum, are fused into 1 bone. SEE: *Illus. below*.

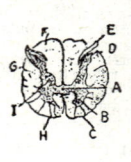

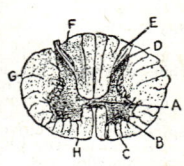

SPINAL COLUMN, CROSS SECTION OF

1. Dorsal portion.
A. Central canal. B. Anterior horns. C. Anterior roots. D. Posterior horns. E. Posterior roots. F. Posterior columns. G. Lateral columns. H. Anterior columns. I. Clarke's columns.
2. Cervical Enlargement.
A. Central canal. B. Anterior horns. C. Anterior roots. D. Posterior horns. E. Posterior roots. F. Posterior columns. G. Lateral columns. H. Anterior columns.

   s. cord. An ovoid column of nervous tissue about 44 cm. long, flattened anteroposteriorly, extending from the medulla to the 2nd lumbar vertebra in the spinal canal. SEE: *Illus.*, p. S-66.

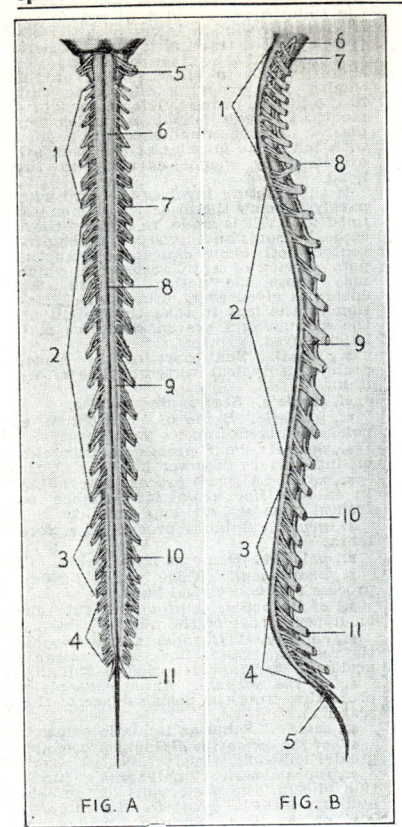

SPINAL CORD.

A. Anterior View of Spinal Cord.
1. Cervical nerves. 2. Thoracic nerves. 3. Lumbar nerves. 4. Sacral nerves. 5. Hypoglossal nerves. 6. Anterior funiculus. 7. Cervical enlargement. 8. Anterior medial fissure. 9. Anterior lateral sulcus. 10. Lumbar enlargement. 11. Coccygeal nerve.

B. Lateral View of Spinal Cord.
1. Cervical portion of spinal cord. 2. Thoracic portion. 3. Lumbar portion. 4. Sacral portion. 5. Filum terminale. 6. Spinal portion of accessory nerve. 7. Cervical enlargement. 8 Eighth cervical nerve. 9. Lateral funiculus. 10. Twelfth thoracic nerve. 11. Fifth lumbar nerve.

In cross section, it does not fill the vertebral space, being surrounded by the pia mater, the cerebrospinal fluid, the arachnoid, and the dura mater, which latter fuses with the periosteum of the inner surfaces of the vertebrae.

The gray substance forms an "H," there being a post. and ant. horn in either half. The ant. horn is composed of motor cells from which the neurons making up the motor portions of the peripheral nerves arise. Sensory neurons enter posteriorly.

The "H" also divides the surrounding white matter into post., lateral and ant. bundles. These serve to connect brain and cord in both directions as well as various portions of the cord itself.

From the s. c. issue all nerves to the trunk and limbs, and it is the center of reflex action containing the conducting paths to and from the brain.

Neoplastic, inflammatory, degenerative and traumatic changes parallel those of the brain. SEE: *brain*.

RS: *albocinereous, amyelinuria, amyelotrophy, anospinal, axion, brain, cerebellospinal, chordoskeleton, chordotomy, ciliospinal, endorrhachis, hydrorrhachis, hydrorrhachitis, medulla, meninges, meningitis, meningocele, meningococcus, myelitis, "myel-" words, oblongata, meningomyelitis, myelitis, "myel-" words, oblongata, syringomyelia, syringomyelitis, syrinx, tabes.*

s. curvature. Abnormal curvature of the spine, frequently constitutional in children.

It may be *angular* (caries), or *lateral* (scoliosis), or *anteroposterior* (kyphosis,* lordosis*).

s. c., angular. Caries of the spine. SYN: *Pott's disease, q.v.*

s. c., lateral. Deviation of spine to one or other side causing a twist of the spine.

s. fluid. The fluid contained within the spinal canal.

It contains 55 to 75 mg. of sugar per 100 cc. when normal. The sugar content is lower than that in the blood.

DIAG: *Cell count*: If normal, 0 to 6 cells per cmm. Increased in all diseased states, several hundred or thousands in meningitis, when fluid becomes opaque.

Lymphocytes found in encephalitis and tuberculous meningitis; polymorphonuclears predominate in septic meningitis and epidemic meningitis.

Bloody fluid: Brain hemorrhages due to arteriosclerosis, high blood pressure, tumors and other causes.

Encephalitis: Sugar content is increased, fluid clear, cell count 100 plus. Forms a spider web clot on standing. SEE: *meningitis*.

Globulin: Absent during health, positive in disease.

Microörganisms: Meningococci, streptococci, pneumococci, tubercle bacilli, and influenza bacilli may be present, any of which may be indicative of meningitis. Epidemic meningitis indicated by Gram-negative, intracellular diplococcus, biscuit-shaped microörganisms. Typhoid bacilli may produce meningeal symptoms in typhoid fever. Long chains of hemolytic, green-producing streptococci enter the meninges through the ear, the lungs being the invading point of pneumococci, influenza bacilli, and pneumobacilli. All these may be found in smears, though sometimes missed and found in cultures.

*Meningitis**: Lower spinal fluid sugar than sugar content of blood; 25 to 15 mg. If suppurative m., spinal fluid is puslike and turbid, but it is clear in tuberculous m., encephalitis and poliomyelitis.

*Poliomyelitis**: Same as in encephalitis, *q.v.*

RS: *anhydromyelia, calcinorrhachia, cerebrospinal fluid.*

s. nerves. Those arising from the spinal cord; 31 pairs, consisting of 8 *cervical*, 12 *dorsal*, 5 *lumbar*, 5 *sacral*, and 1 *coccygeal*, corresponding with the spinal vertebrae. See: *skeleton*.

s. puncture. Puncture of the spinal cavity with a needle to extract the spinal fluid for diagnostic purposes, or to relieve tension aroused by pressure of the fluid, or to induce anesthesia, or to prevent an excess of fluid when a liquid is to be injected.

SITE OF PUNCTURE: To prevent injury of the nerve fibers, the puncture usually made at the juncture bet. the 3rd and 4th lumbar vertebrae. A line drawn posteriorly from the crest of one ilium over the crest of the other will usually pass over the tip of the spinous process of the 4th lumbar vertebra. The point for the needle injection is directly above this line.

BLOOD PRESSURE: The blood pressure drops with the removal of the fluid from the spinal canal. If the puncturing is made for the purpose of lowering the blood pressure, or to remove fluid "under pressure," a manometer should show the reading as the fluid escapes. If 10 mm. of mercury decrease, the withdrawal of the fluid should be discontinued. The dripping of the fluid under normal conditions may be estimated as one drop every 3 to 5 seconds, which is merely a rough estimate. SEE: *cisternal puncture*.

ONP: Drape a small table with a sterile sheet. Doctor's gown and gloves, flat gauze and iodine sponges are placed on the table. Sterile sponges and adhesive plaster should be in readiness. Patient should sit with feet over side of table, arms crossed with elbows on knees and head well forward. After injection of anesthetic patient is slowly placed in dorsal position. Then table is slowly tipped into Trendelenburg position. The patient's head and shoulders must be kept lower than the pelvis.

s. reflex. Any reflex centering in the spinal cord.

spinalgia (spĭ-năl'jĭ-ă) [L. *spina*, thorn, + G. *algos*, pain]. Pain in a vertebra under pressure.

spinalis (spĭ-nā'lĭs). A muscle attached to the spinal process of a vertebra. SEE: *Table of Muscles in Appendix*.

spinant (spī'nănt) [L. *spina*, thorn]. Any agent which increases spinal cord excitability.

spinate (spī'nāt) [L. *spina*, thorn]. Having spines or shaped like a thorn.

spindle (spĭn'dl) [A.S. *spinel*]. A fusiform-shaped body, esp. one in cell nucleus during karyokinesis.

s. cells. Fusiform cells.
s. legged. Having long, thin legs.
s., nuclear. Cone-shaped nucleus during a stage of karyokinesis.

spine (spīn). 1. A sharp process of bone. 2. The spinal column, consisting of 33 vertebrae. Cervical 7, dorsal 12, lumbar 5, sacral 5, coccygeal 4. The bones of the sacrum and coccyx are ankylosed in adult life and counted as one each. SYN: *backbone*.

RS: *cephalorhachidian, cord, spinal, cramp, curvature, rachialgia, rachilysis,* "rach-" words, *scoliosis*.

s., alar, s., angular. Spinous process of the sphenoid bone. SYN: *spina angularis*. [column.
s., dorsal. The backbone or spinal
s., fracture of. A fractured spine is often treated in a plaster jacket with the spine hyperextended to reduce the fracture. A window is cut over the abdomen. If the fracture is high the neck is included in the jacket, which must be short enough to allow flexion of the thighs. The patient is allowed to walk in the jacket, which is left on for 3 or 4 months. A vest is put on under this plaster, and the prominences are padded with felt. The muscles of the back are exercised by weight carrying in the head.

If the fracture involves the cord with paralysis below the injury, a plaster bed lined with felt is made. In nursing these cases, bedsores and cystitis must be prevented, both being dangerous from the point of view of septic absorption, which may cause the patient's death. An enema is given every other day. Traction to the legs to take the weight off the sacrum and prevent bedsores may be employed.

s., hemal. That part of the hemal arch of a typical vertebra that closes it in.
s., Henle's. SEE: *suprameatal s.*
s., ischiatic. Spine of the ischium, a pointed eminence on its post. border.
s., mental. Four prominent tubercles on int. surface of lower jaw.
s., nasal. A sharp process descending in middle line from inf. surface of frontal bone bet. the sup. maxillae.
s., neural. Spinous process of a vertebra.
s., palatine. Same as nasal spine.
s., pharyngeal. Ridge under basilar process of the occipital bone.
s. of the pubes. A prominent tubercle on upper border of the pubis.
s., railway. 1. Chronic meningomyelitis resulting from shock in a railway accident. 2. Traumatic neurasthenia.
s. of the scapula. An osseous plate projecting from the post. surface of the scapula.
s., sciatic. Same as ischiatic spine.
s. of the sphenoid. Spinous process of greater sphenoid wing.
s., suprameatal. A small spine at junction of sup. and post. walls of the ext. auditory meatus. SYN: *Henle's spine*.
s. of the tibia. Eminence projecting upward from the head of the tibia.
s., typhoid. Acute arthritis due to infection causing spinal ankylosis during or following typhoid fever.

spinifugal (spĭ-nĭf'ū-găl) [L. *spina*, thorn, + *fugare*, to flee]. Moving away from the spinal cord.

spinipetal (spī-nĭp'ĕt-ăl) [" + *petere*, to seek]. Moving toward the spinal cord.

spinitis (spī-nī'tĭs) [" + G. *-itis*, inflammation]. Inflammation of the spinal cord. SYN: *myelitis*.

spinobulbar (spī"no-bŭl'bar) [" + G. *bulbos*, a bulb]. Concerning the spinal cord and medulla oblongata.

spinocellular (spī"nō-sĕl'ū-lar) [" + *cellula*, a little chamber]. Pert. to or like prickle cells.

spinocerebellar (spī"nō-sĕr-ē-bĕl'ar) [" + *cerebellum*, little brain]. Concerning spinal cord and cerebellum.

spinocortical (spī"nō-kor'tĭ-kăl) [" + *cortex, cortic-*, rind]. Pert. to the spinal cord and cerebral cortex. SYN: *corticospinal*.

spinoglenoid (spī"nō-glen'oyd) [L. *spina*, thorn, + G. *glēnē*, cavity, + *eidos*, form]. Relating to the spine of scapula and glenoid cavity.

spinoglenoid ligament   S-68   **Spirochaeta vincenti**

s. ligament. Ligament joining spine of the scapula to the border of the glenoid cavity.

spinomuscular (spī″nō-mŭs′kū-lar) [" + *musculus*, muscle]. Pert. to the spinal cord and muscles.

s. segment. Motor cells and nerves in the medulla and spinal cord.

spinoneural (spī″nō-nū′ral) [" + G. *neuron*, nerve]. Pert. to the peripheral nerves and spinal cord.

spinous (spī′nŭs) [L. *spina*, thorn]. Pert. to or resembling a spine.

s. point. Spot over a spinous process very sensitive to pressure.

s. process. Prominence at post. part of each vertebra.

spinthariscope (spĭn-thăr′ĭ-skōp) [G. *spintharis*, spark, + *skopein*, to see]. Apparatus for examining the emanations of radium.

spintherism (spĭn′ther-ĭzm) [G. *spintherizein*, to emit sparks]. Sensation of sparks before the eyes.

spintheropia (spĭn-thĕr-ō′pĭ-ă) [" + *ōps*, eye]. Subjective sensation of sparks before the eyes.

spiradenitis (spi-ra-den-i′tis). A funiculus beginning in coil of a sweat gland. SYN: *hidrosadenitis phlegmonous*.

spiradenoma (spī-răd-en-ō′mă) [G. *speira*, coil, + *adēn*, gland, + *-ōma*, tumor]. Tumor of the sweat glands.

spiral (spī′răl) [G. *speira*, coil]. Coiling like the thread of a screw.

s. bandage. Roller bandage to be applied spirally.

s. canal of the cochlea. One that runs spirally around the modiolus.

s. lamina. A thin plate in the ear. SYN: *lamina spiralis*.

spirem, spireme (spī′rēm, spī-rēm′) [G. *speirēma*, coil]. First stage in karyokinesis or mitotic division in which a wreath of chromatin fibrils forms. SYN: *skein*.

spirilla (spī-rĭl′ă) [L.]. Plural of *spirillum*.

spirillicidal (spī-rĭl″ĭ-sīd′ăl) [L. *spirillum*, coil, + *cidus*, from *caedere*, to kill]. Destroying spirochetes or spirilla.

spirillicide (spī-rĭl′ĭs-īd) [" + *cidus*, from *caedere*, to kill]. Destructive to spirilla.

spirillicidin (spī-rĭl-lĭ-sī′dĭn) [" + *cidus*, from *caedere*, to kill]. A substance developed in blood of patients immunized against spirilla which has the power to destroy them.

spirillolysis (spī-rĭl-lŏl′ĭ-sĭs) [" + G. *lysis*, dissolution]. The destruction of spirilla.

spirillosis (spī-rĭl-ō′sĭs) [" + G. *-ōsis*, condition]. A disease caused by presence of spirilla in the blood.

spirillotropic (spī-rĭl-lō-trŏp′ĭk) [" + G. *tropē*, a turning]. Having an attraction to spirilla.

spirillotropism (spī-rĭl-lŏt′rō-pĭzm) [" + " + *ismos*, condition]. The ability to attract spirilla.

Spirillum (spī-rĭl′ŭm) (pl. *Spirilla*) [L. coil]. A group of more or less spiral-shaped, motile microörganisms, one of which (comma bacillus) causes cholera.

S. buccale. S. from tartar of teeth.

S. cholerae asiaticae. Comma bacillus of epidemic cholera.

S. Milleri. S. from carious teeth.

S. Obermeieri. S. found in relapsing fever.

S. sputigenum. S. in saliva.

S. tyrogenum. S. found in very old cheese resembling that of Asiatic cholera.

S., Vincent's. S. found in Vincent's angina.

spirit (spĭr′ĭt) [L. *spiritus*, breathing]. 1. Any distilled or volatile liquor or a solution of volatile liquid in alcohol. 2. Alcohol.

s., rectified. Alcohol with 16% water.

spir′itual ther′apy [L. *spiritus*, breathing, + G. *therapeia*, treatment]. The application of spiritual knowledge in the treatment of all mental and physical disorders, based upon the assumption that man is a spiritual being living in a spiritual universe; that in proportion to his acceptance of this idea, and in proportion to his success in demonstrating it, he may control the body and the material elements in harmony with a Divine plan.

spirituous (spĭr′ĭt-ū-ŭs) [L. *spiritus*, breathing]. Alcoholic; pert. to alcohol.

spiritus (spĭr′ĭt-ŭs) [L. breathing]. Alcoholic solution of a volatile substance. Usually, 5-10% strength. Thirteen are official. SYN: *spirit*.

s. frumenti. Whisky.

s. juniperi. Gin.

s. myrciae. Bay rum.

s. vini gallici. Brandy.

spirobacteria (spī″rō-băk-tē′rĭ-ă) [G. *speira*, coil, + *baktērion*, little rod]. Curved bacteria, including spirilla, spirochetes, and vibrios.

Spirochaeta (spī″rō-kē′tă) [G. *speira*, coil, + *chaitē*, hair]. A genus of slender, nonflagellated bacteria with spiral filaments.

S. bronchialis. A species in sputum in some nontuberculous forms of bronchitis.

S. icterohaemorrhagiae. Species found in Weil's disease or acute febrile jaundice.

S. morsus muris. The microörganism of rat-bite fever.

S. nodosa. Assumed pathogenic organism of Weil's disease.

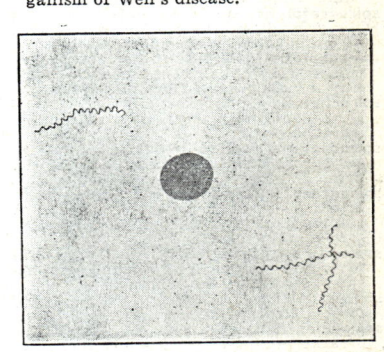

SPIROCHAETA PALLIDA.
Three spirochetes and a red blood cell. Irritation juice from a primary lesion.

S. pallida. Species which is the cause of syphilis. SYN: *Treponema pallidum*.

S. refringens. A species found in gonorrhea and balanitis and in healthy genital organs; apparently nonpathogenic.

S. vincenti. Variety found in Vincent's angina or ulcerative disease of the tonsils.

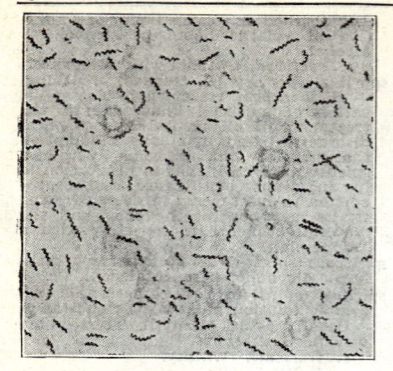

SPIROCHETES IN THE TISSUE, AS SEEN IN THE LIVER IN A CASE OF CONGENITAL SYPHILIS.

spirochetal (spī″rō-kē′tăl) [G. *speira*, coil, + *chaitē*, hair]. Pert. to spirochetes, esp. infections caused by them.

spirochetalytic (spī″rō-kē-tă-lĭt′ĭk) [" + " + *lysis*, dissolution]. Destructive of spirochetes.

spirochete (spī′rō-kēt) [" + *chaitē*, hair]. Any member of the genus *Spirochaeta*.

spirochetemia (spī″rō-kē-tē′mĭ-ă) [" + *aima*, blood]. Spirochetes in the blood.

spirocheticidal (spī″rō-kē-tĭ-sī′dăl) [" + " + L. *cidus*, from *caedere*, to kill]. Destructive to spirochetes.

spirocheticide (spī″rō-kē′tĭs-īd) [" + " + L. *cidus*, from *caedere*, to kill]. Anything which destroys spirochetes.

spirochetolysis (spī″rō-kē-tŏl′ĭ-sĭs) [" + " + *lysis*, dissolution]. The destruction of spirochetes by specific antibodies.

spirochetosis (spī″rō-kē-tō′sĭs) [G. *speira*, coil, + *chaitē*, hair, + *-ōsis*, condition]. Any infection caused by spirochetes.

spirochetotic (spī″rō-kē-tŏt′ĭk) [" + " + *-ōsis*, condition]. Pert. to or marked by spirochetosis.

spirocheturia (spī″rō-kē-tū′rĭ-ă) [" + " + *ouron*, urine]. Spirochetes in the urine.

spirogram (spī′rō-grăm) [L. *spirāre*, to breathe, + G. *gramma*, a mark]. A tracing made by a spirograph of respiratory movements.

spirograph (spī′rō-grăf) [" + G. *graphein*, to write]. Device for recording graphically respiratory movements.

spiroid (spī′royd) [G. *speira*, coil, + *eidos*, form]. Resembling a spiral.

spiroindex (spī″rō-ĭn′dĕks) [L. *spirāre*, to breathe, + *indicāre*, to point out]. The quotient obtained by dividing vital capacity by height.

spiroma (spī-rō′mă) [G. *speira*, coil, + *-ōma*, tumor]. Multiple, benign, cystic epithelioma of the sweat glands. SYN: *spiradenoma*.

spirometer (spī-rŏm′ĕt-ēr) [L. *spirāre*, to breathe, + G. *metron*, measure]. An apparatus consisting of a cylindrical bell immersed in water and so equipped with outlets that gases can be exhaled into it or inhaled out of it while measurements of volume are made.

The following are typical measurements made on normal men by using the spirometer:

Complemental air: 1600 cc., the amount which a subject can still inhale, by a special effort, after a normal inspiration.

Dead air: 150 cc., the air which, taken in through the nose, gets only as far as nasopharynx or trachea and does not reach the lungs.

Minimal air: Less than 1000 cc., that which remains in the lungs after complete collapse, as in pneumothorax.

Reserve air: 2600 cc., the sum of the supplemental and residual air.

Residual air: 1000 cc. that are left in the lungs after a complete expiration.

Supplemental air: 1600 cc. which can still be exhaled after a normal exhalation.

Tidal air: 500 cc., the amount exhaled in a normal inhalation.

spirometry (spī-rŏm′ĕ-trī) [L. *spirāre*, to breathe, + G. *metron*, a measure]. Measurement of air capacity of the lungs.

Spironema (spī-rō-nē′mă) [G. *speira*, coil, + *nēma*, thread]. Another name for a genus of spirochetes. SYN: *Borrelia*.

S. pallida. Causative organism of syphilis. SYN: *Spirochaeta pallida*.

spirophore (spī′rō-fōr) [L. *spirāre*, to breathe, + G. *phoros*, a bearer]. Device for artificial respiration. SYN: *iron lung*.

spirosal (spī′rō-săl). An acid derivative of salicylic acid.

USES: Externally, as an analgesic.

DOSAGE: Diluted with 3 parts alcohol. or 8 parts olive oil, or equal parts by weight of petrolatum.

spiroscope (spī′rō-skōp) [L. *spirāre*, to breathe, + G. *skopein*, to examine]. Device for measuring air capacity of the lungs.

spiroscopy (spī-rŏs′kō-pī) [L. *spirāre*, to breathe, + *skopein*, to examine]. The use of the spiroscope to measure respiratory capacity of the lungs.

spirulina (spī′rū-lī′nă) [L. *spirula*, a twisted shape]. A microörganism coiled and twisted.

spissated (spĭs′ā-ted) [L. *spissāre*, to thicken]. Thickened. SYN: *inspissated*.

spissitude (spĭs′ĭ-tūd) [L. *spissitūdo*, a thickening]. Condition of being inspissated, as a fluid thickened by evaporation almost to a solid; thickness.

spit (spĭt) [A.S. *spittan*, to spit]. 1. Saliva. SYN: *expectoration, sputum, spittle*. 2. To expectorate spittle.

spit′tle [A.S. *spǣtan*]. The digestive fluid of the mouth. SYN: *saliva*.

splanchnapophysis (splăngk-nă-pŏf′ĭ-sĭs) [G. *splagchnon*, viscus, + *apo*, from, + *physis*, shoot]. 1. Any skeletal element connected with the alimentary canal, as the hyoid bone. 2. Outgrowth of a vertebra on opp. side of a vertebral axis, enclosing some viscus.

splanchnectopia (splăngk-nĕk-tō′pĭ-ă) [" + *ektopos*, out of place]. Dislocation of a viscus or of the viscera.

splanchnemphraxis (splăngk-nĕm-frăks′ĭs) [" + *emphraxis*, stoppage]. Obstruction of any internal organ, particularly of the intestine.

splanchnesthesia (splăngk-nĕs-thē′zĭ-ă) [" + *aisthēsis*, sensation]. Visceral sensation.

splanchnesthetic (splăngk-nĕs-thĕt′ĭk) [" + *aisthēsis*, sensation]. Relation to visceral consciousness or sensation.

splanchnic (splăngk′nĭk) [G. *splagchnon*, viscus]. Pert. to the viscera.

s. nerves. Three nerves from the

splanchnicotomy   S-70   **spleen**

thoracic sympathetic ganglia distributed to the viscera.

splanchnicotomy (splăngk-nĭ-kŏt'ō-mĭ) [" + tomē, a cutting]. Section of a splanchnic nerve.

splanchnoblast (splăngk'nō-blăst) [" + blastos, germ]. Incipient rudiment of a viscus. SEE: *anlage, proton.*

splanchnocele (splăngk'nō-sēl) [" + koilos, a hollow]. 1. That part of the celom persisting in the adult, giving rise to the visceral cavities. SYN: *splanchnocoele.* 2. [" + kēlē, hernia]. Protrusion of any abdominal viscus.

splanchnocoele (splăngk'nō-sēl) [" + koilos, a hollow]. Rudimentary embryonic cavity from which the visceral cavities arise.

splanchnodiastasis (splăngk-nō-dī-ăs'tăs-ĭs) [" + diastasis, dilatation]. Displacement or dislocation of a viscus.

splanchnodynia (splăngk-nō-dĭn'ĭ-ă) [" + odynē, pain]. Pain in the abdominal region.

splanchnography (splăngk-nŏg'ră-fĭ) [" + graphein, to write]. Descriptive treatise on anatomy of the viscera.

splanchnolith (splăngk'nō-lĭth) [" + lithos, stone]. An intestinal calculus.

splanchnology (splăngk-nŏl'ō-jĭ) [G. *splagchnon*, viscus, + *logos*, a study]. The study of the viscera.

splanchnopathia (splăngk-nō-păth'ĭ-ă) [" + pathos, disease]. Pathological conditions of the viscera.

splanchnopleure (splăngk'nō-plūr) [" + pleura, a side]. The embryonic layer formed by the union of the visceral layer of the mesoderm with the entoderm. SEE: *somatopleure.*

splanchnoptosia, splanchnoptosis (splăngk-nŏp-tō'sĭ-ă, -sĭs) [" + ptōsis, a dropping]. Prolapse of the viscera. SYN: *abdominal ptosis, enteroptosia, visceroptosia, Glénard's disease.*

splanchnosclerosis (splăngk-nō-sklē-rō'sĭs) [" + sklerōsis, a hardening]. Hardening of any of the viscera through overgrowth of connective tissue.

splanchnoscopy (splăngk-nŏs'kō-pĭ) [G. *splagchnon*, viscus, + *skopein*, to examine]. Examination of the viscera with aid of roentgen rays or transillumination.

splanchnoskeleton (splăngk"nō-skĕl'ĕ-tŏn) [" + skeleton, skeleton]. 1. Any osseous structure in an organ, or the cartilaginous rings of the bronchi and trachea. 2. The visceral skeleton, *i. e.,* the *ribs, sternum, innominate bones,* etc., protecting the viscera.

splanchnotomy (splăngk-nŏt'ō-mĭ) [" + tomē, a cutting]. Dissection of the viscera.

splanchnotribe (splăngk'nō-trīb) [" + tribein, to crush]. An instrument for obliterating the lumen of the intestine temporarily before resection.

splayfoot (splā'foot) [M.E. (dis)plaien, to spread out, + A.S. fōt, foot]. A flatfoot or the deformity flatfoot. SYN: *pes planus, talipes valgus.*

spleen (splēn) [G. splēn]. An oval, vascular, ductless gland situated below the diaphragm in the upper abdominal quarter to the left of the cardiac end of the stomach.

About 200 Gm. in weight. Color, livid reddish purple. Blood forming organ. The spleen is sometimes classed as an endocrine gland. It appears to have some relation to the parathyroids and probably has a part in the calcium metabolism of the body. Its liquid extract is used in the treatment of urticaria. It is desiccated and combined with bone marrow in the treatment of some forms of secondary anemia. The French use it in the treatment of tuberculosis.

RS: *flexure, lien, lienomalacia, "splen-" words.*

PALPATION: Only reliable physical signs are those of enlargement. The tumor presents a smooth, oblong, solid mass felt immediately beneath the integuments extending from the ribs on left side, a little behind the origin of the cartilages; often advancing to the median line in one direction and descending to crest of the ilium in the other, filling the left lumbar region at its upper part. Tumor is usually movable, rounded at its upper portion, and presenting an edge more or less sharp in front, where it is often notched and fissured.

PERCUSSION: In health spleen occupies upper portion of left hypochondriac region; its lower border touches the left kidney, while convex surface occupies concavity of diaphragm. Bounded posteriorly above by lower border of 9th rib; anteriorly by stomach and left colon; inferiorly by free margins of ribs. About 4 in. long and 3 in. wide.

To determine boundaries by percussion patient should lie on right side; its *ant. border* is readily determined because of its relation to the stomach and intestine. *Inferiorly,* where it comes in contact with the kidney, it is difficult and often impossible to determine its boundary. Its *sup. border* corresponds to the line which marks the change from dullness to pulmonary resonance. In disease spleen may be increased or diminished, but can rarely recognize diminution in size during life.

DIFFERENTIAL DIAGNOSIS: Must be differentiated from chronic abscess in abdominal wall, which sometimes occurs in exact position of an enlarged spleen, but is too superficial and too soft to belong to an internal viscus.

Cancerous deposit in cardiac extremity of stomach gives rise to a tumor which, descending from margin of ribs, might be mistaken for enlarged spleen.

The sound elicited by forcible percussion has more or less of a tympanic resonance, while the tumor is harder to the feel than an enlarged spleen. Enlarged left lobe of liver is easily distinguished, as margin of tumor can be traced running to right and not to left as in enlarged spleen. *Cancerous and tubercular enlargements* of the omentum are distinguished from enlarged spleen by fact that they extend across abdomen and cannot be traced backward; they do not ascend behind ribs, and are rough, hard and uneven. Fecal accumulations must be excluded as before mentioned.

Left kidney sometimes enlarges toward left hypochondrium and presents a tumor very nearly in situation of enlarged spleen, but by tracing it back toward the loins find its chief bulk is situated posteriorly; it is more fixed; is not forced downward by a full inspiration; if patient is placed on his hands and knees does not fall forward. In enlargements of kidney, intestine is always pushed forward; this is never the case with the spleen. The rules for diagnosis of ovarian tumors will easily distinguish them from enlarged spleen.

s., accessory. Splenic tissue nodules near the spleen.
s., floating or wandering. An enlarged movable one not protected by the ribs.
s., lardaceous. Enlargement of spleen from lardaceous matter. SEE: *amyloid degeneration*.
s. pulp. The spleen's soft parenchyma.
s., sago. One having appearance of sago* grains.
splenadenoma (splē″nad-en-ō′mă) [G. *splēn*, spleen, + *adēn*, gland, + *-ōma*, tumor]. Enlargement of the spleen caused by hyperplasia of its pulp.
splenalgia (splē-năl′jĭ-ă) [″ + *algos*, pain]. Pain in the spleen. SYN: *splenodynia*.
splenauxe (splē-nawk′sē) [″ + *auxē*, increase]. Enlarged condition or hypertrophy of the spleen. SYN: *splenomegaly*.
splenceratosis (splĕn-sĕr-ă-tō′sĭs) [″ + *keras*, *kerat-*, horn, + *-ōsis*, condition]. Induration of the spleen.
splenculus (splĕn′kŭ-lŭs) [L. *splenculus*, tiny spleen]. An accessory spleen. SYN: *splenulus*.
splenectasia (splē-nĕk-tā′zĭ-ă) [G. *splēn*, spleen, + *ektasis*, dilatation]. Enlargement of the spleen.
splenectasis (splē-nĕk′tă-sĭs) [″ + *ektasis*, dilatation]. Enlargement of the spleen. SYN: *splenectasia*.
splenectomy (splē-nĕk′tō-mĭ) [″ + *ektomē*, excision]. Surgical excision of the spleen.
splenectopia, splenectopy (splē-nĕk-tō′pĭ-ă, -nĕk′tō-pĭ) [″ + *ektopos*, out of place]. Displacement or mobility of the spleen. SYN: *spleen, floating*.
splenelcosis (splē-nĕl-kō′sĭs) [″ + *elkōsis*, ulceration]. Ulceration or abscess of the spleen.
splenemia (splē-nē′mĭ-ă) [″ + *aima*, blood]. 1. Leukemia with splenic hypertrophy. 2. Splenic congestion.
splenemphraxis (splē″nĕm-frăks′ĭs) [″ + *emphraxis*, stoppage]. Congested condition of the spleen.
splenepatitis (splĕn-ĕp-ă-tī′tĭs) [G. *splēn*, spleen, + *ēpar*, *ēpat-*, liver, + *-itis*, inflammation]. Inflammation of both spleen and liver.
splenetic, splenic (splē-nĕt′ĭk, splĕn′ĭk) [G. *splēn*, spleen]. 1. Pert. to the spleen. 2. Suffering with chronic disease of the spleen. 3. Surly, fretful, impatient.
s. flexure. Junction of transverse and descending colon, making a bend on the left side near the spleen.
s. vein. One carrying blood from spleen to the portal vein.
splenicterus (splē-nĭk′tĕr-ŭs) [″ + *ikteros*, jaundice]. Inflammation of spleen associated with jaundice.
splenification (splĕn-ĭf-ĭ-kā′shŭn) [″ + L. *facere*, to make]. Change in a structure whereby it resembles splenic tissue. SYN: *splenization*.
splenitis (splē-nī′tĭs) [″ + *-itis*, inflammation]. Inflamed condition of the spleen.
Comprises acute and chronic hypertrophy, proliferative splenitis and suppurative inflammation, result of acute infectious disease.
SYM: Indefinite or absent, usually little pain or tenderness unless perisplenitis exists. Considerable enlargement may be attended by sense of weight, tension or distress in left hypochondrium, accompanied perhaps by slight dyspnea, sudden pain appearing in gastric region followed by vomiting of pus and blood in course of infectious disease with splenic enlargement which may be due to abscess of spleen.

PROG: Depends upon systemic condition.
TREATMENT: Splenectomy useful in simple hypertrophy, but only 20% of recoveries from operation.
splenium (splē′nĭ-ŭm) [G. *splēnion*, bandage]. 1. A compress or bandage. 2. A structure resembling a bandaged part.
s. corporis callosi. The thickened post. end of the corpus callosum.
splenius (splē′nĭ-ŭs) [G. *splēnion*, bandage]. A flat muscle on either side of back of neck and upper thoracic area. SEE: *muscles, back*, for illustration, Table of Muscles in Appendix.
splenization (splĕn-ĭ-zā′shŭn) [G. *splēn*, spleen]. The change in a tissue, as of the lung, when it resembles splenic tissue.
splenoblast (splē′nō-blăst) [″ + *blastos*, germ]. The mother cell of a splenocyte.
splenocele (splē′nō-sēl) [″ + *kēlē*, mass, hernia]. 1. A hernia of the spleen. 2. A splenic tumor.
splenoceratosis (splē″nō-sĕr-ă-tō′sĭs) [″ + *keras*, *kerat-*, horn, + *-ōsis*, condition]. Induration of the spleen.
splenocleisis (splē″nō-klī′sĭs) [″ + *kleisis*, a closure]. Friction on the surface of the spleen or wrapping with gauze to induce the formation of fibrous tissue.
splenocolic (splē″nō-kŏl′ĭk) [″ + *kolon*, colon]. Pert. to the spleen and colon or reference to a fold of peritoneum bet. the two viscera.
splenocyte (splē′nō-sīt) [″ + *kytos*, cell]. A unicellular leukocyte or lymphocyte of the spleen, which probably originates elsewhere in the body.
splenodiagnosis (splē″nō-dī-ăg-nō′sĭs) [G. *splēn*, spleen, + *dia*, through, + *gnōsis*, knowledge]. Injection of typhoid bacilli extract in the spleen to diagnose typhoid fever.
splenodynia (splē″nō-dĭn′ĭ-ă) [″ + *odynē*, pain]. Pain in the spleen. SYN: *splenalgia*.
splenogenic, splenogenous (splē″nō-jĕn′ĭk, splē-nŏj′ĕn-ŭs) [″ + *gennan*, to produce]. Originating or found in the spleen.
splenography (splē-nog′ră-fĭ) [″ + *graphein*, to write]. A treatise on or a description of the spleen.
splenohemia (splē″nō-hē′mĭ-ă) [″ + *haima*, blood]. Congestion of the spleen. SYN: *splenemia*, 2.
splenohepatomegaly (splē″nō-hĕp″ă-tō-mĕg′ă-lĭ) [″ + *hēpar*, *hēpat-*, liver, + *megas*, *megal-*, large]. Enlargement of both spleen and liver.
splenoid (splē′noyd) [″ + *eidos*, resemblance]. Resembling the spleen.
splenokeratosis (splē″nō-kĕr-ă-tō′sĭs) [G. *splēn*, spleen, + *keras*, horn, + *-ōsis*, condition]. Induration of the spleen.
splenology (splē-nŏl′ō-jĭ) [″ + *logos*, study]. The study of the spleen, its functions and diseases.
splenolysin (splē-nŏl′ĭ-sĭn) [″ + *lysis*, dissolution]. An antibody which destroys splenic tissue.
splenolysis (splē-nŏl′ĭ-sĭs) [″ + *lysis*, dissolution]. Destruction of splenic tissue.
splenoma (splē-nō′mă) [″ + *-ōma*, tumor]. A tumor of the spleen. SYN: *splenocele*.
splenomalacia (splē″nō-măl-ā′sĭ-ă) [″ + *malakia*, softening]. Softening of the spleen.
splenomedullary (splē″nō-mĕd′ŭ-la-rĭ) [″ + L. *medulla*, marrow]. Concerning, or formed by, bone marrow and spleen.
s. leukemia. A disease associated with a great increase in leukocytes per cubic millimeter, hemorrhage into skin and

splenomegalia   S-72   **spodogenous**

from mucous membranes, enlargement of spleen, and changes in bone marrow. SEE: *leukemia*.
splenomegalia, splenomegaly (splē″nō-mĕg-ā′lĭ-ā, -mĕg′ă-lĭ) [G. *splēn*, spleen, + *megas, megal-*, large]. Enlargement of the spleen.
splenomyelogenous (splē″nō-mī-ĕl-ŏj′ĕn-ŭs) [″ + *myelos*, marrow, + *gennan*, to produce]. Originating in the spleen and bone marrow, said of a form of leukemia. SYN: *splenomedullary*.
splenomyelomalacia (splē″nō-mī″ĕl-ō-mă-lā′sĭ-ă) [″ + ″ + *malakia*, softening]. Abnormal softening of the spleen and the bone marrow.
splenoncus (splĕ-nŏng′kŭs) [″ + *ogkos*, tumor]. A splenic tumor or hernia. SYN: *splenocele, splenoma*.
splenonephric (splē″nō-nĕf′rĭk) [″ + *nephros*, kidney]. Relating to the spleen and the kidney. SYN: *lienorenal*.
splenonephroptosis (splē″nō-nĕf-rŏp-tō′sĭs) [″ + ″ + *ptōsis*, a dropping]. Displacement of the spleen and kidney downward.
splenopancreatic (splē″nō-păn-krē-ăt′ĭk) [″ + *pagkreas*, pancreas]. Relating to the spleen and pancreas.
splenoparectasis (splē″nō-pă-rĕk′tă-sĭs) [G. *splēn*, spleen, + *parektasis*, a stretching out]. Abnormal enlargement of the spleen.
splenopathy (splē-nŏp′ă-thĭ) [″ + *pathos*, disease]. Any disorder of the spleen.
splenopexy (splē′nō-pĕks-ĭ) [″ + *pēxis*, fixation]. Artificial fixation of a movable spleen.
splenophrenic ligament (splē″nō-frĕn′ĭk) [″ + *phrēn*, diaphragm]. 1. Pert. to the spleen and diaphragm. 2. Peritoneal fold extending bet. the spleen and diaphragm.
splenopneumonia (splē″nō-nū-mō′nĭ-ă) [″ + *pneumōnia*, inflammation of lung]. Pneumonia with splenization of the lung.
splenoptosis (splē-nop-tō′sĭs) [″ + *ptosis*, a dropping]. Displacement of the spleen downward.
splenorrhagia (splē″nō-rā′jĭ-ă) [″ + *-rrhagia*, from *rhēgnynai*, to burst forth]. Hemorrhage from a ruptured spleen.
splenorrhaphy (splē-nor′ăf-ĭ) [G. *splēn*, spleen, + *rhaphē*, a seam]. Suture of wound of the spleen.
splenotherapy (splē″nō-thĕr′ă-pĭ) [″ + *therapeia*, treatment]. Therapeutic administration of splenic tissue or extract.
splenotomy (splē-nŏt′ō-mĭ) [″ + *tomē*, a cutting]. Incision of spleen.
splenulus (splĕn′ū-lŭs) [L. *splenulus*, a little spleen]. A rudimentary or accessory spleen.
splint (splĭnt) [Middle Dutch *splinte*, a wedge]. An appliance made of bone, wood, metal and/or plaster of Paris, used for the fixation, union, or protection of an injured part of the body. They may be movable or immovable.
   s., **aeroplane**. An appliance usually used on ambulatory patients in the treatment of fractures of the humerus, and it takes its name from the elevated (abducted) position in which it holds the arm suspended in air.
   s., **Agnew's**. A splint for fracture of the patella and metacarpus.
   s., **anchor**. A splint for fracture of the jaw, with metal loops fitting over the teeth and held together by a rod.
   s., **Ashhurst's**. A bracketed splint of wire with a footpiece to cover the thigh and leg after excision of the knee joint.
   s., **Balkan**. One for extension in fracture of the femur.

   s., **banjo traction**. Made out of a steel rod bent to resemble the shape of a banjo, and is used for the treatment of contractures and fractures of the fingers.
   s., **Bavarian**. An immovable dressing in which the plaster is applied bet. 2 layers of flannel.
   s., **Bond's**. A splint for fracture of the lower end of the radius.
   s., **Bowlby's**. One for fracture of shaft of humerus.
   s., **bracketed**. A splint composed of 2 pieces of metal or wood united by brackets.
   s., **Cabot's**. A posterior wire splint.
   s., **Carter's intranasal**. A steel bridge with wings connected by a hinge; used for operation of depressed nasal bridge.
   s., **coaptation**. Small splint adjusted about a fractured limb to produce coaptation of fragments.
   s., **Dupuytren's**. A splint to prevent eversion in Pott's fracture.
   s., **Fox's**. A splint for fractured clavicle.
   s., **Gibson walking**. Modification of Thomas' splint.
   s., **Gordon's**. A side splint for the arm and hand in Colles' fracture.
   s., **Jones' nasal**. A splint for fracture of the nasal bones.
   s., **Kanavel**. One for stiff hands.
   s., **Levis'**. A splint of perforated metal extending from below the elbow to the end of the palm; shaped to fit the arm and hand.
   s., **McIntire's**. A post. splint for leg and thigh like a double inclined plane.
   s., **Sayre's**. One of 3 varieties of splint, for the ankle, for the knee, and for use in hip joint disease.
   s., **Stromeyer's**. A splint of 2 hinged portions which can be fixed at any angle.
   s. **technology**. The scientific study of splints.
   s., **Thomas' knee**. A splint for removing the pressure of the body weight from the knee joint by transferring it to the ischium and perineum.
   s., **Thomas' posterior**. A splint used in hip joint disease. [lower extremity].
   s., **Volkmann's**. One for fracture of
splinter (splĭn′ter) [Middle Dutch *splinte*, a wedge]. 1. A fragment from a fractured bone. 2. A slender, sharp piece of wood piercing the skin.
splinting (splĭnt′ĭng) [Middle Dutch *splinte*, a wedge]. Fixation of a fracture or dislocation with a splint.
split (splĭt) [Middle Dutch *splitten*, to divide]. 1. A longitudinal fissure. 2. Characterized by a deep fissure.
   s. **foot**. Congenital deformity, the division of the toes extending into the metatarsal region.
   s. **hand**. Congenital deformity, the division bet. the fingers extending into the metacarpal region. SYN: *cleft hand*.
   s. **pelvis**. Congenital failure of pubic bones to form a union at the symphysis.
   s. **tongue**. Furrowed tongue. SYN: *cleft tongue*.
splitting (splĭt′ĭng) [Middle Dutch *splitten*, to divide]. A change in a complex substance whereby more simple products are produced chemically. SYN: *hydrolysis*, q.v.
spodiomyelitis (spŏ″dĭ-ō-mī-ō-lī′tĭs) [G. *spodios*, ash colored, + *myelos*, marrow, + *-itis*, inflammation]. Inflammation of spinal cord's anterior cornua. SYN: *poliomyelitis*.
spodogenous (spō-dŏj′ĕn-ŭs) [″ + *gennan*,

spodogenous splenomegaly   S-73   **spontaneous fracture**

to produce]. Caused by waste material.
   s. splenomegaly. Enlargement of the spleen due to degenerated red blood cells.
spodogram (spŏd'ō-grăm). The pattern formed of the ash on microincineration of tissue or other matter.
spodophagous (spō-dŏf'ă-gŭs) [" + phagein, to eat]. Destroying the waste matters in the body; said of scavenger cells.
spondylalgia (spŏn"dĭl-ăl'jĭ-ă) [G. spondylos, vertebra, + algos, pain]. Painful condition of a vertebra.
spondylarthritis (spŏn"dĭl-ar-thrī'tĭs) [" + arthron, joint, + -itis, inflammation]. Inflammation of a vertebra.
spondylarthrocace (spŏn"dĭl-ar-thrŏk'ă-sē) [" + " + kakē, badness]. Tuberculous condition of the vertebrae.
spondyl(e (spŏn'dĭl) [G. spondylos, a vertebra]. A vertebra.
spondylexarthrosis (spŏn"dĭl-ĕks"ar-thrō'sĭs) [" + ex, out, + arthron, joint, + -ōsis, condition]. Displacement of a vertebra.
spondylitis (spŏn-dĭl-ī'tĭs) [" + -itis, inflammation]. Inflammation of one or more vertebrae; esp. tuberculous disease of the vertebrae, Pott's disease.
   s. deformans. Inflammation of the vertebral joints resulting in the outgrowth of bonylike deposits on the vertebrae which may fuse and cause rigid and distorted spine.
   s., Kummell's. Traumatic spondylitis in which the symptoms do not appear until some time after the injury.
   s. rhizomelica. Progressive rigidity of the spine caused by ankylosis of the vertebrae from below upward.
   s. tuberculosa. Tuberculosis of the vertebral joints. SYN: vertebral caries, Pott's disease.
spondylizema (spŏn"dĭl-ĭ-zē'mă) [G. spondylos, vertebrae, + izēma, depression]. Downward settlement of a vertebra caused by the disintegration of the one below it. [a vertebra.
spondylo- [G.]. Combining form meaning
spondylocace (spŏn-dĭ-lŏk'ă-sē) [G. spondylos, vertebrae, + kakē, badness]. Tuberculosis of the vertebrae. SYN: spondylarthrocace.
spondylodiagnosis (spŏn"dī-lō-dī-ăg-nō'sĭs) [" + dia, through, + gnōsis, knowledge]. Diagnosis by means of visceral reflexes obtained by percussion of the vertebrae.
spondylodynia (spŏn"dĭl-ō-dĭn'ĭ-ă) [" + odynē, pain]. Pain in a vertebra.
spondylolisthesis (spŏn"dĭl-ō-lĭs-thē'sĭs) [" + olisthēsis, a slipping]. Forward subluxation of the lower lumbar vertebrae, usually on the sacrum, with consequent pelvic deformity.
spondylolysis (spŏn-dĭ-lŏl'ĭ-sĭs) [" + lysis, a dissolution]. The breaking down of a vertebral structure.
spondylopathy (spŏn"dĭl-ŏp'ă-thĭ) [" + pathos, disease]. Any disorder of the vertebrae.
spondylopyosis (spŏn"dĭl-ō-pī-ō'sĭs) [" + pyōsis, suppuration]. Suppuration with inflammation of the vertebrae.
spondyloschisis (spŏn-dĭl-ŏs'kĭ-sĭs) [G. spondylos, vertebra, + schisis, a cleft]. Congenital fissure of one or more of the vertebral arches. SYN: rhachioschisis.
spondylosis (spŏn-dĭ-lō'sĭs) [" + -ōsis, condition]. Vertebral ankylosis.
   s., rhizomelic. Ankylosis interfering with movements of hips and shoulders.
spondylosyndesis (spŏn"dĭ-lō-sĭn'dĕ-sĭs) ["

+ syndesis, a binding together]. Surgical formation of an ankylosis bet. vertebrae.
spondylotherapy (spŏn"dĭl-ō-thĕr'ă-pī) [" + therapeia, treatment]. Spinal therapeutics; spinal manipulation in the treatment of disease.
spondylotomy (spŏn-dĭl-ŏt'ō-mĭ) [" + tomē, a cutting]. Removal of part of the vertebral column to correct a deformity or facilitate delivery of a fetus.
sponge (spŭnj) [G. spoggia, sponge]. 1. Elastic, porous mass forming internal skeleton of certain marine animals used in surgery to mop up fluids and in bathing. 2. An absorbent pad made of gauze and cotton. 3. Short for sponge bath. Procured dry, loose or on strings or moist, sterilized in jars of 1 or 2 dozen. Do not buy by the pound as they may be loaded with sand.
   s., abdominal. Flat sponges from ½ to 1 in. thick, 3 to 6 in. in diameter, used as packing, to prevent closing or obstruction by intrusion of viscera, as covering to prevent tissue injury, and as absorbents.
   s., artificial. Constructed of antiseptic gauze.
   s. bath. Bathing of the body with a wet sponge.
   s. graft. S. placed in an ulcer to cause granulation.
   s. sterilization. Should be chemical, not by steam or boiling water. Clean or soak in cold water, wrap in linen towel or sack, immerse in 1% hot soda solution, 20 to 30 minutes. Remove, immerse in sack in sterilized water, then preserve in an antiseptic solution.
   s. tent. One impregnated with mucilage of acacia, dried in desired shape, to dilate the os uteri or sinuses by absorbing moisture and expanding.
spongiform (spŭn'jĭ-form) [G. spoggos, sponge, + L. forma, form]. Having the appearance or quality of a sponge.
spongioblast (spŭn'jĭ-ō-blăst) [" + blastos, germ]. 1. An embryonic neuroglia cell of the layer of columnar cells in the neural tube. 2. A modified nerve cell process. [cell]. A neuroglia cell.
spongiocyte (spŭn'jĭ-ō-sīt) [" + kytos,
spongioid (spŭn'jĭ-oyd) [" + eidos, resemblance]. Resembling a sponge. SYN: spongiform.
spongiopilin (spŭn-jĭ-ō-pī'lĭn) [" + pilos, felt]. A loosely woven cotton fabric containing bits of sponge and coated on one side with India rubber, used as a poultice.
spongioplasm (spŭn-jĭ-ō-plăzm) [" + plasma, a thing formed]. Fibrillar network supporting protoplasm. SYN: cytoreticulum.
spongy (spŭn'jĭ) [G. spoggios, sponge]. Resembling a sponge in texture.
   s. body. Spongy portion of the penis surrounding the urethra. SYN: corpus spongiosum.
   s. bone. 1. A turbinate bone. 2. Cancellous bone of a spongy texture.
   s. portion. That part of the urethra within the corpus spongiosum.
spontaneous (spŏn-tā'nē-ŭs) [L. spontaneus, voluntary]. Occurring unaided or without apparent cause; voluntary.
   s. evolution. A rare method by which the fetus is expelled from the uterus while lying in the transverse position. Only possible (a) when the fetus is very small and pelvis large, (b) when fetus is dead.
   s. fracture. Fracture due to the state

spontaneous version   S-74   **sprain**

of the bone and causing little or no injury.
ETIOL: *Fragilitas ossium,* nerve conditions, *i.e., tabes,* secondary malignant growths, *atrophy* in bones of the aged.
s. version. The unaided conversion of a transverse presentation into a vertex or breech presentation.
spoon (spōōn) [A.S. *spōn,* a chip]. Instrument consisting of a small bowl on a handle, used in scooping out tissues, tumors, etc., or in measuring quantities.
s. nail. A nail having a concave outer surface.
sporadic (spō-răd'ĭk) [G. *sporadikos,* scattered]. Occurring occasionally or in scattered instances, as a disease.
RS: *endemic, epidemic, pandemic.*
sporadoneure (spō-răd'ō-nūr) [G. *sporas, sporad-,* scattered, + *neuron,* nerve]. A nerve cell occurring outside of the ganglia or nerve centers in any tissue.
sporangiophore (spō-răn'jĭ-ō-fōr) [G. *sporos,* seed, + *aggeion,* vessel, + *phoros,* a bearer]. BACT: The supporting stalk for a spore sac of certain fungi.
sporangium (spō-răn'jĭ-ŭm) [" + *aggeion,* vessel]. A sac enclosing spores, seen in certain fungi.
spore (spōr) [G. *sporos,* a seed]. Any germ or reproductive element of a plant or protozoan less organized than a true cell.
Sporing is an asexual method of reproduction in many unicellular animals and plants. Certain bacteria also form spores, but more in the nature of a defensive mechanism than for reproduction.
The spores of bacteria are difficult to destroy, as they are very resistant to heat and require prolonged exposure to high temperatures to destroy them.
RS: *apospory, asporogenic, asporous.*
sporicidal (spor-ĭs-ī'dăl) [G. *sporos,* seed, + L. *cidus,* from *caedere,* to kill]. Destructive to spores.
sporicide (spor'ĭs-īd) [" + L. *cidus,* from *caedere,* to kill]. An agent which destroys spores.
sporidium (spor-ĭd'ĭ-ŭm) [L. a little spore]. An embryonic protozoan organism.
sporiferous (spor-ĭf'ĕr-ŭs) [G. *sporos,* seed, + L. *ferre,* to bear]. Producing spores.
sporoblast (spor'ō-blăst) [" + *blastos,* germ]. A secondary cyst within the oöcyst, giving rise to the sporozoite, in certain protozoans.
sporocyst (spor'ō-sĭst) [" + *kystis,* sac]. 1. Sac secreted by certain protozoans prior to spore production. 2. A stage in development of trematode worms in which the int. lining gives off cells, which develop in the cavity.
sporogenesis (spor"ō-jĕn'ĕ-sĭs) [" + *genesis,* production]. Reproduction by spores. SYN: *sporogony.*
sporogenic (spor"ō-jĕn'ĭk) [" + *gennan,* to produce]. Having the ability of developing into spores.
sporogony (spor-ŏg'ō-nĭ) [" + *gonē,* generation]. Reproducing by development of spores. SYN: *sporogenesis.*
sporont (spor'ŏnt) [" + *ontos,* being]. A sexually mature protozoan detached from its host in its sexual cycle.
It produces *anisopores* from which are formed *zygotes* which in turn develop *schizonts, q.v.*
sporophore (spor'ō-fōr) [G. *sporos,* seed, + *phoros,* a bearer]. Part of a plant which bears the seeds.
sporophyte (spor'ō-fīt) [" + *phyton,* plant]. The spore-bearing stage of a plant exhibiting alternation of generation.
sporoplasm (spor'ō-plăzm) [" + *plasma,* a thing formed]. Protoplasm of the ovum.
sporotrichosis (spor"ō-trī-kō'sĭs) [" + *thrix, trich-,* hair, + *-ōsis,* condition]. Infection or mycosis caused by sporotricha affecting the skin and mucosa of the mouth and pharynx.
Sporotrichum (spō-rŏt'rĭ-kŭm) (pl. *Sporotricha*) [" + *thrix, trich-,* hair]. A yeastlike genus of microörganisms.
Of the pathogenic species, one is the causative agent of sporotrichosis.*
Sporozoa (spor"ō-zō'ă) [" + *zōon,* animal]. A class of protozoa, some of which are parasitic and which reproduce by spore formation.
sporozoite (spor"ō-zō'īt) [" + *zōon,* animal]. An elongated, sickle-shaped body formed by division of an oöcyst after fertilization.
In malaria, it is introduced by the bite of a mosquito into an erythrocyte.
sport (spōrt) [O.Fr. *(de) sporter,* to carry away]. An individual organism which spontaneously differs from its parents or from type. SYN: *mutation.*
sporulation (spor-ū-lā'shŭn) [L. *sporula,* little spore]. Production of spores or method of reproduction of unicellular organisms.
sporule (spor'ūl) [L. *sporula,* a little spore]. A spore, or a small one.
spot (spŏt) [M.E. a small bit]. A small area of surface differing from surrounding parts in appearance. SYN: *loculus, macula, papule, pustule.*
s., blind. The optic disk where optic nerve enters the retina.
s., embryonic. Nucleolus of the ovum.
s's., Filatow's, s's., Flindt's. SEE: *Koplik's spots.*
s., germinal. Same as embryonic s.
s., hectic. Bright red s. on cheek from hectic fever.
s., hypnogenic. A point which, when pressed, will throw a susceptible person into hypnosis or sleep.
s., hysterogenic. A point which, upon pressure, will induce in a susceptible subject an attack of hysteroepilepsy.
s., Koplik's. Minute white spots or bluish-white ones on mucous membrane of mouth before appearance of the rash of measles.
s's., rose. Rose-colored maculae of eruption in typhoid fever.
s., yellow. Area surrounding and including the *fovea centralis* in the retina. SYN: *macula lutea.*
spot'ted fe'ver. Popular name for various eruptive fevers: 1. Typhus. 2. Tick fever. 3. Cerebrospinal meningitis.
sprain (sprān) [O.Fr. *espreindre,* to wring]. 1. To wrench a joint. 2. The forcible wrenching of a joint, with partial rupture or other injury of its attachments, and without luxation of bones.
A few fibers may be torn, or tendons or ligaments at the joint may be wrenched or torn. The ankle joint is most often sprained. SEE: *fracture, strain.*
SYM: The signs of a sprain are rapid swelling, heat, and disability; often discoloration and limitation of function, frequently associated with small fractures. The pain is usually great, and is much increased by moving.
TREATMENT: Hot or cold compresses and bandaging; elevate the joint. If recovery proves slow, immobilization of the joint is indicated followed by care-

sprain of back   S-75   **sputum**

ful massage. Very cold water with salt or injections of procaine into injured ligament alleviate the condition quickly.

s. of back. Overstretching of muscles, ligaments or other structures of spinal mechanism, often associated with small fractures.

SYM: Pain, esp. on extreme movements; tenderness; muscle spasm.

F. A. TREATMENT: Have patient lie down on rigid support, do not allow to sit up or walk until fracture is ruled out; intermittent heat, rest, with adhesive strapping, brace, etc.

s. of foot. Usually a fracture or tearing of the ligaments of the foot or ankle.

SYM: Pain, tenderness, swelling, discoloration.

TREATMENT: Sprain is best treated as a fracture, by complete immobilization until proven otherwise by x-ray examination.

s. fracture. The separation of a tendon or ligament from its insertion, taking with it a piece of the bone.

s., riders'. Sprain of the adductor longus muscles of the thigh, resulting from strain in riding horseback.

spray (sprā) [Middle Dutch *sprayen*, to sprinkle]. 1. A jet of fine medicated vapor applied to a diseased part or discharged into the air. 2. An instrument for applying such a spray. SYN: *atomizer*. 3. To discharge fluid in a fine stream.

s. tube. Device for converting liquid into a spray.

spreading (sprĕd'ĭng) [A.S. *sprǣdan*, to strew]. BACT: Noting a growth extending much (several mm. or more) beyond the site of inoculation.

spring (sprĭng) [A.S. *spring*, a rising]. 1. The 1st of the 4 annular seasons. SYN: *vernal season*. 2. A flying back of a body to its original position through its elasticity.

s. conjunctivitis. A form recurring each year in the spring but disappearing with the first frost. SYN: *vernal catarrh*.

s.-finger. Arrested movement of a finger in flexion or extension followed by a jerk. SYN: *trigger finger*.

s. ligament. Int. calcaneoscaphoid ligament of the sole of the foot. It joins the os calcis to the scaphoid bone.

sprue (sprū) [Dutch *sprouw*]. 1. A form of stomatitis with ulcers, due to a fungus. SYN: *thrush*. 2. Tropical disease with chronic diarrhea and digestive disturbances, accompanied by chronic inflammation of the bowel, atrophy of its wall, and ulceration of the mouth. SYN: *psilosis*.

spud (spŭd) [M.E. a knife]. Short, flattened, spadelike blade to dislodge a foreign substance.

spur (spŭr) [A.S. *spora*, a pointed instrument]. A projecting sliver of bone, tissue, or horny outgrowth from the skin.

spurious (spū'rĭ-ŭs) [L. *spurius*, false]. Not true or genuine; adulterated; false.

sputum (spū'tŭm) (pl. *sputa*) [L. *sputum*, from *spuere*, to spit]. Substance ejected from the mouth containing saliva and mucus, and sometimes pus.

Its appearance depends upon the underlying condition as follows:

AMOUNT: *Copious*: This is seen in chronic inflammations of bronchial and pulmonary systems.

Scanty: This obtains in all pulmonary bronchial acute inflammations, and in the early stages of lobar pneumonia, and beginning bronchopneumonia.

COLOR: This depends upon its origin, cause, and amount of decomposition.

CONDITIONS: *Anthracosis* (coal dust): The sputum is black.

Bronchiectasis: The sputum is mucopurulent, and foul if expectoration is infrequent.

Bronchial asthma: Scanty sputum and frothy, later becoming purulent and

**Sputum: Varieties of[1]
The Character and Diseases in Which They Occur**

Variety of Sputum	Character of Sputum	Diseases in Which the Various Types Occur
Mucoid.	Clear, thin, may be somewhat viscid.	Early stages of bronchitis.
Mucopurulent.	Thick, viscid, greenish color, inoffensive, frothy, may have sweetish odor.	Later stages of bronchitis, phthisis, pneumonia.
Purulent.	Thick, viscid yellow; often offensive.	Abscess of lung, empyema, advanced phthisis, bronchiectasis.
Nummular.	Mucopurulent, with small, round, semisolid masses which sink in water.	Advanced phthisis.
Rusty.	Mucopurulent, very viscid and gelatinous; rusty tinge.	Pneumonia.
Prune juice.	Dark brown, offensive, often semisolid.	Later stages of pneumonia, gangrene of lung, new growth of lung.
Red currant jelly.	Blood clots resembling currant jelly.	New growth in lung.
Blood (hemoptysis).	Bright red, frothy, with air bubbles; blood may be in streaks or mixed with sputum, fluid or clotted, or sputum may consist of pure blood.	Phthisis (ulceration of a vessel in a cavity); other diseases of the lung (pneumonia, new growth, gangrene, abscess, bronchiectasis); mitral stenosis; aneurysm rupturing into the bronchial tubes.

[1] Faber's *Nurses' Pocket Encyclopedia*.

grayish, containing eosinophiles.
Bronchitis: The sputum is mucous, later purulent, and in chronic cases, greenish-yellow and thick.
Bronchopneumonia: It is frothy, mucoid, thin, mucopurulent, copious, often with blood, or prune juice in color.
Calcinosis: Shows a sputum containing particles of lime, or chalky deposits such as plaster of Paris.
Empyema: If accompanied by perforations, the sputum resembles that of pulmonary abscess.
Gangrene of lung and putrid bronchitis: The sputum has an obnoxious odor and is purulent, separates on standing into 3 layers containing pus cells, hematoidin crystals and leukocytes.
Lobar pneumonia: It is scanty and viscid, yellowish, and somewhat mucopurulent during early stages, and in later stages, rusty, bloody, tenacious and viscid, esp. near or soon after crisis.
Pulmonary abscess: Usually purulent and fetid with many pus cells, and pieces of lung tissue.
Pulmonary tuberculosis: In early stages, scanty, whitish, or grayish-yellow, frothy and expectorated in small quantities during coughing. Later, when consolidation takes place, it becomes more copious, tenacious and yellowish-gray, and in the late stages, it becomes mucopurulent, musty and fetid, containing fibers and tubercle bacilli, sometimes blood-tinged or mixed with blood.
Pneumonoconiosis: Depends upon the character of dust inhaled.
Siderosis: It contains particles of iron or other metals, and it resembles that of chronic bronchitis. It also contains alveolar cells.
Silicosis: Produces a sputum containing particles of silica, or other stone dusts.
NP: Instruct patients to cough or sneeze into paper napkins, and to expectorate into a sputum box, which should be burned. Cotton and linen handkerchiefs when used should be immersed in boiling water for 20 minutes. Sputum may be disinfected with 5% phenol or 5% formalin by 1 hour's exposure.
Paper sputum cups should be disposed of if there is any evidence of dried sputum on them. Handkerchiefs and gauze should not be used unless disposed of immediately after using. A paper bag should be attached to the bed or the bedside table and the patient instructed how to use it as a receptacle for sputum Paper wipes or squares of cloth, or soft tissues may be used for wiping away the discharge and disposing of in the bag. The bag may be made of newspaper in a conical shape and pinned on, then, as the deposit accumulates, it is removed and another bag replaced. The patient should be instructed to fold the paper well over the material deposited. When removing, the paper should be well folded over and placed in the waste can or burned at once.
RS: *albuminoptysis, albuminoreaction, Charcot-Robin crystals.*
s., bloody. This is seen, of course, in hemorrhages. If the blood is mixed with the sputum the hemorrhage is in the finer bronchioles. Large quantities of blood indicate rupture of larger vessel.
s., currant jelly or **raspberry.** Indicates tumor of a lung. If of a fetid odor, bronchitis.
s., fruity. This precedes rupture of an echinococcus cyst. The sputum may be bloody, mucous, mucopurulent, purulent, serous, frothy and in plugs, or it may contain elastic fibers and fibrinous bronchial casts; also bacteria, tubercles, pneumococci, influenza bacteria, diphtheria bacteria, staphylococci, streptococci, and pneumococci.

s., nummular. Round, coin-shaped, flat forms which sink in water; seen in bronchiectasis and advanced pulmonary tuberculosis.

s., prune juice. Thin, reddish, bloody s. in gangrene, cancer of the lung and certain pneumonias.

s., rusty. This is seen in lobar pneumonia.

s., septicemia. S. acquired from inoculation with organisms in saliva or sputum.

squama (sqwā'mă) (pl. *squamae*) [L. *squama*, a scale]. 1. A thin plate of bone. 2. A scale from the epidermis.

squamoparietal (skwā″mō-pă-rī′ĕ-tăl) ["+ *paries, pariet-*, wall]. Relating to the squamous and parietal bones.

squamosa (skwā-mō′să) [L. *squamōsa*, scaly]. The squamous part of temporal bone.

squamous (skwā′mŭs) [L. *squama*, scale]. Scalelike.
s. bone. Upper anterior portion of temporal bone.
s. cell. Flat, scaly, epithelial cell.
s. epithelium. Flat form of epithelial cells.
s. suture. Line uniting squamosa and parietal bone.

square knot (skwăr). Double knot in which ends and standing parts are together and parallel to each other.
This is used universally because it holds well and because of ease in tying and untying it.
Hold one end in each hand, carry right end over left end and make a loop or simple knot. Now reverse, carry left end over right end and again tie, thus forming a simple symmetrical knot. If this is not done, a false or "granny" knot results which usually slips. To untie, steady the knot, take one end and draw it over knot and then continue pulling this direction until knot slips or jumps, forming 2 half hitches, when it may be slipped off.
s. lobe. 1. The quadrate lobe of the liver. SYN: *lobus quadratus.* 2. A lobe on upper surface of the cerebellum.

squarrose, squarrous (skwăr′ōs, -ŭs) [L. *squarrōsus*, scurfy]. Scurfy or scaly; full of scabs or scales.

squash (skwŏsh) [Algonquin *asquash*, raw]. Av. SERVING (summer and winter): 200-100 Gm. Pro. 0.5-1.00, Fat—0.3, Carbo. 3.5-4.00.
VITAMINS: A+++ for both, B+ both, G+ both
ASH CONST. (summer s. without seeds and winter s.): Ca 0.018-0.019, Mg 0.008-0.011, K 0.150-0.320, Na 0.002-0.004, Fe 0.0006-0.0006.

squat'ting position. One in which patient stoops with knees pressed on abdomen. SYN: *kneeling-squatting position.*

squill (skwĭl) [G. *skilla*]. USP. A drug once popular as an expectorant and diuretic.
DOSAGE: ½ ℳ (0.1 cc.)
s., syrup and **s., compound syrup.** Used to some extent at present.
DOSAGE: 30 ℳ (2 cc.).

squint (skwĭnt) [origin uncertain]. 1. Abnormality in which both the visual axes do not bear toward an objective point

simultaneously. SYN: *strabismus*. 2. To close the eyes partly, as in excess light. 3. To be unable to direct both eyes simultaneously toward a point.
  s., convergent. Condition existing when eyes are turned toward the medial line. SYN: *esotropia*.
  s., divergent. Condition existing when eyes are turned outwards. SYN: *exotropia*.
  s., external. Same as *divergent*.
  s., internal. Same as *convergent*.
Sr. Symb. of *strontium*.
ss. [L.]. Abbr. for *semis*, half.
s. s. & p. enema. A mixture of 1 dram of peppermint added to a soapsuds solution given to relieve flatulence. SEE: *enema*.
s. s. & t. enema. Compound cleaning enema using a mixture of thick liquid soap. SEE: *enema*.
ST. 37. Proprietary germicide and disinfectant. SYN: *caprokol, hexylresorcinol, q.v.*
stab (stăb) [Gaelic *stob*, to pierce]. 1. To pierce with a knife. 2. Inoculum plunged deeply into a solid culture medium with a wire or needle; also, the culture so produced.
  s. culture. Bacterial culture in which organism is introduced into a solid gelatin medium with a wire or needle.
stabile (stā′bĭl) [L. *stabilis*, standing]. Not moving; fixed.
  s. current. An electric current generated by holding stationary electrodes in a fixed position.
stable (stā′bl) [L. *stabilis*, standing]. Firm; steady.
  s. elements. Tissue cells which no longer multiply by mitosis.
staccato speech or **utterance** (stah-kah′tō) [Italian *staccato*, separated]. Jerky pronunciation with words and syllables separated by pauses. SYN: *scanning speech*. SEE: *speech*.
stactometer (stăk-tŏm′ĕt-ĕr) [G. *staktos*, dropping, + *metron*, a measure]. Instrument for counting drops.
stadium (stā′dĭ-ŭm) [G. *stadion*, a measure]. A stage or period, as of a disease.
  s. acmes. The height of a disease.
  s. augmenti. Period of rising temperature or other symptoms.
  s. decrementi. Period of defervescence or decrease of symptoms.
  s. florescentiae. Stage of eruption in an exanthematous disease.
  s. frigoris. Cold stage in intermittent fevers, as malaria.
  s. incrementi. Period of increase of fever or symptoms.
  s. invasionis. Incubative stage of an infectious disease.
  s. sudoris. Sweating stage of a paroxysm of malaria.
staff (stăf) [A.S. *staef*, a stick]. 1. An instrument to be introduced into the urethra and bladder as a guide to a surgical knife. 2. The medical corps attached to a hospital.
  s., attending. Attending physicians and surgeons of a hospital.
  s., consulting. Physicians and surgeons attached to a hospital who may be consulted by members of the attending staff.
  s. of Wrisberg. Prominence of the cuneiform cartilage seen in the normal larynx during examination.
stage (stāj) [O.Fr. *estage*, from L. *stāre*, to stand]. 1. A period in the course of a disease. SYN: *stadium*. 2. The platform of a microscope.

  s., algid. The cold stage or s. of collapse in cholera.
  s., amphibolic. Stage which intervenes bet. acme of a disease and its outcome.
  s., asphyxial. Preliminary stage of Asiatic cholera.
  s., cold. Chill or rigor of a malarial paroxysm.
  s., eruptive. Period in which an exanthem appears.
  s., expulsive. Stage of dilatation of the cervix uteri during which the child is expelled from uterus.
  s., first. Period when the fetal head is molded and the cervix dilated.
  s., hot. Febrile s. in a malarial paroxysm.
  s. of invasion. Period in which a morbific influence precedes the onset of a disease.
  s. of latency. The incubation period of an infectious disease.
  s., preëruptive. Stage following infection and before appearance of eruption.
  s., pyrogenetic. Stage of invasion in a febrile disease.
  s., sweating. The 3rd or terminal s. of malaria during which sweating occurs.
stagnation (stăg-nā′shŭn) [L. *stagnāre*, from *stagnum*, pool]. 1. Cessation of motion. 2. PATH: A stoppage of motion of any fluid in the body, as blood. SYN: *stasis*.
stagnin (stăg′nĭn) [L. *stagnum*, a pool]. A commercial preparation from the spleen of horses, causing coagulation of the blood.
stain (stăn) [M.E. (*di*)*steinen*, from L. *dis*, apart, + *tingere*, to color]. 1. Any discoloration. 2. A pigment used in coloring microscopic objects and tissues. 3. To apply pigment to a tissue or microscopic object.
  s., acid. Stain produced by an acid.
  s., basic. A nonacid (aniline salt) stain.
  s., contrast. One used to color one part of a tissue or cell unaffected when another part is stained by another color.
  s., green. A greenish fungous deposit on the teeth.
  s., neutral. A combination of an acid and a basic stain.
  s., nuclear. A basic stain affecting nuclei.
  s., plasmatic, s., plasmic. One which colors uniformly.
  s's., removal from linen. SEE: *antistain formulary*.
staining (stān′ĭng) [M.E. (*di*)*steinen*, from L. *dis*, apart, + *tingere*, to color]. Process of impregnating a substance, esp. a tissue, with pigments so that its component parts may be visible under a microscope.
  Wright's technic for bloodstains: Five drops of Wright's stain on a dried film and left for 1 minute, then add 5 drops of distilled water, leave for 2 minutes. Gently wash film with distilled water until blue color just disappears and pink color appears. Then dry with blotting paper and mount in balsam. If the stain is good, red cells take a pinkish or copper color and white cells have blue nuclei, with respective granules differentiated.
staircase (stâr′kās) [A.S. *staēger*, to rise, + M.E. *case*, from L. *capsa*, box]. A continuous series of reactions of progressive intensity, a phenomenon seen when a muscle, particularly that of the heart, is stimulated rapidly at regular intervals after a period of rest.

The first few contractions increase in height until a maximum is reached.
SYN: *treppe*.
stalagmometer (stă-lăg-mŏm'ĕ-tĕr) [G. *stalagmos*, dropping, + *metron*, a measure]. Instrument for measuring number of drops in a given amount of fluid.
stamina (stăm'ĭn-ă) [L. *stamina*, fibers]. Inherent force; constitutional energy; strength; endurance.
stammering (stăm'er-ĭng) [A.S. *stamerian*]. Hesitant or faltering speech disorder.
May be due to hesitation, mispronunciation, transposing the letters l, r, or s, and repetition. SEE: *speech*.
RS: *lalling, mytacism*.
  s. of bladder. Interrupted and irregular flow of urine, the muscles acting spasmodically.
standard (stăn'dard) [O.Fr. *estandart*]. That which is established by custom or authority as a model, criterion or rule for comparison of measurement.
  s. solution. A solution of fixed strength, used as a reagent.
stannum (stăn'ŭm) [L.]. Tin; a metallic element. SYMB: Sn. At. wt. 119.
stapedectomy (stă-pē-děk'tō-mĭ) [L. *stapes*, stirrup, + G. *ektomē*, excision]. Excision of the stapes in the ear.
stapedial (stă-pē'dĭ-ăl) [L. *stapes*, stirrup]. Relating to the stapes.
stapediotenotomy (stă-pē"dĭ-ō-těn-ŏt'ō-mĭ) [" + G. *tenōn*, tendon, + *tomē*, a cutting]. Division of the tendon of the stapedius muscle.
stapediovestibular (stă-pē"dĭ-ō-věs-tĭb'ū-lar) [" + *vestibulum*, an antechamber]. Relating to the stapes and vestibule of the ear.
stapedius (stă-pē'dĭ-ŭs) [L. *stapes*, stirrup]. A small muscle of the middle ear inserted in the stapes. SEE: *Table of Muscles in Appendix*.
stapes (stā'pēz) [L. *stapes*, stirrup]. Ossicle in middle ear which articulates with the incus.
The footplate of the stapes fits into oval window. SEE: *ear*.
staphyle (stăf'ĭ-lē) [G. *staphylē*, bunch of grapes]. Pendulous, fleshy mass hanging from the soft palate. SYN: *uvula, q.v.*
staphylectomy (stăf-ĭl-ěk'tō-mĭ) [" + *ektomē*, excision]. Amputation of the uvula. SYN: *staphylotomy, uvulotomy*.
staphyledema (stăf-ĭl-ē-dē'mă) [" + *oidēma*, swelling]. Swelling of the uvula.
staphyline (stăf'ĭ-līn) [G. *staphylē*, a bunch of grapes]. 1. Relating to the uvula. SYN: *uvular*. 2. Resembling a bunch of grapes. SYN: *botryoid*.
staphylinopharyngeus (stăf"ĭ-lĭ"nō-făr-ĭn'-jē-ŭs) [" + *pharygx*, pharynx]. Muscle in undersurface of soft palate which contracts the fauces and elevates back of the tongue. SEE: *Table of Muscles in Appendix*.
staphylinus (stăf-ĭ-lī'nŭs) [G. *staphylē*, a bunch of grapes]. One of 2 muscles which elevate the soft palate and make it tense. SEE: *Table of Muscles in Appendix*.
staphylion (stăf-ĭl'ĭ-ŏn) [G. *staphylion*, little grape]. Craniometric point at median line of posterior border of hard palate.
staphylitis (stăf-ĭl-ī'tĭs) [G. *staphylē*, a bunch of grapes, + *-itis*, inflammation]. Inflammation of uvula.
staphylo- [G.]. Combining form meaning the *uvula*.
staphyloangina (stăf"ĭl-ō-ăn-jī'nă) [G. *staphylē*, bunch of grapes, + L. *angina*, sore throat]. Sore throat due to staphylococcus.
staphylobacterin (stăf"ĭl-ō-băk'tĕr-ĭn) [" + *baktērion*, a little rod]. A staphylococcic bacterial vaccine.
staphylococcemia (stăf"ĭl-ō-kŏk-sē'mĭ-ă) [" + *kokkos*, berry, + *aima*, blood]. The presence of staphylococcus in the blood. SEE: *staphylomycosis*.
Staphylococcus (stăf-ĭl-ō-kŏk'ŭs) [" + *kokkos*, berry]. A class of minute, round organisms found in clusters like bunches of grapes.
A genus of the family Coccaceae producing orange to white pigment. The *S. albus* are white; *S. citreus*, yellow, and *S. aureus*, golden.
  S. albus. Mild form in boils, abscesses, etc.
  S. aureus. Species found in boils, on mucous membranes, in abscesses, and on the skin; also in other suppurative inflammations.
  S. cereus aureus. Species found in nasal mucus in coryza.
  S. cereus flavus. Species found in pus causing yellow color.
  S. pyogenes albus. Form causing suppuration.
  S. pyogenes aureus. A pus-producing form.
  S. viridis flavescens. Species found in lesions of varicella, causing greenish-yellow color.
staphylodialysis (stăf-ĭ-lō-dī-ăl'ĭ-sĭs) [G. *staphylē*, a bunch of grapes, + *dialysis*, a loosening]. Relaxation of the uvula.
staphylohemia (stăf-ĭ-lō-hē'mĭ-ă) [" + *haima*, blood]. Staphylococci in the blood. SYN: *staphylococcemia*.
staphylolysin (stăf-ĭ-lol'ĭ-sĭn) [" + *lysis*, dissolution]. 1. The hemolysin thrown off by a staphylococcus. 2. An antibody producing lysis of staphylococci.
staphyloma (stăf-ĭ-lō'mă) [G. *staphylōma*, grape tumor]. Protrusion of cornea produced by a perforating keratitis.
  s., anterior. Globular enlargement of ant. part of the eye. SYN: *keratoglobus*.
  s. corneae. Thinning and bulging of the cornea.
  s., partial. Extends in one direction displacing the pupil; the remainder of the cornea is clear.
  s., posterior, s. posticum. Bulging of sclera backward.
  s., total. Opaque protuberant, cicatrix found in place of cornea.
  ETIOL: Perforation of cornea. Result: Poor vision, increased tension, rupture of thin scar.
  TREATMENT: Prophylaxis, incision, excision, ablation.
staphylomycosis (stăf"ĭl-ō-mī-kō'sĭs) [G. *staphylē*, a bunch of grapes, + *mykēs*, fungus, + *-ōsis*, condition]. The systemic condition resulting from staphylococci in blood. SYN: *staphylococcemia*.
staphyloncus (stăf-ĭ-long'kŭs) [" + *ogkos*, tumor]. A tumor or enlargement of the uvula.
staphylopharyngeus (stăf"ĭl-ō-far-ĭn'jē-ŭs) [" + *pharygx*, pharynx]. Muscle of soft palate narrowing fauces and occluding nasopharynx. SEE: *Table of Muscles in Appendix*.
staphyloplasty (stăf'ĭ-lō-plăs-tĭ) [" + *plassein*, to form]. Plastic surgery of the uvula or soft palate.
staphyloptosia, staphyloptosis (stăf"ĭ-lŏp-tō'sĭ-ă, -sĭs) [" + *ptōsis*, a dropping]. Relaxation or elongation of the uvula.
SYN: *staphylodialysis*.
staphylorrhaphy (stăf-ĭl-or'ă-fĭ) [" +

rhaphē, a seam]. Suture of a cleft palate.
staphyloschisis (stăf-ĭ-los'kĭ-sĭs) [" + *schisis*, a fissure]. Fissure of the uvula. SYN: *cleft palate*.
staphylotomy (stăf-ĭ-lŏt'ō-mĭ) [" + *tomē*, a cutting]. Amputation of the uvula.
star [A.S. *steorra*]. Any structure resembling a star. SYN: *aster*.
　s., daughter. A figure forming the diaster in mitosis.
　s's. of Verheyen. Star-shaped masses of veins in renal cortex. SYN: *venae stellatae*.
starch [M.E. *starche*, from A.S. *stearc*, stiff]. Noncrystalline carbohydrate of the polysaccharose* group found in plants.
　The polysaccharoses include *vegetable starches*, *animal starch* (glycogen), *celluloses*, *pectins*, *dextrins*, and *gums*, among which it is difficult to make distinctions. All of them are rather easily decomposed, have high molecular weights and yield monosaccharoses on complete hydrolysis.
　Those which the body is able to hydrolyze into hexoses are useful as concentrated energy giving foods. They all must be reduced to simple sugars, except cellulose, before they may be absorbed. What is not needed is stored in the liver as glycogen. They are heat and energy producing foods. In some fruits the starch is changed to sugar when they ripen, while some vegetables (peas and corn) change sugar into starch as their seeds develop.
　The amylases of the saliva and pancreatic juice change starch into dextrin and maltose, the latter changing to glucose in the small intestines. Fatty acids with phosphorus and very small amount of acid radicals are also combined with starch. Starch taken as food is converted into monosaccharides which enter the blood stream; whatever is not immediately needed is stored in the liver and muscles as glycogen.
　Pure starches, having the formula $(C_6H_{10}O_5)n$, if normally metabolized, leave no residue and give rise only to carbon dioxide and water. Starches yield an acid ash.
　RS: *amidin*, *amidulin*, "*amyl-*" *words*, *carbohydrate*, *dextrin*, *dietetics*, *digestion*, *farinaceous*, *glucose*, *glycogen*, *granulose*.
stare (stăr) [A.S. *starian*, to stiffen]. To gaze fixedly at anyone or anything.
starvation (star-vā'shŭn) [A.S. *steorfan*, to die]. The condition of being without food for a long period of time.
　When everything but air and water is

Classification of Starches

Groups

I. Potato Group ....(a) Canna	(b) Potato	(c) Arrowroot
II. Leguminous Group ......(a) Beans	(b) Peas	(c) Lentils
III. Wheat Group ....(a) Wheat	(b) Barley	(c) Rye
IV. Sago Group ....(a) Sago	(b) Cassava	(c) Arum
V. Rice Group ....(a) Rice	(b) Maize	(c) Oats

Starches

Name	From
1. Cornflour	Maize or corn.
2. Arrowroot	Maranta.
3. Cassava	Brazilian arrowroot.
4. Curcuma	East Indian arrowroot.
5. Arum	Portland arrowroot.
6. Tous-les-mois	Canna (West India).
7. Sago	Palm (East India).
8. Inulin	Dahlia tubers.
9. Lichen	Iceland moss.
10. Glycogen	Animal livers.

NOTE: Starch is soluble at 150° F. Only slightly so in cold water.
IODINE acting on starch paste gives a deep blue.
BROMINE acting on starch paste gives an orange-yellow.

The Percentage of Starch in Various Foods

Article	Per cent	Article	Per cent
Acorns	43	Lentils	57
Arrowroot	23	Oatmeal	68
Bananas	22	Potatoes	18
Barley	62	Potatoes, sweet	15
Beans	57	Peas, green	29
Beans, green	29	Peas, dried	55
Bread fruit	14	Peanuts	24
Buckwheat flour	77	Rye flour	78
Chestnuts	42	Rice	79
Cassava (sweet)	31	Wheat flour	75

withheld, the sequence of events is as follows: (a) *Hunger*, beginning about 4 hours after the last meal, accompanied by special activity of the stomach and general restlessness, becoming more acute periodically, esp. at times when meals were customarily taken; (b) *loss of weight;* (c) *utilization of glycogen* stored in liver and muscles; (d) *utilization of stored fat;* (e) *spells of nausea*, and *diminishing acuteness of the sensation of hunger;* (f) *destruction of body protein. The greatest loss of weight is in:* (a) The fatty tissues; (b) the spleen, and (c) the liver. The nervous system loses little and the heart least of all.
stasibasiphobia (stā″sĭ-bā″sĭ-fō′bĭ-á) [G. *stasis*, a standing, + *basis*, step, + *pho-*

stasimorphy

bos, fear]. Delusion of one's inability to stand or walk or fear to make the attempt.

stasimorphy (stăs′ĭ-mor-fī) [" + *morphē*, form]. Deformity resulting from arrested development of a part.

stasiphobia (stă-sĭ-fō′bĭ-ă) [" + *phobos*, fear]. Delusion of one's inability to stand erect or to make the attempt.

stasis (stā′sĭs) [G. *stasis*, halt]. Stagnation of normal flow of fluids, as of the blood, urine, or of the intestinal mechanism.
   s., diffusion. S. with diffusion of lymph or serum.
   s., venous. S. of blood caused by venous congestion.

stat [L.]. Abbr. of statim, immediately.

static (stăt′ĭk) [G. *statikos*, standing]. At rest; in equilibrium; not in motion.
   s. breeze. The brush discharge as used in therapy.
   s. brush. See: *static breeze*.
   s. electricity. Electricity produced by friction.
   s. induced current. The charging and discharging current of a pair of Leyden jars or other condensers which is passed through a patient.
   s. machine. Term applied to certain type of machine for producing high tension direct current.
   s. reflex. One occurring without stimulation.
   s. wave current. The current resulting from the sudden periodic discharge from a patient who has been raised to a high potential by means of an electrostatic generator.

statics (stăt′ĭks) [G. *statikos*, standing]. Study of matter at rest and forces bringing about equilibrium. See: *dynamics*.

statim (stăt′ĭm) [L.]. Immediately; at once.

station (stā′shŭn) [L. *statio*, a standing]. 1. The manner of standing. 2. A stopping place.
   s., aid. One in the army for collecting the wounded in battle.
   s., dressing. A temporary one for wounded soldiers in the field.
   s., rest. A temporary relief station for the sick on a military road or railway.

stationary (stā′shŭn-ar-ĭ) [L. *stationarius*, belonging to a station]. Not moving.
   s. air. Air in lungs after normal expiration.

statometer (stăt-ŏm′ĕt-ẽr) [G. *statos*, standing, + *metron*, a measure]. Instrument for measuring amount of abnormal protrusion of eyeball.

stature (stăt′ŭr) [L. *statura*, size of body]. Natural height of the body.

status (stā′tŭs) (pl. *statuses*) [L. *status*, from *stare*, to stand]. An abnormal state or condition.
   s. arthriticus. Predisposition toward having attacks of gout.
   s. epilepticus. Rapid succession of epileptic attacks without regaining consciousness during the intervals.
   s. lymphaticus. A hyperplastic condition of all lymphatic tissue, the spleen, bone marrow, and thymus, resulting in lowered vitality.
   The thymus enlarges together with lymph glands and lymphoid tissue elsewhere in the body. It is often unsuspected and may cause sudden death.
   Such individuals have a delicate framework, slight musculature, delicate cardiovascular system, low blood pressure, low blood sugar, and lymphocyto-

steariform

sis. They are particularly susceptible to shock and infections, and are frequently weaklings mentally as well as physically.
   Prog: Sudden death possible, esp. in surgical anesthesia. Syn: *lymphatism*.
   s. praesens. The state of a patient under observation.
   s. thymicolymphaticus. Condition resembling *s. lymphaticus*, but with enlarged thymus as primary factor.
   s. thymicus. Same as *s. thymicolymphaticus*.
   s. typhosus. Condition in wasting fevers in which symptoms are stupor; great prostration; coma; vigil or muttering delirium; feeble, frequent pulse; involuntary discharge of urine and feces; sordes, and dry, brownish tongue.
   s. verminosus. Condition due to infestation by worms.
   s. vertiginosus. Persistent condition of vertigo.*

staurion (staw′rĭ-ŏn) [G. *stauros*, across]. Craniometric point where transverse palatine suture crosses the median one.

stauroplegia (staw-rō-plē′jĭ-ă) [" + *plēgē*, a stroke]. Hemiplegia of a part on one side of the body and another part on the other side. Syn: *hemiplegia, crossed*.

steam (stēm) [A.S. *stēam*, vapor]. 1. Invisible vapor into which water is converted at boiling point by heat. 2. Mist formed by condensation of water vapor. 3. Any vaporous exhalation.
   s. tent. A device for inhalation of vapors.
   Various methods of inhaling vapors may be improvised: 1. Tie an old umbrella to the head of the bed, place a pitcher of boiling water in a box alongside of the patient. Vapors tend to fill the umbrella. Solution may be kept hot by placing in a double boiler or wrapping pitcher in an old woolen cloth or newspapers.
   2. Window screens may be used by fastening them about head of bed and then covering with a blanket or sheet lined with newspapers. Solution may be used as above or a steaming teakettle placed alongside of bed with the spout directed under tent.
   3. A rod or rope fastened across head of bed and down to foot of bed. Place a blanket across rod to cover patient and use inhalation as above.
   4. Fasten ropes to all 4 corners of bed, covering with blankets, etc., forming enclosure for patient. Numerous variations will quickly suggest themselves.
   Solutions to be used are about a quart of boiling water to which is added a teaspoonful of compound tincture of benzoin or a teaspoonful of tincture benzoin (this does not contain aloe), a few crystals of menthol or camphor, or a few drops of methyl salicylate. These ingredients are pleasant but have relatively little therapeutic effect. Most of the value is in the water vapor. See: *croup*.

steapsin (stē-ăp′sĭn) [G. *stear*, fat, + *pepsis*, digestion]. A ferment or proteolytic enzyme in the pancreatic juice that splits neutral fat into glycerin and fatty acids.
   The bile salts prepare the fats for the action of steapsin by emulsifying them. Syn: *lipase, pialyn*. See: *enzyme, pancreas*.

stearic acid (stē-ăr′ĭk) [G. *stear*, fat]. A white, fatty acid found in solid animal fats and a few vegetable fats.

steariform (stē-ăr′ĭ-form) [" + L. *forma*, shape]. Resembling fat.

stearin (stē'ăr-ĭn) [G. *stear, steat-*, fat]. $C_3H_5(C_{18}H_{35}O_2)_3$. A white, crystalline solid in animal and vegetable fats; any of the esters of glyceryl and stearic acid, specifically glyceryl tristearate.
One of the commonest fats in the body, esp. the solid ones. It breaks down into stearic acid and glycerol.

stearoconotum (stē"ăr-ō-kŏn-ō'tŭm) [" + *konis*, dust]. An insoluble yellowish fat in brain tissue.

stearodermia (stē"ăr-ō-der'mĭ-ă) [" + *derma*, skin]. Disease of the sebaceous glands of the skin.

stearopten[e (stē-ăr-ŏp'tēn) [" + *ptēnos*, volatile]. A concrete or solid substance obtained from a volatile oil. Ex: *menthol, thymol*.

stearrhea (stē-ăr-ē'ă) [" + *rhoia*, flow]. Excessive secretion of sebum or fat. SYN: *seborrhea, steatorrhea*.

   s. flavescens. S. with yellow sebaceous matter deposited on the skin.

   s. nigricans. S. with black sweat due to presence of indican. SEE: *chromidrosis, chromodermatosis*.

   s. simplex. Excessive discharge of sebum.

steatadenoma (stē-ăt-ăd-en-ō'mă) [" + *aden*, gland, + *-ōma*, tumor]. Tumor of the sebaceous glands.

steatitis (stē-ă-tī'tĭs) [" + *-itis*, inflammation]. Inflammation of adipose tissue.

steato- (stē-ăt-ō) [G.]. Prefix meaning *fatty*.

steatocele (stē-ăt'ō-sēl, stē'ăt-ō-sēl) [G. *stear, steat-*, fat, + *kēlē*, tumor]. Fatty tumor within the scrotum.

steatocryptosis (stē"ăt-ō-krĭp-tō'sĭs) [" + *kryptē*, a sac, + *-ōsis*, disorder]. Any disease of sebaceous glands. SEE: *stearodermia*.

steatogenous (stē-ă-tŏj'ĕn-ŭs) [" + *gennan*, to produce]. Causing fatty degeneration or any sebaceous gland disease.

steatolysis (stē-ăt-ŏl'ĭs-ĭs) [" + *lysis*, dissolution]. Process by which fats are prepared by emulsification into glycerol and free fatty acids for absorption and assimilation.

steatolytic (stē"ăt-ō-lĭt'ĭk) [" + *lysis*, dissolution]. Concerning steatolysis.

steatoma (stē-ăt-ō'mă) [G. *stear, steat-*, fat, + *-ōma*, tumor]. 1. Sebaceous cyst. SYN: *wen*. 2. Benign tumor composed of fat cells. SYN: *lipoma*.
Called a chalazion when on eyelid and meibomian gland.
Smooth, shiny, globular, cutaneous or subcutaneous tumor from pea to orange size arising from sebaceous glands, single or multiple, usually on neck, scalp, back, or scrotum.
ETIOL: Exciting cause unknown. Duct occlusion is causative in some.
PROG: Prolonged irritation may cause suppuration.
TREATMENT: Surgical excision by dissection without perforating sac. Packing in suppurative cases.

   s., Mueller's. Tumor composed of fibrous and fatty tissue. SYN: *lipofibroma*.

steatonecrosis (stē"ăt-ō-nē-krō'sĭs) [" + *nekros*, corpse, + *-ōsis*, condition]. Necrosis of fatty tissue in small patches.

steatopathy (stē-ă-tŏp'ă-thĭ) [" + *pathos*, disease]. Disease of the sebaceous glands of the skin.

steatopygia (stē-ăt-ō-pī'jĭ-ă, -pĭj'ĭ-ă) [" + *pygē*, buttock]. Abnormal fatness of the buttocks.

steatorrhea (stē-ăt-or-rē'ă) [" + *rhoia*, flow]. 1. Increased secretion of sebaceous glands. SYN: *seborrhea*.* 2. Fatty stools, as seen in pancreatic diseases.

steatosis (stē-ăt-ō'sĭs) [" + *-ōsis*, condition]. 1. Fatty degeneration. 2. Disease of the sebaceous glands. 3. Excessive accumulation of fat in the body. SYN: *adiposis,* obesity*.

steatozoon (stē"ăt-ō-zō'ŏn) [" + *zōon*, animal]. A mite found in comedones.

stechiology (stē-kĭ-ŏl'ō-jĭ) [G. *stoicheion*, element, + *logos*, a study]. Sum of what is known of elements and of elementary principles of any branch of science.

stechiometry (stē-kĭ-ŏm'ĕt-rĭ) [" + *metron*, a measure]. 1. The mathematics of chemistry. 2. Measurement of proportion in which elements combine to form compounds.

stegano- [G.]. Combining form meaning *covered*.

stege (stē'jē) [G. *stegos*, roof]. The inner layer of rods of Corti.

stegnosis (stĕg-nō'sĭs) [G. *stegnōsis*, a closing]. 1. Checking of a secretion or discharge. 2. Closing of a passage. SYN: *stenosis*. 3. Constipation. SYN: *costiveness*.

stegnotic (stĕg-nŏt'ĭk) [G. *stegnōsis*, a closing]. Bringing about stegnosis. SYN: *astringent, constipating*.

stellate (stĕl'āt) [L. *stella*, star]. Star-shaped; arranged with parts radiating from a center.

   s. bandage. One wound on the back, crossways.

   s. cells. Nerve cells in the cortex cerebri.

   s. fracture. One with numerous fissures radiating from central point of injury.

   s. ligament. One of the ant. costovertebral ligaments.

   s. veins. Venous plexuses beneath the kidney's capsule. SYN: *stars of Verheyen*.

Stellwag's sign (stĕl'vahg). Widening of palpebral aperture with absence or lessened frequency of winking, seen in Graves' disease.

stem (stĕm) [A.S. *stemm*, trunk]. 1. Any stalklike structure. 2. Offspring. 3. To derive from. 4. To check.

   s., brain. The brain without its fissured portion and cerebrum.

stenion (stĕn'ĭ-ŏn) [G. *stenos*, narrow]. Craniometric point at extremities of the smallest transverse diameter in the temporal region.

steno- [G.]. Combining form meaning *narrow, short*, as *stenosis, stenography*.

stenocardia (stĕn-ō-kar'dĭ-ă) [G. *stenos*, narrow, + *kardia*, heart]. Angina* pectoris.

stenocephaly (stĕn-ō-sĕf'ăl-ĭ) [" + *kephalē*, head]. Narrowness of the cranium in one or more diameters.

stenochoria (stĕn-ō-kō'rĭ-ă) [" + *chōros*, space]. Partial constriction, esp. of the lacrimal duct. SYN: *stenosis*.

stenocompressor (stĕn-ō-kŏm-prĕs'or) [" + L. *compressor*, that which presses together]. An instrument for compressing Stensen's ducts to stop the flow of saliva.

stenocoriasis (stĕn-ō-kō-rī'ăs-ĭs) [" + *korē*, pupil]. Narrowing of pupil of the eye.

Stenon's or **Steno's duct** (stē'nŏn, stē'nō). Excretory duct of the parotid gland. SYN: *Stensen's duct*.

stenopaic, stenopeic (sten-o-pā'ĭk, -pē'ĭk) [G. *stenos*, narrow, + *opē*, opening]. Having a narrow opening.

stenosed (stē-nōst', stĕn'ōzd). Characterized by stenosis; constricted.
stenosis (stĕn-ō'sĭs, stē-nō'sĭs) [G. *stenōsis*, a narrowing]. Constriction or narrowing of a passage or orifice. SYN: stricture.
  VARIETIES: Aortic, mitral, pulmonary, tricuspid, and it may affect the esophagus, pylorus, and vagina. Stenosis of the pylorus is largely confined to children not over 3 years old.
  TREATMENT: In most cases, operation.
  s., aortic. Constriction of the aortic orifice at cardiac base or narrowing of the aorta.
  s., cardiac. Lessened diameter of the conus arteriosus on either side of heart with obstruction to free flow of blood from ventricle into corresponding artery.
  s., cicatricial. S. resulting from any contracted cicatrix.
  s., mitral. S. of mitral valve or orifice of heart, or of both.
  s., pyloric. Obstruction caused by hypertrophy of walls of the pyloric orifice.
stenostegnosis (stē"nō-stĕg-nō'sĭs) [G. *stegnōsis*, a stoppage]. Stenosis or stricture of Stensen's duct.
stenostenosis (stē"nō-stĕn-ō'sĭs) [G. *stenōsis*, a narrowing]. Constriction of Stensen's duct. SYN: stenostegnosis.
stenostomia (stĕn"ō-stō'mĭ-ă) [G. *stenos*, narrow, + *stoma*, mouth]. Narrowing of the mouth.
stenothermal (stĕn"ō-ther'măl) [" + *thermē*, heat]. Resisting only a small change of temperature.
stenothorax (stĕn"ō-thō'răks) [" + *thōrax*, chest]. An unusually narrow thorax.
stenotic (stĕn-ŏt'ĭk) [G. *stenōsis*, a narrowing]. Produced by or characterized by stenosis.
Stensen's duct (stĕn'sĕn). The excretory duct of parotid gland.
  S's. foramina. Incisive foramina of sup. maxillary bone transmitting ant. branches of descending palatine vessels.
step-down transformer. A transformer in which the number of turns of wire in the primary and secondary windings are in such relation as to reduce voltage.
  s.-up t. A transformer in which the number of turns of wire in the primary and secondary windings are in such relation as to increase voltage. SEE: transformer.
stephanion (stē-fā'nĭ-ŏn) [G. *stephanos*, crown]. Point at intersection of sup. temporal ridge and coronal suture.
step'page gait. The high-stepping gait seen in diabetic neuritis of the peroneal nerve and in tabes dorsalis.
  Patient lifts the foot very high in walking to raise the drooping toes from the ground or floor.
sterco- [L.]. Combining form meaning dung, as stercobilin.
stercobilin (stĕr"kō-bī'lĭn) [L. *stercus*, dung, + *bilis*, bile]. A brown pigment derived from the bile giving the characteristic color to feces. SEE: urobilin.
stercoraceous (stĕr-kō-rā'shŭs) [L. *storcoraceus*, like dung]. Having the nature of, pert. to or containing, feces.
stercoral (stĕr'kō-ral) [L. *stercus*, dung]. Pert. to feces. SYN: stercoraceous.
stercoremia (ster-kō-rē'mĭ-ă) [" + G. *aima*, blood]. Toxic state from absorption of poisons in retained feces.
stercorin (ster'kō-rĭn) [L. *stercus*, dung]. Crystallizable reduction product of cholesterol in feces.
stercorolith (stĕr'kō-rō-lĭth) [" + G. *lithos*, stone]. A fecal concretion. SYN: coprolith, fecalith.

stercoroma (ster-kō-rō'mă) [" + G. -*ōma*, tumor]. A fecal tumorlike mass in the rectum. SYN: coproma, fecaloma, scotoma.
stercorous (ster'kŏr-ŭs) [L. *stercus*, stercor-, dung]. Resembling excrement. SYN: stercoral, stercoraceous.
stercus (stĕr'kŭs) [L.]. Feces. SYN: excreta, excrement.
stere (stēr, stār) [Fr. *stère*, from G. *stereos*, solid]. A measure of capacity. SYN: cubic meter, kiloliter.
stereo- [G.]. Combining form meaning solid.
stereoanesthesia (stĕr"ē-ō-ăn-ĕs-thē'zĭ-ă) [G. *stereos*, solid, + *an-*, negative, + *aisthesis*, sensation]. Inability to recognize objects by feeling their form.
stereoarthrolysis (stĕr"ē-ō-ar-thrŏl'ĭ-sĭs) [" + *arthron*, joint, + *lysis*, a loosening]. Surgical formation of a movable new joint in bony ankylosis.
stereochemical (stĕr"ē-ō-kĕm'ĭ-kăl) [" + *chēmeia*, chemistry]. Concerning stereochemistry.
stereochemistry (ster"ē-ō-kĕm'ĭs-trĭ) [" + *chēmeia*, chemistry]. That branch of chemistry dealing with atoms in their space relation.
stereognosis (stĕr-ē-ŏg-nō'sĭs) [" + *gnōsis*, knowledge]. Ability to recognize form of solid objects by touch.
stereometry (stĕr-ē-ŏm'ĕt-rĭ) [" + *metron*, a measure]. The measurement of a solid body or the cubic contents of a hollow body.
stereoörthopter (stĕr"ē-ō-ŏr-thŏp'ter) [" + *orthos*, straight, + *opsis*, vision]. A mirror-reflecting device for treatment of strabismus.
stereophantoscope (stĕr"ē-ō-făn'tō-skōp) [G. *stereos*, solid, + *phantos*, visible, + *skopein*, to examine]. A stereoscopical device with rotating disks for testing vision.
stereophorometer (stĕr"ē-ō-for-ŏm'ĕ-ter) [" + *phoros*, a bearer, + *metron*, a measure]. A prism-refracting device for use in correcting defective vision.
stereophotography (stĕr"ē-ō-fō-tŏg'ră-fĭ) [" + *phōs, phot-*, light, + *graphein*, to write]. Photography which produces effect of solidity or depth of pictures.
stereophotomicrograph (stĕr"ē-ō-fō"tō-mī'-krō-grăf) [" + " + *mikros*, tiny, + *graphein*, to write]. A photograph showing solidity or depth of a microscopical subject.
stereoplasm (stĕr'ē-ō-plăzm) [" + *plasma*, a thing formed]. The solid portion of cell protoplasm.
stereoscope (ster'ē-ō-skōp) [" + *skopein*, to see]. Instrument which creates an impression of solidity or depth of objects seen by combining images of 2 pictures.
stereoscopic, stereoscopical (ster-ē-ō-skŏp'ĭk, -ĭ-kăl) [" + *skopein*, to see]. Pert. to the stereoscope or its use.
  s. vision. Vision in which things have the appearance of solidity and relief as though seen in 3 dimensions.
stereotypy (stĕr-ē-ō-tī'pĭ) [" + *typos*, type]. Repetition of words, posture, or movement without meaning; seen in catatonic partial stupors.
sterile (stĕr'ĭl) [L. *sterilis*, barren]. 1. Free from living microörganisms. SYN: aseptic. 2. Not fertile; unable to reproduce young. SYN: barren.
sterility (stĕr-ĭl'ĭ-tĭ) [L. *sterilitās*, barrenness]. Absence of reproductive power. RS: *acyesis, agenesia, agenesis, aphoria, atocia, dysgenesia, dysgenesis, infecunditas, sterile*.

s., absolute. After 5 years of married life without the use of contraceptives with no ensuing pregnancy.

s., acquired (secondary s.). The failure of further conception after once having given birth to a child.

s., female. Inability to give birth to living young.

s., primary. Condition in which woman has never become pregnant.

s., relative. S. due to causes other than defect of sex organs.

ETIOL. FACTORS: CONGENITAL ABNORMALITIES: Absence or maldevelopment of the uterus tubes, or ovaries; infantile uterus; congenital elongation of the cervix.

ACQUIRED LOCAL CONDITIONS: (a) *Vagina*: Hyperacidity; marked hypertrophy of the vaginal mucous membrane with hiding of the cervix; lacerated vagina with effluvium seminis. (b) *Cervix*: Pinpoint os; sharp angulation; narrowing of the internal os; acute and chronic endocervicitis; polypi occluding the cervical canal; severe lacerations, particularly where the internal os is torn, resulting in precipitate miscarriages before the viability of the child. (c) *Body of the uterus*: Malpositions, particularly retroversion, retroflexion, and hyperanteflexion; fibroids of the uterus which block the canal; diseased endometrium, particularly endometritis. (d) *Fallopian tube*: Chronic salpingo-oöphoritis with closure of the tubal ostium and where the ovary is embedded in adhesions.

GENERAL CONSTITUTIONAL DISEASES: Diabetes mellitus, nephritis, syphilis, some of the blood dyscrasias. About 10% of all marriages are sterile.

Investigation into the cause of sterility includes primarily definite information as to the fertility of the husband. A routine examination for sterility includes a study of the vaginal secretions, a bimanual examination, visualization of the cervix, and in some cases a test for patency of the tubes.

A history of pelvic disorder in the past is of great importance and any information as to the use of strong chemical douches for the purpose of contraception may be vital. In the event that the tubes are found closed, a study of the genital tract by the use of x-ray and lipiodol is indicated.

TREATMENT: The treatment of sterility depends upon the finding and correction of any or all causes of the condition.

sterilization (ster″ĭl-ĭ-zā′shŭn) [L. *sterilis*, barren]. 1. Process of destruction of all microörganisms on a substance by exposure to chemical or physical agents. 2. Process of rendering barren.

RS: *asepsis, autoclave, castration, hands, skin, spay.*

s., discontinuous. Exposure for about an hour on several successive days to 212° F. (100° C.).

s., fractional. S. in which heating is done at separated intervals, so that spores can develop into bacteria and be destroyed.

s., steam, by flowing. Exposure at 212° F. (100° C.) to steam in an unsealed receptacle.

s., steam under pressure. Exposure to steam in an autoclave.

sterilize (ster′ĭl-īz) [L. *sterilis*, barren]. 1. To free from microörganisms. 2. To make barren.

sterilizer (ster′ĭl-ī-zer) [L. *sterilis*, barren]. Oven or appliance for sterilizing.

sterilometer (stĕr-ĭl-ŏm′ĕ-ter) [″ + G. *metron*, a measure]. An apparatus to test the degree of sterilization of any material.

sternal (ster′năl) [G. *sternon*, chest]. Relating to the sternum or breastbone.

sternalgia (stĕr-năl′jĭ-ă) [″ + *algos*, pain]. Pain in the sternum. SYN: *sternodynia.*

sternebra (ster′nē-bră) [″ + L. (*vert*)*ebra*, vertebra]. Segment of the sternum.

sterno- [G.]. Combining form meaning *sternum.*

sternoclavicular (ster″nō-klă-vĭk′ū-lar) [G. *sternon*, breast, + L. *clavicula*, a little key]. Concerning the sternum and clavicle.

sternocleidomastoid (ster″nō-klī-dō-măs′-toyd) [″ + *kleis*, clavicle, + *mastos*, breast, + *eidos*, like]. One of 2 muscles arising from sternum and inner part of clavicle. SEE: *Table of Muscles in Appendix.*

sternocostal (ster″nō-kŏs′tăl) [″ + L. *costa*, rib]. Relating to sternum and ribs.

sternodynia (ster″nō-dĭn′ĭ-ă) [″ + *odynē*, pain]. Pain in the sternum. SYN: *sternalgia.*

sternohyoid (ster″nō-hī′oyd) [″ + *hyoeidēs*, U-shaped]. Muscle from medial end of clavicle and sternum to hyoid bone. SEE: *Table of Muscles in Appendix.*

sternoid (ster′noyd) [″ + *eidos*, resemblance]. Resembling the breastbone.

sternopericardial (ster″nō-per″ĭ-kar′dĭ-al) [″ + *peri*, around, + *kardia*, heart]. Concerning the sternum and pericardium.

sternothyroid (ster″nō-thī′royd) [G. *sternon*, breast, + *thyreos*, shield, + *eidos*, like]. Muscle extending beneath the sternohyoid which depresses the larynx. SEE: *Table of Muscles in Appendix.*

sternotomy (ster-nŏt′ō-mĭ) [″ + *tomē*, a cutting]. The operation of cutting the sternum.

sternotrypesis (ster″nō-trī-pē′sĭs) [″ + *trypēsis*, a boring]. Surgical perforation of the sternum.

sternum (ster′nŭm) [G. *sternon*, breast]. The narrow, flat bone in the median line of the thorax in front. SYN: *breastbone.*

It consists of 3 portions, distinguished as the *manubrium*, the *gladiolus*, and the *ensiform* or *xiphoid appendix.*

RS: *chicken breast, chondrosternal, chondroxiphoid, cleft, gladiolus, ensiform, manubrium, xiphoid process.*

s., cleft. Congenital fissure of the sternum.

sternutament (ster-nū′tăm-ĕnt) [L. *sternutāre*, to sneeze]. A substance causing sneezing.

sternutatio (stĕr-nū-tā′shē-ō) [L. sneezing]. Sneezing.

s. convulsiva. Paroxysmal sneezing, as in hay fever.

sternutation (ster-nū-tā′shŭn) [L. *sternutāre*, to sneeze]. Act of sneezing.

s., convulsive. Spasmodic or paroxysmal sneezing with profusion of watery secretion from the nose.

sternutatory (ster-nū′tă-tō″rĭ) [L. *sternutāre*, to sneeze]. 1. Causing sneezing. 2. An agent causing sneezing. Ex: *quillaja, salicylic acid.*

sterol (stĕr′ŏl) [G. *stereos*, solid, + L. *oleum*, oil]. Any of a class of solid higher alcohols in plants and animals.

Generally colorless, crystalline compounds, nonsaponifiable and soluble in certain organic solvents. Ex: *cholesterol.*

stertor (stĕr′tŏr) [L. *stertor*, a snore]. Snoring or laborious breathing due to

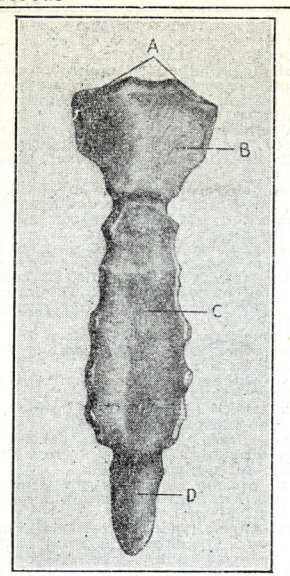

STERNUM, POSTERIOR VIEW.
A. Clavicular facets. B. Manubrium.
C. Body. D. Ensiform cartilage.

obstruction of air passages in the head, seen in certain diseases, as apoplexy.
stertorous (stĕr'tō-rŭs) [L. *stertor*, a snore]. Pert. to laborious breathing provoking a snoring sound.
sterule (stĕr'ūl) [L. *sterilis*, barren]. A glass capsule containing a sterile solution. SYN: *ampoule*.
stetho- [G.]. Combining form meaning the *chest*.
stethogoniometer (stĕth″ō-gō-nĭ-ŏm'ĕt-ĕr) [G. *stēthos*, chest, + *gōnia*, angle, + *metron*, measure]. Device for measuring the curvature of the chest.
stethograph (stĕth'ō-grăf) [" + *graphein*, to write]. Device to record chest movements in respiration.
stethokyrtograph (stĕth″o-kir'tō-grăf) [" + *kyrtos*, bent, + *graphein*, to write]. Device for measuring and recording the dimensions and amount of curves of the chest.
stethometer (stĕth-ŏm'ĕt-ĕr) [" + *metron*, measure]. Device for measuring the chest's expansion during respiration.
stethophonometer (stĕth″ō-fō-nŏm'ĕt-ĕr) [" + *phōnē*, voice, + *metron*, a measure]. Instrument for determining intensity of sound emitted in auscultation.
stethoscope (stĕth'ō-skōp) [G. *stēthos*, chest, + *skopein*, to see]. Instrument used in auscultation to convey to the ear the sounds produced in the body.
Ordinarily, consists of rubber tubing in a Y shape.
 s., **binaural.** S. designed for use with both ears.
 s., **compound.** More than 1 set attached to the same fork and chest piece.
 s., **double.** S. with 2 earpieces and tubes.
 s., **percussion.** Solid cylinder of wood, 1 end wedge-shaped, other enlarged into an earpiece adapted for intercostal use.
 s., **single** or **monaural.** For 1 ear only; rigid or flexible.
stethoscopy (stĕth-ŏs'kō-pĭ) [G. *stēthos*, chest, + *skopein*, to see]. Examination by means of the stethoscope.
stethospasm (stĕth'ō-spăzm) [" + *spasmos*, spasm]. Spasm of the pectoral or chest muscles.
sthenia (sthē'nĭ-ă) [G. *sthenos*, strength]. Normal or unusual strength, the opp. of *asthenia*.
sthenic (sthĕn'ĭk) [G. *sthenos*, strength], Active; strong.
 s. **fever.** One with high temperature; tense, quick pulse, and highly colored urine.
sthenometer (sthĕn-ŏm'ĕ-tĕr) [" + *metron*, a measure]. Device for measuring muscular strength.
sthenometry (sthĕn-ŏm'ĕ-trĭ) [" + *metron*, a measure]. Determination of bodily strength.
sthenopyra (sthĕn″ō-pī'ră) [" + *pyr*, fire]. Fever with a strong, bounding pulse; active delirium, and high temperature. SYN: *sthenic fever*.
stibialism (stĭb'ĭ-ăl-ĭzm) [L. *stibium*, antimony, + G. *-ismos*, condition]. Antimonial poisoning.
stibium (stĭb'ĭ-ŭm) [L.]. Antimony.
stichochrome (stĭk'ō-krōm) [G. *stichos*, row, + *chrōma*, color]. A nerve cell in which the stainable bodies (tigroid mass) are arranged in parallel rows.
stictacne (stĭk-tăk'nē) [G. *stiktos*, pointed, + *aknē*, point]. Acne with red base and black pointed comedo at apex. SYN: *acne punctata*.
stiff neck. Rigidity of neck due to rheumatism or contraction of cervical muscles. SYN: *torticollis, wryneck*.
 s.-n. **fever.** 1. Dengue. 2. Cerebrospinal meningitis.
stigma (stĭg'mă) (pl. *stigmata*) [G. *stigma*, a mark]. 1. A mark or spot on the skin. 2. Spot on ovarian surface where rupture of a graafian follicle will occur. 3. Intercellular cleft in endothelial cells in a capillary. 4. Red spot due to extravasation of blood produced by nervous influence. 5. Mark characterizing a specific disease.
 s. **of degeneration.** Any of the bodily variations from the normal found in numerous instances in degenerate individuals. Some of them are the following: DEGENERATIVE CHANGES: *Face*: May be unusually hairy in the female and abnormally smooth in the male. *Fingers and toes*: May be an extra one, or adherent or webbed. *Forehead*: May be sloping and very low. *Eyes*: May be different in color or set at different levels. *Ears*: Unusual in many ways. *Jaws*: Either may project unusually. *Head*: May be unusually large or small. *Teeth*: May be irregular or project. *Roof of mouth*: May be high and pointed or unusually narrow. Only several of these irregularities may be considered as indicative of defective mentality.
 s., **hysterical.** Spot on skin due to nervous influence.
stigmatic (stĭg-măt'ĭk) [G. *stigma*, mark]. Pert. to or marked with a stigma.
stigmatization (stĭg″măt-ĭ-zā'shŭn) [G. *stigma*, mark]. The formation of stigmata, esp. hysterical s. on the skin.
stigmatodermia (stĭg″măt-ō-der'mĭ-ă) [" + *derma*, skin]. Disease of skin's prickle cell layer.

stigmatometer (stĭg-mă-tŏm'ĕ-tĕr) [" + *metron*, a measure]. Device for testing eye refraction. SYN: *astigmatometer*.

stigmatosis (stĭg-mă-tō'sĭs) [" + *-ōsis*, condition]. A skin disease marked by superficial spots of inflammation.

stilbesterol. SEE: *diethyl s.*

stilet, stilette (stĭl-ĕt') [Fr. *stilette*]. 1. Small, sharp-pointed instrument for probing. 2. Wire used to pass through or stiffen a flexible catheter.

stillbirth (stĭl'birth) [A.S. *stille*, quiet, + M.E. *burth*, birth]. Birth of a dead fetus. [forth]. Dead at birth.

stillborn (stĭl'born) [" + *beran*, to bring

stillicidium (stĭl-ĭ-sĭd'ĭ-ŭm) [L. *stilla*, drop, + *cadere*, to fall]. A dribbling or flowing, drop by drop.

    s. lacrimarum. Watering of the eye. SYN: *epiphora*.

    s. narium. Watery mucus discharged at onset of coryza.

    s. urinae. Urinary incontinence from a distended bladder. SYN: *strangury*.

Stilling's canal (stĭl'ĭng). The hyaloid canal of the vitreous in the eye.

    S's. nucleus. 1. Nucleus containing red ganglion cells found in tegmental region of crus cerebri. 2. Origin of hypoglossal nerve in 4th ventricle.

stimulant (stĭm'ū-lănt) [L. *stimulus*, a goad]. Any agent temporarily increasing functional activity.

    Strong coffee, tea, whiskey, brandy, wine, capsicum, ginger, ammonia applied to the nostrils, cold water dashed alternately over face and chest, atropine, strychnine, electric current, massage, are examples.

    Stimulants may be classified according to the organ upon which they act as follows: Cardiac, bronchial, gastric, cerebral, intestinal, nervous, motor, vasomotor, respiratory, and secretory.

stimulate (stĭm'ū-lāt) [L. *stimulāre*, to goad on]. To increase functional activity of an organ or structure.

stim'ulating en'ema. One given to excite activity in shock or unconscious state. SEE: *enema*.

stimulation (stĭm"ū-lā'shŭn) [L. *stimulāre*, to goad on]. 1. Process of being stimulated. 2. Irritating action of agents on muscles, nerves or sensory end-organs by which activity in a part is evoked.

stimulin (stĭm'ū-lĭn) [L. *stimulus*, a goad]. 1. Substance in fresh gastric juice stimulating gastric glands. 2. A substance in blood serum that increases phagocytic activity.

stimulus (stĭm'ū-lŭs) (pl. *stimuli*) [L. *stimulus*, a goad]. Any agent or factor able to influence directly living protoplasm, as one capable of causing muscular contraction or secretion in a gland, or of initiating an impulse in a nerve.

    RS: *ceptor, chemotaxis, chemotropism, lag phase, latent.*

    s., adequate. One which acts upon nerve terminations in any special organ.

    s., chemical. A stimulus acting by a chemical process.

    s., electric. S. resulting from application of electricity.

    s., heterologous. One acting upon any part of a sensory organ or nerve tract.

    s., homologous. Same as adequate s.

    s., mechanical. S. caused by mechanical means.

    s., thermal. S. caused by application of heat.

sting (stĭng) [A.S. *stingan*, to stick]. 1. Sharp, smarting sensation, as of a wound or astringent. 2. Wound made by a sting; the sharp offensive weapon of an insect, esp. a painful or poisonous wound. SEE: *insect bite.*

stippling (stĭp'lĭng) [Dutch *stippelen*, to spot]. A spotted condition, as in retina in certain ocular diseases or in basophilic red corpuscles.

stirpiculture (stĕr'pĭ-kŭl"tūr) [L. *stirps*, stock, + *cultura*, cultivation]. Scientific breeding of stock or race to improve it.

stirrup, stirrup bone (stĭr'ŭp) [A.S. *stigrāp*, a stirrup]. Stapes of the ears.

stitch (stĭch) [M.E. *stiche*, from A.S. *stice*, a pricking]. 1. A local, sharp, lancinating, or spasmodic pain 2. A single loop of suture material passed through skin or flesh by a needle, to facilitate healing of a wound. 3. To unite skin or flesh with a needle and suture material.

    Some are removed after a few days and other types are absorbed by the body. SYN: *suture.*

    s. abscess. One developing in a suture due to infection.

stock (stŏk) [A.S. *stocc*, a trunk]. The race or line of a family.

    s. culture. Permanent culture of a microörganism reinforced from time to time by fresh media.

    s. vaccine. Vaccine prepared from any strain of the species, but not from patient himself.

Stokes-Adams syndrome (stōks-ăd'ăms). A series of symptoms in those suffering from heart block. Onset is sudden, resembling epilepsy, for which it is sometimes mistaken.

    ETIOL: Due to stoppage or extreme slowness of ventricular contraction.

Stokes' law (stōks). A muscle is frequently a seat of paralysis if lying above an inflamed serous or mucous membrane.

    S's. lens. Device used to diagnose astigmatism.

stoma (stō'mă) (pl. *stomata*) [G. *stoma*, a mouth]. 1. A mouth or small opening or a pore. 2. Artificially created opening bet. 2 passages or body cavities or bet. a cavity or passage and the body's surface. RS: *words containing "stoma."*

stomach (stŭm'ăk) [G. *stomachos*, stomach]. A dilated, saclike, distensible portion of the alimentary canal below the esophagus, 12x4 in., below the diaphragm to right of spleen, partly under the liver.

    It is composed of a *fundus*, or round

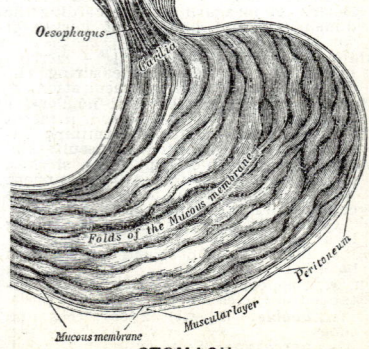

STOMACH.

stomach   S-86   **stomach**

part; a *body*, or middle portion, and pyloric portion which is small end.

It has 2 openings: the upper *cardiac orifice* opens into the esophagus and the lower *pyloric orifice* opens into the duodenum. The stomach is composed of 4 layers: Outer *serous coat* covers almost all of the organ; the *muscular layer* just beneath it is formed of 3 layers of smooth muscle fibers; an outer longitudinal layer; a medial circular layer, and an inner oblique layer. *Submucous layer* is a connecting medium between the muscular and the *mucous layer*, which is the inner lining of the stomach.

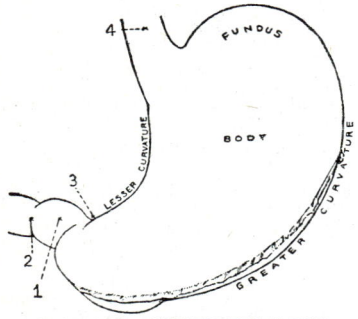

STOMACH, VIEWED FROM THE FRONT.
1. Pyloric canal. 2. Pyloric constriction. 3. Incisura angularis. 4. Esophagus.

The cardiac, fundic (parietal or oxyntic) and pyloric glands of the stomach are composed of columnar and tubular cells which secrete gastric juice containing hydrochloric acid, rennin, pepsin, etc.

FUNCTIONS: It secretes the gastric juice and converts proteids into peptones. In addition to serving strictly as an organ of digestion (SEE: *gastric digestion*), the stomach has the following functions: (1) Acting as a reservoir, it regulates the admission of food to the remainder of the gut; (2) its acid kills a large proportion of the microbes present in most food; (3) it has some power to absorb, SEE: *absorption*; (4) secreting acid, it is important in the acid-base equilibrium of the body; (5) it can excrete some drugs, administered parenterally, into the gastric juice; (6) it acts as a kind of receptor in chemical and nervous mechanisms by which secretion and movement are stimulated in lower parts of the gastrointestinal tract (SEE: *secretagogue* and *reflex, gastrocolic*), and (7) by a special action of gastric juice on foods containing vitamin B_2 it produces a substance which normally prevents pernicious anemia.

S., CANCER OF: VARIETIES: *Colloid, epithelioma, hard cancer or scirrhus, soft cancer or encephaloid*.

SYM: General symptoms of dyspepsia with following characteristic symptoms: Continued pain, often tenderness; vomiting of partially digested food; absence of free hydrochloric acid in gastric juice, and presence of lactic acid after a flour soup test meal; hematemesis or blood in stools, slight in amount and blood altered so it presents a coffee grounds appearance; presence of tumor; loss of flesh and strength; extreme anemia; involvement of superficial lymph glands. When the pylorus is involved symptoms of gastric dilatation will be added.

PROG: Fatal. Duration, 6 months to 2 years.

TREATMENT: Early treatment, surgical. Liquid or semiliquid diet. Rest. Hydrochloric acid and pepsin often required to assist digestion. Constitutional treatment as indicated.

PYLORIC OBSTRUCTION AND DILATATION: Pyloric obstruction increases the resistance offered to the expulsion of food and in its efforts to overcome this the stomach first becomes hypertrophied, then dilated. *Causes of dilatation*: (1) Pyloric obstruction; (2) laxness of walls from simple atony or catarrh; (3) excessive ingestion of food or drink.

SYM: The general symptoms of dyspepsia, together with the following relating to the vomit: Vomiting occurs long after eating, sometimes several hours or days. Amount often excessive, sometimes several quarts; is sour and fermented, and on standing separates into a sediment of undigested food and a turbid, frothy liquid. Ejected fluid rich in torulae and sarcinae, forms of bacteria. Obstinate constipation.

PHYSICAL SIGNS: Bulging over epigastrium; in thin subjects the outline of stomach may be visible. Palpation gives a splashing fremitus.

PERCUSSION: Increased area of gastric tympany.

AUSCULTATION: Splashing sounds often audible at some distance.

MENSURATION: Ordinarily an esophageal sound may be inserted a distance of 60 cm. from the teeth. In dilatation may be inserted 65 to 70 cm.

PROG: Guarded. More favorable in dilatation without obstruction.

TREATMENT: Diet light, nutritious, not bulky, and should be given in small amounts at frequent intervals. Lavage 2 or 3 times weekly. An abdominal support often relieves some of distressing symptoms.

FOREIGN BODIES: These ordinarily should give no concern. Symptoms are usually absent. The patient may be alarmed. Give nothing by mouth. Salts, cathartics, and enemas should under no circumstances be used, inasmuch as they can only make the condition worse.

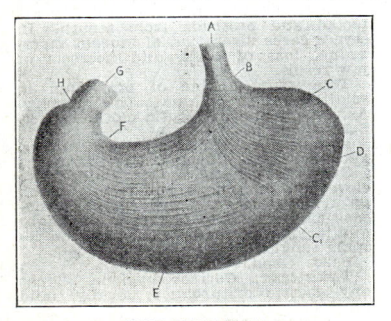

THE STOMACH.
A. Esophagus. B. Cardia. C, C_1. Large cul-de-sac. D. Peak of large cul-de-sac. E. Large curvature. F. Small curvature. G. Duodenum. H. Pylorus.

Such foreign bodies usually pass through the alimentary tract without disturbance. These patients should always be under the care of a doctor.

DIET IN OTHER DISEASES OF STOMACH: *Atony and Hypomobility:* Food is retained longer than normal and if hydrochloric acid is deficient decomposition may occur. Liquids are retained longer than solids. Diet should consist of quickly and easily digested foods, cream, butter, soft cooked vegetables, chicken, fish, scraped beef and moderate amount of milk. Avoid liquids, pastries and rich gravies.

Hypermotility: The stomach empties too rapidly, therefore, diet should be soft and liquid in small amounts and in frequent feedings. Fats delay the emptying of the stomach.

Hyperacidity: Protein to combine with acid, inhibiting its secretion by moderate amt. of fat, and to avoid stimulating secretion of acid. Five small meals, or 3 meals and 2 lunches.

s.-ache. Pain in the stomach. SYN: *gastralgia, gastrodynia, stomachalgia, stomachodynia.*

s., bilocular. SEE: *hourglass stomach.*
s., cardiac. Fundus of the stomach.
s. cough. One caused by reflex action from the stomach.
s., hourglass. One resembling an hourglass, caused by constriction from a band of fibrous exudate.
s., leather bottle. One caused by hypertrophy of the s. walls.
s. pump. Device for removing contents of the stomach by mouth.
s. tooth. A lower canine one during first dentition.
s. tube. One for washing out or feeding the stomach.
s., water-trap. One with the pylorus unusually high, causing slow emptying.

stomach, words pert. to: abdominal cavity; achoresis; achylia gastrica; acidity; anachlorhydria; anadenia; anticardium; atony; atretogastria; bathygastry; bead test; Bouchard's nodules; capotement; cardialgia; cardiodiosis; cardiopyloric; cardiospasm; catastalsis; chlorhydria; cholangiogastrostomy; clapotement; clapotage; digestion; ectasia; endogastritis; feeding, artificial; fractional test meal; gastric juice; gastric lavage; gastric motor meals; "gastr-" words; gavage; hourglass stomach; hunger; lavage; linitis; myxorrhea gastrica; oxyntic glands; pneumatosis; pneumogastric; pylorus; saburra; ulcer; ventriculus.

stomachal (stŭm'ăk-ăl) [G. *stomachos,* stomach]. 1. Relating to the stomach. 2. A gastric tonic.

stomachalgia (stŭm-ăk-ăl'jĭ-ă) [" + *algos,* pain] Pain in the stomach.

stomachic (stō-măk'ĭk) [G. *stomachos,* stomach]. 1. Concerning the stomach. 2. Medicine exciting action of the stomach. SYN: *stomachal.*

stomachoscopy (stŭm-ăk-os'kō-pī) [" + *skopein,* to inspect]. Examination of the stomach. SYN: *gastroscopy.*

stomatalgia (stō-măt-ăl'jĭ-ă) [G. *stoma, stomat-,* mouth, + *algos,* pain]. Pain in the mouth. SYN: *stomatodynia.*

stomatitis (stō-măt-ī'tĭs) [G. *stoma, stomat-,* mouth, + *-itis,* inflammation]. Inflammation of the mouth.

SYM: Heat, pain, increased flow of saliva, fetor of breath, restlessness, languor, disinclination to nurse in infants, sometimes fever. RS: *gangrene, noma, thrush.*

s., aphthous. Formation of tiny ulcers on mucosa of the mouth.

SYM: General symptoms of stomatitis and on inspection numerous small, round vesicles on cheeks, lips and tongue, which soon break and leave little, shallow ulcers with red areola.

PROG: Good.

TREATMENT: For infants, sterilize milk. Nurse at regular intervals. Wash mouth with clean linen cloth. In adults, correct gastric disturbance.

s., catarrhal. Simple stomatitis.

SYM: General symptoms of s. with diffuse red swelling of mucous membrane.

TREATMENT: Good hygienic conditions; cleanse mouth with weak solution of boric acid or chlorate of potassium as a wash.

s., corrosive. S. resulting from use of corrosive substances.

s., diphtheritic. Diphtheria of mucous membranes of the gums or cheeks. SYN: *buccal diphtheria.*

s., follicular. SEE: *aphthous s.*

s., gangrenous. This form seen in debilitated children from 2 to 6 years; usually follows one of the specific fevers, esp. measles and whooping cough.

SYM: General; an inspection shows cheek is affected. Externally, swollen, hard, red and glazed; internally, irregular, sloughing ulcer.

COMPLICATIONS: Perforation, septicemia, lobular pneumonia from aspirated sloughs, and diarrhea from swallowing fetid material.

PROG: Grave. Death common from exhaustion or complications. Recovery often attended with deformity.

TREATMENT: Excision with electrocautery knife early. Nutritious food, good hygiene. As a mouthwash boric acid or peroxide of hydrogen. SYN: *cancrum oris, noma.*

s. materna. S. during pregnancy or lactation.

s., mercurial. This form is seen in artisans who work in mercury; after the administration of very large doses of mercurials, and after small doses where there has been unnatural susceptibility.

PREMONITORY SYMPTOMS: Tenderness of gums, redness near insertion of teeth, metallic taste, increase of saliva.

LATER SYM: Profuse salivation, fetor of breath, redness, swelling and tenderness of gums. Tongue may be similarly affected and protrude from mouth. In severe cases ulceration of mucous membrane, loss of teeth and necrosis of jaw result.

TREATMENT: Iodine of potassium in small doses to eliminate the mercury. Astringent and antiseptic mouthwashes. SEE: *ptyalism.*

s., parasitic. Exciting cause a fungus, *Saccharomyces albicans.* SYN: *thrush.*

SYM: Of general s. with milk-white elevations on tongue and mouth which on removal leave a raw surface. Disease may extend to pharynx, esophagus and larynx. Microscopic examination reveals fungus.

PROG: Good.

TREATMENT: Correct hygiene. Treat any gastric disturbance; locally, mild antiseptic washes.

s., simple. Erythematous inflammation of the mouth occurring in patches on the mucous membranes.

s., ulcerative. Thought by some to be an infectious disease, as it often occurs

stomatitis, vesicular   S-88   **strabismus, accommodative**

in epidemics and attacks both children and adults when congregated and subjected to bad hygienic conditions.
  SYM: Of the general form; gums of lower jaw chiefly affected, are swollen, red and spongy. Linear ulcers soon form and may extend to cheek; gland under jaw swollen. In severe cases loosening of teeth and necrosis of jaw may follow.
  PROG: Guardedly favorable.
  TREATMENT: Correct hygiene; constitutional emetics; antiseptic mouthwashes.
  SYN: *trench mouth.*
  s., vesicular. SEE: *aphthous s.*
stomato- [G.]. Combining form meaning mouth.
stomatodynia (stō″mă-tō-dĭn′ĭ-ă) [G. *stoma, stomat-,* mouth, + *odynē,* pain]. Pain in the mouth. SYN: *stomatalgia.*
stomatodysodia (stō″mă-tō-dĭs-ō′dĭ-ă) [" + *dysōdia,* stench]. Foul odor from the mouth.
stomatogastric (stō″mă-tō-găs′trĭk) [" + *gastēr,* belly]. Concerning the stomach and mouth.
stomatography (stō″mă-tŏg′ră-fĭ) [" + *graphein,* to write]. A treatise on the mouth.
stomatologist (stō″mă-tŏl′ō-jĭst) [" + *logos,* a study]. Specialist in treatment of diseases of the mouth.
stomatology (stō″mă-tol′ō-jĭ) [" + *logos,* a study]. Science of the mouth and teeth and their diseases.
stomatomalacia (stō″mă-tō-mă-lā′sĭ-ă) [" + *malakia,* softening]. Pathological softening of any structures of the mouth.
stomatomy (stō-măt′ō-mĭ) [" + *tomē,* a cutting]. Surgical nicking of the edges of the os uteri to facilitate delivery.
stomatomycosis (stō″mă-tō-mĭ-kō′sĭs) [G. *stoma, stomat-,* mouth, + *mykēs,* fungus, + *-ōsis,* condition]. Any mouth disease resulting from fungi.
stomatonecrosis, stomatonoma (stō″mă-tō-nē-krō′sĭs, -nō′mă) [" + *nekrosis,* death, — + *nomē,* a spreading]. Gangrenous, ulcerative inflammation of the mouth. SYN: *cancrum oris, noma.*
stomatopathy (stō-mă-tŏp′ă-thĭ) [" + *pathos,* disease]. Any mouth disease.
stomatoplasty (stō-măt′ō-plăs″tĭ) [" + *plassein,* to form]. Plastic operation upon the mouth.
stomatorrhagia (stō″mă-tor-rā′jĭ-ă) [" + *-rrhagia,* from *rhēgnynai,* to burst forth]. Hemorrhage from the mouth or gums.
stomatoscope (stō′măt-ō-skōp) [" + *skopein,* to examine]. Instrument for examining the mouth.
stomodaeum, stomodeum (stō″mō-dē′ŭm) [" + *daiein,* to divide]. An invagination of the ectoderm or outer layer of the embryo that forms the mouth cavity.
stone (stōn) [A.S. *stān*]. Hardened mineral matter, as *gallstones.** SYN: *calculus, q.v.*
stool (stōōl) [A.S. *stōl,* a seat]. 1. Evacuation of the bowels. 2. Waste matter discharged from the bowels. SYN: *feces, q.v.*
  COLOR: Iron and bismuth turn the stool black and certain vegetables and berries darken it. Pathological stools are usually grayish or a whitish glistening color, and tarry in hemorrhage or show fresh blood.
  CHARACTER OR NATURE OF STOOLS: *Fatty stools*: These are observed in obstructive jaundice, cancer of the pancreas, pancreatic calculi, and in indigestion or overfeeding in infants.
  Frothy, poorly formed stools: They may indicate a spastic colon, the presence of gas, or intestinal inflammation.
  Lienteric stools: These contain much undigested food and are noted in inflammatory conditions of the stomach and upper bowel.
  Tarry stools: They are indicative of gastric hemorrhage, or may result from swallowing blood from the nose or lungs. They also may denote duodenal ulcer, or ulcer of the intestines, hepatic cirrhosis, or cancer.
  Membranous shreds: They may exist in cancer of the colon, dysentery, relapsing fever, acute proctitis, and in sloughing of intestinal mucosa.
  Mucous stools: Exist in catarrhal or inflamed conditions of the intestines or rectum, in dysentery, enterocolitis, proctitis, impaction, mucous colic, and mucous colitis.
  SHAPE OF: *Cylindrical*: If of small caliber, they may be indicative of prolapsus ani, annular rectal stricture, or intestinal spasms.
  Ribbon-shaped: Indicative of stricture or cancer of the rectum; possibly enlargement of the prostate in males, hemorrhoids, spasm of the lower bowel and anus, prostatic abscess, and prolapsus of the uterus.
  Scybala: Rounded masses or balls of fecal matter or hardened feces, the result of habitual constipation, atony or sacculation (diverticulum) of the colon, gastric ulcer, or dilation, and rectal cancer, or dysentery.
  s., bilious. Yellowish or yellowish-brown discharges in diarrhea becoming darker on exposure. [creatic diseases.
  s., fatty. Fat in the feces, as in pan-
  s., pea soup. Liquid stools of typhoid.
  s., rice water. Watery serum stools with detached epithelium, as in cholera.
stop needle. One with eye at tip and a disk to prevent penetration deeper than desired.
stoppage (stŏp′ăj) [A.S. *stoppian*]. Obstruction of an organ. SEE: *cholestasia.*
stout (stowt) [M.E. stout; bold]. Having a bulky body. SYN: *corpulent.*
stovaine (stō-vā′ĭn). Local anesthetic less toxic than cocaine.
  DOSAGE: ½-¾ gr. (0.02-0.05 Gm.).
stovainization (stō-vă-ĭn-ĭ-zā′shŭn). Induction of local anesthesia with stovaine.
stovarsol (stō′văr-sol). A commercial brand of acetarsone* used in spirochetal infections.
  DOSAGE: 4 gr. (0.25 Gm.).
strabismic (stră-bĭz′mĭk) [G. *strabismos,* a squint]. Pert. to or afflicted with strabismus.
strabismometer (stră-bĭz-mŏm′ĕt-ĕr) [" + *metron,* a measure]. Instrument for determining amount of strabismus.
strabismus (stră-bĭz′mŭs) [G. *strabismos,* a squinting]. Disorder of eye in which optic axes cannot be directed to same object, due to lack of muscular coordination. SYN: *squint.*
  The squinting eye always deviates to the same extent when the eyes are carried in different directions. *Unilateral,* when same eye always deviates. *Alternating,* when either deviates, the other being fixed. *Constant,* when the squint remains permanent. *Periodic,* when eyes are occasionally free from it. Muscles may lead to squint, but prime factor is found in errors of refraction, in hypermetropia or in myopia with or without astigmatism.
  s., accommodative. S. due to disorder of ocular accommodation.

strabismus, alternating   **stratum germinativum**

s., alternating. S. affecting either eye alternately.
s., bilateral. Same as accommodative s.
s., concomitant. Form in which 2 eyes move freely, but retain false relation to each other.
s., convergent (internal squint). The deviating eye turns inwards.
s., deorsum vergens. Vertical strabismus downwards. SYN: *hypotropia.*
s., divergent. Deviating eye turns outwards.
s., intermittent. One recurring at intervals.
s., monolateral. When the squinting eye is always the same.
s., monocular. When the same eye habitually deviates.
s., paralytic. That which is due to paralysis of a muscle. The deviation is present only in the sphere of action of the paralyzed muscle. In paralytic squint the secondary deviation is greater than the primary.
This condition is due to paralysis of one or more ocular muscles and may point to grave cerebral disease or to presence of some constitutional dyscrasia.
This form is recognized by the fact that if a candle or the finger of the surgeon is carried from right to left before the face of the patient the deviating eye fails to follow to its proper limit, and leads us to look for lesions of the 6th nerve in failure of external rectus, of 3rd nerve in failure of internal rectus of either side, of 4th nerve in impairment of superior oblique muscles. In adults this is usually due to syphilitic disease involving the nerve centers or trunks, or to rheumatism.
PROG: In general, guarded.
TREATMENT: Directed to the cause. Use of glasses.
s., spastic. S. due to contraction of an ocular muscle.
s., sursum vergens. Vertical squint upwards. SYN: *hypertropia.*
ETIOL: Defects of fusion faculty, errors of refraction, poor vision in 1 eye, anisometropia.
TREATMENT: Refraction with prescribing of glasses, orthoptic training (training of fusion), operative.
s., vertical. Eye turns upward. The vision is double (diplopia), unless there is unconscious suppression of the image in squinting eye, and expression of face is bizarre and sometimes malign. It is usually the result in childhood of ametropia, or in adult life of central nervous disease.
strabometer (strā-bŏm'ĕt-ẽr) [G. *strabos*, squinting, + *metron*, a measure]. Instrument to ascertain the degree of strabismus.
strabotomy (strā-bŏt'ō-mǐ) [" + *tomē*, a cutting]. Operation for strabismus.
strain (strān) [A.S. *strēon*, begetting]. 1. A stock, said of bacteria or protozoa from a specific source and maintained in successive cultures or animal inoculation. 2. Hereditary streak or tendency. 3. [M.E. *stranen*, from L. *stringere*, to draw tight]. To pass through, as a filter. 4. To injure by making too strong an effort or by excessive use. 5. Excessive use of a part of the body so that it is injured. 6. Injury to muscles from tension due to overuse or misuse. SYN: *sprain.*
F. A. TREATMENT: Apply cold applications and a firm dressing. Immobilize for some time. Adhesive strapping helpful. Operative repair sometimes necessary.
strainer (strān'er) [M.E. *stranen*, from L. *stringere*, to draw tight]. Device used for retaining solid pieces while liquid passes through. SYN: *filter.*
strait (strāt) [M.E. straight, narrow, from L. *strictus*, tight]. A constricted or narrow passage.
s., inferior. The lower outlet of the pelvic canal.
s.-jacket. Shirt with long sleeves laced on patient and fastened to restrain the arms. SYN: *camisole.*
s's. of the pelvis. The inferior and superior openings of the true pelvis.
s., superior. The upper opening or inlet of the pelvic canal.
stramonium (strā-mō'nǐ-ŭm) [L.]. USP. Jamestown weed, Jimson weed. The dried leaves of *Datura stramonium.*
USES: An ingredient in asthma powder for its antispasmodic effect. Local anodyne.
DOSAGE: 1.25 gr. (0.075 Gm.).
POISONING: Related to atropine, *q.v.*
strangalesthesia (strang″ăl-ĕs-thē'zǐ-ă) [G. *strangalizein*, to choke, + *aisthēsis*, sensation]. A girdlelike sensation of constriction. SYN: *zonesthesia.*
strangle (strang'gl) [G. *strangalē*, a halter]. To choke or suffocate or be choked from compression of the trachea.
strangulated (străng'ŭ-lā″tĕd) [L. *strangulāre*, from G. *strangalē*, a halter]. Constricted so that air or blood supply is cut off, as a s. hernia.
strangulation (străng-ŭ-lā'shŭn) [L. *strangulāre*, from G. *strangalē*, a halter]. Compression or constriction of a part, as the bowel or throat, such as causes suspension of breathing or of passage of contents; congestion accompanies condition.
s., internal. Slipping of a coil of the intestine through the diaphragm or an abnormal opening.
strangury (străng'ŭ-rǐ) [G. *stragx, stragg-*, a drop, + *ouron*, urine]. Painful and interrupted urination in drops, produced by spasmodic muscular contraction of urethra and bladder.
strap (străp) [A.S. *stropp*, from G. *strophos*, a cord]. 1. A band, as one of adhesive plaster, used to hold dressings in place or to approximate surfaces of a wound. 2. To bind with strips of adhesive plaster.
strapping (străp'ǐng) [A.S. *stropp*, from G. *strophos*, a band]. 1. Adhesive plaster or other substance used to bind surfaces together or hold dressings in place. 2. Application of adhesive plaster strips on a part so as to give it support or compress it.
stratified (străt'ǐ-fīd) [L. *stratificāre*, to arrange in layers]. In strata or in the form of layers.
s. epithelium. E. in superimposed layers with differently shaped cells in the various layers.
stratiform (străt'ǐ-form) [L. *stratum*, layer, + *forma*, shape]. Arranged in layers, as manner of liquefaction of gelatin stab culture, in which there is liquefaction to the walls of the tube at the top and then downward horizontally.
stratum (strā'tŭm, străt'ŭm) (pl. *strata*) [L. *stratum*, layer]. A layer.
s. corneum. BNA. Horny layer of the skin.
s. germinativum. Innermost layer of epidermis, a row of columnar cells, which divide to replace rest of the epi-

dermis as it wears away. SEE: *prickle cell.*
s. granulosum. A layer of very small cells, or cells containing granules, as that in the skin.
s. granulosum epidermidis. Lozenge-shaped or trapezoid-shaped cells covering the *rete mucosum* and covered by the s. lucidum in the skin.
s. lucidum. A translucent layer of the epidermis.
s. Malpighii. Inner layer of the epidermis. SYN: *rete mucosum, s. germinativum.*
s. mucosum. Same as *s. malpighii.*
s. spinosum. Same as s. malpighii.
s. spongiosum. 1. Spongy layer of the urethra. 2. Medial layer of decidua.
strawberry (straw'bĕr"ĭ) [A.S. *strēawberige*, hay berry]. COMP: Contain little cellulose. Sugar is low. They contain much lime and a salicylic element.
Av. SERVING: 100 Gm. Pro. 1.0, Fat 0.6, Carbo. 6.00.
VITAMINS: A+, B+, C+++.
ASH CONST: Ca 0.041, Mg 0.019, K 0.147, Na 0.050, P 0.028, Cl 0.006, S 0.014, Fe 0.0006.
ACTION: The salicylic element is irritating to many and may result in a skin rash.
straw'berry tongue. The peculiar, redly papillated tongue of scarlatina, *q.v.* SEE: *tongue.*
straw itch (strau). A skin condition accompanied by itching due to working in straw or sleeping on a straw mattress.
streak (strēk) [A.S. *strica*, a line]. A line or stripe. SYN: *stria.*
s. culture. A bacterial culture in streaks.
s., medullary. Deep longitudinal groove on dorsal surface of the embryo which becomes the medullary tube. SYN: *dorsal groove.*
s., meningitic. A red line across the skin formed by drawing a pointed article across it; seen in meningitis and nerve center affections. SYN: *tache cérébrale.*
s., primitive. An opaque band at end of germinal area forming the first signs of the blastoderm in the fertilized ovum.
s. reflex. A white, shining streak along center of retinal vessels.
strephotome (strĕf'ō-tōm) [G. *strephein*, to twist, + *tomē*, a cutting]. Instrument for invagination of a hernial sac.
strepitus (strĕp'ĭt-ŭs) [L. *strepitus*, noise]. A sound or noise, as that heard on auscultation.
strepticemia (strĕp-tĭ-sē'mĭ-ă) [G. *streptos*, twisted, + *aima*, blood]. Streptococci present in the blood stream causing infection. SYN: *streptococcemia.*
strepto- [G.]. Combining form meaning *twisted.*
streptoangina (strĕp"tō-ăn-jī'nă) [G. *streptos*, twisted, + L. *angina*, a choking]. Sore throat with membranous formation due to streptococcus.
streptobacteria (strĕp"tō-băk-tē'rĭ-ă) [" + *baktērion*, a little rod]. Those bacteria which are arranged in chains.
streptobacterin (strĕp"tō-băk'tĕr-ĭn) [" + *baktērion*, a little rod]. A vaccine made from streptococci.
streptococcal (strĕp"tō-kŏk'ăl) [" + *kokkos*, berry]. Caused by or pert. to streptococci.
streptococcemia (strĕp"tō-kŏk-sē'mĭ-ă) [" + " + *aima*, blood]. Presence of streptococci in the blood causing infection.
streptococcic (strĕp"tō-kŏk'sĭk) [" + *kok-*

kos, berry]. Resembling, produced by, or pert. to streptococci.
s. sore throat. Severe epidemic form with membranous formation caused by *Streptococcus haemolyticus.*
streptococcicosis (strĕp"tō-kŏk-sĭ-kō'sĭs) [G. *streptos*, twisted, + *kokkos*, berry, + *-ōsis*, condition]. Any streptococcal infection.
streptococcolysin (strĕp"tō-kŏk-ŏl'ĭ-sĭn) [" + " + *lysis*, dissolution]. A lysin produced by streptococci.
Streptococcus (strĕp"tō-kŏk'ŭs) (pl. *Streptococci*) [G. *streptos*, twisted, + *kokkos*, berry]. A genus of spherical organisms occurring in chains of various lengths.
Most of them are harmless saprophytes, but a few are pathogenic parasites causing suppuration and are grouped generally under the name of *Streptococcus pyogenes.* Pathogenic streptococci can be subdivided into 3 classifications according to their development on cultures of blood agar: *Al-*

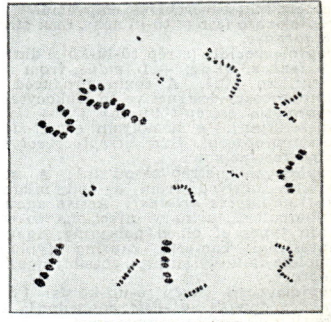

STREPTOCOCCUS.
Cocci of varying size in chains; some in pairs, forming chains. Brain broth culture of infected root of a tooth (focal infection).

pha, or viridans type, which forms a greenish area around the colony; *beta*, or hemolytic type, which forms a clear halo around the colony due to complete breaking down of cells, and the *gamma*, or nonhemolytic type, which causes no apparent change around the colony.
Str. anginosus. Hemolytic variety found in acute pharyngitis.
Str. cardioarthritidis. Variety found in blood and throat secretion cultures in cases of rheumatic fever.
Str. epidemicus. Hemolytic variety seen in throat cultures in cases of epidemic sore throat.
Str. erysipelatis. Organism causing erysipelas, which resembles *Str. pyogenes.*
Str., green. SEE: *Str. viridans.*
Str. haemolyticus, Str., hemolytic. Any of the streptococci causing complete hemolysis of erythrocytes; majority of pathogenic varieties are in this group.
Str. mixtos. SEE: *Str. haemolyticus.*
Str. morbilli. Variety found in cases of measles, the probable cause of that disease.
Str. puerperalis. Species found in puerperal septicemia, which resembles *Str. pyogenes.*
Str. pyogenes. Any of the hemolytic streptococci causing suppurative processes.

Str. scarlatinae. Probable causative agent of scarlet fever.
Str. viridans. Nonhemolytic form producing green colonies on blood agar which frequently is the cause of focal infection, which in turn leads to symptoms of arthritis, neuritis, endocarditis, etc. A form normal in the mouth. Found in the blood of 40 per cent of people after tooth extraction, and in 11 per cent of those with dirty mouths. In 75 per cent of cases, penicillin will kill the germ.

streptocolysin (strĕp″tō-kŏl′ĭ-sĭn) [G. *streptos*, twisted, + *lysis*, dissolution]. A hemolysin produced by streptococci.

streptodermatitis (strĕp″tō-der-mă-tī′tĭs) [" + *derma*, skin, + *-itis*, inflammation]. Inflammation of the skin caused by streptococci.

streptodornase (strĕp″tō-dor′nās). One of the enzymes (*streptokinase* is another) elaborated by hemolytic streptococci, and capable of liquefying fibrinous and purulent exudates. Useful in pneumococcic and tuberculous empyema.

streptokinase (strĕp″tō-kī′nās). SEE: *streptodornase*.

streptoleukocidin (strĕp″tō-lū-kō-sī′dĭn) [" + *leukos*, white, + L. *cidus*, from *caedere*, to kill]. A toxin produced by streptococci destructive to leukocytes.

streptolysin (strĕp-tŏl′ĭ-sĭn) [" + *lysis*, dissolution]. A hemolysin excreted by a streptococcus. SYN: *streptococcolysin, streptocolysin*.

streptomycin (strĕp′tō-mī′sĭn). A substance derived from a soil microbe (*Streptomyces griseus*). Active against tuberculosis, urinary infections, in certain types of blood poisoning, against intestinal bacteria causing typhoid, cholera, and dysentery; possibly against leprosy.

streptomycosis (strĕp″tō-mī-kō′sĭs) [" + *mykes*, fungus, + *-osis*, condition]. Infection caused by streptococci.

streptosepticemia (strĕp″tō-sĕp-tĭ-sē′mĭ-ă) [" + *septikos*, putrid, + *aima*, blood]. Septicemia resulting from streptococcus infection. SYN: *streptococcemia, streptomycosis*.

streptothricosis (strĕp-tō-thrĭ-kō′sĭs) [" + *thrix*, hair, + *-osis*, condition]. Infection caused by a species of Streptothrix.
SYM: Chronic suppurative inflammation.

Streptothrix (strĕp′tō-thrĭks) [" + *thrix*, hair]. A genus of Chlamydobacteriaceae, of which one form is the cause of actinomycosis and another is assumed to be cause of rat-bite fever.

stretcher (strĕch′er) [A.S. *streccan*, to reach]. A litter for carrying the sick, injured or dead.

stretch'ing of contrac'tures. Process performed to loosen contracted ligaments, muscles and adhesions in stiff joints. There should be a slow, steady and gradually increasing pull by the operator or with gradually increasing weights.

stria (strī′a) (pl. *striae*) [L. *stria*, a channel or groove]. A line or band elevated above or depressed below surrounding tissue, or differing in color and texture.
Capillary bleeding occurs, giving the marks a purplish color. Old scars are white. They are commonly seen on the thighs, abdomen, and breasts of pregnant women, but may result from any sudden enlargement due to dropsy, tumors, or excessive obesity.

s., acoustic, s., auditory. One of the horizontal white stripes on floor of the 4th ventricle of the brain.

s. acustica. Same as *s. medullaris*.
s. atrophica. Whitish cicatricial line on the skin caused by stretching, as in pregnancy or obesity.
s. gravidarum. Same as *s. atrophica*.
s. longitudinalis lateralis. One of the longitudinal bands of gray matter, slightly elevated on upper part of the corpus callosum.
s. medullaris. Same as *s., acoustic, s. acustica, s. pinealis*.
s. pinealis. Longitudinal strand of fibers along walls of the 3rd ventricle below the taenia thalami.
s. terminalis. A band of fibers in roof of inf. horn running to floor of body of the lateral ventricle.

striate, striated (strī′āt, strī′āt-ĕd) [L. *stria*, channel]. Striped; marked by streaks or striae.
s. body. Mass of gray and white bands in each cerebral hemisphere. SYN: *corpus striatum*.

striation (strī-ā′shŭn) [L. *stria*, channel]. 1. State of being striped or streaked. 2. One of a series of streaks. SYN: *stria*.

striatum (strī-ā′tŭm) [L. *striatum*, grooved]. The caudate and lentiform nuclei of the brain considered as one. SYN: *corpus striatum*.

stricture (strĭk′chūr) [L. *strictura*, a tightening]. A localized contraction of a tube or canal due to pressure or changes in the wall tissue; may affect the esophagus, ureters and urethra. SEE: *arctation, stenosis*.
s., bridle. One caused by a band across the tube, partially occluding it.
s., cicatricial. One resulting from a scar or wound.
s., functional. One due to muscular spasm.
s., impermeable. One closing the lumen of a tube or canal.
s., irritable. One causing pain when an instrument is passed.
s., spasmodic. Same as *functional s.*
s. of urethra. Most common in men. May be partial or complete.
SYM: Straining to pass urine, esp. at commencement of urination.
ETIOL: Spasm of urethral muscle, congestion of urethra and fibrous formation.

stricturotome (strĭk′chūr-ō-tōm) [L. *strictura*, a contraction, + G. *tome*, a cutting]. Instrument for cutting strictures.

stricturotomy (strĭk-chūr-ŏt′ō-mĭ) [" + G. *tome*, a cutting]. Operation of cutting strictures.

stridor (strī′dōr) [L. a harsh sound]. Harsh sound during respiration; high-pitched and like the blowing of the wind due to obstruction of air passages.
s., congenital or laryngeal. Inspiration at birth or during first 3 weeks giving forth a crowing sound.
s. dentium. Noise from grinding of the teeth.
s. serraticus. Sound of respiration like that of sawing, when heard through a tracheotomy tube.

stridulous (strĭd′ū-lŭs) [L. *stridulus*, harsh, creaking]. Making a shrill grating sound.

string beans. Av. SERVING: 75 Gm. Pro. 1.8, Fat 0.2, Carbo. 5.8.
VITAMINS: $A++$, $B++$, $C++$, $G++$.
ASH CONST: Ca 0.046, Mg 0.025, K 0.247, Na 0.019, P 0.052, Cl 0.024, S 0.030, Fe 0.0011.

strip (strĭp) [A.S. *strȳpan*, to strip off]. To remove all contents from, esp. by gentle pressure, as to strip the seminal vesicles.

strobila (strō-bī'lă) [G. *strobilē*, a twisted plug]. Consecutive segments of body of a tapeworm.

stroke (strōk) [A.S. *strāk*, a going]. 1. A sudden, severe attack of affliction, as apoplexy; a sharp blow. 2. [A.S. *strākian*, a going]. To rub gently in one direction, as in massage. 3. Gentle movement of the hand across a surface.

  s., back. Ventricular recoil of the heart during systole. SYN: *basculation*, 2.

  s. culture. One made by spreading inoculum on surface of the medium. SYN: *smear culture*.

stroma (strō'mă) (pl. *stromata*) [G. *strōma*, a bed]. 1. Foundation supporting tissues of an organ. 2. Spongy, colorless framework of an erythrocyte.

  s. plexus. Ramification of nerves of the cornea.

  s. vitreum. Delicate framework of the vitreous body of the eye.

stromal, stromatic (strō'măl, strō-măt'ĭk) [G. *strōma*, a bed]. Concerning or resembling the stroma of an organ.

stromatolysis (strō″mă-tŏl'ĭ-sĭs) [″ + *lysis*, destruction]. Destruction of the enveloping membrane of a cell without affecting the cell body.

Stromeyer's splint (strō'mī-ĕr). A hinged splint for a joint, which can be fixed at any angle.

stromuhr (strō'moor) [Ger.]. Device for measuring velocity of blood flow. SYN: *rheometer*.

Strongyloides (strŏn-jĭ-loy'dēz) [G. *stroggylos*, round, + *eidos*, form]. A genus of roundworms frequently found in the intestines.

  S. intestinalis. An intestinal roundworm.

strongyloidosis (strŏn″jĭ-loy-dō'sĭs) [″ + ″ + *-ōsis*, condition]. Infestation with Strongyloides.

strongylosis (strŏn-jĭ-lō'sĭs) [G. *stroggylos*, round, + *-ōsis*, condition]. Infestation with Strongylus.

Strongylus (strŏn'jĭ-lŭs) [G. *stroggylos*, round]. A genus of parasitic roundworms.

strontium (strŏn'shĭ-ŭm). A dark, yellowish metal, some of its salts being medicinal.

Strophanthus (strō-făn'thŭs) [G. *strophos*, cord, + *anthos*, flower]. USP. Plant yielding a poisonous, white, crystalline glucoside; used chiefly in the form of alkaloid; strophanthin.

  ACTION AND USES: Similar to digitalis.

  DOSAGE: 1 gr. (0.06 Gm.).

strophulus (strŏf'u-lŭs) [L. *strophulus*, from G. *strophos*, a twisted cord]. An infantile red eruption. SYN: *gum rash, red rash, tooth rash*.

  s. albidus. Small, white nodule below the epidermis. SYN: *milium*.

  s. infantum. Urticaria in infants.

  s. pruriginosus. A form with itching papules.

structural (strŭk'tū-răl) [L. *structūra*, a building]. Pert. to organic structure.

  s. disease. A disease effecting changes in any structure.

struma (strū'mă) [L. a mass]. 1. Tuberculosis of the lymphatics. SYN: *scrofula*. 2. Enlargement of the thyroid gland. SYN: *goiter*.

  s. maligna. Carcinoma of the thyroid gland.

  s. suprarenalis. Fatty tissue tumor of the suprarenals.

  s. vasculosa. Enlargement of the thyroid gland due to dilatation of the blood vessels.

strumectomy (strū-měk'tō-mī) [″ + G. *ektomē*, excision]. Excision of scrofulous glands or of a goiter.

strumiprivus (strū″mĭ-prī'vŭs) [L. *struma*, a mass, + *prīvāre*, to deprive]. Referring to or caused by removal of the thyroid gland. SEE: *cachexia*.

strumitis (strū-mī'tĭs) [″ + G. *-ītis*, inflammation]. Inflammation of a thyroid gland with goiter. SYN: *thyroiditis*.

strumoderma (strū″mō-der'mă) [″ + G. *derma*, skin]. Any tuberculous skin disease. SYN: *scrofuloderma*.

strumous (strū'mŭs) [L. *struma*, a mass]. 1. Affected with scrofula. SYN: *scrofulous*. 2. Affected with goiter.

Strumpell's reflex (strŭm'pĕl). Stroking of thigh and abdomen results in movement of leg on same side accompanied by adduction of corresponding foot.

strychnine (strĭk'nĭn, -nēn, -nĭn) [G. *strychnos*, nightshade]. A poisonous alkaloid obtained from plants, as nux vomica.

It is a marked stimulant, causing the heart to beat more strongly. When taken in small doses for some time the mental powers become sharpened and sensibility intensified. Bowel movements become less sluggish and gastric secretion augmented. The spinal cord is affected in a marked degree, reflex action being increased and the muscle tone improved.

USES: As a tonic in convalescence from weakening diseases, in some nervous conditions, and for the debility caused by excessive overstrain. Contraindicated in diseases connected with overactivity of spinal cord. When heart failure threatens the drug is often used hypodermically. Its stimulating action causes it to be a useful adjunct to purgative medicines.

When the nervous system is depressed owing to poisons or toxins, such as alcohol, lead, tobacco, and diphtheria, it is a much-ordered remedy.

POISONING: The fatal dose of strychnine by mouth is probably between 1 and 2 gr., although much larger doses have been recovered from.

SYM: When swallowed, symptoms usually develop within 15 to 20 minutes. This time element depends largely upon the drug being in solution and the stomach being empty. Given by needle in toxic amounts, the development of symptoms is remarkably prompt. The usual course is, first, a hyperesthesia followed by a modification of the reflexes, especially shown as a tendency for a single stimulus to produce exaggerated reactions and to involve apparently unrelated muscle groups.

If a sufficient amount has been taken, there rapidly develop nervous twitchings followed by convulsions. The seizures are tonic in character, further characterized by cyanosis and opisthotonos, followed by relaxation and exhaustion. The duration of a seizure may be from a few seconds to about a minute. Consciousness may not be lost, so that the tonic contractions may be very painful. They tend to recur in 5 to 15 minutes and may be precipitated by almost any stimulus such as physical contact or unusual noise. In favorable cases, convulsions gradually lessen in severity. Should death occur, it is usually by asphyxiation during one of the early attacks or later by exhaustion following repeated paroxysms.

TREATMENT: Consists in thoroughly

emptying the stomach; best done with a small stomach tube. An ideal chemical antidote is *potassium permanganate*, used in a solution of about 1:2000; about a pint of this left in the stomach. Other measures are keeping patient quiet, free from any disturbing factors, such as noise and confusion. Medication depends upon the administration of antispasmodics. *Barbituric acid salts* are used intravenously, or *chloral hydrate* and *bromides* given by mouth or rectum. Inhalations of *chloroform* have been recommended for controlling a convulsion until the patient can be brought under the influence of other medication. Inhalations of *oxygen* have been used in this condition with apparent benefit. Artificial respiration, especially by the infratracheal method, is sometimes a life saver, but requires the proper apparatus that is not always available. Elimination favored particularly by diuretics.

    s. nitrate. USP. The nitrate of the alkaloid strychnine.
    ACTION AND USES: Same as strychnine sulfate.
    DOSAGE: Same.
    s. sulfate. USP. The sulfate of an alkaloid obtained from nux vomica.
    ACTION AND USES: Stimulant to the spinal cord and respiration.
    DOSAGE: 1/30 gr. (0.002 Gm.).
    POISONING: An extremely bitter alkaloid used as an animal poisoning to destroy pests.
    SYM: Begin shortly after administration. Tightness of chest, a feeling of impending calamity, and shortly violent convulsions with weak, irregular pulse; dilated pupils.
    F. A. TREATMENT: Wash out stomach; anesthesia is given cautiously to diminish convulsions. Tannic acid to precipitate the alkaloid. Sedatives, as barbital, desirable, esp. those varieties that may be given intravenously, as sodium amytal and sodium pentobarbital. SEE: *strychnine*.
    INCOMPATIBILITIES: Potassium iodide.

strychninism (strĭk'nĭn-ĭzm) [G. *strychnos*, nightshade, + *-ismos*, condition]. Chronic strychnine poisoning. SYN: *strychnism*.

strychninomania (strĭk″nĭ-nō-mā'nĭ-ă) [" + *mania*, madness]. Insanity resulting from continued use of strychnine.

strychnism (strĭk'nĭzm). Poisoning from use of strychnine. SYN: *strychninism*.

student's placenta (stū'dĕnt). Retention of the placenta in childbirth because of unskillful manipulation by the obstetrician or midwife.

stump (stŭmp) [M.E. *stumpe*]. Basal part of limb left after amputation.
    s. hallucination. Consciousness of still being possessed of a limb or arm after its amputation.

stun (stŭn) [M.E. *stunein*, to stun]. To render unconscious or stupefied by a blow.

stupe (stūp) [L. *stupa*, tow, from G. *stypē*]. Cloth of flannel wrung out of hot water for a fomentation, often saturated with a counterirritant such as turpentine. SEE: *fomentation*.
    s., opium. 30-60 minims of opium sprinkled over stupe after it has been wrung out.
    s., turpentine. 1-2 drams of turpentine sprinkled evenly over dry flannel before water is poured on.

stupefacient (stū-pē-fā'shĕnt) [L. *stupefaciens*, stupefying]. Causing or that which causes stupor. SYN: *narcotic; soporific*.

stupemania (stū-pē-mā'nĭ-ă) [L. *stupor*, stupor, + G. *mania*, madness]. Insanity with symptoms of stupor.

stupor (stū'por) [L. *stupor*]. 1. Condition of unconsciousness, torpor, or lethargy with suppression of sense or feeling. 2. PSY: A state of lessened responsiveness.
    Stupor occurs in visceral and infectious diseases, melancholia, catatonia, epilepsy, paresis, poisonings, and hysteria. A benign form is seen in manic-depressive psychosis.
    RS: *carotic, catatonia, collapse, coma, lethargy, narcoma, narcose, syncope, unconsciousness*.

stupration, stuprum (stū-prā'shŭn, stū'prŭm) [L. *stuprum*, defilement]. Sexual intercourse with a woman without her consent and by overpowering force, or intimidation. SYN: *rape*.

sturine (stū'rĭn) [L. *sturio*, sturgeon]. Protamine obtained from sperm of sturgeon which has bactericidal action.

stutter (stŭt'er) [M.E. *stutten*, to strike]. To hesitate and repeat or stumble spasmodically in speaking, due to difficulty in pronouncing initial consonants caused by spasm of lingual and palatal muscles.

stuttering (stŭt'er-ĭng) [M.E. *stutten*, to strike]. Defect in speech in which there is stumbling and spasmodic repetition of same syllable. RS: *battarism, mogilalia*.
    s., urinary. Irregular, spasmodic urination. SYN: *stammering* of the bladder*.

sty(e (stī) (pl. *styes* or *sties*) [A.S. *stīgan*, a rising]. A circumscribed inflammation of a sebaceous gland near edge of eyelid ending in suppuration. SYN: *hordeolum*.
    SYM: General edema of lid, pain, localized conjunctivitis.
    TREATMENT: Hot fomentations. When suppuration has taken place, free incision and pressure to evacuate sac. When a succession of styes occurs general system should be built up by constitutional remedies and the ametropia, which is almost always found in these aggravated cases, should be relieved by correcting lenses.
    s., meibomian. Inflammation of a meibomian gland.
    s., Zeissian. Inflammation of one of Zeiss' glands.

styles, stylet (stīles, stī'lĕt) [L. *stylus*, a pointed instrument]. 1. A slender, solid or hollow plug of metal for making permanent a canal after operation or for stiffening or clearing a cannula or catheter. 2. A thin probe.

styliscus (stī-lĭs'kŭs) [G. *styliskos*, pillar]. A slender, cylindrical plug for dilating a channel or for keeping a wound open. SEE: *tent*.

styloglossus (stī-lō-glŏs'ŭs) [G. *stylos*, pillar, + *glōssa*, tongue]. A muscle connecting the tongue and styloid process which raises and retracts the tongue. SEE: *Table of Muscles in Appendix*.

styloid (stī'loyd) [G. *stylos*, pillar, + *eidos*, form]. Resembling a stylus or pointed instrument.
    s. process. 1. A pointed process of the temporal bone, projecting downward, and to which some of the muscles of the tongue are attached. 2. A pointed projection behind the head of the fibula. 3. A protuberance on distal end of radius' outer portion. 4. An ulnar projection on inner side of the distal end.

styloiditis (stī-loyd-ī′tĭs) [G. *stylos*, pillar, + *eidos*, form, + *-itis*, inflammation]. Inflammation of a styloid process.

stylomastoid (stī″lō-măs′toyd) [" + *mastos*, breast, + *eidos*, form]. Concerning the styloid and mastoid processes of the temporal bone.

stylomaxillary (stī″lō-măks′ĭ-lă-rī) [" + L. *maxilla*, jaw]. Concerning the styloid process of the temporal bone and the mandible.

stylopharyngeus (stī″lō-far-ĭn′jē-ŭs) [" + *pharygx*, pharynx]. Muscle connecting the styloid process and pharynx which elevates and dilates the pharynx. SEE: *Table of Muscles in Appendix*.

stylus (stī′lŭs) [L. *stylus*, a pen, from G. *stylos*, a pillar]. 1. A probe or slender wire for stiffening or clearing a canal or catheter. 2. Pointed medicinal preparation in stick form for external application.

stype (stīp) [G. *stypē*, tow]. A pledget or tampon of cotton or other material.

stypsis (stĭp′sĭs) [G. *stypsis*, a steeping in an astringent]. Astringency or the use of an astringent.

styptic (stĭp′tĭk) [G. *styptikos*, contracting]. 1. Contracting a blood vessel; stopping a hemorrhage by astringent action. 2. Anything that checks a hemorrhage. SYN: *astringent, hemostat*.
Ex: *ferrous sulfate, alum, tannic acid*.

stypticin (stĭp′tĭ-sĭn) [G. *styptikos*, contracting]. Proprietary preparation of cotarnine hydrochloride, a yellow, odorless, crystalline powder.
USES: As a hemostatic.
DOSAGE: 1 gr. (0.06 Gm.).

stypven (stĭp′vĕn). Commercial preparation of Russell's viper venom.
The results of recent investigation have proven this to be of value as a hemostatic, used topically to stop bleeding in dental surgery, etc.

sub- [L.]. Combining form meaning *under, beneath, in small quantity*.

subabdominal (sŭb-ăb-dŏm′ĭ-năl) [L. *sub*, beneath, + *abdōmen*, abdomen]. Below the abdomen.

subacetate (sŭb-ăs′ĕt-āt) [" + *acetum*, vinegar]. A basic acetate.

subacromial (sŭb-ă-krō′mĭ-ăl) [" + G. *akron*, point, + *omos*, shoulder]. Under the acromion process.

subacute (sŭb-ă-kūt′) [" + *acutus*, sharp]. Bet. acute and chronic, but with some acute features, said of the course of a disease.

subalimentation (sŭb-ăl-ĭ-mĕn-tā′shŭn) [" + *alimentum*, food]. A state of insufficient nourishment.

subanconeus (sŭb-ăn-kō′nē-ŭs) [" + G. *agkōn*, elbow]. 1. Below the elbow. 2. Muscle beneath the elbow which contracts its post. ligament. SEE: *Table of Muscles in Appendix*.

subaponeurotic (sŭb″ap-ō-nū-rŏt′ĭk) [" + G. *apo*, from + *neuron*, tendon]. Below an aponeurosis.

subarachnoid (sŭb-ă-răk′noyd) [L. *sub*, under, + G. *arachnē*, spider, + *eidos*, form]. Below the arachnoid membrane.
s. space. Space between the pia proper and arachnoid containing the cerebrospinal fluid.

subarcuate (sŭb-ar′kū-āt) [" + *arcuatus*, bow-shaped]. Slightly arched.
s. fossa. Depression beneath the arcuate eminence.

subastragalar (sŭb-ăs-trăg′ă-lar) [" + G. *astragalos*, one of a set of dice]. Beneath the astragalus.

subastringent (sŭb-ăs-trĭn′jĕnt) [" + *astringere*, to contract]. Mildly astringent.

subaural (sŭb-aw′răl) [" + *auris*, ear]. Below the ear.

subcapsular (sŭb-kăp′sū-lar) [" + *capsula*, a little box]. Below any capsule, especially the capsule of the brain, or a capsular ligament.

subcarbonate (sŭb-kar′bŏn-āt) [" + *carbo*, carbon, coal]. A basic carbonate; one having less carbonic acid radical than the normal carbonate.

subcartilaginous (sŭb-kar-tĭl-ăj′ĭn-ŭs) [L. *sub*, beneath, + *cartilāgo*, cartilage]. 1. Beneath a cartilage. 2. Cartilaginous in part.

subchronic (sŭb-krŏn′ĭk) [" + G. *chronos*, time]. Noting a condition bet. subacute and chronic; almost chronic.

subclavian (sŭb-klā′vĭ-ăn) [" + *clavis*, a key]. Under the clavicle or collarbone. SYN: *subclavicular*.
s. artery. Large artery at base of neck.
s. triangle. One of the neck formed by the clavicle, and the omohyoid and sternomastoid muscles.

subclavicular (sŭb-klăv-ĭk′ū-lar) [" + *clavicula*, a little key]. Beneath the clavicle. SYN: *subclavian*.

subclavius (sŭb-klā′vĭ-ŭs) [" + *clavis*, a key]. A tiny muscle from the 1st rib to the undersurface of the clavicle. SEE: *Table of Muscles in Appendix*.

subclinical (sŭb-klĭn′ĭ-kal) [" + G. *klinikos*, pert. to a bed]. Pert. to a period before appearance of typical symptoms of a disease.

subcollateral (sŭb-kō-lăt′ĕr-ăl) [L. *sub*, under, + *con*, with, + *latus, later-*, side]. Below the collateral fissure, indicating a cerebral convolution.

subconjunctival (sŭb-kŏn-jŭnk-tī′văl) [" + *conjunctiva*, a joining]. Beneath the conjunctiva.

subconscious (sŭb-kŏn′shŭs) [" + *conscius*, aware]. Not clearly conscious; pert. to activities of which the mind is not aware or to that which is not cognized through the physical senses; below the threshold of objective consciousness; that which is activated by involuntary processes; intuitional.

subconsciousness (sŭb-kŏn′shŭs-nĕs) [" + *conscius*, aware]. 1. The state of being partially unconscious. 2. Noting of impressions and ideas without conscious knowledge of them. 3. The seat of a hypothetical subconscious mind in which are buried past impressions of objective knowledge. SEE: *subconscious*.

subcontinuous (sŭb-kŏn-tĭn′ū-ŭs) [" + *continuus*, holding together]. Almost continuous; with periods of abatement, but no interruptions to continuity.
s. fever. Fever with periods of remission and exacerbation. SYN: *remittent fever*.

subcoracoid (sŭb-kor′ă-koyd) [" + G. *korakoeidēs*, crowlike]. Beneath the coracoid process.

subcortex (sŭb-kor′tĕks) [" + *cortex*, rind]. White substance of the brain underlying the cortex.

subcortical (sŭb-kor′tĭ-kal) [L. *sub*, under, + *cortex, cortic-*, rind]. Pert. to the region beneath the cerebral cortex.

subcostal (sŭb-kŏs′tăl) [" + *costa*, rib]. Beneath the ribs.

subcostalgia (sŭb-kŏs-tăl′jĭ-ă) [" + " + G. *algos*, pain]. Pain in region over the subcostal nerve.

subcranial (sŭb-krā′nĭ-ăl) [" + G. *kranion*, skull]. Beneath or below the cranium.

subcrepitant (sŭb-krĕp′ĭ-tănt) [" + *crepi-*

tāre, to rattle]. Partially crepitant or crackling in character; noting a râle.

subcrureus (sŭb-krū-rē'ŭs) [" + *crus, crur-,* leg]. Small muscle bet. ant. surface of femoral shaft and synovial membrane of knee joint. SEE: *Table of Muscles in Appendix.*

subculture (sŭb-kŭl'chŭr) [" + *cultūra,* cultivation]. 1. To make a culture of bacteria with material derived from another culture. 2. One made by transferring bacteria from a previous culture to a fresh medium.

subcutaneous (sŭb-kū-tā'nē-ŭs) [L. *sub,* under, + *cutis,* skin]. Beneath or to be introduced beneath the skin. SYN: *hypodermic.*

    s. surgery. Operation performed through a small opening in the skin.

    s. wound. A wound with only a small opening through the skin.

subcuticular (sŭb-kū-tĭk'ū-lar) [" + *cuticula,* little skin]. Beneath the cuticle or epidermis. SYN: *subepidermal.*

subdelirium (sŭb-dē-lĭr'ĭ-ŭm) [" + *dē,* away from, + *lira,* track]. A mild or not continuous delirium.

subdiaphragmatic (sŭb-dī-ă-frăg-măt'ĭk) [" + G. *dia,* across, + *phragma,* wall]. Beneath the diaphragm.

subdural (sŭb-dū'răl) [" + *durus,* hard]. Beneath the dura mater.

    s. space. Space bet. the arachnoid and dura mater.

subencephalon (sŭb-ĕn-sef'ă-lŏn) [" + G. *egkephalos,* brain]. The pons, medulla oblongata, and corpora quadrigemina together. SYN: *hypencephalon.*

subendocardial (sŭb″ĕn-dō-kar'dĭ-ăl) [" + G. *endon,* within, + *kardia,* heart]. Below the endocardium.

subendothelial (sŭb″ĕn-dō-thē'lĭ-ăl) [L. *sub,* under, + G. *endon,* within, + *thēlē,* nipple]. Beneath endothelium.

subendothelium (sŭb″ĕn-dō-thē'lĭ-ŭm) [" + " + *thēlē,* nipple]. A layer bet. the epithelium and basement membrane of the mucosa of the bronchi and intestines. SYN: *Débove's membrane.*

subepidermal (sŭb″ĕp-ĭ-der'măl) [" + G. *epi,* upon, + *derma,* skin]. Beneath the epidermis. SYN: *subcuticular.*

subepithelial (sŭb″ĕp-ĭ-thē'lĭ-ăl) [" + " + *thēlē,* nipple]. Beneath the epithelium.

subfascial (sŭb-făsh'ĭ-ăl) [" + *fascia,* band]. Beneath a fascia.

subfebrile (sŭb-fē'brĭl) [" + *febris,* fever]. Somewhat feverish.

subflavous (sŭb-flā'vŭs) [" + *flavus,* yellow]. Yellowish.

    s. ligament. Yellowish ligament connecting the laminae of the vertebrae. SYN: *ligamentum subflavum.*

subfrontal (sŭb-frŭn'tăl) [L. *sub,* beneath, + *frons, front-,* forehead]. Below a frontal convolution or lobe of the brain.

subglenoid (sŭb-glē'noyd) [" + G. *glēnē,* cavity, + *eidos,* form]. Below the glenoid fossa or glenoid cavity.

subglossal (sŭb-glŏs'ăl) [" + G. *glōssa,* tongue]. Under the tongue. SYN: *hypoglossal, sublingual.*

subglossitis (sŭb-glŏs-sī'tĭs) [" + " + *-itis,* inflammation]. Inflammation of the undersurface or tissues of the tongue.

subgrondation, subgrundation (sŭb-grŏn-dā'shŭn, -grŭn-dā'shŭn) [Fr.]. Depression of one fragment of a broken bone beneath the other, as of the cranium.

subhyoid (sŭb-hī'oyd) [L. *sub,* beneath, + G. *hyoeidēs,* U-shaped]. Beneath the hyoid bone.

subiculum (sū-bĭk'ū-lŭm) [L. *subiculum,* a small support]. A division of hippocampal convolution, composed of a thick layer of myelinated fibers on its surface, and containing the olfactory association centers. SYN: *convolution, uncinate; uncus gyri hippocampi.*

subiliac (sŭb-ĭl'ĭ-ăk) [L. *sub,* under, + *iliacus,* pert. to the hip]. 1. Below the ilium. 2. Pert. to the subilium.

subilium (sŭb-ĭl'ĭ-ŭm) [" + *ilium,* haunch bone]. The lowest part of the ilium.

subimbibitional (sŭb-ĭm-bĭb-ĭsh'ŭn-ăl) [" + *imbibere,* to drink]. Pert. to a condition due to deficient fluid intake.

subinfection (sŭb-ĭn-fĕk'shŭn) [" + *infectio,* a putting into]. 1. Mild infection because of the weakening of the resisting power of the cells against toxic conditions. 2. Condition caused by toxins liberated from bacteria undergoing lysis.

subinflammation (sŭb″ĭn-flăm-ā'shŭn) [" + *inflammatio,* a setting on fire]. Very mild inflammation. SYN: *irritation.*

subinflammatory (sŭb″ĭn-flăm'ă-tō-rī) [" + *inflammatio,* a setting on fire]. Very mildly inflammatory.

subintrant (sŭb-ĭn'trănt) [L. *subintrans,* stealing into]. Having cycles or paroxysms in such rapid succession that they intermingle.

    s. fever. Intermittent fever in which the paroxysms occur so rapidly that one comes on before the previous one has disappeared.

subinvolution (sŭb″ĭn-vō-lū'shŭn) [L. *sub,* beneath, + *involutio,* a turning into]. Imperfect involution; incomplete return of a part to normal dimensions after physiological hypertrophy, as when the uterus following childbirth fails to reduce to normal size. SEE: *uterus.*

subject (sŭb'jĕkt) [L. *subjectus,* thrown or lying under]. 1. A patient undergoing treatment, observation, or experiment. 2. A body used for dissection.

subjective (sŭb-jĕk'tĭv) [L. *subjectivus*]. Arising from or concerned with the individual; not perceptible to an observer. OPP: *objective.*

    s. sensation. A sensation occurring when stimuli due to internal causes excite the nervous system; one not of objective origin.

    s. symptoms. Those which are of internal origin and evident only to the patient.

subjugal (sŭb-jū'găl) [L. *sub,* beneath, + *jugum,* yoke]. Below the malar bone or *os zygomaticum.*

sublatio (sŭb-lā'shĭ-ō) [L. *sublatio,* a taking away]. Removal or detachment of a part.

    s. retinae. Detachment of the retina.

sublethal (sŭb-lē'thăl) [L. *sub,* under, + G. *lēthē,* oblivion]. A little less than lethal; almost fatal.

    s. dose. Dose containing not quite enough toxin to cause death.

sublimate (sŭb'lĭ-māt) [L. *sublimāre,* to elevate]. 1. A substance obtained or prepared by sublimation. 2. To vaporize a solid substance by heat and condense it again without liquefying, for purification. 3. PSY: To overcome the libido by diverting it into nonsexual or higher activities.

sublimation (sŭb-lĭ-mā'shŭn) [L. *sublimatio,* an elevation]. 1. CHEM: To convert a solid into a vapor and condense it again without liquefying to purify it. 2. PSY: Conversion of the libido into nonsexual channels.

    Adequate expression for organic needs, removed from the primitive satisfaction

in such a way that the "herd" regards the outlet as "superior," *i. e.*, best suited to the social interests (demands).
A freudian term pert. to unconscious mental processes whereby the sex instinct finds an outlet through creative mental work.

sublime (sŭb-līm') [L. *sublimāre*, to elevate]. CHEM: To evaporate a substance directly from the solid into the vapor state and condense it again.
Thus, metallic iodine on heating does not liquefy, but forms directly a violet gas.

subliminal (sŭb-lĭm'ĭn-ăl) [L. *sub*, under, + *limen*, threshold]. 1. Below the threshold of sensation; too weak to arouse sensation or muscular contraction. 2. Below the normal consciousness. SYN: *subconscious*.

s. self. PSY: Part of a normal individual's personality in which his mental processes function without consciousness under normal waking conditions.

sublingual (sŭb-lĭng'gwăl) [" + *lingua*, tongue]. Beneath or concerning the area beneath the tongue.

s. gland. The smallest of the salivary glands, located bet. side of tongue and the mandible, one on each side.
It has about 20 ducts opening for the most part directly above the gland.

sublinguitis (sŭb″lĭng-gwī'tĭs) [" + " + G. -*ītis*, inflammation]. Inflammation of the sublingual gland.

sublobular (sŭb-lŏb'ū-lar) [" + *lobulus*, a lobule]. Beneath a lobule.

sublumbar (sŭb-lŭm'bar) [" + *lumbus*, loin]. Below the lumbar region.

subluxation (sŭb″lŭks-ā'shŭn) [" + *luxatio*, dislocation]. A partial or incomplete dislocation.

sublymphemia (sŭb-lĭm-fē'mĭ-ă) [" + *lympha*, clear fluid, + G. *aima*, blood]. Abnormal decrease in lymphocytes in the blood with number of white cells being normal. SYN: *hypolymphemia*.

submammary (sŭb-măm'ă-rĭ) [L. *sub*, under, + *mamma*, breast]. Below the mammary gland.

submaxilla (sŭb-măks-ĭl'ă) [" + *maxilla*, jaw]. The lower jaw or mandible. SYN: *maxilla, inferior*.

submaxillaritis (sŭb-măks-ĭl-ar-ī'tĭs) [" + " + G. -*ītis*, inflammation]. 1. Pert. to the mandible. 2. Inflammation or mumps of the submaxillary gland.

submaxillary (sŭb-măks'ĭl-a-rĭ) [" + *maxillaris*, pert. to the jaw]. Beneath the lower jaw or inferior maxilla.

s. gland. A salivary racemose gland below the angle of the jaw discharging into the mouth, 1/3 the size of the parotid g.

submaxilitis (sŭb-măks-ĭl-lī'tĭs) [" + " + G. -*ītis*, inflammation]. Inflammation of or mumps affecting the submaxillary gland.

submental (sŭb-mĕn'tăl) [" + *mentum*, chin]. Under the chin.

submicron (sŭb-mī'krŏn) [" + G. *mikros*, tiny]. A tiny particle invisible except with the ultramicroscope. SYN: *ultramicron*.

submicroscopical (sŭb″mī-krō-skŏp'ĭ-kal) [L. *sub*, under, + G. *mikros*, tiny, + *skopein*, to examine]. Too minute to be visible under the microscope.

submorphous (sŭb-mor'fŭs) [" + G. *morphē*, form]. Neither completely amorphous nor crystalline, as some calculi.

submucosa (sŭb-mū-kō'să) [" + *mucosus*, mucous]. The layer of areolar connective tissue under a mucous membrane.

submucous (sŭb-mū'kŭs) [" + *mucus*, mucus]. Beneath a mucous membrane.

subnarcotic (sŭb-nar-kŏt'ĭk) [" + G. *narkōtikos*, numb]. Mildly narcotic.

subnasal (sŭb-nā'zăl) [" + *nasus*, nose]. Under the nose.

s. point. Craniometric point at base of nasal spine.

subneural (sŭb-nū'răl) [" + G. *neuron*, nerve]. Beneath the neural axis or the central nervous system.

subnormal (sŭb-nor'măl) [L. *sub*, under, + *norma*, rule]. Below normal.

subnucleus (sŭb-nū'klē-ŭs) [" + *nucleus*, a nut]. 1. One of the secondary nuclei into which the nucleus of a nerve cell divides. 2. An accessory nucleus.

suboccipital (sŭb-ŏk-sĭp'ĭ-tăl) [" + *occiput*, back of head]. Situated below the occiput or occipital bone.

suboperculum (sŭb-ō-per'kū-lŭm) [" + *operculum*, covering]. Portion of occipital convolution overlapping the insula. SEE: *operculum*.

suborbital (sŭb-or'bĭ-tăl) [" + *orbita*, track]. Beneath the orbit.

subpapular (sŭb-păp'ū-lar) [" + *papula*, pimple]. Very slightly papular, as papules elevated being scarcely more than macules.

subpatellar (sŭb-pă-tĕl'ar) [" + *patella*, a pan]. Beneath the patella.

subpeduncular (sŭb″pē-dŭn'kū-lar) [L. *sub*, under, + *pedunculus*, a stem]. Below a peduncle.

s. lobe. Tiny lobe on undersurface of either cerebellar hemisphere. SYN: *flocculus*.

subpericardial (sŭb″pĕr-ĭ-kar'dĭ-ăl) [" + G. *peri*, around, + *kardia*, heart]. Beneath the pericardium.

subperiosteal (sŭb″pĕr-ĭ-ŏs'tē-ăl) [" + *osteon*, bone]. Beneath the periosteum.

s. operation. Bone surgery without removal of the periosteum.

subperitoneal (sŭb″pĕr-ĭ-tō-nē'ăl) [" + G. *peritonaion*, peritoneum]. Beneath the peritoneum.

subpharyngeal (sŭb-făr-ĭn'jē-ăl) [" + G. *pharygx*, pharynx]. Beneath the pharynx.

subphrenic (sŭb-frĕn'ĭk) [" + G. *phrēn*, diaphragm]. Beneath the diaphragm. SYN: *subdiaphragmatic*.

s. abscess. Collection of pus beneath the diaphragm.

subplacenta (sŭb-plă-sĕn'tă) [" + *placenta*, a flat cake]. Part of the decidua directly lining the uterus. SYN: *decidua vera*.

subpleural (sŭb-plū'răl) [L. *sub*, under, + G. *pleura*, a side]. Beneath the pleura.

subpontine (sŭb-pŏn'tĭn, -tīn) [" + *pons*, pont-, bridge]. Below the pons Varolii.

subpreputial (sŭb″prē-pū'shăl) [" + *praeputium*, prepuce]. Under the prepuce.

subpubic (sŭb-pū'bĭk) [" + *pubes*, pubis]. Beneath the pubic arch, as a ligament.

subpulmonary (sŭb-pŭl'mō-na-rĭ) [" + *pulmōn*, lung]. Below the lung.

subretinal (sŭb-rĕt'ĭ-năl) [" + *rētē*, a net]. Beneath the retina.

subscapular (sŭb-skăp'ū-lar) [" + *scapula*, shoulder]. Below the scapula.

subscription (sŭb-skrĭp'shŭn) [L. *subscriptio*, a writing under]. Part of a prescription containing direction to a pharmacist.

subserous (sŭb-sē'rŭs) [L. *sub*, under, + *serum*, whey]. Beneath a serous membrane.

subspinous (sŭb-spī'nŭs) [" + *spina*, thorn]. 1. Beneath any spine. 2. Anterior to or beneath the spinal column.

subspinous dislocation   S-97   **suburethral gland**

s. dislocation. Dislocation with head of the humerus resting below spine of the scapula.

substage (sŭb'stāj) [" + O.Fr. *estage*, a landing]. Attachment to the microscope beneath the stage by which attachments are held in place.

substance (sŭb'stăns) [L. *substantia*, material]. That of which any material thing is composed; matter.

s., agglutinable. S. in red blood corpuscles and bacteria which unites with agglutinin producing specific agglutination.

s., alible. That portion of chyme that nourishes the body.

s., alimentary. Any article of food.

s., alpha. Reticular substance.

s., beta. Tiny body in erythrocytes after staining with azure I.

s., black. Grayish substance in crus cerebri. SYN: *substantia nigra*.

s., chromophilic. Elements of a cell which stain easily.

s., colloid. Jellylike s. in colloid degeneration.

s., cytotoxin. The specific amboceptor and complement in serum which dissolves special cells.

s., depressor. A substance secreted by the pituitary gland which lowers blood pressure.

s., gray. Gray matter of the brain and spinal cord.

s., hemolytic. S. in serum that destroys red blood cells in an added serum. SYN: *alexin*.

s., medullary. 1. White matter of central nervous system. 2. Marrowlike s. of organs, as the kidney.

s., parietal. The matrix of cartilage.

s., prelipoid. Nerve tissue degenerated but not converted into fat.

s., reticular. Threadlike mass in red blood corpuscles after staining. SYN: *alpha s*.

s., sarcous. S. of sarcous elements of a muscle.

s., supporting. Neuroglia, connective tissue, etc., supporting a structure.

s., white. White matter of brain and spinal cord.

s., w., of Schwann. A nerve fiber's medullary sheath.

s., zymoplastic. S. that hastens coagulation of the blood. SYN: *coagulin*.

substantia (sŭb-stăn'shĭ-ă) [L. *substantia*, material]. Substance.

s. alba. White substance of the brain.

s. cinerea. Gray substance of brain and spinal cord.

s. ferruginea. Elongated mass of pigmented cells in the locus caeruleus.

s. gelatinosa. Gray matter of the cord surrounding central canal and capping head of post. horns of spinal cord.

s. grisea. BNA. Gray matter of the spinal cord.

s. nigra. BNA. Black substance in a section of the crus cerebri. SYN: *locus niger*.

s. perforata anterior. BNA. Area on either side of optic chiasm in the olfactory trigone.

s. perforata posterior. BNA. Gray area at base of brain.

s. propria membranae tympani. Fibrous middle layer of drum membrane.

substernal (sŭb-stĕr'năl) [L. *sub*, beneath, + G. *sternon*, chest]. Situated beneath the sternum.

substitution (sŭb-stĭ-tū'shŭn) [L. *substitutio*, a placing under]. 1. CHEM: Displacing an atom (or more than one) of an element in a compound by atoms of another element, equivalently. 2. PSY: The turning from an obstructed desire to one whose gratification is socially acceptable. 3. The turning from an obstructed form of behavior to a more primitive one, as a substitution neurosis.

s. products. Compounds formed by an element or a radical replacing another element or radical in a compound.

s. therapy. Administration of hormone or glandular extract to counteract the deficiency of that gland. SYN: *organotherapy*.

substitutive (sŭb'stĭ-tū-tĭv) [L. *substitutivus*, conditional]. Causing a change or substitution of characteristics.

s. therapy. Treatment to overcome an inflammation of a specific character by exciting an acute nonspecific inflammation.

substrate, substratum (sŭb'strāt, sŭb-strā'tŭm) [L. *substratum*, a strewing under]. 1. An underlying layer or foundation. 2. A base, as of a pigment. 3. The substance acted upon, as by an enzyme. SYN: *zymolyte*. SEE: *enzyme*.

subsultus (sŭb-sŭl'tŭs) [L. *subsultus*, from *sub*, under, + *salire*, to leap]. Any morbid tremor or twitching, as of the tendons; a grave symptom in certain fevers.

s. clonus, s. tendinum. Involuntary twitchings of muscles, esp. of arms and feet, causing movement of tendons, observed in certain febrile conditions.

subsylvian (sŭb-sĭl'vĭ-ăn) [L. *sub*, beneath]. Below the fissure of Sylvius.

subtarsal (sŭb-tar'săl) [" + G. *tarsos*, tarsus]. Below the tarsus.

subthalamic (sŭb-thă-lăm'ĭk) [" + G. *thalamos*, chamber]. Located below the thalamus.

s. nucleus. A small ganglion beneath the optic layer. SYN: *Luy's body*, *hypothalamic nucleus*.

subthalamus (sŭb-thăl'ă-mŭs) [" + G. *thalamos*, chamber]. Prominences and ganglia on ventral side below the thalamus. SYN: *hypothalamus*.

subthyroidism (sŭb-thī'royd-ĭzm) [" + G. *thyreos*, shield, + *eidos*, like, + *-ismos*, condition]. Condition due to lack of activity of the thyroid gland. SYN: *hypothyroidism*.

subtile, subtle (sŭb'tĭl, sŭt'l) [M.E. *sotill*, from L. *subtilis*, woven fine]. 1. Very fine or delicate. 2. Very acute. 3. Mentally acute or crafty or piercing, as sharp. 4. Operating without attracting attention, as subtle poisons.

subtotal (sŭb-tō'tăl) [L. *sub*, beneath, + *totus*, whole]. Just less than total, as subtotal removal of a gland.

subtrochanteric (sŭb-trō-kăn-ter'ĭk) [" + G. *trochantēr*, a runner]. Below a trochanter.

subtuberal (sŭb-tū'bĕr-ăl) [" + *tuber*, a knot]. Located under a tuber.

subtympanic (sŭb-tĭm-păn'ĭk) [" + G. *tympanon*, drum]. Below the tympanum.

sububeres (sŭb-ū'ber-ēz) [" + *ubera*, breast]. Suckling children.

subumbilical (sŭb-ŭm-bĭl'ĭ-kăl) [L. *sub*, beneath, + *umbilicus*, navel]. Below the umbilicus.

s. space. Space within the body cavity below the navel resembling a triangle in shape.

subungual, subunguial (sŭb-ŭng'gwăl, -gwĭ-ăl) [" + *unguis*, nail]. Situated beneath nail of a finger or toe. SEE: *hyponychium*.

suburethral (sŭb-ū-rē'thrăl) [" + G. *ourēthra*, urethra]. Below the urethra.

s. gland. One on either side of the

subvaginal ant. portion of the vagina. SYN: *Bartholin's* or *Duverney's glands, vulvovaginal g.*

subvaginal (sŭb-văj'ĭn-ăl) [" + *vagina*, sheath]. 1. Below the vagina. 2. On inner side of any tubular sheathing membrane.

subvertebral (sŭb-ver'tĕ-brăl) [" + *vertebra*, vertebra]. Beneath or on ventral side of the vertebral column or of a vertebra. SYN: *subspinal*.

subvirile (sŭb-vĭr'ĭl, -vī'rĭl) [" + *virilis*, male]. Of lowered or inferior virility.

subvitrinal (sŭb-vĭt'rĭn-ăl) [" + *vitrina*, vitreous body]. Located beneath the vitreous body.

subvolution (sŭb-vō-lū'shŭn) [" + *volutus*, from *volvere*, to turn]. Method of surgically turning over a flap to prevent adhesions.

subzonal (sŭb-zō'năl) [" + G. *zonē*, a girdle]. Below any zone, such as the *zona pellucida*.

succagogue (sŭk'ăg-ŏg) [L. *succus*, juice, + G. *agōgos*, leading]. Anything inducing glandular secretion, or which stimulates secretion of a gland or of the digestive juice.

succedaneous (sŭk-sē-da'nē-ŭs) [L. *succedaneus*, substituting]. Acting as a substitute or relating to one.

succedaneum (sŭk-sē-dā'nē-ŭm) [L. *succedaneus*, substituting]. A substitute for anything; a remedy used as a substitute.
 s., caput. Serosanguineous infiltration of connective tissue upon presenting part of head of a fetus.

succenturiate (sŭk-sĕn-tū'rĭ-āt) [L. *succenturiāre*, to substitute or supplement]. Serving as a substitute or accessory.
 s. kidney. A suprarenal or adrenal body. [cessory one.
 s. placenta. A supernumerary or ac-

succinylsulfathiazole. 2-(N⁴-succinylsulfanilamido)-thiazole. Member of the sulfonamide family valuable as an antibacterial agent for use in the intestinal tract. White crystalline powder sparingly soluble in alcohol, acetone, and water; readily soluble in aqueous bases, as sodium bicarbonate solution.

succorrhea (sŭk-kor-rē'ă) [L. *succus*, juice, + G. *rhoia*, a flow]. Unnatural increase in secretion of any juice, esp. of a digestive fluid.

succus (sŭk'kŭs) [L. *succus*, juice]. A juice or fluid secretion.
 s. entericus. The intestinal juice of the body. It is alkaline. Sp. gr. 1.010. The secretion of the minute glands lining the small intestine.
 It contains 5 enzymes: Invertin, enterokinase, lactase, maltase, and erepsin.
 s. gastricus. The gastric juice.
 s. pyloricus. An alkaline secretion by the pyloric end of the stomach.

succussion (sŭk-ŭs'shŭn) [L. *succussio*, a shaking]. Shaking of a person to detect the presence of fluid in the bodily cavities by listening for a splashing sound, esp. in the thorax.

suck (sŭk) [A.S. *sūcan*, to suck]. 1. To draw fluid into the mouth, as from the breast. 2. To exhaust air from a tube and thus siphon fluid from a container. 3. That which is drawn into the mouth by sucking.

suck'ing pad. Mass of fat in cheeks, esp. well developed in an infant, aiding it to suck. SEE: *myzesis*.

sucrase (sū'krās) [Fr. *sucre*, sugar]. An enzyme in the intestinal juice which splits cane sugar into glucose and fructose, which are absorbed into the portal circulation. SYN: *invertin*.

sucroclastic (sū-krō-klăs'tĭk) [" + G. *klastos*, destroyed]. Splitting up or hydrolyzing a sugar.

sucrose (sū'krōs) [Fr. *sucre*, sugar]. Saccharose or cane sugar. $C_{12}H_{22}O_{11}$, a disaccharose giving dextrose and levulose on inversion.
 It is split in the intestines by the sucrase of the intestinal juice, resulting in fructose and glucose which are absorbed into the portal blood. Sucrose is apt to ferment in the stomach.
 ACTION: Only a little is retained by the stomach and it is all absorbed in the intestines. The lack of residue tends to cause constipation. The mucous membrane of the stomach is apt to be irritated by too much sugar. It and glucose may also set up fermentation. It is stored by the hepatic cells of the liver in the form of glycogen for future use. No chemical changes take place with the simple sugars, as they are directly absorbed. Any hydrolyzation in the stomach is supposed to be due to regurgitation of intestinal juice. Sugar is superior to starch, which requires more digestion. Sugar stimulates. As a rule, alcoholic drinkers do not care for much sugar, and one of the drink cures is the frequent use of candy. Excessive use causes fermentation.
 USES: Reduction of intracranial pressure, as in brain tumor, brain abscess; also being used as a diuretic.
 DOSAGE: 50 cc. of 50% solution.
 CONTRA: Avoid much sugar in atony, gastric stasis, acne, furunculosis, obesity, liver complaints, and arthritis. In gout it should not be eaten with meat, as acid fermentation sets up and impedes uric acid elimination. A vegetable diet has the opposite effect. Prohibit in diabetes.
 RS: *carbohydrates, disaccharose, fructose, galactose, glucose, lactose, levulose, maltose.*

sucrosemia (sū-krō-sē'mĭ-ă) [Fr. *sucre*, sugar, + *-ōse*, sugar, + G. *aima*, blood]. Sucrose or cane sugar in the blood serum.

sucrosuria (sū-krō-sū'rĭ-ă) [" + " + G. *ouron*, urine]. Sugar in the urine.

suction (sŭk'shŭn) [L. *suctus*, from *sugere*, to suck]. The act of or capacity for sucking up by reduction of air pressure over part of the surface of a substance.
 s., post-tussive. Suction sound over a lung cavity heard on auscultation after a cough.

sudamen (sū-dā'mĕn) (pl. *sudamina*) [L. *sudamen*, sweat]. Noninflammatory eruption from sweat glands characterized by whitish vesicles caused by the retention of sweat in corneous layer of the skin, appearing after profuse sweating or in certain febrile diseases, disappearing by absorption.

sudamina (sū-dăm'ĭn-ă) [L. pl. of *sudamen*, sweat]. Plural of sudamen,* an eruption of vesicles due to retention of sweat in corneous layer of the skin.

sudan (sū-dăn'). A term given to several fat dyes used as stains.
 s. III, s. red III. A powder that colors fatty tissues red, and which stains the fatty covering of the tubercle bacilli.
 s. yellow G. A dye staining fat cells yellow.

sudanophil, sudanophilous (sū-dăn'ō-fĭl, -of'ĭ-lŭs) [*sudan* + G. *philein*, to love]. Staining readily with sudan.

sudanophilia (sū-dăn-ō-fĭl'ĭ-ă) [" + G.

philein, to love]. A condition in which minute fat droplets contained in the leukocytes take a brilliant red stain, probably indicative of suppuration.

sudation (sū-dā'shŭn) [L. *sudatio*, a sweating]. 1. The act of sweating. 2. Excessive perspiration.

sudatoria (sū-dă-to'rĭ-ă) [L. *sudatorius*, sweating]. Excessive sweating. SYN: *ephidrosis, hyperidrosis*.

sudatorium (sū-dă-tō'rĭ-ŭm) [L. *sudatorium*, a sweating room]. 1. A hot air bath or any bath to induce perspiration. 2. A room used to induce sweat baths.

sudokeratosis (sū″dō-ker-ă-tō'sĭs) [L. *sudor*, sweat, + G. *keras, kerat-*, horn, + *-ōsis*, condition]. Circumscribed, horny overgrowths obstructing the sweat ducts.

sudomotor (sū″dō-mō'tōr) [″ + *motor*, a mover]. Pert. to stimulating the secretion of sweat; noting certain nerves.

sudor (sū'dor) [L. *sudor*, sweat]. Secretion from the sweat glands. SYN: *perspiration, sweat*.
RS: *anhydrosis, bromidrosis, chromidrosis, hydrosis, hematidrosis, perspiration, pore, skin, sweat, sudorific, uridrosis*.

s. cruen'tus. Sweating of blood. SYN: *hematidrosis*.

sudoral (sū'dōr-ăl) [L. *sudor* sweat]. Pert. to, caused by, or marked by perspiration.

sudoresis (sū-dō-rē'sĭs) [L. *sudorēsis*, excessive sweating]. Profuse sweating. SYN: *diaphoresis*.

sudoriferous (sū-dor-if'ĕr-ŭs) [L. *sudor*, sweat, + *ferre*, to bear]. Conveying or producing sweat.

s. glands. Sweat-secreting glands of the skin.

sudorific (sū-dōr-ĭf'ĭk) [L. *sudorificus*, producing sweat]. 1. Secreting or promoting the secretion of sweat. 2. Agent which produces sweating. SYN: *diaphoretic*.

sudoriparous (sū-dor-ĭp'ă-rŭs) [L. *sudor*, sweat, + *parēre*, to produce]. Secreting sweat. SYN: *sudoriferous*.

suet (sū'ĕt) [M.E. from L. *sebum*, suet]. Hard fat from the ox or sheep's kidneys and loins, used as the base of certain ointments and as an emollient.

suffocation (sŭf″ō-kā'shŭn) [L. *suffocāre*, to choke]. 1. State of being choked by obstruction of air passages by drowning, smothering, throttling, or inhalation of noxious gases. SYN: *asphyxia*.* Generally from gases. 2. Act of obstructing the air passages.
SYM: Insensibility, breathing slight, face purple and swollen, livid lips. Symptoms not always present.
TREATMENT: Dash cold water in face. Slap chest. Apply ammonia to nostrils. Artificial respiration. RS: *resuscitation, unconsciousness*.

suffumigation (sŭf-ū″mĭ-gā'shŭn) [L. *sub*, beneath, + *fumigātio*, a smoking]. 1. Treatment by application of medicated vapors from below. 2. A vapor so used.

suffusion (sŭf-ū'zhŭn) [L. *suffusio*, a pouring over]. 1. Spreading of a bodily fluid into surrounding tissues. SYN: *extravasation*. 2. Pouring of a fluid over the body as treatment.

sugar (shu'gar) [M.E. *suger*, from L. *saccharum*, from G. *sakcharon*, sugar]. A sweet-tasting carbohydrate belonging to the monosaccharose and disaccharose groups. Crystalline carbohydrates of comparatively low molecular weight and generally having a sweet taste.
CLASSIFICATION: First, as to the number of atoms of simple sugars yielded on hydrolysis by a molecule of the given sugar and, secondly, as to the number of carbon atoms in the molecules of the simple sugars so obtained. Thus, *dextrose* (which see) is a monosaccharide because it cannot be hydrolyzed to a simpler sugar; it is a hexose because it contains 6 carbon atoms per molecule. *Sucrose* is a disaccharide because on hydrolysis it yields 2 molecules, 1 of dextrose and 1 of levulose.

TEST FOR SUGAR IN URINE: Prepare reagents A and B as follows: (a) Dissolve 34.66 Gm. of copper sulfate crystals in water; dilute to 500 cc.; (b) dissolve 173 Gm. of potassium sodium tartrate (Rochelle salt) and 50 Gm. of sodium hydroxide in water and dilute to 500 cc. For the test, first mix, say, 2 cc. of (a) and 2 cc. of (b); add 4 cc. of the urine sample, heat to boiling. The presence of sugar is indicated by the appearance of a red precipitate. Since other substances can reduce Fehling's solution, the results require careful interpretation.

QUANTITATIVE TESTS FOR SUGAR: *Benedict's Method*: Measure 25 cc. of Benedict's reagent into a porcelain evaporation dish. Then add 10 to 20 Gm. of crystallized sodium carbonate. Boil mixture over a Bunsen burner, and pass in urine freely until a white precipitate is formed and blue color of mixture begins to fade, after which run in the urine more slowly (while the fluid is still vigorously boiling) until last remains of color have disappeared. The sugar percentage is calculated by dividing 0.05 by number of cubic centimeters of undiluted urine which has been used. The result is multiplied by 100.

Roberts' Fermentation Test: Based on the fact that specific gravity of urine containing sugar falls when yeast is added. The difference, therefore, bet. fermented and nonfermented urines gives an indication of amount of sugar present.

Fill a 12-oz. bottle with urine and add some yeast. Shake thoroughly, and then lightly plug neck of bottle with absorbent wool. Now fill another 12-oz. bottle with unfermented urine, and cork it lightly. Leave 2 bottles for 24 hr. in a warm room. The specific gravity of both is taken, the difference in degrees showing the number of grains per ounce.

s., beet. A saccharine from beets.
s., cane. Sugar from sugar cane.
s., diabetic. Glucose.
s., fruit. Levulose.
s., grape. Dextrose, glucose.
s., invert. One consisting of 1 molecule of glucose and 1 of fructose.
s., liver. Glycogen.
s., malt. Maltose.
s., milk. Lactose.
DOSAGE: Daily, 1-6 oz. (30-180 Gm.).
s., muscle. Inosite.

sugar, words pert. to: aglycosuric, biose, blood, carbohydrate, dextrose, diabetin, disaccharide, disaccharose, Fehling's tests, fructose, fruit s., galactose, glucide, "gluco-" words, "glyco-" words, hypoglycemia, invert, invertase, lactose, levulose, mannite, melitemia, monosaccharide, monosaccharose, pentose, pentosuria, polysaccharide, polysaccharose, "sacchar-" words, sucrose, xylose.

suggestibility (sŭg-jĕs″tĭ-bĭl'ĭ-tĭ) [L. *suggestus*, suggested]. A condition in which a person responds readily to suggestions or opinions of another.

suggestible (sŭg-jĕs'tĭ-bl) [L. *suggestus*, suggested]. Very susceptible to the opinions or suggestions of others.

suggestion (sŭg-jĕs'chŭn) [L. *suggestio*, from *suggerere*, to supply]. 1. Imparting of an idea in any indirect way. 2. The idea so conveyed. 3. The acceptance or the effect of the statements or actions of one person upon another, depending on the emotional set-up of the recipient and his psychic relationship to the other person.

s., auto-. Self-suggestion as distinguished from that coming from another person, esp. in hypnotic state.
 May produce or cure functional disturbances.

suggestive (sŭg-jĕs'tĭv) [L. *suggestus*, suggested]. Stimulating or pert. to suggestion.

s. medicine. Therapy by suggestion either during consciousness or hypnosis.

s. therapeutics. The practice of treating disease by suggestion or hypnotism.

suggillation (sŭg-jĭl-ā'shŭn) [L. *sugillāre*, to beat black and blue]. A bruise or black and blue mark. SYN: *ecchymosis*.

suicide (sū'ĭ-sīd) [L. *sui*, of oneself, + *cidus*, from *caedere*, to kill]. 1. Act or instance of taking one's own life voluntarily. 2. One who attempts or commits self-murder.

These individuals often have attacks of temporary insanity or mental depression which may be terminated by attempt at suicide. In addition to the usual F. A. Treatment for injuries, kindly interrogation and soothing, tranquil conversation are invaluable. In their after-care, such patients should be watched and kept free from needless questioning or emotional display. Sedatives are useful. SEE: *hysteria*.

MENTAL STATES CONDUCIVE TO: Those with sudden impulses. The depressed. Those with delusions: (a) of persecution; (b) of being ruined; (c) voices suggesting; (d) incurable disease. In melancholia. Schizophrenia. Epilepsy. Confusional states. Alcoholics. Through accidents: (a) Acute delirium; (b) mania; (c) general paralysis.

METHODS RESORTED TO: 1. Hanging. 2. Drowning (in tub or otherwise). 3. Poisoning. 4. Cutting an artery. 5. Burning. 6. Jumping from window. 7. Instruments used: (a) Matches; (b) knives and spoons; (c) glass; (d) cord, rope, suspenders, bedclothing, etc.; (e) harmless articles converted into dangerous tools; (f) nail files. All must be removed if patient is inclined to harm self or others. [to a sulcus.

sulcal (sŭl'kăl) [L. *sulcus*, groove]. Pert.
 s. artery. A tiny branch of ant. spinal artery.

sulcate, sulcated (sŭl'kāt, -ed) [L. *sulcatus*, grooved]. Furrowed or grooved.

sulcus (sŭl'kŭs) (pl. *sulci*) [L. *sulcus*, groove]. A furrow or groove, or slight depression or fissure, esp. of the brain.

s. centralis. BNA. Fissure dividing the frontal and parietal lobes of each cerebral hemisphere. SYN: *fissure of Rolando*.

s., intraparietal. One that separates the inf. from the sup. parietal bones and lobes.

s. praecentralis. BNA. An interrupted one generally parallel with the fissure of Rolando and ant. to it.

s. pulmonalis. Depression on either side of the vertebral column.

s. spiralis cochleae. Groove bet. the labium tympanicum and labium vestibulare.

sulf-, sulfo-. Prefix showing that a compound with this prefix contains sulfurous anhydride or the group SO_3.

sulfabenzamine (sŭl"fă-bĕn'ză-mĭn). A sulfonamide drug effective against anaerobic bacteria which cause gas gangrene. It has some antibacterial action against streptococci, staphylococci, and pneumococci. The trade name is *sulfamylon*.

sulfacetimide (sŭl-fă-sĕt'ĭ-mĭd). A sulfonamide used in treatment of *B. coli*, gonorrhea, and infections of the urinary tract, esp. when resistant to sulfanilamide and sulfathiazole.

sulfadiazine (sŭl"fă-dĭ-ā'zēn). One of a group of diazine derivatives of sulfanilamide, destructive to streptococci, staphylococci and pneumococci.

sulfamerazine (sŭl"fa-mer'ă-zĭn). A sulfur derivative which may be given orally for pneumococci, streptococci, meningococci, and gonococci.

sulfamethazine (sŭl-fă-mĕth'ă-zĭn). A near relative of sulfadiazine. Nausea and vomiting less than with sulfapyridine; solubility good, and damage to kidneys slight.

sulfamethylthiazol (sŭl"fă-mĕth"ĭl-thī-ā'-zōl). A sulfanilamide derivative which is less toxic than sulfapyridine; effective against staphylococcic organisms.

sulfanilamide (sŭl"făn-ĭl'ă-mĭd) (para-amino-benzene-sulfonamide). A white, slightly bitter, crystalline substance from coal tar, the parent of the azo dyes, which has come into use within the past few years, and is regarded by many as an important contribution to our list of effective medicines; however, far too potent to be used indiscriminately.

USES: Primarily in infections due to hemolytic streptococci, but reported to be effective in other infections, such as those due to pneumococci, Types I, II, and III; meningococci; gonococci and septicemia; generalized peritonitis, and puerperal infection; undulant fever; chancroid; typhoid fever; gas gangrene; ulcerative colitis; trachoma; malaria; many skin diseases, and urinary tract infections.

DOSAGE: Calculated on the basis of body weight: 15 gr. (1 Gm.) for each 20 lb. up to 100 lb. The maximum dose seems to have been 75 gr. (5 Gm.) given over a period of 24 hours to a person of average weight, but average dose is 15 gr. every 4 hours for 48 hours, after which dose is lowered.

It is advised to be given with sodium bicarbonate, to help combat acidosis, which is produced by the drug. It is also advised not to administer magnesium sulfate or any drug derived from the benzene series, such as phenacetin, during the treatment. Daily blood counts should be made.

sulfanilyaminoguanidine (sŭl"făn-ĭ-lĭ-ăm-ĭn-ō-gwăn'ĭ-dĭn). A less toxic and an improved product from sulfaguanidine.

sulfanilycyanamide (sŭl"făn-ĭl-ĭ-sī-an'ă-mĭd). A less toxic and improved product from sulfaguanidine.

sulfanilylguanidine (sŭl-făn-ĭl'ĭl-gwan'ĭ-dĭn). Derivative of sulfanilamide having antibacterial activity useful in treating intestinal infections.

sulfanilyl-sulfanilamide (sŭl-făn-ĭl-ĭl-sŭl"-făn-ĭl'ă-mĭd). A sulfanilamide derivative which is less toxic and more effective in the treatment of gonorrhea.

sulfapyridine (sŭl"fă-pĭr'ĭ-dĕn). A sulfanilamide derivative which differs in its chemical structure in that 1 hydrogen atom in the sulfonamide group has been replaced by a basic pyridine group, and is less toxic.

This chemical, recently developed in England, and first introduced in the United States under the name of "Dagenan," was the culmination of a large number of experiments undertaken in an effort to find a drug that was effective against the pneumococcus.

While the importance of sulfapyridine in combating pneumonia seems undisputed, the exact manner in which it acts is not clearly understood. Its value seemingly lies in its ability to inhibit the growth of the pneumococcus in all types. In severe cases it is recommended to be supplemented by specific antiserum. Because of the toxic effects of the drug, it should be under careful usage and close observation of a physician. Make daily blood counts.

USES: Pneumonia, possibly effective against the gonococcus, staphylococcus, meningococcus, and in pertussis complicated by bronchopneumonia.

DOSAGE: It is recommended that the initial dose be sufficient to bring the blood concentration to bet. 3 and 6 mg. per cent of the free drug as promptly as possible, and thereafter sufficient to maintain this concentration. For the average adult it is suggested the first dose be 2 Gm., followed by the same dose within 4 hours; 4 hours later a 3rd dose of 1 Gm., and thereafter 1 Gm. is given until pulse, temperature and respiration have been normal for about 48 hours. The dose then may be reduced to bet. 1 and 3 Gm. daily, for a period of 3 to 5 days.

Nausea and vomiting, which sometimes follow the administration, may be somewhat overcome by powdering the tablets and giving in milk or fruit juice, or by the use of a demulcent such as gelatin, or by the use of smaller doses at more frequent intervals.

sulfapyr'idine so'dium monohy'drate. A soluble salt of sulfapyridine for intravenous use only, as an emergency treatment in pneumonia, where response has not been sufficient by oral administration, or where it is imperative to administer adequate medication at once.

DOSAGE: Calculated on the basis of 0.06 Gm. per kilogram of body weight, and given as a 5% solution in sterile distilled water.

Careful administration to avoid deposition of solution outside vein, since severe irritation results, and wherever possible repeated doses be avoided, although the use of sulfapyridine orally may be continued to insure a satisfactory blood concentration. As with other drugs of this nature, extremely careful usage and close observation of the patient are advised.

sulfarsphenamine (sŭlf″ars-fĕn′ă-mēn). An arsenic compound; 19% arsenic.

USES: Same as for neoarsphenamine, but said to have less reaction.

DOSAGE: Intramuscularly, 0.4-0.5 Gm.

sulfate (sŭl′fāt) [L. *sulphas,* sulfur salt]. A salt or ester of sulfuric acid.

s. iron. Green vitriol; copperas. Fatal in large dosage.
POISONING: Magnesia and diluents.
s. magnesium.*q.v.

sulfathiazole (sŭl″fă-thī-ă′zōl). A sulfanilamide derivative which is less toxic and which can be given in smaller doses.

USES: Effective against all types of pneumonia due to pneumococci. Nausea is mild and infrequent, and fever is reduced gradually over a period of 48 hr.

Sulfathiazole is effective in treatment of infections due to certain strains of staphylococci. In large boils or carbuncles, initial adult dose 4 Gm. (gr. lx), followed by 1 Gm. (gr. xv) every 4 hr., day and night for 5-7 days. In diffuse staphylococcic cellulitis, lymphangitis or acute osteomyelitis, initial dose 4 Gm. (gr. lx), followed by 1.5 Gm. (gr. xxiii) every 4 hr., day and night as long as there is evidence of spreading infection; then 1 Gm. (gr. xv) every 4 hr. day and night; continue as indicated. In staphylococcic bacteriemia, initial adult dose is 4 Gm. (gr. lx) followed by 1.5 Gm. (gr. xxiii) every 4 hr. day and night until temperature has been normal for 48 hr. Then 1 Gm. (gr. xv) every 4 hr. day and night for 14 days, followed by 0.5 Gm. (gr. viii) every 4 hr. day and night for a minimum of 14 days. Relapse may occur if therapy is not sufficiently prolonged. In severe staphylococcic infections in children, dosage is calculated on the basis of 0.2 Gm. (gr. iii) per Kg. of body weight (up to 20 Kg. of weight). This is divided into 6 parts and given at 4-hr. intervals day and night until temperature has been normal for 48 hr. Then reduce each dose one-third and continue treatment at this level for 14 days, when current dose may be reduced one-half. Surgical measures, both supportive and operative, must be used in conjunction with sulfathiazole whenever indicated. Toxic reactions similar to those which occur with sulfanilamide or sulfapyridine therapy should be carefully watched for and administration of the drug reduced or discontinued if necessary.—*The Merck Manual.*

s. microcrystalline. A form of s. in which the crystals are greatly reduced in size. It remains stable in water for many months. A single application in impetigo has cured in a day.

sulfhemoglobin (sŭlf″hĕm-ō-glō′bĭn). Substance formed by action of hydrogen sulfide on blood.

sulfhemoglobinemia (sŭlf″hĕm-ō-glō″bĭn-ē′-mĭ-ă). Persistent cyanotic condition due to sulfhemoglobin in blood.

sulfonal (sŭl′fō-năl). A proprietary hypnotic and sedative.
DOSAGE: 12 gr. (0.75 Gm.).

sulfonalism (sŭl′fō-năl-ĭzm). 1. Sulfonal poisoning and its symptoms. 2. Addiction to sulfonal.

sulfonamides. A family of drugs, including sulfanilamide, sulfapyridine, sulfathiazole, etc. SEE: *Table, pp. S-102-103.*

sulfonethylmethane (sŭl″fŏn-ĕth″ĭl-mĕth′-ăn). USP. Trional. White powder or crystalline substance with a bitter taste.
ACTION AND USES: As a hypnotic.
DOSAGE: 12 gr. (0.75 Gm.).

sulfonmethane (sŭl″fŏn-mĕth′ăn). USP. Crystalline compound with hypnotic and sedative properties. SYN: *sulfonal.*

sulfourea (sŭl″fō-ū-rē′ă) [L. *sulfur,* sulfur, + *urea*]. Urea with oxygen replaced with sulfur. SYN: *thiourea.*

sulfur (sŭl′fŭr) [L.]. SYMB: S. At. wt. 32.064. Sp. gr. 2.07. It is a pale, yellow, crystalline element which burns with a blue flame, producing sulfur dioxide.
ACTION AND USES: Externally, as a parasiticide. A mild purgative. *Germicide*: It is burned to form a gaseous disinfectant and insecticide.
DOSAGE: Each form, 4 Gm. (1 Gm. sulfur ointment, 15% sulfur in benzoinated

TOXIC MANIFESTATIONS OF CERTAIN SULFONAMIDES*

Reactions	Sulfanilamide	Sulfapyridine	Sulfathiazole	Sulfadiazine	Succinylsulfathiazole	Sulfaguanidine**
	The following complications do not necessarily indicate withdrawal of the drug:					
Cyanosis.	Very common, early and late.	Common, early and late.	Uncommon.	Rare.	Not noted.	
Dizziness.	Common.	Common.	Uncommon.	Rare.	Not noted.	
Hemolytic anemia, mild.	3%; occurs early and late.	3%; early and late.	Very rare.	Not reported.	Not noted.	Rare.
Nausea, vomiting	Fairly common.	Fairly common.	Common.	Rare.	Exceedingly rare.	Occasional.
	If the following complications are present, it is advisable to stop the drug and force fluids.					
Acidosis.	1.9%; may occur at any time.	None.	None.	Rare.	Not noted.	
Acute agranulocytosis.	0.1%; occurs 14th to 40th day, common 17th to 25th day.	0.3%; occurs 14th to 40th day, common 17th to 25th day.	Not reported.	Rare.	Not noted.	
Fever.	10%; generally occurs 5th to 9th day, but may occur 1st to 30th.	4%; generally occurs on the 5th to 9th day.	10%; generally occurs on the 5th to 9th day.	Uncommon to 2%.	Not noted.	Has been noted.
Gastrointestinal tract disturbances.	Bleeding rare, diarrhea uncommon.	Rare.	Very rare.	Uncommon.	Not reported except for diarrhea.	
Hematuria.	Not reported.	8%; generally occurs early.	2.5%; early.	1%.	Not noted.	
Hyperleukocytosis.	Generally in presence of acute hemolytic anemia.	Generally occurs in presence of acute hemolytic anemia.	Not reported.	Not reported.	Not noted.	
Painful joints.	Reported.	Not reported.	Have been reported in connection with rash and other manifestations.	Rare.	Not noted.	
Psychoses.	0.6%; occur early.	0.3%; occur early.	Rare.	Rare.	Not noted.	

TOXIC MANIFESTATIONS OF CERTAIN SULFONAMIDES*

Reactions	Sulfanilamide	Sulfapyridine	Sulfathiazole	Sulfadiazine	Succinylsulfathiazole	Sulfaguanidine**
Rash.	1.9%; may take any form, generally 5th to 9th day, may occur 1st to 30th day.	2%; may take any form, generally 5th to 9th day; may occur 1st to 30th day.	5%; nodular type common; may take any form; may occur 5th to 9th day.	Uncommon to 2%.	Exceedingly rare.	
Stomatitis.	Rare.	Not reported.	Not reported.	Not reported.	Not noted.	
If the following complications are present, it is imperative to stop the drug and force fluids:					
Anuria with azo-anemia.	1.8%; occurs 1st to 5th day.	0.3%; generally first 10 days.	0.7%; generally first 10 days.	Anuria not uncommon.	Not noted.	
Hemolytic anemia, acute.	0.6%; may occur early or late.	0.6%; occurs 1st to 5th day.	Very rare.	Rare.	Not noted.	
Hepatitis.	Not reported.	Reported.	Rare.	Not reported.	Not noted.	
Injection of sclerae and conjunctivae.	Not reported.	Not reported.	4%; may occur with rash and fever, 5th to 9th day.	Rare, 0.3%.	Not noted.	Has been reported.
Jaundice.	With acute hemolytic anemia or hepatitis.	With acute hemolytic anemia or hepatitis.	With acute hemolytic anemia or hepatitis.	Not reported.	Not noted.	
Leukopenia with granulocytopenia.	0.3%; early or late.	0.6%; occurs early or late.	1.6%; early or late.	Uncommon.	Not noted.	
Neuritis.	Very rare.	Not seen, but reported.	Rare.	Not reported.	Not noted.	
Ocular and auditory disturbances.	Rare.	Rare.	Very rare.	Not reported.	Not noted.	
Purpura haemorrhagica.	Not seen, but reported.	Not seen, but reported.	Not reported.	Not reported.	Not noted.	

* From *An Outline of the Medical Aspects of the Commonly Used Sulfonamides*, by permission of the copyright owner, Sharp & Dohme, Inc.

**Material for this drug taken from Litchfield, H., and Dembo, L., *Therapeutics of Infancy and Childhood*, F. A. Davis Co., Philadelphia.

sulfur dioxide   S-104   **superinduce**

lard). In the form of alkaline earths it is absorbed by vegetable organisms in the construction of the protein molecule and it is only in the form of protein that it can be utilized by animal life.

FUNCTIONS: Sulfur is a constituent of hair, nails, and bile, and it is excreted in the form of ethereal sulfates. It and its compounds are concerned with oxidation processes and represent a part of protein metabolism.

Sulfur enters the body with the protein foods, since some of the amino acids (cystine, cysteine, and serine) contain sulfur as an essential element. These amino acids, passing through the intestinal wall into the blood, are carried to the liver and probably destroyed there; the sulfur in them is converted into sulfates, which are excreted by the kidneys.

There seems to be a parallel relation bet. sulfur and nitrogen, both derived from protein metabolism in the body. The amount excreted in the urine varies from 0.46 to 0.62. It aids in the ion balance of tissues when oxidized to sulfate and is required for the synthesis of body proteins as cystine or cysteine or their combination. Used as thiosulfate feeding and high protein diets to relieve dermatitis and eczema. A mixed diet contains about 1 Gm. of sulfur in each 100 Gm. of protein.

DEFICIENCY SYM: Dermatitis, imperfect development of hair and nails. Deficiency of cystine or cysteine proteins in diet restricts growth and may be fatal. Tissue oxidation of cystine forms inorganic sulfate if the protein intake is sufficient.

SOURCES: SEE: *names of foods.*

s. dioxide. An irritating gas used in industries to manufacture acids, also used in electrical refrigerators. A bactericide and important disinfectant.

POISONING: SYM: Suffocation from a highly irritating gas which forms sulfuric acid when in contact with moisture of the mouth, eyes, and respiratory passages, with resultant pain, swelling, burning, etc.

TREATMENT: Remove patient from the vitiated atmosphere. Wash affected areas with large amounts of water and weak alkalies, as chalk magnesia, lime water, soapsuds. Follow by bland diet.

sulfurated, sulfureted (sŭl'fū-rā-ted, -rĕt-ĕd) [L. *sulfur*, sulfur]. Combined or impregnated with sulfur.

s. hydrogen. A colorless, inflammable gas of disagreeable odor resulting from decomposition of organic matter containing sulfur; used as a chemical reagent. SYN: *hydrogen sulfide.* H_2S.

sulfuric acid (sŭl-fū'rĭk) [L. *sulfur*, sulfur]. H_2SO_4. A heavy, corrosive, oily, poisonous acid used as an astringent in colic and diarrhea, and in manufacturing processes, as in cleaning metals, batteries.

DOSAGE: (Arom.) 8 gr. (0.5 Gm.); (dil. 10%) 15 gr. (1.0 Gm.).

POISONING: Sometimes accidentally taken by mouth, as it resembles syrup or glycerin.

SYM: Local effects—burning, with destruction of skin. If it strikes eye it may result in blindness. If taken by mouth, intense pain extending from mouth to esophagus and down to stomach, causing marked, excruciating pain; swelling of affected tissues; salivation; painful swallowing; often gasping for breath, and hoarse voice. Mucous membrane has a grayish white coating. There is persistent, painful vomiting. Patient quickly develops shock.

TREATMENT: Dilute acid with large volumes of water. Neutralize acid with soapsuds, milk magnesia, baking soda or other well-diluted alkalies. Follow by soothing substances, as raw eggs.

summation (sŭm-ā'shŭn) [L. *summatio*, an adding]. Cumulative action or effect, as of stimuli.

Thus, an organ reacts to 2 or more weak stimuli as if they were a single strong one.

summer (sŭm'ẽr) [A.S. *sumer*]. The hot season of the year.

s. catarrh. Allergic reaction to grass pollen in early summer. SYN: *rose cold.*

s. cholera, s. complaint, s. diarrhea. Acute form of gastroenteritis with diarrhea, cramps and vomiting. SYN: *cholera morbus, q.v.*

s. itch. Severe bullous eruption occurring in summer.

s. rash. Rash due to perspiration. SYN: *lichen tropicus, prickly heat.*

sunburn (sŭn'burn) [A.S. *sunne*, sun, + *bernan*, to burn]. Dermatitis due to exposure to the actinic rays of the sun. SEE: *burn.*

Sun'day or **Mon'day morn'ing paralysis.** A musculospiral paralysis following excessive use of alcohol.

sunstroke (sŭn'strōk) [A.S. *sunne*, sun, + M.E. *strok*, a blow]. An affection from undue exposure to rays of the sun or excessive heat.

SYM: Extreme prostration, high fever, other symptoms of heatstroke, delirium, collapse, loss of mind, or death. SYN: *insolation, siriasis, thermic fever.* SEE: *aprication, heatstroke, ictus.*

super- [L.]. Combining form meaning *above, beyond, superior.*

superalimentation (sŭp″er-ăl-ĭ-mĕn-tā'-shŭn) [L. *super*, above, + *alimentum*, food]. Therapeutic forcing of food in excess of body needs or appetite.

superalkalinity (sŭp″er-ăl-kă-lĭn'ĭ-tĭ) [" + *alkalinus*, alkaline]. Excessive alkalinity.

superciliary (sŭp-er-sĭl'ĭ-ā-rĭ) [L. *supercilium*, eyebrow]. Pert. to or in the region of an eyebrow.

supercilium (sū-pĕr-sĭl'ĭ-ŭm) [L. *supercilium*, eyebrow]. 1. Eyebrow. 2. A hair of the eyebrow.

super-ego (sŭp″er-ē'gō) [L. *super*, above, + *ego*, I]. An inner, subconscious censor. SEE: *ego.*

superfecundation (sū″pĕr-fē-kŭn-dā'shŭn) [" + *fecundāre*, to fertilize]. Successive fertilization by more than 1 coitus of 2 or more ova formed at the same menstrual period.

superfetation (sū″pĕr-fē-tā'shŭn) [" + *foetus*, fetus]. Supposed fertilization of 2 ova in the same uterus at different menstrual periods within a short interval.

superficial (sū-pĕr-fĭsh'ăl) [" + *facies*, shape]. 1. Confined to the surface. 2. Not thorough; cursory.

s. reflex. One induced by very light stimulus such as stroking skin lightly with soft cotton wad.

superficialis (sū″pĕr-fĭsh-ĭ-ā'lĭs) [L. *superficialis*, superficial]. Superficial; noting a superficial artery, vein, or nerve, or structure near the surface.

superimpregnation (sū″pĕr-ĭm″prĕg-nā'-shŭn) [L. *super*, over, + *impregnatio*, impregnation]. Conception during pregnancy; fertilization by 2 different ovulations. SYN: *superfecundation, superfetation.*

superinduce (sū″pĕr-ĭn-dūs') [" + *in*, into,

superinfection   S-105   **suppuration**

+ *ducere*, to lead]. To bring in over or above that already existing condition or situation.
superinfection (sū″pĕr-ĭn-fĕk′shun) [" + *infectio*, a putting into]. A new infection by the same organism, in addition to a similar one already existing.
superinvolution (sū″pĕr-ĭn-vō-lū′shŭn) [" + *in*, into, + *volutus*, from *volvere*, to roll]. Excessive reduction of the uterus following childbirth to less than its normal size. SYN: *hyperinvolution*.
superior (sū-pē′rĭ-or) [L. comparative of *super*, beyond]. 1. Higher than; situated above something else. 2. Better than. 3. One in charge of others.
superior′ity com′plex. An exaggerated conviction of one's own superiority; a pretense of superiority in order to compensate for supposed inferiority.
superlactation (sū-pĕr-lăk-tā′shŭn) [L. *super*, above, + *lactāre*, to suckle]. Oversecretion of milk, or continuance of lactation beyond normal time.
superlethal (sū″pĕr-lē′thăl) [" + G. *lēthē*, forgetfulness]. Beyond a fatal limit, as a dose that will probably kill.
supermoron (sū″pĕr-mō′rŏn) [" + G. *mōros*, stupid]. One slightly subnormal but above a moron mentally.
supermotility (sū″pĕr-mō-tĭl′ĭ-tĭ) [" + *motilis*, able to move]. Excessive motility in any part. SYN: *hypercinesia*.
supernatant (sū″pĕr-nā′tănt) [" + *natāre*, to float]. Floating on surface, as oil on water. [float]. A supernatant fluid.
supernate (sū-pĕr-nāt′) [" + *natāre*, to
supernumerary (sū″pĕr-nū′mĕr-a-rĭ) [L. *supernumerarius*, above the number]. Exceeding the regular number.
supernutrition (sū″pĕr-nū-trī′shŭn) [L. *super*, above, + *nutritio*, nourishment]. More than normal nutrition.
supersaturated solution (sū″pĕr-săt′ū-rāt″-ĕd) [" + *saturāre*, to sate]. One containing more salt or other substance than it can dissolve at normal temperature.
superscription (sū″pĕr-skrĭp′shŭn) [" + *scriptio*, a writing]. The beginning of a prescription noted by the sign ℞, signifying L. *recipe*, take.
supersecretion (sū″pĕr-sē-krē′shŭn) [" + *secretio*, a separating]. An excess of any secretion.
supersedent (sū″pĕr-sē′dĕnt) [" + *sedere*, to sit]. A remedy which partially cures or prevents a disease.
supersensitiveness (sū″pĕr-sĕn′sĭ-tĭv″nĕs) [" + *sensitivus*, sensitive]. Excessive susceptibility to a foreign protein or pollen. SYN: *hypersensitiveness*.
supersoft (sū″pĕr-sŏft′) [" + A.S. *sōfte*, soft]. Exceptionally soft; noting roentgen rays of extremely long wave length and low penetrating power.
supersphenoid (sū″pĕr-sfē′noyd) [" + G. *sphēn*, wedge, + *eidos*, shape]. Over the sphenoid bone.
supertemporal (sū″pĕr-tĕm′pō-răl) [L. *super*, above, + *tempora*, the temples]. In the upper part above the temporal bone, region, or lobe.
   s. convolution. Convolution bet. sylvian and sup. temporal fissures.
   s. fissure. One ant. and parallel to the sylvian fissure.
supertension (sū″pĕr-tĕn′shŭn) [" + *tensio*, a stretching]. Extremely high tension. SYN: *hypertension*.
supervenosity (sū″pĕr-vē-nŏs′ĭ-tĭ) [" + *venosus*, pert. to a vein]. Incomplete oxidation of the blood; a condition of excessive venosity.
supervention (sū″pĕr-vĕn′shŭn) [L. *super-*

ventio, a coming over]. Additional condition developing besides something already existing, as a complication to an existing disease.
supervirulent (sū″pĕr-vĭr′ū-lĕnt) [L. *super*, above, + *virulentus*, poisonous]. More virulent than usual.
supinate (sū″pĭ-nāt) [L. *supināre*, to lay on the back]. 1. To turn the forearm or hand so that the palm faces upward. 2. To rotate the foot and leg outward. 3. To cause to assume, or to assume, a position of supination.
supination (sū-pĭn-ā′shŭn) [L. *supināre*, to lay on the back]. 1. Turning of the palm or foot upward. 2. Act of lying flat upon the back. 3. Condition of being on the back or having the foot or palm facing upward.
supinator (sū″pĭn-ā′tor) [L.]. A muscle producing the motion of supination of the forearm. SEE: *Table of Muscles in Appendix*.
   s. longus reflex. Flexion of the forearm caused by tapping of the tendon of the supinator longus.
supine (sū-pīn′) [L. *supinus*, bent back; lying on the back]. 1. Of position, lying on the back or with the face upward. 2. Of the hand or foot noting position with the palm or foot facing upward. OPP: *prone*. SEE: *position*.
supplemental (sŭp-lē-mĕn′tăl) [L. *supplementum*, an addition]. Referring to something added to supply a need or to reinforce.
   s. air. The *residual* air of the lungs which, after *tidal* air has been expelled in normal respiration, may be driven out by forced respiration. SEE: *air*.
suppository (sŭp-pŏz′ĭ-tō-rĭ) (pl. *suppositories*) [L. *suppositorium*, that which is placed underneath]. A semisolid, fusible, medicated substance for introduction into the rectum, vagina, or urethra, where it dissolves and is absorbed. Commonly shaped like cylinder or cone and made of soap, glycerinated gelatin or cocoa butter (oil of theobroma).
   s., rectal, anodyne. For local or general effects to reduce pain.
   s., r., astringent. To contract blood vessels and tissues.
   s., r., evacuant. To cause evacuation.
   s., r., specific. Used when specifics cannot be taken by mouth.
suppression (sū-prĕsh′ŭn) [L. *suppressio*, a pressing under]. 1. Repression of the ext. manifestation of a morbid condition. 2. Complete failure of a natural secretion or excretion. OPP: *retention*. 3. PSY: Conscious inhibition of an idea or desire, as distinguished from repression which is considered an unconscious process.
   s. of menses. 1. Amenorrhea in which menstruation ceases after once being established and from some cause other than pregnancy or the climacteric. 2. Any suppression of the menses.
   s. of urine. Suppression of urine resulting from renal conditions.
suppurant (sŭp′ū-rănt) [L. *suppurans*, from *suppurāre*, to cause to suppurate]. 1. Producing, tending to produce, or characterized by pus formation. 2. Agent causing pus formation. SYN: *suppurative*.
suppurate (sŭp′pū-rāt) [L. *suppurāre*, to cause to suppurate]. To form or generate pus.
suppuration (sŭp-ū-rā′shŭn) [L. *suppurātio*, from *sub*, under, + *pus*, *puris*, matter, pus]. 1. The process of pus for-

mation. 2. The discharge produced by suppuration. SYN: *pus.*
One of the terminations of inflammation due to the presence of certain microörganisms called pyogenic* (pus-forming) bacteria. Suppuration does not always obtain even though microörganisms are present in the affected part, as may be the case in erysipelas and acute joint affections where exudate is serous.
The liquefaction of tissues and formation of pus will continue so long as the microörganisms are alive. They cause the death of the leukocytes (white cells) and the cells of the part, liquefying the tissue so that the area becomes filled with a liquid (liquor puris) holding the dead and dying cells. Combination of liquor puris and the dead cells is called "pus."
An abscess may form by the accumulation of this liquid which is indicated by redness, swelling, heat and pain. It will show fluctuation which may be felt by touching it. When the abscess reaches the surface it will burst and discharge its contents.
RS: *abscess, gangrene, inflammation, infection, purulent, pus, pustulant, pustule.*

suppurative (sŭp'ū-rā″tĭv, -rā-tĭv) [L. *suppuratus,* from *suppurāre,* to cause to suppurate]. 1. Producing or associated with generation of pus. 2. Agent producing pus formation.
  s. fever. Pus in the blood causing fever; a form of septicemia. SYN: *pyemia.*
supra- [L.]. Combining form meaning above.
supra-acromial (sū-prā-ăk-rō'mĭ-ăl) [L. *supra,* above, + G. *akron,* point, + *ōmos,* shoulder]. Located above the acromion.
supra-auricular (sū″prā-aw-rĭk'ū-lar) [" + *auricula,* ear]. Located above an auricle.
supracapsulin (sū″prā-kăp'sū-lĭn). Commercial preparation of active principle of medulla of the suprarenals. SYN: *epinephrine.*
supracerebellar (sū″prā-sĕr-ē-bĕl'ar) [L. *supra,* above, + *cerebellum,* little brain]. On or above the upper surface of the cerebellum.
suprachoroid (sū″prā-kō'royd) [" + G. *chorioeidēs,* skinlike]. Upon the outer side of the choroid of the eye.
  s. lam'ina. Connective tissue bet. the sclerotic coats of the eye and the choroid. SYN: *suprachoroidea.*
suprachoroidea (sū″prā-ko-roy'dē-ă) [" + G. *chorioeidēs,* skinlike]. Outermost layer of the choroid. SYN: *suprachoroid lamina.*
supraclavicular (sū″prā-klă-vĭk'ū-lar) [" + *clavicula,* a little key]. Located above the clavicle.
  s. fossa. Depression on either side of neck reaching down behind the clavicle.
  s. point. A stimulation point over the clavicle at which contraction of arm muscles may be produced.
supracommissure (sū″prā-kŏm'ĭ-shŭr) [" + *commissura,* a joining point]. A cerebral commissure ant. to the stalk of the pineal body.
supracondylar (sū″prā-kŏn'dĭl-ar) [" + G. *kondylos,* knuckle]. Above a condyle.
supracostal (sū″prā-kŏs'tăl) [" + *costa,* rib]. Above or beyond the ribs.
supracotyloid (sū″prā-kŏt'ĭ-loyd) [L. *supra,* above, + G. *kotyloeidēs,* cup-shaped]. Above the acetabulum or cotyloid body.
supracranial (sū″prā-krā'nĭ-ăl) [" + G. *kranion,* skull]. On the upper surface of the skull.
supradiaphragmatic (sū″prā-dī″ă-frăg-mat'ĭk) [" + G. *dia,* across, + *phragma,* wall]. Above the diaphragm.
supra-epicondylar (sū″prā-ĕp″ĭ-kŏn'dĭ-lar) [" + G. *epi,* upon, + *kondylos,* knuckle]. Above an epicondyle.
supraglenoid (sū″prā-glē'noyd) [" + G. *glēnē,* cavity, + *eidos,* form]. Above the glenoid cavity or fossa.
  s. tubercle. A rough surface of the scapula above glenoid cavity to which is attached the large head of the biceps muscle.
suprahyoid (sū″prā-hī'oyd) [" + *hyoeidēs,* U-shaped]. Located above the hyoid bone; denoting accessory thyroid glands within the geniohyoid muscle.
  s. muscles. The digastric, geniohyoid, mylohyoid, and stylohyoid muscles.
suprainguinal (sū″prā-ĭn'gwĭn-ăl) [" + *inguinalis,* pert. to the groin]. Above the groin.
supraliminal (sū″prā-lĭm'ĭ-năl) [L. *supra,* above, + *limen, limin-,* threshold]. PSY: 1. Above the threshold of consciousness; conscious. 2. Exceeding the stimulus threshold. SEE: *subliminal.*
supralumbar (sū″prā-lŭm'bar) [" + *lumbus,* loin]. Above the lumbar region.
supramalleolar (sū″prā-mal-lē'ō-lar) [" + *malleolus,* little hammer]. Located above either malleolus.
supramarginal (sū″prā-mar'jĭn-ăl) [" + *margo, margin-,* margin]. Above any border.
  s. convolution, s. gyrus. A cerebral convolution on lateral surface of the parietal lobe above post. part of sylvian fissure.
supramastoid (sū″prā-măs'toyd) [" + *mastos,* breast, + *eidos,* like]. Above the mastoid process of the temporal bone.
  s. crest. A ridge on the temporal bone.
supramaxilla (sū″prā-măks-ĭl'lă) [" + *maxilla,* jaw]. The upper jawbone. SYN: *maxilla.*
supramaxillary (sū″prā-măks'ĭl-lā-rī) [" + *maxillaris,* pert. to the jaw]. 1. Relating to the upper jaw. 2. Located above the upper jaw.
suprameatal (sū″prā-mē-ā'tăl) [L. *supra,* above, + *meatus,* passage]. Above a meatus, esp. the ext. auditory meatus, noting the spine of Henle, a small, bony projection at post. sup. margin of ext. auditory meatus.
  s. triangle. Triangular space bordered by upper half of post. wall of ext. auditory meatus, and the supramastoid crest used to locate the mastoid antrum.
supraoccipital bone (sū″prā-ŏk-sĭp'ĭ-tăl) [" + *occiput,* back of head]. Situated above the occiput, noting a portion of occipital bone above the foramen magnum forming part of occipital bone in the adult but distinct in early childhood.
supraorbital (sū″prā-or'bĭ-tăl) [" + *orbita,* track, circuit]. Located above the orbit.
  s. neuralgia. N. of the supraorbital nerve. SYN: *hemicrania.*
  s. reflex. Contraction of orbicularis palpebrarum with closure of lids resulting from percussion above supraorbital nerve.
  s. ridge. Prominence on frontal bone over eye caused by projection of frontal air sinuses.

suprapelvic (sū″prӑ-pĕl′vĭk) [L. *supra*, above, + *pelvis*, basis]. Located above the pelvis.

suprapontine (sū″prӑ-pŏn′tĭn) [" + *pons, pont-*, bridge]. Located above the pons Varolii.

suprapubic (sū″prӑ-pū′bĭk) [" + *pubis*, pubis]. Above the pubic arch.

 s. cystotomy. Surgical opening of the bladder from just above the symphysis pubis.

 s. reflex. Deflection of linea alba toward stroked side when abdomen is stroked above Poupart's ligament.

suprarenal (sū″prӑ-rē′nӑl) [" + *rēn*, kidney]. 1. Above the kidney. 2. Tiny gland above each kidney. SYN: *adrenal, suprarenal body, s. capsule, s. gland.* 3. Pert. to the suprarenal gland.

 DOSAGE: 4 gr. (0.25 Gm.).

 s. body, s. capsule, s. gland. Small, flat body above each kidney, the left one larger than the right, composed of a cortex and a medulla differing in function and secreting epinephrine. SEE: *medulla, below.*

 Cortex: Function of: In doubt. It influences body growth and development of the sex glands.

 Medulla: Function of: Secretes epinephrine which stimulates the nervous system and the muscles, raises blood pressure and relieves bronchial asthma. SEE: *adrenal.*

suprarenalemia (sū″prӑ-rē-nӑl-ē′mĭ-ӑ) [L. *supra*, above, + *rēn*, kidney, + G. *aima*, blood]. Undue amt. of adrenalin, the suprarenal secretion, in the blood.

suprarenalism (sū″prӑ-rē′nӑl-ĭzm) [" + " + G. *ismos*, condition]. The condition resulting from overactivity of the suprarenal glands.

 Results in adiposity, pigmentation, hirsuties, and in women, amenorrhea.

suprarenalopathy (sū″prӑ-rē-nӑl-ŏp′ӑ-thĭ) [" + " + G. *pathos*, disease]. A disorder due to abnormal functioning of the suprarenal glands.

suprarenogenic (sū″prӑ-rē″no-jĕn′ĭk) [" + " + G. *gennan*, to produce]. Of suprarenal origin.

 s. syndrome. Suprarenalism characterized by adiposity, hirsuties, and pigmentation, and amenorrhea in women.

suprarenoma (sū″prӑ-rē-nō′mӑ) [" + " + G. *-ōma*, tumor]. Suprarenal tissue tumor.

suprarenopathy (sū″prӑ-rē-nŏp′ӑ-thĭ) [" + " + G. *pathos*, disease]. Any disorder of the suprarenal glands.

suprarenotropic (sū″prӑ-rē-nō-trŏp′ĭk) [" + " + G. *tropos*, a turning]. 1. Having an influence on the suprarenal secretion; said of ant. pituitary hormone. 2. Characterized by suprarenal influence on development.

suprascapular (sū″prӑ-skӑp′ū-lar) [L. *supra*, above, + *scapula*, shoulder]. Located above the scapula.

suprasellar (sū″prӑ-sĕl′ar) [" + *sella*, saddle]. Above or over the sella turcica.

suprasonic (sū″prӑ-sŏn′ĭk) [" + *sonus*, sound]. Noting sound with frequencies of vibration above 34,000 per second, probably heard by some animals.

supraspinal (sū″prӑ-spī′nӑl) [" + *spina*, a thorn]. Above a spine.

supraspinous (sū″prӑ-spī′nŭs) [" + *spina*, thorn]. Above any spine.

 s. fossa. A groove above the spine of the scapula.

suprasternal (sū″prӑ-ster′nӑl) [" + G. *sternon*, chest]. Above the sternum. SYN: *episternal.*

suprasylvian (sū″prӑ-sĭl′vĭ-ӑn) [L. *supra*, above, + *sylvian*]. Above the fissure of Sylvius.

 s. convolution. One above the post. limb of the sylvian fissure. SYN: *supramarginal convolution.*

supratrochlear (sū″prӑ-trok′lē-ar) [" + *trochlea*, pulley]. Above a trochlea, esp. that of the humerus.

supravaginal (sū″prӑ-vӑj′ĭ-nӑl) [" + *vagina*, sheath]. Above the vagina or any sheathing membrane.

sura (sū′rӑ) [L. *sura*, calf of the leg]. The calf of the leg.

sural (sū′rӑl) [L. *sura*, calf of the leg]. Relating to the calf of the leg.

suralimentation (sūr-ӑl-ĭm-ĕn-tā′shŭn) [Fr. *sur*, from L. *super*, above, + *alimentum*, nourishment]. Treatment by overfeeding. SYN: *gavage, superalimentation.*

surdity (sūr′dĭ-tĭ) [L. *surditās*, deafness]. Inability to hear. SYN: *deafness.*

surdomute (sūr′dō-mūt″) [L. *surdus*, deaf, + *mutus*, dumb]. 1. A deaf-mute. 2. Deaf and dumb.

surface (sur′fӑs) [Fr. *sur*, from L. *super*, over, + *faciēs*, face]. The outer integument of any body.

 s. tension. Intramolecular attraction inward at the surface of a liquid.

surgeon (sūr′jŭn) [Fr. *chirurgien*, from L. *chirurgus*, from G. *cheir*, hand, + *ergon*, work]. A medical practitioner who specializes in surgery.

 s., dental. A dentist authorized to operate on the mouth and teeth. SYN: *stomatologist.*

 s., house. The chief surgical intern in a hospital.

surgery (sur′jur-ĭ) [M.E. *surgerie*, from G. *cheirourgia*, handwork]. 1. Branch of medicine dealing with manual and operative procedures for correction of deformities and defects, repair of injuries, diagnosis and cure of diseases, relief of suffering and prolongation of life. SYN: *chirurgery, chirurgia.* 2. Surgeon's operating room.

 s., major. Important and serious operations involving risk to life.

 s., minor. Simple, less serious operations.

 s., orificial. Treatment of orifices of the body based on theory that many disorders are due to reflexes at the anus and other orifices.

 s., orthopedic. S. for correction of deformities.

 s., plastic. Repair of parts by transference.

surgical (sūr′jĭk-ӑl) [G. *cheirourgia*, handwork]. Of the nature of or pert. to surgery.

 s. diathermy. The use of high-frequency electrical oscillations in such a way that animal tissues are destroyed.

 s. dressing. Sterile protective covering of gauze or other substance applied to an operative wound. SEE: *chemise.*

 s. fever. Fever following an operation or injury.

 s. kidney. Suppuration of the kidney subsequent to surgery on the genitourinary tract.

 s. neck. Constricted part of shaft of humerus below the tuberosities; commonly the seat of fracture.

surgiology (sūr-jĭ-ŏl′ō-jĭ) [G. *cheirourgia*, handwork, + *logos*, study]. Surgery for experimental purposes in physiology.

surrogate (sūr′rō-gāt) [L. *surrogāre*, to substitute]. Something that replaces another; a substitute.

 PSY: The representation of one whose

identity is concealed from conscious recognition, as in a dream; a figure of importance may represent one's loved one.
sursumduction (sŭr″sŭm-dŭk′shŭn) [L. *sursum*, upward, + *ducere*, to lead]. Elevation, as the power or act of turning an eye upward independently of the other one.
sursumvergence (sŭr″sŭm-vĕr′jĕns) [" + *vergere*, to turn]. An upward turning, as of the eyeballs.
sursumversion (sŭr″sŭm-vĕr′shŭn) [" + *versio*, from *vertere*, to turn]. Process of turning upward; simultaneous movement of both eyes upward.
susceptible (sŭs-sĕp′tĭ-bl) [L. *susceptibilis*, from *suscipere*, to take up]. 1. Having little resistance to a disease or foreign protein. 2. An individual with little resistance to an infectious disease or who is not known to have become immune to one. 3. Easily impressed or influenced.
suscitate (sŭs′sĭ-tāt) [L. *suscitāre*, to rouse]. To arouse to increased activity; to stimulate.
suscitation (sŭs″sĭ-tā′shŭn) [L. *suscitatio*, from *suscitāre*, to rouse]. Act of stimulating to greater activity. SYN: *excitation*.
suspended (sŭs-pĕnd′ĕd) [L. *suspendere*, to hang]. 1. Hanging. 2. Temporarily inactive.
  s. animation. A cessation of the vital functions temporarily.
suspension (sŭs-pĕn′shŭn) [L. *suspensio*, a hanging]. 1. A condition of temporary cessation, as of any vital process. 2. Treatment by immobilization of a part or whole of a patient by hanging in desired position. 3. State of a solid when its particles are mixed with, but not dissolved in, a fluid or another solid; also a substance in this state.
  s., cephalic. Suspension of a patient by the head to extend the vertebral column.
  s. colloid. Solution containing very tiny, solid, dispersed particles. SYN: *suspensoid*.
  s. stability. Degree of speed with which erythrocytes sink to bottom in a mass of citrated blood. SYN: *sedimentation rate*.
  s. of the uterus. The operation of attaching the uterus to the abdominal wall.
suspensoid (sŭs-pĕn′soyd) [L. *suspens*, hanging, + G. *eidos*, form]. A colloid solution in which the dispersed particles are solid, as distinguished from emulsoid. SYN: *suspension colloid*.
suspensory (sŭs-pĕn′sōr-ĭ) [L. *suspensorius*, hanging]. 1. Supporting a part, as a muscle, ligament, or bone. 2. A structure of the body which supports a part. 3. Bandage or sac for supporting or compressing a part, esp. the scrotum.
  s. bandage. A sling for support of the testicles.
suspirious (sŭs-pī′rĭ-ŭs) [L. *suspirāre*, to sigh]. Breathing with apparent effort; sighing.
sustentacular (sŭs-tĕn-tăk′ū-lar) [L. *sustentaculum*, support]. Supporting; upholding.
  s. cell. A supporting cell, esp. a branching connective tissue cell of the spleen.
sustentaculum (sŭs-tĕn-tăk′ū-lŭm) [L. a support]. A supporting structure.
  s. lieni. Phrenocolic ligament which apparently supports the spleen.
  s. tali. A process of the calcaneum which supports part of the astragalus.
susurrus (sū-sŭr′ŭs) [L. a whisper]. A murmur. [a stitch]. Suture.
sutura (sū-tū′ră) (pl. *suturae*) [L. *sutura*, a stitch].
  s. denta′ta. One with interlocking of bones by toothlike processes.
  s. harmo′nia. Simple apposition of 2 contiguous bones.
  s. limbo′sa. Bevelled suture in which opposing margins fit in parallel ridges, as the interparietal surfaces.
  s. no′tha. A false suture with ill-defined projections.
  s. serra′ta. One with deeper and more irregular indentations than a dental s.
  s. squamo′sa. A scalelike suture.
sutural (sū′tū-răl) [L. *sutura*, a stitch]. Relating to a suture.
  s. joint. Articulation bet. 2 bones.
  s. ligament. Fibers uniting opposed bones forming a cranial suture.
suturation (sū″tū-rā′shŭn) [L. *sutura*, a stitch]. Application of sutures; stitching.
suture (sū′tūr) [L. *sutura*, a stitch]. 1. Line of union in an immovable articulation, as those bet. the skull bones; also such an articulation itself. SYN: *synarthrosis*. 2. Operation of uniting parts by stitching them together. 3. The thread or wire or other material used in the operation of stitching parts of the body together. 4. The seam or line of union formed by surgical stitches. 5. To unite by stitching, as *to suture a wound*. SEE: *raphe*.
  s., absorbable. S. undergoing liquefaction or replaced by living tissue.
  s., basilar. The one bet. the occipital bone and sphenoid bone.
  s., bifrontal. SEE: *coronal s.*
  s., biparietal. SEE: *sagittal s.*
  s's., buried. Those completely covered by skin and not involving that structure at all.
  s., button. One in which the threads are passed through buttons on the surface and tied to prevent the thread from cutting.
  s., coaptation. One uniting as distinguished from one intended to relieve tension.
  s., cobbler's. A s. in which the thread has a needle at each end.
  s., continuous. The closure of a wound by means of 1 continuous thread, usually by transfixing first 1 lip and then the other, alternately, from within outward.
  s., coronal. The junction of the frontal and parietal bones.
  s's., cranial. Those s's. bet. the bones of the skull.
  s., dentate. An articulation of long and toothlike processes.
  s., ethmoidofrontal. The one bet. the ethmoid and frontal bones.
  s., ethmoidolacrimal. The one bet. the ethmoid and lacrimal bones.
  s., ethmosphenoid. The one bet. the ethmoid and sphenoid bones.
  s., false. Any form of suture in which one surface is smooth.
  s., figure-of-eight. SEE: *twisted s.*
  s., frontal. An occasional one in the frontal bone from the sagittal s. to root of nose.
  s., frontolacrimal. The one bet. the frontal and lacrimal bones.
  s., frontomalar. The one bet. the frontal and malar bones.
  s., frontomaxillary. The one bet. the frontal bone and sup. maxilla.

s., frontonasal. The one bet. the frontal bone and the alae of the sphenoid bone.
s., frontoparietal. The coronoid suture.
s., frontotemporal. The one bet. the frontal and temporal bones.
s., Glover's. A continuous s. in which the needle is, after each stitch, passed through the loop of the preceding stitch.
s., harelip. SEE: *twisted s.*
s., harmonic. One in which there is simple apposition of bone.
s., horsehair. S. adapted for light, superficial sutures, alternated with heavier ones and for exposed places like the face, where scar tissue is to be avoided. *Dry*, 100 strands in a bunch. *Sterilized*, 50 in a bottle.
s., implanted. A s. formed by placing pins opposite each other on the 2 sides of a wound, and approximating the lips by winding thread or other similar material about the pins.
s., intermaxillary. The s. bet. the sup. maxillae.
s., internasal. The one bet. the nasal bones.
s., interparietal. SEE: *sagittal s.*
s., interrupted. A s. formed by single stitches inserted separately, the needle being usually passed through 1 lip from without inward, and through the other from within outward.
s., jugal. SEE: *sagittal s.*
s., lambdoid. The one bet. the parietal bones and the 2 sup. borders of the occipital bone.
s., Lembert's. An intestinal s.
s., longitudinal. SEE: *sagittal s.*
s., mattress. A continuous s. in which a stitch is taken with a needle, the thread tied, and then needle inserted upon the same side as that from which it emerged and passed in opposite direction through both lips of the wound, the direction of the needle being reversed at each stitch.
s., maxillolacrimal. The one bet. the maxilla and lacrimal bone.
s., maxillopremaxillary. One bet. the premaxillary portion of sup. maxilla and rest of the bone.
s., mediofrontal. SEE: *frontal s.*
s., metopic. SEE: *frontal s.*
s., nasomaxillary. The one bet. the nasal bone and sup. maxilla.
s., nonabsorbable. Silk, silkworm gut, horsehair and wire.
s., occipital. SEE: *lambdoid s.*
s., occipitomastoid. The one bet. the occipital bone and mastoid portion of temporal bone.
s., occipitoparietal. SEE: *lambdoid s.*
s., palatine. One bet. the palate bones.
s., palatine transverse. One bet. the palate processes and sup. maxilla.
s., parietal. SEE: *sagittal s.*
s., parietomastoid. The one bet. parietal bone and mastoid portion of the temporal bone.
s., petrooccipital. The one bet. the petrous portion of the temporal bone and occipital bone.
s., petrosphenoidal. The one bet. petrous portion of the temporal bone and ala magna of sphenoid bone.
s., purse-string. One going in and out around a circular opening, closing when the 2 are drawn taut.
s., quilled, s., quill. An interrupted s. in which a double thread is passed deep into the tissues, even quite below the bottom of the wound, needle being so withdrawn as to leave a loop hanging from 1 lip and the 2 free ends of the thread from the other. A quill, or, more commonly, a piece of bougie, is passed through the loops, which are tightened upon it, and the free ends of each separate thread are tied together over a second quill to bring the deep parts into firm coaptation and to relieve tension.
s., relaxation. A s. that may be loosened to relieve excessive tension.
s., relief. A row of supplementary s's. including the tissues to the extent of 1 or 1½ in. on each side of a fistula or a deep wound, for the purpose of lessening the strain on the coaptation s's.
s., right-angled. A s. used in sewing intestine. The needle is passed in the same direction as the long axis of the incision and the process repeated on the opposite side of the incision, the suture being continuous.
s., Sabatier's. Approximation of an intestinal wound by using cardboard soaked in turpentine oil.
s., sagittal. The suture between the upper margins of the parietal bones.
s., serrated. An articulation by s. in which there is an interlocking of bones by small, fine and delicate projections and indentations.
s., shotted. A s. in which both ends of a wire or silkworm gut are passed through a perforated shot that is then compressed tightly over them.
s., silk. Does not produce suppuration if sterilized. Twisted, braided and floss.
s., silkworm gut. Causes little friction, pliable, does not curl or twist, less liable to produce irritation and sterilizable. Should always be soaked in a sterile solution 30 minutes.
s., sphenoparietal. The one bet. the parietal bone and ala magna of the sphenoid bone.
s., sphenosquamous. Articulation of the great wing of the sphenoid with squamous portion of the temporal bone.
s., sphenotemporal. The one bet. the sphenoid and temporal bones.
s., squamoparietal, s., squamosal. The one bet. the parietal and squamous portion of the temporal bone.
s., squamosphenoidal. One bet. the squamous portion of the temporal bone and great wing of sphenoid.
s., subcuticular. A buried continuous s. in which the needle is passed horizontally under the epidermis into the cutis vera, emerging at the angle of the wound, then in a similar manner passed through cutis vera of opposite side of the wound, and so on until the other angle of the wound is reached.
s., temporooccipital. SEE: *occipitomastoid s.* [temporal and parietal bones.
s., temporoparietal. One bet. the
s., twisted. A s. in which pins are passed through the opposite lips of a wound, at right angles to direction of wound, and material is wound about the pins, crossing them first at one end and then at the other in a figure-of-eight fashion, thus holding the lips of the wound firmly together.
s., uninterrupted. SEE: *continuous s.*
s., wire. Usually silver. Adapted for cases where there is much tension, ends of bones, resection, etc.
s., zygomatic. One bet. zygomatic process of sup. maxilla and temporal bone.

Suzanne's gland (sū-zanz'). A small mucous gland in floor of the mouth, below the alveolingual groove.

swab (swŏb) [Dutch *zwabber*, to wipe]. 1. Cotton or gauze on end of slender stick used for cleansing cavities, applying remedies or for obtaining a piece of tissue or secretion for bacteriological examination. 2. To wipe with a swab, as to *swab a wound*.
  s., test tube. For cleansing tubes, etc.
  s., urethral. Slender rod for holding cotton, used in examinations with speculum, in treating ulcers, removing secretions, etc.
  s., u., male. About 7 in. long.
  s., uterine. For absorbing or wiping away discharges. Slender, flattened wire, plain rod or one with coarse thread on distal end.
swallow (swŏl'ō) [A.S. *swelgan*, to swallow]. To pass into the stomach through the mouth and throat.
swallowing (swŏl'ō-ĭng) [A.S. *swelgan*, to swallow]. 1. A complicated act usually initiated voluntarily but always completely reflexly whereby food is moved from the mouth through the pharynx and esophagus to the stomach. 2. Performance of motions characteristic of swallowing, as in emotion. Movements of the tongue must first get the material into the back of the mouth. Further muscular activity prevents it from returning; the post. nares are closed; the glottis is closed and protected by special mechanisms, and the contraction of the musculi constrictores pharyngis forces the food into the esophagus.
  Movement down the esophagus is accomplished by rapid peristalsis, aided by gravity and by the impetus imparted by the pharyngeal contraction. SEE: *esophagus.*
  RS: *acatoposis, aglutition, air s., aphagia, choking, deglutition, dysphagia.*
  s. reflex. Swallowing induced by stimulation of soft palate.
swallow's nest (swŏl'ŏz). Cerebral depression bet. the uvula and the post. velum. SYN: *nidus hirundinis.*
sweat (swĕt) [A.S. *swāt*, sweat]. 1. The secretion of the sudoriparous glands of the skin. SYN: *perspiration, sudor.* SEE: *glands, Moll's.* 2. Condition of perspiring or of being made to perspire freely, as to order a sweat for a patient. 3. To emit moisture through the skin's pores. SYN: *perspire.* 4. To cause to emit moisture through the pores.
  The perspiration is a colorless, slightly turbid, salty, aqueous fluid, although that from the sweat glands in the axillae, and around the anus, and that of the ceruminous glands have an oily consistency. It contains urea, fatty substances and sodium chloride. This salty, watery fluid is difficult to collect without contamination with sebum.*
  FUNCTION: To cool the body by evaporation, and to rid it of what waste may be expressed through the pores of the skin. The amount per day is about a liter; this figure is subject to extreme variation according to muscular activity and atmospheric conditions.
  PHYS: Perspiration is controlled by the sympathetic nervous system through true secretory fibers supplying the sweat glands.
  s., bloody. S. tinged with blood. SYN: *hematidrosis.*
  s. center. Medullary area controlling sweating.
  s., colored. S. tinged with a pigment. SYN: *chromidrosis.*
  s., fetid. S. with foul odor. SYN: *bromidrosis.*
  s. glands. These are invaginated, epithelial, tubular, coil glands which penetrate the corium* into the subcutaneous fatty tissue and which secrete sweat.
  They are most numerous on the palms of the hands and soles of the feet, averaging about 2300 to the sq. in. or over 2,000,000 to the body.
  s., night. Sweating during the night, a symptom of pulmonary tuberculosis.
  s., profuse. Excessive perspiration. SYN: *hyperidrosis.*
  s., scanty. Abnormally small amount or lack of sweat. SYN: *anidrosis.*
sweat, words pert. to: anaphoresis, antisudoral, antisudorin, bromidrosis, chromidrosis, chylidrosis, diaphoresis, diaphoretic, dyshidria, dysidrosis, ephidrosis, hematidrosis, hidradenitis, hidrorrhea, hidrosis, hydradenitis, hydradenoma, hyphidrosis, hyperidrosis, hypoidrosis, ischidrosis, melanidrosis, perspiration, phosphorhidrosis, sudor, sudorific, sudoriparous, uridrosis.
sweating (swĕt'ĭng) [A.S. *swāt*, sweat]. 1. Act of exuding sweat. 2. Emitting sweat. 3. Causing profuse sweating.
  To induce, paint 2 in. square of skin under each axilla with mixture of equal parts of olive oil and guaiacol solution. Cover with several layers of gauze, then flannel, and hold with adhesive tape. Wrap patient in warm blankets.
  RS: *anhidrosis, bromidrosis, chromidrosis, hydrosis, perspiration, pores, skin, sudor, sudorific, sweat, uridrosis.*
Swedish gymnastics, movements. System of active and passive exercise of the various muscles and joints of the body without using apparatus.
  TYPES: *Active:* Taken by the patient with the assistance or resistance of the operator. *Duplicated active:* Performed by the patient with the operator's assistance. *General active:* Performed by the patient exclusively. *Passive:* All given to the patient by the operator. *General passive:* May be performed while the patient is dressed.
  THE PRINCIPAL MOVEMENTS: 1. *Bending.* 2. *Depression* and *elevation.* 3. *Flexion* and *extension.* 4. *Pressing* and *shaking.* In pressing, the operator uses the tips of his fingers in vertical motion over the principal nerves. In shaking the arm, the operator grasps the hand and shoulder, keeping the arm in an extended position, and shakes as quickly as possible. In shaking the leg, he grasps the foot with one hand and the thigh as high as possible with the other and shakes quickly. These movements are always passive and are principally used in nervous affections. 5. *Pulling.* 6. *Raising.* 7. *Rotation.* This is a rotary movement by which the different joints are brought into motion within their natural limits. Rotation is to lengthen and shorten the veins so as to produce a sucking of their contents, thus stimulating the circulation and assisting the heart in its action. 8. *Separating* and *closing.* 9. *Turning.*
  POSITIONS: The movements may be performed in 5 different positions. Kneeling, lying, sitting, standing, or suspending. These are called ground positions and have many subdivisions. There are 47 derivative positions—about 800 movements in all.
  S. massage. Massage combined with S. gymnastics.
sweet (swĕt) [A.S. *swēte*, sweet]. 1. Pleasing to the taste or smell. SEE: *taste.* 2.

sweetbread   S-111   **symblepharon**

Free from excess of acid, sulfur, or corrosive salts.

sweetbread (swēt′brĕd) [origin uncertain]. The thymus and pancreas glands, esp. of the calf, used as food.
    COMP: Nuclein abundant as well as collagenous substances. Purines are very high.
    AV. SERVING: 115 Gm. Pro. 19.3, Fat 13.9.
    ACTION: Completely digested, but the presence of purines should be considered before recommending them.

swelling (swĕl′ĭng) [A.S. *swellan*, to grow larger]. A morbid enlargement, esp. one appearing on the surface of the body.
    TREATMENT: *Local*: Ice water with salt in it applied to area reduces swelling rapidly.
    RS: *anthorisma, detumescence, node, nodule, turgescence, turgid*.

    s., albuminous. Same as cloudy s.

    s., cloudy. Degeneration of tissues marked by cloudy appearance, swelling, and appearance of tiny albuminoid granules in the cells.

    s., glassy. Starchy degeneration of tissue. SYN: *amyloid degeneration*.

    s., white. Swelling seen in tuberculous arthritis, esp. of the knee.

Swift's disease (swĭft). Condition occurring in very young children characterized by irritability and restlessness; redness and swelling of the hands and feet, esp. on the palms and soles; desquamation; a sensation of tingling or burning; loss of appetite, and the appearance of a rash, mainly on the trunk, and loss of muscle tone. SYN: *acrodynia*.

Swiss chard. AV. SERVING: 100 Gm. Pro. 1.4, Fat 0.2, Carbo. 4.4.

switch, foot. In the application of surgical, high-frequency currents where both hands of the operator are needed, the current is started and cut off by a foot switch.

    s., pole-changing. P.T. A switch by which the polarity of a circuit may be reversed.

swoon (swōōn) [M.E. *swounen*, from A.S. *geswōgen*, in a swoon]. 1. A syncope* or fainting fit. 2. To sink into a fainting fit.

sycoma (sī-kō′mă) [G. *sykon*, fig, + *-ōma*, tumor]. A large, soft wart. SYN: *condyloma*.

sycophancy (sĭk′ō-făn-sĭ) [G. *sykophantēs*, a false adviser]. PSY: Characteristics of one maturely intelligent who has not developed a sense of responsibility and who is more or less dependent upon others.

sycophant (sĭk′ō-fănt) [G. *sykophantēs*, a false adviser]. An adult who, though mature intellectually, lacks a sense of responsibility.

sycosiform (sī-kō′sĭ-form) [G. *sykōsis*, figlike disease, + L. *forma*, shape]. Resembling sycosis.

sycosis (sī-kō′sĭs) [G. *sykōsis*, figlike disease]. Chronic inflammation of hair follicles.
    ETIOL: *Staphylococcus aureus* and *albus* entering through hair follicles, trauma, debility, etc., as predisposing factors.
    SYM: As stated, on hairy regions, and, if severe, may result in alopecia and scarring, characterized by an aggregation of papules and pustules, each of which is pierced by a hair. Pustules show no disposition to rupture but dry to yellow brown crusts; more or less itching and burning. If disease persists may lead to extreme destruction of hair follicles and permanent alopecia.
    PROG: Disease is curable under prolonged treatment; relapses prone to occur.
    TREATMENT: In acute cases soothing applications. In chronic cases crusts should be removed and hairs cut close or preferably shaved; puncture pustule and extract hairs so as to preserve the follicles. Constitutional remedies called for by special conditions.

    s. barbae. Sycosis of the beard, marked by papules and pustules perforated by hairs, and surrounded by infiltrated skin. SYN: *folliculitis barbae*.

    s. tinea. A form due to infection with ringworm commonly affecting the beard.

    s. vulgaris. Same as sycosis.

Sydenham's chorea (sĭd′ĕn-hăm). Simple chorea with only mild convulsive movements.

S's. cough. C. produced in hysteria by spasm of the respiratory muscles.

syllabic utterance (sĭl-ab′ĭk) [G. *syllabē*, a syllable]. A staccato accentuation of syllables, slowly but separately, observed in multiple *sclerosis*. SYN: *scanning speech*.

syllable stumbling (sĭl′ă-bl) [G. *syllabē*, a syllable]. Hesitating utterance (dysphasia) with difficulty in pronouncing certain syllables.

syllabus (sĭl′ă-bŭs) [G. *syllabos*, a collection]. Abstract of a lecture or outline of a course of study or of a book.

syllepsiology (sĭl-lĕp-sĭ-ol′ō-jĭ) [G. *syllēpsis*, conception, + *logos*, study]. The study of conception and pregnancy.

syllepsis (sĭl-ĕp′sĭs) [G. *syllēpsis*, conception]. Conception; impregnation, or pregnancy.

Sylvester's method. Method of artificial respiration by drawing arms of a supine patient out above head, and then bringing them down folded onto the chest, with pressure on the abdomen and ribs to cause expiration.
    This and other methods of artificial respiration should *not* be used for the resuscitation of babies born with asphyxia neonatorum. SEE: *artificial* respiration*.

sylvian aqueduct (sĭl′vĭ-ăn). A narrow canal from 3rd to 4th ventricle. SYN: *aqueduct of Sylvius*.

    s. artery. Middle cerebral artery in the fissure of Sylvius.

    s. fissure. The fissure separating the temporal lobe from the frontal and parietal lobes.

    s. line. One on ext. of cranium marking direction of the sylvian fissure.

sym-, syn- [G.]. Combining form meaning *with, along, together with, beside*.

symbion, symbiont (sĭm′bĭ-ŏn, -ŏnt) [G. *syn*, together, + *bios*, life]. An organism which lives with another to their mutual advantage. SYN: *commensal*.

symbiosis (sĭm-bĭ-ō′sĭs) [G. *symbiōsis*, a living together]. 1. The association of 2 diverse nonparasitic organisms dependent upon each other for existence or where the association is advantageous. 2. PSY: Incorporation of a symptom as a part of one's personality, as delusions of grandeur, seen in paranoia.

symblepharon (sĭm-blĕf′ă-rŏn) [G. *syn*, together, + *blepharon*, eyelid]. Adhesion bet. conjunctivae of lid and eyeball due to injuries, esp. burns from lime, acids, etc.

Also seen in trachoma, pemphigus, and following operations.
SYM: Interference with movement of eyeball, conjunctival irritation.
TREATMENT: Division of cicatricial bands and keeping raw surfaces separated. Mucous membrane grafts.

symbol (sĭm'bŏl) [G. *symbolon*, a sign].
1. A representation of an idea or quality in the form of an object or that which stands for something beside itself.
2. PSY: An object used as an unconscious substitute and which is not connected consciously with the libido, but into which the libido is concentrated.
3. CHEM: A mark or letter representing an atom of an element.

symbolism (sĭm'bŏl-ĭzm) [" + *-ismos*, condition]. PSY: 1. Unconscious substitutive expression of subconscious thoughts of sexual significance in terms recognized by the objective consciousness.
2. An abnormal condition in which everything that occurs is interpreted as a symbol of the patient's own thoughts.

symbolophobia (sĭm-bō-lō-fō'bĭ-ă) [" + *phobos*, fear]. Fear of expressing one's self in words or action that may be interpreted as possessing a symbolic meaning.

Syme's operation (sīm). 1. Amputation of the foot at the ankle joint with removal of the malleoli. 2. Excision of the tongue. 3. External urethrotomy.

symmetric, symmetrical (sĭm-ĕt'rĭk, -rĭ-kl) [G. *symmetrikos*, measuring with]. 1. Exhibiting correspondence in size and shape of parts. 2. CHEM: Denoting an atomic arrangement in a molecule at equal relative intervals.
  s. gangrene. Gangrene affecting corresponding parts simultaneously and similarly. SYN: *Raynaud's disease*, q.v.

symmetromania (sĭm"ĕ-trō-mā'nĭ-ă) [G. *symmetria*, from *syn*, with, + *metron*, a measure]. An abnormal impulse to make symmetrical motions with the arms.

symmetry (sĭm'ĕt-rĭ) [G. *symmetria*, from *syn*, with, + *metron*, a measure]. Correspondence in shape, size, and relative position of parts on opposite sides of a body.

sympathectomy (sĭm-pă-thek'tō-mĭ) [G. *sympathētikos*, suffering with, + *ektomē*, excision]. Partial excision of sympathetic nerve.
  s., chemical. The use of chemicals to destroy part of the sympathetic nerve.
  s., periarterial. Removal of sheath of an artery in which are the sympathetic nerve fibers, used in trophic disturbances.

sympatheoneuritis (sĭm-păth"ē-ō-nū-rī'tĭs) [" + *neuron*, nerve, + *-itis*, inflammation]. Inflammation of the sympathetic nerve.

sympathesis (sĭm-păth'ĕ-sĭs) [G. *syn*, with, + *pathos*, suffering]. The morbid tendencies of the organism as a whole.

sympathetic (sĭm-pă-thĕt'ĭk) [G. *syn*, with, + *pathos*, suffering]. 1. Pert. to a special set of nerves and ganglia, uniting all parts of the body and subjecting them to a common involuntary nerve impulse. SEE: *autonomic system*. 2. Caused by or pert. to sympathy.
  s. irritation. I. of a structure caused by irritation of another related structure.
  s. nerves, s. nervous system. A division of the autonomic* nervous system consisting of a pair of ganglionated cords, 1 on each side of the entire vertebral column, connected with the thoracic and lumbar parts of spinal cord by means of *rami communicantes*, communicating visceral, sensory and preganglionic fibers, distributing to the viscera of the abdomen, and pelvis, the heart and lungs, the peripheral blood vessels, glands and smooth muscles of the skin.
It causes reflex dilatation of the pupil, arterioles, bronchioles, relaxation of the smooth muscle of the stomach and intestines, and acceleration of the heart. Normally, there is a delicate balance bet. the divisions of the autonomic nervous system, so that the insides of the bodies function well.
RS: *nervous system, parasympathetic nervous system, systema*.
  s. ophthalmia. Inflammation of the uveal tract in one eye due to similar inflammation in the other eye.
  s. plexuses. Plexuses formed at intervals by the sympathetic nerves and ganglia.

sympatheticalgia (sĭm-pă-thĕt-ĭ-kal'jĭ-ă) [G. *sympathētikos*, suffering with, + *algos*, pain]. Pain in the cervical sympathetic ganglion.

sympatheticless (sĭm-pă-thĕt'ĭk-lĕs) [" A.S. *lēas*, without]. Noting absence of the abdominal sympathetic chain.

sympatheticoparalytic (sĭm-pă-thĕt"ĭk-ō-par-ăl-ĭt'ĭk) [" + *paralysis*, a loosening at the sides]. Resulting from paralysis of the sympathetic nervous system.

sympatheticopathy (sĭm-pă-thĕt-ĭ-kŏp'ă-thī) [" + *pathos*, disease]. Any condition resulting from disorder of the sympathetic nervous system.

sympatheticotonia (sĭm-pă-thĕt"ĭk-ō-tō'nĭ-ă) [" + *tonos*, tone]. Condition characterized by excessive tone of the sympathetic nervous system with unusually high blood pressure and tendency to vascular spasm. SYN: *sympatheticotonia*.

sympatheticotonic (sĭm-păth-ĕt"ĭk-ō-ton'ĭk) [" + *tonos*, tension]. Marked by increased arterial tone or vasoconstriction due to overaction of the sympathetic nervous system.

sympatheticotripsy (sĭm-pă-thĕt"ĭk-ō-trĭp'sĭ) [" + *tripsis*, a crushing]. Surgical crushing of the sup. cervical ganglion in treatment of mental diseases.

sympathicectomy (sĭm-păth-ĭs-ĕk'tō-mĭ) [G. *sympathētikos*, suffering with, + *ektomē*, excision]. Excision of part of the sympathetic nerve. SYN: *sympathectomy*.

sympathicoblast (sĭm-păth"ĭ-kō-blăst) [" + *blastos*, a germ]. A primitive sympathetic nerve cell. SEE: *sympathoblast*.

sympathicoblastoma (sĭm-păth"ĭk-ō-blăs-tō'mă) [" + " + *-ōma*, tumor]. A tumor made up of sympathicoblasts.

sympathicomimetic (sĭm-păth"ĭk-ō-mĭm-ĕt'ĭk) [" + *mimētikos*, imitating]. Simulating action of adrenalin, said of stimulants of the sympathetic nervous system. SYN: *adrenergic*.

sympathiconeuritis (sĭm-păth"ĭk-ō-nū-rī'tĭs) [" + *neuron*, nerve, + *-itis*, inflammation]. Inflammation of the sympathetic nerves.

sympathicotonia (sĭm-păth"ĭ-kō-tō'nĭ-ă) [" + *tonos*, tone]. Increased tonus of the sympathetic system with marked tendency to vascular spasm and heightened blood pressure. OPP: *vagotonia.*

sympathicotripsy (sĭm-păth"ĭk-ō-trĭp'sĭ) [" + *tripsis*, a crushing]. Crushing of the sup. cervical ganglion in treatment of mental diseases. SYN: *sympatheticotripsy*.

sympathicotropic (sĭm-păth"ĭ-kō-trop'ĭk)

sympathicus   S-113   **symptom**

[" + *tropos*, a turning]. Having a special affinity for the sympathetic nerve.

sympathicus (sĭm-păth'ĭ-kŭs) [G. *sympathētikos*, suffering with]. The sympathetic nervous system. SYN: *systema nervorum sympathicum*.

sympathin (sĭm'păth-ĭn) [G. *syn*, with, + *pathos*, suffering]. An assumed hormone produced in the body by the sympathetic nerves which stimulates cardiac action and parts controlled by the impulses of the sympathetic nervous system.

sympathism (sĭm'păth-ĭzm) [" + " + *-ismos*, condition]. Condition of susceptibility to suggestion. SYN: *suggestibility*.

sympathoblast (sĭm-păth'ō-blăst) [" + *blastos*, germ]. A primitive cell from which arises a sympathetic ganglion cell.

sympathoblastoma (sĭm″păth-ō-blăs-tō'mă) [" + " + " + *-ōma*, tumor]. A malignant tumor made up of sympathetic nerve cells.

sympathoglioblastoma (sĭm″păth-ō-glī″ō-blăs-tō'mă) [" + " + *glia*, glue, + *blastos*, germ, + *-ōma*, tumor]. A tumor made up primarily of sympathoblasts, with scattered neuroblasts and spongioblasts.

sympathogonia (sĭm″păth-ō-gō'nĭ-ă) [" + " + *gonē*, seed]. Primitive cells from which sympathetic cells are derived.

sympathogonioma (sĭm″păth-ō-gō-nĭ-ō'mă) [" + " + " + *-ōma*, tumor]. A tumor containing sympathogonia.

sympathoma (sĭm-păth-ō'mă) [G. *syn*, with, + *pathos*, suffering, + *-ōma*, tumor]. A tumor composed of tissue similar to that of the sympathetic nervous system.

sympathomimetic (sĭm″păth-ō-mĭm-ĕt'ĭk) [" + " + *mimētikos*, imitating]. Capable of stimulating or inhibiting sympathetic nerve endings. SYN: *adrenergic*.

sympathy (sĭm'pă-thĭ) [G. *sympatheia*, from *syn*, with, + *pathos*, suffering]. 1. Relationship bet. 2 organs or parts through which 1 unaffected part is affected or becomes disordered from disease in the other part without actual transmission of morbific cause. 2. Mental influence exerted by one person on another, as in yawning or transmission of hysterical symptoms from one to another.

sympexion (sĭm-pĕks'ĭ-on) [G. *sympēxis*, concretion]. A concretion in the seminal vessels, the thyroid and lymphatic glands.

sympexis (sĭm-pĕks'ĭs) [G. *sympēxis*, concretion]. Term for arrangement of red blood cells in harmony with the laws of surface tension.

symphalangism (sĭm-făl'ăn-jĭzm) [G. *syn*, together, + *phalagx, phalagg-*, phalanx]. 1. Ankylosis of joints of the fingers or toes. 2. Web-fingered or web-toed condition.

symphyseal (sĭm-fĭz'ē-ăl) [G. *symphysis*, a growth together]. Pert. to symphysis.

symphyseotomy (sĭm-fĭz-ē-ŏt'ō-mĭ) [" + *tomē*, incision]. Section of symphysis pubis to enlarge the pelvic diameters during delivery.

symphysiectomy (sĭm-fĭz-ĭ-ĕk'tō-mĭ) [" + *ektomē*, excision]. Section of the symphysis pubis to facilitate delivery.

symphysion (sĭm-fĭz'ĭ-ŏn) [G. *symphysis*, a growth together]. Most ant. point of the alveolar process of the lower jaw.

symphysiotomy (sĭm″fĭz-ĭ-ŏt'ō-mĭ) [" + *tomē*, a cutting]. Section of the symphysis pubis to facilitate delivery by enlarging the pelvic diameters.

symphysis (sĭm'fĭz-ĭs) (pl. *symphyses*) [G. *symphysis*, a growth together]. 1. The joint or point of junction and fusion by fibrocartilage bet. bones originally distinct. 2. Union of any 2 structures. 3. A morbid adhesion.

   s., cardiac. The adhesion of the parietal and visceral layers of the pericardium. SEE: *intervertebral disk*.

   s. of jaw. An ant., median, vertical ridge upon outer surface of lower jaw representing line of union of its 2 halves.

   s. mandibulae. The central line of union of the 2 halves of the mandible.

   s. pubis. The junction of the pubic bones on midline in front; bony eminence under the pubic hair. SEE: *disk, interpubic*.

sympodia (sĭm-pō'dĭ-ă) [G. *syn*, together, + *pous, pod-*, foot]. Condition in which lower extremities are united.

symptom (sĭmp'tŭm) [G. *symptōma*, anything that has befallen one]. Any perceptible change in the body or its functions which indicates disease or the kind or phases of disease.

They may be classified as *objective, subjective, cardinal,* and sometimes as *constitutional*. Another classification considers all symptoms as being subjective, the objective indications being called signs.*

Some of the symptoms affecting different parts are the following:

   ABDOMEN*: May be distended, rigid, flat, flabby, adipose, tympanitic, shiny, enlarged, or bulging in certain areas, and certain discolorations, stripings, or markings. Muscles may be tensed and little affected by pressure. May be cold areas, and various sounds may be heard, such as splashings, roarings, and rumblings (*borborygmus*, also known as *intestinal flatus*). Closely associated with abdominal symptoms is pain. Locate exact area affected, and note nature, time of duration, time when it arises, and any causes that might be responsible.

   Emesis is another condition associated with symptoms pert. to the abdominal region. This may be watery, clear, or containing mucus or undigested food; may be stertorous, bilious, frothy, profuse, purulent, colored from food or medication, and showing blood (hematemesis). It may be sour, or have odor of feces, or garlic, or may be ammoniacal or have odor characteristic of some food or drug. The genital crease may show edema, lesions, discolorations, discharge, malformations, inflammations, infection, or growths.

The patient may complain of abdominal distention, gas, and pain caused by gas, crowding in the region of the heart, and interference with respiration. Heartburn may be present, or gastritis, and regurgitation. Pain may be felt when food enters the stomach, or relieved by eating or shortly after eating. Distention after eating should be noted, or desire to eructate or to expel flatus from the stomach. Colicky pains in the abdomen may be accompanied by pain in the shoulder. Pain at pit of stomach and in lower right quadrant may be indicative of appendicitis. When over lower right ribs or little below, the gallbladder may be suspected.

   BACK*: The dorsal side of the body may reveal edema, deformities, irregularities of the spine, discolorations, eruptions, impaired motion, decubitus, or any condition affecting the skin.

Breath*: May have a fecal odor, a sweet odor, or one of wet hay, an odor of fish, or ammonia, urine, blood, or pus. Respiration may be abdominal or thoracic, and show *dyspnea, orthopnea, apnea,* or it may be normal (*eupnea*).

Chest*: The chest may show abnormalities and deformities. Coughing may be *whooping, hacking, crowing, hoarse, dry,* or *hysterical.* There may or may not be expectoration. A cough may be spasmodic or occur on awakening; during deep sleep it may awaken patient, or it may occur when swallowing food, when in a horizontal position, or when subjected to change of temperatures. If singultus* is present note when it occurs. Sputum may be *mucoid, yellowish, thick, tenacious, ropy, gelatinous, dark green, offensive in odor, copious, streaked with bright or dark blood* (hemoptysis), or it may resemble *cheesy lumps.* It may be clear and watery, scanty, or profuse.

Frequency of coughing and clearing throat should be noted. Patient's respirations may be low pitched, *dyspnea* may be present, inability to expand the lungs or complaints of irritation, sticking pains, or catchy pains on inspiration. There may be an accumulation of phlegm in the air passages, or a tickling in throat. Patient may not be able to take deep inspirations, or may be constantly yawning. There may be migrating, knifelike pains in region of heart or throughout chest. "Heart-consciousness" may be present, or a fluttering feeling about the heart, or cardiac pain. Queer sensations, the loud beating of the heart, friction experienced by action of heart, and heaviness in cardiac region are other symptoms.

Defecation*: Symptoms to observe are the frequency of defecation; the presence of constipation; hemorrhoids; the nature of the feces, such as formation, as ribbon-shaped, soft, semiformed, hard or scybala, cylindrical, and whether watery, liquid, or semiliquid; the color, whether dark brown, light brown, clay-colored, green, yellowish, black, bloody; and whether lienteric, serous, mucous, purulent, tarry, or containing membranous shreds, calculi, or foreign substances. The amount should be noted, as *small, medium, large,* or *copious.* The odor may be characteristic of various conditions: *sour, putrid, offensive,* or *fetid.* The nature of the evacuation should be noted, as *natural, difficult, involuntary,* or *painful.*

Dentition*: Teeth may be irregular, missing, or showing a Hutchinson condition, or affected by caries. There may be a partial or complete denture. Dental hygiene may be good or poor. There may be a loosening of teeth, a film over them, or they may show the presence of sordes.*

Ears*: *Tinnitus aurium,* or ringing in the ears, occurs in certain diseases. Pain in ear, about ears, or swelling under either or both should be noted.

Nose*: May appear *deformed, discolored, edematous,* or *enlarged.* Nostrils may discharge or show obstruction; may be inability to breathe through one or both. Patient may complain of odors not usually manifested as objective symptoms, or for which there is no known cause.

Eyes*: May be staring, or show an excited look, or they may be expressionless. Nystagmus, strabismus, and coma vigil may be indicated. Pupils may be contracted or dilated, or 1 pupil affected. Patient may keep eyes closed constantly, or keep 1 open and the other closed. Eyes may be sunken or protruding. Lacrimation may be present. Eyelids may be edematous, and eyeball soft to the touch. Accommodation may be faulty. Nictating or squinting, or tremor of the eyelids should always be recorded. Blurring of vision is usually associated with other symptoms. Patient may complain of specks dancing before the eyes. These may be red, yellow, green, blue, or black.

Gait*: May be faltering, unsteady, staggering, weakened, swaying, or movements may be stiff, awkward, or unusual; may be total disability or immobility.

General Appearance: The face may show an expression of anxiety, a pinched look, or a "drawn" expression. Patient may have air of apathy, a distorted or a blank look, an emotional expression, a *risus sardonicus,* or sudden lack of all expression.

General Symptoms: Burning sensations may be complained of in various parts of the body, as in the head, throat, arms, chest, or abdomen. They may or may not be accompanied by tenderness. The complaint may be of feeling too hot or too cold without apparent cause, or of having a general feeling of distress.

Anorexia, nausea upon taking food or at the thought of food, or with no reference to food are significant and should be noted; also when nausea obtains, on awakening, when taking fluids, after eating, when changing a position, when taking medication, or in the presence of odors. There always should be an explanation for nausea.

Limbs*: The symptoms pert. to the skin, of course, apply to skin of the limbs. Note if there are deformities, abnormalities, impaired motion, discolorations, sensitivity, varicosities.

Lips*: May be *pale, dry, cyanotic, edematous, drawn, deformed,* out of proportion, motionless and expressionless, *flushed, fissured,* or show other lesions or growths.

Mouth and Gums*: May be pale or ulcerated, highly inflamed and red, infected, discolored, edematous, or abnormal. Pyorrhea or edema may be present. Patient may complain of certain tastes, such as bitter, sweet, salty, sour, fishy, or flat tastes, or an absence of taste. Medication may have much to do with temporary disorders of taste.

Pain*: The exact area affected must be ascertained, and the wording of the patient's complaint of pain must be charted or reported. Note if pain is in nature of a cramp or spasm, if *dull, superficial,* or *deep, remittent, shifting, shooting, lancinating, gnawing, fixed, sharp, inflammatory,* or if there is an absence of pain, especially in conditions in which pain usually occurs. Note whether pain is relieved or increased by pressure, by heat, or by cold, or by other causes. When is pain experienced, how often does the same type of pain recur, and does it awaken the patient from sleep, especially at night? Observe the facial expression during an attack of pain and listen carefully to the patient's description.

Headache: The patient may locate the pain around the eyes and nose, in the center of the forehead above the nose, in 1 or both temples accompanied by throbbing, at the top of the head, or at the base of the brain. It may be felt as a tight, bandlike sensation around the head above the eyes, it may be in the center of the forehead above the eyebrow line or in the upper region of the center forehead, or all over the top of the head, or over 1 or both ears, or back of both ears. Pain may be sharp or dull, or shifting and accompanying head noises, or a roaring in the head may be experienced without pain. Vertigo may be present or a sensation of fainting. Pulsations may perhaps be felt in the occiput or in the temporal region. A patient may be very sensitive to light and sound, and headaches may be accompanied by nausea and vomiting, also by chills. Tenderness or soreness may be associated with rigidity.

POSITIONS AND POSTURES*: An inability to lie down, to arise, or to lie on one side or on the back, or in any special position reveals much to the doctor. Whether lying on the affected or unaffected side is also important to observe. The left leg may be flexed or the right one, or both, or there may be an inclination to lie with the arms above the head.

SKIN*: May appear pale, flushed all over or in spots; may be *cyanotic, jaundiced, shiny, erupted, bruised,* or exhibit dermographia, lesions, growth, or deformities, or be *puffy* and *edematous, ashy, gray,* wet with perspiration, or *discolored.*

THROAT*: May show abnormalities, discoloration, inflammation, diseased tonsils, and presence of adenoids. Dysphagia and hoarseness, or aphonia and other conditions affecting the voice may be present. A lump in the throat (*globus hystericus*), or a dry, scratchy irritation or fullness or pulsations may be present.

TONGUE*: May be coated, clean, smooth, shiny, dry on top and moist on the sides, or dry all over; may look like raw beef or appear *furry, glossy, tremulous,* or sharp pointed. It may be *edematous* or abnormal in size, there may be fissures, the papillae may have disappeared, there may be a *"strawberry-tongue,"* or it may have various colors.

URINE*: It may be blue, milky, pale, lemon, smoky, brick-colored, clear, amber, straw-colored, orange, or some other color. *Hematuria* may be present. *Polyuria* or *oliguria* may be indicated, or there may be frequent urination of small amounts. The odors may be ammoniacal, aromatic, stercorous, or like that of new-mown hay, ripe apples, or violets. There may be retention or suppression, or dribbling, and urination may be painful.

SEE: *Each part or organ in text.*

s's., cardinal. Those pert. to pulse, respiration, and temperature.

s. complex. The entire group of symptoms presenting a clear picture of a disease. SYN: *syndrome.*

s., constitutional, s., general. One caused by or indicating disease of the whole body.

s. of Magendi. Deviation of 1 eye up and out, and the other down, produced by division of the restiform body.

s's., objective. Those that are manifested externally and which are apparent to the observer.

s., pathognomonic. One which unmistakably points out presence of a particular disease.

s's., prodromal. Those which indicate an approaching disease. SYN: *prodrome.**

s's., subjective. Those that have an internal origin and are perceptible to the patient only, including mental symptoms.

s's., withdrawal. Those following sudden withdrawal of a stimulant from an addict, generally excitement and collapse.

symptom, words pert. to: abate, abatement, abeyance, acanesthesia, acedia, acme, amphibolia, anabatic, anabiotic, analepsis, analeptic, anamnesis, anaphylactic shock, anastasis, anathrepsis, anesis, antidromic, antilogia, antipraxis, apogee, apolepsis, apolexis, apostasis, arrhea, assident, assuetude, asthenic body type, astriction, atrophied, autokinesis, Broadbent's sign, Brauch-Romberg's sign, Cardarelli's sign, catastasis, exacerbation, face, facies, girdle symptom, heterocrisis, hippocratic facies, idiopathic, ingravescent, insidious, invasion, kolytic, lysis, malaise, malignant, maximum, Meniere's symptom complex, metabasis, metastable, metastasis, miosis, miotic, Moebius' sign, myurous, nascent, paroxysm, polymorphic, recrudescence, recurrent, relapse, remission, retardation, retrograde, retrogressive changes, Rumpf's symptom, semeiology, semeiosis, sequela, simulation, sign, subjective, supervention, syndrome.

symptomatic (sĭmp-tō-măt'ĭk) [G. *symptōmatikos,* pert. to a symptom]. Of the nature of or concerning a symptom.

symptomatology (sĭmp-tō-mă-tŏl'ō-jĭ) [G. *symptōma,* symptom, + *logos,* a study]. 1. Science of symptoms and indications. SYN: *semeiology.* 2. All of the symptoms of a given disease as a whole.

symptomatolytic (sĭmp"tō-măt"ō-lĭt'ĭk) [" + *lysis,* destruction]. Causing the removal of symptoms.

symp'tom com'plex. All of the symptoms of a disease forming together a picture of it. SYN: *syndrome.*

symptomolytic (sĭmp-tō-mō-lĭt'ĭk) [G. *symptōma,* symptom, + *lysis,* destruction]. Pert. to the removal of symptoms. SYN: *symptomatolytic.*

syn- [G.]. Prefix meaning *joined, together.* SEE: *prefix con.*

synalgia (sĭn-ăl'jĭ-ă) [G. *syn,* with, + *algos,* pain]. Referred or reflex pain felt in a part distant from the site of its origin.

synalgic (sĭn-ăl'jĭk) [" + *algos,* pain]. Pert. to or characterized by referred pain.

synanastomosis (sĭn"an-as"tō-mō'sĭs) [" + *anastomōsis,* a connecting mouth]. The connection of several vessels.

synanthema (sĭn-ăn-thē'mă) [" + *anthein,* to bloom]. Exanthem made up of several different forms of eruption.

synapse, synapsis (sĭn'ăps, sĭn-ăp'sĭs) [G. *synapsis,* from *syn,* with, + *aptein,* to touch]. 1. The minute space or apparent meeting point bet. the terminal arborization of the axon of 1 neuron and the dendrites of another. There is no actual communication, but the synapse functions possibly by either modifying or intensifying the nerve impulse as it passes through. SEE: *nerve.* 2. Process of pairing off of chromosomes from the

male and female pronuclei in the ovum. SYN: *syndesis.*
synaptase (sĭn-ăp'tās) [G. *synaptein,* to join]. A hydrolyzing enzyme found in almonds and certain fungi. SYN: *emulsin.*
synarthrodia (sĭn-ăr-thrō'dĭ-ă) [G. *syn,* with, + *arthron,* joint, + *eidos,* form]. Type of immovable cartilaginous joint without a joint cavity in which bones are separated by only a connective tissue membrane; a fixed articulation. SYN: *synarthrosis.* SEE: *joint.*
synarthrodial (sĭn-ar-thrō'dĭ-ăl) [" + " + *eidos,* form]. Pert. to an immovable articulation bet. bones.
synarthrosis (sĭn″ar-thrō'sĭs) (pl. *synarthroses*) [" + *arthrōsis,* joint]. An immovable joint in which there is no disk of intervening tissue bet. the bones.
RS: *gomphosis, schindylesis, suture, synchondrosis, synostosis.*
syncanthus (sĭn-kăn'thŭs) [G. *syn,* with, + *kanthos,* angle]. Adhesion of eyeball to the structures of the orbit.
synchilia (sĭn-kī'lĭ-ă) [" + *cheilos,* lip]. Adhesion or imperforation (*atresia*) of the lips.
synchiria (sĭn-kī'rĭ-ă) [" + *cheir,* hand]. Disorder of sensibility in which stimulus is referred to the opposite side of the body from that to which it was applied. SYN: *allochiria.* RS: *achiria, dyschiria.*
synchondroseotomy (sĭn-kŏn-drō-sē-ŏt'ō-mĭ) [" + *chondros,* cartilage, + *tomē,* a cutting]. An operation of cutting through the sacroiliac ligaments and closing the arch of the pubes in congenital absence of the ant. wall of the bladder (*exstrophy*).
synchondrosis (sĭn-kŏn-drō'sĭs) [" + *chondros,* cartilage, + *-ōsis,* condition]. An immovable joint having the surfaces bet. the bones connected by cartilages.
synchondrotomy (sĭn-kŏn-drŏt'ō-mĭ) [" + " + *tomē,* a cutting]. 1. Division of articulating cartilage. 2. Section of the symphysis pubis to facilitate childbirth. SEE: *symphyseotomy.*
synchronism (sĭn'krō-nĭzm) [" + *chronos,* time, + *-ismos,* condition]. Occurrence of acts or events simultaneously.
synchronous (sĭn'krŏn-ŭs) [G. *syn,* with, + *chronos,* time]. Occurring simultaneously.
synchysis (sĭn'kĭs-ĭs) [G. *synchysis,* from *syncheein,* to confound]. Fluid state of vitreous of the eye.
s. scintil'lans. Abnormally fluid vitreous, with presence of floating cholesterin crystals.
syncinesis (sĭn-sĭn-ē'sĭs) [G. *syn,* with, + *kinēsis,* motion]. An involuntary movement produced in association with a voluntary one.
s., imitative. Occurs on sound side when movement is attempted on paralyzed side.
s., spasmodic. Occurs on hemiplegic side when muscles of opp. side are voluntarily moved.
synciput (sĭn'sĭp-ŭt) [L.]. Ant. upper half of the cranium. SYN: *sinciput.*
synclitism (sĭn'klĭt-ĭzm) [G. *sygklinein,* to lean together]. Parallelism bet. the planes of the fetal head and those of the maternal pelvis.
synclonus (sĭn'klō-nŭs) [G. *syn,* with, + *klonos,* tumult]. 1. Clonic contraction of several muscles together. 2. A disease marked by muscular spasms.
syncopal (sĭn'kō-păl) [G. *sygkopē,* fainting]. Relating to or marked by syncope.
syncope (sĭn'kō-pē) [G. *sygkopē,* fainting]. A transient form of unconsciousness, during which the person slumps to the ground. SYN: *fainting, swoon.*
No muscular contractions take place and epilepsy can usually be excluded. Some disturbance in cerebral circulation (severe bleeding, low blood pressure) may explain, though many people, young women esp., will faint from excitement, exhaustion, inadequate ventilation, etc.
TREATMENT: Stimulate the heart action, fresh air, treat underlying cause. If seated, depress head bet. knees, compressing abdominal viscera, and stimulating nervous system reflexly as well as the circulation. Remove tight clothing. Apply sudden dash of cold water or cold towel which should be removed immediately. Aromatic spirits of ammonia inhalations for a moment or two, only. Test to see it is not too strong. External heat. When recovered, give hot drinks, strong coffee or tea. Keep lying down. Ten to 20 drops of ammonia by mouth in half a glass of water. Call a physician if recovery is not prompt. SEE: *unconsciousness.*
s. angio'sa. Cardiac spasm due to occlusion of coronary arteries.
s., laryngeal. Brief unconsciousness following coughing and tickling in the throat. SYN: *vertigo, laryngeal.*
s., local. Numbness of a part with sudden blanching, as of the fingers; a symptom of Raynaud's disease or of local asphyxia.
syncytiolysin (sĭn-sĭt-ĭ-ol'ĭ-sĭn) [G. *syn,* with, + *kytos,* cell, + *lysis,* destruction]. A cytolysin that is formed from injections of emulsions of placental tissue.
syncytioma (sĭn-sĭt-ĭ-ō'mă) [" + " + *-ōma,* tumor]. A tumor of the chorion. SYN: *chorioma, deciduoma.*
s. benig'num. A mole.
s. malig'num. A tumor formed of cells from the syncytium and chorion, occurring frequently after abortion or in the puerperium at site of placenta.
syncytium (sĭn-sĭt'ĭ-ŭm) [" + *kytos,* cell]. 1. Multinucleated protoplasmic aggregation of cells without apparent cell outlines. 2. A multinucleated protoplasmic membrane forming outer layer of early chorionic villi.
syndactylism (sĭn-dăk'tĭl-ĭzm) [" + *daktylos,* digit, + *ismos,* condition]. A fusion of 2 or more toes or fingers, usually congenital.
syndectomy (sĭn-dĕk'tō-mĭ) [" + *dein,* to bind, + *ektomē,* excision]. Excision of a circular strip of the conjunctiva around cornea to relieve *pannus.* SYN: *peritomy.*
syndesis (sĭn-dē'sĭs) [" + *desis,* a binding together]. 1. Surgical fixation of a joint. 2. Pairing of chromosomes in pronuclei of the ovum. SYN: *synapse,* 2.
syndesmectomy (sĭn-dĕs-mĕk'tō-mĭ) [" + *desmos,* band, + *ektomē,* excision]. Excision of a section of a ligament.
syndesmectopia (sĭn″dĕs-mĕk-tō'pĭ-ă) [G. *syndesmos,* ligament, + *ektopos,* out of place]. Abnormal position of a ligament.
syndesmitis (sĭn-dĕs-mī'tĭs) [" + *-itis,* inflammation]. 1. Inflammation of a ligament or ligaments. 2. Inflammation of the conjunctiva.
syndesmography (sĭn-dĕs-mŏg'ră-fī) [" + *graphein,* to write]. Treatise on the ligaments.
syndesmology (sĭn-dĕs-mŏl'ō-jī) [" + *logos,* a study]. Study of the ligaments and their disorders.

syndesmoma (sĭn-dĕs-mō'mă) [" + -*ōma*, tumor]. A connective tissue tumor.
syndesmopexy (sĭn-dĕs'mō-pĕks-ĭ) [" + *pēxis*, fixation]. Joining of 2 ligaments or fixation of a ligament in a new place, used in correction of a dislocation.
syndesmoplasty (sĭn-dĕs'mō-plăs-tĭ) [" + *plassein*, to form]. Plastic surgery on a ligament.
syndesmorrhaphy (sĭn-dĕs-mor'ăf-ĭ) [G. *syndesmos*, ligament, + *rhaphē*, a seam]. Repair or suture of a ligament.
syndesmosis (sĭn-dĕs-mō'sĭs) (pl. *syndesmoses*) [" + *-ōsis*, condition]. Articulation in which the bones are united by ligaments. SEE: *joint*.
syndesmotomy (sĭn-dĕs-mŏt'ō-mĭ) [" + *tomē*, a cutting]. Surgical section of ligaments.
syndrome (sĭn'drōm, -drō-mē) [G. *syndromē*, a running together]. A complexus of symptoms. All the symptoms of a disease considered as a whole. The complete picture of a disease.
  s., Adams-Stokes. Bradycardia and intermittent convulsive seizures with loss of consciousness due to organic obstruction of the bundle of His.
  s., Angelucci's. Palpitation, excitable temperament and vasomotor disturbance in spring conjunctivitis.
  s., Fröhlich's. Increase in fat, atrophy of the genitals, transition to feminine type due to lesions of the hypophysis.
  s., Gradenigo's. External rectus paralysis, temporoparietal pain and suppurative otitis media on same side.
  s. of Horner. Contracted pupil, ptosis, enophthalmos and dry, cool face on affected side produced by paralysis of sympathetics.
  ETIOL: Tumors in neck, trauma, apical tuberculosis, tabes, syringomyelia, and neuritis of cervical plexus.
  s., Korsakoff's. A psychosis, ordinarily due to chronic alcoholism, with polyneuritis, disorientation, insomnia, muttering delirium, hallucinations, and a bilateral wrist or foot drop.
  s., Weber's. Paralysis of hypoglossal nerve on one side and of oculomotor nerve on other with paralysis of limbs due to lesion of a cerebral peduncle.
syndromic (sĭn-drom'ĭk) [G. *syn*, with, + *dromos*, a running]. Pert. to or occurring as a syndrome.
synechia (sĭn-ē'kĭ-ă) [G. *synecheia*, continuity]. Adhesion of parts, esp. adhesion of iris to lens and cornea.
  s., annular. Adhesion of the iris to the lens throughout its entire pupillary margin.
  s., anterior. Adhesion of iris to cornea.
  s., posterior. Adhesion of iris to capsule of lens.
  s., total. Adhesion of entire surface of the iris to the lens.
synechotomy (sĭn-ĕk-ŏt'ō-mĭ) [" + *tomē*, a cutting]. Division of a synechia or adhesion.
synecology (sĭn-ē-kŏl'ō-jĭ) [G. *syn*, with, + *oikos*, house, + *logos*, a study]. The study of organisms in relation to their environment in group form.
syneresis (sĭn-ĕr'ĕs-ĭs) [" + *airesis*, a taking]. Contraction of a gel resulting in its separation from the liquid, as a shrinkage by fibrin and other colloidal gels.
synergenesis (sĭn-ĕr-jĕn'ĕ-sĭs) [" + *ergon*, energy, + *genesis*, reproduction]. The theory that each cell contains the protoplasm of every generation of cells derived therefrom.

synergetic (sĭn-ĕr-jĕt'ĭk) [G. *syn*, with, + *ergon*, work]. Exhibiting coöperative action, said of certain muscles; working together. SYN: *synergic*.
synergic (sĭn-ĕr'jĭk) [" + *ergon*, work]. Relating to or exhibiting coöperation, as certain muscles.
synergist (sĭn'ĕr-jĭst) [" + *ergon*, work]. 1. A remedy that stimulates the action of another. SYN: *adjuvant*. 2. A muscle or organ functioning in coöperation with another, as the flexor muscles.
synergy (sĭn'ĕr-jĭ) [" + *ergon*, work]. Action of 2 or more agents or organs coöperating with each other; coöperation. Combined action; coordinated action.
synesthesia (sĭn-ĕs-thē'zĭ-ă) [" + *aisthēsis*, sensation]. 1. A sensation in an area from a stimulus applied to another part. 2. A subjective sensation of another sense than the one being stimulated. SEE: *chromatism, phonism*.
  s. al'gica. Painful synesthesia.
synesthesialgia (sĭn"ĕs-thē-zĭ-ăl'jĭ-ă) [" + " + *algos*, pain]. A painful sensation giving rise to a subjective one of different character. SEE: *synesthesia*.
synezesis (sĭn-ĕ-zē'sĭs) [G. *synizēsis*, a sitting together]. Closure of the pupil.
syngamy (sĭn'gă-mĭ) [G. *syn*, with, + *gamos*, marriage]. Sexual reproduction; cell union, as of gametes in fertilization.
syngenesis (sĭn-jĕn'ĕ-sĭs) [G. *syn*, with, + *genesis*, reproduction]. 1. Reproduction sexually. 2. Doctrine that each sexual cell contains the germs from which all future cells will be derived.
syngignocism (sĭn-jĭg'nō-sĭzm) [" + *gignōskein*, to know]. Hypnotism and its results.
synizesis (sĭn-ĭz-ē'sĭs) [" + *izein*, to sit]. 1. A closure or shutting. 2. Massing of nuclear chromatin prior to maturation division.
  s. pupillae. Closure of the pupil of the eye with loss of vision.
synkaryon (sĭn-kar'ĭ-ŏn) [" + *karyon*, kernel]. A nucleus resulting from fusion of 2 pronuclei.
synkinesis (sĭn-kĭ-nē'sĭs) [" + *kinēsis*, motion]. Involuntary movements in a part when another part is voluntarily moved, as in a paralyzed limb following movements made in an opposite limb.
synneurosis (sĭn-ū-rō'sĭs) [" + *neuron*, sinew, + *-ōsis*, condition]. Synarthrosis in which fibrous connective tissue unites opposing surfaces. SYN: *syndesmosis*.
synocha, synochus (sĭn'ō-kă, -kŭs) [G. *synochos*, lasting]. A fever that is continued.
synococcus (sĭn-ō-kŏk'ŭs) [G. *syn*, with, + *kokkos*, berry]. A coccus often associated with the gonococcus.
synonym (sĭn'ō-nĭm) [" + *onoma*, name]. A word which has the same or very similar meaning as another word.
synoptophore (sĭn-ŏp'tō-for) [" + *ōps, opt-*, sight, + *phoros*, a bearer]. Apparatus for diagnosing and treating strabismus.
synoptoscope (sĭn-ŏp'tō-skōp) [" + " + *skopein*, to examine]. An instrument for diagnosis and treatment of strabismus. SYN: *synoptophore*.
synorchidism, synorchism (sĭn-or'kĭd-ĭzm, -kĭzm) [" + *orchis, orchid-*, testicle, + *-ismos*, condition]. Union or partial fusion of the testicles.
synosteology (sĭn"ŏs-tē-ŏl'ō-jĭ) [" + *osteon*, bone, + *logos*, a study]. The science of joints and articulations.
synosteosis, synostosis (sĭn"ŏs-tē-ō'sĭs, -tō'-

sis) [" + " + -*osis*, condition]. 1. Articulation by osseous tissue of adjacent bones. 2. Union of separate bones by osseous tissue.

synosteotomy (sĭn-ŏs-tē-ŏt'ō-mĭ) [G. *syn*, with, + *osteon*, bone, + *tomē*, a cutting]. Dissection of joints.

synovectomy (sĭn-ō-vĕk'tō-mĭ) [" + L. *ovum*, from G. *ōon*, egg, + G. *ektomē*, excision]. Excision of synovial membrane.

synovia (sĭn-ō'vĭ-ă) [" + L. *ovum*, from G. *ōon*, egg]. A colorless, viscid, lubricating fluid of joints, bursae, and tendon sheaths secreted within synovial membranes.
It contains mucin, albumin, fat, and mineral salts. SEE: *asynovia*.

synovial (sĭn-ō'vĭ-ăl) [G. *syn*, with, + L. *ovum*, from G. *ōon*, egg]. Pert. to synovia, the joint lubricating fluid.
  s. bursa. The mucosa of a bursa.
  s. crypt. Diverticulum of a synovial membrane of a joint.
  s. cyst. Accumulation of synovia in a bursa, s. crypt, or sac of a synovial hernia, causing a tumor.
  s. fluid. Lubricating, clear fluid secreted by the synovial membrane of a joint. SYN: *synovia*.
  s. glands. Folds on synovial membrane secreting synovia. SYN: *haversian glands*.
  s. hernia. Protrusion of a portion of synovial membrane through a tear in the stratum fibrosum of a joint capsule.
  s. ligament. A large synovial fold in a joint.
  s. membrane. One lining the capsule of a joint.
  s. sheath. The mucosa of a tendon sheath.

synovin (sĭn'ō-vĭn) [G. *syn*, with, + L. *ovum*, from G. *ōon*, egg]. A form of mucin found in synovia.

synovioma (sĭn″ō-vĭ-ō'mă) [" + " + G. *-ōma*, tumor]. A tumor arising from a synovial membrane.

synoviparous (sĭn-ō-vĭp'ă-rŭs) [" + " + L. *parēre*, to produce]. Producing or secreting synovia.

synovitis (sĭn-ō-vī'tĭs) [G. *syn*, with, + L. *ovum*, egg, + G. *-itis*, inflammation]. Inflammation of a synovial membrane.
ETIOL: As a result of an aseptic wound, of a subcutaneous injury (contusion or sprain), of the irritation produced by floating cartilage, or of exposure to cold and dampness, simple inflammation may attack the synovial membrane.
SYM: Joint painful, severely so on motion, esp. at night. Swollen, tense; may be fluctuating. At the knee, patella is floated up from condyles, can be readily depressed, to rise again when pressure is taken off. The part is never in full extension, as this produces great suffering. Local heat raised, but skin, which is very sensitive to pressure only at certain points, is neither thickened nor reddened. After a few days, pain lessens, swelling diminishes as the effusion and extravasated blood are absorbed, the limb takes its natural position and recovery follows.
TREATMENT: Joint placed at rest. Cold may be applied locally by ice bag or coil of rubber tubing or by continuous irrigation; or hot applications may be made; or equal pressure as firm as can be comfortably borne. Affected region enveloped in cotton or wool and a bandage, preferably of rubber, put on. If there is great serous distention or large extravasation of blood into the cavity, aspiration may be required under strict asepsis.
  s., chronic. The active congestion largely disappears, but there is an undue amount of fluid in the cavity and the membrane itself is edematous. Later, if disease does not subside, membrane and articular structures become irregularly thickened by plastic exudation and formation of fibrous tissue. Joint is weak, but not esp. painful except on pressure; may not be even then; movements, esp. in extension, are restricted, and generally attended by some grating or creaking. When there is great accumulation of liquid, symptoms are well marked. With the hypodermic needle fluid may be drawn off, which is straw-colored, somewhat viscid, sometimes flocculent and more or less blood stained.
TREATMENT: Varies with amount of fluid present and according to type of arthritis present. When not of long standing and articular fullness not great, rest and pressure, preferably immobilized with plaster-of-Paris. When of long standing, with joint much distended, and impaired usefulness, the condition is called hydrarthrosis or hydrops articuli. If above treatment proves useless, aspirate and inject 3% to 5% solution of carbolic acid after inflammation has gone down entirely.
  s., dendritic. S. with villous growths developing in the sac.
  s., dry. S. without much effusion or no effusion.
  s., fungous. Tuberculosis of a joint. SYN: *arthritis fungosa*.
  s., pannous. Is rarely met with; occurs in tubercular arthritis. The great serous accumulation in the synovial sac will almost certainly be regarded as nontubercular until after aspiration and examination of the fluid.
  s., purulent. S. with purulent effusion within the sac.
  s., serous. S. with nonpurulent, copious effusion.
  s. sicca. Same as *dry* synovitis*.
  s., simple. S. with effusion only slightly turbid if not clear.
  s., tendinous. Inflammation of a tendon sheath.
  s., vaginal. Same as *tendinous* synovitis*.
  s., vibration. S. resulting from a wound near a joint.

synpneumonic (sĭn-nū-mŏn'ĭk) [G. *syn*, with, + *pneumonia*, pneumonia]. Concurrent with pneumonia; complicating pneumonia.

synreflexia (sĭn″rē-flĕks'ĭ-ă) [" + L. *re*, back, + *flexus*, turned]. The relationship existing bet. various reflexes.

syntaxis (sĭn-tăks'ĭs) [" + *taxis*, arrangement]. A junction bet. 2 bones. SYN: *articulation*.

syntenosis (sĭn-tĕn-ō'sĭs) [" + *tenōn*, tendon]. A hinge joint protected by tendons, as a *phalangeal articulation*.

synthermal (sĭn-thĕr'măl) [" + *thermē*, heat]. Having the same temperature.

synthesis (sĭn'thĕs-ĭs) [" + *tithenai*, to place]. 1. CHEM: The union of elements to produce compounds; the process of building up; the opposite of analysis or decomposition. 2. Reuniting of broken or separated structures.
Popularly, synthetic preparation is one made by laboratory methods, esp. of compounds occurring naturally; the

synthetic (sĭn-thĕt′ĭk) [G. *synthetikos*, placed together]. Relating to or made by synthesis; artificially prepared.

syntone (sĭn′tōn) [G. *syn*, with, + *tonos*, tone]. An individual temperamentally responsive to his environment and its social demands. SEE: *syntonic*.

syntonic (sĭn-tŏn′ĭk) [" + *tonos*, tone]. Pert. to a reaction type in which the subject responds strongly to emotional stimuli in harmony with the situation.
The type is exaggerated in maniclike states and in depressions.

syntonin (sĭn′tō-nĭn) [" + *tonos*, tense]. An acid albumin; esp. one formed by the action of dilute hydrochloric acid on muscle during gastric digestion.

syntoxoid (sĭn-tŏks′oyd) [" + *toxikon*, poison, + *eidos*, form]. A toxoid having the same degree of affinity for an antitoxin as the toxin has.

syntripsis (sĭn-trĭp′sĭs) [" + *tripsis*, a crushing]. A comminuted fracture or act causing it.

syntropan (sĭn′trō-păn). Registered trademark for a brand of amprotropine phosphate.
USES: In spastic disorders of gastrointestinal and genitourinary tracts, also experimentally in Parkinsonism.
DOSAGE: 50 mg.

syntropic (sĭn-trŏp′ĭk) [G. *syn*, with, + *tropos*, a turning]. 1. Turned in the same direction, as the ribs. 2. Noting a type characterized by mixing well and easily. SYN: *koinotropic*, q.v.

synulotic (sĭn-ū-lot′ĭk) [" + *oulē*, scar]. 1. An agent stimulating cicatrization. 2. Promoting cicatrization.

syphilelcosis (sĭf-ĭl-ĕl-kō′sĭs) [*syphilis* + G. *elkōsis*, ulceration]. Syphilitic ulceration.

syphilelcus (sĭf-ĭl-ĕl′kŭs) [*syphilis* + G. *elkos*, ulcer]. A syphilitic ulcer.

syphilide (sĭf′ĭl-īd) [Fr.]. Any cutaneous affection of syphilitic origin. SYN: *syphiloderm*.

syphilimetry (sĭf-ĭl-ĭm′ĕt-rī) [*syphilis* + G. *metron*, measure]. Determination of a syphilitic infection's intensity.

syphilionthus (sĭf-ĭl-ĭ-ŏn′thŭs) [" + G. *ionthos*, eruption]. A copper-colored, branny-scaled syphilide.

syphiliphobia (sĭf-ĭl-ĭ-fō′bĭ-ă) [" + G. *phobos*, fear]. Morbid fear of syphilis. SYN: *syphilophobia*.

syphilis (sĭf′ĭl-ĭs) [origin uncertain; possibly from G. *syn*, with, + *philos*, love, or from *Syphilus*, a shepherd in a poem who had the disease]. An infectious, chronic venereal disease resulting in various lesions of structural and cutaneous nature.
ETIOL: *Spirochaeta pallida*.
PRIMARY STAGE SYM: Initial lesion appears 2 to 4 weeks after inoculation, changing from a small red papule to a small ulcer, to a hard chancre. Usually upon prepuce or vulva. Lymph glands enlarge about 2 weeks after appearance of lesion.
Almost positive signs of syphilis are inflammation at mouth of Stensen's duct and enlargement of epitrochlear lymphatic glands.
SECONDARY STAGE SYM: Constitutional symptoms appear in from 6 to 12 weeks after appearance of primary lesion. Continuous fever, 101°, possibly remittent, rarely intermittent. Headache, backache, weakness, sore throat, anemia, skin yellowish (syphilitic cachexia). General enlargement of lymph glands which become indurated. Eruptions of skin, maculae (roseola), syphilide, reddish brown "coppery" spots, continuing for a week or 2, recurring possibly later. On palms and soles esp. are found a scaly syphilide, copper colored. Mucous patches emitting a grayish secretion (contagious) found on the mucous membranes in the groins, navel, axillae, and bet. toes. Tonsils may be ulcerated. Warty growths about the vulva or anus. Loss of hair frequently 3 or 4 months after infection. Periostitis, more painful at night. Tibiae, clavicles and bones of cranium principally affected. Iritis may develop 3 to 6 months after initial lesions. Miscarriage frequent.
TERTIARY STAGE SYM: Appearance of tertiary lesions may appear as soon as 6 months after initial sores; generally several years, however. Diseases of the bone, ankyloid degeneration, syphilomata, cutaneous lesions. Gummata of mucous membranes, bones, periosteum, and muscles may ensue.
TREATMENT: *Penicillin* is now the most prominent agent, although arsenic, bismuth, iodides, mercury, and fever therapy are widely used, principally in conjunction with penicillin. Bismuth, iodides, and mercury are frequently reserved for cases where a slow therapeutic effect is indicated, and fever-therapy is used chiefly in neurosyphilis. Aluminum monostearate may be added to penicillin to prolong the effect.
DOSAGE (American Academy of Dermatology and Syphilology): 1. *Primary, Secondary, Early Latent, or Late Latent Syphilis*: 600,000 units procaine penicillin intramuscularly daily for 10 days. 2. *Late (Cardiovascular) Syphilis*: 1.5 cc. bismuth subsalicylate intramuscularly weekly for 6 to 12 injections, followed by 10,000,000 to 12,000,000 units penicillin over course of 20 days.

s., congenital. S. present at birth.
SYM: May be present at birth or appear in 4 to 8 weeks. Late symptoms may appear at second dentition or at puberty. Hutchinson's teeth, lateral incisors of upper jaw, pegged and central incisors of same jaw having convex sides with crescentric notches on cutting edges are characteristic on the permanent teeth.
Prevention of congenital syphilis can best be effected by recognizing syphilis in the mother and treating her under careful observation.

s. innocen′tium, s. inson′tium. S. not contracted through coition.

s., visceral. Due to pressure of gummata may affect brain, cord, lungs, liver, rectum, heart, kidneys, testicles, or arteries.

syphilis, words pert. to: antiluetic, antivenereal, arsenorelapsing, Biederman's sign, chancre, locomotor ataxia, lues, Ross' bodies, rupia, syphilitic macules, syphilophobia, syphilosis, tabes.

syphilitic (sĭf-ĭl-lĭt′ĭk) [*syphilis*]. Related to, caused by, or affected with syphilis.

s. fever. Rise in temperature in early stage of secondary syphilis.

s. macules. Small red eruptions manifested in secondary syphilis which often cover the entire body.
SYM: Associated with chancre or scar, alopecia, pain in bones, swollen glands, and sore throat.

syphilization (sĭf-ĭl-ĭ-zā'shŭn) [*syphilis*]. Inoculation with the exudate of a chancre to immunize against syphilis.
syphilized (sĭf'ĭl-īzd) [*syphilis*]. Infected with syphilis.
syphilocerebrosis (sĭf″ĭl-ō-sĕr-ē-brō'sĭs) [*syphilis* + L. *cerebrum*, brain, + G. *-ōsis*, condition]. Syphilis of the brain.
syphiloderm, syphiloderma (sĭf-ĭl-ō-derm, sĭf″ĭl-ō-der'mă) [*syphilis* + G. *derma*, skin]. A syphilitic cutaneous disorder.
syphilogenesis, syphilogeny (sĭf″ĭl-ō-jĕn'ē-sĭs, sĭf-ĭl-ŏj'ĕn-ĭ) [*syphilis* + G. *gennan*, to produce, — + *genesis*, production]. The development or origin of syphilis.
syphilographer (sĭf-ĭl-ŏg'ră-fer) [*syphilis* + G. *graphein*, to write]. One who writes about syphilis.
syphilography (sĭf-ĭl-ŏg'ră-fĭ) [*syphilis* + G. *graphein*, to write]. A treatise on syphilis.
syphiloid (sĭf'ĭl-oyd) [*syphilis* + G. *eidos*, form]. 1. Resembling syphilis. 2. A disease akin to syphilis.
syphilologist (sĭf-ĭl-ŏl'ō-jĭst) [*syphilis* + G. *logos*, a study]. A specialist in treatment of syphilis.
syphilology (sĭf-ĭl-ŏl'ō-jĭ) [*syphilis* + G. *logos*, a study]. The study of syphilis and its treatment.
syphiloma (sĭf-ĭl-ō'mă) [*syphilis* + G. *-ōma*, tumor]. A syphilitic tumor.
syphilomania (sĭf-ĭl-ō-mā'nĭ-ă) [*syphilis* + G. *mania*, madness]. Morbid fear of syphilis or inference that one is suffering with it. SYN: *syphilophobia*.
syphilopathy (sĭf-ĭl-ŏp'ă-thĭ) [*syphilis* + G. *pathos*, disease]. Any syphilitic disorder.
syphilophobia (sĭf-ĭl-ō-fō'bĭ-ă) [*syphilis* + G. *phobos*, fear]. Morbid fear of syphilis or delusion of having the disease.
syphilophobic (sĭf″ĭl-ō-fō'bĭk) [*syphilis* + G. *phobos*, fear]. Pert. to or affected with syphilophobia.
syphilophyma (sĭf″ĭl-ō-fī'mă) [*syphilis* + G. *phyma*, a growth]. 1. Any growth or excrescence due to syphilis. 2. Syphiloma of the epidermis.
syphilopsychosis (sĭf″ĭl-ō-sī-kō'sĭs) [*syphilis* + G. *psychē*, soul, + *-ōsis*, condition]. Any mental disease caused by syphilis.
syphilosis (sĭf-ĭ-lō'sĭs) [*syphilis* + G. *-ōsis*, disease]. Generalized syphilitic disease.
syphilotropic (sĭf-ĭl-ō-trŏp'ĭk) [*syphilis* + G. *tropos*, a turning]. Especially susceptible to syphilis.
syphilous (sĭf'ĭl-ŭs) [*syphilis*]. Of the nature of or pert. to syphilis. SYN: *syphilitic*.
syphionthus (sĭf-ĭ-ŏn'thŭs) [*syphilis* + G. *ionthos*, eruption]. The copper-colored patches seen in syphilis.
syphitoxin (sĭf-ĭ-tŏks'ĭn) [*syphilis* + G. *toxikon*, poison]. Antisyphilitic serum.
syrigmophonia (sĭr″ĭg-mō-fō'nĭ-ă) [G. *syrigmos*, a whistle, + *phōnē*, voice]. 1. A sibilant râle. 2. A whistling sound in pronunciation of *s* due to a denture peculiarity.
syringadenoma (sĭr-ĭng-ăd-en-ō'mă) [G. *syrigx*, pipe, + *adēn*, gland, + *-ōma*, tumor]. Tumor of a sweat gland.
syringe (sĭr-ĭnj', sĭr'ĭnj) [G. *syrigx*, pipe]. 1. Instrument for injecting fluids into cavities or vessel. 2. To wash out or introduce fluid with a syringe.
VARIETIES: Antitoxin, antrum, bladder, cocaine, drainage tube, ear, fountain, hemorrhoidal, hydrocele, hypodermic, lacrimal, Luer's, mucous, nasal, urethral, vesical-suction.

syringectomy (sĭr-ĭn-jĕk'tō-mĭ) [G. *syrigx*, pipe, + *ektomē*, excision]. Removal of the walls of a fistula.
syringitis (sĭr-ĭn-jī'tĭs) [" + *-ītis*, inflammation]. Inflammation, eustachian tube.
syringobulbia (sĭr-ĭn-gō-bŭl'bĭ-ă) [G. *syrigx*, pipe, + *bulbos*, a bulb]. Presence of pores in the medulla oblongata, resembling *syringomyelia*.
syringocele (sĭr-ĭn'gō-sēl) [" + *koilia*, a hollow]. The central canal of the myelon or spinal cord.
syringocystadenoma (sĭr-ĭn″gō-sĭs-tad-ĕn-ō'mă) [" + *kystis*, a bladder, + *adēn*, gland, + *-ōma*, tumor]. Adenoma of sweat glands characterized by tiny, hard, papular formations.
syringocystoma (sĭr-ĭn″gō-sĭs-tō'mă) [" + " + *-ōma*, tumor]. Cystic tumor having its origin in ducts of the sweat gland.
syringoid (sĭr-ĭng'oyd) [" + *eidos*, form]. Fistulous. Resembling a tube.
syringoma (sĭr-ĭn-gō'mă) [" + *ōma*, tumor]. Tumor of the sweat glands.
syringomeningocele (sĭr-ĭn″gō-men-ĭn'gō-sēl) [" + *menigx*, membrane, + *kēlē*, hernia]. Meningocele which is similar to a syringomyelocele.
syringomyelia (sĭr-ĭn″gō-mī-ē'lĭ-ă) [G. *syrigx*, tube, + *myelos*, marrow]. The development of cavities within the spinal cord caused by retained fluid within its center. It occurs in early life of the adult and runs a chronic course.
SYM: The cord is gradually stretched tightly, and nerve-fibers to the extremities carrying feeling and movement are destroyed producing numbness and paralysis. Pain and disturbed sensibility prominent features.
TREATMENT: Surgical draining of fluid into spinal-fluid pathway; otherwise unavailing.
syringomyelitis (sĭr-ĭn″gō-mī-ē-lī'tĭs) [" + " + *-ītis*, inflammation]. Inflammation coincident with abnormal dilaion of the central canal of spinal cord.
syringomyelocele (sĭr-ĭn″gō-mī'ĕl-ō-sēl) [" + " + *kēlē*, tumor]. A form of spina bifida in which the cavity of the projecting portion communicates with the central canal of the spinal cord.
syringomyelus (sĭr-ĭn″gō-mī'ĕl-ŭs) [" + *myelos*, marrow]. Abnormal dilatation of central canal of spinal cord.
syringopontia (sĭr-ĭn″gō-pŏn'shĭ-ă) [" + L. *pons*, pont-, bridge]. Cavities in the pons Varolii similar to *syringomyelia*.
syringosystrophy (sĭr-ĭn″gō-sĭs'trō-fĭ) [" + *systrophē*, a twist]. Twisting of the oviduct.
syringotome (sĭr-ĭng'ō-tōm) [" + *tomē*, a cutting]. Instrument for incision of a fistula.
syringotomy (sĭr-ĭn-gŏt'ō-mĭ) [G. *syrigx*, tube, + *tomē*, a cutting]. Operation for cure of fistula by cutting.
syrinx (sĭr'ĭnks) [G. *syrigx*, pipe]. 1. The eustachian tube. 2. Pathological cavity in the spinal cord or brain. 3. A fistula.
syrup (sĭr'ŭp) [L. *syrupus*]. Concentrated solution of sugar in water or aqueous liquid.
They usually do not represent a very high percentage of the active drug. Some are used principally to give a pleasant odor and taste to solutions. There are 18 official syrups.
syssarcosis (sĭs-ar-kō'sĭs) [G. *syn*, with, + *sarkōsis*, flesh condition]. The union of bones by means of muscles; muscular articulation, as of the *hyoid* and *patella*.
systaltic (sĭs-tăl'tĭk) [G. *systaltikos*, con-

tracting]. Contracting and dilating; having a systole. SYN: *pulsating*.

system (sĭs'tĕm) [G. *systēma*, an arrangement]. 1. A grouping of related structures; the whole organism. 2. An interrelationship of organs because of their function.

There are many different systems of the body: (a) Digestive s.; (b) excretory s.; (c) internal secretions; (d) muscular s.; (e) nervous s.; (f) osseous or skeletal s.; (g) respiratory s.; (h) reproductive s., and (i) the vascular or circulatory s.

s., alimentary. The digestive system.

s., autonomic nervous. Part of peripheral nervous system regulating involuntary impulses controlling function of ductless glands, blood vessels, and viscera.

s., central nervous. The brain and spinal cord.

s., circulatory. SEE: *vascular s.*

s., digestive. That of the alimentary tract, its glands and organs.

s., endocrine. That of the ductless glands and their hormones.

s., genitourinary. That of the genitals and urinary organs.

s., muscular. That of the muscles, ligaments, and tendons.

s., nervous. That of the nerves.

s., osseous. That of the bones and cartilages.

s., portal. That of the portal circulation.

s., pulmonary. That of the lungs and air passages.

s., respiratory. SEE: *pulmonary system*.

s., urinary. That of the kidneys, bladder, and appendages.

s., vascular. That of the heart, blood vessels, and lymphatics.

systema (sĭs-tē'mă) [G. *systēma*, an arrangement]. System.

s. nervorum sympath'icum. BNA. The sympathetic nervous system.

systemic (sĭs-tĕm'ĭk) [G. *systēma*, arrangement]. Pert. to a whole body rather than to one of its parts; somatic.

s. circulation. Course of the blood through the general system from left ventricle to right atrium.

s. death. Death of the body as a whole. SYN: *somatic death*.

s. remedies. Remedies which will act on the body as a whole, as a tonic.

systemoid (sĭs'tē-moyd) [G. *systēma*, an arrangement, + *eidos*, form]. 1. Resembling a system. 2. Pert. to tumors made up of several types of tissues.

systole (sĭs'tō-lē) [G. *systolē*, contraction]. That part of the heart cycle in which the heart is in contraction, *i. e.*, the myocardial fibers are tightening and shortening.

It causes the 1st heart sound; the 2nd is *diastole*, q.v. Since the different parts of the heart do not contract at exactly the same time, it is more precise to speak of auricular systole, etc.

RS: *murmur, perisystole.*

s., aborted. One which fails to increase arterial pressure because of mitral regurgitation or insufficient energy.

s., anticipated. One that is aborted because it occurs before the ventricle is filled.

s., arterial. Arterial retraction after a cardiac systole.

s., auricular. An auricular contraction.

s., extra. A premature one occurring in addition to the fundamental rhythm.

s., hemic. One independent and separate systole of one of the ventricles.

s., ventricular. Ventricular contraction.

systolic (sĭs-tŏl'ĭk) [G. *systolē*, contraction]. Pert. to the systole.

s. murmur. A cardiac one during systole. One heard in both systole and diastole.

s. pressure. Blood pressure is expressed in terms of the systolic pressure; the greatest force exerted by the heart and the highest degree of resistance put forth by the arterial walls.

RS: *blood pressure, diastolic p., pulse p., pulse, systole.*

systolometer (sĭs-tō-lŏm'ĕt-ĕr) [" + *metron*, a measure]. Device for determining quality and character of cardiac murmurs.

systremma (sĭs-trĕm'ă) [G. *systremma*, a twist]. Cramp in calf of the leg, the muscles assuming form of a hard ball.

syzygial (sĭz-ĭj'ĭ-ăl) [G. *syzygia*, conjunction]. Pert. to a syzygium.

syzygiology (sĭz-ĭ-jĭ-ŏl'ō-jĭ) [" + *logos*, a study]. Interdependence or interrelationships of the whole as opposed to isolated functions or separate parts.

syzygium (sĭ-zĭj'ĭ-ŭm) [G. *syzygia*, conjunction]. Partial fusion of 2 structures.

syzygy (sĭz'ĭj-ĭ) [G. *syzygia*, yoke]. Fusion of organs, each remaining distinct.

s. bone. An S-shaped bone, such as the *episternum*.

Szabo's test (sah'bō). A test for hydrochloric acid.

Addenda

sleep, physiologic standards. Metabolic rate reduced 10-15% below basal level. Systolic pressure falls 10 to 30 mm. of mercury. Pulse rate slows from 10 to 30 beats. Respiration slowed and typically irregular. Pupils constricted, eyeballs turned upward and outward. Increased sweating. Lacrimal, salivary secretions and volume of urine reduced. Spec. Gray, raised. Newborn sleeps 18-20 hrs. a day; growing child 12-14 hrs., adult 7-9 hrs. Older persons 5-7 hrs.

sleeping pills. They are built on a base of barbituric acid and are habit-forming. The withdrawal, if habitual, impairs the intellect and the emotions become affected. Large doses may induce liver and kidney disorders. The action of *seconal* is quick but brief. *Nembutal* has a slower but longer action. The effect is cumulative, lasting as long as nine days, so repeated doses may become fatal. They should not be taken when alcohol is to be consumed. Cure of the habit is more serious and dangerous than morphine addiction.

T

T. Abbr. for *temperature* and for *tension*. T+ indicates increased tension; T—, diminished tension.

t. Abbr. for *temporal*, and for Latin, *ter*, three times.

T-bandage. Bandage resembling the letter T. SEE: *bandage*.

T-fiber. One given off at right angles from the axis-cylinder process of a nerve cell.

T-wave. One of the waves or elevations in an electrocardiogram due to ventricular activity.

TA. Abbr. for alkaline tuberculin.*

T. A. Abbr. for *toxin-antitoxin*.

tabacism (tăb′ă-sĭzm) [L. *tabacum*, tobacco, + G. *-ismos*, condition]. Chronic tobacco poisoning. SYN: *tabacosis*.

tabacosis (tăb-ă-kō′sĭs) [" + G. *-ōsis*, condition]. Chronic tobacco poisoning, esp. from inhaling tobacco dust.

tabacum (tăb-ăk′ŭm) [L.]. Tobacco.

tabagism (tăb′ăj-ĭzm) [L. *tabacum*, tobacco, + G. *-ismos*, condition]. Tobacco poisoning. SYN: *tabacosis*.

tabatière anatomique (tah-bah-tē-air′ ahn-ah-tō-mĕk′) [Fr. anatomic snuffbox]. Depression at back of hand at base of thumb.

tabefaction (tă-bĕ-făk′shŭn) [L. *tabefacere*, to melt]. A wasting away of the body gradually.

tabella (tă-bĕl′ă) (pl. tabellae) [L. *tabella*, tablet]. A medicated mass of material formed into a small disk.
RS: *disk, lozenge, tablet, troche*.

tabes (tā′bēz) [L. *tabes*, a wasting]. 1. A gradual, progressive wasting in any chronic disease. 2. The final manifestation of syphilis involving particularly the posterior columns of the spinal cord. SYN: *locomotor ataxia*. SEE: *antitabetic, syphilis*.
Tabes causes postural instability, esp. when the eyes are closed, as well as the staggering, wide base gait which gives the disease its common name.
SYM: Motor instability, darting pain in the eyes, swelling of joints, optic atrophy, bladder disturbances, with other evidences of syphilis, usually make the diagnosis easy.
TREATMENT: Antiluetic. Fever treatment now offers new hope.

t., cerebral. Chronic degenerative brain disease with physical and mental deterioration. SYN: *paresis, general*.

t., cervical. T. first affecting the upper extremities.

t., diabetic. Peripheral neuritis, affecting diabetics. May affect spinal cord and simulate tabes dorsalis.

t. dorsalis. Degeneration of posterior columns of the spinal cord. SYN: *locomotor ataxia, tabes*.

t., marantic. T. with great emaciation.

t. mesenterica. Emaciation and general disorder of the functions of nutrition due to engorgement and tubercular degeneration of the mesenteric glands.

t., spasmodic. Lateral sclerosis of spinal cord. SYN: *Little's disease*.

tabetic (tă-bĕt′ĭk) [L. *tabes*, a wasting]. Pert. to or afflicted with tabes or tabes dorsalis.

t. ataxia. Occurs when there are lesions of first order of sensory neurons.

t. crises. Paroxysms of pain or other acute manifestations of episodic character in tabes dorsalis.

t. foot. Twisted foot in locomotor ataxia.

tabetiform (tăb-ĕt′ĭ-form) [L. *tabes*, a wasting, + *forma*, shape]. Resembling or characteristic of tabes.

tabic (tăb′ĭk) [L. *tabes*, a wasting]. Pert. to or affected with tabes or tabes dorsalis. SYN: *tabetic*.

tabid (tăb′ĭd) [L. *tabes*, a wasting]. Pert. to tabes. SYN: *tabetic, tabic*.

table (tā′bl) [L. *tabula*, a board]. 1. A flat-topped structure, as an operating table. 2. A thin, flat plate, as of bone.

t's. of skull. Inner and outer condensed layers of the cranial bone separated by diploe (cancellous bony tissue).

t., vitreous. The inner cranial table.

t's. of weights and measures. SEE: *weights and measures in Appendix*.

tablespoon (tā′bl-spoon). A large spoon containing about 15 cc. or 4 fluidrams.

tablet (tăb′lĕt) [O.Fr. *tablete*, from L. *tabula*, a table]. A small, disklike mass of medicinal powder.

t., coated. Usually made by coating compressed tablets with sugar, chocolate, etc.

t., compressed. Made by forcibly compressing the powdered substances into the desired shape; usually made to contain from 1 to 10 gr. of the active drug.
They are frequently very hard and sometimes not readily soluble.

t., dispensing. Those that contain a comparatively large amount of the active drug, as 1 gr. of strychnine sulfate.
Used by pharmacists and dispensing physicians to avoid the necessity of weighing small amounts of a potent drug in filling prescriptions. There is one official tablet.

t., hypodermic. Usually made as are tablet triturates, frequently containing, in addition, some agents that produce chemical action when water is added, thus causing a rapid disintegration of the mass.

t. triturates. Made by moistening the powder with a volatile liquid, as alcohol, and then molding into shape and allowing the liquid to evaporate.
They seldom contain more than 1 gr. of the active agent. They will usually disintegrate readily and are a very desirable form for administering certain drugs.

taboparalysis (ta″bō-păr-ăl′ĭs-ĭs) [L. *tabes*, a wasting, + *paralysis*, a loosening at the sides]. Tabes associated concurrently with general paralysis.

taboparesis (ta″bō-păr-ē′sĭs, -păr′ĕ-sĭs) [" + G. *paresis*, relaxation]. General paralysis in combination with tabes. SYN: *taboparalysis*.

tabophobia (tā″bō-fō′bĭ-ă) [" + G. *phobos*, fear]. A morbid fear of being afflicted with tabes, a common symptom of neurasthenia.

tabular (tăb′ū-lar) [L. *tabula*, a table]. 1. Resembling a table. 2. Set up in columns, as a *tabulation*.

t. bone. A flat one, or one with 2

tabule

compact bonelike parts with cancellous tissue bet. them.

tabule (tăb'ŭl) [L. *tabula*, table]. A medicated tablet.

tache (tahsh) [Fr. spot]. A colored spot or macule on the skin, as a freckle.

    t. **blanche.** A white spot seen on liver in some infectious diseases.

    t. **bleuâtre** (blu-ăhtr'). A blue spot on skin usually due to bite of cutaneous parasites. SYN: *macula caerulea.*

    t. **cérébrale.** The red line which occurs in meningitis and other nervous disorders, when the fingernail is drawn across the skin, *q.v.*

    t. **de feu.** Reddish area on skin caused by hypertrophy of cutaneous capillaries. SYN: *nevus vascularis.*

tachetic (tăk-ĕt'ĭk) [Fr. *tache*, spot]. Marked by purple or reddish blue patches (*taches*).

tachogram (tăk'ō-grăm) [G. *tachos*, swiftness, + *gramma*, a mark]. A graphic tracing of rate of flow of blood current.

tachography (tăk-ŏg'ră-fĭ) [" + *graphein*, to write]. The recording of the speed of the blood circulation.

tachy- [G.]. Combining form meaning *swift.*

tachycardia (tăk"ĭ-kar'dĭ-ă) [G. *tachys*, swift, + *kardia*, heart]. Abnormal rapidity of heart action.

    t., **constant.** Occurs in some valvular affections, fatty degeneration, compensation failure, pregnancy, nervous disorders, exhaustive diseases, exophthalmic goiter.

    t., **essential.** Rapid, persistent heart action due to functional disturbance.

    t., **extrinsic.** T. caused by factors outside of the heart, as increased metabolism or instability of the nervous system.

    t., **intrinsic.** T. caused by infection, as from rheumatism.

    t., **paroxysmal.** Sudden and abrupt acceleration of cardiac rate, ceasing abruptly.

Due to stimulus of cardiac contraction having its origin at an abnormal point. May go as high as 250 beats per minute. SEE: *arrhythmia, bradycardia.*

    t., **sinus.** Uncomplicated tachycardia when sinus rhythm is faster than 100 beats per minute, as that due to exercise.

tachycardiac (tăk-ĭ-kar'dĭ-ăk) [" + *kardia*, heart]. Pert. to or afflicted with tachycardia.

tachylalia (tăk"ĭ-lā'lĭ-ă) [" + *lalein*, to babble]. Rapid speech.

tachymeter (tăk-ĭm'ĕ-ter) [" + *metron*, a measure]. Instrument for estimating the rapidity of any body in motion.

tachyphagia (tăk"ĭ-fā'jĭ-ă) [" + *phagein*, to eat]. Rapid eating.

tachyphasia (tăk"ĭ-fā'zĭ-ă) [" + *phasis*, speech]. Very rapid or voluble speech. SYN: *tachyphrasia.*

tachyphrasia (tăk"ĭ-frā'zĭ-ă) [" + *phrasis*, speech]. Excessive volubility or rapidity of speech, as seen in mental disorders. SYN: *tachyphasia.*

tachyphrenia (tăk"ĭ-frē'nĭ-ă) [G. *tachys*, swift, + *phrēn*, mind]. Abnormally rapid mental activity.

tachyphylaxis (tăk"ĭ-fĭl-ăk'sĭs) [" + *phylaxis*, protection]. Rapid immunization to a toxic dose of a substance by previously injecting tiny doses of the same substance.

tachypnea (tăk-ĭp-nē'ă) [" + *pnoia*, breath]. Abnormal rapidity of respiration.

    t., **nervous.** Forty or more respirations per minute.

It occurs in hysteria, neurasthenia, etc.

tachypragia (tăk"ĭ-prā'jĭ-ă) [" + *pragein*, to act]. Rapidity of action.

tachypsychia (tăk-ĭ-sī'kĭ-ă) [" + *psychē*, soul]. Rapid action of psychic processes.

tachyrhythmia (tăk-ĭ-rĭth'mĭ-ă) [" + *rhythmos*, rhythm]. Rapid heart action. SYN: *tachycardia.*

    t., **auricular.** Condition in which auricular contractions are extremely rapid, causing impulses to arise in a place other than the sinuauricular node. SYN: *auricular flutter.*

tachysterol(e (tăk"ĭ-stē-rŏl). One of the isomers of ergosterol* obtained by irradiation.

tachysystole (tăk"ĭ-sĭs'tō-lē) [G. *tachys*, swift, + *systolē*, contraction]. Abnormally rapid systole. SEE: *extrasystole.*

tachytrophism (tăk"ĭ-trŏ'fĭzm) [" + *trophē*, nourishment, + *-ismos*, condition]. Accelerated metabolism.

tactile (tăk'tĭl) [L. *tactilis*, tangible, from *tangere*, to touch]. 1. Perceptible to the touch. 2. Pert. to the sense of touch.

This sense is dependent upon end organs in the skin, such as the pacinian corpuscles; from these organs, impulses ascend through various sensory nerves to the white matter of the spinal cord, which conveys them to the brain.

    t. **cell** or **corpuscle.** One in which a sensory nerve fibril terminates.

    t. **papilla.** One of the skin containing a t. cell or corpuscle.

tactometer (tăk-tŏm'ĕt-ĕr) [L. *tactus*, touch, + G. *metron*, a measure]. Instrument for determining acuity of tactile sensitiveness.

tactor (tăk'tor) [L. *tactus*, touch]. A tactile organ, specifically a tactile corpuscle.

tactual (tăk'tū-al) [L. *tactus*, touch]. Relating to the sense of touch. SYN: *tactile.*

tactus (tăk'tus) [L. touch]. Touch.

    t. **eruditus,** *t.* **expertus.** Sensitiveness of touch acquired by long practice, as by a diagnostician or surgeon.

taenia (tē'nĭ-ă) [L. *taenia*, a flat band]. 1. Any bandlike structure. 2. A tapeworm.

    t. **coli.** BNA. One of 3 bands of the large intestines into which muscular fibers are collected, *i. e., t. mesocolica* (mesenteric insertion), *t. libera* (opp. mesocolic band), and *t. omentalis* (at place of adhesion of omentum to transverse colon).

    t. **for'nicis.** One of the upper peduncles of the pineal gland.

    t. **hippocam'pi.** 1. Band on edge of the cornu inferius of lateral ventricle of brain. 2. Outer end of the oviduct. SYN: *corpus fimbriatum.*

    t. **semicircula'ris.** Band on wall of lateral ventricle bet. the corpus striatum and thalamus.

Taenia (tē'nĭ-ă). A genus of tapeworms.

SYM: Often absent. Frequently there are dyspeptic symptoms, colicky pains, loss of flesh, capricious appetite and sometimes reflex nervous phenomena such as vertigo, palpitation, "night terrors," convulsions, itching in the nose and choreic movements.

DIAG: Rests on discovery of the eggs or segments in the stools.

TREATMENT: Light diet for a day or 2 and a saline purge may be taken prior to the administration of anthelmintic. Gilix Mas. a dram of the ethereal extract, in capsules, at bedtime 12 hours after fasting, followed by an ounce of castor oil in the morning or kousso. To 2 drams of powdered flowers of kousso add 4 ounces boiling water, and when cold administer without being strained. Patient should fast day before using the medicine. Worm generally discharged in 24 hours, or pepo semen (pumpkin seed). One or 2 ounces fresh, dry pumpkin seeds, freed from their shells, powder finely and mix in a little milk. Give in morning after fasting 24 hours. Three hours later give an ounce of castor oil. If first dose not sufficient, repeat following morning. Pomegranate bark and Rottlera also good. SEE: *Dibothriophyllum latum*.

T. echinococcus. Species found in dogs' intestines.
Infection from food containing the eggs of this worm from having contaminated hands. It results in hydatid cysts. SEE: *echinococcus*.

T. saginata. Is derived from beef and is 5 or 6 yards in length.

T. solium. Pork tapeworm derived from the hog. Is 2 to 3 yards in length.

T. vulgaris. A broad tapeworm.

tagliacotian operation (tăl-yă-kō'shăn). Plastic operation on the nose in which skin is used from another part of the body. SYN: *rhinoplasty*.

tagma (tăg'mă) (pl. *tagmas, tagmatas*) [G. *tagma*, a thing arranged]. An aggregate of molecules; protoplasm.

tail (tāl) [A.S. *taegel*]. Posterior, long, flexible terminus, as the extremity of the spinal column. SEE: *cauda*.

t. bone. Bone at caudal end of spine. SYN: *coccyx*.

t. fold. An embryonic one enveloping the hindgut.

t. gut. Prolongation of the archenteron in the embryonic caudal extremity.

tailors' cramp or **spasm** (tā'lor). Spasmodic occupational neurosis affecting muscles of the forearm and hand.

Tait's law (tāt). Exploratory laparotomy should be made in every case of obscure abdominal or pelvic disease which is a threat to health or life.

T's. operation. Repair of a torn perineum. SYN: *perineorrhaphy*.

talalgia (tăl-ăl'jĭ-ă) [L. *talus*, heel, + G. *algos*, pain]. Pain in the heel. SYN: *pternalgia*.

Talbot's law (tăl'but). If visual stimuli from a revolving disk are fused and if sensation is uniform, then the intensity is the same as would occur were the same amount of light spread uniformly over the disk.

talc, talcum (tălk, tălk'ŭm) [L. *talcum*, powder]. Powdered soapstone; a soft, soapy powder; native hydrous magnesium silicate used as a dusting powder and as a filter.

talipes (tăl'ĭ-pēz) [L. *talus*, heel, + *pēs*, foot]. A nontraumatic deviation of the foot in the direction of 1 or the other of the 4 lines of movement, or of 2 of these combined. SYN: *clubfoot*.
May have 2 of these combined. Pes cavus, or hollow foot, is sometimes given as *t. cavus*, abnormal curvature of arch.
TREATMENT: Manipulative, mechanical, or both.

t. arcua'tus. Exaggerated normal arch of the foot. SYN: *t. cavus*.

t. calcaneus (flexion). Heel alone touching the ground, the patient walking on inner side of heel. Often follows infantile paralysis of muscle of tendo Achillis.

t. cavus. Same as *t. arcuatus*.

t. equinus (extension). Form with walking on the toes.

t. planus. Flatfoot, splayfoot.

t. valgus (abduction). Form with everted foot.

t. varus (adduction). With inverted foot.

talipomanus (tăl-ĭp-ŏm'ăn-ŭs) [L. *talus*, ankle, + *pēs*, foot, + *manus*, hand]. Deformity of the hand in which it is twisted out of shape. SYN: *clubhand*.

talocalcanean (tā″lō-kăl-kā'nē-ăn) [" + *calcaneum*, heel bone]. Relating to the astragalus and calcaneum. SYN: *astragalocalcanean*.

talocrural (tā″lō-krū'răl) [" + *crus, cruris*, leg]. Relating to the astragalus and leg bones.

talonid (tăl'ō-nĭd) [M.E. *talon*, from L. *talus*, heel]. The crushing region, the post. part of a lower molar tooth.

talus (tā'lŭs) [L. *talus*, ankle]. 1. BNA. The anklebone articulating with the tibia and fibula, and forming the ankle joint. 2. The entire ankle. SYN: *astragalus*.

tambour (tam'boor) [Fr. *tambour*, drum]. A shallow, drum-shaped appliance used in transmitting and registering arterial pulsations, blood pressure, respiratory movements, peristaltic contractions and other slight movements.

tampon (tam'pon) [Fr. *tampon*, plug]. 1. A plug, usually of lint or cotton, for closing a wound or cavity, to absorb secretions, or to arrest hemorrhage. 2. To plug up a wound or cavity with a tampon, as to stop hemorrhage.
MATERIALS: Aseptic cotton, wool, oakum, gauze, etc.
Mikulicz drain or tampon is a capillary drain on a large scale and consists of a square piece of iodoform gauze of requisite size, placed in a cavity and filled with narrow strips of plain gauze until the necessary degree of compression is secured. Used where there is parenchymatous oozing. Serves as a tampon to arrest bleeding and also acts as a capillary drain.
Rectal tampon made of piece of rubber tubing, size of thumb, 12 in. in length, covered with iodoform gauze. Into this tube is inserted a glass cylinder 3 in. in length, over which the rubber tubing should extend 2 in. An umbrella of iodoform gauze, 12x12 in., is fastened to the tube by tying a silk ligature over it at a point corresponding with the glass cylinder. Strips of sterilized gauze are used in packing the space bet. the tube and umbrella or mantle of gauze after the tube has been inserted into rectum.

t., nasal. Soft rubber bulb, dilated with compressed air, for plugging nostrils to stop hemorrhage from the nose.

tamponage, tamponade (tăm-pŏn-ād', tăm'pŏn-āj) [Fr. *tampon*, plug]. To use or make use of a tampon.

tannic acid (tăn'ĭk). Acid extracted from gallnuts. SYN: *tannin, q.v.*

tannigen (tăn'ĭ-jĕn). A brand of acetyltannic acid, which is a diacetic ester of tannic acid.
DOSAGE: 3-10 gr. (0.2-0.6 Gm.).
Acts as an astringent in diarrhea.

tannin (tăn'ĭn). 1. Acid substance found in bark of certain plants and trees or their products, usually from nutgall. Found in coffee and to a greater extent in tea. 2. Any of several substances containing tannin.
ACTION AND USES: Astringent, antidote for various poisons, for burns, and as a

tanning   T-4   **tarsorrhaphy**

hemostatic. It is constipating. It is partly eliminated in the urine as gallic acid.
  DOSAGE: As an antidote, 15 gr. (1.0 Gm.); locally, 1-5% solution; as an ointment, 20%.
  INCOMPATIBILITIES: Salts of iron, gelatin, quinine sulfate. SYN: *tannic acid.**

tanning (tăn'ĭng) [Fr. *tan,* from Breton *tann,* oak]. Exposure of face or body surface to the rays of the sun, thus acquiring a "coat of tan."
  The process is not without danger. SEE: *pigmentation, sunburn.*

tap (tăp) 1. [A.S. *taeppa,* tap]. To puncture or to empty of fluid by paracentesis. 2. [O.Fr. *taper,* of imitative origin]. A slight blow.

tapetum (tă-pē'tŭm) [L. *tapete,* a carpet]. BNA. A layer of fibers from the corpus callosum to each lateral ventricle of the brain and to the temporal lobe.

tapeworm (tăp'wŭrm) [A.S. *taeppe,* a narrow band, + *wurm,* worm]. *Tenia, q.v.* SEE: *cestode, Cestoidea.*
  A flat, tapelike parasite, composed of segments, which attaches itself to the wall of the intestine. SYN: *Taenia.*
  t., armed. The pork tapeworm, *Taenia solinan.*
  t., beef. Common tapeworm found in beef. SYN: *Taenia saginata.*

taphephobia, taphophobia (tăf″ē-fō'bĭ-ă, -ō-fō'bĭ-ă) [G. *taphos,* grave, + *phobos,* fear]. Abnormal fear of being buried alive.

tapinocephalic (tăp″ĭn-ō-sĕf-al'ĭk) [G. *tapeinos,* lying low, + *kephalē,* head]. Pert. to flatness of top of cranium.

tapinocephaly (tăp″ĭn-ō-sĕf'ă-lī) [" + *kephalē,* head]. Flatness of top of the skull.

tapioca (tăp″ĭ-ō'kă) [Portuguese]. COMP: The starchy substance of the cassava plant; a strictly carbohydrate food.
  AV. SERVING: 40 Gm. Pro. 0.2, Fat a trace. Carbo. 35.2.
  ASH CONST: Ca 0.023, P 0.090, Cl 0.018, S 0.029, Fe 0.0016. FUEL VALUE: 30 Gm. = 100 Cal., 1 lb. = 1520 Cal., 100 Gm. = 333 Cal.
  ACTION: Fattening. Easy to digest but leaves little residue.
  TIME FOR DIGESTION: One and two-thirds oz. in 2¾ hr.
  RS: *carbohydrate, starch, sugar.*

tapiroid (tā'pĭr-oyd) [Spanish *tapir,* tapir, + G. *eidos,* form]. Resembling a tapir's snout; said of an elongated cervix uteri.

tapotement (tă-pōt-mon′) [Fr.]. Percussion in massage.
  It is divided into: (a) *Beating* with the clenched hand; used for sciatica and muscular atrophy. (b) *Clapping,* performed with the palm of the hand; used to reach superficial nerves. (c) *Hacking,* with the ulnar border of the hand; used principally around a nerve center and upon the muscles. (d) *Punctuation,* with the tips of the fingers; used principally around the heart and upon the head.
  The strength of the manipulations is a principal point in the massage treatment, and care must be taken not to bruise the patient. As a rule, begin with moderate pressure, ascertaining from the patient his sensation. White petrolatum or some other oleaginous substance should be used to avoid abrading the skin. SEE: *massage.*

tapping (tăp'ĭng) 1. [O.Fr. *taper,* of imitative origin]. Percussion in massage. SYN: *tapotement.* 2. [A.S. *taeppa,* tap].

Removal of fluid from a cavity. SYN: *paracentesis.* SEE: *thoracentesis.*

tarantism (tăr'ăn-tĭzm) [Italian *Taranto,* tarantula, + G. *-ismos,* condition]. A nervous affection marked by stupor, melancholy and uncontrollable dancing mania. [tula.

Popularly attributed to bite of tarantaran′**tula bite.** Treatment the same as for black widow spider* bite, *q.v.*

Tardieu's ecchymoses or spots (tar-dyu′). Subpleural spots of ecchymosis following death by strangulation.

target (tar'gĕt) [O.Fr. *targette*]. 1. PT: The electrode on which cathode rays within an x-ray tube are focused and from which roentgen rays are emitted; usually of a heavy metal such as tungsten. 2. A tiny figure on an ophthalmometer's arm whose image is used to determine the amount of corneal astigmatism. SYN: *mire, q.v.*

Tarnier's sign (tahr-ne-ā′). A sign of coming abortion; the disappearance of angle bet. upper and lower uterine segments in pregnancy.

tarsal (tar'săl) [G. *tarsos,* flat of foot, edge of eyelid]. Pert. to the framework of the eyelid or to the instep.
  t. arches. Those above and below the tarsal cartilages.
  t. bones. The 7 bones of the instep.
  t. cartilages. Layers of cartilage in free edge of each eyelid.
  t. cyst. Small tumor on border of eyelid. SYN: *chalazion.*
  t. glands. Tiny sebaceous follicles at edge of the lid. SYN: *meibomian glands.*

tarsalgia (tar-săl'jĭ-ă) [G. *tarsos,* flat of the foot, + *algos,* pain]. Pain in a tarsus due to flatfoot or shortening of Achilles' tendon. SYN: *podalgia, policeman's disease.* [The tarsal bones.

tarsalia (tar-sā'lĭ-ă) (sing. *tarsale*) [L.].

tarsalis (tar-săl'ĭs) [L.]. One of the tarsal muscles. SEE: *Table of Muscles in Appendix.*

tarsectomy (tar-sĕk'tō-mĭ) [G. *tarsos,* flat of the foot, edge of eyelid, + *ektomē,* excision]. 1. Excision of tarsus or a tarsal bone. 2. Removal of tarsal plate of an eyelid.

tarsitis (tar-sī'tĭs) [" + *-itis,* inflammation]. 1. Inflammation of tarsus of the foot. 2. Inflammation of eyelid's border. SYN: *blepharitis.*

tarso- [G.]. Combining form meaning the *flat of the foot, edge of the eyelid.*

tarsocheiloplasty (tar″sō-kī'lō-plăs-tĭ) [G. *tarsos,* edge of eyelid, flat of the foot, + *cheilos,* lip, + *plassein,* to form]. Plastic surgery of borders of the eyelid.

tarsoclasia, tarsoclasis (tar″sō-klā'sĭ-ă, tar-sŏk'lăs-ĭs) [" + *klasis,* a breaking]. Surgical fracture of the tarsus for correction of clubfoot.

tarsomalacia (tar″sō-mă-lā'sĭ-ă) [" + *malakia,* a softening]. Softening of the tarsal cartilages of the eyes.

tarsometatarsal (tar″sō-mĕt-ă-tar'săl) [" + *meta,* between, + *tarsos,* flat of the foot]. Pert. to the tarsus and the metatarsus.

tarsophyma (tar″sō-fī'mă) [" + *phyma,* a growth]. Any tarsal tumor of the eyelid. SYN: *hordeoleum, sty.*

tarsoplasia, tarsoplasty (tar″sō-plā'zĭ-ă, tar′sō-plăs″tĭ) [" + *plassein,* to form]. Plastic surgery of margin of the eyelid. SYN: *blepharoplasty.*

tarsoptosis (tars-ŏp-tō'sĭs) [" + *ptōsis,* a dropping]. Falling of the tarsus. SYN: *flatfoot.*

tarsorrhaphy (tar-sor'ă-fī) [G. *tarsos,*

tarsotomy   T-5   **tea**

edge of eyelid, flat of the foot, + *rhaphē*, a seam]. The operation of uniting the edges of the lids at the outer commissure for the purpose of reducing the width of the palpebral fissure.

tarsotomy (tar-sŏt'ō-mĭ) [" + *tomē*, a cutting]. 1. Incision of tarsal cartilage of an eyelid. 2. Any surgical incision of the tarsus of the foot.

tarsus (tar'sŭs) (pl. *tarsi*) [G. *tarsos*, a flat structure]. 1. The instep proper with its 7 bones, bet. the tibia and the metatarsus. 2. The condensed connective tissue framework of the eyelids. RS: *cuneiform, scaphoid*.

It forms the proximal segment of the foot. The bones are *astragalus* (or knucklebone), the *calcaneus* (or heel bone), and the *scaphoid*, forming the proximal row; and the *cuboid* and the *internal, middle* and *external cuneiform* bones, forming the distal row, or *tarsalia*. The astragalus articulates with the tibia and fibula; the 4 distal bones, with the metatarsals.

tartar (tar'ter) [G. *tartaron*, dregs]. Calcareous matter deposited upon the teeth.

    t., cream of. Potassium bitartrate.

    t. emetic. A poisonous, white, crystalline salt, the tartrate of potassium and antimony, used in medicine as a diaphoretic, emetic, expectorant, and counterirritant.

    DOSAGE: As *expectorant*, 1/20 gr. (0.003 Gm.); as *emetic*, 1/2 gr. (0.03 Gm.).

    POISONING: SYM: Vomiting severe and sometimes bloody. Abdominal pain, diarrhea, and cramps in legs. Skin is cold and later face becomes cyanotic. Urine suppressed. Delirium and convulsions may occur.

    TREATMENT: If stomach is not emptied by vomiting, use stomach tube. Give strong coffee or tea, or a half teaspoonful of tannic or gallic acid in a half glass of water. Follow with soothing drinks, such as white of an egg in water, barley water or milk. Stimulate if collapse is present. Keep patient warm.

tartaric acid (tar-tar'ĭk). An acid derived from lees of wine and certain plants, occurring in 4 forms. Sometimes used in artificial lemonades or in effervescent drinks and is rarely toxic unless taken in large doses.

tartarization (tar"tar-ĭ-zā'shŭn) [G. *tartaron*, dregs]. Treatment with tartar emetic, esp. in syphilis.

tartarized (tar'tar-īzd) [G. *tartaron*, dregs]. Impregnated with tartaric acid.

taste (tāst) [O.Fr. *taster*, to feel, to taste]. 1. To try or perceive by touch of the tongue. 2. A chemical sense dependent upon sense organs on the surface of the tongue when they are in contact with a substance to ascertain its attributes, the nervous impulses being carried to the brain by the lingual (from the anterior two-thirds of the surface) and the glossopharyngeal (from the posterior third) nerves.

Taste sensation is experienced through stimulation of gustatory nerve endings in the tongue. There are 4 fundamental taste sensations: *sweet, bitter, sour,* and *salt*.

Loss of taste may be due to bilateral disease of chorda tympani nerve and of gustatory fibers of the glossopharyngeal nerve.

RS: *ageusia, agnosia, alliaceous, allotriogeustia, amblygeustia, appetite, cacogeusia, calyculus gustatorii, degustation, dysgeusia, gustation, gustatory,*

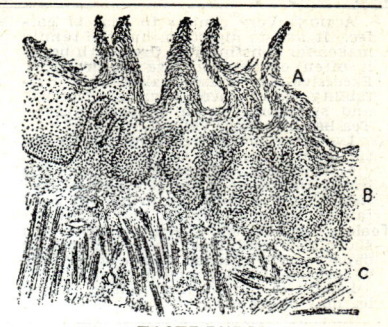

TASTE BUDS.
Tongue, anterior region, man. Cross section. A. Papillae filiformes. B. Deep epithelium. C. Muscular layer.

hypergeusia, hypogeusia, oxygeusia, parageusia, pseudogeusia.

    t. buds. Oval nerve end organs with hairlike processes that project through the central taste pores, principally on the surface of the tongue, but also in various parts of the mouth and throat upon which chemical stimuli have an effect.

    t. cells. Internal cells of a taste bud.

T. A. T. Abbr. for toxin-antitoxin.

taurocholemia (taw"rō-kō-lē'mĭ-ă) [G. *tauros*, a bull, + *cholē*, bile, + *aima*, blood]. Taurocholic acid in the blood.

tauto- [G.] A form meaning *the same*.

tautomeral, tautomeric (taw-tŏm'ĕr-ăl -to-mĕr'ĭk) [G. *tauto*, the same, + *meros*, a part]. Noting certain neurons which send processes to the white matter on the same side of the spinal cord.

tautomerism (taw-tŏm'ĕr-ĭzm) [" + " + *-ismos*, condition]. Phenomenon in which 2 formulae are possible but only one stable substance is obtainable.

tautorotation (taw"tō-rō-tā'shŭn) [" + L. *rotāre*, to turn round]. A change in specific rotation which occurs when a solution of certain sugars stands a while.

Tawara's node (tah-wah'rah). One near the coronary sinus in the right atrium forming beginning of the bundle of His. SYN: *Aschoff's node*.

taxis (tăks'ĭs) [G. *taxis*, arrangement]. Manual replacement of displaced structures.

    t., bipolar. Replacing of a retroverted uterus by drawing down the cervix in the vagina and pressing upward through the rectum.

taxonomy (tăks-ŏn'ō-mĭ) [" + *nomos*, law]. Laws and principles of classification of animals and plants.

T. b. Abbr. for *tubercle bacillus* and for *tuberculosis*.

t. d. s. Abbr. meaning *take 3 times a day*.

Te. Symb. of *tellurium*.

tea (tē). 1. An infusion of a medicinal plant. 2. Leaves of plant *Thea chinensis*, from which a beverage is made.

    COMP: It contains dextrin, gum, nitrogenous extracts, oxalates, phosphate of potassium, and its active principle is thein, a trimethyl xanthine. It contains more tannin (an astringent) than the caffeine of coffee, but there are less of these substances in the black teas than in the green teas. A cup of tea represents one-tenth less of its active principle than a cup of coffee.

tea, Paraguay   T-6   **teeth, milk**

ACTION: Very similar to that of coffee. It assists digestion, but the tannin makes for constipation. Used with beans it often causes digestive disturbances. Excessive use causes palpitation, irritability, nervousness, neuralgia, vertigo, and symptoms of an epileptic nature. Tea has no caloric value.
INCOMPATIBILITIES: Salts of iron, gelatin, quinine sulfate.
t., Paraguay. A tea made from the leaves and stems of the *Ilex paraguaiensis*. It is a stimulating drink and contains volatile oil, tannin, and caffeine.
Teale's amputation. Amputation with short ant. and long post. rectangular flaps used in excision of the lower half of forearm, the leg, or the thigh.
Length of flaps in amputation of the leg may be reversed.

Corti's membrane. SYN: *membrana tectoria*.
tectospinal (těk″tō-spī′năl) [L. *tectum*, roof, + *spina*, thorn]. From the tectum mesencephali to the spinal cord.
t. tract. A tract of white fibers of the spinal cord passing from the tectum of midbrain on 1 side, crossing, and going down through the medulla to the spinal cord.
tectum (těk′tŭm) [L. *tectum*, roof]. Any structure serving as, or resembling, a roof.
t. mesencephali. Roof of the midbrain including the corpora quadrigemina.
teeth (tēth) (sing. *tooth*) [A.S. *tōth*, tooth]. Hard, bony projections in jaws serving as organs of mastication, there being 32 permanent teeth, 16 in each jaw. SEE: *dentition*, *tooth*.

The Teeth

TEMPORARY TEETH: The following is the dental formula for the temporary teeth, with the dates in months of their eruption:

	Mo.	Mo.	Ca.	In.	In.	In.	In.	Ca.	Mo.	Mo.	
Upper ..	2	1	1	2	1	1	2	1	1	2 = 10	⎫ = 20
	24	12	18	9	7	7	9	18	12	24 months.	⎭
Lower ..	2	1	1	2	1	1	2	1	1	2 = 10	

PERMANENT TEETH: Subjoined is the dental formula for the permanent teeth, with the date in years of their eruption:

	Mo.	Pre.Mo.	Ca.	In.	In.	In.	In.	Ca.	Pre.Mo.	Mo.	
Upper	3 2	1 2	1	1	2	1	2	1	1 2	1 2 3 = 16	⎫ = 32
	18 12	6 10	9	11	8	7	7	8 11	9 10	6 12 18 years.	⎭
Lower	3 2	1 2	1	1	2	1	2	1	1 2	1 2 3 = 16	

---

tear (tēr) [A.S. *tēar*,]. A drop of the saline fluid normally secreted by the lacrimal glands to moisten the parts.
RS: *epiphora*, *lacrimal*, *lacrimation*.
t. ducts. The 2 lacrimal* ducts. SEE: *lacrimal*.
t. sac. Upper part of the nasolacrimal duct into which the 2 lacrimal ducts empty. SYN: *saccus lacrimalis*.
tease (tēz) [A.S. *taesan*, to pluck]. To separate a tissue into minute parts with a needle to prepare it for the microscope.
teat (tēt) [M.E. *tete*, from A.S. *tit*, *teat*]. 1. The nipple of the mammary gland. SYN: *papilla mammilla*. 2. Any protuberance resembling a nipple.
teatulation (tēt″ū-lā′shŭn) [A.S. *tit*, teat]. The development of a nipplelike elevation.
technic (těk-něk′) [Fr. from G. *technē*, art]. Details of a procedure or of an operation.
technical (těk′nĭ-kal) [G. *technikos*, skilled]. Requiring technic or special skill.
technician (těk-nĭsh′ăn) [G. *technē*, art]. One skilled in a special art.
techno- [G.]. Combining form meaning *art*, *skill*.
tecno- [G.]. Combining form meaning *child*.
tectocephaly (těk-tō-sěf′ăl-ĭ) [L. *tectum*, roof, + G. *kephalē*, head]. Possession of a boat-shaped cranium. SYN: *scaphocephalism*.
tectonic (těk-tŏn′ĭk) [G. *tektōn*, a builder]. Relating to plastic surgery.
tectorial (těk-tō′rĭ-ăl) [L. *tectum*, roof]. Pert. to a roof or covering. SYN: *tegmental*.
tectorium (těk-tō′rĭ-ŭm) [L. *tectōrium*, a covering]. 1. Any rooflike structure. 2.

t., anterior. Two canine and four incisors in each jaw.
t., auditory. SYN: *Husch′ke's a. teeth*. Minute toothlike projections along the

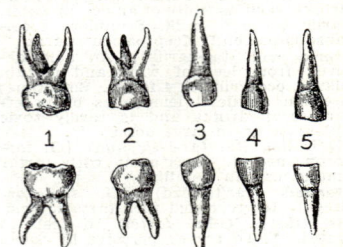

TEETH, DECIDUOUS.
1. Second molar. 2. First molar. 3. Canine. 4. Second incisor. 5. First incisor.

free margin of the labium vestibulare of the cochlea.
t., back. All posterior teeth (to the canines) of the molar series.
t., decid′uous. The milk teeth.
t., Hutchinson's. Lateral incisors of upper jaw when pegged and central incisors of same jaw having convex sides and crescentic notches on their cutting edges; noted only on permanent teeth, indicating hereditary syphilis.
t., malacot′ic. Those which are apt to decay, soft in structure and white in color.
t., mastoid. The supernumerary teeth of the horse.
t., milk. SYN: *deciduous teeth*. The first set of teeth.

t., oral. The anterior teeth.
t., secondary. The permanent teeth erupting about the 6th year and being complete about the 15th year.
t., sclerotic. Yellowish teeth that are naturally hard and not subject to ready decay.
RS: *agomphiasis, alinement, alveolar, alveoli dentales, alveolus, anticarious, apicitis, bicuspid, cacodontia, calcoid, canine, carious, deciduous,* "dent-" *words, detrition, evulsion, Hutchinson's, milk t., occlude, occlusion,* "odont-" *words, orthodontist, sordes, tartar, wisdom t.*

teething (tēth′ĭng) [A.S. *tōth*, tooth]. Eruption of the teeth. SYN: *dentition*.

tegmen (tĕg′mĕn) (pl. *tegmina*) [L. *tegmen*, covering]. A structure that covers a part. [cells.
t. mastoideum. Bony roof of mastoid
t. tympani. BNA. Roof of tympanum separating middle ear from cranial cavity.

tegmental (tĕg-mĕn′tăl) [L. *tegmentum*, covering]. Relating to a tegument or tegmentum; covering.
t. nucleus. Nucleus of gray substance containing red ganglion cells in the cover of the crus cerebri.

tegmentum (tĕg-mĕn′tŭm) [L. *tegmentum*, covering]. Dorsal portion of crus cerebri above the substantia nigra, with fibers running to the cortex.
t. auris. Membrane bet. middle and external ear. SYN: *membrana tympani*.

tegument (tĕg′ū-mĕnt) [L. *tegumentum*, a covering]. 1. The skin; the covering of the body. SYN: *integument*. 2. A covering structure.

tegumental, tegumentary (tĕg″ū-mĕn′tăl, -tă-rĭ) [L. *tegumentum*, a covering]. Concerning a tegument; covering.

Teichmann's crystals (tīk′mahn). Brownish-red crystalline form of hematin hydrochloride, hemin. SYN: *hematin hydrochloride, hemin*.

teichopsia (tī-kŏp′sĭ-ă) [G. *teichos*, wall + *opsis*, vision]. Zigzag lines bounding a luminous area appearing in the visual field causing a temporary blindness in that portion of the eye, sometimes accompanying severe sick headaches and mental or physical strain. SYN: *scotoma, scintillating*.

teinodynia (tī″nō-dĭn′ĭ-ă) [G. *tenōn*, tendon, + *odynē*, pain]. Pain in the tendons. SYN: *tenodynia*. [structure.

tela (tē′lă) [L. *tēla*, web]. Any weblike
t. cellulo′sa. Connective tissue.
t. choroi′dea. Part of the pia mater covering roof of the 3rd and 4th cerebral ventricles.

telalgia (tĕl-ăl′jĭ-ă) [G. *tēle*, far away, + *algos*, pain]. Pain felt at a distance from its stimulus. SYN: *pain, referred*.

telangiectasia, telangiectasis (tel-ăn″jĭ-ĕk-tā′zhĭ-ă, -ĕk′tă-sĭs) [G. *telos*, end, + *aggeion*, vessel, + *ektasis*, dilatation]. Dilatation of capillaries and sometimes of terminal arteries producing an angioma of maculalike appearance, or hyperemic spot.
It may be as a birthmark, or become apparent in young children. In adults probably due to several causes, such as indigestion, gastritis, gallbladder disease, cirrhosis of the liver, exposure to weather, goiter, tuberculosis, and infections. May occur on thighs, nose, or face.
TREATMENT: Finding and removing cause. Coagulation with electric needle; radiotherapy, and cosmetic care.

t. lymphat′ica. Tumor composed of dilated lymph vessels.

telangiectoma (tĕl-ăn-jĭ-ĕk-tō′mă) [" + " + *-ōma*, tumor]. Angioma from dilatation of capillaries or arterioles. SYN: *telangioma*.

telangiitis (tĕl-ăn-jĭ-ī′tĭs) [" + " + *-itis*, inflammation]. Inflammation of the capillaries.

telangioma (tĕl″ăn-jĭ-ō′mă) [" + " + *-ōma*, tumor]. A tumor made up of dilated capillaries or arterioles.

telangiosis (tĕl-ăn-jĭ-ō′sĭs) [" + " + *-ōsis*, condition]. Disease of capillary vessels.

tele-, tel- [G.]. Combining forms meaning *at a distance, far off*.

telecardiogram (tel″ē-kar′dĭ-ō-grăm) [G. *tēle*, distant, + *kardia*, heart, + *gramma*, a writing]. A cardiogram which records at a distance from the patient. SYN: *telelectrocardiogram*.

telecardiography (tĕl″ē-kar″dĭ-og′ră-fĭ) [" + " + *graphein*, to write]. Process of taking telecardiograms.

telecardiophone (tĕl″ē-kar′dĭ-ō-fōn) [" + " + *phōnē*, voice]. A stethoscope will magnify heart sounds so that they may be heard at a distance from patient.

teleceptive (tĕl-ĕ-sĕp′tĭv) [" + L. *-ceptivus*, receiving, from *capere*, to take]. Relating to a teleceptor.

teleceptor (tĕl′ĕ-sĕp-tor) [" + L. *ceptor*, a receiver]. A device that receives stimuli from a distance.

telecinesia (tĕl″ē-sĭn-ē′zĭ-ă) [" + *kinēsis*, movement]. Apparent automatic movement of an object produced without contact with any stimulus or power.

teleo-, tele- [G.]. Combining forms meaning *perfect, complete*.

telecurietherapy (tĕl-ē-kū-rī-thĕr′ă-pĭ) [G. *tēle*, distant, + *curie* + G. *therapeia*, treatment]. Application of radium rays from a distance from a patient.

teledendrite, teledendron (tĕl-ē-dĕn′drĭt, -dĕn′drŏn) [" + *dendron*, a tree]. A terminal dendron. SYN: *telodendron*.

telediastolic (te″lē-dĭ-as-tol′ĭk) [G. *telos*, end, + *diastolē*, a dilatation]. Concerning the last phase of the diastole.

telegony (tĕl-ĕg′ō-nĭ) [G. *tēle*, distant, + *gonē*, offspring]. An alleged theory that the male sperm from a dam's first sexual contact modifies the blood of the female, thus influencing the offspring resulting from mating with another sire.
This is supposed to be due to the absorption of the male sperm by the mucous tissue of the female's genitals, then entering the lymphatics and blood stream.

telelectrocardiogram (tĕl″ē-lĕk″trō-kar′dĭ-ō-grăm) [" + *ēlektron*, amber (electricity), + *kardia*, heart, + *gramma*, a writing]. One taken with a galvanometer attached to the patient by a wire some distance from the instrument. SYN: *telecardiogram*.

telencephalic (tĕl″ĕn-sĕf-al′ĭk) [" + *egkephalos*, brain]. Pert. to the endbrain (telencephalon).

telencephalon (tĕl-ĕn-sĕf′ă-lŏn) [G. *telos*, end, + *egkephalos*, brain]. The embryonic endbrain or ant. division of the prosencephalon from which the cerebral hemispheres are developed.

teleneurite (tĕl-ĕ-nū′rīt) [" + *neuron*, nerve]. The terminal arborization of an axis cylinder.

teleneuron (tĕl-ĕ-nū′rŏn) [" + *neuron*, nerve]. A nerve ending at which an impulse terminates.

teleology (tĕl-ē-ŏl′ō-jĭ) [G. *telos*, end, +

logos, a study]. The belief that everything has a final purpose.

teleomitosis (tĕl″ē-ō-mĭ-tō′sĭs) [G. *teleos*, complete, + *mitos*, a thread, + *-ōsis*, condition]. Completed indirect cell division. SEE: *karyokinesis, mitosis*.

teleorganic (tĕl″ē-or-găn′ĭk) [" + *organon*, organ]. Necessary to organic life. SYN: *vital*.

teleotherapeutics (tĕl″ē-ō-ther-ă-pū′tĭks) [" + *therapeutikē*, treatment]. The use of hypnotic suggestion in the treatment of disease. SYN: *suggestive therapeutics*.

telepathist (tĕl-ĕp′ă-thĭst) [G. *tēle*, distant, + *pathos*, feeling]. One who claims the ability to read the mind of others.

telepathy (tĕl-ĕp′ă-thĭ) [" + *pathos*, feeling]. Supposed communication of one mind with another at a distance without any means known to physical or psychological science. SYN: *thought transference*.

telephase (tĕl′ē-fāz) [G. *telos*, end, + *phasis*, phase]. Final stage of mitosis in which the cytoplasm divides.
RS: *anaphase, centriole, metaphase, prophase*.

teleradiography (tĕl″ē-rā-dĭ-og′ră-fĭ) [G. *tēle*, distant, + L. *radius*, ray, + G. *graphein*, to write]. Radiography with the tube about 2 meters (6½ ft.) from the body.

telergy (tĕl′er-jĭ) [" + *ergon*, work]. 1. Action without conscious exercise of the will. SYN: *automatism*. 2. Hypothetical action of one individual's thoughts upon brain of another by transmission of some unknown form of energy.

teleroentgenography (tĕl″ē-rĕnt″gĕn-ŏg′răf-ĭ) [" + *roentgen* + G. *graphein*, to write]. Radiography in which the tube is about 2 meters (6½ ft.) from the body. SYN: *teleradiography*.

telesthesia (tĕl-ĕs-thē′zĭ-ă) [" + *aisthēsis*, sensation]. An impression received at a distance without normal operation of organs of sense. SYN: *telepathy*.

telesyphilis (tĕl-ĕ-sĭf′ĭl-ĭs) [" + *syphilis*]. 1. Congenital syphilis without lesions. SYN: *metasyphilis*. 2. Any nonsyphilitic condition due to syphilis. SEE: *parasyphilitic*.

telesystolic (tĕl″ē-sĭs-tol′ĭk) [G. *telos*, end, + *systolē*, contraction]. Pert. to the termination of the cardiac systole.

teletherapy (tĕl-ĕ-thĕr′ă-pĭ) [G. *tēle*, distant, + *therapeia*, treatment]. Absent treatment; treatment of disease by telepathy*; method of mental healers.

tellurism (tĕl′ū-rĭzm) [L. *tellus, tellur-*, earth, + G. *-ismos*, condition]. Morbific influence of the soil.

tellurium (tĕl-ū′rĭ-ŭm) [L. *tellus, tellur-*, earth]. SYMB: *Te*. A nonmetallic element used as an electric rectifier and in coloring glass.
POISONING: SYM: Garlic odor of all secretions and excretions. A disagreeable odor to the breath with suppression of perspiration and saliva, resulting in dry skin and mouth. Anorexia, nausea, drowsiness, and weakness often found.
F. A. TREATMENT: Saline cathartics, increase fluid intake, induce perspiration, otherwise treatment is symptomatic.

teloblast (tĕl′ō-blăst) [G. *telos*, end, + *blastos*, germ]. A segmentation cell at the growing end of a germinal band.

telodendron (tĕl-ō-dĕn′drŏn) [" + *dendron*, a tree]. Terminal arborization of the axis cylinder process of a neuron.

telophase (tĕl′ō-fāz) [" + *phasis*, a phase]. The last stage of karyokinesis in which the cytoplasm divides into 2 daughter cells; the last stage in mitosis.*

telotism (tĕl′ō-tĭzm) [" + *-ismos*, process]. The entire performance of a function, as that of one of the senses.

TEM. Abbr. for *triethylene melamine*. SEE: *nitrogen mustard*.

temperament (tĕm′per-ă-mĕnt) [L. *temperamentum*, mixture]. Individual peculiarity of physical and mental organization.

t., bilious. One in which the nutritive system is predominant; usually characterized by dark complexion, muscular activity, energy of action, firmness of purpose, and passionate disposition.

t., choleric. Same as *bilious t.*

t., equal. An equable disposition.

t., lymphatic. Same as *phlegmatic t.*

t., melancholic. One characterized by brooding thoughtfulness, irritability, tenacity of purpose, and obstinacy of disposition.

t., nervous. One in which the nervous organization is exceedingly sensitive, characterized by quick mental action and vivid emotions.

t., phlegmatic. One in which the lymphatic system is supposed to predominate, characterized by mental sluggishness, pale complexion, flabby muscles, and dullness of passionate emotions.

t., sanguine. A temperament characterized by marked physical vitality, irritability, energy of action and liability to nervous exhaustion, light hair, eyes and complexion, good digestion.

temperature (tĕm′per-ă-tūr) [L. *temperatura*, proportion]. 1. Degree of heat of a living body; loosely, body heat above normal. 2. Degree of hotness or coldness of a substance.

(a) Body temperature varies with different organs' areas, and with the time of day. The temperature in the *liver* may be 105.1° F., while that under the *tongue* is 98.6° F.; the temperature under the *arm* at 2 P. M. may be 99.0° F. and at 2 A. M. 96.7° F.; the *rectal* temperature is likely to be 0.5 to 0.75° above the oral.

One of the mechanisms for raising temperature is muscular work (as in shivering); one for lowering it is sweating. The interplay of such processes keeps the body temperature constant.

(b) The sense of temperature is dependent upon the existence of special areas (hot and cold spots) on the skin, from which impulses are carried by sensory nerves to the white matter of the cord and thus ultimately to the brain. Body temperature may be measured by the clinical thermometer placed in the *mouth, axilla,* or *rectum*.

Respiration, Pulse and Temperature Ratio		
Respirations	Pulsations	Temperature
18	80	99° F.
19 (plus)	88	100° F.
21	96	101° F.
23	104	102° F.
25 (minus)	112	103° F.
27	120	104° F.
28 (minus)	128	105° F.
30	136	106° F.

Mouth temperature should not be taken for 10 minutes or more after patient has had hot or cold food or drink;

temperature, absolute   T-9   **temperature scale**

or if coughing, afflicted with dyspnea, if delirious or insane, for at least 3 days after operation, if under 10 years old, or if temperature is below 97° F. or over 100° F.

A temperature under 93° F. except in cholera, when it may be from 85° to 90° F. for several days, or over 107° F., except in intermittent fever, is generally fatal. 108.6° F. indicates almost certain death.

Temperature Indications

107° F. Generally fatal except in intermittent fever.
106° F. Intense fever.
105° F. High fever, dangerous.
104° F. Severe fever.
102° F. Moderate fever.
101° F. Slight fever.
98.6° F. Normal.
98° F. Subnormal.
96° F. Collapse.
94° F. Algid collapse.
93° F. Fatal collapse except in cholera.
t., absolute. T. measured from absolute zero, —273° C.
t., animal. Normal t. of the healthy adult.
t., body. The t. of the body.
t., critical. The t. below which a gas may be converted to liquid form by pressure.
t. curve. Line indicating the fluctuations of t. for a given period.
t., fall of. Extreme weakness.
t., high. More alarming with wet skin than with dry skin.
t., maximum. BACT: T. above which growth will not take place.
t., mean. The average t. for a stated period in a given locality.
t., minimum. BACT: T. below which growth will not take place.
t., normal. T. of the body in health, 98.6° F. (37° C.) in man.
t., optimum. T. at which an operation is best carried out, as the culture of a given organism.
t., rectal. The thermometer should be inserted at least 1½ in. and allowed to remain 3-5 minutes. Do not take following rectal operation or if rectum is diseased.
t., room. T. bet. 65-80° F.
t. sense. Sense responding to heat and cold.
t., subnormal. T. below the normal of 98.6° F.
t., zero. T. at which heat and cold are not felt by a sensory end organ.

Temperature Scale (Approximate)

Degrees Fahrenheit

Alcohol boils	173.1
Acetic acid melts	62.6
Bacillus coli communis dies in 10 minutes	140.0
Bacillus typhosus dies in 10 minutes	136.4
Bacillus acidi lactici dies in 10 minutes	133.0
Bacteria, most die but not all spores	144.0
Bessemer furnace heat	4000.0
Blood heat	98.0
Bread, white, bakes at	464.0
whole wheat, bakes at	430.0
graham, bakes at	400.0
diastase most active	140.0
favorable to fermentation	107.6
Butter melts	91.4
Caramel point	350.0
Casein, hardens slightly	214.0

Degrees Fahrenheit

Climate, highest recorded, South Wales	130.0
Calcutta, average	78.3
New Orleans, average	68.6
Sydney, Australia	63.0
San Francisco	56.6
Rome	59.7
New York	53.8
London	50.3
Berlin	48.5
Greatest cold reported, Boothia	—78.0
Coal ignites	762.0
Cocoa butter melts	86.0
Cream, rises slowly at	50.0
Egg, albumen coagulates, hardens	212.0
coagulation complete	160.0
dissolved albumen rises	160.0
Ether boils	94.8
Fat, boiling point	385.0
Fever, in febrile diseases may go as high as	110.0
almost certain death except in intermittent	108.6
generally fatal except in intermittent	107.0
intense	106.0
high (dangerous)	105.0
severe	104.0
moderate	102.0
slight	101.0
Frying point, highest	400.0
lowest	350.0
Fungus of yeast destroyed	125.0
Germs, Miquel's temperature for destruction of all germs in 1 hour's heating under pressure	221.0
Glucose melts	146.0
Gold melts	1981.0
Ice and salt mixtures	0.0
Lactalbumin coagulated	161.6
Lead melts	600.0
Meats, canned	230.0
roasting, inner temperature	200.0
Meat, connective tissue changes to gelatin	185.0
stewed and boiled, should be dropped and maintained at	180.0
Meats, dissolved albumin rises	160.0
coagulation complete	160.0
Meat coagulation begins	134.0
albumen soluble at	134.0
Microörganisms checked	32.0
destroyed but no spores	154.4
SEE: *germs, bacteria.*	
Milk boils	213.5
scalded	196.0
pasteurized	194.0
household pasteurization	167.0
sterilizes	180.0
lactalbumin coagulates	122.0
freezes	31.1
Olive oil solidifies	30.0
Palmitin melts	143.6
Pasteurization. SEE: *milk.*	
Leed's point, 30 minutes	157.0
Freeman's point, 30 minutes	155.0
Vincent's point, 15 minutes	160.0
Pneumococcus dies in 10 minutes at	126.5
Rennin enzyme destroyed	140.0
Stearin melts	131.0–140.7
Steel melts	2500.0
Storage, beef, fresh, lowest	37.0
beef, fresh, highest	39.0
fish	30.0
fish, fresh, best for	25.0
fish, for cold	15.0
fruits, fresh, highest	39.0
fruits, dried, highest	35.0
fruits, bananas, berries, lemons	36.0
fruits, cranberries	34.0
fruits, cantaloupe, watermelon, apples	32.0

temperature, words pert. to   T-10   tendon, Achilles'

Degrees Fahrenheit

fruits, apples, lowest for	31.0
ham and lard	35.0
meats, brined	35.0
mutton and veal, highest	36.0
mutton and veal, lowest	32.0
oysters in tub	35.0
oysters in shell	40.0
pork, highest	33.0
pork, lowest	30.0
poultry, fresh, best	29.0
vegetables, highest	35.0
Sugar, "crack"	310.0
small "crack"	290.0
hard ball	248.0
soft ball	238.0
feather point	232.0
boil	230.0
large pearl	222.0
pearl	220.0
large thread	217.0
small thread	215.0

TEMPERATURE OF THE BODY.

Temperature, normal body	98.6
blood heat	98.0
subnormal	97.0
subnormal, collapse, dangerous	96.6
collapse, algid, generally fatal except in cholera	94.0
collapse, total. Fatal except in cholera	93.0
may go as low in cholera as	85.0

SEE: *climate, fever.*

Tubercle bacillus, may live an hour at	149.0
Water, boils	212.0
Dead Sea, boils	221.0
simmers	185.0
warm	92-100.0
lowest for hot water	100.0
highest for an emetic	95.0
lowest tepid	95.0
lowest for an emetic	92.0
greatest density	39.2
freezing point	32.0
cold	32-63.0
White wax melts	145.4
Yeast, most favorable to growth	84.0
most favorable for development	66.0
life of, suspended	32.0
killed	212.0
fungus destroyed	125.0

SEE: *thermometer, thermometry.*

temperature, words pert. to: algid, a. stage, algogenic, Baruch's sign, chauffage, cold, enthermic, frigid, frigidity, frigorific, hardening, heat, h. regulation, hyperexis, infant, myothermic, pseudocrisis, respiration, temperature scale, "therm-" words.

temple (tĕm′pl) [O.Fr. from L. *tempora*, pl. of *tempus*, temple]. The region of head in front of ear and over the zygoma.

tempolabile (tĕm″pō-lā′bl) [L. *tempus*, time, + *labilis*, unstable]. Becoming altered spontaneously within a definite time.

temporal (tĕm′por-ăl) [L. *temporalis*, pert. to time; pert. to temples]. 1. Pert. to or limited in time. 2. Relating to the temples.
  t. bone. A bone on both sides of the skull at its base. SYN: *os temporale.* SEE: *Arnold's canal, mastoid, petrosa, petrosal, squamous, styloid process.*
  t. crest. The ridge on frontal bone attaching the temporalis muscle. SYN: *crista temporalis.*
  t. fissure. One on lateral surface of the temporal lobe.
  t. ganglion. A sympathetic one on the ext. carotid artery.
  t. ramus. A branch of the facial nerve in the temporal region.

temporalis (tĕm″pō-rā′lĭs) [L.]. Muscle in temporal fossa which elevates the mandible. SEE: *Muscles, Table of,* in Appendix.

temporo- [L.]. Combining form meaning *temples of the head.*

temporomaxillary (tĕm″por-ō-măks′ĭl-lā-rĭ) [L. *tempus, tempor-*, temple]. Pert. to the temporal and maxillary bones.

temporoöccipital (tĕm″por-ō-ŏk-sĭp′ĭ-tăl) [" + *occipitalis*, pert. to the occiput]. Pert. to the temporal and occipital bones or their regions.

temporosphenoid (tĕm″por-ō-sfē′noyd) [" + G. *sphēn*, wedge, + *eidos*, form]. Pert. to the temporal and sphenoid bones.

tempostabile, tempostable (tĕm″pō-stā′bl) [L. *tempus*, time, + *stabilis*, stable]. Not subject to change chemically in course of time.

temulence (tĕm′ū-lĕns) [L. *temulentia*, intoxication]. Drunkenness; intoxication.

tenacious (tĕ-nā′shŭs) [L. *tenax, tenac-*, holding]. Adhering to; adhesive; retentive.

tenaculum (tĕn-ăk′ū-lŭm) [L. *tenaculum*, a holder]. Sharp, hooklike, pointed instrument with slender shank for grasping and holding a part, as an artery.
  t., abdominal. Longer than others with smaller hook. Sim's, Emmet's, Kelly's, etc.
  t., uterine. Heavier and shorter hook used for manipulating uterus.

tenalgia (tĕn-ăl′jĭ-ă) [G. *tenōn*, tendon, + *algos*, pain]. Pain in a tendon. SYN: *tenodynia.*
  t. crepitans. Inflammation of a tendon sheath which on movement results in a crackling sound. SYN: *tendosynovitis crepitans.*

tenderness (tĕn′dĕr-nĕs) [M.E. *tendre*, from L. *tener*, tender]. Sensitiveness to pain upon pressure, usually cutaneous.

tendinitis (tĕn-dĭn-ī′tĭs) [L. *tendo*, tendon, + G. *-itis*, inflammation]. Inflammation of a tendon. SYN: *tenonitis, 1; tenontitis.*

tendinoplasty (tĕn′dĭ-nō-plăs″tĭ) [" + G. *plassein*, to form]. Plastic surgery of tendons. SYN: *tenontoplasty, tenoplasty.*

tendinosuture (tĕn″dĭn-ō-sū′tūr) [" + *sutura*, a seam]. The suturing of a divided tendon. SYN: *tenorrhaphy.*

tendinous (tĕn′dĭn-ŭs) [L. *tendinōsus*, like a tendon]. Pert. to, composed of, or resembling tendons.
  t. spot. A white thickening of a serous membrane.
  t. synovitis. Inflammation of a tendon's synovial sheath.

tendo (tĕn′dō) (pl. *tendines*) [L. *tendo*, tendon]. A tendon.
  t. Achil′lis. The tendon of the soleus and gastrocnemius muscles inserted into tuberosity of the os calcis. SEE: *leg for Illustration.*
  t. calca′neus. BNA. Same as *t. Achillis.*

tendolysis (tĕn-dŏl′ĭ-sĭs) [" + G. *lysis*, a loosening]. The process of freeing a tendon from adhesions.

tendon (tĕn′dŭn) [L. *tendo*, tendon]. Fibrous connective tissue serving for the attachment of muscles to bones and other parts. SYN: *sinew.*
  RS: *Achilles' jerk, achillobursitis, achillotomy, aponeurotomy, chorda, sinew, "teno-" words.*
  t., Achilles'. The large tendon at lower end of gastrocnemius muscle, inserted into the *os calcis.*
  It is the strongest and thickest one in the body.

t., calcaneous. Achilles* tendon.
t. cells. Certain flat ones in white tissue fiber of tendons.
t. reflex. Reflex act in which a muscle contracts when its tendon is percussed.
t. r., patella. Response to tapping of the quadriceps muscle tendon when patient is sitting with toes pressing on the floor.
t. spindle. Fusiform nerve ending in a tendon.
tendoplasty (tĕn'dō-plăs″tĭ) [L. *tendo*, tendon]. Reparative surgery of an injured tendon. SYN: *tenoplasty, tenontoplasty*.
tendosynovitis (tĕn″dō-sĭn″ō-vī'tĭs) [" + *syn*, with, + L. *ovum*, egg, + G. *-itis*, inflammation]. Inflammation of a sheath of a tendon or the tendon. SYN: *tendovaginitis, tenontothecitis*.
t. crepitans. T. accompanied on movement by a crackling sound.
tendotome (tĕn'dō-tōm) [" + G. *tomos*, a cutting]. Instrument for severing a tendon. SYN: *tenotome*.
tendotomy (tĕn-dŏt'ō-mĭ) [" + G. *tomē*, a cutting]. Division of a tendon. SYN: *tenotomy*.
tendovaginal (tĕn″dō-văj'ĭ-năl) [" + *vagina*, sheath]. Relating to a tendon and its sheath.
tendovaginitis (tĕn″dō-văj″ĭn-ī'tĭs) [" + " + G. *-itis*, inflammation]. Inflamed condition of a tendon and its sheath. SYN: *tenontothecitis*.
tenesmic (tĕn-ĕz'mĭk) [G. *teinesmos*, a stretching]. Pert. to or like tenesmus.
tenesmus (tĕ-nĕz'mŭs) [G. *teinesmos*, a stretching]. Spasmodic contraction of anal or vesical sphincter with pain and persistent desire to empty the bowel or bladder, with involuntary, ineffectual straining efforts.
tenia (tē'nĭ-ă) [L. *taenia*, a flat band]. 1. A flat band of tissue. 2. A genus of tapeworm. SYN: *taenia, q.v.*
teniacide (tē'nĭ-ăs-īd) [" + *cidus*, from *caedere*, to kill]. Destroying or that which destroys tapeworms.
teniafuge (tē'nĭ-ă-fūj) [" + *fugāre*, to put to flight]. Expelling or a drug that expels tapeworms. Ex: *oleoresin of male fern, peletierine tannat*. SYN: *tenifuge*.
teniasis (tē-nī'ăs-ĭs) [" + G. *-iasis*, a condition]. Presence of tapeworms in the body.
tenifuge (tĕn'ĭf-ūj) [" + *fugāre*, to put to flight]. Causing or that which causes expulsion of tapeworms. SYN: *teniafuge*.
tenigue (tĕn-ēg') [L. *tensio*, a stretching, + *fatigare*, to tire]. Tension and fatigue, especially affecting motorists and causing accidents.
ten'nis el'bow. An obscure, insidious, distressing complaint after playing tennis following a period of muscular inactivity of the arm or following a long duration of play.
ETIOL: Sprain of the supinator brevis muscle.
SYM: Slight discomfort, transient weakness of entire arm, with difficulty in handling or grasping things.
F. A. TREATMENT: A splint of adhesive strapping plus a sling. Later, apply heat and massage.
teno- [G.]. Combining form meaning *tendon*.
tenodesis (tĕn-ŏd'e-sĭs) [G. *tenōn*, tendon, + *desis*, a binding]. Suturing of the end of a tendon to a point of attachment.
tenodynia (tĕn-ō-dĭn'ĭ-ă) [" + *odynē*, pain]. Pain in a tendon. SYN: *tenalgia*.
tenomyoplasty (tĕn″ō-mī'ō-plăs″tĭ) [" + *mys, my-*, muscle, + *plassein*, to form]. Reparative operation upon a tendon and muscle. SYN: *tenontomyoplasty*.
tenomyotomy (tĕn″ō-mī-ŏt'ō-mĭ) [" + + *tomē*, a cutting]. Excision of lateral portion of a tendon or muscle.
tenonitis (tĕn-ōn-ī'tĭs) 1. [G. *tenōn*, tendon, + *-itis*, inflammation]. Inflammation of a tendon. SYN: *tenontitis*. 2. [*Tenon* + G. *-itis*, inflammation]. Inflammation of Tenon's capsule.
tenonometer (tē″nō-nŏm'ĕ-ter) [G. *teinein*, to stretch, + *metron*, a measure]. Device for measuring amount of intraocular tension.
Tenon's capsule (tē-non'). A thin connective tissue envelope of the eyeball behind the conjunctiva.
T's. space. One bet. the post. surface of the eyeball and Tenon's capsule.
tenontagra (tĕn-ōn-tā'gră, -tăg'ra) [G. *tenōn, tenont-*, tendon, + *agra*, seizure]. A gouty inflammation of the tendons.
tenontitis (tĕn-ōn-tī'tĭs) [" + *-itis*, inflammation]. Inflammation of a tendon. SYN: *tendinitis, tenositis*.
tenontodynia (tĕn-ōn-tō-dĭn'ĭ-ă) [" + *odynē*, pain]. Pain in a tendon. SYN: *tenalgia, tenodynia*.
tenontography (tĕn-ōn-tŏg'ră-fĭ) [" + *graphein*, to write]. A treatise on the tendons.
tenontology (tĕn-ōn-tŏl'ō-jĭ) [" + *logos*, a study]. The study of the tendons.
tenontomyoplasty (tĕn-ōn″tō-mī'ō-plăs″tĭ) [" + *mys, my-*, muscle, + *plassein*, to form]. Plastic surgery, including muscle and tendon repair, in treatment of hernia. SYN: *tenomyoplasty*.
tenontomyotomy (tĕn-ōn″tō-mī-ŏt'ō-mĭ) [" + " + *tomē*, a cutting]. Cutting of the principal tendon of a muscle, with excision of the muscle in part or in whole. SYN: *myotenotomy*.
tenontoplasty (tĕn-ōn″tō-plăs″tĭ) [G. *tenōn, tenont-*, tendon, + *plassein*, to form]. Plastic surgery of defective or injured tendons. SYN: *tenoplasty*.
tenontothecitis (tĕn-ōn-tō-thē-sī'tĭs) [" + *thēkē*, sheath, + *-itis*, inflammation]. Inflammation of a tendon and its sheath. SYN: *tendosynovitis, tendovaginitis, tenosynovitis*.
t. steno'sans. A chronic form of t. with narrowing of the sheath.
tenophyte (tĕn'ō-fīt) [" + *phyton*, a growth]. A cartilaginous or osseous growth on a tendon.
tenoplasty (tĕn'ō-plăs″tĭ) [" + *plassein*, to form]. Reparative surgery of tendons. SYN: *tenontoplasty*.
tenorrhaphy (tĕn-or'ă-fĭ) [" + *rhaphē*, a seam]. Suturing of a tendon.
tenositis (tĕn-ō-sī'tĭs) [" + *-itis*, inflammation]. Inflammation of a tendon. SYN: *tenontitis*.
tenostosis (tĕn-ŏs-tō'sĭs) [" + *osteon*, bone, + *-ōsis*, condition]. Conversion of a tendon into bony tissue.
tenosuspension (ten-o-sus-pen'shun) [G. *tenōn*, tendon, + L. *suspensiō*, a hanging under]. Suspension of the humerus by a layer of a tendon to the acromion process.
tenosuture (tĕn″ō-sū'tūr) [" + L. *sutura*, a stitch]. Reunion of a divided tendon. SYN: *tenorrhaphy*.
tenosynovitis (tĕn″ō-sĭn-ō-vī'tĭs) [" + *syn*, with, + L. *ovum*, egg, + G. *-itis*, inflammation]. 1. Inflammation of a tendon and its sheath. 2. Inflammation of a tendon sheath.
t. crepitans. Inflammation of a tendon sheath in which a cracking sound is heard on motion.

tenosynovitis hyperplastica   T-12   **tereti-**

ETIOL: May follow puncture wounds, contusions, and lacerations, or from lymphatic extension from an abrasion.
SYM: Pain, finger rigid, excessive tenderness.
Most commonly affects flexor tendons.
TREATMENT: Early drainage, rest.
   t. hyperplastica. Painless swelling of extensor tendons over the wrist joint.
tenotome (těn′ō-tōm) [" + *tomos*, a cutting]. Instrument for section of a tendon.
tenotomist (těn-ŏt′ō-mĭst) [" + *tomos*, a cutting]. Specialist in tenotomy.
tenotomy (těn-ŏt′ō-mĭ) [" + *tomē*, a cutting]. Section of a tendon.
tenovaginitis (těn″ō-văj-ĭn-ī′tĭs) [" + L. *vagina*, sheath, + G. *-itis*, inflammation]. Inflammation of a tendon or a tendon and its sheath. SYN: *tenontothecitis*.
tension (těn′shŭn) [L. *tensio*, a stretching]. 1. Process or act of stretching; state of being strained or stretched. 2. Pressure, as arterial tension. 3. Expansive force of a gas or vapor. 4. PT: A synonym for voltage; thus high tension would mean high voltage.
   Thus, to say that the tension of oxygen in arterial blood is 100 mm. of mercury means that the blood contains as much oxygen as it would absorb if exposed to pure oxygen at a pressure of 100 mm. of mercury long enough to reach equilibrium, or if exposed to a gaseous mixture in which the partial pressure of oxygen was 100 mm. of mercury. This method of expression is very convenient in explaining the direction in which the respiratory gases diffuse within the body.
   t., arterial. That of an artery at height of the pulse wave in pressing against the walls.
   t. of gases. Gas pressure measured in percentages of atmospheric pressure.
   When in solution, gases are measured by gas pressure in surrounding medium sufficient to prevent gas from escaping from the solution.
   t., intraocular. Internal pressure of liquid within eyeball.
   t., surface. Molecular property of film on surface of a liquid to resist rupture, the particles tending to pull inward.
   t., suture. One used to reduce pull of the edges of a wound.
tensiophone (těn′sĭ-ō-fōn) [L. *tensio*, tension, + G. *phōnē*, sound]. Device for obtaining blood pressure readings by auscultation and palpation.
tensor (těn′sor) [L. *tensor*, a stretcher]. A muscle making a part tense. SEE: *Muscles, Table of, in Appendix*.
tent (těnt) [O.Fr. *tente*, from L. *tenta*, stretched out]. 1. To keep open with a tent. 2. Cylindrical rod of absorbable material used to dilate the mouth of any hollow organ or canal, to keep the orifices of a wound open, or to absorb discharges.
   When moist, they swell to twice their ordinary size. Manufactured from sponge, sea angle, elm bark, etc.
   VARIETIES: Plain or waxed, straight or curved. Any size.
tentative (těn′tă-tĭv) [L. *tentativus*, from *tentāre*, to try]. Noting a diagnosis subject to change because of insufficient data; experimental.
tenth cranial nerve. Nerve supplying most of the abdominal viscera, the heart, lungs, and esophagus. SYN: *pneumogastric nerve, q.v.* SEE: *cranial nerves in Appendix*.
tentigo (těn-tī′gō) [L.]. Abnormal sexual desire. SYN: *lasciviousness, lust, nymphomania, satyriasis*.
tentorium (těn-tō′rĭ-ŭm) [L. *tentōrium*, tent]. A tentlike structure or part.
   t. cerebelli. BNA. The process of the dura mater bet. the cerebrum and cerebellum supporting the occipital lobes.
tentum (těn′tŭm) [L. *tentum*, from *tendere*, to stretch]. The penis.
tephromalacia (těf″rō-măl-ā′sĭ-ă) [G. *tephros*, gray, + *malakia*, softening]. Softening of the gray substance of brain or spinal cord.
tephromyelitis (těf″rō-mī-ĕl-ī′tĭs) [" + *myelos*, marrow, + *-itis*, inflammation]. Inflammation of the gray matter of the spinal cord. SYN: *poliomyelitis*.
tephrosis (těf′rō′sĭs) [" + *-osis*, condition]. Incineration; cremation.
tephrylometer (těf-rĭ-lom′ě-ter) [" + *ylē*, matter, + *metron*, a measure]. Device for measuring the thickness of the cerebral cortex, the gray matter of brain.
tepid (těp′ĭd) [L. *tepidus*, lukewarm]. Slightly warm; lukewarm.
   t. bath. One about 86° F. (30° C.).
tepidarium (těp-ĭd-ā′rĭ-ŭm) [L. pert. to a warm bath]. A place for a warm bath.
ter- [L.]. Combining form meaning *thrice*.
teratic (těr-ăt′ĭk) [G. *teratikos*, monstrous]. Pert. to a monster.
terato- [G.]. Combining form meaning a *marvel, prodigy, monster*.
teratoblastoma (těr″ă-tō-blăs-tō′mă) [G. *teras, terat-*, monster, + *blastos*, germ, + *-ōma*, tumor]. A tumor containing embryonic material but which is not representative of all 3 germinal layers. SEE: *teratoma*.
teratoid (těr′ă-toyd) [G. *teras, terat-*, monster, + *eidos*, form]. Resembling a monster.
   t. tumor. Tumor of embryonic remains from all of the germinal layers. SYN: *teratoma*.
teratology (těr-ăt-ŏl′ō-jĭ) [" + *logos*, a study]. Branch of science dealing with the study of monsters.
teratoma (těr-ă-tō′mă) [" + *-ōma*, tumor]. Congenital tumor containing embryonic elements of all 3 primary germ layers, as hair, teeth, etc. SYN: *dermoid*.
teratomatous (ter-ă-tō′mă-tus) [" + *-ōma*, tumor]. Pert. to or resembling a teratoma.
teratophobia (ter″ă-tō-fō′bĭ-ă) [" + *phobos*, fear]. Abnormal fear of giving birth to a monster or of being in contact with one.
teratosis (těr-ă-tō′sĭs) [" + *-osis*, condition]. A monstrosity.
tere (tě′rē) [L. rub]. Rub.
terebinthinate (ter′ě-bĭn′thĭ-nāt) [L. *terebinthus*, turpentine]. Containing or agent containing turpentine.
terebrant, terebrating (ter′ě-brant, -brāt-ing) [L. *terebrāre*, to bore]. Boring or piercing, said of pain.
terebration (ter-ě-brā′shŭn) [L. *terebrāre*, to bore]. 1. The act of boring. SYN: *trephining*. 2. A boring pain.
teres (tě′rēz) [L. *teres*, rounded, polished]. 1. Round and smooth; cylindrical. 2. A rounded muscle.
   t. major. A muscle that draws the arm down and back.
   t. minor. A muscle inserted in the great tuberosity of the humerus, which rotates the humerus outward and abducts it.   [*round*.
tereti- [L.]. Combining form meaning

tergo- [L.]. Combining form, *the back*.
tergum (ter'gŭm) [L.]. The back.
ter in die [L.]. Three times a day.
term (term) [L. *terminus*, a boundary].
1. A limit or boundary. 2. A definite period. 3. Gestation at normal period.
terma (ter'mă) [G. *terma*, limit]. A thin plate in front of the optic chiasm. SYN: *lamina terminalis*.
terminal (ter'mĭn-ăl) [L. *terminus*, a boundary]. 1. An end or extremity. 2. Pert. to or placed at the end. [air sac.
  t. alve'olus. A pulmonary vesicle or
  t. artery. One with no branches, but which splits into capillaries.
  t. dementia. D. following mania or melancholia or other acute insanity.
  t. filum. Slender end of spinal cord.
  t. infection. One appearing in the late stage of another disease; often fatal.
terminology (ter-mĭn-ŏl'ō-jĭ) [L. *terminus*, term, + G. *logos*, word]. The special terms used in any field, as an art or science. SYN: *nomenclature*.
ternary (ter'na-rĭ) [L. *ternarius*, triple]. 1. Threefold; triple; third. 2. Composed of 3 elements.
  t. acid. An inorganic acid containing hydrogen and 2 other elements.
  t. bodies. The fats, proteins, and carbohydrates of any food.
teropterin (ter-ŏp'ter-ĭn). Trade name for sodium pteroyl triglutamate solution. Used for palliation of certain symptoms of malignancy in treatment adjunctive to x-ray, radium, and surgery.
ter'pin hy'drate. USP. White crystalline substance with a turpentine taste made by the interaction of rectified spirits of turpentine, alcohol, and nitric acid.
  ACTION AND USES: As an antiseptic and expectorant.
  DOSAGE (average): 4 gr. (0.25 Gm.).
terra (tĕr'ă) [L.]. Earth; soil.
  t. al'ba. White clay.
  t. fullon'ica. Fuller's earth.
terracing (ter'ăs-ĭng) [O.Fr. *terrace*]. Suturing in several rows through thick tissues in closing a wound.
terramycin hydrochloride (tĕr″ră-mī'sĭn). A chemotherapeutic agent effective in many infectious diseases; in bacterial, rickettsial, and viral-like infections, gonorrhea, and other conditions.
  DOSAGE: From 2 to 3 Gm. daily, in divided doses, every 6 hrs. In severe infections, from 4 to 6 Gm. daily.
terror (ter'or) [L. *terror*, fear]. Very great fear. [esp. of children.
  t., night. Nightmare or night terror,
tertian (ter'shŭn) [L. *tertianus*, pert. to the third]. Occurring every 3rd day.
  t. fever. A malarial fever with paroxysms every other day.
  ETIOL: The sporulation and invasion of a blood parasite in new red blood corpuscles.
  t. fever, double. The paroxysms occur every day, being similar on alternate days. SEE: *quotidian fever*.
tertiarism, tertiarismus (ter'shĭ-ar-ĭzm, -ĭz'mŭs). All the symptoms, collectively, of tertiary syphilis.
tertiary (ter'shĭ-a-rĭ) [L. *tertius*, third]. Third in order or stage.
  t. alcohol. One containing the trivalent group. COH.
  t. syphilis. Third and most advanced stage of syphilis.
tertipara (tĕr-tĭp'ă-ră) [L. *tertius*, third, + *parēre*, to bring forth]. A woman who has given birth to 3 children.
tessellated (tĕs'ĕl-ā-tĕd) [L. *tessella*, a square]. Composed of little squares.

t. epithelium. Pavement epithelium* composed of overlapping squamous cells.
test (test) [L. *testum*, an earthen vessel]. 1. An examination. 2. Method to determine the presence or nature of a substance, or the presence of a disease. 3. A chemical reaction. 4. A reagent or substance used in making a test.
  t., acetone. Test for presence of acetone in the urine; made by adding a few drops of sodium nitroprusside to the urine along with strong ammonia water. Presence of acetone causes formation of a magenta ring at outline of contacts.
  t., Allen-Doisy. Test to determine amount of estrogen content in female blood serum by its reaction on secretions of mice.
  t., Aschheim-Zondek. Test for pregnancy by injecting the patient's urine subcutaneously in immature female mice.
  t., Binet-Simon. Method of ascertaining the mental capacity of children by asking a series of suitable questions. SEE: *Binet age*. [proteins or urea.
  t., biuret. Test for the presence of
  t., Brouha. Test for pregnancy by injecting the urine of the patient into male mice for 8 to 10 days. Positive reaction indicated by hypertrophy and hyperemia of the seminal vesicles.
  t., Chrobak. Cancer is present if probing an eroded cervix produces bleeding and crumbling of the tissue.
  t., Friedman. Test for pregnancy by injecting urine of the patient into unmated mature female rabbits, a positive reaction being indicated by formation of corpora lutea and corpora haemorrhagica.
  t., Gelle's. Test for ear lesions by employing rubber tubing and a tuning fork.
  t., Huhner. Aspiration of vagina within an hour after coitus, to investigate sperm activity.
  t., Kahn's. Precipitation test for syphilis. [as litmus paper.
  t. paper. Paper used in making tests,
  t., pregnancy. Test to determine pregnancy.
  t., Rubin. Test for patency of the fallopian tubes by insufflation with carbon dioxide; used to determine cause of sterility.
  t., Schiller's. Test for cancer of the cervix by painting with iodine solution; since cancer cells do not stain with iodine, they turn white or yellow.
  t., Schneider's. A pregnancy test using female rabbits.
  t., Schwabach's. Test for hearing using tuning forks.
  t. solution. A standard solution used in making a test.
  t. tube. A plain tube of thin glass, closed at 1 end, used for simple tests.
  t., urea balance. Test of the kidney function by measuring intake and output of urea.
  t., Wassermann. Diagnostic test for syphilis based on principle of fixation of complement.
test, words pert. to: albumin, alpha, Babcock's, Benedict's, bensidin, Bercovitz, Bernreuter's, beta, Bourdon's, choloscopy, chromocholoscopy, coagulation time t., Fehling's, fluctuation, group t., heart, Heller's cold t. for albumin, hemoglobin, Kahn, mire, mirror-drill, patch t., precipitin, Rinne, Rothera's, Schick, toleration, Wassermann.
testectomy (tĕs-tĕk'tō-mĭ) [L. *testis*, testicle, + G. *ektomē*, excision]. 1. Removal of a testicle. SYN: *castration*. 2. Removal of a corpus quadrigeminum.

testes (tĕs'tēz) (sing. *testis*) [L.]. Two glandular bodies in the scrotum of the male. The producers of the male germinative cell. SYN: *testicles*.

testicle (tĕs'tĭ-kl) [L. *testiculus*, a little testis]. One of the 2 ovoid male gonads situated in the scrotum which produce spermatozoa and some of the fluid elements of the semen. SYN: *testis, q.v.*

They contain numerous secreting tubules in which spermatozoa are produced, which are gathered from the corpus of Highmore and ejected through the vas* deferens. Testicles are suspended from the spermatic cord. The left one is lower than the right one.

t. compression reflex. Contraction of abdominal muscles following moderate compression of testicle.

t., displaced. A testicle within (abnormally) the inguinal canal, or pelvis.

t., inverted. One reversed in the scrotum so that the epididymis attaches to the ant. instead of post. part of gland.

t., undescended. One or both remain in the inguinal canal or abdominal cavity at birth.

testicond (tes'tĭ-kŏnd) [L. *testis*, testis, + *condere*, to hide]. Having the testicles undescended.

testicular (tĕs-tĭk'ū-lar) [L. *testiculus*, a little testis]. Relating to a testicle.

t. cord. The spermatic cord. SYN: *funiculus spermaticus*.

t. duct. Excretory duct of the testicle. SYN: *vas deferens*.

t. fluid. Semen.

t. therapy. 1. The injections of t. fluid or extracts. 2. T. substances administered by inunction.

testis (tes'tĭs) (pl. *testes*) [L. *testis*, testicle]. 1. A testicle, the male reproductive gland in the scrotum. 2. One of the 2 post. tubercles of the corpus quadrigeminum. SYN: *colliculus inferior*.

They have an internal secretion that influences mental and physical development, which comes from the interstitial cells, or Leydig's cells.

Hyperfunction may cause early maturity, such as dentition, large sexual organs with early functional activity, and growth of hair.

Hypofunction is shown by undeveloped testes, absence of body hair, high-pitched voice, sterility, smooth skin, loss of sex desire, low metabolism, and eunuchoid* or eunuch* type.

RS: *agenitalism, androsterone, apella, castration, chylocele, cremaster, didymis, emasculation, eunuch, eviration, hydrocele, interstitial cell, "orch-" words, sarcocele, scirrhus, scrotum, semen, unsex.*

t., descent of. Change in position of the testis from abdominal cavity to scrotum during fetal life.

testitis (tĕs-tī'tĭs) [L. *testis*, testicle, + *-itis*, inflammation]. Inflammation of a testis. SYN: *orchitis*.

testitoxicosis (tĕs'tĭ-tŏks-ĭ-kō'sĭs) [" + G. *toxikon*, poison, + *-ōsis*, condition]. A toxic state sometimes following ligation of the vas deferens.

test meal. A meal, usually small, of definite quality and composition, given to stimulate gastric secretion and thus furnish material to be withdrawn for examination.

They are given principally to determine: (a) The motility of the stomach, and (b) the functioning of the alimentary tract by determining the character of the food mass after having been acted upon by the digestive secretions.

Today, the test meal is also given to determine the activity and functioning of other organs closely associated with those of digestion. Since the advent of the x-ray and fluoroscope as diagnostic agents the test meal is not so frequently ordered as before. In obtaining results from the test meals, 2 methods are used: (a) The *fractional* method, and (b) the *single specimen* method.

TYPES: (a) One composed of material that determines the character of the gastric contents, and (b) one that determines the motility of the stomach and intestines. A routine examination is conveniently carried out in the following sequence. The first 2 steps must, of course, be modified if the fractional method is adopted:

(1) Give the patient a test meal upon an empty stomach, washing the stomach previously if necessary.

(2) At the height of digestion, usually in 1 hour, remove the contents of the stomach with a stomach tube.

(3) Measure and examine microscopically.

(4) Filter. A suction filter is desirable and may be necessary when much mucus is present.

(5) During filtration, examine microscopically and make qualitative test for (a) free hydrochloric acid, (b) lactic acid.

(6) When sufficient filtrate is obtained, make quantitative estimations of (a) total acidity, (b) free hydrochloric acid, (c) combined hydrochloric acid (if necessary).

(7) Make whatever additional tests

TESTES.
1. Septa. 2. Tunica albuginea. 3. Tunica vaginalis. 4. Spermatic artery. 5. Vas deferens. 6. Vas aberrans. 7. Globus minor.

seem desirable, as for blood, pepsin, or rennin.

OBTAINING THE CONTENTS: Gastric juice is secreted continuously, but quantities sufficiently large for examination are often not obtainable from the fasting stomach. In clinical work, therefore, it is desirable to stimulate secretion with food—which is the natural and most efficient stimulus—before attempting to collect the gastric fluid. Different foods stimulate secretion to different degrees, hence, for sake of uniform results, certain standard test meals have been adopted. The gastric fluid is obtained by aspiration through a tube.

It is important to assure the patient that introduction of the tube cannot possibly be painful and that if he can control the spasm of his throat, he will experience very little choking sensation. The tube should be dipped in warm water just before using, or chilled in ice water in order to reduce possible nausea; the use of glycerin or other lubricant is undesirable. With the patient seated upon a chair, his clothing protected by a large rubber apron (or if these are not on hand, a few towels draped around the upper part of the chest), his head tilted forward, the tip of the tube, held as one would a pen, is introduced far back into the pharynx.

He is then urged to swallow, and the tube is pushed boldly into the esophagus until the colored ring upon it reaches the incisor teeth, thus indicating that the tip is in the stomach. If, now, the patient coughs, or strains as if at stool, the contents of the stomach will usually be forced out through the tube.

Should this fail, the fluid can generally be pumped out by alternate compression of the tube and the bulb. If unsuccessful at first, the attempt should be repeated with the tube pushed a little farther in or withdrawn a few inches, since the distance to the stomach is not the same in all cases. The tube may become clogged with pieces of food, in which case it must be withdrawn, cleaned, and reintroduced.

If, after all efforts, no fluid is obtained, another test meal should be given and withdrawn after a somewhat shorter period, since, owing to excessive motility, the stomach may empty itself in less than the usual time.

Care must be exercised to prevent saliva or vomitus running down the outside of the tube, and mingling with the gastric juice in the basin. As the tube is removed it should be pinched between the fingers so as to save any fluid that may be in it. The stomach tube must be used with great care, or not at all, in cases of gastric ulcer, aneurysm, uncompensated heart disease, and marked arteriosclerosis. Except in gastric ulcer, the danger lies in the retching produced, but the tube can safely be used if the patient takes it easily.

This procedure can be made much easier if one of the newer types of stomach tube is used, of which the Rehfuss tube is best known. The metal tip is placed well back in the patient's pharynx, and he is directed to swallow several times in rapid succession with his lips closed and with his tongue forming a groove for the tube, upon which he sucks bet. swallows. Deep breathing will aid in overcoming nausea.

After it has reached the stomach, indicated by the colored ring reaching the incisor teeth, the heavy tip sinks to the most dependent portion, and as much or as little of the stomach contents as desired may be drawn off by means of an aspirating syringe. A narrow tube of this type is esp. useful for the fractional method of examination described below, as it may be left in place for a long time without serious inconvenience to the patient, particularly if he is induced to read, to take his mind off the procedure that is going on. To prevent its passing on through the pylorus it may be attached to the cheek with adhesive plaster.

THE FRACTIONAL METHOD: With the understanding that there is great variation in the time at which the height of digestion is reached, a method of examination known as the fractional method has come into use. This is carried out as follows:

Insert a Rehfuss stomach tube before breakfast and empty the stomach as much as possible. Remove the tube and give an Ewald test meal, or breakfast, which must be chewed thoroughly.

Reinsert the tube and withdraw 5 cc. of the stomach contents at 15-minute intervals, until the fluid is free from food particles or until the acidity has returned to the same level as was found in the fasting content. The tube is left in place during the whole procedure. By means of the Rehfuss tube a much larger quantity of gastric juice can often be obtained from the fasting stomach than has been thought possible.

ABSORPTIVE POWER OF THE STOMACH: This is a very unimportant function, only a few substances being absorbed in the stomach. It is delayed in most organic diseases of the stomach, esp. in dilatation and carcinoma, but not in neurosis.

MOTOR POWER OF THE STOMACH: This refers to the rapidity with which the stomach passes its contents on into the intestines. It is very important; intestinal digestion can compensate for insufficient or absent stomach digestion only so long as the motor power is good. Motility is impaired to some extent in chronic gastritis. It is esp. deficient in pyloric obstruction caused by malignant or benign new growths; in pyloric spasm, as in hyperchlorhydria, and in atony of the stomach wall which is usually associated with dilatation and gastroptosis.

The best evidence of deficient motor power is the detection of food in the stomach at a time when it should be empty before breakfast in the morning. A special test meal containing easily recognized materials (rice pudding with currants, jam with seeds, or raisins) is sometimes given and removed at the end of 6 or 7 hours. When more than 100 cc. of fluid are obtained with the tube 1 hour after an Ewald breakfast, deficient motility may be inferred.

RS: *Benzidin, Boas, Ewald's, fractional, gastric motor, Hausman's stagnation, Klemperer's, Leube's, Riegel's, Sahli's, Salzer's, Schmidt's and Von Pirquet's test meals.*

testosterone (těs-tŏs'ter-ōn) [L. *testis,* testicle]. A hormonal crystalline substance isolated from bull's testes and prepared synthetically from cholesterol.

t. propionate. The propionic acid ester of testosterone, a much more potent form.

ACTION AND USES: In dysmenorrhea,

gynecomastia, adult eunuchs and eunuchoids, and in adult hypogonadism. Causes erection, growth of penis and prostate to normal size, growth of hair, and psychic changes.
DOSAGE: Minimum effective 3/8 gr. (25 mg.) intramuscularly, 3 times weekly.

tetanic (tē-tăn'ĭk) [G. *tetanikos*, pert. to a stretching]. 1. Pert. to or producing tetanus. 2. Any agent producing tetanic spasms.

t. convulsion. A tonic one with constant muscular contraction.

tetaniform (tē-tan'ĭ-form) [G. *tetanos*, tetanus, + L. *forma*, shape]. Resembling tetanus.

tetanilla (tĕt-ăn-ĭl'lă) [L.]. 1. Mild form of tetany* without rigidity. 2. Twitchings of a limited group of muscular fibers with clonic paroxysmal contractions.

tetanism (tĕt'ăn-ĭzm) [G. *tetanos*, tetanus, + *-ismos*, condition]. Persistent muscular hypertonicity resembling tetanus, esp. in infants.

tetanization (tĕt-ăn-ĭ-zā'shŭn) [G. *tetanos*, tetanus]. The production or condition of tetanic convulsions or symptoms.

tetanize (tĕt'ăn-īz) [G. *tetanos*, tetanus]. To induce tonic muscular spasms.

tetanode (tĕt'ă-nōd) [" + *eidos*, form]. 1. Resembling tetanus. SYN: *tetanoid*. 2. Noting interval bet. recurrent tonic spasms in tetany.

tetanoid (tĕt'ă-noyd) [" + *eidos*, form]. Resembling tetanus. SYN: *tetaniform*.

t. fever. Inflamed condition of membrane of spinal cord and brain. SYN: *cerebrospinal meningitis*.

t. paraplegia. Paralysis of lower extremities due to lateral sclerosis of spinal cord. SYN: *spastic paraplegia*.

tetanomotor (tĕt″ăn-o-mō'tor) [" + L. *motor*, a mover]. Appliance for the production of tetanic motor spasms mechanically by shocking a nerve.

tetanophil, tetanophilic (tĕt'ăn-ō-fĭl, tĕt″ăn-ō-fĭl'ĭk) [" + *philein*, to love]. Possessing an affinity for tetanus toxin.

tetanous (tĕt'ă-nŭs) [G. *tetanos*, tetanus]. Of the nature of or characteristic of tetanus or tetany, as *tetanous serum*.

tetanus (tĕt'ă-nŭs) [G. *tetanos*, tetanus]. 1. An infectious, acute disease due to the toxin of *Bacillus tetani*, in which there is a state of more or less persistent, painful tonic spasm of some of the voluntary muscles. 2. Continuous tonic spasm of a muscle.

Usually begins gradually, but may begin suddenly; may be of brief duration or last some weeks. The first sign is stiffness of the jaw and esophageal muscles and some of the muscles of neck. Soon the jaws become rigidly fixed (trismus, or lockjaw), the voice is altered, muscles of the face contract, producing a wild, excited expression, a compound of bitter laughter and crying (risus sardonicus). The muscles of back, extremities, and penis become tetanic.

If the patient be bent back in a bow, the condition is termed *opisthotonos*; if he be bent to the side, *pleurothotonos*; if he be bent forward, *emprosthotonos*.

The paroxysms are reflex, and are excited by noises, currents of air, and even irritation of bedclothes. The temperature usually rises and may attain remarkable height (113° F.), and continues to rise for a time after death. The pain is great; patient also suffering from hunger, thirst, and want of sleep. The mind is clear. This disease is usually, but not always, fatal, the patient expiring from asphyxia or exhaustion.

RS: *emprosthotonos, lockjaw, opisthotonos, pleurothotonos, posture, risus sardonicus.*

t., anticus. Form in which the body is bowed forward.

t., artificial. Form produced by a drug like strychnine or by mechanical appliance.

t., cephalic. Same as *kopf tetanus*.

t., cerebral. A form produced by inoculating the brain of animals with tetanus antitoxin, marked by epileptiform convulsions and excitement.

t. dorsalis. Tetanus in which the body is bent backward.

t., extensor. That which affects the extensors especially.

t., head. Same as *kopf tetanus*.

t., hydrophobic. Kopf tetanus.

t., idiopathic. That which occurs without any visible lesion.

t., imitative. Hysteria which simulates tetanus.

t., impf. Inoculated tetanus; cultures afford a special form of pathogenic bacillus.

t. infantum. Tetanus of young infants, due to infection of umbilicus.

t., intermittent. A disease characterized by painful tonic and symmetric spasm of muscles of extremities. Occurs after typhoid fever, diarrhea, exposure to cold, rickets, after ingestion of alkaline salts, deficiency of calcium, and excision of the parathyroid gland. May continue for several weeks; usually ends in recovery. SYN: *tetany*.

t., kopf. Form due to a wound of the head, esp. one near the eyebrow. It is marked by trismus, facial paralysis on one side, and pronounced dysphagia; resembles rabies; often fatal. Called also *cephalic tetanus, head tetanus, hydrophobic tetanus.*

t. lateralis. Form in which the body is bent sideways.

t., localized. Tetanic spasm of a single part.

t. neonatorum. Tetanus of very young infants, usually due to infection of navel.

t. paradoxus. Cephalic tetanus in which condition is combined with paralysis of the facial or other cranial nerve.

t., partial. Tetany.

t., posticus. Same as *t. dorsalis*.

t., postoperative. T. which follows an operation.

t., puerperal. T. which occurs in childbed.

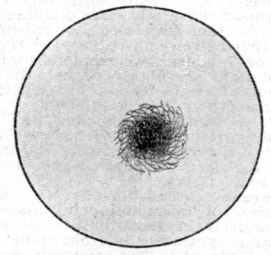

TETANUS BACILLI, GROWTH OF.
In glucose-gelatin, anaerobic. Magnified about ten times. Medusa head type of colony.

t., rheumatic. Form due to exposure to cold and wet.
t., Ritter's. Tetanic contractions at opening of a constant current which has been passing along a nerve for some time; seen in tetany.
t., toxic. Produced by overdose of nux vomica or strychnine.
t., traumatic. T. which follows wound poisoning.
tetany (tĕt′ă-nĭ) [G. *tetanos*, tetanus]. A nervous affection, characterized by intermittent tonic spasms, which are usually paroxysmal and involve the extremities; most frequent in the young; frequently associated with pregnancy or lactation.
  ETIOL: Usually due to parathyroid deficiency. Sometimes excited by exposure, emotional excitement, or one of the infectious fevers; very grave form induced by thyroidectomy and accidental removal of parathyroid glands and by lavage in gastric dilatation.
  SYM: Characterized by nervousness, irritability and apprehension, numbness and tingling of the extremities, cramps of the various muscles, particularly those of the hands, producing a typical accoucheur type of hand and extreme extension of the feet. Cataract is prone to develop in persons afflicted with tetany. Bilateral tonic spasms in arms and legs, jaws rarely involved. Contractions usually paroxysmal and are attended with pain. Electrocontractility of muscles greatly exaggerated. May be slight edema. Sensation not disturbed; mind clear, fever slight or absent.
  PROG: Usually favorable. Attacks following thyroidectomy and lavage sometimes fatal.
  TREATMENT: Parathyroid hormone, injections of calcium for active treatment should be given intramuscularly, and sometimes intravenously or intraspinally. Good hygiene, tonics, electricity, sedatives. Warm or cold baths followed by friction.
  Antitetanic serum most important; should be given as a prophylactic in every wound coming in contact with dirt.
  DIET: Nourish well with beef tea, animal soups, milk, soft eggs, etc. Sometimes necessary to give nutrient enemata.
t., duration. Continuous contraction, esp. in degenerated muscles, in response to a continuous electric current.
t., gastric. Severe t. from stomach disorders accompanied by tonic, painful spasms of extremities.
t., hyperventilation. T. caused by continued forced respiration.
t., latent. T. caused by stimulation.
t., parathyroid. T. due to excision of the parathyroid gland.
t., thyroprival. T. resulting from suspended thyroid function.
tetarcone (tĕt′ar-kōn) [G. *tetartos*, fourth, + *kōnos*, cone]. Fourth or distolingual cusp of an upper molar tooth. SYN: *tetartocone*.
tetartanopia, tetartanopsia (tĕt″ar-tăn-ō′pĭ-ă, -ŏp′sĭ-ă) [″ + *ops*, eye, — + *opsis*, vision]. Symmetrical blindness in the same quadrant of each visual field. SYN: *hemianopsia, quadrant*.
tetartocone (tĕt-ar′tō-kōn) [″ + *kōnos*, cone]. The distolingual cusp of an upper molar tooth. SYN: *tetarcone*.
tethelin (tĕth′ē-lĭn) [G. *tethēlos*, flourishing]. A substance derived from the ant. lobe of the pituitary having an accelerating effect on growth.

tetmil (tĕt′mĭl). Ten millimeters; a unit of measurement.
tetra-, tetr- [G.]. Combining forms meaning *four*.
tetrabasic (tĕt″ră-bā′sĭk) [G. *tetra*, four, + *basis*, base]. Having 4 replaceable hydrogen atoms, said of an acid or acid salt.
tetrablastic (tĕt″ră-blăs′tĭk) [″ + *blastos*, germ]. Having 4 germinal layers, the *ectoderm, endoderm,* and 2 *mesodermic* layers.
tetrabromofluorescein (tĕt″ră-brōm″ō-flū-or-ĕs′ĭn, -ē-ĭn). A dye, $C_{20}H_8Br_4O_5$, obtained from action of bromine on fluorescein, used as a stain in microscopy. SYN: *eosin*.
tetrachlorethylene (tĕt″ră-klor-ĕth′ĭl-ēn). A clear, colorless liquid with a characteristic odor.
  USES: As anthelmintic, resembling in action carbon tetrachloride, but less toxic.
  DOSAGE: 45 ℳ (3 cc.), followed by saline cathartic.
tetracid (tĕ-trăs′ĭd) [G. *tetra*, four, + L. *acidus*, sour]. 1. Able to react with 4 molecules of a monoacid or 2 of a diacid to form a salt or ester, said of a base or alcohol; term disapproved by some authorities. 2. Having 4 hydrogen atoms replaceable by basic atoms or radicals, said of acids. 3. An acid containing 4 acid hydrogen atoms.
Tetracoccus (tĕt″ră-kŏk′ŭs) [″ + *kokkos*, berry]. Genus of micrococcus arranged in groups of 4 by division into 2 planes.
tetracrotic (tĕt″ră-krŏt′ĭk) [″ + *krotos*, a beat]. Noting a pulse or pulse tracing with 4 upward strokes in the descending limb of the wave. SYN: *catatricrotic*.
tetrad (tĕt′răd) [G. *tetras, tetrad-*, number four]. 1. A group of 4 things with something in common. 2. An element having a valency or combining power of 4. 3. A group of 4 similar bodies. 4. A group of 4 parts, said of cells produced by division in 2 planes, or of a chromosome in 4 parts in preparation for 2 mitotic divisions in maturation.
tetragenous (tĕt-răj′ĕn-ŭs) [G. *tetra*, four, + *gennan*, to produce]. Dividing into groups of 4; noting bacteria, as *Micrococcus tetragenus*.
tetragonum (tĕt″ră-gō′nŭm) [L. from G. *tetragōnon*]. Quadrangle.
t. lumba'le. A lumbar quadrangle surrounded by 4 muscles.
tetramastia (tĕt″ră-măs′tĭ-ă) [G. *tetra*, four, + *mastos*, breast]. Condition characterized by presence of 4 breasts. SYN: *tetramazia*.
tetramazia (tĕt″ră-mā′zĭ-ă) [″ + *mazos*, breast]. Condition of having 4 breasts. SYN: *tetramastia*.
tetrameric, tetramerous (tĕt″ră-mĕr′ĭk, tĕt-răm′ĕr-ŭs) [″ + *meros*, a part]. Having 4 parts, or arranged in groups of 4 parts.
tetranopsia (tĕt-ră-nŏp′sĭ-ă) [″ + *an-*, priv. + *opsis*, vision]. Obliteration of visual field by one-quarter.
tetraplegia (tĕt-ră-plē′jĭ-ă) [″ + *plēgē*, a stroke]. Paralysis of both arms and legs.
tetraster (tĕt-răs′ter) [″ + *astēr*, star]. A figure in which there are 4 asters, instead of more commonly 2; occurring abnormally in mitosis.
Tetrastoma (tĕt-răs′tō-mă) [″ + *stoma*, mouth]. A genus of trematode worms found in urine occasionally, having 4 suckers.
tetter (tĕt′ĕr) [A.S. *teter*]. 1. Any of

various vesicular cutaneous diseases, as herpes, ringworm, or eczema. 2. A pimple or blister.
 t., blister. Disease with bullae formation and pigmented spots. SYN: *pemphigus*.
 t., brawny. Excessive discharge from oil glands of scalp. SYN: *seborrhea capitis*.
 t., crusted. Inflammatory skin disease with pustule formation. SYN: *impetigo*.
 t., dry. Inflammatory skin disease with vesiculation and shedding of dry scales. SYN: *eczema, scaly*.
 t., eating. Tuberculous disease of the skin. SYN: *lupus*.
 t., honeycomb. Contagious skin disease with honeycomblike crust formation. SYN: *favus*.
 t., milky. Brawny tetter in infants. SYN: *crusta lactea*.
textiform (těks'tĭ-form) [L. *textum*, web, + *forma*, shape]. Resembling a network, web or mesh.
textoblastic (těks"tō-blăs'tĭk) [L. *textus*, tissue, + G. *blastos*, germ]. Forming adult tissue; regenerative; noting cells.
textoma (těks-tō'mă) [" + G. *-ōma*, tumor]. A tumor made up of completely differentiated tissue cells.
textural (těks'tū-răl [L. *textura*, a weaving]. Concerning the texture or constitution of a tissue.
T fracture. One in which bone splits both longitudinally and transversely.
thalamencephalon (thăl"ăm-ĕn-sĕf'ăl-ŏn) [G. *thalamos*, chamber, + *egkephalos*, brain]. The interbrain; an embryonic structure produced from the post. part of the anterior cerebral vesicle composed of the epithalamus, hypothalamus, and the thalamus. SYN: *diencephalon*.
thalamic (thăl-ăm'ĭk) [G. *thalamos*, chamber]. Pert. to the thalamus.
 t. epilepsy. E. resulting from disease of the thalamus.
 t. syndrome. Sensory disturbances and pain in conjunction with mild hemiplegia.
 ETIOL: Optic thalamus lesion.
thalamo- [G.]. Combining form meaning *chamber, part of brain at which a nerve originates*.
thalamocele, thalamocoele (thăl'ăm-ō-sēl) [G. *thalamos*, chamber, + *koilia*, a hollow]. The 3rd ventricle of the brain.
thalamocortical (thăl"ăm-ō-kor'tĭ-kăl) [" + L. *cortex, cortic-*, rind]. Pert. to the optic thalamus and the cerebral cortex.
thalamolenticular (thăl"ăm-ō-lĕn-tĭk'ū-lar) [" + L. *lenticula*, a small lentil]. Concerning the optic thalamus and the lenticular nucleus.
thalamotomy (thăl-ă-mŏt'ō-mĭ) [G. *thalamos*, chamber, + *tome*, incision]. A psychosurgical procedure for mental illness. A wire electrode is passed down into the thalamus, and a portion about the size of an almond is coagulated. Said to produce fewer unpleasant personality changes than *lobotomy, q.v.*
thalamus (thăl'ă-mŭs) (pl. *thalami*) [G. *thalamos*, chamber]. BNA. The largest subdivision of the diencephalon on either side, consisting chiefly of an ovoid, gray nuclear mass in the lateral wall of the 3rd ventricle.
 The medial and ant. nuclei are phylogenetically the older part or *paleothalamus*, and the lateral part is the *neothalamus*.
 t. opticus. Same as *thalamus*.
thalassophobia (thăl-ăs"sō-fō'bĭ-ă) [G. *thalassa*, sea, + *phobos*, fear]. Abnormal fear of the sea.

thalassotherapy (thăl-ăs"sō-ther'ă-pĭ) [" + *therapeia*, treatment]. Treatment of disease by living at the seaside, by sea bathing, sea voyages, or sea air.
thallinization (thăl-lĕn-ĭ-zā'shŭn) [G. *thallos*, a young shoot]. Treatment with doses of thalline or its salts.
thallium (thăl'lĭ-ŭm) [L. from G. *thallos*, a young shoot]. A rare, lustrous, white metal. Symb. Tl. At. wt. 204.39.
thamuria (thă-mū'rĭ-ă) [G. *thamus*, often, + *ouron*, urine]. Abnormally frequent urination. SYN: *pollakiuria*.
thanato- [G.]. Combining form meaning *death*.
thanatobiological (thăn"ă-tō-bī-ō-lŏj'ĭk-ăl) [G. *thanatos*, death, + *bios*, life, + *logos*, study]. Relating to the processes of life and death.
thanatognomonic (thăn"ăt-ŏg-nō-mŏn'ĭk) [" + *gnōmonikos*, knowing]. Indicative of the approach of death.
thanatoid (thăn'ă-toyd) [" + *eidos*, form]. Resembling death.
thanatology (thăn"ă-tol'ō-jĭ) [" + *logos*, science]. The science of death.
thanatomania (thăn"ă-tō-mā'nĭ-ă) [" + *mania*, madness]. Condition of homicidal or suicidal mania.
thanatometer (thăn-ă-tŏm'ĕt-ĕr) [" + *metron*, a measure]. Instrument for determining occurrence of death by internal temperature.
thanatophobia (thăn"ă-tō-fō'bĭ-ă) [" + *phobos*, fear]. Morbid fear of death.
thanatopsia, thanatopsy (thăn"ă-top'sĭ-ă, thăn'ăt-ŏp"sĭ) [" + *opsis*, view]. Examination of a dead body to determine cause of death. SYN: *autopsy, necropsy*.
thaumato- [G.]. Combining form meaning *wonder, marvel*.
theaism (thē'ă-ĭzm) [L. *thea*, tea, + G. *-ismos*, condition]. Chronic poisoning from excess of tea drinking. SYN: *themism, theism*.
thebaism (thē'bă-ĭzm) [G. *Thebai*, Thebes (opium of)]. Condition produced by opium.
Thebesius' foramina (thē-bē'zĭ-ūs). Orifices of the Thebesius' veins, opening into the right auricle of the heart.
 T's. valve. An endocardial fold at entrance of the coronary sinus into right auricle.
 T's. veins. Venules conveying blood from the myocardium to the auricles or ventricles.
theca (thē'kă) [G. *thēkē*, a box]. A sheath of investing membrane, esp. the synovial sheath of a tendon.
 t. cor'dis. Pericardium, which sheathes the heart.
 t. follic'uli. Outer wall of a graafian follicle.
 t. ten'dinis. Synovial sheath of a tendon.
 t. vertebra'lis. Dura mater of the spinal cord.
thecal (thē'kăl) [G. *thēkē*, a box]. Pert. to a sheath.
 t. abscess. One of the theca of a tendon.
 t. puncture. Puncture of the meningeal sac. SEE: *spinal puncture*.
thecitis (thē-sī'tĭs) [" + *-itis*, inflammation]. Inflammation of the sheath of a tendon.
theco- [G.]. Combining form meaning *sheath, case, envelope*.
thecodont (thē'kō-dont) [G. *thēkē*, box, + *odous, odont-*, tooth]. Having teeth which are inserted in sockets.
thecostegnosia, thecostegnosis (thē"kō-stĕg-nō'sĭ-ă, -nō'sĭs) [" + *stegnōsis*, a

narrowing]. Constriction of a tendon sheath.

theelin (thē'lĭn) [G. *thēlys*, female]. Crystalline estrogenic hormone secreted by the placenta and ovarian follicles and found in the blood and urine of pregnant women.
   USES: Chiefly in menopausal disturbances, functional amenorrhea, and delayed puberty.
   DOSAGE: 0.1-1.0 mg. (1000-10,000 international units).
   SYN: *estrin, estrone, female sex hormone, folliculin, progynon*.

theelol (thē'lŏl) [G. *thēlys*, female]. An estrus-exciting hormone similar to but more active than theelin, found in urine of pregnant women. SYN: *estriol*.

theism (thē'ĭzm) [L. *thea*, tea, + G. *-ismos*, condition]. Chronic poisoning from excess of tea drinking.

thelalgia (thē-lăl'jĭ-ă) [G. *thēlē*, nipple, + *algos*, pain]. Pain in the nipples.

theleplasty (thĕl'ē-plăs"tĭ) [" + *plassein*, to form]. Plastic surgery of the nipple.

thelerethism (thĕl-ĕr'ē-thĭzm) [" + *erethisma*, stimulation]. Erection of the nipple.

thelitis (thē-lī'tĭs) [" + *-itis*, inflammation]. Inflammation of the nipples.

thelium (thē'lĭ-ŭm) [L. from G. *thēlē*, nipple]. 1. A papilla. 2. A nipple. 3. A cellular layer.

thelyblast (thĕl'ĭ-blăst) [G. *thēlys*, female, + *blastos*, germ]. Nucleus of ovum immediately following fertilization. SYN: *feminonucleus*. SEE: *arsenoblast*.

thenad (thē'năd) [G. *thenar*, palm, + L. *ad*, toward]. Toward the palm or thenar eminence.

thenal (thē'năl) [G. *thenar*, palm]. Pert. to the palm or thenar prominence.
   t. aspect. Outer side of the palm.
   t. eminence. Ball of the thumb. SYN: *thenar*.

thenar (thē'nar) [G. *thenar*, palm]. 1. Palm of hand or sole of foot. 2. Fleshy eminence at base of thumb. 3. Concerning the palm.
   t. eminence. One at the base of the thumb.
   t. muscles. Abductor and flexor muscles of the thumb.

Theobroma (thē"ō-brō'mă) [G. *theos*, god, + *brōma*, food]. Plant yielding cacao butter.

theobromine (thē-ō-brō'mēn) [" + *brōma*, food]. A white powder obtained from Theobroma cacao.
   ACTION AND USES: Similar to caffeine, less stimulating to cerebral centers.
   DOSAGE: 5-8 gr. (0.3-0.5 Gm.).
   t. with sodium salicylate. USP. Diuretic. Combination of sodium salicylate and theobromine.
   ACTION AND USES: Same as theobromine but more soluble.
   DOSAGE: 5-10 gr. (0.3-0.6 Gm.).

theocalcin (thē"ō-kăl'sĭn) [" + L. *calx*, lime]. A double salt or mixture of calcium theobromine and calcium salicylate.
   ACTION AND USES: Same as theobromine.
   DOSAGE: 7-15 gr. (0.5-1 Gm.).

theocin (thē'ō-sĭn) [L. *thea*, tea]. A brand of theophylline. USP.
   ACTION AND USES: Same as theophylline.
   DOSAGE: 1½ gr. (0.1 Gm.).
   t. soluble (theocin-sodium acetate). USES: Same as theocin. DOSAGE: 2½ gr. (0.16 Gm.).

theomania (thē-ō-mā'nĭ-ă) [G. *theos*, god, + *mania*, madness]. Religious insanity; esp. that in which patient thinks he is the Deity or is inspired.

theophobia (thē"ō-fō'bĭ-ă) [" + *phobos*, fear]. Abnormal fear of the wrath of God.

theophylline (thē"ō-fĭl'ēn, -ĭn) [L. *thea*, tea, + G. *phyllon*, plant]. USP. A white crystalline powder with action resembling caffeine and theobromine. DOSAGE: 4 gr. (0.25 Gm.).

theotherapy (thē"ō-thĕr'a-pĭ) [G. *theos*, god, + *therapeia*, treatment]. Treatment of disease by spiritual and religious methods.

therapeutic (thĕr-ă-pū'tĭk) [G. *therapeutikos*, treating]. 1. Pert. to results obtained from treatment. 2. Having medicinal or healing properties. 3. A healing agent.
   t. carbons. PT: Carbon electrodes cored or filled with various materials. When burning they emit radiation of various intensities and qualities of ultraviolet, visual, and infrared energy.
   t. exercise. Scientific supervision of bodily movements for curative purposes. SEE: *exercise*.

therapeutics (thĕr"ă-pū'tĭks) [G. *therapeutikē*, treatment]. That branch of medicine concerned with the application of remedies and the treatment of disease. SYN: *therapy, q.v.*
   t., suggestive. Treatment of a condition by using hypnotic suggestion.

therapeutist (thĕr-ă-pū'tĭst) [G. *therapeuein*, to treat medically]. One who practices therapeutics.

therapia sterilisans magna (thĕr"ă-pī'ă stē-rĭl'ĭ-săns măg'nă) [L.]. Ehrlich's method of administering chemical agent which will destroy in 1 large dose all the parasites in the body of a patient without causing serious injury to the patient.

therapy (thĕr'ă-pĭ) [G. *therapeia*, treatment]. Application of remedies in the treatment of disease. SYN: *therapeutics*.
   t., light. Treatment with radiation from the visible spectrum.
   t., maggot. Use of maggots in suppurating wounds of bones and soft tissues to remove necrotic areas.
   t., mental. The use of suggestion in the treatment of disease.
   t., nonspecific. Use of injections of foreign proteins, bacterial vaccines, etc., in treatment of infection to stimulate general cellular activity. SEE: *specific therapy*.
   t., opsonic. Use of bacterial vaccines to elevate the opsonic index of the blood.
   t., physical. Use of physical agents in the treatment of disease, as massage, heat, hydrotherapy, radiation, electricity, and exercise.
   t., serum. Use of injections of blood serum from immunized animals or persons in the treatment of disease. SYN: *serotherapy*.
   t., specific. Administration of a remedy acting directly against the cause of a disease, as arsphenamine or mercury for syphilis, or quinine for malaria.
   t., spiritual. The application of spiritual knowledge in the treatment of disease. SEE: *spiritual therapy*.
   t., substitution. Use of glandular extracts to balance the deficiency of secretion of a gland.
   t., vaccine. Injection of bacteria or their products to produce active immunization against a disease. SYN: *opsonic therapy*.
   t., zone. Mechanical manipulation or stimulation of an area in the same lon-

therapy, words pert. to: actinotherapy, allopathy, bilitherapy, botryotherapeutics, bromatotherapy, cardiotherapy, cardiotrophotherapy, centrotherapy, chiropody, chiropractic, choletherapy, cirsotomy, light, liquid air, mechanotherapy, metrotherapy, occupational, organotherapy, osteopathy, pyretic, radium, rest cure, Rollier technic, serotherapy, solid carbon dioxide, spondylotherapy, substitution, suggestive therapeutics, therapeutics, thermotherapy, ultraviolet, zomotherapy.

theriac, theriaca (thē'rĭ-ăk, thē-rī'ă-kă) [G. *thēriakē*, antidote]. 1. An antidote to poison of venomous animals, esp. a mixture of about 70 drugs pulverized and mixed with honey into an electuary. 2. An opium confection. 3. Molasses.

therm (therm) [G. *thermē*, heat]. A small calory, the amt. of heat required to raise 1 Gm. of water 1° C.

thermacogenesis (thĕr″mă-kō-jĕn′ĕs-ĭs) [" + *genesis*, production]. Production of an increase of body temperature by drug therapy.

thermaerotherapy (thĕr-mā″er-ō-ther′ă-pī) [" + *aēr*, air, + *therapeia*, treatment]. Therapeutic application of hot air.

thermal (ther'măl) [G. *thermē*, heat]. Pert. to heat.
  t. capacity. Heat necessary to raise any body from 0° to 1° C.
  t. death point. Degree of heat that will kill a fluid culture in 10 minutes.
  t. radiation. Heat radiation.
  t. sense. Capacity for recognition of heat and cold. SYN: *thermesthesia*.

thermalgia (thĕr-măl′jĭ-ă) [" + *algos*, pain]. Neuralgia accompanied by intense burning sensation, pain, redness, and sweating of the area involved. SYN: *causalgia*.

thermanalgesia (thĕr″măn-ăl-jē′zĭ-ă) [" + *an-*, priv. + *algēsis*, pain]. Inability to experience reaction to heat because of cerebral lesion.

thermanesthesia (thĕr″măn-ĕs-thē′zĭ-ă) [" + *an-*, priv. + *aisthēsis*, sensation]. Inability to recognize sensations of heat and cold; insensibility to heat changes. It sometimes occurs in syringomyelia. SYN: *thermoanesthesia*.

thermatology (thĕr-mă-tŏl′ō-jī) [" + *logos*, science]. The study of heat in treatment of disease.

thermelometer (thĕr-mĕl-ŏm′ĕt-ĕr) [" + *electric* + G. *metron*, a measure]. An electric thermometer used to indicate temperature changes too slight to be measured on an ordinary thermometer.

thermesthesia (thĕr-mĕs-thē′zĭ-ă) [" + *aisthēsis*, sensation]. Sensitiveness to heat; temperature sense. SYN: *thermoesthesia*.

thermesthesiometer (thĕr″mĕs-thē-zĭ-ŏm′ĕt-ĕr) [G. *thermē*, heat, + *aisthēsis*, sensation, + *metron*, a measure]. Device for determining sensibility to heat.

thermhypesthesia (thĕrm-hī-pĕs-thē′zĭ-ă) [" + *hypo*, under, + *aisthēsis*, sensation]. Lessened sensibility of the temperature sense. SYN: *thermohypesthesia*.

thermic (ther'mĭk) [G. *thermē*, heat]. Pert. to heat.
  t. fever. Sunstroke, collapse and high cutaneous temperature after long exposure to the sun. SYN: *insolation, siriasis*.
  t. sense. The temperature sense; ability to react to heat stimuli. SYN: *thermesthesia, thermoesthesia*.

thermionic rectifier (thĕr″mĭ-ŏn′ĭk) [" + *ion*, going]. PT: A device that converts alternating current into direct current; an electric valve in which the electrons are supplied by a heated electrode.

thermo- [G.]. Combining form meaning *hot, heat*.

thermoalgesia (thĕr″mō-ăl-jē′zĭ-ă) [G. *thermē*, heat, + *algēsis*, pain]. Condition in which pain is caused by application of moderate heat. SYN: *thermalgesia*.

thermoanalgesia (thĕr″mō-ăn-ăl-jē′zĭ-ă) [" + *an-*, priv. + *algēsis*, pain]. Loss of heat sensation. SYN: *thermanalgesia*.

thermoanesthesia (thĕr″mō-ăn-ĕs-thē′zĭ-ă) [" + *an-*, priv. + *aisthēsis*, sensation]. 1. Inability to distinguish bet. heat and cold. 2. Insensibility to heat or temperature changes.

thermobiosis (thĕr″mō-bĭ-ō′sĭs) [" + *biōsis*, a living]. Ability to withstand high temperature.

thermobiotic (thĕr″mō-bĭ-ot′ĭk) [" + *bios*, life]. Able to exist at high temperature.

thermocauterectomy (thĕr″mō-kaw-tĕr-ĕk′tō-mī) [" + *kautērion*, branding iron, + *ektomē*, excision]. Excision by thermocautery.

thermocautery (thĕr″mō-kaw′tĕr-ĭ) [" + *kautērion*, branding iron]. 1. Cautery by application of heat. 2. Cauterizing iron. SEE: *cautery, actual*.

thermocoagulation (thĕr″mō-kō-ăg-ū-lā′shun) [G. *thermē*, heat, + L. *coagulāre*, to clot]. The use of high frequency currents to produce coagulation in checking growths.

thermocouple (thĕr′mō-kŭp-ĕl) [" + L. *copula*, a bond]. Device for measuring slight temperature changes. SYN: *thermopile*.

thermocurrent (thĕr″mō-kŭr′ĕnt) [" + L. *currere*, to run]. Current developed or set in motion by heat; specifically, an electric current. SEE: *thermoelectricity*.

thermodiffusion (thĕr″mō-dĭ-fū′zhun) [" + L. *diffusio*, a pouring apart]. Diffusion of substances by heat.

thermoduric (thĕr″mō-dū′rĭk) [" + L. *durus*, resistant, hard]. Able to live in high temperatures. SEE: *thermophylic*.

thermoelectricity (thĕr″mō-ē-lĕk-trĭs′ĭ-tĭ) [" + *ēlektron*, amber (electricity)]. Electricity generated by heat, as by unequal heating of a circuit of 2 dissimilar metals.

thermoesthesia (thĕr″mō-ĕs-thē′zĭ-ă) [" + *aisthēsis*, sensation]. Ability to recognize temperature differences. SYN: *thermesthesia*.

thermoexcitory (thĕr″mō-ĕk-sī′tō-rī) [G. *thermē*, heat, + L. *excitāre*, to irritate]. Exciting the production of heat in the body.

thermogen (thĕr′mō-jĕn) [" + *gennan*, to produce]. Device for maintaining the temperature of the body during operation.

thermogenesis (thĕr″mō-jĕn′ĕ-sĭs) [" + *genesis*, production]. The production of heat, esp. in the body.

thermograph (thĕr′mō-grăf) [" + *graphein*, to write]. Device for registering variations of heat.

thermohale (thĕr′mō-hāl) [" + L. *halāre*, to breathe]. An electric device for giving inhalations of warmed or medicated air in congestion of the respiratory tract.

thermohyperalgesia (thĕr″mō-hī″pĕr-ăl-gē′zĭ-ă) [" + *hyper*, above, + *algēsis*, pain]. Unbearable pain upon the application of heat.

thermohyperesthesia (thĕr″mō-hī′pĕr-ĕs-thē′zĭ-ă) [G. *thermē*, heat, + *hyper*, above, + *aisthēsis*, sensation]. Exceptional sensitiveness to heat.

thermohypesthesia (thĕr″mō-hī″pĕs-thē′-zĭ-ă) [" + *hypo*, under, + *aisthēsis*, sensation]. Diminished perception of heat.

thermoinhibitory (thĕr″mō-ĭn-hĭb′ĭ-tō″rĭ) [" + L. *inhibere*, to restrain]. Arresting or impeding the generation of bodily heat.

thermolabile (thĕr″mō-lā′bĭl) [" + *labilis*, unstable]. Destroyed or changed easily by heat; unstable. SEE: *heat, latent heat*.

thermolite (thĕr′mō-līt) [G. *thermē*, heat]. A large, carbon, high-power filament lamp used for infrared radiation.

thermology (thĕr-mŏl′ō-jĭ) [" + *logos*, science]. The science of heat.

thermolysis (thĕr-mŏl′ĭs-ĭs) [" + *lysis*, destruction] 1. Loss of heat from the body, as by evaporation. 2. Chemical decomposition by heat.

thermometer (thĕr-mŏm′ĕ-tĕr) [G. *thermē*, heat, + *metron*, a measure]. An instrument for registering heat or cold.

　t., air or gas. One filled with air or gas, the expansion of which registers high temperatures.

　t., alcohol. One containing alcohol.

　t., Celsius. Centigrade t.

　t., Centigrade. Temperature of boiling water at sea level 100° and freezing point 0°, with 100° bet. Generally used in Latin America and in Europe, and in scientific work.

　t., clinical. One for measuring temperature of body and in which the mercury remains stationary at registration point until shaken down.

　t., differential. One recording slight variations.

　t., Fahrenheit. Boiling point 212°, freezing point 32°. Used in English-speaking countries and in Holland.

　t., mercury. One containing mercury.

　t., Reaumur. Used in some parts of Germany and in Russia. Zero is same as 0° C. or same as 32° F., having 80° instead of 100 like the Centigrade t. SEE: *comparative tables*.

　t., spirit. One filled with alcohol instead of mercury for registering low temperatures.

　t. scale. Graduated device on a thermometer to register the temperature.

Comparative Thermometric Scale

	Centigrade	Fahrenheit	Reaumur
Boiling point of water ...	100°	212°	80°
	90°	194°	72°
	80°	176°	64°
	70°	158°	56°
	60°	140°	48°
	50°	122°	40°
	40°	104°	32°
	30°	86°	24°
	20°	68°	16°
	10°	50°	8°
Freezing point of water	0°	32°	0°
	—10°	14°	—8°
	—20°	4°	—16°

CONVERSION: *F. to Centigrade*: Subtract 32 and multiply by 5/9. *C. to Fahrenheit*: Multiply by 9/5 and add 32.

To convert R. into F. *multiply* by 9. *divide* by 4, and *add* 32.

There are 3 major scales, Centigrade, Fahrenheit, and Reaumur in use. The Celsius, no longer used, was the reverse of the *Centigrade*, zero being its boiling point. The *absolute scale*, used for only very low temperatures, based on absolute zero, the point at which the form of motion constituting heat ceases, —459.4° F.

　t., self-registering. One recording variations of temperature.

　t., surface. One for showing temperature of the body's surface.

thermometric (thĕr″mō-mĕt′rĭk) [G. *thermē*, heat, + *metron*, a measure].

Thermometric Equivalents

C	F	C	F	C	F	C	F
0	32	27	80.6	54	129.2	81	177.8
1	33.8	28	82.4	55	131	82	179.6
2	35.6	29	84.2	56	132.8	83	181.4
3	37.4	30	86.0	57	134.6	84	183.2
4	39.2	31	87.8	58	136.4	85	185
5	41	32	89.6	59	138.2	86	186.8
6	42.8	33	91.4	60	140	87	188.6
7	44.6	34	93.2	61	141.8	88	190.4
8	46.4	35	95	62	143.6	89	192.2
9	48.2	36	96.8	63	145.4	90	194
10	50	37	98.6	64	147.2	91	195.8
11	51.8	38	100.4	65	149	92	197.6
12	53.6	39	102.2	66	150.8	93	199.4
13	55.4	40	104	67	152.6	94	201.2
14	57.2	41	105.8	68	154.4	95	203
15	59	42	107.6	69	156.2	96	204.8
16	60.8	43	109.4	70	158	97	206.6
17	62.6	44	111.2	71	159.8	98	208.4
18	64.4	45	113	72	161.6	99	210.2
19	66.2	46	114.8	73	163.4	100	212
20	68	47	116.6	74	165.2		
21	69.8	48	118.4	75	167		
22	71.6	49	120.2	76	168.8		
23	73.4	50	122	77	170.6		
24	75.2	51	123.8	78	172.4		
25	77	52	125.6	79	174.2		
26	78.8	53	127.4	80	176		

Pert. to heat measurement or a thermometer.

thermometry (thĕr-mŏm'ĕt-rĭ) [G. *thermē*, heat, + *metron*, a measure]. Measurement of temperature.

t., clinical. Temperature of body in a state of health ranges between 97.8° and 98.6° F.

Slightly increased by eating, exercising and external heat; reduced about 1½° during sleep. In disease the temperature of body deviates several degrees above and below the average of health. When it moves upwards it is far less dangerous than when it moves downward, particularly in children. Even in adults 1° below the standard of health represents more danger than 2½° above and 2° below more than 4° above, and so on.

In facial erysipelas, acute meningitis, pneumonia, scarlatina, typhus, smallpox, and intermittent fever it sometimes rises as high as 106° or 107° F. In other febrile diseases rarely reaches 104° F. Temperature may reach height of 110° F., as seen in sunstroke, and patient recovers.

The lowest extreme of temperature is sometimes found in cold stage of cholera, when temperature may be very low (90°-85° F.) for several days. Subnormal temperatures below 98° F. are observed in the following conditions:

During convalescence from certain febrile conditions, after pneumonia and typhoid fever, temperature may remain subnormal for several days. In collapse: This may result from shock, from hemorrhage, from action of some tonic agent, from simple heart failure in course of disease or from rupture of a viscus, as the bowel in typhoid, the lung in phthisis or stomach in perforating ulcer. In certain chronic diseases, esp. diabetes, cancer, chronic cardiac, cerebral, and spinal diseases.

In general, for every degree of the thermometer, the pulse rises 10 beats per minute, but rise of temperature to 99½° F. gives more evidence of disease than rising of pulse from 70 to 90 beats per minute. A decrease of heat in the morning is favorable; an increase from night to morning the reverse. If temperature remains above normal after general symptoms denote convalescence. patient is in danger of a relapse or the supervention of some other disease. The range of the increase of heat in different febrile diseases extends to 110° F. and as a rule the amount of increase is a criterion of the intensity of the disease.

Artificial fever induced through diathermy, continuous hot bath, or malarial injections now utilized in some diseases, as general paresis, chronic arthritis, and some forms of asthma.

thermoneurosis (thĕr″mō-nū-rō'sĭs) [G. *thermē*, heat, + *neuron*, nerve, + *-ōsis*, condition]. Elevation of body temperature in hysteria and other nervous conditions.

thermopalpation (thĕr″mō-păl-pā'shŭn) [" + L. *palpāre*, to touch]. Estimation of temperature of the body by palpation at different parts of the body.

thermopenetration (thĕr″mō-pĕn-ĕ-trā'shŭn) [" + L. *penetrāre*, to penetrate]. Application of heat to the deeper tissues of the body by diathermy.

thermophilic (thĕr″mō-fĭl'ĭk) [" + *philein*, to love]. Preferring or thriving best under high temperature, said of bacteria.

thermophobia (thĕr″mō-fō'bĭ-ă) [" + *phobos*, fear]. Abnormal dread of heat.

thermophore (thĕr″mō-fōr) [" + *phoros*, a bearer]. Apparatus for applying heat to a part, consisting of water heater and tubes conveying water to a coil and returning to heater, or salts which produce heat when moistened.

thermophylic (thĕr″mō-fī'lĭk) [" + *phylakē*, guard]. Resistant to destruction by heat, noting certain bacteria.

thermopile (thĕr'mō-pīl) [G. *thermē*, heat, + L. *pila*, pile]. PT: A thermoelectric battery used in measuring small variations in the degree of heat.

It consists of a number of dissimilar metallic plates connected together in which, under the influence of heat, an electric current is produced.

thermoplegia (thĕr″mō-plē'jĭ-ă) [" + *plēgē*, a stroke]. Heatstroke; sunstroke. SYN: *insolation, siriasis*.

thermopolypnea (thĕr″mō-pŏl-ĭp-nē'ă) [" + *polys*, many, + *pnoia*, breath]. Quickened breathing caused by high fever or great heat.

thermoradiotherapy (thĕr″mō-rā″dĭ-ō-thĕr'ă-pĭ) [" + L. *radius*, ray, + G. *therapeia*, treatment]. Application of heat to deep tissues by diathermy. SYN: *thermopenetration*.

thermoresistant (thĕr″mō-rē-zĭs'tănt) [" + L. *resistentia*, resistance]. Able to resist high temperature, but not develop in it, noting bacteria.

thermostabile (thĕr″mō-stā'bl) [" + L. *stabilis*, stationary]. Not changed or destroyed by heat.

thermostat (thĕr″mō-stăt) [G. *thermē*, heat, + *statos*, standing]. An automatic device for regulating the temperature.

thermosteresis (thĕr″mō-stĕ-rē'sĭs) [" + *sterēsis*, deprivation]. The deprivation or loss of heat.

thermosystaltic (thĕr″mō-sĭs-tăl'tĭk) [" + *systellein*, to contract]. Pert. to contraction of the muscles under stimulus of heat.

thermotactic, thermotaxic (thĕr″mō-tăk'tĭk, -tăks'ĭk) [" + *taktikos*, regulating, — + *taxis*, order]. Relating to regulation of the bodily temperature.

thermotaxis (thĕr″mō-tăks'ĭs) [" + *taxis*, arrangement]. 1. Regulation of bodily temperature. 2. Reaction of organisms or of protoplasm in the living body to heat.

thermotherapeutics (thĕr″mō-thĕr-ă-pū'tĭks) [" + *therapeutikē*, treatment]. Use of heat in treatment of disease. SYN: *thermotherapy*.

thermotherapy (thĕr″mō-thĕr'ă-pĭ) [" + *therapeia*, treatment]. PT: The therapeutic application of heat.

thermotolerant (thĕr″mō-tŏl'ĕr-ănt) [G. *thermē*, heat, + L. *tolerāre*, to tolerate]. Able to live normally in high temperature.

thermotonometer (thĕr″mō-tō-nŏm'ĕt-ĕr) [" + *tonos*, tension, + *metron*, a measure]. Device for measuring degree of muscular contraction when under influence of heat.

thermotoxin (thĕr″mō-tŏks'ĭn) [" + *toxikon*, poison]. A poison formed in the tissues by excessive heat.

thesis (thē'sĭs) [G. *thesis*, proposition]. An essay on a given subject offered by a candidate for a collegiate degree.

thiamine chloride (thī'ă-mĭn). Crystalline vitamin B₁ hydrochloride, which may be prepared from rice polishings, yeast, or synthetically.

USES: In conditions resulting from

vitamin B₁ deficiency.
  Dosage: For infants, 50 to 75 international units per day; for adults, 200 to 300 international units per day. Carbohydrates increase the need for it.
thiemia (thī-ē'mĭ-ă) [G. *theion*, sulfur, + *aima*, blood]. Sulfur in the blood.
Thiersch's graft or **method** (tĕrsh). A method of skin grafting using epidermis and a portion of the dermis.
thigh (thī) [A.S. *thīoh*, thigh]. The upper leg above the knee and below the hip. SEE: *hip, pectineus, sartorius*.
  t. bone. The femur.
  t. joint. The hip joint. SYN: *articulatio coxae*.
thigmesthesia (thĭg-mĕs-thē'zĭ-ă) [G. *thigma*, touch, + *aisthēsis*, sensation]. The sense of touch.
thigmocyte (thĭg'mō-sīt) [" + *kytos*, cell]. A blood platelet.
thigmotaxis (thĭg"mō-tăks'ĭs) ["+ *taxis*, arrangement]. Arrangement in which some cells are attracted by contact with solids. SYN: *thigmotropism*.
thigmotropism (thĭg-mŏt'rō-pĭzm) [" + *tropos*, a turning, + *-ismos*, condition]. The attraction exerted by contact with solids over certain cells. SEE: *thigmotaxis*.
thio- [G.]. Prefix denoting *presence of sulfur replacing oxygen*.
thiobismol (thī"ō-bĭz'mol). A compound containing 38% bismuth.
  Uses: In treatment of syphilis.
  Dosage: 3 gr. (0.2 Gm.) intramuscularly.
thiocol (thī'ō-kol) [G. *theion*, sulfur, + *kolla*, glue]. Registered trade-mark for a preparation containing the potassium salt of orthoguaiacol-sulfonic acid.
  Uses: In respiratory disorders.
  Dosage: 5-10 gr. (0.3-0.6 Gm.).
thiogenic (thī-ō-jĕn'ĭk) [G. *theion*, sulfur, + *gennan*, to produce]. Able to convert hydrogen sulfide into higher sulfur compounds, said of bacteria in the water of some mineral springs.
thioneine (thī-ō'nē-ēn) [G. *theion*, sulfur, + *neos*, new]. Crystalline sulfur-containing compound found in ergot and blood.
  Structurally identified as thiolhistidine. It plays an important part in the blood in nutritional processes.
thiopectic, thiopexic (thī-ō-pĕk'tĭk, -pĕks'ĭk) [" + *pēxis*, fixation]. Pert. to the fixation of sulfur.
thiopexy (thī'ō-pĕks-ī) [" + *pēxis*, fixation]. The fixation of sulfur.
thiophil, thiophilic (thī'ō-fĭl, thī-ō-fĭl'ĭk) [" + *philein*, to love]. Thriving in the presence of sulfur or its compounds, as some bacteria.
thiouracil (thī-ō-ū'ră-sĭl). An antithyroid drug used in treatment of hyperthyroidism, thyrotoxicosis, and thyroiditis.
  Dosage: 0.4 Gm. daily in divided doses. After symptoms are controlled and basal metabolic rate is within normal range, dosage should be reduced to 0.1 or 0.2 Gm. daily.
thiourea (thī"ō-ū-rē'ă) [" + *urea*]. Colorless crystalline compound of urea in which sulfur replaces the oxygen.
third cranial nerve. Oculomotor nerve. SEE: *Appendix*.
  t. corpuscle. A blood plate.
  t. intention. Healing of a wound by filling with granulations. SEE: *resolution*.
  t. ventricle. Third ventricle of the brain, a narrow cavity bet. the 2 optic thalami. SYN: *ventriculus tertius*.
thirst. Desire for fluid, esp. for water. This may obtain in fevers and certain other maladies, or it may be entirely lacking in some conditions. The nurse should note whether the intake of fluids allays the patient's thirst.
  RS: *adipsia, adipsous, adipsy, anadipsia, aposia, taste*.
  t., absence of. Adipsia, aposia.
  t., excessive. Polydipsia.
  t., morbid. Dipsosis.
Thiry's fistula (tē'rē). An artificial fistula in a dog's intestines for obtaining intestinal juice for experimental purposes.
Thoma-Zeiss hemocytometer (tō'mă-tsīs hem"ō-sī-tom'ē-ter). Device for counting the blood cells.
Thomsen's disease (thŏm'sĕn). A disease confined to certain families, characterized by tonic spasms of the muscles induced by voluntary movements; usually congenital and transmitted from one generation to another; several of same family commonly affected.
  SYM: Disease appears in early childhood, is manifested by a tonic spasm of the muscles every time they are put in use. In few minutes the rigidity wears away and the movements become free from repeated contractions, the muscles become firm and extremely well developed; under electrical treatment the muscles contract and relax slowly.
  PROG: Incurable.
  TREATMENT: Physical exercise gives improvement.
  SYN: *amyotonia congenita, myotonia congenita*.
thomsonianism (tŏm-sō'nĭ-ăn'ĭzm). An empiric system assuming that only vegetable remedies are of value in treatment.
thoracalgia (thō-ră-kăl'jĭ-ă) [G. *thōrax, thōrak-*, chest, + *algos*, pain]. Pain in the chest wall. SYN: *pleurodynia*.
thoracectomy (thō-ră-sĕk'tō-mī) [" + *ektomē*, excision]. Incision of the chest wall with resection of a portion of rib.
thoracentesis (thō"răs-ĕn-tē'sĭs) [" + *kentēsis*, a puncture]. Tapping through the chest wall for removal of fluids. SYN: *pleurocentesis, q.v.*
  NP: Have patient well supported. Watch for signs of collapse during and following treatment.
thoracic (thōr-ăs'ĭk) [G. *thōrax, thōrak-*, chest]. Pert. to the chest or thorax.
  t. cavity. The pleural cavity, the chest. It contains the trachea, esophagus, lungs and bronchi, the heart and its vessels. It is separated from the abdominal cavity by the diaphragm.
  t. duct. Passage bet. receptaculum chyli and meeting point of left int. jugular and left subclavian veins.
  Absorbed substances carried to the lacteals and blood stream pass to the lymph system and through the t. duct of the lymph system to the vascular system. SEE: *chyle, receptaculum chyli*.
  t. girdle. One formed by the clavicles and scapulae.
  t. limbs. Upper extremities.
  t. spine. The spinal column.
thoraco- [G.]. Combining form meaning *chest, chest wall*.
thoracobronchotomy (thō"răk-ō-brŏn-kŏt'ō-mī) [G. *thōrax, thōrak-*, chest, + *brogchos*, windpipe, + *tomē*, a cutting]. Incision through the thoracic wall into the bronchus.
thoracocautery (thō"răk-ō-kaw'tĕr-ī) [" + *kautērion*, branding iron]. The use of cautery in breaking up pulmonary adhesions to collapse the lung.
thoracoceloschisis (thō"răk-ō-sē-lŏs'kĭ-sĭs) [" + *koilia*, belly, + *schisis*, a fissure].

thoracocentesis   T-24   **thoracomyodynia**

Congenital fissure of the thoracic and abdominal cavities.

thoracocentesis (thō″răk-ō-sĕn-tē′sĭs) [" + *kentēsis*, a puncture]. Tapping of the thorax. SYN: *thoracentesis*.

thoracocyllosis (thō″răk-ō-sĭl-ō′sĭs) [" + *kyllōsis*, crippling]. Deformity of the chest.

thoracocyrtosis (thō″răk-ō-sĭr-tō′sĭs) [" + *kyrtōsis*, curvature]. Excessive curvature of the chest.

thoracodynia (thō″răk-ō-dĭn′ĭ-ă) [" + *odynē*, pain]. Pain in the thorax.

thoracogastroschisis (thō″răk-ō-găs-trŏs′kĭs-ĭs) [G. *thōrax*, *thorak-*, chest, + *gastēr*, belly, + *schisis*, a cleft]. Congenital fissure of abdomen and thorax.

thoracograph (thō-răk′ō-grăf) [" + *graphein*, to write]. Device for recording diagrams of the chest outlines and movements.

thoracolumbar (thō″răk-ō-lŭm′băr) [" + L. *lumbus*, loin]. Pert. to the thoracic *stethometer*. ference of the chest or abdomen. SYN: and lumbar parts of the spine; noting their ganglia and the fibers of the sympathetic nervous system.

thoracolysis (thō″răk-ŏl′ĭs-ĭs) [" + *lysis*, loosening]. The freeing of a lung by

thoracomyodynia (thō″ră-kō-mī″ō-dĭn′ĭ-ă) severing abnormal adhesions bet. it and the chest wall.

thoracometer (thō-răk-ŏm′ĕt-ĕr) [" + *metron*, a measure]. Device for recording variations in respiration of circum-

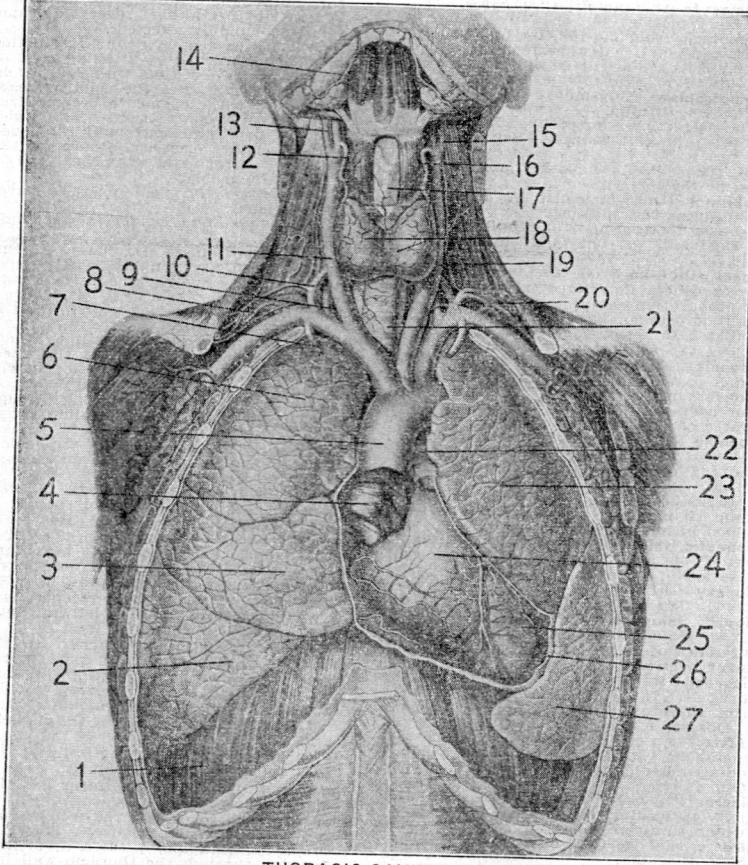

THORACIC CAVITY.

1. Diaphragm. 2. Right lung, lower lobe. 3. Right lung, middle lobe. 4. Right auricle. 5. Aorta. 6. Right lung, upper lobe. 7. Internal mammary artery. 8. Superior scapular artery. 9. Vertebral artery. 10. Inferior thyroid artery. 11. Right common carotid. 12. Right superior thyroid artery. 13. External carotid, left. 14. Facial artery. 15. External carotid, left. 16. Left superior thyroid artery. 17. Thyroid cartilage. 18. Thyroid. 19. Left common carotid. 20. Transverse cervical artery. 21. Trachea. 22. Pulmonary artery. 23. Left lung, upper lobe. 24. Right ventricle. 25. Left ventricle. 26. Pericardium. 27. Left lung, lower lobe.

["+ *mys, my-*, muscle, + *odyně*, pain]. Pain in muscles of the chest wall.
thoracopathy (thō″răk-ŏp′ăth-ĭ) [" + *pathos*, disease]. Any disease of the thorax, thoracic organs, or tissues.
thoracoplasty (thō′ră-kō-plăs″tĭ, thō-ră′kō-plăs″tĭ) [G. *thōrax, thorak-*, chest, + *plassein*, to form]. A plastic operation upon the thorax; removal of portions of the ribs in stages to collapse diseased areas of the lung. SEE: *empyema*.
thoracopneumoplasty (thō″ră-kō-nū′mō-plăs-tĭ) [" + *pneumon*, lung, + *plassein*, to form]. Plastic surgery involving the chest and lung.
thoracoschisis (thō-ră-kŏs′kĭ-sĭs) [" + *schisis*, a cleft]. Congenital fissure of the chest wall.
thoracoscope (thō-ră′kō-skōp, -răk′ō-skōp) [" + *skopein*, to examine]. 1. An instrument used in auscultation to convey the sounds of the chest to the ear. SYN: *stethoscope*. 2. Instrument for inspecting the thoracic cavity which has an electric light and is inserted through an intercostal space.
thoracoscopy (thō″ră-kŏs′kō-pĭ) [" + *skopein*, to examine]. Diagnostic examination of the pleural cavity with an endoscope.
thoracostenosis (thō″ră-kō-stĕn-ō′sĭs) [" + *stenōsis*, a contraction]. Narrowness of the thorax. SYN: *waspwaist*.
thoracostomy (thō-răk-ŏs′tō-mĭ) [" + *stoma*, mouth]. Resection of chest wall to allow room for enlarged heart or for drainage.
thoracotomy (thō″răk-ŏt′ō-mĭ) [G. *thōrax, thorak-*, chest, + *tomē*, a cutting]. Surgical incision of the chest wall.
thorax (thō′răks) (pl. *thoraces* or *thoraxes*) [G. *thōrax*]. That part of the body bet. the base of the neck superiorly and the diaphragm inferiorly. SYN: *chest*.
The surface of the thorax is divided into regions as follows:
ANTERIOR SURFACE: *Supraclavicular*, above the clavicles; *suprasternal*, above the sternum; *clavicular*, over the clavicles; *sternal*, over the sternum; *mammary*, the space bet. the 3rd and 6th ribs on either side; *inframammary*, below the mamma and above the lower border of the 12th rib on either side.
POSTERIOR SURFACE: *Scapular*, over the scapulae; *interscapular*, bet. the scapulae; *infrascapular*, below the scapulae.

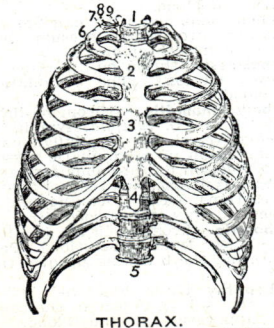

THORAX.
1. First thoracic vertebra. 2. Manubrium. 3. Corpus sterni. 4. Xiphoid processus. 5. Last thoracic vertebra. 6. First rib.

ON SIDES: *Axillary*, above the 6th rib.
RS: *acromiothoracis, cholohemothorax*, "*thorac-*" words.
t., Amazon. A chest with only 1 breast.
t., barrel-shaped. A malformed chest rounded like a barrel seen in pulmonary emphysema.
t., fusiform. A chest deformed by long continued tight lacing.
t. paralyticus. The long, flat chest of patients with constitutional visceroptosis.
t., Peyrot's. A chest that has an obliquely oval, deformed shape, seen in large pleural effusions
t., pigeon. One in which the sternum and ribs anteriorly form a prominent edge or ridge resembling the breastbone of a pigeon.
Thorazine Pg. T-66.
thorium (thō′rĭ-ŭm). SYMB: Th. A metallic element occurring in combination, at. wt. 232.12.
It is antiseptic and radioactive, and it produces mesothorium, radiothorium, and thorium emanation upon disintegration.
Thornwaldt's disease (torn′vahlt). Inflammation of crypt of the pharyngeal tonsil with formation of a pus-containing cyst and nasopharyngeal stenosis.
thoron (thō′rŏn). A gaseous, radioactive element; an emanation or transformation product of thorium.
three-day fever. An epidemic, infectious, eruptive fever due to a parasite transmitted by a mosquito. SYN: *breakbone fever, dandy fever, dengue*.
thremmatology (thrĕm-ă-tŏl′ō-jĭ) [G. *thremma*, nursling, + *logos*, science]. Science of breeding according to the laws of heredity and variation.
threpsology (thrĕp-sŏl′ō-jĭ) [G. *threpsis*, nutrition, + *logos*, study]. Science of nutrition.
threshold (thrĕsh′ōld) [A.S. *therscwold*]. 1. Point at which a psychological or physiological effect begins to be produced. 2. A measure of the sensitivity of an organ or function which is obtained by finding the limiting value of the appropriate stimulus that will give the response.
t., auditory. Minimum audible sound.
t. of consciousness. PSY: Point at which a stimulus is hardly perceived.
t., erythe′ma. Stage in which e. of the skin due to radiation just begins.
t. point. One at which the concentration of glucose begins to pass from the blood into the urine.
t., stim′ulus. Minimal point at which a sensation is aroused.
t. of visual sensation. T. of the minimum vision of an object.
thrill (thrĭl) [M.E. *thrillen*, to pierce]. 1. Abnormal tremor accompanying a vascular or cardiac murmur felt on palpation. SYN: *fremitus*. 2. A tingling or shivering sensation of tremulous excitement, as from pain, pleasure, or horror.
t., aortic. One heard over aortic aperture in lesions of valves.
t., arterial. One heard over an artery.
t., hydatid. Peculiar tremor felt on palpation of a hydatid cyst.
t., presystolic. One sometimes felt over apex of the heart preceding ventricular contraction.
throat (thrōt) [A.S. *throte*]. 1. Cavity from arch of palate to glottis and sup. opening of the esophagus. 2. The front of the neck. SYN: *jugulum*. 3. Any narrow orifice.

throat, sore　　　　　　　　　　T-26　　　　　　　　　　**thrombopenia**

RS: *agranulocytosis, anchone, aphonia clericorum, guttural, jugular, tonsil, tonsillitis.*

FOREIGN BODIES IN: The symptoms depend somewhat on the location and size of the foreign body, and vary from simple discomfort to distressing coughing, difficulty in breathing, retching and cyanosis, and, if not relieved, suffocation resulting in unconsciousness.

TREATMENT: If not causing serious distress, the patient should lie down with the head lower than the body. The common practice of a sudden slap on the back often helps to dislodge bodies in the trachea or throat, and in youngsters it is esp. efficacious when the child is inverted. If this does not succeed, it is possible to introduce a finger through the mouth into the throat, possibly to the larynx, and so dislodge the foreign body. It has been possible in this way to dislodge a bean from the larynx of an unconscious child.

Summon a physician immediately. Make sure to tell him the nature of the case so that he may bring the proper instruments, as it may be necessary for him to open the trachea. Cathartics and enemas are of no value whatever, and may be dangerous.

t., sore. Inflammation of tonsils, larynx, or pharynx. SYN: *odynphagia.*

throb (thrŏb) [M.E. *throbben,* of imitative origin]. 1. A beat or pulsation, as of the heart. 2. To pulsate.

throbbing (thrŏb′ĭng) [M.E. *throbben,* of imitative origin]. Pulsation; a beating; rhythmic movement.

Throckmorton's reflex (thrŏk′mor′tŭn). Extension of great toe and flexion of others when dorsum of foot is percussed in metatarsophalangeal region.

throe (thrō) [A.S. *thrauu,* suffering]. A severe pain or pang, esp. one in childbirth.

thromballosis (thrŏm-băl-ō′sĭs) [G. *thrombos,* a clot, + *alloiōsis,* change]. The condition due to coagulation of the venous blood.

thrombase (thrŏm′bās) [G. *thrombos,* clot, + *ase,* enzyme]. An unstable chemical substance formed in the blood after it is shed and capable of causing the prompt clotting of additional blood by converting fibrinogen into fibrin. SYN: *thrombin.*

thrombasthenia (thrŏm-băs-thē′nĭ-ă) [" + *astheneia,* weakness]. Deficiency of the blood platelets.

thrombectomy (thrŏm-bĕk′tō-mĭ) [" + *ektomē,* excision]. Excision of a thrombus.

thrombin (thrŏm′bĭn) [G. *thrombos,* a clot]. Substance present in blood after it is shed which unites with fibrinogen to form fibrin in blood clotting. SYN: *thrombase.*

thrombo- [G.]. Combining form meaning *clot of blood, curd of milk, lump, piece,* pert. to a thrombus.

thromboangiitis (thrŏm-bō-ăn-jĭ-ī′tĭs) [G. *thrombos,* clot, + *aggeion,* vessel, + *-itis,* inflammation]. Inflammation of inner coat of a blood vessel with clot formation. SEE: *thrombosis.*

t. obliterans. Obliteration by thrombi of the larger veins and arteries of a limb, resulting in gangrene. SYN: *Buerger's disease.*

SYM: Occlusion; thrombosis; excruciating pain in leg or foot, worse at night; cyanotic, clammy cold extremity; diminished sense of heat and cold; gangrene of toes or foot may set in.

thromboarteritis (thrŏm″bō-ar-tē-rī′tĭs) [" + *artēria,* artery, + *-itis,* inflammation]. Inflammation of an artery in connection with thrombosis.

thromboblast (thrŏm′bō-blăst) [" + *blastos,* a germ]. A small basophilic cell, said to be the mother cell of the blood platelet.

thromboclasis (thrŏm-bŏk′lă-sĭs) [" + *klasis,* a breaking]. The breaking up of a thrombus. SYN: *thrombolysis.*

thromboclastic (thrŏm-bō-klăs′tĭk) [" + *klasis,* a breaking]. Pert. to or producing the dissolution of a thrombus. SYN: *thrombolytic.*

thrombocyst, thrombocystis (thrŏm′bō-sĭst, -sĭs′tĭs) [" + *kystis,* a sac]. A membranous sac enveloping a thrombus.

thrombocyte (thrŏm′bō-sīt) [G. *thrombos,* a clot, + *kytos,* cell]. One of the pale disks found in normal blood, 200,000 to 400,000 per c.mm., which aid in coagulation. SYN: *platelet.*

They are much smaller than the corpuscles. SEE: *blood, erythrocyte, leukocyte.*

thrombocytocrit (thrŏm″bō-sī′tō-krĭt) [" + *kytos,* cell, + *krinein,* to separate]. Device for estimating the platelet content of the blood.

thrombocytolysis (thrŏm″bō-sī-tŏl′ĭ-sĭs) [" + " + *lysis,* dissolution]. Dissolution of thrombocytes.

thrombocytopenia (thrŏm″bō-sī′tō-pē′nĭ-ă) [" + " + *penia,* lack]. Abnormal decrease in number of the blood platelets. SYN: *thrombopenia.*

thrombocytopoiesis (thrŏm″bō-sī″tō-poy-ē′sĭs) [" + " + *poiēsis,* production]. The development of blood platelets.

thrombocytozyme (thrŏm-bō-sī′tō-zīm) [" + " + *zymē,* leaven]. An activating substance from thrombocytes which aids in the formation of thrombin.

thrombogen (thrŏm′bō-jĕn) [" + *gennan,* to produce]. A substance believed to be present in blood plasma which is the precursor of thrombin. SYN: *prothrombin.*

thrombogenesis (thrŏm″bō-jĕn′ĕs-ĭs) [G. *thrombos,* a clot, + *genesis,* production]. The formation of a blood clot.

thrombogenic (thrŏm″bō-jĕn′ĭk) [" + *gennan,* to produce]. Producing or tending to produce a clot.

thromboid (thrŏm′boyd) [" + *eidos,* form]. Resembling a thrombus or clot.

thrombokinase (thrŏm-bō-kĭn′ās) [" + *kinēsis,* motion]. A substance liberated from tissues capable of initiating the clotting of blood.

When combined with calcium salt it activates thrombogen, presumably converting it into thrombin.

thrombokinesis (thrŏm″bō-kĭn-ē′sĭs) [" + *kinēsis,* motion]. The coagulation of the blood.

thrombolymphangitis (thrŏm″bō-lĭm-făn-jī′tĭs) [" + L. *lympha,* lymph, + G. *aggeion,* vessel, + *-itis,* inflammation]. Inflammation of a lymphatic vessel due to obstruction by thrombus formation.

thrombolysis (thrŏm-bŏl′ĭ-sĭs) [" + *lysis,* destruction]. The breaking up of a thrombus. SYN: *thromboclasis.*

thrombolytic (thrŏm″bō-lĭt′ĭk) [G. *thrombos,* clot, + *lysis,* dissolution]. Pert. to or causing the breaking up of a thrombus.

thrombopathy (thrŏm-bŏp′ăth-ĭ) [" + *pathos,* disease]. A defect in the coagulation apparatus of the blood. SYN: *hemophilia,* q.v.

thrombopenia (thrŏm-bō-pē′nĭ-ă) [" + *penia,* lack]. Lessening of the number of blood platelets.

thrombophilia (thrŏm-bō-fĭl'ĭ-ă) [" + *philein*, to love]. A tendency to the occurrence of clot formation.

thrombophlebitis (thrŏm-bō-flē-bī'tĭs) [G. *thrombos*, a clot, + *phleps, phleb-*, vein, + *-itis*, inflammation]. Inflammation of a vein associated with formation of a thrombus.

NP: Immobilize the affected limb, elevate it and support with a pillow. The weight of bedclothes should be removed by supporting them on a cradle. Fomentations may be ordered. All applications should be kept in place by a many-tailed bandage made so movement of the limb is prevented in changing dressings. Limb should be kept from pressure and well wrapped to keep it warm. It should be inspected daily to see that skin is in good condition. Light diet to keep blood pressure low. No alcohol or red meats. Constipation and straining at stool must be avoided. No excitement. Keep patient in bed for at least 6 weeks. Limb may have to be bandaged from toes to thigh to keep down swelling.

TREATMENT: Absolute rest to avoid the greatest danger, which is an embolus. Leg elevated so hip and knee are in flexion and heat is applied. Patient must not get up until the temperature has been normal for at least a week; if there have been infarcts, for about 2 weeks.

t. migrans. Slowly advancing thrombophlebitis, which recurs.

t. saltans. T. occurring in the same vein or in a distant one, but not near the original lesion.

thromboplastic (thrŏm"bō-plăs'tĭk) [G. *thrombos*, clot, + *plassein*, to form]. Pert. to or causing acceleration of clot formation in the blood.

thromboplastin (thrŏm"bō-plăs'tĭn) [" + *plassein*, to form]. 1. A substance found in the tissues which accelerates clotting of the blood. 2. Proprietary extract of thromboplastin from cattle brain in physiological salt solution.

USES: Local treatment of hemorrhage.

thrombopoiesis (thrŏm"bō-poy-ē'sĭs) [" + *poiēsis*, production]. The formation of blood platelets.

thrombosed (thrŏm'bōzd) [G. *thrombos*, a clot]. 1. Coagulated; clotted. 2. Denoting a vessel containing a thrombus.

thrombosin (thrŏm-bō'sĭn) [G. *thrombos*, clot]. A substance derived from the cleavage of fibrinogen which can be converted into fibrin.

thrombosinusitis (thrŏm"bō-sī-nū-sī'tĭs) [" + L. *sinus*, cavity, + G. *-itis*, inflammation]. Thrombus formation of a dural sinus.

thrombosis (thrŏm-bō'sĭs) [G. *thrombos*, clot, + *-ōsis*, condition]. The formation of a blood clot or *thrombus*.

RS: *embolus*, "thromb-" *words, angina pectoris*.

It is a solid aggregation formed in circulating blood and such changes constitute *thrombosis*. When a thrombus is detached from its original site and found in another part, it is called a *thrombotic embolus*.* The simpler forms of *thrombi* do not contain clotted blood.

ETIOL: Trauma, esp. following an operation and parturition; cardiac and vascular disorders, obesity, heredity, increasing age, an excess of erythrocytes and of platelets, an overproduction of fibrinogen, and sepsis are predisposing causes.

SYM: *Lungs*: Obstruction of smaller vessels in the lungs causes an infarct manifested by sudden pain in the side of the chest, similar to pleurisy; also the spitting of blood, a pleural friction rub, and signs of consolidation. *Kidneys*: Blood appears in the urine, and small hemorrhagic spots in the skin. *Spleen*: Pain is felt in the left upper abdomen. *Extremities*: If a large artery in one of the extremities, such as the brachial, is suddenly obstructed, the part becomes cold, pale, bluish, and the pulse disappears below the obstructed site. Gangrene of the digits or of the whole limb may ensue. Same symptoms may apply to embolisms, *q.v.*

NP: In thrombosis of a limb rest in bed is essential. Blood pressure must be kept low to prevent movement of a portion of the clot, so patient must remain very quiet. He must not be permitted to move himself; not even the upper portion of his body. Elevate the affected limb on a pillow and steady it with sandbags. Cotton or wool may be wrapped about the limb and held in place by a many-tailed bandage, extending from groin to foot. Any application to the limb must be kept in place by a similar bandage.

If limb is badly swollen watch for pressure sores. Guard against burning with hot water bottle or electric pad. Remember excitement causes a rise in blood pressure and it may dislodge the clot irrespective of body movement. Straining at stool must be avoided, so the bowels should be kept open. No stimulants should be given, although very weak tea or coffee may be taken. All drinks should be cool. From 6 weeks' to 6 months' rest may be necessary according to size of obstructed vessel.

t., atrophic. Marasmic thrombosis.

t., cardiac. Thrombosis of the heart.

t., coagulation. T. due to coagulation of fibrin in a blood vessel.

t., compression. T. due to compression bet. a thrombus and the heart.

t., coronary. T. of the coronary arteries.

SYM: Severe precordial pain extending to right arm, or epigastrium. Dyspnea and restlessness. If patient survives at-

Symptoms	Coronary Thrombosis	Angina Pectoris
Onset	At rest	With effort
Character of pain	Continuous	Paroxysmal
Duration of attack	Hours or days	Seconds or minutes
Patient	Often restless	Remains still
Blood pressure	Falls	Rises
Pulse	Sometimes irregular	Regular
Vomiting	Common	Uncommon
Treatment	Morphia	Amyl nitrite
	Amyl nitrite has no effect	Morphia

thrombosis, dilatation   T-28   **thymotropic**

tack 6 to 18 hr., collapse ensues and recovery is very gradual.

TREATMENT: Anticoagulants; thyroid extract; oxygen; increase of circulation by massage; deep breathing, but only on physician's directions; a mustard plaster twice a day; local applications of hot air; increase water intake, esp. per rectum in postoperative cases. Surgery may be necessary.

DIET: Low protein and carbohydrate diet. Morphine and quinidine sulfate.

NP: Six weeks' to 6 months' rest. Keep patient quiet in bed. Must not move himself. If limb is affected it should be elevated. Do not handle or touch affected vein for fear of dislodging clot. No stimulants; cool drinks, not hot ones. Patient must not strain at stool. Avoid anxiety or annoyance.

t., dilatation. T. due to dilatation of a vein.

t., embolic. T. due to an embolus obstructing a vessel.

t., infective. T. due to bacterial infection.

t., marasmic. T. due to wasting diseases of infancy and old age.

t., placental. Thrombi in the placenta and veins of the uterus.

t., plate. Thrombus formed from an accumulation of blood platelets.

t., puerperal. Coagulation in veins following labor.

t., sinus. T. of a venous sinus.

LATERAL: ETIOL: Associated with middle ear disease. SYM: Sudden rise of temperature with remission, chills, prostration, sweats, headache, mental symptoms, dullness or delirium, high leukocyte count.

CAVERNOUS: Sinus structures involved, edema and venous stasis in and about the eye.

t., traumatic. T. due to a wound or injury of a part.

t., venous. T. of a vein.

thrombostasis (thrŏm-bŏs'tă-sĭs) [G. *thrombos*, clot, + *stasis*, a checking]. Stasis of blood in a part causing or due to formation of thrombus.

thrombotic (thrŏm-bŏt'ĭk) [G. *thrombos*, clot]. Related to, caused by, or of the nature of, a thrombus.

thrombus (thrŏm'bŭs) [G. *thrombos*]. A blood clot obstructing a blood vessel or a cavity of the heart.

Heparin,* an anticoagulant, injected intravenously, is being used in prevention and treatment of this condition.

t., agony. Heart clot formed after prolonged heart failure occurring while patient is dying.

t., antemortem. A clot formed before death in heart or large vessels.

t., ball. A round clot in the heart, esp. in the auricles.

t., lateral. A clot attached to the wall of a vessel, without obstructing its lumen completely.

t., milk. A curdled milk tumor in the female breast due to obstruction in a lactiferous duct.

t., mural. T. which is located on a diseased area of endocardium.

through drainage (thrū). D. by tube passing through a cavity from one surface to another. SEE: *drainage*.

t. illumina′tion. Passage of light through the walls of an organ or cavity, for medical examination. SYN: *transillumination*.

thrush (thrŭsh) [Dutch *tröske*, rotten wood]. Mycotic infection of mouth or throat, esp. in infants and young children, characterized by formation of white patches, ulcer formation, and frequently fever and gastrointestinal inflammation. SYN: *aphtha, sprue, stomatitis, q.v.*

thrypsis (thrĭp′sĭs) [G. *thrypsis*, a breaking in pieces]. A comminuted fracture.

thulium (thū′lĭ-ŭm). A rare metallic element found in combination with minerals. SYMB: *Tm*. At. wt. 169.4.

thumb (thŭm) [A.S. *thūma*, thumb]. The short, thick, first finger on radial side of the hand, having but 2 phalanges and greater freedom of movement than other fingers. SYN: *pollex*.

thylacitis (thī″lă-sī′tĭs) [G. *thylax*, pouch, + *-itis*, inflammation]. Inflammation of the sebaceous glands of the skin.

thymectomy (thī-mĕk′tō-mĭ) [G. *thymos*, thymus, + *-ektomē*, excision]. Surgical removal of the thymus gland.

thymelcosis (thī-mĕl-kō′sĭs) [″ + *elkōsis*, ulceration]. Ulceration of the thymus gland.

thymergastic reaction (thī-mĕr-găs′tĭk) [G. *thymos*, mind, + *ergasia*, work]. Name for psychic disorders most equivalent to manic-depressive or affect psychosis.*

thymic (thī′mĭk) [G. *thymos*, thymus]. Relating to the thymus gland.

t. acid. 1. Acid obtained by heating nucleic acid of thymus gland with water. 2. Thymol, *q.v.*

t. asthma. Spasmodic closing of the glottis followed by a pronounced inspiration. SYN: *laryngismus stridulus*.

t. death. Sudden death in status lymphaticus and thymic asthma.

t. stridor. T. asthma.

thymion (thĭm′ĭ-ŏn) [G. *thymion*, wart]. A wart.

thymitis (thī-mī′tĭs) [G. *thymos*, thymus, + *-itis*, inflammation]. Inflammation of the thymus gland.

thymo- [G.]. Combining form meaning *thymus*.

thymocyte (thī′mō-sīt) [G. *thymos*, thymus, + *kytos*, cell]. A lymphocyte having origin in the thymus gland.

thymokesis (thī″mō-kē′sĭs) [G. *thymos*, thymus]. Abnormal enlargement and persistence of the thymus in the adult.

thymol (thī′mŏl) [G. *thymos*, thyme, + L. *oleum*, oil]. USP. White crystals obtained from oil of thyme.

ACTION AND USES: Antiseptic and anthelmintic.

DOSAGE: Antiseptic, 2 gr. (0.12 Gm.). Anthelmintic, 30 gr. (2 Gm.), div. into 3 doses.

t. iodide. USP. A reddish-brown powder.

USES: As a substitute for iodoform, as a dusting powder in various skin diseases.

thymolysis (thī-mŏl′ĭ-sĭs) [G. *thymos*, thymus, + *lysis*, dissolution]. Dissolution of thymus tissue.

thymolytic (thī″mō-lĭt′ĭk) [″ + *lysis*, dissolution]. Destructive to thymus tissue.

thymoma (thī-mō′mă) [″ + *-ōma*, tumor]. A tumor originating in epithelial tissues of the thymus gland.

thymopathy (thī-mŏp′ă-thī) [G. *thymos*, mind, thymus, + *pathos*, disease]. 1. Any disease of the thymus gland. 2. Any mental disorder.

thymotoxic (thī″mō-tŏks′ĭk) [″ + *toxikon*, poison]. Poisonous to thymus tissue.

thymotrope (thī′mō-trōp) [″ + *tropē*, a turning]. A person exhibiting thymotropism.

thymotropic (thī″mō-trŏp′ĭk) [″ + *tropē*, a turning]. Relating to thymotropism.

thymotropism (thī-mŏt'rō-pĭzm) [" + " + -*ismos*, condition]. The endocrine type in which the thymus influence predominates.

thymus (thī'mŭs) [G. *thymos*]. A lymphoid or ductless glandular organ in the neck and upper part of the thorax behind the manubrium of the sternum, which is included in the endocrine system although it produces no known hormone.

It attains full size at puberty, after which it gradually atrophies so that in adults only remnants remain. Function is unknown. About 2 in. in length, 1½ in. in breadth below and 3 or 4 lines in thickness when full size. At birth weighs about ½ oz.

PATH: Sometimes it is much larger than it should be and is then known as enlarged or persistent thymus. Children having these enlarged structures are particularly susceptible to infections and anesthetics, and are liable to sudden death under the latter. This condition is readily cured by the x-ray.

t., accessory. A lobule isolated from the mass of the thymus gland.

t. persistens hyperplastica. A thymus persisting into adulthood, sometimes hypertrophying.

thymusectomy (thī"mŭs-ĕk'tō-mĭ) [G. *thymos*, thymus, + -*ektome*, excision]. Surgical excision of the thymus.

thypar (thī'păr). Lacking the thyroid and parathyroid glands.

thyrasthenia (thī-răs-thē'nĭ-ă) [G. *thyreos*, shield, (+ *eidos*, form, thyroid), + *astheneia*, weakness]. Neurasthenic condition resulting from deficient thyroid secretion.

thyremphraxis (thī-rĕm-frăks'ĭs) [" + *emphraxis*, stoppage]. Arrested function of the thyroid gland.

thyreocele (thī're̊-ō-sēl) [" + *kele*, a mass]. Enlargement of the thyroid gland. SYN: *goiter*.

thyreoid (thī're-oyd) [" + *eidos*, form]. Thyroid.

thyreoitis (thī-rē-ō-ī'tĭs) [" + -*itis*, inflammation]. Inflammation of the thyroid gland. SYN: *thyroiditis*.

thyrin(e (thī'rĭn) [G. *thyreos*, shield]. The active principle of the thyroid gland's secretion.

thyro-, thyreo- [G.]. Combining forms meaning *oblong, shield, thyroid*.

thyroadenitis (thī"rō-ăd-en-ī'tĭs) [G. *thyreos*, shield, + *aden*, gland, + -*itis*, inflammation]. Inflammation of thyroid gland.

thyroaplasia (thī"rō-ă-plā'zĭ-ă) [" + *a-*, priv. + *plasis*, a molding]. Imperfect development of the thyroid gland.

thyroarytenoid (thī"rō-ă-rĭt'en-oyd) [" + *arytaina*, pitcher, + *eidos*, form]. Relating to the thyroid and arytenoid cartilages.

thyrocardiac (thī"rō-kar'dĭ-ăk) [" + *kardia*, heart]. 1. Pert. to the heart and thyroid gland. 2. A person suffering from thyroid disease complicated by heart disorder.

thyrocarditis (thī"rō-kar-dī'tĭs) [" + " + -*itis*, inflammation]. Any affection of heart muscle occurring with hyperthyroidism, such as auricular fibrillation, tachycardia, etc.

thyrocele (thī'rō-sēl) [" + *kele*, mass]. Enlarged condition of the thyroid gland. SYN: *goiter*.

thyrochondrotomy (thī"rō-kŏn-drŏt'ō-mĭ) [" + *chondros*, cartilage, + *tome*, a cutting]. Surgical incision of thyroid cartilage. SYN: *laryngotomy*.

thyrocricotomy (thī-rō-krī-kŏt'ō-mĭ) [G. *thyreos*, shield, + *krikos*, ring, + *tome*, a cutting]. Tracheotomy; division of the cricothyroid membrane.

thyroepiglottic (thī"rō-ĕp-ĭ-glŏt'ĭk) [" + *epi*, upon, + *glottis*, glottis]. Relating to the thyroid and epiglottis.

thyroepiglottideus (thī"rō-ĕp"ĭ-glŏt-ĭd'ē-ŭs) [" + " + *glottis*, glottis]. Muscle in the thyroid cartilage that depresses the epiglottis.

thyroglobulin (thī"rō-glŏb'ū-lĭn) [" + L. *globulus*, a tiny sphere]. A protein derived from the thyroid gland which contains iodine.

thyrohyal (thī"rō-hī'ăl) [" + *hyoeides*, U-shaped]. 1. Concerning thyroid gland and hyoid bone. 2. Greater cornu of hyoid bone. 3. Embryonic skeletal remnant which becomes one of the major cornu of the hyoid.

thyrohyoid (thī"rō-hī'oyd) [" + *hyoeides*, U-shaped]. Rel. to thyroid cartilage and hyoid bone. SYN: *hyothyroid*.

thyroid (thī'royd) [G. *thyreos*, shield, + *eidos*, form]. 1. Thyroid extract, *q.v.* 2. A gland of internal secretion in the neck, ant. to and partially surrounding the thyroid cartilage and upper rings of the trachea.

It has 3 lobes, 2 lateral and 1 median. It resembles a horseshoe in shape. It controls growth and the rate of metabolism. Hypertrophy of the gland is associated with exophthalmic goiter, and its absence produces cretinism or myxedema.

So far as is known, the thyroid elaborates only 1 hormone, *thyroxine*, a compound rich in iodine. The principal effect of the thyroid hormone is to accelerate the metabolism of all cells and tissues; the rate at which this hormone is discharged into the blood stream regulates the speed at which combustion takes place in the body. This hormone also affects the tone of the autonomic nervous system.

Iodine is a chemical element which enters into the composition of thyroxine. Since it is impossible for the body to manufacture chemical elements, the thyroid cannot make its hormone unless it is supplied with iodine in some form. The amount needed daily is only about 0.001 Gm. SEE: *iodine*.

DOSAGE: 1 gr. (0.06 Gm.).

SYM: *(Deficiency)* May be marked gain in weight and sluggishness. Round face, depression of nose; many folds of skin beneath eyes and jaws; tongue thick, voice guttural, skin dry and cold; hair brittle, falling out easily. Low metabolism, mind and body placid and lazy, all seen in myxedema. Milder forms more common. Fatigue outstanding; brittle or rigid nails, dry skin, shortness of breath, body more or less cold. Impotence may exist. Nervousness, depression, headache and irritability. Increase of cholestrol. Puffiness only in myxedema.

t. cachexia. Exophthalmic goiter.

t. extract. USP. The dried thyroid glands of the ox or sheep.

ACTION AND USES: Used in cases of deficient action of the gland.

DOSAGE: 1-5 gr. (0.06-0.32 Gm.).

ADMINISTRATION: Tablet form by mouth. A large dose may be given for full effect, followed by maintenance dosage. It is more desirable, however, to begin with a small dose and gradually increase until desired effect is produced. It does not exercise its maximum effect

thyroid therapy   T-30   **tic douloureux**

for about 10 days. As it has this cumulative effect dosage should not be increased too rapidly. Thyroid may be necessary all through a patient's life.
t. therapy. Thyroid ext. treatment.
thyroidectomized (thī-roy-děk'tō-mĭzd) [G. *thyreos*, shield, +*eidos*, form, + *-ektomē*, excision]. With the thyroid gland removed.
thyroidectomy (thī-royd-ĕk'tō-mĭ) [" + " + *-ektomē*, excision]. Excision of the thyroid gland.
Post. NP: Patient in sitting position as soon as recovered from anesthesia, head and arms well supported. Watch for edema. Steam inhalations sometimes ordered. Give absolute mental and physical rest as much as possible.
thyroidism (thī'roy-dĭzm) [" + " + *-ismos*, condition]. 1. Poisoning from overdose of thyroid extract or increased secretion of the thyroid gland. 2. Deficiency of thyroid function, as in removal of the gland.
thyroiditis (thī"roy-dī'tĭs) [" + " + *-itis*, inflammation]. Inflammation of the thyroid gland.
thyroidization (thī"roy-dī-zā'shŭn) [G. *thyreos*, shield, + *eidos*, form]. Thyroid extract therapy.
thyroidotomy (thī-royd-ŏt'ō-mĭ) [" + " + *tomē*, a cutting]. Incision of thyroid gland.
thyrointoxication (thī"rō-ĭn-tŏks-ĭ-kā'shŭn) [" + " + L. *in*, into, + G. *toxikon*, poison]. Poisoning from excessive use of thyroid extract or hyperaction of the thyroid gland.
thyrolytic (thī"rō-lĭt'ĭk) [" + " + *lysis*, dissolution]. Causing destruction of thyroid tissue.
thyroncus (thī-rŏng'kŭs) [" + " + *ogkos*, tumor]. Enlarged thyroid gland. Syn: *goiter, struma, thyrocele*.
thyroparathyroidectomy (thī"rō-par-ă-thī-roy-děk'tō-mĭ) [" + " + *para*, beside, + *thyreos*, shield, + *eidos*, form, + *ektomē*, excision]. Surgical removal of the thyroid and parathyroid glands.
thyropenia (thī"rō-pē'nĭ-ă) [" + " + *venia*, lack]. Defective thyroid secretion with no clinical symptoms.
thyrophyma (thī"rō-fī'mă) [G. *thyreos*, shield, + *eidos*, form, + *phyma*, growth]. Neoplasm of the thyroid gland.
thyroprival (thī-rō-prī'văl) [" + L. *privus*, lacking]. Pert. to a condition resulting from loss of function or removal of the thyroid gland.
thyroptosis (thī-rŏp-tō'sĭs) [" + *ptōsis*, a dropping]. Downward displacement of a goitrous thyroid into the thorax.
thyrosis (thī-rō'sĭs) [" + *-ōsis*, condition]. Any condition due to abnormal thyroid action.
thyrotherapy (thī"rō-ther'ă-pĭ) [" + *therapeia*, treatment]. Treatment with thyroid gland extracts.
thyrotome (thī'rō-tōm) [" + *tomos*, a piece]. Knife for cutting the thyroid cartilage.
thyrotomy (thī-rŏt'ō-mĭ) [" + *tomē*, a cutting]. 1. The splitting of the thyroid cartilage anteriorly in midline in order to expose laryngeal structures. Syn: *laryngofissure*. 2. Surgery on the thyroid gland.
thyrotoxic (thī"rō-tŏks'ĭk) [G. *thyreos*, shield, + *toxikon*, poison]. Pert. to, affected by, or marked by toxic activity of the thyroid gland.
thyrotoxicosis (thī"rō-tŏks-ĭ-kō'sĭs) [" + " + *-ōsis*, condition]. The condition of intoxication due to excessive thyroid secretion. Syn: *exophthalmic goiter, q.v.*

Sym: Rapid heart action, tremors, elevated basal metabolism, enlarged gland, exophthalmos, nervous symptoms, and loss of weight.
Before surgery to correct the condition patient must gain weight.
thyrotrope (thī'rō-trōp) [G. *thyreos*, shield, + *tropē*, a turning]. One with tendency to thyroid disorders or thyroid influence of the endocrine system.
thyrotropic (thī"rō-trŏp'ĭk) [" + *tropē*, a turning]. Pert. to or characterized by thyrotropism.
thyrotropin (thī-rŏt'rō-pĭn) [" + *tropē*, a turning]. The anterior pituitary element which influences the thyroid gland.
thyrotropism (thī-rŏt'rō-pĭzm) [" + " + *-ismos*, condition]. That type of endocrine constitution dominated by the effects of thyroid secretion.
thyroxin (thī-rŏks'ĭn) [G. *thyreos*, shield]. USP. Thyroid glands of animals which are used for food by man, dried, powdered, and containing not less than 0.17 or more than 0.23 per cent of iodine.
Action and Uses: Affects metabolism. In cretinism, myxedema, and other cases of deficient thyroid function.
Dosage: Average 1 gr. (0.06 Gm.).
thyroxine (thī-rŏks'ēn) [G. *thyreos*, shield]. The crystalline, active iodine principle (an amino acid derivative) of the thyroid secretion which stimulates the rate of oxidation.
tibia (tĭb'ĭ-ă) [L. *tibia*, shinbone]. The inner and larger bone of the leg bet. the knee and ankle articulating with the femur above and with the astragalus below.
Fracture of: The leg is put in plaster when this bone is broken. If there is much displacement a pin put through the os calcis is incorporated in the plaster and the leg placed in a Braun's splint.
t., Lannelongue's. A syphilitic tibia.
t., saber-shaped. A deformity of the tibia due to gummatous periostitis (syphilitic) in which it curves outward.
tibialis (tĭb-ĭ-ā'lĭs) [L.]. One of 2 muscles of the calf of the leg.
tibioadductor reflex (tĭb"ĭ-ō-ăd-dŭk'tor) [L. *tibia*, shinbone, + *adducere*, to lead to]. Lateral or crossed adduction of leg when tibia is percussed on its inner side.
tibiofemoral (tĭb"ĭ-ō-fem'ō-răl) [" + *femur, femor-*, thigh]. Relating to the tibia and femur.
tibiofibular (tĭb"ĭ-ō-fĭb'ŭ-lar) [" + *fibula*, buckle]. Relating to the tibia and fibula.
tibiotarsal (tĭb"ĭ-ō-tar'săl) [" + G. *tarsos*, flat of the foot]. Relating to the tibia and tarsus.
tic (tĭk) [Fr.]. A spasmodic muscular contraction, most commonly involving the face, head, neck, or shoulder muscles. Syn: *habit spasm*.
The spasms may be tonic* or clonic.* The movement appears purposeful, is often repeated, involuntary, can be inhibited for a short time, only to burst forth with increased severity.
Etiol: Certain of these cases are due to structure changes, many psychogenic, the expression of frustration, and its correlated muscular tension. The former group most commonly encountered in patients who have suffered from lethargic encephalitis. See: *tiqueur*.
t., convulsive. Facial muscle spasm.
t. douloureux (doo-loo-ru'). Degeneration of or pressure on the trigeminal nerve, resulting in neuralgia of that nerve. RF: *neuralgia*. The pain is ex-

tic, facial

cruciating. Usually occurs after forty. Pain is paroxysmal, radiating from angle of the jaw along one of the involved branches. If the first branch, a shocklike pain is felt along the eye and back over the forehead. If it is the middle fiber, the upper lip, nose, and cheek under the eye are affected. If it is the third branch, pain is in the lower lip and outer border of tongue on affected side. Pain is momentary but returns again and again.
  t., facial. Same as *convulsive tic*.
  t., habit. Habitual repetition of a grimace or muscular action.
  t., spasmodic. Tonic contractions and paralysis of muscles of one or both sides of the face.
tick [M.E. *tike*]. Any of the numerous bloodsucking arachnids of the order Acarida. Ixodidae is the hard tick family and Argas the soft. They transmit specific diseases to man and lower animals.
  t. fever. 1. Any infectious disease transmitted by the bite of a tick. 2. African relapsing fever. 3. Specifically, an acute infectious disease transmitted by the bite of a wood tick in the Rocky Mountain region. SYN: *Rocky Mountain spotted fever, spotted fever.*
  ETIOL: A bacillary microörganism (*Dermacentroxenus rickettsi*) transmitted by a tick.
  SYM: *Incubation period:* From the bite to the first symptom, 2-12 days if infection is mild, 3-5 days otherwise. Onset may be gradual or sudden, but generally for a period of 1 or more days; if so, it is preceded by weakness, chilly sensations and then a definite chill.
  Other symptoms are headache in front and back of head, or both; more or less bloodshot eyes with sensitivity to light; eyeballs sore to touch: white coated tongue with red edges; deep, dusky flush on face; pain in muscles, bones, and joints; backache, esp. in lower portion; bronchial cough; nosebleed; constipation, and marked weakness. The skin becomes spotted bet. the 3rd and 5th day after onset. The spots resemble those of measles but differ in distribution. In Rocky Mountain spotted fever spots are apt to be concentrated on the wrist, ankles, and feet, instep, soles, and outer margin of the foot from the small toe, posteriorly. The trunk is usually free from spots. The spots appear to disappear on pressure but later become hemorrhagic, changing to a rust color due to disintegration.
  PRECAUTIONS: If one suspects being infected: (a) Patient must conserve strength; (b) do not use drugs; (c) go to a hospital at the earliest possible moment. If tick is identified on the skin, do not touch with bare hands, but use gloves or a tweezer to remove it. Do not crush it on the skin. *Immediate aid is imperative.*
tickle (tĭk'l) [origin uncertain]. 1. Peculiar sensation caused by titillation or touching, esp. in certain regions, resulting in reflex muscular movements, laughter, or hysteria. 2. To arouse such a sensation by touching a surface lightly.
tickling (tĭk'lĭng) [origin uncertain]. Gentle stimulation of a sensitive surface and its reflex effect, such as involuntary laughter, etc. SYN: *titillation.*
tictology (tĭk-tol'ō-jĭ) [G. *tiktein*, to give birth, + *logos*, science]. Science of managing pregnancy and childbirth. SYN: *obstetrics.*
t. i. d. [L. *ter in die*]. Three times a day.

T-31

tincture

tidal air (tī'dăl). That which is inhaled and exhaled during normal, quiet breathing. SEE: *air, respiration.*
  t. respiration. Cycles of respiratory movements of varying intensity with pauses between them. SYN: *Cheyne-Stokes respiration,* q.v.
tide [A.S. *tid*, time]. Alternate rise and fall; a space of time.
  t., acid. Temporary acidity of urine following fasting.
  t., alkaline. Temporary decrease in acid of urine after eating.
tigretier (tē-grĕt-ē-ā') [Fr.]. A dancing mania or form of tarantism due to bite of a poisonous spider occurring in Tigré, Abyssinia.
tigroid (tī'groyd) [G. *tigroeidēs*, spotted]. Marked like a tiger, a term applied to chromophil corpuscles.
  t. bodies, t. masses. Chromophilic bodies in protoplasm of a nerve cell.
tilmus (tĭl'mŭs) [G. *tilmos*, a plucking]. Delirious picking at the bedclothes by the patient. SYN: *carphology.*
timbre (tĭm'ber, tahn'br) [Fr. a bell to be struck with a hammer]. Resonance quality of a sound by which it is distinguished, other than pitch or intensity, depending upon the number and character of vibrating body's overtones.
time (tīm) [A.S. *tima*, time]. Interval bet. beginning and ending; measured duration. SEE: *biduous, bis in die.* [utes.
  t. bleeding. T. coagulation. 1-3 min
  t., coagulation. Time taken by coagulation of a drop of blood.
  t., prothrombin. That needed for oxalated plasma to clot, measured in seconds, after adding thromboplastin and recalcifying.
  t., reaction. Period bet. application of a stimulus and the response.
tin (tĭn) [A.S.]. SYMB: *Sn.* At. wt. 118.70. A metallic element, used in medicine.
  POISONING: Tin in tinned or soldered containers in the past has occasionally been responsible for poisoning. This is exceedingly rare and for practical purposes need not be considered.
  SYM: Metallic taste, gastrointestinal irritation, nausea, vomiting, cramping, and diarrhea.
  F. A. TREATMENT: Wash out stomach and administer bland or soothing drinks.
tinctorial (tĭnk-tō'rĭ-al) [L. *tinctorius*, dyeing]. Relating to staining or color.
tincture (tĭngk'tūr) [L. *tinctura*, a dyeing]. Diluted alcoholic solutions of nonvolatile substances (tincture of iodine being an exception), 10% being standard strength for powerful drugs and 20% for weaker ones.
  The name of any fluid contained in the tincture other than alcohol is added to the name of the tincture.
  They are the most commonly used class of preparations. They usually contain tannic acid, so, in most instances, cannot be employed with agents that are incompatible with that drug. Those tinctures that contain resinous matter or oils will precipitate with water. Some examples are tinctures of *ginger, benzoin, guaiac,* etc. Tinctures of the most potent drugs usually represent 10% of the crude drug, as tinctures of *opium, digitalis, aconite,* etc. Where more than a fluidram of a 10% tincture would have to be taken to get a dose of the drug, the tincture is usually made to represent 20%, or more, of the agent. The majority of tinctures can be put roughly into 2 groups; those the dose of

tincture iodine   T-32   **tirefond**

which is about 10 minims and those of fluid dram doses. Forty are official.

t. iodine. POISONING: This commonly used antiseptic is sometimes taken by mouth.
DOSAGE: 1½ ℳ (0.1 cc.).
SYM: Very strong irritation of mouth, esophagus, and stomach. Stains membranes dark brown or black. Pain intense, and leads to early vomiting and purging; extreme thirst, often collapse.
TREATMENT: Give large amounts of water, milk and starchy paste; gruels, as boiled rice or arrowroot.

tinea (tĭn'ē-ä) [L. *tinea*, worm]. Any fungous skin disease, esp. ringworm, occurring in various parts of the body, names indicating the part affected, as *T. barbae, T. corporis, T. tonsurans,* etc.
SYM: Superficial or deep types. Superficial is marked by scaling; slight itching; reddish or grayish patches; dry, brittle hair which is easily extracted with hair shaft. Deep type is characterized by flat, reddish, kerionlike tumors, the surface studded with dead or broken hairs or by gaping follicular orifices. Nodules may be broken down in center, discharging pus, etc., through dilated follicular openings.
TREATMENT: Vaccines. Parasiticides for general body surface. That attacking palms and soles is resistant. Fuchsin paint, salicylic and sulfur mixture, avoid soap and water. In tinea cruris, iodine in carbon tetrachloride, salicylic and benzoic acids, iodine. In ringworm of crotch, soothing remedies, antipruritic powders, followed by antiseptics (sod. hyposulfite, carbolized resorcin, iodine, mercuric chloride, formalin), then soothing lotions. In long-standing cases, chrysarobin. Ringworm of scalp is most resistant to treatment. X-rays, total depilation, prevention of new foci, and eradication of those existing, maintaining an aseptic condition of scalp.

t. circinata. On the body—red, slight, elevated, scaly patches, which on examination reveal minute vesicles or papules. New patches spring from the periphery while central portion clears up. Often considerable itching.
PROG: Favorable.
TREATMENT: Constitutional. Mercury, sulfurous acid among best parasiticides.

t. circinata cruris. Tinea about the genitals, esp. on inside of thighs.

t. cruris. Same as *t. circinata cruris.*

t. favosa. An infectious disease of skin, typically on scalp, due to a specific fungus; characterized by peculiar saucer-shaped, sulfur yellow crusts. The fungus is *Achorion schönleinii*. SYN: *favus.*

t. furfuracea. T. with whitish, greasy scales or crusts.

t. inguinalis. SEE: *t. cruris.*

t. intersecto. A rare condition beginning as small, roundish, slightly elevated, itching spots on arms, chest, and back which become brown, with a smooth, tense surface, increasing in size, and coalesce.

t. kerion. A form of *t. tonsurans.*

t. nodosa. Sheathlike, nodular masses in hair of beard and mustache from growth of an unknown fungus. They surround the hairs, which become brittle, and hair may be penetrated by fungus and thus split.

t. sycosis. Begins as a red, scaly patch involving the bearded region; purplish tubercles and pustules form around the opening of the hair, follicles and hairs become lusterless, brittle and loose. Considerable itching.
PROG: Favorable, but unless treated actively may cause permanent loss of hair.
TREATMENT: Affected hairs should be removed and some parasiticide applied. Internal treatment.

t. tonsurans. Observed almost exclusively on scalp of children. Characterized by 1 or more rounded, scaly, elevated, grayish-colored patches through which project dry, brittle, lusterless, broken-off hairs.
PROG: Favorable.
TREATMENT: Parts thoroughly washed with soap and water, affected hairs removed. Any of the above mentioned parasiticides may be employed. General treatment to tone up system.

t. trichophytina. Local infectious disease of skin, produced by the trichophyton fungus. The organism grows in the horny epithelium. The lesions vary according to part of body attacked, and whether the hairs are involved. SYN: *ringworm.*

t. versicolor. A chronic disease excited by a vegetable parasite, the *Microsporon furfur.*
SYM: Disease of adult life. More frequent in the debilitated and uncleanly. Usually appears on front of chest as small, round spots of pale yellow or fawn color, which slowly enlarge, fuse and form slightly elevated, scaly patches. Subjective symptoms absent.
PROG: Favorable.
TREATMENT: Parts should be frequently washed with soap and water, after which a parasiticide may be applied. Corrosive sublimate or some other preparation. SYN: *pityriasis versicolor.*

tingible (tĭn'jĭ-bl) [L. *tingere*, to stain]. Capable of being stained.

tinnitus (tĭn-ī'tŭs) [L. *tinnitus*, a jingling]. A ringing or tinkling sound that is purely subjective.

t. aurium. Ringing, tinkling, buzzing, or other sounds in the ear.
Found in conditions of ext., middle, or inner ear.
ETIOL: Impacted cerumen, myringitis, otitis media, labyrinthitis, Meniere's symptom complex, otosclerosis, hysteria, etc. Also follows overdosage of drugs such as quinine.

t. cere'bri. Noises in the head.

t., nervous. A neurosis; a subjective humming or buzzing sound in nervous people due to disturbance of otic nerve.

t., telephone. Tinnitus resulting from excessive use of the telephone.

tintometer (tĭn-tŏm'ē-ter) [L. *tinctus*, a dyeing, + G. *metron*, a measure]. A scale of different shades of color to determine by comparison the intensity of color of the blood or other fluid.

tintometric (tĭn″tō-mĕt'rĭk) [" + G. *metron*, a measure]. Relating to tintometry.

tintometry (tĭn-tŏm'ē-trĭ) [" + G. *metron*, a measure]. Estimation of a color by comparison with a scale of colors.

-tion. O.E. and L. suffix forming abstract names.

-tious. O.E. suffix forming adjective.

tiqueur (tē-kur') [Fr.]. One afflicted with a tic.

tire (tīr) [A.S. *tyrian*, to tire]. 1. Exhaustion; fatigue. 2. To exhaust or fatigue. 3. To become fatigued.

tirefond (tēr-fon') [Fr.]. Appliance like a corkscrew for raising depressed portions

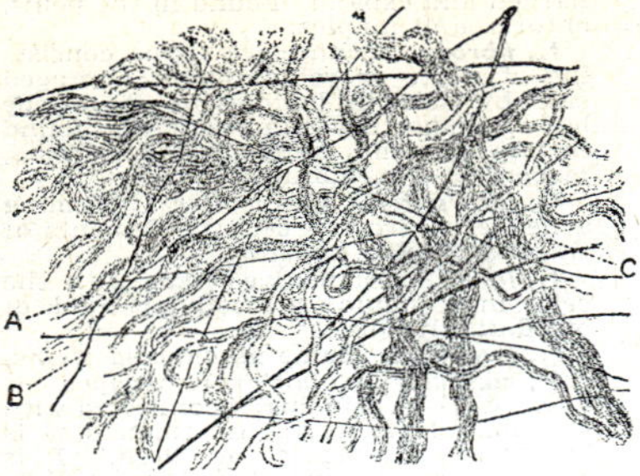

Areolar connective tissue: A. White fiber; B. Elastic fiber; C. Migratory cell.

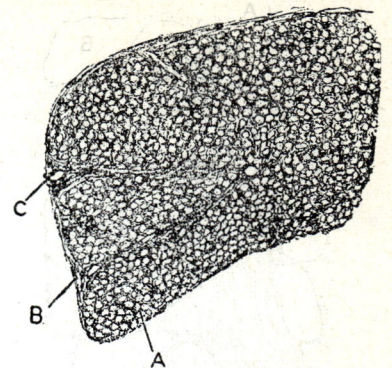

Elastic tissue: Transverse section, ligamentum nuchae: A. Cross section elastic fibers; B. Connective tissue sheath; C. Blood vessel.

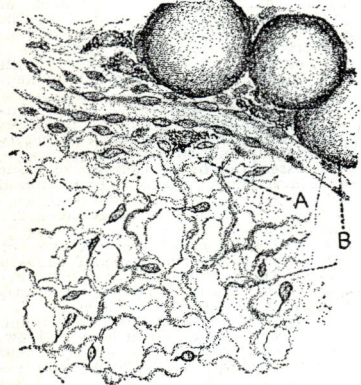

Reticular connective tissue: A. Plasma cells; B. Fat cells.

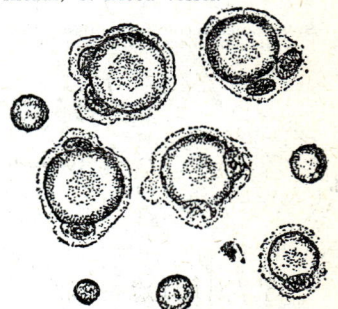

Adipose tissue: Fat cells and fat granules.

TISSUE TYPES.

of bone or for removing foreign bodies.

tires (tīrz). Condition marked by constipation, vomiting, muscular tremors, and pain. SYN: *milk sickness, trembles.*

tisic (tĭz'ĭk) [G. *phthisikos*, wasting]. Pert. to wasting away or emaciation. SYN: *phthisic.*

tissue (tĭsh'ū) [O.Fr. *tissu*, from L. *texere*, to weave]. A collection of similar cells and fibers forming a definite fabric or structure in plants and animals, such as: (a) *Connective t.;* (b) *muscular t.;* (c) *nerve t.;* (d) *epithelial t.*, etc.

Body tissue is built by protein. The amino acids are necessary for tissue repair; 0.6 Gm. of p. will care for 1 kilogram, or 2.2 lb., of body tissue, which is the minimum necessary to maintain the protein at a basal level. One Gm. per kilogram of normal body weight is minimum for children, and 2 to 3 Gm. the maximum.

t., adenoid. Reticular tissue or lymphoid t., which holds lymph cells in the meshes of its network.

t., adipose. Areolar tissue filled with fat cells.

t., areolar. It forms sheaths, insulates and connects. The cells are separated by an irregular network of white and yellow fibers.

t., chromophil. Those tissues which give a chromophil reaction; found in the medulla and sympathetic ganglia.

t., connective. T. which supports and connects other tissues and parts.

They are acted upon by other tissues and are highly vascular with the exception of cartilage. Their characteristics are determined by their intercellular substances. They include: (a) *Adipose t.;* (b) *areolar t.;* (c) *bone or osseous t.;* (d) *cartilage;* (e) *elastic t.;* (f) *embryonic t.;* (g) *fibrous t.;* (h) *liquid t.;* (i) *neuroglia;* (j) *reticular t.*

Connective t. is composed of yellow elastic fibers. It has a few white fibers. Found bet. the adjacent vertebrae, it unites the cartilages of the larynx and helps form the lungs, and is found in the arteries and blood vessels, bronchial tubes and vocal organs.

t., elastic. Part of connective tissue consisting of elastic fibers, or membranes.

t., embryonic. Found in the embryo; a connective tissue in which the cells unite and form a network with closely packed nuclei.

t., epithelial. Cells held together by collagen or a cell cement, arranged to form a membrane or skin covering ex-

tissue, erectile   T-34   **tissue, subserous areolar**

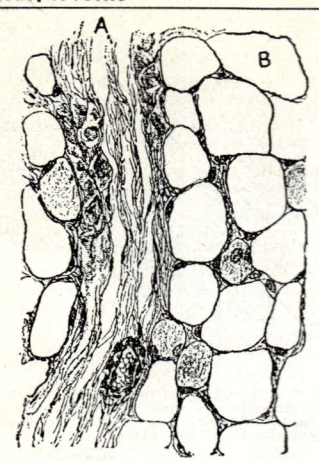

Subcutaneous connective tissue: A. Collagen fibers. B. Fat cells.

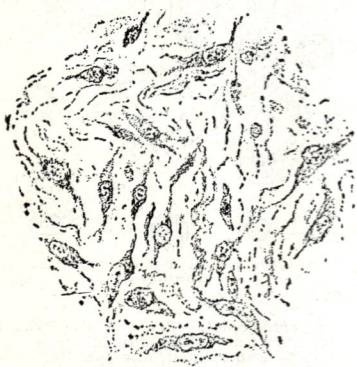

Connective tissue from human umbilical cord.
TISSUE TYPES

ternal surfaces and lining internal ones. It is called *boundary tissue*. It may be squamous, columnar, or modified.

t., erectile. Spongy tissue, the spaces of which fill with blood, causing it to harden and expand. Found in the penis, clitoris, and nipples.

t., fibrous. Connective tissue consisting of white or yellow fibers, arranged side by side in bundles; part of the body's supporting framework, and found in the ligaments, tendons, aponeuroses, fascias, and membranes.

t., interstitial. Connective t. forming a network with the cellular elements of the body. SYN: *stroma*.

t., liquid. Connective tissue with the cells in a liquid intercellular fluid of blood and lymph.

t., lymphoid. Same as *adenoid tissue*.

t., muscular (*voluntary*). Striped or striated tissue principally connected with the bony framework. In animals it is known as "lean meat" or "flesh." It is a cross-striped, muscular tissue, the fibers like a long cylinder with flattened sides and conical ends, enveloped in a delicate sheath, the *sarcolemma*. (*Involuntary*): Smooth or unstriped, or nonstriated, not under control of the will. Principally found in walls of hollow organs, tubes, arteries, and veins.

t., nervous. A mass of nerve cells and their processes supported by neuroglia.

t., neuroglia. Connective tissue containing *glia cells* with many processes intertwining among the cells and nerves of the brain and cord.

t., osseous or bone. Connective tissue with intercellular substance impregnated with phosphate and carbonate of calcium, the mineral substances being 2/3 of the bone's weight.

t., reticular or retiform. A type of connective tissue consisting of delicate fibers forming interlacing networks. Fibers stain selectively with silver stains and are called argyrophil fibers.

It supports lymph nodes and is found in muscular tissue and in bone marrow, the spleen, liver, lungs, kidneys, and mucous membranes of the gastrointestinal tract.

t., simple. T. made up of 1 structural element or slight admixture of others.

t., skeletal. Fibrous, adenoid, adipose, osseous, and cartilaginous tissue.

t., subarachnoid. Trabeculae of fibrous tissue bet. arachnoid and pia, covered with endothelia.

t., subcutaneous. Areolar tissue beneath the corium and becoming part of it.

t., s. adipose. Adipose tissue within subcutaneous tissue.

t., s. areolar. Areolar tissue beneath a mucous membrane connecting it with other parts.

t., subserous areolar. Areolar tissue

Tissue Development

Ectoderm	Mesoderm	Entoderm

1. Epidermis.
2. Epithelium of:
   External and internal ear.
   Nasal cavity.
   Mouth.
   Anus.
   Amnion; chorion.
   Distal part of male urethra.
3. Nervous tissue.
	1. Connective tissues.
	2. Male and female reproductive tracts.
	3. Blood vessels; lymphatics.
	4. Kidneys; ureters; trigone of bladder.
	5. Pleura; peritoneum; pericardium.
		1. Respiratory tract except nose.
		2. Digestive tract except mouth and anus.
		3. Bladder except trigone.
		4. Male urethra, proximal portion.
		5. Female urethra.

attaching serous membranes to parts they invest.

t., trabecular. T., esp. connective tissue, in form of trabeculae often forming a network.

t., white fibrous. Connective t. with white, inelastic fibers, forming tendons, ligaments, and resistant membranes.

t., w. nervous. Nervous tissue of medullated nerve fibers.

t., yellow elastic. Same as *elastic tissue*.

tissue, words pert. to: abirritation, acapnia, adipose, adipositis, adiposity, amyloidosis, antixenic, aponeurosis, areolar, astroglia, biopsy, blastomycosis, bothrenchyma, brawny induration, calcification, calcipexy, cancellous, carnification, carotenosis, cartilage, cataphoric, cellulitis, cellulocutaneous, cerebrin, cerebrose, Chaussier's areola, colliquation, colloid, connective, convolution, degeneration, desmoma, detritus, diploe, dystopic, edema, elastic, elastin, emphysema, enclave, endothelium, epithelium, erosion, fascia, fibrosis, gangrene, "hist-" words, Hodgkin's disease, homeoplasia, hyperplasia, initis, interstitial, keloid, ligament, linea, linitis, malacia, matrix, perichondrium, phlegmon, resolvent, reticular, sarcitis, sarcology, septum, sphacelus, stroma, tease, tendon, trabecula, transpiration, urechysis, uredema.

tissue extract (tĭsh'ū). An insulin-free extract of the pancreas.
  USES: As a vasodilator.
  DOSAGE: 2-5 cc. subcutaneously or intramuscularly.

titanium (tī-tā'nĭ-ŭm) [L.]. A metallic element found in combination in minerals. SYMB: Ti.

titillation (tĭt-ĭl-ā'shŭn) [L. *titillatio*, a tickling]. 1. Act of tickling, as in the throat. 2. State of being tickled. 3. Sensation produced by tickling.

ti'ter [Fr. *titre*]. Standard of strength per volume of volumetric test solution.

titration (tī-trā'shŭn) [Fr. *titre*, a standard]. Determining strength of a solution by use of solutions of known strength.

titrimetric (tī"trĭ-mĕt'rĭk) [" + G. *metron*, a measure]. Employing the process of titration.

titubation (tĭt-ū-bā'shŭn) [L. *titubatio*, a staggering]. A staggering gait, seen in diseases of the cerebellum.

t., lingual. Stuttering, stammering.

Tl. Symb. of *thallium*.

Tn. Symb. of *normal intraocular tension*.

toadstool (tōd'stool). Any of various fungi with an umbrella-shaped cap; popularly a poisonous mushroom.
  POISONING: SYM: Usually come on from 1 to 14 hours after injection, characterized by marked abdominal pain, vomiting and intense diarrhea associated with blood and mucus. Profound weakness comes early and remains. Sometimes perspiration and lacrimation present and occasionally nervous symptoms.
  F. A. TREATMENT: Empty stomach and bowels promptly and completely with gastric lavage and quick acting cathartic and enemata. Atropine is esp. helpful and may be given by any route. Fluid and sodium chloride intake should be increased to point of tolerance. Coffee, tea, and milk are helpful. Charcoal may be given early if available. Treat for shock.

tobacco (tō-băk'ō) [Spanish *tabaco*]. Dried leaves of *Nicotiana tabacum* and other species.
  It is a narcotic containing *nicotine,* *pyridine, picoline,* and *collidin.* SEE: *nicotine*.
  Widely used in forms of cigars, cigarettes, pipe tobacco, snuff, and chewing. During its combustion, various products are given off, the most important being *nicotine, q.v.*

t. heart. Disturbance of function of heart from use of tobacco.

t., Indian. Lobelia.

tobaccoism (tō-băk'ō-ĭzm) [" + G. *-ismos*, condition]. Modbid state due to excessive use of tobacco.

tocodynamometer (tō"kō-dī-năm-ŏm'ĕ-ter) [G. *tokos*, birth, + *dynamis*, power, + *metron*, a measure]. Device for estimating expulsive force of uterine contractions in childbirth.

tocogony (tō-kŏg'ō-nĭ) [" + *gonē*, seed]. Parental generation as opposed to abiogenesis.

tocograph (tŏk'ō-graf) [" + *graphein*, to write]. A device for estimating and recording the force of uterine contractions.

tocology (tō-kŏl'ō-jĭ) [" + *logos*, science]. Science of parturition and obstetrics.

tocomania (to"kō-mā'nĭ-ă) [" + *mania*, madness]. Puerperal insanity.

tocometer (tō-kŏm'ĕt-ĕr) [" + *metron*, a measure]. Device for estimating expulsive force of the uterus in labor. SYN: *tocodynamometer*.

tocophobia (tō"kō-fō'bĭ-ă) [" + *phobos*, fear]. Abnormal fear of childbirth.

tocus (tō'kŭs) [L. from G. *tokos*, birth]. Parturition; childbirth.

toe (tō) [A.S. *tā*]. A digit of the foot.
  RS: acroataxia, acrodynia, bunion, camptodactylia, clavus, dactyl, dactylus, digit, gout, hallex, hallus, metatarsus.

t. clonus. Contraction of the big toe in sudden extension of the first phalanx.

t., dislocations of. These are treated essentially same as dislocations of the fingers, *q.v.*

t. drop. Inability to lift the toes.
  DISEASES: Thromboangiitis obliterans, gangrene, deformities, rashes, bromidrosis.

t. reflex. When great toe is strongly flexed all muscles below knee become tense.

toilet (toy'lĕt) [Fr. *toilette*, a little cloth]. Cleansing of a wound after operation or of an obstetrical patient.

toko- [G.]. Combining form meaning birth.

tolerance (tŏl'ĕr-ăns) [L. *tolerantia*, tolerance]. Capacity for enduring a poison, or a food or drug which may be harmful if taken in excess; power of resistance to such, or point at which such resistance ends; amount of a drug or food which may be so tolerated.

t. test. Master's exercise tolerance test for circulatory efficiency consists in ascending and descending 2 steps a variable number of times and in a given period. Blood pressure and pulse readings are estimated for age and result.

tolu balsam (tō-loo') [Sp.]. USP. A resin-like substance obtained from a tree grown in South America.
  USES: In compound tincture of benzoin. As a flavor for expectorants in the form of syrup of tolu balsam.
  DOSAGE: Of the syrup, 1-2 drams (4-8 cc.).

tomato and **tomato juice.** AV. SERVING: 125-120 Gm. Pro. 1.1-1.2, Fat 0.5-0.1, Carbo. 4.1-4.3. VITAMINS (for both): A+++, B++, C+++, G+ to ++, and + for juice.
  ASH CONST. (tomatoes and juice): Ca

0.011-0.006, Mg 0.010-0.010, K 0.275-0.310, Na 0.010-0.015, P 0.026-0.015, Cl 0.034-0.055, S 0.014, Fe 0.00044. Second figure represents "juice."
A base forming food; alkaline potentially 5.6 cc. per 100 Gm., 24.5 cc. per 100 Cal.
ACTION: Antitoxic and laxative.

-tome [G.]. Combining form meaning *a cutting, a cutting instrument.*

tomentum, tomentum cerebri (tō-men'tum ser'ē-brī) [L.]. Network of numerous minute blood vessels bet. the cerebral surface of the pia mater and cortex cerebri.

Tomes' fibers, fibrils (tōmz). Processes from the odontoblasts which enter the tubules of dentine.

tomomania (tō″mō-mā'nĭ-ă) [G. *tomē*, a cutting, + *mania*, madness]. 1. Tendency of a surgeon to resort to unnecessary surgical operations. 2. Abnormal desire to be operated upon.

tomotocia (tō″mō-tō'sĭ-ă) [" + *tokos*, birth]. Cesarean section delivery by incising the uterus.

tonaphasia (tō-nă-fā'zhĭ-ă) [L. *tonus*, from G. *tonos*, a stretching, + *a-*, priv, + *phasis*, speech]. Inability to remember a tune due to cerebral lesion. SYN: *amusia, vocal.*

tone (tōn) [L. *tonus*, from G. *tonos*, a stretching]. 1. PHYS: That state of a body or any of its organs or parts in which the functions are healthy and performed with due vigor. 2. Normal tension or responsiveness to stimuli, as of arteries or muscles, seen particularly in involuntary muscle (such as the sphincter of the urinary bladder). 3. A musical or vocal sound.

t. deafness. Inability to detect differences in musical sounds. SYN: *amusia.*

t., muscle. Contractile tension in muscle. SEE: *tonus.*

tongue (tŭng) [A.S. *tunge*]. The organ of speech and taste.
ANAT: It connects at the base with the hyoid bone, epiglottis, ant. pillars of the soft palate, and with the pharynx. The geniohyoglossus runs from base to tip connecting it with the hyoid bone and mandible. The *frenum linguae* is a fold of mucous membrane on the undersurface. It has numerous mucous or lingual glands.
Arteries: Lingual, tonsillar, or facial a.
Muscles: The sup., inf. lingualis, transversus linguae, and verticalis linguae.
Nerves: Lingual of inf. maxillary, glossopharyngeal, and hypoglossal.
Septum: This is a vertical fibrous partition from the hyoid bone to the tip extending through the muscular portion.

CHARACTERISTICS AND DIAGNOSIS

t., beefy. Occurs in chronic inflammation of the bowels, liver, or mucous surfaces.

t., clearing of. If it clears slowly, commencing at tip and edges, leaving natural appearance, permanent recovery may be expected. If fur comes off in patches, leaving smooth, red surface, recovery will be slow. If fur disappears rapidly, leaving glassy, cracked surface, it is unfavorable.

t., furred. This occurs in nearly all fevers.
Brown fur: Nervous prostration, putrefaction; a bad indication; deeper the color the worse the omen. If dry with fissures, condition is grave. Circumscribed furring often indicates local disturbance, as from a jagged tooth, or from tonsillitis.
Light fur: If moist, simple irritation of stomach.
Heavy fur: Great disturbance; serious trouble.
Unilateral furring: May result from disturbed innervation, as in condition affecting the 2nd and 3rd branches of the 5th nerve. Has been noted in neuralgia of those branches and in fractures of the skull involving the foramen rotundum.
Yellow fur: Liver derangement.
FISSURES: May be normal. Causes obscure. If deep and inflamed, may be due to syphilitic infection, or dissecting glossitis, a broken tooth, chronic dysentery, hepatic disease, or diabetes mellitus.
PAIN: Occurs in local lesions, fissures, glossitis, malignancies, and pernicious anemia.
PROTRUSION: This occurs with very sick patients, as in advanced typhoid fever and toxemia. The tongue is tremulous in early typhoid and in meningitis. In chorea it is thrust out suddenly and at once withdrawn. If it is protruded very slowly or if left exposed after being shown, it is a sign of great exhaustion, congestion, or other pressure on the brain.
SCARS: These may be the result of injury or bulbar palsy causing ulceration and resulting in scars.
SHARP-POINTED T: Observed in irritation and inflammation of the brain, smoker's tongue, leukoplakia.
SPASM: Occurs in multiple sclerosis, general paresis, melancholia, and in stuttering.
TREMBLING: With tongue immobile, indicates torpor of brain.
TREMULOUS: In all acute diseases of evil import, but no particular significance in chronic nervous disorders.
TREMORS: Noted in asthenia, alcoholism, bulbar palsy, Graves' disorder, and in hemiplegia it is turned toward the paralyzed side if face is affected. If turned toward the unaffected side, it denotes lesion of the medulla.
COLOR OF TONGUE: *Black coating*: Glossophytia; may be due to stain or presence of microphytes. In dysentery, indicates exhaustion, mortification, death. In jaundice, denotes organic disease of liver. In smallpox, is unfavorable sign.
Bluish: Denotes impeded circulation. Interference with respiration. Heart disease, asthma, cyanosis.
Dark-brown: Malignant fever, Addison's disease.
Gray-coated and flabby t: With an oval bare spot in center, which is red and glossy, sometimes seen in children; indicative of gastrointestinal catarrh.
Lead colored: Found in cholera and mortification of lungs and stomach; with thrush, it denotes death.
Pale: Indicates severe anemia; the tongue appears smaller than normal.
Red: Redness along center indicates intestinal irritation. An early sign in typhoid fever. If glassy, very unfavorable.
Red, cracked t: Points to kidney trouble.
Bright red t: Indicates inflammation of gastric or intestinal mucous membrane, glossitis, stomatitis.
Clean, red t: With papillae prominent,

or a white-coated tongue with papillae projecting through the fur, indicates scarlatina.

Red tip and edges, or having red, dry streak in center typical of typhoid and gastric fever.

Scarlet t: Acute in inflammation usually of the stomach, if red along edges and tip.

Strawberry t: White fur through which project bright red and prominent papillae. Seen in early stage of scarlet fever.

White coating: This denotes gastric derangement.

Yellow, with thick fur covering the tongue indicates biliary derangement.

SIZE: *Macroglossia*, or large tongue, is generally congenital, or may result from inflammation of lymphatics, Ludwig's angina, glossitis, actinomycosis, acromegaly, myxedema. If localized, may be due to gumma, carcinoma, foot and mouth disease, and local trauma.

Microglossia, small tongue, atrophy due to hemorrhage, in anemia, emaciation, convalescence from typhoid. These conditions are temporary.

POSITION AND CONDITIONS: If thick and flabby, showing imprints of the teeth, indicates gastric and nervous irritation.

Thrust to one side: Indicates hemiplegia if continually held in this position.

t., smoker's. Disease with white patch and fissure formation on tongue. SYN: leukoplakia.

tongue tie (tŭng′ tī). This is a congenital shortening of the frenum.
SYM: Interference in sucking and in articulation.
TREATMENT: Surgical.

tongue, words pert. to: circumballate papillae, cleft, frenulum, "gloss-" words, hypoglossal, lingua, macroglossia, microglossia, ranula, strawberry, sublingual, s. gland.

tonic (tŏn′ĭk) [G. *tonikos*, pert. to tone]. 1. Pert. to or characterized by tension or contraction, esp. muscular tension. 2. Restoring tone. 3. A medicine that increases strength and tone.
They are subdivided according to action, as *cardiac, general*, etc. Ex: *iron, arsenic, digitalis*.

t. spasm. A persistent, involuntary, firm or violent muscular contraction. SEE: *clonic*.

tonicity (tō-nĭs′ĭ-tĭ) [G. *tonos*, tone]. 1. Property of possessing tone, esp. muscular tone. 2. State of normal tension or partial contraction of muscle fibers while at rest. SYN: *tone*.

tonisator (tō″nĭ-sa′tor). Instrument giving both the interrupted galvanic and faradic current with a sinusoidal wave superimposed.

tonoclonic (tŏn″o-klŏn′ĭk) [G. *tonos*, tone, + *klonos*, tumult]. Both tonic and clonic, said of muscular spasms.

tonofibrils (tŏn-ō-fī′brĭls) [" + L. *fibrilla*, fibril]. Fibrils seen in cells, particularly in epithelial cells.

tonograph (tŏn′ō-grăf) [" + *graphein*, to write]. Device for recording blood pressure.

tonometer (tŏn-ŏm′ĕ-ter) [" + *metron*, a measure]. Instrument for measuring the intraocular tension or blood pressure.

tonometry (tŏn-ŏm′ĕ-trĭ) [" + *metron*, a measure]. The measurement of tension of a part, as intraocular tension.

tonophant (tŏn′ō-fănt) [" + *phainein*, to show]. Device for visualizing sound waves.

tonoplast (tŏn′ō-plăst) [" + *plastos*, a thing formed]. An intracellular body. SYN: *vacuole*.

tonoscope (tŏn′ō-skōp) [" + *skopein*, to examine]. A device for examining interior of the skull or brain by means of sound.

tonsil (tŏn′sĭl) [L. *tonsilla*, almond]. 1. Any mass of lymphoid tissue. 2. Either of a pair of masses of lymphoid tissue bet. anterior and posterior pillars of the fauces.
RS: *adenoid, a. tissue, adenoidectomy, "amygdal-" words, quinsy*.
FUNCTION: Acts as filter to protect body from invasion of bacteria, and aids in the formation of white cells.

t., cerebellar. One of a pair of cerebellar lobules on either side of the uvula projecting from inf. surface of cerebellum.

t., laryngeal. Lymphoid tissue on the ventricular band.

t., Luschka's. Same as *pharyngeal t*.

t., pharyngeal. Lymphoid tissue on post. sup. wall of pharynx. SEE: *adenoid*.

t., nasal. Lymphoid tissue on the nasal septum.

t., sublingual. One behind the faucial pillars.

tonsilla (tŏn-sĭl′ă) [L. *tonsilla*, almond]. Tonsil.

t. pharyngea. BNA. Lymphoid mass on post. wall of the nasopharynx.

tonsillar (tŏn′sĭ-lar) [L. *tonsilla*, almond]. Pert. to a tonsil, esp. the faucial or palatine t.

tonsillectomy (tŏn-sĭl-ĕk′tō-mĭ) [" + G. *ektome*, excision]. Surgical removal of the tonsils.

OPER. NP: Patient is placed in dorsal position with head extended and covered with a sterile sheet up to neck in usual manner; over sterile sheet, at neck, place a sterile towel.

Immediately following operation patient is turned on side or face down, so that vomitus or blood is not inhaled, and ice compress is placed around throat. It is important for nurse to test suction apparatus before operation. Cold water should be flushed through the suction tip into bottle after operation to prevent stoppage through clotting of blood.

DIET: No acid, highly seasoned, or hot foods; beef and fruit juices to be avoided. Milk and cream, iced tea, coffee, cocoa, custard, junket, gelatin, strained cereals, little sugar.

tonsillitis (tŏn-sĭl-ī′tĭs) [L. *tonsilla*, almond, + G. *-itis*, inflammation]. Inflammation of faucial tonsils.

t., acute catarrhal. Associated with an acute nasopharyngitis. Tonsils reddened and enlarged. Posterior pillars edematous and injected.
SYM: Soreness of throat as well as underlying nasopharyngeal discomfort.
TREATMENT: Same as that of acute rhinitis in addition to frequent hot, medicated gargles.

t., acute follicular. Inflammation of tonsils with islands of exudate on the surface of the tonsils representing crypts filled with débris and pus.
SYM: Malaise, fever, chills, sore throat and pain on swallowing.
TREATMENT (general): Catharsis, force fluids, rest in bed, anodynes. (Local): Hot medicated gargles. Topical applications are of questionable value.

t., herpetic. Herpes on the tonsil.

t., mycotic. T. due to fungi.

t., parenchymatous. Inflammation of all of the faucial tonsil.

tonsillitis, pustular   T-38   **torso**

t., pustular. T. with pustular formations.

t., superficial. Inflammation of membrane covering the tonsil.

t., suppurative. T. with high fever, suppuration, pain, etc. SYN: *quinsy, q.v.*

t., ulcerative. Plaut-Vincent's angina, syphilis, tuberculosis, agranulocytic angina, blood dyscrasias, fungi, as Leptothrix.

DIET (in general): Ice to suck, meat juice, white of egg, and lemon water. Where swallowing is possible, begin with milk, raw eggs, etc.

tonsillolith (tŏn'sĭl-ō-lĭth) [L. *tonsilla*, almond, + G. *lithos*, stone]. A concretion within a tonsil. SYN: *amygdalolith.*

tonsillomycosis (tŏn″sĭl-lō-mī-kō'sĭs) [" + G. *mykēs*, fungus, + *-osis*, condition]. A fungous infection of the tonsil.

tonsilloöidiosis (tŏn″sĭl-lō-oy-dĭ-ō'sĭs) [" + *Oidium* + G. *-osis*, condition]. Infection of a tonsil with the fungus Oidium.

tonsilloscopy (tŏn″sĭl-los'kŏ-pĭ) [" + G. *skopein*, to examine]. Inspection of the tonsils.

tonsillotome (tŏn'sĭl-ō-tōm) [" + G. *tomē*, a cutting]. Sliding knife for excision of enclosed soft tissue.

tonsillotomy (tŏn-sĭl-ŏt'ō-mĭ) [" + G. *tomē*, a cutting]. Excision of the tonsils. SEE: *amygdalotomy.*

tonus (tō'nŭs) [L. from G. *tonos*, tone]. That partial, steady contraction of muscle which determines tonicity or firmness. SYN: *tone, tonicity.*

Particularly, a condition of contractile tension in muscle which exists independently of voluntary innervation.

t., neurogenic. Tonic muscular contraction caused by constant sensory impulses into the cord and brain.

t., reflex. Assumption that muscular tonus is due to reflex from flow of sensory impulses into the central nervous system.

tooth (tooth) (pl. *teeth*) [A.S. *tōth*]. One of the conical hard structures in the upper and lower jaws used for mastication.

A tooth is not bone but dentine encased in cement and covered with enamel. Its *root* (radix) is inserted in the *alveolus*, gum covers its *neck*, and the exposed portion is its *crown*. The *pulp cavity* is in the center and it contains a substance like jelly. Blood vessels and nerves find entrance through a canal at apex of the root. SEE: *dentition, teeth.*

topectomy (tō-pĕkt-ō-mĭ). Excision of the cerebral lobe or lobes. Also a psychosurgical procedure for mental illness, in which small areas of the frontal lobes are removed on both sides of the brain in the superior convexity.

topesthesia (to-pes-the'zĭ-ă) [G. *topos*, place, + *aisthēsis*, sensation]. Ability through tactile sense to determine any part that is touched.

tophaceous (tō-fā'shŭs) [L. *tophaceus*, sandy]. 1. Relating to a tophus. 2. Sandy, gritty.

tophus (tō'fŭs) (pl. *tophi*) [L. *tophus*, porous stone]. 1. Deposit of sodium biurate in tissues near a joint in gout. 2. A salivary calculus. 3. Tartar on the teeth.

t. syphilit'icus. A syphilitic node on the tibia or periosteum of the cranium.

tophyperidrosis (tŏf″ĭp-ĕr-ĭd-rō'sĭs) [G. *topos*, place, + *hyper*, above, + *idrōsis*, perspiration]. Excessive sweating in local areas.

top'ical [G. *topos*, place]. Pert. to a definite area; local.

topoalgia (tō-pō-ăl'jĭ-ă) [" + *algos*, pain]. Localized pain; common in neurasthenia following emotional upsets.

topoanesthesia (tō″pō-ăn-ĕs-thē'zĭ-ă) [" + *an-*, priv. + *aisthesis*, sensation]. Loss of ability to recognize the location of a tactile sensation.

topognosia, topognosis (tō-pŏg-nō'sĭ-ă, -sĭs) [" + *gnosis*, knowledge]. Recognition of the location of a tactile sensation. SYN: *topesthesia.*

topographic (top-ō-grăf'ĭk) [" + *graphein*, to write]. Pert. to description of special regions.

topography (tō-pŏg'ră-fĭ) [" + *graphein*, to write]. Description of a part of the body.

toponarcosis (tō″pō-nar-kō'sĭs) [" + *narkōsis*, stupor]. Local anesthesia.

toponeurosis (tō″pō-nū-rō'sĭs) [G. *topos*, place, + *neuron*, nerve, + *-osis*, condition]. Neurosis of a limited area.

topophobia (tō-pō-fō'bĭ-ă) [" + *phobos*, fear]. A fear of psychoneurotic origin in relation to a particular locality.

topothermesthesiometer (top″ō-ther-mĕs-thē-zhĭ-ŏm'ē-ter) [" + *thermē*, heat, + *aisthēsis*, sensation]. Device for measuring local temperature sense.

torantil (tō-răn'tĭl). A biologically standardized histamine destroying enzyme, obtained from the mucosa of the small intestines and kidneys of hogs.

USES: In hay fever, some forms of dermatitis, serum sickness, and allergic conditions.

DOSAGE: Varies according to the condition, from 10 to 20 units 3 times a day.

torcular Herophili (tor'kŭ-lar her-of'ĭl-ī) [L. *Herophilus*' wine press]. Expanded end of the sup. longitudinal sinus in a depression on inner surface of the occipital bone.

tormen (tor'mĕn) (pl. *tormina*) [L. *tormen*, a twisting]. Griping pain in the bowels.

tormina (tor'mĭn-ă) (sing. *tormen*) [L. twistings]. Intestinal colic with griping pains.

Tornwald's disease (torn'valdt). Purulent inflammation of Luschka's tonsil.

torose, torous (tō'rōs, -rŭs) [L. *torosus*, full of muscle]. Knobby or bulging; tubercular.

torpent (tor'pĕnt) [L. *torpens*, numbing]. 1. Medicine which modifies irritation. 2. Not capable of active functioning; dormant.

torpid (tor'pĭd) [L. *torpidus*, numb]. Not acting vigorously; sluggish.

torpidity (tor-pĭd'ĭ-tĭ) [L. *torpidus*, numb]. Sluggishness; inactivity.

torpor (tor'por) [L. *torpor*, numbness]. Abnormal inactivity; dormancy; numbness; apathy.

t. intestino'rum. Constipation.

t. peristal'ticus. Atonic constipation.

torrefaction (tor-e-făk'shŭn) [L. *torrefactio*, parching]. The act of drying or parching.

torrefy (tor'ĕ-fī) [L. *torrefacere*, to parch]. To parch or dry by heat.

torsion (tor'shŭn) [L. *torsio*, a twisting]. 1. Act of twisting or condition of being twisted. 2. Formerly, a griping pain. SEE: *ileus.* 3. Rotation of the vertical meridians of the eye.

torsive (tor'sĭv) [L. *torsio*, a twisting]. Twisted, as in a spiral.

torso (tor'sō) [Italian]. The trunk of the body.

torsoclusion (tor-sŏk-lū'zhun) [" + L. *occlusio*, a shutting out]. 1. Acupressure in combination with torsion to stop a bleeding vessel. 2. Malocclusion characterized by rotation of a tooth on its long axis.

torticollis (tor-tĭk-ŏl'ĭs) [L. *tortus*, twisted, + *collum*, neck]. Stiff neck caused by spasmodic contraction of neck muscles drawing the head to one side with chin pointing to the other side. Congenital or acquired. SYN: *wryneck*.

ETIOL: Result of scars, disease of cervical vertebrae, adenitis, tonsillitis, rheumatism, enlarged cervical glands, retropharyngeal abscess, cerebellar tumors. It may be spasmodic (clonic) or permanent (tonic). The latter type may be due to Pott's disease.

The muscles affected are principally those supplied by the spinal accessory nerve.

t., intermittent. Same as *spasmodic t.*
t., fixed. Abnormal position of head due to organic shortening of the muscles.
t., ocular. T. from inequality in sight of the two eyes.
t., rheumatic. Same as *symptomatic t.*
t., spasmodic. T. with recurrent but transient contractions of muscles of neck and esp. of the sternocleidomastoid.
t., spurious. T. from caries of the cervical vertebrae.
t., symptomatic. Rheumatic stiff neck.

tortipelvis (tor"tĭ-pĕl'vĭs) [L. *tortus*, twisted, + *pelvis*, basin]. Muscular contractions distorting the spine and hip. SYN: *dystonia musculorum deformans*.

toruloid (tor'ū-loyd) [L. *torulus*, a little bulge, + G. *eidos*, form]. BACT: Beaded; noting an aggregate of colonies like those seen in the budding of yeast.

torulosis (tor-ū-lō'sĭs) [Torula + G. -ōsis, condition]. Infestation with Torula or yeast cells.

torulus (tor'ū-lŭs) [L. *torulus*, a little elevation]. A very small elevation. SYN: *papilla*.
t. tac'tilis. A tactile cutaneous elevation on palms and soles.

touch (tŭtsh) [O.Fr. *touchier*]. 1. To perceive by the tactile sense; to feel with the hands, to palpate. 2. The sense by which pressure on the skin or mucosa is perceived; the tactile sense. 3. Examination with the hand. SYN: *palpation*.

Various disorders may disturb or impair the tactile sense or the ability to feel normally. There are a number of words pert. to sensation and its modifications, a few of the more important ones being listed as follows: *algesia, -algia, anesthesia, dysesthesia, -dynia, esthesia, esthesioneurosis, hyperesthesia, paresthesia.*

t., abdominal. Palpation of the abdomen.
t., double. Vaginal and rectal examination made at same time.
t., rectal. Digital exploration of the rectum.
t., vaginal. Digital exploration of the vagina.
t., vesical. Digital exploration of the bladder.

touch, words pert. to: amblyaphia, anaphia, anaptic, ankyglossia, asterognosis, atopognosis, delire de toucher, dysaphia, hallucinations, haphephobia, haptic, polyesthesia, stereognosis, tactile.

tour de maitre (toor deh mātr) [Fr. the master's turn]. A method of introducing a catheter or sound into the male bladder or into the uterus.

Tourette's disease (too-rĕt'). Convulsive tic, with echolalia and coprolalia, associated with motor incoördination.

Tournay's sign (toor-nā'). Dilatation of the pupil of the eye on unusually strong lateral fixation.

tourniquet (tŭr'nĭ-kĕt) [Fr. a turning]. Any constrictor used on an extremity to make pressure over an artery and to control bleeding; also used to distend veins for aspiration or intravenous injections.

Tourniquets are made more effective by placing a firm object such as a padded stone or a padded piece of wood over an artery to concentrate pressure at that point. A figure-of-eight knot pulled tight is also an excellent method for making firm such an object.

Tourniquet should never be left in place too long. Ordinarily, it should be released from 12 to 18 minutes to determine whether bleeding has ceased. If it has, leave tourniquet loosely in place so that it may be retightened if necessary. If not retighten at once.

Arterial hemorrhage: Apply bet. the wound and the heart, close to the wound, placing a hard pad over point of pressure. Should be discontinued not later than 1 hour and a tight bandage substituted under the loosened tourniquet.

Venous hemorrhage: Place below bleeding point, but close to the wound. The tourniquet should remain in place with periodic momentary loosening until released by a physician.

The tourniquet should remain in place until released by a physician.

Tousey method (tow'zē). Painless removal of cutaneous tumors without anesthesia by electrocoagulation.

tow (tō) [A.S. *tow*, a weaving]. Coarse fibers of flax, used for surgical dressings.

towelette (tow-ĕl-ĕt') [M.E. *towele*, towel]. A small towel for surgical or obstetrical use.

toweling, towelling (tow'ĕl-ĭng) [M.E. *towele*, a towel]. Friction with a coarse towel.

toxalbumin (tŏks"ăl-bū'mĭn) [G. *toxikon*, poison, + L. *albumen*, white of egg]. A poisonous albumin or protein.

toxalbumose (tŏks-ăl'bū-mōs) [" + L. *albumen*, white of egg]. A poisonous albumose.

toxamin (tŏks'ăm-ĭn) [" + *amine*]. One of a class of injurious substances said to be present in grain food, which are harmful unless overpowered by vitamins.

toxanemia (tŏks"ă-nē'mĭ-ă) [" + *an-*, priv. + *aima*, blood]. Anemia due to a hemolytic poison.

toxemia (tŏks-ē'mĭ-ă) [G. *toxikon*, poison, + *aima*, blood]. Distribution throughout body of poisonous products of bacteria growing in a focal or local site, thus producing generalized symptoms.

SYM: Constitutional disturbances, rigors, increased temperature, diarrhea, vomiting, pulse and respiration quickened or depressed, prostration.

In *tetanus*, the nervous system is esp. affected; in *diphtheria*, nerves and muscles.

t. of pregnancy. Series of conditions affecting women in pregnancy.
ETIOL: Disordered metabolism causing circulating toxins which are unknown.
FORMS: Simple vomiting, pernicious vomiting (hyperemesis gravidarum), acute yellow atrophy of the liver, nephritic toxemia, low reserve kidney, preëclampsia, and eclampsia.

toxenzyme (tŏks-ĕn'zīm) [G. *toxikon*, poison, + *en*, in, + *zymē*, leaven]. A poisonous enzyme.

toxic (tŏks'ĭk) [G. *toxikon*, poison]. Pert. to, resembling or caused by poison. SYN: *poisonous*.

    t. unit. Smallest dose of a toxin fatal to a guinea pig of standard weight in 3-4 days. Also, smallest amount of scarlet fever toxin necessary to produce a positive skin test reaction in a susceptible person.

toxicant (tŏks'ĭ-kănt) [G. *toxikon*, poison]. 1. Poisonous; toxic. 2. Any poison, esp. one from alcohol.

toxicide (tŏks'ĭ-sīd) [" + L. *cidus*, from *caedere*, to kill]. 1. Destructive to toxins. 2. A chemical antidote for poisons.

toxicity (tŏks-ĭs'ĭ-tĭ) [G. *toxikon*, poison]. The condition of being poisonous.

toxico- [G.]. Combining form meaning *poison*.

toxidermitis (tŏks″ĭ-der-mī'tĭs) [G. *toxikon*, poison, + *derma*, skin, + *-itis*, inflammation]. Any inflammatory skin disease due to poisoning. SYN: *toxicodermatitis*.

toxiferous (tŏks-ĭf'ĕr-ŭs) [" + L. *ferre*, to carry]. Containing a poison. SYN: *poisonous*.

toxigenic (tŏks″ĭ-jĕn'ĭk) [" + *gennan*, to produce]. Producing toxins or poisons.

toxignomic (tŏks-ĭg-nŏm'ĭk) [" + *gnomikos*, knowing]. Having the toxic action peculiar to a poison.

toxin (tŏks'ĭn) [G. *toxikon*, poison]. Poisonous substance or compound of vegetable, animal, or bacterial origin.

    RS: *anatoxin, apotoxin, biotoxin, cardiolysin, endotoxin, exotoxin, pyrotoxin*.

    t., bacterial. T. produced by bacteria.

    t., endo-. Toxin produced in the body

The Best-Known Toxins

Species	Type of Toxin
Corynebacterium diphtheriae	Exotoxin
Clostridium tetani	Exotoxin
Clostridium botulinum	Exotoxin
Clostridium welchii	Exotoxin*
Streptococcus pyogenes	Exotoxin*
Staphylococcus aureus	Exotoxin*
Bacterium dysenteriae (Shiga)	Intermediate
Bacterium typhosum	Endotoxin
Vibrio cholerae	Endotoxin
Neisseria meningitidis	Endotoxin
Neisseria gonorrhoeae	Endotoxin

*Atypical exotoxins, with a high heat resistance.

toxicoderma (tŏks″ĭ-kō-der'mă) [G. *toxikon*, poison, + *derma*, skin]. Any skin disease resulting from a poison.

toxicogenic (tŏks-ĭk-ō-jĕn'ĭk) [" + *gennan*, to produce]. Caused by, or producing, a poison.

toxicohemia (tŏks″ĭ-ko-hē'mĭ-ă) [" + *haima*, blood]. Blood poisoning. SYN: *toxemia*.

toxicoid (tŏks'ĭ-koyd) [" + *eidos*, resemblance]. Of the nature of a poison.

toxicology (tŏks-ĭ-kŏl'ō-jĭ) [" + *logos*, science]. The science of poisons, their nature, effects, and antidotes.

toxicomania (tŏks″ĭ-kō-mā'nĭ-ă) [" + *mania*, madness]. Abnormal craving for narcotics, intoxicants, or poisons.

toxicopathic (tŏks″ĭ-kō-păth'ĭk) [" + *pathos*, disease]. Pert. to any condition caused by a poison.

toxicopathy (tŏks″ĭ-kop'ă-thĭ) [G. *toxikon*, poison, + *pathos*, disease]. Any disease caused by a poison.

toxicopexic (tŏks″ĭ-kō-pĕks'ĭk) [" + *pēxis*, fixation]. Relating to neutralization of poison.

toxicophobia (tŏks″ĭk-ō-fō'bĭ-ă) [" + *phobos*, fear]. Abnormal fear of being poisoned by any medium: food, gas, water, drugs, etc.

toxicophylaxin (tŏks″ĭ-kō-fĭ-lăks'ĭn) [" + *phylaxis*, protection]. Any antitoxin which counteracts bacterial poisons.

toxicosis (tŏks-ĭ-kō'sĭs) [" + *-ōsis*, condition]. A diseased condition resulting from poisoning. SYN: *toxicopathy*.

    t., endogen'ic. Disease due to poisons generated within the body. SYN: *autointoxication*.

    t., exogen'ic. Any disease resulting from a poison not generated in the body.

    t., retention. T. from retained products which normally are excreted as formed.

of the bacterium and freed only after its destruction.

    t., exo-. T. excreted during life of the bacterium.

    t., extracellular. Same as *exotoxin*.

    t., fatigue. Substance deposited by body fluids in tissues after muscular exertion, said to be the cause of fatigue.

    t., intracellular. Same as *endotoxin*.

toxin-antitoxin (tŏks″ĭn-ăn″tĭ-tŏks'ĭn) [G. *toxikon*, poison, + *anti*, against, + *toxikon*]. Diphtheria toxin with its antitoxin in a nearly neutral mixture, the diphtheria toxin being about 85% neutralized.

Used for immunization against diphtheria. Also known as *T. A. T. mixture*.

toxinemia (tŏks″ĭn-ē'mĭ-ă) [" + *aima*, blood]. Blood poisoning. SYN: *toxemia*.

toxinfection (tŏks-ĭn-fĕk'shŭn) [" + L. *infectio*, a putting into]. Infection caused by toxins or other poisons.

toxinicide (tŏks-ĭn'ĭs-ĭd) [" + L. *cidus*, from *caedere*, to kill]. That which is destructive to toxins.

toxinosis (tŏks-ĭn-ō'sĭs) [" + *-ōsis*, condition]. Disease due to a toxin.

toxipathy (tŏks-ĭp'ă-thĭ) [" + *pathos*, disease]. Any disease due to poison.

toxiphobia (tŏks″ĭ-fō'bĭ-ă) [" + *phobos*, fear]. Abnormal fear of being poisoned.

toxiphoric (tŏks-ĭ-for'ĭk) [G. *toxikon*, poison, + *phoros*, a bearer]. Having affinity for or carrying a toxin.

toxis (tŏks'ĭs) [G. *toxikon*, poison]. Condition of being poisoned; poisoning. SYN: *toxicosis*.

toxitabellae (tŏks-ĭ-tăb-ĕl'ē) [" + L. *tabella*, tablet]. Poisonous tablets.

toxitherapy (tŏks″ĭ-ther'ă-pĭ) [" + *therapeia*, treatment]. Use of toxins in treatment of disease.

toxoalexin (tŏks″ō-ăl-ĕks'ĭn) [" + *alexein*,

toxogenin

to ward off]. An alexin which counteracts bacterial toxins.

toxogenin (tŏks″ŏj′ĕn-ĭn) [" + *gennan*, to produce]. Hypothetical substance in the blood caused by injection of antigens, innocuous in itself, but causing anaphylaxis upon addition of fresh antigen.

toxoid (tŏks′oyd) [" + *eidos*, form]. A toxin treated so as to destroy its toxicity, but still capable of inducing formation of antibodies on injection. SEE: *Ehrlich's side-chain theory.*

t., alum-precipitated. T. of diphtheria or tetanus precipitated with potashalum.

t., diphtheria. Diphtheria toxin detoxified by formaldehyde treatment.

toxolysin (tŏks-ŏl′ĭ-sĭn) [" + *lysis*, dissolution]. Substance destroying toxins. SYN: *antitoxin, toxicide.*

toxomucin (tŏks″ō-mū′sĭn) [" + L. *mucus*, mucus]. Specific toxic albuminoid from cultures of tubercle bacilli.

toxon, toxone (tŏks′ŏn, -ōn) [G. *toxikon*, poison]. A bacterial toxin with lessened activity, producing paralysis and delayed death.

toxonoid (tŏks′ō-noyd) [" + *eidos*, form]. A nontoxic substance with a weak affinity for antitoxin.

toxonosis (tŏks″ō-nō′sĭs) [" + *-ōsis*, condition]. A disease caused by poisoning. SYN: *toxicosis, toxinosis.*

toxopeptone (tŏks-ō-pĕp′tōn) [" + *peptón*, digesting]. A protein derivative produced by action of a toxin on peptones.

toxopexic (tŏks″ō-pĕks′ĭk) [" + *pēxis*, fixation]. Pert. to the neutralization of a toxin.

toxophil(e (tŏks′ō-fĭl, -fīl) [" + *philein*, to love]. Having a special affinity for toxins, said of certain haptophore groups.

toxophore, toxophorous (tŏks′ō-fōr, tŏks-ŏf′ōrŭs) [G. *toxikon*, poison + *phoros*, a bearer]. Producing the combination of a toxin with the cells of an organism. SEE: *Ehrlich's side-chain theory.*

toxophore group (tŏks′ō-for) [" + *phoros*, a bearer]. Poison-bearing group of a toxin. SEE: *Ehrlich's side-chain theory.*

toxophylaxin (tŏks-ō-fī-lăks′ĭn) [" + *phylaxis*, protection]. A defensive protein that neutralizes bacterial poisons. SYN: *toxicophylaxin.*

toxosozin (tŏks″ō-sō′zĭn) [" + *sōzein*, to save]. A normal defensive protein that neutralizes bacterial poisons. SEE: *sozin.*

t.p.r. Abbr. for *temperature, pulse,* and *respiration.*

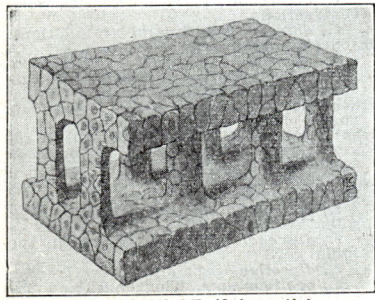

TRABECULAE (Schematic).
Pillarlike or beamlike arrangements of cells within an organ. Sometimes they are bathed in tissue fluid, but sometimes the spaces between trabeculae are filled in with other cell types.

T-41

trachelism, trachelismus

trabecula (tră-bĕk′ū-lă) (pl. *trabeculae*) [L. *trabecula*, a little beam]. Fibrous cord of connective tissue, serving as supporting fiber by forming septum extending into an organ from its wall or capsule. SEE: *Illus., this page.*

t. carneae. BNA. Thick muscular tissue bands attached to inner walls of the ventricles of the heart.

trabs, trabs cerebri (trăbz ser′ē-brī) [L. *trabs*, a beam]. Arched band of white fibers connecting the cerebral hemispheres. SYN: *corpus callosum.*

trace (trās) [Fr. *tracer*, from L. *tractus*, a drawing]. 1. A very small quantity. 2. A mark.

t. elements. Organic elements normally found in minute traces in foods and tissues, such as fluorine, copper, manganese, zinc, nickle, aluminum, silicon, bromine, and other physiologically rare minerals.

t., primitive. Pale white streak in germinal area indicating beginning of development of the blastoderm. SYN: *primitive streak.*

trachea (trā′kē-ă) (pl. *tracheae*) [G. *tracheia*, rough]. A cylindrical cartilaginous tube, 4½ inches long, from the larynx to the bronchial tubes. SYN: *windpipe.*

It extends from the sixth cervical to the fifth dorsal vertebra. Here it divides into 2 bronchi, 1 for each lung. It is lined with mucous membrane. Its inner surface is lined with ciliated epithelium.

tracheaectasy (trā″kē-ă-ĕk′tă-sĭ) [G. *tracheia*, rough + *ektasis*, dilatation]. Dilatation of the trachea.

tracheal (trā′kē-ăl) [G. *tracheia*, rough]. Pertaining to the trachea.

t. tugging. Pulsation of the larynx or downward pull of the trachea, symptomatic of thoracic aneurysm.

trachealgia (trā″kē-ăl′jĭ-ă) [" + *algos*, pain]. Pain in the trachea.

trachealis (trā-kē-ā′lĭs) [L.]. Unstriped muscular fibrous membrane connecting with the tracheal rings.

tracheitis (trā-kē-ī′tĭs) [G. *tracheia*, rough + *-itis*, inflammation]. An inflammation of the trachea.

It may be acute or chronic and may be associated with bronchitis and laryngitis.

NP: It is necessary to keep patient in bed, as the condition may spread and give rise to bronchial complications. As the middle aged are more apt to be afflicted, cardiac strain from constant coughing and loss of sleep must be avoided. Inflammation of the chest must be guarded against. Pulse and temperature must be carefully checked and recorded. Camphorated oil may be rubbed on the chest, which is then covered with warm wool. Lemonade should be within reach of the patient as constant small sips will help relieve irritation from coughing. Diet should be light.

trachelagra (trā-kĕl-ăg′ră) [G. *trachēlos*, neck + *agra*, seizure]. Rheumatic condition of neck muscles resulting in torticollis.

trachelectomopexy (trā″kĕl-ĕk-tom″ō-pĕks′ĭ) [" + *ektome*, a cutting out + *pexis*, fixation]. Fixation of uterine neck with partial excision.

trachelectomy (trā-kĕl-ĕk′tō-mĭ) [" + *ektomē*, excision]. Amputation of the cervix uteri.

trachelematoma (trā″kĕl-ĕ-mă-tō′mă) [" + *haima*, blood + *-ōma*, tumor]. A hematoma situated on the neck.

trachelism, trachelismus (trā′ke-lĭzm, trā-

ke-lĭz'mŭs) [" + -ismos, condition]. Backward spasm of the neck, sometimes preceding an epileptic attack.
trachelitis (tră-kē-lī'tĭs) [" + -itis, inflammation]. Inflammation of mucous membrane of the cervix uteri. SYN: cervicitis.
trachelo [G.]. Combining form, meaning neck.
trachelobregmatic (tră″kē-lō-brĕg-măt'ĭk) [G. trachelos, neck, + bregma, front of the head]. Pert. to the neck and the bregma.
trachelocystitis (tră″kĕl-ō-sĭs-tī'tĭs) [" + kystis, bladder, + -itis, inflammation]. Inflammation of neck of bladder.
trachelodynia (tră″kē-lō-dĭn'ĭ-ă) [" + odyne, pain]. Pain in the neck.
trachelology (tră″ke-lŏl'ō-jī) [" + logos, study]. Scientific study of the neck, its diseases and injuries.
trachelomastoid (tră″ke-lō-măs'toyd) [" + mastos, breast, + eidos, form]. A muscle of the neck. SEE: Muscles, Table of, in Appendix.
trachelomyitis (tră″ke-lō-mī-ī'tĭs) [" + mys, my-, muscle, + -itis, inflammation]. Inflammation of muscles of neck.
trachelopexy (tră-kel-ō-pĕks'ī) [" + pexis, fixation]. Surgical fixation of the cervix uteri to an adjacent part.
tracheloplasty (tră'kel-ō-plas″tĭ) [G. trachēlos, neck, + plassein, to form]. Plastic surgery of the cervix uteri.
trachelorrhaphy (tră-kel-or'ă-fī) [" + rhaphē, seam]. Suturing of a torn cervix uteri.
trachelos (tra'ke-lŏs) [G. trachēlos, neck]. Neck.
trachelotomy (tră-kel-ŏt'ō-mĭ) [" + tome, a cutting]. Incision of the cervix of the uterus.
tracheo- [G.]. Combining form meaning trachea, windpipe.
tracheoaerocele (tră″kē-ō-ā'er-ō-sēl) [G. tracheia, rough, + aēr, air, + kēlē, hernia.] Hernia or cyst of trachea containing air.
tracheobronchoscopy (tră″kē-ō-brŏng-kŏs'kō-pī) [" + brogchos, tube, + skopein, to examine]. Inspection of the trachea and bronchi through a bronchoscope.
tracheocele (tră'kē-ō-sēl) [" + kēlē, hernia]. 1. Protrusion of mucous membrane through the wall of the trachea. 2. Enlargement of the thyroid gland. SYN: goiter.
tracheoesophageal (tră″-kē-ō-ē-so-faj'ē-ăl) [" + oisophagos, esophagus]. Pert. to the trachea and the esophagus.
tracheolaryngotomy (tră″kē-ō-lăr-ĭn-gŏt-ō-mĭ) [" + larygx, larynx, + tome, a cutting]. Incision into larynx and trachea.
tracheopathia, tracheopathy (tră″kē-ō-păth'ĭ-a, -op'ă-thī) [" + pathos, disease]. Diseased condition of the trachea.
tracheopharyngeal (tră″kē-ō-far-in'jē-ăl) [" + pharygx, pharynx]. Pert. to both the trachea and pharynx.
tracheophonesis (tră″kē-ō-fōn-ē'zhĭ-ă) [G. tracheia, rough, + phōnēsis, a sounding]. Cardiac auscultation at the sternal notch.
tracheophony (tră-kē-ŏf'ō-nĭ) [" + phōnē, a sound]. Sound heard over the trachea in auscultation.
tracheoplasty (tră'kē-ō-plăs″tĭ) [" + plassein, to form]. Plastic operation on the trachea.
tracheopyosis (tră″kē-ō-pī-ō'sĭs) [" + pyon, pus, + -ōsis, condition]. Tracheitis with suppuration.
tracheorrhagia (tră-kē-or-ā'jĭ-ă) [" + rhēgnŭnai, to burst forth]. Tracheal hemorrhage.
tracheoschisis (tră-kē-ŏs'kĭs-ĭs) [" + schisis, a cleft]. Fissure of the trachea.
tracheoscopy (tră-kē-ŏs'kō-pī) [" + skopein, to examine]. Inspection of interior of trachea, by means of reflected light.
tracheostenosis (tră″kē-ō-sten-ō'sĭs) [" + stenōsis, a narrowing]. Contraction or narrowing of lumen of the trachea.
tracheotome (tră'kē-ō-tōm) [G. tracheia, rough, + tome, a cutting]. Instrument used in opening of trachea.
tracheotomy (tră-kē-ŏt'ō-mĭ) [" + tome, a cutting]. Operation of cutting into the trachea usually for insertion of tube to overcome tracheal obstruction.
 NP: Temperature of tracheotomy room must be not less than 80° F. and atmosphere should be saturated with steam. The outer tube should not be removed by nurse, but inner one should be removed every hour or oftener if so directed by physician. The movable or inner tube should be washed in a solution of salt water (1 dram of salt to quart of water) or boric acid and swabbed out with a sterilized cotton mop. Before replacing inner tube, the tube remaining in trachea should also be cleaned to remove mucus that collects in and around tube. Never leave patient alone. SEE: diphtheria.
 t. tube. T. to insert into opening made in tracheotomy.
trachitis (tră-kī'tĭs) [G. tracheia, rough, + -itis, inflammation]. Inflammation of the trachea. SYN: tracheitis.
trachoma (tră-kō'mă) [G. trachōma, roughness]. A chronic contagious form of conjunctivitis, noted by hypertrophy of conjunctiva, formation of follicles with subsequent cicatricial changes.
 ETIOL: Infected secretion from another trachomatous eye; the specific organisms have not been isolated.
 COMPLICATIONS: Pannus, ptosis, corneal ulcers.
 Sequelae: Trichiasis, entropion, ectropion, symblepharon, corneal opacities, staphyloma, blindness.
 TREATMENT: Copper sulfate application, silver nitrate, grattage, excision of tarsus, x-ray, radium. Combination of sulfanilamide and neoprontosil in small doses for about 3 weeks produces cure.
 t., brawny. T. with general lymphoid infiltration without granulation of the conjunctiva.
 t. deformans. Vulvitis with cicatricial contractions.
 t., diffuse. T. with large granulations.
trachychromatic (tră″kĭ-krō-mat'ĭk) [G. trachys, rough, + chrōma, color]. Pert. to a nucleus with very deeply staining chromatin.
trachyphonia (tră-kĭ-fō'nĭ-ă) [" + phōnè, voice]. Roughness of the voice.
tract (trăkt) [L. tractus, a track]. A region or area longer than its breadth, serving a special purpose.
 t., alimentary. The canal or passage from the mouth to the anus.
 t., ascending. Afferent white fibers in spinal cord.
 t., descending. Efferent fibers in the spinal cord.
 t., digestive. SEE: alimentary tract.
 t., genitourinary. The genital and urinary organs.
 t., habenular. White fibers from the habenula to the red nucleus.
 t., intermediolateral. Olivospinal tracts of the spinal cord.
 t., Monakow's. Same as rubrospinal t.

t., motor. Descending tract of an impulse from the brain to a muscle.
t., olfactory. Central portion of the olfactory lobe of the brain.
t., ophthalmic, t., optic. Fibers bet. the visual centers and optic chiasm.
t., pyramidal. Any of columns of motor fibers in the spinal cord which are continuations of pyramids in the medulla.
t., respiratory. The respiratory organs in continuity.
t., rubrospinal. Fibers from the red nucleus to the gray matter of the spinal cord.
t., sensory. Any tract of fibers conducting sensation to the brain.
tractellum (trăk-tel'lŭm) [L., a pulling organ]. An ant. locomotor protozoan flagellum.
traction (trăk'shŭn) [L. *tractio*, a drawing]. 1. Process of drawing or pulling. 2. Contraction, as of a muscle.
t., axis. Traction in line with the long axis of a course through which a body (fetus) is to be drawn.
tractus (trăk'tŭs) (pl. *tractūs*) [L., a tract.] A tract or path.
tragacanth (trag'ă-kănth) [G. *tragakantha*, a goat thorn]. USP. The dried gummy exudation from a plant grown in Asia, used in the form of mucilage as a greaseless lubricant, and as an application for chapped skin.
tragal (trā'găl) [G. *tragos*, goat]. Relating to the tragus.
tragicus (trăj'ĭk-ŭs) [L.]. Muscle on the outer surface of the tragus. SEE: *Muscles, Table of, in Appendix.*
tragomaschalia (trag″ō-măs-kăl'ĭ-ă) [G. *tragos*, goat, + *maschale*, axilla]. Odorous perspiration (bromidrosis) of the axilla.
tragophonia, tragophony (trăg″ō-fō'nĭ-ă, -of'ō-nĭ) [" + *phōnē*, voice]. A bleating sound heard in auscultation at level of fluid in hydrothorax. SYN: *egophony.*
tragopodia (trăg-ō-pō'dĭ-ă) [" + *pous, pod-*, foot]. Knock-knee.
tragus (trā'gŭs) [G. *tragos*, goat]. 1. Cartilaginous tonguelike projection in front of the ext. meatus of the ear. 2. One of the hairs at the entrance of the ext. auditory meatus.
trajector (tra-jĕk'tor) [L. *trajectus*, thrown across]. Device for determining approximate location of a bullet in a wound.
trance (trăns) [L. *transitus*, a passing over]. A sleeplike state, as in deep hypnosis, appearing also in hysteria and in some spiritualistic mediums, with limited sensory and motor contact with the ordinary surroundings, and with subsequent amnesia of what has occurred during the state.
t., coma. Hypnotic lethargy.
t., death. Trance simulating death.
t., induced. Hypnotic or somnambulistic t.
t., somnambulistic. T. with anesthesia, or catalepsy, or paralysis induced by hypnotism. [*beyond, through.*
trans- [L.]. Prefix meaning *across, over,*
transanimation (trans″ăn-ĭ-mā'shŭn) [L. *trans*, across, + *anima*, breath]. Resuscitation of a stillborn infant.
transaudient (trăns″aw'dĭ-ent) [" + *audīre*, to hear]. Permeable to sound waves.
transcalent (trăns-kā'lĕnt) [" + *calere*, to be hot]. Permeable to heat rays. SYN: *diathermanous.*
transection (trăn-sĕk'shŭn) [" + *sectio*, a cutting]. A cutting made across a long axis; a cross section.
transfer, transference (trans'fer, trans-fer'ĕns) [L. *trans*, across, + *ferre*, to bear]. 1. PSY: Transmission of any affect from one idea to another, or from one object or person to another, unconscious identifications being the activating motive. 2. State in which the symptoms of one area are transmitted to a similar area on the other side, as in hysteria.
t. neuroses. Compulsion neuroses and hysteria.
t. situation. The emotional state of a patient existing bet. him and his physician during psychoanalysis.
Either affection or distrust is transferred by the patient to the physician, although such feelings are not related to reality.
t., thought. Transference of one's thoughts to another. SYN: *telepathy.*
transfix (trăns-fĭks') [L. *trans*, across, + *fīgere*, to fix]. To pierce through or impale with a sharp instrument.
transfixion (trăns-fĭk'shŭn) [" + *fīgere*, to fix]. Maneuver in performing an amputation.
transforation (trăns″for-ā'shŭn) [" + *forāre*, to pierce]. The perforation of the fetal skull at the base in craniotomy.
transforator (trăns″fo-rā-tor) [" + *forāre*, to pierce]. Instrument for perforating fetal skull.
transformation (trăns″for-mā'shŭn) [" + *formatio*, a forming]. 1. Change of shape or form. SYN: *metamorphosis.* 2. Change of one tissue into another. 3. Degeneration.
transformer (trăns-form'er) [L. *trans*, across, + *formāre*, to form]. PT: A stationary induction apparatus to change electrical energy at one voltage and current to electrical energy at another voltage and current through the medium of magnetic energy, without mechanical motion.
It consists of a primary and a secondary winding placed on a core built up of thin sheets of steel, called laminations. These windings are ordinarily insulated one from the other (see autotransformer).
The primary winding receives the energy from the supply circuit, and the secondary receives the energy by induction from the primary. The electromotive force induced in the secondary winding depends on the number of turns in that winding and is approximately equal to the primary voltage multiplied by the ratio of secondary turns to primary turns. A device of this nature can, of course, be used only with alternating current.
transfusion (trăns-fū-zhŭn) [L. *trans*, across, + *fusio*, a pouring]. 1. Injection of the blood of one person into the blood vessels of another. SEE: *blood transfusion.*
2. Injection of saline or other solutions into a vein for a therapeutic purpose. SEE: *donor.*
t., direct. Transfer of blood directly from one person to another.
t., indirect. T. of blood from a vessel to the patient.
t., subcutaneous. Infusion of saline solution or other fluid beneath the skin.
t., venous. T. direct from a vein of a donor into a vein of patient.
transic (trăn'sĭk) [L. *transitus*, a passing over]. Relating to a trance.
transiliac (trăns-ĭl'ĭ-ăk) [L. *trans*, across, + *iliacus*, pert. to a haunch bone]. Extending bet. the 2 ilia.
transillumination (trăns″ĭl-lū″mĭ-nā'shŭn)

transition

[L. *trans*, across, + *illumināre*, to enlighten]. Inspection of a cavity or organ by passing a light through its walls.
When pus or lesion or degeneration is present, the reflection of light is diminished or absent.

transition (trănz-ĭ'shŭn) [L. *transitio*, a going across]. Passage from one state or position to another, or from one part to another part. SEE: *transitional*.

transitional (trănz-ĭsh'ŭn-ăl) [L. *transitio*, a going across]. Marked by or relating to a transition.

 t. douche. One using alternately hot and cold water.

 t. tumor. A benign one which, if it recurs after removal, may become malignant.

transitionals (trănz-ĭsh'ŭn-ăls) [L. *transitio*, a going across]. Mononuclear leukocytes, characterized by their large size, often 3 times as large as a red cell.
Commonly slightly irregular and found in from 2 to 4% of a normal differential. The nucleus is oval, lobulated or a horseshoe, and stains an even dirty blue color. Protoplasm likewise stained a dirty blue tint. It has neutrophilic granules which take a lilac shade.

translucent (trăns-lū'sĕnt) [L. *trans*, across, + *lucens*, shining]. Not transparent but permitting passage of light.

transmigration (trăns"mĭ-grā'shŭn) [" + *migratio*, migration]. The passage of cells, as of the blood, through a membranous septum. SYN: *diapedesis*.

 t., external. Transfer of an ovum from an ovary to an opp. tube through the pelvic cavity.

 t., internal. Transfer of an ovum through the uterus to the opposite oviduct.

transmissible (trăns-mĭs'ĭ-bl) [L. *transmissio*, a sending across]. Capable of being carried from one person to another, as an infectious disease.

transmission (trăns-mĭsh'ŭn) [L. *transmissio*, a sending across]. Transfer of anything, as a disease or hereditary characteristics.

 t., duplex. Passage of impulses through a nerve trunk in both directions.

transmutation (trăns-mū-tā'shŭn) [L. *transmutātio*, a changing across]. A transformation or change, as of one species into another.

transparent (trăns-păr'ĕnt) [L. *trans*, across, + *parere*, to appear]. 1. Transmitting light rays so that objects are visible through the substance. 2. Pervious to radiant energy. SEE: *clearing agent*.

transpirable (trăns-pī'ră-bl) [" + *spirāre*, to exhale]. Permitting excretion through the skin or membranes, as perspiration.

transpiration (trăns-pī-rā'shŭn) [" + *spiratio*, exhalation]. 1. Act of exhaling water, gas, or vapor through the skin or a membrane. SEE: *perspiration*. 2. Substance exhaled.

 t., cutaneous. Giving off sweat from pores of the skin. SYN: *perspiration*.

 t., pulmonary. Escape of watery vapor from the blood to the air in the lungs.

transplantation (trăns-plăn-tā-shŭn) [" + *plantāre*, to plant]. The taking of a portion of living tissue from its normal position in the body or from the body of another person and uniting it with like tissue in another place, to lessen defect or remedy deformity or injury. SEE: *autotransplantation, graft*.

transportation of the injured. ONE-MAN CARRIES: *Carrying in arms*: Patient is picked up in both arms as a child.
 One-arm assist: Patient's arm is placed about neck of bearer and bearer's arms are placed about waist, thus assisting patient to walk.
 Chair carry: SEE: *chair stretcher*.
 Chair stretcher: Any ordinary firm chair should be tested. Patient is placed seated upon it tilted back. One bearer grasps back of the chair and the other the legs of the chair (either the front or rear, depending on the construction of the chair). Both bearers face in the same direction. Patient's head rests either on chest or back of the head bearer. Turn 2 chairs to the ground; overlap the backs and tie or wire them together, using the legs as handles.
 Double loop: A sheet is rolled on its long axis, tied and placed over the shoulder of both bearers. Patient sits on the long loop and rests his back against a short upper loop with the bearers supporting him. The weight is thus distributed on shoulders of both bearers.
 Fireman's drag: Patient's wrists are crossed and tied with tie, belt, etc. Bearer kneels astride patient, places his head under patient's wrists and walks on all fours dragging patient beneath him.
 Fireman's lift: Bearer grasps patient's left wrist with right arm; places patient's head under left armpit drawing patient's body over his left shoulder. Left arm should encircle both thighs, then lift patient. Patient's wrist is transferred to bearer's left hand, thus leaving 1 hand free to remove obstacles or to open doors, etc.
 Four-handed basket seat: Each bearer grasps his own wrist and then grasps partner's free wrist. Patient sits upon this support.
 Pack-strap carry: Patient lies on bearer's back. Patient's right arm is brought over bearer's right shoulder and held by his left hand. Left arm is brought over left shoulder and held by his right hand. Patient is thus carried on the back with arms resembling pack straps.
 Pickaback carry: This is the pack strap carry only bearer supports patient's knees in flexed position. This leaves patient practically in a sitting position astride bearer's back.
 Ring carry: A cravat or folded towel is rolled and tied to form a small ring. Bearer grasps this ring and allows patient to sit upon it. One free arm is used to support patient.
 Saddle-back carry: Bearer places arm under patient's armpit around his back and grasps it around armpit. Patient's body is across bearer's back. Rescuer's free arm grasps both thighs, allowing patient to rest across patient's back as a saddle.
 Shirt-tail carry: Bearer grasps patient's coat, blouse, or shirt tail, twists it to make a handle and brings it over his shoulder thus carrying patient back to back.
 TWO-MAN CARRIES: *Six- or eight-man carry*: This is done as the 3-man carry except 3 or 4 bearers are on each side of patient, thus dividing weight more uniformly.
 Three - handed basket seat: Bearer grasps his own wrist, partner grasps the other wrist and leaves 1 arm free for supporting patient.
 Three- or four-man carry: The little carry used by emergency squads. Three men kneel on one side of patient, place

their hands under him and lift him up. The head bearer supports head and shoulders, center bearer lifts waist and hips, and third bearer lifts both lower extremities. If a fourth man is available, he should help steady patient while he is being lifted.

Triangular or greater arm sling, or brachiocervical sling: Place triangle on chest with 1 end over the sound shoulder, the point at elbow of affected side. Fold the base. Flex injured arm outside of triangle above the horizontal. Carry other end upward outside of arm back over shoulder of affected side. Tie to side of neck with square knot. Bring point anteriorly around back of elbow and fasten to ascending base or tie forming a cup at elbow. (In this bandage the weight is taken from entire length of forearm.)

Two-handed seat: Bearers kneel on either side of patient. Each passes 1 arm around back (under armpits) and other arm under knees and lifts him carefully. Patient is in a sitting position.

Wheel chair, improvised: Fastening casters to ordinary chair: Tie on a broom handle or similar stick for footrest by placing chair legs on parallel boards and fastening roller skates, wheels, etc.

Fastening as rocker to roller skates: Remove legs from an old chair and fasten to frame of a baby carriage, or play wagon.

t. by vehicle. Ambulances are desirable if available and usually contain appropriate stretchers. When not obtainable, stretchers may be made with poles, chairs or ladders. SEE: *stretchers.* When entering or leaving an airplane one must remember that patient must be tied to the stretcher.

t. by automobile. This is difficult. One bearer should be in the car and 1 or 2 outside to assist patient. A small chair-stretcher can sometimes be used with advantage. A door or ladder slung across the open windows or from front to rear seats may be used. The large rear seat can be used, a stretcher being placed diagonally and supported at 1 end by the seat and the other end on a box or folded blankets.

transposition (trăns-pō-zĭ'shŭn) [L. *trans,* across, + *positio,* a placing]. 1. A transfer of position from one spot to another. SEE: *metathesis.* 2. Displacement of an organ, esp. a viscus, to the opposite side. 3. Transplantation of a flap of tissue without severing it entirely from its original position until it has united in the new position.

transsegmental (trăns"sĕg-mĕn-tăl) [" + *segmentum,* a cutting]. Extending across or beyond a segment as of a limb.

transseptal (trăns-sĕp'tăl) [" + *saeptum,* septum]. Across a septum.

transtemporal (trăns-tĕm'pōral) [" + *temporalis,* pert. to a temple]. Crossing the temporal lobe of the cerebrum.

transthalamic (trăns"thăl-ăm'ĭk) [" + *thalamos,* chamber]. Passing across the optic thalamus.

transthermia (trăns-thĕr'mĭ-ă) [" + *therme,* heat]. Production of heat in the deep tissues by electric currents. SYN: *diathermy, medical, thermopenetration.*

transthoracic (trăns-thō-răs'ĭk) [" + *thorax,* chest]. Across the thorax.

transthoracotomy (trăns"thō-răk-ŏt'ō-mĭ) [L. *trans,* across, + *thorax,* chest, +

tome, a cutting]. The operation of incising across the thorax.

transudate (trăns'ū-dăt) [" + *sudare,* to sweat]. A substance which has passed through the pores of tissues or textures, as blood serum.

transudation (trăns-ū-dā'shŭn) [" + *sudatio,* a sweating]. 1. Oozing of a fluid through pores or interstices, as of a membrane. 2. The substance so passed. A transudate has a low specific gravity, very few cells, and traces of albumin.

transurethral (trăns"ū-rē'thrăl) [" + *ourethra,* urethra]. Pert. to an operation performed through the urethra.

transvaginal (trăns-văj'ĭn-ăl) [" + *vagina,* sheath]. Through the vagina.

transverse (trăns-vĕrs') [L. *transversus,* turned across]. Lying across; crosswise.

t. fora'men. Canal in each transverse process of a cervical vertebra for the arteries and veins.

transversectomy (trăns-vĕr-sĕk'tō-mĭ) [" + G. *ektome,* excision]. Excision of a transverse vertebral process.

transversospinalis (trăns-vĕr"sō-spī-nā'lĭs) [L. *transversus,* turned across, + *spina,* thorn]. Semispinalis capitus, s. cervicis. SEE: *Muscles, Table of, in Appendix.*

transversus (trăns-vĕr'sŭs) [L. turned across]. 1. Any of several small muscles. SEE: *Muscles, Table of, in Appendix.* 2. Lying across the long axis of a part or organ.

transvestism, transvestitism (trăns-vĕst'ĭzm, -ĭ-tĭzm) [L. *trans,* across, + *vestitus,* clothed, +G. *-ismos,* condition]. A sexual perversion in which men prefer to dress as women, or women dress as men. SYN: *eonism, q.v.*

Dr. Mary Walker and Rosa Bonheur were notable examples. Although the practice is against the law of most states, modern trends are making it more or less common. The dominancy of women is now encouraging the practice and possibly increasing the feminism of the male.

trapezium (tră-pē'zĭ-ŭm) [G. *trapezion,* a little table]. 1. First bone of the second carpal row. SYN: *os multangulum majus.* 2. A bundle of transverse fibers in dorsal part of pons Varolii.

trapezius (tră-pē'zĭ-ŭs) [L.]. Large muscle of back and neck.

trapezoid (trăp'ĕ-zoyd) [G. *trapezoeidēs,* table-shaped]. Shaped like a table.

t. bone. One of the carpal bones of the wrist, bet. the trapezium and magnum. SYN: *os multangulum minus.*

Trapp-Hässer formula (trăp-hă'sĕr). To estimate the grains of solids in urine, multiply last 2 figures of the sp. gr. by 2.33, which gives the solids in 1000 cc.

tras'entin. Spasmolytic agent similar to atropine, but lacking its undesirable properties.

trauma (traw'mă) (pl. *traumata* or *traumas*) [G. *trauma,* wound]. An injury or a wound.

t., psychic. A painful, emotional experience, which may cause a neurosis.

traumatic (traw-măt'ĭk) [G. *trauma,* wound]. 1. Caused by or relating to an injury. 2. Causing the healing of wounds. 3. A drug promoting healing.

t. fever. One following an injury.

traumatin (traw'măt-ĭn) [G. *trauma,* wound]. Plant substance which helps the healing of injured tissues.

traumatism (traw'mă-tĭzm) [" + *-ismos,* condition]. 1. Morbid condition of system due to an injury or wound. 2. Incorrectly, a trauma.

traumatology (traw-mă-tŏl′ō-jĭ) [" + *logos*, science]. The science of wounds and their care.

traumatopnea (traw″mă-tŏp-nē′ă) [" + *pnoiē*, breath]. Passage of air in and out of a wound in the chest wall.

treatment (trēt′mĕnt) [M.E. *treten*, to handle]. Management, medical or surgical care of a patient.

t., active. Treatment directed specifically toward cure of a disease.

t., expectant. Relief of symptoms as they arise. [of health.

t., hygienic. Application of the laws

t., preventive, prophylactic. T. directed to prevention of disease.

t., specific. T. directed to the cause of a disease.

t., suprasonic. The use of sound vibrations in small doses to create heat-friction in cells. They have an analgesic, spasmolytic, and anti-inflammatory and bactericidal effect. Favorable results have been had in neuritis, bursitis, arthritis, myalgia, leg ulcers, bronchial asthma, prostatitis, and Dupuytren's contracture. SEE: *suprasonic*.

t., surgical. T. by means of operation.

trematode (trĕm′ăt-ōd) [G. *trēmatōdēs*, full of holes]. 1. A parasitic worm, a fluke. 2. Pert. to a parasitic worm. SEE: *cercaria*.

tremelloid, tremellose (trĕm′el-oyd, -ĕl-ōs) [L. *tremere*, to tremble, + G. *eidos*, resemblance]. Gelatinous.

tremogram (trĕm′ō-grăm) [L. *tremere*, to shake, + G. *gramma*, a mark]. Graphic representation made by a tremograph.

tremograph (trĕm′ō-grăf) [" + *graphein*, to write]. Device for recording tremors.

tremolabile (trē″mō-lā′bĭl) [" + *labilis*, unsteady]. Easily destroyed or inactivated by shaking; said of a ferment.

tremophobia (trĕm″ō-fō′bĭ-ă) [" + G. *phobos*, fear]. Abnormal fear of trembling.

tremor (trĕm′or, trē′mor) [L. *tremor*, a shaking]. A quivering, esp. continuous quivering of a convulsive nature.

A rhythmic to and fro movement of a part which does not change the relationship of the affected segment to the rest of the body. SEE: *amyostasia*. Tremors are rhythmic and fail to cause gross movement of the part.

Tremors may be classified as *involuntary*, *static*, *dynamic*, *kinetic*, *hereditary*, and *hysteric*. Pathologic tremors are independent of the will. The trembling may be fine or coarse, rapid or slow, may appear on movement (intention tremor) or improve when the part is employed. Often due to organic disease; trembling may express an emotion (*e. g.*, fear). [cause. SEE: *subsultus*.

TREATMENT: Varies with underlying

t., alcoholic. The visible t. exhibited by alcoholics.

t., continuous. One that resembles tremors of paralysis agitans.

t., fibrillary. One caused by consecutive contractions of separate muscular fibrillae, rather than of a muscle or muscles. [tary motion has ceased.

t., forced. T. continuing after volun-

t., hysterical. Due to the instability of nervous impulse seen in hysteria.

t., intention. T. when voluntary motion is attempted.

t., intermittent. One common to paralyzed muscles in hemiplegia when attempting voluntary movement.

t., muscular. Slight oscillating muscular contractions in rhythmical order.

t., volitional. Trembling of limbs or of body when making a voluntary effort; in connection with multiple sclerosis and other nervous diseases.

tremulous (trĕm′ū-lŭs) [L. *tremulāre*, to tremble]. Trembling or shaking.

trench mouth. Infection of tonsils and floor of the mouth with Vincent's bacillus, characterized by inflammation, ulceration, and painful swelling. SYN: *ulceromembranous angina, Vincent's angina, q.v.*

trend, psychiatric. Benign or malignant emotional interests and urges, revealed by postures, gestures, actions, speech.

Trendelenburg position (trĕn-dĕl′ĕn-burg). The bed or table is raised from the foot, greatly elevating the knees, the legs projecting on an extended leg rest.

In this position the abdominal organs are pushed up toward the chest by grav-

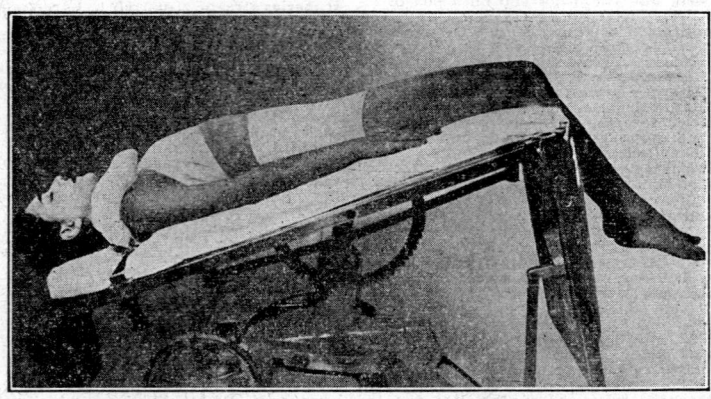

Posed by Professional Model—Photo by Whitaker. Courtesy of Mount Vernon Hospital.
TRENDELENBURG POSITION.
Shoulder braces on table prevent patient from slipping.

trepan   T-47   **triad**

ity. The legs are elevated at an angle of 45°. The head is lower than the hips and legs. The foot of the bed may be elevated by resting upon blocks or pins.

This position is assumed in some abdominal surgery, in case of shock, or low blood pressure. In surgical cases, the legs and feet hang over the end of the table.

trepan (trē-păn') [G. *trypanon*, a borer]. 1. To perforate the skull with a trepan to relieve brain from pressure. 2. An instrument resembling a carpenter's bit for incision of the skull. SYN: *trephine*.

trephination (trĕf-ĭn-ā'shŭn) [Fr. *tréphine*, a bore]. Process of cutting out a piece of bone with the trephine.

trephine (trē-fīn') [Fr. *tréphine*, a bore]. 1. To perforate with a trephine. 2. A cylindrical saw for cutting circular piece of bone out of skull. SEE: *trepan*.

trephocyte (trĕf'ō-sīt) [G. *trephein*, to nourish, + *kytos*, cell]. Any cell supplying nutritive substances to the tissues.

trephone (trĕf'ōn) [G. *trephein*, to nourish]. Hypothetical growth-promoting substance in the blood serum, used by cells as food material.

trepidant (trĕp'ĭ-dănt) [L. *trepidans*, trembling]. Marked by tremor.

trepidation (trĕp-ĭ-dā'shŭn) [L. *trepidatio*, a trembling]. 1. Fear, anxiety. 2. Trembling movement, esp. when involuntary.

Treponema (trĕp-ō-nē'mă) [G. *trepein*, to turn, + *nēma*, thread]. A genus of spirochetes, parasitic in man, with undulating or rigid bodies.

   T. pallidum. Causative organism of syphilis. SYN: *Spirochaeta pallida*.

treponemiasis (trĕp″ō-nē-mī'ă-sĭs) [G. *trepein*, to turn, + *nēma*, thread, + *iasis*, infection]. Infestation with Treponema.

treponemicidal (trĕp″ō-nē-mĭ-sī'dăl) [" + L. *cidus*, from *caedere*, to kill]. Destructive to Treponema.

treppe (trĕp'eh) [Ger. *treppe*, staircase]. Increase in height of contractions when the heart or a muscle is stimulated rapidly at regular intervals. SYN: *staircase effect*, *q.v.*

tresis (trē'sĭs) [G. *trēsis*, perforation]. Perforation.

tri- [G.]. Combining form meaning *three*.

triad (trī'ăd) [G. *trias*, three]. 1. Any 3 things having something in common. 2. A trivalent element. 3. Trivalent.

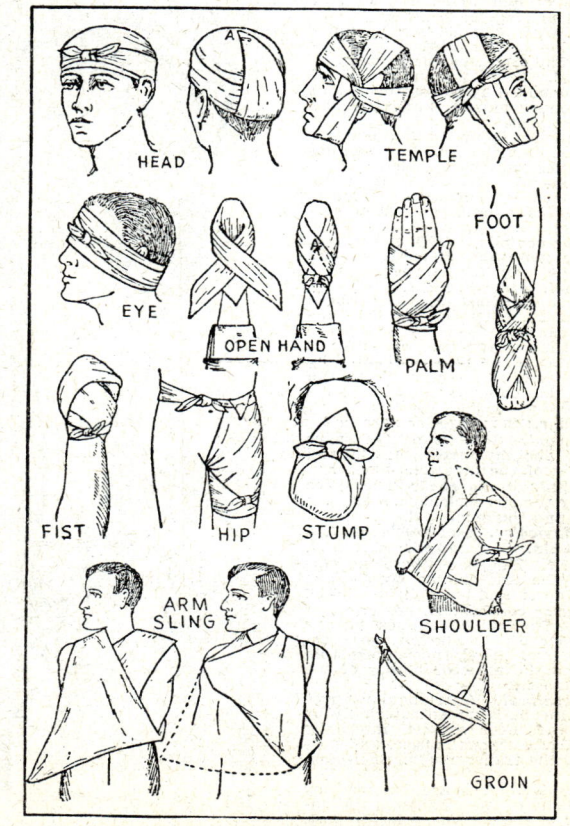

TRIANGULAR BANDAGES.

triakaidekaphobia (trī″ăk-ĭ-děk-ă-fō′bĭ-ă) [" + *kai*, and, + *deka*, ten, + *phobos*, fear]. Superstition regarding the number 13.

trial case (trī′ăl kās). An optician's box containing trial lenses.

  t. frame. Spectacle frame for holding lenses for testing one's vision.

triangle (trī′ăng-l) [L. *tres*, three, + *angulus*, angle; *triangulum*]. A figure or area formed by 3 angles and 3 sides.

  t., anterior, of the neck. The space bounded by the middle line of the neck, the ant. border of the sternocleidomastoid, and a line running along the lower border of the mandible and continued to the mastoid process of the occipital bone.

  t., carotid, inferior. The space bounded by the middle line of the neck, the sternomastoid and the ant. belly of the omohyoid muscle.

  t., carotid, superior. The space bounded by the ant. belly of the omohyoid muscle, the post. belly of the digastricus and the sternomastoid.

  t., cephalic. A t. on the anteroposterior plane of the skull formed by lines joining the occiput and forehead and chin, and 1 uniting the 2 latter.

  t., facial. A t. bounded by lines uniting the basion and the alveolar and nasal points, and 1 uniting the 2 latter.

  t., femoral. T. on the inner part of the thigh, bounded by the sartorius and adductor longus muscle, and above by inguinal ligament.

  t., frontal. A t. bounded by the maximum frontal diameter and lines joining its extremities and the glabella.

  t., Hesselbach's. The interval in the groin bounded by Poupart's ligament, edge of rectus muscle, and deep epigastric artery.

  t., inferior occipital. Of Welcker, a t. having the bimastoid diameter for its base and the inion for its apex.

  t., inguinal. See: *femoral t.*

  t., lumbocostoabdominal. The space bounded in front by the obliquus abdominis externus, above by the lower border of the serratus posticus inferior and the point of the 12th rib, behind by the outer edge of the erector spinae, and below by the obliquus abdominis internus.

  t., muscular. See: *inferior carotid t.*

  t., mylohyoid. The triangular space formed by the mylohyoid muscle and the 2 bellies of the digastric muscle.

  t., occipital, of the neck. The space bounded by the sternocleidomastoid, the trapezius, and the omohyoid.

  t., omoclavicular. See: *subclavian t.*

  t., omohyoid. See: *superior carotid t.*

  t. of Petit. The space above the hipbone, bet. the ext. oblique muscle, the latissimus dorsi, and int. oblique muscle.

  t., posterior cervical; t., posterior, of the neck. The space bounded by the upper border of the clavicle, the posterior border of the sternocleidomastoid muscle, and the anterior border of the trapezius muscle.

  t., pubourethral. A triangular space in the perineum, bounded externally by the ischiocavernous muscle, internally by the bulbocavernous muscle, and posteriorly by the transversus perinei muscle.

  t., subclavian. A space bounded by the post. belly of the omohyoid, the upper border of the clavicle, and the post. margin of the sternocleidomastoid.

  t., submaxillary. The space between the lower border of the inf. maxilla, the parotid gland, and the mastoid process of the temporal bone above, the post. belly of the digastric and the stylohyoid below, and the middle line of the neck in front.

  t., supraclavicular. See: *subclavian t.*

triangular bandage. One folded diagonally. When folded the several thicknesses afford some support.

  t. ligament. 1. L. having 3 sides or angles. 2. One of the urethra attached to Poupart's ligament.

  t. nucleus. Upper part of the cuneate fasciculus in the medulla oblongata. Syn: *nucleus, cuneate.*

triangularis (trī-ăng-ū-lā′rĭs) [L.]. A muscle of the chin. See: *Muscles, Table of, in Appendix.*

tribadism (trĭb′ăd-ĭzm) [G. *tribein*, to rub, + *-ismos*, condition]. A form of perversion in which women seek sexual gratification from one of their own sex.

tribromoethanol (trī-brō-mō-eth′an-ōl). USP. Syn. for *avertin.*

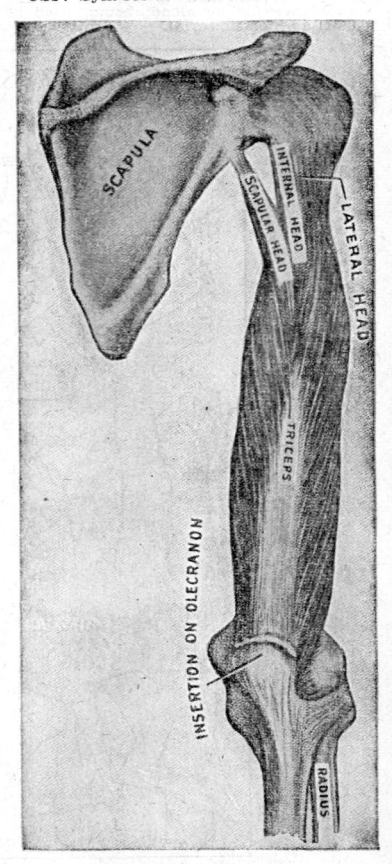

TRICEPS MUSCLE.

triceps (trī'sĕps) [L. *trēs*, three, + *caput*, head]. A muscle arising by 3 heads with a single insertion. SEE: *Muscles, Table of, in Appendix*.
 t. reflex. Sharp extension of forearm resulting from tapping of triceps tendon while arm is held loosely in bent position.
trichangiectasia, trichangiectasis (trik″ăn-ji-ĕk-ta′zĭ-ă, -ĕk′tă-sĭs) [G. *thrix, trich-*, hair, + *aggeion*, vessel, + *ektasis*, dilatation]. Dilatation of capillaries. SYN: *telangiectasia*.
trichauxe, trichauxis (trĭk-awk′sē, -sĭs) [" + *auxē*, increase]. Excessive growth of hair. SYN: *hypertrichosis*.
trichi-, tricho- [G.]. Combining forms meaning *hair*.
trichiasis (trĭk-ī′ăs-ĭs) [G. *trichiasis*, hair condition]. 1. Presence of hairlike filaments in the urine. 2. Inversion of eyelashes so that they rub against the cornea, causing a continual irritation of the eyeball.
 SYM: Photophobia, lacrimation, and feeling of foreign body in eye.
 TREATMENT: Epilation, electrolysis and operation, such as correcting the underlying entropion with which this condition is usually associated.
Trichina (trĭk-ī′nă) [G. *trichinos*, of hair]. A nematoid, parasitic worm usually found in the intestinal tract of certain lower animals and man.
Trichinella (trĭk-ĭn-ĕl′ă) [G. *trichinos*, of hair]. A genus of nematode worms. SYN: *Trichina*.
 T. spira′lis. The adult nematode causing trichinosis.
trichinellosis (trĭ-kĭ-nel-lo′sĭs) [" + *-ōsis*, condition]. Disease caused by *Trichinella spiralis*. SYN: *trichinosis, q.v.*
trichinization (trĭk″ĭn-ĭ-zā′shŭn) [G. *trichinos*, of hair]. Infestation with trichinae.
trichinophobia (trĭk″ĭn-ō-fō′bĭ-ă) [" + *phobos*, fear]. Abnormal fear of developing trichiniasis.
trichinoscope (trĭk-ī′nŏ-skōp) [" + *skopein*, to examine]. Magnifying glass used to discover trichinae in meat.
trichinosis (trĭk-ĭn-ō′sĭs) [G. *trichinos*, of hair, + *-ōsis*, condition]. Disease caused by the ingestion of *Trichina spiralis* into the system through eating raw or insufficiently cooked pork.
 SYM: Sometimes lacking. When large numbers have been ingested, gastrointestinal symptoms develop in a few days. These are pain, nausea, vomiting and serous diarrhea.
 In from 1 to 2 weeks muscular symptoms develop, muscles become swollen, firm, extremely painful; movement is inhibited, and dyspnea results from involvement of respiratory muscles. Edema, esp. of face, is a prominent symptom. Profuse sweating sometimes observed and high fever commonly present. Blood shows an eosinophilia.
 PROG: Depends on number of worms ingested. Majority recover.
 TREATMENT: Prevent by thoroughly cooking all pork products. In first stage use purgatives. After migration, when the living embryos have left stomach and gone into the muscles, employ opium, warm fomentations and stimulants.
trichinous (trĭk′ĭn-ŭs) [G. *trichinos*, of hair]. Infested with trichinae.
trichitis (trĭk-ī′tĭs) [G. *thrix, trich-*, hair, + *-itis*, inflammation]. Inflammation of hair bulbs.
trichlorethylene (trī″klor-ĕth′ĭl-ēn). A colorless liquid (CHCl:CCl$_2$).
 USES: In trigeminal neuralgia.
 DOSAGE: 20-25 drops by inhalation, 6 or 7 breaths.
 CAUTION: Must be kept away from open flame. May cause watery eyes and other unpleasant symptoms.
trichobacteria (trĭk″ō-băk-tē′rĭ-ă) [G. *thrix, trich-*, hair, + *baktērion*, rod]. Filamentous or flagellate bacteria.
trichobezoar (trĭk″ō-bē′zō-ar) [" + Persian *bezoar*]. A hair ball or concretion in the intestine or stomach.
trichocardia (trĭk-ō-kar′dĭ-ă) [" + *kardia*, heart]. Pericardial inflammation with elevations resembling hair. SYN: *cor hirsutum, hairy heart, shaggy pericardium*.
trichocephaliasis (trĭk″ō-sĕf-ăl-ī′ă-sĭs) [" + *kephalē*, head]. Infestation with Trichocephalus.
Trichocephalus (trĭk-ō-sĕf′ăl-ŭs) [" + *kephalē*, head]. A genus of parasitic worms infesting the colon.
 T. dis′par. A common, harmless, intestinal parasite of the cecum.
trichoclasia, trichoclasis (trĭk″ō-klā′zĭ-ă, -ok′lăs-ĭs) [" + *klasis*, a breaking]. Brittleness of the hair. SYN: *trichorrhexis*.
trichocryptosis (trĭk″ō-krĭp-tō′sĭs) [" + *kryptos*, concealed]. Any disease of the hair follicles.
trichoepithelioma (trĭk″ō-ĕp″ĭ-thē-lĭ-ō′mă) [G. *thrix, trich-*, hair, + *epi*, upon, + *thēlē*, nipple, + *-ōma*, tumor]. A benign skin tumor originating in the hair follicles.
trichoesthesia (trĭk″ō-ĕs-thē′zĭ-ă) [" + *aisthēsis*, sensation]. 1. Sensation felt when a hair is touched. 2. A paresthesia causing a sensation of the presence of a hair on a mucous membrane or on the skin.
trichoesthesiometer (trĭk″ō-ĕs-thē-zĭ-ŏm′ĕ-ter) [" + " + *metron*, a measure]. Device for testing sensibility of the scalp by means of the hair.
trichogen (trĭk′ō-jĕn) [" + *gennan*, to produce]. An agent stimulating growth of hair.
trichogenous (trĭk-ŏj′ĕn-ŭs) [" + *gennan*, to produce]. Promoting hair growth.
trichoglossia (trĭk-ō-glŏs′sĭ-ă) [" + *glōssa*, tongue]. Hairy condition of the tongue.
trichoid (trĭk′oyd) [" + *eidos*, resemblance]. Hairlike.
trichokyptomania (trĭk″ō-kĭp″tō-mā′nĭ-ă) [G. *thrix, trich-*, hair, + *kyptos*, crooked, + *mania*, madness]. Abnormal desire to break off the hair or beard with the fingernail. SYN: *trichorrhexomania*.
trichology (trĭk-ŏl′ō-jĭ) [" + *logos*, a study]. Study of the hair and its care and treatment.
trichoma (trĭk-ō′mă) [G. *trichōma*, hairiness]. 1. Inversion of 1 or more eyelashes. SYN: *entropion*. 2. Matted, verminous, encrusted state of the hair. SYN: *plica polonica*.
trichomatosis (trĭk-ō-mă-tō′sĭs) [" + *-ōsis*, condition]. Entangled, matted hair due to fungous disease of scalp and want of cleanliness. SYN: *plica polonica*.
trichomatous (trĭk-ō′mă-tŭs) [G. *trichōma*, hairiness]. Of the nature of, or affected with trichoma.
Trichomonas (trĭk-ŏm′ō-năs) [G. *thrix, trich-*, hair, + *monas*, unit]. Genus of flagellate parasitic protozoa.
 T. hom′inis. Species in human intestines sometimes causing diarrhea and bacillary dysentery.
 T. vaginalis. Vaginitis caused by a species of T. in secretions of the va-

trichomoniasis gina; sometimes found in the male urethra. SEE: *colpitis*.

trichomoniasis (trĭk″ō-mō-nī′ăs-ĭs) [" + " + *-iasis*, infection]. Infestation with a parasite of genus Trichomonas.

trichomycosis (trĭk-ō-mī-kō′sĭs) [" + *mykēs*, fungus, + *-ōsis*, condition]. Any disease of the hair due to a fungus.

 t. nodosa. Disease marked by nodule formations on the hair shafts. SYN: *piedra*.

trichonosis, trichonosus (trĭk-ō-nō′sĭs, -ŏn′-ō-sŭs) [" + *nosos*, disease]. Any diseased condition of the hair.

trichopathophobia (trĭk″ō-păth-ō-fō′bĭ-ă) [" + *pathos*, disease, + *phobos*, fear]. Morbid fear of hair on the face experienced by women, or any abnormal anxiety regarding hair.

trichopathy (trĭk-ŏp′ăth-ĭ) [" + *pathos*, disease]. Any disease of the hair.

trichophagia, trichophagy (trĭk-ō-fā′jĭ-ă, -of′ă-jĭ) [" + *phagein*, to eat]. The habit of swallowing hair.

trichophobia (trĭk-ō-fō′bĭ-ă) [G. *thrix*, *trich-*, hair, + *phobos*, fear]. Abnormal dread of hair or of touching it.

trichophytic (trĭk″ō-fĭt′ĭk) [" + *phyton*, growth]. 1. Relating to Trichophyton. 2. Promoting hair growth.

Trichophyton (trĭk-ŏf′ĭt-ŏn) [" + *phyton*, growth]. A parasitic fungus on the hair causing ringworm.

 T. ton'surans. The fungus responsible for ringworm.

trichophytosis (trĭk″ō-fī-tō′sĭs) [" + " + *-ōsis*, condition]. Infestation with trichophyton fungi; mostly in children.

trichoptilosis (trĭk″ŏp-tĭl-ō′sĭs) [" + *ptilon*, feather, + *-ōsis*, condition]. 1. The splitting of hairs at their ends, giving them a featherlike appearance. 2. Disease of hair marked by development of nodules along the hair shaft at which point it splits off. SYN: *trichorrhexis nodosa*.

trichorrhea (trĭk-or-ē′ă) [" + *rhoia*, a flow]. Rapid falling of the hair.

trichorrhexis (trĭk″ō-rĕks′ĭs) [" + *rhēxis*, a breaking]. Condition in which the hair splits. SYN: *fragilitas crinium, trichoschisis*.

 t. nodo'sa. Longitudinal splitting of hair at nodules formed on the shaft. SYN: *clastothrix, trichoclasia*.

trichorrhexomania (trĭk″ō-rĕks″ō-mā′nĭ-ă) [" + " + *mania*, madness]. The abnormal habit of breaking off the hair with the fingernails.

trichoschisis (tri-kos′kis-is) [G. *thrix*, *trich-*, hair, + *schisis*, a fissure]. Splitting of the hairs.

trichoscopy (trĭk-ŏs′kō-pĭ) [" + *skopein*, to examine]. Inspection of the hair.

trichosis (trī-kō′sĭs) [" + *-ōsis*, condition]. Any disease of the hair or its abnormal growth or development in an abnormal place.

 t. dec'olor. Any abnormal coloring or lack of coloring of the hair. SYN: *canities*.

 t. seto'sa. Coarse hair.

Trichosporon (trī-kŏs′pŏ-rŏn) [" + *sporos*, a seed]. A genus of fungi causing trichomycosis nodosa.

trichosporosis (trĭk″ō-spō-rō′sĭs) [" + " + *-ōsis*, condition]. Infestation of the hair with Trichosporon.

trichosyphilis, trichosyphilosis (trĭk″ō-sĭf′-ĭ-lĭs, -sĭf″ĭl-ō′sĭs) [" + *syphilis* + *-ōsis*, condition]. Any hair disease arising from a syphilitic condition.

Trichothecium (trĭk″ō-thē′sĭ-ŭm) [" + *thēkē*, a box]. A genus of mold fungi causing disease of the hair.

 T. ro'seum. A species of mold fungus found in certain cases of inflammation of the eardrum (mycomyringitis).

trichotillomania (tri-ko-til-o-ma′nĭ-ă) [G. *thrix, trich-*, hair, + *tillein*, to pull, + *mania*, madness]. The unnatural impulse to pull out one's own hair.

trichotomy (trī-kŏt′ō-mĭ) [G. *tricha*, threefold, + *tomē*, a cutting]. Division into three parts.

trichotoxin (trĭk″ō-tŏks′ĭn) [G. *thrix, trich-*, hair, + *toxikon*, poison]. An antibody or cytotoxin which destroys ciliated epithelial cells.

trichotrophy (trī-kŏt′rō-fĭ) [" + *trophē*, nourishment]. Nutrition of the hair.

trichroic (trī-krō′ĭk) [G. *treis*, three, + *chroa*, color]. Presenting 3 different colors from 3 different aspects.

trichroism (trī′krō-ĭzm) [" + " + *-ismos*, condition]. Quality of showing a different color from each of 3 positions.

trichromatic (trī″krō-măt′ĭk) [" + *chroma*, color]. Relating to or able to see the 3 primary colors; noting normal color vision.

trichromic (trī-krō′mĭk) [" + *chrōma*, color]. Pert. to normal color vision or ability to see the 3 primary colors. SYN: *trichromatic*.

trichuriasis (trĭk″ū-rī′ă-sĭs) [G. *thrix, trich-*, hair, + *oura*, tail]. Presence of worms of genus Trichuris in the colon, or in the ileum. SYN: *trichocephaliasis*.

Trichuris (trī-kū′rĭs) [" + *oura*, tail]. A genus of Trematoda.

 T. trichiur'ia. The whipworm. SYN: *Trichocephalus dispar*.

tricipital (trī-sĭp′ĭ-tăl) [L. *tres, tria*, three, + *caput*, head]. Three-headed, as the triceps muscle.

tricornic, tricornute (trī-kor′nĭk, -nūt) [" + *cornu*, horn]. Having 3 horns or cornua.

tricrotic (trī-krŏt′ĭk) [G. *treis*, three, + *krotos*, a beat]. Having 3 beats, as the downward stroke of the sphygmographic tracing.

tricrotism (trī′krŏt-ĭzm) [" + " + *-ismos*, condition]. Condition of being tricrotic.

tricuspid (trī-kŭs′pĭd) [L. *tres, tria*, three, + *cuspis*, a point]. 1. Pert. to the tricuspid valve. 2. Having 3 points or cusps. 3. A tooth having 3 cusps.

 t. area. Lower portion of body of sternum where sounds of right atrioventricular orifice are best heard.

 t. murmur. One caused by stenosis of the tricuspid valve or by its incompetency.

 t. orifice. Right atrioventricular cardiac aperture.

 t. tooth. One with a crown having three cusps.

 t. valve. Right atrioventricular valve. SYN: *valvula tricuspidalis*.

trident, tridentate (trī′dĕnt, trī-dĕn′tāt) [L. *trēs, tria*, three, + *dens, dent-*, tooth]. Having three prongs.

tridermic (trī-der′mĭk) [G. *treis*, three, + *derma*, skin]. Developed from the ectoderm, endoderm, and mesoderm.

tridermoma (trī″dĕr-mō′mă) [" + " + *-ōma*, tumor]. A teratoid growth containing all three germ layers.

trielcon (trī-ĕl′kŏn) [" + *elkein*, to draw]. Instrument with 3 branches for removing foreign substances from wounds.

triethylene melamine. Commonly abbr. *TEM*. One of the nitrogen mustard compounds. SEE: *nitrogen mustard*.

trifacial (trī-fā′shăl) [L. *trēs, tria*, three,

trifacial neuralgia   T-51   **tritanopia**

+ *facialis*, facial]. Pert. to the 5th pair of cranial nerves. SYN: *trigeminal*.
t. neuralgia. N. of 1 of the branches of the 5th cranial nerve; often severe. SYN: *tic douloureux*.
trifid (trī'fĭd) [L. *trifidus*, split thrice]. Split into 3; having 3 clefts.
trigeminal (trī-jĕm'ĭn-ăl) [L. *trēs, tria*, three, + *geminus*, twin]. Pert. to the trigeminus or 5th cranial nerve.
t. cough. A reflex cough from irritation of the trigeminal nerve terminations in respiratory upper passages.
t. neuralgia. Facial neuralgia. SYN: *tic* douloureux*.
t. pulse. One with longer or shorter interval after each 3 beats because the 3rd beat is an extra systole. SYN: *pulsus trigeminus*.
trigeminus (trī-jĕm'ĭ-nŭs) [" + *geminus*, twin]. The 5th cranial nerve or trifacial n.
FUNCT: Sensation, motion, taste.
ORIG: Floor of 4th ventricle and oblongata.
DIST: Surface of face, tongue, and teeth.
BRS: Divides into 3 portions: ophthalmic, sensory; sup. maxillary, sensory; inf. maxillary, sensory, motor, and a lingual nerve of sense of taste. The most difficult of all cranial nerves to trace. SEE: *cranial nerves*.
trig'ger finger. State in which flexion or extension is arrested temporarily, but finally completed with a jerk.
trigonal (trĭg'ō-năl) [G. *trigōnon*, a three-cornered figure]. Triangular; pert. to a trigone.
trigone (trī'gōn) [G. *trigōnon*, a three-cornered figure]. A triangular space, esp. one at the base of the bladder. SYN: *trigonum*.
trigonitis (trī-gō-nī'tĭs) [" + *-itis*, inflammation]. Inflammation of trigone of bladder confined to its mucous membrane.
trigonocephalic (trī"gō-nō-sef-ăl'ĭk) [" + *kephalē*, head]. Having a head shaped like a triangle.
trigonum (trī-gō'nŭm) [L. from G. *trigōnon*, a three-cornered figure]. Any triangular area. SYN: *trigone*.
trilabe (trī'lāb) [G. *treis*, three, + *labē*, a handle]. Three-pronged forceps for removing foreign substances from the bladder. SEE: *lithotrite*.
trill (trĭl) [Italian *trillare*, probably imitative]. A tremulous sound, esp. in vocal music, made by vibration of 1 speech organ against another.
trimanual (trī-măn'ū-ăl) [L. *trēs, tria*, three, + *manualis*, by hand]. Performed with three hands, as an obstetrical maneuver.
trimensual (trī-mĕn'shū-ăl) [" + *mensualis*, monthly]. Occurring quarterly or every 3 months.
trimorphous (trī-mor'fŭs) [G. *treis*, three, + *morphē*, form]. Having 3 different forms, as the larva, pupa, and image of certain insects, or certain crystals.
trineuric (trī-nū'rĭk) [" + *neuron*, nerve]. Having 3 axis cylinders.
trinitrophenol (trī-nī-trō-fē'nōl). USP. Picric acid, a yellow crystalline powder, explosive when heated.
ACTION AND USES: An astringent and antiseptic. Used chiefly in the treatment of burns as a saturated solution.
triorchid, triorchis (trī-or'kĭd, -kĭs) [G. *treis*, three, + *orchis*, testicle]. One having 3 testicles.
triorchidism (trī-or'kĭd-ĭzm) [" + " +

-ismos, condition]. The condition of having 3 testicles.
tripara (trĭp'ă-ră) [L. *trēs, tria*, three, + *parēre*, to bear]. A woman who has had 3 children in separate pregnancies. SYN: *tertipara*.
tripeptid(e (trī-pĕp'tīd) [G. *treis*, three, + *peptōn*, digested]. Product of combination of 3 amino acids formed during proteolytic digestion.
triphalangia (trī-fă-lan'jĭ-ă) [" + *phalagx, phalagg-*, phalanx]. Deformity marked by presence of 3 phalanges in a thumb or great toe.
triphasic (trī-fā'sĭk) [" + *phasis*, phase]. Consisting of 3 phases or stages, said of electric currents.
triphthemia (trĭf-thē'mĭ-ă) [G. *triphthos*, waste, + *aima*, blood]. Waste products in the blood.
Tripier's amputation (trĭp-ē-ā'). Amputation of a foot with part of the calcaneus removed.
triplegia (trī-plē'jĭ-ă) [G. *treis*, three, + *plēgē*, stroke]. Hemiplegia with paralysis of 1 limb on the other side of the body.
triplet (trĭp'lĕt) [L. *triplus*, threefold]. 1. One of 3 persons born of the same mother from 1 pregnancy. SEE: *Hellin's law*. 2. A combination of 3 of a kind.
triplex (trī'plĕks, trĭp'lĕks) [L. *trēs, tria*, three, + *plexus*, folded]. Triple; threefold.
triploia (trĭp-lō'pĭ-ă) [G. *triploos*, triple, + *opsis*, vision]. Condition in which 3 images are visioned of the same object.
triquetrous (trī-kwē'trŭs) [L. *triquetrus*, triangular]. Triangular.
t. bone. 1. A wormian bone. 2. The Cuneiform bone of the carpus.
triradial, triradiate (trī-rā'dĭ-ăl, -ra'dĭ-āt) [L. *trēs, tria*, three, + *radius*, ray]. Radiating in 3 directions.
t. lines. The embryonic stars of the lens.
t. sulcus. The orbital fissure. SYN: *sulcus orbitalis*.
trismoid (trĭz'moyd) [G. *trismos*, trismus, + *eidos*, form]. 1. Of the nature of trismus. 2. A form of trismus nascentium; once thought to be due to pressure on occiput during delivery.
trismus (trĭz'mŭs) [G. *trismos*]. Tonic spasm of muscles of the jaw seen in inflammation of the mouth at the angle of the jaw. SYN: *lockjaw*.
A mild form of tetanus when the contractions are limited to the group of muscles about neck and face.
t. capistra'tus. Adhesion of cheeks to the gums; congenital.
t. nascentium. A form attacking infants within 2 weeks of birth, due to infection through the navel. Generally fatal. Also called 9-day fits. SEE: *tetanus*.
t. neonatorum. SEE: *t. nascentium*.
t. sardon'icus. Facial muscle spasm producing a grinning expression.
trisodarsin (trī-sō-dar'sĭn). An antisyphilitic drug esp. good in congenital cases.
DOSAGE: 0.45-0.6 Gm.
trisplanchnic (trī-splănk'nĭk) [G. *treis*, three, + *splagchna*, viscera]. Pert. to the 3 visceral cavities, the *skull, thorax*, and *abdomen*.
t. nervous system. Sympathetic nervous system.
tristichia (trī-stĭk'ĭ-ă) [" + *stichos*, row]. The presence of 3 rows of eyelashes.
tristimania (trĭs-tĭm-ā'nĭ-ă) [L. *tristis*, sad, + *mania*, madness]. Melancholia.
trisulcate (trī-sŭl'kāt) [L. *trēs, tria*, three, + *sulcus*, groove]. Having 3 grooves or furrows.
tritanopia (trī-tăn-ō'pĭ-ă) [G. *tritos*, third,

triticeous

+ *an-*, priv. + *opsis*, vision]. Color blindness in which blue and yellow appear gray.
triticeous (trĭt-ĭsh'ŭs) [L. *triticeus*, of wheat]. Shaped like a grain of wheat.
  t. cartilage, t. nodule. A cartilaginous nodule in the thyrohyoid ligament.
triticeum (trĭt-ĭs'ē-ŭm) [L.]. A nodule in the thyrohyoid ligament.
tritium (trĭsh'ĭ-ŭm) [L.]. The mass 3 isotope of hydrogen; triple-weight hydrogen.
tritotoxin (trī"tō-tŏks'ĭn) [G. *tritos*, third, + *toxikon*, poison]. A toxin, according to Ehrlich, which is the 3rd or lowest in order of toxicity.
triturable (trĭt'ū-ră-bl) [L. *triturāre*, to pulverize]. Susceptible of being powdered.
triturate (trĭt'ū-rāt) [L. *triturāre*, to pulverize]. 1. To reduce to a fine powder by rubbing. 2. A finely divided substance made by rubbing.
trituration (trĭt-ū-rā'shŭn) [L. *triturātio*, a rubbing to powder]. Powdered preparation containing 10% of the active drug and 90% of sugar of milk. None are official.
trivalent (trī-vā'lĕnt, trĭv'ăl-ĕnt) [L. *tres*, *tria*, three, + *valens*, powerful]. Combining with or replacing 3 hydrogen atoms.
trocar (trō'kar) [Fr. *troisquarts*, three-quarters]. Instrument with a triangular tip used for aspiration or removal of fluids from cavities.
trochanter (trō-kăn'ter) [G. *trochantēr*, a runner]. Either of the 2 bony processes below the neck of the femur.
  The greater trochanter is located at the lateral side; the lesser trochanter at the medial.
  t. major. BNA. A thick process at upper end of the femur projecting upward externally to union of neck and shaft.
  t. minor. BNA. A conical tuberosity upon inner and post. surface of upper end of femur, at junction of shaft and neck.
  t. tertius. The gluteal ridge of the femur when it is unusually prominent.
trochanterian, trochanteric (trō"kăn-tē'rĭ-ăn, trō-kăn-ter'ĭk) [G. *trochantēr*, a runner]. Relating to a trochanter.
troche (trō'kē) [G. *trochē*, a round object]. Solid, discoid, or cylindrical mass consisting chiefly of medicinal powder, sugar, and mucilage.
  They are intended to be used by placing them in the mouth and allowing them to remain until, through slow solution or disintegration, their purpose of mild medication is effected. They are not often prescribed. None are official. SYN: *lozenge*.
trochin (trō'kĭn) [G. *trochos*, a wheel]. The lesser tuberosity of the head of the humerus. SYN: *tuberculum minus*.
trochiter (trŏk'ĭt-er) [G. *trochos*, a wheel]. Greater tuberosity of the head of the humerus.
trochlea (trŏk'lē-ă) (pl. *trochleae*) [L. *trochlea*, pulley]. 1. A structure having the function of a pulley; a ring or hook through which a tendon or muscle projects. 2. The articular smooth surface of a bone upon which glides another bone.
trochlear nerve. Patheticus or 4th cranial nerve.
  FUNCT: Motor.
  ORIG: Floor of aquaeductus cerebri.
  DIST: Sup. oblique muscle of lip.

BRS: Recurrent terminal. SEE: *cranial nerves*.
trochlearis (trō-klē-ā'rĭs) [L.]. Sup. oblique muscle of the eye. SEE: *Muscles, Table of, in Appendix*.
trochocardia (trō"kō-kar'dĭ-ă) [G. *trochos*, a wheel, + *kardia*, heart]. Rotary displacement of the heart on its axis.
trochocephalia, trochocephaly (trō"kō-se-fā'lĭ-ă, -sĕf'ă-lĭ) [" + *kephalē*, head]. Roundheadedness, a deformity due to premature union of frontal and parietal bones.
trochoid (trō'koyd) [" + *eidos*, resemblance]. Rotating or revolving, noting an articulation.
trochoides (trō-koy'dēz) [G. *trochoeidēs*, wheellike]. A pivot or rotary joint.
trombidiiasis, trombidiosis (trŏm-bĭ-dī-ī'ă-sĭs, -bĭd-ĭ-ō'sĭs). Infestation with the *Trombidium irritans*.
Trombidium (trŏm-bĭd'ĭ-ŭm) [L.]. A genus of red mites, some of which attack man.
  T. irritans. The harvest mite which is a semiparasite.
Trommer's test (trŏm'er). Test for sugar in the urine.
tromomania (trŏm"ō-mā'nĭ-ă) [G. *tromos*, a trembling, + *mania*, madness]. Delirium tremens.
tropesis (trō-pē'sĭs) [G. *tropē*, a turning]. An inclination to action possessed by all substances.
troph-, tropho- [G.]. Combining forms meaning *nourishment*.
trophedema (trō-fē-dē'mă) [G. *trophē*, nourishment, + *oidēma*, a swelling]. A permanent, localized edema of the extremities.
trophema (trō-fē'mă) [" + *aima*, blood]. Nutrient blood of the uterine mucosa.
trophesy (trof'ĕ-sĭ) [G. *trophē*, nourishment]. Deficient nutrition of a part from failure of nerve regulating nutrition. SYN: *trophoneurosis*.
trophic (trŏf'ĭk) [G. *trophē*, nourishment]. Concerned with nourishment.
  Applied particularly to a type of efferent nerves believed to control the growth and nourishment of the parts they innervate. SEE: *autotrophic*.
  t. center. One of the centers of the sympathetic system whence the nutrition of nerve fiber is supposed to be controlled.
  t. nerve. One regulating nutritive functions of a part.
  t. neurosis. Disorder due to injury of the trophic nerves of a part. SYN: *trophoneurosis*.
trophoblast (trŏf'ō-blăst) [G. *trophē*, nourishment, + *blastos*, germ]. The outer epiblastic layer that establishes relations with the uterus and is supposedly concerned with nutrition.
trophoblastoma (trof"ō-blăs-tō'mă) [" + *-ōma*, tumor]. A neoplasm due to excessive proliferation of chorionic epithelium. SYN: *chorioepithelioma*.
trophoderm (trŏf'ō-derm) [" + *derma*, skin]. A layer of cells on the ext. surface of the ectoderm of the blastodermic vesicle which brings about ovular implantation in the uterus and nourishment.
trophology (tro-fŏl'ō-jĭ) [" + *logos*, a science]. The science of nutrition.
trophoneurosis (trŏf"ō-nū-rō'sĭs) [" + *neuron*, nerve, + *-ōsis*, condition]. Any trophic disorder due to defective function of the nerves concerned with nutrition of the part.
  t., disseminated. Thickening and hardening of the skin. SYN: *sclerema*, *scleroderma*.

trophoneurosis, facial T-53 **trypsinogen**

t., facial. Progressive facial atrophy.
t., muscular. Muscular changes in connection with nervous disorders.
trophoneurotic (trŏf″ō-nū-rŏt′ĭk) [" + *neuron*, nerve]. Relating to a trophoneurosis.
trophonosis (trŏf″ō-nō′sĭs) [" + *nosos*, disease]. Any disease of metabolism or nutrition, or condition resulting from them.
trophonucleus (trŏf″ō-nū′klē-ŭs) [G. *trophē*, nourishment, + L. *nucleus*, kernel]. Protozoan nucleus concerned with vegetative functions in metabolism and not reproduction. SYN: *macronucleus*.
trophopathia, trophopathy (trŏf″ō-path′-ĭ-ă, trof-op′ă-thĭ) [" + *pathos*, disease]. 1. Any disorder of the nutrition. 2. A trophic disease.
trophoplast (trŏf′ō-plăst) [" + *plassein*, to form]. A granular body of specialized protoplasm in a cell. SYN: *plastid*.
trophospongia (trŏf″ō-spŭn′jĭ-ă) [" + *spoggia*, sponge]. 1. A deeply staining, delicate, intracellular network of certain cells which is probably instrumental in nutritive circulation. 2. The outer layer of the trophoblast which is a vascular, spongy, mucous membrane.
trophotaxis (trŏf″ō-tăks′ĭs) [" + *taxis*, arrangement]. The adaptation or selectivity and repulsion to nutrients by organic cells. SYN: *trophotropism*.
trophotherapy (trŏf″ō-ther′ă-pĭ) [" + *therapeia*, treatment]. The therapeutic use of foods. SYN: *dietotherapy*.
trophotonos (trŏf-ŏt′ŏn-ŏs) [" + *tonos*, tension]. A rigid state of contractile tissue resulting from trophic disorder.
trophotropism (trŏf-ot′rō-pĭzm) [G. *trophē*, nourishment, + *tropē*, a turning, + *-ismos*, condition]. Attraction and repulsion of cells to nutritive substances. SYN: *trophotaxis*.
trophozoite (trŏf″ō-zō′ĭt) [" + *zōon*, animal]. A sporozoan nourished by its host during its growth stage.
tropical (trŏp′ĭ-kăl) [G. *tropikos*, turning]. Pert. to the tropics.
t. anemia. A., or merely pallor without blood changes, in northerners traveling in the tropics.
t. lichen. Prickly heat, acute inflammation of the sweat glands.
tropism (trō′pĭzm) [G. *tropē*, a turn, + *-ismos*, condition]. Reaction of living organisms involuntarily toward or away from light, darkness, heat, cold, or other stimuli.
tropistic action (trō-pĭs′tĭk) [G. *tropē*, a turn]. Directional response of an organism to certain ext. influences. SYN: *tropism*.
t. a., chemio-. Influence of chemicals on the organism.
tropometer (trŏp-om′ĕ-ter) [G. *tropē*, a turn, + *metron*, a measure]. 1. Device for measuring the rotation of the eyeballs. 2. Instrument for measuring torsion in long bones.
Trousseau's disease (trū-sō′). 1. Generalized hypertrophy of lymphatic glands. 2. Gastric vertigo.
T's. spots. Streaking of the skin with the fingernail, seen in meningitis and other cerebral diseases. SYN: *meningitic streak*.
T's. symptom. Spasmodic muscular contractions indicative of tetany, on pressing the principle vessel and nerve of the limb.
troy weight (troi). A system of weighing gold, silver, precious metals, and jewels, and in making philosophical experiments. 5,760 gr. equal 1 lb.

24 grains (gr.) equal.....1 pennyweight
20 pennyweights equal.....1 ounce (oz.)
12 oz. equal................1 pound (lb.)
RS: *apothecaries, avoirdupois, household measures, metric system in Appendix*.
true (trū) [A.S. *trēowe*, faithful]. Not false; real; genuine.
t. pelvis. Portion below the iliopectineal line.
t. ribs. The 7 upper ones on each side with cartilages articulating directly with the sternum. SYN: *costa vera*. SEE: *ribs*.
truncal (trŭng′kăl) [L. *truncus*, trunk]. Relating to the trunk.
truncate (trŭng′kăt) [L. *truncāre*, to cut off]. 1. Cut across at right angles to the long axis. 2. To cut off; to amputate.
trunk (trŭnk) [L. *truncus*, trunk]. 1. The body exclusive of the head and limbs. SYN: *torso*. 2. Main stem of a lymphatic, nerve, or blood vessel.
truss (trŭs) [O.Fr. *trousser*, to bundle]. Device for holding a hernia in its place.
trypanocide, trypanocidal (trĭp′ăn-ō-sīd, trĭp″ăn-ō-sī′dăl) [G. *trypanon*, a borer, + L. *cidus*, from *caedere*, to kill]. 1. Destructive to trypanosomes. 2. An agent which kills trypanosomes. SYN: *trypanosomicide*.
trypanolysis (trĭp-an-ŏl′ĭ-sĭs) [" + *lysis*, dissolution]. The dissolution of trypanosomes.
Trypanoplasmia (trĭ″păn-ō-plăz′mă) [" + *plasma*, a thing formed]. A genus of protozoan parasites resembling trypanosomes.
Trypanosoma (trĭ″păn-ō-sō′mă) [G. *trypanon*, a borer, + *sōma*, a body]. A genus of parasite, flagellate protozoa found in the blood.
T. bru′cei. The cause of tsetse fly disease.
T. gambien′se. The parasite of sleeping sickness.
trypanosomal (trĭp-ăn-ō-sō′măl) [" + *sōma*, body]. Pert. to trypanosomata.
trypanosome (trĭ′pan-ō-sōm). Any protozoan of the Trypanosoma genus.
t. fever. Sleeping sickness.
trypanosomiasis (tri-pan-o-sō-mī′ă-sĭs) [" + " + *-iasis*, infection]. A disease caused by trypanosomes.
trypanosomic (trĭ-păn-ō-sō′mĭk) [" + *sōma*, body]. Pert. to trypanosomes.
trypanosomicide (trĭ-păn-ō-sō′mĭ-sīd) [" + " + L. *cidus*, from *caedere*, to kill]. Destructive to trypanosomes.
trypanosomid(e (trĭ-pan′ō-sō-mĭd) [" + *sōma*, body]. A skin eruption in any disease caused by a trypanosome.
tryparsamide (trĭp-ars′ă-mĭd, -mĭd). An arsenic compound containing about 25% arsenic. [sleeping sickness.
USES: Chiefly in neurosyphilis and
DOSAGE: 15-45 gr. (1-3 Gm.) intravenously preferably.
trypesis (trĭp-ē′sĭs) [G. *trypēsis*, a boring]. An incision of the skull to reduce pressure by removing a disk of bone. SYN: *trephining*.
trypsin (trĭp′sĭn) [G. *tripsis*, a rubbing]. A proteolytic ferment of pancreatic fluid. The digestive products of trypsin are *proteoses, peptones, peptides, polypeptides,* and *amino acids*. It is derived from tripsinogen of the pancreatic juice. SEE: *enzyme, pancreas*.
DOSAGE: Intracut., 3-10 ɱ (0.2-0.6 cc.).
trypsinized (trĭp′sĭ-nīzd) [G. *tripsis*, a rubbing]. Subjected to action of trypsin, thus having antitryptic power abolished.
trypsinogen (trĭp-sĭn′ō-jĕn) [" + *gennan*, to produce]. The proenzyme, or inactive

tryptic   T-54   **tuberculin**

form of trypsin found in pancreatic juice, believed to be activated when mixed in the intestine with the enterokinase of the *succus entericus*.

tryptic (trĭp'tĭk) [G. *tripsis*, a rubbing]. Relating to trypsin.

tryptolysis (trĭp-tŏl'ĭ-sĭs) [" + *lysis*, dissolution]. The splitting up of tryptone.

tryptone (trĭp'tōn) [G. *tryptōn*, a rubbing]. Peptone formed by action of trypsin.

tryptonemia (trĭp″tō-nē'mĭ-ă) [" + *aima*, blood]. Tryptones in the blood.

tryptophan(e (trĭp'tō-făn). An amino acid in proteins needed for tissue repair and growth; a product of tryptic digestion.

  t. test. One to determine presence of tryptophan in gastric juice, the presence of which indicates cancer.

tryptophanuria (trĭp-tō-fă-nū'rĭ-ă) [*tryptophan* + G. *ouron*, urine]. Tryptophan in the urine.

tsetse fly (tsĕt'sē) [South African]. One that carries the infective protozoan of trypanosomiasis.

tub (tŭb) [Middle Dutch *tubbe*]. 1. A receptacle for bathing. 2. The use of the cold bath. 3. To treat by using a cold bath.

tubal (tū'băl) [L. *tuba*, tube]. Pert. to a tube, esp. the fallopian tube.

  t. nephritis. Inflammation of kidney tubules.

  t. pregnancy. Pregnancy in one of the oviducts.

tubatorsion (tū″bă-tor'shŭn) [" + *torsio*, a twisting]. The twisting of an oviduct.

tube (tūb) [L. *tuba*, a tube]. A long, hollow, cylindrical structure.

  t., cathode-ray. A vacuum tube with a thin window at the end opposite the cathode to allow the cathode rays to pass outside. More generally, any discharge tube in which the vacuum is fairly high.

  t., Coolidge. A kind of hot cathode tube, which is so highly exhausted that the residual gas plays no part in the production of the cathode stream, and which is regulated by variable heating of the cathode filament.

  t., Crookes'. One with an exhausted vacuum, used in obtaining roentgen rays.

  t., drainage. A glass or rubber tube which, when inserted into a cavity, drains away its fluid contents.

  t., electric. Hollow glass or metal receptacles wired for electricity.

  t., esophageal. Same as *stomach t.*

  t., eustachian. The tube passing from the throat to the middle ear.

  t., fallopian. One of 2 oviducts.

  t., hot-cathode. A vacuum tube in which the cathode is electrically heated to incandescence and in which the supply of electrons depends on the temperature of the cathode.

  t., h.-c. roentgen-ray. A vacuum roentgen-ray tube in which the electron stream is supplied by a heated cathode. The cathode stream may be regulated by varying the current through the cathode filament.

  t., intubation. A tube for passing into the larynx to facilitate breathing.

  t., Leonard. SEE: *cathode-ray tube*.

  t., oscillator vacuum. Method of producing alternating current. Current produced by this is a continuous sine wave current in contradistinction to the damped harmonic wave of spark gap diathermy machine.

  t., stomach. A rubber tube, 16 in. in length, for introducing food or other fluid into the stomach.

  t., tracheotomy. A tube for inserting into the trachea.

tube feeding diet. Milk, cream, eggs, glucose, orange juice or tomato juice, strained spinach, vitamin concentrates, other constituents added when ordered.

tuber (tū'ber) (pl. *tubers, tubera*) [L. *tuber*, a swelling]. A swelling or enlargement.

tubercle (tū'ber-kl) [L. *tuberculum*, a little swelling]. 1. The lesion of tuberculosis. 2. Elevation of a bone for the attachment of a ligament or muscle. 3. Large, circumscribed, solid elevation of skin or mucosa from size of a large pea to that of a hazelnut.

  They are seen in erythema nodosum multiformes, lupus vulgaris, syphilis, keloid, neurofibromatosis, tenia sycosis, and leprosy. SEE: *chloroformin*.

  t., adductor. That part of femur to which is attached the tendon of the adductor magnus.

  t. bacillus. Organism causing tuberculosis.

  t., deltoid. One in clavicle for attachment of deltoid muscle.

  t., genial. One on either side of lower jawbone.

  t., genital. The fetal structure that becomes the clitoris, or the penis.

  t., lacrimal. One on upper jawbone.

  t., laminated. The cerebellar nodule.

  t., Lisfranc's. T. for scalenus anticus muscle on the 1st rib.

  t., miliary. A small tubercle resembling a millet seed; the lesion of tuberculosis.

  t., zygomatic. One on the zygoma at junction of ant. root.

tubercular (tū-ber'kū-lar) [L. *tuberculum*, a little swelling]. 1. Relating to or marked by nodules. 2. Incorrectly pert. to tuberculosis. 3. Person with tuberculosis. SEE: *torose*.

  t. syphilide. Cutaneous gummata.

tuberculase (tū-ber'kū-lās) [L. *tuberculum*, a little swelling]. An extract of tubercle bacilli used for immunizing against tuberculosis.

tuberculate, tuberculated (tū-ber'kū-lāt, -lāt″ed) [L. *tuberculum*, a small swelling]. Covered with nodules. SYN: *tubercular*.

tuberculation (tū-ber″kū-lā'shŭn) [L. *tuberculum*, a little swelling]. The formation of tubercles.

tuberculid(e (tū-ber'kū-lĭd, -lĭd) [L. *tuberculum*, a small nodule]. A tuberculous cutaneous eruption due to toxins of tuberculosis.

tuberculigenous (tū-ber-kū-lĭj'ĕn-ŭs) [" + G. *gennan*, to produce]. Causing or predisposing to tuberculosis.

tuberculin (tū-ber'kū-lĭn) [L. *tuberculum*, a little swelling]. A culture of tubercle bacillus to be used for active immunization or for diagnostic purposes in tuberculosis. SEE: *anticutin, antiphthisin, autotuberculin*.

  METHODS: (1) *Subcutaneous Injection*: A small quantity of tuberculin is subcutaneously injected. In tuberculous patients this results in a reaction: (a) A general reaction of fever and malaise; (b) a local reaction of inflammation at the site of injection, and (c) in cases with a focus of disease, a focal reaction also, characterized by increase in the symptoms at the focus of disease; for example, if this be in the lung, by increased cough and sputum; if of a joint, by the signs of inflammation in the joint.

(2) *Ophthalmic Reaction of Calmette*: A drop of a weak solution of tuberculin is placed in the lower conjunctival sac; in tuberculous persons this is followed by conjunctivitis. This test is rarely used, as the inflammation so set up may prove difficult to control.

(3) *Moro's Test*: Ointment containing tuberculin is rubbed into the skin of the forearm, or some other part, simple ointment being rubbed into the skin of the opposite forearm. A positive reaction is shown by signs of inflammation occurring in the test forearm only, within 24 hr. of the inunction.

(4) *Von Pirquet's Test*: The skin of 3 areas on 1 forearm is sterilized. On 1 area a small quantity of tuberculin is placed; on the 2nd area a small quantity of tuberculin, previously heated to destroy the toxin, is similarly placed; the 3rd area is not covered. All 3 areas are then lightly scarified with a sterile instrument. The reaction is considered positive when the inflammatory changes appear only on the area on which unheated tuberculin was placed.

(5) *Mantoux's Test*: This is similar to Von Pirquet's test, see note above, as it is a skin test, but instead of having the tuberculin placed on the skin, in the Mantoux test dilute tuberculin is injected intradermally and, if the reaction is positive, a few hours later redness and swelling appear over the area injected. This test is usually found to give a positive reaction in persons who have lived in crowded cities, but in those who have spent their childhood and adolescence in the country or by the sea in sparsely populated areas it may be found to be negative.—*Pearce.*

t., alkaline. Substance obtained from tubercle bacilli by extracting with 1/10 normal soda solution.

tuberculinization (tū-ber″kū-lĭ-nĭ-zā′shŭn) [L. *tuberculum*, a small nodule]. Treatment or diagnosis with tuberculin.

tuberculinose (tū-ber′kū-lĭn-ōs) [L. *tuberculum*, a small nodule]. A form of tuberculin.

tuberculitis (tū-ber″kū-lī′tĭs) [" + G. -*itis*, inflammation]. Inflammation of any tubercle.

tuberculization (tū-ber″kū-lĭ-zā′shŭn) [L. *tuberculum*, a little swelling]. 1. The formation of tubercles. 2. Therapeutic use of tuberculin. SYN: *tuberculinization*.

tuberculocele (tū-ber′kū-lō-sēl) [" + G. *kēlē*, a mass]. Tuberculosis of a testicle.

tuberculocide (tū-ber′kū-lō-sīd) [" + *cidus*, from *caedere*, to kill]. Destroying tubercle bacilli.

tuberculoderma (tū-ber″kū-lō-der′mă) [" + G. *derma*, skin]. A tuberculous lesion of the skin. SYN: *tuberculide*.

tuberculofibroid (tū-ber″kū-lō-fī′broyd) [" + *fibra*, fiber, + G. *eidos*, form]. Denoting fibroid degeneration of tubercles.

tuberculofibrosis (tū-ber″kū-lō-fī-brō′sĭs) [" + " + G. -*ōsis*, condition]. 1. Chronic pulmonary inflammation with formation of fibrous tissue. 2. Interstitial pneumonia.

tuberculoid (tū-ber′kū-loyd) [" + G. *eidos*, resemblance]. Resembling tuberculosis or a tubercle.

tuberculoidin (tū-ber-kū-loy′dĭn) [" + G. *eidos*, form]. A form of tuberculin treated with alcohol.

tuberculol (tū-ber′kū-lol) [L. *tuberculum*, a little swelling]. Tuberculin which is free from secondary products.

tuberculoma (tū-ber-kū-lō′mă) [" + G. -*ōma*, tumor]. 1. A tuberculous abscess. 2. Any tuberculous neoplasm.

tuberculomania (tū-ber″kū-lō-mā′nĭ-ă) [" + G. *mania*, madness]. Abnormal certainty that one has tuberculosis.

tuberculomucin (tū-ber″kū-lō-mū′sĭn) [" + *mucus*, mucus]. A mucinlike substance prepared from old cultures of tubercle bacilli.

tuberculoöpsonic index (tū-ber″kū-lō-ŏp-sŏn′ĭk) [" + G. *opsōnein*, to prepare food for]. Opsonic index in tuberculous infection.

tuberculophobia (tū-ber″kū-lō-fō′bĭ-ă) [" + G. *phobos*, fear]. An abnormal fear of becoming affected with tuberculosis.

tuberculosis (tū-ber″kū-lō′sĭs) [L. *tuberculum*, a little swelling, + G. -*ōsis*, disease]. An infectious disease marked by the formation of tubercles in any tissue, due to the presence of the tubercle bacillus.

t., acute general. An acute infectious disease excited by the tubercle bacillus, characterized anatomically by the simultaneous formation of miliary tubercles in many parts of the body.

SYM: Debility, loss of flesh and strength; fever, 102° to 104° F., irregular, marked by evening exacerbations and morning remissions; cough; hurried respirations; a brown, fissured tongue; weak, rapid pulse; enlargement of spleen; delirium; stupor. Tubercle bacilli rarely found in expectoration or in the blood. Duration, from 2 to 4 weeks.

When lungs are chiefly affected, there are dyspnea, marked cough, mucopurulent and bloody expectorations, cyanosis, sibilant and subcrepitant râles, and perhaps areas over which bronchial breathing is heard.

When meninges are chiefly affected there are intense headache, convulsive seizures, photophobia, delirium, facial palsies, stupor, coma, and Cheyne-Stokes breathing. Tubercles may be detected on the retina.

When intestines and peritoneum are affected there are pain, tenderness, abdominal distention, and diarrhea.

PROG: Generally fatal.

TREATMENT: Palliative. Diet of milk, eggs and broth. Stimulants are indicated; control high fever by applications of cold. Remedies to suit special form of case.

t. cutis. Tuberculosis of the skin of various forms marked by warty growths, pustules, and brownish patches. SYN: *scrofuloderma*.

t. c. orificialis. Secondary to tuberculosis of internal organs and attacks integument contiguous to mucous outlet, beginning with yellowish miliary tubercles which break down to form rounded or oval, sluggish, granulating, painless ulcers.

t. c. vulgosa. Patches of soft, "apple-butterlike" tubercles which ultimately undergo absorption but which may break down and ulcerate, healing with more or less scarring. Progresses slowly by formation of more patches. Deformity may be great from scarring and cicatrization.

PROG: Extremely chronic, resistant to treatment, prone to relapse and recur. Cancer may develop in cicatrices.

TREATMENT: Hygienic regimen. Cod-liver oil, arsenic, hypophosfites internally. Tuberculin. Locally, x-rays, radium, helio- and phototherapy. Antiseptics. SYN: *lupus vulgaris*.

t., pulmonary. A specific, inflammatory disease of the lungs, caused by the tubercle bacillus, characterized anatomically by a cellular infiltration, which subsequently caseates, softens and leads to ulceration of lung tissues. Manifested clinically by wasting, exhaustion, fever, and cough.

Acute: Resembles pneumonia and is marked by chill; high fever; rapid pulse; dyspnea; sputum at first rusty, then purulent; flushed face; profuse sweats, and the signs of consolidation. Instead of ending 9th day by crisis, as an ordinary pneumonia, the symptoms grow rapidly worse, signs of softening appear, the sputum shows bacilli and elastic fibers, and death results in a few weeks to months.

Fibroid: A disease of long duration. Gradual loss of strength and abundant mucopurulent expectoration, which is at times fetid from being retained in dilated bronchi. Dyspnea, sweating, and fever are slight. There is marked retraction on affected side from shrinking of the fibrous tissue; with this exception, physical signs are similar to those of *ulcerative t.*

Chronic Ulcerative: SYM: Outset usually insidious and marked by pallor; gastric disturbance; loss of flesh and strength; by a dry, hacking cough, esp. noted in the morning.

From some undue exposure, the cough is aggravated and so to this obstinate "cold" the disease is attributed. In some cases symptoms appear abruptly with hemorrhage or an acute pleurisy. Slight fever and acceleration of pulse are early symptoms of great diagnostic import. Temperature marked by evening exacerbation, during which face is flushed, eyes bright, mind animated. Later, cough becomes troublesome, expectoration more abundant.

In well developed cases expectoration is greenish in color, is in coin-shaped plugs, is heavy and sinks in water, is often blood-streaked and contains bacilli and fibers of elastic tissue.

Tuberculosis in itself is not a painful disease, but the associated dry pleurisy causes much suffering. Hemoptysis occurs at all stages, but profuse hemorrhages occur late. Blood is bright red, frothy, and mixed with mucus. Profuse sweating troublesome in advanced cases. Final stage characterized by extreme emaciation, weakness, pallor, high remittent or intermittent fever, and edema of feet. Mind clear and hopeful to the end.

INSPECTION: Chest usually long and flat; spaces above and below clavicles are sunken; scapular prominent; ribs oblique. May be flattening or less expansion over one apex.

PALPATION: Diminished expansion and increased vocal fremitus.

PERCUSSION: Dullness as a rule; noted earliest above or below clavicles, in supraspinous fossae, bet. the scapulae, or in front near sternal border. A cavity yields tympany or a "cracked pot" resonance.

AUSCULTATION: In early stage respiration may be inaudible over affected area. Later, breathing harsh, expiration prolonged, high pitched. Vocal resonance increased. Cracking râles are usually audible and are so produced by liquid in small tubes. If not present, coughing will usually develop then. Over large cavities may detect cavernous or amphoric breathing. Pectoriloquy and large, gurgling râles.

PROG: Guarded.

TREATMENT: Preventive. Sputa of consumptives should be received in suitable vessels, containing antiseptic solutions and subsequently be destroyed. Tuberculous mothers should not nurse their children. The healthy should not sleep in apartments occupied by those affected. Streptomycin, artificial pneumothorax, phrenicotomy, thoracoplasty when indicated.

PERSONAL HYGIENE: Good food; fresh air; frequent bathing; avoidance of exposure; graduated exercise; residence in an elevated locality; a dry, well-ventilated house; plenty of sleep and recreation. Abundance of fresh air, simple living, and sleeping out of doors where possible. Warm clothing, protection overhead from storms. Some regulated exercise. Constitutional remedies.

DIET: No forced or overfeeding. Protein, 1 to 1.5 Gm. for kg. of normal body weight with from 35 to 40 Calories per kg. of normal body weight for bed patients, and from 40 to 45 for moderately active patients. Fats, carbohydrates, minerals, and vitamins. Little cellulose if digestive tract is affected. If patient is weak, bland foods and semisolids. Daily allowance: Milk, 3 to 5 pt., with or bet. meals; meat, 3 to 6 oz.; bacon, 1 to 2 oz.; eggs, 1 to 2; butter, 1 to 2½ oz.; bread, 8 to 12 oz.; sugar, 1 to 3 oz.; potatoes, 3 to 4 oz.; fresh vegetables, 2 to 3 oz.; milk-pudding, 5 oz.; cream, 3 oz. Liver should be included frequently. Green, leafy vegetables should be used regularly, and ripe fruit.

RS: *antitulase, atylosis, carreau, phthisis, scrofula, spes phthisica, tuberculin.*

tuberculotherapy (tū-ber″kū-lō-ther′ă-pĭ) [L. *tuberculum*, a little swelling, + G. *therapeia*, treatment]. The treatment of tuberculosis, esp. with meat of cattle affected with tuberculosis in an attempt at immunization.

tuberculotoxoidin (tū-ber″kū-lō-tŏks-oy′-dĭn) [" + G. *toxikon*, poison, + *eidos*, form]. A preparation of nontoxic, immunizing tubercle bacilli.

tuberculotropic (tū-ber″kū-lō-trop′ĭk) [" + G. *tropē*, a turning]. Combining with tubercle bacilli.

tuberculous (tū-ber′kū-lŭs) [L. *tuberculum*, a little swelling]. Relating to or affected with tuberculosis, or conditions marked by infiltration of a specific tubercle, as opposed to the term tubercular, referring to nonspecific tubercle.

tuberculum (tū-ber′kū-lŭm) (pl. *tubercula*) [L. a little swelling]. A small knot or nodule.

t. acus′ticum. Dorsal nucleus of the cochlear nerve.

t. ma′jus hu′meri. BNA. Larger tuberosity of the humerus at upper end of its lateral surface giving attachment to infraspinatus, supraspinatus, and teres minor muscles.

t. mi′nus hu′meri. BNA. The projection at proximal end of humerus' ant. surface giving attachment to subscapularis muscle.

tuberin (tu′ber-ĭn) [L. *tuber*, a swelling]. A simple protein; a globulin in potatoes.

tuberositas (tū-ber-ŏs′ĭt-ăs) (pl. *tuberositates*) [L. a nodule]. A projection, nodule, or prominence.

tuberosity (tū-ber-ŏs′ĭ-tĭ) [L. *tuberositas*, tuberosity]. 1. An elevated round process of a bone. 2. A tubercle or nodule.

tuberous (tū'ber-ŭs) [L. *tuber*, a swelling]. Resembling a nodular or knotty mass.
   t. root. A thickened primary root. Ex: *aconite, jalap*.
   t. sclero'sis. A localized or diffuse fibrosis of the brain often associated with grave mental deterioration and epilepsy, showing adenoma sebaceum, esp. about the face, and often tumors elsewhere in the body, notably the kidneys and viscera. SEE: *sclerosis*.

tubo- [L.]. Combining form meaning *tube*.

tuboabdominal (tū″bō-ăb-dŏm'ĭn-ăl) [L. *tuba*, tube, + *abdominalis*, pert. to the abdomen]. Pert. to the fallopian tubes and the abdomen.
   t. pregnancy. Ectopic gestation with embryo partly in tube and partly in the abdominal cavity.

tuboligamentus (tū″bō-lĭg-ă-měn'tŭs) [" + *ligamentum*, a band]. Pert. to the fallopian tube and broad ligament of the uterus.

tuboövarian (tū″bō-ō-vā'rĭ-ăn) [" + *ovarium*, egg holder]. Pert. to the fallopian tube and the ovary.

tuboövariotomy (tū″bō-ō-vā-rĭ-ŏt'ō-mĭ) [" + " + G. *tomē*, a cutting]. Excision of ovaries and oviducts. SYN: *salpingoöthecotomy*.

tuboperitoneal (tū″bō-pěr-ĭ-tō-nē'ăl) [" + G. *peritonaion*, peritoneum]. Relating to the oviduct and peritoneum.

tuborrhea (tū-bor-rē'ă) [" + G. *rhoia*, a flow]. Discharge from the eustachian tube.

tubotympanal (tū″bō-tĭm'pă-năl) [" + G. *tympanon*, a drum]. Relating to the tympanum of the ear and the eustachian tube.

tubouterine (tū″bō-ū'těr-ĭn) [" + *uterinus*, pert. to the uterus]. Relating to the oviduct and the uterus.

tubular (tū'bū-lar) [L. *tubularis*, like a tube]. Relating to or having the form of a tube or tubule.
   t. breathing. Bronchial breathing.
   t. gestation. Ectopic pregnancy in the fallopian tube.
   t. membrane. Connective tissue sheath of a primary bundle of nerve fibers or of a funiculus. SYN: *perineurium*.

tubule (tū'būl) [L. *tubulus*, a tubule]. A small tube or canal.
   t., collecting. T. in renal medulla which is part of the discharging tubule.
   t., excretory. The uriniferous tubules in medullary portion of kidneys.
   t., junctional. Short part of a uriniferous t. connecting with a collecting t.
   t's., seminal. Epithelial lined tubes (1/150-1/200 in. in diam.) forming the major portion of the testis.
   t., uriniferous. Minute canals forming the glandular substance of the kidney, originating in Bowman's capsules and emptying into pelvis of kidney.

tubulodermoid (tū″bū-lō-der'moyd) [L. *tubulus*, tubule, + G. *derma*, skin, + *eidos*, form]. A dermoid tumor due to the persistent embryonic tubular structure.

tubulus (tū'bū-lŭs) (pl. *tubuli*) [L. a tubule]. A tubule; a small tube.

Tuffnell's method (tŭf'něl). The treatment of int. aneurysm by low diet, with little liquid, rest, and potassium iodide.

tug'ging. A dragging or pulling.
   t., tracheal. An indication of thoracic aneurysm.
   SYM: A sense of downward pulling of larynx with cardiac systole when thyroid cartilage is gently raised bet. the finger and thumb.

tularemia (too-lăr-ē'mĭ-ă) [*Tularé*, part of California where disease was first discovered, + G. *aima*, blood]. Deer fly fever transmitted to man from rodents and rabbits bitten by a blood-sucking insect infected with *Pasteurella tularensis* or by direct contact.
   SYM: Three days after infection headache, chilliness, vomiting, aching pains, and fever. Site of infection develops into an ulcer. Glands at elbow or in armpit become enlarged, tender, and painful; later may develop into an abscess. Sweating, loss of weight, and debility.

tulase (tū'lās). Von Behring's tuberculin for treatment of tuberculosis.

tumefacient (tū-mē-fā'shĕnt) [L. *tumefaciens*, producing swelling]. Producing or tending to produce swelling; swollen.

tumefaction (tū″mē-făk'shŭn) [L. *tumefactio*, a swelling]. 1. A swelling. 2. Act of swelling or the state of being swollen.

tumor (tū'mor) [L. *tumor*, a swelling]. 1. A swelling or enlargement. 2. A neoplasm, abnormal prominence of a part not due to inflammation with no physiological function.
   TYPES OF TUMORS: *Myeloid Sarcomata, Giant Celled S*: Consist of elements formed chiefly of protoplasm containing 2 or more nuclei, up to 20 or even 50; with a varying number of round, spindle, or mixed cells. Vary in consistence from that of jelly to that of muscle. More frequently occurs on lower jaw, femur, and tibia.
   Round Celled Sarcomata: Usually soft, vascular, rapidly growing, become large, and early give rise to metastatic deposits in distant parts and in viscera. Occur in periosteum, bone, lymphatic glands, subcutaneous tissue, testicle, eye, ovary, uterus, lung, kidneys; though may occur wherever fibrous tissue exists.
   Glioma: Grows from the connective tissue of nerve centers and its basic substance resembles that structure. Occurs in retina and brain.
   Melanotic Sarcoma: In which cells may be either of round or spindle variety. Is the most malignant form.
   Spindle-cell Sarcoma: Cells vary much in size, from small oat-shaped cells to greatly elongated bodies with long, fine, tapering extremities. Chiefly in bones.
   Endotheliomata: Attack in different forms the testicle, pia mater, pleura, and peritoneum.
   Acinous or Spheroidal-celled Carcinoma: (1) Hard, spheroidal-celled (scirrhus or chronic c.). SEE: *scirrhus*. (2) Soft, spheroidal celled (encephaloid, or acute c.); resembles brain tissue in appearance and consistence. Occurs in testicle, liver, bladder, kidney, ovary, fundus oculi, more rarely in the breast.
   Colloid Carcinoma: Really one of preceding varieties which has undergone mucoid degeneration, and so distended the alveoli they may be seen by naked eye. Occurs in stomach, intestine, omentum, ovary.
   Epithelial Carcinoma: (1) The squamous-celled epitheliomata which always spring from skin or mucous membranes, or their glands, esp. at junctions of mucous and cutaneous surfaces. Are not encapsulated. Commence as wart-like growth, flattened tubercle, or fissure, ulceration in all these forms setting in early. (2) Cylindrical or columnar-celled. Less common form of carcinoma. Originates from either the cylindrical surface epithelium of a mu-

cous membrane, or of its glands, closely imitating these structures in microscopic appearance. These growths form indurated, infiltrating masses in the walls of organs attacked, producing considerable stenosis of lumen, of hollow viscera; as rectum and small intestinal obstruction. Occur in uterus and intestinal tract. (3) Tumors composed of epiblastic, hypoblastic, and mesoblastic elements.

Warty or Villous Growth (Papillomata): Resemble in their structure hypertrophied papillae of skin—or mucous membrane. These include condylomata and mucous tubercles. Occur about anus and genitals, or in mouth and throat. Warts and warty growths on skin of hands and genitalia, and mucous surface of larynx. Villous growths, bladder, rectum, and larynx.

Teratoma: Tumors containing bone, hair, teeth, etc., situated in ovaries or testicles.

t., connective tissue (chondroma). Composed of some variety of connective tissue, forming hard, elastic, slowly growing tumors, often nodular or lobulated. Occurs on bones, salivary glands, testicle, etc.

t., fatty (lipoma). Consists of adipose tissue, identical with normal fat. Innocent—grows slowly. May reach large size. Adults—do not recur after removal. Occur on shoulders, back, nates. Diffuse form, under chin.

t., fibrous (fibroma). Consisting of fibrous tissue. May be dense and firm as a tendon, or soft as areola tissue. Innocent—commonly possess distinct capsule. May occur wherever fibrous tissue is found in any of its forms.

t., glandular (adenoma). Innocent growths originate only from preëxisting glandular tissue which they imitate. Two forms: Acinous and tubular. Do not infiltrate the connective tissue. Acinous occur in mammae, lip, ovary, testes, prostate, thyroid, parotid, lacrimal gland, cutaneous and sebaceous glands. Tubular, in intestine, esp. in rectum.

t., lymphatic (vessel) (lymphangioma). Lymphatic vessels are subject to dilatations and varicosities of every degree and extent. To such dilatations in general the term lymphangiectasis is applied, but when by their size, confluence and aggregation they form tumors the term lymphangiomata may be substituted. Occurs on inside of thigh, genitals, ant. wall of abdomen.

t., mucous (myxomata). Resemble the whartonian jelly of the umbilical cord and vitreous humor of the eye. Grows slowly; large size; innocent, not returning if completely removed. Mucoid softening may attack other forms of tumors. Occurs most frequently in nasal cavities, mammary gland, intermuscular spaces, and submucous and subserous spaces.

t., muscular (myomata). Only those of congenital origin are composed of striated muscle elements (rhabdomyoma), but even in these, the bulk of tumor not composed of muscle cells — new growths made up in part of smooth, nonstriated muscle cells. Occurs in uterus and in prostate, in combination with fibromata.

Classification of Tumors

Benign	Malignant
Generally encapsulated (not invasive). Slow growing. Do not metastasize. Do not interfere with health.	Not encapsulated (invasive). Rapidly growing. Metastasize. Detrimental to health and life.

I. Connective Tissue Tumors
A. *Benign*:
   (a) Fibroma, composed of fibrous tissue.
   (b) Chondroma, composed of cartilage.
   (c) Osteoma, composed of bone.
   (d) Lipoma, composed of fat.
B. *Malignant*:
   Sarcoma, a cellular tumor composed of any connective tissue cells in disorderly arrangement.

II. Muscle Tissue Tumors
Benign:
   Myoma, composed of smooth muscle tissue.

III. Epithelial Tumors
A. *Benign*:
   (a) Papilloma, composed of surface epithelium.
   (b) Adenoma, composed of glandular epithelium.
B. *Malignant*:
   (a) Epithelioma, composed of squamous epithelial cells in disorderly arrangement.
   (b) Carcinoma, composed of glandular epithelial cells in disorderly arrangement.

IV. Endothelial Tumors
A. *Benign*:
   (a) Hemangioma, composed of blood vessels.
   (b) Lymphangioma, composed of lymph vessels.
B. *Malignant*:
   Endothelioma, composed of endothelial cells in disorderly arrangement.

V. Pigmented Tumors
A. *Benign*:
   Nevus, a pigmented mole.
B. *Malignant*:
   Melanoma, pigmented tumor derived from moles.

t., nerve (neuromata). True neuromata other than the bulbous ends of cut nerves, made up of nerve fibers themselves, are rare. Usually made up of amyelenic fibers, *i. e.*, fibers that have no myelin within the sheath.
t., osseous (osteomata). Formed of true bone—almost solely of either cancellous or compact bone. Occurs on tibia, fibula, humerus, great toe, cranial and nasal sinuses. Compact form grows from cranium; great density, scarcely be cut by any instrument.
t., vascular (angiomata). Neoplasms composed of blood vessels, either arteries, veins, or capillaries, or in which blood is contained in cavernous spaces, not true blood vessels. Angiomata of nose are rare—must be distinguished from simple varicose condition of mucous membrane which is common. Occurs mostly in males during adolescence. Epistaxis frequent, profuse, and persistent. SEE: *nevus* and *varix*.
tumor, words pert. to: angiofibroma; angiolipoma; argentaffinoma; astroblastoma; astrocytoma; calor; carcinosarcoma; celioma; celioncus; cementoma; cephalematocele; ceroma; cholangioma; chondroangioma; chondrofibroma; chondrolipoma; chondrosarcoma; chorioadenoma; chorioangioma; chorioepithelioma; choristoma; chromaffinoma; chylangioma; dolor; "-oma" and "-oncus," words ending in; rubor; swelling; tumefaction.
tumoraffin (tū'mor-ăf-ĭn) [L. *tumor*, a swelling, + *affinis*, related]. Having an affinity for tumor cells. SYN: *oncotropic*.
tumultus (tū-mŭl'tŭs) [L.]. Over or disturbed action.
t. cordis. Irregular heart action with palpitation.
t. sermo'nis. Extreme stuttering due to pathologic cause.
tuna fish (tū'nă). Pro. 26.6. Fat 11.4. FUEL VALUE: 100 Gm. equal 208 Cal.
tungsten arc (tŭng'stĕn). Lamp with tungsten electrodes for production of ultraviolet radiation. SEE: *lamp, tungsten*.
tunic (tū'nĭk) [L. *tunica*, a sheath]. An investing membrane.
tunica (tū'nĭ-kă) (pl. *tunicae*) [L. *tunica*, a sheath]. An enveloping or covering membrane.
t. adnata. The conjunctival lining of the eyeball.
t. adventitia. BNA. Outer coat of an artery or any tubular structure.
t. albuginea. The white fibrous coat of the eye, testicle, ovary, or spleen.
t. externa. Outer coat of an artery.
t. interna. SEE: *t. intima*.
t. intima. Lining coat of an artery.
t. media. Middle muscular coat of an artery.
t. propria. BNA. Deep portion of the corium containing blood vessels, nerves, glands, and hair follicles.
t. vaginalis. Serous lining of the testicles.
tunnel anemia (tŭn'ĕl). A disease due to ankylostoma, and resembling idiopathic anemia.
t. disease. Paralytic and apoplectic symptoms in those working under high atmospheric pressure. SYN: *caisson disease*.
turbidimeter (tŭr-bĭ-dĭm'ĕ-ter) [L. *turbidus*, disturbed, + G. *metron*, a measure]. Device for estimating degree of turbidity of a fluid.
turbidimetry (tŭr-bĭ-dĭm'ĕ-trĭ) [" + G. *metron*, a measure]. Estimation of the turbidity of a liquid.

turbidity (tŭr-bĭd'ĭ-tĭ) [L. *turbiditas*, turbidity]. 1. BACT: Quality of not having translucent appearance of liquid due to growth of microörganisms. 2. Having flaky or granular particles suspended in a clear liquid giving it a cloudy appearance. SEE: *clarificant*.
turbinal (tŭr'bĭ-năl) [L. *turbō, turbin-*, a whirl]. 1. Spiral; scroll-like. 2. A turbinated bone; any 1 of the 3 bones situated in the lateral wall of the nose. *Inferior, middle,* and *superior* turbinates.
turbinated (tŭr'bĭ-nā"tĕd) [L. *turbō, turbin-*, a whirl]. Top- or cone-shaped.
t. bones. The 3 spiral, bony projections upon the outer walls of each nasal fossa.
turbinectomy (tŭr-bĭn-ĕk'tō-mĭ) [" + G. *ektomē*, excision]. Excision of a turbinated bone.
NP: Patient in a sitting position. Ice packs may be ordered.
turbinotome (tŭr-bĭn'ō-tōm) [" + G. *tomē*, a cutting]. Instrument for excision of a turbinated bone.
turbinotomy (tŭr-bĭn-ŏt'ō-mĭ) [" + G. *tomē*, incision]. Surgical incision of a turbinated bone.
Türck's zone (turk). One in intestinal wall in which microörganisms penetrating from the lumen are destroyed.
turgescence (tur-jĕs'ĕns) [L. *turgescens*, swelling]. Swelling or enlargement of a part.
turgescent (tur-jĕs'ĕnt) [L. *turgescens*, swelling]. Swelling; inflated.
turgid (tur'jĭd) [L. *turgidus*, swollen]. Swollen; bloated.
turgor (tur'gor) [L. *turgor*, a swelling]. 1. Normal tension in a cell. 2. Distention, swelling.
t. vita'lis. Normal fullness of the capillaries and blood vessels.
tur'key. AV. SERVING: 230 Gm. Pro. 48.5, Fat 52.7, Carbo. 0.0.
VITAMINS: A— to +, B+.
FUEL VALUE: 100 Gm. equal 294 Cal.
turning (turn'ĭng) [A.S. *turnian*, to turn]. Process of manually changing position of fetus in utero to permit normal delivery. SYN: *version*.
tur'nip (yellow and tops or greens). COMP: Their carbohydrates are in the form of sugar but no starch.
(Second set of figures for *greens*.)
AV. SERVING: 120-100 Gm. Pro. 1.6-2.9, Fat 0.2-0.4, Carbo. 7.3-5.4.
VITAMINS: A— to +—, A+++, B both++, C both+++.
ASH CONST: Ca 0.064-0.347, Mg 0.017-0.028, K 0.338-0.307, Na 0.056-0.082, P 0.046-0.049, Cl 0.041-0.168, S 0.065-0.069, Fe 0.005-0.
A base-forming food; alkaline potentiality, 2.7 cc. per 100 Gm., 6.8 cc. per 100 Cal.
ACTION: Slightly stimulating and flatulent.
TIME FOR DIGESTION: Boiled, 4 hr.
turpentine (tur'pĕn-tĭn) [G. *terebinthos*, turpentine tree]. Oleoresin obtained from the pine tree.
A mixture of terpenes and other hydrocarbons obtained from pine trees used externally in liniments and counter irritants; by mouth as an anthelmintic. The source of oil of turpentine or "spirits of turpentine."
ACTION AND USES: Antiseptic, anthelmintic, and diuretic.
DOSAGE: Internally, of the rectified oil, 5 minims (0.3 cc.).
POISONING: May occur from inhalation.

SYM: Warm or burning sensation in the gullet and stomach, followed by cramping, vomiting, and diarrhea. Pulse and respiration become weak, slow, and irregular; irritation of urinary tract and central nervous system resembling alcoholic intoxication.
  F. A. TREATMENT: Gastric lavage, soothing drinks, and stimulants. Increase fluid intake.

turunda (tu-run'dă) [L.]. 1. A surgical tent, drain, or tampon. 2. A suppository.

tussal (tŭs'ăl) [L. *tussis*, cough]. Relating to a cough. SYN: *tussive*.

tussis (tŭs'ĭs) [L. *tussis*, a cough]. A cough, as bronchial tussis, senile tussis, etc.
  t. convulsi'va. Pertussis* or whooping cough.
  t. stomacha'lis. Reflex cough from irritation of the mucosa of the stomach.

tussive (tŭs'ĭv) [L. *tussis*, cough]. Relating to a cough. SYN: *tussal*.

tutamen (tū-tā'mĕn) (pl. *tutamina*) [L. *tutāmen*, protection]. Any protective structure.
  t. cerebri. The scalp, cranium, and cerebral meninges.
  t. oculi. The eyebrows, eyelids, and eyelashes.

tutocain (tū'tō-kăn). A local anesthetic used both locally and hypodermically.

twelfth cranial nerve. One of a pair of cranial nerves distributing to the base of the tongue. SEE: *hypoglossal nerve*, and *Table of Nerves in Appendix*.

twilight sleep (twī'lĭt slēp). A state of partial anesthesia and hypoconsciousness in which pain sense has been greatly reduced by the injection of morphine and scopolamine.
  Patient responds to pain, but afterward memory of pain is dulled or effaced, as following childbirth. SEE: *labor*.
  t. state. PSY: One in which consciousness is disordered, making possible actions subsequently forgotten.
  Evidenced in hysteria, epilepsy, and dementia precox.

twin (twĭn) [A.S. *twinn*]. One of 2 children developed within the uterus at the same time from the same impregnation. SEE: *Hellin's law*.
  RS: *biovular, dizygotic, enzygotic, fetus papyraceous, identical*.
  t's., dizygotic. Those from 2 separate ova fertilized at the same time.
  t's., identical. Twins of the same sex developed from the same ovum having 2 nuclei, both of which have been impregnated, or resulting from a splitting of the blastodermic vesicle, thus forming two embryos.
  I. twins usually resemble each other so closely that they hardly may be distinguished from each other.

twinge (twĭnj) [A.S. *twengan*, to pinch]. A sudden, keen pain.

twitch (twĭch) [M.E. *twicchen*]. 1. A simple, quick, spasmodic contraction of a muscle. 2. To jerk convulsively. SEE: *myokymia, myopalmus*.

two-four-six enema. An enema with a double portion of the ingredients of the one-two-three enema; often given for flatulence as well as evacuation.

tylion (tĭl'ĭ-ŏn) [G. *tyleion*, knot]. Point at middle of ant. edge of the sulcus chiasmatis.

tyloma (tī-lō'mă) [G. *tylos*, knot, + *-ōma*, tumor]. A callosity.

tylosis (tī-lō'sĭs) [" + *-ōsis*, condition]. 1. A callosity. SYN: *tyloma*. 2. Formation of a callus.

tympanal (tĭm'păn-ăl) [G. *typanon*, drum]. Relating to the tympanum. SYN: *tympanic*.

tympanectomy (tĭm-păn-ĕk'tō-mĭ) [" + *ektomē*, excision]. Excision of the tympanic membrane.

tympanic (tĭm-păn'ĭk) [G. *tympanon*, drum]. 1. Pert. to the tympanum. 2. Resonant.
  t. bone, ring, or **plate.** The wall surrounding the tympanum and supporting t. membrane.
  t. membrane. Membrane closing cavity of the middle ear. SEE: *tympanum*.

tympanism (tĭm'păn-ĭzm) [G. *tympanon*, drum, + *-ismos*, condition]. Abdominal inflation from gas. SYN: *tympanites*.

tympanites (tĭm-păn-ī'tēz) [G. *tympanitēs*, distention]. Gaseous distention of the abdomen.

tympanitic (tĭm-păn-ĭt'ĭk) [G. *tympanitēs*, distention]. 1. Pert. to or characterized by tympanites. 2. Resonant. SYN: *tympanic*.
  t. resonance. A sound produced by percussion over an air- or gas-filled cavity.

tympanitis (tĭm-păn-ī'tĭs) [G. *tympanon*, drum, + *-itis*, inflammation]. Inflammation of the middle ear. SYN: *otitis media*.

tympano- [G.]. Combining form meaning *eardrum, tympanum of the ear*.

tympanohyal (tĭm"păn-ō-hī'ăl) [G. *tympanon*, drum, + *hyoeidēs*, U-shaped]. 1. Pert. to the hyoid arch and the tympanum. 2. A small, fetal cartilage, part of the hyoid arch, which later fuses with the styloid process.

tympanomastoiditis (tĭm"păn-ō-măs-toy-dī'tĭs) [" + *mastos*, breast, + *eidos*, form, + *-itis*, inflammation]. Inflammation of the tympanum and mastoid cells.

tympanotomy (tĭm"păn-ŏt'ō-mĭ) [" + *tomē*, a cutting]. Incision of the membrana tympani. SYN: *myringotomy*.

tympanous (tĭm'păn-ŭs) [G. *tympanon*, a drum]. Marked by abdominal distention with gas.

tympanum (tĭm'păn-ŭm) [G. *tympanon*]. The eardrum; the cavity of the middle ear containing the ossicular chain, *epitympanum, mesotympanum*, and *hypotympanum*.
  RELATIONS: *Roof* (tegmen tympani), middle cranial fossa; *floor*, jugular bulb; *lateral wall*, tympanic membrane; *medial wall*, cochlea and vestibule, facial nerve; *anterior wall*, internal carotid artery—entrance of eustachian tube, tensor tympani muscle; *posterior wall*, antrum, mastoid cells and facial nerve.
  Sometimes incorrectly refers to the tympanic membrane.
  RS: *aerotympanal, attic, atticitis, myringa, myringitis, myringodermatitis, tegmen tympani, tympanic membrane, tympanites, tympany*.

tympany (tĭm'pă-nĭ) [G. *tympanon*, drum]. 1. Abdominal distention with gas. 2. Tympanic resonance on percussion.
  It is a clear hollow note like that of a drum having no vesicular quality. It indicates a pathologic condition of the lung or of a cavity.

type (tīp) [G. *typos*, type]. The general character of a person, a disease, or substance.
  RS: *Aztec, koinotropic, sexual psychopathy, syntonic, syntropic*.
  t., asthenic. One who is slender with

a long chest that is flat and who has poor muscular development.
t., pyknic. One with a rounded body, thick shoulders, large chest, short neck, and broad head.
t., vagotonic. One with deficient adrenal stimulus, slow pulse, low blood pressure, and high sugar tolerance.
t., vesanic. Functional insanity due to no evident external cause.
typembryo (tĭ-pĕm'brĭ-ō) [G. *typos*, type, + *embryon*, embryo]. An embryo in that stage of development when its structural type may be recognized.
typhemia (tī-fē'mĭ-ă) [G. *typhos*, stupor, + *aima*, blood]. Typhoid bacilli in the blood. SYN: *typhoid bacillemia*.
typh fever (tĭf). Name for all low fevers of typhus and typhoid type.
typhinia (tī-fĭn'ĭ-ă) [G. *typhos*, stupor]. Disease marked by recurrent periods of fever, chills, vomiting, and neuromuscular pains. SYN: *relapsing fever*.
typhization (tī-fĭ-zā'shŭn). 1. Typhus or typhoid infection. 2. Inoculation with typhoid vaccine.
typhlatonia, typhlatony (tĭf-lă-tō'nĭ-ă, -lăt'ō-nĭ) [G. *typlon*, cecum, + *tonos*, tone]. Deficient motor activity of the cecum.
typhlectasis (tĭf-lĕk'tă-sĭs) [" + *ektasis*, dilatation]. Cecal distention.
typhlectomy (tĭf-lĕk'tō-mĭ) [" + *ektomē*, excision]. Excision of the cecum. SYN: *cecectomy*.
typhlenteritis (tĭf-lĕn-ter-ī'tĭs) [" + *enteron*, intestine, + *-itis*, inflammation]. Inflammation of the cecum. SYN: *typhlitis*.
typhlitis (tĭf-lī'tĭs) [" + *-itis*, inflammation]. Inflammation of the cecum. Clinically cannot be distinguished from appendicitis. Treatment similar.
typhlodicliditis (tĭf″lō-dĭk-lĭ-dī'tĭs) [" + *diklis*, door, + *-itis*, inflammation]. Inflammation of the ileocecal valve.
typhloempyema (tĭf″lō-ĕm-pī-ē'mă) [" + *en*, in, + *pyon*, pus, + *aima*, blood]. An abdominal abscess following typhlitis.
typhoenteritis (tĭf″lō-ĕn-ter-ī'tĭs) [G. *typhlon*, cecum, + *enteron*, intestine, + *-itis*, inflammation]. Inflammation of the cecum. SYN: *typhlenteritis, typhlitis*.
typhlolexia (tĭf″lō-lĕks'ĭ-ă) [G. *typlos*, blind, + *lexis*, speech]. Inability to recognize written words. SYN: *word blindness*.
typhlology (tĭf-lŏl'ō-jĭ) [" + *logos*, study]. Study of blindness, its causes and effects.
typhlopexy (tĭf'lo-pĕks″ĭ) [G. *typhlon*, cecum, + *pēxis*, fixation]. Suturing of a movable cecum to the abdominal wall.
typhlosis (tĭf-lō'sĭs) [G. *typhlos*, blind, + *-ōsis*, condition]. Blindness.
typhlostenosis (tĭf-lō-stĕn-ō'sĭs) [G. *typhlon*, cecum, + *stenōsis*, a narrowing]. Stenosis or stricture of the cecum.
typhlostomy (tĭf-lŏs'tō-mĭ) [" + *stoma*, opening]. Establishment of a permanent cecal fistula.
typhlotomy (tĭf-lŏt'ō-mĭ) [" + *tomē*, a cutting]. Incision of the cecum.
typhloureterostomy (tĭf″lō-ū-rē″ter-ŏs'tō-mĭ) [" + *ourētēr*, ureter, + *stoma*, opening]. Implantation of a ureter in the cecum.
typho- [G.]. Combining form *pert. to fever*, *typhoid*.
typhobacillosis (tī″fō-băs-ĭl-ō'sĭs) [G. *typhos*, stupor, + L. *bacillus*, little stick, + G. *-ōsis*, condition]. Poisoning due to toxins produced by the *Bacillus typhosus*.
typhogenic (tĭ″fō-jĕn'ĭk) [" + *gennan*, to produce]. Causing typhus or typhoid fever.
typhohemia (tĭ″fō-hē'mĭ-ă) [" + *haima*, blood]. Degeneration of the blood due to presence of bacilli.
typhoid (tī'foyd) [G. *typhos*, stupor, + *eidos*, form]. Resembling typhus.
t. fever. An acute, infectious disease characterized by definite lesions in Peyer's patches, mesenteric glands, and spleen accompanied by fever, headache, and abdominal symptoms.
ETIOL: Causative organism Eberth's bacillus, generally referred to as the *bacillus typhosis*. May occur at any age. Common in early adult life and esp. prevalent during fall and early winter. It may be transmitted by infected water or milk supplies. Well water in country districts sometimes contaminated through the soil from outhouses. Human carriers, particularly when food handlers, may be responsible for spread of infection. Body discharges from active or convalescent cases may be the means of infecting others.
INCUBATION: Two to 3 weeks.
SYM: *Early*: Headache, general weakness, indefinite pains, nosebleed; constipation may occur.
Within a few days to a week the temperature may reach a maximum of 104° to 105° F. and during this time, or up to the 10th day, rose spots can usually be seen, particularly on the abdomen, though they may be observed on the chest and back. They disappear on pressure and usually come out in crops during a period of several days. Abdominal tenderness develops and with it, generally, distention.
During following weeks fever is characterized by marked daily remissions, evening temperature being from 1° to 3° F. higher than the morning. In the young, the temperature often rises very abruptly. When the diurnal remissions are slight, a protracted case is forecast. As defervescence advances, the temperature becomes more irregular. Remissions are more decided and not infrequently a higher temperature is recorded in the morning. Hurried respiration, slight cough, and bronchial râles are common. Pulse is usually slow in comparison with the temperature, and is dicrotic. Heart sounds often feeble, expression dull and heavy, cheeks somewhat flushed, conjunctivae clear, pupils dilated. Tongue tremulous; at first red at tip and edges, and covered posteriorly with a whitish fur.
In severe cases, tongue becomes dry, brown and fissured, and sordes collect on teeth. Gastric symptoms not common, but obstinate. Vomiting sometimes develops and becomes a serious complication. Abdomen tympanitic, tenderness on palpation, esp. in iliac fossa. Diarrhea generally present, though not a constant symptom. Discharges vary from 3 to 6 or more a day; thin, offensive, yellowish. Stupor, muttering, delirium, twitching of the tendons, carphologia, and coma vigil may be present. Urine usually shows albumin. Retention common.
White blood count demonstrates a leukopenia. Convalescence marked by anemia, falling of hair, often desquamation. The patient gives evidence of having suffered from a protracted illness that has produced general enfeeblement of mind and body.
VARIETIES: *Absorptive*: Abrupt onset

typhoid fever

with severe symptoms, but convalescence follows within a few days.

Mild form: Moderate fever with marked remissions, diarrhea slight, nervous symptoms often absent, rash usually present and often abundant.

Ambulatory type: Symptoms mild and often disregarded by patient, who refuses to go to bed. However, grave symptoms may suddenly develop and even death from intestinal perforation may follow.

Typhoid of children: Rash often absent, fever rises abruptly, cerebral symptoms may be sufficiently marked to suggest meningitis.

RELAPSES: These are common in typhoid. There may be a complete repetition of all symptoms experienced during primary attack, but they are usually of shorter duration.

RECRUDESCENCE: This is a sudden, temporary elevation of temperature occurring during convalescence, and is not associated with a return of other symptoms. It may be due to constipation, excitement, or irritating food.

COMPLICATIONS: Pneumonia, periostitis, parotitis, deafness, myocarditis, nephritis. Bedsores may also come under this classification. An abrupt fall of several degrees in temperature is suggestive of intestinal hemorrhage or perforation. Hemorrhage takes place in from 3 to 5% of all cases and usually occurs during 3rd or 4th week. Hemorrhage is a fatal complication in from 30 to 40%. Intestinal perforation most common during the 2nd or 3rd week, and is said to occur in from 5 to 6% of cases. More frequent in males than in females.

DIFFERENTIAL DIAG: Paratyphoid, pneumonia, dysentery, meningitis, smallpox, appendicitis. Diagnostic points of value will be the presence of a leukopenia, the Widal test, blood culture and examination of feces for presence of causative organism.

PROG: Should always be guarded, no matter how mild the case appears to be. Fatality rate varies in different epidemics. In private practice, it may be less than 5%; in hospital practice it sometimes exceeds 10%. Hemorrhages in any form, together with excessive diarrhea, are unfavorable omens.

TREATMENT: *Preventive*: Safeguards adopted for the supply of drinking water in large cities and the more or less general pasteurization of milk are probably chief factors in the great reduction of typhoid fever in well-governed communities. Active immunization is a factor in reduction of mortality. Individual immunity can ordinarily be established by means of 3 injections of antityphoid vaccine given at weekly intervals.

Treatment of the active case: General care, isolation of patient, and disinfection of all discharges are of primary importance. Those caring for the typhoid patient should be immunized against the disease. All precautions applicable to such infections must be adopted. Articles in contact with the patient must be sterilized or disinfected before being handled by other persons

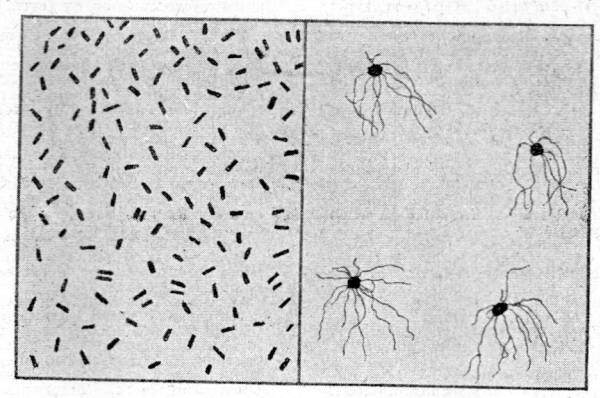

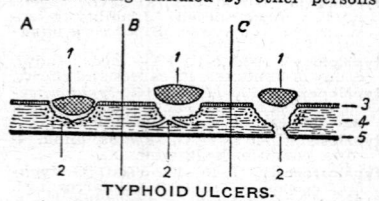

TYPHOID BACILLI.
Left, smear from a culture; right, stain for flagella (higher magnification).

TYPHOID ULCERS.
A. In Peyer's patch. 1. Slough in ulcer. 2. Lymphoid tissue. B. Erosion of blood vessel, with separation of slough, causing hemorrhage. 1. Slough separated. 2. Eroded artery. C. Perforation of ulcer through peritoneum. 1. Slough separated. 2. Peritoneal perforation. 3. Mucous membrane. 4. Muscle layer. 5. Peritoneum.

than the immediate attendant. It is necessary to guard against development of bedsores. Since delirium is not infrequent, patient may require constant watching to prevent his leaving the bed, which might result in fatal consequences. The mouth should be kept as clean as possible to prevent development of sordes.

TYPHOID FEVER

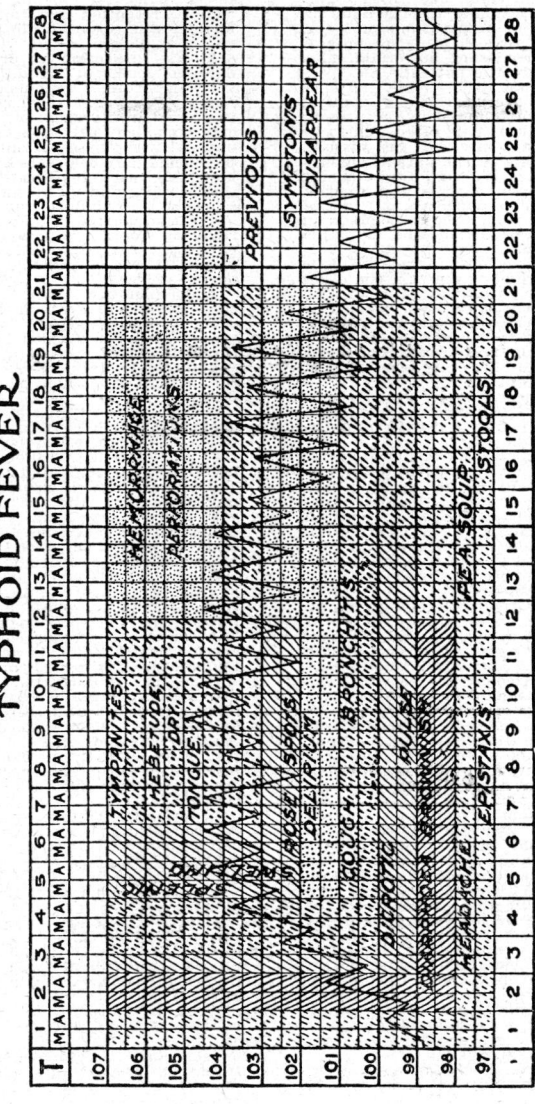

typhoid fever

DIET: In the early stages, diet may be largely liquid, including plenty of water and milk given in from 2 to 4 pints in the 24-hour period. This is usually best administered in small quantities at intervals of 2 to 3 hours, and the addition of lime water in preparations of ½ oz. of lime water to each 2 oz. of milk is advisable. Koumiss or buttermilk may be acceptable to the patient.

The starvation diet, which was once so common in the treatment of typhoid fever, is seldom followed in the present day. Nevertheless, it is often well to be cautious during onset of the disease, gradually adding to the patient's nourishment until it is found that he may be placed on a soft diet without danger. When this can be done, a great loss of weight, which used to be so common in typhoid fever patients, may be, to a large extent, avoided.

Ice bags and cold sponging are little used at the present time. On the other hand, sponging with tepid water, or with alcohol, is sometimes used when the temperature has reached unusual heights. In case of severe hemorrhage or intestinal perforation, nothing short of surgical interference offers any possibility of saving the patient's life.

NP: The objectives are: (a) *To support the patient's strength;* (b) *to lessen toxemia,* and (c) *to prevent complications.*

Quiet is essential; visitors, excitement, and noise are not conducive to quiet or peace of mind. Bright lights, heavy bedclothing, and everything that might irritate the patient should be avoided. An airy, well-ventilated room is essential. The bed must be comfortable and protection provided in case of incontinence. If the patient becomes emaciated an air bed may be necessary.

Position of patient: Usually he lies on one side with knees drawn up, so if sores are apt to develop the knees should be wrapped in wool to prevent chafing when together. Extra pillows are permissible if desired by the patient. The patient should make no muscular effort while the bed is being made.

Care of the mouth: Frequent soft swabs and bland lotions should be used, as sordes gather on the teeth and the mouth is dry, brown, and fissured. Keeping the mouth moist cannot be overemphasized.

Care of the skin: A morning and night cleansing bath should be given. In the meantime, tepid sponging will remove perspiration, and help maintain the function of the skin and also assist in elimination. As the secretion of the skin carries infection, water used for bathing should be disposed of and the basin disinfected. The patient's hands should be kept scrupulously clean to prevent them from being contaminated with excreta. Ointment should be used to protect the skin in cases of incontinence. At regular intervals washing with hot water is necessary if ointment has been used, to prevent the pores from becoming filled up.

Headache and backache: A severe frontal headache may last from 10 to 14 days from inception of the fever. The light should be shaded and cold compresses applied. The legs and back should be supported with pillows.

Restlessness: This may induce sleeplessness. A change of position; a sponge bath; taking off a cover if the patient is hot, or adding one if cold; washing the face, and brushing the hair will do much to rest the patient.

Urine: This should be measured and tested daily for albumin. Watch for sign of retention due to atony of the bladder's muscular wall in the latter weeks of illness.

Stools: Inspection for presence of undigested food, for blood, and flatus is very important. Frequency should be noted. Four or 5 movements per day is normal in diarrhea, but 8 to 12 indicate complications. Constipation is not unusual with these patients and a simple enema may be ordered, but it should be small, with temperature not more than 98° F., and given with a catheter, allowing the fluid to run very gently. When complicated by hemorrhages, and frequent stools, the patient may be too exhausted to use a bedpan, in which case the excreta should be received on pads.

Abdominal distention: This may become a dangerous complication; in any event it is distressing. Water may be given but not sweetened lemonade, and the diet may have to be reduced to prevent excessive fermentation. Change of the patient's position may relieve the flatus.

Bathing: Baths, their nature, and frequency should be left to the discretion of the physician; otherwise routine care, such as cleansing and sponge baths, may be used unless contraindicated.

Delirium: This is usually of the low muttering type, and the patient stares with a fixed gaze upon the ceiling and plucks on the bedclothing. Utensils and other articles should not be left within his reach and *he must not be left alone*.

Charting: A 4-hour chart should be kept of temperature, pulse, and respiration, although the pulse should be taken much more frequently than this. In the 3rd week, the temperature should be taken every 2 hours. A sudden drop in temperature indicates hemorrhage.

Disinfection: The usual methods of disinfection should be observed in handling all excreta and secretions, linens, and utensils. Disinfection for the nurse is also very important.

t. state. Condition in many diseases marked by profound prostration and other symptoms like those of typhus or typhoid fever.

t., walking. T. fever with mild general constitutional symptoms, the patient being able to be up and to walk. SYN: *ambulatory typhoid.*

typhoidal (tī-foy'dăl) [G. *typhos,* stupor, + *eidos,* resemblance]. Resembling typhoid.

typhoidette (tī-foy-dĕt') [Fr.]. A mild form of typhoid fever.

typhoin (tī'fō-ĭn) [G. *typhos,* stupor]. A preparation of dead typhoid bacilli introduced hypodermically in typhoid fever as a vaccine.

typholysin (tī-fŏl'ĭ-sĭn) [" + *lysis,* dissolution]. A lysin destructive to typhoid bacilli.

typhomalarial (tī'fō-mă-lā'rĭ-ăl) [" + Italian *malaria,* bad air]. Having symptoms of both typhoid and malarial fever.

typhomania (tī-fō-mā'nĭ-ă) [" + *mania,* madness]. Muttering delirium characteristic of typhoid fever and typhus.

typhonia (tī-fō'nĭ-ă) [G. *typhos,* stupor]. The delirium in typhoid or typhus fever.

typhophor (tī'fō-fŏr) [" + *phoros,* a bearer]. A typhoid carrier.*

typhopneumonia (tī″fō-nū-mō′nĭ-ă) [" + *pneumōnia*, inflammation of lungs]. 1. Pneumonia occurring in typhoid fever. 2. Pneumonia with typhoid symptoms.

typhose (tī′fōs) [G. *typhos*, stupor]. Having the appearance of typhoid fever, esp. when its symptoms appear in some forms of syphilis with pyrexia.

typhosepsis (tī″fō-sĕp′sĭs) [" + *sēpsis*, putrefaction]. The general poisoning which occurs in typhoid fever.

typhosis (tī-fō′sĭs) [" + *-ōsis*, condition]. A morbid condition with symptoms similar to those of typhoid or typhus fever.

typhosus (tī-fō′sŭs) [G. *typhos*, stupor]. Pert. to typhoid or typhus fever.

typhous (tī′fŭs) [G. *typhos*, stupor]. Pert. to typhus fever.

typhus, typhus fever (tī′fŭs) [G. *typhos*, stupor]. An acute, contagious disease manifested by great prostration, a petechial rash, marked by nervous symptoms and high fever. SYN: *jail fever, ship fever*. There are several forms: endemic (murine typhus), epidemic, and scrub typhus.

dark red, subcuticular mottling. Bowels are constipated, urine is scanty, high-colored, and often albuminous.

COMPLICATIONS: Bronchopneumonia more frequent than lobar, hypostatic congestion of lungs, nephritis, and parotid abscess.

DIFFERENTIAL DIAG: Typhoid fever, hemorrhagic smallpox, Henoch's purpura, epidemic meningitis of fulminating type, and ulcerative endocarditis may have to be considered.

PROG: Mortality often high. Disease esp. severe in advanced years and in alcoholics. Fatality rate 12% to 20%.

TREATMENT: *Preventive*: Absolute cleanliness, sterilization of clothing, and the use of apparel to prevent infestation of the body louse. The delousing camps, so common during the late war, were examples of the precautions necessary to prevent its spread. Patient must be isolated. Absolute rest necessary, and a liquid diet. For *specific* therapy, aureomycin, chloromycetin, and terramycin are said to be equally effective. PABA

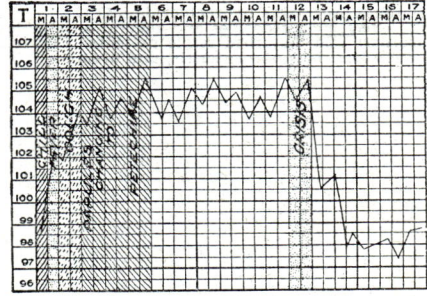

TYPHUS

ETIOL: *Endemic* typhus is caused by the *Rickettsia typhi*, and is transmitted to man by the rat flea. *Epidemic* typhus is caused by the *R. prowazekii*, and is transmitted to man by the louse. *Scrub* typhus (tsutsugamushi disease) is caused by the *R. tsutsugamushi*, and is transmitted to man by mites.

Epidemic typhus is particularly prevalent amid unsanitary conditions. It often develops on shipboard, in army camps, and where living conditions are unfavorable and congestion is marked. The disease is rare in the United States, infection being found principally at the seaboard as a result of imported cases.

INCUBATION: Ten to 14 days.

SYM: Onset sudden. Severe headache, pain in back and limbs, extreme prostration. Fever rises rapidly, often reaching 104° to 105° F. in from 2 to 3 days. Remains high for about 10 days, when it falls by crisis. Pulse rapid, weak, often dicrotic. Tongue tremulous, may be covered with whitish fur; in bad cases becomes black and rolled up like a ball in back of mouth. Face dusky, conjunctivae injected, pupil contracted, headache, stupor, delirium, subsultus tendinum, carphologia.

From 4th to 5th day, bluish spots appear over body, esp. on abdomen. These are petechial in character and do not disappear on pressure. The extent of eruption is indicative of severity of attack. Sometimes there is a diffuse,

(paraäminobenzoic acid) is also useful. Sulfonamides are contraindicated, and penicillin has no antirickettsial effect.

t. petechial. True typhus fever.

t. recur'rens. Relapsing fever.

t. sid'erans. Malignant t., quickly fatal.

typical (tĭp′ĭ-kăl) [G. *typikos*, pert. to type]. Having the characteristics of, pert. to, or conforming to, a type or condition or group.

typ'ing of blood. Determination of agglutination in the blood of donor and recipient before blood transfusion. SEE: *blood transfusion*.

typo- [G.]. Combining form meaning a *type*.

typology (tī-pŏl′ō-jī) [G. *typos*, type, + *logos*, a study]. The study of types, as of blood or constitutional types.

typoscope (tī′pō-skōp) [" + *skopein*, to examine]. Device to aid patients with amblyopia and cataract in reading.

tyrannism (tīr′ăn-ĭzm) [G. *tyrannos*, tyrant, + *-ismos*, condition]. Abnormal tendency to exercise cruelty. SYN: *sadism, q.v.*

ty reflex (tī). Sudden reflex grasping of mother's body by infant when startled.

tyremesis (tī-rĕm′ē-sĭs) [G. *tyros*, cheese, + *emesis*, vomiting]. Infant vomiting of curdy or cheesy substances.

tyriasis (tīr-ī′ăs-ĭs) [" + *-iasis*, infection]. 1. Hypertrophy of skin and connective tissue with induration due to obstruc-

tion of the lymphatics. Syn: *elephantiasis.* 2. Baldness. Syn: *alopecia.*
tyrogenous (tī-rŏj'ĕn-ŭs) [" + *gennan*, to produce]. Having origin in cheese or produced by it.
tyroid (tī'royd) [" + *eidos*, form]. Caseous; cheesy. [caseous tumor.
tyroma (tī-rō'mă) [" + *-oma*, tumor]. A
tyromatosis (tī-rō-mă-tō'sĭs) [" + " + *-osis*, condition]. Cheesy degeneration. Syn: *caseation.*
tyrosinase (tī-rō'sĭn-ās) [G. *tyros*, cheese]. A ferment that acts on tyrosine.
tyrosine (tī'rō-sēn) [G. *tyros*, cheese]. An amino acid formed in decomposition of protein.
tyrosinuria (tī-rō-sĭn-ū'rĭ-ă) [" + *ouron*, urine]. Tyrosine in the urine.
tyrosis (tī-rō'sĭs) [" + *-osis*, condition]. 1. Curdling of milk. 2. Vomiting of cheesy substance by infants. Syn: *tyremesis.** 3. Cheesy degeneration. Syn: *tyromatosis.*

tyrothricin (tī-roth'rĭ-sĭn). A bacterial substance isolated from a soil bacterium; used in local affections externally. Gramicidin obtained from it is less toxic.
Tyrothrix (tī'rō-thrĭks) [" + *thrix*, hair]. A genus of bacteria (Schizomycetes) causing coagulation of casein.
tyrotoxin (tī"rō-tŏks'ĭn) [" + *toxikon*, poison]. Any toxic product of milk or cheese due to a bacillus.
tyrotoxism (tī-rō-tŏks'ĭzm) [" + " + *-ismos*, condition]. Poisoning produced by a milk product or by cheese.
tyroxin (tī-rŏks'ĭn) [G. *tyros*, cheese]. A decomposition product of albumin.
Tyrrel's fascia (tĭr'ĕl). An illy-defined fibromuscular layer from the middle aponeurosis of the perineum, behind the prostate gland. Syn: *rectovesical fascia.*
Tyson's glands (tī'sŭn). Sebaceous glands at base of glans penis which secrete a sebaceous substance, *smegma.**

Addendum
Thorazine (thor-ă-zīn) (chlorpromazine hydrochloride SKF).
It has a synergistic effect upon sedatives and general anesthetics, a quieting effect in neuropsychiatric disorders and disturbed senile patients. Controls nausea and vomiting, due to cancer, cholecystitis, gastroenteritis, and uremia.

U

U. 1. Chem. symbol of *uranium*. 2. Abbr. for *unit*.
uarthritis (ū″ar-thrī′tĭs) [G. *arthron*, joint, + *-itis*, inflammation]. Gout supposed to result from excess of uric acid. SYN: *arthritis urica*.
uaterium (wă-tē′rĭ-ŭm). A medical preparation to be used in the ear.
uberous (ū′bĕr-ŭs) [L. *uber*, udder]. Prolific; fruitful; fertile.
uberty (ū′bĕr-tĭ) [L. *uber*, udder]. Fruitfulness; fertility.
Uffelmann's test (oof′ĕl-mahn). Gastric test for hydrochloric acid or lactic acid.
Uhthoff's sign (oot′hof). The nystagmus which occurs in multiple disseminated sclerosis.
ulalgia (ū-lăl′jĭ-ă) [G. *oulon*, gum, + *algos*, pain]. Pain in the gums.
ulatrophia (ū″lăt-rō′fĭ-ă). Shrinking of gums; recession of the gums.
ulcer (ŭl′ser) [L. *ulcus*, *ulcer-*, ulcer]. An open lesion upon the skin or mucous membrane of the body, with loss of substance, accompanied by formation of pus.
Simple ulcers may result from trauma, caustics, or intense heat or cold. They may accompany varicose veins in the aged. SEE: *Table*, p. U-2.
In syphilis, they are deep seated, having an offensive secretion; in epithelioma, they appear late in life with a single center and a thickened, infiltrated edge with a scanty, bloody secretion; in lupus vulgaris, they appear early in life, but they are superficial.
RS: *abscission 3, anabrosia, anthracosis, aphtha, argema, carcinelcosis, carcinomelcosis, chalarosis, dieresis, duodenal u., helicoid, peptic, phagedena, rodent u., slough, stomach, vomicose.*
  u., amputating. One which destroys tissue to the bone by encircling the part.
  u., atonic. A chronic ulcer.
  u., callous. A chronic u. with indurated, elevated edges and no granulations, which does not heal.
  u., duodenal. An ulcer on the mucosa of the duodenum, due to the action of the gastric juice.
  u., erethistic. One with an inflamed, red, painful surface.
  u., follicular. A tiny ulcer having its origin in a lymph follicle and affecting a mucous membrane.
  u., fungous. One in which the granulations protrude above edges of wound and bleed easily.
  u., gastric. SEE: *peptic u.*
  u., healthy. One u. which tends toward healing, its surface being soft and smooth with tiny red granulations.
  u., indolent. Nearly painless u. usually found on leg, characterized by indurated and elevated edge, and nongranulating base.
  u., peptic. An ulcer of the mucosa of the duodenum or stomach.
  TREATMENT: Protein diet; colloidal aluminum hydroxide relieves pain promptly and ulcer heals rapidly. SEE: *peptic ulcer.*
  u., perforating. An ulcer which permeates the entire thickness of the part, as the foot.

  u., phagedenic. An ulcer which sloughs particles, spreading rapidly and disintegrating the tissues.
  u., rodent. A deeply infiltrating ulcer which slowly eats away the bones and soft tissues; commonly affects the upper part of the face.
  u., round. SEE: *peptic ulcer.*
  u., serpiginous. A creeping ulcer which heals in 1 part and extends to another.
  u., simple. A local ulcer with no severe inflammation or pain.
  u., specific. An ulcer caused by a specific disease, as syphilis or lupus.
  u., stercoral. 1. Ulcer caused by pressure from impacted feces. 2. Ulcer through which feces escapes.
ulcerate (ŭl′sĕr-āt) [L. *ulcerāre*, to ulcerate]. To produce or become affected with an ulcer.
ulcerated (ŭl′sĕr-ā″tĕd) [L. *ulcerāre*, to ulcerate]. Of the nature of an ulcer or affected with one.
  u. sore throat. Putrid sore throat, a gangrenous inflammation.
  u. tooth. Suppuration of the alveolar periosteum with ulceration of gum surrounding the decaying root of a tooth.
ulceration (ŭl″sĕr-ā′shŭn) [L. *ulcerāre*, to ulcerate]. Suppuration taking place on a free surface, as on the skin or on a mucous membrane.
A termination of inflammation.
ulcerative (ŭl′sĕr-ā-tĭv) [L. *ulcerāre*, to form ulcers]. Pert. to or causing ulceration.
  u. scrof′uloderma. Progressive fatal skin disease with hard, red, ulcerating tumors.
ulceromembranous (ŭl″sĕr-ō-mĕm′brăn-ŭs) [" + *membrana*, membrane]. Pert. to ulceration and formation of a membrane.
  u. tonsillitis. Tonsillitis that ulcerates and develops a membranous film.
ulcerous (ŭl′sĕr-ŭs) [L. *ulcerāre*, to ulcerate]. Pert. to or affected with an ulcer.
ulcus (ŭl′kŭs) (pl. *ulcera*) [L.]. Ulcer.
  u. cancro′sum. 1. Cancerous ulcer which eats away the tissues. SYN: *rodent ulcer*. 2. Same as *u. durum*.
  u. durum. Lesion of syphilis. SYN: *chancre.*
  u. indura′tum. Same as *u. durum*.
  u. tuberculo′sum. Tuberculosis of the skin. SYN: *lupus.*
  u. ventric′uli. Gastric ulceration.
  u. vul′vae acu′tum. Nonvenereal, rapidly spreading ulceration of the vulva of about 2 weeks' duration associated with presence of *Bacillus crassus*.
ulectomy (ū-lĕk′tō-mĭ) 1. [G. *oulē*, scar, + *ektomē*, excision]. Excision of scar tissue, esp. in secondary iridectomy. 2. [G. *oulon*, gum]. Removal of gum tissue, as in pyorrhea alveolaris. SYN: *gingivectomy.*
ulemorrhagia (ū-lē-mor-ā′jĭ-ă) [G. *oulon*, gum, + *haimorrhagia*, bleeding]. Bleeding from the gums.
ulerythema (ū-lĕr-ĭ-thē′mă) [G. *oulē*, scar, + *erythēma*, redness]. An erythematous disorder with atrophic scar formation. SEE: *lupus erythematosus.*

U-1

Ulcers, Commoner: Classification of (After Chiene)[1]

Type of Ulcer	Healing	Weak	Callous	Irritable	Inflamed	Syphilitic	Tubercular
SURFACE	Smooth and healing.	Raised and flabby granulations.	Granulations absent or pale and ill-formed.	Congested, red, no granulations.	Sloughing irregular, no granulations.	Circular or irregular.	Pale, unhealthy granulations.
EDGES	Smooth and regular.	Smooth and healthy.	Raised, firm, hard, dense, white.	Dark red, irregular.	Sharp and turned outwards, irregular and undermined.	Steep and sharp cut, dull red, undermined.	Pale, bluish, thin, undermined.
SURROUNDINGS	Healthy.	Usually healthy.	Pigmented, indurated, eczematous.	Normal. Tender spots.	Dusky, swollen and inflamed, skin brawny.	Smooth, glistening, pigmented, old cicatrices.	Enlarged glands; purplish, old cicatrices.
DISCHARGE	Sweet pus or serum.	Watery, copious.	Scanty, offensive.	Scanty, thin, serous.	Serous, bloody, putrid.	Breaking down débris.	Thin, yellowish-green, scanty débris.
PAIN	Absent.	Absent.	Inconsiderable.	Intense.	Severe constitutional fever.	None.	None.
CICATRIZATION	All round.	None.	None.	None.	None.	Often in center.	None.
TREATMENT	Rest and cleanliness, skin grafting.	Removal of cause, elevation, stimulating lotions or caustics.	Rest, elevation, antiseptics, ointments, strapping, excision of the whole ulcer followed by skin grafting of the raw surface. Amputation.	Improve general health, opiates, caustics locally, operation to divide nerve.	Rest, elevation, soothing applications; constitutional.	Iodide of potash and mercury internally, poultices, followed by black wash. Intravenous injection of salvarsan.	Pare edges, scrape base, iodoform. Tonics.

[1] From *Faber's Nurses Encyclopedia*.

u. ophryog'enes. Folliculitis of eyebrows.
SYM: Falling out of hair and scarring.
uletic (ū-lĕt'ĭk) [G. *oulon,* gum]. Pert. to the gums.
uletomy (ū-lĕt'ō-mĭ) [G. *oulē,* scar, + *tomē,* a cutting]. Incision of a scar to relieve tension. SYN: *cicatricotomy.*
uliginous (ū-lĭj'ĭn-ŭs) [L. *uliginosus,* wet]. Muddy; slimy.
ulilampe (ū'lĭ-lămp). Low pressure glow tube in uviol glass tube used abroad for therapeutic purposes. SEE: *uviol.*
ulitis (ū-lī'tĭs) [G. *oulon,* gum, + *-itis,* inflammation]. Inflammation of the gums.
u., interstitial. Inflammation of connective tissue of gums about the necks of the teeth.
ulna (ŭl'nă) [L. *ulna,* elbow]. The inner and larger bone of the forearm, bet. the wrist and the elbow, on the side opposite that of the thumb.
It articulates with the head of the radius and humerus above and with the radius below.
RS: *coronoid process, cubital, cubitus, olecranon process.*
ulnad (ŭl'năd) [" + *ad,* toward]. In the direction of the ulna.
ulnar (ŭl'nar) [L. *ulna,* elbow]. 1. Relating to the ulna, or to nerve or artery named from it. 2. Cuneiform carpal bone. SYN: *ulnare.*
ulnare (ŭl-nā'rē) [L.]. The 3rd or cuneiform bone of the carpus.
ulnaris (ŭl-nā'rĭs) [L.]. A muscle on ulnar side of the forearm. SEE: *Muscles, Table of, in Appendix.*
ulnocarpal (ŭl"nō-kar'păl) [L. *ulna,* elbow, + G. *karpos,* wrist]. Relating to the carpus and ulna, or to the ulnar side of the wrist.
ulnoradial (ŭl"nō-rā'dĭ-ăl) [" + *radius,* spoke of a wheel]. Relating to the ulna and radius, as their ligaments and articulations.
ulocace (ū-lŏk'ă-sē) [G. *oulon,* gum, + *kakē,* badness]. Ulcerative inflammation of the gums.
ulocarcinoma (ū"lō-kar-sĭn-ō'mă) [" + *karkinos,* cancer, + *-ōma,* tumor]. Carcinoma of the gums.
uloglossitis (ū"lō-glos-ī'tĭs) [" + *glossa,* tongue, + *-itis,* inflammation]. Inflammation of the gums and tongue.
uloid (ū'loyd) [G. *oulē,* scar, + *eidos,* resemblance]. 1. Scarlike. 2. A scarlike lesion caused by subcutaneous degeneration.
u. cicatrix. Same as *uloid, 2.*
uloncus (ū-lŏn'kŭs) [G. *oulon,* gum, + *ogkos,* mass]. Swelling or tumor of the gums. SEE: *epulis.*
ulorrhagia (ū-lor-ā'jĭ-ă) [" + *-rrhagia,* bleeding]. Bleeding from the gums.
ulorrhea (ū-lor-rē'ă) [" + *rhoia,* a flow]. Slow bleeding from the gums.
ulosis (ū-lō'sĭs) [G. *oulē,* scar, + *-ōsis,* condition]. Formation of scar tissue. SYN: *cicatrization.*
ulotic (ū-lŏt'ĭk) [G. *oulē,* scar]. Causing cicatrization. SYN: *cicatricial.*
ulotomy (ū-lŏt'ō-mĭ) 1. [" + *tomē,* a cutting]. The cutting of scar tissue to relieve deformity or tension. 2. [G. *oulon,* gum]. Incision of the gums.
ulotrichous (ū-lŏt'rĭk-ŭs) [G. *oulos,* woolly, + *thrix, trich-,* hair]. Having short, woolly hair, as a negro.
ulotropsis (ū"lō-trop'sĭs) [G. *oulon,* gum, + *tropsis,* nutrition]. Revitalization of the gums by massage.
ultex (ŭl'tĕks). A bifocal glass in which the near section is ground with the spherical curved.
ultimate (ŭl'tĭm-ăt) [L. *ultimus,* last]. Final or last.
u. analysis. Resolution of a substance into its constituent elements.
ultimum moriens (ŭl'tĭ-mŭm mō'rĭ-ĕns) [L. last thing dying]. 1. The right auricle, last part of the body to die, said to contract after the heart has ceased to beat. 2. Upper portion of the trapezius muscle, which frequently is not involved in progressive muscular atrophy.
ultra- [L.]. Prefix meaning *beyond, excess.*
ultrabrachycephalic (ŭl"tră-brăk"ĭ-sē-făl'-ĭk) [L. *ultra,* beyond, + G. *brachys,* short, + *kephalē,* head]. Having a cephalic index of 90 or over.
ultrafiltration (ŭl"tră-fĭl-trā'shŭn) [" + *filtrum,* a filter]. Filtration of a colloidal substance in which the dispersed particles, but not the liquid, are held back.
ultraligation (ŭl"trā-lī-gā'shŭn) [" + *ligāre,* to bind]. Ligation of a blood vessel beyond the origin of a branch.
ultramicrobe (ŭl"tră-mī'krōb) [" + G. *mikros,* tiny, + *bios,* life]. A microorganism too small to be visible by the ordinary microscope.
ultramicroscope (ŭl"tră-mī'krō-skōp) [" + " + *skopein,* to examine]. Microscope by which objects invisible through an ordinary microscope may be seen by means of powerful side illumination.
ultramicron (ŭl"tră-mī'krŏn) [" + G. *mikros,* small]. A particle so tiny that it can be seen only through the ultramicroscope. SYN: *submicron.*
ultramicroscopical (ŭl"tră-mĭk-rō-skŏp'ĭ-kăl) [" + " + *skopein,* to examine]. Too small to be seen with aid of an ordinary microscope.
ultramicroscopy (ŭl"tră-mī-krŏs'kō-pī) [" + " + *skopein,* to examine]. The use of the ultramicroscope for scientific purposes.
ultraprophylaxis (ŭl"tră-prō-fĭl-ăks'ĭs) [L. *ultra,* beyond, + G. *pro,* before, + *phylaxis,* protection]. Prevention of diseased or abnormal offspring by regulating the marriage of the unfit.
ultratherm (ŭl'tră-therm) [" + G. *thermē,* heat]. A short wave diathermy machine.
ultratoxon (ŭl"tră-tŏks'ŏn) [" + *toxikon,* poison]. A toxon of a very low degree of toxicity.
ultraviolet (ŭl"tră-vī'ō-lĕt) [" + *violet*]. Beyond the visible spectrum at its violet end, said of rays. SEE: *infrared.*
u. therapy. Treatment with ultraviolet radiation. SEE: *heliotherapy, light therapy.*
ultravirus (ŭl"tră-vī'rŭs) [" + *virus,* poison]. A virus which is filtrable but which can be demonstrated by inoculation test. SEE: *filtrable virus.*
Ultzmann's test (oolts'mahn). A solution test for bile pigments in the urine.
The fluid will show bright green if bile pigments are present.
umbilical (ŭm-bĭl'ĭ-kăl) [L. *umbilicus,* navel]. Pert. to the umbilicus.
u. cord. The attachment connecting the fetus with the placenta, artificially severed at birth of the child.
It leaves a depression on the abdomen of the child called the navel or *umbilicus,** where the cord was attached to the fetus. It contains 2 arteries and 1 vein protected by Wharton's jelly, through which the embryo receives from the mother its blood supply and nourishment.
Cord should not be cut or tied until

umbilical fissure   U-4   **unconsciousness, words pert. to**

umbilical vessels have ceased pulsating. This gives the infant a better red blood cell count. SEE: *cord, Wharton's jelly.*
    u. fissure. Portion of hepatic longitudinal fissure in which the umbilical vein is lodged. [the umbilicus.
    u. hernia. A hernia in the region of
    u. souffle. A hissing sound said to arise from the u. cord.
    u. vesicle. That part of the embryonic yolk sac leading from the umbilicus.
umbilicate (ŭm-bĭl'ĭ-kāt) [L. *umbilicātus*, dimpled]. Pert. to or shaped like the navel, noting a bacterial colony with a central depression resembling an umbilicus.
umbilication (ŭm-bĭl-ĭ-kā'shŭn) [L. *umbilicātus*, dimpled]. 1. A depression resembling a navel. 2. Formation at apex of a pustule or vesicle of a pit or depression.
umbilicus (ŭm-bĭ-lī'kŭs, -bĭl'ĭ-kŭs) (pl. *umbilici*) [L. a pit]. A depressed point in the middle of the abdomen; the scar which marks the former attachment of the umbilical cord to the fetus.
    RS: *angiolysis; cord, umbilical; funic; f. souffle; funiculus; funis; hydromphalus; mesogastrium; navel; "omphal-" words; varicomphalus; Wharton's jelly.*
umbo (ŭm'bō) [L. boss]. Projecting center of a round surface.
    u. tympani. Shallow, funnel-shaped area on drum membrane at the tip of the manubrium where malleus is attached.
umbrascopy (ŭm-brăs'kō-pĭ) [L. *umbra*, shadow, + G. *skopein*, to view]. Use of shadows in refraction of the eye or use of roentgen rays. SYN: *skiascopy.*
un- [A.S.]. Prefix meaning *back, reversal, annulment of, not.*
uncia (ŭn'sĭ-ă) [L. *uncia*, the twelfth part of a whole]. An ounce, or an inch.
unciform (ŭn'sĭ-form) [L. *uncus*, hook, + *forma*, shape]. Hook-shaped.
    u. bone. Hook-shaped bone on ulnar side of distal row of the carpus. SYN: *os hamatum.*
    u. fasciculus. Bundle of fibers connecting frontal cerebral lobes with the temporosphenoid ones.
    u. process. 1. Long, thin lamina of bone from orbital plate of the ethmoid articulating with the inf. turbinate. 2. Hook at ant. end of hippocampal gyrus. 3. Hooked end of unciform bone.
uncinariasis (ŭn-sĭ-na-rī'ă-sĭs) [L. *uncus*, hook]. Hookworm disease. SYN: *ankylostomiasis*, q.v.
    u. of skin. Vesicular dermatitis generally of the feet from invasion by the *Uncinaria duodenale*.
Uncinaria (ŭn-sĭn-ā'rĭ-ă) [L. *uncus*, a hook]. A genus of nematode worms infesting man and lower animals.
uncinate (ŭn'sĭn-āt) [L. *uncinātus*, hooked]. Hook-shaped; hooked.
    u. convolution. An occipital lobe convolution near temporal lobe.
    u. epilepsy. Form of e. occurring in disease of uncinate area of the temporal lobe.
    u. gyrus. SEE: *u. convolution.*
uncinatum (ŭn-sĭ-nā'tŭm) [L. *uncus*]. The unciform bone of the hand. SYN: *os hamatum.*
uncipressure (ŭn'sĭ-prĕsh-ur) [L. *uncus*, hook, + *pressura*, a pressing]. Pressure by means of hooks to arrest hemorrhage.
un"condi'tioned re'flex. Any reflex not the result of special training.
unconscious (ŭn-kŏn'shŭs) [A.S. *un*, not, + L. *conscius*, conscious]. 1. In a state unaccompanied by conscious experience, as in a faint. 2. PSY: Excluded from consciousness by repression. 3. Repository of previous experiences in life of the individual and of the historical past of the race.
    As a noun, the term has been used in place of the "subconscious" as a storehouse of repressed or forgotten concepts and urges which still have potential energy and which may be brought to light by psychoanalysis.
    CAUSES OF UNCONSCIOUS STATES: Among them are the following: Alcoholism; apoplexy; asphyxia; asphyxia, choking; asphyxia, drowning; asphyxia, foreign bodies; asphyxia, gases; asphyxia, suffocation; collapse; coma; convulsions; epilepsy; freezing; head concussions; head injuries; head fractures; heart attacks; hemorrhages; hemorrhages, external; hemorrhages, internal; hysteria; thermoreactions; thermoreactions, burns; thermoreactions, frostbites; thermoreactions, heatstroke, thermoreactions, heat exhaustion; poisoning; shock; syncope; uremia.
    TO MOVE AN UNCONSCIOUS PATIENT FROM STRETCHER TO BED: *Method I:* 1. Fold draw sheet in half lengthwise and place it across center of stretcher, pleating the excess and tucking the ends under for about 6 in. before patient is put on stretcher. 2. When patient is on stretcher this sheet should be under the buttocks. 3. Place stretcher parallel with bed and as close as you can get it. Get 3 other people to help you. 4. Have one person at patient's head, one at feet, one at side, and one at far side of bed. The ones at the sides take firm hold of the ends of the draw sheet and all 4 lift together, the person at the far side pulling the draw sheet toward her.
    Method II: 1. This takes 3 people. 2. Place stretcher at right angles to the foot of the bed. Patient's head at end nearest bed. 3. Standing side by side the 3 people put their arms under patient, lift him, and swing him around onto the bed.
unconsciousness (ŭn-kŏn'shŭs-nĕs) [A.S. *un*, not, + L. *conscius*, aware]. State of being insensible or without conscious experiences.
    Unconsciousness physiologically occurs in sleep, pathologically in coma, epilepsy, etc. SEE: *Table, p. U-5.*
    SYM: Patient unable to swallow; eyes do not react, insensible to surroundings. The cause varies considerably.
    Coma is commonly due to alcoholism, fainting, shock, hemorrhage, sunstroke, poisoning, electric shock, apoplexy, skull fracture, uremia, epilepsy, or to diabetes. Decide probable cause before treating.
    If face is flushed, or if hemorrhage is present or suspected, do not lower head and do not give stimulants. In all other instances, it is desirable to lower head and shoulders, loosen clothing and keep patient warm. Turn head to one side to prevent vomit, if any, from being drawn into lungs. Loosen clothing. Fresh air and, if necessary, artificial respiration. Look for fractures, paralysis. Test pulse, respiration, odor of breath, condition of skin and pupils of eyes. See *diagnosis* under these subjects. Make a diagnosis prior to further treatment.
unconsciousness, words pert. to: aochlesia, aphrenia, aphronia, apoplexy, apopsychia, asphyctic, asphyxial, asphyxiation, catalepsy, collapse, coma, fainting, gas, shock, sleep, stupor, syncope, trance, twilight sleep.

Unconsciousness, Common Causes of

Causes	Onset	General Condition	Pupils	Pulse	Respiration	Muscles	Temperature	Special Points
Acute alcoholism.	Gradual.	Can be roused.	Dilated.	Full.	Deep, slightly stertorous.	Twitching.	Below normal.	Odor in breath, face is flushed.
Apoplexy.	Sudden.	Cannot be roused.	Unequally dilated and fixed.	Slow, full, and tense.	Slow, stertorous.	One side paralyzed.	Below normal.	Face dusky.
Compression.	Gradual.	Cannot be roused.	Pin point at first, then dilated, fixed, and unequal.	Slow and full.	Slow, irregular, and stertorous.	Paralysis of certain groups.	First below normal, later above.	
Concussion.	Sudden.	Can be roused.	Equal, and react to light.	Slow and weak.	Slow, irregular, and shallow.	Relaxed and flaccid.	Below normal.	
Diabetes.	Gradual.	Cannot be roused.	Normal.	Slow.	Slow, deep, and sighing.	Relaxed.	Below normal.	Dry skin, odor of acetone in breath, sugar and acetone in urine.
Insulin.	Fairly sudden.	Gradually deepening coma, preceded by excitement.	Normal.	Weak and rapid.		Relaxed, twitching in advanced stages.		Sweating.
Epilepsy.	Preceded by fits.	Cannot be roused.	Variable.	Becoming less rapid.	Noisy or stertorous.	Relaxed.	Raised.	
Opium.	Gradual.	Cannot be roused.	Pin point.	Slow.	Labored, irregular, stertorous, and slow.	Relaxed.		Face pallid, skin sweating.
Uremia.	Sudden or gradual.	Cannot be roused.	Usually contracted.	Hard.		Frequent convulsions.	Below normal.	Tonguefurred, breath foul.

From *Faber's Nurses Encyclopedia.*

unction (ŭnk′shŭn) [L. *unctio*, ointment]. 1. The application of an ointment. 2. Substance used for anointing. Syn: *unguent*.

unctuous (ŭnk′chŭ-ŭs) [L. *unctus*, an ointment]. Oily; greasy.

uncus (ŭn′kŭs) [L. *uncus*, hook]. Any structure that is hook-shaped.
  u. gyri hippocampi. BNA. Hooked ant. end of the hippocampal gyrus.

undertoe (ŭn′dẽr-tō) [A.S. *under*, beneath, + *tā*, toe]. Condition of displacement of the great toe underneath the others.

undifferentiation (ŭn-dĭf-ẽr-ĕn-shĭ-ā′shŭn) [A.S. *un*, not, + L. *differens*, bearing apart]. Alteration in cell character to a more embryonic type or toward a malignant state. Syn: *anaplasia*.

undine (ŭn′dĭn). A small glass flask used for irrigating the conjunctiva and in removal of a cataract.

undinism (ŭn′dĭn-ĭzm). Awakening of the libido by running water, as by urination or at sight of urine.

undulant (ŭn′dŭ-lănt) [L. *undulatus*, wavy]. Rising and falling like waves, or moving like them.
  u. fever. One of long duration due to the *Brucella melitensis*.
  Sym: Febrile paroxysms lasting a week or more which are repeated. Enlarged spleen, sweating, painful swelling of joints.

undulate (ŭn′dŭ-lāt) [L. *undulatus*, wavy]. Wavy; having a wavy border with shallow sinuses, said of bacterial colonies.

undulation (ŭn-dŭ-lā′shŭn) [L. *undulatus*, wavy]. A continuous wavelike motion or pulsation.

un′finished cough. A cough frequently caused by, and typical of, aneurysm of the aortic arch.

ung. [L.]. Abbr. of *unguentum*, ointment.

ungual (ŭng′gwăl) [L. *unguis*, nail]. Pert. to or resembling the nails. Syn: *unguinal*.
  u. bone. The thin, platelike lacrimal bone.
  u. phalanx. Terminal phalanx of each finger and toe.
  u. tuberosity. Spatula-shaped extremity of the terminal phalanx which supports the nails of fingers and toes.

unguent (ŭng′gwĕnt) [L. *unguentum*, ointment]. A lubricant or salve for sores, burns, etc. Syn: *ointment*.

unguentum (ŭn-gwĕn′tŭm) [L. *unguentum*, ointment]. 1. Fatty, soft, solid preparation intended to be applied to the skin by inunction. Sixteen ointments are official.
  2. Simple ointment, usually a compound of lard and yellow wax or occasionally wool fat, white wax, and white petroleum. Syn: *ointment, q.v.*

ungues (ŭng′gwēz) (sing. *unguis*) [L.]. The nails. See: *unguis*.

unguinal (ŭng′gwĭn-ăl) [L. *unguis*, nail]. Relating to or resembling a nail or an unguis.

unguis (ŭng′gwĭs) (pl. *ungues*) [L. *unguis*, nail]. 1. A finger- or toenail. See: *onyx*. 2. The lacrimal bone. 3. Pus mass in cornea. 4. A white prominence on floor of the lateral ventricle's post. horn. Syn: *hippocampus minor*.

ungula (ŭn′gū-lā) [L. *ungula*, claw]. Instrument for removal of dead fetus.

uni- [L.]. Combining form meaning *one*.

unicellular (ū″nĭ-sĕl′ū-lar) [L. *unus*, one, + *cellula*, a little box]. Having only 1 cell.

uniceptor (ū′nĭ-sĕp′tor) [″ + *ceptor*, a receiver]. A receptor occurring in blood serum having only a single combining group.

unicorn (ū′nĭ-korn) [″ + *cornū*, horn]. Having a single cornu or horn.
  u. uterus. A uterus with but 1 horn perfectly formed.

unicornous (ū-nĭ-kor′nŭs) [″ + *cornū*, horn]. Having but 1 horn or cornu.

unidirectional (ū″nĭ-dĭ-rĕk′shŭn-ăl) [″ + *directio*, a going straight]. Flowing in only one direction, as an electric current in a circuit.

uniglandular (ū″nĭ-glăn′dū-lar) [″ + *glandula*, a little kernel]. Pert. to or having only one gland.

unigravida (ū″nĭ-grăv′ĭ-dă) [″ + *gravida*, pregnant]. Woman who is pregnant for the first time.

unilateral (ū″nĭ-lăt′ẽr-al) [L. *unus*, one, + *latus*, later-, side]. Affecting or occurring on only one side.

unilocular (ū″nĭ-lŏk′ū-lar) [″ + *loculus*, a little place]. Having but one cavity.

uninuclear, uninucleate(d (ū″nĭ-nū′klē-ar, -ăt, -ā-tĕd) [″ + *nucleus*, a kernel]. Having only one nucleus.

uniocular (ū″nĭ-ok′ū-lar) [″ + *oculus*, eye]. Pert. to or having only one eye.

union (ūn′yŭn) [L. *unio*, oneness, union]. 1. Act of joining 2 or more things into 1 part, or state of being so united. 2. Growing together of severed or broken parts, as of bones or lips of a wound. See: *healing*.
  u. of granulations. A healing by third-intention with wound filling up with granulations.
  u., non-. Failure to unite, as a fractured bone.
  u., secondary. A healing by second-intention with adhesion of granulating surfaces.
  u., vicious. Union of ends of a broken bone in such a way as to cause deformity.

unioval (ū″nĭ-ō′văl) [L. *unus*, one, + *ovum*, egg]. Developed from 1 ovum, as identical twins.

unipara (ū-nĭp′ă-ră) [″ + *parere*, to bring forth]. A woman who has had only 1 child.

uniparous (ū-nĭp′ă-rŭs) [″ + *parere*, to bring forth]. 1. Having produced but 1 child. 2. Giving birth to 1 offspring at a time.

unipolar (ū″nĭ-pō′lar) [″ + *polus*, pole]. 1. Having, produced by, or acting by, only 1 pole, as a nerve cell, the branches of which project from only 1 side. 2. At 1 extremity of a cell only. See: *mono-terminal*.

unipotent (ū-nĭp′ō-tent) [″ + *potentia*, power]. Having power in 1 way only, as a cell capable of producing cells of only 1 order. Syn: *unipotential*.

unipotential (ū″nĭ-pō-tĕn′shăl) [″ + *potentia*, power]. Able in 1 way only, as able to give rise to cells of 1 order only; said of certain cells.

unit (ū′nĭt) [L. *unus*, one]. 1. One of anything. 2. A determined amount adopted as a standard of measurement.
  u., Allen-Doisy. See: *mouse and rat unit*.
  u., amboceptor. The smallest amount of amboceptor required in the presence of which a given quantity of red blood corpuscles will be dissolved by an excess of complement.
  u., Angström's. An internationally adopted unit of measurement of wave length, 1/10,000,000 of a millimeter, or 1/254,000,000 of an inch.
  u., antigen. Smallest quantity of an-

unit, antitoxic U-7 **uraniscoplasty**

tigen required to fix 1 unit of complement, preventing hemolysis.
u., antitoxic. The amt. of antitoxin needed to neutralize 100 times the least fatal dose of standard toxin that will kill a guinea pig weighing 250 Gm.
u., British thermal. The amt. of heat necessary to raise 1 pound of water at 39° F. one degree.
u., candlepower. SEE: *light unit.*
u. of capacity. Capacity of a condenser which gives a difference of potential of 1 volt when charged with 1 coulomb. SYN: *curie; farad; u., zlumen.*
u., cat. The amount of a drug per kg. of weight of animal just sufficient to kill a cat when injected intravenously slowly and continuously.
u., complement. Smallest quantity of complement required for hemolysis of a given amount of red blood corpuscles with 1 amboceptor unit present.
u., electrical. SEE: *ampere, ohm, volt, watt, etc.*
u., Hampson. An x-ray unit of measurement, ¼ the erythema dose.
u., hemolytic. The amount of inactivated immune serum which causes complete hemolysis of 1 cc. of a 5% emulsion of washed red blood corpuscles, in the presence of complement.
u., Holzknecht. An x-ray unit of measurement, 1/5 the erythema dose. ABBR: *H.*
u., immunizing. SEE: *antitoxic unit.*
u., international, of vitamin A. The vitamin activity of 0.6 mg. of the international standard carotene.
u., i., of vitamin B. The vitamin activity of 10 mg. of the international standard absorption product.
u., i., of vitamin C. The vitamin activity of 0.05 mg. of the international standard levo-ascorbic acid.
u., i., of vitamin D. The vitamin activity of 1 mg. of the international standard solution of irradiated ergosterol (0.025 mg. crystalline vitamin D).
u., Kienböck. Measurement of x-ray dosage, 1/10 the erythema dose.
u., light. A foot-candle, or the amount of light 1 ft. from a standard candle.
u., Mache. Unit of measurement of radium emanation. ABBR: *M. u.*
u., mouse. Least amount of estrus-producing hormone which induces, in a spayed mouse, a characteristic desquamation of the vaginal epithelium.
u., physical. SEE: *coulomb, erg, dyne, household measures, metric system, apothecaries' s., avoirdupois s., Troy weight.*
u., radiation. SEE: *Angström u., Mache u.*
u., rat. Greatest dilution of an estrus-producing hormone which will cause desquamation and cornification of vaginal epithelium during 1st day, if given to a mature spayed rat in 3 injections, 1 every 4 hours.
u., toxic. 1. Lowest dose of diphtheria toxin which in 3-4 days will kill a guinea pig weighing 250 Gm. 2. The amount of scarlet fever toxin that gives a positive reaction in susceptible persons when injected intradermally or no reaction in immune individuals.
u., X-radiation. The international unit is the quantity of X-radiation which, when the secondary electrons are fully utilized, and the wall effect of the chamber is avoided, produces in 1 cc. of atmospheric air at 0° C. and 76 cm. mercury pressure, such degree of conductivity that 1 electrostatic unit of charge is measured at saturation current. Designated by the small letter "r."
u., x-ray. SEE: *Kienböck u.*
unitarian (u-nĭ-tā'rĭ-an) [L. *unitarius*]. Composed of a single unit.
u. theory. That of Bordet that assumes only 1 alexin or complement in the serum of an animal, despite the fact that the alexins in different species differ.
unitary (ū'nĭ-tā-rĭ) [L. *unitarius*]. Relating to a unit. SYN: *unitarian.*
uniterminal (ū″nĭ-ter'mĭn-ăl) [L. *unus*, one, + *terminus*, end]. Having only 1 terminal. SEE: *monoterminal.*
univalent (ū″nĭ-vā'lĕnt, ū-nĭv'ă-lĕnt) [" + *valens*, to be powerful]. 1. Possessing the power of combining or replacing 1 atom of hydrogen. 2. Single, noting a chromosome which lacks or fails to unite with a synaptic mate.
universal (ū″nĭ-ver'săl) [L. *universalis*, combined into one whole]. General.
u. joint. One movable in any direction, as a ball and socket joint.
unofficial (ŭn-of-ish'ăl) [A.S. *un*, not, + L. *officialis*, doing work]. Not listed by the pharmacopeia.
unorganized (ŭn-or'găn-īzd) [" + L. *organizāre*, to form a structure]. 1. Not organized into an organic structure. 2. Without the characteristics of a living organism; inorganic.
u. ferment. A chemical ferment, one that is not a living organism. SYN: *enzyme.* SEE: *ferment.*
unsaturated (ŭn-săt'ū-rāt″ĕd) [" + L. *saturāre*, to sate]. 1. Capable of dissolving or absorbing to a greater degree. 2. Not combined to the greatest possible extent.
u. compound. One capable of combining with additional elements or compounds, as any member of the hydrocarbon series. SEE: *saturated compound.*
Unschuld's sign (oon'shoolt). Cramps frequently felt in the calves of the legs, an early sign in diabetes.
unsex (ŭn-sĕks′) [A.S. *un*, not, + L. *sexus*, sex]. To castrate; to spay or excise the ovaries.
unstriated (ŭn-strī'āt-ĕd) [" + *strĭātus*, striped]. Unstriped, as smooth muscle fiber.
unwell (ŭn-wĕl') [" + *wel*]. 1. Sick; ill; indisposed. 2. Menstruating.
upsiloid (ŭp'sĭ-loyd) [G. *upsilon*, letter U, + *eidos*, form]. Shaped like the letter U or V.
urachal (ū'ră-kăl) [G. *ourachos*, fetal urinary canal]. Relating to the urachus.
urachus (ū'răk-ŭs) [G. *ourachos*, fetal urinary canal]. Fibrous cord from the bladder to umbilicus, the remnant of part of the duct of the allantois of the embryo.
uracrasia (ū-ră-krā'sĭ-ă) [G. *ouron*, urine, + *akrasia*, incontinence]. 1. A disordered condition of urine. 2. Inability to retain the urine. SYN: *enuresis.*
uracratia (ū-ră-krā'shĭ-ă) [G. *ouron*, urine, + *akratia*, incontinence]. Incontinence of the urine. SYN: *enuresis.*
uragogue (ū'ră-gog) [" + *agogos*, leading]. Increasing the secretion of urine. SYN: *diuretic.*
uranalysis (ū″răn-ăl'ĭs-ĭs) [" + *ana*, apart, + *lysis*, a loosening]. Chemical analysis of the urine.
uranisconitis (ū-răn-ĭs″kon-ī'tĭs) [G. *ouraniskos*, palate, + *-itis*, inflammation]. Inflammation of the palate.
uraniscoplasty (ū-răn-ĭs'kŏ-plăs″tī) [" + *plassein*, to form]. Operation for repair

of cleft palate. SYN: *uranoplasty, uranorrhaphy.*
uraniscorrhaphy (ū-răn-ĭs-kor'ră-fĭ) [" + *rhaphē*, a seam]. Operation for suturing of a cleft palate. SYN: *uraniscoplasty.*
uraniscus (ū-răn-ĭs'kŭs) [G. *ouraniskos*, palate]. Palate, or roof of mouth.
uranism (ū'răn-ĭzm) [G. *ouranos*, heaven, + *-ismos*, condition]. Unnatural sex relations bet. males. SYN: *urningism, q.v.*
uranist (ū'răn-ĭst) [G. *ouranos*, heaven]. A male homosexual. SYN: *urning.**
uranium (ū-rā'nĭ-ŭm) [G. *ouranos*, sky]. SYMB: U. Primary radioactive element, the parent of radium and other radio-elements.
u. unit. A measure of radioactivity, uranium being taken as 1.
uranoplasty (ū'răn-ō-plăs"tĭ) [G. *ouranos*, palate, + *plassein*, to form]. Operation for cleft palate. SYN: *uraniscoplasty.*
uranorrhaphy (ū-răn-or'ră-fĭ) [" + *rhaphē*, a seam]. Operation for suture of a cleft palate. SYN: *uraniscorrhaphy.*
uranoschisis (ū-răn-ŏs'kĭs-ĭs) [" + *schisis*, a fissure]. Cleft palate.
uranostaphyloplasty (ū"răn-ō-stăf'ĭl-ō-plăs"tĭ) [" + *staphylē*, uvula, + *plassein*, to form]. Operation for correction of a defect of the soft and hard palates.
uranostaphylorrhaphy (ū"răn-ō-stăf-ĭl-or"ă-fĭ) [" + " + *rhaphē*, a seam]. Operation for repair of cleft of hard and soft palates.
uraroma (ū-ră-rō'mă) [G. *ouron*, urine, + *aroma*, spice]. Aromatic, spicy odor of the urine.
urarthritis (ū"rar-thrī'tĭs) [uric acid + G. *arthron*, joint, + *-itis*, inflammation]. Gouty inflammation of the joints.
urate (ū'rāt) [G. *ouron*, urine]. Combination of uric acid with a base; a salt of uric acid.
Urates in urine insignificant unless excessive. Urates can be dispersed by boiling the urine. SEE: *antiuratic.*
uratemia (ū"ră-tē'mĭ-ă) [" + *aima*, blood]. Urates, esp. sodium urate, in the blood.
uratic (ū-răt'ĭk) [G. *ouron*, urine]. Relating or made up of urates.
uratolysis (ū-ră-tŏl'ĭ-sĭs) [" + *lysis*, dissolution]. Decomposition of urates.
uratolytic (ū-ră-tō-lĭt'ĭk) [" + *lysis*, dissolution]. Capable of dissolving urates.
uratoma (ū-ră-tō'mă) [" + *ōma*, a mass]. A concretion composed of urates. SYN: *tophus.*
uratosis (ū-ră-tō'sĭs) [" + *-ōsis*, condition]. Morbid condition of the body, due to the deposit of urates in the tissues and circulating fluids.
uraturia (ū-ră-tū-rĭ'ă) [" + *ouron*, urine]. Excess of urates in the urine. SYN: *lithuria.*
urceiform (ûr-sē'ĭ-form) [L. *urceus*, pitcher, + *forma*, shape]. Pitcher shaped.
urea (ū-rē'ă) [G. *ouron*, urine]. The diamide of carbonic acid, a crystalline solid having the formula $CO(NH_2)_2$; found in blood, lymph, and urine. SYN: *carbamide.*
It is the chief nitrogenous constituent of urine and final product of protein metabolism in the body, and carrying off about 6/7 of the nitrogen excreted and 2 to 6% ammonium salts.
It is without odor and is colorless, appearing as white prismatic crystals, and forming salts with acids. Its excess is one of the causes of *uremia, q.v.* The amount excreted per day varies from 20-70 Gm., or about an ounce (32 Gm.) on the average. The amount of excreted urea is less on a low protein diet. From 8 to 10 Gm. per day may be excreted on a low protein diet of 50 Gm. per day.
USES: As a diuretic.
DOSAGE: 8-60 gr. (0.5-4.0 Gm.).
INCOMPATIBILITIES: Chloral hydrate, lead acetate.
INCREASED UREA: Observed in (a) fevers and loss of weight; (b) in increased protein intake; (c) following a large intake of water or beer; (d) during and after parturition.
DECREASED UREA: Observed in (a) reduced elimination; (b) low protein intake; (c) pregnancy; (d) gain in weight.
U. CONCENTRATION TEST: Performed for estimating renal efficiency.
It depends upon fact that when healthy kidneys are presented with an extra amount of urea in blood, they will excrete an equal amount of urea into urine.
Method: The patient urinates, and is then given a solution of 15 Gm. of urea in 2 or 3 oz. of water to drink. After 1 hr. patient urinates again, and also after the 2nd hr. The 2 specimens are then tested for the amount of urea, which should rise above 2%.
RS: *anazoturia, azoturia, urine, uremia.*
ureagenetic (ū-rē"ă-jĕn-ĕt'ĭk) [urea + G. *genesis*, production]. Pert. to or producing urea.
ureal (ū-rē'ăl) [urea from G. *ouron*, urine]. Relating to or containing urea.
ureameter (ū-rē-ăm'et-er) [urea + G. *metron*, a measure]. Device for determining amount of urea in urine.
ureametry (ū-rē-ăm'ĕt-rĭ) [urea + G. *metron*, a measure]. Determination of amt. of urea in urine.
ureapoiesis (ū-rē"ă-poy-ē'sĭs) [urea + G. *poiēsis*, formation]. Formation of urea.
urease (ū'rē-ās) [urea, from G. *ouron*, urine]. An enzyme which accelerates hydrolysis of urea into ammonium carbonate and hippuric acid into glycocoll and benzoic acid.
It is found in alkaline fermentation of urine, produced by many microörganisms, and is also found in seeds, as the soybean.
It is used in determining the amount of urea in blood or in urine.
urecchysis (ū-rĕk'ĭs-ĭs) [G. *ouron*, urine, + *ekchysis*, a pouring out]. Effusion of urine into areolar tissue.
uredema (ū-re-dē'mă) [" + *oidēma*, a swelling]. Urine in the subcutaneous tissues distending them.
uredo (ū-rē'dō) [L. *uredo*, a blight]. 1. Burning sensation in the skin. 2. Skin disorder marked by smooth, white elevations which itch severely. SYN: *hives, urticaria, q.v.*
ureide (ū'rē-īd) [urea from G. *ouron*, urine]. Any compound of urea in which acid radicals have taken the place of 1 or more of its hydrogen atoms.
urein(e (ū-rē'ĭn) [G. *ouron*, urine]. An oily substance isolated from urine supposed to cause symptoms of uremia.
urelcosis (ū-rĕl-kō'sĭs) [" + *elkōsis*, ulceration]. Ulceration of the urinary organs.
uremia (ū-rē'mĭ-ă) [G. *ouron*, urine, + *aima*, blood]. Toxic condition from urinary constituents in the blood.
ETIOL: Result of disturbed kidney metabolism seen in nephritis and due to suppression or deficient secretion of urine from any cause.
SYM: Nausea, vomiting, headache, dizziness, dimness of vision, coma or convulsions. urinous odor of breath, and

uremia, chronic perspiration. Stupor, stertorous respiration. No change in pupillary reaction; dry skin; hard, rapid pulse; elevated blood pressure; scanty urine containing casts and albumin. There is a reduction of urea, and presence of tube casts in uremic coma. SEE: *coma, uremic.*

u., chronic. Visual disturbance, headache, dizziness, anorexia, low heart action, vomiting, scanty urine, retention of nitrogenous products in the blood.

uremic (ū-rē'mĭk) [G. *ouron,* urine, + *aima,* blood]. Pert. to or caused by uremia.

uremide (ū're-mīd) [" + *aima,* blood]. The skin lesions of uric acid poisoning.

uremigenic (ū-rē-mĭ-jĕn'ĭk) [" + " + *gennan,* to produce]. Caused by uremia or producing it.

ureometer (ū"rē-ŏm'ĕt-ĕr) [G. *ouron,* urine, + *metron,* a measure]. Appliance used to determine the amt. of urea in urine. SYN: *ureameter.*

ureometry (ū-rē-ŏm'ĕt-rĭ) [" + *metron,* a measure]. Estimation of amt. of urea in urine.

ureopoiesis (ū-rē"ō-poy-ē'sĭs) [" + *poiēsis,* formation]. Formation of urea. SYN: *ureapoiesis.*

ureosecretory (ū-rē-ō-sē'kre-tōr-ĭ) [" + L. *secretus,* secreted]. Relating to the secretion of urea.

urerythrin (ūr-er'ĭ-thrĭn) [" + *erythros,* red]. A red pigment in the urine in rheumatic and certain other fevers. SYN: *uroerythrin.*

uresiesthesia, uresiesthesis (ū-rē"sĭ-ĕs-thē'-zĭ-ă, -sĭs) [G. *ourēsis,* urination, + *aisthēsis,* sensation]. The normal inclination to void urine.

uresis (ū-rē'sĭs) [G. *ourēsis,* urination]. The excretion of urine. SYN: *urination.*

ureter (u're-ter, ū-rē'tĕr) [G. *ourētēr,* ureter]. One of 2 tubes carrying urine from the kidney to the bladder, beginning with the pelvis of the kidney, and emptying into the base of the bladder. They are each from 12 to 16 inches long and about the size of a goose quill. The ureter has 3 coats, mucous, muscular, and fibrous.

RS: *autonephrectomy, kidney, urelcosis, "uret-"* words.

ureteralgia (ū-rē-ter-ăl'jĭ-ă) [G. *ourētēr,* ureter, + *algos,* pain]. Pain in the ureter.

uretercystoscope (ū-rē"tĕr-sĭs'tō-skōp) [" + *kystis,* bladder, + *skopein,* to examine]. A cystoscope combined with a ureteral catheter.

ureterectasis (ū-rē"-ter-ĕk'tă'sĭs) [" + *ektasis,* dilatation]. Dilatation of the ureter.

ureterectomy (ū-rē"tĕr-ĕk'tō-mĭ) [" + *ektomē,* excision]. Excision of a ureter.

ureteritis (ū-rē"-tĕr-ī'tĭs) [" + *-itis,* inflammation]. Inflammation of the ureters.

ureterocele (ū-rē"tĕr-ō-sēl) [" + *kēlē,* hernia]. Hernia of the ureter or hernia containing the ureter.

ureterocolostomy (ū-rē"tĕr-ō-kō-lŏs'tō-mĭ) [" + *kōlon,* colon, + *stoma,* passage]. The implantation of the ureter into the colon.

ureterocystoneostomy (ū-rē"tĕr-ō-sĭst"ō-nē-ŏs'tō-mĭ) [G. *ourētēr,* ureter, + *kystis,* bladder, + *neos,* bladder, + *stoma,* passage]. Formation of a passage bet. a ureter and the bladder. SYN: *ureterocystostomy, ureteroneocystostomy.*

ureterocystostomy (ū-rē"tĕr-ō-sĭs-tŏs'tō-mĭ) [" + *kystis,* bladder, + *stoma,* pas-

U-9 **ureterosigmoidostomy**

sage]. Artificial formation of a passage bet. a ureter and the bladder.

ureterodialysis (ū-rē"tĕr-ō-dī-ăl'ĭ-sĭs) [" + *dialysis,* a separation]. Rupture of one of the ureters.

ureteroenterostomy (ū-rē"tĕr-ō-ĕn-ter-ŏs'-tō-mĭ) [" + *enteron,* intestine, + *stoma,* passage]. Formation of a passage bet. a ureter and the intestine.

ureterography (ū-rē"tĕr-ŏg'ră-fĭ) [" + *graphein,* to write]. X-ray photography of the ureter after injection of some opaque substance into it.

ureterolith (ū-rē'ter-ō-lĭth) [" + *lithos,* stone]. A stone or calculus in the ureter.

ureterolithiasis (ū-rē"ter-ō-lĭth-ī'ăs-ĭs) [" + " + *-iasis,* condition]. Development of a calculus in the ureter.

ureterolithotomy (ū-rē"ter-ō-lĭth-ŏt'ō-mĭ) [" + *tomē,* a cutting]. Surgical incision for removal of a calculus from ureter.

ureterolysis (ū-rē"ter-ŏl'ĭ-sĭs) [G. *ourētēr,* ureter, + *lysis,* loosening]. 1. Rupture of the ureter. SYN: *ureterodialysis.* 2. Paralysis of the ureter. 3. The process of loosening adhesions around the ureter.

ureteroneocystostomy (ū-rē"ter-ō-nē"ō-sĭs-tŏs'tō-mĭ) [" + *neos,* new, + *kystis,* bladder, + *stoma,* passage]. Surgical formation of a passage bet. the ureter and the bladder. SYN: *ureterocystostomy.*

ureteroneopyelostomy (ū-rē"ter-ō-nē"ō-pī-ĕ-lŏs'tō-mĭ) [" + " + *pyelos,* pelvis, + *stoma,* passage]. Excision of a portion of the ureter with attachment of the ureter to a new aperture in the renal pelvis.

ureteronephrectomy (ū-rē"ter-o-nef-rĕk'-tō-mĭ) [" + *nephros,* kidney, + *ektomē,* excision]. Removal of a kidney and its ureter.

ureteropathy (ū-rē-ter-ŏp'ă-thĭ) [" + *pathos,* disease]. Any diseased condition of the ureter.

ureterophlegma (ū-rē"ter-ō-flĕg'mă) [" + *phlegma,* phlegm]. Mucous accumulation in the ureter.

ureteroplasty (ū-rē'ter-ō-plăs"tĭ) [" + *plassein,* to form]. Plastic surgery of the ureter.

ureteroproctostomy (ū-rē"ter-ō-prŏk-tŏs'-tō-mĭ) [G. *ourētēr,* ureter, + *prōktos,* anus, + *stoma,* passage]. Formation of a passage from the ureter to the anus.

ureteropyelitis (ū-rē"ter-ō-pī-ĕl-ī'tĭs) [" + *pyelos,* pelvis, + *-itis,* inflammation]. Inflammation of the pelvis of the kidney and a ureter.

ureteropyeloneostomy (ū-rē"ter-ō-pī'ĕl-ō-nē-ŏs'tō-mĭ) [" + " + *neos,* new, + *stoma,* passage]. Artificial formation of a new passage from pelvis of kidney to ureter. SYN: *ureteroneopyelostomy.*

ureteropyelonephritis (ū-rē"ter-ō-pī'ĕl-ō-nef-rī'tĭs) [" + " + *nephros,* kidney, + *-itis,* inflammation]. Inflammation of the renal pelvis and the ureter.

ureteropyeloplasty (ū-rē"ter-ō-pī'ĕl-o-plăs"tĭ) [" + " + *plassein,* to mold]. Plastic surgery of the ureter and renal pelvis.

ureteropyosis (ū-rē"tĕr-ō-pī-ō'sĭs) [" + *pyon,* pus, + *-ōsis,* condition]. Suppurative inflammation within a ureter.

ureterorrhagia (ū-rē"ter-or-rā'jĭ-ă) [" + *-rrhagia,* from *rhēgnunai,* to burst forth]. Hemorrhage from the ureter.

ureterorrhaphy (ū-rē"ter-or'ră-fĭ) [G. *ourētēr,* ureter, + *rhaphē,* a seam]. Suture of the ureter, as for fistula.

ureterosigmoidostomy (ū-rē"ter-ō-sĭg-

ureterostenosis   U-10   **urethritis, specific**

moyd-ŏs'tō-mĭ) [" + *sigma*, letter S, + *eidos*, shape, + *stoma*, passage]. Surgical implantation of the ureter into the sigmoid flexure.

ureterostenosis (ū-rē″ter-ō-stĕn-ō'sĭs) [" + *stenōsis*, a narrowing]. Stricture of a ureter.

ureterostomy (ū-rē″ter-ŏs'tō-mĭ) [" + *stoma*, passage]. Formation of a permanent fistula for drainage of a ureter.

ureterotomy (ū-rē″ter-ŏt'ō-mĭ) [" + *tomē*, a cutting]. Incision or surgery of the ureter.

ureteroureterostomy (ū-rē″ter-ō-ū-rē″ter-ŏs'tō-mĭ) [G. *ourētēr*, ureter, + *ourētēr*, ureter, + *stoma*, passage]. 1. Formation of a connection from 1 ureter to the other. 2. Reëstablishment of a passage bet. the ends of a divided ureter.

ureterovaginal (ū-rē″ter-ō-vǎj'ĭ-nǎl) [" + L. *vagina*, sheath]. Relating to a ureter and the vagina, noting a fistula connecting them.

ureterovesical (ū-rē″ter-ō-vĕs'ĭ-kǎl) [" + L. *vesica*, bladder]. Pert. to a connection bet. the ureter and the bladder.

ureterovesicostomy (ū-rē″ter-ō-vĕs″ĭ-kŏs'-tō-mĭ) [" + " + G. *stoma*, passage]. Reimplantation of a ureter into the bladder.

urethra (ū-rē'thrǎ) [G. *ourēthra*, urethra]. A membranous canal for the external discharge of urine from the bladder to the *meatus urinarius* and in the male also for an outlet for the seminal fluids. It is from 8 to 10 inches long in the male and 1½ inches long in the female. It has 3 coats, mucous, submucous, and muscular.

In the male it is divided into 3 portions, *prostatic*, where it passes through the prostate gland; *membranous*, a short, narrow section, and *cavernous* or *spongy*, which lies in the corpus spongiosum.

    u. **mulie'bris.** BNA. The female urethra.

    u. **viri'lis.** BNA. The male urethra.

urethra, words pert. to: aerourethroscopy; anaspadias; ankylurethria; atreturethria; blennurethria; bulb; bulbourethral glands; corpus spongiosum; gleet; habenula urethralis; hypospadias; ligament, Carcasonne's; meatus urinarius; Skene's glands; urelcosis; "urethr-" words.

urethral (ū-rē'thrăl) [G. *ourēthra*, urethra]. Relating to the urethra.

    u. **caruncle.** Small, fleshy growth from wall of the urethra. Very sensitive.

urethralgia (ū-rē-thrǎl'jĭ-ǎ) [G. *ourēthra*, urethra, + *algos*, pain]. Urethral pain; pain in the urethra.

urethratresia (ū-rē-thrǎ-trē'zĭ-ǎ) [" + *atrēsis*, imperforation]. Occlusion, or imperforation of the urethra.

urethrectomy (ū-rē-thrĕk'tō-mĭ) [" + *ektomē*, excision]. Surgical excision of the urethra or part of it.

urethremphraxis (ū-rē-thrĕm-frǎk'sĭs) [" + *emphraxis*, obstruction]. Urethral obstruction. SYN: *urethrophraxis*.

urethreurynter (ū-rē-thrū-rĭn'ter) [" + *eurynein*, to dilate]. Appliance for dilating the urethra.

urethrism, urethrismus (ū'rē-thrĭzm, ū″rē-thrĭz'mŭs) [" + *-ismos*, condition]. Irritability or spasm of the urethra.

urethritis (ū-re-thrī'tĭs) [G. *ourēthra*, urethra, + *-itis*, inflammation]. Inflammation of the urethra.

    u., **anterior.** Inflammation of that portion of the urethra ant. to the ant. layer of the triangular ligament.

    u., **gonococcal.** U. caused by gonococcus.

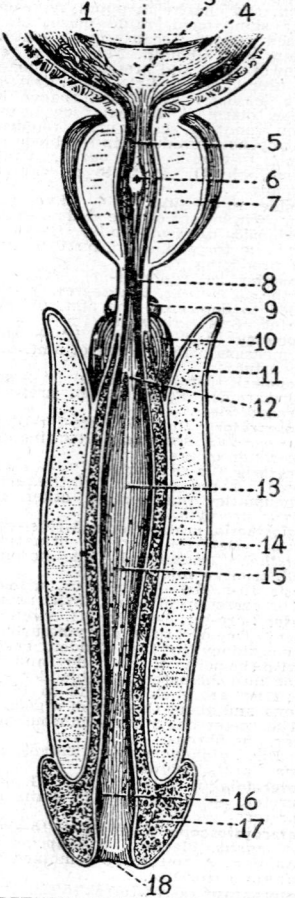

URETHRA, INTERIOR OF MALE, SHOWING THE FLOOR

1. Bell's muscle. 2. Interureteric ridge. 3. Internal trigone. 4. Left ureteric opening. 5. Crest. 6. Opening of utricle. 7. Prostate gland in section (showing prostatic portion of urethra). 8. Membranous portion of urethra. 9. Bulbourethral gland of left side. 10. Left half of bulb of urethra. 11. Left crus penis. 12. Openings of ducts of bulbourethral glands. 13. Spongy portion of urethra. 14. Left corpus cavernosum. 15. Urethral glands and lacunae. 16. Fossa terminalis. 17. Left half of glans penis. 18 Orifice of urethra.

    u., **posterior.** Inflammation of membranous and prostatic portions of the urethra.

    u., **simple.** Catarrhal inflammation of the urethra. SYN: *blennorrhea*.

    u., **specific.** Urethritis occurring in gonorrhea.

urethritis venerea

u. vene′rea. SEE: *urethritis, specific.*
urethro- [G.]. Combining form meaning *urethra.*
urethrocele (ū-rē′thrō-sēl) [G. *ourēthra,* urethra, + *kēlē,* hernia]. 1. Pouchlike protrusion of the urethral wall in the female. 2. Thickening of connective tissue around the urethra in the female.
urethrocystitis (ū-rē″thrō-sĭs-tī′tĭs) [" + *kystis,* bladder, + *-itis,* inflammation]. Inflammation of urethra and bladder.
urethrography (ū-rē-thrŏg′rȧ-fĭ) [" + *graphein,* to write]. X-ray photography of the urethra, after the injection of an opaque medium.
urethrometer (ū-rē-thrŏm′et-er) [" + *metron,* a measure]. Instrument for measuring diameter of urethra or lumen of a stricture.
urethropenile (ū-rē″thrō-pē′nĭl) [" + L. *penis,* penis]. Relating to the urethra and penis.
urethroperineal (ū-rē″thrō-pĕr-ĭ-nē′ȧl) [" + *perinaion,* perineum]. Relating to the urethra and perineum.
urethroperineoscrotal (ū-rē″thrō-pĕr-ĭ-nē″-ō-skrō′tȧl) [" + " + L. *scrotum,* pouch]. Relating to the urethra, perineum, and scrotum.
urethrophraxis (ū-rē-thrō-frȧks′ĭs) [G. *ourēthra,* urethra, + *phrassein,* to obstruct]. Urethral obstruction. SYN: *urethremphraxis.*
urethrophyma (ū-rē-thrō-fī′mȧ) [" + *phyma,* growth]. A neoplasm in the urethra.
urethroplasty (ū-rē′thrō-plȧs″tĭ) [" + *plassein,* to mold]. Reparative surgery of the urethra.
urethrorectal (ū-rē″thrō-rĕk′tȧl) [" + L. *rectus,* straight]. Relating to the urethra and the rectum.
urethrorrhagia (ū-rē″thror-ā′jĭ-ȧ) [" + *-rrhagia,* from *rhēgnunai,* to burst forth]. Hemorrhage from urethra.
urethrorrhaphy (ū-rē-thror′ȧf-ĭ) [" + *rhaphē,* a seam]. Suture of the urethra, as a urethral fistula.
urethrorrhea (ū-rē″thror-ē′ȧ) [" + *rhoia,* a flow]. Morbid discharge from the urethra.
urethroscope (ū-rē′thrō-skōp) [G. *ourēthra,* urethra, + *skopein,* to examine]. Device for examining interior of urethra.
urethroscopic (ū-rē″thrō-skŏp′ĭk) [" + *skopein,* to examine]. Relating to the urethroscope or urethroscopy.
urethroscopy (ū-rē-thrŏs′kō-pĭ) [" + *skopein,* to examine]. An examination of the mucous membrane of the urethra with a urethroscope.
urethrospasm (ū-rē′thrō-spȧzm) [" + *spasmos,* a spasm]. Spasmodic stricture of the urethra.
urethrostaxis (ū-rē″thrō-stȧks′ĭs) [" + *staxis,* a dropping]. Oozing of blood from the urethral mucous membrane.
urethrostenosis (ū-rē″thrō-sten-ō′sĭs) [" + *stenōsis,* a narrowing]. Stricture of the urethra.
urethrostomy (ū-rē-thrŏs′tō-mĭ) [" + *stoma,* opening]. Formation of a permanent fistula opening into the urethra by perineal section and fixation of membranous urethra in perineum.
urethrotome (ū-rē′thrō-tōm) [G. *ourēthra,* urethra, + *tomē,* a cutting]. An instrument for incision of urethral stricture.
urethrotomy (ū-rē-thrŏt′ō-mĭ) [" + *tomē,* a cutting]. Incision of a urethral stricture.
urethrovaginal (ū-rē″thrō-vȧj′ĭ-nȧl) [" + L. *vagina,* sheath]. Pert. to the urethra and vagina.

uridrosis

uretic (ū-ret′ĭk) [G. *ourētikos,* pert. to urine]. 1. Pert. to urine. 2. Pert. to or stimulating the flow of urine. 3. That which stimulates the flow of the urine. SYN: *diuretic.*
urginin (ŭr′jĭn-ĭn). A proprietary mixture of 2 glucosides derived from squill. USES: As a cardiac stimulant similar to digitalis. DOSAGE: From 1-3 mg. per day, depending on the severity.
uric (ū′rĭk) [G. *ouron,* urine]. Of or pert. to urine.
 u. acid. A crystalline acid in the urine, a metabolism product of nuclein. It is a common constituent of urinary and renal calculi, and gouty concretions. OUTPUT: Bet. 0.5 and 1 Gm. per day on ordinary mixed diet. Uric acid must be excreted, as it cannot be destroyed within the body. Kidney "stones" are concretions of uric acid crystals. Eating of vegetables increases the power of dissolving uric acid, as do the base-forming elements.
 INCREASED ELIMINATION: Observed in: (1) Ingestion of proteins; (2) gout; (3) leukemia; (4) acute articular rheumatism; (5) after exercise, and (6) the ingestion of nitrogenous foods.
 DECREASED ELIMINATION: Observed in: (a) Nephritis; (b) chlorosis; (c) lead poisoning; (d) protein-free diet. Other primary products are the presence of chlorides, phosphates, sulfates, sulfur, indican, oxalates, creatinine, cystine, and hippuric acid. SEE: *urea.*
 u. a., endogenous. Uric acid derived from purines undergoing metabolism from the nucleoprotein of body tissues.
 u. a., exogenous. Uric acid derived from those purines from food made up of free purines and nucleoproteins.
 SEE: *urate, uratosis, uraturia.*
uricacidemia (ū″rĭk-ȧs-ĭd-ē′mĭ-ȧ) [G. *ouron,* urine, + L. *acidus,* sour, + G. *aima,* blood]. Excess uric acid in the blood and the condition produced thereby.
uricaciduria (ū″rĭk-ȧs-ĭd-ū′rĭ-ȧ) [" + " + G. *ouron,* urine]. Excessive amount of uric acid in the urine.
uricase (ū′rĭ-kāz) [G. *ouron,* urine, + *ase,* enzyme]. A hydrolytic enzyme capable of changing uric acid into allantoin.
uricemia (ū-rĭ-sē′mĭ-ȧ) [" + *aima,* blood]. Uric acid in the blood. SYN: *uricacidemia.*
uricocholia (ū″rĭk-ō-kō′lĭ-ȧ) [" + *cholē,* bile]. Uric acid in the bile.
uricolysis (ū-rĭk-ŏl′ĭs-ĭs) [" + *lysis,* dissolution]. The decomposition of uric acid.
uricolytic (ū″rĭk-ō-lĭt′ĭk) [" + *lysis,* dissolution]. Decomposing uric acid into urea.
 u. index. The amt. of uric acid converted into allantoin.
uricometer (ū-rĭk-ŏm′ē-tēr) [" + *metron,* a measure]. Apparatus for quantitative estimation of uric acid in the urine.
uricopoiesis (ū″rĭk-ō-poy-ē′sĭs) [" + *poiēsis,* formation]. The development of uric acid.
uricoxydase (ū″rĭk-oks′ĭ-dās) [G. *ouron,* urine, + *oxys,* sharp, + *ase,* enzyme]. An enzyme capable of oxidizing uric acid.
uridrosis (ū-rĭd-rō′sĭs) [G. *ouron,* urine, + *idrōsis,* a sweating]. The presence of urea in the sweat.
 Evaporation may show white scales, the crystals of urinary solids.

uridrosis crystallina   U-12   **urine**

   u. crystalli'na. White powder of uric acid deposited on the skin.
uriesthesis (ū-re-ĕs-thē'sĭs) [" + *aisthēsis*, sensation]. Normal desire to void urine.
urina (ū-rī'nă) [L.]. Urine.
   u. cibi. Urine voided after a full meal.
   u. cruenta. Bloody urine.
   u. galactodes. Urine of a milky color.
   u. hysterica. Watery, pale urine following hysteria.
   u. jumentosa. Cloudy urine.
   u. potus. U. voided after drinking.
   u. sanguinis. U. on arising in morning uninfluenced by food or drink.

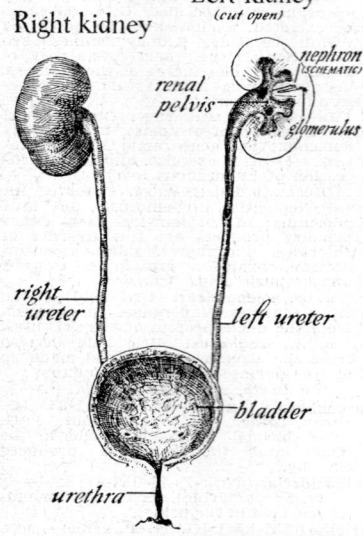

ENTIRE URINARY TRACT
Copyright 1939, *R. N.—A Journal for Nurses.*

urinal (ū'rĭn-ăl) [L. *urina*, urine]. 1. A vessel for the urine. 2. A toilet for the male consisting of a vessel attached to a wall.
urinalysis (ū-rĭn-ăl'ĭs-ĭs) [L. *urina*, urine, + G. *ana*, apart, + *lysis*, a loosening]. Analysis of the urine.
urinary (ū'rĭn-a"rĭ) [L. *urina*, urine]. Pert. to, secreting, or containing urine.
   u. bladder. Receptacle for urine before it is voided. SEE: *bladder.*
   u. calculi. Concretions formed in the urinary passages.
   They contain urates, calcium, oxalate, calcium carbonate, phosphates, and cystine.
   u. casts. Casts of kidney tubules passed in the urine.
   u. organs. The structures concerned with the secretion and excretion of urinary products, consisting of the 2 *kidneys*, 2 *ureters*, the *bladder*, and the *urethra.*
   u. pigments. Urochrome, urobilin, uroerythrin, and hematoporphyrin.
   u. reflex. Desire to void resulting from accumulation of urine in bladder.

   u. sediments. Substances found in standing urine, *i. e.*, water, phosphates, uric acid, calcium oxalate, calcium carbonate, calcium phosphate, magnesium and ammonium phosphate; more rarely, cystine, tyrosine, xanthine, hippuric acid, hematoidin.
   u. stammering. Temporary interruptions in voiding urine.
   u. stuttering. Same as *u. stammering.*
   u. system. Kidneys, ureters, bladder, and urethra.
urinate (ū'rĭn-āt) [L. *urināre*, to discharge urine]. To discharge the urine.
urination (ū-rĭn-ā'shŭn) [L. *urinātio*, a discharging of urine]. The act of voiding urine.
   Although this act is somewhat under voluntary control, it is accomplished chiefly by the action of involuntary muscles. The musculus sphincter vesicae relaxes, while the general musculature of the wall of the urinary bladder contracts to force out its contents.
   INCREASED FREQUENCY: Seen in polyuria; nervous excitement; irritation of bladder, urethra, or urinary meatus; disease of spinal cord; enlarged prostate in male; pregnancy in female; beer drinking; interstitial nephritis; diabetes; phimosis; adenoids, and intestinal worms in children.
   DECREASED FREQUENCY: After sweating, diarrhea, or bleeding; in anuria, oliguria, uremia, brain disease, drug poisoning, coma, and parenchymatous nephritis. SEE: *urine.*
urination, words pert. to: aconuresis, acraturesis, anisuria, bacilluria, bladder, bradyuria, catheterization, chaudepisse, diuresis, diuretic, dysuria, enuresis, kidney, melanuria, micturate, micturition, nocturia, nycturia, oliguria, polyuria, strangury, uracratia, urea, "ureč-" words, uric acid, "urin-" words, void.
urine (ū'rĭn) [L. *urina*, from G. *ouron*, urine]. The fluid secreted from the blood by the kidneys, stored in the bladder, and discharged, usually voluntarily, by the urethra.
   It is conveyed to the bladder by 2 ureters from the kidneys. In health, urine is of amber color, slightly acid reaction (about 30%), and it has a peculiar odor, with a bitter, saline taste, frequently depositing a precipitate of phosphates when fresh, but esp. on standing, and having a specific gravity that varies bet. 1.001 and 1.026.
   The greater the amt. excreted, the lower is the specific gravity. The normal amt. of nonprotein nitrogen is from 25-35 mg. per 100 cc. of blood.
   The daily output is equally variable, being adapted to the amt. of water taken in, and to the amt. lost by evaporation from the respiratory and cutaneous surfaces.
   In addition to urea (35 grams excreted per day, the most important end product

Normal Amount Voided and Specific Gravity		
Time	cc.	Specific Gravity
8–10 A. M.	153	1.016
10–12 A. M.	156	1.019
12– 2 P. M.	194	1.012
2– 4 P. M.	260	1.014
4– 6 P. M.	114	1.020
6– 8 P. M.	238	1.010
8– 9 A. M.	375	1.020
	1490	

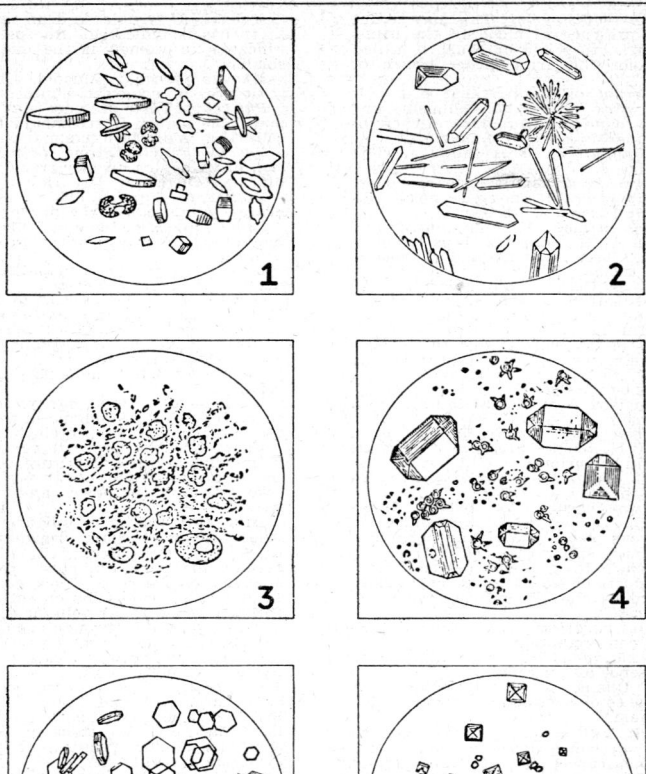

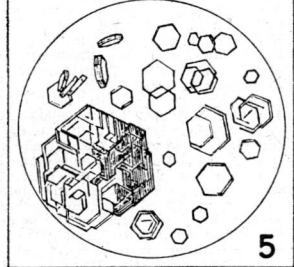

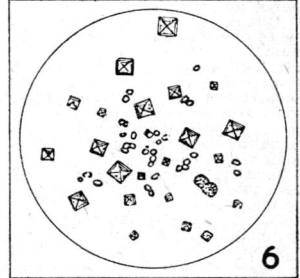

URINARY PRODUCTS

1. Various forms of uric acid crystals. 2. Crystals of hippuric acid. 3. Mucus deposited from urine. 4. Urinary sediment of triple phosphates (large, prismatic crystals) and urate of ammonium, from urine which had undergone alkaline fermentation. 5. Crystals of cystin. 6. Crystals of calcium oxalate.

of protein metabolism), urine contains inorganic salts, pigments, and other end products of protein and mineral metabolism.

Diagnosis

COLOR OF URINE: Normal urine is amber color. Its color is imparted by urobilin,* a pigment mainly derived from bilirubin* in the bile. This pigment is found in more than normal quantities in fever, and it may be indicative of blood destruction. The effect of food and medication must be considered before concluding that the color of the urine reflects a pathological condition.

Black: Melanuria. Malignant pigmented tumor, melanotic cancer or carbolic acid poisoning.

Bile-colored: Seen in jaundice.

Blue: This may result from methylene blue or the presence of indigo.

Colorless urine: This is known as achromaturia.

Milky urine: May be due to chyluria, lipuria, or pus.

Orange-red urine: It may indicate the presence of pyridine dyes.

Pale urine: This indicates an excess of water and contra in high fevers. It is found in conditions causing polyuria.

Red or reddish color: This may be due to the presence of blood in the urine, hematuria, to senna or rhubarb, which may color the urine either brown or orange.

CONDITION OF URINE: *Acid urine*: It shows pink or pinkish sediment, and may be found in tuberculosis of the kidneys, acidosis, and pyelonephritis.

Alkaline urine: This shows a white sediment.

Bacteria in urine: It appears cloudy.

Bloody urine: It shows a smoky sediment, and is reddish-brown.

Pus in urine: This is mucoid and shows a white sediment. It is found in cystitis, severe vomiting, and obstructive gastric ulcers.

ODOR OF URINE: *Ammoniacal*: This may result from decomposition products.

Aromatic urine: This is the odor of a normal urine.

Fecal odor: This is due to fistulous communication bet. the intestinal and urinary tracts.

Fishy odor: Cystitis.

New-mown hay odor: Indicative of diabetes.

Overripe apple odor: Indicative of acetonuria, or the presence of acetone bodies in the urine.

Violet odor: This may be caused by turpentine.

URINARY PRODUCTS IN DISEASE: *Albumin*: Due to nephritis and inflammation of mucous membrane of any portion of the urinary apparatus.

Acetone: Its presence represents the by-products of excessive fat metabolism excreted by the kidneys and known as ketonuria.

Animal parasites: Rare, found as result of contamination.

Bacteria: They have no significance in the absence of pus cells.

Bile: Bile in the urine indicates retention due to obstruction of flow above the duodenum.

Blood: Indicates hemorrhagic nephritis, calculi, congestion of a kidney, renal carcinoma, tuberculosis of kidney, chronic infections, and certain drugs.

Casts: These indicate renal disease. A few hyaline casts in the aged denote slight damage to the kidneys. Casts are found in large numbers in nephritis. The less acute the disease, the finer are the granular casts.

Crystals: Acid urine produces crystals, calcium oxalate, and urates; alkaline urine, ammonium biurate and phosphates. Crystals have little significance, excepting leucine and tyrosine crystals which indicate yellow atrophy of the liver, or phosphorus poisoning, or other serious liver damage.

Cylindroids: They have no special significance.

Diacetic acid: Indicates deficient carbohydrate metabolism of an advanced stage. It is preceded by the presence of acetone.

Epithelial cells (squamous): If in large numbers from urinary bladder and ureters they indicate inflammation of these parts; *renal epithelial cells of kidney*: Serious damage to the same.

Fat droplets: Indicate fatty degeneration of kidneys and lipemia.

Indican: It has small significance but is seen in intestinal putrefaction and constipation.

Lipoids, double refractile: Epstein's lipoidal nephrosis.

Mucus: If visible and in quantity, urethritis is indicated. No special significance in women if the quantity is small.

Mucous threads: Mucoid, ribbonlike structures of no great significance.

Pus cells: Their presence may be normal if not many. If accompanied by red cells, they indicate inflammation.

Red blood cells: Stones or inflammation of kidney or urinary tract. No significance during menstruation of women.

Sediment: Pinkish due to excess of urates, white, caused by phosphates.

Sugar (glucose): Denotes faulty carbohydrate metabolism as seen in diabetes mellitus,.

Urea:* This is the principal end product of protein metabolism.

Yeasts and molds: Result of contamination. SEE: *urinary conditions*.

EXCRETION: *Increased in*: Fevers, esp. if weight is lost, after pregnancy, during parturition, after the intake of large quantities of liquid and after protein intake.

Diminished in: Pregnancy, convalescence with gain in weight, in disease of the liver, and in low protein intake.

URINARY CONDITIONS: *Difficult urine*: Found in urethral stricture, enlarged prostate, atony and impairment of the bladder's muscular power, and in gonorrhea.

DIAG: *Diminished u.* (oliguria): Valvular disease of heart, degeneration of cardiac muscles. Scanty in all fevers, accompanies acute and chronic and parenchymatous nephritis, obstruction of return venous circulation of kidney, thrombosis of renal vein or inf. vena cava, loss of fluids through hemorrhages, vomiting or diarrhea, obstruction or pressure upon ureter, lead poisoning, hysteria, or melancholia.

Frequent u: Excess of urea (azoturia) or of uric acid and urates (lithuria). Reflex of renal calculus in ureter; pyelitis. May precede attack of ague, accompany angina pectoris or prove a symptom of sunstroke.

Strangury: Painful and spasmodic. May be indicative of cystitis, neuralgia, tuberculosis, cancer or ulceration of bladder, urethritis, urethral stricture, hypertrophied, cancerous or inflamed prostate, prolapsus of uterus, pelvic peritonitis and abscess, metritis, cancer of cervix, dysmenorrhea, vesical tenesmus. Pain and burning often caused by the concentrated or acid urine. May be a symptom of acute nephritis.

Incontinence: (a) Paralysis or relaxation of sphincters or (b) contraction of longitudinal muscular layer of bladder. Paralysis of both a and b, retention, incontinence and dribbling are results. All forms of coma, shock, sunstroke and some forms of insanity, typhoid, typhus. Injuries to spinal cord and tumors of same and lesions; transverse myelitis, spinal meningitis, locomotor ataxia, paralysis. Reflex excitability of nervous system. Local irritation. Cystitis, phimosis, vesical calculus, meatus contracted, ascarides, diabetic or too concentrated urine. Relaxation of vesical sphincters. Hydrocyanic acid poisoning.

Increased u. (polyuria): May be indicative of chronic interstitial nephritis, diabetes (mellitus or insipidus), amyloid disease of kidney; reabsorption of effusions, functional disease of nervous system, as hysteria, neurasthenia, migraine, etc. Persistent in bulbar, cerebellar and

Significance of Changes in Urine

Normal	Abnormal	Significance
1000-1500 cc. (96% H_2O)		Depends upon water and fluid foods consumed, exercise, temperature, kidney function, etc.
	High (polyuria)	Diabetes mellitus, diabetes insipidus, nervous diseases, certain types of chronic nephritis (kidney disorder), diuretics (drugs as caffeine, calomel, digitalis, causing increased urinary excretion).
	Low (oliguria)	Acute nephritis, heart disease, fevers, eclampsia, diarrhea, vomiting.
	None (anuria)	Uremia (urinary substances in blood), acute nephritis, metal poisoning, e. g., due to bichloride of mercury.

Color

Normal	Abnormal	Significance
Yellow to amber		Depends upon concentration of pigment (urochrome).
	Pale	Diabetes insipidus, granular kidney, due to a very dilute urine.
	Milky	Fat globules, pus corpuscles in genitourinary infections.
	Reddish	Blood pigments, drugs, or food pigments.
	Greenish	Bile pigment, associated with jaundice.
	Brown-black	Poisoning (mercury, lead, phenol), hemorrhages.

Transparency

Normal	Abnormal	Significance
Clear		No significance.
Cloudy on standing		Precipitation of mucin from urinary tract. Not pathological.
Turbid		Precipitation of calcium phosphate. Not pathological.
	Milky	Presence of fat globules. Pathological.
	Turbid	Presence of pus as result of inflammation of urinary tract. Pathological.

Odor

Normal	Abnormal	Significance
Faintly aromatic		No significance.
	Pleasant (sweet)	Acetone, associated with diabetes mellitus.
	Unpleasant	Decomposition or ingestion of certain drugs or foods.

Specific Gravity

Normal	Abnormal	Significance
1.015 to 1.025 sp. gr.		Ordinarily, sp. gr. inversely proportional to volume.
	Low	Dilution, if volume is large, otherwise nephritis.
	High	Concentrated if volume is small; otherwise if volume is large and light colored, diabetes mellitus. Acute nephritis.

Acidity

Normal	Abnormal	Significance
Acid (slight)		Diet of acid-forming foods (meats, eggs, prunes, wheat, etc.) overbalancing the base-forming foods (vegetables and fruits).
	High acidity	Acidosis, diabetes mellitus, many pathological disorders (fevers, starvation).
	Alkaline	Putrefying bacteria change urea into ammonium carbonate. Infection or ingestion of alkaline compounds.

Urine: Examination of[1]

Table Giving the More Important Characters of the Urine in Some of the Commoner Diseases.

	Names of Diseases	Condition of Urine
I.	Gastric Catarrh	Quantity normal; high colored; sp. gr. often raised; acid. Urates, oxalates, or phosphates may be deposited.
II.	Jaundice	Urine greenish-brown in color, frothy; acid reaction; contains bile. Quantity and sp. gr. usually normal.
III.	Heart and Lung Disease	Urine often diminished, dark in color, acid; high sp. gr. Urates deposited; albumin often present.
IV.	Fevers, General and Special	Quantity nearly always diminished, high colored, usually acid; high sp. gr.; urates. May be albumin, blood and tube casts. Urea usually increased in amount.
V.	Diabetes Mellitus	Quantity increased, pale, usually acid, sweet odor; high sp. gr. Sugar in greater or less quantity. Sometimes diacetic acid and(or) acetone amount of urea usually increased.
VI.	Acute Nephritis	Quantity diminished. Urine may be suppressed. Sp. gr. at first raised, then lowered. Albumen; sometimes blood, tube casts; sometimes urates, urea diminished.
VII.	Chronic Nephritis	Urine increased in quantity, pale; sp. gr. low. Albumin in small amount, or absent; no blood; a few tube casts.
VIII.	Chronic Cystitis	Quantity not usually altered, turbid, often alkaline and offensive. Mucus and pus (muco-pus) often present.
IX.	Acute Gout	Quantity usually diminished, high colored; sp. gr. raised. Abundant deposit of urates.

[1] From *Faber's Nurses Encyclopedia*.

spinal tumors, locomotor ataxia and meningitis.
Obstructive *u*: Result of occlusion of one or both ureters.
Painful urination: Dysuria.* Vesical tenesmus. There is a persistent desire to urinate.
Retention:* Almost same diseases and injuries of cord producing incontinence. All forms of coma, typhoid, in peritonitis, and hysteria, atony, prostatic enlargement; urethral stricture, urethritis, cystitis or tumors of bladder or calculus in urethra.
Suppression (anuria): Failure of kidneys to secrete the urine or failure to reach the bladder if secreted may be found in acute nephritis or congestion, renal abscess, last stages of chronic nephritis. Inhalation of ether, lead, phosphorus, cantharides or turpentine poisoning, may occur in connection with Asiatic cholera, cholera infantum or cholera morbus, gastrointestinal perforations, shock or collapse. Typhoid or yellow fever, pernicious malaria, acute yellow atrophy of liver, hysteria.
SEDIMENT, HOW TO OBTAIN: The examination should be made quickly after urine is voided by centrifuging for 3 minutes, or by placing some urine in a glass with a conical base, allowing organic matter to settle by gravity. If sediment from a 24-hour specimen is to be examined, entire urine should be shaken vigorously before portions are placed in either the centrifuge tube or the sediment glass.
urine, words pert. to: acathectic; acetone; a. bodies; a., tests for; acetonuria; achromaturia; acidaminuria; acromaturia; adrenaluria; albiduria; albinuria; albuminaturia; albuminorrhea; albuminuria; albumosuria; alkalinuria; alkaliretic; alkaptone; alkaptonuria; allantoinuria; allotriuria; alloxuria; Almen's test; aminosuria; ammoniuria; amylosuria; amyluria; anisuria; antidiuresis; antidiuretic; anuresis; anuria; arabinosuria; ardor urinae; azoturia; baruria; Bence-Jones albumose; Benedict's test; bilirubinuria; bladder, urinary; b. stammering; b. percussion; blennuria; blood, test for; brick dust; calcariuria; carbohydraturia; carboluria; carbonuria; cast; ceramuria; cerebrosuria; chlorides, test for; chloriduria; chloruremia; chloruria; cholerytrin; choleuria; choluria; chondroituria; chromaturia; chyluria; clap threads; diacetic acid test; epithelium; erythruria; Esbach's method; galactosuria; galacturia; glucose; glycosuria; Haines formula; Heller's test; hemoglobinuria; hippuria; hyaline casts; hydruria; incontinence; ischuria; jumentous; ketonuria; ketosis; kidney; lactosuria; lipuria; lithuria; lithium; melanuria; mucus; myosinuria; oliguresis; oxaluria; pentosuria; polyduria; pus; pyuria; residual; residuum; retention; Rothera's test; secretion; tyrosinuria; uraturia; urea; urechysis; uredema; uremia; ureter; uric acid urinalysis; "uro-" words.
urinemia (ū-rĭn-ē'mĭ-ă) [L. *urina*, urine, + G. *aima*, blood]. Contamination of the blood with urinary constituents. SYN: *uremia, q. v.*
uriniferous (ū-rĭn-ĭf'ĕr-ŭs) [" + *ferre*, to bear]. Carrying urine.
u. tubules. Small tubes of the kidneys for passage of kidney products.
uriniparous (ū-rĭn-ĭp'ăr-ŭs) [" + *parere*, to bear]. Producing or secreting urine.
urinogenital (ū"rĭn-ō-jĕn'ĭt-ăl) [" + *genitalia*, genitals]. Pert. to the genital and urinary organs. SYN: *urogenital.*
urinogenous (ū"rĭn-ŏj'ĕn-ŭs) [" + G. *gennan*, to produce]. 1. Producing urine. 2. Originating in urine. SYN: *urogenous.*
urinoglucosometer (ū"rĭn-ō-glū"kŏs-ŏm'ĕ-tĕr) [" + G. *glukus*, sweet, + *metron*, a measure]. Apparatus for estimating amt. of glucose in the urine.
urinology (ū-rĭn-ŏl'ō-jĭ) [" + G. *logos*, study]. Scientific study of the urine. SYN: *urology.*
urinoma (ū"rĭn-ō'mă) [L. *urina*, urine, + G. *-ōma*, mass]. A cyst containing urine.
urinometer (ū-rĭn-ŏm'ĕt-ĕr) [" + G. *metron*, a measure]. Device for determining urine's specific gravity.
urinometry (ū"rĭn-ŏm'ĕt-rĭ) [" + G. *metron*, a measure]. Determination of specific gravity of the urine.
urinophil (ū'rĭn-ō-fĭl) [" + G. *philein*, to love]. Capable of existing in the urine.
urinoscopy (ū-rĭn-ŏs'kō-pĭ) [" + G. *skopein*, to examine]. Examination of the urine.
urinose, urinous (ū'rĭn-ōs, ū'rĭn-ŭs) [L. *urina*, urine]. Having the characteristics of, or containing urine.
urisolvent (ū"rĭ-sŏl'vĕnt) [" + *solvens*, dissolving]. Dissolving uric acid or causing it to be dissolved.
urning (oorn'ĭng) [Ger.]. One exhibiting and conscious of sexual inversion. SYN: *homosexual, uranist.* SEE: *urningism.*
urningism, urnism (oorn'ĭng-ĭzm, oorn'ĭzm) [Ger.]. Perversion in which sexual desire is only for one of the same sex. SYN: *lesbianism, sapphism, tribadism, amor lesbicus, homosexualism, q. v.*
Lesbianism is a term applied only to the female sex. The opposite sex has no interest for urnings, but seems to inhibit the normal sexual act. Sexual hyperesthesia and paraesthesia are often present. Passionate love and deification of the object of affection are common. Such perversion may be congenital, but in many instances it is the result of acquired habits. SEE: *uranism.*
uro- [G.]. Combining form meaning *pert. to urine.*
uroacidimeter (ū"rō-ăs-ĭ-dĭm'ĕ-tĕr) [G. *ouron*, urine, + L. *acidus*, sour, + G. *metron*, a measure]. An apparatus for measuring the degree of acidity of the urine.
Urobacillus (ū"rō-bă-sĭl'ŭs) [" + L. *bacillus*, a little rod]. A rod-shaped organism found in urine or decomposing urine.
urobilin (ū"rō-bī'lĭn) [" + L. *bilis*, bile]. A derivative of the bile pigments of yellow color found in urine.
It may be indicative of the activity of blood destruction and is found in more than normal quantities in fever.
u. jaundice. J. said to be result of urobilin in the blood.
urobilinemia (ū"rō-bĭ"lĭn-ē'mĭ-ă) [" + G. *aima*, blood]. Urobilin in blood.
urobilinicterus (ū"rō-bĭ-lĭn-ĭk'tĕr-ŭs) [" + G. *ikteros*, jaundice]. Jaundice resulting from urobilinemia. SYN: *urobilin-jaundice.*
urobilinogen (ū-rō-bĭ-lĭn'ō-jĕn) [" + " + G. *gennan*, to produce]. A chromogen in urine which gives rise to urobilin on oxidation.
urobilinogenemia (ū"rō-bĭ"lĭn-ō-jĕn-ē'mĭ-ă) [" + " + " + *aima*, blood]. Urobilinogen in the blood.
urobilinuria (ū"rō-bĭ"lĭn-ū'rĭ-ă) [" + " + G. *ouron*, urine]. Excess of urobilin in the urine.
urocele (ū'rō-sēl) [G. *ouron*, urine, +

urocheras   U-18   **uropoietic**

kēlē, hernia]. Effusion of urine into the scrotum.

urocheras (ū-rŏk'ĕr-ăs) [" + *cheras*, gravel]. Sand in the urine. SYN: *uropsammus*.

urochesia (u-rō-kē'zĭ-ă) [" + *chezein*, to defecate]. A discharge of urine through the anus.

urochrome (ū'rō-krōm) [" + *chrōma*, color]. A yellow coloring matter in urine, assumed to be closely related to urobilin, which probably gives urine its color.

uroclepsia (ū-rō-klĕp'sĭ-ă) [" + *kleptein*, to steal]. Involuntary and unconscious discharge of urine.

urocrisia (ū'rō-krĭz'ĭ-ă) [" + *krinein*, to judge]. 1. A diagnosis by inspection of the urine. 2. Change (generally favorable) which supervenes in the crisis of a disease accompanied by copious urination.

urocrisis (ū-rŏk'rĭs-ĭs) [" + *krisis*, crisis]. 1. A crisis marked by excessive urination. 2. Examination of the urine. 3. Pain in bladder in locomotor ataxia.

urocriterion (ū"rō-krī-tē'rĭ-ŏn) [G. *ouron*, urine, + *kriterion*, a test]. A symptom observed in the inspection of urine which indicates the diagnosis.

urocyanogen (ū"rō-sī-ăn'ō-jĕn) [" + *kyanos*, blue, + *gennan*, to produce]. A blue pigment in urine, esp. in cholera patients.

urocyanosis (ū"rō-sī-ăn-ō'sĭs) [" + " + *-ōsis*, condition]. Blue discoloration of the urine. SYN: *indicanuria*.

urocyst (ū'rō-sĭst) [" + *kystis*, bladder]. The urinary bladder.

urocystitis (ū"rō-sĭs-tī'tĭs) [" + " + *-itis*, inflammation]. Inflammation of the urinary bladder.

urodialysis (ū"rō-dī-ăl'ĭs-ĭs) [" + *dialysis*, a separation]. A partial and temporary suppression of the urine.

    u. neonatorum. U. when occurring in children.

    u. senum. Urodialysis in the aged.

uroedema (ū"rō-ē-dē'mă) [" + *oidēma*, a swelling]. Extravasation of urine distending the tissues. SYN: *uredema*.

uroerythrin (ū-rō-ĕr'ĭth-rĭn) [G. *ouron* + *erythros*, red]. A reddish pigment of urine with acid reaction found in rheumatism and other diseases.

urofuscohematin (ū"rō-fŭs"kō-hĕm'ăt-ĭn) [" + L. *fuscus*, brown, + G. *haima*, blood]. A red-brown pigment in urine in some diseases.

urogaster (ū"rō-găs'tĕr) [" + *gaster*, belly]. The urinary intestine or urinary tract of the embryo.

urogenital (ū"rō-jĕn'ĭ-tăl) [" + L. *genitalia*, genitals]. Pert. to the urinary organs and the genitalia.

    u. ducts. Embryonic ducts of the mesonephron; the wolffian duct and duct of Müller.

    u. sinus. Ant. part of the cloaca into which the urogenital ducts open in the embryo.

urogenous (ū-rŏj'ĕn-ŭs) [" + *gennan*, to produce]. 1. Producing urine. 2. Originating in urine.

uroglaucin (ū"rō-glaw'sĭn) [" + *glaukos*, green]. Indigo blue, a pigment sometimes occurring in the urine, assumed to be result of chromogen oxidation, as in *scarlatina*.

urogram (ū'rō-grăm) [" + *gramma*, a mark]. An x-ray photograph of any part of the urinary tract.

urography (ū-rŏg'ră-fĭ) [G. *ouron*, urine, + *graphein*, to write]. Roentgenography of any part of the urinary tract, after introduction of an opaque medium.

urogravimeter (ū"rō-grăv-ĭm'ĕt-ĕr) [" + L. *gravis*, heavy, + G. *metron*, a measure]. Apparatus for estimating sp. gr. of urine. SYN: *urinometer*.

urohematin (ū"rō-hĕm'ăt-ĭn) [" + *haima, haimat-*, blood]. Pigment in urine, considered as identical with hematin,* which alters color of urine in proportion to degree of oxidation.

urohematoporphyrin (ū"rō-hĕm"ăt-ō-por'-fĭr-ĭn) [" + " + *porphyra*, purple]. Iron-free hematin in urine when hemolysis occurs.

urolith (ū'rō-lĭth) [" + *lithos*, stone]. A concretion in the urine.

urolithiasis (ū"rō-lĭth-ī'ăs-ĭs) [" + " + *iasis*, condition]. Formation of urinary calculi. SEE: *calculus, renal*.

urolithology (ū"rō-lĭth-ŏl'ō-jĭ) [" + " + *logos*, a study]. Science dealing with urinary calculi.

urologic (ū-rō-lŏj'ĭk) [G. *ouron*, urine, + *logos*, study]. Pert. to urology.

urologist (ū-rŏl'ō-jĭst) [" + *logos*, a study]. One who specializes in the practice of urology.

urology (ū-rŏl'ō-jĭ) [" + *logos*, a study]. The science dealing with the urine and diseases of the urogenital organs.

urolutein (ū"rō-lū'tē-ĭn) [" + L. *luteus*, yellow]. A yellow pigment seen in the urine.

uromancy (ū'rō-măn-sĭ) [" + *manteia*, divination]. Diagnosis of disease by inspection of urine.

urometer (ū-rŏm'ĕt-ĕr) [" + *metron*, a measure]. Instrument for determining specific gravity of urine. SYN: *urinometer*.

uroncus (ū-rŏn'kŭs) [" + *ogkos*, a mass]. A swelling or cyst containing urine.

uronephrosis (ū"rō-nĕf-rō'sĭs) [G. *ouron*, urine, + *nephros*, kidney, + *-ōsis*, condition]. Dilatation of renal structures from obstruction of renal pelvis and tubules with urine. SYN: *hydronephrosis*.

uronology (ū-rŏn-ŏl'ō-jĭ) [" + *logos*, a study]. The science of urine and genitourinary diseases. SYN: *urology*.

urononcometry (ū"rŏn-ŏn-kŏm'ĕ-trĭ) [" + *ogkos*, mass, + *metron*, a measure]. Measurement of amt. of urine voided in 24 hours.

uronophile (ū-rŏn'ō-fīl) [" + *philein*, to love]. Developing best in a culture containing urine, noting a microörganism.

uropathy (ū-rŏp'ă-thĭ) [" + *pathos*, disease]. Any disease affecting the urinary tract.

    u., obstructive. Any disease resulting from obstruction of the urinary tract.

uropenia (ū-rō-pē'nĭ-ă) [" + *penia*, a lack]. Lack of urinary secretion.

urophanic (ū-rō-făn'ĭk) [" + *phainein*, to appear]. Appearing in the urine.

urophein, urophaein (ū"rō-fē'ĭn) [G. *ouron*, urine, + *phaios*, gray]. Gray pigment in urine said to cause its characteristic odor.

urophosphometer (ū"rō-fŏs-fŏm'ĕ-tĕr) [" + L. *phosphas*, phosphorus]. Device for estimating amt. of phosphorus in the urine.

uroplania (ū"rō-plā'nĭ-ă) [" + *planē*, a wandering]. Condition in which urine is present or discharged from parts other than the urinary organs.

uropoiesis ((ū"rō-poy-ē'sĭs) [" + *poiēsis*, production]. Secretion of urine by the kidneys.

uropoietic (ū"rō-poy-ĕt-ĭk) [" + *poiein*, to

uropsammus form]. Concerned in the formation of urine, or uropoiesis.
uropsammus (ū″rō-săm'ŭs) [" + *psammos*, sand]. Gravel in urine.
uroptysis (ū-rŏp'tĭs-ĭs) [" + *ptysis*, a spitting]. Urination through the mouth.
uropyonephrosis (ū″rō-pī-ō-nĕf-rō'sĭs) [G. *ouron*, urine, + *pyon*, pus, + *nephros*, kidney, + *-ōsis*, condition]. Urine and pus in the renal pelvis.
uropyoureter (ū″rō-pī″ō-ū-rē'tĕr) [" + + *ourētēr*, ureter]. Mass of urine and pus in the ureter.
urorosein (ū″rō-rō'zē-ĭn) [" + L. *roseus*, rosy]. A rose-colored pigment in urine, which is increased in certain diseases. SYN: *urorrhodin*.
urorrhagia (ū-ror-ā'jĭ-ă) [" + *-rrhagia*, a flowing]. Excessive secretion of urine. SYN: *polyuria*.
urorrhea (ū-ror-ē'ă) [" + *rhoia*, a flow]. Involuntary flow of urine. SYN: *enuresis*.
urorrhodin (ū-rō-rō'dĭn) [" + *rhodon*, rose]. A rose-colored pigment in the urine. SYN: *urorosein, q.v.*
urorrhodinogen (ū-rō-rō-dĭn″ō-jĕn) [" + + *gennan*, to produce]. A chromogen of the urine which, when decomposed, forms urorrhodin.
urorubin (ū-rō-rū'bĭn) [G. *ouron*, urine, + L. *ruber*, red]. A red pigment obtained from urine, by treatment with hydrochloric acid.
urorubrohematin (ū″rō-rū″brō-hĕm'ă-tĭn) [" + " + G. *haima, haimat-*, blood]. A reddish pigment occasionally found in the urine in some chronic diseases.
urosaccharometry (ū″rō-săk-ăr-ŏm'ĕ-trĭ) [" + *sakcharon*, sugar, + *metron*, a measure]. Determination of amt. of sugar in the urine.
urosacin (ū-rō'sa-sĭn) [G. *ouron*, urine]. A red pigment in the urine. SYN: *urorrhodin*.
uroscheocele (ū-rŏs'kē-ō-sēl) [G. *ouron*, urine, + *oscheon*, scrotum, + *kēlē*, mass]. Swelling of scrotum from extravasation of urine into scrotal sac. SYN: *urocele*.
uroschesis (ū-rŏs'kĕs-ĭs) [" + *schesis*, a holding]. 1. Suppression of urine. 2. Retention of the urine.
uroscopy (ū-rŏs'kō-pĭ) [" + *skopein*, to examine]. 1. Examination of the urine. 2. Diagnosis by examination of the urine.
uroselectan (ū″rō-sĕ-lĕk'tăn) [G. *ouron*, urine]. A pyridine derivative for intravenous pyelography.
urosemiology (ū″rō-sē-mĭ-ŏl'ō-jĭ) [" + *sēmeion*, sign, + *logos*, study]. Examination of the urine as an aid to diagnosis.
urosepsin (ū-rō-sĕp'sĭn) [" + *sēpsis*, putrefaction]. A septic poison formed from decomposition of urine in the tissues.
urosepsis (ū-rō-sĕp'sĭs) [" + *sēpsis*, putrefaction]. Septic poisoning due to retention and absorption of urinary products in the tissues.
urosin (ū'rō-sĭn) [G. *ouron*, urine]. A proprietary uric acid solvent.
urosis (ū-rō'sĭs) [" + *-ōsis*, disease]. Any disease of the urinary organs.
urospectrin (ū-rō-spĕk'trĭn) [" + L. *spectrum*, image]. A pigment derived from normal urine when shaken with acetic ether.
urostealith (ū″rō-stē'ă-lĭth) [" + *stear*, fat, + *lithos*, stone]. A fatty substance in some urinary calculi.
urotherapy (ū″rō-thĕr'ă-pĭ) [" + *therapeia*, treatment]. Therapeutic subcutaneous injection of the patient's urine.
urotoxia (ū-rō-tŏks'ĭ-ă) [" + *toxikon*, poison]. 1. Urinary systemic poisoning. 2. Toxicity of the urine. 3. The toxic unit of urine which is amt. needed to kill 1 kilogram of living matter. SYN: *urotoxy*.
urotoxic (ū″-rō-tŏks'ĭk) [" + *toxikon*, poison]. Pert. to poisonous substances in the urine or poisoning by urine.
u. **coefficient**. Number of urotoxias (in 24 hr.) formed by a person, about 0.4 for each kilogram of body weight.
urotoxicity (ū″rō-tŏks-ĭs'ĭ-tĭ) [G. *ouron*, urine, + *toxikon*, poison]. The toxic character of the urine.
urotoxin (ū″rō-tŏks'ĭn) [" + *toxikon*, poison]. The toxic principle of the urine.
urotoxy (ū'rō-tŏks″ĭ) [" + *toxikon*, poison]. Amount of urine required to kill an animal weighing 1 kilogram; unit of toxicity of urine. SYN: *urotoxia*.
urotropin (ū-rŏt'rō-pĭn). A proprietary uric acid solvent.
DOSAGE: 5 gr. (0.3 Gm.).
uroureter (ū″rō-ū-rē'tĕr, -ū-rē'tĕr) [" + *ourētēr*, ureter]. Distention of the ureter with urine, due to stricture or obstruction. SYN: *hydrometer*.
urous (ū'rŭs) [G. *ouron*, urine]. Having the nature of urine.
uroxanthin (ū″rō-zăn'thĭn) [" + *xanthos*, yellow]. Yellow coloring matter of the urine; an indigo-forming substance.
uroxin (ū-rŏk'sĭn) [" + *oxys*, sharp]. A derivative of alloxan.*
urticaria (ŭr-tĭ-kā'rĭ-ă) [L. *urtica*, nettle]. An inflammatory affection, characterized by the eruption of pale, evanescent wheals, which are associated with severe itching. SYN: *hives, nettle rash*. SEE: *allergy*.
ETIOL: Contact with an ext. irritant, as the nettle rash, physical agents, foods, insect bites, serum sickness, pollens, drugs, neurogenic factors.
SYM: Sudden general eruption of papules or wheals associated with intense itching. Each lesion lasts a few hours, and is succeeded by new ones in other places.
TREATMENT: Subcutaneous administration of ½ to 1 cc. of adrenalin, or epinephrine in oil. In chronic cases, daily injection of 1 Gm. of sodium or calcium thiosulfate or 10 cc. of strontium bromide solution. Locally, carbolized lotions and lukewarm baths containing a handful of bran or oatmeal in a bag, or ½ cup of cornstarch and ½ cup of baking soda. Alcohol sponges.
u. **bullo'sa**. Eruption of temporary vesicles with infusion of fluid under the epidermis.
u. **confer'ta**. U. with lesions in groups.
u. **endem'ica,** *u.* **epidem'ica**. U. caused by caterpillar hairs.
u. **facti'tia**. Wheals following slight irritation of the skin. SYN: *autographism*. [SYN: *angioneurotic edema*.
u. **gigan'tea**. U. with very large wheals.
u. **haemorrhagica**. U. with lesions infiltrated with blood.
u. **maculo'sa**. A chronic form of u. with red-colored lesions.
u. **mariti'ma**. U. due to salt water bathing.
u. **medicamento'sa**. U. due to certain drugs.
u. **papulosa**. In this form the wheal is followed by a lingering papule which is attended by considerable itching. Most commonly observed in debilitated children.
PROG: Unfavorable. In some cases tends to become chronic.

TREATMENT: Remove cause. If from gastric irritation, treat the stomach. When there is constipation, a saline laxative may prove very efficient. To allay itching and burning, apply hot water to affected parts, or give warm bath and dry without rubbing. Suitable diet. Regular habits.
u. per′stans. U. in which wheals remain.
u. pigmentosa. An eruption of wheals which are itchy and persistent and which leave behind a yellowish or brownish pigmentation. Observed in young children. Runs a chronic course of months or years.
TREATMENT: In general, constitutional. Search out and remove exciting cause. In case of foodstuff, an emetic if it has not passed the stomach, otherwise a saline cathartic or sometimes a mercurial purge followed by a saline. In chronic types isolation of offending cause is more difficult. Remove focal infection, keep elimination open. Sodium bicarbonate, locally, ephedrine, calcium, pilocarpine, etc., have been employed. Locally, antipruritics.
u. subcuta′nea. U. without wheals but persistent itching.
u. vesiculo′sa. Same as *u. bullosa*.
urticarial, urticarious (ŭr-tĭk-ā-rī-ăl, ŭr-tĭk-ā′rĭ-ŭs) [L. *urtica*, a nettle]. Pert. to urticaria.
urtication (ŭr-tĭk-ā′shŭn) [L. *urtica*, a nettle]. 1. Flogging of a part with nettles to induce counterirritation. 2. Burning or itching sensation. 3. Eruption of itching wheals. SYN: *urticaria*.
U. S. P., U. S. Phar. Abbr. for *United States Pharmacopeia*.
U. S. P. H. S. Abbr. for *United States Public Health Service*.
ustilaginism (ŭs-tĭl-ăj′ĭn-ĭzm) [L. *ustulatus*, scorched]. Poisoning caused by Ustilago, a moldlike fungus.
ustion (ŭs′chŭn) [L. *ustio*, a burning]. 1. Cauterization with actual cautery. 2. Incineration.
ustulation (ŭs-tū-lā′shŭn) [L. *ustulāre*, to scorch]. Roasting, parching, or drying of a moist substance.
ustus (ŭs′tŭs) [L.]. Burned. SEE: *calcination*.
uteralgia (ū-tĕr-ăl′jĭ-ă) [L. *uterus*, womb, + G. *algos*, pain]. Uterine pain.
uterectomy (ū-tĕr-ĕk′tō-mĭ) [" + G. *ektomē*, excision]. Removal of uterus through the abdomen or vagina. SYN: *hysterectomy, q.v.*
uterine (ū′tĕr-ĭn, -ĭn) [L. *uterinus*, pert. to the womb]. Pert. to the uterus.
u. cake. The placenta.
u. glands. The tubular glands in the endometrium.
u. milk. A milky, white substance bet. the gravid uterus and the placental villi.
u. souffle (soof′fl). Vascular sound in the pregnant uterus heard with stethoscope.
u. tubes. Small tubes attached to either side of the uterus, and leading from the region of the ovary. SYN: *fallopian tubes*.
uteritis (ū-tĕr-ī′tĭs) [L. *uterus*, womb, + G. *-itis*, inflammation]. Inflammation of the uterus.
uteroabdominal (ū″tĕr-ō-ăb-dŏm′ĭn-ăl) [" + *abdominalis*, pert. to abdomen]. Pert. to both the uterus and abdomen.
uterocele (ū-tĕr′ō-sēl) [" + G. *kēlē*, hernia]. Hernia containing the uterus.
uterocervical (ū″tĕr-ō-sĕr′vĭ-kăl) [" + *cervix*, neck]. Relating to the uterus and the cervix.
uterocystostomy (ū″tĕr-ō-sĭs-tŏs′tō-mĭ) [" + G. *kystis*, bladder, + *stoma*, mouth]. Formation of a passage bet. the uterine cervix and the bladder.
uterofixation (ū″tĕr-ō-fĭks-ā′shŭn) [" + *fīxātio*, a fixing]. Fixation of a displaced uterus. SYN: *hysteropexy*.
uterogenic (ū″tĕr-ō-jĕn′ĭk) [" + G. *gennan*, to produce]. Developed in the uterus.
uterogestation (ū-tĕr-ō-jĕs-tā′shŭn) [L. *uterus*, womb, + *gestātio*, a carrying]. Pregnancy in the uterus; normal pregnancy.
uterography (ū″tĕr-ŏg′ră-fī) [" + G. *graphein*, to write]. Roentgenography of the uterus.
uterolith (ū′tĕr-ō-lĭth) [" + G. *lithos*, stone]. A uterine concretion.
uterologist (ū″tĕr-ŏl′ō-jĭst) [" + G. *logos*, a study]. One who specializes in the practice of gynecology and obstetrics.
uterology (ū-tĕr-ŏl′ō-jĭ) [" + G. *logos*, a study]. Gynecology combined with obstetrics.
uteromania (ū″tĕr-ō-mā′nĭ-ă) [" + G. *mania*, madness]. Pathological sexual desire in a woman. SYN: *nymphomania*.
uterometer (ū″tĕr-ŏm′ĕt-ĕr) [" + G. *metron*, a measure]. Device for measuring the uterus and for determining its position.
uteroövarian (ū″tĕr-ō-ō-vā′rĭ-ăn) [L. *uterus*, womb, + *ovarium*, ovary]. Relating to the uterus and ovary.
uteropexia, uteropexy (ū″tĕr-ō-pĕks′ĭ-ă, ū′tĕr-ō-pĕks-ĭ) [" + G. *pexis*, fixation]. Fixation of the uterus to the abdominal wall. SYN: *hysteropexy*.
uteroplacental (ū″tĕr-ō-plă-sen′tăl) [" + *placenta*, a flat cake]. Relating to the placenta and uterus.
uteroplasty (ū″tĕr-ō-plăs′tĭ) [" + G. *plassein*, to form]. Reparative operation upon the uterus.
uterosacral (ū″tĕr-ō-sā′krăl) [" + *sacralis*, pert. to the sacrum]. Relating to the uterus and sacrum.
uterosalpingography (ū″tĕr-ō-săl-pĭng-ŏg′-ră-fī) [" + G. *salpigx*, tube, + *graphein*, to write]. Visualization of the interior of the uterus and fallopian tubes by x-ray.
uterosclerosis (ū″tĕr-ō-sklē-rō′sĭs) [" + G. *sklērōsis*, a hardening]. Uterine sclerosis.
uteroscope (ū′tĕr-ō-skōp) [L. *uterus*, womb, + G. *skopein*, to examine]. Device for viewing the uterine cavity.
uterotome (ū′tĕr-ō-tōm) [" + G. *tomē*, a cutting]. An instrument used for uterotomy. SYN: *hysterotome*.
uterotomy (ū-tĕr-ŏt′ō-mĭ) [" + G. *tomē*, a cutting]. Incisions of the uterus.
uterotonic (ū″tĕr-ō-tŏn′ĭk) [" + G. *tonos*, tone]. Giving muscular tone to the uterus.
uterotractor (ū″tĕr-ō-trăk′tor) [" + *tractor*, a drawer]. An instrument for making traction on the cervix uteri.
uterotubal (ū″tĕr-ō-tū′băl) [" + *tuba*, tube]. Relating to the uterus and the oviducts.
uterovaginal (ū″tĕr-ō-văj′ĭ-năl) [" + *vagina*, sheath]. Relating to the uterus and vagina.
uterovesical (ū″tĕr-ō-vĕs′ĭ-kăl) [" + *vesica*, bladder]. Relating to the uterus and bladder.
uterus (ū′tĕr-ŭs) [L. *uterus*, womb]. The organ of gestation. SYN: *womb*.
ANAT: A muscular, hollow, pear-shaped structure of the female. It is partly

covered by peritoneum, the cavity lined by mucous membrane which is the *endometrium*.

Fully developed uterus is approximately 3 inches long, 2 inches wide, and 1 inch in thickness, situated in the pelvis. The uterus is partly abdominal and partly vaginal.

The organ is divided into a body, or upper part, and cervix, or lower part. The upper part of the body is called the *fundus* and the ends of the fundus to which the tubes are attached are called the *cornual ends*. The cavity of the uterus is triangular in shape, with the base of the triangle in the fundal portion. The canal of the cervix is long and narrow, and is constricted at the upper end by the internal os and at the lower end by the external os.

The largest portion of the uterus is made up of musculature which is longitudinal and circular. The outer covering of the uterus is peritoneum with the exception of that part upon which the bladder rests and the vaginal portion of the cervix. The inner lining of the body of the uterus varies in form and histological structure with the period of life in which it is studied, the prepuberty stage, the actively menstruating stage and the menopausal stage each having its own characteristics.

The uterus is situated in the midpelvis approximately halfway bet. the sacrum and the *symphysis pubis*. It is supported in this position by the 2 broad ligaments, the round ligaments, the uterosacral ligaments, and the ligaments attached to bladder. The uterus is normally anteflexed. The blood supply of the uterus is derived from the uterine and ovarian arteries.

POSITIONS: *Anteflexion*: Bending forward. *Anteversion*: Forward displacement of fundus towards pubis, while cervix is tilted up towards sacrum. *Retroflexion*: Bending backward, at junction of body and cervix. *Retroversion*: Inclination backward with retention of normal curve; opposed to anteversion.

AUSCULTATION: After the 4th month of gestation if uterus contains a living fetus 3 distinct sounds may be heard. *Fetal heart sounds*: Consist of a succession of short, rapid, double pulsations varying in frequency from 120 to 140 per minute. First sound is short, feeble, and obscure, while the 2nd, the one usually heard, is loud and distinct; sounds like ticking of a watch wrapped in a napkin. Sound is usually transmitted over space of 3 or 4 inches square. Location is determined by position of fetus. Generally, when maximum intensity is on level of, or above umbilicus, a breech presentation; when low down in front on left side, 1st position; low in front on right side, in 2nd position. During labor examinations, if made, should be bet. uterine contractions. In protracted labors is of value in indicating the time for manual or instrumental interference to save life of child.

Sounds: Irregularity and feebleness of sound are the most threatening to the life of the child.

Funic souffle: A sound usually heard at a point quite remote from the uterine bruit. It is short, blowing in character, and corresponds in pregnancy with the fetal pulsation. Supposed to depend upon obstruction to the transmission of blood through the umbilical arteries, as from twirling or knotting of the funis, or from ext. pressure. Is not a constant or even frequent sound, the conditions of production being rarely met with.

Uterine bruit: This sound is single, intermitting and in character a combination of blowing and hissing sounds. Increases in intensity up to the period of labor. Believed to depend upon rapid passage of blood from the arteries into the distended venous sinuses of the uterus. Synchronous with maternal pulse, subject to same variations, and is always heard before the pulsations of the fetal heart; area over which is audible varies, greatest point of intensity in median line a little above pubes.

After 5th month, at latest and inferior borders of uterus, next at fundus. Not a positive proof of pregnancy, as is sometimes heard in uterine and ovarian tumors. Does not prove fetus alive, as it is sometimes heard after its death.

PALPATION: During pregnancy: In 3rd month, if walls of abdomen are not too thick, by placing patient upon her back, with head raised and thighs flexed, and pressing points of fingers gently downward and backward above the pubes, a hard, round tumor will be found on the median line, rising out of the pelvis. In 2 or 4 weeks later the increase is much more strongly marked. As pregnancy advances, the tumor loses more and more of its hardness, and becomes more and more elastic, like a cyst filled with water. In doubtful cases where decided enlargement of abdomen is present, exploration *per vaginum* becomes of great importance.

"Touch," or really internal palpation, signifies the means by which knowledge is obtained of internal conditions by vaginal or anal examination with the finger. By vaginal touch may be able to diagnose the stage of gestation, stage of parturition, or whether the woman is in that state, the progress of labor, the presentation and position of the child, the position of uterus—tenderness or prolapse of the ovaries, etc. May be practiced with the woman standing, lying on either side, or back. The sensation of the tip of cervix of unimpregnated uterus to the touch is like that imparted to the finger by touching the tip of the nose, firm and cartilaginous; of the impregnated, like that of touching the lips. Feels soft like velvet, but deeper, beyond the softness, is a hardness, as of board.

PERCUSSION: Unimpregnated uterus is inaccessible to touch externally, or to percussion. In pregnancy at end of 2nd month a dull sound on percussion just above pubes indicates the enlarging uterus; later, as uterus increases in volume and rises into abdomen, able, by oval tumor felt, in hypogastrium and by circumscribed area of dullness corresponding to situation of the tumor, to establish strong presumptive evidence of pregnancy. This presumption becomes strengthened if the area of dullness increases with the regularity proper to gestation. Palpation and percussion, however, are not sufficient to determine whether the enlargement is due to pregnancy or to some morbid deposit in its wall or cavity, as fibrous tumors, etc. After the 5th month both these methods are inf. to auscultation.

PROLAPSE: Rigid cleanliness, regular elimination, frequent douching.

INVERSION: Raise foot of table or bed;

apply ext. heat. Hot vaginal douches if immediate reduction not possible. Maintain proper posture in bed.

U., TUMORS OF: (a) May cause sterility, abortion, or obstruct labor. (b) May become infected or twisted on their attachments. (c) Myomata possible, but not common in young women. (d) Fibroids common beyond 30 and in negro race. (e) Subserous tumors do not affect pregnancy. May bar labor. (f) May disappear following labor. (g) Interstitial and submucous type may interfere with pregnancy and produce abortion.

EFFECTS UPON LABOR: (a) Usually have no effects. (b) If low, may cause malpresentation or impossible labor. (c) Labor pains weak and inefficient. (d) Often severe pains and rupture of uterus. (e) Submucous tumors may protrude before or after birth. (f) Placenta may be retained. (g) Tumor may be infected postpartum. (h) Knee-chest position helps patient, if tumor is in pelvis. (i) If in fundus, delivery is through vagina; if not, cesarean section may be needed. (j) Control hemorrhage by packing.

UTERUS, CANCER OF: (a) Extremely rare in pregnancy; growth increases with pregnancy. (b) May produce sterility or abortion, hemorrhage, sepsis. (c) Detected by size, intermittent bleeding, purulent discharge.

UTERUS, RUPTURE OF, IN PREGNANCY: (a) Rare but serious. (b) Etiology: weakness of uterine wall, or obstruction. (c) Scars may be cause of weakness of wall. (d) May be spontaneous or traumatic. (e) Child and amniotic sac may be expelled into peritoneal cavity. (f) Spontaneous rupture may occur without warning. (g) Abdominal pains, shock, hemorrhage may occur. (h) Child easily palpated. (i) Active movements of child which cease with death ensuing. (j) Obstruction usually precedes symptoms. (k) Combat shock and hemorrhage; salt solutions, etc.

SUBINVOLUTION: The lack of involution of the uterus following childbirth. It is manifested by a large uterus and a con-

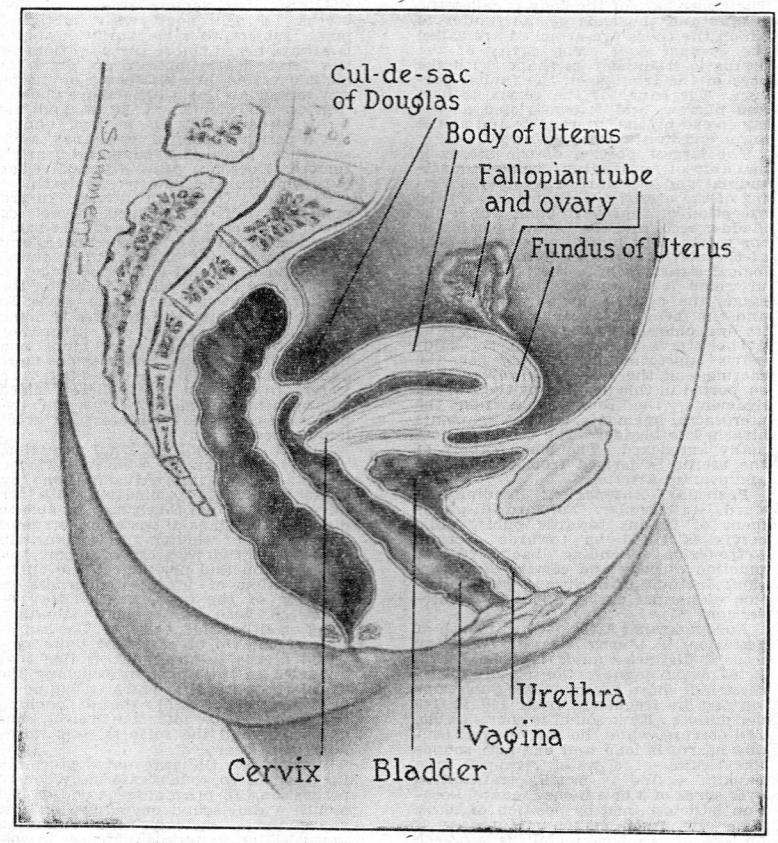

THE UTERUS AND OTHER FEMALE PELVIC ORGANS.

tinuation of lochia rubra beyond the usual time. The factors in its causation are usually puerperal infection, multiparity, overdistention of the uterus by multiple pregnancy or polyhydramnios, lack of lactation, malposition of the uterus, and retained secundines. Involution is aided by being certain that the placenta is intact at the time of delivery, and the use of ecbolics to cause contraction of the uterus. Reposition of the uterus should be practiced when malposition is discovered.
u. acollis. Uterus without a cervix.
u. arcuatus. Uterus with a depressed arched fundus.
u. bicornis. Uterus in which the fundus is divided into 2 parts.
u. biforis. Uterus in which the ext. os is divided into 2 parts by a septum.
u. bilocularis. Uterus in which the cavity is divided into 2 parts by a partition.
u. cordiformis. A heart-shaped uterus.
u. didelphys. Double uterus.
u. gravid. Pregnant uterus.
u. septus. SEE: *u. bilocularis.*
u. unicornis. Uterus that is only one-half developed and has only 1 horn.
uterus, words pert. to: adenomyometritis; anteposition; anterversion; basculation; bicornuate; blennometritis; caduca; cervicitis; cervix; descensus uteri; dihysteria; dimetria; endocervical; endocervix; "endometr-" words; eversion; exometritis; fistula; flooding; follicle, nabothian; fundus; gravid; hematocolpometra; hematometra; hydrometra; hydrophysometra, hydrorrhea gravidarum; hyperinvolution; "hyster-" words; idiometritis; in utero; inversion; involution; leukorrhea; lithometra; lochia; lochiopyra; lochiorrhagia; lochiorrhea; lochiotritis; matrix; mesometritis; metacyesis; "metr-" words; myometritis; myometrium; os uteri; parauterine; perimetritis; perimetrium; physometra; physohydrometra; pyometra; pyometritis; retroflexion; retroversion; subinvolution; suspension; taxis, bipolar; tubouterine; uterine; uterocele; venter; version; womb.
utricle (ū′trĭk-l) [L. *utriculus*, a little bag]. One of 2 sacs of the membranous labyrinth in the bony vestibule of the inner ear.
The utricle communicates with the 3 semicircular canals by 5 openings and is part of the otolith apparatus.
u. of the urethra. The prostatic vesicle of the male.
u. of vestibule. Vestibular cavity connecting with the semicircular canals.
utricular (ū-trĭk′ū-lar) [L. *utriculus*, a little bag]. 1. Pert. to the utricle. 2. Uterine; pert. to the uterus. 3. Like a bladder.
utriculitis (ū-trĭk-ū-lī′tĭs) [" + G. *-itis,* inflammation]. Inflammation of the internal ear, or of the utriculus prostaticus.
utriculoplasty (ū-trĭk′ū-lō-plăs″tĭ) [" + G. *plassein,* to form]. Reduction of the uterus by excision of a longitudinal, wedge-shaped section.
utriculosaccular (ū-trĭk″ū-lō-săk′ū-lar) [" + *sacculus,* a small cavity]. Pert. to the utricle and saccule of the labyrinth.
u. duct. A duct uniting the utricle and saccule.
utriculus (ū-trĭk′ū-lūs) [L. *utriculus,* a little bag]. 1. The larger membranous sac in the vestibule of the labyrinth (in the *recessus ellipticus*), from which the semicircular duct arises. 2. Same as *u. prostaticus.* SYN: *utricle.*

u. masculi′nus, u. prostat′icus. BNA. Very small pouch in the prostate gland opening into the urethra, the analogue of the vagina and uterus.
utriform (ū′trĭ-form) [L. *uter, utri-,* a skin bag, + *forma,* shape]. Having a shape like a leather bottle.
uvea (ū′vē-ă) [L. *uva,* grape]. The 2nd or vascular coat of the eye lying immediately beneath the sclera.
It consists of iris, ciliary body and choroid, forming pigmented layer.
uveal (ū′vē-ăl) [L. *uva,* grape]. Pert. to the middle coat of the eye, or uvea.
u. tract. Pigmented layer of the eye.
SYN: *uvea.*
uveitic (ū-vē-ĭt′ĭk) [L. *uva,* grape, + G. *-itis,* inflammation]. Marked by or pert. to uveitis.
uveitis (ū-vē-ī′tĭs) [" + G. *-itis,* inflammation]. Inflammation of the iris, ciliary body and choroid, the entire uveal tract.
uveoplasty (ū′vē-ō-plăs″tĭ) [" + G. *plassein,* to form]. Reparative operation on the uvea.
uveoparotitis (ū″vē-ō-păr-ō-tī′tĭs) [" + G. *para,* near, + *ous, ot-,* ear, + *-itis,* inflammation]. Parotitis with uveitis.
uviarc (ū′vĭ-ark). Trade name of a mercury quartz lamp, *q.v.*
uviform (ū′vĭ-form) [L. *uva,* grape, + *forma,* shape]. Shaped like or resembling a bunch of grapes, or a grape.
uviofast (ū′vĭ-ō-făst). Unaffected by ultraviolet radiation.
uviol (ū′vĭ-ŏl). Glass which is unusually transparent to ultraviolet rays.
u. lamp. Electric l. with uviol glass globe. [rays therapeutically.
uviolize (ū′vē-ō-līz). To use ultraviolet
uvioresistant (ū″vĭ-ō-rē-zĭs′tănt). Resistant to effects of ultraviolet rays. SYN: *uviofast.* [to effects of ultraviolet rays.
uviosensitive (ū″vĭ-ō-sĕn′sĭ-tĭv). Sensitive
uvula (ū′vū-lă) [L. *uvula,* a little grape]. 1. Tiny projection on inf. vermiform cerebellar process bet. the amygdalae. 2. Small, soft structure hanging from free edge of soft palate in midline above the root of the tongue. It is composed of muscle, connective tissue and mucous membrane.
RS: *cion, cionitis, cionotomy, staphyle.*
u. of cerebellum. Projection on inf. vermiform process of cerebellum in front of pyramid and bet. the amygdalae.
u. vesicae. BNA. Post. portion of *caput galli* projecting into the prostatic urethra, or into the bladder in old men, marking the prostatic middle lobe.
uvulaptosis (ū″vū-lăp-tō′sĭs) [" + G. *ptōsis,* a dropping]. A relaxed condition of the uvula. SYN: *uvuloptosis.*
uvular (ū′vū-lar) [L. *uvula,* little grape]. Pert. to the uvula.
uvularis (ū-vū-lā′rĭs) [L.]. The azygos uvulae muscle. SEE: *Muscles, Table of, in Appendix.*
uvulatome (ū′vū-lă-tōm) [L. *uvula,* little grape, + *tome,* a cutting]. Instrument for removal of uvula.
uvulatomy (ū-vū-lăt′ō-mĭ) [" + G. *tome,* a cutting]. Excision of the uvula.
uvulitis (ū″vū-lī′tĭs) [" + G. *-itis,* inflammation]. Inflammation of the uvula.
uvuloptosis (ū-vū-lŏp-tō′sĭs) [" + G. *ptōsis,* a dropping]. Relaxed condition of the palate.
uvulotome (ū′vū-lo-tōm) [" + G. *tome,* a cutting]. Instrument for performing uvulotomy. SYN: *uvulatome.*
uvulotomy (ū-vū-lŏt′ō-mĭ) [" + G. *tome,* a cutting]. Amputation of the uvula.

V

V. Abbr. of *vision, visual acuity, Vibrio*, and for *volt*. SYMB. for *vanadium*.

vaccigenous (văk-sĭj′ĕn-ŭs) [L. *vaccinus*, pert. to a cow, + G. *gennan*, to produce]. Producing vaccine. SYN: *vaccinogenous*.

vaccin (văk′sĭn) [L. *vaccinus*, pert. to a cow]. Any substance for inoculation against disease. SYN: *vaccine*.

vaccina (văk-sī′nă) [L. *vaccinus*, pert. to a cow]. A disease resulting from inoculation with cowpox virus.

Papules form about 3rd day after vaccination which change to umbilicated vesicles and then to pustules. They dry and form scabs which fall about the 21st day. SEE: *Paschen bodies*.

vaccinal (văk′sĭn-ăl) [L. *vaccinus*, pert. to a cow]. Relating to vaccine or to vaccination.

v. fever. A mild fever that may follow vaccination.

vaccinate (văk′sĭn-āt) [L. *vaccinus*, pert. to a cow]. 1. To inoculate with cowpox vaccine to prevent or mitigate an attack of smallpox. 2. To inoculate with any vaccine to produce immunity against disease.

vaccination (văk-sĭn-ā′shŭn) [L. *vaccinus*, pert. to a cow]. 1. Inoculation against smallpox. 2. Inoculation with bacterial vaccine as a preventive measure.

Vaccination against smallpox was introduced by Edward Jenner in 1796.

TIME OF PERFORMANCE: In normal infant of good health, about 4th month, unless definite exposure to smallpox is known, when vaccination should be performed regardless of age. It is advisable to undertake vaccination about every 5 years.

METHOD: *Site of selection*: Usually, the left arm, just above point of insertion of deltoid. Not advisable to vaccinate on leg, as secondary infections are much more likely to develop. If vaccination is performed on the leg, the outer muscles at the midthird is the proper point for inoculation. The skin should be cleansed with soap and water, then rendered aseptic by sponging with 95% alcohol and allowed to dry. The vaccine lymph is expelled from the capillary tube by means of a small rubber bulb, and a sterile needle is selected for the purpose of abrading the epidermis through the drop of vaccine. This may be readily accomplished by the multiple pressure method which consists of simply tapping the skin repeatedly with end of needle until the epidermis is denuded over an area no longer than the diameter of the shaft of an ordinary match. Cross scratching or vertical scratching with needle is totally unnecessary and often produces a needlessly large scar. Following inoculation, the area involved should be allowed to dry or protected from contact with clothing. Celluloid shields, or any appliance which encircles the arm and causes constriction not only inadvisable, but many times proves to be dangerous, inasmuch as possibilities of secondary infection are promoted by such appliances.

SYM: From the 3rd to the 5th day following inoculation, a papule should develop. This is surrounded by a red areola. By 6th to 7th day, the papule is converted into a pearly vesicle, the center of which becomes depressed. The surrounding tissue may be red and tender with considerable infiltration. From 10th to 12th day, the vesicle becomes a pustule, when there may be some swelling and tenderness of the axillary glands, as well as elevation of temperature. From 12th to 25th day, the pustule passes through the stage of desiccation and scab drops off, leaving a pitty scar at its former site. A potent vaccine should always produce a reaction in a susceptible individual. The fact that the vaccination does not take in one who has never been successfully vaccinated, or who has never had smallpox, does not indicate that such an individual is immune.

RS: *arm-to-arm v., autovaccination, autovaccine, vaccina, vaccine, vaccinella, variola*.

v., arm-to-arm. V. in which virus is taken from arm of one person and injected into arm of another.

v., bovine. V. with vaccine lymph of a calf.

v. rash. One sometimes following vaccination.

vaccinationist (văk″sĭn-ā′shŭn-ĭst) [L. *vaccinus*, pert. to a cow]. One who upholds the efficacy of vaccination.

vaccinator (văk′sĭn-ā″tor) [L. *vaccinus*, pert. to a cow]. 1. One who vaccinates. 2. An instrument for vaccinating.

vaccine (văk′sēn) [L. *vaccinus*, from *vacca*, a cow]. 1. Pert. to vaccine or vaccination. 2. Substance containing virus of cowpox in a form for vaccination against smallpox. 3. Any substance for preventive inoculation, esp. a bacterial preparation. SEE: *bacterine*.

Vaccines are made in 3 general classes: (1) Those with living organisms; (2) those with killed bacteria, and (3) those with the toxins or other products thrown off by bacteria during growth. An example of the 1st class is smallpox vaccine where the living virus is used.

Examples of the 2nd class are vaccines used to protect human beings against typhoid fever, rabies, and whooping cough. Vaccines of this class have been prepared for use in preventing several other diseases including pneumonia, cholera, dysentery, undulant fever, and plague, but they are less reliable as preventives against these.

In the 3rd class comes toxoid used in the prevention of diphtheria and tetanus.

FUNCTION: To stimulate the development in the body of specific defensive mechanism which results in more or less permanent protection against a disease. An attack of smallpox or diphtheria, for example, usually leaves the recovered patient permanently immune to those diseases. As a result of infection, the body succeeds in building up its own defenses, so that a new infection causes no illness. A successful vaccine does the same thing without the risk of illness.

vaccine, aqueous   V-2   **vaginal hysterectomy**

v., aqueous. V. employing physiological salt solution as the vehicle.
v., autogenous. Bacterial v. taken from the individual to be inoculated.
v., bacterial. Preparation of bacteria in saline solution or in oil injected into the body to induce immunity to same species of bacteria or their toxins.
v., BCG (Calmette - Guérin bacillus). Substance used in prophylactic vaccination of infants against tuberculosis with virulence reduced by repeated cultures on glycerinated ox bile.
v., corresponding. SEE: *stock vaccine*.
v., humanized. Vaccine obtained from vaccinia vesicles in human beings.
v., oil. V. prepared with oil as the vehicle. SEE: *aqueous vaccine*.
v. point. A bone or quill coated with vaccine lymph at its tip.
v., polyvalent. V. made from several strains of the same species of bacterium.
v. rash. One due to vaccination.
v., sensitized. V. made more active by treatment of the bacteria with their specific immune serum. SYN: *serobacterin*.
v., stock. Bacterial v. made from same species as that causing the infection, but not autogenous.
v. therapy. Treatment of a disease by inoculation with a vaccine specific for that disease.
v. virus. An emulsion containing substance from pustules of vaccinia used for inoculation.
vaccinella (văk-sĭn-ĕl′ă) [L. *vaccinus*, pert. to a cow]. A secondary eruption sometimes following vaccination, but not conferring immunity.
vaccinia (văk-sĭn′ĭ-ă) [L. *vaccinus*, pert. to a cow]. A contagious disease resulting from inoculation with cowpox virus.
    Papules form about 3rd day after vaccination which change to umbilicated vesicles about the 5th day and then, at end of 1st week, to umbilicated pustules surrounded by a red areola. They dry and form scabs, which fall about the 2nd week, leaving a white, pitted depression.
    Inoculation with this virus confers upon man more or less immunity against smallpox.
    RS: *vaccination, variola, varicella*.
vacciniform (văk-sĭn′ĭ-form) [L. *vaccinus*, pert. to a cow, + *forma*, shape]. Of the nature of vaccinia or cowpox.
vaccinin (văk′sĭn-ĭn) [L. *vaccinus*, pert. to a cow]. The inoculable element by which cowpox is transmitted.
vacciniola (văk-sĭn-ĭ-ō′lă) [L. diminutive of *vaccinia*, from *vaccinus*, pert. to a cow]. Secondary general eruption after local eruption from vaccine.
vaccinization (văk″sĭn-ĭ-zā′shŭn) [L. *vaccinus*, pert. to a cow]. Vaccination by repeated inoculations until the virus has no effect.
vaccinogenous (văk″sĭn-ŏj′ĕn-ŭs) [" + G. *gennan*, to produce]. Producing vaccine or pert. to its production.
vaccinosyphilis (văk″sĭn-ō-sĭf′ĭl-ĭs) [L. *vaccinus*, pert. to a cow, + *syphilis*]. Syphilis following inoculation conveyed by impure vaccine or a contaminated instrument.
vaccinotherapeutics, vaccinotherapy (văk″-sĭn-ō-thĕr-ă-pū′tĭks, -thĕr′ă-pĭ) [" + G. *therapeutikē*, treatment, — + G. *therapeia*, treatment]. Treatment by injection of bacterial vaccines.
vacuolation (văk-ū-ō-lā′shŭn) [L. *vacuolum*, a tiny empty space]. Formation of vacuoles.

vacuole (văk′ū-ōl) [L. *vacuolum*, a tiny empty space]. 1. A clear space in cell protoplasm filled with fluid or air. 2. A very small space in any tissue; source of a lymphatic vessel. SEE: *cytoplasm*.
vacuolization (văk″ū-ō-lĭz-ā′shŭn) [L. *vacuolum*, a tiny space]. The formation of vacuoles. SYN: *vacuolation*.
vacuum (văk′ū-ŭm) [L. *vacuum*, empty]. A space exhausted of its air content.
v. treatment. Insertion of a limb in a partial vacuum.
v. tube. A vessel of insulating material (usually glass) provided with metal electrodes, which has been so highly evacuated that the residual gas does not affect the current passing bet. metal electrodes projecting from the outside.
vag′abond's disease. Discoloration of skin caused by exposure and scratching due to presence of lice.
vagal (vā′găl) [L. *vagus*, wandering]. Pert. to the vagus nerve.
v. attack. A condition of dyspnea, cardiac distress, a fear of impending death, and a sinking sensation assumed to be the result of vasomotor spasm.
v. nervous system. The autonomic* nervous system, which controls the viscera, ductless glands, blood vessels, and organs containing involuntary muscle.
vagina (vă-jī′nă) (pl. *vaginae, vaginas*) [L. *vagina*, sheath]. 1. A sheathlike part. 2. A musculomembranous tube which forms the passageway bet. the uterus and the external orifice.
    ANAT: It is divided into 4 walls, 2 lateral, 1 ant., and 1 post. In the uppermost part, the cervix divides the vagina into 4 *fornices*, the 2 lateral, the anterior and the posterior. It is about 2½ inches along the ant. wall and 3¾ inches along the post. wall.
    The bladder is situated on the ant. wall of the vagina and the rectum is behind the post. wall. In a nulliparous woman all walls approximate each other, making an H shape. The vagina is lined by mucous membrane made up of squamous epithelium. It is surrounded by fascias which allow for easy distensibility. The blood supply of the vagina is furnished from the inferior vesical, inferior hemorrhoidal, and uterine arteries.
    FUNCTION: A passage for the intromission of the penis, the reception of the semen, and for the discharge of the menstrual flow; also, for the delivery of the fruits of pregnancy.
v., bulb of. Small erectile body on each side of the vaginal vestibule. SYN: *bulbi vestibuli*.
v. cordis. Sac investing the heart. SYN: *pericardium*.
v. femoris. Fascia lata of the thigh.
v. oculi. Sheath investing the eyeball forming its socket. SYN: *Tenon's capsule*.
vagina, words pert. to: aerocoly, bulbi vestibuli, "colp-" words, Duverney's gland, "elytr-" words, endocolpitis, enterocele, esthiomene, fistula, fornix, fourchette, gynatresia, hematocolpometra, hydrocolpos, hymen, kysthoptosis, leukorrhea, lochiocolpos, pachycolpismus, pachyvaginitis, paravaginal, pronaus, supravaginal, transvaginal, "vagin-" words.
vaginal (văj′ĭn-ăl) [L. *vagina*, sheath]. Pert. to the vagina or to any enveloping sheath.
v. hysterectomy. Excision of uterus through vagina.

vaginalectomy (văj″ĭn-ăl-ĕk'tō-mĭ) [" + G. *ektomē*, excision]. Excision of the tunica vaginalis. SYN: *vaginectomy*.
vaginalitis (văj-ĭn-ăl-ī'tĭs) [L. *vagina*, sheath, + G. *-itis*, inflammation]. Inflammation of *tunica vaginalis testis*.
vaginate (văj'ĭn-āt) [L. *vagina*, sheath]. Sheathed.
vaginectomy (văj-ĭn-ĕk'tō-mĭ) [" + G. *ektomē*, excision]. Resection of tunica vaginalis.
vaginicoline (văj-ĭn-ĭk'ō-lĭn) [" + *colere*, to dwell]. Living in the vagina, as microörganisms.
vaginismus (văj-ĭn-ĭz'mŭs) [L.]. Painful spasm of vagina from contraction of the vaginal walls preventing coitus.
It may indicate neurotic aversion to the act. Extraordinary hyperesthesia of nerve supply to mucous membrane of vagina at or near site of the hymen, resulting in spasmodic constriction of sphincter vaginae muscle, preventing coitus.
SYM: Extreme sensitiveness. Spasmodic closure of vaginal orifice on slightest touch. In severe cases, sterility.
TREATMENT: Perfect rest. Coition prohibited. Bathing with tepid water. General constitutional treatment. Diet strictly guarded. All use of tea, coffee, spirituous liquors, stimulants of all kinds, and spices, positively prohibited.
v., mental. V. resulting from repugnance to cohabitation.
v., posterior. V. due to contraction of the levator ani muscle.
vaginitis (văj-ĭn-ī'tĭs) [L. *vagina*, sheath, + G. *-itis*, inflammation]. 1. Inflammation of a sheath. 2. Inflammation of vagina.
At first acute; unless promptly treated assumes chronic form. Erysipelatous and erythematous inflammation may cause intensely red, painful, elevated, more or less extensive patches.
v. adhaesiva. Inflammation with mucous membrane exfoliation causing adhesions and partial obliteration of the vaginal lumen.
v., diphtheritic. V. with membranous exudate.
v., emphysematous. V. with gas in connective tissues.
v., glandular. V. when the follicles alone seem affected, when mucous membrane shows no traces of change and when secretion appears more copious and of a yellowish-white or grayish color.
v., granular. V. with infiltrated cells and enlarged papillae. The most common form of v.
v., papulous. Vagina and neck of womb covered with papulae or follicles more or less developed or resembling fleshy granulations.
v., pustulous. May result from appearance of pustules in persons affected with pustulous affections of the skin.
v. senilis. Same as *v. adhaesiva*, *q.v.*
v. testis. Inflammation of the tunica vaginalis of the testis.
v., trichomonas. V. due to infection with Trichomonas.
v., vesicular. V. from extension of eczema from vulva to the vagina.
SYM: Feeling of heat and burning in vagina and vulva; feeling of aching and sense of weight in perineum; frequent desire to urinate; pain and throbbing in pelvic region of abdomen; profuse leukorrhea, which may be purulent, offensive and acrid; excoriation of vulva and external adjacent parts. In chronic cases same set of symptoms exist but lesser degree.
TREATMENT: Mild antiseptic douches or, better still, sterilized water as hot as can be borne should be used for cleanliness and relief. The system in general should be treated. Cause ascertained and removed.
vaginoabdominal (văj″ĭn-ō-ăb-dŏm'ĭn-ăl) [L. *vagina*, sheath, + *abdominalis*, abdominal]. Relating to the vagina and abdomen.
vaginocele (văj'ĭn-ō-sēl) [" + G. *kēlē*, hernia]. Vaginal hernia. SYN: *colpocele*.
vaginodynia (văj″ĭn-ō-dĭn'ĭ-ă) [" + G. *odynē*, pain]. Pain in the vagina.
vaginofixation (văj″ĭn-ō-fĭks-ā'shŭn) [" + *fixātio*, a fixing]. 1. Process of rendering the vagina immovable. 2. Attachment of uterus to vaginal peritoneum.
vaginogenic (văj″ĭn-ō-jĕn'ĭk) [" + G. *gennan*, to produce]. Developed in the vagina.
vaginography (văj-ĭn-ŏg'ră-fĭ) [" + G. *graphein*, to write]. The taking of x-ray pictures of the vagina.
vaginolabial (văj″ĭn-ō-lā'bĭ-ăl) [" + *labium*, lip]. Relating to the vagina and the labia. SYN: *vaginovulvar*, *vulvovaginal*.
vaginometer (văj-ĭn-ŏm'ĕ-tĕr) [L. *vagina*, sheath, + G. *metron*, a measure]. Device for measuring the length and expansion of the vagina.
vaginomycosis (văj″ĭn-ō-mī-kō'sĭs) [" + G. *mykēs*, fungus, + *-ōsis*, disease]. A fungous infection (mycosis) of the vagina.
vaginoperineal (văj″ĭn-ō-pĕr-ĭ-nē'ăl) [" + G. *perinaion*, perineum]. Relating to the vagina and perineum.
vaginoperineorrhaphy (văj″ĭn-ō-pĕr-ĭ-nē-or'ăf-ĭ) [" + " + *rhaphē*, a sewing]. Repair of a perineal laceration in the vagina. SYN: *colpoperineorrhaphy*.
vaginoperineotomy (văj″ĭn-ō-pĕr-ĭn-ē-ŏt'-ō-mĭ) [" + " + *tomē*, a cutting]. Separation of the vagina and perineum.
vaginoperitoneal (văj″ĭn-ō-pĕr-ĭ-tō-nē'ăl) [" + G. *peritonaion*, peritoneum]. Relating to the vagina and peritoneum.
vaginopexy (vă-jĭ'nō-pĕk″sĭ) [" + G. *pēxis*, fixation]. Fixation of the vagina. SYN: *colpopexy*.
vaginoplasty (vă-jĭ'nō-plăs″tĭ) [L. *vagina*, sheath, + G. *plassein*, to form]. Reparative surgery on the vagina.
vaginoscope (văj'ĭn-ō-skōp) [" + G. *skopein*, to examine]. Instrument for inspection of the vagina.
vaginoscopy (văj-ĭn-ŏs'kō-pĭ) [" + G. *skopein*, to examine]. Visual examination of the vagina.
vaginotome (văj-ĭ'nō-tōm) [" + G. *tomē*, a cutting]. An instrument for making an incision in the vaginal walls.
vaginotomy (văj-ĭn-ŏt'ō-mĭ) [" + G. *tomē*, a cutting]. Incision of vagina.
vaginovesical (văj″ĭn-ō-vĕs'ĭk-ăl) [" + *vesica*, bladder]. Relating to the vagina and the bladder. SYN: *vesicovaginal*.
vaginovulvar (văj″ĭn-ō-vŭl'var) [" + *vulva*, a covering]. Pert. to the vulva and vagina.
vagitis (văj-ī'tĭs) [L. *vagus*, wandering, + G. *-itis*, inflammation]. Inflammation of the vagus, the 10th cranial nerve.
vagitus (vă-jī'tŭs) [L. *vagire*, to squall]. First cry of newlyborn infant.
v. uterinus. Crying of the fetus before birth when membrane has been ruptured permitting passage of air into the uterus.
v. vaginalis. Cry of a child or infant with head still in the vagina.

vagogram (vā'gō-grăm) [L. *vagus*, wandering, + G. *gramma*, a mark]. Tracing of variations of the vagus nerve made by an electrical device.

vagolysis (vā-gŏl'ĭ-sĭs) [" + G. *lysis*, a loosening]. Process of loosening the esophageal branches of the vagus nerve for relief of cardiospasm.

vagomimetic (vā"gō-mĭm-ĕt'ĭk) [" + G. *mimētikos*, imitating]. Resembling action of stimulated vagus nerve.

vagosympathetic (vā"gō-sĭm-pă-thĕt'ĭk) [" + G. *sympathētikos*, suffering with]. The cervical sympathetic and the vagus nerves considered together.

vagotomy (vā-gŏt'ō-mĭ) [" + G. *tomē*, a cutting]. Section of the vagus nerve.

vagotonia (vā-gō-tō'nĭ-ă) [L. *vagus*, wandering, + G. *tonos*, tone]. Hyperirritability of vagus nerve resulting in a condition marked by spastic tendency in smooth muscles, fatigue, nervousness, and vasomotor instability.

vagotonic (vā"gō-tŏn'ĭk) [" + G. *tonos*, tone]. Pertaining to vagotonia.

v. type. Type characterized by deficient suprarenal activity.

SYM: Lowered blood pressure, slow pulse, high sugar tolerance, skin pale and cool, localized sweating, and oculocardiac reflex.

vagotropic (vā"gō-trŏp'ĭk) [" + G. *tropos*, a turning]. Acting upon the vagus nerve.

vagotropism (vā-gŏt'rō-pĭzm) [" + " + *-ismos*, condition]. Affinity for the vagus nerve, as a drug.

vagrant (vā'grănt) [L. *vagrans*, from *vagāre*, to wander]. 1. Wandering from place to place, as the leukocytes. 2. A vagabond.

v's. disease. Cutaneous discoloration and irritation caused by filth and body lice. SYN: *vagabond's disease*.

vagus (vā'gŭs) (pl. *vagi*) [L. *vagus*, wandering]. The pneumogastric or 10th cranial nerve.

It is a mixed nerve having motor and sensory functions and a wider distribution than any of the cranial nerves.

v. pneumonia. P. caused by trauma of the pneumogastric nerve.

v. pulse. A slow pulse caused by the slowing action of the heart due to inhibition of the vagus nerve. SEE: *vagotomy*, *vagotonia*.

valence, valency (vā'lĕns, -lĕn-sĭ) [L. *valens*, powerful]. 1. Property of an element or radical combining with or replacing other elements or radicals in definite proportion. 2. Degree of the combining power or replacing power of an element or radical, the hydrogen atom being unit of comparison.

The number indicates how many atoms of hydrogen can unite with 1 atom of another element.

SEE: *artiad*, *atomicity*.

valetudinarian (văl-e-tū-dĭn-ā'rĭ-ăn) [L. *valetudinarius*, pert. to ill health]. 1. Sickly; ailing. 2. One subject to frequent illness, or feebleness. SYN: *invalid*.

valgus (văl'gŭs) [L. *valgus*, bowlegged]. 1. Clubfoot in which the foot is bent outward. 2. Bowlegged or knock-kneed. 3. One with knock-knees or bowlegs. SYN: *talipes* valgus*.

valine (văl'ēn, vā'lēn). An amino acid derived from protein decomposition. $C_5H_{11}NO_2$.

vallate (văl'āt) [L. *vallātus*, walled]. Having a rim around a depression.

vallecula (văl-lĕk'ŭ-lă) [L. *vallecula*, a depression]. A depression or crevice.

v. cerebel'li. BNA. A deep fissure on inf. surface of the cerebellum.

v. ova'ta. A depression in the liver in which rests the gallbladder.

v. syl'vii. A depression marking beginning of the fissure of Sylvius.

v. un'guis. Fold of skin in which the proximal and lateral edges of the nails are imbedded.

Vallet's mass (văl-ā'). Mass of ferrous carbonate, containing 36% ferrous carbonate.

USES: In simple anemia.

DOSAGE: 3-5 gr. (0.2-0.3 Gm).

valley of the cerebellum (văl'ē). Hollow on inf. surface of cerebellum. SYN: *vallecula cerebelli*.

vallum unguis (văl'um ŭng'gwĭs). BNA. Fold of skin overlapping the nail.

Valsalva's sinuses (văl-săl'vă). Pouches of the aortic and pulmonary arteries behind the flaps of the semilunar valves.

valvate (văl'vāt) [L. *valva*, valve]. Pert. to or provided with valves. SYN: *valvular*.

valvotomy (văl-vŏt'ō-mĭ) [L. *valva*, valve, + G. *tomē*, a cutting]. Surgical cutting of a valve, esp. one of the rectum.

valve (vălv) [L. *valva*, a fold]. Any one of various structures for temporarily closing an orifice or passage, or for allowing movement of fluid in 1 direction only.

v., aortic. The semilunar valve preventing regurgitation at the entrance of the aorta to the heart, composed of 3 segments.

v., bicuspid. Valve closing orifice bet. left cardiac auricle and ventricle.

v., ileocecal. Valve bet. ileum and large intestine to prevent regurgitation of intestinal contents; composed of 2 membranous folds.

v., mitral. Cardiac valve bet. the left auricle and ventricle. SYN: *bicuspid valve*.

v., pulmonary. Valve composed of 3 cusps separating pulmonary artery and right ventricle.

v., pyloric. Prominent circular membranous fold at pyloric orifice of the stomach.

v., semilunar. Valve bet. heart and the aorta and valve bet. the heart and the pulmonary artery.

v., tricuspid. Valve bet. the right cardiac auricle and ventricle.

v. tube. An electric valve consisting of a vacuum tube having for 1 electrode a hot filament.

v. of Varolius. SEE: *ileocecal valve*.

valvula (văl'vū-lă) [L. *valvula*, a tiny fold]. A valve, specifically a small valve.

v. bicuspidalis. BNA. Valve bet. left cardiac auricle and ventricle.

v. coli. BNA. Valve bet. ileum and large intestine.

v. pylori. BNA. Prominent mucosal fold at pyloric entrance of the stomach.

v. semilunaris. BNA. Valve separating heart and aorta and heart and pulmonary artery.

v. tricuspidalis. Valve bet. the right auricle and ventricle of the heart.

valvulae conniventes (văl'vū-lē kon-nĭ-věn'-tēs) [L.]. Circular membranous folds projecting into lumen of small intestine; they do not disappear on distention of bowel, and act by retarding passage of the food along the bowel; they also provide a greater absorbing area. SYN: *plicae circulares*.

valvular (văl'vū-lar) [L. *valvula*, a small fold]. Relating to or having a valve. SYN: *valvate*.

valvulitis (văl-vū-lī'-tĭs) [" + G. *-itis*, inflammation]. Inflammation of a valve, especially a cardiac valve. SYN: *dicliditis*.

valvulotome (văl'vū-lō-tōm) [" + G. *tomē*, a cutting]. An instrument for incising a valve.

valvulotomy (văl-vū-lŏt'ō-mĭ) [" + G. *tomē*, a cutting]. Process of cutting through a valve, as a too rigid rectal fold. SYN: *valvotomy*.

vanadium (văn-ā'dĭ-ŭm). A light gray metallic element. SYMB: V. At. wt. 50.95.

van Buren's disease (văn bū'rĕn). Induration of the corpora cavernosa.

van den Bergh's test. A direct or indirect test to detect the presence of bilirubin in blood serum in assumed cases of obstructive jaundice or impaired liver functioning.

vanillism (văn-ĭl'lĭzm). Irritation of the skin, mucous membranes and conjunctiva sometimes experienced by workers handling vanilla.

van Swieten's solution (văn swē'ten). Mercuric chloride 1, alcohol 100, distilled water 900.

vapor (vā'por) [L. *vapor*, smoke]. 1. Gaseous state of any substance. 2. Medicinal substance for administration in form of inhaled vapor.
  v. bath. Exposure of body to hot vapor.
  v. cabinet. Cabinet in which to give vapor baths.
  v. douche. Treatment with a jet of hot vapor.
  SEE: *halitus, nebulization*.

vaporium (vā-pō'rĭ-ŭm) [L. *vaporium*]. Apparatus for applying hot or cold or medicated vapors.

vaporization (vā"por-ĭ-zā'shŭn) [L. *vapor*, smoke]. 1. The conversion of a liquid or solid into vapor. 2. Therapeutic use of a vapor.

vaporizer (vā'por-īz-ĕr) [L. *vapor*, smoke]. Device for converting liquids into a vapor spray.

vaporole (vā'pō-rōl). 1. An ampule or capsule of glass containing a single dose of a volatile drug for inhalation. 2. Trade name of a glass ampule.

vaporous (vā'por-ŭs) [L. *vapor*, smoke]. Consisting of, pert. to, or producing vapors.

Vaquez's disease (vă-kā'). Continuous excessive erythrocyte formation by the diseased bone marrow with enlargement of the spleen.

varicella (var-ĭ-sel'ă) [L. *varicella*, a tiny spot]. An acute, highly contagious disease characterized by an eruption that makes its appearance in crops and passes through successive stages of macules, papules, vesicles, and crusts. SYN: *chickenpox*.
  ETIOL: May occur at any age, though far less common in adults than in children. Epidemics most frequent in winter and spring. One attack nearly always confers immunity.
  INCUBATION: 4 to 27 days.
  SYM: *Onset:* There may be but slight elevation of temperature, followed within 24 hours by appearance of the eruption after which time temperature usually rises still further. Eruption first appears on back and chest, crops continuing to make their appearance for a period of from 2 to 3 days on an average.
  Each crop requires about 36 hours to pass through the several stages. Because of this, in the same general locality, macules, papules, vesicles and crusts may be found side by side. Lesions are superficial and rupture very easily.
  They have a tendency to be ovoid and on the chest their distribution is often particularly marked along the course of the intercostal nerves. Some, though possibly few, scars nearly always remain as evidence of a chickenpox attack. The extremities are relatively free as compared with the trunk.
  COMPLICATIONS: Secondary infections, due to scratching, which may result in abscess formation, or at times development of erysipelas or even septicemia. Occasionally lesions in the vicinity of the larynx may cause edema of the glottis and threaten the life of the patient. Encephalitis is a rare complication.
  DIFFERENTIAL DIAG: Confusion bet. this disease and smallpox is responsible for the chief importance given chickenpox. Impetigo, dermatitis herpetiformis, herpes zoster, and furunculosis may require consideration.
  PROG: Always favorable except in a very severe type which is described as varicella gangraenosa. In this variety, gangrene may develop about the site of the lesions.
  TREATMENT: Isolation. Restrain the hands in the case of infants or young children in order that the lesions may not be scratched. Use of calamine lotion locally may alleviate irritation. Ordinarily, no internal remedies are necessary. The usual duration of the disease is from 2 to 3 weeks. Cases usually classed as contagious until the skin is free of all crusts. Except in those cases suffering from one of the few complications that may occur, a soft diet for the first few days and a general diet later will be found suitable.

varices (var'ĭs-ēz) (Sing. *varix*) [L. *varicēs*, dilated veins]. Enlarged twisted veins.

variciform (văr-ĭs'ĭ-form) [L. *varix, varic-*, a twisted vein, + *forma*, shape]. Resembling a varix. SYN: *varicose*.

varicoblepharon (văr-ĭ-kō-blĕf'ă-ron) [" + G. *blepharon*, eyelid]. Varicose tumor of the eyelid.

varicocele (văr'ĭ-kō-sēl) [L. *varix, varic-*, a twisted vein, + G. *kēlē*, hernia]. Enlargement of the veins of the spermatic cord (spermatic plexus), occurring in adolescents and young men, most commonly on the left side. SYN: *cirsocele*.
  SYM: Vessels on affected side of scrotum are full, feeling like a bundle of worms, sometimes purplish in color. Dull ache along the cord. Testis oversensitive, slight dragging sensation in groin, hypochondriacal outlook, defective morale.
  TREATMENT: Sexual hygiene. Suspensory. Surgery if insisted upon and to patient's benefit.

varicocelectomy (văr-ĭ-kō-sē-lĕk'tō-mĭ) [L. *varix, varic-*, twisted vein, + G. *kēlē*, hernia, + *ektomē*, excision]. Excision of portion of scrotal sac with ligation of the dilated veins to relieve varicocele.

varicography (văr-ĭ-kŏg'ră-fĭ) [" + G. *graphein*, to write]. X-ray photography of varicose veins.

varicomphalus (văr-ĭk-ŏm'făl-ŭs) [" + G. *omphalos*, navel]. Varicose tumor of the navel.

varicophlebitis (văr"ĭ-kō-flē-bī-tĭs) (" + G. *phleps, phleb-*, vein, + *-itis*, inflammation]. Phlebitis combined with varicose veins.

varicose (văr'ĭ-kōs). Pert. to varices; distended, swollen, noting veins.

v. veins. Enlarged twisted veins most commonly found on leg and thigh.
ETIOL: Congenitally defective venous valves, pregnancy, occupations requiring standing positions, and obesity.
SYM: Pain in feet and ankles, swelling, ulcers on skin. Severe bleeding, if a vein is injured.
F. A. TREATMENT: Elevation of extremity and gentle pressure over wound will always stop bleeding. The use of a tourniquet is undesirable. Sterile dressing should be held in place with a firm bandage. Patient should not be permitted to walk for some time.
General: Occlusion of the dilated veins. Sometimes, surgery.
RS: *cirsenchysis, cirsodesis, cirsomphalos, cirsotomy.*
varicosity (văr-ĭ-kŏs'ĭ-tĭ) [L. *varix, varic-*, vein]. 1. Condition of being varicose. 2. A swollen, twisted vein. SYN: *varix.*
varicotomy (văr-ĭ-kŏt'ō-mĭ) [" + G. *tomē*, a cutting]. Excision of a varicose vein.
varicula (văr-ĭk'ū-lă) [L. *varicula*, a tiny dilated vein]. A small varix, esp. a varicose dilation of the veins of mucous membrane covering ant. surface of the eye.
varietism (vă-rī'ĕt-ĭzm) [L. *varietas*, variety + G. *ismos*, condition]. Plural love relations; generally on the part of the male. SEE: *polyandry.*
variola (vă-rī'ō-lă) [*variola*, a small spot]. An acute contagious disease characterized by a prodromal stage during which the constitutional symptoms are usually severe, and followed by an eruption which passes through the successive stages of macules, papules, vesicles, pustules, and crusts. SYN: *smallpox.*
ETIOL: Causative organism not definitely known. More common during colder seasons. No age exempt. May occur in utero. No preference as to sex. Acquired chiefly by direct contact with patient. May also be spread through the handling of articles contaminated by the patient. Susceptibility practically universal in those unprotected by proper vaccination, or before a first attack of smallpox, although second attacks have been reported.
INCUBATION: Seven to 14 days. Occasionally longer; average time, 10 to 12 days.
SYM: Onset abrupt with chill or chilliness. Headache usually frontal, intense lumbar pains, elevation of temperature, which may rise to 104° or higher, nausea, or more frequently, vomiting. Fever remains high until evening of 3rd or morning of 4th day, when it falls sharply, often to normal.
With drop in temperature, the eruption makes its appearance, coming out first as a rule, about the face, and soon afterward on extremities and to lesser extent on trunk. Eruption is of same character in any one general location, in this respect differing markedly from eruption of chickenpox.
About 2nd day of eruption, the macules become papular, and from 3rd to 5th day these papules become vesicles. The vesicles increase in size and from 7th to 8th day, well developed pustules are present, having appearance of being deep-seated and areola may, or may not, be markedly evident.
The fever of suppuration, so commonly referred to, which is generally anticipated at the time pustules develop, is not always present in the discrete type of smallpox. From 8th to 11th day, desiccation occurs and by end of 21st day in the average discrete case the skin is likely to be free of crusts. The customary observation that smallpox papules when found on the palmar or plantar surfaces feel like shot underneath the skin is a fact to which too much importance is commonly attached.
Preceding eruption of smallpox, a leukocytosis is not present. However, albuminuria may be noted. It may always be expected that the lesions will predominate on the head and extremities, the trunk being relatively free in the discrete type.
The lesions of smallpox, being deepseated, do not rupture easily, for two reasons. First, the smallpox lesion is not single celled, but multilocular. Second, because of a deeper invasion, there is a thicker protective covering. It is because of the first of these reasons that the smallpox lesion does not collapse when pricked by a needle. If properly treated, the majority of discrete cases will show little evidence of the disease some months after recovery.
Pitting is not an inevitable misfortune in all cases, but depends principally on extent to which the true skin is involved. However, though pitting does not occur, marked pigmentation may exist at the sites of the lesions and continue to attract attention for many weeks following recovery from an acute attack.
Prodromal rashes sometimes make their appearance before the true eruption of smallpox, and when present, may be mistaken for either measles or scarlet fever. These rashes, which may develop soon after the onset, bear no significance to the severity of the attack which is to follow. Several other types are described and often classified under one heading—the malignant. Of these, the principal ones are the confluent and the hemorrhagic.
COMPLICATIONS: Abscesses, iritis, conjunctivitis, cervical adenitis, nephritis, and pneumonia are among the more common ones.
DIFFERENTIAL DIAG: Although smallpox may be suspected because of known exposure, a definite diagnosis cannot be established prior to appearance of the eruption. After the eruption, chickenpox is the disease which is most constantly confused with smallpox. The presence or absence of a vaccination scar may carry some weight in making a decision. However, distribution of the lesions which predominate on the trunk in chickenpox, as well as milder constitutional symptoms should be an aid in diagnosing. Pustular syphilis, impetigo contagiosa, and various drug eruptions may require consideration.
PROG: In modified and discrete smallpox, the outcome may be considered favorable in practically all instances. In confluent smallpox, recovery is always doubtful and in the hemorrhagic types, death is almost inevitable.
TREATMENT: *Prophylactic:* Successful vaccination against smallpox is an absolute preventive. However, this should always be repeated in the presence of an epidemic or when knowledge of recent exposure is possessed.
General: Absolute isolation of patient in a cool, well-ventilated room. If there are many lesions on mucous membranes a liquid diet may be essential. In the discrete type, patient need not be lim-

ited as to diet, unless there is some contraindication. Plenty of water, fruit juices and vegetables should be given. Milk is often soothing as well as nourishing in those cases in which the throat symptoms are severe. Cathartics or laxatives as indicated.

Closest attention should be given to the eyes. For washing the eyes a saturated boric acid solution and sometimes the addition of some silver salt as well. It is not advisable to use ointments on the skin before desiccation is complete, as such treatment only blocks the surface and increases likelihood of abscess formation.

The itching commonly associated with smallpox is seldom complained of; when present, calomine lotion may be applied. In the confluent type, weak iodine baths, or weak permanganate tubbings are often necessary not merely for cleansing skin but for purpose of acting as a deodorant.

Patients suffering from delirium must be properly restrained in order that no personal injury develops because of their mental condition. In such patients, sedatives are a necessity. Other internal remedies may be indicated in smallpox to meet such necessities as arise. During convalescence, tonics are frequently of value.

v., black. Same as *hemorrhagic v.*

v., coherent. V. in which pustules are not confluent,* but coalesce at edges.

v., confluent. V. in which pustules run together. In confluent smallpox, the onset may be no different than in the discrete variety.

However, as eruption develops, lesions are so numerous that their presentation may be mistaken for measles. As this eruption progresses, the lesions enlarge until destroyed by breaking down of their walls and so pustular material flows together into small pools.

The temperature does not show the same remission as in the discrete type, the toxemia is much more profound, the throat symptoms are likely to be unusually severe, and swallowing may be practically impossible.

Lesions frequently develop on the conjunctiva, or even on the cornea itself, resulting in the destruction of sight. Death may be due directly to profound toxemia, or to a complicating anemia. Delirium of a violent character is common in these cases, which frequently die between the 7th and 12th day of eruption. Death, however, is not inevitable, and if patient recovers, severe pitting is likely to remain.

v., discrete. V. when pustules are distinct.

v., hemorrhagic. V. with hemorrhage into the vesicles.

In the hemorrhagic type, following customary onset, an extensive eruption of skin may develop, suggestive of scarlet fever. Profuse subconjunctival hemorrhages, profuse hemorrhages from nose and mouth may develop and patient die within 24 to 48 hours with no prior loss of consciousness. In some cases of hemorrhagic smallpox, there may be seen only a few, or sometimes many spots, followed by death within 24 hours of their appearance. In still a 3rd type of the hemorrhagic variety lesions progress in the customary manner until pustular stage is reached, when hemorrhages take place in the lesions. Cases of this kind are not necessarily fatal in comparison with the 2 preceding hemorrhagic varieties mentioned.

v., malignant. A fatal form of hemorrhagic v., *q.v.*

v., modified. Type of the disease commonly called varioloid. Case of modified smallpox seen in patients who have been vaccinated some years previously, but have not retained a complete immunity to the disease.

As a result, the infection is usually mild as to number and character of lesions, though at times the onset is somewhat severe.

variolate (văr'ĭ-ō-lāt) [L. *variola*, a tiny mark]. 1. To vaccinate with smallpox virus. 2. Having lesions like those of smallpox.

variolation, variolization (văr-ĭ-ō-lā'shŭn, văr-ĭ-ō-lĭ-zā'shŭn) [L. *variola*, a tiny spot]. Inoculation with smallpox.

varioloid (văr'ĭ-ō-loyd) [" + G. *eidos*, form]. 1. Resembling smallpox. 2. Pert. to varioloid. 3. A mild but contagious type of smallpox in those who have had smallpox or have been vaccinated.

variolous (văr-ĭ'ō-lŭs) [L. *variola*, a tiny mark]. Relating to smallpox.

varix (vā'rĭks) [L. *varix*, a dilated twisted vein]. 1. A tortuous dilatation of a vein. 2. Less commonly, dilatation of an artery or lymph vessel.

v., aneurysmal. A direct communication bet. an artery and a varicose vein without an intervening sac.

v. lymphaticus. Dilatation of lymphatic vessel.

v., turbinal. Permanent dilatation of veins of turbinate bodies.

TREATMENT: Palliative support by rubber bandage or rubber stocking. Internal remedies to remove underlying cause. Surgical measures may be resorted to in all forms.

varolian (vă-rō'lĭ-ăn). Relating to the pons Varolii.

v. bend. Ant. extension of hindgut on its ventral surface in the fetus.

varus (vā'rŭs) [L. *varus*, bent inward]. 1. Turned inward; bowlegged. 2. A condition in which a clubfooted person walks on outer border of the foot. SYN: *talipes varus*. 3. Any eruption of papules on the face. SYN: *acne*.

v. com'edo. A blackhead.

vas (văs) (pl. *vasa*) [L. *vas*, vessel]. A vessel or duct.

v. aberrans. 1. A narrow tube varying in length from 1½ to 14 inches, occasionally found connected with the lower part of the canal of the epididymis or with the commencement of the vas deferens. 2. Vestige of the biliary ducts sometimes found in the liver.

v. capillare. BNA. A capillary blood vessel.

v. deferens. The excretory duct of the testis, the continuation of the epididymis, terminating at *ductus ejaculatorius* at prostatic urethra. SYN: *ductus deferens*.

RS: *Ampullitis, cord, spermatic, deferentitis*.

v. lymphaticum. BNA. One of the vessels carrying the lymph.

v. prominens. BNA. Blood vessel on the cochlea's accessory spiral ligament.

v. spirale. A large blood vessel beneath the tunnel of corti in the basilar membrane.

vasa (vā'să) (sing. *vas*) [L. *vas*, vessel].

v. afferen'tia. 1. Arteries carrying blood to a structure. 2. The lymphatic vessels entering a gland.

vasa brevia   V-8   **vasomotor spasm**

v. bre'via. Branches of the splenic artery going to greater curvature of the stomach.
v. efferen'tia. 1. Lymphatics which leave a gland. 2. Veins carrying blood away from a part. 3. Excretory ducts of the testis.
v. prae'via. The blood vessels of the cord presenting before the fetus.
v. rec'ta. 1. Tubules which become straight prior to entering the mediastinum testis. 2. Straight collecting tubules of the kidney.
v. vaso'rum. BNA. Tiny blood vessels which are distributed to walls of larger veins and arteries.
v. vortico'sa. Stellate veins of the choroid, carrying blood to the sup. ophthalmic vein.
vasal (vā'săl) [L. *vas*, vessel]. Relating to a vas or vessel.
vasalium (văs-ā'lĭ-ŭm) (pl. *vasalia*) [L. *vasalium*]. Tissue peculiar to vascular organs.
vascular (văs'kŭ-lăr) [L. *vasculum*, a small vessel]. Pert. to or composed of blood vessels.
v. reflex. Constriction or dilation of vascular trunk or area resulting from mental or physical irritation.
v. system. The heart, blood vessels, lymphatics and their parts considered collectively.
It includes the pulmonary and portal systems.
v. tuft. One of the vascular processes on the chorion in the fetus at an early stage of development. SYN: *villi, chorionic*.
v. tumor. One containing dilated blood vessels. SYN: *angioma, telangioma*.
vascularization (văs"-kŭ-lă-rĭ-zā'shŭn) [L. *vasculum*, a tiny vessel]. Development of new blood vessels in a structure.
vascularize (văs'kŭ-lă-rīz) [L. *vasculum*, a tiny vessel]. To become vascular by development of new blood vessels.
vasculitis (văs-kŭ-lī'tĭs) [" + *-itis*, inflammation]. Inflammation of a vessel. SYN: *angeitis*.
vasculum (văs'kŭ-lŭm) [L. a small vessel]. A tiny vessel.
v. aber'rans. A tube with a blind end occasionally connected with the vas deferens or the epididymis. SYN: *vas aberrans*.
vasectomy (văs-ĕk'tō-mĭ) [L. *vas*, vessel, + G. *ektomē*, excision]. Removal of all or a segment of the vas deferens.
vasifactive (văs-ĭ-făk'tĭv) [" + *facere*, to make]. Forming new vessels.
vasiform (văs'ĭ-form) [" + *forma*, shape]. Resembling a tubular structure or vas.
vas'o- [L.]. Combining form meaning *a vessel*, as a blood vessel.
vasoconstrictive (văs"ō-kŏn-strĭk'tĭv) [L. *vas*, vessel, + *constrictus*, bound]. Causing constriction of the blood vessels.
vasoconstrictor (văs"ō-kŏn-strĭk'tor) [" + *constrictor*, a binder]. 1. Causing constriction of blood vessels. 2. That which constricts or narrows the caliber of blood vessels, as a drug or a nerve.
vasocorona (văs"ō-kor-ō'nă) [" + *corona*, a crown]. The system of peripheral vessels of the spinal cord sending branches inward.
vasodentine (văs"ō-dĕn-tēn) [" + *dentinus*, pert. to a tooth]. Modified dentine provided with blood capillaries.
vasodepression (văs"ō-dē-prĕsh'ŭn) [" + *depressio*, a pushing down]. Vasomotor depression or collapse.
vasodepressor (văs"ō-dē-prĕs'or) [" + *de-pressor*, that which pushes down]. 1.

Having a depressing influence on the circulation. 2. An agent which depresses circulation.
vasodilatation (văs"ō-dĭl-ă-tā'shŭn) [" + *dilatare*, to widen]. Dilatation of lumen of blood vessels.
v., reflex. Formation of a red mark on the skin, which turns white quickly when rubbed firmly by a penholder.
vasodilatin (văs"ō-dī-lā'tĭn) [L. *vas*, vessel, + *dilatare*, to widen]. A vasodilator substance said to be present in organic extracts, which depresses nerves and blood vessels.
vasodilator (văs"ō-dī-lā'tor) [" + *dilatare*, to widen]. 1. Causing relaxation of the blood vessels. 2. A nerve or drug which dilates the blood vessels.
vaso-epididymostomy (văs"ō-ĕp"ĭ-dĭd-ĭ-mōs'tō-mĭ) [" + G. *epi*, upon, + *didymos*, testicle, + *stoma*, passage]. Formation of a passage bet. the vas deferens and the epididymis.
vasofactive (văs"ō-făk'tĭv) [" + *facere*, to make]. Forming new blood vessels. SYN: *vasifactive, vasoformative*.
vasoformative (văs"ō-for'mă-tĭv) [" + *formare*, to form]. Forming new blood vessels. SYN: *vasofactive*.
vasoganglion (văs"ō-găng'glĭ-ŏn) [" + G. *gagglion*, knot]. Mass of blood vessels. SYN: *rete*.
vasogen (văs'ō-jĕn). Commercial ointment base used as a vehicle for remedies for skin diseases.
vasography (văs-ŏg-ră-fī) [L. *vas*, vessel, + *graphein*, to write]. X-ray photography of the blood vessels.
vasohypertonic (văs"ō-hī-pĕr-tŏn'ĭk) [" + G. *hyper*, over, + *tonikos*, pert. to tension]. Causing or that which causes constriction of blood vessels. SYN: *vasoconstrictor*.
vasohypotonic (văs"ō-hī-pō-tŏn'ĭk) [" + G. *hypo*, under, + *tonikos*, pert. to tension]. Relaxing or that which relaxes blood vessels. SYN: *vasodilator*.
vasoinhibitor (văs"ō-ĭn-hĭb'ĭ-tor) [" + *inhibere*, to restrain]. An agent that depresses vasomotor nerve.
vasoinhibitory (văs"ō-ĭn-hĭb'ĭ-tor-ĭ) [" + *inhibere*, to restrain]. Restricting vasomotor activity.
vasoligation (văs"ō-lī-gā'shŭn) [" + *ligare*, to bind]. Ligation of a vessel, specifically the vas deferens.
vasomotion (văs"ō-mō'shŭn) [" + *motio*, a moving]. Change in caliber of a blood vessel.
vasomotor (văs"ō-mō'tor) [L. *vas*, vessel, + *motor*, a mover]. 1. Pert. to the nerves having muscular control of the blood vessel walls.
The circulatory arranged fibers of the muscles of arteries and veins can contract or relax; the affected region is accordingly either blanched or flushed. The former effect can commonly be produced by stimulating sympathetic fibers, which are consequently called vasoconstrictor; certain other nerves on stimulation cause vasodilation, examples being the nervus chorda tympani and the nervi erigentes.
A vasomotor reflex is one in which the stimulus, *e. g.*, a horrifying sight, results in a change in vasomotor stage, *e. g.*, pallor. SEE: *vasoconstrictor, vasodilator*.
v. catarrh. An allergic acute nasal catarrh. SYN: *hay fever*.
v. epilepsy. E. with vasomotor changes in the skin.
v. nerves. Those which cause either contraction or dilation of blood vessels.
v. spasm. Spasm of smaller arteries.

vasomotory (văs″ō-mō′tor-ĭ) [L. *vas*, vessel, + *motor*, a mover]. Controlling changes in the size of the blood vessels. SYN: *vasomotor*.

vasoneurosis (văs″ō-nū-rō′sĭs) [" + G. *neuron*, nerve, + -*ōsis*, condition]. A neurosis affecting blood vessels; a disorder of the vasomotor system. SEE: *angioneurosis*.

vasoörchidostomy (văs″ō-or-kĭd-ŏs′tō-mĭ) ["+G. *orchis, orchid*-, testicle, + *stoma*, mouth]. Surgical connection of the epididymis to the severed end of the vas deferens.

vasoparesis (văs″ō-par-ē-sĭs, -păr-ē′sĭs) [" + G. *paresis*, relaxation]. Partial paralysis or weakness of the vasomotor nerves.

vasopressin (văs″ō-prĕs′ĭn). A post. pituitary lobe hormone.
It stimulates intestinal muscles and raises blood pressure. SEE: *oxytocin, pitressin*.

vasopuncture (văs′ō-pŭnk-chŭr) [L. *vas*, vessel, + *punctura*, a piercing]. Puncture of the vas deferens.

vasorelaxation (văs″ō-rē-lăks-ā′shŭn) [" + *relaxāre*, to loosen]. Lessening of vascular pressure.

vasorrhaphy (văs-or′ă-fĭ) [" + G. *rhaphē*, a seam]. Surgical suture of the vas deferens.

vasosection (văs′-ō-sĕk′shŭn) [" + *sectio*, a cutting]. Surgical division of the vasa deferentia.

vasosensory (văs″ō-sen′sō-rĭ) [" + *sensōrius*, pert. to sensation]. Distributing sensory filaments to the blood vessels.

vasospasm (văs″ō-spăzm) [" + G. *spasmos*, a spasm]. Spasm of any vessel, esp. of a blood vessel. SYN: *angiospasm, vasoconstriction*.

vasostimulant (văs″ō-stĭm′ū-lănt) [" + *stimulāre*, to goad]. Exciting vasomotor action.

vasostomy (va-zos′to-mĭ) [L. *vas*, vessel, + G. *stoma*, mouth]. Surgical procedure of making an opening into the vas deferens.

vasothrombin (văs″ō-thrŏm′bĭn) [" + G. *thrombos*, a clot]. Thrombin derived from the intima of blood vessels.

vasotomy (văs-ŏt′ō-mĭ) [" + G. *tomē*, a cutting]. Incision of the vas deferens.

vasotonic (văs″ō-tŏn′ĭk) [" + G. *tonikos*, pert. to tone]. Pert. to the tone of a vessel.

vasotribe (văs′ō-trĭb) [" + G. *tribein*, to crush]. Pressure forceps used for controlling hemorrhages. SYN: *angiotribe*.

vasotripsy (văs′ō-trĭp-sĭ) [" + G. *tripsis*, a crushing]. Arrest of hemorrhages with a strong forceps by crushing an artery. SYN: *angiotripsy*.

vasotrophic (văs″ō-trof′ĭk) [" + G. *trophē*, nourishment]. Affecting the nutrition by change in caliber of blood vessels.

vasovesiculectomy (văs″ō-vĕs-ĭk-ū-lĕk′tō-mĭ) [" + *vesicula*, tiny sac, + G. *ektomē*, excision]. Excision of the vas deferens and seminal vesicles.

vasovesiculitis (văs″ō-vĕs-ĭk-ū-lī′tĭs) [" + *vesicula*, tiny sac, + G. -*itis*, inflammation]. Inflammation of the vas deferens and seminal vesicles.

Vater's ampullae (fäh′ter). Dilatation at junction of common bile duct and pancreatic duct, just before they empty into the duodenum.
V.'s corpuscles. Ovoid end organs of nerves supplying the skin. SYN: *pacinian corpuscles*.

veal (vēl) [ME *veel*]. COMP: Poor in fat and myosin and inferior to beef. Overburdened with xanthines and nuclein. More or less toxic.
v. cutlet (cooked). AV. SERVING: 230 Gm. Pro. 22.7; fat 2.7.

Veal (Nutrients)

	Pro.	Fat	Fuel Value	Calories
Breast	20.3	11.0	100 Gm.	178
Forequarters	20.0	8.0	100 Gm.	151
Hindquarters	20.7	8.3	100 Gm.	156
Side	20.2	8.1	100 Gm.	153

ASH: Ca 0.058, Mg 0.118, K 1.694, Na 0.421, P 1.078, Cl 0.378, S 1.146, Fe 0.015.
VITAMINS: A— to +, B+.
Fifteen milligrams of iron per 100 Gm. of protein ascribed to meats is too high for veal.
ACTION: It resists the action of the gastric juice and is less digestible than beef.

vection (vĕk′shŭn) [L. *vectio*, a carrying]. Carrying of disease germ from the sick to well persons.
v., circumferen′tial. Transference through an intermediate host.
v., ra′dial. Direct transference of disease germs from one individual to another.

vectis (vĕk′tĭs) [L. *rectis*, pole]. A curved lever for making traction on the presenting part of the fetus.

vector (vĕk′tor) [L. *vector*, a carrier]. A living carrier of disease germs from the sick to a well person. SEE: *vection*.
v., circumferen′tial. One carrying infection from the sick to the well.

vectorial (vĕk-tō′rĭ-ăl) [L. *vector*, a carrier]. Relating to a vector.

vegetable (vĕj′ĕt-ă-bl) [O. Fr. from L. *vegetus*, active]. 1. Pert. to plants. 2. A herbaceous plant cultivated for food. They supply necessary bulk and are rich in mineral and vitamin value. Five average servings of vegetables and fruit per day are supposed to supply sufficient cellulose, or four if a whole wheat cereal is used. Vegetables give low intestinal reduction value and are conducive to favorable intestinal flora. SEE: *names of vegetables*.
v., green. ACTION: They promote intestinal hygiene.
CONTENTS: Vegetables in general are valuable for their mineral content and for their cellulose. *Copper* is estimated at 1.2 milligrams per kilo for leafy vegetables, and 0.7 milligram per kilo for nonleafy ones. They are deficient in fat, which should be made up by adding milk, cream, butter in their preparation. SEE: *names of minerals*.

Purines in Vegetables		
	Per Cent	Grains in Lb.
Asparagus	.021	1.50
Beans	.063	4.16
Onions	.009	.06
Oatmeal	.053	3.45
Peameal	.039	2.54
Potatoes	.002	.14

DIET: The question of a vegetarian diet is a debatable one, there being good arguments on both sides. The argument of the vegetarian that meat should be

avoided on account of its toxic principles seems to be offset by the fact that purines and xanthic bodies are present in vegetables as well as in meat. Probably the rational diet should be made up of a small quantity of meat with vegetables predominating. [0.95.
NUTRIENTS: Pro. 0.83, Fat 0.90, Carbo.
ACTION: Vegetables for the most part are base-forming foods. They increase the dissolving of uric acid, and cause diminishing of ammonia content. They stimulate the entire system, esp. the stomach, intestines, kidneys, skin, and generative organs. They are antiscorbutic, prevent scurvy, constipation, rheumatism, diabetes, purpura, anemia, and they render the blood and urine alkaline.

The green parts of all vegetables are esp. good for anemia and chlorosis. Fibrous vegetables should be avoided in hyperacidity. Vegetable foods cause fermentation, increasing peristalsis, and they are hurried through the system without proper time for absorption.

LOSS IN COOKING: (a) The more water a vegetable absorbs, the less will be the nutritive values as they are diluted by the water.
(b) Boiling lessens the nutritive value, esp. vegetables without skins, as the salts are absorbed by the water.
(c) The average loss in cooking vegetables is about one-third; of this loss, 0.5 per cent is protein, 30 to 50 per cent is carbohydrates and about 50 per cent salts. Baked vegetables lose their juice through absorption by heated air.

CHEMICAL CHANGES: 1. Dry heat changes starch to dextrin. 2. Heat and acid or a ferment change dextrin to dextrose. 3. In germinating grain, starch is changed to dextrin and dextrose. 4. Dextrose in fermentation turns to alcohol and carbon dioxide. 5. Raw starch is not digestible. All starches must be changed to sugars before they can be absorbed in the system. SEE: *classification of sugars.*

vegetarian (vĕj-ē-tā′rĭ-ăn) [L. *vegetabilis*, quickening]. One who eats no animal products, but who lives on vegetables.

vegetarianism (vĕj-ē-tā′rĭ-ăn-Izm) [" + G. -*ismos*, condition]. The belief and practice of eating vegetables and fruits, only.

Time for Cooking Vegetables

Asparagus	30–45 min.
Beans, dried, boiled	2 hours
Beans, dried, baked	4–10 hours
Beans, string, boiled	45–60 min.
Beans, old	1–1½ hours
Bean soup, simmer	2 hours

Some beans require longer cooking than others. Hard water makes it necessary to boil beans and roots longer because the lime in the water is deposited upon the vegetable, making it harder for the water to penetrate.

Beets, boiled, if young, 2-3 hours; if old	3–4 hours
Brussels sprouts, boiled	15–25 min.
Cabbage, boiled, if young	25–60 min.
Cabbage, fried	30–45 min.

Cooking too long renders it bitter.

Carrots	30–45 min.
Cauliflower, boiled	20–30 min.
Chard, boiled	30 min.
Celery, boiled	30 min.
Cereals—Oats	4 hours
Quaker Oats	2 hours
Wheat, steam cooked	20 min.
Cream of Wheat	45 min.
Corn Meal	3–4 hours
Rice, boiled, 30 min.; steamed	45–60 min.
Corn, boiled, 5–7 min.; baked	30 min.

Corn in the ear should be boiled just long enough to set the milk. Too long boiling makes it hard.

Eggplant, boiled, 20 min.; Baked	15 min.

Fry until brown.

Kohlrabi, boiled	30–50 min.
Macaroni, boiled 20–60 min.; baked	1 hour
Onions, boiled	30–60 min.
Onions, fried	30–45 min.
Onions, baked	30 min.
Parsnips, boiled	30–45 min.

Fry until brown.

Peas, boiled	20–30 min.

Old peas require longer boiling.

Potatoes, boiled	20–30 min.
Potatoes, baked (according to size)	30–60 min.
Potatoes, fried, raw	30–45 min.
Potatoes, sweet, boiled	15–25 min.

New potatoes take longer to boil than old ones. Medium sized, 45 min. to 1 hour to boil.

Rice, boil until tender or about	20–30 min.
Salsify, boiled	30–45 min.
Spaghetti, boiled, until tender or about	15–30 min.
Tomatoes, boiled	20–30 min.
If canned, boil	12–20 min.
Tomatoes, fried	20–30 min.
Tomatoes, baked	30 min.
Tapioca, boiled	1 hour
Turnips, boiled	30–45 min.
Spinach	15–30 min.
Squash, baked	1 hour
Squash, summer, steamed 1 hour; baked	20 min.

Percentage Loss of Nutrients of Boiled Vegetables		
	Carbohydrates In Raw Vegetables	Carbohydrates After boil'g and strain'g
Asparagus	3.30	1.60
Cauliflower	2.10	1.40
Cabbage, savoy	6.00	2.70
Cabbage, turnip	3.09	2.43
Cabbage, winter	6.75	3.20
Spinach	2.97	0.85

vegetation (vĕj-ē-tā′shŭn) [L. *vegetātio*, animation]. A morbid luxurious outgrowth on any part, esp. wartlike projections made up of collections of fibrin in which are enmeshed white and red blood cells; sometimes seen on denuded areas of the endocardium covering the valves of the heart.

vegetative (vĕj′ē-tā″tĭv) [L. *vegetāre*, to animate). 1. Having the power to grow, as plants. 2. Functioning involuntarily. 3. Quiescent, passive, noting a stage of development.
  v. nervous system. The sympathetic* nervous system.
  v. pole. Area at end of ovum containing nutritive matter.

vehicle (vē′ĭ-kl) [L. *vehiculum*, that which carries]. A substance used as a medium for the administration of medicine, as syrup in liquid preparations. SYN: *menstruum*.

veil (vāl) [L. *velum*, a covering]. 1. Any veillike structure. 2. A piece of the amniotic sac occasionally covering the face of a newborn infant. SYN: *caul*. 3. Slight obscuration of the voice.
  v., acquired. Slight imperfection of the voice due to strain or exposure.
  v., uterine. Device for covering the cervix uteri to prevent impregnation.

vein (vān) [L. *vena*]. Vessel carrying dark red (unaerated) blood to the heart, except for pulmonary veins.
Veins have 3 coats. They differ from arteries in their larger capacity and greater number; also in their thinner walls, larger and more frequent anastomoses and presence of valves which prevent backward circulation. They consist of 2 sets, *superficial* or *subcutaneous* and the *deep* veins with frequent communications. The former do not usually accompany an artery, as do the latter. The systemic veins consist of 3 groups: Those entering the heart through the (a) *superior vena cava*, (b) those through the *inferior vena cava*, and (c) those through the *coronary sinus*. Blood from the capillary plexuses enters the right auricle of the heart. SEE: *circulation, Table of Veins in Appendix*.

vein, words pert. to: basilic, cava, innominate, intravenous, janitrix, jugular, phlebectomy, phlebitis, phlebogram, phlebotomy, phlegmasia alba dolens, portal, thrombophlebitis, thrombus, "varic-" words, varix, vascular, vasoconstrictor, vasodilator, vasomotor, vasoparesis, vena, vena cava, venesection, venosity, venovenostomy, venule, venous.

velamen (vĕl-ā′mĕn) (pl. *velamina*) [L. *velamen*, veil]. Any covering membrane.
  v. nativum. The skin covering the body.
  v. vul′vae. Abnormal elongation of the nymphae. SYN: *Hottentot apron*.

velamentous (vĕl-ă-mĕn′tŭs) [L. *velamen*, veil]. Expanding like a veil, or sheet.

velamentum (vĕl-ă-mĕn′tŭm) (pl. *velamenta*) [L. *velamentum*, a cover]. A membranous covering.

velar (vē′lar) [L. *velum*, a veil]. Pert. to a veil or veillike structure.

vellication (vĕl-ĭk-ā′shŭn) [L. *vellicāre*, to twitch]. Spasmodic twitching of muscular fibers.

velocity (vē-lŏs′ĭt-ĭ) [L. *velocitas*, swiftness]. Rate of speed of an object or process. In the following table some commonly known velocities are stated in metric units (meters per second) for comparison with certain data of physiological interest:
Speed of blood in fastest arteries, 0.3 m. per sec.
Light, 299,877.000 meters.
Nervous impulse, 80.
Sound in air, 331.
Pulse wave in arteries, 9.
Walking (3 miles per hour), 1.3.

velosynthesis (vĕl-o-sĭn′thĕs-ĭs) [L. *velum*, veil, + G. *synthesis*, a placing together]. Suture of a cleft palate, particularly the soft palate. SYN: *staphylorrhaphy*.

Velpeau's bandage (vĕl-pō′). A bandage for the shoulder. SEE: *bandage*.

V's deformity. D. seen in Colles'* fracture in which lower fragment is displaced backward.

velum (vē′lŭm) [L. *velum*, veil]. Any veillike structure.
  v. palati′num. BNA. The soft palate.

vena (vē′nă) (pl. *venae*) [L. *vena*, vein]. A vein. SEE: *Table of Veins in Appendix*.

venenation (vĕn-ē-nā′shŭn) [L. *venenum*, poison]. 1. Condition of being poisoned. 2. Act of poisoning.

venene (vē-nēn′) [L. *venenum*, poison]. Toxic substance in snake venom.

veneniferous (vĕn-ē-nĭf′ĕr-ŭs) [" + *ferre*, to carry]. Transmitting or carrying poison.

venenific (vĕn-ē-nĭf′ĭk) [" + *facere*, to make]. Producing poison.

venenous (vĕn′ĕn-ŭs) [L. *venenum*, poison]. Poisonous.

venepuncture (vĕn′ĕ-pŭnk″chŭr) [L. *vena*, vein, + *punctura*, a piercing]. Puncture of a vein to withdraw blood or inject a remedy.

venereal (vē-nē′rē-ăl) [L. *venereus*, from *Venus*, goddess of love]. Pert. to or resulting from sexual intercourse.
  v. bubo. Enlarged gland in the groin, the result of a venereal disease.
  v. collar. Mottled condition of the neck seen occasionally in syphilis.
  v. disease. One acquired ordinarily as a result of sexual intercourse with an individual who is afflicted.
  The diseases are gonorrhea, syphilis and chancroid, Vincent's infection of the genitals known as the fourth venereal disease, and the fifth venereal disease, venereal lymphogranuloma.
  v. sore, v. ulcer. Chancroid.
  v. wart. Moist reddish elevations on genitals and anus. SYN: *verruca acuminata, condyloma*.

venereologist (vē-nēr″ē-ŏl′ō-jĭst) [L. *venereus*, venereal, + G. *logos*, a study]. A doctor who specializes in the treatment of venereal diseases.

venereology (vē-nēr″ē-ŏl′ō-jĭ) [" + G. *logos*, a study]. The scientific study and treatment of venereal diseases.

venereophobia (vē-nēr″ē-ō-fō′bĭ-ă) [" + G. *phobos*, *fear*]. Abnormal fear of venereal disease. SYN: *cypridophobia*.

venery (věn′ěr-ĭ) [L. *Venus*, *Vener*-, Venus, goddess of love]. Sexual intercourse. SYN: *coitus*.

venesection (věn″-ē-sěk′shŭn) [L. *vena*, vein, + *sectio*, a cutting]. Opening of a vein for withdrawal of blood.

venin(e (věn′ĭn) [L. *venenum*, poison]. Toxic substance in snake venom.

venin-antivenin (věn″ĭn-ăn″tĭ-věn′ĭn). Vaccine to counteract snake poison.

veniplex (věn′ĭ-plěks) [L. *vena*, vein, + *plexus*, a braid]. A plexus of veins.

venipuncture (věn″ĭ-pŭnk′chŭr) [" + *punctura*, a piercing]. Puncture of a vein for any purpose.

venisection (věn″ĭ-sěk′shŭn) [" + *sectio*, a cutting]. Opening of a vein for blood abstraction. SYN: *phlebotomy*.

venisuture (věn-ĭ-sū-chŭr) [" + *sutura*, a stitch]. Suture of a vein. SYN: *phleborrhaphy*.

venoauricular (vē″nō-aw-rĭk′ū-lar) [L. *vena*, vein, + *auricula*, auricle]. Relating to the vena cava and the auricle.

venoclysis (vē-nŏk′lĭ-sĭs) [" + G. *klysis*, injection]. The continuous injection of medicinal or nutrient fluid intravenously. SYN: *phleboclysis*.

venogram (vē′nō-grăm) [" + G. *gramma*, a writing]. 1. A roentgenogram of the veins. SYN: *phlebogram*. 2. A tracing of the venous pulse.

venography (vē-nŏg′ră-fĭ) [" + G. *graphein*, to write]. 1. Roentgenography of veins. 2. The making of a tracing of the venous pulse.

venom (věn′ŏm) [L. *venenum*, poison]. A poison excreted by some animals, such as insects or snakes, and transmitted by bites or stings.

venoperitoneostomy(vē″nō-pěr″ĭ-tō-nē-ŏs′-tō-mĭ) [L. *vena*, vein, + G. *peritonaion*, peritoneum, + *stoma*, passage]. Attachment of the cut end of the saphenous vein into the cavity of the peritoneum.

venopressor (vē′nō-prěs′or) [" + *pressor*, that which squeezes]. Pert. to venous blood pressure and its supply to the right side of the heart.

venosclerosis (vē″nō-sklē-rō′sĭs) [" + G. *sklērōsis*, a hardening]. Sclerosis of veins. SYN: *phlebosclerosis*.

venosity (vē-nŏs′ĭ-tĭ) [L. *vena*, vein]. 1. Condition in which there is an excess of venous blood in a part causing venous congestion. 2. Deficient aeration of venous blood.

venostasis (vē-nŏs′tă-sĭs) [" + G. *stasis*, a standing]. Abstraction of blood from the circulation by compression of veins in an extremity. SYN: *phlebostasis*.

venostat (vē′nō-stăt) [" + G. *statikos*, standing]. Appliance for performing venous compression.

venotomy (vē-nŏt′ō-mĭ) [L. *vena*, vein, + G. *tomē*, a cutting]. Incision of a vein.

venous (vē′nŭs) [L. *vena*, vein]. Pert. to the veins or blood passing through them.
  v. blood. The dark blood in the veins.
  v. hum. Murmur heard upon auscultation over larger veins of the neck.
  v. hypere′mia. Excess of venous blood in a part. SYN: *venosity*.
  v. sinus. Cerebral sinus.

venovenostomy (vē-nō-vē-nŏs′tō-mĭ) [L. *vena*, vein, + *vena*, vein, + G. *stoma*, mouth]. Formation of an anastomosis of a vein into a vein.

vent (věnt) [O. Fr. *fente*, slit]. An opening in any cavity, esp. one for excretion.

venter (věn′ter) [L. *venter*, belly]. 1. The abdomen. SYN: *belly*. 2. Any of the greater body cavities. 3. The uterus. 4. The hollowed part of a muscle or other structure.

ventilation (věn-tĭl-ā′shŭn) [L. *ventilāre*, to air]. 1. Circulation of air or amt. of fresh air in a room and withdrawal of foul air. 2. Oxygenation of blood. 3. PHYS: The amt. of air inhaled per day. This can be estimated by spirometry, multiplying the tidal air by the number of respirations per day. An average figure is 10,000 liters. This must not be confused with the total amt. of oxygen consumed, which is on the average only 490 liters. 2000 cu. ft. of air per hr. are necessary to maintain health. Inspired air contains *carbon dioxide*, 4.38%; *oxygen*, 16.02%, and *nitrogen*, 79%. SEE: *air*, *humidity*, *respiration*.
  v., exhaustion. Forcible withdrawal of air from a room.
  v., ple′num. Forcible introduction of air into a room.

ventose (věn′tōs) [L. *ventōsus*, windy]. Distended with gas. SYN: *flatulent*.

ventouse (vahn-tooz′) [Fr.]. A glass for cupping.

ven′trad [L. *venter*, belly, + *ad*, toward]. Toward the ventral aspect, opp. to *dorsad*.

ventral (věn′trăl) [L. *ventralis*, pert. to the belly]. Pert. to the ant. or front side of the body. Opp. of *dorsal*.*
  v. aspect. Ant. or inf. view; toward the belly.
  v. hernia. One through the abdominal wall.

ventricle (věn′trĭk-l) [L. *ventriculus*, a little belly]. 1. A small cavity. 2. One of 2 lower chambers of the heart, which propel blood into the arteries. The right v. forces it into the pulmonary artery and the lungs; the left, through the aorta. At each beat, each ventricle pumps more than 6 oz. of blood.
  RS: *Arantius'*, *aula*, *aulatela*, *carneous columns*.
  v., aortic. Left v. of the heart.
  v. of the brain. Five cavities filled with cerebrospinal fluid.
  v. of the larynx. The space bet. the true and false vocal cords.
  v. of Morgagni. Space bet. true and false cords extending laterally to the thyroid cartilage.
  v. of the myelon. Central canal of spinal cord.
  v., prolapse of. Seen in tuberculosis and syphilis.

ventricornu (věn-trĭ-kor′nū) [L. *venter*, belly, + *cornu*, horn]. The ant. ventral horn of gray matter of the spinal cord.

ventricornual (věn″trĭ-kor′nū-ăl) [" + *cornu*, horn]. Relating to the ventricornu.

ventricose (věn′trĭ-kōs) [L. *ventricōsus*, big-bellied]. 1. Inflated on 1 side. 2. Corpulent.

ventricular (věn-trĭk′ū-lar) [L. *ventriculus*, a little belly]. Pert. to a ventricle.
  v. aqueduct. Canal connecting 3rd and 4th cerebral ventricles. SYN: *aquaeductus Sylvii*.
  v. bands. The false vocal cords or folds of mucous membrane parallel or above the vocal bands.
  v. ligament. A false vocal band.
  v. muscle. The thyreoepiglottideus.
  v. septum. S. between ventricles of the heart.

ventriculin (věn-trĭk′ū-lĭn). Desiccated,

ventriculography   V-13   vernal

defatted hog stomach used in primary anemia.
DOSAGE: From 20-30 Gm. daily.
ventriculography (vĕn-trĭk-ū-lŏg'rā-fĭ) [L. *ventriculus*, a little belly, + G. *graphein*, to write]. An x-ray process used for localization of cerebral tumors, following the injection of air into the cerebral ventricles.
ventriculometry (vĕn-trĭk″ū-lŏm'ĕ-trĭ) [" + G. *metron*, a measure]. The measurement of the intraventricular cerebral pressure.
ventriculonector (vĕn-trĭk″ū-lŏ-nĕk'tor) [" + *nector*, a joiner]. Muscular band connecting auricles and ventricles of the heart. SYN: *atrioventricular bundle.*
ventriculoscopy (vĕn-trĭk″ū-lŏs'kō-pĭ) [" + G. *skopein*, to examine]. Examination of the ventricles of the brain with an endoscope.
ventriculus (vĕn-trĭk'ū-lŭs) [L. a little belly]. BNA. 1. The stomach. 2. A ventricle of the brain or heart.
ventricumbent (vĕn-trĭ-kŭm'bĕnt) [L. *venter*, belly, + *cumbere*, to lie]. Lying on the belly. SYN: *prone.*
ventriduct (vĕn'trĭ-dŭkt) [" + *ductus*, leading]. To draw toward the abdomen.
ventrimeson (vĕn-trĭ-mĕs'ŏn) [" + G. *mesos*, middle]. The median line on the ventral surface of the body.
ventripyramid (vĕn″trĭ-pir'ă-mĭd) [" + G. *pyramis*, pyramid]. An ant. pyramid of the medulla oblongata.
ventrocystorrhaphy (vĕn-trō-sĭs-tor'ă-fĭ) [" + G. *kystis*, sac, + *rhaphē*, a seam]. Suture of a cyst to the abdominal wall to permit drainage.
ventrofixation (vĕn″trō-fĭks-ā-shŭn) [" + *fixāre*, to fix]. The suture of a displaced viscus to the abdominal wall.
ventrohysteropexy (vĕn″trō-hĭs'tĕr-ŏ-pĕks″ĭ) [" + G. *hystera*, uterus, + *pēxis*, fixation]. Attachment of the uterus to the abdominal wall.
ventroscopy (vĕn-trŏs'kō-pĭ) [L. *venter*, belly, + G. *skopein*, to examine]. Examination of the abdominal cavity by illumination. SYN: *celioscopy.*
ventrose (vĕn'trōs) [L. *venter*, belly]. Having a belly or swelling like one.
ventrosuspension (vĕn″trō-sŭs-pĕn'shŭn) [" + *suspensio*, a hanging]. Fixation of displaced uterus to abdominal wall.
ventrotomy (vĕn-trŏt'ō-mĭ) [" + G. *tomē*, a cutting]. Incision into abdominal cavity. SYN: *celiotomy, laparotomy, q.v.*
ventrovesicofixation (vĕn″trō-vĕs-ĭ-kō-fĭks-ā'shŭn) [" + *vesica*, bladder, + *fixāre*, to fix]. Suture of uterus to abdominal wall and bladder. SYN: *hysterocystopexy.*
venula (vĕn'ū-lă) [L. little vein]. Venule.
venule (vĕn'ūl) [L. *venula*, little vein]. A veinlet, a tiny vein continuous with a capillary.
venus (vē'nŭs) [L. *Venus*, goddess of love]. Sexual intercourse. SYN: *copulation.*
   v.'s collar. Pigmentation around the neck in eruption due to syphilis.
verbigeration (vĕr-bĭj-ĕr-ā'shŭn) [L. *verbigerāre*, to chatter]. Uncontrollable repetition of phrases, absence of coherent thought combined with voluble speech, seen in insanity.
verbomania (vĕr″bō-mā'nĭ-ă) [L. *verba*, word, + G. *mania*, madness]. The flow of talk in some forms of psychosis.
verdigris (vĕr'dĭg-rĭs) [O.Fr.]. 1. Mixture of basic copper acetates. 2. Deposit of copper carbonate upon copper and bronze vessels.
   POISONING: TREATMENT: Same as for copper sulfate.
Vergas' ventricle (vĕr'gă). Cleftlike space bet. the callosum and fornix of the brain.
vergency (vĕr'jĕn-sĭ) [L. *vergere*, to turn].
1. Any turning movement about the eyes.
2. The reciprocal of the focal distance of a lens taken as a measure of the divergence or convergence of rays.
Verheyen's stars (fĕr-hī'ĕn). Starlike venous plexuses on surface of the kidney below its capsule.
verjuice (vĕr'jŭs) [Fr. *verd*, green, + *jus*, juice]. Acid juice from unripe fruit.
vermicidal (vĕr″mĭ-sĭ'dăl) [L. *vermis*, worm, + *cidus*, from *caedere*, to kill]. Destroying worms parasitic in the intestines.
vermicide (vĕr'mĭ-sīd) [" + *cidus*, from *caedere*, to kill]. 1. Destroying worms. 2. An agent that will kill intestinal worms. Ex: *santonin, oil of chenopodium.*
vermicular (vĕr-mĭk'ū-lăr) [L. *vermicularis*, like a worm]. Resembling a worm.
   v. appendix. The vermiform appendix.
   v. movements. The wormlike movements of peristalsis.
   v. pulse. Small, rapid one resulting in wormlike feeling in the fingers.
vermiculation (vĕr-mĭk″-ū-lā'shŭn) [L. *vermiculāre*, to wriggle]. A wormlike motion, as in the intestines. SEE: *peristalsis.*
vermiculose, vermiculous (vĕr-mĭk'ū-lōs, vĕr-mĭk'ū-lŭs) [L. *vermicularis*, wormlike]. 1. Infested with worms or larvae. 2. Wormlike.
vermiform (vĕr'mĭ-form) [L. *vermis*, worm, + *forma*, shape]. Contoured like a worm.
   v. appendix. A small tube about the size of a goose quill opening into the cecum and closed at its other end.
   Its inflammation is called *appendicitis.**
vermifugal (vĕr-mĭf'ū-găl) [" + *fugāre*, to put to flight]. Expelling worms from the intestines.
vermifuge (vĕr'mĭ-fūj) [" + *fugāre*, to put to flight]. 1. Expelling worms. 2. Agent for expelling intestinal worms. SYN: *vermicide.*
vermilion (vĕr-mĭl'yŭn) [L. *vermilium*]. Red mercuric sulfide.
   v. border. Junction of mucous membrane of the lips with the skin.
   v. poisoning. Poisoning is slower and less marked, but resembles mercuric chloride, *q.v.*
vermin (vĕr'mĭn) [L. *vermis*, worm]. Parasitic insects and animals, such as mice, lice, bedbugs.
   v. killers. POISONING: SEE: *arsenic, strychnine, phosphorus* and *fluorides*, which are the principal poisonous ingredients.
   F. A. TREATMENT: Wash out stomach. Administer saline cathartic and soothing or demulcent drinks.
vermination (vĕr-mĭn-ā'shŭn) [L. *vermis*, worm]. Vermin or worm infestation.
verminosis (vĕr-mĭn-ō'sĭs) [" + G. *-ōsis*, condition]. Infestation with vermin.
verminous (vĕr'mĭn-ŭs) [L. *vermis*, worm]. Pert. to or infested with worms.
vermiphobia (vĕr-mĭ-fō'bĭ-ă) [" + G. *phobos*, fear]. An abnormal fear of being infestated with worms.
vermis (vĕr'mĭs) [L. *vermis*, worm]. 1. A worm. 2. Median connecting lobe of the cerebellum.
   v. cerebel'li. BNA. Same as vermis, 2.
vermography (vĕr-mŏg'ră-fĭ) [" + G. *graphein*, to write]. Roentgenography of the vermiform appendix.
vernal (vĕr'năl) [L. *vernalis*, pert. to

vernal catarrh — vertebra

spring]. Occurring in or pert. to the spring.
 v. catarrh. A chronic form of conjunctivitis occurring usually in spring and remaining until cool weather. SEE: *catarrh vernal.*
 v. fever. Malarial fever.
Vernes' test (värn). A blood test for syphilis.
vernix (vĕr'nĭks) [L.]. Varnish.
 v. caseo'sa. A sebaceous deposit covering the fetus due to secretion of skin glands. Most abundant in creases and flexor surfaces. Consists of exfoliations of outer skin layer, lanugo, and secretions of sebaceous glands.
 After birth, rub the skin with olive oil and it will disappear. SEE: *sebum.*
verodigen (vē-rō'dĭj-ĕn). A purified digitalis principle.
 DOSAGE: 1/80 gr. (0.0008 Gm.).
veronal (vĕr'ō-năl). USP. A brand of barbital, a white crystalline substance.
 USES: As a hypnotic.
 DOSAGE: 5 gr. (0.3 Gm.).
 v. sodium. A brand of soluble barbital.
veronalism (vĕr'ō-năl-ĭzm). Addiction to the use of veronal and the resultant symptoms.
verruca (vĕr-rū'kă) (pl. *verrucae*) [L. *verruca*, wart]. Elevation of the skin, small, circumscribed, formed by hypertrophy of the papillae and of various forms according to location. SYN: *wart.*
 ETIOL: Essential cause not known. Believed to be autoinoculable with bruise or trauma as predisposing factor in localization.
 PROG: Essentially benign, particularly in children and young adults. In elderly with long-standing dry seborrhea, lesions have potential malignancy.
 TREATMENT: Removal with sharp spoon under local anesthesia, touching base with iodine. If elevated, clip off with sharp scissors and touch with iodine. Negative galvanism, cauterization with zinc chloride, formalin, trichloracetic acid, liquor potassii, acid nitrate of mercury, freezing with carbon dioxide snow, fulguration and, if multiple, x-rays.
 Injections of bismuth salicylate into a muscle have been tried very successfully. Ordinary warts may be removed by electrolysis, excision or caustics. Venereal warts should be bathed in some antiseptic solution and dusted with iodoform or boric acid. Constitutional remedies.
 v. acuminata. A pointed reddish moist wart about the genitals and the anus, seen in gonorrhea. SYN: *venereal wart.*
 Develops near mucocutaneous junctures, forming pointed, tufted, or pedunculated, pinkish or purplish projections of varying lengths and consistence.
 Venereal warts should be bathed in an antiseptic solution and dusted with iodoform or boric acid.
 v. digitata. Form seen on face and scalp, possibly serving as starting point of cutaneous horns, forming several filiform projections with horny caps closely grouped on a comparatively narrow base which in turn may be separated from skin surface by slightly contracted neck.
 v. filiformis. Small threadlike growths on neck and eyelids covered with smooth and apparently normal epidermis.
 v. plana. Flat oily wart, pigmented, on backs of old people. [feet.
 v. plantaris. Warts on the soles of the
 v. senilis. SEE: *v. plana.*
 v. simplex. V. vulgaris, *q.v.*
 v. vulgaris. Common warts, usually on backs of hands and fingers.

verruciform (vĕr-ū'sĭ-form) [L. *verruca*, wart, + *forma*, shape]. Wartlike.
verrucose, verrucous (vĕr'rū-kōs, vĕr-rū'kŭs) [L. *verrucōsus*, wartlike]. Wartlike, with raised portions.
versicolor (vĕr'sĭ-kŭl"er) [L. *versicolor*, of changing colors]. 1. Having many shades or colors. 2. Changeable in color.
version (ver'shŭn) [L. *versio*, a turning].
 1. Condition of uterus in which its axis is deflected from the normal position without being bent on itself. SEE: *anteversion, lateroversion, retroversion.* 2. Process of turning the fetus in the uterus to facilitate delivery.
 v., cephalic. Turning of fetus so that the head presents.
 v., pelvic. Manipulation of a cross presentation until it is changed to a pelvic presentation.
 v., podalic. Manipulation of fetus by the feet so that the breech presents.
 v., spontaneous. V. of fetus by uterine muscular contraction without artificial assistance.

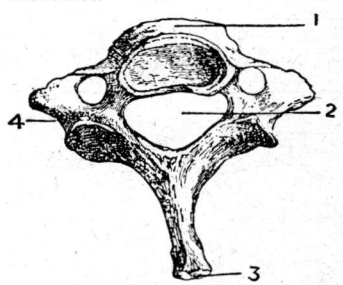

TYPICAL VERTEBRA
1. Body. 2. Vertebral foramen. 3. Spinous process. 4. Transverse process.

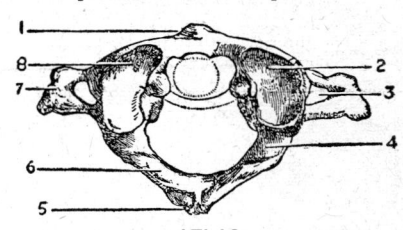

ATLAS
1. Anterior tubercle. 2. Lateral mass. 3. Foramen transversarium. 4. Groove for vertebral artery. 5. Posterior tubercle. 6. Posterior arch. 7. Transverse process. 8. Superior articular surface.

vertebra (ver'tē-bră) (pl. *vertebrae*) [L. *vertebra*]. Any one of the 33 bony segments of the spinal column.
 The vertebrae comprise 7 cervical, 12 thoracic dorsal, 5 lumbar, 5 sacral, and 4 coccygeal.
 Each vertebra is composed of (a) a body, or centrum, forming the main part of the spine; (b) 4 articulating processes (zygapophyses*), by which it is joined to the next vertebra. These are sometimes called oblique processes—the upper ones the ascending oblique, the lower, the descending oblique processes; (c) a spinous process which projects directly backward, those of the different verte-

Vertebrae

Regional Characteristics of Vertebrae	Cervical	Dorsal	Lumbar
Body (transverse section)	Elliptical	Heart-shaped. 2 demi-facets for heads of ribs	Kidney-shaped
2 pedicles			
2 laminae			
2 transverse processes	2 roots. Vertebral foramen. 2 tubercles.	Facet for tubercle of rib	Long and slender
Spinous process	Bifid	Long, slender and overlapping	Short, heavy, horizontal, with tubercles
2 sup. articular processes	Face upward	Face backward	Face inward
2 inf. articular processes	Face downward	Face forward	Face outward
Extra tubercles			2 mammillary, 2 accessory
Neural canal (caliber)	Largest	Smallest	Intermediate

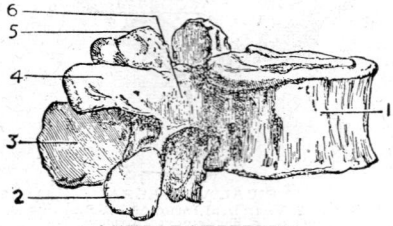

LUMBAR VERTEBRA
1. Body. 2. Inferior articular process. 3. Spinal process. 4. Transverse process. 5. Inferior articular process. 6. Pedicle.

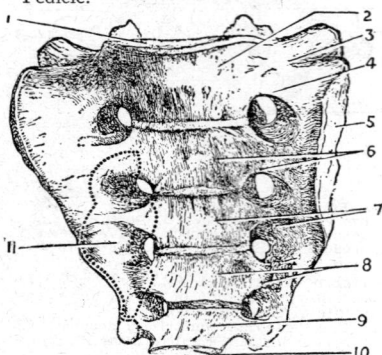

SACRUM
1. Superior articular process. 2. Body of first sacral vertebra. 3. Ala. 4. First anterior sacral foramen. 5. Lateral articular process. 6. Body and foramen of second sacral vertebra. 7. Body and foramen of third sacral vertebra. 8. Body and foramen of fourth sacral vertebra. 9. Body of fifth vertebra. 10. Inferior articular process. 11. Attachment of the piriformis muscle.

brae forming, with their points, the ridge of the back; (d) 2 transverse processes, which stand out at right angles, or laterally, from the body of the vertebra, and in the thoracic region articulate with the ribs.
RS: *acantha, anapophysis, anticlinal, atlas, axis, cervical v., lamina, spondyle, spondylitis, spondylotherapy.*
v., basilar. The lowest of the lumbar vertebrae.
v., cervical. The 7 vertebrae of the neck.
v., coccygeal. The rudimentary vertebrae of the coccyx.
v., cranial. The segments of the skull and facial bones, by some regarded as homologous with vertebrae.
v. dentata. The 2nd cervical vertebra. SYN: *axis.*
v., thoracic. The 12 vertebrae which connect the ribs and form part of the post. wall of the thorax. SYN: *dorsal v.*
v., false. One of the segments of the sacrum and the coccyx.
v., lumbar. The 5 vertebrae bet. the dorsal vertebrae and the sacrum.
v. magnum. The sacrum.
v., odontoid. Same as *v. dentata.*
v. prominens. The 7th cervical vertebra.
v., sacral. The 5 fused segments forming the sacrum.
v., sternal. The segments of the sternum.
v., thoracic. SEE: *dorsal vertebra.*
v., true. The vertebrae which remain unfused through life.
vertebral (ver'tē-brăl) [L. *vertebra*]. Pert. to a vertebra or the vertebral artery.
v. arch. Sup. loop of the vertebra enclosing the neural canal. SYN: *neural arch.*
v. canal. Vertebral foramen.
v. column. Spinal column.
v. foramen. 1. The hollow space enclosed by a vertebral arch. 2. A vertebrarterial foramen.
v. groove. The groove bet. the transverse and spinous processes of the spine.
v. ribs. The lower 2, or floating ribs.

vertebrarium (ver″tē-brā′rĭ-ŭm) [L.]. The spinal column.
vertebrarterial (ver″tē-brar-tē′rĭ-ăl [L. *vertebra* + G. *artēria*, artery]. Pert. to a vertebra and an artery.
v. foramen. A foramen in the transverse processes of the cervical vertebrae for passage of the vertebral artery.
vertebrate, vertebrated (ver′tē-brāt, ver′-tē-brā-tĕd) [L. *vertebra*]. Having or resembling a vertebral column.
vertebrectomy (ver-tē-brĕk′tō-mĭ) [" + G. *ektomē*, excision]. Excision of a vertebra or part of one.
vertebrochondral (ver″tē-brō-kŏn′drăl) [" + G. *chondros*, cartilage]. Denoting the false ribs (8th, 9th, 10th) connected with a vertebra at 1 end and the costal cartilages at the other.
vertebrocostal (ver″tē-brō-kŏs′tăl) [" + *costa*, rib]. Pert. to a vertebra and a rib. SYN: *costovertebral*.
vertebromammary (ver″tē-brō-măm′mă-rĭ) [" + *mammarius*, pert. to a breast]. Pert. to the vertebral and mammary area.
v. diameter. The anteroposterior diameter of the thorax.
vertebrosternal (ver″tē-brō-ster′năl) [" + G. *sternon*, chest]. Pert. to a vertebra and the sternum.
vertex (ver′tĕks) [L. *vertex*, summit]. The top of the head. SYN: *crown*.
v. cordis. Apex of the heart.
v. presentation. Presentation in labor of vertex of the fetal skull.
vertical (ver′tĭk-ăl) [L. *vertex*, vertic-, summit]. 1. Pert. to or situated at the vertex. 2. Directed up or down at right angles to the plane of the body or part of the earth's surface.
verticillate (ver-tĭs′ĭl-āt, -tĭs-ĭl′āt) [L. *verticillus*, a little whirl]. Arranged like the spokes of a wheel or a whorl.
vertiginous (ver-tĭj′ĭn-ŭs) [L. *vertigo, vertigin-*, a turning round]. Pert. to or afflicted with vertigo.
vertigo (ver′tĭg-ō, ver-tī′gō) [L. *vertigo*, a turning round]. Sensation of dizziness, a whirling motion of oneself or of ext. objects.
Denotes cerebral anemia or congestion; reflex irritation, as in gastric disturbances, eyestrain, uterine disease, constipation and diseases of middle ear; organic disease of the brain and cord; toxic substances in the blood; epilepsy, hysteria, unknown causes. SEE: *antidinic*.
v., auditory, v., aural. V. due to disease of the ear.
v., cerebral. V. due to brain disease.
v., epileptic. V. attending an epileptic attack or following it.
v., essential. V. from an unknown cause.
v., gastric. V. from gastric disturbance.
v., hysterical. V. accompanying hysteria.
v., labyrinthine. V. due to disease of labyrinth of the ear. SYN: *Ménière's disease*.
v., laryngeal. V. accompanying laryngeal spasm.
v., lithemic. V. experienced in gout or lithemia.
v., objective. V. when objects seen appear to be moving when stationary.
v., ocular. V. caused by disease of the eye.
v., organic. V. from a brain lesion.
v., peripheral. V. from disturbance distant from the brain.

v., subjective. V. in which patient seems to be turning or rotating.
v., toxic. V. from presence of a toxin in the body.
verumontanitis (ver″ū-mŏn-tăn-ī′tĭs) [L. *verumontānum*, mountainous ridge, + G. *-itis*, inflammation]. Inflammation of the verumontanum. SYN: *colliculitis*.
verumontanum (ver″ū-mŏn-tā′nŭm) [L. *verumontānum*, mountainous ridge]. An elevation on the floor of the prostatic portion of the urethra where the seminal ducts enter.
vesalianum (vĕs-a-lĭ-ā′nŭm). One of the sesamoid bones in the tendon of origin of the gastrocnemius muscle, and another on outer border of foot in the angle bet. the cuboid and fifth metatarsal.
Vesalius, foramen of (vĕs-ā′lĭ-ŭs). One in base of the skull transmitting an emissary vein.
V., vein of. Small vein giving from the cavernous sinus passing through Vesalius' foramen.
vesania (vē-sā′nĭ-ă) [L.]. Mental derangement without coma or fever. SYN: *insanity*.
Any well-defined psychosis without structural pathology of the functional group.
vesanic (vĕs-ăn′ĭk) [L. *vesania*, insanity]. Pertaining to insanity.
vescette (vĕs-ĕt′) [Fr.]. Commercial tablet made of compressed effervescent salts.
vesica (vĕs-ī′kă) [L. *vesica*, a bladder]. A bladder.
v. fellea. BNA. The gallbladder.
v. prostat′ica. A minute pouch in the prostatic urethra, remnant of müllerian duct. SYN: *utriculus prostaticus*.
v. urinaria. BNA. The urinary bladder.
vesical (vĕs′ĭk-ăl) [L. *vesica*, a bladder]. Pert. to or shaped like a bladder.
v. reflex. Inclination to urinate, caused by moderate bladder distention.
vesicant (vĕs′ĭk-ănt) [L. *vesicāre*, to blister]. 1. Blistering; causing or forming blisters. 2. Agent used to produce blisters. They are much less severe than escharotics. SYN: *epispastic*.
They draw the deeper fluids to the surface in the form of blisters.
Used in joint affections, for neuralgia and in the inflammation of internal organs. They must not be used over acutely inflamed areas, or on infants, or the aged as they may be absorbed and thus weaken the patient.
They are used also in acute pleurisy and in pneumonia, along the vertebral column in abdominal pain and pleurodynia,* for chronically inflamed glands, bronchitis in children and in erysipelas. They are also applied over the sacrum in vesical paralysis.
Cantharides, iodine, and iodine ointment are the principal vesicants.
vesication (vĕs-ĭ-kā′shŭn) [L. *vesicāre*, to blister]. 1. Process of blistering. 2. A blister.
vesicatory (vĕs′ĭk-ă-tor″ĭ) [L. *vesicāre*, to blister]. 1. Causing or pert. to blisters. 2. Agent causing blisters. SYN: *vesicant*.
vesicle (vĕs′ĭ-kl) [L. *vesicula*, a little bladder]. 1. A small sac or bladder containing fluid. 2. A blisterlike small elevation on the skin from the size of a pinhead to that of a split pea, containing serous fluid.
Vesicles may be round, transparent, opaque, or dark elevations of the skin, sometimes containing seropurulent or bloody fluid.
They are seen in *sudamina* as the

result of sweat which cannot escape from the layers of the skin; in *herpes*, mounted on an inflammatory base, having no tendency to rupture but associated with burning pain. In *herpes zoster* they follow the line of the nerve trunks. They are also seen in *dermatitis venenata*, as the result of poison ivy or oak, and accompanied by great itching, in *dermatitis herpetiformis* or *multiformis*, in *impetigo contagiosa*, occurring especially in children in discrete form, flat and umbilicated, filled with straw-color fluid with no tendency to break. They dry up, forming yellow crusts with little itching; also seen in *vesicular eczema, miliaria* (prickly heat or heat rash), in *chickenpox, smallpox*, and in *scabies*.
RS: *chiropompholyx, herpes, miliaria*.
v., allantoic. Int. cavity of the allantois.
v., auditory. That portion of the cerebral v. from which the ext. ear is formed.
v., blastodermic. Sac developed from the blastoderm.
v., cerebral. Expansion of neural embryonic canal from which the brain develops.
v., compound. V. with more than 1 cavity.
v., germinal. Nucleus of the ovum.
v., graafian. The ovarian structure containing the ovum.
v., seminal. One of the 2 membranous, sacculated tubes situated at the base of the bladder, bet. it and the rectum, serving as a reservoir for the semen and having a secretion of its own.
v., umbilical. Portion of embryonic yolk sac outside the body cavity.
vesico- [L.]. Combining form meaning *bladder*.
vesicocele (ves'ĭk-ō-sēl) [L. *vesica*, bladder, + G. *kēlē*, hernia]. Hernia of bladder. SYN: *cystocele*.
vesicocervical (vĕs″ĭk-ō-ser'vĭ-kăl) [" + *cervix*, neck]. Relating to the urinary bladder and cervix uteri.
vesicoclysis (vĕs-ĭk-ŏk'lĭs-ĭs) [" + G. *klysis*, a washing out]. Injection of fluid into the bladder.
vesicofixation (ves″ĭk-ō-fĭks-ā'shŭn) [" + *fixātio*, a fixing]. Attachment of the uterus to the bladder or the bladder to the abdominal wall.
vesicoprostatic (vĕs″ĭk-ō-prŏs-tăt'ĭk) [" + G. *prostatēs*, prostate]. Relating to the bladder and prostate.
vesicopubic (vĕs″ĭk-ō-pū'bĭk) [" + *pubis*, pubis]. Pert. to the bladder and the os pubis.
vesicospinal (vĕs″ĭk-ō-spī'năl) [" + *spina*, a thorn]. Relating to the urinary bladder and spinal cord.
vesicotomy (vĕs-ĭ-kŏt'ō-mĭ) [L. *vesica*, a bladder, + G. *tomē*, a cutting]. Incision of the bladder.
vesicouterine (ves″ĭk-ō-ū'ter-ĭn) [" + *uterinus*, pert. to the womb]. Pert. to the urinary bladder and the uterus.
vesicovaginal (vĕs″ĭk-ō-văj'ĭ-năl) [" + *vagina*, a sheath]. Pert. to the urinary bladder and vagina.
vesicula (vĕs-ĭk'ū-lă) (pl. *vesiculae*) [L. *vesicula*, a tiny bladder]. A small bladder, or vesicle.
v. seminalis. BNA. Tiny reservoir of semen at base of the bladder. SYN: *vesicle, seminal, q.v.*
vesicular (vĕs-ĭk'ū-lar) [L. *vesicula*, a tiny bladder]. Pert. to vesicles or small blisters.

v. breathing. Murmur heard in normal breathing.
v. column, v. cylinder. Ganglion cells at base of post. horn of spinal cord.
v. eczema. E. accompanied by formation of vesicles.
v. emphysema. Pulmonary emphysema.
v. erysipelas. A form of erysipelas that develops vesicles on the inflamed surface.
v. fever. 1. Condition marked by vesicular eruption; rise in temperature, slight; localized pain. 2. Skin disease marked by formation of vesicles. SYN: *pemphigus*.
v. murmur. The normal sound of respiration heard on auscultation. Same as *v. breathing*.
v. râle. The crepitant râle, a crackling sound heard at end of inspiration.
v. resonance. Percussion sound heard over the normal lung.
vesiculase (vĕs-ĭk'ū-lās) [L. *vesicula*, tiny bladder]. An enzyme in prostatic fluid said to coagulate semen.
vesiculation (vĕs-ĭk-ū-lā'shŭn) [L. *vesicula*, a tiny bladder]. Formation of vesicles or state of having or forming them.
vesiculectomy (vĕs-ĭk″ū-lĕk'tō-mĭ) [" + G. *ektomē*, excision]. Partial or complete excision of a vesicle, particularly a seminal vesicle.
vesiculiform (vĕs-ĭk'ū-lĭ-form) [" + *forma*, shape]. Having the shape of a vesicle.
vesiculitis (vĕs-ĭk″ū-lī'tis) [" + G. *-itis*, inflammation]. Inflammation of a vesicle, particularly the seminal vesicle.
vesiculocavernous (vĕs-ĭk″ū-lō-kăv'ĕr-nŭs) [" + *cavernōsis*, hollow]. Vesicular and cavernous.
vesiculogram (vĕs-ĭk'ū-lō-grăm [" + G. *gramma*, a mark]. An x-ray picture of the seminal vesicles.
vesiculography (vĕs-ĭk″ū-lŏg'ră-fĭ) [" + G. *graphein*, to write]. X-ray photography of the seminal vesicles.
vesiculopapular (vĕs-ĭk″ū-lō-păp'ū-lăr) [L. *vesicula*, a tiny bladder, + *papula*, a pimple]. Composed of vesicles and papules.
vesiculopustular (vĕs-ĭk″ū-lō-pŭs'tū-lăr) [" + *pustula*, pustule]. Having both vesicles and pustules.
vesiculotomy (vĕs-ĭk″ū-lŏt'ō-mĭ) [" + G. *tomē*, a cutting]. Division of a vesicle, as a seminal vesicle.
vesiculotympanic (vĕs-ĭk″ū-lō-tĭm-păn'ĭk) [" + G. *tympanon*, drum]. Vesicular and tympanic.
vespajus (vĕs-pā'jŭs). Follicular, suppurative inflammation of the hairy part of the scalp.
vessel (vĕs'ĕl) [O. Fr. from L. *vascellum*, a little vessel]. A tube, duct, or canal to convey the fluids of the body. SYN: *vas*.
RS: *anastomose, anastomosis, angiitis, angiodystrophia, arrosion, atresic, atretic, capreolary, capreolate, endothelial, intima, rhegma, vas, vascular*.
v.'s, absorbent. The lacteals, lymphatics and capillaries of the intestines.
v.'s, blood. Arteries, veins, and capillaries.
v.'s, chyliferous. V.'s arising in the villi of the intestinal walls carrying chyle and terminating in the thoracic duct. [lymph.
v.'s, lymphatic. Vessels conveying
v.'s, nutrient. Those supplying interior of the bones.
v., radicular. Branch of a vertebral artery supplying cerebral nerve root.

vestibular (vĕs-tĭb′ū-lăr) [L. *vestibulum*, vestibule]. Pert. to a vestibule.
 v. bulbs. Two sacculated collections of veins, lying on either side of the vagina beneath the bulbocavernosus muscle, connected anteriorly by the *pars intermedia*, and through this strip of cavernous tissue communicating with the erectile tissue of the clitoris.
 Injury during labor may give rise to troublesome bleeding. The vestibular bulbs are the homologues of the male corpus spongiosum. SEE: *vestibule, Bartholin's glands, vagina.*
vestibule (vĕs′tĭb-ūl) [L. *vestibulum*, vestibule]. A small space or cavity at the beginning of a canal, such as the aortic v.
 v. of ear. The middle part of the inner ear, behind the cochlea, and in front of the semicircular canals; it contains the utriculus and sacculus.
 v. of larynx. The portion of the larynx above the vocal cords.
 v. of nose. The anterior part of the nostrils containing the vibrissae.
 v. of pharynx. The fauces.
 v. of vulva. An almond-shaped space bet. the lines of attachment of the labia minora. At the ant. angle the *clitoris* is situated; the post. boundary is the *fourchette*. The vestibule appears approximately 4 or 5 cm. long and 2 cm. in greatest width when the labia minora are separated. Four major structures open into vestibule: The *urethra anteriorly*, the *vagina posteriorly*, and the two *extretory ducts of the glands of Bartholin*, laterally. The covering membranes are pink in color and constructed of delicate stratified squamous epithelium. Collections of cavernous tissue are disposed beneath the integument. SEE: *vestibular bulbs, Bartholin's glands, vagina.*
vestibulitis (vĕs-tĭb-ū-lī′tĭs). A dermatitis of the nasal vestibule; common in diabetics.
vestibulotomy (vĕs-tĭb″ū-lŏt′ō-mĭ) [L. *vestibulum*, vestibule, + G. *tomē*, a cutting]. Surgical incision into the vestibule of the inner ear.
vestibulourethral (vĕs-tĭb″ū-lŏ-ū-rē-thrăl) [″ + G. *ourēthra*, urethra]. Relating to the vestibule of the vulva and the urethra.
vestibulum (vĕs-tĭb′ū-lŭm) (pl. *vestibula*) [L. *vestibulum*, vestibule]. Vestibule.
 v. vagi′nae. BNA. Space behind glans clitoridis bet. labia minora enveloping vagina, urethra, and Bartholin's glands.
vestige (vĕs′tĭj) [L. *vestigium*, footstep]. A small degenerate or incompletely developed structure which has been more fully developed in the embryo or in a past generation.
vestigial (vĕs-tĭj′ĭ-ăl) [L. *vestigium*, a footstep]. Of the nature of a vestige. SYN: *rudimentary*.
 v. fold. A fibrous band of the pericardium, a remnant of the obliterated left innominate vein.
vestigium (vĕs-tĭj′ĭ-ŭm) [L. a footstep]. Vestige. [passage in the body.
via (vī′ă) (pl. *viae*) [L. *via*, path]. Any
 v. prima. First channel for passage of food, the alimentary canal.
 v. secunda. The lacteals and blood vessels, the second path for entrance of nutriment into the body.
viability (vī-ă-bĭl′ĭ-tĭ) [L. *vita*, life, + *habilis*, fit]. Ability to live, grow and develop.
viable (vī′ă-bl) [L. *vita*, life, + *habilis*,

fit]. Capable of living, as a 7 months' fetus.
vial (vī′ăl) [G. *phialē*, a drinking cup]. A small glass bottle for medicines or chemicals.
vibex (vī′bĕks) (pl. *vibices*) [L. *vibex*, mark of a blow]. A linear subcutaneous extravasation of blood.
vibices (vĭb-ī′sēz) (sing. *vibex*) [L. *vibices*, marks of a blow]. A form of macula, appearing as long narrow purple spots under the skin; hemorrhagic lesions.
 ETIOL: Linear subcutaneous effusions of blood. Occur in malignant fevers.
vibratile (vī′bră-tĭl) [L. *vibrāre*, to shake]. Adapted to or used in vibratory motion; moving to and fro. SEE: *vibratory.*
vibration (vī-brā′shŭn) [L. *vibrāre*, to shake]. 1. A to and fro movement. SYN: *oscillation*. 2. Therapeutic shaking of the body, a form of massage.
 Consists of a quick motion of the fingers or the hand vertical to the body or use of a mechanical vibrator.
vibrator (vī′brā-tor) [L. *vibrator*, a shaker]. Device for causing artificial vibration of body or its parts.
 v., mechanical. Machine driven by hand or motor to give general shake-up of part desired.
 v., ossicle. Instrument for breaking up aural adhesions.
vibratory (vī′bră-tō″rĭ) [L. *vibrator*, a shaker]. Having a vibrating or oscillatory movement.
Vibrio (vĭb′rĭ-ō) [L. from *vibrāre*, to shake]. A genus of short, rigid, motile bacteria, shaped like an "S" or a comma.
 V. chol′erae asiat′icae, V. com′ma. The spirillum of Asiatic cholera.
 V. Fink′leri. Same as *V. proteus.*
 V. pro′teus. A species in the feces of patients with cholera nostras and cholera infantum.
 V. sputig′enus. A species found in sputum septicemia.
vibrion septique (vē-brē-on′sĕp-tĕk) [Fr., septic vibrio]. Bacillus causing malignant edema.
vibrissae (vī-brĭs′ē) (sing. *vibrissa*) [L. *vibrissa*, that which shakes]. Stiff hairs within the nostrils at the ant. nares.
vibrometer (vī-brŏm′ĕt-ĕr) [L. *vibrāre*, to shake, + G. *metron*, a measure]. Device for the treatment of deafness which produces rapid vibrations of the membrana tympani.
vibrotherapeutics (vī″brō-thĕr-ă-pū′tĭks) [″ + G. *therapeutikē*, treatment]. The therapeutic application of vibration.
vicarious (vī-kā′rĭ-ŭs) [L. *vicarius*, substitute]. Taking the place of another; pert. to assumption of the function of 1 organ by another.
 v. menstruation. Menstruation through some other channel than the vagina, as hemorrhage from the nose, from the breast, or eyes, or in form of a leukorrhea at menstrual period.
 v. respiration. Increased r. in 1 lung when the other is lessened or abolished.
vicious (vĭsh′ŭs) [L. *vitiōsus*]. Faulty, defective.
 v. cicatrix. One causing a deformity.
 v. union. Deformity caused by improper uniting of ends of a fractured bone.
Vicq d'Azyr's bundle (vĭk-dă-zēr′). Mass of nerve fibers from the optic thalamus to the corpus albicans.
vidian artery (vĭd′ĭ-ăn). Branch of int. maxillary artery passing through the vidian canal.
 v. canal. Sphenoidal foramen for vidian nerve and artery.

v. nerve. A branch from the sphenopalatine ganglion. SEE: *Nerves, Table of, in Appendix.*

vigil (vĭj'ĭl) [L. *vigil*, awake]. Insomnia; wakefulness.

v., coma. Condition of muttering delirium in which patient is partially conscious and not completely comatose. SEE: *vigilambulism.*

vigilambulism (vĭj-ĭl-ăm'bū-lĭzm) [L. *vigil*, awake, + *ambulāre*, to walk, + G. *-ismos*, condition]. The secondary state of dual or multiple personality, occurring in a state resembling somnambulism, but not during sleep.

According to Charcot, an attack of transformed hysteria producing a primary state in which the subject is normal, and a secondary state, in which vigilambulism takes place, during which all the automatic acts of life continue to take place, but during which the victim assumes a personality entirely unlike the normal personality, each living 2 distinct existences, 1 of them always ignorant of the other, or both ignorant of each other. The secondary state appears to be analogous to hysteric somnambulism.

vigintinormal (vī-jĭn″-tĭ-nor'măl) [L. *viginti*, twenty, + *norma*, rule]. Consisting of one-twentieth of what is normal, as a solution.

Vigo plaster (vē'gō). A plaster containing mercury, turpentine, wax, lead plaster, and other materials.

Villate's solution (vē-lăt'). Preparation for injection into carious bones of zinc and copper sulfate, and lead subacetate.

villi (vĭl'ī) (sing. *villus*) [L. *villus*, tuft of hair]. Tiny projections from a surface. SEE: *villus.*

v., chorionic. Tiny branching processes of surface of chorion which become vascular and help to form the placenta.

villiferous (vĭl-ĭf'ĕr-ŭs) [" + *ferre*, to bear]. Having villi, or tufts of hair.

villikinin (vĭl-ĭk'ĭn-ĭn) [" + G. *kinein*, to move]. A hormone supposed to stimulate the intestinal villi.

villoma (vĭl-lō'mă) [" + G. *-ōma*, tumor]. A tumor of the papillae of the mucous surfaces. SYN: *papilloma.*

villose, villous (vĭl'ōs, vĭl'ŭs) [L. *villus*, tuft of hair]. Pert. to or furnished with villi or with fine hairlike extensions.

villositis (vĭl-ōs-ī'tĭs) [L. *villus*, tuft of hair, + G. *-itis*, inflammation]. A bacterial disease causing inflammation of the placental villi.

villosity (vĭl-ŏs'ĭ-tĭ) [L. *villus*, tuft of hair]. 1. Condition of being furnished with villi. 2. Proliferation of a membrane. SYN: *villus.*

villus (vĭl'ŭs) (pl. *villi*) [L. *villus*, tuft of hair]. One of the short vascular hairlike processes found on certain membranous surfaces.

The villi of the small intestine contain the beginning of the lacteals surrounded by a plexus of capillaries. They assist in absorption and secretion. SEE: *villose, villous.*

v., chorionic. Tiny vascular projections on the chorionic surface which help to form the placenta. SEE: *chorion.*

Vincent's angina (vĭn'sĕnts ăn-jī'nă). Painful ulceromembranous disease of the tonsils and pharynx. SYN: *trench mouth.* SEE: *Borrelia vincenti.*

ETIOL: Fusiform bacillus.

SYN: Painful swelling of lymphatic nodes, inf. of tonsils extending to floor of mouth. Membranous exudate, later ulceration; fever.

vinculum (vĭn'kū-lŭm) [L. *vinculum*, a band]. A uniting band or bundle. SYN: *frenulum, frenum, ligament.*

v. ten'dinum. 1. BNA. Tendinous, slender filaments connecting the phalanges with the flexor tendons. 2. The ringlike ligament of the ankle or wrist.

vinegar (vĭn'ē-găr) [M.E. *vinegre*, from Fr. *vin*, wine, + *aigre*, sour]. The product of the fermentation of cider, wine, or beer used as a condiment.

AV. SERVING: 5 Gm.

ASH CONST: Ca 0.016, Mg 0.008, K 0.165, P 0.013, Na 0.017, Fe 0.0003. No sodium or chlorine. SYN: *acetum.* SEE: *condiments.*

vinethene (vĭn'ĕth-ēn). Proprietary general anesthetic, acting rapidly, but of short duration.

USES: Chiefly in dentistry and minor surgery.

vinous (vī'nŭs) [L. *vinum*, wine]. Containing or of the nature of wine.

vinum (vī'nŭm) [L. *vinum*, wine]. Wine. The medicated wines are solutions of medicinal substances in wine. They are not often prescribed. None are official.

vioform (vī'ō-form). An almost odorless substitute for iodoform.

USES: As a dusting powder for application to wounds, ulcers, etc., and against amebiasis.

DOSAGE: Internally 4 gr. (0.25 Gm.).

violence (vī'ō-lĕns) [L. *violentia*]. The use of force or physical compulsion.

It may be expected in: *Acute delirious mania. Epileptics:* Especially when planned by 2 or more patients. *Epileptic furor:* These cases have no memory of their violent attacks. *General paralytics:* If their delusions are properly handled, violence may be averted. *Systematized delusional psychosis:* Generally they hold in check attacks of violence within the institution, but more apt to yield to such violence outside of the hospital. *Schizophrenia:* Some cases may become violent.

Many attacks of violence may be averted by recognizing warning signs and by knowing the patient.

violet (vī'ō-lĕt) [ME. *violett*, from L. *viola*, violet]. One of the colors of the spectrum resembling purple.

v. blindness. Inability to see violet tints.

viomycin (vī-ō-mī'sĭn). An antibiotic that exerts a suppressive effect against tubercle bacilli. Effective against streptomycin-resistant organisms. Not suitable for routine use, since renal irritation, vestibular impairment, and deafness may result.

viosterol (vī-ŏs'tĕr-ōl). A solution of irradiated ergosterol in vegetable oil.

USES: Same as cod-liver oil.

AVERAGE INFANT DOSE: 5 drops.

viraginity (vĭr-ăj-ĭn'ĭ-tĭ) [L. *virāgo*, a manlike woman]. Presence in a woman of masculine qualities and sexual tendencies.

virgin (vĭr'jĭn) [L. *virgo*, a maiden]. 1. A woman (or man) who has had no sexual contact. 2. Uncontaminated; fresh; new. SEE: *virginity.*

virginal (vĭr'jĭn-ăl) [L. *virgo*, a maid]. Relating to a virgin or to virginity.

v. membrane. The membrane occluding the ext. orifice of the vagina. SYN: *hymen.*

virginity (vĭr-jĭn'ĭt-ĭ) [L. *virginitas*, maidenhood]. The state of being a virgin; not having sustained sexual relations with the opposite sex.

PRESUMPTIVE EVIDENCE OF: Distinct,

regular, intact hymen with orifice of small dimensions scarcely allowing tip of finger to penetrate, the hymen being well stretched when thighs are separated; labia majora no more than slightly separated; small clitoris, labia minora in contact, narrow vagina, and intact fourchette and fossa navicularis. Such a condition is not always a proof of virginity, however, as the male seminal fluid can penetrate through the hymenal opening with resultant pregnancy.
viricidal (vĭ-rĭ-sī'dăl) [L. *virus*, poison, + *cidus*, from *caedere*, to kill]. Destructive to or inhibiting a virus. SYN: *virucidal*.
virile (vĭr'ĭl) [L. *virilis*, masculine]. Having characteristics of a mature male. SYN: *masculine*.
   v. reflex. 1. Sudden downward movement of penis when the prepuce or gland of a completely relaxed penis is pulled upward. 2. Contraction of bulbocavernous muscle on percussing dorsum of penis. 3. Contraction of bulbocavernous muscle resulting from compression of glans penis.
virilescence (vĭr-ĭl-ĕs'ĕns) [L. *virilis*, masculine]. The acquisition of masculine characteristics by an aged female.
virilia (vĭr-ĭl'ĭ-ă) [L. *virilia*, male genitalia]. The male generative organs.
virilism (vĭr'ĭl-ĭzm) [L. *virilis*, masculine, + G. *-ismos*, condition]. Presence or development of male secondary characteristics in a woman.
   v., prosopopilary. V. with growth of hair on face of a woman.
virility (vĭr-ĭl'ĭ-tĭ) [L. *virilitas*, masculinity]. 1. The state of possessing masculine qualities. 2. Normal power of procreation in the male sex.
viripotent (vĭr-ĭp'ō-tĕnt) [L. *vir*, man, + *potens*, able]. 1. Sexually mature, noting male sex. 2. Marriageable, applied only to a female. SYN: *nubile*.
virology (vīr-ŏl'ō-jī) [L. *virus*, poison, + G. *logos*, study]. The phase of biology dealing with viruses and virus diseases.
virose, virous (vī'rōs, vī'rŭs) [L. *virus*, poison]. Having poisonous qualities or effects. SYN: *poisonous*.
virtual (vĭr'tū-ăl) [L. *virtus*, excellence]. Being in effect, but not in fact; potential.
   v. cautery. Application of caustics to a part.
virucidal (vĭ-rŭ-sī'dăl) [L. *virus*, poison, + *cidus*, from *caedere*, to kill]. Destructive of a virus.
virulence (vĭr'ū-lĕns) [L. *virulentia*, a stench]. 1. Relative power possessed by organisms to produce disease. 2. Property of being virulent; venomousness, as of a disease. SEE: *attenuation*, *avirulent*.
virulent (vĭr'ū-lĕnt) [L. *virulentus*, full of poison]. 1. Very poisonous. 2. Infectious; able to overcome the host's defensive mechanism; distinguished from toxic and pathogenic.
viruliferous (vĭr-ū-lĭf'ĕr-ŭs) [L. *virus*, poison, + *ferre*, to bear]. Conveying or producing a virus.
virulin (vĭr'ū-lĭn) [L. *virus*, poison]. A constituent of virulent bacteria making it possible to resist phagocytic action.
virus (vī'rŭs) [L. *virus*, poison). 1. The specific living morbid principle by which an infectious disease is transmitted. 2. The fluid exudate from vesicles of vaccinia used for vaccination.
   v., attenuated. A virus so treated that it is less pathogenic.
   v., dehumanized. Vaccine obtained by the inoculation of a heifer with virus from a human being.

   v. diseases. Smallpox, chickenpox, measles, mumps, the common cold, poliomyelitis, rabies, epidemic encephalitis, and v. pneumonia.
   v., filtrable. A virus causing infectious disease, the essential elements of which are so tiny that they retain infectivity after passing through a filter of the Berkefeld* type.
   v., neurotropic. Those that seek out the nerves.
vis (vĭs) (pl. *vires*) [L. *vis*, force]. Force, strength, energy, power.
   v. afron'te. Force that attracts.
   v. formati'va. Energy resulting in development of new tissue.
   v. medica'trix natu'rae. The healing power of nature.
viscera (vĭs'ĕr-ă) (sing. *viscus*) [L. *viscus*, *viscer-*, viscus]. Internal organs, esp. the abdominal.   [*nic*.
   RS: *celosomia*, *evisceration*, *splanch-*
viscerad (vĭs'ĕr-ăd) [" + *ad*, toward]. Toward the viscera.
visceral (vĭs'sĕr-ăl) [L. *viscus*, *viscer-*, viscus]. Pert. to viscera.
   v. arches. The 4 depressions of lateral walls of the embryonic cervical region.
   v. cavity. Body cavity containing the viscera.
   v. clefts. The fissures separating the visceral arches.
   v. crisis. Severe paroxysmal pain in any of the viscera in tabes dorsalis.
   v. skeleton. The pelvis, ribs and sternum enclosing the viscera.
visceralgia (vĭs-ĕr-ăl'jĭ-ă) [L. *viscus*, *viscer-*, viscera, + G. *algos*, pain]. Neuralgia of any of the viscera.
visceralism (vĭs'ĕr-ăl-ĭzm) [" + G. *-ismos*, condition]. The idea that disease originates in the viscera.
viscerimotor (vĭs-ĕr-ĭ-mō'tor) [" + *motor*, a mover]. Conveying motor impulses to a viscus.
viscerogenic (vĭs"ĕr-ō-jĕn'ĭk) [" + G. *gennan*, to produce]. Originality in the viscera, noting reflexes.
visceroinhibitory (vĭs"ĕr-ō-ĭn-hĭb'ĭ-tō-rĭ) [" + *inhibere*, to restrain]. Checking the action of the viscera.
visceromotor (vĭs"ĕr-ō-mō'tor) [" + *motor*, a mover]. Conveying motor impulses to the viscera. SYN: *viscerimotor*.
visceroparietal (vĭs"ĕr-ō-pă-rī'ĕ-tăl) [" + *paries*, *pariet-*, wall]. Relating to the viscera and the abdominal wall.
visceroperitoneal (vĭs"ĕr-ō-pĕr"ĭ-tō-nē'ăl) [L. *viscus*, *viscer-*, viscus, + G. *peritonaion*, peritoneum]. Relating to the abdominal viscera and peritoneum.
visceropleural (vĭs"ĕr-ō-plū'răl) [" + G. *pleura*, a side]. Relating to the thoracic viscera and the pleura. SYN: *pleurovisceral*.
visceroptosis (vĭs-ĕr-ŏp-tō'sĭs) [" + G. *ptosis*, a dropping]. Downward displacement of a viscus. SEE: *Glénard's disease*.
viscerosensory (vĭs"ĕr-ō-sĕn'sō-rĭ) [" + *sensorius*, sensory]. Noting sensation caused by visceral disorder.
visceroskeletal (vĭs"ĕr-ō-skĕl'ĕt-ăl) [" + G. *skeleton*, skeleton]. Relating to the visceral skeleton.
viscerosomatic (vĭs"ĕr-ō-sō-măt'ĭk) [" + G. *sōma*, body]. Relating to the viscera and the body.
viscid (vĭs'ĭd) [L. *viscidus*, sticky]. Adhering, glutinous, sticky.
   BACT: Said of a growth that follows the needle when it is touched to the culture and withdrawn. The sediment rises in a coherent whirl when the liquid culture is shaken.

viscidity (vĭs-ĭd′ĭ-tĭ) [L. *viscidus*, sticky]. The property of being viscid or sticky. SYN: *viscosity*.

viscosimeter (vĭs-kŏs-ĭm′ĕt-ĕr) [L. *viscosus*, sticky, + G. *metron*, a measure]. Device for estimating the viscosity of a fluid, esp. of blood.

viscosity (vĭs-kŏs′ĭ-tĭ) [L. *viscosus*, sticky]. State of being sticky or gummy.

   v., specific. The internal friction of a fluid, measured by comparing the rate of flow of the liquid through a tube with that of some standard liquid, or by measuring the resistance to rotating paddles.

viscous (vĭs′kŭs) [L. *viscosus*, sticky]. Sticky, gummy, gelatinous.

viscus (vĭs′kŭs) (pl. *viscera*) [L. *viscus*, viscus]. Any internal organ enclosed within a cavity, such as the thorax or abdomen. SEE: *viscera*.

visile (vĭz′ĭl) [L. *visum*, seeing]. 1. Pert. to vision. 2. Readily recalling what is seen, more than that which is audible or motile.

vision (vĭzh′ŭn) [L. *visio*, a seeing]. 1. Act of viewing external objects. SYN: *sight*. 2. Sense by which light and color are apprehended. 3. An imaginary sight.

   Visual hallucinations, esp. frequent in toxic and febrile deliria, rarely verbal. Probably because of the elaborate nature of a visual perception involving perspective, color, complexity, mobility, hallucinations of sight tend to be less convincing than those of hearing.

   v., achromatic. Complete color blindness.

   v., binocular. Visual sensation which is produced when the images fall on symmetrical points of each retina.

   v., central, v., direct. Vision with the fovea centralis.

   v., day. Condition in which patient sees better during the day than at night, found in peripheral lesions of the retina, such as retinitis pigmentosa.

   v., double. Seeing of one object as two. SYN: *diplopia*.

   v., field of. The space within which an object can be seen while the eye remains fixed on some one point.

   v., half. Blindness in one or both eyes for half of the visual field. SYN: *hemianopia*.

   v., indirect, v., peripheral. Vision with the retina outside of the macular field.

   v., multiple. Seeing of one object as two or more. SYN: *polyopia*.

   v., night. Condition in which patient sees better after dusk, found in lesions of the macula.

vision, words pert. to: aberration, chromatic, accommodation, aftercataract, afterimage, ambiopia, amblyopia, ametropia, anopsia, astigmatic, astigmatism, autophony, amphodiplopia, amplitude of accommodation, ananthinopsy, anopsia, anotropia, asthenope, asthenopic, bifocal, caligation, caligo, chloropia, chloropsia, chromatopsia, convergence, cyanopia, chromopsia, diplopia, erythropsia, farpoint, farsightedness, field, fogging, gerontopia, glare, halation, hypermetropia, hypometropia, ianthinopia, image, macropsia, metamorphosis, micropsia, mire, monoblepsia, mucae volitantes, myometrium, myope, myopia, nyctalopia, nyetamblyopia, nyctotyphlosis, ocular, oculist, orthophrenia, oxyblepsia, polyopia, second sight, scintillation, scotoma, spintherism, strabismus, vergency, visile, visual, xanthopsia.

visual (vĭzh′ū-ăl) [L. *visio*, a seeing]. 1. Pert. to vision. 2. One whose learning and memorizing processes are largely of a visual nature.

   v. angle. Angle bet. line of sight and the extremities of object seen.

   v. axis. The line of vision, from object seen through the pupil's center to macula lutea.

   v. cone. The cone whose vertex is at the eye and whose generating lines touch the boundary of a visible object.

   v. field. The area within which objects may be seen when the eye is fixed.

   v. line. The visual axis. [optic axes lie.

   v. plane. The plane in which both

   v. point. Center of vision.

   v. purple. A purple pigment in retinal rods. SYN: *rhodopsin*.

visuoauditory (vĭzh″ū-ō-aw′dĭ-tor-ĭ) [L. *visio*, a seeing, + *auditorius*, pert. to hearing]. Relating to sight and hearing, as connecting nerve fibers bet. auditory and visual centers.

visuognosis (vĭzh-ū-ŏg-nō′sĭs) [″ + G. *gnosis*, knowledge]. The recognition and appreciation of what is seen.

visuometer (vĭzh-ū-ŏm′ĕ-tĕr) [″ + G. *metron*, a measure]. Device for ascertaining the range of vision.

visuopsychic (vĭzh″ū-ō-sī′kĭk) [″ + G. *psyche*, soul]. Both visual and psychic noting cerebral area involved in apprehension of visual sensations.

visuosensory (vĭzh″ū-ō-sĕn′sō-rĭ) [″ + *sensorius*, sensory]. Relating to the recognition of visual impressions.

vi′tagens. 1. Like vitamins. They are substances essential to health, but unlike vitamins, they enter into tissue as structural building units.

vitaglass (vī′tă-glăs). Window glass containing quartz for transmitting the ultraviolet antirachitic rays of sunlight.

vital (vī′tăl) [L. *vitalis*, pert. to life]. Pert. to or characteristic of life.

   v. capacity. Volume of air that can be expelled following full inspiration.

   v. center. Respiratory center in medulla. [all life depends.

   v. principle. The energy upon which

   v. signs. Respiration, pulse, and temperature.

   v. statistics. A record of births, marriages, disease, and deaths in an area.

vitalism (vī′tăl-ĭzm) [L. *vitalis*, pert. to life, + G. *-ismos*, condition]. The opinion that a vital force neither chemical nor mechanical is responsible for bodily functions.

vitalist (vī′tăl-ĭst) [L. *vitalis*, pert. to life]. One who believes in vitalism.

vitalistic (vī-tăl-ĭs′tĭk) [L. *vitalis*, pert. to life]. Relating to vitalism.

vitality (vī-tăl′ĭ-tĭ) [L. *vitalitas*]. 1. Principle of life. 2. Animation, action. SYN: *strength*. 3. State of being alive.

vitals (vī′tălz) [L. *vita*, life]. Organs of the body, esp. the heart, liver, lungs, and brain, essential to life.

vitamers (vī′tă-mers). Compounds which differ in structure from vitamins but which exert vitaminlike function.

vitameter (vi-tam′e-ter). Device for assaying vitamins.

vitamin(e (vī′tă-mĭn, -mēn) [L. *vita*, life, + *amine*]. Any of a group of accessory organic substances existing in most foods in minute amts. in their natural state, needed in the diet for metabolism, the absence of which results in malnutrition and specific deficiency diseases.

   Their effects are out of proportion, as judged from the viewpoint of caloric content to the small quantities required.

   Some unknown substance in the stomach seems to be necessary to activate

vitamin A

the vitamins. Without it they seem ineffectual. The complexity of their chemistry and the difficulties of nutritional experimentation necessitate continual revision of the knowledge of vitamins. No vitamin can take the place of any other vitamin but they are more or less associated with each other and with proteins, carbohydrates, and mineral salts, these substances remaining unutilized without the aid of other vitamins. They do not furnish energy.

vitamin A (fat soluble). Evidently manufactured in the body from *carotin,* which is supposed to be responsible for this vitamin in green vegetables, carrots, egg yolk, and butter.

ACTION: Promotes healthy functioning of nasal cavities, eyes and ears, sinuses, the respiratory and urinary tracts, and of intestinal flora, and resistance to disease, esp. anemia and xerophthalmia.* It is associated with and an aid to vit. B in the endocrine and digestive systems, and with vits. C and D in the formation of bone and teeth. Its absence causes damage to the digestive glands. Yeast or lipocaic necessary for full absorption of Vit. A.

STABILITY: Resists boiling for some time if not exposed to oxidation. Quite stable to heat but not to continued high temperatures (above 100° C.). Vit. A is present in most canned fruits and vegetables.

VIT. A DEFICIENCY DISORDERS: Interference with growth, reduced resistance to infections, interference with calcium metabolism and development of bone, teeth, and cartilage, and with nutrition of cornea; tendency to edema, increase of uric acid, unhealthy tissues and interference with blood building; responsible for deposit of oxalates and phosphates in urinary tract; anemia, development of respiratory infections, interference with intestinal flora, and induces infections of ear and nasal cavities.

VIT. A FOODS: Butter, and butter fat in milk and cod liver oil are rich sources, as are yolk of eggs. Green leafy and yellow vegetables and some fruits; prunes, pineapples, oranges, limes, cantaloupes, liver; kidney and to a much lesser extent, muscle meat, dates, avocados, apples, figs, grapes, and bananas; then heart.

Recommended Daily Allowances for Vitamin A

International Units

Man (70 kg.); woman (56 kg.)	5000
Pregnancy, latter half	6000
Lactation	8000
Children:	
Under 1 year	1500
1 to 3 years	2000
4 to 6 years	2500
7 to 9 years	3500
10 to 12 years	4500
12 to 15 years	5000
16 to 20 years	6000

vitamin A₁. Form found in the eye tissues of marine fish.

vitamin A₂. A compound found in the livers of fresh-water fish. Similar in properties to vitamin A but with different absorption spectrum in the ultraviolet.

vitamin B complex (water soluble). An antineuritic and beriberi vitamin composed of many factors. The original vitamin B, containing all factors found in a wide range of natural foods, particularly rich sources.

vitamin B₁

B₁ or F or thiamine deficiency leads to beriberi, and B₂ or G, riboflavin and nicotinic acid, are factors associated with pellagra. B₆ or pyridoxine*; its deficiency manifestations have not been well established. Symptoms may include nervousness, insomnia, weakness, abdominal cramps, and muscle stiffness. H, a B factor called *biotin,* is a powerful cellular stimulant.

ACTION: Affects growth, appetite, lactation, gastrointestinal, nervous and endocrine systems; aids in marasmus and lymphocytosis, stimulates appetite, reduces sugar content in diabetes, stimulates biliary action, aids in tuberculosis, and is necessary for carbohydrate metabolism.

Only grain-made yeast that is at once dried preserves its potency, containing more vit. B potencies than butter contains vit. A potencies. Advertised fresh yeast does not contain enough in 60 ½ Gm. tablets to be of any value. Vit. B is associated more directly with the intestinal tract absorption and growth.

B₁, *thiamine,* for growth and nutrition. B₂, *riboflavin,* for growth and a healthy nervous system. Relieves body swelling in disease. 750-1000 units daily aid gastrointestinal disease. *Nicotinic acid,* accompanied by diet adequate in all nutritional factors, stimulates recovery from pellagra.

Although not destroyed by ordinary cooking, it may be destroyed by excessive heating for 2-4 hours. Soda in cooking aids destruction. Riboflavin and nicotinic acid are more stable than thiamine; are not destroyed by heat or oxidation.

VIT. B DEFICIENCY DISORDERS: Beriberi, pellagra, digestive disturbances, enlargement of liver, reduction of pancreas, affects the thyroid, causes degeneration of sex glands, reduces catalysis of tissues, affects the nervous system, deranges the endocrines; induces edema, affects the heart, liver, spleen and kidneys; enlarges the adrenals and deranges function of the pituitary and salivary glands, and cause of some disorders in diabetes. Polyneuritis, gastrointestinal disorders, achlorhydria, anorexia, and failure of lactation have been attributed to deficiency of B₁.

SOURCES OF VIT. B FACTORS: *Thiamine:* Whole grains, wheat embryo, brewer's yeast, legumes, nuts, egg yolk, fruits and vegetables.

Riboflavin: Brewer's yeast, liver, meat, especially pork, fish, poultry, eggs, and milk; green vegetables.

Nicotinic Acid: Brewer's yeast, liver, meat, poultry, and green vegetables.

Pyridoxine: Rice, bran, yeast.

Folic Acid: Leafy, green vegetables, organ meats, lean beef and veal, wheat cereals.

STABILITY: Long-continued cooking or high temperature destroys and soda in cooking aids its destruction. Not destroyed by ordinary cooking or heat.

vitamin Bc. *Folic acid, q.v.*

vitamin Bc conjugate. *Folic acid, q.v.*

vitamin BT. Found in the meal worm and in human flesh. Same as *carnitine.*

vitamin Bx. *Paraäminobenzoic acid, q.v.*

vitamin B₁. Thiamine, thiamine hydrochloride. Growth promoting. Necessary for carbohydrate metabolism and normal development. Helps to prevent beriberi and lack of appetite from vit. B deficiency; helpful in alcoholic neuritis,

pregnancy, and pellagra. Increases quantity and quality of milk in lactation.
SYN: *aneurin, antineuritic, antiberiberi factor, torulin.*

Recommended Daily Allowances for Vitamin B₁ (Thiamine)
Mg.
Adults 1.5–3.0
(1500-3000 micrograms)
Children 0.6–1.5
(600-1500 micrograms)
Pregnant women 1.8–2.3
(1800-2300 micrograms)

vitamin B₂. Riboflavin. Found in milk, eggs, lean meat, yeast, and in some leafy vegetables.
VIT. B₂ DEFICIENCY DISORDERS: Cheilosis, glossitis. SYN: *antipellagra v., lactoflavin, oroflavin, hepatoflavin, vitamin G.* SEE: *vitamin G.*

vitamin B₃. A heat-labile factor needed for growth and weight in pigeons. Found in yeast, grain, liver, and malt.

vitamin B₄. An undetermined factor in wheat germ, dried grass, yeast, and liver.

vitamin B₅. An undetermined heat-stable factor.

vitamin B₆. Pyridoxine. Found in rice, bran, and yeast. SYN: *antidermatitis v.*

vitamin B₈. Adenylic acid.

vitamin B₁₀, B₁₁. Folic acid compounds affecting chicks.

vitamin B₁₂. An animal protein factor. A red crystalline substance isolated from liver. Effective in pernicious anemia, sprue, and nutritional macrocytic anemia. A few micrograms daily produce remission in pernicious anemia. Added to an all-vegetable diet, it brings such a diet up to par with an animal-protein diet.

vitamin B₁₄. A crystalline compound isolated from human urine. It has high cell-proliferating activity in bone-marrow cultures. The effect upon certain suspensions of neoplastic cells is inhibitory.

vitamin C. Ascorbic acid. This vitamin is associated with vits. A and D and calcium and phosphorus balance in development of bone.

Only small amts. if any are stored in the body.

STABILITY: Destroyed easily by heat in the presence of oxygen, as in open-kettle boiling. Less affected by heat in an acid medium; otherwise stable.

Necessary for pregnant and nursing women, in certain disturbances of stomach and bowel, diseases of the liver. Aids in growth, weight gain, improved appetite, blood-building. Essential in infant feeding. Accepted for correction and prevention of scurvy.

At least 100 mg. per day is the optimum requirement, and this amt. given in lead poisoning improves the general health and blood picture with decrease in amt. of lead in urine.

VIT. C DEFICIENCY DISORDERS: Scurvy, imperfect prenatal skeletal formation; defective teeth, pyorrhea, anorexia, anemia, undernutrition, injury to bone, cells, and blood vessels.

VIT. C FOODS: Raw cabbage, young carrots, orange juice, lettuce, celery, onions, tomatoes, radishes and small amts. in potatoes. Citric fruits are esp-rich in this vitamin. Strawberries are about as rich a source as tomatoes, apples, pears, apricots, plums, peaches, and pineapples. Rutabagas are also rich in this vitamin. SYN: *cevitamic acid, antiscorbutin, scorbutanin, antiscorbutic*

factor. SEE: *antiscorbutic.*

Recommended Daily Allowances for Vitamin C
Mg.
Infants 10–50
Children 20–100
Adults 30–100

vitamin conversion tables. For vitamins A, B₁, B₂, and C:

Vitamin A:
1 international unit = 2 Sherman units
= 0.6 microgram of carotene

Vitamin B₁:
1 international unit = 3 micrograms
= 0.003 mg.
= 2 Sherman units

Vitamin B₂:
1 mg. = 333 Sherman-Bourquin units
= 100 micrograms

Vitamin C:
1 mg. = 20 international units
= 2 Sherman units

vitamin D. Vitamin concerned with bone formation; derived from plants, food and from the sun and ultraviolet rays.

ACTION: Related to utilization of calcium and phosphorus in blood and bone building. It is called the antirachitic vitamin because deficiency of it interferes with calcium and phosphorous utilization, which in turn causes rickets.* Exposure to the sun or ultraviolet ray synthesizes this vitamin in the body. Necessary for most efficient absorption of calcium and phosphorus. A specific in treatment of infantile rickets, spasmophilia (infantile tetany), and softening of bone; valuable also in prevention. Important in normal growth and mineralization of skeleton and teeth.

One large dose of 600,000 international units cures convulsions and helps cure rickets.

VIT. D DEFICIENCY DISORDERS: Imperfect skeletal formation, bone diseases, rickets, caries. Its use without vits. A, B and C is harmful and it increases infection if there is a deficiency of vit. A.

VIT. D FOODS: Milk, cod-liver oil, salmon and cod livers, egg yolk, butter fat, ergosterol activated by sunlight or the ultraviolet ray possesses vit. D potency. A teaspoon of cod liver oil is required by the USP to contain at least 312 units of vit. D, and emulsion of cod liver oil is required to contain not less than 50 per cent of cod liver oil, or 156 units of vit. D.

STABILITY: Not affected by oxidation or by heat unless over 100° C. or long-continued cooking.

Recommended Daily Allowances for Vitamin D
International Units
Infants artificially fed 300–800
Infants breast fed 300–400
Children 300–800
Adults 300–400
Pregnant and lactating women .. 300–800

vitamin E (fat soluble). Tocopherol. A vitamin concerned with sterility. Necessary for the maturation and differentiation of certain cells. More than 150 compounds exhibit vit. E activity.

ACTION: Metabolism of excess fats.

VIT. E DEFICIENCY DISORDERS: Lack of fertility or reproductive powers, habitual abortion, amenorrhea, and uterine hypoplasia, but it is associated therein with vits. A and B. Late maturity, infrequent ovulation.

VIT. E FOODS: It is found in muscle, fat, spleen, heart and pancreas; also in the seeds and leaves of plants, in nuts,

yellow beef, oil, wheat-germ and lettuce leaf. It is low in corn and olive oil, flaxseed oil, but higher in cotton oil. SYN: *antisterility v.*
vitamin F. A formerly used term for essential fatty acids.
vitamin G (B_2) (water soluble). Riboflavin. A vitamin needed for growth and a healthy nervous system.
Affects the gastrointestinal tract and skin. A part of complex of vit. B. Differentiation of sources of B and G not yet determined. The *B complex*, combination of B and G vitamins, is found in most foods, yeast, milk, egg yolks, fresh muscle and esp. liver; less in fruits and vegetables and whole-grain cereals.
VIT. G FOODS: As above.
STABILITY: Not affected by heat unless long continued or over 100° C.
VIT. G DEFICIENCY DISORDERS: Lowering of resistance to infectious diseases. Stunting of growth in the young. Lowering of general tone and premature aging and unwholesomeness of skin. Loss of hair. Dermatitis and probably pellagra. The B_2-G factor is missing in pellagra.
SEE: *riboflavin, nicotinic acid.*
vitamin H. A factor in the B group called biotin.* It is a powerful cellular stimulant found in animal tissues. It, with *avertin*,* a depressant found in white of eggs, acts as a gyroscope to maintain cellular, chemical equilibrium. Lack of this equilibrium may be the cause of disease. The two factors need to be balanced in the body.
vitamin H'. *Paraäminobenzoic acid, q.v.*
vitamin K. An antihemorrhagic factor whose activity is associated with compounds derived from naphthoquinone. Vit. K is from alfalfa; vit. K_2 from fishmeal; vit. K_3 is synthesized as menadione sodium bisulfite USP. Vit. K aids blood coagulation, and is necessary for formation of prothrombin. Its deficiency prolongs blood-clotting time and causes hemorrhages.
ACTION: Practically eliminates prolonged bleeding in operations and in biliary tract of jaundiced patients. Bile salts necessary for its absorption.
VIT. K SOURCES: Found in fats, fishmeal, oats, wheat, rye and afalfa. Synthesized from coal tar, and is 4 times as potent as the natural. SYN: *antihemorrhagic v., prothrombin factor.*
vitamin L. A vitamin found to be necessary for lactation in rats.
vitamin loss. Commercial canning destroys from 50 to 85 per cent of vit. C. In peas, lima beans, spinach, and asparagus. The wheat embryo is removed from wheat flour in milling. As the wheat embryo is rich in vits. B_1, E, and G, these vitamins are lost by removal. Apple pie and freshly prepared applesauce retain only from 20 to 30 per cent of the vit. C value of the apple. Pickling, salting, curing, or fermenting usually causes complete loss of vit. C. Pasteurization, unless special precautions are observed, causes a loss of from 30 to 60 per cent of vit. C.
vitamin M. Folic acid, *q.v.* A member of the vitamin B complex, found in green, leafy vegetables, some meats, and wheat cereals. Used in treatment of sprue, and certain anemias.
vitamin P. Associated in citrus fruits with vit. C.
ACTION: Helps prevent scurvy, and is effective in diseases marked by increased capillary permeability. Helps prevent bleeding, prevents black and blue marks following blows.

VIT. P FOODS: Found in lemon and lime juice, grapefruit, oranges and red peppers. SYN: *citrin, permeability v.*
vitamin P-P. Nicotinic acid, *q.v.*
vitamin T. Found in vegetable oils and in egg yolk, it increases blood platelet count in humans, and is effective in purpura.
vitamin U. One assumed to be necessary for the growth of the chick.
vitamin units. These are shown in the accompanying tabulation, p. V-25.
vitamin X. The name once applied to vit. P.
vitaminoid (vī′tăm-ĭn-oyd) [L. *vita*, life, + *amine*, + G. *eidos*, resemblance]. Of the nature of vitamin.
vitaminology (vī″tăm-ĭn-ŏl′ō-jĭ) [" + " + G. *logos*, a study]. The science dealing with vitamins.
vita sexualis (vī′tă sĕks-ū-ā′lĭs) [L. sexual life]. The sex life.
vitellary (vĭt′ĕl-ă-rĭ) [L. *vitellus*, yolk of an egg]. Pert. to the vitellus. SYN: *vitelline.*
vitellin (vī-tĕl′ĭn) [L. *vitellus*, yolk of egg]. A protein which can be extracted from egg yolk and contains lecithin. SEE: *nucleoprotein, ovovitellin.*
vitelline (vī-tĕl′ēn) [L. *vitellus*, yolk of egg]. Pert. to the yolk of an egg or the ovum.
v. duct. The pedicle by which the umbilical vesicle is attached to the intestine of the embryo.
v. membrane. Membrane that surrounds the ovum.
v. veins. Veins from yolk sac to heart and portal vein in the embryo.
vitellus (vĭ-tĕl′ŭs) [L. *vitellus*, yolk of egg]. The protoplasmic contents of the ovum. The yolk of the egg with its germinal (*v. format′ivus*) and nutritive portion (*v. nutriti′vus*). SEE: *cleavage nucleus.*
vitiation (vĭsh″ĭ-ā′shŭn) [L. *vitiāre*, to corrupt]. Injury, contamination, impairment of use.
vitiligo (vĭt-ĭl-ī′gō) [L. *vitilīgō*, tetter]. An acquired cutaneous affection characterized by milk-white patches, surrounded by areas of normal pigmentation.
More common in tropics and in the colored race.
SYM: Milk-white spots appear on body and grow very slowly; borders reveal increase of normal pigment. Apart from absence of pigment, skin is normal. Condition probably results from disturbed innervation.
PROG: Unfavorable; disease usually persists through life.
TREATMENT: Constitutional remedies. Local stimulants as electricity, blisters, etc. SYN: *leukoderma.*
vitiligoidea (vĭt-ĭl-ĭg-oyd′ē-ă) [L. *vitilīgō*, tetter, + G. *eidos*, appearance]. Disease marked by formation of tiny yellow patches or nodules on the skin, as on the eyelids. SYN: *xanthoma.*
vitium (vĭsh′ĭ-ŭm) (pl. *vitia*) [L. *vitium*, fault]. A fault, defect, or vice.
v. cordis. An organic heart lesion.
vitodynamic (vī″tō-dī-năm′ĭk) [L. *vita*, life, + G. *dynamis*, force]. Relating to vital force.
vitreocapsulitis (vĭt″rē-ō-kăp-sū-lī′tĭs) [L. *vitreus*, glassy, + *capsula*, capsule, + G. *-itis*, inflammation]. Inflammation of the vitreous humor. SYN: *hyalitis.*
vitreous (vĭt′rē-ŭs) [L. *vitreus*, glassy]. 1. Glassy. 2. Pert. to the vitreous body. SEE: *pseudoglioma.*
v. body. A transparent jellylike mass

Definition of Vitamin Units

Vitamin	Sherman	U.S.P. A.D.M.A.	International Units 1934	Equivalents
A	The Sherman-Munsell unit is that amount of the vitamin which, when fed daily, just suffices to support a rate of gain of 3 grams per week in a standard test animal (rat) during an experimental feeding period of 4 to 8 weeks.	The Sherman-Munsell unit was included in the Tenth Revision of the U.S. Pharmacopoeia and is referred to as U.S.P.X. Sherman vitamin A unit. The American Drug Mfg. Assoc. also adopted this unit. For this purpose it is designated as A.D.M.A. vitamin A unit. In the U.S. Pharmacopoeia the International Unit 1934 is referred to as vitamin A unit U.S.P. Revised 1934.	The International unit is the activity of 0.6 gamma of Betacarotene. This amount of Betacarotene has the same biological activity as 1 gamma of the original International Standard Carotene.	One U.S.P.X. Sherman or A.D.M.A. vitamin A unit approximates 0.7 International units. Two vitamin A units U.S.P. Revised 1934 equal 1 International unit.
B	The Sherman-Chase unit is that amount of the vitamin which, when fed daily, will induce a gain of 3 grams per week in a standard test animal during a test period of 4 to 8 weeks.		The International unit is the antineuritic activity of 10 milligrams of an international standard adsorption product of rice polishings prepared by the Seidell method.	Two Sherman units equal 1 International unit.
C	The Sherman unit is that amount which, when fed daily, will just suffice to protect a 300-gram guinea pig from scurvy during a period of 90 days.		The International unit is the activity of 0.05 milligram levo-ascorbic acid. This amount of ascorbic acid has the same biological activity of 0.1 cc. lemon juice.	One Sherman unit equals 15 International units.
G	The Sherman-Bourquin unit is that amount of vitamin G which, when fed daily to young rats, will give an average gain of 3 grams per week during 8 weeks in addition to any appreciable gain in the group of control test animals on the vitamin G free ration.			
D	The Steenbock unit is the *total* amount of vitamin D which will produce a narrow line of calcium deposit in the rachitic metaphyses of distal ends of the radii and ulnae of standard rachitic rats in a period of 10 days.	The A.D.M.A. unit is the average *daily* amount (of vitamin D) required to produce recalcification. The average daily dose is understood to be the total amount of vitamin D given divided by the length of the test period, 10 days. In the U.S. Pharmacopoeia, the International Unit 1934 is referred to as U.S.P. Revised 1934 unit.	The International unit is the activity of 1 milligram of the International Standard solution of irradiated ergosterol, equal to .000025 milligram (.025 gamma) crystalline vitamin D. This amount fed daily for 8 days to rachitic young rats will produce a wide line of calcium deposits in the metaphyses of the long bones.	One Steenbock unit equals 3.3 International units. By definition, 1 Steenbock unit equals 10 A.D.M.A. units. One U.S.P. Revised 1934 unit equals 1.00 International unit. One A.D.M.A. unit equals 0.27 International Unit.

(Courtesy of The Williams and Wilkins Company, from *Applied Dietetics* by Frances Stern.)

that fills the cavity of the eyeball, enclosed by the hyaloid membrane.
v. chamber. The portion of the cavity of the eyeball behind the lens.
v. degeneration. Retrogressive change of a part into a translucent shining substance, esp. of a blood vessel wall.
v. humor of the ear. The endolymph.
v. membrane. 1. Inner one of the choroid. 2. One of hair follicles bet. outer root sheath and internal layer.
v. table. The inner layer of compact tissue belonging to most of the bones of the cranium.
vitriol (vĭt′rē-ol) [L. *vitriolum*]. A sulfate of any of various metals.
v., blue. Copper sulfate, *q.v.*
v., green. Ferrous sulfate, *q.v.*
v., oil of. Sulfuric acid, *q.v.*
v., white. Zinc sulfate, *q.v.*
vitropression (vĭt″rō-prĕsh′ŭn) [L. *vitrum*, glass, + *pressio*, a squeezing]. Method of temporarily eliminating redness of the skin caused by hyperemia by pressure with a glass slide on the skin for purpose of studying any lesions or discolorations.
vitrum (vĭt′rŭm) [L. *vitrum*, glass]. Glass. *In vitro* is an expression meaning, in a test tube or in glass.
Vitus' dance, St. (vī′tŭs). A functional nervous disorder causing muscular spasms. SYN: *chorea, q.v.*
vivi- [L.]. Combining form meaning alive.
vividiffusion (vĭv-ĭ-dĭf-ū′zhŭn) [L. *vivus*, alive, + *diffusio*, a pouring apart]. Dialysis of the blood of a living animal by removing it from an artery, passing it through tubes and back into a vein, without exposure to air.
vivification (vĭv-ĭ-fĭ-kā′shŭn) [" + *facere*, to make]. 1. Trimming of the surface layer of a wound to aid union of tissues. 2. Transformation of protein food through assimilation into the living matter of cellular organisms.
viviparous (vĭv-ĭp′ăr-ŭs) [" + *parēre*, to bear young]. Developing young within the body, the young being expelled and born alive, the opposite of *oviparous*.
vivipation (vĭv-ĭp-ā′shŭn) [" + *parēre*, to bear young]. A form of generation in which the ovum matures in the womb.
viviperception (vĭv″ĭ-pĕr-sĕp′shŭn) [" + *perceptio*, a seeing through]. The study of the vital processes of a living body without vivisection.
vivisect (vĭv′ĭ-sĕkt) [" + *sectio*, a cutting]. To dissect a living animal for experimental purposes.
vivisection (vĭv″ĭ-sĕk′shŭn) [L. *vivus*, alive, + *sectio*, a cutting]. Cutting of or operation upon a living animal for physiological investigation and the study of disease. SEE: *biotomy, callisection*.
vivisectionist (vĭv″ĭ-sĕk′shŭn-ĭst) [" + *sectio*, a cutting]. One who practices or believes in vivisection.
vivisector (vĭv-ĭs-ĕk′tor) [" + *sector*, a cutting]. One who practices vivisection.
vivisectorium (vĭv-ĭs-ĕk-tō′rĭ-ŭm) [" + *sectio*, a cutting]. A place where vivisection is performed.
Vleminckx's solution (flĕm′ĭnks). A solution of sulfurated lime.
USES: In various skin diseases.
DOSAGE: Externally diluted with 5 to 10 volumes of water.
vo′cal. Pert. to the voice.
v. area. That portion of glottis bet. the vocal cords.
v. cords. Four mucous membranous folds in int. of the larynx. SEE: *chorditis nodosa*.

v. frem′itus. Chest-wall vibration felt on palpation while patient is speaking.
v. process. That of the arytenoid cartilage to which are attached the vocal cords.
v. res′onance. Sound heard in auscultation of lung while patient is speaking.
v. signs. Indication of disease by changes in the voice.
voice (voys) [L. *vox, voc-*, voice]. Sound uttered by human beings, produced by vibration of the vocal cords.
voice, words pert. to: *amphoricity, amphoriloquy, amphorophony, anepia, apsithyria, apsithurea, arytenoid, Baccelli's sign, cacophonia, caverniloquy, heterophonia, hoarseness, mogiphonia, paraphonia, phonation, resonance, rhinolalia, rhinophonia, trachyphonia*.
voices (voys′ĕs). Verbal, auditory hallucinations. SYN: *phoneme*.
void (voyd) [O. Fr. *voider*, to empty]. To evacuate the bowels or bladder.
vola (vō′lă) [L.). The sole of foot or palm of the hand.
v. manus. Palm of hand.
v. pedis. Sole of foot.
volar (vō′lăr) [L. *vola*, palm, sole]. Relating to the palm, or sole of foot.
volatile (vol′ă-tĭl) [L. *volatilis*, from *volāre*, to fly]. CHEM: Easily vaporized or evaporated.
Examples of volatile liquids are ether (boiling point, 34.5° C.) and ethyl chloride (b. p. 12.2° C.).
volatilization (vŏl″ă-tĭl-ĭ-zā′shŭn) [L. *volatilis*, from *volāre*, to fly]. Conversion of a solid or liquid into a vapor.
volition (vō-lĭsh′ŭn) [L. *volitio*, will]. The act or power of willing or choosing.
Volkmann's contracture (fōlk′mahn). Degeneration, contracture, and atrophy of a muscle resulting from long-continued interference with normal circulation by bandage or elastics, or from exposure to cold or injury of an artery.
volley (vŏl′ē) [L. *volāre*, to fly]. A series of artificially induced rapid muscular contractions.
volsella (vŏl-sĕl′ă) [L. *volsella*, a tweezer]. Forceps with sharp pointed hooks at end of each blade.
volt (vŏlt). An electrical unit of pressure, the electromotive force required to produce 1 ampere of current through a resistance of 1 ohm.
voltage (vŏlt-āj). Electromotive force or difference in potential expressed in volts.
v., effective. Voltage of high frequency machine when patient is in the electrical circuit.
It is that voltage which is the driving force of the diathermy current.
v., load. Same as *effective voltage*.
v., no-load. Voltage produced by high frequency apparatus while the patient is not connected in the circuit.
v., peak. Two types of diathermy voltage: (1) Peak voltage, highest instantaneous value which it reaches in its course. (2) SEE: *effective voltage*.
v., roentgen ray. Quality of x-rays is a function of the voltage at which they are generated. The lower the voltage the larger the proportion of rays of long wave length (soft rays of low power of penetration) and the higher the voltage the greater the proportion of rays of short wave length (penetrating rays).
voltaic pile (vŏl-tā′ĭk). Alternate disks of 2 dissimilar metals, as copper and zinc separated by strips of cloth wet with acid for producing electrical current.

voltaism   V-27   **vomiting**

First means of generating a constant flow of current. Invented by Volta.

voltaism (vŏl'tă-ĭzm). Electricity produced by chemical decomposition in a battery. SYN: *galvanism.*

voltameter (vŏl-tăm'ĕt-ĕr) [*volt*, + G. *metron*, a measure]. Device for measuring force of a current in volts.

voltmeter (vŏlt'mē-tĕr) [*volt*, + G. *metron*, a measure]. A meter calibrated to measure electromotive force in volts.

Voltmeters are connected in parallel with the circuit or resistance over which the potential drop is to be measured.

Voltolini's disease (vŏl-tō-lē'nē). Primary labyrinthitis in children with symptoms of meningitis, and subsequently a staggering gait and deaf-mutism.

volubil′ity [L. *volubilitas*, flow of discourse]. PSY: Excessive fluency of speech.

vol′ume in′dex. An expression of average size of individual red blood cells, normally about I; indices below this indicate abnormally small red cells; above, abnormally large ones. The volume index is found by dividing the percentage of red cells into the hematocrit* percentage. SEE: *color index.*

volumetric (vŏl″ū-mĕt′rĭk) [L. *volūmen*, a volume, + G. *metron*, a measure]. Pert. to measurement of volume.

volumette (vŏl-ū-mĕt′) [Fr.]. Device for administering predetermined dosages of fluid, repeatedly.

volumination (vŏl-ū″mĭn-ā′shŭn) [L. *volūmen*, a volume]. Increase in size of bacteria produced by action of serum.

volumometer (vŏl″ū-mŏm′ĕ-tĕr) [" + G. *metron*, a measure]. Apparatus for measuring volume or changes in volume.

voluntary (vŏl′ŭn-tā-rĭ) [L. *voluntas*, will]. Pert. to or under control of the will.

    v. muscles. Voluntary muscles are generally attached to the skeleton, are innervated by myelinated nerves coming directly from the brain or spinal cord, and under the microscope are seen to consist of long cylindrical fibers bearing crosswise striations.

Voluntary, striped, striated, cross-striated, and skeletal are practically synonymous when applied to muscle.

    v. nervous system. Brain and spinal cord and their nerves and end organs controlling voluntary movements.

voluntomotory (vŏl″ŭn-tō-mō′tō-rĭ) [L. *voluntas*, will, + *motor*, a mover]. Relating to voluntary motor influence.

voluptuous (vō-lŭp′tū-ŭs) [L. *voluptas*, pleasure]. 1. Pert. to, arising from, or provoking consciously or otherwise, sensual desire, usually applied to the female sex. 2. Given to sensualism.

volupty (vŏl′ŭp-tĭ) [O. Fr. *volupté*, pleasure]. Sexual pleasure.

volute (vō-lūt′) [L. *volutus*, rolled]. Spiral, rolled up. SYN: *convoluted.*

volvulosis (vŏl-vū-lō′sĭs). Disease characterized by cutaneous or subcutaneous elastic fibrous tumors due to infestation with the worm *Oncocerca volvulus.*

volvulus (vŏl′vū-lŭs) [L. *volvere*, to roll]. A twisting of the bowel upon itself causing obstruction.

ETIOL: Prolapsed mesentery predisposing cause. Usually occurs at sigmoid flexure in middle-aged men.

PROG: Grave.

vomer (vō′mĕr) [L. *vomer*, plowshare]. The plow-shaped bone which forms the lower and post. portion of the nasal septum, articulating with the ethmoid, splenoid, the 2 palate bones, and 2 sup. axillary bones.

vomerine (vō′mĕr-ĭn) [L. *vomer*, plowshare]. Pert. to the vomer.

vomerobasilar (vō″mĕr-ō-băs′ĭl-ar) [" + *basilaris*, pert. to a base]. Concerning the vomer and the basilar region of the cranium.

    v. canal. Canal occurring at junction of sphenoid bone and vomer.

vomica (vŏm′ĭk-ă) [L. *vomica*, ulcer]. 1. A cavity in the lungs, as from suppuration. 2. Sudden and profuse expectoration of putrid, purulent matter.

vomicose (vŏm′ĭk-ōs) [L. *vomica*, ulcer]. Marked by many ulcers; ulcerous; purulent.

vomit (vŏm′ĭt) [L. *vomere*, to vomit]. 1. Matter ejected from stomach through the mouth. 2. To yield up gastric and intestinal contents through the mouth.

PHYS: The act is usually reflex involving coördinated activity of both voluntary and involuntary muscles. A certain position is assumed, the glottis is closed, the diaphragm and abdominal muscles contract, and the cardiac sphincter of the stomach relaxes while antiperistaltic waves course over the duodenum, stomach and esophagus.

RS: *bloody melena, nausea, vomiting.*

    v., bilious. Bile forced back into the stomach and ejected with vomited matter.

    v., black. Vomit containing blood acted on by the gastric juice. Seen in worst form of yellow fever.

    v., coffee-ground. Bloody vomit of gastric malignancy.

After Sears.

DIAGRAM ILLUSTRATING THE MECHANISM OF VOMITING

1. Focal causes act here. 2. Toxic causes act here. 3. Nervous causes act here. A. Diaphragm and abdominal muscles. B. Efferent nerve. C. Higher centers of brain. D. Vomiting center in medulla. E. Afferent nerve. F. Stomach and other abdominal organs.

vomiting (vŏm′ĭt-ĭng) [L. *vomere*, to vomit]. Ejection through the mouth of the gastric contents. SYN: *emesis.*

Emesis may result from:

1. Toxins from ptomaines, drugs, uremia and specific fevers.

2. Centric diseases, as cerebral tumors and meningitis. This form often is un-

accompanied by nausea and it does not relieve associated headache.
3. Diseases of the stomach, such as ulcer, cancer, dilatation, dyspepsia, etc.
4. Reflex from pregnancy, uterine or ovarian disease, irritation of the fauces, worms, biliary colic.
5. Intestinal obstruction.
6. Disturbed cerebral circulation, as in swinging, car- and seasickness.
7. Nervous affections, as hysteria and migraine.
8. Periodic vomiting may be in itself a neurosis or associated with the gastric crises of locomotor ataxia.
9. Esophageal vomiting results from obstruction, and the vomitus* is alkaline in reaction.

TREATMENT: The doctor may order ice, white of egg in lemon water, milk and lime water in equal parts in teaspoonful doses, champagne, brandy and soda, or effervescing drinks, such as Seidlitz powder. In severe cases no liquids should be given for 24 hours.

Place small amt. of salt on tongue when nauseated. Fluids in large quantities, esp. ginger ale.

In pregnancy: The diet should be dry and high in carbohydrates and water and liquids should be taken only bet. meals and in small quantities. Do not construe this to mean that all pregnant women should be subjected to this regimen, as it is only intended for women subject to emesis.

POSTOPERATIVE: NP. At first sign restrict fluids for ½ hr., then resume in gradually increasing amts. In certain cases (gastric) record *time, color, amt.*, whether *regurgitant* or *projectile*. Save specimen for examination. Wash mouth frequently. Take specimen of urine, if vomiting is persistent. (May be due to acidosis. If so, alkalis and glucose may be given.) Magnesia, ½ oz., with 6-8 oz. water; ½ teaspoonful at time may be given. Odor, *ammoniacal, fecal, garlic*, etc., should be charted. Fecal v. indicates intestinal obstruction. SEE: *hematemesis.*

POISONS: Emesis may result from taking arsenic, aconite, antimony, barium, colchicum, cantharides, copper, corrosive alkalis, acids, digitalis, iodine, mercury, phenol, phosphorus, veratrum, wood alcohol, food poisons, and zinc.

TREATMENT: Same as for vomiting.
RS: *anabole, anacatharsis, anagoge, antemesis, antiemetic, cyclic v., emesis, emetic, hyperemesis, poison retch, tyremesis, vomit, vomitous.*

v., cyclic. Recurring paroxysms of vomiting.
v., dry. Nausea without vomitus.
v., incoercible. Uncontrollable vomiting.
v., pernicious. Severe vomiting of pregnancy.
v. of pregnancy. That of morning sickness.
v., projectile. Ejection of vomitus with great force.
v., stercoraceous. Vomiting of fecal matter.
vomito negro (vŏm′ĭt-ō nā′grō) [Sp.] Vomit containing blood darkened by gastric secretion. SYN: *black vomit.*
vomitory (vŏm′ĭ-tō-rĭ) [L. *vomitōrius*, pert. to vomit]. 1. Causing vomiting. 2. An agent inducing emesis. 3. A vessel to receive ejecta.
vomiturition (vŏm″ĭ-tū-rĭsh′ŭn) [L. *vomitus*, vomit]. Repeated ineffective efforts to vomit. SYN: *retching.*

vomitus (vŏm′ĭt-ŭs) [L. *vomitus*, vomiting]. 1. Act of ejecting matter from the stomach through the mouth. 2. Material ejected from the stomach by vomiting.

NATURE OF VOMITUS: *Bilious*: Green or greenish-yellow, containing bile, appears after frequent and violent vomiting; if early in the act of vomiting, it may be grass-green; a symptom of peritonitis which also precedes fecal vomiting in intestinal obstruction.

Fecal: This is indicative of intestinal obstruction, general peritonitis, and abnormal communication bet. the intestines and stomach. [soning.

Garlic odor: Denotes phosphorous poi-
Hematemesis: The vomiting of blood. If bright and fluid it has not been long in the stomach; otherwise, it has the appearance of coffee-grounds, reddish-brown, or it forms in clots. This may indicate, also, rupture of aneurysms into the stomach or esophagus, or various esophageal veins; gastric ulcer, cirrhosis of liver, enlarged spleen, carcinoma of the stomach. It is not necessarily fatal.

It may result from swallowed blood, straining in vomiting, injuries in the epigastric region (rarely possible). It may occur in vicarious menstruation, gastritis, corrosive poisoning, in the presence of strong alkalis or acids, or it may result from anemia, leukemia, Hodgkin's disease and it is sometimes present in chronic nephritis, scurvy, purpura haemorrhagica, acute yellow atrophy of the liver, and in malarial fevers.

Ammoniacal odor: Indicates uremia.
Profuse: The ejection of large quantities of frothy fermented material is highly significant of gastric dilatation.
Purulent: This may result from the rupture of an abscess into the esophagus or stomach.
Watery and mucous: From an empty stomach this may denote gastric catarrh. Vomiting of excessive acid gastric juice occurs in migraine, hysteria, locomotor ataxia, gastric ulcer, movable kidney and exophthalmic goiter.

Without nausea, distress, or other phenomena: This may occur in certain neuroses of the stomach, in hysteria, uremia, brain disease, as from a tumor, or as a precursor of apoplexy. The vomitus may be colored by certain fruits, by wine, coffee, cocoa, soups and bile. SEE: *blennemesis, cholemesis.*

v. mari′nus. Seasickness.
v. matuti′nus. Morning vomiting of chronic gastric catarrh.
von Graefe's sign (fŏn grā′fēz). Failure of lid to move downward promptly with eyeball, the lid moving tardily and jerkily; seen in exophthalmic goiter.
von Leube motor test meal (fŏn loy′be). Soup, 400 cc.; beef, 200 Gm.; water, 200 cc. If at end of 6 hours a gastric lavage fails to show a residue, the motility of the stomach is normal.
v. L.'s test meal. Clear soup, 200 cc.; beefsteak, 200 Gm.; bread, 50 Gm.; water, 200 cc. The stomach contents are expressed in 6 hours. This is a gastric test meal.
Von Pirquet's test (fŏn pēr′kä). A diagnostic test for tuberculosis, in which a little tuberculin is applied to a scarified area of the skin of the arm.

A positive reaction is seen if a red papillary eruption appears at the site of inoculation.
Von Recklinghausen's disease (fŏn rĕk′lĭng-how″zĕn). 1. Multiple neurofibromata

occurring on the skin along the course of the nerves; associated with marked cutaneous pigmentation. 2. Generalized fibrocystic disease of the bones. SYN: *molluscum fibrosum.*

Voorhees' bag (voor'ēz). An inflatable rubber bag for dilating the cervix uteri to induce labor.

voracious (vō-rā'shŭs) [L. *vorāre*, to devour]. Having an insatiable or ravenous appetite.

Voronoff's method (vo'rŏn-ŏf). Attempt to rejuvenate by transplantation of the testis of a young anthropoid ape into the male.

vortex (vor'tĕks) (pl. *vortices*) [L. *vortex,* a whirlpool]. A spiral arrangement of the cardiac muscular fibers.

vorticose (vor'tĭk-ōs) [L. *vortex, vortic-,* a whirlpool]. Whirling.

vox (vŏks) (pl. *voces*) [L. *vox*]. Voice.
   v. choler'ica. The suppressed voice of last stages of cholera.

voyeur (voi-ūr') [Fr. one who sees]. One whose erotic stimulus is derived from looking at sexual objects or situations, such as watching others during coitus.

vril (vrĭl) [L. *virilis*, masculine]. The initial energy with which man is supposed to be endowed from birth and which makes it possible for him to reach full maturity and to reproduce his kind; also applied to all living organisms.

vuerometer (vū″ĕr-ŏm'ĕt-ĕr) [Fr. *vue,* sight, + G. *metron,* a measure]. Apparatus for measuring distance bet. the eyes.

vulgaris (vŭl-gā'rĭs) [L. *vulgaris,* common.] Ordinary.

vulnerable (vŭl'nĕr-ă-bl) [L. *vulnerāre,* to wound]. Easily injured or wounded.

vulnerary (vŭl'nĕr-ār-ĭ) [L. *vulnerāre,* to wound]. 1. Pert. to wounds. 2. A remedy used to heal wounds.

vulnerate (vŭl'nĕr-āt) [L. *vulnerāre,* to wound]. To wound.

vulnus (vŭl'nŭs) (pl. *vulnera*) [L. *vulnus,* wound]. A wound or injury.

vulsella, vulsellum (vŭl-sĕl'ă, vŭl-sĕl'ŭm) [L. *vulsella,* tweezers]. A forceps with a hook on each blade. SYN: *volsella.*

vulva (vŭl'vă) (pl. *vulvae*) [L. *vulva,* a covering]. The ext. female genitalia lying beneath the mons veneris consisting of the labia majora, labia minora, and clitoris.
   v. cerebri. A small opening leading from third ventricle of brain into the infundibulum.
   v. tuberculoma. An ulcerative feature of tuberculosis of the vulva.
   v., tuberculosis of. A condition of the v. due to tuberculous infection, not to be confused with tuberculous disease of the v., which is the rarest form of genital tuberculosis. SEE: *vulvar.*
   v., vestibule of. The portion immediately behind the mouth of the vagina.

vulvar (vŭl'var) [L. *vulva,* covering]. Relating to the vulva.

vulvectomy (vŭl-vĕk'tō-mĭ) [" + G. *ektomē,* excision]. Excision of the vulva.

vulvismus (vŭl-vĭz'mŭs) [" + G. *-ismos,* condition]. Painful spasm of the vagina. SYN: *vaginismus.*

vulvitis (vŭl-vī'tĭs) [L. *vulva,* covering, + G. *-itis,* inflammation]. Inflammation of the vulva.
   ETIOL: This condition usually exists as a part of an inflammation of the vagina and the etiological factors are the same. Besides these conditions vulvitis is produced by highly acid urine, and urine containing acetone bodies, as in diabetes mellitus.
   SYM: Swelling, heat, redness, severe pain, remarkable excitement of sexual passion where clitoris is involved. Inflammation of the glands of Bartholin will declare itself by the appearance of a painful tense oval swelling, low down on inner aspect of the vulva at entrance of vagina. In the phlegmonous forms of vulvitis increased local swelling and pain and more marked constitutional reaction are present. Suppuration and gangrene shown by usual signs.
   TREATMENT: Rest, removal of exciting cause, cleanliness. Parts may be irrigated with a warm solution of borax and labia kept separated by fold of soft absorbent fabric. *Deep suppuration*: Incision. Constitutional treatment.
   v., leukoplakic. Atrophy and wrinkling of the vulva with discoloration.

vulvo- (L.). Combining form meaning *a covering, the vulva.*

vulvocrural (vŭl″vō-krŭ'răl) [L. *vulva,* covering, + *cruralis,* pert. to the leg]. Relating to the vulva and the thigh.

vulvopathy (vŭl-vŏp'ă-thĭ) [" + G. *pathos,* disease]. Any disorder of the vulva.

vulvouterine (vŭl″vō-ū'tĕr-ĭn) [" + *uterīnus,* pert. to the uterus]. Relating to the vulva and uterus.

vulvovaginal (vŭl″vō-văj'ĭn-ăl) [" + *vagina,* a sheath]. Pert. to the vulva and vagina.
   v. glands. Small glands on either side of the vulvar orifice. SEE: *Bartholin's glands.*

vulvovaginitis (vŭl″vō-văj″ĭn-ī'tĭs) [" + " + G. *-itis,* inflammation]. Inflammation of both the vulva and vagina at the same time, or of the vulvovaginal glands.

W

W. Chemical symbol for *tungsten*.
Wachendorf's membrane (vahk'ĕn-dōrf'). 1. A thin vascular membrane occluding the pupil in the fetus. SYN: *membrana pupillaris*. 2. The outer membrane ensheathing a cell.
Wachsmuth's mixture (vahks'moot). Mixture of 5 parts of chloroform and 1 of oil of turpentine for general anesthesia.
wafer (wā'fer) [ME. *wafre*]. 1. A thin sheet of flour paste used to enclose a medicinal dose of powder. 2. A flat vaginal suppository.
Wagner's corpuscles (vahg'ner). The oval-shaped end organs of certain nerve fibers. SYN: *tactile corpuscles*.
W.'s spot. Germinal spot in an ovum.
Wagstaffe's fracture (wăg'stăf). One with separation of the internal malleolus.
waist (wāst) [ME. *wast*, growth]. Small part of body bet. thorax and hips. SEE: *cincture sensation*.
wakefulness (wāk'fŭl-nĕs) [A.S. *wacan*, to wake]. State marked by inability to sleep. SYN: *insomnia*.
Walcheren fever (vahl'kha-ren). A severe type of malarial fever found in Holland.
Walcher's position (vahl'ker). The patient assumes the dorsal-recumbent position with the legs hanging down over the end of the table from just above the knees, the legs fairly well separated. Used to enlarge the pelvic diameters in delivery.
walking (wauk'ĭng) [A.S. *wealcan*, to turn]. Act or manner of movement on foot without running, as for exercise.
RS: *abasia, a. paralytic, a. statica, akathisia, astasia, a. abasia, atremia, basophobia, claudication, dysbasia, gait*.
w. apparatus. Apparatus to aid walking of patients with weak or paralyzed leg muscles.
w. typhoid. Typhoid fever in which the symptoms are mild so that the patient is ambulatory.
wall (wawl) [L. *vallum*, a wall]. A limiting structure or partition often forming an enclosure, as the abdominal wall.
wallerian degeneration (wŏl-ē'rĭ-ăn). Degeneration of a nerve fiber severed from its trophic center.
walleye (wawl'ī). 1. Eye in which iris is light-colored or white. 2. Leukoma or dense opacity of cornea. 3. Squint in which both visual axes diverge. SYN: *divergent strabismus*.
wall-plate (wawl'plāt). Apparatus for furnishing low tension and low frequency current.
walnut (wawl'nŭt) [A.S. *wealhhnutu*, a foreign nut]. Black and English. A tree and its nuts of the Juglans genus.
AV. SERVING: 35 Gm. each. Pro. 9.7 and 6.4, Fat 19.7 and 22.5, Carbo. 3.5 and 4.1.
VITAMINS: Eng., A+, B++ for both. Black, C+.
ASH CONST: Eng. Ca 0.089, Mg 0.134, K 0.332, P 0.328, Cl 0.040, S 0.172, Fe 0.0021.
wan'dering. Moving about; not fixed.
w. abscess. One that burrows and comes to the surface at a point distant from its origin.
w. cell. A leukocyte which moves about the substance of an organ.

w. kidney, w. spleen. Dislocated floating kidney or spleen.
Wangensteen's method (wăng'ĕn-stēn). Technic for relieving postoperative distention, nausea and vomiting and certain cases of mechanical bowel obstruction. It involves use of an intranasal catheter in combination with a suction siphonage apparatus. SEE: *decompression, distention*.
ward (ward) [A.S. *weard*, a guarding]. A large room or hall in a hospital.
w., accident. One reserved for accident cases.
w., isolation. One for isolation of those suspected of being affected with an infectious disease.
w., psychopathic. One in a general hospital for temporary reception of mental cases.
Wardrop's disease (war'drŏp). Acute inflammation of matrix of the nail in scrofulous children. SYN: *onychia maligna*.
W.'s operation. Ligation of an artery for aneurysm at a distance beyond the sac.
warehousemen's itch (wār'hows-mĕnz ĭtsh). Eczema of hands from touching irritating substances.
war gases. There are at least 4 classes of these gases: (1) Suffocating gases; (2) irritating gases; (3) vesicants, and (4) general poisons or toxic gases. Some of these are explosive.
Mustard Gas: A vesicant causing blisters and vesicles. Its chemical name is *Dichlorethyl sulfide*.
Suffocating Gases: These are made up of chlorine compounds.
Tear Gases: These are of 2 types: benzyl bromide and ammonia compounds, and arsines or the sternutatory type.
Toxic Gases: These are of the hydrocyanic acid type. SEE: *gas*.
warm-blooded. Having a high and constant body temperature. SYN: *homothermal*.
wart (wort) [A.S. *wearte*]. A circumscribed cutaneous elevation resulting from hypertrophy of the papillae and epidermis. SYN: *verruca, q.v.*
RS: *condyloma, keratosis seborrheica, sycoma, venereal, verrucose*.
w., seborrheic. Patch of corneous hypertrophy on face of the aged.
w., senile. SEE: *seborrheic wart*.
w.'s, venereal. Vegetating growths upon skin, esp. on the mucocutaneous juncture of the genitals, having an offensive discharge. SYN: *verruca acuminata*.
warty (war'tĭ) [A.S. *wearte*]. Relating to or covered with warts.
wash (wash) [A.S. *wascan*, to wash]. 1. To bathe with a fluid, as an injured part. 2. A lotion.
washerwomen's itch (wash'ĕr-wŭm"ăn). Eczema of the hands of laundry workers.
wash-leath'er skin. A trophic change in the skin in which silver drawn across it leaves a black mark.
wasp sting. Sting from a wasp, which causes a general urticaria. SEE: *hornet sting*.
Wassermann-fast (vas'ĕr-mahn). Indicat-

W-1

Wassermann reaction

ing a positive reaction shown by a Wassermann test which continues after repeated antisyphilitic medication.
W. reaction. Serum complement fixation test as a diagnosis of syphilis.
The results are designated as 1, 2, 3, and 4 plus, the intensity of the reaction usually corresponding to the severity of the infection. The disease may still exist with a negative reaction. Several such reactions would indicate its absence. Several years after treatment and after last "negative" is obtained should pass before cure is definitely accepted.
waste (wăst) [L. *vastāre*, to devastate]. 1. To shrink in physical bulk or strength, as from disease. 2. Loss by breaking down of bodily tissue. 3. Refuse material no longer useful to an organism.
w. products. Carbon dioxide, organic and inorganic salts, water, dead skin, hair, nails, undigested foods.
w. p.'s, metabolic. Soluble salts in the form of nitrogenous salts (urea) and inorganic salts (sodium chloride); gas in form of carbon dioxide, and liquid in the form of water.
They are excreta, removed by the process of elimination, *q.v.*
wasting (wăst′ĭng) [L. *vastāre*, to devastate]. Enfeebling; causing loss of strength or size; emaciating. SEE: *marasmus.*
w. palsy or **paralysis.** Chronic disease marked by gradual atrophy of muscular tissue with paralysis. SYN: *progressive muscular atrophy.*

foundation and prevent sagging; it should be refilled every fortnight.
w.-borne. Disease spread by germs in drinking water or bath water.
w. on brain. Disease marked by abnormal increase in cerebral fluid. SYN: *hydrocephalus.*
w. brash. Gastric burning pain with eructations. SYN: *heartburn.*
w.-cure. Use of water in treatment. SYN: *hydrotherapy.*
w.-hammer pulse. Pulse marked by quick powerful beat, collapsing suddenly. SYN: *Corrigan's pulse, q.v.* RS: *pulse.*
w., heavy. Water incapable of supporting life containing the mass 2 isotope of hydrogen.
w.-pox. True chickenpox or varicella, *q.v.*
water balance diet. Water content of diet is calculated to individual prescription. The water content of foods as well as beverages is calculated as part of the fluid allowance given in the diet prescription.
water cress (waw′tĕr krĕs). Av. SERVING: 20 Gm. Pro., 0.2; Fat, 0.2; Carbo., 0.8.
VITAMINS: A+++, B++, C+++, G++ to +++.
ASH CONST: Ca, 0.187; Mg, 0.034; K, 0.287; Na, 0.099; P, 0.005; Cl, 0.061; S, 0.107; Fe, 0.0019.
watermelon (waw′tĕr-mĕl″ŏn). Av. SERVING: 240 Gm. Pro. 0.9, Fat 0.4, Carbo 16.0.
VITAMINS: A+, B+, C++, G+.

Water Exchange

Available		Excreted	
Intake (diet water as such)...	5394 Gm.	As urine	1948 Gm.
Endogenous (oxidation less hydrated water in body protein or fat that is set free on oxidation)	1052	As feces .... As vapor	446 3804
	6446 Gm.		6198 Gm.

The retention of water by the body was 6446 — 6198 = 248 Gm.

water (waw′tẽr) [A.S. *waeter*]. 1. A solution in water of a volatile substance. 2. The urine. 3. H_2O, hydrogen and oxygen, a tasteless, clear odorless fluid, constituting bet. 75% and 90% of all tissues.
It freezes at 32° F. (0° C.) and boils at 212° F. (100° C.).
Its evaporation helps prevent the body from experiencing a temperature above normal.
Increased intake raises the blood pressure and secretion of urine; decrease causes thirst. A greater proportion is found in the young. It is important to supply fluid for the secretions, for metabolic purposes, and as an aid in elimination and temperature control.
The large intestines absorb more of it than the small ones, little being absorbed in the stomach. 95% of the urine is water, varying according to conditions. It is lost through the kidneys, skin, lungs, and alimentary canal.
RS: *a. b. c. process, albumen w., anhydrous, aqua, aqueous, Baruch's law, dehydration, deliquescent, dropsy, exsiccosis, fever, humidity, hydrate, hydrogen, hygric, hygroma, orrhorrhea, skin, urinary system.*
w.-bed. A rubber mattress, filled 3 parts full with warm water (temp. 100° F.); must not be too full or it will be hard. Fracture boards are placed across the wire mattress to produce a firm

ASH CONST: Ca 0.011, Mg 0.003, K 0.073, Na 0.008, P 0.003, Cl 0.008, S 0.007. A base-forming fruit, alkaline potentiality 2.7 cc. per 100 Gm.; 8.9 cc. per 100 cal. SEE: *cantaloupe, melon.*
waters (waw′tĕrs). Common term for the amniotic fluid surrounding the fetus.
w., bag of. Sac enclosing liquor amnii surrounding the fetus. SYN: *amniotic sac.*
watt (wŏt). A unit of electric power equal to work done at rate of 1 joule per second or work represented by current of 1 ampere under a pressure of 1 volt.
Its mechanical equivalent is 107 ergs per second; or 0.7376 foot-pounds per seconds.
In direct current circuits, the wattage equals current in amperes multiplied by the drop in voltage. In alternating current circuits, the wattage equals the effective current in amperes multiplied by the effective voltage and the cosine of the angle of their phase difference.
w.-hour. An electrical unit of work or energy. It is equal to the wattage multiplied by the time in hours. Its mechanical equivalent is 2655 foot-pounds.
wattage (wŏt′ăj). The consumption of electricity measured in watts.
wattmeter (wŏt′mē-tĕr) [*watt* + G. *metron*, a measure]. Device for measuring consumption of an electric current.
wave (wāv) [A.S. *wafian*, to wave]. 1. A

wave, hertzian   W-3   **Wernicke's syndrome**

disturbance of the equilibrium of a body or medium propagated from point to point with a continuous motion through a closed curve. 2. An undulating or vibrating motion.
w., hertzian. Electromagnetic radiations used in radio and wireless transmission.

Hertzian Waves	1,000,000 A.U.	To several kilometers	
Infrared rays	7,700 " "	" 150,000	A.U.
Visible rays	3,900 " "	" 7,700	" "
Ultraviolet rays	136 " "	" 3,900	" "
Roentgen rays	1.4 " "	" 136	" "
Gamma rays	0.01 " "	" 1.4	" "

w. length. The distance bet. corresponding points in 2 adjacent waves; e. g., bet. 2 crests.
In therapeutic radiations it is stated in angstroms* (A.U.) or millimicrons.
w., pulse. Elevation of the pulse noted by the finger or in curve graphically recorded by the sphygmograph.
w.'s, Traube-Hering. Rhythmical fluctuations in arterial pressure due to disturbance of the respiratory center.
wax (wăks) [A.S. *weax*]. 1. A substance secreted by bees. SYN: *cera*. 2. Anything having the physical properties of, or resembling beeswax. 3. Earwax. SYN: *cerumen*. SEE: *ceroplasty*.
waxing kernels (wăks'ĭng kẽr'nĕls). Enlarged lymph glands, forming small tumors, seen esp. in children.
waxy (wăks'ĭ) [A.S. *weax*, wax]. Resembling or pert. to wax.
w. cast. Dense, highly refractile urinary cast.
They have clean-cut contours, sometimes irregular curves and notches. Obtained in severe chronic renal disease.
w. degeneration. Amyloid degeneration seen in wasting diseases.
weak (wēk) [ME. *weik*, from Old Norse *veiker*]. Deficient in strength of body; infirm.
RS: *asthenia, atony, cardiasthenia, enervation, ergasthenia, fatigue, lassitude, lipothmia, vitiate.*
wean (wēn) [A.S. *wenian*, to accustom]. To accustom to loss of breast milk by substitution of other nourishment.
weaning brash (wēn'ĭng brăsh). Severe diarrhea sometimes attacking infants just weaned.
weasand (wē'zănd) [A.S. *wāesand*]. Esophagus or windpipe; loosely, the throat.
webbed (wĕbd) [A.S. *webb*, a fabric]. Having a membrane connecting adjacent structures, as the duck's feet.
w. fingers, w. toes. Two or more toes or fingers connected by a membrane.
weber (wē'bẽr). 1. Ampere. 2. Coulomb. Both uses are obsolete.
Weber's syndrome (wĕb'er). Palsy of 3rd cranial nerve on 1 side and hemiplegia on the other side.
ETIOL: Lesion of *crus cerebri*.
weeping (wēp'ĭng) [A.S. *wēpan*, to lament]. 1. Shedding tears. 2. Moist, dripping.
w. eczema. Dermatitis with eruption of vesicles exuding serum.
w. sinew. Circumscribed cystic swelling of a tendon sheath.
Weidel's reaction (vī'dĕl). Test for presence of xanthine bodies or uric acid.
Weigert's law (vī'gẽrt). Loss or destruction of organic elements is usually followed by excessive production during reparative process.
weight (wāt) [A.S. *gewiht*]. 1. The property of matter which causes it to fall to the earth by gravitation. 2. Amt. of such a tendency.
Weight of the body progressively increases in pathological obesity; and progressively decreases in Addison's disease, cancer, chronic diarrhea, chronic suppurations, diabetes, hysteria, anorexia, fevers, lactation when prolonged, marasmus, obstruction of pylorus or thoracic duct, tuberculosis, ulcer of stomach.
RS: *abarognosis, barognosis measure, molecular, Tables in Appendix, Troy.*

Weight and Height Ratio			
Lbs.	H.	Lbs.	H.
115	5 ft. 0 in.	155	5 ft. 8 in.
120	5 " 1 "	160	5 " 9 "
125	5 " 2 "	165	5 " 10 "
130	5 " 3 "	170	5 " 11 "
135	5 " 4 "	175	6 " 0 "
140	5 " 5 "	180	6 " 1 "
145	5 " 6 "	185	6 " 2 "
150	5 " 7 "	190	6 " 3 "

w., atomic. W. of an atom of elementary substances compared with that of oxygen, which is taken as 16.
w., molecular. W. of a molecule of substance compared with hydrogen being equal to the sum of weights of its constituent atoms.
weights and measures. SEE: *apothecaries' m., avoirdupois, measures, metric system, Tables in Appendix, Troy w., unit.*
Weil's disease (vīl, wīl). An acute infectious febrile disorder, caused by a spirochete.
It is a specific infection accompanied by muscular pains, fever, jaundice, and enlargement of liver and spleen.
TREATMENT: Rest in bed, liquid diet, remedies indicated for special manifestations.
Weir Mitchell's treatment (wēr mĭt'shĕl). Rest in bed, massage, nourishing diet and isolation for hysteria and neurasthenia.
Welch's bacillus (wĕlsh). Rod-shaped organism, nonmotile, encapsulated organism, frequently causing gas gangrene. SYN: *Bacillus aerogenes capsulatus.*
wen (wĕn) [A.S. *wenn*]. A cyst resulting from the retention of secretion in a sebaceous gland. SYN: *steatoma*.
SYM: One or more rounded or oval elevations, varying in size from a pea to a large walnut; slowly appears on scalp, face or back; painless, rather soft; contains a yellowish-white caseous mass.
TREATMENT: Sac and contents should be carefully dissected out. SEE: *sebaceous gland.*
Werlhof's disease (verl'hof). Form of progressive purpura marked by hemorrhages from the mucous membranes and severe prostration. SYN: *purpura haemorrhagica.*
SYM: Large reduction of blood platelets, spontaneous hemorrhages into and from tissues, enlargement of spleen, marked prostration.
Wernicke's syndrome (ver'nĭk-ē). Condition of old age frequently seen, marked by loss of memory and disorientation

with confabulation. SYN: *presbyophrenia*, q.v.

Westphal's nucleus (věst'fahl). Small bulbar one post. to and above nucleus of the 4th cranial nerve.

W's. phenom'enon, W's. sign. Loss of the knee jerk, the patellar reflex.

wet (wět) [A.S. *wǣt*]. Soaked with moisture.

    w. brain. Increased amt. of cerebrospinal fluid with edema of the meninges, due to alcoholism.

    w. cup. A cupping glass used after scarification.

    w. dream. Nocturnal seminal emission during a sex dream.

    w. nurse. A woman who gives suck to another's child.

    w. pack. A form of bath, given by wrapping patient in hot or cold wet sheets, covered with a blanket, used esp. to reduce fever.

whartonitis (hwar″ton-ī′tĭs) [*Wharton* + G. *-itis*, inflammation]. Inflammation of Wharton's duct in the submaxillary gland.

Wharton's duct (hwar′ton). That of the sublingual gland (2 in. long) opening into the mouth at side of the *frenum linguae*.

    W's. jelly. A gelatinous basic substance in the umbilical cord.

wheal (hwēl) [A.S. *hwele*]. More or less round and evanescent elevation of the skin, white in center with pale red periphery, accompanied by itching.

Seen in urticaria, insect bites, anaphylaxis, angineurotic edema. SYN: *pomphus*.

wheat (hwēt) [A.S. *hwǣte*]. COMP: NUTRIENTS (entire and cracked): Pro. 13.8 and 11.1, Fat 1.9 and 1.7, Carbo. 71.9 and 75.5.

    VITAMINS: A+, B++, E+, G+.

    ASH CONST. (whole): Ca 0.045, Mg 0.133, K 0.473, Na 0.039, P 0.423, Cl 0.068, S 0.181, Fe 0.0050.

An acid-forming food; potential acidity 12 cc. per 100 cal. Wheat flour 9 cc. per 100 Gm.

RS: *bread, cereal, crackers, oatmeal, rye*.

STRUCTURE OF A GRAIN OF WHEAT: 1. Husk or outer coat. Removed before grinding. 2. Bran coats removed in making white flour contains the mineral substances. 3. Gluten. Contains the fat and protein. 4. Starch. The center of the kernel.

ACTION: See bread for a comparison of flours made from wheat and other cereals. Boiled whole wheat is a most excellent food. Time required for digestion: Cracked, 2 hours.

WHEAT PREPARATIONS AND PASTES: Macaroni, vermicelli, noodles, etc., are made from flour and water, molded, dried, and slightly baked. They are easy to digest and not over 10% of nitrogen content is lost.

Composition: In macaroni, vermicelli, spaghetti, noodles, the food value is lower than 2 cereals and breads. Their ash is acid and phosphates of soda are too high.

Action: They are easy on intestinal digestion.

wheeze (hwēz) [M.E. *whesen*, to hiss]. 1. A sound made by air as it passes with difficulty through the glottis and fauces in difficult respiration. 2. To breathe noisily or with effort.

wheezing (hwē′zĭng) [M.E. *whesen*, to hiss]. Noisy and difficult breathing.

whelk (hwělk) [A.S. *hwylca*, a suppuration]. A wheal; a protuberance on the face, as a nodule or tubercle.

whey (hwā) [A.S. *hwaeg*]. The liquid left after milk has been coagulated by the aid of rennet.

It is diuretic, laxative, and mineralizing.

    AV. SERVING: 325 Gm. Pro. 2.3, Fat 0.7, Carbo. 11.4.

    VITAMIN: G+++.

    ASH CONST: Ca 0.044, Mg 0.008, K 0.157, Na 0.038, P 0.035, Cl 0.119, S 0.009.

SEE: *buttermilk, milk*.

whipworm (hwĭp′worm) [named from its shape]. A round worm often parasitic in the human intestines. SEE: *Trichocephalus dispar*.

whirl (hwĭrl) [M.E. *whirlen*]. To revolve rapidly; to feel giddiness.

whirlbone (hwĭrl′bōn). 1. The kneecap. SYN: *patella*. 2. The head of the femur.

whisky, whiskey (hwĭs′kē). A distilled alcoholic liquor made from grain. SYN: *spiritus frumenti*.

whisper (hwĭs′pẽr) [A.S. *hwisprian*]. 1. Speech without voice; a low, sibilant sound. 2. To utter in a low, nonvocal sound.

    w., cavernous. Direct transmission of a whisper through a cavity in auscultation.

white (hwīt) [A.S. *hwīt*]. 1. The achromatic color of highest brilliance. 2. Of the color of milk.

    w. cell, w. corpuscle. The leukocyte. SEE: *blood, corpuscle*.

    w. gangrene. G. due to local anemia.

    w. leg. Phlebitis of femoral vein marked by white swelling of the leg. SYN: *phlegmasia alba dolens*.

    w. line. White tendinous attachment of abdominal oblique and transverse muscles. SYN: *linea* alba*.

    w. precipitate. SEE: *ammoniated mercury*.

    w. matter, w. substance. Any nervous structure composed of white medullated nerve fibers.

    w. softening. Stage of softening of any substance in which the affected area has become white and anemic.

    w. swelling. Tuberculous arthritis. SEE: *gonatocele*.

whites (hwīts). A thick, whitish vaginal discharge. SYN: *leukorrhea*, q.v.

white fish. COMP: NUTRITIVES: E. P. Pro. 22.9, Fat 6.5. FUEL VALUE: 100 Gm. equals 149 cal.

White's operation (hwīt). Castration for relief of enlarged prostate.

whitlow (hwĭt′lō) [origin uncertain]. Suppurative inflammation at the end of a finger or toe. SYN: *felon, panaris, paronychia*, q.v.

It may be deep seated, involving the bone and its periosteum, or superficial, affecting parts of the nail.

wholesome (hōl′sŭm) [M.E. *holsum*]. Promoting physical well-being.

whoop (hoop) [O.Fr. *houper*, to whoop]. The sonorous and convulsive inspiratory crow following a paroxysm of whooping cough.

whooping cough (hoop′ĭng kawf). An acute infectious disease with recurrent spasms of coughing ending in a whooping inspiration. SYN: *pertussis*, q.v.

SEE: *bex convulsiva, chin cough*.

whorl (hwŭrl) [M.E. *wharle*, whirl of a spindle]. 1. Spiral arrangement of cardiac muscular fibers. SYN: *vortex*. 2. A type of fingerprint in which the central papillary ridges turn through at least 1 complete circle.

whortleberry (hwur'tl-bĕr"ĭ) [A.S. *horte, whortleberry*]. Av. SERVING: 100 Gm. Pro. 0.7, Fat 3.0, Carbo. 10.3. ASH CONST. (whole): Ca 0.031, Mg 0.021, K 0.261, Na 0.021, P 0.042.

Widal's reaction or **test** (vē-dal'). An agglutination test for typhoid fever.

wild cherry (*prunus virginiana*). USP. The dried bark of the plant, used principally in the form of the syrup as a vehicle for cough medicine.
  DOSAGE: 2½ drams (10 cc.).

Wilde's cords (wīld). Fibrous bands which cross the callosum transversely.

W's. incision or **operation**. Incision behind the auricle for relief of mastoid abscess.

will (wĭl) [A.S. *willa*]. Power of controlling one's actions or emotions.
  RS: *acrasia, bulesis, volition, voluntary.*

Willis' bands (wĭl'ĭs). Those crossing the sup. longitudinal sinus, transversely.
  W. circle. The intercommunications established at the base of the brain bet. the branches of the basilar and internal carotid arteries.

Wilson's disease (wĭl'sun). A rare disease of degeneration of corpus striatum and cirrhosis of the liver, characterized by tremulous distortion of the muscles (increased by activity), dysarthria, dysphagia, and emotionalism.
  It begins in the limbs and spreads to the voluntary muscles, but the intrinsic eye muscles are exempted. Excitement and attention increase the rhythmic tremors. Hypertrophic cirrhosis of liver during adolescence. Pyramidal tract symptoms absent.

Wimshurst machine (wĭmz'hurst). A type of influence machine to produce static current.

Winckel's disease (vĭn'kĕl). A fatal disease of the newborn characterized by profuse hemorrhages, hematuria, jaundice, enlarged spleen, and punctiform hemorrhages upon the skin. SEE: *Buhl's disease.*

windage (wĭnd'ăj). Compression of air by passage of a missile near the body causing injury of an internal organ by the external concussion.

windpipe (wĭnd'pīp). Passage for breath from the larynx to the lungs. SYN: *trachea, q.v.*

wine (wīn) [L. *vinum*, wine]. 1. Fermented grape juice or fermented juice of any fruit. 2. Solution of a medicinal substance in wine. SYN: *vinum.*
  ASH CONST. (average): Ca 0.009, Mg 0.010, K 0.104, Na 0.008, P 0.015, Cl 0.011, S 0.015, Fe 0.0003.

wink (wĭnk) [A.S. *wincian*]. 1. To close and open the eyelids quickly. 2. Act of closing and opening the eyelids quickly. SEE: *mication, nictitation.*

win'ter itch. Itching occurring only in the winter. SYN: *pruritus hiemalis.*

Winternitz's ablutions (vĭn'ter-nĭts). Patient sits on edge of bathtub, back exposed. Cold water from hose is allowed to flow down back while the back is rubbed vigorously.

Wirsung, duct of (vēr'soong). Excretory duct of the pancreas. SYN: *pancreatic duct.*

wisdom tooth (wĭz'dŏm). The hindmost or last molar tooth on each side of the jaw, which may appear as late as the 25th year.

witches' milk (wĭtsh'es). Milk secreted by the newly born infant's breast, stimulated by the lactating hormone circulating in the mother.

witherings (wĭth'ĕr-ĭngs). Tumor due to fatty degeneration and absorption of epithelial cells. SYN: *scirrhus, atrophic.*

wolffian body (wool'fĭ-ăn). An embryonic organ on each side of the vertebral column. SYN: *mesonephros.* SEE: *archinephron, embryo, paroöphoron, parovarium.*
  w. cyst. One of the broad ligaments of the uterus.
  w. duct. The mesonephric canal that joins post. end of the intestine. SEE: *epoöphoron.*
  w. tubules. Small tubes joining the wolffian duct at right angles.

wom'an [A.S. *wimmann*, wife man]. An adult female person. SEE: *misogyny.*

womb (woom) [A.S. *wamb*]. Female organ for protection and nourishment of the fetus. SYN: *uterus, q.v.*

wood alcohol (wud al'kŏ-hŏl). Alcohol obtained by distillation from wood.
  It is a poisonous substance and frequently causes loss of sight. SEE: *methyl alcohol.*

Wood's filter. A screen that absorbs visible rays but allows a portion of the ultraviolet rays to be transmitted.

wood tick. Parasite which bites man and produces wheals with itching central punctures causing spotted or Rocky Mountain spotted* fever.

woolsorter's disease (wool'sor-ter). A pulmonary form of anthrax which develops in those who handle wool contaminated with *Bacillus anthrax.*

word blindness. Inability to comprehend written words; a form of aphasia, *q.v.*
  w. salad. The use of words with no apparent meaning attached to them or to their relations one with another; usually found in schizophrenia.

work (wurk) [A.S. *worc*]. For definition, SEE: *erg.* For comparison of various energy units, SEE: *calorie, unit.*

worm (werm) [A.S. *wyrm*]. 1. An invertebrate, cylindrical animal of the group *Vermes.* 2. Any small, limbless, creeping animal. 3. Median portion of the cerebellum. 4. Any wormlike structure.
  RS: *ankylostomiasis, anthelmintic, ascariasis, ascaris, distoma, distomiasis, helminthiasis, hookworm disease, leech, lumbricus, nematode, oxyuriasis, oxyuricide, tenia, teniacide, teniafuge, trichina, trichinosis, uncinariasis, vermicide, vermicular, vermifuge.*
  w. abscess. A. resulting from lodgment of a worm in the body.
  w. fever. Fever due to irritation caused by worms in the intestinal canal.

worms (werms). Any disorder due to the presence of parasitic worms in the body.
  TYPES: *Tape w., tenia, nematodes. Ascaris lumbricoides* (roundworm). Pale pink in color, resemble earthworms in form.
  Inhabits small intestines, occasionally migrates into stomach, bile ducts, and larynx.
  TREATMENT: Santonin, wormseed oil. Spigelia.
  Oxyuris vermicularis (seatworm, pinworm). Occupies colon and rectum. Produces intense itching of anus, worse at night; may migrate to vagina and cause vaginitis or pruritus, and lead to masturbation.
  TREATMENT: An injection of water followed by the injection of 2 to 3 ounces of an infusion of quassia chips. May be detected by smearing anus and vulva with lard.
  Ankylostomum duodenale. A small worm not uncommon in Egypt and north

of Europe. Inhabits small intestines.
Trichocephalus dispar (whipworm). Small worm, thick at one end, threadlike at other.
Filaria sanguinis hominis. Small, threadlike worm most commonly seen in the tropics. Adult worm occupies the lymphatics; embryos find way into blood current.

wormian bones (wur'mĭ-ăn). Small, irregular bones in the course of the cranial sutures.

worsted test (wus'tĕd). Matching of the differently colored skeins of worsted yarn to detect color blindness. SYN: *Holmgren's test.*

wound (woond) [A.S. *wund*]. Break in the continuity of soft parts from violence or trauma of tissues.
TREATMENT: Crude cod-liver oil applied to ulcers, wounds, and burns in which there has been a loss of 1 or more layers of the skin, has proved very effective as a healing, sterile, and antiseptic remedy. Cellophane* used as a wound dressing is singularly free of infection and doesn't crack. Allantoin is esp. useful in nonhealing wounds and ulcers. The applications should be followed with the use of a plaster of Paris bandage to insure rest of the part. Toxins are thus rendered harmless, and the growth of bacteria checked. Ulcers should first be cleansed before using the oil. Felons and infections of tendons and bedsores may also be treated in this manner.

w., abdominal. Frequently sustained; ordinarily involves structure of abdominal wall.
In such instances, it may be treated as ordinary wounds. Where a cavity has been opened, and esp. if viscera have been exposed, they should be kept sterile and moist with a sterile normal salt solution prepared by dissolving a teaspoonful of salt in pint of boiling water, or use the clearest water at hand, because allowing viscera to dry destroys them.
Such injuries are not accompanied by much bleeding; ordinarily associated shock is marked. Treat additionally as for internal injuries, *q.v.*

w., bullet. A puncture wound from a bullet. Usually there is a small point of entrance; if the bullet left the body a larger point of exit; it is associated with injuries of bone, tendon, blood vessels, etc.
SYM: Depend on site, speed, and character of bullet.
F. A. TREATMENT: Antitetanic serum. Antiseptic to wound and dressing. Treat complications and shock.

w., cellulitis of. When wounds have been closed without drainage, esp. in such cases as appendicitis, local inflammation of the wound may occur.
SYM: Elevation of temperature from 4th to 7th day with tenderness. Inspect dressing and chart.
TREATMENT: Evacuation of the abscess; hot wet dressings.

w., contused. A bruise. It may be caused by a blunt instrument.
The skin need not necessarily be broken, but injury of the tissues under skin, leaving skin unbroken, causes more or less change in the normal musculature. The blood vessels underneath skin being ruptured causes discoloration. If extravasated blood becomes encapsulated it is termed *hematoma**; if it is diffused, an *ecchymosis.** More or less shock depending on the extent of the contusion.
TREATMENT: Cold compresses, pressure, and rest of part with elevation. When acute stage is over (6 to 24 hours) soapsuds application, massage with camphorated oil, exposure to a 60 watt electric light with continued rest and elevation are prescribed. Aseptic drainage may be indicated.

w., crushing. If bleeding, apply cold cloths; if not, gently mold to proper shape, apply cloth dipped in warm water, and keep warm. If bone is fractured, apply splint.

w., fish-hook. Imbedded fish hooks are notably difficult to remove. Push the hook through, then cut off barb with an instrument. These injuries frequently become infected, so carefully saturate with an antiseptic and cover with a dressing, and observe for several days.

w., gunshot. Penetrating or perforating wound which may contain a foreign body, as a bullet.
F. A. TREATMENT: Should be conservative. Apply antiseptic, sterile dressing; treat hemorrhage. If large vessels are torn, antitetanic serum to prevent lockjaw. *Do not probe.*

w., incised. A clean-cut wound.
Caused by a keen cutting instrument. There are no jagged edges. Any sharp cut in which the tissues are not severed is an incised wound. It may be either an aseptic or infected w., depending on circumstances which caused it.
An *aseptic* wound, or one occurring under surgical conditions, should heal if conditions are favorable and no contaminations due to pathogenic organisms or foreign material enter into it. During healing process, area of the wound must be kept aseptic. The skin must be cleansed with antiseptic solution and covered securely with sterile dressings, preventing external contact with microörganisms. A clean wound should be left alone. The dressings should be changed only often enough to keep wound clean. There should be no squeezing or pulling of its edges.

w., lacerated. A torn wound.
It provides many avenues for infection. It is *not* a clean wound. The edges are ragged. May be caused by many kinds of implements, and the implement may be covered with any kind of pathogenic bacteria. These may be of a violent nature causing tetanus, or only a slight abscess. The infiltration of bacteria may cause any stage of a septic condition. In dealing with such wounds, all possibilities should be taken into consideration.
TREATMENT: The wound should be cleansed with antiseptic solution and ragged edges trimmed off, if too ragged. Some doctors advise that wet dressings be applied. The patient should be given tetanus antitoxin. The wound should never be sealed. It is well to hold it open with some form of drain from a piece of sterile silkworm gut or a rubber drain.

w., open. Contusion where skin is also broken, such as a gunshot w., incised w., or lacerated w.

w., perforating. One in which the vulnerating body both enters and emerges from the cavity.

w., poisoned. This may be classed as a lacerated wound, or a punctured wound, depending on tearing of tissue.
The poisoned wound may be caused by a diseased animal, as a snake or a

dog, or some of the wild animals, such as the coon or the squirrel.

TREATMENT: A poisoned wound should be treated the same as a punctured wound. Cauterize with silver nitrate; wet dressings should be applied. The animal, if possible, should be put under observatioz.

w., punctured. One made by sharp-pointed instrument, such as a dagger, an ice pick, or needle. The chief danger is from thrombosis and possible release of emboli. A puncture wound never gives access to int. of wound. Tetanus germs thrive in such a wound, as they live in darkness and progress rapidly without air. Inspect instrument that caused the wound. The puncture should be found and, if possible, squeezed until the blood flows.

TREATMENT: Tetanus antitoxin at once and apply moist dressings. If the patient does not respond, the punctured wound should be incised.

w., subcutaneous. Include all which are unaccompanied by break in skin. As contusions.

w. tearing off parts. If completely severed, treat same as lacerated wound. A few drops of carbolic acid should be used in water for washing wounds. Watch for shock. If parts are not completely severed, gently bring into position, apply splints where necessary, and bandage until surgical aid is obtainable. Watch for shock.

wound, words pert. to: agglutination; anastole; aneroplasty; antiseptic; autorrhaphy; avivement; Carrel-Dakin treatment; cicatrix; cicatrization; Dakin's solution; epulosis; gas gangrene; granulation; healing; ichor; incise; injury; intention, first, second, and third; lacerated; laceration; lesion; resolution; slough; suture; toilet; transportation; trauma; vulnerable; vulnerary; vulnerate; vulnus.

Wrisberg's ansa (vrĭz'bĕrk). Loop made by anastomosis of right pneumogastric and great splanchnic nerves with right semilunar ganglion.

W's. cartilage. Cuneiform cartilage of the larynx.

W's. ganglion. One often found in superficial cardiac plexus.

W's. nerve. 1. Small branch of the brachial plexus. 2. Small int. cutaneous nerve bet. facial and auditory nerves.

wrist (rĭst) [A.S.]. The joint bet. hand and arm; the carpus, consisting of 8 bones.

RS: *armilla, carpagra, carpal, carpale, carpopedal spasm, carpoptosis, carpus, jerk, skeleton, trapezoid.*

w. clonus. Irregular convulsive movements of the hand due to inability to control the muscles that bend the wrist backward.

w. clonus reflex. Lateral clonic movements of hand occurring when hand is held down at arm's length in extreme extension.

w.-drop. A dropping of the hand caused by paralysis of extensor muscles of fingers and wrist.

A flexion deformity due to paralysis of the forearm extensors. The most common cause is lead poisoning, though any paralysis of these muscles will produce the condition; also arsenic intoxication or brachial nerve pressure. SYN: *carpoptosis.*

NP: It may be avoided in fractures by exercising the hands whenever possible and by keeping them at right angles with the adjacent part.

w. joint. Joint formed by the radius and the first row of carpal bones.

wri'ter's cramp. An occupational disability due to excessive writing.

The writer is able to use the fingers for any other purpose; will find that grasping a pen will immediately, or shortly, result in a painful muscular contraction, entirely preventing writing. The nature of the disability is uncertain.

SYM: Sense of weight fatigue or actual pain in affected muscles. Soon the fingers are seized with a tonic or clonic spasm whenever the pen is grasped. Sometimes, when in use, hand becomes seat of a decided tremor. In a third form the chief phenomena are excessive weakness and fatigue, which disappear soon as pen is laid aside.

PROG: Guardedly favorable. Disease obstinate, but cure generally follows protracted rest.

TREATMENT: Absolute rest is essential element. Improve general health. Massage, electricity, and passive movements.

SYN: *graphospasm.* SEE: *agraphia.*

writing hand. Position seen in paralysis agitans marked by contraction of muscle of the hand.

The fingers assume the position similar to holding a pen.

wryneck (rĭ'nĕk). Contracted state of 1 or more muscles of the neck, producing an abnormal position of the head. SYN: *loxia, torticollis.*

It is occasionally acute, due to cold or trauma; more commonly chronic and is then spastic in character and dependent upon nerve irritation. Has been produced by habitual malposition of the head assumed because of existing ocular defect. May be congenital.

When acute, generally passes away under influence of rest, heat, and time. Chronic may require friction, electricity, or stretching, section or removal of a portion of spinal accessory nerve. May be little benefit from any treatment.

Wunderlich's curve (voon'dĕr-lĭk). The fever curve typical of typhoid fever.

X. 1. Abbr. of *Kienböck's unit.* 2. Roman numeral 10. 3. Symb. of *reactance.*
Xe. Chemical symbol for *xenon.*
xanthelasma (zăn-thĕl-ăz'mă) [G. *xanthos,* yellow, + *elasma,* plate]. 1. Yellow. 2. Flat or slightly raised yellowish tumor occurring in elderly persons, found most frequently on the upper and lower lids, esp. near the inner canthus. SYN: *xanthoma.*
xanthelasmoidea (zăn-thel-ăz-moy'dē-ă) [" + " + *eidos,* resemblance]. Chronic disease of childhood marked by wheals and followed by brownish-yellow patches. SYN: *urticaria pigmentosa.*
xanthematin (zăn-thĕm'ă-tĭn) [" + *haima, haimat-,* blood]. A yellow substance derivable from hematin when treated with nitric acid.
xanthemia (zăn-thē'mĭ-ă) [" + *haima,* blood]. Yellow pigment in the blood. SYN: *carotinemia.*
xanthic (zăn'thĭk) [G. *xanthos,* yellow]. 1. Yellow. 2. Pert. to xanthine.
   x. calculus. A urinary concretion containing xanthine.
xanthin(e (zăn'thĭn, -thēn) [G. *xanthos,* yellow]. A nitrogenous extractive contained in muscle tissue, liver, spleen, pancreas, and other organs, and in the urine, formed during the metabolism of nucleoproteins.
   Through the action of certain enzymes it becomes further converted into uric acid, and as such is passed into the urine.
   x. bases. Nitrogenous substances resulting from splitting up of nucleins. SEE: *purine bases.*
xanthinuria (zăn-thĭn-ū'rĭ-ă) [G. *xanthos,* yellow, + *ouron,* urine]. Excretion of large amounts of xanthine in the urine.
xanthochromia (zăn″thō-krō'mĭ-ă) [" + *chrōma,* color]. Yellow discoloration, as of the skin in patches or of the cerebrospinal fluid, resembling jaundice.
xanthochroous (zăn-thok'rō-ŭs) [" + *chroa,* color]. Having a yellowish or light complexion.
xanthocyanopia, xanthocyanopsia (zăn″thō-sī-ăn-ō'pĭ-ă, -ŏp'sĭ-ă) [" + *kyanos,* blue, + *opsis,* sight]. A form of color blindness in which yellow and blue are distinguishable, but not red and green.
xanthoderma (zăn″thō-der'mă) [" + *derma,* skin]. Yellowness of the skin.
xanthodont, xanthodontous (zăn'thō-dŏnt, zăn-thō-dŏn'tŭs) [" + *odous, odont-,* tooth]. Having yellow teeth.
xanthokyanopy (zăn″thō-kĭ-ăn'ō-pī) [" + *kyanos,* blue, + *opsis,* sight]. Partial blindness for color, yellow and blue only being discerned. SYN: *xanthocyanopia.*
xanthoma (zăn-thō'mă) [G. *xanthos,* yellow, + *-ōma,* tumor]. Flat, slightly elevated, soft, rounded, chamois-covered plaque or nodule, usually on the eyelids.
   They may occur in patches of yellowish macule on orbital regions, confined to middle life or later, and to the female sex, consisting of a degenerative process involving fibers of the orbicularis muscle.
   TREATMENT: Carbon dioxide snow, carbon arc light.
   SEE: *vitiligoidea.*

   x. diabeticorum. Cutaneous disease associated with diabetes mellitus.
   x. mul'tiplex. Xanthomas all over the body.
   x. palpebra'rum. X. affecting the eyelids.
   x. tuberosum. A form which may appear on the neck, shoulders, trunk, or extremities, consisting of small, elastic, and yellowish-colored nodules.
   TREATMENT: Excision, electrolysis, or caustics. Constitutional.
xanthomatosis (zăn-thō-mă-tō'sĭs) [G. *xanthos,* yellow, + *-ōma,* tumor]. General eruption of xanthomas. SYN: *xanthoma multiplex.*
xanthomelanous (zăn″thō-mĕl'ăn-ŭs) [" + *melas, melan-,* black]. Having black hair and an olive skin.
xanthopathy (zăn-thŏp'ă-thī) [" + *pathos,* disease]. Yellowish pigmentation of the skin. SYN: *xanthochromia, xanthoderma.*
xanthophane (zăn'thō-fān) [" + *phanein,* to appear]. A yellow pigment in the retinal cones.
xanthoplasty (zăn-thō-plăs'tĭ) [" + *plassein,* to form]. Yellow color of the skin. SYN: *xanthoderma.*
xanthoproteic (zăn″thō-prō-te'ĭk) [" + *prōtos,* first]. Derived from or pertaining to xanthoprotein.
   x. reaction. Deep orange color produced by adding ammonia and heating proteids with nitric acid; a test for protein.
xanthoprotein (zăn″thō-prō'tē-ĭn) [" + *prōtos,* first]. Yellowish substance produced by heating proteids with nitric acid.
xanthopsia (zăn-thŏp'sĭ-ă) [G. *xanthos,* yellow, + *opsis,* sight]. Condition in which objects appear yellow.
xanthopsin (zăn-thŏp'sĭn) [" + *opsis,* sight]. Visual yellow, the visual purple produced by light acting on rhodopsin.
xanthopsis (zăn-thŏp'sĭs) [" + *opsis,* appearance]. Yellow pigmentation seen in cancers.
xanthopsydracia (zăn″thŏp-sĭ-drā'shĭ-ă) [" + *psydrax,* pustule]. Skin disease marked by the formation of yellow pustules or pimples on the skin.
xanthosarcoma (zăn″thō-sar-kō'mă) [" + *sarx, sark-,* flesh, + *-ōma,* tumor]. Giant cell sarcoma of tendon sheaths containing xanthoma cells.
xanthosis (zăn-thō'sĭs) [" + *-ōsis,* condition]. A yellowish pigmentation, esp. seen in degenerating tissues and malignancies.
   x. diabet'ica. Yellowish skin seen in diabetics.
xanthous (zăn'thŭs) [G. *xanthos,* yellow]. Yellow.
xanthuria (zăn-thū'rĭ-ă) [" + *ouron,* urine]. Excretion of an excess of xanthine in the urine. SYN: *xanthinuria.*
x chromosome. A chromosome which probably carries sexual characteristics and passes whole into the daughter cell. SYN: *chromosome, accessory.*
x-disease. General malaise with disturbances of digestion, cardiac action, respiration, with extreme sensitiveness to cold.
x-element. Aggregate of accessory chromo-

xenogenous

somes, paired or unpaired with group of varying size or shape known as the y-element.
xenogenous (zĕn-ŏj'ĕn-ŭs) [G. *xenos*, strange, host, + *gennan*, to produce]. 1. Caused by a foreign body. 2. Originating in the host, as a toxin resulting from stimuli applied to cells of the host.
xenomenia (zĕn-ō-mē'nĭ-ă) [G. *xenos*, strange, + *mēniaia*, menses]. Menstruation from a part of the body other than the normal one. SYN: *vicarious menstruation*.
xenon (zē'non) [G. *xenos*, strange]. A gaseous element in the atmosphere. At. wt. 131.3. SYMB: Xe.
xenoparasite (zĕn″ō-păr'ă-sīt) [G. *xenos*, host, + *parasitos*, a parasite]. One that may become pathogenic if the resistance of the host has been weakened.
xenophobia (zĕn″ō-fō'bĭ-ă) [G. *xenos*, stranger, + *phobos*, fear]. Abnormal reluctance to meeting strangers.
xenophonia (zĕn″ō-fō'nĭ-ă) [G. *xenos*, strange, + *phōnē*, voice]. Alteration in accent and intonation of a person's voice due to defect of speech.
xenophthalmia (zĕn-ŏf-thăl'mĭ-ă) [" + *ophthalmia*, inflammation of the eye]. Inflammation of the eye caused by a foreign body.
xeransis (zē-răn'sĭs) [G. *xēros*, dry]. Loss of moisture in tissues or drugs brought about gradually. SYN: *siccation*.
xerantic (zē-răn'tĭk). Causing dryness. SYN: *siccant, siccative*.
xerasia (zē-rā'sĭ-ă) [G. *xēros*, dry]. Disease of the hair in which there is abnormal dryness, followed by brittleness, and eventually loss.
xero- (zē″rō-) [G.]. Prefix meaning *dry*.
xerocheilia (zē″rō-kī'lĭ-ă) [G. *xeros*, dry, + *cheilos*, lip]. Dryness of the lips; a type of cheilitis.
xeroderma (zē-rō-der'mă) [G. *xēros*, dry, + *derma*, skin]. Roughness and dryness of the skin; mild ichthyosis.
 x. pigmento'sum. A rare disease of the skin starting in childhood marked by disseminated pigment discolorations, ulcers, cutaneous and muscular atrophy and death. SYN: *Kaposi's disease*.
xerodermatic (zē″rō-der-măt'ĭk) [G. *xēros*, dry, + *derma*, skin]. Relating to xeroderma.
xeroma (zē-rō'mă) [" + -*ōma*, mass]. An abnormally dry state of the conjunctiva. SYN: *xerophthalmia*.
xeromenia (zē-rō-mē'nĭ-ă) [" + *mēniaia*, menses]. The occurrence of the usual disturbances during menses without menstrual flow.
xeromycteria (zē-rō-mĭk-tē'rĭ-ă) [" + *myktēr*, nose]. Dryness of the nasal passages.
xeronosus (zē-rŏn'ō-sŭs) [" + *nosos*, disease]. Dryness of the skin.
xerophagia (zē-rō-fā'jĭ-ă) [" + *phagein*, to eat]. The eating of dry food only.
xerophthalmia (zē-rŏf-thăl'mĭ-ă) [G. *xēros*, dry, + *ophthalmos*, eye]. Conjunctival dryness with keratinization of epithelium following chronic conjunctivitis and in disease due to deficiency of Vitamin A.
xerosis (zē-rō'sĭs) [G. *xēros*, dry, + -*ōsis*, condition]. 1. Abnormal dryness of skin, mucous membranes, or of the conjunctiva. 2. Normal sclerosis of tissues in the aged.
xerostomia (zē-rō-stō'mĭ-ă) [" + *stoma*, mouth]. Dryness of the mouth.
 It occurs in diabetes, hysteria, paralysis of facial nerve involving chorda tympani, acute infections, some types of neuroses, and is induced by certain drugs such as nicotine and atropine; all arresting salivary secretion. SEE: *ptyalism*.
xerotes (zē'rō-tēz) [G. *xērotēs*, dryness]. Dryness of the body; dryness.
xerotocia (zē-rō-tō'shĭ-ă) [G. *xēros*, dry, + *tokos*, birth]. Dry labor.
xerotic (zē-rŏt'ĭk) [G. *xēros*, dry]. Dry; characterized by dryness.
xerotripsis (zē″rō-trĭp'sĭs) [" + *tripsis*, a rubbing]. Dry friction.
xiphi-, xipho- (zĭf-ĭ-, -ō-) [G.]. Prefixes pert. to the *xiphoid cartilage*.
xiphisternum (zĭf-ĭ-ster'nŭm) [G. *xiphos*, sword, + *sternon*, chest]. The pointed process of the lower end of the sternum. SYN: *xiphoid cartilage*.
xiphocostal (zĭf″ō-kŏs'tăl) [" + L. *costa*, rib]. Relating to the xiphoid cartilage and the ribs.
 x. ligament. One connecting the xiphoid cartilage to the cartilage of the 8th rib.
xiphodynia (zĭf-ō-dĭn'ĭ-ă) [" + *odynē*, pain]. Pain in the ensiform cartilage.
xiphoid (zĭf'oyd) [G. *xiphos*, sword, + *eidos*, process]. Sword-shaped, ensiform.
 x. process. The lowest portion of the sternum, a sword-shaped cartilaginous process supported by bone.
 It has no ribs attached to it, but some of the abdominal muscles are attached to it. It ossifies in the aged.
xiphoiditis (zĭf-oyd-ī'tĭs) [" + " + -*itis*, inflammation]. Inflammation of the ensiform or xiphoid cartilage.
x-knee. Knock-knee.
xoanthropy (zō-ăn'thrō-pĭ) [G. *zōon*, animal, + *anthropos*, man]. Monomania in which one believes himself to be an animal.
X-radiation unit. SYMB: *r*. Amt. of x-radiation which, when the secondary electrons are fully utilized, and wall effect of the chamber is avoided, produces in 1 cc. of atmospheric air at 0° C. and 76 cm. mercury pressure such degree of conductivity that 1 electrostatic unit of charge is measured at saturation current.
x-ray. 1. Any of the radiations of an extremely short wave length, emitted primarily as result of sudden change in velocity of a moving electric charge and as the result of atomic changes of target due to this impact. 2. A photograph obtained by use of x-rays.
 Properties of x-rays include penetration through various thicknesses of all solids, production of secondary x-rays by impinging on material bodies and action on photographic plates and fluorescent screens.
 RS: *cathodograph, cholecystogram, ray, ray,* roentgen*.
 x. dermatitis. Cutaneous inflammation due to exposure to x-rays.
 x. unit. Unit of x-ray dosage equal to 1/10 the erythema dose.
xylenin (zī'lē-nĭn) [G. *xylon*, wood]. A toxic substance extracted by xylene from tubercle bacilli.
xylo- (zī-lō-) [G.]. Prefix pert. to or derived *from wood*.
xylol (zī'lŏl) [G. *xylon*, wood]. A commercial mixture of the 3 xylenes (ortho, meta, and para dimethylbenzene).
 It is a liquid, boiling at about 140° C., used as a cleaning agent and solvent, and it has been given in smallpox and syphilis.

xylose (zī'lōs) [G. *xylon*, wood]. Wood sugar, a crystalline, nonfermentable pentose.
xylotherapy (zī"lō-ther'ă-pĭ) [G. *xylon*, wood, + *therapeia*, treatment]. Therapeutic application of certain woods to the body.
xyrospasm (zī'rō-spăzm) [G. *xyron*, razor, + *spasmos*, spasm]. Occupational neurosis of the fingers seen in barbers.
xysma (zĭz'mă) [G. *zysma*, filings]. In diarrhea, flocculent pseudomembranous matter sometimes seen in stools.
xyster (zĭs'ter) [G. *xystēr*, a scraper]. A surgeon's rasp, used mainly for scraping bones. SYN: *raspatory*.
xystus (zĭs'tŭs) [G. *xystos*, scraped]. Scraped lint.

Y

Y. Symb. of element *yttrium*.
yaghourt (yah-ghoort'). Milk curdled by a ferment possessing an active lactic acid bacillus, *B. bulgaricus*, used in Bulgaria.
Y-angle. Angle bet. line uniting lambda and inion and radius fixus.
yard [A.S. *gyrd*, a rod]. 1. A measure of 3 feet or 36 inches. 2. The penis.
yatren (yăt'rĕn). Commercial brand of chiniofon, *q.v.*
yava skin (yah'va skĭn). A form of elephantiasis due to the excessive use of kava. SEE: *elephantiasis.*
yawn [A.S. *gānian*, to yawn]. 1. To open the mouth involuntarily, as in drowsiness or fatigue. 2. Involuntary act of gaping, accompanied by attempts at inspiration, excited by drowsiness.
yawning (yawn'ĭng) [A.S. *gānian*, to yawn]. Deep inspiration, gaping induced by drowsiness or fatigue. SYN: *oscitation.*
yaws (yawz) [Cariban]. An infectious tropical disease. SYN: *frambesia.*
  SYM: Febrile disturbances, rheumatism, eruption of tubercles with a caseous crust on hands, feet, face, and external genitals.
Yb. The symb. for *ytterbium.*
Y bacil'lus. A dysentery bacillus.
Y car'tilage. The cartilage uniting the 3 pelvic bones at bottom of the acetabulum early in life.
y chromosome. An accessory chromosome in male cells supposed to be the male determining principle in fertilization. SEE: *chromosome, heredity.*
yeast (yēst) [A.S. *gist*]. 1. A substance composed of aggregated cells (Saccharomyces) of minute unicellular sac fungi. 2. A commercial product composed of meal impregnated with living yeast.
  Yeasts are in some instances pathogenic. They are used to produce fermentation, as in beer; to leaven bread, and as a remedy.
  An excellent source of Vits. B and G. Vits. A and C lacking.
  FUEL VALUE (compressed): 90 Gm. = 100 cal. 1 lb. = 506 cal., 100 Gm. = 111 cal.
  ACTION: No amount of fresh or dried yeast, aside from brewer's yeast, can be consumed that will contribute any appreciable quantity of vitamins or other principles.
  y. enema. One quart of warm water and ½ cake of yeast, thoroughly mixed and given very warm.
yelk (yelk). Variant of yolk.
yellow (yĕl'ō) [A.S. *geolu*]. 1. One of the primary colors resembling that of a ripe lemon. 2. Colored yellow, as the skin in disease.
  y. fever. An acute infectious disease characterized by jaundice, epigastric tenderness, vomiting, hemorrhages, and a febrile course consisting of 2 paroxysms.
  ETIOL: Hot climate, warm season, salt water, bad drainage, and overcrowding favor epidemics. Disease spread by mosquitos.
  PERIOD OF INCUBATION: A few hours to a week.
  SYM: *First Stage:* Disease begins with a chill followed by pain in head, back, and limbs. Temperature rises rapidly till it reaches its maximum, 103° to 105° F. Face flushed, conjunctivae injected, pupils small, tongue coated, epigastrium tender, stomach irritable and unretentive, bowels constipated, urine scanty and albuminous. This stage lasts from a few hours to several days.
  It is followed by a marked fall in temperature and an improvement in general symptoms. At this time convalescence may begin or patient may pass into second febrile paroxysm.
  Second Stage: Fever rises to its original height, skin becomes yellow, vomiting persistent, and ejected matter may contain dark blood (black vomit). Hemorrhages sometimes occur from other mucous membranes. Pulse rapid, but not proportionate to the fever. Urine becomes very scanty and contains albumen and casts. Death frequently results from exhaustion or uremia, though recovery may follow the gravest symptoms.
  DURATION: From a few hours to a week.
  PROG: Always grave. Mortality, 7 to 10%. In severe epidemics, 20 to 70%.
  TREATMENT: Absolute rest; cool, well-ventilated room; liquid diet. Pain in back and limbs may be relieved by hot water bags, high fever by applications of cold. Internal remedies to suit individual cases. Charcoal taken internally, ½ teaspoonful of the crude powder 2 or 3 times per day of great value as a prophylactic.
  y. softening. A stage of softening of the brain marked by fatty degeneration and yellow discoloration.
  y. spot. 1. Yellowish nodule at ant. end of vocal cord. 2. Center of the retina, the point of clearest vision. SYN: *macula lutea.*
  y. vision. Condition in which objects seem yellow in color. SYN: *xanthopsia.*
yerba (yĕr'ba) [Sp.]. An herb.
  y. maté (mah'tā). Paraguay tea.
Yersin's serum (yer-san'). An antitoxic serum for the plague.
-yl [G.]. Suffix signifying, in chemistry, a *radical.*
-ylene [G.]. Suffix denoting, in chemistry, a *bivalent hydrocarbon radical.*
Y ligament. A y-shaped band covering the upper and front portions of the hip joint. SYN: *iliofemoral ligament.*
yoghurt (yŏg'hert). Curdled milk containing lactic acid.
  Acts as intestinal antiseptic; lessens fermentation. Useful in arthritis and cecal obstructions. It contains only 2 lactic ferments, *i. e.*, a streptococcus bacillus and a streptobacillus. Much used in Bulgaria. SEE: *milk.*
yolk (yōk) [M.E. *yolke*, from A.S. *geolca*]. The contents of the ovum; sometimes only the nutritive portion. SYN: *vitellus.** SEE: *zona pellucida, z. radiata.*
  y. cavity. One within a yolk.
  y. cells, y. granules. The granulations composing the yolk.
  y. sac. Membranous sac surrounding food yolk in the embryo.

Y-1

y. stalk. The umbilical duct connecting the yolk sac with the embryo.
y. of wool. Crude wool fat.
Young-Helmholtz theory (yŭng-hĕlm'hōlts). Belief that color vision depends on 3 different sets of retinal fibers responsible for perception of red, green, and violet.
The loss of either red, green, or violet as color perceptive elements in the retina causes an inability to perceive a primary color or any color of which it forms a part.
Young's rule (yŭng). A dose for children is arrived at by adding 12 to the age and dividing the result by the age, making the quotient the denominator of a fraction, the numerator of which is 1. The proportion of the adult dose to be given the child is represented by the fraction.
youth (yūth) [A.S. *geoguth*]. Period bet. childhood and maturity.
y. s. Abbr. for *yellow spot* of the retina.
ytterbium (ĭ-tur'bĭ-ŭm). A rare metallic element. SYMB: Yb. At. wt. 173.5.
yttrium (ĭt'rĭ-ŭm). A metallic element. SYMB: Y. At. wt. 88.92.
Yvon's coefficient (ē'vŏn). The ratio bet. the amount of urea and phosphates in the urine.
Y's. tests. One for presence of acetanilide and the other for alkaloids in urine.

Z

Zaglas' ligament (zah′glahz). The part of the post. sacroiliac ligament from post. sup. spinous process of ilium to side of sacrum.

Zahn's lines or ribs (zahn). Transverse whitish marks on the free surface of a thrombus made by the edges of the lamellae of blood platelets.

Zander apparatus (zan′der). Mechanical means for massage and exercise designed by Zander about 1857.

Zang's space (zang). One bet. the 2 lower tendons of the sternomastoid muscle in the supraclavicular fossa.

zaranthan (zar-an′than) [Hebrew]. Scirrhous hardening of the breast.

zein (zē′ĭn) [G. *zeia*, a kind of grain]. A protein obtained from maize. [lysine.
It is deficient in tryptophane and

zeismus (zē-ĭz′mŭs) [G. *zea*, a kind of grain]. Pellagra believed to be due to excessive diet of corn or corn products.

Zeiss' gland (zīs). One of the sebaceous glands at free edges of eyelids.

zeist (zē′ĭst). A person who believes that pellagra is the result of a diet of maize.

zelotypia (zē-lō-tĭp′ĭ-ă) [G. *zēlos*, zeal, + *typtein*, to strike]. 1. Morbid or monomaniacal zeal in the interest of any project or cause. 2. Insane jealousy.

Zenker's degeneration, zenkerism (zĕng′-kĕr, -ĭzm). A glassy or waxy, hyaline degeneration of skeletal muscles in acute infectious diseases, esp. in typhoid.

zeoscope (zē′ō-skōp) [G. *zein*, to boil, + *skopein*, to view]. Device for determining the alcoholic content of a liquid by means of its boiling point.

zero (zē′rō) [Italian *zero*, from Arabic *sifr*, a cipher]. 1. Figure corresponding to nothing. 2. The point from which the graduation of a scale commences.
On the centigrade and Réaumur scales the zero (0°) is the temperature of melting ice. On the Fahrenheit it is 32° lower. To obtain this fixed point the thermometer is immersed in melting ice, and when the mercury column ceases to fall, the level at which it remains is fixed as 0° on the C. and R. scales, and as 32° on the F. scale. SEE: *thermometer*.

zestocausis (zĕs″tō-kaw′sĭs) [G. *zestos*, boiling hot, + *kausis*, a burning]. Cauterization with heated steam.

Ziehl-Neelsen method. One for staining *B. tuberculosis*.

zinc (zĭnk) [L. *zincum*]. A bluish-white, crystalline, metallic element. SYMB: Zn. At. wt. 65.38. Sp. gr. 7-7.2. It boils at 930° C. (1706° F.). It is found as a carbonate and silicate, known as *calamine*, as a sulfide, and as a blende.
FUNCTION: Promotes normal growth and tissue respiration.
DEFICIENCY SYM: Retarded growth.
SOURCES: SEE: *names of foods*.

   z. ac′etate. USP. White, pearly crystals.
ACTION AND USES: Astringent and antiseptic. Used chiefly in eye solutions, in 1/10 to 5/10%. [powder.

   z. chlo′ride. USP. White granular
ACTION AND USES: Antiseptic, astringent, and escharotic.

   z. ointment. An ointment consisting of 20% of zinc oxide mixed with petrolatum or a lard base, used in treating skin diseases. [der.

   z. ox′ide. USP. Very fine white powACTION AND USES: Slightly antiseptic and astringent. Used chiefly in the form of ointment, 20%.
DOSAGE: 2-5 gr. (0.12-0.3 Gm.).

   z. salts. A bluish-white metal used to make various containers and also to "galvanize" iron to prevent rust. The most commonly used compounds are zinc oxide as a pigment for paints, in ointments, and in chloride and sulfate which resemble epsom salts and have thus been accidentally administered. The salts are used also as a wood preservative, in soldering, and in medicine to neutralize tissue, and in dilute solutions as an astringent and emetic.
POISONING: SYM: Metallic taste with prompt burning of mouth, throat, esophagus, and stomach; violent vomiting, often bloody; increased salivation; painful diarrhea, and coma. If patient recovers, nervous complications are frequent.
F. A. TREATMENT: Wash out stomach and treat as for sulfuric acid.

   z. stearate. USP. Very fine, smooth powder.
USES: A nonirritating antiseptic and astringent for burns, scalds, abrasions.

   z. sul′fate. USP. White, transparent crystals.
ACTION AND USES: Externally, astringent and styptic. Internally, as an emetic.
DOSAGE: As an emetic, 15 gr. (1 Gm.).

Zinn's ligament (zĭn). Connective tissue giving attachment to the rectus muscles of the eyeball.

   Z., zonule of. Suspensory ligament of lens of the eye. SYN: *zonula ciliaris*.

zirconium (zĭr-kō′nĭ-ŭm). A metallic element found only in combination. SYMB: Zr. At. wt. 91.22.

Zn. Chemical symb. for *zinc*.

zoanthropy (zō-ăn′thrō-pĭ) [G. *zōon*, animal, + *anthropos*, man]. Delusion that one is an animal.

zoetic (zō-ĕt′ĭk) [G. *zōē*, life]. Pert. to life. SYN: *vital*.

zoetrope (zō′e-trōp) [" + *tropos*, turning]. Instrument in which pictures of objects viewed are apparently moving.

zomidin (zō′mĭd-ĭn) [G. *zōmos*, broth]. A component of meat extract.

zomotherapy (zō″mō-ther′ă-pĭ) [" + *therapeia*, treatment]. Therapeutic administration of a meat diet or meat juice.

zona (zō′nă) [L. *zona*, a girdle]. 1. A band or girdle. 2. An acute inflammatory disease, characterized by groups of small vesicles mounted on inflammatory bases, associated with neuralgic pain and following the distribution of certain nerve trunks. SYN: *herpes zoster*.
Commonly depends on a peripheral neuritis. Injury, exposure to cold and damp clothes predispose to it.
SYM: Clusters of vesicles appear on any part of body, but are most frequently observed along the course of the intercostal nerves. Sharp neuralgic pain precedes and accompanies the eruption. The fluid in the vesicles soon becomes

turbid, dries up, and forms yellowish-brown crusts which fall off in a few days.
PROG: Favorable.
TREATMENT: Constitutional. Build up whole system. Good hygiene. Nourishing food.
   z. **ciliaris.** Ciliary processes taken together. SYN: *corona ciliaris.*
   z. **facia′lis.** Herpes zoster of the face.
   z. **granulo′sa.** A layer of cells lining the graafian follicle from which the corpus luteum develops.
   z. **pellucida.** Inner, thick, solid, membranous envelope of the ovum.
   It is pierced by many radiating canals, giving it a striated appearance.
   z. **radiata.** SEE: *zona pellucida.*
zonal (zō′năl) [L. *zona,* girdle]. Pert. to a zone.
   z. **stratum.** A layer of white fibrous layers on the ventricular surface of the thalamus.
zonary (zō′nar-ĭ) [L. *zona,* a girdle]. Pert. to or shaped like a zone.
   z. **placenta.** One arranged in the form of a broad ring around the chorion.
Zondek-Aschheim test (zŏn′dĕk ahsh′hīm). A test for pregnancy. SEE: *test, Aschheim-Zondek.*
zone (zōn) [L. *zona,* a girdle]. A small zone or belt.
   z′s., erotogenic. Areas of the body which when stimulated produce erotic desires.
   These areas include the breasts, lips, genital and anal regions, the buttocks, and sometimes the special senses which excite the libido, such as the smell of certain perfumes.
   z. **therapy.** Therapeutic stimulation of a part, mechanically, in the same longitudinal zone as the diseased area.
   z. **of Zinn.** Suspensory ligament of crystalline lens of eye.
zonesthesia (zŏn-ĕs-thē′zĭ-ă) [G. *zōnē,* girdle, + *aisthēsis,* sensation]. A sensation, as of a cord constricting the body. SYN: *cincture sensation.*
zonifugal (zō-nĭf′ŭ-găl) [L. *zona,* a band, + *fugere,* to flee]. Passing outward from within any zone or area.
zoning (zō′nĭng) [L. *zona,* a band]. The occurrence of a stronger fixation of complement in a lesser amount of suspected serum; a phenomenon occasionally observed in diagnosing syphilis by complement fixation method.
zonipetal (zō-nĭp′ĕt-ăl) [L. *zona,* a band, + *petere,* to seek]. Passing from without into a zone or area of the body.
zonula (zŏn′ū-lă) [L. *zonula,* a tiny zone]. A small zone. SYN: *zonule.*
   z. **ciliaris.** BNA. Suspensory ligament of the crystalline lens.
zonular (zŏn′ū-lar) [L. *zonula,* a tiny band]. Pert. to a zonula.
   z. **cataract.** One with opacity limited to certain layers of the lens.
   z. **fibers.** Interlacing ones of the zonula ciliaris.
   z. **spaces.** Those bet. fibers of ligament of the lens.
zonule (zŏn′ūl) [L. *zonula,* a tiny band]. A small band or area. SYN: *zonula.*
   z. **of Zinn.** Suspensory ligament of the crystalline lens. SYN: *zonula ciliaris.*
zonulitis (zŏn-ū-lī′tĭs) [″ + G. -*itis,* inflammation]. Inflammation of Zinn's zonule.
zoöbiology (zō″ō-bī-ŏl′ō-jĭ) [G. *zōon,* animal, + *bios,* life, + *logos,* study]. The study of animal life.
zoöchemistry (zō″ō-kĕm′ĭs-trĭ) [″ + *chēmeia,* chemistry]. Chemistry of solids and fluids in animal tissues.

zoödermic (zō″ō-der′mĭk) [″ + *derma,* skin]. Performed with the skin of an animal, said of a method of skin grafting.
zoödynamics (zō″ō-dī-năm′ĭks) [″ + *dynamis,* power]. Science dealing with the vital powers of animals.
zoögenous (zō-ŏj′ĕn-ŭs) [″ + *gennan,* to produce]. Derived or acquired from animals.
zoögeny, zoögony (zō-ŏj′ĕn-ĭ, -ŏn-ĭ) [″ + *gennan,* to produce, — + *gonē,* offspring]. The generation of animals.
zoöglea (zō″ō-glē′ă) [″ + *gloios,* sticky]. A stage in development of certain organisms in which colonies of microbes are embedded in a gelatinous matrix.
zoögraft (zō′ō-grăft) [G. *zōon,* animal, + L. *graphium,* a grafting knife]. A graft of tissue obtained from an animal.
zoögrafting (zō″ō-grăft′ĭng) [″ + L. *graphium,* a grafting knife]. Use of animal tissue in grafting on a human body.
zoöid (zō′oyd) [″ + *eidos,* resemblance]. 1. Resembling an animal. 2. A form resembling an animal; an organism produced by fission. 3. An animal cell which can move or exist independently.
zoölogy (zō-ŏl′ō-jĭ) [″ + *logos,* a study]. The science of animal life.
zoönomy (zō-ŏn′ō-mĭ) [″ + *nomos,* law]. Laws of animal life. SYN: *zoöbiology.*
zoönosis (zō-ŏn′ō-sĭs) [″ + *nosos,* disease]. Any disease acquired from an animal or an animal parasite.
zoöparasite (zō″ō-par′ă-sīt) [″ + *parasitos,* parasite]. An animal parasite.
zoöpathology (zō″ō-păth-ŏl′ō-jĭ) [G. *zōon,* animal, + *pathos,* disease, + *logos,* a study]. Science of the diseases of animals.
zoöphagous (zō-ŏf′ăg-ŭs) [″ + *phagein,* to eat]. Living upon animal food.
zoöphilism (zō-ŏf′ĭl-ĭzm) [″ + *philein,* to love, + -*ismos,* condition]. Abnormal love of animals.
zoöphobia (zō″o-fō′bĭ-ă) [″ + *phobos,* fear]. Abnormal fear of animals.
zoöphyte (zō′ō-fīt) [″ + *phyton,* plant]. A plantlike animal; any of numerous invertebrate animals resembling plants in appearance or mode of growth.
zoöplasty (zō″ō-plăs-tĭ) [″ + *plassein,* to form]. Transplantation of animal tissue to man.
zoöprecipitin (zō″ō-prē-sĭp′ĭ-tĭn) [″ + L. *praecipitāre,* to cast down]. A precipitin formed from repeated animal protein injections.
zoöpsychology (zō″ō-sī-kŏl′ō-jĭ) [G. *zōon,* animal, + *psychē,* soul, + *logos,* study]. Psychology of animals.
zoösis (zō-ō′sĭs) [″ + -*osis,* disease]. Any disease caused by animal agents, as a parasite. SYN: *zoönosis.*
zoösmosis (zō″ōz-mō′sĭs) [″ + *osmos,* impulsion]. Process of passage of living protoplasm into the tissues from blood vessels.
zoösperm (zō′ō-sperm) [″ + *sperma,* seed]. Mature male germ cell. SYN: *spermatozoon, q.v.*
zoöspore (zō′ō-spōr) [″ + *sporos,* seed]. Any spore moving by means of flagella.
zoötomy (zō-ŏt′ō-mĭ) [″ + *tomē,* a cutting]. Science dealing with the anatomy of the lower animals.
zoötoxin (zō″ō-tŏks′ĭn) [″ + *toxikon,* poison]. Any toxin or poison produced by an animal, as *snake venom.*
zoster (zŏs′ter) [G. *zōstēr,* girdle]. Acute inflammatory disease with vesicles

grouped in the course of cutaneous nerves. SYN: *herpes zoster, zona.*
z. auricula'ris. Herpes zoster of the ear.
z. ophthal'micus. Herpes affecting the ophthalmic nerve.
zosteriform (zŏs-tĕr'ĭ-form) [" + L. *forma*, shape]. Resembling herpes zoster. SYN: *zosteroid.*
zosteroid (zŏs'ter-oyd) [" + *eidos*, form]. Resembling herpes zoster. SYN: *zosteriform.*
zwieback (swī'băk). Av. SERVING: 5 Gm. Pro. 0.5, Fat 0.5, Carbo. 3.7.
zygal (zī'găl) [G. *zygon*, yoke]. Yoked.
z. fissure. A cerebral fissure consisting of 2 pairs of branches connected by a stem.
zygapophysis (zī-găp-ŏf'ĭs-ĭs) [" + *apo*, from, + *physis*, growth]. One of the articular processes of the neural arch of a vertebra.
zygion (zĭj'ĭ-ŏn) [G. *zygon*, yoke]. Craniometrical point on the zygoma at either end of bizygomatic diameter.
zygocyte (zī'gō-sīt) [G. *zygon*, a yoke, + *kytos*, cell]. A cell formed by the union of 2 gametes. SYN: *zygote.*
zygodactyly (zī'gō-dăk'tĭl-ĭ) [" + *daktylos*, digit]. Fusion of 2 or more fingers or toes. SYN: *syndactylism.*
zygolabialis (zī"gō-lă-bĭ-ā'lĭs) [L.]. The zygomaticus minor muscle. SEE: *Table of Muscles in Appendix.*

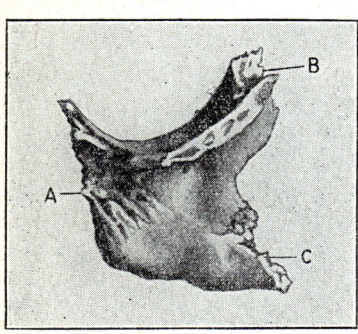

ZYGOMA
A. Maxillary process. B. Frontal process. C. Zygomatic process.

zygoma (zī-gō'mă) [G. *zygōma*, cheekbone]. 1. BNA. The long arch that joins zygomatic processes of the temporal and malar bones on the sides of the skull. 2. The malar bone.
zygomatic (zī"gō-măt'ĭk) [G. *zygōma*, cheekbone]. Pert. to the zygoma.
z. arch. The formation on each side of the cheeks of the zygomatic process of each malar bone articulating with the zygomatic process of the temporal bone.
z. bone. Bone on either side of the face below the eye. SYN: *malar bone.*
z. process. 1. A thin projection from the temporal bone bounding its squamous portion. 2. A part of the malar bone helping to form the zygoma.
z. reflex. Movement of lower jaw toward percussed side when zygoma is percussed.
zygomaticoauricularis (zī"gō-măt"ĭk-ō-aw-rĭk"ū-lā'rĭs) [L.]. Muscle which draws the pinna of the ear forward. SEE: *Table of Muscles in Appendix.*
zygomaticum (zī"gō-măt'ĭk-ŭm) [L.]. The zygomatic bone.
zygomaticus (zī-gō-mat'ĭk-ŭs) [L.]. A muscle which draws the upper lip upward and outward. SEE: *Table of Muscles in Appendix.*
zygomaxillary (zī"gō-măks'ĭl-ar-ĭ) [G. *zygoma*, cheekbone, + L. *maxilla*, jaw]. Pert. to the cheekbone and upper jaw.
z. point. A craniometrical point marked at the lower end of the zygomatic suture.
zygon (zī'gŏn) [G. *zygon*, yoke]. The bar connecting the 2 pairs of branches of a zygal fissure in the cerebrum.
zygoneure (zī'gō-nŭr) [" + *neuron*, nerve]. A nerve cell connecting other nerve cells.
zygosis (zī-gō'sĭs) [" + *-ōsis*, condition]. Fusion of the nuclei of 2 unicellular organisms in sexual union.
zygote (zī'gōt) [G. *zygōtos*, yoked]. Cell produced by union of 2 gametes. SYN: *zygocyte.*
zygotoblast (zī-gō'tō-blăst) [" + *blastos*, a germ]. Any germ originating within a zygote.
zymase (zī'mās) [G. *zymē*, leaven, + *ase*, enzyme]. Any of a group of enzymes* which, in the presence of oxygen, convert certain carbohydrates into carbon dioxide and water or, in absence of oxygen, into alcohol and carbon dioxide or lactic acid.
They are found in yeast, bacteria, and higher plants and animals. SEE: *ferment.*
zyme (zīm) [G. *zymē*, leaven]. A ferment; a disease-producing ferment, as the morbific principle of a zymotic disease.
zymic (zī'mĭk) [G. *zymē*, leaven]. 1. Pert. to or due to fermentation or a ferment. 2. Denoting an anaerobic microörganism.
zymin (zī'mĭn) [G. *zymē*, leaven]. 1. A pancreatic preparation. 2. A ferment. SYN: *zyme.*
zymocyte (zī'mō-sīt) [" + *kytos*, cell]. An organism causing fermentation.
zymogen (zī'mō-jĕn) [" + *gennan*, to produce]. 1. A substance that develops into a chemical ferment or enzyme.
It exists in an inactive form antecedent to the active enzyme. SYN: *proenzyme.* SEE: *pepsinogen, trypsinogen.* 2. A bacterium which produces or is converted into an enzyme.
zymogene (zī'mō-gēn) [" + *gennan*, to produce]. Microbe causing fermentation.
zymogenic (zī-mō-jĕn'ĭk) [" + *gennan*, to produce]. 1. Causing a fermentation. 2. Pert. to or producing a zymogen.
zymohydrolysis (zī"mō-hī-drŏl'ĭ-sĭs) [" + *hydōr*, water, + *lysis*, dissolution]. Decomposition brought about by a ferment. SYN: *zymosis.**
zymoid (zī'moyd) [" + *eidos*, resemblance]. 1. Resembling an enzyme or ferment. 2. An enzyme that can unite with the substratum, but not decompose it.
zymologic (zī-mō-lŏj'ĭk) [G. *zymē*, leaven, + *logos*, a study]. Relating to zymology.
zymologist (zī-mŏl'ō-jĭst) [" + *logos*, a study]. One who specializes in study of ferments.
zymology (zī-mŏl'ō-jī) [" + *logos*, a study]. The science of fermentation.
zymolysis (zī-mŏl'ĭ-sĭs) [" + *lysis*, a dissolution]. Changes produced by an enzyme; action of enzymes. SYN: *fermentation, zymosis.**
zymolyte (zī'mō-līt) [" + *lysis*, dissolution]. Substance upon which a ferment acts. SYN: *substrate.*

zymolytic (zī-mō-lĭt′ĭk) [" + *lytikos*, dissolved]. Causing fermentation; fermentative.

zymoma (zī-mō′mă) [G. *zymoein*, to cause to ferment]. Any ferment.

zymometer (zī-mŏm′et-er) [G. *zymē*, leaven, + *metron*, a measure]. Device for measuring fermentation. SYN: *zymosimeter*.

Zymonema (zī-mō-nē′mă) [" + *nēma*, thread]. A genus of fungi.

zymonematosis (zī″mō-nē-măt-ō′sĭs) [" + " + *-osis*, condition]. Infestation with Zymonema. SYN: *blastomycosis*.

zymophore (zī′mō-fōr) [" + *phoros*, a bearer]. Noting the atomic group bearing the ferment.

zymophoric, zymophorous (zī-mō-fōr′ĭk, -mŏf′or-ŭs) [" + *phoros*, bearing]. Having fermentative properties.

zymophyte (zī′mō-fīt) [" + *phyton*, growth]. A microörganism causing fermentation.

zymoplastic (zī-mō-plăs′tĭk) [G. *zymē*, leaven, + *plassein*, to form]. Producing a ferment.

zymoscope (zī′mō-skōp) [" + *skopein*, to examine]. Device for determining zymotic power of yeast.

zymose (zī′mōs) [" + *ose*, sugar]. An enzyme that changes a disaccharide into a monosaccharide, such as cane sugar into invert sugar. SYN: *invertin*.

zymosimeter (zī-mōs-ĭm′ĕt-ĕr) [" + *metron*, a measure]. Device for determining amount of fermentation.

zymosis (zī-mō′sĭs) [G. *zymōsis*, fermentation]. 1. Fermentation. 2. Process by which an infectious disease is supposed to develop. 3. An infectious disease.

   z. gas′trica. Organic acid in the stomach.

zymosthenic (zī-mŏs-thĕn′ĭk) [G. *zymē*, leaven, + *sthenos*, strength]. Increasing the power and activity of an enzyme.

zymotic (zī-mŏt′ĭk) [G. *zymē*, leaven]. Relating to or produced by fermentation.

   z. disease. Any epidemic, endemic, or contagious disease capable of being induced or produced by some morbific agent or element incident to process or condition of fermentation.

   z. papilloma. Contagious skin disease characterized by reddish sores on the face and hands, feet and ext. genitals. SYN: *yaws*.

   z. principle. A specific matter or element that of itself propagates a zymotic disease, as the zymotic principle of smallpox or syphilis.

   z. theory. The hypothesis that a poisonous particle, either atmospheric or communicated by contact, acts as a ferment to produce certain diseases.

Appendix

Appendix

Index to Appendix

Abbreviations, medical	App. 14-15
Anatomical and physiological emergencies	App. 89-116
Anatomy and physiology	App. 33-76
Apothecaries' weight	App. 6
Arteries, table of	App. 58-63
Avoirdupois weight	App. 6
Blood, physiological standards	App. 11
Calorie portion tables	App. 78-84
Cerebrospinal fluid, physiological standards	App. 11
Circular measure	App. 6
Conversion tables, metric system	App. 4
Convulsions	App. 90-91
Cranial nerves	App. 53-57
Cubic measure	App. 6
Dietetics	App. 77-88
Dislocations	App. 92-94
Dry measure	App. 6
Elements, physical constants	App. 9-10
Emergencies, physiological	App. 89-116
Energy, units of	App. 8
Equivalents, English, Latin and Greek	App. 24-27
Equivalents, measures and weights	App. 7
Food tables	App. 78-84
Fractures	App. 95-96
Greek and Latin singulars and plurals	App. 28
Household measures and weights	App. 7
Joints	App. 44
Latin and Greek nomenclature	App. 16-31
Latin and Greek singulars and plurals	App. 28
Latin medical words	App. 16-22
Latin numerals	App. 29
Liquid measure	App. 6
Long measure	App. 6
Medical abbreviations	App. 14-15
Metric system	App. 4-5
Muscles of the body	App. 34-43
Nerve plexuses	App. 51-52
Nerves, cranial	App. 53-57
Nerves, table of	App. 45-50
Numerals, Latin	App. 29
Nutrients, daily allowance	App. 85
pH, table of	App. 8
Physical constants of the elements	App. 9-10
Physiological emergencies	App. 89-116
Physiological standards	App. 11
Plexuses, nerve	App. 51-52
Poisons and poisoning	App. 97-110
Prefixes and suffixes	App. 30-31
Singulars and plurals, Greek and Latin	App. 28
Solutions, percentage	App. 8
Suffocations	App. 111
Symbols	App. 12
Temperature, units of	App. 8
Time, units of	App. 8
Troy weight	App. 6
Unconsciousness	App. 112-114
Veins	App. 64-76
Vitamin tables	App. 86-88
Weights and measures	App. 6
Wounds	App. 115-116

Units of Measurement

Metric System

Scale	Table		Grams		Grains
Myria.	1 Myriagram	=	10,000	=	154,323.5
Kilo.	1 Kilogram	=	1,000.	=	15,432.35
Hecto.	1 Hectogram	=	100.	=	1,543.23
Deca.	1 Decagram	=	10.	=	154.323
Unit.	1 Gram	=	1.	=	15.432
Deci.	1 Decigram	=	.1	=	1.5432
Centi.	1 Centigram	=	.01	=	.15432
Milli.	1 Milligram	=	.001	=	.01543

The Arabic numerals are used with the symbol after the quantity, as 10 Gm., or 3 ml., etc. Portions of a measure are always expressed decimally. Grams should always be abbreviated with a capital initial, as Gm. A drop (gtt) of water is sometimes considered equivalent to a minim (m) but should not be used without physician's instructions.

CONVERSION TABLES (for measures most commonly used in the United States)

Lengths	Cm.	Inches	Feet	Yards	Meters
1 centimeter.	1.000	0.394	0.0328	0.01094	0.0100
1 inch.	2.54	1.000	0.0833	0.0278	0.0254
1 foot.	30.48	12.00	1.000	0.333	0.305
1 yard.	91.4	36.00	3.000	1.000	0.914
1 meter.	100.0	39.4	3.28	1.094	1.000
1 kilometer.	100000.	39400.	3280.	1094.	1000.
1 mile.	160903.	63360.	5280.	1760.	1609.

Volumes	Cc.	Fl. drams	Cu. in.	Fl. oz.	Quarts	Liters
1 cubic centimeter.	1.000	0.270	0.0610	0.0338	0.001057	0.001000
1 fluid dram.	3.70	1.000	0.226	0.1250	0.00391	0.00370
1 cubic inch.	16.39	4.43	1.000	0.554	0.0173	0.01639
1 fluid ounce.	29.6	8.00	1.804	1.000	0.03125	0.0296
1 quart.	946.	255.	57.75	32.0	1.000	0.946
1 liter.	1000.	270.	61.0	33.8	1.056	1.000

Weights	Gr.	Gm.	Ap. oz.	Lb.	Kilos
1 grain (gr.).	1.000	0.0648	0.00208	0.0001429	0.0000648
1 gram (Gm.).	15.43	1.000	0.03215	0.002205	0.001000
1 apothecary ounce.	480.	31.1	1.000	0.06855	0.0311
1 avoirdupois pound.	7000.	454.	14.58	1.000	0.454
1 kilogram.	15432.	1000.	32.15	2.205	1.000

RULES FOR CONVERTING ONE SYSTEM TO ANOTHER

To Convert Grains, Drams, and Ounces into Grams or CC.:

Divide the number of grains by 15.
Multiply the number of drams by 4.
Multiply the number of ounces by 30.
The result = the number of grams or cc.

To Convert from the Metric System

Milligrams to grains: Multiply by 0.0154.
Grams to grains: Multiply by 15.
Grams to drams: Multiply by 0.257.
Grams to ounces: Multiply by 0.0311.

To Convert into Metric Fluid Measures

Minims to cubic millimeters: Multiply by 63.
Minims to cubic centimeters: Multiply by 0.06.

To Convert Metric Fluid Measures

Cubic millimeters to minims: Divide by 63 (or multiply by 0.016).
Cubic centimeters to minims: Multiply by 16.
Cubic centimeters to fluid ounces: Divide by 30 (or multiply by 0.033).
Liters to pints (U.S.): Multiply by 2.1.
Liters to pints (Imperial): Multiply by 1.76.

To Convert Centigrade Degrees to Fahrenheit Degrees

Multiply the number of centigrade degrees by 9/5 and add 32 to the result.
Example: 55°C. × 9/5 = 99 + 32 = 131° F.

To convert Fahrenheit degrees to centigrade degrees: Subtract 32 from the number of centigrade degrees and multiply the difference by 5/9.
Example: 243° F. − 32 = 211 × 5/9 = 117.2°

TABLES OF DATA

The Arabic numerals are used with the symbol after the quantity, as 10 Gm., or 3 ml., etc. Portions of a measure are always expressed decimally. Grams should always be abbreviated with a capital initial, as Gm. A drop (gtt) of water is sometimes considered equivalent to a minim (m) but should not be used without physician's instructions.

UNITS OF LENGTH

	Millimeters	Centimeters	Inches	Feet	Yards	Meters
1 mm. =	1.00	0.100	0.0394	0.00328	0.0011	0.0010
1 cm. =	10.0	1.00	0.394	0.0328	0.0109	0.0100
1 in. =	25.4	2.54	1.00	0.0833	0.0278	0.0254
1 ft. =	304.8	30.48	12.00	1.00	0.333	0.305
1 yd. =	914.	91.4	36.0	3.00	1.000	0.914
1 m. =	1000.	100.	39.4	3.28	1.094	1.00

1μ = 1 mu = 1 micron = 0.001 millimeter. One mm. = 1000 μ.
1 km. = 1 kilometer = 1000 meters = 0.6215 mile.
1 mile = 5280 feet = 1.609 kilometers.

UNITS OF VOLUME

	Cubic Centimeters	Fluid Drams	Cubic Inches	Fluid Ounces	Quarts	Liters
1 cc. =	1.00	0.270	0.0610	0.0338	0.00106	0.00100
1 fl. ʒ =	3.70	1.000	0.226	0.1250	0.00391	0.00370
1 cu. in. =	16.39	4.43	1.000	0.554	0.0173	0.01639
1 fl. ℥ =	29.6	8.00	1.804	1.000	0.03125	0.0296
1 qt. =	946.	255.	57.75	32.00	1.000	0.946
1 L. =	1000.	270.	61.0	33.8	1.056	1.000

1 cubic millimeter = 0.001 cubic centimeter; 1 cc. = 1000 cu. mm.
1 gallon = 4 quarts = 8 pints = 3.78 liters.
1 pint = 473 cc.

UNITS OF WEIGHT

	Grains	Grams	Apothecary Ounces	Pounds Avoirdupois	Kilograms
1 gr. =	1.000	0.0648	0.00208	0.0001429	0.000065
1 Gm. =	15.43	1.000	0.03215	0.002205	0.001000
1 ℥ =	480.	31.1	1.000	0.06855	0.0311
1 lb. =	7000.	454.	14.58	1.000	0.454
1 Kg. =	15432.	1000.	32.15	2.205	1.000

1γ = 1 gamma = 1 microgram = 0.001 milligram; 1000 γ = 1 mg.
1 mg. = 1 milligram = 0.001 Gm.; 1000 mg. = 1 Gm.
1 grain = 64.8 mg.; 1 mg. = 0.0154 grain.

Weights and Measures

ENGLISH

APOTHECARIES' WEIGHT

20 grains = 1 scruple
8 drams = 1 ounce
3 scruples = 1 dram
12 ounces = 1 pound

The ounce and pound in this are the same as in Troy Weight.

AVOIRDUPOIS WEIGHT

$27\frac{11}{32}$ grains = 1 dram
16 ounces = 1 pound
2000 pounds = 1 short ton
1 oz. Troy = 480 gr.
1 lb. Troy = 5760 grains
16 drams = 1 ounce
100 pounds = 1 cwt.
2240 pounds = 1 long ton
1 oz. Avoirdupois = $437\frac{1}{2}$ grains
1 lb. Avoirdupois = 7000 grains

CIRCULAR MEASURE

60 seconds = 1 minute
30 degrees = 1 sign
60 minutes = 1 degree
90 degrees = 1 quadrant

4 quadrants = 12 signs, or 360 degrees = circle

CUBIC MEASURE

1728 cubic inches = 1 cubic foot
2150.42 cubic inches = 1 standard bushel
1 cubic foot = about four-fifths of a bushel
27 cubic feet = 1 cubic yard
231 cubic inches = 1 standard gallon
128 cubic feet = 1 cord (wood)

40 cubic feet = 1 ton

DRY MEASURE

2 pints = 1 quart   8 quarts = 1 peck   4 pecks = 1 bushel

LIQUID MEASURE

4 gills = 1 pint
4 quarts = 1 gallon
$31\frac{1}{2}$ gallons = 1 barrel
2 pints = 1 quart
2 barrels = 1 hogshead

Barrels and hogsheads vary in size.

LONG MEASURE

12 inches = 1 foot
40 rods = 1 furlong
3 feet = 1 yard
8 furlongs = 1 stat. mile
$5\frac{1}{2}$ yards = 1 rod
3 miles = 1 league

TROY WEIGHT

24 grains = 1 pwt.   20 pwts. = 1 ounce   12 ounces = 1 pound

Used for weighing gold, silver, and jewels.

App. 6

MEASURES AND WEIGHTS EQUIVALENTS

General Measures: Approximate Equivalents: 60 gtt. = 1 teaspoonful. = 4 cc. or ml. = 60 minims, = 60 grains. = 1 dram. = ⅛ ounce.

RS: avoirdupois m., apothecaries m., bushel, metric m., Troy weight, unit of measures.

HOUSEHOLD MEASURES AND WEIGHTS

1 teaspoon equals	⅛ fl. oz. or 1 dr.
4 teaspoons equal	1 tablespoon
1 dessertspoon equals	⅓ fl. oz. or 2⅔ dr.
1 tablespoon equals	½ fl. oz or 4 dr.
4 tablespoons equal	½ gill or 1 wineglass
16 tablespoons (liquid) equal	1 cup
12 tablespoons (dry) equal	1 cup
1 cup (ordinary) equals	8 fl. oz.
1 tumbler or glass equals	8 fl. oz. or ½ pt.
1 wineglass equals	2 fl. oz.
16 fl. oz. equal	1 lb.
4 gills equal	1 lb.
1 pint equals	1 lb.

ARTICLES

Butter—1 pint, packed equals............1 lb.
    piece, size of an egg, equals............2 oz.
    2 cups, packed, equal............1 lb.
    1 tablespoon equals............½ oz.
Chocolate—1 square equals............1 oz.
Coffee—4⅓ cups equal............1 lb.
Cornmeal—2⅔ cups equal............1 lb.
Eggs (large)—9 equal............1 lb.
Flour—1 quart equals............1 lb.
    4 cups equal............1 lb. or 1 qt.
    4 tablespoons equal............1 oz.
    Graham—4½ cups equal............1 lb.
    entire wheat—3⅞ cups equal............1 lb.
    pastry—4 cups equal............1 lb.
Meat—Fine chopped, 2 cups equal............1 lb.
Oatmeal—2⅔ cups equal............1 lb.
Oats, Rolled—4¾ cups equal............1 lb.
Rice—1⅞ cups equal............1 lb.
Rye, Meal—4⅓ cups equal............1 lb.
Sugar, brown—2⅔ cups equal............1 lb.
    1 quart equals............1 lb. 10 oz.
    confectioner's—3½ cups equal............1 lb.
    granulated—2 cups equal............1 lb.
    1 quart equals............1 lb. 9 oz.
    powdered—2⅔ cups equal............1 lb.
    1 quart equals............1 lb. 7 oz.
    coffee "A"—1 quart equals............1 lb. 8 oz.
Water—1 pint equals............1 lb.
    1 cup equals............8 oz.

Miscellaneous

UNITS OF TIME

1 σ = 1 sigma = 0.001 second; 1000 σ = 1 second.

UNITS OF TEMPERATURE

Given a temperature on the Fahrenheit scale; to convert it to Centigrade, subtract 32 and multiply by 5/9. Given a temperature on the Centigrade scale; to convert it to Fahrenheit, multiply by 9/5 and add 32.

UNITS OF ENERGY

1 gram-centimeter = 981 ergs.
1 foot-pound = 13,600,000 ergs = 13,800 gram-centimeters.
1 Calorie = 42,600,000 gram-centimeters = 3080 foot-pounds.

TABLE OF pH

In trying to understand the following pH table, one need not be concerned about the intricate mathematical *theory* implied in the symbol "*p*H." If one concerns oneself with the *facts* one will find them simple and satisfying. One need only imagine oneself confronted with three beakers containing (*a*) a weakly acid solution, (*b*) pure water, (*c*) a weakly alkaline solution. If now one is given a fourth, unknown, solution and tests it with litmus paper, phenolphthalein, and other indicators, one finds it possible to place the unknown in one of four places in the series, thus:

(1)	Un	Ac		W	—	Al
(2)		Ac	Un	W	—	Al
(3)		Ac	—	W	Un	Al
(4)		Ac	—	W	—	Al	Un

Its position will depend on whether it is (1) strongly acid, (2) weakly acid, (3) weakly alkaline, or (4) strongly alkaline.

Now the *p*H scale is simply a series of numbers by which one states where a given solution would stand in a series of solutions arranged according to acidity (or alkalinity). At one extreme lies an alkaline solution made by dissolving 4 Gm. of sodium hydroxide in water to make a liter of solution; at the other is a solution containing 3.65 Gm. of hydrogen chloride per liter. Half-way between lies pure water, which is neutral. All other solutions can be arranged on this scale, and their acidity or alkalinity can be stated by giving the numbers that indicate their relative positions.

Tenth-normal HCl	1.00
Gastric juice	*1.4	Litmus is red in this range
Urine	*6.0
Water	7.00
Blood	7.45
Bile	7.5	Litmus is blue in this range.
Pancreatic juice	8.5
Tenth-normal NaOH	13.00

Thus if one is told that the *p*H of a certain solution is 5.3, one can tell at once that it falls between gastric juice and urine on the above scale, is moderately acid, and will turn litmus red. The body fluids marked by asterisks above vary rather widely in *p*H, and typical figures have been used for the sake of definiteness. Urine samples obtained from normal people may have *p*H's anywhere between 4.8 and 7.5.

PREPARATION OF PERCENTAGE SOLUTIONS

When the metric system is used the preparation of percentage solutions is simple: a 1 per cent solution contains 1 Gm. in 100 cc.; a 0.1 per cent solution contains 0.1 Gm. (or 100 milligrams) per 100 cc.

When the apothecaries' system is used the following are helpful:

4.6 grains to the ounce, or 2.5 drams to 32 ounces; or 3.25 drams to 40 ounces, all make a 1 per cent solution.

To Prepare a Dilute Solution From One Which Is Stronger:

E. g. To make 80 per cent alcohol from 95 per cent: Dilute 80 cc. of the 95 per cent alcohol to 95 cc. with distilled water.

Rule: Dilute a volume equal to the per cent desired to a volume equal to the per cent used.

SEE: *Dosage*, in vocabulary.

Table of Physical Constants of the Elements

Element	Symbol	Valence	Atomic Number	Atomic Weight	Specific Gravity or Density	Melting Point °C	Boiling Point °C
Actinium	Ac	3	89	227			
Aluminum	Al	3	13	26.97	2.70	658.7	1800.0
Americium	Am		95	241			
Antimony	Sb	3, 5	51	121.76	6.68	630.0	1635.0±8°
Argon	A	0	18	39.944	1.782	−189.2	−185.7
Arsenic	As	3, 5	33	74.91	5.73	500.0*	615.0
Astatine	At	1, 3, 5, 7	85	210			
Barium	Ba	2	56	137.36	3.5	850.0	1140.0
Berkelium	Bk		97	243 (?)			
Beryllium	Be, Gl	2	4	9.02	1.85	1350.0	1530.0
Bismuth	Bi	3, 5	83	209.00	9.78	271.0	1450.0
Boron	B	3	5	10.82	2.5	2000.0	2550.0*
Bromine	Br	1, 3, 5, 7	35	79.916	3.12	−7.2	58.8
Cadmium	Cd	2	48	112.41	8.65	320.9	778.0
Calcium	Ca	2	20	40.08	1.54	810.0	1439.0±5°
Californium	Cf		98	244 (?)			
Carbon	C	2, 3, 4	6	12.01	1.88–3.5	3500.0*	4200.0
Cerium	Ce	3, 4	58	140.13	6.90	640.0	1400.0
Cesium	Cs	1	55	132.91	1.87	28.5	670.0
Chlorine	Cl	1, 3, 5, 7	17	35.457	1.56	−101.6	−34.6
Chromium	Cr	2, 3, 6	24	52.01	7.1	1615.0	2200.0
Cobalt	Co	2, 3	27	58.94	8.9	1480.0	2900.0
Columbium	Cb, Nb	3, 5	41	92.91	8.4	1950.0	3300.0
Copper	Cu	1, 2	29	63.57	8.93–8.95	1083.0	2310.0
Curium	Cm	3	96	242			
Dysprosium	Dy	3	66	162.46			
Erbium	Er	3	68	167.2	4.77(?)		
Europium	Eu	2, 3	63	152.0		1100–1200	
Fluorine	F	1	9	19.00	1.11	−223.0	−187.0
Francium	Fa		87	224			
Gadolinium	Gd	3	64	156.9			
Gallium	Ga	2, 3	31	69.72	5.91	29.75	2000±150°
Germanium	Ge	4	32	72.60	5.36	958.0	2700 volatilizes
Gold	Au	1, 3	79	197.2	19.32	1063.0	2600.0
Hafnium	Hf	4	72	178.6	13.3	2207.0	3200.0
Helium	He	0	2	4.003	0.177	−272.2	−268.9
Holmium	Ho	3	67	163.5			
Hydrogen	H	1	1	1.0081	0.07	−259.0	−252.8
Illinium	Il	3(?)	61	146 (?)			
Indium	In	3	49	114.76	7.28	155.0	1450.0
Iodine	I	1, 3, 5, 7	53	126.92	4.93	113.5	183.0
Iridium	Ir	3, 4	77	193.1	22.42	2440±15° C.	4400.0
Iron	Fe	2, 3	26	55.84	7.865	1535.0	3000.0
Krypton	Kr	0	36	83.7	3.708	−157.0	−152.9
Lanthanum	La	3	57	138.92	6.15	885±5° C.	1800.0
Lead	Pb	2, 4	82	207.21	11.35	327.5	1620.0
Lithium	Li	1	3	6.94	0.534	186.0	1336.0
Lutecium	Lu	3	71	175.0			
Magnesium	Mg	2	12	24.32	1.74	651.0	1110.0
Manganese	Mn	2, 3, 4, 6, 7	25	54.93	7.2	1260.0	1900.0
Mercury	Hg	1, 2	80	200.61	13.595	−38.89	356.9
Molybdenum	Mo	3, 4, 6	42	95.95	10.2	2620.0	3700.0
Neodymium	Nd	3	60	144.27	6.95	840.0	
Neon	Ne	0	10	20.183	0.9002	−248.67	−245.9
Neptunium	Np	3, 4, 5, 6	93	237			
Nickel	Ni	2, 3	28	58.69	8.90	1452.0	2900.0
Nitrogen	N	3, 5	7	14.008	0.808	−209.9	−195.8
Osmium	Os	2, 3, 4, 8	76	190.2	22.48	2700.0	4450.0
Oxygen	O	2	8	16.00	1.14	−218.4	−183.0
Palladium	Pd	2, 4	46	106.7	11.40	1555.0	2200.0
Phosphorus	P	3, 5	15	31.02	1.82–2.20	44.1	280.0
Platinum	Pt	2, 4	78	195.23	21.45	1755.0	4050.0
Plutonium	Pu	3, 4, 6	94	239			
Polonium	Po		84	210.0 (?)			
Potassium	K	1	19	39.096	0.86	62.3	760.0
Praseodymium	Pr	3	59	140.92	6.5	940.0	
Protoactinium	Pa		91	231.0			
Radium	Ra	2	88	226.05	5.0	960.0	1140.0
Radon	Rn	0	86	222.0	9.73	−71.0	−61.8
Rhenium	Re		75	186.31	20.53	3440.0	

*Element sublimes unless under pressure.

Physical Constants — App. 10

Element	Symbol	Valence	Atomic Number	Atomic Weight	Specific Gravity or Density	Melting Point °C	Boiling Point °C
Rhodium	Rh	3	45	102.91	12.5	1985±15° C.	2500.0
Rubidium	Rb	1	37	85.48	1.53	38.4	700.0
Ruthenium	Ru	3, 4, 6, 8	44	101.7	12.2	2450.0	4150.0
Samarium	Sm	3	62	150.43	7.7–7.8	1300–1400	
Scandium	Sc	3	21	45.10	2.5 (?)	1200.0	2400.0
Selenium	Se	2, 4, 6	34	78.96	4.47–4.80	217.0	688.0
Silicon	Si	4	14	28.06	2.42	1420.0	2600.0
Silver	Ag	1	47	107.88	10.50	960.5	1950.0
Sodium	Na	1	11	22.997	0.971	97.5	880.0
Strontium	Sr	2	38	87.63	2.6	752.0	1150.0
Sulfur	S	2, 4, 6	16	32.06	1.957, 2.07	112.8, 119.0	444.6
Tantalum	Ta	5	73	180.88	16.6	2850.0	4100.0
Technetium	Tc		43	99			
Tellurium	Te	2, 4, 6	52	127.61	6.24	452.0	1390.0
Terbium	Tb	3	65	159.2			
Thallium	Tl	1, 3	81	204.39	11.85	303.5	1650.0
Thorium	Th	4	90	232.12	11.2	1845.0	3000.0
Thulium	Tm	3	69	169.4			
Tin	Sn	2, 4	50	118.7	6.55	231.9	2270.0
Titanium	Ti	3, 4	22	47.90	4.5	1800.0	3000.0
Tungsten	W	6	74	183.92	19.3	3370.0	4727.0
Uranium	U	4, 6	92	238.07	18.68	1850.0	
Vanadium	V	3, 5	23	50.95	5.87	1715.0	3400.0
Xenon	Xe	0	54	131.3	3.06	—112.0	—107.1
Ytterbium	Yb	3	70	173.04		1800.0	
Yttrium	Y	3	39	88.92	5.51	1490.0	2500.0
Zinc	Zn	2	30	65.35	7.14	419.4	907.0
Zirconium	Zr	4	40	91.22	6.4	1700.0	2900.0

TERMINOLOGY CHANGES

Alabamine, *astatine;* argentum, *silver;* aurum, *gold;* cuprum, *copper;* cyclonium, *illinium;* ferrum, *iron;* florentium, *illinium;* glucinum, *beryllium;* hydrargyrum, *mercury;* kalium, *potassium;* masurium, *technetium;* natrium, *sodium;* niobium, *columbium;* niton, *radon;* plumbum, *lead;* promethium, *illinium;* stabium, *antimony;* stannum, *tin;* virginium, *francium;* wolfranium, *tungsten;* zincum, *zinc.*

Physiological Standards, Average Normal

Blood

(Expressed in mg. per 100 cc. of whole blood unless otherwise stated)

Acetone bodies, total (as acetone)	0.5-1.0.
Albumin (serum)	4-5 Gm. %.
Amylase (serum or plasma)	70-200 Somogyi units.
Ascorbic acid (reduced)	0.6-2.5.
Bilirubin (serum)	0.1-0.5.
Bleeding time	2-3 minutes.
Calcium, total (serum)	9-11.
	4.5-5.5 mEq./l.
Carbon dioxide content:	
Arterial	45-55 vol. %.
Venous	50-60 vol. %.
	22-27 mEq./l.
Chlorides (as sodium chloride) (plasma or serum)	450-520.
Cholesterol, total (plasma or serum)	140-180.
Coagulation time	2-8 minutes.
Creatine	3-7.
Creatinine	1-2.
Glucose	70-120.
Hemoglobin	100%.
Hydrogen-ion concentration	pH 7.3-7.5.
Icterus index (serum)	4-6 units.
Iodine, total	3-13 micrograms %.
Iron, inorganic (serum)	0.005-0.18.
Lactic acid	5-20.
Lipids, total (serum)	400-800.
Magnesium (serum)	1-3.
Nitrogen, nonprotein	24-40.
Oxygen capacity	16-24 vol. %.
Phosphorus, inorganic (serum)	2.5-4.5.
Platelets	200,000-400,000 per cu. mm.
Potassium (serum)	16-22.
Red cells	5,000,000 per cu. mm.
Average diameter	7.1-7.5 microns.
Reticulocytes	Less than 1%.
Sodium (serum)	310-335.
Specific gravity	1.055.
Plasma	1.052-1.063.
Sugar	80-110.
Sulfates, inorganic (as sulfur) (serum)	0.9-1.5.
Urea	20-35.
Urea nitrogen	10-15.
Uric acid	2-4.
Water	77-81%.
White cells	6000-10,000 per cu. mm.
Neutrophil polymorphs	50-70%.
Lymphocytes	20-40%.
Monocytes	2-8%.
Eosinophil polymorphs	1-4%.
Basophil polymorphs	0.5-1%.

Cerebrospinal Fluid

Character	Clear; colorless; no coagulum.
Pressure	100-200 mm. of water.
Specific gravity	1.006-1.008.
Globulin (Pandy test)	Nil.
Total protein	15- 40 mg. per 100 cc.
Sugar	50- 60 mg. per 100 cc.
Nonprotein nitrogen	20- 40 mg. per 100 cc.
Chlorides	720-750 mg. per 100 cc.
Cells	0-5 (lymphocytes).
Colloidal gold reaction	Negative.

Symbols

♏. Minim.
℈. Scruple.
ʒ. Dram.
f ʒ. Fluid dram.
℥. Ounce.
f ℥. Fluid ounce.
O. Pint.
℔. Pound.
℞. Recipe; take.
M̅. Misce; mix.
āā, āa. Of each.
A, Å. Angstrom unit.
C′. Complement.
c̄, c. [*L. cum.*]. With
E₀. Electroaffinity.
F₁. First filial generation.
F₂. Second filial generation.
L+. Limes death.
L₀. Limes zero.
mμ. Millimicron, micromillimeter.
μg. Microgram.
mEq. Milliequivalent.
mg. Milligram.
mg.%. Milligrams per cent.
QO₂. Oxygen consumption.
m-. Meta-.
o-. Ortho-.
p-. Para-.
s̄s, ss. [*L. semis*]. One-half.
′. Foot; minute; primary accent; univalent.
″. Inch; second; secondary accent; bivalent.

‴. Line (1/12 inch); trivalent.
μ. Micron.
μμ. Micromicron.
+. Plus; excess; acid reaction; positive.
—. Minus; deficiency; alkaline reaction; negative.
±. Plus or minus; either positive or negative; indefinite.
#. Number; following a number; pounds.
÷. Divided by.
×. Multiplied by; magnification.
=. Equals.
>. Greater than; from which is derived.
<. Less than; derived from.
√. Root; square root; radical.
∛. Square root.
∛. Cube root.
∞. Infinity.
:. Ratio; "is to."
::. Equality between ratios; "as."
*. Birth.
†. Death.
°. Degree.
%. Per cent.
σ. 1/1000 of a second.
π. 3.1416—ratio of circumference of a circle to its diameter.
☐, ♂. Male.
○, ♀. Female.
⇌. Denotes a reversible reaction.
#. Number.

Abbreviations, Prefixes, Suffixes

and

Latin and Greek Nomenclature

Principal Medical Abbreviations

Abbreviation	Latin	English Definition
a or āā	ana (Greek)	of each
a. c.	ante cibos	before meals
ad.	ad	to; up to
ad lib.	ad libitum	as desired
alt. dieb.	alternis diebus	every other day
alt. hor.	alternis horis	every other hour
alt. noc.	alternis noctus	every other night
aq.	aqua	water
aq. com.	aqua communis	common water
aq. dest.	aqua destillata	distilled water
aq. tep.	aqua tepida	tepid water
arg.	argentum	silver
av.	(French)	avoirdupois
bib.	bibe	drink
b. i. d.	bis in die	twice a day
b. i. n.	bis in noctus	twice a night
c	cum	with
C.	Centrigradus	centigrade
C.	congius	gallon
cap.	capsula	capsule
cc.	(French)	cubic centimeter
cg.	(French)	centigram
cm.	(French)	centimeter
comp.	compositus	compound
cong.	congius	gallon
def.	defaecatio	defecation
Dil., dil.	dilue	dilute
dr.	drachma	dram or drams
elix.	(Arabic)	elixir
emp.	emplastrum	a plaster
et	et	and
ext.	extractum	extract
F.		Fahrenheit (proper name)
Fld.	fluidus	fluid
fl. dr.	fluidrachma	fluid dram
fl. oz.	fluidus uncia	fluid ounce
Ft., ft.	fiat	let there be made
Gm.	gramme (French)	gram
gr.	granum	grain
Gtt., gtt.	guttae	drops
H.	hora	hour
h.n.	hac nocte	tonight
hor. interm.	horis intermediis	at intermediate hours
h.s.	hora somni	at bedtime or hour of sleep
hypo	Greek: under	hypodermically
inf.	infusum	infusion
l.		liter
Lb.	libra	pound
liq.	liquor	liquid; fluid
M.	(French)	meter
m.	minimum	minim
mEq.		milliequivalent
mg.		milligram
mist.	mistura	mixture
ml.		milliliter
mm.	(French)	millimeter
n.b.	nota bene	note well
no.	numero	number
non rep.	non repetatur	don't repeat
noxt.	nocte; noxte	at night
O.	octarius	pint
ol.	oleum	oil
omn. hor.	omni hora	every hour
omn. noct.	omni nocte	every night
os.	os; ora	mouth
oz.	uncia	ounce
p.c.	post cibum	after food; after meals
per.		through or by
pil.	pilula	pill
p.o.	per os	by mouth
p.r.n.	pro re nata	as needed; as desired
pt.	(French; pinte)	pint
pulv.	pulvis	powder
Q.h.	quaque hora	every hour
Q.2h.		every two hours

App. 14

Medical Abbreviations

Abbreviation	Latin	English Definition
q.₃h.		every three hours
q.i.d.	quater in die	four times a day
Q.s.	quantum sufficiat	a sufficient quantity
qt.	quartina	quart
quotid.	quotidie	every day
Q.v.	quantum vis	as much as you will
℞	recipe	take
rep.	repatatur	let it be repeated
s	sans	without
S.	signa	mark
S.c.	sub cutis	subcutaneously
Sig.	signetur	let it be marked
Sol.	solutio	solution
solv.	solve	dissolve
s.o.s.	si opus sit	if occasion require, if necessary
spt.	spiritus	spirit
sp. gr.	gravitus-heavy	specific gravity
ss.	semis	half
stat.	statim	immediately
syr.	syrupus	syrup
T.	temperatura	temperature
tab.	tabella	tablet
t.i.d.	ter in die	three times a day
t.i.n.	ter in nocte	three times a night
tr., tinct.	tinctura	tincture
ung.	unguentum	ointment
Ur.	urina	urine
vin	vinum	wine
vol. %.		volume per cent
Wt.		weight
w/v.		weight by volume

SEE: *Symbols*, p. App. 12.

A Glossary of Latin Medical Words

NOTE: Latin words which have become a part of the general medical vocabulary are listed in alphabetical order in the text.

abacus, -ī. *m.* Shelf.
abdōminālis, -e. Abdominal.
abdūcēns, -ntis. Leading or drawing from (the median line); applied, also, to 6th pair of cranial nerves.
aberrāns, -ntis. Wandering.
abstractum, -ī. *n.* Abstract.
accessōrius, -a. -um. Accessory.
accidō, -ere, -cidī. Occur; happen.
ācer, ācris, ācre. Sharp; severe.
acervulus, -ī. *m.* (Lit., little heap), acervulus.
acētābulum, -ī. *n.* (Lit., vinegar cup), the bony, cuplike cavity of the hip joint; acetabulum.
acētās, -ātis. *m.* Acetate.
acētum, -ī. *n.* Vinegar.
acidum, -ī. *n.* Acid.
acinus, -ī. *m.* A terminal compartment or secreting portion of a gland; acinus.
acusticus, -a, -um. Auditory.
acūtus, -a, -um. Acute.
adeps, adipis. *m.* and *f.* Fat; lard.
adjūtor, -ōris. *m.* Helper; assistant.
adjuvō, -āre, -jūvī, -jūtus. Aid; assist.
adsum, -esse, -fuī. Be present.
aeger, -gra, -grum. Sick.
aegrōtus, -a, -um. Sick.
āēr, āëris. *m.* Air.
aeternus, -a, -um. Eternal.
aether, -is. *m.* Ether.
āla, -ae. *f.* Wing.
ālāris, -e. Winglike; alar.
albicāns, -ntis. Whitening; white.
albūgineus, -a, -um. White.
albulus, -a, -um. Whitish.
albus, -a, -um. White.
alcoholicus, -a, -um. Alcoholic.
aliquandō. Sometimes.
alius, -a, -ud. Other.
aloina, -ae. *f.* Aloin.
alter, -tera, -terum. Other.
altus, -a, -um. High.
alūmen, -inis. *n.* Alum.
alvus, -ī. *f.* Belly, or its contents.
amārus, -a, -um. Bitter.
amīcus, -ī. *m.* Friend.
āmissiō, -ōnis. *f.* Loss.
āmissus, -ūs. *m.* Loss.
ammōnium, -ī. *n.* Ammonium.
amygdala, -ae. *f.* Almond.
anaestheticus, -a, -um. Producing insensibility; anesthetic.
anastomoticus, -a, -um. Anastomosing.
ānellus, -ī. *m.* Ring.
angulus, -ī. *m.* Angle.
anima, -ae. *f.* Breath; life.
anīsum, -ī. *n.* Anise.
annulāris, -e. Ringlike; annular.
annulus, -ī. *m.* Ring.
anterius, -a, -um. Anterior.
antīcus, -a, -um. Foremost.
antidōtum, -ī. *n.* Antidote.
antimōnium, -ī. *n.* Antimony.
antimōniālis, -e. Of antimony; antimonial.
antipyreticus, -a, -um. Reducing the temperature; antipyretic.
antisepticus, -a, -um. Destroying germ life; antiseptic.
antitrāgus, -ī. *m.* A conical eminence opposite the tragus, *q.v.*; antitragus.
antīquus, -a, -um. Ancient.
aperiēns, -ntis. Laying open; laxative; aperient.
appellō, -āre, -āvī, -ātus. Call.
aptē. Aptly.
apud. Near.
aqua, -ae. *f.* Water.
aqueductus, -ūs. *m.* A canal; aqueduct.
aquōsus, -a, -um. Watery.
arbor, -oris. *f.* Tree.
arceō, -ēre, -uī, -tus. Ward off.
arcuātus, -a, -um (arcus, a bow). Curved like a bow.
arcus, -ūs. *m.* A bow; arch.
āreola, -ae. *f.* Small area (especially around the nipple).
argentum, -ī. *n.* Silver.
arōmaticus, -a, -um. Aromatic.
arsenicum, -ī. *n.* Arsenic.
arsenis, -itis. *m.* Arsenite.
artēria, -ae. *f.* Artery.
articulāris, -e. Articular.
articulō, -āre, -āvī, -ātus. Articulate.
artus, -ūs. *m.* Joint.
ascendēns, -ntis. Ascending.
asepticus, -a, -um. Free from putrefactive matter; aseptic.
asper, -a, -um. Rough.
astrictus, -a, -um. Bound up.
astūtus, -a, -um. Shrewd; artful.
atropina, -ae. *f.* Active principle of belladonna; atropine.
attollēns, -ntis. Raising up; elevating.
attrahēns, -ntis. Drawing to or towards.
auditōrius, -a, -um. Auditory.
aurantium, -ī. *n.* Orange.
auricula, -ae. *f.* (dim., **auris**). Auricle.
auris, -is. *f.* Ear.
axis, -is. *m.* (Lit., that about which a body turns), 2nd cervical vertebra; axis.
azygos. (Gr.) Without a fellow.
balneum, -ī. *n.* Bath.
basilāris, -e. Basilar.
basis, -is. *f.* Base.
bene. Well.
benignus, -a, -um. Mild; benign; not malignant.
berberis, -idis. *f.* Barberry.
bibō, -ere, bibī. Drink.
bicarbonās, -ātis. *m.* Bicarbonate.
biceps, -cipitis. Two-headed.
bifidus, -a, -um. Cleft.
biliaris, -e. Pert. to or conveying bile; biliary.
bīnī, -ae, -a. Two each.
bismuthum, -ī. *n.* Bismuth.
bitartrās, -ātis. *m.* Bitartrate.
bonus, -a, -um. Good.
borās, -ātis. *m.* Borate.
brachiālis, -e. Of the arm; brachial.
brachium, -ī. *n.* Arm.
brevis, -e. Short.
brōmidum, -ī. *n.* Bromide.
būbula, -ae. *f.* Beef.
būccinātor, -ōris. *m.* The trumpeter muscle; buccinator.
bulbus, -ī. *m.* Bulb.
caecus, -a, -um. Blind.
calamus, -ī. *m.* Reed.
calcaneum, -ī. *n.* The heelbone (os calcis).
calcium, -ī. *n.* Calcium.
calidus, -a, -um. Hot.
callōsus, -a, -um. Hard, tough.
calor, -ōris. *m.* Heat.
calumba, -ae. *f.* Calumba.
calvārium, -ī. *n.* The skullcap.
calx, -cis. *f.* Lime.
calyx, -icis. *f.* Cup; calyx.
camphora, -ae. *f.* Camphor.
camphorātus, -a, -um. Camphorated.
canāliculus, -ī. *m.* Small duct or canal.

Latin Medical Words — App. 17

canālis, -is. *m.* Canal.
canīnus, -a, -um. Of a dog, canine.
canis, -is. *m.* and *f.* Dog.
cānitiēs, -ēī. *f.* A gray color, hoariness.
cannabis, -is. *f.* Hemp.
cantharis, -idis. *f.* Spanish fly.
canthus, -ī. *m.* The corner or angle of the eye.
capiō, -ere, cēpī, captus. Take.
capitulum, -ī. *n.* Dim. (caput), a knob or protuberance of bone received into a concavity of another bone.
capsicum, -ī. *n.* Cayenne pepper; capsicum.
capsula, -ae. *f.* A small box; capsule.
carbō, -ōnis. *m.* Carbon; coal; charcoal.
carbolicus, -a, -um. Carbolic.
carbonās, -ātis. *m.* Carbonate.
cardamōmum, -ī. *n.* Cardamom.
careō, -ēre, -uī, -itus. Need; want.
carneus, -a, -um. Fleshy.
carpus, -ī. *m.* Wrist.
cartilāginōsus, -a, -um. Cartilaginous.
cartilāgo, -inis. *f.* Cartilage.
caruncula, -ae. *f.* (Dim., **carō**, flesh), a little piece of flesh; caruncle.
cataplasma, -atis. *n.* Poultice; cataplasm.
catharticus, -a, -um. Cathartic.
cauda, -ae. *f.* Tail.
caudātus, -a, -um. Having a tail; caudate.
causa, -ae. *f.* Cause.
causō, -āre, -āvī, -ātus. Cause.
cavernōsus, -a, -um. Hollow; cavernous.
cavitās, -ātis. *f.* Cavity.
cavus, -a, -um. Hollow.
celeriter. Quickly.
centrālis, -e. Central.
centrum, -ī. *n.* Center.
cephalalgia, -ae. *f.* Headache.
cērātum, -ī. *n.* Waxed dressing; cerate.
cerātus, -a, -um. Waxed.
cerevisa, -ae. *f.* Beer.
certus, -a, -um. Sure; certain.
cēterus, -a, -um. Other.
charta, -ae. *f.* Medicated paper.
chartula, -ae. *f.* Small paper (powder).
chirāta, -ae. *f.* Chirata.
chīrurgia, -ae. *f.* Surgery.
chīrurgus, -ī. *m.* Surgeon.
chlōral. *n.* Chloral.
chlōrās, -ātis. *m.* Chlorate.
chlōridum, -ī. *n.* Chloride.
chlōrōformum, -ī. *n.* Chloroform.
choledochus, -ī. *m.* Holding or receiving bile.
chorda, -ae. *f.* Cord.
chronicus, -a, -um. Chronic.
chylum, -ī. *n.* Chyle.
cibus, -ī. *m.* Food.
cicātrōsus, -a, -um. Full of scars, scarred.
ciliāris, -e. Ciliary.
cinchōna, -ae. *f.* Cinchona.
cinchonīna, -ae. *f.* Cinchonine.
cinereus, -a, -um. Ash-colored.
cinnamōmum, -ī. *n.* Cinnamon.
circulāris, -e. Circular.
circulātiō, -ōnis. *f.* Circulation.
circulus, -ī. *m.* Circle.
circum. Around.
circumdō, -dare, -dedī, -datus. Surround.
citō. Promptly; quickly.
citrās, -ātis. *m.* Citrate.
clārus, -a, -um. Clear, distinguished.
claudus, -a, -um. Lame.
clāvus, -ī. *m.* A corn, usually on the toes.
cludō, -ere, -sī, -sus. Shut; close.
cochlea, -ae. *f.* (Lit., snail shell), spiral cavity of the internal ear; cochlea.
cochleāre, -is. *n.* Spoon.
codeina, -ae. *f.* An alkaloid of opium; codeine.
coeliacus -a, -um. Relating to the stomach; celiac.
colicus, -a, -um. Of or pert. to the colon.
collateriālis, -e. Collateral.
collum, -ī. *n.* Neck.

colocynthis, -idis. *f.* Colocynth.
color, -ōris. *m.* Color.
cōlum, -ī. *n.* Large intestine; colon.
columna, -ae. *f.* Column.
comes, -itis. *m.* Companion.
commissūra, -as. *f.* A joining; commissure.
communicāns, -ntis. Communicating.
commūnis, -e. Common.
compōnō, -ere, -posuī, -positus. Compound.
conarium, -ī. *n.* (From Gr. κῶνος, a cone), a synonym for the pineal gland; conarium.
concha, -ae. *f.* (Lit., a shell), hollow part of the external ear; concha.
confectiō, -ōnis. *f.* Confection.
conium, -ī. *n.* Poison hemlock; conium.
coniveō, -āre, -nīvī. Blink; half close.
coniectūra, -ae. *f.* Guess.
contineō, -ēre, -tinuī, -tentus. Contain.
contrāhō, -ere, -xī, -ctus. Draw together; contract.
contusiō, -ōnis. *f.* Bruise.
cōnus, -ūs. *m.* Cone.
convalescō, -ere, -valuī. Recover health.
cor, cordis. *n.* Heart.
cornicula, -ae. *f.* Dim. (**cornus**), little horn.
cornu, -ūs. *n.* Horn; horn-shaped process.
corōna, -ae. *f.* Crown.
corōnārius, -a, -um. Encircling like a crown; coronary.
corpus, -oris. *n.* Body.
corrōsivus, -a, -um. Corrosive.
corrugātor, -ōris. *m.* A muscle which wrinkles; corrugator.
cortex, -icis. *m.* and *f.* Bark; rind; external layer; cortex.
costa, -ae. *f.* Rib.
craniālis, -e. Cranial.
crās. *adv.* Tomorrow.
crassus, -a, -um. Gross; large.
creasōtum, -ī. *n.* Creasote.
crēber, -bra, -brum. Frequent.
crēdō, -ere, -credidī, -creditus. Trust; believe.
crēta, -ae. *f.* Chalk.
cribriformis, -e. Sievelike; cribriform.
cribrōsus, -a, -um. Having holes like a sieve.
crista, -ae. *f.* Crest; comb of a cock (gallus).
crūrālis, -e. Of the leg; crural.
crūreus, -a, -um. Of the leg.
crūs, crūris. *n.* The leg.
crusta, -ae. *f.* Crust.
cubēba, -ae. *f.* Cubeb.
cubitum, -ī. *n.* Elbow.
cuboideus, -a, -um. Cubelike; cuboid.
cum. With.
cuneiformis, -e. Wedge-shaped; cuneiform.
cūra, -ae. *f.* Care.
cūrō, -āre, -āvī, -ātus. Treat; cure.
cutis, -is. *f.* Skin.
decem. Ten.
deciduus, -a, -um. That falls off.
decoctum, -ī. *n.* Decoction.
deferēns, -ntis. Bearing away.
defessus, -a, -um. Tired; wearied.
deformāns, -ntis. Deforming.
deformitās, -ātis. *f.* Deformity.
demonstrō, -āre, -āvī, -ātus. Show; prove.
dēns, dentis. *m.* Tooth.
dentātus, -a, -um. Toothed; dentate.
depressor, -ōris. *m.* That which depresses; depressor.
descendēns, -ntis. Descending.
dexter, -tra, -trum. Right.
diabēticus, -a, -um. Diabetic (*subst.*, one having diabetes).
diabolus, -ī. *m.* Devil.
dīcō, -ere, -dixī, dictus. Say.
diēs, -ēī. *m.* Day.
difficilis, -e. Difficult.
digitus, -ī. *m.* Finger (**digitus pedis**, a toe).
dīlātor, -ōris. *m.* That which dilates; dilator.

Latin Medical Words — App. 18 — Latin Medical Words

dilūtus, -a, -um. Dilute.
dimidius, -a, -um. Half.
discipulus, -ī. *m.* A learner; pupil; student.
diū. For a long time.
diureticus, -a, -um. Diuretic.
dividō, -ere, -vīsī, -vīsus. Divide.
dō, dare, dedī, datus. Give.
doctus, -a, -um. Learned.
dolor, -ōris. *m.* Pain.
dolōrōsus, -a, -um. Painful.
domicilium, -ī. *n.* Abode.
dorsālis, -e. Of the back; dorsal.
dorsum, -ī. *n.* Back.
dosis, -is. *f.* Dose.
drachma, -ae. *f.* Dram.
ductus, -ūs. *m.* Duct.
dulcis, -e. Sweet.
duo, duae, du. Two.
dūrus, -a, -um. Hard.
dyspepticus, -a, -um. Dyspeptic (*subst.*, a dyspeptic).
edō, -ere, -ēdī, -ēsus. Eat.
efferēns, -ntis. Bearing out or away; efferent.
effervescēns, -ntis. Boiling up.
elegāns, -ntis. Elegant.
ēluviēs, -ēī. *f.* Discharge.
emeticus, -a, -um. Causing vomiting; emetic.
ēminentia, -ae. *f.* Eminence.
emō, -ere, -ēmī, emptus. Buy.
empiricus, -ī. *n.* Quack; empiric.
emplastrum, -ī. *n.* Plaster.
ensiformis, -e. Sword-shaped; ensiform.
eō, īre, īvī, itus. Go.
epilepsia, -ae. *f.* Epilepsy.
epiploicus, -a, -um. Relating to the epiploön (omentum).
equinus, -a, -um. Of a horse; equine.
ergota, -ae. *f.* Ergot.
errō, -āre, -āvī, -ātus. Wander; err.
ērudītus, -a, -um. Learned; educated; erudite.
et. And.
et-et. Both-and.
ethmoidālis, -e (ήθμός, a sieve), ethmoid.
etiam. Even.
euonymus, -ī. *m.* Wahoo; Euonymus.
eupatōrium, -ī. *n.* Boneset; eupatorium.
excessus, -ūs. *m.* Departure.
excīdō, -ere, -īdī, -īsus. Cut out; excise.
excitō, -āre, -āvī, -ātus. Excite.
expectātiō, -ōnis. *f.* Expectation.
experimentum, -ī. *n.* Experiment.
expressiō, -ōnis. *f.* Expression.
exsiccātus, -a, -um. Dried out.
exsudō, -āre, -āvī, -ātus. Sweat out; exude.
externus, -a, -um. External.
extractum, -ī. *n.* Extract.
faciēs, -ēī. *f.* Face; countenance.
faciō, -ere, fēcī, factus. Make.
falx, -cis. *f.* Sickle (a sickle-shaped process).
familia, -ae (or -as). *f.* Family.
fasciculus, -ī. *m.* A small bundle of fibers.
febrifuga, -ae. *f.* Agent that reduces fever; febrifuge.
febris, -is. *f.* Fever.
fēmina, -ae. *f.* Woman.
femorālis, -e. Of the thigh; femoral.
fenestra, -ae. *f.* Window; an opening in the wall of the tympanum.
ferē. Almost.
ferrum, -ī. *n.* Iron.
fibrilla, -ae. *f.* Filament; fibril.
fibrōsus, -a, -um. Fibrous.
fidēs, -eī. *f.* Faith; trustworthiness.
fīdus, -a, -um. Faithful; trustworthy.
filia, -ae. *f.* Daughter.
filius, -ī. *m.* Son.
filix, -icis. *f.* Fern.
fimbria, -ae. *f.* Fringe.
fimbriātus, -a, -um. Fringed; fimbriated.
finiō, -īre, -īvī, -itus. End; finish.

fīō, fierī, factus. Be made.
fissūra, -ae. *f.* Cleft; fissure.
flavus, -a, -um. Yellow.
flexilis, -e. Flexible.
flōs, flōris. *m.* Flower.
fluidus, -a, -um. Fluid.
flūmen, -inis. *n.* River.
fluō, -ere, fluxī, fluxus. Flow.
fluor, -ōris. *m.* Flux; flow.
foetidus, -a, -um. Offensive; fetid.
folium, -ī. *n.* Leaf.
folliculus, -ī. *m.* A small secretory sac; follicle.
fons, -ntis. *m.* Fountain; spring.
formō, -āre, -āvī, -ātus. Form.
fornicātus, -a, -um. Arched.
fornix, -icis. *m.* Arch; vault; fornix.
fortis, -e. Strong; brave.
fossa, -ae. *f.* Ditch; depression; fossa.
fovea, -ae. *f.* Small pit; depression.
fractus, -a, -um. Broken.
fragilitās, -ātis. *f.* Brittleness.
frēnum, -ī. *n.* A bridle; a membranous fold; frenum.
frigidus, -a, -um. Cold.
fructus, -ūs. *m.* Fruit.
frumentum, -ī. *n.* Corn; grain.
frustum, -ī. *n.* Piece; bit.
functiō, -ōnis. *f.* Execution; normal action; function.
fuscus, -a, -um. Brown.
fūsiformis, -e. Spindle-shaped; fusiform.
gallus, -ī. *m.* Cock.
ganglioniformis, -e. Ganglionlike.
gelsemium, -ī. *n.* Gelsemium; yellow jasmine (root).
gemellus, -a, -um. Paired; twin.
gena, -ae. *f.* The cheek.
geniōhyoglossus, -ī. *m.* Muscle attached to chin, hyoid bone and tongue.
gentiāna, -ae. *f.* Gentian.
genu, -ūs. *n.* Knee.
genus, generis. *n.* Kind.
germinātivus, -a, -um. Germinative; germinal.
glabrus, -a, -um. Smooth.
glaciēs, -ēī. *f.* Ice.
globus, -ī. *m.* Globe.
glomerulus, -ī. *m.* Small ball, or tuft of vessels; glomerule.
glūteus, -a, -um (γογλστό, the buttock), of the buttock; gluteal.
glycerīnum, -ī. *n.* Glycerin.
glyceritum, -ī. *n.* Glycerite.
glycyrrhiza, -ae. *f.* Licorice.
gracilis, -e. Slender; graceful.
granulōsus, -a, -um. Granular.
granum, -ī. *n.* Grain.
grātus, -a, -um. Agreeable; pleasing.
gubernāculum, -ī. *n.* (Lit., a helm), applied to fetal cord directing descent of testes; gubernaculum.
gummi. Gum.
gustō, -āre, -āvī, -ātus. Taste.
gutta, -ae. *f.* Drop.
gyrus, -ī. *m.* Circle; ring; convolution (of the brain).
habeō, -ēre, -uī, -itus. Have.
habitō, -āre, -āvī, -ātus. Inhabit.
hallex, -icis, or **hallux, -ucis.** *f.* The great toe.
harmonia, -ae. *f.* Harmony, "suture of harmony."
helix, -icis. *f.* (ξυέι , a tendril), outer ring of the external ear; helix.
hemisphericus, -a, -um. Hemispherical.
hēpar, hepatis. *n.* (Gr.) Liver.
herba, -ae. *f.* Herb.
herī. Yesterday.
hiātus, -ūs. *m.* Opening; aperture.
hīc, haec, hoc. This.
hilāris, -e. Cheerful.
hilus, -ī. *m.* Small fissure or depression.

Latin Medical Words — App. 19

hippocampus, -ī. *m.* (Lit., sea horse), applied to 2 convolutions of brain (major and minor); hippocampus.
homo, -inis. *m.* Man.
horribilis, -e. Horrible.
hūmānus, -a, -um. Human.
hūmor, -ōris. *m.* Fluid; humor.
hydrargyrum, -ī. *n.* Mercury.
hydrastis, -is. *f.* Golden seal (root); hydrastis.
hyoideus, -a, -um. Hyoid.
Hyoscyamus, -ī. *m.* Henbane; Hyoscyamus.
īdem, eadem, idem. Same.
ignārus, -a, -um. Ignorant.
iliacus, -a, -um. Of or pert. to the flanks or ilium; iliac.
ille, illa, illud. He; she; it.
immōbilis, -e. Immovable.
immōbilitas, -ātis. *f.* Immobility.
impar, -is. Without a mate or fellow.
impediō, -īre, -īvī, -ītus. Hinder; check; prevent.
imperītus, -a, -um. Unskilled.
impūrus, -a, -um. Impure.
īmus, -a, -um. Lowest.
incisūra, -ae. *f.* Groove or notch.
Indicus, -a, -um. Indian.
infans, -ntis. *m.* and *f.* Infant.
inflammātiō, -ōnis. *f.* Inflammation.
infraspinātus, -a, -um. Beneath the spine (of the scapula); infraspinate.
infūsum, -ī. *m.* Infusion.
ingressus, -ūs. *m.* Entrance.
innominātus, -a, -um. Unnamed; innominate.
intermittō, -ere, -mīsī, -missus. Intermit.
internōdium, -ī. *n.* Space between 2 joints; internode.
internus, -a, -um. Inner.
interpositus, -a, -um. Placed between.
intertragicus, -a, -um. Between the tragus and antitragus.
intestīnum, -ī. *n.* Intestine.
intumescentia, -ae. *f.* An enlargement; intumescence.
inveniō, -īre, -vēnī, -ventus. Find; discover.
inversiō, -ōnis. *f.* Inversion.
iodidum, -ī. *n.* Iodide.
ipecacuanha, -ae. *f.* Ipecac.
ipse, ipsa, ipsum. Himself; herself; itself.
iris, iridis. *f.* Iris.
is, ea, id. He; she; it.
iter, itineris. *n.* Way; passageway.
jecur, jecinoris. *n.* Liver.
jūcundē. *adv.* Happily; pleasantly.
jūglans, juglandis. *f.* Walnut.
jugulāris, -e. Jugular.
jūniperus, -ī. *f.* Juniper tree.
juvenis, -is. *m.* and *f.*, *adj.* and *subst.* Young; a youth.
labium, -ī. *n.* Lip.
lacer, -a, -um. Lacerated; mutilated.
lacrima, -ae. *f.* Tear.
lacrimālis, -e. Pert. to tears; lacrimal.
lactās, -ātis. *m.* A salt of lactic acid; lactate.
lactiferus, -a, -um. Milk-bearing; lactiferous.
lacus, -ūs. *m.* Lake; basin; reservoir.
lamella, -ae. *f.* Dim. (lamina), layer.
lamina, -ae. *f.* Thin plate; layer.
lāna, -ae. *f.* Wool.
lassus, -a, -um. Weary.
laterālis, -e. Lateral.
lātus, -a, -um. Broad.
laudō, -āre, -āvī, -ātus. Praise.
lavandula, -ae. *f.* Lavender.
lavō, -āre, -āvī, -ātus or **lavi, lautus.** Wash.
laxātor, -ōris. *m.* A muscle that loosens; relaxer.
legō, -ere, -lēgī, lectus. Bring together; collect.

leniō, -īre, -īvī, -ītus. Calm; soothe; assuage.
lenticulāris, -e. Lentil-shaped (double-convex); lenticular.
lentus, -a, -um. Sticky.
letifer, -a, -um. Deadly.
levis, -e. Light.
lienālis, -e. Of the spleen.
ligamentōsus, -a, -um. Ligamentous.
ligamentum, -ī. *n.* Ligament.
lignum, -ī. *n.* Wood.
limbus, -ī. *n.* Border; band; fringe.
limitāns, -ntis. Limiting.
limon, -ōnis. *f.* Lemon.
linea, -ae. *f.* Line.
lingua, -ae. *f.* Tongue.
linguālis, -e. Of the tongue; lingual.
linimentum, -ī. *n.* Liniment.
linum, -ī. *n.* Flax.
liquidus, -a, -um. Liquid.
lobulus, -ī. *m.* Lobule.
lobus, -ī. *m.* Lobe.
longitudinālis, -e. Longitudinal.
longus, -a, -um. Long.
lotiō, -ōnis. *f.* Wash; lotion.
lucidus, -a, -um. Clear; transparent.
lumbālis, -e. Of the loins; lumbar.
lumbus, -ī. *m.* Loin.
lūnula, -ae. *f.* Small crescent; lunula.
lupulīna, -ae. *f.* Yellow powder from the scales of the hop; lupulin.
luteus, -a, -um. Yellow.
luxatiō, -ōnis. *f.* Dislocation.
lympha, -ae. *f.* Chyle; lymph.
mācerō, -āre, -āvī, ātus. Soak; macerate.
magister, -trī. *m.* Teacher; master.
magnus, -a, -um. Large; great.
māla, -ae. *f.* The cheekbone.
malignus, -a, -um. Malignant.
malus, -a, -um. Bad.
mandibulum, -ī. *n.* A jaw.
māne. *n.* Morning.
manūbrium, -ī. *n.* (Lit., a handle, hilt); upper part of sternum; manubrium.
manus, -ūs. *f.* Hand.
massa, -ae. *f.* Mass.
masticō, -āre, -āvī, -ātus. Chew.
mastoideus, -a, -um. Nipplelike; mastoid.
mater, -tris. *f.* Mother.
māteria, -ae. *f.* Materials.
māternus, -a, -um. Maternal.
matrix, -icis. *f.* Source; origin.
maxilla, -ae. *f.* Jawbone; jaw.
meātus, -ūs. *m.* Opening; passage.
mediānus, -a, -um. Middle; median.
medicāmen, -inis. *n.* Drug.
medicāmentārius, -a, -um. Medicated.
medicāmentum, -ī. *n.* Drug.
medicātus, -a, -um. Medicated.
medicīna, -ae. *f.* Medicine.
medicus, -ī. *m.* Physician; doctor.
medius, -a, -um. Middle.
membrāna, -ae. *f.* Membrane.
membrum, -ī. *n.* Member.
memoria, -ae. *f.* Memory.
mentha, -ae. *f.* Mint.
mentum, -ī. *n.* Chin.
mesentericus, -a, -um. Of the mesentery; mesenteric.
metus, -ūs. *m.* Fear.
mīles, -itis. *m.* Soldier.
minerālis, -e. Mineral.
misceō, -ēre, miscuī, mixtus. Mix.
miser, -a, -um. Poor; wretched.
mistūra, -ae. *f.* Mixture.
mītis, -e. Mild.
mitto, -ere, mīsī, missus. Send.
mobilis, -e. Movable.
mobilitās, -ātis. *f.* Mobility.
modiolus, -ī. *m.* (Lit., a small measure), hollow cone in the cochlea of the ear; modiolus.
molāris, -e (mola, mill), a term applied to the grinder teeth; molar.
molliō, -īre, -īvī, -ītus. Soften; mitigate.

mollis, -e. Soft.
molitiēs, -ēī. *f.* Softness.
mons, -ntis. *m.* Mountain.
montānus, -a, -um. Of a mountain; mountain (*adj.*).
monticulus, -ī. *m.* Dim. (**mons**), small eminence.
morbus, -ī. *m.* Disease.
mordeō, --ēre, momordī, morsus. Bite.
moritūrus, -a, -um. About to die.
morphīna, -ae. *f.* Morphine.
morrhua, -ae. *f.* A genus of fishes, including the cod; cod.
mors, mortis. *f.* Death.
morsus, -ūs. *m.* Bite.
mortārium, -ī. *n.* Mortar.
mōtor, -ōris. *m.* That which moves; mover.
moveō, -ēre, mōvī, mōtus. Move.
mox. Presently; soon; directly.
mucilāgō, -inis. *f.* Mucilage.
mucōsus, -a, -um. Mucous.
mulceō, -ere, mulsi, mulsus. Soothe; allay.
multifidus, -a, -um. Many-clefted.
multus, -a, -um. Much; many.
muriāticus, -a, um. Muriatic.
musculus, -ī. *m.* Muscle.
mūtātiō, -ōnis. *f.* Change.
myristica, -ae. *f.* Nutmeg.
myrtiformis, -e. Shaped like the myrtle-leaf or berry; myrtiform.
nāris, -is. *f.* Nostril.
nāsus, -ī. *m.* Nose.
natō, -āre, -āvī, -ātus. Swim; float.
natūra, -ae. *f.* Nature.
nauta, -ae. *m.* Sailor.
naviculāris, -e. Boat-shaped; navicular.
neglectus, -a, -um. Neglected.
nēmō, -inis. *m.* and *f.* No one.
nervus, -ī. *m.* Nerve.
nescio, -īre, -īvī, -ītus. Not know; be ignorant of.
neurilemma, -atis. *n.* Nerve sheath.
nictitāns, -ntis. Winking.
nil. Nothing.
nimium. Too often.
nisi. Unless.
nitrās, -ātis. *m.* Nitrate.
nitricus, -a, -um. Nitric.
nitrōsus, -a, -um. Nitrous.
nōmen, -inis. *n.* Name.
nōminō, -āre, -āvī, -ātus. Name.
nōn. Not.
nondum. Not yet.
nōnus, -a, -um. Ninth.
nosco, -ere, nōvī, nōtus. Learn; know.
novem. Nine.
novus, -a, -um. New.
nox, noctis. *f.* Night.
nucha, -ae. *f.* Nape of neck.
nullus, -a, -um. No; none.
numerus, -ī. *m.* Number.
nunc. Now.
oblīquus, -a, -um. Oblique.
oblongātus, -a, -um. Oblong.
octō. Eight.
oculus, -ī. *m.* Eye.
officīna, -ae. *f.* Office.
officinālis ,-e. Officinal.
oleorēsīna, -ae. *f.* Oleoresin.
oleum, -ī. *n.* Oil.
olfactōrius, -a, -um. Olfactory.
omentum, -ī. *n.* Epiploön; omentum.
omnis, -e. Every; all.
operculum, -ī. *n.* (Lit., a cover or lid), applied to a group of convolutions in the cerebrum, between the 2 divisions of the fissure of Sylvius.
ophthalmicus, -a, -um. Of the eye; ophthalmic.
oppōnēns, -ntis. Opposing.
opticus, -a, -um. Optic.
opus, operis. *n.* Work.
orbita, -ae. *f.* (**orbis**, a circle), the cavity which lodges the eye; orbit.
ordō, -inis. *m.* Row.

orificium, -ī. *n.* Opening.
orior, -īrī, ortus. Arise.
ōs, ōris. *n.* Mouth.
os, ossis. *n.* Bone.
ossiculum, -ī. *n.* Small bone.
ostium, -ī. *n.* An opening.
ovālis, -e. Egg-shaped; oval.
oxalās, -ātis. *m.* A salt of oxalic acid; oxalate.
oxidum, -ī. *n.* Oxide.
palātum, -ī. *n.* Palate.
palpēbra, -ae. *f.* Eyelid.
pālus, -ūdis. *f.* Marsh; swamp.
pancreāticus, -a, -um. Pancreatic.
papillāris, -e. Resembling or covered with papillae; papillary.
pār, paris. *n.* A pair.
parasiticus, -a, -um. Parasitic.
pariēs, -iētis. *m.* Wall.
parō, -āre, -āvī, -ātus. Prepare.
pars, partis. *f.* Part.
partus, -ūs. *m.* Parturition; childbirth.
parvus, -a, -um. Small.
pater, -tris. *n.* Father.
pathēticus, -a, -um. That which moves the passions; a name given to the 4th pair of nerves.
patria, -ae. *f.* Fatherland; country.
paucus, -a, -um. Few.
pectinātus, -a, -um. Resembling the teeth of a comb; pectinate.
pectineus, -a, -um. Comblike.
pectiniformis, -e. Comblike.
pectus, pectoris. *n.* Breast; bosom.
pellūcidus, -a, -um. Transparent.
pensō, -āre, -āvī, -ātus. Weigh.
pepsīnum, -ī. *n.* Pepsin.
percolō, -āre, -āvī, -ātus. Filter; strain.
perforō, -āre, -āvī, -ātus. Bore through; perforate.
periculōsus, -a, -um. Dangerous.
perītus, -a, -um. Skilled.
peronēus, -a, -um. ($\kappa \epsilon \rho \acute{o} \nu \eta$, fibula), relating to the fibula; peroneal.
persōna, -ae. *f.* Person.
perspirātōrius, -a, -um. Relating to perspiration; perspiratory.
pēs, pedis. *m.* Foot.
petō, -ere, -īvī, -ītus. Seek.
petrolātum, -ī. *n.* Petrolatum; vaseline.
petrōsus, -a, -um. Rocklike; petrous.
pharmacopoeia, -a. *f.* Pharmacopoeia.
phiala, -ae. *f.* Vial.
philosophus, -ī. *m.* Philosopher.
phosphās, -ātis. *m.* A salt of phosphoric acid; phosphate.
phrenicus, -a, -um. Of the diaphragm; phrenic.
physostigma, -atis. *n.* Calabar bean; physostigma.
piger, -gra, -grum. Lazy.
pigmentum, -ī. *n.* Pigment.
pilula, -ae. *f.* Pill.
pilus, -ī. *m.* Hair.
pineālis, -e. Resembling a pine cone; pineal.
pinna, -ae. *f.* (Lit., feather), pavilion of the ear; pinna.
piper, piperis. *n.* Pepper.
piperītus, -a, -um. Pepper, peppery.
pistillum, -ī. *n.* Pestle.
pituitārius, -a, -um. (**pituita**, phlegm or mucus), pituitary (applied to a reddish-gray body occupying the *sella Turcica* of the sphenoid bone, from a former erroneous belief that it discharged mucus into the nostrils).
pius, -a, -um. Tender.
pix, picis. *f.* Pitch.
plantāris, -e. Relating to the sole of the foot; plantar.
plānus, -a, -um. Flat; level; smooth.
plexus, -a, -um. Network; plexus.
plica, -ae. *f.* Fold.

plumbum, -ī. *n.* Lead.
poculum, -ī. *n.* Cup.
pollex, -icis. *f.* The thumb.
pomum, -ī. *n.* Apple.
pons, pontis. *m.* Bridge.
popies, poplitis. *m.* Ham of the knee; popliteal space.
poplitēus, -a, -um. Relating to the ham; popliteal.
populus, -ī. *m.* People.
portō, -āre, -āvī, -ātus. Carry.
portiō, -ōnis. *f.* Portion.
porus, -ī. *m.* Channel; canal.
post. Behind; after
posteā. Afterward
posticus, -a, -um. Hindmost.
potēns, -ntis. Powerful.
potiō, -ōnis. A drink; draught.
potō, -āre, -āvī, -ātus. Drink.
potus, -ūs. *m.* Drink.
praeparō, -āre, -āvī, -ātus. Prepare.
praeparatiō, -ōnis. *f.* Preparation.
praeputium, -ī. *n.* Foreskin; prepuce.
praescrībō, -ere, -scripsī, -scriptus. Prescribe.
praescriptum, -ī. *n.* Prescription.
praesēns, -ntis. Present.
praestāns, -ntis. Excellent.
pressiō, -ōnis. *f.* Pressure.
primus, -a, -um. First.
princeps, -ipis. The first; chief; principal.
privō, -āre, -āvī, -ātus. Deprive.
prō. For; in behalf of.
processus, -ūs. *m.* A prominence; process.
profundus, -a, -um. Deep.
pronātor, -ōris. *m.* A muscle which turns the palm of the hand downward; pronator.
properō, -āre, -āvī, -ātus. Hasten.
proprius, -a, -um. One's own; special; proper.
prudēns, -ntis. Prudent.
pterygium, -ī. *n.* An eye disease; pterygium.
publicus, -a, -um. Public.
puella, -ae. *f.* Girl.
pugnō, -āre, -āvī, -ātus. Fight.
pulcher, -chra, -chrum. Beautiful.
pulmo, -ōnis. *m.* Lung.
pulmonālis, -e. Of the lungs; pulmonary.
pulverō, -āre, -āvī, -ātus. Powder; pulverize.
pulvis, pulveris. *m.* Powder.
punctum, -ī. *n.* Point.
puniō, -īre, -īvī, -ītus. Punish.
pūpilla, -ae. *f.* Pupil (of eye).
pupillāris, -e. Pupillary; applied to a delicate membrane which covers the pupil of the eye in the fetus.
purgātivus, -a, -um. Purgative.
purificātus, -a, -um. Purified.
pūrus, -a, -um. Pure.
pyramidālis, -e. Pyramidal.
pyramis, -idis. *f.* Pyramid.
pyriformis, -e. Pear-shaped; pyriform.
quadrātus, -a, -um. Four-sided; square.
quadriceps, -cipitis. Four-headed.
quadrigeminus, -a, -um. Fourfold; four.
quaestiō, -ōnis. *f.* Question.
quam. Than.
quartus, -a, -um. Fourth.
quatuor. Four.
quatuordecim. Fourteen.
que. And.
quinīna, -ae. *f.* Quinine.
quis, quae, quid. Who; which; what.
quondam. Formerly.
quoque. Also.
quot. How many.
radiālis, -e. Of the radius; radial.
radiātus, -a, -um. Radiated.
rādix, -īcis. *f.* Root.
ramus, -ī. *m.* Branch.
rārō. Rarely.

rārus, -a, -um. Rare.
recens. Recently.
recipiō, -ere, -cēpī, -ceptus. Take.
recreō, -āre, -āvī, -ātus. Refresh.
rectus, -a, -um. Straight.
reductio, -ōnis. *f.* A bringing back.
reflexus, -a, -um. Turned back; reflected.
relevō, -āre, -āvī, -ātus. Relieve.
remedium, -ī. *n.* Remedy.
removeō, -ēre, -mōvī, -mōtus. Remove.
remittō, -ēre, -misī, -missus. Send back; remit.
rēn, rēnis. *m.* (usually pl.), kidney.
rēnalis, -e. Of the kidney; renal.
reperiō, -īre, -perī, -pertus. Find.
reprimō, -ēre, -pressī, -pressus. Check; repress.
requiesco, -ēre, -ēvī, -ētus. Rest.
rēs, reī. *f.* Thing.
rēsina, -ae. *f.* Resin.
rēspīrātiō, -ōnis. *f.* Respiration.
rēte, -is. *n.* Net.
reticulāris, -e. Like a net; reticular.
retrāhēns, -ntis. Drawing back; retracting.
rheumatismus, -ī. *m.* Rheumatism.
ricinus, -ī. *m.* (Lit., a tick, which the seeds resemble), the castor oil plant (**Ricinus communis**).
rima, -ae. *f.* Slit; cleft.
rogō, -āre, -āvī, -ātus. Ask.
rosa, -ae. *f.* Rose.
rostrum, -ī. *n.* Beak.
rotundus, -a, -um. Round.
ruber, -bra, -brum. Red.
rubor, -ōris. *m.* Redness.
rūga, -ae. *f.* A wrinkle; fold.
rumex, -icis. *m.* and *f.* Sorrel.
sabulum, -ī. *n.* Sand.
saccharātus, -a, -um. Saccharated.
saccharum, -ī. *n.* Sugar.
sacciformis, -e. Saclike.
saccus, -ī. *m.* A sack or bag.
saepe. Often.
sal, -is. *m.* and *f.* Salt.
salicīnum, -ī. *n.* Salicin.
salicylās, -ātis. *m.* Salicylate.
salix, -icis. *f.* Willow.
sānābilis, -e. Curable.
sanguis, -guinis. *m.* Blood.
sānitās, -ātis. *f.* Healing.
sānō, -āre, -āvī, -ātus. Heal; cure.
sapientia, -ae. *f.* Wisdom.
sapō, -ōnis. *m.* Soap.
sartōrius, -ī. *m.* The tailor's muscle; sartorius.
scāla, -ae. *f.* Ladder.
scalēnus, -a, -um. Of unequal sides.
scaphoideus, -a, -um. Boat-shaped; scaphoid.
schola, -ae. *f.* (Lit., leisure given to learning), school.
scientia, -ae. *f.* Knowledge; science.
scilla, -ae. *f.* Squill.
sciō, -īre, -īvī, -ītus. Know.
scrībō, -ēre, scripsī, scriptus. Write.
scriptōrius, -a, -um. Of a writer; writer's.
secundus, -a, -um. Second.
sed. But.
sēdes, -is. *f.* Seat.
segmentum, -ī. *n.* Segment.
sella, -ae. *f.* Saddle.
sēmicirculāris, -e. Semicircular.
sēmiellipticus, -a, -um. Semielliptical.
sēmilunāris, -e. Semilunar.
sēmimembranōsus, -a, -um. Semimembranous.
seminālis, -e. Seminal.
sēmis, sēmissis. *m.* Half.
sēmitendinōsus, -a, -um. Semitendinous.
senectus, -tūtis. *f.* Old age.
senex, senis. *m.* Old man.
senilitās, -ātis. The feebleness of old age; senility.
sentiō, -īre, -sī, -sus. Feel.

septem. Seven.
sequestrum, -ī. *n.* A portion of dead bone; sequestrum.
sermō, -ōnis. *m.* Conversation.
serrātus, -a, -um. Notched like a saw; serrated.
servus, -ī. *m.* Servant; assistant.
sesamoideus, -a, -um. Like a sesame seed; sesamoid (applied to a bone developed in a tendon).
seu. Whether.
signō, -āre, -āvī, -ātus. Write; direct.
simplex, -icis. Simple.
similō, -āre, -āvī, -ātus. Simulate.
sināpis, -is. *f.* Mustard.
sitis, -is. *f.* Thirst.
solitārius, -a, -um. Solitary.
somnificus, -a, -um. Sleep-producing.
somnus, -ī. *m.* Sleep.
sopor, -ōris. *m.* Deep sleep.
spectrum, -ī. *n.* Image.
spēs, spei. *f.* Hope.
sphenoideus, -a, -um. Wedge-shaped; sphenoid.
spina, -ae. *f.* (A thorn), a process on the surface of a bone; the backbone.
spinālis, -e. Spinal.
spinōsus, -a, -um. Spiny.
spirālis, -e. Spiral.
spiritus, -ūs. *m.* Spirit.
splēnius, -a, -um. Resembling the spleen; applied to a muscle of the back and neck.
spongiōsus, -a, -um. Spongy.
squamōsus, -a, -um. Scaly; squamous.
stapēdius, -ī. *m.* A muscle acting upon the stapes; stapedius.
stertor, -ōris. *m.* Snoring.
stomachālis, -e. Stomachic.
stomachus, -ī. *m.* Stomach.
stramōnium, -ī. *n.* Jamestown weed; stramonium.
stria, -ae. *f.* Stripe; stria.
striātus, -a, -um. Striped; striated.
struō, -ere, -xī, -ctus. Arrange.
strychnina, -ae. *f.* Strychnine.
subacetās, -ātis. *m.* Subacetate.
subanconeus, -a, -um. Under the elbow.
subitō. Suddenly.
subitus, -a, -um. Sudden.
sublimis, -e. Deep.
submuriās, -ātis. *m.* Submuriate.
subnitras, -ātis. *m.* Subnitrate.
subscapulāris, -e. Under the scapula; subscapular.
substantia, -ae. *f.* Substance.
subsultus, -ūs. *m.* A jumping; a twitching.
succus, -ī. *m.* Juice.
sudor, -ōris. *m.* Sweat.
sulcus, -ī. *m.* Furrow.
sulphonal. Sulfonal.
sulphās, -ātis. *m.* Sulfate.
sulphuricus, -a, -um. Sulfuric.
sum, esse, fui. Be.
sūmō, -ere, -psi, -ptus. Take.
supercilium, -ī. *n.* Eyebrow.
superficiālis, -e. Superficial.
superficiēs, -ēī. *f.* Surface.
supraspinātus, -a, -um. Above the spine (of scapula); supraspinate.
suppositōrium, -ī. *n.* Suppository.
suspensōrium, -ī. *n.* That which suspends.
suspensōrius, -a, -um. Suspensory.
sustentaculum, -ī. *n.* A prop; support.
sutūra, -ae. *f.* Seam; suture.
sympatheticus, -a, -um. Sympathetic.
symptōma, -atis. *n.* Symptom.
synoviālis, -e. Synovial.
tabacum, -ī. *n.* Tobacco.
taenia, -ae. *f.* A band. **t. semicirculāris.** A layer in the cerebrum; also, a genus of intestinal worms; the tapeworm.
talus, -ī. *m.* The heel.
tam. So.

tapētum, -ī. *n* (**tapēte,** carpet, tapestry), a lining membrane; also, the radiating fibers of the *corpus callōsum.*
taraxacum, -ī. *n.* Dandelion (root); taraxacum.
tarsus, -ī. *m.* Ankle.
tartaricus, -a, -um. Tartaric.
tartrās, -ātis. *m.* Tartrate.
tegō, -ere, -xī, -ctum. Cover; protect.
tectōrium, -ī. *n.* A covering.
tectōrius, -a, -um. Protecting; covering.
temporālis, -e. Temporal.
tempus, -oris. *n.* Time.
tenax, -ācis. Holding fast; tenacious.
tendineus, -a, -um. Tendinous.
tendō, -ere, tetendī, tentus. Stretch; reach.
tendō, -dinis. *m.* Tendon.
teneō, -ēre, -uī, -tus. Keep; hold.
tener, -a, -um. Delicate; tender.
tensor, -ōris. *m.* Stretcher; tensor.
tentō, -āre, -āvī, -ātus. Test; try.
tentōrium, -ī. *n.* A tent; covering.
tenuis, -e. Thin; small.
tepidus, -a, -um. Lukewarm.
terebinthina, -ae. *f.* Turpentine.
teres, -etis. Rounded; smooth.
tergum, -ī. *n.* Back.
terminus, -ī. *m.* End.
tertius, -a, -um. Third.
theobrōma, -ātis. *n.* Cacao (food of the gods).
thoracicus, -a, -um. Thoracic.
thyroideus, -a, -um. Having the shape of an oblong shield; thyroid.
tiglium, -ī. *n.* The specific name of the croton oil plant.
tinctūra, -ae. *f.* Tincture.
tonicus, -a, -um. Tonic.
tonsilla, -ae. *f.* Tonsil.
torcular, -āris. *n.* A wine press.
tracheālis, -e. Tracheal.
tractō, -āre, -āvī, -ātus. Handle.
tragus, -ī. *m.* (τράγος, a goat), small nipple in front of external auditory meatus; so called because sometimes covered with hair; tragus.
transversālis, -e. Transverse.
transversus, -a, -um. Transverse.
trapezoideus, -a, -um. Like a trapezium; trapezoid.
trauma, -atis. *n.* Injury; wound.
trēs, tria. Three.
triangulāris, -e. Triangular.
triceps, -ipitis. Three-headed.
trigeminus, -a, -um. Three-fold.
trigīnta. Thirty.
trigōnum, -ī. *n.* Triangle.
triquetrus, -a, -um. Three-cornered; triangular.
trochiscus, -ī. *m.* Troche.
tuba, -ae. *f.* (Trumpet), tube.
tuber, -eris. *n.* Swelling; protuberance.
tuberculum, -ī. *n.* A protuberance; tubercle.
tubulus, -ī. *m.* Small tube.
tubus, -ī. *m.* Tube.
tunica, -ae. *f.* Coat; covering.
tussiō, -ire, -īvī, -itus. Cough.
tūtāmen, -minis. *n.* Means of defense; a protection.
tūtō. Safely.
tympanicus, -a, -um. Of the tympanum; tympanic.
ubi. Where.
ulna, -ae. *f.* Larger bone of forearm; ulna.
ulnāris, -e. Of the ulna; ulnar.
uncia, -ae. *f.* Ounce.
unciformis, -e. Hooked.
uncinātus, -a, -um. Hooked; uncinate.
unguentum, -ī. *n.* Ointment.
unguis, -is. *m.* Nail.
ūnus, -a, -um. One.
urbānus, -a, -um. Of the city; urbane.
urīna, -ae. *f.* Urine.

uriniferus, -a, -um. Urine-bearing; uriniferous.
usque. Continuously; constantly.
uterīnus, -a, -um. Of the uterus; uterine.
ūtilis, -e. Useful.
uvula, -ae. *f.* Dim. (**uva**, bunch of grapes), a small appendix or tubercle; uvula.
uxor, -ōris. *f.* Wife.
vaginālis, -e. Sheathlike; vaginal.
valeriānās, -ātis. *m.* Valerianate.
valetūdō, -inis. *f.* Health.
validus, -a, -um. Strong; sturdy; healthy.
valvula, -ae. *f.* Valve.
vās, vāsis. *n.* Vessel.
vasculōsus, -a, -um. Vascular.
vasculum, -ī. *n.* Small vessel.
vastus, -a, -um. Extensive; large.
vegetābilis, -e. Vegetable.
vehiculum, -ī. *n.* Vehicle.
vel. Either.
vēlum, -ī. *n.* Veil.
vēna, -ae. *f.* Vein.
vendō, -ēre, vendidī. Sell.
veneficus, -ī. *m.* Poisoner.
venēnum, -ī. *n.* Poison.
venōsus, -a, -um. Venous.
venter, -tris. *m.* Belly.
ventriculus, -ī. *m.* Dim. (**venter**), ventricle.
vērātrum, -ī. *n.* Hellebore; veratrum.
vermiformis, -e. Wormlike.
veru, -ūs. *n.* A spit (for roasting upon); used only in the term **verumontanum**, a longitudinal ridge in the floor of the male urethra.
verus, -a, -um. True.

vesīca, -ae. *f.* Urinary bladder.
vesicatōrium, -ī. *n.* Blister.
vesicula, -ae. *f.* Vesicle.
vesiculāris, -e. Full of vesicles or cells; vesicular.
vestibulāris, -e. Relating to the vestibule of the ear; vestibular.
vetus, veteris. Old.
vigilō, -āre, -āvī, -ātus. Watch.
vigintī. Twenty.
villus, -ī. *m.* Tuft of hair; villus.
vinculum, -ī. *n.* Link; chain.
vīnum, -ī. *n.* Wine.
vir, virī. *m.* Man.
viridis, -e. Green.
vīs, vīs, pl. **vīres, -ium.** *f.* Force; power.
viscus, -eris. *n.* Any internal organ of the body.
visiō, -ōnis. *f.* Vision.
visus, -ūs. *m.* Vision.
vīta, -ae. *f.* Life.
vitellus, -ī. *m.* Yolk.
vitreus, -a, -um. Resembling glass; vitreous.
vocālis, -e. Vocal.
vocō, -āre, -āvī, -ātus. Call.
vola, -ae. *f.* Palm of the hand (sole of the foot).
vorticōsus, -a, -um. Resembling an eddy or whirlpool.
vulnerō, -āre, -āvī, -ātus. Wound.
vulnus, vulneris. *n.* A wound.
vultus, -ūs. *m.* Countenance.
zincum, -ī. *n.* Zinc.
zingiber, -eris. *n.* Ginger.
zōna, -ae. *f.* Zone; belt.
zōnula, -ae. *f.* Little zone, or belt; zonule.

(*See also prescriptions*)

English, Latin and Greek Equivalents

acid. Acidum.
ague. Febris.
and. Et.
arm. Brachium. Gr., brachion.
artery. Arteria.
attachment. Adhaesio.
back. Tergum; dorsum.
backbone. Spina.
backward. Retro.
bath. Balneum.
beef. Bubula.
belly. Venter; abdomen.
bend. Flexus.
bile. Bilis. Gr., chole.
bladder. Vesica.
bleed. Fluere.
blind. Obscurus.
blister. Pustulo; vesicatorium.
bloat. Tumeo.
blood. Sanguis. Gr., haima, aima.
blood vessel. Vena.
body. Corpus. Gr., soma.
boiling (up). Effervescens.
bone. Os. Gr., osteon.
bony. Osseus.
bowels. Intestina; viscera.
bow-legged. Valgus.
brain. Cerebrum. Gr., egkephalon.
breach. Ruptura.
breast. Mamma. Gr., mastos.
breath. Halitus.
bubble. Pustula.
bulb. Bulbus.
buttock. Clunis. Gr., gloutos.
calcareous. Calci similis.
canal. Canalis.
cartilage. Cartilago. Gr., chondros.
catarrh. Coryza.
cavity. Caverna.
change. Mutatio.
chest. Thorax. Gr., thorax.
chin. Mentum. Gr., geneion.
choke. Strangulo.
clavicle. Clavicula.
confinement. Puerperium.
congestion. Conglobatio.
consumption. Phthisis, pulmonaria.
convulsion. Convulsio.
cord. Corda.
corn. Callus-clavus.
cornea. Cornu. Gr., keras.
costive. Astrictus.
cough. Tussio.
countenance. Vultus.
cramp. Spasmus.
crisis. Dies crisimus.
cup. Poculum.
cure. Sano.
curvature. Curvatura.
cuticle. Cuticula.
daily. Diurnus.
dandruff. Furfures capitas.
day. Dies.
dead. Mortuus; defunctus.
deadly. Lethalis.
deafness. Surditas.
decompose. Dissolvo.
dental. Dentalis.
depression. Depressio.
digestive. Digestorius; pepticus.
dilute. Dilutus.
discharge. Eluvies; effluens.
disease. Morbus.
dorsal. Dorsalis.
dose. Potio.
dram. Drachma.
drink. Bibo; potis.
dropsy. Hydrops; opis.

drug. Medicamentum.
duct. Ductus.
dysentery. Dysenteria.
ear. Auris. Gr., ous.
eat. Edo.
egg. Ovum.
elbow. Cubitum. Gr., agkon.
embryo. Partus immaturus.
emission. Emissio.
entrails. Viscera.
epidemic. Epidemus.
epilepsy. Morbus comitalis; epilepsia.
epileptic. Epilepticus.
erection. Erectio.
erotic. Amatorius.
eunuch. Eunuchus.
every. Omnis.
excrement. Excrementum.
excretion. Excrementum; excretio.
exhalation. Exhalatio.
exhale. Exhalo.
expel. Expello.
expire. Expiro.
external. Externus.
extract. Extractum.
eye. Oculus. Gr., ophthalmos.
eyeball. Pupula.
eyebrow. Supercilium.
eyelid. Palpebra.
eyetooth. Dens caninus.
face. Facies.
faculty. Facultas.
faint. Collabor.
fat. Adeps. Gr., lipos.
feature. Lineomentum.
febrile. Febriculosus.
fecundity. Fecunditas.
feel. Tactus.
fever. Febris.
film. Membranula.
filter. Percolo.
finger. Digitus. Gr., dactylos.
fistula. Fistula putris.
fit. Accessus.
flesh. Carnis. Gr., sarx.
fluid. Fluidus.
food. Cibus.
foot. Pes, pedis. Gr., pous.
forearm. Brachium.
forehead. Frons.
freckle. Lentigo.
gall. Bilis.
gangrene. Gangraena.
gargle. Gargarizo.
gland. Glandula.
gleet. Ichor.
gout. Morbus articularis; (in feet), podagra.
grain. Granum.
gravel. Calculus.
grinder tooth. Dens maxillaris.
gullet. Gula.
gum. Gingiva (of mouth).
gut. Intestinum.
hair. Capillus. Gr., thrix.
half. Dimidius.
hand. Manus. Gr., cheir.
harelip. Labrum fissum.
haunch. Clunis.
head. Caput. Gr., kephale.
heal. Sano.
healer. Medicus.
healing. Salutaris.
health. Sanitas.
healthful. Salutaris; saluber.
healthy. Sanus.
hear. Audio.
hearing. Auditio; (sense of) auditus.

App. 24

English, Latin and App. 25 **Greek Equivalents**

heart. Cor. Gr., kardia.
heart burning. Redundatio stomachi.
heat. Calor; v. a. calefacio.
hectic. Hecticus.
heel. Calx, talus.
hirsute. Hirsutus.
homeopathic. Homeopathicus.
hysterics. Hysteria.
illness. Morbus.
incisor. Dens acutus.
infant. Infans; puerilis.
infect. Inficio.
infectious. Contagiosus.
infirm. Infirmus; debilis.
inflammation. Inflammatio; (of lungs) inflammatio pulmonaria.
injection. Injectio.
insane. Insanus.
intellect. Intellectus.
intercourse. Congressus.
internal. Intestinus.
intestine. Intestinum. Gr., enteron.
itch. Scabies.
itching. Pruritus.
jaw. Maxilla.
joint. Artus. Gr., arthron.
jugular vein. Vena jugularis.
kidney. Ren. Gr., nephros.
knee. Genu. Gr., gonu.
kneepan. Patella.
knuckle. Condylus.
labor. Partus.
labyrinth. Labyrinthus.
lacerate. Lacero.
larynx. Guttur.
lateral. Lateralis.
leech. Sanguisuga.
leg. Tibia.
leprosy. Leprosus.
ligament. Ligamentum. Gr., syndesmos.
ligature. Ligatura.
limb. Membrum.
lime. Calx.
listen. Ausculto.
liver. Jecur. Gr., hepar, epar.
livid. Lividus.
loin. Lumbus. Gr., lapara.
looseness. Laxitas.
lotion. Lotio.
lukewarm. Tepidus.
lung. Pulmo. Gr., pneumon.
lymph. Lympha.
mad. Insanus.
malady. Morbus.
male. Masculinus.
malignant. Malignus.
maternity. Conditio matris.
medicine. (Remedy) Medicamentum.
medicated. Medicatus.
milk. Lac.
mind. Animus.
mix. Misceo.
mixture. Mistura.
moist. Humidus.
molar. Dens molaris.
month. Mensis.
monthly. Menstruus.
morbid. Morbidus.
mouth. Os. Gr., stoma.
mucous. Mucosus.
muscle. Musculus. Gr., mys.
mustard. Sinapis.
nail. Unguis.
navel. Umbilicus. Gr., omphalos.
neck. Cervix; collum. Gr., trachelos.
nerve. Nervus. Gr., neuron.
nipple. Papilla.
no, none. Nullus.
normal. Normalis.
nose. Nasus. Gr., rhis, ris.
nostril. Naris.
not. Non.
nourish. Nutrio.
nourishment. Alimentus.
now. Nunc.

nudity. Nudatio.
nurse. Nutrix.
obesity. Obesitas.
ocular. Ocularis.
oculist. Ocularis medicus.
oil. Oleum.
ointment. Unguentum.
operator. Manus curatio.
opiate. Medicamentum somnificum.
optics. Optice.
orifice. Foramen.
pain. Dolor.
palate. Palatum.
palm. Palma.
parasite. Parasitus.
part. Pars.
patient. Patiens.
pectoral. Pectoralis.
pedal. Pedale.
phlegm. Pituita.
pill. Pilus.
pimple. Pustula.
plaster. Emplastrum.
poison. Venenum.
poultice. Cataplasma.
powder. Pulvis.
pregnant. Gravida.
prepare. Paro.
prescribe. Praescribo.
prescription. Praescriptum.
puberty. Pubertas.
pubic bone. Os pubis. Gr., pecten.
pulverize. Pulvero.
pupil. Pupilla.
purgative. Purgativus.
putrid. Putris.
quinsy. Cynanche; angina.
rash. Exanthema.
recover. Convalesco.
recumbent. Recubans.
recur. Recurro.
redness. Rubor.
remedy. Remedium.
respiration. Respiratio.
rheum. Fluxio.
rib. Costa.
rigid. Rigidus.
ringing. Tinnitus.
rupture. Hernia.
saliva. Sputum.
sallow. Salix.
salt. Sal.
salve. Unguentum.
sane. Sanus.
scab. Scabies.
scalp. Pericranium.
scaly. Squamosus.
scar. Cicatrix.
sciatica. Ischias.
scruple. Scrupulum.
seed. Semen.
senile. Senilis.
serum. Sanguinis pars equosa.
sheath. Vagina.
shin. Tibia.
shock. Concussio; (of electricity), ictus electricus.
short. Brevis.
shoulder. Humerus. Gr., omos.
shoulder blade. Scapula.
shudder. Tremor.
sick. Aegrotus.
side. Latus.
sinew. Nervus.
skeleton. Sceletos.
skin. Cutis. Gr., derma.
skull. Cranium. Gr., kranion.
sleep. Somnus.
smallpox. Variola.
smell. Odoratus.
soap. Sapo.
socket. Cavum.
soft. Mollis.
solid. Solidus.
solution. Dilutum.

soporific. Soporus.
sore. Ulcus.
spasm. Spasmus.
spinal. Dorsalis; spinalis.
spine. Spina.
spirit. Spiritus.
spittle. Sputum.
spleen. Lien.
spoon. Cochleare.
sprain. Luxatio.
stomach. Stomachus. Gr., gaster.
stone. Calculus.
stricture. Strictura.
sugar. Saccharum.
suture. Sutura.
swallow. Glutio.
sweat. Sudor. Gr., idros.
symptom. Symptoma.
system. Systema.
tail. Cauda.
take. Sumo.
tapeworm. Taenia.
taste. Gustatus.
tear. Lacrima.
teeth. Dentes.
tendon. Tendo. Gr., tenon.
testicle. Testis. Gr., orchis.
thigh. Femur.
throat. Fauces. Gr., pharygx.
throb. Palpito.
thumb. Pollex.

tongue. Lingua. Gr., glossa.
tonsil. Tonsilla.
tooth. Dens. Gr., odous.
troche. Trochiscus.
tube. Tuba.
twin. Geminus.
twitching. Subsultus.
ulcer. Ulcus.
unless. Nisi.
urine. Urina.
uterine. Uterinus.
vaccine. Vaccinum.
vagina. Vagina. Gr., kolpos.
valve. Valvula.
vein. Vena. Gr., phleps.
vertebra. Vertebra. Gr., spondylos.
vessel. Vas.
wash. Lavo.
water. Aqua.
wax. Cera.
waxed dressing. Ceratum.
weary. Lassus.
wet. Humidus.
windpipe. Arteria aspera.
wine. Vinum.
woman. Femina.
womb. Uterus. Gr., hystera; ystera.
worm. Vermis.
wound. Vulnus.
wrist. Carpus. Gr., karpos.
yolk. Luteum.

Latin and Greek Medical Words

LATIN EQUIVALENTS

COLORS
blue. Caeruleus; cyaneus; lividus.
black. Niger; nigra; nigrum.
brown. Fulvus.
crimson. Coccum; coccineus.
green. Viridis.
gray. Cinereus.
lemon. Citreum.
pink. Rosaceus.
purple. Purpura; purpureus.
red. Ruber.
scarlet. Coccineus.
violet. Violaceus.
white. Albus.
yellow. Flavus; luteus; croceus.

QUALITIES
bitter. Acerbus.
chill. Friguscolum.
cold. Frigidus.
dry. Aridus.
dull. Stupidus; hebes.
faintness. Languor.
fat. obesus; pinguis.
heat. Calor; ardor; fervor.
short. Brevis.
sour. Acidus.
sweet. Dulcis.
tall. Longus; celsus; procerus.
thick. Densus.
heavy. Gravis; ponderosus.
hot. Calidus; fervens; candens.
light. Levis.
liquid. Liquidus.
moist. Humidus; uvidus.
sharp. Acutus.
thin. Tenuis; macer.
warm. Calidus.
warmth. Calor.
weary. Lassus; languidus; fatigatus.
wet. Humidus.

METALS
gold. Aurum; aureus.
silver. Argentum; argenteus.
copper. Cuprum; cuprinus.
iron. Ferrum; ferreus.
tin. Stannum; plumbum album.

TIME
Words expressing periods of time.
afternoon. Post-meridiem.
age. Aetas; maturas; adultus; impubis.
autumn. Autumnus.
birth. Partus; natales.
breakfast. Prandium.
child. Infans; puer, filius.
day. Dies.
daily. Diurnus.
date. Status dies.
dawn. Prima lux.
death. Mors.
dinner. Cena.
evening. Vesper.
hour. Hora.
infant. Infans.
maturity. Maturitas; aetas matura.
meal. Epulae.
midnight. Media nox.
midsummer. Media aestas.
moment. Punctum.
month. Mens.
monthly. Menstruus.
morning. Matutinum.
night. Nox, noctis.
noon. Meridies.
old. Antiquus.
puberty. Pubertas.
second. Secundum.
spring. Ver; veris.
summer. Aestas.
sunrise. Solis ortus.
sunset. Solis occasus.
supper. Cena.
time. Tempus.
winter. Hiems, hiemis.
year. Annus.
young. Parvus; infans.
youth. Adolescentia.

RELATIONSHIP
aunt. Amita; matertera.
brother. Frater.
child. Infans.
cousin. Consobrinus.
father. Pater; paterfamilias.
husband. Maritus.
infant. Infans.
grandfather. Avus.
grandmother. Avia.
granddaughter. Neptis.
grandson. Nepos.
mother. Mater.
nephew. Fratris or sororis filius or sororis nepos.
niece. Fratris or sororis filia.
sister. Soror.
uncle. Patruus; avunculus.
widow. Vidua.
widower. Viduus.
wife. Uxor.

NUMERALS
SEE: Latin Numerals, in Appendix. (Roman Numerals.)

Greek and Latin Singulars and Plurals

Singular	Plural	Singular	Plural
addendum	addenda	focus	foci
aden	adena	fornix	fornices
adenoma	adenomata	fossa	fossae
ala	alae	glans	glandes
albacans	albacantes	gonad	gonades
amygdala	amygdalae	gonococcus	gonococci
antenna	antennae	gyrus	gyri
antiad	antiades	ilium	ilia
antrum	antra	keratosis	keratoses
apertura	aperturae	labium	labia
apex	apices	lamina	laminae
aponeurosis	aponeuroses	loculus	loculi
appendix	appendices	locus	loci
aqua	aquae	medium	media
arcus	arcus	mucosa	mucosae
ascaris	ascarides	naevus	naevi
ascus	asci	nodus	nodi
atrium	atria	nox	noxa
axis	axes	os	ora
bacillus	bacilli	ovum	ova
bacterium	bacteria	papilla	papillae
bronchus	bronchi	pathema	pathemata
bulla	bullae	pes	pedes
bursa	bursae	petechia	petechiae
cactus	cacti	pilula	pilulae
cadaver	cadavera	polypus	polypi
calcaneum	calcanea	ramus	rami
calculus	calculi	septum	septa
calix	calices	sequestrum	sequestra
cantharis	cantharides	serosa	serosae
canthus	canthi	spasmus	spasmi
cornu	cornua	spectrum	spectra
corpus	corpora	speculum	specula
crisis	crises	sperma	spermata
cuniculus	cuniculi	stoma	stomata
dens	dentes	sudamen	sudamina
diagnosis	diagnoses	sulcus	sulci
diaphoreticus	diaphoretici	tarsus	tarsi
diastema	diastemata	tela	telae
digitus	digiti	tinctura	tincturae
dorsum	dorsi	toxicosis	toxicoses
echolatus	echolati	typha	typhae
enema	enemata	ulcus	ulcera
ensis	enses	varix	varices
epididymis	epididymides	vas	vasa
esthesis	estheses	vesicula	vesiculae
fibroma	fibromata	vis	vires
filix	filices	viscus	viscera
filum	fila	vomica	vomicae
flagellum	flagella	zygoma	zygomata

Numerals, Latin

Cardinals

1. ūnus
2. duo
3. trēs
4. quattuor
5. quīnque
6. sex
7. septem
8. octō
9. novem
10. decem
11. ūndecim
12. duodecim
13. tredecim
14. quattuordecim
15. quīndecim
16. sēdecim
17. septendecim
18. duodēvigintī
19. ūndēvigintī
20. vigintī
21. { vigintī ūnus, or ūnus et vigintī
22. { vigintī duo, or duo et vigintī
28. duodētrigintā
29. ūndētrigintā
30. trigintā
40. quadrāgintā
50. quīnquāgintā
60. sexāgintā
70. septuāgintā
80. octōgintā
90. nōnāgintā
100. centum
101. { centum ūnus, or centum et ūnus
102. { centum duo, or centum et duo
200. ducentī
300. trecentī
400. quadringentī
500. quīngentī
600. sēscentī, or sexcentī
700. septingentī
800. octingentī
900. nōngentī
1,000. mīlle
2,000. duo mīllia
10,000. decem mīllia
100,000. centum mīllia

Ordinals

1st. prīmus
2nd. secundus
3rd. tertius
4th. quartus
5th. quīntus
6th. sextus
7th. septimus
8th. octāvus
9th. nōnus
10th. decimus
11th. ūndecimus
12th. duodecimus
13th. tertius decimus
14th. quartus decimus
15th. quīntus decimus
16th. septus decimus
17th. septimus decimus
18th. duodēvicēsimus
19th. ūndēvicēsimus
20th. vīcēsimus
21st. { vīcēsimus prīmus, or prīmus et vīcēsimus
22nd. { vīcēsimus secundus, or duo et vīcēsimus
28th. duodētrīcēsimus
29th. ūndētrīcēsimus
30th. trīcēsimus
40th. quadrāgēsimus
50th. quīnquāgēsimus
60th. sexāgēsimus
70th. septuāgēsimus
80th. octōgēsimus
90th. nōnāgēsimus
100th. centēsimus
101st. { centēsimus prīmus, centēsimus et prīmus
102nd. { centēsimus secundus, centēsimus et secundus
200th. ducentēsimus
300th. trecentēsimus
400th. quadringentēsimus
500th. quīngentēsimus
600th. sēscentēsimus
700th. septimgentēsimus
800th. octingentēsimus
900th. nōngentēsimus
1,000th. mīllēsimus
2,000th. bis mīllēsimus
10,000th. deciēs mīllēsimus
100,000th. centiēs mīllēsimus

Prefixes and Suffixes

a-, an. Negative.
a-, ab-, abs-. Away from.
ad-, -ad. Toward.
-aemia. Blood.
aer-. Air.
-aesthesia. Sensation.
-algesia, algia. Suffering; pain.
algi-. Pain.
all-. Other.
amb-. Both; on both sides.
amph-. Around; on both sides.
ana-, an-. Up.
angio-. Relating to blood or lymph vessels.
ante-. Before.
anti-. Against.
apo-. From; opposed.
-ase. Enzyme.
aut-, auto-. Self.
bi, bis-. Twice; double.
brachy-. Short.
brady-. Slow.
cac-, caco-. Bad; evil.
cat, cata, cath-. Down.
-cele. A tumor; a cyst; a hernia.
cent-. Hundred.
cephal-. Relating to a head.
chrom-, chromo-. Color.
-cide. Causing death.
circum-. Around.
co, com, con-. Together.
contra-. Against.
cyst-, -cyst. Bag; bladder.
-cyte. A cell.
dacry-. Tears.
dactyl-. Fingers.
de-. From; not.
deca-. Ten.
deci-. Tenth.
demi-. Half.
dent-. Relating to the teeth.
derma-. The skin.
di-. Double; apart from.
dia-. Through; between; asunder.
dipla, diplo-. Double.
dis-. Negative; double; apart; absence of.
-dynia. Pain.
dys-. Difficult; bad.
ec, ecto-. Out; on the outside.
-ectomy. A cutting out.
ef, es, ex, exo-. Out
-emesis. Vomiting.
-emia. Blood.
en-. In, into.
endo-. Within.
entero-. Relating to the intestine.
ento-. Within.
epi-. Upon.
-esthesia. Sensation.
eu-. Well.
ex-, exo-. Out.
extra-. On the outside; beyond.
fore-. Before; in front of.
-form. Form.
-fuge. To drive away.
galact, galacto-. Milk.
gaster, gastro-. The stomach; the belly.
-gene, -genesis, -genetic, -genic. Production; origin; formation.
glosso-. Relating to the tongue.
-gog, gogue. To make flow.
-gram. A tracing; a mark.
-graphy. A writing; a record.
hem, hemato-. Relating to the blood.
hemi-. Half.
hepa-, hepar-, hepato-. Liver.
hetero-. Other; indicating dissimilarity.
holo-. All.

homo, homeo-. Same; similar.
hydra, hydro-. Relating to water.
hyp, hyph, hypo-. Under.
hyper-. Over; above; beyond.
hypo-. Under.
-iasis. Condition; pathological state.
idio-. Peculiar to the individual or organ.
ileo-. Relating to the ileum.
in-. In; into; not.
infra-. Beneath.
inter-. Between.
intra, intro-. Within.
-ism. Condition; theory.
iso-. Equal.
-itis. Inflammation.
-ize. To treat by special method.
juxta-. Near.
karyo-. Nucleus; nut.
kata-, kath-. Down.
kera-. Horn; indicates hardness.
kinesi-. Movement.
-kinesis. Motion.
lact-. Milk.
laparo-. The loin; relating to the loin or abdomen.
laryng, laryngo-. The larynx.
latero-. Side.
lepto-. Small; soft.
leuco, leuko-. White.
-lite, -lith. A stone; a calculus.
lith-. A stone.
-logia, -logy. Science of; study of.
-lysis. Setting free; disintegration.
macro-. Large; long; big.
mal-. Bad; poor; evil.
med-, medi-. Middle.
mega, megal-. Large; great.
-megalia or **megaly.** Large; great; extreme.
melan-, melano-. Black.
mes-, meso-. Middle.
meta-. Beyond; over; between; change, or transposition.
-meter. Measure.
metra, metro-. The uterus.
micro-. Small.
mio-. Less; smaller.
mono-. Single.
multi-. Many.
my, myo-. Muscle.
myel, myelo-. Marrow.
myxa, myxo-. Mucus.
neo-. New.
nephr, nephra, nephro-. Kidney.
neu, neuro-. Nerve.
niter, nitro-. Nitrogen.
non-, not-. No.
nucleo-. A nucleus.
ob-. Against.
oculo-. The eye.
-ode, oid. Form; shape; resemblance.
odont-. A tooth.
-oid. Form; shape; resemblance.
oligo-. Few.
-oma. A tumor.
omo-. Shoulder.
o-. An egg; ovum.
oophoron-. Ovary.
opisth-. Backward.
orchid-. Testicle.
ortho-. Straight; normal.
os-. A mouth; a bone.
-osis. Condition; disease; intensive.
oste, osteo-. A bone.
-ostomosis, ostomy. To furnish with a mouth or an outlet.
-otomy. Cutting.
oxy-. Sharp; acid.

Prefixes and Suffixes

pachy-. Thick.
pan-. All; entire.
para-. Alongside of.
path-, -path, -pathy. Disease; suffering.
-penia. Lack.
per-. Excessive; through.
peri-. Around.
-phobia. Fear.
-phylaxis. Protection.
-plasm. To mold.
-plastic. Molded; indicates restoration of lost or badly formed features.
-plegia. A stroke.
plur. More.
pneu-. Relating to the air or lungs.
poly-. Much; many.
post-. After.
pre-. Before.
pro-. Before; in behalf of.
proto-. First.
pseud, pseudo-. False.
psych-. The soul; the mind.
py-, pyo-. Pus.
re-. Back; again.
retro-. Backward.
-rhage, -rhagia. Hemorrhage; flow.
-rhaphy. A suturing or stitching.
-rhea. To flow; indicates discharge.
sacchar-. Sugar.
sacro-. Sacrum.
salping, salpingo-. A tube; relating to a fallopian tube.
sarco-. Flesh.
sclero-. Hard; relating to the sclera.
-sclerosis. Dryness; hardness.
-scopy. To see.
semi-. Half.
-stomosis, stormy. To furnish with a mouth or outlet.
sub-. Under.
super, supra-. Above.
syn-. With; together.
tele. Distant; far.
tetra-. Four.
thio-. Sulfur.
thyro-. Thyroid gland.
-tomy. Cutting.
trans-. Across.
tri-. Three.
tropho-. Relating to nutrition.
-trophic. Relating to nourishment.
uni-. One.
-uria. Relating to the urine.
urino, uro-. Relating to the urine or urinary organs.
vaso-. A vessel.
venter, ventro-. The abdomen.
xanth-. Yellow.

Anatomy and Physiology

Muscles of the Body with Their Action, Origin and Insertion

Number of muscles in the body, 659; 327 are in pairs and 5 are single muscles. Gray gives a total of 682; Dutton 652. Some authorities list as separate muscles what others regard as portions of adjacent muscles.

HEAD AND FACE (37 MUSCLES)

attolens aurem (ăt-ol'ĕnz aw'rĕm). ACTION: Elevates pinna (ear). ORIGIN: Occipitofrontalis aponeurosis. INSERTION: Pinna of ear superiorly. INNERVATION: Facial.

attrahens aurem (ăt'ra-hĕnz aw'rĕm). ACTION: Advances pinna (ear). ORIGIN: Lateral cranial aponeurosis. INSERTION: Helix of ear anteriorly. INNERVATION: Facial.

auricularis anterior (aw-rĭk"ū-lā'rĭs ăn-tēr'ĭ-or). SAME AS: *attrahens aurem*.

auricularis posterior (aw-rĭk"ū-lā'rĭs pŏs-tēr'ĭ-or). SAME AS: *retrahens aurem*.

auricularis superior (aw"rĭk"ū-lā'rĭs sū-pēr'ĭ-or). SAME AS: *attolens aurem*.

buccinator (bŭk'sĭn-ā"tor). ACTION: Compresses cheek, retracts angle of mouth. ORIGIN: Alveolar process of maxilla, pterygomaxillary ligament, buccinator ridge of mandible. INSERTION: Orbicularis oris. INNERVATION: Facial.

caninus (kā-nī'nŭs). SAME AS: *levator anguli oris*.

choroideus (kō-roy'dē-ŭs). SAME AS: *ciliaris*.

ciliaris (sĭl-ĭ-ā'rĭs). ACTION: Alters shape of crystalline lens in accommodation. ORIGIN: 1. *Longitudinal*: Junction of cornea and sclera. 2. *Circular*: Fibers forming a circle. INSERTION: 1. External layers of choroid. 2. Ciliary process. INNERVATION: Ciliary (oculomotor).

compressor narium (kŏm-prĕs'or nā'rĭ-ŭm). ACTION: Narrows nostril. ORIGIN: Nasal aponeurosis, superior maxilla above incisive fossa. INSERTION: Fellow muscle and canine fossa, fibrocartilage of nose. INNERVATION: Facial.

compressor narium minor (kŏm-prĕs'or nā'rĭ-ŭm mī'nor). ACTION: Narrows nostril. ORIGIN: Alar cartilage of nose. INSERTION: Skin at end of nose. INNERVATION: Facial.

compressor nasi (kŏm-prĕs'or nā'sī). SAME AS: *compressor narium*.

corrugator supercilii (kŏr'ū-gā-tor sū-pĕr-sĭl'ĭ-ī). ACTION: Draws eyebrows down and in. ORIGIN: Inner end of superciliary ridge of frontal bone. INSERTION: Orbicularis palpebrarum. INNERVATION: Facial.

depressor alae nasi (dē-prĕs'or ā'lē nā'sī). ACTION: Contracts nostril. ORIGIN: Incisive fossa of superior maxillary bone. INSERTION: Septum and ala of nose. INNERVATION: Facial.

depressor anguli oris (dē-prĕs'or ăng'ū-lī ō'rĭs). ACTION: Depresses angle of mouth. ORIGIN: External oblique line of mandible. INSERTION: Angle of mouth. INNERVATION: Facial.

depressor labii inferioris (dē-prĕs'or lā'bĭ-ī ĭn-fē'rĭ-ō-rĭs). ACTION: Depresses lower lip. ORIGIN: External oblique line of the mandible. INSERTION: Lower lip and orbicularis oris. INNERVATION: Facial.

dilator naris anterior (dī-lā'tor nā'rĭs ăn-tēr'ĭ-or). ACTION: Dilates apertures of

nostril. ORIGIN: Cartilage of ala of nose. INSERTION: Border of ala. INNERVATION: Facial.

dilator naris posterior (dī-lā'tor nā'rĭs pŏs-tēr'ĭ-or). ACTION: Dilates apertures of nostril. ORIGIN: Nasal notch of superior maxilla and the sesamoid cartilages. INSERTION: Integument of margin of nostril. INNERVATION: Infraorbital branch of facial.

epicranius (ĕp-ĭ-krā'nĭ-ŭs). ACTION: Moves scalp and wrinkles forehead. ORIGIN: Superior curved line of occiput and angular process of frontal bone. INSERTION: Aponeurosis which covers the vertex of skull. INNERVATION: Facial.

frontalis (frŏn-tā'lĭs). ACTION: Pulls scalp forward and wrinkles forehead. ORIGIN: Frontal bone above supraorbital line. INSERTION: Galea aponeurotica. INNERVATION: Facial.

levator anguli oris (lē-vā'tor ăng'ū-lī ō'rĭs). ACTION: Elevates angle of mouth. ORIGIN: Canine fossa of maxilla. INSERTION: Angle of mouth and orbicularis oris. INNERVATION: Facial.

levator labii inferioris (lē-vā'tor lā'bĭ-ī ĭn-fē'rĭ-ō'rĭs). ACTION: Elevates lower lip and wrinkles skin of chin. ORIGIN: Incisive fossa of mandible. INSERTION: Integument of chin or lower lip. INNERVATION: Facial.

levator labii superioris (lē-vā'tor lā'bĭ-ī sū-pē"rĭ-ō'rĭs). ACTION: Elevates and extends upper lip. ORIGIN: Lower margin of orbit, malar bone. INSERTION: Upper lip. INNERVATION: Facial; infraorbital branch.

levator labii superioris alaeque nasi (lē-vā'tor lā'bĭ-ī sū-pē"rĭ-ō'rĭs ā-lē'kwē nā'sī). ACTION: Elevates upper lip, dilates nostril. ORIGIN: Nasal process of maxilla. INSERTION: Cartilage of ala of nose and upper lip. INNERVATION: Facial; infraorbital branch.

levator menti (lē-vā'tor mĕn'tī). SAME AS: *levator labii inferioris*.

levator palpebrae superioris (lē-vā'tor păl'pē-brē sū-pē"rĭ-ō'rĭs). ACTION: Raises upper eyelid. ORIGIN: Lesser wing of the sphenoid bone. INSERTION: Upper tarsal cartilage. INNERVATION: Oculomotor.

masseter (mă-sē'ter). ACTION: Mastication. ORIGIN: Zygomatic arch and malar process of superior maxilla. INSERTION: Angle, ramus, and coronoid process of mandible. INNERVATION: Trigeminal; mandibular branch.

mentalis (mĕn-tā'lĭs). SAME AS: *levator labii inferioris*.

nasalis (nā-sā'lĭs). SAME AS: *compressor narium and depressor alae nasi*.

obliquus inferior (ŏb-lī'kwŭs ĭn-fē'rĭ-or). ACTION: Rotates eyeball up and out. ORIGIN: Orbital plate of superior maxillary bone. INSERTION: Sclerotic coat at right angles to insertion of rectus externus just below it. INNERVATION: Oculomotor.

App. 34

Muscles of the Body

obliquus superior (ŏb-lĭ'kwŭs sū-pē'rĭ-or). ACTION: Rotates eyeball down and out. ORIGIN: Above optic foramen. INSERTION: By a tendon through trochlea to the sclerotic coat. INNERVATION: Trochlear.

occipitalis (ŏk-sĭp"ĭ-tā'lĭs). ACTION: Draws scalp back. ORIGIN: Superior curved line of occipital bone. INSERTION: Galea aponeurotica. INNERVATION: Facial.

occipitofrontalis (ŏk-sĭp"ĭ-tō-frŏn-tā'lĭs). SAME AS: *epicranius*.

orbicularis oculi (or-bĭk"ū-lā'rĭs ŏk'ū-lī). ACTION: Closes eyelid, wrinkles forehead vertically, compresses lacrimal sac. ORIGIN: 1. (*Pars lacrimalis*.) Lacrimal bone. 2. (*Pars orbitalis*.) Frontal processes of maxilla and frontal bone. 3. (*Pars palpebralis*.) Inner canthus. INSERTION: 1. Joins palpebral portion. 2. Encircles orbit to orbit. 3. Outer canthus. INNERVATION: Facial.

orbicularis oris (or-bĭk"ū-lā'rĭs ō'rĭs). ACTION: Closes mouth. ORIGIN: Nasal septum and canine fossa of mandible by accessory fibers. INSERTION: Buccinator and adjacent muscles surrounding mouth. INNERVATION: Facial.

orbicularis palpebrarum (or-bĭk"ū-lā'rĭs păl-pē-brā'rŭm). SAME AS: *orbicularis oculi* (*Pars palpebralis*).

orbitalis (or-bĭ-tā'lĭs). A rudimentary muscle crossing the infraorbital groove and sphenomaxillary fissure, united with periosteum of the orbit.

orbitopalpebralis (or"bĭ-tō-păl"pē-brā'lĭs). SAME AS: *levator palpebrae superioris*.

procerus (prō-sē'rŭs). SAME AS: *pyramidalis nasi*.

pterygoideus externus (tĕr-ĭ-goyd"ē-ŭs ĕkster'nŭs). ACTION: Brings jaw forward. ORIGIN: 1. Outer plate of pterygoid, palate bone, tuberosity of maxilla. 2. Great wing of sphenoid. INSERTION: Neck of condyle of mandible. INNERVATION: External pterygoid from trigeminus.

pterygoideus internus (tĕr-ĭ-goyd'ē-ŭs ĭnter'nŭs). ACTION: Closes jaw by raising and advancing it. ORIGIN: Pterygoid fossa of sphenoid bone. INSERTION: Inner surface of angle of mandible. INNERVATION: Internal pterygoid from trigeminus.

pyramidalis nasi (pĭ-răm"ĭ-dā'lĭs nā'sī). ACTION: Draws skin of forehead down. ORIGIN: Bridge of nose. INSERTION: Skin over root of nose. INNERVATION: Facial.

quadratus labii inferioris (kwăd-rā'tŭs lā'bĭ-ī ĭn-fē"rĭ-ō'rĭs). SAME AS: *depressor labii inferioris*.

quadratus labii superioris (kwăd-rā-tŭs lā'bĭ-ī sū-pēr"ĭ-ō'rĭs). Composed of *levator labii superioris alaeque nasi*, *levator labii superioris*, *zygomaticus minor*.

quadratus menti (kwăd-rā'tŭs mĕn'tī). SAME AS: *quadratus labii inferioris*.

rectus externus or **lateralis** (rĕk'tŭs ĕkster'nŭs, lăt-ĕr-ā'lĭs). ACTION: Rotates eyeball outward. ORIGIN: Margin of sphenoidal fissure and outer margin of optic foramen. INSERTION: Sclerotic coat. INNERVATION: Abducens.

rectus inferior (rĕk'tŭs ĭn-fē'rĭ-or). ACTION: Rotates eyeball downward. ORIGIN: Lower margin of optic foramen. INSERTION: Sclerotic coat. INNERVATION: Oculomotor.

rectus internus or **medialis** (rĕk'tŭs ĭnter'nŭs, mē-dĭ-ā'lĭs). ACTION: Rotates eyeball inward. ORIGIN: Lower margin of optic foramen. INSERTION: Sclerotic coat. INNERVATION: Oculomotor.

rectus superior (rĕk'tŭs sū-pē'rĭ-or). ACTION: Rotates eyeball upward. ORIGIN: Upper margin of optic foramen. INSERTION: Sclerotic coat. INNERVATION: Oculomotor.

retrahens aurem (rĕt'ră-hĕns aw'rĕm). ACTION: Retracts pinna (ear). ORIGIN: Mastoid process of temporal bone. INSERTION: Root of auricle. INNERVATION: Facial.

risorius (rĭ-sō'rĭ-ŭs) (*laughing muscle*). ACTION: Draws angle of mouth outward and compresses cheek. ORIGIN: Fascia over masseter muscle. INSERTION: Angle of mouth. INNERVATION: Facial; buccal branch.

Santorini's (săn-tō-rĭ'nĭs). SAME AS: *risorius*.

temporalis (tĕm-pō-rā'lĭs). ACTION: Mastication. ORIGIN: Temporal fossa and temporal fascia. INSERTION: Coronoid process of lower jaw. INNERVATION: Trigeminal; mandibular branch.

tensor tarsi (tĕn'sor tar'sī). ACTION: Compresses puncta and lacrimal sac. ORIGIN: Crest of the lacrimal bone. INSERTION: The tarsal cartilages of the eye by 2 slips. INNERVATION: Facial.

triangularis (trī-ăng"gū-lā'rĭs). SAME AS: *depressor anguli oris*.

zygomaticus major (zī-gō-măt'ĭ-kŭs mā'jor). ACTION: Draws upper lip backward, upward and outward. ORIGIN: Malar bone, zygomatic arch. INSERTION: Angle of mouth. INNERVATION: Facial.

zygomaticus minor (zī-gō-măt'ĭ-kŭs mī'nor). ACTION: Draws the upper lip up and out. ORIGIN: Malar bone behind the maxillary arch. INSERTION: Angle of mouth, orbicularis oris. INNERVATION: Facial.

EAR (9)

helicis major and minor (hĕl'ĭ-sĭs mā'jŏr, mī'nŏr). ACTION: Tighten the skin of auditory canal. ORIGIN: Tuberosity on helix. INSERTION: Rim of helix. INNERVATION: Auriculotemporal and posterior auricular.

incisurae helicis or **santorini** (ĭn-sī-zū'rē hĕl'ĭ-sĭs, săn-tō-rĭ'nĭ). SAME AS: *intertragicus*.

intertragicus (ĭn"tĕr-trā'jĭ-kŭs). ACTION: Dilates concha. ORIGIN: Anterior part of cartilaginous canal of ear. INSERTION: Opposite side at larger auricular fissure. INNERVATION: Posterior auricular.

laxator tympani major (lăks-ā'tor tĭm'păn-ī mā'jor). ACTION: (Not muscular.) Probably helps to relax membrana tympani. ORIGIN: Spinous process of sphenoid and cartilaginous eustachian tube. INSERTION: Neck of malleus. INNERVATION: Tympanic.

laxator tympani minor (lăks-ā'tor tĭm'păn-ī mī'nor). ACTION: (Not muscular.) Probably helps to relax membrana tympani. ORIGIN: Back of external meatus (ligamentum mallei posticum to some anatomists). INSERTION: Handle of malleus and processus brevis. INNERVATION: Tympanic.

obliquus auriculae (ŏb-lĭ'kwŭs aw-rĭk'ū-lē). ORIGIN: Conch of the ear. INSERTION: Fossa of antihelix. INNERVATION: Auricular and temporal.

stapedius (stă-pē'dĭ-ŭs). ACTION: Depress base of the stapes. ORIGIN: Interior of pyramid. INSERTION: Into neck of stapes. INNERVATION: Facial; tympanic branch.

tensor tympani (tĕn'sor tĭm'păn-ī). ACTION: To draw the membrana tympani tense. ORIGIN: Temporal tube, eustachian tube and canal. INSERTION: Handle of malleus. INNERVATION: Otic ganglion.

tragicus (trā'jĭ-kŭs). ORIGIN: Outer part

of tragus. INSERTION: Outer portion of tragus. INNERVATION: Temporal and posterior auricular.
transversus auriculae (trăns-vĕr'sŭs aw-rĭk'ū-lē). ACTION: Retracts helix. ORIGIN: Cranial surface of auricle. INSERTION: Circumference of pinna. INNERVATION: Auricularis magnus and posterior auricular.

NECK (32)

amygdaloglossus (ăm-ĭg″dă-lō-glŏs'ŭs). ACTION: Lifts edge of tongue. ORIGIN: Pharyngeal aponeurosis over tonsil. INSERTION: Continuous with palatoglossus.
azygos uvulae (ăz'ĭ-gŏs ū'vū-lē). SAME AS: *uvulae.*
cephalopharyngeus (sĕf″ă-lō-făr-ĭn-jē'ŭs). SAME AS: *constrictor pharyngis superior.*
circumflexus palati (sĭr-kŭm-flĕks'ŭs păl-ā'tī). SAME AS: *tensor veli palatini.*
constrictor isthmi faucium (kŏn-strĭk'tor ĭs'mī fo'shĭ-ŭm). SAME AS: *glossopalatinus.*
constrictor pharyngis inferior (kŏn-strĭk'-tor făr-ĭn'gĭs ĭn-fēr'ĭ-ŏr). ACTION: Narrows the pharynx, as in swallowing. ORIGIN: Sides of cricoid and thyroid cartilages. INSERTION: Posterior of pharyngeal wall. INNERVATION: Pharyngeal plexus.
constrictor pharyngis medius (kŏn-strĭk'tor făr-ĭn'gĭs mē'dĭ-ŭs). ACTION: Narrows pharynx, as in swallowing. ORIGIN: Both cornua of hyoid bone and stylohyoid ligament. INSERTION: Middle of posterior pharyngeal wall. INNERVATION: Pharyngeal plexus.
constrictor pharyngis superior (kŏn-strĭk'-tor făr-ĭn'gĭs sū-pēr'ĭ-ŏr). ACTION: Narrows pharynx, as in swallowing. ORIGIN: Internal pterygoid plate, pterygomandibular ligament, jaw, side of tongue. INSERTION: Posterior pharyngeal wall. INNERVATION: Pharyngeal plexus.
digastricus (dī-găs'trĭ-kŭs) *(anterior).* ACTION: Depresses jaw. ORIGIN: Inferior maxillary near symphysis. INSERTION: Lower border of mandible. INNERVATION: Mylohyoid branch from 3rd division of trigeminus.
digastricus (dī-găs'trĭk-ŭs) *(posterior).* ACTION: Elevates and helps to fix hyoid. ORIGIN: Digastric groove of mastoid. INSERTION: Lower border of mandible by anterior belly. INNERVATION: Facial.
genioglossus (jē-nī″ō-glŏs'ŭs). ACTION: Protrudes and retracts tongue, elevates hyoid. ORIGIN: Mental spine of inferior maxilla. INSERTION: Hyoid and bottom of tongue. INNERVATION: Hypoglossal.
geniohyoglossus (jē-nī″ō-hī″ō-glŏs'ŭs). SAME AS: *genioglossus.*
geniohyoideus (jē-nī″ō-hī-oyd'ē-ŭs). ACTION: Elevates and advances hyoid and helps to depress jaw. ORIGIN: Mental spine of inferior maxilla. INSERTION: Hyoid. INNERVATION: Hypoglossal.
glossopalatinus (glŏs″ō-păl-ă-tī'nŭs). ACTION: Elevates back of tongue and constricts fauces. ORIGIN: Undersurface of soft palate. INSERTION: Side of tongue. INNERVATION: Pharyngeal plexus.
hyoglossus (hī″ō-glŏs'ŭs). ACTION: Depresses side of tongue and retracts tongue. ORIGIN: Cornua and body of hyoid. INSERTION: Side of tongue. INNERVATION: Hypoglossal.
hyopharyngeus (hī″ō-făr-ĭn-jē'ŭs). SAME AS: *constrictor pharyngis medius.*
laryngopharyngeus (lăr-ĭn″gō-făr-ĭn-jē'-ŭs). SAME AS: *constrictor pharyngis inferior.*
latissimus colli (lăt-ĭs′ĭ-mŭs kŏlī). SAME AS: *platysma.*

levator palati (lē-vā'tor păl'ă-tī). SAME AS: *levator veli palatini.*
levator veli palatini (lē-vā'tor vē'lī păl″ă-tī'nī). ACTION: Elevates soft palate. ORIGIN: Petrous portion of temporal bone and cartilaginous eustachian tube. INSERTION: Aponeurosis of soft palate. INNERVATION: Pharyngeal plexus.
lingualis (lĭng-gwā'lĭs). ACTION: Elevates sides and center of tongue. ORIGIN: Undersurface of tongue. INSERTION: Edge of tongue. INNERVATION: Hypoglossal.
longus capitis (lŏng'ŭs kăp'ĭ-tĭs). ACTION: Twists or bends the neck. ORIGIN: Transverse processes of 3rd to 6th cervical vertebrae. INSERTION: Occipital bone, basilar process. INNERVATION: Cervical plexus.
longus cervicis (lŏng'ŭs sĕr'vī-sĭs). SAME AS: *longus colli.*
longus colli (lŏng'ŭs kŏl'ī). ACTION: Twists and bends neck forward. ORIGIN: 3 parts: 1. Transverse processes of 3rd to 5th cervical vertebrae. 2. Bodies of 1st to 3rd dorsal vertebrae. 3. Bodies of 3rd dorsal to 5th cervical vertebrae. INSERTION: 1. Anterior tubercle of atlas. 2. Transverse processes of 5th and 6th cervical vertebrae. 3. Bodies of 2nd to 4th cervical vertebrae. INNERVATION: Anterior cervical.
mylohyoideus (mī″lō-hī-oyd'ē-ŭs). ACTION: Elevates floor of mouth and hyoid, depresses jaw. ORIGIN: Mylohyoid line of mandible. INSERTION: Body of hyoid and raphe. INNERVATION: Mylohyoid from 3rd division of trigeminus.
omohyoideus (ō″mō-hī-oyd'ē-ŭs). ACTION: Depresses hyoid. ORIGIN: Upper border of scapula. INSERTION: Hyoid bone. INNERVATION: Upper cervical through ansa hypoglossi.
palatoglossus (păl″ă-tō-glŏs'ŭs). SAME AS: *glossopalatinus.*
palatopharyngeus (păl″ă-tō-făr-ĭn-jē'ŭs). SAME AS: *pharyngopalatinus.*
pharyngopalatinus (făr-ĭng″gō-păl-ă-tī'-nŭs). ACTION: Narrows fauces and shuts off nasopharynx. ORIGIN: Soft palate. INSERTION: Thyroid cartilage and aponeurosis of the pharynx. INNERVATION: Pharyngeal plexus.
platysma (myoides) (plă-tĭz'mă mī-oyd'-ēs). ACTION: Wrinkles skin of neck and chest; depresses jaw and lower lip. ORIGIN: Clavicle, acromion and fascia over deltoid, and pectoralis major. INSERTION: Lower border of mandible, risorius and opposite platysma. INNERVATION: Cervical branch of facial.
rectus capitis anterior (rĕk'tŭs kăp'ĭ-tĭs ăn-tēr'ĭ-or). ACTION: Turns and inclines the head. ORIGIN: Base of atlas. INSERTION: Occipital bone, basilar process. INNERVATION: First and 2nd cervical.
rectus capitis anticus major (rĕk'tŭs kăp'ĭ-tĭs ăn-tī'kŭs mā'jor). SAME AS: *longus capitis.*
rectus capitis anticus minor (rĕk'tŭs kăp'ĭ-tĭs ăn-tī'kŭs mī'nor). SAME AS: *rectus capitis anterior.*
rectus capitis lateralis (rĕk'tŭs kăp'ĭ-tĭs lătĕr-ā'lĭs). ACTION: Inclines head laterally and supports it. ORIGIN: Transverse process of atlas. INSERTION: Jugular process of occipital bone. INNERVATION: Suboccipital.
salpingopharyngeus (săl-pĭn″gō-făr-ĭn-jē'-ŭs). ACTION: Elevates nasopharynx. ORIGIN: Eustachian tube close to nasopharynx. INSERTION: Posterior portion of the palatopharyngeus. INNERVATION: Internal spinal accessory.
scalenus anterior (anticus) (skā-lē'nŭs ăn-

tĕr'ĭ-or). ACTION: Elevates 1st rib. ORIGIN: Transverse processes of 3rd to 6th cervical vertebrae. INSERTION: Tubercle of 1st rib. INNERVATION: Cervical plexus.
scalenus medius (skā-lē'nŭs mē'dĭ-ŭs). ACTION: Elevates 1st rib. ORIGIN: Transverse processes of 2nd to 6th cervical vertebrae. INSERTION: First rib. INNERVATION: Cervical plexus.
scalenus posterior (posticus) (skā-lē'nŭs pŏs-tĕr'ĭ-ŏr). ACTION: Elevates 2nd rib. ORIGIN: Transverse processes of 4th to 6th cervical vertebrae. INSERTION: Second rib. INNERVATION: Cervical and brachial plexus.
sphenosalpingostaphylinus (sfē"nō-săl-pĭn"- gō-stăf-ĭ-lī'nŭs). SAME AS: *tensor veli palatini*.
sternocleidomastoideus (stĕr"nō-klī-dō- măs-toyd'ē-ŭs). ACTION: Rotates and depresses head. ORIGIN: By 2 heads, from sternum and clavicle. INSERTION: Mastoid process and outer part of superior curved line of occipital bone. INNERVATION: Spinal accessory.
sternohyoideus (stĕr"nō-hī-oyd'ē-ŭs). ACTION: Depresses hyoid bone. ORIGIN: Manubrium sterni and 1st costal cartilage. INSERTION: Body of hyoid bone. INNERVATION: Upper cervical through ansa hypoglossi.
sternomastoideus (stĕr"nō-măs-toyd'ē-ŭs). SAME AS: *sternocleidomastoideus*.
sternothyroideus (stĕr"nō-thī-royd'ē-ŭs). ACTION: Depresses larynx. ORIGIN: Sternum and 1st costal cartilage. INSERTION: Side of thyroid cartilage. INNERVATION: Upper cervical through ansa hypoglossi.
styloglossus (stī"lō-glŏs'ŭs). ACTION: Retracts and elevates tongue. ORIGIN: Styloid process. INSERTION: Side of tongue. INNERVATION: Hypoglossal.
stylohyoideus (stī"lō-hī-oyd'ē-ŭs). ACTION: Fixes hyoid, drawing it up and back. ORIGIN: Styloid process. INSERTION: Body of hyoid bone. INNERVATION: Facial.
stylopharyngeus (stī"lō-făr-ĭn-jē'ŭs). ACTION: Elevates and dilates pharynx. ORIGIN: Styloid process. INSERTION: Thyroid cartilage and side of pharynx. INNERVATION: Glossopharyngeal.
tensor palati (tĕn'sŏr păl-ā'tī). SAME AS: *tensor veli palatini*.
tensor veli palatini (tĕn'sŏr vē'lī păl"ă-tī'- nī). ACTION: Stretches soft palate. ORIGIN: Spine of sphenoid, scaphoid fossa of internal pterygoid process and eustachian tube. INSERTION: Posterior border of hard palate and aponeurosis of soft palate. INNERVATION: Otic ganglion.
tetragonus (tĕt-ră-gō'nŭs). SAME AS: *platysma*.
thyrohyoideus (thī-rō-hī-oyd'ē-ŭs). ACTION: Elevates larynx. ORIGIN: Side of thyroid cartilage. INSERTION: Cornu and body of hyoid bone. INNERVATION: Hypoglossal.
uvulae (ū'vū-lē). ACTION: Elevates the uvula. ORIGIN: Posterior nasal spine. INSERTION: Forms large part of uvula. INNERVATION: Pharyngeal plexus.

LARYNX AND EPIGLOTTIS (8)

aryteno-epiglottideus inferior (ăr-ĭ-tē"nō- ĕp-ĭ-glŏt-ĭd'ē-ŭs ĭn-fēr'ĭ-or). ACTION: Compresses sacculus laryngis. ORIGIN: Arytenoid cartilage. INSERTION: Epiglottis, anterior. INNERVATION: Recurrent laryngeal.
aryteno-epiglottideus superior (ăr-ĭ-tē"nō- ĕp-ĭ-glŏt-ĭd'ē-ŭs sū-pēr'ĭ-or). ACTION: Narrows laryngeal opening. ORIGIN: Tip of arytenoid cartilage. INSERTION: Aryteno-epiglottidean folds. INNERVATION: Recurrent laryngeal.
arytenoideus (ăr-ĭ-tē-noyd'ē-ŭs). ACTION: Narrows rima glottidis. ORIGIN: Base of arytenoid cartilage. INSERTION: Apex of opposite arytenoid cartilage. INNERVATION: Recurrent laryngeal.
crico-arytenoideus lateralis (krī"kō-ăr-ĭ- tē-noyd'ē-ŭs lăt-ĕr-ā'lĭs). ACTION: Narrows glottis. ORIGIN: Upper border of arch of cricoid cartilage. INSERTION: Muscular process of arytenoid. INNERVATION: Recurrent laryngeal.
crico-arytenoideus posterior (posticus) (krī"kō-ăr-ĭ-tē-noyd'ē-ŭs pŏs-tĕr'ĭ-or). ACTION: Opens glottis. ORIGIN: Back of cricoid cartilage. INSERTION: Muscular process of arytenoid. INNERVATION: Recurrent laryngeal.
cricothyroideus (krī"kō-thī-royd'ē-ŭs). ACTION: Tightens vocal cords. ORIGIN: Anterior surface of cricoid cartilage. INSERTION: Thyroid cartilage. INNERVATION: Superior laryngeal.
thyro-arytenoideus (thī"rō-ăr-ĭ-tē-noyd'- ē-ŭs). ACTION: Relaxes vocal cords. ORIGIN: Thyroid cartilage. INSERTION: Arytenoid cartilage. INNERVATION: Recurrent laryngeal.
thyro-epiglotticus (thī"rō-ĕp-ĭ-glŏt'ĭk-ŭs). ACTION: Depresses epiglottis. ORIGIN: Thyroid cartilage. INSERTION: Epiglottis and sacculus laryngis. INNERVATION: Recurrent laryngeal.

BACK (83)

accessorius ad sacrolumbalem (ăk"sĕs-sō'- rĭ-ŭs ăd să"crō-lŭm-bā'lĕm). SAME AS: *iliocostalis dorsi*.
biventer cervicis (bī-vĕn'ter sĕr'vĭ-sĭs). SAME AS: *spinalis capitis*.
cervicalis ascendens (sĕr-vĭ-kā'lĭs ă-sĕn'- dĕns). SAME AS: *iliocostalis cervicis*.
complexus (kŏm-plĕks'ŭs). SAME AS: *semispinalis capitis*.
erector spinae (ē-rĕk'tor spī'nē). SAME AS: *sacrospinalis*.
extensor coccygis (ĕks-tĕn'sor kŏks-ĭj'ĭs). ACTION: Extends coccyx. ORIGIN: Last segment of sacrum. INSERTION: Tip of coccyx. INNERVATION: Sacral branches.
iliocostalis cervicis (ĭl"ĭ-ō-kŏs-tā'lĭs sĕr'- vĭ-sĭs). ACTION: Extends cervical spine. ORIGIN: Angle of middle and upper ribs. INSERTION: Middle cervical vertebra. INNERVATION: Branches of cervical.
iliocostalis dorsi (ĭl"ĭ-ō-kŏs-tā'lĭs dor'sī). ACTION: Keeps dorsal spine erect. ORIGIN: Angles of 12th to 7th ribs. INSERTION: Sixth to 1st ribs and 7th cervical vertebra. INNERVATION: Branches of dorsal.
iliocostalis lumborum (ĭl"ĭ-ō-kŏs-tā'lĭs lŭm- bō'rŭm). ACTION: Extends lumbar spine. ORIGIN: With sacrospinalis. INSERTION: In angles of 5th to 12th ribs. INNERVATION: Branches of dorsal and lumbar.
interspinalis (ĭn"tĕr-spī-nā'lĭs). A series. ACTION: Supports and extends vertebral column. ORIGIN: Undersurface of spine of 1 vertebra. INSERTION: Spine of vertebra above. INNERVATION: Branches of spinal.
intertransversalis (ĭn-tĕr-trăns-vĕr-sā'lĭs). (4 sets.) ACTION: Supports and flexes vertebral column. ORIGIN: Between transverse processes of contiguous vertebrae. INNERVATION: Posterior branches of spinal.
intertransversarius (ĭn"tĕr-trăns-vĕr-sā'- rĭ-ŭs). SAME AS: *intertransversalis*.
latissimus dorsi (lăt-ĭs'ĭ-mŭs dor'sī). ACTION: Adducts and rotates arm. ORIGIN: Lower thoracic and lumbar vertebrae, sacrum and tip of iliac crest. INSER-

TION: Bicipital groove of humerus. INNERVATION: Brachial plexus.
levator (anguli) scapulae (lē-vā′tor ăng′ū-lī skăp′ū-lē). ACTION: Elevates posterior angle of scapula. ORIGIN: Transverse processes of 4 upper cervical vertebrae. INSERTION: Superior edge of scapula. INNERVATION: Dorsal scapular from bronchial plexus.
longissimus capitis (lŏn-jĭs′ĭ-mŭs kăp′ĭ-tĭs). ACTION: Keeps head erect, draws it backward or to 1 side. ORIGIN: Upper thoracic and lower and middle cervical vertebrae. INSERTION: Mastoid process. INNERVATION: Branches of cervical.
longissimus cervicis (lŏn-jĭs′ĭ-mŭs sĕr′vĭ-sĭs). ACTION: Extends cervical spine. ORIGIN: Upper thoracic vertebrae. INSERTION: Ribs and upper lumbar and thoracic vertebrae. INNERVATION: Lower cervical and upper dorsal.
longissimus dorsi (lŏn-jĭs′ĭ-mŭs (dor′sī). ACTION: Extends spinal column. ORIGIN: Transverse processes of lumbar and dorsal vertebrae. INSERTION: Lowest ribs and lumbar and dorsal vertebrae. INNERVATION: Lumbar and dorsal.
multifidus (mŭl-tĭf′ĭd-ŭs). ACTION: Rotates spinal column. ORIGIN: Sacrum, iliac spine, lumbar, cervical, and dorsal vertebrae. INSERTION: Laminae and spinous processes of next 4 vertebrae above. INNERVATION: Posterior spinal branches.
multifidus spinae (mŭl-tĭf′ĭd-ŭs spī′nē). SAME AS: *multifidus*.
obliquus capitis inferior (ŏb-lī′kwŭs kăp′ĭ-tĭs ĭn-fēr′ĭ-or). ACTION: Rotates head. ORIGIN: Spine of axis. INSERTION: Transverse process of atlas. INNERVATION: Suboccipital.
obliquus capitis superior (ŏb-lī′kwŭs kăp′ĭ-tĭs sū-pēr′ĭ-or). ACTION: Rotates head. ORIGIN: Transverse process of atlas. INSERTION: Occipital bone. INNERVATION: Suboccipital.
rectus capitis posterior (posticus) major (rĕk′tŭs kăp′ĭ-tĭs pŏs-tēr′ĭ-or mā′jor). ACTION: Rotates and draws head backward. ORIGIN: Spine of axis. INSERTION: Inferior curved line of occipital bone. INNERVATION: Suboccipital.
rectus capitis posterior (posticus) minor (rĕk′tŭs kăp′ĭ-tĭs pŏs-tēr′ĭ-or mī′nor). ACTION: Rotates and draws head backward. ORIGIN: Posterior tubercle of atlas. INSERTION: Inferior curved line of occipital bone. INNERVATION: Suboccipital.
rhomboideus major (rŏm-boy′dē-ŭs mā′jor). ACTION: Elevates scapula. ORIGIN: Spinous processes of first 4 or 5 thoracic vertebrae. INSERTION: Vertebral border of scapula below spine. INNERVATION: Dorsal scapular.
rhomboideus minor (rŏm-boy′dē-ŭs mī′nor). ACTION: Retracts and elevates scapula. ORIGIN: Spinous processes of 6th and 7th cervical vertebrae and 1st thoracic vertebra. INSERTION: Border of scapula above spine. INNERVATION: Dorsal scapular.
rotator spinae (rō-tā′tor spī′nē). ACTION: Rotates the vertebral column. ORIGIN: Transverse processes of 2nd to 12th dorsal vertebrae. INSERTION: Lamina of next vertebra above. INNERVATION: Posterior branches of spinal.
sacrococcygeus posticus (sā′krō-kŏk-sĭj′ē-ŭs pŏs-tī′kŭs). SAME AS: *extensor coccygis*.
sacrolumbalis (sā′krō-lŭm-bā′lĭs). SAME AS: *iliocostalis lumborum*.
sacrospinalis (sā′krō-spī-nā′lĭs). ACTION: Extends vertebral column. ORIGIN: Sacrum, lumbar vertebrae, iliac crest. INSERTION: Iliocostalis and longissimus dorsi. INNERVATION: Posterior branches of spinal.
semispinalis capitis (sĕm″ĭ-spī-nā′lĭs kăp′ĭ-tĭs). ACTION: Rotates and draws head backward. ORIGIN: Transverse processes of upper 5 or 6 thoracic and lower 4 cervical vertebrae. INSERTION: Occipital bone, between inferior and superior curved line. INNERVATION: Suboccipital and branches of cervical.
semispinalis cervicis (sĕm″ĭ-spī-nā′lĭs sŭr′vĭ-sĭs). ACTION: Erects cervical spine. ORIGIN: Transverse processes of 2nd to 5th cervical vertebrae. INSERTION: Spines of 2nd to 5th cervical vertebrae. INNERVATION: Cervical branches.
semispinalis colli (sĕm″ĭ-spī-nā′lĭs kŏ′lī). SAME AS: *semispinalis cervicis*.
semispinalis dorsi (sĕm″ĭ-spī-nā′lĭs dor′sī). ACTION: Erects vertebral column. ORIGIN: Transverse processes of 5th to 11th dorsal vertebrae. INSERTION: Spines of first 4 dorsal and 6th and 7th cervical vertebrae. INNERVATION: Brs. of dorsal.
semispinalis thoracis (sĕm″ĭ-spī-nā′lĭs thō-rā′sĭs). SAME AS: *semispinalis dorsi*.
serratus posterior (posticus) inferior (sĕr-ā′tŭs pŏs-tēr′ĭ-or ĭn-fēr′ĭ-or). ACTION: Draws ribs back and downward. ORIGIN: Spines of 2 lower thoracic and 2 upper lumbar vertebrae. INSERTION: Last 4 ribs. INNERVATION: Intercostal.
serratus posterior (posticus) superior (sĕr-ā′tŭs pŏs-tēr′ĭ-or sū-pēr′ĭ-or). ACTION: Possibly elevates the ribs. ORIGIN: Spines of 2 lower cervical and 2 upper thoracic vertebrae. INSERTION: Angles of 2nd to 5th ribs. INNERVATION: Intercostal.
spinalis capitis (spī-nā′lĭs kăp′ĭ-tĭs). ORIGIN: Inconstant; from spines of upper dorsal and lower cervical vertebrae. INSERTION: Blends with the semispinalis capitis.
spinalis cervicis (spī-nā′lĭs sĕr′vĭ-sĭs). ACTION: Extends cervical spine. ORIGIN: Spines of 5th, 6th, and 7th cervical vertebrae. INSERTION: Third and 4th cervical vertebrae. INNERVATION: Branches of cervical.
spinalis dorsi (spī-nā′lĭs dor′sī). ACTION: Erects spinal column. ORIGIN: Spines of first 2 lumbar and last 2 thoracic vertebrae. INSERTION: Spines of middle and upper thoracic vertebrae. INNERVATION: Dorsal branches.
splenius capitis (splē′nĭ-us kăp′ĭ-tĭs). ACTION: Rotates and extends head. ORIGIN: Ligamentum nuchae, 7th cervical and first 3 dorsal vertebrae. INSERTION: Mastoid process and superior curved line of occiput. INNERVATION: Cervical.
splenius cervicis (splē′nĭ-us sĕr′vĭ-sĭs). ACTION: Rotates and flexes head and neck. ORIGIN: Spines of 3rd to 5th cervical. INSERTION: Transverse processes of 1st and 2nd cervical vertebrae. INNERVATION: Cervical.
splenius colli (splē′nĭ-us kŏl′ī). SAME AS: *splenius cervicis*.
supraspinalis (sū-prā-spī-nā′lĭs). Series. ACTION: Help support head and neck. ORIGIN: Apex of spines in cervical area. INSERTION: To similar summits. INNERVATION: Cervical branches.
suspensorius duodeni (sŭs-pĕn-sō′rĭ-ŭs dū″ō-dē′nī). Wide, flat band of unstriped muscle attached to the left crus of diaphragm and continuous with the muscular coat of the duodenum at its point of junction with the jejunum.
trachelomastoid (trā″kĕ-lō-măs′toyd). SAME AS: *longissimus capitis*.

Muscles of the Body

transversalis colli (trăns″vĕr-sā′lĭs kŏl′ī). SAME AS: *longissimus cervicis*.
trapezius (tră-pē′zĭ-ŭs). ACTION: Draws head back and to the side, rotates scapula. ORIGIN: Superior curved line of occipital, spinous processes of last cervical and all dorsal vertebrae. INSERTION: Clavicle, acromion, base of spine of scapula. INNERVATION: Spinal accessory and cervical plexus.

ABDOMEN (8)

cremaster (krē-măs′tĕr). ACTION: Raises testicle. ORIGIN: Midportion of Poupart's ligament. INSERTION: Cremasteric fascia and pubic bone. INNERVATION: Genitocrural.
obliquus externus abdominis (ŏb-lī′kwŭs ĕks-tĕr′nŭs ăb-dŏm′ĭ-nĭs). ACTION: Contracts abdomen and viscera. ORIGIN: Lower 8 ribs. INSERTION: Iliac crest, Poupart's ligament, linea alba, pubic crest. INNERVATION: Lower thoracic.
obliquus internus abdominis (ŏb-lī′kwŭs in-tĕr′nŭs ăb-dŏm′ĭ-nĭs). ACTION: Compresses viscera, flexes thorax forward. ORIGIN: Iliac crest, Poupart's ligament, lumbar fascia. INSERTION: Few lowest ribs, linea alba, pubic crest. INNERVATION: Lower thoracic.
pyramidalis (pĭ-răm-ĭ-dā′lĭs). ACTION: Tightens linea alba. ORIGIN: Pubic crest. INSERTION: Linea alba. INNERVATION: Last thoracic.
quadratus lumborum (kwăd-rā′tŭs lŭm-bō′-rŭm). ACTION: Flexes trunk laterally and forward. ORIGIN: Iliac crest, iliolumbar ligament, lower lumbar vertebrae. INSERTION: Twelfth rib and the upper lumbar vertebrae. INNERVATION: Upper lumbar.
rectus abdominis (rĕk′tŭs ăb-dŏm′ĭ-nĭs). ACTION: Compresses abdomen. ORIGIN: Pubis. INSERTION: Cartilage of 5th to 7th ribs. INNERVATION: Branches of lower thoracic.
sphincter pylori (sfĭnk′tĕr pĭ-lō′rī). A thickening of middle circular layer of the gastric musculature surrounding the pyloris.
transversalis abdominis (trăns″vĕr-sā′lĭs ăb-dŏm′ĭ-nĭs). SAME AS: *transversus abdominis*.
transversus abdominis (trăns″vĕr′sŭs ăb-dŏm′ĭ-nĭs). ACTION: Compresses abdomen, flexes thorax. ORIGIN: Lumbar fascia, 7th to 12th costal cartilages, Poupart's ligament, iliac crest. INSERTION: Xiphoid cartilage, linea alba, pubic crest and iliopectineal line. INNERVATION: Lower thoracic.

PERINEUM (14)

accelerator urinae (ăk-sĕl-ĕ-rā′tŏr ū-rī′-nē). SAME AS: *bulbocavernosus*.
bulbocavernosus (bŭl-bō-kă-vĕr-nō′sŭs). ACTION: Constricts bulbous urethra in male; in female constricts urethra. ORIGIN: Central point of perineum. INSERTION: Undersurface of bulb, spongy and cavernous part of penis; root of clitoris. INNERVATION: Pudic.
coccygeus (kŏk-sĭj′ē-ŭs). ACTION: Supports coccyx, closes pelvic outlet. ORIGIN: Ischial spine. INSERTION: Coccyx. INNERVATION: Third and 4th sacral.
compressor urethrae (kŏm-prĕs′ŏr ū-rē′-thrē). SAME AS: *sphincter urethrae membranaceae*.
constrictor urethrae (kŏn-strĭk′tŏr ū-rē′-thrē). SAME AS: *sphincter urethrae membranaceae*.
corrugator cutis ani (kor-ū-gā′tŏr kū′tĭs ā′nī). ACTION: Corrugates skin of anus.

ORIGIN: Submucous tissue, interior of anus. INSERTION: Subcutaneous tissue on opposite side of anus. INNERVATION: Sympathetic.
depressor urethrae (dē-prĕs′ŏr ū-rē′thrē). ACTION: Depresses urethra. ORIGIN: Ramus of ischium near the transversus perinei profundus. INSERTION: Fibers of constrictor vaginae.
erector clitoridis (ē-rĕk′tŏr klĭ-tŏr′ĭ-dĭs). SAME AS: *ischiocavernosus*.
erector penis (ē-rĕk′tŏr pē′nĭs). SAME AS: *ischiocavernosus*.
ischiocavernosus (ĭs″kĭ-ō-kă-vĕr-nō′sŭs). ACTION: Maintains erection of penis or clitoris. ORIGIN: Tuberosity of ischium and great sacrosciatic ligament. INSERTION: Corpus cavernosum of clitoris or penis. INNERVATION: Perineal.
ischiococcygeus (ĭs″kĭ-ō-kŏk-sĭj′ē-ŭs). SAME AS: *coccygeus*.
levator ani (lē-vă′tŏr ā′nī). ACTION: Supports rectum and pelvic floor, aids in defecation. ORIGIN: Pubis, pelvic fascia, ischial spine. INSERTION: Rectum, coccyx and fibrous raphe of perineum. INNERVATION: Sacral and perineal.
sphincter ani externus (sfĭnk′tĕr ā′nī ĕks-tĕr′nŭs). ACTION: Closes anus. ORIGIN: Ring of fibers surrounding anus. INSERTION: Coccyx and central point of perineum. INNERVATION: Hemorrhoidal.
sphincter ani internus (sfĭnk′tĕr ā′nī ĭn-tĕr′nŭs). ACTION: Contracts rectum and anus, but not voluntarily. ORIGIN: Muscular ring of rectal fibers above canal. INSERTION: ..... INNERVATION: Hemorrhoidal.
sphincter tertius of Hyrth (sfĭnk′tĕr tĕr′-shĭ-ŭs of hirth) (single). ACTION: Constricts rectum. ORIGIN: From sacrum, encircles rectum about 4 in. above anal orifice. INSERTION: Denied by most anatomists, demonstrated by Hyrth, Nealton and others.
sphincter urethrae membranaceae (sfĭnk′-tĕr ū-rē′thrē mĕm-brā-nā′sē-ē). ACTION: Constricts membranous urethra. ORIGIN: Ramus of pubis. INSERTION: Behind and in front of urethra. INNERVATION: Pudic.
sphincter vaginae (sfĭnk′tĕr vă-jī′nē). SAME AS: *bulbocavernosus*.
sphincter vesicae (sfĭnk′tĕr vĕs′ĭ-kē). ACTION: Shuts off internal orifice of urethra. ORIGIN: Near urethra orifice of bladder. INNERVATION: Vesical.
transversus perinei profundus (trăns-vĕr′-sŭs pĕr-ĭ-nē′ī prō-fŭn′dŭs). ACTION: Assists compressor urethrae. ORIGIN: Ramus of ischium. INSERTION: Central tendon. INNERVATION: Pudic.
transversus perinei superficialis (trăns-vĕr′sŭs pĕr-ĭ-nē′ī sū″pĕr-fĭsh-ĭ-ā′lĭs). ACTION: Tenses central tendon. ORIGIN: Ramus of ischium. INSERTION: Central point of perineum. INNERVATION: Pudic.

THORAX (46)

diaphragma (dī″ă-frăg′mă). ACTION: Increases chest capacity. ORIGIN: Ensiform cartilage, 7th to 12th ribs, arcuate ligaments and lumbar vertebrae. INSERTION: Central tendon. INNERVATION: Phrenic.
infracostalis (ĭn″frā-kŏs-tā′lĭs). SAME AS: *subcostalis*.
intercostales externus (ĭn″tĕr-kŏs-tā′lĭs ĕks-tĕr′nŭs). ACTION: Probably expands chest. ORIGIN: Lower border of rib. INSERTION: Upper border of rib below. INNERVATION: Intercostal.
intercostalis internus (ĭn″tĕr-kŏs-tā′lĭs ĭn-tĕr′nŭs). ACTION: Probably expands

Muscles of the Body App. 40 **Muscles of the Body**

chest in expiration. ORIGIN: Lower border of rib. INSERTION: Upper border of rib below. INNERVATION: Intercostal.

levator costae (lē-vā'tōr kŏs'tē). ACTION: Raises ribs. ORIGIN: Last cervical and 11th thoracic vertebrae. INSERTION: Into rib next below. INNERVATION: Intercostal.

subcostalis (sŭb-kŏs-tā'lĭs). ACTION: Raises ribs. ORIGIN: Inconstant; inner surface of the ribs. INSERTION: Inner surface of one of ribs just below. INNERVATION: Intercostal.

transversus thoracis (trăns-vĕr'sŭs thōr-ā'-sĭs). ACTION: Narrows the chest. ORIGIN: Xiphoid cartilage and sternum. INSERTION: Costal cartilages, 2nd to 6th ribs. INNERVATION: Intercostal.

triangularis sterni (trī"ăn-gū-lā'rĭs stĕr'-nī). SAME AS: *transversus thoracis*.

SHOULDER (10)

deltoideus (dĕl-toy'dē-ŭs). ACTION: Raises arm and rotates it. ORIGIN: Clavicle, acromion process and spine of scapula. INSERTION: Shaft of humerus. INNERVATION: Circumflex.

infraspinatus (ĭn"fră-spī-nā'tŭs). ACTION: Rotates arm back and out. ORIGIN: Infraspinous fossa of scapula. INSERTION: Great tuberosity of humerus. INNERVATION: Suprascapular.

pectoralis major (pĕk-tō-rā'lĭs mā'jōr). ACTION: Adducts and rotates arm. ORIGIN: Sternum, clavicle, and cartilages of 1st to 6th ribs. INSERTION: Bicipital ridge of humerus. INNERVATION: Anterior thoracic.

pectoralis minor (pĕk-tō-rā'lĭs mī'nōr). ACTION: Draws down scapula and point of shoulder, raises ribs. ORIGIN: Third to 5th ribs. INSERTION: Coracoid process of scapula. INNERVATION: Anterior thoracic.

serratus anterior (sĕr-ā'-tŭs ăn-tēr'ĭ-ōr). ACTION: Elevates ribs, rotates scapula. ORIGIN: Upper 8 or 9 ribs. INSERTION: Angles and dorsal border of scapula. INNERVATION: Posterior thoracic.

serratus magnus (sĕr-ā'tŭs măg'nŭs). SAME AS: *serratus anterior*.

subclavius (sŭb-klā'vĭ-ŭs). ACTION: Draws clavicle down and forward or elevates the 1st rib. ORIGIN: First rib and its cartilage. INSERTION: Undersurface of clavicle. INNERVATION: Subclavian from brachial plexus.

subscapularis (sŭb-skăp-ū-lā'rĭs). ACTION: Rotates humerus inward and lowers it. ORIGIN: Subscapular fossa. INSERTION: Lesser tuberosity of humerus. INNERVATION: Subscapular.

supraspinatus (sūp-ră-spī-nā'tŭs). ACTION: Abducts and raises arm. ORIGIN: Supraspinous fossa of scapula. INSERTION: Greater tuberosity of humerus. INNERVATION: Suprascapular.

teres major (tē'rēz mā'jor). ACTION: Rotates arm inward, draws it down and back. ORIGIN: Axillary border of scapula. INSERTION: Anterior surface of upper portion of humerus. INNERVATION: Lower subscapular.

teres minor (tē'rēz mī'nor). ACTION: Rotates arm outward. ORIGIN: Axillary border of scapula. INSERTION: Greater tubercle of humerus. INNERVATION: Circumflex.

ARM (6), FOREARM (20)

abductor pollicis longus (ăb-dŭk'tōr pŏl'ĭ-sĭs lŏn'gŭs). ACTION: Abducts and helps to extend thumb. ORIGIN: Dorsal surface of radius, ulna and interosseous membrane. INSERTION: Base of 1st metacarpal. INNERVATION: Radial.

anconeus (ăn-kō'nē-ŭs). ACTION: Extends forearm. ORIGIN: Lateral epicondyle of humerus. INSERTION: Olecranon and posterior surface of ulna. INNERVATION: Radial (musculospiral).

biceps brachii (bī'sĕps brā'kĭ-ī). ACTION: Flexes and supinates forearm. ORIGIN: 1. Short head from coracoid process. 2. Long head from scapula above glenoid fossa. INSERTION: Bicipital tuberosity of radius. INNERVATION: Musculocutaneous.

brachialis (anticus) (brā"kĭ-ā'lĭs (ăn-tī'-kŭs)). ACTION: Flexes forearm. ORIGIN: Lower half of anterior surface of humerus. INSERTION: Coronoid process of ulna. INNERVATION: Musculocutaneous and musculospiral.

brachioradialis (brā"kĭ-ō-rā"dĭ-ā'lĭs). ACTION: Flexes and supinates forearm. ORIGIN: Supracondylar ridge of humerus. INSERTION: Styloid process of radius. INNERVATION: Musculospiral.

coracobrachialis (kor-ă-kō-brā"kĭ-ā'lĭs). ACTION: Raises and adducts arm. ORIGIN: Coracoid process of scapula. INSERTION: Middle of inner border of humerus. INNERVATION: Musculocutaneous.

coracoradialis (kor"ă-kō-rā"dĭ-ā'lĭs). ACTION: Flexes and adducts arm. ORIGIN: Coracoid process of scapula. INSERTION: Middle 3rd of humerus. INNERVATION: Musculocutaneous.

extensor carpi radialis brevis (brevior) (ĕks-tĕn'sōr kar'pī rā"dĭ-ā'lĭs brē'vĭs (brē'vĭ-ōr)). ACTION: Extends and abducts wrist. ORIGIN: External condyloid ridge of humerus. INSERTION: Base of 3rd metacarpal. INNERVATION: Musculospiral.

extensor carpi radialis longus (longior) (ĕks-tĕn'sōr kar'pī rā"dĭ-ā'lĭs lŏng'gŭs (lŏn'gĭ-ōr)). ACTION: Extends and abducts wrist. ORIGIN: External condyloid ridge of humerus. INSERTION: Base of 2nd metacarpal. INNERVATION: Musculospiral.

extensor carpi ulnaris (ĕks-tĕn'sōr kar'pī ŭl-nā'rĭs). ACTION: Extends and abducts wrist. ORIGIN: Lateral epicondyle of humerus. INSERTION: Base of 5th metacarpal. INNERVATION: Radial (dorsal interosseous).

extensor digiti quinti proprius (ĕks-tĕn'sōr dĭj'ĭ-tī kwĭn'tī prō'prī-ŭs). ACTION: Extends little finger. ORIGIN: External epicondyle of humerus. INSERTION: Dorsum of 1st phalanx of little finger. INNERVATION: Radial (dorsal interosseous).

extensor digitorum communis (ĕks-tĕn'sōr dĭj-ĭ-tō'rŭm kŏm-mū'nĭs). ACTION: Extends fingers and wrist. ORIGIN: External epicondyle of humerus. INSERTION: Second and 3rd phalanges. INNERVATION: Radial (dorsal interosseous).

extensor indicis proprius (ĕks-tĕn'sōr ĭn'-dĭ-sĭs prō'prī-ŭs). ACTION: Extends index finger. ORIGIN: Dorsal surface of ulna and interosseous membrane. INSERTION: First tendon of extensor communis digitorum. INNERVATION: Radial (musculospiral).

extensor metacarpi pollicis (ĕks-tĕn'sōr mĕt"ă-kar'pī pŏl'ĭ-sĭs). SAME AS: *abductor pollicis longus*.

extensor minimi digiti (ĕks-tĕn'sōr mĭn'ĭm-ī dĭj'ĭ-tī). SAME AS: *extensor digiti quinti proprius*.

extensor pollicis brevis (ĕks-tĕn'sōr pŏl'ĭ-sĭs brē'vĭs). ACTION: Extends thumb and abducts 1st metacarpal. ORIGIN: Dorsal surface of radius. INSERTION: Base of 1st phalanx. INNERVATION: Radial.

extensor pollicis longus (ĕks-tĕn'sōr pŏl'ĭ-sĭs lŏng'gŭs). ACTION: Extends terminal phalanx of thumb. ORIGIN: Dorsal sur-

Muscles of the Body

face of ulna. INSERTION: Base of 2nd phalanx of thumb. INNERVATION: Radial.
extensor primi internodii pollicis (ĕks-tĕn'sŏr prī'mī ĭn"tĕr-nō'dĭ-ī pŏl'ĭ-sĭs). SAME AS: *extensor pollicis brevis.*
extensor secundi internodii pollicis (ĕks-tĕn'sŏr sē-kŭn'dī ĭn"tĕr-nō'dĭ-ī pŏl'ĭ-sĭs). SAME AS: *extensor pollicis longus.*
flexor carpi radialis (flĕks'ŏr kar'pī rā"dĭ-ā'lĭs). ACTION: Flexes and abducts wrist. ORIGIN: Internal condyle of humerus. INSERTION: Base of 2nd metacarpal. INNERVATION: Median.
flexor carpi ulnaris (flĕks'ŏr kar'pī ŭl-nā'rĭs). ACTION: Flexes and adducts wrist. ORIGIN: 1. Medial condyle of humerus. 2. Olecranon process and posterior border of ulna. INSERTION: Pisiform bone and 5th metacarpal. INNERVATION: Ulnar.
flexor digitorum profundus (flĕks'ŏr dĭj-ĭ-tō'rŭm prō-fŭn'dŭs). ACTION: Flexes the phalanges. ORIGIN: Upper ¾ of shaft of ulna. INSERTION: Terminal phalanges of fingers. INNERVATION: Ulnar and median.
flexor digitorum sublimis (flĕks'ŏr dĭj-ĭ-tō'rŭm sŭb-lĭ'mĭs). ACTION: Flexes middle phalanges. ORIGIN: 1. Internal condyle of humerus. 2. Coronoid process of ulna. 3. Outer border of radius. INSERTION: Second phalanx of each finger. INNERVATION: Median.
flexor pollicis longus (flĕks'ŏr pŏl'ĭ-sĭs lŏng'gŭs). ACTION: Flexes thumb. ORIGIN: Anterior surface of middle 3rd of radius. INSERTION: Terminal phalanx of thumb. INNERVATION: Median (volar interosseous).
palmaris longus (păl-mā'rĭs lŏng'gŭs). ACTION: Tightens palmar fascia, flexes wrist. ORIGIN: Internal condyle of humerus. INSERTION: Annular ligament and palmar fascia. INNERVATION: Median.
pronator quadratus (prō-nā'tŏr kwăd-rā'tŭs). ACTION: Pronates forearm. ORIGIN: Lower 4th of ulna. INSERTION: Lower 4th of radius. INNERVATION: Volar interosseous.
pronator teres (prō-nā'tŏr tē'rēz). ACTION: Pronates forearm. ORIGIN: 1. Internal condyle of humerus. 2. Coronoid process of ulna. INSERTION: Lateral surface of shaft of radius. INNERVATION: Median.
radiocarpus (rā"dĭ-ō-kar'pŭs). SAME AS: *flexor carpi radialis.*
subanconeus (sŭb-ăn-kō'nē-ŭs). ACTION: Tightens posterior ligament of elbow. ORIGIN: Lower portion of humerus. INSERTION: Posterior ligament of elbow joint. INNERVATION: Radial (musculo-spiral).
supinator (sū"pĭ-nā'tŏr). ACTION: Supinates forearm. ORIGIN: External condyle of humerus, oblique line of ulna. INSERTION: Outer surface of radius. INNERVATION: Radial (dorsal interosseous).
supinator longus (sū"pĭ-nā'tŏr lŏng'gŭs). SAME AS: *brachioradialis.*
supinator radii brevis (sū"pĭ-nā'tŏr rā'dĭ-ī brē'vĭs). SAME AS: *supinator.*
triceps brachii (trī'sĕps brā'kĭ-ī). ACTION: Extends forearm and arm. ORIGIN: 1. Long or middle head from infraglenoid tubercle of scapula. 2. Outer or external head from posterior surface of humerus below great tubercle. 3. Inner or internal head from humerus below radial groove. INSERTION: Olecranon process of ulna. INNERVATION: Radial (musculospiral).

HAND (20)

abductor digiti quinti (ăb-dŭk'tŏr dĭj'ĭ-tī kwĭn'tī). ACTION: Abducts little finger. ORIGIN: Pisiform bone and ligaments. INSERTION: Inner side of 1st phalanx of little finger. INNERVATION: Ulnar, palmar branch.
abductor indicis (ăb-dŭk'tŏr ĭn'dĭ-sĭs). SAME AS: *interosseous dorsalis manus.*
abductor minimi digiti (ăb-dŭk'tŏr mĭn'ĭ-mī dĭj'ĭ-tī). SAME AS: *abductor digiti quinti.*
abductor pollicis brevis (ăb-dŭk'tŏr pŏl'ĭ-sĭs brē'vĭs). ACTION: Abducts thumb. ORIGIN: Ridge of trapezium and anterior annular ligament. INSERTION: Outer side of 1st phalanx of thumb. INNERVATION: Median.
abductor pollicis longus (ăb-dŭk'tŏr pŏl'ĭ-sĭs lŏng'gŭs). ACTION: Abducts and assists in extending thumb. ORIGIN: Posterior surfaces of radius and ulna. INSERTION: Outer side of base of 1st metacarpal. INNERVATION: Radial.
adductor pollicis (ăd-dŭk'tŏr pŏl'ĭ-sĭs). ACTION: Adducts thumb. ORIGIN: Third metacarpal bone. INSERTION: Inner side of base of 1st phalanx of thumb. INNERVATION: Ulnar.
flexor brevis minimi digiti (flĕks'ŏr brē'vĭs mĭn'ĭ-mī dĭj'ĭ-tī). SAME AS: *flexor digiti quinti brevis.*
flexor digiti quinti brevis (flĕks'ŏr dĭj'ĭ-tī kwĭn'tī brē'vĭs). ACTION: Flexes 1st phalanx of little finger. ORIGIN: Unciform bone. INSERTION: First phalanx of little finger. INNERVATION: Ulnar.
flexor minimi digiti (flĕks'ŏr mĭn'ĭ-mī dĭj'ĭ-tī). SAME AS: *opponens minimi digiti.*
flexor ossis metacarpi minimi digiti (flĕks'ŏr ŏs'ĭs mĕt"ă-kar'pī mĭn'ĭ-mī dĭj'ĭ-tī). SAME AS: *opponens minimi digiti.*
flexor ossis metacarpi pollicis (flĕks'ŏr ŏs'ĭs mĕt"ă-kar'pī pŏl'ĭ-sĭs). SAME AS: *opponens pollicis.*
flexor pollicis brevis (flĕks'ŏr pŏl'ĭ-sĭs brē'vĭs). ACTION: Flexes 1st phalanx of thumb. ORIGIN: Transverse carpal ligament, metacarpal bone. INSERTION: Base of 1st phalanx of thumb. INNERVATION: Median, ulnar.
interosseus dorsalis manus (ĭn"tĕr-ŏs'ē-ŭs dŏr-sā'lĭs mā'nŭs). Four. ACTION: Abduct and adduct fingers. ORIGIN: Sides of metacarpal bones. INSERTION: First phalanges. INNERVATION: Ulnar.
interosseus palmaris (ĭn"tĕr-ŏs'ē-ŭs păl-mā'rĭs). SAME AS: *interosseus volaris.*
interosseus volaris (ĭn"tĕr-ŏs'ē-ŭs vō-lā'rĭs). Three. ACTION: Adducts index finger, abducts ring and little fingers. ORIGIN: Metacarpal bones laterally. INSERTION: Ulnar side of index finger, and radial sides of ring and little fingers. INNERVATION: Ulnar.
lumbricalis manus (lŭm-brĭ-kā'lĭs mā'nŭs). Four. ACTION: Flexes 1st and extends 2nd and 3rd phalanges. ORIGIN: Tendon of flexor digitorum profundus. INSERTION: First phalanx and extensor tendon. INNERVATION: Median and ulnar.
opponens digiti quinti (ŏp-pō'nĕns dĭj'ĭ-tī kwĭn'tī). ACTION: Flexes and adducts little finger. ORIGIN: Unciform bone; annular ligament. INSERTION: Fifth metacarpal bone. INNERVATION: Ulnar.
opponens minimi digiti (ŏp-pō'nĕns mĭn'ĭ-mī dĭj'ĭ-tī). SAME AS: *opponens digiti quinti.*
opponens pollicis (ŏp-pō'nĕns pŏl'ĭ-sĭs). ACTION: Flexes and adducts thumb. ORIGIN: Trapezium and annular ligament. INSERTION: First metacarpal bone. INNERVATION: Median.
palmaris brevis (păl-mā'rĭs brē'vĭs). ACTION: Wrinkles skin on inner side of hand. ORIGIN: Central portion of palmar aponeurosis. INSERTION: Skin of ulnar side of hand. INNERVATION: Ulnar.

Muscles of the Body

HIP (12), THIGH (12), LOWER EXTREMITY (3)

adductor brevis (ăd-dŭk'tŏr brē'vĭs). ACTION: Flexes and adducts thigh. ORIGIN: Ramus of pubis. INSERTION: Upper portion of linea aspera of femur. INNERVATION: Obturator.

adductor longus (ăd-dŭk'tŏr lŏng'gŭs). ACTION: Adducts thigh. ORIGIN: Pubic crest and symphysis. INSERTION: Middle of linea aspera of femur. INNERVATION: Obturator.

adductor magnus (ăd-dŭk'tŏr măg'nŭs). ACTION: Adducts thigh and rotates it outward. ORIGIN: Ramus of ischium and pubis. INSERTION: Linea aspera of femur and internal epicondyle. INNERVATION: Sciatic and obturator.

articularis genu (ar-tĭk″ū-lā'rĭs jē'nū). ACTION: Elevates capsule of knee joint. ORIGIN: Lower quarter of anterior surface of femoral shaft. INSERTION: Synovial membrane of knee joint. INNERVATION: Femoral.

biceps femoris (bī'sĕps fĕm'ō-rĭs). ACTION: Flexes knee and rotates it outward. ORIGIN: 1. Short head from linea aspera. 2. Long head from ischial tuberosity. INSERTION: Head of fibula; lateral condyle of tibia. INNERVATION: Short head, peroneal; long head, tibial.

crureus (krū'rē-ŭs). SAME AS: *vastus intermedius*.

gemellus inferior (jē-mĕl'ŭs ĭn-fēr'ĭ-ōr). ACTION: Rotates thigh outward. ORIGIN: Ischial tuberosity. INSERTION: Great trochanter. INNERVATION: Sacral.

gemellus superior (jē-mĕl'ŭs sū-pēr'ĭ-ōr). ACTION: Rotates thigh outward. ORIGIN: Ischiospine. INSERTION: Great trochanter. INNERVATION: Sacral.

gluteus maximus (glū'tē-ŭs măks'ĭ-mŭs). ACTION: Extends thigh. ORIGIN: Superior curved iliac line and crest, coccyx and sacrum. INSERTION: Fascia lata and femur below great trochanter. INNERVATION: Inferior gluteal.

gluteus medius (glū'tē-ŭs mē'dĭ-ŭs). ACTION: Abducts and rotates thigh. ORIGIN: Lateral surface of ilium. INSERTION: Great trochanter. INNERVATION: Superior gluteal.

gluteus minimus (glū'tē-ŭs mĭn'ĭ-mŭs). ACTION: Abducts and extends thigh. ORIGIN: Lateral surface of ilium. INSERTION: Great trochanter. INNERVATION: Superior gluteal.

gracilis (grăs'ĭ-lĭs). ACTION: Flexes and adducts leg, adducts thigh. ORIGIN: Pubic and ischial ramus. INSERTION: Medial surface of shaft of tibia. INNERVATION: Obturator.

iliacus (ĭ-lī'ă-kŭs). ACTION: Flexes and rotates thigh. ORIGIN: Margin of iliac fossa. INSERTION: Lesser trochanter. INNERVATION: Lumbar plexus.

obturator externus (ŏb-tū-rā'tŏr ĕks-tĕr'nŭs). ACTION: Rotates thigh outward. ORIGIN: Margin of thyroid foramen and obturator membrane. INSERTION: Digital fossa of great trochanter. INNERVATION: Obturator.

obturator internus (ŏb-tū-rā'tŏr ĭn-tĕr'nŭs). ACTION: Rotates thigh outward. ORIGIN: Pubes, ischium, obturator foramen. INSERTION: Inner surface of great trochanter. INNERVATION: Sacral.

pectineus (pĕk-tĭn'ē-ŭs). ACTION: Flexes and adducts thigh. ORIGIN: Pubic spine; iliopectineal line. INSERTION: Pectineal line of femur. INNERVATION: Obturator and femoral.

piriformis (pĭ-rĭ-fŏr'mĭs). ACTION: Rotates thigh outward. ORIGIN: Margins of anterior sacral foramina and great sacrosciatic notch of ilium. INSERTION: Upper margin of great trochanter. INNERVATION: Sciatic plexus.

psoas major (magnus) (sō'ăs mā'jŏr, măg'nŭs). ACTION: Flexes thigh, adducts and rotates it medially. ORIGIN: Last dorsal and all of the lumbar vertebrae. INSERTION: Lesser trochanter of femur. INNERVATION: Lumbar plexus.

psoas minor (parvus) (sō'ăs mī'nŏr, par'vŭs). ACTION: Tenses iliac fascia. ORIGIN: Twelfth dorsal and 1st lumbar vertebrae. INSERTION: Iliac fascia and iliopectineal tuberosity. INNERVATION: Lumbar plexus.

pyriformis (pĭ-rĭ-fŏr'mĭs). SAME AS: *piriformis*.

quadratus femoris (kwăd-rā'tŭs fĕm'ō-rĭs). ACTION: Rotates thigh outward. ORIGIN: Ischial tuberosity. INSERTION: Intertrochanteric ridge. INNERVATION: Sciatic.

quadriceps extensor femoris (kwăd'rĭ-sĕps ĕks-tĕn'sŏr fĕm'ō-rĭs). SAME AS: *quadriceps femoris*.

quadriceps femoris (kwăd'rĭ-sĕps fĕm'ō-rĭs). ACTION: Extends leg. ORIGIN: By 4 heads, rectus femoris, vastus internus, vastus externus and crureus. INSERTION: Patella and tibial tuberosity. INNERVATION: Femoral.

rectus femoris (rĕk'tŭs fĕm'ō-rĭs). ACTION: Extends leg. ORIGIN: Iliac spine, upper margin of acetabulum. INSERTION: Common tendon of quadriceps femoris. INNERVATION: Anterior crural.

sartorius (sar-tō'rĭ-ŭs). ACTION: Flexes and crosses legs. ORIGIN: Anterior superior iliac spine. INSERTION: Tibial tuberosity. INNERVATION: Femoral.

semimembranosus (sĕm'ĭ-mĕm-brā-nō'sŭs). ACTION: Flexes and rotates leg. ORIGIN: Ischial tuberosity. INSERTION: Inner tibial tuberosity. INNERVATION: Tibial.

semitendinosus (sĕm'ĭ-tĕn-dĭ-nō'sŭs). ACTION: Flexes and rotates leg, extends hip. ORIGIN: Ischial tuberosity. INSERTION: Shaft of tibia below internal tuberosity. INNERVATION: Tibial.

subcrureus (sŭb-krū'rē-ŭs). SAME AS: *articularis genu*.

tensor fasciae latae (tĕn'sŏr făs'ĭ-ē lā'tē). ACTION: Tenses the fascia lata. ORIGIN: Dorsum of ilium. INSERTION: Iliotibial band of fascia lata. INNERVATION: Superior gluteal.

tensor vaginae femoris (tĕn'sŏr vă-jī'nē fĕm'ō-rĭs). SAME AS: *tensor fasciae latae*.

vastus externus (lateralis) (văs'tŭs ĕks-tĕr'nŭs, lăt-ĕr-ā'lĭs). ACTION: Extends knee. ORIGIN: Linea aspera to great trochanter. INSERTION: Common tendon of quadriceps femoris. INNERVATION: Anterior crural.

vastus intermedius (văs'tŭs ĭn″tĕr-mē'dĭ-ŭs). ORIGIN: Upper part of anterior surface of shaft of femur. INSERTION: Common tendon of quadriceps femoris.

vastus internus (medialis) (văs'tŭs ĭn-tĕr'nŭs, mē-dĭ-ā'lĭs). ACTION: Extends leg, draws patella in. ORIGIN: Linea aspera of femur. INSERTION: Common tendon of quadriceps femoris. INNERVATION: Anterior crural.

LEG (13)

extensor digitorum longus (ĕks-tĕn'sŏr dĭj'ĭ-tō'rŭm lŏng'gŭs). ACTION: Extends toes, flexes foot. ORIGIN: External tuberosity of tibia. INSERTION: Second and 3rd phalanges of toes. INNERVATION: Peroneal.

extensor hallucis longus (ĕks-tĕn'sŏr hăl-ū'sĭs lŏng'gŭs). ACTION: Extends great toe. ORIGIN: Front of tibia and inter-

Muscles of the Body

osseous membrane. INSERTION: Terminal phalanx of great toe. INNERVATION: Anterior tibial.
extensor proprius hallucis (ĕks-tĕn'sōr prō'prĭ-ŭs hăl-ū'sĭs). SAME AS: *extensor hallucis longus.*
flexor digitorum longus (flĕks'ōr dĭj-ĭ-tō'rŭm lŏng'gŭs). ACTION: Flexes phalanges and extends toes. ORIGIN: Posterior surface of tibia. INSERTION: Terminal phalanges of 4 lesser toes. INNERVATION: Tibial.
flexor hallucis longus (flĕks'ōr hăl-ū'sĭs lŏng'gŭs). ACTION: Flexes great toe and extends foot. ORIGIN: Lower portion of shaft of fibula. INSERTION: Distal phalanx of great toe. INNERVATION: Posterior tibial.
gastrocnemius (găs-trŏk-nē'mĭ-ŭs). ACTION: Flexes foot and leg. ORIGIN: External and internal femoral condyles. INSERTION: By tendo Achillis into os calcis. INNERVATION: Tibial.
peroneus brevis (pĕr-ō-nē'ŭs brē'vĭs). ACTION: Extends and abducts foot. ORIGIN: Midportion of shaft of fibula. INSERTION: Base of 5th metatarsal bone. INNERVATION: Peroneal.
peroneus longus (pĕr-ō-nē'ŭs lŏng'gŭs). ACTION: Extends, abducts and everts foot. ORIGIN: Upper fibula and external condyle of tibia. INSERTION: By tendon to internal cuneiform and 1st metatarsal bone. INNERVATION: Peroneal.
peroneus tertius (pĕr-ō-nē'ŭs tĕr'shĭ-ŭs). ACTION: Flexes tarsus. ORIGIN: Lower part of fibula. INSERTION: Fifth metatarsal bone. INNERVATION: Deep branch of peroneal.
plantaris (plăn-tā'rĭs). ACTION: Extends foot. ORIGIN: External supracondyloid ridge of femur. INSERTION: Inner border of tendo Achillis and internal annular ligament of ankle. INNERVATION: Tibial.
popliteus (pŏp'lĭt-ē-ŭs). ACTION: Flexes leg, rotates it inward. ORIGIN: External condyle of femur. INSERTION: Posterior surface of tibia. INNERVATION: Tibial.
soleus (sō'lē-ŭs). ACTION: Extends and rotates foot. ORIGIN: Upper shaft of fibula, oblique line of tibia. INSERTION: by tendo Achillis to os calcis. INNERVATION: Tibial.
tibialis anterior (anticus) (tĭb-ĭ-ā'lĭs ăn-tēr'ĭ-ōr, ăn-tī'kŭs). ACTION: Elevates and flexes foot. ORIGIN: Upper tibia, interosseous membrane and intermuscular septum. INSERTION: Internal cuneiform and 1st metatarsal. INNERVATION: Peroneal.
tibialis posterior (posticus) (tĭb-ĭ-ā'lĭs pŏs-tēr'ĭ-ōr, pŏs-tī'kŭs). ACTION: Extends tarsus and inverts foot. ORIGIN: Shaft of fibula and tibia. INSERTION: Tuberosity of scaphoid, 2nd to 4th metatarsal, internal cuneiform. INNERVATION: Tibial.

FOOT (20)

abductor digiti quinti (ăb-dŭk'tōr dĭj'ĭ-tī kwĭn'tī). ACTION: Abducts and flexes the little toe. ORIGIN: Outer tuberosity of calcaneus, plantar fascia and intermuscular septum. INSERTION: External side of 1st phalanx of little toe. INNERVATION: Lateral plantar.
abductor hallucis (ăb-dŭk'tōr hăl-ū'sĭs). ACTION: Abducts great toe. ORIGIN: Inner tuberosity of os calcis, plantar fascia. INSERTION: Inner side, 1st phalanx of great toe. INNERVATION: Internal plantar.
abductor minimi digiti (ăb-dŭk'tōr mĭn'ĭ-mī dĭj'ĭ-tī). SAME AS: *abductor digiti quinti.*
adductor hallucis (ăd-dŭk'tōr hăl-ū'sĭs).

Muscles of the Body

ACTION: Adducts great toe. ORIGIN: Tarsal terminations of middle metatarsal bones. INSERTION: Base of 1st phalanx of great toe. INNERVATION: External plantar.
adductor obliquus hallucis (ăd-dŭk'tōr ŏb-lī'kwŭs hăl-ū'sĭs). SAME AS: *adductor hallucis.*
adductor transversus hallucis (ăd-dŭk'tōr trăns-vĕr'sŭs hăl-ū'sĭs). SAME AS: *adductor hallucis.*
extensor digitorum brevis (ĕks-tĕn'sōr dĭj-ĭ-tō'rŭm brē'vĭs). ACTION: Extends toes. ORIGIN: Dorsal surface of os calcis. INSERTION: To 1st phalanx of great toe and the tendons of extensor digitorum longus. INNERVATION: Deep peroneal.
flexor accessorius digitorum (flĕks'ōr ăk-sĕ-sō'rĭ-ŭs dĭj-ĭ-tō'rŭm). SAME AS: *quadratus plantae.*
flexor brevis minimi digiti (flĕks'ōr brē'vĭs mĭn'ĭ-mī dĭj'ĭ-tī). SAME AS: *flexor digiti quinti brevis.*
flexor digiti quinti brevis (flĕks'ōr dĭj'ĭ-tī kwĭn'tī brē'vĭs). ACTION: Flexes the little toe. ORIGIN: Base of metatarsal of little toe and sheath of peroneus longus. INSERTION: Outer side of base of 1st phalanx of little toe. INNERVATION: External plantar.
flexor digitorum brevis (flĕks'ōr dĭj'-ĭ-tō'rŭm brē'vĭs). ACTION: Flexes toe. ORIGIN: Os calcis and plantar fascia. INSERTION: Second phalanges of lesser toes. INNERVATION: Internal plantar.
flexor hallucis brevis (flĕks'ōr hăl-ū'sĭs brē'vĭs). ACTION: Flexes great toe. ORIGIN: Internal surface of cuboid and middle and external cuneiform bones. INSERTION: Sides of base of 1st phalanx of great toe. INNERVATION: Internal and external plantar.
interosseus dorsalis pedis (ĭn"tĕr-ŏs'ē-ŭs dōr-sā'lĭs pē'dĭs). Four. ACTION: Adduct 2nd toe; abduct 2nd, 3rd, and 4th toe. ORIGIN: Shafts of adjacent metatarsal bones. INSERTION: First phalanges of lesser toes. INNERVATION: External plantar.
interosseus plantaris (ĭn"tĕr-ŏs'ē-ŭs plăn-tā'rĭs). Three. ACTION: Adduct 3 outer toes. ORIGIN: Third, 4th, and 5th metatarsal bones. INSERTION: First phalanx of corresponding toe. INNERVATION: External plantar.
lumbricalis (lŭm-brĭ-kā'lĭs). Four. ACTION: Flex the 1st and extend the 2nd and 3rd phalanges. ORIGIN: Tendons of flexor digitorum longus. INSERTION: First phalanx and extensor tendon. INNERVATION: External and internal plantar.
pronator pedis (prō-nā'tōr pē'dĭs). SAME AS: *quadratus plantae.*
quadratus plantae (kwăd-rā'tŭs plăn'tē). ACTION: Assists flexor digitorum longus. ORIGIN: Inferior surface of os calcis by 2 heads from outer and inner borders. INSERTION: Tendons of flexor digitorum longus. INNERVATION: External plantar.
tibioaccessorius (tĭb"ĭ-ō-ăk-sĕs-sō'rĭ-ŭs). SAME AS: *quadratus plantae.*
transversus pedis (trăns-vĕr'sŭs pē'dĭs). ACTION: Adducts great toe. ORIGIN: Inferior metatarsophalangeal ligaments and transverse metatarsal ligaments. INSERTION: Outer side of base of 1st phalanx of great toe. INNERVATION: External plantar.

GENERAL

arrectores pilorum (ăr-rĕk-tō'rēz pī-lō'rŭm). ACTION: Elevates hairs of skin. ORIGIN: Papillary layer of skin. INSERTION: Hair follicles. INNERVATION: Sympathetic.

Principal Joints

Joints and Ligamentous Attachments	Variety	Ligaments
Sternoclavicular	Arthrodial	Capsular.
Acromioclavicular	Arthrodial	Capsular.
Coracoclavicular	Syndesmosis	Conoid and trapezoid. Coracoacromial (overhangs shoulder).
Shoulder	Enarthrosis	Capsular, coracohumeral and glenoid.
Elbow	Ginglymus	Anterior, posterior, internal and external lateral.
Superior radioulnar	Trochoides	Orbicular.
Inferior radioulnar	Trochoides	Anterior and posterior radioulnar and triangular fibrocartilage.
Wrist, radius and cart. with scaphoid, semi-ulnar and cuneiform	Ginglymus	Anterior, posterior, internal and external lateral.
Trapezium, scaphoid Unciform, pisiform		Anterior annular ligament.
Radius, ulna, cuneiform. Pisiform		Posterior annular ligament.
Carpal	Arthrodial	Interosseous and capsular.
Sacroiliac	Amphiarthrosis	Anterior and posterior sacroiliac.
Sacroischial		Greater and lesser sacrosciatic.
Hip	Enarthrosis	Capsular, with three thickenings (iliofemoral, ischiofemoral, pubofemoral). Cotyloid, transverse, ligamentum teres.
Knee	Condyloid (in limited motion) Ginglymus (in flexion)	Anterior. Internal lateral (going down three inches on tibia). External lateral (having a long and short slip). Posterior (ligament of Winslow). Two semilunar. Two coronary. Two crucial. Two alaria. Capsular, mucosum. Patellar and transverse.
Sup. tibiofibular	Arthrodial	Capsular, anterior and posterior superior tibiofibular.
Inf. tibiofibular	Syndesmosis	Transverse, interosseous, anterior and posterior inferior tibiofibular.
Ankle	Ginglymus	Capsular, anterior, posterior, internal lateral (deltoid) (internal mall. to scaphoid, calcaneum and astragalus), external lateral (three slips, external mall. to astragalus, to sustentaculum tali, digital fossa to astragalus).
Calcaneocuboid	Arthrodial	Inferior calcaneocuboid (long and short plantar), capsular.
Calcaneoscaphoid		"Spring ligament." Artics. with astragalus.
Occipitoatlantal	Condyloid	
Atlantoaxial (odontoid)	Trochoides	Transverse.
Occipitoaxial		Anterior occipitoaxial, two lateral occipitoaxial.
Intervertebral (bodies)	Symphysis	Intervertebral disks, anterior and posterior common ligaments.
Spines		Supraspinous, ligament nuchae.
Laminae		Ligament subflava.
Articular processes	Arthrodial	Capsular.
Vertebrocostal (rib-heads)	Arthrodial	Capsular, intervertebral, stellate.
Vertebrocostal (rib tubercles and necks)	Arthrodial	Capsular, anterior middle and posterior costotransverse.
Jaws	Ginglymus	Capsular, external lateral, internal lateral.

Table of Nerves[1]

Name	B. N. A. Equivalent	Origin	Function	Distribution
Abducent............	N. Abducens.	Fasciculus teres.	Motor.	External oblique muscle of eye.
Auditory.............	N. Acusticus.	Cochlea.	Special sense of hearing.	Temporal lobes.
Auricular—				
Anterior...........	N. Auricularis, anterior.	Mandibular div. of trigeminal.	Sensory.	Skin of pinna.
Great..............	N. Auricularis, magnus.	Second and third cervical through cervical plexus.	Sensory.	Side of neck and ear.
Inferior............		Auriculotemporal.	Sensory.	Lobule of ear.
Posterior..........	N. Auricularis, posterior.	Facial.	Motor.	Retrahens aurem and occipitofrontalis.
Auriculotemporal......	N. Auriculotemporalis.	Mandibular div. of trigeminal.	Sensory.	Side of scalp.
Buccal...............	N. Buccalis.	Facial.	Motor.	Buccinator and orbicularis oris.
Buccal, long..........	N. Buccinatorius.	Mandibular div. of trigeminal.	Sensory.	Cheek.
Calcaneus, internal...	N. Calcaneus medialis.	Posterior tibial.	Sensory.	Sole of foot.
Chorda tympani......	N. Chorda tympani.	Facial.	Motor.	Submaxillary gland.
Ciliary, long..........	NN. Ciliares longi.	Nasal branch of ophthalmic div. of trigeminal.	Sensory and motor.	Cornea, iris and ciliary body.
Ciliary, short.........	NN. Ciliares, breves.	Ciliary ganglion.	Sensory and motor.	Cornea, iris and ciliary body.
Circumflex...........	N. Axillaris.	Posterior cord of brachial plexus.	Motor and sensory.	Deltoid, teres minor, shoulder joint, and overlying skin.
Coccygeal............	N. Coccygeus.	Spinal cord.	Motor and sensory.	Coccygeus muscle and skin over coccyx.
Cochlear.............	N. Cochlearis.	Auditory.	Special sense of hearing.	Cochlea.
Colli, superficialis....	N. Cutaneous, colli.	Second and third cervical through cervical plexus.	Sensory.	Skin of neck and throat.
Crural, anterior.......	N. Lumbo-inguinalis.	Genitocrural.	Sensory.	Skin of upper part of thigh.
Crural, anterior.......	N. Femoralis.	Second, third and fourth lumbar through lumbar plexus.	Motor and sensory.	Iliacus, pectineus, sartorius, quadriceps extensor, skin of thigh and inner aspect of leg.
Cutaneous, internal...	N. Cutaneus, antibrachii medialis.	Inner cord of brachial plexus.	Sensory.	Skin of inner aspect of forearm.
Cutaneous, lesser internal (of Wrisberg)...........	N. Cutaneus, brachii medialis.	Inner cord of brachial plexus.	Sensory.	Skin of inner aspect of upper arm.
Dental, anterior, superior...		Maxillary div. of trigeminal.	Sensory.	Superior incisors and canine teeth.

[1] From *Appleton's Medical Dictionary*, Courtesy Appleton Century Company.

TABLE OF NERVES—Continued

Name	B. N. A. Equivalent	Origin	Function	Distribution
Dental, inferior		Mandibular div. of trigeminal.	Sensory and motor.	Teeth of lower jaw, mylohyoid muscle and skin of chin.
Dental, middle, superior		Maxillary div. of trigeminal.	Sensory.	Superior bicuspid teeth.
Dental, posterior, superior		Maxillary div. of trigeminal.	Sensory.	Superior molar teeth.
Descendens hypoglossi (or noni)	N. Descendens hypoglossi.	Hypoglossal.	Motor.	Sternohyoid, sternothyroid, omohyoid.
Digastric		Facial.	Motor.	Stylohyoid and posterior belly of digastric muscle.
Facial	N. Facialis.	Floor of fourth ventricle.	Motor.	Muscles of expression.
Frontal	N. Frontalis	Ophthalmic div. of trigeminal.	Sensory.	Skin of forehead.
Genital		Genitocrural.	Motor.	Cremaster muscle and round ligament.
Genitocrural		First and second lumbar through lumbar plexus.	Sensory and motor.	Cremaster and skin of groin and upper part of thigh.
Glossopharyngeal	N. Glossopharyngeus.	Floor of fourth ventricle.	Motor, sensory and special sense.	Muscles and mucous membrane of pharynx, posterior third of tongue.
Gluteal, inferior	N. Gluteus, inferior.	2nd and 3rd sacral through sacral plexus.	Motor.	Gluteus maximus.
Gluteal, superior	N. Gluteus, superior.	2nd and 3rd sacral through sacral plexus.	Motor.	Gluteus medius and minimus, tensor fasciae femoris.
Hypogastric	N. Ramus cutaneus, anterior.	Iliohypogastric.	Motor and sensory.	Muscles and skin of abdominal wall.
Hypoglossal	N. Hypoglossa.	Floor of 4th ventricle.	Motor.	Thyrohyoid, hyoglossus, geniohyoid, styloglossus, and palatoglossus.
Iliac	N. Ramus cutaneus lateralis.	Iliohypogastric.	Sensory.	Skin of gluteal region.
Iliohypogastric	N. Iliohypogastricus.	1st lumbar through lumbar plexus.	Sensory and motor.	Muscles and skin of hypogastrium.
Ilio-inguinal	N. Ilio-inguinalis.	1st lumbar through lumbar plexus.	Sensory and motor.	Internal oblique muscle and skin of groin.
Incisive		Inferior dental.	Sensory.	Lower incisor and canine teeth.
Infraorbital	N. Infraorbitalis.	Maxillary div. of trigeminal nerve.	Sensory.	Skin of cheek and lower eyelid.
Infratrochlear	N. Infratrochlearus.	Nasal.	Sensory.	Skin of lower eyelid and side of nose.
Intercostal	NN. Intercostales.	Thoracic nerves.	Sensory and motor.	Muscles and skin of back thorax and upper abdomen.
Intercostohumeral	N. Intercostobrachialis.	2nd or 3rd intercostal.	Sensory.	Skin of axilla.

App. 46

TABLE OF NERVES—Continued

Name	B. N. A. Equivalent	Origin	Function	Distribution
Interosseous, anterior	N. Interosseus valaris.	Median.	Motor.	Deep flexor and pronator muscles of forearm.
Interosseous, posterior	N. Interosseus dorsalis.	Musculospiral.	Motor and sensory.	Muscles and skin of back of forearm and wrist.
Lacrimal	N. Lacrimalis.	Ophthalmic div. of trigeminal.	Sensory.	Lacrimal gland and conjunctiva.
Laryngeal, inferior or recurrent	N. Recurrens.	Vagus.	Motor.	Muscles of larynx.
Laryngeal, superior	N. Laryngeus, superior.	Vagus.	Sensory and motor.	Mucous membrane of larynx; arytenoid and cricothyroid muscles.
Lingual	N. Lingualis.	Mandibular branch of trigeminal.	Sensory.	Mucous membrane of anterior two-thirds of tongue.
Lumbar	NN. Lumbales.	Spinal cord.	Motor and sensory.	Loins and front of lower abdomen and thigh through lumbar plexus.
Mandibular	N. Mandibularis.	Trigeminal.	Sensory and motor.	Teeth and skin of lower jaw and cheek; muscles of mastication.
Masseteric	N. Massetericus.	Mandibular div. of trigeminal.	Motor.	Masseter muscle.
Maxillary	N. Maxillaris.	Trigeminal.	Sensory.	Nasal pharynx, palate, teeth of upper jaw and skin of cheek.
Median	N. Medianis.	Internal and external cords of brachial plexus.	Motor and sensory.	Pronators and flexors of forearm, two external lumbricales, thenar muscles, skin of palm of outer three and a half fingers.
Mental	N. Mentalis.	Inferior dental.	Sensory.	Skin of lower lip and chin.
Musculocutaneous	N. Musculocutaneus.	External cord of brachial plexus.	Motor and sensory.	Flexors of upper arm and skin of external aspect of forearm.
Musculocutaneous of leg	N. Peroneus superficialis.	External popliteal.	Motor and sensory.	Peroneal muscles, skin of external aspect of lower leg and foot.
Musculospiral	N. Radialis.	Posterior cord of brachial plexus.	Motor and sensory.	Extensors of entire arm and hand, skin of back of forearm.
Mylohyoid	N. Mylohyoideus.	Inferior dental.	Motor.	Mylohyoid and anterior belly of digastric muscles.

App. 47

TABLE OF NERVES—Continued

Name	B. N. A. Equivalent	Origin	Function	Distribution
Nasal (nasociliary)	N. Nasociliaris.	Ophthalmic div. of trigeminal.	Sensory.	Ciliary ganglion, iris conjunctiva, ethmoid cells, mucous membrane and skin of nose.
Nasopalatine	N. Nasopalatinus.	Meckel's ganglion.	Sensory.	Mucous membrane of nose and palate.
Obturator	N. Obturatorius.	3rd, 4th and 5th lumbar through lumbar plexus.	Motor and sensory.	Adductors of thigh, hip and knee joints and skin of inner aspect of thigh.
Occipital, greater	N. Occipitalis, major.	2nd cervical.	Motor and sensory.	Muscles of back of neck, skin over occiput.
Occipital, lesser	N. Occipitalis, minor.	2nd cervical through cervical plexus.	Sensory.	Skin behind ear and on back of scalp.
Oculomotor	N. Oculomotorius.	Floor of aqueduct of Sylvius.	Motor.	Levator palpebrae superioris, superior, internal and inferior recti, and inferior oblique muscles of eye.
Olfactory	NN. Olfactorii.	Olfactory lobe.	Special sense of smell.	Upper turbinates and ethmoid plate.
Ophthalmic	N. Ophthalmicus.	Trigeminal.	Sensory.	Lacrimal gland, conjunctiva, skin of forehead, skin and mucous membrane of nose.
Optic	N. Opticus.	Corpora quadrigemina.	Special sense of sight.	Retina.
Orbital	N. Zygomaticus.	Maxillary div. of trigeminal.	Sensory.	Skin of temple.
Palatine, posterior	N. Palatinus, posterior.	Meckel's ganglion.	Motor.	Levator palati, and azygos uvulae muscles.
Pectineal	N. Perinei.	Anterior crural.	Motor.	Pectineus muscle.
Perineal	N. Perinei.	Internal pudic.	Motor and sensory.	Muscles and skin of perineum.
Phrenic	N. Phrenicus.	Third and fourth cervical.	Motor.	Diaphragm.
Pneumogastric	N. Vagus.	Floor of fourth ventricle.	Motor and sensory.	Pharynx, larynx, heart, lungs, stomach.
Popliteal, external	N. Peroneus communis.	Great sciatic.	Motor and sensory.	Extensor muscles of lower leg and foot and overlying skin.
Popliteal, internal	N. Tibialis.	Great sciatic.	Motor and sensory.	Flexors of lower leg and foot and overlying skin.
Pterygoid, external	N. Pterygoideus, externus.	Mandibular div. of trigeminal.	Motor.	External pterygoid muscle.
Pterygoid, internal	N. Pterygoideus, internus.	Mandibular div. of trigeminal.	Motor.	Internal pterygoid muscle.
Pudendal		Small sciatic.	Sensory.	Skin of perineum and genitalia.

TABLE OF NERVES—Continued

Name	B. N. A. Equivalent	Origin	Function	Distribution
Pudic	N. Pudendus.	3rd, 4th and 5th sacral through sacral plexus.	Motor and sensory.	Muscles and skin of perineum and genitalia.
Radial	N. Radialis, ramus superficialis.	Musculospiral.	Sensory.	Back of hand and outer three and a half digits.
Sacral	NN. Sacrales.	Spinal cord.	Motor and sensory.	Muscles and skin of loins and lower extremities.
Saphenous, external or short	N. Suralis.	Internal popliteal.	Sensory.	Skin of foot and fifth toe.
Saphenous, internal or long	N. Saphenus.	Anterior crural.	Sensory.	Skin of inner aspect of knee, leg, ankle and dorsum of foot.
Sciatic, great	N. Ischiadicus.	2nd, 3rd and 4th sacral through sacral plexus.	Motor and sensory.	Flexor muscles of thigh, leg and foot, skin of calf and sole.
Sciatic, small	N. Cutaneus femoris, posterior.	Sacral plexus.	Sensory.	Skin of perineum and back of thigh.
Sphenopalatine		Maxillary div. of trigeminal.	Sensory.	Meckel's ganglion.
Spinal accessory	N. Accessorius.	Floor of fourth ventricle and cervical cord.	Motor.	Sternomastoid and trapezius muscles.
Stapedial		Facial.	Motor.	Stapedius muscle.
Stylohyoid		Facial.	Motor.	Stylohyoid and posterior belly of digastric muscle.
Suboccipital	N. Suboccipitalis.	Posterior div. of first cervical.	Motor.	Complexus oblique and rectus muscles of back of neck.
Subscapular, inferior	N. Subscapularis, inferior.	Posterior cord of brachial plexus.	Motor.	Teres major.
Subscapular, middle	N. Thoracodorsalis.	Posterior cord of brachial plexus.	Motor.	Latissimus dorsi.
Subscapular, superior	N. Subscapularis, superior.	Posterior cord of brachial plexus.	Motor.	Subscapularis.
Superficial cervical	N. Cutaneus colli.	Cervical plexus.	Sensory.	Skin of front of neck.
Supraacromial	NN. Supraclaviculares, posterior.	Cervical plexus.	Sensory.	Skin over shoulder.
Supraorbital	N. Supraorbitalis.	Frontal.	Sensory.	Skin of forehead.
Suprascapular	N. Suprascapularis.	5th and 6th cervical.	Motor.	Supraspinatus and infraspinatus.
Suprasternal	NN. Supraclavicularis anteriores.	Cervical plexus.	Sensory.	Skin over top of sternum.
Supratrochlear	N. Supratrochlearis.	Frontal.	Sensory.	Skin of upper eyelid and root of nose.
Temporal, external anterior	N. Temporalis.	Mandibular div. of trigeminal.	Motor.	Temporal muscle.
Thoracic, external anterior	N. Thoracalis, anterior.	External cord of brachial plexus.	Motor.	Pectoralis major.
Thoracic, internal anterior	N. Thoracalis, anterior.	Internal cord of brachial plexus.	Motor.	Pectoralis minor and major.
Thoracic, long, external, respiratory or posterior	N. Thoracalis, longus.	5th, 6th and 7th cervical.	Motor.	Serratus magnus.

App. 49

TABLE OF NERVES—Continued

Name	B. N. A. Equivalent	Origin	Function	Distribution
Thoracic, spinal	NN. Thoracales.	Spinal cord.	Motor and sensory.	Muscles and skin of thorax.
Tibial anterior	N. Peroneus profundus.	External popliteal.	Motor and sensory.	Extensor muscles of foot and foot, skin of dorsum of foot.
Tibial posterior	N. Tibialis.	Internal popliteal.	Motor and sensory.	Flexor muscles of foot and toes, skin of sole.
Trigeminal	N. Trigeminus.	Floor of 4th ventricle.	Sensory and motor.	Skin of face, tongue, teeth and muscles of mastication.
Trochlear	N. Trochlearis.	Floor of aqueduct of Sylvius.	Motor.	Superior oblique muscle of eye.
Tympanic	N. Tympanicus.	Glossopharyngeal.	Sensory.	Tympanum, eustachian tube and structures of middle ear.
Ulnar	N. Ulnaris.	Inner cord of brachial plexus.	Motor and sensory.	Flexor carpi ulnaris, flexor profundus digitorum, elbow and wrist joints, skin of 5th and inner half of 4th fingers and hypothenar eminence.
Vidian	N. Canalis pterygoidei.	Facial.	Sensory.	Meckel's ganglion.

App. 50

Nerve Plexuses of the Sympathetic and Cerebrospinal Systems

aortic (ā-or'tĭk) (*abdominal*). ORIGIN: Semilunar, lumbar ganglia, renal and solar plexuses. LOCATION: Sides and front of aorta. DISTRIBUTION: Inferior mesenteric, spermatic and hypogastric plexus. Filaments to inferior vena cava. (*thoracic*). ORIGIN: Thoracic ganglia of sympathetic nerve, cardiac plexus. LOCATION: Surrounding the thoracic aorta. DISTRIBUTION: Solar plexus, aorta.

*****brachial** (brā'kĭ-ăl). ORIGIN: Anterior branches of 5th, 6th, 7th, 8th, cervical, and greater part of 1st dorsal nerves. LOCATION: Lower part of neck to axilla. DISTRIBUTION: Sixteen branches of suprascapular, subscapular, rhomboid, median, ulnar, musculospiral, posterior thoracic, musculothoracic, circumflex, musculocutaneous nerves.

cardiac (kar'dĭ-ăk) (*great or deep*). ORIGIN: Cardiac nerves of cervical ganglion of sympathetic and vagus. LOCATION: In front of bifurcation of trachea. DISTRIBUTION: Pulmonary, coronary and cardiac plexuses. (*superficial or anterior*). ORIGIN: Left superior cardiac nerve, branch of vagus and filaments of deep cardiac plexus. LOCATION: Beneath arch of aorta. Front of right pulmonary artery. DISTRIBUTION: Coronary and pulmonary plexuses.

carotid (kăr-ŏt'ĭd) (*external*). ORIGIN: Pharyngeal plexus, superior cardiac nerve and superior cervical ganglion. LOCATION: Around external carotid artery. DISTRIBUTION: External carotid artery and its branches. (*internal*). ORIGIN: Asymptomatic plexus. LOCATION: Surrounding internal carotid artery. DISTRIBUTION: Tympanic plexus, sphenopalatine ganglion, abducens and oculomotor nerves, the cerebral vessels and the ciliary ganglion.

cavernous (kăv'ĕr-nŭs). ORIGIN: 3rd to 6th cranial nerves and ophthalmic ganglion. LOCATION: Cavernous sinus. DISTRIBUTION: Wall of internal carotid artery.

celiac (sē'lĭ-ăk). ORIGIN: Solar plexus, branches from lesser splanchnic and vagus nerves. LOCATION: Behind stomach, in front of aorta at level of origin of celiac artery. DISTRIBUTION: Coronary, hepatic, pyloric, gastroduodenal, gastroepiploic and splenic plexuses. SYN: *solar plexus*.

*****cervical** (ser'vĭ-kăl). ORIGIN: Anterior branches of first 4 cervical nerves. LOCATION: Beneath sternocleidomastoid muscle opposite first 4 cervical vertebrae. DISTRIBUTION: Cutaneous, muscular and communicating rami.

*****coccygeal** (kŏk-sĭj'ē-ăl). ORIGIN: Fourth and 5th sacral and the coccygeal nerves. LOCATION: Dorsal surface of coccyx and caudal end of sacrum. DISTRIBUTION: Anococcygeal nerves.

cystic (sĭs'tĭk). ORIGIN: Hepatic plexus. LOCATION: At gallbladder. DISTRIBUTION: Gallbladder.

esophageal (ē-sō-făj'ē-ăl). ORIGIN: Vagus nerve, thoracic sympathetic ganglia. LOCATION: Around the esophagus. DISTRIBUTION: Esophagus.

gastric (găs'trĭk). ORIGIN: Celiac plexus and continuations of esophageal plexuses. LOCATION: Gastric artery. DISTRIBUTION: Abdominal viscera.

hemorrhoidal (hĕm"ō-roy'dăl). ORIGIN: Pelvic and inferior mesenteric plexuses. LOCATION: Rectum and sides of rectum. DISTRIBUTION: Rectum.

hepatic (hē-păt'ĭk). ORIGIN: Celiac plexus, left vagus, right phrenic. LOCATION: Accompanies hepatic artery. DISTRIBUTION: Liver.

hypogastric (hī"pō-găs'trĭk). ORIGIN: Aortic plexus and lumbar ganglia. LOCATION: Promontory of sacrum. DISTRIBUTION: Pelvic plexus.

*****lumbar** (lŭm'bar). ORIGIN: First 4 lumbar nerves. LOCATION: Psoas muscle. DISTRIBUTION: Iliohypogastric, ilioinguinal, genitocrural, external cutaneous, obturator, accessory, and anterior crural nerves.

Meissner's (mīs'nĕrs). ORIGIN: Superior mesenteric plexus (controls secretions of the bowels). LOCATION: Submucous coat of small intestines. DISTRIBUTION: Intestinal walls.

mesenteric (mĕs-ĕn-tĕr'ĭk). ORIGIN: Celiac plexus and left side of aortic plexus. LOCATION: Surrounding the inferior and superior mesenteric arteries. DISTRIBUTION: Descending colon, sigmoid, rectum, intestines.

myenteric (mī-ĕn-tĕr'ĭk). ORIGIN: Sympathetic system (controls peristalsis). LOCATION: Between the circular and longitudinal coats of small intestines. DISTRIBUTION: Intestinal walls.

ophthalmic (ŏf-thăl'mĭk). ORIGIN: Internal carotid plexus. LOCATION: Around ophthalmic artery and optic nerve. DISTRIBUTION: Optic region.

pancreatic (păn-krē-ăt'ĭk). ORIGIN: Splenic plexus. LOCATION: Near pancreas. DISTRIBUTION: Filaments to pancreas.

pancreaticoduodenal (păn-krē-ăt"ĭ-kō-dū"ō-dē'năl). ORIGIN: Hepatic plexus. LOCATION: Near head of pancreas. DISTRIBUTION: Filaments to pancreas and duodenum.

pelvic (pĕl'vĭk). ORIGIN: Hypogastric plexus, 2nd to 4th sacral nerves, 1st and 2nd sacral ganglia (pelvic brain). LOCATION: Side of rectum and bladder. DISTRIBUTION: Viscera of pelvis, pelvic plexus.

phrenic (frĕn'ĭk). ORIGIN: Solar plexus, semilunar ganglia. LOCATION: Accompanies phrenic artery to diaphragm. DISTRIBUTION: Diaphragm and suprarenal capsules.

prostatic (prŏs-tăt'ĭk). ORIGIN: Hypogastric plexus. LOCATION: Vesical arteries. DISTRIBUTION: Bladder.

pulmonary (pŭl'mō-nā"rĭ). ORIGIN: Anterior and posterior pulmonary branches of vagus and sympathetic nerves. LOCATION: Root of lungs, front and back. DISTRIBUTION: Root of lungs.

pyloric (pī-lor'ĭk). ORIGIN: Hepatic plexus.

---

* Plexuses of central nervous system.

App. 51

Nerve Plexuses

LOCATION: Near pylorus. DISTRIBUTION: Filaments to pylorus.
renal (rē'năl). ORIGIN: Solar and aortic plexuses and semilunar ganglia. LOCATION: Renal artery. DISTRIBUTION: Kidneys, posterior vena cava, spermatic plexus.
*sacral (sā'krăl). ORIGIN: Anterior branch of 4th and 5th lumbar and 1st, 2nd, 3rd, and 4th sacral nerves. LOCATION: Front of sacrum on piriformis muscle. DISTRIBUTION: Muscular, pudic, superior gluteal, great and small sciatic nerves.
solar (sō'lar) (*epigastric*). ORIGIN: Splanchnics and right vagus. LOCATION: Back of stomach. DISTRIBUTION: Semilunar ganglia, phrenic, suprarenal, renal, spermatic, celiac, superior mesenteric, and aortic plexuses. Called *abdominal brain*. SYN: *celiac plexus*.
spermatic (spĕr-măt'ĭk) (*ovarian*). ORIGIN: Aortic plexus. LOCATION: Accompanies spermatic vessels to testes or ovaries. DISTRIBUTION: Testes or ovaries.
splenic (splĕ'nĭk). ORIGIN: Celiac plexus, left semilunar ganglion, right vagus nerve. LOCATION: Accompanies splenic artery. DISTRIBUTION: Spleen, pancreatic plexus, left gastroepiploic plexus.

suprarenal (sū-prā-rē'năl). ORIGIN: Diaphragmatic, solar and renal plexuses. LOCATION: Around suprarenal capsules. DISTRIBUTION: Filaments to medulla of suprarenal capsules.
thyroid (thī'royd) (*inferior*). ORIGIN: Middle cervical ganglion. LOCATION: Around external carotid and inferior thyroid arteries. DISTRIBUTION: Larynx, pharynx, thyroid gland. (*superior*). ORIGIN: Superior laryngeal and cardiac nerves. LOCATION: Around the thyroid gland. DISTRIBUTION: Thyroid region.
uterine (ū'tĕr-ĭn). ORIGIN: Pelvic plexus. LOCATION: Accompanies uterine arteries. DISTRIBUTION: Cervix and lower part of uterus.
vaginal (văj'ĭ-năl). ORIGIN: Pelvic plexus. LOCATION: Vaginal walls. DISTRIBUTION: Vagina.
vertebral (vĕrt'ĕ-brăl). ORIGIN: First part thoracic ganglion, upper cervical nerves. LOCATION: Surrounding basilar and vertebral arteries. DISTRIBUTION: Vertebral and cerebellar regions.
vesical (vĕs'ĭ-kăl). ORIGIN: Pelvic plexus. LOCATION: Accompanies vesical arteries. DISTRIBUTION: Vesicula seminalis, vas deferens.

* Plexuses of central nervous system.

A. Cranial Nerves

Ref.	Cranial Nerve Supply to the	No.	Name of Nerve	Div. of Nerve
A	CHEEK—Tongue, teeth, ear and muscles of mastication	5th	Trigeminus or Trifacial	2nd
A 1			Great Sensory Nerve of head and face	3rd
B	EYE—Retina	2nd	Optic	
B 1	Muscles of Orbit (rectus, et al.) and motor filaments to Iris	3rd	Oculomotor	
B 2	" " (Supr. oblique)	4th	Trochlear or Pathetieus	
B 3	Conjunctiva, Laerimal gland and eyelids	5th-7th	Trigeminus and Facial	
B 4	Muscle of Orbit (external rectus)	6th	Abducent	
B 5	Eyeball	3rd-6th	Oculomotor and Trigeminus	1st div. of 6th
C	EAR—Tympanum	9th	Glossopharyngeal	1st Div. Branches of
C 1	External	5th	Trigeminus	
C 2	Muscles External, also Parotid Gland	7th	Facial	3rd
C 3	External	10th	Pneumogastrie or Vagus	
C 4	Middle	9th	Glossopharyngeal	
C 5	Internal	8th	Auditory	
D	EXPRESSION—(Muscles of face, lips, etc.)	7th	Facial (Great Motor Nerve of Face Muscles)	
E	ESOPHAGUS	10th	Pneumogastrie	
F	FOREHEAD—(Eyes and nose)	5th	Trigeminus	1st
G	FACE—Muscles of mastication, ear, cheek, tongue, teeth	5th	Trigeminus	2nd
G 1	" ear, cheek, tongue, taste, teeth	5th	Trigeminus	3rd
H	HEART	10th	Pneumogastrie	
I	INTESTINES	10th	Pneumogastrie	
J	LIVER	10th	Pneumogastrie	Left Pneumogastric
K	LARYNX—Voice	10th	Pneumogastrie	
K 1		11th	Accessory Spinal	
L	LUNGS	10th	Pneumogastrie	2nd
M	NOSE—Smell	1st	Olfactory	
M 1	Mucous membrane	5th	Trigeminus	1st
M 2	" and lip	7th	Facial	
N	PALATE—Muscles	7th	Facial	
N 1	Hard and soft (gums, tonsils and nose)	5th	Trigeminus	2. Meekel's Ganglion
O	PHARYNX	10th	Pneumogastrie	also Meekel's Ganglion
O 1		9th	Glossopharyngeal	
O 2		11th	Accessory Spinal	2nd
P	STOMACH	10th	Pneumogastrie	
Q	SPLEEN	10th	Pneumogastrie	Right Pneumogastric
R	TEETH—Upper (4 incisors, 2 canine, 4 bicuspids, 6 molars)	5th	Trigeminus	2nd
R 1	Lower (4 " 2 " 4 " 6 ")	5th	Trigeminus	3rd
S	TONSILS	9th	Glossopharyngeal	
S 1		5th	Trigeminus	
T	TONGUE—(Papillae)	5th	Trigeminus	2nd
T 1	Muscles	7th	Facial	3rd
T 2	Taste	9th	Glossopharyngeal	
T 3	Muscles	12th	Hypoglossal	
T 4	Circulation and secretion of Sub. Max. glands	7th	Facial	

Ref. Numbers Refer to Parts Supplied

App. 53

A. CRANIAL NERVES (Continued)

Ref.	Name of Division	Function of Nerve	Principal Arteries
A	Superior Maxillary	Sensory[2]	Cheek—†Facial
B 1	Inferior	Sensory, Motor and Taste[2]	Eye—13 brs. from Int. Carotid
B 2		Special Sense of Sight	‟ ‡Infraorbital, from Ex. Carotid
B 3	Ophthalmic	Motor entirely	
B 4		5th Sensory[2] and 7th Motor[1]	
B 5		Motor entirely	
C 1	Also branches from Sympathetic	3rd Motor, 5th Sensory and Nutrition[3]	
C 2	Inferior Maxillary	Motor[4]	Ear—Post. †Auricular (Br. Ext. Car.)
C 3		Sensory[2]	‟ Ant. ‡Auricular (Br. Temporal)
C 4	Auricular branch	Motor[1]	‟ ‡Auricular, ‡Posterior and ‡Ant.
C 5		Sensory[4]	Deep Auricular, ‡Tympanic
D		Special Sense of Hearing	‡Stylomastoid, Petrossal, ‡Vidian
E	Esophageal branch	Motor	Int. Auditory
F	Ophthalmic	Motor and Sensory[3]	Face—†Facial
G	Superior Maxillary	Sensory[2]	Esophageal—*Esophageal
G 1	Inferior Maxillary	Sensory, Motor and Taste[2]	(See Head)
H	Sup. Laryngeal branch	Motor and Sensory[3]	Face—†Facial
I	Gastric branch	Motor and Sensory[3]	
J	Gastric branch	Motor and Sensory[3]	
K	Laryngeal branch	Motor and Sensory[3]	
K 1		Motor[5]	
L	Pulmonary branch	Motor and Sensory[3]	
M 1	Ophthalmic	Special Sense of Smell	Nose—‡Lateralis Nasi, ‡Nasal
M 2		Sensory[2] and Motor[1]	Nasal Br. of Ophthalmic
N 1		Motor[1]	
N 2	Superior Maxillary	Sensory[2]	Palate—‡Dorsalis ‡Linguae (†lingual)
O 1	Pharyngeal branch	Sensory and Motor[3]	Pharynx—Asc'd †Pharyngeal
O 2		Sensory and Motor[4]	‟ ‟
P		Motor[5]	
Q	Gastric branch	Motor and Sensory[3]	Stomach—*Gastric
R	Gastric branch	Motor and Sensory[3]	Spleen—*Splenic
R 1	Superior Maxillary	Sensory[2]	Teeth—‡Inf. dental, ‖Sup. dental,
S	Inferior Maxillary	Sensory[2]	‡Alveolar
S 1	Meekel's Ganglion	Sensory[2]	Tonsils—‡Dorsalis linguae, †asc'd Ph.
T 1	Inf. Maxillary (gustatory branch)	Sensory, Motor and Taste[2]	‡Asc'd palat., ‡tonsilar, (†facial)
T 2		Motor[1]	Tongue—‡Lingual (Ext. Carotid)
T 3	Lingual branch	Motor entirely	‡Submental (†facial)
T 4	Chorda Tympani (§Br. of 7th)	Circulation and Secretion of Tongue	Asc'd †Pharyngeal (Ext. Carotid)

Ref. Numbers Refer to Parts Supplied

App. 54

B. The Twelve Pairs of Cranial Nerves

No.	Name	Div.	Branches	Function and Distribution*	Remarks
1	Olfactory		20	M	Its bulb is a lobe of the Cerebrum
2	Optic		None	B	
3	Oculomotor		Filaments	B1-B5	Great motor nerve of 5 of 7 muscles of eye
4	Trochlear or Patheticus		None	B2	Smallest cranial nerve
5	Trigeminus or Trifacial (Three Twins)	1st	Ophthalmic	B3-B5-F-M1	The great Sensory nerve of the head and face
5	Trigeminus or Trifacial (Three Twins)	2nd	Superior Maxillary	A-G-N1-R-S1	
5	Trigeminus or Trifacial (Three Twins)	3rd	Inferior Maxillary	A1-C2-G1-R1-T	
6	Abducent		Filaments	B4	(Leading from)
7	Facial or Portio Dura (Hard Portion)			C1-D-M2-N-F1-F4-B3	Great motor nerve of Facial Muscles
8	Auditory or Portio Mollis, of 7 (Soft Portion)			C5	
9	Glossopharyngeal			C-C4-O1-S-T2	Tongue and throat nerve
10	Pneumogastric (Vagus or Par Vagum)		12	C3-E-H-I-J-K-L-O-P-Q	Wandering nerve
11	Accessory Spinal	1 Ext.	Spinal portion		
11	Accessory Spinal	2 Int.	Accessory portion	K1-O2	Accessory to the Pneumogastric
12	Hypoglossal			T3	Hypoglossal (Under the tongue)

*To find the Function and Distribution of the Cranial Nerves, reference is given to Table "A" and "B."

B. CRANIAL NERVES (Continued)

No.	Function	Origin	Exit
1	Special Sense Smell	Frontal lobe, optic thalamus deeply and island of Reil, by three roots	Exit by 20 branches through the cribriform plate to the schneiderian membrane of nose
2	Special Sense Sight	Optic thalamus, corpora geniculata and corpora quadrigemina or optic lobes, which communicate with cerebrum and cerebellum	Through optic foramen to retina
3	Motor	Floor of aqueduct of Sylvius and inner surface of crus cerebri	Sphenoidal fissure to eye muscles
4	Motor of superior oblique mus. of eye	Valve of Vieussens, a thin plate of nervous matter above the fourth ventricle	Sphenoidal fissure to sup. oblique muscle of eye
5	Sensory	Superficial origin in, side of pons Varolii by two roots. Deep origin cerebellum and medulla oblongata and floor of fourth ventricle	1st Br. sphenoidal fissure and supraorbital foramen 2nd Br. foramen rotund and intraorbital foramen
	Sensory, Motor, Taste		3rd Br. foramen ovale and mental foramen
6	Motor of external rectus of eye	Fourth ventricle, deep origin posterior part of medulla oblongata	Sphenoidal fissure, between the two heads of the external rectus muscle
7	Motor	Floor of fourth ventricle	Internal auditory meatus through aqueductus Fallopii and stylomastoid foramen
8	Special Sense Hearing	Restiform body of 4th ventricle	Internal auditory meatus through the internal auditory canal
9	Mixed, Sensory, Motor, Taste	Medulla oblongata. Deeply from floor of fourth ventricle	Jugular foramen to back of tongue, middle ear, tonsils, pharynx and meninges
10	Mixed, Sensory and Motor	Medulla oblongata. Deeply from floor of fourth ventricle	Jugular foramen
11	Motor	Without cavity of cranium, lateral tract of spinal cord as low as the sixth cervical nerve	Enters cranium through the foramen magnum, uniting with the accessory portion which originates within the cranium and both make their exit through jugular foramen
	Motor	Within the cavity of the cranium, medulla oblongata deeply, near floor of 4th ventricle	
12	Motor	Medulla oblongata deeply from floor of 4th ventricle	Anterior condyloid foramen

EXPLANATION TABLES A AND B. CRANIAL NERVES

1st Pair—Olfactory, Special Sense of Smell.
2d " Optic, Special Sense of Sight.
3rd " Oculomotor, Great Motor of Eye, supplies five of the seven eye muscles.
4th " Trochlear or Pathetieus, motor of superior oblique muscle of eye.
2§5th " Trigeminus or Trifacial, great sensory nerve of head and face; divides into three portions, viz.: 1st Ophthalmic Sensory; 2nd Supr. Max. Sensory; 3rd Inf. Sensory, Max. Motor and a lingual nerve of the sense of taste. Most difficult of all the cranial nerves to trace.
6th Pair—Abducent, Motor of External Rectus of Eye.
‡7th " Facial or Portio Dura, great motor nerve of face muscles; exclusively motor at its origin, but it subsequently receives fibers from the (5th) Trigeminus, which give it some sensory function.
§Some anatomists claim that the Chorda Tympani nerve is a branch of the Sympathetic system.
8th Pair—Auditory, or Portio Mollis of 7th, Special Sense of Hearing.
‡9th " Glossopharyngeal, in part a special nerve of taste, nerve of sensation, and also contains motor fibers.
³‖10th " Pneumogastric, Vagus or Par Vagum, (a mixed nerve) at its origin it is exclusively sensory, but lower down it is also motor and capable of providing both for sensation and motion in organs to which distributed.
‡11th " Accessory Spinal, considered to be exclusively motor, but some authorities claim for it sensory fibers.
Accessory portion joins the vagus, to which it supplies its motor and some of its cardioinhibitory fibers.
Spinal portion supplies the trapezius and sternomastoid muscles.
12th " Hypoglossal, exclusively motor.

*Branches of the aorta. †Branches of branches of the aorta. ‡Branches of branches of branches of the aorta. ‖Branches of branches of branches of branches of the aorta

App. 57

Table of Arteries[1]

Name of Artery	Origin	Distribution	Branches
Acromial.	Acromiothoracic.	Deltoid muscle.	
Acromiothoracic.	Axillary.	Side of thorax and part of arm.	Acromial, clavicular, pectoral.
Adipose.	Capsular arteries, small branches of thoracic aorta.	Adipose tissue of heart.	
Afferent.	Interlobular of kidneys.	Glomeruli.	
Alar thoracic.	Axillary.	Glands and tissue of the axilla.	
Alveolar.	Internal maxillary.	Molar and bicuspid teeth.	
Anastomotic, of the arm.	Brachial.	Elbow.	Anterior and posterior.
Anastomotic, of the sciatic.	Sciatic.	External rotator muscles of thigh.	Branches of gluteal artery.
Anastomotic, of the thigh.	Femoral.	Knee.	Superficial and deep.
Angular.	Facial.	Lacrimal sac.	Infraorbital.
Aorta. See: *aorta*, in vocabulary.			
Appendicular.	Ileocolic.	Mesentery of the vermiform appendix.	
Articular, middle, of knee.	Popliteal.	Crucial ligaments and joint.	
Articular, superior, external of knee.	Popliteal.	Femur and knee joint.	
Articular, superior, internal.	Popliteal.	Knee joint. Vasti.	
Ascending.	External circumflex.	Gluteal muscles and hip joint.	
Auditory, external.	Internal maxillary.	Tympanum.	
Auditory, internal.	Basilar.	Internal ear.	
Auricular.	Occipital.	Auricle.	
Auricular, anterior, inferior.	Temporal.	Auricle.	
Auricular, deep.	Internal maxillary.	Tympanum and external auditory meatus.	
Auricular, left.	Left coronary artery.	Left auricle; pulmonary artery.	
Auricular, posterior.	Fifth branch of external carotid.	Back of auricle and part of neck.	Parotid, muscular, stylomastoid, auricular, and mastoid.
Auricular, right.	Right coronary artery.	Right auricle, septum, and aorta.	
Axillary.	Subclavian.	Brachial and seven branches.	Superior thoracic, acromiothoracic, long thoracic, alar thoracic, subscapular, ant. and post. circumflex.
Azygos (of knee).	Popliteal.	Crucial ligament, knee joint.	
Azygos.	External plantar.	Articulations of tarsus.	Into branches of external plantar.
Azygos.	Internal plantar.	Joints on inner side of foot.	
Azygos (of elbow).	Superior profunda.	Posterior part of elbow joint.	Anastomotica magna and interosseous recurrent.
Azygos (of shoulder).	Suprascapular.	Shoulder joint.	
Basilar.	Right and left vertebral.	Brain.	Transverse, internal auditory, anterior cerebellar, superior cerebellar, posterior cerebral.

[1] From *Appleton's Medical Dictionary*, Courtesy, Appleton Century Company.

App. 58

TABLE OF ARTERIES—Continued

Name of Artery	Origin	Distribution	Branches
Bicipital	Anterior circumflex.	Long tendon of biceps and shoulder joint.	
Brachial	Axillary.	Arm and forearm.	Superior and inferior profunda, anastomotica magna, nutrient, muscular, radial, and ulnar.
Brachiocephalic	See: *Innominate a.*		
Bronchial, inferior	Thoracic aorta.	Bronchi and lungs.	
Bronchial, superior	Arch of aorta.	Bronchi.	
Buccal	Internal maxillary.	Muscles and integument of the cheek.	
Bulb, artery of	Internal pudic.	Erectile tissue of the corpus spongiosum.	
Calcanean, external	Posterior peroneal.	Outer side of foot and heel.	Anastomosing with external malleolar, external plantar and tarsal arteries.
Calcanean, inferior	External plantar.	External plantar muscles.	
Calcanean, internal	Posterior tibial and peroneal.	Inner side of heel and sole.	
Calcanean, middle	Posterior tibial.	Outer and back surface of os calcis.	
Capsular	See: *Suprarenal.*		
Carotid, common	Innominate (right); arch of aorta (left).	External and internal carotid.	
Carotid, external	Common carotid.	Front and back of neck, face, side of head, meninges, middle ear, thyroid, tongue, tonsils.	Internal maxillary, superior thyroid, lingual, facial, occipital, posterior auricular, superficial temporal.
Carotid, internal	Common carotid.	Brain, nose, orbit, internal ear, and forehead.	Anterior and middle cerebral, ophthalmic, tympanic, vidian, pituitary, gasserian, meningeal, communicating, anterior choroid.
Carpal	Radial.	Lower radius and wrist.	Anterior carpal rete.
Carpal	Ulnar.	Carpus.	Posterior carpal rete.
Cecal, anterior	Inferior mesenteric.	Front part of cecum.	
Cecal, posterior	Posterior mesenteric.	Back part of cecum.	
Celiac axis	Abdominal aorta.	Esophagus, stomach, duodenum, gallbladder, liver, pancreas, spleen.	Gastric, hepatic, splenic.
Cerebellar (three)	Basilar and vertebral.	Cerebellum.	Inferior and superior vermiform and hemispheral.
Cerebral, anterior and middle	Internal carotid.	Cerebrum.	
Cerebral, posterior	Basilar.	Cerebrum.	
Cervical, ascending	Inferior thyroid.	Neck.	
Cervical, deep	Superior intercostal.	Neck.	
Cervical, superficial	Transverse cervical.	Muscles of back of neck.	Muscular, spinal.
Cervical, transverse	Thyroid axis.	Posterior cervical and scapular regions.	Muscular, spinal.

App. 59

TABLE OF ARTERIES—Continued

Name of Artery	Origin	Distribution	Branches
Circumflex, anterior	Axillary.	Pectoralis major, biceps, shoulder joint.	Bicipital and pectoral.
Circumflex, posterior	Axillary.	Deltoid, teres minor, triceps, shoulder joint.	Acromial, articular, muscular, nutrient.
Coronary, left	Left anterior sinus of Valsalva.	Heart.	Left auricular, anterior interventricular, left marginal, terminal.
Coronary, right	Right anterior sinus of Valsalva.	Heart.	Right auricular, preventricular, right marginal, posterior interventricular, tranvserse.
Digital	External plantar.	Outer side second to fifth toes.	
Digital, palmar	Superficial palmar arch.	Sides of fingers.	
Dorsalis pedis	Anterior tibial.	Foot.	Tarsal, metatarsal, dorsalis hallucis, communicating.
Epigastric	External iliac.	Abdominal wall, femoral ring and cremaster.	Cremasteric, pubic, muscular, and terminal branches.
Facial	External carotid.	Pharynx and face.	Inferior palatine, tonsillar, glandular, muscular, submental, mesenteric, buccal, inferior labial, coronary of lips, lateralis nasi, angular.
Femoral	External iliac.	Lower part of abdominal wall, genitals, upper thigh.	
Gastric	Celiac axis.	Liver, esophagus, stomach.	Cardiac, esophageal, gastric and hepatic.
Gastroduodenal	Hepatic.	Duodenum, liver, pancreas, stomach.	Gastroepiploic, pancreaticoduodenal, pyloric.
Gluteal	Internal iliac.	Gluteal muscles.	Deep and superficial gluteal.
Hepatic	Celiac axis.	Duodenum, liver, pancreas, stomach.	Gastroduodenal, pancreatic, subpyloric, terminal.
Iliac, common	Abdominal aorta.	Peritoneum.	Peritoneal, ureteric, external and internal iliac.
Iliac, external	Common iliac.	Lower limb.	Deep epigastric, circumflex, femoral.
Iliac, internal	Common iliac.	Pelvic and generative organs, inner thigh.	Anterior and posterior trunk.
Iliac, inferior (anterior trunk)	Internal iliac.	Pelvic and generative organs of thigh.	Vesical, uterine, vaginal, obturator, sciatic, internal pudic, middle hemorrhoidal.
Iliac, inferior (posterior trunk)	Internal iliac.	Muscles of hip and sacrum.	Gluteal, iliolumbar and lateral sacral.
Innominate	Arch of aorta.	Right side of head and right arm.	Right common carotid, right subclavian.
Intercostal, superior	Subclavian.	Neck and upper thorax.	Deep cervical, first intercostal, arteria aberrans.
Interosseous	Ulnar.	Deep muscles of the forearm.	Anterior and posterior interosseous.
Laryngeal, superior	Superior thyroid.	Muscles and mucous membrane of larynx.	
Lingual	External carotid.	Tongue.	Hyoid, dorsalis linguae, sublingual, ranine.
Mammary, internal	Subclavian.	Thorax.	Superior phrenic, mediastinal, pericardiac, sternal, anterior intercostal, perforating, lateral intercostal, superior epigastric.

App. 60

TABLE OF ARTERIES—Continued

Name of Artery	Origin	Distribution	Branches
Maxillary, internal	External carotid.	Structures indicated in names of branches.	Middle and small meningeal, inferior dental, deep temporal, tympanic, pterygoid, masseteric, buccal, posterior palatine, vidian, pterygopalatine, sphenopalatine, alveolar, infraorbital.
Mediastinal, anterior	Internal mammary.	Superior and anterior mediastinums, thymus gland.	
Meningeal (four)	Ascending pharyngeal and posterior ethmoid.	Dura mater.	
Mesenteric, inferior	Abdominal aorta.	Descending colon, sigmoid flexure, rectum.	Colica sinistra, sigmoid, superior hemorrhoidal.
Mesenteric, superior	Abdominal aorta.	Small intestine, colon, cecum, ileum.	Inferior pancreaticoduodenal, colica media, colica dextra, ileocolic, vasa intestinae tenuis.
Musculophrenic	Internal mammary.	Diaphragm, 5th and 6th intercostal spaces, muscles of abdomen.	Phrenic, anterior intercostals, muscular.
Nasal	Ophthalmic.	Lacrima sac, integuments of nose.	Lacrima land transverse nasal.
Obturator	Internal iliac.	Pelvis and thigh.	Iliac, vesical, pubic, external and internal pelvic.
Occipital	External carotid.	Muscles of neck and scalp, meninges.	Muscular, auricular, meningeal, cranial branches, princeps cervicis.
Ophthalmic	Internal carotid.	Eye, adjacent structures, part of face.	Lacrimal, supraorbital, central of retina, ciliary, muscular, posterior and anterior ethmoid, palpebral, nasal, frontal.
Palmar arch (deep)	Radial.	Palm and fingers.	Perforating, palmar interosseous, recurrent.
Palmar arch (superficial)	Ulnar.	Palm and fingers.	Digital, cutaneous, muscular.
Pharyngeal, ascending	External carotid.	Pharynx soft palate, tympanum, meninges.	Meningeal, palatine, pharyngeal, prevertebral, tympanic.
Phrenic, superior	Internal mammary.	Diaphragm, pericardium pleura.	
Plantar arch	External plantar.	Anterior part of foot and toes.	Anastomotic, calcaneal, cutaneous, posterior perforating, plantar arch.
Plantar, external	Posterior tibial.	Sole and toes.	Anastomotic, articular, cutaneous, muscular, superficial digital.
Plantar, internal	Posterior tibial.	Inner side of foot.	
Popliteal	Femoral.	Knee and leg.	Cutaneous, superior and inferior muscular, superior external and internal articular, inferior external and interior articular, azygos articular, anterior and posterior tibial.
Profunda (deep femoral)	Femoral.	Thigh.	External and internal circumflex, three perforating.

TABLE OF ARTERIES—Continued

Name of Artery	Origin	Distribution	Branches
Profunda, inferior	Brachial.	Triceps, elbow joint.	Articular, ascending, cutaneous, muscular, nutrient.
Profunda, superior	Brachial.	Humerus, muscles and skin of arm.	
Pterygopalatine	Internal maxillary.	Pharynx, eustachian tubes, sphenoidal cells.	Eustachian, pharyngeal, sphenoid.
Pudic, external	Common femoral.	Skin and integument above pubes and external genitalia.	
Pudic, internal	Internal iliac, anterior trunk.	Generative organs.	Inferior hemorrhoidal, superficial and transverse perineal, muscular, artery of the bulb, of the corpus cavernosum, dorsalis penis.
Pulmonary	Right ventricle.	Lungs.	Right and left pulmonary.
Pyloric, superior	Hepatic.	Pyloric end of stomach.	
Radial	Brachial.	Forearm, wrist, hand.	Radial recurrent, muscular, anterior and posterior carpal, superficial volar, metacarpal, dorsalis pollicis, dorsalis indicis, deep palmar arch.
Renal	Abdominal aorta.	Kidney.	Inferior suprarenal, capsular, ureteral.
Scapular, dorsal	Subscapular.	Muscles of infraspinous fossa.	Infrascapular.
Scapular, posterior	Transverse cervical.	Muscles of scapular region.	Supraspinous and infraspinous, muscular, subscapular.
Sciatic	Internal iliac, anterior trunk.	Muscles and viscera of pelvis.	Coccygeal, inferior gluteal, muscular, anastomotic, articular cutaneous, vesical, rectal, etc.
Spermatic	Abdominal aorta.	Scrotum and testis.	Cremasteric, epididymal, testicular, ureteral.
Sphenopalatine	Internal maxillary.	Pharynx, nose and sphenoid cells.	Nasal, pharyngeal, ascending septal, sphenoid.
Spinal, anterior	Vertebral.	Spinal cord.	
Spinal, lateral	Vertebral.	Vertebrae and spinal canal.	
Spinal, posterior	Vertebral.	Spine.	
Splenic	Celiac axis.	Pancreas, great curvature of stomach, spleen.	Gastric, left gastroepiploic, splenic branches, small and large pancreatic.
Subclavian	Right—Innominate. Left—Arch of aorta.	Neck, thorax, arms, brain, meninges.	Vertebral, internal mammary, superior intercostal, thyroid axis.
Subscapular	Axillary.	Subscapularis, teres major, latissimus dorsi, serratus magnus, axillary glands.	Dorsal and infrascapular.
Suprarenal, inferior	Renal.	Suprarenal body.	
Suprarenal, middle	Aorta.	Suprarenal bodies.	
Suprarenal, superior	Phrenic.	Suprarenal bodies.	
Suprascapular	Thyroid axis.	Muscles of shoulder.	Inferior sternomastoid, nutrient, suprasternal, acromial, articular, supraspinous, and infraspinous.

TABLE OF ARTERIES—Continued

Name of Artery	Origin	Distribution	Branches
Temporal	External carotid.	Forehead, parotid gland, masseter muscle, ear.	Anterior auricular, middle, anterior and posterior temporal, transverse facial.
Thoracic, acromial	Axillary.	Muscles of shoulder, chest and arm.	Acromial, clavicular, humeral, pectoral.
Thoracic, alar	Axillary.	Axillary glands.	
Thoracic, long	Axillary.	Pectoral muscles, mammary and axillary glands.	
Thyroid axis	Subclavian.	Shoulder, neck, thorax, spine, cord.	Inferior thyroid, suprascapular, transverse cervical.
Thyroid, inferior	Thyroid axis.	Esophagus, larynx, muscles of neck.	Ascending cervical, esophageal, inferior laryngeal, muscular, tracheal.
Thyroid, superior	External carotid.	Omohyoid, sternohyoid, sternothyroid, thyroid gland.	Hyoid, sternomastoid, superior laryngeal, cricothyroid.
Tibial, anterior	Popliteal.	Leg.	Posterior and anterior tibial, recurrent, muscular, internal and external malleolar.
Tibial, posterior	Popliteal.	Leg, heel and foot.	Communicating, cutaneous, calcanean, internal and external plantar, malleolar, medullary, muscular, peroneal.
Ulnar	Brachial.	Forearm, wrist and hand.	Anterior and posterior ulnar, recurrent, common interosseous, muscular, nutrient, carpal, palmar arch.
Uterine	Branch of internal iliac.	Uterus.	Azygos, cervical, vaginal.
Vertebral	Subclavian.	Neck and cerebrum.	Anastomotic, lateral spinal, muscular, posterior cerebellar, posterior meningeal, posterior and anterior spinal.
Vesical, inferior	Internal iliac, anterior trunk.	Bladder, prostate, seminal vesicles, vagina.	
Vesical, superior	Internal iliac, anterior trunk.	Bladder.	Deferentia, ureteric.
Vidian	Internal maxillary.	Roof of pharynx, eustachian tube, tympanum.	Eustachian, pharyngeal, tympanic.

App. 63

Table of Veins

Name	Description	Origin	Distribution
Alveolares superior and inferior (superior and inferior dental veins)	Veins supplying teeth and jaws. Anastomose with pterygoid plexuses.	Capillaries of teeth canals and gums.	Through jaws to structures of teeth. Between surfaces of maxillae below alveolar processes to v. facialis anterior at angle of jaw.
Angularis (angular vein)	Short superficial vein in nasal region.	Union of vv. nasofrontalis, frontalis, and supraorbitalis at root of nose.	From root of nose laterally to below eye.
Anonyma (innominate veins)	Paired veins without valves. Flow together to form vena cava superior.	Union of vv. jugularis interna and subclavia.	From sternoclavicular articulation to 1st right costal cartilage where they flow together to form vena cava superior.
Articulares genus (articular veins of knee)	Vein of knee.	Tissues of region of knee and m. articularis genu.	Tissues of region of knee to v. poplitea.
Articulares mandibulae (articular veins of mandible).	Deep veins of region of jaw; form large plexus lateral to ear. Anastomose with pterygoid plexus.	Plexus surrounding joint of jaw and tissues of external auditory canal region.	Region of jaw and adjacent structures diagonally downward to v. facialis posterior.
Auditivae internae (internal auditory)	Paired 2 from each ear. Arise in internal ear, pass through meatus acusticus internus. Drain blood from labyrinth.	From internal ear through meatus acusticus internus to sinus transversus or sinus petrosus inferior.	Empty into sinus transversus or sinus petrosus inferior.
Auriculares anteriores (anterior auricular veins)	Small veins of external ear structures.	Capillaries of tissues of external ear.	From tissues of external ear to v. facialis posterior in front of ear.
Auricularis posterior (posterior auricular vein)	Superficial vein of posterior skull region.	Capillaries of tissues of posterior portion of skull and mastoid emissarium.	From tissues of occipital region behind ear diagonally downward below ear to v. jugularis externa.
Axillaris (axillary vein)	Portion of large venous trunk from upper extremity in axillary region. Receives veins from arms and adjacent structures.	Union of deep brachial veins at lower margin of m. pectoralis major.	Region of axilla to clavicle.
Azygos (azygos vein)	Single vein draining blood from intercostal spaces, esophagus, bronchi, and mediastinal structures. Anastomoses freely with v. hemiazygos which flows into it.	Continuation of v. lumbalis ascendens dextra at diaphragm.	From level of diaphragm up posterior thoracic wall on right of vertebral bodies to v. cava superior.
Basilica (basilic vein)	Large superficial vein on medial and lateral aspect of arm and forearm. Anastomoses freely with v. cephalica.	Dorsum of hand at ulnar end of arcus venosus dorsalis.	Tissues of hand diagonally across back of hand to anterior surface of arm above elbow to upper 3rd of arm to flow into vv. brachiales.
Basivertebrales (basivertebral veins)	Veins of bodies of vertebrae.	Capillaries of vertebral bodies.	From body of each vertebra to venous plexuses of spinal column.
Brachiales (brachial veins)	Two large deep veins of upper arm.	Union of vv. ulnares and radialis at elbow.	From elbow on each side of forearm in deep tissues to unite to form v. axillaris.

Table of Veins — App. 65

Name	Description	Origin	Distribution
Bronchiales anteriores (anterior bronchiole veins)	Veins of bronchi.	Capillaries of bronchi.	From bronchi to anonyma separately or in common with other thoracic viscera.
Bronchiales posteriores (posterior bronchial veins)	Veins of posterior bronchial walls.	Capillaries of bronchial walls.	From tissues of bronchi to v. azygos at level of 4th to 6th thoracic vertebrae.
Bulbi urethrae (artery of bulb)	Corresponds to v. bulbi vestibuli in female.	Tissues of bulbus urethrae and muscles in region of trigone.	From tissues above rectum to trigone diagonally lateral to v. pudenda interna.
Canaliculi cochleae (vein of cochlear canal)	Vein of inner ear structures.	From capillaries of cochlea.	From cochlea through the canaliculus cochlea to bulbus v. jugularis superioris and jugularis interna.
Cava inferior (inferior vena cava)	Large venous trunk carrying blood from lower extremities, abdomen and trunk to right atrium. Branches from abdominal viscera flow into it.	Union of vv. iliacae communes in front of 4th or 5th lumbar vertebra.	Along posterior abdominal wall through liver and diaphragm diagonally upward in thorax to right atrium.
Cava superior (superior vena cava)	Large single venous trunk without valves, draining blood from upper part of body.	Union of two v. anonyma.	From first right costal cartilage downward to right atrium.
Cephalica (cephalic vein)	Superficial vein of arm and forearm. Anastomoses freely with v. basilica.	Dorsum of hand at radial end of arcus venosus dorsalis.	Tissues of hand, arm and forearm. Extends up lateral region of arm and forearm to v. axillaris at level of clavicle.
Cerebri externae and internae (superficial and inferior cerebral or Galen veins)	Have no valves. Collect blood from cerebral tissue.	From superficial tissues of cerebral surface and inferior substance of cerebrum.	From cerebrum through subarachnoid connective tissue of third ventricle to point where they flow together near the interventricular foramen.
Cerebri magna (magnus Galeni)	Large vein formed by union of vv. cerebri internae.	Capillaries of cerebrum.	From region of splenium corporis callosi forward to vena rectus.
Cervicalis profunda (deep cervical vein)	Deep vein of neck. Corresponds to arteria cervicalis profunda.	Plexus vertebralis posterior.	Posterior to v. jugularis interna to level of 7th cervical vertebra where it flows into vertebralis.
Circularis (circular sinus)	A blood channel in the region of the sella turcica.	Border of sella turcica.	Between 2 venae cavernosae.
Circumflexae femoris laterales (lateral circumflex femoral veins)	Veins of deep tissues of lateral aspect of thigh.	Capillaries of muscles in lateral region of thigh.	Laterally between m. rectus femoris and vastus intermedia diagonally upward to v. profunda femoris.
Circumflexae femoris mediales (internal circumflex veins)	Veins of medial and dorsal aspect of thigh and hip. Anastomose with v. glutaea.	Capillaries of tissues of knee joint and muscles of thigh.	From muscles of medial region of thigh upward beneath m. quadratus femoris to v. profunda femoris at its union with v. femoralis.
Circumflexa ilium profunda (deep circumflex iliac vein)	Vein of deep structures in iliac region.	Capillaries of deep muscles of upper portion of thigh and lower portion of abdomen.	From deep tissues from anterior superior spine of ileum along inner surface of pelvic brim to v. iliaca externa.
Circumflexa ilium superficialis (superficial circumflex iliac vein)	Superficial vein in lateral iliac region.	Capillaries of superficial tissues of lateral aspect of region of hip joint.	From superficial tissues from anterior iliac crest diagonally downward to flow into v. femoralis just before it enters external femoral ring.
Colica dextra (right colic vein)	Vein of ascending colon. Usually two.	Capillaries of walls of ascending colon.	From tissues of ascending colon through mesentery to v. mesenterica superior.

Table of Veins — App. 66

Name	Description	Origin	Distribution
Colica media (middle colic vein)	Vein of transverse colon.	Capillaries of walls of transverse colon.	From tissues of transverse colon through mesentery to v. mesenterica superior.
Colica sinistra (left colic vein)	Vein of descending colon. Anastomoses freely with vv. sigmoideae.	Capillaries of wall of descending colon.	From tissues of descending colon through mesentery laterally upward to v. mesenterica inferior.
Comitans lateralis	Vein of region of knee.	Capillaries of region of knee.	From tissues of leg and knee upward on either side of v. poplitea to flow into it.
Comitans medalis	Vein of region of knee.	Capillaries of region of knee.	From tissues of knee and leg upward to v. poplitea.
Cordis anteriores (anterior coronary veins)	Small veins of right ventricle.	Tissues of right ventricle.	From right ventricles near apex upward to flow directly into right atrium.
Cordis magna (coronary or great cardiac vein)	Large vein of anterior portion of ventricles.	Tissues of ventricles in region of apex.	From apex in anterior longitudinal sulcus upward to coronary sulcus left to right atrium through coronary sinus.
Cordis media (middle coronary vein)	Large vein of posterior portion of ventricles.	Capillaries of ventricles and ventricular septum.	From apex of heart along ventricles in longitudinal sulcus upward from apex to right atrium through coronary sinus.
Cordis parva (small or rt. cardiac vein)	Small vein of right atrium and ventricle.	Capillaries of right auricle and ventricle.	From branches in right auricle and ventricle along coronary sulcus to right atrium through coronary sinus.
Coronaria ventriculi (coronary vein of stomach)	Vein of stomach. Anastomoses with vv. gastroepiploica and pylorica.	Capillaries of upper portion of stomach.	From right or left along lesser curvature of stomach to vv. portae or lienalis near pylorus.
Costoaxillaris (costoaxillary vein)	Vein draining blood from middle portion of first 6th or 7th intercostal spaces.	Capillaries of upper intercostal spaces and veins.	From middle portion of upper 6 vv. intercostales to v. thoracoepigastrica.
Cutaneae abdominis et pectoris (subcutaneous abdominal and thoracic veins)	Veins in subcutaneous tissues of abdomen and thorax wall.	Capillaries of superficial tissues of body wall.	Throughout subcutaneous tissue of body wall by anastomoses to veins of neck, axilla and anterior abdominal wall.
Cystica (cystic vein)	Vein of gallbladder.	Capillaries of gallbladder.	From tissues of gallbladder downward to v. portae just below its entrance into liver.
Deferentiales	Veins of testes.	Capillaries of testes.	From testes along ductus deferens to plexus vesicalis.
Digitales communes pedis (common digital veins of foot)	Short veins on back of foot.	Union of vv. digitalis pedis dorsalis and intercapitulares.	From base of toes to venous arches of back of foot.
Digitales dorsales propriae (dorsal digital veins of hand)	Superficial veins of back of fingers. Anastomose freely with each other.	Capillaries of superficial tissues of fingers.	From tissues of fingers proximally along fingers dorsally to hand, uniting to form vv. digitales volares communes.
Digitales pedis dorsales (dorsal digital veins of foot)	Veins of toes on dorsal surface.	Capillaries of toes.	From tissues of toes to vv. digitales communes pedis at base of toes.
Digitales plantares (plantar digital veins)	Veins of toes on plantar surface.	From capillaries of toes.	Along plantar surface of toes to foot to become vv. metatarseae plantares.
Digitales volares communes (common digital vein of palm)	Superficial veins of palm of hand.	Capillaries of tissues of palm of hand.	From base of fingers to superficial venous arches of palm.

Table of Veins

Name	Description	Origin	Distribution
Digitales volares propriae (palmar digital veins of hand)	Superficial veins of palmar surface of fingers. Anastomose freely with each other and dorsal veins.	Capillaries of superficial tissues of palmar surface of fingers.	Tissues of fingers along fingers to dorsal veins by vv. intercapitulares.
Diploicae (diploic veins)	Thin walled tubes in canals between the inner and outer skull surface. They have no valves except at mouth of vessels, form a network through the skull and are variable in distribution. Named from regions they drain.	Bony tissue between internal and external skull surfaces.	From bones of skull to venae durae matres and external veins of skull.
Dorsalis penis (dorsal vein of penis)	Large vein of penis along midline of dorsum.	Tissue of penis.	Along dorsum of penis upward to pelvis between symphysis pubes and urogenital trigon into plexus pudendalis in front of bladder.
Dorsales penis cutaneae (superficial veins of penis)	Small veins of skin of penis.	Capillaries of skin of penis.	From superficial tissues of penis laterally upward to v. pudendis externa.
Ductus venosus	Vein in liver functioning in fetal circulation, connecting v. umbilicalis and v. cava inferior.	V. umbilicalis.	From v. umbilicalis transversely through liver to v. cava inferior.
Duodenales (duodenal veins)	Veins of duodenum.	Walls of duodenum.	From duodenum by anastomoses to vv. iliocolica, colica media, and mesenterica superior.
Epigastricae superiores (superior epigastric veins)	Double veins of upper anterior abdominal wall. Anastomose freely with v. epigastrica inferior.	Capillaries of upper anterior abdominal wall.	From tissues of anterior abdominal wall along inner surface of m. rectus abdominis upward through diaphragm to form v. mammaria interna with v. musculophrenica.
Epigastrica inferior (inferior epigastric vein)	Vein of lower anterior abdominal wall. Tributaries drain blood from paraumbilical veins and superficial tissues of testes.	Capillaries of internal surface of lower anterior abdominal wall.	From internal surface of lower abdominal wall along m. rectus abdominus, diagonally across abdominal wall to flow into v. iliaca externa.
Epigastrica superficialis (superficial epigastric veins)	Veins draining blood from superficial regions of lower half of anterior abdominal wall.	Superficial tissues of lower portion of anterior abdominal wall.	From superficial tissues of abdominal wall, downward with many anastomoses diagonally to v. femoralis just outside entrance to external femoral ring.
Facialis anterior (anterior facial)	Superficial vein of face. Corresponds to arteria maxillaris externa. Drains blood from most of smaller superficial facial veins.	From union of vv. angularis and nasales externae at medial angle of eye.	Beneath superficial muscles of face. Diagonally across face from nose to angle to jaw where it flows into v. facialis communis.
Facialis communis (common facial vein)	Large vein of face beneath platysma.	Union of vv. facialis anterior and posterior.	From convergence of vv. faciales at angle of jaw to v. jugularis interna at level of hyoid bone.
Facialis posterior (posterior facial vein)	Deep vein of face. Branches drain deep structures of face.	Union of vv. temporalis superficialis and media.	From origin in front of ear downward through parotid gland behind ramus of mandible to angle of jaw where it forms v. jugularis interna.
Femoralis (femoral vein)	Large vein of thigh.	Continuation of v. poplitea.	From posterior region of knee through m. abductor magna upward beneath m. sartorius across thigh through femoral ring to become v. iliaca externa.

Table of Veins

Name	Description	Origin	Distribution
Femoropoplitea (femoropopliteal vein)	Small superficial vein of dorsum of thigh and knee. Anastomoses with v. saphena magna.	Capillaries of superficial tissues in posterior region of knee.	From laterodorsal superficial tissues of knee transversely across and above knee through muscles to flow into v. poplitea.
Frontalis (frontal veins)	Superficial vein of skull, anastomosing with temporalis.	Capillaries of anterior region of scalp.	Anterior region of scalp down anterior midline diagonally across forehead to left of root of nose where it forms v. angularis.
Gastricae breves (short gastric veins)	Short veins of fundus of stomach, usually 3 to 5.	Capillaries of fundus of stomach.	From capillaries of fundus of stomach in gastrosplenic ligament to v. lienalis.
Gastroepiploica dextra (right gastroepiploic vein)	Vein of lower portion of stomach.	Capillaries of stomach.	Along lower portion of greater curvature of stomach to unite with v. gastroepiploica sinistra. Flows into v. mesenterica superior.
Gastroepiploica sinistra (left gastroepiploic vein)	Large vein of upper portion of stomach.	Capillaries of stomach.	Along greater curvature of stomach between it and spleen, unites with v. gastroepiploica dextra. Flows into v. lienalis.
Glutaea inferior (inferior gluteal vein)	Vein of lower region of hip. Anastomoses freely with v. glutaea superior.	Capillaries, gluteal and adjacent muscles.	From tissues of hip through pelvic wall to inner surface, to flow into v. hypogastrica.
Glutaea superior (superior gluteal vein)	Vein of upper region of hip. Anastomoses freely with v. glutaea inferior.	Capillaries of gluteal and adjacent muscles.	From tissues of hip through pelvic wall to inner surface to flow into v. hypogastrica.
Haemorrhoidales externae (external hemorrhoidal veins)	A plexus of veins on outer surface of rectum.	From internal plexus of rectum and veins of adjacent structures.	From outer surface of rectum to vv. pudendae internae, hypogastrica and mesenterica inferior by numerous branches.
Haemorrhoidales inferiores (inferior hemorrhoidal veins)	Veins of lower region of rectum and anus.	From plexus haemorrhoidalis externus of outer wall of rectum.	From region of anus diagonally lateral beneath m. glutaea to v. pudendae internae.
Haemorrhoidales internae (internal hemorrhoidal veins)	A plexus of veins in submucosa of rectum.	Tissues of rectum.	From inner wall of rectum through tissues of rectum by numerous branches to external plexus.
Haemorrhoidales mediae (middle hemorrhoidal veins)	Veins of middle region of plexus haemorrhoidalis externa.	Plexus haemorrhoidalis externa and tissues of bladder, prostate and seminal vesicles.	From plexus of outer rectal wall laterally to v. hypogastrica.
Haemorrhoidalis superior (superior hemorrhoidal vein)	Largest vein of region of rectum.	Capillaries of rectum and plexus on lower anterior lateral surface of rectum.	Posterior to rectum upward through mesorectum to flow into v. mesenterica inferior.
Hemiazygos (hemiazygos vein)	Single vein of lower left thoracic wall. Drains blood from intercostal veins. Anastomoses with v. azygos.	Continuation of v. lumbalis ascendens sinistra above diaphragm.	From diaphragm along left of vertebral bodies to v. azygos at 6th to 7th intercostal space.
Hemiazygos accessoria (accessory hemiazygos vein)	Drains blood from intercostal spaces above level of 6th to 7th intercostal space.	Capillaries of upper intercostal spaces.	From upper intercostal spaces along left margin of bodies of vertebrae to level of 6th to 7th intercostal space where it enters v. hemiazygos.
Hepaticae (hepatic veins)	Short, large veins from liver to v. cava inferior. Vary in number from 2 to 4.	Tissues of liver.	From lobes of liver to v. cava inferior, just below inferior surface of diaphragm.

Table of Veins — App. 69

Name	Description	Origin	Distribution
Hypogastrica (internal iliac or hypogastric vein)	Large, short vein draining blood from pelvis.	Convergence of veins of internal pelvic organs and structures.	From posterior pelvic wall upward and anterior to v. iliaca externa at brim of pelvis.
Ileocolica (ileocolic vein)	Vein of mesentery of ascending colon.	Capillaries of intestine in region of union of ileum and colon.	From region of lower portion of ascending colon and ileum through mesentery to unite with vv. colicae dextrae to flow into v. mesenterica superior.
Iliaca communis (common iliac vein)	Large vein draining blood from pelvis and leg. Flow together to form v. cava inferior.	Union of vv. hypogastrica and iliaca externa.	Diagonally across pelvis from lateral region to meet in posterior midline.
Iliaca externa (external iliac vein)	Large vein from leg along anterior portion of rim of true pelvis. A continuation of v. femoralis.	V. femoralis, at its entrance into pelvis.	From v. femoralis behind inguinal ligament diagonally upward and backward to unite with v. hypogastrica to form v. iliaca communis.
Iliaca interna (see v. hypogastrica)			
Iliolumbalis (iliolumbar vein)	Vein of lower abdominal wall. Anastomoses to form collateral circulation with v. lumbalis ascendens.	Capillaries of tissues of body wall in lumbar regions.	From walls of false pelvis diagonally across inner surface of ilium to flow into v. hypogastrica or v. iliaca communis.
Intercapitulares (intercapitular veins)	Veins of hand in tissues between fingers.	Veins of fingers and tissues between fingers.	Connect between bases of fingers volar and dorsal veins of hand.
Intercavernous anterior and posterior (anterior and posterior intercavernous sinuses)	Unpaired blood channels connecting two cavernous sinuses, forming with them the circular sinus.	Layers of dura mater in region of hypophysis.	Anterior is in front and beneath hypophysis. Posterior is behind and beneath hypophysis.
Intercostales (intercostal veins)	Veins of intercostal spaces.	Capillaries of intercostal spaces.	From intercostal spaces to region along lower margin of ribs to vv. mammaria interna, azygos and costoaxillaris.
Intervertebrales (intervertebral veins)	Veins accompanying spinal nerves. Permit collateral circulation of venous plexuses of spinal cord.	From plexuses of spinal column.	Between vertebrae and between internal and external venous plexuses of spinal column.
Jugularis anterior (anterior jugular vein)	Superficial vein of anterior region of neck. Pair anastomose freely with other and adjacent veins.		From chin upon superficial muscles laterally downward across neck to v. jugularis externa or subclavia.
Jugularis externa (external jugular vein)	Large superficial vein in lateral region of neck. Main branches are vv. occipitalis and jugularis anterior.	From union of facialis posterior and auricularis posterior.	Below ear across sternocleidomastoid muscle beneath platysma down neck to v. subclavia.
Jugularis interna (internal jugular vein)	Largest vein of head and neck. Receives veins from face, neck, thyroid and larynx. With jugulares externa and anterior corresponds to arteria carotis communis.	Arises from capillaries of brain and regions of pharynx and neck, as direct continuation of v. transversus.	From foramen jugulare, where it connects with bulbus v. jugularis superioris downward on lateral wall of pharynx to junction with v. subclavia to form v. anonyma.
Labiales posteriores (labial veins)	Correspond to vv. scrotales posteriores.	Tissues of labia.	From labia to v. pudenda interna.

Table of Veins — App. 70

Name	Description	Origin	Distribution
Labiales (superior and inferior) (superior and inferior labial veins)	Superficial veins of the lips. Anastomose with each other.	Capillaries of lips.	Tissues of lip to facialis anterior.
Lienalis (splenic vein)	Large vein draining blood from spleen and part of stomach.	Capillaries of spleen.	From spleen transversely across abdomen to head of pancreas where it forms v. portae with v. mesenterica.
Lingualis (lingual vein)	Vein of tongue corresponding to arteria lingualis. Anastomoses with vv. pharyngeae and thyreoidea superior.	From tongue along lower jaw to facialis. Capillaries of tongue and sublingual regions.	From tongue along lower jaw to vv. facialis or thyreoideae superiores.
Lumbales (lumbar veins)	Four or five veins of abdominal walls. Anastomose freely with each other.	Capillaries of walls of abdominal cavity.	From somatic tissues of abdomen posteriorly to v. cava inferior at various levels.
Lumbalis ascendens (ascending lumbar vein)	Vein parallel to v. cava inferior connecting lumbar veins.	Vv. Lumbales.	Along lateral border of spinal column through abdomen flowing into v. iliaca communis and continuing in thorax on right as v. azygos and on left as v. hemiazygos.
Mammaria interna (internal mammary)	Deep vein of chest draining blood from intercostal spaces. Double in the region m. transversus covered by m. transversus thoracis and single above it.	Union of vv. epigastricae superiores and musculophrenicae.	Between 7th and 10th ribs, lateral margin of inner aspect of sternum, beneath pleura, behind cartilages of the 1st to 7th rib to v. anonyma dextra at its junction with anonyma sinistra.
Mediana antebrachii (median antebrachial vein)	Superficial vein of forearm running between vv. cephalica and basilica. Anastomoses with them.	Tissues of hand and forearm.	From superficial veins of hand up forearm to v. basilica below elbow.
Mediana cubiti	Short vein of forearm for collateral circulation between vv. basilica and cephalica.	Tissues of forearm.	From v. cephalica below elbow diagonally across forearm to v. basilica at elbow.
Mediastinales anteriores (anterior mediastinal veins)	Veins of mediastinal region. May flow together or flow into veins of other viscera.	Capillaries of mediastinal viscera.	From mediastinal region to v. anonyma.
Mediastinales posteriores (posterior mediastinal veins)	Drain blood from posterior mediastinal structures.	Capillaries of mediastinal structures.	From posterior mediastinal structures to v. azygos at level of 9th to 11th thoracic vertebrae.
Meningeae (meningeal veins)	Multiple veins. Numerous in the dura mater of brain, anastomosing freely with each other. Usually accompany arteries with 2 veins for each artery.	Meninges of brain.	From meninges to sagittalis superior, sinus cavernosus and internal maxillary vein.
Mesenterica inferior (inferior mesenteric vein)	Large vein from mesentery of colon. Receives veins from region of rectum.	Capillaries of colon and rectum.	Through mesentery of colon upward to v. lienalis or v. mesenterica superior.
Mesenterica superior (superior mesenteric vein)	Large vein from small intestine which flows into v. portae.	Capillaries of mesentery of small intestines.	From mesentery of small intestines upward to head of pancreas to unite with v. lienalis to form v. portae.
Metacarpeae dorsales (dorsal metacarpal veins)	Superficial veins of back of hand. Anastomose freely with each other.	Capillaries of hand.	Superficial tissues of hand along metacarpal bones to venous arches of back of hand.

Table of Veins — App. 71

Name	Description	Origin	Distribution
Metacarpeae volares (palmar metacarpal veins)	Deep veins on both sides of hand. Anastomose with each other.	Capillaries of hand.	Deep tissues of palm of hand along metacarpal bone to palmar arches.
Metatarseae dorsales pedis (dorsal metatarsal veins)	Deep veins of back of foot.	Capillaries of deep structures of foot.	Along metatarsal bones toward ankle, uniting to form vv. tibiales anteriores.
Metatarseae plantares (plantar metatarsal veins)	Deep veins of solar aspect of foot.	Deep tissues of foot and vv. digitales plantares.	Along metatarsal bones to ankles and plantar venous arches.
Musculophrenicae (musculophrenic veins)	Veins of thoracic surface of diaphragm and lower thoracic wall.	Capillaries of thoracic surface of diaphragm and lower intercostal veins.	Along thoracic surface of diaphragm upward lateral to sternum to unite with vv. epigastricae superiores to form v. mammaria interna.
Nasales externae (external nasal veins)	Superficial veins of lower portion of nose.	Capillaries of lower portion of nose.	From tissue of nose to v. anterior facialis which they enter just below the eye.
Nasofrontalis (nasofrontal vein)	Short vein on each side of bridge of nose.	Capillaries in anterior of orbital cavity and region of frontal bone.	Between vv. supraorbitalis and angularis.
Obturatoria (obturator vein)	Vein draining blood from region of acetabulum and obturator foramen.	Capillaries of region of articulation of femur into pelvis.	Tissues of region of acetabulum and obturator foramen. Diagonally upward through tissues of region to enter pelvis on lateral aspect, diagonally backward and upward across pelvic wall to v. hypogastrica or iliaca externa.
Occipitalis (occipital vein)	Superficial vein of occipital region. Anastomoses with posterior vertebral plexus.	Capillaries of occipital region.	From superficial tissue of occipital region, and posterior vertebral plexus downward behind ear to v. jugularis externa below ear.
Oesophageae (esophageal veins)	Veins of esophagus.	Capillaries of esophagus.	From esophagus to v. azygos at level of 8th to 10th thoracic vertebrae.
Ophthalmica inferior (inferior ophthalmic vein)	Paired veins of floor of orbital cavity. Anastomose with superior ophthalmic veins.	Capillaries of lacrimal sac and eyelids.	From anterior of orbit between medial and interior wall of orbit to cavernous sinus.
Ophthalmica superior (superior ophthalmic vein)	Paired veins of orbital cavity. Have no valves. Anastomose with facial vein and inferior ophthalmic vein.	Capillaries of region of ethmoid and lacrimal bones, eyelids and ocular bulb.	From medial palpebral commissure of eye to cavernous sinus.
Ovarica (ovarian vein)	Vein of ovary.	Capillaries of ovaries and uterine tube and adjacent structures which form plexus around artery.	From plexus around artery upward from ovary across pelvic brim to become v. spermatica interna.
Palatina (palatine vein)	Deep vein of face corresponding to arteria palatina ascendens.	Capillaries of deep tissues of neck.	Deep tissues along ramus of jaw to v. facialis anterior at angle of jaw.
Palpebrales inferiores (inferior palpebral veins)	Veins of region of lower eyelid.	Capillaries of region of lower eyelid.	From region of lower eyelid to v. facialis anterior.
Palpebrales superiores (superior palpebral veins)	Veins of region of upper eyelid.	Capillaries of region of upper eyelid.	From region of upper eyelid to v. facialis anterior.
Pancreaticae (pancreatic veins)	Veins of pancreas.	Capillaries of pancreas.	From capillaries of tissues of pancreas by short veins which flow into v. lienalis at intervals.

Name	Description	Origin	Distribution
Pancreaticoduodenalis (pancreaticoduodenal vein)	Vein from duodenum and head of pancreas. Anastomoses freely with gastric veins.	Capillaries of duodenum and portions of pancreas.	Along duodenum between it and pancreas, upward to v. mesenterica superior just below its union with v. lienalis.
Parotidea anterior (anterior parotid vein)	Vein of parotid gland.	Capillaries of parotid gland.	From tissues of parotid gland to v. facialis anterior which it enters above angle of jaw.
Parotidea posterior (posterior parotid vein)	Vein of posterior portion of parotid gland.	Capillaries of posterior portion of parotid gland.	Posterior portion of parotid gland, interior to ear upward to union of v. temporalis superficialis with v. facialis posterior.
Parumbilicales (paraumbilical veins)	Small veins in region of umbilicus connecting superficial and deep veins.	Superficial tissues of region of umbilicus.	From superficial veins in umbilical region by anastomoses with vv. epigastricae to liver substance.
Pericardiacae (pericardial veins)	Veins of pericardium.	From capillaries of pericardium.	From pericardium to v. anonyma or to other veins of viscera which empty into it.
Peronaea (peroneal vein)	Deep vein of leg.	Veins of ankle and capillaries of tissues of leg.	From venous plexus in region of heel upward along lateral region of deep tissue to flow into v. tibialis posterior below knee.
Petrosus inferior (inferior petrosal sinus)	Paired blood channels in dura mater in temporal region.	Groove between petrous portion of temporal bone and basilar portion of occipital.	From petrous portion of temporal bone to superior jugular vein at its bulb.
Petrosus superior (superior petrosal sinus)	Paired blood channels in dura mater in temporal regions.	From region of petrous portion of temporal bone in the attached margin of tentorium cerebelli.	Between vena cavernosus and vena transversus.
Pharyngeae (pharyngeal veins)	Veins of pharyngeal region. Vary in number, from the plexus pharyngeus. Anastomose with veins of external ear, deep muscles of pharynx, palate and dura mater.	From plexus on outer pharyngeal surface.	From capillaries of pharyngeal region to v. jugularis interna or its adjacent branches at various levels.
Phrenica inferior (inferior phrenic)	Vein of abdominal surface of diaphragm.	Tissues of diaphragm.	Throughout abdominal surface of diaphragm to v. cava superior just below cava hiatus of diaphragm.
Phrenicae superiores (superior phrenic veins)	Paired veins of anterior wall of thorax, corresponding to arteriae pericardiacophrenicae.	Capillaries of pericardium.	From diaphragm through thoracic cavity in front of root of lung on pericardium to v. anonyma.
Plantares laterales (lateral plantar veins)	Veins of sole of foot.	Venous arches of sole of foot.	Along lateral margin of sole of foot upward to form vv. tibiales posteriores with vv. plantares mediales.
Plantares mediales (medial plantar veins)	Veins of sole of foot.	Venous arches of sole of foot.	Along medial aspect of sole of foot upward to form vv. tibiales posteriores with vv. plantares laterales.
Poplitea (popliteal vein)	Large vein in posterior region of knee. Has parallel median and lateral concomitants.	Union of vv. tibiales.	From vv. tibiales below knee in middorsal line upward to become femoral vein as it enters m. adductor.
Portae (portal vein)	Collects blood from digestive tract and conveys it to the liver. Terminates in capillary formation in liver	Union of vv. mesenterica superior and lienalis.	From head of pancreas upward posterior to bile ducts to hilum of liver to divide into right and left branch to liver.

Table of Veins

Name	Description	Origin	Distribution
Profundae clitoridis (deep veins of clitoris)	Vein of clitoris.	Tissues of clitoris.	From clitoris to v. pudenda interna.
Profundae penis (deep veins of penis)	Vein of corpora cavernosa of penis. Branches anastomose freely with each other.	Capillaries of penis.	Above penis in crus penis. Flows into v. dorsalis penis at root of penis.
Profunda femoris (deep femoral vein)	Deep vein of thigh.	Capillaries of muscles of thigh.	From midregion of thigh upward beneath anterior muscles to v. femoralis.
Pudendae externae (external pudic veins)	Veins draining blood from superficial regions of medial aspect of upper thigh.	Capillaries of superficial tissues of lower abdomen, scrotum or labia.	Superficial tissues of lower abdomen and scrotum or labia, transversely across upper region of thigh to v. femoralis.
Pudenda interna (internal pudic vein)	Vein of pelvic floor draining blood from pelvic walls and penis or clitoris.	From anastomoses with v. dorsalis penis or clitoridis below symphysis pubis.	From trigonum urogenitale along pelvic wall backwards and upwards to flow into v. hypogastrica.
Pylorica (pyloric vein)	Small vein of pyloric region of stomach. Anastomoses with other gastric veins.	Capillaries of pyloric portion of stomach.	Along lesser curvature of stomach to v. portae near pylorus.
Radialis (radial vein)	Large deep vein on radial side of forearm.	Palmar arches of hand.	Palmar arches of hand along lateral side of forearm in deep tissues to unite with v. ulnaris at elbow to form vv. brachiales.
Rectus (straight sinus)	Single blood channel in layers of dura mater connecting superior and inferior sagittal sinuses.	At point of attachment of falx cerebri to tentorium cerebelli.	Between superior and inferior venous channel at base of skull.
Renales (renal veins)	Veins of kidney. Receive blood from veins of ureter. The v. spermatica interna flows into v. renalis on left.	From capillaries of kidneys by fusion of small vessels near hilum of kidney.	From hilus of kidney transversely across posterior abdominal wall to v. cava inferior.
Rete dorsale manus (dorsal venous rete of hand)	A network of veins on dorsal surface of hand at wrist.	Veins of dorsal surface of hands.	From vv. metacarpeae dorsales, flowing together and multiple anastomoses at wrist, becoming vv. basilica and cephalica.
Rete dorsale pedis (dorsal venous rete of foot)	A network of veins on back of foot at ankle.	Veins of dorsal surface of foot.	From vv. digitales pedis dorsales by multiple anastomoses to network of veins of ankle.
Sacralis lateralis (lateral sacral vein)	Vein of posterior pelvic wall. Forms plexus with v. sacralis media.	Capillaries of tissues of posterior pelvic wall.	From tissues of posterior wall upward laterally on pelvic surface of sacrum to flow into v. hypogastrica or iliaca communis.
Sacralis media (middle sacral vein)	Large vein of posterior pelvic wall. Forms plexus with v. sacralis lateralis.	Capillaries of tissues of posterior wall.	From tissues of pelvic wall in sacral region upward along sacrum in middle line to flow into v. hypogastrica or iliaca communis.
Sagittalis inferior (inferior longitudinal sinus)	Single blood channel between layers of dura mater at the base of the falx cerebri.	From regions of superior dura mater and skull.	Entire length of inferior free margin of falx cerebri.
Sagittalis superior (superior longitudinal sinus)	Single blood channel between layers of dura mater in sagittal plane. Triangular in shape.	Region of falx cerebri and anterior portion of skull cavity.	From crista galli of ethmoid bone along sagittal sulcus of frontal, parietal, and occipital bones into transverse sinus.

Table of Veins

Name	Description	Origin	Distribution
Saphena magna	Large superficial vein of leg and thigh. Longest in body.	Capillaries of superficial tissues of leg and thigh and veins of foot.	Along medial aspect of leg from ankle upward across knee and thigh to enter femoral ring to flow into v. femoris.
Saphena parva (short saphenous vein)	Large superficial vein of back of leg.	Superficial veins of foot and capillaries of tissues of leg.	From ankle upward in middorsal line to above knee. Flows into v. saphena magna.
Scrotales anteriores (anterior scrotal veins)	Superficial veins of anterior region of scrotum.	Capillaries of superficial tissues of scrotum.	From anterior of scrotum transversely across thigh to v. pudenda externa.
Scrotales posteriores (posterior scrotal veins)	Veins of scrotum. Correspond to vv. labiales in female.	Capillaries of scrotum, posterior portion.	From scrotum upward laterally in perineum to pudenda interna in pelvic floor.
Sigmoideae (sigmoid veins)	Small veins of region of sigmoid flexure of colon.	Capillaries in region of sigmoid flexure.	Tissues of sigmoid colon through mesentery to v. mesenterica inferior.
Spermatica interna (spermatic vein)	Consists of 2 or 3 anastomosing vessels surrounding a. spermatica. Receives veins from ureters, peritoneum and kidney capsule.	From testicular vein in male and ovarian vein in female.	From brim of pelvis upward along posterior abdominal wall to v. cava inferior on right and v. renalis on left.
Sphenopalatina (sphenopalatine vein)	Vein draining deep structures of face and skull in nasal region.	Capillaries of deep nasal regions.	From nasal cavity through sphenopalatine foramen to pterygoid plexus in front of ear.
Sphenoparietalis (sphenoparietal sinus)	Paired blood channels of dura mater, from sphenoparietal region.	Capillaries of anterior temporal vein of diploë, middle meningeal and ophthalmomeningeal vein.	Each side of skull, behind coronal suture, to anterior end of sinus cavernosus.
Stylomastoidea (stylomastoid vein)	Corresponds to arteria stylomastoideus from middle and inner ear.	Capillaries of mastoid region and middle ear structures.	From mastoid and middle ear through stylomastoid foramen into facial canal behind ear to v. facialis posterior.
Subclavia (subclavian vein)	Large venous trunk to upper extremity. A continuation of v. axillaris in region of clavicle. Main tributaries are vv. transversa scapulae and coli.	V. axillaris and veins flowing into it from adjacent regions.	Beneath clavicle across first rib, to form v. anonyma with v. jugularis interna.
Submentalis (submental vein)	Superficial vein of under portion of chin. Anastomoses with v. lingualis and palatina.	Capillaries of region of chin.	From tissues of chin diagonally across chin to flow into v. facialis anterior or facialis communis below angle of jaw.
Supraorbitalis (supraorbital vein)	Vein of upper portion of orbital cavity.	Capillaries and superficial tissues in region of eye.	From superficial tissues of region of eye through supraorbital foramen along lateral wall of orbital cavity to nose where it joins v. nasofrontalis.
Suprarenalis (suprarenal vein)	Vein of adrenal glands.	Capillaries of adrenal glands.	From tissues of adrenal glands to v. cava inferior on right and vv. renales on left.
Temporalis media (median temporal vein)	Superficial vein of lateral portion of skull. Anastomoses with vv. temporalis superficialis and supraorbitalis.	Lateral superficial plexus of skull.	From lateral superficial tissues of skull transversely downward from level of lateral canthus of eye through temporal muscle to join v. temporalis superficialis in front of ear.
Temporalis superficialis (superficial temporal vein)	Vein of superficial tissues of skull. Anastomoses freely with v. frontalis.	Superficial plexus of roof of skull.	Tissues of roof of skull diagonally downward to join vv. temporalis media in front of ear.

Table of Veins

Name	Description	Origin	Distribution
Testicularis (testicular vein)	Vein of testes.	Capillaries of testes and epididymis which form close plexus around artery.	From tissues of testes and epididymis and plexus from veins of these organs through inguinal canal to become v. spermatica interna.
Thoracalis lateralis (long thoracic vein)	Long vein of lateral and anterior chest wall.	Capillaries of muscles in anterior chest and mammary glands.	Tissues of anterior chest muscles to v. axillaris with v. transversa colli.
Thoracoepigastrica (thoracoepigastric vein)	Superficial vein of trunk to permit collateral circulation between veins of arms and legs and trunk.	V. femoralis in inguinal region, and capillaries of superficial tissues of trunk.	Lateral wall of body from v. femoralis to v. thoracalis lateralis in axillary region below its union with v. axillaris.
Thymicae (veins of thymus)	Veins of thymus gland.	From capillaries of thymus gland.	From thymus gland to v. anonyma.
Thyreoidea ima (thyroid ima)	Large, short vein from plexus thyreoideus.	Plexus of thyroid.	From middle portion of plexus thyreoideus downward anterior to trachea to v. anonyma sinistra.
Thyreoideae inferiores (inferior thyroid veins)	Paired veins from plexus thyreoideus. Anastomose freely with thyreoideae superiores.	Plexus thyreoideus and regions of trachea, esophagus and larynx.	From thyroid plexus to v. jugularis interna at junction with subclavia.
Thyreoideae superiores (superior thyroid veins)	Two veins from superior portion of thyroid. Receive blood from vv. sternocleidomastoidea and laryngea.	Capillaries of thyroid.	From tissues of thyroid to v. jugularis interna at level of larynx, or to v. facialis communis.
Tibiales anteriores (anterior tibial veins)	Deep veins of anterior aspect of leg.	From union of vv. metatarseae dorsales pedis and capillaries of tissues of leg.	From dorsum of foot upward beneath m. tibialis anterior upward to knee, passing backward to flow into v. poplitea.
Tibiales posteriores (posterior tibial veins)	Deep veins of back of leg.	Union of vv. plantares and laterales and mediales in region of heel and capillaries of deep tissues of leg.	From ankle upward in median portion of deep tissues of posterior aspect of leg to flow into v. poplitea below knee.
Transversa colli (transverse cervical vein)	Drains blood from supraspinous region of scapula and neck.	Capillaries of supraspinous region of scapula and neck.	From supraspinous region of scapula diagonally across shoulder to v. axillaris with transversa scapulae.
Transversa faciei (transverse facial vein)	Superficial facial vein running directly upon masseter muscle and behind parotid gland.	Capillaries of middle portion of face.	From tissues of middle portion of face, transversely across face to v. facialis posterior in front of ear.
Transversa scapulae (transverse scapular vein)	Large vein of dorsal surface of scapula.	Capillaries of tissues of dorsal surface of scapula.	From tissues of dorsal scapular surface, two trunks on each side of scapular spine across shoulder to v. subclavia.
Transversus (lateral sinus)	Paired blood channels between layers of dura mater of base of skull. Cylindrical in shape.	Posterior region of skull cavity.	From internal occipital protuberance medially and inferiorly into internal jugular vein at jugular foramen.
Ulnaris (ulnar vein)	Large deep vein of medial side of forearm.	From palmar arches of hand.	From palmar arches of hand upward in deep tissues along ulnar side of forearm to form v. brachialis with v. radialis at elbow.
Umbilicalis (umbilical vein)	Vein carrying arterial blood from placenta to fetus.	Placental tissues.	Along umbilical cord through umbilicus to liver and ductus venosus.

Table of Veins

Name	Description	Origin	Distribution
Urethrales (urethral veins)	Veins of corpus cavernosum urethrae.	Capillaries of urethra and adjacent regions.	From structures of urethra to plexus pudendalis behind symphysis pubis to v. pudenda interna.
Uterinae (uterine veins)	Veins carrying blood from uterus.	From tissues of uterus through plexus uterovaginalis.	From lateral margin of uterus in plexus uterovaginalis laterally to v. hypogastrica.
Uterovaginales (uterovaginal veins)	Plexus of veins around vagina at lateral margin of uterus.	Tissues of vagina and uterus.	From lower regions of uterus and vagina by multiple anastomoses to plexus pudendalis and v. ovarica.
Vertebrales externi anteriores and posteriores (anterior and posterior external vertebral plexuses)	Plexuses on external surfaces of spinal column.	From tissues of vertebrae from vv. intercostales and intervertebrales along anterior and posterior aspects of spinal column. Branches flow into vv. vertebrales interni.	From branches from tissues of spinal column and cord longitudinally in canal.
Vertebrales interni (internal vertebral veins)	Plexuses of veins running within spinal canal, the length of the canal.	Capillaries of vertebrae and tissues of spinal cord.	From foramen magnum. Empty into v. occipitalis and plexus basilaris superiorly and vv. sacrales inferiorly.
Vertebralis (vertebral vein)	Vein draining blood from plexus venosi vertebrales, v. occipitalis, deep muscles of neck and plexus vertebralis externi. Corresponds to cervical portion of arteria vertebralis.	From vena occipitalis and capillaries of veins of spinal canal and deep muscles of neck.	Foramen magnum downward lateral to arteria vertebralis through foramina transversaria of 1st, 6th or 7th cervical vertebra to external jugularis externa.
Vesicales (vesicular veins)	Veins of urinary bladder.	Tissues of bladder and plexus vesicalis.	From plexus vesicalis at base of bladder to v. pudenda interna.

Dietetics

Food Tables[1]

100 CALORIE PORTION TABLE

Foodstuffs	Weight Gm.	Weight Oz.	P., Gm.	F., Gm.	C., Gm.	Water, Gm.	P., Cal.	F., Cal.	C., Cal.	Vitamins A	Vitamins B	Vitamins C	Calcium (Ca), Gm.	Phosphorus (P), Gm.	Iron (Fe), Gm.
Breads, etc.:															
Rye, 1 thick slice	38.3	1.35	3.44	0.23	20.40	14.12	14.1	2.1	83.7	*	++	*	0.009	0.58	0.0006
White, 1 thick slice	37.1	1.31	3.37	0.59	19.75	13.10	13.8	5.6	81.0	+to++	++	—to++	0.010	0.035	0.00034
Whole wheat, 1 thick slice	39.7	1.40	3.85	0.36	19.83	15.25	15.8	3.4	81.2	++	++	—to++	0.020	0.072	0.00065
Zwieback, 3 pieces	23.2	0.82	2.27	2.30	17.09	1.34	9.3	21.4	70.0	—	—to+	—	0.006	0.026	0.00023
Flour, white, pastry, 3 tbs.	27.7	0.83	3.41	0.30	20.20	3.63	14.0	2.8	82.8	—	—	—			
Flour, whole wheat, 2¾ tbs.	27.1	0.95	3.74	0.52	19.50	3.10	15.3	4.1	80.0	+	++	—	0.009	0.025	0.0007
Cereals, dry:															
Cornflakes, 1½ cups	27.1	0.96	1.49	0.41	21.95		6.1	3.8	90.2	++	++	—	0.005	0.052	0.00055
Cornmeal, 2⅜ cups	27.4	0.97	2.52	0.52	20.70		10.4	4.8	84.9	—	—	—			0.00025
Cornstarch, 3 tbs.	27.1	0.96	—	—	24.4				100	—	—	—			
Farina, 2 tbs.	26.9	0.97	2.86	0.37	20.50	3.06	11.7	3.4	84.0	—	—to+	—	0.006	0.035	0.00022
Grapenuts, 3 tbs.	26.3	0.95	3.03	0.26	20.20		12.4	2.0	85.4	—	—	—			
Macaroni, 1¼ cups	27.2	0.96	3.59	0.26	20.25	2.72	14.7	2.3	83.0	—	—to+	—	0.006	0.039	0.0003
Oatmeal, 2¼ tbs.	24.8	0.88	4.00	1.64	16.75		16.4	15.3	68.7	—to+	++	—	0.017	0.099	0.00096
Puffed rice, 1⅝ cups	26.2	0.93	2.16	0.07	21.9	2.80	8.9	0.6	90.0	—	—	—	0.003	0.027	0.00025
Rice, raw, 2 tbs.	27.8	0.97	2.22	0.08	22.0	1.81	9.1	0.7	90.2	+	++	—	0.011	0.089	0.0012
Shredded wheat, 1 biscuit	26.8	0.95	2.7	0.37	20.78	3.42	11.1	3.5	85.4	—	—	—	0.006	0.025	0.0004
Tapioca, pearl, 2½ tbs.	27.5	0.97	0.11	0.03	24.18	2.18	0.5	0.3	99.2	—	—	—			
Graham crackers, 6 or 7 small	23.3	0.82	2.33	2.19	17.18	3.14	9.6	20.4	70.4	+	++	—	0.005	0.024	0.0004
Soda crackers, 5	23.5	0.83	2.30	2.14	17.20	1.26	9.4	19.6	70.5	—	—	—			
						1.39									

— indicates that the food contains no appreciable amount of the vitamin.
* indicates that evidence is lacking or appears insufficient.
+ indicates that the food contains the vitamin.
++ indicates that the food is a good source of the vitamin.
+++ indicates that the food is an excellent source of the vitamin.
e.p. edible portion. a.p. as purchased.

[1]Boynton, *Cyclopedia of Medicine, Surgery, and Specialties*, F. A. Davis Company.

100 CALORIE PORTION TABLE—Continued

Foodstuffs	Weight Gm.	Weight Oz.	P., Gm.	F., Gm.	C., Gm.	Water, Gm.	P., Cal.	F., Cal.	C., Cal.	Vitamins A	Vitamins B	Vitamins C	Calcium (Ca), Gm.	Phosphorus (P), Gm.	Iron (Fe), Gm.
Dairy Products:															
Butter, 1 tbs.	12.6	0.45	0.13	10.70	—	1.38	0.5	99.5	—	+++	—	*	0.002	0.002	0.00003
Cheese, American, 1¼ in. cube.	22.0	0.73	6.30	7.85	0.66	6.94	25.0	73.0	2.0	++	*	*	0.204	0.154	0.00028
Cheese, cottage, 5½ tbs.	89.0	3.12	18.50	0.89	3.80	64.10	76.0	8.3	15.6	+	*	*			
Cheese, full cream, 1½ in. cube.	23.0	0.82	5.95	7.85	0.55	7.86	24.2	73.0	2.2	++	*	—			
Cream, "20 per cent," 4 tbs.	51.4	1.81	1.28	9.50	2.31	37.74	5.2	88.4	9.5	+++	++	— to +			
Cream, "40 per cent," 2 tbs.	25.3	0.90	0.57	10.12	0.76	12.28	2.3	94.2	3.1	+++	++	— to +	0.022	0.017	0.00008
Milk:															
Buttermilk, 1½ cups.	275	9.70	8.30	1.29	13.20	250	34	12	54	+	++	— to +	0.289	0.266	0.0007
Condensed, sweetened, 1½ tbs.	30	1.06	2.4	2.5	16.2	8.1	10	23	67	+++	++	+	0.177	0.138	0.00036
Evaporated, unsweetened, 3¾ tbs.	59.0	2.08	5.8	5.4	6.3	40.25	24	50	26	+++	+++	— to	0.311	0.245	0.00064
Skim, 1⅛ cups.	255	9.4	9.0	0.75	13.7	231	37	7	56	+	+++	— to	0.167	0.129	0.00033
Whole, scant ⅔ cup.	140	4.9	4.6	5.6	7.0	122	18.9	51.7	28.6	+++	+++	— to			
Fats:															
Cottonseed oil, 1 tbs.	10.7	0.5	—	10.7	—	—	—	100	—	—	—	—			
Crisco, 1 tbs.	11.3	0.4	—	10.7	—	—	—	100	—	— to +	—	—			
Lard, 1 tbs.	11.3	0.4	—	10.7	—	—	—	100	—	— to ++	—	—			
Oleo, 1 tbs.	12.9	0.42	0.15	10.6	—	0.7	0.6	99.5	—	— to +	—	—			
Fish:															
Haddock, e. p., generous serving.	135.5	4.8	23.3	0.4	—	111	95.7	3.8	—	— to +	+ to	*	0.025	0.267	0.0013
Oysters, a. p., ⅔ cup.	197	7	11.83	2.56	6.52	174	48.7	23.8	26.8	++ to +	++	— to +	0.103	0.305	0.0087
Salmon, canned, ½ cup.	49.7	1.76	10.82	6.02	—	31.6	44.3	56.0	—	+	*	*	0.011	0.124	0.0006

100 CALORIE PORTION TABLE—Continued

Foodstuffs	Weight Gm.	Weight Oz.	P., Gm.	F., Gm.	C., Gm.	Water, Gm.	P., Cal.	F., Cal.	C., Cal.	Vitamins A	Vitamins B	Vitamins C	Minerals Calcium (Ca), Gm.	Minerals Phosphorus (P), Gm.	Minerals Iron (Fe), Gm.
Fruits:															
Apples, fresh, 1 large	157	5.6	0.63	0.78	22.1	132	2.6	7.3	90.5	+	+	++	0.011	0.019	0.0005
Apricots, dried, 7 halves	35.1	1.24	1.65	0.35	21.9	10.3	6.8	3.3	90	+	+	++	0.023	0.041	0.0005
Banana, 1 small	99	3.5	1.28	0.6	21.7	74	5.3	5.5	89	+ to ++			0.009	0.031	0.0006
Blackberries, canned, 1 cup	168	6.0	2.2	1.7	18.3	145	9.0	15.6	75.2				0.029	0.057	0.001
Cantaloupe, e. p., average serving	245	8.9	1.47	—	22.8	222	6.4	—	93.4	++	+++	+*	0.041	0.037	0.0007
Cherries, canned, ⅔ cup	109	3.9	1.21	0.11	23.1	84	4.9	1.0	94.5	++*	++*	+*	0.020	0.034	0.0004
Cranberries, a. p., 2 cups	245	7.5	0.84	1.26	20.8	188	3.4	11.7	85.4	+	++	+*	0.038	0.027	0.0012
Dates, dried, e. p., 4 or 5	28.1	1.0	0.6	0.8	22.0	4.4	2.5	7.5	90.2				0.018	0.016	0.0008
Figs, dried, a. p., 1½ or 2	30.8	1.1	1.32	0.1	22.8	5.8	5.4	0.8	93.6				0.050	0.035	0.0009
Grapes, e. p., 1 medium bunch	100.5	3.6	1.3	1.6	19.3	77.7	5.4	15.0	79.3	+	+	+	0.019	0.031	0.0003
Grapefruit, ½	207	7.3	1.7	0.44	21.7	181	6.9	4.1	88.5	+++	+++	++++	0.043	0.041	0.0006
Lemons, e. p., 3 large	221	7.8	2.2	1.5	18.8	197	9.1	14.3	77.0	+++	+++++	++++	0.080	0.049	0.0013
Oranges, e. p., 1 large	189	6.7	1.5	0.38	21.8	164	6.2	3.5	89.8	++ to ++	++ to +++	++ to +++	0.085	0.040	0.0004
Peaches, canned, 3 halves	206	7.3	1.4	0.21	22.25	182	5.9	2.0	91.5	++	+	++	0.033	0.049	0.0006
Peaches, fresh, e. p., 2 large	239	8.5	1.7	0.24	22.4	213	6.8	2.2	91.8	+ to ++	+*	+	0.038	0.057	0.0007
Pears, canned, 3 halves	128	4.5	0.38	0.38	23.1	104	1.6	3.5	94.5	++*	+*	— to +	0.019	0.033	0.0004
Pears, fresh, 1 large	154	5.4	0.92	0.77	21.7	129	3.8	7.2	89	*	+++	+	0.023	0.040	0.0005
Pineapple, canned, 1 slice	63.5	2.24	0.25	0.44	23.1	39.2	1.0	4.1	94.8	++	+++	++			
Pineapple, fresh, 2 in. slice	227	8.0	0.9	0.7	21.8	201	3.7	6.3	89.5	++	+++	++	0.041	0.063	0.0011
Prunes, dried, e. p., 3 or 4	32.4	1.14	0.7	—	23.7	7.2	2.8	—	97.2		++	—	0.017	0.034	0.001
Raisins, ¼ cup	31.4	1.1	0.72	0.94	21.5	4.6	3.0	8.7	88.1	—	+	—	0.020	0.041	0.0007

App 80

100 CALORIE PORTION TABLE—Continued

Foodstuffs	Weight Gm.	Weight Oz.	P., Gm.	F., Gm.	C., Gm.	Water, Gm.	P., Cal.	F., Cal.	C., Cal.	Vitamins A	Vitamins B	Vitamins C	Calcium (Ca), Gm.	Phosphorus (P), Gm.	Iron (Fe), Gm.
Fruits (continued):															
Raspberries, black, 1¼ cups	146	5.2	2.5	1.5	18.4	123	10.2	13.6	75.7	*	*	+++	0.190	.0131	0.004
Rhubarb, e. p., 1 quart diced	423	15	2.5	3.0	15.3	399	10.4	27.5	62.7	*	*	+	0.103	0.070	0.002
Strawberries, e. p., 1½ cups	252	8.9	2.5	1.5	18.6	227	10.3	14.0	76.2	+	+	+++	0.035	0.010	0.00030
Watermelon, e. p., large serving, ½ cup	324	11.4	1.3	0.65	21.7	300	5.3	6.0	89.0		+to+++	+	0.011	0.011	
Grape juice, ½ cup	132	4.7	0.52	—	24.2	106	2.1	—	99.0						
Orange juice, 1 cup	233	8.2	—	—	24.4	—	—	—	100	++	+++	+++	0.067	0.037	0.00046
Meat:															
Beef, liver, e. p., average serving	75.1	2.66	15.3	3.4	1.3	53.5	62.8	31.4	5.3	+to+++	++	*	0.009	0.165	0.002
Loin medium fat, e. p., small serving	38.1	1.35	7.05	7.7	—	23.2	28.9	71.2	—	+	+	—to+	0.004	0.077	0.001
Round medium fat, e. p., small serving	47.8	1.7	9.7	6.5	—	31.2	39.7	60.4	—	+	+	—to+	0.006	0.104	0.0015
Lamb, leg. e. p., small serving	43	1.5	8.25	7.1	—	27.4	33.8	66	—	—to+	+	*	0.005	0.089	0.0012
Pork, bacon, medium fat, e. p., 2 or 3 slices cooked	15	0.53	1.48	10.1	—	3.0	6.1	93.7	—						
Ham, fresh, e. p., small serving	30.2	1.06	4.62	8.72	—	15.1	19.0	81.2	—	—to+	++	*	0.003	0.050	0.0007
Ham, smoked, e. p., boneless, small serving	30.6	1.08	4.56	8.73	—	12.2	18.7	81.2	—	—to++	++	—			
Sausage, a. p., 1 small	21.4	0.76	2.8	9.4	0.24	8.6	11.4	87.7	1.0	—to++	++	—			
Veal, cutlet, average serving	64.4	2.27	13.1	5.0	—	45.5	53.6	46.1	—	—to+	+	—	0.008	0.141	0.0019

100 CALORIE PORTION TABLE—Continued

Foodstuffs	Weight Gm.	Weight Oz.	P., Gm.	F., Gm.	C., Gm.	Water, Gm.	P., Cal.	F., Cal.	C., Cal.	Vitamins A	Vitamins B	Vitamins C	Calcium (Ca), Gm.	Phosphorus (P), Gm.	Iron (Fe), Gm.
Miscellaneous:															
Eggs, whites	181	6.4	23.5	0.36	—	156	96.5	3.4	—	—	—	*	0.021	0.025	0.0002
Whole, e. p., 1¼	63	2.2	9.32	6.62	—	42.45	38.2	61.6	—	—	+to++	*	0.042	0.113	0.0019
Yolks, 1½	26.6	0.94	4.18	8.87	—	13.15	17.1	82.5	—	+++	+++	*	0.036	0.139	0.0023
Gelatin, 3 tbs.	27.3	0.96	24.3	0.03	—	—	99.8	0.3	—						
Mayonnaise, 1 tbs.	11.3	0.40	0.14	10.7	0.03	—	0.6	99.5	0.1						
Soup, celery, canned, ¾ cup	182	6.4	3.8	5.1	9.1	161	15.6	47.2	32.3				0.065	0.054	
Soup, tomato, canned, 1 cup	245	8.7	4.4	2.2	13.7	220	18.1	25.1	56.3				0.088	0.073	
Nuts:															
Almonds, e. p., 10 to 15	14.9	0.53	3.14	8.21	2.58	0.72	12.9	77.1	10.5	+++	+++	*	0.036	0.070	0.0006
Peanuts, e. p., 20 to 25	17.7	0.63	4.57	6.85	4.33	1.63	18.8	63.6	17.7	+++	+++	*	0.013	0.071	0.0004
Peanut butter, a. p., 2 tbs.	15.9	0.56	4.66	7.40	2.70	1.09	19.1	68.8	11.1		+++	*			
Walnuts, e. p., 10 to 15	13.8	0.45	2.30	8.77	2.23	0.35	9.4	81.6	9.1	++	++	*	0.012	0.050	0.0003
Poultry:															
Fowl, ½ serving	43.4	1.5	8.37	7.07	—	27.8	34.3	65.7	—	—to+	+	*	0.005	0.090	0.0012
Sugar:															
Granulated, 1⅞ tbs, 5 tps.	24.4	0.86	—	—	24.4	—	—	—	100	—	—	—			
Vegetables:															
Asparagus, fresh, 20 large stalks	435	15.4	7.85	0.87	14.4	410	32.2	8.1	59.1	++	+++	*	0.109	0.017	0.0044
Beans, baked, canned, 1⅞ cups	75	2.7	5.1	1.9	15.1	51.6	21	18	62	+	++	*			
Beans, dried, 2 tbs.	28.2	1.0	6.35	0.51	16.8	3.6	26.1	4.7	69.1	*	++	*	0.45	1.33	0.002

App. 82

100 CALORIE PORTION TABLE—Continued

Foodstuffs	Weight Gm.	Weight Oz.	P., Gm.	F., Gm.	C., Gm.	Water, Gm.	P., Cal.	F., Cal.	C., Cal.	Vitamins A	Vitamins B	Vitamins C	Calcium (Ca), Gm.	Phosphorus (P), Gm.	Iron (Fe), Gm.
Vegetables (continued):															
Beans, fresh, string, 2¾ cups	232	8.1	5.4	0.70	17.4	207	22.1	6.5	71.4	++	++	++	0.107	0.121	0.0026
Beans, dried, lima, 2 tbs.	27.9	0.8	5.05	0.42	18.3		20.8	3.8	75.7	+	+	+	0.022	0.086	0.002
Beets, fresh, e. p., 3 to 5	211	7.4	3.4	0.21	20.5	185	13.8	2.0	84				0.556	0.075	0.0012
Cabbage, e. p., 1 small, 5 cups	313	11.2	5.0	0.94	17.4	284	20.4	8.8	71.5	+++	+++	+++	0.141	0.091	0.0034
Carrots, e. p., 5 medium	215	7.6	2.4	0.89	19.7	190	10	8	82	+++	+++	+++	0.120	0.099	0.0013
Cauliflower, a. p., 1 small	312	11	5.6	1.6	15.1	288	23	15	62	+	+++	+++	0.384	0.190	0.0019
Celery, e. p., 4 to 5 small bunches	540	19	5.6	0.54	19.0	510	24	5	71	— to +	+++	*	0.421	0.199	0.0027
Corn, green, e. p., ½ cup	100	3.54	2.8	1.2	19.0	75.4	11.5	11.2	78	+	+++	+	0.006	0.103	0.0008
Eggplant, ¾	350	12	4.15	1.07	17.8	325	17	10	73	+	+++	—	0.039	0.119	0.0018
Lentils, dried, 2½ tbs.	28	1.0	7.2	0.28	16.6	2.4	29.4	2.6	68	+ to ++	+++		0.030	0.123	0.0018
Lettuce, e. p., 2 heads	505	18	6.1	1.5	14.7	479	24.9	14.2	60.3	++	+++	+++	0.217	0.212	0.0002
Mushrooms, e. p., 20 to 25 small	216	7.5	7.6	0.9	14.7	190	31	8	60.2	— to ++	++		0.037	0.231	0.0012
Onions, e. p., 5 medium	202	7.15	3.23	0.61	20.0	177	13.2	5.6	81.9	— to ++	++	+*	0.069	0.091	0.0009
Parsnips, e. p., 2 to 3	151	5.35	2.42	0.76	20.4	125	9.9	7	83.5	— to ++	— to ++	++	0.089	0.115	0.0017
Peas, green, ⅓ cup	97.6	3.45	6.85	0.5	16.5	73	28.2	4.5	67.5	++	+++++	++	0.027	0.124	
Potato, boiled, 1 medium	103	3.4	2.6	0.10	21.7	78	10.5	0.93	87.8	++	++++	+++	0.017	0.058	0.0015
Potato, raw, 1 medium	118	4.16	2.6	0.12	21.7	92	10.6	1.1	89	++ to ++	++++	+++	0.015	0.036	0.0004
Potato, sweet, ½ medium	79.6	2.81	1.43	0.57	21.8	54.9	5.9	5.3	89	++					
Rutabagas	238	8.4	3.1	0.48	20.2	212	12.7	4.4	83	+++	+	+ to +++	0.176	0.133	
Sauerkraut, 1¼ cups	363	12.8	6.15	1.83	13.8	322	25.2	17.2	56.6			+++++			
Spinach, cooked, 2 cups	174	6.15	3.7	7.1	4.5	156	15	66.3	18.5	+++	++	+ to +++		0.280	
Spinach, fresh, a. p.	412	14.6	8.7	1.24	13.4	380	35.4	11.5	54.8	+++	++	++	0.276		0.0148

App. 83

100 CALORIE PORTION TABLE—Continued

Foodstuffs	Weight Gm.	Weight Oz.	P., Gm.	F., Gm.	C., Gm.	Water, Gm.	P., Cal.	F., Cal.	C., Cal.	Vitamins A	Vitamins B	Vitamins C	Calcium (Ca), Gm.	Phosphorus (P), Gm.	Iron (Fe), Gm.
Vegetables (continued):															
Squash	211	7.5	3.0	1.1	19.3	186	12.3	9.8	79	++	*	*	0.038	0.061	0.0013
Tomato, canned, a. p., 1¾ cups	178	6.3	5.2	0.86	17.3	167	21.3	8	70.8	++	++	++ to +++			
Tomato, fresh, a. p., 5 small	433	15.3	3.9	1.73	16.9	408	16	16.1	69.1	++ to +	++	+++	0.048	0.113	0.0017
Turnip, 2 cups, diced	245	8.65	3.2	0.48	19.9	220	13	4.5	81.5		++	+++	0.157	0.118	0.0012

CHART OF RECOMMENDED DAILY ALLOWANCES FOR SPECIFIC NUTRIENTS[1]

References to Table on Page App. 85

These are tentative allowances toward which to aim in planning practical dietaries. They can be met by a good diet of natural foods; this will also provide other minerals and vitamins, the requirements for which are less well known.

* Per Kg.

① 1 mg. thiamine = 333 I.U.; 1 mg. ascorbic acid = 20 I.U. (1 I.U. = 1 U.S.P. unit).

② Less may be required if provided as vitamin A; greater if obtained as provitamin carotene.

③ Infant needs increase from month to month; Amounts given are for approx. 6–18 mos. Amounts

protein and calcium needed are less if from breast milk.

④ Vitamin D undoubtedly necessary for older children and adults. If not available from sunshine, should be provided probably up to minimal amounts recommended for infants.

⑤ Allowances based on middle age for each group (as 2, 5, 8, etc.) and for moderate activity.

---

[1] Committee on Foods and Nutrition of the National Research Council.

Chart of Recommended Daily Allowances for Specific Nutrients
COMMITTEE ON FOODS AND NUTRITION OF THE NATIONAL RESEARCH COUNCIL

	Calories	Protein	Calcium	Iron	Vitamin A ②	Thiamine (B₁)①	Ascorbic Acid (C)①	Ribo-flavin	Nicotinic Acid	Vitamin D
		gms.	gms.	mgs.	I.U.	mgs.	mgs.	mgs.	mgs.	I.U.
Man (70 Kg.)										
Fairly active	3000	70	0.8	12	5000	1.8	75	2.7	18	③
Very Active	4500					2.3		3.3	23	
Sedentary	2500					1.5		2.2	15	
Woman (56 Kg.)										
Fairly active	2500	60	0.8	12	5000	1.5	70	2.2	15	③
Very active	3000					1.8		2.7	18	
Sedentary	2100					1.2		1.8	12	
Pregnancy (Latter half)	2500	85	1.5	15	6000	1.8	100	2.5	18	400-800
Lactation	3000	100	2.0	15	8000	2.3	150	3.0	23	400-800
Children to 12 yrs.										
Under 1 year④	100*	3–4*	1.0	6	1500	0.4	30	0.6	4	400-800
1 to 3 years	1200	40	1.0	7	2000	0.6	35	0.9	6	
4 to 6 years⑤	1600	50	1.0	8	2500	0.8	50	1.2	8	
7 to 9 years	2000	60	1.0	10	3500	1.0	60	1.5	10	
10 to 12 years	2500	70	1.2	12	4500	1.2	75	1.8	12	
Children over 12										
Girls 13 to 15 years	2800	80	1.3	15	5000	1.4	80	2.0	14	③
16 to 20 years	2400	75	1.0	15	5000	1.2	80	1.8	12	③
Boys 13 to 15 years	3200	85	1.4	15	5000	1.6	90	2.4	16	③
16 to 20 years	3800	100	1.4	15	6000	2.0	100	3.0	20	③

See notes on page App. 84.

App. 85

Vitamin Tables (Summary)

Vitamin	Mode of Action	Result of Deficiency	Characteristics	Good Sources	Daily Req. I. U.
VITAMIN A Carotene $(C_{20}H_{28})_2$ A yellow pigment, found in certain foods. When these foods are eaten, it is converted into vitamin A. $(C_{20}H_{28})HOH$ 'Vitamin A is the only vitamin so far discovered which is a product solely of animal metabolism from precursors which are metabolic products only of plants." *Chemistry of Vitamin A.* L. S. Palmer, Ph.D. J.A.M.A., 5/20/38.	Promotes growth, appetite, digestion. Aids in maintaining health and vigor. Important rôle in visual organs.	*Mild:* Retards growth. Respiratory infections of several types. Disturbed gastrointestinal tract. Skin dries, shrivels, thickens, sometimes pustule formation. *Severe:* Xerophthalmia, a characteristic eye disease, and other local infections.	Fat soluble Not destroyed by ordinary cooking temperatures. Is destroyed by high temperatures when oxygen is present. Marked capacity for storage in the liver.	Animal fats butter cheese cream egg yolk whole milk. Fish liver oil. Fruits Liver Vegetables 1. green leafy, esp. escarole, kale, parsley 2. yellow esp. carrots. *Artificial:* Concentrates in several forms. Irradiated fish oils.	*Adults:* Liberal allowance: 6300. *Growing youth:* 6000. *Small children:* 4500.
VITAMIN B Factors that have been identified: B₁ Thiamine $(C_{12}H_{16}N_4OS$, a base) antiberiberi, antineuritic in man, antipolyneuritis in birds. B₂—See: vitamin G B₃ ⎫ B₄ ⎬ Isolated but relationship not clear. B₅ ⎭ B₆ antidermatitis.	Important role in carbohydrate metabolism. Promotes tonicity of digestive tract. Promotes appetite. Helps maintain healthy nerves.	*Mild:* Loss of appetite. Impaired digestion of starches and sugars. Colitis Constipation or diarrhea. Emaciation. *Severe:* Nervous disorders of various types. Loss of co-ordinating power of muscles. Beriberi Paralysis in man. Polyneuritis in pigeons.	Water soluble Not readily destroyed by ordinary cooking temperature. More readily destroyed in alkaline medium than in acid. Limited capacity for storage in the body.	Widely distributed in plant and animal tissues but seldom occurs in high concentration, exception is brewer's yeast. Other good sources are: Whole grain cereals Peas, Beans Organs, glandular—heart, liver, kidney Many vegetables and fruits Nuts *Artificial:* Concentrates from yeast Rice polishings. Wheat germ.	*Adults:* 250-300 Recommended: 400. *Growing youth:* 400. Recommended: 500-600.

Vitamin	Mode of Action	Result of Deficiency	Characteristics	Good Sources	Daily Req. I. U.
VITAMIN C Ascorbic acid ($C_6H_8O_6$). Cevitamic acid.	Essential for normal growth; for nutrition of bone, teeth, gums. Increased resistance to infections. Antiscurvy.	*Mild:* Lowered vitality, resistance to infections, affects structure of fibrous tissues. Susceptibility to dental caries, pyorrhea and bleeding gums. *Severe:* Hemorrhage Anemia Scurvy	Water soluble. Easily destroyed by oxidation, heat hastens the process. Lost in cookery unless container is airtight; more readily affected in alkaline than in acid medium. Lost in storage if exposed to air, less lost at low temperature. Retained in canning if process excludes air (as commercial canning); in quick freezing process. Stored in the body to a limited extent.	Abundant in most fresh fruits and vegetables, especially citrus fruit and juices, tomato and orange. *Artificial:* Ascorbic acid. Cevitamic acid.	*Adults:* 75-100. *Growing youth:* Recommended: 100. The infant diet is likely to be deficient in vitamin C unless orange or tomato juice or other form is added.
VITAMIN D Ergosterol exposed to ultraviolet light. "Calciferol" ($C_{28}H_{44}O$).	Regulates the utilization of calcium and phosphorus in the development of bones and teeth. Normalizes blood. Antirachitic. Some authorities think its greatest benefits are in the first 21 years of life.	*Mild:* Interferes with utilization of calcium and phosphorus in bone and teeth formation. Irritability Weakness *Severe:* Rickets, may be common in young children, rare in adults.	Fat soluble. Relatively stable to heat and oxidation, although slowly lost in storage. Stored in liver. Often associated with vitamin A.	Butter Egg yolk Fish liver oils Fish having fat distributed through the flesh, salmon, tuna fish, herring, sardines Liver Oysters Yeast and foods irradiated with ultraviolet light. Formed in the skin by exposure to sunlight. Artificially prepared eight forms to date.	Depends upon climate, season, mode of life (amount of time spent in sunlight).
Vitamin E This vitamin, associated with fats and oils, is of sterol nature.	Necessary for fertility in certain animals and human beings.	Young embryo fails to develop.	Fat soluble. Very stable in high temperature, acid and alkali media. Iron salts in food tend to destroy it. Extra amounts do not increase fertility. Stored in body tissues.	Found in nearly all types of food. Highest in wheat and corn germ, water cress, lettuce, fresh beef fat, and glandular organs. *Artificial:* Wheat germ.	A diet of reasonable variety is apparently adequate protection against deficiency.

Vitamin	Mode of Action	Result of Deficiency	Characteristics	Good Sources	Daily Req. I. U.
Vitamin G Vitamin G is a term applied to all unidentified water soluble, nutritional factors present in yeast, liver, etc. Riboflavin Nicotinic acid.	Promotes growth and vigor. Improves general tone of skin and alimentary canal. With other substances it protects against pellagra, black tongue, etc. Thought to improve certain kinds of cataract.	No specific disease is known to be due to a shortage.	Water soluble. Resistant to heat, freezing and oxidation. Good capacity for storing in the body.	Widely distributed in both plant and animal foods. Most vegetables and fruits, eggs, milk, meat. *Artificial:* Concentrate from yeast and whey powder.	Not likely to be deficient in the diet.

(Courtesy of The Williams and Wilkins Company, from *Applied Dietetics* by Frances Stern.)

Vitamin	Mode of Action	Source
VITAMIN H	A powerful stimulant of cellular activity. A Vitamin B complex.	A tissue substance.
VITAMIN K Complex (K₁ and K₂)	Practically eliminates prolonged bleeding in operations and in biliary tract in jaundice.	Alfalfa, fats, oats, wheat, rye and fish meal. Synthesized from coal tar.
VITAMIN L	Necessary for lactation in rats.	
VITAMIN P (Citrin)	Helps prevent scurvy. Effective in diseases with increased capillary permeability. Helps prevent bleeding, and black and blue marks.	Lemons, limes, grapefruit, oranges and red peppers.
VITAMIN T	Increases blood platelet count in humans, effective in purpura.	Egg yolk, vegetable oils.

Anatomical and Physiological

Emergencies

Convulsions

Type	History	Clonic or Tonic	Pulse	Breathing	Color	Muscles	Pupils	Pathology	Treatment
1. Epilepsy.	Previous history of "fits" occurring principally at night. Patient gets an "aura."	Generalized clonic type.	Pulse is rapid.	Respirations are rapid, deep and stertorous.	Blue. Patient may become very cyanotic.	Rigid in tonic and in clonic origin.	Pupils are contracted and occasionally of unequal size.	Deficient oxygenation of brain areas. Increased cerebral edema and intracranial pressure. Great accumulation of lactic acid within tissues.	Prevent the patient from injuring himself or from falling. Place on floor with pillow, etc. Use no stimulant.
2. Eclampsia.	Occurs in toxemia of pregnancy in ante partum and post partum stages.	Prolonged tonic convulsions are characteristic with the whole body in a state of rigidity. Both tonic and clonic types may occur.	Pulse is rapid and becomes thready.	Respirations are rapid and shallow.	Blue. Patient may become very cyanotic.	Rigidity of the body sets in. Extremities are flexed. General tonic spasm of body may be followed by clonic spasm for approximately 4 minutes.	Pupils may be dilated and may be of unequal size.	Hypertension. Degeneration of kidney and liver. Rapid gain of weight.	Control convulsions. Give proper antenatal care for toxemia of pregnancy. Control of diet, elimination and prevention of hypertension.
3. Apoplexy.	Usually sequel to cerebral hemorrhage. May be result of vascular disease. Occurs usually after age of 40 years.	Usually tonic. May be limited to different areas, or to one side of the body.	Pulse is strong and of a bounding quality.	Respirations are deep and stertorous.	Red. Skin has a florid and flushed appearance.	Spastic in tonic usage with hemiplegia. One side of body shows paralysis. Other is normal.	Pupils are unequal in size.	Hemorrhage in intracranial areas. Arteriosclerosis.	Keep the patient absolutely quiet with an icecap to head. No stimulants.
4. Hysteria.	Usually onset is not sudden. Is accompanied by laughter and crying. Seizure may be more prolonged than epilepsy.	May be of the stimulation types and take on those of epilepsy. Usually are of the tonic nature.	Pulse is normal. Shows no definite changes unless slightly rapid due to excitement.	Respirations may become rapid.	No change in color of skin.	Rigidity or relaxed as the victim wishes to demonstrate.	Pupils are normal and react to light. Muscles of eye resist when forced opening is attempted.	Patient seldom loses consciousness. May fall but not in an area where an injury may follow. Highly reactive to suggestion.	Inhalation of NH₄OH. Ice water dashed upon the face. Seizure is over usually when the audience disappears.

App. 90

CONVULSIONS—Continued

Type	History	Clonic or Tonic	Pulse	Breathing	Color	Muscles	Pupils	Pathology	Treatment
5. Cerebrospinal Meningitis	May be primary condition or may be some complicated disease.	Spasm is of Opisthotonic character (body in arched position). Extremities continually rigid.	Characteristic very slow pulse.	Respirations are of Cheyne-Stokes nature.	Pupuric eruption. Face is flushed with elevated temp. Skin hot and dry.	Rigidity and arching of body. Legs and arms are too rigid to return to normal position.	Photophobia or supersensitive to light, with strabismus of simple or complicated forms.	Inflammation of the spinal cord. Opisthotonos.	Spinal tap. Specific sera. Symptomatic treatment. Keep quiet.
6. Tetanus.	After injury—deep wound—and entrance of tetanus bacillus. Gunshot wound.	Tonic convulsions to coma. Clonic.	Rapid pulse to weak (from the toxin of bacteria).	Rapid. Labored to irregular.	Cyanotic in convulsions.	Constant rigidity. Trismus may not appear for 24 hrs. after symptoms.	Pupils may be unequal. Eyes are fixed.	Toxin unites with cells and nerve fibers to the point of degeneration in brain and the medulla.	Antitoxin.
7. Catalepsy.	Tendency to hold any position by maintaining flexibility in definite period. Form of muscular anesthesia in which position of part of body is apparently unknown or unfelt.	Tonic with a prolonged stage of sustained immobility in muscles after placed.	Pulse is weak but perceptible.	Respirations shallow. Labored.	No definite change in color.	Fixed and rigid. Muscles will maintain any position for an indefinite period.	No dilatation. Eyes stare. Nonreactive to light.	Catatonic manifestations. Injury from convulsions.	Provide rest. Careful watching of patient to see that no injurious effect may come from prolonged fatigue.
8. Uremic Convulsions.	Condition is usually accompanied by chronic or acute nephritis or chronic cardiac conditions. Marked edema noted.	Clonic (mild) to severe forms of muscle jerking.	Pulse rapid weak. Muscles are rigid (tends to imperceptibility).	Respirations are slow and stertorous	Skin is pale, dry, scaly and has waxy appearance.	Tonic and clonic.	Pupils may be "pin point."	Arterial hypertension Albuminuria suppression of urine. Visual disturbance. Detached retina.	Measures to reduce high blood pressure. Diaphoretic and diuretic medicaments. Bed rest.
9. Diabetic Convulsions.	Diabetes mellitus hyperglycemia acidosis	Clonic and Tonic	Pulse rapid weak to irregular.	Deep breathing, rapid with extreme effort.	Dry skin. Very soft, cyanotic in convulsion.	Tonic and clonic.	Eye balls soft. Cataracts are frequent.	Generalized arteriosclerosis. Kidneys are enlarged. Degeneration in islets of Langerhans.	Use of insulin. Diabetic diet. Care of skin. Bed rest.

Dislocations

Type	History	Pathology	Muscles	Complications	Treatment	Strapping and Support	Differentiation
1. Neck.	Caused by violent twists or fall upon the head or diving into pool.	Bilateral dislocation. Severs spinal cord. Death follows. Nerve injury caused by tension or displacement. Permanent Torticollis and limited neck motion.	Torticollis. Muscles spastic on uninjured side. Injured side are relaxed.	Severance of cord. Pressure on cord. causing predisposal to recurrence of dislocation, permanent torticollis, paralysis death.	Keep patient in recumbent position in hyperextension of the neck. Reduction by leverage and not by manual traction. Keep traction by collar or plaster cast.	Reduction done by leverage. Application of plaster or rigid collar which must be worn until recovery of the ligaments to prevent recurrence.	Unilateral dislocation produces torticollis with head tilted on side and chin rotated away from displaced vertebrae. Reduction aids in complete disappearance of torticollis.
2. Back.	Sudden and violent twisting of the back—thrown from a horse or from lifting too great a load.	Cervical dislocation—Paraplegia may occur. Respiratory failure or ascending myelitis. Dorsal dislocation. Urinary infection.	Affected side relaxed; uninjured side spastic. Muscle spasm holds back in rigidity with severe pain when any movement is made.	Damage to cord. Incomplete paraplegia. Failure to replace results in kyphosis deformity. Weakness and arthritis.	Do not allow patient to sit up or to be turned. Prepare patient for cast and brace. Control the pain. Watch for decubitus.	Treat as for fracture. Transport in prone position on rigid stretcher. Keep the body in hyperextension with cast or brace.	Compression fracture of first lumbar vertebrae is the most common injury of the spine. Decided excursion of the ilium (noted when the back is extended or flexed is corrected. No crepitus. Discoloration, swelling, and persistent pain in muscle.
3. Shoulder.	ANTERIOR force was from behind—head of the humerus lies just below the coracoid process. POSTERIOR. Direct force upon the flexed elbow. Head of humerus is placed in front and lower than the axilla.	Rupture of tendon. Injury to circumflex nerve or brachial plexus. Disability. Injury to axillary vessels. Greater tuberosity (coracoid). Acromion processes fractured.	Muscle tension in the bicep muscle. Triceps muscle immobilized, may be slightly rigid.	Chronic arthritis. Cartilage displacement. Complete loss of function. Recurrences if a repeated injury or improper or inadequate mobilization after the first injury.	Kocher method of Replacement. Keep the 1. Flex elbow to a right angle and against body with elbow against body. Rotate arm outward until forearm points away from body. 2. Keep elbow and arm (lower arm) flexed to upper. Raise elbow forward until it reaches a right angle position to the long axis (or horizontal) of the body. 3. Arm is directed obliquely inward and the hand placed on the opposite shoulder so that reduction or replacement is complete. Immobilize by sling. X-ray is necessary.	Dislocation of shoulder is corrected when the hand (unassisted) can be placed upon the opposite shoulder. Repeated recurrence of dislocation of the shoulder may be common.
4. Elbow.	In childhood between ages 8 to 12 years. Child falls upon the outstretched hand. Produces hyperextension of the elbow.	Elbow swollen. Held midway between flexion and extension. Head of radius is felt rotating behind humerus.	Tension in biceps muscle. Muscle ossification at the elbow.	Arthritis in joint. Muscle tissue ossification. Recurrence of dislocation.	Apply splint. Immobilize elbow until replacement can be made. Treat symptomatically.	Supinate the forearm. Make traction forward and downward on the forearm until radius and ulna slip back into position.	The ability to acutely flex the elbow when dislocation is satisfactorily reduced.

App. 92

DISLOCATIONS—Continued

Type	History	Pathology	Muscles	Complications	Treatment	Strapping and Support	Differentiation
5. Wrist.	Caused by the hyperextended hand or by severe blows upon the dorsal portion of the wrist.	Dislocation of Semilunar bone. Flexion of the wrist is blocked by displaced bone. Usually results in a permanently weak wrist.	Muscles of back of hand tense. Usually marked swelling in area of the sprain.	Permanent pain, weakness and limitation of motion. Flexion limited. Displaced bones may have to be removed by surgical methods.	Surgical removal of displaced bone if unable to replace it. Support by splint or strapping.	Apply traction upon hand. Put firm pressure of the thumb upon the displaced bone.	Flexion of the wrist with slight limitations of motion and manifestation of weakness will indicate satisfactory reduction of the wrist.
6. Hand.	Most frequent in thumb due to forced hyperextension of the thumb or finger.	Head of metacarpal bone is wedged between flexor tendons (may necessitate an operation).	Marked muscle tension.	Deformity and permanent disability unless successful reduction is made.	Hyperextend the phalanx or thumb and then flex it. Use adhesive strapping.	Hyperextension of thumb as local pressure is made—thereby replacement is effected. Very early reduction is necessary.	Displacement of the thumb is the most frequent injury of the hand. Swelling, discoloration, and deformity (without point tenderness) are present.
7. Hip.	If posterior by indirect violence upon head of femur. If anterior by violent hyperabduction.	Injury to capsular and surrounding tissues of capsule of the acetabulum.	Posterior dislocation—hip is held rigidly flexed. Adduction, inward rotation and flexion of the thigh. Anterior dislocation—hip is immovable in abduction and external rotation. Knee flexed.	Torn tendons and ligaments. Fracture of the neck of femur.	1. Symptomatic for discomforts. 2. Splinting—since fracture is frequently a sequel. 3. Shock treatment. 4. Preparation for reduction of the dislocation.	Board or rigid splint. Keep limb in slight elevation unless fracture is imminent.	Reduction will be complete when flexion with extension and adduction of the thigh are possible.
8. Knee.	After violent fall or force upon knee.	Torn ligaments. Traumatized muscles of patellar and popliteal area. Loss of synovial fluid after rupture of bursa.	Rigid with pain. May include slight to marked swelling. Ecchymosis—slight or marked.	Disability and deformity. Permanently stiffened knee when synovial fluid is lost.	Splint as for fracture of femur and lower leg. Symptomatic (to relieve discomfort). Treat for shock.	Board or rigid splint. Keep knee and limb in slight elevation unless fracture is present.	The depression adjacent to the patella is diminished and complete flexion of the knee is restored.

DISLOCATIONS—Continued

Type	History	Pathology	Muscles	Complications	Treatment	Strapping and Support	Diferentiation
9. Ankle.	From violence of undue weight or twisting upon the knee.	Production of scar tissue and contractures, which produce prolonged restriction of motion. Usually a short period of disability and then satisfactory recovery.	Rigid with pain. May include swelling and discoloration (may be delayed).	Fractures—Minor or Major as determined by accident. Temporary or permanent disability.	Hot and cold compresses. Gentle massage on adjoining area.	Allow no use (fracture may be present). X-ray for fracture. Immobilize the foot and ankle on a pillow or a rigid splint.	Satisfactory reduction is made when the ankle can be dorsiflexed within a right angle.
10. Foot.	Force of violent nature upon plantar flexor of foot. Misstepping.	May include a compound dislocation of the ankle. Slight to increased amount of trauma and strain upon all soft tissue of foot.	Tense; and including marked swelling and discoloration.	Fracture of ankle. Weakness of muscles of plantar arch.	Hot and cold applications and reduction of swelling. Slight massage. Watch for ecchymosis.	Pillow splint or rigid splint as for fractures. Watch for swelling and cyanosis in part.	Satisfactory reduction is made when the displaced astralgus (projecting on the back of the foot) has been leveled.
11. Clavicle.	May be due to a heavy blow or fall upon the side of the shoulder.	Posterior dislocation causes pressure on structures at base of neck; Rupture of sternoclavicular ligament.	Muscles are hyperextended. Fatigue results if prolonged.	Increased deformity and insecurity of movement of shoulder. Prolonged disability.	Symptomatic treatment. Slight massage. Adhesive strapping. Sling for four weeks.	In recumbent position with small narrow sand bag between scapulae. Posterior Dislocation—press shoulders backward. Make traction on arm as it is held abducted at right angle—Clavical returns to position.	Complete reduction corrects the deformity at the sternoclavicular joint, no crepitus is present. Stretched ligaments and torn muscles are manifested by swelling, discoloration, and generalized pain. Shoulder has secure movement.
12. Jaw.	The too wide opening of the mouth, for example in yawning, laughing or eating.	Capsule of Glenoid fossa is too loose. Muscles are soft. Tissues aid in chronic displacement. Jaw becomes locked beneath maxillary prominence.	Muscles spastic. Later become fatigued.	Embarrassment in the unexpected recurrence. Trauma and fatigue in muscles. Predisposes infection.	Symptomatic treatment. Replacement by pressure of operators thumbs upon molars until normal placement in the mandibular cavity.	Replacement. Jaw bandage (supporting).	Anterior dislocation manifests partly opened and locked jaws with the teeth projecting forward. Complete reduction will restore the jaw for normal occlusion.

Fractures

Type	History	Pathology	Complications	Hemorrhage	Color of Area	Treatment	Transportation
1. Simple	Fall or accident.	A complete fracture with no fragments compounding.	Pressure on the blood supply. Malunion. Osteomyelitis.	Subcutaneous or capillary.	Slight to marked increase in ecchymosis.	Splint before preparation for transportation. Reduction (depending upon skill of operator).	In splint.
2. Compound	Fall or accident.	Injury where either one or both fragments are through the skin.	Infection. Hemorrhage. Shock.	May or may not include hemorrhage.	Slight to marked increase in ecchymosis.	Immediate debridement in hospital. Further treatment elective.	Cover with sterile dressing. Maintain traction. (Thomas splint.)
3. Greenstick	Fall or accident. (In children.)	Fracture is incomplete but there is bowing of the bone.	Complete fracture. Deformity.	Probably no hemorrhage will occur.	Discoloration may be slight. It may be marked.	Splint for preparation for transportation. Reduction of the curvature and place in cast.	Splint.
4. Comminuted	Injury due to crushing blow.	Bone is broken into two or more fragments.	Malunion. Infection.	Hemorrhage will occur in area of injury.	In area of deeper bones. Discoloration is delayed.	Splint before transportation. Replacement of fracture. Occasionally requires open reduction.	Splint and traction.
5. Impacted	Crushing force causing fracture. Fragments telescoped.	One fragment is jammed into another.	Deformity. Loss of function. Pain. Osteomyelitis.	Hemorrhage will occur in area of injury.	Discoloration according to extent of bone injury—it may be delayed.	Traction must be made while reduction and proper cast is fitted to hold extremity in place.	Splint and traction.
6. Transverse and 7. Spiral	Sudden twisting violence exerted upon extremity.	Fracture line across the bone. Fracture through the bone or around it.	Malfunction. Loss of function. Cuts of blood supply. Infection of bone.	Hemorrhage frequently occurs around area of fracture.	Same as compound fracture.	According to the site. Splint and traction.	Traction and immobilization.
a. Fracture of Skull	From a fall, or blow upon the skull.	In Vault with little or no intracranial trauma. Linear fracture may be overlooked. In Base serious compression in brain. Conous sion injury to vital cranial nerves.	Concussion. Paralysis of limbs of the body. Infection of brain. Compression of brain.	Clots on the brain. Extent and nature determined by location of injury. Dangers of pressure up on the brain.	Linear fractures may be slight and overlooked. Bleeding (bright) from mouth and ears.	Place in dorsal recumbent position. Watch for infection. Allow skull base fractures to bleed. Limit fluids.	Place on rigid stretcher. Keep flat. Keep patient quiet.
b. Fracture of Neck	Diving into pools. Auto wrecks. Accidents.	Break extends through body of vertebrae or the laminae.	Death. Paralysis (total or partial).	No hemorrhage noted in the tissues.	No change in color of the skin.	Keep neck in hyperextension. Place rolled blanket under shoulders. Minor fracture needs traction for 5-6 weeks. Major (with cord injury) need collar for 10-12 months.	Patient must not move the neck under any consideration. Keep neck and head hyperextended. Restrain if necessary. Rigid stretcher or improvision for rigidity.

FRACTURES—Continued

Type	History	Pathology	Complications	Hemorrhage	Color of Area	Treatment	Transportation
c. Fracture of Back	Occurs after jack-knife fall and other accidents.	Usually crushing body of vertebrae.	Paralysis and Shock (depending upon the location of the fracture).	No hemorrhage in surrounding tissues.	No change in color of the skin.	Extreme care in preparation and transportation. Rigid support. Place in hyperextension for 8 weeks. Body cast.	Place and secure in prone position. Keep patient in hyperextension. Restrain if necessary. Rigid stretcher or improvision.
d. Fracture of Coccyx	Falling into sitting position.	Fracture may be from sacral region or from tip of coccyx.	Constant pain. Abscesses. Osteomyelitis.	No hemorrhage in surrounding tissues.	No change in color of the skin.	Hot sitz bath. Rest in bed. If not cured then operate (coccygectomy).	Carry patient on rigid stretcher. Keep in dorsal recumbent position.
e. Fracture of Pelvis	From a blow or crushing force.	Bone impairment. Involvement of sacral nerves. Paralysis, torn ligaments and lacerated muscles.	Rupture of bladder and rectum. Deformity and shortening of limb. Sprain of pelvic joints.	Same as in compound fracture. Discoloration may be delayed.	Same as in compound fracture if compound. Otherwise delayed.	Keep in dorsal recumbent position. After reduction keep prone. Reduction of fragments. Symptomatic treatment.	On rigid stretcher in dorsal recumbent position. Keep body extended.
f. Fracture of Femur or Thigh	Epiphyseal separation in endocrine subjects. Twisting violence in lower parts.	Bone and nerve injury. Paralysis and permanent disability.	Deformity and shortening of the limb, where an endocrine disturbance is present. Severance of nerves and blood vessels. Paralysis and gangrene.	Same as in compound fracture. Discoloration may be delayed.	Same as in fracture of Pelvis.	Splint to leg and body. Keep patient flat. Provide and retain traction. Watch for shock.	Use rigid stretcher. Keep leg in traction until ready for reduction.
g. Fracture of Hip	Usually found in elderly people.	Fracture through neck or through trochanter or both.	Loss of function. Deformity shortening.	Hemorrhage but not in large amounts.	Ecchymosis but it may be delayed.	Traction (Russell). Smith Peterson Nail.	Place in Thomas Splint as improvised.
h. Fracture of Ankle (Potts Fracture)	From a sudden or forceful wrenching of the lower end of tibia and fibula.	Fracture of the lower ends of the fibula and tibia. Foot is displaced outward. Impairment of tissues, vessels, etc., from trauma.	Dislocations and sprains may occur simultaneously.	Same as in compound fracture. Discoloration.	Slight or marked areas of ecchymosis.	Immobilize immediately by pillow splint or rigid splint.	Keep limb well supported with slight elevation.
i. Fracture of Humerus	Result of a twisting force or blow upon upper arm.	Injury to the osseous structures. Trauma and lacerations of tissues, muscles, etc., if compound fracture.	Severance of nerves and blood vessels. Temporary deformity.	Slight—increased if compound fracture.	Slight or marked areas of discoloration.	Immobilize immediately by splint or sling (weight of forearm usually provides the necessary traction).	Keep arm in sling or splint.
j. Fracture of Forearm and Colles Fracture	Result of a twisting force upon the lower arm or wrist or from violence exerted upon the arm in preventing the body from falling.	Fracture and displacement of distal end of the radius. Tip of styloid process of ulna broken off. Backward displacement of radius.	Dislocations and sprains may be included. Trauma and swelling of tissues.	Slight—increased if fracture is not immediately immobilized.	Slight to marked.	Rigid splint, arm support with a sling.	Place in a sling after splinting.

App. 96

Poisons and Poisoning

Drug or Poison	"Lethal Dose" (Minimal)†	Symptoms of Poisoning	Emergency Measures	Supportive and Follow Up Treatment	Pathology
Acetanilid.	5-10 gr.	1. Skin cold and clammy and temperature subnormal. Cyanosis noted. 2. Profuse diaphoresis. 3. Respirations shallow, slow dyspneic. 4. Heart weaker with collapse and death.	1. Empty stomach by a gastric lavage. 2. Artificial respiration. 3. Oxygen by respirator. 4. Stimulants: Caffein; digitalis; ammonia. Antidote—Oxygen.	1. Keep patient in recumbent position. Keep quiet. 2. External heat. 3. Stimulants as needed. 4. Blood transfusion as emergency; or as is necessary.	Affects heat center. Temperature subnormal. Formation of methemoglobin which depresses the cerebral and medullary centers. Mental sluggishness.
Acetone.	6 oz.				
Anilin.	6 drams.				
Antipyrine.	15-30 gr.				
Acids (Corrosive). Acetic. Hydrochloric. Nitric. Phosphoric. Sulfuric.	1 dr. to 4 dr. 2 drams. * 1 dram.	1. Mouth and throat whitish, swollen and burning with pain. 2. Dysphagia, nausea and increased thirst, "Coffee ground" vomitus. 3. Pupils contracted. 4. Pulse weak, rapid. 5. Swelling, blistering of mouth, pharynx with increased edema and closure. 6. Respirations shallow and labored.	1. Counteragents or use antagonists such as magnesia, milk of magnesia, lime water, soda bicarbonate, soap solution. 2. Demulcents and vegetable oil (olive oil). Albumin: White of egg. Antidote—Alkalies and sodium or potassium carbonate.	1. Keep the patient at rest. Apply external heat. 2. Morphine for discomfort. 3. Atropine for excessive secretion. 4. Avoid the use of alkaline carbonates and chalk which liberate CO2 and produce marked distention. 5. When poisons are corrosive avoid stomach tube treatments. Caustics—use acetic acid with equal parts of water. No emetics—no lavages.	Lips and tongue are soft and corroded. Tissues will tear under gentle manipulation. Ulcers and contractions of the gastroenteric areas.
Acids, Cont'd. Boric (Boracic Acid).	*	1. Patient complains of headache with nausea, vomiting, diarrhea. 2. Skin is cold, clammy, diaphoresis. 3. Fine bright red rash. 4. Muscular weakness, cardiac failure and collapse.	Gastric lavage.	Provide therapy for the symptoms as they develop. Treat for shock.	Excessive damage to kidney tissues.
Acids, Cont'd. Carbolic. Cresol. Creosote. Lysol. Phenol.	1 dram to 4 drams. * 1 dram.	1. Mouth and upper respiratory tract are corroded. Dysphagia is present. 2. Coffee ground vomitus. 3. Pulse is rapid, weak, respirations are shallow and labored.	1. Gastric lavage with caution. 2. Magnesium or sodium sulfate. 3. Milk, white of egg, soap solution lime water. Avoid alcohol and glycerine. 4. Artificial respiration to supply oxygen if necessary. Antidote—Sodium or magnesium sulfate as gavage and instillation.	1. Keep patient quiet and in recumbent position. 2. Apply external heat and keep cold compresses on head. 3. Treat for shock. 4. Morphine for pain. 5. Stimulants—Caffein, strychnine. 6. Treat edema with atropine sulfate.	1. Shrunken patches about the mouth. 2. Destruction of lining of gastrointestinal tract. 3. Paralysis of respiratory tract.

*Not determined.
†"Lethal Dose," from De Re Medicina, pages 280 to 291, Eli Lilly Co., Indianapolis, Indiana.

App. 97

POISONS AND POISONING—Continued

Drug or Poison	"Lethal Dose" (Minimal)‡	Symptoms of Poisoning	Emergency Measures	Supportive and Follow Up Treatment	Pathology
Acids, Cont'd. Carbonic Acid.	*	Poison in smaller amounts.	1. Artificial respiration. 2. Introduction of oxygen by respirator. Antidote—Oxygen.	1. Continue giving oxygen. Keep patient in fresh air if weather permits. 2. Treat for shock—external heat and massage of limbs. 3. Stimulants—Caffein, ammonia.	Overstimulates respiratory center.
Acids, Cont'd. Hydrocyanic (Prussic Acid).	1 grain to 2 grains.	1. Poison in smaller amounts. 2. Headache, mental confusion and weakness. Pulse weak, slow and imperceptible. Respirations forced, labored, dyspneic. 4. Pupils dilated. Eyes glassy and bulging. Larger amount of Poison: Patient has convulsions and death follows due to paralysis of heart and respiratory center.	Rapid team work. 1. Empty stomach by lavage immediately with hydrogen peroxide 3% or potassium permanganate 1 to 500. Antidote—Hydrogen peroxide lavage of potassium permanganate. Inhalation amyl nitrite.	1. Artificial respiration started immediately. 2. Amyl nitrite inhalations. 3. Keep patient in recumbent position and apply external heat. Shock treatment. 4. Very careful supervision for recurrence of symptoms. 5. Treatment. Repetition if necessary if patient shows signs of collapse.	Depressant action upon the protoplasm retards oxidation process. Blood retains its bright arterial color in the veins.
Acids, Cont'd. Oxalic Acid.	½ dram to 2 drams.	1. Severe gastrointestinal irritation and intense pain in upper gastrointestinal tract. Intense thirst and vomiting. 2. Pulse weak, thready. Pupils dilated. 3. Skin cold and cyanotic. 4. Muscles of face twitching. 5. Convulsions, coma and collapse and death.	Avoid lavages. Induce vomiting. Give lime in any form immediately. Intravenous doses of calcium chloride. Antidote—Magnesia or chalk.	1. Keep patient quiet and in recumbent position. 2. Give salts of sodium and avoid potassium—since soluble oxalates are formed. 3. Avoid alkalies and alkaline carbonates or bicarbonates because soluble poisons will be formed.	Stomach tissues blacken, after extensive venous engorgement. Peritonitis. Pleuritis.
Aconite. Aconitine.	4 grains. 1/10 grain.	1. Tingling sensation in the mouth and upper gastrointestinal tract with excessive flow of saliva. 2. Patient is very restless, dizzy or staggering. 3. Pulse is slow, and later irregular, very rapid. 4. Respirations are slow, shallow, irregular. 5. Skin is cold and cyanotic. 6. Pupils contracted and then dilated—eyes staring. 7. Patient is syncopic and lies in prostration, coma until death.	1. Wash stomach with tannic acid taken by mouth. 2. No emetics or lavages unless specified. Antidote—Tannic acid gr. 10 to 30 put in water or charcoal.	1. Keep patient flat in bed. 2. Artificial respiration and oxygen if necessary. 3. External heat to body and ice compresses to head. 4. Mustard plaster for acute pain in epigastrium. 5. Continue stimulants as directed. 6. Catharsis of Mg. SO_4—to drastic purging. 7. Close observation.	Depresses respiratory center. Respiratory failure.

* Not determined.
‡ "Lethal Dose," from De Re Medicina, pages 280 to 291, Eli Lilly Co., Indianapolis, Indiana.

App. 98

POISONS AND POISONING—Continued

Drug or Poison	"Lethal Dose" (Minimal)‡	Symptoms of Poisoning	Emergency Measures	Supportive and Follow Up Treatment	Pathology
Alcohol, Ethyl. Acute.	3½ ounces to 7 ounces.	Face is red, bloated, lips are cyanotic. Skin becomes red and bloated with veins enlarged. Delirium: Dilated pupils, mental excitement. Rapid pulse—Shallow rapid respiration. Subnormal temperature. Coma and convulsive seizures.	Antidote — Apomorphine if patient is irritable. Gastric lavage. Stimulating emetic. Aromatic spirits of ammonia. Coffee enemata.	1. "Moderate drinking is the nursery of inebriety."† 2. Sobering up patient. Keep the patient aroused. Infusion. Stimulants if necessary. Artificial respiration.	Depression of the respiratory and circulatory system.
Chronic in Delirium Tremens.		Complications are: Gastritis, chronic nephritis; cirrhosis of liver; arteriosclerosis; coma of alcoholism differentiated from others by history, absence of paralysis, subnormal temperature. Patient can be aroused. Odor of liquor.	Carbon dioxide and oxygen to stimulate respiration and hasten elimination of alcoholic products from lungs. Rouse the patient. Caffrin and strychnine. Antidote—Apomorphine	Bed rest after alcohol is removed.	Acute hepatic necrosis leading to lethal effects (after drunken bout).
Alcohol, Methyl.	1 ounce to 2 ounces.	Exhilaration accompanied by headache, muscular weakness, nausea, vomiting and abdominal pain. Delirium with visual disturbance to blindness. Pulse is weak and rapid. Respirations slow and dyspneic, unconsciousness, coma with cyanosis. Death from respiratory paralysis.	Gastric lavage. Alkalies by mouth and intravenously. Oxygen inhalations. Keep the body warm. Treat for shock. Antidote — Sodium bicarbonate.	Bed rest. Treat for shock (external heat). Stimulants as necessary.	Partial to complete blindness (if patient survives poison effect) due to atrophy of the optic nerve.
Aldehydes. Formalin. Formaldehyde.	1 ounce.	Pain in epigastrium, nausea and vomiting, intense anxiety. Pulse: Weak and rapid, coma to collapse.	Gastric lavage. R. Ammon. acetate sol. 2 tablespoons, aromatic spirits of ammonia 1 teaspoon, household ammonia (1%) 10 to 20 drops. Dilute with cold water. Egg white—stimulants. Antidote— Ammon. acetate sol. 2 tablespoons.	Bed rest. Shock treatment. Stimulants as needed.	Irritating to eyes. Destroys outer skin layers.
Alkalies. Lye. Potash. Caustic Soda. Ammonia. Lime.	½ dram to 4 drams.	Severe pain in mouth, difficulty in swallowing, gastrointestinal symptoms of pain and purging. Expression—apprehensive. Shock symptoms. Pulse is rapid and weak.	Diluted vinegar and lemon juice. Avoid gastric lavage. Olive oil by mouth. Give milk and egg white. Stimulants to prevent shock. Antidote—Weak acetic acid.	Morphine as analgesic. Fluids by hypodermoclysis. Use of bougies to prevent esophageal stricture. If in eye, wash with boric acid.	Corrosive effect upon tissues of upper respiratory tract. Lye damages esophagus; produces stricture.

‡ "Lethal Dose" from De Re Medicine, Eli Lilly and Co., Indianapolis, Indiana.
† Merck Manual of Therapeutics and Materia Medica, Rahway, New Jersey.

POISONS AND POISONING—Continued

Drug or Poison	"Lethal Dose" (Minimal)‡	Symptoms of Poisoning	Emergency Measures	Supportive and Follow Up Treatment	Pathology
Animal poisons. Venoms.	*	Vary in terms of type, or snake and area of bite. On area where bitten: Swelling, discoloration and sloughing of skin. Symptoms of uremia may be delayed.	Keep patient quiet. Tourniquet applied above the bite. Incision and suction for aspiration of venom, from the muscles. Antidote—Aspiration of venom.	Constant watching for areas increasing in swelling. Continue with incision and aspiration of venom.	Poisonous substance. Hematoxic—Causes: 1. Destruction of red blood cells. 2. Sloughing of the skin. Neurotoxic—Causes paralysis of vital centers in the brain. Respiratory paralysis produces death.
Anesthetics. Chloroform. Ether.	*	Stertorous to rapid and shallow respirations. Pulse weak, slow and feeble. Skin: Cold, pale and clammy if chloroform; cyanotic if ether; pupils are dilated. Cardiac and respiratory failure (pulse is weak and very rapid).	Evacuate stomach (if swallowed). Demulcents and sodium bicarbonate solution. Ammonia by inhalation (if poison was inhaled). Antidote—Demulcents and sodium bicarbonate.	Lower head, pull tongue forward. Stimulants for prostration. Alternate hot and cold water douched upon the face.	Blood pressure is lowered. Respiratory center is depressed. Congestion of lungs, bronchi and kidney. Delayed jaundice and degeneration of the heart.
Antimony.	¾ grain to 1½ grains.	Burning heat—constriction in throat. Pain in abdomen—vomiting. Skin: Cold and clammy with rash resembling the lesions of eczema. Supression of urine, pulse feeble, rapid, irregular to imperceptible. Respirations slow and shallow.	Solution of warm tannic acid as emetic until free emesis. Strong tea and tannin. Egg white, milk. Magnesium oxide. Antidote—Tannic acid (warm, weak).	Artificial respirations. Stimulants, saline solutions (rectally or intravenously). Respiratory and circulatory stimulants. External heat for shock.	Inflammation of gastric tract. Destructive ulceration of epiglottis, pharynx, chronic poisoning — inflammation of liver and kidneys.
Arsenic: Arsenious acid. Fowler's solution. "Paris green." Rough on Rats.	1 grain to 1½ grains.	Burning pain in esophagus. Abdominal pain, nausea, vomiting and diarrhea. Persistent headache. Pains around the joints of the extremities. Redness of eyes with edema of eyelids, coryza. Supersensitiveness of the extremities to nerve stimulus.	Sodium thiosulfate. Gastric lavage for the complete removal of poison. Demulcents (milk, eggs, olive oil in water (1 to 4). Ferric hydroxide and magnesium. Sodium thiosulfate by intravenous or by mouth. Morphine after all acute symptoms have subsided. Antidote—Ferric hydroxide.	Supportive and symptomatic. Keep patient in recumbent position. Flush body with fluids by mouth or intravenously. Treat for shock. Avoid collapse—use strychnine, caffein, etc., give bismuth, chalk or opium for the severe diarrhea. For paralysis of the extremities—give deep massage by electric vibrator.	Lessens combination of body tissues with oxygen . . . the patient becomes stouter. Produces paralysis of the extensor muscles of the extremities. Hence—drop foot and drop hands.

* Not determined.
‡ "Lethal Dose" from De Re Medicina, Eli Lilly and Co., Indianapolis, Indiana.

App. 100

POISONS AND POISONING—Continued

Drug or Poison	"Lethal Dose" (Minimal)‡	Symptoms of Poisoning	Emergency Measures	Supportive and Follow Up Treatment	Pathology
Atropine. Belladonna. Hyoscyamus. Stramonium.	1 grain.	"Mouth is dry (thirst is intensified). Skin flushed and dry. Headache, nausea, vomiting, diarrhea. Respiration slow, rapid, and stertorous. Pulse slow to rapid and feeble. Headache, dizziness, weakness. Temperature elevation. Cyanosis and cold extremities in fatal cases. If scopolamine, skin is cyanotic and patient becomes comatose. Pupils are widely dilated. Delirium to belladonna jag."	Emetics or gastric lavage. Stimulants of strong coffee or strychnine. Morphine not except for poisoning by scopalamine. Artificial respiration if necessary. Antidote—Weak tannic acid.	Ice cap to head for the delirious cases. Watch for coma. Artificial respiration if necessary. Catheterize patient.	Paralysis of respiratory centers. Lessens secretion of all secretory glands (nerve endings of the sympathetic controls the secretion of sweat. Blood vessels are dilated (increases the flush or color in the face).
Barbiturates.	15 grains.	"Headache—mental confusion, ataxia; twitching of muscles, ptosis, sleep at first quiet, then deepening rapidly into coma; respiration at first slow and quiet, then noisy; moderately dilated pupils, absence of corneal reflex; nystagmus; hippus (rapid, spasmodic change in size of pupil), occasionally temperature rises; may be skin eruptions. Cyanosis, anuria, collapse. Respiration stertorous, irregular. Pulse in severe cases small, soft and irregular. Blood pressure low, death from respiratory failure within a few hours exceptional."	Gastric lavage of 2% potassium permanganate. Picrotoxin gr. 1/10 for spastic muscles. Strychnine gr. 1/8, hypodermoclysis saline. Antidote—Magnesium sulfate.	Oxygen and carbon dioxide inhalations if necessary for cyanosis. Body fluids.	Pulmonary edema. Acidosis. Depression of the respiratory center. Chronic mental depression. Anxiety neurosis. Cardiac disorders. Speech disturbance.
Barium.	15 grains.	Nausea, vomiting, abdominal cramps, diarrhea, swallowing and speech inhibitions. Muscular weakness to paralysis of extremities. Cold sweats, headache, dizziness, convulsions. Pulse rapid, tense, becoming weaker. "Blue line on gums" not always present.	Lavage with magnesium sulfate or sodium sulfate. Aluminum sulfate. Use of emetics. Morphine gr. 1/4 and atropine gr. 1/120 to relieve pain. Antidote—Magnesium or sodium sulfate.	Clear the stomach of all poison by lavages or emetics. Treat symptomatically. Keep the patient warm (shock treatment).	Paralysis of respiratory center. Overstimulates the heart. Contracts the muscles of small blood vessels and those muscles in the sphincter of the bladder and the intestines.
Benzine.		See Solvents.			

‡ "Lethal Dose" from De Re Medicina, Eli Lilly and Company, Indianapolis, Indiana.
† Merck Manual of Therapeutics and Materia Medica.

POISONS AND POISONING—Continued

Drug or Poison	"Lethal Dose" (Minimal)‡	Symptoms of Poisoning	Emergency Measures	Supportive and Follow Up Treatment	Pathology
Benzol.		See Solvents.			
Belladonna.		See Atropine.			
Botulism.		See Food Poisoning.			
Bromides.	*	Sudden eruption of reddish blots over body. Loss of appetite. Constipation. Drowsiness with slow and stammering speech. Very sluggish mental reaction. Memory is poor. Slow, uncertain gait.	Sodium chloride—by gavage. Catharsis of saline to purge thoroughly. Antidote—Sodium chloride.	Continuous reduction of bromides from body by perspiration. Force fluids. Warm continuous baths.	Acne eruption, bullae and pustules. Mucus membranes inflamed, softened and loosened. Depresses entire nervous system. Exhaustion and heart failure.
Cannabis. American Hemp. Indian Hemp. Marihuana.	*	Exhilaration or a pleasurable intoxication to drowsiness and muscular weakness of the legs. Pupils are dilated. Pulse is rapid. Respirations slow.	Atropine by hypodermic. Amyl nitrite if necessary. Strychnine is necessary. Treat for shock. Antidote—Tannic acid.	Cold compresses to head. Continue artificial respirations. External heat as is necessary.	Over-stimulates the nervous system to delirium with inability to suppress mental desire for drug. Sexual desires increased. Respiratory depressant. Produces heart failure.
Cantharides.	¼ ounce.	Burning pain increases to blisters, swelling in tongue, throat and stomach. Nausea, vomiting and intense thirst. Diarrhea (sanguineously streaked), tenesmus. Pain in back with pain in bladder, urethra and strangury. Heart stimulated to depressed. Patient is delirious. Has comatose and convulsive indications. Syncope to comatose and collapse.	Gastric lavage. Demulcents (except oil). Morphine gr. ¼ for pain. Treat for shock. Antidote—Demulcents.	External heat continuously. Anesthetics if convulsive. Treat conditions of acute nephritis and cystitis.	Softens and destroys mucosa of gastroenteric areas. Injures kidney tissues. Produces severe gastroenteritis; nephritis; cystitis, urethritis.
Carbon Tetrachloride.		See Solvents.			
Chloral Hydrate. Chloralamide.	20 grains.	Nausea, vomiting and headache with relaxation of muscles. Temperature lowered with cyanosis and cold, clammy extremities. Pulse slower and weak. Respiration slow and irregular. Asphyxia to coma and collapse. Pupils may become "pin point."	Gastric lavage solution of potassa—½ to 2 fluid drams every hour to decompose the chloral hydrate in the blood. Picrotoxin intravenously. Antidote—Tannic acid.	Lavage of strong tea or coffee. Agitation (or shaking to arouse the patient).	"Wheals." (mental depression). Very sudden weakness of the heart to paralysis of the heart; causing death.

* Not determined.
‡ "Lethal Dose" from the De Re Medicina, Eli Lilly and Company, Indianapolis, Indiana.

POISONS AND POISONING—Continued

Drug or Poison	"Lethal Dose" (Minimal)‡	Symptoms of Poisoning	Emergency Measures	Supportive and Follow Up Treatment	Pathology
Chloroform.	1 ounce.	Pulse slow and weak. Respirations stertorous, shallow and irregular. Pupils are dilated. Skin cold, clammy and pale. Blood pressure lowers to cardiac failure.	If swallowed—gastric lavage. Lower the head and open mouth (pull tongue forward to allow air passage). Antidote—Artificial respiration.	Douche the face with alternating hot and cold sponges or towels. Artificial respiration.	Paralytic sensations. Produces nephritis, hepatitis. Depresses respiratory center. Heart failure.
Cocaine and its substitutes.	½ grain to 15 grains.	Stimulation followed by depression. Nausea, vomiting, and dryness and numbness of throat. Loss of ability to see and hear. Respirations labored with clonic and tonic convulsions. Pulse slow to rapid. Blood pressure lowers. Patient becomes cyanotic, delirious and comatose. Sudden collapse.	Oxygen—Artificial respiration. Morphine as necessary. Sodium phenobarbital to be given. For collapse use caffeine, strychnine. Antidote—Tannic acid.	Ice cap to head. Keep patient quiet (flat on back) to control nervous tension. External heat. Artificial respiration.	Medulla is temporarily stimulated to depressed. Heart muscle is depressed to extent of heart failure.
Codeine.		See Opium.			
Conium. Coniine (Poison Hemlock).	± 2 grains.	Very definite weakness of the legs with staggering increased to inability. Pulse slow, rapid and feeble. Respiration first rapid and deep to slow and labored. Convulsions to coma and paralysis.	Artificial respirations. Potassium iodide grains x preceding gastric lavage. Demulcents. Shock treatment. Antidote—Tannic acid.	Dorsal recumbent position. External heat. Deep massage to limbs.	Brain meninges and lungs show congestion. Hyperemia of mucous membrane esophagus and stomach.
Copper Sulfate (Blue vitriol). Subacetate. (Verdigris). Acetoarsenite. Paris Green.	5 drams.	Nausea, vomiting and diarrhea accompanied by severe abdominal pain with bloody stools. Pulse weak and soft. Respirations shallow and labored. Skin cold and clammy. Delirium to unconsciousness. Coma and death.	Solution—Potassium ferrocyanide (5 grain doses as a gastric lavage). Demulcents—milk, egg, magnesia. Morphine gr. ¼ for pain. Treat for shock. Antidote — Potassium ferrocyanide.	Artificial respiration if necessary. Strong coffee. External heat.	Congestion, swelling and softening of mucous membrane of stomach and bowels. Ulceration of colon. Kidneys are swollen, liver soft and fatty.
Corrosive Sublimate.		See Mercury.			
Creosote.		See Acids, Carbolic.			

‡ "Lethal Dose" from De Re Medicina, Eli Lilly and Company, Indianapolis, Indiana.

POISONS AND POISONING—Continued

Drug or Poison	"Lethal Dose" (Minimal)‡	Symptoms of Poisoning	Emergency Measures	Supportive and Follow Up Treatment	Pathology
Croton Oil.	20 gtt.	Patient complains of severe abdominal pain—vomiting, diarrhea, prostration. Pulse weak and thready. Respiration shallow and rapid. Burning in mouth, throat and stomach more intense.	Lavage freely with water, milk. Use emetics. Demulcents as desired. Treat for shock. Antidote—Demulcents.	Force fluids. Application of heat to the abdomen. External heat. Shock treatment.	Mucous membrane of the stomach and intestines is swollen, reddened and partially detached.
Cyanide.		Use Hydrocyanic Acid, etc.			
Digitalis.	40 grains.	Headache, dizziness, nausea, vomiting with abdominal pain and diarrhea. Excessive muscular weakness. Vision disturbed with dilated to contracted pupils. Eyeballs protruding. Pulse slow and regular (at rest); pulse changes to rapid and weak (on rising). Skin pale and cold, extremities clammy. Lethargy, delirium and coma.	Gastric lavage of tannic acid. Saline catharsis. Tincture of aconite. Artificial respiration. Treat for shock. Antidote—Tannic acid.	Keep patient flat in bed. Artificial respiration as is needed. Symptomatic treatments. Keep body warm.	Stimulation of the medullary—cardio inhibitory center slows the heart action, passes into fibrillary contractions and ceases to beat (culminating effect upon the heart).
Ergot.	12 grains.	Vomiting, diarrhea, thirst, tingling in the feet and cramps in extremities. Skin—burning, itching and tingling as well as cold. Dizziness, visual disturbance and dilated pupils. Hemorrhage (pregnancy), weakness to convulsions.	Treat for shock. Emetics—gastric lavage purges with castor oil or magnesium sulfate. Amyl nitrite (by inhalation). Nitroglycerine (type), caffein and strychnine as stimulants. Antidote—Tannic acid.	Keep patient warm and quiet. Massage extremities. External heat. Treat for shock.	Persistent contraction of small blood vessels (in chronic ergot poisoning). Acute ergot poisoning very rare.
Eserine.		See Physostigmine.			
Food Poisoning (Ptomaine). Botulism.	*	Symptoms appear 18 to 36 hours after ingestion of food. Headache, dizziness and inhibition of swallowing or speaking. Intense thirst. Abdominal pain, diarrhea and great prostration.	Emetics and gastric lavage until stomach is emptied of all poison. Purging with magnesium sulfate. Strychnine or digitalis given as stimulants. Antidote—Specific antitoxin (if early).	Preventive treatment (cook all preserved food just before eating). Proper sealing of canned food. Symptomatic treatment. Artificial respiration if necessary.	Acts upon central nervous system. Hemorrhages in the spinal cord and ganglion. Paralysis of muscles of the eyes. Progressive paralysis of muscles of the chest. Cardiac failure.

* Not determined.
‡ "Lethal Dose" from De Re Medicina, Eli Lilly and Company, Indianapolis, Indiana.

App. 104

POISONS AND POISONING—Continued

Drug or Poison	"Lethal Dose" (Minimal)‡	Symptoms of Poisoning	Emergency Measures	Supportive and Follow Up Treatment	Pathology
Food Poisoning, Salmonella Group.	*	Rise in temperature with symptoms as given above.	Gastric lavage. Purging use of magnesium sulfate and castor oil. Antidote—Gastric lavage.	Symptomatic treatments.	May produce an acute appendicitis.
Staphylococcus group.		Symptoms as above. Additional rise in temperature.	Same as above.	Symptomatic treatments.	Death is usually due to cardiac failure.
Gas: Carbon Monoxide. Illuminating Gas. Automobile Exhaust Gas.	*	Symptoms vary. 1. Concentration of gas. 2. Time exposure. Concentrated—death immediately. Low concentration — headache (throbbing of temples), dizziness. Respiration accelerated and stertorous. Pulse weak and irregular. Skin dusky, lips cyanotic or cherry red.	Get patient into fresh air. Artificial respiration. Oxygen inhalations + CO_2. Stimulants. Cardiac respiratory. Normal saline infusions. Shock treatment. Antidote—Oxygen.	Plentiful supply of O_2. Keep patient in open. Artificial respiration. Transfusion in 1 hour for best effect.	Respiratory paralysis. Lungs, brain and abdominal viscera deeply congested.
Hydrocyanic Acid. Prussic Acid. Cyanides. Fumigating Gas. Bitter Almonds. Choke Berries.	1 grain to 2 grains.	Large doses, immediate death. Smaller doses, headache, mental confusion. Pulse slow and not perceptible. Respiration very dyspneic; eyes dilated, pupils with protruding balls, glassy. Breath — characteristic odor. Asphyxia to convulsions, unconsciousness, coma, paralysis, stupor to respiratory failure and death.	Rapid work. Keep patient in fresh air. Artificial respiration immediately. Gastric lavage. Hydrogen peroxide. Give amyl nitrite as inhalation every 2 to 3 min. for 15 seconds to 20 seconds. Antidote—Oxygen.	Artificial respiration and oxygen, recumbent position. External heat.	Interference with the oxidative processes within the body. (Inability of cells of body to use the O_2 necessary for maintenance of life.)
Hyoscyamus.		See Atropine.			
Iodine.	1 dram.	Patient describes burning pain in throat and stomach. Acute gastrointestinal pain and intense thirst. Vomiting, diarrhea (may be blood streaked), anuria or strangury, albumin or blood in urine. Skin—cold, clammy, cyanotic. Pulse—rapid, feeble. Respirations—dyspneic and shallow. Convulsive manifestations. Twitchings, collapse.	Solution of starch: prompt and frequent administration of demulcents—starch, barley water, gruel. Gastric lavage and emetics. Stimulants are necessary. Morphine gr. ¼ for pain. Antidote—Starch solution, or barley water.	Counteract with starch—and emptying stomach of poison. Force fluids. Saline hypodermoclysis. Inclusion of alkalies to antagonize renal suppression and dehydration. Keep patient quiet.	Irritation and swelling within throat, esophagus and stomach. Loss of electrolytes by vomiting, tends to support dehydration and suppression or urine.

* Not determined.
‡ "Lethal Dose" from De Re Medicina, Eli Lilly and Co., Indianapolis, Indiana.

POISONS AND POISONING—Continued

Drug or Poison	"Lethal Dose" (Minimal)†	Symptoms of Poisoning	Emergency Measures	Supportive and Follow Up Treatment	Pathology
Lead Salts. Lead Acetate. White Lead.	300 grs.	Dryness in throat with burning pain in stomach. Severe pain in abdomen. Diarrhea follows constipation. Muscular weakness and paralysis of the limbs. Skin cyanotic (face) and cold. (Blue line on the gums). Delayed severe anemia.	Gastric lavage and emetics. Purgation, morphine, atropine, as ordered for pain. Demulcents: Milk and egg white. Chloral hydrate for relaxation of muscles during convulsions. Antidote—Magnesium or sodium sulfate.	Keep patient quiet. Flush system of the poisons by large ingestions of water. Treat for shock.	Gastrointestinal inflammation. Liver and kidney damage when lead has not been removed early by the gavage. If albuminuria has been present the kidneys have become atrophied and contracted.
Mercury. Corrosive Sublimate. Bichloride.	3 grains to 5 grains.	Patient complains of metallic taste in mouth and burning of mouth and throat. Abdominal pain and cramps with nausea, vomiting, diarrhea and bloody stools. Urine scanty with albumin. Collapse after severe pain and effect of diarrhea. Pulse: Rapid, weak. Respirations, slow and shallow. Skin cold and clammy. Face is pinched and apprehensive.	Lavage (egg white, milk, flour), Lavage of 3% sodium formaldehyde. Sulfoxylate. Stimulants (caffeine, strychnine, atropine). Morphine gr. ¼ for pain. Shock treatment. Antidote—Demulcents.	Rapid treatment. Colonic irrigations for colitis. Repeat hyposulf'ate and continue with gastric lavage to release all of poisonous metal. Keep patient warm. Treat for shock.	Ulcerations of gums, mouth and loosening of teeth. Paralysis of extremities. "Hand drop".—"Foot drop" produces a progressive peripheral nephritis. Nerve lesion. Restriction of the myelin.
Mushroom Muscarine.	*	Patient vomits violently, severe diarrhea. Very apprehensive, severe abdominal pain. Pulse weak and slow. Resp. labored and slow. Delirium, stupor and convulsions.	Tincture Belladonna min. xx. Gastric lavage and emetic. Artificial respiration if necessary. Atropine gr. 1/120 hypo. Antidote—Tannic acid in lavage.	Evacuation of stomach. Stimulants as necessary. External heat O₂ as inhalations if necessary.	Stenosis of bronchial tubes. Produces pulmonary edema. Congestion and hemorrhage in stomach and the intestines.
Morphine.		See Opium.			
Nicotine. Black Leaf 40.	1 minim to 4 minims.	"Patient becomes excited is confused and restless. Abdominal cramps with nausea, salivation, vomiting and diarrhea to prostration. Skin pale, cold, clammy. Pulse slow to rapid. Respirations: Rapid and dyspneic. Larger doses; this order is reversed. Tremors: Palpitation of heart. Pupils contracted and then dilated. Headache, vertigo, collapse, coma." From the Merck Manual of Materia Medica and Therapeutics.	Gastric lavage and emetics. Strychnine gr. 1/30-1/20. Nitrous Ether 1 tsp. to 2 tsp. Treat for shock. Antidote—Tannic acid lavage.	Artificial respiration if necessary. Cold applications to the head. Symptomatic treatment. Keep patient warm.	Paralysis of respiratory center. Paralysis of the central nervous system.

*Not determined.
†"Lethal Dose" from De Re Medicina, Eli Lilly and Company, Indianapolis, Indiana.

App. 106

POISONS AND POISONING—Continued

Drug or Poison	"Lethal Dose" (Minimal)†	Symptoms of Poisoning	Emergency Measures	Supportive and Follow Up Treatment	Pathology
Nitrites. Amyl Nitrite. Nitroglycerine. Spirits of Niter.	*	Face is flushed then diminished. Intense throbbing of the head. Dizziness and faintness and excessive muscular relaxation and tremors. Pupils are dilated. Pulse weak and rapid. Stupor follows the period of excitement.	Stimulants if necessary. Apomorphine chloride gr. 1/10. Alternate hot and cold douches upon the chest. Antidote—Cardiac and respiratory stimulants.	Keep patient in reclining position.	Paralysis of respiratory and circulatory centers.
Nux Vomica.		See Strychnine.			
Opium and Codeine. Heroin. Laudanum. Morphine. Paregoric.	3 grains to 4 grains. 1 grain to 2 grains.	Mental excitement to weariness, sleepiness. Respirations slow and shallow. Pulse rapid and forceful to slower. As in comatose condition can be aroused with much difficulty. Pulse may change to rapid and feeble. Pupils are pin point. Skin is pale, cold and clammy with cyanosis. Convulsions to coma and collapse.	Tannic acid and emetics. Atropine sulfate gr. 1/150. Stimulants. Strychnine gr. 1/30-1/20. Caffeine if necessary. Oxygen inhalations. Antidote—Potassium permanganate 5% to 1%.	Keep the patient awake by walking when condition is permissible. Alternate hot and cold douches to the chest for arousing the patient. Hot drinks. Catheterize bladder. Keep the patient warm.	Depresses the nervous system and relaxes the convulsive state in such conditions as tetanus. Produces lung congestion.
Paris Green.		See Arsenic.			
Petroleum. Kerosene. Gasoline. Benzene.	*	Suggestive of mild alcoholic poisoning. Depression, headache, nausea, feeling of constriction in throat, diarrhea, extreme thirst. If severe, convulsions and sometimes death.	Gastric lavage. Emetic. Remove to fresh air if fumes are inhaled. Remove clothing, if contacting the liquid. Antidote—Emetics and lavage.	Symptomatic stimulation, oxygen, external heat, artificial respiration.	Small hemorrhages in G. I. tract and lung. Some hemolysis has been found.
Phosphorus. Rat and roach paste. Matches.	1 to 3 grains.	Usually appear after several hours. Jaundice, odor of garlic on breath which is luminous in the dark.	Gastric lavage with ½% copper sulfate, sol. potassium permanganate sol. 1-1000 or dilute hydrogen peroxide. Repeat lavage frequently. Magnesium sulfate, oil of furpentine: 1 tsp. in 1 pt. water. Antidote—Lavage of potassium permanganate solution 1%.	Intravenous dextrose and calcium salts will aid in protecting liver from damage. Morphine and symptomatic stimulation with caffeine, oxygen if necessary. Turpentine as cathartic given for several days.	Fatty degeneration of liver, kidney and heart.

* Not determined.
† "Lethal Dose" from De Re Medicina, Eli Lilly and Company, Indianapolis, Indiana.

App. 107

POISONS AND POISONING—Continued

Drug or Poison	"Lethal Dose" (Minimal) ‡	Symptoms of Poisoning	Emergency Measures	Supportive and Follow Up Treatment	Pathology
Physostigmine. Calabar bean. Eserine. Ordeal bean.	2 to 3 grains. 6 beans.	Contracted pupils. Salivation and perspiration. Muscular weakness, muscular twitching. Vomiting, pain in stomach, dyspneic; pulse slow.	Gastric lavage. Atropine 1/40 to 1/60 gr. Magnesium sulfate intravenously. Antidote—Gastric lavage and atropine sulfate gr. 1/40 to 1/60 gr. (as antagonist).	Keep body warm, stimulate with strychnine, digitalis and ammonia.	Lungs distended and edematous. Hyperemia of brain. Mucous membranes of tongue, pharynx, stomach, lower portion of trachea swollen.
Picrotoxin. Cocculus Indicus.	*	Weakness, confusion, increased salivation, nausea, vomiting and diarrhea, drowsiness, cold, profuse diaphoresis and unconsciousness.	Gastric lavage, emetics, chloroform. Intravenous barbiturates to control convulsions.	Symptomatic stimulation, artificial respiration. Inhalations of CO_2 and O_2. Hot mustard baths.	No characteristic lesions have been found in man.
Pilocarpine. Jaborandi.	2 grains.	Great weakness, profuse salivation, diaphoresees, and lacrimation. Twitchings of muscles starting at lower extremities and extending upwards. Contracted pupils. Danger symptoms, slow, irregular, weak pulse, rapid, difficult breathing accompanied by rales.	Lavage, tannic acid, stimulants, caffeine. Heart Antidote—Tannic acid, atropine as antagonist.	External heat to body. Artificial respiration.	Increases secretion of secretory glands, except breasts, liver and kidneys, edema of lungs. Excreted rapidly within 24 hours by kidneys.
Ptomaines.		See Food Poisoning.			
Silver Salts, Lunar caustic, Nitrite.	30 grains.	Pain in throat and stomach. Bloody stools. Vertigo disturbance, respiration and coma.	Gastric lavage or emetic with large quantities of table salt and water. Antidote—Sodium chloride.	Eggs and milk for demulcent effect. Morphine; stimulants if necessary.	Deposits of metallic silver under the skin in chronic poisoning, white stains, turning dark on exposure on lips, mouth and mucous membrane of digestive tract. Gastrointestinal inflammation present.
Solvents: Benzol. Tolul. Xylol.	*	In mild cases resembles early alcoholic intoxication. If exposure is great, delirium followed by loss of consciousness, convulsions and death.	Remove patient to fresh air, remove clothing if it contains solvent. If ingested, gastric lavage with warm water, artificial respirations; $O_2 + CO_2$ inhalations. Antidote—Artificial respiration and O_2.	Recumbent posture, stimulate with caffeine, combat anemia with blood transfusions. Liver extracts parenterally. Frequent blood counts.	Leukocytes destroyed. Damage to bone marrow. Lymph glands and spleen. Paralysis of respiratory center.

* Dosage undetermined.
‡ "Lethal Dose" from De Re Medicina, Eli Lilly and Company, Indianapolis, Indiana.

POISONS AND POISONING—Continued

Drug or Poison	"Lethal Dose" (Minimal)‡	Symptoms of Poisoning	Emergency Measures	Supportive and Follow Up Treatment	Pathology
Carbon tetrachloride.	1 dram.	Nausea, unconsciousness, convulsions.	Remove patient to fresh air. If ingested, wash stomach with warm water. Artificial respiration, $O_2 + CO_2$ inhalation. Antidote—Artificial respiration and O_2.	Stimulate symptomatically, maintain free catharsis, force fluids, high carbohydrate diet, dextrose and calcium salts intravenously.	Damage to heart, liver necrosis.
Stramonium.		See Atropine.			
Strophanthus. Ouabain.	*	Vomiting, double vision, headache, irregular pulse, convulsions.	Gastric lavage of tannic acid solution. Magnesium sulfate. Control convulsions with sedatives intravenously. Antidote—Tannic acid.	Horizontal position, artificial respiration, sedatives.	Increases contraction of heart muscle has no cumulative effect.
Strychnine. Nux Vomica. Brucine.	½ to 1 grain.	Stiffness of muscles, twitching of face and arms, sudden tetanic convulsions of entire body, face, lips, cyanotic, pulse slow and strong. Face fixed in a grin. Death in 1 to 3 hours.	Gastric lavage with potassium permanganate, iodine, tannic acid, apomorphine by hypo as emetic, control of convulsions with chloroform or ether inhalations, barbiturates, intravenously. Antidote—Lavage of potassium permanganate solution.	Quiet, dark room, no drafts. Artificial respiration if indicated. Ringer's solution intravenously. Dextrose intravenously. Frequent catheterization.	Stimulation of spinal cord, congestion of brain, upper part of spinal cord enclosing membranes. Congestion frequently found in liver, kidney and mucous membrane of stomach.
Sulfonal.	30 grains.	See Barbiturates.			
Tobacco.		See Nicotine.			
Turpentine.	2 ounces.	Sensation of warmth in throat and stomach followed by abdominal pain, vomiting and diarrhea. Pulse weak, respiration slow and irregular, nervous irritation suggestive of alcohol intoxication, convulsions, coma and death.	Gastric lavage and demulcents. Antidote—Tannic acid demulcents.	Morphine if large dose taken. Symptomatic stimulation.	Irritation of kidneys with hematuria and albuminuria and sometimes complete suppression of urine.

* Dosage undetermined.
‡ "Lethal Dose" from De Re Medicina, Eli Lilly and Company, Indianapolis, Indiana.

POISONS AND POISONING—Continued

Drug or Poison	"Lethal Dose" (Minimal) ‡	Symptoms of Poisoning	Emergency Measures	Supportive and Follow Up Treatment	Pathology
Veratrum. Veratrine. V. Viride.	1 dram. (fluid extract).	Prickling and burning in mouth, intense burning pain in stomach, extreme thirst, followed by salivation, marked nausea, severe, persistent vomiting and violent purging and extreme abdominal colic. Respiration, gasping shallow. Blood pressure lowered. Death due to respiratory failure or cardiac failure.	Gastric lavage with warm water or tannic acid. Antidote—Tannic acid.	Flat on back, head lower than feet. External stimuli, continued strychnine and digitalis for respiratory and cardiac failure.	Paralysis of vagus nerve.
Zinc Salts: Chloride. Sulfate.	90 grains. ± 4 drams.	Violent vomiting, purging, followed by prostration, increased salivation.	Large quantities of warm water, tannic acid solution to evacuate stomach. Lavage with soda bicarbonate solution. Follow with lime water, soap, milk or mucilaginous drinks.	Recumbent position, external heat to body. Morphine for pain, treat shock, stimulate with caffeine, strychnine, atropine.	Stricture of esophagus, pylorus, destruction of glandular structure of stomach. Ulceration and perforation of stomach.

* Dosage undetermined.
‡ "Lethal Dose" from De Re Medicina, Eli Lilly and Company, Indianapolis, Indiana.

App. 110

Suffocations

Type	History	Pathology	Symptoms and Color	Pulse	Breathing	Muscles	Pupils	Complications	Treatment
1. Drowning	Victim removed from body of water.	Waterlogging of lungs, and asphyxia are present.	Patient is unconscious. Color is gray and changing to blue (cyanosis).	When pulse is perceptible it is rapid and may be shallow.	If respirations are present the patient may gasp occasionally or very irregularly.	Muscles will be relaxed and body is very limp.	Pupils are dilated.	Fracture of neck. Heart failure. Suffocation, shock and collapse.	Artificial respiration. Oxygen—Treat for shock. Heart stimulants.
2. Gas Poisoning	Victim rescued from room with escaping gas from open jet or—victim overcome in closed garage.	Changes in the blood chemistry and then anemia is present. Respiratory paralysis which leads to death.	Patient unconscious. Color of the typical cherry red or pallor and cyanosis (carbon monoxide).	Pulse is rapid and may be irregular.	Respirations are usually slow but may be rapid and shallow very early after the exposure to gas.	Muscles are relaxed. Body is limp.	This varies with the type of gas poisoning.	Respiratory failure. Depletion of O_2 supply in the blood.	Artificial respiration. Oxygen. Shock treatment.
3. Choking	Edema of larynx. Diseases of the larynx. Foreign bodies are aspirated into the larynx.	Trauma of larynx.	Patient in a state of apprehension. Color—cyanotic.	Pulse is rapid due to exertion.	Respirations are very rapid or patient may gasp occasionally.	Muscles may be voluntarily contracted.	Pupils are dilated.	Pneumonia. Sinusitis. Complete obstruction of the bronchi. Lung abscess.	Manual removal or encourage coughing by slap on back.
4 Strangulation and Hanging	Patient usually found during or after the act. Very definite signs of violence will be noted.	Fracture of cervical vertebrae. Suffocation. Trauma of Medulla by odontoid process of axis.	Unconscious or dead. Living patient is in a state of excitement or desperation. Color—cyanotic if body is long deceased.	Pulse may be perceptible. Pulse may be absent.	No respirations or respirations are very rapid or patient may gasp occasionally.	Muscles may be voluntarily contracted.	Pupils are dilated. Unequal if there is cerebral injury.	Fracture of neck. Suffocation. Contusions on neck.	Release pull of rope by placing chair under patient's feet, cut rope. Oxygen therapy. Artifical respiration Treat for shock.

App. 111

Unconsciousness

Type	History	Color	Pupils	Muscles	Pulse	Breathing	Reflexes	Complications	Treatment
1. Shock	This condition is a result of a blow or damage to the nervous system.	Skin cold, temperature subnormal. Skin is an ashen gray to cyanotic color.	Pupils are dilated.	Muscles are relaxed.	Pulse is rapid and becomes thready and feeble.	Respirations are rapid and shallow.	Reflexes diminished (not significant).	Respiratory and circulatory embarrassment to collapse and death.	Elevate foot of bed. Keep body warm. Transfusions usually indicated for depression of vascular system.
2. Bleeding	Victim of a trauma causing bright red spurting or welling bleeding. Bleeding after an operation.	Skin shows pallor which grows progressively worse to a yellow or greenish tinge.	Pupils are dilated.	Muscles are relaxed.	Pulse is rapid and becomes thready.	Respirations are rapid and shallow. Air hunger is evident.	Reflexes diminished.	Shock. Anemia. Heart failure. Death.	Digital pressure and tourniquet. Pad in joint. Keep patient quiet. Treat for shock. Transfusion if necessary.
3. Drowning	Victim is found unconscious in body of water. May have a fractured neck or skull.	Skin is cold and clammy and cyanotic.	Pupils are dilated.	Muscles are relaxed, unless death, then rigidity of rigor mortis.	If pulse is perceptible it will be rapid, weak or very irregular.	No respirations. Occasional gasp if alive.	Reflexes abolished.	Heart failure. Shock—Pneumonia—aspiration of foreign material.	Resuscitation. Schafer (or prone pressure). Keep body warm. Stimulating drinks when conscious.
4. Gases	Victim rescued from a mine, a burning building, or room with open gas jet. Overcome in garage or car.	Skin is cyanotic and changing to the characteristic color, usually cherry red. (Carbon monoxide.)	Eyes fixed. Pupils are usually fully dilated. Varies with types of gas.	If alive, muscles are relaxed. If dead, rigor mortis.	Pulse is weak, slow and irregular.	Respirations irregular and jerky to only an occasional gasp.	Reflex abolished.	Respiratory failure. Asphyxia. Collapse.	Place the patient in the open air. Give oxygen and resuscitation. (Prone pressure) Treat for shock.
5. Hanging	Victim is found hanging with constriction of the neck.	Skin is pale and face is cyanotic.	Pupils are dilated and unequal if cerebral injury.	Muscles are relaxed. Varies with the level of tenure.	If strangulation is incomplete pulse is rapid, weak and irregular. If complete, pulse is absent.	Respirations have ceased or an occasional gasp is observed.	Reflexes are abolished.	Respiratory and circulatory failure. Fracture of neck.	Release the patient—out the rope. Artificial respirations. Treat for shock and possible fracture of neck.
6. Obstruction in throat	Victim has aspirated a foreign body or respiratory tract is obstructed by edema or disease.	Skin is cyanotic.	Pupils are dilated.	Sternal retraction. Muscles are tense with effort in trying to breathe and to remove obstruction.	Pulse is rapid and very weak.	Respirations are deep and labored.	Reflexes are increased.	Asphyxia; pulmonary infection; shock.	Remove obstruction. Respiratory stimulant or give artificial respiration. Treat for shock. Tracheotomy if indicated.

App. 112

UNCONSCIOUSNESS—Continued

Type	History	Color	Pupils	Muscles	Pulse	Breathing	Reflexes	Complications	Treatment
7. Electric Shock	Victim is found after coming in contact with a "live wire."	Skin is pale, cold and clammy.	Pupils unequal if severe shock.	Muscles are tense.	Weak and imperceptible pulse.	Respirations cease suddenly.	Muscle reflex is increased.	Low voltage affects heart action, makes resuscitation impossible. High voltage affects the resp. center in medulla and patient may be resuscitated.	Release the patient from current with care. Artificial respiration by prone pressure.
8. Concussion	Head injury caused by fall or blow upon the head.	Skin pale, cold and clammy. Varies with degree of pathology.	Pupils are dilated. Varies with degree and area of injury.	Muscles may be spastic.	Pulse rate usually shows a slight increase. May be weak and rapid.	Respirations are usually deep.	Muscle reflex is increased.	Shock in severe cases. Paralysis of limbs may occur.	Bed rest. Keep patient flat and warm.
9. Epilepsy	History reveals the previous nocturnal occurrences of "fits" or spells with or without aura.	Pallor to flush followed by cyanosis — may be slight and gradually increased to marked cyanosis.	Pupils are unequal. Eyes rolling.	Muscles may be spastic. Tonic type of convulsions is followed by the clonic type.	Pulse is usually rapid.	Respirations are deep and stertorous.	Reflex is increased.	Injuries in falling or biting the tongue. Patient may react violently (fighting others).	Bed rest. Prevent falling or biting tongue. Sedative—luminal.
10. Drunkenness	History of fondness of alcohol; victim is unable to cope with the amount of intoxicants taken.	Color varies. Face may be flushed, skin is moist, relaxed and cool.	Pupils are usually dilated, but are equal.	Muscles are relaxed body and limbs are limp.	Pulse is strong and slow.	Respirations are slow, deep, stertorous, accompanied by characteristic "lip blowing," and cheyne stokes type of breathing.	Reflex is usually increased.	Cerebral hemorrhage (injections of MgSO₄ tend to reduce the edema throughout the body). Pneumonia.	Keep the body warm. If conscious give emetic. Gastric lavage. Give hot coffee or aromatic spirits of ammonia.
11. Stroke (Apoplectic)	Patient has history of arteriosclerosis and is usually past 40 years of age.	Skin is injected. May be cyanotic or ashen gray. Hot and dry to flushed (elevation of temperature).	Pupils vary, may be dilated, often unequal. In deep coma are inactive.	Muscles of the involved side (hemiplegia) are usually spastic with a facial palsy.	Pulse is slow, full with increased tension.	Respirations are slow, loud, usually deep.	Reflexes are diminished on one side.	Pneumonia—injury from falling.	Rest and absolute quiet with head of bed elevated and feet lowered. Ice cap to head. Cathartic if needed. No stimulants.
12. Narcotic Poisoning	History of addiction or idiosyncrasy for the drug.	Skin is ashen gray, cyanotic and cold.	Pupils are contracted to "pin point."	Muscles are relaxed.	Pulse usually slow but varies with type of drug poisoning.	Respirations slow, irregular, stertorous.	Reflex is diminished.	Addiction to drug or production of a marked sensitivity to a drug.	Removal of the drug by emetics or lavage. Use of antidotes. Specific counteractives.

App. 113

UNCONSCIOUSNESS—Continued

Type	History	Color	Pupils	Muscles	Pulse	Breathing	Reflexes	Complications	Treatment
13. Acid and Alkali Poisoning.	History of accidental or intentional poisoning.	Clammy skin. Skin pale; face cyanotic.	Eyes sunken, staring. Pupils are dilated.	Tense. Patient in convulsion.	Rapid, feeble pulse.	Shallow, rapid, labored, irregular.	Reflexes are increased.	Corrosion of mucous membranes. Ulcers of stomach. Gastrites jaundice.	For acids — Milk of magnesia, egg albumin, lime water, no chalk or alkaline carbonate. For Alkalies—Neutralize with acetic acid (vinegar).
14. Mineral Poisoning.	History of accidental or suicidal poisoning.	Skin is cold and clammy, pallor.	Eyes fixed, staring. Pupils are dilated.	Tense, convulsive to relaxed when in stupor.	Rapid, feeble to imperceptible.	Respirations are shallow, rapid, labored.	Reflexes are increased.	Nephritis. Liver degeneration. Colitis.	Gastric lavage—Emetics.
15. Heat Exhaustion	Victim is overcome by the degree of heat in surrounding field of work and loss of sodium chloride through perspiration.	Skin is pale and cool with a subnormal temperature.	Pupils are moderately contracted.	Muscles are tense. Muscle cramps.	Pulse is rapid and may become weak.	Respirations shallow with rigidity of the chest muscles.	Reflexes are increased.	Shock.	Treat for shock (keep body warm). Give salt by mouth, and intravenous injections.
16. Sun Stroke	Victim has been exposed to intense degree or a prolonged period of heat from sun.	Skin is flushed (red) and hot when touched.	Pupils are dilated.	Muscles are relaxed.	Rapid and weak.	Respirations may be shallow and gasping or deep and slow.	Reflexes increased.	Suppressed diaphoresis and paralysis for prolonged period. Paralysis of vasomotor centers within medilla. Paralysis of heart, collapse and death.	Remove patient to cool area. Cold application to head and body. Keep in cold, wet sheet. Continue to lower body temperature. No stimulants.
17. Freezing	Victim is found after period of exposure to intense cold or prolonged period of exposure to the cold.	Frostbite—Skin is cold, pale and blanched. Frozen—Skin is livid and later cyanotic, then turns to purplish or greenish black.	Pupils are dilated.	Muscles are tense and become very rigid.	Pulse is rapid and weak.	Breathing is slower and deeper. Patient falls into very deep slumber.	Reflexes are not discernible.	Pneumonia— certain damage due to mechanical destruction of the cells, sloughing and gangrene of the part previously frozen.	Gradual warming of the parts. Slight massage of extremities for better circulation. Elevation of parts. Treatment of the dry gangrene.
18. Fainting	History of fatigue or shock or horrible sight or "light headedness."	Skin of face and the lips are blanched. Body is cold and clammy.	Pupils are regular.	Muscles are completely relaxed.	Pulse is rapid and thready.	Respirations are rapid and shallow.	Reflexes are slightly increased.	Shock is usually a serious complication. Body injury and fracture if patient falls.	Apply cold water to face, head and chest. Lower patient's head. Lift body by heels (to control brain anemia). Give aromatic spirits of ammonia.

App. 114

Wounds

Type	History	Pathology	Symptoms and Color	Complications	Treatment	Transportation	Points of Identification
1. Contusions.	History of blow or fall.	A bruise (hematoma) or petechial area with underlying injury.	Skin surface is rough, the area includes a large or small hematoma (depending upon the extent of injury).	Destruction of underlying tissue if hematoma is not aspirated early. Infection if skin is punctured or probed.	Alternate ice and warm applications to area of injury. Gentle massage of surrounding tissues not involved in injury.	Cover area with loose fitting triangle. Keep the part well elevated if possible.	Skin is not broken. Tissues underlying skin may be slightly or very markedly crushed.
2. "Brush Burns" or Abrasions.	Area of injury has been subjected to rapid passing object or body thrown against rough surface. Ex—skidding on wet grass.	Skin, mucous membranes show niches in skin. Top surface effaced with remaining surface dotted with small drops of blood.	Skin discolored. Top surface peeled off with fine beadlike dots of blood. Skin may also be loaded with dirt and refuse.	Complications include infection developments. Recovery may show very rough unsightly scars.	Carefully brush away all loose dirt and debris. Cleanse the wound with soap and water. Use antiseptic solutions, ointment, and apply dressings.	Use loose applications of sterile dressings held in place by loose fitting triangle.	Top surface of the skin is brushed completely away, or remains very lightly attached to the area.
3. Lacerations.	History of an accident wherein sharp instruments have cut (lacerated) the area of the body.	Jagged or torn and roughened edges of tissues. May include evulsion of certain parts.	Injury has produced area of deep or shallow degree with opening from between two raw or bleeding surfaces of the skin.	Infection may develop. Septicemia may follow. Wound usually heals with very unsightly scar.	Remove the large debris and dirt. Clean the wound by water dripping from sterile cloth or use soap and warm water, antiseptics and sterile dressings. Use mild antiseptics.	Cover the area of injury with loose application of dressings held by triangle or cravat bandage. Edges of wound may be united with flamed strip of adhesive tape.	Wound edges are jagged and irregular. Wound may contain amount of debris or dirt, and usually is infected.
4. Puncture.	Object may be still probing tissues, or patient may have been lifted from a rusty nail or thorn.	Tissues are pierced; small opening through the tissues (excellent course or inlet for infection).	Area usually manifests no bleeding. Trauma of tissues is usually evident.	Infection of the anaerobic type (Tetanus bacillus) infection—and septicemia.	Early indications of antitoxin. Probe the wound very carefully to enlarge bore for irrigation with antiseptic solutions.	Cover the area with sterile dressings and triangle or cravat bandage.	Puncture site is very small. Object is usually withdrawn with fair amount of ease.

App. 115

WOUNDS—Continued

Type	History	Pathology	Symptoms and Color	Complications	Treatment	Transportation	Points of Identification
Stab.	History of injury during a brawl or duel. Accident of fall or thrust upon blunt or heavy pointed object.	Size of hole in the tissues varies with the size of the instrument. Foreign material and pathogenic bacteria of anaerobic nature are introduced.	Evidence of the instrument that was used—such as knife, ice pick, etc. Victim shows pallor syncope and later collapse.	Internal hemorrhage collapse of the lung. Pulmonary hemorrhage. Infection of body by anaerobic organisms —(Tetanus bacillus).	Cleanse and irrigate the wound when possible. Irrigation and inclusion of antiseptic drain or wet dressings. Early use of antitetanic sera.	Keep patient very quiet with head and chest slightly elevated. Treat for shock. If chest is involved then watch T.P.R. and blood pressure.	Large puncture site and very deep. Victim may still be pinned by the force of the blow.
5. Gun Shot.	History of an accident in care of a gun or pistol, etc. Victim of aimed shot or assailant.	Wound of single outer puncture site with deep injury (twisting and tearing of tissue) by buck shot, etc.	Aperture is small. Powder burns are occasionally found.	Shock, internal hemorrhage. Tetanus bacillus infection.	Early use of antitetanus sera. Cleanse and irrigate when possible. Wet antiseptic dressings. Debridement when necessary.	Keep patient very quiet. Head slightly lower than body. Treat for shock. Watch T.P.R. and blood pressure when hemorrhaging.	Puncture site. Deep wound shows characteristic twisting of the deeper tissues.
6. Poisoned.	History of bite of a rabid human, animal or reptile. Or the sting or bite of poisonous insect. Occasionally no history.	Tissue degeneration at site of wound. Muscular paralysis. Venom has a very drastic effect upon respiratory nerve centers.	Human—shape of denture, change of disposition. Dog—lacerated wound. Rabid disposition. Snake—two fang wound. Insect—elevated wheal with itching or burning sensation and pain or single or double red dot.	Infection introduced pathogenic organisms. Venom of toxic nature depresses victim. Death if too long delay in treatment.	1. Observe the victim. Enclose the dog. 2. Pasteur treatment if deemed necessary. 3. Apply tourniquet, Incision and suction as swelling rises. 4. Neutralize acid of "sting" with alkalies. 5. Treat for shock, respiratory stimulants for snake or insect venom.	Avert apprehension. Keep patient quiet. Keep muscles of the area elevated and at rest.	1. Shape of denture. 2. Odor of colon bacillus about the wound (human bite). 3. Two fang puncture. Small red dot or presence of stinger.

App. 116

A Sourcebook of Canadian

MEDIA
Law

Second Edition

Robert Martin & G. Stuart Adam

CARLETON LIBRARY SERIES #181

Carleton University Press
Ottawa, Canada
1994

©Carleton University Press, Inc. 1994
Carleton Library Series # 181
Printed and Bound in Canada

Canadian Cataloguing in Publication Data

Martin, Robert, 1939-

    A sourcebook of Canadian media law

2nd. ed.
(The Carleton library ; 181)
ISBN 0-88629-238-7 (bound).—
    ISBN 0-88629-231-X (pbk.)

1. Freedom of the press—Canada. 2. Freedom of information—Canada. 3. Freedom of speech—Canada. I. Adam, G. Stuart (Gordon Stuart), 1939-   II. Title. III. Series.

KE4422.M37 1994   342.71'0853   C94-900437-5

Carleton University Press
160 Paterson Hall
Carleton University
1125 Colonel By Drive
Ottawa, Ontario
K1S 5B6
(613) 788-3740

Distributed in Canada by:

Oxford University Press Canada
70 Wynford Drive
Don Mills, Ontario
M3C 1J9
(416) 441-2941

Cover Design: First Image
Typeset by: Howarth & Smith Typesetting & Printing Limited

Acknowledgements:

Carleton University Press gratefully acknowledges the support extended to its publishing programme by the Canada Council and the financial assistance of the Ontario Arts Council.

The Press would also like to thank the Department of Communications, Government of Canada, and the Government of Ontario through the Ministry of Culture, Tourism and Recreation, for their assistance.

To

Ivan and Dawson,

Mark, Julia and Sara

The Carleton Library Series

A series of original works, new collections and reprints of source material relating to Canada, issued under the supervision of the Editorial Board, Carleton Library Series, Carleton University Press Inc., Ottawa, Canada.

General Editor
  Michael Gnarowski

Editorial Board
  Syd F. Wise (Chair and History)
  Bruce Cox (Anthropology and Sociology)
  W. Irwin Gillespie (Economics)
  Robert J. Jackson (Political Science)
  Peter Johansen (Journalism)
  Iain Wallace (Geography)

TABLE OF CONTENTS

Preface to Second Edition xvii
Preface to First Edition xix
Acknowledgements xxiii

Chapter One: Freedom of Expression and the Canadian Constitution.. 1

1.1 The Law and the Mass Media 1
    1.1.1 The Meaning of Freedom of Expression 1
1.2 The Structure of the Constitution 5
1.3 The Judiciary.. 6
    1.3.1 E. Jacqueline R. Castel and Omeela K. Latchman, *The Practical Guide to Canadian Legal Research* (Toronto: Carswell Thomson Professional Publishing, 1993), pp. 12-19..................................... 6
    1.3.2 The Supreme Court of Canada 11
    1.3.3 Andrew Heard, *Canadian Constitutional Conventions: The Marriage of Law and Politics* (Toronto: Oxford University Press, 1991), pp. 118-120; 121-123; 134-139... 11
1.4 Federalism and Freedom of Expression 21
    1.4.1 *The Constitution Act, 1867* 23
    1.4.2 *Re Alberta Legislation*, [1938] 2 D.L.R. 81 (S.C.C.) 27
    1.4.3 *Switzman v. Elbling and Attorney-General of Quebec*, [1957] S.C.R. 285 (S.C.C.) 34
    1.4.4 *Re Nova Scotia Board of Censors and McNeil* (1978), 84 D.L.R. (3d) 1 (S.C.C.) 42
    1.4.5 *Gay Alliance Toward Equality v. Vancouver Sun* (1979), 97 D.L.R. (3d) 577 (S.C.C.) 47
    1.4.6 *Attorney-General of Quebec v. Irwin Toy Ltd., Moreau et al., Intervenors* (1989), 58 D.L.R. (4th) 577 (S.C.C.) 60
    1.4.7 Peter Hogg, *Constitutional Law of Canada*, 3rd ed. (Scarborough: 1992), pp. 774-777... 67
1.5 The *Canadian Charter of Rights and Freedoms* and Freedom of Expression .. 71
    1.5.1 The *Canadian Charter of Rights and Freedoms, Part One, Constitution Act*, 1982.. 72
        1.5.1.1 F.L. Morton, *Morgentaler v. Borowski: Abortion, the Charter and the Courts* (Toronto: 1992), pp. 294-314 78
    1.5.2 The Meaning of Expression 94
        1.5.2.1 *Koumoudouros v. Municipality of Metropolitan Toronto* (1984), 8 C.R.R. 179 (Ont. H.C.).. 94

1.5.2.2 *Attorney-General of Québec v. Irwin Toy Ltd.* (1989), 58 D.L.R. (4th) 577 (S.C.C.) 95
1.5.2.3 A Note on Advertising and Free Expression 106
1.5.2.4 *R. v. Keegstra*, [1990] 3 S.C.R. 697 (S.C.C.).................... 108
1.5.2.5 *Retail, Wholesale and Department Store Union, Local 580 v. Dolphin Delivery Ltd.*, [1986] 2 S.C.R. 573..................... 111
1.5.2.6 *The Queen v. Committee for the Commonwealth of Canada et al.* (1991), 77 D.L.R. (4th) 385 (S.C.C.) 114
1.5.2.7 *International Fund for Animal Welfare Inc. v. The Queen* (1986), 30 C.C.C. (3d) 80 (F.C.T.D.)....................................... 118
1.5.2.8 *Re Information Retailers Association of Metropolitan Toronto Inc. and Municipality of Metropolitan Toronto* (1985), 52 O.R. (2d) 449 (Ont. C.A.)... 119
1.5.3 Applying Section One 120
1.5.3.1 "Prescribed by Law"... 120
1.5.3.1.1 *Re Ontario Film and Video Appreciation Society and Ontario Board of Censors* (1983), 41 O.R. (2d) 583 (Div. Ct.) 120
1.5.3.1.2 *Re Ontario Film and Video Appreciation Society and Ontario Board of Censors* (1984), 45 O.R. (2d) 80 (Ont. C.A.) 121
1.5.3.1.3 *An Act to Amend the Theatres Act*, S.O. 1984, c. 56 122
1.5.3.1.4 O. Reg. 56/85. Regulation to Amend Regulation 931 of Revised Regulations of Ontario, 1980, Made Under the *Theatres Act* .. 122
1.5.3.1.5 *Osborne v. Canada (Treasury Board)* (1991), 82 D.L.R. (4th) 321 (S.C.C.) 123
1.5.3.2 "Reasonable and Demonstrably Justified in a Free and Democratic Society" 126
1.5.3.2.1 *Attorney-General of Quebec v. Irwin Toy Ltd.* (1989), 58 D.L.R. (4th) 577 (S.C.C.) 126
1.5.3.2.2 *R. v. Keegstra*, [1990] 3 S.C.R. 697 (S.C.C.)................ 135
1.6 Should Journalists Enjoy Special Legal Status? 138
1.6.1 *MacLeod et al. v. Canadian Armed Forces (Chief, Defence Staff)*, [1991] 1 F.C. 114 (F.C.T.D.) 138
1.6.2 Stephen Bindman, "Court Rulings Tightening Muzzle on Media," *The London Free Press*, 13 March 1993, p. E5 146
1.6.3 A Note on Litigation and Journalism 148
1.7 Two Essays on the Freedom of the Press 149
1.7.1 G. Stuart Adam, "The Charter and the Role of the Media: A Journalist's Perspective," in *The Media, the Courts and the Charter*, eds. Philip Anisman and Allen M. Linden (Toronto: Carswell, 1986).............. 149
1.7.2 Robert Martin, "Press Councils: Watchdogs with No Bite," *Bulletin of the Centre for Investigative Journalism*, No. 29 (1986), p. 30.............. 167

Chapter Two: Security, the Public Order and Democratic Institutions: Legal Limitations to Protect the State's Rights, Prerogatives and Responsibilities, Part I 171

2.1 Legitimacy and the Scope of State Power 171

2.2 National Security 172
   2.2.1 Emergencies 172
      2.2.1.1 *Emergencies Act*, S.C. 1988, c. 29. 172
      2.2.1.2 Note on the *War Measures Act* 183
   2.2.2 Official Secrets... 194
      2.2.2.1 *Official Secrets Act*, R.S.C. 1985, c. O-5 194
      2.2.2.2 Walter Tarnopolsky, "Freedom of the Press," in *Newspapers and the Law* (Ottawa: Ministry of Supply and Services Canada, 1981), pp. 19-21 198
      2.2.2.3 Law Reform Commission of Canada, *Crimes Against the State*, Working Paper 49 (Ottawa: 1986), pp. 30, 33-34 201

2.3 Access to Information 202
   2.3.1 *Access to Information Act*, R.S.C. 1985, c. A-1 202
      2.3.1.1 *The Information Commissioner v. The Minister of Employment and Immigration* (1986), 3 F.C. 63 (F.C.T.D.)....................... 209
      2.3.1.2 David Scheidermann, "The Access to Information Act: A Practical Review" (1987), *Advocates Quarterly* 7, p. 474 211
      2.3.1.3. Canadian Daily Newspaper Publishers Association, *What Newsrooms Need to Know* (Toronto: 1984) 225
   2.3.2 Provincial Access to Information Statutes.......................... 230

2.4 Public Order and Criminal Libel...................................... 233
   2.4.1 *Criminal Code*, R.S.C. 1985, c. C-46.............................. 236
      2.4.1.1 *Boucher v. The King*, [1950] 1 D.L.R. 657 (S.C.C.) 237
      2.4.1.2 Law Reform Commission of Canada, *Crimes Against the State*, Working Paper 49 (Ottawa: 1986), pp. 32, 35-36 247
   2.4.2 *Criminal Code*, R.S.C. 1985, c. C-46.............................. 248
      2.4.2.1 *R. v. Georgia Straight Publishing Ltd.* (1969), 4 D.L.R. (3d) 383 (B.C.Co.Ct.)... 252
      2.4.2.2 Robert Martin, "Law Reform Commission of Canada, Working Paper 35: Defamatory Libel, (1984), *University of Western Ontario Law Review* 22, p. 249 256

Chapter Three: Judicial Proceedings: Legal Limitations to Protect the State's Rights, Prerogatives and Responsibilities, Part II 259

3.1 Introduction... 259

3.2 The Principle of Openness.. 260
   3.2.1 *Re Southam Inc. and the Queen (No. 1)* (1983), 41 O.R. (2d) 113 (Ont. C.A.) 260
   3.2.2 *R. v. Robinson* (1983), 41 O.R. (2d) 764 (Ont. H.C.) 272
   3.2.3 Cameras, Video Recorders and Audio Recorders in the Courtroom 274
      3.2.3.1 Ontario *Courts of Justice Act*, R.S.O. 1990, c. C.43 274
      3.2.3.2 *R. v. Rowbotham (No. 3)* (1976), 2 C.R. (3d) 241 (Ont. Co.Ct.) 275

x TABLE OF CONTENTS

        3.2.3.3 *R. v. Squires* (1989), 69 C.R. (3d) 337, at pp. 339; 342; 343; 345-357; 358-360 277
        3.2.3.4 Law Reform Commission of Canada, *Public and Media Access to the Criminal Process*, Working Paper 56 (Ottawa: Minister of Supply and Services Canada, 1987) 290
    3.2.4 Sparing Parties from Embarrassment 292
        3.2.4.1 *Re Regina and an Unnamed Person* (1985), 22 C.C.C. (3d) 284 (Ont. C.A.) 292
3.3 Contempt of Court 294
    3.3.1 General Considerations 294
        3.3.1.1 *Attorney-General v. Leveller Magazine Ltd. and Others*, [1979] A.C. 440 (H.L.) 294
        3.3.1.2 *Criminal Code*, R.S.C. 1985, c. C-46 301
        3.3.1.3 *R. v. Kopyto* (1988), 24 O.A.C. 81 (Ont. C.A.) 301
    3.3.2 Scandalising the Court 302
        3.3.2.1 Robert Martin, "Criticising the Judges," 28 *McGill Law Journal* 1, pp. 13-20 302
        3.3.2.2 *Re Nicol*, [1954] 3 D.L.R. 690 (B.C.S.C.) 304
        3.3.2.3 *R. v. Kopyto* (1988), 24 O.A.C. 81 (Ont. C.A.) 311
    3.3.3 The Sub-Judice Rule 318
        3.3.3.1 Robert Martin, "Contempt of Court: The Effect of the Charter," in *The Media, the Courts and the Charter*, ed. Philip Anisman and Allen M. Linden (Toronto: Carswell, 1986), pp. 208-210 318
        3.3.3.2 Statutory Sub-Judice 320
            3.3.3.2.1 Sexual Offence 320
                3.3.3.2.1.1 *Criminal Code*, R.S.C. 1985, c. C-46 320
                3.3.3.2.1.2 *R. v. Canadian Newspapers Company Limited and Interveners*, [1988] 2 S.C.R. 122 (S.C.C.) 324
            3.3.3.2.2 Young Offenders 327
                3.3.3.2.2.1 *Young Offenders Act*, R.S.C. 1985, c. Y-1 327
                3.3.3.2.2.2 *Southam v. R.* (1934), 42 C.R. (3d) 336, at 354-360 (Ont. H.C.) 329
            3.3.3.2.3 Preliminary Inquiries 334
                3.3.3.2.3.1 *Criminal Code*, R.S.C. 1985, c. C-46 334
                3.3.3.2.3.2 *R. v. Banville* (1983), 45 N.B.R. (2d) 134 (Q.B.) 335
                3.3.3.2.3.3 *Criminal Code*, R.S.C. 1985, c. C-46 339
            3.3.3.2.4 Bail Hearings 339
                3.3.3.2.4.1 *Criminal Code*, R.S.C. 1985, c. C-46 339
            3.3.3.2.5 Jury Trials 340
                3.3.3.2.5.1 *Criminal Code*, R.S.C. 1985, c. C-46 340
        3.3.3.3 Common Law Sub-Judice 341
            3.3.3.3.1 *Attorney-General v. Times Newspapers Ltd.*, [1973] 3 All E.R. 54 (H.L.) 341
            3.3.3.3.2 *Zehr v. McIsaac et al.* (1982), 39 O.R. (2d) 237 (Ont. H.C.) ... 351
            3.3.3.3.3 *Bellitti v. Canadian Broadcasting Corp.* (1973), 2 O.R. 232 (Ont. H.C.) 356

  3.3.3.3.4 *Bielek v. Ristimaki* (1979), (Ont. H.C.) in Stuart Robertson, *Courts and the Media* (Toronto: Butterworth, 1981), pp. 287-292 359
  3.3.3.3.5 *Re Church of Scientology of Toronto v. The Queen (No. 6)* (1986), 27 C.C.C. (3d) 193 (Ont. H.C.).................. 364
  3.3.3.3.6 *C.B.C. v. Keegstra* (1986), 35 D.L.R. (4th) 76 (Alta. C.A.).... 365
  3.3.3.3.7 *C.B.C. v. Dagenais et al.* (1992), 12 O.R. (3d) 239 (Ont. C.A.) 368
  3.3.3.3.8 Stuart Robertson, *Courts and the Media* (Toronto: Butterworth, 1981), p. 25 374
 3.3.4 Disobeying an Order of a Court 375
  3.3.4.1 *Criminal Code*, R.S.C. 1985, c. C-46 375
  3.3.4.2 Wilfred H. Kesterton, *The Law and the Press in Canada* (Toronto: 1976), pp. 32-39 376
  3.3.4.3 John Sawatsky, "John Sawatsky Stakes Out the High Ground," (1988), *Bulletin of the Centre for Investigative Journalism* 11, No. 29 382
  3.3.4.4 *Re Legislative Privilege* (1978), 83 D.L.R. (3d) 161 (Ont. C.A.) ... 387
  3.3.4.5 *Moysa v. Alberta Labour Relations Board*, [1989] 1 S.C.R. 1572 (S.C.C.) 390
  3.3.4.6 *Attorney-General v. Mulholland; Attorney-General v. Foster*, [1963] 2 W.L.R. 658 (C.A. Eng.)...................................... 394
  3.3.4.7 *Re Legislative Privilege* (1978), 83 D.L.R. (3d) 161 (Ont. C.A.) ... 400
 3.3.5 Procedure in Contempt Cases 400
  3.3.5.1 Robert Martin, "Contempt of Court: The Effect of the Charter," in *The Media, the Courts, and the Charter*, ed. Philip Anisman and Allen M. Linden (Toronto: Carswell, 1986)..................... 400
 3.3.6 Reforming the Law 401
  3.3.6.1 Robert Martin, "An Open Legal System," (1985), 25 *University of Western Ontario Law Review* 169 401

3.4 Dealing with Material that Might Become Evidence in a Judicial Proceeding . 403
 3.4.1 *Criminal Code*, R.S.C. 1985, c. C-46............................. 404
 3.4.2 Harold Levy, "What Should We Do When the Cops Arrive?" *Content* 95, 1979... 407
 3.4.3 *C.B.C. v. Attorney-General for New Brunswick et al.* (1991), 85 D.L.R. (4th) 57 (S.C.C.)... 413
 3.4.4 Taking Photographs or Videotaping against the Instructions of the Police 423

Chapter Four: Legal Limitations Protecting Social Values and Social Groups 425

4.1 Introduction 425
4.2 Blasphemy.. 426
 4.2.1 *Criminal Code*, R.S.C. 1985, c. C-46............................. 426
 4.2.2 *R. v. Rahard* (1935), 65 C.C.C. 344 (Que.S.C.) 427
 4.2.3 *R. v. Gay News Ltd.*, [1979] 1 All E.R. 898 (H.L.).................. 433

4.2.4 *R. v. Chief Metropolitan Stipendiary Magistrate, ex parte Choudhury,*
[1991] L.R.C. (Const) 278 (Q.B.)(U.K.) 440
4.3 Expressions of Racism 445
    4.3.1 *Criminal Code,* R.S.C. 1985, c. C-46 445
    4.3.2 *R. v. Buzzanga and Durocher* (1979), 101 D.L.R. (3d) 488 (Ont. C.A.) .. 447
    4.3.3 *R. v. Keegstra,* [1990] 3 S.C.R. 697 (S.C.C.). 459
    4.3.4 *R. v. Andrews and Smith,* [1990] 3 S.C.R. 870 (S.C.C.) 459
    4.3.5 Law Reform Commission of Canada, *Hate Propaganda,* Working Paper 50 (Ottawa: 1986), pp. 39-41 460
    4.3.6 *Criminal Code,* R.S.C. 1985, c. C-46 462
    4.3.7 *R. v. Zundel* (1992), 16 C.R. (4th) 1 (S.C.C.) 463
    4.3.8 *Canadian Human Rights Act,* R.S.C. 1985, c. H-6 470
        4.3.8.1 J.P. Boyer, *Political Rights: The Legal Framework of Elections in Canada* (Toronto: Butterworth, 1981), pp. 308-309 470
        4.3.8.2 *Canada (Human Rights Commission) v. Taylor,* [1990] 3 S.C.R. 892 (S.C.C.) 471
    4.3.9 Television Regulations S.O.R. 87-49 477
        4.3.9.1 *Regina v. Buffalo Broadcasting Co. Ltd.* (1977), 36 C.P.R. (2d) 170 (Sask. Magistrates' Ct.) 477
    4.3.10 *Ontario Human Rights Code,* R.S.O. 1990, c. H-19 489
4.4 Obscenity 491
    4.4.1 *Criminal Code,* R.S.C. 1985, c. C-46 491
    4.4.2 Law Reform Commission of Canada, *Limits of Criminal Law; Obscenity: A Test Case, Working Paper* 10 (Ottawa: Information Canada, 1975), pp. 39-49 494
    4.4.3 Bill C-239. An Act to Amend the Criminal Code, First Reading, 31 October 1977 500
    4.4.4 Standing Committee on Justice and Legal Affairs, "The Third Report to the House (Report on Pornography)" 22 March, 1978, pp. 7-10. 501
    4.4.5 Bill C-19. An Act to Amend the Criminal Code, ss. 159(8), 163.1 503
    4.4.6 Canada, Special Committee on Pornography and Prostitution Report (1985) (Fraser Report) 504
    4.4.7 Bill C-114. An Act to Amend the Criminal Code, s. 138 510
    4.4.8 Bill C-54. An Act to Amend the Criminal Code, ss. 1, 2 510
    4.4.9 *Criminal Code,* R.S.C. 1985, c. C-46 as am. S.C. 1993, c. 46. 513
        4.4.9.1 *R. v. Butler* (1992), 89 D.L.R. (4th) 449 (S.C.C.) 513
        4.4.9.2 *Popert et al. v. R.* (1981), 19 C.R. (3d) 393 (Ont. C.A.) 537
    4.4.10 *Canada Post Corporation Act,* R.S.C. 1985, c. C-10 541
        4.4.10.1 *Luscher v. Deputy Minister, Revenue Canada, Customs and Excise* (1985), 45 C.R. (3d) 81 (F.C.A.) 542
    4.4.11 *Customs Tariff,* R.S.C. 1970, c. C-41 as am. S.C. 1984-85, c. 12 545
    4.4.12 A Note on Provincial Movie Censorship Laws 545

Chapter Five: Legal Limitations Arising from Private Rights 555

5.1 Introduction 555

5.2 Defamation 556
   5.2.1 Anne Skarsgard, "Freedom of the Press," (1980-81), *Saskatchewan Law
          Review* 45, pp. 296-99 556
   5.2.2 The Plaintiff's Case 559
          5.2.2.1 Defamatory 559
                   5.2.2.1.1 *Brannigan v. S.I.U.* (1964), 42 D.L.R. (2d) 249 (B.C.S.C.).... 559
                   5.2.2.1.2 *Thomas v. C.B.C.*, [1981] 4 W.W.R. 289 (N.W.T.S.C.)........ 562
                   5.2.2.1.3 *Murphy v. LaMarsh* (1970), 73 W.W.R. 114 (B.C.S.C.)....... 569
                   5.2.2.1.4 *Vogel v. C.B.C.* (1982), 21 C.C.L.T. 105 574
          5.2.2.2 Reference to the Plaintiff 574
                   5.2.2.2.1 *E. Hulton and Co. v. Jones*, [1910] A.C. 22 (H.L.)........... 574
                   5.2.2.2.2 *Booth et al. v. B.C.T.V.* (1983), 139 D.L.R. (3d) 88 (B.C.C.A.) 577
                   5.2.2.2.3 *Planned Parenthood Federation v. Fedorik* (1982), 135 D.L.R.
                              (3d) 714, at 718 (Nfld. S.C.T.D.) 583
                   5.2.2.2.4 *Whitaker v. Huntington* (1981), 15 C.C.L.T. 19, at 21-22
                              (B.C.S.C.) 584
                   5.2.2.2.5 *Stark v. Toronto Sun* (1983), 42 O.R. (2d) 791, at 794-795
                              (Ont. H.C.) 585
                   5.2.2.2.6 *Manitoba Defamation Act*, R.S.M. 1987, c. D20............. 586
          5.2.2.3 Publication 586
                   5.2.2.3.1 *Ontario Libel and Slander Act*, R.S.O. 1990, c. L.12. 586
                   5.2.2.3.2 *Basse v. Toronto Star Newspapers Ltd. et al.* (1984), 37 C.P.C.
                              213, at 216-217 (Ont. H.C.)............................... 588
                   5.2.2.3.3 *Farrell v. St. John's Publishing Co.* (1986), 58 Nfld. & P.E.I.R.
                              66 (Nfld. C.A.) 589
   5.2.3 The Defendant's Case 590
          5.2.3.1 Justification 590
                   5.2.3.1.1 Anne Skarsgard, "Freedom of the Press," (1980-81),
                              Saskatchewan Law Review 45, pp. 302-303 591
                   5.2.3.1.2 Robert Martin, "Does Libel Have a 'Chilling Effect' in
                              Canada?" (1990), *Studies in Communications* 4, pp. 143-163,
                              at pp. 146-148.. 591
                   5.2.3.1.3 *Brannigan v. S.I.U.* (1964), 42 D.L.R. (2d) 249 (B.C.S.C.).... 593
                   5.2.3.1.4 *Baxter v. C.B.C.* (1974), 30 N.B.R. (2d) 102 (N.B.C.A.)...... 595
                   5.2.3.1.5 *Munro v. Toronto Sun* (1982), 21 C.C.L.T. 261 (Ont. H.C.) ... 599
                   5.2.3.1.6 *Gordon v. Caswell* (1984), 33 Sask. R. 202 (Q.B.)........... 599
                   5.2.3.1.7 *Ontario Libel and Slander Act*, R.S.O. 1990, c. L.12. 601
          5.2.3.2 Fair Comment 602
                   5.2.3.2.1 Alexander Stark, *Dangerous Words* (Toronto: Ryerson Institute
                              of Technology, 1985), p. 15.............................. 602
                   5.2.3.2.2 *Pearlman v. C.B.C.* (1982), Man. L.R. (2d) 1 (Man. Q.B.).... 602
                   5.2.3.2.3 Anne Skarsgard, "Freedom of the Press," (1980-81),
                              Saskatchewan Law Review 45, pp. 307-316 603
                   5.2.3.2.4 *Vander Zalm v. Times Publishers* (1980), 18 B.C.L.R. 210
                              (B.C.C.A.)... 612

TABLE OF CONTENTS

5.2.3.2.5 *Farrell v. St. John's Publishing Co.* (1986), 58 Nfld. & P.E.I.R. 66 (Nfld. C.A.) 621
5.2.3.2.6 *Pound v. Scott* (1973), 4 W.W.R. 403 (B.C.S.C.) 621
5.2.3.2.7 *Mack v. North Hill News Ltd.* (1964), 44 D.L.R. (2d) 147 (Alta. S.C.) 628
5.2.3.2.8 *Ontario Libel and Slander Act*, R.S.O. 1990, c. L.12. 629
5.2.3.2.9 *Cherneskey v. Armadale Publishers* (1979), 90 D.L.R. (3d) 321 (S.C.C.) 629
5.2.3.2.10 Robert Martin, "Libel and Letters to the Editor," (1983), *Queen's Law Journal* 188 641
5.2.3.2.11 *Masters v. Fox* (1978), 85 D.L.R. (3d) 64 (B.C.S.C.)......... 647
5.2.3.2.12 *Vogel v. C.B.C.* (1982), 21 C.C.L.T. 105 (B.C.S.C.).......... 655
5.2.3.3 Privilege... 656
  5.2.3.3.1 *Shultz v. Porter and Block Brothers Ltd.* (1979), 9 A.R. 381 (Alta. S.C.) 656
  5.2.3.3.2 Absolute Privilege 657
    5.2.3.3.2.1 *Ontario Libel and Slander Act*, R.S.O. 1990, c. L.12. 657
    5.2.3.3.2.2 *Tedlie v. Southam*, [1950] 4 D.L.R. 415 (Man. K.B.)..... 658
  5.2.3.3.3 Qualified Privilege 666
    5.2.3.3.3.1 Anne Skarsgard, "Freedom of the Press," (1980-81), *Saskatchewan Law Review* 45, pp. 303-307 666
    5.2.3.3.3.2 Qualified Privilege Under Statute 669
      5.2.3.3.3.2.1 *Ontario Libel and Slander Act*, R.S.O. 1990, c. L.12. 669
      5.2.3.3.3.2.2 *Cook v. Alexander and Others*, [1973] 3 All E.R. 1037 (C.A.) 672
      5.2.3.3.3.2.3 *Hefferman v. Regina Daily Star*, [1930] 3 W.W.R. 656 (Sask. K.B.) 679
    5.2.3.3.3.3 Qualified Privilege Under Common Law 682
      5.2.3.3.3.3.1 *Banks v. Globe and Mail* (1961), 28 D.L.R. (2d) 343 (S.C.C.) 682
      5.2.3.3.3.3.2 *Stopforth v. Goyer* (1978), 4 C.C.L.T. 265 (Ont. H.C.)... 690
      5.2.3.3.3.3.3 *Stopforth v. Goyer* (1979), 23 O.R. (2d) 696 (Ont. C.A.)... 697
      5.2.3.3.3.3.4 *Parlett v. Robinson* (1986), 30 D.L.R. (4th) 247 (B.C.C.A.)..................................... 698
      5.2.3.3.3.3.5 *Camporese v. Parton* (1983), 150 D.L.R. (3d) 208 (B.C.S.C.) 705
      5.2.3.3.3.3.6 *Hill v. Church of Scientology of Toronto* 1994, unreported (Ont. C.A.)......................... 712
  5.2.3.3.4 Malice 715
    5.2.3.3.4.1 *Shultz v. Porter and Block Brother Ltd.* (1979), 9 A.R. 381 (Alta. S.C.) 715
    5.2.3.3.4.2 *Farrell v. St. John's Publishing Co.* (1986), 58 Nfld. & P.E.I.R. 66 (Nfld. C.A.).............................. 717

5.2.3.3.4.3 *Vogel v. C.B.C.* (1982), 21 C.C.L.T. 105, at 132, 133 and 193	720
5.2.3.4 Consent	721
5.2.3.4.1 *Syms v. Warren* (1976), 71 D.L.R. (3d) 558 (Man. Q.B.)	721
5.2.3.5 The Charter and Libel	726
5.2.3.5.1 *Hill v. Church of Scientology of Toronto* 1994, unreported (Ont. C.A.)	726
5.2.4 Remedies	738
5.2.4.1 Damages	739
5.2.4.1.1 General Considerations	739
5.2.4.1.1.1 *Munro v. Toronto Sun* (1982), 21 C.C.L.T. 261 (Ont. H.C.)	739
5.2.4.1.1.2 *Walker and Walker Brothers Quarries Ltd. v. CFTO Ltd. et al.* (1987), 19 O.A.C. 10 (Ont. C.A.)	739
5.2.4.1.1.3 Julian Porter, Q.C., "Tangents," *Canadian Lawyer*, April 1981, p. 24	740
5.2.4.1.1.4 *Snyder v. Montreal Gazette Ltd.* (1988), 49 D.L.R. (4th) 17 (S.C.C.)	742
5.2.4.1.1.5 *Hill v. Church of Scientology of Toronto* 1994, unreported (Ont. C.A.)	747
5.2.4.1.2 Factors Related to the Plaintiff	748
5.2.4.1.2.1 *Barltrop v. C.B.C.* (1978), 25 N.S.R. (2d) 637 (N.S.C.A.)	748
5.2.4.1.2.2 *Leonhard v. Sun Publishing* (1956), 4 D.L.R. (2d) 514 (B.C.S.C.)	752
5.2.4.1.3 Factors Related to the Defendant	754
5.2.4.1.3.1 *Vogel v. C.B.C.* (1982), 21 C.C.L.T. 105 (B.C.S.C.)	754
5.2.4.1.3.2 *Baxter v. C.B.C.* (1980), 30 N.B.R. (2d) 102 (N.B.C.A.)	755
5.2.4.1.3.3 *Westbank Band of Indians v. Tomat* (1992), 10 C.C.L.T. (2d) 1 (B.C.C.A.)	755
5.2.4.1.3.4 *Munro v. Toronto Sun* (1982), 21 C.C.L.T. 261 (Ont. H.C.)	759
5.2.4.1.3.5 *Vogel v. C.B.C.* (1982), 21 C.C.L.T. 105 (B.C.S.C.)	759
5.2.4.1.3.6 *Hill v. Church of Scientology of Toronto* 1994, unreported (Ont. C.A.)	764
5.2.4.1.3.7 *Walker Brothers Quarries Ltd. v. CFTO Ltd. et al.* (1987), 19 O.A.C. 10 (Ont. C.A.)	765
5.2.4.1.4 Apology	766
5.2.4.1.4.1 *Ontario Libel and Slander Act*, R.S.O. 1990, c. L.12	766
5.2.4.1.4.2 *Teskey v. Canadian Newspapers Co.* (1989), 68 O.R. (2d) 737 (Ont. C.A.)	770
5.2.4.1.4.3 *Hoste v. Victoria Times Publishing Co.* (1989), 1 B.C.R. (PT 2) 365 (B.C.S.C.)	777
5.2.4.1.4.4 *Brannigan v. S.I.U.* (1964), 42 D.L.R. (2d) 249 (B.C.S.C.)	777
5.2.4.1.4.5 John G. Fleming, "Retraction and Reply; Alternative Remedies for Defamation," (1978), *University of British Columbia Law Review* 12, p. 15	778

        5.2.4.2   Injunctions..   784
           5.2.4.2.1   *Canada Metal Co. Ltd. v. C.B.C.* (1974), 44 D.L.R. (3d) 329
                      (Ont. H.C.)   784
           5.2.4.2.2   Robert Martin, "Interlocutory Injunctions in Libel Actions,"
                      (1982), *University of Western Ontario Law Review* 20, p. 12 ..   790
     5.2.5   Procedural Issues   796
        5.2.5.1   Time Limits..   796
           5.2.5.1.1   *Ontario Libel and Slander Act*, R.S.O. 1990, c. L.12.........   796
           5.2.5.1.2   *Grossman v. C.F.T.O.* (1983), 139 D.L.R. (3d) 618 (Ont. C.A.)   797
           5.2.5.1.3   *Crown Liability Act*, R.S.C. 1985, c. C-50, as am. S.C. 1990,
                      c. 8, s. 29   798
           5.2.5.1.4   *Ontario Libel and Slander Act*, R.S.O. 1990, c. L.12.........   798
        5.2.5.2   Legal Aid...   799
           5.2.5.2.1   *Ontario Legal Aid Act*, R.S.O. 1990, c. L.9................   799
        5.2.5.3   Juries   800
           5.2.5.3.1   *Ontario Libel and Slander Act*, R.S.O. 1990, c. L.12.........   803
           5.2.5.3.2   *McLoughlin v. Kutasy* (1979), 26 N.R. 242 (S.C.C)..........   804
           5.2.5.3.3   *Burnett v. C.B.C. (No. 2)* (1981), 48 N.S.R. (2d) 181 (S.C.T.D.)   805
           5.2.5.3.4   *Crown Liability Act*, R.S.C. 1985, c. C-50, as am. S.C. 1990,
                      c. 8, s. 31   806
        5.2.5.4   Libel Insurance   806
           5.2.5.4.1   *Ontario Libel and Slander Act*, R.S.O. 1990, c. L.12.........   806
        5.2.5.5   Offer to Settle   807
        5.2.5.6   Consolidation of Actions and Security for Costs.................   809
           5.2.5.6.1   *Ontario Libel and Slander Act*, R.S.O. 1990, c. L.12.........   809
5.3   Privacy...   811
  5.3.1   The Charter..   811
     5.3.1.1   *The Canadian Charter of Rights and Freedoms*   811
     5.3.1.2   *R. v. Nicolucci and Papier* (1985), 22 C.C.C. (3d) 207 (Que. S.C.) .   812
  5.3.2   Privacy at Common Law..   812
     5.3.2.1   *Robbins v. C.B.C.* (1957), 12 D.L.R. (2d) 35 (Que. S.C.)..........   812
     5.3.2.2   *Krouse v. Chrysler Canada* (1973), 1 O.R. (2d) 225 (Ont. C.A.) ...   820
     5.3.2.3   *Burnett v. The Queen in Right of Canada* (1979), 23 O.R. (2d) 109
              (Ont. H.C.)..   821
     5.3.2.4   *Motherwell v. Motherwell* (1976), 73 D.L.R. (3d) 62 (Alta. S.C.)...   822
     5.3.2.5   *Capan v. Capan* (1981), 14 C.C.L.T. 191 (Ont. H.C.)   836
     5.3.2.6   *Saccone v. Orr* (1982), 19 C.C.L.T. 37 (Ont. Co.Ct.)   839
     5.3.2.7   Annotation to *Saccone v. Orr*   844
     5.3.2.8   *P.F. v. Ontario et al.* (1989), 7 C.C.L.T. 231 (Ont. D.C.)   847
     5.3.2.9   Note on Photographs and Rights of Privacy   849
  5.3.3   Privacy Statutes   855
     5.3.3.1   Notes on Provincial Privacy Acts   855
     5.3.3.2   *Privacy Act*, R.S.C. 1985, c. P-21   856
     5.3.3.3   *Silber and Value Industries Ltd. v. British Columbia Television
              Broadcasting System Ltd., Hicks and Chu*, [1986] 2 W.W.R. 609
              (B.C.S.C.)   864

PREFACE TO SECOND EDITION

More than five years have passed since the first edition was published and it is three years since the appearance of the revised edition. We are grateful that both these earlier editions sold out and were generally well received by journalism educators and even some lawyers.

In preparing this edition, we have removed material which has become out of date or has been superceded. We have added a great deal of new and topical material including commentaries and transitional notes, and decisions of the Supreme Court of Canada on such issues as pornography, journalistic privilege and hate propaganda. Chapter One has been expanded to provide greater detail and background on the Constitution of Canada. At the same time, we have attempted to edit more tightly material which has survived from the first edition.

Having used the book for our own teaching, we are persuaded that the structure which we adopted for the first edition is ideal. It is unchanged.

The book's primary purpose is to introduce students to the legal system and, more specifically, to the laws affecting the workings of the mass media. Our book is informed by a belief in the rule of law and a belief that intelligent and critical journalism is essential to the health of democracy.

R.M.
G.S.A.
July, 1994

PREFACE TO FIRST EDITION

The study of law has been recognized for centuries as a basic intellectual discipline in European universities. However, only in recent years has it become a feature of undergraduate programs in English-Canadian universities. Traditionally, legal learning has been viewed in such institutions as the special preserve of lawyers, rather than a necessary part of the intellectual equipment of an educated person. Happily, the older and more continental view of legal education is establishing itself in a number of Canadian universities and some have even begun to offer undergraduate degrees in law.

If the study of law is beginning to establish itself as part and parcel of a general education, its aims and methods should appeal directly to journalism educators. Law is a discipline which encourages responsible judgment. On the one hand, it provides opportunities to analyze such ideas as justice, democracy and freedom. On the other, it links these concepts to everyday realities in a manner which is parallel to the links journalists forge on a daily basis as they cover and comment on the news. For example, notions of evidence and fact, of basic rights and public interest are at work in the process of journalistic judgment and production just as in courts of law. Sharpening judgment by absorbing and reflecting on law is a desirable component of a journalist's intellectual preparation for his or her career.

But the idea that the journalist must understand the law more profoundly than an ordinary citizen turns on an understanding of the established conventions and special responsibilities of the news media. Politics or, more broadly, the functioning of the state, is a major subject for journalists. The better informed they are about the way the state works, the better their reporting will be. In fact, it is difficult to see how journalists who do not have a clear grasp of the basic features of the Canadian Constitution can do a competent job on political stories.

Furthermore, the legal system and the events which occur within it are primary subjects for journalists. While the quality of legal journalism varies greatly, there is an undue reliance amongst many journalists on interpretations supplied to them by lawyers. While comment and reaction from lawyers may enhance stories, it is preferable for journalists to rely on their own notions of significance and make their own judgments. These can only come from a well-grounded understanding of the legal system.

Finally, the study of law requires an understanding of freedom of expression. The law is full of traps for the unwary. Neither being prosecuted for contempt of court nor getting sued for defamation is attractive. Some reporters end up in trouble. However, what seems to happen most often is that the fear of unpleasant legal consequences results in stories never being broadcast or published. The trepidation of the reporter or editor or publisher is generally reinforced by the caution of the lawyer.

The study of law cannot be viewed as providing the reporter with the skills necessary to be a legal advisor. But it should be possible to equip the reporter with sufficient legal knowledge to enable him or her to exploit the possibilities which the law provides. In this fashion, the working journalist comes to possess the tools necessary to ensure the most ample freedom of expression.

This book is devoted primarily to the latter task although, as will be seen, the method of presentation reflects a dedication to the broader intellectual goals of legal education.

Our primary aim is to equip journalists with the technical knowledge to recognize and interpret the laws that affect their work. This sourcebook contains an inventory of the statutes and case law which circumscribe journalistic practice. Official Secrets, contempt, criminal and civil libel, obscenity, racism and privacy are some of the subjects described and discussed in what follows. However, in addition to equipping apprentice journalists with an understanding of rules and warning signs, we have other goals in mind. We have sought to use the necessity that journalism students master specific legal rules as an opportunity to explore law as an organized system of judgment and intellectual discrimination. In other words, the method of presentation reflects an ambition to elevate the study of law beyond the memorizing of statutory rules to a level of intellectual exploration which reflects the general aims of university legal education.

Finally, we have sought to show how freedom of expression is incorporated into the Canadian legal system. This has been achieved through the book's structure. We have organized the materials in a manner which shows how the Canadian legal tradition has absorbed and expressed the ideas of freedom of expression, press and media.

Accordingly, Chapter One explores the Canadian Constitution and features cases involving freedom of speech and the press from before and after the adoption of the *Canadian Charter of Rights and Freedoms* in 1982. The chapter concludes with an exploration of the Canadian theory of freedom of expression.

Chapters Two to Five explore the legal limitations, sanctioned by Section 1 of the Charter, on freedom of expression. Section 2(b) declares that freedom of expression, press and media are fundamental freedoms that Canadians possess.

Section 1 says that these fundamental freedoms may be subject to reasonable limitations prescribed by law which can be demonstrably justified in a free and democratic society. Such limitations on free expression may be grouped into three broad categories. Chapter Two is concerned with the limitations which protect the state's rights, obligations and prerogatives such as the obligation to maintain secrets and public order. Chapter Three, which represents a continuation of the same theme, looks at the limitations protecting the judicial system. Chapter Four is concerned with legal limitations intended to protect certain social values. Thus, the law prohibits forms of obscenity and seeks to protect minority groups against racist attacks. Chapter Five is concerned with limitations intended to protect individuals against attacks on their reputations. The law of civil defamation is its principal subject.

Media law embraces elements from criminal, civil and even administrative law. It is complex and extraordinarily rich. However, what makes it especially important is that its study reveals both the character and limitations of Canadian democracy.

>	Robert Martin
>	Professor of Law
>
>	G. Stuart Adam
>	Professor of Journalism
>	Chair, Centre of Mass Media Studies
>
>	The University of Western Ontario
>
>	September, 1988
>	(Revised, December, 1993)

ACKNOWLEDGEMENTS

This sourcebook is the product of the work of many people over many years.

Several of these people are current and former students — in both the Faculty of Law and the Graduate School of Journalism — at the University of Western Ontario.

The first edition of this book owed much to the work of Shelley Appleby-Ostroff, Eve Donner, Karen Douglas, Natham Golas, Kathryn Hazel, D. James Newland, Lynda Rogers, and Michael Rumball.

For the second edition we are grateful to Elaine Crossland and Maureen Dennison for their dedicated, skillful and cheerful efforts.

Special thanks go, again, to Kathleen Adair of the Faculty of Law at Western Ontario, who has been assisting with the growth of this work since 1976, and to Cheryl Cadrin at Carleton University Press who ably supervised the completion of this edition.

We thank the Dean of Graduate Studies at Carleton for making funds available to assist in the preparation of this edition. The Support of the Ontario Law Foundation has been crucial for many years.

Finally, the authors gratefully acknowledge and thank:

The editors of Butterworths and Mr. Stuart Robertson for permission to reproduce p. 25 of *Courts and the Media*, by Stuart Robertson (Toronto: 1981); and Mr. Patrick Boyer for permission to reproduce pp. 308-309 of *Political Rights: The Legal Framework of Elections in Canada* (Toronto: Butterworths, 1981);

The Canadian Daily Newspaper Publishers Association for permission to reproduce "What Newsrooms Need to Know," CDNPA (Toronto: 1984);

The publisher of *Canadian Lawyer* for permission to reproduce an excerpt from "Tangents" by Julian Porter, *Canadian Lawyer*, April 1981, p. 24;

The editor of Carleton University Press for permission to reproduce pp. 32-39 of *The Law and the Press in Canada*, by Wilfren H. Kesterton (Toronto: McClelland and Stewart in association with the Institute of Canadian Studies, Carleton University, 1976);

xxiv ACKNOWLEDGEMENTS

The editors of Carswell, a division of Thomson Canada Limited, for permission to reprint the court chart from *The Practical Guide to Canadian Legal Research* by Jacqueline R. Castel and Omeela K. Latchman (Toronto: 1993) pp. 12-19, and for their permission and the permission of Prof. Peter Hogg to reprint p. 774 of *Constitutional Law of Canada* (Third Edition) by Peter Hogg (Scarborough: 1992); and for their permission to reproduce excerpts from the annotation to *Saccone v. Orr* (1982), 19 C.C.L.T. 37 by John Irvine, the annotation to *Luscher v. Deputy Minister, Revenue Canada, Customs and Excise* (1985), 45 C.R. (3d) 81 by Don Stuart; and for their permission and the permission of Prof. H.R.S. Ryan for permission to reproduce his annotation to *R. v. Zundel* (1992), 16 C.R. (4th) 1 (S.C.C.).

The executive director of the Centre for Investigative Journalism (now the Canadian Association of Journalists) and Mr. John Sawatsky for permission to reprint "John Sawatsky Stakes Out the High Ground" in *Bulletin* of the Centre for Investigative Journalism, 11, 1986;

The editor of *content for Canadian Journalists* and Mr. Harold Levy for permission to reproduce "What Should We Do When the Cops Arrive?" (1979), *Content* 95;

The Minister of Supply and Services Canada for permission to reproduce "Freedom of the Press" by Walter Tarnopolsky in *Newspapers and the Law* 1981, ix, 19-21;

The former Law Reform Commission of Canada for permission to reprint excerpts from Working Paper #49, *Crimes against the State* (1986), pp. 30, 33-36; Working Paper #56, *Public and Media Access to the Criminal Process*, (1986), pp. 89-91; Working Paper #50, *Hate Propaganda* (1986), pp. 39-41; and Working Paper #10, *Limits of Criminal Law; Obscenity, a Test Case* (1975), pp. 39-49;

The chairman of the Ryerson School of Journalism for permission to reprint an excerpt from Alexander Stark's *Dangerous Words*;

The editor of the *Saskatchewan Law Review* and Ann Skarsgard for permission to reproduce excerpts from "Freedom of the Press (1980-81), *Sask. L. R.*, pp. 296-99, 302, 307-16.

The editor of the *University of British Columbia Law Review* and John G. Fleming for permission to reproduce "Retraction and Reply: Alternative Remedies for Defamation" (1978), 12 U.B.C.L. *Rev.* 15.

The editor of *Lawyers Weekly* for permission to reproduce an excerpt from "No Cameras in Court", by Patricia Chisolm, *Ontario Lawyers Weekly*, 20 January 1984;

The publishers of Canada Law Book Inc. and Prof. David Scheiderman for permission to reprint "The Access to Information Act: A Practical Review," by David Scheiderman (1987), 7 *Advocates Quarterly* 474;

Oxford University Press for permission to reprint pp. 118-120, 121-123 and 134-139 from *Canadian Constitutional Conventions: The Marriage of Law and Politics* (Toronto: 1991) by Andrew Heard;

McClelland and Stewart for permission to reprint an excerpt from *Morgentaler v. Borowski; Abortion, the Charter and the Courts* (Toronto; 1992), pp. 294-314;

And the editors of Southam News for permission to reprint "Court Rulings Tightening Muzzle on Media" by Stephen Bindman, *The London Free Press*, 13 March 1993.

CHAPTER ONE

Freedom of Expression and the Canadian Constitution

1.1 The Law and the Mass Media

1.1.1 The Meaning of Freedom of Expression

John Milton asked in his pamphlet *Areopagitica*, published in England in 1644, for "the liberty to know, to utter and to argue freely, according to conscience, above all liberties".[1] Freedom of expression continues to be directed towards these goals. The democratic tradition recognizes the right to know, to speak and to express opinions without first seeking the permission of authorities and without the risk that the law will be used to forbid or punish the exercise of the right. The understanding is that free expression is so fundamental to democratic societies that it can be limited only for clear and pressing reasons. There cannot be democracy if the right to criticize is not secure; nor can there be democracy if governments possess the power to define the meaning of events and values. Accordingly, the notion of freedom of expression in liberal democracies includes the belief that the state has no right to abrogate this fundamental freedom.

The constitutions of the United States, Canada and Great Britain reflect in different ways these beliefs. The constitution of the United States includes the First Amendment which says that Congress may not pass a law "abridging the freedom of speech, or of the press". Section 2(b) of the *Canadian Charter of Rights and Freedoms* declares that "freedom of thought, belief, opinion and expression, including freedom of the press and other media of communication" is a fundamental freedom. Both Canada and the United States have established rights in their constitutions which are protected by the courts. By contrast, the largely unwritten British constitution posits liberties or conventions protected by Parliament. The British Parliament has traditionally recognized liberties, including liberty of the press.

The distinction between the right to know, on the one hand, and the rights to utter and express opinions on the other may be blurred. But it can be usefully maintained in order to consider the work of journalists. People who make their living as reporters are exercising the right to know. They are exercising the right to know what goes on in Parliament, or in the courts, or in public institutions generally on behalf of a public which is distant from the centres of political and public action. Although the journalist may be actively exercising the right to know, his or her rights are the same as those of the ordinary citizen. The knowledge communicated by the journalist is one element in forming the political consciousness of citizens.

The right to know — that is, the right to gather information — is one thing; the rights to pass it on and express opinions about it are another. There have been occasions in, for example, the United States where individuals have been silenced by political pressure or by law itself. The blacklisted Hollywood producers and writers in the period during which Senator Joseph McCarthy was at the height of his influence were denied the exercise of both rights.[2] The South African journalist, Donald Woods, who was placed under banning orders when he was the editor of the *East London Disptach* in 1977 was similarly denied the rights to utter or express opinions. He had published an account of the death of the African nationalist Steven Biko at the hands of the security police.[3] Banning orders silence individuals. They deprive them of the right to utter and there have been many legal instruments developed over the years for such purposes. Banning powers were incorporated into Alberta's *Act to Ensure the Publication of Accurate News and Information* which was ruled unconstitutional by the Supreme Court of Canada in 1938.[4]

The right to express radical opinions has led to the most dramatic events in the development of the democratic tradition. As late as the early eighteenth century an English printer's apprentice was executed for publishing a document in which it was argued that the Pretender's claim to the throne was legitimate.[5]

Attempts by the state to punish the expression of radical opinions has continued. Section 98 of the old Canadian *Criminal Code* was used until 1935 to prosecute Communists. The Quebec Padlock law (An *Act to Protect the Province Against Communistic Propaganda*) was enacted under the Duplessis government in Quebec in 1937 and enforced for 20 years until the Supreme Court of Canada ruled it unconstitutional in 1957. That act made it an offence to publish and circulate communist opinions.[6]

While there have always been powerful advocates of the notion of freedom of expression — from John Milton to George Orwell who said in his essay, "The Prevention of Literature" that the debate over freedom of the press is a debate about the "desirability of telling lies" — none has attacked the idea of law itself.[7] The early advocates of freedom may have attacked the law of seditious libel, but they would have accepted at the same time a notion that originated with the eighteenth-century British jurist Mansfield who said freedom of the press means freedom "subject to the consequence of the law".[8] In the twentieth century, we would say we ought to be free to speak and publish and broadcast without prior restraint, subject to the laws (or at least some of the laws) with which this book is concerned.

However, the consensus on what social harms should be the concern of the laws has shifted considerably. For example, in the seventeenth and eighteenth centuries when printing and publishing were coming of age, the British government used the law of seditious libel to protect itself from critics in the belief that if the public did not believe that government was good, neither the government nor the institutions of state could survive. To those in power, it was reasonable to limit political speech to safe or, at the most, mildly critical utterances and to punish everything else.

The limitations in the twentieth century on the exercise of the rights to utter, know and argue, must, in the words of the Canadian Constitution, be reasonable. Section 1 of the Canadian Charter says that is guarantees are "subject only to such reasonable limits prescribed by law as can be demonstrably justified in a free and democratic society". Attempts are made to justify the limitations in the laws of civil and criminal libel, or contempt of court, by referring to such harms — for example, the possible loss of reputation arising from libel, or the assumed peril to human lives because of incitements to riot, or the fear that an accused person may be denied a fair trial because of the publication, before the trial, of possibly prejudicial material.

Just as there are several variants of democratic theory, there are several ways in which freedom of expression has been justified. The dominant theory is part and parcel of liberal democratic theory in which the analytic starting point is the individual. The theory puts the individual citizen into the foreground and, in a manner of speaking, subordinates the rights of the state and society to the will or desires and, ultimately, the freedom of the individual. Much of legal theory in the common law jurisdictions is based on the philosophical method and arguments of the British philosophers Jeremy Bentham and James and John Stuart Mill.[9]

But many people are not comfortable with an approach to freedom of expression which takes the individual as its analytical starting point. Other democratic approaches are possible. They include a collectivist or socialist conception in which freedom of expression is viewed as a necessary pre-condition to the realization of important collective values and aims. Such an approach sees freedom of expression not merely as a commodity possessed by individuals, but as an essential pre-condition to the creation and maintenance of democracy itself.

The Canadian tradition has absorbed and confirmed the political and democratic values embedded in both traditions. For example, Chief Justice Lyman Duff said in the *Alberta Press Act* case that the "right to free public discussion of public affairs . . . is the breath of life for parliamentary institutions.[10] In that case, the court did not offer constitutional protection to freedom of expression on the basis of a notion of individual rights. Rather the court was seeking to protect the social institution of parliamentary democracy. It affirmed that parliamentary democracy could not function without free expression.

But there is a broader sense in which freedom of expression may be considered. Democracy is not solely a matter of parliaments and elections. A democratic society must not only permit, but encourage, the widest possible participation of all its members in its economic, social and cultural affairs. The creation of the means and the institutions to make this possible constitutes an obligation affecting society as a whole. Freedom of expression is, once again, essential to these processes.

While individualist justifications for freedom of expression are the norm in Canadian society, pressing the individualistic approach too far may have a contradictory effect. By focussing on the individual, the notion may develop that freedom of expression has to do largely, or exclusively, with the proprietary rights of the individual owners of newspapers, or radio or television stations.

There is a sense in which this issue commanded the attention of the Kent Royal Commission, which studied Canada's newspaper industry in 1980-81.[11] The commissioners noted, for example, that the right of the editor of the newspaper to express his opinions was subordinated in law to the right of the owners and publishers to hire and fire. It has been noted elsewhere that there are occasions when a journalist's right to free expression may be subordinated to codes of professional conduct and thereby to freedom of the press itself. An example would occur when an employer reprimands a journalist for engaging in political activity such as joining a political party or making partisan speeches. Journalists may denounce the government in newspaper columns, but they may not, according to some employment codes, join and campaign for political parties.[12]

Freedom of expression is, then, an idea which may be considered in more than one way and from differing philosophical starting points. However, regardless of the philosophical underpinnings, it is everywhere seen to be fundamental to the political architecture of a genuine democracy.

Endnotes

1. "Areopagitica: A Speech for the Liberty of Unlicensed Printing to the Parliament of England (1644)" in George Sabine, ed., *John Milton, Areopagitica and of Education with Autobiographical Passages from other Prose Works* (Chicago, 1985), p. 49.
2. See, for example: Richard H. Rovere, *Senator Joe McCarthy*, (New York, 1959), and Victor S. Navarky, *Naming Names* (New York, 1980).
3. Donald Woods, *Biko* (New York, 1978), and *Asking for Trouble: Autobiography of a Banned Journalist* (London, 1980).
4. The judgment in this reference is reprinted in section 1.4.2.
5. See Laurence William Hanson's *Government and the Press, 1695-1763* (Oxford, 1967).

6. The judgment of the Supreme Court is reprinted in section 1.3.3.
7. Orwell's essay may be found in *The Complete Works of George Orwell* (London, 1986), p. 327.
8. T.B. Howell, *A Complete Collection of State Trials*, Vol. XXI (London, 1813), p. 1040.
9. John Stuart Mill, *On Liberty* (London, 1974).
10. That decision is reported in full in section 1.3.2 of the text.
11. *Report of the Royal Commission on Newspapers* (Ottawa, 1981), Vol. 1.
12. See "Political Activity and The Journalist: A Paradox" by Andrew MacFarlane and Robert Martin, *Canadian Journal of Communication*, Vol. 10, No. 2, 1984, pp. 1-35.

1.2 The Structure of the Constitution

The three principal components of the Canadian Constitution are the unwritten conventions and practices inherited from the United Kingdom, the *Constitution Act*, 1867 or, as it used to be called, *The British North America Act, 1867*, and the *Constitution Act, 1982*.

That the inspiration for Canadian political and legal practices is British may be inferred from the utterance in the preamble to the *Constitution Act, 1867*, that Canada is to have a constitution "similar in principle" to that of the United Kingdom. The statement means that fundamental principles of British democracy such as the supremacy of Parliament, the freedom of the press, and the rule of law protected by an independent judiciary are basic to Canada's Constitution.

However, from the beginning Canada was a federal rather than a unitary state and, accordingly, the *Constitution Act, 1867*, established principles of federalism by defining the jurisdictional limits within which the federal Parliament and provincial legislatures could make laws.

The *Constitution Act, 1867*, served as the principal constitutional document from 1867 until 1982 when a new element was added to the constitutional structure. In that year the U.K. Parliament enacted the *Canada Act, 1982*. One of its purposes was to give to Canadian institutions the ownership, so to speak, of the Canadian Constitution. Until 1982, the *B.N.A. Act* had remained an act of Westminster and as a result could only be amended there. The curious legal anomaly of the Parliament of one modern sovereign state acting as the custodian of the constitution of another modern sovereign state was ended when the *Canada Act* was passed.

The *Canada Act* also permitted the incorporation into Canada's legal foundations of a set of declarations on the basic rights of Canadian citizens. These declarations are contained in the *Canadian Charter of Rights and Freedoms* which puts in statutory form values which have long been part of the democratic tradition.

1.3 The Judiciary

1.3.1 E. Jacqueline R. Castel and Omeela K. Latchman, *The Practical Guide to Canadian Legal Research* **(Toronto: Carswell Thomson Professional Publishing, 1993), pp. 12-19**

CANADIAN COURT SYSTEM

The following is an overview in two parts of the Canadian court system from the beginning of British settlement to date. The first part shows the Courts of the Provinces, with courts currently in existence in bold face; the second shows the federal courts, with a brief description of their jurisdictions. It is provided for reference when assessing the weight to be given to any given case, and for aid when the case law deals with procedural issues which may depend upon the court structures in existence at the time. All footnotes can be found at the end of this section.

Jurisdiction	Justices, Magistrates and Provincial Courts[1]	County and District Courts	Surrogate and Probate Courts	Provincial Superior Courts Trial Division[2]	Courts of Appeal[3]	Family and Youth Courts	Admiralty Courts[4]
Alberta	Justice of the Peace (1835-) Magistrates' Court (1918-1978) Provincial Court (Civil Division) (1978-) Provincial Court (Criminal Division) (1978-) Provincial Court (Small Claims Division) (1978-)	District Court (1907-1978)	Surrogate Court (1967-)	Supreme Court Trial Division (1907-1978) Court of Queen's Bench (1978-)	Supreme Court Appeal Division (1919-)	Provincial Court (Family Division) (1978-) Provincial Court (Youth Division) (1978-)	
British Columbia	Justice of the Peace (1935-) Small Debt Court (1895-1969) Provincial Court (1969-)	Vancouver Island District Court (1853-1867) British Columbia County Court (1859-1990)		Supreme Court of Vancouver Island (1853-1870) Supreme Court of British Columbia (1859-)	Supreme Court en banc (1972-1906) Court of Appeal (1909-)		Vancouver Island Vice-Admiralty Court (1849-1891) British Columbia Vice-Admiralty Court (?-1866)
Manitoba	Justices of the Peace (1835-) Magistrates' Court (1916-1972) Provincial Court (1972-)	County Court (1872-1984)	Surrogate Court (1881-1984)	General Court of Assiniboia (1935-1872) Court of Queen's Bench (1872-)	Supreme Court en banc (1872-1906) Court of Appeal (1906-)	Provincial Court (Family Division) (1984-)	
New Brunswick	Justices of the Peace (1786-) Parish Court (1876-1942) Magistrates' Court (1942-1969) Provincial Court (1969-)	Inferior Court of Common Pleas (1785-1867) County Court (1867-1979)	Probate Court (1786-)	Supreme Court (1785-1909) Law only until 1854 Court of Chancery (1838-1854) Equity Supreme Court (Queen's Bench Division) (1909-1966) Law only Supreme Court (Chancery Side) (1909-1966) Equity Court of Queen's Bench (1966-)	Supreme Court en banc (1785-1909) Supreme Court (Chancery Division) (1909-1966) Court of Appeal (1966-)	Court of Divorce and Matrimonial Causes (1860-1948) Court of Queen's Bench (Family Division) (1978-)	Vice-Admiralty Court (1787-1891)
Newfoundland	Justices of the Peace (1728-) Stipendiary Magistrates (1858-1974) District Courts (1869-1949) Provincial Court (1974-)	District Court (1949-1986)		Supreme Court (1793-)	Supreme Court en banc (1793-1986) Court of Appeal (1986-)	Unified Family Court (1978-)	Vice-Admiralty Court (1743-1891)

Jurisdiction	Justices, Magistrates and Provincial Courts[1]	County and District Courts	Surrogate and Probate Courts	Provincial Superior Courts Trial Division[2]	Courts of Appeal[3]	Family and Youth Courts	Admiralty Courts[4]
Nova Scotia	Justices of the Peace (1727-) Civil Court (1727-1749) Municipal Court (1895-1958) **Provincial Court (1958-)**	County Court of the City of Halifax (1749-1752) Inferior Court of Common Pleas (1752-1841) Court of Sessions (1841-1876) **County Court (1876-)**	Probate Court (1759-1897)	Governor in Council (1721-1749) General Court (1749-1754) Supreme Court (1754-) Law only until 1857, and from 1864-1884 Court of Chancery (1825-1857) (1864-1884) Equity Supreme Court of Cape Breton (?-1820) Law only	Supreme Court en banc (1754-1966) **Supreme Court Appellate Division (1966-)**	Divorce Court (1866-1948) **Family Court (1963-)**	Vice-Admiralty Court (1739-1891)
Ontario*	Justices of the Peace (1764-) Magistrates' Court (1849-1968) Provincial Court (Criminal Division) (1968-1990) Court of Requests (1792-1841) Division Court (1841-1970) Small Claims Court (1970-1984) Provincial Court (Civil Division) (1984-1990) General [Quarter] Sessions of the Peace (1777-1984) **Ontario Court of Justice (Provincial Division) (1990-) Ontario Court of Justice (General Division); Small Claims Court (1990-)**	District Court (1794-1849), (1984-1990) County Court (1849-1984)	Surrogate Court (1793-1990) Probate Court (1793-1858)	Court of Common Pleas (1788-1794) Law only Supreme Court (Queen's Bench Division) (1794-1913) Law only Supreme Court (Chancery Division) (1837-1913) Equity Supreme Court (Common Pleas Division) (1849-1913) Law only Supreme Court (Exchequer Division) (1903-1913) Law only Supreme Court (High Court of Justice) (1913-1990) **Supreme Court in Bankruptcy (1913-) Jurisdiction conferred by Bankruptcy Act (Federal) Ontario Court of Justice (General Division) (1990-)**	Court of Error and Appeal (1849-1881) Court of Appeal (1881-1913) Divisional Courts of Appellate Division (1913-1931) **Court of Appeal (1931-)** Divisional Court (1881-1913) **(1972-)**	Provincial Court (Family Division) (1968-1990) **Unified Family Court of Hamilton-Wentworth (1976-) Ontario Court of Justice (Provincial Division) (1990-)**	Maritime Court (1877-1891)

Jurisdiction	Justices, Magistrates and Provincial Courts[1]	County and District Courts	Surrogate and Probate Courts	Provincial Superior Courts Trial Division[2]	Courts of Appeal[3]	Family and Youth Courts	Admiralty Courts[4]
P.E.I.	**Justices of the Peace (1773-)** Small Debt Commissioners (1832-1873) Stipendiary Magistrates (?-1974) **Provincial Court (1974-)**	County Court (1873-1975)	Probate Court (1772-1937)	**Supreme Court Trial Division (1770-) Law** only until 1975 Court of Chancery (1848-1975) Equity	Supreme Court *en banc* (1770-1987) Court of Appeal (Equity) (1869-1975) Equity **Supreme Court Appeal Division (1987-)**	Supreme Court (Family Division) (1975-)	
Québec	**Juge de paix (1764-)** Cours des Sessions de la Paix (1777-1988) Cours des Requêtes (1770-1793) Juge provincial (1794-1843) Cour du Banc du Roi en "terme inférieur" (1794-1849) Cour de Circuit (1794-1953) Cour des Commissaires (1807-1839), (1843-1963) Cour des Magistrats (1869-1965) Cour provinciale (1965-1988) **Cour du Québec (1988-)**			Cour du Banc du Roi (1764-1777) Common Law Cour du Banc du Roi (1777-1794) Criminal Law only Cour des plaids communs (1764-1794) Cour du Banc du Roi (1794-1849) **Cour Supérieure (1849-)**	Cour d'Appel (1843-1849) Cour du Banc de la Reine (1849-1965) **Cour d'Appel (1967-)** Cour de Révision (1864-1920)	Tribunal de la jeunesse (1980-1988) **Cour de Québec (1988-)**	Cour de Vice-Admirauté (1764-1891)
Saskatchewan	**Justices of the Peace (1873-)** Magistrates' Court (1913-1978) **Provincial Court (1978-)**	District Court (1907-1981)	Surrogate Court (1907-)	Supreme Court (1907-1918) **Court of Queen's Bench (1918-)**	Supreme Court *en banc* (1907-1915) **Court of Appeal (1915-)**	**Unified Family Court (1978-)**	
Northwest Territories	**Justices of the Peace (1873-)** Stipendiary Magistrates (1873-1887), (1907-1956) **Territorial Court (1978-)**			Supreme Court (1978-) (1887-1907) Territorial Court (1956-1978)	Prior to 1960, appeals to Alberta Supreme Court Appeal Division **Court of Appeal (1960-)**		
Yukon Territory	**Justices of the Peace (1873-) Territorial Court (1983-)**			Territorial Court (1898-1985) **Supreme Court (1983-)**	Prior to 1960, appeals to British Columbia Court of Appeal **Court of Appeal (1960-)**		

Federal Courts

Although matters arising under federal law are in general dealt with by the Superior Courts of the Provinces, there are a number of exceptions to this general rule which are dealt with by a separate structure of federal Courts.

Subject Matter	Original Jurisdiction	Appeal Jurisdiction
Intellectual Property Admirialty [6]Litigation involving the Crown in right of Canada, concurrent with provincial Superior Courts Appeals from Federal Tribunals under the *Income Tax Act* and *Estate Tax Act*	Exchequer Court of Canada (1875-1970) **Federal Court Trial Division (1970-)** [5]**Tax Court of Canada (1983-)**	**Federal Court of Appeal (1970-)**
Appeals from Federal Tribunals under the *Citizenship Act* [6]Review of Federal Tribunals under s. 18 of the *Federal Court Act* relief in the nature of injunction, prerogative remedies or declaration References from Federal Tribunals under s. 18.1 of the *Federal Court Act*.	**Federal Court Trial Division (1970-)**	**Federal Court of Appeal (1970-)**
Appeals from Federal Tribunals under other specific statutes [6]Review of Federal Tribunals listed in s. 28 of the *Federal Court Act*, judicial review of quasi-judicial tribunals	**Federal Court of Appeal (1970-)**	
Appeals from Courts Martial	Court Martial Appeal Board (1950-1959) **Court Martial Appeal Court (1959-)**	

*The Courts of Justice Amendment Act, 1989 made the following changes in the Ontario court system:

1) the Court of Appeal is confirmed as the final court of appeal for the province and is separated from the High Court;
2) a new superior court is established, known as the Ontario Court of Justice, composed of two divisions — the General Division and the Provincial Division;
3) the Ontario Court (General Division) combines the jurisdiction formerly exercised by the High Court, the District Court and the surroage courts. The Divisional Court is continued as

a branch of the Ontario Court (General Division). The Small Claims Court is also a branch of the Ontario Court (General Division);
4) the Ontario Court (Provincial Division) combines the jurisdiction formerly exercised by the Provincial Court (Criminal Division), the Provincial Court (Family Division) and the Provincial Offences Court;
5) the Unified Family Court is established as a superior court but is otherwise not changed.

[1] In addition to the courts listed above, some of the older provinces have municipal and local courts of a magistrates' level in the more major cities.

[2] Except where otherwise noted, all Courts have jurisdiction over both law and equity.

[3] The Supreme Court of Canada is the final court of appeal from judgments of all provincial and federal courts. All of the older colonies had appeals to the govenor in Council (in the Maritimes, called the Court of Error and Appeal, not to be confused with the Ontario court of the same name). These died out when the Privy Council began to accept appeals from lower courts.

[4] When Great Britain handed its admiralty jurisdiction over to Canada in 1891, the Exchequer Court assumed the admiralty jurisdiction which remains with the Federal Court.

[5] Pursuant to the *Tax Court Amendment Act*, R.S.C. 1985 (4th Supp.), c. 51 the Tax Court of Canada has exclusive original jurisdiction to hear and determine references and appeals on matters involving the *Income Tax Act* and certain other Acts. Appeals from decisions of the Tax Court of Canada go directly to the Federal Court of Appeal and not to the Federal Court, Trial Division.

[6] Jurisdictions given reflect the amendments to the *Federal Court Act* — the *Federal Court Amendment Act*, S.C. 1990, c. 8, to which Royal Assent was given on March 29, 1990 and which is to come into force on proclamation.

1.3.2 The Supreme Court of Canada

The Supreme Court of Canada was not established by the *Constitution Act, 1867*, but instead, section 101 of the Act gave Parliament the authority to create a "General Court of Appeal for Canada." The Mackenzie government introduced legislation in 1875 to establish the Supreme Court, but did not make it the final court of appeal for Canada. Section 47 of the Act allowed appeals to the Judicial Committee of the Privy Council in the United Kingdom. In a move towards national autonomy, this avenue of appeal was abolished in 1949, making the Supreme Court of Canada the highest court in the Canadian judicial system.

The Supreme Court of Canada is an appeal court dealing exclusively with disputed questions of law. The Court selects which cases it will hear on the basis of their public importance. Occasionally the Supreme Court will hear reference cases directed to it by the government of Canada as authorized by section 55 of the *Supreme Court Act* (R.S.C. 1985, c. S-26). While the Court has a complement of nine judges, it is rare to find a decision rendered by the full court. Only a quorum of five judges is required to decide a case, but most often the Court sits in panels of seven judges.

1.3.3 Andrew Heard, *Canadian Constitutional Conventions: The Marriage of Law and Politics* (Toronto: Oxford University Press, 1991), pp. 118-120; 121-123; 134-139

An independent judiciary is a fundamental element of liberal democracy. The rule of law necessary to democracy is obtainable only through a judiciary that is free from overt political pressures and remains neutral and impartial between parties and issues.[1] With the federal division of powers the Canadian courts must also play an essential role as umpire in disputes of jurisdiction between the national and provincial governments. As Chief Justice Brian Dickson has pointed out, this role 'requires that the umpire be autonomous and completely independent of the parties involved in federal-provincial disputes.'[2] It is crucial that the judiciary be viwed, both individually and collectively, as impartial in resolving disputes that come to the courts for resolution. In essence this independence is ensured by protecting the judiciary from direction by any level of government, and by preventing the off-bench excursion of judges into political debates.

The independence of the Canadian judiciary was achieved through a mixture of positive law and constitutional convention. The basis of judicial independence has existed in England since the *Act of Settlement* in 1701 and was gradually applied to colonial judges in British North America.[3] This protection was formally embodied in s. 99(1) of the *Constitution Act, 1867*, which provides that judges hold office during 'good behaviour'. For the most part, however, the independence of the judiciary has been assured in Canada by the respect that has been accorded to the constitutional conventions prohibiting the executive from interfering in judicial decisions, as well as to those limiting the activities of judges. But as Mr. Justice Gerald Le Dain wrote in an 1985 decision of the Supreme Court of Canada, '... while tradition reinforced by public opinion may operate as a restraint upon the exercise of power in a manner that interferes with judicial independence, it cannot supply essential conditions of independence for which specific provision of law is necessary.'[4] Since 1968 statutory measures have introduced across the country the progressive institution of judicial councils, created to remove the executive from the initial investigation of complaints against judges. At present a national Canadian Judicial Council exists, as well as eleven other provincial and territorial councils; only Prince Edward Island has yet to create a council.

The Quebec provincial *Charter of Human Rights and Freedoms*, enacted in 1975, added a further statutory guarantee of judicial independence. Article 23 provides: 'Every person has the right to a full and equal, public and fair hearing by an independent and impartial tribunal, for the determination of his rights and obligations or of the merits of any charge brought against him.'[5]

A broad declaration of judicial independence would have been included in the *Constitution Act, 1982* had the ill-fated Bill C-60 been enacted after its introduction by the Trudeau government in 1978. Section 100 of that Bill stated: 'The principle of the independence of the judiciary under the rule of law and in consonance with the supremacy of law is a fundamental principle of the Constitution of Canada.'

The range of constitutional protection was extended much further during the 1980s. In the 1982 Constitution Act, the Charter of Rights and Freedoms declared in s. 11(d) that anyone charged with an offence has the right 'to be presumed innocent until proven guilty according to law in a fair and public hearing by an independent and impartial tribunal.' In *Valente v. The Queen*, where a provincial court judge refused to hear a case on the grounds that he could not act independently of the executive, the Supreme Court of Canada interpreted this section and outlined three elements constituting 'a standard that reflects what is common to, or at least at the heart of, the various approaches to the essential conditions of judicial independence in Canada.'[6] In the unanimous judgment of the Court, Mr. Justice Le Dain wrote that the first element of this independence lies in security of tenure, 'whether until an age of retirement, for a fixed term, or for a specific adjudicative task, that is secure against interference by the executive or other appointing authority in a discretionary or arbitrary manner.'[7] Financial security was delcared to be the second essential condition of judicial independence. And as Le Dain wrote: 'The essence of such security is that the right to salary and pension should be established by law and not subject to arbitrary interference by the executive in a manner that could affect judicial independence.'[8] The judgment then went on to state that the administrative independence of the courts comprises the third essential element. This independence is satisfied by judicial control over 'the assignment of judges, sittings of the courts and court lists — as well as matters of allocation of rooms and direction of the administrative staff engaged in carrying out these functions . . .'[9]

The most important manner in which the independence of the judiciary is achieved lies in the freedom of judges to decide the outcome of individual cases without any pressure from outside the courts. It is inherent in the rule of law that a case be decided on its particular merits, according to the law that applies to the situation at hand.[10] Judges must be able to make their decisions without fear that they will be sued, dismissed, demoted, removed from the court roster, or have their pay reduced. As long as judges fulfil their duties, act within the law, and do not behave in some fashion that brings the courts into fundamental disrepute, they should have no concern for retribution because of the disposition of a case. Furthermore, the independence of the judiciary has to be protected from attempts by either the legislature, the executive, or private parties to direct the outcome of a case.

. . . . .

As Mr. Justice Le Dain declared in *Valente*, security of tenure is the first requirement of an independent judiciary. The most blunt pressure the executive or legislature can exert on the judiciary is to remove a judge who makes a decision contrary to their interests. Since the *Act of Settlement* was passed in 1701, English judges have enjoyed statutory protection from arbitrary removal, and this security of tenure has since been extended to the Canadian judiciary. This protection was embodied in s. 99(1) of the *Constitution Act, 1867*, which provides that 'the Judges of the Superior Courts shall hold office during good behaviour, but shall be removable by the Governor General on Address of the

Senate and House of Commons.' There is some question about whether this provision creates two methods of removal: one by executive action for misbehaviour, and another by parliamentary resolution for any reason.[11] However, it is generally assumed by contemporary Canadian authorites that s. 99(1) creates only one method of removal: by parliamentary resolution for misbehaviour.[12] William R. Lederman has cited the English method of removing judges for misbehaviour by the Crown's applying to a Queen's Bench judge for dismissal by writ of *scire facias*, but this common-law means of removal seems to have been superseded in Canada by statutory provisions, as it is no longer mentioned by any authority.[13]

The protection afforded by s. 99(1) of the 1867 *Constitution Act*, however, extends only to superior court judges; it does not embrace county or provincial court judges. Under the federal *Judges Act*, county court judges are removable by the Governor in Council after a recommendation to do so from the Canadian Judicial Council. The statutory provisions relating to provincially appointed judges vary from province to province. Nevertheless, almost all judges are covered by the guarantees of secure tenure, which Le Dain declared to be an essential feature of judicial independence under s. 11(d) of the Charter: '... that the judge be removable only for cause and that cause be subject to independent review and determination by a process at which the judge is afforded a full opportunity to be heard.'[14] Thus most Canadian judges are protected from ever been summarily removed by the government of the day.

Although judges should be shielded from removal simply because the politicians or public disagree with the policies enforced by the judge, there must always be some mechanism to remove individuals from the bench who behave in such an unacceptable manner that the judiciary is brought into disrepute. It would be fair to paraphrase the Supreme Court of Canada's ruling on cabinet secrecy[15] in terms that apply to the independence of the judiciary: '... the purpose of judicial independence is to promote its proper functioning, not to facilitate improper conduct by the jduges.' In order to ensure that the misbehaviour for which judges may be constitutionally removed does not simply comprise going against government policy, every Canadian jurisdiction except Prince Edward Island has set up judicial councils to deal with complaints raised against individual judges and to recommend whether they should be removed; several provinces also provide that a judicial hearing may either replace or supplement the judicial council's inquiry. In PEI a judge of the Supreme Court conducts a formal investigation of complaints against a provincial court judge.[16]

Considering the number of people who have held judicial office, a surpising few have actually been removed from the bench. Not one member of a superior court has actually been formally dismissed, although four recommendations for removal have reached at least the stage of a parliamentary petition; on two of these occasions, however, the judges resigned.[17] Only four judges from county and district courts have been removed since Confederation.[18] Unfortunately no comprehensive historical figures are available for provincially appointed judges, but there do not appear to have been many instances of removal before the early 1980s.[19]

There does, however, seem to have been increasing attention paid to the behaviour of judges in the 1980s. Perhaps the advent of the Charter of Rights heightened the public awareness of judicial behaviour in response to the added responsibilities of the courts. Judge Paul Thériault, of the New Brunswick Provincial Court, was removed in 1989 after pleading guilty to refusing the breathalyzer.[20] In 1988 the Chief Justice of the Manitoba Provincial Court, Harold Gyles, lost that position, while remaining as an ordinary judge of that court, after being acquitted of criminal charges in a traffic-ticket-fixing scandal; two other judges were given suspended sentences and resigned in this same affair.[21] Judge Raymond Barlett, of the Nova Scotia Family Court, was fired in 1987 — a first in that province — after upbraiding women who appeared before him for not being subservient to their husbands, as he declared the Bible required.[22] Several provincial court judges have resigned either after their removal has been recommended or in anticipation of a judicial council investigation. Judge Lloyd Henriksen, of the Ontario Provincial Court, resigned in 1985 after being recommended for dismissal, as did Judge Ronald MacDonald in Nova Scotia in 1989. One Quebec and two Ontario provincial court judges resigned during 1989-90 before formal investigations were held by respective judicial councils.

. . . . .

A vital contribution to the independence of the judiciary is made in the initial selection and appointment of jurists to serve on the bench.[23] Given the security of tenure and wide immunities of serving judges, it is critical that careful choices are made in staffing the judiciary. The appointment procedures across the country have come under much criticism because of the wide latitude governments have had in choosing new judges.[24] The main concern has been the extent to which political patronage has influenced the selection of judges; in the Maritime Provinces particular problems have been seen with respect to both federal appointments and provincially appointed judges.[25] Patronage poses three obvious problems: there is concern that partisans will favour their former political colleagues; that unsuitable individuals can be appointed to the bench because of their political connections; and that well-qualified candidates may never be appointed because they support the wrong party. These objections are compounded when one party has been in office for an extended period. A study by Peter Russell and Jacob Ziegel of the appointments made by the Mulroney government during its first term in office has revealed an alarming degree of political overtones. They found that 48 per cent of all the judges appointed in this period were known Conservative Party supporters, while only 7.1 per cent were known Opposition party supporters. The portion of Tory supporters soared to over 70 per cent of the judges appointed in Saskatchewan, Manitoba, and the

Maritimes.[26] In a study I have made of the 32 provincial judges appointed by the Nova Scotia Conservatives between 1979 and mid-1990, not one publicly identifiable Liberal was appointed and the only NDP partisan was an MLA who was appointed on the eve of a general election.

A related weakness could be perceived in the promotion of judges from one level of court to a higher bench. However, there appears to be little evidence that judges have tried to curry favour in order to be promoted, or that judges who have been elevated have favoured the government in their decisions. In fact there is merit in providing appellate courts with judges who have gained adjudicating experience in trial-level courts.[27] At present the federal government has an informal practice of consulting with both the Chief Justice and the Attorney General of the province involved before elevating any judge.[28] Unfortunately the research done by Russell and Ziegel casts an ominous shadow by revealing that 45.3 per cent of judges promoted by the first Mulroney government had once been Tory party supporters, while only 17.2 per cent had been known Opposition party supporters before their initial appointments to the bench.[29]

Fortunately there appears to be an increasing tendency among provincial governments to move to a more impartial selection process, which limits the discretion of the executive and establishes some means for assessing the professional qualifications of potential candidates. An important role has been given to the judicial councils in British Columbia, Alberta, Saskatchewan, Newfoundland, and the two Territories.[30] Since 1978 separate nominating committees have existed in Quebec to make an initial recommendation on candidates for judicial appointment, and a central nominating commission was also established in Ontario in 1988. Although few jurisdictions require it by statute, most appointments are now made only from lists of nominees approved by the judicial councils and nominating commissions.

The federal government has also changed its appointment procedures with the institution of committees in each province and territory to screen candidates and place them on a list of qualified persons from which the Minister of Justice will choose new appointees.[31] A similar procedure was also adopted in Nova Scotia in 1989, although that committee may also distinguish between qualified and highly qualified candidates. The difficulty with this arrangement is that the committees merely screen out the incompetent candidates and are unable to recommend which candidates are best suited to judicial careers. As a result, the ministers still have an unfettered discretion to choose, and there is no impediment to the continued play of partisan considerations in the actual selection of judges. The first six appointments made to the Nova Scotia Provincial Court under the new system all involved known government partisans; one person had not even been in the courtroom for twenty years before his appointment, and had practised real-estate law for much of this time.

Some developments in the appointment of judges, especially in Ontario, have gone a long way to promoting the institutional independence of the judiciary. It is to be hoped that the range of discretion remaining to the executive in other jurisdictions will be similarly restricted. Once the influence of partisan politics has been overcome, more attention can be focused on the experience, knowledge, and capabilities of candidates for judgeships. Too little attention has been paid to the attributes appointing authorities should look for in new judges, but an ability to approach issues with an open mind, and the self-discipline to examine competing claims dispassionately, are just two essential qualities. Judicial independence relies to a great extent on the personal qualities of those appointed to the bench.

The independence of the Canadian judiciary relies increasingly on entrenched constitutional provisions as well as on statute and case law. Nevertheless constitutional conventions continue to play an important role in modifying these legal rules. Although basic procedures for the removal of judges — preventing the summary removal of most judges — now exist in all jurisdictions in Canada, the essential reasons justifying any removal are still largely determined by informal understandings of the substance of impermissible behaviour. Furthermore, the interference by the executive or legislature in the determination of specific cases before the courts is prohibited largely by convention. Finally, the restrictions placed on the private and public behaviour of judges that prevent their off-bench intrusion into the political arena are also determined by convention.

The entrenchment of the principle of judicial independence in the Charter of Rights, however, has provided the impetus for a further spread of positive law to regulate this important aspect of the Canadian constitution. With the Supreme Court of Canada's decisions in *Beauregard* and *Valente*, we have had clear signals that the judiciary are fully prepared to chart the course to be followed in ensuring their own independence. I believe that these decisions foreshadow a potential shift in the political role of the judiciary, especially with respect to what control the elected representatives of the public may have held over it.

The independence of the judiciary essentially evolved in Britain during the eighteenth and nineteenth centuries. Its essence lay in the legal security of tenure of judges, as well as in the conventional prohibition against executive interference in the resolution of cases before the bar. However, elected politicians still remained in overall control. The doctrine of the sovereignty of Parliament ensured that the legislature could amend or overturn any decisions that ran counter to the general will of the electorate. Furthermore, the whole body politic retained control, through Cabinet and Parliament, over the general level of financial and administrative resources to be allocated to the justice system.

In Canada, however, with the indication by the courts that their financial and administrative independence are essential ingredients of any judicial independence, there is now the potential for a political battle to emerge between the judiciary and the other branches of government over just what resources are to be made available to the courts. This danger is well illustrated by the Quebec judges who boycotted their courtrooms in 1989 over their salaries, and by those Ontario judges who previously threatened strike action. One can foresee that the courts may eventually decide that their independence can be assured only when the judges are in control over the full range of physical and human resources involved in the judicial process. As Judge François Beaudoin, president of the Conference des juges du Québec, said: 'When you are reduced to begging for a decent salary, how can you be truly independent?'[32]

A long-term difficulty lies in the complete freedom of judges to interpret as they wish provisions of the Constitution relating to judicial independence. In its interpretation of s. 100 of the 1867 *Constitution Act* in *Beauregard*, the Supreme Court of Canada has already placed its own restrictions on the clear language giving Parliament the right to set salaries. The Court has also interpreted the Charter of Rights so that its provisions do not apply *in toto* to the judiciary — despite the fact that some sections make sense only if the courts are so included.[33] Furthermore, this freedom of interpretation with respect to the judicial function is seen in the Supreme Court of Canada's persistent willingness to restrict, for the benefit of the courts, the very clear language of legislation providing that 'any matter' may be put to the courts by executives as reference questions.[34]

The Canadian constitution has now effectively placed the courts as the ultimate definers of the requirements of judicial independence. And it is possible that the courts will gather to themselves, through constitutional interpretation, overall control of finanacial matters relating to the courts. But as a Vice-Chancellor of Britain has written:

> However important the system of justice may be, its demands have to be weighed against the competing demands of other public services. The question of how the available national resources are to be divided between the various functions of government is essentially a political question. Therefore, in the last resort, the amount of the total legal budget must be determined politically and controlled by Parliament.[35]

The essential protection against a judicial usurpation of the right of the legislative and executive branches of government to control the overall finances of the judiciary lies in the possibility of introducing amendments to the formal Constitution to overturn explicitly such interpretations made by the courts. Furthermore, s. 33 of the 1982 *Constitution Act* provides the legislature with the legal, though fading, power to enact legislation notwithstanding the provisions in the Charter concerning judicial independence. Even so, politicians would face considerable political resistance in trying to overturn pronouncements by appellate courts relating to the requirements of judicial independence. Survey research has indicated a fundamental reverence of the judiciary among Canadians. A 1989 Gallup Poll revealed that 59 per cent of the respondents had either 'a great deal' or 'quite a lot' of confidence in the Supreme Court of Canada, while only 33 per cent felt the same about the House of Commons.[36] In addition, a national survey conducted on public attitudes towards the Charter of Rights in Canada has revealed that more than 60 per cent of Canadians prefer the courts to be the final arbiters, rather than the legislatures, when a law is found to offend the Charter.[37]

Because of this veneration of the judiciary, it is extremely doubtful that a government would be able to exercise its ultimate legal option to overturn a court's declaration on judicial independence.

In the end, the independence of the judiciary and its place within the overall framework of Canadian government must depend on a respect for the constitutional conventions that modify the formal provisions of the constitution. So long as the executives and legislatures do not encroach on the courts in such a manner that the judiciary fear the loss of their essential independence in adjudication, the couts will no doubt continue to respect the rules that restrict their basic activities in resolving legal disputes. By the same token the judiciary must respect the rules that essentially limit judges to adjudication and exclude them from open political debate; if they do not, they risk the imposition of new laws that could restore the primacy of elected politicians over the appointed judicial branch of government. The Charter of Rights, however, has brought with it an increasingly political dimension to litigation that expands the reach of the judiciary.[38] It may become more important than ever in the future to appreciate the present conventions supporting judicial independence if judicial power ever challenges fundamentally the activities of the other branches of government.

Endnotes

1. For several critical views of the rule of law, see Allan C. Hutchinson and Patrick Monahan, eds., *The Rule of Law: Ideal or Ideology*, Toronto: Carswell, 1987.
2. *R. v. Beauregard*, [1986] 2 S.C.R. 56 at 72.
3. J.R. Mallory, *The Structure of Canadian Government* (rev. ed.), Toronto: Gage, 1984, pp. 314-19.
4. *Valente v. The Queen*, [1985] 2 S.C.R. 673 at 702.
5. *Charter of Human Rights and Freedoms*, S.Q. 1975, c. 6.
6. *Valente v. The Queen*, [1985] 2 S.C.R. 673 at 694.
7. *Ibid.*, at 698.
8. *Ibid.*, at 704.
9. *Ibid.*, at 709. For further discussions on administrative independence, see Jules Deschênes, *Masters in their Own House*, Ottawa: Canadian Judicial Council, 1981, pp. 140-60.
10. For modern discussions on the rule of law, see E.C.S. Wade and A.W. Bradley, *Constitutional and Administrative Law* (10th ed.), London: Longmans, 1985, ch. 6; Henri Brun and Guy Tremblay, *Droit Constitutionnel*, Cowansville: Editions Yvon Blais, 1982, pp. 476-82; F.L. Morton, ed., *Law, Politics and the Judicial Process in Canada*, Calgary: University of Calgary Press, 1984, ch. 1.

11. Such a two-pronged interpretation is favoured with respect to similar wording in British statutes by Harry Street and Rodney Brazier, eds., *De Smith's Constitutional and Administrative Law* (5th ed.), London: Penguin, 1987, p. 388.
12. Peter W. Hogg, *Constitutional Law of Canada* (2nd ed.), Toronto: Carswell, 1985, p. 139; J.R. Mallory, *The Structure of Canadian Government* (rev. ed.), Toronto: Gage, 1984, p. 318; Ronald I. Cheffins and Ronald N. Tucker, *The Constitutional Process in Canada* (2nd ed.), Toronto: McGraw-Hill Ryerson, 1976, p. 98.
13. William R. Lederman, 'The Independence of the Judiciary', *Canadian Bar Review* 34 (1956), 769 at pp. 786-7.
14. *Valente v. The Queen*, [1985] 2 S.C.R. 673 at 698.
15. *Carey v. Ontario*, [1986] 2 S.C.R. 637 at 673.
16. See Deschênes, op. cit., pp. 173-7; Peter H. Russell. *The Judiciary in Canada: The Third Branch of Government*, Toronto: McGraw-Hill Ryerson, 1987, pp. 178-81.
17. Gerald L. Gall, *The Canadian Legal System* (2nd ed.), Toronto: Carswell, 1983, p. 187.
18. *Ibid.*, pp. 187-8. The most recent instances occurred in 1933, and none have been removed since.
19. Gall lists only three examples of removal, in Ontario, and four instances in three provinces where provincial judges have resigned before they could be removed. *Ibid.*, pp. 188-9.
20. Toronto: *Globe and Mail*, 19 May 1989, p. A10.
21. Toronto: *Globe and Mail*, 20 August 1988, p. A4.
22. Toronto: *Globe and Mail*, 16 January 1987, p. A1.
23. For a comprehensive discussion on the appointment of judges, see Russell, op. cit., ch. 5.
24. Dawson, op. cit., pp. 403-4; Russell, op. cit., ch. 5; Mallory, op. cit., p. 332; Canadian Bar Association Committee on the Appointment of Judges in Canada, *The Appointment of Judges in Canada*, Ottawa: The Canadian Bar Foundation, 1985, ch. 6.
25. *Ibid.*, p. 57.
26. Peter H. Russell and Jacob S. Ziegel, 'Federal Judicial Appointments: An Appraisal of the First Mulroney Government's Appointments', paper presented to the Annual Meeting of the Canadian Political Science Association, Laval, Quebec, June 1989, p. 50 (on microfilm).
27. Russell, op. cit., pp. 135-7; Canadian Bar Association Committee, 'The Independence of the Judiciary', p. 44.
28. Department of Justice, op. cit., p. 13.

29. Russell and Ziegel, op. cit., p. 52.
30. See Russell, op. cit., pp. 127-9.
31. For a description of the federal system of appointment, see Department of Justice, op. cit., pp. 7-13.
32. Toronto: *Globe and Mail*, 12 July 1989, p. A4.
33. *Retail, Wholesale & Department Store Union, Local 580 et al. v. Dolphin Delivery*, [1986] 2 S.C.R. 573. For a concise criticism of this judgment, see Peter W. Hogg, 'The Dolphin Delivery Case: The Application of the Charter of Rights', *Saskatchewan Law Review* 51 (1987), p. 273.
34. John McEvoy, 'Separation of the Powers and the Reference Power: Is there a Right to Refuse?', *Supreme Court Law Review* 10 (1988), p. 428.
35. Nicolas Browne-Wilkinson, 'The Independence of the Judiciary in the 1980s', *Public Law* (1988), p. 54.
36. *Gallup*, Toronto: Gallup Canada Inc., 9 February 1989, p. 2.
37. Peter H. Russell, 'Canada's Charter of Rights and Freedoms: A Political Report', *Public Law* (1988), p. 398.
38. Michael Mandel, *The Charter of Rights and the Legalization of Politics in Canada*, Toronto: Wall & Thompson, 1989.

1.4 Federalism and Freedom of Expression

The *British North America Act* defined and gave legal sanction to Canada's political system and institutions. The Senate, the House of Commons, the offices of the Governor General and Lieutenants Governor, the legislatures of the federating provinces and the judiciary were authoritatively described.

Because Canada was to be a federation, the Act divided power between the federal Parliament and the provincial legislatures. Section 91 of the Act conferred on Parliament a general power to "make Laws for the Peace, Order and good Government of Canada" and enumerated 29 hearings under which the Parliament of Canada had "exclusive legislative authority". The headings were extensive and varied. They included such items as trade and commerce, postal services, marriage and divorce, money and banking, and criminal law.

Section 92 conferred on the legislatures the exclusive right to legislate in areas defined by 16 headings including direct taxation, municipal institutions, local works, property and civil rights and, as section 16 said, "Generally, all Matters of a merely local or private Nature in the Province".

The location of the boundary between the two jurisdictional territories may seem obvious from a plain reading of the document. It was carefully drafted. However, the legislative practices and ambitions of both levels of government led to disputes. It became the responsibility of the courts to draw that boundary. Constitutional law in Canada from 1867 until 1982, when the *Constitution Act, 1982* was approved, was composed mainly of the record of the adjudications by the Supreme Court of Canada and, until 1949, the Judicial Committee of the Privy Council, on the practical ambiguities of the *British North America Act*.

Until 1949 Canadian appeals could be taken to the Judicial Committee. Historians and constitutional lawyers in Canada have concluded from their studies that that court tilted the balance of power in the direction of the provincial legislatures and away from Parliament. However, as influential as the Judicial Committee once was, the procedures governing judicial review in cases involving sections 91 and 92 were established mainly by the Supreme Court of Canada. Typically, the Court would examine "the pith and substance" or "true intent" of contested legislation and then align it under the appropriate heading within section 91 or 92. If, for example, the legislature of a province passed a bill which appeared to regulate banks (sections 91(15) and (16)) but claimed that it was an appropriate exercise of the power to regulate property or a purely local matter (sections 92(10) and (13)), the Court would examine the bill and decide under which of the headings it properly belonged.

Curiously, the *Alberta Press Act* case which led to the first and perhaps most influential discussion in the Supreme Court of freedom of the press involved such issues. The Court ruled in 1938 that a bill to regulate part of the contents of Alberta's newspapers was not constitutional or *ultra vires* because it was interpreted to be part and parcel of an attempt by the province to impose a Social Credit economic scheme. The Court concluded that the legislative methods of constructing the scheme led to bills which invaded the jurisdiction of Parliament established in section 91. The Court went on to rule that "ancillary and dependent" legislation such as the *Press Act* was also unconstitutional.

Put differently, the pathway to the issue of freedom of expression in constitutional law under the *B.N.A. Act* required a first step around jurisdictional obstacles. The old statute did not provide for a direct and unambiguous legal route, although in the Quebec Padlock Law case, which was heard in the Supreme Court in 1957, the Court had an easier time of it.

The legislature of Quebec passed an *Act Respecting Communistic Propaganda* in 1937. When a case involving that statute was finally heard in the Supreme Court 20 years later, the Court ruled that the province had disguised its true purpose of making expressions of communist sentiment a crime — section 91(27) granted the right to pass criminal law to Parliament — by claiming a right to regulate the use of buildings under section 92(13) and 92(16). The Government of Quebec had simply padlocked houses and buildings in which left-wing propaganda was being produced and argued that their regulation of such buildings was akin to the regulation of brothels. The Court rejected that claim and located the statute's purpose and application in the federal parliament's jurisdiction. It was, accordingly, *ultra vires* the power of the legislature.

The *Alberta Press Act* case and the case of the Quebec Padlock Law demonstrate that the Court's power to rule on questions of freedom of expression under the *B.N.A. Act* was circumscribed. In order to rule on such questions the

Court had to deal first with the issue of jurisdiction. The *ratio* — that is, the reason for the decision in both cases — was necessarily based on a conclusion about the location of the boundary dividing the jurisdictions of the levels of government. The expressions from the bench about the importance of freedom of the press were uttered as *dicta* or non-binding observations. Still, the statements by Justices Rand and Duff in the *Alberta Press Act* and Quebec Padlock Law cases remain highly influential.

Although the *Canadian Charter of Rights and Freedoms* extends the scope of judicial review to substantive questions involving fundamental freedoms and civil liberties, the question of jurisdiction remains important. If, for example, the terms of a statute limiting freedom of the press were contested, the judges would ask first if the statute were legally enacted. In other words, before addressing questions of value, the Court would ask if Parliament, or a legislature, possessed the power to enact the disputed statute. The terms of the *Constitution Act, 1867*, remain an important source of constitutional law.

1.4.1 The *Constitution Act, 1867*

WHEREAS the Provinces of Canada, Nova Scotia and New Brunswick have expressed their Desire to be federally united into One Dominion under the Crown of the United Kingdom of Great Britain and Ireland, with a Constitution similar in Principle to that of the United Kingdom:

And whereas such a Union would conduce to the Welfare of the Provinces and promote the Interests of the British Empire:

And whereas on the Establishment of the Union by Authority of Parliament it is expedient, not only that the Constitution of the Legislative Authority in the Dominion be provided for, but also that the Nature of the Executive Government therein be declared:

And whereas it is expedient that Provision be made for the eventual Admission into the Union of other Parts of British North America:

91. It shall be lawful for the Queen, by and with the Advice and Consent of the Senate and House of Commons, to make Laws for the Peace, Order, and good Government of Canada, in relation to all Matters not coming within the Classes of Subjects by this Act assigned exclusively to the Legislatures of the Provinces; and for greater Certainty, but not so as to restrict the Generality of the foregoing Terms of this Section, it is hereby declared that (notwithstanding anything in this Act) the exclusive Legislative Authority of the Parliament of Canada extends to all Matters coming within the Classes of Subjects next hereinafter enumerated; that is to say, —

1. Repealed.
1A. The Public Debt and Property.
2. The Regulation of Trade and Commerce.
2A. Unemployment insurance.

3. The raising of Money by any Mode or System of Taxation.
4. The borrowing of Money on the Public Credit.
5. Postal Service.
6. The Census and Statistics.
7. Militia, Military and Naval Service, and Defence.
8. The fixing of and providing for the Salaries and Allowances of Civil and other Officers of the Government of Canada.
9. Beacons, Buoys, Lighthouses, and Sable Island.
10. Navigation and Shipping.
11. Quarantine and the Establishment and Maintenance of Marine Hospitals.
12. Sea Coast and Inland Fisheries.
13. Ferries between a Province and any British or Foreign Country or between Two Provinces.
14. Currency and Coinage.
15. Banking, Incorporation of Banks, and the Issue of Paper Money.
16. Savings Banks.
17. Weights and Measures.
18. Bills of Exchange and Promissory Notes.
19. Interest.
20. Legal Tender.
21. Bankruptcy and Insolvency.
22. Patents of Invention and Discovery.
23. Copyrights.
24. Indians, and Lands reserved for the Indians.
25. Naturalization and Aliens.
26. Marriage and Divorce.
27. The Criminal Law, except the Constitution of Courts of Criminal Jurisdiction, but including the Procedure in Criminal Matters.
28. The Establishment, Maintenance, and Management of Penitentiaries.
29. Such Classes of Subjects as are expressly excepted in the Enumeration of the Classes of Subjects by this Act assigned exclusively to the Legislatures of the Provinces.

And any Matter coming within any of the Classes of Subjects enumerated in this Section shall not be deemed to come within the Class of Matters of a local or private Nature comprised in the Enumeration of the Classes of Subjects by this Act assigned exclusively to the Legislatures of the Provinces.

92. In each Province the Legislature may exclusively make Laws in relation to Matters coming within the Classes of Subject next hereinafter enumerated; that is to say, —
1. Repealed.
2. Direct Taxation within the Province in order to the raising of a Revenue for Provincial Purposes.

3. The borrowing of Money on the sole Credit of the Province.
4. The Establishment and Tenure of Provincial Offices and the Appointment and Payment of Provincial Officers.
5. The Management and Sale of the Public Lands belonging to the Province and of the Timber and Wood thereon.
6. The Establishment, Maintenance, and Management of Public and Reformatory Prisons in and for the Province.
7. The Establishment, Maintenance, and Management of Hospitals, Asylums, Charities, and Eleemosynary Institutions in and for the Province, other than Marine Hospitals.
8. Municipal Institutions in the Province.
9. Shop, Saloon, Tavern, Auctioneer, and other Licences in order to the raising of a Revenue for Provincial, Local, or Municipal Purposes.
10. Local Works and Undertakings other than such as are of the following Classes: —
    (*a*) Lines of Steam or other Ships, Railways, Canals, Telegraphs, and other Works and Undertakings connecting the Province with any other or others of the Provinces, or extending beyond the Limits of the Province;
    (*b*) Lines of Steam Ships between the Province and any British or Foreign Country;
    (*c*) Such Works as, although wholly situate within the Province, are before or after their Execution declared by the Parliament of Canada to be for the general Advantage of Canada or for the Advantage of Two or more of the Provinces.
11. The Incorporation of Companies with Provincial Objects.
12. The Solemnization of Marriage in the Province.
13. Property and Civil Rights in the Province.
14. The Administration of Justice in the Province, including the Constitution, Maintenance, and Organization of Provincial Courts, both of Civil and of Criminal Jurisdiction, and including Procedure in Civil Matters in those Courts.
15. The Imposition of Punishment by Fine, Penalty, or Imprisonment for enforcing any Law of the Province made in relation to any Matter coming within any of the Classes of Subjects enumerated in this Section.
16. Generally all Matters of a merely local or private Nature in the Province.

Non-Renewable Natural Resources, Forestry Resources and Electrical Energy

92A. (1) In each province, the legislature may exclusively make laws in relation to

(a) exploration for non-renewable natural resources in the province;

(b) development, conservation and management of non-renewable natural resources and forestry resources in the province, including laws in relation to the rate of primary production therefrom; and

(c) development, conservation and management of sites and facilities in the province for the generation and production of electrical energy.

(2) In each province, the legislature may make laws in relation to the export from the province to another part of Canada of the primary production from non-renewable natural resources and forestry resources in the province and the production from facilities in the province for the generation of electrical energy, but such laws may not authorize or provide for discrimination in prices or in supplies exported to another part of Canada.

(3) Nothing in subsection (2) derogates from the authority of Parliament to enact laws in relation to the matters referred to in that subsection and, where such a law of Parliament and a law of a province conflict, the law of Parliament prevails to the extent of the conflict.

(4) In each province, the legislature may make laws in relation to the raising of money by any mode or system of taxation in respect of

(a) non-renewable natural resources and forestry resources in the province and the primary production therefrom, and

(b) sites and facilities in the province for the generation of electrical energy and the production therefrom.

whether or not such production is exported in whole or in part from the province, but such laws may not authorize or provide for taxation that differentiates between production exported to another part of Canada and production not exported from the province.

(5) The expression "primary production" has the meaning assigned by the Sixth Schedule.

(6) Nothing in subsections (1) to (5) derogates from any powers or rights that a legislature or government of a province had immediately before the coming into force of this section.

93. In and for each Province the Legislature may exclusively make Laws in relation to Education, subject and according to the following Provisions: —

(1) Nothing in any such Law shall prejudicially affect any Right or Privilege with respect to Denominational Schools which any Class of Persons have by Law in the Province at the Union:

(2) All the Powers, Privileges, and Duties at the Union by Law conferred and imposed in Upper Canada on the Separate Schools and School Trustees of the Queen's Roman Catholic Subjects shall be and the same are hereby extended to the Dissentient Schools of the Queen's Protestant and Roman Catholic Subjects in Quebec:

(3) Where in any Province a System of Separate or Dissentient Schools exists by Law at the Union or is thereafter established by the Legislature of the Province, an Appeal shall lie to the Governor General in Council from any Act or Decision of any Provincial Authority affecting any Right or Privilege of the Protestant or Roman Catholic Minority of the Queen's Subjects in relation to Education:

(4) In case any such Provincial Law as from Time to Time seems to the Governor General in Council requisite for the due Execution of the Provisions of this Section is not made, or in case any Decision of the Governor General in Council on any Appeal under this Section is not duly executed by the proper Provincial Authority in that Behalf, then and in every such Case, and as far only as the Circumstances of each Case require, the Parliament of Canada may make remedial Laws for the due Execution of the Provisions of this Section and of any Decision of the Governor General in Council under this Section.

133. Either the English or the French Language may be used by any Person in the Debates of the Houses of the Parliament of Canada and of the Houses of the Legislature of Quebec; and both those Languages shall be used in the respective Records and Journals of those Houses; and either of those Languages may be used by any Person or in any Pleading or Process in or issuing from any Court of Canada established under this Act, and in or from all or any of the Courts of Quebec.

The Acts of the Parliament of Canada and of the Legislature of Quebec shall be printed and published in both those Languages.

1.4.2 *Re Alberta Legislation*, [1938] 2 D.L.R. 81 (S.C.C.)

SIR LYMAN P. DUFF, C.J.C.:— The three Bills referred to us are part of a general scheme of legislation and in order to ascertain the object and effect of them it is proper to look at the history of the legislation passed in furtherance of the general design.

It is no part of our duty (it is, perhaps, needless to say) to consider the wisdom of these measures. We have only to ascertain whether or not they come within the ambit of the authority entrusted by the constitutional statutes (the *British North America Act* and the *Alberta Act*) to the Legislature of Alberta and our responsibility is rigorously confined to the determination of that issue. As Judges, we do not and cannot intimate any opinion upon the merits of the legislative proposals embodied in them, as to their practicability or in any other respect. . . .

We now turn to Bill No. 9.

This Bill contains two substantive provisions. Both of them impose duties upon newspapers published in Alberta which they are required to perform on the demand of "the Chairman," who is, by the interpretation clause, the Chairman of "the Board constituted by s. 3 of the *Alberta Social Credit Act*."

The Board, upon the acts of whose Chairman the operation of this statute depends, is, in point of law, a non-existent body (there is, in a word, no "board" in existence "constituted by section 3 of the *Alberta Social Credit Act*") and both of the substantive sections, ss. 3 and 4, are, therefore, inoperative. The same, indeed, may be said of ss. 6 and 7 which are the enactments creating sanctions. It appears to us, furthermore, that this Bill is a part of the general scheme of Social Credit legislation, the basis of which is the *Alberta Social Credit Act*; the Bill presupposes, as a condition of its operation, that the *Alberta Social Credit Act* is validly enacted; and, since that Act is *ultra vires*, the ancillary and dependent legislation must fall with it.

This is sufficient for disposing of the question referred to us but, we think, there are some further observations upon the Bill which may properly be made.

Under the constitution established by the *B.N.A. Act*, legislative power for Canada is vested in one Parliament consisting of the Sovereign, an upper house styled the Senate, and the House of Commons. Without entering in detail upon an examination of the enactments of the Act relating to the House of Commons, it can be said that these provisions manifestly contemplate a House of Commons which is to be, as the name itself implies, a representative body; constituted, that is to say, by members elected by such of the population of the united Provinces as may be qualified to vote. The preamble of the statute, moreover, shows plainly enough that the constitution of the Dominion is to be similar in principle to that of the United Kingdom. The statute contemplates a Parliament working under the influence of public opinion and public discussion. There can be no controversy that such institutions derive their efficacy from the free public discussion of affairs, from criticism and answer and counter-criticism, from attack upon policy and administration and defence and counter-attack; from the freest and fullest analysis and examination from every point of view of political proposals. This is signally true in respect of the discharge by Ministers of the Crown of their responsibility to Parliament, by members of Parliament of their duty to the electors and by the electors themselves of their responsibilities in the election of their representatives.

The right of public discussion is, of course, subject to legal restrictions; those based upon considerations of decency and public order, and others conceived for the protection of various private and public interests with which, for example, the laws of defamation and sedition are concerned. In a word, freedom of discussion means, to quote the words of Lord Wright in *James v. Commonwealth of Australia*, [1936] A.C. at p. 627, "freedom governed by law."

Even within its legal limits, it is liable to abuse and grave abuse, and such abuse is constantly exemplified before our eyes; but it is axiomatic that the practice of this right of free public discussion of public affairs, notwithstanding its incidental mischiefs, is the breath of life for parliamentary institutions.

We do not doubt that (in addition to the power of disallowance vested in the Governor General) the Parliament of Canada possesses authority to legislate for the protection of this right. That authority rests upon the principle that the powers requisite for the protection of the constitution itself arise by necessary implication from the *B.N.A. Act* as a whole (*Fort Frances Pulp & Paper Co. v. Manitoba Free Press Co.*, [1923] 3 D.L.R. 629); and since the subject matter in relation to which the power is exercised is not exclusively a provincial matter, it is necessarily vested in Parliament.

But this by no means exhausts the matter. Any attempt to abrogate this right of public debate or to suppress the traditional forms of the exercise of the right (in public meeting and through the press) would, in our opinion, be incompetent to the Legislatures of the Provinces, or to the Legislature of any one of the Provinces, as repugnant to the provisions of the *B.N.A. Act*, by which the Parliament of Canada is established as the legislative organ of the people of Canada under the Crown, and Dominion legislation enacted pursuant to the legislative authority given by those provisions. The subject matter of such legislation could not be described as a provincial matter purely; as in substance exclusively a matter of property and civil rights within the Province, or a matter private or local within the Province. It would not be, to quote the words of the judgment of the Judicial Committee in *Great West Saddlery Co. v. The King*, 58 D.L.R., at p. 26, legislation "directed solely to the purposes specified in s. 92;" and it would be invalid on the principles enunciated in that judgment and adopted in *Caron v. The King*, [1924] 4 D.L.R. 105, at pp. 109-10.

The question, discussed in argument, of the validity of the legislation before us, considered as a wholly independent enactment having no relation to the *Alberta Social Credit Act*, presents no little difficulty. Some degree of regulation of newspapers everybody would concede to the Provinces. Indeed, there is a very wide field in which the Provinces undoubtedly are invested with legislative authority over newspapers; but the limit, in our opinion, is reached when the legislation effects such a curtailment of the exercise of the right of public discussion as substantially to interfere with the working of the parliamentary institutions of Canada as contemplated by the provisions of the *B.N.A. Act* and the statutes of the Dominion of Canada. Such a limitation is necessary, in our opinion, "in order," to adapt the words quoted above from the judgment in *Bank of Toronto v. Lambe*, "to afford scope" for the working of such parliamentary institutions. In this region of constitutional practice, it is not permitted to a Provincial Legislature to do indirectly what cannot be done directly. *Great West Saddlery Co. v. The King*, 58 D.L.R., at p. 6.

Section 129 of the *B.N.A. Act* is in these words: —

"129. Except as otherwise provided by this Act, all Laws in force in Canada, Nova Scotia or New Brunswick at the Union, and all Courts of Civil and Criminal Jurisdiction, and all legal Commissions, Powers, and Authorities, and all Officers, Judicial, Administrative, and Ministerial, existing therein at the Union, shall continue in Ontario, Quebec, Nova Scotia, and New Brunswick respectively, as if the Union had not been made; subject nevertheless (except with respect to such as are enacted by or exist under Acts of the Parliament of Great Britain or of the Parliament of the United Kingdom of Great Britain and Ireland,) to be repealed, abolished, or altered by the Parliament of Canada, or by the Legislature of the respective Province, according to the Authority of the Parliament or of that Legislature under this Act."

The law by which the right of public discussion is protected existed at the time of the enactment of the *B.N.A. Act* and, as far as Alberta is concerned, at the date on which the *Alberta Act* came into force, the 1st of September, 1905. In our opinion (on the broad principle of the cases mentioned which has been recognized as limiting the scope of general words defining the legislative authority of the Dominion) the Legislature of Alberta has not the capacity under s. 129 to alter that law by legislation obnoxious to the principle stated.

The legislation now under consideration manifestly places in the hands of the Chairman of the Social Credit Commission autocratic powers which, it may well be thought, could, if arbitrarily wielded, be employed to frustrate in Alberta these rights of the Crown and the people of Canada as a whole. We do not, however, find it necessary to express an opinion upon the concrete question whether or not this particular measure is invalid as exceeding the limits indicated above.

The answer to the question concerning this Bill is that it is *ultra vires*.

. . . . .

CANNON, J.: . . . The third question put to us is the following:

Is Bill No. 9, entitled *"An Act to ensure the Publication of Accurate News and Information"* or any of the provisions thereof and in what particular or particulars or to what extent *intra vires* of the Legislature of the Province of Alberta?

The order-in-council represents that it has been and is the avowed object of the present Government of the Province of Alberta to inaugurate in the said Province a "new economic order" upon the principles or plan of the theory known as the "Social Credit;" and that the said Government has since secured the enactment of several statutes more or less related to the policy of effectuating the said object. The preamble of the bill, which I will hereafter call the Press bill recites that it is "expedient and in the public interest that the newspapers published in the Province should furnish to the people of the Province statements made by the authority of the Government of the Province as to the true and exact objects of the policy of the Government and as to the hindrances to or difficulties in achieving such objects to the end that the people may be informed with respect thereto."

Section 3 provides that any proprietor, editor, publisher or manager of any newspaper published in the Province shall, when required to do so by the Chairman of the Board constituted by s. 3 of the *Alberta Social Credit Act*, publish in that newspaper any statement furnished by the Chairman which has for its object the correction or amplification of any statement relating to any policy or activity of the Government of the Province published by that newspaper within the next preceding 21 days.

And s. 4 provides that the proprietor, etc., of any newspaper upon being required by the Chairman in writing shall within 24 hours after the delivery of the requirement "make a return in writing setting out every source from which any information emanated, as to any statement contained in any issue of the newspaper published within sixty days of the making of the requirement and the names, addresses and occupations of all persons by whom such information was furnished to the newspaper and the name and address of the writer of any editorial, article or news item contained in any such issue of the newspaper."

Section 5 denies any action for libel on account of the publication of any statement pursuant to the Act.

Section 6 enacts that in the event of a proprietor, etc., of any newspaper being guilty of any contravention of any of the provisions of the Act, the Lieutenant-Governor-in-Council, upon a recommendation of the Chairman, may by order prohibit, (*a*) the publication of such newspaper either for a definite time or until further order; (*b*) the publication in any newspaper of anything written by any person specified in the order; (*c*) the publication of any information emanating from any person or source specified in the order.

Section 7 provides for penalties for contraventions or defaults in complying with any requirement of the Act.

The policy referred to in the preamble of the Press Bill regarding which the people of the Province are to be informed from the Government standpoint, is undoubtedly the Social Credit policy of the Government. The administration of the Bill is in the hands of the Chairman of the Social Credit Board who is given complete and discretionary power by the Bill. "Social Credit," according to s. 2(*b*) of c. 3, 1937, 2nd sess., of the *Alberta Social Credit Amendment Act* is "the power resulting from the belief inherent within society that its individual members in association can gain the objectives they desire;" and the objectives in which the people of Alberta must have a firm and unshaken belief are the monetization of credit and the creation of a provincial medium of exchange instead of money to be used for the purposes of distributing to Albertans loans without interest, per capita dividends and discount rates to purchase goods from retailers. This free distribution would be based on the unused capacity of the industries and people of the Province of Alberta to produce goods and services, which capacity remains unused on account of the lack or absence of purchasing power in the consumers in the Province. The purchasing power would equal or absorb this hitherto unused capacity to produce goods and services by the issue of Treasury Credit certificates against a Credit Fund or provincial credit account established by the Commission each year representing the monetary value of this "unused capacity" — which is also called "Alberta credit."

It seems obvious that this kind of credit cannot succeed unless every one should be induced to believe in it and help it along. The word "credit" comes from the Latin: *credere*, to believe. It is, therefore, essential to control the sources of information of the people of Alberta, in order to keep them immune from any vacillation in their absolute faith in the plan of the Government. The Social Credit doctrine must become, for the people of Alberta, a sort of religious dogma of which a free and uncontrolled discussion is not permissible. The Bill aims to control any statement relating to any policy or activity of the Government of the Province and declares this object to be a matter of public interest. The Bill does not regulate the relations of the newspapers' owners with private individual members of the public, but deals exclusively with expressions of opinion by the newspapers concerning government policies and activities. The pith and substance of the Bill is to regulate the press of Alberta from the viewpoint of public policy by preventing the public from being misled or deceived as to any policy or activity of the Social Credit Government and by reducing any opposition to silence or bring upon it ridicule and public contempt.

I agree with the submission of the Attorney-General for Canada that this bill deals with the regulation of the press of Alberta, not from the viewpoint of private wrongs or civil injuries resulting from any alleged infringement or privation of civil rights which belong to individuals, considered as individuals, but from the viewpoint of public wrongs or crimes, i.e., involving a violation of the public rights and duties to the whole community, considered as a community, in its social aggregate capacity.

Do the provisions of this Bill, as alleged by the Attorney-General for Canada, invade the domain of criminal law and trench upon the exclusive legislative jurisdiction of the Dominion in this regard?

The object of an amendment of the criminal law, as a rule, is to deprive the citizen of the right to do that which, apart from the amendment, he could lawfully do. Sections 130 to 136 of the *Criminal Code* deal with seditious words and seditious publications; and s. 133 (as amended by 1930 (Can.), c. 11, s. 2) reads as follows:—

"No one shall be deemed to have a seditious intention only because he intends in good faith,—

"(*a*) to show that His Majesty has been misled or mistaken in his measures; or

"(*b*) to point out errors or defects in the government or constitution of the United Kingdom, or of any part of it, or of Canada or any province thereof, or in either House of Parliament of the United Kingdom or of Canada, or in any legislature, or in the administration of justice: or to excite His Majesty's subjects to attempt to procure, by lawful means, the alteration of any matter in the state; or,

"(*c*) to point out, in order to their removal, matters which are producing or have a tendency to produce feelings of hatred and ill-will between different classes of His Majesty's subjects."

It appears that in England, at first, criticism of any Government policy was regarded as a crime involving severe penalties and punishable as such; but since the passing of Fox's *Libel Act* in 1792, the considerations now found in the above article of our *Criminal Code* that it is not criminal to point out errors in the Government of the country and to urge their removal by lawful means have been admitted as a valid defence in a trial for libel.

Now, it seems to me that the Alberta Legislature by this retrograde Bill is attempting to revive the old theory of the crime of seditious libel by enacting penalties, confiscation of space in newspapers and prohibitions for actions which, after due consideration by the Dominion Parliament, have been declared innocuous and which, therefore, every citizen of Canada can do lawfully and without hindrance or fear of punishment. It is an attempt by the Legislature to amend the *Criminal Code* in this respect and to deny the advantage of s. 133(A) to the Alberta newspaper publishers.

Under the British system, which is ours, no political party can erect a prohibitory barrier to prevent the electors from getting information concerning the policy of the Government. Freedom of discussion is essential to enlighten public opinion in a democratic State; it cannot be curtailed without affecting the right of the people to be informed through sources independent of the Government concerning matters of public interest. There must be an untrammelled publication of the news and political opinions of the political parties contending for ascendancy. As stated in the preamble of the *British North America Act*, our constitution is and will remain, unless radically changed, "similar in principle to that of the United Kingdom." At the time of Confederation, the United Kingdom was a democracy. Democracy cannot be maintained without its foundation: free public opinion and free discussion throughout the nation of all matters affecting the State within the limits set by the *Criminal Code* and the common law. Every inhabitant in Alberta is also a citizen of the Dominion. The Province may deal with his property and civil rights of a local and private nature within the Province; but the Province cannot interfere with his status as a Canadian citizen and his fundamental right to express freely his untrammelled opinion about Government policies and discuss matters of public concern. The mandatory and prohibitory provisions of the Press Bill are, in my opinion, *ultra vires* of the Provincial Legislature. They interfere with the free working of the political organization of the Dominion. They have a tendency to nullify the political rights of the inhabitants of Alberta, as citizens of Canada, and cannot be considered as dealing with matters purely private and local in that Province. The Federal Parliament is the sole authority to curtail, if deemed expedient and in the public interest, the freedom of the press and the equal rights in that respect of all citizens throughout the Dominion. These subjects were matters of criminal law before Confederation, have been recognized by Parliament as criminal matters and have been expressly dealt with by the *Criminal Code*. No Province has the power to reduce in that Province the political rights of its citizens as compared with those enjoyed by the citizens of other Provinces of Canada. Moreover, citizens outside the Province of Alberta have a vital interest in having full information and comment, favourable and unfavourable, regarding the policy of the Alberta Government and concerning events in that Province which would, in the ordinary course, be the subject of Alberta newspapers' news items and articles.

I would, therefore, answer the question as to Bill No. 9 in the negative.

1.4.3 *Switzman v. Elbling and Attorney-General of Quebec*, [1957] S.C.R. 285 (S.C.C.)

KERWIN, C.J.: This appeal was brought by John Switzman pursuant to leave granted by the Court of Queen's Bench (Appeal Side) for the Province of Quebec from its judgment [[1954] Que. Q.B. 421] confirming that of the Superior Court cancelling and annulling a certain lease between the plaintiff, Freda Elbling, and the defendant Switzman and maintaining the intervention of the Attorney-General of the Province of Quebec and declaring *An Act to Protect the Province against Communistic Propaganda*, R.S.Q. 1941, c. 52, to be *intra vires* of the Legislature of the Province of Quebec. It is quite true that if no *lis* exists between parties this Court will decline to hear an appeal, even though leave has been granted by a provincial Court of Appeal: *Coca-Cola Co. of Can. Ltd. v. Mathews*, [1944] S.C.R. 385, [1945] 1 D.L.R. 1, where the earlier cases are collected. While, in the present case, it is suggested that the time has elapsed when the appellant had any interest in the lease to him from Freda Elbling, and therefore as between those two parties it is argued that there was nothing left in dispute except the questions of costs, the intervention of the Attorney-General of the Province of Quebec, pursuant to Art. 114 of the Quebec Code of Civil Procedure, raises an issue between him and the present appellant as to the constitutionality of the statute mentioned....

Section 1 provides: "This Act may be cited as *Act* Respecting Communistic Propaganda."

Sections 3 and 12 read:

3. It shall be illegal for any person, who possesses or occupies a house within the Province, to use it or allow any person to make use of it to propagate communism or bolshevism by any means whatsoever.

12. It shall be unlawful to print, to publish in any manner whatsoever or to distribute in the Province any newspaper, periodical, pamphlet, circular, document or writing whatsoever propagating or tending to propagate communism or bolshevism.

Sections 4 to 11 provide that the Attorney-General, upon satisfactory proof that an infringement of s. 3 has been committed, may order the closing of the house; authorize any Peace Officer to execute such order and provide a procedure by which the owner may apply by petition to a Judge of the Superior Court to have the order revised. Section 13 provides for imprisonment of anyone infringing or participating in the infringement of s. 12. In my opinion it is impossible to separate the provisions of ss. 3 and 12.

The validity of the statute was attacked upon a number of grounds, but, in cases where constitutional issues are involved, it is important that nothing be said that is unnecessary. In my view it is sufficient to declare that the Act is legislation in relation to the criminal law over which, by virtue of head 27 of s. 91 of the *B.N.A. Act*, the Parliament of Canada has exclusive legislative authority. The decision of this court in *Bédard v. Dawson & A.-G. Que.*, [1923] S.C.R. 681, 4 D.L.R. 293, 40 Can. C.C. 404, is clearly distinguishable. As Mr. Justice Barclay points out, the real object of the Act here under consideration is to prevent propagation of Communism within the Province and to punish anyone who does so — with provisions authorizing steps for the closing of premises used for such object. The *Bédard* case was concerned with the control and enjoyment of property. I am unable to agree with the decision of Greenshields C.J. in *Fineberg v. Taub* (1939), 77 Que. S.C. 233, [1940] 1 D.L.R. 114, 73 Can. C.C. 37. It is not necessary to refer to other authorities, because, once the conclusion is reached that the pith and substance of the impugned Act is in relation to criminal law, the conclusion is inevitable that the Act is unconstitutional.

The appeal should be allowed . . .

TASCHEREAU, J. (dissenting) (translation): . . . There can be no doubt that by virtue of s. 91 of the *B.N.A. Act* (head 27), criminal law is a matter within the federal authority, and upon which it has exclusive power to legislate. And in a case such as this, the theory of the "unoccupied field" cannot find its application, and cannot justify a provincial Legislature to assume a right which is barred by the Constitution itself; *Fisheries Case [A.-G. Can. v. A.-G. Ont., Que. & N.S.]*, [1898] A.C. 700 at 715; *Reference re Debt Adjustment Act, 1937 (Alta.), A.-G. Alta. v. A.-G. Can.*, [1943] A.C. 356 at 370, 2 D.L.R. 1 at 8-9.

The appellant contends that this legislation is exclusively within the domain of the criminal law, and that consequently it is without the legislative competency of the provincial authority. I would willingly agree with him, if the Legislature had enacted that Communism was a crime punishable by law, because there would then be clearly an encroachment on the federal domain, which would make the legislation *ultra vires* of the Province. But such is not the case that we have before us. The Legislature did not say that any act constituted a crime, and it did not confer the character of criminality upon the Communistic doctrine. If the provincial Legislature has no power to create criminal offences, it has the right to legislate to prevent crimes, disorders, as treason, sedition, illegal public meetings, which are crimes under the *Criminal Code*, and to prevent conditions calculated to favour the development of crime. In order to achieve its aims, I entertain no doubt that it may validly legislate as to the possession and use of property, as this is exclusively within the domain of civil law, and is by virtue of s. 92 of the *B.N.A. Act* (head 13) within the provincial competency . . .

I am clearly of opinion that if a Province may validly legislate on all civil matters in relation to criminal law, *that if it may enact laws calculated to suppress conditions favouring the development of crime*, and control properties in order to protect society against any illegal uses that may be made of them, if it has the undeniable right to supervise brokers in their financial transactions in order to protect the public against fraud, if, finally, it has the right to impose civil incapacities as a consequence of a criminal offence, I cannot see why it could not also have the power to enact that all those who extol doctrines, calculated to incite to treason, to the violation of official secrets, to sedition, etc., should be deprived of the enjoyment of the properties from where are spread these theories, the object of which is to undermine and overthrow the established order.

Experience, and it is within our power to take judicial notice of it, teaches us that Canadians, less than 10 years ago, in violation of their oath of allegiance, did not hesitate for the sake of Communism, to reveal official secrets and thus imperil the security of the state. The suppression of the spreading of these subversive doctrines by civil sanctions is, to my mind, as important as the suppression of disorderly houses. I remain convinced that the domain of criminal law, exclusively of federal competency, has not been encroached upon by the impugned legislation, and that *the latter merely establishes civil sanctions for the prevention of crime and the security of the country.*

It has also been contended that this legislation constituted an obstacle to the liberty of the press and the liberty of speech. I believe in those fundamental liberties: they are undeniable rights which, fortunately, the citizens of this country enjoy, but these liberties would cease to be a right and become a privilege, if it were permitted to certain individuals to misuse them in order to propagate dangerous doctrines that are necessarily conducive to violations of the established order. These liberties, which citizens and the press enjoy of expressing their beliefs, their thoughts and their doctrines without previous authorization or censure, do not constitute absolute rights. They are necessarily limited and must be exercised within the bounds of legality. When these limits are overstepped, these liberties become abusive, and the law must then necessarily intervene to exercise a repressive control in order to protect the citizens and society.

The same reasoning must serve to meet the objection raised by the appellant, to the effect that the impugned law is an obstacle to the free expression of all individuals, candidates in an election. Destructive ideas of social order and of established authority by dictatorial methods, do not have more rights in electoral periods than in any other times. In the minds of many, this law may appear rigid (it is not within my province to judge of its wisdom), but the severity of a law adopted by a competent power, does not brand it with unconstitutionality . . .

RAND, J.: The first ground on which the validity of s. 3 is supported is head 13 of s. 92 of the *B.N.A. Act*, "Property in the Province" and Mr. Beaulieu's contention goes in this manner: by that head the Province is vested with unlimited legislative power over property; it may, for instance, take land without compensation and generally may act as amply as if it were a sovereign state, untrammelled by constitutional limitation. The power being absolute can be used as an instrument or means to effect any purpose or object. Since the objective accomplishment under the statute here is an act on property, its validity is self-evident and the question is concluded.

I am unable to agree that in our federal organization power absolute in such a sense resides in either Legislature. The detailed distribution made by ss. 91 and 92 places limits to direct and immediate purposes of provincial action. Under head 13 the purpose would, in general, be a "property" purpose either primary or subsidiary to another head of the same section. If such a purpose is foreign to powers vested in the Province by the Act, it will invade the field of the Dominion. For example, land could not be declared forfeited or descent destroyed by attainder on conviction of a crime, nor could the convicted person's right of access to provincial Courts be destroyed. These would trench upon both criminal law and citizenship status. The settled principle that calls for a determination of the "real character", the "pith and substance", of what purports to be enacted and whether it is "colourable" or is intended to effect its ostensible object, means that the true nature of the legislative act, its substance in purpose, must lie within s. 92 or some other endowment of provincial power. That a power ostensibly as here under a specific head cannot be exercised as a means directly and immediately to accomplish a purpose not within that endowment is demonstrated by the following decisions of the Judicial Committee: *Union Colliery Co. of B.C. Ltd. v. Bryden*, [1899] A.C. 580 holding that legislative power in relation to employment in a coal mine could not be used as a means of nullifying the civil capacities of citizenship and, specifically, of persons qualifying under head 25 of s. 91, Naturalization and Aliens; *Reference re Validity of Section 5(a) of Dairy Industry Act, Can. Federation of Agriculture v. A.-G. Que.*, [1951] A.C. 179 [1950] 4 D.L.R., 689, holding that the Dominion, under its power in relation to criminal law, could not prohibit the manufacture of margarine for the purpose of benefiting in local trade one class of producer as against another. The heads of ss. 91 and 92 are to be read and interpreted with each other and with the provisions of the statute as a whole, and what is then exhibited is a pattern of limitations, curtailments and modifications of legislative scope within a texture of interwoven and interacting powers.

In support of the legislation on this ground, *Bédard v. Dawson*, [1923] S.C.R. 681, 4 D.L.R. 293, 40 Can. C.C. 404, was relied on. In that case the statute provided that it should be illegal for the owner or occupier of any house or building to use or allow it to be used as a disorderly house; and procedure was provided by which the Superior Court could, after a conviction under the Criminal Code, grant an injunction against the owner restraining that use of it. If the use continued, the Court could order the building to be closed for a period of not more than one year.

This power is seen to have been based upon a conviction for maintaining a public nuisance. Under the public law of England which underlies that of all the Provinces, such an act was not only a matter for indictment but in a civil aspect the Court could enjoin its continuance. The essence of this aspect is its repugnant or prejudicial effect upon the neighbouring inhabitants and properties.

On that view this Court proceeded in *Bédard* . . .

That the scene of study, discussion or dissemination of views or opinions on any matter has ever been brought under legal sanction in terms of nuisance is not suggested. For the past century and a half in both the United Kingdom and Canada, there has been a steady removal of restraints on this freedom, stopping only at perimeters where the foundation of the freedom itself is threatened. Apart from sedition, obscene writings and criminal libels, the public law leaves the literary, discursive and polemic use of language, in the broadest sense, free.

The object of the legislation here, as expressed by the title, is admittedly to prevent the propagation of Communism and Bolshevism, but it could just as properly have been the suppression of any other political, economic or social doctrine or theory; and the issue is whether that object is a matter "in relation to which" under s. 92 the Province may exclusively make laws. Two heads of the section are claimed to authorize it: head 13, as a matter of "Civil Rights", and head 16, "Local and Private Matters".

Mr. Tremblay in a lucid argument treated such a limitation of free discussion and the spread of ideas generally as in the same category as the ordinary civil restrictions of libel and slander. These obviously affect the matter and scope of discussion to the extent that it trenches upon the rights of individuals to reputation and standing in the community; and the line at which the restraint is drawn is that at which public concern for the discharge of legal or moral duties and government through rational persuasion, and that for private security, are found to be in rough balance.

But the analogy is not a true one. The ban is directed against the freedom or civil liberty of the actor; no civil right of anyone is affected nor is any civil remedy created. The aim of the statute is, by means of penalties, to prevent what is considered a poisoning of men's minds, to shield the individual from exposure to dangerous ideas, to protect him, in short, from his own thinking propensities. There is nothing of civil rights in this; it is to curtail or proscribe these freedoms which the majority so far consider to be the condition of social cohesion and its ultimate stabilizing force.

It is then said that the ban is a local matter under head 16; that the social situation in Quebec is such that safeguarding its intellectual and spiritual life against subversive doctrines becomes a special need in contrast with that for a general regulation by Parliament. A similar contention was made in the *Reference re Saskatchewan Farm Security Act, 1944, Section 6*, [1947] S.C.R. 394, 3 D.L.R. 689, affirmed in the Judicial Committee [*sub nom. A.-G. Sask. v. A.-G. Can.*], [1949] A.C. 110, 2 D.L.R. 145. What was dealt with there was the matter of interest on mortgages and a great deal of evidence to show the unique vicissitudes of farming in that Province was adduced. But there, as here, it was and is obvious that local conditions of that nature, assuming, for the purpose of the argument only, their existence, cannot extend legislation to matters which lie outside of s. 92.

Indicated by the opening words of the preamble in the Act of 1867, reciting the desire of the four Provinces to be united in a federal union with a Constitution "similar in Principle to that of the United Kingdom", the political theory which the Act embodies is that of parliamentary Government, with all its social implications, and the provisions of the statute elaborate that principle in the institutional apparatus which they create or contemplate. Whatever the deficiencies in its workings, Canadian Government is in substance the will of the majority expressed directly or indirectly through popular assemblies. This means ultimately government by the free public opinion of an open society, the effectiveness of which, as events have not infrequently demonstrated, is undoubted.

But public opinion, in order to meet such a responsibility, demands the condition of a virtually unobstructed access to and diffusion of ideas. Parliamentary Government postulates a capacity in men, acting freely and under self-restraints, to govern themselves; and that advance is best served in the degree achieved of individual liberation from subjective as well as objective shackles. Under that Government, the freedom of discussion in Canada, as a subject-matter of legislation, has a unity of interest and significance extending equally to every part of the Dominion. With such dimensions it is *ipso facto* excluded from head 16 as a local matter.

This constitutional fact is the political expression of the primary condition of social life, thought and its communication by language. Liberty in this is little less vital to man's mind and spirit than breathing is to his physical existence. As such an inherence in the individual it is embodied in his status of citizenship. Outlawry, for example, divesting civil standing and destroying citizenship, is a matter of Dominion concern. Of the fitness of this order of Government to the Canadian organization, the words of Taschereau J. in *Brassard v. Langevin* (1877), 1 S.C.R. 145 at 195 should be recalled: "The object of the electoral law was to promote, by means of the ballot, and with the absence of all undue influence, the free and sincere expression of public opinion in the choice of members of the Parliament of Canada. This law is the just sequence to the excellent institutions which we have borrowed from England, institutions which, as regards civil and religious liberty, leave to Canadians nothing to envy in other countries."

Prohibition of any part of this activity as an evil would be within the scope of criminal law, as ss. 60, 61 and 62 of the *Criminal Code* dealing with sedition exemplify. Bearing in mind that the endowment of parliamentary institutions is one and entire for the Dominion, that Legislatures and Parliament are permanent features of our constitutional structure, and that the body of discussion is indivisible, apart from the incidence of criminal law and civil rights, and incidental effects of legislation in relation to other matters, the degree and nature of its regulation must await future consideration; for the purposes here it is sufficient to say that it is not a matter within the regulation of a Province.

Mr. Scott, in his able examination of the questions raised, challenged also the validity of ss. 4 *et seq.* which vest in the Attorney-General the authority to adjudicate upon the commission of the illegal act under s. 3 and to issue the order of closure; but in view of the conclusions reached on the other grounds, the consideration of this becomes unnecessary.

I would, therefore, allow the appeal, set aside the judgments below, dismiss the action and direct a declaration on the intervention that the statute in its entirety is *ultra vires* of the Province. The appellant will be entitled to the costs of the action in the Superior Court against the respondent Elbling and the costs occasioned by the intervention in all courts against the Attorney-General.

CARTWRIGHT, J.: The question in this appeal is whether c. 52 of R.S.Q. 1941, formerly c. 11 of the Statutes of Quebec, 1937, entitled *An Act to Protect the Province against Communistic Propaganda*, hereinafter referred to as the Act, is *intra vires* of the Legislature. The relevant circumstances and the nature of the arguments addressed to us sufficiently appear in the reasons of other members of the Court.

In my opinion the Act is invalid *in toto*, as being in pith and substance legislation in relation to the criminal law, a matter assigned by s. 91, head 27, of The B.N.A. Act to the exclusive legislative authority of the Parliament of Canada.

The nature and purpose of the legislation clearly appear from the words of the Act. The propagation of Communism or Bolshevism is regarded as an evil and such propagation, by any means whatsoever in a house within the Province and by any writing whatsoever elsewhere in the Province, is forbidden under punitive sanctions.

The circumstance that the penalty prescribed for a breach of the provisions of s. 3 is the closing of a house within the Province has not the effect of making the enactment one in relation to property and civil rights in the Province, and I find myself unable to relate the Act to any provincial purpose falling within heads 13 or 16 of s. 92 of the *B.N.A. Act*. The purpose and effect of the Act are to make criminal the propagation of Communism or Bolshevism which the Legislature in the public interest intends to prohibit. It is legislation in relation to what is conceived to be a public evil not in relation to civil rights or local matters.. . .

ABBOTT, J.: . . . The first question to be determined is whether the impugned legislation, in pith and substance, deals with the use of real property or with the propagation of ideas. As Mr. Scott put it to us in his very able argument: (1) the *motive* of this legislation is dislike of Communism as being an evil and subversive doctrine, motive of course, being something with which the courts are not concerned; (2) the *purpose* is clearly the suppression of the propagation of Communism in the Province and (3) one *means* provided for effecting such suppression is denial of the use of a house.

In my opinion the Act does not create two illegalities which are separate and independent, as was suggested to us by Mr. Beaulieu, it creates only one, namely, the propagation of Communism in the Province. Both s. 3 and s. 12 are directed to the same purpose, namely, the suppression of Communism, although different means are provided to achieve that end. The whole Act constitutes one legislative scheme and in my opinion its provisions are not severable.

Since in my view the true nature and purpose of the *Padlock Act* is to suppress the propagation of Communism in the Province, the next question which must be answered is whether such a measure, aimed at suppressing the propagation of ideas within a Province, is within the legislative competence of such Province.

The right of free expression of opinion and of criticism, upon matters of public policy and public administration, and the right to discuss and debate such matters, whether they be social, economic or political, are essential to the working of a parliamentary democracy such as ours. Moreover, it is not necessary to prohibit the discussion of such matters, in order to protect the personal reputation or the private rights of the citizen. That view was clearly expressed by Duff C.J.C. in *Re Alberta Legislation*, [1938] S.C.R. 100 at 132-4, 2 D.L.R. 81 at 107-8, ...: [For Duff's words, see s. 1.34.2.]

The *Canada Elections Act*, R.S.C. 1952, c. 23, the provisions of the *B.N.A. Act* which provide for Parliament meeting at least once a year and for the election of a new Parliament at least every 5 years, and the *Senate and House of Commons Act*, R.S.C. 1952, c. 249, are examples of enactments which make specific statutory provision for ensuring the exercise of this right of public debate and public discussion. Implicit in all such legislation is the right of candidates for Parliament or for a Legislature, and of citizens generally, to explain, criticize, debate and discuss in the freest possible manner such matters as the qualifications, the policies, and the political, economic and social principles advocated by such candidates or by the political parties or groups of which they may be members.

This right cannot be abrogated by a provincial Legislature, and the power of such Legislature to limit it, is restricted to what may be necessary to protect purely private rights, such as for example provincial laws of defamation. It is obvious that the impugned statute does not fall within that category. It does not, in substance, deal with matters of property and civil rights or with a local or private matter within the Province and in my opinion is clearly *ultra vires*. Although it is not necessary, of course, to determine this question for the purposes of the present appeal, the Canadian Constitution being declared to be similar in principle to that of the United Kingdom, I am also of opinion that as our constitutional Act now stands, Parliament itself could not abrogate this right of discussion and debate. The power of Parliament to limit it is, in my view, restricted to such powers as may be exercisable under its exclusive legislative jurisdiction with respect to criminal law and to make laws for the peace, order and good Government of the nation.

For the reasons which I have given, I would allow the appeal . . .

1.4.4 *Re Nova Scotia Board of Censors and McNeil* (1978), 84 D.L.R. (3d) 1 (S.C.C.)

RITCHIE, J.: The respondent's application was for a declaration that certain sections of the *Theatres and Amusements Act*, R.S.N.S. 1967, c. 304, as amended, and certain Regulations made thereunder were *ultra vires* and beyond the legislative competence of the Province of Nova Scotia.

The exciting cause of the application appears to have been the exercise by the Nova Scotia Amusements Regulation Board (hereinafter referred to as "the Board") of the authority which the Act purports to confer on it, to prevent a film entitled "Last Tango in Paris" from being exhibited in the theatres of Nova Scotia.

It is the statutory provisions purporting to authorize the Board to regulate and control the film industry within the Province of Nova Scotia according to standards fixed by it, which are challenged by the respondent on the ground that the citizens of Nova Scotia are thereby denied, on moral grounds, their right to exercise their freedom of choice in the viewing of films and theatre performances which might otherwise be available to them, and it is further alleged that the legislation constitutes an invasion of fundamental freedoms...

In all such cases the Court cannot ignore the rule implicit in the proposition stated as early as 1878 by Mr. Justice Strong in *Severn v. The Queen*, 2 S.C.R. 70 at p. 103, that any question as to the validity of provincial legislation is to be approached on the assumption that it was validly enacted...

When the Act and the Regulations are read as a whole, I find that to be primarily directed to the regulation, supervision and control of the film business within the Province of Nova Scotia, including the use and exhibition of films in that Province. To this end the impugned provisions are, in my view, enacted for the purpose of reinforcing the authority vested in a provincially appointed Board to perform the task of regulation which includes the authority to prevent the exhibition of films which the Board, applying its own local standards, has rejected as unsuitable for viewing by provincial audiences. This legislation is concerned with dealings in and the use of property (*i.e.*, films) which take place wholly within the Province and in my opinion it is subject to the same considerations as those which were held to be applicable in such cases as *Shannon et al. v. Lower Mainland Dairy Products Board et al.*, [1938] 4 D.L.R. 81, [1938] A.C. 708, [1938] 2 W.W.R. 604; *Home Oil Distributors Ltd. et al. v. A.-G. B.C.*, [1940] 2 D.L.R. 609, [1940] S.C.R. 444, and *Caloil Inc. v. A.-G. Can. et al.* (1971), 20 D.L.R. (3d) 472, [1971] S.C.R. 543, [1971] 4 W.W.R. 37...

It will be seen that, in my opinion, the impugned legislation constitutes nothing more than the exercise of provincial authority over transactions taking place wholly within the Province and it applies to the "regulating, exhibition, sale and exchange of films" whether those films have been imported from another country or not.

We are concerned, however, in this appeal with a decision of the Appeal Division of the Supreme Court of Nova Scotia in which the majority quite clearly struck down the legislation as *ultra vires* on the sole ground that it was concerned with morality and as such constituted an invasion of the criminal law field reserved to the exclusive legislative authority of Parliament under s. 91(27) of the *British North America Act, 1867*...

Although no reasons were given by the board for the rejection of "Last Tango in Paris", all members of the Appeal Division, were satisfied that its exhibition was prohibited on moral grounds and under all the circumstances I think it to be apparent that this was the case. In any event, I am satisfied that the Board is clothed with authority to fix its own local standards of morality in deciding whether a film is to be rejected or not for local viewing.

Simply put, the issue raised by the majority opinion in the Appeal Division is whether the Province is clothed with authority under s. 92 of the *British North America Act, 1867* to regulate the exhibition and distribution of films within its own boundaries which are considered unsuitable for local viewing by a local board on grounds of morality or whether this is a matter of criminal law reserved to Parliament under s. 91(27)...

Under the authority assigned to it by s. 92(27), the Parliament of Canada has enacted the *Criminal Code*, a penal statute the end purpose of which is the definition and punishment of crime when it has been proved to have been committed.

On the other hand, the *Theatres and Amusements Act* is not concerned with creating a criminal offence or providing for its punishment, but rather in so regulating a business within the Province as to prevent the exhibition in its theatres of performances which do not comply with the standards of propriety established by the Board.

The areas of operation of the two statutes are therefore fundamentally different on dual grounds. In the first place, one is directed to regulating a trade or business where the other is concerned with the definition and punishment of crime; and in the second place, one is preventive while the other is penal.

As the decision of the Appeal Division depends upon equating morality with criminality, I think it desirable at this stage to refer to the definitive statement made by Lord Atkin in this regard in the course of his reasons for judgment in *Proprietary Articles Trade Ass'n v. A.-G. Can.*, [1931] 2 D.L.R. 1 at pp. 9-10, 55 C.C.C. 241, [1931] A.C. 310 at p. 324, where he said:

> Morality and criminality are far from co-extensive; nor is the sphere of criminality necessarily part of a more extensive field covered by morality — unless the moral code necessarily disapproves all acts prohibited by the State, in which case the argument moves in a circle. It appears to their Lordships to be of little value to seek to confine crimes to a category of acts which by their very nature belong to the domain of "criminal jurisprudence"...

I share the opinion expressed in this passage that morality and criminality are far from co-extensive and it follows in my view that legislation which authorizes the establishment and enforcement of a local standard of morality in the exhibition of films is not necessarily "an invasion of the federal criminal field" as Chief Justice MacKeigan thought it to be in this case...

As I have already said, however, I take the view that the impugned legislation is not concerned with criminality. The rejection of films by the Board is based on a failure to conform to the standards of propriety which it has itself adopted and this failure cannot be said to be "an act prohibited with penal consequences" by the Parliament of Canada either in enacting the *Criminal Code* or otherwise. This is not to say that Parliament is in any way restricted in its authority to pass laws penalizing immoral acts or conduct, but simply that the provincial Government in regulating a local trade may set its own standards which in no sense exclude the operation of the federal law.

There is, in my view, no constitutional barrier preventing the Board from rejecting a film for exhibition in Nova Scotia on the sole ground that it fails to conform to standards of morality which the Board itself has fixed notwithstanding the fact that the film is not offensive to any provision of the *Criminal Code*; and, equally, there is no constitutional reason why a prosecution cannot be brought under s. 163 of the *Criminal Code* in respect of the exhibition of a film which the Board of Censors has approved as conforming to its standards of propriety...

It will be seen that in my view the impugned legislation "has for its true object, purpose, nature and character" the regulation and control of a local trade and that it is therefore valid provincial legislation...

As I have said, I take the view that the legislation here in question is, in pith and substance, directed to property and civil rights and therefore valid under s. 92(13) of the *British North America Act, 1867* but there is a further and different ground on which its validity might be sustained. In a country as vast and diverse as Canada, where tastes and standards may vary from one area to another, the determination of what is and what is not acceptable for public exhibition on moral grounds may be viewed as a matter of a "local and private nature in the Province" within the meaning of s. 92(16) of the *British North America Act, 1867*, and as it is not a matter coming within any of the classes of subject enumerated in s. 91, this is a field in which the Legislature is free to act...

As I indicated at the outset, I have taken note of the lengthy judgment of Mr. Justice Macdonald in the Appeal Division in which he finds that the impugned legislation is *ultra vires* as infringing on the fundamental freedoms to which he refers, which include freedom of association; of assembly; of speech; of the press; of other media in the dissemination of news and opinion; of conscience and of religion.

Mr. Justice Macdonald's approach appears to me to be illustrated by the following comment which he makes after referring to censorship legislation relating to morals in other provinces [at p. 55]:

The foregoing criteria are of the usual "sex, morals and violence" type that are normally associated with film censorship. In the present case, however, the censorship criterion, being left to the *Board* to determine, *could* be much wider and encompass political, religious and other matters. In my opinion censorship relating to party politics cannot be tolerated in a free society where unfettered debate on political issues is a necessity, subject, of course, to the criminal law, particularly those provisions of the Criminal Code, relating to sedition, treason and incitement to crime.

(The emphasis is added.)

It is true that no limitations on the authority of the board are spelled out in the Act and that it might be inferred that it *could* possibly affect some of the rights listed by Macdonald, J.A., but having regard to the presumption of constitutional validity to which I have already referred, it appears to me that this does not afford justification for concluding that the purpose of the Act was directed to the infringement of one or more of those rights. With the greatest respect, this conclusion appears to me to involve speculation as to the intention of the Legislature and the placing of a construction on the statute which is nowhere made manifest by the language employed in enacting it.

For all these reasons, I would allow this appeal, set aside the judgment of the Appeal Division of Nova Scotia and substitute for the declaration made thereunder a declaration that Regulation 32 made pursuant to the *Theatre and Amusements Act* of Nova Scotia is null and void.

LASKIN, C.J.C. (dissenting):—...What is involved, as I have already noted, is an unqualified power in the Nova Scotia Board to determine the fitness of films for public viewing on considerations that may extend beyond the moral and may include the political, the social and the religious. Giving its assertion of power the narrowest compass, related to the film in the present case, the Board is asserting authority to protect public morals, to safeguard the public from exposure to films, to ideas and images in films, that it regards as morally offensive, as indecent, probably as obscene.

The determination of what is decent or indecent or obscene in conduct or in a publication, what is morally fit for public viewing, whether in films, in art or in a live performance is, as such, within the exclusive power of the Parliament of Canada under its enumerated authority to legislate in relation to the criminal law. This has been recognized in a line of cases in which, beginning with the seminal case of *A.-G. Ont. v. Hamilton Street R. Co.*, [1903] A.C. 524 (where it was said that it is the criminal law in the widest sense that falls within exclusive federal authority), the criminal law power has been held to be as much a brake on provincial legislation as a source of federal legislation...

It is beside the point to urge that morality is not co-extensive with the criminal law. Such a contention cannot of itself bring legislation respecting public morals within provincial competence. Moreover, the federal power in relation to the criminal law extends beyond control of morality, and is wide enough to embrace anti-social conduct or behaviour and has, indeed, been exercised in those respects.

Films have been held to fall within s. 159 of the *Criminal Code*, dealing with obscene publications: see *R. v. Fraser et al.* (1965), 51 D.L.R. (2d) 408, [1966] 1 C.C.C. 110, 52 W.W.R. 712; affirmed 59 D.L.R. (2d) 240, [1967] 2 C.C.C. 43, [1967] S.C.R. 38; *R. v. Goldberg and Reitman* (1971), 4 C.C.C. (2d) 187, [1971] 3 O.R. 323; *Daylight Theatre Co. Ltd. v. The Queen* (1973), 48 D.L.R. (3d) 390, 17 C.C.C. (2d) 451, 24 C.R.N.S. 368. Indeed, the very film, "Last Tango in Paris", out of which this case arose, was the subject of a prosecution under s. 159 which was unsuccessful: see *R. v. Odeon Morton Theatres Ltd. et al.* (1974), 45 D.L.R. (3d) 224, 16 C.C.C. (2d) 185, [1974] 3 W.W.R. 304. I draw attention as well to s. 163 of the *Criminal Code* dealing with the presentation or giving of immoral, indecent or obscene performances, entertainments or representations, and it seems to me that if films are within s. 159 they are a *fortiori* within s. 163...

This is not the case where civil consequences are attached to conduct defined and punished as criminal under federal legislation, as in *McDonald v. Down*, [1939] 2 D.L.R. 177, 71 C.C.C. 179; affirmed [1941] D.L.R. 799, 75 C.C.C. 404 (Ont. C.A.), but rather a case where a provincially authorized tribunal itself defines and determines legality, what is permissible and what is not. This, in my view, is a direct intrusion into the field of criminal law. At best, what the challenged Nova Scotia legislation is doing is seeking to supplement the criminal law enacted by Parliament, and this is forbidden: see *Johnson v. A.-G. Alta.*, [1954] 2 D.L.R. 625 at p. 636, 108 C.C.C. 1, [1954] S.C.R. 127 at p. 138, *per* Rand, J. (see also *St. Leonard v. Fournier, supra*, at p. 320).

It was contended, however, by the appellant and by supporting intervenants that the Nova Scotia Board was merely exercising a preventive power, no penalty or punishment being involved, no offence having been created. It is true, of course, that no penalty or punishment is involved in the making of an order prohibiting the exhibition of a film, but it is ingenuous to say that no offence is created when a licensee who disobeyed the order would be at risk of a cancellation of his licence and at risk of a penalty and any one else who proposed to exhibit the film publicly would likewise be liable to a penalty. Indeed, the contention invites this Court to allow form to mask substance and amounts to an assertion that the provincial Legislature may use the injunction or prohibitory order as a means of controlling conduct or performances or exhibitions, doing by prior restraint what it could not do by defining an offence and prescribing *post facto* punishment.

It does not follow from all of the foregoing that provincial legislative authority may not extend to objects where moral considerations are involved, but those objects must in themselves be anchored in the provincial catalogue of powers and must, moreover, not be in conflict with valid federal legislation. It is impossible in the present case to find any such anchorage in the provisions of the Nova Scotia statute that are challenged, and this apart from the issue of conflict which, I think, arises in relation to ss. 159 and 163 of the *Criminal Code*. What is asserted, by way of tying the challenged provisions to valid provincial regulatory control, is that the Province is competent to licence the use of premises, and entry into occupations, and may in that connection determine what shall be exhibited in those premises. This hardly touches the important issue raised by the present case and would, if correct, equally justify control by the Province of any conduct and activity in licensed premises even if not related to the property aspect of licensing, and this is patently indefensible. Moreover, what is missing from this assertion by the appellant is a failure to recognize that the censorship of films takes place without relation to any premises and is a direct prior control of public taste.

It is not enough to save the challenged prohibitory provisions of the Nova Scotia statute, if they are otherwise invalid, that they are part of a legislative scheme which embraces licensing of theatres and of motion picture projectionists. As I have already noted, the provisions now challenged go beyond the licensing provisions and engage the public directly.

For all the foregoing reasons I would dismiss this appeal and answer the constitutional question in the negative.

MARTLAND, J., concurs with RITCHIE, J.

JUDSON, J., concurs with LASKIN, C.J.C.

SPENCE, J., concurs with LASKIN, C.J.C.

PIGEON, J., concurs with RITCHIE, J.

DICKSON, J., concurs with LASKIN, C.J.C.

BEETZ and DE GRANDPRÉ, JJ., concur with RITCHIE, J.

Appeal allowed in part.

1.4.5 *Gay Alliance Toward Equality v. Vancouver Sun* (1979), 97 D.L.R. (3d) 577 (S.C.C.)

APPEAL from a judgment of the British Columbia Court of Appeal, 77 D.L.R. (3d) 487, [1977] 5 W.W.R. 198, allowing an appeal from a judgment of MacDonald, J., [1976] W.W.D. 160, holding that a board of inquiry under the *Human Rights Code of British Columbia*, 1973 (B.C.) (2nd Sess.), c. 119, did not err in deciding that the respondent newspaper failed to show reasonable cause for refusing to print an advertisement submitted by the appellant.

MARTLAND, J.: The issues in this appeal arise in respect of the application of the provisions of s. 3 [since am. 1974, c. 114, s. 6(a)] of the *Human Rights Code of British Columbia*, 1973 (B.C.) (2nd Sess.), c. 119. That section appears under a heading "Discriminatory Practices" and it read at the relevant time as follows:

> 3(1) No person shall
> (a) deny to any person or class of persons any accommodation, service, or facility customarily available to the public; or

(b) discriminate against any person or class of persons with respect to any accommodation, service, or facility customarily available to the public, unless reasonable cause exists for such denial or discrimination.

(2) For the purposes of subsection (1),
(a) the race, religion, colour, ancestry, or place of origin of any person or class of persons shall not constitute reasonable cause; and
(b) the sex of any person shall not constitute reasonable cause unless it relates to the maintenance of public decency...

The Act established a commission, the British Columbia Human Rights Commission. It provided for the appointment of a director, who is the chief executive officer of the Commission. When the director receives a complaint alleging a contravention of the Act, he is required to investigate and endeavour to effect a settlement of the alleged contravention. If he is unable to settle an allegation, provision is made for the appointment of a board of inquiry which investigates the allegation. The board of inquiry, if it is of the opinion that an allegation is justified, may order a person who has contravened the Act to cease such contravention and may order such person to make available to the person discriminated against such rights, opportunities, or privileges as, in the opinion of the board, he was denied. The board is also empowered to direct the payment of compensation and to make orders as to costs.

An appeal is given from a decision of the board of inquiry to the Supreme Court on any question of law or jurisdiction or any finding of fact necessary to establish its jurisdiction that is manifestly incorrect. The rules under the *Summary Convictions Act*, R.S.B.C. 1960, c. 373, governing appeals by way of stated case are made applicable.

A complaint was filed by an individual complainant on behalf of the appellant, the Gay Alliance Toward Equality, hereinafter referred to as "Alliance", alleging that the respondent, the Vancouver Sun, hereinafter referred to as "Sun", had refused to publish an advertisement promoting the sale of subscriptions to "Gay Tide" in the classified advertising section of the Sun newspaper in violation of s. 3 of the Act. The Sun advised the Alliance by letter that the advertisement was "not acceptable for publication in this newspaper".

The Sun's refusal to print the advertisement was because it promoted subscriptions to "Gay Tide". "Gay Tide" is a publication which reflects the purposes of the Alliance, *i.e.*, to establish recognition for the thesis that homosexuality is a valid and legitimate form of human sexual and emotional expression in no way harmful to society or the individual and completely on a par with heterosexuality.

A board of inquiry was constituted to consider the complaint of the Alliance. After conducting a hearing, the board found that there had been a violation of s. 3 of the *Human Rights Code*.

From this decision the Sun appealed. A case was stated by the board as required under the Act. The stated case referred to the facts previously mentioned. Paragraphs 10, 11 and 12 of the stated case are as follows:

10. The refusal by the Appellant to publish the advertisement in question was stated to be the result of a policy which the paper has in its advertising department (as distinct from its editorial department) to avoid any advertising material dealing with homosexuals or homosexuality, and the Appellant argued that this policy was justified on three grounds:

(1) That homosexuality is offensive to public decency and that the advertisement would offend some of its subscribers;

(2) That the Code of Advertising Standards, a code of advertising ethics subscribed to by most of the daily newspapers in Canada includes the following section:

"Public decency — no advertisement shall be prepared, or be knowingly accepted which is vulgar, suggestive or in any way offensive to public decency."

and that the advertisement in question did not conform to the standards therein set out; and

(3) That the Appellant newspaper had a duty to protect the morals of the community.

11. This Board of Inquiry found that the central theme of the Appellant's argument was that the policy in question was predicated on a desire to protect a reasonable standard of decency and good taste.

12. Assessing all the evidence offered on the question of the cause or motivation behind the Appellant's refusal to publish the Respondent's advertisement, the majority of the Board of Inquiry found the inevitable conclusion to be that the real reason behind the policy was not a concern for any standard of public decency, but was, in fact, a personal bias against homosexuals and homosexuality on the part of various individuals within the management of the Appellant newspaper. Board Member Dr. Dorothy Smith dissented on this point and held that there was no evidence whatsoever on which the Board could make such a finding; and that, in particular there was no evidence to rebut the Appellant's repeated statements that its policy was predicated on a desire to protect a reasonable standard of decency and good taste.

The questions of law stated in the stated case are as follows:

The appellant desires to question the finding that a violation did take place on the grounds that the said Judgment was erroneous in point of law or in excess of jurisdiction, the questions submitted being:

1. Was the Board of Inquiry correct in law in holding that pursuant to Section 3(1) of the Human Rights Code of British Columbia that classified advertising was a service or facility customarily available to the public.

2. Was the Board of Inquiry correct in law in holding that the Appellant herein denied to any person or class of persons any accommodation, service or facility customarily available to the public or discriminated against any person or class of persons with respect to any accommodation service or facility customarily available to the public pursuant to Section 3(1) of the Human Rights Code of British Columbia.

3. Was the Board of Inquiry correct in law in holding that pursuant to Section 3(1) of the Human Rights Code of British Columbia that the Appellant herein did not

have reasonable cause for the alleged denial and did not have reasonable cause for the alleged discrimination.

Sun's appeal to a Judge of the Supreme Court of British Columbia was dismissed [[1976] W.W.D. 160], but its appeal to the Court of Appeal succeeded by a majority decision [77 D.L.R. (3d) 487, [1977] 5 W.W.R. 198]. It is from that judgment that the present appeal, with leave, has been brought to this Court.

The following excerpts from the judgments of Branca, J.A., and Robertson, J.A., who comprised the majority in the Court of Appeal, state the basis upon which they were of the opinion that Sun's appeal should be allowed.

Per Branca, J.A. [at p. 494]:

> The Board concluded that having assessed all of the evidence that it was a personal bias on the part of various individuals, within the management of the advertising department of the newspaper, which was the real reason motivating the refusal to publish and not a genuine concern on the part of the newspaper for any standard of public decency. It seems to me that the real question for determination was not whether certain individuals within management had a bias against homosexuals or homosexuality which may have motivated the policy, but whether or not the resultant policy dealing with public decency even though motivated by a bias on the part of certain individuals constituted a reasonable cause for the refusal to publish. In other words, despite the fact that certain individuals may have had that bias and that bias might well have motivated the refusal, the vital question remained: did the resultant policy of the newspaper furnish reasonable cause within the meaning of those words as used in s. 3 of the *Human Rights Code* which in the event might constitute a lawful ground for refusal.

Per Robertson, J.A. [at p. 496]:

> It is my view that the words in s. 3(1) of the Code, "unless reasonable cause exists" require the application of an objective test: Does such a cause exist? It is wrong in law to substitute for this the subjective test that the Board applied: What motivated the person who denied or discriminated and was this motivation reasonable cause for the denial or discrimination? To put it another way: If reasonable cause does in fact exist, the person discriminated against cannot claim the benefit of s. 3, even though the other person did not know of the existence of the cause; conversely, if reasonable cause does not in fact exist, the other person cannot justify his act of discrimination by a genuine belief that a reasonable cause did exist.
>
> Of course, in applying the Code the "cause" must be considered in relation to the person and the circumstances. Also, it must be borne in mind that the members of majorities have rights and sensibilities. I do not think that it is the intention of the Code that these are generally to be ignored for the benefit of those who are different. The words "unless reasonable cause exists" make this abundantly clear.
>
> If the grounds upon which the Board reached its decision are to be gathered from the stated case alone, it appears from para. 12 that the Board went wrong, in that it applied the wrong test, that of motivation, and gave no effect to the evidence referred to in para. 10(1), that the advertisement would offend some of the newspaper's subscribers, which in addition would, of course, result in a loss of subscribers and afford reasonable cause for declining to accept the business.

The first two questions of law stated in the stated case raise a serious issue as to the extent to which the discretion of a newspaper publisher to determine what he wishes to publish in his newspaper has been curtailed by the *Human Rights Code*. Is his decision not to publish some item in his newspaper subject to review by a board of inquiry set upon under the Act, with power, if it considers his decision unreasonable, to compel him to publish that which he does not wish to publish?

The Supreme Court of the United States, in 1974, in *Miami Herald Publishing Co. v. Tornillo*, 418 U.S. 241, had to consider whether a Florida statute violated the First Amendment's guarantee of freedom of the press. This statute granted to a political candidate the right to equal space in a newspaper to answer criticism and attacks on his record by a newspaper. This right is somewhat similar to that defined in s. 3 of Bill No. 9 entitled "An Act to ensure the Publication of Accurate News and Information", which had been reserved by the Lieutenant-Governor of Alberta, and which was under consideration in this Court: see *Reference re Alberta Legislation*, [1938] 2 D.L.R. 81, [1938] S.C.R. 100 [affd [1938] 4 D.L.R. 433, [1939] A.C. 117 *sub nom. A.-G. Alta. v. A.-G. Can.*, [1938] 3 W.W.R. 337 (P.C.) (the *Alberta Press* case)].

The Supreme Court of the United States held that the statute under consideration was a violation of the First Amendment. In the course of his reasons for judgment, Chief Justice Burger, who delivered the opinion of the Court, said that the statute failed to clear the barriers of the First Amendment because of its intrusion into the function of editors. He went on to say at p. 258:

> A newspaper is more than a passive receptacle or conduit of news, comment, and advertising. The choice of material to go into a newspaper, and the decisions made as to limitations on the size and content of the paper, and treatment of public issues and public officials — whether fair or unfair — constitute the exercise of editorial control and judgment. It has yet to be demonstrated how governmental regulations of this crucial process can be exercised consistent with First Amendment guarantees of a free press as they have evolved at this time.

The *Canadian Bill of Rights*, s. 1(*f*), recognizes freedom of the press as a fundamental freedom.

While there is no legislation in British Columbia in relation to freedom of the press, similar to the First Amendment or to the *Canadian Bill of Rights*, and while there is no attack made in this appeal on the constitutional validity of the *Human Rights Code*, I think that Chief Justice Burger's statement about editorial control and judgment in relation to a newspaper is of assistance in considering one of the essential ingredients of freedom of the press. The issue which arises in this appeal is as to whether s. 3 of the Act is to be construed as purporting to limit that freedom.

Section 3 of the Act refers, in paras. (a) and (b), to "service...customarily available to the public". It forbids the denial of such a service to any person or class of persons and it forbids discrimination against any person or class of persons with respect to such a service, unless reasonable cause exists for such denial or discrimination.

In my opinion the general purpose of s. 3 was to prevent discrimination against individuals or groups of individuals in respect of the provision of certain things available generally to the public. The items dealt with are similar to those covered by legislation in the United States, both federal and state. "Accommodation" refers to such matters as accommodation in hotels, inns and motels. "Service" refers to such matters as restaurants, bars, taverns, service stations, public transportation and public utilities. "Facility" refers to such matters as public parks and recreational facilities. These are all items "customarily available to the public". It is matters such as these which have been dealt with in American case law on the subject of civil rights.

The case in question here deals with the refusal by a newspaper to publish a classified advertisement, but it raises larger issues, which would include the whole field of newspaper advertising and letters to the editor. A newspaper exists for the purpose of disseminating information and for the expression of its views on a wide variety of issues. Revenues are derived from the sale of its newspapers and from advertising. It is true that its advertising facilities are made available, at a price, to the general public. But Sun reserved to itself the right to revise, edit, classify or reject any advertisement submitted to it for publication and this reservation was displayed daily at the head of its classified advertisement section.

The law has recognized the freedom of the press to propagate its views and ideas on any issue and to select the material which it publishes. As a corollary to that, a newspaper also has the right to refuse to publish material which runs contrary to the views which it expresses. A newspaper published by a religious organization does not have to publish an advertisement advocating atheistic doctrine. A newspaper supporting certain political views does not have to publish an advertisement advancing contrary views. In fact, the judgments of Duff, C.J.C., Davis and Cannon, JJ., in the *Alberta Press* case, previously mentioned, suggest that provincial legislation to compel such publication may be unconstitutional.

In my opinion the service which is customarily available to the public in the case of a newspaper which accepts advertising is a service subject to the right of the newspaper to control the content of such advertising. In the present case, the Sun had adopted a position on the controversial subject of homosexuality. It did not wish to accept an advertisement seeking subscription to a publication which propagates the views of the Alliance. Such refusal was not based upon any personal characteristic of the person seeking to place that advertisement, but upon the content of the advertisement itself.

Section 3 of the Act does not purport to dictate the nature and scope of a service which must be offered to the public. In the case of a newspaper, the nature and scope of the service which it offers, including advertising service, is determined by the newspaper itself. What s. 3 does is to provide that a service which is offered to the public is to be available to all persons seeking to use it, and the newspaper cannot deny the service which it offers to any particular member of the public unless reasonable cause exists for so doing.

In my opinion the Board erred in law in considering that s. 3 was applicable in the circumstances of this case. I would dismiss the appeal with costs.

RITCHIE, SPENCE AND PIGEON, JJ., concur with MARTLAND, J.

DICKSON, J. (dissenting): Counsel for the Vancouver Sun strongly contended for the traditional right of editorial control over newspaper content, including advertising. English law is remarkably bereft of guidance on the subject of editorial control over advertising. But in the United States, the common law is clear. Perhaps the best statement of the law is found in *Approved Personnel Inc. v. The Tribune Co.* (1965), 177 So. 2d 704 (Dist. C.A. Fla.) at p. 706:

> In the absence of any statutory provisions to the contrary, the law seems to be uniformly settled by the great weight of authority throughout the United States that the newspaper publishing business is a private enterprise and is neither a public utility nor affected with the public interest. The decisions appear to hold that even though a particular newspaper may enjoy a virtual monopoly in the area of its publication, this fact is neither unusual nor of important significance. The courts have consistently held that in the absence of statutory regulation on the subject, a newspaper may publish or reject commercial advertising tendered to it as its judgment best dictates without incurring liability for advertisements rejected by it.

In "Annotation — Right of Publisher of Newspaper or Magazine, in Absence of Contractual Obligation, to Refuse Publication of Advertisement", by E.L. Kellett, 18 A.L.R. 3d 1286 at pp. 1287-8, the following summary is provided:

> With the exception of one case, it has universally been held that in the absence of circumstances amounting to an illegal monopoly or conspiracy, the publisher of a newspaper or magazine is not required by law to accept and publish an advertisement, even where the advertisement is a proper one, and the regular fee for publication has been paid or tendered....
>
> The reasons for refusing to compel publication of an advertisement are that at common law a newspaper is strictly a private enterprise, is not a business clothed or affected with a public interest as is a public utility, innkeeper, or railroad, and that newspaper publishers are accordingly free to contract and deal with whom they please in conformity with the inherent right of every person to refuse to maintain trade relations with any individual.

In the British Royal Commission on the Press, 1947-49, Report (Cmd. 7700, 1949), there is a brief discussion of the "right of newspapers to reject advertisements" at p. 144:

> We have received evidence that some newspapers refuse all advertisements of a particular class. This is a different matter. We consider that a newspaper has a right to refuse advertisements of any kind which is contrary to its standards or may be objectionable to its readers. This right, however, should not be exercised arbitrarily.

I think it would be correct to state that a newspaper has a right to reject advertising at common law.

Apart from the common law position, counsel for the Vancouver Sun also cast his argument in terms of press freedom. This raises issues which have not been satisfactorily resolved, either in Canada, in Britain or in the United States. These issues which can be defined broadly as (1) the content of the term "freedom of the press"; (2) the distinction between "political" and "commercial" speech; and (3) the vexed issue of access to the press. The discussion which follows is not for the purpose of resolving any constitutional issue. There is no constitutional challenge to s. 3(1) of the *Human Rights Code of British Columbia*. I wish merely to sketch the broad and important judicial background to the question posed in the case at bar.

As a starting point, I can do no better than quote from the British Royal Commission on the Press, Final Report (Cmd. 6810, 1977), pp. 8-9:

> Freedom of the press carries different meanings for different people. Some emphasize the freedom of proprietors to market their publications, others the freedom of individuals, whether professional journalists or not, to address the public through the press; still others stress the freedom of editors to decide what shall be published. These are all elements in the right to freedom of expression. But proprietors, contributors and editors must accept the limits to free expression set by the need to reconcile claims which may often conflict. The public, too, asserts a right to accurate information and fair comment which, in turn, has to be balanced against the claims both of national security and of individuals to safeguards for their reputation and privacy except when these are overridden by the public interest. But the public interest does not reside in whatever the public may happen to find interesting, and the press must be careful not to perpetrate abuses and call them freedom. Freedom of the press cannot be absolute. There must be boundaries to it and realistic discussion concerns where those boundaries ought to be set.
>
> We define freedom of the press as that degree of freedom from restraint which is essential to enable proprietors, editors and journalists to advance the public interest by publishing the facts and opinions without which a democratic electorate cannot make responsible judgments.

Later in their report, the Commissioners discuss legal constraints on the press and make the following general comment which, save for the freedom of the press assured by the *Canadian Bill of Rights*, is equally applicable to Canada (at p. 183):

> This country is unlike many others in having no laws which relate specifically to the press. There is no constitutional guarantee of the freedom of the press, as there is in the United States, and no judicial surveillance of the contents of the newspapers, as there is in Sweden. Nevertheless, there are areas of general law which relate predominantly, and in some cases almost exclusively, to the activities of the press. In important ways, legal provisions help to maintain the delicate balance between freedom of the press and the public interest.

In Canada, as in Britain, much of the protection of the freedom of the press must derive from the interpretation of the "general law" rather than from a constitutional guarantee, and from the interpretation of statutes such as the British Columbia *Human Rights Code* as they may affect the press. While admittedly the *Alberta Press* case, *Reference re Alberta Legislation*, [1938] 2 D.L.R. 81, [1938] S.C.R. 100 [affd [1938] 4 D.L.R. 433, [1939] A.C. 117 *sub nom. A.-G. Alta. v. A.-G. Can.*, [1938] 3 W.W.R. 337 (P.C.)], dealt with the constitutional validity of the "Alberta Press bill", as it was termed, the comments of Chief Justice Duff and Mr. Justice Cannon in that case are important in defining the notion of freedom of the press in the Canadian context.

In the United States, freedom of the press rests upon the First Amendment, which reads:

> Congress shall make no law respecting an establishment of religion, or prohibiting the free exercise thereof; or abridging the freedom of speech, or of the press, or the right of the people peaceably to assemble, and to petition the Government for redress of grievances.

The framers of the United States Constitution linked freedom of speech in the First Amendment to freedom of the press to provide an effective forum for such expression: "Conflict Within the First Amendment: A Right of Access to Newspapers", 48 N.Y.U.L.R. 1200 (1973). In the result, there would appear to be general agreement in Britain, Canada, and the United States, as to the "free public discussion" rationale for freedom of the press.

Within the First Amendment in the United States two issues have been much discussed: whether the First Amendment mandates equal protection for "commercial" as opposed to "political" speech, and whether the First Amendment not only protects expression once it comes to the fore, but also serves to ground an affirmative right of access to the media. In response to these issues two trends can be discerned in the American cases. The first is the obliteration of any meaningful distinction between "political" and "commercial" speech within the First Amendment. The second is the rejection of a right of access to the press based upon the First Amendment.

The so-called "commercial speech" doctrine finds its origin in the case of *Valentine v. Crestensen* (1942), 316 U.S. 52 at p. 54, where Mr. Justice Roberts, on behalf of the Court, stated unequivocally: "We are equally clear that the Constitution imposes no such restraint [the First Amendment] on government as respects purely commercial advertising." I do not intend any detailed canvas of the American authorities other than to say that the "commercial" exception appeared to retain its virility as recently as the case of *Pittsburgh Press Co. v. Pittsburgh Commission on Human Relations* (1973), 413 U.S. 376, but the ambit of that case was shortly thereafter cut down in *Bigelow v. Virginia* (1975) 421 U.S. 809, and further narrowed the following year in *Virginia State Board of Pharmacy v. Virginia Citizens Consumer Council Inc.* (1976) 425 U.S. 748, where the Court struck down the restrictions on prescription drug advertising found in Virginia law as violating the First Amendment. Nor has this wave receded: see *Bates v. State Bar of Arizona* (1977), 97 S. Ct. 2691, where State bar restrictions on advertising by lawyers were struck down.

A separate line of cases has upheld the view that the First Amendment serves no affirmative function, *i.e.*, it does not mandate any right of access, however limited, to the media: see *Chicago Joint Board, Amalgamated Clothing Workers of America A.F.L.-CLO v. Chicago Tribune Co.* (1969), 307 F. Supp. 422 (N.D. Ill); affd 435 F.2d 470 (7th Cir.); *certiorari* denied 402 U.S. 973. Any doubts, so far as the United States is concerned, as to a right of access to newspapers, would appear to be settled by the Supreme Court in *Miami Herald Publishing Co. v. Tornillo* (1974), 418 U.S. 241. The newspaper had refused to print Tornillo's replies to editorials critical of his candidacy for State office and Tornillo brought suit seeking injunctive and declaratory relief under Florida's "right of reply" statute. That statute provided that:

> ...if a candidate for nomination or election is assailed regarding his personal character or official record by any newspaper, the candidate has the right to demand that the newspaper print, free of

cost to the candidate, any reply the candidate may make to the newspaper's charges. The reply must appear in as conspicuous a place and in the same kind of type as the charges which prompted the reply, provided it does not take up more space than the charges. Failure to comply with the statute constitutes a first-degree misdemeanour.

While the Circuit Court held the statute unconstitutional as an infringement on the freedom of the press under the First and Fourteenth Amendments, the Florida Supreme Court found no such violation, free speech being enhanced and not abridged by the statute, which furthered the "broad societal interest in the free flow of information to the public". This view was rejected by the Supreme Court on the ground that it constituted interference by the Government with the exercise of editorial control and judgment, and hence with First Amendment guarantees of a free press. See also *Columbia Broadcasting System Inc. v. Democratic National Committee* (1973), 412 U.S. 94.

Before leaving the American cases it is, I think, appropriate to note that these cases were decided in light of a strong First Amendment constitutional underpinning, and legislation such as that found in the British Columbia *Human Rights Code* was not in issue. Our limited jurisprudence, to which I will shortly refer, would appear to accept a greater degree of regulation in respect of newspaper advertising than is apparent in the United States.

Although freedom of the press is one of our cherished freedoms, recognized in the *quasi*-constitutional *Canadian Bill of Rights*, the freedom is not absolute. Publishers of newspapers are amenable to civil and criminal laws which bear equally upon all businessmen and employers, generally, in the community, for example, those regulating labour relations, combines, or imposing non-discriminatory general taxation. False and misleading advertising may properly be proscribed. In *Cowen et al. v. A.-G. B.C. et al.*, [1941] 2 D.L.R. 687, [1941] S.C.R. 321, the central question was whether a 1939 amendment to the British Columbia *Dentistry Act*, which barred any person not registered under the Act from practising or offering to practise dentistry in the Province, was limited to acts within the Province, and press freedom was not raised. The result of the decision, however, was the maintenance of an injunction to prevent the publication of certain advertisements in a daily newspaper. In *Benson & Hedges (Canada) Ltd. et al. v. A.-G. B.C.* (1972), 27 D.L.R. (3d) 257, 6 C.P.R. (2d) 182, [1972] 5 W.W.R. 32 (B.C.S.C.), an Act, the effect of which was "to prohibit advertising by any person of tobacco products", was upheld, although press freedom does not appear to have been in issue or argued. In *R. v. Telegram Publishing Co. Ltd.* (1960), 25 D.L.R. (2d) 471, 129 C.C.C. 209, [1960] O.R. 518 sub nom. *R. v. Toronto Magistrates, Ex p. Telegram Publishing Co.* (Ont. H.C.), Mr. Justice Schatz held that a section of the *Liquor Control Act* of Ontario prohibiting the publication of any announcement concerning liquor was not an encroachment on the freedom of the press, or upon freedom of speech.

Newspapers occupy a unique place in western society. The press has been felicitously referred to by de Toqueville as "the chief democratic instrument of freedom". Blackstone wrote, "The liberty of the press is indeed essential to the nature of a free state." Jefferson went so far as to assert, "Were it left for me to decide whether we should have a government without newspapers, or newspapers without a government, I should not hesitate a moment to prefer the latter." There is a direct and vital relationship between a free press and a free society. The right to speak freely, publish freely, and worship freely, are fundamental and indigenous rights, but it is "freedom governed by law", as Lord Wright observed in *James v. Commonwealth of Australia*, [1936] A.C. 578 at p. 627. In the *Alberta Press* case, *supra*, we find these words of Sir Lyman P. Duff, C.J.C., at p. 108 D.L.R., p. 134 S.C.R.:

> Some degree of regulation of newspapers everybody would concede to the Provinces. Indeed, there is a very wide field in which the Provinces undoubtedly are invested with legislative authority over newspapers; but the limit, in our opinion, is reached when the legislation effects such a curtailment of the exercise of the right of public discussion as substantially to interfere with the working of the parliamentary institutions of Canada...

Governments in Canada have generally respected press independence and have followed a policy of non-intervention.

There is an important distinction to be made between legislation designed to control the editorial content of a newspaper, and legislation designed to control discriminatory practices in the offering of commercial services to the public. We are dealing in this case with the classified advertising section of a newspaper. The primary purpose of commercial advertising is to advance the economic welfare of the newspaper. That part of the paper is not concerned with freedom of speech on matters of public concern as a condition of democratic polity, but rather with the provision of a "service or facility customarily available to the public" with a view to profit. As such, in British Columbia a newspaper is impressed with a statutory obligation not to deny space or discriminate with respect to classified advertising, unless for reasonable cause. It should be made clear that the right of access with which we are here concerned has nothing to do with those parts of the paper where one finds news or editorial content, parts which can in no way be characterized as a service customarily available to the public. The effect of s. 3 of the British Columbia *Human Rights Code* is to require newspapers within the Province to adopt advertising policies which are not in violation of the principles set out in the *Code*.

I turn now to the stated case, paras. 10, 11, and 12 of which read:

> 10. The refusal by the Appellant to publish the advertisement in question was stated to be the result of a policy which the paper has in its advertising department (as distinct from its editorial department) to avoid any advertising material dealing with homosexuals or homosexuality, and the Appellant argued that this policy was justified on three grounds:
>
> (1) That homosexuality is offensive to public decency and that the advertisement would offend some of its subscribers;
>
> (2) That the Code of Advertising Standards, a Code of Advertising Ethics subscribed to by most of the daily newspapers in Canada includes the following section:

"Public decency — no advertisement shall be prepared, or be knowingly accepted which is vulgar, suggestive or in any way offensive to public decency." and that the advertisement in question did not conform to the standards therein set out; and

(3) That the Appellant newspaper had a duty to protect the morals of the community:

11. This Board of Inquiry found that the central theme of the Appellant's argument was that the policy in question was predicated on a desire to protect a reasonable standard of decency and good taste.

12. Assessing all the evidence offered on the question of the cause or motivation behind the Appellant's refusal to publish the Respondent's advertisement, the majority of the Board of Inquiry found the inevitable conclusion to be that the real reason behind the policy was not a concern for any standard of public decency, but was, in fact, a personal bias against homosexuals and homosexuality on the part of various individuals within the management of the Appellant newspaper. Board Member Dr. Dorothy Smith dissented on this point and held that there was no evidence whatsoever on which the Board could make such a finding; and that, in particular there was no evidence to rebut the Appellant's repeated statements that its policy was predicated on a desire to protect a reasonable standard of decency and good taste.

It seems clear from the foregoing that the Vancouver Sun in its advertising department, as distinct from its editorial department, had a particular policy. That policy was to avoid any advertising material dealing with homosexuals or homosexuality. The paper advanced three grounds as constituting reasonable cause, the "central theme" of which was a "desire to protect a reasonable standard for decency and good taste".

In its main factum, the respondent newspaper contended that the board failed to address itself to the only question posed by the statute, "did reasonable cause exist?", and instead substituted a determination as to motive for refusing the advertisement. Although the stated case leaves something to be desired in terms of clarity, there does not seem to be any doubt that the board rejected the three grounds advanced on the part of the paper in justification of its refusal to publish the advertisement. A majority of the board also found that the real reason for the refusal to publish was a personal bias against homosexuals and homosexuality on the part of various individuals within the management of the newspaper. The paper, therefore, had failed to establish reasonable cause. Much was made of the word "motivation" and "the real reason behind the policy". These words do not give any particular trouble. We need not indulge in nice appraisal based upon casuistic distinctions between the meaning of "cause" and "motive", words which are virtually synonymous.

I have earlier adverted to the matter of reasonable cause. "Reasonableness" is normally a question of fact. The most recent authoritative affirmation of that statement is from Lord Hailsham, L.C., in *Re W. (An Infant)*, [1971] A.C. 682 at p. 699:

FREEDOM OF EXPRESSION AND THE CANADIAN CONSTITUTION 59

> And, be it observed, "reasonableness," or "unreasonableness," where either word is employed in English law, is normally a question of fact and degree and not a question of law so long as there is evidence to support the finding of the court.

Whatever else it may have done, the board of inquiry in the case at bar found the fact of "reasonable cause" adversely to the respondent newspaper. From that finding, there is a very limited right of appeal provided by s. 18 of the British Columbia *Human Rights Code*. The section reads in part:

> 18. An appeal lies from a decision of a board of inquiry to the Supreme Court upon
> (a) any point or question of law or jurisdiction; or
> (b) any finding of fact necessary to establish its jurisdiction that is manifestly incorrect,

The jurisdiction of the board of inquiry is not challenged. Insufficiency of evidence was not even argued in this Court or in the Courts below.

Counsel for the Sun argued that the *Human Rights Code* does not purport to be, and should not be employed as, an instrument to compel a newspaper to accept advertisements which it can reasonably be said will harm its reputation and standing. If the paper had taken that position before the board and had established adverse economic impact, the board's conclusions might well have been different. What counsel is really asking this Court to do is make new findings of fact. This we cannot undertake unless there is no evidence to support the board's findings or unless those findings are perverse. In my view, Mr. Justice MacDonald expressed the legal position correctly when he said:

> Whether particular circumstances amount to reasonable cause for denial or discrimination under s. 3 is purely a question of fact. It must be decided as a matter of law, under a proper definition of the phrase "reasonable cause". The only restraints which the law places upon the triers of fact are the provisions of s. 3(2). They may not find the race, religion, colour, ancestry, or place of origin of any person or class of persons reasonable cause unless it relates to the maintenance of public decency or to the determination of premiums or benefits under contracts of insurance. What the appellant's submission does is to take some elements — what it submits are the circumstances of its case — and ask the Court to find that, as a matter of law, they must constitute reasonable cause. But it is really an invasion of the area of fact. If the appellant's submission is sound, how long is the list of different plausible circumstances which the court would be bound to find constituted reasonable cause?

In an alternative argument, counsel submitted that, if the board did address itself to whether reasonable cause for the refusal existed on an objective basis, then the board erred in failing to construe the term "reasonable cause" solely in relation to the characteristics of the person tendering the advertisement. The argument, as I understand it, would limit the Code to unreasonable refusals based upon the characteristics of the persons seeking the public service. It was said the board erred in considering the text of the advertisement which gave rise to the denial of service. The paper, at most, discriminated against the idea of a thesis of homosexuality, and it is no offence to discriminate against ideas. A number of American authorities based on the First Amendment, to which I have earlier referred, were relied upon. The argument is an interesting one but, for the reasons given by the Chief Justice, whose judgment in draft I have had the advantage of reading, I would reject the argument.

I would only add in concluding that I do not think a newspaper, or any other institution or business providing a service to the public, can insulate itself from human rights legislation by relying upon "honest" bias, or upon a statement of policy which reserves to the proprietor the right to decide whom he shall serve.

I am unable to find in the stated case any convincing proof that the board of inquiry misunderstood the evidence or misdirected itself in law. I note again that there has been no constitutional challenge on the ground that interference with the right of a newspaper to control its content is an attempt to abrogate the rights of a free press and is, consequently, outside the legislative jurisdiction of the Province of British Columbia.

I would allow the appeal, set aside the judgment of the British Columbia Court of Appeal and restore the judgment of MacDonald, J., and the order of the board of inquiry, with costs throughout.

BEETZ, J., concurs with MARTLAND, J.

ESTEY, J., concurs with DICKSON, J.

PRATTE, J., concurs with MARTLAND, J.

[LASKIN, C.J.C. also dissented]

Appeal dismissed.

1.4.6 *Attorney-General of Quebec v. Irwin Toy Ltd., Moreau et al., Intervenors* **(1989), 58 D.L.R. (4th) 577 (S.C.C.)**

[Sections 248 and 249 of Quebec's *Consumer Protection Act* prohibited commercial advertising directed at persons under thirteen years of age. In the excerpt from the S.C.C.'s reasons which follows, the Court addressed two issues: whether these provisions were *ultra vires* and whether they could apply to television advertising. The Court's analysis of the Charter arguments raised in the case is reproduced later in this chapter.]

Per Dickson, C.J.C. and Lamer and Wilson, J.J.: [McIntyre and Beetz, J.J. concurred with the majority's analysis on these issues but dissented from the result reached regarding the challenge based on the Charter.]

Four separate issues emerge from the argument in this court with respect to the validity or operative effect of ss. 248 and 249 of the *Consumer Protection Act*: (a) whether these provisions are distinguishable, in so far as their constitutional characterization is concerned, from the challenged provision of the advertising regulations under the *Consumer Protection Act* that was characterized by this court in *Kellogg's, supra,* as having a valid provincial purpose; (b) whether, as contended by Pathonic, their effect on a television broadcast undertaking is such as to render them, despite the judgment of the court in *Kellogg's,* inoperative in so far as television advertising is concerned; (c) whether they are practically and functionally incompatible with the regulatory scheme put into place by the Canadian Radio-television and Telecommunications Commission (CRTC) pursuant to the *Broadcasting Act*, R.S.C. 1970, c. B-11; and (d) whether they amount to any invasion of the federal criminal law power. We discuss each of these issues in turn.

A. *The constitutional characterization of ss. 248 and 249*

In *Kellogg's*, the challenged provision was s. 11.53 of Division XI-A, entitled "Advertising intended for children", of the general regulations (O.C. 1408-72) adopted pursuant to the authority conferred on the Lieutenant-Governor in Council by s. 102(*o*) of the *Consumer Protection Act*, S.Q. 1971, c. 74, to make regulations "to determine standards for advertising goods, whether or not they are the object of a contract, or credit, especially all advertising intended for children". Section 11.53 of the regulations provided:

> 11.53 No one shall prepare, use, publish or cause to be published in Quebec advertising intended for children which:
>
> . . . . .
>
> (*n*) employs cartoons;

The Kellogg companies were charged with breaches of this provision in connection with certain television advertisements and an injunction was sought against them to restrain further infractions. An injunction was granted by the Superior Court, [1974] Que. S.C. 498, but an appeal from this judgment was allowed by a majority of the Court of Appeal (Tremblay, C.J.Q. and Montgomery, J.A.), [1975] Que. C.A. 518, who held that since the content of television broadcasting fell within exclusive federal jurisdiction provincial legislation with respect to such content was inoperative, citing the judgment of this court in *Commission du Salaire Minimum v. Bell Telephone Co. of Canada* (1966), 59 D.L.R. (2d) 145, [1966] S.C.R. 767, in support of this conclusion. Turgeon J.A., dissenting, applied the distinction between legislation in relation to a matter and legislation incidentally affecting a matter. He held the challenged regulation and the law under which it was adopted to be within provincial jurisdiction although it might incidentally affect a matter within federal jurisdiction.

Martland, J., with whom Ritchie, Pigeon, Dickson, Beetz and de Grandpré, JJ. concurred, held that the challenged provision validly applied to television advertising because it was part of a general regulation of advertising for children that had a valid provincial purpose and its effect on a television broadcast undertaking was a merely incidental one. Laskin, C.J.C., dissenting, with whom Judson and Spence, JJ. concurred, was of the view that the challenged provision could not validly apply to prevent an advertiser from advertising its products on television because in such application it encroached on a matter within exclusive federal jurisdiction, the content of television broadcasting.

Like Turgeon, J.A. in the Court of Appeal, Martland, J. applied the distinction between legislation in relation to a matter and legislation which incidentally affects a matter, citing the judgment of the court in *Carnation Co. Ltd. v. Quebec Agricultural Marketing Board* (1968), 67 D.L.R. (2d) 1, [1968] S.C.R. 238, as an analogous application of this distinction. He held that the challenged provision was aimed at certain kinds of advertising by advertisers and not at the operation of a television broadcast undertaking. He said at pp. 322-3:

> In my opinion this Regulation does not seek to regulate or to interfere with the operation of a broadcast undertaking. In relation to the facts of this case it seeks to prevent Kellogg from using a certain kind of advertising by any means. It aims at controlling the commercial activity of Kellogg. The fact that Kellogg is precluded from using televised advertising may, incidentally, affect the revenue of one or more television stations but it does not change the true nature of the regulation. In this connection the case of *Carnation Co. Ltd. v. Quebec Agricultural Marketing Board* . . . is analogous.

Martland, J. stressed the fact that the regulation was being applied and the injunction sought against Kellogg and not against a television station. He reserved his opinion as to whether the regulation could be validly applied against a television station. He said at p. 323:

> Whether the Regulation could be applied to the television station itself or whether an injunction against Kellogg would bind such station does not arise in this case and I prefer to express no opinion with respect to it.

The disputed regulation in *Kellogg's*, as Martland, J. observed, sought to prevent the advertiser "from using a certain kind of advertising by any means." It was concerned with a certain kind of advertising content but it applied to all advertising media employing such content. Moreover, it had a limited application to advertising content, merely prohibiting the use of cartoons, but otherwise permitting children's advertising. It was thus a provision of general application in pursuit of the legislative object which Martland, J. characterized as "to protect children in Quebec from the harmful effect of the kinds of advertising therein prohibited" (p. 321). It was aimed at all children's advertising employing cartoons, not at television advertising as such nor at the television broadcaster. The implication of the distinction emphasized by Martland, J. between application to the advertiser and application to a broadcast undertaking is that provincial legislation of general application with respect to advertising content would only be considered to encroach on exclusive federal jurisdiction with respect to broadcast content to the extent it was applied to a broadcast undertaking, that is, to the control over content exercised by such an undertaking rather than by an advertiser.

In the case at bar the respondent contended that the challenged provisions of the *Consumer Protection Act*, when read together with the regulations to which they are made expressly subject and considered in the light of the evidence of their practical effect, exhibit a different purpose or object from that of the regulation that was in issue in *Kellogg's*. The respondent contends that when the challenged provisions are seen in the context of the regulations and the evidence it is clear that they are aimed essentially and primarily at television as a medium of children's advertising, a matter within exclusive federal jurisdiction. In support of this contention the respondent emphasizes the relative importance of the prohibition of television advertising directed to persons under 13 years of age, as indicated by the evidence and the extent of the exemptions provided by the regulations for other forms of children's advertising. The respondent contends that the trial judge was in error in taking judicial notice of the existence and relative importance of other forms of children's advertising. There is no doubt that the evidence adduced by the respondent at trial and the s. 1 and s. 9.1 materials submitted by the Attorney-General of Quebec show that television advertising is by any measure the most important form of children's advertising. It is indisputably, however, not the only form as the exemptions indicate. Moreover, the genuine concern with the other forms of children's advertising is indicated by the extent to which the exempted forms are made subject to the content requirements of s. 91 of the regulations. The Attorney-General of Quebec submitted that television advertising, because of its massive penetration and ease of access for children, did not lend itself to as precise regulation as other forms of communication and must therefore be the subject of a particular regime. The respondent argued that this was an admission that the prohibition in s. 248 of the Act was primarily directed at television advertising. We take it to have been in justification of a prohibition in the case of television advertising rather than a concession that the challenged provisions as modified by the regulations are aimed primarily at such advertising. The Attorney-General of Quebec noted that there are other forms of children's advertising subject to the prohibition. On the whole, despite the fact that the relative impact on television advertising is much greater than it was in *Kellogg's*, we are of the opinion that ss. 248 and 249 of the Act, as modified by or completed by the regulations, can also be said to be legislation of general application enacted in relation to consumer protection, as in *Kellogg's*, rather than a colourable attempt, under the guise of a law of general application, to legislate in relation to television advertising. In other words, the dominant aspect of the law for purposes of characterization is the regulation of all forms of advertising directed at persons under 13 years of age rather than the prohibition of television advertising which cannot be said to be the exclusive or even primary aim of the legislation. In effect, we agree with Hugessen, A.C.J.S.C. on the general significance for the purposes of characterization of the legislation of the fact that other forms of advertising directed to persons under 13 years, whatever be their relative importance, are not exempted from the prohibition. The existence of such other forms of children's advertising was not seriously challenged but rather their significance from the constitutional point of view in attempting to ascertain the dominant aspect of the legislation. The existence of such other forms of children's advertising did not rest entirely on the judicial notice taken by the trial judge, who said that even if there was not evidence of such other forms he would be prepared to take judicial notice of them. The relative importance of television advertising and the other forms of children's advertising subject to exemption and prohibition is not in our opinion a sufficient basis for a finding of colourability. There is no suggestion that the legislative or regulatory concern with these other forms of children's advertising is a mere pretense or facade for a primary, if not exclusive, purpose of regulating television advertising. It is not the relative importance of these other forms of advertising but the *bona fide* nature of the legislative concern with them that is in issue on the question of colourability.

B. *The effect of ss. 248 and 249 on broadcasting undertakings*

The interveners Pathonic, as we understood their argument, did not contend, as did the respondent, that the challenged provisions of the *Consumer Protection Act* were distinguishable on their face in respect of the characterization of their purpose or object from the provision of the regulations that was considered in *Kellogg's*. They contended that the challenged provisions were rendered *ultra vires* or inoperative because of their effect on a television broadcast undertaking. They submitted that the prohibition of television advertising affected a vital part of the operation of such an undertaking and impaired the undertaking. The interveners suggested that what distinguished *Kellogg's* from the case at bar was the presence of a television undertaking in the proceedings. The presence of the interveners in the proceedings does not, of course, make the challenged provisions ones that are being applied to a television undertaking. What the interveners really suggest is that had a television broadcast undertaking been represented in *Kellogg's* to establish the effect of a regulation of television advertising on such an undertaking, the court might have come to a different conclusion.

Recently, in *Bell Canada v. Que. (Commission de la santé et sécurité du travail)* (1988), 51 D.L.R. (4th) 161, [1988] 1 S.C.R. 749, 85 N.R. 285 (*Bell Canada 1988*), Beetz, J., writing for the court, reviewed the principles of constitutional interpretation applicable to the regulation of federal undertakings. He distinguished between situations in which (1) a provincial law would, if applied to a federal undertaking, affect a vital part of its operations and (2) the effect of the provincial law on a federal undertaking, whether applied to it directly or not, would impair its operations (at p. 244):

> The impairment test is not necessary in cases in which, without going so far as to impair the federal undertaking, the application of the provincial law affects a vital part of the undertaking...
>
> . . . . .
>
> In order for the inapplicability of provincial legislation rule to be given effect, it is sufficient that the provincial statute which purports to apply to the federal undertaking affects a vital or essential part of that undertaking, without necessarily going as far as impairing or paralyzing it.

The federal government has exclusive jurisdiction as regards "essential and vital elements" of a federal undertaking, including the management of such an undertaking, because those matters form the "basic, minimum and unassailable content" of the head of power created by operation of s. 91(29) and the exceptions in s. 92(10) of the *Constitution Act, 1867*. No provincial law touching on those matters can apply to a federal undertaking. However, where provincial legislation does not purport to apply to a federal undertaking, its incidental effect, even upon a vital part of the operation of the undertaking, will not normally render the provincial legislation *ultra vires*.

The case of *A.-G. Man. v. A.-G. Can.*, [1929] 1 D.L.R. 369, [1929] A.C. 260, [1929] 1 W.W.R. 136 (P.C.), upon which Pathonic relied a great deal in its submissions, provides a counter-example to this last statement and illustrates the doctrine of impairment. The legislation there in issue, the Manitoba *Municipal and Public Utility Board Act*, S.M. 1926, c. 33, s. 162, provided that:

> 162. No person, firm, or corporation shall sell, or offer to agree to sell, or directly or indirectly attempt to sell, in Manitoba, any shares, stocks, bonds or other securities of or issued by any company unless the company has first been approved by the Board as one the securities of which are permitted to be sold in Manitoba and a certificate to that effect . . . [is] issued by the Board.

The Act exempted block sales of securities by companies to brokers but did regulate the sale of those securities by brokers to the public. In this sense, as Pathonic submitted, s. 162 did not apply to the companies themselves but applied, rather, to brokers. The issue before the Privy Council was whether s. 162 was *ultra vires* the province in so far as it purported to apply to the sale of the shares of a federally incorporated company.

In concluding that the province did not have jurisdiction to enact s. 162, Viscount Sumner, who delivered the judgment of their Lordships, considered the effect of the provision on federally incorporated companies (at p. 373):

> An artificial person, incorporated under the powers of the Dominion with certain objects, invested by these powers with capacities to trade in pursuit of those objects and with the status and capacities of a Dominion incorporation, is . . . liable in the most ordinary course of business to be stillborn from the moment of incorporation, sterilized in all its functions and activities, thwarted and interfered with in its first and essential endeavours to enter on the beneficial and active employment of its powers, by the necessity of applying to a provincial executive for permission to begin to act and to raise its necessary capital, a permission which may be subjected to conditions or refused altogether according to the view, which in their discretion that executive may take of the plans, promises and prospects of a creation of the Dominion.

Despite the fact that s. 162 did not apply to federally incorporated companies, it succeeded, indirectly, in impairing their operation. That consequence was sufficient to render the provision *ultra vires* the Province of Manitoba.

Although the impairment doctrine was developed in cases concerning the federal power to incorporate companies, Beetz, J., in *Bell Canada 1988*, identified the relevance of this doctrine to the regulation of federal undertakings (at p. 246):

> [T]he transposition of the concept of impairment from the field of federally incorporated companies to that of federal undertakings may be valid in cases in which the application of provincial legislation to federal undertakings in fact impairs the latter, paralyzes them or destroys them.

As the *A.-G. Man. v. A.-G. Can.* case makes clear, the concept of impairment extends not only to the direct application of provincial legislation but also to the indirect effect of that legislation. Thus, where provincial legislation applied to a federal undertaking affects a vital part of that undertaking or, though not applied directly to a federal undertaking, has the effect of impairing its operation, the legislation in question is *ultra vires*.

There is no doubt that television advertising is a vital part of the operation of a television broadcast undertaking. The advertising services of these undertakings therefore fall within exclusive federal legislative jurisdiction. It is well established that such jurisdiction extends to the content of broadcasting: *Re C.F.R.B. and A.-G. Can. (No. 2)* (1973), 38 D.L.R. (3d) 335, [1973] 3 O.R. 819, 14 C.C.C. (2d) 345 (C.A.); *Capital Cities Communications Inc. v. C.R.T.C.* (1977), 81 D.L.R. (3d) 609, 36 C.P.R. (2d) 1, [1978] 2 S.C.R. 141, and advertising forms a part of such content. However, ss. 248 and 249 of the *Consumer Protection Act* do not purport to apply to television broadcast undertakings. Read together with s. 252, it is clear that ss. 248 and 249 apply to the acts of an advertiser, not to the acts of a broadcaster. Nor did Pathonic contend that ss. 248 and 249 applied to television broadcasters. Indeed, it went so far as to submit that the Province of Quebec was unable to regulate the advertising practices of television broadcasters because signals coming from outside the province and received directly by the public or redistributed by a cable company could not be subject to the standards of the *Consumer Protection Act*. While this submission demonstrates that the Quebec government can only achieve partial success in controlling commercial advertising aimed at children, it also demonstrates that a province can aim to regulate provincial advertisers without applying its regulations to television broadcasters situate in the province. Therefore, the provisions in question do not trench on exclusive federal jurisdiction by purporting to apply to a federal undertaking and, in so doing, affecting a vital part of its operation.

Do the provisions nevertheless have the effect of impairing the operation of a federal undertaking? The interveners adduced evidence showing the importance of advertising revenues in the operation of a television broadcast undertaking and that the prohibition of commercial advertising directed to persons under 13 years of age affected the capacity to provide children's programmes. This is not a sufficient basis on which to conclude that the effect of the provisions was to impair the operation of the undertaking, in the sense that the undertaking was "sterilized in all its functions and activities". The most that can be said, as in *Kellogg's* (at p. 323), is that the provisions "may, incidentally, affect the revenue of one or more television stations". Nor can it be said that the provisions have the potential to impair the operation of a broadcast undertaking. Interpreted strictly, as under the Application Guide for sections 248 and 249 (Advertising intended for children under 13 years of age) produced by the Office de la protection du consommateur (October 8, 1980), products and services aimed exclusively at children "may not, for all practical purposes, be advertised during children's programs (unless the message is presented so that it cannot, in any way, arouse a child's interest)". Even if it were true, as Pathonic submitted, that applied this way, the provisions prevent the production of programmes aimed at children since they remove potential funding for those programmes — a contention which was denied by the Attorney-General of Quebec, who insisted that advertisers were always free to aim their message at adults rather than children, and which must also be considered in light of the explicit acceptance in the *Application Guide for sections 248 and 249* (at p. 9) of educational advertising aimed at children produced by private companies — this would only demonstrate that the legislation constrains business decisions both for those who produce advertisements and for those who carry them. It should also be noted that Pathonic is subject to a parallel, though somewhat less stringent, requirement under the terms of the Broadcast Code for Advertising to Children (Canadian Association of Broadcasters, rev. 1982), which code is incorporated by reference as a condition of Pathonic's licence to carry on a broadcasting transmitting undertaking granted by the CRTC (at p. 3):

Pre-schoolers
Children of pre-school age often are unable to distinguish between program content and actual promotions. Therefore, any commercials scheduled for viewing during the school-day morning hours must be directed to the family, parent, or an adult, rather than to children.

Pathonic did not claim that such a limit on the conduct of its business had or could have the effect of disrupting its operations. Nor do we find that ss. 248 and 249 have or could have that effect.

1.4.7. Peter Hogg, *Constitutional Law of Canada*, 3rd ed. (Scarborough: 1992), pp. 774-777

Restraints on legislative power that are derived only from the federal distribution of powers are incomplete, in that a law which is denied to one level of government will be open to the other level of government. For example, when Ontario's *Lord's Day Act* was held to be unconstitutional, on the ground that the observance of days of religious significance was a matter of criminal law,[1] the federal Parliament enacted a *Lord's Day Act* that was held to be constitutional for precisely the reason that had defeated it as a provincial measure.[2] Only under a bill of rights can the courts consider the question whether any legislative body should be able to impose Christian days of religious observance upon a pluralistic society.[3]

In the absence of a bill of rights, when a law abridging a civil liberty is challenged, the issue is "which jurisdiction should have power to work the injustice, not whether the injustice should be prohibited completely".[4] The theory that there are some "injustices" that should be "prohibited completely" is, of course, the impulse to adoption of a bill of rights. Indeed, some judges have professed to find in the *Constitution Act, 1867* an "implied bill of rights". In the *Alberta Press* case (1938),[5] where the Supreme Court of Canada held that a province could not require newspapers to give the government a right of reply to criticism of provincial policies, Duff, C.J.'s opinion could be read as suggesting that the *Constitution Act, 1867* impliedly forbade both the Legislatures and the Parliament from curtailing political speech.[6] In *Switzman v. Elbling* (1957),[7] where the Court held that a province could not prohibit the use of a house to propagate communism, Rand, J. left open the possibility that Parliament as well as the Legislatures might be incompetent to curtail political speech;[8] but Abbott, J. went further, saying explicitly that "Parliament itself could not abrogate this right of discussion and debate".[9] Abbott, J.'s obiter dictum was an unequivocal expression of the implied bill of rights theory.

The implied bill of rights theory was forgotten, or at least was never mentioned, by the Supreme Court of Canada from 1963 until 1978, when the Court decided the *Dupond* case (1978).[10] In that case, Beetz, J., for the majority, said that none of the fundamental freedoms that were inherited from the United Kingdom "is so enshrined in the Constitution as to be beyond the reach of competent legislation". This seemed to have given the theory its quietus. However, like freeway proposals and snakes, the theory does not die easily. Since the adoption of the Charter of Rights in 1982, it has been revived in a number of obiter dicta, the clearest of which was uttered by Beetz, J., who had been so dismissive of the theory in *Dupond*. In the *OPSEU* case (1987),[11] his lordship for the majority quoted with evident approval the dicta in the *Alberta Press* case and *Switzman v. Elbling*, and said that "quite apart from Charter considerations, the legislative bodies in this country must conform to these basic structural imperatives and can in no way override them". In context, it is clear that by "basic structural imperatives" he meant the political freedoms, including freedom of expression, that were necessary to preserve "the essential structure of free parliamentary institutions".

Two reasons have been suggested in the dicta as supporting the existence of an implied bill of rights. The first is the language of the preamble to the *Constitution Act, 1867*, which refers to "a Constitution similar in principle to that of the United Kingdom". The reasoning here is that civil liberties that were enjoyed in the United Kingdom in 1867 were intended to be enjoyed in Canada as well. The difficulty with this reasoning is that the central feature of the Constitution of the United Kingdom, and of its Parliament, was in 1867, and still is, parliamentary sovereignty: any of the civil liberties, including freedom of political speech, can be abolished by the Parliament at Westminster at any time. In the United Kingdom, the tradition of respect for civil liberties is not reflected in the law of the Constitution. It therefore seems likely that "a Constitution similar in principle to that of the United Kingdom" would not contain implied guarantees of civil liberties.

A second reason which has been offered in favour of an implied bill of rights is the *Constitution Act, 1867*'s establishment of representative parliamentary institutions. The reasoning here is that free political speech is "the breath of life of parliamentary institutions", and therefore the establishment of such institutions must be implicitly accompanied by a guarantee of the conditions that are necessary to the effective functioning of the institutions. This is a stronger argument,[12] but it is subject to a similar difficulty to the argument based on the preamble. When the Canadian Constitution established parliamentary institutions on the Westminster model, the plausible assumption would be that they were intended to exercise powers of the same order as those of the Parliament at Westminster, and, of course, those powers included the power to curtail civil liberties, including freedom of political speech. Any limitations on legislative power, such as those entailed by the federal system, could be expected to be expressed, or at least very clearly implied. This seems especially clear with respect to a bill of rights. The framers of the Constitution had the United States Constitution before them; it was their only useful precedent. They followed its federal character, but they deliberately did not copy its bill of rights.[13]

The conventional wisdom is that legislative powers are exhaustively distributed in Canada. As has been explained in chapter 12, Parliamentary Sovereignty,[14] while there are undoubted exceptions to exhaustive distribution, the principle is certainly inconsistent with the theory of an implied bill of rights. It seems to me that it is the principle of exhaustive distribution that is more faithful to the history and text of the *Constitution Act, 1867*. We have noticed that the adoption of the Charter of Rights in 1982 seems to have provoked the Supreme Court of Canada into a renewal of its lagging faith in the implied bill of rights.[15] This is surely a perverse reaction. Since s. 2 of the Charter explicitly guarantees freedom of expression, it is now even harder to argue that an implicit guarantee is to be derived from the *Constitution Act, 1867*.[16]

Endnotes

1. *A.G. Ont. v. Hamilton Street Ry.*, [1903] A.C. 524.
2. *Lord's Day Alliance of Can. v. A.-G. B.C.*, [1959] S.C.R. 497.
3. After the adoption of the Canadian Bill of Rights in 1960, the Lord's Day Act was unsuccessfully challenged under the Bill: *Robertson and Rosetanni v. The Queen*, [1963] S.C.R. 651; and, after the adoption of the Charter of Rights in 1982, the Act was successfully challenged under the Charter: *R. v. Big M Drug Mart*, [1985] 1 S.C.R. 295.
4. Weiler, "The Supreme Court and the Law of Canadian Federalism" (1973), 23 U. Toronto L.J. 307, 344, although Weiler points out that the Supreme Court of Canada has occasionally used federalism as a surreptitious bill of rights, allocating jurisdiction to that level of government which has not exercised it in order to invalidate a law which it really believes should not be enacted at all.
5. *Re Alta. Statutes*, [1938] S.C.R. 100; this case is discussed in ch. 40, Expression, under heading 40.1, "Distribution of powers."

6. *Ibid.*, 133-134. This passage was quoted with approval in *Saumur v. City of Quebec*, [1953] 2 S.C.R. 299 by Rand, J. at 331, Kellock, J. at 353-354 and Locke, J. at 373-374; and Kellock, J. at 354 and Locke, J. at 363 each suggested the possibility of an implied bill of rights.
7. [1957] S.C.R. 285; this case is discussed in ch. 40, Expression, under heading 40.1, "Distribution of powers."
8. *Ibid.*, 307.
9. *Ibid.*, 328. He cautiously repeated the proposition in *Oil, Chemical and Atomic Wkrs. v. Imperial Oil*, [1963] S.C.R. 584, 600.
10. *A.G. Can. and Dupond v. Montreal*, [1978] 2 S.C.R. 770, 796; this case is discussed in ch. 40, Expression, under heading 40.1, "Distribution of powers." The quoted dictum was quoted with approval by Estey, J. for the Court in *A.G. Can. v. Law Society of B.C.*, [1982] 2 S.C.R. 307, 364.
11. *OPSEU v. Ont.*, [1987] 1 S.C.R. 2, 57 *per* Beetz, J.; 25 *per* Dickson, C.J. is to the same effect. Other implied bill of rights dicta are to be found in *Fraser v. Public Service Staff Relations Bd.*, [1985] 2 S.C.R. 455, 462-463 *per* Dickson, C.J.; *RWDSU v. Dolphin Delivery*, [1986] 2 S.C.R. 573, 584 *per* McIntyre, J.
12. It can be buttressed by the suggestion in *Re Initiative and Referendum Act*, [1919] A.C. 935, 945, that the establishment in the *Constitution Act* of representative parliamentary institutions guarantees the existence of those institutions. It is conceivable that this argument could be pushed so far as to guarantee freedom of political discussion: see Russell, "The Political Role of the Supreme Court of Canada in its First Century" (1975), 53 Can. Bar Rev. 576, 592; although the ironic result would be that the establishment of institutions in a written constitution radically distinguishes the institutions from those upon which they were modelled!
13. The implied bill of rights is supported by Scott, note 1, above, 18-21; Schmeiser, note 1, above, 203 (but compare 15) and Gibson, "Constitutional Amendment and the Implied Bill of Rights" (1967), 12 McGill L.J. 497; and is opposed by Laskin, "An Inquiry into the Diefenbaker Bill of Rights" (1959), 37 Can. Bar Rev. 77, 103 and Weiler, note 52, above, 344.
14. The implied bill of rights is supported by Scott, note 1, above, 18-21; Schmeiser, note 1, above, 203 (but compare 15) and Gibson, "Constitutional Amendment and the Implied Bill of Rights" (1967), 12 McGill L.J. 497; and is opposed by Laskin, "An Inquiry into the Diefenbaker Bill of Rights" (1959) 37 Can. Bar Rev. 77, 103 and Weiler, note 4, above, 344.
15. Note 11, above.
16. Such an argument would normally be pointless since the explicit guarantee could be relied upon. Note, however, that s. 2 of the Charter is subject to

the power of override in s. 33, while the implied bill of rights (if it exists) would not be subject to override.

1.5 The *Canadian Charter of Rights and Freedoms* and Freedom of Expression

The Charter combines ancient civil liberties such as those enshrined in writs of Habeas Corpus and the *Magna Carta* with modern notions of human rights.

As noted above, sections 1 and 2 are especially important to students of media law. Section 2(b) declares that "freedom of thought, belief, opinion and expression, including freedom of the press and other media of communication" are amongst the freedoms fundamental to the organization of Canadian society. Section 1 guarantees these freedoms and the other rights set out in the Charter subject to "such reasonable limits prescribed by law as can be demonstrably justified in a free and democratic society."

The rest of the Charter guarantees democratic rights (such as the right to vote) in sections 3-5; mobility rights in section 6; legal rights (such as the right to be tried for an offence within a reasonable length of time) in sections 7-14; equality rights (such as the right to the equal benefit of the law without discrimination) in section 15; and linguistic and educational rights in sections 23 and 24. Sections 25 to 31 add some important qualifiers — for example, section 31 says that nothing in the Charter "extends the legislative powers of any body or authority", and section 32 describes the sphere within which the Charter operates by saying that it applies to all matters of government in Canada.

The Charter has substantially expanded the scope of judicial review in Canada. Under the *Constitution Act, 1867*, the courts were empowered to determine if Parliament or the legislatures were acting within their respective jurisdictions. A decision by a court that a statute passed by Parliament usurped the authority of a provincial legislature would mean that the statute was a nullity, of no force. By contrast, the Charter confers on the courts the additional and extraordinary power to examine whether contested legislation conforms to the values and declarations in the Charter. The autonomy and power of each level of government have been diminished to the extent that the legislation each passes must in the end conform to the substantive standards contained in the Charter. Section 52 of the *Constitution Act, 1982* makes this clear by declaring that "The Constitution of Canada is the supreme law of Canada, and any law that is inconsistent with the provisions of the Constitution is, to the extent of the inconsistency, of no force and effect."

Section 52 means that judicial review now embraces the whole field of fundamental freedoms, civil liberties and human rights.

Since the Charter was proclaimed, the Supreme Court of Canada has made it clear that its provisions will be made to apply only to the state and its institutions. If, for example, a statute contains provisions which are deemed to be unjustifiable encroachments on freedom of expression, the Court will strike them down. If, on the other hand, a private individual, such as a publisher, interferes with a journalist's right to free expression, a court is unlikely to interfere. Similarly, in defamation cases involving private individuals, neither a journalist nor a private citizen is likely to benefit from the Charter.

Canada's Constitution acquired some of the characteristics of the U.S. Constitution when the scope of judicial review was expanded so drastically, The Supreme Court of Canada began to exercise powers long held by the Supreme Court of the United States, this despite the fact that Canada purports to be a parliamentary democracy rather than a republic. Parliamentary democracies are marked by an acceptance of a basic constitutional rule that Parliament is supreme. The Canadian version of that principle, until 1982, was that Parliament was supreme in its domain and the provincial legislatures were supreme in theirs. From another perspective, then, the Charter represents another step in the Americanization of our institutions.

The extent to which the notion of parliamentary supremacy survives in our constitution is found in section 33 of the *Constitution Act, 1982*, which says "Parliament or the legislature of a province may expressly declare . . . that (an) Act . . . shall operate notwithstanding the provisions included in Section 2 (fundamental freedoms) or sections 7 to 15 (legal rights) . . ." If such an act is passed, the enabling declaration will lapse after five years. In other words, statutes which are in conflict with the terms of the Charter, but which rely upon the notwithstanding provision in section 33 will either disappear from the statute books in five years or be debated and renewed.

Finally, parts II to V of the *Constitution Act, 1982*, contain declarations of rights of the aboriginal people of Canada, principles governing the management of regional disparities and procedures for amending the Constitution. While these parts of the Constitution are important, they do not directly affect questions of freedom of expression or of the press.

1.5.1 The *Canadian Charter of Rights and Freedoms, Part One, Constitution Act, 1982*

Whereas Canada is founded upon principles that recognize the supremacy of God and the rule of law:

Guarantee of Rights and Freedoms

1. The *Canadian Charter of Rights and Freedoms* guarantees the rights and freedoms set out in it subject only to such reasonable limits prescribed by law as can be demonstrably justified in a free and democratic society.

Fundamental Freedoms

2. Everyone has the following fundamental freedoms:

(*a*) freedom of conscience and religion;
(*b*) freedom of thought, belief, opinion and expression, including freedom of the press and other media of communication;
(*c*) freedom of peaceful assembly; and
(*d*) freedom of association.

Democratic Rights

3. Every citizen of Canada has the right to vote in an election of members of the House of Commons or of a legislative assembly and to be qualified for membership therein.

4. (1) No House of Commons and no legislative assembly shall continue for longer than five years from the date fixed for the return of the writs of a general election of its members.

(2) In time of real or apprehended war, invasion or insurrection, a House of Commons may be continued by Parliament and a legislative assembly may be continued by the legislature beyond five years if such continuation is not opposed by the votes of more than one-third of the members of the House of Commons or the legislative assembly, as the case may be.

5. There shall be a sitting of Parliament and of each legislature at least once every twelve months.

Mobility Rights

6. (1) Every citizen of Canada has the right to enter, remain in and leave Canada.

(2) Every citizen of Canada and every person who has the status of a permanent resident of Canada has the right
   (*a*) to move to and take up residence in any province; and
   (*b*) to pursue the gaining of a livelihood in any province.

(3) The rights specified in subsection (2) are subject to
   (*a*) any laws or practices of general application in force in a province other than those that discriminate among persons primarily on the basis of province of present or previous residence; and
   (b) any laws providing for reasonable residency requirements as a qualification for the receipt of publicly provided social services.

(4) Subsections (2) and (3) do not preclude any law, program or activity that has as its object the amelioration in a province of conditions of individuals in that province who are socially or economically disadvantaged if the rate of employment in that province is below the rate of employment in Canada.

Legal Rights

7. Everyone has the right to life, liberty and security of the person and the right not to be deprived thereof except in accordance with the principles of fundamental justice.

8. Everyone has the right to be secure against unreasonable search or seizure.

9. Everyone has the right not to be arbitrarily detained or imprisoned.

10. Everyone has the right on arrest or detention
    (a) to be informed promptly of the reasons therefor;
    (b) to retain and instruct counsel without delay and to be informed of that right; and
    (c) to have the validity of the detention determined by way of *habeas corpus* and to be released if the detention is not lawful.

11. Any person charged with an offence has the right
    (a) to be informed without unreasonable delay of the specific offence;
    (b) to be tried within a reasonable time;
    (c) not to be compelled to be a witness in proceedings against that person in respect of the offence;
    (d) to be presumed innocent until proven guilty according to law in a fair and public hearing by an independent and impartial tribunal;
    (e) not to be denied reasonable bail without just cause;
    (f) except in the case of an offence under military law tried before a military tribunal, to the benefit of trial by jury where the maximum punishment for the offence is imprisonment for five years or a more severe punishment;
    (g) not to be found guilty on account of any act or omission unless, at the time of the act or omission, it constituted an offence under Canadian or international law or was criminal according to the general principles of law recognized by the community of nations;
    (h) if finally acquitted of the offence, not to be tried for it again and, if finally found guilty and punished for the offence, not to be tried or punished for it again; and
    (i) if found guilty of the offence and if the punishment for the offence has been varied between the time of commission and the time of sentencing, to the benefit of the lesser punishment.

12. Everyone has the right not to be subjected to any cruel and unusual treatment or punishment.

13. A witness who testifies in any proceedings has the right not to have any incriminating evidence so given used to incriminate that witness in any other proceedings, except in a prosecution for perjury or for the giving of contradictory evidence.

14. A party or witness in any proceedings who does not understand or speak the language in which the proceedings are conducted or who is deaf has the right to the assistance of an interpreter.

Equality Rights

15. (1) Every individual is equal before and under the law and has the right to the equal protection and equal benefit of the law without discrimination and,

in particular, without discrimination based on race, national or ethnic origin, colour, religion, sex, age or mental or physical disability.

(2) Subsection (1) does not preclude any law, program or activity that has as its object the amelioration of conditions of disadvantaged individuals or groups including those that are disadvantaged because of race, national or ethnic origin, colour, religion, sex, age or mental or physical disability.

Official Language of Canada

16. (1) English and French are the official languages of Canada and have equality of status and equal rights and privileges as to their use in all institutions of the Parliament and government of Canada.

(2) English and French are the official languages of New Brunswick and have equality of status and equal rights and privileges as to their use in all institutions of the legislature and government of New Brunswick.

(3) Nothing in this Charter limits the authority of Parliament or a legislature to advance the quality of status or use of English and French.

17. (1) Everyone has the right to use English or French in any debates and other proceedings of Parliament.

(2) Everyone has the right to use English or French in any debates and other proceedings of the legislature of New Brunswick.

18. (1) The statutes, records and journals of Parliament shall be printed and published in English and French and both language versions are equally authoritative.

(2) The statutes, records and journals of the legislature of New Brunswick shall be printed and published in English and French and both language versions are equally authoritative.

19. (1) Either English or French may be used by any person in, or in any pleading in or process issuing from, any court established by Parliament.

(2) Either English or French may be used by any person in, or in any pleading in or process issuing from, any court of New Brunswick.

20. (1) Any member of the public in Canada has the right to communicate with, and to receive available services from, any head or central office of an institution of the Parliament or government of Canada in English or French, and has the same right with respect to any other office of any such institution where

    (*a*) there is a significant demand for communications with and services from that office in such language; or

    (*b*) due to the nature of the office, it is reasonable that communications with and services from that office be available in both English and French.

(2) Any member of the public in New Brunswick has the right to communicate with, and to receive available services from, any office of an institution of the legislature or government of New Brunswick in English or French.

21. Nothing in sections 16 to 20 abrogates or derogates from any right, privilege or obligation with respect to the English and French languages, or either of them, that exists or is continued by virtue of any other provision of the Constitution of Canada.

22. Nothing in sections 16 to 20 abrogates or derogates from any legal or customary right or privilege acquired or enjoyed either before or after the coming into force of this Charter with respect to any language that is not English or French.

Minority Language Educational Rights

23. (1) Citizens of Canada
   (*a*) whose first language learned and still understood is that of the English or French linguistic minority population of the province in which they reside, or
   (*b*) who have received their primary school instruction in Canada in English or French and reside in a province where the language in which they received that instruction is the language of the English or French linguistic minority population of the province,
have the right to have their children receive primary and secondary school instruction in that language in the province.

(2) Citizens of Canada of whom any child has received or is receiving primary or secondary school instruction in English or French in Canada, have the right to have all their children receive primary and secondary school instruction in the same language.

(3) The right of citizens of Canada under subsections (1) and (2) to have their children receive primary and secondary school instruction in the language of the English or French linguistic minority population of a province
   (*a*) applies wherever in the province the number of children of citizens who have such a right is sufficient to warrant the provision to them out of public funds of minority language instruction; and
   (*b*) includes, where the number of those children so warrants, the right to have them receive that instruction in minority language educational facilities provided out of public funds.

Enforcement

24. (1) Anyone whose rights or freedoms, as guaranteed by this Charter, have been infringed or denied may apply to a court of competent jurisdiction to obtain such remedy as the court considers appropriate and just in the circumstances.

(2) Where, in proceedings under subsection (1), a court concludes that evidence was obtained in a manner that infringed or denied any rights or freedoms

guaranteed by this Charter, the evidence shall be excluded if it is established that, having regard to all the circumstances, the admission of it in the proceedings would bring the administration of justice into disrepute.

General

25. The guarantee in this Charter of certain rights and freedoms shall not be construed so as to abrogate or derogate from any aboriginal, treaty or other rights or freedoms that pertain to the aboriginal peoples of Canada including
    (*a*) any rights or freedoms that have been recognized by the Royal Proclamation of October 7, 1763; and
    (*b*) any rights or freedoms that now exist by way of land claims agreements or may be so acquired.

26. The guarantee in this Charter of certain rights and freedoms shall not be construed as denying the existence of any other rights or freedoms that exist in Canada.

27. This Charter shall be interpreted in a manner consistent with the preservation and enhancement of the multicultural heritage of Canadians.

28. Notwithstanding anything in this Charter, the rights and freedoms referred to in it are guaranteed equally to male and female persons.

29. Nothing in this Charter abrogates or derogates from any rights or privileges guaranteed by or under the Constitution of Canada in respect of denominational, separate or dissentient schools.

30. A reference in this Charter to a Province or to the legislative assembly or legislature of a province shall be deemed to include a reference to the Yukon Territory and the Northwest Territories, or to the appropriate legislative authority thereof, as the case may be.

31. Nothing in this Charter extends the legislative powers of any body or authority.

Application of Charter

32. (1) This Charter applies
    (*a*) to the Parliament and government of Canada in respect of all matters within the authority of Parliament including all matters relating to the Yukon Territory and Northwest Territories; and
    (*b*) to the legislature and government of each province in respect of all matters within the authority of the legislature of each province.

(2) Notwithstanding subsection (1), section 15 shall not have effect until three years after this section comes into force.

33. (1) Parliament or the legislature of a province may expressly declare in an Act of Parliament or of the legislature, as the case may be, that the Act or a provision thereof shall operate notwithstanding a provision included in section 2 or sections 7 to 15 of this Charter.

(2) An Act or a provision of an Act in respect of which a declaration made under this section is in effect shall have such operation as it would have but for the provision of this Charter referred to in the declaration.

(3) A declaration made under subsection (1) shall cease to have effect five years after it comes into force or on such earlier date as may be specified in the declaration.

(4) Parliament or the legislature of a province may re-enact a declaration made under subsection (1).

(5) Subsection (3) applies in respect of a re-enactment made under subsection (4).

1.5.1.1 F. L. Morton, *Morgentaler v. Borowski: Abortion, the Charter and the Courts* (Toronto: 1992), pp. 294-314

The abortion trilogy illustrates how much and how fast the Charter of Rights has changed Canadian politics. Less than twenty-five years ago, the federal government enacted major reforms to the abortion law. During this long and controversial process, there was never once a suggestion to use a court challenge to try to influence the process of abortion law reform. Interest-group use of litigation was perceived as an illegitimate attempt to do an "end run" around "responsible government." From start to finish, the 1969 reform was entirely a government-parliamentary matter.

Within six years, this had begun to change. Encouraged by the American Supreme Court's 1973 abortion decision, *Roe v. Wade*, Henry Morgentaler set out on a one-man crusade of civil disobedience to challenge Canada's abortion law. The Supreme Court of Canada thought so little of his *Roe*-inspired "right to privacy" argument that they rejected it *during* oral argument, told the Crown that it need not even reply, and subsequently sent Henry Morgentaler to prison. Eleven years later, the same man was back in the same court challenging the same law, only this time his arguments were based on the Charter of Rights and this time he won. The Supreme Court declared Canada's abortion law unconstitutional. What had been unthinkable in the sixties, and impossible in the seventies, became a reality in the eighties.

Morgentaler's ultimate victory was remarkable not just because it changed the abortion law, but because it cut against the grain of the Canadian legal tradition. In 1975, the year that the Supreme Court sent Morgentaler to prison, Kenneth McNaught, one of Canada's foremost historians, wrote that in Canada attempts to use the courts as an instrument for political change had rarely succeeded and were generally regarded as illegitimate, not least because they smacked of Americanism. From the rebellion of 1837 to the hanging of Louis Riel to the FLQ crisis of 1970, McNaught traced a common strand of Canadian commitment to the beliefs that "order must underlie liberty" and "resort to violence, no matter how just the cause, must be decisively condemned." This belief in "ordered liberty" was still vital on the eve of the adoption of the Charter, as was evident in Justice Hugessen's 1974 sentencing of Morgentaler in Montreal. In sentencing him to eighteen months in prison, Hugessen declared that Morgentaler's "massive and public flouting of the law ... set at risk the entire fabric upon which our society is founded" and represented the actions not of a "democrat" but an "anarchist."

Only a decade later, the continued accuracy of this analysis became doubtful, suggesting still deeper changes in the Canadian polity. Government funding of interest groups and test cases contradicted the view that the use of the courts to pursue social change was illegitimate, while Morgentaler showed that it was even possible to succeed. Nor does civil disobedience evoke the automatic disapproval it once did. It was perhaps predictable that Morgentaler's example would be followed by pro-life activists. But public flouting of the law by large corporations, as in the Sunday closing controversies in Ontario and Alberta, was something novel. As for the tradition of not tolerating the political use of illegal violence, government responses to the Oka and Kanewake confrontations of 1990 suggested this, too, was changing. Collectively, these changes represented a waning of British influence and a waxing of American ideas and practices. There is a growing amount of evidence, both empirical and anecdotal, to support such a thesis.

The Canadian abortion cases cannot be explained by the Charter alone. The wording of the Charter was purposely silent on the topic of abortion and the right to privacy. The abortion trilogy can only be properly understood in the context of developments beyond the courtroom and the Charter. Like the acquittal of Dorothea Palmer in the 1937 contraception trial, Morgentaler's victory was as much an effect of social change as it was a cause. It reflected the emergence of feminism as a major force in Canadian politics.

Judges, of course, deny this, at least when they have their robes on. They like to compare their exercise of judicial review to a carpenter's use of a square: hard, precise, and impersonal. Both the majority and dissenting judgments in *Morgentaler* wrote that their task was simply "to measure the content of s. 251 against the Charter." This was also how Justice Estey explained the Court's decision to the public: we measured the abortion law by the Charter, "like a tailor measures a sleeve. It didn't fit, so we threw it back to parliament." In cases like the abortion trilogy, this type of talk cannot be taken seriously by non-lawyers, and in fact is not even taken seriously by lawyers when they are *entre nous*.

In practice a constitution functions more like a sponge than a carpenter's square, absorbing the never-ending shifts in political opinion and social values from one generation to the next. The medium of adaptation is judges, especially Supreme Court judges. The growth of feminist influence in Canadian political, educational, and legal elites was a necessary pre-condition for the *Morgentaler* decision. The Charter provided Morgentaler a new lever, but its successful use was contingent on a more receptive legal and political environment.

There was almost no feminist input into the 1969 abortion law reform. In 1975 there was a feminist presence but little influence. By 1986, when Morgentaler returned to the Supreme Court, this situation had changed dramatically. In 1982 the first woman justice, Bertha Wilson, was appointed to the Supreme Court of Canada. Wilson went on to write the feminist perspective on abortion into her concurring opinion in the *Morgentaler* decision. In 1987 a second woman, Claire L'Heureux-Dubé, was appointed to the Court. During this same twenty-year period, the number of women in Canadian law schools went from less than 10 per cent to almost half.

Stung by their lack of success under the 1960 *Bill of Rights*, feminists worked to influence the drafting of the 1982 Charter of Rights and then mobilized public support for its adoption. Aware that constitutional rights are neither self-interpreting nor self-actualizing, feminists put in place the various institutional means that would be necessary to actualize the potential of their Charter blueprint for sexual equality. The National Action Committee on the Status of Women helped to organize LEAF to conduct strategic litigation of women's rights under the Charter. Feminists were also active in the creation of the Court Challenges Program (CCP) in 1985, a $9 million fund to pay for equality (and language) rights litigation. LEAF in turn became the single largest recipient of CCP funding, including funding for its interventions in the *Borowski* and *Daigle* cases. (The feminist orientation of the CCP was confirmed by its rejection of funding requests from REAL Women in both these cases.)

These changes within the legal world reflected parallel changes in the larger political landscape. Feminists converted their legal defeats of the seventies into political victories. They persuaded Parliament to amend the *Indian Act* to end the disabilities that previously attached to Indian women. Parliament was also persuaded to amend the *Unemployment Insurance Act* to cover all pregnancy-related unemployment. While political elites still resisted many feminist policy proposals, they had become careful not to offend feminist sensibilities, for fear of bad public relations and political backlash.

Nor were the emergence of feminism and the abortion issue limited to Canada or even North America. Both emerged as new factors in the politics in most Western industrial democracies during the same period. Between 1965 and 1984, seventeen of twenty European and North American nations liberalized their abortion laws. The social conditions that gave rise to both the movement and the issue—industrialization and the mechanization of physical labour, urbanization, the displacement of the industrial and farm sectors by the service sector of the economy, and the commercial availability of the birth control pill — were common to all seventeen societies. In other words, Canada would have had an abortion reform movement (and opposition) without either Henry Morgentaler or the Charter of Rights. What the latter two did was to give abortion politics in Canada a peculiarly legalistic character, unlike any other democracy except the United States.

The emergence of feminism as a force in Canadian politics has been part of a larger reorientation of political conflict in Canada and other Western democracies. Feminism is only one of a cluster of new political issues that cut across the old class-based lines of political cleavage. These new "social issues," as they are sometimes called, also include environmental protection, state promotion of cultural pluralism and equal status for minorities educational policy, disarmament and peace issues, and a more permissive sexual morality, including abortion.

These issues have been collectively described as the politics of "post-materialism" because they do not track along the same lines of class conflict (or labour-management) that characterized politics in the industrial (or "materialist") democracies from the mid-nineteenth to the mid-twentieth centuries. The politics of post-materialism is concerned not so much with the redistribution of wealth between capital and labour as with the social issues. The post-materialist agenda tends to divide old allies and bring old adversaries together. The abortion issue, for example, has driven pro-lifers like Borowski and Shumiatcher out of the NDP. Similarly, the environmental movement has united old adversaries such as unions and management in the west coast timber, lumber, and pulp industries.

These new concerns are most prevalent outside the working classes. Seymour Martin Lipset has observed that in post-war Western democracies, the most dynamic agent of social change has not been Marx's industrial proletariat but a new "oppositionist intelligentsia," drawn from and supported by the well-educated, more affluent strata of society.

> The reform elements concerned with postmaterialist or social issues largely derive their strength not from the workers and the less privileged, the social base of the Left in industrial society, but from segments of the well educated and affluent, students, academics, journalists, professionals and civil servants.

In Canada, the Charter has served as a lightning rod for many groups of the post-materialist or New Left. The connection of the Charter and post-materialism was evident in the conflict over the 1987 Meech Lake Accord. The Accord was originally conceived by the Mulroney government and the other nine provincial governments as a means to "bring Quebec back into the constitutional family." This was to be achieved by an omnibus constitutional amendment that would have recognized Quebec's status as a "distinct society" and its right to "protect and promote" this distinctiveness. In the end, the Accord was defeated by an *ad hoc* coalition of groups who said the Meech Lake Accord betrayed both the Charter and the groups it protected. Deborah Coyne, a leader of the Meech opposition, described her organization, the Canadian Coalition on the Constitution, as follows:

> The Charter's appeal to our non-territorial identities — shared characteristics such as gender, ethnicity and disability — is finding concrete expression in an emerging new power structure in

society.... This power structure involves new networks and coalitions among women, the disabled, aboriginal groups, social reform activists, church groups, environmentalists, ethnocultural organizations, just to name a few. All these new groups have mobilized a broad range of interests that draw their inspiration from the Charter and the Constitution...

Given the outcome of Meech Lake, the power of this coalition of "Charter Canadians," as Alan Cairns has described them, cannot be doubted. Together with some improbable allies, the Charter Canadians achieved what was unimaginable only a decade earlier: the defeat of a constitutional amendment that enjoyed the support of all eleven first ministers and of the leaders of both opposition parties. While this coalition was initially spontaneous, it is now as entrenched in Canada's unwritten constitution as the Charter is in the formal Constitution. Indeed, each is the reflection of the other.

The Meech Lake affair may be seen as two different constitutions battling for control of the Canadian state. One is the old constitution, with its roots in Confederation. The other dates only from 1982. The old constitution is the constitution of governments, federalism, and French-English dualism. Since this constitution belongs to the governments, its guardians believe it may be appropriately changed by the governments — by first ministers' conferences. Under it, constitutional politics is mainly a process of bargaining among political elites. Implicitly, this old constitution has always recognized the special status of Quebec. Meech Lake merely made this explicit through the "distinct society" clause.

The new constitution is the constitution of the Charter. It is concerned with individuals and their rights and freedoms. It is also concerned with group rights, but not in the old sense of only the French and English. The new constitution is multicultural and asserts the equal status of ethnic Canadians and aboriginals with the two founding peoples. Since this new constitution belongs to "the people," it should not be amended without their participation and consent. Charter Canadians objected to Meech Lake not only because of its content, but also because they were excluded from the closed and private process that produced it.

The Charter is, of course, uniquely Canadian, but the various social movements that have rallied around it are not. These social movements would certainly be present in Canada without the Charter. They would not, however, have gone so far so fast. The Charter has conferred the status and the institutional means to influence public policy more effectively. Because of the symbiotic relation these groups have with the Charter and the legalized form of politics it supports, I have elsewhere described these groups as the "Court Party."

The opposite, however, is not true. Without a Court Party, the Charter and the Supreme Court would not have attained their new prominence. Post-materialism provided the political *zeitgeist* that breathed life and energy into the Charter by providing the army of true believers who lifted it out of the inert pages of the statute books and made it a vital force, and the courts powerful new actors, in Canada's political process. Some have described this as the "Charter Revolution."

From the perspective of post-materialism, however, the Charter has been not so much the cause as the means by which the Court Party has pursued this revolution.

The abortion trilogy illustrates as well as any three cases could a new dimension in Canadian politics — the "politics of rights." The adoption of the Charter did not (with several important exceptions) create new rights so much as it created a new way of making decisions about rights in which courts have played a more central and authoritative role. The Charter has created a new forum: courts; a new set of decision-makers: judges; and a new resource: not votes or money but simply the "right argument." Interest groups who "lose" in the traditional arenas of electoral, legislative, and administrative politics can now turn to the courts for a second kick at the can. This is the politics of rights, "the [new] forms of political activity made possible by the presence of [constitutional] rights."

Interest-group litigation has been encouraged by both the Court and the government since 1982. The government's Court Challenges Program has funded hundreds of language and section 15 equality cases since its creaton in 1985. Since one of the criteria for funding is the likelihood that the case will have "consequences for a number of people," interest group seeking to make strategic use of Charter litigation have been the primary beneficiaries of the program. It has been estimated that over 80 per cent of the litigation grants go to interest groups.

The Supreme Court itself has encouraged interest group use of Charter litigation through a variety of procedural rulings and decisions. Its 1981 decision in *Borowski* broadening the rules of standing made it easier for interest groups to get their feet in the door of the local courthouse. The Court's liberal interpretations of "mootness" culminating in the second *Borowski* decision made it easier for litigants (except for Borowski) to stay in the courts even after their disputes ceased to exist. Finally, the Supreme Court's "open door" policy for interveners has made it easy for groups who were not involved in the earlier stages of a Charter case to participate in the final appeal.

Nothing, however, has encouraged Charter litigation more than the Court's willing embrace of the noninterpretivist approach to assigning meaning to Charter rights. The effective sundering of constitutional law from constitutional text has maximized the discretion of judges, thereby giving almost all interest groups at least the hope of winning a test case on the back of a plausible interpretation of a Charter right, regardless of its original or intended meaning. Individuals and interest groups representing every ideological stripe — from the National Citizens' Coalition to the Canadian Union of Public Employees, from the Canadian Jewish Congress to anti-Semite Jim Keegstra — have flocked to the courts to claim the protection and assistance of the Charter. In the Supreme Court's first 100 Charter decisions, at least sixty-three interest groups were present as litigants or interveners in seventeen cases.

The *Morgentaler* and *Borowski* cases are particularly telling examples of how the judicially induced malleability of the Charter's meaning can elicit constitutional challenges based on diametrically opposed interpretations of the same Charter section. How could section 7 of the Charter protect both a right to life and a right to abortion? The answer, of course, was that it protected neither, at least not explicitly. Both Morgentaler and Borowski claimed that these rights were "implied" by the broad contours of "life, liberty, and security of the person ... [and] the principles of fundamental justice." When freed from the constraints of fidelity to original understanding, judges can and do create new rights that were not intended, or even were purposely excluded, as in the case of abortion.

Many Charter experts, following the lead of Justice Lamer's opinion in the *B.C. Motor Vehicle Reference*, have minimized the significance of judicial fidelity to the original or intended meaning of constitutional language by characterizing it as an American idiosyncrasy. This "Canadian school" likes to subsume all constitutional law — the Charter, as well as federalism — under the benign shade of Lord Sankey's "living tree." Like most appeals to nationalism, this argument generates more heat than light. The issues underlying the interpretivist/noninterpretivist debate involve constitutional logic, not nationality. The debate is not one-sided, and it is a mistake not to take it seriously.

It is one thing to adopt the interpretivist version of the "living tree" imagery, thereby allowing judges to adapt the constitution to new factual situations. It is quite another to give judges a free hand to create new constitutional rules while working with the same old facts. The first adds new meaning, but the second changes the original meaning. The former is necessary to preserve constitutionalism over time. The latter challenges the very logic of a "written constitution." What is the point of "carving in [constitutional] stone," so to speak, the "binding" rules of a nation's politics, if judges are immediately free to amend the meaning intended by those rules. If flexibility and adaptability to social change are the most important virtues of a constitution, why did Canada ever abandon the "unwritten constitution" inherited from Great Britain, the ultimate in "living tree" constitutionalism.

Even if one accepts the legitimacy of non-interpretivist rewriting of the constitution, it would still seem more appropriate in the case of an old constitutional provision than a very recent one. After all, the standard justification of non-interpretivism is that living generations should not be bound by the constitutional decisions of dead ones. This argument is not without problems, but to the extent that it is valid, it surely applies more strongly to such documents as the *Constitution Act, 1867* than to the 1982 Charter. At the time the Court heard the Morgentaler appeal, the Charter was less than five years old and the appeal turned on Charter provisions where the intent of the framers was as clear as such things ever get.

In any case, the Supreme Court has been inconsistent on the issue of original intent. When it has suited their purposes — in cases like *Quebec Protestant*

School Board Association, Alberta Labour Reference, and of course *Daigle* — the judges have been quick to hide behind the intent of the framers. This was not surprising. Indeed, it is how judicial review is supposed to work in theory. Judicial fidelity to original intent can enhance the authority of the Court's decision by making it clear, especially to the losing side, that the Court's decision is not based on the policy preferences of the judges but on the constitution itself. With its decision in the *B.C. Motor Vehicle Reference*, however, the Supreme Court denied itself this important support. Once the Court said in both word and deed that the framers' intent should receive only "minimal weight" in interpreting the meaning of a Charter right, future appeals to it tend to be viewed as opportunistic attempts to justify the desired result. Rather than evoking public acceptance of the Court's decisions, these sporadic appeals tend to inspire cynicism about the judges and ultimately about the entire Charter enterprise.

The *Morgentaler* and the *Borowski* cases illustrated the "politics of rights" writ large. Neither man represented the lonely individual who, wronged by the system, humbly came before the Supreme Court asking for redress. For both, the use of the courts was a calculated political choice. It was a choice based on repeated rejections by political parties and public opinion polls. Both were represented by some of Canada's best and most expensive legal talent. Their legal expenses — over a quarter of a million dollars each — were mostly picked up by the pro-choice and pro-life movements who causes they championed.

The abortion trilogy also reveals different ways to use the Charter to influence public policy. The first is to challenge directly the validity of an existing law, the path chosen by both Morgentaler and Borowski. The debate over Bill C-43 reveals a second: to invoke the principles of the Charter (and the no-so-veiled threat of future litigation) to shape public policy *during* the legislative process. When the first tactic succeeds in invalidating a policy, the second tactic may suffice to prevent its reintroduction in some amended form. The claim that a bill violates the Charter can be used to stigmatize the bill and mobilize opinion (within cabinet, caucus, or the public at large) against it. The more credible the claim, the less likely the government is to proceed with the bill.

This perspective also discloses the closer relationship between the courthouse and the legislative assembly under the Charter. Interest-group use of Charter litigation may be understood as legal battles in a larger political war. The objective of the litigants is not to enforce the law of the Charter but to use the Charter to change the law of the government. The Supreme Court's final rulings provided the winners with new resources with which to return to the larger political struggle. Legal defeat does not necessarily mean political defeat: consider Morgentaler's ultimate victory in Quebec in the seventies. Nor does legal victory ensure political victory: consider the apparent success of the pro-life movement in the United States to limit if not reverse *Roe v. Wade* in the *Webster* case. With these caveats in mind, however, success in the judicial arena is always preferable. In the Canadian abortion cases of the 1980s, the success of the pro-choice parties has helped them achieve their policy objectives for the foreseeable future.

This is the new Canadian version of the "politics of rights." The various rights enumerated in the Charter become "political resources of unknown value in the hands of those who want to alter the course of public policy." Judicial pronouncements notwithstanding, the Charter is not so much the cause as the means through which such change is sought. Individuals and interest groups can recast their policy goals in the rhetoric of rights and then take them to the courts to be "enforced." Whether they succeed depends largely on how the judges exercise their considerable discretion to interpret the Charter.

Lawyers are trained to think about winning cases in terms of the "right argument." Cases like the abortion trilogy suggest that often it is more a question of the "right judge." The Court's unreserved (and inconsistent) embrace of noninterpretivism has maximized the judges' discretion to the point that they appear to be able to reach almost any result they want. This was certainly the appearance given by the four different judgments delivered in the Court's *Morgentaler* decision. Only one justice out of seven declared a constitutional right to abortion. The other four members of the majority coalition found only procedural violations of the Charter, and they were further divided on the seriousness of these violations. The two dissenters said there was no constitutional violation.

This division of the Court was not caused by technical disagreements over a narrow point of law. Rather, it reflected a growing division on the Court between two different theories of Charter review, two different conceptions of the proper role of the judge. During its first two years of Charter cases (1984-85), the Supreme Court was unanimous in 87 per cent (thirteen out of fifteen) of its decisions. In 1986, this figure dropped to 55 per cent and has remained at about 64 per cent ever since. During the same timeframe, unanimity in non-Charter decisions remained constant at above 80 per cent. The fractured *Morgentaler* decision accurately reflected the growing division of the Court.

One wing of the Court, exemplified by Justice Wilson, adopted an activist, noninterpretivist approach to applying the Charter. As evidenced by her opinion in *Morgentaler*, Justice Wilson was inclined to read in new and even unintended meaning to the broadly worded principles of the Charter, and she was not reluctant to strike down parliamentary enactments that failed to meet her vision of the Charter. The other wing of the Court was best exemplified by Justice McIntyre's judicial self-restraint and interpretivist approach to applying the Charter. The Charter, McIntyre wrote, was not "an empty vessel to be filled with whatever meaning we might wish." The McIntyre approach attempted to minimize judicial discretion by limiting Charter rights to their "original meaning," as disclosed (when possible) by the intent of the framers, and as a result was usually more differential to Parliament's policy decisions.

These two different approaches to interpreting the Charter led to very different results. A study of the Supreme Court's first 100 Charter decisions revealed that the judges had very different "voting records" on Charter cases. Predictably, Justice Wilson had the highest percentage of votes supporting individuals' Charter claims, 53 per cent, while Justice McIntyre had one of the lowest, 23 per cent. The Court average was 35 per cent.

The contrast between McIntyre and Wilson was still more stark when the number and "directionality" of their dissenting and concurring opinions were taken into account. The decision to write a concurring or dissenting opinion indicates a judge's dissatisfaction or disagreement with the majority opinion. Repeated use of concurring and dissenting opinions indicates that a judge is outside the mainstream of the court. Significantly, Justices Wilson and McIntyre wrote the most dissenting opinions, yet never dissented together. Not only did they depart from the majority most frequently, but they did so in opposite directions. In each of her thirteen dissents, Wilson supported the individual's Charter claim. McIntyre supported the Crown in ten of his eleven dissents. Twenty-eight of Wilson's thirty-one concurring and dissenting opinions supported a broader interpretation of the Charter than the majority. (*Morgentaler* was one of these.) In all sixteen of his dissenting and concurring opinions, McIntyre supported a narrower interpretation of the Charter.

These statistics confirm what most Charter experts already knew: the meaning of the Charter, and thus the "existence" of a right, can vary from one judge to another. In many Charter cases, the policy preferences (conscious or otherwise) of a judge combined with his or her judicial philosophy are more likely to determine the outcome than the text of the Charter. Different judges "find" different rights. To put this point in context, if the justices of the Supreme Court had been as fond of fetuses as they were of bilingualism, Joe Borowski would probably be on the lecture circuit and Henry Morgentaler out of business.

A version of this previously heretical view was actually voiced by Justice Estey, *after* he retired from the Court, in an interview with the *Globe and Mail*.

> Justice Estey said it worries him that Canadians still do not realize how decisions vary according to the personality of each judge. As the misconception is gradually corrected, he said, people may lose respect and faith in the institution....People think a court is a court is a court. But it is elastic. It is always sliding.

In fact, it is less likely that people will lose respect for the court than that they will simply want to know more about a judicial nominee before he or she is appointed. As the political implications of this fact are recognized by affected political actors and interest groups, there will be growing pressure to appoint the "right kind of judge" to Canadian appeal courts.

To most Canadians, the political controversies sparked by the recent nominations of Robert Bork (1987) and Clarence Thomas (1991) to the United States Supreme Court were politically repugnant. They were perceived as transparent attempts to control the meaning of American constitutional law by controlling the appointment of Supreme Court judges. Such attempts at "court-packing" appear to strike at the foundations of judicial independence and thus the "rule of law" tradition. For better or for worse, however, the Canadian Supreme Court's relatively activist and noninterpretivist approach to the Charter is likely to encourage a growing politicization of the judicial appointment process in Canada.

"Where power rests, there influence will be brought to bear." This was written in the 1950s by a leading American political scientist to explain American lobbyists' concentration on administrative agencies. In the 1980s, this analysis provided an equally compelling explanation for the new attention being paid to judicial appointments to the American Supreme Court. There is no *a priori* reason to assume that this axiom does not apply equally to Canadian democracy, and events in the wake of *Morgentaler* revealed a new attitude toward judicial appointments. Angela Costigan, counsel for Choose Life Canada, a national pro-life lobby group, criticized the decision as "the expression of personal opinion by the judges," and indicated that in the future her group would try to influence the appointment of judges who shared its position. Norma Scarborough, president of the Canadian Abortion Rights League, responded by declaring that while her group had never tried to influence judicial appointments in the past, it would, if necessary, in the future. "We are going to protect our position as much as possible," she declared.

When Justice William Estey announced his intention to resign from the Supreme Court two months after the *Morgentaler* decision, the search for his replacement immediately attracted the attention of pro-life and pro-choice groups. The *Globe and Mail* reported that "activists in the abortion debate and representatives of ethnic communities are lobbying hard....Many members of the ruling PC Party's right-wing...are putting pressure on PM Mulroney to appoint a conservative judge." Member of Parliament James Jepson, one of the most outspoken pro-life Tory backbenchers, explained the importance of the new Supreme Court appointment: "We now have a chance to put men and women on the bench with a more conservative point of view." While emphasizing that he had never lobbied for a judicial appointment before, Jepson continued:

> But this one seems to have caught the people's attention. Unfortunately, with the Charter that Trudeau left us, we legislators do not have final power. It rests with the courts.... You have seen the battling in the United States for the [most recent] Supreme Court nominee. Well, it doesn't take a rocket scientist to see we have the same situation here now.

In the end, the pro-life lobbying had no apparent effect on the government's appointment of Toronto lawyer John Sopinka to fill Estey's seat on the Court. But Jepson's comments represented a sharp break with past Canadian practice and were not an isolated incident. The year before, when the Mulroney government appointed former Manitoba Premier Sterling Lyon, an outspoken critic of the Charter, to the Manitoba Court of Appeal, Charter groups protested and called for some form of public scrutiny of nominees prior to appointment. Demands for public screening of judicial candidates are not likely to disappear as political elites become more sophisticated in their understanding of the connection between the "right argument" and the "right judge."

These developments are consistent with the judicial appointment practices of other democracies with written constitutions and judicial review. Attention to the politics and judicial philosophies of would-be Supreme Court judges is also consistent with democratic norms of legitimacy. Most Canadians are no longer willing to accept the spectacle of an unelected Senate blocking government policy. (Even the pro-choice *Globe and Mail* criticized the Senate's defeat of Bill C-43.) The more the Supreme Court exercises its new power under the Charter, the more Canadians are going to want to know something about the backgrounds of their future constitutional rulers *before* they take office. To take just one example, when Bertha Wilson was appointed to the Supreme Court in 1982, no one noticed that five years earlier she had chaired a policy committee of the United Church that strongly endorsed liberal reform of the abortion law. It seems unlikely that this type of information would go unnoticed any longer. For better or for worse, the relationship between courts and politics is a two-way street. The more that judges influence the political process, the more political actors will seek to influence the selection of judges.

While the empowerment of judges under the Charter has inevitably drawn more attention to the judicial appointment process, the presence of the section 33 "legislative override" or "notwithstanding" clause may mitigate the more excessive forms of court-packing witnessed in recent American politics. The legislative override is unique to the Canadian constitution and provides an alternative means to deal with what a government views as an unacceptable or mistaken judicial interpretation of the Charter. Rather than using the blunt instrument of judicial appointment—which can leave its ideological imprint on the Court for years and even decades—section 33 allows a legislature to remove surgically, as it were, the effect of an unacceptable Charter decision without permanently "disfiguring" the composition of the Court. It seems unlikely, for example, that the more extreme examples of court-packing in American politics—President Roosevelt's in the 1930s and President Reagan's in the 1980s—would have been considered necessary if something like the section 33 legislative override had been available.

Many Canadian commentators consider this the vice, not the virtue, of section 33—that it will make it *too* easy for governments to override Charter decisions. For evidence, these critics point to the best-known and most controversial use of section 33 to date: the Quebec government's decision to reinstate its "French-only" public signs law following the Supreme Court's ruling that this policy violated the Charter right to freedom of expression. In the uproar that followed Quebec's use of the legislative override, even Prime Minister Mulroney declared that the Charter was "not worth the paper it was written on" so long as section 33 remained intact, and vowed to work for its removal.

These kinds of blanket condemnations of section 33 are premised on a view of constitutional rights and judicial review that is more mythical than real. The section 33 critics tend to think of constitutional rights as judicially enforceable moral rules and draw a sharp distinction between the realm of rights and the realm of politics. Politics is characterized as the realm of self-interest, driven by will and ruled by compromise. Rights are portrayed as the realm of justice, governed by reason and discerned by impartial judges. The beauty of the Charter, according to this view, is that it lifts questions of rights out of the grimy give and take of party politics and into a sphere where independent judges, exercising reason, not will, can define and defend rights against the excesses of majority-rule democracy.

The politics of rights, as illustrated by the abortion trilogy, serves as an antidote to this "myth of rights." While the dichotomy of rights and interest certainly animates the enterprise of constitutional rights, in practice it is impossible to keep them distinct. As the abortion trilogy illustrates, both individual and collective self-interest are usually present in Charter litigation; nor are reason and consideration of principle absent from the deliberations of Parliament. The extensive development of interest-group litigation under the Charter, encouraged in part by the Court's own decisions, ensures that political interests will find their way into the courtroom. When judges determine what is or is not a "reasonable limitation" on a Charter right by sifting and weighing social facts, the distinction between judging and legislating is also blurred. As Chief Justice Antonio Lamer observed on the tenth anniversary of the Charter, determining what constitutes "reasonable limitation" on a right is "to make what is essentially what used to be a political call." At the same time, the existence of Charter precedents, combined with the threat of future litigation, ensures that legislators take into account the same appeals to moral principles and fairness that are heard in court.

In sum, the differences between courts and legislatures, while important, are not as absolute as the critics of section 33 tend to claim. Both must fashion law from an impure compound of interest and right. Both must exercise practical judgment. Neither is infallible. From this perspective, just as judicial review serves as a check on legislative decision-making, so section 33 provides a check on judicial decision-making. It is in this sense that Peter Russell has described and defended section 33 as providing a form of "legislative review of judicial review."

The value of this contribution to institutional "checks and balances" is not just that it negatively blocks the "mistakes" of the other branch. It can also stimulate a creative and productive dialogue between the two different branches of government, each with its respective strengths and weaknesses. It would be just as perverse to require elected governments to acquiesce passively in every judicial pronouncement as it would be to encourage judges to approve meekly every legislative act. The latter would defeat the very purpose of judicial review, while the former would undermine any meaningful form of democratic self-government.

Mutual persuasion, not coercion, is the medium of exchange appropriate to the challenge of giving concrete meaning to constitutional rights. Everyone recognizes the government's obligation in constitutional litigation to try to persuade the Court of the rightness and reasonableness of its legislation. Less obvious but no less real is the obligation of the Court to persuade the government of the rightness and reasonableness of its judgments. Indeed, the obligation to persuade is ultimately more incumbent on the Court than the government. Courts can coerce individuals, but, "possessing neither the purse nor the sword," they cannot coerce governments.

In the end, no constitutional court can hold out forever against sustained popular opposition. American history is littered with the metaphorical corpses of Supreme Court majorities who tried to block sustained political majorities. Recent developments in France confirm that this is not an American idiosyncrasy. Democracies do not tolerate for long courts that get too far ahead or too far behind public opinion. This does not mean that a constitutional court cannot lead or brake public opinion, but its success depends on its ability to persuade.

In Canada, section 33 institutionalizes and thereby formalizes this relationship between democracy and judicial review. In so doing, it creates the framework for a constitutional dialogue, not just between courts and governments, but also between political parties. The legislative override cannot be decreed by an order-in-council. Section 33 requires legislation, and legislation requires three readings and parliamentary debate. This ensures ample opportunity for opponents to criticize the government both inside and outside the legislative chambers. Moreover, any use of section 33 expires five years from the date it is proclaimed—the maximum time permitted between elections in Canada. This means that before a legislative override can be re-enacted, general elections must be held, thereby providing the opportunity for opposition parties to mobilize public opinion and to force the government to defend publicly its use of the override power.

Government by argument and persuasion is very much what parliamentary democracy is all about. A parliament is, after all, a place where people *parler* — or talk. In a liberal democracy—that is, in a society committed not just to conducting its affairs by majority rule, but also to respecting individuals and minorities—such talk will include talk about rights. In the most global sense, this "rights talk" is what the adoption of the Charter of Rights has brought to Canada.

As today's university students (most of whom came of age politically *after* 1982) must be constantly reminded, the Charter did not bring rights to Canada. Canada was very much a free and democratic society prior to 1982. Its many imperfections notwithstanding, the Canadian record on human rights and civil liberties prior to 1982 would easily rank in the top ten in the world, and arguably ahead of the United States, which already had a constitutional bill of rights. What Canada did not have, however, was "rights talk." British constitutionalism and the belief in "ordered liberty" cast their long shadows over both the thought and speech of Canadian politics. "Peace, order and good government" were the trump cards of Canadian political rhetoric. Our ancestors enjoyed rights—or liberties, as they preferred to call them—but they did not talk a great deal about them. A decade after the adoption of the Charter, rights talk is all about us. Via the media, rights talk has spilled out of the courtrooms and into the surrounding social environment, permeating political discourse and behaviour.

The advent of rights talk to Canadian politics holds out both promise and peril. For most Canadians the positive contribution of rights talk is more obvious. It is an antidote to positivism, the idea that might makes right. It leavens democratic discourse by pointing to standards of justice that transcend "the will of the people." The appeal to rights can be used to challenge coercive assertions of self-interest and power. It reminds both governments and citizens that there is more to self-government than self-interest. Rights talk provides a rhetorical sword and a legal shield to groups and individuals who find themselves the target of majoritarian malice or government oppression.

Rights talk, however, also has its down side. This has recently been explored by Mary Ann Glendon, drawing on American political experience. The assertion of rights is often grounded in immediate self-interest, fuelled by the inarticulate but powerful sense that "I have a right to do what I want." This kind of moral relativism is the very opposite of the traditional view of rights as standards of right and wrong that exist independently of individual or collection opinion. Motivated by selfishness and moral relativism, rights talk can contribute to a "hyper-individualism" that erodes the social and political fabric.

Rights talk tends to carry the adversarial character of the courtroom into society at large, threatening to create natural adversaries out of those who were previously considered natural friends: parents and children, husbands and wives, teachers and students. Since rights talk can express only self-interest, any inequality in these relationships is automatically presumed to prejudice the interest of the dependent party. The possibility of a mutually beneficial common interest or altruistic behaviour is denied. In this respect, Glendon argues that rights talk represents only half of the political equation. Rights talk, she suggests, provides an incomplete political vocabulary, because it cannot express the equally important concepts of personal, civic, and collective responsibilities.

Glendon reports that rights talk has also negatively influenced public debate and behaviour in contemporary American politics. She argues that rights talk has tended to inflate political claims with a moral absolutism, encouraging unrealistic expectations and making mutual understanding and political compromise more difficult. Rights-talk "promotes mere assertion over reason-giving" and can become "the language of no compromise," writes Glendon. "The winner takes all and the loser has to get out of town. The conversation is over.".

Glendon argues that abortion policy and politics in America illustrate the negative aspects of judicialized politics and rights talk. While almost all of the European countries she studied had liberalized their abortion laws, most still provided some form of protection for the fetus. Typically, the abortion law was part of a broader family policy that included birth control, alternatives to abortion, and economic support for low-income or single-parent families. While an abortion could be rather easily obtained in these countries, the legislative framework sent out a message that it was not to be considered just another form of birth control and that there was public support for alternatives. Contrary to the "accepted wisdom" in the United States, compromise on abortion was "not only possible but typical." How had the European democracies been able to achieve what appeared impossible in the United States? Through the consensus-building made possible in the legislative process, concluded Glendon. In the U.S., by contrast, the Supreme Court's *Roe v. Wade* decision had "shut down the legislative process of bargaining, education, and persuasion on the abortion issue."

How much of Glendon's analysis applies to abortion politics in Canada? It is important to remember that *Morgentaler*, unlike *Roe v. Wade*, did not shut the door on legislative regulation of abortion. Thus the central criticisms made of *Roe* are not applicable to *Morgentaler* and the Supreme Court of Canada. Still, the fate of Bill C-43 suggests that the polarizing effects of rights talk is at work in the Canadian body politic. As noted in the preceding chapter, the Mulroney government's attempt to fashion a new abortion policy represented a compromise. It said that abortion was still wrong in principle but available in practice. It was neither pro-choice nor pro-life. It also clearly followed the constitutional requirements articulated by four of the five judges in the *Morgentaler* majority. Notwithstanding these characteristics, it was defeated on the combined strength of the pro-choice and pro-life factions in the Senate, neither of whom would accept such a compromise.

While this outcome was not dictated by the Supreme Court's decision in *Morgentaler*, it was facilitated by it. After the decision, the rights talk inspired by the Charter encouraged moralistic confrontation and discouraged compromise. In the end, the pro-choice and pro-life extremes united to defeat a compromise abortion policy that had the support of the political middle. Canada thus joined, indeed surpassed, the United States as the only Western democracy not to provide at least symbolic support for the unborn child, while still respecting a woman's freedom to choose. Ironically, Canada's new "non-policy" goes even further than Dr. Henry Morgentaler thinks appropriate. Morgentaler believes there is no justification to abort a healthy and viable fetus in a non-threatening pregnancy after the twenty-fourth week of a pregnancy. If rights talk has carried public policy even further than the chief protagonist for the pro-choice side thinks appropriate, this is surely evidence that it has not served Canadians well in this instance.

While the abortion trilogy represents only a thin slice of the Charter pie, it is a rich and revealing one. We must be careful about making conclusive judgments on the Charter based on the study of a single set of cases, but we can learn a great deal about the politics of rights. Whether one thinks that the Supreme Court made the right or wrong choices in these cases is less important than the realization that the judges were indeed making choices and not simply "applying the law of the Charter." To understand this is to begin to understand the Charter. A country can take its constitution out of politics, but it cannot take the politics out of the constitution. For this very reason, constitutional law is much too important to be left solely in the hands of lawyers and judges.

1.5.2 The Meaning of Expression

In order to determine whether a guarantee set out in the Charter has been infringed or denied, a court must define the boundaries of the guarantee. What sort of activity is encompassed within a particular guarantee and what is not?

More precisely, what is meant by "expression"? Are all forms of expression protected? Are some forms of expression not protected and, if so, which ones? In the first years after the Charter's adoption, there was division and uncertainty over these questions. The contexts in which the issue arose were concrete. Courts were asked whether the following forms of expression were protected: commercial advertising, communications in public places between prostitutes and potential clients, hate propaganda, and obscenity.

1.5.2.1 *Koumoudouros v. Municipality of Metropolitan Toronto* (1984), 8 C.R.R. 179 (Ont. H. C.)

EBERLE, J.: ...The applicants' submissions that nude burlesque dancing is an expression, even an artistic expression, that is guaranteed to them by the guarantee of "freedom of expression" in the Charter, raises what is to me a most interesting question: is the Charter dealing with "artistic" expression at all when it guarantees "freedom of expression"? The close linking in s. 2(b) of the Charter of the freedoms of thought, belief, opinion and expression, suggests rather that freedom of expression refers to the freedom of communication of ideas and opinions among the citizens of Canada, so that, in broad terms, those citizens may continue to live in the free and democratic society referred to in s. 1 of the Charter. Furthermore, s. 2(b) goes on, after providing for "freedom of expression", with the following words "including freedom of the press and other media of communication"; these words reinforce the view that the thrust of s. 2(b) is in the political and governmental domain, a domain in which the freedoms of thought, belief, opinion and expression are inseparable from a free and democratic society. Further, it must not be forgotten that the Charter is found in the *Constitution Act, 1982*, which is one of Canada's principal constitutional documents, concerned with the fundamental political and governmental structures of the nation.

Nevertheless, in these cases it is not necessary, and is indeed unwise, to attempt to determine the precise ambit of freedom of expression. It is preferable to decide them on the basis of evidence in the record. The sales figures found at pp. 100-104, when taken with the evidence already referred to, put the matter in perspective, and emphasize the intimate connection between exposed female pubic areas and the dollar volume of liquor sales in the applicants' premises.

Therefore, assuming, without deciding, that "expression", in the Charter includes "artistic" expression, the conclusion from the evidence is clear that the right claimed in these cases is not a right to freedom of artistic expression but the right to expose performers' pubic areas for the purpose of stimulating liquor sales. I find it difficult to accept that the framers of the Charter had any such right in mind and the whole tenor and effect of the language in the Charter belies such a right.

The question to be decided is a question of constitutionality, not of taste; and I am satisfied that the "freedom of expression" guaranteed by the Charter does not include the public exposure of female pubic areas for the primary purpose of selling larger quantities of liquor. Accordingly the requirement of opaque clothing in cl. 28(2) of the by-law does not infringe upon the "freedom of expression" guaranteed by s. 2(b) of the Charter.

In the result, therefore, the applications fail upon all grounds and must be dismissed with costs.

SIROIS, J. concurs with EBERLE, J.

Applications dismissed.

1.5.2.2 *Attorney-General of Québec v. Irwin Toy Ltd.* **(1989), 58 D.L.R. (4th) 577 (S.C.C.)**

DICKSON, C.J.C., LAMER AND WILSON, JJ.: This appeal raises questions concerning the constitutionality, under ss. 91 and 92 of the *Constitution Act, 1867* and ss. 2(b) and 7 of the *Canadian Charter of Rights and Freedoms*, of ss. 248 and 249 of the *Quebec Consumer Protection Act*, S.Q. 1978, c. 9 (R.S.Q., c. P-40.1), respecting the prohibition of television advertising directed at persons under 13 years of age.

The appeal is by leave of this court from the judgment of the Quebec Court of Appeal (Kaufman and Jacques JJ.A., Vallerand J.A. dissenting) on September 18, 1986, 32 D.L.R. (4th) 641, 14 C.P.R. (3d) 60, [1986] R.J.Q. 2441, 3 Q.A.C. 285, 26 C.R.R. 193, 1 A.C.W.S. (3d) 311, allowing an appeal from the judgment of Hugessen A.C.J. of the Superior Court for the District of Montreal on January 8, 1982, [1982] Que. S.C. 96, which dismissed the respondent's action for a declaration that ss. 248 and 249 of the *Consumer Protection Act* were *ultra vires* the legislature of the Province of Quebec and subsidiarily that they were inoperative as infringing the Quebec *Charter of Human Rights and Freedoms*, R.S.Q. 1977, c. C-12.

The relevant provisions of the *Consumer Protection Act* are ss. 248, 249 and 252, which provide:

248. Subject to what is provided in the regulations, no person may make use of commercial advertising directed at persons under thirteen years of age.

249. To determine whether or not an advertisement is directed at persons under thirteen years of age, account must be taken of the context of its presentation, and in particular of
- (a) the nature and intended purpose of the goods advertised;
- (b) the manner of presenting such advertisement;
- (c) the time and place it is shown.

The fact that such advertisement may be contained in printed matter intended for persons thirteen years of age and over or intended both for persons under thirteen years of age and for persons thirteen years of age and over, or that it may be broadcast during air time intended for persons thirteen years of age and over does not create a presumption that it is not directed at persons under thirteen years of age.

252. For the purpose of sections 231, 246, 247, 248 and 250, "to advertise" or "to make use of advertising" means to prepare, utilize, distribute, publish or broadcast an advertisement, or to cause it to be distributed, published or broadcast.

The relevant provisions of the *Regulation respecting the application of the Consumer Protection Act*, R.R.Q., c. P-40-1, r. 1, are ss. 87 to 91 in Division II of Chapter VII, entitled "Advertising directed at children," which provide:

87. For the purposes of the Division, the "child" means a person under 13 years of age.

88. An advertisement directed at children is exempt from the application of section 248 of the Act, under the following conditions:
- (a) it must appear in a magazine or insert directed at children;
- (b) the magazine or interest must be for sale or inserted in a publication which is for sale;
- (c) the magazine or insert must be published at intervals of not more than 3 months; and
- (d) the advertisement must meet the requirements of section 91.

89. An advertisement directed at children is exempted from the application of section 248 of the Act if its purpose is to announce a programme or show directed at them, provided that the advertisement is in conformity with the requirements of section 91.

90. An advertisement directed at children is exempt from the application of section 248 of the Act, if it is constituted by a store window, a display, a container, a wrapping or a label or if it appears therein, provided that the requirements of paragraphs *a* to *g, j, k, o* and *p* of section 91 are met.

91. For the purposes of applying sections 88, 89 and 90, an advertisement directed at children may not:
- (a) exaggerate the nature, characteristics, performance or duration of goods or services;
- (b) minimize the degree of skill, strength or dexterity or the age necessary to use goods or services;
- (c) use a superlative to describe the characteristics of goods or services or a diminutive to indicate its cost;

(d) use a comparative or establish a comparison with the goods or services advertised;
(e) directly incite a child to buy or to urge another person to buy goods or services or to seek information about it;
(f) portray reprehensible social or family lifestyles;
(g) advertise goods or services that, because of their nature, quality or ordinary use, should not be used by children;
(h) advertise a drug or patent medicine;
(i) advertise vitamin in liquid, powdered or tablet form;
(j) portray a person acting in an imprudent manner;
(k) portray goods or services in a way that suggests an improper or dangerous use thereof;
(l) portray a person or character known to children to promote goods or services, except;
> i. in the case of an artist, actor or professional announcer who does not appear in a publication or programme directed at children;
>
> ii. in the case provided for in section 89 where he is illustrated as a participant in a show directed at children.

For the purposes of this paragraph, a character created expressly to advertise goods or services is not considered a character known to children if it is used for advertising alone;
(m) use an animated cartoon process except to advertise a cartoon show directed at children;
(n) use a comic strip except to advertise a comic book directed at children;
(o) suggest that owning or using a product will develop in a child a physical, social or psychological advantage over other children of his age, or that being without the product will have the opposite effect;
(p) advertise goods in a manner misleading a child into thinking that, for the regular price of those goods, he can obtain goods other than those advertised.

Sections 3 and 9.1 of the Quebec *Charter of Human Rights and Freedoms* provide:

3. Every person is the possessor of the fundamental freedoms, including freedom of conscience, freedom of religion, freedom of opinion, freedom of expression, freedom of peaceful assembly and freedom of association.

9.1 In exercising his fundamental freedoms and rights, a person shall maintain a proper regard for democratic values, public order and the general well-being of the citizens of Québec.

In this respect, the scope of the freedoms and rights, and limits to their exercise, may be fixed by law.

Sections 1, 2(b) and 7 of the *Canadian Charter of Rights and Freedoms* provide:

1. The *Canadian Charter of Rights and Freedoms* guarantees the rights and freedoms set out in it subject only to such reasonable limits prescribed by law as can be demonstrably justified in a free and democratic society.

2. Everyone has the following fundamental freedoms:

b. freedom of thought, belief, opinion and expression, including freedom of the press and other media of communication;

7. Everyone has the right to life, liberty and security of the person and the right not to be deprived thereof except in accordance with principles of fundamental justice.

A. The Ford and Devine Appeals

Although the issue relating to freedom of expression in this appeal was argued together with the *Ford* and *Devine* appeals, it is important to emphasize that, unlike in the present case, the two latter cases involved government measures restricting one's choice of language. As the court stated in *Ford* (at p. 604):

> Language is so intimately related to the form and content of expression that there cannot be true freedom of expression by means of language if one is prohibited from using the language of one's choice. Language is not merely a means or medium of expression; it colours the content and meaning of expression.

Having determined that freedom of expression prevents prohibitions against using the language of one's choice, the question became whether, in the court's words (at p. 618) "a commercial purpose removes the expression ... from the scope of protected freedom." Thus, while choice of language was the principal matter in those appeals, the commercial element to the expression in issue raised an ancillary question. As the court made clear at the end of its discussion concerning freedom of expression (at p. 619):

> Although the expression in this case has a commercial element, it should be noted that the focus here is on choice of language and on a law which prohibits the use of a language. We are not asked in this case to deal with the distinct issue of the permissible scope of regulation of advertising (for example to protect consumers) where different governmental interests come into play, particularly when assessing the reasonableness of limits on such commercial expression pursuant to s. 1 of the Canadian Charter or to s. 9.1 of the Quebec Charter.

The instant case concerns the regulation of advertising aimed at children and thus raises squarely the issues which are not treated in *Ford*. Whereas it was sufficient in *Ford* to reject the submission that the guarantee of freedom of expression does not extend to signs having a commercial message, this case requires a determination whether regulations aimed solely at commercial advertising limit that guarantee. This, in turn, requires an elaboration of the conclusion already reached in *Ford* that there is no sound basis on which to exclude commercial expression, as a category of expression, from the sphere of activity protected by s. 2(b) of the Canadian Charter and s. 3 of the Quebec Charter.

B. The First Step: Was the Plaintiff's Activity Within the Sphere of Conduct Protected by Freedom of Expression?

Does advertising aimed at children fall within the scope of freedom of expression? This question must be put even before deciding whether there has been a limitation of the guarantee. Clearly, not all activity is protected by freedom of expression, and governmental action restricting this form of advertising only limits the guarantee if the activity in issue was protected in the first place. Thus, for example, in *Reference re Public Service Employee Relations Act (Alta.)* (1987), 38 D.L.R. (4th) 161, [1987] 1 S.C.R. 313, 51 Alta. L.R. (2d) 97; *P.S.A.C. v. Canada* (1987), 38 D.L.R. (4th) 249, [1987] 1 S.C.R. 424, 87 C.L.L.C. ¶14,022, and *R.W.D.S.U. v. Saskatchewan* (1987), 38 L.D.R. (4th) 277, [1987] 1 S.C.R. 460, [1987] 3 W.W.R. 673, the majority of the court found that freedom of association did not include the right to strike. The activity itself was not within the sphere protected by s. 2(d); therefore the government action in restricting it was not contrary to the Charter. The same procedure must be followed with respect to an analysis of freedom of expression; the first step to be taken in an inquiry of this kind is to discover whether the activity which the plaintiff wishes to pursue may properly be characterized as falling within "freedom of expression." If the activity is not within s. 2(b), the government action obviously cannot be challenged under that section.

The necessity of this first stop has been described, with reference to the narrower concept of "freedom of speech," by Frederick Schauer in his work entitled *Free Speech: A Philosophical Enquiry* (Cambridge: Cambridge University Press, 1982), at p. 92:

> We are attempting to identify those things that one is free (or at least more free) to do when a Free Speech Principle is accepted. What activities justify an appeal to the concept of freedom of speech? These activities are clearly something less than the totality of human conduct and ... something more than merely moving one's tongue, mouth and vocal chords to make linguistic noises.

"Expression" has both a content and a form, and the two can be inextricably connected. Activity is expressive if it attempts to convey meaning. That meaning is its content. Freedom of expression was entrenched in our Constitution and is guaranteed in the Quebec Charter so as to ensure that everyone can manifest their thoughts, opinions, beliefs, indeed all expressions of the heart and mind, however unpopular, distasteful or contrary to the mainstream. Such protection is, in the words of both the Canadian and Quebec Charters, "fundamental" because in a free, pluralistic and democratic society we prize a diversity of ideas and opinions for their inherent value both to the community and to the individual. Free expression was for Cardozo, J. of the United States Supreme Court "the matrix, the indispensable condition of nearly every other form of freedom" (*Palko v. Connecticut*, 302 U.S. 319 (1937) at p. 327); for Rand, J. of the Supreme Court of Canada, it was "little less vital to man's mind and spirit than breathing is to his physical existence" (*Switzman v. Elbling* (1957), 7 D.L.R. (2d) 337 at p. 358, 117 C.C.C. 129, [1957] S.C.R. 285). And as the European Court stated in the *Handyside Case*, Eur. Court H.R., decision of April 29, 1976, Series A., No. 24, at p. 23, freedom of expression:

> ...is applicable not only to "information" or "ideas" that are favourably received or regarded as inoffensive or as a matter of indifference, but also to those that offend, shock or disturb the State

or any sector of the population. Such are the demands of that pluralism, tolerance and broad-mindedness without which there is no "democratic society."

We cannot, then, exclude human activity from the scope of guaranteed free expression on the basis of the content or meaning being conveyed. Indeed, if the activity conveys or attempts to convey a meaning, it has expressive content and *prima facie* falls within the scope of the guarantee. Of course, while most human activity combines expressive and physical elements, some human activity is purely physical and does not convey or attempt to convey meaning. It might be difficult to characterize certain day-to-day tasks, like parking a car, as having expressive content. To bring such activity within the protected sphere, the plaintiff would have to show that it was performed to convey a meaning. For example, an unmarried person might, as part of a public protest, park in a zone reserved for spouses of government employees in order to express dissatisfaction or outrage at the chosen method of allocating a limited resource. If that person could demonstrate that his activity did in fact have expressive content, he would, at this stage, be within the protected sphere and the s. 2(b) challenge would proceed.

The content of expression can be conveyed through an infinite variety of forms of expression: for example, the written or spoken word, the arts, and even physical gestures or acts. While the guarantee of free expression protects all content of expression, certainly violence as a form of expression receives no such protection. It is not necessary here to delineate precisely when and on what basis a *form* of expression chosen to convey a meaning falls outside the sphere of the guarantee. But it is clear, for example, that a murderer or rapist cannot invoke freedom of expression in justification of the form of expression he has chosen. As McIntyre, J., writing for the majority in *R.W.D.S.U. v. Dolphin Delivery Ltd.* (1986), 33 D.L.R. (4th) 174 at p. 187, [1986] 2 S.C.R. 573, 9 B.C.L.R. (2d) 273, observed in the course of discussing whether picketing fell within the scope of s. 2(b):

> Action on the part of the picketers will, of course, always accompany the expression, but not every action on the part of the picketers will be such as to alter the nature of the whole transaction and remove it from Charter protection for freedom of expression. That freedom, of course, would not extend to protect threats of violence or acts of violence.

Indeed, freedom of expression ensures that we can convey our thoughts and feelings in non-violent ways without fear of censure.

The broad, inclusive approach to the protected sphere of free expression here outlined is consonant with that suggested by some leading theorists. Thomas Emerson, in his article entitled "Toward a General Theory of the First Amendment", 72 Yale L.J. 877 (1963), notes (at p. 886) that:

> ...the theory of freedom of expression involves more than a technique for arriving at better social judgments through democratic procedures. It comprehends a vision of society, a faith and a whole way of life. The theory grew out of an age that was awakened and invigorated by the idea of a new society in which man's mind was free, his fate determined by his own powers of reason, and

his prospects of creating a rational and enlightened civilization virtually unlimited. It is put forward as a prescription for attaining a creative, progressive, exciting and intellectually robust community. It contemplates a mode of life that, through encouraging toleration, scepticism, reason and initiative, will allow man to realize his full potentialities. It spurns the alternative of a society that is tyrannical, conformist, irrational and stagnant.

D.F.B. Tucker in his book *Law, Liberalism and Free Speech* (Totowa, New Jersey: Rowman & Allanheld, 1985) describes what he calls a "deontological approach" to freedom of expression as one in which "the protected sphere of liberty is delineated by interpreting an understanding of the democratic commitment" (p. 35). It is upon precisely this enterprise that we have embarked.

Thus, the first question remains: Does the advertising aimed at children fall within the scope of freedom of expression? Surely it aims to convey a meaning, and cannot be excluded as having no expressive content. Nor is there any basis for excluding the form of expression chosen from the sphere of projected activity. As we stated in *Ford*, at p. 618:

> Given the earlier pronouncements of this court to the effect that the rights and freedoms guaranteed in the Canadian Charter should be given a large and liberal interpretation, there is no sound basis on which commercial expression can be excluded from the protection of s. 2(*b*) of the Charter.

Consequently, we must proceed to the second step of the inquiry and ask whether the purpose or effect of the government action in question was to restrict freedom of expression.

It bears repeating that in *Ford*, the discussion of commercial expression ended at this first stage. The court had already found that the aim of ss. 58 and 69 of the *Charter of the French Language* was to prohibit the use of one's language of choice. The centrality of choice of language to freedom of expression transcends any significance that the context in which the expression is intended to be used might have. It was therefore unnecessary in that case to inquire further whether the restriction of commercial expression limited freedom of expression.

C. The Second Step: Was the Purpose or Effect of the Government Action to Restrict Freedom of Expression?

Having found that the plaintiff's activity does fall within the scope of guaranteed free expression, it must next be determined whether the purpose or effect of the impugned governmental action was to control attempts to convey meaning through that activity. The importance of focusing at this stage on the purpose and effect of the legislation is nowhere more clearly stated than in *R. v. Big M Drug Mart Ltd.* (1985), 18 D.L.R. (4th) 321 at p. 350, 18 C.C.C. (3d) 385, [1985] 1 S.C.R. 295, where Dickson, J. (as he then was), speaking for the majority, observed:

> In my view, both purpose and effect are relevant in determining constitutionality; either an unconstitutional purpose or an unconstitutional effect can invalidate legislation. All legislation is animated by an object the legislature intends to achieve. This object is realized through the impact

produced by the operation and application of the legislation. Purpose and effect respectively, in the sense of the legislation's object and its ultimate impact, are clearly linked, if not indivisible. Intended and actual effects have often been looked to for guidance in assessing the legislation's object and thus, its validity.

Moreover, consideration of the object of legislation is vital if rights are to be fully protected. The assessment by the courts of legislative purpose focuses scrutiny upon the aims and objectives of the legislature and ensures they are consonant with the guarantees enshrined in the Charter. The declaration that certain objects lie outside the legislature's power checks governmental action at the first stage of unconstitutional conduct. Further, it will provide more ready and more vigorous protection of constitutional rights by obviating the individual litigant's needs to prove effects violative of Charter rights. It will also allow courts to dispose of cases where the object is clearly improper, without inquiring into the legislation's actual impact.

Dickson, J. went on to specify how this inquiry into purpose and effects should be carried out (at pp. 351-2):

In short, I agree with the respondent that the legislation's purpose is the initial test of constitutional validity and its effects are to be considered when the law under review has passed or, at least, has purportedly passed the purpose test. If the legislation fails the purpose test, there is no need to consider further its effects, since it has already been demonstrated to be invalid. Thus, if a law with a valid purpose interferes by its impact, with rights or freedoms, a litigant could still argue the effects of the legislation as a means to defeat its applicability and possibly its validity. In short, the effects test will only be necessary to defeat legislation with a valid purpose; effects can never be relied upon to save legislation with an invalid purpose.

If the government's purpose, then, was to restrict attempts to convey a meaning, there has been a limitation by law of s. 2(b) and a s. 1 analysis is required to determine whether the law is inconsistent with the provisions of the Constitution. If, however, this was not the government's purpose, the court must move on to an analysis of the effects of the government action.

a. Purpose

When applying the purpose test to the guarantee of free expression, one must beware of drifting to either of two extremes. On the one hand, the greatest part of human activity has an expressive element and so one might find, on an objective test, that an aspect of the government's purpose is virtually always to restrict expression. On the other hand, the government can almost always claim that its subjective purpose was to address some real or purported social need, not to restrict expression. To avoid both extremes, the government's purpose must be assessed from the standpoint of the guarantee in question. Just as the division of powers jurisprudence of this court measures the purpose of government action against the ambit of the heads of power established under the *Constitution Act, 1867*, so too, in cases involving the rights and freedoms guaranteed by the Canadian Charter, the purpose of government action must be measured against the ambit of the relevant guarantee. It is important, of course, to heed Dickson, J.'s warning against a "theory of shifting purpose" (*Big M Drug Mart*, at p. 353): "Purpose is a function of the intent of those who drafted and enacted the legislation at the time, and not of any shifting variable." This is not to say that the degree to which a purpose remains or becomes pressing and substantial cannot change over time. In *Big M Drug Mart*, Dickson, J.'s principal concern was to avoid characterizing purposes in a way that shifted over time. But it is equally true that the government cannot have had one purpose as concerns the division of powers, a different purpose as concerns the guaranteed right or freedom, and a different purpose again as concerns reasonable and justified limits to that guarantee. Nevertheless, the same purpose can be assessed from different standpoints when interpreting the division of powers, limitation of a guarantee, or reasonable limits to that guarantee.

If the government's purpose is to restrict the content of expression by singling out particular meanings that are not be to conveyed, it necessarily limits the guarantee of free expression. If the government's purpose is to restrict a form of expression in order to control access by others to the meaning being conveyed or to control the ability of the one conveying the meaning to do so, it also limits the guarantee. On the other hand, where the government aims to control only the physical consequences of certain human activity, regardless of the meaning being conveyed, its purpose is not to control expression. Archibald Cox has described the distinction as follows (Freedom of Expression (Cambridge, Mass.: Harvard University Press, 1981), at pp. 59-60:

> The bold line ... between restrictions upon publication and regulation of the time, place and manner of expression tied to content, on the one hand, and regulation of time, place, or manner of expression regardless of content, on the other hand, reflects the difference between the state's usually impermissible effort to suppress "harmful" information, ideas, or emotions and the state's often justifiable desire to secure other interests against interference from the noise and the physical intrusion that accompany speech, regardless of the information, ideas, or emotions expressed.

Thus, for example, a rule against handing out pamphlets is a restriction on a manner of expression and is "tied to content," even if that restriction purports to control litter. The rule aims to control access by others to a meaning being conveyed as well as to control the ability of the pamphleteer. To restrict this form of expression, handing out pamphlets, entails restricting its content. By contrast, a rule against littering is not a restriction "tied to content." It aims to control the physical consequences of certain conduct regardless of whether that conduct attempts to convey meaning. To restrict littering as a "manner of expression" need not lead inexorably to restricting content. Of course, rules can be framed to appear neutral as to content even if their true purpose is to control attempts to convey a meaning. For example, in *Saumur v. A.-G. Que.* (1962), 37 D.L.R. (2d) 708 (Que. C.A.); affirmed 45 D.L.R. (2d) 627, [1964] S.C.R. 252, a municipal by-law forbidding distribution of pamphlets without prior authorization from the chief of police was a colourable attempt to restrict expression.

If the government is to assert successfully that its purpose was to control a harmful consequence of the particular conduct in question, it must not have aimed to avoid, in Thomas Scanlon's words ("A Theory of Freedom of Expression," in Dworkin, ed., *The Philosophy of Law* (London: Oxford University Press, 1977), at p. 161):

...a) harms to certain individuals which consist in their coming to have false beliefs as a result of those acts of expression; b) harmful consequences of acts performed as a result of those acts of expression, where the connection between the acts of expression and the subsequent harmful acts consists merely in the fact that the act of expression led the agents to believe (or increased their tendency to believe) these acts to be worth performing.

In each of Scanlon's two categories, the government's purpose is to regulate thoughts, opinions, beliefs or particular meanings. That is the mischief in view. On the other hand, where the harm caused by the expression in issue is direct, without the intervening element of thought, opinion, belief, or a particular meaning, the regulation does aim at a harmful physical consequence, not the content or form of expression.

In sum, the characterization of government purpose must proceed from the standpoint of the guarantee in issue. With regard to freedom of expression, if the government has aimed to control attempts to convey a meaning either by directly restricting the content of expression or by restricting a form of expression tied to content, its purpose trenches upon the guarantee. Where, on the other hand, it aims only to control the physical consequences of particular conduct, its purpose does not trench upon the guarantee. In determining whether the government's purpose aims simply at harmful physical consequences, the question becomes: does the mischief consist in the meaning of the activity or the purported influence that meaning has on the behaviour of others, or does it consist, rather, only in the direct physical result of the activity.

b. Effects

Even if the government's purpose was not to control or restrict attempts to convey a meaning, the court must still decide whether the effect of the government action was to restrict the plaintiff's free expression. Here, the burden in on the plaintiff to demonstrate that such an effect occurred. In order so to demonstrate, a plaintiff must state her claim with reference to the principles and values underlying the freedom.

We have already discussed the nature of the principles and values underlying the vigilant protection of free expression in a society such as ours. They were also discussed by the court in *Ford* (at pp. 617-9), and can be summarized as follows: (1) seeking and attaining the truth is an inherently good activity; (2) participation in social and political decision-making is to be fostered and encouraged; and (3) the diversity in forms of individual self-fulfilment and human flourishing ought to be cultivated in an essentially tolerant, indeed welcoming, environment not only for the sake of those who convey a meaning, but also for the sake of those to whom it is conveyed. In showing that the effect of the government's action was to restrict her free expression, a plaintiff must demonstrate that her activity promotes at least one of those principles. It is not enough that shouting, for example, has an expressive element. If the plaintiff challenges the effect of government action to control noise, presuming that action to have a purpose neutral as to expression, she must show that her aim was to convey a meaning reflective of the principles underlying freedom of expression. The precise and complete articulation of what kinds of activity promote these principles is, of course, a matter for judicial appreciation to be developed on a case-by-case basis. But the plaintiff must at least identify the meaning being conveyed and how it relates to the pursuit of truth, participation in the community, or individual self-fulfilment and human flourishing.

c. Sections 248 and 249

There is no question but that the purpose of ss. 248 and 249 of the Consumer Protection Act was to restrict both a particular range of content and certain forms of expression in the name of protecting children. Section 248 prohibits, subject to regulation, attempts to communicate a commercial message to persons under 13 years of age. Section 249 identifies factors to be considered in deciding whether the commercial message in fact has that prohibited content. At first blush, the regulations exempting certain advertisements transform the prohibition into a "time, place or manner" restriction aiming only at the form of expression. According to ss. 88 to 90 of the *Regulation respecting the application of the Consumer Protection Act*, an advertisement can be aimed at children if: (1) it appears in certain magazine or inserts directed at children; (2) it announces a programme or show directed at children; or (3) it appears in or on a store window, display, container, wrapping, or label. Yet, even if all advertising aimed at children were permitted to appear in the manner specified, the restriction would be tied to content because it aims to restrict access to the particular message being conveyed. However, the regulations in question do more than just restrict the manner in which a particular content must be expressed. They also restrict content directly. Section 91 provides that even where advertisements directed at children are permitted, such advertisements must not, for example, "use a superlative to describe the characteristics of goods or services" or "directly incite a child to buy or to urge another person to buy goods or services or to seek information about it". Furthermore, it is clear from the substantial body of material submitted by the Attorney-General of Quebec as well as by the intervener, Gilles Moreau, president of the Office de la protection du consommateur, that the purported mischief at which the Act and regulations were directed was the harm caused by the message itself. In combination, therefore, the Act and the regulations prohibit particular content of expression. Such as prohibition can only be justified if it meets the test under s. 1 of the Canadian Charter and s. 9.1 of the Quebec Charter.

d. Summary and Conclusion

When faced with an alleged violation of the guarantee of freedom of expression, the first step in the analysis is to determine whether the plaintiff's activity falls within the sphere of conduct protected by the guarantee. Activity which (1) does not convey or attempt to convey a meaning, and thus has no *content* of expression or (2) which conveys a meaning but through a violent *form* of expression, is not within the protected sphere of conduct. If the activity falls within the protected sphere of conduct, the second step in the analysis is to determine whether the purpose or effect of the government action in issue was to restrict freedom of expression. If the government has aimed to control attempts to convey a meaning either by directly restricting the content of expression or by restricting a form of expression tied to content, its purpose trenches upon the guarantee. Where, on the other hand, it aims only to control the physical consequences of particular conduct, its purpose does not trench upon the guarantee. In determining whether the government's purpose aims simply at harmful physical consequences, the question becomes: does the mischief consist in the meaning of the activity or the purported influence that meaning has on the behaviour of others, or does it consist, rather, only in the direct physical result of the activity. If the government's purpose was not to restrict free expression, the plaintiff can still claim that the effect of the government's action was to restrict her expression. To make this claim, the plaintiff must at least identify the meaning being conveyed and how it relates to the pursuit of truth, participation in the community, or individual self-fulfillment and human flourishing.

In the instant case, the plaintiff's activity is not excluded from the sphere of conduct protected by freedom of expression. The government's purpose in enacting ss. 248 and 249 of the *Consumer Protection Act* and in promulgating ss. 87 to 91 of the *Regulation respecting the application of the Consumer Protection Act* was to prohibit particular content of expression in the name of protecting children. These provisions therefore constitute limitations to s. 2(b) of the Canadian Charter and s. 3 of the Quebec Charter. They fall to be justified under s. 1 of the Canadian Charter and s. 9.1 of the Quebec Charter.

1.5.2.3 A Note on Advertising and Free Expression

While the courts have in the past suggested that only Parliament may legislate to restrict freedom of expression, it has traditionally been accepted that the provinces may make laws about advertising. In *A.G. Canada v. Law Society of British Columbia* (1982), 137 D.L.R. (3d) 1, Estey, J., speaking for the Supreme Court of Canada said:

> The freedom of expression with which the court is here concerned of course has nothing to do with the elective process and the operations of our democratic institutions, the House of Commons and the provincial legislature. We are indeed speaking about the right of economic free speech, the right to commercial advertising. it can hardly be contended that the province by proper legislation could not regulate the ethical, moral and financial aspects of a trade or profession within its boundaries. (pp. 44-45)

For similar statements, see *R. v. Telegram Publishing Co.* (1960), 25 D.L.R. (2d) 471; and *Benson and Hedges Ltd. v. A.G. British Columbia* (1972), 27

D.L.R. (3d) 257. Post-Charter cases have adopted a similar approach holding that "expression" in section 2(b) does not include advertising or commercial speech. See *Klein and Law Society of Upper Canada; Re Dvorak and Law Society of Upper Canada* (1985), 50 O.R. (2d) 118 (Div. Ct.); *Grier v. Alberta Optometric Association and Council of Management of Alberta Optometric Association* (1985), 5 W.W.R. 436 (Alta. Q.B.); and *R. v. Prof. Technology of Canada Ltd.* (1986), 7 C.R.D. 525.100-01 (Alta. Prov. Ct.). Although not expressed in these terms, the distinction is similar in some respects to that made by U.S. courts between "political" or "core" speech and "commercial" speech. The effect of this distinction has been that commercial speech does not attract the same degree of protection under the First Amendment as does political speech. (See *Valentine v. Chrestensen*, 316 U.S. 52 (1942).) Recent decisions have cast doubt on this distinction. (See *Virginia State Board of Pharmacy v. Virginia Citizens Consumer Council*, 425 U.S. 748 (1976).)

As we have seen, the Supreme Court of Canada has decided that advertising is "expression". See *A.G. of Québec v. Irwin Toy Ltd.* (1989), 58 D.L.R. (4th) 577.

Advertising in Canada is regulated under both federal and provincial laws.

Federal law is extensive. The *Competition Act* (R.S.C. 1985, c. C-34) seeks to limit false or misleading advertising. The *Broadcasting Act* (S.C. 1991, c. 11) imposes restrictions, not on advertisers, but on broadcasters.

The various sets of regulations made under the *Broadcasting Act* (see, for example, the Television Regulations, S.O.R. 87-49) lay down detailed rules concerning advertising. The *Food and Drug Act* (R.S.C. 1985, c. F-27) deals with advertisements for food and drugs. The *Trade Marks Act* (R.S.C. 1985, c. T-13) deals in part with comparative advertising.

The *Textile Labelling Act* (R.S.C. 1985, c. T-10) and the *Consumer Packaging and Labelling Act* (R.S.C. 1985, c. C-38) both seek to limit false or misleading labelling. The *Criminal Code* (R.S.C. 1985, c. C-46) contains a number of provisions that affect advertising.

Provincial laws are similarly extensive. For example, in Ontario, the *Business Practices Act* (R.S.O. 1990, c. B.18) and the *Consumer Protection Act* (R.S.O. 1990, c. C.31) both deal with false or misleading advertising. The *Election Finances Act* (R.S.O. 1990, c. E.7), s. 37, deals with broadcast advertising during provincial elections.

On 13 November 1891 the Carbolic Smoke Ball Company inserted the following advertisement in various English newspapers:

> £100 reward will be paid by the Carbolic Smoke Ball Company to any person who contracts the increasing epidemic of influenza, colds, or any disease caused by taking cold, after having used the ball three times daily for two weeks according to the printed directions supplied with each ball. £100 is deposited with the Alliance Bank, Regent Street, shewing our sincerity in the matter.

On the strength of this advertisement a woman bought a smoke ball and used it three times a day for a period of two months. She then contracted influenza. She was able to recover £100 from the company (*Carlill v. Carbolic Smoke Ball Company*, [1938] 1 Q.B. 256). Despite this decision, the tradition of the courts has been to regard advertising claims as "mere puffs" that is, as statements that do not give rise to contractual obligations.

The contemporary approach to the control of false and misleading advertising relies on regulation by the state rather that private litigation.

Comparative advertising seems popular today. The legal risk involved is that by saying nasty things about your competitors' products you may be laying yourself open to civil proceedings. The obscure tort in question is called "slander of goods". See *Frank Flaman Wholesale Ltd. v. Firman* (1982), 20 C.C.L.T. 246.

1.5.2.4 *R. v. Keegstra*, [1990] 3 S.C.R. 697 (S.C.C.)

DICKSON, C.J.: Having reviewed the *Irwin Toy* test, it remains to determine whether the impugned legislation in this appeal — s. 319(2) of the *Criminal Code* — infringes the freedom of expression guarantee of s. 2(b). Communications that wilfully promote hatred against an identifiable group without doubt convey a meaning, and are intended to do so by those who make them. Because *Irwin Toy* stresses that the type of meaning conveyed is irrelevant to the question of whether s. 2(b) is infringed, that the expression covered by s. 319(2) is invidious and obnoxious is beside the point. It is enough that those who publicly and wilfully promote hatred convey or attempt to convey a meaning, and it must therefore be concluded that the first step of the *Irwin Toy* test is satisfied.

Moving to the second stage of the s. 2(b) inquiry, one notes that the prohibition is s. 319(2) aims directly at words — in this appeal, Mr. Keegstra's teachings — that have as their content and objective the promotion of racial or religious hatred. The purpose of s. 319(2) can consequently be formulated as follows: to restrict the content of expression by singling out particular meanings that are not to be conveyed. Section 319(2) therefore overtly seeks to prevent the communication of expression, and hence meets the second requirement of the *Irwin Toy* test.

In my view, through s. 319(2) Parliament seeks to prohibit communications that convey a meaning; namely, those communications that are intended to promote hatred against identifiable groups. I thus find s. 319(2) to constitute an infringement of the freedom of expression guaranteed by s. 2(b) of the Charter. Before moving on to see whether the impugned provision is nonetheless justified under s. 1, however, I wish to canvass two arguments made in favour of the position that communications intended to promote hatred do not fall within the ambit of s. 2(b). The first of these arguments concerns an exception mentioned in *Irwin Toy* concerning expression manifested in a violent form. The second relates to the impact of other sections of the Charter and international agreements in interpreting the scope of the freedom of expression guarantee.

Beginning with the suggestion that expression covered by s. 319(2) falls within an exception articulated in *Irwin Toy*, it was argued before this Court that the wilful promotion of hatred is an activity the form and consequences of which are analogous to those associated with violence or threats of violence. This argument contends that Supreme Court of Canada precedent excludes violence and threats of violence from the ambit of s. 2(b), and that the reason for such exclusion must lie in the fact that these forms of expression are inimical to the values supporting freedom of speech. Indeed, in support of this view it was pointed out to us that the court in *Irwin Toy* stated that "freedom of expression ensures that we can convey our thoughts and feelings in non-violent ways without fear of censure" (p. 97). Accordingly, we were urged to find that hate propaganda of the type caught by s. 319(2), insofar as it imperils the ability of target group members themselves to convey thoughts and feeling in non-violent ways without fear of censure, is analogous to violence and threats of violence and hence does not fall within s. 2(b).

The proposition in *Irwin Toy* that violent expression is not afforded protection under s. 2(b) has its origin in a comment made by McIntyre, J. in *Dolphin Delivery Ltd.*, in which he stated that the freedom of expression guaranteed picketers would not extend to protect violence or threats of violence (p. 558). Restricting s. 2(b) in this manner has also been mentioned in more recent Supreme Court of Canada decisions, in particular by Lamer, J. in *Reference re ss. 193 and 195.1(1)(c) of the Criminal Code (Man.)* and by a unanimous Court in *Royal College of Dental Surgeons*. It should be emphasized, however, that no decision of this Court has rested on the notion that expressive conduct is excluded from s. 2(b) where it involves violence.

Turning specifically to the proposition that hate propaganda should be excluded from the coverage of s. 2(b), I begin by stating that the communications restricted by s. 319(2) cannot be considered as violence, which on a reading of *Irwin Toy* I find to refer to expression communicated directly through physical harm. Nor do I find hate propaganda to be analogous to violence, and through this route exclude it from the protection of the guarantee of freedom of expression. As I have explained, the starting proposition in *Irwin Toy* is that all activities conveying or attempting to convey meaning are considered expression for the purposes of s. 2(b); the content of expression is irrelevant in determining the scope of the Charter provision. Stated at its highest, an exception has been suggested where meaning is communicated directly via physical violence. This form of meaning is extremely repugnant to the values of free expression and thus justifies such an extraordinary step. Section 319(2) of the *Criminal Code* prohibits the communication of meaning that is repugnant, but the repugnance stems from the content of the message as opposed to its form. For this reason, I am of the view that hate propaganda is to be categorized as expression so as to bring it within the coverage of s. 2(b).

As for threats of violence, *Irwin Toy* spoke only of restricting s. 2(b) to certain *forms* of expression stating at p. 970 that:

> [w]hile the guarantee of free expression protects all content of expression, certainly violence as a form of expression receives no such protection. It is not necessary here to delineate precisely when and on what basis a form of expression chosen to convey a meaning falls outside the sphere of the guarantee. But it is clear, for example, that a murderer or rapist cannot invoke the freedom of expression in justification of the form of expression he has chosen.

While the line between form and content is not always easily drawn, in my opinion threats of violence can only be so classified by reference to the content of their meaning. As such, they do not fall within the exception spoken of in *Irwin Toy*, and their suppression must be justified under s. 1. As I do not find threats of violence to be excluded from the definition of expression envisioned by s. 2(b), it is unnecessary to determine whether the threatening aspects of hate propaganda can be seen as threats of violence, or analogous to such threats, so as to deny it protection under s. 2(b).

The second matter that I wish to address before leaving the s. 2(b) inquiry concerns the relevance of other Charter provisions and international agreements to which Canada is a party in interpreting the coverage of the freedom of expression guarantee. It has been argued in support of excluding hate propaganda from the coverage of s. 2(b) that the use of ss. 15 and 27 of the Charter—dealing respectively with equality and multiculturalism—and Canada's acceptance of international agreements requiring the prohibition of racist statements make s. 319(2) incompatible with even a large and liberal definition of the freedom (see, e.g., Irwin Cotler, "Hate Literature," in Rosalie S. Abella and Melvin L. Rothman, eds., *Justice Beyond Orwell* (1985) p. 117, at pp. 121-22). The general tenor of this argument is that these interpretive aids inextricably infuse each constitutional guarantee with values supporting equal societal participation and the security and dignity of all persons. Consequently, it is said that s. 2(b) must be curtailed so as not to extend to communications that seriously undermine the equality, security and dignity of others.

Because I will deal extensively with the impact of various Charter provisions and international agreements when considering whether s. 319(2) is a justifiable limit under s. 1, I will keep my comments here to a minimum. Suffice it to say that I agree with the general approach of Wilson, J. in *Edmonton Journal*, where she speaks of the danger of balancing competing values without the benefit of a context. This approach does not logically preclude the presence of balancing within s. 2(b); one could avoid the dangers of an overly abstract analysis simply by making sure that the circumstances surrounding both the use of the freedom and the legislative limit were carefully considered. I believe, however, that s. 1 of the Charter is especially well suited to the task of balancing, and consider this Court's previous freedom of expression decisions to support this belief. It is, in my opinion, inappropriate to attenuate the s. 2(b) freedom on the grounds that a *particular* context requires such; the large and liberal interpretation given the freedom of expression in *Irwin Toy* indicates that the preferable course is to weigh the various contextual values and factors in s. 1.

I thus conclude on the issue of s. 2(b) by finding that s. 319(2) of the *Criminal Code* constitutes an infringement of the Charter guarantee of freedom of expression, and turn to examine whether such an infringement is justifiable under s. 1 as a reasonable limit in a free and democratic society.

1.5.2.5 Retail, Wholesale and Department Store Union, Local 580 v. Dolphin Delivery Ltd., [1986] 2 S.C.R. 573

McINTYRE, J.: As has been noted above, the only basis on which the picketing in question was defended by the appellants was under the provisions of s. 2(b) of the Charter which guarantees the freedom of expression as a fundamental freedom. Freedom of expression is not, however, a creature of the Charter. It is one of the fundamental concepts that has formed the basis for the historical development of the political, social and educational institutions of western society. Representative democracy, as we know it today, which is in great part the product of free expression and discussion of varying ideas, depends upon its maintenance and protection.

The importance of freedom of expression has been recognized since early times: see John Milton, *Areopagitica; A Speech for the Liberty of Unlicenc'd Printing, to the Parliament of England* (1644), and as well John Stuart Mill, "On Liberty" in *On Liberty and Considerations on Representative Government* (Oxford 1946), at p. 14:

> If all mankind minus one were of one opinion, and only one person were of the contrary opinion, mankind would be no more justified in silencing that one person, than he, if he had the power, would be justified in silencing mankind.

And, after stating that "All silencing of discussion is an assumption of infallibility", he said, at p. 16:

> Yet it is as evident in itself, as any amount of argument can make it, that ages are no more infallible than individuals; every age having held many opinions which subsequent ages have deemed not only false but absurd; and it is as certain that many opinions now general will be rejected by future ages, as it is that many, once general, are rejected by the present.

Nothing in the vast literature on this subject reduces the importance of Mill's words. The principle of freedom of speech and expression has been firmly accepted as a necessary feature of modern democracy. The courts have recognized this fact. For an American example, see the words of Holmes, J. in his dissent in *Abrams v. United States* (1919), 250 U.S. 616 at p. 630:

> Persecution for the expression of opinions seems to me perfectly logical. If you have no doubt of your premises or your power and want a certain result with all your heart you naturally express your wishes in law and sweep away all opposition . . . . But when men have realized that time has upset many fighting faiths, they may come to believe even more than they believe the very foundations of their own conduct that the ultimate good desired is better reached by free trade in ideas—that the best test of truth is the power of the thought to get itself accepted in the

competition of the market, and that truth is the only ground upon which their wishes safely can be carried out.

Prior to the adoption of the Charter, freedom of speech and expression had been recognized as an essential feature of Canadian parliamentary democracy. Indeed, this Court may be said to have given it constitutional status. In *Boucher v. The King*, [1951] S.C.R. 265, Rand, J., who formed a part of the majority which narrowed the scope of the crime of sedition, said, at p. 288:

> There is no modern authority which holds that the mere effect of tending to create discontent or disaffection among His Majesty's subjects or ill-will or hostility between groups of them, but not tending to issue in illegal conduct, constitutes the crime, and this for obvious reasons: Freedom in thought and speech and disagreement in ideas and beliefs, on every conceivable subject, are of the essence of our life. The clash of critical discussion on political, social and religious subjects has too deeply become the stuff of daily experience to suggest that mere ill-will as a product of controversy can strike down the latter with illegality. A superficial examination of the word shows its insufficiency: what is the degree necessary to criminality? Can it ever, as mere subjective condition, be so? Controversial fury is aroused constantly by differences in abstract conceptions; heresy in some fields is again a mortal sin; there can be fanatical puritanism in ideas as well as in morals; but our compact of free society accepts and absorbs these differences and they are exercised at large within the framework of freedom and order on broader and deeper uniformities as bases of social stability. Similarly in discontent, affection and hostility: as subjective incidents of controversy, they and the ideas which arouse them are part of our living which ultimately serve us in stimulation, in the clarification of thought and, as we believe, in the search for the constitution and truth of things generally.

In *Switzman v. Elbling*, [1957] S.C.R. 285, where this Court struck down Quebec's padlock law, Rand, J. again spoke strongly on this issue. He said, at p. 306:

> But public opinion, in order to meet such a responsibility, demands the condition of a virtually unobstructed access to and diffusion of ideas. Parliamentary government postulates a capacity in men, acting freely and under self-restraints, to govern themselves; and that advance is best served in the degree achieved of individual liberation from subjective as well as objective shackles. Under that government, the freedom of discussion in Canada, as a subject-matter of legislation, has a unity of interest and significance extending equally to every part of the Dominion. With such dimensions it is *ipso facto* excluded from head 16 as a local matter.
>
> This constitutional fact is the political expression of the primary condition of social life, thought and its communication by language. Liberty in this is little less vital to man's mind and spirit than breathing is to his physical existence. As such an inherence in the individual it is embodied in his status of citizenship.

In the same case, Abbott, J. said, at p. 326:

> The right of free expression of opinion and of criticism, upon matters of public policy and public administration, and the right to discuss and debate such matters, whether they be social, economic or political, are essential to the working of a parliamentary democracy such as ours.

He went on to make extensive reference to the words of Duff, C.J. in *Reference re Alberta Statutes*, [1938] S.C.R. 100, at pp. 132-33, strongly supporting what could almost be described as a constitutional position for the concept of freedom of speech and expression in Canadian law, and then said, at p. 328:

Although it is not necessary, of course, to determine this question for the purposes of the present appeal, the Canadian constitution being declared to be similar in principle to that of the United Kingdom, I am also of opinion that as our constitutional Act now stands, Parliament itself could not abrogate this right of discussion and debate. The power of Parliament to limit it is, in my view, restricted to such powers as may be exercisable under its exclusive legislative jurisdiction with respect to criminal law and to make laws for the peace, order and good government of the nation.

It will be seen at once that Professor Peter W. Hogg, at p. 713 in his text, *Constitutional Law of Canada* (2nd ed. 1985), is justified in his comment that:

Canadian judges have always placed a high value on freedom of expression as an element of parliamentary democracy and have sought to protect it with the limited tools that were at their disposal before the adoption of the Charter of Rights.

The Charter has now in s.2(b) declared freedom of expression to be a fundamental freedom and any questions as to its constitutional status have therefore been settled.

The question now arises: Is freedom of expression involved in this case? In seeking an answer to this question, it must be observed at once that in any form of picketing there is involved at least some element of expression. The picketers would be conveying a message which at a very minimum would be classed as persuasion, aimed at deterring customers and prospective customers from doing business with the respondent. The question then arises. Does this expression in the circumstances of this case have Charter protection under the provisions of s.2(b), and if it does, then does the injunction abridge or infringe such freedom?

The appellants argue strongly that picketing is a form of expression fully entitled to Charter protection and rely on various authorities to support the proposition, including *Reference re Alberta Statutes, supra; Switzman v. Elbling, supra*; the American cases of *Thornhill v. Alabama*, 310 U.S. 88 (1940) (*per* Murphy, J., at p. 95); *Milk Wagon Drivers Union v. Medowmoor Dairies*, 312 U.S. 287 (1941), (*per* Black, J., at p. 302), and various other Canadian authorities . They reject the American distinction between the concept of speech and that of conduct made in picketing cases, and they accept the view of Hutcheon, J.A. in the Court of Appeal, in adopting the words of Freedman, C.J.M. in *Channel Seven Television Ltd. v. National Association of Broadcast Employees and Technicians*, [1971] 5 W.W.R. 328, that "Peaceful picketing falls within freedom of speech".

The respondent contends for a narrower approach to the concept of freedom of expression. The position is summarized in the respondent's factum:

4. We submit that constitutional protection under section 2(b) should only be given to those forms of expression that warrant such protection. To do otherwise would trivialize freedom of expression generally and lead to a downgrading or dilution of this freedom.

Reliance is placed on the view of the majority in the Court of Appeal that picketing in a labour dispute is more than mere communication of information. It is also a signal to trade unionists not to cross the picket line. The respect accorded to picket lines by trade unionists is such that the result of the picketing would be to damage seriously the operation of the employer, not to communicate any information. Therefore, it is argued, since the picket line was not intended to promote dialogue or discourse (as would be the case where its purpose was the exercise of freedom of expression), it cannot qualify for protection under the Charter.

On the basis of the findings of fact that 1 have referred to above, it is evident that the purpose of the picketing in this case was to induce a breach of contract between the respondent and Supercourier and thus to exert economic pressure to force it to cease doing business with Supercourier. It is equally evident that, if successful, the picketing would have done serious injury to the respondent. There is nothing remarkable about this, however, because all picketing is designed to bring economic pressure on the person picketed and to cause economic loss for so long as the object of the picketing remains unfulfilled. There is, as I have earlier said, always some element of expression in picketing. The union is making a statement to the general public that it is involved in a dispute, that it is seeking to impose its will on the object of the picketing, and that it solicits the assistance of the public in honouring the picket line. Action on the part of the picketers will, of course, always accompany the expression, but not every action on the part of the picketers will be such as to alter the nature of the whole transaction and remove it from Charter protection for freedom of expression. That freedom, of course, would not extend to protect threats of violence or acts of violence. It would not protect the destruction of property, or assaults, or other clearly unlawful conduct. We need not, however, be concerned with such matters here because the picketing would have been peaceful. I am therefore of the view that the picketing sought to be restrained would have involved the exercise of the right of freedom of expression.

1.5.2.6 *The Queen v. Committee for the Commonwealth of Canada et al.* (1991), 77 D.L.R. (4th) 385 (S.C.C.)

Respondents L and D were at an airport telling passers-by about the respondent committee and its goals and recruiting members when they were asked by an RCMP officer to cease their activities. The airport's assistant manager confirmed to them that such political propaganda activities were not permitted, as ss. 7(a) and 7(b) of the *Government Airport Concession Operations Regulations* prohibited the conducting of any business or undertaking, commercial or otherwise, and any advertising or soliciting at an airport, except as authorized in writing by the Minister. The trial judge granted respondents' action for a declaration that appellant had not respected their fundamental freedoms. The Federal Court of Appeal affirmed the judgment. This appeal is to determine whether ss. 7(a) and 7(b) of the *Regulations* are inconsistent with the freedom of expression guaranteed in s.2(b) of the *Canadian Charter of Rights and Freedoms*, and if so, whether they are a reasonable limit under s. 1 of the Charter.

HELD: The appeal should be dismissed; respondents' freedom of expression was infringed.

LAMER, C.J. AND SOPINKA, J.: The government's right of ownership, as a consequence of its special nature, cannot of itself authorize an infringement of the freedom guaranteed by s. 2(b) of the Charter. When a person claims that his freedom of expression was infringed while he was trying to express himself in a place owned by the government, the interests at issue must be examined; namely, the interest of the individual wishing to express himself in a place suitable for such expression and the interest of the government, which must ensure effective operation of the place owned by it. An individual will thus only be free to communicate in such a place if the form of expression he uses is compatible with the principal function or intended purpose of the place and does not have the effect of depriving the citizens as a whole of the effective operation of government services and undertakings. If the expression takes a form that contravenes the function of the place, such a form of expression will not fall under s. 2(b). It is only after the complainant has proved that his form of expression is compatible with the function of the place that the justifications which may be put forward under s. 1 of the Charter can be analysed.

In this case, respondents' activities at the airport benefited from the protection of s. 2(b) of the Charter. The distribution of pamphlets and discussion with certain members of the public are in no way incompatible with the airport's's primary function, that of accommodating the needs of the travelling public. An airport is a thoroughfare, which in its open areas or waiting areas can accommodate expression without the effectiveness or function of the place being in any way threatened. There was thus a limitation on the freedom of expression enjoyed by respondents when the airport manager ordered them to cease their activities. However, in the absence of a limit prescribed by law, this limitation cannot be justified under s. 1 of the, Charter. The language of ss. 7(a) and 7(b) of the *Regulations*, analysed in the context of the section and of the *Regulations* as a whole, prohibits only undertakings of a commercial nature and does not cover political propaganda. Section 7 is accordingly not applicable in this case. The limitation imposed on respondents' freedom of expression arose from the action taken by the airport manager, a government official, who ordered them to cease their activities. Although this action was based on an established policy or internal directive, it cannot be concluded from this that there was a "law" which could be justified under s. 1 of the Charter. The government's internal directives or policies differ essentially from statutes and regulations in that they are generally not published and so are not known to the public. Moreover, they are binding only on government officials and may be amended or cancelled at will.

LA FOREST, J.: Freedom of expression, while it does not encompass the right to use any and all government property for purposes of disseminating views on public matters, does include the right to use streets and parks which are dedicated to the use of the public, subject to reasonable limitation to ensure their continued use for the purposes to which they are dedicated. This should include areas of airports frequented by travelers and members of the public. The blanket prohibition against the use of such areas for the purpose of the expression of views violated the freedom of expression guaranteed by s. 2(b) of the Charter, and is not justifiable under s. 1. Section 7 of the *Regulations* does not cover political activities, but in prohibiting expression of political views at the airport. the officials were exercising the Crown's legal right to manage its property, and the prohibition was thus prescribed by law.

L'HEUREUX DUBÉ, J.: Section 7 of the *Regulations* has the effect of restricting political expression, even if that is not its purpose, and thus breaches s. 2(b) of the Charter Where a restriction on expressive activity is content-neutral. the government must demonstrate that the restriction is not an unreasonable restriction on the time, place and manner of the expressive activity. This must be demonstrated under s. 1 of the Charter.

Although the expressive activity took place on government property, the government cannot have complete discretion to treat its property as would a private citizen. If members of the public had no right whatsoever to engage in expressive activity on government-owned property, little opportunity would exist to exercise their freedom of expression. While s. 2(b) of the Charter does not provide a right of access to all government property, some property will be constitutional open to the public. This analysis is properly dealt with under s. 1 of the Charter. A number of factors are helpful to determine whether the restrictions by the government have been applied to property which is a "public arena" These factors include: the traditional openness of such property for expressive activity; whether the public is ordinarily admitted to the property as of right; the compatibility of the property's purpose which such activity; the impact of the property's availability on the achievement of s. 2(b)'s purposes; the property's's symbolic significance for the message being communicated; and the availability of other public arenas in the vicinity. The "traditional" component of the public arena analysis must appreciate the "type" of place historically associated with public discussion, and should not be restricted to the actual places themselves. Bus, train and airport.terminals, which draw large numbers of travelers, are contemporary crossroads or modern thoroughfares and should thus be accessible to those seeking to communicate with the passing crowds. Similarly, while the symbolism of a courthouse lawn or Parliament Hill is self-evident, streets and parks have also acquired special significance as places where one can address one's fellow citizens on any number of matters, and the same holds true for airport terminals. The non-security zones within airport terminals are thus properly regarded as public arenas, and the government cannot simply assert property rights, or claim that the expression is unrelated to an airport's function, in order to justify the restriction.

Section 7 of the *Regulations* is too vague and does not constitute a limit "prescribed by law" and thus cannot be saved under s. 1 of the Charter. Section

7(a) prohibits "any business or undertaking, commercial or otherwise" at the airport. It has failed to offer an intelligible standard which would enable a citizen to regulate his or her conduct. The *Regulation* can be read as an attempt to eradicate all types of expression or, more narrowly, to exclude only certain types of expression, and thus creates confusion. This does not allow fundamental freedoms to be fully exercised. The plenary discretion given to the Minister may also create a vague standard which does not accord with the requirement in s. 1 of the Charter that a limit on a right or freedom be "prescribed by law."

Section 7 of the *Regulations* is also overbroad and thus does not impair freedom of expression as little as possible. The *Regulation* applies not only to the activity at issue but also to virtually all conceivable activity involving freedom of expression at airports.

Although some objectives would be reasonable in justifying restrictions on expression in an airport, the time, place and manner of the restrictions are not reasonable in the context and circumstances of this case. They bear no rational connection to the government's possible objectives and are broad to the point of being unintelligible. Section 7 of the *Regulation* does not, for the same reason pass the proportionality test. Its impairment, far from being minimal, could not be greater.

MCLACHLIN, J.: The test for the constitutional right to use government property for public expression should be based on the values and interests at stake and should not be confined to the characteristics of particular types of government property. This test should reflect the concepts traditionally associated with free expression and should extend constitutional protection to expression on some but not all government property. The analysis under s. 2(b) of the Charter should be primarily definitional, and the test should be sufficiently generous to ensure that valid claims are not excluded for want of proof.

The test for whether s. 2(b) applies to protect expression in a particular forum depends on the class into which the restriction at issue falls. Section 2(b) of the Charter, would usually be infringed if the government's purpose was to restrict the content of expression by limiting the forums in which it can be made. A content-neutral restriction, however, may not infringe freedom of expression at all. Section 2(b) of the Charter should apply if it were established that the expression (including its time, place and manner) promoted one of the purposes underlying the guarantee of free expression: the seeking and obtaining of truth; participation in social and political decision-making; and the encouragement of diversity in forms of individual self-fulfillment by cultivating a tolerant, welcoming environment for the conveyance and reception of ideas. A link must be established between the use of the forum for public expression and at least one of these purposes if the protection of s. 2(b) of the Charter is to apply.

The policy of the airport officials of prohibiting all political propaganda was content-neutral; it was aimed at the consequences of such expression rather than the particular messages communicated. The restriction had the effect of limiting expression, and the expression in question promoted one of the purposes of the guarantee of free expression, namely participation in political or social issues in the community. The government's action thus constituted a limitation of respondents' rights under s. 2(b) of the Charter.

The limitation of respondents' rights is not justifiable under s. 1 of the Charter. The words "advertise" and "solicit", s. 7(b) of the *Regulations* are broad enough to cover non-commercial publicity and solicitation, and respondents conduct thus falls within the regulation. Even if it did not, the act of the airport officials in preventing respondents from handing out leaflets and soliciting members of the public constitutes a limit prescribed by law because the officials were acting pursuant to the Crown's legal rights as owner of the premises. The government's objective in imposing the limit is not of sufficient importance to warrant overriding a Charter right, since there is nothing in the function or purpose of an airport which is incompatible with respondents' conduct. Further, the means chosen to attain the objective are neither reasonable nor proportionate to respondents' interest in conveying their message pursuant to their right under s. 2(b) of the Charter. The practice of airport authorities of preventing all "political propaganda activities constitutes a blanket exclusion of political solicitation in the airport unrelated to concerns for its function and devoid of safeguards to protect against over-reaching application. The limitation is over-broad and hence not saved by s. 1.

GONTHIER, J.: While in agreement with the several elements put forward by Lamer, C.J. and L'Heureux-Dubé, J. pertinent to a determination of the extent of freedom of expression on government property, the application of ss. 1 and 2(b) of the Charter should be structured as outlined by McLachlin, J. The reasons of L'Heureux-Dubé, J. as to the application of s. 7 of the *Regulations* to the conduct of the respondents were agreed with.

CORY, J.: Notwithstanding agreement with the reasons of Lamer, C.J. in so far as they deal with the use of government-owned property by members of the public for the purpose of expressing themselves on various issues, the impugned *Regulation* contravenes s. 2(b) and cannot be saved by s. 1 of the Charter, as found by L'Heureux-Dubé, J.

Courts have also recognized that free expression must be viewed as a process.

1.5.2.7 *International Fund for Animal Welfare Inc. v. The Queen* (1986), 30 C.C.C. (3d) 80 (F.C.T.D.)

McNAIR, J. The regulations subjected to attack in the present lawsuit are the following provisions of the *Seal Protection Regulations*, C.R.C. 1978, c.833, viz:

11. (2) No person shall use a helicopter or other aircraft in searching for seals unless he has an aircraft sealing license issued by the Minister.

(3) An aircraft sealing license may be issued only in respect of an aircraft registered in Canada under Part 11 of the *Air Regulations* made pursuant to the *Aeronautics Act*.

(5) Except with the permission of the Minister, no person shall
  (*a*) land a helicopter or other aircraft less than 1/2 nautical mile from any seal that is on the ice in the Gulf Area or Front Area; or
  (*b*) operate a helicopter or other aircraft over any seal on the ice at an altitude of less than 2,000 feet, except for commercial flights operating on scheduled flight plans.

(6) No person shall, unless he is the holder of a license or a permit, approach within half a nautical mile of any area in which a seal hunt is being carried out [enacted SOR/78-167].

The first issue concerns the constitutional validity of the above mentioned provisions of the *Seal Protection Regulations*, which the plaintiffs have challenged in their action by invoking s.2(b) of the Charter. The question thus raised for determination is whether the regulations deny to the plaintiffs their guaranteed right of freedom of expression within the meaning of s.2(b) of the Charter. This right, it is contended, must be seen to include "freedom to seek, receive and impart information and ideas of all kinds", whether by the written or spoken word or photography or whatever other media of communication might be chosen. Although I.F.A.W. is unquestionably a redoubtable protester, the gist of the case is not concerned with the right to protest per se. The plaintiffs' evidence is that they have never deliberately interfered with the sealers. Their avowed objective is access to information rather than altercation and confrontation.

On the issue of constitutionality, it is the plaintiffs' contention that the impugned provisions of the *Seal Protection Regulations* violate their right of free access to information contrary to s.2(b) of the Charter. It is further contended that the regulatory prohibitions against landing or flying an aircraft in proximity to any seal on the ice have the effect of rendering meaningless any licence or permit to approach within half a nautical mile of an area where a seal hunt is being carried out. The plaintiffs also submit that I.F.A.W. is a member of the media. I cannot accept this last-mentioned submission. The defendants contend, on the other hand, that the right of freedom of expression is limited to the dissemination of ideas and beliefs in the expressible sense and does not comprehend the broader aspect of access to information as the fountainhead for the formulation and expression of those ideas and beliefs.

An expansive and purposive scrutiny of s.2(b) leads inevitably, in my judgment, to the conclusion that freedom of expression must include freedom of access to all information pertinent to the ideas or beliefs sought to be expressed, subject to such reasonable limitations as are necessary to national security, public order, public health or morals, or the fundamental rights and freedoms of others.

1.5.2.8 *Re Information Retailers Association of Metropolitan Toronto Inc. and Municipality of Metropolitan Toronto* (1985), 52 O.R. (2d) 449 (Ont.C.A.)

HOULDEN, CORY and ROBINS, JJ. A.: Freedom of expression is a fundamental freedom protected by s.2(b) of the Charter. The protection applies to all phases of expression from writer, artist and photographer through to distributor and retailer and on to reader and viewer: *R. v. Videoflicks Ltd. et al.* (1984), 48 O.R. (2d) 395 at p. 431, 14 D.L.R. (4th) 10 at p. 46, 15 C.C.C. (3d) 353 (C.A.); *Re Ontario Film & Video Appreciation Society and Ontario Board of Censors* (1984), 45 O.R. (2d) 80n, 5 D.L.R. (4th) 766n, 38 C.R. (3d) 271 (C.A.). The freedom to distribute and sell is as essential to the exercise of the freedom as the freedom to publish, for without the means of disseminating expression, the publication would be of little value. Non-obscene "adult books and magazines", no matter how tasteless or tawdry they may be, are entitled to no less protection than other forms of expression; the constitutional guarantee extends not only to that which is pleasing, but also to that which to many may be aesthetically distasteful or morally offensive; it is indeed often true that "one man's vulgarity is another's lyric".

1.5.3 Applying Section One

1.5.3.1 "Prescribed by Law"

1.5.3.1.1 *Re Ontario Film and Video Appreciation Society and Ontario Board of Censors* (1983), 41 O.R. (2d) 583 (Div. Ct.)

J. HOLLAND, BOLAND and LINDEN, JJ: The next issue is whether the limits placed on the applicant's freedom of expression by the board of censors were "prescribed by law". It is clear that statutory law, regulations and even common law limitations may be permitted. But the limit, to be acceptable, must have legal force. This is to ensure that it has been established democratically through the legislative process or judicially through the operation of precedent over the years. This requirement under-scores the seriousness with which courts will view any interference with the fundamental freedoms.

The Crown has argued that the board's authority to curtail freedom of expression is prescribed by law in the *Theatres Act*, ss.3, 35 and 38. In our view, although there has certainly been a legislative grant of power to the board to censor and prohibit certain films, the reasonable limits placed upon that freedom of expression of film-makers have not been legislatively authorized. The Charter requires reasonable limits that are prescribed by law; it is not enough to authorize a board to censor or prohibit the exhibition of any film of which it disapproves. That kind of authority is not legal for it depends on the discretion of an administrative tribunal. However dedicated, competent and well-meaning the board may be, that kind of regulation cannot be considered as "law". It is accepted that law cannot be vague, undefined, and totally discretionary; it must be ascertainable and understandable. Any limits placed on the freedom of expression cannot be left to the whim of an official; such limits must be articulated with some precision or they cannot be considered to be law.

There are no reasonable limits contained in the statute or the regulations. The standards and the pamphlets utilized by the Ontario Board of Censors do contain certain information upon which a film-maker may get some indication of how his film will be judged. However, the board is not bound by these standards. They have no legislative or legal force of any kind. Hence, since they do not qualify as law, they cannot be employed so as to justify any limitation on expression, pursuant to s.1 of the Charter. We draw comfort in this conclusion from the views of Professor Beckton, in *The Canadian Charter of Rights and Freedoms: Commentary* (1982), p. 107 (Tarnopolsky & Beaudoin, editors), where she wrote:

> Clearly statutes which create censorship boards without specific criteria would be contrary to the guarantees of free expression, since no line is drawn between objectionable and non-objectionable forms of expression. Now standards will have to be created to measure the limits to which obscene expressions may be regulated.

This does not mean that the censorship scheme set out in the *Theatres Act* is invalid. Clearly the classification scheme by itself does not offend the Charter. Nor do we find that ss.3, 35 and 38 are invalid, but the problem is that standing alone they cannot be used to censor or prohibit the exhibition of films because they are so general, and because the detailed criteria employed in the process are not prescribed by law. These sections, in so far as they purport to prohibit or to allow censorship of films, may be said to be "of no force or effect", but they may be rendered operable by the passage of regulations pursuant to the legislative authority or by the enactment of statutory amendments, imposing reasonable limits and standards.

1.5.3.1.2 *Re Ontario Film and Video Appreciation Society and Ontario Board of Censors* (1984), 45 O.R. (2d) 80 (Ont. C.A.)

MACKINNON, A.C.J.O.: We would go further than the Divisional Court on this issue. In our view, s.3(2)(a), rather than being of "no force or effect", is *ultra vires* as it stands. The subsection allows for the complete denial or prohibition of the freedom of expression in this particular year and sets no limits on the Ontario Board of Censors. It clearly sets no limit, reasonable or otherwise, on which an argument can be mounted that it falls within the saving words of s.1 of the Charter: "subject only to such reasonable limits prescribed by law". Further, like the Divisional Court, we conclude that s.3(2)(b) and ss.35 and 38 cannot be interpreted and applied in their present form to support the censorship of film although they have a valid role to play otherwise. As pointed out by the Divisional Court, there is no challenge in these proceedings to the system of film classification, to the general regulation of theatres and projectionists and other matters dealt with in the statute and regulations.

Note: In response to the Ontario Court of Appeal decision the legislature amended the *Theatres Act*.

1.5.3.1.3 *An Act to Amend the Theatres Act*, S.O. 1984, c. 56

35. (1) Before the exhibition or distribution in Ontario of a film, an application for approval to exhibit or distribute and for classification of the film shall be made to the Board.

(2) After viewing a film, the Board, in accordance with the criteria prescribed by the regulations, may refuse to approve the film for exhibition or distribution in Ontario.

(3) The Board, having regard to the criteria prescribed by the regulations, may make an approval conditional upon the film being exhibited in designated locations and on specified dates only.

(4) Except as otherwise provided, for the purpose of exercising a power under clause 3(5)(a) or (d), three members of the Board constitute a quorum.

(5) Where a film has been submitted for approval and classification under subsection (1), the person submitting the film, on payment of the prescribed fee, may appeal the Board's decision by submitting the film for reconsideration by a panel of the Board and that panel, after viewing the film, shall make a decision on its approval and classification.

(6) A decision by a panel of the Board under subsection (5) as to classification is final.

(7) The panel referred to in subsection (5) shall be composed of at least five members, none of whom had participated in a previous decision on the film.

(8) A person who has appealed under subsection (5) may appeal the Board's decision as to approval to the Divisional Court in accordance with the rules of court and, where there is an appeal, the Minister is entitled to be heard.

(9) An appeal under subsection (8) may be made on question of law or fact or both and the Court may affirm or may rescind the decision of the Board and may direct the Board to take any action that the Board may take and as the Court considers proper.

35a. (1) Where the chairman of the Board is of the opinion that the criteria prescribed by regulation respecting subject-matter or content in films have changed since a film was originally approved and classified and that the film may not be entitled to the approval or classification determined at the time of the original decision, the chairman may require that the film be submitted for reconsideration by the Board.

(2) Where a film is submitted for reconsideration under subsection (1), the provisions of section 35 apply with necessary modifications except that no fees shall be charged.

38. (1) No person shall exhibit, distribute or offer to distribute or cause to be exhibited, distributed or offered for distribution in Ontario any film that has not been approved by the Board.

(2) No person shall exhibit or cause to be exhibited in Ontario any film that has been approved by the Board subject to any conditions except in accordance with those conditions.

39. No person shall alter or cause to be altered, for the purpose of exhibition or distribution in Ontario, any film from its state as approved by the Board.

1.2.3.1.4 O. Reg. 56/85. Regulation to Amend Regulation 931 of Revised Regulations of Ontario, 1980, Made Under the *Theatres Act*

21. (1) In exercising its authority under sections 3 and 35 of the Act, the Board shall consider the film in its entirety and take into account the general character and integrity of the film.

(2) After viewing a film, the Board may refuse to approve a film for exhibition or distribution in Ontario where the film contains,

 (*a*) a graphic or prolonged scene of violence, torture, crime, cruelty, horror or human degradation:

 (*b*) the depiction of the physical abuse or humiliation of human beings for purposes of sexual gratification or as pleasing to the victim:

 (*c*) a scene where a person who is or is intended to represent a person under the age of sixteen years appears,

  (i) nude or partially nude in a sexually suggestive context, or

  (ii) in a scene of explicit sexual activity;

 (*d*) the explicit and gratuitous depiction of urination, defecation or vomiting;

 (*e*) the explicit depiction of sexual activity;

 (*f*) a scene depicting indignities to the human body in an explicit manner;

 (*g*) a scene where there is undue emphasis on human genital organs; or

 (*h*) a scene where an animal has been abused in the making of the film.

(3) In this section, "sexual activity" means acts, whether real or simulated, of intercourse or masturbation, and includes the depiction of genital, anal or oral-genital connection between human beings or human beings and animals, and anal or genital connection between human beings by means of objects. O. Reg. 56/85, s.2.

1.5.3.1.5 *Osborne v. Canada (Treasury Board)* **(1991), 82 D.L.R. (4th) 321 (S.C.C.)**

Section 33 of the *Public Service Employment Act*, R.S.C. 1985, c. P-33 (formerly s. 32 of the *Public Service Employment Act*, R.S.C. 1970, c. P-32), prohibits federal public servants from "engaging in work" for or against a candidate or political party, subject to s. 33(2) which provides an exception for attending a political meeting or contributing money to a candidate or party. The respondents, one of whom was a candidate for election to Parliament at the time the action was brought and the others of whom were public servants who wished to work on his behalf, brought actions against the appellant Public Service Commission for declarations that s. 33 of the Act was void by reason of its conflict with the guarantee of freedom of expression found in s. 2(b) of the *Canadian Charter of Rights and Freedoms* and the guarantee of freedom of association found in s. 2(d) of the Charter. The Federal Court, Trial Division dismissed the actions. The Federal Court of Appeal allowed the respondents' appeals and granted declarations that s. 33(1) of the Act is of no force and effect except as it applies to a deputy head.

On further appeal by the appellant commission to the Supreme Court of Canada, held, Stevenson, J. dissenting, the appeal should be dismissed and the Federal Court of Appeal's orders that s. 33(1) is of no force and effect except as it applies to a deputy head should stand.

SOPINKA, J. (CORY and McLACHLIN, JJ. concurring):

(a) *Limit prescribed by law*

The respondents contend that s. 33 of the Act is so vague that it contains no intelligible standard to enable the appellant to resort to the justificatory provisions of s. 1. This argument succeeded in the Court of Appeal. To support their position, the respondents refer the court to the annual report of the appellant in which it was acknowledged that it had "considerable difficulty" in administering s. 33 of the Act. The respondents submit, further, that a limitation that is so unclear in its application as to require extensive guidelines in the form of non-authoritative views such as are contained in "Dialogue Express", the bulletin of the appellant setting out guidelines of permissible conduct, is *ipso facto* not a limit prescribed by law.

Vagueness can have constitutional significance in at least two ways in a s. 1 analysis. A law may be so uncertain as to be incapable of being interpreted so as to constitute any restraint on governmental power. The uncertainty may arise either from the generality of the discretion conferred on the donee of the power or from the use of language that is so obscure as to be incapable of interpretation with any degree of precision using the ordinary tools. In these circumstances, there is no "limit prescribed by law" and no s.1 analysis is necessary as the threshold requirement for its application is not met. The second way in which vagueness can play a constitutional role is in the analysis of s. 1. A law which passes the threshold test may, nevertheless, by reason of its imprecision, not qualify as a reasonable limit. Generality and imprecision of language may fail to confine the invasion of a Charter right within reasonable limits. In this sense vagueness is an aspect of overbreadth.

This court has shown a reluctance to disentitle a law to s. 1 scrutiny on the basis of vagueness which results in the granting of wide discretionary powers. Much of the activity of government is carried on under the aegis of laws which of necessity leave a broad discretion to government officials: see *R. v. Jones* (1986), 31 D.L.R. (4th) 569, 28 C.C.C. (3d) 513, [1986] 2 S.C.R. 284; *United States of America v. Cotroni* (1989), 48 C.C.C. (3d) 193, [1989] 1 S.C.R. 1469, 42 C.R.R. 101, and *R. v. Beare* (1988), 55 D.L.R. (4th) 481, 45 C.C.C. (3d) 67, [1988] 2 S.C.R. 387. Since it may very well be reasonable in the circumstances to confer a wide discretion, it is preferable in the vast majority of cases to deal with vagueness in the content of a s. 1 analysis rather than disqualifying the law *in limine*. In this regard, I adopt the language of McLachlin, J. in *Canada (Human Rights Commission) v. Taylor* (1990), 75 D.L.R. (4th) 577 at pp. 621-2, [1990] 3 S.C.R. 892, 117 N.R. 191:

> That is not to say that the alleged vagueness of the standard set by the provision is irrelevant to the s.1 analysis. For reasons discussed below, I am of the opinion that the difficulty in ascribing a constant and universal meaning to the terms used is a factor to be taken into account in assessing whether the law is "demonstrably justified in a free and democratic society". But I would be reluctant to circumvent the entire balancing analysis of the s.1 test by finding that the words used

were so vague as not to constitute a "limit prescribed by law", unless the provision could truly be described as failing to offer an intelligible standard. That is not the case here.

Irwin Toy Ltd. v. Quebec (Attorney-General), supra, is an apt illustration of this approach which is particularly apposite to this case. At issue in this case were ss. 248 and 249 of the *Consumer Protection Act* which prohibited commercial advertising directed at persons under the age of 13. It was argued that the sections could not be saved pursuant to s. 1 because the provisions were "confusing and contradictory", because they provided insufficient guidance to the courts in determining whether advertising was directed towards children, and because the legislation provided too much scope for discretion to promulgate regulations. The majority opinion written conjointly by Dickson, C.J.C., Lamer and Wilson, JJ. rejected out of hand the "regulations" argument. In dealing with the "insufficient guidance" argument, the court remarked (at p. 617):

> Absolute precision in the law exists rarely, if at all. The question is whether the legislature has provided an intelligible standard according to which the judiciary must do its work. The task of interpreting how that standard applied in particular instances might always be characterized as having a discretionary element, because the standard can never specify all the instances in which it applies. On the other hand, where there is no intelligible standard and where the legislature has given a plenary discretion to do whatever seems best in a wide set of circumstances, there is no "limit prescribed by law".

Ultimately, it was held that the impugned provisions of the *Consumer Protection Act* were satisfactory since they could be given a "sensible interpretation" and did not confer a discretion on the courts to ban whichever advertisements they pleased. The fact that guidelines were published by the Office de la protection du consommateur to assist in the administration of the Act did not necessarily indicate that the courts had no intelligible standard to abide by.

Applying the foregoing to this case, I cannot conclude that s. 33 is couched in such vague or general language that it does not contain an intelligible standard. The words "engage in work", while capable of very wide import, are ordinary simple words in the English language that are capable of interpretation. The same is true of the French version which refers to *"travailler."* They undoubtedly present considerable difficulty in application to a specific situation, as the Report of the Commission attests, but difficulty of interpretation cannot be equated with the absence of any intelligible standard: see *R. v. Rowley* (1986), 31 C.C.C. (3d) 183, 25 C.R.R. 375, 43 M.V.R. 290 (B.C.C.A.), and *Montreal (City) v. Arcade Amusements Inc.* (1985), 18 D.L R. (4th) 161, [1985] 1 S.C.R. 368, 29 M.P.L.R. 220. The language of a. 33 does not create a standard which leaves it to the Commission to ban whatever activity they please, to paraphrase the words used in *Irwin Toy, supra.* I therefore conclude that a 33 does constitute a limit prescribed by law and it is necessary to proceed to a s. 1 analysis.

In *R. v. Oakes, supra,* at p. 227, Dickson, C.J.C. explained that to establish a reasonable limit two central criteria must be satisfied: first, the government objective must be "of sufficient importance to warrant overriding a constitutionally protected right or freedom" and secondly, the means chosen must be reasonable and demonstrably justifiable in a free and democratic society. It is necessary to test s. 33 against these basic criteria of constitutional validity.

1.5.3.2 "Reasonable and Demonstrably Justified in a Free and Democratic Society"

1.5.3.2.1 *Attorney-General of Quebec v. Irwin Toy Ltd.* (1989), 58 D.L.R. (4th) 577 (S.C.C.)

DICKSON, C.J.C., LAMER AND WILSON, JJ.: It is now well established that the onus of justifying the limitation of a right or freedom rests with the party seeking to uphold the limitation, in this case the Attorney-General of Quebec, and that the analysis to be conducted is that set forth by Dickson, C.J.C. in *R. v. Oakes*.

A. Pressing and Substantial Objective

The first part of the test involves asking whether the objective sought to be achieved by the impugned legislation relates to concerns which are "pressing and substantial in a free and democratic society." Dickson, C.J.C. explained this requirement in *Oakes* at p. 227:

> First, the objective, which the measures responsible for a limit on a Charter right or freedom are designed to serve, must be "of sufficient importance to warrant overriding a constitutionally protected right or freedom": *R. v. Big M Drug Mart Ltd., supra*, at p. 430 C.C.C., p.366 D.L.R., p. 352 S.C.R. The standard must be high in order to ensure that objectives which are trivial or discordant with the principles integral to a free and democratic society do not gain s. 1 protection. It is necessary, at a minimum, that an objective relate to concerns which are pressing and substantial in a free and democratic society before it can be characterized as sufficiently important.

Because we have already found that the plaintiff's activity falls within the sphere of conduct protected by freedom of expression and that the purpose of the legislation is to prohibit particular content of expression in the name of protecting children, it is far from onerous to require that the concern underlying the restrictive legislation be a pressing and substantial one. Without such a high standard of justification, enshrined rights and freedoms would be stripped of most of their value.

In our view, the Attorney-General of Quebec has demonstrated that the concern which prompted the enactment of the impugned legislation is pressing and substantial and that the purpose of the legislation is one of great importance. The concern is for the protection of a group which is particularly vulnerable to the techniques of seduction and manipulation abundant in advertising. In the words of the Attorney-General of Quebec (translation), "children experience most manifestly the kind of inequality and imbalance between producers and consumers which the legislature wanted to correct." The material given in evidence before this court is indicative of a generalized concern in Western societies with the impact of media, and particularly but not solely televised advertising, on the development and perceptions of young children. (For example: Canadian Radio-Television and Telecommunications Commission, Decision 79-320, April 30, 1979, Renewal of the Canadian Broadcasting Corporation's Television and Radio Network Licences (1979)113 *Can. Gaz.*, Part I, 3082, Canadian Association of Broadcasters, *Broadcast Code for Advertising to Children (op. cit.)*; Canadian Broadcasting Corporation, *Commercial Acceptance Policy Guideline*, see in particular "The CBC and Children's Advertising;" National Associations of Broadcasters, *Television Code* (21st ed., 1980), see in particular "Responsibility Towards Children;" Organization for Economic Cooperation and Development (OECD), *Advertising Directed at Children: Endorsements in Advertising* (1982); and J.J. Boddewyn, *Advertising to Children: Regulation and Self-regulation in 40 Countries* (New York; International Association Inc., 1984). Broadly speaking, the concerns which have motivated both legislative and voluntary regulation in this area are the particular susceptibility of young children to media manipulation, their inability to differentiate between reality and fiction and to grasp the persuasive intention behind the message, and the secondary effects of exterior influences on the family and parental authority. Responses to the perceived problems are as varied as she agencies and governments which have promulgated them. However, the consensus of concern is high.

In establishing the factual basis for this generally identified concern, the Attorney-General relied heavily upon the U.S. Federal Trade Commission (FTC) Final Staff Report and Recommendation, "In the Matter of Children's Advertising" which contains a thorough review of the scientific evidence on the subject as at 1981. The report emerged from a rule-making proceeding initiated by the FTC. The report's assessment both of children's cognitive ability to evaluate television advertising directed at them and of the possible remedies to mitigate the adverse effects of such advertising are relevant here. One of its principal conclusions is that young children (two to six) cannot distinguish fact from fiction or programming from advertising and are completely credulous when presented with advertising messages (at pp. 34-5):

> In summary, the rule-making record establishes that the specific cognitive abilities of young children lead to their inability to fully understand child-oriented television advertising, even if they grasp some aspects of it. They place indiscriminate trust in the selling message. They do not correctly perceive persuasive bias in advertising, and their life experience is insufficient to help them counter-argue. Finally, the content, placement and various techniques met in child-oriented television commercials attract children and enhance the advertising and the product As a result, children are not able to evaluate adequately child-oriented advertising.

The report thus provides a sound basis on which to conclude that television advertising directed at young children is *per se* manipulative. Such advertising aims to promote products by convincing those who will always believe.

It is reasonable to extend this conclusion in two ways. First, it can be extended to advertising in other media. For example, the OECD Report, discussed children's advertising in all media including television, although the greatest body of evidence focuses on the persuasive force of television advertising. Second, it can be extended to advertising aimed at older children (7-13). The Attorney-General filed a number of studies reaching somewhat different conclusions about the age at which children generally develop the cognitive ability to recognize the persuasive nature of advertising and to evaluate its comparative worth. The studies suggest that at some point between age seven and adolescence, children become as capable as adults of understanding and responding to advertisements. The majority in the Court of Appeal interpreted this evidence narrowly and found that it only justified the objective of regulating advertising aimed at children six or younger, not the regulation of advertising aimed at children between the ages of seven and thirteen. They concluded, and we agree, that the evidence was strongest with respect to the younger age category, Opinion is more divided when children in the older age category are involved. But the legislature was not obliged to confine itself solely to protecting the most clearly vulnerable group. It was only required to exercise a renewable judgment in specifying the vulnerable group.

As Dickson, C.J.C. noted in *R. v. Edwards Books & Art Ltd.*, commenting on the legislative decision to exempt businesses having seven or fewer employees from a Sunday closing rule:

> I might add that I do not believe there is any magic in the number seven as distinct from, say, 5, 10, or 15 employees as a cut-off point for eligibility for the exemption. In balancing the interests of retail employees to a holiday in common with their family and friends against the s. 2(a) interests of those affected the legislature' engaged in the process envisaged by s. 1 of the Charter. A "reasonable limit" is one which, having regard to the principles enunciated in *Oakes*, it was reasonable for the legislature to impose. The courts are not called upon to substitute judicial opinions for legislative ones as to the place at which to draw the line.

The same can be said of evaluating competing credible scientific evidence and choosing 13, as opposed to ten or seven, as the upper age limit for the protected group here in issue. Where the legislature mediates between the competing claims of different groups in the community, it will inevitably be called upon to draw a line marking where one set of claims legitimately begins and the other fades away without access to complete knowledge as to its precise location. If the legislature has made a reasonable assessment as to where the line is most properly drawn, especially if that assessment involves weighing conflicting scientific evidence and allocating scarce resources on this basis, it is not for the court to second guess. That would only be to substitute one estimate for another. In dealing with inherently heterogeneous groups defined in terms of age or a characteristic analogous to age, evidence showing that a clear majority of the group requires the protection which the government has identified can help to establish that the group was defined reasonably. Here, the legislature has mediated between the claims of advertisers and those seeking commercial information on the one hand, and the claims of children and parents on the other. There is sufficient evidence to warrant drawing a line at age 13, and we would not presume to re-draw the line. We note that in *Ford*, at pp.6268, the court also recognized that the government was afforded a margin of appreciation to form legitimate objectives bases on somewhat inconclusive social science evidence.

In sum, the objective of regulating commercial advertising directed at children accords with a general goal of consumer protection legislation, *viz*, to protect a group that is most vulnerable to commercial manipulation. Indeed, that goal is reflected in general contract doctrine (see, for example, *Civil Code of Lower Canada*, arts. 987 and 1001 to 1011 respecting contracts with minors). Children are not as equipped as adults to evaluate the persuasive force of advertising and advertisements directed at children would take advantage of this. The legislature reasonably concluded that advertisers should be precluded from taking advantage of children both by inciting them to make purchases and by inciting them to have their parents make purchases. Either way, the advertiser would not be able to capitalize upon children's credulity. The s. 1 and s. 9.1 materials demonstrate, on the balance of probabilities, that children up to the age of 13 are manipulated by commercial advertising and that the objective of protecting all children in this age group is predicated on a pressing and substantial concern. We thus conclude that the Attorney-General has discharged the onus under the first part of the *Oakes* test.

B. Means Proportional to the Ends

The second part of the s.1 test involves balancing a number of factors to determine whether the means chosen by the government are proportional to its objective. As Dickson, C.J.C. stated in *Edwards Books*, at p. 41:

Secondly, the means chosen to attain those objectives must be proportional or appropriate to the ends. The proportionality requirement, in turn, normally has three aspects the limiting measures must be carefully designed, or rationally connected, to the objective; they must impair the right as little as possible; ant their effect must not so severely trench on individual or group rights that the legislative objective, albeit important, is nevertheless, outweighed by the abridgement of rights.

i) **Rational Connection**

There can be no doubt that a ban on advertising directed to children is rationally connected to the objective of protecting children from advertising. The government measure aims precisely at the problem identified is the s. 1 and s. 9.1 materials. It is important to note that there is no general ban on the advertising of children's products, but simply a prohibition against directing advertisements to those unaware of their persuasive intent. Commercial advertisements may clearly be directed at the true purchasers—parents or other adults. Indeed, non-commercial educational advertising aimed at children is permitted. Simply put, advertisers are prevented from capitalizing on the inability of children either to differentiate between fact and fiction or to acknowledge and thereby resist or treat with some skepticism the persuasive intent bestind the advertisement. In the present case, we are of the opinion that the evidence does establish the necessary rational connection between means and objective. In *Ford*, by contrast, no rational correction was established between excluding all languages other than French from signs in Quebec and having the reality of Quebec society communicated through the "visage linguistique."

ii) Minimal Impairment

We turn now to the requirement that "the means, even if radonauy connected to the objective ... should impair 'as little as possible' the right or freedom to question;" *Oakes* at p. 227. We would note that in this context, the standard of proof is the civil standard, that is, proof on the balance of probabilities. Furthermore, as Dickson, C.J.C. observed in *Oakes* at p. 226:

> Within the broad category of the civil standard, there exist different degrees of probability depending on the nature of the case: see Sopinka and Lederman, *The Law of Evidence in Civil Cases* (Toronto, 1974), p. 385. As Lord Denning explained in *Bater v. Bater*, [1950] 2 All ER. 458 at p. 459 (C.A.):
>
>> "The case may be proved by a preponderance of probability, but there may be degrees of probability within that standard. The degree depends on the subject-matter. A civil court, when considering a charge of fraud, will naturally require a higher degree of probability than that which it would require if considering whether negligence were established. It does not adopt so high a degree as a criminal court, even when considering a charge of a criminal nature, but still it does require a degree of probability which is commensurate with the occasion."

This observation is particularly relevant to the "minimal impairment" branch of the *Oakes* proportionality test. The party seeking to uphold the limit must demonstrate on a balance of probabilities that the means chosen impair the freedom or right in question as little as possible. What will be "as little as possible" will of course vary depending on the government objective and on the means available to achieve it. As the Chief Justice wrote in *Oakes*, at p. 227:

> Although the nature of the proportionality test will vary depending on the circumstances, in each case courts will be required to balance the interests of society with those of individuals and groups.

Thus, in matching means to ends and asking whether rights or freedoms are impaired as little as possible, a legislature mediating between the claims of competing groups will be forced to strike a balance without the benefit of absolute certainty concerning how that balance is best struck. Vulnerable groups will claim the need for protection by the government whereas other groups and individuals will assert that the government should not intrude. In *Edwards Books*, Chief Justice Dickson expressed an important concern about the situation of vulnerable groups (at p. 49):

> In interpreting and applying the Charter I believe that the courts must be cautious to ensure that it does not simply become an instrument of better situated individuals to roll back legislation which has as its object the improvement of the condition of less advantaged persons.

When striking a balance between the claims of competing groups, the choice of means, like the choice of ends, frequently will require an assessment of conflicting scientific evidence and differing justified demands on scarce resources. Democratic institutions are meant to let us all share in the responsibility for these difficult choices. Thus, as courts review the results of the deliberations, particularly with respect to the protection of vulnerable groups, they must be mindful of the legislature's representative function. For example, when "regulating industry or business it is open to the legislature to restrict its legislative reforms to sectors in which there appear to be particularly urgent concerns or to constituencies that seem especially needy" (*Edwards Books*, at p. 44).

In other cases, however, rather than mediating between different groups, the government is best characterized as the singular antagonist of the individual whose right has been infringed. For example, in justifying an infringement of legal rights enshrined in ss. 7 to 14 of the Charter, the state, on behalf of the whole community, typically will assert its responsibility for prosecuting crime whereas the individual will assert the paramountcy of principles of fundamental justice. There might not be any further commending claims among different groups. In such circumstances, and indeed whenever the government's purpose relates to maintaining the authority and impartiality of the judicial system, the courts can assess with some certainty whether the "least drastic means" for achieving the purpose have been chosen, especially given their accumulated experience in dealing with such questions: see *The Sunday Times v. United Kingdom* (1979), 2 E.H.R.R. 245 at p. 276. The same degree of certainty may not be achievable in cases involving the reconciliation of claims of competing individuals or groups or the distribution of scarce government resources.

In the instant case, the court is called upon to assess competing social science evidence respecting the appropriate means for addressing the problem of children's advertising. The question is whether the government had a reasonable basis, on the evidence tendered, for concluding that the ban on all advertising directed at children impaired freedom of expression as little as possible given the government's pressing and substantial objective.

The strongest evidence for the proposition that this ban impairs freedom of expression as little as possible comes from the FTC Report. Because the report found that children are not equipped to identify the persuasive intent of advertising, content regulation could not address the problem. The report concluded that the only effective means for dealing with advertising directed at children would be a ban on all such advertising because "[a]n informational remedy would not eliminate nor overcome the cognitive limitations that prevent young children from understanding advertising" (p. 36). However, the report also concluded that such a ban could not be implemented either on the basis of audience composition data or on the basis of a definition of "advertising directed at children." It thus counselled against a ban (at p. 2):

132   A SOURCEBOOK OF CANADIAN MEDIA LAW

> [T]he record establishes that the only effective remedy would be a ban on all advertisements oriented toward young children, and such a ban, as a practical matter, cannot be implemented.

The report gave two reasons why a ban could not be implemented on the basis of audience composition data First, according to the report, viewing audiences were not so sufficiently segmented that one could implement a total ban on advertising during time periods when, on the basis of television ratings, programming is directed at young children. Only one network programme was identified as attracting a viewing audience composed, over 30%, by young children. Second, if the percentage were relaxed to, say, 20%, a total ban on advertising would catch too many non-children and would still fail to catch all programmes frequently watched by young children (at pp.39-41):

> The data indicate that if either at 50% or a 30% audience cutoff figure is used (i.e. when young children constitute 50% or 30% of the actual viewing audience), advertising on only one network program (Captain Kangaroo) would be affected. Advertising on more programs would be included in a ban only if the cutoff figure were lowered to 20%. However, the staff believes that utilizing a 20% cutoff figure would not be advisable because the use of such a low cutoff figure would affect the viewing of the 80% of the audience who are not young children and who do not have their cognitive limitations ...
>
> Staff believes that implementing a ban utilizing a 20% figure would not be advisable because the ban's scope would still be underinclusive from the standpoint of advertising affected and the proportion of the child's total television viewing affected... Further analysis of viewing data for young children (two to five) indicates more specifically that if a 20% cutoff figure were used, advertising on only 24 network programs would be affected, 22 of which are shown on Saturday or Sunday mornings. The use of a 20% figure would not include advertising on child-oriented programs shown during other time periods. Only 13% of a young child's weekly viewing of television occurs on weekend mornings.

Because the FTC Report focussed on the effect of advertising aimed at *young* children (2-6) and proceeded on the basis that advertising directed at *older* children (7-13) did not pose a problem, it concluded, reasonably enough, that no definition could distinguish adequately between advertising directed at young children and advertising directed at older children (at pp. 44-5):

> [The preliminary] Staff Report suggested a definition of "advertising directed to children" based on program design. A remedy based on this definition would ban advertising "in or adjacent to programs that have been designated as children's programs using some *a priori* judgments." The major and inherent drawback to this definition is that it does not distinguish between programs designed for younger children and those designed for older children ...
>
> The lack of specificity in categorizing children's programs as being primarily for two-six years old appears to coincide with the industry's practice of not directing advertisements solely to young children. For instance, CBS stated: "while certain advertisers who use television may wish to address young views, they rarely, if ever, limit their appeal to the young children alone."

Sections 248 and 249 preserve the rationale for a ban contained in the FTC Report at the same time as overcoming the practical limitations suggested therein. The sections contemplate a larger age group than that envisaged by the FTC Report, and always allow advertising aimed at adults, thereby avoiding the difficulties identified in the report both with a ban based on audience composition and with a ban based on the definition of "advertising directed to children. *"The Guidelines for the application of sections 248 and 249* help to illustrate this. They specify a number of time periods during the day when, based on Bureau of Broadcast Measurements (BBM) statistics, over 15% of the audience is made up of children aged 2 to 11. It was possible to arrive at these time periods despite the FTC's arguments precisely because a larger target group was specified. Furthermore, using this larger target group, it was possible for the Office de la protection du consommateur to identify products and advertising methods aimed at children. in this way, the 15% cut-off does not serve to justify a ban on all advertising (as the 20% cut-off discussed by the FTC was designed to do). By specifying categories of (1) products, (2) advertisements and (3) audience, the guidelines allow for a sophisticated appraisal of when an advertisement is aimed at children. These three categories are drawn directly from s. 249 and their elaboration by the office is an attempt to perform the same balancing test required of the courts. Three categories of products are specified: (1) those aimed exclusively at children (toys, and certain candies and foods); (2) those having a large attraction for children (certain cereals, desserts and games); and (3) those aimed at adults. Four categories of advertisements are specified: (1) those not likely to interest children; (2) those not designed to interest children; (3) those directed only partly to children; and (4) those aimed mainly at children. Three categories of audience are specified: (1) children compose over 15%; (2) children compose between 5% and 15%; and (3) children compose less than 5%. On this basis, the guidelines set forth a table according to which different kinds of advertisements for the various product categories will be permitted depending upon audience composition. There is a system of pre-clearance run by a committee of the office which helps advertisers to determine whether any given commercial is subject to the ban.

While ss. 248 and 249 do not incorporate all the details included in the guidelines, they do put into place the framework for a practicable ban on advertising directed at children. The courts, rather than the Office de la protection du consommateur, are left with the final word as to whether, for example, the strictest limit on advertising should apply where children compose over 15% of the audience rather than for example, 20%. But if a ban is the only effective means to achieve the legislative objective, and if such a ban can only be implemented using a flexible balancing test, the legislature cannot be faulted for leaving that balancing to the courts. Indeed, this should help to ensure that minimal impairment of free expression is a constant factor in the application of the law.

Of course, despite the FTC Report's conclusions to the contrary, the respondent argued that a ban was not the only effective means for dealing with the problem posed by children's advertising. In particular, it pointed to the self-regulation mechanism provided by the Broadcast Code for Advertising to Children as an obvious alternative and emphasized that Quebec was unique among industrialized countries in banning advertising aimed at children (see Boddewyn). The latter assertion must be qualified in two respects. First, as of 1984, Belgium, Denmark, Norway and Sweden did not allow any commercials on television and radio. Second, throughout Canada, as in Italy, the public network does not accept children's commercials (except, in the case of the CBC, during "family programmes"). Consequently, Quebec's ban on advertising aimed at children is not out of proportion to measures taken in other jurisdictions. Nor is legislative action to protect vulnerable groups necessarily restricted to the least common denominator of actions taken elsewhere. Based on narrower objectives than those pursued by Quebec, some governments might reasonably conclude that self-regulation is an adequate mechanism for addressing the problem of children's advertising. But having identified advertising aimed at persons under 13 as *per se* manipulative, the legislature of Quebec could conclude, just as reasonably, that the only effective statutory response was to ban such advertising.

In sum the evidence sustains the reasonableness of the legislature's conclusion that a ban on commercial advertising directed to children was the minimal impairment of free expression consistent with the pressing and substantial goal of protecting children against manipulation through such advertising. While evidence exists that other less intrusive options reflecting more modest objectives were available to the government, there is evidence establishing the necessity of a bam to meet the objectives the government had reasonably set. This court will not, in the name of minimal impairment, take a restrictive approach to social science evidence and require legislatures to choose the least ambitious means to protect vulnerable groups. There must nevertheless be a sound evidentiary basis for the government's conclusions. In *Ford*, there was no evidence of any kind introduced to show that the exclusion of all languages other than French was necessary to achieve the objective of protecting the French language and reflecting the reality of Quebec society. What evidence was introduced established, at most, that a marked preponderance for the French language in the "visage linguistique" was proportional to that objective. The court was prepared to allow a margin of appreciation to the government despite the fact that less intrusive measures, such as requiring equal prominence for the French language, were available. But there still had to be an evidentiary basis for concluding that the means chosen were proportional to the ends and impaired freedom of expression as little as possible. In *Ford*, that evidentiary basis did not exist.

iii) Deleterious Effects

There is no suggestion here that the effects of the ban are so severe as to outweigh the government's pressing and substantial objective. Advertisers are always free to direct their message at parents and other adults. They are also free to participate in educational advertising. The real concern animating the challenge to the legislation is that revenues are in some degree affected. This only implies that advertisers will have to develop new marketing strategies for children's products. Thus, there is no prospect that "because of the severity of the deleterious effects of [the] measure on individuals or groups, the measure will not be justified by the purposes it is intended to serve" (*Oakes*, at p. 228). The final component of the proponionality test is easily satisfied. In *Ford*, by contrast, the Attorney-General of Quebec underscored the importance of the "visage linguistique" for francophone identity and culture and yet the effect of the measure taken was to prohibit the public manifestation of the identity and culture of non-francophones.

1.5.3.2.2 *R. v. Keegstra*, [1990] 3 S.C.R. 697 (S.C.C.)

DICKSON, C.J. AND WILSON, L'HEUREUX-DUBÉ AND GONTHIER, JJ.: Section 319(2) of the *Code* constitutes a reasonable limit on freedom of expression. Parliament's objective of preventing the harm caused by hate propaganda is of sufficient importance to warrant overriding a constitutional freedom. Parliament has recognized the substantial harm that can flow from hate propaganda and, in trying to prevent the pain suffered by target group members and to reduce racial, ethnic and religious tension and perhaps even violence in Canada, has decided to suppress the willful promotion of hatred against identifiable groups. Parliament's objective is supported not only by the work of numerous study group, but also by our collective historical knowledge of the potentially catastrophic effects of the promotion of hatred. Additionally, the international commitment to eradicate hate propaganda and Canada's commitment to the values of equality and multiculturalism in ss. 15 and 27 of the Charter strongly buttress the importance of this objective.

Section 319(2) of the *Code* is an acceptably proportional response to Parliament's valid objective. There is obviously a rational connection between the criminal prohibition of hate propaganda and the objective of protecting target group members and of fostering harmonious social relations in a community dedicated to equality and multiculturalism. Section 319(2) serves to illustrate to the public the severe reprobation with which society holds messages of hate directed towards racial and religious groups. It makes that kind of expression less attractive and hence decrees acceptance of its content. Section 319(2) is also a means by which the values beneficial to a free and democratic society, in particular, the value of equality and the worth and dignity of each human person can be publicized.

Section 319(2) of the *Code* does not unduly impair freedom of expression. This section does not suffer from overbreadth or vagueness; rather, the terms of the offence indicate that s. 319(2) possesses definitional limits which act as safeguards to ensure that it will capture only expressive activity that is openly hostile to Parliament's objective, and will thus attack only the harm at which the prohibition is targeted. The word "willfully" imports into the offence a stringent standard of *mens rea* which significantly restricts the reach of s. 319(2) by necessitating the proof of either an intent to promote hatred or knowledge of the substantial certainty of such a consequence. The word "hatred" further reduces the scope of the prohibition. This word, in the context of s. 319(2), must be construed as encompassing only the most severe and deeply felt form of opprobrium Further, the exclusion of private communications from the scope of s. 319(2), the need for the promotion of hatred to focus upon an identifiable group and the presence of the s. 319(3) defences, which clarify the scope of s. 319(2), all support the view that the impugned section creates a narrowly confined offence. Section 319(2) is not an excessive impairment of freedom of expression merely because the defence of truth in s. 319(3)(a) does not cover negligent or innocent error as to the truthfulness of a statement. Whether or not a statement is susceptible to classification as true or false, such error should not excuse an accused who has willfully wed a statement in order to promote hatred against an identifiable group. That the legislative line is drawn so as to convict the accused who is negligent or even innocent regarding the accuracy of his statements is perfectly acceptable. Finally. while other non-criminal modes of combating hate propaganda exist, it is eminently reasonable to utilize more than one type of legislative tool in working to prevent the spread of racist expression and its resultant harm. To send out a strong message of condemnation both reinforcing the values underlying s. 319(2) and deterring the few individuals who would harm target group members and the larger community by communicating hate propaganda, will occasionally require use of the criminal law.

The effects of s.319(2) are not of such a deleterious nature as to outweigh any advantage gleaned from the limitation of s. 2(b). The expressive activity at which s. 319(2) is aimed constitutes a special category, a category only tenuously connected with the values underlying the guarantee of freedom of expression. Hate propaganda contributes little to the aspirations of Canadians or Canada in either the quest for truth, the promotion of individual self-development or the protection and fostering of a vibrant democracy where the participation of all individuals is accepted and encouraged. Moreover, the narrowly drawn terms of s. 319(2) and its defences prevent the prohibition of expression lying outside of this narrow category. Consequently, the suppression of hate propaganda represents an impairment of the individual's freedom of expression which is not of a most serious nature.

LA FOREST, SOPINKA AND McLACHLIN, JJ. (dissenting): Section 319(2) of the *Code* does not constitute a reasonable limit upon freedom of expression. While the legislative objectives of preventing the promotion of hatred, of avoiding racial violence and of promoting equality and multiculturalism are of sufficient importance to warrant overriding the guarantee of freedom of expression, s. 319(2) fails to meet the proportionality test.

Section 319(2) does, to some degree, further Parliament's objective. However, the rational connection between s. 319(2) and its goals is tenuous, as there is not a strong and evident connection between the criminalization of hate propaganda and its suppression. Section 319(2) may in fact detract from the objectives it is designed to promote by deterring legitimate expression. Law-abiding citizens, who do not wish to run afoul of the law, could decide not to take the chance in a doubtful case. Creativity and the beneficial exchange of ideas could be adversely affected. At the same time, it is unclear that s. 319(2) provides an effective way of curbing hatemongers. Not only does the criminal process attract extensive media coverage and confer on the accused publicity for his dubious causes, it may even bring him sympathy.

Section 319(2) of the *Code* does not interfere as little as possible with freedom of expression. Section 319(2) is drafted too broadly, catching more expressive conduct than can be justified by the objectives of promoting social harmony and individual dignity. The term "hatred" in s. 319(2) is capable of denoting a wide range of diverse emotions and is highly subjective, making it difficult to ensure that only cases meriting prosecution are pursued and that only those whose conduct is calculated to dissolve the social bonds of society are convicted. Despite the requirement of "willful promotion," people who make statements primarily for non-nefarious reasons may also be convicted under s. 319(2). A belief that what one says about a group is true and important to political and social debate is quite compatible with, and indeed may inspire, an intention to promote active dislike of that group. Such a belief is equally compatible with foreseeing that promotion of such dislike may stem from one's statements. The absence of any requirement that actual hum or incitement to hatred be shown further broadens the scope of s. 319(2), and it is unclear, in practice, if the s. 319(3) defences, including the defence of truth, significantly narrow the ambit of s. 319(2). Moreover, not only is the category of speech caught by s. 319(2) defined broadly, the application of the definition of offending speech, i.e., the circumstances in which the offending statements are prohibited, is virtually unlimited. Only private conversations are exempt from state scrutiny. Given the vagueness of the prohibition of expression in s.319(2), there is again a danger that the legislation may have a chilling effect on legitimate activities important to our society by subjecting innocent persons to constraints born out of a fear of the criminal process. Finally, the prohibition is effected through the criminal law which is the severest our society can impose and this is arguably unnecessary given the availability of alternate and more appropriate and effective remedies.

Any questionable benefit conferred by s. 319(2) of the *Code* is outweighed by the significant infringement on the guarantee of freedom of expression. Section 319(2) does not merely regulate the form or tone of expression, it strikes directly at its content. It is capable of catching not only statements like those at issue in this case, but works of art and the intemperate statement made in the heat of social controversy. While few may actually be prosecuted to conviction under s. 319(2) and imprisoned, many fall within the shadow of its broad prohibition. Section 319(2) touches on the vital values upon which s. 2(b) of the Charter rests: the value of fostering a vibrant and creative society through the marketplace of ideas; the value of the vigorous and open debate essential to democratic government and preservation of our rights and freedoms; and the value of a society that fosters the self-actualization and freedom of its members. An infringement of this seriousness can only be justified by a countervailing state interest of the most compelling nature. However, the claims of gains to be achieved at the cost of the infringement of free speech represented by s. 319(2) are tenuous. Indeed, it is difficult to see how s. 319(2) fosters the goals of social harmony and individual dignity.

1.6 Should Journalists Enjoy Special Legal Status?

This is a fundamental question and one we will return to throughout this book. The following material seeks to raise the question in a preliminary fashion.

1.6.1 *MacLeod et al. v. Canadian Armed Forces (Chief, Defence Staff)*, [1991] 1 F.C. 114 (F.C.T.D.)

JOYAL, J.: The issues raised in these applications were heard on September 26, 1990. By the time the proceedings had concluded, the issues had, in a sense, become moot. I was nevertheless asked to rule on them. I did so rule and delivered brief oral reasons. What follows are my more detailed written reasons for the disposition I made of the case. These reasons are written in the context of the circumstances as they existed at the date of hearing.

The Parties

The plaintiffs Ian MacLeod and Ann McLaughlin are journalists for the Ottawa Citizen and the Montreal Gazette respectively. The plaintiff Southam Inc. owns both newspapers. These plaintiffs apply for interlocutory relief on terms which will be explored later in these reasons.

Concurrently, the plaintiffs, of Canadian Civil Liberties Association and its counsel Alan Borovoy, apply for similar relief. The issues being the same and no objection being taken as to standing of the last-named plaintiffs, the two applications were heard together on common evidence.

The defendants, as their several titles imply, are senior commanders of the Canadian Armed Forces. The Attorney General of Canada is also named for good measure.

The Background

The applications arise as a result of events which have occurred at Mohawk Indian Reserves near Oka and Chateauguay, Quebec during the last three months. On July 11, 1990, the provincial police force, the Sûreté du Quebec, unsuccessfully tried to dismantle a barricade near Oka. The barricade had been erected by Mohawks in order to protest and to prevent the proposed development of a golf course by the Municipality of Oka on land to which the Mohawks claimed title. To maintain this barricade, self-defined armed Warriors joined the local Mohawk band. Eventually, the Province of Quebec called in the services of the Canadian Armed Forces to dismantle this barricade, as well as several other barricades which had been erected by the natives and Warriors at Oka and Chateauguay. The Canadian Armed Forces began to dismantle the barricades on August 27, 1990 and by September 3rd, they had gained control of the final Mohawk barricade at Oka. On that same date, some fifty Indians, including Warriors, men, women and children, retreated into a detoxification centre at the Kanesatake Reserve at Oka. The Canadian Armed Forces surrounded the centre and erected a razor wire perimeter. From that date on, there was a veritable standoff between the warriors and natives within the perimeter and the besieging Canadian Armed Forces. Women and children in the compound made it imperative that armed assault be avoided if at all possible. Several journalists, among them the plaintiffs MacLeod and McLaughlin, stayed at the treatment centre and eleven of them are still behind the perimeter with the Mohawks there. It is the situation of those journalists which forms the object of the present applications for interlocutory injunctions.

The Plaintiffs' Position

The policy of the Canadian Armed Forces has been to break the impasse and accordingly, security measures were taken to isolate the people within the compound and bring the siege to an end. Given the presence of women and children, however, the defendants allowed food and other essential supplies to pass through the perimeter, albeit in a controlled fashion. There were obvious humanitarian and compassionate grounds for that policy. According to the plaintiffs, up until September 11, 1990, the defendants allowed the delivery of food and supplies to the journalists directly and separately from the food and supplies which were being delivered to the natives inside the centre. However, on September 12th, the delivery of supplies, such as notepads, batteries, tape and film, was stopped. Then, on September 14, 1990, the defendants decided to halt *separate* delivery of food and other necessaries of life to the journalists inside the treatment centre. Instead, deliveries of food, clothing and other supplies were to be ordered in bulk by "hot line" and to be delivered once a day to the compound to be distributed among all of the occupants, including the journalists.

The plaintiffs argue that the defendants' refusal to permit separate delivery of food and supplies to the journalists inside the centre infringes upon the latter's right to freedom of expression and freedom of the press, as is guaranteed by section 2(b) of the *Canadian Charter of Rights and Freedoms*. Subsidiarily, the plaintiff Southam Inc. claims that the defendants' actions infringe the plaintiff's right to life, liberty and security of the person, as is guaranteed by section 7 of the Canadian Charter. More specifically, the plaintiffs argue that the journalists are being forced to rely upon the good will of the Warriors inside the compound with respect to the proper distribution of food. This reliance threatens their objectivity and independence in reporting on matters as they arise at Oka.

The plaintiffs also allege that the food being delivered is insufficient to feed the number of people there. As a result, the journalists are receiving only leftovers from the natives and their health is there being jeopardized. Furthermore, the Canadian Armed Forces have denied the plaintiffs access to the tools of their trade, so that it has become very difficult for the journalists to file their stories to their publishers. As a result, the plaintiffs believe that their basic freedoms and rights as guaranteed by the Charter are being infringed.

The Defendants' Position

The defendants argue that, whatever trials and tribulations might be visited on the journalists, the exigencies of the siege have nothing specifically to do with the presence of these journalists in the compound. The defendants' policy is to bring the standoff to an end and to leave no alternative to the Warriors and other natives but to evacuate the compound.

The defendants are fettered in achieving this purpose by the presence of women and children in the compound. To take by assault or storm would put these people at grave risk and would certainly be counter to the defendants' objective of resolving the conflict peacefully.

Furthermore, humanitarian and compassionate grounds preclude the defendants from simply starving the insurgents out. Again the presence of women and children, effectively controlled by armed Warriors, imposes this restriction on the defendants.

The defendants see no reason why the journalists in the compound should be treated differently from the natives. The journalists are there because it suits the Warriors' purpose to have them there. The journalists' conditions in terms of food and necessaries might be difficult to bear but if food is to be provided on humanitarian grounds, there is no reason why there should be special treatment for the journalists.

The defendants further state that since the adoption of stricter measures on September 11th and September 14th, the journalists have continued to file their stories to the media. It cannot therefore be argued that the actions of the defendants result in an embargo on news stories to the outside world giving rise to a Charter challenge.

The Issue

The issue, therefore, is whether the refusal of the defendants and of those under their control to allow separate delivery of food and other supplies to the journalists within the treatment centre, as well as their refusal to allow delivery of additional film, tape, batteries and other tools of the trade to these journalists, violates the freedom of the press as is guaranteed by section 2(b) of the *Canadian Charter of Rights and Freedoms*. The narrower issue is whether, in the light of all the circumstances of the case, an interlocutory injunction should issue at this time.

It is trite law that in order to succeed in their applications for an interlocutory injunction the plaintiffs must demonstrate that:

(a) there is a serious question to be tried;
(b) the plaintiffs will suffer irreparable harm unless the injunction is granted; and
(c) the balance of convenience favours the plaintiffs.

A final criterion. which was formulated by Lord Diploclc in *N.W.L. Ltd. v. Woods*, is that the issuance of the interlocutory injunction must not have the effect of finally disposing of the action before the trial takes place.

The Findings

On the basic facts and circumstances giving rise to these proceedings, there is no serious conflict in the evidence submitted by the parties. In making findings, therefore, it should not be necessary for me to refer to any specific piece of evidence or to attribute such evidence to any one of the several parties.

Admittedly, the role normally exercised by journalists is one which is fundamental to a free and democratic society. This is the role which the plaintiffs have voluntarily undertaken by maintaining their vigil in the compound and by continually filing their stories. In so doing, the plaintiffs are exercising their right to stay there in spite of the fact that as the critical standoff situation evolves at the compound, the conditions which they have to bear become increasingly onerous and difficult.

Yet these are conditions which are not the result of coercion, of imprisonment or of detention, lawful or otherwise. On the contrary, the defendants have repeatedly invited the journalists to leave the compound and have not hidden their displeasure at their continued presence there. In the context of the standoff itself, the Court would be loathe to express any views on the propriety or impropriety of the defendants' attitude towards these journalists. There is a limit to the kind of curial arrogance which might justify critical comment. I can only observe that the standoff has lasted 70 days and, so far, the measures taken by the defendants have not provoked serious violence.

Until September 11, 1990, both the natives and the plaintiffs were given access to necessaries of life. The plaintiffs were furnished with these necessaries directly by their employer. From that date onward, however, the defendants decreed that deliveries of food, clothing, medical supplies and other necessaries would be ordered on the "hot line" and delivered once a day to the compound to be shared by all the occupants, including the journalists.

The delivery of these necessaries is obviously a humanitarian gesture in regard to the women and children in the compound. Of necessity, however, that humanitarian gesture also ensures to the benefit of the armed Warriors, and unless the plaintiffs be treated with less than minimum hospitality, to the benefit of the plaintiffs as well. The plaintiffs concede that at all times their presence in the compound is on sufferance. They are there only so long as the Warriors want them there and only so long as the Warriors find the presence of the journalists to be to their advantage. The Warriors, in my view, are not suffering the plaintiffs' presence in the centre on the ground that by doing otherwise, they would violate section 2(b) of the Charter.

It is clear that the defendants' policy is to treat the journalists, the Warriors and the women and children indiscriminately with respect to the supply of food and necessaries. As the plaintiffs state, they are not now getting their fair share of necessaries and are denied the technical supplies required of their trade. This, they suggest, amounts to an oblique or indirect method of stifling access to information from the compound and is tantamount to an actual prohibition by the defendants of the coverage of events occurring at Oka and as such constitutes a denial of Charter rights.

The question may now be expressed as to whether or not the policy imposed by the defendants on the plaintiffs raises a triable issue justifying the intervention of the Court by way of interlocutory relief at this stage of the proceedings. In assisting in such determination, consideration must of necessity be given to some judicial pronouncements dealing with such fundamental principles of Canadian law as freedom of the press and freedom of information.

The Law

In *Re Canadian Newspaper Co. and Isaac*, a coroner allowed a witness to testify at an inquest anonymously. Canadian Newspaper Co. brought an application for a declaration that the coroner's order violated section 2(b) of the Canadian Charter and to require disclosure of the name of the witness. Mr. Justice Campbell decided that there was some basis in law on which the coroner could have made the order and that no public interest would be served by requiring that the name of the witness be published. With respect to the rights of the press, he stated:

> The right of the press under Charter s. 2(b) is no greater than the right of the public to know what goes on in the courts and in public hearings such as inquests.
> ... The right to publish what has already been compelled and disclosed is different from the right to compel a disclosure that has not been made to the trier of fact. The Charter does not give the press or the public the right to insist that the coroner compel into evidence any fact. The press has a right to report the inquest, not to control its conduct.

I conclude therefore that there has been no infringement of the Charter guarantee of freedom of the press.

Although Mr. Justice Hughes and Mr. Justice Austin did not agree that the coroner's order could be justified in law, they too felt that the application should be dismissed on the ground that to require disclosure of the name of the witness, after he had acted upon the promise of anonymity, would bring the administration of justice into disrepute.

In that decision, therefore, the press was held to have no greater right than other members of the public to compel disclosure of information.

Counsel for the defendants also brought to my attention two decisions of the United States Supreme Court which more clearly illustrate the principle that the press is to be treated on an equal footing with other members of the public in general.

The first of those cases is *Pell v. Procunier*, where prison inmates and journalists challenged the constitutionality of a prison regulation prohibiting face-to-face interviews with inmates specifically chosen by the media. It also prohibited interviews which an inmate initiated himself. The majority of the Supreme Court held that the regulation did not violate either the inmates' First Amendment rights or the right of the media to freedom of the press.

Justice Stewart, on behalf of the majority of the Court, cited from an earlier Supreme Court decision, *Branzburg v. Hayes*, which had indicated that the press did not have a constitutional right of special access to information not available to the general public and that:

> Newsmen have no constitutional right of access to the scenes of crime or disaster when the general public is excluded.

The learned Justice then applied that principle to the facts before him:

> The First and Fourteenth Amendments bar government from interfering in any way with a free press. *The Constitution does not, however, require government to accord the press special access to information not shared by members of the public generally.* It is one thing to say that a journalist is free to seek out sources of information not available to members of the general public, that he is entitled to some constitutional protection of the confidentiality of such sources, cf. Branzburg v. Hayes, and that government cannot restrain the publication of news emanating from such sources. Cf. New York Times Co. c. United States. *It is quite another thing to suggest that the Constitution imposes upon government the affirmative duty to make available to journalist's sources of information not available to members of the public generally. That proposition finds no support in the words of the Constitution or in any decision of this Court.* Accordingly, since S. 415.0771 does not deny the press access to sources of information available to members of the general public, we hold that it does not abridge the protections that the First and Fourteenth Amendments guarantee.

The issue was much the same in *Saxbe v. Washington Post Co.*, where a Policy Statement prohibited face-to-face interviews by newsmen with individually designated prison inmates. Mr. Justice Stewart, again speaking for a majority of the Court, first noted that the inmates' families, attorneys and religious counsel were accorded liberal visitation privileges; members of the public at large were not allowed to enter prisons and interview consenting inmates. This policy was applied evenly to all prospective visitors, including journalists. Applying the decision in Pell he concluded that it was:

... unnecessary to engage in any delicate balancing of such penal considerations against the legitimate demands of the First Amendment. For it is apparent that the sole limitation imposed on news gathering by Policy Statement 1220.1 A is no more than particularized application of the general rule that nobody may enter the prison and designate an inmate whom he would like to visit, unless the prospective visitor is a lawyer, clergyman, relative, or friend of that inmate. This limitation on visitations is justified by what the Court of Appeals acknowledged as 'the truism that prisons are institutions where public access is generally limited,' 161 U.S. App. D.C., at 80, 494 F.2d, at 999. *In this regard, the Bureau of Prisons visitation policy does not place the press in any less advantageous position than the public generally.* Indeed, the total access to federal prisons and prison inmates that the Bureau of Prisons accords to the press far surpasses that available to other members of the public.

Mr. Justice Stewart then quoted from *Pell* to the effect that the government has no affirmative duty to make available to journalists sources of information not available to members of the general public. Accordingly, the Policy Statement did not abridge the freedom of the press guaranteed by the First Amendment.

Although U.S. authorities are not determinative whenever dealing with a Charter issue, they have often been quoted whenever there is an absence of Canadian judicial precedents on point. In essence, the cases I have cited deny the existence of special status to journalists on constitutional grounds. No express stipulation is found in American law which would directly or by inference confer such a stalus on them. Neither do find any under the Charter. On the contrary, the decision of the Ontario Divisional Court in *Re Canadian Newspaper Co. and Isaac* is confirmative, in my view, that journalists have no more right to information, or to disclosure or even to access to information than the ordinary citizen.

The Conclusion

If journalists are to be treated as ordinary citizens and if they enjoy no special status to obtain information denied to others, it would follow, in my view, that under conditions of siege and in a compound defended by armed Warriors who effectively control the journalists' conduct, their status would not impose on the defendants a special affirmative duty of care in a manner the plaintiffs have claimed. The defendants have not forced the plaintiffs to enter into or to remain in the compound. Nor have the defendants, by threats or otherwise, stopped them from leaving. On the contrary, they have urged the plaintiffs to leave. Irrespective of journalistic duties or ethics, the plaintiffs are remaining on the scene voluntarily and their liberty to leave the compound at any time is no more restricted than the liberty of anyone else, women, children and armed Warriors alike, from leaving the compound.

In such circumstances, it is my view that the principle applied in both U.S. and Canadian jurisprudence is applicable to the issue before me. Freedom of the press as a concept does not confer any special status on media people. Should a journalist in quest of news put himself in a dangerous situation he has no greater right to protection than his neighbour. If he should decide to file stories "Behind

Warrior Lines" as the plaintiff MacLeod so headnoted his articles in the *Ottawa Citizen*, it does not create a concomitant duty to people in front of the same lines to provide him with special treatment. If a journalist, in the centre of an armed confrontation, feels it his professional duty to remain there, he cannot impose on any person, an obligation to do all that would be necessary to keep him there. If a journalist freely and voluntarily hazards the security of his person to fulfill his functions, I know of no principle of law granting him immunity from the consequences of his conduct. Finally, if as stated in *Branzburg v. Hayes* a journalist has no constitutional right of access to scenes of crime or disaster when the general public is excluded, I should fail to see how he might gain constitutional prolection when he voluntarily remains in a compound under siege.

I should not venture any further than is necessary along this line of thinking. I am not called upon today to decide the merits of the case but rather to ascertain if the plaintiffs present a serious question to be tried and, if so, whether injunctive orders at this stage are warranted.

I must conclude that on the evidence before me, and on the state of the law made available to me, the plaintiffs have failed to show me that on the basis of a Charter right to freedom of the press, the defendants thereby owe a special duty of care towards the plaintiffs. I cannot accept they should enjoy immunity or other special status. They cannot expect nor do they have a right to receive special treatment except at the invitation of whomsoever, like the Warriors, might be enjoying or tolerating their presence.

It is true that journalists in the compound did enjoy some semblance of privilege in having their needs filled separately by their employer and having deliveries accepted separately through checkpoints. In my view, that kind of privilege does not make a right which should now be encapsulated within the right conferred on paragraph 2(b) of the Charter in particular or within the rights and freedoms conferred on the Charter generally.

In any event, the evidence discloses that since September 11, information has been continually fed by the journalists to their newspapers for the purpose of fulfilling the purported insatiable need of the public for information on the current crisis. It is admired of course that the policy adopted by the defendants makes that purpose more difficult to maintain. Such difficulties, however, are inherent in the circumstances which have developed at Oka. To subscribe to the defendants' policy the characteristics of a violation such as I have been invited to find would go far beyond the purpose and object of that particular Charter right.

Touching briefly upon the evidence of the plaintiffs that the current system of food allocation is such as to create shortages of food to individual journalists, I can only observe that this is a matter more properly addressed to the Warriors than to the defendants. in closing, I would only refer to the remarks of Mr. Justice Beetz in *A.G. Manitoba v. Metropolitan Stores Ltd.*:

> "In short, I conclude that in a case where the authority of a law enforcement agency is constitutionally challenged, no interlocutory injunction or stay should issue to restrain that

authority from performing its duties to the public unless, in the balance of convenience, the public interest is taken into consideration and given the weight it should carry. Such is the rule where the case against the authority of the law enforcement agency is serious for if it were not, the question of granting interlocutory relief should not even arise. But that is the rule also even when there is the rule also even when there is a *prima facie* case against the enforcement agency, such as one which would require the coming into play of s. 1 of the *Canadian Charter of Rights and Freedoms.*"

If such is the case when an applicant has succeeded in demonstrating a *prima facie* case, then a *fortiori* this Court should be even more loathe to intervene in the exercise of government policy of this nature when an applicant has been unable to make out a serious case.

The journalists in the compound might be deserving of admiration and respect for the fortitude they have shown during a long siege. Nevertheless, on the basis of the facts and the law put before me, the plaintiffs have not made out a serious issue to be tried and the applications for injunctive relief are hereby dismissed.

This is not a matter for costs.

1.6.2 Stephen Bindman, "Court Rulings Tightening Muzzle on Media," *The London Free Press*, 13 March 1993, p. E5

OTTAWA — Freedom of the press in Canada is under attack.

A spate of disturbing recent legal developments — court rulings, new bureaucratic rules and a proposed new gag law — threaten the ability of journalists to do their jobs.

The guarantee of freedom of the press in the *Charter of Rights and Freedoms*, far from improving the journalistic lot, may have actually given judges and bureaucrats a new tool to muzzle the free flow of information.

Consider these developments:

Gag Orders: Judges have been granting injunctions blocking television broadcasts or the publication of stories in recent months with increasing regularity. Although such gag orders are supposed to be rare, there have been a number of high-profile cases in recent months

In December, the CBC was prohibited from airing the acclaimed TV mini-series, "The Boys Of St. Vincent", in large parts of Central Canada. The fictitious series, which chronicled sexual and physical abuse of boys at a Newfoundland Catholic orphanage, was banned in Ontario and parts of Quebec after the Ontario court of appeal ruled the film could prejudice the criminal trials of four Christian Brothers. The network is seeking to appeal to the Supreme Court of Canada.

The CBC was also prevented from broadcasting the videotaped testimony of a one-time blood donor alleged to have transmitted the AIDS virus. The man's evidence was made for use in a lawsuit by a woman who claims she contracted AIDS from a blood transfusion, but an Ontario judge ruled the testimony could only be used for the trial later this year. The CBC did not fight the gag.

A British Columbia judge banned the *Financial Times* of Canada from publishing information obtained from a court registry file dealing with a dispute over the division of property after the breakup of an industrialist's marriage. Under B.C. court rules, such information is supposed to be inaccessible to the public. Another judge later overturned the injunction.

During the referendum campaign, one of Quebec Premier Robert Bourassa's top advisers obtained an injunction preventing the news media from publishing details of an eavesdropped cellular phone conversation in which she accuses the premier of "caving in" during the negotiations.

The injunction was lifted after the transcripts were published by several newspapers outside Quebec and were well-circulated in the province by fax machine.

A Montreal weekly, *Voir*, was ordered to stop publishing any further articles on a marketing company and its business practice. The company is suing the newspaper.

Tape Seizures: Despite a 1991 Supreme court ruling—or because of it — police forces have been turning more often to journalists as a tool in criminal investigations.

In February, the RCMP seized CBC videotapes which had sparked an investigation into allegations that residents of a southern Alberta treatment facility for autistic adults were abused by staff members The Mounties seized both aired and unaired material. The network is challenging, the search warrant.

Following a May, 1992, windowsmashing riot along downtown Yonge Street, Toronto police seized hundreds of rolls of film and videotape from nine media outlets. A judge later upheld the seizure.

Canadian National Railways is seeking a court order to obtain footage shot by an independent film-maker of events leading up to a railway blockade by an Indian band in B.C. CN wants the tape for a civil suit against the Gitwangak band.

Toronto lawyer Paul Schabas recently wrote that the Supreme Court ruling — which said newsrooms were not immune from searches, but suggested police seek other sources first—means the press can now "be used quite freely by the police and others to help serve their investigative needs and to fill in any gaps."

Court Exhibits: Two provinces, relying erroneously on another top-court ruling, have imposed new restrictions on public and media access to court exhibits.

In Saskatchewan, new rules state that access to exhibits and even court transcripts, while a public right before, during and after a trial, is subject to ensuring witnesses, those found not guilty, "or those vulnerable to the court process, do not have their privacy rights violated or find themselves subject to harassment."

In case of doubt, the reporter will have to file a written request explaining the reason for seeking the court record and for what purpose it will be used. A judge will have the final say.

In Ontario, reporters will now need a judge's permission to see criminal court exhibits and will have to file a written request explaining what the information will be used for.

TV Cameras: The Supreme Court has ruled provincial and federal legislatures have the constitutional right to ban television cameras from their chambers.

Although most provincial legislatures now have some form of television coverage, the ruling means provinces will be allowed to change the rules at will, without having to consult with the media and without considering the charter's free-press guarantee.

Ontario's top court has also upheld a provincial law which prohibits filming or photographing people entering or leaving courtrooms.

The court of appeal, in a 3-2 ruling, said the no-cameras rule was necessary to preserve the "calm, dignified atmosphere" of courthouses. The case will likely be appealed to the Supreme Court.

Cellular Phones: A bill now before Parliament would make it a crime punishable by up to two years in prison and a $5,000 fine to disclose to anyone even the existence of a cellular phone conversation. It would also be a crime to use or disclose the contents of such a conversation without the consent of one of the parties.

It would also be against the law to intercept a cellular call "maliciously or for gain" without the consent of one of the parties. It is unclear whether journalists who intercept a call using a legal scanner are included in the definition of "for gain,"; although clearly it would be against the Criminal Code to use the information in a story, no matter how important.

The bill, introduced by former justice minister Kim Campbell, has not yet been given second reading in the Commons.

"What the bill does is suppress information using a highly intrusive and sweeping gag law," *Lawyers Weekly* Ottawa correspondent Cristin Schmitz wrote in a recent analysis. "Journalists and all citizens would be vulnerable to prosecution for activities which have never been considered to be immoral or unethical."

Note: Stephen Bindman is a former President of the Canadian Association of Journalists and an employee of the Southam Corporation.

1.6.3 A Note on Litigation and Journalism

The Southam company, as well as some of the individual newspapers, in particular the Edmonton *Journal* and the Ottawa *Citizen*, which are part of the Southam chain, has been very active in using the Charter in litigation. The ostensible purpose of this litigation has been to remove what were perceived as legal fetters on the ability of journalists to do their work. Many of the results of that litigation can be found in this Sourcebook. (See items 1.6.1, 3.2.1 and 3.3.4.5.) Southam has challenged limits on the access of reporters to various judicial proceedings, to Senate committee hearings, and to RCMP disciplinary tribunals. It has argued that reporters should be privileged to the extent of not being required to reveal information about sources to courts or tribunals. Is has attempted to use the Charter as a means of placing the law of civil libel on a constitutional footing. Some of this litigation has been successful; much of it has not. Southam has obviously spent a substantial amount of money on bringing Charter-based claims before the courts.

By the end of 1990 a certain disenchantment had begun to set in and Southam was re-thinking its position. It appears the corporation has decided to be more selective about the issues it actually takes to court. Furthermore. there is a sense that, since any legal victory won by Southam presumably benefits everyone in the Canadian media, it should not have to cover all the expenses involved.

More important is the question whether this is a sensible way to use the funds of a media corporation. Does spending money on litigation produce better journalism? Would it make more sense to eschew litigation and use the money saved to hire more reporters and provide them with better resources?

1.7 Two Essays on the Freedom of the Press

1.7.1 G. Stuart Adam, "The Charter and the Role of the Media: A Journalist's Perspective," in *The Media, the Courts and the Charter*, eds. Philip Anisman and Allen M. Linden (Toronto: Carswell, 1986)

> *Give me the liberty to know, to utter, and to argue freely according to conscience above all liberties.*
>
> John Milton, *Areopagitica**

1. Introduction

Generations of journalists have been told — some fewer may have learned through study — that John Milton's defence of liberty of the press is the best and most persuasive document on the subject in the English language. The reputation of that short pamphlet, published in 1644 in the hope that England's Long Parliament would rescind its *Licensing Act*, is deserved. A modern reader can only be impressed by Milton's powers of logic and argument, his vision, his mastery of the language and his self-confidence. These qualities combine in the pamphlet to produce a remarkable example of intellectual craftsmanship. It may not have been the first time that a writer asked for the liberties to know, to publish without prior restraint, and to express opinions freely, but it is certainly the standing point for any modern discussion in English of the sources of and the meaning we give to the cluster of liberties which provide a backdrop to that great democratic phrase, "freedom of the press".

Canada's law now recognizes these liberties and, in a manner of speaking, has turned them into rights. In fact, the *Charter of Rights and Freedoms* which was annexed to the Constitution in 1982 goes further than to say they are ordinary rights. It declares significantly and solemnly in section 2(b) of the "supreme law" of Canada that freedom of thought, belief, opinion and expression, "including freedom of the press and other media of communication" are fundamental freedoms.[1]

The legal consequences of this powerful declaration will no doubt be manifold, but the most basic and important consequence will surely be (or ought to be) that when the press's freedom is at issue, a presumption arising out of the law will favour unimpeded freedom. The system of free expression will expand and cases for limiting that freedom will be recognized only when the goals are both narrowly and sharply defined. If the legal consequences are not these, then we will have failed to understand properly what Milton and other writers on intellectual freedom have taught us. We will have used the Charter for mischief rather than for freedom — at least that is the sense of this paper's argument.

We will also have failed to appreciate the extent to which the exercise of these rights, more often by journalists, writers and broadcasting producers than by other citizens, provides a foundation for democratic society. A theme explored later in the text suggests that the principal function of journalism and journalists is to connect citizens to one another and to their major social and political institutions. If this view of journalism is accepted, then the exercise by journalists of these fundamental rights of expression should be seen as an important source of a process which, in a manner of speaking, is the *sine qua non* of democratic life.

It should be noted at the outset, then, that journalists see themselves as specially associated with the exercise and defence of these rights. One could say that a journalist has a professional stake, as well as a citizen's interest, in the manner in which the Charter is interpreted. Accordingly, I propose to analyze some of the documents in which the idea of intellectual freedom was initially expounded and to show that an important part of the social and political vision Milton and others presented is still valid and provides a basis for the meaning we should give to the Charter.

The order of business is as follows. I shall make some preliminary observations about the nature of freedom and the role of journalism. I shall then analyze Milton's essay and relate its central features to subsequent developments in democratic theory. Thirdly, I shall provide examples of pre-Charter judgments in Canadian law which, I think, can usefully guide the interpretation of section 2(b). In the process I shall attempt to demonstrate the importance of intellectual freedom to journalists and their work and thereby illustrate the relationship between the Charter and the role of the media.

2. Preliminary Observations

It is useful to note as a preliminary matter that Milton's use of the term, "liberty," is not entirely accidental. The idea of freedom reflected in our constitutional and intellectual history has emphasized liberties over rights. Very generally, liberties have been secured in the face of parliamentary authority; rights are within the domain of the courts. In other words, pre-Charter parliamentarians were traditionally expected to safeguard the liberties of citizens to speak freely, to assemble or to vote, but they retained a power in principle to alter or modify the manner in which those liberties were expressed in law. By contrast, the notion of rights is more legal than political. It is now up to the courts as much as the legislatures to define and safeguard the freedoms of expression. The impact of this distinction may be emphasized unduly, but it should be recognized that in general terms the power of the parliamentarians has been diminished by the Charter and the arguments for liberties have become arguments for rights.[2]

It is also important to recognize that the freedom that is generally claimed for journalists is or ought to be as connected to notions of democratic responsibility as to notions of natural right. In fact, the idea of freedom is no more important to the operations and idea of democracy than the values, although they may differ in important ways, which promote individual and collective responsibility. It is arguable, for example, that the idea of freedom, sacred as it might be, is itself dependent on the force and breadth of an "empirical" tradition in our popular culture. (Although science provides a more familiar context for "empiricism," I am using the concept here to suggest a popular rendering that the English editor, C.P. Scott, might have had in mind when he said, "comment is free, but facts are sacred".)[3] In this respect, the freedom we celebrate makes sense when the notion of empiricism permeates the popular culture and is expressed in journalism itself.

This is not to say that freedom need always be justified with reference to the attachment most people have to facts and inductive methods of reasoning,[4] but rather that empirical standards are recognized as primary in the adjudication of ideas and in the maintenance of the social and political order. Freedom of expression, in this light, is relied upon to produce forms of truth. Democracy extends the forum within which judgment occurs.

The idea of empiricism can be linked, despite prevailing academic fashions,[5] to the role of journalism and the media generally. To the extent that journalism is orchestrated by an empirical tradition, the media circulate facts which can be discussed in the light of different values. Put a little differently, the media are as important for the facts they circulate as they are for the values they promote.

Acceptance of this view of the role of the media should make it easier to live with the freedom claimed for it, but only if one is free of nostalgia or utopianism. The media constitute a system in a complex society and that system hovers over ordinary lives just as political, judicial and commercial institutions do. The media's achievement is to democratize society, not to perfect it as Milton's ideas on liberty might encourage us to believe. Nevertheless, there is an important thread of understanding that comes from Milton which, with patience, can be connected to the manner in which we structure modern communications.

3. Milton's Liberty

There is a strong possibility that John Milton would have been unenthusiastic about the Charter. He was opposed to the codification of virtue or of value if it meant endangering genuine understanding. A primary aim of Milton was to ensure that purity and wisdom came from individual acts of understanding rather than from obedience and habit. In Milton's eyes, our new document might put understanding at risk.[6] He observed:

> [O]ur faith and knowledge thrives by exercise ... Truth is ... a streaming fountain; if her waters flow not in perpetual progression, they sicken into a muddy pool of conformity and tradition. A man may be a heretic in the truth; and if he believe things only because his pastor says so, or the Assembly so determines, without knowing other reason, though his belief be true, yet the very truth he holds is heresy.[7]

While Milton might have had reservations about the Charter of Rights, it is certain that modern liberals continue to have difficulty swallowing some of the things he had to say, for, not surprisingly, Reformation theology and politics dominated his language and thinking. There is also every chance that modern conservatives would object to his reckless use of the divine to defend something so manifestly earthbound as the press. As will be seen, Milton linked without embarrassment human thought and behaviour to divine purpose. He was writing about God's plan. While such convictions might offend modern readers, it should be recalled that they would have been easy for a seventeenth-century reader to accept. *Areopagitica* was published when the competition for souls amongst the wings of the Christian church was at its height and religious ideas were universally, although not uniformly, affirmed.

Still, there is much that is left after the Protestant dogmatism. The starting point for an understanding of *Areopagitica* is the frame of reference that Milton and other serious advocates of freedom have adopted. It is clear that he was not arguing for a system of free expression without limits. Milton was opposed to a licensing system that empowered 20 censors to examine and approve publications for circulation. His most important short-run goal was to convince parliamentarians of the day that a board of censorship was incompatible with the welfare of a nation of free men. At the same time, he forthrightly approved of the application of the law after publication to material which was seditious or blasphemous. He said, for example, that he denied not "but that it is of greatest concernment in the church and commonwealth, to have a vigilant eye how books demean themselves as well as men; and thereafter to confine, imprison, and do sharpest justice on them as malefactors."[8] And drawing on his classical scholarship to illustrate his ideas, he observed that in ancient Athens the magistrates were concerned with two kinds of writings, "those either blasphemous and atheistical, or libellous."[9]

Although the scope of sedition and blasphemy were only partially developed in his text, it is clear that Milton was hoping for a strong measure of wisdom and restraint in their application. In this respect he said, "but here the great art lies, to discern in what the law is to bid restraint and punishment and in what things persuasion only is to work."[10] Thus Milton's ideas of freedom include a structure or a frame of reference in which laws continue to operate even if censorship boards do not. Unhappily, there was a deep vein of intolerance running through his pamphlet as religious values were considered in relation to the laws. But there was nevertheless an incipient trust in the power of persuasion as a substitute for the use of the law and a belief that the law should be used for limited purposes.

In this latter respect Milton's pamphlet on freedom can be compared to all great liberal essays on the subject. The freedom that is so vigorously justified presumes the existence and persistence of law, but a law deprived of the power of prior restraint. The purposes to which law may be applied after publication are the questions to which legislators and philosophers have returned and about which we continue to fight. Happily, Milton's arguments are of assistance in this latter combat, for they can be used not only to demolish the practice of censorship, but also to justify shrinking the power of the law. To understand how requires a deeper interrogation of his text.

The first quarter of *Areopagitica* contains an attack on the Church of Rome for its alleged role in developing the idea of censorship and indexing. Despite the obvious energy Milton put into this part of his presentation, he was wise enough to recognize that his historical reflections did not in themselves provide a reason for rejecting censorship. As he wrote, "some will say, that though the inventors were bad, the thing for all that may be good."[11] The sense of his position was simply that a good Protestant would be wise to look skeptically upon any "fruit" of the Church of Rome.[12] He was suggesting a prudential skepticism and, further, that the return to licensing was a betrayal of the Reformation. But at the same time he admitted that the rules of good argument forced him to make the case on its merits. It is in the balance of his text that Milton showed his real strength and developed the ideas which moderns can more safely consider.

After disposing of the Church of Rome, Milton presented three interwoven, but distinctive, sets of claims. The first concerned essentially practical questions bearing on the effectiveness of licensing. The second and third addressed the evil effects of licensing measured against Reformation notions of rationality and virtue.

Milton said that licensing "conduces nothing to the end for which it was framed."[13] It does not put a stop to seditious or blasphemous writing. Those who want to take the risks and circulate their material will do so regardless of the licenser. "Do we not see, not once or oftener, but weekly — that continued Court libel against the Parliament and City . . . dispersed among us, for all licensing can do?"[14] In any event schismatical ideas do not need to be circulated through the press; they may be passed on mouth-to-mouth and a licenser is impotent to stop them. Moreover licensing actually leads to a result opposite to the one intended. Milton argued that forbidding certain ideas from being circulated gives them a significance they would not otherwise possess: "instead of suppressing sects and schisms, it raises them and invests them with a reputation."[15]

He added parenthetically that if censorship was intended to cultivate manners and virtue in English society, it would only be consistent to regulate other activities in the same manner. In a mocking tone, he wrote:

> If we think to regulate printing, thereby to rectify manners, we must regulate all recreations and pastimes, all that is delightful to man. No music must be heard, no song be set or sung, but what is grave and Doric.. . . . Who shall be the rectors of daily rioting? And what shall be done to inhibit the multitude that frequent those houses where drunkenness is sold and harbored?[16]

Finally, Milton declared that if the licensing system was to be used to cultivate manners and improve thought, its effectiveness would be dependent on the quality of the licenser. He put the case this way: If a licensing system is to improve society, then it is important that the licenser be "above the common measure, both studious, learned and judicious."[17] But how could it be so, Milton asked. The work is tedious, "an unpleasing journey-work" which could have only one result, namely, that the licenser would be "either ignorant, imperious and remiss, or basely pecuniary."[18]

In short, there was a compelling case, based primarily on practical considerations, for putting licensing aside. But the real force of Milton's argument derived from his exposition of the conditions that ought to circumscribe moral and rational life. In this respect, he put aside the part of his argument based on the inability of the scheme to achieve its goals and emphasized the positive evils it would cause. The essence of his argument was that licensing is destructive of reason and virtue, the two qualities men of God and justice should be interested in cultivating.

At the core of this and several collateral claims were utterly individualistic and rationalistic images of man and mind. Milton said that individuals are capable of investigating and arriving at the nature of truth unaided by priests or politicians and an enlightened society is one which takes the faculty of reason and gives it a life in individuals. Not to do so is an "undervaluing and vilifying of the whole nation."[19]

> [T]o distrust the judgment and the honesty of one who hath but a common repute in learning and never yet offended, as not to count him fit to print his mind without a tutor and examiner, lest he should drop a schism, or something of corruption, is the greatest displeasure and indignity to a free and knowing spirit that can be put upon him.[20]

But granting freedom to such individuals was not merely a matter of recognizing and allowing for the conditions of human dignity. There was a theological and, one could say, utilitarian justification as well. According to Milton, the intellectual power possessed by an individual, however modest, was almost literally a fragment of the divine. The God of Milton's imagination was a God of Reason and the venue of this reason was man's mind. Thus, to discourage independent thought through licensing was to deprive society of Reason itself. He wrote, who kills a man kills a reasonable creature, God's image; but he who destroys a good book, kills reason itself, kills the image of God, as it were, in the eye ... a good book is the precious lifeblood of a master spirit, embalmed and treasured up on purpose to a life beyond.[21]

Although he enshrined reason in the minds of independent men, Milton did not at the same time overlook evil and irrationality. Falsehood and vice were in man's mind just as truth and virtue were. But his faith was such that the growth of rationality and virtue could only occur in the face of falsehood and evil. He did not believe, for example, that a "cloistered virtue" or a virtue proceeding from obedience were virtues at all. Virtue could only come into being when it was enacted independently by individuals who could also choose to do evil. Thus, the dominion of rationality and virtue, a dominion that was guaranteed in faith, would only come about through the interplay of opposing forces in the marketplace of ideas.

The marketplace concept was implied early in the *Areopagitica* in a passage declaring that "all opinions, yea errors, known, read or collated, are of main service and assistance toward the speedy attainment of what is truest."[22] Much later in the text, it received fuller treatment:

And though all the winds of doctrine were let loose to play upon the earth, so Truth be in the field, we do injuriously by licensing and prohibiting to misdoubt her strength. Let her and Falsehood grapple; who ever knew Truth put to the worse, in a free and open encounter? Her confuting is the best and surest suppressing.[23]

It made no difference to the principle that reason and virtue were distinct concepts. Where good and evil were the entangled elements, the marketplace operated in much the same way:

Good and evil we know in the field of this world grow up together almost inseparably; and the knowledge of good is so involved and interwoven with the knowledge of evil; and in so many cunning resemblances hardly to be discerned, that those confused seeds which were imposed upon Psyche as an incessant labor to cull out and sort asunder, were not more intermixed.[24]

He concluded this last passage with the question "what wisdom can there be to choose what continence to forbear without the knowledge of evil?"[25]

Milton went further in the substance of the argument and rhetoric of persuasion. He wrote prophetically, convinced that he possessed direct knowledge of God's will. He claimed, for example, "God is decreeing to begin some new and great period in his church, even to the reforming of reformation itself."[26] But all the arguments, based on the theology and philosophy of his brand of low-church Protestantism led inevitably to the claim he laid out in the opening passages of the text, namely, that licensing "would be primely to the discouragement of all learning and the stop of truth, not only by disexercising and blunting our abilities in what we know already, but by hindering and cropping the discovery that might be yet further made, both in religious and civil wisdom."[27]

The cadence to the argument resonates in the mind of every good liberal as does his conclusion: "Give me liberty to know, to utter and to argue freely according to conscience, above all liberties."[28]

4. Milton's Successors: The Mills

Milton's legacy is comprised partly of his arguments and partly of his blueprint for social and political organization. The arguments can be resurrected when the state or a school board suggests that movies or literature or magazines are dangerous. We are likely to say under such circumstances that censorship or harsh laws are administered by fools, that bad causes are given publicity when the law is applied carelessly to them or that undesirable material and habits of mind are only driven underground when censored. In our more optimistic moods we might also link social and intellectual progress to the rights we exercise as free individuals. Many of us still believe that an open and free system of expression is likely to produce a more humane future and that a system of expression which allows for the circulation only of "good" ideas is hardly free. But it is harder for us to forge the links that were evident to Milton and his intellectual descendants. Imperialism, the wars, sociology and Freud have taken their toll.

But despite the difficulty of uncritical acceptance of such beliefs, we do recognize the importance and centrality of our individuality and if the rights we claim for ourselves are less easily linked to a progressive and benign future, they at least represent our certainty that it is not for the state to tell us what and how to think. Accordingly, the second part of Milton's legacy emphasizes our individuality and the role reason plays in our lives and the life of society. We can say, therefore, that he helped to make it inevitable that later writers would argue that the state should be small or limited in its power to supervise and monitor matters of the mind.

As it turned out the blueprint for linking the individual to a limited state was the achievement of writers who wrote under his influence through the eighteenth and into the nineteenth century. Among the writers who came late in the day were James Mill and his son, John Stuart. James Mill's writing on the press is an especially important example of the impulse of this radical liberal tradition which looked suspiciously on the power of the state. It could be said that he and Bentham anticipated the Orwellian nightmare in which the state supervises all thought. Thus, they tried to ensure that the state had practically no power of legal control over language. I say practically "no power" because it is limited power they would confer. It is important to recall that they also bear the marks of the other side of this tradition, namely, that the law is still a necessary device and that the exercise of free speech and free press, although it should occur in the widest possible arena, should still be circumscribed by some legal limitations.

Once again, how much law and with what effect would remain a matter of debate. But the presumptions that arise in the wake of the notion of the sovereign individual are clear. One is that the individual is a citizen, a kind of minigovernor; the other is that the state cannot use its power to usurp his "citizenship".

In the domain of politics, the organizational elements were put directly by James Mill:

> The point of greatest importance to [governments] is, to keep the people at large from complaining, or from knowing or thinking that they have any ground of complaint. If this object is fully attained, they may then, without anxiety, and without trouble, riot in the pleasures of misrule.[29]

In his view the method of preventing governors from "rioting in the pleasures of misrule" was to install a system of reporting and commenting on the activities of government with the rights to report and comment limited by a very restricted concept of seditious libel and by the law of civil defamation. The rest would be free territory.

> The end which is sought ... by allowing anything to be said in censure of the government, is, to ensure the goodness of the government.... If the goodness of government could be ensured by any preferable means, it is evident that all censure of the government ought to be prohibited. All discontent with the government is only good, in so far as it is a means of removing real cause of discontent....
>
> So true it is, however, that the discontent of the people is the only means of removing the defects of vicious governments, that the freedom of the press, the main instrument of creating discontent, is, in all civilized countries, among all but the advocates of misgovernment, regarded as an indispensable security, and the greatest safeguard of the interests of mankind.[30]

But there was more required than Milton, eighteenth-century writers[31] the elder Mill had provided. On no occasion were these elements drawn more carefully than by John Stuart Mill in his essay, *On Liberty*, published in 1859.

John Stuart Mill's view of the individual was, of course, modern, secular and optimistic. For example, he said: "the source of everything respectable in man either as an intellectual or as a moral being [is that] his errors are corrigible. He is capable of rectifying his mistakes, by discussion and experience. Not by experience alone. There must be discussion, to show how experience is to be interpreted."[32] His most important aim was to convince his fellow Britons that they should encourage, on a society-wide scale, opportunities for all individuals to grow intellectually. "There have been," he wrote, "great individual thinkers in a general atmosphere of mental slavery. But there never has been, nor ever will be, in that atmosphere an intellectually active people."[33] He returned to this theme several times because it underlined a foundational assumption of his work, that there was no goal or aim in life higher than that of developing in individuals the capacity to be self-sufficient and creative. He said:

> It really is of importance, not only what men do, but also what manner of men they are that do it. Among the works of man, which human life is rightly employed in perfecting and beautifying ... is man himself.[34]

He went on to say that human nature "is not a machine to be built after a model and set to do exactly the work prescribed for it, but a tree, which requires to grow and develop itself on all sides...." And to underline the point he asked: "for what more or better can be said of any condition of human affairs than that it brings human beings themselves nearer to the best thing they can be?"[35]

One part of the method of achieving his goal included establishing a system of free expression. But Mill argued that to secure such a system there had to be a limit on the sacred democratic principle of majority rule. Although the notion that the "people have no need to limit their power over themselves, might seem axiomatic, when popular government was a thing only dreamed about, or read of",[36] in real life or in the light of such serious aims as the cultivation of genuine human growth and the attendant benefits to all of society, it would be necessary to protect individuals, especially in their thoughts, from the majority.

> The limitation . . . of the power over individuals loses none of its importance when the holders of power are regularly accountable to the community. . . . Protection . . . against the tyranny of the magistrate is not enough: there needs to be protection against the tyranny of the prevailing opinion and feeling; against the tendency of society to impose . . . its own ideas and practices as rules of conduct on those who dissent from them. . . .[37]

In other words, the system could not be democratic if a democratic principle could be used to usurp the individual rights on which the system was dependent. Moreover, the methods necessary to protect individuals from the power of legislatures were also necessary with respect to the tyranny of convention and consensus in society at large.

Although his views reflect some of Milton, the later Mill substituted humankind and secular wisdom for the divine. In Mill's view humankind has an obligation to initiate the process of human development and to perpetuate its good effects. The start is education. Not to educate, in John Stuart Mill's view, was "a moral crime"[38] against individuals and society. Not to allow freedom of expression after individuals have been educated would equally be a moral crime because freedom of expression is the means of perpetuating the good effects of education. The press thus assumes the task of promoting discussion and the interpretation of experience in the interests of strong and growing individual citizens. A warning and a prescription in the concluding paragraph of the essay reflects these premises:

> [A] State which dwarfs its men, in order that they may be more docile instruments in its hands even for beneficial purposes — will find that with small men no great thing can really be accomplished; and that the perfection of machinery to which it has sacrificed everything will in the end avail it nothing, for want of the vital power which, in order that the machine might work more smoothly, it has preferred to banish.[39]

The writings summarized above represent important chapters in the history of democratic theory and, more particularly, in the development of a theory of intellectual freedom. They addressed the rights and prerogatives of the citizen to speak, to know and to argue. The building began with Milton in the middle of the seventeenth century and an ending of sorts came with John Stuart Mill in the middle of the nineteenth century. The achievement of these writers and those that came between was to put individuals into the foreground of society and politics and to connect them to the business of society, not as property holders as Locke and others might have done, but as living intellects. This celebration and promotion of the development of individual minds was accompanied by the idea that both the state and organized society could dangerously usurp the freedom which alone could guarantee the general welfare.

No danger would be more forbidding in their eyes than the danger that came from the power in society that possessed, as Max Weber would say later, a monopoly on the means of violence. The state would inevitably want to control thought, but all it should be allowed is the right, for radically limited and well defined purposes, to outlaw certain occasions of speech. Their commitment to freedom did not represent a departure from a belief in the importance and necessity of law. But it did include a fundamental distrust of the uses to which law might be turned. Put differently, their primary goal was to ensure that meaning, understanding and moral life would be the product of discussion and persuasion rather than of power and compulsion. The promise was a better life.

5. Milton's Successors: The Supreme Court's Pre-Charter Decisions

As everyone knows, the Supreme Court's opportunities to illuminate and discuss the meaning of freedom of expression before the enactment of the Charter were few in number. Judicial review in Canadian constitutional history has involved primarily adjudication of jurisdictional disputes between the federal and provincial powers. Civil liberties have generally been on the margins of the Supreme Court's work.

The contrast between American and Canadian law in this respect is striking. Courts in the United States have turned the First Amendment's provisions forbidding the abridgement of freedom of the press into a fully elaborated philosophy. By contrast, justices on Canada's Supreme Court have only hesitatingly elaborated a theory, and then only within the rather limited framework provided by the *British North America Act*.[40] Still, if Canadians were looking for a Canadian version of the "liberal" theory of freedom in the *dicta* of Supreme Court justices, they could find it. The series of judgments in which the "Implied Bill of Rights" was developed included judgments on the press and the underpinnings of those judgments can be aligned to the vision that originates with Milton.

The cases include the *Alberta Press Reference*,[41] *Saumur v. City of Quebec and Attorney-General of Quebec*, the Jehovah's Witnesses case,[42] and *Switzman v. Elbling* and *Attorney-General of Quebec*, the *Padlock Act* case.[43] The judges who were prominent in formulating and expressing theory include Duff, Cannon, Rand and Abbott.

The background to these judgments need not be described here, nor is it necessary to provide the full detail of them.[44] It will suffice to note first, that a major point of reference in these judgments, as in all pre-Charter judgments, was the matter of jurisdiction; secondly, while three of these judges insisted the federal Parliament alone had the power to regulate so-called "original" freedoms,[45] a fourth argued that the real sense of his brother judges' opinions was that neither the federal Parliament nor the provincial legislatures had the power to abrogate these freedoms.[46] Mr. Justice Abbott argued in the *Switzman* case that both levels of government were, as has now become the case under the Charter, subject to the provisions of a theory of freedom.[47]

Mr. Justice Duff's *dicta* in the *Alberta Press* case paved the way. He premised a right of free expression on the preamble of the *British North America Act* which declared that the Constitution of Canada was to be "similar in principle to that of the United Kingdom". On the basis of this declaration, he said that the right of "public discussion is ... subject to legal restrictions ... but it is axiomatic that the practice of this right of free public discussion of public affairs ... is the breath of life for parliamentary institutions."[48] In the same case, Mr. Justice Cannon added that freedom "of discussion is essential to enlighten public opinion in a democratic State; it cannot be curtailed without affecting the right of the people to be informed through sources independent of the Government concerning matters of public interest." He also relied on the preamble of the *British North America Act* and reprimanded the government of Alberta for trying to pass a law which, he said, had a kinship to the law of seditious libel. He concluded the "federal Parliament is the sole authority to curtail ... the freedom of the press and the equal rights in that respect of all citizens throughout the Dominion."[49]

In the *Saumur* case Mr. Justice Rand spoke to the limitations on freedom of expression and affirmed that freedom of expression is the very touchstone of the democratic system.

> The *Confederation Act* recites the desire of the three provinces to be federally united into one Dominion "with a constitution similar in principle to that of the United Kingdom." Under that constitution, government is by parliamentary institutions, including popular assemblies elected by the people at large in both provinces and Dominion: government resting ultimately on public opinion reached by discussion and the interplay of ideas. If that discussion is placed under license, its basic condition is destroyed: the government, as licensor, becomes disjoined from the citizenry. The only security is steadily advancing enlightenment, for which the widest range of controversy is the sine qua non.[50]

He returned to this theme in the *Switzman* case where he said that in a democracy "public opinion ... demands the condition of a virtually unobstructed access to and diffusion of ideas."[51] But Mr. Justice Abbott went further and emancipated Rand's view from the jurisdictional terms of the *British North America Act* and from the doctrine of parliamentary supremacy itself. He said:

> This right cannot be abrogated by a provincial Legislature, and the power of such Legislature to limit it, is restricted to what may be necessary to protect purely private rights, such as for example provincial laws of defamation. It is obvious that the impugned statute does not fall within that category. It does not, in substance, deal with matters of property and civil rights or with a local or private matter within the Province and in my opinion is clearly *ultra vires*. Although it is not necessary ... to determine this question for the purposes of the present appeal, the Canadian Constitution being declared similar in principle to that of the United Kingdom, am also of opinion that as our constitutional Act now stands, Parliament itself could not abrogate this right of discussion and debate. The power of Parliament to limit it is, in my view, restricted to such

powers as may be exercisable under its exclusive legislative jurisdiction with respect to criminal law and to make laws for the peace, order and good government of the nation.[51a]

Although Mr. Justice Abbott's liberalism may seem naive in retrospect, it is not without a foundation in logic. His logic derives from an understanding that "original" or "axiomatic" freedoms, as freedom of the press and of expression have been characterized,[52] require that all governments in a democracy be subordinated in one way or another to them. Of course Abbott's position was not accepted as a matter of constitutional law or convention.

The Charter, however, seems to express such a position subject to section 33 which returns the notion of parliamentary and legislative supremacy to the politicians.[53] Perhaps, it is better — although a bit precious — to say the notion of freedom of expression is more axiomatic than it once was. Still, long before the Charter our judges adopted a theory of freedom of expression arising out of the tenets of historic liberalism. It is useful at this point to restate its central features in language which reflects our understanding of the ever-lurking threats to free expression and which may guide the use of the Charter.

What Milton, the Mills and the Canadian justices had in common, although they expressed it differently and with different goals in mind, is the belief that certain liberties or rights must be secure if a recognizably democratic system or process is to occur. For example, there cannot be a democracy without a right to oppose; nor can there be a democracy if governments possess the power to define the meaning of events and values or if governments are not themselves governed by rules. Accordingly, a fundamental rule out of which democracies are constructed is the rule that requires speech to be free. No government possesses the right to abrogate this fundamental freedom. Put a little differently, governance in democracies is circumscribed by an ideal of free expression. This limit on the power of governments reflects an understanding that the majorities they represent can, without violating other democratic rules, destroy the very rights on which the whole system turns. To give full licence to the idea of majority rule without providing a limit to it could in the end be a denial of democracy itself.

The image or analogy that best suits this line of thinking comes more from architecture than from philosophy. This is not to deny that philosophical questions are important in the resolution of the conundra of democratic theory, but rather to acknowledge that we build systems of politics and governance just as we build buildings. As a consequence, the fundamental freedoms may be seen as the foundations on which the democratic system rests. Since freedom of expression is a foundation, it may be seen as a means rather than as an end, as a starting point for democratic life rather than a goal or an end for which the political process or the regulatory machinery of the state can ordinarily be used.

The steps that make it possible for "liberals" to advocate or approve freedom of expression include the reasons already reviewed. Most importantly and directly they include: (1) a distrust of the narrow and self-serving uses to which politicians can turn the machinery of state; (2) a belief that virtue and progress are more likely to come from individual choice than from compulsion; (3) a belief that the activities of state, conceived in the broadest political as well as in a narrow governmental sense, are the public's business; and (4) a belief that the public can be trusted. With respect to this last point, it does not follow that no judgment or sanction should be imposed on heresies or "evil" speech. Rather it is believed that in order for genuine freedom to occur, the court of public opinion rather than the courts of law should be used to censure and condemn in most cases. At the same time, there is a belief that certain interests must be protected against abuses of free expression. For the justices, consistent with the traditions of their intellectual forebears, this protection entailed approval of the laws of defamation and contempt, and probably official secrets and seditious libel, in which palpable and immediate harms to the operations of state, the public order or private welfare could be measured. Thus, Mr. Justice Rand spoke of the "circumscription of ... liberties" by civil and public law aimed at punishing "consequential incidents". Concerns over incitement and the protection of the administration of justice have also figured prominently in the justifications of these limitations.

Even if it sounds occasionally as if absolute freedom is being espoused, the fact is that limitations have been explicitly defended in the very tradition that advocates the widest measure of freedom. However, the central feature of the tradition is the belief that limitations can only be imposed for the narrowest of reasons and then only in the face of a powerful presumption that they are made in the face of a fundamental freedom on which the whole edifice of democracy rests.[54]

6. Conclusion

In the late twentieth century it is not as easy as it once was to relate a traditional treatment of freedom of the press to the activities of journalists and journalism. Journalistic activity has always been looked upon by some individuals or groups with suspicion and fear. In the nineteenth century, when James Mill wrote his essay on the press, the social and political elites wanted to limit and control it, no doubt because they wanted "to riot in the pleasures of misrule".[55] That James Mill thought so is no surprise. Nor is it a surprise that genuine democrats such as Mill would identify with the career and welfare of an upstart institution which was challenging those very elites. Faith in the press as an instrument for achieving good works began when the democratic spirit took hold in our culture and challenged established power.[56]

But now that phase of the democratic revolution is over. To some degree the press is an established institution or even part of an establishment. It has become, therefore, harder to believe that the press possesses and acquits the same democratic mandate it once did. Members of our current reform movement are sometimes tempted to suspect that the press — especially in light of the scope of the Thomson and Southam empires — is not a genuinely democratic institution, and they sometimes join other groups in discrediting it.[57]

The word "media" also complicates the application of the traditional freedom to journalists, for it directs attention to institutions in which most journalists work rather than to the journalists themselves. Such institutions may be very large and notwithstanding profound differences in function, they have some of the characteristics of major commercial and industrial enterprises. They employ thousands of people, many of whom are not journalists, and they spread their products randomly and opportunistically like any good business. The large size of these media institutions makes them seem factory-like or bureaucratic and their number puts their products and activities in the foreground of modern life and experience and makes it inevitable that they are subject to close scrutiny and criticism. It is, in short, more difficult to see their growth and security as part and parcel of a "democratic" establishment.

The fact that journalists have their own agenda for covering society's stories and issues exaggerates these difficulties. The operations and practices of the news media probably confuse members of the public and seem to them only remotely, if at all, connected to the difficult chore of supporting the democratic edifice. Finally, journalists are not as able as other professional groups such as lawyers and doctors to camouflage their errors in judgment. Like the politicians whose work they so carefully monitor, their limitations and errors, and their courage and acumen, are public events.

Still, it is important to continue to recognize that there is much to be gained by conferring on journalists a wide measure of freedom to practise their craft as they see fit and it is no more absurd to connect their work to democracy than to connect the work of lawyers to the attainment of justice.

The right or the liberty of free expression is conferred on citizens. It is they who are entitled to know what is going on about them and what the government is doing on their behalf. Equally, they have the right as citizens to "utter and to argue freely". If citizens have these liberties, then journalists possess them as well. It is hard to imagine it being otherwise. That some citizens exercise these rights and freedoms more vigorously than others is consistent with the division of labour in complex societies. This is not to make a virtue of the size and complexity of our society, but rather to recognize, perhaps even tragically, the inevitability of such divisions and specialization.

Put a little differently, the division of labour in a complex society makes it inevitable that specialists will emerge in the areas of communication and culture. In this respect, society's writers, including all who make their living as journalists, are on the receiving end of a delegation whereby, in a political sense especially, fundamental rights of free expression are handled by them on behalf of the members of the public who are more distant from centres of political and other action.

The exercise of these rights by journalists in a complex society brings the democratic process into being. Journalists and writers, not just those employed by the mass media, start the process of discussion and judgment by conveying and commenting on the news. They flood the air with stories and opinions covering an enormous range of political and social events. In a rough way the ideal that guides their work is that there is a public which is interested in what they say. That the law permits them a wide territory within which to practise their craft is consistent with the aims of democracy. The more freedom, the more discussion, the more democracy.

But to say the process begins with journalists and journalism is obviously different than saying it ends with them. Just as the conferral of these rights and liberties on citizens and journalists makes the quality and character of the process indeterminate, their exercise leads to outcomes that are also indeterminate. Public discussion begins where journalists sign off. Political, religious and moral discussion in society at large, as well as gossip about the trivial and the ephemeral, take as points of reference some of the contents of the media. For political and governmental discussion the relationship between the media and the public is both vital and profound.

That the communication of relevant information and evaluation of it could be arranged and done better and with better effects is obvious. But to conclude that it is never done well is to fail to examine carefully what the best of our journalists are able to achieve under difficult circumstances. To say conversely that journalists carry the full burden of responsibility for democracy is also to miss the point. In a developed society such as ours, we give a life to the ideal of freedom of expression, and to some degree to democracy, by conferring rights on citizens and by encouraging journalists especially to implement them. This is how we Canadians do it.

Accordingly, the journalist's perspective on the Charter and the role of the media is that democracy is the issue. The ability of journalists to practise their craft turns on the manner in which the rights of freedom are secured in law or tradition. Citizens need these rights to be citizens of a democracy; creative people such as journalists need them in order to be genuinely and safely creative. These are not differences in kind so much as differences in degree. But they explain why journalists see themselves as being specially associated with the defence of these rights.

Endnotes

* "Areopagitica: A Speech for the Liberty of Unlicensed Printing to the Parliament of England (1644)", in George Sabine, ed. *John Milton, Areopagitica and of Education with Autobiographical Passages from other Prose Works* (1951), p. 49.
1. *Constitution Act, 1982*, Sched. B of the *Canada Act, 1982* (U.K.), c. 11, s. 52.
2. Although the balancing process required under s. 1 of the Charter provides a middle ground between "liberties" and "rights", it will be determined by

the courts, see Anisman, "Application of the Charter A Structural Approach," *supra*, at pp. 21-22.

3. Quoted in J.A. Hammond, *C.P. Scott of the Manchester Guardian* 96 (1934).

4. For an interesting exploration of this idea see Park "News as a Form of Knowledge," in R. Turner, ed., *Robert Park on Social Control and Collective Behaviour* 33 (1967).

5. The most influential recent essays and studies concentrate on structural or cultural factors such as the patterns of ownership or conservative ideology which, it is alleged, dominate the content of modern journalism. On the issue of ownership see, for example, *Report of the Royal Commission on Newspapers* (Kent Commission) (1981), Vol.I and Lorend Ghiglione, ed., *The Buying and Selling of America's Newspapers* (1984). Cultural and ideological analyses of the press may be found in J. Porter, *The Vertical Mosaic* (1964), W. Clement, *The Canadian Corporate Elite* (1975); and R. Miliband, *The State in Capitalist Society* (1973).

6. I owe this idea to Prof. T. K. Rymes of the Department of Economics, Carleton University. I am grateful to him and to Professors Roger Bird and Anthony Westell of the School of Journalism for their helpful comments on this part of the paper.

7. G. Sabine, *op. cit.*, note at 37.

8. *Ibid.*, at 5.

9. *Ibid.*, at 7.

10. *Ibid.*, at 25.

11. *Ibid.*, at 13.

12. *Ibid.*, at 14.

13. *Ibid.*, at 22.

14. *Ibid.*, at 26.

15. *Ibid.*, at 37.

16. *Ibid.*, at 23-24.

17. *Ibid.*, at 28.

18. *Ibid.*, at 28.

19. *Ibid.*, at 32.

20. *Ibid.*, at 29.

21. *Ibid.*, at 6.

22. *Ibid.*, at 16.

23. *Ibid.*, at 50.

24. *Ibid.*, at 17-18.

25. *Ibid.*, at 18.
26. *Ibid.*, at 44.
27. *Ibid.*, at 5.
28. *Ibid.*, at 49.
29. James Mill, *Essays on Government, Jurisprudence, Liberty of the Press, and Law of Nations*, 1825 16 (Reprint ed. 1967).
30. *Ibid.*, at 18.
31. In the eighteenth century, some expert legal thinkers such as Lord Camden and Thomas Erskine, a few major political thinkers such as David Hume, Edmund Burke and Thomas Paine, and many politicians, publicists and journalists offered their ideas on the liberty of the press to the English public. Among the latter were Daniel Defoe, Jonathan Swift, Joseph Addison, Lord Bolingbroke, John Wilkes and John Almon and the authors who wrote under such pseudonyms as Cato, Candor and Junius. For a summary and interpretation of their essays and others see G. Stuart Adam, *The Press and Its Liberty, Myth and Ideology in Eighteenth-Century English Politics*, Ph D. thesis, Queen's University, Kingston, 1978.
32. Gertrude Himmelfarb, ed., *John Stuart Mill, On Liberty* 79-80 (1984).
33. *Ibid.*, at 95.
34. *Ibid.*, at 123.
35. *Ibid.*, at 128.
36. *Ibid.*, at 61-62.
37. *Ibid.*, at 62-63.
38. *Ibid.*, at 176.
39. *Ibid.*, at 187.
40. Now the *Constitution Act, 1867*. Canadian courts have also addressed issues involving freedom of the press in the context of libel and other laws, but have not promoted the concept in these non-constitutional areas, see Beckton "Freedom of the Press in Canada: Prior Restraints," *infra*, at pp. 127-37; see also Grant, "Criminal Investigation," *infra*, at pp. 269-73.
41. *Ref. re Alberta Statutes*, [1938] S.C.R. 100 (S.C.C.).
42. *Saumur v. Quebec*, [1953] 2 S.C.R. 299 (S.C.C.).
43. *Switzman v. Elbling and A.G. Que.*, [1957] S.C.R. 285 (S.C.C.).
44. For a discussion of these decisions see, e.g., P. Hogg, *Constitutional Law of Canada* 706-709 (2d ed. 1985).
45. See *Alberta Statutes, supra*, note 41 at 132-35 (Duff, C.J.) and 142-47 (Cannon, J.), *Saumur, supra*, note 42 at 328-34 (Rand, J.); *Switzman, supra* note 43 at 302-307 (Rand, J.).
46. See *supra*, note 43 at 325-28 (Abbott, J.).

47. *Ibid.*
48. *Supra*, note 41 at 133.
49. *Ibid.*, at 146.
50. *Supra*, note 42 at 330. See generally Price, "Mr. Justice Rand and the Privileges and Immunities of Canadian Citizens," 16 *U.T. Fac. L. Rev.* 16 (1958).
51. *Supra*, note 43 at 306.
51a. *Ibid.*, at 328.
52. See *supra*, note 41 at 133 ("axiomatic," *per* Duff, C.J.); *supra*, note 42 at 329 ("original," *per* Rand, J.).
53. See, e.g., Anisman, *supra*, note 2, at pp. 5-6.
54. The Charter therefore reflects this tradition in that the freedom is subject to restrictions that meet the test of s. 1, see *ibid.*
55. See *supra*, note 29.
56. For an interesting analysis of important developments in the nineteenth century, see W. Wickwar, *The Struggle for Freedom of the Press*, 1819-1832 (1928).
57. See *supra*, note 5, especially the reference to the *Report of the Royal Commission on Newspapers*. The Commission's proposals included a Newspaper Act which was vigorously opposed by the publishers and senior editors of Canada's newspapers.

1.7.2 Robert Martin, "Press Councils: Watchdogs with No Bite," *Bulletin of the Centre for Investigative Journalism*, No. 29 (1986), p. 30.

Canadian law and policy on broadcasting began with the 1929 Report of the Royal Commission on Radio Broadcasting. Its central recommendation was that broadcasting should be a "public service" and, for that reason, subject to regulation by the state. This was accepted by the government of R.B. Bennett and has remained at the core of Canadian broadcasting policy ever since. The federal Broadcasting Act continues this policy, stating that broadcasting frequencies are "public property."

The approach to newspapers, however, has been different. Newspapers are simply another form of private property, which has a number of consequences: since newspapers are private property, their owners are free, apart from limitations imposed by law, to run them as they please.

Owners, and those who manage newspapers on their behalf, have absolute discretion to determine what they will or will not print. This principle was upheld by the Supreme Court of Canada in the 1930s and again in the 1970s. In both cases the court held that a provincial law could not be used to force a newspaper to publish material against the owner's wishes. This also means the owner and management can decide what stories are to be covered and what positions the newspaper will take on question of public interest.

Owners have, within provincial employment laws, absolute authority over hiring and firing. This includes the authority to dismiss journalists who express uncongenial opinions in the pages of the newspaper or even outside the workplace.

Also, owners have authority over all financial matters affecting their newspapers. This means the crucial authority to decide how much or how little money will be spent on hiring and keeping editorial staff. Even more important, it encompasses the authority to decide how newspaper profits shall be disposed of. Will profits be reinvested in improving the newspaper or, as often happens where newspapers are part of conglomerate corporate empires, will they be used to finance other corporate ventures?

Finally, owners have complete freedom to dispose of newspapers. They can sell them to whomsoever they choose or simply kill them.

Newspaper owners have the same rights as the owners of soap factories or used car lots. Difficulties arise because some people in this country believe there are significant social difference between newspapers and detergent or used cars. Such beliefs are only stated publicly when something especially outrageous occurs.

Something the federal government perceived to be outrageous occurred in the summer of 1980. The Southam and Thomson chains made a trade-off. Southam folded the Winnipeg *Tribune* and Thomson did the same for the Ottawa *Journal*. This left both Winnipeg and Ottawa as one-newspaper towns. A degree of public concern was expressed. The government of Canada set up a Royal Commission to look into newspapers. Whatever interest there is today in press councils arose largely in response to the recommendations of this commission.

The commission was chaired by Tom Kent. Kent began this career as a journalist in the U.K., before moving to Canada where he headed Lester Pearson's version of the war on poverty in the mid-1960s. Before undertaking the Royal Commission he was dean of management studies at Dalhousie University. He has, despite the views of some newspaper owners, an abiding faith in capitalism.

The Kent Commission made its report in 1981. It recommended limitations on the proprietary rights of newspaper owners and Kent was roundly vilified on editorial pages from sea to sea. The commission's recommendations were portrayed as a monstrous scheme to destroy freedom of expression and freedom of the press in Canada. It appeared that the country's fearless and outspoken editors and journalists were to be subjected to a stultifying regime of bureaucratic control.

The reality was different. Kent proposed the enactment of a *Canada Newspapers Act*. The Act would have sought to inhibit further concentration of newspaper ownership. It would have guaranteed a degree of independence for newspaper editors against owners. Advisory committees were to be set up to permit members of the community to express their views about the local newspaper.

Draft legislation was prepared. But as the hysteria of editorial page denunciations of Kent and all his works mounted, the government lost its nerve. The draft bill went nowhere and the report was quickly forgotten. So if the Kent Commission came to naught, what is its significance in a discussion of press councils? Newspaper owners apparently decided that, having torpedoed the Kent Commission, they would have to make some symbolic concession. I surmise that they wished to give the appearance of limiting their ownership rights and of recognizing the legitimacy of the public interest in the content of newspapers. So they decided to join press councils. The Kent Commission had made it easier for owners. Its report contained this admonition:

"We think that newspapers which do not become enthusiastically involved in the establishment and operation of press councils are exceedingly shortsighted."

The Ontario Press Council was formed in 1972, with eight newspapers as members. They were the *Toronto Star*, the *London Free Press* and a number of Southam papers. Membership grew slowly, with only one daily and a few weeklies joining before 1981. But 1981 was, as the Press Council put it in its Annual Report for 1981, a "Record Year for Growth", One daily and nine weeklies joined. The Annual Report for 1982 stated "Council Membership Booms". The number of dailies belonging to the Press Council increased from 10 to 32. This included the *Globe and Mail* and some other Thomson papers. Membership among weeklies jumped from 14 to 49. Eighteen more dailies joined the council in 1983 and by the beginning of 1985 all 42 English-language daily newspapers in Ontario were members.

The activity was not confined to Ontario. As the Ontario Council stated in its 1982 Annual Report:

"The press council movement got into high gear across Canada in late 1982."

Today there are press council in Québec, Manitoba, Alberta, and B.C., as well as the Atlantic Press Council.

This is all, no doubt, wonderful. But to return to where we started, the burgeoning of press councils has in no way altered the proprietary rights of newspaper owners.

The Ontario Press Council is a voluntary body. A member newspaper may withdraw at any time and although the council investigates complaints, it has no enforcement powers. A member newspaper is obliged to publish the council's decision in an adjudication, but there is no authority to make binding orders against newspapers. There is no provision for expelling a member newspaper from the council.

If the unlimited proprietary rights of newspaper owners give rise to legitimate concerns, then press councils, whatever their other merits may be, simply do not address those concerns.

CHAPTER TWO

Security, the Public Order and Democratic Institutions:
Legal Limitations to Protect the State's Rights, Prerogatives and Responsibilities, Part I

2.1 Legitimacy and the Scope of State Power

The freedom of expression in the *Constitution Act, 1982*, is not, strictly speaking, the product of positive law. Although now sanctioned by the "supreme law of Canada", the fundamental freedoms have been understood historically as areas of human behaviour and action with which the State may not interfere. Put differently, there has been an historical understanding in liberal democracies that the State cannot enact statutes to create such freedoms; they are presumed to exist outside the domain of the legislated order. The State's responsibilities begin at the point where the exercise of such freedoms threatens an equally fundamental social interest. As will be seen in the cases, there is a practical notion in law of "balancing" the benefits of freedom against the benefits of protecting certain social or state interests with which the freedoms may be in conflict. As a consequence, the notion of "reasonable limits" expressed in section 1 of the Charter appears to legitimate an extensive range of restrictive laws. The limits may relate to the State's obligation to protect national security, prevent riots or the disruption of the legislative and legal processes; they may protect public morality by creating criminal penalties or administrative procedures to prevent the distribution of certain kinds of pornographic or violent material; they might protect minority groups from hate propagandists; or, finally, they might protect individuals from defamation.

The broad categories to which limitations are related — state rights, social values and groups, and individuals — are well established in the Canadian legal system although the debate on the substance of the second set of restrictions remains vigorous. But regardless of how some Canadians may regard obscenity or hate propaganda, few would challenge the notion that legislation can legitimately be used to protect certain interests — for example, bona fide state secrets. The *Official Secrets Act* is justified generally as an expression of the permission the Charter grants through section 1 to Parliament to legislate a "limit" on freedom of expression. Whether the way in which the Act is written or applied is reasonable is another matter.

This chapter is concerned with the statutory limitations on freedom of expression which protect some of the State's rights, prerogatives and responsibilities. The items for analysis include national security, and public order and safety.

2.2 National Security

2.2.1 Emergencies

The *War Measures Act*, which was invoked during both World Wars and again in October, 1970, during the so-called FLQ crisis, was repealed in 1988 and replaced by the *Emergencies Act*.

There are four levels of emergency distinguished in the new act: a Public Welfare Emergency caused by a natural disaster, disease, industrial accident or pollution; a Public Order Emergency caused by a "serious" threat to the security of Canada; an International Emergency caused by acts in which Canada is entangled "of intimidation or coercion or the real or imminent use of serious force or violence"; and a War Emergency which "means war or other armed conflict, real or imminent, involving Canada or any of its allies that is so serious as to be a national emergency". The following provisions may be noted.

2.2.1.1 *Emergencies Act*, S.C. 1988, c. 29

WHEREAS the safety and security of the individual, the protection of the values of the body politic and the preservation of the sovereignty, security and territorial integrity of the state are fundamental obligations of government;

AND WHEREAS the fulfilment of those obligations in Canada may be seriously threatened by a national emergency and, in order to ensure safety and security during such an emergency, the Governor in Council should be authorized, subject to the supervision of Parliament, to take special temporary measures that may not be appropriate in normal times;

AND WHEREAS the Governor in Council, in taking such special temporary measures, would be subject to the *Canadian Charter of Rights and Freedoms* and the *Canadian Bill of Rights* and must have regard to the *International Covenant on Civil and Political Rights*, particularly with respect to those fundamental rights that are not to be limited or abridged even in a national emergency;

NOW THEREFORE, Her Majesty, by and with the advice and consent of the Senate and House of Commons of Canada, enacts as follows:

3. For the purposes of this Act, a "national emergency" is an urgent and critical situation of a temporary nature that

(*a*) seriously endangers the lives, health or safety of Canadians and is of such proportions or nature as to exceed the capacity or authority of a province to deal with it, or

(b) seriously threatens the ability of the Government of Canada to preserve the sovereignty, security and territorial integrity of Canada and that cannot be effectively dealt with under any other law of Canada.

5. In this Part,

"declaration of a public welfare emergency" means a proclamation issued pursuant to subsection 6(1);

"public welfare emergency" means an emergency that is caused by a real or imminent

    (a) fire, flood, drought, storm, earthquake or other natural phenomenon,
    (b) disease in human beings, animals or plants, or
    (c) accident or pollution

and that results or may result in a danger to life or property, social disruption or a breakdown in the flow of essential goods, services or resources, so serious as to be a national emergency.

6. (1) When the Governor in Council believes, on reasonable grounds, that a public welfare emergency exists and necessitates the taking of special temporary measures for dealing with the emergency, the Governor in Council, after such consultation as is required by section 14, may, by proclamation, so declare.

(2) A, declaration of a public welfare emergency shall specify

    (a) concisely the state of affairs constituting the emergency;
    (b) the special temporary measures that the Governor in Council anticipates may be necessary for dealing with the emergency; and
    (c) if the direct effects of the emergency do not extend to the whole of Canada, the area of Canada to which the direct effects of the emergency extend.

7. (1) A declaration of a public welfare emergency is effective on the day on which it is issued, but a motion for confirmation of the declaration shall be laid before each House of Parliament and be considered in accordance with section 58.

(2) A declaration of a public welfare emergency expires at the end of ninety days, unless the declaration is previously revoked or continued in accordance with this Act.

8. (1) While a declaration of a public welfare emergency is in effect, the Governor in Council may make such orders or regulations with respect to the following matters as the Governor in Council believes, on reasonable grounds, are necessary for dealing with the emergency:

    (a) the regulation or prohibition of travel to, from or within any specified area where necessary for the protection of the health or safety of individuals;
    (b) the evacuation of persons and the removal of personal property from any specified area and the making of arrangements for the adequate care and protection thereof;

(c) the requisition, use or disposition of property;
(d) the authorization of or direction to any person, or any person of a class of persons, to render essential services of a type that that person, or a person of that class, is competent to provide and the provision of reasonable compensation in respect of services so rendered;
(e) the regulation of the distribution and availability of essential goods, services and resources;
(f) the authorization and making of emergency payments;
(g) the establishment of emergency shelters and hospitals;
(h) the assessment of damage to any works or undertakings and the repair, replacement or restoration thereof;

16. In this Part,

"declaration of a public order emergency" means a proclamation issued pursuant to subsection 17(1);

"public order emergency" means an emergency that arises from threats to the security of Canada and that is so serious as to be a national emergency;

"threats to the security of Canada" has the meaning assigned by section 2 of the *Canadian Security Intelligence Service Act*.

Declaration of a Public Order Emergency

17. (1) When the Governor in Council believes, on reasonable grounds, that a public order emergency exists and necessitates the taking of special temporary measures for dealing with the emergency, the Governor in Council, after such consultation as is required by section 25, may, by proclamation, so declare.

(2) A declaration of a public order emergency shall specify
(a) concisely the state of affairs constituting the emergency;
(b) the special temporary measures that the Governor in Council anticipates may be necessary for dealing with the emergency; and
(c) if the effects of the emergency do not extend to the whole of Canada, the area of Canada to which the effects of the emergency extend.

18. (1) A declaration of a public order emergency is effective on the day on which it is issued, but a motion for confirmation of the declaration shall be laid before each House of Parliament and be considered in accordance with section 58.

(2) A declaration of a public order emergency expires at the end of thirty days unless the declaration is previously revoked or continued in accordance with this Act.

19. (1) While a declaration of a public order emergency is in effect, the Governor in Council may make such orders or regulations with respect to the following matters as the Governor in Council believes, on reasonable grounds, are necessary for dealing with the emergency:

(*a*) the regulation or prohibition of
   (i) any public assembly that may reasonably be expected to lead to a breach of the peace,
   (ii) travel to, from or within any specified area, or
   (iii) the use of specified property;
(*b*) the designation and securing of protected places;
(*c*) the assumption of the control, and the restoration and maintenance, of public utilities and services;
(*d*) the authorization of or direction to any person, or any person of a class of persons, to render essential services of a type that that person, or a person of that class, is competent to provide and the provision of reasonable compensation in respect of services so rendered; and
(*e*) the imposition
   (i) on summary conviction, of a fine not exceeding five hundred dollars or imprisonment not exceeding six months or both that fine and imprisonment, or
   (ii) on indictment, of a fine not exceeding five thousand dollars or imprisonment not exceeding five years or both that fine and imprisonment
for contravention of any order or regulation made under this section.

(2) Where a declaration of a public order emergency specifies that the effects of the emergency extend to only a specified area of Canada, the power under subsection (1) to make orders and regulations, and any powers, duties or functions conferred or imposed by or pursuant to any such order or regulation, may be exercised or performed only with respect to that area.

(3) The power under subsection (1) to make orders and regulations, and any powers, duties or functions conferred or imposed by or pursuant to any such order or regulation, shall be exercised or performed
(*a*) in a manner that will not unduly impair the ability of any province to take measures, under an Act of the legislature of the province, for dealing with an emergency in the province; and
(*b*) with the view to achieving, to the extent possible, concerted action with each province with respect to which the power, duty or function is exercised or performed.

27. In this Part,

"declaration of an international emergency" means a proclamation issued pursuant to subsection 28(1);

"international emergency" means an emergency involving Canada and one or more other countries that arises from acts of intimidation or coercion or the real or imminent use of serious force or violence and that is so serious as to be a national emergency.

28. (1) When the Governor in Council believes, on reasonable grounds, that an international emergency exists and necessitates the taking of special temporary measures for dealing with the emergency, the Governor in Council, after such consultation as is required by section 35, may, by proclamation, so declare.

(2) A declaration of an international emergency shall specify

(*a*) concisely the state of affairs constituting the emergency; and

(*b*) the special temporary measures that the Governor in Council anticipates may be necessary for dealing with the emergency.

29. (1) A declaration of an international emergency is effective on the day on which it is issued, but a motion for confirmation of the declaration shall be laid before each House of Parliament and be considered in accordance with section 58.

(2) A declaration of an international emergency expires at the end of sixty days unless the declaration is previously revoked or continued in accordance with this Act.

30. (1) While a declaration of an international emergency is in effect, the Governor in Council may make such orders or regulations with respect to the following matters as the Governor in Council believes, on reasonable grounds, are necessary for dealing with the emergency:

(*a*) the control or regulation of any specified industry or service, including the use of equipment, facilities and inventory;

(*b*) the appropriation, control, forfeiture, use and disposition of property or services;

(*c*) the authorization and conduct of inquiries in relation to defence contracts or defence supplies as defined in the *Defence Production Act* or to hoarding, overcharging, black marketing or fraudulent operations in respect of scarce commodities, including the conferral of powers under the *Inquiries Act* on any person authorized to conduct such an inquiry;

(*d*) the authorization of the entry and search of any dwelling-house, premises, conveyance or place, and the search of any person found therein, for any thing that may be evidence relevant to any matter that is the subject of an inquiry referred to in paragraph (c), and the seizure and detention of any such thing;

(*e*) the authorization of or direction to any person, or any person of a class of persons, to render essential services of a type that that person, or a person of that class, is competent to provide and the provision of reasonable compensation in respect of services so rendered;

(*f*) the designation and securing of protected places;

(*g*) the regulation or prohibition of travel outside Canada by Canadian citizens or permanent residents as defined in the *Immigration Act, 1976* and of admission into Canada by other persons;

(*h*) the removal from Canada of persons, other than Canadian citizens, permanent residents as defined in the *Immigration Act, 1976* and persons, not being persons described in paragraph 19(1)(c), (e), (f) or (g) of that Act, who are finally determined under that Act to be Convention refugees;

(*i*) the control or regulation of the international aspects of specified financial activities within Canada;

(*j*) the authorization of expenditures for dealing with an international emergency in excess of any limit set by an Act of Parliament and the setting of a limit on such expenditures;

(*k*) the authorization of any Minister of the Crown to discharge specified responsibilities respecting the international emergency or to take specified actions of a political, diplomatic or economic nature for dealing with the emergency; and

(*l*) the imposition

(i) on summary conviction, of a fine not exceeding five hundred dollars or imprisonment not exceeding six months or both that fine and imprisonment, or

(ii) on indictment, of a fine not exceeding five thousand dollars or imprisonment not exceeding five years or both that fine and imprisonment

for contravention of any order or regulation made under this section.

(2) The power under subsection (1) to make orders and regulations, and any powers, duties or functions conferred or imposed by or pursuant to any such order or regulation,

(*a*) shall be exercised or performed

(i) in a manner that will not unduly impair the ability of any province to take measures, under an Act of the legislature of the province, for dealing with an emergency in the province, and

(ii) with the view to achieving, to the extent possible, concerted action with each province with respect to which the power, duty or function is exercised or performed; and

(*b*) shall not be exercised or performed for the purpose of censoring, suppressing or controlling the publication or communication of any information regardless of its form or characteristics.

37. In this Part,

"declaration of a war emergency" means a proclamation issued pursuant to subsection 38(1);

"war emergency" means war or other armed conflict, real or imminent, involving Canada or any of its allies that is so serious as to be a national emergency.

38. (1) When the Governor in Council believes, on reasonable grounds, that a war emergency exists and necessitates the taking of special temporary measures for dealing with the emergency, the Governor in Council, after such consultation as is required by section 44, may, by proclamation, so declare.

(2) A declaration of a war emergency shall specify the state of affairs constituting the emergency to the extent that, in the opinion of the Governor in Council, it is possible to do so without jeopardizing any special temporary measures proposed to be taken for dealing with the emergency.

39. (1) A declaration of a war emergency is effective on the day on which it is issued, but a motion for confirmation of the declaration shall be laid before each House of Parliament and be considered in accordance with section 58.

(2) A declaration of a war emergency expires at the end of one hundred and twenty days unless the declaration is previously revoked or continued in accordance with this Act.

40. (1) While a declaration of a war emergency is in effect, the Governor in Council may make such orders or regulations as the Governor in Council believes, on reasonable grounds, are necessary or advisable for dealing with the emergency.

(1.1) The power under subsection (1) to make orders and regulations may not be exercised for the purpose of requiring persons to serve in the Canadian Forces.

(2) The Governor in Council may make regulations providing for the imposition

   (*a*) on summary conviction, of a fine not exceeding five hundred dollars or imprisonment not exceeding six months or both that fine and imprisonment, or
   (*b*) on indictment, of a fine not exceeding five thousand dollars or imprisonment not exceeding five years or both that fine and imprisonment

for contravention of any order or regulation made under subsection (1).

(3) The power under subsection (1) to make orders and regulations, and any powers, duties or functions conferred or imposed by or pursuant to any such order or regulation, shall be exercised or performed with the view to achieving, to the extent possible, concerted action with each province with respect to which the power, duty or function is exercised or performed.

41. Parliament may revoke a declaration of a war emergency in accordance with section 58 or 59.

42. The Governor in Council may, by proclamation, revoke a declaration of a war emergency effective on such day as is specified in the proclamation.

43. (1) At any time before a declaration of a war emergency would otherwise expire, the Governor in Council, after such consultation as is required by section 44, may, by proclamation, continue the declaration for such period, not exceeding one hundred and twenty days, as is specified in the proclamation if the Governor in Council believes, on reasonable grounds, that the emergency will continue to exist.

(2) Before issuing a proclamation continuing a declaration of a war emergency, the Governor in Council shall review all current orders and regulations made under section 40 to determine if the Governor in Council believes, on reasonable grounds, that they continue to be necessary or advisable for dealing with the emergency and shall revoke or amend them to the extent that they do not so continue.

(3) A declaration of a war emergency may be continued more than once pursuant to subsection (1).

(4) A proclamation continuing a declaration of a war emergency is effective on the day on which it is issued, but a motion for confirmation of the proclamation shall be laid before each House of Parliament and be considered in accordance with section 60.

Consultation

44. Before the Governor in Council issues or continues a declaration of a war emergency, the lieutenant governor in council of each province shall be consulted with respect to the proposed action to the extent that, in the opinion of the Governor in Council, it is appropriate and practicable to do so in the circumstances.

Effect of Expiration or Revocation

45. (1) Where, pursuant to this Act, a declaration of a war emergency expires, all orders and regulations made pursuant to the declaration expire on the day on which the declaration expires.

(2) Where, pursuant to this Act, a declaration of a war emergency is revoked, all orders and regulations made pursuant to the declaration are revoked effective on the revocation of the declaration.

(3) Where, pursuant to this Act, a proclamation continuing a declaration of a war emergency is revoked after the time the declaration would, but for the proclamation, have otherwise expired, the declaration and all orders and regulations made pursuant to the declaration are revoked effective on the revocation of the proclamation.

57. In this Part,

"declaration of emergency" means a proclamation issued pursuant to subsection 6(1), 17(1), 28(1) or 38(1);

"Parliamentary Review Committee" means the committee referred to in subsection 62(1);

"sitting day", in respect of a House of Parliament, means a day on which that House is sitting.

58. (1) Subject to subsection (4), a motion for confirmation of a declaration of emergency, signed by a Minister of the Crown, together with an explanation of the reasons for issuing the declaration and a report on any consultation with the lieutenant governors in council of the provinces with respect to the declaration, shall be laid before each House of Parliament within seven sitting days after the declaration is issued.

(2) If a declaration of emergency is issued during a prorogation of Parliament or when either House of Parliament stands adjourned, Parliament or that House, as the case may be, shall be summoned forthwith to sit within seven days after the declaration is issued.

(3) If a declaration of emergency is issued at a time when the House of Commons is dissolved, Parliament shall be summoned to sit at the earliest opportunity after the declaration is issued.

(4) Where Parliament or a House of Parliament is summoned to sit in accordance with subsection (2) or (3), the motion, explanation and report described in subsection (1) shall be laid before each House of Parliament or that House of Parliament, as the case may be, on the first sitting day after Parliament or that House is summoned.

(5) Where a motion is laid before a House of Parliament as provided in subsection (1) or (4), that House shall, on the sitting day next following the sitting day on which the motion was so laid, take up and consider the motion.

(6) A motion taken up and considered in accordance with subsection (5) shall be debated without interruption and, at such time as the House is ready for the question, the Speaker shall forthwith, without further debate or amendment, put every question necessary for the disposition of the motion.

(7) If a motion for confirmation of a declaration of emergency is negatived by either House of Parliament, the declaration, to the extent that it has not previously expired or been revoked, is revoked effective on the day of the negative vote and no further action under this section need be taken in the other House with respect to the motion.

59. (1) Where a motion for the consideration of the Senate or the House of Commons to the effect that

(*a*) a declaration of emergency under Part I or II be revoked either generally or with respect to any area of Canada, or

(*b*) a declaration of emergency under Part III or IV be revoked,

signed by not less than ten members of the Senate or twenty members of the House of Commons, as the case may be, is filed with the Speaker, that House of Parliament shall take up and consider the motion within three sitting days after it is filed.

(2) A motion taken up and considered in accordance with subsection (1) shall be debated without interruption for not more than ten hours and, on the expiration of the tenth hour or at such earlier time as the House is ready for the question, the Speaker shall forthwith, without further debate or amendment, put every question necessary for the disposition of the motion.

(3) If a motion debated in accordance with subsection (2) is adopted by the House, the declaration, to the extent that it has not previously expired or been revoked, is revoked in accordance with the motion, effective on the day specified in the motion, which day may not be earlier than the day of the vote adopting the motion.

60. (1) A motion for confirmation of a proclamation continuing a declaration of emergency and of any orders and regulations named in the motion pursuant to subsection (3), signed by a Minister of the Crown, together with an explanation of the reasons for issuing the proclamation, a report on any consultation with the lieutenant governors in council of the provinces with respect to the proclamation and a report on the review of orders and regulations conducted before the issuing of the proclamation, shall be laid before each House of Parliament within seven sitting days after the proclamation is issued.

(2) A motion for confirmation of a proclamation amending a declaration of emergency, signed by a Minister of the Crown, together with an explanation of the reasons for issuing the proclamation and a report on any consultations with the lieutenant governors in council of the provinces with respect to the proclamation, shall be laid before each House of Parliament within seven sitting days after the proclamation is issued.

(3) A motion for confirmation of a proclamation continuing a declaration of emergency shall name the orders and regulations in force on the issuing of the proclamation that the Governor in Council believed, on reasonable grounds, continued at that time to be necessary or, in the case of a proclamation issued pursuant to subsection 43(1), advisable, for dealing with the emergency.

(4) Where a motion is laid before a House of Parliament as provided in subsection (1) or (2), that House shall, on the sitting day next following the sitting day on which the motion was so laid, take up and consider the motion.

(5) A motion taken up and considered in accordance with subsection (4) shall be debated without interruption and, at such time as the House is ready for the question, the Speaker shall forthwith, without further debate or amendment, put every question necessary for the disposition of the motion.

(6) If a motion for confirmation of a proclamation is negatived by either House of Parliament, the proclamation, to the extent that it has not previously expired or been revoked, is revoked effective on the day of the negative vote and no further action under this section need be taken in the other House with respect to the motion.

(7) If a motion for confirmation of a proclamation continuing a declaration of emergency is amended by either House of Parliament by the deletion therefrom of an order or regulation named in the motion pursuant to subsection (3), the order or regulation is revoked effective on the day on which the motion, as amended, is adopted.

61. (1) Subject to subsection (2), every order or regulation made by the Governor in Council pursuant to this Act shall be laid before each House of Parliament within two sitting days after it is made.

(2) Where an order or regulation made pursuant to this Act is exempted from publication in the *Canada Gazette* by regulations made under the *Statutory Instruments Act*, the order or regulation, in lieu of being laid before each House of Parliament as required by subsection (1), shall be referred to the Parliamentary Review Committee within two days after it is made, or if the Committee is not then designated or established, within the first two days after it is designated or established.

(3) Where a motion for the consideration of the Senate or the House of Commons to the effect that an order or regulation laid before it pursuant to subsection (1) be revoked or amended, signed by not less than ten members of the Senate or twenty members of the House of Commons, as the case may be, is filed with the Speaker, that House of Parliament shall take up and consider the motion within three sitting days after it is filed.

(4) A motion taken up and considered in accordance with subsection (3) shall be debated without interruption and, at such time as the House is ready for the question, the Speaker shall forthwith, without further debate or amendment, put every question necessary for the disposition of the motion.

(5) If a motion debated in accordance with subsection (4) is adopted by the House, a message shall forthwith be sent from that House informing the other House that the motion has been so adopted and requesting that the motion be concurred in by that other House.

(6) Where a request for concurrence in a motion is made pursuant to subsection (5), the House to which the request is made shall take up and consider the motion within three sitting days after the request is made.

(7) A motion taken up and considered in accordance with subsection (6) shall be debated without interruption and, at such time as the House is ready for the question, the Speaker shall forthwith, without further debate or amendment, put every question necessary for the disposition of the motion.

(8) If a motion taken up and considered in accordance with subsection (6) is concurred in, the order or regulation is revoked or amended in accordance with the motion, effective on the day specified in the motion, which day may not be earlier than the day of the vote of concurrence.

62. (1) The exercise of powers and the performance of duties and functions pursuant to a declaration of emergency shall be reviewed by a committee of both Houses of Parliament designated or established for that purpose.

(2) The Parliamentary Review Committee shall include at least one member of the House of Commons from each party that has a recognized membership of twelve or more persons in that House and at least one senator from each party in

the Senate that is represented on the committee by a member of the House of Commons.

(3) Every member of the Parliamentary Review Committee and every person employed in the work of the Committee shall take the oath of secrecy set out in the schedule.

(4) Every meeting of the Parliamentary Review Committee held to consider an order or regulation referred to it pursuant to subsection 61(2) shall be held in private.

(5) If, within thirty days after an order or regulation is referred to the Parliamentary Review Committee pursuant to subsection 61(2), the Committee adopts a motion to the effect that the order or regulation be revoked or amended, the order or regulation is revoked or amended in accordance with the motion, effective on the day specified in the motion, which day may not be earlier than the day on which the motion is adopted.

(6) The Parliamentary Review Committee shall report or cause to be reported the results of its review under subsection (1) to both Houses of Parliament at least once every sixty days while the declaration of emergency is in effect and, in any case,

(*a*) within three sitting days after a motion for revocation of the declaration is filed under subsection 59(1);

(*b*) within seven sitting days after a proclamation continuing the declaration is issued; and

(*c*) within seven sitting days after the expiration of the declaration or the revocation of the declaration by the Governor in Council.

63. (1) The Governor in Council shall, within sixty days after the expiration or revocation of a declaration of emergency, cause an inquiry to be held into the circumstances that led to the declaration being issued and the measures taken for dealing with the emergency.

(2) A report of an inquiry held pursuant to this section shall be laid before each House of Parliament within three hundred and sixty days after the expiration or revocation of the declaration of emergency.

2.2.1.2 Note on the *War Measures Act*

In 1914, Parliament passed the first *War Measures Act*, which vested in the Governor-in-Council — the Cabinet in other words — substantial powers to enact binding regulations related to the security, defence, peace, order and welfare of Canada. War had been declared by King George V on behalf of the British Empire on Germany on 4 August 1914, and on Austro-Hungary on 12 August 1914.

Section 6 of the bill granted the Governor-in-Council the power to authorize,

...such acts and things, and to make from time to time such orders and regulations, as he may by reason of the existence of real or apprehended war, invasion, or insurrection deem necessary or advisable for the security, defense, peace, order, and welfare of Canada; and for greater certainty, but not so as to restrict the generality of the foregoing terms, it is hereby declared that the powers of the Governor in Council shall extend to all matters hereinafter enumerated...[1]

Six enumerated items included, first,

(a) censorship and the control and suppression of publications, writings, maps, plans, photographs, communications and means of communication;[2]

The *War Measures Act* was given royal assent on August 22. The provisions of s.6, as well as other sections were, by s.3, to be in force only during a state of war, invasion, or insurrection, real or apprehended Section 4 stated that a proclamation by His Majesty, or under the authority of the Governor-in-Council, would be conclusive evidence that war, invasion, or insurrection, real or apprehended, existed and had existed for any period of time stated. It was declared, accordingly, that war had existed since August 4, and that it would be deemed to exist until the Governor-in-Council by a proclamation published in *The Canada Gazette* declared that war no longer existed.

During the whole of the First World War, and for most of the year after it ended the individual and communicative freedoms of many Canadians were limited by executive orders made pursuant to the *War Measures Act*. A large number of ethnic publications, some English-language publications, and, at the end of the war, many publications on the left of the political spectrum were banned.

On 12 September 1914 an Order-in-Council was issued, under the provisions of s.6 of the *War Measures Act*, prohibiting the publication or communication of military information, if the information was calculated to be, or might be directly or indirectly useful to the enemy. A criminal conviction was possible under the order whether or not the information was intended to be useful to the enemy. A test of *mens rea* was not required.

On September 24 an Order-in-Council was issued to provide for the censorship of telephone and telegraphic communication. The Secretary of State became responsible for enforcing this order on 1 November 1915.

The powers of censorship granted to the Postmaster General under the Act were enlarged by another Order-in-Council on 6 November 1914. This order granted the Postmaster General the authority to deny the privileges of the mails and to prevent the circulation or possession of any publication or material he believed,

...contains, has contained or is in the habit of containing articles...bearing directly or indirectly on the present state of war, or on the causes thereof, contrary to the actual facts, and tending directly or indirectly to influence the people of Canada against the cause of the United Kingdom...or in favour of the enemy...[3].

Seventy publications were prohibited by the terms of this order. They were predominantly German-language publications, although they included Russian,

Hungarian, Ukrainian, Croatian, Finnish, Rutherian (a Ukrainian dialect), Yiddish, Syrian, and Hindu publications. Some English-language publications were also banned. The publications prohibited by warrant of the Postmaster General included:

1. Lincoln Freie Press, German-language weekly, Lincoln, Nebraska (withheld 26 June, 1915).
2. The Gaelic American, weekly newspaper, New York, N.Y. (withheld 11 September, 1915).
3. Abendpost, German-language daily, Chicago, Ill. (withheld 25 September, 1915).
4. The King, The Kaiser and Irish Freedom, a book by James McGuire (8 November, 1915).
5. Szabadsag (Liberty), Hungarian daily, Cleveland, Ohio (13 November, 1915).
6. American Independant, weekly, San Francisco (31 January, 1916).
7. Buffalo Volksfreund, German weekly, Buffalo, N.Y. (26 September, 1916).
8. Boston American, weekly, Boston, Mass. (11 November 1916).
9. Narodna Wola, Rutherian tri-weekly, Scanton, Pa. (18 December, 1916).
10. Der Wanderer, German weekly, St. Paul, Minn. (18 December, 1916).

Many of these publications belonged to the American Association of Foreign Language Newspapers, and it was widely believed that the Association was funded by the German and Austrian governments. English-language publications banned under this order included newspapers published by the Hearst syndicate. Some of the papers in the Hearst chain were critical of the British war effort and opposed to American involvement in the war.

In January, 1917, the several orders regarding censorship were collectively repealed and replaced by Consolidated Orders Respecting Censorship, 1917.[4] Besides reaffirming existing powers of censorship, the order further defined objectionable matter. The Chief Press Censor could withold from public consumption material which contained military or strategic information; material that commented unfavourably on the causes or operations of the war, or was intended or likely to cause disaffection to the Crown or to interfere with the success of the armed forces; material purporting to describe or actually describing any secret session of Parliament, or of any meeting of the Cabinet; and any matter dealing with a confidential government document. The writing, printing, publication, posting, circulation or possession of any material considered to belong to a prohibited category became a criminal offense punishable by imprisonment for up to five years and/or a fine of up to $5,000 Any copies of such publications, as well as printing presses, plant and machinery used in their printing, publication, or circulation would be seized.

Between February, 1917 and June, 1918, 81 publications were prohibited. The banning orders were largely directed towards non-English-speaking Canadians, although English-language publications were also seized. Some works prohibited under the consolidated orders included:

1. America's Relations to The Great War, a book by John Williams Burgess, formerly Dean of the Faculties of Political Science, Philosophy, and Pure Science, and professor of constitutional and international law, Columbia University, New York (withheld 7 February 1917).
2. The European War of 1914, Its Causes, Purposes and Probable Results, by John Williams Burgess (withheld 7 July 1917).
3. The Vampire of the Continent, a book by Count Ernest Zu Reventlow, translated from the German, published by The Jackson Press, New York, 1916 (7 February 1917).
4. The New World, a weekly published by The Fatherland Corporation, New York (20 February 1917).
5. The Jewish Morning Journal (The Morgan Journal), a daily newspaper published by the Jewish Press Pub. Co., New York (20 February 1917. Prohibition withdrawn 26 July 1917).
6. Oregon Deutches Zeitung, daily German-language newspaper, Portland, Oregon (20 February 1917).
7. The Minneapolis Freie Presse-Herold, weekly German-language newspaper, Minneapolis, Minn. (20 February 1917)
8. Velykoye Europayskaye Viny (The Great European War), Ukrainian magazine, New York (28 March, 1917).
9. Philadelphia Demokrat, German-language daily newspaper, Philadelphia, Penn (28 March 1917)
10. Blaetter Und Bluten, a book in German, St. Louis, Mo. (18 April 1917).

One other supposed threat to the war effort was the Temperance Movement. The Censor's office, like all other branches of government, encouraged recruitment. Anything that could conceivably interfere with such efforts was subject to censorship and, as a consequence, a number of publications issued by the Temperance Movement were prohibited in the belief that they discouraged enlistment. The Temperance publications condemned the use of alcohol by Canadian troops and claimed that the liquor business was Britain's most dangerous enemy. Whether the purpose of these publications was to attack the Canadian forces or the drink trade was debated in the House of Commons and as a consequence Temperance literature was suppressed after September 1917.

However, the government's fear of information damaging to its recruiting efforts persisted. On 28 March 1918, a protest erupted in Quebec in opposition to the *Military Service Act*. As a consequence, an Order-in-Council was issued on April 16 saying it was illegal to publish, publicly express, or circulate information likely to have an objectionable effect. The effect of a publication rather than its subject matter determined whether an offense had been committed. Publishers could commit an offense without defying a specific prohibition order. A charge against a publication could be made at a local level by a Provincial Attorney General or Municipal Crown Attorney. These new regulations were never used to ban the Quebec nationalist press, although they were inspired by nationalist sentiment, and there was only one reported criminal case concerning a charge of breach of the order.[5]

Sedition charges were laid during the First World War under the Criminal Code. In *R. v. Trainor*[6] a man was convicted of sedition because while sitting in a drug store he said he approved of the sinking of the Lusitania. An appeal was allowed. The Alberta judge remarked that "(t)here had been more prosecutions for seditious words in Alberta in the past two years than in all the history of England for over one hundred years, and England has had numerous and critical wars in that time".

At the close of the war, Canada was confronted with a serious movement of anti-capitalist opinion. The Russian Revolution had made communism a world force, frightening the supporters of the existing system. The Consolidated Orders Respecting Censorship, 1918[7] was substantially the same as the 1917 consolidation except that it increased the emphasis on the prevention of undesirable information and opinion. An Order Respecting Enemy Publications[8] was also issued, followed by the Unlawful Associations order, 1918[9]. Under the terms of the Enemy Publications order, it became an offense to publish, import, or possess any publication printed in an enemy language unless the material was of a literary, scientific, religious or artistic character and did not contain objectionable manner. An enemy language was that of any country at war with Great Britain or in whole or in part occupied by a state at war with Great Britain. Enemy languages included German, Hungarian, Bulgarian, Turkish, Romanian, Russian, Ukrainian, Finnish, Srian, Croatian, Rutherian and Livonian (Latvian). Organizations outlawed by the Unlawful Associations order included:

The Industrial Workers of the World
The Russian Social Democratic Party
The Russian Revolutionary Group
The Russian Social Revolutions
The Russian Workers Union
The Ukrainian Revolutionary Group
The Ukrainian Social Democratic Party
The Social Democratic Party
The Social Labour Party
Group of Social Democrats of Bolsheviki
Group of Social Democrats of Anarchists
The Workers International Union
Chinese Nationalist League

Chinese Labour Association
The Finnish Social Democratic Party
The Revolutionary Socialist Party of North America

The government also directed its efforts against a perceived Bolshevik menace rather than the threat of enemy propaganda. Under the Consolidated Orders Respecting Censorship, 1918, examples of banned publications were:

1. The Morning messenger, English-language journal, Winnipeg, Manitoba (withheld 15 June 1918).
2. The Labour Defender, an English-language by-weekly pub. by the 1. W. W. Defense Committee, New York (10 July 1918).

All publications by the Industrial Workers of the World were prohibited by 2 October 1918.

3. To The Young Workers, a pamphlet in Russian by A. Karelyn, pub. by The Union of Russian Workmen, New York (21 September 1918).
4. Rabotchyj Narod (The Working People), newspaper, Winnipeg, Manitoba (21 September 1918).
5. The Canadian Forward, a monthly in English, edited by Isaac Bainbridge, Toronto, Ontario (2 October 1918).
6. The Western Clarion, a monthly in English, pub. by the Socialist Party of Canada, Vancouver, B.C. (5 October 1918).

The *Unlawful Associations Order* was repealed in April of 1919 and replaced by s.99 of the *Criminal Code*.[1] The government's power to create such orders and regulations under the *War Measures Act* ceased with the issuance of the *Treaty of Peace (Germany) Order, 1920*.

. . . . .

The 1914 *War Measures Act* was consolidated with little change in the Revised Statutes of 1927. By 1938, when hopes for peace had faded, an Interdepartmental Committee on Emergency Legislation was created to examine the legal capacity of the Ministry to take additional measures to protect the state in the event of war.[11] Some months later the committee announced:

> Pursuant to our terms of reference we have surveyed the position as regards the legislation which would be required in the event of grave emergency and we have reached the conclusion that little in the way of special legislation in Parliament will be required. Under the provisions of the War Measures Act, Chapter 206, Revised Statutes of Canada. 1927, the Governor in Council may do and authorize such acts and things, and make from time to time such orders and regulations as he may by reason of real or apprehended war, invasion or insurrection deem necessary or advisable for the security, defence, peace, order and welfare of Canada;. . .It is clear, therefore. that this statute confers upon the Executive ample authority to take pretty well whatever action might be found to be necessary to meet the exigencies of war or other emergency.[12]

On 1 September 1939, the *War Measures Act* was renewed by proclamation and made retroactive to August 25. The legality of the Act had already been affirmed by the courts.[13] The Defence of Canada regulations were drawn up by an interdepartmental committee during the spring of 1939, and were approved by Cabinet. On September 3, under the *War Measures Act*, they were instituted.[14]

Despite the fact that Parliament met from September 7 through September 13 the regulations were not discussed. Parliament did not meet again for ordinary business until 16 May 1940. During the following winter and election campaign, the opposition parties attacked Mr. King and his colleagues as autocratic and dictatorial. A select committee on the Defence of Canada regulations was created on 13 June 1940. The regulations established new prohibitions enforceable by the courts and conferred extraordinary powers on the executive who were made immune from judicial review. New limits were imposed on freedom of speech and the press by regulation 39. The original rule stated:

39. No person shall by word of mouth: —
a) spread reports or make statements, false or otherwise, intended or likely to cause disaffection to His Majesty or to interfere with the success of His Majesty's forces or of the forces of any allied or associated Powers or to prejudice His Majesty's relations with foreign powers, or
b) spread reports or make statements, false or otherwise, intended or likely to prejudice the recruiting, training, discipline, or administration of any of His Majesty's forces.

Some weeks later, regulation 39A was included. It provided:

39A. No person shall print, make, publish, issue, circulate or distribute any book, card, letter, writing, print, publication or document of any kind containing any material, report or statement,
a) intended or likely to cause disaffection to His Majesty or to interfere with the success of His Majesty's forces or of the forces of any allied or associated powers, or to prejudice His Majesty's relations with foreign powers;
b) intended or likely to prejudice the recruiting, training, discipline or administration of any of His Majesty's troops; or
c) intended or likely to be prejudicial to the safety of the State or the efficient prosecution of the war.[15]

It was later added that it would be a defence against such a prosecution to prove that the accused had intended not to aid or comfort the enemy, but merely to participate in the ordinary political processes.[16] Regulation 39B(2) provided that it was a defence to prove that the accused intended in good faith merely to criticize or point out errors or defects in the government, legislature, or administration of justice. However, the view of the court in one of the few reported cases under this regulation appeared to withdraw the protection afforded by the section.[17] The defendant was a high school teacher who, during a current events discussion in his classroom, expressed pacifist opinions. The court examined his teaching technique and found that students were encouraged to accept no point of view at face value. There was no evidence to show that any student was influenced by the defendant's contributions to the discussion and that his statements were either intended or likely to interfere with the prosecution of the war. However, the court claimed that the intention of the regulations was to compel individuals to maintain silence or speak in the unconquerable spirit by which troops in action must be moved if they are to win.

The first restrictions on association were made by the execution of regulation 39C on 8 June 1940. Any association, society, group or organization which the Governor-in-Council declared to be illegal became so upon notice published in *The Canada Gazette*. Any person associated with such an organization became guilty of an offense. Guilty persons could be those who attended a meeting of an illegal organization, spoke publicly in advocacy of the organization, or distributed literature of an illegal organization. Outlawed groups were not just German or fascist. By 8 June 1940 the following societies had been declared illegal:

The Auslands Organization of the National Sozialistische Deutsche Arbeitpartei
The Deutsche Arbeitsfront
The Canadian Society for German Culture
The National Unity Party
The Canadian Union of Fascists
The Communist Party of Canada
The Young Communist League of Canada
The Canadian Labour Defence League
The League for Peace and Democracy
The Ukrainian Labour Farmer Temple Association
The Finnish Organization of Canada
The Russian Workers and Fanners Club
The Polish People's Association
The Canadian Ukrainian Youth Federation

The Ukrainian Labour Farmer Temple Association was declared illegal on the theory that it was being used for anti-war propaganda by the Communist Party. So far as the published expressions of the Association's periodicals go there appeared to be no basis for this belief. One hundred and eight pieces of property, mostly halls and meeting places in more Canadian cities, towns and villages, were seized by the R.C.M.P. under the authority of the Custodian of Alien Enemy Property Act and sold, many at fire sale prices and often to a rival Ukrainian society. On 12 June 1940, more groups were banned:

Italian Fascio Abroad
O.V.R.A., Opere Voluntere Repressione Anti-Fascislo (national Organization for the Repression of Anti-Facism)
Dopolavoro (After Work Organization).
Associazione Combattenti Italiani (Italian War Veterans' Association)

The Jehovah's Witnesses were banned on 4 July 1940. In one case arising out of the ban, a Jehovah's Witness was convicted for making statements prejudicial to the safety of the State. He had complained about the expulsion of his children from school for refusing to salute the flag or sing the national anthem. His letter to the school administration explained why his religion quashed the conviction and held that what the accused wrote was neither intended or likely to affect the prosecution of the war, nor was it addressed to the general public.

The following groups were banned on 29 August 1940:

The Workers and Farmers Publishing Association
The Road Publishing Company
The Croatian Publishing Company
The Polish People's Press
The Serbian Publishing Association
The Finnish Society of Toronto

In further recognition of the ban on Jehovah's Witnesses, on 19 January 1941, the Watch Tower Bible and Tract Society and the International Bible Students' Association were also declared illegal.

Regulations 39 and 39A had a chilling effect on the ordinary complaints and grumblings of many Canadians. Between three to four hundred prosecutions had been initiated by the winter of 1941. The courts, who were often zealous in returning convictions, commonly sentenced offenders to six months imprisonment for prohibited oral utterances. The Minister of Justice explained in the House that,

> Some joyous friend may imbibe a little too much liquor in a tavern and think it smart, for instance, to say that the Germans are better soldiers than the British, or something like that. Such a man should not be treated as a real enemy who is plotting against the state. There the summary conviction (carrying a lighter maximum sentence) applies. But when a case is serious the prosecution should be by way of indictment, and I believe that the choice should be left to the Minister of Justice or the attorney general.[18]

Regulation 15 of the *Defence of Canada Regulations* empowered the Secretary of State to make orders,

> ...for preventing or restricting the publication in Canada of matters as to which he is satisfied that the publication, or, as the case may be, the unrestricted publication, thereof would or might be prejudicial to the safety of the State or the efficient prosecution of the war.

The suppression of material deemed to be hazardous to state security was widespread. By 27 March 1941, 325 periodicals had been suppressed or banned. The quantity of outlawed publications and some reported cases suggest that prosecution under these regulations was not limited to those reasonably understood to be a threat to the war effort. Most of the newspapers banned were foreign-language papers:

1. Gudok (The Canadian Whistle), Russian published in Winnipeg, Manitoba (withheld 28 March 1940).
2. Hlas L'Udu, Slovak, published by Hlas L'Udu Publishing Association, Toronto (withheld 6 July 1940).
3. Jiskra, Czech, published in Toronto (withheld 31 July 1940).
4. Glos Pracy, Polish, published by the Polish People's Press, Toronto (withheld 17 August 1940).

5. Der Zeg, Yiddish (withheld 17 August 1940).

Left-wing publications were outlawed. *The Clarion*, a Communist Party newspaper with a circulation of approximately 12,000 was banned along with nine other publications. The *Canadian Tribune* of Toronto, a successor to the banned *Clarion* was suspended for three weeks. The Communist Party of Canada was outlawed under regulation 39C. Regulation 21, which dealt with the internment of citizens of Canada to forestall acts of assistance to the enemy, was used to prosecute John A. (Pat) Sullivan, at the time considered to be the leading member of the Party.[19]

The House of Commons eventually decided to review the Defence of Canada regulations by selecting a committee composed of representatives from each party in proportion to their membership in the House. They were to inspect the provisions and operations of the regulations. Three years of meetings were held *in camera*. Criticism came chiefly from members of the C.C.F., who claimed that the regulations were too vague and contained inadequate safeguards against error. T.C. Douglas argued that newspapers could be suppressed without a hearing under regulation 15. He stated that organizations such as Jehovah's Witnesses and Technocracy Incorporated (banned 30 June 1941), whose subversive tendencies were not self-evident, had been outlawed under regulation 39C without any adequate explanation.[20] C.C.F. leader M.J. Coldwell said that the committee had two approaches to the regulations. "Some took the view that the regulations and final decisions should be administrative matters. Whilst the majority in both years took that view, a minority was of the opinion that the procedure should more nearly approximate a judicial procedure, and that at least the final decisions ought not be left to the minister and his advisers. Because what I may call the administrative view prevailed, to that extent I was not able to approve the report.[21]

The committee suggested the addition of the words "have knowingly in his possession in quantity" to regulation 39A. This was adopted by the Privy Council on 12 September 1940.[22]

In *R. v. Money* the possession of three or four copies of an illegal publication was ruled not sufficient for a conviction.[23] Furthermore, a bookstore or library which possessed works believed likely to be prejudicial to the safety of the state was not to be convicted if the number of copies was limited.[24]

The report of the committee concerning outlawed organizations was not welcomed by the government. Its main suggestion was that certain organizations cease to be illegal. These groups were the Communist Party of Canada, the Ukrainian Farmer Temple Association, the Finnish Organization of Canada, Technocracy Incorporated and the various Jehovah's Witnesses organizations. The recommendation that Jehovah's Witnesses and Technocracy Incorporated be dropped from the regulation 39C list was expressed unanimously by the committee. The Jehovah's Witnesses were viewed simply as an over-zealous religious organization and not a danger to the war effort. No member of the

House moved the acceptance of the report when it was tabled and the government did not heed its advice. The Minister of Justice moved that the committee be appointed again in 1943. A member complained that "there is little use in setting up a committee of responsible members of this House to deal with questions of this kind if the government or Parliament is not going to give [more] consideration to its report than was given to the report made by the committee of last year".[25] The Minister was asked what harm would be done by removing the Communist Party from the 39C list. He replied that to propagate doctrines espoused by members of the Communist Party constituted sedition under the Criminal Code and the organization must remain outlawed.

In 1943, in spite of vigorous protests by the C.C.F., the new committee busied itself with matters concerned with naturalization and deportation and did not discuss the Defence of Canada regulations. On 14 October 1943, the Ukrainian Labour Farmer Temple Association, the Finnish Organization of Canada, Technocracy Incorporated and the Jehovah's Witnesses groups were once again legal. The emergency powers available during wartime were exercised for a certain time after the war for the sake of an orderly transition from war to pace. Regulations 15, 39, 39A, 39B and 39C were revoked on 16 August 1945.

The remarks of Mr. Coldwell in the House of Commons, 20 May 1940, may be cited as indicative of criticism against the extreme censorship powers contained in the Defence of Canada regulations: "We are prepared to support the struggle against aggression and for the preservation of democratic institutions, but we insist that democratic institutions be respected and safeguarded in our own country. . . Ever since the outbreak of war we have been governed by decree, largely in secrecy."[26]

Endnotes

1. *An Act to confer certain powers upon the Governor-in-Council and to amend the Immigration Act*, S.C. 1914, c. 6, s.6.
2. *Ibid.*, s.6(a).
3. P.C. 94, November 6, 1914, s.1.
4. P.C. 146, January 17, 1917.
5. *R. v. Watson* (1918), 15 O.W.N. 417 (S.C.O.).
6. [1917] 1 W.W.R. 415 (Alta. C.A.)
7. P.C. 1241, May 22, 1918.
8. P.C. 2381, September 25, 1918.
9. P.C. 2384, September 28, 1918.
10. *Statutes of Canada*, 1919.
11. Established by P.C. 531, March 14, 1938.

12. Report of the Interdepartmental Committee on Emergency Legislation, July, 1939.
13. *Fort Frances Pulp and Power Co. v. Manitoba Free Press Co.*, [1923] A.C. 695.
14. P.C. 2483, September 3, 1939.
15. P.C. 2891, September 27, 1939.
16. P.C. 146, January 14, 1940.
17. *R. v. Coffin*, [1940] 2 W.W.R. 592 (Alta. Pol. Ct.)
18. House of Commons Debates, Hansard, 1940 at p. 745.
19. *Ex parte Sullivan*, [1941] 1 D.L.R. 676.
20. Mr. T.C. Douglas 19:2, pp. 1188, 1189, March 3, 1941.
21. Mr. M.J. Coldwell 19:2, p. 3658, June 9, 1941.
22. P.C. 4750, September 12, 1940.
23. [1941] 1 W.W.R. 93 (B.C. Pol. Ct.).
24. *R. v. Ravenor*, [1941] 1 W.W.R. 191.
25. Mr. Angus MacInnis 9:4, p. 606, February 22, 1943.
26. Mr. M.J. Coldwell 9:1, p. 51, May 20, 1940.

2.2.2 Official Secrets

2.2.2.1 *Official Secrets Act*, R.S.C. 1985, c. O-5

3. (1) Every person is guilty of an offence under this Act who, for any purpose prejudicial to the safety or interests of the State,

(*a*) approaches, inspects, passes over, or is in the neighbourhood of, or enters any prohibited place;

(*b*) makes any sketch, plan, model or note that is calculated to be or might be or is intended to be directly or indirectly useful to a foreign power; or

(*c*) obtains, collects, records, or publishes, or communicates to any other person any secret official code word, or pass word, or any sketch, plan, model, article, or note, or other document of information that is calculated to be or might be or is intended to be directly or indirectly useful to a foreign power.

(2) On a prosecution under this section, it is not necessary to show that the accused person was guilty of any particular act tending to show a purpose prejudicial to the safety or interests of the State, and, notwithstanding that no such act is proved against him, he may be convicted if, from the circumstances of the case, or his conduct, or his known character as proved, it appears that his purpose was a purpose prejudicial to the safety or interests of the State; and if any sketch, plan, model, article, note, document or information relating to or used in any prohibited place, or anything in such a place, or any secret official

code word or pass word is made, obtained, collected, recorded, published or communicated by any person other than a person acting under lawful authority, it shall be deemed to have been made, obtained, collected, recorded, published or communicated for a purpose prejudicial to the safety or interests of the State unless the contrary is proved.

(3) In any proceedings against a person for an offence under this section, the fact that he has been in communication with, or attempted to communicate with, an agent of a foreign power, whether within or outside Canada, is evidence that he has, for a purpose prejudicial to the safety or interests of the State, obtained or attempted to obtain information that is calculated to be or might be or is intended to be directly or indirectly useful to a foreign power.

(4) For the purpose of this section, but without prejudice to the generality of the foregoing provision
   (*a*) a person shall, unless he proves the contrary, be deemed to have been in communication with an agent of a foreign power if
      (i) he has. either within or outside Canada, visited the address of an agent of a foreign power or consorted or associated with such agent, or
      (ii) either within or outside Canada, the name or address of, or any other information regarding such an agent has been found in his possession, or has been supplied by him to any other person, or has been obtained by him from any other person;
   (*b*) "an agent of a foreign power" includes any person who is or has been or is reasonably suspected of being or having been employed by a foreign power either directly or indirectly for the purpose of committing an act, either within or outside Canada, prejudicial to the safety or interests of the State, or who has or is reasonably suspected of having, either within or outside Canada, committed, or attempted to commit, such an act in the interests of a foreign power; and
   (*c*) any address, whether within or outside Canada, reasonably suspected of being an address used for the receipt of communications intended for an agent of a foreign power, or any address at which such an agent resides, or to which he resorts for the purpose of giving or receiving communications, or at which he carries on any business, shall be deemed to be the address of an agent of a foreign power, and communications addressed to such an address to be communications with such an agent.

4. (1) Every person is guilty of an offence under this Act who, having in his possession or control any secret official code word, or pass word, or any sketch, plan, model, article, note, document or information that relates to or is used in a prohibited place or anything in such a place, or that has been made or obtained in contravention of this Act, or that has been entrusted in confidence to him by any person holding office under Her Majesty, or that he has obtained or to which he has had access while subject to the Code of Service Discipline within the meaning of the *National Defence Act* or owing to his position as a person who holds or has held office under Her Majesty, or as a person who holds or has held a contract made on behalf of Her Majesty, or a contract the performance of which in whole or in part is carried out in a prohibited place, or as a person who is or has been employed under a person who holds or has held such an office or contract,

    (*a*) communicates the code word, pass word, sketch, plan, model, article, note, document or information to any person, other than a person to whom he is authorized to communicate with, or a person to whom it is in the interest of the State his duty to communicate it;

    (*b*) uses the information in his possession for the benefit of any foreign power or in any other manner prejudicial to the safety or interests of the State;

    (*c*) retains the sketch, plan, model, article, note, or document in his possession or control when he has no right to retain it or when it is contrary to his duty to retain it or fails to comply with all directions issued by lawful authority with regard to the return or disposal thereof; or

    (*d*) fails to take reasonable care of, or so conducts himself as to endanger the safety of the sketch, plan, model, article, note, document, secret official code word or pass word or information.

(2) Every person is guilty of an offence under this Act who, having in his possession or control any sketch, plan, model, article, note, document or information that relates to munitions of war, communicates it directly or indirectly to any foreign power, or in any other manner prejudicial to the safety or interests of the State.

(3) Every person who receives any secret official code word, or pass word, or sketch, plan, model, article, note, document or information, knowing, or having reasonable ground to believe, at the time when he receives it, that the code word, pass word, sketch, plan, model, article, note, document or information is communicated to him in contravention of this Act, is guilty of an offence under this Act, unless he proves that the communication to him of the code word, pass word, sketch, plan, model, article, note, document or information was contrary to his desire.

(4) Every person is guilty of an offence under this Act who

    (*a*) retains for any purpose prejudicial to the safety or interests of the State any official document, whether or not completed or issued for use, when he has no right to retain it, or when it is contrary to his duty to retain it, or fails to comply with any directions issued by any Government department or any person authorized by such department with regard to the return or disposal thereof; or

    (*b*) allows any other person to have possession of any official document issued for his use alone, or communicates any secret official code word or pass word so issued, or, without lawful authority or excuse, has in his possession any official document or secret official code word or pass word issued for the use of some person other than himself, or on obtaining possession of any official document by finding or otherwise, neglects or fails to restore it to the person or authority by whom or for whose use it was issued, or to a police constable.

7. (1) Where it appears to the Minister of Justice that such a course is expedient in the public interest, he may, by warrant under his hand, require any person who owns or controls any telegraphic cable or wire, or any apparatus for wireless telegraphy, used for the sending or receipt of telegrams to or from any place out of Canada, to produce to him, or to any person named in the warrant, the originals and transcripts, either of all telegrams, or of telegrams of any specified class or description, or of telegrams sent from or addressed to any specified person or place, sent to or received from any place out of Canada by means of any such cable, wire, or apparatus and all other papers relating to any such telegram as aforesaid.

(2) Every person who, on being required to produce any such original or transcript or paper as aforesaid, refuses or neglects to do so is guilty of an offence under this Act, and is for each offence, liable on summary conviction to imprisonment, with or without hard labour, for a term not exceeding three months, or to a fine not exceeding two hundred dollars, or to both imprisonment and fine.

8. Every person who knowingly harbours any person whom he knows, or has reasonable grounds for supposing, to be a person who is about to commit or who has committed an offence under this Act, or knowingly permits to meet or assemble in any premises in his occupation or under his control any such persons, and every person who, having harboured any such person, or permitted any such persons to meet or assemble in any premises in his occupation or under his control, wilfully omits or refuses to disclose to a senior police officer any information that it is in his power to give in relation to any such person, is guilty of an offence under this Act.

9. Every person who attempts to commit any offence under this Act, or solicits or incites or endeavours to persuade another person to commit an offence, or aids or abets and does any act preparatory to the commission of an offence under this Act, is guilty of an offence under this Act and is liable to the same punishment, and to be proceeded against in the same manner, as if he had committed the offence.

10. Every person who is found committing an offence under this Act, or who is reasonably suspected of having committed, or having attempted to commit, or being about to commit, such an offence, may be arrested without, a warrant and detained by any constable or police officer.

11. (1) If a justice of the peace is satisfied by information on oath that there is reasonable ground for suspecting that an offence under this Act has been or is about to be committed, he may grant a search warrant authorizing any constable named therein, to enter at any time any premises or place named in the warrant, if necessary by force, and to search the premises or place and every person found therein, and to seize any sketch, plan, model, article, note or document, or anything that is evidence of an offence under this Act having been or being about to be committed, that he may find on the premises or place or on any such person, and with regard to or in connection with which he has reasonable ground for suspecting that an offence under this Act has been or is about to be committed.

(2) Where it appears to an officer of the Royal Canadian Mounted Police not below the rank of superintendent that the case is one of great emergency and that in the interest of the State immediate action is necessary, he may by a written order under his hand give to any constable the like authority as may be given by the warrant of a justice under this section.

14. (1) For the purposes of the trial of a person for an offence under this Act, the offence shall be deemed to have been committed either at the place in which the offence actually was committed, or at any place in Canada in which the offender may be found

(2) In addition and without prejudice to any powers that a court may possess to order the exclusion of the public from any proceedings if, in the course of proceedings before a court against any person for an offence under this Act or the proceedings on appeal, application is made by the prosecution, on the ground that the publication of any evidence to be given or of any statement to be made in the course of the proceedings would be prejudicial to the interest of the State, that all or any portion of the public shall be excluded during any part of the hearing. the court may make an order to that effect, but the passing of sentence shall in any case take place in public.

15. (1) Where no specific penalty is provided in this Act, any person who is guilty of an offence under this Act shall be deemed to be guilty of an indictable offence and is, on conviction, punishable by imprisonment for a term not exceeding fourteen years; but such person may, at the election of the Attorney General, be prosecuted summarily in the manner provided by the provisions of the Criminal Code relating to summary convictions, and, if so prosecuted, is punishable by a fine not exceeding five hundred dollars, or by imprisonment not exceeding twelve months, or by both.

2.2.2.2 Walter Tarnopolsky, "Freedom of the Press," in Newspapers and the Law (Ottawa: Ministry of Supply and Services Canada, 1981), pp. 19-21

Before discussing the Canadian *Official Secrets Act*, a consideration of the United Kingdom experience is enlightening. The first *Official Secrets Act* in the United Kingdom was enacted in 1889, apparently in reaction to a publication by a newspaper of the particulars of a secret treaty negotiated between England and

Russia which was given to it by the government clerk whose job it was to copy the document. The government tried to prosecute the clerk for removing a state document, but was not successful because no document was stolen. An attempt was made to fill the gap by passing the Act, which made it a crime, *inter alia*, for a person wrongfully to communicate information which had been obtained while working as a civil servant. The Act used the standard criminal law approach of placing the burden of proof on the prosecution and defining the offences with considerable particularity.

Subsequently, in 1909, a German secret service officer came to London and openly admitted recruiting people for an espionage system for all of England. The government was advised that there was no offence for which he could be arrested. The result was the passing of a new *Official Secrets Act* in 1911, by which the onus of proof was shifted strongly against the accused. The Act made it a felony for any purpose prejudicial to the safety or interest of the state for anyone to approach any military or naval installation or other prohibited place, or to obtain or communicate information, or make a sketch or note, which might help an enemy. The Act also made it a misdemeanor for a person, having any information mentioned, or information entrusted in confidence by an officer of the Crown, or which was obtained as a Crown servant, to communicate that information to an unauthorized person, or to retain a sketch or other document, without any right to do so. Also, anyone receiving such document or information could be found guilty unless he proved that the communication to him was contrary to his desire. In the light of wartime experience, a new Act was enacted in 1920. Among other amendments, the new Act made it a felony to do any act preparatory to the commission of a felony under the Act.

It is particularly worthy of note that *Official Secrets Acts* are deliberately intended to cover more than just protection of national or state security; they are framed so widely as to cover all kinds of official information unrelated to security.

Soon after the enactment of the *Official Secrets Act* of 1911, the government of the United Kingdom sought means of clarifying the position of the press with respect to publication of sensitive information. The solution was to set up, in 1912, a committee (now known as the Services, Press and Broadcasting Committee) consisting of a majority of press and broadcasting members, along with the permanent secretaries (deputy ministers) of the various defence ministries. The object of the Committee is to let the press know unofficially when an offence could be committed under the *Official Secrets Acts* without risk of prosecution. What is involved are what are known as the "D" Notices.

The "D" Notice, which relates to defence matters "the publication of which would be prejudicial to the national interest", indicates what the government is willing to have the communications media publish or broadcast on security matters and what it does not wish the media to use, with the unofficial assurance that there will be no prosecution under the Acts as long as the press and broadcasting bodies comply. The system worked secretly and informally. On the one hand a minister could ignore the Committee; on the other, the press could ignore the "D" notice. It was not until 1961 when George Blake, an agent both for the British and the Russians, was convicted under the *Official Secrets Acts* that existence of the Committee first came to public notice.

In Canada we do not have "D" Notice arrangements, but we do have an *Official Secrets Act*. In fact, the first one was enacted in 1890, just a year after the *United Kingdom Act*. It was passed at the request of the United Kingdom and was almost verbatim copy. Two years later, the provisions of the Canadian Act were transferred to the first Canadian Criminal Code, where they remained until the enactment of a new *Official Secrets Act* in 1939. However, both the 1889 and 1911 *Official Secrets Acts* of the United Kingdom had specifically applied not just to the United Kingdom but to the overseas Dominions as well. Since the 1920 Act was specifically devised not to apply to the Dominions, and since Canada did not have an *Official Secrets Act* in the 20th century until 1939, the 1911 Act of the United Kingdom and the Canadian Criminal Code provisions were in force in this country. When the 1939 Act was drafted, it was in effect a combination of the 1911 and 1920 *United Kingdom Acts*.

The *Official Secrets Act* is somewhat difficult to read, in that the attempt has been to cast a wide enough net while not being too vague. Essentially it covers two distinct, if somewhat similar, activities: spying (Section 3), and wrongful communication of government information, or leakage (Section 4).

It is Section 4 which is of main concern to the press. Rather than quote its terms, which can be consulted in the statute books, it would be more instructive to quote the description of the "catch-all" nature of this section provided by the United Kingdom Franks Committee on the *Official Secrets Act* of 1911:

> The leading characteristic of this offence is its catch-all quality. It catches all official documents and information. It makes no distinctions of kind. and no distinctions of degree. All information which a Crown servant learns in the course of his duty is "official" for the purposes of section 2. whatever its nature, whatever its importance, whatever its original source. A blanket it thrown over everything; nothing escapes. The section catches all Crown servants as well as all official information. Again, it makes no distinctions according to the nature or importance of a Crown servant's duties. All are covered. Every Minister of the Crown, every civil servant, every member of the Armed Forces, every police officer, performs his duties subject to section 2.

What is equally important for the press is that Subsection (3) of Section 4 provides that:

> Every person who receives any...information, knowing, or having reasonable ground to believe, at the time when he receives it, that the...information is communicated to him in contravention of this Act, is guilty of an offence under this Act unless he proves that the communication to him of the...information was contrary to his desire.

Professor Friedland reports that of the 21 prosecutions under the 1939 *Official Secrets Act*, some 17 were concerned with the Gouzenko affair, just after the Second World War. Since then there have been only four. Two of these were concerned with Section 3, the espionage section, and so are not relevant to our topic. The third was the recent *Treu* case which, although under the leakage of information section (Section 4), is also not relevant since it concerned retaining classified documents and failing to take reasonable care of such documents. The fourth case is of direct concern because it involved the Toronto *Sun*. The *Sun* had published a document which had outlined suspected Russian spying activities in Canada, and which had been designated as "top secret". Charges were brought against both the publisher and the editor under Section 4 of the Act. However, at the preliminary inquiry stage, Judge Waisberg of the Ontario Provincial Court concluded that earlier disclosures had "brought the document, now 'shopworn' and no longer secret, into the public domain". He concluded that the document, even if it had ever been secret, was no longer so.

Although the approach taken by Judge Waisberg may be welcome to the press, there may be some question whether higher courts, if the case had been appealed, would have upheld such an interpretation; that is, it is not an offence to publish information, merely because some parts of it had been improperly leaked. It is interesting to note that the United Kingdom White Paper, in proposing amendments to the Act following the Franks Committee report, recommended that although the "mere receipt of protected information" should not be a criminal offence, communication by the recipient should be.

2.2.2.3 Law Reform Commission of Canada, *Crimes Against the State*, Working Paper 49 (Ottawa: 1986), pp. 30, 33-34

The worst examples of complexity and excess detail, however, are to be found in the *O.S.A.*, an Act which can fairly be condemned as one of the poorest examples of legislative drafting in the statute books. The Act only deals with leakage — and espionage-related offences: section 3, the spying offence proper, contains a long list of proscribed conduct; section 4 deals at length with wrongful communication or use of information, and then sets out three additional specific offences; sections 5, 6, 8 and 9 create further spying-related offences. All of these provisions are long-winded, some with sentences of over one hundred and fifty words in length, and many are incomprehensible. The O.S.A. devotes several pages and over a thousand words to espionage-related offences whereas the *Criminal Code* manages to say perhaps all that needs to be said about the offence of spying in one short paragraph (s.46(2)(b)). Despite all the detail and complexity, the O.S.A. espionage offences are no more precise than paragraph 46(2)(b) of the *Code*; indeed, their exact scope remains unclear.[1]

. . . . .

Finally there are specific problems of uncertainty that arise only in the O.S.A. Two examples will suffice. Foremost is the difficulty in ascertaining whether the Act is meant to apply only to secret and official information or to any kind of information. The statute itself offers conflicting possibilities. Legislative history suggests that the Act was not meant to be limited to secret and official information and that the words "secret official" were not meant to qualify the entire list of items protected, but only "code word" and "password." On the other hand, the title of the Act and the fact these two words appear at the beginning of the list of items ("secret official code word, or password, or any sketch, plan, model, article, or note, or other document or information") covered in the Act, suggest that only secret official information was meant to be protected by the Act. It is an indication of the uncertainty as to the intended meaning of the *O.S.A.* that the Quebec Court of Appeal held that it applied to secret and official information only, whereas the Franks Committee concluded that the English Act had much wider application, with the words "secret and official" only qualifying "code word or password," and not the other items listed. Clearly, this is a matter of such critical importance that it should only be settled by Parliament, not the courts.

The last (and equally unresolvable) example of the problem of uncertainty is found in section 8 of the *O.S.A.* which rather cryptically makes it an offence to "willfully omit or refuse to disclose to a senior police officer" certain information that one has about suspected spies. The phrase "willfully omit . . . to disclose" is ambiguous. Does it impose an affirmative duty to seek out and inform the senior police officer, or is one only bound to disclose information if one is actually being questioned? Clearly, such an exceptional duty to inform the police about suspected criminals should be worded in unequivocal language, so that people can know the extent of their criminal liability.

NOTE: The O.S.A. presented no serious impediments to the prosecution of Morrison (Long Knife). Because of the strong evidence against him he had confessed his crime in a television interview. On January 23, 1986, he pleaded guilty to violating O.S.A. paragraph 3(1)(c). See also *Re Regina and Morrison* (1984), 47 O.R. (2d) 185 (Ont. H.C.), appeal dismissed October 17, 1984.

2.3 Access to Information

2.3.1 *Access to Information Act*, R.S.C. 1985, c. A-1

2. (1) The purpose of this Act is to extend the present laws of Canada to provide a right of access to information in records under the control of a government institution in accordance with the principles that government information should be available to the public, that necessary exceptions to the right of access should be limited and specific and that decisions on the disclosure of government information should be reviewed independently of government.

(2) This Act is intended to complement and not replace existing procedures for access to government information and is not intended to limit in any way access to the type of government information that is normally available to the general public.

4. (1) Subject to this Act, but notwithstanding any other Act of Parliament, every person who is (*a*) a Canadian citizen, or

(*b*) a permanent resident within the meaning of the Immigration Act. 1976, has a right to and shall, on request, be given access to any record under the control of a government institution.

(2) The Governor in Council may, by order, extend the right to be given access to records under subsection (1) to include persons not referred to in that subsection and may set such conditions as the Governor in Council deems appropriate.

(3) For the purposes of this Act, any record requested under this Act that does not exist but can, subject to such limitations as may be prescribed by regulation, be produced from a machine readable record under the control of a government institution using computer hardware and software and technical expertise normally used by the government institution shall be deemed to be a record under the control of the government institution.

10. (1) Where the head of a government institution refuses to give access to a record requested under this Act or a part thereof, the head of the institution shall state in the notice given under paragraph 7(a)

(*a*) that the record does not exist, or

(*b*) the specific provision of this Act on which the refusal was based or, where the head of the institution does not indicate whether a record exists, the provision on which a refusal could reasonably be expected to be based if the record existed,

and shall state in the notice that the person who made the request has a right to make a complaint to the Information Commissioner about the refusal.

13. (1) Subject to subsection (2), the head of a government institution shall refuse to disclose any record requested under this Act that contains information that was obtained in confidence from

(*a*) the government of a foreign state or an institution thereof;

(*b*) an international organization of states or an institution thereof;

(*c*) the government of a province or an institution thereof; or

(*d*) a municipal or regional government established by or pursuant to an Act of the legislature of a province or an institution of such a government.

(2) The head of a government institution may disclose any record requested under this Act that contains information described in subsection (1) if the government, organization or institution from which the information was obtained

(*a*) consents to the disclosure; or

(*b*) makes the information public.

14. The head of a government institution may refuse to disclose any record requested under this Act that contains information the disclosure of which could reasonably be expected to be injurious to the conduct by the Government of Canada of federal provincial affairs, including. without restricting the generality of the foregoing, any such information

(a) on federal-provincial consultations or deliberations; or

(b) on strategy or tactics adopted or to be adopted by the Government of Canada relating to the conduct of federal-provincial affairs.

15. (1) The head of a government institution may refuse to disclose any record requested under this Act that contains information the disclosure of which could reasonably be expected to be injurious to the conduct of international affairs, the defence of Canada or any state allied or associated with Canada or the detection, prevention or suppression of subversive or hostile activities, including, without restricting the generality of the foregoing, any such information

(a) relating to military tactics or strategy, or relating to military exercises or operations undertaken in preparation for hostilities or in connection with the detection, prevention or suppression of subversive or hostile activities;

(b) relating to the quantity, characteristics, capabilities or deployment of weapons or other defence equipment or of anything being designed, developed, produced or considered for use as weapons or other defence equipment;

(c) relating to the characteristics, capabilities, performance, potential, deployment, functions or role of any defence establishment, of any military force, unit or personnel or of any organization or person responsible for the detection, prevention or suppression of subversive or hostile activities;

(d) obtained or prepared for the purpose of intelligence relating to

(i) the defence of Canada or any state allied or associated with Canada, or

(ii) the detection, prevention or suppression of subversive or hostile activities;

(e) obtained or prepared for the purpose of intelligence respecting foreign states, international organizations of states or citizens of foreign states used by the Government of Canada in the process of deliberation and consultation or in the conduct of international affairs;

(f) on methods of, and scientific or technical equipment for, collecting, assessing or handling information referred to in paragraph (a) or (e) or on sources of such information;

(g) on the positions adopted or to be adopted by the Government of Canada, governments of foreign states or international organizations of states for the purpose of present or future international negotiations;

(h) that constitutes diplomatic correspondence exchanged with foreign states or international organizations of states or official correspondence exchanged with Canadian diplomatic missions or consular posts abroad; or

(i) relating to the communications or cryptographic systems of Canada or foreign states used

(ii) for the defence of Canada or any state allied or associated with Canada, or

(iii) in relation to the detection, prevention or suppression of subversive or hostile activities.

16. (1) The head of a government institution may refuse to disclose any record requested under this Act that contains

(*a*) information obtained or prepared by any government institution, or part of a government institution, that is an investigative body specified in the regulations in the course of lawful investigations pertaining to

(i) the detection, prevention or suppression of crime, or

(ii) the enforcement of any law of Canada or a province, if the record came into existence less than twenty years prior to the request;

(*b*) information relating to investigative techniques or plans for specific lawful investigations;

(*c*) information the disclosure of which could reasonably be expected to be injurious to the enforcement of any law of Canada or a province or the conduct of lawful investigations, including, without restricting the generality of the foregoing, any such information

(i) relating to the existence or nature of a particular investigation,

(ii) that would reveal the identity of a confidential source of information, or

(iii) that was obtained or prepared in the course of an investigation; or

(*d*) information the disclosure of which could reasonably be expected to be injurious to the security of penal institutions.

(2) The head of a government institution may refuse to disclose any record requested under this Act that contains information that could reasonably be expected to facilitate the commission of an offence, including, without restricting the generality of the foregoing, any such information

(*a*) on criminal methods or techniques;

(*b*) that is technical information relating to weapons or potential weapons; or

(*c*) on the vulnerability of particular buildings or other structures or systems, including computer or communication systems, or methods employed to protect such buildings or other structures or systems.

(3) The head of a government institution shall refuse to disclose any record requested under this Act that contains information that was obtained or prepared by the *Royal Canadian Mounted Police* while performing policing services for a province or a municipality pursuant to an arrangement made under section 20 of the Royal Canadian Mounted Police Act, where the Government of Canada has, on the request of the province or the municipality agreed not to disclose such information.

(4) For the purposes of paragraphs (1)(*b*) and (c), "investigation" means an investigation that

(*a*) pertains to the administration or enforcement of an Act of Parliament;

(b) is authorized by or pursuant to an Act of Parliament; or

(c) is within a class of investigations specified in the regulations.

17. The head of a government institution may refuse to disclose any record requested under this Act that contains information the disclosure of which could reasonably be expected to threaten the safety of individuals.

18. The head of a government institution may refuse to disclose any record requested under this Act that contains

(a) trade secrets or financial, commercial, scientific or technical information that belongs to the Government of Canada or a government institution and has substantial value or is reasonably likely to have substantial value;

(b) information the disclosure of which could reasonably be expected to prejudice the competitive position of a government institution;

(c) scientific or technical information obtained through research by an officer or employee of a government institution, the disclosure of which could reasonably be expected to deprive the officer or employee of priority of publication; or

(d) information the disclosure of which could reasonably be expected to be materially injurious to the financial interests of the Government of Canada or the ability of the Government of Canada to manage the economy of Canada or could reasonably be expected to result in an undue benefit to any person, including, without restricting the generality of the foregoing, any such information relating to

(i) the currency, coinage or legal tender of Canada,

(ii) a contemplated change in the rate of bank interest or in government borrowing,

(iii) a contemplated change in tariff rates, taxes, duties or, any other revenue source,

(iv) a contemplated change in the conditions of operation of financial institutions,

(v) a contemplated sale or purchase of securities or of foreign or Canadian currency, or

(vi) a contemplated sale or acquisition of land or property.

Personal Information

19. (1) Subject to subsection (2), the head of a government institution shall refuse to disclose any record requested under this Act that contains personal information as defined in section 3 of the *Privacy Act*.

(2) The head of a government institution may disclose any record requested under this Act that contains personal information if

(a) the individual to whom it relates consents to the disclosure;

(b) the information is publicly available; or

(c) the disclosure is in accordance with section 8 of the *Privacy Act*.

Third Party Information

20. (1) Subject to this section, the head of a government institution shall refuse to disclose any record requested under this Act that contains
   (*a*) trade secrets of a third party;
   (*b*) financial, commercial, scientific or technical information that is confidential information supplied to a government institution by a third party and is treated consistently in a confidential manner by the third party;
   (*c*) information the disclosure of which could reasonably be expected to result in material financial loss or gain to, or could reasonably be expected to prejudice the competitive position of, a third party; or
   (*d*) information the disclosure of which could reasonably be expected to interfere with contractual or other negotiations of a third party.

(2) The head of a government institution shall not, pursuant to subsection (1), refuse to disclose a part of a record if that part contains the results of product or environmental testing carried out by or on behalf of a government institution unless the testing was done as a service to a person, a group of persons or an organization other than a government institution and for a fee.

(3) Where the head of a government institution discloses a record requested under this Act, or a part thereof, that contains the results of product or environmental testing, the head of the institution shall at the same time as the record or part thereof is disclosed provide the person who requested the record with a written explanation of the methods used in conducting the tests.

(4) For the purposes of this section, the results of product or environmental testing do not include the results of preliminary testing conducted for the purpose of developing methods of testing.

(5) The head of a government institution may disclose any record that contains information described in subsection (1) with the consent of the third party to whom the information relates.

(6) The head of a government institution may disclose any record requested under this Act, or any part thereof, that contains information described in paragraph (1)(b), (c) or (d) if such disclosure would be in the public interest as it relates to public health, public safety or protection of the environment and, if such public interest in disclosure clearly outweighs in importance any financial loss or gain to, prejudice to the competitive position of or interference with contractual or other negotiations of a third party.

Operations of Government

21. (1) The head of a government institution may refuse to disclose any record requested under this Act that contains
   (*a*) advice or recommendations developed by or for a government institution or a Minister of the Crown,

(b) an account of consultations or deliberations involving officials or employees of a government institution, a Minister of the Crown or the staff of a Minister of the Crown,

(c) positions or plans developed for the purpose of negotiations carried on or to be carried on by or on behalf of the Government of Canada and considerations relating thereto, or

(d) plans relating to the management of personnel or the administration of a government institution that have not yet been put into operation,

if the record came into existence less than twenty years prior to the request.

(2) Subsection (1) does not apply in respect of a record that contains

(a) an account of, or a statement of reasons for, a decision that is made in the exercise of a discretionary power or an adjudicative function and that affects the rights of a person; or

(b) a report prepared by a consultant or adviser who was not, at the time the report was prepared, an officer or employee of a government institution or a member of the staff of a Minister of the Crown.

22. The head of a government institution may refuse to disclose any record requested under this Act that contains information relating to testing or auditing procedures or techniques or details of specific tests to be given or audits to be conducted if such disclosure would prejudice the use or results of particular tests or audits.

23. The head of a government institution may refuse to disclose any record requested under this Act that contains information that is subject to solicitor-client privilege.

Statutory Prohibitions

24. (1) The head of a government institution shall refuse to disclose any record requested under this Act that contains information the disclosure of which is restricted by or pursuant to any provision set out in Schedule 11.

(2) Such committee as may be designated or established under section 75 shall review every provision set out in Schedule 11 and shall, within three years after the coming into force of this Act or, if Parliament is not then sitting, on any of the first fifteen days next thereafter that Parliament is sitting, cause a report to be laid before Parliament on whether and to what extent the provisions are necessary.

25. Notwithstanding any other provision of this Act, where a request is made to a government institution for access to a record that the head of the institution is authorized to refuse to disclose under this Act by reason of information or other material contained in the record, the head of the institution shall disclose any part of the record that does not contain, and can reasonably be severed from any part that contains, any such information or material.

General

26. The head of a government institution may refuse to disclose any record requested under this Act or any part thereof if the head of the institution believes on reasonable grounds that the material in the record or part thereof will be published by a government institution, agent of the Government of Canada or Minister of the Crown within ninety days after the request is made or within such further period of time as may be necessary for printing or translating the material for the purpose of printing it.

27. (1) The head of a government institution may refuse to disclose any record requested under this Act

(*a*) during the first year after the coming into force of this Act, in the case of a record that was in existence more than three years before the coming into force of this Act;

(*b*) during the second year after the coming into force of this Act, in the case of a record that was in existence more than five years before the coming into force of this Act; and

(*c*) during the third year after the coming into force of this Act, in the case of a record that was in existence more than five years before the coming into force of this Act where, in the opinion of the head of the institution, to comply with a request for the record would unreasonably interfere with the operations of the government institution.

(2) Subsection (1) does not apply in respect of any record that is available to the public at the Public Archives at the time this Act comes into force.

2.3.1.1 *The Information Commissioner v. The Minister of Employment and Immigration* (1986), F.C. 63 (F.C.T.D.)

JEROME, A.C.J.: This application under paragraph 42(1)(a) of the *Access to Information Act* [S.C. 1980-81-82-83, c. 111, Schedule I] came on for hearing at Ottawa, Ontario, on November 27, 1985. The facts are not in dispute and are contained in a Statement of Agreed Facts dated July 15, 1985, which reads, in part:

> 1. On May 23, 1984, the Employment and Immigration Commission received a request pursuant to the *Privacy Act* from D.F., a Canadian Citizen, requesting as follows:
>> "I request full access to and disclosure of the immigration file relating to my sponsorship of my wife's application for permanent residence status in Canada. The Canadian Immigration Commission file number at the Vancouver office for the part of this file held there is 5133-15-6763. The Canadian Consulate General, Immigration Affairs, file number for that part of this file held in Seattle is 6054-B0138-5657. My wife's name is P.F."
>
> 2. By letter dated July 13, 1984, the said D.F. was given all personal information relating to him. Personal information relating to P.F. was exempted from disclosure pursuant to section 26 of the *Privacy Act*.
>
> 3. On May 23, 1984, the Employment and Immigration Commission received a request pursuant to the *Privacy Act* from P.F. requesting as follows

> "I request full access to and disclosure of the immigration file and record. The Canadian Immigration Commission file number at the Vancouver office for the part of this file held there is 5133-15-6763. The Canadian Consulate General, Immigration Affairs, file number for the part of this file held in Seattle is 6054-B0138-5657. Access is requested to the whole of the records and files at these offices, including all correspondence, memoranda, and all other documentary material relating to myself, my immigration matters, my application for permanent residence, and the issues of my marital status in Canada, and whether I have been previously married in the Philippines."

4. By letter dated July 13, 1984, P.F. was denied access to the personal information requested by her on the basis that she was not a Canadian Citizen or Permanent Resident as required by subsection 12(1) of the *Privacy Act*.

5. On May 23, 1984, the Employment and Immigration Commission received a request pursuant to the *Access to Information Act* from D.F. requesting as follows:

> "The record of which and to which access is requested is the immigration file relating to my sponsorship of the application for permanent residence by my wife, P.F. The Canadian Immigration Commission file number at the Vancouver office for the part of the record there is 5133-15-6763 . The Canadian Consulate General, Immigration Affairs, file number for the part of the record being held by that office in Seattle is 6054-B01385657. Access is requested to the whole of the record at these offices', including all correspondence, memoranda, and all other documentary material relating to myself, my sponsorship of my wife's application, the related immigration matters, and the allegation being made by the Canadian Immigration Commission that my marriage to my wife is defective or void in some way due to her alleged previous marriage."

6. By letter dated July 13, 1984, the said D.F. was notified that the information he requested constituted personal information which should be accessed under the *Privacy Act*, and that, since he had submitted a request under the *Privacy Act*, he would receive all personal information to which he was entitled in response to his *Privacy Act* request.

It is not disputed that the record in issue contains personal information as defined in section 3 of the *Privacy Act* [S.C. 1980-81-82-83, c.111, Schedule 11] nor that the individual to whom that information relates has consented to its disclosure. Nevertheless, counsel contends that since subsection 19(2) provides that the head of a government institution may disclose personal information, it establishes with equal force a discretion not to disclose even though the conditions of subsection 19(2) have been met.

I reject the argument for two reasons: first, as a question of law, it is contrary to principles of statutory interpretation; second, it represents an approach that runs directly against the very purpose for which this legislation was enacted, as stated in the express provisions of the statute and confirmed in jurisprudence.

In terms of statutory interpretation, when legislators intend to create an obligation to do something, they use the word "shall". When they intend instead to establish a discretion or a right to do it, they use the word "may". Had the legislators intended here to repose residual discretion in the head of the government institution not to disclose information, even though the conditions of section 19(2) had been met, that appropriate and precise language would have been used. Of course, the Act does not establish the discretion not to disclose in such circumstances (in which case the respondent's argument might have had merit). The language chosen expresses the intent to establish a discretion to release personal information under certain circumstances. Those conditions having been fulfilled, it becomes tantamount to an obligation upon the head of the government institution to do so, especially where the purpose for which the statute was enacted is, as here, to create a right of access in the public. In support of the argument to the contrary, counsel for the respondent relied upon the decision of the Supreme Court of Canada in *Maple Lodge Farms Ltd. v. Government of Canada*, [1982] 2 S.C.R. 2. However, in the judgment in the Federal Court of Appeal [[1981] 1 F.C. 500]. delivered by Le Dain J., and affirmed in the Supreme Court of Canada, the following significant passage appears [at page 508]:

> 7. On May 23, 1984, the Employment and Immigration Commission received a request pursuant to the *Access to Information Act* from the Complainant, Gerald G. Goldstein. That request is the request referred to in the Affidavit of Douglas W. McGibbon.
> 8. The said Gerald G. Goldstein is a barrister and Solicitor practicing in the Province of British Columbia who represents the said P.F.

Together with his request for access, the complainant submitted a document signed by P.F. consenting to the release to the complainant of documents and information relating to her immigration matters. On July 13, 1984 the respondent informed the complainant that the information which he sought could not be obtained under the *Access to Information Act* because it was personal information about another person. A complaint was lodged with the Information Commissioner who, following an investigation, recommended that the information be released. The respondent subsequently provided the complainant with access to documents consisting of 5 pages, but refused to disclose in excess of 200 pages of documents.

. . . . .

To repeat, the purpose of the *Access to Information Act* is to codify the right of access to information held by the government. It is not to codify the government's right of refusal. Access should be the normal course. Exemptions should be exceptional and must be confined to those specifically set out in the statute. In the present case, the applicant was quite properly informed that the information sought could not be obtained except by a Canadian citizen or a resident and could not involve disclosure of personal information about another person without their consent. Once those conditions were met, and they were here, the information should have been disclosed.

2.3.1.2 David Schneidermann, "The Access to Information Act: A Practical Review" (1987), *Advocates Quarterly*, vol. 7, 474

The *Access to Information Act* grants the right to every person who is a Canadian citizen or a permanent resident to apply for and, subject to the Act, be given access to any record under the control of a government institution.[1]

Corporations would appear to have no such right and must act through agents who are Canadian citizens or permanent residents in order to obtain access to information. Other than the prerequisites of citizenship or permanent residency, there is no screening procedure for requests for information. Accordingly, information can be obtained for any purpose and by anyone acting through an appropriate agent.

The Act makes no specific mention of the form of request to be supplied to the government institution other than that it be made in writing and provide sufficient detail "to enable an experienced employee of the institution with a reasonable effort to identify the record".[2] The Government of Canada has made available, through public agencies such as post offices, "Access to Information Request Forms". The *Access to Information Act Regulations* provide that a request under the Act must be made by completing an Access to Information Request Form or, alternatively, by a written request that provides sufficient detail to enable identification of a record by the appropriate officer.[3]

Pursuant to the requirement in s. 5 of the Act, and in order to facilitate one's ability to provide sufficient detail in a request for information, the Treasury Board has published an Access Register. The Access Register is an index of departments of the federal government indicating the nature of matters governed by each department and the specific agencies under each department's control. The Register also describes the types of government records under the control of each department and its agencies. The Access Register is a revealing document which makes easier the difficult task of determining under whose administrative control any one governmental function lies. Thus its use will lie beyond formulating requests for information. The Access Register has been criticized for its vague and broad descriptions of the contents of records under the control of government institutions.[4] Because of these broad descriptions, requests for information have at times yielded volumes of records and high fee estimates.[5] As a result, its usefulness as a tool for initiating requests under the Act is in some doubt and will have to undergo review and revision.

Each request for information must be accompanied by an application fee of $5.[6] A further fee of $0.25 per photocopy is required to be paid upon the information being furnished to the party requesting. Other reproduction fees are chargeable depending on the form of reproduction requested.[7] The Access to Information Request Form asks that the requesting party indicate what fees he authorizes to be charged. No search of a record will be completed until that authorization is given. Fees may be charged for copies made of a record[8] or for every hour in excess of five hours "reasonably required" to search for or prepare a record for disclosure[9] or for a record produced from a machine readable record.[10] Where fees are charged other than for copies, the head of the government institution[11] may require payment of a deposit before search or production is made.[12]

Once the written request and required fee is received by a government institution, where appropriate; the applicant will be notified of the estimate of total costs; the amount of deposit required to be paid, if any; he will be informed that he may personally examine records free of charge; that he may specify parts of the record to be produced[13] and that he may complain about unreasonable fees to the Information Commissioner.[14]

The Act makes provision for the waiver of fees or any other amounts required to be paid.[15] The Treasury Board Interim Policy Guide published for the use by civil servants in applying the Act and available to the public, suggests that waiver, reduction or refund of a fee by the head of a government institution should be decided by assessing whether the information sought is normally available without charge and "the degree to which a general public benefit is obtained through release of the information".[16] This test effectively allows the head of a government institution complete discretion in determining whether fees should be waived. The Treasury Board has reported that, of the requests for information received by government institutions, fees have been waived for approximately 30% of requests.[17] This high percentage may simply be a reflection of the policy to waive fees in instances where the fee is too small to warrant initiating collection procedures.

One Ken Rubin made requests for information from several government institutions without submitting a $5 filing fee with each request.[18] As a result, his requests were not considered applications within the terms of the Act by those government institutions. Mr. Rubin petitioned three Ministers to the Federal Court of Canada, Trial Division respecting their failure to consider his application, claiming that the filing fee requirement was not enforced uniformly by all departments.[19] As the Act expressly authorizes the filing fee, Jerome A.C.J. refused Mr. Rubin's application.

Exempted Information

The Act specifically exempts from disclosure records containing many types of information held by government institutions. Sections 13 to 27 of the Act provide broad descriptions of those records exempt from disclosure. The Act distinguishes between information of which a head of a government institution is required to refuse disclosure and information of which he has a discretion to refuse disclosure. Among the records of the former class are records containing information obtained in confidence from other governments or international organizations[20] personal information as defined in the *Privacy Act*[21] and records which contain trade secrets and other confidential commercial information.[22] Any record containing information obtained or prepared by the R.C.M.P., in certain circumstances, must also be protected from disclosure.[23]

Among the class of records also prohibited from disclosure are records restricted by a series of statutes listed in Sch. 11 of the Act.[24] It is likely that any record previously restricted from public access by statute remains restricted by virtue of Sch. II of the Act. It is cumbersome to expect an applicant to consult these statutes prior to initiating a request and, therefore, it would be prudent to make application and, as with all other exemptions, patiently await the government's decision regarding whether the record is exempted under the Act.

Among the records of which the head of a government institution has a discretion to refuse disclosure are records containing information which could reasonably be expected to be injurious to the conduct of federal/provincial affairs by the Government of Canada,[25] the conduct of international affairs or the defence of Canada or any allied or associated state or to the "detection, prevention or suppression of subversive or hostile activities".[26] Information obtained or prepared in the course of criminal investigation or the enforcement of any law, federal or provincial, if less than 20 years old, or relating to law enforcement or criminal methods or techniques[27] may also be protected from disclosure by the head of a government institution. As well, information which could reasonably be expected to threaten the safety of an individual or would likely injure the financial or other economic interests of the Government of Canada may also be protected from disclosure.[28]

The Act expressly provides that it does not apply to confidential Cabinet material and proceeds to list examples of types of Cabinet information excluded from the operation of the Act.[29] A similar provision is contained in the *Privacy Act*.[30] The exception does not apply to confidential Cabinet material in existence for more than 20 years, and discussion papers, where decisions in respect of those discussion papers have been made public or four years have passed since decisions in respect of those discussion papers were made.[31]

Of particular concern to practitioners will be the mandatory third party exemptions contained in the Act, exempting trade secrets and other confidential commercial information.[32]

The third party exemptions are designed to protect disclosure of confidential information submitted by corporations or individuals in the course of many governmental inquiries. The exemptions are designed to facilitate the submission of information which, if otherwise disclosed, would likely injure a third party submitter's economic interests. Although the exemption is mandatory, the information is subject to disclosure if the third party supplier of the information consents[33] or if disclosure would be in the public interest as it relates to public health, safety or protection of the environment and the public interest clearly outweighs in importance the impact to the third party if disclosure is made.[34] The exemptions contained in s. 20(1)(b) of the Act pertaining to records containing financial, commercial, scientific or technical information, that are confidential and treated consistently in a confidential manner by a third party and those contained in s. 20(1)(d) of the Act pertaining to information the disclosure of which could reasonably be expected to interfere with contractual or other negotiations of a third party, were sought to be relied upon by the third-party applicant in *Re Maislin Industries Ltd. and Minister for Industry, Trade and Commerce, Regional Economic Expansion*[35] in order to prevent disclosure by the Minister.

Jerome A.C.J. dismissed Maislin's application for review of the Minister's decision to disclose a portion of the government record regarding the granting of $34 million in loan guarantees by the Government of Canada in favour of Maislin Industries Ltd. The court was of the view that the information in issue was not confidential in its nature and had not been treated in a confidential manner by Maislin Industries Ltd. Some of the information was admittedly available in Maislin Industries Ltd.'s annual financial reports. As for the balance of the information, Jerome A.C.J. held that the application failed to persuade him, by any of the objective standards to which he had referred, that the information was confidential in its nature.[36]

The test adopted by Jerome A.C.J. to determine whether information is confidential in its nature does not leap out at the reader even upon a careful reading of his reasons for judgment. The only test referred to by him is that contained in *National Parks & Conservation Assn v. Morton*,[37] a case cited by counsel for the respondents.[38] In *National Parks*, Tamm J. interpreted exemption No. 4 of the *Freedom of Information Act*[39] as follows:[40]

> "To summarize, a commercial or financial matter is *'confidential'* for purposes of the exemption if disclosure of the information is likely to have either of the following effects: (1) to impair the Government's ability to obtain necessary information in the future; or (2) to cause substantial harm to the competitive position of the person from whom the information was obtained."

The exemption contained in s. 20(1)(c) of the Act, not the subject of commentary in *Maislin*, exempts from disclosure information which, if disclosed, could reasonably be expected to result in material financial loss or gain to, or to prejudice the "competitive position" of, a third party. Other than the fact that s. 20(1)(c) does not require that to qualify for the exemption the information be confidential, the second branch of this test falls directly within the scope of s. 20(1)(c) of the Act. With all due respect, the second branch of this test is therefore of no aid in interpreting the confidential information provision contained in s. 20(1)(b) of the Act.

The first branch of the test has been the subject of strong criticism in the United States.[41] Standing alone, this branch of the test has no application to types of information which have been voluntarily submitted to government or for which a government institution has the power to compel submission. Accordingly, this test is wholly inadequate as a means of testing the confidentiality of information under the *Access to Information Act*.

A wholly subjective test, dependent upon the intentions of the submitter and receiver of the information, would be inadequate as a means of determining confidentiality.[42] An appropriate test might be that advocated by James T. O'Reilly regarding exemption No. 4 of the *Freedom of Information Act*.[43] He adopts as a definition of confidential information that type of information expressly excluded by the Restatement of Tort's definition of trade secrets: "information as to single or ephemeral events in the conduct of the business, as, for example, the amount of terms of a secret bid of a contract . . .". To this may be added compilations of information such as computer programs regarding a business, processes and programs regarding suppliers or customers of a business and lists of employees.[44] As well, in order to determine the confidentiality of the information it "must be judged in the light of the usage and practices of the particular industry or trade concerned".[45]

It would appear that the mandatory third party exemptions are vague and in need of legislative clarification. The exemptions are multitudinous and may even be inclusive of each other. For instance, it is likely only in rare circumstances that confidential commercial information sought to be disclosed does not satisfy the test contained in s. 20(1)(c) of the Act, preventing disclosure of information which could reasonably be expected to result in material financial loss or gain to, or prejudice.the competitive position of, a third party. It would be reasonable to expect that confidential commercial information if disclosed will, at the very least, always prejudice the competitive position of the owner of that information.

Jerome, A.C.J. referred to a further qualification for confidential information protected from disclosure pursuant to s. 20(1)(b). The information must have been kept confidential by both parties, the third party submitter and the government institution that received the information. The statute makes no mention of this requirement.

If confidential information is available from other sources to which the public has access than it would be expected that a government institution would not protect that information from disclosure. But government institutions should not be granted the discretion to determine confidentiality by disclosing information through other channels. Needless to say, the courts should not sanction unauthorized disclosure of confidential information by government agencies.

In instances where a government institution has disclosed confidential information through other channels, the court should weigh the effect of further disclosure before allowing disclosure pursuant to the Act. The court should distinguish between those instances where information, while available in the public domain through government, is not so well-known that further protection will benefit the third party submitter and those instances where information is, in a sense, too public to qualify as confidential.[46] Instances of government disclosure through newspaper accounts, press releases and ministerial budgets may disclose confidential information but justify protection from further disclosure pursuant to the Act. If the disclosed portion is sufficiently severable from the undisclosed, the latter should be protected from disclosure if otherwise exempt.

There will be circumstances, such as those existing in *DMR & Associates v. Minister of Supply & Services*,[47] where future disclosure of information by government through information sessions to bidding competitors would justify disclosure of commercial information through the Act. Jerome A.C.J. found it inappropriate to restrain disclosure where it seemed "not only possible but quite likely[48] that the applicant's competitors would have access to the allegedly confidential information.

The Decision and Process for Review

The Act confers upon the heads of government institutions the role of administering requests for disclosure. Within 30 days after a request for disclosure is made[49] or, if circumstances require a greater amount of time[50], the head of the government institution must give written notice of his decision. If access to a record is not granted he must state in his written notice that the record does not exist or the specific provision of the Act upon which the refusal is based.[51] The head of a government institution is not required to indicate whether a requested record exists[52] and, where he fails to do so in the written notice, he must indicate in the notice "the provision on which a refusal could reasonably be expected to be based if the record existed".[53] Jurisprudence to date suggests that the head of the government institution will be bound by the grounds of refusal asserted in his notice of refusal.[54]

Where a statutory exemption applies, the head of the institution is required to disclose any part of a record that does not contain and can be reasonably severed from the exempted information.[55]

In instances where third party information is intended to be disclosed, the head of an institution must notify the third party of this intention within 30 days after the request for access is received.[56] Within 20 days after the notice is given, the third party is given an opportunity to make written representations, or oral representations if so granted by the head of an institution, regarding disclosure.[57] Within 30 days after notice, and if the third party has been granted the opportunity to make representations, he must make a decision regarding disclosure and notify the parties in writing of his decision.[58] Interestingly, an applicant is not entitled to receive a copy of the notice provided to the third party, nor is an applicant entitled to reply to the representations made by a third party to the head of an institution.

The Office of Information Commissioner is established under the Act to receive and investigate complaints regarding refusals, fees, time-limits within which a decision regarding disclosure is to be made and the official language of the record disclosed.[59] The Information Commissioner has herself described her mandate as that of an ombudsman.[60] Complaints may be submitted by authorized individuals on behalf of a complainant.[61] The complaint must be made in writing and made no later than one year from the time a request for a record was received by the head 6 of the government institution.[62]

The Information Commissioner is granted broad powers of investigation regarding complaints.[63] The incumbent is Inger Hansen. She is obliged to give a reasonable opportunity to complainants, third parties and the head of government institutions to make representations during the course of the investigation but no party has the right to be present during an investigation or to have access to or comment on representations made to the Commissioner by any other person.[64]

Any findings and recommendations made by the Information Commissioner are reported to all parties concerned. Those recommendations need not be acted upon by the heads of government institutions as no means of enforcement exists under the Act.[65] Should the head of the government institution not give access to a record when recommended to do so by the Information Commissioner, the complainant's only recourse is the right to apply for review of the decision to the Federal Court of Canada, Trial Division.

Unlike the powers of the Privacy Commissioner, her counterpart under the *Privacy Act*, the Information Commissioner is not specifically empowered to review information contained in exempt banks in order to determine whether a record is properly designated as exempt.[66]

The party making the request for information, after receiving an answer to his complaint from the Information Commissioner, and third parties are entitled to have decisions reviewed in the Federal Court of Canada, Trial Division. Applications to review refusals of disclosure must be made within 45 days after the time the results of an investigation by the Information Commissioner are reported to the complainant or such further time as the court may order.[67] A request for review by a third party must be filed within 20 days after notice is given of the decision made by the head of a government institution to disclose a record or where the Information Commissioner has recommended disclosure.[68]

Applications for review should be commenced by notice of motion.[69] The motion is required to be supported by an affidavit setting out the facts upon which the motion is based,[70] although this had to be directed to be done by the court in *Maislin*[71] and, with respect to the existence of exempt information under the *Privacy Act*, in *Ternette*.[72]

The hearing of an application for review is conducted in a summary manner[73] and is not a *de novo* review of the Minister's decision.[74] The Act is unclear in regard to the test to be generally applied by a court in applications for review. The Act does provide a hint in regard to the scope of review by providing that, in proceedings for review initiated by a person who has been refused access to a record or by the Information Commissioner, the burden of proof is upon the head of the government institution to establish that the head of an institution "is authorized to refuse disclosure".[75] This would suggest that the test to be applied by the Federal Court in proceedings other than review proceedings initiated by a third party is to determine whether information is authorized to be exempt from disclosure. There is no mention in the Act of the burden of proof to be applied in third party proceedings. Furthermore, such a test would appear to be inadequate in instances where the head of an institution has the discretion of deciding whether a record may be disclosed.

The court has indicated the direction it will likely take in instances where the head of a government institution refuses disclosure pursuant to an exemption which grants a discretion to refuse disclosure. In *Information Com'r v. Min. of Employment & Immigration*,[76] a person expressly authorized disclosure of a record containing personal information regarding that person. The effect of that authorization was to grant to the Minister the discretion, pursuant to the Act,[77] to disclose that personal information to the requesting party. The Minister declined to release the personal information which decision was reviewed by the Information Commissioner who recommended disclosure. When this recommendation was not followed by the respondent Minister, the Information Commissioner initiated an application for judicial review pursuant to the Act.

Jerome, A.C.J. allowed the application by the Information Commissioner to compel disclosure as the approach taken by the respondent Minister was directly in conflict with the purpose of the legislation. Jerome A.C.J. stated that the purpose of the Act was not to codify the right of refusal but the right of access and that access should be granted in the normal course. Exemptions, if relied upon by a head of an institution, must be exceptional and confined to those instances specifically enumerated in the statute. Once the statutory conditions in question have been met, disclosure should occur in the normal course. Although the judgment can be confined to only those instances where the Act enumerates conditions required to be met before the head of an institution may exercise his discretion to grant access, Jerome A.C.J.'s reasons apply with equal force to all the discretionary exemptions contained in the Act.

In instances where disclosure is refused on the basis of injury to the conduct of federal/provincial affairs, international affairs, the defence of Canada or the detection, prevention or suppression of subversive or hostile activities, to law enforcement or the security of penal institutions or to the financial interests of the Government of Canada, the court, on review, may determine only whether the head of the institution had reasonable grounds on which to refuse disclosure.[78]

In instances where review is initiated by a third party the burden of proof will lie on the party resisting disclosure.[79] The Associate Chief Justice has stated, on at least two occasions,[80] that in applying that burden of proof "public access ought not to be frustrated by the courts except upon the clearest grounds so that doubt ought to be resolved in favour of disclosure".[81] This would suggest that a party resisting disclosure must satisfy a criminal standard of proof. That burden of proof would appear to be difficult to apply in instances where the court need only determine whether the head of an institution has reasonable grounds on which to refuse disclosure. The court has yet to consider that burden of proof in such instances.

Considering the similar provisions contained in the *Privacy Act*, Strayer J. has held that the general power of review of the Federal Court entitles the court to review the alleged exempt information to determine whether the information was properly included in that bank of exempted information.[82] Strayer J. did not go on to say whether the same scope of review existed for information concerning national security, etc., where the court is required to determine whether "reasonable grounds" existed to refuse disclosure.

An open court-room would appear to be an ill-suited place for hearing an application to prevent disclosure of exempted information. The *Access to Information Act* addresses this issue in s. 47 by providing that the Court of Review shall take every reasonable precaution to avoid disclosure of information which the head of a government institution would be authorized to refuse to disclose, including, when appropriate, receiving representations *ex parte* or conducting hearings *in camera*. In *Maislin* the court found it appropriate to conduct the hearing *in camera* and to restrict attendance at the hearing to counsel for the parties.

For those applications regarding national security matters, Parliament has seen fit to make mandatory *in camera* proceedings. Applications for review by requesters or the Information Commissioner regarding a record which has been denied disclosure on the basis of ss. 13(1)(*a*) or (*b*) and 15, relating, in part, to the government or institution of a foreign state, the defence of Canada or any allied state or the "detection, prevention or suppression of subversive or hostile activities", must be heard in camera and, if requested by the head of the government institution, be heard in Ottawa and by government representations made *ex parte*.[83]

The Act is silent on the issue of whether the contents of a record sought to be disclosed ought to be disclosed to the requesting party. Whether an application for review is initiated by the requesting party or third party, the former must be given an opportunity to know the case that needs to be met. This can only be accomplished though some form of disclosure of the exempted record.

In *Reyes v. Secretary of State*,[84] where the Federal Court considered the analogous provisions of the *Privacy Act* regarding in camera proceedings, Jerome, A.C.J. directed that the investigation sought to be disclosed by Mr. Reyes regarding the investigation and assessment of his citizenship application be appended to an affidavit, placed in a sealed envelope and filed with the court. Before the court would review the record *ex parte* Jerome, A.C.J. invited counsel for the applicant to suggest specific questions which would be asked of deponents during the *ex parte* hearing.

Parliament has seen fit to exclude the attendance of client or counsel in "national security" matters. In all other instances the requesting party, or solely his counsel as in *Maislin Industries Ltd.*,[85] may hear representations made by other parties concerning potentially confidential information. In *Maislin Industries Ltd.* Jerome, A.C.J., having examined the full text of the study, allowed disclosure of the record in issue to Mr. Hunter's counsel on his undertaking of non-disclosure, even to his client. Jerome, A.C.J. concluded that this kind of determination will vary with the circumstances of each case.

One can reasonably conclude that in circumstances concerning national security matters, no disclosure of the record will be available to counsel for the requesting party.[86] However, without some form of disclosure counsel cannot argue intelligently whether the information falls within any of the exempted categories. It can be reasonably forseen that, in instances where disclosure of exempted information is required in the public interest as it relates to public health, safety or protection of the environment,[87] expert evidence regarding those subjects must be adduced. Certainly the public interest requires a more rigorous inquiry into the nature of a document which will otherwise be exempt from disclosure pursuant to the third party exemptions, than the kind of inquiry that will result where counsel for the requesting party receives no particulars regarding the contents of the exempted document.

A minimum standard of disclosure ought to be instituted by the Federal Court of Canada. A reasonable standard was that adopted by Wilkey, C.J. in *Vaughn v. Rosen*,[88] where the Chief Justice ordered an index of the document sought to be disclosed to be provided to the requesting party and the court.[89] The particulars of the index should be sufficient to inform the requesting party and the court of the nature of the document while keeping confidential the matters sought to be disclosed. The judge, in each instance, should have an opportunity to fully review the record and may be amend the index to ensure its accuracy and completeness.[90]

A last area of concern to the practitioner is the matter of costs. Any successful party to an application for review is entitled to costs unless the court otherwise orders.[91] Where a complainant or the Information Commissioner has appealed a refusal to disclose and the court is of the opinion that an important new principle has been raised in relation to the Act, the court must order that costs be awarded in favour of the applicant even if unsuccessful.[92] It is fair to presume that in appropriate cases where a third party applicant has unsuccessfully applied for review and has raised an important new principle in relation to the Act, the court would exercise its discretion pursuant to s. 53(1) and make an order for costs in favour of the third party.

If the Information Commissioner has appealed a decision to refuse disclosure of a record or otherwise appears on behalf of a complainant who has applied for review, a complainant need not likely worry about the matter of costs

Endnotes

1. *Access to Information Act*, s. 4(1).
2. *Ibid.*, s. 6.
3. SOR/85-395, s. 1.
4. Toronto, *Globe and Mail*, January 4, 1985.
5. See *Main Brief to House of Commons Standing Committee on Justice and Legal Affairs from Office of the Information Commissioner*, May 7, 1986.
6. *Access to Information Act*, s. 11; SOR/83-507, s. 7(1)(a).

7. See SOR/83-507 s.7(1)(b).
8. *Access to Information Act*, s. 11(1)(b).
9. *Ibid.*, s. 11(2).
10. *Ibid.*, s. 11(3).
11. *Ibid.*, s. 3 defines "head" in respect of a government institution to mean, in the case of a department or ministry, the minister or, in any other case, a person designated by Order in Council.
12. *Ibid.*, s. 11(4).
13. SOR/83-507, s. 5.
14. Treasury Board, *Interim Policy Guide* Part 11, p. 15. In certain circumstances, the head of the government institution may specify that the applicant may only examine the record personally or that only a copy of the record will be provided to the applicant. See SOR/83-507, s. 8, as amended by SOR/85-395, s. 2.
15. *Access to Information Act*, s. 11(6).
16. Treasury Board, *Interim Policy Guide*, Part 11, pp. 22-3.
17. Treasury Board of Canada, *Report to the Standing Commitee on Justice and Legal Affairs on the Access to Information Act and the Privacy Act*, March, 1986.
18. Mr. Rubin is a self-proclaimed "public interest researcher". See Toronto, *Globe and Mail*, January 4, 1985.
19. *Rubin v. Min. of Employment and Immigration Canada*, unreported, F.C.T.D., No. T-194-85, Jerome A.C.J. October 4, 1985.
20. *Access to Information Act*, s. 13(1).
21. *Ibid.*, s. 19(1).
22. *Ibid.*, s. 20(1).
23. *Ibid.*, s. 16(3), as amended by S.C. 1983-84, c. 21, s. 70(2).
24. *Ibid.*, s. 24 and see *An Act to enact the Access to Information Act and the Privacy Act (to amend the Federal Court Act and the Canada Evidence Act and to amend certain other Acts in consequence thereof)*, S.C. 1980-81-82-83, c. 111, ss. 6 to 9 and SOR/85-751.
25. *Access to Information Act*, s. 14.
26. *Ibid.*, s. 15.
27. *Ibid.*, s. 16(1) and (2).
28. *Ibid.*, ss. 17 and 18.
29. *Ibid.*, s. 69(1). See the comments of Jerome A.C.J. in *Auditor General of Canada v. Minister of Energy, Mines and Resources* (1985), 23 D.L.R. (4th) 210 at pp. 226-7, [1985] 1 F.C. 719 at pp. 741-2 (T.D.).
30. S.C. 1980-81-82-83, c. 111 (Schedule II), s. 70.

31. *Access to Information Act*, s. 69(3).
32. For those concerned with the circumstances required to qualify for third party exemptions in s. 20(1), it is best to refer to the Treasury Board *Interim Policy Guidelines*. The Guidelines will be most useful when making representations to the government institution regarding disclosure pursuant to s. 28(5) and (6).
33. *Access to Information Act*, s. 20(5).
34. *Ibid.*, s. 20(6).
35. (1984), 10 D.L.R. (4th) 417, [1984] 1 F.C. 939, 80 C.P.R. (2d) 253 (T.D.).
36. *Ibid.*, at p. 424 D.L.R., p. 947 F.C.
37. 498 F. 2d 765 (1974).
38. See reference in *Maislin, supra*, footnote 36, at p. 421 D.L.R., p. 944 F.C.
39. U.S.C. para. 552: "Trade secrets and commercial or financial information obtained from a person and privileged or confidential."
40. See reference in *Maislin*, at p. 421 D.L.R., p. 944 F.C.
41. See, for instance, Patten, "Developments in the Protection of Commercial Information" 38 Fed. B.J. 141 (1979), at p. 143; and O'Reilly, *Federal Information Disclosure*, Vol. 1 para. 14.08.
42. However, see the commentary of K.C. Davis in, "The Information Act: A preliminary Analysis" 34 U. Chi. L. Rev. 761 (1967), who advocates the exemption of information submitted to government on the good raith understanding that it will remain confidential
43. Cited in McCarthy and Kornweiler, "Maintaining the Confidentiality of Confidential Business Information submitted to the Federal Government" (1980), 36 Bus. Law 57 at p. 61.
44. As to such types of confidential information, see *R. v. Stewart* (1983), 149 D.L.R. (3d) 583 at p.599, 5 C.C.C. (3d) 481 at p. 497, 42 O.R. (2d) 225 (C.A.), *per* Cory, J.A. For an interesting discussion of Maislin and the test for confidential information, see P.G. Capriolo, "Confidentiality and the Protection of Third Party Business Information" (1985), 10 C.B.L.J. 463.
45. *Per* Megarry V.C. in *Thomas Marshall (Exports) Ltd. v. Guinle*, [1978] 3 All E.R. 193 (Ch.), at p. 210.
46. See A.M. Tetterborn, "Breach of Confidence, Secrecy and the Public Domain", 11 Anglo-Am. L. Rev. 273 (1982), at p. 279.
47. (1984), 11 C.P.R. (3d) 87 (F.C.T.D.).
48. *Ibid.*, at p. 91.
49. *Access to Information Act*, s. 7.
50. *Ibid.*, s. 9.
51. *Ibid.*, s. 10(1).

52. *Ibid.*, s. 10(2).
53. *Ibid.*, s. 10(1)(b).
54. This was so held by Strayer, J. while considering the identical provisions in the *Privacy Act* in *Ternette v. Solicitor-General of Canada* (1984), 10 D.L.R. (4th) 587 at pp. 594-5, [1984] 5 W.W.R. 612 at pp. 620-1, [1984] 2 F.C. 486 (T.D.).
55. *Access to Information Act*, s. 25. In the *Maislin* case the Minister for, Industry, Trade and Commerce chose to sever and disclose portions of the study upon which the loan guarantee was based. It was this decision that was ultimately appealed to the Federal Court of Canada, Trial Division.
56. *Ibid.*, s. 28(1).
57. *Ibid.*, s. 28(5) and (6).
58. *Ibid.*, s. 28(5)(b).
59. *Ibid.*, s. 30(1).
60. *Supra*, footnote 5, at p. 5.
61. *Access to Information Act*, s. 30(2).
62. *Ibid.*, s. 31.
63. *Ibid.*, s. 36.
64. *Ibid.*, s. 35(2).
65. *Ibid.*, s. 37(5).
66. *Privacy Act, supra*, footnote 30, s. 36. For a discussion of this provision, see *Ternette v. Solicitor-General of Canada* (1984), 10 D.L.R. (4th) 587, [1984] 5 W.W.R. 612, [1984] 2 F.C. 486 (F.C.T.D.).
67. *Access to Information Act*, s. 41.
68. *Ibid.*, s. 44.
69. Federal Court Rule 319(1), C.R.C. 1978, c. 663.
70. *Ibid.*
71. *Re Maislin Industries Ltd. and Minister for Industry, Trade and Commerce, Regional Economic Expansion* (1984), 10 D.L.R. (4th) 417, [1984] 1 F.C. 939, 80 C.P.R. (2d) 253 (T.D.).
72. *Ternette v. Solicitor General of Canada, supra*, footnote 66.
73. *Access to Information Act*, s. 45.
74. This is in contrast to the *Freedom of Information Act* 5, U.S.C. p. 662 (1976) where the party requesting disclosure has means of *de novo* review. The third party has no status at such a hearing or a means of review even if the information falls within an exempted category; see *Chrysler Corp. v. Brown*, 441 U.S. 281 (1979).
75. *Access to Information Act*, s. 48.
76. (1986), 11 C.P.R. (3d) 81 (F.C.T.D.).

77. *Access to Information Act*, s. 19(2)(a).
78. *Ibid.*, s. 50.
79. See *Re Maislin Industries Ltd. and Minister for Industry Trade and Commerce Regional Economic Expansion* (1984), 10 D.L.R. (4th) 417, [1984] 1 F.C. 939, 80 C.P.R. (2d) 253 (T.D.); *DMR & Associates v. Minister of Supply & Services* (1984), 11 C.P.R. (3d) 87 (F.C.T.D.).
80. *Maislin, ibid.; Reyes v. Secretary of State* (1984), 9 Admin. L.R. 296 (F.C.T.D.).
81. *Maislin, ibid.*, at p. 420 D.L.R. p. 943 F.C.; *Reyes, ibid.*, at p. 299.
82. *Ternette v. Solicitor-General of Canada* (1984), 10 D.L.R. (4th) 587, [1984] 5 W.W.R. 612, [1984] 2 F.C. 486 (T.D.).
83. *Access to Information Act*, s. 52.
84. *Supra*, footnote 80.
85. *Supra*, footnote 79.
86. See, for instance, *Reyes, supra*, footnote 80.
87. *Access to Information Act*, s. 20(6).
88. 484 F.2d 820 (1973).
89. *Ibid.*, p. 825.
90. Such a procedure would seem to be in conflict with the discretion accorded to heads of government institutions pursuant to s. 10(2) of the *Access to Information Act* which provides that they are not required to indicate to a requester whether a record exists upon a request for information. It is submitted that such a provision makes no sense in the context of an application for review before the Federal Court. This provision should be confined to the initial step of the access request when the head of a government institution refuses to give access to a record and considers it necessary, in the public or private interest, to not indicate whether the record exists.
91. *Access to Information Act*, s. 53(1).
92. *Access to Information Act*, s. 53(2).

2.3.1.3. Canadian Daily Newspaper Publishers Association, *What Newsrooms Need to Know* (Toronto: 1984)

How FOI works

1. Any Canadian citizen or landed immigrant can request information from a federal government body. Cabinet may extend the right to citizens of other lands.

2. The information cannot be a Cabinet document (see Cabinet System reference) and there are five mandatory exemptions and 12 discretionary exemptions (more on these later). The right exists to seek a judicial review of a request for the discretionary exemptions if the government refuses to disclose information sought.

3. The head of a government institution or his designate (access coordinator is the technical term must, within 30 days after receiving a formal request, either produce the information sought, or give the reasons for denial in writing. The government can request an extension of 30 days if it decides a search is complicated, if long consultation is necessary or if a third party must be told of the request.

4. Anyone refused access to information has the right to appeal to the Information Commissioner to review and assess the request. He has power similar to an auditor-general, and can enter any government office, call any witness, and study all documents and information except those of Cabinet. He can recommend that the information be released or withheld.

5. If the government refuses to comply with an Information Commissioner recommendation for release of what is sought, or if he agrees with the refusal, the matter can be taken to the Federal court within 45 days after the commissioner reports. The court has the final say.

What's available

1. Under the act, the federal government must provide on a yearly basis, a publication or index containing:

(a) A description of the organization and responsibilities of each federal government institution, including federal crown corporations, embracing details on the programs and functions of each division or branch of the institutions;

(b) A detailed description of all classes of records under the control of each government institution;

(c) A description of all manuals used by employees of each government institution in administering or carrying out any of the programs or activities concerned with their jobs.

(d) Each government institution must furnish the address of the Access Coordinator to whom request for information should be sent.

2. The index also includes a citizen's guide outlining basic rights under the act, instructions on how to use the index and make requests (with sample entries and requests), guidance on existing information and channels of information, and descriptions of where to go to get it.

3. At least twice a year, an updating bulletin is to be posted.

4. According to the act, these indices and bulletins should be found in government buildings, libraries, and post offices.

How to use FOI

1. Based on the experiences of users of FOI in the United States, which has a more liberal act than in Canada (its law was passed in 1966), it would seem a reporter, researcher or scholar should first contact the government institution's press officer, who may readily agree to supply all or part of the documents requested.

In the face of refusal here, the government institution's Access Coordinator should be approached. He may be persuaded to provide the documents sought without the need to file a formal access-to-information request.

The right to an independent review should be borne in mind. (The government must prove why the information should not be disclosed and the head of the government institution may feel that this isn't worth the trouble or potential cost. If the government institution loses in court, it has to pay.)

2. If the informal approach doesn't work, consult the index posted at a government office, post office or library and fill out an application form. It asks for subject, title, author and date of the document sought and specific decisions, meetings, or whatever else you hope it contains.

3. Be reasonably specific. It's not essential to provide an exact description of document and its precise location but a request should have sufficient detail to ensure a government employee familiar with the subject can locate the record with a reasonable amount of effort.

It's wise to send formal requests to several government institutions if you are unsure which one has the information sought. However, the index should help narrow the search.

Costs for FOI

1. Each search request should cost no more than $25, the fee set to cover government costs. However, should the staff search time exceed five hours, or should the volume of photocopying exceed standards yet do be set, the rate may be higher.

2. The government may waive or refuse fees.

3. Appeal can be lodged with the information commissioner if it's felt the fees are too high. He can waive the fee or seek redress.

FOI does not apply to the Cabinet system

The price that was paid for freedom of information legislation in Canada was the federal government's insistence on total exemption of Cabinet documents from access. The government retains absolute privilege on Cabinet confidences.

Section 69(1) of the *Access to Information Act* reads:

"This Act does not apply to confidences of the Queen's Privy Council for Canada, including, without restricting the generality of the foregoing. . . ."

While you still may have access to Cabinet data through normal journalistic channels such as leaks, the "confidences" include: memoranda to Cabinet, discussion papers containing background explanations, analyses of problems or policy options, Cabinet agenda and minutes, communications between ministers, briefing papers and draft legislation.

The phrase "without restricting the generality of. . ." is, in critics' minds, a dangerous one which a Cabinet minister or Clerk of the Privy Council could apply to just about any document on the grounds that it is a Cabinet document.

The documents exempt from access are those of the Queen's Privy Council of Canada. In other words, anything to do with the Cabinet, Prime Minister's Office, and their committees and anyone who was a Cabinet minister.

The limits of this exemption will likely be settled in the courts. That is, a person can seek to determine in court if a document is indeed a Cabinet document.

Exemptions which may be subject to federal court review

Mandatory exemptions

There are five mandatory exemptions in the act, but there is nothing preventing the request for a judicial review to force disclosure of the information.

The following are summaries of the five sections of the Act which include the phrase "shall refuse to disclose", the operative phrase for the mandatory exemptions:

Section 12. (1) . . .information obtained in confidence from a government of a foreign state or institution, a group of allied states such as NATO, and a provincial or municipal government.

Section 16. (2) . . .information that was obtained or prepared by the RCMP while performing contract police duties for a province or municipality where the federal government has, on the request of the province or municipality, agreed not to disclose such information.

Section 19. (1) . . .any record requested under the act that contains personal information as defined in Section 3 of the *Privacy Act*—i.e. race, ethnic origin, color, religion, age, marital status; education, medical, criminal or employment records; address, fingerprints, or blood type; personal opinions or views of the individual; and private correspondence by the individual to government.

Section 20. (1) . . .any record requested that contains trade secrets of a third party; financial, scientific or technical information that is confidential information supplied by a third party; information that could "reasonably" be expected to interfere with contractual or other negotiations of a third party and which could be expected to result in material financial loss or gain to, or prejudice the competitor's position of, a third party. In other words, a businessman could not steal a competitor's secret information that has to be filed with Ottawa because of some law.

Section 24. (1) . . .any information which is already prohibited by statute against disclosure. There are sections of 33 other acts which override Bill C-43's provisions (e.g., sections 178.14 and 178.2 of the Criminal Code which relate to information in an affidavit sworn before a judge for permission to use a wiretap).

Discretionary Exemptions

There are 12 discretionary exemptions which contain the operative phrase "may refuse to disclose. . ." Many, no doubt, will be tested under judicial review. These are:

Section 14. . .information which could "reasonably" be expected to be injurious to federal-provincial relations such as disclosure of strategies, tactics, consultations, or deliberations.

Section 15. (1). . .information the disclosure of which could "reasonably" be expected to be injurious to the conduct of international affairs, the defence of Canada or any state allied or associated with Canada, various intelligence activities, defence equipment development or use, and diplomatic correspondence.

Section 16. (1). . .any record containing information that is part of law enforcement, including detection, prevention or suppression of a crime. Two examples are the identity of confidential source and information injurious to the security of penal institutions.

Section 16. (2). . .information that could "reasonably" facilitate the commission of a crime, such as a blueprint explaining how to break into a secure building.

Section 17. . .information that could "reasonably" be expected to threaten the safety of individuals.

Section 18. . .much economic information, including any trade secrets or other government financial, commercial. scientific or technical information of substantive value information that could prejudice the competitive position of a government institution, scientific or technical information obtained through research by an officer or employee of a government institution; information that could be "materially injurious" to the financial interests of Canada such as information relating to Canada's currency; a contemplated change in the bank interest rate or in government borrowing; contemplated changes in tariff rates, duties or any other revenue source contemplated changes in the conditions of operation of financial institutions contemplated sale or acquisition of land or property.

Section 21. (1) ...is quite vague, but may preclude any account of internal discussions, advice, or negotiations within the past 20 years concerning government employees, their ministers and the ministers' staff, as well as plans that relate to new institutions.

Section 23 ...information subject to solicitor-client privilege.

Section 26 ...if the information is "reasonably" expected to be released within 90 days after request is made for access. Additional time may be allowed for translation or printing.

2.3.2 Provincial Access to Information Statutes

Legislative provisions providing access to information and protecting the privacy of personal information differ from province to province. Seven provinces have enacted statutes which touch on these issues. The provinces of Manitoba, New Brunswick, Newfoundland and Nova Scotia have legislation dealing exclusively with access to government information. (The *Freedom of Information Act*, S.M. 1985-86, c. 6; *Right to Information Act*, S.N.B. 1978, c. R-10.3; *Freedom of Information Act*, R.S.N. 1990, c. F-25; *Freedom of Information Act*, S.N.S. 1990, c. 11) Ontario, Quebec and Saskatchewan have enacted broader legislative schemes which encompass the protection of privacy as well. (*Freedom of Information and Protection of Privacy Act*, R.S.O. 1990, c. F.31; An *Act Respecting Access to Documents Held by Public Bodies and the Protection of Personal Information*, S.Q. 1982, c. 30; *Freedom of Information and Protection of Privacy Act*, S.S. 1990-91, c. F-22.01) The legislature of British Columbia has passed similar provisions which have as yet to be proclaimed in force. (*Freedom of Information and Protection of Privacy Act*, S.B.C. 1992, c. 61) Finally, the Yukon territory enacted a short statute in 1983 which provides public access to government information through a territorial archivist.

Section 1 of Ontario's *Freedom of Information and Protection of Privacy Act* summarizes the aims of most access to information legislation:

1. The purposes of this Act are,
    (*a*) to provide a right of access to information under the control of institutions in accordance with the principles that,
        (i) information should be available to the public,
        (ii) necessary exemptions from the right of access should be limited and specific, and
        (iii) decisions on the disclosure of government information should be reviewed independently of government;
    (*b*) to protect the privacy of individuals with respect to personal information about themselves held by institutions and to provide individuals with a right of access to that information.

All the provincial legislation seeks to achieve one or both of these objectives. There are, however, significant differences among the acts.

Most of the statutes provide that any "person" has the right of access to government information. This means that any individual or corporation may request information from the government.

Newfoundland is the exception. The Newfoundland act restricts eligibility to Canadian citizens and landed immigrants. To qualify for access rights, the Canadian citizen must have a permanent home in the province. The landed immigrant, on the other hand, need not have a permanent connection with the province. Corporations may request information in Newfoundland so long as they were incorporated in Canada and conduct business within the province.

Access legislation specifies who must disclose information upon request. Some of the provincial statutes stipulate that a "government institution" or "department" must disclose. Quebec stands alone in specifying that a "public body" falls within the provisions of the act. While the definition section of each act may help to narrow the field, acts such as the one passed in New Brunswick often provide a definitive list of the government departments and affiliates covered by the provisions. For the other provincial acts, one may generally assume that government departments and ministries are covered by the legislation. A government body that regards itself as exempt from the provisions may refuse a request for information. Under these circumstances a requester may ask for a review of the decision. This will be discussed further below.

The general rule is that the access to information legislation establishes the right of access for any person to government-held information. However, there are some specific exemptions that affect a government's disclosure obligation. Disclosure may be denied if releasing the requested information would disclose personal information about another person. The government may also deny an access request if disclosure would prejudice business negotiations or cause financial loss, or would be detrimental to the administration of the criminal justice system, or breach a confidential matter protected by law.

Court records are not accessible through access legislation since many of the provincial statutes, such as those of Quebec and Saskatchewan, explicitly exempt courts from the scope of their respective acts. On the other hand, tribunals and other such quasi-judicial bodies generally fall within the scope of the access legislation. One must note, however, that *in camera* proceedings of provincial tribunals are handled differently in the different provinces. Manitoba, Ontario and Saskatchewan allow access to tribunal records since the access legislation supercedes the confidentiality provisions of other statutes. In the Atlantic provinces, however, the tribunal records fall within the exemption disclosure provisions.

Access disputes are resolved by specific appeal processes once sufficient grounds for review are established. A review of the request for information will take place if the information was not provided and if the institution: denied the existence of the information; only partially supplied the information requested; refused the entire request; or did not respond to the request within the specified time limit given in the applicable act. A requester must make an application for a review to either a judge, an ombudsman or other official as designated by the relevant provincial access statute.

In Ontario and Saskatchewan a requester would apply to the Information Commissioner. The Ontario Commissioner has the power to delegate the review process to a subordinate officer. In Quebec, any one of three members of the Commission d'accès à l'information may hear the application for review. The Ombudsman functions as the reviewing officer in Manitoba and New Brunswick. In Newfoundland and Nova Scotia a requester may appeal to a judge of the Trial Division of the Supreme Court. One must note that in Saskatchewan, a review will not take place if the request is viewed as one not made in good faith. The Saskatchewan Commissioner may also refuse a request for information if he or she feels that "...disclosure could threaten the safety or the physical or mental health of an individual." (S.S. 1990-91, c. F-22.01, s.21)

There are two types of review processes: one which is primarily investigative and the other which is adjudicative. Manitoba, New Brunswick and Saskatchewan have adopted the former approach which requires the reviewing officer to hear the appeal and recommend corrective action if this is deemed necessary. The latter approach, followed by the other provinces (New Brunswick, Newfoundland, Nova Scotia, Ontario and Quebec), gives the reviewing officer the authority to direct the government department or agency to disclose the requested information.

Disclosure of third party information is usually subject to review, upon request of a third party, before it is released. However, in New Brunswick, Nova Scotia and Manitoba, the respective legislatures have passed unique procedures applicable to this situation. In New Brunswick, third parties do not have the standing to object to disclosure. In Nova Scotia the scope for third party proceedings is very restricted. Therefore, the judge of the Supreme Court must balance the confidentiality interest of the third party against the public interest in distributing the information. Where the public interest is deemed to be paramount, the information would be released despite the concerns expressed by the third party. Similar to the New Brunswick legislation, the Manitoba act does not provide that third parties may obtain a review of a decision already made. However, the Manitoba legislature included a procedure requiring that third parties be given notice of disclosure based on the public interest criterion and a chance to object to a proposed disclosure. When such a situation arises, a requester may chose one of two avenues: leave the disclosure to the discretion of the government institution with the hope that it will not be dissuaded by third party objections; or the requester may make an application to the Court of Queen's Bench for a judicial order requiring disclosure.

On occasion, information may be improperly released by government authorities. In such cases, the government may incur civil or criminal liability. Indeed, the injured person or party may seek redress for damages suffered. The Manitoba,

Newfoundland and Saskatchewan access statutes have general immunity provisions, protecting the government and government officials from liability if disclosure was made in good faith. While the Ontario act only provides protection for government officials, the government itself may still be liable for the actions of its employees. The Nova Scotia act contains protective provisions with regard to criminal liability.

Where no provision exists to protect from liability, actions may be brought on the basis of breach of confidentiality, negligence, if the information was carelessly released, or breach of a contractual duty to keep the information confidential. In circumstances where information is released contrary to provisions imposed by statute, criminal as well as civil liability may arise. The Quebec Act makes it a specific offence to knowingly disclose information protected by statute. (S.Q. 1982, c. A-2.1, s. 159).

There are only three provinces in Canada which have attempted to deal with the issue of access to municipal records and protecting the privacy of personal information found there. Quebec's legislation specifies that local bodies fall within the legislative scheme. (*An Act Respecting Access to Documents Held by Public Bodies and the Protection of Personal Information*, S.Q. 1982, c. 30, s.2.2(a)(v)) The Saskatchewan legislature passed The *Local Authority Freedom of Information and Protection of Privacy Act*, S.S. 1990-91, c. L-27.1, in June, 1991, but it has not been proclaimed in force. Ontario has legislation in force on this point, the *Municipal Freedom of Information and Protection of Privacy Act*, R.S.O. 1990, c. M.56, which is very similar to its legislation dealing with provincial government records.

Provincial Access to Information Statutes

Manitoba	*The Freedom of Information Act*, S.M. 1985-86, c. 6
New Brunswick	*Right to Information Act*, S.N.B. 1978, c. R-10.3
Newfoundland	*Freedom of Information Act*, R.S.N. 1990, c. F-25
Nova Scotia	*Freedom of Information Act*, S.N.S. 1990, c. 11
Ontario	*Freedom of Information and Protection of Privacy Act*, R.S.O. 1990, c. F. 31
Quebec	*An Act Respecting Access to Documents Held by Public Bodies and the Protection of Personal Information*, S.Q. 1982, c. 30
Saskatchewan	*Freedom of Information and Protection of Privacy Act*, S.S. 1990-91, c. F-22.01

NOTE: Detailed information can be found in:
McNairn, Colin H.H. and Woodbury, Christopher D., *Government Information: Access and Privacy* (Toronto: Carswell, 1992).

2.4 Public Order and Criminal Libel

Criminal libel embraces a range of offences against the state and the public order. Technically, it includes seditious libel, defamatory libel, blasphemous libel and obscene libel. The first two of these are included in this chapter because of the manner in which they might still be used to protect institutions of state such as the legislatures, Parliament or the courts.

Although each has played an important role in limiting freedom of expression, the law of seditious libel has played the most central role in the emergence of free political expression. As that law has declined in importance there has been a corresponding growth in toleration for political opposition.

The law of seditious libel used to have two functions. The first of these was to punish incitements to riot or incitements to commit acts which would disturb the public order. The current Canadian hate propaganda law expresses some of the spirit of the traditional law in the sections referring to advocating genocide or the killing of a group defined by ethnic, linguistic or racial characteristics.

The modern law of seditious libel continues to restrict speech which incites riots, but as will be seen in the *Boucher* case, the Supreme Court of Canada has interpreted the law so as to broaden free expression by requiring a disturbance or a crime against the state as a planned outcome of the seditious words.

The second function of the law of seditious libel, as with its civil counterpart, was to protect the reputation of state institutions. In its earlier incarnations, the law incorporated a belief that opinions—however calmly and deliberately expressed—which condemned the established political and social order were dangerous. The notions of treason and seditious libel were blurred for most of the seventeenth and eighteenth centuries. There was a belief, often expressed by eighteenth-century judges, that if the people were allowed to read material which would predispose them to dislike governing institutions, then the whole social and political order would eventually collapse.

That idea has not completely disappeared and if the vestiges of it are no longer serious parts of the modern law of seditious libel, expressions of it may be found here and there in twentieth-century Canadian history. For example, section 98 of the old Criminal Code prohibited membership in certain organizations including the Communist Party. A parallel sentiment was expressed in the case of *Switzman v. Elbling and the Attorney-General of Quebec* in which the Quebec Padlock law was at issue. That law prohibited the circulation of Communist material in Quebec from 1937 until 1957 when it was finally ruled *ultra vires* by the Supreme Court of Canada.

As will be seen below, the part of the law of contempt of court called "scandalizing the court" is equally a vestige of the old notion of seditious libel. That law renders criminal disrespectful and aggressively expressed condemnations of judges or the courts.

That the law of seditious libel has been central to the history of English and Canadian democracy can be seen by a consideration of the manner in which the law changed between the seventeenth century and the twentieth. During the seventeenth and eighteenth centuries in England it was a crime to promote disaffection against the Monarch and his or her heirs, the Government, Parliament, the administration of justice, the Constitution or the State. It was, for example, libelous in the eighteenth century to argue that the Glorious Revolution of 1688 and the end of the Stuart monarchy were unhappy events.

The law of seditious libel has gone through four distinctive phases. The first involved licensing. Printing came of age in the seventeenth century and for most of it there was a licensing act in place to prevent seditious (or blasphemous) libel from being committed. Those in power in England were so afraid of the effects of printing that they set up a licensing authority which empowered political and church authorities to examine all materials published for public circulation. These authorities exercised what the Americans now call 'prior restraint' . (We continue to examine films for obscene content in all Canadian provinces.) The end of licensing in 1695 marked the beginning of a second stage which lasted until 1792 when *Fox's Libel Act* was passed.

Stage two is a period during which the law was severely applied, but was constantly challenged and to some degree modified. The modifications came partly as a result of changes in attitude toward the importance and danger of seditious libel, but more so because the various oppositions to the ministries of the eighteenth century were able to challenge and eventually remove a set of legal instruments and devices associated with policing and prosecuting printers and writers.

When *Fox's Libel Act* was passed in 1792 the last trace of the special methods of applying the law, which had been conceived and elaborated during the licensing period, was removed. Until that act was passed, juries had very little to do in trials for libel. They could establish that the authorities had brought the right person to trial—that for example, the accused actually wrote or published the material alleged to be criminal—and they could also rule on the meaning of the words. But it was the judge alone who decided whether the materials were libellous. *Fox's Libel Act* changed the role of juries and gave them the right to rule on the larger question of libel.

The third stage is marked by the absence of special legal instruments. From 1792 on, there was just a law—seriously and severely applied, but supported by conventional means of police and prosecution. It was sometimes harshly applied, especially in the period just before 1832. There was much radical publishing during that period and as a consequence many prosecutions. This stage of the law's evolution lasted through the nineteenth century and into the twentieth.

If rough measures are taken, the fourth stage is the period during the twentieth century when the law becomes relatively innocuous—when, for example, it becomes impossible to libel the State (with the exception of the courts). When the lawmakers had absorbed the idea that the State and its officials had to earn their reputations rather than compel them, the legal system expressed finally an idea which had had support in the eighteenth century. Still, it should be recognized that states are tempted occasionally to restore some of the ideas contained in the traditional law of seditious libel. They are sometimes tempted to criminalize political opinions, the purposes of which are to alter radically the political system or social order.

2.4.1 *Criminal Code*, R.S.C. 1985, c. C-46

59. (1) Seditious words are words that express a seditious intention.

(2) A seditious libel is a libel that expresses a seditious intention.

(3) A seditious conspiracy is an agreement between two or more persons to carry out a seditious intention.

(4) Without limiting the generality of the meaning of the expression "seditious intention", every one shall be presumed to have a seditious intention who
   (*a*) teaches or advocates, or
   (*b*) publishes or circulates any writing that advocates, the use, without the authority of law, of force as a means of accomplishing a governmental change within Canada.

60. Notwithstanding subsection 59(4), no person shall be deemed to have a seditious intention by reason only that he intends, in good faith,
   (*a*) to show that Her Majesty has been misled or mistaken in her measures;
   (*b*) to point out errors or defects in
      (i) the government or constitution of Canada or a province,
      (ii) the Parliament of Canada or the legislature of a province,
      (iii) the administration of justice in Canada,
   (*c*) to procure, by lawful means, the alteration of any matter of government in Canada; or
   (*d*) to point out, for the purpose of removal, matters that produce or tend to produce feelings of hostility and ill-will between different classes of persons in Canada.

61. Every one who
   (*a*) speaks seditious words,
   (*b*) publishes a seditious libel, or
   (*c*) is a party to a seditious conspiracy,
is guilty of an indictable offence and is liable to imprisonment for fourteen years.

62. (1) Every one who willfully
   (*a*) interferes with, impairs or influences the loyalty or discipline of a member of a force,
   (*b*) publishes, edits, issues, circulates or distributes a writing that advises, counsels or urges insubordination, disloyalty, mutiny or refusal of duty by a member of a force, or
   (*c*) advises, counsels, urges or in any manner causes insubordination, disloyalty, mutiny or refusal of duty by a member of a force,
is guilty of an indictable offence and is liable to imprisonment for five years.

(2) In this section, "member of a force" means a member of
   (a) the Canadian Forces, or
   (b) the naval, army or air forces of a state other than Canada that are lawfully present in Canada.

2.4.1.1. *Boucher v. The King*, [1950] 1 D.L.R. 657 (S.C.C.)

RAND, J. (dissenting in part):—This appeal arises out of features of what, in substance, is religious controversy, and it is necessary that the facts be clearly appreciated. The appellant, a farmer, living near the Town of St. Joseph de Beauce, Quebec, was convicted of uttering a seditious libel. The libel was contained in a four-page document published apparently at Toronto by the Watch Tower Bible & Tract Society, which I take to be the name of the official publishers of the religious group known as the Witnesses of Jehovah. The document was headed "Quebec's Burning Hate for God and Christ and Freedom Is the Shame of all Canada": it consisted first of an invocation to calmness and reason in appraising the matters to be dealt with in support of the heading; then of general references to vindictive persecution accorded in Quebec to the Witnesses as brethren in Christ; a detailed narrative of specific incidents of persecution; and a concluding appeal to the people of the Province, in protest against mob rule and gestapo tactics, that through the study of God's Word and obedience to its commands, there might be brought about a "bounteous crop of the good fruits of love for Him and Christ and human freedom". At the foot of the document is an advertisement of two books entitled "Let God be True" and "Be Glad, Ye Nations", the former revealing, in the light of God's Word, the truth concerning the Trinity, Sabbath, prayer, etc., and the latter, the facts of the endurance of Witnesses in the crucible of "fiery persecution".

The incidents, as described, are of peaceable Canadians who seem not to be lacking in meekness, but who, for distributing, apparently without permits, Bibles and tracts on Christian doctrine; for conducting religious services in private homes or on private lands in Christian fellowship; for holding public lecture meetings to teach religious truth as they believe it of the Christian religion; who, for this exercise of what has been taken for granted to be the challengeable rights of Canadians, have been assaulted and beaten and their Bibles and publications torn up and destroyed, by individuals and by mobs; who have had their homes invaded and their property taken; and in hundreds have been charged with public offences and held to exorbitant bail. The police are declared to have exhibited an attitude of animosity toward them and to have treated them as the criminals in provoking by their action of Christian profession and teaching, the violence to which they have been subjected; and public officials and members of the Roman Catholic Clergy are said not only to have witnessed these outrages but to have been privy to some of the prosecutions. The document charged that the Roman Catholic Church in Quebec was in some objectionable relation to the administration of justice and that the force behind the prosecutions was that of the priests of that Church.

The conduct of the accused appears to have been unexceptionable; so far as disclosed, he is an exemplary citizen who is at least sympathetic to doctrines of the Christian religion which are, evidently, different from either the Protestant or the Roman Catholic versions: but the foundation in all is the same, Christ and his relation to God and humanity.

The crime of seditious libel is well known to the common law. Its history has been thoroughly examined and traced by Stephen, Holdsworth and other eminent legal scholars and they are in agreement both in what it originally consisted and in the social assumptions underlying it. Up to the end of the 18th century it was, in essence, a contempt in words of political authority or the actions of authority. If we conceive of the governors of society as superior beings, exercising a divine mandate, by whom laws, institutions and administrations are given to men to be obeyed, who are, in short, beyond criticism, reflection or censure upon them or what they do implies either an equality with them or an accountability by them, both equally offensive. In that lay sedition by words and the libel was its written form.

But constitutional conceptions of a different order making rapid progress in the 19th century have necessitated a modification of the legal view of public criticism; and the administrators of what we call democratic government have come to be looked upon as servants bound to carry out their duties accountably to the public. The basic nature of the common law lies in its flexible process of traditional reasoning upon significant social and political matter; and just as in the 17th century the crime of seditious libel was a deduction from fundamental conceptions of government, the substitution of new conceptions, under the same principle of reasoning called for new jural conclusions: *Bourne v. Keane*, [1919] A.C. 815.

As early as 1839 in *Reg. v. Collins*, 9 Car. & P. 456 at pp. 460-1, 173 E.R. 910, Littledale J., in his charge to the jury, laid it down that "you are to consider whether.... [they] meant to excite the people to take the power into their own hands, and meant to excite them to tumult and disorder.... the people have a right to discuss any grievances that they have to complain of, but they must not do it in a way to excite tumult", which Stephen, in vol. 2 of his *History of the Criminal Law* at p. 375, sums up: "In one word, nothing short of direct incitement to disorder and violence is a seditious libel. " Coleridge J. in *R. v. Aldred* (1909), 22 Cox C.C. I, at p. 3, used these words: "The man who is accused may not plead the truth of the statements that he makes as a defence to the charge, nor may be plead the innocence of his motive; that is not a defence to the charge. The test is not either the truth of the language or the innocence of the motive with which he publishes it, but the test is this: was the language used calculated, or was it not, to promote public disorder or physical force?" ((1941), 85 Sol. Io., 251). The language used must, obviously, be related to the particular matters in each case complained of.

This development is to be considered also in the light of the practice in administering the law of seditious words followed after *Fox's Libel Act* of 1792. The jury in such cases by its right under the statute to bring in a general verdict, must, in addition to the publication of the libel and its meaning have found a seditious intention. That meant more than the issue of the writing knowing what it contained. The Act was interpreted as requiring the libel to have been published with an *illegal* intention. The word "intention" was not always clearly differentiated from indirect purpose or motive, but if the intention, as envisaging immediate or proximate response, regardless of a remote object of whatever nature, was illegal, the libel was seditious.

Stephen suggests a theoretical continuity of the law by taking that Act to have made material those consequential allegations such as of ill-will, disaffection, etc., with which the early indictments were liberally encumbered, but which were looked upon as formal or assumed as necessary effects of the libel otherwise seditious. But if that is sound, then we must have regard to the sense which they then bore; and it would seem to be clear that they signified feelings and attitudes toward established authority.

The definition of seditious intention as formulated by Stephen, summarized, is, (1) to bring into hatred or contempt, or to excite disaffection against, the King or the Government and Constitution of the United Kingdom, or either House of Parliament, or the administration of justice; or (2) to excite the King's subjects to attempt, otherwise than by lawful means, the alteration of any matter in Church or State by law established; or (3) to incite persons to commit any crime in general disturbance of the pace; or (4) to raise discontent or disaffection amongst His Majesty's subjects; or (5) to promote feelings of ill-will and hostility between different classes of such subjects. The only items of this definition that could be drawn into question here are that relating to the administration of justice in (1) and those of (4) and (5). It was the latter which were brought most prominently to the notice of the jury, and it is with an examination of what in these days their language must be taken to mean that I will chiefly concern myself.

There is no modern authority which holds that the mere effect of tending to create discontent or disaffection among His Majesty's subjects or ill-will or hostility between groups of them, but not tending to issue in illegal conduct, constitutes the crime, and this for obvious reasons. Freedom in thought and speech and disagreement in ideas and beliefs, on every conceivable subject, are of the essence of our life. The clash of critical discussion on political, social and religious subjects has too deeply become the stuff of daily experience to suggest that mere ill-will as a product of controversy can strike down the latter with illegality. A superficial examination of the word shows its insufficiency. What is the degree necessary to criminality? Can it ever, as mere subjective condition, be so? Controversial fury is aroused constantly by differences in abstract conceptions; heresy in some fields is again a mortal sin; there can be fanatical puritanism in ideas as well as in morals; but our compact of free society accepts and absorbs these differences and they are exercised at large within the framework of freedom and order on broader and deeper uniformities as bases of social stability. Similarly in discontent, disaffection and hostility: as subjective incidents of controversy, they and the ideas which arouse them are part of our living which ultimately serve us in stimulation, in the clarification of thought and, as we believe, in the search for the constitution and truth of things generally.

Although Stephen's definition was adopted substantially as it is by the Criminal Code Commission of England in 1880, the latter's report, in this respect, was not acted on by the Imperial Parliament, and the *Criminal Code* of this country, enacted in 1891, did not incorporate its provisions. The latter omits any reference to definition except in s. 133 to declare that the intention includes the advocacy of the use of force as a means of bringing about a change of Government and by s.133A, that certain actions are not included. What the words in (4) and (5) must in the present day be taken to signify is the use of language which, by inflaming the minds of people into hatred, ill-will, discontent, disaffection, is intended, or is so likely to do so as to be deemed to be intended, to disorder community life, but directly or indirectly in relation to Government in the broadest sense: Phillimore J. in *R. v. Antonelli & Barberi* (1905), 70 J.P. 4 at p. 6, "seditious libels are such as tend to disturb the government of this country." That may be through tumult or violence, in resistance to public authority, in defiance of law. This conception lies behind the association which the word is given in C.S.L.C. 1861, c. 10, s. 1(1), dealing with illegal oaths: "To engage in any seditious, rebellious, or treasonable purpose"; and the corresponding s.131(a)(i) of the *Code:* "To engage in any mutinous or seditious purpose."

The baiting or denouncing of one group by another or others without an aim directly or indirectly at Government, is in the nature of public mischief: *R. v. Leese & Whitehead* (*The Times*, September 22, 1936, cited in 85 Sol. Jo. 252); and incitement to unlawful acts is itself an offence.

This result must be distinguished from an undesired reaction provoked by the exercise of common rights, such as the violent opposition to the early services of the Salvation Army. In that situation it was the hoodlums who were held to be the lawless and not the members of the Army: *Beatty v. Gillbanks* (1882), 9 Q.B.D. 308. On the allegations in the document here, had the Salvationists been arrested for bringing about by unlawful assembly a breach of the pace and fined, had they then made an impassioned protest against such treatment of law-abiding citizens, and had they thereupon been charged with seditious words, their plight would have been that of the accused in this case.

These considerations are confirmed by s.133A of the *Code*, which is as follows:

"133A. No one shall be deemed to have a seditious intention only because he intends in good faith.—

"(a) to show that His Majesty has been misled or mistaken in his measures; or

"(b) to point out errors or defects in the government or constitution of the United Kingdom, or of any part of it, or of Canada or any province thereof, or in either House of Parliament of the United Kingdom or of Canada, or In any legislature, or in the administration of justice; or to excite His Majesty's subjects to attempt to procure, by lawful means, the alteration of any matter in the state; or,

"(c) to point out, in order to their removal, matters which are producing or have a tendency to produce feelings of hatred and ill-will between different classes of His Majesty's subjects."

This, as is seen, is a fundamental provision which, with its background of free criticism as a constituent of modem democratic Government, protects the widest range of public discussion and controversy, so long as it is done in good faith and for the purposes mentioned. Its effect is to eviscerate the older concept of its anachronistic elements. But a motive or ultimate purpose, whether good or believed to be good is unavailing if the means employed is bad; disturbance or corrosion may be ends in themselves, but whether means or ends, their character stamps them and intention behind them as illegal.

The condemned intention lies then in a residue of criticism of Government, the negative touchstone of which is the test of good faith by legitimate means toward legitimate ends. That claim was the real defence in the proceedings here but it was virtually ignored by the trial Judge. On that failure, as well as others, the Chief Justice of the King's Bench and Galipeault, J. have rested their dissent, and with them I am in agreement.

But a further question remains. In the circumstances, should the appellant be subjected to a second trial? Could a jury, properly instructed and acting judicially have found, beyond a reasonable doubt, a seditious intention in circulating the document? In the heading is the chief source of resentment but there are also statements, such as the insinuation of the part played by the Church in judicial administration and the role of some of the clergy in the prosecutions, which offend likewise. Now these allegations are inferences and conclusions drawn from the facts and incidents presented in detail which the accused was ready with evidence to prove, and it is obvious that they and the matters from which they are deduced, must be read together. When it is said that Quebec hates Christ, it is hate *sub modo*; it means that to persecute is to hate, and that to hate those who follow and love Him, *i.e.* the Witnesses, for what they do in His service, is to hate Him. Only in that manner can the real intention evidenced by the document be appreciated.

The writing was undoubtedly made under an aroused sense of wrong to the Witnesses; but it is beyond dispute that its end and object was the removal of what they considered iniquitous treatment. Here are conscientious professing followers of Christ who claim to have been denied the right to worship in their own homes and their own manner and to have been jailed for obeying the injunction to "teach all nations". They are said to have been called "a bunch of crazy nuts" by one of the Magistrates. Whatever that means, it may from his standpoint be a correct description; I do not know; but it is not challenged that, as they allege, whatever they did was done peaceably, and, as they saw it, in the way of bringing the light and peace of the Christian religion to the souls of men and women. To say that is to say that their acts were lawful. Whether, in like circumstances, other groups of the Christian Church would show greater forbearance and earnestness in the appeal to Christian charity to have done with such abuses, may be doubtful. The Courts below have not, as, with the greatest respect, I think they should have, viewed the document as primarily a burning protest and as a result have lost sight of the fact that, expressive as it is of a deep indignation, its conclusion is an earnest petition to the public opinion of the Province to extend to the Witnesses of Jehovah, as a minority, the protection of impartial laws. No one would suggest that the document is intended to arouse French-speaking Roman Catholics to disorderly conduct against their own Government, and to treat it as directed, with the same purpose, towards the Witnesses themselves in the Province, would be quite absurd: in relation to Courts, it is, to use the language of s.133A, pointing out, "in order to their removal", what are believed to be "matters which are producing or have a tendency to produce feelings of hatred and ill-will between different classes of His Majesty's subjects" . That some of the expressions, divorced from their context, may be extravagant and may arouse resentment, is not, in the circumstances, sufficient to take the intention of the writing as a whole beyond what is recognized by s.133A as lawful.

Where a conviction is set aside, this Court must dispose of the appeal as the justice of the case requires; and where the evidence offered could not, under a proper instruction, have supported a conviction, the accused must be discharged: *Schwartzenhauer v. The King*, [1935] 3 D.L.R. 711, S.C.R. 367, 64 Can. C.C. I; *Manchuk v. The King*, [1938] 3 D.L.R. 693, S.C.R. 341, 70 Can. C.C. 161; *Savard & Lizotte v. The King*, [1946] 3 D.L.R. 468, S.C.R. 20, 85 Can. C.C. 254.

I would therefore, allow the appeal, set aside the conviction, and order judgment of acquittal to be entered.

ESTEY, J. (dissenting in part):—This is an appeal under s.1023 of the *Code* on questions of law raised in the dissenting opinions of the learned Judges in the Court of King's Bench (Appeal Side) of the Province of Quebec [95 Can. C.C. 119]. The appellant was convicted of seditious libel in that he did on or about December 11, 1946, at St. Joseph "dans le district de Beauce", distribute a pamphlet entitled "La haine ardente du Quebec, pour Dieu, pour le Christ, et pour la liberte, est un sujet de honte pour tout le Canada". Upon appeal this conviction was affirmed, Letourneau, C.J. and Galipault, J. dissenting.

The pamphlet consists of four pages entitled as aforesaid which the appellant admitted he had read and distributed. The main issue is, therefore, whether the appellant had a seditious intention in distributing and thereby publishing the pamphlet.

There were several points raised in the dissenting opinions but it will be sufficient to continue the discussion to two of them, namely, that the learned trial Judge in charging the jury (a) did not sufficiently define " seditious intention", (b) did not adequately explain to the jury the place and meaning of "reasonable doubt".

A "seditious libel" is defined in s.133 of the *Code* the material part of which reads:

"133(1) Seditious words are words expressive of a seditious intention.

"(2) A seditious libel is a libel expressive of a seditious intention."

A "seditious intention" is not defined in either s. 133 or in any other part of the Code and we must therefore look to the common law. It will there be found that the definition in Stephen's "Digest of the Criminal Law", 5th ed., p. 70, and described by the Commissioners who prepared the draft of the English Code to be "as accurate a statement of the existing law as we can make", is generally accepted.

This is set out in s. 102 of the draft Code:

"A seditious intention is an intention to bring into hatred or contempt, or to excite disaffection against the person of Her Majesty, or the Government and Constitution of the United Kingdom or of any part of it as by law established, or either House of Parliament, or the administration of justice; or to excite Her Majesty's subjects to attempt to procure otherwise than by lawful means the alteration of any matter in Church or State by law established; or to raise discontent or disaffection amongst Her Majesty's subjects; or to promote feelings of ill-will and hostility between different classes of such subjects:

"Provided that no one shall be deemed to have a seditious intention only because he intends in good faith to show that Her Majesty has been misled or mistaken in her measures; or to point out errors or defects in the Government or Constitution of the United Kingdom or of any part of it as by law established, or in the administration of justice, with a view to the reformation of such alleged errors or defects; or to excite Her Majesty's subjects to attempt to procure by lawful means the alteration of any matter in Church or State by law established; or to point out in order to their removal matters which are producing or have a tendency to produce feelings of hatred and ill will between different classes of Her Majesty's subjects.

"Seditious words are words expressive of or intended to carry into execution or to excite others to carry into execution a seditious intention."

While the foregoing definition has never been enacted as part of our *Criminal Code*, the proviso was enacted in our first Code in 1892 as part of s.123 (1892, c.29) and was deleted by an amendment in 1919 [c.46, s.4] and re-enacted in 1930 and is now s.133A (1930, c. 11, s.2).

The learned trial Judge did not discuss a "seditious intention" in the terms of or in terms similar to those in the foregoing definition more than to say that a seditious intention is one "to provoke feelings of ill-will and hostility between different classes of His Majesty's Subjects," and expressed it in French as follows: "Le Libelle sedi tieux c'est la publication ou la distribution d'un pamphlet, ou d'un ecrit injurieux, blessant, et qui peut provoquer de la haine et de la discorde parmi les differentes classes de sujets de Sa Majeste."

However vague and indefinite the words "ill-will and hostility" may be when read as part of the foregoing definition of sedition, they are certainly more so when, as in this case, they were stated to the jury as separate and apart therefrom.

Cave J. in *Reg. v. Burns* (1886), 16 Cox C.C. 355, referred to the foregoing definition as somewhat vague and general and particularly that person reading "ill will and hostility between different classes of Her Majesty's subjects". This vague and general character is further emphasized in *Law of the Constitution*, Dicey, 9th ed., p. 244, where, after pointing out that the law permits publication of statements indicating "the Crown has been misled, or that the government has committed errors... and, in short, sanctions criticism of public affairs which is *bona fide* intended to recommend the reform of existing institutions by legal methods", the learned author concludes: "But any one will see at once that the legal definition of a seditious libel might easily be so used as to check a great deal of what is ordinarily considered allowable discussion, and would if rigidly enforced be inconsistent with prevailing forms of political agitation."

The foregoing emphasizes the importance of intention and the necessity of a trial Judge explaining to a jury, in such a ease as here, the meaning of "intention to promote feelings of ill-will and hostility between different classes" of His Majesty's subjects as an essential in the offence of sedition.

In determining whether a seditious intention is present in a particular case, the language of Fitzgerald J. in *Reg. v. Sullivan* (1868), 11 Cox C.C. 44, at p. 45, adopted by Cave J. in *Reg. v. Burns*, 16 Cox C.C. at p. 361, is pertinent: "'Sedition has been described as disloyalty in action, and the law considers as seditious all those practices which have for their object to excite discontent or disaffection, to create public disturbances, or to lead to civil war; to bring into hatred or contempt the Sovereign or the Government, the laws or constitution of the Realm, and generally all endeavours to promote public disorder.'"

Stephen's *History of the Criminal Law of England*, vol. 2, p. 375: "In one word, nothing short of direct incitement to disorder and violence is a seditious libel."

Reg. v. Burns, supra, and other authorities rather indicate that an intention to incite something less than violence is sufficient, and that the offence of sedition is committed if it be established that the parties charged intentionally incited ill-will and hostility between different classes of citizens in such a manner as may be likely to cause public disorder or disturbance. It will be recognized that one may freely and forcefully express his views within the limits defined by the law. Those engaged in campaigns or controversies of a public nature may cause feelings of hatred and ill-will but it does not at all follow that those taking part therein and causing these feelings are acting with a seditious intention. The essential, without which there cannot be sedition, is the presence of a seditious intention as above defined and which is a fact to be determined on the evidence adduced in each case.

It is therefore important to determine whether there was any evidence which in law would support a verdict of guilty which in this case, would include a finding that the appellant in distributing this pamphlet acted with a seditious intention.

The Crown asked the jury to find the intention of the accused from the language of this four-page pamphlet. Nine excerpts from it were specifically embodied in the indictment. These, however, cannot be read separate and apart, but rather their meaning and effect must be determined by reading and construing them in relation to the statements in the pamphlet as a whole.

The pamphlet is entitled, as already stated, "La haine ardente du Quebec, pour Dieu, pour le Christ, et pour la liberte, est un sujet de honte pour tout le Canada". In the first paragraph the reader is requested to "calmly and soberly and with clear mental faculties reason on the evidence presented in support of the above-headlined indictment". Then follows a recitation of facts and circumstances in support of the conclusions that the witnesses of Jehovah are ill-treated and their freedom to worship according to the tenets of their religion denied; and that this condition exists because members of the judiciary, police and groups of citizens are directed and controlled by the priests of the Roman Catholic Church. All of which the pamphlet declares to be contrary to the principles of Christianity and that "such blind course will lead to the ditch of destruction. To avoid it turn from following men and traditions, and study and follow the Bible's teaching; that was Jesus' advice". This is the appeal made to all who read this pamphlet. It does not disclose an intention, nor reading the pamphlet as a whole can it be concluded that it is calculated to incite persons or classes of persons to acts or conduct leading to public disorder or disturbance. On the contrary, the pamphlet stresses the view that if the plea therein contained is acted upon the existent ill-will and hatred will disappear and the interference complained of will no longer exist. In these circumstances it is difficult to conclude that the appellant in distributing and publishing this pamphlet was doing so with a seditious intention.

We are not, however, left in this case with respect to a seditious intention to the construction of the pamphlet alone. The appellant gave evidence on his own behalf. He explained that he was a minister of the Witnesses of Jehovah, that hatred and ill will already existed against Jehovah's Witnesses and that he had read the pamphlet and distributed it, as he explained (translation):

"A. In the desire to make known the things contained in the pamphlet in order to have the persecutions undergone by the Witnesses of Jehovah changed so that men of good will may know the things.... not in order to stir up hatred or trouble as the Witnesses just said that there had been no stirring up... Q. When you distributed that, what was the object? A. With the object that people would see that the world after having come to know of what is in this pamphlet, might see to it that the Government and the authorities should take the means to correct these things and that there should be no more persecutions, it was truly with that object so that men of good-will might have the vision to preach peace and live in peace whereas you see them speak of hatred all the time."

The appellant specifically denied that he had any intention of creating public disorder; on the contrary he stated that he desired to establish pace between the Roman Catholics and the Witnesses of Jehovah. He stated: "I have studied it, read it and have seen the facts."

Apart from this general declaration, he deposed that it was his own child, eleven years of age, referred to in the pamphlet who, because of her religious views, was expelled from her school.

The learned trial Judge in the course of his charge suggested that the distribution of this pamphlet was a ludicrous or strange way to effect a reconciliation. The conduct of the appellant may not only, in the opinion of the learned trial Judge, but of many others, be ludicrous or strange. That, however, is quite apart from the question whether the appellant had, upon the whole of the evidence, a seditious intention.

The good faith of the appellant in distributing this pamphlet was directly in issue under s.133A(c). He, in the course of his evidence as above indicated, adopted as true the statements in the pamphlet. The truth of the pamphlet is not a defence to a charge of sedition but if the facts set out in the pamphlet are untrue, evidence to that effect would have gone far to have shown the appellant did not act in good faith. No such evidence was adduced.

The conduct on the part of any group in Canada which denies to or even interferes with the right of the members of any religious body to worship is a matter of public concern. The pamphlet, in the conception of the appellant as he deposed, discusses such an interference. He pledged his oath that it sets forth facts and circumstances which establish this interference with respect to the rights of the Witnesses of Jehovah to worship in the Province of Quebec and that hatred and ill-will exist toward them. He believed the plea set forth in the pamphlet would remove that hatred and ill-will and the interference would cease. He therefore, as he deposed, in good faith and for that purpose published and distributed the pamphlet. No evidence was introduced to contradict any of these factors and therefore the evidence here adduced brings this position of the appellant within the provisions of s.133A already quoted.

The facts as set forth in the pamphlet may be inaccurately stated, even incorrect and the comments unjustified. The statements in it may be objectionable, even repugnant to some and provoke ill-will and hatred. That, however, is not sufficient. It still remains to be proved as a fact that the accused acted with a seditious intention. Under s.133A that intention does not exist if the appellant's conduct was within that section and he was acting in good faith. The evidence of good faith on behalf of the defence is consistent with the intent and purpose of the pamphlet as therein expressed and no evidence has been adduced to the contrary. The onus rested upon the Crown throughout to prove beyond a reasonable doubt that the accused acted with a seditious intention and this record does not disclose any evidence that would properly sustain a verdict that the accused possessed such an intention.

The appeal should be allowed, the conviction quashed and a judgment and verdict of acquittal directed to be entered.

New trial ordered.

2.4.1.2. Law Reform Commission of Canada, *Crimes Against the State*, Working Paper 49 (Ottawa: 1986), pp. 32, 35-36

The seditious offences in sections 60, 61 and 62 [now sections 59, 60 and 61] provide yet another example of uncertainty in the *Code*. For example, the three offences of speaking seditious words, publishing a seditious libel and being a party to a seditious conspiracy, each require that there be a "seditious intention," but this phrase is not defined. Subsection 60(4) tells us what will be presumed to be a seditious intention and section 61 tells us what will not be treated as a seditious intention, and yet nowhere in the *Code* is there a conclusive definition of what is in fact a seditious intention. Instead we have to turn to the common law to find its meaning, but the common law definition is also vague and uncertain.

. . . . .

The offence of sedition provides another example of an outdated and unprincipled law. The original aim of the crime of sedition was to forbid criticism and derision of political authority, and as Fitzjames Stephen pointed out, the offence was a natural concomitant of the once prevalent view that the governors of the State were wise and superior beings exercising a divine mandate and beyond the reproach of the common people. With the coming of age of parliamentary democracy in the nineteenth century, government could no longer be conceived as the infallible master of the people, but as their servant, and subjects were seen to have a perfect right to criticize and even dismiss their government. Indeed it is essential to the health of a parliamentary democracy such as Canada that citizens have the right to criticize, debate and discuss political, economic and social matters in the freest possible manner. This has already been recognized by our courts and now the *Canadian Charter of Rights and Freedoms* provides additional guarantees of political freedom of expression (see ss.2, 3). Is it not odd then that our *Criminal Code* still contains the offence of sedition which has as its very object the suppression of such freedom? In the *Boucher* case, the Supreme Court of Canada tries to deal with this inconsistency by taking a narrow view of the common law definition of a seditious intention. Applying their narrow definition, there no longer seems to be a need for a separate offence of sedition, because the only conduct that would be proscribed by it could just as well be dealt with as incitement . . ., conspiracy . . ., contempt of court, or hate propaganda . . . . Clearly, legislative revision is in order as well.

2.4.2 *Criminal Code*, R.S.C. 1985, c . C-46

297. In sections 303, 304 and 308, "newspaper" means any paper, magazine or periodical containing public news, intelligence or reports of events, or any remarks or observations thereon, printed for sale and published periodically or in parts or numbers, at intervals not exceeding thirty-one days between the publication of any two such papers, parts or numbers, and any paper, magazine or periodical printed in order to be dispersed and made public, weekly or more often, or at intervals not exceeding thirty-one days, that contains advertisements, exclusively or principally.

298. (1) A defamatory libel is matter published, without lawful justification or excuse, that is likely to injure the reputation of any person by exposing him to hatred, contempt or ridicule, or that is designed to insult the person of or concerning whom it is published.

(2) A defamatory libel may be expressed directly or by insinuation or irony
   (*a*) in words legibly marked upon any substance, or
   (*b*) by any object signifying a defamatory libel otherwise than by words.

299. A person publishes a libel when he
   (*a*) exhibits it in public,
   (*b*) causes it to be read or seen, or
   (*c*) shows or delivers it, or causes it to be shown or delivered, with intent that it should be read or seen by the person whom it defames or by any other person.

300. Every one who publishes a defamatory libel that he knows is false is guilty of an indictable offence and is liable to imprisonment for five years.

301. Every one who publishes a defamatory libel is guilty of an indictable offence and is liable to imprisonment for two years.

302. (1) Every one commits an offence who, with intent
   (*a*) to extort money from any person, or
   (*b*) to induce a person to confer upon or procure for another person an appointment or office of profit or trust,
publishes or threatens to publish or offers to abstain from publishing or to prevent the publication of a defamatory libel.

(2) Every one commits an offence who, as the result of the refusal of any person to permit money to be extorted or to confer or procure an appointment or office of profit or trust, publishes or threatens to publish a defamatory libel.

(3) Every one who commits an offence under this section is guilty of an indictable offence and is liable to imprisonment for five years.

303. (1) The proprietor of a newspaper shall be deemed to publish defamatory matter that is inserted and published therein, unless he proves that the defamatory matter was inserted in the newspaper with out his knowledge and without negligence on his part.

(2) Where the proprietor of a newspaper gives to a person general authority to manage or conduct the newspaper as editor or otherwise, the insertion by that person of defamatory matter in the newspaper shall, for the purposes of subsection (1), be deemed not to be negligence on the part of the proprietor unless it is proved that

> (*a*) he intended the general authority to include authority to insert defamatory matter in the newspaper, or
>
> (*b*) he continued to confer general authority after he knew that it had been exercised by the insertion of defamatory matter in the newspaper.

(3) No person shall be deemed to publish a defamatory libel by reason only that he sells a number or part of a newspaper that contains a defamatory libel, unless he knows that the number or part contains defamatory matter or that defamatory matter is habitually contained in the newspaper.

304. (1) No person shall be deemed to publish a defamatory libel by reason only that he sells a book, magazine, pamphlet or other thing, other than a newspaper that contains defamatory matter if, at the time of the sale, he does not know that it contains the defamatory matter.

(2) Where a servant, in the course of his employment, sells a book, magazine, pamphlet or other thing, other than a newspaper, the employer shall be deemed not to publish any defamatory matter contained therein unless it is proved that the employer authorized the sale knowing that

> (*a*) defamatory matter was contained therein, or
>
> (*b*) defamatory matter was habitually contained therein, in the case of a periodical.

305. No person shall be deemed to publish a defamatory libel by reason only that he publishes defamatory matter

> (*a*) in a proceeding held before or under the authority of a court exercising judicial authority, or
>
> (*b*) in an inquiry made under the authority of an Act or by order of Her Majesty, or under the authority of a public department or a department of the government of a province.

306. No person shall be deemed to publish a defamatory libel by reason only that he (*a*) publishes to the Senate or House of Commons or to a legislature, defamatory matter contained in a petition to the Senate or House of Commons or to the legislature, as the case may be,

(*b*) publishes by order or under the authority of the Senate or House of Commons or of a legislature, a paper containing defamatory matter, or

(*c*) publishes, in good faith and without ill will to the person defamed, an extract from or abstract of a petition or paper mentioned in paragraph (a) or (b).

307. (1) No person shall be deemed to publish a defamatory libel by reason only that he publishes in good faith, for the information of the public, a fair report of the proceedings of the Senate or House of Commons or a legislature, or a committee thereof, or of the public proceedings before a court exercising judicial authority, or publishes, in good faith, any fair comment upon any such proceedings.

(2) This section does not apply to a person who publishes a report of evidence taken or offered in any proceeding before the Senate or House of Commons or any committee thereof, upon a petition or bill relating to any matter of marriage or divorce, if the report is published without authority from or leave of the House in which the proceeding is held or is contrary to any rule, order or practice of that House.

308. No person shall be deemed to publish a defamatory libel by reason only that he publishes in good faith, in a newspaper, a fair report of the proceedings of any public meeting if

(*a*) the meeting is lawfully convened for a lawful purpose and is open to the public,

(*b*) the report is fair and accurate,

(*c*) the publication of the matter complained of is for the public benefit, and

(*d*) he does not refuse to publish in a conspicuous place in the newspaper a reasonable explanation or contradiction by the person defamed in respect of the defamatory matter.

309. No person shall be deemed to publish a defamatory libel by reason only that he publishes defamatory matter that, on reasonable grounds, he believes is true, and that is relevant to any subject of public interest, the public discussion of which is for the public benefit.

310. No person shall be deemed to publish a defamatory libel by reason only that he publishes fair comments

(*a*) upon the public conduct of a person who takes part in public affairs, or

(*b*) upon a published book or other literary production, or on any composition or work of art or performance publicly exhibited, or on any other communication made to the public on any subject, if the comments are confined to criticism thereof.

311. No person shall be deemed to publish a defamatory libel where he proves that the publication of the defamatory matter in the manner in which it was published was for the public benefit at the time when it was published and that the matter itself was true.

312. No person shall be deemed to publish a defamatory libel by reason only that he publishes defamatory matter
    (*a*) on the invitation or challenge of the person in respect of whom it is published, or
    (*b*) that it is necessary to publish in order to refute defamatory matter published in respect of him by another person,
if he believes that the defamatory matter is true and it is relevant to the invitation, challenge or necessary refutation, as the case may be, and does not in any respect exceed what is reasonably sufficient in the circumstances.

313. No person shall be deemed to publish a defamatory libel by reason only that he publishes, in answer to inquiries made to him, defamatory matter relating to a subject-matter in respect of which the person by whom or on whose behalf the inquiries are made has an interest in knowing the truth or who, on reasonable grounds, the person who publishes the defamatory matter believes has such an interest, if
    (*a*) the matter is published, in good faith, for the purpose of giving information in answer to the inquiries,
    (*b*) the person who publishes the defamatory maker believes that it is true,
    (*c*) the defamatory matter is relevant to the inquiries, and
    (*d*) the defamatory matter does not in any respect exceed what is reasonably sufficient in the circumstances.

314. No person shall be deemed to publish a defamatory libel by reason only that he publishes to another person defamatory matter for the purpose of giving information to that person with respect to a subject-matter in which the person to whom the information is given has, or is believed on reasonable grounds by the person who gives it to have, an interest in knowing the truth with respect to that subject matter if
    (*a*) the conduct of the person who gives the information is reason able in the circumstances,
    (*b*) the defamatory matter is relevant to the subject-matter, and
    (*c*) the defamatory matter is true, or if it is not true, is made without ill-will toward the person who is defamed and is made in the belief, on reasonable grounds, that it is true.

315. No person shall be deemed to publish a defamatory libel by reason only that he publishes defamatory matter in good faith for the purpose of seeking remedy or redress for a private or public wrong or grievance from a person who has, or who on reasonable grounds he believes has the right or is under an obligation to remedy or redress the wrong or grievance, if (*a*) he believes that the defamatory matter is true,

(*b*) the defamatory matter is relevant to the remedy or redress that is sought, and

(*c*) the defamatory matter does not in any respect exceed what is reasonably sufficient in the circumstances.

316. (1) An accused who is alleged to have published a defamatory libel may, at any stage of the proceedings, adduce evidence to prove that the matter that is alleged to be defamatory was contained in a paper published by order or under the authority of the Senate or House of Commons or a legislature.

(2) Where at any stage in proceedings referred to in subsection (1) the court, judge, justice or magistrate is satisfied that matter alleged to be defamatory was contained in a paper published by order or under the authority of the Senate or House of Commons or a legislature, he shall direct a verdict of not guilty to be entered and shall discharge the accused.

(3) For the purpose of this section a certificate under the hand of the Speaker or clerk of the Senate or House of Commons or a legislature to the effect that the matter that is alleged to be defamatory was contained in a paper published by order or under the authority of the Senate, House of Commons or legislature, as the case may be, is conclusive evidence thereof.

Verdicts

317. Where, on the trial of an indictment for publishing a defamatory libel, a plea of not guilty is pleaded, the jury that is sworn to try the issue may give a general verdict of guilty or not guilty upon the whole matter put in issue upon the indictment, and shall not be required or directed by the judge to find the defendant guilty merely on proof of publication by the defendant of the alleged defamatory libel, and of the sense ascribed thereto in the indictment, but the judge may, in his discretion, give a direction or opinion to the jury on the matter in issue as in other criminal proceedings, and the jury may, on the issue, find a special verdict.

2.4.2.1 *R. v. Georgia Straight Publishing Ltd.* **(1969), 4 D.L.R. (3d) 383 (B.C. Co. Ct.)**

MORROW, Co. Ct. J.:—The accused stand charged for,

That they the said Georgia Straight Publishing Ltd., and Daniel McLeod and Robert Cummings at the City Vancouver, County of Vancouver, Province of British Columbia, between the 10th day of July 1968 and the 10th day of August, 1968, unlawfully without lawful justification or excuse did publish a defamatory libel of and concerning Magistrate Lawrence Eckhardt on Page 6 of the *Georgia Straight*, Volume 2, dated July 26—August 8 and numbered 23 in the words. "Eckhardt, Magistrate Lawrence—The Pontius Pilate Certificate of Justice—(Unfairly maligned by critics, Pilate upheld the highest traditions of a judge by placing law and order above human considerations and by helping to clear the streets of Jerusalem of degenerate non-conformists.) The Citation reads: "To Lawrence Eckhardt, who, by closing his mind to justice, his eyes to fairness, and his ears to equality, has encouraged the belief that the law is not only blind, but also deaf, dumb and stupid. Let history judge your actions—then appeal", designed to insult the said Magistrate Lawrence Eckardt, contrary to the form of the Statute in such case made and provided and against the peace of our Lady the Queen her Crown add Dignity.

The indictment was preferred under s.251 of the Canadian *Criminal Code* which reads:

> 251. Every one who publishes a defamatory libel is guilty of an indictable offence and is liable to imprisonment for two years.

When the hearing opened, counsel agreed on all of the facts with the exception of "publication" by Cummings; exs. I and 4 set out the admissions.

Exhibit 2 was the certificate of incorporation of Georgia Straight Publishing limited.

Exhibit 3, being p. 6 of the *Georgia Straight*, contained the article complained of.

Exhibit 5 is a copy of the judgment of His Worship Magistrate Eckhudt wherein one Persky was convicted of "loitering" under Order in Council 104 being B.C. Reg. 10/63, which regulation was made pursuant to the provisions contained in s.49 of the *Department of Public Works Act*, R.S.B.C. 1960, c. 109.

Exhibit 6 is an editorial taken from the Vancouver Province of April 10,1968; it is entitled "Mr. Bonner End This Nonsense".

Exhibit 7 is the decision of Seaton, J., dismissing the appeal by way of stated case of the said Persky; therein, in effect, he ruled that the Magistrate had acted correctly in disposing of the matter as he did.

The prosecution relief on the admissions and the exhibits.

The defence called one witness, the accused, Robert Howard Cummings; he is a journalist employed by the accused Georgia Straight Publishing Limited and is the author of the article in question, the purpose of which, in his words was a "spoof, joke, satire or piece of humour along the lines of the 'City Town Fool Award' "; he was, he claimed, satirizing the Establishment; in ex. 3 he awarded the "Order of the Abundant Flatulence" to several individuals and specifically he awarded Magistrate Eckhudt the "Pontius Pilate Certificate of Justice" using the words contained in the indictment.

In direct examination he outlined how the police had made selective arrests of nonconformists and stressed the fact that the regulation under which the authorities proceeded was discriminatory and that the Magistrate agreed it was; it was on the basis of that decision he made the award.

The said Cummings testified that the accused McLeod was the editor and publisher of the paper which is virtually a one-man company. In cross-examination he said he had been with the paper over a year and wrote articles steadily. As to the title, "Order of Abundant Flatulence", in his words, this meant "super abundance of gas in the intestinal tract or pomposity" and he was trying to take pomposity out of the Establishment. The defence argued along five lines:

(1) There is no evidence as to publication against the accused Cummings.
(2) There was no intent to insult.
(3) The words are not defamatory.
(4) If they are defamatory, the accused are entitled to the protection of s. 259 of the *Criminal Code* which reads:

> No person shall be deemed to publish defamatory libel by reason only that he publishes defamatory manner that, on reasonable grounds, he believes is true, and that is relevant to any subject of public interest, the public discussion of which is for the public benefit.

(5) If the words are defamatory, the accused are entitled to the benefit of s. 260 of the *Code* which reads:

> No person shall be deemed to publish a defamatory libel by reason only that he publishes fair comments
> (a) upon the public conduct of a person who takes part in public affairs...

As to the first line of argument there can be no doubt there was publication under s. 249(b); in his own evidence Cummings admitted he was the author of the article which appeared on p. 6 and the paper was distributed; he is a journalist and it would be odd, indeed, if he did not intend his writings to be read; he also falls within s. 21 of the *Code* (Parties to Offence—Common Intent). As to the second defence, nowhere in s.248 does the word "intent" appear; the definition has two puts; the latter reads or that is designed to insult the person of or concerning whom it is published". If it had been the decision of Parliament to use the word "intent" it would have done so as has been done in many other sections; instead of the word "intent" the section uses the word "designed"; this word simply means "to put together" or "purpose".

As regards the third, fourth and fifth defences, these seem to overlap and will be considered together. The defence emphasized that because the regulation or law was bad the words should be taken to mean criticism against the law rather than against the Magistrate. I disagree as the article is directed against the Magistrate, not the law.

A perusal of p. 6 of ex. 3 indicates how far the accused went; there is a sketch of the award in question which I consider to be in very bad taste, particularly the description of it; the "Order of the Abundant Flatulence" is described in detail in column one; in so far as Magistrate Eckhudt is concerned, he should have been praised for drawing the attention of the authorities to a law that he did not feel could be enforced generally; instead, he was accused of having "closed his mind to justice, his eyes to fairness and his ears to equality" which words are insulting.

I am grateful to counsel for giving me the many authorities they did. I have read them all; the following have been helpful: *Salmond on Torts*, 14th ed., dealing with privilege and privileged reports, at p. 198, the author has this to say:

> The statement is judged by the standard of an ordinary, right-thinking member of society. Hence the test is an objective one, and it is no defence to say that the statement was not intended to be defamatory or uttered by way of a joke.

See *Capital and Counties Bank, Ltd. v. Henry & Sons* (1882), 7 App. Cas. 741; again, at p. 222, under the heading "Privilege" the author has this to say:

> The cases in which privilege exists are. generally speaking, those in which there is some just occasion for publishing defamatory matter in the public interest or in the furtherance or protection of the rights or lawful interests of individuals. In such cases the exigency of the occasion amounts to a lawful excuse for the attack so made upon the plaintiff's reputation. The right of free speech is allowed wholly or partially to prevail over the right of reputation.

In regard to this last quotation, the difficulty the accused find themselves in is the fact that they have defamed the Magistrate rather than making an attack on the law which they had a right to do.

Candler v. Crane Christmas & Co., [1951] 1 All E.R. 426 at pp. 431 and 442.

This case was put forth by the defence to indicate the great conflict there has been in trying to resolve the issue at bar. It was contended one of the reasons the statements made were not defamatory was that it was directed against a bad law rather than against a bad Judge. The defence quoted from the judgment at p. 431 quoting Denning, L.J., but he was dissenting.

In addition the case is distinguishable from the case at bar as the accused were not commenting on the law but rather commenting on the fact that the Magistrate had acted improperly. The comments were not proved to be true and they were unfair and they could not be classed as a discussion for the public benefit; ss.259 and 260 do not help them.

The Queen v. Gray, [1900] 2 Q.B. 36 at p. 40. Here the headnote reads [paraphrased]:

> The publication in a newspaper of an article containing a scandalous abuse of a judge with reference to his conduct as a judge in a judicial proceeding which has terminated is contempt of court, punishable by the court on summary process.

Hoare v. Silverlock (1848), 12 Q.B. 624 at p. 632, 116 E.R. 1004. The headnote reads [paraphrased]:

> This case revolves around the fable of "The Frozen Snake"; the verdict found the plaintiff entitled to judgment since the jury may have understood the words, :'frozen snake" to charge the plaintiff with ingratitude to friends; it is no objection in arrest of judgment that the words are not explained by innuendo.

In the case at bar, innuendo is not involved as the words, taken in their ordinary meaning, are very clear.

Gatley on Libel and Slander, 6th ed., is authority for the proposition that innuendo must be pleaded but no innuendo is necessary in the case at bar as the words are defamatory in their common use.

"Pilate (Pontius Pilate)": this word is defined in the *Oxford Dictionary* as a term of reproach.

R. v. Unwin, [1938] 1 D.L.R. 529 at pp. 530-1, 69 C.C.C. 197 at pp. 199-200, [1938] 1 W.W.R. 339. The accused was tried before Ives, J., and a jury on a charge in two counts:

(1) the publishing of a defamatory libel knowing it to be false;
(2) the publishing of a defamatory libel.

The writing complained of was a printed leaflet headed "Bankers' Toadies" followed by the words, *inter alia*, "God made Bankers' Toadies, just as He made snakes, slugs, snails and other creepy-crawly, treacherous and poisonous things. NEVER therefore, abuse them—just exterminate them!" On the reverse side, under the heading "Bankers' Toadies", were the names of nine citizens of Edmonton and the institutions with which they are associated and underneath their names were the words, in larger type, "Exterminate Them". The jury returned a verdict of guilty on the first count and the accused was sentenced to three months' imprisonment. On appeal, it was held the leaflet was beyond question defamatory of the persons named; this was a private prosecution and during the course of the judgment in the Appellate Division, Harvey, C.J.A., at pp. 532-3 D.L.R., pp. 201-2 C.C.C., had this to say:

> It is further objected that the jury should have been directed that if they considered that the private prosecutor who by the way in the notice of objection is described as "General Griesbach," was bringing the prosecution to vindicate his own private character, there should be no conviction and he should be left to his civil rights. It is stated in Russell on Crimes, 9th ed., p. 695, that the disposition of the Courts is to discourage criminal prosecutions launched merely to extract apologies or vindicate private character leaving the party libelled to civil remedies, and it is stated in the same work at p. 698 that:—'a scandal published of three or four persons is punishable on the complaint of one or more, or all of them." Of course there could have been nine separate civil actions for this libel but the purpose of the prosecution one gathers from the evidence was not so much for the redress of private wrongs as to punish for the wrong done the public. There certainly is nothing in the case that would warrant conclusion that civil proceedings would be an appropriate remedy.

The appeal and application for leave to appeal from the sentence was dismissed on all respects.

The penal provisions relating to criminal libel were, I believe, inserted in the Code to apply against people who make the type of statements made in the case at bar; I agree that public discussion should not be muzzled but invective does not advance the truth and I feel the accused have fallen within the definition following s.247. The defence contended that the paper was merely a college type of periodical but there was no evidence as to this.

There have been few cases of defamatory libel in our Courts but the words of Harvey, C.J.A., in *R. v. Unwin* seem to be apropos; it is unfortunate the accused did not apply their undoubted talents in a constructive sense. I find all accused guilty as charged.

2.4.2.2. Robert Martin, "Law Reform Commission of Canada, Working Paper 35: Defamatory Libel," (1984), *University of Western Ontario Law Review*, vol. 22, p. 249

The *Criminal Code* contains a number of unusual prohibitions. These are the result of particular historical circumstances which no longer obtain. Few

Canadians today would, I imagine, regard the playing of three-card monte or the possession of crime comics as acts likely to undermine the social order. Yet both are crimes. Criminal libel is another of these anachronistic survivals.

The crime of libel originated in England in the 17th century. This was a time when the state was not sensitive to the importance of freedom of speech. Criminal libel was pure and simple, an instrument of repression.

Canada inherited criminal libel along with the rest of the general English criminal law. The *Criminal Code* of Canada recognizes three categories of criminal libel-seditious libel, blasphemous libel, and defamatory libel. None of these offences looms very large. The Supreme Court of Canada effectively disposed of sedition in 1950. Blasphemy seems moribund, although in England the House of Lords has recently attempted to revive it. Canadians—not many, it is true—continue to be prosecuted for defamatory libel and some are convicted.

The Law Reform Commission of Canada is in the process of carrying out a general review of our criminal law. As part of this exercise, the Commission has published a *Working Paper* on defamatory libel. It is unfortunate that the Commission did not study the whole field of criminal libel. That is, however, the only point where I wish to take issue. The *Working Paper* is a thorough, careful study. It is well documented, systematically organized, and clearly written. Its recommendations are straightforward and sensible. All of which is a convoluted way of saying that I like the *Working Paper* a lot and agree with it completely.

The purport of the Law Reform Commission's argument is that the offence of defamatory libel is neither necessary nor desirable in late 20th century Canada. I will attempt to summarize the argument.

The Court of Star Chamber created the offence of defamatory libel, in part at least, to discourage duelling. Since duelling is not widely perceived as a major social issue in Canada today, this fact alone would lead one to question the utility of maintaining the offence. But there is more.

The Commission believes that the tort of defamation provides both protection for reputation and a means of seeking redress against character assassins. The Commission thinks this should be enough. It is disturbed by the fact that statements or expressions which would not give rise to tortuous liability might, nonetheless, be regarded as criminal. The *Working Paper* notes that mere insults can amount to defamatory libel, that publication to the victim alone is sufficient, and that truth is not a complete defence.

The Commission notes further that the offence of defamatory libel is badly expressed in the *Criminal Code* and that it is "... defective because it is not a full *mens rea* offence".

The effect of the *Canadian Charter of Rights and Freedoms* is addressed. Not only does the offence appear to deny the fundamental freedom of expression, it seems in a number of respects to be inconsistent with the presumption of innocence.

There is no social policy justification, the Law Reform Commission believes, for keeping defamatory libel in the *Criminal Code*. A number of dubious arguments in support of this are surveyed and quickly, and properly, dismissed. The lack of enthusiasm for the offence in a number of other Commonwealth states is mentioned.

At the end of its analysis, the Commission asks the right question, the only question:

> If there were no previously existing crime of libel, would it be necessary to create one now?

The answer, by this point, is obvious. And the *Working Paper's* main recommendation is equally clear and direct.

> There should be no offence of defamation in the new *Criminal Code* or elsewhere.

Bravo!

The broader issue raised by this Working Paper is important. The issue is this. In a democratic society are there circumstances in which mere words, with nothing more, should properly be the subject of a criminal prosecution? The Commission was faced with this question in its *Report* on Contempt of Court and made a mess of it. The people who drafted the *Criminal Law Reform Bill* of 1984 had the good sense to pay no attention to the Commission's recommendations. But now that it seems to have got itself back on track, the Law Reform Commission of Canada might consider tackling the complicated and difficult issue of freedom of speech and the criminal law.

CHAPTER THREE

Judicial Proceedings: Legal Limitations to Protect the State's Rights, Prerogatives and Responsibilities, Part II

3.1 Introduction

The courts are public institutions. Their business is public business. Accordingly, there is a tradition in common law countries that the courts will remain open to the public and, subject to certain rules, what happens in them may be fully described in the media. The Constitution of Canada contains expressions of these principles. They are implied in the guarantees of freedom of the press in section 2(b) of the Charter, and explicit in section 11(d) which says that a person charged with an offence has the right "to be presumed innocent until proven guilty in a fair and public hearing by an independent and impartial tribunal". Those provisions speak to the public's right to know and to the rights of an accused person. The quality of justice is assumed to be related to the principle of openness.

However, there are a number of rules that apply to reporting the activities of courts and judges which journalists must know in detail. These rules have emerged from the courts themselves or have been legislated. They deliberately restrict freedom of expression. The justification for the rules is that they are supposed to provide a balance between free expression and the rights of individuals to fair trials. In fact, the rules are a haphazard and random collection of restrictions.

Technically, the law includes both statutory limitations on freedom of expression — the prohibitions on publishing the names of young offenders or victims of sexual crimes are examples — and the uncodified law of criminal contempt. The law of contempt can be considered alongside the several statutory rules since the latter serve the same purpose and are similarly inspired.

The purpose of the law of contempt is said to be the protection of the administration of justice. There are two types: *in facie* contempt, which means in the face of the court or in the courtroom itself; and *ex facie* contempt, or a contempt which occurs outside the court. A decision by a journalist to disobey an order by a judge to reveal the sources on which he or she based a story could lead to a citation for an *in facie* contempt. Some journalists have refused to obey such orders on the grounds that to do so would require breaking promises they made in order to gather the information in the first place.

Ex facie contempt includes "scandalizing the court" or criticising it or a judge by suggesting in vigorous language that justice has been thwarted or corrupted. Saying a judge is stupid or corrupt could earn a journalist a citation for contempt. Another *ex facie* contempt could occur if a judge ordered that certain materials or facts not be published during a proceeding and a journalist proceeded to do so anyway.

The law of contempt also empowers a judge to cite a journalist for breaching the sub-judice rule. When a charge has been laid and the matter is formally within the court's jurisdiction, public discussion is then restricted to contemporaneous and accurate reports of the facts or proceedings. Editorials which urge or predict a particular finding are viewed as usurping the court's authority. Publishing the criminal record of a defendant could prejudice the court's view of him or her, prevent a fair trial, and thereby be in contempt of court. It would be contrary to the *sub judice* rule to broadcast or publish an assumption that a defendant was guilty.

Technical breaches of the *sub judice* rule or other parts of the law of contempt will not lead inevitably to a prosecution. The timing and character of the breach, the size of the community, the place of publication or broadcast or whether the matter is to be decided by a judge or a judge and jury can all have a bearing. In the latter case, it is believed that juries are easier to prejudice than judges and that judges in the highest courts are the most difficult to prejudice.

3.2 The Principle of Openness

3.2.1. *Re Southam Inc. and the Queen (No. 1)* (1983), 41 O.R. (2d) 113 (Ont. C.A.)

How the issue arose

On June 11th a reporter employed by the respondent Southam Inc. attended with counsel at the Provincial Court (Family Division) in Ottawa presided over by His Honour Judge Guzzo. They were advised that reporters or other members of the general public were not permitted to be present during the hearing of proceedings under the *Juvenile Delinquents Act*. Counsel for the respondent thereupon made an application to Judge Guzzo requesting that the public and, in particular, representatives of the media, be permitted to be present at such hearings.

After hearing submissions, Judge Guzzo was of the view that the Attorneys-General of Ontario and Canada should be served with notice of the respondent's application before he considered the submissions made. The application was, accordingly, adjourned to permit respondent's counsel time to research the matter further. The respondent did not renew this particular application but the same reporter once again, on June 15th attempted to enter Judge Guzzo's courtroom. Upon being advised that the reporter was not a witness in the proceedings involving a juvenile delinquent, Judge Guzzo directed her to leave the courtroom.

The respondent then moved before the learned motions court judge for an order "in the nature of mandamus compelling His Honour Judge Guzzo of the Provincial Court (Family Division) to permit the applicants to be present during the hearings of proceedings held in Provincial Court (Family Division) in Ottawa pursuant to the *Juvenile Delinquents Act*, R.S.C. 1970, c.J-3". It was, we were advised, a general motion to "open the Juvenile Court" not related to any specific proceedings. The application was made pursuant to "the provisions of Sec. 24 of the *Constitution Act 1982*". Initially, in its appellant's statement, the Crown argued that the respondent did not have status to bring the application and that the Supreme Court of Ontario was not "a court of competent jurisdiction" within the meaning of that phrase found in s.24(1) of the Charter. However, as already noted that position was not pressed during the argument, the Crown agreeing that the application was properly before Mr. Justice Smith. Counsel also agreed that the Crown has a right of appeal in the instant case under s.28 of the *Judicature Act*. R.S.O. 1980, c.223. It is not necessary, accordingly, for me to consider these two questions further.

During the course of the argument in the court below the respondent altered its application in regard to the relief it sought and asked for a declaration that s. 12(1) of the *Juvenile Delinguents Act* was ultra vires. The motions court judge granted the declaration requested.

The argument which was made before us and which found favour with the motions court judge was that the exclusion of the public from such trials offends "freedom of expression, including freedom of the press", guaranteed by the Charter.

The sections of the Charter to which we were referred are the following:

Rights and freedoms in Canada

1. The *Canadian Charter of Rights and Freedoms* guarantees the rights and freedoms set out in it subject only to such reasonable limits prescribed by law as can be demonstrably justified in a free and democratic society.

Fundamental freedoms

2. Everyone has the following fundamental freedoms:

. . . . .

(*b*) freedom of thought, belief, opinion and expression, including freedom of the press and other media of communications;

Other rights and freedoms not affected by Charter

26. The guarantee in this Charter of certain rights and freedoms shall not be construed as denying the existence of any other rights or freedoms that exist in Canada.

We were also referred to s.52 of the *Constitution Act, 1982* which establishes the supremacy of the Constitution of Canada, including the Charter, over other laws, and provides the basis for judicial review of legislation in Canada:

52. (1) The Constitution of Canada is the supreme law of Canada, and any law that is inconsistent with the provisions of the Constitution is, to the extent of the inconsistency, of no force or effect.

This section gives to the court the necessary power to make the requested declaration if there is found to be the required inconsistency. The basic question is whether the trial of children in camera is a breach of freedom of "opinion and expression, including freedom of the press and other media communication". Following the wording in some American authorities the motions court judge held that freedom of expression and of the press are "adjuncts" to the concept of the openness of our judicial system and the right of access to the courts.

Is free access to the courts a fundamental right or freedom?

Section 2(b) of the Charter

There can be no doubt that the openness of the courts to the public is one of the hallmarks of a democratic society. Public accessibility to the courts was and is a felt necessity; it is a restraint on arbitrary action by those who govern and by the powerful. The most recent and comprehensive review of principle in this area of the law was made by Dickson J. in his reasons for the majority in A.-G. N.S. *et al.* v. *MacIntyre* (1982), 65 C.C.C. (2d) 129, 132 D.L.R. (3d) 385, 40 N.R. 181.

In this case, a television journalist applied for an order requiring a justice of the peace to make available to him for inspection, search warrants and information in his possession. A Supreme Court Judge allowed the application and held that the journalist, as a member of the general public, was entitled to inspect executed search warrants and supporting informations. The Nova Scotia Court of Appeal dismissed the appeal from that judgment and did not restrict the right of access to only executed warrants. The Supreme Court dismissed the appeal but restricted the right of access, as had the Supreme Court Judge, to executed search warrants.

In the course of his reasons, Dickson J. said (pp. 144-5 C.C.C., pp. 400-1 D.L.R., pp. 188-9 N.R.):

> The question before us is limited to search warrants and informations. The response to that question, it seems to me, should be guided by several broad policy considerations, namely, respect for the privacy of the individual, protection of the administration of justice, implementation of the will of Parliament that a search warrant be an effective aid in the investigation of crime, and finally, a strong public policy in favour of "openness" in respect of judicial acts. The *rationale* of this last-mentioned consideration has been eloquently expressed by Bentham in these terms:
>
>> "In the darkness of secrecy, sinister interest, and evil in every shape have full swing. Only in proportion as publicity has place can any of the checks applicable to judicial injustice operate. Where there is no publicity there is no justice. Publicity is the very soul of justice.

It is the keenest spur to exertion and surest of all guards against improbity. It keeps the judge himself while trying under trial."

The concern for accountability is not diminished by the fact that the search warrants might be issued by a Justice *in camera*. On the contrary. this fact increases the policy argument in favour of accessibility. Initial secrecy surrounding the issuance of warrants may lead to abuse, and publicity is a strong deterrent to potential malversation.

In short, what should be sought is maximum accountability and accessibility but not to the extent of harming the innocent or of impairing the efficiency of the search warrant as a weapon in society's never ending fight against crime.

And, at pp. 145-6 C.C.C., pp. 401-2 D.L.R., p. 190 N.R.:

It is now well established, however, that covertness is the exception and openness the rule. Public confidence in the integrity of the Court system and understanding of the administration of justice are thereby fostered. As a general rule the sensibilities of the individuals involved are no basis for exclusion of the public from judicial proceedings. The following comments of Laurence J. in *R. v. Wright*, 8 T.L.R. 293, are apposite and were cited with approval by Duff J. in the *Gazette Printing Co. v. Shallow* (1909), 41 S.C.R. 339, at p. 359:

" 'Though the publication of such proceedings may be to the disadvantage of the particular individual concerned, yet it is of vast importance to the public that the proceedings of courts of justice should be universally known. The general advantage to the country in having these proceedings made public more than counterbalances the inconveniences to the private persons whose conduct may be the subject of such proceedings.' "

The leading case is the decision of the House of Lords in *Scott v. Scott*, [1913] A.C. 417. In the later case of *McPherson v. McPherson*, [1936] A.C. 177 at p. 200, Lord Blanesburgh, delivering the judgment of the Privy Council. referred to "publicity" as the "authentic hall mark of judicial as distinct from administrative procedure".

It is, of course, true that *Scott v. Scott* and *McPherson v. McPherson* were cases in which proceedings had reached the stage of trial whereas the issuance of a search warrant takes place at the pre-trial investigative stage. The cases mentioned, however, and many others which could be cited, establish the broad principle of openness in judicial proceedings, whatever their nature, and in the exercise of judicial powers. The same policy considerations upon which is predicated our reluctance to inhibit accessibility at the trial stage are still present and should be addressed at the pre-trial stage.

And, at pp. 146-7 C.C.C., pp. 402-3 D.L.R., p. 191 N.R.:

Ex parte applications for injunctions, interlocutory proceedings, or preliminary inquiries are not trial proceedings, and yet the open court' rule applies in these cases. The authorities have held that subject to a few well-recognized exceptions, as in the case of infants, mentally disordered persons or secret processes, all judicial proceedings must be held in public. The editor of Halsbury's Laws of England, 4th ed., vol. Io, para. 705, p. 316, states the rule in these terms:

"In general, all cases, both civil and criminal, must be heard in open court, but in certain exceptional cases, where the administration of justice would be rendered impracticable by the presence of the public, the court may sit in camera.'

At every stage the rule should be one of public accessibility and concomitant judicial accountability; all with a view to ensuring there is no abuse in the issue of search Warrants, that once issued they are executed according to law, and finally that any evidence seized is dealt with according to law. A decision by the Crown not to prosecute, notwithstanding the finding of evidence appearing to establish the commission of a crime may, in some circumstances, raise issues of public importance.

In my view, curtailment of public accessibility can only be justified where there is present the need to protect social values of superordinate importance. One of these is the protection of the innocent.

He concluded that the effective administration of justice would be frustrated if individuals were permitted to be present when the warrants were issued and that the exclusion of the public from the proceedings attending the actual issuance of the warrant was justified. However, once the warrant has been executed, the need for concealment virtually disappears and "The curtailment of the traditionally uninhibited accessibility of the public to the working of the Courts should be undertaken with the greatest reluctance" (pp. 148-9 C.C.C., pp. 404-5 D.L.R., p. 193 N.R.).

In the instant case, counsel for the Crown argued strenuously that public access to the courts was not a specific or fundamental right guaranteed by the Charter and therefore s.24(1) could not be invoked as it had no application to the question. Further, he argued, that being so, there was no need to resort to s. 1 and determine whether s.12(1) imposed "reasonable limits . . . as can be demonstrably justified in a free and democratic society".

It is true that public accessibility to the courts is not spelled out in terms as part of the fundamental freedoms. Counsel argued that "freedom of the press" is limited by s.2(b) itself, in that it is but part of freedom of thought, belief, opinion and expression. I do not believe that it is appropriate to use the word "limited" in connection with s.2(b) although I do accept that freedom of the press refers to the dissemination of expression of thought, belief or opinion through the medium of the press. If anything, the words "freedom of expression" would seem to have a wider or larger connotation than the words "freedom of the press".

Counsel for the Crown pointed out that the wording in the Charter with regard to "freedom of the press" differs significantly from that in the First Amendment to the United States Constitution. The First Amendment reads, in part:

> Congress shall make no law . . . abridging the freedom of speech or of the press; or the right of the people peaceably to assemble . . .

It can be seen that the reference is to freedom of the press, *simpliciter*, unlike the Charter which includes freedom of the press in freedom of thought, belief, opinion and expression. However, whether the American case-law on freedom of the press is of persuasive authority is of small moment in the instant case as the respondent is relying on s.2(b) as guaranteeing to the general public free access to the courts as an integral part of the fundamental freedom of opinion and expression. It is not an issue of "freedom of the press" *per se*.

In *Richmond Newspapers, Inc. et al. v. Commonwealth of Virginia et al.*, 100 S. Ct. 2814, 48 L.W. 5008 (1980), the Supreme Court of the United States considered for the first time the narrow question of whether the right of the public and the press to attend criminal trials was guaranteed under the United States Constitution. One Stevenson had been indicted for murder, three abortive trials had taken place and he was being tried in the same court for a fourth time. At the opening of that trial, counsel for the accused moved that it be closed to the public and the prosecutor stated that he had no objection. The trial judge thereupon ordered the court-room cleared. Richmond Newspapers subsequently moved to intervene and ultimately took the issue to appeal.

In delivering the lead judgment of the court, Chief Justice Burger reviewed at some length the Anglo-American history of criminal trials. This review emphasized that from time immemorial, judicial trials have been held in open court, to which the public have free access. He concluded that "from this unbroken, uncontradicted history, supported by reasons as valid today as in centuries past, we are bound to conclude that a presumption of openness inheres in the very nature of a criminal trial under our system of justice" (p. 2825). He went on to say (p. 2826):

> The First Amendment, in conjunction with the Fourteenth, prohibits governments from "abridging the freedom of speech or of the press; or the right of the people peaceably to assemble, and to petition the government for a redress of grievances". These expressly guaranteed freedoms share a common core purpose of assuring freedom of communication on matters relating to the functioning of government. Plainly it would be difficult to single out any aspect of government of higher concern and importance to the people than the manner in which criminal trials are conducted.

As stated, counsel for the Crown submits that the right of public access to the courts does not fall under the fundamental freedoms guaranteed by the Charter. I do not agree. The Charter as part of a constitutional document should be given a large and liberal construction. The spirit of this new "living tree" planted in friendly Canadian soil should not be stultified by narrow technical, literal interpretations without regard to its background and purpose; capability for growth must be recognized: *Re s.24 of B.N.A. Act; Edwards et al. v. A.-G. Can. et al.*, [1930] 1 D.L.R. 98 at pp. 1078, [1930] A.C. 124 at p. 136, [1929] 3 W.W.R. 479. Although said in a very different connection, it is apposite here: "For the letter killeth but the spirit giveth life."

Trials of juveniles are not criminal trials as such and the enforcement process is "specially adapted to the age and impressibility of juveniles and fundamentally different, in pattern and purpose, from the one governing in the case of adults": *A.-G. B.C. v. Smith*, [1969] 1 C.C.C. 244 at p. 251, [1967] S.C.R. 702 at p. 710, 65 D.L.R. (2d) 82 at p. 88. Nevertheless, serious criminal matters are heard by juvenile courts, matters in which there is a public interest and concern, and in which in many cases, it is acknowledged by the Crown, no necessary interest of the juvenile is served by the exclusion of the public from such hearings.

It is true, as argued, that free access to the courts is not specifically enumerated under the heading of fundamental freedoms but, in my view, such access, having regard to its historic origin and necessary purpose already recited at length, is an integral and implicit part of the guarantee given to everyone of freedom of opinion and expression which, in terms, includes freedom of the press. However the rule may have had its origin, as Mr. Justice Dickson pointed out, the "openness" rule fosters the necessary public confidence in the integrity of the court system and an under standing of the administration of justice. The respondent has established that its right, as a member of the public, under s. 2(b) of the Charter has, *prima facie*, been infringed.

Is s.12(1) a reasonable limit as can be demonstrably justified in a free and democratic society?

Section 1 of the Charter

I turn now to the last question to be answered: is the exclusion of the public under s. 12(1) a reasonable limit prescribed by law as can be demonstrably justified in a free and democratic society (to quote the relevant words of s.1 of the Charter)? As a subsidiary consideration, the standard as formed by Mr. Justice Dickson would have to be met, namely: "[C]urtailment of public accessibility can only be justified where there is present the need to protect social values of superordinate importance." A preliminary question which has to be determined is: upon whom is the burden of establishing that the limit in issue is a reasonable one demonstrably justifiable in a free and democratic society?

"Onus" or "burden" of proof under s. 1

The Crown takes the initial position that the freedoms granted under s.2 of the Charter, guaranteed by s. 1, are conditioned, qualified or limited rights by virtue of the wording of s.1 which qualifies the rights and freedoms by making them subject to reasonable limits on a particular basis. The onus or burden, the argument goes, is on him who is asserting that his particular freedom has been infringed or breached to establish that the limit imposed by the law being attacked, is an unreasonable limit which cannot be demonstrably justified in a free and democratic society.

It appears to me that that position and the reasoning supporting it is strained and inappropriate to the clear wording of the two sections. Section 2 states that everyone has the named fundamental freedoms. Section 1 guarantees those rights and, although the rights are not absolute or unrestricted, makes it clear that if there is a limit imposed on these fundamental rights by law, the limits must be reasonable and demonstrably justified in a free and democratic society. The wording imposes a positive obligation on those seeking to uphold the limit or limits to establish to the satisfaction of the court by evidence, by the terms and purpose of the limiting law, its economic, social and political background, and, if felt helpful, by references to comparable legislation of other acknowledged free and democratic societies, that such limit or limits are reasonable and demonstrably justified in a free and democratic society. I cannot accept the proposition urged upon us that, as the freedoms may be limited ones, the person who establishes that, *prima facie* his freedom has been infringed or denied must then take the further step and establish. on the balance of probabilities, the negative, namely, that such infringement or limit is unreasonable and cannot be demonstrably justified in a free and democratic society. In some cases, of course, the frivolous nature of the claim to protection of a freedom or right and of the submissions made in support will be immediately apparent and it will not take great effort to determine that the claim to a guaranteed freedom or right is not tenable under the Charter and under the circumstances. But that is not this case.

As part of his submission in connection with the alleged onus or burden on the respondent, counsel for the Crown pointed out that under s.24(1) the applicant initiates the proceeding and, accordingly, the usual rules should apply, namely, that if at the end of the hearing the court is undecided and matters are left in balance, then the application must fail. He argued that the onus has always been on an applicant claiming that a Legislature has exceeded in legislation or a portion thereof, its legislative jurisdiction or competence. He submitted that, under the "presumption of constitutionality", there is a clear evidentiary burden on the applicant which includes establishing that the limit is not a reasonable one and that it is not demonstrably justified in a free and democratic society. It does not appear to me that the so-called "presumption of constitutionality" assists in this type of case. There is no conflict here between two legislative bodies, federal and provincial, claiming jurisdiction over a particular legislative subject-matter. This rather is a determination whether a portion of a law is inconsistent with the provisions of the Constitution, the supreme law of Canada. This supreme law was enacted long after the *Juvenile Delinquents Act* and there can be no presumption that the legislators intended to act constitutionally in light of legislation that was not, at that time, a gleam in its progenitor's eye. In any event, like Chief Justice Deschenes, I am of the view that the complete burden of proving an exception under s. 1 of the Charter rests on the party claiming the benefit of the exception or limitation: *Quebec Ass'n of Protestant School Boards et al. v. A .-G. Que. et al. (No. 2)* (1982), 140 D.L.R. (3d) 33 at p. 59.

Is the limit a "reasonable limit" as can be demonstrably justified in a free and democratic society?

It is agreed that the limit in the instant case is "prescribed by law".

The learned motions court judge, in the course of his reasons, stated [70 C.C.C. (2d) 257 at p. 262, 38 O.R. (2d) 748 at p. 754 *sub nom. Reference re Constitutional Validity of s.12 of Juvenile Delinquents Act*, 141 D.L.R. (3d) 341 at p. 347]: "That the courts possess an inherent jurisdiction to forbid access [to the courts] in certain narrow instances, is beyond dispute." If that were so I would have very little difficulty in giving effect to the respondent's position. However, a statutory court such as the provincial court (family division) has no inherent jurisdiction but has only that jurisdiction which is specifically conferred on it by statute. Both counsel before us agreed that the motions court judge was in error in this regard.

However, counsel for the respondent sought to support the position that a family court judge had a discretion under the *Juvenile Delinquents Act* to close his court by arguing that such a discretion was given under ss. 12(2) and 36(1) of that Act. Section 12(2), quoted, beginning as it does with the words, "Such trials", refers back to s.12(1), the section under attack. That section directs that trials of children shall be held *in camera* and s.(2) is a permissive section dealing with the location of the trials to be held *in camera*. Section 12(1) is absolute in its terms and s. 12(2) was not intended to give and does not give an additional discretionary power to the judge to exclude the public which, in view of the wording of s.12(1), would be quite unnecessary.

Section 36(1) reads:

36. (1) Every juvenile court has such and like powers and authority to preserve order in court during the sittings thereof and by the like ways and means as now by law are or may be exercised and used in like cases and for the like purposes by any court in Canada and by the judges thereof, during the sittings thereof.

The power given to the juvenile court to preserve order and cite for contempt of court has no relevance to a discretionary power to exclude the public in order to protect the interests of the child and advance the perceived purpose and object of juvenile hearings. A juvenile judge could not use this subsection to exclude the public (and the press as part of the public) at the beginning of a hearing when there is no prospect of nor concern for disorder.

We are accordingly left in the unhappy position of it being all or nothing. If s. 12(1) is allowed to stand, so long as the present Act is in existence the public is excluded from every such hearing; if s. 12(1) is struck down the public, until further amendment, can attend all such hearings without regard to any other interests. There is no halfway house such as now exists in similar legislation actual and contemplated, where the court is given a discretion to exclude the public in the best interests of the child and ultimately of the public. The choice, accordingly, at present has to be made between the two absolutes.

The purpose of the legislation under review is effectively set out in ss.3(2) and 38 of the Act:

3. (2) Where a child is adjudged to have committed a delinquency he shall be dealt with, not as an offender, but as one in a condition of delinquency and therefore requiring help and guidance and proper supervision.

. . . . .

38. This Act shall be liberally construed in order that its purpose may be carried out, namely, that the care and custody and discipline of a juvenile delinquent shall approximate as nearly as may be that which should be given by his parents, and that as far as practicable every juvenile delinquent shall be treated, not as criminal, but as a misdirected and misguided child, and one needing aid, encouragement, help and assistance.

As the motions court judge pointed out, the *Young Offenders Act*, 1980-81-82 (Can.), c. 110 (which will replace the *Juvenile Delinquents Act*), enacted but not yet proclaimed in force, is now based on the principle of responsibility and accountability (s.3(1)). Under that Act hearings are open to the public with the court having the power under certain conditions or circumstances to exclude any or all members of the public from the proceedings, with certain exceptions. It is not an automatic exclusion as under the present legislation.

Section 39 of the *Young Offenders Act* reads:

39. (1) Subject to subsection (2), where a court or justice before whom proceedings are carried out under this Act is of the opinion

(*a*) that any evidence or information presented to the court or justice would be seriously injurious or prejudicial to

(i) the young person who is being dealt with in the proceedings,

(ii) a child or young person who is a witness in the proceedings,

(iii) a child or young person who is aggrieved by or the victim of the offence charged in the proceedings, or

(*b*) that it would be in the interest of public morals, the maintenance of order or the proper administration of justice to exclude any or all members of the public from the court room,

the court or justice may exclude any person from all or part of the proceedings if the court or justice deems that person's presence to be unnecessary to the conduct of the proceedings.

(2) A court or justice may not, pursuant to subsection (1), exclude from proceedings under this Act

(*a*) the prosecutor;

(*b*) the young person who is being dealt with in the proceedings, his parent, his counsel or any adult assisting him pursuant to subsection 11(7);

(*c*) the provincial director or his agent; or

(*d*) the youth worker to whom the young person's case has been assigned.

(3) The youth court, after it has found a young person guilty of an offence, or the youth court or the review board, during a review of a disposition under sections 28 to 33, may, in its discretion, exclude from the court or from a hearing of the review board, as the case may be, any person other than

(*a*) the young person or his counsel,

(*b*) the provincial director or his agent,

(*c*) the youth worker to whom the young person's case has been assigned, and

(*d*) the Attorney General or his agent,

when any information is being presented to the court or the review board the knowledge of which might, in the opinion of the court or review board, be seriously injurious or seriously prejudicial to the young person.

When and if the *Young Offenders Act* in its present form will be proclaimed in force cannot be predicted.

Counsel for the appellant, although candidly acknowledging that not every hearing under the *Juvenile Delinquents Act* would call for the exclusion of the public, argued that to give effect to the declared purpose of the Act, it was necessary to close all juvenile court hearings to the public and this is a reasonable limit on the rights of the public to be present at trials. He pointed out that in smaller municipalities the presence of friends and curious neighbours could have a chilling and inhibiting effect on the evidence of the child and parents or guardian. The court might not have the necessary full information to be able to reach a proper understanding in order to give the necessary aid, encouragement and protection to the child. He, in substance, argued the grounds that give to the court under the proposed legislation (s.39) the discretionary power to exclude members of the public. The difference is that the reasoning is used to support the reasonableness of mandating the total exclusion of the public in all cases, not to support the use of a discretionary power.

Counsel submitted that the interests of the public are protected in that s. 12(3) gives to the court the discretion to allow for the publication of the identity of the child. Further, it was suggested that the offensive aspects of a "private" trial are ameliorated by other parts of the governing Act. For example, there is no prohibition against speaking to those who were in attendance at the hearing nor against securing a transcript of the proceedings. The parents or guardians must be served with notice of any charge of delinquency and may be present and be heard (ss.10 and 22(4)). The child's probation officer must be present in the court in order to represent the interests of the child when the case is heard (s.31); the juvenile court committee, being a committee of citizens, may be present at any session of the juvenile court (ss.27 and 28). The child is entitled to be represented by counsel. All these are factors which, counsel for the appellant argues, establish that s.12(1), in the context of the Act, does not truly deprive the public of the right of access to the courts, and therefore it is a reasonable limit on s.2(b) of the Charter.

While the argument is superficially an attractive one, it does not meet the basic objection under the Charter respecting the arbitrary nature of the operation of the section. Further, the examples of public access to the proceedings recited above (some of which are indirect at best) raise with even greater clarity and emphasis the question of the necessity and reasonableness of an absolute bar in all cases. It can be seen that under the *Young Offenders Act* although the court is given the discretionary power to exclude all members of the public, it cannot exclude the young offender, his parents, his counsel or his youth worker (probation officer). Such representation of the public does not, in my view, satisfy the required fundamental freedom of expression as earlier reviewed, or reasonably qualify the arbitrary nature of the absolute effect of the present section.

Counsel for the appellant argued that, in any event, the limit imposed on the fundamental freedom was a *reasonable limit demonstrably justified in a free and democratic society* (emphasis added). In support of his position he pointed out that the section had been on the Canadian statute books since 1908 without objection, and that Canada was a free and democratic society. It seems to me that this reasoning, by itself, has little to do with the requirements of s.1 of the Charter. If the fact that an Act had been on our statute books without challenge for a period of years was determinative of the question an issue raised by s.1, no statute or section of a statute in existence prior to the Charter coming into force could be effectively challenged.

We are left, at present, to a certain extent wandering in unexplored terrain in which we have to set up our own guide-posts in interpreting the meaning and effect of the words of s.1 of the Charter. In determining the reasonableness of the limit in each particular case, the court must examine objectively its argued rational basis in light of what the court understands to be reasonable in a free and democratic society. Further, there is, it appears to me, a significant burden on the proponent of the limit or limits to demonstrate their justification to the satisfaction of the court. As I said earlier that may be easily done in a number of cases.

In determining whether the limit is justifiable, some help may be derived from considering the legislative approaches taken in similar fields by other acknowledged free and democratic societies. Presumably this may also assist in determining whether the limit is a reasonable one. It may be that some of the rights guaranteed by the Charter do not have their counterpart in other free and democratic societies and one is sent back immediately to the facts of our own society. In any event I believe the court must come back, ultimately, having derived whatever assistance can be secured from the experience of other free and democratic societies, to the facts of our own free and democratic society to answer the question whether the limit imposed on the particular guaranteed freedom has been demonstrably justified as a reasonable one, having balanced the perceived purpose and objectives of the limiting legislation, in light of all relevant considerations, against the freedom or right allegedly infringed.

. . . . .

In England, no person shall be present at any sitting of a juvenile court except, *inter alia*, "bona fide representatives of newspapers or news agencies" and "such other persons as the court may specially authorize to be present": see the *Children and Young Persons Act*, 1933 (U.K.), c. 12, s.47.

I should note that in all the cases where the media is allowed to be present, there is, similar to s. 12(3) of the *Juvenile Delinquents Act*, a ban on the publication of the name of the child or anything that might lead to his identification. The court, however, is given the discretion to lift the ban.

If any majority approach can be identified from the review of comparable legislation, it is that juvenile courts are given the discretion to exclude members of the public depending upon its view of the circumstances. There are comparatively few jurisdictions where the prohibition of access is absolute with no discretion left to the hearing judge to determine whether it is appropriate and necessary to exclude all or any of the public.

As I stated earlier, I think it is necessary to view the reasonableness of the absolute ban in light of the purpose of the ban as balanced against the fundamental right guaranteed by the Charter.

Although there is a rational basis for the exclusion of the public from hearings under the *Juvenile Delinquents Act*, I do not think an absolute ban in all cases is a reasonable limit on the right of access to the courts, subsumed under the guaranteed freedom of expression, including freedom of the press. The net which s.12(1) casts is too wide for the purpose which it serves. Society loses more than it protects by the all-embracing nature of the section. As stated earlier, counsel for the Attorney-General was quick to acknowledge (and very fairly so) that not every juvenile court proceeding would require the barring of public access. An amendment giving jurisdiction to the court to exclude the public from juvenile court proceedings where it concludes, under the circumstances, that it is in the best interests of the child or others concerned or in the best interests of the administration of justice to do so would meet any residual concern arising from the striking down of the section. As Mr. Justice Martin said in *R. v. Oakes* (released February 2, 1983, unreported) [since reported 2 C.C.C. (3d) 339, 40 O.R. (2d) 660] we are not entitled to rewrite the statute under attack when considering the applicability of the provisions of the Charter. Parliament can give the necessary discretion to the court to be exercised on a case-to-case basis which, in my view, would be a prospective reasonable limit on the guaranteed right and demonstrably justifiable. The protection of social values of "superordinate importance" referred to by Dickson J. in A.-G. N.S. *et al. v. MacIntyre* (1982), 65 C.C.C. (2d) 129, 132 D.L.R. (3d) 385, 26 C.R. (3d) 193, does not require, in my view, an absolute bar in all cases of the public, including the press, from juvenile court proceedings.

The appellant in the present case has not demonstrably justified the limit imposed by s.12(1) as a reasonable one in this free and democratic society and, accordingly, the appeal is dismissed.

Appeal dismissed.

Note: The *Juvenile Delinquents Act* is no longer law. See section 3.3.3.2.2. for relevant provisions of the *Young Offenders Act*.

3.2.2 *R. v. Robinson* (1983), 41 O.R. (2d) 764 (Ont. H.C.)

BOLAND, J. (orally): — This is an application pursuant to s.24(1) of the *Canadian Charter of Rights and Freedoms* to continue the temporary order prohibiting the broadcast and publication of the name, address and other information that would identify the applicant who has been charged with murder under s.218 of the *Criminal Code*.

Section 2(b) of the Charter provides everyone with specific fundamental freedoms including:

> (*b*) freedom of thought, belief, opinion and expression, including freedom of the press and other media of communication.

Section 11 (d) provides that

> **11.** Any person charged with an offence has the right
>
> . . . . .
>
> (*d*) to be presumed innocent until proven guilty according to law in a fair and public hearing by an independent and impartial tribunal.

Section 1 guarantees these rights and freedoms "subject only to such reasonable limits prescribed by law as can be demonstrably justified in a free and democratic society".

Section 24(1) states:

24. (1) Anyone whose rights or freedoms, as guaranteed by this Charter, have been infringed or denied may apply to a court of competent jurisdiction to obtain such remedy as the court considers appropriate and just in the circumstances.

The issue surfaced on March 27, 1983, when the applicant was charged with murder. The following afternoon his counsel obtained a temporary publication ban from Mr. Justice Osler, on the name, address and any other information that would identify the accused. The application was based on the premise that the right of the accused to be presumed innocent as guaranteed by the Charter would be infringed if his name and address were published or broadcast. The order was served on the media and Mr. Justice Osler arranged for his temporary order to be reviewed on the merits on April 5, 1983.

Counsel for the applicant contended there was a confrontation between the freedom of the press and the public's "right to know" *and* the individual's right to be presumed innocent until proven guilty, the right to a fair trial and the right to security of the person. He argued that free press and fair trial cannot coexist as absolutes.

Counsel for the media urged the court to find the temporary order infringes or denies the fundamental freedom of expression, including freedom of the press as guaranteed by the Charter and was not a reasonable limit prescribed by law as can be demonstrably justified in a free and democratic society.

Having reviewed the material, I would like to emphasize that there was no suggestion of contempt raised on the application and there is no evidence of irresponsible reporting on the part of the media. I am satisfied that the publication of the name of the applicant, who has been charged with murder, would not infringe or deny his right to be presumed innocent and his right to a fair trial.

The presumption of innocence referred to in s. 11 (d) of the Charter is a presumption in favour of an accused which operates at trial and gives rise to the burden of proof beyond a reasonable doubt which rests upon the Crown throughout the trial. That presumption does not create a right in an accused person to undermine the statutory power to secure fingerprint identification or affect the conduct of a bail hearing or remain anonymous until after trial. Such a right would have to be based on statutory or common law.

The right to a fair trial is fundamental to our system of justice. There is nothing new about this concept. Moreover there are numerous procedural safeguards to ensure the accused a fair trial in the face of pre-trial publicity such as the juror's oath, the trial judge's instructions to the jury with respect to the media, the rights of the accused in jury selection, the screening of jurors by the trial judge, the criminal standard of proof and possibly a change of venue.

Furthermore, the essential quality of the criminal process in a democracy is the absence of secrecy. From the information to the acquittal or conviction, our judicial process is characterized by public access. The public has the right to be informed and the media has a duty to advise the public what is happening in our courts. Openness prevents abuse of the judicial system and fosters public confidence in the fairness and integrity of our system of justice. The press is a positive influence in assuring fair trial.

Parliament is supreme as a lawmaking body and the traditional role of the judiciary is to interpret the law. Where Parliament has concluded that the public interest dictates that the names of persons involved in the judicial process be withheld from the public, Parliament has created specific statutory prohibitions. For example, the *Criminal Code* provides when the name of the complainant in cases of sexual assault is not to be published and provides similar prohibitions with respect to the names of children and wire-taps. Parliament has not seen fit to legislate such a right in favour of an adult accused and such a right is not supported by the Charter.

On the other hand, freedom of the press is a fundamental freedom guaranteed by the Charter. If a free press is to fulfill its function it requires access to information that should be public and it requires freedom to print without prior restraint. Prior restraint should only be imposed on the press in extraordinary circumstances. There are no extraordinary circumstances in this case and I find there is no right provided by the Charter that has been infringed or denied.

For these reasons I am not continuing the order and the application is dismissed.

Application dismissed.

3.2.3 Cameras, Video Recorders and Audio Recorders in the Courtroom

3.2.3.1 Ontario *Courts of Justice Act*, R.S.O. 1990, c. C.43

136. (1) Subject to subsections (2) and (3), no person shall,
  (*a*) take or attempt to take a photograph, motion picture, audio recording or other record capable of producing visual or aural representations by electronic means or otherwise,
    (i) at a court hearing,
    (ii) of any person entering or leaving the room in which a court hearing is to be or has been convened, or
    (iii) of any person in the building in which a court hearing is to be or has been convened where there is reasonable ground for believing that the person is there for the purpose of attending or leaving the hearing;
  (*b*) publish, broadcast, reproduce or otherwise disseminate a photograph, motion picture, audio recording or record taken in contravention of clause (a); or
  (*c*) broadcast or reproduce an audio recording made as described in clause (2) (b). 1984, c. 11, s. 146 (1); 1988, c. 69, s. 1 (1).

(2) Nothing in subsection (1),

(*a*) prohibits a person from unobtrusively making handwritten notes or sketches at a court hearing; or

(*b*) prohibits a solicitor, a party acting in person or a journalist from unobtrusively making an audio recording at a court hearing, in the manner that has been approved by the judge, for the sole purpose of supplementing or replacing handwritten notes. 1984, c. 11, s. 146 (2); 1988, c. 69, s. 1 (2).

(3) Subsection (1) does not apply to a photograph, motion picture, audio recording or record made with authorization of the judge,

(*a*) where required for the presentation of evidence or the making of a record or for any other purpose of the court hearing;

(*b*) in connection with any investitive, naturalization, ceremonial or other similar proceeding; or

(*c*) with the consent of the parties and witnesses, for such educational or instructional purposes as the judge approves. 1984, c. 11, s. 146 (3).

(4) Every person who contravenes this section is guilty of an offence and on conviction is liable to a fine of not more than $25,000 or to imprisonment for a term of not more than six months, or to both. 1984, c. 11, s. 146 (4); 1989, c. 72, s.18, *part.*

3.2.3.2 *R. v. Rowbotham (No. 3)* (1976), 2 C.R. (3d) 241 (Ont. Co.Ct.)

3rd November 1976. BORINS Co. Ct. J. (orally): — Gentlemen, I had occasion to speak to you briefly in chambers with respect to the situation that has caused me to reconvene the court in this case, and I think that for the purposes of the record, it would be appropriate if I briefly outlined what occurred.

On Monday, 1st November, at about 4:45 p.m. the sheriff came into my office to advise me that there was a photographer loitering in the vicinity of my car in the parking area to the west of the court house, and this person advised the sheriff that he was there to take a photograph of me. The sheriff accompanied me to my car at about 5:00 p.m. and there was a man there with a camera. The sheriff told him that he was not to take a photograph of me, and I told this person the same thing. After I had told him not to take a photograph of me, he did so, or appeared to do so. The camera made a clicking sound. The sheriff identified himself. He requested that this person accompany us into the court house, which he did. He came into my office and identified himself as Chris Rennie. He said that he had been instructed to take a photograph of the prosecutor in this case, and the two undercover officers involved in this case, and of the judge in this case. When I asked him who gave him these instructions, he said that he was working for a magazine in the United States called "High Times". However, he was unable to tell me who the editor of the magazine is, or he did not want to tell me who the editor of the magazine is, and I advised him that in my opinion he was acting in an irresponsible manner, doing what he did. I told him that a responsible journalist would have asked permission to take my photograph and presumably he would be governed by whatever my response to the request would have been.

To say that this young man acted in a flippant, rude manner would be an understatement.

The sheriff asked him to surrender his camera to him. He was about to do so, then asked if it would be acceptable if he surrendered the film. He said that it would be. The film is now in the custody of the sheriff, and as stated to Chris Rennie, the film would not be destroyed. However, I indicated to him that he would have to apply to the court if he wished to have the film returned to him.

Yesterday, 2nd November, Maedel Co. Ct. J. advised me at about 2:30 p.m. that there were two people with cameras just outside of the south-west door, the judge's entrance to the court house, and that they had apparently taken a photograph of Gord Russell, one of the sheriff's officers. It was at that stage that I determined the court ought to be reconvened today so that I could advise you formally of what has occurred so that the matter could be placed on the record.

The legislature of this province has recently enacted a section of the *Judicature Act*, R.S.O. 1970, c.228, s.68a [en. 1974, c.81, s.3], which prohibits the taking of photographs, motion pictures, or other records capable of producing visual representations by electronic means at a judicial proceeding, or of a person entering or leaving the court room in which the judicial proceeding is to be or has been convened, or of any person in the precincts of the building in which the judicial proceeding is to be or has been convened. The legislature has provided rather severe penalties for anyone in contravention of this section. If he is convicted of the offence contrary to this section, a fine of not more than $10,000, or imprisonment for a term of not more than six months, or both, represent the penalties which the legislature, in its view, feels is appropriate. However, the section does not cover the taking of photographs outside the court house. The "precincts of the building" are defined in s.68a(1)(c) as being "the space enclosed by the walls of the building", so that it would appear that this section does not relate to what occurred on 1st November or 2nd November.

It is my view that a trial judge in any trial occupies a special role, and he is to be free of harassment both in and out of the court room. I should add that on Monday, 1st November, after Mr. Rennie gave the film to the sheriff, he left my office. I remained in the building for about ten minutes. When I left to go home, he was there outside the court house. He approached my car after I begun entering it and begun shouting at me from a distance of two or three feet away, that I was abusing the freedom of the press. Freedom of the press is certainly a relevant term, as I indicated earlier. The press has an obligation to be responsible. It has been my experience that the press in this jurisdiction and in Metropolitan Toronto have always conducted themselves in a responsible manner.

Whether the failure to comply with the request of a trial judge outside the court room constitutes a contempt of court is another matter upon which I do not care to express myself at the present time. There is certainly a matter of public interest involved. In my view, those persons who are responsible for the enforcement of law are entitled to do so free from harassment and interference which may fall short of a criminal offence as defined in the *Criminal Code*.

So that a similar situation such as I have described does not occur, I feel that I must make an order in this case, and I do so with considerable regret, because I do value the freedom of the press, and responsible reporting and responsible journalism. However, if it exceeds the bounds of responsible journalism, I feel that such an order as the one I am about to make is required.

Order

The following order is, therefore, made:

No person shall take, or attempt to take any photograph, motion picture, or other record capable of producing visual representations by electronic means or otherwise, of any person in any way involved in the case of Regina and Robert Wilson Rowbotham and others, either inside the Peel County Court House, or outside the Peel County Court House, or publish, broadcast, reproduce, or otherwise disseminate any photo graph, motion picture, or record taken or made in contravention of this order.

This order is meant to complement the provisions of s.68a of the *Judicature Act*.

3.2.3.3 *R. v. Squires* (1989), 69 C.R. (3d) 337, at pp. 339; 342; 343; 345-357; 358-360

MERCIER D.C.J.:- Catherine Squires appeals her conviction for taking motion pictures or other records capable of producing visual representation by electronic means of persons leaving the room in which judicial proceedings had been convened, contrary to s. 67(2)(a) of the *Judicature Act*, R.S.O. 1980, c. 223.

The facts are not in issue. The accused admitted having filmed per sons leaving the courtroom where a preliminary hearing was being held and, in effect, admitted having contravened the provisions of s. 67(2)(a) of the *Judicature Act*. The appeal is really from the decision of the learned trial judge rejecting the accused's contention that the provisions of s. 67 of the Ontario *Judicature Act* constitute an infringement of a protected right under the Charter, specifically s. 2(b), which infringement does not fall within reasonable limits demonstrably justifiable in a free and democratic society, under s. 1 of the Charter.

. . . . .

Does s. 67 of the *Judicature Act* infringe on the freedom of the press, bestowed by s. 2(b) of the Charter? (Section 67 was in essentially the same terms as section 136 of the *Courts of Justice Act*.)

. . . . .

With the greatest of respect to the learned trial judge, contrary to his finding on this point, I am of a view that it does.

I agree that the burden of proving this is borne by the appellant.

As indicated by the learned trial judge, the Attorney General explained to the legislature that s. 67 of the *Judicature Act* was necessary because the general power of a judge over proceedings before him did not appear to include any authority over the photographing and televising of activities associated with judicial proceedings, and that a form of control was needed to codify the practice that had grown up.

I would take it from this that, without this law, it was the view of the Attorney-General that photographing and televising of judicial proceedings could not be controlled.

The trial judge was of the opinion that the purpose intended to be served by s. 67 was to ensure:

a) dignity and decorum in the courtroom and the courthouse,

b) that a person charged with an offence will receive a fair trial and, generally, the proper administration of justice and due enforcement of the law, and

c) the protection of the rights, dignity and privacy of trial participants.

While I agree that such was the purpose of s. 67, these are matters which one could argue are reasons justifying restrictions on the right to film, pursuant to s. 1.

Since s. 67 deals exclusively with the question of photographing or filming in the courtroom or courthouse, why would it be required, if no one had an existing or arguable right to do so?

. . . . .

It is, I believe, settled law that s. 2(b) of the Charter grants free access to the courts as a fundamental right or freedom. The question is: Is this free access limited to the right to be present and report what goes on, or does it include the right to record what goes on, and if so, is the manner of recording limited in any way?

Counsel for the Attorney General of Ontario argues very forcefully that s. 2(b) constitutionally protects the dissemination of information but it does not provide constitutional protection in the gathering of information. He cites three authorities in support of this proposition.

1) *R. v. Thomson Newspapers Ltd.*, an unreported decision of Anderson J. of the High Court of Ontario, 8th December 1983 [11 W.C.B. 436].

In that case the court was dealing with the question of the right of the media to film exhibits filed at trial. Anderson J. states:

> A clear line must be drawn between the right of access to the court engaged by members of the public, including members of the press, and the right to *intervene* in any way in the process and conduct of a trial. [the emphasis is mine]

In my view, filming in a Courtroom is not intervening in the process and conduct of a trial. Anderson J. does seem to state, however, that the rights of the press are different and may be greater than those of the general public. He states:

> I directed that those documents be made available as part of a usage and convention ... of providing to the members of the press some limited accommodations which are not available to members of the public generally.

I do not see this as a decision which is in any way binding upon me in this case.

2) *Lorne v. R.* (1985), 46 C.R. (3d) 322, 21 C.C.C. (3d) 436 (Que. C.A.).

Video cassettes of the crime from cameras in the National Assembly focused the attention of the Quebec Court of Appeal. The court ruled that cassettes should not be publicly shown pending the disposition of the appeal. The court stated that a temporary prohibition did involve a violation of the rights or freedoms as guaranteed by the Charter. Still, the guarantee to freedom of expression, including the press, in s. 2(*b*) of the Charter is subject to reasonable limitations under s. 1. It held that, although the temporary prohibition on the broadcasting of the tapes limited freedom of expression, it did so in a manner permitted by s. 1.

The court did not find that the press did not have a right to the cassettes. It held the temporary prohibition was justified under s. 1 of the Charter.

Madame Justice L'Heureux-Dube, in dissent, said the right to consult a document includes the right to take notes and to copy or photocopy that document. The news media have the right to make copies of the tapes and to broadcast them. The guarantee to freedom of expression, including freedom of the press and other media, as guaranteed by s. 2(b) of the Charter, required the prosecution to demonstrate that the prohibition order was essential to secure the right of the accused to a fair trial, should a new trial be ordered.

The majority of the court did not seem to disagree with those statements of principle. They only disagreed as to whether the tapes could be withheld from public dissemination before the appeal had been dealt with, and determined that, if they were, it could only be done pursuant to s. 1 of the Charter.

The *Lortie* case, if it establishes anything, establishes, in my view, that the media have a right to make copies of exhibits. Inferentially, then, they have a right to film a trial pursuant to s. 2(b) of the Charter. Such a right can only be limited if the limitations are justified pursuant to s. 1.

3) Royal Commission of Enquiry re Judge Henriksen

That decision applies only to its own particular facts. It was an inquiry, not a trial. Mr. Justice Houlden dealt with press coverage where a particular individual happened to be a judge. Would television coverage be damaging to him and to the public if he should continue as a judge? The learned justice decided on the particular facts of that case and does not appear to have considered s. 2(b) of the Charter as being relevant in that case.

The learned trial judge states that at common law the right of access to judicial proceedings is a fundamental right, but is only a presumptive right. It is a right only to attend in court, observe and listen to the proceedings and to report thereon. Representatives of the press and other media of communication possess the right of access merely in their capacity as members of the general public.

With respect, I disagree. If the members of the press only have access in their capacity as members of the public, why would the words "including freedom of the press and other media of communication" have been added to s. 2(b) of the

Charter? Surely. members of the press and other media of communication would be included in "everyone".

Since the press and other media are specifically mentioned, it has to be for a purpose. They cannot be mere surplusage. It has been recognized by the courts that the media do receive special attention. Reporters are often guaranteed space in the courtroom, special tables are made available for them, etc. This is because it is of paramount importance that not only should the public be entitled to attend, it should be entitled to know what goes on in our courts when they cannot attend. The media, in effect, represents the public very often in courtrooms and is therefore not there just as a member of the public. The reporter is present in his own right and in our right.

The learned trial judge said that if the media had a right to televise judicial proceedings and thus bring its equipment into the courtroom, there would be a corresponding duty on the province to provide appropriate accommodation. He objects to this because of the expense involved.

Quite apart from the fact that it is far from certain that such consequences would necessarily follow, I cannot agree that one should determine whether a freedom is guaranteed by postulating on the potential costs involved. A freedom is a freedom, and should be guaranteed at whatever cost. If freedoms are not to be guaranteed, because it would be expensive to do so, then there is no freedom. If freedoms are to be guaranteed only when there is no cost, then there is no guarantee of freedom, only costs are guaranteed. Freedoms exist or they do not. If they do exist they can be limited but the limitation must be justified. That is the purpose of s. 1 of the Charter.

The Crown has argued, and the trial judge agreed, that the "freedom of the press and other media of communication" given by s. 2(b) of the Charter is the right to *disseminate* information, not a right to *gather* that information.

With the greatest of respect to the learned trial judge and to the learned counsel, that would only put a superficial gloss on the words of s. 2(b) of the Charter. To say that you cannot be limited in the dissemination of information without justifying such limitation pursuant to s. 1 of the Charter, but that you can be limited in gathering the information you wish to disseminate, or at least in the manner of gathering that information, without any obligation to justify those limitations, renders that right meaningless. The information to be disseminated, if it is to achieve the purpose intended, i.e., to ensure openness of trials and to keep the public properly informed as to what transpires in courtrooms, must, as much as possible, be accurate. If the print media were not allowed to take notes, and were called upon to rely exclusively on their memory of what transpired in a courtroom, reporting accuracy would surely decline and probably — drastically. Logically, if the manner of gathering the information is not protected by s. 2(b), a law could be passed preventing the taking of notes in a courtroom. without having to justify it pursuant to s. 1.

Parallel with the special meaning of the words "including members of the press and other media of communication" as a whole, some specific meaning must also be attributed to the words "and other media of communication". Again, they are there for a reason. If they were intended only to refer to the traditional rights of the press to attend and take notes, it would not be necessary to specify "other media of communication", as they would obviously qualify as "members of the press". The addition of those words, in my view, is an indication by Parliament that it indeed had in mind the "living tree" doctrine as espoused by MacKinnon A.C.J.O. when it adopted the *Constitution Act, 1982*. Those words can only mean that it was intended such other media could gather their information, in whatever way was required, to enable them to best fulfill their duty of properly reporting or disseminating the information. For the television media, that is filming. It is an integral part of the gathering of information and its dissemination by that particular medium. Who is to say what other types of news gathering and dissemination may be devised in the future? Will those all be restricted to the taking of notes, regardless of whether that method cannot possibly permit that medium to do properly what it is required to do? To state the question is to answer it. Any restriction of those rights ought to require justification That is the purpose of s. 1; it allows limitations on freedoms, but only if they can be justified.

The learned trial judge disagrees with the appellant's argument that the right to film is absolute subject only to an objecting party post facto satisfying the "heavy onus" under s. 1 of the Charter see p. 345.

If the limitations are reasonable the onus can be met. The fact that the onus shifts once a right is guaranteed does not justify denying the existence of that right.

The learned trial judge finds, as I do. that the media's right of access to the courts does not carry with it any right to intervene in any way in the conduct of a trial. But he goes on to find [at p. 348] that in the context of this case that means "it does not include a right to bring photographic and television cameras and broadcast equipment into a court and televise the proceedings in the court". He repeats his earlier finding that " 'freedom of expression' confers a right merely to 'publish' or 'broad cast' information lawfully obtained, in other words, a right of dissemination of material and not a right of news gathering as such."

With respect, that is not my view of what "intervene" means in this context. I see it as meaning "to come between so as to prevent or modify the result" or to "interpose oneself in a lawsuit", and not as meaning "come in as something extraneous". These are all definitions of "intervene" in the *Concise Oxford Dictionary.*

If the latter was the definition adopted by the courts, that would exclude everyone and everything from the courtroom, and obviously that was not what was intended. The courts intended that, however access to them is exercised by the media, they do not have the right to do so in a manner that would prevent or modify the result of a trial, nor could they interpose themselves into any lawsuit.

To simply set up and watch and listen to proceedings is not intervening. That is what cameras do once set up; they watch and listen and record the goings-on. If the media do in fact have free access to the courts and if they have a duty to record and disseminate the information as accurately as possible, that is what they must be allowed to do. Any limitations on these rights ought to be required to be justified pursuant to s. 1 of the Charter.

It is my view that the authorities I have dealt with, and others which I have been referred to and which I have perused, but do not intend to comment on individually, have decided the following:

1) Section 2(b) grants to the media free access to the courts as a fundamental right.

2) That right includes the right to gather information as well as to disseminate it.

3) The words "to the press and other media of communication" do grant to the media something more than the right granted the general public.

4) Filming is an integral part of television reporting, and that medium should be entitled to use its cameras as part of its access, as the printed media ought to be entitled to use photography in their access.

5) Where these rights conflict with rights to fair trial, decorum in the courtroom, rights to privacy, etc., they may be limited, but such interference must be shown to exist and the limitation must therefore be justified, under s. 1 of the Charter.

I therefore conclude that the *Canadian Charter of Rights and Freedoms* does confer upon the media a constitutional right under s. 2(b) to televise or photograph judicial proceedings in court, and that the provisions of s. 67 of the Ontario *Judicature Act* do constitute a violation of a protected right under the Charter.

If s. 2(b) confers on the media a constitutional right to film or photograph in the courtroom, does it do likewise for the courthouse?

The learned trial judge was "unable to find any justification in the evidence for allowing the media to photograph people who are present in the courthouse for the purpose of attending judicial proceedings, either by still photography for publication in the (print) press or by television camera for broadcast". He found [at p. 366] that "to allow the practice would constitute a substantial threat to the dignity and integrity of judicial proceedings." He concluded his findings in this respect by stating "to allow free access to photograph persons in the courthouse who are there for the purpose of attending judicial proceedings would not assist in any way in deciding any of the issues before the court or serve any short term or long term educational function."

While I do not disagree with those findings they should apply, in my view, in determining whether s. 67 of the *Judicature Act* imposes reasonable limits on the freedom of the press and other media of communication as can be demonstrably justified in a free and democratic society, under s. 1 of the Charter.

The learned judge has dealt with this issue on the basis that there is no prima facie right on the part of the media to photograph or film in the courthouse, under s. 2(b) of the Charter. This follows logically from his similar finding with respect to filming in the courtroom.

For the same reasons given with respect to filming in the court rooms, I find that there is a prima facie right on the part of the media to film or photograph within the confines of the courthouse and that any restrictions on these rights must be justified under s. 1 of the Charter.

I would find it difficult to conclude that there was no right to film or photograph in the corridors of any public building, although I could well see that some restrictions might lawfully be imposed on these rights in certain circumstances, which restrictions would have to be justified.

In particular, with respect to the courthouse in which this appeal has been argued, there are many rooms available where filming and/or photography could take place without in any way disturbing the calm and serene atmosphere one should be entitled to expect in a courthouse.

There is in fact in this building a room commonly called "the marriage room", where wedding ceremonies are performed regularly and photographing and filming therein, and in the corridors leading to that room, take place as a matter of course.

Filming and photographing has taken place in the halls of this court house on certain official functions and social occasions.

Section 67 of the *Judicature Act* does not purport to prohibit this sort of filming. It forbids only the filming "of any person entering or leaving the room in which the judicial proceeding is to be or has been convened" and "of any person in the precincts of the building in which the judicial proceeding is to be or has been convened where there is reasonable ground for believing that such person is there for the purpose of attending or leaving the proceeding".

This, in my view, is a restriction on the prima facie right of the media to photograph or film in the courthouse and must be justified under s. 1 of the Charter.

Are the infringements on media rights imposed by s. 67 of the Judicature Act justifiable pursuant to s. 1 of the Charter?

To determine this we must first look at the objects of the section. 1 agree with the learned trial judge that s. 67 aims at:

1) protecting the interests of the parties and the public in ensuring fair trials,

2) protecting the rights, dignity and privacy of trial participants. and

3) ensuring order and decorum in the courtrooms and within the precincts of the courthouse.

We must then determine if the legislation serves societal interests of superordinate importance and in doing so we must assess if a valid governmental objective is served by the limitation of the right to film and if the limitation imposed by s. 67 is restricted to that which is necessary for the attainment of that objective.

As Mr. Justice Dickson wrote in *R. v. Big M Drug Mart Ltd.*, [1985] 1 S.C.R. 295, [1985] 3 W.W.R. 481, 37 Alta. L.R. (2d) 97, 18 C.C.C. (3d) 385, 18 D.L.R. (4th) 321 at 366, 13 C.R.R. 64, 85 C.L.L.C. 14,023, 60 A.R. 161, 58 N.R. 81:

> Principles will have to be developed for recognizing which government objectives are of sufficient importance to warrant overriding a constitutionally protected right or freedom. Once a sufficiently significant government interest is recognized then it must be decided if the means chosen to achieve this interest are reasonable . . . The court may wish to ask whether the means adopted to achieve the end sought do so by impairing as little as possible the right or freedom in question.

Does s. 67 serve societal interests of superordinate importance?

The right to a fair trial is a societal interest of superordinate importance. The "raison d'etre" of courthouses is to provide facilities where members of the public may have differences between them tried, where society may have persons alleged to have committed crimes tried, and where persons who have been charged with the commission of criminal offences can expect due process.

The learned trial judge held that the right to a fair trial is a constitutional right which is to be given priority over any competing interest under s. 2(b). The appellant alleges that he erred. I cannot agree. Within the confines of the courthouse, there can be no more important right than that to a fair trial. Any other freedom or right which competes with the right to a fair trial within the confines of a building erected for the purpose of ensuring that right must be subordinate.

Contrary to the submissions of counsel for the appellant, I am of the view that the guaranteed right to a fair trial is paramount to the fundamental freedom of the press and other media of communication, certainly within the confines of a courthouse and probably anywhere.

This paramount right, therefore, justifies some limitation of any other freedom which might affect it negatively. The government objective to ensure fair trials is of sufficient importance to warrant overriding the constitutionally protected freedom of the press and other media of communication if it is established that it can interfere with that objective.

The respondent has the onus of establishing that such is the case. The trial judge found that the respondent has satisfied that onus.

The evidence adduced by the appellant, including the reports and surveys which the trial judge refused to admit and which I have nevertheless read and considered, establishes that television in the courtroom does not always have a negative effect on a trial.

It indicates that no decision has ever been reversed on the basis that the proceedings were televised. Witnesses testifying at this trial, who had some experience with televising proceedings, had not received complaints from anyone that the televising of the proceedings had in any way interfered with their testimony or behaviour.

The respondent's evidence, on the other hand, established that persons who had participated in televised proceedings had either actually been advised of adverse reaction by witnesses and jurors or had them selves been adversely affected by the presence of television cameras in the courtroom.

The learned trial judge preferred the evidence of the respondent's witnesses, but not because of the credibility of the various witnesses. Their opinion stemmed from actual reactions seen or felt by them as opposed to what really amounts to impressions described by the witnesses of the appellant.

The evidence does establish that televising judicial proceedings can and does interfere with fair trials.

It is not necessary for me to go over the evidence in detail, as it has been thoroughly canvassed by the learned trial judge and I agree with his conclusions.

One might quibble on the emphasis placed on the evidence of certain witnesses as opposed to others. The totality of the evidence, nonetheless, makes one thing clear. The television media have testified that operating without a camera is for them like operating without a pencil would be for the print media. I accept this. The fact remains, apt analogies apart, that cameras in the courtroom and in the courthouse can sometimes be so disruptive as to seriously affect the right to a fair trial.

The evidence has established that cameras in the courtroom can have a negative effect on witnesses and jurors which could lead to an unfair trial. It is true that "The general advantage to the country in having these proceedings made public more than counterbalances the inconvenience to the private persons whose conduct may be the subject of such proceedings", as stated by Lawrence J. in *R. v. Wright, supra*. The right of a person to a fair trial is, however, more than an inconvenience.

Moreover, one must consider that many witnesses and all jurors are in court because they are obliged to be there and consequently they ought to be entitled to reasonable privacy and/or protection. If they are to have no say in whether they are to be filmed, witnesses may not be so willing to step forward and this would obviously have a deleterious effect on trials. Jurors might well be reluctant to serve and look for excuses not to, or be less attentive to the evidence than to the cameras. The evidence does establish that the presence of cameras in courtrooms can have an effect on witnesses and on jurors, and I accept the learned trial judge's view on these.

While I also accept that cameras in the courtrooms could affect the conduct of counsel and judges as well, I am less concerned with this aspect of the question, as I feel certain that with time and experience these problems could be resolved.

I do agree that there was evidence on which the court below could find that filming in court could conflict with the accused's right to a fair trial in certain cases, and this possibility must be taken seriously. There should, therefore, be rules established as to how and when cameras are to be used.

Were the means adopted (s. 67 of the *Judicature Act*) to achieve this interest (right to a fair trial) reasonable? Do they achieve the end sought by impairing as little as possible the freedom of the press?

Section 67(2)(a)(i) prohibits the taking of photographs or motion pictures, etc., at a judicial proceeding. As the evidence establishes that such filming can adversely affect a fair trial, this limitation is obviously reasonable, and as it does not prohibit the representatives of the media from doing anything other than what has been found to be disruptive. it impairs their freedom as little as possible.

Section 67(2)(a)(ii) prohibits the taking of photographs or motion pictures of any person entering or leaving the room in which a judicial proceeding is to be or has been convened.

As the evidence establishes that witnesses and/or jurors can be intimidated by such filming or photographing, thus affecting their willingness to testify or act as jurors, this limitation too is reasonable, and as it only pertains to photographing or filming those persons as they enter or leave the room and can be permitted if the persons consent and the judge authorizes it, it does not impair the media's freedom more than is necessary.

Section 67(2)(a)(iii) prohibits the taking of photographs or motion pictures of any person in the courthouse where there is reasonable ground for believing that such person is there for the purpose of attending or leaving the proceeding.

The same reasons exist for this prohibition as exist for the prohibition against filming in the courtroom or of persons entering or leaving the courtroom and it is, therefore, a reasonable restriction to achieve the objective sought, and again, as it only prohibits such filming without the consent of the persons concerned and the authorization of the judge, it does not unduly impair the media's rights.

The purpose of forbidding the filming of persons entering or leaving a courtroom or anywhere in the courthouse, when such persons are there to attend or leave the proceedings, is to ensure proper decorum within the courthouse and to assure the participants' right to a fair trial. For the same reason that they might well not wish to be filmed in the courtroom, witnesses and jurors would not wish to be filmed elsewhere in the building.

As to decorum and peace and quiet within the corridors of the court house, these are important factors which must be protected.

I have indicated that in this courthouse it might well be possible to regulate filming in certain areas without disrupting the judicial process or the decorum that should surround it, but this is not the case in all court houses. It is impossible to legislate different rules of conduct for each courthouse. Consequently, the legislation must ensure that the right to a fair trial is never compromised by filming in courthouses, and this is what these subsections attempt to do.

If the media were granted the unfettered right to film in the corridors of the courthouse, the evidence clearly establishes that it would be quite obtrusive and could be intimidating to the participants, witnesses and/or jurors. It is one thing to have a reporter try to speak to you - you can simply avoid him or her - but it-is quite another thing to be filmed as you attempt to avoid the reporter. If the participant accepts to be filmed, and the judge is satisfied there is an area where this can be done without disrupting proceedings or destroying decorum, s. 67 of the *Judicature Act* permits filming. Under existing circumstances this appears to me, as it did to the trial judge, to be a reasonable limit on the rights of the media to film as guaranteed under s. 2(b) of the Charter.

Section 67(2)(b) naturally follows from subs. (2)(a) and need not be commented on further.

Section 67(3) is actually permissive but it, of course, must be read in conjunction with subs. (2).

Paragraphs (a) and (b) thereof need not be commented upon, as they simply permit photographing and filming in the circumstances set out therein.

Paragraph (c), while permitting the photographing and filming with the consent of the parties and witnesses, requires that it be for such educational or instruction purposes as may be approved by the judge.

For the reasons already gives it is obvious that if the judge authorizes such filming, and the parties and witnesses agree, the proceedings would not be disrupted nor adversely affected and the prohibitions would become unnecessary. I would question whether it is necessary in those circumstances to confine the electronic media to educational or instructional purposes. If the parties and witnesses agree, and a satisfying arrangement can be devised whereby the judge was satisfied that filming in the courtroom or elsewhere in the building could be allowed without fear of disrupting the proceedings or of affecting the trial, I do not see why it would be necessary to restrict such filming "to such educational or instructional purposes as may be approved by the judge." The learned trial judge was of the opinion that news purposes and educational purposes are not mutually exclusive. He, therefore, felt the presiding judge could determine that a purpose of reporting news may also be regarded as an educational purpose in certain circumstances.

While it is true that in given circumstances news purposes could be deemed to be educational purposes, one can imagine circumstances where news purposes would not be accepted by the trial judge as incorporating any educational or instructional purpose. Therefore, the legislators felt that filming in the courtroom would not be objectionable if done with the consent of the parties and witnesses, as it seems to have in legislating para. (c) of subs. (3) of s. 67 of the *Judicature Act*, I see no reason why it would have to be only for educational or instructional purposes approved by the judge. The judge's authorization for filming is already required by the provisions of subs. (3) and that is sufficient for him to exercise the control he should have over what goes on in his courtroom.

While I find that portion of para. (c) to be inconsistent with the Charter and of no force and effect, it does it necessarily follow that I must, therefore, declare the whole of s. 67, or even the whole of subs. (3)(c) thereof, invalid.

. . . . .

It is really a question of determining, in any given situation, if the remainder of the legislation can survive after the offending portion has been removed.

In my view, this is the case in the present circumstance and the of fending words "for such educational or instructional purposes as may be approved by the judge" should be severed from para. (c) of subs. (3) of s. 67 of the *Judicature Act*.

The remaining words of s. 67 of *Judicature Act*, while violating the constitutional right of freedom of the press guaranteed by s. 2(b) of the Charter, are justified pursuant to s. 1 of the Charter, as they fall within reasonable limits demonstrably justified in a free and democratic society.

The trial judge and I have been asked to deal with this constitutional question within the framework of a charge laid pursuant to s. 67 of the *Judicature Act*. This trial does not really pertain to a finding of guilt or innocence of the accused on the basis of whether or not the evidence establishes beyond a reasonable doubt that she did commit the offence with which she was charged, but to a decision as to whether the law which the accused is alleged to have offended is constitutionally valid.

While one would prefer this sort of decision be made by higher authority, this court, as the one below, has a duty to make a finding on the constitutional issue as it is pertinent to the accused's right to defend herself.

As Mr. Justice Dickson stated in *R. v. Big M Drug Mart*, at p. 336:

> Any accused . . . may defend a criminal charge by arguing that the law under which the charge is brought is constitutionally invalid.

Thus, although this is a matter which, in my opinion, would better be addressed by a committee of competent persons having expertise and experience in the field, who would report to the Attorney General and through him to the legislature, with a view of setting out a valid set of rules as to how the televising of trials could be restricted, the trial judge, as I, must make a determination as to whether s. 67 of the *Judicature Act* is a denial of the freedom of the press, and if so, whether the restriction imposed by it can be justified under s. 1 of the Charter. in order to determine the guilt or innocence of the accused on the charge we are dealing with.

While I have come to a different conclusion from that of the learned trial judge with respect to the constitutional right of the media, pursuant to s. 2(b) of the Charter, I am in general agreement with his findings in considering whether the Crown has established that s. 67 of the *Judicature Act* falls within reasonable limits demonstrably justifiable in a free and democratic society.

Specifically, I agree with the trial judge's findings that the televising of judicial proceedings has a strong tendency to affect adversely the fact finding process and, hence, to influence the results of the proceedings. I find, as did the trial judge, the discussion as to the social values of televising in the courtroom to be inconclusive. I feel the subject ought to be studied more extensively in a less focused milieu than that of a trial.

I have, in these reasons, indicated that the evidence establishes that photographing or filming in a courtroom can adversely affect a trial and I have emphasized the effect it could have on witnesses and jurors.

I have also indicated that s. 67 of the *Judicature Act* permits filming with the consent of the parties and the authorization of the judge and, where those circumstances exist, the media would be allowed to film without requiring that such filming be solely for educational or instructional purposes.

I am conscious of the fact that this would appear to ignore the jurors' right to refuse to be filmed if the parties and witnesses agree to it and, while I would feel better if the legislation had included jurors as persons whose consent was required in para. (c) of s. 67(3) of the Judicature Act, I cannot add restrictions which the legislators did not see fit to impose, although I can sever some in proper circumstances.

I take it that the legislators left it up to the judge to protect the interest of the jurors in requiring his authorization in addition to the consent of the parties and the witnesses.

In summary, therefore, I find:

1) While I would have admitted in evidence certain documentation proffered by accused's counsel, the trial judge's refusal to receive it in no way prejudiced the appellant's position.

2) As an appellate court, I would not be bound by the findings of the trial judge based on his preference of the evidence of certain expert witnesses over others, as credibility is not in issue.

3) Section 67 of the *Judicature Act* does infringe on the freedom of the press, bestowed by s. 2(b) of the Charter, with respect to televising in the courtroom.

4) It likewise infringes on the freedom of the press, bestowed by s. 2(b) of the Charter, with respect to filming in the courthouse.

5) The infringements imposed by s. 67 of the *Judicature Act* are justified as being reasonable limits demonstrably justifiable in a free and democratic society under s. 1 of the Charter, with the exception of the words "for such educational or instructional purposes as may be approved by the judge", in para. (c) of subs. (3) thereof, which are severed and declared to be of no effect.

In the circumstances the appeal will be dismissed and the conviction of the accused is maintained.

There was also an appeal as to the sentence. Neither counsel made oral submissions with respect to same. While I would not have judged the accused's conduct as severely as did the trial judge, I can find no error of principle in the fine imposed and the appeal as to sentence will be dismissed.

Appeal dismissed.

3.2.3.4 Law Reform Commission of Canada, *Public and Media Access to the Criminal Process, Working Paper 56* (Ottawa: Minister of Supply and Services Canada, 1987)

Electronic Media Coverage

23. (1) Electronic media coverage should be permitted in relation to appeals in criminal cases.

(2) Use of audio recorders should be permitted in criminal proceedings as a substitute for, or in addition to, handwritten notes.

(3) A national experiment with electronic media coverage of criminal trials should be conducted with a view to studying comprehensively the impact of the presence of video and still cameras and audio recorders on witnesses, counsel, judges and jurors.

Commentary

There is much speculation about whether the presence of television cameras affects the fact finding process. There is no reason to suspect, in our opinion, that electronic media coverage of appeals would in any way interfere with those proceedings, so long as the court was able to maintain an atmosphere of decorum conducive to a proper hearing on the matters before it. Technology that is presently available would, we believe, allow appellate courts to proceed in a dignified fashion. Thus, in Recommendation 23(1), we suggest that there be no limit placed on electronic media coverage of criminal appeals. Where a publication ban is in force, the electronic media would, of course, be bound by it along with the other media.

Recommendation 23(2) suggests that use of audio recorders be permitted in criminal proceedings. Audio recorders constitute a means for ensuring the accuracy of statements and testimony made in legal proceedings. A recent study revealed "a high level of serious error" was discovered in an analysis of quotations published by the print media in relation to the trial of Colin Thatcher. Use of audio recorders was recommended by the study's author to improve this situation. Use of audio recorders in court by the media was also recommended by the New South Wales Law Reform Commission. It found that use of recorders did not constitute a nuisance or interfere with proceedings. That Commission recommended, however, that recordings be broadcast to the public only with leave of the court. Audio recordings may be made of legal proceedings in the United Kingdom again only with leave of the court. Recordings may not be broadcast. Our proposal would merely permit recorders to be used to obtain statements and testimony made in a criminal proceeding with complete accuracy. We do not recommend at this time that recordings be broadcast. Any recommendation regarding the broadcast of recorded proceedings should await the results of the experiment we propose in Recommendation 23(3). While it may seem incongruous to permit audio recorders to be used in criminal proceedings, but not to allow recordings to be broadcast, it is our view that any impact that the introduction of recorders would be likely to have on the process would relate to the participants' knowledge that their comments could ultimately be broadcast. This may result in nervousness or self-consciousness on their part which should be studied along with the impact of video recording and broadcasts.

Recommendation 23(3) reflects our hesitancy to make a definitive recommendation supporting or opposing blanket electronic media coverage. We believe that a meaningful decision on this issue can only follow a comprehensive study for a significant period of time in various parts of the country. The guidelines for the experiment would have to be generated in consultation with many groups, such as the Canadian Judicial Council, the Canadian Bar Association, provincial law societies, Crown attorneys, law professors, the police and social scientists. Guidelines for the media have already been proposed by the Radio Television News Directors Association and could form the basis for media activity during the experiment. Comparative studies of the effects of audio, as opposed to video, recording ought to form part of the experiment, as should a comparison of electronic with conventional media coverage. The data should be carefully analyzed by social science experts and the conclusions widely circulated. In the absence of clear evidence that electronic media coverage has a significantly greater impact on participants than present media activity, electronic media should be given access to criminal trials on the same footing as other media.

Technology now permits unobtrusive audio or video recording. No special lighting is required; sound can be transmitted through the courts' own sound recording system; only one video camera is necessary to serve all media outlets. The effectiveness of the present technology has been borne out in electronic media coverage of the Royal Commission of Inquiry into Certain Deaths at Hospital for Sick Children and Related Matters (the Grange Commission). Both the Commission's counsel and its Commissioner have been persuaded, after months of experience with intensive electronic media activity, that the media's presence had no adverse impact. Rather, according to Justice Grange, the introduction of television into courtrooms would perform a valuable public benefit:

> I do not want [television] in all courts at all times. I do, however, think it should be tried in some courts at some times under controlled conditions. The reason is simple. The public must know what goes on in our courts and the only way they can get a proper conception is the way they get their conception of all our institutions, i.e. through television. And the ignorance of the public of our system and the way it runs (as opposed to some other system or some totally imaginary systems) is appalling.

We concur with this opinion in principle. However, doubts about the impact of electronic media coverage on the trial process will always linger in the absence of a satisfactory empirical study. This study should, therefore, precede the introduction of electronic media on a scale beyond what is now permitted.

3.2.4 Sparing Parties from Embarrassment

3.2.4.1 *Re Regina and an Unnamed Person* (1985), 22 C.C.C. (3d) 284 (Ont. C.A.)

ZUBER J.A.: — This is an appeal by Southam Inc. and the Brockville Recorder and Times Limited from an order made by Keith J. prohibiting the publication or broadcast of the identity of a female person. An appreciation of the issues requires only a brief outline of the facts.

On May 1, 1984, a 17-year-old woman was charged in the provincial court (criminal division) at Brockville with two offences: infanticide, contrary to s.216 of the *Criminal Code*, and neglect to obtain assistance in childbirth contrary to s.226 of the *Criminal Code*. While these charges generated some publicity, the 17-year-old woman was not identified.

On June 13, 1984, counsel for the young woman brought an application before Mr. Justice Keith in Motions Court in Ottawa seeking prohibition of the publication of the identity of the young woman. Both of the appellants were served with notice of the application and both appeared before the learned judge and made submissions.

The basis of the application was simply that the unnamed young woman would suffer embarrassment and possibly detrimental effects with respect to employment. It was also said that members of her family would also suffer embarrassment and detrimental effects with respect to employment.

On this basis the order was made:

(1) prohibiting the broadcast or publication of the identity of the young woman who was the subject of the charges;
(2) directing that the criminal proceedings be held in camera (excepting only representatives of the media), and
(3) providing that this order not be the subject of any time limit

... there is no statutory basis for the order in this case. The respondent and the Attorney-General argue that the authority to make the order in this case proceeds from the inherent jurisdiction of a judge of the High Court.

The term "inherent jurisdiction" is one that is commonly and not always accurately used when arguments are made with respect to the jurisdictional basis upon which a court is asked to make a particular order. The inherent jurisdiction of a superior court is derived not from any statute or rule of law but from the very nature of the court as a superior court: (see, generally, I. H. Jacob, "The Inherent Jurisdiction of the Court", *Current Legal Problems* 23 (1970). Utilizing this power, superior courts, to maintain their authority and to prevent their processes from being obstructed or abused, have amongst other things punished for contempt of court, stayed matters that are frivolous and vexatious and regulated their own process. The limits of this power are difficult to define with precision but cannot extend to the creation of a new rule of substantive law.

In *R. v. McArthur* (1984), 13 C.C.C (3d) 152, 10 C.R.R. 220, Dupont J. made an order prohibiting the publication of the names of witnesses who were to testify at trial. Dupont J. was the trial judge. It was his view that if the identity of the witnesses were published, the witnesses (who were inmates of the penitentiary) might be deterred from testifying. With respect, I think that such an order was properly within the inherent jurisdiction of the court to protect the trial that was being conducted. In the case at hand, Keith J. was of course not protecting the integrity of any matter that was otherwise before him.

It appears, as well, that a superior court has power under its inherent jurisdiction to render assistance to inferior courts to enable them to administer justice fully and effectively: see *Jacob, supra*, p. 48. However, in the case at hand, there is nothing in the material to suggest that either the provincial court or the county court required assistance from the High Court in order that they might fully and effectively administer justice. The order in this case was made not to protect the process before the court but simply to protect the accused and her family from embarrassment and other potential losses that might flow from identification.

The respondents rely heavily upon the judgment of Linden J. in *R. v. P.* (1978), 41 C.C.C (2d) 377, 3 C.R. (3d) 59. In that case, the accused had been acquitted on a charge of soliciting for the purpose of prostitution. The Crown appealed to the High Court by way of stated case. The accused sought to avoid embarrassment to his wife and children and applied to Linden J. of the High Court for an order prohibiting the publication of his identity. Linden J. said at p. 378:

> It falls to this Court to determine whether the interests of the public is best served by protecting the identity of this individual or whether it would be preferable to permit the public to know not only the details of the offence, but also the name of the person involved. The Court is invited to make this order pursuant to its inherent jurisdiction and pursuant to s.768(1)(d) of the *Criminal Code* which reads as follows:
>
>> "768(1) Where a case is stated under this Part, the superior court shall hear and determine the grounds of appeal and may
>>
>> . . . . .
>>
>> make
>>
>> (*d*) any other order in relation to the matter that it considers proper, and . . ."

Linden J. then proceeded to deal with the merits of the matter and made the order asked for. Linden J., however, did not further discuss the issue of jurisdiction. Nor did he say whether he found power under s.768(1) or in his inherent jurisdiction. Later, Steele J. was asked to continue the order made by Linden J.: *R. v. P.* (1978), 43 C.C.C. (2d) 197, 3 C.R. (3d) 62. Steele J. held that he had the power to continue the order but declined to do so. In *Re Regina and Several Unnamed Persons* (1983), 8 C.C.C. (3d) 528, 4 D.L.R. (4th) 310, 44 O.R. (2d) 81, O'Brien J. was asked to prohibit publication of the identity of an accused person in a proceeding in a court other than the High Court. The basis of the application was similar to the basis of the application in the case at hand —

embarrassment and possible loss of employment. O'Brien J. accepted the premise that he had inherent jurisdiction to make such an order but declined to do so.

To the extent that these cases support the premise that a High Court Judge can issue a non-publication order respecting matters pending before other courts where no case is made out to show that those other courts require the assistance of a superior court so that justice can be fully and effectively administered, I must respectfully disagree with them. Other than the decision by Linden J. and the approvals by way of *obiter* that followed, I have been unable to discover any principle or any case which supports the proposition that there is inherent jurisdiction in the High Court to make the order in the case at hand. In my respectful view, the order which is the subject of this appeal has little, if anything, to do with protecting the process of the court. What the respondents seek in this case is the creation of a discretionary right of privacy to be extended to those caught up in the criminal process. I conclude that Keith J. was without jurisdiction to make the order which is the subject of this appeal. In the result, the appeal is allowed and the order of Keith J. is set aside and the application for the non-publication order is dismissed.

Appeal allowed.

3.3 Contempt of Court

3.3.1 General Considerations

3.3.1.1 *Attorney-General v. Leveller Magazine Ltd. and Others*, [1979] A.C. 440 (H.L.)

LORD DIPLOCK. My Lords, in November 1977 three defendants, two of whom were journalists, had been charged with offences under the *Official Secrets Act*. Committal proceedings against them were being heard before the Tottenham Magistrates' Court acting as examining justices. The proceedings extended over a considerable number of days. On the first day, on the application of counsel for the prosecution, some of the evidence was heard in camera pursuant to section 8 (4) of the *Official Secrets Act* 1920. On the third day, November 10, counsel for the prosecution made an application that the next witness whom he proposed to call should, for his own security and for reasons of national safety, be referred to as "Colonel A" and that his name should not be disclosed to anyone. The magistrates, upon the advice of their clerk, ruled, correctly but with expressed reluctance, that this would not be possible and that although the witness should be referred to as "Colonel A," his name would have to be written down and disclosed to the court and to the defendants and their counsel. The prosecution decided not to call that witness and the proceedings were adjourned.

The hearing was resumed four days later on November 14. The prosecution called, instead of "Colonel A," another witness. Counsel for the prosecution applied for him to be referred to as "Colonel B," and that his name be written down and shown only to the court, the defendants and their counsel. This was said to be necessary for reasons of national safety; risk to "Colonel B's" own security was not relied on. Counsel for the defendants raised no objection to the course proposed; the magistrates assented to it and the witness then gave evidence in open court. He was throughout referred to as "Colonel B"; his real name was never mentioned. For the purposes of the proceedings for contempt of court with which the Divisional Court and now your Lordships have been concerned, it must be taken, although initially there was conflicting evidence as to this, that the magistrates gave no express ruling or direction other than that the witness was to be referred to in court as "Colonel B" and not by his real name and that his real name was to be written down and disclosed only to the court, the defendants and their counsel.

In the course of the cross-examination of "Colonel B" questions were put the effect of which was to elicit from him (1) the official name and number of the army unit to which he belonged and (2) the fact that his posting to it was recorded in a particular issue of "Wire," the magazine of the Royal Corps of Signals which is obtainable by the public. These answers enabled his identity to be discovered by anyone who cared to follow up this simple clue. The line of questioning which elicited this information was pursued without objection from counsel for the prosecution, the witness or the magistrates; and the answers which made his identity so easy to discover were included in the colonel's deposition read out to him in open court before he signed

In the issue of "Peace News" for November 18 these two pieces of information about "Colonel B" elicited in open court were published; and in the issue for December 16, the name of "Colonel B" was disclosed and an account was given of his military career. In the January and March 1978 issues of another magazine, "The Leveller," the name of "Colonel B" was published. Finally, in the issues of the "Journalist" for March and April 1978 published by the National Union of Journalists, "Colonel B" was again identified by name.

All this occurred before the trial of the defendants at the Central Criminal Court began.

On March 22, 1978, the Attorney-General brought in the Divisional Court proceedings for contempt of court against Peace News Ltd. and Leveller Magazine Ltd. and persons responsible for the publication in those periodicals of the articles which published the real name of "Colonel B"; and on April 18, 1978, he brought similar proceedings against the National Union of Journalists in respect of the articles appearing in the "Journalist." In each of these proceedings the statement filed pursuant to R.S.C., Ord. 52, r.2 contained an allegation that at the committal proceedings in the Tottenham Magistrates' Court on November 14, 1978, not only had the magistrates permitted "Colonel B" not to disclose his identity but their chairman had also given an express direction in open court that no attempt should be made to disclose the identity of "Colonel B." Before the three motions, which were heard together, came on for hearing, an affidavit by the clerk to the Tottenham Magistrates' Court was filed, denying that any such explicit direction had been given by the chairman of the magistrates and stating that the reason why such a direction was not given was because he had advised the magistrates that they had no power to do so. In view of this evidence the hearing of the motions proceeded on the basis that no explicit direction had been given to those present at the hearing that no attempt should be made to disclose the identity of "Colonel B"; and that what had happened at the committal proceedings in relation to the witness being referred to only as "Colonel B" was as I have already stated it.

My Lords, it is not disputed that the disclosure of "Colonel B's" identity by the appellants was part of a campaign of protest against the Official Secrets Act. It was designed, no doubt, to ridicule the notion that national safety needed to be protected by suppression of the colonel's name. The only question for your Lordships is whether in doing what they did the appellants were guilty of contempt of court.

The Divisional Court found contempt of court established against all appellants but made orders only against the National Union of Journalists and the two companies. The National Union of Journalists was fined £200, Peace News Ltd. and Leveller Magazine Ltd. were each fined £500. Against these orders these appeals are now brought to this House.

In the judgment of the Divisional Count delivered by Lord Widgery C.J. it is pointed out that contempt of court can take many forms. The publication by the appellants of the witness's identity after the magistrates had ruled that he should be referred to in their court only as "Colonel B" was held by the Divisional Court to fall into a class said to be exemplified in *Attorney-General v. Butterworth*, [1963] 1 Q.B. 696 and *Reg. v. Socialist Worker Printers and Publishers Ltd., Ex parte Attorney-General*, [1975] Q.B. 637 and variously described in the course of the judgment as "a deliberate flouting of the court's authority," "a flounding or deliberate disregard outside the court [of the court's ruling]," a "deliberate intention of frustrating the arrangement which the court had made to preserve Colonel B's anonymity" and finally a "deliberate flouting of the court's intention." I do not think that any of these ways of describing what the appellants did is sufficiently precise to lead inexorably to the conclusion that what they did amounted to contempt of court. Closer analysis is needed.

The only "ruling" that the magistrates had in fact given was that the witness should be referred to *at the hearing in their court* as "Colonel B" and that his name must be written down and shown to the court, the defendants and their counsel but to no one else. That it was also the only ruling that they intended to give is apparent from the fact that they had been advised by their clerk that it was the only ruling that they had power to give, however much they might have preferred to give a wider one. None of the appellants committed any breach of this ruling. What they did, and did deliberately, outside the court and after the conclusion of "Colonel B's" evidence in the committal proceedings, was to take steps to ensure that this anonymity was not preserved.

My Lords, although criminal contempts of court make take a variety of forms they all share a common characteristic: they involve an interference with the due administration of justice either in a particular case or more generally as a continuing process. It is justice itself that is flouted by contempt of court, not the individual court or judge who is attempting to administer it.

Of those contempts that can be committed outside the courtroom the most familiar consist of publishing, in connection with legal proceedings that are pending or imminent, comment or information that has a tendency to pervert the course of justice, either in those proceedings or by deterring other people from having recourse to courts of justice in the future for the vindication of their lawful rights or for the enforcement of the criminal law. In determining whether what is published has such a tendency a distinction must be drawn between reporting what actually occurred at the hearing of the proceedings and publishing other kinds of comment or information; for prima facie the interests of justice are served by its being administered in the full light of publicity.

As a general rule the English system of administering justice does require that it be done in public: *Scott v. Scott*, [1913] A.C. 417. If the way that courts behave cannot be hidden from the public ear and eye this provides a safeguard against judicial arbitrariness or idiosyncrasy and maintains the public confidence in the administration of justice. The application of this principle of open justice has two aspects: as respects proceedings in the court itself it requires that they should be held in open court to which the press and public are admitted and that, in criminal cases at any rate, all evidence communicated to the court is communicated publicly. As respects the publication to a wider public of fair and accurate reports of proceedings that have taken place in court the principle requires that nothing should be done to discourage this.

However, since the purpose of the general rule is to serve the ends of justice it may be necessary to depart from it where the nature or circumstances of the particular proceeding are such that the application of the general rule in its entirety would frustrate or render impracticable the administration of justice or would damage some other public interest for whose protection Parliament has made some statutory derogation from the rule. Apart from statutory exceptions, however, where a court in the exercise of its inherent power to control the conduct of proceedings before it departs in any way from the general rule, the departure is justified to the extent and to no more than the extent that the court reasonably believes it to be necessary in order to serve the ends of justice. A familiar instance of this is provided by the "trial within a trial" as to the admissibility of a confession in a criminal prosecution. The due administration of justice requires that the jury should be unaware of what was the evidence adduced at the "trial within a trial" until after they have reached their verdict; but no greater derogation from the general rule as to the public nature of all proceedings at a criminal trial is justified than is necessary to ensure this. So far as proceedings in the courtroom are concerned the trial within a trial is held in open court in the presence of the press and public but in the absence of the jury. So far as publishing those proceedings outside the court is concerned any report of them which might come to the knowledge of the jury must be withheld until after they have reached their verdict; but it may be published after that. Only premature publication would constitute contempt of court.

In the instant case the only statutory provisions that have any relevance are section 8(4) of the *Official Secrets Act* 1920 and section 12(1)(c) of the *Administration of Justice Act* 1960. Both deal with the giving of evidence before a court sitting in camera. They do not apply to the evidence given by "Colonel B" in the instant case. Their relevance is thus peripheral and I can dispose of them shortly.

Section 8(4) of the Act of 1920 applies to prosecutions under that Act and the *Official Secrets Act* 1911. It empowers but it does not compel a court to sit to hear evidence in private if the Crown applies for this on the ground that national safety would be prejudiced by its publication. Section 12(1) of the Act of 1960 defines and limits the circumstances in which the publication of information relating to proceedings before any court sitting in private is of itself contempt of court. The circumstance defined in section 12(1)(c) is

> "where the court sits in private for reasons of national security during that part of the proceedings about which the information in question is published; . . ."

So to report evidence in camera in a prosecution under the *Official Secrets Act* would be contempt of court.

In the instant case the magistrates would have had power to sit in camera to hear the whole or part of the evidence of "Colonel B" if this had been requested by the prosecution; and although they would not have been bound to accede to such a request it would naturally and properly have carried great weight with them. So would the absence of any such request. Without it the magistrates, in my opinion, would have had no reasonable ground for believing that so drastic a derogation from the general principle of open justice as is involved in hearing evidence in a criminal case in camera was necessary in the interests of the due administration of justice.

In substitution for hearing "Colonel B's" evidence in camera which it could have asked for the prosecution was content to treat a much less drastic derogation from the principle of open justice as adequate to protect the interests of national security. The witness's evidence was to be given in open court in the normal way except that he was to be referred to by the pseudonym of "Colonel B" and evidence as to his real name and address was to be written down and disclosed only to the court, the defendants and their legal representatives.

I do not doubt that, applying their minds to the matter that it was their duty to consider — the interests of the due administration of justice — the magistrates had power to accede to this proposal for the very reason that it would involve less derogation from the general principle of upon justice than would result from the Crown being driven to have recourse to the statutory procedure for hearing evidence in camera under section 8(4) of the *Official Secrets Act* 1920; but in adopting this particular device which on the face of it related only to how proceedings within the courtroom were to be conducted it behaved the magistrates to make it clear what restrictions, if any, were intended by them to be imposed upon publishing outside the courtroom information relating to those proceedings and whether such restrictions were to be precatory only or enforceable by the sanction of proceedings for contempt of court.

My Lords, in the argument before this House little attempt was made to analyse the juristic basis on which a court can make a "ruling," "order" or "direction" — call it what you will — relating to proceedings taking place before it which has the effect in law of restricting what may be done outside the courtroom by members of the public who are not engaged in those proceedings as parties or their legal representatives or as witnesses. The Court of Appeal of New Zealand in *Taylor v. Attorney-General*, [1975] 2 N.Z.L.R. 675 was clearly of opinion that a court had power to make an explicit order directed to and binding on the public ipso jure as to what might lawfully be published outside the courtroom in relation to proceedings held before it. For my part I am prepared to leave this as an open question in the instant case. It may be that a "ruling" by the court as to the conduct of proceedings can have binding effect as such within the courtroom only, so that breach of it is not ipso facto a contempt of court unless it is committed there. Nevertheless where (1) the reason for a ruling which involves departing in some measure from the general principle of open justice within the courtroom is that the departure is necessary in the interests of the due administration of justice and (2) it would be apparent to anyone who was aware of the ruling that the result which the ruling is designed to achieve would be frustrated by a particular kind of act done outside the courtroom, the doing of such an act with knowledge of the ruling and of its purpose may constitute a contempt of court, not because it is a breach of the ruling but because it interferes with the due administration of justice.

So it does not seem to me to matter greatly in the instant case whether or not the magistrates were rightly advised that they had in law no power to give directions which would be binding as such upon members of the public as to what information relating to the proceedings taking place before them might be published outside the courtroom. What was incumbent upon them was to make it clear to anyone present at, or reading an accurate report of, the proceedings what in the interests of the due administration of justice was the result that was intended by them to be achieved by the limited derogation from the principle of open justice within the courtroom which they had authorized, and what kind of information derived from what happened in the courtroom would if it were published frustrate that result.

There may be many cases in which the result intended to be achieved by a ruling by the court as to what is to be done in court is so obvious as to speak for itself; it calls for no explicit statement. Sending the jury out of court during a trial within a trial is an example of this; so may be the common ruling in prosecutions for blackmail that a victim called as a witness be referred to in court by a pseudonym (see *Reg. v. Socialist Worker Printers and Publishers Ltd., Ex parte Attorney-General*, [1975] Q.B. 637); but, in the absence of any explicit statement by the Tottenham magistrates at the conclusion of the colonel's evidence that the purpose of their ruling would be frustrated if anything were published outside the courtroom that would be likely to lead to the identification of "Colonel B" as the person who had given evidence in the case, I do not think that the instant case falls into this class.

The ruling that the witness was to be referred to in court only as "Colonel B" was given before any of his evidence had been heard and at that stage of the proceedings it might be an obvious inference that the effect intended by the magistrates to be achieved by their ruling was to prevent his identity being publicly disclosed. As I have already pointed out however the evidence that he gave in open court in cross-examination did in effect disclose his identity to anyone prepared to take the trouble to consult a particular issue (specified in the evidence) of a magazine that was on sale to the public. This evidence was elicited without any protest from counsel for the prosecution; no application was made that this part of the evidence should be heard in camera; no suggestion, let alone request, was made to members of the press present in court that it should not be reported; and once it was reported the witness's anonymity was blown.

In these circumstances whatever may have been the effect intended to be achieved by the magistrates at the time of their initial ruling, this, as it seems to me, had been abandoned with the acquiescence of counsel for the Crown, by the time that "Colonel B's" evidence was over. I see no grounds on which a person present at or reading a report of the proceedings was bound to infer that to publish that part of the colonel's evidence in open court that disclosed his identity would interfere with the due administration of justice so as to constitute a contempt of court. Indeed the natural inference is to the contrary and it may not be without significance that no proceedings were brought against "Peace News" in respect of the issue of November 18 in which this evidence was published, without actually stating what would be found to be the colonel's name if the particular issue of "Wire" were consulted. But if there was no reason to suppose that publication of this evidence would interfere with the due administration of justice, how could it reasonably be supposed that to take the final step of publishing the name itself made all the difference?

My Lords, I would allow these appeals upon the ground that in the particular and peculiar circumstances of this case the disclosure of "Colonel B's" identity as a witness involved no interference with the due administration of justice and was not a contempt of court.

Editor's note: Contempt of court is unique in Canadian criminal law in that it is nowhere given statutory definition.

3.3.1.2 *Criminal Code*, R.S.C. 1985, c . C-46

9. Notwithstanding anything in this Act or any other Act, no person shall be convicted or discharged under section 736

(*a*) of an offence at common law,

(*b*) of an offence under an Act of the Parliament of England, or of Great Britain, or of the United Kingdom of Great Britain and Ireland, or

(*c*) of an offence under an Act or ordinance in force in any province, territory or place before that province, territory or place became a province of Canada,

but nothing in this section affects the power, jurisdiction or authority that a court, judge, justice or provincial court judge had, immediately before the 1st day of April 1955, to impose punishment for contempt of court.

10. (1) Where a court, judge, justice or magistrate summarily convicts a person for a contempt of court committed in the face of the court and imposes punishment in respect thereof, that person may appeal

(*a*) from the conviction, or

(*b*) against the punishment imposed.

(2) Where a court or judge summarily convicts a person for a contempt of court not committed in the face of the court and punishment is imposed in respect thereof, that person may appeal

(*a*) from the conviction, or

(*b*) against the punishment imposed.

(3) An appeal under this section lies to the court of appeal of the province in which the proceedings take place, and, for the purposes of this section, the provisions of Part XVI apply, *mutatis mutandis.*

3.3.1.3 *R. v. Kopyto* (1988), 24 O.A.C. 81 (Ont. C.A.)

CORY, J.A.: The common law offence of contempt of court is thus preserved by s.8. There are two types of conduct which come within the scope of criminal contempt. Firstly, there is contempt in the face of the court. This type of offence encompasses any word spoken or act done in or in the precinct of the court which obstructs or interferes with the due administration of justice or is calculated to do so. It would include assaults committed in the court, insults to the court made in the presence of the court, interruption of court proceedings, a refusal of a witness to be sworn or, after being sworn. refusal to answer. Secondly, the offence may be committed by acts which are committed outside the court. Contempt not in the face of the court includes words spoken or published or acts done which are intended to interfere or are likely to interfere with the fair administration of justice. Examples of that type of contempt are publications which are intended or are likely to prejudice the fair trial or conduct of a criminal or civil proceeding or publications which scandalize or otherwise lower the authority of the court, and acts which would obstruct persons having duties to discharge in a court of justice.

3.3.2 Scandalising the Court

How much public criticism of judges and the courts is permissible?

3.3.2.1 Robert Martin, "Criticising the Judges," 28 *McGill Law Journal* 1, pp. 13-20

1. Scandalising the Court

Having established a general context, I will turn now to an analysis of a specific aspect or branch of the law of contempt of court — scandalising the court. Scandalising the court is that portion of the criminal law which is brought to bear to punish individuals who say nasty things about courts or judges. This form of contempt is now unknown in England; there has not, it appears, been a successful prosecution for fifty years. It is unfortunately, alive and well in Canada.

The law of contempt generally is supposed to protect against interference with the due administration of justice. Scandalising the court seeks to sanction, in the classic definition, "any act done or writing published calculated to bring a court or a judge of the court into contempt or lower his authority". Such statements may involve either (a) scurrilous abuse of a judge or court, or (b) imputing improper motives to a judge or court. We have on the highest judicial authority that scandalising the court is not intended to prevent criticism of judges or the courts. Thus Lord Atkin stated in *Ambard v. A.-G. Trinidad and Tobago*:

> But whether the authority and position of an individual judge, or the due administration of justice, is concerned, no wrong is committed by any member of the public who exercises the ordinary right of criticising, in good faith, in private or public, the public act done in the seat of justice. The path of criticism is a public way: the wrong headed are permitted to err therein: provided that members of the public abstain from imputing improper motives to those taking part in the administration of justice, and are genuinely exercising a right of criticism, and not acting in malice or attempting to impair the administration of justice, they are immune. Justice is not a cloistered virtue: she must be allowed to suffer the scrutiny and respectful, even though outspoken, comments of ordinary men.

What I propose to do now is to look at the Canadian cases, sort them, more or less, into the two recognised categories of scandalising the court, assess the results of the decisions, and note some technical problems.

a. *Scurrilous Abuse*

It is not easy to define scurrilous abuse. Canadians have been found guilty under this rubric for: describing the judge and jury at a murder trial as being themselves murderers and, to boot, torturers; saying that a judicial decision was "silly" and could not have been made by a sane judge, calling a court a "mockery of justice"; writing of a particular proceeding that "the whole thing stinks from the word go"; accusing a court of "intimidation" and "iron curtain" tactics; and vowing with respect to a particular magistrate, "if that bastard hears the case I will see to it that he is defrocked and debarred". The people who made these statements were: a columnist in a major urban daily newspaper; a federal cabinet minister; the editor of a university student newspaper; a municipal politician; a reporter for an urban daily; and a provincial cabinet minister. On the other hand, a columnist for a large urban daily who described a coroner's inquest as "one of the worst examples of idiocy by public officials that I've ever seen" was acquitted. The cases do not suggest any clear standard for determining what is or is not scurrilous abuse. Courts have convicted on the basis of language which they found "vulgar, abusive, and threatening" or which exceeded the "bounds of temperate and fair criticism" . The New Brunswick Court of Queen's Bench recently advanced the extraordinary assertion that criticism which was "ungentlemanly" was contemptuous. In order to amount to scurrilous abuse it appears that the statement in question must identify a particular judge or court. Beyond that, the crucial factor seems to be the literary taste of the presiding judge. If the judge finds the words used excessive then there will likely be a conviction.

b. *Impuring Improper Motives*

Imputing improper motives is a concept that should be susceptible to more precise definition. What appears to be involved here is an allegation of partiality, bias or prejudice. The cause or origin of the alleged improper motive is irrelevant. The allegation may be directed at the judiciary as a whole, at a particular court or group of judges, at a specific, named judge, or at a jury. Contempts of this nature are viewed with considerable disfavour by the Canadian judiciary. Such statements are seen as undermining the reputation for integrity and fairness upon which, it is claimed, the independence of the judiciary is based. The extreme sensitivity of the judges in such matters is illustrated in *Re Duncan*. Lewis Duncan was a lawyer, a Q.C. in fact, arguing an appeal before the Supreme Court of Canada in 1957. Duncan suspected that one member of the Court was prejudiced against him. It was Duncan's belief that this prejudice originated with a personal incident thirty years earlier and that it had been demonstrated in two previous cases before the Supreme Court of Canada in which he had been involved. There was some dispute as to what Duncan actually said to the court, but the essence was that he did not want Locke J. to be a member of the panel hearing his client's appeal and that he did not believe the administration of justice would be served if Locke J. remained on the panel. Accordingly, he requested that Locke J. withdraw. Kerwin C.J.C., speaking for himself and six other judges (not including Locke J.) had no hesitation in holding that Duncan's remarks were contemptuous. Duncan was ordered to pay a fine of $2,000 or, failing that, to serve sixty days in jail. This fine was one of the largest ever imposed in a Canadian contempt case.

c. *General Considerations*

Some general questions remain to be answered with respect to scandalising the court. First, is truth a defence? This issue is unlikely to use where the statements in question amount to scurrilous abuse, since truth or falsity has little to do with a statement being abusive or not. However, where improper motives on the part of a judge have been suggested, can the accused contemnor seek to prove the truth of such allegations? If I have written that judge X accepts bribes, can I escape punishment by proving that judge X is on the take? The answer is unequivocal *no*. There is no Canadian case directly on point, but all the commentators, having made appropriate disclaimers, agree that truth is not a defence. Secondly, is *mens rea* required? The question should be rephrased since, it will be remembered, the burden of proof is on the accused. Can the accused escape liability by establishing the absence of *mens rea*, that is to say, by showing that the statement in question was not intended to interfere with the due administration of justice? The answer here is clear. It is — *no*.

Finally, what is the range of punishment that is allowed in such cases? The most common punishment is a fine. In 1963, the publisher of *The Division Court Reporter*, a periodical which alleged partiality and corruption on the Division Court bench, was fined $4.000, or about $12,000 in 1982 dollars. This is the largest fine in a reported case. In 1969, the writer of an article in a student newspaper which described the courts as "simply the instruments of the corporate elite" was sentenced to ten days imprisonment without the option of paying a fine. Occasionally, the contemnor may be ordered to apologise to the court. This may be imposed either in conjunction with, or independently of, a fine.

3.3.2.2 *Re Nicol*, [1954] 3 D.L.R. 690 (B.C.S.C.)

CLYNE J.: — Two weeks ago the owners, proprietors and printers of the Vancouver Province, its publisher Mr. A. W. Moscuella, its editor-in-chief Mr. H. H. C. Anderson, and Mr. Eric Nicol appeared before me to answer a charge of contempt of Court and to show cause why they should not be committed for a contempt said to have been contained in an article written by Mr. Nicol which was published by the Province on the 20th of last month.

The contempt charged in this case is of an unusual character. It is not a contempt arising out of the disobedience to the orders of the Court, nor does it arise from interference with the fair trial of a cause which is pending before the Courts. The offence which is alleged consists in the publication, after the conclusion of a trial, of remarks which are said to be derogatory of the Court and calculated to bring the Court and the administration of justice into contempt and disrepute. As contempts of this nature are fortunately rare and as the jurisdiction to punish this type of contempt should be exercised with scrupulous care and only when the case is clear, I reserved the matter for consideration: see *R. v. Gray*, [1900] 2 Q.B. 36. Speaking for myself, I consider that it is a jurisdiction which should be exercised, not in vindication of the character of any individual, nor in retort to any personal affront, but only in the public interest when the Court then becomes bound to exercise it: *R. v. Davison* (1821), 4 B. & Ald. 329, 106 E.R. 958.

The facts are that on Thursday, Much 18th, William Gash was found guilty by a jury of the murder of Frank Pitsch and was sentenced to be hanged on June 22nd next. On Saturday, Much 20th, the Vancouver Province published an article written by Mr. Nicol in which he pictured himself as being tried after death before God for the murder of William Gash, the man convicted of the murder of Pitsch, and pleading guilty to killing him by hanging on June 22, 1954. In the second paragraph of the article he uses these words: "Although I did not myself spring the trap that caused my victim to be strangled in cold blood, I admit that the man who put the rope around his neck was in my employ. Also serving me were the 12 people who planned the murder, and the judge who chose the time and place and caused the victim to suffer the exquisite torture of anticipation." He then proceeds to elaborate his confession and addresses to his Maker a plea for mercy in his own behalf.

Counsel for the newspaper has urged that there was no intention to cast any slur upon the Court but that the article was written to express opposition to capital punishment and in particular to capital punishment by hanging. From the extravagant language used by the writer there can be no doubt that it was written in opposition to capital punishment. It is to be noted, however, that the article goes much further than a discussion of capital punishment and indicates that in the writer's opinion society is responsible for having caused William Gash to commit murder. It continues in this vein:

"And I know that the society to which I belong, and which has killed this man, may have provoked him and may provoke others to the same crime. Hunger, temptation, worldly desires — can I say that I am innocent of all responsibility for these incitements to kill?

"I know that I cannot. In a society where all of us enjoyed what most of us enjoy, no man would kill another. Society is what I, and my accomplices, have made it, and one of the things we have made it is a death-trap for William Gash. No, Your Honour, I never said that William Gash was paying his debt to society. What did he owe to us, that we should drive him to murder, then commit him to the hell of the death chamber?"

The facts of the case of *R. v. Gash* were fully reported in the press. At the time Gash committed the crime with which he was charged he was 19 years of age. He came from what appeared to be a respectable, hard-working family. He married when he was eighteen and has one child. He was not working at the time of the murder. His wife and child had been living with him at his father's home, but had gone to live with her people, his father having apparently been unwilling to continue to support his son and his son's family. There was no apparent reason why Gash should not have obtained work. He was strong and healthy and there was no suggestion at trial that he was not of average intelligence. He had enough skill in wood-working to have taught this subject as a voluntary worker at a recreational centre where he also had some reputation as a good boxer. He had done casual work from time to time but did not appear to be active in his search for employment and was spending his time frequenting a public golf course. There is no doubt that he wanted money, but apparently he was unwilling to work for it. About 6 weeks before the murder he told a friend that he intended to rob an acquaintance by the name of Pitsch who was known to carry a good deal of money upon his person, and several weeks later he communicated his intention to another friend. He invited them to join with him in the enterprise and described the weapon which he intended to use and eventually did use to render his victim unconscious. When asked by one of his friends what he would do if the unfortunate man recognized him, he explained he would have to kill him.

I have mentioned these facts because I conceive that, if the jury's verdict had been perverse, the newspaper would have had a perfect right to criticize it. The time for appeal has now expired and I feel free to comment upon the jury's finding. Under no stretch of imagination could the verdict be said to have been perverse and in fact defence counsel in his address made no attempt to offer a defence in law but confined himself to a plea for compassion, mainly on account of the offender's youth, to which the jury acceded by adding as a rider to its verdict a very strong recommendation for mercy. In these circumstances, and in spite of the fact that in order to obtain money Gash preferred to kill rather than to work, Mr. Nicol states that society had driven him to murder.

It is clear, therefore, that in writing the article Mr. Nicol not only was seeking to express his opposition to capital punishment but he was also presenting an argument against a man's individual responsibility for his acts. There is no doubt that in a great number of cases environment has much to do with causes of crime, but in the present case it does not appear that the accused was lacking in the ordinary advantages which are available to the youth of this country. He was not suffering from hunger as Mr. Nicol's article appears to indicate, nor was the crime committed in the heat of passion nor under the influence of any temptation other than the desire to steal money. The only thing suggested by his counsel in his plea to the jury for compassion was that the accused's father had been unnecessarily harsh to him in refusing to continue to support him with his wife and child. On the evidence it appears that the murder of Pitsch had been coldly premeditated by Gash for some time and robbery appears to have been the only motive for the killing. Under the circumstances it is difficult to understand why any blame should be attached to society for the actions of the accused, or why society should be accused of making "a death trap for William Gash".

Counsel for the Crown argues that in seeking to relieve the accused from any moral responsibility for the crime and in blaming society at large, the writer of the article and the Vancouver Province are attempting to undermine the administration of justice. He argues that the article tends to encourage individuals to do wrong with an easy conscience in the belief that it is the state and not the individual who is ultimately responsible and he suggests that in the case of a number of young people who happen to be familiar with the facts of this particular crime the article is likely to have very deleterious effects.

The philosophy underlying this article is very familiar. It denies the individual's responsibility for his actions and by the same token it denies the individual's freedom of choice and the exercise of free-will. It blames society for the wrongs committed by individuals because it says by reason of social or economic pressures the individual is unable to do otherwise. It affords the individual the means of escaping the moral consequences of any wrongful act by enabling him to say: "Because of the influences which have surrounded me from my birth I have become the sort of person that I am, and I am not responsible for those conditions which have moulded my character." It is the materialistic philosophy of determinism which is very popular in some quarters of the world-to-day and which emphasizes the importance of causes and minimizes the importance of the choice by the individual between good and evil. In its last result it elevates the importance of the state at the expense of the individual and leaves to the state the acceptance of responsibility for both good and evil.

Whatever opinion may be held as to the moral conceptions involved in this article, it is no part of the duty or function of the Court to deal with a question of ethics in an application of this kind. The newspaper is free to express its views upon questions of morality and it is for its readers to decide whether or not they agree with them. It is free to express its views upon the workings of our penal system and it is free to say whether or not it believes that men should be punished for their crimes or whether they should be excused by reason of some external or internal conditioning. Our Courts have been astute to protect the freedom of speech and, from the point of view of contempt proceedings, the morality of the article is irrelevant and it is for those who read to decide for themselves if the philosophy expressed therein is pernicious or not.

Whether or not contempt has been committed in this case must depend upon the construction to be put upon the paragraph in which the reference is made to the jury as being "the twelve people who planned the murder". Counsel for the newspaper has suggested rather faintly that the article should not be read with specific reference to the Gash trial or to the Gash jury. This contention must be definitely rejected. As counsel for the Crown has pointed out, the article consists of eleven paragraphs and in eight of those paragraphs the name of Gash appears. The murder of Pitsch by Gash received considerable publicity in the press and there can be no question that anyone reading the article would most certainly consider that the article had direct reference to the case of William Gash and to the jury who tried him. In pursuing his allegory Mr. Nicol has inextricably involved the facts of this case in the web of his fantasy.

Counsel for the newspaper states that the article was written in the form of an allegory, and, in a somewhat tepid apology printed the day before these proceedings came on for hearing the Vancouver Province stated that the object of the column was to express the opposition of Mr. Nicol to execution by hanging and that in order to dramatize the subject Mr. Nicol mentioned the Gash murder case. The writer of the apology overlooks the fact that the Gash case was "mentioned" in eight paragraphs out of eleven, and that the verb "to mention" hardly does justice to the exaggerated and heavy-handed use which Mr. Nicol made of the case. The tenor of the apology is to the effect that the article should not be construed as a contempt, but if it were capable of such interpretation it was to be regretted. It does not explain why it was necessary for Mr. Nicol, in order to adorn his allegory with a moral, to refer to the jurors as persons planning to commit murder. It does not explain why Mr. Nicol's ingenuity was insufficient to accomplish his ends without branding twelve innocent people as criminals.

It was not necessary for counsel to point out the particular literary form in which the article was written, in view of the fact that whatever type of symbolism a writer chooses to use is irrelevant to the issue in cases of this kind. Allegories have frequently been used as vehicles of criticism or abuse but the point to be decided here is whether the words are in fact abusive and whether they have been unjustifiably applied to the members of the jury while promoting their functions as such.

The word "murderer" is a term of opprobrium and, even when it is used in circumstances where actual killing is not implied, it nevertheless carries a connotation of evil intent. To plan or conspire to commit murder is a criminal act. The use of words imputing a criminal offence is actionable *per se* because they expose to public shame the person against whom they are directed and a newspaper has no greater licence to defame than any ordinary member of the public. The fact that a public issue is involved such as the question of capital punishment does not justify or excuse the application of defamatory words to those discharging public duties. Long ago Sir James Mansfield C.J. held that to call a man a murderer and an assassin was not to be excused merely by the fact that he was a candidate for Parliament: *Harwood v. Astley* (1804), 1 Bos. & P.N.R. 47, 127 E.R. 375, see also *Pankhurst v. Hamilton* (1887), 3 T.L.R. 500. Regardless of the purpose which Mr. Nicol had in mind when he wrote the article, his reference to the members of the Gash jury as being "the twelve persons who planned the murder" amounts in my view to a gratuitous insult. It would have been quite easy for Mr. Nicol to have accomplished his purpose without making remarks of this kind.

I have considered whether it might be sufficient to leave the individual members of the jury to assert whatever rights which they may have against Mr. Nicol and the publishers of the Province in the civil Courts, but I have reached the conclusion, upon the strength of the authorities cited to me by Crown counsel, that the Court cannot permit juries to be accorded this sort of treatment during the course of an Assize. The men and women who serve upon our juries are performing one of the most onerous and important functions in the life of a free society. It is a duty which is far from pleasant, especially in a murder case. It is quite possible that members of the jury sitting upon the Gash case may have held similar views to those of Mr. Nicol in regard to capital punishment. However, it is no part of the jury's duty to decide the punishment which is to be meted out to a convicted person. All the jury is required to do is to reach a decision upon the facts. Each juror is sworn to bring in a true verdict upon the facts, and if the facts are such that the crime is proved beyond reasonable doubt and the members of the jury are unanimous in that opinion then they have no other course upon their oaths but to bring in a verdict of guilty. This is often a most painful duty and the distress in having to find a youth of 19 years of age guilty of murder was apparent upon the faces of some of the jurors who tried the Gash case. However, these men discharge their duty honestly as do other men and women who serve upon juries in Canada and the Court would be derelict in its duty if it did not protect them from the degradation of being referred to as criminals. I have no hesitation in finding that the remarks concerning the jury as published in the Province were insulting and, contemptuous in the sense of that word as used by Lord Russell of Killowen C.J. in, *R. v. Gray*, [1900] 2 Q.B. 36, as approved in *Amhard v. A.-G. Trinidad*, [1936] A.C. 322, and in *Perera v. The King*, [1951] A.C. 482.

There is another aspect of the article which must also be taken into consideration, and that is the effect which it may have upon future juries. The last Assize at Vancouver continued for 3 months and the next Assize is starting in a few weeks. Members of the community serve upon juries at these long Assizes at a good deal of inconvenience to themselves and it would not be surprising if they should express unwillingness to serve if they are to be exposed to undeservedly shameful epithets cast upon them by a newspaper. No doubt members of juries at following Assizes who are called upon to sit in murder cases will have in mind that if they bring in verdicts of guilty they will run the risk of being described as persons who have planned a murder or worse and for that reason this type of newspaper comment must be stopped. It may well be that Mr. Nicol, in his anxiety to assert his own opinions in regard to punishment for crime, hoped that by writing this article he would discourage juries from bringing in verdicts of guilty in capital cases, and it is quite conceivable that the article might have that result. Counsel for the Vancouver Province stated that in his opinion the words of the article would have no effect upon jurors, but he might have come to a different conclusion if he had heard the vigorous protests addressed to me through the Sheriff of the county by members of the jury, at the Assize which has just been finished. There could have been no possible objection to Mr. Nicol raising in his column a strenuous objection to capital punishment and urging that clemency be extended to William Gash, and this he could have done effectively without descending to vilification of the Gash jury. To say that he did not intend to cast any slur upon the Court or jury begs the question, as what must be considered on this phase of the matter is the effect of the article upon the minds of the public and of future juries. From this aspect, the article can be said to obstruct the administration of justice in that it is calculated to interfere with future juries and to deter them from carrying out their duties in reaching true verdicts upon the facts as presented to them. I cannot escape the conclusion that the effect of the writing and publishing of the article is such as "to bring a Court. ... into contempt, or ... to obstruct or interfere with the due course of justice or the lawful process of the Courts": *R. v. Gray*, [1900] 2 Q.B. at p. 40; *Izuora v. The Queen*, [1953] A.C. 327 at p. 334.

It is also necessary for me to deal with the reference to "the judge who chose the time and place and caused the victim to suffer the exquisite torture of anticipation". If these words could be construed in the light of a personal affront. I should pay no attention to them. The test which should be applied is whether or not they discredit the Court as such and bring the administration of justice into disrepute. They clearly have reference to the interval of 3 months between the date of sentence, Much 18th, and the date set for execution, June 22nd, which is mentioned in the opening paragraph of the article. The mischief here is the inference, to one unfamiliar with the processes of the law, that the Judge in fixing the date of execution caused and intended to cause the convicted man "the exquisite torture of anticipation". Few people are aware of the fact that in sentencing a man to death the Court always postpones the date of execution in order to give the convicted man time to appeal to the Court of Appeal, and then, if his appeal is rejected, time to appeal to the Supreme Court of Canada, and then, if both appeals fail, still to leave ample time for an application for clemency to the Governor-General in Council, when the most careful consideration is always given to the circumstances of the case by the Governor-General and his advisers before it is decided whether the death penalty should be exacted or clemency exercised. It is important that the mind of the public should not be affected by any insidious idea that the Judge who presided at the Gash trial exercised his choice of an execution date for the purpose of causing the convicted man additional suffering by having to wait in anticipation of the sentence being carried out. Nothing of course, could be further from the truth. It is discreditable to the administration of justice that any false suggestion should be made to the public that the sentences of the Court involve any idea of torture and the words are contemptuous in that they carry with them an imputation of improper motives on the part of the Judge who imposed the sentence: see *Ambard v. A.-G. Trinidad*, [1936] A.C. at p. 335.

Mr. Nicol and the publishers of the Vancouver Province have every right in the world to express their views on capital punishment, but in denouncing capital punishment they have chosen to include in their denunciation those who are charged with the duty of carrying out the law as it exists. If Mr. Nicol and his employers wish to change the law their broadsides should be directed to Parliament, and they have in their possession a powerful medium for expressing their opinions. But they should not, and must not, seek to inflame public opinion against the Courts, and the article read as whole is undoubtedly inflammatory.

There is no question of freedom of the press involved here. The press can and should criticize a law which it believes to be wrong. The press is at liberty to criticize a judge or a jury if a Judge or jury should act improperly, for, as Lord Atkin said in the *Ambard* case [p. 335], "Justice is not a cloistered virtue". The business of the Courts is transacted in public and it is important that what goes on in the Courts should be reported by the press so that the public should know and should be able to judge whether its system of justice is being administered fairly and properly. No wrong is committed by anyone who criticizes the Courts or a Judge in good faith, but it is of vital importance to the public that the authority and dignity of the Courts should be maintained and that when criticism is offered it should be legitimate. To refer to the jurors in this case as criminals and to describe the Judge as causing exquisite torture is calculated to lower the dignity of the Court and to destroy public confidence in the administration of justice, and a practice of this kind must be stopped and stopped immediately in the public interest. I find the parties guilty of contempt and if it were not for the fact that the Vancouver Province possesses a long and respected background in this community and that an apology, even though inept, has been made, I would impose severe penalties. Taking those factors into consideration, I impose a fine of $250 upon the author of the article and a fine of $2,500 upon the publishers and proprietors of the Vancouver Province and they must pay the costs of these proceedings.

Note: Several members of the jury in the Gash case sued Nicol and his newspaper civilly for libel and were successful. See *MacKay v. Southam Co. Ltd.* (1955), 1 D.L.R. (2d) 1 (B.C.C.A.).

3.3.2.3 *R. v. Kopyto* (1988), 24 O.A.C. 81 (Ont. C.A.)

CORY, J.A.: Harry Kopyto was convicted of contempt of court by scandalizing the court. This appeal is brought from that conviction.

Factual Background

For a number of years the appellant acted as the lawyer for his friend, Mr. Dowson. Mr. Dowson was from 1961 to 1972 the Executive Secretary and subsequently Chairman of the League for Socialist Action. Allegations have been made that the R.C.M.P. had investigated the activities of the League and Mr. Dowson in an improper manner.

The appellant on behalf of Dowson, brought an action for defamation. The alleged defamation was contained in a summary of the R.C.M.P. investigation of the League that was read by the Attorney General in the Legislature. The claim was struck down by the Federal Court of Appeal . . .

The appellant, again on behalf of Dowson, also sought to have criminal charges brought against members of the R.C.M.P. for purportedly forging letters during their investigation of the League. The legal proceedings involving these charges also had a long and unsuccessful history.

On May 11, 1982 the appellant, still acting for Dowson, instituted civil proceedings in the Small Claims Court against members of the R.C.M.P. The allegation was made that the defendants had conspired to injure Dowson and had made injurious false statements about him. This action too gave rise to a number of well-publicized proceedings. Eventually a truncated version of the case came before Judge Zuker. The decision was reserved. On December 12, 1985, carefully considered reasons were delivered by Judge Zuker. He dismissed the plaintiff's claim, in part on the grounds that the action was not brought within the statutorily prescribed limitation period.

Following the release of the reasons a reporter from the Globe and Mail called the appellant seeking his comments on the judgment. The appellant indicated that he would call the reporter back after he had read the reasons. On the next day, December 17, 1985, the appellant called the reporter. He gave a long statement, portions of which were included in an article published in the Globe and Mail on December 18, 1985, and which form the subject matter of the charge against him.

The appellant admitted that the Globe and Mail quoted him correctly. The quotations read as follows:

This decision is a mockery of justice. It stinks to high hell. It says it is okay to break the law and you are immune so long as someone above you said to do it.

Mr. Dowson and I have lost faith in the judicial system to render justice.

We're wondering what is the point of appealing and continuing this charade of the courts in this country which are warped in favour of protecting the police. The courts and the RCMP are sticking so close together you'd think they were put together with Krazy Glue.

The Decision at Trial on the Charge of Contempt of Court

The learned trial judge gave careful, complete and detailed reasons for his conclusion that the appellant was guilty of the offence of contempt of court by scandalizing the court. He observed that there was no doubt about the appellant's sincerity or the bona fides of his desire to correct what the appellant perceived to be a social injustice. He rejected the appellant's contention that the remarks had referred to "systemic bias" and that they had not been intended to malign Judge Zuker. He found the appellant's statements to be "a vitriolic unmitigated attack on the trial judge" and, as well, "a blatant attack on all judges of all courts". The appellant's words, he observed, went far beyond criticism and demonstrated an intention to vilify.

The trial judge also concluded that the offence of scandalizing the court did not constitute an infringement of s.2(b) of the *Canadian Charter of Rights and Freedoms* which guarantees freedom of expression. Furthermore, he determined that even if the offence did constitute an infringement of s.2(b), it was a justifiable limitation under s. 1 of the *Charter*.

. . . . .

The courts play an important role in any democratic society. They are the forum not only for the resolution of disputes between citizens but also for the resolution of disputes between the citizen and the state in all its manifestations. The more complex society becomes the greater is the resultant frustration imposed on citizens by that complexity and the more important becomes the function of the courts. As a result of their importance the courts are bound to be the subject of comment and criticism. Not all will be sweetly reasoned. An unsuccessful litigant may well make comments after the decision is rendered that are not felicitously worded. Some criticism may be well founded, some suggestions for change worth adopting. But the courts are not fragile flowers that will wither in the hot heat of controversy. Rules of evidence, methods of procedure and means of review and appeal exist that go far to establishing a fair and equitable rule of law. The courts have functioned well and effectively in difficult times. They are well-regarded in the community because they merit respect. They need not fear criticism nor need they seek to sustain unnecessary barriers to complaints about their operations or decisions.

. . . . .

In my view, statements of a sincerely held belief on a matter of public interest, even if intemperately worded, so long as they are not obscene or criminally libelous, should, as a general rule, come within the protection afforded by s.2(b) of the *Charter*. It would, I think, be unfortunate if freedom of expression on matters of public interest so vital to a free and democratic society was to be unduly restricted. The constitutional guarantee should be given a broad and liberal interpretation. The comment of the appellant came within the ambit of that protection. This, I believe, must be the conclusion, whether the two step procedure described in *R. v. Oakes* is followed or the approach to s.2(b) set forth in *R. v. Zundel* is adopted.

It remains to be determined whether the offence of contempt by scandalizing the court is a constitutionally permissible limit on the protection afforded the appellant's words.

3. If the Words are "Protected" by s.2(b) of the Charter does the Offence of Contempt by Scandalizing the Court Constitute a Constitutionally Permissible Limit on that Protection?

It is incumbent upon the Crown to establish, on a balance of probabilities, that the limitation on freedom of expression imposed by the offence of scandalizing the court meets the requirement of s. 1 of the *Charter*; That section reads:

> 1. *The Canadian Charter of Rights and Freedoms* guarantees the rights and freedoms set out in it subject only to such reasonable limits prescribed by law as can be demonstrably justified in a free and democratic society.

A s.1 analysis can usefully be divided into three parts: first, is the limit a reasonable limit? Second, is the limit prescribed by law? Third, can the limit be demonstrably justified in a free and democratic society?

. . . . .

It was conceded by counsel for the intervenant and I am satisfied that the first criterion was met in that the objective of protecting the administration of justice was of sufficient importance to warrant overriding a constitutionally protected right or freedom. However, in my view, the second criterion has not been satisfied. Without requiring any proof of the matter the offence *assumes* that the words which are the subject-matter of the charge will bring the court into contempt or lower its authority. This I take to be an unwarranted and questionable assumption, and leads me to conclude that the offence has not been "carefully designed to achieve the objective in question". By undertaking the proceedings the prosecution must be taken as alleging that the words spoken by the accused which were "calculated to bring the administration of justice into disrepute" will in fact have such an effect. If this is not the basis of the charge then the measure adopted is arbitrary, unfair or based upon irrational considerations. If the essence of the charge is, as it must be, that the words spoken do, bring the court into contempt, then it would not be unreasonable to require the prosecution to prove that this is in fact the effect of those words. This requirement is lacking in the offence of scandalizing the court as it is presently known.

It may be helpful in considering this issue to recall that when dealing with contempt cases arising out of statements made pertaining to cases that are pending or under consideration, the courts have always required proof that the statements constituted a serious danger to the administration of justice. That is to say that the Crown must show that such statements put the function of the courts in serious question. In *Attorney General v. Times Newspaper Ltd.*, Lord Denning. M.R., in the Court of Appeal (reversed in the result by the House of Lords) stated:

> I regard it as of the first importance that the law which I have just stated should be maintained in its full integrity. We must not allow 'trial by newspaper' or 'trial by television' or trial by any medium other than the courts of law. But, in so stating the law, I would emphasise that it applies only 'when litigation is pending and is actively in suit before the court'. To which I would add that there must appear to be *'a real and substantial danger of prejudice'* to the trial of the case or to the settlement of it.
>
> (Emphasis added).

This was essentially the test laid down by the European Court later in that same case. That requirement should also be an essential condition of the offence of scandalizing the court, as it would go some distance towards ensuring that the offence "impairs 'as little as possible' the right or freedom in question". In the absence of such a requirement the limitation imposed by the offence cannot meet the proportionality test as it is both arbitrary and irrational, based as it is on the unproved assumption that the comment will lower the authority of the court. I am confident that the public, if not the media, will take into account the source of the comment before deciding that the court should be regarded with contempt or its authority lowered.

Furthermore, there is some question as to what mens rea is required to prove the offence of scandalizing the court. It has been said that the words themselves can constitute the offence. Yet it would seem reasonable to require the Crown to prove that the accused either intended to cause disrepute to the administration of justice or was reckless as to whether that disrepute would follow in spite of the reasonable foreseeability of that result from the words used. Anything less would also seem to be contrary to the proportionality test as it applies too arbitrary a standard.

In light of the conclusion that the offence of scandalizing the court is not a reasonable limitation on freedom of expression it is not necessary to consider whether the offence is prescribed by law as required by s.1 of the *Charter*. If it had been I would have concluded that *R. v. Cohn, supra*, makes it clear that it is.

Conclusion

I am of the view that the offence of contempt by scandalizing the court does not constitute or impose a reasonable limitation upon the guaranteed right of freedom expression provided by s.2(b) of the *Charter*. As the words spoken by the appellant are protected by s.2(b) and the offence of scandalizing the court is not a constitutionally permissible limit on that protection, the conviction must be set aside.

HOULDEN, J.A.: Montgomery J., found that the appellant's statements constituted a vitriolic, unmitigated attack upon Judge Zuker. He also found that they were made with intent to vilify, that they were a blatant attack on all judges of all courts in Canada, and that they implied bias on the part of all judges. Notwithstanding these findings, there is no doubt that what was said by the appellant was an "expression" within the meaning of s.2(b).

In *R. v. Zundel*, we held that freedom of expression is not absolute. In determining the limits of freedom, the court observed that it is necessary to first determine the regulated area; the freedom is then what exists in the unregulated area. The court did not find it necessary to define the limits of the unregulated area where freedom of expression is supreme. It held that the offence created by s. 177 of the *Code* of spreading falsehoods knowingly was the antithesis of seeking truth through free exchange of ideas. In finding that the conduct covered by s. 177 did not fall within the unregulated area, the court said:

> It would appear to have no social or moral value which would merit constitutional protection. Nor would it aid the working of parliamentary democracy or further self-fulfillment. In our opinion an offence falling within the ambit of s. 177 lies within the permissibly regulated area which is not constitutionally protected. It does not come within the residue which comprises freedom of expression guaranteed by s.2(b) of the *Charter*.

The determination of whether statements that may constitute contempt by scandalizing the court fall within the regulated or unregulated area is a difficult one. As the Supreme Court of Canada pointed out in *Retail, Wholesale and Department Store Union, Local 580 et al. v. Dolphin Delivery Ltd.*:

> The principle of freedom of speech and expression has been firmly accepted as a necessary feature of modern democracy.

Before conduct is placed in the regulated area, I believe that a court should be satisfied that it is clearly antithetical to the freedom conferred by s.2(b); the regulated area must, if freedom of expression is to have meaning, be very narrow in scope. Expression of opinion about the conduct of judges or courts after a case has been decided, no matter how vitriolic, scurrilous or vilifying are not, in my judgment, antithetical to the freedom of expression conferred by s.2(b) of the *Charter*, and hence, should not be placed in the regulated area. I am not to be taken as suggesting that "freedom of expression" would preclude a civil action for defamation by the judge, but only that it would preclude proceedings for committal for contempt of court.

. . . . .

The inclusion of contempt by scandalizing the court in the regulated area could lead to orthodoxy, and orthodoxy, in my opinion, is neither essential nor desirable for the proper functioning of our judicial system. Courts and judges should be subject to criticism, no matter how extreme; they will function better as a result of it.

Since the statements made by the appellant are protected by s.2(b) of the *Charter* it is necessary to turn to s. 1 of the *Charter* to see if the law proscribing contempt by scandalizing the court is a reasonable limit demonstrably justifiable in, a free and democratic society. For s. 1 to be applicable, the limit must be "prescribed by law". Ms. Codina argued that the law as to scandalizing the court was too vague and uncertain to be such a limit. With respect, I do not agree. This branch of the law has been clearly defined by both English and Canadian courts. A person would have no difficulty in ascertaining the law and regulating his conduct accordingly. The law of contempt of court by scandalizing the court is, therefore, a limit prescribed by law.

The onus of proving that the law of contempt by scandalizing the court is a reasonable limit under s. 1 is, of course, upon the Crown. This is not a case, however, where evidence is required, the elements of the s. 1 analysis being "obvious or self-evident": *R. v. Oakes*.

The criteria for the application of s. 1 have been clearly defined by Dickson, C.J.C. in *R. v. Oakes*. First, the objective of the prescribed law must relate to concerns which are pressing and substantial and which are of sufficient importance to warrant overriding the constitutionally protected freedom. The objective of this branch of the law is perhaps best summed up in Borrie & Lowe's *Law of Contempt*.

> The necessity for this branch of contempt lies in the idea that without well-regulated laws a civilised community cannot survive. It is therefore thought important to maintain the respect and

dignity of the court and its officers, whose task it is to uphold and enforce the law because without such respect, public faith in the administration of justice would be undermined and the law itself would fall into disrepute.

In my opinion, this objective is of sufficient importance to satisfy the first condition of *R. v. Oakes* for the application of s. 1.

Second, once a sufficiently significant objective has been identified, the party having the onus must show that the means chosen to protect that objective are reasonable and demonstrably justified. This involves a "proportionality test". There are three components of this test: (a) the means adopted must be rationally connected to the objective; (b) the means adopted should go no further than is required to achieve the objective; and (c) there must be a proportionality between the effect of the means adopted and the objective.

It is the second component of the proportionality test which causes me concern in this case. The present law assumes that if any act is done or writing is published calculated to bring the court or a judge of a court into contempt or to lower his authority, then it is necessary to curtail freedom of expression and to penalize the offender. Mr. Doherty submitted that this went a great deal further than was required to achieve the objective of the prescribed law. With respect, I agree with this submission.

Freedom of speech and expression were well recognized rights in Canada prior to the *Charter*. In *Retail Wholesale and Department Store Union, Local 580 v. Dolphin Delivery Ltd.*, McIntyre, J., quoted with approval the following passage from Hogg, *Constitutional Law of Canada* (2nd Ed. 1985):

> Canadian judges have always placed a high value on freedom of expression as an element of parliamentary democracy and have sought to protect it with the limited tools that were at their disposal before the adoption of the *Charter of Rights*.

The freedom guaranteed by s. 2(b) of the *Charter* should not be limited to any greater extent than is absolutely essential. As Lord Morris of Borth-Y-Gest said in *Attorney General v. Times Newspapers Ltd.*:

> But as the purpose and existence of courts of laws is to preserve freedom within the law for all well disposed members of the community, it is manifest that the courts must never impose any limitations on free speech or free discussion or free criticism beyond those which are absolutely necessary.

In my judgment, the restraint imposed by the existing law of contempt by scandalizing the court is not proportionate to the objective sought to be attained.

GOODMAN, J.A.: In my opinion the application of the *Charter* to the common law now places a limitation on freedom of expression and opinion as they relate to the administration of justice from utterances or statements which consist of assertions of facts which are false and are known to be false by the person making the assertion or are recklessly made by such person. It also places such limitation on those freedoms where the utterances consist of an expression of an opinion which is not honestly and sincerely held. That limitation and consequently the offence of contempt is constitutionally valid, however, only where the utterance or statement is found to result in a clear, significant and imminent or present danger to the fair and effective administration of justice. In that case it meets the test of proportionality and becomes a reasonable limitation prescribed by law which can be demonstrably justified in a free and democratic society. The limitation and consequently the offence of contempt will not be constitutionally valid where such utterances are calculated to bring the administration of justice into disrepute even if it is proven that they in fact do unless the clear and present danger test is also met.

I agree with the statement of my brother Houlden that our judiciary and courts are strong enough to withstand criticism after a case has been decided no matter how outrageous or scurrilous that criticism may be. That reflects the present state of affairs having regard to the circumstances which exist in Canada today. It would require an extreme combination of unusual circumstances at the present time to suffice to convince a court that utterances or statements constitute a real, significant and imminent or present danger to the fair and effective administration of justice. The utterances with which the court is concerned in the present case, having regard to all the circumstances, fall far short of meeting the test. Nevertheless, in my opinion, the offence of contempt for utterances and statements made outside of the court remains a constitutionally valid offence subject to strict proof of the fulfillment of the prescribed conditions necessary for the commission thereof.

Note: The Court of Appeal overturned Kopyto's conviction by a majority of three to two. The dissenting judgments have been omitted.

3.3.3 The Sub-Judice Rule

3.3.3.1 Robert Martin, "Contempt of Court: The Effect of the Charter," in ed Philip Anisman and Allen M. Linden *The Media, the Courts and the Charter*, (Toronto: Carswell, 1986), pp. 208-210

The *sub judice* rule seeks to control the publication of information which might affect the outcome of judicial proceedings. It has been said that the *sub judice* rule merely postpones, but does not prevent, the publication of certain information. This distinction would not be accepted by a journalist, since the newsworthiness of information is often a function of its timeliness.

Both the ambit of the *sub judice* rule and the justification for it were enunciated by Lord Reid in *A.G. v. Times Newspapers*:

> The law on this subject is and must be founded entirely on public policy. It is not there to protect the private rights of parties to a litigation or prosecution. It is there to prevent interference with the administration of justice and it should in my judgment be limited to what is reasonably necessary for that purpose. Public policy generally requires a balancing of interests which may conflict. Freedom of speech should not be limited to any greater extent than is necessary but it cannot be allowed where there would be real prejudice to the administration of justice.

As a definition of the rule this is elegant, but not very precise. What information will, if published, cause real prejudice to the administration of justice? The honest answer is that no one really knows for sure. Similarly, at what point does the *sub judice* rule begin to apply and at what point does it cease to? Here again there is uncertainty. After careful analysis, for example, Stuart Robertson can only state that "the closer the publication time of the offensive communications is to the time of the trial, the greater is the risk; of interfering with the legal proceeding".

This vagueness has an unfortunate effect on journalists, an effect which seriously inhibits freedom of expression. Contempt of court is a crime. People, generally, prefer to avoid being convicted of crimes. This natural desire is reinforced when the definition of the crime is vague. And the circumspection thereby induced is further reinforced by the caution of lawyers. The result is stories of which the following is a not unduly exaggerated example:

> Stout balding Mr. John Jones, cashier to a firm of textile converters, was missing yesterday from his home in Cemetery Avenue, Openshaw.
>
> Round the corner on Funeral Street. Mr. Henry Brown said he had not seen his blonde attractive wife Marnie since the weekend.
>
> A director of the firm which employs Mr. Jones said yesterday that the firm's books would have been due for audit next week. Mr. Jones was also the treasurer of the local Working Men's Holiday Fund.
>
> Neighbours described Mrs. Brown as a gay girl. It is understood that she and Mr. Jones were close friends.
>
> At a flat in Southpool, stout balding Mr. Arthur Smith said he had never heard of Mr. Jones of Openshaw. Blonde attractive Mrs. Dolly Smith said she had never been known as Mamie Brown. Early yesterday police were seeking to interview a stout, bald-headed man who they believed could be of assistance to them in their inquiries into a case of fraudulent conversion.
>
> A man accompanied police to Southpool police station. Blows were exchanged in Southpool's High Street after a man ran at high speed along the street. Police ran at high speed along the street after a man.
>
> Later a man was detained. A man will appear in court today.

If we turn to the justification for the rule we realize that we are being asked to accept it as a matter of faith. There is no empirical basis upon which it can be determined that the publication of a particular piece of information does or does not constitute an interference with the administration of justice. The concerns that are usually expressed with respect to pre-trial publicity tend to focus on the effect such publicity may have on the reputations of individuals, in particular the accused in a criminal proceeding, and on questions of good taste. These may both be significant matters, but neither has anything to do with whether there will or will not be a fair trial.

Does pre-trial publicity actually influence anybody? The following statement of Quigley J. in the Alberta Court of Queen's Bench is interesting. He was replying to the argument advanced by counsel for James Keegstra that the publicity surrounding the case had been such that it might be impossible to find a panel of impartial jurors.

You know, I don't buy that argument. I don't buy the argument that people in high places or the newspapers or television necessarily have the influence that you're ready to give them. As a matter of fact, you know, there's another school of thought that they used to teach us when I was younger, that you — you only believed about 10 percent of what you read but, you know, I don't think the general public in the populace of Alberta are such that they're led by the nose by any particular politician or any person in so-called high places or led by people in low places, or that those with less education, more education, lack the ordinary good will that most people have. So, you know, to assume that that is a conclusion, is not one that this Court would — would take. I've been sitting in these courts now for 27 years. So I've seen juries act and I've seen many things happen that shores up the fact that I'm not so quick to draw the conclusion that because people in high places say something, or [a] newspaper writes an editorial for or against something, that ordinary people don't just use that as one factor when they come to a conclusion of how they're going to view a certain matter.

Or take the view which Monnin C.J.M. expressed recently with respect to a highly publicized murder trial.

The mere fact that a previous trial, ending in no verdict, has been reported at length in the media should not ordinarily provide a case of probable bias or prejudice on the part of the jurors at the second trial for the same offence. It is most unfair to prospective jurors and contrary to the jury system to assume that since these prospective jurors may have some prior knowledge of the Case by virtue of the media they are probably biased or prejudiced.

If these judges are right and in the absence of any evidence to the contrary, I am inclined to believe they are, much of the justification for the *sub judice* rule falls away. But the matter becomes even stranger when we consider the application of the rule to proceedings before appellate courts. It is clear that the rule does not apply to appellate proceedings with equal rigour. The reason for this is straightforward. Many trials take place before juries. Juries are composed of ordinary human beings who are, presumably, susceptible to being swayed by what they read or hear or see in the media. But there are no juries in appellate courts, only judges, and judges can be relied upon to be sufficiently detached not to be caught up in media-inflamed public passions. I raise the point here to draw attention to the judicial presumptuousness which underlies much of the law of contempt of court.

Finally, one should note that certain aspects of the *sub judice* rule have been codified. Thus, we find in the Criminal Code, for example, prohibitions on reporting certain information with respect to preliminary inquiries, bail hearings, sexual offence proceedings and so on. These statutory prohibitions have the virtue of being reasonably clear and precise.

3.3.3.2 Statutory Sub-Judice

3.3.3.2.1 Sexual Offence

3.3.3.2.1.1 *Criminal Code*, R.S.C. 1985, c . C-46

166. (1) A proprietor, editor, master printer or publisher commits an offence who prints or publishes (*a*) in relation to any judicial proceedings any indecent maker or indecent medical, surgical or physiological details, being maker or details that, if published, are calculated to injure public morals;

(*b*) in relation to any judicial proceedings for dissolution of marriage, nullity of marriage, judicial separation or restitution of conjugal rights, any particulars other than

(i) the names, addresses and occupations of the parties and witnesses,

(ii) a concise statement of the charges, defences and countercharges in support of which evidence has been given,

(iii) submissions on a point of law arising in the course of the proceedings, and the decision of the court in connection therewith, and

(iv) the summing up of the judge, the finding of the jury and the judgment of the court and the observations that are made by the judge in giving judgment.

(2) Nothing in paragraph (1)(b) affects the operation of paragraph (1)(a).

(3) No proceedings for an offence under this section shall be commenced without the consent of the Attorney General.

(4) This section does not apply to a person who

(*a*) prints or publishes any matter for use in connection with any judicial proceedings or communicates it to persons who are concerned in the proceedings,

(*b*) prints or publishes a notice or report pursuant to directions of a court, or

(*c*) prints or publishes any matter

(i) in a volume or part of a genuine series of law reports that does not form part of any other publication and consists solely of reports of proceedings in courts of law, or

(ii) in a publication of a technical character that is *bona fide* intended for circulation among members of the legal or medical professions.

. . . . .

271. (1) Every one who commits a sexual assault is guilty of

(*a*) an indictable offence and is liable to imprisonment for ten years; or

(*b*) an offence punishable on summary conviction.

272. Every one who, in committing a sexual assault,

(*a*) carries, uses or threatens to use a weapon or an innitation thereof,

(*b*) threatens to cause bodily harm to a person other than the complainant,

(*c*) causes bodily harm to the complainant, or

(*d*) is a party to the offence with any other person,

is guilty of an indictable offence and is liable to imprisonment for fourteen years.

273. (1) Every one commits an aggravated sexual assault who, in committing a sexual assault, wounds, maims, disfigures or endangers the life of the complainant.

(2) Every one who commits an aggravated sexual assault is guilty of an indictable offence and is liable to imprisonment for life.

276. (1) In proceedings in respect of an offence under section 151, 152, 153, 155, or 159, subsection 160(2) or (3) or section 170, 171, 172, 173, 271, 272 or 273, evidence that the complainant has engaged in sexual activity, whether with the accused or with any other person, is not admissible to support an inference that, by reason of the sexual activity, the complainant

(a) is more likely to have consented to the sexual activity that forms the subject-matter of the charge; or

(b) is less worthy of belief.

(2) In proceedings in respect of an offence referred to in subsection (1), no evidence shall be adduced by or on behalf of the accused that the complainant has engaged in sexual activity other than the sexual activity that forms the subject-matter of the charge, whether with the accused or with any other person, unless the judge, provincial court judge or justice determines, in accordance with the procedures set out in sections 276.1 and 276.2, that the evidence

(a) is of specific instances of sexual activity;

(b) is relevant to an issue at trial; and

(c) has significant probative value that is not substantially outweighed by the danger of prejudice to the proper administration of justice.

(3) In determining whether evidence is admissible under subsection (2), the judge, provincial court judge or justice shall take into account

(a) the interests of justice, including the right of the accused to make a full answer and defence;

(b) society's interest in encouraging the reporting of sexual assault offences;

(c) whether there is a reasonable prospect that the evidence will assist in arriving at a just determination in the case;

(d) the need to remove from the fact-finding process any discriminatory belief or bias;

(e) the risk that the evidence may unduly arouse sentiments of prejudice, sympathy or hostility in the jury;

(f) the potential prejudice to the complainant's personal dignity and right of privacy;

(g) the right of the complainant and of every individual to personal security and to the full protection and benefit of the law; and

(h) any other factor that the judge, provincial court judge or justice considers relevant.

276.1 (1) Application may be made to the judge, provincial court judge or justice by or on behalf of the accused for a hearing under section 276.2 to determine whether evidence is admissible under subsection 276(2).

(2) An application referred, to in subsection (1) must be made in writing: and set out

(a) detailed particulars of the evidence that the accused seeks to adduce,

(b) the relevance of that evidence to an issue at trial, and a copy of the application must be given to the prosecutor and to the clerk of the court.

(3) The judge, provincial court judge or justice shall consider the application with the jury and the public excluded.

(4) Where the judge, provincial court judge or justice is satisfied

(a) that the application was made in accordance with subsection (2),

(b) that a copy of the application was given to the prosecutor and to the clerk of the court at least seven days previously, or such shorter interval as the judge, provincial court judge, or justice may allow where the interests of justice so require, and

(c) that the evidence sought to be adduced is capable of being admissible under subsection 276(2).

the judge, provincial court judge or justice shall grant the application and hold a hearing under section 276.2 to determine whether the evidence is admissible under subsection 276(2).

276.2 (1) At a hearing to determine whether evidence is admissible under subsection 276(2), the jury and the public shall be excluded.

(2) The complainant is not a compellable witness at the hearing.

(3) At the conclusion of the hearing, the judge, provincial court judge or justice shall determine whether the evidence, or any part thereof, is admissible under subsection 276(2) and shall provide reasons for that determination, and

(a) where not all of the evidence is to be admitted, the reasons must state the part of the evidence that is to be admitted;

(b) the reasons must state the factors referred to in subsection 276(3) that affected the determination, and

(c) where all or any part of the evidence is to be admitted, the reasons must state the manner in which that evidence is expected to be relevant to an issue at trial.

(4) The reasons provided under subsection (3) shall be entered in the record of the proceedings or, where the proceedings are not recorded, shall be provided in writing.

276.3 (1) No person shall publish in a newspaper, as defined in section 297, or in a broadcast, any of the following:

(a) the contents of an application made under section 276.1;

(b) any evidence taken, the information given and the representations made at an application under section 276.1 or at a hearing under section 276.2;

(c) the decision of a judge, provincial court judge or justice under subsection 276.1(4), unless the judge, provincial court judge or justice, after taking into account the complainant's right of privacy and the interests of justice, orders that the decision may be published; and

(d) the determination made and the reasons provided under section 276.2 unless

(i) that determination is that evidence is admissible, or

(ii) the judge, provincial court judge or justice, after taking into account the complainant's right of privacy and the interests of justice, orders that the determination and reasons may be published.

(2) Every person who contravenes subsection (1) is guilty of an offence punishable on summary conviction.

276.4 Where evidence is admitted at trial pursuant to a determination made under section 276.2, the judge shall instruct the jury as to the uses that the jury may and may not make of that evidence.

. . . . .

486. (1) Any proceedings against an accused shall be held in open court, but where the presiding judge, provincial court judge or justice, as the case may be, is of the opinion that it is in the interest of public morals, the maintenance of order or the proper administration of justice to exclude all or any members of the public from the court room for all or part of the proceedings, he may so order.

(2) Where an accused is charged with an offence mentioned in section 274 and the prosecutor or the accused makes an application for an order under subsection (1), the presiding judge, Provincial Court judge or justice, as the case may be, shall, if no such order is made, state, by reference to the circumstances of the case, the reason for not making an order.

(3) Where an accused is charged with an offence mentioned in section 274, the presiding judge, Provincial Court judge or justice may, or if application is made by the complainant or prosecutor, shall, make an order directing that the identity of the complainant and any information that could disclose the identity of the complainant shall not be published in any newspaper or broadcast.

3.3.3.2.1.2 *R. v. Canadian Newspapers Company Limited and Interveners*, [1988] 2 S.C.R. 122 (S.C.C.)

Dickson, C.J.C. stated the following constitutional questions:

1. Does section 442(3) [now 486(3)] of the *Criminal Code*, R.S.C. 1970, c. C-34, infringe or deny:

   (a) the freedom of the press guaranteed in s. 2(b) of the *Canadian Charter of Rights and Freedoms?* or
   (b) the right so be presumed innocent until proven guilty according to law in a fair and public hearing guaranteed in s. 11(d) of the *Canadian Charter of Rights and Freedoms*; and if so,

2. Is section 442(3) [Now 486(3)] of the *Criminal Code*, R.S.C. 1970, c. C-34, justified on the basis of s. 1 of the *Canadian Charter of Rights and Freedoms?*

Both courts below held that s. 442(3) infringes the freedom of the press guaranteed by s. 2(b) of the Charter. In this Court, appellant conceded that point. Freedom of the press is indeed an important and essential attribute of a free and democratic society, and measures which prohibit the media from publishing information deemed of interest obviously restrict that freedom. Therefore, the main issue before us is whether the impugned provision can be salvaged under s. 1 of the *Charter*, which states:

1. The *Canadian Charter of Rights and Freedoms* guarantees the rights and freedoms set out in it subject only to such reasonable limits prescribed by law as can be demonstrably justified in a free and democratic society.

The test to be applied has been set out in *R. v. Oakes*, [1986] 1 S.C.R. 103, and restated in *R. v. Edwards Books and Art Ltd.*, [1986] 2 S.C.R. 713. In order to justify a limitation of a *Charter* right in a free and democratic society, two requirements must be met. The first one is related to the importance of the legislative objective which the limitation is designed to achieve. In the present case, the impugned provision purports to foster complaints by victims of sexual assault by protecting them from the trauma of wide-spread publication resulting in embarrassment and humiliation. Encouraging victims to come forward and complain facilitates the prosecution and conviction of those guilty of sexual offenses. Ultimately, the overall objective of the publication ban imposed by s. 442(3) is to favour the suppression of crime and to improve the administration of justice. This objective undoubtedly bears on a "pressing and substantial concern" and respondent conceded that it is of sufficient importance to warrant overriding a constitutional right. The first requirement under s. 1 is thus satisfied and we must now turn to the second part of the *Oakes* test.

To determine whether the means chosen in furtherance of the recognized objective are reasonable and demonstrably justified, a proportionality test balancing the various interests involved must be applied. The proportionality requirement has three aspects: the existence of a rational link between the means and the objective, a minimal impairment on the right or freedom asserted and a proper balance between the effects of the limiting measures and the legislative objective. As to the first aspect, respondent conceded that there is a rational connection between s. 442(3) and the objective it is designed to serve, and I agree.

Respondent contended that s. 442(3) cannot be justified because a mandatory ban on publication is not a measure that impairs freedom of the press as little as possible. It submitted that only a provision which gives to the trial judge a discretion to determine if publication is appropriate in the circumstances of the case would satisfy the second criterion of the proportionality test. Respondent also argued that appellant had failed to adduce any evidence demonstrating that a mandatory ban impairs the right as little as possible. The Court of Appeal agreed, but this was predicated upon the fact that the only evidence brought forward by the Attorney General of Canada was the testimony of Doreen Carlo Boucher, the co-ordinator of a rape crisis center. The Court further held that this witness had testified that she was aware of some instances where a rape was imagined and the alleged victim wanted to humiliate a person. With respect, the Court of Appeal, probably as a result of an oversight, failed to consider other material that was before the Court. Indeed, contrary to what Howland C.J.O. wrote, Carole Boucher's testimony was not the only evidence adduced before the trial judge, as the Attorney General also tendered in evidence various studies and reports on sexual assaults and other criminal offences. Moreover, with respect, the Court of Appeal misread what Carole Boucher said. While acknowledging that there may be cases whereby the person charged with the offence is falsely accused, the witness never stated that these false allegations were intended to humiliate the accused. During cross-examination, Carole Boucher answered:

Q. So it is quite conceivable that there are cases whereby the real victim is the person accused by the alleged victim.
A. Yes, I could say yes to that.
Q. Therefore you have been exposed to cases where an alleged victim wanted to humiliate a person —

A. — Well *I don't know whether the intention was to humiliate the person*, but the proportion that we have had is very small in proportion to the actual rapes.
Q. Oh I agree.
A. But there has been a small percentage, not only here but in other centres. [Emphasis added.]

When considering all of the evidence adduced by appellant, it appears that, of the most serious crimes, sexual assault is one of the most unreported. The main reasons stated by those who do not report this offence are fear of treatment by police or prosecutors, fear of trial procedures and fear of publicity or embarrassment. Section 442(3) is one of the measures adopted by Parliament to remedy this situation, the rationale being that a victim who fears publicity is assured, when deciding whether to report the crime or not, that the judge must prohibit upon request the publication of the complainant's identity or any information that could disclose it. Obviously, since fear of publication is one of the factors that influences the reporting of sexual assault, certainty with respect to non-publication *at the time of deciding whether to report* plays a vital role in that decision. Therefore, a discretionary provision under which the judge retains the power to decide whether to grant or refuse the ban on publication would be counterproductive, since it would deprive the victim of that certainty. Assuming that there would be a lesser impairment of freedom of the press if the impugned provision were limited to a discretionary power, it is clear, in my view, that such a measure would not, however, achieve Parliament's objective, but rather defeats it.

With respect, there seems to be a certain inconsistency in respondent's position. While it concedes the importance of the objective and the existence of a rational link between that objective and s. 442(3), respondent argues that the judge should retain a discretion. It is difficult to reconcile these submissions, because once these concessions are made, one is forced to admit that an absolute ban on publication is the only means to reach the desired objective. Respondent goes even further by contending that a case-by-case approach should be adopted to ensure that publication will not be banned, except where the social values competing with freedom of the press are of superordinate importance. If we were to adopt this submission, the legislative objective embodied in s. 442(3) would never be met, because publication would be the rule and a sexual assault victim could rarely predict whether the circumstances of the case would be viewed as an exception warranting a non-publication order. As a result, while it might impair less the freedom of the press, the discretionary ban is not an option as it is not effective in attaining Parliament's pressing goal.

While freedom of the press is nonetheless an important value in our democratic society which should not be hampered lightly, it must be recognized that the limits imposed by s. 442(3) on the media's rights are minimal. The section applies only to sexual offence cases, it restricts publication of facts disclosing the complainant's identity and it does not provide for a general ban but is limited to instances where the complainant or prosecutor requests the order or the court considers it necessary. Nothing prevents the media from being present at the hearing and reporting the facts of the case and the conduct of the trial. Only information likely to reveal the complainant's identity is concealed from the public. Therefore, it cannot be said that the effects of s. 442(3) are such an infringement on the media's rights that the legislative objective is outweighed by the abridgement of freedom of the press.

Respondent further argued that s. 442(3) has a potential chilling effect on the media because in any given case it is difficult to ascertain what evidence could disclose the identity of the complainant. There is thus a risk that the press will choose not to publish any meaningful report on some trials. In my view, it is sufficient to say that media people are certainly competent enough to determine which information is subject to the ban; if not, the judge in his or her order can clarify the matters which cannot be published.

3.3.3.2.2 Young Offenders

3.3.3.2.2.1 *Young Offenders Act,* R.S.C. 1985, c. Y-1

16. (1) At any time after an information is laid against a young person alleged to have, after attaining the age of fourteen years, committed an indictable offence referred to in section 553 of the *Criminal Code* but prior to adjudication, a youth court may, on application of the young person or his counsel, or the Attorney General or his agent, after affording both parties and the parents of the young person an opportunity to be heard, if the court is of the opinion that, in the interest of society and having regard to the needs of the young person, the young person should be proceeded against in ordinary court, order that the young person be so proceeded against in accordance with the law ordinarily applicable to an adult charged with the offence.

17. (1) Where a youth court hears an application for a transfer to ordinary court under section 16, it shall

(*a*) where the young person is not represented by counsel, or

(*b*) an application made by or on behalf of the young person or the prosecutor, where the young person is represented by counsel,

make an order directing that any information respecting the offence presented at the hearing shall not be published in any newspaper or broadcast before such time as,

(*c*) an order for a transfer is refused or set aside on review and the time for all reviews against the decision has expired or all proceedings in respect of any such review have been completed; or

(*d*) the trial is ended, if the case is transferred to ordinary court.

(2) Every one who fails to comply with an order made pursuant to subsection (1) is guilty of an offence punishable on summary conviction.

(3) In this section, "newspaper" has the meaning set out in section 297 of the *Criminal Code.*

Protection of Privacy of Young Persons

38. (1) Subject to this section, no person shall publish by any means any report,
- (*a*) of an offence committed or alleged to have been committed by a young person unless an order has been made under s. 16 with respect thereto, or
- (*b*) of a hearing, adjudication, disposition or appeal concerning a young person who committed or is alleged to have committed an offence

in which the name of the young person, a child or a young person who is a victim of the offence or a child or a young person who appeared as a witness in connection with the offence, or in which any information serving to identify such person or child, is disclosed.

(1.1) Subsection (1) does not apply in respect of the disclosure of information in the course of the administration of justice where it is not the purpose of the disclosure to make the information known in the community.

(1.2) A youth court judge shall, on the ex parte application of a peace officer, make an order permitting any person to publish a report described in subsection (1) that contains the name of a young person, or information serving to identify a young person, who has committed or is alleged to have committed an indictable offence, if the judge is satisfied that
- (*a*) there is reason to believe that the young person is dangerous to others; and
- (*b*) publication of the report is necessary to assist in apprehending the young person.

(1.3) An order made under subsection (1.2) shall cease to have effect two days after it is made.

(1.4) The youth court may, on the application of any person referred to in subsection (1), make an order permitting any person to publish a report in which the name of that person, or information serving to identify that person, would be disclosed, if the court is satisfied that the publication of the report would not be contrary to the best interests of that person.

(2) Every one who contravenes subsection (1)(a) is guilty of an indictable offence and is liable to imprisonment for not more than two years; or
- (*b*) is guilty of an offence punishable on summary conviction.

(3) Where an accused is charged with an offence under paragraph (2)(a), a provincial court judge has absolute jurisdiction to try the case and his jurisdiction does not depend on the consent of the accused.

39. (1) Subject to subsection (2), where a court or justice before whom proceedings are carried out under this Act is of the opinion
- (*a*) that any evidence or information presented to the court or justice would be seriously injurious or seriously prejudicial to
    - (i) the young person who is being dealt with in the proceedings,
    - (ii) a child or young person who is a witness in the proceedings,
    - (iii) a child or young person who is aggrieved by or the victim of the offence charged in the proceedings, or
- (*b*) that it would be in the interest of public morals, the maintenance of order or the proper administration of justice to exclude any or all members of the public from the court room, the court or justice may exclude any person from all or part of the

proceedings if the court or justice deems that person's presence to be unnecessary to the conduct of the proceedings.

(2) Subject to section 650 of the *Criminal Code* and except where it is necessary for the purposes of subsection 13(6) of this Act, a court or justice may not, pursuant to subsection (1), exclude from proceedings under this Act
> (*a*) the prosecutor;
> (*b*) the young person who is being dealt with in the proceedings, his parent, his counsel or any adult assisting him pursuant to subsection 11(7);
> (*c*) the provincial director or his agent; or
> (*d*) the youth worker to whom the young person's case has been assigned.

(3) The youth court, after it has found a young person guilty of an offence, or the youth court or the review board, during a review of a disposition under sections 28 to 32, may, in its discretion, exclude from the court or from a hearing of the review board, as the case may be, any person other than
> (*a*) the young person or his counsel,
> (*b*) the provincial director or his agent,
> (*c*) the youth worker to whom the young person's case has been assigned, and
> (*d*) the Attorney General or his agent, when any information is being presented to the court or the review board the knowledge of which might, in the opinion of the court or review board, be seriously injurious or seriously prejudicial to the young person.

(4) The exception set out in paragraph (3)(a) is subject to subsection 13(6) of this Act and section 577 of the *Criminal Code*.

3.3.3.2.2.2 *Southam v. R.* (1934), 42 C.R. (3d) 336, at 354-360 (Ont. H.C.)

HOLLAND, J.:

Reasonable Limit

Counsel for the applicant placed great emphasis on the fact that the expert witnesses agreed that the absolute ban provided for in s.38(1) was not "necessary", and he argued that the limit could therefore not be considered "reasonable and demonstrably justifiable". Counsel for the Attorney General of Canada countered this by arguing that he did not have to prove that the legislation was necessary or perfect or even the best answer to the problem. He said he only had to prove that the legislation has a "rational basis" and is "in furtherance of a reasonable state object", and relied on the following cases:

In *Re Southam Inc., supra*, MacKinnon A.C.J.O. said at p. 424:

We are left, at present, to a certain extent wandering in unexplored terrain in which we have to set up our own guideposts in interpreting the meaning and effect of the words of s. 1 of the Charter. In determining the reasonableness of the limit in each particular case, the court must examine objectively its argued rational basis in light of what the court understands to be reasonable in a free and democratic society.

In *R. v. T.R.* (1984), 10 C.C.C. (3d) 481, 7 D.L.R. (4th) 205, 52 A.R. 149 at 156 (Q.B.):

"Section 12(3) [of the Juvenile Delinquents Act], to a moderate extent, is inconsistent with s.2(b) of the *Charter*. But in my view the limit upon freedom of the press which is imposed by s.12(3) is a reasonable one and is demonstrably justified in a free and democratic society. This is one of those cases in which, without any evidence or very much in the way of information as to what is done in other free and democratic societies, the court can conclude as a matter of reasoning that such a limit is 'reasonable' in the sense that it is in furtherance of a reasonable state object (already referred to) and that it is demonstrably justified."

In *Nat. Citizens' Coalition Inc. — Coalition Nat. des Citoyens Inc. v. A.G. Can.*, [1984] 5 W.W.R. 436 at 449-50, 32 Alta. L.R. (2d) 249 (Q.B.), Medhurst J., speaking for the court, said:

"McDonald J. considered the meaning of reasonable limit in *Reich [Reich v. Alta. College of Physicians & Surgeons* (1984), 31 Alta. L.R. (2d) 205 (Q.B.)] and concluded after a review of the relevant authorities that it meant having a rational basis. At p. 18 he said:

" 'In my opinion, the words "reasonable limits" as used in s. 1 mean "capable of being supported as a rational means of achieving a rational objective".' "

In *R. v. D.*, Ont. H.C., 12th June 1984 (not yet reported), Osborne J. put it in the following way:

"There is, however, one somewhat dominant, analytical common denominator emerging from those cases. In *Global [Re Global Communications Ltd. and A.G. Can.* (1984), 44 O.R. (2d) 609, 38 C.R. (3d) 209 (sub nom. *Re Smith; Global Communications Ltd. v. California*), 10 C.C.C. (3d) 97, 5 D.L.R. (4th) 634, 2 O.A.C. 21 (C.A.)], Thorson J.A. put it this way at p. 614:

> " 'I think the time has come when the issue ought to be decided from the broader perspective of the presumed policy object of the legislation here in question, standing back if need be from what the cases have said on the subject.'
>
> "McKinnon A.C.J.O. said in *Southam* [supra] at p. 134:
>
> " 'The net which s.12(1) casts is too wide for the purpose which it serves. Society loses more than it protects by the all-embracing nature of the section.'

"It is quite apparent that in both *Global* and *Southam* emphasis was placed upon the policy objectives of the legislation alleged to infringe the Charter right in issue."

A consideration of whether a limit on a guaranteed freedom is reasonable involves a balancing of the competing interests, so that what is lost by the limitation can be compared with what is gained by the legislation.

As the Court of Appeal said in *Rauca*, supra, at p. 241:

"In approaching the question objectively, it is recognized that the listed rights and freedoms are never absolute and that there are always qualifications and limitations to allow for the protection of other competing interests in a democratic society. A readily demonstrable example of this is 'freedom of speech' which is limited or qualified by the laws of defamation, obscenity, sedition, etc. Lord Reid pointed out in *Attorney-General v. Times Newspapers Ltd.*, [1974] A.C. 273 at p. 294:

> " 'Public policy generally requires a balancing of interests which may conflict. Freedom of speech should not be limited to any greater extent than is necessary but it cannot be allowed where there would be real prejudice to the administration of justice.' "

The freedom at issue here is the freedom of expression, including freedom of the press. In the context of s.38(1) this involves the freedom to publish, and in the context of s.39(1)(a) it involves access to the courts. To be balanced against the value of that freedom is the value to society and to involved youths of protecting young people involved in youth court proceedings from the damaging effects of publicity.

Freedom of the Press

In *Gay Alliance Toward Equality v. Vancouver Sun; B.C. Human Rights Comm. v. Vancouver Sun*, [1979] 2 S.C.R. 435, [1979] 4 W.W.R. 118, 10 B.C.L.R. 257, 97 D.L.R. (3d) 577, Dickson J. in dissent enunciated the following definition of "freedom of the press" at p. 598 [quoting from the British Royal Commission on the Press, Final Report (1977), p. 9]:

"We define freedom of the press as that degree of freedom from restraint which is essential to enable proprietors, editors and journalists to advance the public interest by publishing the facts and opinions without which a democratic electorate cannot make responsible judgments."

The value of access to the courts has been held by the Supreme Court of Canada to be so important to society that its curtailment "can only be justified where there is present the need to protect social values of *superordinate importance*": *MacIntyre v. A.G. N.S.*, [1982] 1 S.C.R. 175, 26 C.R. (3d) 193 at 213, 65 C.C.C. (2d) 129, 132 D.L.R. (3d) 385, 49 N.S.R. (2d) 609, 96 A.P.R. 609, 40 N.R. 181.

In *Re Southam Inc. and R.*, *supra*, MacKinnon A.C.J.O. for the Ontario Court of Appeal said the following about free access to the courts at p. 418:

> ... in my view, such access, having regard to its historic origin and necessary purpose already recited at length, is an integral and implicit part of the guarantee given to everyone of freedom of opinion and expression which, in terms, includes freedom of the press. However the rule may have had its origin, as Mr. Justice Dickson pointed out, the 'openess' rule fosters the necessary public confidence in the integrity of the court system and an understanding of the administration of justice.

The aim of s.38(1) and s.39(1)(a) is the protection of young people from harmful effects which publicity may have on them. A corollary to this is the protection of society, since, on the evidence of the experts, most young offenders are one-time offenders only and the less harm on them from their experience with the criminal justice system the less likely they are to commit further criminal acts. Thus it can be said that the legislation is also aimed at rehabilitation of the young person.

The declaration of principles in s.3 of the YOA helps in ascertaining the aim of the legislation and points to the importance of special treatment for young people. While I have previously set these out, it is well worth mentioning them again. Section 3(1)(a) declares that young persons must bear responsibility for their actions, although they should not in all circumstances be held accountable or suffer the same consequences for their behaviour as adults, and s.3(1)(b) recognizes that society must be afforded protection from illegal behaviour. Section 3(1)(c) is particularly important:

"(c) young persons who commit offences require supervision, discipline and control, but, because of their state of dependency and level of development and maturity, they also have special needs and require guidance and assistance."

This was essentially the thrust of the evidence from the expert witnesses, with the obvious result that children should be treated differently from adults and that the criminal justice system should, in some ways, operate differently for children than for adults. Where there is good reason for a young person to be tried in adult court, the trial may be transferred under s.16 of the YOA.

The introduction to the YOA, 1982 — Highlights booklet describes the YOA [at p. 1] as "one of the most significant pieces of social policy legislation to have been passed in recent years". While this may well be indisputable, the good to be gained by having the legislation in place must be weighed against the loss to the press in particular and society in general from the limited denial of a freedom. In examining this question, it is necessary to look at s.38(1) and s.39(1)(a) separately.

Section 38(1)

Section 38(1) of the YOA is absolute and, in the words of MacKinnon A.C.J.O. in *Re Southam Inc. and R., supra* [p. 421]: "We are accordingly left in the unhappy position of it being all or nothing. " In *Re Southam*, the Court of Appeal was considering s. 12(1) of the JDA, which provided that trials of all juveniles were to be held in camera. In striking down s. 12(1) as not being a reasonable limit on the rights of access to the courts, MacKinnon A.C.I.O. said at p. 429:

> The net which s. 12(1) casts is too wide for the purpose which it serves. Society loses more than it protects by the all-embracing nature of the section. As stated earlier, counsel for the Attorney-General was quick to acknowledge (and very fairly so) that not every juvenile court proceeding would require the barring of public access.

Counsel for the applicant relied on this decision and I must say that at first blush it does seem to deny the validity of a total ban, particularly where it has been conceded that the total ban is not necessary. However, on closer examination I believe that the differences between s.12(1) of the JDA and s.38(1) of the YOA are important. In s.12(1) of the JDA, the effect of the total ban reached further than mere accessibility to the courts, since it also resulted in an effective ban on the publication of *any* details of the court proceedings. If the press is not allowed to be present, it can hardly report on what happened at the proceeding.

Section 38(1) does not contain an absolute ban, and consequent denial of freedom of the press, in the same way. The press is entitled to be present (subject to s.39(1)(a)) and can publish everything except the identity of a young person involved. Admittedly, there may be other information which the press cannot publish because it may tend to reveal the identity of a young person, but the essence of the provision is that the press is entitled to publish all details except one. Counsel for the Attorney General of Canada termed the identification of the young person a "sliver of information", and submitted that this is not an essential detail for the making of responsible judgment by a democratic electorate (to meet the test in *Gay Alliance, supra*).

In my view, based on the evidence which I heard from expert witnesses, the protection and rehabilitation of young people involved in the criminal justice system is a social value of the "subordinate importance" which justifies the abrogation of fundamental freedom of expression, including freedom of the press, to the extent effected by s.38(1) of the YOA. Section 38(1) is, in my view, a reasonable limitation on that freedom.

Section 39(1)(a)

This provision gives to the youth court judge the discretion to exclude any member of the public if, in his or her opinion, any of the criteria set out in the section are met. Thus, the section does not impose an absolute ban, as did s.12(1) of the JDA.

When the Court of Appeal decided *Re Southam Inc. and R., supra*, the YOA had been enacted but not yet proclaimed. Section 39(1)(a) was proclaimed at it was set out in *Re Southam*, with the addition of the word "seriously" before the word "prejudicial". At pp. 429-30 MacKinnon A.C.J.O. said:

"An amendment giving jurisdiction to the court to exclude the public from juvenile court proceedings where it concludes under the circumstances, that it is in the best interests of the child or others concerned or in the best interests of the administration of justice to do so would meet any residual concern arising from the striking down of the section. As Mr. Justice Martin said in *R. v. Oakes* (released February 2, 1983, unreported) (since reported, 145 D.L.R. (3d) 123, 2 C.C.C. (3d) 339, 409 O.R. (2d) 660), we are not entitled to rewrite the statute under attack when considering the applicability of the provisions of the Charter. Parliament can give the necessary discretion to the court to be exercised on a case-to-case basis which, in my view, would be a prospective reasonable limit on the guaranteed right and demonstrably justifiable."

While these statements by MacKinnon A.C.J.O. were clearly obiter and therefore not strictly binding upon me, I feel that I must given them great weight and that they are indicative of the view that the Court of Appeal would take on the constitutionality of s. 39(1)(a) . Admittedly, the Court of Appeal did not hear evidence and full argument on s.39(1)(a), but it is my opinion that the evidence I have heard strengthens the view expressed by the Court of Appeal.

Again, I hold that the interests of society in the protection and rehabilitation of young people involved in youth court proceedings is a value of such superordinate importance that it justifies the discretion given to a youth court judge under s.39(1)(a). Section 39(1)(a) is, in my view, a reasonable limitation on freedom of expression, including freedom of the press.

Having made those decisions, I am aware that I have not referred to legislation of other free and democratic societies. I have considered the legislation for the United Kingdom, the United States and the Commonwealth which were put before me, and they indicate that there is a range of legislation acceptable in other free and democratic societies. In my view, ss.38(1) and 39(1)(a) are within the acceptable range.

In any event, I do not need to rely on legislation in other jurisdictions. While I accept that in some circumstances it may be helpful, I adopt the words of Osborne, J. in *R. v. D.*, supra:

"The fact that this legislation is not mirrored in other free and democratic societies may cause one to pause, but, it seems to me, not stop. This is a Canadian solution to a problem that I am sure exists in all jurisdictions. The Canadian solution is not to be rejected because others have seen fit not to follow the path chosen by Parliament in order to better protect the victims of alleged sexual assault."

3.3.3.2.3 Preliminary Inquiries

3.3.3.2.3.1 *Criminal Code*, R.S.C. 1985, c. C-46

537. (1) A justice acting under this Part may

(*h*) order that no person other than the prosecutor, the accused and their counsel shall have access to or remain in the room in which the inquiry is held, where it appears to him that the ends of justice will be best served by so doing;

"539. (1) Prior to the commencement of the taking of evidence at a preliminary inquiry, the justice holding the inquiry

(*a*) *may*, if application therefor is made by *the prosecutor, and*
(*b*) shall, if application therefor is made by *any of the accused*,

make an order directing that the evidence taken at the inquiry shall not be published in any newspaper or broadcast before such time as, *in respect of each of the accused*,

(*c*) *he* is discharged; or
(*d*) if *he is* ordered to stand trial, the trial is ended."

(2) Where an accused is not represented by counsel at a preliminary inquiry, the justice holding the inquiry shall, prior to the commencement of the taking of evidence at the inquiry, inform the accused of his right to make application under subsection (1).

(3) Every one who fails to comply with an order made pursuant to subsection (1) is guilty of an offence punishable on summary conviction.,

(4) In this section, "newspaper" has the same meaning as it has in section 297.

3.3.3.2.3.2 *R. v. Banville* **(1983), 45 N.B.R. (2d) 134 (Q.B.)**

HOYT, J. [orally]: This is an appeal from both the conviction entered against and sentence imposed upon Beurmond Banville by Provincial Court Judge James D. Harper for not complying with an order made by another Provincial Court Judge in which he prohibited the publication of evidence at a preliminary inquiry contrary to s.467(3) [Now 539(1)] of the *Criminal Code* of Canada.

Judge Harper's decision is reported in (1982), 41 N. B .R. (2d) 114; 107 A.P.R. 114. The facts are given in detail by him and I do not propose to repeat them here in such detail.

Briefly, Mr. Banville, a reporter for the Bangor Daily News, a daily newspaper printed in Bangor, Maine with general circulation in eastern and northern Maine, attended a preliminary inquiry which was held on February the 15th, 1982, in the Provincial Court in Edmundston, Madawaska County, New Brunswick. The presiding judge, upon the request of defence counsel and using the provisions of s.467(1) of the *Criminal Code*, made an order prohibiting the publication of evidence taken at the preliminary inquiry in the following terms:

> Be the order of this court that all of the evidence advanced in this preliminary hearing be banned from being published in any mode of media until the conclusion of this particular matter.

That order was made in open court with Mr. Banville present and in addition he was personally warned by the presiding judge and counsel for the Crown and the defence.

Mr. Banville filed a story which included some of the prohibited material. The story was published in the February 16th, 1982 issue of the Bangor Daily News. In all some 56 or 57 copies of that issue of the paper were distributed in Canada with 17 of those copies being distributed in Edmundston where the trial of the accused eventually occurred. Also some of the papers were delivered to Clair, which like Edmundston, is in the County of Madawaska from which county the jury was selected.

Mr. Banville, as I said, was charged under s.467(3) of the *Criminal Code* and upon conviction by Judge Harper was fined $200.00. In Mr. Banville's appeal from his conviction he presses some 8 grounds of appeal. They are:

> (a) The learned trial judge erred in law in finding that the *Constitution Act*, 1981, which proclaimed as law, a *Canadian Charter of Rights and Freedoms*, is not retroactive in its aspects and has no bearing on the present case.
>
> (b) The learned trial judge erred in law in finding that s.1 of the *Charter* fully justifies the existence of s.467 of the *Criminal Code* of Canada, R.S.C. 1970, c.C-34.

(c) The learned trial judge erred in law in failing to consider the applicability of s.1(f) of the *Canadian Bill of Rights* (1960) to the present case.

(d) The learned trial judge erred in law in holding that "the actual geographical area of publication is of no legal import" when s. 5(2) of the *Criminal Code* prohibits a conviction in Canada for an offence committed outside of Canada.

(e) The learned trial judge erred in law in finding the appellant guilty of the offence charged on the basis of s.21 of the *Criminal Code* when there was no proof of the commission of the principal offence within Canada.

(f) The learned trial judge erred in law in finding that the appellant "published" in his capacity as reporter.

(g) The learned trial judge erred in law in finding that the court had jurisdiction over the offence when there was no evidence of the commission of the offence in Canada.

(h) The learned trial judge erred in law in his application of the legal principle "de minimis non curat lex."

The first 3 grounds of appeal deal with the *Canadian Charter of Rights and Freedoms* which came into force on April the 17th, 1982, as part of the *Constitution Act* of 1982.

Briefly, the appellant contends that s. 2(b) of the *Charter* has retrospective effect and strikes down s.467(1) of the *Criminal Code* as it places a restriction on the freedom of the press. To support this argument, he says that s. 1(f) of the *Bill of Rights* codified this previously although unwritten freedom.

My view is that, in some applications, the *Charter* does have retrospective application. In *R. v. Davidson* (1982), 40 N.B.R. (2d) 702; 105 A.P.R. 702, I held that articles seized as a result of a police search before April 17th, 1982, could be rejected at a trial held after that date if their seizure brought the administration of justice into disrepute. I might say that to date this appears to be a minority view. *R v. Potma*, 7 W.C.B. 365, appears to be the more generally accepted view. Here, however, there is nothing of a continuing nature, as there was in both *Davidson* and *Potma*, which stretches over April 17th, 1982. There was no evidence tainted by the *Charter*. Thus, the *Charter* has no application. The offence, if there was one, was complete on February the 16th, 1982.

However, should I have found that the *Charter* did have application, I must think that s.467(1) of the *Criminal Code* is not a restraint on freedom of the press, which cannot be demonstrably justified in a free and democratic society.

First of all, the section does not prevent an open trial, one which may be attended by reporters and the general public, nor does it prohibit the publication of evidence given at the preliminary inquiry. It only defers its publication until the accused is either discharged or his trial is ended. If the media wish to publish or broadcast evidence given at the preliminary inquiry, at that time there is no sanction. It may not be as newsworthy but the public's right to know is preserved and protected.

Secondly, the mere fact that Parliament enacts a procedure which is apparently contrary to the *Charter* does not mean that such enactment is thus demonstrably justified in a free and democratic society. As Mr. Justice Smith said in *Re S.12 of the Juvenile Delinquents Act*, 8 W.C.B. 206:

> In my view, sovereignty of Parliament has been dealt a mild blow.

There he struck down s. 12(1) of the *Juvenile Delinquents Act*, R.S.C. 1970, c.J-3, which provides for the trials of children to take place without publicity.

Here freedom of the press is said to be interfered with by s.467(1) because the publication of evidence given at a preliminary inquiry is delayed. The purpose of the section is to insure that the accused receive the fairest possible trial or as is said in s.11(d) of the *Charter of Rights*:

> Any person charged with an offence has the right to be presumed innocent until proven guilty according to law in a fair and public hearing by an independent and impartial tribunal.

Thus, we appear to have 2 competing interests, freedom of the press and a fair and public trial before an independent and impartial tribunal. If there is such a conflict, and I am not certain that delay in reporting evidence of a preliminary inquiry is essential to the maintenance of a well-informed public opinion, then the concept of freedom of the press must, in my view, give way to the overriding obligation to insure that an individual have a fair trial before an independent and impartial tribunal. I find it difficult to accept that our democratic institutions are threatened if the public, including potential jurors, are delayed, not denied, but delayed in finding out that, for example,

> ... hairs found at the scene are consistent with a standard said to come from the accused's body.

In *Re C.B.R.*, 8 W.C.B. 206, Mr. Justice Smith dealt with an application to quash the order of a judge prohibiting the publication of a motion for a change of venue in a criminal trial. He dismissed the application, and although I have not had the benefit of reading his reasons, the report that I have just cited says:

> ... the Charter did not contemplate that an accused's rights should be whittled down in the name of a general concept of freedom of the press, a weighing process being required with the right to a fair trial being paramount — In the circumstances, the court was not persuaded that a temporary ban in the circumstances of the case was an unreasonable exercise of the trial judge's discretion.

I realize that there is a danger that each individual case can be rationalized on its merits, thus losing sight of the general principle. If s.467(1) was permissive rather than mandatory, the section would perhaps be easier to justify, as was the last case that I mentioned. The judge was exercising a discretion in prohibiting the publication of a motion for a change of venue and he made the order, which was upheld by Mr. Justice Smith, after hearing arguments of counsel. In dealing with blanket proscriptions, such as s.467(1), as I said, there is a danger that each case can be rationalized on its own merits and thus losing sight of the general principle. However, if there is a conflict between the two competing concepts, and I am not sure that there is, but if there is, the individual's right to a fair trial before an independent and impartial tribunal must prevail. Thus, I reject the argument that the *Charter of Rights and Freedoms*, even if it had retrospective effect, strikes down s.467(1) of the *Criminal Code*.

Grounds 4 to 7 of the appellant relate to the jurisdiction of Canadian Courts over this offense. Judge Harper carefully considered this argument, as well as the *Charter* argument, and I do not disagree with his finding. Mr. Hanson suggested that Judge Harper may have found Mr. Banville guilty as an accessory in aiding in the offense which occurred in the United States . . . I do not understand that to be Judge Harper's decision. At pages 121 and 122 of the report he says, after quoting s.21 of the *Criminal Code*:

> It is beyond argument that publication of the evidence complained of would have been impossible if it had been reported by the defendant in the first instance. It follows, therefore, that if an offense occurred he is a party to it and, therefore, guilty of it.

Mr. Banville wrote the story on February 15th, after he had knowledge of the order. Thus, he was the person who actually committed the offense. The publication was complete, in my view, when the story was made available to the public in Edmundston, to be precise, the following day.

Mr. Hanson argues that a reporter does not publish a newspaper. That is so. But s.467(1) does not prohibit the publication of a newspaper. It prohibits the evidence taken at the preliminary inquiry from being published in a newspaper. The reporter, particularly one who knows of the ban, becomes guilty when his story is printed and circulated in Canada — if it contains evidence taken at the inquiry. I distinguish between publication and printing.

The final ground of appeal against the conviction is that the offense is so trivial as not to be worthy of notice. I agree with Judge Harper whom after reviewing the authorities, said at page 127:

> The degree of such breach is of no consequences in coming to a decision upon whether or not the defendant is guilty of the charge, nor is his notice of any import. Once the breach of the court order is established by the prosecution the probable or improbable results of the failure of the defendant to abide the order are of no significance only insofar as sentence is concerned.

Initially I was not disposed to tinker with the sentence imposed by Judge Harper. If I may say so, he approached the task of sentencing with great sensitivity. Little harm was done and Mr. Banville voluntarily returned to Canada to face his trial. His defense was conducted with dignity. However, he was aware of the possible consequences should the story be published.

However, I am of the view that this is an appropriate situation for a discharge. I feel that it would be clearly in the best interests of the accused, having regard to the nature and place of his employment, and not contrary to the public interest by ordering a discharge.

I allow the appeal against the sentence and direct that the accused be discharged absolutely. In the result, the appeal against conviction is dismissed and the appeal against sentence is allowed with the substitution of an absolute discharge.

Appeal against conviction dismissed; appeal against sentence allowed.

3.3.3.2.3.3 *Criminal Code*, R.S.C. 1985, c. C-46

542. (1) Nothing in this Act prevents a prosecutor giving in evidence at a preliminary inquiry any admission, confession or statement made at any time by the accused that by law is admissible against him.

(2) Every one who publishes in any newspaper, or broadcasts, a report that any admission or confession was tendered in evidence at a preliminary inquiry or a report of the nature of such admission or confession so tendered in evidence unless
   (*a*) the accused has been discharged, or
   (*b*) if the accused has been ordered to stand trial, the trial has ended (as am. S.C. 1985, c.19, s.101(2)).

is guilty of an offence punishable on summary conviction.

(3) In this section "newspaper" has the same meaning that it has in section 297.

3.3.3.2.4 Bail Hearings

3.3.3.2.4.1 *Criminal Code*, R.S.C. 1985, c. C-46

515. (1) Subject to this section, where an accused who is charged with an offence other than an offence listed in section 427 is taken before a justice, the justice shall, unless a plea of guilty by the accused is accepted, order, in respect of that offence, that the accused be released upon his giving an undertaking without conditions, unless the prosecutor, having been given a reasonable opportunity to do so, shows cause, in respect of that offence, why the detention of the accused in custody is justified or why an order under any other provision of this section should be made and where the justice makes an order under any other provision of this section, the order shall refer only to the particular offence for which the accused was taken before the justice.

(10) For the purposes of this section, the detention of an accused in custody is justified only on either of the following grounds, namely:
   (*a*) on the primary ground that his detention is necessary to ensure his attendance in court in order to be dealt with according to law; and
   (*b*) on the secondary ground (the applicability of which shall be determined only in the event that and after it is determined that his detention is not justified on the primary ground referred to in paragraph (a)) that his detention is necessary in the public interest or for the protection or safety of the public, having regard to all the circumstances including any substantial likelihood that the accused will, if he is released from custody, commit a criminal offence or an interference with the administration of justice.

Note: In *R. v. Morales* the Supreme Court of Canada found the phrase "in the public interest" in s. 515(10) to be an unjustifiable limit on a Charter guarantee. (1983), 144 N.R. 176.

517. (1) Where the prosecutor or the accused intends to show cause under section 515, he shall so state to the justice and the justice may, and shall upon application by the accused, before or at any time during the course of the proceedings under that section, make an order directing that the evidence taken, the information given or the representations made and the reasons, if any, given or to be given by the justice shall not be published in any newspaper or broadcast before such time as

(*a*) if a preliminary inquiry is held, the accused in respect of whom the proceedings are held is discharged, or

(*b*) if the accused in respect of whom the proceedings are held is tried or ordered to stand trial, the trial is ended.

(2) Every one who fails without lawful excuse, the proof of which lies upon him to comply with an order made under subsection (1) is guilty of an offence punishable on summary conviction.

(3) In this section, "newspaper" has the same meaning as it has in section 297.

Note: The validity of this provision was upheld by the Ontario Court of Appeal in *Re Smith* (1984), 38 C.R. (3d) 209.

THORSON, J.A. observed at p. 228:

> ... The right to a fair trial is a fragile right. It is quite capable of being shattered by the kind of publicity that can attend a bail hearing and, once shattered, it may, like Humpty Dumpty, be quite impossible to put back together again. Often the proceedings at a bail hearing do not enact any particular media notice, but when they do, as they have in this case the risk of prejudice to the accused in the manner of his or her subsequent trial can be severe in the absence of a mechanism such as that provided in s.457.2(1) for minimizing that prejudice by means of a time-limited restraint on what can be published or broadcast about the hearing. In my opinion it is no answer at all that the need for such a mechanism might be avoided if only our legal system were otherwise and adopted a different approach altogether to the safeguarding of a fair trial for the accused. As has been said in other words elsewhere by this court, ultimately our courts must come back to our own free and democratic society in applying the test in this regard which s. 1 of the Charter requires us to apply.

3.3.3.2.5 Jury Trials

3.3.3.2.5.1 *Criminal Code*, R.S.C. 1985, c. C-46

648. (1) Where permission to separate is given to members of a jury under subsection 647(1), no information regarding any portion of the trial at which the jury is not present shall be published, after the permission is granted, in any newspaper or broadcast before the jury retires to consider its verdict.

(2) Every one who fails to comply with subsection (1) is guilty of an offence punishable on summary conviction.

(3) In this section, "newspaper" has the same meaning as it has in section 297.

649. Every member of a jury who, except for the purpose of

(*a*) an investigation of an alleged offence under subsection 127(2) in relation to a juror, or

(*b*) giving evidence in criminal proceedings in relation to such an offence, discloses any information relating to the proceedings of the jury when it was absent from the courtroom that was not subsequently disclosed in open court is guilty of an offence punishable on summary conviction. 1972, c.13, s.49.

Note: The main source for reporters covering a trial is the lawyers involved. In its *Communique* dated March 22 and 23, 1984, the Law Society of Upper Canada stated that: "The Society has received complaints from the judiciary and others concerning the growing frequency of press interviews by counsel involved in court proceedings and shares this concern. The profession is reminded of the language of Commentary 18(a) to Rule 13 of the Rules of Professional Conduct and should be aware that any interview with the media about court proceedings invites the inference that it was given to publicize the lawyer and carries the danger of being a contempt of court. The Society intends to institute discipline proceedings where appropriate to ensure that the rule is observed. " The Supreme Court of Ontario invalidated this restriction in *Re Klein and Law Society of Upper Canada; Re Dvorak and Law Society of Upper Canada* (1985), 50 O.R. (2d) 118.

3.3.3.3 Common Law Sub-Judice

3.3.3.3.1 *Attorney-General v. Times Newspapers Ltd.*, [1973] 3 All E.R. 54 (H.L.)

LORD REID. My Lords, in 1958 Distillers Co. (Biochemicals) Ltd. began to make and sell in this country a sedative which contained a drug thalidomide which had been invented and used in Germany. This product was available on prescription and was consumed by many pregnant women having been said to be quite safe for them. But soon there were cases of babies being born with terrible deformities. As such deformities do occasionally occur naturally, it took a little time to prove that these deformities were caused by the action of thalidomide in the unborn child at a certain stage of pregnancy. As soon as this was realised Distillers withdrew their product in 1961.

The matter attracted some publicity and the question arose whether Distillers were legally liable to pay damages in respect of these deformed children. Distillers denied liability and the first action against them was begun in 1962. Further publicity resulted in some 70 actions having been raised before 1968.

Claimants were faced by two difficulties. First there was a highly debatable legal question whether a person can sue for damage done to him before his birth. And secondly, an attempt to prove negligence by Distillers in putting this drug on the market would require long and expensive enquiries. The claimants combined to negotiate with Distillers and early in 1968 a settlement was reached by which Distillers agreed to pay to each claimant 40 percent of the damages which he or she would recover if successful in establishing liability. Regarded from a purely legal point of view this appears to have been a very reasonable compromise.

Two cases were then tried by agreement to establish the proper measure of damages and ultimately 65 cases were settled, Distillers paying about a million pounds in all. But more cases gradually came to light. Leave to serve writs was now necessary and the first orders granting leave were made in July 1968. By February 1969, 248 writs had been served. A few more followed. And there were many cases where claims had been made but no writs served. It may be that there are still some cases where claims will be made. In all there appear to be more than 400 outstanding claims not covered by the 1968 settlement.

Distillers proposed to settle these claims by setting up a trust fund of over 3 million. But they made it a condition of any settlement that all claimants should agree to accept it. The great majority agreed but five refused to do so. One parent at least refused because payments out of the trust fund were to be based on need, and his financial position was such that his child would get no benefit from such a settlement.

An attempt was made to compel these five to agree by having the Official Solicitor appointed to look after the interests of their children. But the Court of Appeal, in April 1972, reinstated these five parents (*Re Taylor's Application*). In June 1972 Distillers made some new proposals but they were not accepted. There were then 389 claims outstanding and there seemed little prospect of an early settlement.

The editor of the Sunday Times took a keen interest in this matter. He collected a great deal of material and on 24th September 1972 that newspaper published a long and powerful article. Two general propositions were argued at some length: first whether those who put such drugs on the market ought to be absolutely liable for damage done by them, and secondly that in such cases the currently accepted method of assessing damages is inadequate. But the sting of the article lay in the following paragraph:

> Thirdly, the thalidomide children shame Distillers. It is appreciated that Distillers have always denied negligence and that if the cases were pursued, the children might end up with nothing. It is appreciated that Distillers' lawyers have a professional duty to secure the best terms for their clients. But at the end of the day what is to be paid in settlement is the decision of Distillers, and they should offer much, much more to every one of the thalidomide victims. It may be argued that Distillers have a duty to their shareholders and that, having taken account of skilled legal advice, the terms are just. But the law is not always the same as justice. There are times when to insist on the letter of the law is as exposed to criticism as infringement of another's legal rights. The figure in the proposed settlement is to be £3.25m., spread over 10 years. This does not shine as a beacon against pre-tax profits last year of £64.8 million and company assets worth £421 million. Without in any way surrendering on negligence, Distillers could and should think again.

Distillers immediately brought this to the attention of the Attorney-General maintaining that it was in contempt of court. The Attorney-General decided to take no action. But this did not in any way prevent Distillers from bringing the matter before the court if they chose to do so. However they took no action.

I agree with your Lordships that the Attorney-General has a right to bring before the court any matter which he thinks may amount to contempt of court and which he considers should in the public interest be brought before the court. The party aggrieved has the right to bring before the court any matter which he alleges amounts to contempt but he has no duty to do so. So if the party aggrieved failed to take action either because of expense or because he thought it better not to do so, very serious contempt might escape punishment if the Attorney-General had no right to act. But the Attorney-General is not obliged to bring before the court every prima facie case of contempt reported to him. It is entirely for him to judge whether it is in the public interest that he should act.

The editor of the Sunday Times had in mind to publish a further article of a different character. As a result of communications between him and the Attorney-General regarding the article of 24th September, he sent the material for the further article to the learned attorney and this time the Attorney-General took the view that he should intervene. By a writ of 12th October 1972 he claimed an injunction against the respondents, who own the Sunday Times, restraining them from publishing the proposed article. The Divisional Court granted an injunction but the Court of Appeal on 16th February 1973 discharged the injunction. The Attorney-General now appeals to this House.

Before dealing with the arguments submitted to your Lordshlps I find it necessary to set out some general considerations which must govern the whole subject of contempt of court. It appears never to have come before this House; there is no recent review of the subject in the Court of Appeal; and the circumstances of cases which arise in practice are generally not such as to require any detailed analysis of the law. I cannot disagree with a statement in a recent report of Justice on the Law and the Press that the main objection to the existing law of contempt is its uncertainty I think that we must try to remove that reproach at least with regard to those parts of the law with which the present case is concerned.

The law on this subject is and must be founded entirely on public policy. It is not there to protect the private rights of parties to a litigation or prosecution. It is there to prevent interference with the administration of justice and it should in my judgment be limited to what is reasonably necessary for that purpose. Public policy generally requires a balancing of interests which may conflict. Freedom of speech should not be limited to any greater extent than is necessary but it cannot be allowed where there would be real prejudice to the administration of justice.

In *Ambard v. Attorney-General for Trinidad and Tobago* Lord Atkin said:

> But whether the authority and position of an individual judge or the due administration of justice is concerned. no wrong is committed by any member of the public who exercises the ordinary right of criticising in good faith in private or public, the public act done in the seat of justice. The path of criticism is a public way: the wrong headed are permitted to err therein: provided that members of the public abstain from imputing improper motives to those taking part in the administration of justice, and are genuinely exercising a right of criticism and not acting in malice or attempting to impart the administration of justice, they are immune. Justice is not a cloistered virtue: she must be allowed to suffer the scrutiny and respectful even though outspoken comments of ordinary men.

I think that these words have an application beyond the particular type of contempt in that case.

Discussion of questions of contempt generally begin with the observations of Lord Hardwicke L.C. in *The St. James's Evening Post Case*. Dealing with a case where there had been gross abuse of litigants he said:

> Nothing is more incumbent upon courts of justice, than to preserve their proceedings from being misrepresented; nor is there any thing of more pernicious consequence, than to prejudice the minds of the public against persons concerned as parties in causes, before the cause is finally heard.

And later:

> There are three different sorts of contempt. One kind of contempt is, scandalizing the court itself. There may be likewise a contempt of this court, in abusing parties who are concerned in causes here. There may be also a contempt of this court, in prejudicing mankind against persons before the cause is heard. There cannot be any thing of greater consequence, than to keep the streams of justice clear and pure, that parties may proceed with safety both to themselves and their characters.

I do not think that Lord Hardwicke L.C. intended this to be a universally applicable definition, although it has too often been treated as if it were. It is a good guide but it must be supplemented in cases of a type which he did not have in mind.

We are particularly concerned here with "abusing parties" and "prejudicing mankind" against them. Of course parties must be protected from scurrilous abuse; otherwise many litigants would fear to bring their cases to court. But the argument of the Attorney-General goes far beyond that. His argument was based on a passage in the judgment of Buckiey J. in *Vine Products Ltd. v. Mackenzie & Co. Ltd.*:

> It is a contempt of this court for any newspaper to comment on pending legal proceedings in any way which is likely to prejudice the fair trial of the action. That may arise in various ways. It may be that the comment is likely in some way or other to bring pressure to bear on one or other of the parties to the action, so as to prevent that party from prosecuting or from defending the action, or encourage him to submit to terms of compromise which he otherwise might not have been prepared to entertain, or influence him in some other way in his conduct in the action, which he ought to be free to prosecute or to defend, as he is advised, without being subject to such pressure.

I think that this is much too widely stated. It is true that there is some authority for it but it does not in the least follow from the observations of Lord Hardwicke L.C. and it does not seem to me to be in accord with sound public policy. Why would it be contrary to public policy to seek by fair comment to dissuade Shylock from proceeding with his action? Surely it could not be wrong for the officious bystander to draw his attention to the risk that, if he goes on, decent people will cease to trade with him. Or suppose that his best customer ceased to trade with him when he heard of his lawsuit. That could not be contempt of court. Would it become contempt if, when asked by Shylock why he was sending no more business his way, he told him the reason? Nothing would be more likely to influence Shylock to discontinue his action. It might become widely known that such pressure was being brought to bear. Would that make any difference? And though widely known must the local press keep silent about it? There must be some limitation of this general statement of the law.

And then suppose that there is in the press and elsewhere active discussion of some question of wide public interest, such as the propriety of local authorities or other landlords ejecting squatters from empty premises due for demolition. Then legal proceedings are begun against some squatters, it may be by some authority which had already been criticised in the press. The controversy could hardly be continued without likelihood that it might influence the authority in its conduct of the action. Must there then be silence until that case is decided? And there may be a series of actions by the same or different landlords. Surely public policy does not require that a system of stop and go shall apply to public discussion.

I think that there is a difference between direct interference with the fair trial of an action and words or conduct which may affect the minds of a litigant. Comment likely to affect the minds of witnesses and of the tribunal must be stopped for otherwise the trial may well be unfair. But the fact that a party refrains from seeking to enforce his full legal rights in no way prejudices a fair trial whether the decision is or is not influenced by some third party. There are other weighty reasons for preventing improper influence being brought to bear on litigants, but they have little to do with interference with the fairness of a trial. There must be absolute prohibition of interference with a fair trial but beyond that there must be a balancing of relevant considerations.

I know of no better statement of the law than that contained in the judgment of Jordan C.J. in *Re Truth and Sportsman Ltd., ex parte Bread Manufacturers Ltd.*:

> It is of extreme public interest that no conduct should be permitted which is likely to prevent a litigant in a court of justice from having his case tried free from all matter of prejudice. But the administration of justice, important though it undoubtedly is, is not the only matter in which the public is vitally interested; and if in the course of the ventilation of a question of public concern matter is published which may prejudice a party in the conduct of a law suit, it does not follow that a contempt has been committed. The case may be one in which as between competing matters of public interest the possibility of prejudice to a litigant may be required to yield to other and superior considerations. The discussion of public affairs and the denunciation of public abuses, actual or supposed, cannot be required to be suspended merely because the discussion or the denunciation may, as an incidental but not intended by-product, cause some likelihood of prejudice to a person who happens at the time to be a litigant. It is well settled that a person cannot be prevented by process of contempt from continuing to discuss publicly a matter which may fairly be regarded as one of public interest, by reason merely of the fact that the matter in question has become the subject of litigation, or that person whose conduct is being publicly criticised has become a party to litigation either as plaintiff or as defendant, and whether in relation to the matter which is under discussion or with respect to some other matter.

Guidance with regard to the dividing line between comment about a litigant which is permissible and that which involves contempt, is to be found in the judgment of Maugham J. in *Re William Thomas Shipping Co. Ltd.* The company had suffered severely from the prevailing depression and debenture holders sought liquidation. Sir Robert Thomas, the governing director, gave a statement to a Liverpool newspaper which it published. The debenture holders sought an order on the ground that the statement was in contempt of court. Maugham J. rejected an argument that the statement might influence the judge dealing with the proceedings for liquidation. But he went on to consider whether it is a contempt "to abuse the parties concerned in a pending case or matter by injurious misrepresentations". He held that there was contempt for that reason but added:

> I am not saying that if Sir Robert Thomas had fairly stated the result of the evidence on which the Court made the order for the appointment of a receiver and manager, and had in a temperate manner expressed his opinion that another course ought to have been taken by the plaintiff, the Court would have thought fit to interfere or could properly have interfered.

So the dividing line there drawn was between comment containing injurious misrepresentation which was contempt and fair and temprate criticism which would not have been. That is emphasised by the last paragraph of his judgment where he deals with the newspaper. Their fault was that they were in too much of a hurry and published a statement of a most misleading character. I must follow that Maugham J. thought that if a newspaper published fair and temprate criticism of a litigant, it is in general entitled to do so.

I would compare with that case the decision of Talbot and Macnaghten JJ. in *Re South Shields (Thames Street) Clearance Order 1931*. The corporation had made a clearance order and the owners of property affected by it had taken the matter before the court. An article was published suggesting that the owners by their appeal were keeping the tenants out of new houses and hindering the progress of housing in the borough. The owners contended that this was contempt of court as tending to deter them and others from coming before the court. They relied on the *William Thomas Shipping Co.* case. But it was held that this would be an extension of the law of contempt beyond anything that could justify it. No reasons are given in the very brief report of the case but I think that the ground of judgment must have been that the article complained of did not go beyond fair and temperate comment on the owners' action. If the argument of the Attorney-General in the present case were right, I think that the case would have been wrongly decided. But it appears to me to have been rightly decided.

So I would hold that as a general rule where the only matter to be considered is pressure put on a litigant, fair and temprate criticism is legitimate, but anything which goes beyond that may well involve contempt of court. But in a case involving witnesses, jury or magistrates, other considerations are involved: there even fair and temperate criticism might be likely to affect the minds of some of them so as to involve contempt. But it can be assumed that it would not affect the mind of a professional judge.

In some recent cases about influencing litigants the court has accepted the law as stated in the passage from the judgment of Buckley J. in the *Vine Products* case, but has held that there is no contempt unless there is a serious risk that the litigant will be influenced. Perhaps this was an attempt to mitigate the extreme consequences of that view of the law, but I think this test is most unsatisfactory. First, when considering whether the risk is serious do you consider the particular litigant so that what would be contempt if he is easily influenced would not be contempt if the particular litigant is so strong minded as not to be easily influenced? That would not seem right but if you have to imagine a reasonable man in the shoes of that litigant the test becomes rather unreal. And then are you to take that one comment alone or are you to consider the cumulative effect if others are free to say and probably will say the same kind of thing?

I think that this view of the law caused the court to give wrong reasons for reaching a correct decision in *Attorney General v. London Weekend Television*. The respondent company had produced a television programme about the thalidomide tragedy on 8th October 1972. So far as I can judge from the report it seems to have had much the same object and character as the Sunday Times article of 24th September. If the view which I take about that article is correct then I think that for similar reasons the television programme was not in contempt of court.

But the court, following the judgment of the Divisional Court in the present case, held that the programme bore many of the badges of contempt and only dismissed the application on the ground that they were unable to say that the programme "would result in the creation of a *serious* [their italics] risk" that the course of justice would be interfered with. They had said earlier "We find that the spoken words on this programme did not have that impact which the producer might have hoped that they would have had on the viewers". So the company only escaped because of their inefficiency. I cannot believe that the law could be left in such an unsatisfactory state.

I think, agreeing with Cotton L.J. in his judgment in *Hunt v. Clarke*, that there must be two questions: first, was there any contempt at all? and, secondly, was it sufficiently serious to require or justify the court in making an order against the respondent? The question whether there was a serious risk of influencing the litigant is certainly a factor to be considered in what course to take by way of punishment, as is the intention with which the comment was made. But it is I think confusing to import this into the question whether there was any contempt at all or into the definition of contempt.

I think the true view is that expressed by Lord Parker C.J. in *R. v. Duffy, ex parte Nash*, that there must be a real risk as opposed to a remote possibility. That is an application of the ordinary de minimis principle. There is no contempt if the possibility of influence is remote. If there is some but only a small likelihood, that may influence the court to refrain from inflicting any punishment. If there is a serious risk some action may be necessary. And I think that the particular comment cannot be considered in isolation when considering its probable effect. If others are to be free and are likely to make similar comments that must be taken into account.

The crucial question on this point of the case is whether it can ever be permissible to urge a party to a litigation to forego his legal rights in whole or in part. The Attorney-General argues that it cannot and I think that the Divisional Court has accepted that view. In my view it is permissible so long as it is done in a fair and temperate way and without any oblique motive. The Sunday Times article of 24th September 1972 affords a good illustration of the difference between the two views. It is plainly intended to bring pressure to bear on Distillers. It was likely to attract support from others and it did so. It was outspoken. It said "There are times when to insist on the letter of the law is as exposed to criticism as infringement of another's legal rights" and clearly implied that that was such a time. If the view maintained by the Attorney-General were right I could hardly imagine a clearer case of contempt of court. It could be no excuse that the passage which I quoted earlier was combined with a great deal of other totally unobjectionable material. And it could not be said that it created no serious risk of causing Distillers to do what they did not want to do. On the facts submitted to your Lordships in argument it seems to me to have played a large part in causing Distillers to offer far more money than they had in mind at that time. But I am quite unable to subscribe to the view that it ought never to have been published because it was in contempt of court. I see no offence against public policy and no pollution of the stream of justice by its publication.

Now I must turn to the material to which the injunction applied. If it is not to be published at this time it would not be proper to refer to it in any detail. But I can say that it consists in the main of detailed evidence and argument intended to show that Distillers did not exercise due care to see that thalidomide was safe before they put it on the market.

If we regard this material solely from the point of view of its likely effect on Distillers I do not think that its publication in 1972 would have added much to the pressure on them created, or at least begun, by the earlier article of 24th September. From Distillers' point of view the damage had already been done. I doubt whether the subsequent course of events would have been very different in their effect on Distillers if the matter had been published.

But to my mind there is another consideration even more important than the effect of publication on the mind of the litigant. The controversy about the tragedy of the thalidomide children has ranged widely but as yet there seems to have been little, if any, detailed discussion of the issues which the court may have to determine if the outstanding claims are not settled. The question whether Distillers were negligent has been frequently referred to but so far as I am aware there has been no attempt to assess the evidence. If this material were released now it appears to me to be almost inevitable that detailed answers would be published and there would be expressed various public prejudgments of this issue. That I would regard as very much against the public interest.

There has long been and there still is in this country a strong and generally held feeling that trial by newspaper is wrong and should be prevented. I find for example in the report of Lord Salmon's committee dealing with the law of contempt with regard to Tribunals of Inquiry a reference to the 'horror' in such a thing. What I think is regarded as most objectionable is that a newspaper or television programme should seek to persuade the public, by discussing the issues and evidence in a case before the court, whether civil or criminal, that one side is right and the other wrong. If we were to ask the ordinary man or even a lawyer in his leisure moments why he has that feeling, I suspect that the first reply would be — well look at what happens in some other countries where that is permitted. As in so many other matters, strong feelings are based on one's general experience rather than on specific reasons, and it often requires an effort to marshall one's reasons. But public policy is generally the result of strong feelings, commonly held, rather than of cold argument.

If the law is to be developed in accord with public policy we must not be too legalistic in our general approach. No doubt public policy is an unruly horse to ride but in a chapter of the law so intimately associated with public policy as contempt of court we must not be too pedestrian. It is hardly sufficient to ask what Lord Hardwicke L.C. meant in 1742 when he referred to prejudicing mankind against parties before a cause is heard.

There is ample authority for the proposition that issues must not be prejudged in a manner likely to affect the mind of those who may later be witnesses or jurors. But very little has been said about the wider proposition that trial by newspaper is intrinsically objectionable. That may be because if one can find more limited and familiar grounds adequate for the decision of a case it is rash to venture on uncharted seas.

I think that anything in the nature of prejudgment of a case or of specific issues in it is objectionable not only because of its possible effect on that particular case but also because of its side effects which may be far reaching. Responsible 'mass media' will do their best to be fair, but there will also be ill-informed, slapdash or prejudiced attempts to influence the public. If people are led to think that it is easy to find the truth disrespect for the processes of the law could follow and, if mass media are allowed to judge, unpopular people and unpopular causes will fare very badly. Most cases of prejudging of issues fall within the existing authorities on contempt. I do not think that the freedom of the press would suffer, and I think that the law would be clearer and easier to apply in practice if it is made a general rule that it is not permissible to prejudge issues in pending cases.

In my opinion the law was rather too narrowly stated in *Vine Products Ltd. v. Mackenzie & Co. Ltd.* There the question was what wines could properly be called sherry and a newspaper published an article which clearly prejudged the issue. In my view that was technically in contempt of court. But the fault was so venial and the possible consequences so trifling that it would have been quite wrong to impose punishment or I think even to require the newspaper to pay the costs of the applicant. But the newspaper ought to have withheld its judgment until the case had been decided.

There is no magic in the issue of a writ or in a charge being made against an accused person. Comment on a case which is imminent may be as objectionable as comment after it has begun. And a 'gagging' writ ought to have no effect. But I must add to prevent misunderstanding that comment where a case is under appeal is a very different matter. For one thing it is scarcely possible to imagine a case where comment could influence judges in the Court of Appeal or noble and learned Lords in this House. And it would be wrong and contrary to existing practice to limit proper criticism of judgments already given but under appeal.

Now I must deal with the reasons which induced the Court of Appeal to discharge the injunction. It was said that the actions had been dormant or asleep for several years. Nothing appears to have been done in court but active negotiations for a settlement were going on all the time. No one denies that it would be contempt of court to use improper pressure to induce a litigant to settle a case on terms to which he did not wish to agree. So if there is no undue procrastination in the negotiations for a settlement I do not see how in this context action can be said to be dormant.

Then it was said that there is here a public interest which counterbalances the private interests of the litigants. But contempt of court has nothing to do with the private interests of the litigants. I have already indicated the way in which I think that a balance must be struck between the public interest in freedom of speech and the public interest in protecting the administration of justice from interference. I do not see why there should be any difference in principle between a case which is thought to have news value and one which is not. Protection of the administration of justice is equally important whether or not the case involves important general issues.

Some reference was made to the debate in the House of Commons. It was not extensively referred to in argument. But so far as I have noticed there was little said in the House which could not have been said outside if my view of the law is right.

If we were only concerned with the effect which publication of the new material might now have on the mind of Distillers I might be able to agree with the decision of the Court of Appeal though for different reasons. But I have already stated my view that wider considerations are involved. The purpose of the law is not to prevent publication of such material but to postpone it. The information set before us gives us hope that the general lines of a settlement of the whole of this unfortunate controversy may soon emerge. It should then be possible to permit this material to be published. But if things drag on indefinitely so that there is no early prospect either of a settlement or of a trial in court then I think that there will have to be a wakening of the public interest in a unique situation.

As matters stand at present I think that this appeal must be allowed.

3.3.3.3.2 *Zehr v. McIsaac et al.* (1982), 39 O.R. (2d) 237 (Ont.H.C.)

O'Driscoll, J.: —

I Type of application

The applicant seeks a conviction and committal against each person named as a respondent and a conviction and fine as against the corporate respondent as the result of an article published on p. 5 of the newspaper *The Globe and Mail* on Tuesday February 9, 1982. It is alleged that McIsaac was the author of the contemptuous statements which were reported by Makin and his editor-in-chief, Doyle, and published by the corporate respondent.

The application fails as against all respondents.

II History

1. Steven Wayne Zehr, the applicant, was charged with raping a female "X" at the City of Barrie on November 14, 1978. He was tried at the Barrie Assizes by Callon J. and a jury and convicted.

2. Zehr launched an appeal from his conviction to the Ontario Court of Appeal. On June 23, 1980, that court (Howland C.J.O., Brooke and Thorson JJ.A.), quashed the conviction and ordered a new trial: 54 C.C.C. (2d) 65.

3. On March 2, 1981, the Attorney-General for Ontario preferred a two count indictment against Zehr:

(1) that Zehr raped a female "X" at the City of Barrie on November 14, 1978, and

(2) that Zehr raped a female "Y" at the City of Barrie on October 6, 1980.

4. On March 24, 1981, Labrosse J. ordered that Zehr be tried separately on each count and traversed the trial to the next sittings at Barrie, Ontario.

5. On May 25, 1981, at the new trial at the Barrie Assizes conducted by Grange J. with a jury, Zehr was arraigned on count No. I — that he did rape the female "X" at the City of Barrie on November 14, 1978; Zehr pleaded not guilty; the trial proceeded and on June 11, 1981, the jury rendered a verdict of "not guilty" on count No. 1. The Crown did not appeal the verdict of not guilty rendered at the new trial of count.

On June 11, 1981, Grange J. ordered that count No. 2 (the charge of rape with regard to female "Y") be traversed to the September Assizes at Barrie, Ontario.

6. On July 13, 1981, Griffiths J. granted Zehr judicial interim release.

7. An order was made for a change of venue from Barrie to Toronto.

8. On September 17, 1981, on consent, a trial date was set for November 30, 1981, with regard to count No. 2.

9. At Toronto, on December 1, 1981, before Craig J. and a jury, Zehr was arraigned on count No. 2 — that he did rape the female "Y" at the City of Barrie on October 6, 1980; Zehr pleaded not guilty and the trial proceeded.

On December 14, 1981, the jury returned a verdict of "guilty as charged" on count No. 2. Zehr was remanded in custody to February 8, 1982, to await sentence.

10. On January 12, 1982, Zehr filed a notice of appeal from his conviction for rape on count No. 2, which appeal is still pending.

11. Prior to February 8, 1982, the Crown had served Zehr with notice that it would proceed against him as a dangerous offender under Part XXI of the *Criminal Code*, R.S.C. 1970, c.C-34 (s.688(b)).

12. On February 8, 1982, Craig J. heard submissions concerning psychiatric assessments of Zehr; at that time Crown counsel John McIsaac, advised Craig J.:

> You'd also be hearing about a circumstance involving a female by the name of "X". There will be a lengthy argument by my friend in relation to the admissibility of this testimony.

On the same day, February 8, 1982, Craig J., after hearing evidence from Dr. Russell Fleming, further remanded Zehr in custody until March 22, 1982.

13. On February 9, 1982, the article in question appeared in *The Globe and Mail* on p. 5:

Fed up with Deciding on Confining Criminals Indefinitely, MD Says
by KIRK MAKIN

A director at the Penetanguishene Mental Health Centre says he is fed up with being asked to decide whether criminals should be designated dangerous offenders and thus incarcerated indefinitely.

The courts should stop foisting the question on psychiatrists and instead make the dangerous offender designation automatic if a crime is repeated a certain number of times, said Russell Fleming, director of the centre's forensic science unit.

The designation is seldom used but carries serious consequences. If a person is designated a dangerous offender, he is incarcerated undefinitely in a penal or mental institution and is on mandatory supervision for the rest of his life if he is released.

"It's like a life sentence," Dr. Fleming said in an interview yesterday. "Potentially, they can be kept forever."

He said his unit is asked to assess four or five candidates for dangerous offender status every year. The National Parole Board first reviews dangerous offenders after three years and every two years after that.

The courts "shouldn't ask us to get involved in this adversarial nonsense where a Crown attorney shops around for a right-wing psychiatrist to say the man should go (to an institution), while the defence shops around for a left-wing psychiatrist to say he shouldn't," Dr. Fleming said.

"I've never said this in court, but frankly I feel it's never a palatable experience," he said. "You have to make a decision on whether someone is or is not going to do it again. It makes much more sense to hinge it on something reasonable, like the number of previous convictions.

"You could devise a system where you get one free rape with a sentence of two years less a day at the most, a five-year penitentiary term for the second rape and dangerous offender status after the third."

Robert Ash, a Crown attorney in the Judicial District of York, said in an interview that he "can appreciate Dr. Fleming's frustration," but his office must retain psychiatrists to testify about the sanity of accused people in order to get a neutral opinion.

"There are psychiatrists who can be retained by defence counsel who will pretty well say whatever the defence wants them to say. We have to check to see exactly what's happening."

Jerry Cooper, a psychiatrist who often appears as a defence witness, said Dr. Fleming's reference to shopping around for psychiatrists is silly.

"I don't know of any psychiatrist so desperate he has to hire out. ... If a defence lawyer gets an opinion adverse to his case, why should he just take my opinion?

"We just give out opinions and the lawyer decides. If a neurosurgeon said he had to open your head up, wouldn't you get a second opinion? I can be wrong, you know. Dr. Fleming can be wrong, too. We're not gods."

He said it would be destructive to justice if psychiatrists could not testify in dangerous offender applications. "It's a sentence that's worse than life imprisonment. There are guys who were put there 15 years ago who are still there."

Dr. Fleming's remarks came after he testified in the Supreme Court of Ontario concerning a Crown application to have a convicted rapist designated a dangerous offender.

A 24-year-old man with a long record of breaking and entering was convicted in December of raping a woman while holding a knife to her throat.

He had one previous rape conviction, but the Ontario Court of Appeal ordered another trial at which the man was found not guilty.

"We and the police are satisfied he has done it twice anyway," John McIsaac, the Crown attorney handling the case, said in an interview. Persuading the judge hearing the dangerous-offender application that the man could commit another rape will be tough because of the successful appeal, he said. "But I'm going to try and revive it.

"Fortunately for the victims, they went along with him when he produced the knife. But if the next lady panics, we'll be investigating a murder, not a rape."

Dr. Fleming testified that his unit could not conduct a psychiatric assessment of the man now because it is filled to capacity. "There's simply too much at stake to do it in a hurry."

14. On March 22, 1982, Zehr was further remanded to May 10, 1982, on the dangerous offender application.

15. On May 10, 1982, at Toronto, the dangerous offender application commenced before Craig J. Crown counsel filed what was marked before me as ex. No. 3 (Crown submission on the admissibility of evidence) and submitted that on the Part XXI application, the Crown should be allowed to introduce the evidence it called at the trial of Zehr when it alleged that he raped the female "X" although the jury had acquitted Zehr of that offence (count No. 1).

16. On May 11, 1982, Craig J. ruled that the proposed evidence regarding female "X" on Count No. I was inadmissible (ex. No. 4).

17. On May 17, 1982, Craig J. dismissed the Crown's application under Part XXI, s.688(b) of the *Criminal Code*; on the same date Craig J. sentenced Zehr to five years on the conviction of rape on count No. 2 of the indictment and ordered a five-year prohibition under s.98(1) [rep. & sub. 1976-77, c.53, s.3] of the *Criminal Code*.

IV The case against Makin, Doyle and the publisher, the corporate defendant

Counsel for these respondents admits that Makin was the newspaper reporter, Doyle the editor-in-chief of *The Globe and Mail* and that the corporate defendant was the publisher of the article.

At the request of counsel for the Attorney-General and over the objections of counsel for the applicant, I permitted four exhibits to be filed by counsel for the Attorney General:

(a) Exhibit No. 1 — a certified copy of the two count indictment against Zehr preferred by the Attorney-General of Ontario;

(b) Exhibit No. 2 — a partial transcript of submissions made to Craig J. on February 8, 1982;

(c) Exhibit No. 3 — Crown submissions filed before Craig J. on May 10, 1982

(d) Exhibit No. 4 — Craig J.'s ruling regarding the proposed evidence on the dangerous offender application that concerned count No. 1 in the indictment.

Counsel for the newspaper respondents submits that the article in question is not a contempt of court because:

1. the article in question does not name Zehr either directly or indirectly;
2. the article was published on February 9, 1982; the dangerous offender hearing was held on May 10, 1982, some three months later;
3. the *Criminal Code* required that Craig J., and he alone, be the judge to hear the Part XXI, s.688(b) application because Craig J. had been the trial judge on the trial of count No. 2.
4. The most appropriate forum for this motion was before Craig J. at the opening of the Part XXI, s.688(b) application. No such application was made to Craig J., the only person who could possibly have been prejudiced by the article in question.
5. On May 10, 1982, Craig J. heard the Crown's allegations that Zehr raped the female "X" — indeed the Crown's written submissions, ex. No. 3, deal exclusively with those allegations.
6. The article in question appeared on p. 5 of *The Globe and Mail*; the portions of the article that are attacked are the 16th, 17th, 18th and 19th paras. of a 20-para. article.
7. There is no allegation that any of these respondents intended to subvert the course of justice.

V. What is the test, what are the rules against which the impugned article is to be measured?

(i) *R. v. Payne and Cooper*, [1896] 1 Q.B. 577, 74 L.T. 351 at 352, *per* Lord Russell C.J.:

> That this summary power is most salutary no one can doubt, and it is a power which the court will not hesitate to use where there is any attempt to interfere with the administration of justice. But it is an arbitrary power, and, therefore, it ought to be used only in cases where the needs of justice call for its exercise. The learned counsel seems to think that every libel upon a person under trial is a contempt, but this is not necessarily so. To justify the exercise of this summary power something must have been published which was intended or clearly calculated to prejudice the fair trial of the charge or action.

per Wright J. [at p. 353 L.T.]:

I agree entirely in what the Lord Chief Justice has said. As is pointed out by Cotton, L.J., in *Re O'Malley, Hunt v. Clarke* (1889), 61 L.T. 343, in all cases of this kind there are two questions involved. The first is: Is the publication of such a nature as to be calculated to interfere with a fair trial? If it is not so calculated, we have nothing to do with it. But even if it is calculated to interfere with a fair trial there is a second question. Is it a proper case for such an application? The rule laid down in *Re O'Malley, Hunt v. Clarke* (supra) for answering this is that such an application should not be made except in serious cases.

(ii) *R. v. Duffy et al.; Ex parte Nash*, [1960] 2 Q.B. 188, [1960] 2 All E.R. 891, Lord Parker C.J. at p. 896 All E.R.:

The question always is whether a judge would be so influenced by the article that his impartiality might well be consciously, or even unconsciously, affected. In other words, was there a real risk, as opposed to a remote possibility, that the article was calculated to prejudice a fair hearing?

(iii) *A.-G. v. Times Newspapers Ltd.*, [1974] A.C. 273, [1973] 3 All E.R. 54 at 63-64 (H.L.) *per* Lord Reid:

I think agreeing with Cotton L.J. in his judgment in *Hunt v. Clarke* (1889), 58 L.J.Q.B. 490, that there must be two questions: first, was there any contempt at all? and secondly, was it sufficiently serious to require or justify the court in making an order against the respondent? The question whether there was a serious risk of influencing the litigant is certainly a factor to be considered in what course to take by way of punishment, as is the intention with which the comment was made. But it is I think confusing to import this into the question whether there was any contempt at all or into the definition of contempt.

I think the true view is that expressed by Lord Parker C.J. in *R. v. Duffy, ex parte Nash*, [1960] 2 All E.R. 891 at 896, [1960] 2 Q.B. 188 at 200, that there must be "a real risk as opposed to a remote possibility". That is an application of the ordinary de minimis principle. There is no contempt if the possibility of influence is remote. If there is some but only a small likelihood, that may influence the court to refrain from inflicting any punishment. If there is a serious risk some action may be necessary. And I think that the particular comment cannot be considered in isolation when considering its probable effect. If others are to be free and are likely to make similar comments that must be taken into account.

(iv) *Meriden Britannia Co. Ltd. v. Walters* (1915), 34 O.L.R. 518 at 521, 25 D.L.R. 167, 24 C.C.C. 364, *per* Boyd C.:

The apprehension of detriment must be of a tangible character, plainly tending to obstruct or prejudice the due administration of justice in the particular case pending. Regard must be had to all the surrounding circumstances: the manner of trial, the time of publication, the causes leading to the publication, and the tenour of what is published.

(v) *R. v. Duffy, per* Lord Parker C.J. pp. 894-95 All E.R.:

In the present case there is no suggestion of any such intention, and the sole question is whether the article when published on May 10 was in all the circumstances calculated to interfere or calculated really to interfere with the hearing of the appeal, should one be brought. Looking at it in that way and in the absence of authority, we should have thought that the answer was plainly: "No". Even if a judge who eventually sat on the appeal had seen the article in question and had remembered its contents, it is inconceivable that he would be influenced consciously or unconsciously by it. A judge is in a very different position to a juryman. Though in no sense superhuman, he has by his training no difficulty in putting out of his mind matters which are not evidence in the case. This indeed happens daily to judges on Assize. This is all the more so in the case of a member of the Court of Criminal Appeal . . .

(vi) *Re Depoe et al. and Lamport et al.*, [1968] 1 O.R. 185, 66 D.L.R. (2d) 46, [1968] 2 C.C.C. 209 at 213, (H.C.J.).

The defendant Lamport was then a controller of the City of Toronto; on the day after the arrest of certain "hippies" he expressed his hope to the press that the courts would treat those people seriously on their charges of disturbing the peace.

Per Donohue J. at p. 189 O.R.:

> The statements taken at their worst imply an assumption of the guilt of the accused and an attempt on the part of Mr. Lamport to prescribe a certain punishment for the offence.
>
> It is to be remembered that the alleged offences will be tried not by juries but necessarily by a Magistrate. The Magistrates are professional Judges and I cannot conceive that any of them would be affected by Mr. Lamport's opinion as to the guilt of the accused. Likewise, in the matter of punishment for the offence it is inconceivable that Mr. Lamport's views would exert the slightest influence.

VI Conclusions

When I consider the type and tenor of the article, the lead on the article, the position of the article in the newspaper (p. 5), the absence of Zehr's name from the article, the absence of any sensationalism in connection with the article, the date of the article in relation to the date of the hearing, the fact that only one person, Craig J., was qualified to hear the proposed application under s.688(b) of the *Criminal Code*, that in court on May 10, 1982, Craig J. heard that Zehr had been charged, convicted and on a new trial had been found not guilty of the rape of the female "X", and considering the fact that Craig J. would have seen the two-count indictment as of the date of arraignment on December 1, 1981, 1 am led to the inevitable conclusion that "no judge would be so influenced by the article that his impartiality might be consciously or even unconsciously affected"; there was no real risk that the article was calculated to prejudice a fair hearing.

VII Result

The application is dismissed as against Makin, Doyle and the corporate defendant.

3.3.3.3.3 Bellitti v. Canadian Broadcasting Corp. (1973), 2 O.R. (2d) 232 (Ont.H.C.)

ZUBER, J. (orally): — This is an application to continue an injunction issued by Mr. Justice Fraser on November 6th, 1973.

Earlier this year, Mr. Bellitti, the applicant, was arrested and charged with three narcotic offences and was tried together with others before His Honour Judge Honsberger and a jury in the City of Toronto. The applicant Bellitti was convicted of conspiracy to import heroin and was acquitted on the other two charges. He is to be sentenced on November 12, 1973. He has appealed his conviction and it is said that he may independently also appeal the sentence.

On November 6th of this year, Mr. Fay, counsel for Mr. Bellitti, became aware that the Canadian Broadcasting Corporation was, in his words, "about to televise a documentary concerning the trial". On that basis an application was made to Mr. Justice Fraser who issued the order now before me. The order restrains the CBC from "communicating to the public in any form any of the proceedings before His Honour Judge Honsberger and the jury".

Clearly, the CBC has the right to freedom of the press, which is a variation of the liberty enjoyed by all of us as freedom of speech. It is obvious as well that this right is not an absolute right, but ends where such things as defamation, sedition, obscenity and contempt of Court begin. The problem in discerning the border, however, is frequently a difficult one and involves the balancing of competing public interests such as the freedom of speech and of the press and the public interest in the proper administration of justice. In this case, it is argued that the broadcast of this programme would constitute a contempt of Court. Contempt can take many forms, but in this case the point in issue is that this broadcast would constitute an interference with the administration of justice or, in other words, would prejudice a fair trial.

In my view, the argument to continue the injunction in its present form is completely untenable. Justice is administered in public and it is in the public interest that the proceedings be freely reported, save only those specific instances where prohibition of publicity is provided by statute. It is only when publication or broadcast departs from factual reporting and expresses comments or opinions and those comments or opinions interfere with the administration of justice or prejudice a fair trial that the broadcast or publication will constitute contempt of Court. The injunction, as it presently stands, would prohibit simple reporting and it seems to me obvious that this injunction cannot stand. The more particular question that faces us is whether an injunction in more modified terms should stand, that is, should the CBC be enjoined from broadcasting the specific programme which is the subject of this application on the grounds that it will interfere with the administration of justice or prejudice a fair trial.

In the affidavit material filed, the programme is simply described as "a documentary concerning the trial of the applicant". That bald assertion is not helpful. So, with the consent of counsel and in the presence of all of us, the film was shown. The film was entitled "Flour of the Poppy". It purported to show the facts disclosed at trial. This was done pictorially by showing places, vehicles, houses and so forth; the movements of people were depicted pictorially by the utilization of actors, but I pause to observe that with the exception of one or two minor instances there was no dialogue between the actors. A narrator described the events. It is said by counsel that this pictorial portrayal represents nothing more than the evidence that was given at trial. There is no material before me that suggests anything to the contrary. This pictorial representation related the facts upon which the prosecution was based. Later there was disclosure of the fact of arrest and trial and pictures were shown of the Metropolitan Toronto Court

House, the empty interior of a court-room in that building and so forth. The narrator announced the length of the trial, I believe the name of the presiding Judge and the verdict of the jury and perhaps the length of time that it took them to reach a verdict.

The film also showed in another segment the process of growing poppies and producing heroin and the profits to be made. The film also showed a police officer who commented upon the shortage of police and there was some speculation as to whether or not activity of a similar sort was still going on undetected, but this was of a general nature. Specifically, there was no comment made or opinion expressed as to whether or not the verdict of the jury was right or wrong. There was no comment or opinion expressed, as I saw and heard the film, as to the sentence that should be given. In my opinion, there was no undue dramatization or emphasis of the matter which would indirectly operate on the mind of whoever pronounces sentence.

Since the jury has already reached a verdict of guilty, the question of the interference with the administration of justice or the issue of prejudice, as I understand the argument of the applicant, relates to three areas. Obviously the exhibition of this film can hardly prejudice the minds of the jurors who have now been discharged.

The first issue to be looked at is whether or not the exhibition of this film will interfere with the administration of justice in so far as it concerns the duty yet to be performed by Judge Honsberger in the pronouncing of sentence. As I have already stated, there is no comment in the film by way of directly or indirectly urging a high sentence or a low sentence. There is nothing in the film, as I saw it and heard it, that attempts to characterize the accused as a person who might deserve either a high or a low sentence. The maximum view that can be taken of this film is that simply because it is a pictorial representation rather than a printed account, it might have some extra impact. I cannot believe that this would make any difference to the mind of a professional Judge.

The second point raised by the applicant is the effect of the film on the pending appeal. As I have mentioned, I found nothing in the nature of comment in the film. However, even if any of the statements in the programme could be construed as comments, there is no prejudice to the appeal.

In *Attorney-General v. Times Newspapers Ltd.*, [1973] 3 All E.R. 54 at p. 65, Lord Reid said: "... it is scarcely possible to imagine a case where comment could influence judges in the Court of Appeal ...", and Lord Simon stated at p. 83: "... any comment on pending appellate proceedings could only rarely be intrinsically an interference with the due course of law."

I subscribe to those views.

The third argument raised by the applicant relates to the effect of this film on jurors selected in a new trial, if that situation should arise. It is clear at once that all of this is largely speculative, hinged on the success of the appeal and on the fact that there may be a new trial, which is not the inevitable result of a successful appeal. This argument that a subsequent jury would accept this pictorial representation as fact and would thereby in some way be prejudiced in their assessment of the evidence at the subsequent trial, taken to its logical conclusion would lead to the prohibition of reporting any trial. A second trial always creates the possibility that the jurors in the second trial may be prejudiced by knowing something of the first one, either by having been present at the trial or having simply read the newspaper accounts. This problem is simply met and sorted out in the jury selection process. It seems to me that anyone seeing this programme would be in no different position with respect to service on a subsequent jury, if that eventuality arises, than would anyone who had either been at the trial or read newspaper accounts of it.

The fact that a new trial is only a possibility, and the fact that a person who watches this programme is really in no different position than those who either saw the trial or read about it, lead me to the conclusion that there is no real risk of prejudicing a fair trial or interfering with the administration of justice.

The application to continue the injunction is dismissed and the injunction dissolved.

A number of procedural arguments were raised by the CBC, upon which I express no opinion. It is not necessary for me to deal with them in view of the disposition that I have made of the matter on the merits.

Note: Recent decisions suggest that subjudice may have some application to proceedings before appellate courts. See, for example, *Lortie v. R.* (1985), 46 C.R. (3d) 322.

3.3.3.3.4 *Bielek v. Ristimaki* (1979), (Ont.H.C.) in Stuart Robertson, *Courts and the Media* (Toronto: Butterworth, 1981), pp. 287-292

HENRY, J.: Now, this matter now comes before me at the end of an aborted trial in the action Hendrick R. Bielek v. Albert J. Ristimaki, which commenced on Monday last, June 18th, and has continued in one form or another until today, June 21st. Yesterday, after hearing an application by counsel for the defendant arising out of the publication of a press report in the Timmins Daily Press of June 19th, which included a specific reference to the amount of $500,000 being claimed by the plaintiff for libel and slander, which information was not conveyed to the jury and was therefore not mentioned in their presence in the court. The application was that I, should proceed without a jury and discharge the jury. As I found, I am not authorized to do that in the absence of a waiver of the right to a trial by jury in a defamation action, which is prescribed by the *Judicature Act* [R.S.O. 1970, c.228, as am.]. On the basis of the facts before me and as I indicate in my reasons, because the publication in the press of the amount of the damages claimed must be assumed to find its way in one form or another to one or more members of the jury, I made the decision at what was an early stage of the trial which had proceeded to the point where only the plaintiff had been examined in chief, to abort the trial, declare a mistrial, and discharge the jury.

Because this matter arose out of the press report that I have mentioned, I called for the attendance of representatives and counsel for the newspaper, and for the attendance of the reporter who wrote the report. All are now before me with their counsel Mr. G.C. Evans, Q.C., who acts on behalf of the newspaper, Thomson Publications, and who is also acting for Mr. Peter Black, the reporter, and Mr. Gregory Reynolds, the editor of the Timmins Daily Press. I have heard evidence called by Mr. Evans from both Mr. Black and from Mr. Reynolds, and I have heard the submissions of Mr. Evans on my request that he now show cause why one or more of those persons should not be found in contempt of this court. I may say that I have had great assistance from Mr. Evans, as well as from other counsel, although other counsel did not take part in this particular proceeding.

I find that the press report in question was published in the June 19th issue of the Timmins Daily Press, and that it contained the offending information about the amount of $500,000 claimed by the plaintiff in his pleadings against the defendant. There is no doubt, as Mr. Evans has quite properly conceded, that publication of this information in the circumstances was wrong. It is in evidence, and it was submitted to me by counsel, that this publication was primarily the result of inexperience on the part of a young reporter. I might say that the reporter, Mr. Black, acknowledges that. The information in question concerning the amount of damages claimed was not placed in evidence before the jury and is in no way before them to his knowledge. It is also in evidence that he was asked by his editor, Mr. Reynolds, whether the information in the report was all placed before the court in the presence of the jury, and that he assured his editor that this was so. In this of course, he was quite wrong, but I do not think that in telling his editor that he was actuated in any way by malice, or an attempt to say something which to his knowledge was not true. The amount of damages claimed was published contrary to the well-known rule in the conduct of trials before juries that information of any kind whatever that takes place in the courtroom in the absence of the jury ought not to be published in the news media during the currency of the trial. There is, of course, no obstacle to its publication at a later stage, and I emphasize that, because this is not a muzzle on the press — it is not to keep the public from knowing what happened; it is merely a rule of fairness and convenience to assure that the jury will not read for example of matters that are discussed in a voir dire which ought not to be brought to the attention of the jury and for which purpose the jury are excluded. As I say, that rule is well-known to reporters and editors generally in my experience, and there is no doubt about that before me. I find that the reporting of that figure so far as the reporter, Mr. Black is concerned, was deliberate although mistaken. The editor, Mr. Reynolds, has made an apology to the court orally when in the witness box for the course that was taken. The result of what happened is a mistrial and if I may put the matter bluntly, is, in this particular case, a subversion of the system of justice. The parties and the public have been put to considerable expense for the period of the trial which turned out to be abortive, and therefore that expense, and the time of those concerned, both of the parties, and witnesses, and counsel, has been to no avail. I might describe those costs and expenses perhaps in well-known terms as "costs thrown away."

In my opinion, it is the obligation of press reporters and their editors who control the publication of news in the media, whether the press or the electronic media, to ensure that what is published are matters that may be revealed, and also to ensure that they know the rules governing trials which specify what matters ought not to be published in the course of a trial. I emphasize that the responsibility is on a free but responsible press to be informed about those matters as part of their professional expertise. They are, after all, professionals and are, in my judgment, to be held accountable as such. In short they must know what they are doing when what they do may affect the rights of other people. This is only another way of saying that in a democratic regime, characterized by, among other things, a free press, the freedom conferred on the press (to use the well-known phrase appearing in Canada at least in the Alberta Press case) is freedom governed by law. The press is not free to invade the rights of others, and the liberties of others without being held to account in accordance with law. So, I say that surely it is incumbent upon those who publish, certainly professionally, to exercise a duty to inform themselves fully as professional people, as to what they may and may not publish, and particularly the time at which publication may be made. I accordingly find, and I do so beyond a reasonable doubt, that the newspaper, the Timmins Daily Press, as a corporation, is in contempt of this court for the action which has been taken. There can be no question that in our democratic society a free press is a fundamental pillar of our polity. It is also fundamental to the fair and impartial administration of justice by an independent judiciary. That a free press be at liberty to comment on and to publish proceedings in the courts, both the right of the public to know and the duty of in this case the professional press to report what is going on in a court, as well as in other parts of society, is so fundamental that it need not be further restated. Equally fundamental is.the right of the citizen to bring his complaints before the courts to have a fair and impartial adjudication of his dispute with another citizen carried out and resolved in accordance with the principles which have been laid down over many many years in the common law courts to ensure the proper enforcement of those rights and to give the citizen his day in court. The right of free speech, and the right of the citizen that I have described, to a fair and impartial trial has been won at great cost and with great pain over the years and over, at times apparently, insurmountable odds against the executive and against powerful agencies in the state, whether public or private. The courts have, in our democratic society, been the organs which have established and maintained those rights. It is the right of every citizen to a trial by a jury in criminal and civil cases, and particularly in a defamation action, but that right, so far, from being supported and maintained by a free press, can be impaired and subverted by untutored or irresponsible exercise of the right to publish. The most important role of the press in respect of trials in our courts is to inform the public of what is happening and to monitor the system by close and informed scrutiny, and fair and responsible comment and criticism. It is not the role of the press to conduct itself in a way which will impair the effective and fair work of the judicial system, but the line must be drawn as here, where the right of the parties to a fair trial by jury is impaired or destroyed by an improper disclosure; indeed a disclosure at an inopportune time. The information may be published; that is it is not to be withheld from the public, but it ought not to be published at a time when justice may be impaired. In other words it's a question of timing, and one of the problems the press faces in these days is the timing of its news releases, which I think experience has shown, sometimes takes priority over the fairness of the publication at that particular time. Except in rare cases the public may ultimately be told all the information that is available. The question arises that the statement of claim from which the offending information was taken, is a public document. It is true that any press reporter is at liberty to go to the registrar's office and be shown the file which is a public document, except to the extent that portions of it may be, for good and sufficient reason by order of the court, sealed. That is not the case here, and those cases are indeed rare. Moreover there has been much publicity at an earlier stage concerning the damages asked of one-half million dollars in this case, but that publicity occurred some time ago, in November, 1977. Generally speaking there is no inhibition on the press reporting factual information at an early stage, although that is a matter which must be dealt with with caution, but if that information were still fresh in the minds of the public the court might feel it necessary to change the venue, but as is well known, the passage of time tends to make memories dim, and it frequently occurs that even where there has been wide publicity at a much earlier stage, a court does not consider that a fair trial will be impaired, for the very simple reason that it is not freshly brought into the minds of a jury panel, or the jury themselves if the press conducts itself properly. I should add that neither the judge nor the counsel could put the offending information about the amount of damages claimed to the jury in the court room without giving rise to a mistrial, and the press cannot be above that. The parties and the public in this case have been put to the expanse of this abortive trial. In my opinion the press, who caused this situation, ought to be held accountable to the parties at least for the consequences of the improper report.

There is already an apology on behalf of the corporation involved, but I think it necessary to go beyond that. The contempt of the corporation, Thomson Newspapers, may in this case, be purged by payment to the two parties of their costs thrown away by the declaration of the mistrial arising out of the conduct of the press. The amount in question I am prepared to fix at $2500 to each party. The contempt will be purged if payment is made by Thomson Newspapers, or the Timmins Daily Press of the amount of $2500 to the solicitor for each party. That payment, in order to purge the contempt, is to be made on or before June 30th, 1979. In default of such payment being made I impose a fine upon the corporate newspaper of $7500, which fine shall be paid by cheque into the office of the Registrar of this Court in Toronto.

I turn now to the case of the reporter, Mr. Black. For the above reasons I find with some regret, that Mr. Black is in contempt of this court as is his employer, but he may purge that contempt by filing a written apology with this court. This apology may be made by letter addressed to The Registrar of the Supreme Court of Ontario, in Cochrane, to be forwarded to Toronto. No other penalty will be imposed.

I have also considered the position of the editor, Mr. Reynolds, and I do not propose to find him in contempt in view of the circumstances. He was given an incorrect assurance by his reporter that the facts were all facts placed before the jury, and that matter is therefore closed.

I add, in a general way, that in my opinion the course of responsible journalism (if I may use that phrase) is to know and inform the reporting staff of what matters, even those contained in public documents or in previous media reports, must not be published in circumstances that may come to the knowledge of the jury, or of a jury panel summoned for the assize at which a trial will take place. I give by way of example of such information only, and it's clearly not exhaustive, the one before me; namely general damages claimed, which, as is well known, can be quite misleading; payment of money into court by a defendant as part of the conduct of the pretrial proceedings; and the fact that an insurance company, or some other indemnifier is going to pay any damages assessed against a defendant. Those, as I say, are not exhaustive, but they are examples we will find. Pleadings generally, unless they have been read to the jury, or proved by evidence at the trial, if published may not necessarily be fatal, but their publication does create the grave risk of alleging what a reporter may think are facts that are never in fact proved before the jury. In other words I think I should make it plain that public documents such as pleadings, that may come into the hands of a reporter, should be treated with the greatest caution because they may contain allegations which ought not to be known to the jury, whose task it is to decide the case only on the evidence placed before them as all jurors are firmly told by the trial judge. Usually the general facts upon which the case will be tried are disclosed in the opening address of counsel for the plaintiff to the jury. That, being made in open court is the source of the information from which press reports may properly be derived in most circumstances.

Those are my reasons gentlemen. I don't think there is anything I need to add. I will endorse on the record what I have just said, and perhaps I can do that in the lunch hour and read it to you gentlemen.

Gentlemen I believe I can now dispose of the matter of the change of venue. I intend to change the venue because if nothing else the publicity that has been during this week given to the issue that is being raised will be in people's minds in this community of some knowledge it might be difficult for them to have forgotten. I wouldn't say that it would not be possible to get a jury who hadn't heard of it, but in view of the nature of the question that gave rise to the mistrial, which is an extremely simple one, a simple fact might very well remain in people's minds over the course of the summer, so in the result therefore I have decided that I should change the venue to Bracebridge. I have looked at not only the state of the list there, but the state of the list in the other centres as well and I may simply say to you that although that assize will not start until the beginning of October, that the list is extremely short and there are only about two days' work ahead of you; and indeed the trial judge may be able to bring you on right away; that's up to him, so the venue will be changed then to the Fall Assize in Bracebridge. It starts October the 9th. There are two civil jury cases on the list which are forecast for two days total, and I think that probably it's up to counsel to speak to the trial judge and he of course will have to tell you whether he can bring you on at once, or wait for those two.

Now, gentlemen I endorse the following:

> Venue is changed to Bracebridge. Set down for trial at the assize comrnencing October 9th. 1979. The case is peremptory for the defendant. Any preliminary motions at the outset of trial to be on proper notice to the other party and the costs of this motion I would propose gentlemen, to reserve for the trial judge.

. . . . .

I think I would be remiss gentlemen, if I didn't say, when leaving the courtroom, to Mr. Black's superior, Mr. Reynolds, who is here, Mr. Reynolds I have put a considerable amount of blame on Mr. Black because he was the reporter on the firing line. I tried to make it plain to him that I thought he was not properly instructed and I think in that sense, in the instruction of reporters who go out to report a sophisticated thing like a jury trial, it isn't sufficient to send them out and give them one rule of thumb. I wouldn't like it to be thought that I was criticizing Mr. Black in the carrying out of his job. I think if he did anything wrong it was because he was not properly instructed.

Finding of contempt made; change of venue ordered

3.3.3.3.5 *Re Church of Scientology of Toronto v. The Queen (No. 6)* (1986), 27 C.C.C. (3d) 193 (Ont.H.C.)

WATT, J.: It would plainly appear that simple fear of embarrassment, whether of a witness or an accused person, is not a sufficient basis upon which to found a blanket prohibition enjoining in perpetuity publication of the identity of an accused or of the identity or evidence of a witness, actual or proposed. It would seem clear that the purpose of any order prohibiting publication, of whatever length and in whatever terms, is to protect the integrity of the court's process not merely to minimize the embarrassment of those changed with or giving evidence of crime.

It is, indeed, almost a commonplace where several accused jointly indicted are together presented for trial at a jury sittings that, upon a plea of guilty being entered by one or more accused upon arraignment before the presiding judge, to direct that there be no publication of the fact of such plea, the "facts" tendered in support of it, representations made and reasons given at the conclusion of the plea proceedings until the conclusion of the proceedings pending against the co-accused. Such orders are made and equally salutary whether the offence charged is listed in s.427 of the *Criminal Code* or otherwise and whether the plea is preceded by re-election for trial by judge alone or consent to trial by judge alone by the accused who enters the plea of guilty. It would generally not seem to be thought that an order suspending publication is necessary in the event that all remaining accused are to be tried by judge alone or provincial court judge. It is assumed that in such cases the presiding judge is less likely to be affected by the publication of such information. For jurisdictional purposes, in my view, it matters not whether the judge to whom the application is made is, in circumstances like the present, sitting under Part XVI of the *Criminal Code* or whether he or she is presiding at a jury sittings whose procedure is regulated by Part XVII of the *Criminal Code*. The court is none the less a court of record and the fairness of the pending trials ought equally to be their concern. It is absolutely critical that if an order for non-publication is to be made that it be made in the plea of guilty proceedings, for in the event that it should not there be made it will be of no avail if left to the judge presiding in the jury trial thereafter taking place as the damage occasioned by such publicity may well, by then, have been done.

III Conclusion

It is, accordingly, my respectful view that, as a court of record, a provincial court judge, acting under Part XVI in receiving a plea of guilty tendered by one of several accused jointly charged has authority to entertain an application, on behalf of another or other accused jointly charged, for an order suspending publication of such matters disclosed in the proceedings upon the plea of guilty as may reasonably be said, if published, to impair the appearance of fairness in subsequent proceedings taken against such co-accused.

3.3.3.3.6 *C.B.C. v. Keegstra* (1986), 35 D.L.R. (4th) 76 (Alta. C.A.)

KERANS, J.A.: — In this case the appellant Canadian Broadcasting Corporation proposed to broadcast a television drama in Alberta on December 8, 1985. The story was set in Ontario and involved a teacher who advocated anti-Semitism in the class-room. An injunction against publication was sought by the respondent Keegstra, who stands convicted in Alberta of wilfully promoting hatred of an identifiable group. He was convicted by a jury in July, 1985. The particulars in that case were that he allegedly promoted hatred of Jews when he taught school.

Keegstra had filed a notice of appeal of that conviction and the matter was before this court but not yet heard. That situation obtains today.

On December 6, 1985, Keegstra issued a statement of claim against the appellant sounding in defamation and made an emergent application that very Friday in Queen's Bench Chambers. The matter came on in such a rush that most material was hand-written. His counsel saw a videotape of the proposed show but the judge did not.

Notwithstanding the allegation of defamation, the judgment of the learned chambers judge does not deal with that subject. He seems rather to have approached the matter as an application for a *quia timet* injunction against a feared *sub judice* contempt in terms of the pending appeal in the criminal case involving Mr. Keegstra and any new trial which this court might order. The learned chambers judge enjoined the appellant and the appellant appealed.

The case was argued before us this morning on the issue of administration of justice, not defamation, notwithstanding obvious procedural irregularities. We have noticed, for example, that the order has no relevance to the statement of claim, that the application probably should have been heard by this court as an aspect of the pending appeal, and that the prosecutor or the Attorney-General of Alberta should have been heard. We put these procedural difficulties down to the rush of events on December 6, 1985, although we must observe the parties do not explain why they were not corrected in the 10 months they took to prepare themselves for this appeal. Notwithstanding our grave misgivings about the validity of the order on procedural grounds, we will deal with the case therefore on its merits because both parties invite us to do so.

The learned chambers judge found that:

> The play appears to be a thinly-guised characterization of the plaintiff, Keegstra, in this action.

and that Alberta viewers would find "an association" with him. Mr. Christie, counsel for Mr. Keegstra, says that this is an acceptance of his argument that the play is a vilification of Mr. Keegstra. We disagree. The learned chambers judge says only:

> ... it characterizes a person presently before the courts ... in an unfavourable manner which might influence proceedings ...

For the purposes of this appeal, it is not necessary for us to agree or disagree that this play unfairly "characterizes" Mr. Keegstra.

The learned chambers judge enjoined broadcast because he said the play was a possible contempt. He says: "I must say better not to publish than be damned later." While perhaps a prudent rule for self-restraint, this is, with respect, the wrong test for the granting of an injunction against a proposed publication on the ground that it might interfere with the administration of justice. The test rather is this: is there a real and substantial risk that a fair trial will be impossible in the circumstances of the case if publication is allowed? Not every act which might be criminal can be enjoined: see *A.-G. Alta. v. Plantation Indoor Plants Ltd.*

(1982), 133 D.L.R. (3d) 741, 65 C.C.C. (2d) 544, 34 A.R. 348 (C.A.). Thus, it is possible that an attempt to interfere with the course of justice might be criminal because intentional and yet not enjoined because ineffectual: see *A.-G. v. Times Newspapers Ltd.*, [1973] 3 All E.R. 54 at p. 74 (Lord Diplock). We take this almost to be common ground. Mr. Christie points to the decision in *Re Regina and Lortie* (1985), 21 C.C.C. (3d) 436, [1985] Que. C.A. 451, 46 C.R. (3d) 322, but we do not consider this to be authority to the contrary. Nor do we retreat from what was said by Chief Justice Harvey in *Hatfield v. Healy* (1911), 3 Alta. L.R. 327, 18 W.L.R. 512. The law has many means to protect the right of an accused person to a fair trial. The first is the jury selection process itself, which permits the challenge of a prospective juror who is not indifferent as between the accused and the Crown. Another important protection is to change the venue of the trial when the judge is of the view that an entire local population is inflamed against the accused. Yet another is to delay the trial. Yet another is a warning to the jury about the need impartially to judge the accused. The rules about *sub judice* contempt are simply yet another means to assure a fair trial. They are, however, only invoked when the others likely will not be effective. Thus, for example, the contempt power is more readily invoked *during* a trial, after a jury is chosen, because it is then almost the only weapon remaining in the judicial arsenal to assure justice for all. That was the case in *Hatfield v. Healy*.

The risk to the administration of justice posed by the publication here involves many contingencies: that Mr. Keegstra win his appeal, that this court decide that a new trial be ordered, that potential jurors will have seen this programme, that they will have been inflamed against Mr. Keegstra by it, that they remain so at the time of jury selection, that they will not be successfully challenged during the jury selection process, and that a fair array of potential jurors could not then be found.

It is important, we think, at this point to stress these facts: the appellant wanted to publish this programme on December 8, 1985. As we have said, Mr. Keegstra's appeal had then only just been launched. It has not yet been heard, and if a new trial were to be ordered by this court it would (because it will take more than a week) not commence according to the standard practice in Queen's Bench for at least six months. It is even now not likely that any new trial would occur before 1988. Remembering all this, it is our judgment that nothing said for the respondent here, nor anything in the material before us, persuades us that there was any real or substantial risk of the realization of at least the last two possibilities just mentioned, that prejudiced jurors could not be challenged for cause nor a disinterested array found. Thus, the risk of an interference with the course of justice is not real or substantial.

This is not to say that the courts will hesitate later to intervene in some way if Mr. Christie's fears are justified and the showing stirs a debate in Alberta which so inflames the public that a fair trial might be impossible. We simply say that he has not persuaded us on the material before us today that publication of this programme on December 8, 1985, would have produced those dire consequences.

Mr. Christie says in his factum:

> The film is really a piece of propaganda which creates an emotionally powerful mix of fact and fiction to create maximum damage to the reputation of the accused while his case is still before the courts. It is skillfully fabricated to even include and refute some of his counsel's arguments at trial into the early stages of this story, which does not itself include a trial. The process is designed for maximum prejudicial impact with no legal responsibility.

These are serious allegations. They should be the subject of investigation. No doubt the Attorney-General of Alberta will cause appropriate inquiries to be made if the programme is indeed shown in Alberta. We will say no more about that except to urge upon the appellant that Mr. Christie and the Attorney-General of Alberta should be given adequate notice of any publication.

In the result, because the requirements for an injunction of this sort have not been made out on application of the correct test, we allow the appeal and vacate the order made.

We wish to emphasize that this is not an order permitting publication. The Canadian Broadcasting Corporation publishes at its risk. We have simply said that publication of this programme on December 8, 1985, would not have interfered with the due administration of justice. This being so, we do not reach the issue whether the rule here invoked is a reasonable limit on free speech in a free and democratic society.

Appeal allowed.

3.3.3.3.7 *C.B.C. v. Dagenais et al.* (1992), 12 O.R. (3d) 239 (Ont.C.A.)

DUBIN, C.J.O.: — This is an appeal by Canadian Broadcasting Corporation from the judgment of Madam Justice Gotlib restraining it from broadcasting the program "The Boys of St. Vincent" anywhere in Canada and from publishing in any media any information relating to the proposed broadcast program, until the completion of the criminal trials of the four respondents, and prohibiting the publication of the fact of the application before her or any other material relating to it.

At the commencement of the appeal, leave was granted to the National Film Board of Canada and John Newton Smith and to Thomson Newspapers Company Limited, to be added as intervener appellants. At the conclusion of the argument, because of the urgency of the matter, the court announced its judgment, with reasons to follow.

Facts

The respondents are members of a Catholic religious order known as the Christian Brothers, and are either former Christian Brothers or present Christian Brothers. They are all charged with physical and sexual abuse that allegedly took place in Catholic training schools where the respondents were teachers and the victims young boys who were in their care. At the time of the hearing before Madam Justice Gotlib and before us, the trial of one of the respondents was in progress in L'Orignal. The other three respondents are scheduled to be tried, one in L'Orignal in February, and the other two in Oshawa, one in April and the other between May and July.

The Canadian Broadcasting Corporation proposed to broadcast a four-hour mini-series entitled, "The Boys of St. Vincent". The broadcast was to be in two two-hour segments, one on Sunday evening, December 6, 1992, and the other on the following evening.

The court was not invited to see the film and must assume that the appellants did not feel it would advance their cause by showing it. However, we had before us a great deal of information of the details of the film from persons who had viewed it and with respect to which there is no conflict. The parties were content that we proceed on that basis.

At the beginning of each episode there is a disclaimer that, although the work has been inspired by recent events in Newfoundland and elsewhere in Canada, it is a work of fiction. However, the material discloses that the facts depicted in the mini-series "The Boys of St. Vincent" parallel and are strikingly similar to the allegations upon which charges have been brought against the respondents.

A member of the bar who had viewed the film described it by way of overview as follows. The film was divided into two parts. The first part covers a certain time period in which physical and sexual abuses were inflicted upon children residing in an orphanage run by a lay division of brothers. The second part takes place fifteen years later when a brother and a former brother are engaged in criminal trials and a public inquiry looks into allegations of a cover-up at the orphanage.

During the film, the audience follows the story of two orphans who are sexually and/or physically assaulted by the brothers of the lay religious order. At one point in the first half of the film, the police have most of the orphans bussed to the police station to give statements. It is evident that all of these orphans have been abused. As each one is dictating his statement, the audience sees flashbacks of the actual abuse. There are graphic scenes of young boys naked and involved in sexual activity with brothers, and an older boy forced to his knees to perform fellatio on a brother. In the film, it is also clear that there is a cover-up of this abuse by the church and high ranking members of the government.

In the second part of the film the audience witnesses the trials of a superintendent and another brother. The lawyers representing the brother and former brother are portrayed as being cruel and insensitive. They are also portrayed as treating the victims in a seemingly heartless and unnecessary manner. Because the audience has witnessed all the actual physical and sexual assaults, the contention of the defence lawyers seems ridiculous and misleading. The audience is left with the feeling that the victims, no matter what problems there may be with their testimony, should be believed because all their problems are due to the abuse inflicted upon them by the brothers.

The mini-series had been given a great deal of pre-airing publicity and had been exhibited to film critics.

In Maclean's Magazine, December 7, 1992, the reviewer stated, in part, as follows:

> *The drama's timeliness is indisputable.* In April, Douglas Kenny, the ninth Irish Christian Brother involved in the Mount Cashel scandal to be charged with sexual offences, was sentenced to five years in jail. *In Ontario, several Christian Brothers are currently on trial,* the result of more than 200 assault and sexual assault charges against 28 current and former members of the lay order who had worked at two reform schools . . .

(Emphasis added).

The following was stated in the entertainment section of the Toronto *Star* on November 29, 1992:

> Smith's movie is a dramatized, *loosely* fictionalized drama about the sexual and physical abuse of young boys in a Catholic orphanage in Newfoundland in the mid-1970s, and the public inquiry and trials 15 years later that lead to the conviction of several Catholic brothers, and of the particularly vicious orphanage superintendent, Peter Lavin (Czerny).
>
> Yes, it's the Mount Cashel saga, with echoes of other cases recently prosecuted in Ontario, in Canada's Western provinces, and in the United States. *Direct references are thinly veiled,* and Smith and his producers at the NFB and CBC are careful to include a disclaimer assuring viewers that this is not a re-enactment of any specific series of events, nor a portrayal of real people.
>
> Each of those cases was so similar, however, even to the degree of government disinterest in legitimate complaints, that they are almost interchangeable. Given recent revelations, The Boys of St. Vincent takes on the semblance of a modern morality play; its plot points and characters are ubiquitous, almost part of contemporary folk lore . . .

(Emphasis added).

In the *Globe & Mail*, Broadcast Week, December 5 to 11,1992, the proposed mini-series was described in part as follows:

> This four hour CBC/NFB mini-series is a work of fiction inspired by the scandal of Mount Cashel and the terrible abuse suffered by children in orphanages and residential schools in Ontario and the West. Directed by John N. Smith, who has established a tradition of alternative, reality-based films for the NFB, *the drama explores both the intricate intensities of life in a religious-run institution and the aftermath for both the abused and the abusers. The first two hours of the series are among the most startling ever seen on Canadian television* . . .

(Emphasis added).

That the mini-series, "The Boys of St. Vincent", parallels the facts upon which the charges have been brought against the respondents was conceded by the appellant Canadian Broadcasting Corporation. It states in its factum, in part, as follows:

> All of the Applicants are either former Christian Brothers or Christian Brothers who are charged with events involving physical or sexual abuse at Catholic training schools where they were teachers.
>
> In the film, which is set in Newfoundland, it seems that the majority of the brothers are abusing children, that there is a cover up of this abuse by the church, and that the brother around

which the story is set lies to a psychiatrist by saying that the children are lying. The lawyers representing the brother are seen as cruel and insensitive.

Although the work is aired as fictional and commences with a clear disclaimer to that effect, there are parallels between the mini-series and the facts upon which the charges have been brought against the accused persons.

There has already been widespread and substantial publicity regarding Mount Cashel in Ontario, Newfoundland and elsewhere.

(Emphasis added).

In deciding to restrain the hearing of the mini-series until after the trial of the four respondents had been concluded, the learned motions court judge stated in part as follows:

> I, too, have great faith in the jury system, as indicated in the cases, and by counsel before me. Juries are not stupid. They come, for the most part, from a variety of sophisticated backgrounds, and can understand and follow instructions from a judge. What we have here, however, is, in the particular charges against the four applicants, a highly explosive and inflammatory issue to be decided by, in effect, four separate juries in four separate courts.
>
> There has already been wide-spread publicity, and I take judicial notice of the large amount of publicity involving the Mount Cashel charges, and other educational institutions operated by the Christian Brothers, both in Ontario Newfoundland, and elsewhere. It may well be that in future trials . . . potential jurors will have to be challenged for cause as to, first of all, their contact with publications already available, and secondly, if they have seen or read the material that pertains to other trials of a similar nature whether or not they feel that they can render an impartial verdict. I see, however, no need to add fuel to the fire, particularly in view of the imminent dates for trial of the three remaining accused persons. Those trials will be concluded, for the most part, by the & 11 of 1993.

and concluded as follows:

> *In all, I am satisfied that the harm that would be caused by the showing of this particular film before the jury trials of the three remaining accused persons would be such that the possibility of impartial jury selection virtually anywhere in Canada would be seriously compromised.* For that reason, I grant an interim injunction restraining the Canadian Broadcasting Corporation from broadcasting the TV programme, "The Boys of St. Vincent", and from publishing further media information relating to the proposed broadcast until such time as the three remaining criminal trials are completed.

(Emphasis added).

Conclusion

In this appeal, the court is called upon to determine how best to balance two fundamental values in our society, *i.e.*, freedom of expression, and the right of an accused to a fair trial. This is not a new issue. Nor is it a contest between the media and the court. Indeed, what is often overlooked when this issue is discussed is that it was the common law courts and not Parliament or the Legislative Assemblies that first recognized the importance of freedom of expression and the crucial role of the press in informing the public in a free and democratic society. Thus, in the absence of any legislation, and long before the *Canadian Charter of Rights and Freedoms*, it was the common law courts that held freedom of expression, including freedom of the press, to be a fundamental freedom, defended it, and gave it almost a constitutional status.

In the same way, it was the common law courts that first recognized, as a fundamental legal right, the right of are accused to a fair trial, and again, in the absence of any legislation by Parliament or the Legislative Assemblies, and it was the common law courts that assured public access to its proceedings, including access by the press, as an aid to assuring the accused a fair trial. These two values were in many respects complementary.

However, where there was a conflict between the two values, the courts have persistently held that the right to a fair trial is paramount. This view was echoed by McRuer C.J.H.C. in *Steiner v. Toronto Star Ltd.*, [1956] O.R. 14, 114 C.C.C. 117 (H.C.J.), at p. 17 O.R., p. 120 C.C.C., where he stated:

> In considering a case of this kind there are two interests involved — the freedom of the press and the right of an accused person to have a fair and unprejudiced trial before the tribunal having legal jurisdiction to try him. In many cases the press renders great public service by the publication of reports of events surrounding the commission of a crime or an alleged crime and it is *no function of the Courts to act as censors of the press, but it is the function of the Courts scrupulously to preserve the right of the individual to have a fair trial and to see that there shall not be any trespass of this right by the publication of reports that are calculated to interfere with it.*

(Emphasis added).

In *R. v. Begley* (1982), 38 O.R. (2d) 549, 2 C.R.R. 50 (H.C.J.), Smith J. noted, to the same effect, as follows, at p. 552 O.R., p. 53 C.R.R.:

> Even before the Charter, the right to a fair trial under the British system of justice was very vigilantly and jealously guarded by the courts. Fear of prejudice was always in the forefront of their concerns. *And when the two interests, namely the freedom of the press and the right of an accused person to have a fair and unprejudiced trial, competed one with the other, the second was invariably held to be paramount.*

(Emphasis added).

Freedom of expression, including freedom of speech, and the right to a fair trial, have now been given constitutional status by having been entrenched in the *Canadian Charter of Rights and Freedoms*. However, where there is a conflict between these two values, or indeed a conflict between any of the values enunciated in the *Charter*, the court is again called upon to balance them, and as was the case before the *Charter*, if there is a conflict between freedom of expression and a fair trial, then the right to a fair trial is held to be paramount.

In discussing the need to balance values entrenched in the *Charter*, Chief Justice Dickson wrote, in *Fraser v. Public Service Staff Relations Board*, [1985] 2 S.C.R. 455 at pp. 467-68,19 C.R.R. 152 at pp. 160-61:

> On the other side, however, it is equally obvious that free speech or expression is not in absolute, unqualified value. Other values must be weighed with it. Sometimes these other values supplement, and build on, the value of speech. But in other situations there is a collision. When that happens the value of speech may be cut back if the competing value is a powerful one. Thus, for example, we have laws dealing with libel and slander, sedition and blasphemy. *We also have*

> laws imposing restrictions on the press in the interests of, for example, ensuring a fair trial or protecting the privacy of minors or victims of sexual assaults.

(Emphasis added).

The circumstances here are unique. As noted earlier, the four respondents are either former Christian Brothers or present Christian Brothers who have been charged with physical and sexual assault of young boys in their care. The trial of one of the respondents was in progress at the time of these proceedings and the other trials are imminent. The film "The Boys of St. Vincent", as noted earlier, parallels the facts upon which the charges have been brought against the respondents. The complainants, young boys, are all portrayed as being truthful; the accused liars, the defence lawyers insensitive and cruel. The first two hours of the series was said to be simply amongst the most startling ever seen on television. It is well known that showing a drama portrayed in this way on television has a much more powerful and lasting impact upon the viewer than the printed word. The prejudicial effect on a potential juror is apparent.

It is to be observed that the order under appeal with respect to the airing of the film does not purport to censor the film or to ban its being aired. It directs that the airing be postponed until the trials of the four respondents are completed, to avoid the risk of denying the four respondents a fair trial.

It is not unusual for the media to be required to postpone publication in the interests of a fair trial. For example, the evidence given on a preliminary hearing is not permitted to be published until after trial, nor is evidence taken on a *voir dire* permitted to be published during the trial. As Smith J. noted in *R. v. Begley, supra*, at p. 552 O.R., pp. 53-54 C.R.R.:

> Freedom of the press being a fundamental freedom, guaranteed in 9.1 of the Charter, and also a hallmark of a democratic society, requires access which will only yield to another right or freedom on the test of what is a reasonable limit prescribed by law in the circumstances of each case. The right to publish will usually follow. Its temporary suspension, however, may be justified for a variety of good reasons. The cases are replete with examples and statutory provisions permitting it are not rare.

However, even in the case of a postponement, as opposed to a permanent banning, no injunction should be granted unless there is a real and substantial risk that a fair trial would be impossible in the circumstances of the case if the program was to be aired as proposed. No one contested the proposition that if there was such a risk, the right to a fair trial is paramount.

What was submitted, however, was that there were other remedies less drastic than injunctive relief to protect the rights of the respondents, such as a challenge for cause or relying on the trial judge instructing the jury to decide the case only on the evidence that is heard in the courtroom.

The learned motions court judge concluded that such procedures would not be effective. There had already been widespread publicity of similar conduct alleged against other Christian Brothers in Newfoundland and elsewhere, and the matter had received such widespread attention that, in the view of the learned motions court judge, it would make it difficult for the four respondents to be tried by jurors who had not been tainted by such publicity. As I read her reasons, she concluded that by showing the film now, before the trials of the four respondents had been concluded, there was a real and substantial risk that it would be impossible to empanel an impartial jury. If the film had been shown when proposed, and the judge presiding over the trials of the four respondents were of like mind, the charges would be stayed and the respondents discharged without a trial. It is in the public interest, and in the interest of victims of crime, that those charged with criminal offences should be tried according to law and, if found not guilty, discharged, and if found guilty, sentenced.

The risk of denying the respondents a fair trial far outweighs any inconvenience which the appellant, Canadian Broadcasting Corporation, may suffer by not airing the film when it proposed to do so. No pressing need was shown why the film had to be aired before the conclusion of the four trials. The film will still be timely when it is shown at a later date and the interests of justice dictate postponing its airing rather than running the risk attendant upon showing it at the time proposed.

In order to assure the four respondents a fair trial, the learned motions court judge had a broad discretion and I cannot say that she erred in the exercise of her discretion in directing that the airing of the film be postponed.

However, I think, with respect, that she erred in directing that the airing of the film be postponed throughout Canada and should have limited the postponement of the showing of the film to the Province of Ontario and the appellant's television station in Montreal, the signal of which reached L'Orignal.

I also think the motions court judge erred by prohibiting the publishing in any media of any information relating to the proposed broadcast of the program until the completion of the criminal trials of the four respondents, as well as banning publication of the fact of the proceedings before her.

In the result, the appeal was allowed in part by varying the judgment of Madam Justice Gotlib as follows:

(1) limiting the scope of the injunction restraining the CBC from broadcasting the program "The Boys of St. Vincent" to the Province of Ontario and by CBMT-TV in Montreal, and by deleting the prohibition against publishing in any media any information relating to the proposed broadcast of the program until the completion of the criminal trials of the four applicants;
(2) deleting the prohibition against publication of the proceedings.

In all other respects the appeal was dismissed.

Appeal allowed in part.

3.3.3.3.8 Stuart Robertson, *Courts and the Media* (Toronto: Butterworths, 1981), p. 25

Members of the media breach the sub judice rule when they interfere, or potentially interfere, with the court's handling of a legal proceeding. The following is a list of the ways the media have been found to have interfered with the courts' processes.

(a) reporting that the accused has given a confession or admission before it is entered as evidence in open court;
(b) prejudging or urging a particular result in the legal proceeding;
(c) advising parties involved in a legal proceeding, thereby discouraging them from pursuing their interests;
(d) reporting that the accused in a criminal proceeding has a criminal record, or that the accused engages in criminal activities or consorts with criminals;
(e) reporting the identity of the accused when the identity is an issue in the proceeding;
(f) reporting the contents of court documents;
(g) reporting on one proceeding in such a way as to prejudice another action;
(h) breaching court orders;
(i) carrying on a media investigation while a related criminal matter is proceeding.

3.3.4 Disobeying an Order of a Court

If a journalist is subpoenaed as a witness at a judicial proceeding and refuses to answer a question properly put, the refusal can amount to that form of contempt known as disobeying an order of the court. The refusal to reveal such information will be dealt with either summarily as a contempt or as an offence under a specific section of the *Criminal Code*.

3.3.4.1 *Criminal Code*, R.S.C. 1985, c. C-46

545. (1) Where a person, being present at a preliminary inquiry and being required by the justice to give evidence,
   (*a*) refuses to be sworn,
   (*b*) having been sworn, refuses to answer the questions that are put to him,
   (*c*) fails to produce any writings that he is required to produce, or
   (*d*) refuses to sign his deposition,
without offering a reasonable excuse for his failure or refusal, the justice may adjourn the inquiry and may, by warrant in Form 16, commit the person to prison for a period not exceeding eight clear days or for the period during which the inquiry is adjourned, whichever is the lesser period.

(2) Where a person to whom subsection (1) applies is brought before the justice upon the resumption of the adjourned inquiry and again refuses to do what is required of him, the justice may again adjourn the inquiry for a period not exceeding eight clear days and commit him to prison for the period of adjournment or any part thereof, and may adjourn the inquiry and commit the person to prison from time to time until the person consents to do what is required of him.

(3) Nothing in this section shall be deemed to prevent the justice from sending the case for trial upon any other sufficient evidence taken by him.

3.3.4.2 Wilfred H. Kesterton, *The Law and the Press in Canada* (Toronto: 1976), pp. 32-39

Probably no incident in recent times has aroused so much Canadian debate on the subject of confidentiality of sources as a 1969 event. Early that year the CBC public affairs show, "The Way It Is," prepared a film report on the city of Montreal. As part of this offering, John Smith, a member of the CBC unit, interviewed a man who claimed to be an FLQ terrorist. The man told Smith that it was his job to teach others how to make and set off bombs. Feeling that this sort of information was important to authorities concerned with protecting life and property, the CBC told the police. But the corporation did not name the man who had been interviewed because Smith had promised not to disclose his identity.

Smith was soon summoned to appear before the Montreal Fire Commission, the body chosen to investigate the bombings which had been taking place. By now Smith had come to believe the interview had been a hoax. Believing also that it was necessary to protect his sources, Smith refused to be sworn before the Fire Commission. Lawyers Marcel Beauchemin and Marcel Cote asked Fire Commissioner John McDougall to cite the CBC reporter-researcher for contempt of the hearing.

Summoned again, Smith again refused to be sworn. In doing so he read from a prepared text which said, "I know full well that the law obliges me to answer the questions of this Commission ... but nevertheless I will not testify." He contended that "it is the job of the journalist to inform his public of the state of society" and that he "is continuously privy to confidential information." He maintained that giving assurances that information divulged confidentially will be so treated was as much a part of the journalist's function as it was a lawyer's. "If my refusal to testify is illegal," he said, "then it is illegal to have a free press and an informed public, because a press cannot be free and a public cannot be informed if journalists cannot give assurances ... confidentiality will be kept confidential."

Reaction to the Smith incident was sharp and categorical. Predictably, many journalists condemned the sentencing and imprisonment of the CBC reporter-interviewer. Some editors and commentators demanded shield laws to protect journalists from having to divulge the sources of the stories they write or broadcast. Some claimed that denial of confidentiality might lead to the state of affairs existing in South Africa. They were afraid that an insistence on disclosure might help to bring about a situation in which papers could not print anything detrimental to the government. Others, believing that Canada should follow the example of the American shield law states, raised the question of whether courts should not be required to show that a matter was in the public interest before they could compel a journalist to reveal his sources.

The Toronto *Globe and Mail* editorialized about Bill 79, the Fire Investigations Act under which Smith had been summoned to the Commission hearing. The editorial said, "Bill 79 has ... harshly bruised the legitimate rights of John Smith." It contended that "Bill 79 springs, not just from the dark waters through which Quebec is now passing, but from the style in which Canadian law, both inside and outside Quebec, has evolved." It also quoted approvingly — and attempted to apply to the Smith case — the words of Justice Oliver Wendell Holmes, in reference to another, American court: "To declare that the government may commit crimes in order to secure the arrest of private individuals — this would bring terrible retribution. Against that pernicious doctrine, this court should resolutely set its face. "

Was the John Smith case as significant as such commentators seemed to think? Was it a *cause célèbre*? Did it pose a real threat to the freedom of Canada's mass media? Should the journalist be given the blanket right to preserve the anonymity of the sources of his reports? Attempts made by many media professionals to answer such questions were not reassuring. Many editorial writers made errors in their assessment of the John Smith affair. Many were singularly uninformed about the law of the press in the area of contempt of court and the revealing of sources. Many seemed unaware of any underlying philosophy designed to reconcile the interests of the journalist with the interests of the society he serves.

Some critics of the Smith imprisonment made the issue of revealing of sources unnecessarily confusing by coupling it with an account of what the police were reported to have done to the prisoner. As Warren Davis described it, on the CBC television program, "The Way It Is, " " [Smith] is then shackled, chained at the ankle, handcuffed to a guard and taken to Bordeaux jail, where, before a group of watching guards, he is stripped, given forms to sign, and in prison clothes put in a solitary cell in the punishment block, the hole." With similar emphasis Doug Collins asked whether the Oliver Wendell Holmes stricture previously quoted did not apply "if, under the Fire Investigation Act, they can hold people ... without right of consulting counsel." On the same program, other panelists hastened to point out that they too did not approve of any denial of the right of an arrested person to receive the advice of his solicitor at any time. But they were equally firm in pointing out that the iniquitous things which were alleged to have happened to Smith were an issue quite separate from his refusal to testify. Quite clearly it is possible to condemn the rather high-handed treatment which Smith was reported to have received and still favor the requirement that the journalist name his sources in appropriate situations.

Some critics made the mistake of regarding the Montreal incident as introducing a new threat, one perhaps unique to Quebec. In doing so they showed ignorance of Canadian contempt citation precedents. The fact is, of course, that Wigmore's four canons, discussed earlier in this chapter, apply equally throughout

Canada. People knowledgeable in the law thought it a mistake to regard the Quebec contretemps as unique. The Quebec legislation was not a piece of isolated legislation, they said, since there were a similar act at the federal level and an Inquiry Act in each of the provinces. They called attention to the fact that any Supreme Court judge could commit reporters for refusal to disclose. Indeed, some felt that any Supreme Court judge in Canada might have imposed a longer sentence than the Montreal Five Investigation Commission did.

Many journalists, in a spontaneous reaction to a situation about which they were not too knowledgeable, seemed to regard the controversy as a contest between an all embracing requirement of disclosure under all circumstances and a complete and absolute protection of journalists under all circumstances. As a result they conceived the defenselessness of the journalist to be far greater than it actually is; and they called for an absolute protection which could not, under the free press-fair trial philosophy which prevails in Canada, be justified. The fact is that the media enjoy a degree of protection far greater than generally realized. As has been indicated earlier, it is also true that to grant the media the absolute privilege of keeping their sources secret might produce injustices that would outweigh any hardships imposed on the press by the requirement to name sources.

Related to the average journalist's ignorance about his obligation to disclose was a comparable ignorance about the previously discussed privileges of others involved with the law: husband and wife; solicitor and client; penitent and priest; doctor and patient. Such faulty knowledge was typified by John Smith when he claimed for the journalist the lawyer's privilege of confidentiality on the grounds that such confidentiality was as essential to the journalist's function as it was to the lawyer's. In doing so he showed no awareness of the difference between the lawyer-client and journalist-informant relationships — a difference which has already been examined.

There was still another facet of the John Smith affair about which commentators and editorialists were not too clear. Many discussed the CBC journalist's citation for contempt as though he had been punished for refusing to name sources, when, in point of fact, his offence had been to decline to answer any questions put to him by the Commission. Both Hyliard Chappell and Bruce Phillips on the "Something Else" program commented more knowledgeably. They were exceptional in realizing, as not too many journalist commentators did, that what Smith had done was, in fact, to say, "I refuse to give any evidence whatsoever;" they felt that Smith should have accepted the summons and then decided what answers to give after the questions were put. As Bruce Phillips commented, "It's pretty hard for him to defend not turning up at the hearing at all. If, on the other hand, he went and they demanded disclosure of sources he would have been on an entirely different wicket. He doesn't even know ... for sure ... what questions were going to be put to him. I think it's better to go to court and make a case there.

In his statement to justify his refusal to testify before the Montreal Fire Commission, John Smith protested that he was being required to reveal sources *even though he had not been charged with a criminal offence.* In doing so he implied that the requirement of disclosure was an exceptional one. The *Globe and Mail* editorial previously cited and Doug Collins in the program already referred to also gave the impression that they thought it remarkable that Smith should be so dealt with even though he was not arraigned under criminal proceedings. Yet there was nothing abnormal in what the Fire Commissioner had done, as was illustrated by the previously considered Blair Fraser, Jacqueline Skois and Marie Torre cases, three earlier precedents which did not involve criminal prosecutions.

Perhaps the most influential journalist to speak out against the treatment of the CBC staffer and in favor of protection of sources was Gerard Pelletier. Interviewed by Patrick Watson, the Secretary of State took the view that under appropriate conditions, the most notable being that the privileged reporter be a *bona fide* journalist investigating stories in the performance of his professional duties, "the public interest will be best served" by granting him immunity. Mr. Pelletier made it clear that he felt that the decision for or against disclosure should be in the hands of the press rather than of the judiciary. The decisiveness of his answer was perhaps partially accounted for by the form used by Watson in one of his questions. After describing a hypothetical situation in which, through interview, a newspaper had learned that someone had been responsible for separatist violence, the CBC interviewer asked, "You would not feel obligated to go to the police and say, 'Here's how we got this story'?" Naturally enough, perhaps, Pelletier remarked in the course of his answer, ". . . we are not police informers, we are informers of the public . . ." Yet the picture thus conjured up hardly represents the disclosure vs. anonymity issue. There is a world of difference between (on the one hand) running to the police every time the press gets information that might conceivably affect public security, and (on the other) writing news stories based on such information and being willing to divulge sources on those rare occasions when the journalist is summoned to appear before a properly constituted court or commission.

An objection to the Pelletier assessment of the disclosure question is that it leaves it to the journalist exclusively to weigh the countervailing considerations of public and press interest, and to decide whether sources are to be divulged. Part of the argument against the granting of such a privilege arises out of the uncertainty of the status of journalism. It is not a profession, has no code of ethics, is not subject to self-regulation as is the case with law or medicine, and in Canada is just beginning to face the gentle and by no means ubiquitous scrutiny of press councils. Both its failure to achieve professional status and the unwisdom of setting up press councils with anything more than the power to admonish derives from the nature of the freedom it claims. It is a platitude that freedom of the press is no different in kind or degree than the freedom to which any citizen in the country is entitled. It might be argued that both the working journalist and the casual "man in the street" correspondent should be subject to the same type of Press Council supervision. The same line of reasoning suggests that if the press were granted the privilege of unvarying confidentiality so too should any member of the public be granted that privilege.

Mr. Chappell stated an opinion widely held by thoughtful students of the question when he said that he could not see how the privilege of confidentiality could be granted to the journalist without granting the same privilege to doctors, psychiatrists, social workers, probation officers and religious people. To extend the privilege that far, he thought, would seriously impair the ability of the courts to function. Others have made the same point about stockbrokers, accountants, detectives and officials of banks and trust companies, for which the right of confidentiality has sometimes been claimed.

Several commentators have expressed scepticism of the press in claiming privilege. They contend that if the journalist can repeat stories but conceal their source, he can invent stories and use privilege to conceal the pretense. They feel that the real motive for privilege is not zeal for the public good, but the desure for prestige or readership attention. Mr. Chappell felt that under the guise of confidentiality the newspaper might perpetrate a simple hoax. Desmond Morton, Osgoode Hall law school professor, considered the public interest not to be served by keeping confidentiality. He called attention to the fact that newspapers publish for a wide variety of reasons, one of which is to sell copies and make money, and that many journals, while speaking of the public interest at a high level of abstraction, were really concerned with their own private interest of trying to get a headline. While conceding that there might be occasions when such headlines might incidentally serve the public interest where a creative piece of journalism was involved, he felt that all too often such stories were only marginal to the public interest. Thus he did not believe journalism was justified in asking for a *generalized* (italics mine) protection when the value of non-disclosure was by no means proved.

All four legal authorities interviewed by Patrick Watson on the program, "The Way It Is," (Morton; Maxwell Cohen, dean of the McGill Law School; Michel Cote, legal adviser to the Montreal Police Department; and Joseph Sedgwick, a distinguished practising lawyer with 46 years' experience) refused to accept Watson's suggestion that the law should require the court to show that it was in the public interest before it could compel a journalist to reveal his sources. Even Maxwell Cohen, who seemed most aware of the journalist's watch-dog role in exposing public acts to public scrutiny, felt that, in terms of Wigmore's fourth canon, "... the onus is really on the journalists to prove that they are on balance hampered in their job by the general duty to disclose."

When Watson persisted and questioned what public interest would be served by putting Smith in jail, Morton replied readily that Smith's punishment fulfilled the *pour encourager les autres* principle. He felt that what was done to Smith would encourage reporters not to rely on their unnamed sources but to go out and verify their information with evidence they could expose to public scrutiny.

Mr. Sedgwick supplemented the Morton answer by saying that, unless contumacious journalists were to be punished for defiance of the courts, the courts would be effectively amending the law, and that they would be implying that journalists have a protection which they do not, in fact, have.

All four legal authorities were at pains to point out that the law lays no heavy hand on the press through indiscriminate contempt citations. They firmly rejected Watson's implications that the fact that two *La Presse* reporters had just been excused from testifying in a Montreal trial indicated that the treatment of John Smith had somehow gone beyond what was right and proper. Mr. Sedgwick felt that "In the case of Mr. Smith it was thought that the public interest demanded that he should disclose [his source]. In the case of the two *La Presse* reporters it was thought that it didn't." He took this to show that the law as it stands is able to settle such questions with wisdom and discretion.

While there seemed to be a consensus that the power to punish contempt was needed to check irresponsibility and to protect the private and public interest, Professor Cohen at least showed an awareness of journalism's praiseworthy role in combatting government secrecy. He said, "Where you are dealing with an enormously complex series of relationships of the state to the individual, and where the state is still in many respects highly secrecy-oriented . . . journalism becomes a kind of countervailing power to unloosen the congealed secrecies that don't make the democratic process perhaps as loose-limbed as it ought to be. " He believed that one of the prices society should be prepared to pay might be an increase in the area of insecurity resulting from an increased confidentiality of sources. But he felt that any changes in this direction should be made with "a certain sense of the other price we're paying for it, namely that you may be providing new privileges, the total consequences of which you cannot foresee." It is less a matter of irony and more an illustration of the intricacy of the revealing of sources question that journalists should claim the privilege of secrecy in order to help them thwart government secrecy.

Canadian joumalists seem aware that the laws of contempt hold hazards. Bruce Phillips perhaps typified such a viewpoint when he said, speaking of the John Smith case, "I'm quite prepared to live with [the] situation and refuse to divulge sources and take the consequences. My view is that Smith and any other newspaperman worth his salt would behave that way. If he is given information in confidence he has his own bond upon it, and unless it is something affecting the security of the country or a matter of that character, he has no choice if he wishes to go on being a journalist except to defend the confidence that he has been given . . . I think the press is able to take care of itself in cases like this. I think that we've got to accept the fact there are going to be situations where the court's requirement for information is going to directly conflict with the reporter's obligation to his source of information . . . Sometimes [journalists] are going to land in jail because of it, but it wouldn't be the first time a journalist went to jail."

Journalists who did go to jail under the conditions described by Mr. Phillips would at least have been dealt with under the well-understood concept of "due process" of law, with the requirement to divulge being exacted only by a properly constituted court or commission. If the Alberta Press Act of 1937 had not been ruled *ultra vires* the government itself would have been empowered to compel disclosure without the journalist enjoying any of the protections built into the procedures which make up "due process." One of its harsh terms was that it would have required any newspaper "to name within twenty-four hours sources of any statement" made by that paper "within sixty days of the making of an order so to do." Failure to comply would have brought dire punishments. Journalists all across Canada recognized in the Bill a genuine threat to freedom and reacted with anger. Both the principles involved in the successful fight against the enactment and the public reaction to the measure made the affair a true Canadian *cause célèbre*.

By the Alberta Press Bill yardstick, the John Smith affair was not a *cause célèbre*.

3.3.4.3 John Sawatsky, "John Sawatsky Stakes Out the High Ground," (1988), *Bulletin of the Centre for Investigative Journalism* 11, No. 29

I didn't think the Crown would go through with it — use the media to prosecute a former Mountie for espionage.

But it did happen. I was subpoenaed to testify in the Long Knife case.

For years I had vaguely expected to experience something like this: sooner or later the needs of the media to expose events for the public good would collide with the desires of the courts. The Long Knife story happened to be the case.

Back in the 1950s the KGB slipped into Canada an Intelligence Officer who, posing as a Canadian photographer in Montreal named David Soboloff, fell in love with a Canadian woman (the wife of a Canadian soldier, just to make things a little more interesting). Soboloff defected and the RCMP turned him into a double agent.

At the same time a Mountie, later given the code name Long Knife, fell deeply and unmanageably into debt, and sold the Soboloff secret to the Russians for an envelope full of cash. Soboloff soon returned to Moscow not knowing he had been betrayed. Soboloff never came back and the RCMP couldn't figure out how it had lost its number one agent.

Long Knife was eventually discovered and in January 1958 confessed to his Mountie superiors, who prosecuted him not for treason but for passing bad cheques. He was convicted and dismissed from the force. The RCMP never told its minister. Everything was covered up.

Publication of *For Services Rendered* in November 1982 exposed the whole affair but identified the treacherous Mountie only by the name Long Knife. At the same time CBC-TV's *The Fifth Estate* with Eric Malling filmed an interview of Long Knife in disguise. About a week later the *Winnipeg Free Press* published a story identifying Long Knife as former RCMP Corporal James Morrison and quoted Morrison acknowledging his role.

Mounties Finally Act

The RCMP, too embarrassed to prosecute Long Knife in 1958, was now too embarrassed *not* to prosecute. They raided my house, the CBC, Doubleday Canada Ltd., the *Winnipeg Free Press* as well as Morrison's home, arrested him and charged him with three counts of treason under the Official Secrets Act.

Malling and I were subpoenaed at the preliminary hearing in November 1983. refused to answer a number of questions. Malling answered but skillfully avoided betraying Long Knife's identity.

Legal challenges delayed the trial until this year. One of the first things Justice Coulter Osborne did when the trial finally did start on Monday morning, last January 20, was to dismiss the jury until Wednesday while the defence and prosecution argued about which evidence was admissible. On Tuesday, with the jury still absent and with the press barred from publishing the proceedings, I was called.

Sources not Revealed

I tried to be as helpful as possible until the questions required me to identify sources. At that point I replied frequently: "I object to answering that question. The answer to that question is privileged. If I were to answer that question I would breach an express undertaking of confidentiality and violate and undermine an historical and ethical standard of my profession."

I felt it important to state my position without apology. I wanted the court to know that I was not asking for mercy but claiming a right. Whether the judge would accept this claim or find me in contempt would have to await the return of the jury when I would testify all over again.

The jury returned the next morning and the Crown put me on notice for 2 P.M. Thursday.

My lawyer and I were busily lining up witnesses to help fight the expected contempt citation. Pierre Berton, Barbara Frum, Jock Ferguson and Walter Stewart waited in the wings. So did Nick Hills, June Callwood, Michael Enright and Peter Calamai. Some of these people contorted their schedules to clear time for a flight to Ottawa.

Pleaded Guilty

Just before noon Thursday, as I was leaving for the Parliamentary Press Gallery en route to court, a phone call came in. Earlier that morning. Morrison surprised the court by pleading guilty to one of the three espionage counts. (In return the Crown dropped the other two). The case had suddenly ended just hours before the showdown.

In one sense I was disappointed. Freedom of the press under the *Charter of Rights and Freedoms* has yet to be interpreted and this case represented an excellent opportunity for a ruling favorable to the media. Clearly the Crown had abused its authority, having in the name of RCMP first covered up the story and then, when finally forced to act, compelled journalists to be *de facto* agents of the prosecution when virtually all the journalists' information originated from RCMP filing cabinets. The press had acted in the public interest and, on balance, the Crown had acted against it. It is hard to think of a better opportunity to have entrenched the media's privilege to protect sources.

. . . . .

At the moment, the media does not have the protection it deserves. Until that time arrives, those who cannot stand the heat of honoring commitments should not become involved with them in the first place.

Sawatsky's Notes

NOTE: While John Sawatsky still believed that he would be asked to divulge his sources and thereby cited for contempt in the Long Knife trial, he prepared the following notes to be read into the court record. They express carefully the perspective of many thoughtful journalists on the exercise of the law of contempt when journalists refuse to comply with a court order to betray confidences and reveal the names of sources. The information in this case was covered up and Sawatsky stated persuasively that he had acted honourably and in the interests of justice when he researched and then published the facts. A justification for escaping the sanctions of the law of contempt in this case is that he performed a very important public duty relating directly to the standards of justice in Canada.

As noted earlier, the accused changed his plea and Sawatsky was not asked by the Court to testify.

Reasons for Refusing to Divulge Sources

John Sawatsky

I would like to explain my position to the court. I want to make it clear that my position in no ways suggests lack of respect for the court or anybody appearing before this court. I believe the court has a vital responsibility in seeing that justice is done.

Society must assist the court in carrying out its duties and I do not seek an unqualified exemption. If, as a citizen, I witness an accident and the court issues me a subpoena I would see it as my duty to give conscientious testimony and generally do what I reasonably can to assist the legal process. I would do so even in my role as a journalist when I have been a third-party witness. In fact my cooperation goes further as it clearly has here already today. I have made a genuine effort to answer questions as fully as I can. However I cannot provide source-sensitive information when the sources have been promised anonymity.

My role as a journalist is to put information on the public record. I have specialized in areas where little documentary material has been available to the public. Consequently most of my information comes from oral sources — who sometimes used to be convinced into talking — and this from time to time puts me into a position of being responsible for their anonymity. Such undertakings have enabled me to reveal stories that have served the public interest and would otherwise never have been revealed. Non-attribution is the basis on which some people talk to me and my ability to serve the public interest hinges directly on this trust.

The court's probing causes me two major concerns.

First, the court wants me to breach an express undertaking of confidentiality and violate and undermine an historic ethical practice of my profession. I believe it is wrong for the court to make this demand. Some people have entrusted their careers in my hands. If I discard this commitment I break my personal word and dishonour a fundamental rule of journalism, a rule that is virtually an oath. I feel I simply have no discretion here.

That is the ethical side. There is also a practical side. In reality the court is requiring me to sacrifice my livelihood. If I betray sources I cannot continue to function as a journalist. This is no philosophical issue. It is a continual reality for me. I conduct several long, probing interviews a week and I am only as good as the respect and confidence I receive. If I fail this responsibility here today, people will stop trusting me and my effectiveness will evaporate. Trust is hard to earn and easy to lose and I've spent years earning the trust of others. The court is asking me not only to answer a question but to forsake a career of 15 years.

As I said earlier, I see a duty to cooperate with the court. But ethically and practically the consequences of betraying sources are worse than any penalty the court is likely to impose. I cannot comply with the court's demand. I want to make it clear I feel obligated to stand firm to the end.

I was able to write *For Services Rendered* only because people trusted me. I first learned of the Long Knife case in October or November of 1977 while researching my first book, *Men in the Shadows*. I tried but could not flesh out the story. So I dropped it. As far as I was concerned the Long Knife investigation was over and dead. Unexpectantly, my career changed course and I found myself writing a second RCMP book, which turned out to be *For Services Rendered*. By this time *Men in the Shadows* was published and some key people saw how carefully I protected sources. THAT was when the Long Knife investigation got back on track. I mention this to illustrate the direct correlation between the level of trust in me and my ability to reveal the Long Knife story. The Long Knife case is only one example.

This trust has carried over into my current research into lobbying. One lobbyist volunteered [that] he was talking to me because of the way I had obviously treated sources in my RCMP books.

Let me provide a hypothetical example of how an overreaching court can harm the public interest. If an influence peddler told me he was bribing the government I think everybody agrees the practice should be exposed and halted. No influence peddler will describe his activities if he believes I will become the Crown's star witness against him. Otherwise he might as well confess to the police. I would be a de facto policeman. The press would be crippled because, not surprisingly, sources would treat us as policemen rather than joumalists.- Everybody would suffer, including the court. Without an effective press, ciminal cases that otherwise would have been exposed would never reach the court. The court cannot act on cases it never hears. So in the end our system of justice and — all society — would be damaged.

My role, which I take very seriously, is to inform the public so that the public can make independent and enlightened decisions for better or for worse. I'm not so much interested in what decision the public makes so long as it has access to as many facts as possible. Once I become an agent of the court, the police, or any other institution my role is compromised.

I take this stand not only for myself. I have given this matter considerable thought recently and have discussed it with colleagues. They agree I have no alternative. One colleague said: "John, you're doing this for all of us. Otherwise we couldn't function either."

It is impossible for a free society to operate without a free press. The role of the press must be respected and allowed to flourish. I realize the court has a job to do. I hope the court acknowledges that the media also have a crucial job to do.

Statement to be delivered if cited for contempt of court

John Sawatsky

I'm being cited for being in contempt of court. I take issue with that allegation. Let's step back and take a broader look at my so-called "contempt". I agree that the administration of justice in society is fundamentally important and that the court system must be able to work and, furthermore, that people who set out to frustrate the working of the court are in contempt. But even a narrow view — one that gives no weight to my responsibility to uphold the ability of a free press to perform its duty — must conclude that my actions, in total, have not inhibited the administration of justice but, in fact, have assisted it.

The trial that is being heard here today is based on events that occurred more than 25 years ago. Most of the facts known today were known by officials in positions of appropriate authority shortly after they happened and yet the evidence was not referred to the Department of Justice or to the courts. This was not the result of oversight. The decision to withhold information was a conscious decision taken by the top officers of the RCMP. In my opinion, this decision to withhold evidence is an obstruction of justice amounting to contempt.

In contrast, my actions have been consistent and clear and all directed toward exposing the events — to break the cover-up that prior to 1982 had blocked the case from reaching court. The court would not be hearing this case if the knowledge of events had continued to rest solely in the hands of the RCMP. That is why I say when you look at the whole context — and look at it fairly — my involvement has served to help the court to see that justice is done in society. Frankly, I don't see how you can justly find contempt against someone who uncovered the facts in the first place. It seems to me that the court's right to cite contempt should be reserved for those who originally conspired to frustrate the legal process.

Also, I think you have to look at motive. I think all sides agree that my position is not a device to hide skeletons or escape unethical behaviour. I have acted honourably both as journalist and citizen. In fact if I was less honourable — if I was a defendant who had performed some heinous crime I could exercise my right not to take the stand. That, in my layman's view, is contempt: frustrating the administration of justice by withholding information for selfish reasons. If I acted in that manner my position would be contemptuous and immoral but entirely lawful. I now find myself being very moral but seemingly not lawful. I realize this is not an easy matter for the court because other issues are involved. But it demonstrates the need for the court to look at motive and if the court examines motive it will conclude that my motive has been to correct injustice and not cause it.

There is good reason not to challenge somebody in my circumstances. Courts recognize the role of the press. A court will not allow witnesses in the same trial to sit in the courtroom for the very good reason that they should not hear what other witnesses say. But witnesses can read a newspaper and learn who said what. If the court pursued its interests narrowly it would prohibit press coverage of multi-day trials. But the court realizes that society has many interests to protect in addition to supporting the administration of justice. In this instance the court has concluded that freedom of the press takes precedence over the needs of the justice system.

It works the other way as well. The press may be barred from reporting evidence in preliminary hearings and in some kinds of trials the press must withhold names of victims. In these instances other interests are put ahead of the public's need to know. So neither the court nor the press always has everything it would ideally like. Both institutions acknowledge each other's interest and attach public good to it. So we're not talking about absolutes here. The court and the press have conflicting interests and try to accommodate each other. Yet both institutions have certain boundaries the other must not cross. For me — and I believe for the rest of the press as well-source protection is one of these inviolate boundaries. At this stage I must stop compromising and start defending my territory.

The court itself recognizes cases where confidences must remain sacred. The most notable example is the lawyer-client relationship. Why are lawyers not required to reveal everything about their clients? This would open a tremendous source of information for the court's benefit. Chances are that all kinds of unsavoury criminals who now get off would be convicted. This avenue, nevertheless, has been put off limits — and for good reason. Merely the threat of a subpoena to a defence lawyer would — for reasons that need no explaining — sabotage the lawyer's ability to defend the client. In very practical terms, the system would not work. The court, in its wisdom, recognizes the principle that a trial must exempt certain sources of information.

Court probing into journalistic sources — if successful — would also undermine a journalist's ability to function. In the same way that clients would stop confiding in their lawyers, sources would stop talking to reporters.

Why are lawyers exempted and not journalists? The legal profession — be they the Canadian Bar Association, the lawyers in the Department of Justice or judges-molds the law with a vested interest. The legal community is saying: "We'll exempt ourselves but not you." It is discriminatory and unfair.

There is one other issue I feel needs to be raised and that has to do with conflict of interest. I raise it only because I believe it touches directly on the ability of justice to prevail. With respect, your honour, I don't think you should be even presiding when adjudicating between two institutions when one of the institutions happens to be your own. On issues such as these you cannot possibly be an independent arbitrator no matter how good a judge you are nor how hard you attempt to be impartial. I am a traditionalist who believes that reporters should report and not advocate and I go to considerable lengths to practice this philosophy. Yet when it comes to freedom of the press, I acknowledge myself to be an advocate. Furthermore, I don't think I would be a good person to adjudicate a dispute between a newspaper and someone who complained of unfair coverage. I could probably do a fair analysis of the issues-but whose issues? Between my views on the need for public disclosure and the complainant's concern about the dangers of defamation, the complainant and I probably would not agree on what the appropriate issues were. I am an advocate for an effective and diligent press. I think judges are advocates for judicial authority. In fact I believe judges would be remiss if they were not because judges must protect their ability to carry out their responsibilities. The problem is that when judicial interests come into conflict with press interests a judge is no longer a disinterested party. A judge's ability to be unbiased is in question just as a journalist's bias must be questioned on a press complaint.

I am raising a fundamental issue — one so fundamental that its resolution should be left to society. When the legitimate needs of the press come into conflict with the legitimate needs of the court, the decision should rest with a jury. Not a jury of experts — because this is more a fundamental issue than a technical one — but a jury of citizens from all walks of life. By citing me for contempt you are de facto acting as a plaintiff. I do not think one gets fair process when the plaintiff and the judge are the same person.

I know what the law says. You have the lawful right to find me in contempt of court for not answering specific questions but you have no moral right to do so. In fact you would be abusing your moral authority. Society has entrusted a lot of authority in you and society expects you to handle this responsibility not only lawfully but wisely. Society also gives broad powers to the police. A police officer is able to stop a car and for no good reason cause the operator considerable distress while remaining entirely within the law. Customs inspectors at border points possess awesome powers which can be employed at any time. But these powers are reserved for critical situations. Society extends broad powers to certain agents but they were never meant to be blank cheques.

The case is even more compelling with judges. If the police overstep their moral authority the victim can appeal to a body of non-policemen. But when judges overstep their moral authority I must appeal to another judge. Given the fact that you have tremendous authority, and that there are fundamental rights involved, and that realistically there is no appeal, I believe the best public service the court could perform is by proceeding only with extraordinary caution. And, I believe, when all factors are taken into consideration, extraordinary caution in this case compels the court not to proceed with a contempt citation.

3.3.4.4 *Re Legislative Privilege* (1978), 83 D.L.R. (3d) 161 (Ont. C.A.)

LACOURCIERE, J.A.:

The common law has recognized certain types of communications which are privileged, subject to certain exceptions, and not subject to judicially enforced disclosure. The exempted classes include communications between solicitor and client; communications between husband and wife; communications concerning the deliberations of a jury; and, finally, communications with Government and Government of officials. We are not concerned with the first three classes, which respectively rest upon social policy to promote freedom of consultation with legal advisers in the defence of legal rights, the need to preserve mutual trust and confidence in domestic relations and the obvious necessity in the administration of justice of preserving the secrecy of jury deliberations. The privilege respecting Government documents creates an exclusion which is limited to the requirements of the public interest in maintaining the confidentiality of its internal communications. We adopt the apt words of Lord Simon of Glaisdale in *D. v. National Society for Prevention of Cruelty to Children*, [1977] 2 W.L.R. 201 at pp. 221-2:

> The various classes of excluded relevant evidence may for ease of exposition be presented under different colours. But in reality they constitute a spectrum, refractions of the single light of a public interest which may outshine that of the desirability that all relevant evidence should be adduced to a court of law.

An extension of the so-called Crown privilege has been accorded, in the public interest, to protect from disclosure the identity of police informers. The *rationale* for this extension was clearly the importance to the public of the detection of crimes, and the necessity of preserving the anonymity of police informers to maintain the sources of information. This necessity has generally outweighed the public interest of full disclosure of relevant facts to the adjudicating tribunal. This privilege, however, is not absolute and is subject to one important exception, stated by Lord Diplock in *D. v. N.S.P.C.C., supra*, at p. 207:

> By the uniform practice of the judges which by the time of *Marks v. Beyfus*, 25 Q.B.D. 494 had already hardened into a rule of law, the balance has fallen upon the side of non-disclosure except where upon the trial of a defendant for a criminal offence disclosure of the identity of the informer could help to show that the defendant was innocent of the offence. In that case, and it that case only, the balance falls upon the side of disclosure.

The House of Lords in D. v. N.S.P.C.C., *supra*, extended the protection for the non-disclosure of police informants to protect the identity of an informant to the National Society for the Prevention of Cruelty to Children.

It is clear that the classes of evidence which give rise to privileged communications have foundations in social policy in which the general liability of every person to give testimony upon all facts inquired of in a Court gives way to more important social considerations

3.3.4.5 *Moysa v. Alberta Labour Relations Board*, [1989] 1 S.C.R. 1572 (S.C.C.)

SOPINKA, J.: The issue in this case is the right of the appellant, a journalist, to refuse to answer relevant questions in a proceeding before the Alberta Labour Relations Board. The refusal was grounded in part on an alleged right to protect sources of information on the basis of a qualified privilege either at common law or under s. 2(b) of the *Canadian Charter of Rights and Freedoms*. The appellant's claim arose in the following manner.

In 1985, an organizing drive by Alberta Food and Commercial Workers Union, Local 401, was ongoing at the Hudson Bay Company in St. Albert. On February 23 of that year, an article written by the appellant entitled "Union Eyes Major Stores" was published in the *Edmonton Journal*. The article referred to the union's organizing efforts at several department stores in the Edmonton and St. Albert area though it did not name the particular stores. Approximately one week later, the Hudson Bay Company terminated the employment of six employees at the St. Albert store.

As a result of these firings, allegations of unfair labour practices were directed against the Hudson Bay Company and formed the subject matter of the Labour Relations Board hearing. The Union claimed that the employees were fired due to their organizing activities. The appellant was summoned to attend pursuant to s. 13 of the *Labour Relations Act*, R.S.A. 1980, c.L-1.1. The Union proposed to ask her under oath whether she had spoken with someone at the Hudson Bay Company before witting the article and, if so, what the details were of that conversation. The appellant objected to being compelled to testify.

The Labour Relations Board first determined that it possessed the necessary jurisdiction and power to compel the appellant to be sworn and give oral testimony. As well, the evidence that the appellant might give was determined to be relevant. Then in its decision of October 24,1985, the Board held that neither the common law nor the *Charter* protected the appellant from being sworn and from being compelled to answer questions at a Board hearing.

In determining that the appellant could not rely upon any common law privilege, the Board considered the appellant's argument that a qualified privilege not to testify might be recognized on the basis of four criteria outlined by Wigmore (8 *Wigmore on Evidence*, 2285 (McNaughton rev. 1961)). These four factors were discussed by this Court in *Slavutych v. Baker*, [1976] 1 S.C.R. 254. They are the following (at p. 260):

(1) The communications must originate in a confidence that they will not be disclosed.
(2) This element of *confidentiality must be essential* to the full and satisfactory maintenance of the relation between the parties.
(3) The *relation* must be one which in the opinion of the community ought to be sedulously *fosterred*.
(4) The *injury* that would inure to the relation by the disclosure of the communications must be *greater than the benefit* thereby gained for the correct disposal of litigation.

The Board held that Wigmore's four criteria were not satisfied in this case. The Board was of the view that the element of confidence was not part of the maintenance of a continuing relationship between the appellant and her source and that the injury resultant from disclosure would not be greater than the benefit.

The Board then proceeded to consider the alleged right to a qualified privilege for reporters under s. 2(b) of the *Charter*. The Board examined the decision of the United States Supreme Court in *Branzburg v. Hayes*, 408 U.S. 665 (1972), which considered whether the guarantee of the freedom of the press under the First Amendment to the American Constitution permits a reporter to refuse to answer questions before a grand jury. White J. for the majority (speaking for four members of the Court) held that the First Amendment accords a reporter no privilege against appearing before a grand jury and answering questions as to either the identity of his or her news sources or information which he or she has received in confidence. In a concurring opinion, Powell J. agreed in the result, but held that each claim of privilege should be judged on its particular facts by striking a balance between the freedom of the press and the obligation of all citizens to give relevant testimony.

The Labour Board was of the opinion that Powell J. had identified two criteria that need be demonstrated before the government could compel a journalist to testify. The perceived evidence must b crucial to whomever seeks it and the evidence also must be relevant. The Board felt that this was the appropriate test under s. 2(b) of the *Charter*. However, on the facts presented before the Board, it was held that the evidence sought from the appellant was crucial to the Union's allegation of unfair labour practices and was also relevant. Further, the Board heard that if there is a third requirement that the information not be available from an alternative source it, too, had been satisfied. Therefore the Board concluded that the appellant could be compelled to testify.

The appellant filed a notice of motion before the Alberta Court of Queen's Bench for an order in the nature of *certiorari*, seeking to quash the October 24, 1985 decision of the Labour Relations Board. On May 9,1986, MacCallum J. dismissed the motion on the grounds that the appellant had no privilege, either under the common law or under s. 2(b) of the *Charter*, to refuse to testify before the Board (1986), 45 Alta. L.R. (2d) 37, 71 A.R. 70, D.L.R. (4th) 140, 25 C.R.R. 346. The appellant's appeal to the Alberta Court of Appeal was dismissed by McLung J.A. who agreed with the reasoning of MacCallum J. that there was no privilege under either the common law or under s. 2(b) of the *Charter*: (1987), 52 Alta. L.R. (2d) 193, 78 A.R. 118, 43 D.L.R. (4th) 159.

After leave to appeal to this Court was granted on December 3, 1987, [1987] 2 S.C.R. viii, the following constitutional questions were set on March 30, 1988 pursuant to Rule 32 of the Supreme Court Rules:

1. Does requiring a journalist witness to disclose communications form a source violate s. 2(b) of the *Canadian Charter of Rights and Freedoms?*
2. Does requiring a journalist witness to disclose communications to some other person violate s. 2(b) of the *Canadian Charter of Rights and Freedoms?*
3. If the answer to either questions 1 or 2 is in the affirmative, can compulsive disclosure be justified under s. 1 of the *Canadian Charter of Rights and Freedoms?*

The appellant does not suggest that there is in Canada an absolute right for journalists to claim a privilege not to testify in relation to matters discussed with journalists' sources. Rather, the appellant contends that she should not have been compelled to testify before the Labour Relations Board because she fell within the scope of a qualified testimonial privilege under either common law principles or s. 2(b) of the *Charter*. Even if such a qualified testimonial privilege exists in Canada this appeal must be dismissed as the appellant here does not fall within any of the possible tests which have been proposed as establishing the conditions necessary to justify a refusal to testify.

The appellant argued that the four criteria cited by Wigmore and referred to with approval by Spence J. in *Slavutych v. Baker*, at p. 260, provide a guide for the operation of a privilege against the disclosure of communications. The Board examined this submission and held that the injury resulting from disclosure was not greater than the benefit and the evidence was relevant, proper, and necessary to administer the *Labour Relations Act*. As well, the Board held that an element of confidence was not part of the continuing relationship between the appellant and the managers at the Hudson Bay Company store in St. Albert. Accordingly, the appellant failed to satisfy several of the necessary criteria propounded by Wigmore. Therefore, even if a qualified form of privilege exists, the appellant's claim on the facts of this case must fail. The Board did not err in dismissing the claim of privilege on this ground.

It is also worth noting that the Labour Board suggests that the Union was primarily interested in the information that the appellant *gave to* the Company officials concerning the organizing efforts. This information would not come within the ambit of any qualified privilege with respect to information *received from* sources.

The appellant also argued that s. 2(b) of the *Charter* includes the right of the press to seek and receive as well as impart information. The appellant contends that if journalists are compelled to disclose sources then they will lose access to information as new sources "dry up." This hindrance on the ability of the press to gather information is said to violate s. 2(b). The discussion of this issue in the courts below resulted in the three constitutional questions being stated. Despite the importance of ascertaining the extent of the s. 2(b) rights I am of the opinion that the disposition of this appeal does not require that the constitutional questions be answered.

Section 2(b) of the *Charter* provides:

2. Everyone has the following fundamental freedoms:
(*b*) Freedom of thought, belief, opinion and expression including freedom of the press and other media of communication;

In oral argument counsel for the appellant stated that he was not asserting a special constitutional privilege for members of the press beyond that which is available to everyone generally under the right to freedom of expression. However, it was argued that s. 2(b) was violated when the appellant was required to testify before the Labour Relations Board and was not permitted by the Board to avail herself of a claim of qualified privilege. The appellant's argument is premised on s. 2(b) according the same protection of the gathering of news as it extends to the dissemination of news. The appellant contends that the ability to gather news is hindered by the failure to extend testimonial privilege to journalists in situations such as the appellant's.

Even if I assume for the moment that the right to gather the news is constitutionally enshrined in s. 2(b) the appellant has not demonstrated that compelling journalists to testify before bodies such as the Labour Relations Board would detrimentally affect journalists' ability to gather information. No evidence was placed before the Court suggesting that such a direct link exists. While judicial notice may be taken of self-evident facts, I am not convinced that it is indisputable that there is a direct relationship between testimonial compulsion and a "drying-up" of news sources as alleged by the appellant. The burden of proof that there has been violation of s. 2(b) rests on the appellant. Absent any evidence that there is a de between the impairment of the alleged right to gather information and the requirement that journalists testify before the Labour Relations Board, I cannot find that there has been a breach of s. 2(b) in this case.

In addition, the Labour Relations Board held that the relationship between the appellant and the persons she spoke with at the Hudson Bay Company was not one based on confidence. The protection of confidence was neither sought nor given. The Board also held that the evidence was crucial, relevant and was not available from alternative sources. As well, the Board concluded that the appellant would fail in her claim for qualified privilege based on the test proposed by Powell J. in *Branzburg v. Hayes*. Therefore, in my opinion, even if this Court were to adopt Powell J.'s approach to a qualified privilege, on the facts of this case no possible violation of s. 2(b) has been made out.

Disposition

In these circumstances I am of the opinion that the Board did not err in law in ordering the appellant to answer the questions posed. This does not mean that I necessarily agree that a journalist is entitled to a qualified privilege when asked to testify about sources of information. The record in this case simply does not justify such a conclusion. Furthermore, the factual basis does not raise for determination the constitutional questions which were posed. There are no facts to support the contention that the gathering of information by the media would be threatened in the absence of *Charter* protection.

In the result, the appeal is dismissed with costs.

3.3.4.6 *Attorney-General v. Mulholland; Attorney-General v. Foster*, [1963] 2 W.L.R. 658 (C.A.Eng.)

LORD DENNING M.R. These are appeals by two journalists, Brendan Joseph Mulholland and Reginald William Foster, against sentences which have been passed upon them by Gorman J. A tribunal of inquiry was inquiring into matters which Parliament had required to be investigated. The chairman of the tribunal in pursuance of the statute, certified to the High Court that they had refused to answer the questions to which the tribunal had legally required an answer. After hearing the case and a claim of privilege which the journalists had put forward, the judge found each of them guilty as if he had been guilty of a contempt of court and passed sentence accordingly.

I need not go into the statute or the facts in great detail. It appears that allegations were made in some newspapers which reflected gravely on persons in high places and on naval officers and civil servants in the Admiralty. The articles clearly imported that there had been neglect of duty on their part in not discovering a spy who was in their midst. In making these allegations the newspapers were exercising the undoubted freedom which belongs to them. They are entitled to expose wrongdoing and to criticise the Government and anyone else, no matter how high and powerful he may be. But these were allegations which could not be overlooked. Coming from newspapers with such great influence for good or ill, they demanded investigation. If well founded, the security arrangements at the Admiralty needed complete overhaul and those at fault would have to pay the penalty for their neglect. So Parliament decided that there should be an investigation. It set up a tribunal to inquire into the matter as of urgent public importance. In the course of the inquiry the journalists responsible for these articles were asked to give the source of their information and they refused to answer.

Now, was this a question which they could legally be required to answer? That depends on two questions. First, was it relevant and necessary in this sense, that it was a question that ought to be answered to enable proper investigation to be made? Secondly, if it was, have the journalists a privilege in point of law to refuse to answer? Under the statute any witness before the tribunal is entitled to the same immunities and privileges as if he were a witness before the High Court. I turn to consider these two points in order, remembering that the certificate of the tribunal is not binding on the courts. The judge before whom it comes must inquire into the matters afresh to see if an offence has been committed.

So far as Mr. Mulholland is concerned, these were the three passages in the newspaper as to which he was asked his source. One was a passage in an article which asserted that "colleagues of his in the admiralty called Vassall 'Auntie' to his face." Another passage in another article was this, that "a girl typist "in the Admiralty office where he worked and decided that no "15-a-week clerk could possibly live the way he did honestly," and the third passage was that "it was the sponsorship of two "high ranking officials which led to Vassall avoiding the strictest "part of the Admiralty's security vetting." Mr. Mulholland was asked what were the sources of that information and he declined to give the source. He said he would not inquire from the source as to whether he was willing that it should be divulged. The chairman of the tribunal, Lord Radcliffe, directed him to answer and he declined.

Was the question relevant to the inquiry? Was it one that the journalist ought to answer? It seems to me that if the inquiry was to be as thorough as the circumstances demanded, it was incumbent on Mr. Mulholland to disclose to the tribunal the source of his information. The newspapers had made these allegations. If they made them with a due sense of responsibility (as befits a press which enjoys such freedom as ours) then they must have based them on a trustworthy source. Heaven forbid that they should invent them! And if they did get them from a trustworthy source, then the tribunal must be told of it. How otherwise can the tribunal discover whether the allegations are well founded or not? The tribunal cannot tell unless they see for themselves this trustworthy source, this witness who is the foundation of it all. The tribunal must, therefore, be entitled to ask what was the source from which the information came.

It is said that the tribunal had access to other sources of information which might make it unnecessary for the newspapers to disclose their source: and that the newspapers do not know of these other sources because so much of the proceedings were held in camera. I am not in the least impressed by this argument. Even if the tribunal did have access to other sources of information, nevertheless it is still necessary for the tribunal to know whence the newspapers got their information so as to confirm, contradict or complete these other sources. The root cause of the whole inquiry was the information which the newspapers published, and it is their sources which must be tracked down so as to see whether they are trustworthy or not. Once the source of the information is ascertained, the tribunal are better able to see whether it is such as to implicate or exculpate those concerned at the Admiralty.

I hold, therefore, that so far as Mulholland is concerned, these questions were both relevant and necessary to the inquiry which the tribunal had in hand.

So far as Foster is concerned, the case is rather different. We were invited by Mr. Cusack to take a special course with him on the ground that the questions were not relevant. The part of the article on which he was questioned was this: "Why did the "spy-catchers fail to notice Vassall, who sometimes wore women's clothes on West End trips?" When Foster was asked on that matter, he said he was not responsible for the word "wore." He said: "I was informed that Vassall was known to have "bought women's clothing in the West End." Then he was further asked whether he could remember the source of the information and he said he could not remember the particular source, the particular person; there were a number of people to be considered in these inquiries. But then he was asked: "If you cannot remember the names of your informants, can you remember the type of source from which your information came, and I added the specific question, did it come from a shop? (A.) It did not come from a shop. (Q.) How do you know it did not come from a shop? He was pressed on that question: did he know the type of source? He refused to answer as a matter of principle questions as to the type of source from which it came."

It was said by Mr. Cusack on his behalf that his case is different from Mr. Mulholland's. Here is a case of a man who did not remember the actual source. All he refused to give was the type of source. It was said that later Vassall himself gave evidence to the tribunal that he bought women's clothes in the West End. Why then was it necessary for this question to be pressed, at all events at this stage, when the later evidence has been given? I seems to me that the answer is simply this: the fact that Vassall bought women's clothes is not the whole point. The point is: did those about him in the Admiralty know it before he was arrested, and ought they to have reported it? Were they guilty of a neglect of duty? On that point the type of source is a relevant question which could be asked and was asked. It could and might have led to further inquiries which would have more nearly pinpointed the actual source so that it could be tracked down by the tribunal.

I feel that in Foster's case also the answer must be that the question was relevant and one that ought to be answered for the proper purposes of the inquiry.

But then it is said (and this is the second point) that however relevant these questions were and however proper to be answered for the purpose of the inquiry, a journalist has a privilege by law entitling him to refuse to give his sources of information. The journalist puts forward as his justification the pursuit of truth. It is in the public interest, he says, that he should obtain information in confidence and publish it to the world at large, for by so doing he brings to the public notice that which they should know. He can expose wrongdoing and neglect of duty which would otherwise go unremedied. He cannot get this information, he says, unless he keeps the source of it secret. The mouths of his informants will be closed to him if it is known that their identity will be disclosed. So he claims to be entitled to publish all his information without ever being under any obligation, even when directed by the court or a judge, to disclose whence he got it. It seems to me that the journalists put the matter much too high. The only profession that I know which is given a privilege from disclosing information to a court of law is the legal profession, and then it is not the privilege of the lawyer but of his client. Take the clergyman, the banker or the medical man. None of these is entitled to refuse to answer when directed to by a judge. Let me not be mistaken. The judge will respect the confidences which each member of these honourable professions receives in the course of it, and will not direct him to answer unless not only it is relevant but also it is a proper and, indeed, necessary question in the course of justice to be put and answered. A judge is the person entrusted, on behalf of the community, to weigh these conflicting interests — to weigh on the one hand the respect due to confidence in the profession and on the other hand the ultimate interest of the community in justice being done or, in the case of a tribunal such as this, in a proper investigation being made into these serious allegations. If the judge determines that the journalist must answer, then no privilege will avail him to refuse.

This seems to me the explanation of the cases on interrogatories to which we have been referred. The courts will not as a rule compel a newspaper in a libel action to disclose before the trial the source of its information. The reason is because, on weighing the considerations involved, the balance is in favour of exempting the newspaper from disclosure. The person who is defamed has his remedy against the newspaper and that is enough, without letting him delve round to see who else he can sue. It may rightly be said, as Buckley L.J. said in *Adam v. Fisher*, that the public has an interest to see that the newspapers are not compelled to disclose their source of information; unless, I would add, the interests of justice so demand. But that rule is not a rule of law; it is only a rule of practice which applies in those particular cases. It is made more general now and applies not only to newspapers but to other persons in the particular circumstances covered by R.S.C., Ord. 31, r.1A. It seems to me that whenever a case arises when the interests of justice or of the public require that there should be disclosure and the judge so rules, the newspapers must disclose the source of their information; they have no privilege in law to refuse.

I need not go through the authorities on this matter; they are few enough. The only cases that I have discovered where a journalist raised this question in our common law jurisdictions are three. The first was in the Parnell Inquiry Commission. On February 20, 1889, Mr. McDonald, the managing editor of The Times, was asked by Mr. Asquith: "(Q.) Do you not know who the writer of the article was? (A.) I do indirectly, not directly." (Q.) Who was it then? (A.) I do not know that I am bound to tell you. (Q.) I ask you a question? (A.) The conductors and the editor of The Times would be responsible for the statements contained in the paper, and I consider that that being so, counsel are not entitled to demand or to force from the conductors of The Times the names of the contributors. (Mr. Asquith, of counsel:) I know of no, such privilege. (Sir Charles Russell, leading him:) The question is whether there is any such privilege as is claimed. (The President, Sir James Hannen, with whom sat Day J. and A. L. Smith J.:) There is no such privilege as that suggested by the witness. (Sir Charles Russell:) Then we are entitled to an answer to our question." Then after further discussion there was the ruling by the President. He said to Mr. Asquith: "You are entitled to ask him as to specific statements which are made in some of these articles and to ascertain from him who is the writer, if he knows it. If he does not, you must take it that you have exhausted all the information you can get from this source." That is reported in The Times newspaper of Wednesday, February 20, 1889.

The next case in our common law- jurisdictions is an Irish case: *O'Brennan v. Tully.* In that case the editor of a newspaper was called as a witness and was asked about the name of a writer of an anonymous letter. He was asked: "Who was the writer of the letter? (A.) I promised the writer of the letter that I would refuse to disclose his name." Hanna J. said: You must disclose it in this court. (The witness:) I am sorry, sir, I promised I would not disclose it. (Hanna J.:) You are sworn to tell the truth; you must disclose it," and he ordered him to do it and the editor refused. The judge found him guilty of contempt of court and fined him £25.

The remaining case is a decision of the High Court of Australia in 1941, *McGuinness v. Attorney-General of Victoria*, where a Royal Commission was appointed to inquire into a question whether there had been bribery of members of the Victorian Parliament. A journalist was asked what was the source of his information. He refused to give it and he was held guilty of an offence against the Act and he was fined the sum of £15. The question whether a journalist was privileged or not was fully argued and considered by the High Court of Australia and it was unanimously held that there was no such privilege. The judgments of the court, particularly of Rich J. and Dixon J., are well worthy of study.

It seems to me, therefore, that the authorities are all one way. There is no privilege known to the law by which a journalist can refuse to answer a question which is relevant to the inquiry and is one which, in the opinion of the judge, it is proper for him to be asked. I think it plain that in this particular case it is in the public interest for the tribunal to inquire as to the sources of information. How is anyone to know that this story was not a pure invention. if the journalist will not tell the tribunal its source? Even if it was not invention. how is anyone to know it was not the gossip of some idler seeking to impress? It may be mere rumour unless the journalist shows he got it from a trustworthy source. And if he has got it from a trustworthy source (as I take it on his statement he has, which I fully accept), then however much he may desire to keep it secret, he must remember that he has been directed by the tribunal to disclose it as a matter of public duty, and that is justification enough.

I have no doubt that the journalist ought to have answered the questions put to them. These were questions they were legally required to answer and they have no privilege to refuse.

I would dismiss the appeal on the points of principle accordingly.

DONOVAN, L.J. I agree. I add a few words only about the need for some residual discretion in the court of trial in case where a journalist is asked in the course of the trial for the source of his information. While the journalist has no privilege entitling him as of right to refuse to disclose the source, so I think the interrogator has no absolute right to require such disclosure. In the first place the question has to be relevant to be admissible at all: in the second place it ought to be one the answer to which will serve a useful purpose in relation to the proceedings in hand — I prefer that expression to the term "necessary." Both these matters are for the consideration and, if need be, the decision of the judge. And over and above these two requirements, there may be other considerations, impossible to define in advance, but arising out of the infinite variety of fact and circumstance which a court encounters, which may lead a judge to conclude that more harm than good would result from compelling a disclosure or punishing a refusal to answer.

For these reasons I think it would be wrong to hold that a judge is tied hand and foot in such a case as the present and must always order an answer or punish a refusal to give the answer once it is shown that the question is technically admissible. Indeed, I understood the Attorney-General to concur in this view, namely, that the judge should always keep an ultimate discretion. This would apply not only in the case of journalists but in other cases where information is given and received under the seal of confidence, for example, information given by a patient to his doctor and arising out of that relationship. In the present case, where the ultimate matter at stake is the safety of the community, I agree that no such consideration as I have mentioned, calling for the exercise of a discretion in favour of the appellants, arises, and that accordingly their appeals fail and must be dismissed.

DANCKWERTS, L.J. I agree and I am bound to say that I thought the law was perfectly clear on the principal point which has been argued in these appeals.

LORD DENNING, M.R. That is the argument on the point of principle. We still have the question as to the punishment.

Argument was then heard on the terms of imprisonment imposed.

LORD DENNING, M.R. We feel that this is a case where the law was clearly declared by Gorman J. He gave Mr. Mulholland and Mr. Foster an opportunity to reveal their source of information and they have not done so. We have anxiously considered the sentences of six months and three months respectively which he passed on Mr. Mulholland and Mr. Foster, and after full consideration we have felt unable to adopt the view that the sentences are disproportionate to the serious nature of the offence.

3.3.4.7 *Re Legislative Privilege* (1978), 83 D.L.R. (3d) 161 (Ont.C.A.)

Weatherson, J.A.:

Thus, although the law does not recognize a privilege to refuse to disclose confidential communications between priest and penitent, or doctor and patient, it has for many years been the practice of Judges to ask counsel not to press the question, and such request has always, or almost always, been acceded to. The same concern would he had for communications made to social workers or others in efforts towards marriage reconciliation, or in proceedings involving the welfare of children. In all these cases the Court should give great weight to the fact of confidentiality, and, if the evidence is not vital to the due administration of justice, decline to compel disclosure.

Note: The so-called "newspaper rule" holds that a media defendant in a libel action may refuse to reveal, *prior to trial*, sources of information forming the basis of the alleged libel. See *Reid v. Telegram Pubishing* (1961), 28 D.L.R. (2d) 6; *Drabinsky v. Maclean-Hunter Ltd.* (1980), 108 D.L.R. (3d) 390; *Hatfield v. Globe and Mail* (1983), 41 O.R. (2d) 218; and *McInnes v. University Students' Council of the University of Western Ontario et al.* (1985), 48 O.R. (2d) 542.

3.3.5 Procedure in Contempt Cases

3.3.5.1 Robert Martin, "Contempt of Court: The Effect of the Charter," in *The Media, the Courts and the Charter*, ed. Philip Anisman and Allen M. Linden (Toronto: Carswell, 1986)

The procedure followed in contempt cases is unusual. It denies many of the rights which we assume to be associated with criminal procedure. One can do no better than to quote the observation which Harold Laski made in 1928:

> A procedure stands self-condemned when it applies methods and ideas against which the whole of Anglo-American constitutional history has been a considered and masterful protest.

As is typical of the law of contempt of court generally, there exists substantial confusion as to precisely the procedure to be followed. I am not so foolhardy as to imagine I could resolve this confusion. Some general observations will suffice.

Contempt proceedings, regardless of the technical rubric under which we seek to subsume them, are show cause proceedings. This means that the person imagined to have committed the contempt is required to establish his innocence. The task is not made easier by the fact that in certain contempt cases the accused may not be able to call witnesses. Furthermore, it is implicit in the nature of show cause proceedings that the accused, if he is to have any hope of escaping conviction, will be compelled to testify.

There is no legal rule to prevent the judge before whom a contempt is supposed, to have occurred or at whom apparently contemptuous remarks were directed from hearing the proceeding. Questions of *mens rea* are tangential. If, for example, the alleged contempt consists in a breach of the subjudice rule, the accused will not be permitted to adduce evidence that he did not intend any interference with the due administration of justice. The court is concerned with whether the material is apt to, or has a tendency to, interfere with the administration of justice, and not with the actual intention of the accused. It has, however, been held that the presiding judge must be satisfied beyond a reasonable doubt of the guilt of the accused before convicting.

A particularly odious provision of the current law is that a person who is accused of having scandalized the court by imputing improper motives to a judge is not allowed to attempt to prove the truth of his allegations. There is no provision for a jury trial in contempt prosecutions. Since contempt is a common law crime there is no stipulated maximum punishment which may be awarded. The punishment for a common law crime is a matter within the discretion of the presiding judge.

3.3.6 Reforming the Law

3.3.6.1 Robert Martin, "An Open Legal System," (1985), 25 *U.W.O. Law Review* 169

In 1982 the Law Reform Commission of Canada produced a *Report* on contempt of court. This *Report* was a disaster. The only useful portions of the *Report* were those dealing with procedure in contempt cases. The Commission advocated that the law of contempt be codified. It recommended that, except for two special instances, proceedings in contempt matters should be by way of indictment. An accused contemnor would, therefore, have all the procedural rights associated with ordinary criminal proceedings. Further, where a contempt was directed at a named judge, that judge was not to be permitted to hear the subsequent prosecution. And, fourthly, the maximum punishment for the various offences suggested by the Commission's draft bill was to be two years imprisonment.

The effect of the substantive recommendations in the *Report* would have been to make the law even more restrictive than it now is.

Scandalising was to be replaced by "affront to judicial authority", defined as follows: Everyone commits an offence who "(a) affronts judicial authority by any conduct calculated to insult a court, or (b) attacks the independence, impartiality or integrity of a court". While the existing scurrilous abuse is a nebulous standard, "conduct calculated to insult a court" is hardly an improvement. Indeed, the Law Reform Commission itself had no idea what this phrase meant. The only example vouchsafed was that under this definition "slurring a judge *qua* judge" would be an offence. Attacking the independence, impartiality or integrity of a court, which the Commission grandly characterised as " self-explanatory", is vastly broader than imputing improper motives. The Commission rejected the notion that truth should be a defence to this charge.

The only justification advanced in support of this continued sheltering of judges from public criticism was the tired and inaccurate statement that judges may not reply publicly to criticism directed to them.

Turning to the *sub judice* rule, one can say in the Commission's favour that it attempted once again to introduce a degree of precision into a dangerously vague area of the law.

When does the *sub judice* rule begin to operate? The Law Reform Commission itself noted the problem in its 1977 Working Paper on contempt. The draft bill in the *Report* stated that the proposed new offence of interfering with judicial proceedings would apply to proceedings which were "pending". "Pending" was defined in civil matters as the period beginning when a matter is set down for trial and ending when the trial is terminated; in criminal matters the period would run from the laying of an information or the proffering of an indictment until a verdict, order, or sentence is pronounced. One effect of this is that *sub judice* would not apply to appellate proceedings.

The substantive re-definition of the *sub judice* rule was the disturbing element. The new offence would be committed by anyone who "publishes or causes to be published anything he knows or ought to know may interfere with [pending judicial] proceedings". The English decision in *A.G. v. Times Newspapers Ltd.* was much criticised as unduly limiting freedom of the press. The European Court of Human Rights strongly disapproved of the view taken by the House of Lords, and, indeed, the European Court's decision is one of the few instances when a national law that infringed a right guaranteed by the European Convention on Human Rights was held not to be "necessary in a democratic society". The standard that the House of Lords thought to be appropriate was rejected by the European Court as an undue restriction on freedom of expression. But that standard is substantially less restrictive than the one proposed by the Law Reform Commission of Canada. There is a significant difference between interfering with freedom of speech only where there is "real prejudice to the administration of justice" and attempting to prevent publication of material that one ought to know may interfere with judicial proceedings. Fortunately, the *Report* seems to have been rejected by the Government of Canada.

The omnibus Criminal Law Reform Bill which was introduced in Parliament in 1984 contained provisions for reform of the law of contempt of court. These were more encouraging. The existing common law was to be supplanted by statutorily-defined offences, all of which, presumably, would have attracted the procedural protections of both the Charter and the Criminal Code. Maximum penalties were specified. A judge was not to be able to preside at the trial of an offence which related to him or to a proceeding over which he had presided.

The *sub judice* rule was to be re-defined as follows:

> Every one who knowingly makes or causes to be made any publication that creates a substantial risk that the course of justice in any particular civil or criminal proceeding pending at the time of the publication will be seriously impeded or prejudiced is guilty of ...

This was something of an improvement. It seems that *means rea* was required. More important, the language, "substantial risk" that a "particular" proceeding will be "seriously impeded or prejudiced", suggests that some concrete evidence, rather than mere supposition, of impeding or prejudicing would be required. "Pending" was defined. The defences of "fair and accurate report", borrowed from libel law, and "discussion in good faith of public affairs" were created.

Scandalising the court was to involve:

> Every one who without lawful justification or excuse, wilfully makes or causes to be made any publication of a false, scandalous or scurrilous statement calculated to bring unto disrepute a court or judge in his official capacity.

This provision could have gone much farther. Still, it did make clear that *mens rea* was required and that the offence did not embrace statements made about judges in their non-official capacities. More important, a defence of truth and public benefit was created.

The Bill died with the government that introduced it. The current Government of Canada has introduced proposals for criminal law reform, but these proposals do not touch contempt of court.

My own views on the directions reform should take are as follows.

The offence of scandalising the court has no place in the law of a democratic state and should be abolished. With respect to *sub judice*, there should be specific provisions in the *Criminal Code* which state precisely the sorts of information which may not be published about judicial proceedings and the time period within which such information is not to be published. A number of prohibitions of this nature now appear in the Code. In drafting such provisions there should be a bias in favour of openness.

3.4 Dealing with Material that Might Become Evidence in a Judicial Proceeding

> The material in this sub-section is not, strictly speaking, part of the law of contempt. It raises questions about the rights and duties of journalists with respect to material in their possession which the State may seek to use as evidence in proceedings before the courts.

3.4.1 *Criminal Code*, R.S.C. 1985, c. C-46

139. (1) Every one who wilfully attempts in any manner to obstruct, pervert or defeat the course of justice in a judicial proceeding,

  (*a*) by indemnifying or agreeing to indemnify a surety, in any way and either in whole or in part, or

  (*b*) where he is a surety, by accepting or agreeing to accept a fee or any form of indemnity whether in whole or in part from or in respect of a person who is released or is to be released from custody,

is guilty of

  (*c*) an indictable offence and is liable to imprisonment for two years, or

  (*d*) an offence punishable on summary conviction.

(2) Every one who wilfully attempts in any manner other than a manner described in subsection (1) to obstruct, pervert or defeat the course of justice is guilty of an indictable offence and is liable to imprisonment for ten years.

(3) Without restricting the generality of subsection (2), every one shall be deemed wilfully to attempt to obstruct, pervert or defeat the course of justice who in a judicial proceeding, existing or proposed,

  (*a*) dissuades or attempts to dissuade a person by threats, bribes or other corrupt means from giving evidence;

  (*b*) influences or attempts to influence by threats, bribes or other corrupt means, a person in his conduct as a juror; or

  (*c*) accepts or obtains, agrees to accept or attempts to obtain a bribe or other corrupt consideration to abstain from giving evidence, or to do or to refrain from doing anything as a juror.

487. (1) A justice who is satisfied by information upon oath in Form 1, that there is reasonable ground to believe that there is in a building, receptacle or place

  (*a*) anything on or in respect of which any offence against this Act or any other Act of Parliament has been or is suspected to have been committed,

  (*b*) anything that there is reasonable ground to believe will afford evidence with respect to the commission of an offence against this Act or any other Act of Parliament, or

  (*c*) anything that there is reasonable ground to believe is intended to be used for the purpose of committing any offence against the person for which a person may be arrested without warrant,

may at any time issue a warrant under his hand authorizing a person named therein or a peace officer

  (*d*) to search the building, receptacle or place for any such thing and to seize it, and

  (*e*) subject to any other Act of Parliament, to, as soon as practicable, bring the thing seized before, or make a report in respect thereof to, the justice or some other justice for the same territorial division in accordance with section 489.1.

(2) Where the building, receptacle, or place in which anything mentioned in subsection (1) is believed to be is in some other territorial division, the justice may issue his warrant in like form modified according to the circumstances, and the warrant may be executed in the other territorial division after it has been endorsed, in Form 25, by a justice having jurisdiction in that territorial division.

(3) A search warrant issued under this section may be in the form set out as Form 5 in Part XXV, varied to suit the case.

(4) An endorsement that is made on a warrant as provided for in subsection (2) is sufficient authority to the peace officers or such persons to whom it was originally directed and to all peace officers within the jurisdiction of the justice by whom it is endorsed to execute the warrant and to deal with the things seized in accordance with section 489.1 or as otherwise provided by law.

487.1 (1) Where a peace officer believes that an indictable offence has been I committed and that it would be impracticable to appear personally before a justice to make application for a warrant in accordance with section 258 or 487, the peace officer may submit an information on oath by telephone or other means of telecommunication to a justice designated for the purpose by the chief judge of the provincial court having jurisdiction in the matter.

(2) An information submitted by telephone or other means of telecommunication shall be on oath and shall be recorded verbatim by the justice who shall, as soon as practicable, cause to be filed with the clerk of the court for the territorial division in which the warrant is intended for execution the record or a transcription thereof, certified by the justice as to time, date and contents.

(3) For the purposes of subsection (2), an oath may be administered by telephone or others means of telecommunication.

(4) An information on oath submitted by telephone or other means of telecommunication shall include

(*a*) a statement of the circumstances that make it impracticable for the peace officer to appear personally before a justice;

(*b*) a statement of the indictable offence alleged, the place or premises to be searched and the items alleged to be liable to seizure;

(*c*) a statement of the peace officer's grounds for believing that items liable to seizure in respect of the offence alleged will be found in the place of premises to be searched; and

(*d*) a statement as to any prior application for a warrant under this section or any other search warrant, in respect of the same matter, of which the pace officer has knowledge.

(5) A justice referred to in subsection (1) who is satisfied that an information on oath submitted by telephone or other means of telecommunication

(*a*) is in respect of an indictable offence and conforms to the requirements of — subsection (4),

(*b*) discloses reasonable grounds for dispensing with an information presented personally and in writing, and

(*c*) discloses reasonable grounds, in accordance with paragraph 443(1)(a), (b) or (c) or subsection 240(1), as the case may be, for the issuance of a warrant in respect of an indictable offence,

may issue a warrant to a pace officer conferring the same authority respecting search and seizure as may be conferred by a warrant issued by a justice before whom the peace officer appears personally pursuant to subsection 240(1) or 443(1), as the case may be, and may require that the warrant be executed within such time period as the justice may order.

(6) Where a justice issues a warrant by telephone or other means of telecommunication,
   (a) the justice shall complete and sign the warrant in Form 5.1, noting on its face the time, date and place of issuance;
   (b) the peace officer, on the direction of the justice, shall complete, in duplicate, a facsimile of the warrant in Form 5.1, noting on its face the name of the issuing justice and the time, date and place of issuance; and
   (c) the justice shall, as soon as practicable after the warrant has been issued, cause the warrant to be field with the clerk of the court for the territorial division in which the warrant is intended for execution.

(7) A pace officer who executes a warrant issued by telephone or other means of telecommunication, other than a warrant issued pursuant to subsection 240(1), shall, before entering the place or premises to be searched or as soon as practicable thereafter, give a facsimile of the warrant to any person present and ostensibly in control of the place or premises.

(8) A peace officer who, in any unoccupied place or premises, executes a warrant issued by telephone or other means of telecommunication, other than a warrant issued pursuant to subsection 240(1), shall, on entering the place or premises or as soon as practicable thereafter, cause a facsimile of the warrant to be suitably affixed in a prominent place within the place or premises.

(9) A peace officer to whom a warrant is issued by telephone or other means of telecommunication shall file a written report with the clerk of the court for the territorial division in which the warrant was intended for execution as soon as practicable but within a period not exceeding seven days after the warrant has been executed, which report shall include
   (a) a statement of the time and date the warrant was executed or, if the warrant was not executed, a statement of the reasons why it was not executed;
   (b) a statement of the things, if any, that were seized pursuant to the warrant and the location where they are being held; and
   (c) a statement of the things, if any, that were seized in addition to the things mentioned in the warrant and the location where they are being held, together with a statement of the peace officer's grounds for believing that those additional things had been obtained by, or used in, the commission of an offence.

(10) The clerk of the court with whom a written report is filed pursuant to subsection (9) shall, as soon as practicable, cause the report, together with the information on oath and the wurunt to which it pertains, to be brought before a justice to be dealt with, in respect of the things seized referred to in the report, in the same manner as if the things were seized pursuant to a warrant issued, on an information presented personally by a peace officer, by that justice or another justice for the same territorial division.

(11) In any proceeding in which it is material for a court to be satisfied that a search or seizure was authorized by a warrant issued by telephone or other means of telecommunication, the absence of the information on oath, transcribed and certified by the justice as to time, date and contents, or of the original warrant, signed by the justice and carrying on its face a notation of the time, date and place of issuance, is, in the absence of evidence to the contrary. proof that the search or seizure was not authorized by a warrant issued by telephone or other means of telecommunication.

487.2 (1) Where a search warrant is issued under section 487 or 487.1 or a search is made under such a warrant, every one who publishes in any newspaper or broadcasts any information with respect to

    (*a*) the location of the place searched or to be searched, or

    (*b*) the identity of any person who is or appears to occupy or be in possession or control of that place or who is suspected of being involved in any offence in relation to which the warrant was issued,

without the consent of every person referred to in paragraph (b) is, unless a change has been laid in respect of any offence in relation to which the warrant was issued, guilty of an offence punishable on summary conviction.

Note: In *Canadian Newspapers Ltd. v. Attorney-General for Canada* (1986) 32 D.L.R. (4th) 233 the Ontario High Court of Justice held that this section was an unjustifiable limit on freedom of expression.

3.4.2 Harold Levy, "What Should We Do When the Cops Arrive?" *Content* 95, 1979

Freedom of Expression in Canada is being subvened on many fronts Nowhere is the trend more evident than in the area of freedom of the press, both print and broadcast.

In the United States, a similar tendency toward subversion of a free press has occasioned an intense, concerned and often acrimonious debate.

But in Canada all is peaceful. True, the press is agonizing, but more over the latest Margaret Trudeau escapade or Joe Clark gaffe than over its own freedom.

And Canadians blithely coast along, apparently unconcerned or unaware that Canadian joumalists have never had those rights which their U.S. counterparts are so distraught about losing.

FACT: Canadian journalists have always been compellable witnesses. No legal privilege has ever been recognized between joumalists and their sources, just as no legal privilege attaches to communications between members of Parliament and their constituents, doctors and their patients, or even priests and their parishioners. And that's always been the law.

FACT: Parliament has not built into the search warrant process special protections to be applied when a news service is the object of the search.

The same provisions of the Criminal Code apply, whether the place sought to be searched is a newspaper or an outhouse.

Unfortunately, under Canadian law, all that stands between the government and the confidential sources of the reporter is a justice of the pace issuing a search warrant — and that's not much protection at all.

The only concern of the justice of the pace who issues the warrant is whether there is reasonable ground to believe that the search will yield evidence with respect to the commission of an offence.

Those experienced with the system suspect that the justice of the peace often acts as a "rubber stamp" for the police, issuing warrants in a routine fashion on the skimpiest of evidence and without a hearing.

FACTS: There is no requirement in law whatsoever, where the object of the search is a newspaper or a news room, that prior notice and a hearing be given in connection with the issuance of search warrants. Nor is there any requirement, where the newspaper is not suspected of a crime, that the state restrict itself to the subpoena process.

Such requirements would eliminate raids by the police on the offices of the media and would allow the courts to make the decision on the relevance and admissibility of the materials desired.

FACT: Police and government officials can legally tap journalists' telephones.

They are not limited to searching for or subpoenaing the long-distance telephone records of reporters and news organizations. In Canada's wire-tap legislation, The Protection of Privacy Act — better described as the *Invasion of Privacy Act* — there are no special provisions protecting the press. And under the *Official Secrets Act*, the federal solicitor-general can entirely by-pass the judicial process and on his own unreviewable authority order the interception of a journalist's communications. Although the number of interceptions carried out under the act must be disclosed, there is no way to know whether the communications of journalists has been intercepted by executive order.

FACT: The federal government is expected to reintroduce legislation, which died with the last session of Parliament, giving its solicitor-general the power to intercept anyone's mail, including mail to or from journalists, on his own order and without application to the court.

IN SUM, by failing to recognize the very special role of the press in a democratic society, successive Canadian governments have given their own investigators and law enforcement officials vast powers which make it easy to investigate, inhibit, discourage and disrupt the press, while at the same time, by intimidating sources and creating an "iron curtain" of secrecy under the *Official Secrets Act*, making it difficult for the press to investigate the government.

If you think that these powers have not been widely used or are not being used more and more frequently or likely will not be used against you, they have a look at our Dossier Noir on page 38 and keep in mind that this is just a partial list of offences against the press.

If you're still not convinced, then ask somebody with the Fredericton *Daily Gleaner* or Montreal's *Quebec-Presse* or *Radio-Canada* or *The Toronto Sun* or the *CBC* or *Global* television or *The London Free Press* or *The Vancouver Sun* or the Trail, B.C. *Times*. They've all experienced police raids.

With such raids becoming ever more frequent, you might well ask what you can do to protect your independence. If so, turn to the next two pages and find out what you can do when the police arrive in your newsroom.

1. Ask to see the warrant

BEFORE THE POLICE come to your door, they will have obtained a search warrant from a justice of the peace, authorizing a search of the specified documents, to be conducted within a particular time period.

The officers are obligated by law to produce the warrant upon request and may only execute it by day unless the justice authorizes execution by night.

2. Check the warrant for defects.

IT IS DIFFICULT for a layperson to make a decision on whether a search warrant is legally valid — and it is risky as well. Even an experienced lawyer might well be unable to predict whether a court would, at a subsequent date, declare a warrant to be valid in law or not.

In an interview for this article, *The Vancouver Sun's* Allan Fotheringham, whose newspaper is very experienced in such matters, said that, when the police arrive, they should be told to "get the hell out" until a lawyer can be summoned to determine the validity of the warrant.

He recognizes, however, that not all publications have the services of a lawyer at hand and that employees of the paper might find themselves in a dilemma if the police politely refuse and insist on entering to conduct their search.

Nonetheless it can be worthwhile to examine the warrant for obvious defects. If the warrant appears patently defective in that (1) it does not name or describe the premises to be searched or (2) does not contain a time limit within which the search is to be conducted or (3) does not detail the offence which the search is expected to reveal or (4) does not give details of the grounds on which the warrant was sought, you can stall the police by threatening to expose the defectiveness of the warrant to legal counsel and to instruct counsel to take steps against the police.

3. Let them search.

IF THE WARRANT appears a lawful one, those on the premises are obliged to stand aside and permit the search.

If you do not permit the police to enter in a voluntary manner, they are authorized to use reasonable force to effect an entry in order to conduct the search.

If you use force to impede their entry, you could be charged with obstructing the police.

Although the *Criminal Code* contains a procedure which requires the prosecution to make available copies of the material seized, it may well be advisable to seek permission to list the various items being removed or to photocopy on the premises prior to removal.

4. Say as little as possible.

THERE IS NO obligation whatsoever on any person in the premises to speak to the police or answer any questions put by the police during the course of the search. This was well understood by *Toronto Sun* editor Peter Worthington when

RCMP officers visited him in search of a letter known to be in his possession and addressed to a high-ranking officer of the Security Service.

Worthington's comments, made in an interview for *Content*, are most instructive in regards to handling the police when they are searching for a single item.

The Mounties initially asked me to co-operate by voluntarily furnishing the letter to them, so that they would not have to obtain a search warrant. I refused to co-operate and, in fact, they had a search warrant with them all the time . . . It is well-known that newspaper offices are not the neatest places in the world. They looked everywhere — under pictures and behind desks. Finally, four or five hours later, they got around to the top drawer of my desk and almost missed the letter. It was a very confusing scene. I think it was Bob Johnson, then with the CBC, who said, "I don't know if they will find a letter in this mess — but they may lose a Mountie."

5. Protect sensitive material

WHERE THE POLICE have in fact entered the premises and are intent on seizing an easily locatable item which may contain names or information of a confidential nature, an effective technique is to insist that the item be placed in an envelope which is then to be sealed and marked for the attention of either the justice of the peace who issued the warrant or the sheriff of the county in which the premises are located.

The value of this tactic is that the information must be kept confidential, beyond the scrutiny of the police, until a hearing can be held as to its admissibility in evidence at a future date.

6. Use cooperation to your own advantage:

ACCORDING TO Toronto lawyer Clayton C. Ruby, who is counsel to a television network, it is quite common for the police to request the co-operation of the station being searched.

In his view, there is little to lose in co-operating with regard to film which has been aired.

He has, however, advised his network to refuse to co-operate with regard to the outs. To co-operate puts the station in the position of acting as agents of the state in enforcing the law, a role inconsistent with the independence of a free press.

In Ruby's experience, the purpose of the police in obtaining the outs is usually to assist in identifying individuals who participated in a particular demonstration or disturbance.

Needless to state, where the network co-oprates by turning over film that has been aired, it should be duplicated so that the police will not have the only copy.

Clayton Ruby cautions that, although there is no obligation imposed upon anyone to answer questions posed by the police or to assist in any way, this is not to say that total non-coopration is advisable — only that it is important that the media should make their own decisions about co-operating.

What to do *before* the police arrive.

Safeguard notes and outs

EVERY JOURNALIST must have a personal solution for safeguarding crucial notes. Clayton Ruby cautions that it is necessary to retain outs and reporters' notes in case of libel suits or allegations of inaccuracy and, therefore, does not advise his clients to destroy these materials. He cautions as well that, if you destroy material which you have been notified may be evidence in legal proceedings, you may be committing the crime of obstructing the course of justice.

However, in Ruby's view,

"It is foolish for the TV stations and the newspapers to keep their "outs" and reporters' notes in such a way that any fool with a search warrant can walk in and find them. Such material should be filed in ways which suit the convenience of the newspapers or TV stations, as opposed to the police."

In the long run, however, prudence and common sense rather than paranoia is called for.

Learn about the law

RUBY ALSO RECOMMENDS that the press and other media should retain counsel to hold meetings with staff on the subject of the rights and obligations of journalists so that they can evaluate situations as they arise and can react in an informed way.

Protect your subscribers

ONE OF THE WORST features of the 1977 raid conducted by the police on the offices of the Pink Triangle Press was the seizure of a list of subscribers to *The Body Politic*.

Such evidence could have little value in a prosecution for mailing indecent matter, since all that is required to evidence the mailing of a periodical is a standard form from Canada Post and a copy of the issue in question. And, in fact, none of the material seized in the raid was introduced at trial.

The police could find pretexts for conducting raids on all sorts of publications expressing views different from those of the majority, thus exposing the subscribers to political harassment.

An effective method of protecting the subscription list involved the keeping of circulation documents off the premises with the use of a "fulfillment" house which utilizes computers equipped with magnetic taps.

According the Rolf Brauch, the president of Brauch-Neville Associates Ltd., a fulfillment house is not a Japanese brothel — it is rather a service which assists the publisher by maintaining the circulation list and preparing the labels which are usually then affixed at the printers and mailed. The two principle concerns identified by Brauch are those of continuity and confidentiality.

Continuity is easily assured by maintaining a back-up tap containing the names of the subscribers. Thus, even if the police raided the fulfillment house and were able to identify a tape or a portion of a tap and seize it, the publisher would be left with a back-up tape and would thus be assured that the next issue could be readily mailed.

In order to ensure confidentiality, Brauch suggests that the customer be recorded in the firm's records under a pseudonym such as *Garden-Club* News.

The police would be confronted by a forest of racks containing hundreds of magnetic reels each containing between 300,000 and 600,000 names.

This method works because there is no obligation in law requiring anyone to assist the police by telling them where the original circulation documents are located or on which tape the subscription list is to be found.

An advantage of the system suggested by Brauch, is that not only are continuity and security preserved, but there is no extra cost to the customer.

What really boggles the mind is that it should be necessary in a free society for the media to have to indulge in such subterfuge in order to counter the unwarranted and unjustifiable intrusion of the state.

Fight fire with fire

THE MEDIA HAVE a great advantage in that they can use their own facilities to report incidents of harassment by the police.

Back in 1972, when the Times of Trail, B.C. was visited by RCMP officers who questioned company employees about a series of articles describing routine activities of the local RCMP detachinent, ME Herb Legg called upon the federal solicitor-general and provincial attorney-general to investigate whether members of the RCMP would return and highlighted the harassment on the front page.

There are numerous examples of such selective police harassment, but few are as odious as the actions of former Kitchener police chief Sidney Brown, who denied reporters with the Kitchener-Waterloo Record access to the Waterloo Regional Police Headquarters and access to further investigation information after photographs were published in the newspaper showing members of the force's tactical squad standing guard over a group of Henchmen Motorcycle Club members after a raid on their clubhouse. One of the pictures showed cyclists kneeling with their hands cuffed behind their backs under the waiting fangs of an angry-looking German shepherd.

Because of the intensive public pressure generated by the newspaper and the support of other media, the police chief had to retreat and the threatened criminal charges against employees of the paper in connection with the photographs were not pursued.

The lesson stemming from all of these incidents and so many others, is that the media must make the facts known whenever such harassment occurs.

3.4.3 C.B.C. v. Attorney-General for New Brunswick et al. (1991), 85 D.L.R. (4th) 57 (S.C.C.)

CORY, J.: — This appeal is concerned with the factors that should be taken into account by a justice of the peace when determining whether to issue a warrant to search the premises of a media organization that is not implicated in the crime under investigation. Specifically, the court must determine whether freedom of the press, as protected by s. 2(b) of the *Canadian Charter of Rights and Freedoms*, requires that a justice of the peace, before issuing a warrant to search media offices, be satisfied that no reasonable alternative source of the information exists.

Factual Background

In early September of 1988, demonstrations were held in the Kedgewicks-St-Quentin regions of New Brunswick to protest the policies of the Fraser Co., a large pulp and paper concern. On September 10th, during one of those protests, Molotov cocktails were thrown at a company guardhouse, setting it on fire.

While the police had turned out in force during much of the demonstration, only a handful were present when the guardhouse was ignited. Among the remaining officers were identification specialists. As well, a number of police informers were circulating among the crowd to help identify any wrongdoers. As might be expected, members of the media were on the scene, including reporters of the Canadian Broadcasting Corporation (the C.B.C.) who recorded much of the protest on video tape.

Officer Marcel Ouellette of the Royal Canadian Mounted Police (the R.C.M.P.) swore an information in support of an application for a search warrant to seize from the C.B.C. tapes, films and video cassettes recording the events of September 9 and 10, 1988, at St. Quentin. Officer Ouellette described the material to be seized as follows:

> Tapes, and/or films and/or videocassettes and/or portions of films or video tapes commonly known as "outs" or "out-takes", the latter being portions of tape or videocassette from a lengthier film or videocassette and not subsequently used for transmission by the facility of Radio-Canada...

In his information, Officer Ouellette explained that while other sources of information existed, they, for various reasons, either provided insufficient evidence or else were unavailable or unwilling to testify. It was set out in this way in the information:

(4) THAT all three informants have expressed fear for their own physical safety which I do verily believe is reasonable in the circumstances in view of the high tensions surrounding the disputes with Fraser Inc., such apprehension in the view of your dependent is aptly justified. All three informants live within the area.

(10) THAT as a result of the information conveyed to me by Constables FORTIN and GLADU earlier referred to which I do verily believe I have reasonable grounds to believe that the information contained in the said film or portions thereof will afford relevant evidence for the prosecution of a criminal offence evidence which would not otherwise be available due to:
- (a) The considerable confusion at the scene;
- (b) The limited number of R.C.M.P. officers available at the time for identification purposes;
- (c) The darkness and general visibility problems at the time preventing easy eye witness identification by the Royal Canadian Mounted

(11) THAT alternative sources of information have been exhausted, such as the use of informants as earlier referred to, the informants having made it very clear to your deponent that they do not dare come forward and testify in court of law.

(12) THAT despite considerable investigation effort in the area, no eye witnesses are prepared to come forward and describe the events and give evidence against the participants in the attempted and actual criminal activities.

(13) THAT as the result of the three paragraphs above, your deponent does have reason to believe and does believe that there are no other means available to the police for obtaining evidences for the proper determination of possible charges.

The information did not reveal that police identification experts were also present at the scene. Relying upon the information of Officer Ouellette, a justice of the peace issued the requested search warrant on October 26, 1988. The following day, three R.C.M.P. officers attended at the offices of the C.B.C. in Moncton. The officers and officials from the C.B.C. agreed to place the video tapes in question in a sealed envelope to be held by Judge McIntyre of the Provincial Court pending the outcome of these proceedings.

On December 22, 1988, the C.B.C. brought an application to quash the warrant and to order the return of the seized tapes. On April 7, 1989, Daigle J. quashed the warrant. On December 22, 1989, the Court of Appeal allowed the Crown's appeal and upheld the issuance of the warrant.

Relevant Legislation

Section 487 (formerly s. 443) of the *Criminal Code* provides:

487. (1) A justice who is satisfied by information on oath in Form 1 that there are reasonable grounds to believe that there is in a building, receptacle or place

. . . . .

(*b*) anything that there is reasonable ground to believe will afford evidence with respect to the commission of an offence against this Act or any other Act or Parliament . . .

. . . . .

may at any time issue a warrant under his hand authorizing a person named therein or a peace officer

(*d*) to search the building, receptacle or place for any such thing and to seize it, and

(e) subject to any other Act of Parliament, to, as soon as practicable bring the thing seized before, or make a report in respect thereof to, the justice or some other justice for the same territorial division in accordance with section 489.1.

Requirements for obtaining a search warrant and the discretion of the issuing officer

Section 487 of the *Criminal Code* sets out the only requirements which must be met for the Issuance of a search warrant. They are but two. It must be demonstrated that reasonable grounds exist to believe: (1) that there is in a building, receptacle or place; (2) something that will afford evidence with respect to the commission of an offence against the *Code* or any other Act of Parliament.

The section, by the use of the word "may", recognizes that the justice of the peace has a discretion to determine whether to issue the warrant. The two decisions referred to above, one by the British Columbia Supreme Court and the other by the Supreme Court of Canada, have discussed the nature of this discretion.

1. *Re Pacific Press Ltd. and The Queen*

In *Pacific Press*, journalists had observed individuals picketing and then occupying the premises in which the Restrictive Trade Practices Commission was to hold an inquiry. The obstruction of an inquiry constitutes an offence under s. 41 of the *Combines Investigation Act*, R.S.C. 1970, c. C-23. Combines Investigation officers contacted the editor of "The Vancouver Sun", asking for information as to the identity of the individuals involved in the picketing and occupation. The editor refused to provide this information.

Combines officers then applied for a search warrant in order to obtain the desired information from "The Vancouver Sun" and "The Province", both of which were owned by Pacific Press Limited. The warrants were issued and served the next day. The search was conducted in the area where newspapers were being prepared for publication. Some 77 pieces of paper, a number of handwritten notes and 69 frames of negative film were seized together with a reporter's private "contact book" which contained a list of the names and addresses of people who acted as sources of information for the newspapers. In considering the application of Pacific Press Ltd. to quash the warrant, Nemetz C.J.B.C. observed, at p. 489 that "[t]here is little doubt that the search disrupted the operation of the newspapers and delayed the preparation and publication of both newspapers that day".

Nemetz C.J.B.C. found that there was a defect in the search warrant for "The Province" which rendered it invalid. He then addressed the issue of whether, because "The Vancouver Sun" was a press organization, a justice of the peace could issue a warrant in the absence of proof that no reasonable alternative to the search existed as a means of obtaining the desired evidence. In considering this question, Nemetz C.J.B.C. adopted a passage from the judgment of Lord Denning in *Senior v. Holdsworth, Ex p. Independent Television News Ltd.*, [1976] 1 Q.B. 23, which recognizes the news media as occupying a "special position" in relation to search warrants and, in particular, recognizes the difficult and careful balancing required when freedom of the press rights collide with the state interest in investigating and prosecuting clime through the use of search warrants.

Expressing his agreement with this view, Nemetz C.J.B.C. concluded at pp. 494-5:

> Where, then, does the matter stand in Canada? Counsel for the petitioner submits that Parliament has accorded the free press a special place under the *Canadian Bill of Rights*. Accordingly, he argues, ss. 1(f) and 2, must be taken into consideration and weighed by the Justice of the Peace before he exercises his judicial discretion to grant the issuance of a search warrant against an organ of the free press of this country. A *fortiori*, he says, this fact is to be weighed in cases where the premises of the newspaper are not the premises of those persons accused of the crime. I agree with this submission. Furthermore, he submits, it was wrong, in the circumstances, to attempt to render the press an investigative arm of the State when other means of obtaining the names of the persons involved in the melee at the combines hearing may have been available. In particular, counsel points to the fact that many persons other than the newspaper people were in attendance at the combines office on the days in question and the material does not show whether these other people were approached to establish the identity of the participants in the fracas.
>
> The issuing of any search warrant is a serious matter, especially when its issuance against a newspaper may have, as it did, the effect of impeding its publication. To use the words of my distinguished predecessor in *United Distillers Ltd.* (1948), 88 C.C.C. 338, [1947] 3 D.L.R. 900, the Justice of the Peace "should have reasonable information before him to entitle him to judicially decide whether such warrant should issue or not". In my opinion, no such reasonable information was before him since there was no material to show:
> 1. whether a reasonable alternative source of obtaining the information was or was not available, and
> 2. if available, that reasonable steps had been taken to obtain it from that alternative source.

2. *Descoteaux v. Mierzwinski, supra*

In *Descoteaux v. Mierzwinski*, this court considered whether a search which was said to impinge upon solicitor-client privilege was permitted under what is now s. 487 of the *Criminal Code*. In that case, Mierzwinski had allegedly lied to a lawyer at a legal aid clinic with respect to his finances. At issue was the validity of a search warrant to search the offices of the clinic to find the form upon which Mierzwinski made his financial declaration. Lamer J., as he then was, writing for the court, found that since it was the financial declaration itself which was alleged to be fraudulent, it was not subject to solicitor-client privilege.

In the course of his reasons, Lamer J. discussed the jurisdiction of a justice of the peace to issue a search warrant and noted that the jurisdiction did not, in any way, depend on the nature of the premises to be searched. That is to say, a search could be authorized of any premises within a residence, lawyer's office or media organization.

Lamer J. observed, however, that a justice of the peace could lose jurisdiction if sufficient protection were not given to the fundamental right of freedom of the press. At pp. 411-2 C.C.C., pp. 616-7 D.L.R., he held:

> The justice of the peace, in my view, has the authority, where circumstances warrant. to set out execution procedures in the search warrant; I would even go so far as to say that he has the right to refuse to issue the warrant in special circumstances, such as those found in *Re Pacific Press Ltd. and the Queen, supra.*
>
> That case involved a search of a newspaper office for information gathered by the newspaper staff. Neither the newspaper staff nor the newspaper itself were accused of having been involved in the commission of an offence. In view of the special situation of a newspaper in light of ss. 1(f) and 2 of the *Canadian Bill of Rights*, R.S.C. 1970, App. III, Nemetz C.J. of the British Columbia Supreme Court quashed the search warrant issued by the justice of the peace ...
>
> . . . . .
>
> It could be advanced that the two conditions set out by Nemetz C.J. should be met before a warrant is issued whenever a search is sought to be conducted, under s. 443(1)(b), of premises occupied by an innocent third party which are not alleged by the information to be connected in any way with the crime. It is not necessary for purposes of this appeal to decide that point. *It is sufficient to say that in situations such as the one in Re Pacific Press Ltd., where the search would interfere with rights as fundamental as freedom of the press, and, as in the case at bar, a lawyer's client's right to confidentiality, the justice of the peace may and should refuse to issue the warrant if these two conditions have not been met, lest he exceed the jurisdiction he had ab initio.*

(Emphasis added).

From this I take it that if the failure to meet these two conditions would interfere with the freedom of the press, this could result in a loss of jurisdiction. Such a failure would not necessarily result in an automatic loss of jurisdiction. It must not be forgotten that in the *Pacfic Press* case, the search significantly interfered with the operations of the newspaper resulting in a delay in publication of the news. Today that same situation would require a court to take into consideration ss. 8 and 24 of the Charter.

The decisions in both *Descoteaux and Pacific Press* recognized that a justice of the peace has a discretion to determine whether to issue a search warrant. In exercising this discretion a balance must be struck between the interests of the state in investigating and prosecuting crime and the privacy interests of the individual or body whose premises the state wishes to search. Both cases indicate that a proper balancing of these interests must involve a consideration of the effects of the search on both the ability of the police to proceed with their investigation and on the ability of those being searched to carry out their functions.

In *Pacific Press*, the search disrupted the operation of a corporation which was not implicated in the crime being investigated and delayed the publication of its newspaper. These factors weighed heavily in the determination that the search warrant was not valid. Perhaps the only circumstance which could have counterbalanced and outweighed the serious interference with the operations of the media organization was a demonstrated necessity to obtain the information. This necessity could have been demonstrated by establishing that:

1. no other reasonable alternative source of obtaining the information was available, or
2. if an alternative source were available, that reasonable steps had been taken to obtain the information from the alternative source and that they had been proved unsuccessful.

Because these two factors were not demonstrated on the information placed before the justice of the peace, Nemetz C.J.B.C., on balancing all of the factors involved, held that the search warrant should be quashed.

The balancing of interests is essential to the entire process involved in the issuance of search warrants. As Lamer J. noted in *Descoteaux*, the various interests must not only be considered in determining whether a warrant should be issued, but also in determining the form the warrant should take. He wrote at p. 412 C.C.C., p. 617 D.L.R.:

> Moreover, even if the conditions are met, the justice of the peace *must* set out procedures for the execution of the warrant that reconcile protection of the interests this right is seeking to promote with protection of those the search power is seeking to promote, and limit the breach of this fundamental right to what is strictly inevitable.

(Emphasis in original).

The Constitutional Protection of Freedom of Expression

Any search of premises is certain to be disquieting and upsetting. The invasion of privacy rights which a search entails is an important concern for all members of a democratic society. Some searches are obviously more intrusive and upsetting than others For example, the search of a residence is likely to have graver consequences than a search of commercial premises which may be subject to statutory regulation and inspection. Because of its intrusive nature, a warrant to search any premises must only be issued when a justice of the peace is satisfied that all the statutory requirements have been met. In those situations where all the statutory prerequisites have been established, the justice of the peace should still consider all of the circumstances in determining whether to exercise his or her discretion to issue a warrant. It is not a step that can be taken lightly. This is particularly true when a warrant is sought to search the offices of a news media organization, where the consequences are likely to be disruptive of the media's role of gathering and publishing news.

The media have a vitally important role to play in a democratic society. It is the media that by gathering and disseminating news, enable members of our society to make an informed assessment of the issues which may significantly affect their lives and well being. The special significance of the work of the media was recognized by this court in *Edmonton Journal v. Alberta (Attorney-General)* (1989), 64 D.L.R. (4th) 577 at pp. 609-10, [1989] 2 S.C.R. 1326, 41 C.F.C. (2d) 109. The importance of that role and the manner in which it must be fulfilled gives rise to special concerns when a warrant is sought to search media premises.

The constitutional protection of freedom of expression afforded by s. 2(b) of the Charter does not, however; import any new or additional requirements for the issuance of search warrants. What it does is provide a backdrop against which the reasonableness of the search may be evaluated. It requires that careful consideration be given not only to whether a warrant should issue but also to the conditions which might properly be imposed upon any search of media premises.

Whether the search of a media office can be considered reasonable will depend on a number of factors including the nature of the objects to be seized, the manner in which the search is to be conducted and the degree of urgency of the search. It is of particular importance that the justice of the peace consider the effects of the search and seizure on the ability of the particular media organization in question to fulfil its function as a news gatherer and news disseminator. If a search will impede the media from fulfilling these functions and the impediments cannot reasonably be controlled through the imposition of conditions on the execution of the search warrant, then a warrant should only be issued where a compelling state interest is demonstrated. This might be accomplished by satisfying the two factors set out by Nemetz C.J.B.C. in Pacific Press: namely, that there is no alternative source of information available or, if there is, that reasonable steps have been taken to obtain the information from that source. Alternatively, the search might be justified on the grounds of the gravity of the offence under investigation and the urgent need to obtain the evidence expected to be revealed by the search.

The balancing of interests is always a difficult and delicate task. In this case, for example, the throwing of Molotov cocktails at a building not only damaged the property but constituted a potential threat to the lives and safety of others. The investigation of a serious and violent crime was of importance to the state. Further, in light of the ongoing demonstrations, some urgency in conducting the search must be recognized. On the other hand, the objects sought to be seized were the product of the research and investigation of a media organization. It was important that the continuing work of the media should not be unduly impeded. The factors to be weighed with regard to issuing a warrant to search any premises will vary with the circumstances presented. This is as true of searches of media offices as of any other premises. It seems to me, however, that where the media have fulfilled their role by gathering the news and publishing it, there would seem to be less to be said for refusing to make that material available to the police. At that point, the media have given to the public, by way of picture or print, evidence of the commission of a crime. The media, like any good citizen, should not be unduly opposed to disclosing to the police the evidence they have gathered with regard to that crime.

For example, if a private citizen took pictures of a crime being committed and posted those pictures on a public notice board, the public could quite properly expect that those pictures and the negatives would, upon request, be delivered to the police. This is so as it is in the best interests of all members of the community to see that crimes are investigated and prosecuted. Should the private citizen fail to do so, the police would be expected to take steps to obtain a warrant to search the citizen's premises for the negatives and copies of the photographs. Once the media have published the information, the same principles might well apply to them.

The media argue that the issuance of a search warrant would have the effect of "drying up" their sources of information. In my view, that argument is seriously weakened once the media have placed the information in the public domain. They can then no longer say, in effect: "I know that a crime was committed; I have relevant information that could assist in its investigation and prosecution, but I'm not going to assist you towards that end." Once the information has been made public, it becomes difficult to contend there would be a "chilling effect" on the media sources if that information were also disclosed to the police. At that point, it is unlikely that the police would want more than the video tape itself. With the tape in their possession, the police would usually have no interest in identifying the media's informant whose tip led to the making of the film. Should it be necessary, appropriate steps might be taken by the media to have the court determine what protection could properly be obtained. The police themselves might very well be interested in protecting the identity of a media informant in many cases.

Counsel for the C.B.C. submits that the two factors referred to in *Pacific Press* should, pursuant to ss. 2(b) and 8 of the Charter, be made mandatory conditions for the issuance of any warrant for the search of premises of media organizations. In essence, the C.B.C. submits that these two factors ought to be separated from all others that have to be considered in determining the reasonableness of a search. It is said that they should be made constitutional prerequisites of any search of media offices, where the media are not implicated in the crime under investigation.

In my view, the assessment of the reasonableness of a search cannot be said to rest only upon these two factors. Rather all factors should be evaluated in light of the particular factual situation presented. The factors which may be vital in assessing the reasonableness or one search may be irrelevant in another. Simply stated, it is impossible to isolate two factors from the numerous considerations which bear on assessment of the reasonableness of a search and label them as conditional prerequisites. The essential question can be put in this way: taking into account all the circumstances and viewing them fairly and objectively can it be said that the search was a reasonable one?

It is the over-all reasonableness of a search which is protected by s. 8 of the Charter. Certainly the potentially damaging effect of a search and seizure upon the freedom and the functioning of the press is highly relevant to the assessment of the reasonableness of the search. Yet neither s. 2(b) nor s. 8 of the Charter require that the two factors set out in *Pacific Press* must always be met in order for a search to be permissible and constitutionally valid. It is essential that flexibility in the balancing process be preserved so that all the factors relevant to the individual case may be taken into consideration and properly weighed.

. . . . .

Summary of Factors to be Considered on the Issuance of a Search Warrant and Review of a Search Warrant

It may be helpful to summarize the factors to be considered by a justice of the peace on an application to obtain a warrant to search the premises of a news media organization together with those factors which may be pertinent to a court reviewing the issuance of a search warrant.

(1) It is essential that all the requirements set out in s. 487(1)(b) of the *Criminal Code* for the issuance of a search warrant be met.

(2) Once the statutory conditions have been met, the justice of the peace should consider all of the circumstances in determining whether to exercise his or her discretion to issue a warrant.

(3) The justice of the peace should ensure that a balance is struck between the competing interests of the state in the investigation and prosecution of crimes and the right to privacy of the media in the course of their news gathering and news dissemination. It must be borne in mind that the media play a vital role in the functioning of a democratic society. Generally speaking, the news media will not be implicated in the crime under investigation. They are truly an innocent third party. This is a particularly important factor to be considered in attempting to strike an appropriate balance, including the consideration of imposing conditions on that warrant.

(4) The affidavit in support of the application must contain sufficient detail to enable the justice of the peace to properly exercise his or her discretion as to the issuance of a search warrant.

(5) Although it is not a constitutional requirement, the affidavit material should ordinarily disclose whether there are alternative sources from which the information may reasonably be obtained and, if there is an alternative source, that it has been investigated and all reasonable efforts to obtain the information have been exhausted.

(6) If the information sought has been disseminated by the media in whole or in part, this will be a factor which will favour the issuing of the search warrant.

(7) If a justice of the peace determines that a warrant should be issued for the search of media premises, consideration should then be given to the imposition of some conditions on its implementation so that the media

organization will not be unduly impeded in the publishing or dissemination of the news.
(8) If, subsequent to the issuing of a search warrant, it comes to light the authorities failed to disclose pertinent information that could well have affected the decision to issue the warrant, this may result in a finding that the warrant was invalid.
(9) Similarly, if the search itself is unreasonably conducted, this may render the search invalid.

Application of These Principles to this Case

The *Criminal Code*, by means of s. 487, does no more than require that a justice of the peace, before issuing a search warrant, be satisfied that there are reasonable grounds to believe that something which will afford evidence with respect to the commission of a crime will be found in the described building, receptacle or place. In the present case, Officer Ouellette's information was sufficient to meet these requirements. There is no evidence in this case that the search impeded the media in their function of gathering and disseminating the news. In these circumstances, the search was a reasonable one under s. 8 of the Charter, notwithstanding any deficiencies in the information with respect to alternate sources. But, in the alternative, Officer Ouellette declared in his information that all reasonable sources of the information sought had been pursued but none were available. In this regard, it is of considerable significance that there was a specific finding that there was no bad faith involved on the part of the police.

In light of this finding, it is safe to accept the information as one sworn in good faith. It follows that there is nothing nefarious in the failure to mention the presence at the scene of the, identification officers. That same finding makes it appropriate to assume that these officers could not be considered an alternative source of information. If they could, the police would surely prefer to use their own witnesses and photographs or video tapes in the preparation of their cases. In any event, the finding that there was no bad faith is of critical importance to my conclusions.

Ouellette's information, therefore, directly addressed the concerns expressed by Nemetz C.J.B.C. in *Pacific Press* in declaring that no alternative source of information was available. It must be assumed that the identification officers who were present at the scene could not be of assistance.

It would have been preferable if the presence of police identification officers at the scene had been set out in the information, together with the explanation as to why the officers were unable to supply the information sought by the police. However, as I have said, it must be assumed that the information was drawn and presented in good faith. This can be the only conclusion to be drawn, in light of the finding of Daigle J. that there was no bad faith involved on the part of the police. The statement that "there [were] no other means available to the police for obtaining evidence" must be accepted at face value. That statement should be taken as a short form of saying that the evidence sought was not available from the identification officers. While the police were required to provide an accurate description of the relevant facts, they were not obliged to describe every minute step taken in the course of the investigation. In sum, the information provided the justice of the peace with sufficient evidence to issue a search warrant. There is nothing in the record to indicate that the justice of the peace improperly exercised her discretion. In the circumstances, it should be accepted that the warrant was validly Issued.

Disposition

In the result, the appeal should be dismissed.

3.4.4 Taking Photographs or Videotaping against the Instructions of the Police

Although photographers have a right to take photographs, such activity may become criminal if done against instructions of the police. Under s.129(a) of the *Criminal Code* it is an offence to resist or wilfully obstruct "a public officer or peace officer in the execution of his duty or any person lawfully acting in aid of such an officer." The offence of obstructing a police officer in the execution of his duty consists of three essential elements:

(1) there was an obstruction of the police officer;
(2) the obstruction affected the police officer in the execution of the duty he was then executing; and
(3) the person obstructing did so wilfully in the sense of intentionally and without lawful excuse.

(*R. v. Westlie* (1971), 2 C.C.C. (2d) 315 (B.C.C.A.); *R. v. Tortolano, Kelly and Cadwell* (1975), 28 C.C.C. (2d) 562 (Ont. C.A.); *R. v. Kalnins* (1978), 41 C.C.C. (2d) 524 (Ont. Co. Ct.); and *R. v. Sandford* (1980), 62 C.C.C. (2d) 89 (Ont. Prov. Ct.)).

In discussing the first two elements, the court in *Tortolano, Kelly and Cadwell* said that it is the purpose of the obstruction, not its result, that goes to the offence under s.129(a). Accordingly, an officer's duty need not be completely frustrated for a s. 129(a) charge to made out. The fact that the obstruction did not prevent the officer from executing his duty is, therefore, no defence to a charge of obstructing a peace officer in the execution of his duty. Further, at the time of the obstruction, the officer need not be engaged in the performance of a specific duty in order to support a conviction under s. 118(a) (*Westlie*). And in determining whether the obstruction was "wilful", as required by the third element of the offence, it has been suggested that the court must take all the circumstances of the matter into consideration (*Sandford*).

Press photographers have been convicted pursuant to s. 129(a) in a couple of cases. In *Knowlton v. R.* (1973), 10 C.C.C. (2d) 377, the Supreme Court of Canada upheld the conviction of a photographer who tried to enter an area which had been cordoned off as a security measure during a visit to Vancouver by a foreign dignitary. A peace officer warned the photographer that he could not enter the area, but the photographer forcefully insisted on his right to do so and attempted to enter notwithstanding the warning. And in *Kalnins*, the Ontario County Court held that a charge under s. 129(a) was made out against a press photographer who attempted to take pictures of a psychiatric patient being taken to the hospital by police. Although asked by the officer not to take any pictures, the accused insisted that it was his right to do so. The presence of the photographer greatly upset the patient, making it impossible initially for the ambulance attendants to remove the patient's stretcher from the ambulance.

In *Sandford*, however, a press photographer was found not guilty of a s.129(a) offence when he continued to take pictures of an accident scene although repeatedly told by police officers to get off the roadway to make way for the emergency crew still working at the scene. The charge was dismissed in that case because the judge was not satisfied that the obstruction was "wilfull".

CHAPTER FOUR

Legal Limitations Protecting Social Values and Social Groups

4.1 Introduction

The laws protecting religious belief, minority groups and morality belong conceptually to criminal libel. Just as the law of seditious libel was used historically to protect the legitimacy (or the reputation) of the State and its institutions, the law of blasphemous libel has been used to protect the name of the Divine. Just as the law of seditious libel was used to prohibit incitements to riot, modern hate propaganda law is intended to prevent incitements which could harm racial or ethnic groups. The laws relating to obscene libel exist partly to promote standards of conduct and belief, but also to protect women and children from exploitation and harm.

However, debate continues about the content and rigour of such laws. This is, in part, because the social harms which the prohibited acts cause are not always easy to establish and, in part, because our social perceptions seem to be constantly changing. For example, advocates of liberalizing the practices governing the production and showing of explicit erotic material made substantial gains in the 1960s.

One part of this trinity of moral prohibition may have been put to rest. Although the *Criminal Code* of Canada continues to prohibit blasphemous libel, there have been no reported cases since 1935. That blasphemy has ceased to be regarded as a crime reflects the process of secularization in which a substantial percentage of Canada's population profess neither a belief in God nor an attachment to a particular doctrinal tradition. It also reflects the norm, now rarely challenged, that regardless of the desirability or extent of such beliefs, the law in a pluralistic state cannot be legitimately used to enforce them. In other words, an idea that John Milton promoted in the seventeenth century has taken hold — namely, that individuals should be persuaded rather than compelled to believe one doctrine or another.

The idea that persuasion rather than compulsion is the best remedy to harms caused by words has haunted the career of the law prohibiting expressions of race hatred. That law, which dates from the early sixties, makes it a crime to advocate genocide or to promote hatred towards an identifiable group. But neither offence may be prosecuted without the consent of the Attorney-General of a province and the part of the law that applies to statements promoting race hatred includes provisions which establish defences to the charge and make it difficult to secure a conviction. As a consequence, there have been few charges brought under these sections of the *Criminal Code*.

To avoid the restrictions in the hate propaganda sections of the *Criminal Code* which make it difficult both to bring a charge and secure a conviction, the Crown proceeded against Ernst Zundel in 1985 under section 177 (now s.181). This makes it a crime to publish a statement which is known to be false and which can cause injury or mischief to a public interest. Zundel had published pamphlets that said the Holocaust, the murder of European Jews by the Nazis during the Second World War, did not occur and that the statement that six million Jews died in death camps was a lie promulgated by Zionists. It should be noted that the resort to s.177 suggests great reluctance on the part of the State to enforce the hate propaganda prohibitions.

If there has been hesitation in the area of hate propaganda, there has been confusion and continued debate in the areas of obscenity and pornography. As recently as 1962, the Supreme Court of Canada was asked to determine if *Lady Chatterley's Lover*, was obscene. The Court determined that it was not and followed the wording of the 1959 amendments to the *Criminal Code*, rather than the classical common-law test of obscenity.

The new wording in the code allowed for a defence that countenanced both literary or artistic merits and community standards. However, the law has been subject to a debate because it has been variously interpreted across Canada and, in the opinion of some, has allowed for the circulation of films and videos which promote violence against women and children. In the meantime, the judges have devoted themselves to redefining the law to bring it into line with contemporary concerns. The courts have both modernized and clarified the law — something Parliament has significantly failed to achieve.

Although these elements of the law affect freedom of expression in a fundamental way, they are not centrally important to the operations of newspapers and other news agencies. It is fair to say that producers of films and authors of fiction are more likely to face problems than are the news media.

4.2 Blasphemy

4.2.1 *Criminal Code*, R.S.C. 1985, c . C-46

296. (1) Every one who publishes a blasphemous libel is guilty of an indictable offence and is liable to imprisonment for two years.

(2) It is a question of fact whether or not any matter that is published is a blasphemous libel.

(3) No person shall be convicted of an offence under this section for expressing in good faith and in decent language, or attempting to establish by argument used in good faith and conveyed in decent language. an opinion upon a religious subject.

4.2.2 R. v. Rahard (1935), 65 C.C.C. 344 (Que. S.C.)

PERRAULT, C.J.S.C: — The indictment based upon s.198 of the *Criminal Code* states that the accused the Rev. Victor Rahard, while a minister of the Anglican Church situated at the corner of Cartier & Sherbrooke Sts., in Montreal, published upon posters, a writing constituting blasphemous libel.

This case raises a very difficult and important question. Furthermore, I believe this is the first time that the question of blasphemous libel has been brought before our Canadian Courts under such circumstances.

Moreover, it must be understood that this does not involve a question of religious doctrine, but solely a legal question, that is, the application of s.198 of the *Cr. Code*. This section must be interpreted and it must be decided whether the writing published constitutes blasphemous libel.

In all justice to the defence and in order to better place the dispute before you I will reproduce the entire writing from which the present action arose.

"The Canadian Catholic Church, Anglican rite.

"Sermon by an old monk.

"The seven commandments of the Church of Rome.

"If Christ returned to visit all His churches, He could still chase the merchants from the temple crying: 'My house is a house of prayer and you have made it a den of thieves.' (St. Matthew, c.xxi, v.13.)

"Judas and the Roman priest. . . . The Mass.

"So Christ is sold. Judas sold Christ but did not kill Him, the priests attempt to sell Him and immolate Him. Judas sold Christ for a large sum of money; the Roman priests sell Him every day and even three times.

"Judas repented and threw his money away; the Roman priests do not repent and keep the money. Now what do you think of the papist religion?

"Christ has condemned the commandments of men whatever they may be when He said to the Pharisees: 'It is in vain that they honour Me teaching maxims and human ordinances; (Matthew, c.xv, v.3.)

"The Roman Church is not content with the commandments of God. She wished to have her own commandments for the satisfaction of her ambition and the prosperity of her shop."

"First of all it should be observed that these commandments be a false name. It is not the commandments of the Church that they should have been called but commandments of the Roman clergy.

"These human commandments are not of God nor of universal morality nor of the conscience. They bind no one and their transgression may be considered as an act of enfranchisement in regard to usurped authority."

The indictment reproduced is in writing; the accused, the Rev. Victor Rahard assumes full and complete responsibility for the writing and its publication. He admits having on August 12, 1933, affixed it to the property of his church, the length of Sherbrooke St. in the eastern put of the City of Montreal in full view of passers by and especially of Roman Catholics and French Canadians who compose at least three-quarters of the population of the City of Montreal.

The facts are therefore established and are admitted by the parties; only a question of law remains. In his admission (ex. Da.) the Rev. Victor Rahard declares that he is a priest of the Anglican Church in Canada, that his ecclesiastical superiors have conferred upon him the charge of the church known by the name of Church of the Redeemer, situated upon Sherbrooke St. East where he has the right to preach the doctrine of his church.

Upon the argument the Crown maintained the following proposition; s. 198 of the *Cr. Code* interpreted literally as well as in spirit gives every freedom of opinion upon any religious subject whatever; as it gives every latitude to the expression of this opinion in writing or otherwise, provided that this publication is made in good faith and in agreeable language, in such a manner as not to offend either by its terms or expressions the feelings of others who are not of the same opinion or point of view and finally to keep from disturbing the public peace through offensive or injurious terms.

In short to insure the public peace among His Majesty's subjects is the object of all the provisions of the *Cr. Code*.

On the other hand the defence maintains the following propositions: —

1. Blasphemy is a crime by English common law which exists only in an attack against the Divinity or Christianity in general; and the writing attacks neither the Divinity or Christianity.

2. By believing that the writing was directed against the Divinity or Christianity in general, the accused would be protected by s.198 of the *Cr. Code* because he attempted to establish in good faith and in decent language an opinion upon the question of religious doctrine.

3. That more particularly the statement he made regarding the Mass was part of the teaching of the Church of England; that in his capacity of priest he has the right to teach, just as he has the right to discuss, the question of whether belief in the Mass is well founded or not; for it is a question of controversy between the Roman and the Protestant Church.

4. That considering the place and the circumstances of the publication of this writing, criminal intent on the put of the accused could not be inferred.

At the outset I declared that this was not a question of doctrine but solely a question of law. Besides this Court is not called upon to determine the right of the accused to preach in his own church the religious doctrine which he deems fit, which right is not debated any more than his liberty of opinion. But could he, without contravening s.198 of the *Cr. Code*, publish the writing reproduced above in the terms and expressions used? That is the question which the Court has to decide.

This s. 198 of the *Cr. Code* placed under Part V, under the rubrics "offences against religion. morals and public convenience" does not define blasphemous libel but contains the simple statement that blasphemous libel constitutes an offence and is a question of fact. Nevertheless the section contains the following provision: — "Provided that no one is guilty of a blasphemous libel for expressing in good faith and in decent language, or attempting to establish by arguments in good faith and conveyed in decent language, any opinion whatever upon any religious subject."

Hence it is to be noted that our Code speaks of a religious subject and not only of Divinity or of Christianity in general, but in order to understand and know the essential elements constituting the offence of criminal libel the common law must be resorted to. It is a principle of our Criminal law (s. 16) that the English common law is applicable in our country although the subject is not specially mentioned in our Code. See Annotation, 48 Can. C.C., at p. 4.

"The common law jurisdiction as to crime is still operative notwithstanding the Criminal Code, but subject to the latter prevailing where there is a repugnancy between the common law and the Code" (*Rex v. Cole* (1902), 5 Can. C.C. 330).

The Supreme Court of Canada accepted this interpretation in *Brousseau v. The King* (1917), 29 Can. C.C. 207, at p. 209, 39 D.L.R. 114, at p. 115: — "The criminal common law of England is still in force in Canada, except in so far as repealed either expressly or by implication."

But the English common law in regard to a blasphemous libel has been varied with the ages. With the times and a new understanding of freedom of opinion, the doctrine and jurisprudence has attached significance to the intention of the author, to the terms used by him and to the circumstances rather than to the subject treated.

In Odgers on Libel and Slander, 5th ed., p. 498, it is said: — "It is the malicious intent to insult the religious feelings of others by profanely scoffing at all they hold sacred, which deserves and receives punishment."

And at p. 467: — "It is sufficient to prove a publication to the prosecutor himself, provided the obvious tendency of the words be to provoke the prosecutor and excite him to break the pace."

Blasphemy which otherwise was under the jurisdiction of the Ecclesiastical Courts, has come under the jurisdiction of the Civil Courts in order, the authors say, to prevent a disturbance of the peace. In the year 1676 in *Taylor's Case*, I Vent. 293, 86 E.R. 189, the English Courts sanctioned the axiom which, since that time, has often been invoked: "Christianity is parcel of the laws of England," and the following syllogism arose: "To disparage any put of the law of England is a crime. Christianity is a part of the law of England, therefore to disparage Christianity is a crime."

But later Lord Coleridge in the case of *Reg. v. Ramsay* (1883), 15 Cox C.C. 231, at p. 235, declared: — "I think that these old cases can no longer be taken to be a statement of the law at the present day. It is no longer true in the sense in which it was true when these *dicta* were uttered, that 'Christianity is part of the law of the land.'"

And further on he adds — "The principles of law remain, and it is the great advantage of the common law that its principles do remain; but then they have to be applied to the changing circumstances of the times. This may be called by some retrogression, but I should rather say it is progression — the progress of human opinion."

This case was decided in 1883 and established the following principle: — "The mere denial of the truth of the Christian religion, or of the Scriptures, is not enough, per se, to constitute a writing and blasphemous libel, so as to render the writer or publisher indictable. But indecent and offensive attacks on Christianity or the Scriptures, or sacred persons or objects, calculated to outrage the feelings of the general body of the community, do constitute the offence of blasphemy, and render writers or publishers liable at common law to criminal prosecution."

This doctrine was maintained in the more recent decision of *Rex v. Gott* (1922), 16 Cr. App. R. 86. It decided as follows:

"The essence of the crime consists in the publication of words concerning the Christian religion so scurrilous and offensive as to pass the limits of decent controversy and to be calculated to outrage the feelings of any sympathiser with Christianity. In considering whether these limits have been passed the circumstances in which the words are published should be taken into account. The limits of decent controversy would certainly be passed if the circumstances in which the words were published were such that the publication was likely to lead to a breach of the peace."

Folkard in his *Law of Slander and Libel*, 7th ed., p. 361, interpreting the case of *Rex v. Woolston* (1729), 1 Bun. K.B. 162, 94 E.R. 112, declares: — "It may be observed, that all the recorded instances of prosecution for blasphemy, subsequent to *Woolston's case*, have been for publication of indecent, scoffing, and opprobrious language against natural or revealed religion; and that in most of such cases, the jury have been directed to look both to the matter and manner of the publication in order to decide on its blasphemous quality; and in those cases where the defendants have been convicted, the judges, in the remarks they have made upon the mischievous tendency of the offence, have, usually, founded their reasons for the punishment awarded, more upon the offensive manner of the publication in the particular instances, than upon the matter itself; and all have cautiously avoided laying down any general prohibitory rule."

It may be noted that the English jurisprudence attaches more importance to the intention of the author and the terms in which he expresses his opinion than to the subject treated and because of the danger of disturbing the public peace. This doctrine was expressed by Starkie in his work on the *Law of Slander and*

Libel, 3rd ed., p. 590: — "It is the mischievous abuse of this state of intellectual liberty which calls for penal censure. The law visits not the honest errors, but the malice of mankind. A wilful intention to pervert, insult, and mislead others, by means of licentious and contumelious abuse applied to sacred subjects, or by wilful misrepresentations or wilful sophistry, calculated to mislead the ignorant and unwary, is the criterion and test of guilt. A malicious and mischievous intention, or what is equivalent to such an intention, in law, as well as in morals, — a state of apathy and indifference to the interests of society, — is the broad boundary between right and wrong. If it can be collected from the circumstances of the publication, from a display of offensive levity, from contumelious and abusive expressions applied to sacred persons or subjects, that the design of the author is to occasion that mischief to which the matter which he publishes immediately tends, to destroy or even to weaken men's sense of religious or moral obligations, to insult those who believe by casting contumelious abuse and ridicule upon their doctrines, or to bring the established religion and form of worship into disgrace and contempt, the offence against society is complete."

And in regard to this doctrine of Starkie, Lord Coleridge in *Reg v. Ramsay*, 15 Cox C.C., at p. 236, states: — "It is my duty to lay down the law on the subject as I find it laid down in the best books of authority, and in 'Starkie on Libel,' it is there laid down as, I believe, correctly."

Odgers, *ubi supra*, p. 408, says: — "This view of our law against blasphemy was strongly advocated by that eminent lawyer, the late Mr. Starkie ... This is the view adopted by the Judges in the House of Lords in *Shore v. Wilson*, 9 Ct. & Fin. 355 [8 E.R. 450]. This is the view expressed in the admirable address of the late Chief Justice Coleridge to the jury in the case of *R. v. Ramsey and Foote*."

See Odgers, 5th ed., p. 478. This author expresses the same doctrine as Starkie: —

"The intent to shock and insult believers, or to pervert or mislead the ignorant and unwary, is an essential element in the crime. *Actus non facit reum nisi mens sit rea.* The existence of such an intent is a question of fact for the jury, and the *onus* of proving it lies on the prosecution. The best evidence of such an intention is usually to be found in the work itself. If it is full of scurrilous and opprobrious language, if sacred subjects are treated with offensive levity, if indiscriminate abuse is employed instead of argument, then a malicious design to wound the religious feelings of others may be readily inferred. . . . This would tend to show that he did not write from conscientious conviction, but desired to pervert and mislead the ignorant; or at all events that he was criminally indifferent to the distinctions between right and wrong."

Our s.198 of the *Cr. Code* has been interpreted in a profound article by E. J. Murphy, K.C., representing the Crown in the case of *Rex v. Sterry*. He states as follows (48 Can. C.C., at p. 22): — "The question is, is the language used calculated and intended to insult the feelings and the deepest religious convictions of the great majority of the persons amongst whom we live? If so, they are not to be tolerated. . . . We must not do things that are outrageous to the general feeling of propriety among the persons amongst whom we live."

Rex v. Pilon (unreported) June 15, 1934, judgment of Wilson, J.; *Rex v. St. Martin* (1933), 40 Rev. de Jur. 411, Lacroix, J.S.P.; *Reg. v. Pelletier* (1900), 6 Rev. Leg. 116.

Hence it follows that s.198 of the *Cr. Code* must be interpreted to mean that it is permitted to express any opinion whatever upon a religious subject in a public document if this opinion is expressed in good faith and in decent language since anyone may support his opinion by arguments expressed in good faith and in decent language.

I believe it has been shown that that is not only our Canadian law but the most recent English doctrine and jurisprudence as well.

Let us apply these principles to the present case. It is certain that the document published August 12, 1933, deals with a religious subject.

Has the Rev. Victor Rahard expressed his opinion upon this religious question in good faith and in decent language? He wrote and published that the Roman Church is not satisfied with the commandments of God; that it wished to have its own commandments for the satisfaction of its own ambition and the prosperity of its shop. In other words the church to which a Roman Catholic goes to pray, where he has been baptized, where he fulfils his religious duties and where at the end of his life his body will be taken before its final rest in the cemetery, is a place of commerce. And what kind of trade?

And in order that there might be no mistake as to the meaning which the accused attaches to the word shop, he declares as follows: — "If Christ should return to visit all His churches He could still chase the merchants from the temples by crying 'My house is a house of prayer and you have made it a den of thieves.'"

Furthermore he compares the Roman priest to Judas saying: — "Although Judas sold Christ he did not kill Him while the priests attempt to sell Him and immolate Him; the Roman priests sell Him for a few cents and do not repent but keep the money." And he concludes by saying: — "Now what do you think of the papist religion?"

I maintain that these terms are offensive and injurious to the Roman Catholics and of such a nature that they may lead to a disturbance of the public peace.

Where in the above quoted words can be found an argument expressed in good faith or in decent language to sustain the opinion of the accused? The bad faith of the accused is more than manifest. This writing is posted the length of Sherbrooke St. in a place frequented above all by the Roman Catholic and French Canadian population, and in order to give more force and authority to the statements which he made in this writing, he places at its head the words "Sermon by an old monk."

What could be the impression upon a Catholic population of these words "Sermon by an old monk" may easily be understood.

If we apply the English doctrine which I have cited above, that is to say, taking into account the circumstances of the publication as well as the terms and expressions used by the accused, we have evidence of bad faith on the part of the accused.

I will repeat what was said by Mr. Murphy in his article in 48 Can. C.C., at p. 22: — "The question is, is the language used calculated and intended to insult the feelings and the deepest religious convictions of the great majority of the persons amongst whom we live? If so, they are not to be tolerated. ... We must not do things that are outrageous to the general feeling of propriety among the persons amongst whom we live."

At the hearing of the case the accused, by this counsel, made a motion to quash on the ground of the nullity of the indictment because no intent was alleged therein. I do not believe that it is necessary to allege specially the intent in the indictment. Intent results from facts. Furthermore the indictment declares that the Rev. Victor Rahard published a blasphemous writing on August 12, 1933. And s.198 of the *Cr. Code* states that a blasphemous writing constitutes a criminal offence.

Hence it follows that the fact that the indictment alleges that the accused published a blasphemous writing was sufficient to include all the elements of the offence.

What is it which constitutes a blasphemous writing? That is a question of fact left to the appreciation either of the Judge or jury. That is the import of s. 198 of the *Cr. Code*. As a result the motion to quash is dismissed and the accused is declared guilty.

4.2.3 *R. v. Gay News Ltd.*, [1979] 1 All E.R. 898 (H.L.)

The appellants, the editor and publishers of a newspaper for homosexuals, published in the newspaper a poem accompanied by a drawing illustrating its subject-matter which purported to describe in explicit detail acts of sodomy and fellatio with the body of Christ immediately after His death and to ascribe to Him during His lifetime promiscuous homosexual practices with the Apostles and with other men. The appellants were charged with the offence of blasphemous libel. The particulars of the offence alleged that the appellants unlawfully and wickedly published or caused to be published a blasphemous libel concerning the Christian religion, namely 'an obscene poem and illustration vilifying Christ in His life and in His crucifixion'. The trial judge directed the jury that in order to secure the conviction of the appellants for publishing a blasphemous libel it was sufficient if they took the view that the publication complained of vilified Christ in His life and crucifixion and that it was not necessary for the Crown to prove an intention other than an intention to publish that which in the jury's view was a blasphemous libel. The appellants were convicted. They appealed to the Court of Appeal contending that a subjective intent on the part of the appellants to shock and arouse resentment among Christians had to be proved by the prosecution and that the judge had misdirected the jury. The Court of Appeal dismissed their appeal and they appealed to the House of Lords.

. . . . .

VISCOUNT DILHORNE. My Lords, the appellants, Denis Lemon and Gay News Ltd., were tried at the Central Criminal Court on an indictment which contained the following count:

> 'Statement of Offence
> 'Blasphemous Libel.
> 'Particulars of Offence
> 'Gay News Limited and Denis Lemon on a day or days unknown between the 1st day of May and 30th day of June 1976 unlawfully and wickedly published or caused to be published in a newspaper called *Gay News* No. 96 a blasphemous libel concerning the Christian religion namely an obscene poem and illustration vilifying Christ in His life and in His crucifixion.'

After a trial which lasted for seven days they were found guilty by a majority verdict of ten to two. They appealed to the Court of Appeal (Criminal Division) on a number of grounds. Their appeal against conviction was dismissed and they now appeal with the leave of this House, the Court of Appeal having certified that a point of law of general public importance was involved, namely the question:

> Was the learned trial Judge correct (as the Court of Appeal held) first in ruling and then in directing the jury that in order to secure the conviction of the appellants for publishing a blasphemous libel (1) it was sufficient if the jury took the view that the publication complained of vilified Christ in His life and crucifixion and (2) it was not necessary for the Crown to establish any further intention on the part of the appellants beyond an intention to publish that which in the jury's view was a blasphemous libel?

By their verdict the jury showed that they were satisfied that the publication complained of, a poem by a Professor James Kirkup and a drawing published alongside it, vilified Christ in His life and crucifixion and were blasphemous. That finding has not been challenged in this appeal, nor could it have been with the slightest prospect of success.

Gay News Ltd. publishes a newspaper for homosexuals called *Gay News* of which Denis Lemon is the editor. He holds the majority of the shares in that company. The jury's conclusion that they published the poem and the drawing was not challenged.

The only question to be decided in this appeal is what mens rea has to be established to justify conviction of the offence of publishing a blasphemous libel. The choice does not, in my opinion, lie between regarding the offence as one of strict liability or as one involving mens rea, for, as was said by Stephen in 1883 in his *History of the Criminal Law of England*:

> It is undoubtedly true that the definition of libel, like the definitions of nearly all other crimes, contains a mental element the existence of which must be found by a jury before a defendant can be convicted, but the important question is, What is that mental element? What is the intention

which makes the act of publishing criminal? Is it the mere intention to publish written blame, or is it an intention to produce by such a publication some particular evil effect?

He said that he knew of no authority for saying that the presence of any specific intention other than the intent to publish was necessary before Fox's *Libel Act* 1792. During the course of the proceedings in Parliament on the Bill which became that Act, a number of questions were put to the judges. In their answer to one of them they said:

> The crime consists in publishing a libel. A criminal intention in the writer is no part of the definition of libel at the common law. "He who scattereth firebrands, arrows, and death," which, if not a definition, is a very intelligible description of a libel, is *eâ ratione* criminal; it is not incumbent on the prosecutor to prove his intent, and on his part he shall not be heard to say, "Am I not in sport?"

In the *Dean of St. Asaph* case Erskine had argued that it had to be proved that the dean had had a seditious intent. That argument was rejected in that case as it was by the judges in their answer to Parliament. Prior to 1792 on a charge of publishing a seditious libel, the only questions left to the jury were (1) did the matter published bear the meaning ascribed to it in the indictment or information and (2) was it published by the defendant? It was for the judges to rule whether the matter published, bearing the sense ascribed to it, was seditious, that being regarded as a question of law (see *R. v. Shipley*). I do not doubt that the same procedure was followed when the charge was of publishing any other form of criminal libel.

It thus appears that prior to 1792 the specific intent of the accused was not an ingredient of the offence. Why was that? It is, I think, only explicable on the ground that the evil sought to be prevented by treating the publication of a libel as a criminal offence was the dissemination of libels. The mischief lay in the scattering of firebrands in the form of libels, and, if what was published was held to be seditious, the person who published it or was responsible for its publication was guilty. It mattered not, if what had been published was seditious, that he had no seditious intent (see *R. v. Shipley*).

The next question for consideration is, was the definition of a criminal libel altered later, either by Fox's *Libel Act* 1792 or in the course of the development of the common law, so that on a charge of publishing a seditious or a blasphemous libel proof that the defendant had a seditious or blasphemous intent, as the case might be, was essential to establish guilt?

Fox's *Libel Act* was 'An Act to remove Doubts respecting the Functions of Juries in Cases of Libel'. Its preamble stated that doubts had arisen whether on a trial 'for the making or publishing any libel' the jury could give their verdict 'upon the whole matter put in issue' and its first section provided that they might do so and that they should not be directed to find a defendant guilty merely on proof of publication by him and of the sense ascribed to the matter published in the indictment or information.

Parke B. in *Parmiter v. Coupland* said that the Act was declaratory and put prosecutions for libel on the same footing as other criminal cases. While the Act allowed a trial judge to tell the jury his opinion of the publication, after 1792 it was for the jury to decide what its character was.

I can see nothing in this Act "to remove Doubts respecting the Functions of Juries" to justify the conclusion that it made a change in the definition of the offence of publishing a criminal libel. It does not mention intent, and if it had been the desire of Parliament to give statutory authority to the argument of Erskine in *R. v. Shipley* and to reject the opinion of the judges as to the ingredients of the offence, I regard it as inconceivable that the Act would have taken the form it did. Stephen, however, regarded it as having enlarged "the old definition of a seditious libel by the addition of a reference to the specific intentions of the libeller — to the purpose for which he wrote", and said that the Act assumed that the specific intentions of the defendant were material. I must confess my inability to find in the Act any basis for either conclusion. Professor Holdsworth in his *History of English Law* recognised that the view that 'the crime was not so much the intentional publication of matter bearing the seditious or defamatory meaning ... as its publication with a seditious or malicious intent' began to appear in the 18th century. He did not attribute this to Fox's *Libel Act* but to the practice of filling indictments 'with averments of every sort or bad intention on the part of the defendant', averments which in Stephen's opinion were surplusage.

The conclusion to which I come is that if any change in the definition of the offence occurred after 1792 it did not result from Fox's *Libel Act*.

Stephen also asserted that since that Act the law had ever since been administered on the supposition that the specific intentions of the defendant were material. My examination of the cases since 1792 leads me to think that that is not so and Professor Holdsworth said that the view that the publication had to be with a seditious or malicious intent was "not finally got rid of till the nineteenth century". I infer from what he said that he thought that that view was erroneous.

It was not until 1967 by the *Criminal Justice Act*, s.8, that it was enacted that a court or jury should not be bound in law to infer that an accused intended or foresaw a result of his actions by reason only of its being a natural and probable result of those actions but that whether he intended or foresaw that result had to be decided by reference to all the evidence drawing such inferences from the evidence as appeared proper. If the conclusion was reached that a particular publication was blasphemous and it was proved that the defendant had published it, it could be presumed under the old law that he had done so with intent to blaspheme. In many cases it may be that the existence of such an intent was undeniable but the fact that a man might be presumed to have such an intent or had that intent does not in my opinion lead to the conclusion that the existence of such an intent was an essential element in the crime, though it may account for a reference being made in some cases in the course of a summing-up to the accused's intent (see, for instance, *R. v. Hone, R. v. Richard Carlile, R. v. Moxon, R. v. Holyoake*).

In this appeal we are not, as I see it, concerned with how such an intent is to be established or its existence rebutted but whether it is an element in the offence. So with great respect to my noble and learned friend, Lord Diplock, I do not think that the terms of the *Criminal Evidence Act* 1898 and of s.8 of the *Criminal Justice Act* 1967 have any relevance to the question to be decided. If in a prosecution for the publication of a blasphemous libel the accused's intent to blaspheme has to be proved, the 1898 Act enables him to give evidence that he had no such intent and the 1967 Act gives guidance as to the proof of such an intent.

What I regard as of great significance is that in none of what I regard as the leading cases on the publication of a blasphemous libel is there to be found any direction to the jury telling them that it had to be proved that the defendant intended to blaspheme, and I have not found in any decided case any criticism of the omission to do so.

In *R. v. Mary Ann Carlile*, in an intervention, Best, J. told the defendant that he would be happy to hear anything that she might urge to show that the publication was not a blasphemous libel and that she was not the publisher. It is not without significance that he said nothing about her intent particularly in view of the fact that in *R. v. Richard Carlile*, tried only a short time before, the direction to the jury had referred to the accused's intent.

A case of more importance is *R. v. Hetherington*. Hetherington was prosecuted for publishing a blasphemous libel, it being alleged that such a libel had been sold from his shop by his employee. He was convicted. It was not suggested that it had to be shown that he had any blasphemous intent, nor, it is to be noted, that the employee had any such intent. It sufficed to show that what was published was a blasphemous libel and that he was responsible for its publication. This vicarious criminal liability is wholly inconsistent with an intent to engage in blasphemy being regarded at that time as an ingredient of the offence.

Two years later Parliament changed the law, not by enacting that proof of such an intent was necessary for a conviction but by s.7 of Lord Campbell's *Libel Act* 1843 providing that, on a trial for the publication of a libel where the publication was by the act of a person other than the defendant but with his authority, it was competent for the defendant to prove that the publication was made without his authority, consent or knowledge, and that the publication did not arise from want of care or caution on his part. As Stephen observes by virtue of this Act the "negligent publication of a libel by a bookseller who is ignorant of its contents" suffices to render him guilty and the fact that he may be found guilty if negligent is wholly inconsistent with the existence of any necessity to show that he intended to blaspheme. Again it may be noted that the intention of the person actually responsible for the publication was not relevant. If proof of such an intent was and is necessary, this Act did not serve any useful purpose.

I now come to the first of the two cases which I regard as the leading cases in this field. Prior to *R. v. Bradlaugh* there had been very considerable controversy about what constituted blasphemy. In the 18th century and before it appears to have been thought that any attack or criticism, no matter how reasonably expressed, on the fundamental principles of the Christian religion and any discussion hostile to the inspiration and perfect purity of the Scriptures was against the law. That was Stephen's view but in this case it was rejected by Lord Coleridge, C.J. who told the jury that he thought the law had been accurately stated in Starkie on *Slander and Libel* in the following terms:

> The wilful intention to insult and mislead others by means of licentious and contumelious abuse offered to sacred subjects, or by will misrepresentations or wilful sophistry, calculated to mislead the ignorant and unwary, is the criterion and test of guilt A malicious and mischievous intention. or what is equivalent to such an intention, in law, as well as morals — a state of apathy and indifference to the interests of society — is the broad boundary between right and wrong.

At first sight the citation of this passage by Lord Coleridge, C.J. might appear to give support to the view that such an intent on the part of the accused had to be proved but it is to be noted that Lord Coleridge, C.J. began his summing-up by telling the jury that there were two questions to be considered, first, whether the publications in question were blasphemous libels and, secondly, whether, assuming them to be so, Mr. Bradlaugh was guilty of publishing them. He did not at any time tell the jury that they had to consider Mr. Bradlaugh's intent, an astonishing omission if he regarded it necessary to prove that he had a blasphemous intent, and the passage he cited from Starkie was cited by him as providing the test for determining whether or not the publication itself was blasphemous.

This, to my mind, is shown beyond doubt by the fact that, after citing Starkie, he said:

> That I apprehend to be a correct statement of the law, and if you think the broad boundary between right and wrong that is laid down in the passage, has been overpast in the articles which are the subject-matter of this indictment, then it will be your duty to answer the first question ... against the defendant.

And by his saying at the end of his summing-up:

> It is a question, first of all, whether these things are not in any point of view blasphemous libels, whether they are not calculated and intended to insult the feelings and the deepest religious convictions of the great majority of the persons amongst whom we live; and if so they are not to be tolerated any more than any other nuisance is tolerated. We must not do things that are outrages to the general feeling of property among the persons amongst whom we live. That is the first thing. Then the second thing is: Is Mr. Bradlaugh made out to have joined in the publication of these?

"To say that the crime lies in the manner and not in the matter appears to me an attempt to evade and explain away a law which has no doubt ceased to be in harmony with the temper of the times" was Stephen's view, but since 1883 it has been accepted that it is the manner in which they are expressed that may constitute views expressed in a publication a blasphemous libel and this passage from Starkie has been relied on as providing the test for determining whether the publication exceeds that which is permissible. It is the intention revealed by the publication that may lead to its being held to be blasphemous. There was nothing in Lord Coleridge, C.J.'s summing-up to support the view that there was a third question for the jury to consider, namely the intent of the accused.

This case was followed by *R. v. Ramsay and Foote*, a case greatly relied on by the appellants, a case of great importance and also tried by Lord Coleridge, C.J. Again he told the jury that there were two questions for them to consider:

> First, are these publications in themselves blasphemous libels? Secondly, if they are so, is the publication of them traced home to the defendants so that you can find them guilty?

He went on to say: "The great point still remains, are these articles within the meaning of the law blasphemous libels?"

Again he cited the passage from Starkie, not as indicating that it must be shown that the accused had an intention to blaspheme but as providing the test for determining whether the articles exceeded the permissible bounds. Again Lord Coleridge, C.J. gave no direction to the jury as to the intent of the accused, an omission which I regard as of great significance.

Lord Coleridge, C.J.'s approach in this case was followed by Phillimore, J. in *R. v. Boulter*.

While it may be that the development of the law as to seditious libel has now taken a different course, in *R. v. Aldred*, in the course of his summing-up on a charge of publishing a seditious libel, Coleridge, J. told the jury that the accused could not plead the innocence of his motive as a defence to the charge, telling them that —

> The test is not either the truth of the language or the innocence of the motive with which he published it, but the test is this: was the language used calculated, or was it not, to promote public disorder or physical force or violence in a matter of State?

and if the language was calculated to promote public disorder —

> ... then, whatever his motives, whatever his intentions, there would be evidence on which a jury might, on which I should think a jury ought, and on which a jury would decide that he was guilty of a seditious publication.

This direction was not followed in *R. v. Caunt* a seditious libel case tried in 1947. The transcript of that case shows that counsel agreed that a man published a seditious libel if he did so with a seditious intent and Birkett, J. so directed the jury.

It is not necessary in this appeal to decide whether Birkett, J.'s direction was right or unduly favourable to the accused and whether *R. v. Aldred* was rightly decided for we are only concerned with blasphemous libel.

The last case to which I need refer is *R. v. Gott*. Avory, J. in his summing-up cited the passage I have cited from the end of Lord Coleridge, C.J.'s summing-up in *R. v. Bradlaugh*. He did not tell the jury that it was necessary to prove that the defendant had a blasphemous intent. He said nothing about the accused's intent. The case went to appeal but his omission to do so was not a ground of appeal or the subject of adverse comment by the Court of Criminal Appeal.

In the light of the authorities to which I have referred and for the reasons I have stated, I am unable to reach the conclusion that the ingredients of the offence of publishing a blasphemous libel have changed since 1792. Indeed, it would, I think, be surprising if they had. If it be accepted, as I think it must, that that which it is sought to prevent is the publication of blasphemous libels, the harm is done by their intentional publication, whether or not the publisher intended to blaspheme. To hold that it must be proved that he had that intent appears to me to be going some way to making the accused judge in his own cause. If Mr. Lemon had testified that he did not regard the poem and drawing as blasphemous, that he had no intention to blaspheme and it might be, that his intention was to promote the love and affection of some homosexuals for Our Lord, the jury properly directed would surely have been told that unless satisfied beyond reasonable doubt that he intended to blaspheme they should acquit, no matter how blasphemous they thought the publication. Whether or not they would have done so on such evidence is a matter of speculation on which views may differ.

The question we have to decide is a pure question of law and my conclusions thereon do not, I hope, evince any distrust of juries. The question here is what is the proper direction to give to them, not how they might act on such a direction, and distrust, which I do not have, of the way a jury might act, does not enter into it.

My Lords, for the reasons I have stated in my opinion the question certified should be answered in the affirmative. Guilt of the offence of publishing a blasphemous libel does not depend on the accused having an intent to blaspheme but on proof that the publication was intentional (or, in the case of a bookseller, negligent (Lord Campbell's *Libel Act* 1843)) and that the matter published was blasphemous.

I would dismiss these appeals.

4.2.4 R. v. Chief Metropolitan Stipendiary Magistrate, ex parte Choudhury, [1991] L.R.C. (Const) 278 (Q.B.)(U.K.)

WATKINS, L.J.: On 13 March 1989 the Chief Metropolitan Stipendiary Magistrat, sitting at Bow Street Magistrates' Court, refused to grant the applicant, Abdul Hussain Choudhury, summonses he had applied for against Salman Rushdie, the author, and Viking Publishing Co Ltd (Viking Penguin), the publishers of a book entitled *The Satanic Verses*, alleging the commission of the offences of blasphemous libel and seditious libel at common law.

The draft summonses in respect of blasphemy accuse Salman Rushdie and Viking Penguin of, between 1 January 1988 and 31 January 1989, unlawfully and wickedly publishing or causing to be published in a book entitled *The Satanic Verses* a blasphemous libel concerning Almighty God (Allah), the supreme deity common to all the major religions of the world, the Prophet Abraham and his son Ishmael, Muhammad (Pbuh) the Holy Prophet of Islam, his wives and companions and the religion of Islam and Christianity, contrary to common law.

The draft summonses in respect of sedition accuse them both of, between the same dates, unlawfully and wickedly publishing or causing to be published in the book a seditious libel in that it raised widespread discontent and disaffection among her Majesty's subjects, contrary to common law.

The relief the applicant seeks is an order of certiorari to quash the decision of the magistrate and an order of mandamus directing him to issue the summonses in the form applied for.

Leave to move this court was granted by the single judge on 19 June 1989 following an oral hearing and consideration of documents. In granting that leave Nolan, J said of the courts of this country:

> They are not concerned with the question of whether the proposed defendants are blasphemous according to Moslem law. They are concerned to establish the scope of the English criminal law. Whatever the outcome of these proceedings may be, the fundamental rule of English law is that the peace must be preserved. I know that this is fully understood by your own very responsible clients. It would be a great tragedy if the continuation of this argument in court were taken by others as a sign that demonstrations and the like, which might lead to breaches of the law, would give assistance; in fact they will be counter-productive.

The arguments on all sides of this application have been presented with skill, objectivity and restraint and there has been, as far as this court is aware, no unseemly conduct either in the court or outside it by any person.

The Satanic Verses is a book, said to be a novel, published by Viking Penguin in 1988. In that year the book won the Whitbread Prize for Literature. It has been translated into 15 different languages.

The book has achieved considerable notoriety. It has been banned, so we were told by Mr. Azhar, counsel for the applicant, in all Muslim countries, in South Africa, China and India. He said that there had been demonstrations abroad against the book in which people had died, notably in Bombay, which is Mr. Rushdie's place of birth, in Lahore and in Kashmir, that Muslims have demonstrated against the book in the United Kingdom (there are two million of that faith here) and that Muslims, otherwise of good character, have been arrested and convicted of offences against public order arising out of those demonstrations, in particular where the demonstrations by Muslims against the book have encountered groups demonstrating in favour of the book.

There can be little doubt that the contents of the book have deeply offended many law-abiding Muslims who are United Kingdom citizens.

Mr. Robertson, Q.C. for Mr. Rushdie sought to explain the author's purpose in writing the book. The book is a fictional story, he said, of two men, each of whom is divided in himself. The division in one man is between his attraction to life in the East and his attraction to life in the West. In the other the division is spiritual: a division between the desire to believe and the inability to believe in God. The first man survives by returning to the East where his roots are, whereas the second does not survive because of his inability to return to religious belief. The second man, called Gibreel, finally kills himself.

Gibreel dreams of the conversion of Jahilia (the city of Mecca) to Islam by Mahound (the Prophet Muhammad). In those parts of the books relating to Gibreel there appear passages which are set out as particulars of blasphemy in the information which was laid before the magistrate, of which the applicant and Moulanay Zaki Ahmed, who with the applicant laid the information, both complain.

The particulars can be summarised under six headings. Firstly, God is described as "The Destroyer of Man". Secondly, the book vilifies the prophet Abraham, who is, as "Ibrahim", a prophet revered by Muslims, by recounting the story of Abraham, Hagar and Ishmail, their son and commenting adversely on Abraham's behaviour towards Hagar and Ishmail. Thirdly, the book refers to Muhammad as Mahound, which is a word having the meaning of a devil, and that elsewhere in the book Muhammad is called "a conjurer", a "magician" and "a false prophet". Fourthly, the book grossly vilifies and profoundly insults the wives of Muhammad by calling some whores after their names. Muslims hold the prophet's wives in the highest esteem as mothers of the faithful. Fifthly, the book vilifies the close companions of Muhammad (calling them "some sort of bums from Persia" and "clowns") whereas the Koran recounts that they were men of high moral character and righteousness. Sixthly, the book vilifies and ridicules the teachings of Islam as containing too many rules and as seeking to control every aspect of day-to-day life. Moreover, insult is added to injury by the liberal use of an offensive four letter word.

Mr. Robertson pointed out that those passages form part of Gibreel's dreams and are, for the most part, words spoken by characters in the book who appear in Gibreel's dreams, some of whom have not been converted to Islam at the moment they make the utterances to which objection is taken.

That appears to be so, but, in our opinion, a statement will not necessarily be prevented from being a blasphemous libel simply because the statement is put into the mouth of a character, even a disreputable character, in a novel.

Mr. Robertson made the point that even if the law of blasphemy extended to cover Islam, a proposition he contests, when read in their context and properly understood the passages complained of are not blasphemous inasmuch as they do not amount, as is alleged by the applicant, to a scurrilous and insulting attack by the author on that religion. Generally speaking, the whole of those passages of the book complained of form part, he reiterated, of a dream or nightmare sequence of a fictional character. Nothing there is meant to be, nor should be taken to be, the views of the author. As to the specific complaints in the information, Mr. Robertson made the following assertions.

(1) It is not blasphemous to describe God as the destroyer of men. While God is portrayed in scripture and the Koran as merciful and compassionate, he is also described, especially in the Old Testament and the book of Revelation, as an avenging and destructive God, particularly towards unbelievers and the enemies of the Jews.

(2) The story of Abraham and Hagar is not one which reflects credit on Abraham, whether it is told in the Old Testament or the Koran. Abraham is not seen as without fault, either by the Judaic, Islamic or Christian religions. The comment in words underlined in the information, though strong, is not unjustified. It cannot be blasphemous to say that pilgrims gather to worship and spend.

(3) In relation to the complaint concerning Muhammad, the name Mahound is a name used by Christians for the prophet, though it appears to be used in a derogatory sense. Anyway, most of these matters complained of came from the mouth of a character in the book who is a drunken apostate. They cannot reasonably be taken to be the views of the author.

(4) The passage in which the whores in the brothel assume the names of the prophet's wives cannot reasonably be taken to be derogatory or insulting of the wives, who were expressly said to be chaste. Rather it is a reflection on the perverted lusts of those in a decadent society such as Jahilia was portrayed to be before it submitted to the Islam faith.

(5) As for the references to the companions of the prophet, these words came from the mouth of a decadent hack poet, who is hired by the ruler of Jahilia to denigrate Mahound and his companions. If a fictional work were written about the times of Christ, it could not, Mr. Robertson submitted, be blasphemous to put into the mouth of an opponent of Christ calumnies on the apostles; indeed it is clear that they were derided by such people as being simple ignorant fishermen.

(6) It is not blasphemous to criticise the religion of Islam on the basis that there are too many rules sought to be laid down for the conduct of everyday life. Although this passage complained of is in strong language, it does not amount to vilifying Islam.

Since the magistrate did not refuse to grant a summons on the grounds that the passages complained of did not amount to a scurrilous attack on Islam, he never considered Mr. Robertson's points. He decided the matter on the basis that the offence of blasphemy relates only to Christianity. Therefore, we need not comment on Mr. Robertson's submissions save only to emphasise that neither respondents accept, indeed they strenuously deny, that the book is an attack on Islam, scurrilous or otherwise.

Mr. Azhar for the applicant submitted that the passages complained of are blasphemous inasmuch as they amount to a scurrilous attack on Christianity. The magistrate found as a fact that that is not so. Unless, in our view, that finding is perverse or unsupported by any evidence, it cannot, as we shall later explain, be reversed by this court.

The main issue for us in respect of blasphemy is whether it is an offence at common law solely against Christianity. Did the magistrate take a correct view of the law of England and Wales?

In 1914 the Attorney General, Sir John Simon, was asked to advise the Home Office on the current state of the law. In the course of his opinion he said:

> It seems certainly to be the fact that no offence is committed if the religious beliefs which are attacked are not those of the Church of England; this seems a gross anomaly.

With that comment we entirely agree; but the anomaly arises from what Lord Scarman called "the chains of history", the origins of the law in the ecclesiastical courts, and the fact that the Anglican religion is the established law of the country. Perhaps more important, and certainly more recent, are the views of the Law Commission set out in *Offences against Religion and Public Worship* (Working Paper no 79 (1981)). At para 6.9, p 82 they report:

> Another shortcoming - or at any rate an anomaly - in the present law of blasphemy is the narrow scope of its protection. As we have seen, it is clear that that protection does not extend beyond the Christian religion, but it is less clear whether in the law of England and Wales it also protects the tenets of Christian denominations other than the established Church. Having regard to the authorities, it seems probably that at most other denominations are protected only to the extent that their fundamental beliefs are those which are held in common with the established Church.

See also para 3.2 where reference is made to Alderson B.'s dictum in *R. v. Gathercole* (1838), Lew CC 237 at 254, 168 ER 1140 at 114;.

We have no doubt that as the law now stands it does not extend to religions other than Christianity.

Can it in the light of the present conditions of society be extended by the courts to cover other religions? Mr. Azhar submits that it can and should be on the grounds that it is anomalous and unjust to discriminate in favour of one religion. In our judgment, where the law is clear it is not the proper function of this court to extend it; particularly is this so in criminal cases, where offences cannot be retrospectively created. It is in that circumstance the function of Parliament alone to change the law. This was the view of Lord Scarman in the passage already quoted. In *Knuller (Publishing Printing and Promotions) Ltd v DPP*, [1972] 2 All E.R. 898, [1973] A.C. 435 the House of Lords repudiated the suggestion that the court had any such power. There Lord Reid said ([1972] 2 All E.R. 898 at 905, [1973] A.C. 435 at 457):

> In upholding the decision in *Shaw's* case [*Shaw v DPP*, [1961] 2 All ER 446, [1962] AC 220] we are, in my view, in no way affirming or lending any support to the doctrine that the courts still have some general or residual power either to create new offences or so to widen existing offences as to make punishable conduct of a type hitherto not subject to punishment.

Lord Simon said ([1972] 2 All E.R. 898 at 932, [1973] A.C. 435 at 490):

> Thirdly, in this connection, it has been suggested that the speeches in *Shaw's* case indicated that the courts retain a residual power to create new offences. I do not think they did so. Certainly, it is my view that the courts have no more power to create new offences than they have to abolish those already established in the law; both tasks are for Parliament.

The mere fact that the law is anomalous or even unjust does not, in our view, justify the court in changing it, if it is clear. If the law is uncertain, in interpreting and declaring the law the judges will do so in accordance with justice and to avoid anomaly or discrimination against certain classes of citizens; but taking that course is not open to us, even though we may think justice demands it, for the law is not, we think, uncertain.

There have been a number of attempts in the past to change the law in Parliament. When Professor Kenny entered Parliament in 1885 he introduced a Bill abolishing the common law offence of blasphemy and replacing it with a statutory offence penalising intentional insults to religious feelings based on the *Indian Penal Code*. In 1889 it was dropped in favour of Bradlaugh's Bill, drafted by Stephen, abolishing all laws relating to blasphemy and not replacing them. But it was not carried. Similar Bills were introduced in 1923 and 1925. When the government introduced an amendment to one of them to include the statutory offence of outraging religious convictions, the Bill was dropped. In 1985 the majority of the Law Commission recommended abolition of the offence of blasphemy.

We think it right to say that, were it open to us to extend the law to cover religions other than Christianity, we should refrain from doing so. Considerations of public policy are extremely difficult and complex. It would be virtually impossible by judicial decision to set sufficient clear limits to the offence, and other problems involved are formidable. These are considered at length in *Criminal Law: Offences against Religion and Public Worship* (Law Com. No. 145 (1985)). We need only mention a few briefly.

Among other matters consideration would have to be given to the kinds of religions to be protected and to how religion is to be defined (see for an illustration of this problem *Church of the New Faith v Comr for Pay-roll Tax (Victoria)* (1983), 49 ALR 65, in which it was held that Scientology was a religion)

Although an English jury may be expected, or certainly was in the last century, to understand the tenets of Christianity, this would not be so with other religions. There would be a need for expert evidence no doubt for both prosecution and defence. If different sects of the same religion had differing views and the published material scandalised one sect and not another, how would the matter be decided? Since the only mental element in the offence is the intention to publish the words complained of, there would be a serious risk that the words might, unknown to the author, scandalise and outrage some sect or religion.

In any event, in the light of the majority opinion of the Law Commission in favour of abolition of the offence, it would, in our judgment, be wholly wrong to extend the law, even if, which we do not, we had the power to do so.

4.3 Expressions of Racism

4.3.1 *Criminal Code*, R.S.C. 1985, c. C-46

318. (1) Every one who advocates or promotes genocide is guilty of an indictable offence and is liable to imprisonment for five years.

(2) In this section "genocide" means any of the following acts committed with intent to destroy in whole or in part any identifiable group, namely:

    (*a*) killing members of the group, or

    (*b*) deliberately inflicting on the group conditions of life calculated to bring about its physical destruction.

(3) No proceeding for an offence under this section shall be instituted without the consent of the Attorney General.

(4) In this section "identifiable group" means any section of the public distinguished by colour, race, religion or ethnic origin.

319. (1) Every one who, by communicating statements in any public place, incites hatred against any identifiable group where such incitement is likely to had to a breach of the peace, is guilty of

    (*a*) an indictable offence and is liable to imprisonment for two years; or

    (*b*) an offence punishable on summary conviction.

(2) Every one who, by communicating statements, other than in private conversation, wilfully promotes hatred against any identifiable group is guilty of

    (*a*) an indictable offence and is liable to imprisonment for two years; or

    (*b*) an offence punishable on summary conviction.

(3) No person shall be convicted of an offence under subsection (2)

    (*a*) if he establishes that the statements communicated were true;

    (*b*) if, in good faith, he expressed or attempted to establish by argument an opinion upon a religious subject;

    (*c*) if the statements were relevant to any subject of public interest, the discussion of which was for the public benefit, and if on reasonable grounds he believed them to be true; or

    (*d*) if, in good faith, he intended to point out, for the purpose of removal, matters producing or tending to produce feelings of hatred towards an identifiable group in Canada.

(4) Where a person is convicted of an offence under section 318 or subsection (1) or (2) of this section, anything by means of or in relation to which the offence was committed, upon such conviction, may, in addition to any other punishment imposed, be ordered by the presiding magistrate or judge to be forfeited to Her Majesty in right of the province in which that person is convicted, for disposal as the Attorney General may direct.

(5) Subsections 199(6) and (7) apply mutatis mutandis to section 318 or subsection-(1) or (2) of this section.

(6) No proceeding for an offence under subsection (2) shall be instituted without the consent of the Attorney General.

(7) In this section

"communicating" includes communicating by telephone, broadcasting or other audible or visible means;

"identifiable group" has the same meaning as it has in section 318;

"public place" includes any place to which the public have access as of right or by invitation, express or implied;

"statements" includes words spoken or written or recorded electronically or electromagnetically or otherwise, and gestures, signs or other visible representations.

320. (1) A judge who is satisfied by information upon oath that there are reasonable grounds for believing that any publication, copies of which are kept for sale or distribution in premises within the jurisdiction of the court, is hate propaganda, shall issue a warrant under his hand authorizing seizure of the copies.

(2) Within seven days of the issue of the warrant, the judge shall issue a summons to the occupier of the premises requiring him to appear before the court and show cause why the matter seized should not be forfeited to Her Majesty.

(3) The owner and the author of the matter seized and alleged to be hate propaganda may appear and be represented in the proceedings in order to oppose the making of an order for the forfeiture of the said matter.

(4) If the court is satisfied that the publication is hate propaganda, it shall make an order declaring the matter forfeited to Her Majesty in right of the province in which the proceedings take place, for disposal as the Attorney General may direct.

(5) If the court is not satisfied that the publication is hate propaganda, shall order that the matter be restored to the person from whom it was seized forthwith after the time for final appeal has expired.

4.3.2 *R. v. Buzzanga and Durocher* (1979), 101 D.L.R. (3d) 488 (Ont. C.A.)

MARTIN, J.A.: The appellants Robert Buzzanga and Jean Wilfred Durocher, after a trial at Windsor before His Honour Judge J. P. McMahon, sitting without a jury, were convicted on an indictment charging them with wilfully promoting hatred against an identifiable group, namely, the French Canadian public in Essex County by communicating on or about January 12, 1977, at Windsor, statements contained in copies of a handbill entitled "Wake Up Canadians Your Future Is At Stake!", contrary to s.281.2(2) [enacted R.S.C. 1970, c.11 (1st Supp.), s.1] of the *Criminal Code*. [The relevant section is now 319-ed.]

Following the conviction of the appellants, the learned trial Judge suspended the passing of sentence and directed that they be released on probation for a period of two years. The appellants now appeal against their convictions and the appellant Durocher also appeals, in the alternative, against the sentence imposed upon him, on the ground that the learned trial Judge erred in not granting him a conditional or absolute discharge.

This case is somewhat incongruous in that the appellants identify with Frenchspeaking Canadians against whom they are alleged to have wilfully promoted hatred.

The Factual Background

The appellant Durocher was born in Windsor, and is bilingual. His early education was received in a French-language public school, a bilingual high school and a French oblate seminary. He attended the University of Windsor for three years where he formed a bilingual theatre group which produced plays designed to show the harmony between the official languages of Canada. He was subsequently employed by the Essex County Board of Education and taught French. In August, 1976, he commenced to work for the Association Canadian Francais de L'Ontario (hereafter, LACFO), an organization funded by the Secretary of State. His role in that organization. as he perceived it, was to stimulate and assist the French-speaking community of Essex County with respect to political, social and cultural matters, and in particular, in relation to the issue of the construction of a French-language secondary school.

The appellant Buzzanga was born of Italian parents in Egypt where he learned the French language. He said he went to France, but did not "fit in" and immigrated to Canada where he felt that he could achieve a sense of personal identity. He testified that he embraced the culture of the French Canadian people and identified himself with their aspirations for preserving their culture. He completed his education in Quebec and took courses at Laval University leading to a degree in French literature, but did not obtain a degree. He was employed for a time by the Canadian Broadcasting Corporation, and afterwards as a teacher at St. Bernard's school in Amherstberg. He became a director of LACFO in 1972.

There had been a movement for some time for the construction in Essex County of a French-language high school. The appellant Durocher testified that there had been an agreement between the Ministry of Education and the Essex County School Board for the construction of a French-language high school, under the terms of which the Essex County Board of Education received a grant of $500,000 to renovate two English-language schools and the Ministry of Education agreed to pay 95% of the cost of constructing a French-language high school. He testified that the Ministry subsequently reduced the grant rate from 95% to 77% of the cost of the proposed French-language high school, and the board decided not to build the school, although it had received and spent the grant to renovate the two English-language schools.

Eventually, the Essex County Board of Education was required by the *Essex County French-language Secondary School Act*, 1977 (Ont.), c.5, to construct the school. In the meantime, however, the French-speaking community, according to the testimony of the appellant Durocher, was "quite upset" by the position taken by the board of education.

There was a great deal of opposition, not entirely confined to the English-speaking community of Essex County, to the construction of the French-language high school. One of the strongest opponents of the construction of the high school was the Essex County Ratepayers Association, the chairman of which was Wilfred Fortowsky.

There was to be an election in the month of December, 1976, of members of the Essex County Board of Education. An action committee was formed by LACFO which set up an election office to inform the Francophone community of the stand taken by school-board candidates on the high school issue. The action committee compiled a list of the candidates whom they endorsed, but most of the candidates rejected the endorsement.

The list itself became an issue in the election and the appellant Durocher was accused of being an outside agitator sent in to stir up trouble in the francophone community of Essex County. The appellants were angered by the issue created by the action committee's endorsement of a list of candidates, and by the candidates' rejection of the endorsement. They were, of course, disappointed when the majority of candidates elected to the school board were persons who opposed the construction of the French-language high school.

After the election, the appellant Durocher began to organize a dinner-dance that "was designed as a political evening to engender protest against the treatment of Francophones and to put pressure on the government and the school board to react favourably to the school issue".

On January 5, 1977, Durocher issued a press release which read:

The Essex County Action Committee for a French-language High School
On January 29. 1977. approximately 1000 French-speaking ratepayers of Essex County and the Province of Ontario will assemble at 6 PM at Windsor's Cleary auditorium for a festive dinner-dance. What have we to celebrate? It was 65 years ago that the Provincial Government passed the infamous "Regulation 17" which forbade the teaching of the French language in Ontario. Today the same principle holds true in Essex County re the teaching of that language on the secondary level. We will celebrate 65 years of injustice. It was 8 years ago that the Francophones of Essex County actively began to fight for a French-language high school. We will celebrate 8 years of struggle. It has been 2 years since the Provincial Government has guaranteed the grants to cover construction of said school. We will celebrate 2 years of promises. It has been 1 year since the Essex Board of Education broke its promise to build said school after having spent the 1/2 million dollar "conditional grant" given them by the Provincial Government to secure that promise. We will celebrate 1 year of treachery. It was Lord Durham who said that the French-Canadians were a people without history & without culture and that they should & would be assimilated. It was a local Essex County politician who said last year that the Francophones of Essex County should accept assimilation and that our tax dollars should not be spent to prevent it. We will celebrate the perpetuation of racism and bigotry in Canadian history But we will also act. On January, 29, 1977, the Action Committee For A French-Language High School will exhort its fellow compatriots to take action, to no longer tolerate their status of second-class citizens, to openly and publicly condemn those "Canadians" who deny us our rights and thereby undermine the very foundations of our country and place its future in jeopardy. We invite all English-speaking medias of Ontario and Canada to come and cover this event at the Cleary Auditorium, to leave something of Canadian history and to witness the celebration of people who will not accept cultural and linguistic genocide.
Jean W. Durocher
Spokesman,
Essex County Action Committee
For A French-Language High School.

At about the same time, the appellants began preparing for dissemination the following document, the distribution of which is the subject of the charge:

WAKE UP CANADIANS
YOUR FUTURE IS AT STAKE!

IT IS YOUR TAX DOLLARS THAT SUBSIDIZE THE ACTIVITIES OF THE FRENCH MINORITY OF ESSEX COUNTY .

DID YOU KNOW THAT THE ASSOCIATION CANADIAN FRANÇAIS DE L'ONTARIO HAS INVESTED SEVERAL HUNDREDS OF THOUSANDS OF DOLLARS OF YOUR TAX MONEY IN QUEBEC?
AND THAT NOW THEY ARE STILL DEMANDING 5 MILLION MORE OF YOUR TAX DOLLARS TO BUILD A FRENCH LANGUAGE HIGH SCHOOL?
YOU ARE SUBSIDIZING SEPARATISM WHETHER IN QUEBEC OR ESSEX COUNTY.
DID YOU KNOW THAT THOSE OF THE FRENCH MINORITY WHO SUPPORT THE BUILDING OF THE FRENCH LANGUAGE HIGH SCHOOL ARE IN FACT A SUBVERSIVE GROUP AND THAT MOST FRENCH CANADIANS OF ESSEX COUNTY ARE OPPOSED TO THE BUILDING OF THAT SCHOOL?
WHO WILL RID US OF THIS SUBVERSIVE GROUP IF NOT OURSELVES?
IF WE GIVE THEM A SCHOOL, WHAT WILL THEY DEMAND NEXT . . . INDEPENDENT CITY STATES? CONSIDER THE ETHNIC PROBLEM OF THE UNITED STATES AND TAKE HEED.
WE MUST STAMP OUT THE SUBVERSIVE ELEMENT WHICH USES HISTORY TO JUSTIFY ITS FREELOADING ON THE TAXPAYERS OF CANADA, NOW.
THE BRITISH SOLVED THIS PROBLEM ONCE BEFORE WITH THE ACADIANS, WHAT ARE WE WAITING FOR. . . ?

The statement was composed by the appellant Durocher whose facility with the English language was greater than that of Buzzanga.

The appellant Durocher testified that the francophone community seemed to be "fed up" with the issue of the French-language high school and was becoming apathetic. He said that although economics was the stated reason for not building the school, this was merely an excuse and the real reason was prejudice. The appellant Buzzanga shared Durocher's feeling in this respect.

Both appellants testified as to their purpose in preparing and distributing the pamphlets. The appellant Durocher testified that his purpose was to show the prejudice directed towards French Canadians and expose the truth about the real problem that existed with respect to the French-language school. He said that the statement was largely composed from written material he had seen and from experiences he had had although the paragraph: WHO WILL RID US OF THIS SUBVERSIVE GROUP, IF NOT OURSELVES?" was pure theatrics and has its origin in the quotation "Who will rid me of this meddlesome priest", attributed to Henry II. He testified in some detail as to the origin of various parts of the document and endeavoured to show that it reflected statements contained in such sources as letters to the editor of the Windsor *Star*, a document alleged to have been circulated by a member of the Essex County Ratepayers Association, a paid advertisement published in several newspapers, a book entitled *Bilingual Today, French Tomorrow*, and the like. He said that he thought the pamphlet would be a catalyst that would bring a quick solution to the problem of the French-language school by provoking a Government reaction and thereby put pressure on the school board. He thought that by stating these things people would say: "This is ridiculous. " A fair reading of his evidence is that he did not want to promote hatred against the "French people", for to do so would be to promote hatred against himself.

The appellant Buzzanga, too, said that he wanted to expose the situation, to show the things that were being said so that intelligent people could see how ridiculous they were. The pamphlet was intended as a satire. He wanted to create a furor that would reach the "House of Commons" and compel the Government to do something what would compel the opposing factions on the school question to reopen communications. He said it was not his intention "to raise hatred towards anyone".

The appellant Buzzanga arranged for the printing and distribution of the document. He placed the order for the printing of the document in the name of Wilfred Fortowsky, the president of the Essex County Ratepayers Association, but asked the printer to delete the name of Mr. Fortowsky when he picked up the material, leaving, however, the name of the Essex County Ratepayers Association on the order form. Neither Mr. Fortowsky nor the Essex County Ratepayers Association were, of course, aware that their names had been so used.

The appellant Buzzanga procured two 16-year-old boys, Martin Foley and Kevin Seguin, to distribute the handbills. Martin Foley testified that the appellants picked up Seguin and him in Buzzanga's car and drove them around while he and Seguin distributed the handbills. The appellants told them not to say anything about it and not to let anyone see them delivering the handbills. The handbills were distributed in apartment buildings, office buildings, a church and at the University of Windsor; the remainder were thrown in a snow bank at the Essex County Education Centre.

Apparently, the two youths were later questioned by Kevin Seguin's mother about their involvement and, a day or two later, Martin Foley called the appellant Buzzanga and asked him if the papers that he and Kevin Seguin had distributed were "French hate literature papers". He testified that the appellant Buzzanga said: "Don't say anything or I'll kill you, and tell Kevin that too." He later met both the appellants who were angry because they thought Kevin had told his mother, and he testified that the appellant Buzzanga said that if Kevin were there he would "run him over". The appellant Buzzanga denied making these statements but, in any event, it is clear that these extravagant statements, if made by the appellant Buzzanga, were neither intended nor understood by Foley to be serious threats to harm him or Kevin Seguin. The appellants then obtained some other documents for Foley to give to Mrs. Seguin to convince her that the youths were not involved in the distribution of the pamphlets which form the basis of the charge. Foley gave the papers, with which he had been supplied by the appellants, to Mr. Seguin but afterwards told him the truth.

The appellants testified that it had been their intention to come forward and acknowledge the authorship of the pamphlet but when the police investigation commenced they remained silent as a result of legal advice.

Father Claude Vincent of the Department of Sociology of the University of Windsor, a witness of eminent qualifications, testified that all persons belong to an ethnic group. He said that the Canadian Government Census assumes the existence of ethnic groups and that for census purposes a person's ethnic group is traced through the father. He testified that the term French Canadian represents the type of ethnic group. It has a distinct sense of identity, distinct sense of history, a common culture, a continuing tradition and, above all else, a consciousness of kind. He said that there is an identifiable French Canadian culture or community in Essex County. Within the term "culture" are subsumed the ideas of language, religion and history. He said that the more opposition there is to a particular group, the stronger the "in-group" solidarity becomes. It is, I think, clear that one of the purposes of the appellants in preparing and distributing the pamphlet was to "rally" the French-speaking community on the French-language secondary school issue.

Grounds of Appeal

Although additional grounds of appeal were advanced, only the following grounds of appeal require discussion. The first and principal ground of appeal was that the learned trial Judge misdirected himself with respect to the meaning of the word "wilfully" in the expression "wilfully promotes hatred" in s.281.2(2) of the Code by holding that "wilfully" meant intentionally as opposed to accidentally . . .

The threshold question to be determined is the meaning of "wilfully" in the term "wilfully promotes hatred" in s.281.2(2) of the *Criminal Code*. It will, of course, be observed that the word "wilfully" modifies the words "promotes hatred", rather than the words "communicating statements".

The word "wilfully" has not been uniformly interpreted and its meaning to some extent depends upon the context in which it is used. Its primary meaning is "intentionally", but it is also used to mean "recklessly": see Glanville Williams, *Criminal Law, The General Part*, 2nd ed. (1961), pp. 51-2; Glanville Williams, *Textbook of Criminal Law* (1978), p. 87; Smith and Hogan, *Criminal Law*, 4th ed. (1978), pp. 104-5. The term "recklessly" is here used to denote the subjective state of mind of a person who foresees that his conduct may cause the prohibited result but, nevertheless, takes a deliberate and unjustifiable risk of bringing it about: see Glanville Williams, *Textbook of Criminal Law*, pp. 70 and 76; Smith and Hogan, *Criminal Law*, 4th ed., pp. 52-3.

The word "wilfully" has, however, also been held to mean no more than that the accused's act is done intentionally and not accidentally. In *R. v. Senior*, [1899] 1 Q.B. 283, Lord Russell of Killowen, C.J., in interpreting the meaning of the words "wilfully neglects" in s. 1 of the *Prevention of Cruelty to Children Act*, 1894 (U.K.), c.41, said at pp. 290-1: "'Wilfully' means that the act is done deliberately and intentionally, not by accident or inadvertence, but so that the mind of the person who does the act goes with it."

On the other hand, in *Rice v. Connolly*, [1966] 2 Q.B. 414, where the accused was charged with wilfully obstructing a constable in the execution of his duty,

Lord Parker, L.C.J., said at p. 419: " 'Wilful' in this context not only in my judgment means 'intentional' but something which is done without lawful excuse ...".

In *Willmott v. Atack*, [1976] 3 All E.R. 794, the appellant was convicted on a charge of wilfully obstructing a peace officer in the execution of his duty. A police officer, acting in the execution of his duty, arrested a motorist who struggled and resisted. The appellant, who knew the motorist, intervened with the intention of assisting the officer but, in fact, his conduct obstructed the officer. The Queen's Bench Divisional Court quashed the conviction and held that it was not sufficient to prove the appellant intended to do what he did, and which resulted in an obstruction, but that the prosecution must prove that the appellant intended to obstruct the officer.

The judgment of the Court of Criminal Appeal of Queensland in *R. v. Burnell*, [1966] Qd. R. 348, also illustrates that, depending on its context, the word "wilfully" may connote an intention to bring about a proscribed consequence. In that case the appellant was charged with arson in having set fire to a shed. Section 461 of the Queensland *Criminal Code* provides that "... any person who wilfully and unlawfully sets fire to ... any building or structure is guilty of a crime ...". The accused had deliberately set fire to some mattresses in a shed whereby the shed was set on fire. The trial Judge instructed the jury that "wilfully" connoted no more than a willed and voluntary act as distinguished from the result of an accident or mere negligence. The Queensland Court of Criminal Appeal, in setting aside the conviction, held that in the context of the section "wilfully" required proof that the accused did an act which resulted in setting fire to the building with the intention of bringing about that result. Gibbs, J. (with whom Douglas, J., concurred), said at p. 356:

> Under s.461 it is not enough that the accused did the act which resulted in setting fire to the building foreseeing that his act might have that effect but recklessly taking the risk; it is necessary that the accused did the act which resulted in setting fire to the building with the intention of bringing about that result.

Mr. Manning conceded that in some cases the element of wilfulness is supplied by recklessness but he contended that in its context in s.281.2(2) of the *Criminal Code* "wilfully" means with the intention of promoting hatred. In the course of his argument, Mr. Manning stressed the definition of "wilfully" contained in s.386(1) of the *Code*, which reads:

> 386(1) Every one who causes the occurrence of an event by doing an act or by omitting to do an act that it is his duty to do, knowing that the act or omission will probably cause the occurrence of the event and being reckless whether the event occurs or not, shall be deemed, for the purposes of this Part, wilfully to have caused the occurrence of the event.

Mr. Manning emphasized that s. 386(1) provides that wilfully is to have the meaning specified in that section for the purposes of Part IX of the *Code*. He argued with much force that the state of mind specified in s.386(1) is recklessness and that where Parliament intends to extend the meaning of wilfully to include recklessness it does so expressly. In *R. v. Rese*, [1968] 1 C.C.C. 363 at p. 366, [1967] 2 O.R. 451 at p. 454, 2 C.R.N.S. 99, Laskin, J.A. (as he then was), referred to the definition now contained in s.386(1) as an extended meaning of "wilfully".

As previously indicated, the word "wilfully" does not have a fixed meaning, but I am satisfied that in the context of s. 281.2(2) it means with the intention of promoting hatred, and does not include recklessness. The arrangement of the legislation proscribing the incitement of hatred, in my view, leads to that conclusion.

Section 281.2(1), unlike s.281.2(2), is restricted to the incitement of hatred by communicating statements *in a public place* where such incitement is likely to lead to a breach of the peace. Although no mental element is expressly mentioned in s.281.2(1), where the communication poses an immediate threat to public order, *mens rea* is, none the less, required since the inclusion of an offence in the *Criminal Code* must be taken to import *mens rea* in the absence of a clear intention to dispense with it: see *R. v. Prue; R. v Baril* (1979), 46 C.C.C. (2d) 257 at pp. 260-1, 96 D.L.R. 577 at pp. 580-1, 8 C.R. (3d) 68 at p. 73. The general *mens rea* which is required and which suffices for most crimes where no mental element is mentioned in the definition of the crime, is either the intentional or reckless bringing about of the result which the law, in creating the offence, seeks to prevent and, hence, under s.281.2(1) is either the intentional or reckless inciting of hatred in the specified circumstances.

The insertion of the word "wilfully" in s.281.2(2) was not necessary to import *mens rea* since that requirement would be implied in any event because of the serious nature of the offence: see *R. v. Prue, supra*. The statements, the communication of which are proscribed by s.281.2(2), are not confined to statements communicated in a public place in circumstances likely to lead to a breach of the peace and they, consequently, do not pose such an immediate threat to public order as those falling under s.281.2(1); it is reasonable to assume, therefore, that Parliament intended to limit the offence under s.281.2(2) to the intentional promotion of hatred. It is evident that the use of the word "wilfully" in s.281.2(2), and not in s.281.2(1), reflects Parliament's policy to strike a balance in protecting the competing social interests of freedom of expression on the one hand, and public order and group reputation on the other hand. . . .

I conclude, therefore, that the appellants "wilfully" (intentionally) promoted hatred against the French Canadian community of Essex County only if: (a) their conscious purpose in distributing the document was to promote hatred against that group, or (b) they foresaw that the promotion of hatred against that group was certain or morally certain to result from the distribution of the pamphlet, but distributed it as a means of achieving their purpose of obtaining the French-language high school.

Whether the Trial Judge Misdirected Himself as to the Meaning of Wilfully?

The learned trial Judge in comprehensive reasons first considered whether the document objectively promoted hatred and concluded that the cumulative effect of the document rendered it a communication that promoted hatred against the French-speaking community of Essex County. He then said:

> It is, however, incumbent upon the Crown to prove beyond a reasonable doubt that the two accused wilfully promoted such hatred. In other words, has the Crown established the necessary element of *mens rea*. In considering the meaning to be given to the word "wilfully" in this section the Court must distinguish between what has been described by learned writers as primary and secondary intent: or to phrase it in a more understanding way, the distinction between intent and motive. I have earlier discussed the purpose or motive as explained by the accused themselves. They wished to create a situation that would require the intervention of senior levels of Government and result in the construction of the high school. It is in evidence that the handbill was, in fact, shown to a mediator representing the Minister of Education who was in this area attempting to resolve the school issue. It is, of course, a matter of judicial notice that the Province did pass special legislation requiring the construction of the school. It is extremely doubtful, however, that this document played any part in the formulation of that decision. It was also their desire to unify the French Canadian community. As Father Vincent stated, opposition from outside often cements an ethnic group and tends to strengthen people rather than weaken them.
>
> This is what the Court would refer to as the purpose or motive of the accused.
>
> Wilful in this section, however, means intentional as opposed to accidental. Miss Susan Moylan who testified for the accused was involved in the early discussions between the accused in the preparation of the handbill. She testified that the document was not to create strong feelings but to create strong actions and strong reactions. How one can do the latter without the former is beyond the comprehension of this Court. The accused themselves testified they wished to create controversy, furor and an uproar. What better way of describing active dislike, detestation, enmity or ill will, The motives of the accused may or may not be laudable. The means chosen by the accused was the wilful promotion of hatred.

Mr. Manning contended before us that the learned trial Judge erred in his interpretation of the meaning of "wilfully". He said that the trial Judge, in concluding that the document, viewed objectively, promoted hatred, separated the word "wilfully" from the words "promotes hatred" and, consequently, fell into error in only considering the question whether the document was distributed intentionally as opposed to accidentally, when the offence charged was committed only if the appellants' purpose in distributing the document was to promote hatred. Mr. Manning said that the trial Judge was concerned only with the effect of the document, whereas if he had "looked for" an intention to promote hatred, he would have come to a different conclusion with respect to the appellants' guilt. Mr. Hunt for the Crown did not dispute that the central issue in the case is whether the appellants, when they distributed the pamphlet, intended to promote hatred. He contended, however, that the trial Judge found that the appellants intended to promote hatred as a means of accomplishing their purpose.

Despite Mr. Manning's able argument I am not persuaded that the learned trial Judge fell into the error of detaching the word "wilfully" from the words "promotes hatred" and applied it only to the distribution of the pamphlet. I am of the view, however, that the learned trial Judge erred in holding that "wilfully" means only "intentional as opposed to accidental". Although, as previously indicated, "wilfully" has sometimes been used to mean that the accused's act, as distinct from its consequences, must be intended and not accidental (as in *R. v.*

Senior, [1899] 1 Q.B. 283), it does not have that meaning in the provisions under consideration.

The learned trial Judge's view of the meaning of "wilfully" inevitably caused him to focus attention on the intentional nature of the appellants' conduct, rather than on the question whether they actually intended to produce the consequence of promoting hatred. I observe that even if, contrary to the view which I have expressed, recklessness satisfies the mental element denoted by the word "wilfully", recklessness when used to denote the mental element attitude which suffices for the ordinary *mens rea*, requires actual foresight on the part of the accused that his conduct may bring about the prohibited consequence, although I am not unmindful that for some purposes recklessness may denote only a marked departure from objective standards. Where the prosecution, in order to establish the accused's guilt of the offence charged, is required to prove that he intended to bring about a particular consequence or foresaw a particular consequence, the question to be determined is what was in the mind of this particular accused, and the necessary intent or foresight must be brought home to him subjectively: see *R. v. Mulligan* (1974), 18 C.C.C. (2d) 270 at pp. 274-5, 26 C.R.N.S. 179; affirmed 28 C.C.C. (2d) 266, [1977] 1 S.C.R. 612, 66 D.L.R. (3d) 627.

What the accused intended or foresaw must be determined on a consideration of all the circumstances, as well as from his own evidence, if he testifies, as to what his state of mind or intention was.

Since people are usually able to foresee the consequences of their acts, if a person does an act likely to produce certain consequences it is, in general, reasonable to assume that the accused also foresaw the probable consequences of his act and if he, nevertheless, acted so as to produce those consequences, that he intended them. The greater the likelihood of the relevant consequences ensuing from the accused's act, the easier it is to draw the inference that he intended those consequences. The purpose of this process, however, is to determine what the particular accused intended, not to fix him with the intention that a reasonable person might be assumed to have in the circumstances, where doubt exists as to the actual intention of the accused. The accused's testimony, if he gives evidence as to what was in his mind, is important material to be weighed with the other evidence in determining whether the necessary intent has been established. Indeed, Mr. Justice Devlin, in his charge to the jury in *R. v. Adams* (*The Times*, April 10, 1957), said that where the accused testified as to what was in his mind and the jury "thought he might be telling the truth", they would "have the best evidence available on what was in his own mind". The background of the appellants and their commitment to preserving the French Canadian culture was, of counsel relevant to the credibility of their denial that they intended to promote hatred against the French-speaking community of Essex County. The appellants' evidence as to their state of mind or intention is not, of course, conclusive.

In some cases the inference from the circumstances that the necessary intent existed may be so strong as to compel the rejection of the accused's evidence that he did not intend to bring about the prohibited consequence. The learned trial Judge did not, however, state that he disbelieved the appellants' evidence that they did not intend to promote hatred. He appears to have treated the appellants' testimony that they wished to create "controversy, furor and an uproar" as a virtual admission that they had the state of mind requisite for guilt.

I am, with deference to the learned trial Judge, of the view that an intention to create "controversy, furor and an uproar" is not the same thing as an intention to promote hatred, and it was an error to equate them. I would, of course, agree that if the appellants intentionally promoted hatred against the French-speaking community of Essex County as a means of obtaining the French-language high school, they committed the offence charged. The appellants' evidence, if believed, does not, however, as the learned trial Judge appears to have thought, inevitably lead to that conclusion. The learned trial Judge, not having disbelieved the appellants' evidence, failed to give appropriate consideration to their evidence on the issue of intent and, in the circumstances, his failure so to do constituted self-misdirection.

In view of the conclusion which I have reached it is necessary to refer only briefly to the other grounds of appeal which we regard as requiring discussion.

The Exemption under s.281.2(3)(d)

Mr. Rosenberg contended that there was an evidentiary base for the application of the exemption under s.281.2(3)(d) of the *Criminal Code* and that the learned trial Judge erred in holding that it was not available to the appellants.

The learned trial Judge said:

> Counsel have submitted, however, that the accused are entitled to the statutory exemption in para. (d). An accused cannot be found guilty "if, in good faith, he intended to point out, for the purpose of removal, manners producing or tending to produce feelings of hatred towards an identifiable group in Canada".
>
> If the accused had produced a document, for example, which pointed out, that in their view, these statements were being made in Essex County and that the public should be aware of it then clearly they would be within the exemption. The exemption also works for the protection of the media, who in the course of editorial comment would be required for the purpose of removal to repeat such statements. The Parliament, in enacting this section, included the words "in good faith". Were the accused acting in good faith when Mr. Buzzanga used the name of Mr. Fortowsky in placing the order with the printer? Were the accused acting in good faith when they instructed young Foley and Seguin to deceive their parents? Were the accused acting in good faith when their stated objective was to deceive elected Members of Parliament and Ministers of the Crown? Surely not.

Mr. Rosenberg submitted that the requirement in s.281.2(3)(d) of "good faith" means no more than the accused "honestly" or "genuinely" intended to point out for the purpose of removal, matters producing or tending to produce feelings of hatred towards an identifiable group. He argued that if the appellants otherwise came within it, the exemption was available to them, notwithstanding that they did not act in an open and "above-board" manner. I accept Mr. Rosenberg's submission that the appellants' devious conduct did not, as a matter of law, exclude them from the exemption under s.281.2(3)(d). I also accept that the exemption under s.281.2(3)(d) is not, as a matter of law, limited to cases where the communication on its face expressly states that the matters producing or tending to produce feelings of hatred are pointed out for the purpose of removing them. The appellants' devious conduct and the character of the pamphlet were, however, relevant items of evidence to be weighed in determining whether the appellants came within the exemption. If the appellants were properly found to have wilfully promoted hatred as alleged, I would not readily have interfered with a finding that they had not brought themselves within the exemption.

The exemption contained in s.281.2(3)(d) is, in my view, provided out of abundant caution, and where a person has "wilfully" promoted hatred, the cases in which the exemption may successfully be invoked must be comparatively rare.

The persons referred to in the Pamphlet

Dr. Bernhard Harder, who has a doctorate in English literature and linguistics, testified on behalf of the defence. The substance of his testimony was that from the point of view of linguistics the "subversive" group or element referred to in the pamphlet is the French minority who support the building of the French-language high school and not the French Canadian community in Essex County.

Counsel for the appellants, on the basis of the evidence, argued that even if the pamphlet promoted hatred, it promoted hatred only against the French minority who supported the building of the high school and not the French Canadian public in Essex County as alleged in the indictment, and the charge, as laid, was not proved.

I have serious reservations as to the admissibility of this evidence: see *Phipson on Evidence*, 12th ed. (1976), pp. 504-5. In any event, I agree with the trial Judge that the meaning of the document is to be gathered from its entirety, and the construction that would be placed upon it by the average person into whose hands it fell. I would not give effect to this ground of appeal.

Conclusion

I have concluded that the self-misdirection with respect to the meaning of the word "wilfully", and the failure to appreciate the significance of the appellants' evidence on the issue of intent require a new trial. The outrageous conduct of the appellants in preparing and distributing this deplorable document was evidence to be weighed in determining their intent, but in the peculiar circumstances of this case I am not satisfied that the inferences to be drawn from it are such as to inevitably lead to a conclusion that they had the requisite intent or that the trial Judge would inevitably have reached that conclusion but for his self-misdirection.

In the result, I would allow the appeal, set aside the convictions and order new trials.

Appeal allowed; new trial ordered.

4.3.3 *R v. Keegstra*, [1990] 3 S.C.R. 697 (S.C.C.)

See above pages.

4.3.4 *R. v. Andrews and Smith*, [1990] 3 S.C.R. 870 (S.C.C.)

Facts

The appellants belonged to the Nationalist Party of Canada. a white nationalist political organization. Mr. Andrews was the party leader and Mr. Smith its secretary. Both were members of the party's central committee. the organization responsible for publishing and distributing the bi-monthly *Nationalist Reporter*. This publication constitutes the primary subject-matter of the prosecution and was subscribed to by 43 individuals and 50 groups, clubs or organizations.

Pursuant to a search warrant, 89 materials were seized from the home of the appellants. Included in these materials were copies of the *Nationalist Reporter*, letters written by subscribers, subscription lists and mimeographed sticker cards containing such messages as "Nigger go home", "Hoax on the Holocaust", "Israel stinks" and "Hitler was right. Communism is Jewish". The ideology expressed by the material was summarized as follows by counsel for the appellants:

... the material argues that God bestowed his greatest gifts only on the "White people"; that if it were God's plan to create one "coffee-coloured race of 'humanity' it would have been created from Genesis"; and that therefore all those who urge a homogeneous "race-mixed planet" are, in fact, working against God's will. In forwarding the opinion that members of minority groups are responsible for increases in the violent crime rate, it is said that violent crime is increasing almost in proportion to the increase of minority immigrants coming into Canada. A high proportion of violent crimes are committed by blacks. America is being "swamped by coloureds who do not believe in democracy and harbour hatred for white people." The best way to end racial strife, an excerpt opines, is by a separation of the races "through a repatriation of non-whites to their own lands where their own race is the majority ... The "Nationalist Reporter" also promulgated the thesis that Zionists had fabricated the "Holocaust Hoax" and that because Zionists dominate financial life and resources, the nation cannot remain in good health because the "alien community's interests" are not those of the majority of the citizens either culturally or economically.

Cory, J.A. in the Ontario Court of Appeal, referring specifically to the contents of the *Nationalists Reporter* and other publications of the Nationalist Party, characterized this material as "rubbish and offal", and stated that the writings were "malodorous. malicious and evil".

On January 28, 1985, the appellants were charged under s. 319(2) of the *Criminal Code* with unlawfully communicating statements, other than in private conversation, which wilfully promote hatred against an identifiable group. After trial in the District Court of Ontario by the Honourable Judge E. Wren, the appellants were convicted on December 9, 1985. They were sentenced four days later, Mr. Andrews receiving twelve months incarceration and Mr. Smith being sentenced to seven months. As already mentioned, the appeal to the Court of Appeal was dismissed, although the terms of incarceration for Messrs. Andrews and Smith were reduced to three months and one month respectively.

4.3.5 Law Reform Commission of Canada, *Hate Propaganda*, Working Paper 50 (Ottawa: 1986), pp. 39-41

There is no easy solution to the problem of spreading hatred. Even among civil libertarians who believe strongly in protecting freedom of speech, opinion is divided as to whether these crimes are necessary.

These proposals may not meet with overwhelming approval from the public. On the one hand, visible minorities may regard with dismay the decision to retain, for the revised offence of fomenting hatred, the *mens rea* requirement of intent or purpose and all the existing defences. On the other hand, civil libertarians may be disappointed that we did not advocate abolition of the offence of wilfully promoting hatred, and indeed may shudder at the proposal to expand the definition of "identifiable group" to protect those groups enumerated specifically in subsection 15(1) of the Charter. Both sides may argue that the Commission has failed to act boldly and imaginatively on an important social issue.

Nonetheless, the proposals made here are entirely consistent with our view that, while the criminal law should uphold fundamental values, it should nonetheless be applied with restraint.

Admittedly, the very existence of these crimes of fomenting hatred is open to two fundamental objections. First, they encroach upon freedom of expression in an unjustifiable manner. In other words, restricting freedom of expression for some restricts freedom of expression for all. Second, they may not do what they are expected to do. After all, the Weimar Republic had crimes of hate propaganda; yet Hitler still came to power.

The crimes proposed in this Paper, however, infringe upon freedom of expression in a justifiable manner by ensuring that only the most serious kinds of hatred are caught by the criminal law. Moreover, these crimes will do what they are expected to do, in two ways: first, by underlining the fundamental values of equality and dignity; second, by deterring others from engaging in such activity.

Admittedly, too, the restricted definition of these crimes is open to the fundamental objection that they do not propose adequate legal controls on the propagation of hatred.

The issue here, however, is to what extent the *criminal law* must be used to combat fomenting hatred against identifiable groups. Given its coercive and brutal nature, criminal law must be used with restraint. It should be used as the last resort, not the first. Of course, our society can use other means to deal with the spreading of hatred. The work of human rights commissions is all-important in helping to eliminate attitudes which support discrimination. Perhaps a more effective way to deal with fomenting hatred would be to ensure that these commissions play a stronger role in combatting such attitudes. But the role of the criminal law must be limited to preventing the most harmful hatreds being aimed at clearly socially important groups. Otherwise, in the name of fighting hatred, our society runs the risk of creating unjustifiable repression.

The crimes dealing with hate propaganda should be amended or altered in the following manner.

Recommendations

General

Groups

1. All these crimes should protect those groups identifiable on the basis of race, national or ethnic origin, colour, religion, sex, age or mental or physical disability.

Placement

2. The definition of "identifiable group" should be removed from the offence of advocating genocide and put into a separate definition section.

3. These crimes should be placed in our new Code in a chapter on Offences against Society.

Specific Offences

Genocide

4. (1) Whether there should be a crime of genocide in our new Code should not be resolved by this Paper, but should be deferred for future consideration.

(2) The crime of advocating or promoting genocide should be retained. However, the crime should be modified to catch "advocating, promoting, or urging" genocide. Also, any recommendation concerning the requirement of the Attorney General's consent should await the results of a forthcoming Commission Working Paper on the Powers of the Attorney General.

Publishing False News

5. Section 177, the crime of publishing false news, should be abolished. Any new offence designed to deal with causing public alarm should be defined in a precise enough manner to prevent its being used to prosecute hatemongers.

Crimes of Promoting or Inciting Hatred in Section 281.2

6. (1) Both crimes should be amended to catch clearly any means by which hatred is fomented.

(2) The crime of inciting hatred in a public place where such incitement is likely to lead to a breach of the peace should be redefined in the following manner:

Any person who intentionally [purposely] and publicly foments hatred in a public place where it is likely to cause harm to a person or damage to property commits a crime. ["Public place" would continue to be defined as including any place to which the public have access as of right or by invitation, express or implied.]

(3) The crime of wilfully promoting hatred, other than in private conversation, against any identifiable group, should be redefined in the following manner:

    (*a*) Any person who intentionally [purposely] and publicly foments hatred against any identifiable group commits a crime.

    (*b*) No person shall be convicted if he or she

        (i) uses the truth and proves such truth;

        (ii) in good faith, expresses an opinion upon a religious subject;

        (iii) uses anything which, on reasonable grounds, he or she believes to be true and which was relevant to any subject of public interest, the discussion of which was for the public benefit; or

        (iv) in good faith, intended to point out, for the purpose of removal, matters producing or tending to produce feelings of hatred towards an identifiable group in Canada.

    (*c*) Any recommendation concerning the requirement of the Attorney General's consent should await the results of a forthcoming Commission Working Paper on the Powers of the Attorney General.

Forfeiture Provisions

7. In accordance with a recommendation made in our Report on *Search and Seizure*, section 281.3, dealing with *in rem* proceedings for seizure and forfeiture of hate propaganda, should be taken out of the *Code* and put into federal regulatory legislation.

It is open to question whether subsections 281.2 [now s.320] (4) and (5), which govern the forfeiture of material after conviction for a hate propaganda offence, belong among these crimes or among provisions dealing with sentencing.

4.3.6 *Criminal Code*, R.S.C. 1985, c. C-46

181. Every one who wilfully publishes a statement, tale or news that he knows is false and that causes or is likely to cause injury or mischief to a public interest is guilty of an indictable offence and is liable to imprisonment for two years.

Note: In the case of *R. v. Kirby* (1970), 1 C.C.C. (2d) 286, the Quebec Court of Appeal quashed a conviction under this section. In this case the accused had published and distributed a parody of the Montreal *Gazette*. The headline story was entitled "Mayor Shot by Dope-enraged Hippie" and was accompanied by a photo of Jean Drapeau. The Court stated that while the statement was knowingly false, as well as being "stupid, pointless and in bad taste", it could not be said to be likely to cause injury or mischief to the public interest. The reasons given for this conclusion included that satire and parody have a long tradition ranging from Chaucer and Swift to Punch and the *New Yorker*, that the parody could be readily distinguished &from the *Gazette* upon inspection, and that Mayor Drapeau himself appeared unconcerned.

4.3.7 *R. v. Zundel* (1992), 16 C.R. (4th) 1 (S.C.C.)

Z published a booklet entitled "Did Six Million Really Die?" which purported to provide evidence that the Holocaust is a myth perpetrated by an international Jewish conspiracy to obtain reparations for Jews and support for Israel. He was charged with the offence of spreading false news contrary to s. 181 [formerly s.177] of the Code. To obtain a conviction under this provision, it must be established that the accused published a false statement, tale, or news; that he knew the statement was false; and that the statement caused or is likely to cause injury or mischief to a public interest.

At trial, by application of the doctrine of judicial notice, the jury was charged that the "mass murder and extermination of Jews in Europe by the Nazi regime" was an historical fact which no reasonable person could dispute. The jury was also charged that the "maintenance of racial and religious tolerance" is a matter of public interest in Canada. The question of knowledge of falsity was left to the jury as a question of fact. Z was convicted and he appcaled lo the Court of Appeal on numerous grounds. The appeal was dismissed. Leave to appeal to the Supreme Court was granted only in respect of the constitutionality of s. 181, which was challenged as an infringement of freedom of expression contrary to s. 2(b) of the *Charter*, and on the basis of vagueness contrary to s. 7 of the *Charter*.

MCLACHLIN, J. (LA FOREST, L'HEUREUX-DUBÉ and SOPINKA, JJ. concurring): Section 181 infringes the fundamental freedom of thought, belief, opinion, and expression, as guaranteed by s. 2(b) of the *Charter* and cannot be saved by s. 1. Section 2(b) is to be given a broad, purposive interpretation. The purpose of the guarantee is to permit free expression to promote truth, political or social participation, and self-fulfilment. It serves to protect the right of the minority to express its views no matter how unpopular. All communications which convey or attempt to convey meaning are protected by s. 2(b) unless the physical form by which the communication is made, for example a violent act, excludes protection. The content of the communication should not be considered in order to ensure that unpopular statements are given protection. Accordingly, the communication of hate propaganda is protected by s. 2(b). The falsity of the publication in issue in this case does not remove it from the ambit of s. 2(b) protection. A deliberate lie does not constitute an illegitimate form of expression. A violent act is excluded from protection by reason of the physical form in which the message is communicated, not its content. While a deliberate lie does not serve to promote any of the values which underlie s. 2(b), it cannot be said that all deliberate lies have no value. In some situations, exaggeration or even clear falsification may serve some useful social purpose or foster political participation or self-fulfillment. Moreover, one cannot assume that falsity can be identified with sufficient accuracy to make it a fair criterion for the denial of constitutional protection. Freedom of expression protects both the meaning which the publisher intends to communicate and the meaning understood by the reader. Where complex social and historical facts are involved, it may be difficult to determine whether the particular meaning assigned to a statement is true or false. As well, a statement that is true on one level for one person may be false on another level for a different person. Rather than use falsity as a criterion for denying constitutional protection, it is preferable to leave arguments relating the value of a deliberate falsehood to its prejudicial effect to be dealt with under s. 1.

Assuming, without deciding, that s. 181 is not so vague that it cannot be considered a "limit prescribed by law", s. 1 requires that the intrusion of rights represented by the impugned legislation be weighed against the state's interest in maintaining the legislation. The objective of the legislation cannot be considered pressing and substantial and, thus, is not of sufficient importance to justify overriding the constitutional guarantee of freedom of expression. The court must look at the intention of Parliament when the provision was enacted or amended. It cannot assign new objectives to accord with a perceived current utility. While the interpretation of an objective may vary over time as our understanding of a detrimental impact changes, it is not permissible to invent a new and different purpose. The false news provision can be traced to an English statute of 1275, the purpose of which was to preserve political harmony by preventing slanders against the monarch and the nobility. It was abolished in England in 1887 and does not survive in the United States. It was enacted in Canada in 1892 as part of the first Canadian *Criminal Code*. It is not possible to say with any assurance what Parliament had in mind when chose to retain the false news provision as part of our criminal law. No documentation, debates or comments exist to explain its retention. Furthermore, the decision to move the provision from the "Sedition" section to the "Nuisance" section in the 20th century suggests that Parliament no longer saw it as serving a political purpose. It is not permissible to characterize its current purpose as a concern for attacks on religious, racial or ethnic minorities and call this simply a shift in emphasis from the original objective. Also, it cannot be argued that the legislative objective is the protection of the public interest from harm because this broad formulation would apply to all provisions of the Code. Justification under s. 1 requires a specific purpose which is so pressing and substantial as to be capable of overriding the *Charter's* guarantees. Here, Parliament has identified no social problem, much less one of pressing concern. To suggest what the objective of s. 181 is to combat hate propaganda or racism is to go beyond its history and its wording, and adopt a "shifting purpose". Other provisions deal with hate propaganda more fairly and more effectively. The rejection of any pressing and substantial concern underlying s. 181 is supported by the fact that it has been so rarely used in Canada and appears to have no direct counterpart in other free and democratic countries.

Even if one assumes that the preservation of social harmony is the relevant objective and that it is pressing and substantial, the provision cannot satisfy the proportionality aspect of s. 1. The breadth of the section goes much further than necessary to achieve that aim by encompassing a vast territory carved out by its vague and broad wording. The phrase "statement, tale or news" engages the debate between fact and opinion. The phrase "injury or mischief to a public interest" is undefined and virtually unlimited. It is not permissible to redefine "public interest" by equating it with the rights and freedoms protected by the *Charter*. To do so is to create a new offence, hitherto unknown to criminal law. The danger of the breadth of s. 181 is not only that it may criminalize a vast penumbra of statements, but also that it will inhibit worthy minority groups or individuals from saying what they want to say. Overbreadth is the fatal flaw of s. 181. Section 181 fails the tests of minimal impairment and proportionality by which the criminalization of hate propaganda under s. 319(2) was upheld. It is no answer to say that prosecutorial discretion will protect against undue impingement on the free expression of facts and opinions.

CORY and IACOBUCCI, JJ. (dissenting) (GONTHIER, J. concurring): Section 181, while it infringes freedom of expression, can be saved by s. 1 of the *Charter*. The sphere of expression protected by s. 2(b) has been broadly defined to encompass all content of expression irrespective of the particular meaning sought to be conveyed unless the expression is conveyed in a physically violent form. While Z deliberately published lies which were damaging to members of the Jewish community, even statements on the extreme periphery must be brought within the protective ambit of s. 2(b). The purpose of s. 181 it to restrict free expression and, hence, it constitutes an infringement of freedom of expression.

In order to determine whether s. 181 can be justified under s. 1, a careful balancing of a number of factors must be considered. Section 181 cannot be said to be so vague so as not to qualify as a limit "prescribed by law". It provides clear guidelines of conduct so that a citizen knows that he or she is at risk if a false statement is wilfully published with the knowledge that it is false. The term "public interest", while undefined, can be defined by the courts. In the context of s. 181, the "public interest" should be interpreted in light of *Charter* values. Accordingly, the "public interest" encompassed by s. 181 should be confined to those rights recognized in the *Charter* as being fundamental to Canadian democracy including, for example, the rights enacted in ss. 7, 15 and 27. If the Crown can establish beyond a reasonable doubt that the rights protected by those sections are likely to have been seriously damaged by the wilful publication of statements known to be false, it will have satisfied this part of the provision.

The aim of s. 181 is to prevent the harm caused by the wilful publication of injurious lies. This has the effect of protecting the vulnerable in society and, as such, is a pressing and substantial concern. There is a pressing and substantial need to protect the groups identifiable under s. 15 of the *Charter*. The serious harm wreaked by hate propaganda can be demonstrated by the publication at issue in this case. Holocaust denial has pernicious effects upon Canadians who suffered, fought and died as a result of the Nazi campaign of racial bigotry. It is the foulest of falsehoods and the essence of cruelty to lie about the indescribable suffering and death of Jews at the hands of the Nazis. Similar provisions in other free and democratic countries support the conclusion that the objective is of sufficient importance to warrant justifying an infringement of freedom of expression. Viewed in the light of ss. 15 and 27 of the *Charter*, it can be seen that s. 181 has a very useful and important role to play in Canadian society. Over the years, the purpose of s. 181 and its predecessors has evolved from protecting the "great persons of the realm" to protecting vulnerable social groups from the harm caused by false speech. In a multicultural society, the sowing of dissension through the publication of known falsehoods cannot be tolerated. This analysis does not run afoul of the shifting purpose caveat. Section 181 was always aimed at protection from the harm of false speech. The aim has been maintained; only its emphasis has been shifted. This is permissible since it is consistent with a shift in values that inform the public interest, especially the values encompassed by equality and multiculturalism.

With respect to proportionality, a commitment to the fostering of free speech is directly related to the prohibition of deliberate lies which foment racism. There is no risk of losing a kernel of truth when the speech in question must be known even by its source to be false. The argument that truth is in the eye of the beholder supports protection of false speech under s. 2(b) but does not render state intervention unjustiflable when the speech threatens the dignity of the target group and promotes discrimination. Self-fulfilment and human flourishing can never be achieved by the publication of statements known to be false. Furthermore, intentional and harmful falsehoods repudiate democratic values by denying respect and dignity to certain members of society. Section 181 is rationally connected to the suppression of deliberate and injurious lies. Section 181 does not unduly infringe freedom of expression and satisfies the minimal impairment test. The provision is not overly broad nor does it produce a chilling effect on expression. Given the elements of s. 181, it is not an easy task to obtain a conviction. For an acquittal, there need only be a reasonable doubt with regard to the wilful publication of the statements presented as truth, or the falsity of the statements, or the knowledge of falsity. Moreover, there can be no confusion between opinions and statements of fact. The provision only applies to a statement, tale, or news which, taken as a whole and understood in context, conveys an assertion of fact. This means an expression which is verifiable through empirical proof or disproof. It must be made in a linguistic context in which it will be understood as fact rather than opinion. Statements like the pamphlet in issue, which are disguised as the reasoned product of scholarly investigation, make specific claims about discrete historical incidents which are verifiable through an examination of reliable historical documents. The presence of existing hate propaganda legislation in s. 319 of the Code should not weigh for or against the validity of s. 181. An overlap of provisions is not fatal. The government may legitimately employ a variety of measures to achieve its objectives. Finally, the prohibition of the wilful publication of what are known to be deliberate lies is proportional to the importance of protecting the public interest in preventing the harms caused by false speech and thereby promoting racial and social tolerance in a multicultural democracy.

Annotation

The success of Zundel's *Charter* challenge to his conviction at his new trial on a charge of wilfully publishing a statement or tale that he knew was false and that was likely to cause mischief to the public interest in social and religious tolerance is not in itself surprising. What was surprising was the narrow majority, the length of the reasons for judgment, particularly those of the minority, and the tendency of the writers of both reasons to stray from relevant issues.

The charge was brought under s. 181, (formerly s. 177), of the *Criminal Code* [R.S.C. 1985, c. C46], which purports to create an offence of wilfully publishing a statement, tale or news that the publisher knows to be false and that causes or is likely to cause injury or mischief to any public interest. The majority held that s. 181 infringes the freedom of expression affirmed by s. 2(b) of the *Charter* and is not saved by s. 1 as a reasonable limit prescribed by law that can be demonstrably justified in our free and democratic society.

Simply put, the majority held, correctly in my view, that the phrase "likely to cause injury or mischief" to such a vaguely described concept as a public interest does not satisfy the accepted requirement of a defined, pressing and substantial objective of importance sufficient to justify overriding the protected freedom. Failure to satisfy the other criteria of justification under s. 1 flows, in this case, from the impossibility of imposing reasonable limits on the meaning of "public interest" although the majority demolished the opposing arguments under the other criteria of the *Oakes* test as well.

The Ontario Court of Appeal had answered this attack, on Zundel's appeal from his first conviction at (1987), 56 C.R. (3d) 1, 18 O.A.C. 161, 58 O.R. (2d) 129, 31 C.C.C. (3d) 97, 35 D.L.R. (4th) 338, 29 C.R.R. 349, at pp. 31-33 (C.R.). It began with a general statement that if a person's conduct clearly falls within the prescription of a statute, that person cannot complain of the vagueness of the statute as applied by others. The court relied on knowledge of the publisher of the falsehood of the statement, the absence of social or moral value in false statements, and an assertion based on earlier judicial recognition that maintenance of racial and religious harmony is "certainly a matter of public interest in Canada. The accused and those who administer the law would have a reasonable opportunity to know what was covered by s. 177 and act accordingly". On this argument, Zundel should have known that he was violating s. 177 "upon instinct", as Falstaff said he had recognized the disguised Prince Hal at Gad's Hill, in *Henry IV,* Part 1.

The minority in the Supreme Court gave a different answer.

"Section 181 cannot be said to be vague. It provides clear guidelines of conduct. The citizen knows that to be at risk under this section, he or she must wilfully publish a false statement knowing it to be false. Further, the publication of those statements must injure or be likely to injure the public interest.

. . . . .

The fact that the term is undefined by the legislation is of little significance. There are many phrases and words contained in the *Criminal Code* which have been interpreted by the courts."

Among examples given by the minority are "obscene", "indecent", "immoral" and "scurrilous". It would be a bold assertion to say that the courts have done well in defining these terms. Others also unsatisfactorily defined could be added. Legislatures have been compelled frequently to correct judicial misinterpretation of statutes. In any case, the obligation of defining the meaning of a vague and unlimited term should not be unnecessarily thrust upon the courts, and accused persons should not be compelled to wait until the courts trying them have defined the term to learn whether their conduct came within the offence.

The minority reasons add that the phrase "public interest" is mentioned 224 times in federal statutes: it must be interpreted in its context; in s. 181, the public interest must be confined to those rights recognized in the *Charter* as being fundamental to Canadian democracy. For example, the wilful publication of statements which are known to be false, that seriously injure a group identifiable under s. 15 of the *Charter*, would tear at the very fabric of Canadian society. It follows that the wilful publication of such lies would be contrary to the public interest.

This argument is buttressed by reference to the Holocaust and to Canada's obligations under the International Covenant on Civil and Political Rights and the International Convention on the Elimination of All Forms of Racial Discrimination, both of which condemn national, racial or religious hatred. Section 27's stress on multicultural values is brought in, as it was in *R. v. Keegstra*, [1990] 3 S.C.R. 697,1 C.R. (4th) 129, 77 Alta. L.R. (2d) 193, [1991] 2 W.W.R. 1, 61 C.C.C. (3d) 1,117 N.R. 1,114 A.R. 81, 3 C.R.R. (2d) 193.

There follows a lengthy defence of s. 181 by the four accepted criteria for justification of a restriction on a *Charter* freedom. The argument is based in part on the theory that freedom of expression is designed for reasoned debate, in part on the unworthiness of false statements of alleged fact wilfully published with knowledge of the falsehood, and in part on the inadequacy of the hate propaganda offences to afford full protection to racial, religious or other *Charter* recognized minority groups.

All these arguments are based on the assumption that the challenge of want of definition of "public interest" has been defeated. Unfortunately for the argument that assumption is unfounded. Nowhere in s. 181 do we learn that the interest protected is racial and religious tolerance. Still less do we find in it a requirement that the protected interest must be a *Charter* right or freedom. That proposition is an arbitrary assumption by the minority. According to its terms, the offence could be related to any of the 224 public interests mentioned in federal legislation and many others, few, if any, of which are of sufficient pressing importance to override freedom of expression. The whole argument misses the mark.

I would have been happier if the reasons for the majority had not begun with irrelevant criticisms of the course of the trial and the judge's charge, and had not become enmeshed in a lengthy discussion of fact versus opinion. The writer conveyed the impression that she thought that the occurrence of the Holocaust was a subject of debate. I find that proposition incomprehensible. In any event, it would have been better to admit for the purpose of the argument that the Holocaust had occurred and that the assertion published by Zundel, that it was a fiction created by the Jews of the world to extort vast sums of money from the Federal Republic of Germany was false, to Zundel's knowledge. The majority's reasons would not have been affected by that assumption, since it was part of the argument that some lies are protected by s. 2(b).

Both the majority and the minority lost their way for a while in tracing the derivation of offences of false news from the *Statute of Westminster* of 1275. The precursor of s. 181 in the Canadian *Criminal Code* of 1892 was defined in terms different from those of any predecessor. It must be interpreted on its own terms.

These remarks aside, the reasons of the majority constitute a masterly refutation of all efforts to justify s. 181 under all accepted criteria In particular, any effort to limit freedom of expression to true statements or reasoned debate must be rejected, unless some clearly defined objective of sufficient and pressing importance justifying infringement on the *Charter* freedom is stated. If that requirement is met, the other criteria must be examined. Otherwise, the inquiry must stop.

If an offence designed to protect interests protected by the *Charter* is enacted, to implement the interpretation of "public interest" by the minority, we must ask why the remedies provided for by s. 24(1) of the *Charter*, do not provide adequate protection for those suffering from infringement on their *Charter* rights or freedoms by publication of harmful falsehoods.

A further question that must be asked in any event, is whether the hate propaganda offences and sedition adequately cover the field of justifiable restriction on freedom of expression in this context. The reasons of the minority in this case draw heavily on incitement of hatred, although asserting a need for broader coverage. It is not clear that Zundel would have been convicted under s. 319(2) of the Code, but he might have been. A broader restriction enforced by criminal sanctions would appear not to be justified.

In my comment on Zundel's first trial, 44 C.R. (3d) 334, at pp. 343-349, I suggested that the sanctions of the criminal law are not appropriate means of protecting members of threatened minority groups from harmful publications. I invited consideration of the remedy of an injunction to prevent publication of a group libel in a restrictively defined situation, modelled after s. 19(1) of the Manitoba *Defamation Act*, R.S.M. 1987, c. D20, C.C.S.M., c. D20. The prosecution and conviction of Zundel have enabled him to parade himself in public as a martyr, and have gained enormous publicity for his publications. The public impact of an application for an injunction would stir up less undeserved sympathy for him.

H.R.S. Ryan
Faculty of Law
Queen's University
Kingston, Ontario

4.3.8 *Canadian Human Rights Act*, R.S.C. 1985, c. H-6

13. (1) It is a discriminatory practice for a person or a group of persons acting in concert to communicate telephonically or to cause to be so communicated, repeatedly, in whole or in part by means of the facilities of a telecommunication undertaking within the legislative authority of Parliament, any matter that is likely to expose a person or persons to hatred or contempt by reason of the fact that that person or those persons are identifiable on the basis of a prohibited ground of discrimination.

(2) Subsection (1) does not apply in respect of any matter that is communicated in whole or in part by means of the facilities of a broadcasting undertaking.

(3) For the purposes of this section, no owner or operator of a telecommunication undertaking communicates or causes to be communicated any matter described in subsection (1) by reason, only that the facilities of a telecommunication undertaking owned or operated by that person are used by other persons for the transmission of such matter.

4.3.8.1 J.P. Boyer, *Political Rights: The Legal Framework of Elections in Canada* (Toronto: Butterworth, 1981), pp. 308-309

These lessons appear to have been learned by governments and courts which have been called on to deal with the Western Guard Party in Canada. The Western Guard is a neo-fascist political organization with very few members but which, through its occasional public rallies and its taped telephone messages, made an impact on the public. Instead of seeking a law to make the Western Guard an unlawful organization generally, specific charges were brought against the leader and the party for identifiable breaches of the existing and adequate law. Thus, John Ross Taylor and the Western Guard Party were taken to court by the Canadian Human Rights Commission, on the grounds that the Party's telephone messages in Toronto in 1979 were violations of s.13(1) of the *Canadian Human Rights Act*.

Taylor and the Western Guard were brought before the Federal Court of Canada for having disobeyed the order of the Canadian Human Rights Commission to cease their discriminatory practice of using the telephone to communicate repeatedly tape-recorded messages. The order, dated July 20, 1979, was entered in the judgment book of the Federal Court of Canada, and was founded on the provisions of s.13(1) of the *Canadian Human Rights Act*.

The section makes it a "discriminatory practice" for a person or group of persons acting in concert to communicate telephonicly or to cause to be communicated, repeatedly, any matter that is likely to expose a person or persons to hatred or contempt "by reason of the fact that that person or those persons are identifiable on the basis of a prohibited ground of discrimination". The basis for the order was that a Human Rights Tribunal, appointed by the Commission to inquire into complaints against the recorded telephone messages of the Western Guard, had looked at transcriptions of the telephone messages and found that they exposed persons to hatred or contempt merely on the basis that those persons were Jewish. It ordered the respondents to cease this discriminatory practice.

The Federal Court observed that the Canadian Human Rights Commission was a relatively new institution created by Parliament to extend the present laws in Canada that proscribe discrimination and that protect the privacy of individuals, and that its mandate is strong and significant. "It is therefore very important, at this early stage", stated the Court, "that its mission be taken seriously by all, including would-be merchants of racial discrimination."

The Court found that John Ross Taylor had shown no intention to obey the Commission's order and no repentance for his violations of the law, and sentenced him to one year imprisonment, although the sentence was suspended "as long as he, or the Western Guard Party of which he is the Leader, do not use telephone communications for the dissemination of hate messages, or any messages the subject matter of which has been dealt with in the judgment of the Human Rights Tribunal". The Western Guard Party itself was fined $5,000, a sentence which was also suspended and would only take effect if the order of the Commission was further disobeyed. The order was disobeyed, and in June 1980 Mr. Justice Alan Walsh of the Federal Court of Canada ordered Taylor imprisoned and the Party fined. The appeal by Taylor against this order was dismissed.

4.3.8.2 *Canada (Human Rights Commission) v. Taylor*, [1990] 3 S.C.R. 892 (S.C.C.)

Upon his release, Mr. Taylor and the Western Guard Party resumed the telephone message service, and on May 12,1983, the Human Rights Commission filed a second application with the Federal Court. This application alleged that the appellants had breached the order of the Tribunal by taping four messages between the dates of June 22, 1982, and April 20,1983, and again sought an order of committal against Mr. Taylor and the Party. Since the first order of committal, however, the *Charter* had come into effect, and the appellants thus relied on the *Charter* in filing a notice of motion challenging the validity of s. 13(1) of the *Canadian Human Rights Act* as contrary to the freedom of expression.

Jerome, A.C.J. of the Federal Court, Trial Division dealt with both the Commission's applications for committal and the appellants' attempt to have s. 13(1) struck down as unconstitutional. On August 15,1984, he made the committal order sought by the Commission and gave oral reasons dismissing the appellant's motion as to the constitutionality of s. 13(1). Written reasons on the *Charter* issue were released on December 20, 1984: [1984], 6 C.H.R.R.D/2595.

The appellants sought to overturn the decision of Jerome, A.C.J. in the Federal Court of Appeal, but their appeal was dismissed by reasons dated April 22, 1987: [1987] 3 F.C. 593. It is from the ruling of the Federal Court of Appeal that they now appeal to this Court.

DICKSON, C.J.: Beginning with the constitutional issues raised by this appeal, the pivotal challenge is to s. 13(1), for a ruling that the section is unconstitutional will necessarily render invalid any order made to cease and desist telephonic communications. I will thus look first to the question of s. 13(1)'s validity under s. 2(b) of the *Charter*, an inquiry that can be divided into two parts: i) does the impugned provision infringe the constitutional guarantee of free expression; and ii) if so, is it nonetheless justified as a reasonable limit in a free and democratic society under s. 1?

The initial step in determining whether s. 13(1) violates the *Charter* is to decide whether the sphere of the freedom entrenched in s. 2(b) extends to telephone communications likely to expose persons to hatred or contempt by reason of identification on the basis of race or religion. According to *Attorney General of Quebec v. Irwin Toy Ltd.*, [1989] 1 S.C.R. 927, an activity that conveys or attempts to convey a meaning is generally considered to have expressive content within the meaning of s. 2(b). The s. 2(b) guarantee is infringed if it can be shown that either: i) the purpose of the impugned government regulation is to restrict expressive activity; or ii) the regulation has such an effect and the activity in question supports the principles and values upon which the freedom of expression is based.

Applying the *Irwin Toy* approach to the facts of this appeal, I have no doubt that the activity described by s. 13(1) is protected by s. 2(b) of the Charter. Indeed, the point is conceded by the respondent Commission. To begin with, it is serf-evident that this activity conveys or attempts to convey a meaning, the medium in issue to my mind being susceptible to no other use. Indeed, I find it impossible to conceive of an instance where the "telephonic communication of matter" (to paraphrase the language of s. 13(1)) could not be said to involve a conveyance of meaning. The inescapable conclusion is that the activity affected by s. 13(1) constitutes "expression" as the term is envisioned by s. 2(b).

As for the *Irwin Toy* requirement that the purpose or effect of the impugned regulatory measure be to restrict expressive activity, it is clear that Parliament's aim in passing s. 13(1) is to constrain expression communicated by telephone, for the section operates to prohibit directly messages likely to expose certain persons or groups of persons to hatred or contempt. The desire of the government in enacting s. 13(1) being to restrict expression by singling out for censure particular conveyances of meaning, the second requirement of *Irwin Toy* is met, necessarily leading to the conclusion that s. 2(b) is infringed.

Though having decided that the freedom of expression is breached by s. 13(1), before moving on to the s. 1 analysis I should make brief reference to an argument emanating from several of the interveners in support of excluding hate propaganda entirely from the scope of s. 2(b). This argument posits that the expression prohibited by the section is the very antithesis of the values supporting the freedom of expression guarantee and therefore is not deserving of protection under s. 2(b). It should be manifest from my comments in *Keegstra*, however, that I cannot accept this argument. The approach taken in *Irwin Toy* depends upon a large and liberal interpretation of the s. 2(b) freedom, and the gravamen of this approach is the refusal to exclude certain expression because of content. As Lamer J. said in *Reference re ss. 193 and 195.1(1)(c) of the Criminal Code (Man.)*, [1990] I S.C.R. 1123, on this point speaking for the entire Court, "s. 2(b) of the *Charter* protects all content of expression irrespective of the meaning or message sought to be conveyed" (p. 1181). Aside from those instances where only the effect (as opposed to the purpose) of government regulation impinges upon the conveyance of meaning, the more refined and searching analysis of the restricted expression is better done in the context of s.1.

It is also suggested by certain interveners, however, that despite the reluctance of the Court to enter into a discussion of content in defining the scope of s. 2(b), *Irwin Toy* excludes violence and threats of violence from the ambit of the freedom of expression guarantee. As the communications prohibited by s. 13(1) are said to be analogous to these excluded forms of communication, we are urged to place them outside the sphere of protected expression. For the reasons I gave in *Keegstra*, however, the exception suggested in *Irwin Toy* speaks only of physical forms of violence, and extends neither to analogous types of expression nor to mere threats of violence. As the messages dealt with by s. 13(1) do not involve the direct application of physical violence, I cannot find that they fall within any exception that might exist under *Irwin Toy*. It is this purpose — the promotion of equal opportunity unhindered by discriminatory practices based on, *inter alia*, race or religion — that informs the objective of s . 13(1). In denoting the activity described in s. 13(1) as a discriminatory practice, Parliament has indicated that it views repeated telephonic communications likely to expose individuals or groups to hatred or contempt by reason of their being identifiable on the basis of certain characteristics as contrary to the furtherance of equality.

In seeking to prevent the harms caused by hate propaganda, the objective behind s. 13(1) is obviously one of pressing and substantial importance sufficient to warrant some limitation upon the freedom of expression. It is worth stressing, however, the heightened importance attached to this objective by reason of international human rights instruments to which Canada is a party and ss. 15 and 27 of the *Charter*.

That the values of equality and multiculturalism are enshrined in ss. 15 and 27 of the *Charter* further magnify the weightiness of Parliament's objective in enacting s. 13(1). These *Charter* provisions indicate that the guiding principles in undertaking the s. 1 inquiry include respect and concern for the dignity and equality of the individual and a recognition that one's concept of self may in large part be a function of membership in a particular cultural group. As the harm flowing from hate propaganda works in opposition to these linchpin Charter principles, the importance of taking steps to limit its pernicious effects becomes manifest.

As I have stated above, s. 13(1) of the *Canadian Human Rights Act* promotes the ends sought by Parliament, and consequently evinces a rational connection to those ends. This conclusion does not settle the matter of proportionality, however, for a legislative measure may go some way towards securing a pressing and substantial objective yet do so in a manner that limits a *Charter* right or freedom requires a court to ensure that a challenged measure minimally impairs the right or freedom at stake, and to my mind the criticisms levelled at s. 13(1) by the CCLA are best addressed at this point in the proportionality inquiry. I therefore direct my attention to the question of minimal impairment.

I find it helpful to address the question of whether s. 13(1) minimally impairs the freedom of expression by examining in turn the arguments marshalled by the appellants and the CCLA in support of striking down the section. One of the strongest of these arguments is the complaint that the phrase "hatred or contempt" used in s. 13(1) is overbroad and excessively vague. Specifically, it is said that the wide range of meanings available for both "hatred" and "contempt" extend the scope of the section to cover expression not causing the harm which Parliament seeks to prevent. Additionally, the appellants contend that the process of determining whether a particular communication is likely to expose persons to "hatred or contempt" is necessarily subjective, leaving open the possibility that in deciding whether a complaint is well-founded the Tribunal will fall into the error of censuring expression simply because it is felt to be offensive.

When considering the scope of the phrase "hatred or contempt," it is worthwhile mentioning that the nature of human rights legislation militates against an unduly narrow reading of s. 13(1). As was stated by Lamer J. in *Insurance Corp. of British Columbia v. Heerspink*, [1982] 2 S.C.R. 145, at p. 158, a human rights code "is not to be treated as another ordinary law of general application. It should be recognized for what it is: a fundamental law." I therefore do not wish to transgress the well-established principle that the rights enumerated in such a code should be given their full recognition and effect through a fair, large and liberal interpretation. At the same time, however, the purposive definition to be given a human rights code cannot extend so far as to permit the limitation of a *Charter* right or freedom not otherwise justified under s. 1.

In my view, there is no conflict between providing a meaningful interpretation of s. 13(1) and protecting the s. 2(b) freedom of expression, so long as the interpretation of the words "hatred" and "contempt" is fully informed by an awareness that Parliament's objective is to protect the equality and dignity of all individuals by reducing the incidence of harm-causing expression.

To the extent that the section may impose a slightly broader limit upon freedom of expression than does s. 319(2) of the *Criminal Code* I am of the view that the conciliatory bent of a human rights statute renders such a limit more acceptable than would be the case with a criminal provision.

In sum, the language employed in s.13(1) of the *Canadian Human Rights Act* extends only to that expression giving rise to the evil sought to be eradicated and provides a standard of conduct sufficiently precise to prevent the unacceptable chilling of expressive activity. Moreover, as long as the Human Rights Tribunal continues to be well aware of the purpose of s. 13(1) and pays heed to the ardent and extreme nature of feeling described in the phrase "hatred or contempt," there is little danger that subjective opinion as to offensiveness will supplant the proper meaning of the section.

While words in s. 13(1) such as "hatred" and "contempt" can be read consistently with both the intent of Parliament to eradicate hate propaganda and a minimal impairment of s. 2(b) of the *Charter* the appellants argue that no sympathetic interpretation can remedy the overbreadth created by reason of the section's lack of an intent requirement. The focus of s. 13(1) is solely upon likely effects, it being irrelevant whether an individual wishes to expose persons to hatred or contempt on the basis of their race or religion. This inconsequentiality of intent is said to impinge seriously and unnecessarily upon the freedom of expression, and indeed in my reasons in *Keegstra* particular emphasis is placed upon the stringent intent requirement in savings 319(2) of the *Criminal Code* under s. 1 of the *Charter*. The argument of the CCLA referred to above in discussion of "rational connection" is thus revisited, the gist of this intervener's submission being that individuals oblivious to the consequences of their communications, or even intending to reduce the incidence of discrimination, may be caught by s. 13(1).

The preoccupation with effects, and not with intent, is readily explicable when one considers that systemic discrimination is much more widespread in our society than is intentional discrimination.

The chill placed on open expression in such a context will ordinarily be less severe than that occasioned where criminal legislation is involved, for attached to a criminal conviction is a significant degree of stigma and punishment, whereas the extent of opprobrium connected with the finding of discrimination is much diminished and the aim of remedial measures is more to compensate and protect the victim.

In sum, it is my opinion that the absence of an intent component in s. 13(1) raises no problem of minimal impairment when one considers that the objective of the section requires an emphasis on discriminatory effects. Moreover, and this is where I am perhaps jumping ahead to the "effects" component of the proportionality test, the purpose and impact of human rights codes is to prevent discriminatory effects rather than to stigmatize and punish those who discriminate. Consequently, in this context the absence of intent in s. 13(1) does not impinge so deleteriously on the s. 2(b) freedom of expression so as to make intolerable the challenged provision's existence in a free and democratic society.

It is said in response by the appellants, however, that a finding of discrimination may affect an individual very severely indeed, an excellent case in point being the one-year term of imprisonment imposed on Mr. Taylor in the Federal Court, Trial Division. While I would have difficulty defending human rights provisions from a s. 2(b) attack if they exposed a discriminator to imprisonment despite a lack of intent, it must be remembered that Mr. Taylor's jail sentence was the result of a contempt order.

Although I have found the absence of an intent requirement in s.13(1) to be constitutionally acceptable, the section evinces yet another feature which is said to give it a fatally broad scope. In contrast to s. 319(2) of the Criminal Code. s. 13(1) provides no defences to the discriminatory practice it describes, and most especially does not contain an exemption for truthful statements. Accepting that the value of truth in all facets of life, including the political, is central to the s. 2(b) guarantee, the question becomes whether a restriction on freedom of expression is excessive where it operates to suppress statements that are either truthful or perceived to be truthful.

In *Keegstra*, I dealt in considerable detail with hate propaganda and the defence of truth, though in relation to the criminal offence of willfully promoting hatred against an identifiable group. It was not strictly necessary in that appeal to decide whether or not this defence was essential to the constitutional validity of the impugned criminal provision, but I nevertheless offered an opinion of the matter. stating (at pp. 9091):

> The way in which I have defined the s. 319(2) offence, in the context of the objective sought by society and the value of the prohibited expression, gives me some doubt as to whether the *Charter* mandates that truthful statements communicated *with an intention to promote hatred* need to be excepted from criminal condemnation. Truth may be used for widely disparate ends, and I find it difficult to accept that circumstances exist where factually accurate statements can be used for no other purpose than to stir up hatred against a racial or religious group. It would seem to follow that there is no reason why the individual who intentionally employs such statements to achieve harmful ends must *under the Charter* be protected from criminal censure (Emphasis in original).

For the reasons given in the above quotation, I am of the view that the *Charter* does not mandate an exception for truthful statements in the context of s. 13(1) of the *Canadian Human Rights Act*.

As the preceding discussion shows, the freedom of expression is not unnecessarily impaired by s. 13(1) of the *Canadian Human Rights Act*. The terms of the section, in particular the phrase "hatred or contempt," are sufficiently precise and narrow to limit its impact to those expressive activities that are repugnant to Parliament's objective of promoting equality in society. That no special provision exists to emphasize the importance of minimally impairing the freedom of expression does not create in s. 13(1) an overly wide or loose scope, for both its purpose and the common law's traditional desire to protect expressive activity permit an interpretation solicitous of this important freedom.

Though it is true that the absence of an intent requirement under s. 13(1) may take the section wider in scope than the criminal provision upheld in *Keegstra*, this particular distinction is made necessary by the important objective of the *Canadian Human Rights* Act of eradicating systemic discrimination. Moreover, intent is far from irrelevant when imposing incarceration sanctions on an individual by way of a contempt order, subjective awareness of the likely effect of one's messages being a necessary precondition for the issuance of such an order by the Federal Court. A similar point can be made regarding the lack of defences offered under the Act, though as I have noted it is quite conceivable that the full panoply of defences is not constitutionally required in even a criminal provision. Finally, by focusing on "repeated" telephonic messages, s. 13(1) directs its attention to public, larger-scale schemes for the dissemination of hate propaganda, the very type of phone use that most threatens the admirable aim underlying the *Canadian Human Rights Act*.

4.3.9 Television Regulations S.O.R. 87-49

5. (1) A licensee shall not broadcast;
 (*a*) anything in contravention of the law;
 (*b*) any abusive comment or abusive pictorial representation that, when taken in context, tends or is likely to expose an individual or a group or class of individuals to hatred or contempt on the basis of race, national or ethnic origin, colour religion, sex, age or mental or physical disability;
 (*c*) any obscene or profane language or pictorial representation; or
 (*d*) any false or misleading news.

4.3.9.1 *Regina v. Buffalo Broadcasting Co. Ltd.* (1977), 36 C.P.R. (2d) 170 (Sask. M.Ct.)

BENCE, J.M.C.: — The defendant company is charged that on or about November 18, 1976, at Regina, in the Province of Saskatchewan, it did broadcast an abusive comment on a race contrary to s.29(1) of the *Broadcasting Act*, R.S.C. 1970, c.B-11, and the Regulations thereto. To this charge a plea of not guilty was entered and on the day fixed for trial counsel for the defendant company made a preliminary objection to the wording of the charge. As s.732(1) of the *Criminal Code* provides that such objection can only be made with leave once a plea has been entered that leave was granted: there being no objection on the part of the prosecutor. Mr. Gerein pointed out that there were no particulars as to the abusive comment, as to what race and as to the Regulation offended. Mr. Merchant then specified the following particulars:

> Between 9:05 a.m. on the date alleged in a poem and comments on a poem about the Pakistani race contrary to Regulation 5(1)(b).

The trial proceeded on the basis that the charge contained these particulars.

Defence counsel admitted that the letters CKRM constituted the call sign of Buffalo Broadcasting Company Ltd. There was testimony from a radio monitor analyst with the Canadian Radio-Television Commission that the Commission received a letter of complaint from a citizen living in Saskatchewan with respect to the broadcast in question and CKRM was required to send to the Commission an air check of all programming broadcast on November 18th from 9:00 a.m. to 12:00 noon. CKRM sent a cassette tape which was received by this witness and it was played in Court for the period mentioned in the charge. A typewritten transcript of that portion was entered in evidence. Mr. Gerein agreed that the tape, as played, was accurate. The citizen who made the complaint was called and testified that the tape played in Court was verbatim as he recalled the incident. No defence evidence was adduced and this constituted the evidence except for the filing of some documents including a certified true copy of the certificate of incorporation of the defendant company and of the licence granted to the defendant on June 13, 1975, for the call sign CKRM.

The portion of the broadcast giving rise to this was as follows:

ANNOUNCER #1: I don't know if I should read this poem or not. See what you think of the first verse of it.

ANNOUNCER #2: I'll let you know if it s offensive or not.

ANNOUNCER #1: I come to Canada poor and broke, Get on bus, see Manpower bloke, Kind man treat me really swell there Send me down to see the Welfare, Welfare say: come down no more We send the cash out to your door Norman Levy make you wealthy Medical Plan will make you healthy.
How's that sound?

ANNOUNCER #2: I see that yeah. I'll go with that.

ANNOUNCER #1: Six months on dole get plenty money Thanks to working man, real dummy Write to friends in Pakistan Tell them to come as fast as can They all come in rags and turbans I buy big house in suburbans They come with me. we live together Only one thing bad — the weather Fourteen families living in, Neighbours' patience wearing thin. Finally whites must move away I buy their house too, I say: Find more Pakis, house I rent More in garden, live in tent.
Is that good?

ANNOUNCER #2: Remember friends, smoke a pack a day.

ANNOUNCER #1: Send for family, they all trash They all draw more welfare cash Everything is going good Soon we own the neighbourhood Now on quiet summer nights Go to temple, watch the fights. We have hobby, it called breeding Baby bonus keep us feeding.

	How we doing so far?
ANNOUNCER #2:	Pretty good. (unintelligible)
ANNOUNCER #1:	Two years later, big bank roll Still go to Manpower, still draw dole Kids need dentist, wife needs pills We get free, we got no bills White man good, he pay all year To keep the welfare running here Bless all white men, big and small For paying tax to keep us all.
	(Laughter) This is good.
ANNOUNCER #2:	Did you write this?
ANNOUNCER #1:	We thank Canada, damn good place Too damn good for white man race If they don't like coloured man, Plenty room, back in Pakistan.
	(Laughter) That's not all.
ANNOUNCER #2:	Oh, you're kidding.
ANNOUNCER #1:	That's it yeah.
ANNOUNCER #1:	That's good.
ANNOUNCER #2:	Did you write that? Or is it . . .
ANNOUNCER #1:	No . . . Canada damn good place Too darn good for white man race If they no like colored man . . .
ANNOUNCER #2:	Drive a cab in Pakistan.
ANNOUNCER #1:	Hey, that's cute. Do you like that?
ANNOUNCER #2:	That's good . . . if Mary wrote that . . .
ANNOUNCER #1:	I don't know if she wrote it or not but . . .
ANNOUNCER #2:	Certainly is funny.
ANNOUNCER #1:	That's good. Good morning.
LADY CALLER:	Good morning.
ANNOUNCER #1:	How are ya?
LADY CALLER:	Pretty good.
ANNOUNCER #1:	That's good. What's your name?
LADY CALLER:	Carol Campbell.
ANNOUNCER #1:	Carol Campbell.
LADY CALLER:	Yeah.
ANNOUNCER #2:	Carol the Barrel, they call her.
LADY CALLER:	(laughs) Thanks.
ANNOUNCER #1:	Did you hear the poem, Carol?
LADY CALLER:	Yes, I did. I thought that was really good.

ANNOUNCER #1:   Kind of funny, isn't it, eh?
LADY CALLER: Uh, huh, that's for sure.

The Broadcasting Act provides:

Broadcasting Policy for Canada

3. It is hereby declared that
  (*a*) broadcasting undertakings in Canada make use of radio frequencies that are public property and such undertakings constitute a single system, herein referred to as the Canadian broadcasting system, comprising public and private elements.
  (*b*) the Canadian broadcasting system should be effectively owned and controlled by Canadians so as to safeguard, enrich and strengthen the cultural, political, social and economic fabric of Canada:
  (*c*) all persons licensed to carry on broadcasting undertakings have a responsibility for programs they broadcast but the right to freedom of expression and the right of persons to receive programs, subject only to generally applicable statutes and regulations, is unquestioned:
  (*d*) the programming provided by the Canadian broadcasting system should be varied and comprehensive and should provide reasonable, balanced opportunity for the expression of differing views on matters of public concern, and the programming provided by each broadcaster should be of high standard, using predominantly Canadian creative and other resources;
  (*e*) all Canadians are entitled to broadcasting service in English and French as public funds become available;
  (*f*) there should be provided, through a corporation established by Parliament for the purpose, a national broadcasting service that is predominantly Canadian in content and character;
  (*g*) the national broadcasting service should
    (i) be a balanced service of information, enlightenment and entertainment for people of different ages, interests and tastes covering the whole range of programming in fair proportion,
    (ii) be extended to all parts of Canada. as public funds become available,
    (iii) be in English and French, serving the special needs of geographic regions, and actively contributing to the flow and exchange of cultural and regional information and entertainment, and
    (iv) contribute to the development of national unity and provide for a continuing expression of Canadian identity:
  (*h*) where any conflict arises between the objectives of the national broadcasting service and the interests of the private element of the Canadian broadcasting system, it shall be resolved in the public interest but paramount consideration shall be given to the objectives of the national broadcasting service
  (*i*) facilities should be provided within the Canadian broadcasting system for educational broadcasting; and
  (*j*) the regulation and supervision of the Canadian broadcasting system should be flexible and readily adaptable to scientific and technical advances;

and that the objectives of the broadcasting policy for Canada enunciated in this section can best be achieved by providing for the regulation and supervision of the Canadian broadcasting system by a single independent public authority.

Objects of the Commission

15. Subject to this Act and the *Radio Act* and any directions to the Commission issued from time to time by the Governor in Council under the authority of this Act, the Commission shall regulate and supervise all aspects of the Canadian Broadcasting system with a view to plementing the broadcasting policy enunciated in section 3 of this Act.

Powers of the Commission

16. (1) In furtherance of its objects, the Commission. on the recommendation of the Executive Committee, may

(*a*) prescribe classes of broadcasting licences;

(*b*) make regulations applicable to all persons holding broadcasting licences, or to all persons holding broadcasting licences of one or more classes.

(i) respecting standards of programs, and the allocation of broadcasting time for the purpose of giving effect to paragraph 3(d),

(ii) respecting the character of advertising and the amount of time that may be devoted to advertising,

(iii) respecting the proportion of time that may be devoted to the broadcasting of programs, advertisements or announcements of a partisan political character and the assignment of such time on an equitable basis to political parties and candidates.

(iv) respecting the use of dramatization in programs, advertisements or announcements of a partisan political character,

(v) respecting the broadcasting times to be reserved for network programs by any broadcasting station operated as pan of a network,

(vi) prescribing the conditions for the operation of broadcasting stations as part of a network and the conditions for the broadcasting of network programs,

(vii) with the approval of the Treasury Board, fixing the schedules of fees to be paid by licensees and providing for the payment thereof,

(viii) requiring licensees to submit to the Commission such information regarding their programs and financial affairs or otherwise relating to the conduct and management of their affairs as the regulations may specify, and

(ix) respecting such other matters as it deems necessary for the furtherance of its objects; and

(*c*) subject to this Part, revoke any broadcasting licence other than a broadcasting licence issued to the Corporation.

(2) A copy of each regulation or amendment to a regulation that the Commission proposes to make under this section shall be published in the *Canada Gazette* and a reasonable opportunity shall be afforded to licensees and other interested persons to make representations with respect thereto.

29. (1) Every licensee who violates the provisions of any regulation applicable to him made under this Part is guilty of an offence and is liable on summary conviction to a fine not exceeding twenty-five thousand dollars for a first offence and not exceeding fifty thousand dollars for each subsequent offence.

(2) Every licensee who violates the provisions of section 28 is guilty of an offence and is liable on summary conviction to a fine not exceeding five thousand dollars.

(3) Every person who carries on a broadcasting undertaking without a valid and subsisting broadcasting licence therefor, or who, being the holder of a broadcasting licence, operates a broadcasting undertaking as part of a network other than in accordance with the conditions of such licence, is guilty of an offence and is liable on summary conviction to a fine not exceeding one thousand dollars for each day that the offence continues.

The *Radio (A.M.) Broadcasting Regulations*, SOR164-49, provide:

Broadcasting Generally

5. (1) No station or network operator shall broadcast
   (*a*) anything contrary to law;
   (*b*) any abusive comment on any race or religion;
   (*c*) any obscene, indecent or profane language:
   (*d*) any false or misleading news;
   (*e*) any program on the subject of birth control unless that program is presented in a manner appropriate to the medium of broadcasting;
   (*f*) any program on the subject of venereal diseases unless that program is presented in a manner appropriate to the medium of broadcasting;
   (*g*) any advertising content in the body of a news broadcast and for the purpose of this section, a summary is deemed to be a part of the body of the broadcast;
   (*h*) except with the consent in writing of a representative of the Commission, any appeal for donations or subscriptions in money or kind on behalf of any person or organization other than
      (i) a church or religious body permanently established in Canada and serving the area covered by the station,
      (ii) a recognized charitable institution or organization,
      (iii) a university, or
      (iv) a musical or artistic organization whose principal aim or object is not that of monetary gain;
   (*i*) any program involving a lottery or similar scheme that is prohibited by the *Criminal Code*: [rep. & sub. SOR70-286]
   (*j*) any program reconstructing or simulating the direct description of any sport or other event through a description prepared from wired reports or other indirect source of information unless assurance has been given in writing to a representative of the Commission that source material will not be obtained directly or indirectly from a broadcast of the event, and
      (i) a reconstructed broadcast shall not be broadcast until after the conclusion of the event if an actuality broadcast of the event is available in the area,
      (ii) a reconstructed broadcast shall be identified at the beginning and end thereof as having been so prepared, and if it is more than fifteen minutes in length, it shall be identified at the end of each fifteen-minute period, and

(iii) the form of such announcement shall be:
"This program is a reconstructed broadcast of .... (name of event) ....",
"This program has been a reconstructed broadcast of .... (name of event) ....,
or some suitable variation of these forms; or [am. SOR65-519, s.1(1)]

(k) any telephone interview or Conversation, or any part thereof, with any person unless

(i) the person's oral or written consent to the interview or conversation being broadcast was obtained prior to such broadcast, or

(ii) the person telephoned the station for the purpose of participating in a broadcast. [rep. & sub. SOR/70-256, s.3]

(1) (a) [Revoked SOR70-256, s.3; effective January 18, 1971]

(2) The value of articles or money to be awarded in any single contest sponsored in whole or in part by or on behalf of the station shall not exceed five thousand dollars, and no station shall broadcast more than one such contest per month.

(3) Subsection (2) does not apply to a contest

(a) in which the value of articles or money to be awarded is one hundred dollars or less; or

(b) which are wholly sponsored by or wholly paid for by any advertiser or group of advertisers.

Mr. Gerein raised several points in his defence of the company. Firstly, he submitted that the word "abusive" is not applicable to this particular type of situation; that to abuse a thing is to misuse it or to take something and use it for a wrong purpose. Secondly, that a comment is a statement about something else; to read off a literary work (and I do not think Mr. Gerein was intending to class this as such) is not comment. He suggested that if a person criticizes something he comments on it. Further, he submitted that the poem in question was not a statement about the Pakistani people in general but about only one person and it was a statement of fact not a comment. He referred to the fact that only one person testified that it was offensive and according to the transcript in evidence one person thought it was good. He pointed out that there was no evidence of a Pakistani finding it abusive. Then he dealt with the matter of proof that a race was involved. He suggested that there was no proof that Pakistani are a race and no judicial notice of that can be taken. He said the United Nations (Charter) does not acknowledge the existence of a race and suggested race is a scientific myth. He argued that the race is Indian and there is nothing in texts or otherwise to suggest that Pakistani make up a race. Mr. Gerein submitted that the CRTC did not have jurisdiction to pass s.5(1)(b); that it exceeds any of the powers given in s.16 of the *Broadcasting Act* and nothing in the Act gives the CRTC the right to censor any particular programme. He cited *National Indian Brotherhood et al. v. Juneau et al. (No. 3)*, [1971] F.C. 498, and *R. v. CKOY Ltd.* (1976), 28 C.P.R. (2d) 1, 70 D.L.R. (3d) 662, 30 C.C.C. (2d) 314 (Ont. C.A.) [reversing 19 C.P.R.

(2d) 1, 25 C.C.C. (2d) 333, 9 O.R. (2d) 549 (Ont. H.C.J.)]. His final point was that s.29 creates the offence for breach of the Regulations. He submitted that there was no evidence that on November 18, 1976, the defendant company was a licensee. He cited *R. v. Empire Hotel Co. Ltd.* (1971), 4 C.C.C. (2d) 97, [1971] 5 W.W.R. 106, where Disbery, J. held that a certificate that the company had been granted a licence for the current year did not prove that on the date in question the hotel was licensed.

On the merits of this charge I would have no hesitation in holding that the broadcasting of this poem was an abusive comment about the Pakistani race and within the mischief aimed at by s. 5(1)(b). I went to a rather old dictionary that I have — Cassells *New English Dictionary* published in 1946. The three words — abuse, comment and race — which Mr. Gerein felt were inappropriate to the present situation — were defined as follows:

> *Abuse* — (verb) to put to an improper use, misuse, to reproach coarsely, to use in an illegitimate sense, to pervert the meaning of, to maltreat, act cruelly to; to violate, to deflower: to deceive.
> (noun) improper treatment or employment; misuse; a corrupt practice or custom insulting or scurrilous language; perversion from the proper meaning; violation.

There seems to me little doubt that the content of this poem was insulting and scurrilous and to use it was to maltreat and act cruelly to another.

> *Comment* — (noun) A remark, a criticism; a note interpreting or illustrating a, work or portion of a work.

I do not think that either of these words — abuse or comment — can be interpreted as narrowly as Mr. Gerein would have me do. In my opinion the poem itself may be described as a comment. In addition, there were clearly comments in the poem.

> *Race* — a group or division of persons, animals or plants sprung from a common stock; a particular ethnical stock (as the Caucasian, mongolian. etc.); a subdivision of this, a tribe, nation or group of people, distinguished by less important differences; a clan, a family, a house; a genus, species, stock, strain or variety, of plants or animals, persisting through several generations; lineage, pedigree, descent; a class of persons or animals differentiated from others by some common characteristic; a peculiar quality, a strong flavour, as of wine; natural disposition.

I did not think that the definition of the words — comment or abuse — would change much over the years but being a bit in doubt as to the word "race" I checked it with a more modern dictionary — the *Shorter Oxford English Dictionary* (1973) and I could find little difference. Again, the word "race" is wider than the interpretation sought by Mr. Gerein and would, on this definition, in my opinion, clearly include the term "Pakistani". In Jowitt's *Dictionary of English Law* under Pakistan the following appears:

> The Indian Independence Act, 1947, set up two independent Dominions in India known respectively as India and Pakistan. Both were independent republics which accepted the Crown as the symbol of the free association of the independent nations who are members of the

Commonwealth. This did not, however, imply allegiance to the Crown or affect the sovereignty of the republic. Pakistan is no longer a member of the Commonwealth. See *Pakistan Act*, 1973: *Pakistan Act* 1974. See Gledhill, *Pakistan*.

Under s. 11 of the *Interpretation Act*, R.S.C. 1970, c.I-23:

11. Every enactment shall be deemed remedial, and shall be given such fair, large and liberal construction and interpretation as best ensures the attainment of its objects.

At the same time, this Regulation being a penal provision must be strictly interpreted and any doubt must be resolved in favour of the accused. These apparently contradictory propositions have to be nicely balanced but I have no hesitation in saying that on common sense interpretation of s.5(1)(b) the defendant company broadcast an abusive comment in the sense of an insulting or scurrilous remark about the Pakistani race. While the poem purports to speak of an individual it is clearly aimed, in my opinion, at all members of the Pakistani race or the Pakistani people generally.

I turn now to the two technical objections raised by Mr. Gerein. First, that there was no proof that the defendant is a licensee and that s.29 makes it an offence for a licensee to broadcast and contravene the Regulations. The situation is very similar to that facing the Crown in *R. v. Empire Hotel Co. Ltd., supra*, cited by Mr. Gerein. There the company was charged that it on June 6, 1970, at Elrose in the Province of Saskatchewan permitted a person under the age of 19 years to be in an outlet contrary to the *Liquor Licensing Act*, R.S.S. 1965, c.383. Section 138(4) [am. 1970, c.8, s.32(13)(d)] thereof reads:

138. (4) No licensee or any employee of a licensee shall suffer or permit a person apparently or to the knowledge of the licensee, or of the employee, under the age of nineteen years to enter, be in or remain in the outlet.

The Crown filed a certificate that declared that the defendant had been licensed under the *Liquor Licensing Act* in March, 1970, and unless sooner cancelled or revoked it would continue to be licensed for a period of one year from the date of issue. Disbery, J., held there was no admissible evidence that the defendant was a licensee on the material date and the conviction was quashed on appeal. I note that the charge in that case did not allege that the defendant was a licensee as is the case here. If it is not alleged then does the Crown have to prove it? No objection was taken to the charge prior to the plea nor was any objection taken on this point when leave was granted to object to the charge on other grounds after the plea of not guilty was entered. In my opinion, the Crown was under no obligation to prove that the defendant company was a licensee. See *R. v. Cote*, judgment dated February 7, 1977 — Supreme Court of Canada [reported 73 D.L.R. (3d) 752, 33 C.C.C. (2d) 353, [1978]1 S.C.R. 8] reversing the Saskatchewan Court of Appeal [reported 21 C.C.C. (2d) 474, [1975] W.W.D. 59] — a decision in which it was held that a charge which omitted an essential ingredient was valid as no objection was taken before the plea. In any event I would hold that there was some evidence before me that the defendant company was licensed

— certainly the defendant company was carrying on the broadcasting business on the date alleged with the knowledge and consent of the CRTC as if it did hold a licence — the Latin phrase — *Omnia praessurnuntur legitime facta donec probetim in contrarium* — all things are presumed to have been legitimately done, until the contrary is proved — would appear to apply and common sense would dictate that I so hold on the basis that it is a reasonable inference from the evidence adduced that the defendant did hold such a licence at the time and it would be unreasonable to permit the defendant to plead as a defence that it might have been committing another offence. The objection that the CRTC did not have the authority to pass s.5(1)(b) presents, in my opinion, a greater problem. In *R. v. CKOY Ltd., supra*, the accused radio station was charged with breach of s.5(1)(k) of the *Radio (A.M.) Broadcasting Regulations of the Broadcasting Act* which prohibits the broadcasting of any telephone interview unless the person interviewed has called the station for the purpose of participating in the broadcast or has consented to the interview being broadcast. At trial the charge was dismissed on the basis that the Regulation was outside the regulatory powers granted by the CRTC. An appeal by the Crown was dismissed but on further appeal to the Court of Appeal of the Province of Ontario the appeal was allowed and the case was remitted to the trial Judge to enter a conviction.

In considering the question of whether or not there was power to make the particular Regulation in that case, Mr. Justice Evans said [at pp. 5-6 C.P.R., p. 667 D.L.R.]:

> I do not conceive it to be the function of the Court to evaluate and balance the competing factors, favourable or unfavourable, which the implementation of the particular Regulation may create; that, in my view, is the responsibility cast upon the Commission. The Court looks at the Regulation in an objective manner and asks whether the Commission in promulgating this Regulation exceeded the statutory authority vested in it. This does not mean that the Commission has unlimited power to pass Regulations. Section 15 provides the restriction, "... the Commission shall *regulate* and *supervise* all aspects of the Canadian broadcasting system with a view to implementing the *broadcasting policy enunciated* in section 3 of this Act" If s.5(1)(k) reasonably falls within s.3 then it is *intra vires* the Commission.
>
> It is obvious from the broad language of the Act that Parliament intended to give to the Commission a wide latitude with respect to the making of Regulations to implement the policies and objects for which the Commission was created.

Both Mr. Justice Evans and Mr. Justice Brooke referred to s. 16(1)(b)(i) of the *Broadcasting Act* and held that that section allows the Commission to regulate "respecting standards of programs ..." while s.3(d) requires that "the programming provided ... should be of high standard ..." and then held that the impugned Regulation is to prohibit an undesirable broadcasting technique, one which does not reflect the high standard of programming which the Commission must by regulation of licensees, endeavour to maintain. Reference was made to freedom of speech and freedom of the press being curtailed but the two Judges held that the Regulation protects the freedom of speech by protecting the privacy of the individual and is consistent with the other freedom. Mr. Justice Brooke added [at p. 10 C.P.R., p. 672 D.L.R.]:

The purpose of the section of the Regulation cannot be attacked on that basis and so long as it is the maintenance of the high standard of broadcasting in accordance with its objects, the Commission has the power to enact it.

The difficulty of this question is apparent in that the Court of Appeal members split two to one and there is now an appeal pending in the Supreme Court of Canada. Mr. Justice Dubin. who dissented, referred to *National Indian Brotherhood et al. v. Juneau et al.* (No. 3). This case was also cited by Mr. Gerein as I have indicated above. The facts of that case were that some time in March, 1970, the CTV Network screened the film entitled "The Taming of the Canadian West" which according to the National Indian Brotherhood and others is blatantly racist, historically inaccurate and slanderous to the Indian race and culture. Various avenues were explored including a request that the CRTC conduct a formal investigation. Eventually this was denied and this ruling came on an application for an order forcing the CRTC to hold and conduct a public inquiry. The application was dismissed by Walsh, J., and he made certain observations with respect to the *Broadcasting Act* which Dubin, J.A., referred to in his dissenting judgment and Mr. Gerein used in his argument. These, in part, were as follows [at p. 12 C.P.R., p. 675 D.L.R.]:

> Reading the Act as a whole and in particular the sections to which I have referred, I find it difficult to conclude that Parliament intended to or did give the Commission the authority to act as a censor of programmes to be broadcast or televised. If this had been intended, surely provision would have been made somewhere in the Act giving the Commission authority to order an individual station or a network, as the case may be, to make changes in a programme deemed by the Commission, after an inquiry, to be offensive or to refrain from broadcasting same. Instead of that, it appears that its only control over the nature of programmes is by use of its power to revoke, suspend or fail to renew the licence of the offending station.

and at p. 13 C.P.R., p. 676 D.L.R.:

> This seems to impose a sort of self-censorship on the individual licensees which is, in practice, not very effective and does not prevent them from producing from time to time programmes which are in poor taste or offensive to a substantial number of viewers. So long as they do not infringe on laws relating to slander, libel or obscenity, they are apparently on safe ground as there is nothing in the Act which gives the CRTC the right to act as censor of the contents of any individual programme.

And at p. 10 C.P.R., p. 673 D.L.R., Dubin, J.A., said:

> I have had the advantage of reading the judgments of my learned brothers, both of whom have concluded that the above-cited Regulation has been validly enacted by the Commission. With deference, I do not agree. It is trite to say that there must be a clear grant of legislative authority before a Commission such as the Canadian Radio-Television Commission like the one in issue here, particularly where a breach of the Regulation is, by the Act, created an offence. [I think something is missing from the statement such as the words "make a Regulation" following the word "Commission".]

And he added [at p. 12 C.P.R., pp. 674-5 D.L.R.]:

> As my brothers have observed, the Regulation in issue purports to strike down an undesirable broadcasting technique. The fact that the object of the Regulation may very well be a laudatory

one is quite irrelevant. The broadcast in issue in this case may have been one of considerable public interest, or may have been one which was quite offensive, but the Regulation in question here would prohibit it, whatever quality it may have, if no consent is obtained to it being broadcast. It is only one step removed to contemplate the Regulation ordering that no such interview could be broadcast without the consent of the Commission itself. It could then equally be said that the Commission was thereby seeking to establish a high standard of programming, but looked at in that way it cannot be anything other than a form of censorship.

As was the case in *R. v. CKOY Ltd.*, the only provisions of s. 16(1)(b) which set out the power of the Commission to make regulations of this nature, are subpara. (i) respecting standards of programmes and subpara. (ix) respecting such other matters as it deems necessary for the furtherance of its objects. One would have thought Parliament would have been more specific if it intended to give the power in question. The whole of subpara. 16(1)(b)(i) must be considered. It reads:

> (i) respecting standards of programs and the allocation of broadcasting time for the purpose of giving effect to paragraph 3(d),

Section 3(d) reads:

> (d) the programming provided by the Canadian broadcasting system should be varied and comprehensive and should provide reasonable, balanced opportunity for the expression of differing views on matters of public concern, and the programming provided by each broadcaster should be of high standard. using predominantly Canadian creative and other resources;

The Commission side-stepped the responsibility in the *National Indian Brotherhood* case and I cannot help thinking that Walsh, J., and Dubin, J.A., are correct when they say that there is nothing in the *Broadcasting Act* which gives the CRTC the right to act as censor of the contents of any individual programme. I quote from the judgment of Walsh, J., at pp. 515-6 of the report cited, *supra*:

> Section 3(c) of the Act, under the heading "Broadcasting Policy for Canada" sets forth: 3. It is hereby declared that
>
> . . . . .
>
> (c) all persons licensed to carry on broadcasting undertakings have a responsibility for programs they broadcast but the right to freedom of expression and the right of persons to receive programs, subject only to generally applicable statutes and regulations, is unquestioned;
>
> This seems to impose a sort of self-censorship on the individual licensees which is, in practice, not very effective and does not prevent them from producing from time to time programmes which are in poor taste or offensive to a substantial number of viewers. So long as they do not infringe on laws relating to slander, libel or obscenity, they are apparently on safe ground as there is nothing in the Act which gives the CRTC the right to act as censor of the contents of any individual programme. It is apparent in the manner in which the Commission handled this complaint that it does not intend to act as such. The revocation, suspension or failure to renew a licence is such a serious matter that it is not a course the Commission is likely to adopt save for grave and repeated offences, and it would appear that it is reluctant to use this power as a threat to compel the individual licensees or, in the present case, a broadcasting chain, to alter or withhold a programme with respect to which complaints have been received. The most it was prepared to do in the present case was to attempt to bring the parties together in the hope that they, themselves,

might find a satisfactory solution to their controversy. I therefore find that under the existing law the decision of the Executive Committee that it would not be in the public interest to hold a public hearing was an administrative one which it was entitled to make. It is not for the Court to comment on whether or not the CRTC should be given more powers of control over the subject-matter of programmes broadcast or televised by its licensees as this is a decision which Parliament alone can make but, at present, it is evident that the powers given to it in this field are very limited and ineffective.

In *R. v. CKOY Ltd.* the Court of Appeal of Ontario was dealing with a much different regulatory power. Mr. Justice Evans, however, appears to agree with Walsh, J., and Dubin J.A., with respect to the power of censorship because he said, at p. 6 C.P.R., p. 668 D.L.R., of the report cited above:

> The right of prohibition in s.5(k)(i) is not to be confused with censorship. The Commission does not attempt to censor the content of the conversation or to deny the right of freedom of expression.

Mr. Justice Evans applied this test [at p. 6 C.P.R., p. 667 D.L.R.]: "If s.5(1)(k) reasonably falls within s.3 then it is *intra vires* the Commission." In my view s.5(1)(b) of the Regulations does not reasonably fall within ss.3 and 16 of the Act so that it is *ultra vires* and this prosecution cannot be maintained.

While the programme or portion of it we are concerned with here was in jocular vein and while there have been many races and nationalities that have been made the butt of jokes, in my view, this "poem" went far beyond those we have been accustomed to hearing. But if there is to be this regulatory provision where is the line to be drawn? It is much like trying to draw lines as to what is obscene and what is not and one can visualize the difficulties that would be encountered. If the broadcaster is not prepared to impose a sort of self-censorship as suggested by Mr. Justice Walsh then the CRTC can refuse to renew its licence or appropriate statutory provisions can give it power to do so. The charge is dismissed.

Charge dismissed.

Note: The decision of the Supreme Court of Canada in *CKOY Ltd. v. Her Majesty The Queen*, [1979] 1 S.C.R. 2 casts doubt on this decision.

4.3.10 *Ontario Human Rights Code*, R.S.O. 1990, c. H-19

Part I
Freedom from Discrimination

1. Every person has a right to equal treatment with respect to services, goods and facilities, without discrimination because of race, ancestry, place of origin, colour, ethnic origin, citizenship, creed, sex, sexual orientation, age, marital status, family status or handicap. 1981, c. 53, s. 1; 1986, c. 64 s. 18 (1).

2.— (1) Every person has a right to equal treatment with respect to the occupancy of accommodation, without discrimination because of race, ancestry, place of origin, colour, ethnic origin, citizenship, creed, sex, sexual orientation, age, marital status, family status, handicap or the receipt of public assistance. 1981, c. 53; s. 2 (1); 1986, c. 64, s. 18 (2).

(2) Every person who occupies accommodation has a right to freedom from harassment by the landlord or agent of the landlord or by an occupant of the same building because of race, ancestry, place of origin, colour, ethnic origin, citizenship, creed, age, marital status, family status, handicap or the receipt of public assistance. 1981, c. 53, s. 2 (2).

3. Every person having legal capacity has a right to contract on equal terms without discrimination because of race, ancestry, place of origin, colour, ethnic origin, citizenship, creed, sex, sexual orientation, age, marital status, family status or handicap. 1981, c. 53, s. 3; 1986, c. 64, s. 18 (3).

4.—(1) Every sixteen or seventeen year old person who has withdrawn from parental control has a right to equal treatment with respect to occupancy of and contracting for accommodation without discrimination because the person is less than eighteen years old.

(2) A contract for accommodation entered into by a sixteen or seventeen year old person who has withdrawn from parental control is enforceable against that person as if the person were eighteen years old. 1986, c. 64 s. 18(4).

5.—(1) Every person has a right to equal treatment with respect to employment without discrimination because of race, ancestry place of origin, colour, ethnic origin, citizenship, creed, sex, sexual orientation, age, record of offences, marital status, family status or handicap. 1981, c. 53, s. 4 (1), 1986 c. 64, s. 18 (5).

(2) Every person who is an employee has a right to freedom from harassment in the workplace by the employer or agent of the employer or by another employee because of race, ancestry, place of origin, colour, ethnic origin, citizenship, creed, age, record of offences, marital status, family status or handicap. 1981, c. 53, s. 4 (2).

6. Every person has a right to equal treatment with respect to membership in any trade union, trade or occupational association or self-governing profession without discrimination because of race, ancestry, place of origin, colour, ethnic origin, citizenship creed, sex, sexual orientation, age, marital status, family status or handicap. 1981, c. 53 s. 5; 1986, c. 64, s. 18 (6).

7.—(1) Every person who occupies accommodation has a right to freedom from harassment because of sex by the landlord or agent of the landlord or by an occupant of the same building.

(2) Every person who is an employee has a right to freedom from harassment in the workplace because of sex by his or her employer or agent of the employer or by another employee.

(3) Every person has a right to be free from,
   (*a*) a sexual solicitation or advance made by a person in a position to confer grant or deny a benefit or advancement to the person where the person making the solicitation or advance knows or ought reasonably to know that it is unwelcome; or
   (*b*) a reprisal or a threat of reprisal for the rejection of a sexual solicitation or advance where the reprisal is made or threatened by a person in a position to confer, grant or deny a benefit or advancement to the person. 1981, c. 53, s. 6.

8. Every person has a right to claim and enforce his or her rights under this Act, to institute and participate in proceedings under this Act and to refuse to infringe a right of another person under this Act, without reprisal or threat of reprisal for so doing. 1981, c. 53, s. 7.

9. No person shall infringe or do, directly or indirectly, anything that infringes a right under this Part. 1981, c. 53, s. 8.

13.—(1) A right under Part I is infringed by a person who publishes or displays before the public or causes the publication or display before the public of any notice, sign symbol, emblem, or other similar representation that indicates the intention of the person to infringe a right under Part I or that is intended by the person to incite the infringement of a right under Part I.

(2) Subsection (1) shall not interfere with freedom of expression of opinion. 1981 c. 53, s. 12.

Note: A Manitoba prohibition similar to s.13 has been held not to apply to the editorial content of a newspaper. See *Re Warren and Chapman* (1985), 11 D.L.R. (4th) 474. In Saskatchewan a similar provision has been held to apply to an advertising display outside a commercial establishment. See *Re Iwasyk* (1977), 80 D.L.R. (3d) 1 (Sask. Q. B.).

4.4 Obscenity

4.4.1 *Criminal Code*, R.S.C. 1985, c. C-46

Offences Tending to Corrupt Morals

163. (1) Every one commits an offence who

(*a*) makes, prints, publishes, distributes, circulates, or has in his possession for the purpose of publication, distribution or circulation any obscene written matter, picture, model, phonograph record or other thing whatsoever, or

(*b*) makes, prints, publishes, distributes, sells or has in his possession for the purpose of publication, distribution or circulation, a crime comic.

(2) Every one commits an offence who knowingly, without lawful justification or excuse,

(*a*) sells, exposes to public view or has in his possession for such a purpose any obscene written matter, picture, model, phonograph record or other thing whatsoever,

(*b*) publicly exhibits a disgusting object or an indecent show,

(*c*) offers to sell, advertises, publishes an advertisement of, or has for sale or disposal any means, instructions, medicine, drug or article intended or represented as a method of causing abortion or miscarriage, or

(*d*) advertises or publishes an advertisement of any means, instructions, medicine, drug or article intended or represented as a method for restoring sexual virility or curing venereal diseases or diseases of the generative organs.

(3) No person shall be convicted of an offence under this section if the public good was served by the acts that are alleged to constitute the offence and if the acts alleged did not extend beyond what served the public good.

(4) For the purposes of this section it is a question of law whether an act served the public good and whether there is evidence that the act alleged went beyond what served the public good, but it is a question of fact whether the acts did or did not extend beyond what served the public good.

(5) For the purposes of this section the motives of an accused are irrelevant.

(7) In this section, "crime comic" means a magazine, periodical or book that exclusively or substantially comprises matter depicting pictorially
  (a) the commission of crimes, real or fictitious, or
  (b) events connected with the commission of crimes, real or fictitious, whether occurring before or after the commission of the crime.

(8) For the purposes of this Act, any publication a dominant characteristic of which is the undue exploitation of sex, or of sex and any one or more of the following subjects, namely, crime, horror, cruelty and violence, shall be deemed to be obscene.

164. (1) A judge who is satisfied by information on oath that there are reasonable grounds for believing that any publication or representation, copies of which are kept for sale or distribution in premises within the jurisdiction of the court, is obscene or a crime comic within the meaning of section 163 or is child pornography within the meaning of section 163.1 shall issue a warrant authorizing seizure of the copies.

(2) Within seven days of the issue of the warrant; the judge shall issue a summons to the occupier of the premises requiring him to appear before the court and show cause why the matter seized should not be forfeited to Her Majesty.

(3) The owner and the maker of the matter seized unclear subsection (1) and alleged to be obscene, a crime comic or child pornography, may appear and be represented in the proceedings in order to oppose the making of an order for the forfeiture of the matter.

(4) If the court is satisfied that the publication or representation referred to in subsection (1) is obscene, a crime comic or child pornography, it shall make an order declaring the matter forfeited to Her Majesty in right of the province in which the proceedings take place, for disposal as the Attorney General may direct.

(5) If the court is not satisfied that the publication or representation referred to in subsection (1) is obscene, a crime comic or child pornography, it shall order that the matter be restored to the person from whom it was seized forthwith after the time for final appeal has expired.

(6) An appeal lies from an order made under subsection (4) or (5) by any person who appeared in the proceedings
  (a) on any ground of appeal that involves a question of law alone,
  (b) on any ground of appeal that involves a question of fact alone, or
  (c) on any ground of appeal that involves a question of mixed law and fact,
as if it were an appeal; against conviction or against a judgment or verdict of acquittal, as the case may be, on a question of law alone under Part XXI and sections 673 to 696 apply *mutatis mutandis*.

(7) Where an order has been made under this section by a judge in a province with respect to one or more copies of a publication or representation, no proceedings shall be instituted or continued in that province under section 163 or 163.1 with respect to those or other copies of the same publication or representation without the consent of the Attorney General.

(8) In this section "court" means a county or district court or, in the Province of Quebec, the provincial court, the court of the sessions of the peace, the municipal court of Montreal and the municipal court of Quebec;
  "(*a.1*) in the Provinces of New Brunswick, Manitoba, Alberta and Saskatchewan, the Court of Queen's Bench,"

"crime comic" has the same meaning as it has in section 163

"judge" means a judge of a court.

165. Every one commits an offence who refuses to sell or supply to any other person copies of any publication for the reason only that such other person refuses to purchase or acquire from him copies of any other publication that such other person is apprehensive may be obscene or a crime comic.

166. (1) A proprietor, editor, master printer or publisher commits an offence who prints or publishes

(*a*) in relation to any judicial proceedings any indecent matter or indecent medical, surgical or physiological details, being matter or details that, if published, are calculated to injure public morals;

(*b*) in relation to any judicial proceedings for dissolution of marriage, nullity of marriage, judicial separation or restitution of conjugal rights, any particulars other than

(i) the names, addresses and occupations of the parties and witnesses,

(ii) a concise statement of the charges, defences and counter-charges in support of which evidence has been given,

(iii) submissions on a point of law arising in the course of the proceedings, and the decision of the court in connection therewith, and

(iv) the summing up of the judge, the finding of the jury and the judgment of the court and the observations that are made by the judge in giving judgment.

(2) Nothing in paragraph (1)(b) affects the operation of paragraph (1)(a).

(3) No proceedings for an offence under this section shall be commenced without the consent of the Attorney General.

(4) This section does not apply to a person who

(*a*) prints or publishes any matter for use in connection with any judicial proceedings or communicates it to persons who are concerned in the proceedings;

(*b*) prints or publishes a notice or report pursuant to directions of a court; or

(*c*) prints or publishes any matter

(i) in a volume or part of a *bona fide* series of law reports that does not form part of any other publication and consists solely of reports of proceedings in courts of law, or

(ii) in a publication of a technical character that is *bona fide* intended for circulation among members of the legal or medical professions.

167. (1) Every one commits an offence who, being the lessee, manager, agent.or person in charge of a theatre, presents or gives or allows to be presented or given therein an immoral, indecent or obscene performance, entertainment or representation.

(2) Every one commits an offence who takes part or appears as an actor, performer, or assistant in any capacity. in an immoral, indecent or obscene performance, entertainment or representation in a theatre.

168. Every one commits an offence who makes use of the mails for the purpose of transmitting or delivering anything that is obscene, indecent, immoral or scurrilous, but this section does not apply to a person who makes use of the mails for the purpose of transmitting or delivering anything mentioned in subsection 166(4).

169. Every one who commits an offence under section 163, 165, 166, 167 or 168 is guilty of
   (*a*) an indictable offence and is liable to imprisonment for two years, or
   (*b*) an offence punishable on summary conviction.

For many years these provisions have been regarded as unsatisfactory. Various attempts, largely unsuccessful, have been made to reform them.

4.4.2 Law Reform Commission of Canada, *Limits of Criminal Law; Obscenity: A Test Case, Working Paper* 10 (Ottawa: Information Canada, 1975), pp. 39-49

... In practical terms, however, how far does it make sense to use the criminal law against any act causing harm or running counter to our values? Take for example our test case of obscenity. How far should we use criminal law against obscenity? Even if obscenity offends, results in harm and threatens some of our values, do we really need to bring in the whole machinery of the criminal law?

The use of criminal law, we pointed out, imposes a cost. The convicted offender who is punished and the citizen who is forbidden to do the act prohibited both suffer a cost. One cost is a reduction of their freedom. Of course if the act in question is quite obviously a serious wrong, like murder, we are not worried by this loss of liberty. With Justice Holmes we reply: "your freedom to shake your fist ends where my chin begins". On the other hand, the less serious the act, the more concern for freedom — one reason among others why acts in no way wrong shouldn't be prohibited by criminal law and perhaps why even some immoral acts aren't in fact prohibited by it.

After all, in Canada as in many countries, an act can be wrong without being criminal. Here attention always focuses on fornication, homosexuality and lesbianism. But these are poor examples. We don't all agree that such things are wrong. Besides we can find much better examples of non-criminal wrongful acts. Two spring to mind: *lying and breaking promises*.

To tell a serious lie is clearly wrong. By this we mean a serious lie where there are no justifying or excusing circumstances. It is wrong because it militates against the truth-telling value, a value which we saw was necessary to society. Why hasn't lying, then, been made a crime? It has been, but only in certain circumstances: (1) where the lie amounts to fraud and (2) where it amounts to perjury. Short of cases where there is a danger of pecuniary loss or miscarriage of justice, liars are left to the informal sanctions of social intercourse.

The same with breaking promises. Again, breaking one's promise is clearly wrong. And here again by this we mean breaking a serious promise where there are no justifying or excusing factors. It is wrong because it militates against the highly useful social practice of promising. All the same, it hasn't generally been made a crime. At most the promise-breaker may be liable for breach of contract. And where he isn't even liable in contract, he too is left to the more informal sanctions of society.

One reason for not invoking criminal law in both these cases is the loss of liberty involved. This might well be too high a price to pay. All the more so, because of two extra factors. One is that lies and breaking promises range from very serious conduct down to relatively trivial behaviour and we wouldn't want every item of such trivial behaviour to set in motion the whole panoply of police, prosecutors, courts and prison officers. The other factor is that criminal law isn't the only way of bolstering truth and promising — there are other informal and possibly more effective social sanctions in reserve.

Another reason for not involving criminal law in such matters is the financial cost. We simply can't afford to take the criminal justice sledgehammer to every nut. Criminal law is a blunt and costly instrument best reserved for large targets — for targets constituting "clear and present danger" — which justify the monetary expense involved. Prosecute every simple lie or breach of promise and the game isn't worth the candle. How does this apply to obscenity?

Is it worth using criminal law against obscenity? Quite obviously obscenity itself won't ever be as significant a target for the criminal law as murder, say, or rape or robbery. Equally obviously, however, it isn't utterly without significance. Public obscenity clearly has significance — it annoys, disgusts, offends. As such it merits just as much and just as little place within the criminal law as other species of nuisance. Loud noises, nauseating smells and so on aren't anything like as serious as murder. But still they do make life less tolerable and so we use the criminal law against them to a limited degree. Society thinks the cost is worth it. So may it be with public, or involuntary, obscenity.

But what about private, or voluntary, obscenity? "A problem left to itself", said the playwright N. F. Simpson, "dries up or goes wrong. Fertilize it with a solution and you'll hatch dozens". What problems might we hatch by trying to fertilize voluntary obscenity with a criminal law solution?

First, in order to prevent a person's private voluntary enjoyment of obscenity, we should be calling in law enforcement agents to invade his privacy and freedom. By this we should ourselves be contravening some of those very values which we are trying to protect by preventing obscenity. In order to foster freedom, privacy and human dignity, we should in fact be invading the offender's own privacy, dignity, and freedom — his freedom of speech, of expression and of living his life in his own way, as well as his freedom to be secure in his own home from the interventions of the authorities.

Of course there's nothing self-contradictory about this. It could be argued that the threat obscenity poses to these values and to the value regarding violence is such as to justify this invasion. Some indeed will say that the danger that voluntary consumption of obscenity will lead to Manson murders is sufficient justification. But is it? How clear and obvious is the danger? Obvious enough for us to want to deal with it by risking another danger — the danger of all our homes being open to entry, search and seizure on mere suspicion of obscenity? Obvious enough for us to want to divert law enforcement resources on to this potential harm and away from actual harms such as murder, rape and robbery? Is that the sort of society we want?

The art of politics, however, — and law is ultimately a branch of politics — is the art of the possible, the art of the practical. And is it really practical to use the criminal law against voluntary obscenity simply on account of the conflict between obscenity and our taboo on violence? Not that there may not be other and better reasons for using the law against voluntary obscenity. After all, mightn't it be in the voluntary consumer's own best interest to use the law against him? Mightn't we be justified in using the law to protect him from himself?

But is it ever right to save a person from himself? Of course it is. A person might harm himself through ignorance, error or mistake: to stop him drinking something which, unknown to him, is poison is obviously justifiable — he would want us to. Or again, a person might harm himself through weakness of will or loss of self control: to stop him drinking himself blind on wood alcohol is clearly justifiable — he'd surely thank us afterwards. In both these cases the person we protect against himself will in general — though not at the moment of being protected — put his long-term welfare before his short-term preference.

But what if he prefers a moment of bliss to a lifetime's welfare? Of course he might not fully appreciate what is involved: he may have got his priorities wrong just now, but later come to see things as we do. But suppose, despite maturity, he just orders his priorities a different way. Suppose he really sets more store on a moment's ecstasy than on a long and healthy life. He's merely out of step with us, that's all. "If a man doesn't keep pace with his companions", said Thoreau, "perhaps it is because he hears a different drummer: let him step to the music which he hears, however measured or far away" . Different people, different preferences. In the ultimate analysis each man must choose his own priorities: no one can choose them for him.

This isn't so with children. Children are a special case. We rightly stop toddlers playing with few for their own good. Why can't we say the same about obscenity? For even though ultimately people should choose their own priorities and make their own commitments, they need maturity to do so. Children don't yet have this maturity, and exposure to obscenity could possibly prevent them reaching it. Free choice requires protection against influences militating against it: early brain-washing into some creed could rule out a full and free religious commitment later: early exposure to addictive drugs could preclude a freer choice of lifestyle in maturity; and early exposure to obscenity could possibly foreclose a person's options afterwards. So a limited paternalism is not at odds with liberty; in fact it serves to buttress it.

Unlimited paternalism is a different matter. Treating children as children is one thing, treating adults as children quite another. On this point we agree with John Stuart Mill that a man's own good, either physical or moral, is not a sufficient warrant for exercising power over him against his will. With Montesquieu we hold that, "changing people's manners and morals mustn't be done by changing the law".

But may there not still be a reason for using the criminal law against voluntary obscenity? May it not be justifiable in order to prevent overall decline in values?

As we saw earlier, it isn't impossible that widespread obscenity could cause decline in general values. This helps to make it justifiable to use the law to prohibit involuntary public obscenity and exposure of children to obscenity. Would it also make it justifiable to go further and outlaw private, voluntary, obscenity?

This brings us back to the notion of shared values and morality as the cement that binds society together. So important are these values that they have to be protected. Indeed Devlin once suggested that acts contravening and therefore threatening such values are acts akin to treason.

At the root of the analogy is the claim that a society is entitled to protect itself against change and dissolution. Yet is a society entitled to use the criminal law to resist change? If it's entitled to use it to combat treason, why shouldn't it be similarly entitled to use it to combat change due to declining values?

But why is society entitled to use the force of criminal law against treason? A paradigm case of treason is the use of force to overthrow the government or constitution. Why is this a crime? After all the new government or constitution might be an improvement. Even in Canada the constitution can't be perfect, otherwise why hold conferences to try and alter it? On the other hand, the new one might be worse. Or lots of people might consider it worse. And they of course would never have been consulted.

There is an obvious moral difference, then, between forcibly changing the government or constitution and doing this by peaceful means — by persuading society itself to change its institutions. Violent attack on these institutions, then, is rightly a crime, while non-violent attempts to bring about political changes are not. "Like may be repelled with like", says common law principle. Violent attacks can justifiably be met with force — the force of the criminal law. Non-violent advocacy of change can justifiably be met only with counter-argument in favour of the status quo. Society can justifiably use the criminal law to stop itself *being changed* but not to stop itself changing.

What light does this throw on society's right to use the criminal law to stop decline in moral values? If obscenity brings about decline by changing moral values, are society and its values simply changing or are they being changed? In one sense neither, in another both. Our moral values aren't being changed by force — indeed it is hard to imagine how they could be. And yet we're not just being asked to change them. Public obscenity, after all, tramples on values many hold and forces us, unless we yield our right to frequent public places, to see and become used to seeing obscenity; and this may lessen our sensitivity and may undermine our present values. To this extent society is entitled to use the criminal law against obscenity. But if the spectator has an option and consumes it willingly, society has less right to use the criminal law, for here the victim of obscenity is changing his values himself — another aspect of the argument that adults should be free to choose obscenity if they want.

But what if their voluntary consumption of obscenity weakens the values of society as a whole? Now is society entitled to use the criminal law against this risk? It depends how great the risk is to essential values. Suppose we could prove indubitably that individual consumption of pornography would thoroughly undermine the principle against violence. In that event it would be time to use the criminal law against such individual consumption. But that time hasn't arrived. The threat to the anti-violence principle — and we don't deny that there may be one — is uncertain, hard to assess and still a matter for speculation. A wholly clear and present danger hasn't been proved.

A further objection to using the criminal law against private consumption of obscenity by adults is the risk of increasing its profitability. Forbidden fruit, if not sweeter, is always dearer. Illegalising it adds an extra cost. It could be that those with most to lose from the legalising of obscenity may be the dealers who supply it. Certainly there is some evidence of this from Denmark.

Lastly, one final snag. Use criminal law against obscenity and perhaps we obscure the real problem. To take an analogy, our criminal law has concerned itself with non-medical use of drugs, but may not the real problem be the overall use of drugs in the modern "chemical" society? So with obscenity. The law concerns itself with "undue exploitation of sex", but may not the real problem be something else — our society's reluctance to be open and direct in dealing with sexual matters? Sex is a basic human drive but also something calling for maturity.

Obscenity, however, is immaturity. Obscenity is at odds with personal growth. At best, as in a dirty joke or filthy postcard. it is, as Orwell pointed out, a sort of mental rebellion against a conspiracy to pretend that human nature has no baser side. At worst, it is, as D. H. Lawrence said, an attempt "to insult sex, to do dirt on sex". Neither obscenity nor the law relating to it helps towards a maturer view of sex.

... So should obscenity be against the criminal law? In our view, yes, and no. Public obscenity — like other nuisances that give offence — can rightly be the subject of the criminal law. Private obscenity — which causes little, if any, harm and which doesn't threaten significantly — on the whole cannot. That's not to say that it can't be the subject of other types of law.

Criminal law, after all, is only one weapon in the arsenal of the law. Others are administrative regulation, customs laws, planning laws and finally tax laws. What may and what may not be published might best be dealt with by administrative control — a technique that is particularly appropriate perhaps to television and radio. Again, in so far as the pornography industry isn't homegrown, customs regulation is an obvious method of dealing with the problem. Or, if we accept that some obscenity is here to stay, mightn't a sensible approach be to use city planning to mark out certain areas for obscenity and to keep the rest obscenity-free? Or finally, if obscenity, like alcohol, is going to be always with us, why not use our tax laws to do two things — to siphon off some of the excess profit from the industry and at the same time to apply a measure of discouragement to the trade?

These questions, however, are outside the scope of this Working Paper. How far our objectives are best achieved by criminal or civil law techniques, how far criminal law enforcement against obscenity should allow for local varying standards, how far the present legal definition of obscenity should remain or be replaced by something else and where precisely the line between public and private should be drawn — all these are matters calling for more detailed legal and empirical research than is called for by this inquiry which, though focussing on obscenity, does so primarily as a test case to illuminate the general question of the proper scope and ambit of the criminal law. Such an inquiry rather serves to indicate the proper goals or objectives of criminal law in connection with the specific problem of obscenity, and so to indicate in general the reaches and the limits of the criminal law.

What, therefore, are our justified objectives with obscenity? As we have said public obscenity can rightly be a crime. Public obscenity then should remain an offence. In practical terms this means continued prohibition against lurid posters, advertisements, magazines and so on being shown in public. It also means restricting what can be broadcast and televised.

Private obscenity too can rightly be a crime, as we have said, when it comes to children. In practice this means that things like the Ottawa peep-show discussed earlier remain against the law. It doesn't mean of course that children won't ever get obscenity. They will — just as they get cigarettes and alcohol and other things we try to guard them from. But retaining the criminal law may still have effect. In effect it will serve at least to keep obscenity out of the classroom and restrict it to the playground — and this can have two results: it may help to limit the amount of obscenity that children are exposed to, and it will give underlining support to the general view that obscenity is not for public consumption.

Apart from this, however, private obscenity in our view should no longer be a crime. In this context the criminal law can't properly be used either to save the individual or society from itself. Individuals should be free to choose their own life-style and society should be free to change. In practical terms this would mean considerable change. It would mean decriminalizing much obscenity. In detail it would mean that pornography stores, pictures and so on carefully restricted to "adults only" would be allowed.

On the other hand decriminalizing — "legalizing", as it is sometimes called-would not imply condoning. Chamfort spoke truly when he said: "It is easier to make things legal than legitimate". In any case, voluntary consumption of obscenity could still be wrong in the civil law: contracts, for instance, to put on obscene displays for private consumption could still be contrary to public policy and so illegal. Besides, voluntary obscenity could still be dealt with, and surely better dealt with, by less formal sanctions, which after all are cheaper, and not only in monetary terms. The formal sanctions of the criminal law are in many ways too expensive.

In short, we must always bear in mind the price we pay for using criminal law. That price — in terms of suffering, loss of liberty and financial cost — sets limits to the proper use of criminal law. Acts of violence, acts of terror and acts causing serious distress can justifiably fall within that law. So too, occasionally, can obscenity when it gives serious offence and causes real annoyance by threatening fundamental values. This after all is what the criminal law is for — dealing. with acts that threaten or infringe essential or important values.

Restrict the criminal law to these kinds of acts and we may hope that even in a world where we get nothing for nothing, at least we won't get nothing for our penny too.

4.4.3 Bill C-239
An Act to Amend the Criminal Code, First Reading, 31 October 1977

1. Subsection 159(8) of the *Criminal Code* is repealed and the following substituted therefor:

"(8) In this Act,
"obscene thing" includes any explicit representation or detailed description of a sexual act and any pictorial representation tending to solicit partners for a sexual act;
"sexual act" means

    (*a*) masturbation,
    (*b*) any act of sado-masochism, and
    (*c*) any act of anal, oral or vaginal intercourse;

whether alone or with or upon another person, animal, dead body or inanimate object, and includes an attempted or simulated sexual act."

2. The said Act is further amended by adding thereto, immediately after section 166 thereof, the following new section:

"**166.1** (1) Every one commits an offence who photographs, produces, publishes, imports, exports, distributes, sells, advertises or displays in a public place anything that depicts a child performing a sexual act or assuming a sexually suggestive pose while in a state of undress.

(2) Every one who commits an offence under this section is guilty of
    (*a*) an indictable offence and is liable to imprisonment for two years, or
    (*b*) an offence punishable on summary conviction and is liable to a fine in the discretion of the court.

(3) Every one convicted of an offence under this section is liable to forfeit to the Crown any matter or thing, or part thereof, to which the offence relates.

(4) In this section,

"child" means a person who is or appears to be under the age of sixteen years."

Note: Bill C-239 was withdrawn after first reading and the subject-matter was referred to the Standing Committee on Justice and Legal Affairs.

4.4.4 Standing Committee on Justice and Legal Affairs, "The Third Report to the House (Report on Pornography)," 22 March 1978, pp. 7-10

The present definition of obscenity is vague and imprecise. It has led to confusion and dismay in the minds of the public, retailers, distributors, police officers, Crown prosecutors, defence lawyers, judges, and juries. This uncertainty in the law of obscenity is one of the factors causing the character of the sexually explicit material to change drastically in the past ten years. It has become more widely-disseminated and more easily available throughout the country.

Obscenity must be redefined in the *Criminal Code* to deal with the current situation. Much of this sexually explicit material depicts, describes, and advocates acts and simulated acts of violence, exploitation, subjugation, and humiliation. It promotes values and behaviour which are unacceptable in a society committed to egalitarian, consensual, mutual and non-violent human relationships. Most troubling of all has been the recent influx and availability of sexually explicit material involving children in suggestive situations either alone or with other children, adults, animals or objects. This kind of material is unacceptable in a civilized society and should be denounced and prohibited. Since the effective enforcement of the obscenity provisions of the *Criminal Code* is dependent upon a clear definition, it is essential that s. 159(8) *Cr.C.* be amended to make it evident what type of sexually explicit material will not be tolerated in this country.

Recommendation 4: Section 159(8) of the *Criminal Code* should be amended to define obscenity more clearly and to include sexually explicit material involving children within that definition in the following or similar terms:

"159. (8) For the purposes of this Act, a matter or thing shall be deemed to be obscene where

(*a*) a dominant characteristic of the matter or thing is the undue exploitation of sex, crime, horror, cruelty or violence, or the undue degradation of the human person; or

(*b*) the matter or thing depicts or describes a child

(i) engaged or participating in an act or simulated act of masturbation, sexual intercourse, gross indecency, buggery or bestiality, or

(ii) displaying any portion of its body in a sexually suggestive manner.

159. (9) In this section,

"child" means a person who is or appears to be under the age of sixteen years."

The community standards controversy is one that has raged throughout this country since 1959 when the present definition of obscenity was adopted. Canada is a country whose strength is in its diversity — many values and concerns differ from one place to another. The appreciation and acceptance of sexually explicit materials is no exception to this general principle. One of the most common complaints heard about the present idea of community standards in the case law is that although they may express some vague country-wide level of tolerance or acceptance they are not necessarily reflective of local or regional feeling. Since it appears that real community standards are local in nature, they should be determined by the inhabitants of the region, township, city, town, or village where an obscenity prosecution is undertaken. This is best done by trying obscenity cases before a judge and jury. As was seen earlier, the role of experts in obscenity trials has led to undesirable results, and in our view they should not be permitted to testify in such cases. The purpose of having a jury is to let a representative group of the community itself express the standards of the community as the jurors see and feel them, and the use of expert witnesses is inconsistent with such a purpose.

Recommendation 5: Section 498 of the *Criminal Code* should be amended to permit the Attorney General to override an accused's option for mode of trial, and request a trial by jury in cases where the prosecution is taken under s. 159 in the following or similar terms:

"498. The Attorney General may, notwithstanding that an accused elects under sections 464, 484, 491 or 492 to be tried by a judge or magistrate, as the case may be, require the accused to be tried by a court composed of a judge and jury, unless the alleged offence is one that is punishable with imprisonment for less than five years, and where the Attorney General so requires, a judge or magistrate has no jurisdiction to try the accused under this Part and a magistrate shall hold a preliminary inquiry unless a preliminary inquiry has been held prior to the requirement by the Attorney General that the accused be tried by a court composed of a judge and jury."

Recommendation 6: The testimony or evidence of expert witnesses as to community standards should under no circumstances be permitted during the trial of a person who has been charged with a criminal offence under s. 159. This should be done by adding ss.10 to s.159 in the following or similar terms:

"159. (10) Where an accused is tried for an offence under this section, no opinion evidence is admissible with respect to community standards in order to prove that any matter or thing is or is not obscene, any law or practice to the contrary notwithstanding."

The most unacceptable of the sexually explicit material so easily available is that involving infants and children. Many of these young people are what are commonly called "runaways" who have fled from troubled family situations and who have been enticed into the worlds of prostitution and drug abuse. Their participation in the production of this type of sexually explicit material is frequently incidental to these other parts of their lives. The consequence of the exploitation of children in such ways is often tragic both for these young people themselves and for their families. It is therefore necessary to deal severely with those who procure and entice children and young people for the purposes of prostitution and the production of sexually explicit material.

Recommendation 7: Section 166 of the *Criminal Code* should be amended to make the procurement of children for the purposes of prostitution or to participate in the production of sexually explicit materials criminal offences punishable by ten years imprisonment in the following or similar terms:

"166. (1) Every one commits an offence who
   (*a*) procures a child to engage in or to assist any person to engage in a sexually explicit act, or
   (*b*) orders, is party to, or knowingly receives the avails of the defilement, seduction or prostitution of a child.

(2) Every one who commits an offence under this section is guilty of an indictable offence and is liable to imprisonment for ten years.

(3) In this section,
"child" means a person who is under the age of sixteen years; and
"sexually explicit act" includes any act or simulated act of masturbation, sexual intercourse, gross indecency, buggery or bestiality, or the display of any portion of one's body in a sexually suggestive manner."

The easy accessibility of both acceptable and unacceptable sexually explicit material was vividly brought to the attention of the Committee during its hearing of evidence. This often takes the form of theatrical advertising, as well as book or magazine displays in neighbourhood retail outlets. Many members of the community where this type of material is publicly displayed find it offensive and have expressed the wish to have it controlled. The Committee has been impressed by the evidence presented to it showing the easy availability of sexually explicit material to young people. Where sexually explicit material is available to the adult members of Canadian society, this should be done through the adoption of discreet advertising, display and sales policies. Under no circumstances should such material be made visible or available to those who are not adults.

Recommendation 8: Provincial, regional, municipal and local authorities should adopt the necessary licensing, zoning, and child protection legislation, regulations, and by-laws to ensure that acceptable sexually explicit material is advertised, displayed, and sold discreetly to adults and under no circumstances to children or young people.

4.4.5 Bill C-19
An Act to Amend the Criminal Code, ss. 159(8), 163.1

In 1984 a Criminal Reform Bill was introduced in Parliament. This Bill would have replaced s.159(8) of the *Criminal Code* with the following:

"(8) For the purposes of this Act, any *matter or thing* obscene where a dominant characteristic of the *matter or thing* is the undue exploitation of any one or more of the following subjects, namely, sex, violence, crime, horror or cruelty, *through degrading representations of* a male or female person or in any other manner

(9) Where a court convicts a person of an offence under this section, it shall make an order declaring the matter or thing by means of or in relation to which the offence was committed forfeited to Her Majesty in right of the province in which the proceedings took place, for disposal as the Attorney General may direct."

It would also have added a new s.163.1:

"**163.1** Where any film or videotape is presented, published or shown in accordance with a classification or rating established for films or videotapes pursuant to the law of the province in which the film or videotape is presented, published or shown, no proceedings shall be instituted under section 159 or 163 in respect of such presentation, publication or showing or in respect of the possession of the film or videotape for any such purpose without the personal consent of the Attorney General."

4.4.6 Canada, Special Committee on Pornography and Prostitution Report (1985) (Fraser *Report*)

1. Criminal Code

Recommendation 1

The term "obscenity" should no longer be used in the *Criminal Code*, and the heading "Offences Tending to Corrupt Morals" should also be removed.

Recommendation 2

New criminal offences relating to "pornography" should be created, with care being exercised to ensure that the definition of the prohibited conduct, material or thing is very precise.

Recommendation 3

The federal government should give immediate consideration to studying carefully the introduction of criminal sanctions against the production or sale or distribution of material containing representations of violence without sex.

Recommendation 4

There should be no sanctions introduced respecting material that is 'disgusting' even though our proposed repeal of section 159 would remove the existing offence related to a disgusting object.

Recommendation 5

Controls on pornographic material should be organized on the basis of a three-tier system. The most serious criminal sanctions would apply to material in the first tier, including a visual representation of a person under 18 years of age, participating in explicit sexual conduct, which is defined as any conduct in which vaginal, oral or anal intercourse, bestiality, necrophilia, masturbation, sexually violent behaviour, lewd touching of the breasts or the genital parts of the body, or the lewd exhibition of the genitals is depicted. Also included in tier one is material which advocates, encourages, condones, or presents as normal the sexual abuse of children, and material which was made or produced in such a way that actual physical harm was caused to the person or persons depicted.

Less onerous criminal sanctions would apply to material in the second tier. Defences of artistic merit and educational or scientific purpose would be available. The second tier consists of any matter which depicts or describes sexually violent behaviour, bestiality, incest or necrophilia. Sexually violent behaviour includes sexual assault, and physical harm depicted for the apparent purpose of causing sexual gratification or stimulation to the viewer, including murder, assault or bondage of another person or persons, or self-infliction of physical harm.

Material in the third tier would attract criminal sanctions only when it is displayed to the public without a warning as to its nature or sold or made accessible to people under 18. In tier three is visual pornographic material in which is depicted vaginal, oral, or anal intercourse, masturbation, lewd touching of the breasts or the genital parts of the body or the lewd exhibition of the genitals, but no portrayal of a person under 18 or sexually violent pornography is included.

Recommendation 6

The provinces and the municipalities should play a major role in regulation of the visual pornographic representations that are not prohibited by the *Criminal Code* through film classification, display by-laws and other similar means. The provinces should not, however, attempt to control such representations by means of prior restraint.

Recommendation 7

Section 159 of the *Criminal Code* should be repealed, and replaced with the following provision:

159(1)(*a*) Everyone who makes, prints, publishes, distributes, or has in his possession for the purposes of publication or distribution. any visual pornographic material which was made or produced in such a way that actual physical harm was caused to the person or persons depicted, is guilty of an indictable offence and liable to imprisonment for five years.

(*b*) Everyone who sells, rents, offers to sell or rent, receives for sale or rent or has in his possession for the purpose of sale or rent any visual pornographic material which was made or produced in such a way that actual physical harm was caused to the person or persons depicted is guilty

(i) of an indictable offence and is liable to imprisonment for two years, or

(ii) of an offence punishable on summary conviction and is liable to a fine of not less than $500 and not more than $2,000 or to imprisonment for six months or to both.

(*c*) "visual pornographic material" includes any matter or thing in or on which is depicted vaginal, oral or anal intercourse, sexually violent behaviour, bestiality, incest, necrophilia, masturbation. lewd touching of the breasts or the genital parts of the body, or the lewd exhibition of the genitals.

159(2)(a) Everyone who makes, prints. publishes, distributes or has in his possession for the purposes of publication or distribution any matter or thing which depicts or describes:

    (i) sexually violent behaviour;
    (ii) bestiality;
    (iii) incest, or
    (iv) necrophilia

is guilty of an indictable offence and liable to imprisonment for five years.

    (b) Everyone who sells, rents, offers to sell or rent, receives for sale or has in his possession for the purpose of sale or rent any matter or thing which depicts or describes:

    (i) sexually violent behaviour;
    (ii) bestiality;
    (iii) incest, or
    (iv) necrophilia

is guilty

    (i) of an indictable offence and is liable to imprisonment for two years, or
    (ii) of an offence punishable on summary conviction and is liable to a fine of not less than $500 and not more than 51,000 or to imprisonment for six months or to both.

    (c) Everyone who displays any matter or thing which depicts

    (i) sexually violent behaviour;
    (ii) bestiality;
    (iii) incest; or
    (iv) necrophilia

in such a way that it is visible to members of the public in a place to which the public has access by right or by express or implied invitation is guilty of

    (i) an indictable offence and is liable to imprisonment for two years, or
    (ii) an offence punishable on similars conviction and is liable to a fine of not less than $500 and not more than 51000 or lo imprisonment for six months or to both.

(d) Nobody shall be convicted of the offence in subsection (2)(a) who can demonstrate that the matter or thing has a genuine educational or scientific purpose.

(e) Nobody shall be convicted of the offence in subsection (2)(b) who can demonstrate that the matter or thing has a genuine educational or scientific purpose, and that he sold, rented, offered to sell or rent or had in his possession for the purpose of sale of rent the matter or thing for a genuine education or scientific purpose.

(f) Nobody shall be convicted of the offences in subsections (2)(a) and (2)(b) who can demonstrate that the matter or thing is or is part of a work of artistic merit.

(g) Nobody shall be convicted of the offence in subsection (2)(c) who can demonstrate that the matter or thing

    (i) has a genuine educational or scientific purpose; or
    (ii) is or is part of a work of artistic merit, and

(iii) was displayed in a place or premises or a part of premises to which access is possible only by passing a promnent warning notice advising of the nature of the display therein,

(*h*) In determining whether a matter or thing is or is not part of a work of artistic merit the court shall consider the impugned material in the context of the whole work of which it is a part in the case of a book, film, video recording or broadcast which presents a discrete story. In the case of a magazine or any other composite or segmented work the court shall consider the impugned material in the context of the specific feature of which it is a part.

159(3)(*a*) Everyone who displays visual pornographic material so that it is visible to members of the public in a place to which the public has access by right or by express or implied invitation is guilty of an offence punishable on summary conviction.

(*b*) No one shall be convicted of an offence under subsection (1) who can demonstrate that the visual pornographic material was displayed in a place or premises or a part of premises to which access is possible only by passing a prominent warning notice advising of the display therein of visual pornographic material.

(*c*) For purposes of this section "visual pornographic material" includes any matter or thing in or on which is depicted vaginal, oral or anal intercourse, masturbation, lewd touching of the breasts or the genital parts of the body, or the lewd exhibition of the genitals, but does not include any manner or thing prohibited by subsections (1) and (2) of this section.

159(4) In any proceedings under section 159(1)(a) and (b), 159(2)(a) and (b), and 104, where an accused is found guilty of the offence the court shall order the offending matter or thing or copies thereof forfeited to Her Majesty in the Right of the Province in which proceedings took place, for disposal as the Attorney General may direct.

159(5) It shall not be a defence to a charge under sections 159(1)(a) and 159(2)(a) that the accused was ignorant of the character of matter or thing in respect of which the charge was laid.

159(6) Nobody shall be convicted of the offences in sections 159(1)(b) and 159(2)(b) who can demonstrate that he used due diligence to ensure that there were no representations in the matter or thing which he sold, rented, offered for sale or rent, or had in his possession for purposes of sale or rent, which offended the section.

159(7) Where an offence under this section committed by a body corporate is proved to have been committed with the consent or connivance of, or to be attributable to any neglect on the part of, any director, manager, secretary or other similar officer of the body corporate or any person who was purporting to act in any such capacity, he as well as the body corporate shall be guilty of the offence and shall be liable to be proceeded against and punished accordingly.

159(8) For purposes of this section, "sexually violent behaviour" includes
(i) sexual assault,
(ii) physical harm. including murder, assault or bondage of another person or persons, or self-infliction of physical harm, depicted for the apparent purpose of causing sexual gratification to or stimulation of the viewer.

Recommendation 8

Section 160 of the Code, allowing forfeiture proceedings to be brought, as an alternative to a criminal charge, should be retained in the Code but its application should be limited to tier one and tier two material.

Recommendation 9

To clarify the law on this point, section 160 should be amended to make it clear that the onus rests on the Crown under this section to prove beyond a reasonable doubt that the material comes within either tier one or tier two.

Recommendation 10

Section 161 of the Code should be amended as follows:

161. Everyone who refuses to sell or supply to any other person copies of any publication for the reason only that such other person refuses to purchase or acquire from him copies of any other publication that such other person is apprehensive may offend section 159(1) or section 159(2) of the Code is guilty of an indictable offence and is liable to imprisonment for two years.

Recommendation 11

Section 162 of the Code should be repealed.

Recommendation 12

Section 164 of the Code should be repealed and replaced by:

164(1) Everyone who makes use of the mails for the purpose of transmitting or delivering any matter or thing which:

(a) depicts or describes a person or persons under the age of 18 years engaging in sexual conduct,

(b) advocates, encourages, condones, or presents as normal the sexual abuse of children is guilty of an indictable offence and liable to imprisonment for ten years.

(2) Everyone who makes use of the mails for the purpose of transmitting or delivering any matter or thing which:

(a) by virtue of its character gives reason to believe that actual physical harm was caused to the person or persons depicted, or

(b) depicts or describes:
   (i) sexually violent behaviour,
   (ii) bestiality,
   (iii) incest, or
   (iv) necrophilia

is guilty of an indictable offence and liable to imprisonment for five years.

(3) Everyone who makes use of the mails for the purpose of transmitting or delivering unsohcited visual pornographic material to members of the public is guilty of an offence punishable on summary conviction.

(4) Nobody shall be convicted of the offence in subsection (2)(b) who can demonstrate that the matter or thing mailed

(i) has and is being transmitted or delivered for a genuine educational or scientific purpose, or

(ii) is or is part of a work of artistic merit.

(5) It shall not be a defence to a charge under subsections (1) and (2) of this section that the accused was ignorant of the character of the matter or thing in respect of which the charge was laid.

(6) For purposes of this section "visual pornographic material" includes any matter or thing in or on which is depicted vaginal, oral or anal intercourse, masturbation, sexually violent behaviour, incest, bestiality, necrophilia, lewd touching of the breasts or the genital parts of the body, or the lewd exhibition of the genitals.

Recommendation 13

Section 165 of the *Criminal Code* should be repealed.

Recommendation 14

Section 163 of the Code should be repealed and replaced by:

163(1) Everyone who, being the owner, operator, lessee, or manager, agent or person in charge of a theatre or any other place in which live shows are presented, presents or gives or allows to be presented or given therein a performance which advocates, encourages, condones or presents as normal the sexual abuse of children is guilty of an indictable offence and liable to imprisonment for ten years.

(2) Everyone who, being the owner, operator, lessee. manager, agent or person in charge of a theatre or any other place in which live shows are presented, presents or gives or allows to be presented or given therein a performance which

(*a*) involves actual physical harm is being caused to a person participating in the performance, or

(*b*) represents:
(i) sexually violent behaviour
(ii) bestiality;
(iii) incest; or
(iv) necrophilia

is guilty of an indictable offence and liable to imprisonment for five years.

(3) Everyone who, being the owner, operator, lessee, manager, agent or person in charge of a theatre or any other place in which live shows are presented, presents or gives, or allows to be presented or given therein without appropriate warning a performance in which explicit sexual conduct is depicted is guilty of an offence punishable on summary conviction.

(4) It shall not be a defence to a charge under subsections (1) and (2) that the accused was ignorant of the character of the production.

(5) Nobody shall be convicted of the offence under subsection (2)(b) who can demonstrate that

(i) the performance is or is pan of work of artistic merit; and

(ii) the performance was presented or given in a place or premises or a part of premises to which access is possible only by passing a prominent warning notice advising of the nature of the performance.

(6) For purposes of subsection 3 it shall be sufficient to establish that an appropriate warning was given that the performance was presented or given in a place or premises or

a part of premises to which access is possible only by passing a prominent warning notice advising of the nature of the performance.

(7) For purposes of subsection 3 "explicit sexual conduct" includes vaginal, oral or anal intercourse, masturbation, lewd touching of the breasts or the genital parts of the body, or the lewd exhibition of the genitals.

Recommendation 15

The provinces and the municipalities should play a major role in regulation of live performances involving sexual activity that are not prohibited by the *Criminal Code* through licensing, zoning and other similar means.

Recommendation 16

Section 170 of the *Criminal Code* should be amended to add the following provision:

This section has no application to a theatre or other place licensed to present live shows.

4.4.7 Bill C-114
An Act to Amend the Criminal Code, s. 138

In 1986, Bill C-114 was the result of further efforts to amend the legislation concerning obscenity and pornography. The following excerpt from that bill focusses on the attempt to redefine the offence of pornography.

1. Section 138 of the *Criminal Code* is amended by adding thereto, in alphabetical order within the section, the following definitions:

" "degrading pornography" means any pornography that shows defecation, urination, ejaculation or expectoration by one person onto another, lactation, menstruation, penetration of a bodily orifice with an object, one person treating himself or another as an animal or object, an act of bondage or any act in which one person attempts to degrade himself or another;

"pornography" means any visual matter showing vaginal, anal or oral intercourse, ejaculation, sexually violent behaviour, bestiality, incest, necrophilia, masturbation or other sexual activity;

"pornography that shows physical harm" means any pornography that shows a person in the act of causing or attempting to cause actual or simulated permanent or extended impairment of the body of any person or of its functions;

"sexually violent behaviour" includes sexual assault and any behaviour shown for the apparent purpose of causing sexual gratification to or stimulation of the viewer, in which physical pain is inflicted or apparently inflicted on a person by another person or by the person himself."

4.4.8 Bill C-54
An Act to Amend the Criminal Code, ss. 1, 2

In 1987, Bill C-54 was introduced in Parliament in a further effort to amend *Criminal Code* legislation dealing with pornography.

1. Section 138 of the *Criminal Code* is amended by adding thereto, in alphabetical order within the section, the following definitions:

" "erotica" means any visual matter a dominant characteristic of which is the depiction, in a sexual context or for the purpose of the sexual stimulation of the viewer, of a human sexual organ, a female breast or the human anal region;

"pornography" means

(*a*) any visual matter that shows

(i) sexual conduct that is referred to in any of subparagraphs

(ii) to (vi) and that involves or is conducted in the presence of a person who is, or is depicted as being or appears to be, under the age of eighteen years, or the exhibition, for a sexual purpose, of a human sexual organ, a female breast or the human anal region of, or in the presence of, a person who is, or is depicted as being or appears to be, under the age of eighteen years,

(ii) a person causing, attempting to cause or appearing to cause, in a sexual context, permanent or extended impairment of the body or bodily functions of that person or any other person

(iii) sexually violent conduct, including sexual assault and any conduct in which physical pain is inflicted or apparently inflicted on a person by that person or any other person in a sexual context,

(iv) a degrading act in a sexual context, including an act by which one person treats that person or any other person as an animal or object, engages in an act of bondage, penetrates with an object the vagina or the anus of that person or any other person or defecates, urinates or ejaculates onto another person, whether or not the other person appears to be consenting to any such degrading act, or lactation or menstruation in a sexual context,

(v) bestiality, incest or necrophilia, or

(vi) masturbation or ejaculation not referred to in subparagraph

(iv), or vaginal, anal or oral intercourse, or

(*b*) any matter or commercial communication that incites, promotes, encourages or advocates any conduct referred to in any of subparagraphs (a)(i) to (v);"

2. Sections 159 to 165 of the said Act are repealed and the following substituted therefor:

159. (1) Every person who deals in pornography is guilty of an offence.

(2) For the purposes of this section, a person deals in pornography if the person imports, makes, prints, publishes, broadcasts, distributes, possesses for the purpose of distribution, sells, rents, offers to sell or rent, receives for sale or rental, possesses for the purpose of sale or rental or displays, in a way that is visible to a member of the public in a public place, the pornography.

(3) Every person who commits the offence refined to in subsection (1) with respect to any matter referred to in subparagraph (a)(i) or (ii) of the definition "pornography" in section 138 or any matter or communication referred to in paragraph (b) of that definition, if the matter or communication is in relation to conduct referred to in either of those subparagraphs, is guilty of an indictable offence and is liable to imprisonment for a term not exceeding ten years.

(4) Every person who commits the offence referred to in subsection (1) with respect to any matter referred to in any of subparagraphs (a)(iii) to (v) of the definition "pornography" in section 138 or any matter or communication referred to in paragraph (b) of that definition, if the matter or communication is in relation to conduct referred to in any of those subparagraphs, is guilty

(a) of an indictable offence and is liable to imprisonment for a term not exceeding five years; or

(b) of an offence punishable on summary conviction.

(5) Every person who commits the offence referred to in subsection (1) with respect to any matter referred to in subparagraph (a)(vi) of the definition "pornography" in section 138 is guilty

(a) of an indictable offence and is liable to imprisonment for a term not exceeding two years; or

(b) of an offence punishable on summary conviction.

159.1 (1) Where an accused is charged with an offence under section 159, other than an offence that is in relation to conduct referred to in subparagraph (a)(i) or (ii) of the definition "pornography" in section 138 or any matter or communication referred to in paragraph (b) of that definition, if the matter or communication is in relation to conduct referred to in either of those subparagraphs, the court shall find the accused not guilty if the accused establishes, on a balance of probabilities, that the matter or communication in question has artistic merit or an educational, scientific or medical purpose.

(2) Where a court finds an accused not guilty by reason of the defence of artistic merit set out in subsection (1), the court shall declare that the matter or communication that formed the subject-matter of the alleged offence is not pornography.

159.2 (1) Every person who

(a) uses, induces, incites, coerces or agrees to use a person who is under the age of eighteen years to participate in the production of any matter referred to in subparagraph (a)(i) of the definition "pornography" in section 138 or any matter. or communication referred to in paragraph (b) of that definition and that involves a person referred to in subparagraph (a)(i) of that definition, or

(b) depicts a person as being under the age of eighteen years in such matter or communication

is guilty of an indictable offence and is liable to imprisonment for a term not exceeding ten years.

(2) Every person who, knowingly, without lawful justification or excuse, possesses any matter referred to in subparagraph (a)(i) of the definition "pornography" in section 138 or any matter or communication referred to in paragraph (b) of that definition and that involves a person referred to in subparagraph (a)(i) of that definition is guilty of an offence punishable on summary conviction.

In 1993 Parliament actually enacted amending legislation. The legislation, S.C. 1993, c. 46, made minor changes in section 163 of the *Criminal Code*. The main changes sought to create a new category of obscenity called "child pornography". Amendments were made to include "child pornography" within the forfeiture provisions of section 164. A new section was added to the *Criminal Code* to define "child pornography" and create an offence in relation to it.

4.4.9 *Criminal Code*, R.S.C. 1985, c. C-46, as am. S.C. 1993, c. 46

163.1 (1) In this section, "child pornography" means a photographic, film, video or other visual representation, whether or not it was made by electronic or mechanical means, that shows a person who is or is depicted as being under the age of eighteen years and is engaged in or is depicted as engaged in explicit sexual activity.

(2) Every person who makes, prints, publishes or possesses for the purpose of publication any child pornography is guilty of

> (*a*) an indictable offence and liable to imprisonment for a term not exceeding ten years; or
>
> (*b*) an offence punishable on summary conviction.

(3) Every person who distributes or sells any child pornography is guilty of

> (*a*) an indictable offence and liable to imprisonment for a term not exceeding ten years; or
>
> (*b*) an offence punishable on summary conviction.

(4) Every person who possesses any child pornography is guilty of

> (*a*) an indictable offence and liable to imprisonment for a term not exceeding five years; or
>
> (*b*) an offence punishable on summary conviction.

(5) It is not a defence to a charge under subsection (2) that the accused believed that a person shown in the representation that is alleged to constitute child pornography was or was depicted as being eighteen years of age or more unless the accused took all reasonable steps to ascertain the age of that person and took all reasonable steps to ensure that, where the person was eighteen years of age or more, the representation did not depict that person as being under the age of eighteen years.

(6) Where the accused is charged with an offence under subsection (2), (3) or (4), the court shall find the accused not guilty if the representation that is alleged to constitute child pornography has artistic merit or an educational, scientific or medical purpose.

(7) Subsections 163(3) to (5) apply, with such modifications as the circumstances require, with respect to an offence under subsection (2), (3) or (4).

4.4.9.1 *R. v. Butler* (1992), 89 D.L.R. (4th) 449 (S.C.C.)

SOPINKA, J.: — This appeal calls into question the constitutionality of the obscenity provisions of the *Criminal Code*, R.S.C. 1985, c. C-46, s. 163. They are attacked on the ground that they contravene s. 2(b) of the *Canadian Charter of Rights and Freedoms*. The case requires the court to address one of the most difficult and controversial of contemporary issues, that of determining whether, and to what extent, Parliament may legitimately criminalize obscenity. I propose to begin with a review of the facts which gave rise to this appeal, as well of the proceedings in the lower courts.

1. Facts and proceedings

In August, 1987, the appellant, Donald Victor Butler, opened the Avenue Video Boutique located in Winnipeg, Manitoba. The shop sells and rents "hard core" video tapes and magazines as well as sexual paraphernalia. Outside the store is a sign which reads:

> Avenue Video Boutique; a private members only adult video/visual club.
> Notice: if sex oriented material offends you, please do not enter.
> No admittance to persons under 18 years.

On August 21, 1987, the City of Winnipeg police entered the appellant's store with a search warrant and seized all the inventory. The appellant was charged with 173 counts in the first indictment: three counts of selling obscene material contrary to s. 159(2)(a) of the *Criminal Code*, R.S.C. 1970, c. C-34 (now s. 163(2)(a)), 41 counts of possessing obscene material for the purpose of distribution contrary to s. 159(1)(a) (now s. 163(1)(a) of the *Criminal Code*), 128 counts of possessing obscene material for the purpose of sale contrary to s. 159(2)(a) of the *Criminal Code* and one count of exposing obscene material to public view contrary to s. 159(2)(a) of the *Criminal Code*.

On October 19, 1987, the appellant reopened the store at the same location. As a result of a police operation a search warrant was executed on October 29, 1987, resulting in the arrest of an employee, Norma McCord. The appellant was arrested at a later date.

A joint indictment was laid against the appellant doing business as Avenue Video Boutique and Norma McCord. The joint indictment contains 77 counts under s. 159 (now s. 163) of the *Criminal Code*: two counts of selling obscene material contrary to s. 159(2)(a), 73 counts of possessing obscene material for the purpose of distribution contrary to s. 159(1)(a), one count of possessing obscene material for the purpose of sale contrary to s. 159(2)(a) and one count of exposing obscene material to public view contrary to s. 159(2)(a).

The trial judge convicted the appellant on eight counts relating to eight films. Convictions were entered against the co-accused McCord with respect to two counts relating to two of the films. Fines of $1,000 per offence were imposed on the appellant. Acquittals were entered on the remaining charges.

The Crown appealed the 242 acquittals with respect to the appellant and the appellant cross-appealed the convictions. The majority of the Manitoba Court of Appeal allowed the appeal of the Crown and entered convictions for the appellant with respect to all of the counts, Twaddle and Helper, JJ.A. dissenting.

3. Issues

The following constitutional questions are raised by this appeal:

> 1. Does s. 163 of the *Criminal Code* of Canada, R.S.C., 1985, c. C-46, violate s. 2(b) of the *Canadian Charter of Rights and Freedoms?*

2. If s. 163 of the *Criminal Code of Canada*, R.S.C., 1985, c. C-46, violates s. 2(b) of the *Canadian Charter of Rights and Freedoms*, can s. 163 of the *Criminal Code of Canada* be demonstrably justified under s. 1 of the *Canadian Charter of Rights and Freedoms* as a reasonable limit prescribed by law?

4. *Analysis*

The constitutional questions, as stated, bring under scrutiny the entirety of s. 163. However, both lower courts as well as the parties have focused almost exclusively on the definition of obscenity found in s. 163(8). Other portions of the impugned provision, such as the reverse onus provision envisaged in s. 163(3) as well as the absolute liability offence created by s. 163(6), raise substantial Charter issues which should be left to be dealt with in proceedings specifically directed to these issues. In my view, in the circumstances, this appeal should be confined to the examination of the constitutional validity of s. 163(8) only.

Before proceeding to consider the constitutional questions, it will be helpful to review the legislative history of the provision as well as the extensive judicial interpretation and analysis which have infused meaning into the bare words of the statute.

A. *Legislative History*

Parliament's first attempt to criminalize obscenity was in s. 179 of the *Criminal Code*, 1892, S.C. 1892, c. 29, which provided in part as follows:

179. Every one is guilty of an indictable offence and liable to two years' imprisonment who knowingly, without lawful justification or excuse —
    (*a*) publicly sells, or exposes for public sale or to public view, any obscene book, or other printed or written matter, or any picture, photograph, model or other object, *tending to corrupt morals*; or
    (*b*) publicly exhibits any *disgusting object or indecent show*;
    (*c*) offers to sell, advertises, publishes an advertisement of or has for sale or disposal any medicine, drug or article intended or represented as a means of preventing conception or causing abortion. (Emphasis added.)

In 1949 [by S.C. 1949, c. 13 s. 1], Parliament repealed the successor to s.179 and substituted it with the following provision:

207.(1) Every one who is guilty of an indictable offence and liable to two years' imprisonment who
    (*a*) makes, prints, publishes, distributes, circulates, or has in possession for any such purpose any obscene written matter, picture, model or other thing whatsoever; or
    (*b*) makes, prints, publishes, distributes, sells or has in possession for any such purpose, any crime comic.
(2) Every one is guilty of an indictable offence and liable to two years' imprisonment who knowingly, without lawful justification or excuse

(a) sells, exposes to public view or has in possession for any such purpose any obscene written matter, picture, model or other thing whatsoever;
(b) publicly exhibits any disgusting object or any indecent show; or
(c) offers to sell, advertises, publishes an advertisement of, or has for sale or disposal any means, instructions, medicine, drug or article intended or represented as a means of preventing conception or causing abortion or miscarriage or advertises or publishes an advertisement of any means, instructions, medicine, drug or article for restoring sexual virility or curing venereal diseases or diseases of the generative organs.

The *Criminal Code* did not provide a definition of any of the operative terms, "obscene", "indecent" or "disgusting". The notion of obscenity embodied in these provisions was based on the test formulated by Cockburn, C.J. in *R. v. Hicklin* (1868), L.R. 3 Q.B. 360 at p. 371:

> ... I think the test of obscenity is this, whether the tendency of the matter charged as obscenity is to deprave and corrupt those whose minds are open to such immoral influences, and into whose hands a publication of this sort may fall.

The focus on the "corruption of morals" in the earlier legislation grew out of the English obscenity law which made the court the "guardian of public morals". As Charron, D.C.J. stated in *R. v. Fringe Product Inc.* (1990), 53 C.C.C. (3d) 422 at pp. 441-2, 46 C.R.R. 154 (Ont. Dist. Ct.):

> When one looks at the legislative history of the obscenity provisions of the *Code*, it is clear that when the English Court of King's Bench first asserted itself in this field following the demise of the Star Chamber in 1641, it did so as the guardian of public morals: *R. v. Sidley* (1663),1 Sid. 168, 82 E.R. 1036. The crime of publishing an obscene libel was created in 1727 in the case of *R. v. Curl* (1727), 2 Stra. 788, 93 E.R. 849, when the court accepted the argument that publishing an obscene libel tended to corrupt the morals of the King's subjects and as such was against the peace of the King and government.

The current provision, which is the subject of this appeal, entered into force in 1959 in response to the much criticized former version (*Criminal Code*, S.C. 1953-54, c. 51, s. 150). Unlike the previous statutes, ss. (8) provided a statutory definition of "obscene":

> 150.(8) For the purposes of this Act, any publication a dominant characteristic of which is the undue exploitation of sex, or of sex and any one or more of the following subjects, namely, crime, horror, cruelty and violence, shall be deemed to be obscene.

As will be discussed further, the introduction of the statutory definition had the effect of replacing the *Hicklin* test with a series of rules developed by the courts. The provision must be considered in light of these tests.

B. *Judicial Interpretation of s. 163.(8)*

The first case to consider the current provision was *R. v. Brodie* (1962),132 C.C.C. 161, 32 D.L.R. (2d) 507, [1962] S.C.R. 681. The majority of this court found in that case that D. H. Lawrence's novel, *Lady Chatterley's Lover*, was not obscene within the meaning of the *Code*. The *Brodie* case laid the groundwork for the interpretation of s. 163.(8) by setting out the principal tests which should govern the determination of what is obscene for the purposes of criminal prosecution. The first step was to discard the *Hicklin* test.

(a) *Section 163.(8) to be Exclusive Test*

In examining the definition provided by s-s. (8), the majority of this court was of the view that the new provision provided a clean slate and had the effect of bringing in an "objective standard of obscenity" which rendered all the jurisprudence under the *Hicklin* definition obsolete. In the words of Judson, J. (at p. 179):

> I think that the new statutory definition does give the Court an opportunity to apply tests which have some certainty of meaning and are capable of objective application and which do not so much depend as before upon the idiosyncrasies and sensitivities of the tribunal of fact, whether judge or jury. We are now concerned with a Canadian statute which is exclusive of all others.

Any doubt that s. 163.(8) was intended to provide an exhaustive test of obscenity was settled in *Dechow v. The Queen, supra*.

. . . . .

In the *Dechow* case, the majority ascribed a liberal meaning to the term "publication", and found that the sex devices in question were "publications" as the accused had made such objects "publicly known" and had produced and issued such articles for public sale. Furthermore, in *R. v. Germain, supra*, La Forest, J., with whom a majority of the court agreed on this point, held that the word "obscene" must be given the same meaning whether the articles are publications under s. 159.(1) (now s. 163.(1)) or matter covered by s. 159.(2)(a) (now s. 163.(2)(a)). As a consequence, it is now beyond dispute that s. 163.(8) provides the exhaustive test of obscenity with respect to publications and objects which exploit sex as a dominant characteristic and that the common law test of obscenity found in the *Hicklin* decision is no longer applicable.

(b) *Tests of "Undue Exploitation of Sex"*

In order for the work or material to qualify as "obscene", the exploitation of sex must not only be its dominant characteristic, but such exploitation must be "undue". In determining when the exploitation of sex will be considered "undue", the courts have attempted to formulate workable tests. The most important of these is the "community standard of tolerance" test.

(i) *"Community standard of tolerance" test*

In *Brodie*, Judson, J. accepted the view espoused notably by the Australian and New Zealand courts that obscenity is to be measured against "community standards".

. . . . .

The community standards test has been the subject of extensive Judicial analysis. It is the standards of the community as a whole which must be considered and not the standards of a small segment of that community such as the university community where a film was shown . . .

. . . . .

With respect to expert evidence, it is not necessary and is not a fact which the Crown is obliged to prove as part of its case.

In *R. v. Dominion News & Gifts Ltd.,* [1963] 2 C.C.C. 103 Freedman, J.A. (dissenting) emphasized that the community standards test must necessarily respond to changing mores:

> Community standards must be contemporary. Times change, and ideas change with them. Compared to the Victorian era this is a liberal age in which we live. One manifestation of it is the relative freedom with which the whole question of sex is discussed. In books, magazines, movies, television, and sometimes even in parlour conversation, various aspects of sex are made the subject of comment, with a candour that in an earlier day would have been regarded as indecent and intolerable. We cannot and should not ignore these present-day attitudes when we face the question whether [the subject materials] are obscene according to our criminal law.

Our court was called upon to elaborate the community standards test in *R. v. Towne Cinema Theatres Ltd.* (1985), 18 C.C.C. (3d) 193 at p. 205, 18 D.L.R. (4th) 1, [1985] 1 S.C.R. 494. Dickson, C.J.C. reviewed the case-law and found:

> The cases all emphasize that it is a standard of *tolerance*, not taste, that is relevant. What matters is not what Canadians think is right for themselves to see. What matters is what Canadians would not abide other Canadians seeing because it would be beyond the contemporary Canadian standard of tolerance to allow them to see it.
>
> Since the standard is tolerance, I think the audience to which the allegedly obscene material is targeted must be relevant. The operative standards are those of the Canadian community as a whole, but since what matters is what other people may see, it is quite conceivable that the Canadian community would tolerate varying degrees of explicitness depending upon the audience and the circumstances.

(Emphasis in original.)

Therefore, the community standards test is concerned not with what Canadians would not tolerate being exposed to themselves, but what they would not tolerate *other* Canadians being exposed to. The minority view was that the tolerance level will vary depending on the manner, time and place in which the material is presented as well as the audience to whom it is directed. The majority opinion on this point was expressed by Wilson, J. in the following passage (at p. 215):

> It is not, in my opinion, open to the courts under s. 159.(8) of the *Criminal Code* to characterize a movie as obscene if shown to one constituency but not if shown to another . . . In my view, a movie is either obscene under the *Code* based on a national community standard of tolerance or it is not. If it is not, it may still be the subject of provincial regulatory control.

(ii) *"Degradation or dehumanization" test*

There has been a growing recognition in recent cases that material which may be said to exploit sex in a "degrading or dehumanizing" manner will necessarily fail the community standards test. Borins, Co. Ct. J. expressed this view in *R. v.*

Doug Rankine Co. Ltd. (1983), 9 C.C.C. (3d) 53 at p. 70, 36 C.R. (3d) 154 (Ont. Co. Ct.):

> ... films which consist substantially or partially of scenes which portray violence and cruelty in conjunction with sex, particularly where the performance of indignities degrade and dehumanize the people upon whom they are performed, exceed the level of community tolerance.

Subsequent decisions, such as *R. v. Ramsingh* (1984), 14 C.C.C. (3d) 230, 29 Man. R. (2d) 110 (Q.B.), and in *R. v. Wagner* (1985), 43 C.R. (3d) 318, 36 Alta. L.R. (2d) 301 (Q.B.), held that material that "degraded" or "dehumanized" any of the participants would exceed community standards even in the absence of cruelty and violence. In *R. v. Ramsingh, supra*, Ferg, J. described in graphic terms the type of material that qualified for this label. He states on p. 239:

> They are exploited, portrayed as desiring pleasure from pain, by being humiliated and treated only as an object of male domination sexually, or in cruel or violent bondage. Women are portrayed in these films as pining away their lives waiting for a huge male penis to come along, on the person of a so called sex therapist, or window washer, supposedly to transport them into complete sexual ecstasy. Or even more false and degrading one is led to believe their raison d'etre is to savour semen as a life elixir, or that they secretly desire to be forcefully taken by a male.

Among other things, degrading or dehumanizing materials place women (and sometimes men) in positions of subordination, servile submission or humiliation. They run against the principles of equality and dignity of all human beings. In the appreciation of whether material is degrading or dehumanizing, the appearance of consent is not necessarily determinative. Consent cannot save materials that otherwise contain degrading or dehumanizing scenes. Sometimes the very appearance of consent makes the depicted acts even more degrading or dehumanizing.

This type of material would, apparently, fail the community standards test not because it offends against morals but because it is perceived by public opinion to be harmful to society, particularly to women. While the accuracy of this perception is not susceptible of exact proof, there is a substantial body of opinion that holds that the portrayal of persons being subjected to degrading or dehumanizing sexual treatment results in harm, particularly to women and therefore to society as a whole.

. . . . .

It would be reasonable to conclude that there is an appreciable risk of harm to society in the portrayal of such material. The effect of the evidence on public opinion was summed up by Wilson, J. in Towne Cinema, supra, as follows (at pp. 217-8):

> The most that can be said, I think, is that the public has concluded that exposure to material which degrades the human dimensions of life to a subhuman or merely physical dimension and thereby contributes to a process of moral desensitization must be harmful in some way.

In *Towne Cinema*, Dickson, C.J.C. considered the "degradation" or "dehumanization" test to be the principal indicator of "undueness" without specifying what role the community tolerance test plays in respect of this issue. He did observe, however, that the community might tolerate some forms of exploitation that caused harm that were nevertheless undue. The relevant passages appear at pp. 202-3:

> There are other ways in which exploitation of sex might be "undue". Ours is not a perfect society and it is unfortunate but true that the community may tolerate publications that cause harm to members of society and therefore to society as a whole. Even if, at certain times, there is a coincidence between what is not tolerated and what is harmful to society, there is no necessary connection between these two concepts. Thus, a legal definition of "undue" must also encompass publications harmful to members of society and therefore, to society as a whole.
>
> Sex-related publications which portray persons in a degrading manner as objects of violence, cruelty or other forms of dehumanizing treatment, may be "undue" for the purpose of s. 159(8). No one should be subject to the degradation and humiliation inherent in publications which link sex with violence, cruelty, and other forms of dehumanizing treatment. It is not likely that at a given moment in a society's history, such publications will be tolerated . . .
>
> However, as I have noted above, there is no necessary coincidence between the undueness of publications which degrade people by linking violence, cruelty or other forms of dehumanizing treatment with sex, and the community standard of tolerance. Even if certain sex-related materials were found to be within the standard of tolerance of the community, it would still be necessary to ensure that they were not "undue" in some other sense, for example in the sense that they portray persons in a degrading manner as objects of violence, cruelty, or other forms of dehumanizing treatment. (Emphasis in original.)

In the reasons of Wilson, J. concurring in the result, the line between the mere portrayal of sex and the dehumanization of people is drawn by the "undueness" concept. The community is the arbiter as to what is harmful to it. She states (at pp. 217-8):

> As I see it, the essential difficulty with the definition of obscenity is that "undueness" must presumably be assessed in relation to consequences. It is implicit in the definition that at some point the exploitation of sex becomes harmful to the public or at least the public believes that to be so. It is therefore necessary for the protection of the public to put limits on the degree of exploitation and, through the application of the community standard test, the public is made the arbiter of what is harmful to it and what is not. The problem is that we know so little of the consequences we are seeking to avoid. Do obscene movies spawn immoral conduct? Do they degrade women? Do they promote violence? The most that can be said, I think, is that the public has concluded that exposure to material which degrades the human dimensions of life to a subhuman or merely physical dimension and thereby contributes to a process of moral desensitization must be harmful in some way. It must therefore be controlled when it sets out of hand, when it becomes "undue".

(iii) *"Internal necessities test" or "artistic defence"*

In determining whether the exploitation of sex is "undue", Judson, J. set out the test of "internal necessities" in *Brodie, supra* (at p. 181):

> What I think is aimed at is excessive emphasis on the theme for a base purpose. But I do not think that there is undue exploitation if there is no more emphasis on the theme than is required in the serious treatment of the theme of a novel with honesty and uprightness. That the work under attack is a serious work of fiction is to me beyond question. It has none of the characteristics that are often described in judgments dealing with obscenity — dirt for dirt's sake, the leer of the sensualist, depravity in the mind of an author with an obsession for dirt, pornography, an appeal

to a prurient interest, etc. The section recognizes that the serious-minded author must have freedom in the production of a work of genuine artistic and literary merit and the quality of the work, as the witnesses point out and common sense indicates, must have real relevance in determining not only a dominant characteristic but also whether there is undue exploitation.

As counsel for the Crown pointed out in his oral submissions, the artistic defence is the last step in the analysis of whether the exploitation of sex is undue. Even material which by itself offends community standards will not be considered "undue", if it is required for the serious treatment of a theme. For example, in *R. v. Odeon Morton Theatres Ltd. and United Artists Corp.* (1974), 16 C.C.C. (2d) 185, 45 D.L.R. (3d) 224, [1974] 3 W.W.R. 304 (Man. C.A.), the majority of the Manitoba Court of Appeal held that the film "Last Tango in Palis" was not obscene within the meaning of the *Code*. To determine whether a dominant characteristic of the film is the undue exploitation of sex, Freedman, C.J.M. noted that the courts must have regard to various things — the author's artistic purpose, the manner in which he or she has portrayed and developed the story, the depiction and interplay of character and the creation of visual effect through skilful camera techniques (at p. 194). Freedman, C.J.M. stated that the issue of whether the film is obscene must be determined according to contemporary community standards in Canada. Relevant to that determination were several factors: the testimony of experts, the classification of "Restricted" which made the film unavailable to persons under 18 years of age and the fact that the film had passed the scrutiny of the censor boards of several provinces.

Accordingly, the "internal necessities" test, or what has been referred to as the "artistic defence", has been interpreted to assess whether the exploitation of sex has a justifiable role in advancing the plot or the theme, and in considering the work as a whole, does not merely represent "dirt for dirt's sake" but has a legitimate role when measured by the internal necessities of the work itself.

(iv) *The relationship of the tests to each other*

This review of jurisprudence shows that it fails to specify the relationship of the tests one to another. Failure to do so with respect to the community standards test and the degrading or dehumanizing test, for example, raises a serious question as to the basis on which the community acts in determining whether the impugned material will be tolerated. With both these tests being applied to the same material and apparently independently, we do not know whether the community found the material to be intolerable because it was degrading or dehumanizing, because it offended against morals or on some other basis. In some circumstances a finding that the material is tolerable can be overruled by the conclusion by the court that it causes harm and is therefore undue. Moreover, is the internal necessities test dominant so that it will redeem material that would otherwise be undue or is it just one factor? Is this test applied by the community or is it determined by the court without regard for the community? This hiatus in the jurisprudence has left the legislation open to attack on the ground of vagueness and uncertainty. That attack is made in this case. This lacuna in the interpretation of the legislation must, if possible, be filled before subjecting the legislation to Charter scrutiny. The necessity to do so was foreseen by Wilson, J. in *Towne Cinema* when she stated (at p. 218):

> The test of the community standard is helpful to the extent that it provides a norm against which impugned material may be assessed but it does little to elucidate the underlying question as to why some exploitation of sex falls on the permitted side of the line under s.159(8) and some on the prohibited side. No doubt this question will have to be addressed when the validity of the obscenity provisions of the Code is subjected to attack as an infringement on freedom of speech and the infringement is sought to be justified as reasonable.

Pornography can be usefully divided into three categories: (1) explicit sex with violence, (2) explicit sex without violence but which subjects people to treatment that is degrading or dehumanizing, and (3) explicit sex without violence that is neither degrading nor dehumanizing. Violence in this context includes both actual physical violence and threats of physical violence. Relating these three categories to the terms of s. 163.(8) of the *Code*, the first, explicit sex coupled with violence, is expressly mentioned. Sex coupled with crime, horror or cruelty will sometimes involve violence. Cruelty, for instance, will usually do so. But, even in the absence of violence, sex coupled with crime, horror or cruelty may fall within the second category. As for category (3), subject to the exception referred to below, it is not covered.

Some segments of society would consider that all three categories of pornography cause harm to society because they tend to undermine its moral fibre. Others would contend that none of the categories cause harm. Furthermore there is a range of opinion as to what is degrading or dehumanizing: see *Pornography and Prostitution in Canada: Report of the Special Committee on Pornography and Prostitution* (1985) (the Fraser Report), vol. 1, at p. 51. Because this is not a matter that is susceptible of proof in the traditional way and because we do not wish to leave it to the individual tastes of judges, we must have a norm that will serve as an arbiter in determining what amounts to an undue exploitation of sex. That arbiter is the community as a whole

The courts must determine as best they can what the community would tolerate others being exposed to on the basis of the degree of harm that may flow from such exposure. Harm in this context means that it predisposes persons to act in an antisocial manner as, for example, the physical or mental mistreatment of women by men, or, what is perhaps debatable, the reverse. Antisocial conduct for this purpose is conduct which society formally recognizes as incompatible with its proper functioning. The stronger the inference of a risk of harm the lesser the likelihood of tolerance. The inference may be drawn from the material itself or from the material and other evidence. Similarly, evidence as to the community standards is desirable but not essential.

In making this determination with respect to the three categories of pornography referred to above, the portrayal of sex coupled with violence will almost always constitute the undue exploitation of sex. Explicit sex which is degrading or dehumanizing may be undue if the risk of harm is substantial. Finally, explicit sex that is not violent and neither degrading nor dehumanizing is generally tolerated in our society and will not qualify as the undue exploitation of sex unless it employs children in its production.

If material is not obscene under this framework, it does not become so by reason of the person to whom it is or may be shown or exposed nor by reason of the place or manner in which it is shown. The availability of sexually explicit materials in theatres and other public places is subject to regulation by competent provincial legislation. Typically such legislation imposes restrictions on the material available to children: see *Nova Scotia Board of Censors v. McNeil* (1978), 84 D.L.R. (3d) 1, [1978] 2 S.C.R. 662, 25 N.S.R. (2d) 128.

The foregoing deals with the interrelationship of the "community standards test" and "the degrading or dehumanizing" test. How does the "internal necessities" test fit into this scheme? The need to apply this test only arises if a work contains sexually explicit material that by itself would constitute the undue exploitation of sex. The portrayal of sex must then be viewed in context to determine whether that is the dominant theme of the work as a whole. Put another way, is undue exploitation of sex the main object of the work or is this portrayal of sex essential to a wider artistic, literary, or other similar purpose? Since the threshold determination must be made on the basis of community standards, that is, whether the sexually explicit aspect is undue, its impact when considered in context must be determined on the same basis. The court must determine whether the sexually explicit material when viewed in the context of the whole work would be tolerated by the community as a whole. Artistic expression rests at the heart of freedom of expression values and any doubt in this regard must be resolved in favour of freedom of expression.

C. *Does s. 163 violate s. 2(b) of the Charter?*

The majority of the Court of Appeal in this case allowed the appeal of the Crown on the ground that s. 163 does not violate freedom of expression as guaranteed under s. 2(b) of the Charter. Huband, J.A. (at p. 230), applied the first step of the test set out in *Irwin Toy, supra*, as follows:

> In this case, it is unnecessary to proceed beyond the first step because the materials are devoid of a "meaning". That word, as it is employed in the majority reasons in the *Irwin Toy* case, leads to the realm of ideas, opinions thoughts, beliefs, or feelings. Expression for economic purposes is included because commercial expression conveys meaning. But the majority judgment in the *Irwin Toy* case acknowledges [at p. 607] that "... *some human activity is purely physical and does not convey or attempt to convey meaning*". *I think that is true of the materials in this case.*

(Emphasis added.)

In my view, the majority of the Manitoba Court of Appeal erred in several respects in its application of the test enunciated in *Irwin Toy*. First, Huband, J.A. misinterpreted the distinction between purely physical activity and activity having expressive content. The subject-matter of the materials in this case is clearly "physical", but this does not mean that the materials do not convey or attempt to convey meaning such that they are without expressive content. An example of the "purely physical" activity alluded to in *Irwin Toy* was that of parking a car which, if performed as a day-to-day task, cannot be said to have expressive content. Such purely physical activity may be distinguished from that form of activity which we are concerned with in the present appeal which, while indeed "physical", conveys ideas, opinions, or feelings. As Twaddle, J.A. noted (at pp. 237-8):

> The subject matter of the material under review ... is sexual activity. Such activity is part of the human experience ... The depiction of such activity has the potential of titillating some and of informing others. How can images which have such effect be meaningless?
>
> . . . . . .
>
> In my view, the content of a video movie, the content of a magazine and the imagery of a sexual gadget are all within the freedom of expression.

Secondly, the majority of the Court of Appeal erred in failing to properly draw the distinction between the content of the materials and the form of expression. Huband, J.A. wrote (at p. 230):

> Concerning the form of the activity, it falls within an area which has been criminalized as an offence relating to public morality — an area identified by Lamer, J. in his reasons for decision in *Reference re ss. 193 and 195.1(1)(c), supra*, as one where the form might well be unprotected by the Charter. *The form consists of the undue exploitation of sex, the degradation of human sexuality. In my view, the form of the activity is not one which the Charter was designed or intended to protect.* Thus, in terms of both content and form the activity properly falls within the regulated area of freedom of expression. (Emphasis added.)

The form of activity in this case is the medium through which the meaning sought to be conveyed is expressed, namely, the film, magazine, written matter, or sexual gadget. There is nothing inherently violent in the vehicle of expression, and it accordingly does not fall outside the protected sphere of activity.

In light of our recent decision in *R. v. Keegstra* (1990), 61 C.C.C. (3d) 1, [1990] 3 S.C.R. 697, 1 C.R. (4th) 129, the respondent, and most of the parties intervening in support of the respondent, do not take issue with the proposition that s. 163 of the *Criminal Code* violates s. 2(b) of the Charter. In *Keegstra*, we were unanimous in advocating a generous approach to the protection afforded by s. 2(b) of the Charter. Our court confirmed the view expressed in *Reference re: ss. 193 and 195.1(1)(c) of Criminal Code* (1990), 56 C.C.C. (3d) 66, [1990] 1 S.C.R. 1123, 77 C.R. (3d) 1 (the *"Prostitution Reference"*), that activities cannot be excluded from the scope of the guaranteed freedom on the basis of the content or meaning being conveyed. McLachlin, J. wrote (at p. 97):

> As this court has repeatedly affirmed, the content of a statement cannot deprive it of the protection accorded by s. 2(b), no matter how offensive it may be. The content of Mr. Keegstra's statements was offensive and demeaning in the extreme; nevertheless, on the principles affirmed by this court, that alone would appear not to deprive them of the protection guaranteed by the Charter.

With respect, the majority of the Court of Appeal did not sufficiently distance itself from the content of the materials. In assessing the purpose of the legislation, the majority stated (at pp. 230-1):

> The purpose of s. 163 of the *Code* is not to interfere with the free exchange of ideas and opinions, and not to suppress the attempt to convey a message or a meaning. The intent of the legislation is to bar the distribution or sale of prurient materials devoid of a redeeming meaning.

Meaning sought to be expressed need not be "redeeming" in the eyes of the court to merit the protection of s. 2(b) whose purpose is to ensure that thoughts and feelings may be conveyed freely in non-violent ways without fear of censure.

In this case, both the purpose and effect of s. 163 is specifically to restrict the communication of certain types of materials based on their content. In my view, there is no doubt that s. 163 seeks to prohibit certain types of expressive activity and thereby infringes s. 2(b) of the Charter.

Before turning to consider whether this infringement is justified under s. 1 of the Charter, I wish to address the argument advanced by the Attorney-General of B.C. that in applying s. 2(b), a distinction should be made between films and written works. It is argued that by its very nature, the medium of the written word is such that it is, when used, inherently an attempt to convey meaning. In contrast, British Columbia argues that the medium of film can be used for a purpose "not significantly communicative". In its factum, British Columbia maintains that if the activity captured in hard core pornographic magazines and video tapes is itself not expression, the fact that they are reproduced by the technology of a camera does not magically transform them into "expression": the appellant cannot hide behind the label "film" to claim protection for the reproduction of activity the sole purpose of which is to arouse or shock.

In my view, this submission cannot be maintained. This position is not far from that taken by the majority of the Court of Appeal, that the depiction of purely physical activity does not convey meaning. First, I cannot agree with the premise that purely physical activity, such as sexual activity, cannot be expression. Secondly, in creating a film, regardless of its content, the maker of the film is consciously choosing the particular images which together constitute the film. In choosing his or her images, the creator of the film is attempting to convey some meaning. The meaning to be ascribed to the work cannot be measured by the reaction of the audience, which, in some cases, may amount to no more than physical arousal or shock. Rather, the meaning of the work derives from the fact that it has been intentionally created by its author. To use an example, it may very well be said that a blank wall in itself conveys no meaning. However, if one deliberately chooses to capture that image by the medium of film, the work necessarily has some meaning for its author and thereby constitutes expression. The same would apply to the depiction of persons engaged in purely sexual activity.

I would conclude that the first constitutional question should be answered in the affirmative.

D. *Is s. 163 justified under s. 1 of the Charter?*

(a) *Is s. 163 a Limit Described by Law?*

The appellant argues that the provision is so vague that it is impossible to apply it. Vagueness must be considered in relation to two issues in this appeal: (1) is the law so vague that it does not qualify as "a limit prescribed by law", and (2) is it so imprecise that it is not a reasonable limit. Dealing with (1), the test is whether the law "is so obscure as to be incapable of interpretation with any degree of precision using the ordinary tools": *Osborne v. Canada (Treasury Board)* (1991), 82 D.L.R. (4th) 321 at p. 339, [1991] 2 S.C.R. 69, 91 C.L.L.C. 14,026. Put another way, does the law provide "an intelligible standard according to which the judiciary must do its work" (*Irwin Toy, supra,* at p. 617; adopted in *Osborne v. Canada (Treasury Board), supra,* at p. 340).

In assessing whether s.163(8) prescribes an intelligible standard, consideration must be given to the manner in which the provision has been judicially interpreted. Accordingly, in the *Prostitution Reference, supra,* the majority reached the conclusion that words such as "acts of indecency" were capable of constituting a limit prescribed by law. Lamer, J. (as he then was) stated (at p. 90):

> Also, as the Ontario Court of Appeal has held in *R. v. LeBeau* (1988), 41 C.C.C. (3d) 163 at p. 173, 62 C.R. (3d) 157, 4 U.C.B. (2d) 102, "the void for vagueness doctrine is not to be applied to the bare words of the statutory provision but, rather, to the provision as interpreted and applied in judicial decisions".
>
> The fact that a particular legislative term is open to varying interpretations by the courts is not fatal. As Beetz, J. observed in *R. v. Morgentaler* (1988), 37 C.C.C. (3d) 449 at p. 505, 44 D.L.R. (4th) 385, [1988] 1 S.C.R. 30 "[f]lexibility and vagueness are not synonymous". Therefore the question at hand is whether the impugned sections of the *Criminal Code* can be or have been given sensible meanings by the courts.

Standards which escape precise technical definition, such as "undue", are an inevitable part of the law. The *Criminal Code* contains other such standards. Without commenting on their constitutional validity, I note that the terms "indecent", "immoral" or "scurrilous", found in ss. 167, 168, 173 and 175, are nowhere defined in the *Code*. It is within the role of the judiciary to attempt to interpret these terms. If such interpretation yields an intelligible standard, the threshold test for the application of s. 1 is met. In my opinion, the interpretation of s. 163(8) in prior judgments which I have reviewed, as supplemented by these reasons, provides an intelligible standard.

(b) *Objective*

The respondent argues that there are several pressing and substantial objectives which justify overriding the freedom to distribute obscene materials. Essentially, these objectives are the avoidance of harm resulting from antisocial attitudinal changes that exposure to obscene material causes and the public interest in maintaining a "decent society". On the other hand, the appellant argues that the objective of s. 163 is to have the state act as "moral custodian" in sexual matters and to impose subjective standards of morality.

The obscenity legislation and jurisprudence prior to the enactment of s. 163 were evidently concerned with prohibiting the "immoral influences" of obscene publications and safeguarding the morals of individuals into whose hands such works could fall. The *Hicklin* philosophy posits that explicit sexual depictions, particularly outside the sanctioned contexts of marriage and procreation, threatened the morals or the fabric of society (Clare Beckton, "Freedom of Expression (s. 2(b))", in Tarnopolsky and Beaudoin (eds.), *The Canadian Charter of Rights and Freedoms: Commentary* (1982), at p. 105. In this sense, its dominant, if not exclusive, purpose was to advance a particular conception of morality. Any deviation from such morality was considered to be inherently undesirable, independently of any harm to society. As Judson, J. described the test in *Brodie, supra* (at p. 181):

> [The work under attack] has none of the characteristics that are often described in judgments dealing with obscenity — dirt for dirt's sake, the leer of the sensualist, depravity in the mind of an author with an obsession for dirt pornography, an appeal to a prurient interest, etc.

I agree with Twaddle, J.A. of the Court of Appeal that this particular objective is no longer defensible in view of the Charter. To impose a certain standard of public and sexual morality, solely because it reflects the conventions of a given community, is inimical to the exercise and enjoyment of individual freedoms, which form the basis of our social contract. D. Dyzenhaus, "Obscenity and the Charter: Autonomy and Equality" (1991), 1 C.R. (4th) 367 at p. 370, refers to this as "legal moralism", of a majority deciding what values should inform individual lives and then coercively imposing those values on minorities. The prevention of "dirt for dirt's sake" is not a legitimate objective which would justify the violation of one of the most fundamental freedoms enshrined in the Charter.

On the other hand, I cannot agree with the suggestion of the appellant that Parliament does not have the right to legislate on the basis of some fundamental conception of morality for the purposes of safeguarding the values which are integral to a free and democratic society. As Dyzenhaus, *ibid.*, writes (at p. 376) "Moral disapprobation is recognized as an appropriate response when it has its basis in *Charter* values."

As the respondent and many of the interveners have pointed out, much of the criminal law is based on moral conceptions of right and wrong and the mere fact that a law is grounded in morality does not automatically render it illegitimate. In this regard, criminalizing the proliferation of materials which undermine another basic Charter right may indeed be a legitimate objective.

In my view, however, the overriding objective of s. 163 is not moral disapprobation but the avoidance of harm to society. In *Towne Cinema*, Dickson, C.J.C. stated (at p. 204): "It is harm to society from undue exploitation that is aimed at by the section, not simply lapses in propriety or good taste."

The harm was described in the following way in the Report on Pornography by the Standing Committee on Justice and Legal Affairs (MacGuigan Report) (1978) (at p. 18:4):

> The clear and unquestionable danger of this type of material is that it reinforces some unhealthy tendencies in Canadian society. The effect of this type of material is to reinforce male-female stereotypes to the detriment of both sexes. It attempts to make degradation, humiliation, victimization, and violence in human relationships appear normal and acceptable. A society which holds that egalitarianism, non-violence, consensualism, and mutuality are basic to any human interaction, whether sexual or other, is clearly justified in controlling and prohibiting any medium of depiction, description or advocacy which :violates these principles.

The appellant argues that to accept the objective of the provision as being related to the harm associated with obscenity would be to adopt the "shifting purpose" doctrine explicitly rejected in *R. v. Big M Drug Mart Ltd.* (1985), 18 C.C.C. (3d) 385, 18 D.L.R. (4th) 321, [1985] 1 S.C.R. 295. This court concluded in that case that a finding that the *Lord's Day Act* has a secular purpose was not possible given that its religious purpose, in compelling sabbatical observance, has been long-established and consistently maintained by the courts. The appellant relies on the words of Dickson, J. (as he then was) stated (at p. 417):

> ... the theory of a shifting purpose stands in stark contrast to fundamental notions developed in our law concerning the nature of "Parliamentary intention". Purpose is a function of the intent of those who drafted and enacted the legislation at the time, and not of any shifting variable.
>
> . . . . .
>
> While the effect of such legislation as the *Lord's Day Act* may be more secular today than it was in 1677 or in 1906, such a finding cannot justify a conclusion that its purpose has similarly changed. In result, therefore, the *Lord's Day Act* must be characterized as it has always been, a law the primary purpose of which is the compulsion of sabbatical observance.

I do not agree that to identify the objective of the impugned legislation as the prevention of harm to society, one must resort to the "shifting purpose" doctrine. First, the notions of moral corruption and harm to society are not distinct, as the appellant suggests, but are inextricably linked. It is moral corruption of a certain kind which leads to the detrimental effect on society. Secondly, and more importantly, I am of the view that with the enactment of s. 163, Parliament explicitly sought to address the harms which are linked to certain types of obscene materials. The prohibition of such materials was based on a belief that they had a detrimental impact on individuals exposed to them and consequently on society as a whole. Our understanding of the harms caused by these materials has developed considerably since that time; however, this does not detract from the fact that the purpose of this legislation remains, as it was in 1959, the protection of society from harms caused by the exposure to obscene materials.

. . . . .

A permissible shift in emphasis was built into the legislation when, as interpreted by the courts, it adopted the community standards test. Community standards as to what is harmful have changed since 1959.

This being the objective, is it pressing and substantial? Does the prevention of the harm associated with the dissemination of certain obscene materials constitute a sufficiently pressing and substantial concern to warrant a restriction on the freedom of expression? In this regard, it should be recalled that in *Keegstra, supra,* this court unanimously accepted that the prevention of the influence of hate propaganda on society at large was a legitimate objective. Dickson, C.J.C. wrote with respect to the changes in attitudes which exposure to hate propaganda can bring about (at p. 37):

> ... the alteration of views held by the recipients of hate propaganda may occur subtly, and is not always attendant upon conscious acceptance of the communicated ideas. Even if the message of hate propaganda is outwardly rejected, there is evidence that its premise of racial or religious inferiority may persist in a recipient's mind as an idea that holds some truth, an incipient effect not to be entirely discounted ...
>
> The threat to the self-dignity of target group members is thus matched by the possibility that prejudiced messages will gain some credence, with the attendant result of discrimination, and perhaps even violence, against minority groups in Canadian society.

This court has thus recognized that the harm caused by the proliferation of materials which seriously offend the values fundamental to our society is a substantial concern which justifies restricting the otherwise full exercise of the freedom of expression. In my view, the harm sought to be avoided in the case of the dissemination of obscene materials is similar. In the words of Nemetz, C.J.B.C. in *R. v. Red Hot Video Ltd.* (1985), 18 C.C.C. (3d) 1 at p. 8, 45 C.R. (3d) 36, 15 C.R.R. 206 (B.C.C.A.), there is a growing concern that the exploitation of women and children, depicted in publications and films can, in certain circumstances, lead to "abject and servile victimization". As Anderson, J.A. also noted in that same case, if true equality between male and female persons is to be achieved, we cannot ignore the threat to equality resulting from exposure to audiences of certain types of violent and degrading material. Materials portraying women as a class as objects for sexual exploitation and abuse have a negative impact on "the individual's sense of self-worth and acceptance".

In reaching the conclusion that legislation proscribing obscenity is a valid objective which justifies some encroachment of the right to freedom of expression, I am persuaded in part that such legislation may be found in most free and democratic societies. As Nemetz, C.J.B.C. aptly pointed out in *R. v. Red Hot Video, supra,* for centuries democratic societies have set certain limits to freedom of expression. He cited (at p. 5) the following passage of Dickson, J.A. (as he then was) in *R. v. Great West News Ltd., supra,* at p. 309:

> ... all organized societies have sought in one manner or another to suppress obscenity. The right of the state to legislate to protect its moral fibre and well-being has long been recognized, with roots deep in history. It is within this frame that the Courts and Judges must work.

The advent of the Charter did not have the effect of dramatically depriving Parliament of a power which it has historically enjoyed. It is also noteworthy that the criminalization of obscenity was considered to be compatible with the

Canadian Bill of Rights. As Dickson, J.A. stated in *R. v. Prairie Schooner News Ltd., supra*, at p. 271:

> Freedom of speech is not unfettered either in criminal law or civil law. *The Canadian Bill of Rights* was intended to protect, and does protect, basic freedoms of vital importance to all Canadians. It does not serve as a shield behind which obscene matter may be disseminated without concern for criminal consequences. The interdiction of the publications which are the subject of the present charges in no way trenches upon the freedom of expression which the *Canadian Bill of Rights* assures.

The enactment of the impugned provision is also consistent with Canada's international obligations (*Agreement for the Suppression of the Circulation of Obscene Publications and the Convention for the Suppression of the Circulation of and Traffic in Obscene Publications*).

Finally, it should be noted that the burgeoning pornography industry renders the concern even more pressing and substantial than when the impugned provisions were first enacted. I would therefore conclude that the objective of avoiding the harm associated with the dissemination of pornography in this case is sufficiently pressing and substantial to warrant some restriction on full exercise of the right to freedom of expression. The analysis of whether the measure is proportional to the objective must, in my view, be undertaken in light of the conclusion that the objective of the impugned section is valid only in so far as it relates to the harm to society associated with obscene materials. Indeed, the section as interpreted in previous decisions and in these reasons is fully consistent with that objective. The objective of maintaining conventional standards of propriety, independently of any harm to society, is no longer justified in light of the values of individual liberty which underlie the Charter. This, then, being the objective of s. 163, which I have found to be pressing and substantial, I must now determine whether the section is rationally connected and proportional to this objective. As outlined above, s.163(8) criminalizes the exploitation of sex and sex and violence, when, on the basis of the community test, it is undue. The determination of when such exploitation is undue is directly related to the immediacy of a risk of harm to society which is reasonably perceived as arising from its dissemination.

(c) *Proportionality*

(i) *General*

The proportionality requirement has three aspects:

(1) the existence of a rational connection between the impugned measures and the objective;
(2) minimal impairment of the right or freedom, and
(3) a proper balance between the effects of the limiting measures and the legislative objective.

In assessing whether the proportionality test is met, it is important to keep in mind the nature of expression which has been infringed. In the *Prostitution Reference, supra*, Dickson, C.J.C. wrote (at pp. 73-4):

> When a Charter freedom has been infringed by state action that takes the form of criminalization, the Crown bears the heavy burden of justifying that infringement. Yet, the expressive activity, as with any infringed Charter right should also be analysed in the particular context of the case. Here, the activity to which the impugned legislation is directed is expression with an economic purpose. It can hardly be said that communications regarding an economic transaction of sex for money lie at, or even near, the core of the guarantee of freedom of expression.

The values which underlie the protection of freedom of expression relate to the search for truth, participation in the political process, and individual self-fulfilment. The Attorney-General for Ontario argues that of these, only "individual self-fulfilment", and only in its most base aspect, that of physical arousal, is engaged by pornography. On the other hand, the civil liberties groups argue that pornography forces us to question conventional notions of sexuality and thereby launches us into an inherently political discourse. In their factum, the B.C. Civil Liberties Association adopts a passage from R. West, "The Feminist-Conservative Anti-Pornography Alliance and the 1986 Attorney General's Commission on Pornography Report", 4 *Am. Bar Found. Res. Jo.* 68 (1987), at p. 696:

> Good pornography has value because it validates women's will to pleasure. It celebrates female nature. It validates a range of female sexuality that is wider and truer than that legitimated by the non-pornographic culture. Pornography when it is good celebrates both female pleasure and male rationality.

A proper application of the test should not suppress what West refers to as "good pornography". The objective of the impugned provision is not to inhibit the celebration of human sexuality. However, it cannot be ignored that the realities of the pornography industry are far from the picture which the B.C. Civil Liberties Association would have us paint. Shannon, J., in *R. v. Wagner, supra*, described the materials more accurately when he observed (at p. 331):

> Women, particularly, are deprived of unique human character or identity and are depicted as sexual playthings, hysterically and instantly responsive to male sexual demands. They worship male genitals and their own value depends upon the quality of their genitals and breasts.

In my view, the kind of expression which is sought to be advanced does not stand on equal footing with other kinds of expression which directly engage the "core" of the freedom of expression values.

This conclusion is further buttressed by the fact that the targeted material is expression which is motivated, in the overwhelming majority of cases, by economic profit. This court held in *Rocket v. Royal College of Dental Surgeons of Ontario* (1990), 71 D.L.R. (4th) 68 at p. 79, [1990] 2 S.C.R. 232, 47 C.R.R. 193, that an economic motive for expression means that restrictions on the expression might "be easier to justify than other infringements".

I will now turn to an examination of the three basic aspects of the proportionality test.

(ii) *Rational connection*

The message of obscenity which degrades and dehumanizes is analogous to that of hate propaganda. As the Attorney-General of Ontario has argued in its factum, obscenity wields the power to wreak social damage in that a significant portion of the population is humiliated by its gross misrepresentations.

Accordingly, the rational link between s. 163 and the objective of Parliament relates to the actual causal relationship between obscenity and the risk of harm to society at large. On this point, it is clear that the literature of the social sciences remains subject to controversy. In *Fringe Product Inc., supra*, Charron, D.C.J. considered numerous written reports and works and heard six days of testimony from experts who endeavoured to describe the status of the social sciences with respect to the study of the effects of pornography. Charron, D.C.J. reached the conclusion that the relationship between pornography and harm was sufficient to justify Parliament's intervention. This conclusion is not supported unanimously.

The recent conclusions of the Fraser Report, *ibid.*, could not postulate any causal relationship between pornography and the commission of violent crimes, the sexual abuse of children, or the disintegration of communities and society. This is in contrast to the findings of the MacGuigan Report, *ibid.*

While a direct link between obscenity and harm to society may be difficult, if not impossible, to establish, it is reasonable to presume that exposure to images bears a causal relationship to changes in attitudes and beliefs. The Meese Commission Report, *ibid.*, concluded in respect of sexually violent material (vol. 1, at p. 326):

> ... the available evidence strongly supports the hypothesis that substantial exposure to sexually violent materials as described here bears a causal relationship to antisocial acts of sexual violence and, for some subgroups, possibly to unlawful acts of sexual violence.
>
> Although we rely for this conclusion on significant scientific empirical evidence, we feel it worthwhile to note the underlying logic of the conclusion. The evidence says simply that the images that people are exposed to bear a causal relationship to their behaviour. This is hardly surprising. What would be surprising would be to find otherwise, and we have not so found. We have not, of course, found that the images people are exposed to are a greater cause of sexual violence than all or even many other possible causes the investigation of which has been beyond our mandate. Nevertheless, it would be strange indeed if graphic representations of a form of behaviour, especially in a form that almost exclusively portrays such behaviour as desirable, did not have at least some effect on patterns of behaviour.

In the face of inconclusive social science evidence, the approach adopted by our court in *Irwin Toy* is instructive. In that case, the basis for the legislation was that television advertising directed at young children is *per se* manipulative. The court made it clear that in choosing its mode of intervention, it is sufficient that Parliament had a *reasonable basis* (at p. 626):

> In the instant case, the court is called upon to assess competing social science evidence respecting the appropriate means for addressing the problem of children's advertising. The question is whether the government had a reasonable basis, on the evidence tendered, for

concluding that the ban on all advertising directed at children impaired freedom of expression as little as possible given the government's pressing and substantial objective.

And at p. 623: "... the court also recognized that the government was afforded a margin of appreciation to form legitimate objectives based on somewhat inconclusive social science evidence".

Similarly, in *Keegstra, supra*, the absence of proof of a causative link between hate propaganda and hatred of an identifiable group was discounted as a determinative factor in assessing the constitutionality of the hate literature provisions of the *Criminal Code*. Dickson, C.J.C. stated (at pp. 58-9):

> First, to predicate the limitation of free expression upon proof of actual hatred gives insufficient attention to the severe psychological trauma suffered by members of those identifiable groups targeted by hate propaganda. Secondly, it is clearly difficult to prove a causative link between a specific statement and hatred of an identifiable group.

McLachlin, J. (dissenting) expressed it as follows (at pp. 118-9):

> To view hate propaganda as "victimless" in the absence of any proof that it moved its listeners to hatred is to discount the wrenching impact that it may have on members of the target group themselves ... Moreover, it is simply not possible to assess with any precision the effects that expression of a particular message will have on all those who are ultimately exposed to it.

The American approach on the necessity of a causal link between obscenity and harm to society was set out by Burger, C.J. in *Paris Adult Theatre I v. Slaton*, 413 U.S. 49 at pp. 60-1(1972): "Although there is no conclusive proof of a connection between antisocial behaviour and obscene material, the legislature ... could quite reasonably determine that such a connection does or might exist."

I am in agreement with Twaddle, J.A. who expressed the view that Parliament was entitled to have a "reasoned apprehension of harm" resulting from the desensitization of individuals exposed to materials which depict violence, cruelty, and dehumanization in sexual relations.

Accordingly, I am of the view that there is a sufficiently rational link between the criminal sanction, which demonstrates our community's disapproval of the dissemination of materials which potentially victimize women and which restricts the negative influence which such materials have on changes in attitudes and behaviour, and the objective.

Finally, I wish to distinguish this case from *Keegstra*, in which the minority adopted the view that there was no rational connection between the criminalization of hate propaganda and its suppression. As McLachlin, J. noted, prosecutions under the *Criminal Code* for racist expression have attracted extensive media coverage. The criminal process confers on the accused publicity for his or her causes and succeeds even in generating sympathy. The same cannot be said of the kinds of expression sought to be suppressed in the present case. The general availability of the subject materials and the rampant pornography industry are such that, in the words of Dickson, C.J.C. in *Keegstra*, "pornography is not dignified by its suppression". In contrast to the hate-monger who may succeed, by the sudden media attention, in gaining an audience, the prohibition of obscene materials does nothing to promote the pornographer's cause.

(iii) *Minimal impairment*

In determining whether less intrusive legislation may be imagined, this court stressed in the *Prostitution Reference, supra,* that it is not necessary that the legislative scheme be the "perfect" scheme, but that it be appropriately tailored *in the context of the infringed right* (at p. 75). Furthermore, in *Irwin Toy, supra,* Dickson, C.J.C., Lamer and Wilson, JJ. stated (at pp. 629-30):

> While evidence exists that other less intrusive options reflecting more modest objectives were available to the government, there is evidence establishing the necessity of a ban to meet the objectives the government had reasonably set. This court will not, in the name of minimal impairment, take a restrictive approach to social science evidence and require legislatures to choose the least ambitious means to protect vulnerable groups.

There are several factors which contribute to the finding that the provision minimally impairs the freedom which is infringed.

First, the impugned provision does not proscribe sexually explicit erotica without violence that is not degrading or dehumanizing. It is designed to catch material that creates a risk of harm to society. It might be suggested that proof of actual harm should be required. It is apparent from what I have said above that it is sufficient in this regard for Parliament to have a reasonable basis for concluding that harm will result and this requirement does not demand actual proof of harm.

Secondly, materials which have scientific, artistic or literary merit are not captured by the provision. As discussed above, the court must be generous in its application of the "artistic defence". For example, in certain cases, materials such as photographs, prints, books and films which may undoubtedly be produced with some motive for economic profit, may none the less claim the protection of the Charter in so far as their defining characteristic is that of aesthetic expression, and thus represent the artist's attempt at individual fulfilment. The existence of an accompanying economic motive does not, of itself, deprive a work of significance as an example of individual artistic or self-fulfilment.

Thirdly, in considering whether the provision minimally impairs the freedom in question, it is legitimate for the court to take into account Parliament's past abortive attempts to replace the definition with one that is more explicit. In *Irwin Toy* our court recognized that it is legitimate to take into account the fact that earlier laws and proposed alternatives were thought to be less effective than the legislation that is presently being challenged The attempt to provide exhaustive instances of obscenity has been shown to be destined to fail (Bill C-54, 2nd Sess., 33rd Part.). It seems that the only practicable alternative is to strive towards a more abstract definition of obscenity which is contextually sensitive and responsive to progress in the knowledge and understanding of the phenomenon to which the legislation is directed. In my view, the standard of "undue exploitation" is therefore appropriate. The intractable nature of the problem and the impossibility of precisely defining a notion which is inherently elusive makes the possibility of a more explicit provision remote. In this light, it is appropriate to question whether, and at what cost, greater legislative precision can be demanded.

Fourthly, while the discussion in this appeal has been limited to the definition portion of s. 163, I would note that the impugned section, with the possible exception of s-s. (1) which is not in issue here, has been held by this court not to extend its reach to the private use or viewing of obscene materials. *R. v. Rioux*, [1970] 3 C.C.C. 149, 10 D.L.R. (3d) 196, [1969] S.C.R. 599, unanimously upheld the finding of the Quebec Court of Appeal that s. 163.(2) (then s. 150(2)) does not include the private viewing of obscene materials. Hall, J. affirmed the finding of Pratte, J. (at pp. 151-2, translation):

> "If exposing to 'public view' is mentioned in s-s. (2)(a), it is because the legislator intended that this and, not a private showing, should constitute a crime.
>
> "I would therefore say that showing obscene pictures to a friend or projecting an obscene film in one's own home is not in itself a crime nor is it enough to establish intention of circulating them nor help to prove such an intention."

This court also cited with approval the words of Hyde, J. (at p. 152):

> "Before I am prepared to hold that private use of written matter or pictures within an individual's residence may constitute a criminal offence, I require a much more specific text of law than we are now dealing with. It would have been very simple for Parliament to have included the word 'exhibit' in this section if it had wished to cover this situation."

Accordingly, it is only the public distribution and exhibition of obscene materials which is in issue here.

Finally, I wish to address the arguments of the interveners, Canadian Civil Liberties Association and Manitoba Association for Rights and Liberties, that the objectives of this kind of legislation may be met by alternative, less intrusive measures. First, it is submitted that reasonable time, manner and place restrictions would be preferable to outright prohibition. I am of the view that this argument should be rejected. Once it has been established that the objective is the avoidance of harm caused by the degradation which many women feel as "victims" of the message of obscenity, and of the negative impact exposure to such material has on perceptions and attitudes towards women, it is untenable to argue that these harms could be avoided by placing restrictions on access to such material. Making the materials more difficult to obtain by increasing their cost and reducing their availability does not achieve the same objective. Once Parliament has reasonably concluded that certain acts are harmful to certain groups in society and to society in general, it would be inconsistent, if not hypocritical, to argue that such acts could be committed in more restrictive conditions. The harm sought to be avoided would remain the same in either case.

It is also submitted that there are more effective techniques to promote the objectives of Parliament. For example, if pornography is seen as encouraging violence against women, there are certain activities which discourage it —

counselling rape victims to charge their assailants, provision of shelter and assistance for battered women, campaigns for laws against discrimination on the grounds of sex, education to increase the sensitivity of law enforcement agencies and other governmental authorities. In addition, it is submitted that education is an under-used response.

It is noteworthy that many of the above suggested alternatives are in the form of *responses* to the harm engendered by negative attitudes against women. The role of the impugned provision is to control the dissemination of the very images that contribute to such attitudes. Moreover, it is true that there are additional measures which could alleviate the problem of violence against women. However, given the gravity of the harm, and the threat to the values at stake, I do not believe that the measure chosen by Parliament is equalled by the alternatives which have been suggested. Education, too, may offer a means of combating negative attitudes to women, just as it is currently used as a means of addressing other problems dealt with in the *Code*. However, there is no reason to rely on education alone. It should be emphasized that this is in no way intended to deny the value of other educational and counselling measures to deal with the roots and effects of negative attitudes. Rather, it is only to stress the arbitrariness and unacceptability of the claim that such measures represent the sole legitimate means of addressing the phenomenon. Serious social problems such as violence against women require multi-pronged approaches by government. Education and legislation are not alternatives but complements in addressing such problems. There is nothing in the Charter which requires Parliament to choose between such complementary measures.

(iv) *Balance between effects of limiting measures and legislative objective*

The final question to be answered in the proportionality test is whether the effects of the law so severely trench on a protected right that the legislative objective is outweighed by the infringement. The infringement on freedom of expression is confined to a measure designed to prohibit the distribution of sexually explicit materials accompanied by violence, and those without violence that are degrading or dehumanizing. As I have already concluded, this kind of expression lies far from the core of the guarantee of freedom of expression. It appeals only to the most base aspect of individual fulfilment, and it is primarily economically motivated.

The objective of the legislation, on the other hand, is of fundamental importance in a free and democratic society. It is aimed at avoiding harm, which Parliament has reasonably concluded will be caused directly or indirectly, to individuals, groups such as women and children, and consequently to society as a whole, by the distribution of these materials. It thus seeks to enhance respect for all members of society, and non-violence and equality in their relations with each other.

I therefore conclude that the restriction on freedom of expression does not outweigh the importance of the legislative objective.

5. *Conclusion*

I conclude that while s. 163(8) infringes s. 2(b) of the Charter, freedom of expression, it constitutes a reasonable limit and is saved by virtue of the provisions of s. 1. The trial judge convicted the appellant only with respect to materials which contained scenes involving violence or cruelty intermingled with sexual activity or depicted lack of consent to sexual contact or otherwise could be said to dehumanize men or women in a sexual context. The majority of the Court of Appeal, on the other hand, convicted the appellant on all charges.

While the trial judge concluded that the material for which the accused were acquitted was not degrading or dehumanizing, he did so in the context of s. 1 of the Charter. In effect, he asked himself whether, if the material was proscribed by s. 163(8), that section would still be supportable under s. 1. In this context, he considered the government objectives of s. 163(8) and measured the material which was the subject of the charges against this objective. The findings at trial were therefore made in a legal framework that is different from that outlined in these reasons. Specifically, in considering whether the materials were degrading or dehumanizing, he did not address the issue of harm. Accordingly, it would be speculation to conclude that the same result would have been obtained if the definition of obscenity contained in these reasons had been applied. The test applied by the majority of the Court of Appeal also differed significantly from these reasons. I therefore cannot accept their conclusion that all of the materials are obscene. Accordingly, I would allow the appeal and direct a new trial on all charges. I note, however, that I am in agreement with Wright, J.'s conclusion that, in the case of material found to be obscene, there should only be one conviction imposed with respect to a single tape. I would answer the constitutional questions as follows:

> *Question 1.* Does s. 163 of the *Criminal Code of Canada*, R.S.C., 1985 c. C-46, violate s. 2(b) of the *Canadian Charter of Rights and Freedoms?*

Answer: Yes.

> *Question 2.* If s. 163 of the *Criminal Code* of Canada, R.S.C., 1985 c. C-46, violates s. 2(b) of the *Canadian Charter of Rights and Freedoms* can s. 163 of the *Criminal Code* of Canada be demonstrably justified under s. 1 of the *Canadian Charter of Rights and Freedoms* as a reasonable limit prescribed by law?

Answer: Yes.

4.4.9.2 *Popert et al v. R.* (1981), 19 C.R. (3d) 393 (Ont. C.A.)

ZUBER, J.A.: — The appellants were charged that in 1977 they made use of the mails for the purpose of transmitting indecent, immoral or scurrilous matter contrary to s.164 of the *Criminal Code*, R.S.C. 1970, c.C-34. The case was tried in the Provincial Court before Harris, Prov. J., who acquitted the appellants [45 C.C.C. (2d) 385].

The Crown appealed to Ferguson, Co. Ct. J., who disagreed with Harris, Prov. J. on a number of legal issues. He set aside the acquittal and ordered a new trial [51 C.C.C. (2d) 485]. The appellants appeal to this court seeking a reversal of Ferguson, Co. Ct. J.'s order and a restoration of the verdict of acquittal.

The Facts

The facts in this case are disarmingly simple. The appellants Popert, Jackson and Hannon are all officers of the corporate appellant, Pink Triangle Press, which publishes a newspaper entitled *The Body Politic*. The December 1977-January 1978 issue of this publication (Ex. 1), which is the subject of this prosection, was sent through the mails to subscribers in Canada and the United States. The subscribers, it is conceded, are homosexuals. The publication addresses itself to that readership.

Exhibit I contains an article entitled "Men Loving Boys Loving Men". The central figures of this article are apparently fictional characters named Peter, Barry and Simon. The article describes the relationship of these men with young boys, and particularly acts of buggery and gross indecency, and concludes that "they ... deserve our praise, our admiration and our support".

It is appropriate to mention at this point that no issue is taken in this court as to whether the personal appellants were insulated from criminal responsibility by the corporate appellant.

While the facts are not complicated, they have spawned a number of troublesome legal issues. Both of the learned judges who have thus far dealt with this case have responded to the problems by the delivery of detailed written reasons.

Harris, Prov. J. placed the acquittal of the appellants on four grounds. These grounds are:

(a) Section 164 is not aimed at the distribution by mail of magazines or journals to subscribers;

(b) There is insufficient evidence to establish a community standard;

(c) The word "immoral" in s. 164, being undefined, does not establish an acceptable area for a lawful action; and

(d) Exhibit 1, as a whole or in part, is not indecent.

On the hearing of this appeal, Mr. Ruby argued (and I agree) that it was not necessary that Harris, Prov. J. be right on every issue. A single valid reason for acquittal is sufficient and if one can be found the acquittal should be restored. I propose to deal in turn with each of the four reasons for acquittal.

(a) The purpose of s.164

Section 164 of the *Criminal Code* is as follows:

164. Every one commits an offence who makes use of the mails for the purpose of transmitting or delivering anything that is obscene, indecent, immoral or scurrilous, but this section does not apply to a person who makes use of the mails for the purpose of transmitting or delivering anything mentioned in subsection 162(4).

(Note: The section is now s. 168, R.S.C. 1985, c. C-46.)

Harris, Prov. J. was of the view that this section was not designed to catch the kind of distribution of mailed material that occurred in this case, but was designed to catch the sick individual who, rather than indulging in obscene telephone calls, indulges in obscene, indecent, immoral or scurrilous mailing.

I find no basis for such a restriction on this section. By its own plain words, it applies to *everyone* who makes use of the mails in the manner prohibited by the section.

(b) *Community standards*

It is apparent that the real issue in this case is whether the article "Men Loving Boys Loving Men" published in *The Body Politic* is immoral or indecent. (I leave aside the term "scurrilous" as having no application to the facts of this case.)

The determination of what is immoral or indecent is to be determined by a judge, not by reference to his own standards of indecency or immorality but by reference to a community standard. I defer, for the moment, the exact nature of the community standards test. The learned trial judge, however, was of the opinion that there rested on the Crown an obligation to produce evidence and prove a community standard. In his reasons for judgment he said at p. 400:

"... in this case the trial Judge must determine on the evidence what is the community standard of acceptance of material that is or may be indecent, immoral or scurrilous."

And, at p. 403:

"I am of the opinion that all in all the evidence adduced from the majority of both Crown and Defence witnesses establishes nothing which really assists the Court in ascertaining the limits of community tolerance ..."

And at p. 411:

"In the result, therefore, I, having found ... that there is insufficient evidence to establish a community standard. ... it follows that each of the accused is not guilty of this charge ..."

In my view, the learned trial judge was in error. The reference to a community standard imports an objective test into the ascertainment of indecency and immorality and, while evidence with respect to community standards is admissible and sometimes helpful, it is not a fact which the Crown is obliged to prove as a part of its case: see *R. v. Prairie Schooner News Ltd.* (1970), 75 W.W.R. 585, 12 Cr. L.Q. 462, 1 C.C.C. (2d) 251 (Man. C.A.); *R. v. Great West News Ltd.*, 10 C.R.N.S. 42, 72 W.W.R. 354, [1970] 4 C.C.C. 307 (Man. C.A.).

(c) Immoral

In turning his attention to the word "immoral" as used in s. 164, Harris, Prov. J. expressed the view that he could find no legally enforceable meaning in the term "immoral" and, as a result, Ex. I could not be legally immoral. I concede that the term "immoral" is a word of imprecise meaning and that it may be difficult to apply. However, the problem is not unique. Often the law, whether a product of case law or statute, expresses itself in imprecise terms such as "reasonable", "undue", and "dangerous" . It is through such words that the values of the community find expression in the courtroom. It is the function of the courts to work as best as they can with the tools in hand. In my view, the learned trial judge was wrong in simply finding no meaning in this word.

(d) Indecent

As his final reason for acquittal, Harris, Prov. J. held that using the "ordinary meaning" of the word "indecent" he could not find that Ex. 1 was indecent. It is at this point that Mr. Ruby presents his most forceful argument. It is his position that if Harris, Prov. J. was right in finding that the material was not indecent then, in the circumstances of this case, neither could the impugned material be immoral. Further, the errors with respect to other issues then become unimportant and the Crown's case must fail.

I begin by observing that Ferguson, Co. Ct. J. did not, as he might have done, simply disagree with Harris, Prov. J. as to the assessment of the publication. Instead, he dealt with certain matters of law involved in the determination of whether or not Ex. 1 was indecent.

In his approach to the issue of indecency, Harris, Prov. J. began by dealing with the publication as a whole. This was an error. It was the specific article that was the focus of this case. In some instances an otherwise indecent part of a single work, such as a novel, may be redeemed by the artistic necessity to maintain the integrity of a plot or story line. Exhibit 1 is not a single work. It is a newspaper containing a variety of material that has no connection with the impugned article. In *R. v. Penthouse Internat. Ltd.* (1979), 46 C.C.C. (2d) 111 (Ont. C.A.), Weatherston, J.A. dealt with a magazine and said at p. 117:

"Each page must be looked at more or less in isolation from the others, for it is but rarely that a reader of a magazine will start at the beginning and read through to the end. Offensive passages or pictorial presentations in a magazine cannot be saved merely by surrounding them with profound articles on foreign policy."

That principle applies here.

In his concluding paragraph, however, the trial judge stated that he found that the term "indecent" did not apply either to Ex. I as a whole or *the article therein primarily objected to by the Crown*. In this conclusion, as well, there was error in law. In dealing with the term "indecent", he purported to apply "the ordinary meaning" of the term. He had earlier found insufficient evidence to establish a community standard and, as a result, discarded that concept. I agree with Ferguson, Co. Ct. J. that the trial judge's conclusion, reached upon a test which ignored the community standards test, must be open to doubt. I further agree with Ferguson, Co. Ct. J. that, as a result of the legal errors which occurred, the verdict of acquittal is vitiated and, as a result, the order directing a new trial must stand.

There remains, however, one further issue. In directing a new trial, Ferguson Co. Ct. J. directed his attention to the community standards test to be applied in determining whether the impugned material is either indecent or immoral. He came to the conclusion that the appropriate measure of the terms "immoral" or "indecent" was the community standard of immorality or indecency. He rejected the community standard of tolerance as the appropriate test in determining the application of these terms.

In cases dealing with obscenity, it is now accepted that the appropriate test is the community standard of tolerance: see *R. v. Penthouse Internat. Ltd., supra; R. v. Sudbury News Service Ltd.* (1978), 18 O.R. (2d) 428, 39 C.C.C. (2d) 1 (C.A.); and *R. v. Prairie Schooner News Ltd., supra.* In my respectful view, the same test should be applied in determining whether material is immoral or indecent. In *R. v. Prairie Schooner News Ltd.*, Dickson, J.A. (as he then was) said at p. 269:

> In the *Great West News* case, we referred to contemporary standards of tolerance. I have no doubt, as Dr. Rich testified, and as the judge agreed, a distinction can be made between private taste and standard of tolerance. It can hardly be questioned that many people would find personally offensive, material which they would permit others to read. Parliament, through its legislation on obscenity, could hardly have wished to proscribe as criminal that which was acceptable or tolerable according to current standards of the Canadian community.

Although those words were written within the context of the case dealing with obscenity, in my view they apply with equal validity to the terms "indecent" and "immoral" in this case. Further, the advantage of a consistent test in the application of these various terms is not insignificant.

For the foregoing reasons this appeal is dismissed.

Appeal dismissed.

Note: A new trial was held, as ordered. At this trial the accused were acquitted again. The Crown again appealed to the County Court which ordered another new trial. The accused appealed this ruling to the Court of Appeal, which again upheld the County Court. The third trial has yet to be held.

4.4.10 *Canada Post Corporation Act*, R.S.C. 1985, c. C-10

Use of Mails for Unlawful Purposes

43. (1) Where the Minister believes on reasonable grounds that any person
   (*a*) is, by means of the mails,
      (i) committing or attempting to commit an offence, or

542   A SOURCEBOOK OF CANADIAN MEDIA LAW

(ii) aiding, counselling or procuring any person to commit an offence, or
(b) with intent to commit an offence, is using the mails for the purpose of accomplishing his object,

the Minister may make an order (in this section . . . called an "interim prohibitory order") prohibiting the delivery, without the consent of the Minister, of mail addressed to or posted by that person (in this section . . . called the "person affected").

4.4.10.1 *Luscher v. Deputy Minister, Revenue Canada, Customs and Excise* (1985), 45 C.R. (3d) 81 (F.C.A.)

Annotation

Before the advent of the Charter, void for uncertainty was a well-recognized ground of challenge to by-law offences (see, for example, *Harrison v. Toronto* (1982), 39 O.R. (2d) 721, 31 C.R. (3d) 244, 19 M.P.L.R. 310, 140 D.L.R. (3d) 309 (H.C.)), but our courts had recoiled from its availability in the case of other types of criminal sanction. In *R. v. Pink Triangle Press* (1979), 45 C.C.C. (2d) 385 (Ont. Prov. Ct.) Harris, Prov. J. held that the undefined term "immoral" in s. 164 of the *Criminal Code* was so "ambiguous and indefinite" (p. 407) that it had "no legally enforceable meaning" (p. 408). This decision was, however, soon reversed (51 C.C.C. (2d) 485 (Co. Ct.)) and on further appeal the Ontario Court of Appeal (19 C.R. (3d) 393 (sub nom. *Popert v. R.*), 58 C.C.C. (2d) 505) confirmed that the trial judge had erred. On behalf of the court Zuber, J.A. agreed that the meaning of "immoral" was imprecise but observing that the courts often had to interpret imprecise terms such as "reasonable", "undue" and "dangerous", held at p. 398 that the courts had "to work as best they can with the tools in hand".

Now various Courts of Appeal have held that a Charter right or freedom cannot be subject to a reasonable limit prescribed by law under s. 1 if that law is too vague. In adopting in this context the complex United States doctrine of "void for vagueness", our courts have now opened a "Pandora's box of constitutional concepts": see Mansell's annotation to *Ont. Film & Video Appreciation Soc. v. Ont. Bd. of Censors* (1983), 34 C.R. (3d) 74, at p. 74. The ruling of the Divisional Court of the Ontario Supreme Court in *Ont. Film & Video Appreciation Soc. v. Ont. Bd. of Censors* (1983), 41 O.R. (2d) 583, 34 C.R. (3d) 73 at 83, 147 D.L.R. (3d) 58, 5 C.R.R. 373, was *obiter* — as it was held that a non-binding set of guidelines promulgated by pamphlet were not capable of being law, a decision that was confirmed by the Ontario Court of Appeal, 45 O.R. (2d) 80, 38 C.R. (3d) 271, 5 D.L.R. (4th) 766, 7 C.R.R. 120, 2 O.A.C. 388. Now, however, there is express authority for the void for vagueness approach to the concept of reasonable limits in the decisions of the British Columbia Court of Appeal in *R. v. Red Hot Video Ltd.*, ante, p. 36, and *R. v. Robson*, ante, p. 68, also 31 M.V.R. 220, and by the Federal Court of Appeal in *Luscher*. The rulings that our existing obscenity laws are not too vague — express in *Red Hot Video* and obiter in

Luscher — now seem ironic in view of the level of complexity characterizing the Supreme Court of Canada judgments in *Towne Cinema Theatres Ltd. v. R.*, ante, p. 1 also [1984] 4 W.W.R. 1.

Don Stuart

HUGESSEN, J.: The principal thrust of the appeal to this court is not against the decision of the deputy minister, which was confirmed by Anderson, Co. Ct. J., but against the legislation under which that decision was reached. The appellant argues that tariff item 99201-1 is an infringement upon the freedoms protected by s.2(*b*) of the *Canadian Charter of Rights and Freedoms* and, as such, inoperative as not being saved by the excepting words of s.1. The appellant does not argue that Parliament could not prohibit or regulate the importation of material of this sort, commonly described as "smut", but rather that the prohibition as drawn in the legislation is invalid. I am in agreement with that submission.

Tariff item 99201-1, read in conjunction with s. 14 of the *Customs Tariff*, prohibits the importation of:

> Books, printed paper, drawings, paintings, prints, photographs or representations of any kind of a treasonable or seditious, or of an immoral or indecent character.

Section 2(b) of the Charter enshrines and protects as "fundamental" freedoms:

> (*b*) freedom of thought, belief, opinion and expression, including freedom of the press and other media of communication.

That a prohibition whose first object is "books" is prima facie an infringement of the freedoms protected by s.2(b) appears to me to be a proposition not requiring demonstration.

No freedom, however, can be absolute and those guaranteed by the Charter are no exception. They are, by s. 1, subject to:

> 1 ... such reasonable limits prescribed by law as can be demonstrabiy justified in a free and democratic society.

That text, in its turn, makes it clear enough that the task of demonstrating the justification for a limitation of a protected freedom falls upon government: see *Re Southam Inc. and R.* (1983), 41 O.R. (2d) 113, 34 C.R. (3d) 27, 33 R.F.L. (2d) 279, 3 C.C.C. (3d) 515, 146 D.L.R. (3d) 408, 6 C.R.R. I (C.A.); *Re Germany (Fed. Republic) and Rauca* (1983), 41 O.R. (2d) 225, 34 C.R. (3d) 97 (sub nom. *R. v. Rauca*), 4 C.C.C. (3d) 385, 145 D.L.R. (3d) 638, 4 C.R.R. 42 (C.A.).

. . . . .

What has to be determined today is whether the words of tariff item 99201-1, together with any judicial gloss which has been placed on them; are sufficiently clear to constitute a "reasonable limit prescribed by law".

The first observation to be made in this regard is that the words "immoral" and "indecent" are nowhere defined in the legislation. This at once serves to distinguish the provisions of tariff item 99201-1 from the obscenity provisions of the *Criminal Code*, which contains in s.159(8) words which might be thought to give to those provisions sufficient certainty and particularity.

Secondly, the words "immoral" and "indecent" are highly subjective and emotional in their content. Opinions honestly held by reasonable people will vary widely. The current public debate on abortion has its eloquent and persuasive adherents on both sides arguing that their view alone is moral, that of their opponents immoral. Standards of decency also vary even (or perhaps especially) amongst judges. The case of *R. v. P.*, 3 C.R.N.S. 302, 63 W.W.R. 222, [1968] 3 C.C.C. 129 (Man. C.A.), provides an interesting example of a learned and articulate debate between the present Chief Justices of Canada and Manitoba respectively as to whether an act of heterosexual fellatio performed in private (such as Ex. I herein depicts, amongst other things) was grossly indecent. (The case was, of course, decided prior to the enactment of the present s.158 of the *Criminal Code*, by which Parliament legislated an end to the controversy.)

While obscenity under the *Criminal Code* is, by statutory definition, limited to matters predominantly sexual, there is no such limitation upon the concepts of immorality or indecency, and this is so notwithstanding the judicial gloss which has carried over into the test for immorality or indecency the test of community standards of tolerance. As stated by Lord Reid in *Knuller v. D.P.P.*, [1973] A.C. 435 at 458, [1972] 3 W.L.R. 143, 56 Cr. App. R. 633 (H.L.):

> Indecency is not confined to sexual indecency: indeed it is difficult to find any limit short of saying that it includes anything which an ordinary decent man or woman would find to be shocking, disgusting and revolting.

While it is, of course, true that the judicial overlay of the community standards of tolerance test has done something to reduce the inherent subjectivity of the words "immoral" and "indecent", this has, if anything, had the effect of increasing their uncertainty. Community standards themselves are in a constant state of flux and vary widely from place to place within the country. Yet the courts are obliged to apply a contemporary and nationwide standard.

. . . . .

I would add that it is, of course, no answer to the argument that a limitation on freedom is so vague as to be unreasonable to say that this publication or that is so immoral or indecent that it clearly falls afoul of the prohibition. One might as well argue that the Tale of Peter Rabbit was clearly not immoral or indecent and could therefore be admitted. Even the most defective provision is unlikely to be so vague as not to permit the placing of some cases on one side of the line or the other. What is significant is the size and importance of the grey area between the two extremes. Vagueness or uncertainty, like unreasonableness, are not themselves absolutes but tests by which the courts must measure the acceptability of limits upon Charter-protected freedoms.

Finally, let it be quite clear that what the Charter protects in s.2(b) is not acts or deeds but thought, expression and depiction. While the activities shown in the subject magazine are probably, as far as one can determine, legal, it would make no difference if they were crimes. The depiction of murder, real or imagined, is protected by s.2(b), but that does not mean that the Charter has declared open season for assassination.

I conclude that, insofar as it prohibits the importation of matters of immoral or indecent character, tariff item 99201 - 1 is not a reasonable limitation upon the freedoms guaranteed by s.2(b) of the Charter and is of no force or effect.

4.4.11 *Customs Tariff*, R.S.C. 1970, c. C-41, as am. S.C. 1984-85, c. 12

1. Tariff item 99201-1 of Schedule C to the *Customs Tariff* is repealed and the following substituted therefor:

"99201-1 Books, printed paper, drawings, paintings, prints, photographs or representations of any kind

(*a*) of a treasonable or seditious character;

(*b*) that are deemed to be obscene under subsection 159(8) of the *Criminal Code*; or

(*c*) that constitute hate propaganda within the meaning of subsection 281.3(8) of the *Criminal Code*."

2. Tariff item 99201 - 1, as enacted by section 1, shall cease to have effect on June 30, 1986.

In 1993 the following item was added to the *Customs Tariff* by S.C. 1993, c. 46.

9968 Photographic, film, video or other visual representations, whether or not made by mechanical or electronic means, that are child pornography within the meaning of section 163.1 of the *Criminal Code*.

4.4.12 A Note on Provincial Movie Censorship Laws

All the provinces and the territories, except Prince Edward Island, have passed legislation dealing with the exhibition of films. In 1986, Prince Edward Island repealed the *Entertainments Act*, R.S.P.E.I. 1974, c.E-7. See the following: *Amusements Act*, R.S.A. 1980, c.A-41; *Motion Picture Act*, S.B.C. 1986, c.17; *Amusements Act*, R.S.M. 1987, c.A70; *Theatres, Cinematographs and Amusements Act*, R.S.N.B. 1973 c.T-5; *The Censoring of Moving Pictures Act*, R.S.N. 1990, c.C-5; *Theatres and Amusements Act*, R.S.N.S. 1989, c.466; *Theatres Act*, R.S.O. 1990, c.T-6; *Cinema Act*, R.S.Q. 1984, c.18-1; *Film and Video Classification Act*, R.S.S. 1984-85-86, c.F-13.2; *Motion Pictures Ordinance*, C.O.Y.T. 1978, c.M-10; *Motion Pictures Act*, R.S.N.W.T. 1988, c.M-15. The provisions of the above Acts that deal specifically with censorship of films will be highlighted in the following note.

1. Alberta

The *Amusements Act*, R.S.A. 1980, c.A-41 is typical of the other provincial film censorship laws. A censor, or board of censors, of up to three persons, with the power to "permit or prohibit the exhibition of any film in Alberta" may be appointed by the Lieutenant Governor in Council (sections 9 and 10(1)). Any film which the censor permits to be exhibited must bear his/or her stamp of approval (s.12). A film not bearing such a stamp may be seized and confiscated (s.16). Under s. 15(1), "any film to be exhibited by or on behalf of an educational organization" may be exempt from censorship. And an appeal from the censor's decision is provided for in s. 10(2).

The Lieutenant Governor in Council may make various regulations including "prescribing that all or any of the advertising or other matter be submitted to the censor and not be used within Alberta except with his or their approval" (s.23(m)(iii)).

Anyone who contravenes "the Act or regulations is guilty of an offence and liable to a fine of not more than $200 and in default of payment to imprisonment for a term not exceeding 6 months" (s.22).

2. British Columbia

The appointment of a "film classification director, together with other employees" is not specifically stated in the *Motion Picture Act*. The director is appointed under the *Public Service Act*. Of the various powers given to the director in s. 5, "the director shall, before approving a motion picture submitted under section 2 (1) or 3 (1), remove or require the removal of, by erasure or otherwise, any portion of it . . . "(s.5(3)). Section 5(6) provides that "where the director reviews a motion picture . . . he shall, unless he takes action under subsection (3) or (4) . . . approve the motion picture, and . . . where the motion picture is intended to be exhibited in a theatre, classify the motion picture in accordance with the regulations made under section 14 (c)" Further, section 7 provides that "[t]he director may require that advertising material contain . . . words describing the classification of the motion picture, and . . . other comments that the director considers advisable".

Before any film is publicly exhibited or displayed in a movie theatre in British Columbia it must first be submitted to the director for approval (s.2(1)) unless an exemption is available under ss. 1, 2 (6) or 4 (1) . Section 1 provides that the definition of a "motion picture distributor" "does not include . . . a public library . . . a university . . . an educational institution approved by the Minister of Education where the films is distributed for educational purposes . . . the government of British Columbia, or . . . the government of Canada" . Section 2 (6) provides that "[t]his section does not apply to the exhibition of a motion picture for educational purposes . . . to a university or at another educational institution approved by the Minister of Education, or . . . under the auspices of the government of British Columbia or Canada" . Section 4 (1) states that " [t]he director may, in the public interest, exempt from section 2 a non-profit cultural organization, membership of which is by annual subscription and is limited to persons who are not less than 18 years of age, where the director considers that the organization has as its objects the encouragement and appreciation of motion pictures as a medium of art, information or education, subject to any conditions contained in the exemption"...

Section 2 (4) provides that " [b]efore a motion picture distributor distributes a motion picture for the purpose of exhibition in a theatre, he shall attach, in a manner determined by the director, a certificate or some other evidence of approval, satisfactory to the director, to the film or film casing and to all copies of the motion picture that are intended for exhibition" . The director may also " impose conditions on his approval of a motion picture submitted under section 2 (1) including conditions . . . that any advertising material in connection with the exhibition of the motion picture be submitted to the director for approval" (s. 5 (7) (c)) . Any "decision, order or prohibition of the director" may be appealed (s. 11(1)) .

Under s. 13 the Lieutenant Governor in Council may make various "regulations including regulations

(c) prescribing a classification scheme, for the purposes of section 5(6), that he considers necessary for motion pictures that are exhibited in theatres,

. . . . .

(g) respecting the use and display of advertising material in connection with motion pictures or their exhibition".

Section 13(2) states that "[a] person who . . . contravenes an order of the director made under this Act or under the regulations . . . commits an offence and is liable to a fine of not more than $10 000 or to imprisonment for not more than 6 months, or to both".

In addition, the director may suspend or cancel the licence held by a person who contravenes the Act, the regulations or an order of the director, or is convicted of an offence under the Act (s.8(2)).

3. Manitoba

The Lieutenant Governor in Council may appoint a film classification board of "not fewer than sixteen members" under s. 14 of the *Amusements Act*, R.S.M. 1987, c.A-70. The board is empowered to classify all films prior to their exhibition in the province and to control and regulate the advertising of films (s.23 as amended by S.M. 1991-92, c.7). Before they are exhibited, all films must be inspected and classified by the board (s.42(1)). Under s. 36, the board may review any film at any time, cancel the original certificate of classification and issue a new one. Any film exhibited or brought into Manitoba for exhibition that does not bear the board's classification or does not comply with the Act or regulations in some other way may be seized and confiscated (s.51(1)(f)). An appeal lies from any ruling or decision of the board (s.39(1)).

The Lieutenant Governor in Council may make regulations under s. 52(f) (as amended by S.M. 1991-92, c.7) governing the advertising of film; and s. 53(m) (as amended by S.M. 1991-92, c.7) generally, for the purpose of giving effect to the purposes of the Act.

Section 44 lays out the general penalty for contravention of the act or regulations:

> Every person who wilfully
>
> (*a*) contravenes any provision of this Act or the regulations; or
>
> (*b*) hinders or misleads a person authorized to carry out an investigation or inspection under this Act; or
>
> (*c*) furnishes false information to a person referred to in clause (b); or
>
> (*d*) withholds, conceals or destroys anything relevant to the subject matter of an investigation under this Act; or
>
> (*e*) hinders or prevents the board from effectively carrying out its duties and powers under this Act; or
>
> (*f*) fails, refuses or neglects to comply with a decision or order of the board;
>
> is guilty of an offence, and in addition to any other penalty provided by this Act, is liable, on summary conviction, to a fine not exceeding $5,000. and to such costs as may be awarded by the court.

4. Newfoundland

In its entirety, the *Censoring of Moving Pictures Act*, R.S.N. 1990, c.C-5 provides:

1. This Act may be cited as the *Censoring of Moving Pictures Act*.

2. (1) The Lieutenant-Governor in Council may appoint a board consisting of 3 persons, to be called the board of censors.

(2) A majority of members of the board of censors shall be a quorum.

3. (1) The board of censors, or a member of the board, may enter a building or place where an exhibition of moving pictures is carried on for the purpose of inspecting and passing upon the fitness for public exhibition of a moving or stationary picture, films or slides used or displayed in that building or place.

(2) A person hindering or obstructing a member of the board of censors in the performance of his or her duty under subsection (1) shall on summary conviction be liable to a fine not exceeding $100, or, in default of payment, to imprisonment for a period not exceeding 2 months.

4. (1) A quorum of the members of the board of censors present at an exhibition may, by oral or written notification to the proprietor of that exhibition or to the person operating the projection machine at the exhibition, summarily prohibit the exhibition of a moving or stationary picture, film or slide which they consider to be injurious to the morals of the public, or against the public welfare, or offensive to the public.

(2) The proprietor or operator exhibiting a film or slide referred to in subsection (1) after the receipt of the notification, is guilty of an offence against this Act, and is liable on

summary conviction, for each offence, to a fine not exceeding $100, or, in default of payment, to imprisonment for a period not exceeding 2 months.

5. Nova Scotia

Pursuant to s. 5(1) of the *Theatres and Amusements Act*, R.S.N.S. 1989, c.466 the Governor in Council may set up an Amusements Regulation Board, consisting of one or more people. The Board

> may, in accordance with the criteria prescribed by the regulations, permit or prohibit ... the use of exhibition in the Province, or in any part or parts thereof, for public entertainment of any film (s.5(2)(a));

and

> classify a film (s.5(3)(a)).

Regulations may be made by the Governor in Council under s. 4 (1):

> (*b*) regulating and licensing or prohibiting
> (i) any performance or performances in a theatre or theatres,
> (ii) any amusement or amusements or recreation or recreations in a place or places of amusement, and
> (iii) any amusement or amusements or recreation or recreations for participating or indulging in which, by the public or some of them, fees are charged by any amusement owner;
> (*c*) prescribing criteria in accordance with which the Board may exercise its powers.

General penalties for contravention of the Act are provided for in s. 26 (1).

> Where the Board is satisfied after due inquiry that any film exchange or theatre owner has violated this Act or any regulations made hereunder the Board may:
> (*a*) revoke or cancel any licence of such film exchange;
> (*b*) revoke or cancel any licence of such theatre owner; or
> (*c*) attach to any of such licences such terms, conditions or restrictions as it deems advisable.

And an additional penalty of up to one year in prison will be imposed where a violation of the Act or the regulations causes "either directly or indirectly to any person either bodily injury or loss of life" (s. 15) .

Section 13 also provides that it is a summary conviction offence, punishable as an offence under the *Consumer Protection Act*, to violate or fail to comply with any provision of the Act, the regulations, or an, order or direction given under the Act or the regulations.

6. Ontario

Major amendments were made to the *Theatres Act*, R.S.O. 1980, c.498 in 1984 (S.0. 1984, c.56) and these were carried through to the *Theatres Act*, R.S.O. 1990, c.T-6. Pursuant to s. 3 (1) of the Act, the "Board of Censors" became the

"Ontario Film Review Board", consisting of such persons "as the Lieutenant Governor in Council may appoint". The Board is given power, under s. 3 (7) of the Act:

(*a*) subject to the regulations, to approve, prohibit and regulate the exhibition and distribution of film in Ontario;
(*b*) when authorized by the person submitting film for approval, to remove from the film any portion that it does not approve of for exhibition or distribution;
(*c*) subject to the regulations, to approve, prohibit or regulate advertising in Ontario in connection with any film or the exhibition or distribution thereof;

Before a film may be exhibited in Ontario, an application for approval to exhibit and for classification of the film must be made to the Board (s. 33(1)). The Board, after viewing a film, may, "in accordance with the criteria prescribed by the regulations", refuse to approve the film for exhibition in Ontario (s. 33(2)) or "make an approval conditional upon the film being exhibited in designated locations and on specified dates only" (s. 33(3)). Any film not approved by the Board is not to be exhibited (s. 37(1)) and once approved, a film is not to be altered (s. 38). The Board's approval of a film is to be indicated "in the manner prescribed by the regulations" (s. 35). A sample of advertising matter intended for public display in connection with a film or its exhibition must first be approved by the Board (s. 39(1)) and so stamped (s. 39(6)). The Board's decision on approval and classification may be reviewed (s. 33(5)) or appealed (s. 33(8)). Section 34(1) of the 1990 Act also provides:

(1) Where the chair of the Board is of the opinion that the criteria prescribed by regulation respecting subject-matter or content in films have changed since a film was originally approved and classified and that the film may not be entitled to the approval or classification determined at the time of the original decision, the chair may require that the film be submitted for reconsideration by the Board.

(2) Where a film is submitted for reconsideration under subsection (1), section 33 applies with necessary modifications except that no fees shall be charged.

Regulations may be made under s. 60(1):

9. prohibiting and regulating the use, distribution or exhibition of film or any type of class thereof;
10. prohibiting and regulating the use and display of any advertising matter in connection with any film or exhibition thereof;
33. exempting any theatre, film exchange, projector, film or person or any class or type thereof from any provision of this Act or the regulations;
34. prescribing criteria on which the Board may exercise its powers under sections 3, 33 and 39 including prescribing the film or advertising content or subject matter that the Board may refuse to approve;

. . . . .

Every person who "knowingly fails to comply with any order, direction or other requirement made under" the *Theatres Act*, or contravenes any of its provisions or regulations is guilty of an offence and may be fined up to $25,000 or to imprisonment for a term of not more than one year, or sentenced to both (s.61(1)).

7. Prince Edward Island

The *Entertainments Act*, R.S.P.E.I. 1974, c.E-7 was repealed in 1986. Sections dealing with video were enacted in the *Films Act*, R.S.P.E.I. 1988, c.F-8, but are specifically stated to be not applicable to theatres. The sections of the old Act dealing with censorship were not retained; however, the *Films Act* accepts, for the purposes of video classifications, those classifications as determined by the Nova Scotia Classification Board.

8. Quebec

The "Regie du Cinema" is established under. s.123 of the *Cinema Act*, R.S.Q. 1984, c.18.1, to be composed of three members (s.124). The functions of the Regie include classifying films "according to the segments of the total audience to which they are directed" (s.135(1)). Every print of every film intended for exhibition to the public must be stamped by the Regie showing the classification assigned to the film (s.82) before it may be exhibited (s.76). Any film not stamped or any print of a film used in contravention of the Act or any of the regulations may be seized (s.176). The Regie's decisions may be reviewed or appealed pursuant to ss.149-166.

Of the several regulations the Regie may make, s. 167(2) empowers it to "establish standards and conditions for the exhibition of a stamp, the posting up and the exhibition of the classification of a film, including any information or warning that must appear thereon".

The general offences and penalties provision (s. 178, as amended by 1986, c.58) states:

> Any person who infringes section 76, 86, 87, 90, 92, 98, 99, 100, 102, 111, 114, 118, 120, 121, 122 or 177 or a regulation made under this chapter is guilty of an offence and liable to a fine of not less than $175 nor more than $1,400 in the case of an individual and not less than $700 nor more than $2,800 in the case of a corporation or partnership and, for a subsequent offence within two years, to a fine of not less than $325 nor more than $7,000 in the case of an individual and not less than $1,400 nor more than $13,975 in the case of a corporation or partnership.

9. Saskatchewan

The *Film and Video Classification Act*, R.S.S. 1984-85-86, c.F-13.2 provides for the continuation of the three-member Saskatchewan Film Classification Board (s.3(1)). The board is empowered, under s.4(1) to:

> (*a*) approve or disapprove films that are intended for exhibition or distribution in Saskatchewan;
>
> (*b*) require the exhibitor, retail distributor or wholesale distributor, as the case may be, who intends to exhibit or distribute a film approved by the board to remove any portion of the film that the board does not approve of.

Section 9 provides that no exhibitor, retail distributor or wholesale distributor or a film, shall exhibit or distribute the film, as the case may be, unless:

> (a) the board has approved the film and classified or approved a classification for the film; and
> (b) where the board has approved a film subject to certain portions of the film being removed from the film, unless the portions of the film that the board has required to be removed are removed.

Section 13(1) (as amended by 1988-89, c.42) states:

> This Act does not apply to:
> (a) a film owned or sponsored by:
>   (i) a church or religious society, where the film is designed for purposes of worship or religious instruction; or
>   (ii) a university, school or other educational institution for which the minister responsible for the administration of the *Education Act* is responsible, where the film is designed for educational purposes;
> (b) films designed for the purpose of advertising, demonstrating or instructing in the use of commercial or industrial products; or
> (c) any other films or classes of films, persons or classes of persons or advertising associated with films that may be exempted in the regulations or by the board pursuant to clause 3(3)(b).

Section 3(3)(b) states:

> The board may ... exempt in accordance with the criteria to be prescribed in the regulations and, subject to any terms and conditions that the board considers appropriate, any person, class of persons, film or class of films from all or any provision of this Act or the regulations;

The board may require that the person proposing to distribute a film ensure that the film and any advertising associated with the film display the classification for that film given or approved by the board and any additional information that the board may require (s.6(1)(b)).

Under s. 7, an unapproved film may be seized and confiscated. Section 11(1) sets up an appeal committee to consider and determine appeals from the board's decisions.

The Lieutenant Governor in Council may make the following regulations "for the purpose of carrying out the provisions of this Act according to their intent (s.18): .

. . . . .

> (d) prescribing the terms and conditions under which films may be sold, leased, exchanged or exhibited;
>   (i) respecting any other matter or thing that may be necessary for the carrying out of the provisions of this Act.

The general penal provision (s. 14) states:

> A person who violates any provision of this Act or the regulations or any decision of the board, for which no penalty is otherwise provided, is guilty of an offence and

liable on summary conviction to a fine of not more than $2,000 and, in the case of a continuing offence, to a further fine of $100 for every day during which the offence continues.

10. Northwest Territories

The censorship provisions are contained in s. 18 of the *Motion Pictures Act* which states:

18.(1) The Commissioner may, generally or in any particular case, require that films or slides be submitted to an officer for approval before they are exhibited.

(2) The Commissioner or an officer, as the case may be, may, in that person's discretion, prohibit the exhibition of a film or slide to prevent the use of dialogue and pictures depicting criminal or immoral scenes or that are otherwise injurious to public morals or opposed to public welfare.

(3) Where the Commissioner or an officer has ordered that a film or slide is prohibited from exhibition, no person shall exhibit that film or slide.

The Commissioner may also make regulations, including those "governing the classification and censorship of films or slides" (s.21(d)).

The general penalty for violation of any provision of the ordinance or regulations is a fine of up to $200, three months in jail, or both (s. 20).

11. Yukon Territory

The *Motion Pictures Ordinance*, C.O.Y.T. 1978, c.M-10 does not contain any specific provisions on the censorship of films.

CHAPTER 5

Legal Limitations Arising from Private Rights

5.1 Introduction

While many of the limitations on freedom of expression are found in the criminal law, some are also found in the civil law of the provinces.

The most important part of the provincial law affecting freedom of expression and, more particularly, the freedom of journalists is the law of civil defamation. The common law and provincial defamation statutes confer on individuals a right to sue journalists or others who publish or broadcast material which unjustifiably damages their reputation.

Defamation encompasses the two sub-categories of libel and slander. Since libel is the part of the law which directly affects journalists, the materials on defamation in this chapter will focus entirely on it. There is, in addition, a short section on the right to privacy which, like defamation, reflects a respect for individual rights that may limit the right to publish information.

Libel is a part of the law of torts. Just as individuals can sue for damages when someone's negligence has led to an injury to their person, they may sue for injury to their reputation. A libel is an unjustified statement, published or broadcast, that subjects a person to hatred, ridicule or contempt or, put differently, it is a false statement to a person's discredit. It is a strict liability tort. Whether or not the injury to reputation was intended, the injuring party is held responsible. The law is complex and journalists must understand its complexity. Much that they write or broadcast pertains to reputation.

A defamation suit begins when a person notifies an alleged defamer that he or she is going to sue. There are a number of stages in the procedure, but if the matter gets to court, the plaintiff must prove that the matter is defamatory, that it refers to the plaintiff, and that it has been published.

The defendant must defend the allegedly libelous statement. The defendant can choose one or a combination of four lines of defence. The first of these is justification. The defendant argues that the statement about the plaintiff is true. If the truth of the statement can be proved, there is a complete defence. This defence should demonstrate to journalists that their standards for publishing material related to reputation should be the same as the standards of evidence recognized by a court.

A second defence is fair comment, in which the defendant demonstrates that the defamatory statements are not allegations of fact, but honestly expressed opinions based on facts that are true. Thirdly, a journalist may plead that the matter was published on an occasion of privilege. There are provisions in most libel and slander acts that provide a guide to occasions of privilege. Finally, there is a defence of consent. A journalist may publish a defamatory statement if the person defamed consents to its publication.

Journalists should recognize that they and their editors and publishers may be responsible for damaging an individual's reputation and could pay a healthy sum in damages to that person. In 1982, the Canadian Broadcasting Corporation was required to pay the Deputy Attorney-General of the Province of British Columbia $125,000, plus costs, for declaring that he had used his position improperly to interfere in the judicial process on behalf of friends.

The law also embraces a notion of privacy, although it is very limited and, so far, cautiously interpreted. It is still generally the law in Canada that you can publish anything you like about another person as long as it is true.

5.2 Defamation

5.2.1 Anne Skarsgard, "Freedom of the Press," (1980-81), *Saskatchewan Law Review* 45, pp. 296-99

In *Parmiter v. Coupland* Parke, J. defined defamation as "a publication, without justification or lawful excuse, which is calculated to injure the reputation of another by exposing him to hatred, contempt or ridicule." This classical formulation of the tort is misleading in two respects. Firstly, it does not make clear the fact that defamation is a *false* statement about the plaintiff. Secondly, the words "calculated to injure" convey the impression that defendant's intention is relevant. Defamation is a strict liability tort and good faith is no defence. Said Scrutton, L.J. in *Tourner v. National Provincial and Union Bank of England*:

> I do not myself think this ancient formula is sufficient in all cases, for words may damage the reputation of a man as a business man, which no one would connect with hatred, ridicule or contempt.

In *Youssoupoff v. Metro-Goldwyn Mayer Pictures Ltd.* he quoted with approval Cave, J. in *Scott v. Sampson*:

> The law recognizes in every man a right to have the estimation in which he stands in the opinion of others unaffected by false statements to his discredit.

And in *Sim v. Stretch* Lord Atkin formulated the modern test for determining whether a statement is defamatory: Would the words tend to lower the plaintiff in the estimation of right-thinking members of society generally?

Fleming agrees that feelings of disapprobation are not necessary to the tort provided that the words cause the plaintiff to be shunned and avoided. This definition takes into account the fact that an attribution of misfortune such as an allegation that a man is insane or that a woman had been raped has a tendency to lower a person's standing in the community even though it does not arouse feelings of animosity in the minds of decent people.

The interest protected by the tort is an individual's reputation described as "perhaps the most dearly prized attribute of civilized man." What is the meaning of the word "reputation"? In popular parlance a person's reputation is what other peoples say or think of him, maybe what image they hold of him. But does a person actually have a public image or is this "image" only a statistical conclusion drawn from numerous individual images? No doubt a person's wife, employer, subordinate and friends all have different images of him. In other words, "reputation" is a legal fiction used by the courts to describe a variety of interpersonal relations that have been damaged as a result of the defamatory statement.

The idea that a person's reputation is valuable and should not be harmed with impunity has been recognized for a very long time. The law of Moses forbade slandering anyone, especially a person in authority, and in Ancient Rome, by the law of the Twelve Tables, anybody who slandered another "by words or defamatory verses" was to be beaten with a club.

Roman law distinguished written defamation (*malum carmen* and *famous libellus*) from oral defamation (*injuria verbalis*), which was a less serious tort. This distinction was not made in the common law until the end of the eighteenth century. Until that time in our law both libel and slander could involve either spoken or written statements, but they were entertained in different courts, slander at first only in ecclesiastical courts and later also in civil courts, whereas libel was primarily a criminal action of sedition and was entertained in the Star Chamber.

The Church tried slander actions because of its jurisdiction over sin. If a person's reputation was sufficiently evil, he was put "on his trial". If he was acquitted, it was those who had defamed him who had committed a sin and were put on trial in their turn. If convicted, the defamers were required to do penance and were sometimes even excommunicated.

As civil courts gained influence, the doctrine developed that the ecclesiastical courts could not try sin if there was also a civil cause of action. By the sixteenth century this doctrine was applied to slander imputing a common law crime. Because most common law crimes involved trespass to the person which is actionable *per se* without proof of damages, the false allegation that someone had committed such a crime became actionable *per se* also, and general damages could be recovered. Later the class of slander actionable *per se* was increased to include not just slander imputing a common law crime, but also imputations of a "hideous disease" and injury to business reputation. The former was probably included because the Church, by administering the last rites to those who were about to enter a leper colony, relinquished its jurisdiction over lepers, while an injury to one's reputation in one's trade or calling was deemed temporal in nature and therefore removed from the Church's jurisdiction.

The Star Chamber had jurisdiction over libel until its abolition in 1641, at which time libel actions were transferred to the same common law courts which had previously taken over slander jurisdiction from the church courts. Unfortunately the consolidation of defamation actions in one court did not result in a more unified body of law. The Roman distinction between spoken defamations actionable as slander and written defamations actionable as libel was revived, an accident of history that has contributed towards making our present day law of defamation needlessly complicated, irrational and often unfair.

The distinction between libel and slander is an important one. Libel is a crime as well as a tort, whereas slander is a tort only. Of more practical importance, as criminal prosecution for libel is rare, is the fact that only libel is actionable without proof of special damage, because damage is presumed. Special damage is harm flowing directly from the act which is either economic loss or is capable of pecuniary assessment. Normally slander, a less serious tort, is not actionable without proof of special damage. However, there are four exceptions to this rule. Slander accusing the plaintiff of being charged with a crime, an imputation that the plaintiff is, at present, infected with a "loathsome disease", slandering the plaintiff with respect to his trade or profession, and attacks on the plaintiff's chastity are actionable per se, without proof of damage.

Said Lord Mansfield in *Thorley v. Lord Kerry*:

> An action for a libel may be brought on words written, when the words, if spoken, would not sustain it.

Although the distinction between the spoken and the written word is important, there is a further test for distinguishing libel from slander, and that is the test of performance. Libel is published in a "permanent" form. For example, a statue, a cartoon, an effigy, even chalk marks on a wall are observed through the sense of sight and published in a permanent form and are therefore libels if defamatory. In this context "permanent" does not mean that the form will endure for a long time, but that it is not transient like the spoken word or a gesture.

This distinction was easy enough to make two hundred years ago, but the advent of the electronic media of communication, has posed many problems. How does one classify defamatory statements broadcast over the radio or television? Would a spontaneous defamatory statement broadcast live and untaped over radio or television be classified as slander, and would the same statement become libel if read or memorized from a script or if it was taped and thus available in permanent form? But if the rationale behind the distinction between permanent and transitory forms is the fact that the former is capable of wider circulation, should defamation on radio and television be treated as libel? Or should we distinguish between broadcasts for general reception and those for only a limited audience, such as broadcasts on amateur shortwave radio frequencies, police, fire or taxi radio frequencies, or closed-circuit television?

There are no uniform answers to these questions. Legislation providing that defamatory words in a broadcast constitute libel has been introduced in Ontario, England and Australia, whereas the Canadian *Uniform Defamation Act* enacted so far only in Alberta, Manitoba and the Yukon abolishes the distinction between libel and slander and makes all defamation actionable without proof of damage.

Such legislation, if introduced in the other Canadian provinces, would remedy the unwarranted preferred position of the electronic media over the press under the strict common law rule. In the remainder of this paper we shall assume that the defamation, whether published in the press or on the radio or television, is libelous. (Such an assumption is supported by the facts. In many cases of radio or television defamation either there is a script or else the program has been taped.)

Note: For a full and careful statement of the law, see Raymond E. Brown, *The Law of Defamation in Canada* (Toronto, 1987), 2 vols.

5.2.2 The Plaintiff's Case

As in all civil proceedings, the burden of proof in a defamation action rests with the plaintiff, the person who claims to have been defamed. The plaintiff is required to establish a *prima facie* case, that is, to satisfy the court that the essential elements of a defamation action are present.

More precisely, the plaintiff must prove three things:
a. that the material complained of is defamatory;
b. that it refers to the plaintiff; and
c. that it was published.

5.2.2.1 Defamatory

5.2.2.1.1 *Brannigan v . S.I.U.* (1964), 42 D.L.R. (2d) 249 (B.C.S.C.)

HUTCHESON, J.: In this action the plaintiff seeks to recover damages for libel.

The plaintiff is a seaman living in the City of Vancouver, in the Province of British Columbia, and is a member of the union known as the Canadian Brotherhood of Railway Transport and General Workers. This union is generally referred to as the C.B.R.T. and I will use that designation.

The defendant is a union known as the Seafarers' International Union of Canada. I will refer to it as the S.I.U.

The plaintiff has been a seaman since 1937. At that time he became a member of the Canadian Seamen's Union. That union was outlawed and, according to the evidence, by reason of its being Communist-dominated. The plaintiff came to British Columbia in 1952 and at that time became a member of the West Coast

Canadian Seamen's Union. Later the West Coast Canadian Seamen's Union was merged with the S.I.U. and, on that taking place, the plaintiff became a member of the latter union. In 1959 he left the S.I.U. The circumstances of his leaving, as I understand it, were that there was a strike by the Marine Workers' Union, who had established a picket line, and the plaintiff received instructions from a dispatcher of the S.I.U. to remain at his work which involved his crossing the picket line. The plaintiff did not believe that he should cross the picket line and he refused to carry out his instructions. This resulted in his being expelled from the S.I.U. Following his expulsion from the S.l.U. he was instrumental in forming in the City of Vancouver the C.B.R.T. Local 400. Upon the formation of that local he held for a time the post of financial secretary but, finding that he did not have the necessary educational qualifications, he ceased to hold that office. As I have already mentioned, he is presently a member of the C.B.R.T.

The defendant publishes and distributes what is referred to in the pleadings as a newspaper and which is known as the *"Canadian Sailor"*. This paper is distributed among the members of the S.l.U. and is sent to other unions and to companies and,generally speaking, to any person or corporation who may ask to be placed upon the mailing list . The circulation of this publication on August 23, 1961, was at least 15,000, according to the evidence.

In the issue of the *Canadian Sailor* of August 23, 1961, under the heading "C.B.R.T. Official Waves Red Flag" there is a photograph of a parade and particularly of two men in that parade carrying between them a banner upon which are the words "Communist Party of Canada". Below that picture appear these words: "Positive proof that the C.B.R.T. is Commie tinged is the picture shown here. It is a picture of the May Day parade in Vancouver in 1961, and the Commie pictured on right is none other than the Financial Secretary of the Vancouver local of the C.B.R.T. WILLIAM BRANNIGAN."

Roderick B. Heinekey, the vice-president of the S.l.U. in charge of the Pacific Coast, was examined for discovery and upon his examination agreed that the word "Commie" in the caption under the photograph means "Communist" and that the William Brannigan referred to therein is the plaintiff.

It is not disputed that the person pictured on the right is the plaintiff nor is it disputed that it was erroneously stated that (a) it is a picture of the May Day parade in Vancouver in 1961, and (b) that William Brannigan was the financial secretary of the Vancouver local of the C.B.R.T. The picture is a picture of the May Day parade in Vancouver in the year 1960 at which time William Brannigan had ceased to be the financial secretary of the Vancouver local of the C.B.R.T.

In his evidence the plaintiff stated that the placard he was carrying did have words upon it. While he cannot remember the exact wording of the placard, which was not composed by him but was given to him to carry, he thinks it was to the effect, "Canada Needs More Ships" or "Canada Needs More Jobs" but he is definite in his sworn testimony that the wording on the sign had nothing to do with Red countries or Communist countries and that he was not nor to his knowledge was any one in his group giving support to the Communist party.

Other than denials of publication and circulation, the defences pleaded on behalf of the defendant may be summarized as follows:

(a) neither the words nor the photograph were reasonably capable of causing injury to the plaintiff or his character, credit or reputation or capable of bringing him into public scandal, odium or contempt;

(b) the issue of *Canadian Sailor* of December 13, 1961, contained a public apology intended to correct any errors contained in the issue of the *Canadian Sailor* of which the plaintiff complains;

(c) The words complained of are true in substance and in fact, and

(d) that the plaintiff marched in the May Day parade at some distance behind a banner bearing the words "Communist Party of Canada" and in so far as the words referring to the plaintiff and of which the plaintiff complains consist of expressions of opinion, they are fair comment on a matter of public interest.

I find that the article published on August 23, 1961, taken as a whole, both the picture and the accompanying printed statements, is clearly a statement that the plaintiff was, as of the date of the publication, a Communist.

While noting the difficulty of giving an exhaustive definition of libel, the learned authors of *Gatley on Libel & Slander*, 5th ed., p. 16 state:

> Any written or printed words which tend to lower a person in the estimation of right-thinking men, or cause him to be shunned or avoided, or expose him to hatred, contempt, or ridicule, constitute a libel.

This statement is, in my view, supported by the decided cases.

Having in mind, as I must, the time, place and circumstances under which the statement was made, I am of the opinion that it was defamatory of the plaintiff to publish of him that he was a Communist. With respect, I find confirmation of this view in the words of O'Halloran, J.A., who stated at pp. 178-9 of his judgment in *Martin v. Law Society of B.C.*, [1950] 3 D.L.R. 173:

> Labour Unions, Universities, and other public bodies have publicly sought and are still seeking to rid themselves of men and women professing Communist beliefs. It has come to be universally accepted in the Western nations that it is dangerous to our way of life to allow a known Communist or Communist sympathizer to remain in a position of trust or influence.

And those of Robertson, J.A., at p. 192:

> Every one knows that many Trade Unions are expelling Communists from their organizations. I think that neither the Government of Canada, nor that of the United States, nor that of England knowingly would employ a Communist.

See also *Burns et al. v. Associated Newspapers, Ltd.* (1925), 42 T.L.R. 37; *Dennison et al. v. Sanderson*, [1946] 4 D.L.R. 314, [1946] O.R. 601.

The plaintiff was a member of a trade union and had been active in the organization of the local to which he belongs.

5.2.2.1.2 *Thomas v. C.B.C.*, [1981] 4 W.W.R. 289 (N.W.T.S.C.)

DISBERY, J.: The defendant Sanders prepared and assisted other CBC employees in the preparation of four news stories concerning the drilling operations at K 91 and an explosion that occurred on the drillship Explorer I, for broadcasting over the radio facilities of CBC. Such were all broadcast within a period of approximately 19 hours. The plaintiff alleges that the said broadcasts defamed him. Transcripts of the four broadcasts, admitted by the defendants to be true and correct transcripts thereof, were filed as part of Ex. P75 and are pleaded verbatim in para. 7 of the amended statement of defence. I will now set forth these broadcasts seriatim and, inter alia, the extent of the defendant Sanders' participation in them.

The First Broadcast

The first broadcast was made on 3rd February 1977 about 5:30 p.m. as part of CBC's regular daily news program "CBC Mackenzie News" for reception by the public in the Northwest Territories and other nearby northern areas. The broadcast was as follows:

> (CBC) CBC News has learned that Dome Petroleum required a substantial amendment to its drilling authority at the Explorer I site last summer. The amendment authorized by lower level officials in the Department of Indian Affairs and Northern Development resulted in the company having unexpected problems from the gas pressure from the bottom of the well. These pressure problems could have led to the explosion of Explorer I which killed one drill worker. Larry Sanders has the story.
>
> (Sanders) The original drilling authority approved by the federal cabinet last April required Dome to secure its drill pipe and casing with cement before it entered any high pressure zones that might contain oil. Because they did not start drilling until early August, to meet this requirement would have meant Dome would not have been able to reach any substantial depth since securing the casing with cement all the way down takes much more time. By the end of August Explorer I had drilled to 4,000 feet and had secured the casing with cement. Dome wanted to drill down to 10,000 feet right away so they applied for an amendment to the drilling authority to stop the cementing at the 4,000 foot level. The amendment was approved without any long examination by Maurice Thomas the supervisor of the Oil and Gas Division in Yellowknife. Mr. Thomas says he approved the amendments because Dome did not expect any high pressure gas or oil until at least 12,000 feet. But by September 10th they had reached just below 10,000 feet and unexpectedly hit water and gas at very high pressure. Because they did not expect to hit pressure at that depth they had great difficulty controlling the well from that point on. Gas and water flowed continually from the bottom and Mr. Thomas says Dome tried plugging it at different depths for four weeks without any success. Mr. Thomas says after the explosion of October 12th they finally sealed off the well at the top and left it for the winter. If the amendment to the drilling authority had not been approved they would not have had any of these problems. Securing the casing with cement all the way down to 10,000 feet would also likely have prevented the gas problems which led to the explosion that killed data engineer, George Ross MacKay. None of these facts were presented to the inquest jury last month which found that Mr. MacKay's death was an industrial accident. More information will likely come to light when the federal advisory committee on offshore drilling makes it [sic] preliminary report public in a tour of the North starting February 14th. Until then government officials here will not say whether they will allow such an amendment to Dome's drilling authority in next summer's operations. But the government

officials do admit that if Dome had encountered oil instead of gas, the environmental catastrophe for the Beaufort Sea would have been public long before now. Larry Sanders, CBC News, Ottawa.

(CBC) The reaction to the new information about Dome's drilling operation last summer is already coming in. The Committee for Original People's Entitlement has called again on the federal government to hold a public inquiry into the whole operation. Bob Delury, a biologist for COPE, says the additional information proves that the government is not able to regulate Dome effectively, nor is the company able to regulate itself. Wally Firth says the amendment is a betrayal of public faith since Dome was able to change the rules for drilling once they were in operation. Mr. Firth says he supports COPE's call for an independent inquiry before Dome can proceed this summer with more drilling. Vince Steen the vice president of ITC said the credibility of government monitors should be questioned. Mr. Steen says independent inspectors who are not so close to Dome should be authorized to keep track of the operations from the ship.

The defendant Sanders, hereinafter referred to as "Sanders" for brevity's sake, was the author of the first two paragraphs. The first or lead-in paragraph was spoken by the program's newscaster. Sanders himself spoke the second paragraph. The final paragraph was spoken by the newscaster. The initials "ITC" appearing in the third paragraph designate the Inuit Tapirisat Canada or Eskimo Brotherhood. This third paragraph was not written by Sanders but he provided the information therefor to the newsroom. . .

The Statement of Claim

The *Defamation Ordinance* (hereafter referred to as "the Ordinance") by s.4 enacts as follows:

> 4. In an action for defamation the plaintiff may allege that the matter complained of was used in a defamatory sense, specifying the defamatory sense without alleging how the matter was used in that sense, and the pleading shall be put in issue by the denial of the alleged defamation; and, where the matters set forth, with or without the alleged meaning, show a cause of action, the pleading is sufficient.

By this salutary enactment this court is no longer plagued by many former precedents as to the sufficiency of statements of claim where an innuendo is raised together with the pleading of extrinsic facts in support thereof. Several such precedents were considered by the court in *Grubb v. Bristol United Press*, [1963] 1 Q.B. 309, [1962] 2 All E.R. 380 (C.A.).

After identifying the parties in its first three paragraphs, the plaintiff's statement of claim in paras. 4 and 5 alleges the making of the said four broadcasts by the defendants. Paragraph 6 alleges that the broadcasts referred to the plaintiff either "by name or by reference as the government official who was responsible for the issuing of a Drilling Authority and amendments to the Drilling Authority to Dome Petroleums Ltd." to drill K 91.

Paragraph 7 alleges that certain of the statements that the plaintiff complains of as defamatory were made by the defendants in each and every one of the four broadcasts.

Paragraphs 8 to 11 inclusive, give particulars, broadcast by broadcast, of specific words, phrases, clauses and sentences which were included in and form part of such broadcasts considered separately and which the plaintiff complains, directly or by innuendoes naturally arising therefrom, defamed him. Paragraphs 12 to 16, inclusive, of the statement of claim read as follows

"12. By the use of the words in the four preceding paragraphs the Defendants meant, and were understood to mean:

"(a) that the Plaintiff permitted the amendment to the Drilling Authority without careful consideration and sufficient examination of the facts, and was thereby negligent and incompetent in the performance of his duties as Regional Oil and Gas Conservation Engineer;

"(b) that the Plaintiff permitted the amendment without regard to the safety of the drilling operation and to the consequences to the environment, and was thereby negligent and incompetent in the performance of his duties as Regional Oil and Gas Conservation Engineer;

"(c) that the amendment authorized by the Plaintiff caused the subsequent problems in the drilling operations;

"(d) that the amendment authorized by the Plaintiff caused the explosion which resulted in the death of George Ross MacKay;

"(e) that the Plaintiff improperly authorized the amendment;

"(f) that the amendment authorized by the Plaintiff was contrary to government regulations;

"(g) that the Plaintiff was under the control and influence of the Operator, and failed to perform his duties as Regional Oil and Gas Conservation Engineer in an independent and impartial manner;

"(h) that the Plaintiff engaged in an improper scheme to withhold or suppress evidence from the coroner's inquest;

"13. The Plaintiff says that the defamatory meanings alleged in the immediately preceding paragraph are the natural and ordinary meanings of the words in paragraphs 8, 9, 10 and 11, or alternatively, that taken in the context of the whole of each of the said radio broadcasts, and by reason of the other statements published on the said radio broadcasts, that the words in paragraphs 8, 9, 10 and 11 have the meanings, and were understood to have the meanings alleged in the immediately preceding paragraph.

"14. The words published on the said radio broadcasts were calculated to have and had the effect of disparaging the Plaintiff and exposing him to public scandal and contempt.

"15. By the use and publication of the said words the Defendants have imputed to the Plaintiff a lack of fitness, incompetence, negligence and impropriety in the conduct of his duties as a government official.

"16. The Plaintiff says that the amendment authorized by the Plaintiff did not cause the subsequent 'problems' in the drilling operations, nor did the said amendment cause the explosion which resulted in the death of George Ross MacKay."

The defendants in their joint statement of defence denied the defamations alleged by the plaintiff, and by virtue of s.4 of the Ordinance such allegations were put in issue in this action.

It is common ground that in the area served by the regional program "CBC Mackenzie News" on 3rd and 4th February there were approximately 24,700 persons resident. It is also common ground that on said 4th February the national program, "The World at Eight", had an actual audience of approximately 540,000 listeners, including, of course, listeners in the Territories.

The First Broadcast

I now turn to a consideration of the first broadcast made at 5:30 p.m. on 3rd February, and as to whether the plaintiff was defamed therein and thereby. I have adopted and applied the following authorities and statements as to what constitutes a defamatory imputation.

Gatley on Libel and Slander, 7th ed. (1974), pp. 13-14, para. 31, states as follows:

> The gist of the torts of libel and slander is the publication of matter (usually words) conveying a defamatory imputation. A defamatory imputation is one to a man's discredit, or which tends to lower him in the estimation of others, or to expose him to hatred, contempt or ridicule, or to injure his reputation in his office, trade or profession, or to injure his financial credit. The standard of opinion is that of right-thinking persons generally. To be defamatory an imputation need have no actual effect on a person's reputation; the law looks only to its tendency. A true imputation may still be defamatory, although its truth may be a defence to an action brought on it; conversely untruth alone does not render an imputation defamatory.

Tallis, J., adopted and applied this excerpt in *England v. C.B.C.*, [1979] 3 W.W.R. 193 at 206, 97 D.L.R. (3d) 472 (N.W.T.S.C.).

In *Cherneskey v. Armadale Publishers Ltd.*, *supra*, Ritchie, J. with Laskin, C.J.C., Pigeon and Pratte, JJ. concurring, at p. 623, approved the following excerpt from Gatley, 7th ed., pp. 4-5, para. 4, where the learned author said:

> Any imputation which may tend "to lower the plaintiff in the estimation of right-thinking members of society generally," ... or "to expose him to hatred, contempt or ridicule," is defamatory of him.

This excerpt was applied by Tallis, J. in *England v. C.B.C.*, *supra*, at p. 207 together with the immediately following sentence, namely:

> An imputation may be defamatory whether or not it is believed by those to whom it is published.

I have also adopted and applied the following authorities as to what constitutes a defamatory imputation made with respect to a person's profession, trade or occupation, or with respect to the carrying out by the holder of a public or private office of the duties and responsibilities pertaining thereto.

In *England v. C.B.C.* Tallis, J. said at p. 208:

> "Learned counsel for the defendants cited the following excerpt from Gatley on Libel and Slander, 7th ed., pp. 31-32, paras. 57 and 58, where he said:
>
> " 'Any imputation which may tend to injure a man's reputation in a business, employment, trade, profession, calling or office carried on or held by him is defamatory. To be actionable, words must impute to the plaintiff some quality which would be detrimental, or the absence of some quality which is essential, to the successful carrying on of his office, profession or trade. The mere fact that words tend to injure the plaintiff in the way of his office, profession or trade is insufficient. If they do not involve any reflection upon the personal character, or official, professional or trading reputation of the plaintiff, they are not defamatory.
>
> " 'It is defamatory to impute to a man in any office any corrupt, dishonest or fraudulent conduct or other misconduct or inefficiency in it, or any unfitness or want of ability to discharge his duties, and this is so whether the office be public or private, or whether it be one of profit, honour or trust. Thus, it has been held defamatory to charge a parish overseer with oppressive conduct towards the poor of the parish, or a vestry clerk with having misappropriated or misapplied the parish moneys, or a mayor of a borough, though retired from office, with ignorance of his duties, partiality and corruption.' "

Learned counsel for the defendants cited the following excerpts from *Odgers on Libel and Slander*, 6th ed. (1929), to be found at pp. 25 and 46 respectively:

> It is libellous to impute to a member of any profession, that he does not possess the skill or technical knowledge necessary for the proper practice of such profession, or that he had been guilty of any discreditable conduct in his profession . . .
>
> . . . they must be shown to have been spoken of the plaintiff in relation thereto, and to be such as would prejudice him therein . . . They must impeach either his skill or knowledge or attack his conduct therein. His special office or profession need not be expressly named or referred to, if the charge made be such as must necessarily affect him in it. And in determining whether the words used would necessarily so affect the plaintiff, regard must be had to the mental and moral requirements of the office he holds or the profession or trade he carries on. Where integrity and ability are essential to the due conduct of the plaintiff's office or profession, words impugning his integrity or ability are clearly actionable for they then imply if he is unfit to continue therein.

The first of the main facts that the plaintiff must prove to succeed in this action so far as the first broadcast is concerned is that he was identified to the listeners as the person whose conduct was attacked in the course of the broadcast in a defamatory way. As Ritchie, J. in *Skyes v. Fraser*, [1974] S.C.R. 526, [1973] 5 W.W.R. 484 at 495, 39 D.L.R. (3d) 321, affirming [1971] 3 W.W.R. 161, which affirmed [1971] I W.W.R. 246, said:

> . . . there are two questions to be determined at the outset. The first is a question of law as to whether the statement complained of can, having regard to its language, be regarded as capable of referring to the respondent.

The transcript, ante, proves that the plaintiff was named four times in the course of the broadcast. He was further identified during the broadcast as being the supervisor in Yellowknife of the oil and gas division of the federal Department of Indian Affairs and Northern Development and a low level official of that department. Not only were the words used "capable of referring to the plaintiff" but they specifically designated him by name.

The plaintiff's next task is to satisfy the court that the words that were used in the said broadcast were themselves, per se, capable of conveying a meaning tending to defame the plaintiff, either by forthrightly saying so or by a reasonable inference flowing therefrom. The alleged slander must be found in what is so said or inferred therefrom.

In *Grubb v. Bristol United Press Ltd.*, *supra*, Holroyd Pearce, L.J. said, at p. 390:

> Thus, there is one cause of action for the libel itself, based on whatever imputations or implications can reasonably be derived from the words themselves, and there is another different cause of action, namely, the innuendo, based not merely on the libel itself but on an extended meaning created by a conjunction of the words with something outside them. The latter cause of action cannot come into existence unless there is some extrinsic fact to create the extended meaning. This view is simple and accords with common sense.

In *England v. C.B.C.*, *supra*, Tallis, J. [p. 205] approved the following excerpt from *Gatley on Libel and Slander*, 6th ed., p. 68, para. 120, where the learned author said:

It is well settled that the question whether words which are complained of are capable of conveying a defamatory meaning is a question of law, and is therefore one calling for the decision of the court. If the words are so capable, then it is a question for the jury whether the words do, in fact, convey a defamatory meaning.

The law has long settled upon and established the touchstone to be used by Her Majesty's judges in determining whether or not words used by a defendant and alleged to be libellous or slanderous were capable of conveying to the persons to whom they were published a meaning defamatory of the plaintiff.

In *Rubber Improvement v. Daily Telegraph*, supra, Lord Reid said, at p. 259:

> The leading case is *Capital & Counties Bank v. Henty* (1882), 7 App. Cas. 741 at 745 (H.L.). In that case Lord Selborne, L.C. said: "The test, according to the authorities, is, whether under the circumstances in which the writing was published, reasonable men, to whom the publication was made, would be likely to understand it in a libellous sense.

And Lord Devlin in the same case, said, at p. 277:

> My Lords, the natural and ordinary meaning of words ought in theory to be the same for the lawyer as for the layman, because the lawyer's first rule of construction is that words are to be given their natural and ordinary meaning as popularly understood. The proposition that ordinary words are the same for the lawyer as for the layman is as a matter of pure construction undoubtedly true. But it is very difficult to draw the line between pure construction and implication, and the layman's capacity for implication is much greater than the lawyer's. The lawyer's rule is that the implication must be necessary as well as reasonable. The layman reads in an implication much more freely; and unfortunately, as the law of defamation has to take into account, is especially prone to do so when it is derogatory.

It therefore becomes my duty to determine if the words that were spoken in the first broadcast, upon being given their natural and ordinary meaning as understood by average, right-thinking and reasonable persons, *could* convey to such persons who heard the broadcast a derogatory meaning tending to defame the plaintiff.

In *Rubber Improvement v. Daily Telegraph*, at p. 258, Lord Reid said:

> What the ordinary man would infer without special knowledge has generally been called the natural and ordinary meaning of the words.

And at p. 259:

> In *Nevill v. Fine Arts & Gen. Ins. Co.*, [1897] A.C. 68 at 72, 73 (H.L.), Lord Halsbury said: '. . . what is the sense in which any ordinary reasonable man would understand the words of the communication so as to expose the plaintiff to hatred, or contempt or ridicule . . . it is not enough to say that by some person or another the words *might* be understood in a defamatory sense.' These statements of the law appear to have been generally accepted and I would not attempt to restate the general principle.
>
> In this case it is, I think, sufficient to put the test in this way. Ordinary men and women have different temperaments and outlooks. Some are unusually suspicious and some are unusually naive. One must try to envisage people between these two extremes and see what is the most damaging meaning they would put on the words in question.

See also *Jones v. Bennett* (1967), 59 W.W.R. 449 at 454-55, reversed 63 W.W.R. 1, which was reversed [1969] S.C.R. 277, 66 W.W.R. 419, 2 D.L.R. (3d) 291; and *Lawson v. Burns*, [1975] 1 W.W.R. 171, 56 D.L.R. (3d) 240 (B.C.).

Divesting myself of such professional legal knowledge and skill in the interpretation of words and the application of legal rules pertaining thereto that I have acquired over the years, and summoning to my aid such common sense as I possess, I have figuratively replayed the broadcast by reading the transcript thereof. Average, ordinary, right-thinking reasonable men and women, hereafter referred to as "average ordinary persons", who listened to this broadcast heard, inter alia, that the plaintiff was the supervisor of the oil and gas division in Yellowknife; and that he had "approved without any long examination" "a substantial amendment" to the drilling authority held by Dome Petroleum for the drilling of K 91. The listeners further heard the amendment described as a "betrayal of public faith" and that "the government is not able to regulate Dome effectively". The listeners further heard that the drilling operations, as authorized by the amendment approved by the plaintiff, resulted in the company encountering gas pressure problems from the bottom of the well; and that such problems "could have led to the explosion of Explorer I which killed one drill worker", and that if the amendment had not been approved by the plaintiff the company would not have had the pressure problems or the explosion that killed the drill worker.

Read as a whole, the broad and general import of the words spoken in this broadcast were capable, per se, of conveying to an average ordinary person hearing it a defamatory imputation that the plaintiff had improperly performed the duties of his public office of supervisor of the federal oil and gas division of the department by approving a "substantial amendment" without giving proper consideration to the potential dangers such might engender, and that as a result of his misconduct the explosion that killed MacKay later occurred. Furthermore in carrying on his office as such supervisor, the plaintiff was not able to "regulate Dome effectively" and thus was unfit to hold that office. I have no difficulty in finding that the words spoken in the first broadcast were capable of defamatory meanings with reference to the plaintiff.

The plaintiff pleads and his counsel submits that, in addition to the two defamatory meanings I have just mentioned and found the broadcast to be capable of, the broadcast is also capable of additional other defamatory meanings. Be that as it may, nothing would be gained by my cataloguing such additions to a broadcast already found by me to be pregnant with such capabilities, other than to be able to say that the broadcast was a little more pregnant by reason of such additional capabilities.

Sitting without a jury as the trier of the facts, it becomes my duty at this point to decide if, under the circumstances in which the words were spoken, the words used in the broadcast, upon being given their natural and ordinary meanings as understood by average ordinary persons, conveyed to such persons who heard them derogatory imputations that were not only capable of but did, *in fact*, defame the plaintiff.

The broadcast identified the plaintiff by name four times. The average ordinary person would, in my opinion, infer from the broadcast, not merely that the plaintiff had failed to carry out his duties as such supervisor in a competent manner, but that his conduct had been so wrong that it had amounted to "a betrayal of public faith". It was said in the broadcast that the attacked amendment and the plaintiff's approval of it were not disclosed to the coroner's jury at the inquest into MacKay's death, thereby implying that the plaintiff had participated in a "cover up" of the amendment and his approval. The broadcast also said that the plaintiff had participated in the breaking of drilling regulations by Dome Petroleum. I repeat the grounds and reasons that I have given above in finding this broadcast to have been capable of conveying defamatory imputations to the persons who heard it. In this broadcast what had been called "the sting" of the slander by some judges was the tying together of the plaintiff's conduct with the explosion and death of MacKay, thereby imputing that the death resulted from the plaintiff's wrongful conduct. The authorities are clear that all these derogatory imputations must be viewed cumulatively in order to determine what the real impact of the broadcast would have been upon the average ordinary listener. In my opinion, the cumulative impact of these derogatory imputations did defame the plaintiff both in his professional occupation as a petroleum engineer and also in his office as regional conservation engineer, one of whose duties was to supervise the drilling operations of K 91. The effect of hearing the "sting" might well lower the plaintiff in the estimation of average ordinary persons and even expose him to their hatred, contempt or ridicule.

5.2.2.1.3 *Murphy v. LaMarsh* (1970), 73 W.W.R. 114 (B.C.S.C.)

WILSON, C.J.S.C — The plaintiff Murphy was formerly employed as a radio newsman in the press gallery at Ottawa reporting for his radio station the doings of Parliament and the Government of Canada and general political news, including the public and private actions of politicians who were in the public eye.

The defendant Julia (more usually called Judy) LaMarsh is the author of, and the defendant McClelland and Stewart Limited is the publisher of, a book of political reminiscences called *Memoirs of a Bird in a Gilded Cage*, first published in 1968.

The first edition of this book, 10,000 copies, contained statements about the plaintiff which he says are defamatory and upon which this lawsuit is based. It is necessary to cite the impugned passage in full, from pp. 151, 152 and 153:

> A brash young radio reporter, named Ed Murphy (heartily detested by most of the Press Gallery and the members), had somehow learned that Maurice Lamontagne (then Secretary of State, and a long-time friend and adviser of the Prime Minister) had purchased furniture but had not paid for it. It sounded like an odd enough situation but what made it appear sinister was the fact that the furniture had been purchased from Futurama Galleries, a Montreal firm which was owned by a couple of gamblers, named Sefkind, who had disappeared in the wake of the Quebec Government's inquiry into bankruptcy. Futurama Galleries had gone into bankruptcy with Lamontagne's debt still showing on its books, and no payments had been made for furniture nor interest in over two years. Again, the hue and cry was raised over what might be — or might have been. A minister might have so compromised himself by being party to such an unusual "credit"

arrangement that he could be pressured into paying off the debt by trading some special treatment from the Government for his debtors or their associates. What that "special treatment" might be was never specified, but it must be granted that it isn't inconceivable that there could be some.

Maurice Lamontagne has a very lively, young-seeming wife, who likes nice things. As a university economist, I doubt that he had ever earned much money. He certainly had not while he was a full-time adviser to Pearson, in Opposition, when he began to buy his furniture. As a minister, his salary was, of course, much improved, but there were many demands upon it (although not so many as upon most Quebec ministers, who were expected to be pretty lavish with constituents' wedding presents and other similar gifts at Christmas or graduations; his wealthy predecessor in the riding of Outremont-St. John, now Senator Romuald Bourque continued to look after the riding as though he were still its member, leaving Lamontagne free of those usual financial commitments). However, Maurice and his wife, Jeannette, liked to live comfortably and to entertain their friends well. He furnished a home in Ottawa for them, buying all his furniture from Futurama, then noted for the type and quality of furniture they sold. It would not, I think, be unusual for any firm to extend credit, even in such large amounts, for any reasonable period of time. After all, a minister's income is fairly assured. and fairly substantial (although unlike a private business arrangement, everyone knows what a minister is paid), and no minister could permit word to get around that he wasn't paying his bills, so men in public life are normally fairly good credit risks. (That is the way I bought my own furniture for my Ottawa apartment, entirely on credit, even as a private member of Parliament, and I paid it off without any difficulty to myself or worry to my Ottawa suppliers. The difference in Lamontagne's case, of course, is that most people pay regularly until their balance is paid, and the public, which buys furniture most often upon credit arrangements, knows that heavy interest is ordinarily charged.) In Lamontagne's case, when the firm went bankrupt and the manner became public, over two years after his first purchases, he had not paid anything. The exposure of the matter was, of course, acutely embarrassing, because it drew attention to his personal financial situation (completely, when he gave a statement of the whole sorry deal to the press and the House), and no one likes to have to do that. But Lamontagne considered that there was not much else to be concerned about, and he felt, and I think still feels, that he was hounded out of office for doing something that was not reprehensible. For he was indeed hounded out. Although the Prime Minister appeared to stand by him for nearly a year, until he had run again and been re-elected in late 1965, gaining some personal vindication, Pearson had been trying to force his resignation during much of that period. Rene Tremblay was caught in the furniture scandal too, although perfectly innocently. He had also bought furniture from Futurama in November, 1963, but he had not received full delivery at first and refused to pay the balance until full delivery might be made. He did pay the whole account only three months later, in February 1964. There could be no supportable suggestion that he had compromised himself.

In subsequent editions (25,000 copies) the words "heartily detested by most of the Press Gallery and the members" were deleted and they are also omitted from a paperback edition of which 50,000 copies are being circulated by another publisher.

The passage just cited ("heartily detested by most of the Press Gallery and the members") is alleged to be libellous. The plaintiff also claims that the latter part of the extract cited, considered in its context, imputes to the plaintiff a disreputable action, the hounding of Mr. Lamontagne out of office, and is therefore libellous.

Miss LaMarsh was Member of Parliament for Niagara Falls from 1960 to 1968 and was, from 1963 to 1968, a Minister in a Government headed by Mr.

Lester Pearson as Prime Minister and consisting of members of the Liberal political party.

Miss LaMarsh's memoirs were her publisher tells me, expected to be a lively and colourful account of her political career. A good deal of the book fits readily into that definition and if Mr. Murphy's head is left bloody it is not the only one.

The first question is whether or not it is libel to say of a man in Mr. Murphy's occupation that he was "heartily detested" by most of his colleagues and by most Members of Parliament.

Plaintiff's counsel has not argued that the word "brash" is defamatory. I have given some thought to this conception — that the word "brash" is the governing word in the sentence and that the words "heartily detested by most of the Press Gallery and the members" are only inserted to reflect the reaction of those persons to Mr. Murphy's brashness. I have come to the conclusion that this interpretation of what Miss LaMarsh has said will not stand analysis — the statement, in parenthesis, that Mr. Murphy was heartily detested is an independent clause, emphasized by the parenthesis, and not clearly related to the quality of brashness. I do not say that brashness cannot arouse detestation. "Brash", in Canada bears, I think, more the American meaning stated in *Webster's Dictionary*, 1966 of "bumptious", "tactless", "loudly assertive", rather than the English meaning given in the *Oxford Dictionary* of "bold", "rash" or "impudent". But I do not think Miss LaMarsh has asserted that Mr. Murphy is detested because of his brashness; I think she has merely said he is detested by majorities of two groups of people.

These are the people best placed to know and value him, his associates in the press gallery and the Members of Parliament with whom he must associate and about whom he writes.

Ordinarily a libel is more specific than the one alleged here. A shameful action is attributed to a man (he stole my purse), a shameful character (he is dishonest), a shameful course of action (he lives on the avails of prostitution), a shameful condition (he has the pox). Such words are considered defamatory because they tend to bring the man named, according to the classic definition, into hatred, contempt or ridicule. The more modern definition, given by Lord Atkin, in *Sim v. Stretch* 52 T.L.R. 669, 80 Sol. J. 703, [1936] 2 All E.R. 1237, at 1240, is words tending "to lower the plaintiff in the estimation of right-thinking members of society generally." Perhaps "words likely to cause a man to be detested" might also, although not an all inclusive definition, fit into the class of defamatory words.

The difference between this and other cases I have read or tried is that no shameful action or characteristic or condition is directly attributed to Mr. Murphy. It is only said of him that he is heartily detested. A fairly careful search of authority has revealed to me no case in which the libel alleged has been couched in such terms — an allegation of bad repute without some direct supporting charge of wrongdoing or bad character.

It is obvious that any decision as to whether or not such words as were used here are libellous must be approached with care. Under proper circumstances I think it must generally be open to writers to express of certain persons opinions as to their popularity or unpopularity, perhaps to say they are by some classes of people liked or disliked. The words used, the circumstances, the person who comments, the person upon whom the comment is made, must all be considered. It may be permissible, for instance, in certain circumstances, to say of a politician that he is losing his popularity, even though such words will certainly not help him in his career and may well hurt him.

The first thing to consider is the nature of the operative word "detested" and this was much discussed at the trial. The *Oxford Dictionary* gives to the word "detests" the meanings "hate", "abominate", "abhor", "dislike intensely". *Webster's Dictionary*, I think, is more up to date in its definitions when it says, "Detest indicates very strong aversion but may lack the actively hostile malevolence associated with hate."

I would say, for instance, that Hamlet hated, or thought he ought to hate Claudius, the murderer of his father and the defiler, as Hamlet thought, of his mother but that he detested Polonius as a sycophant and a tedious moralizing bore ("These tedious old fools": Act II, Scene 2).

But "detest" remains a strong word. While it may express the feeling one has toward a boor, a bore or a braggart, it may also express the feeling one has toward an unscrupulous reporter, a reporter whose actions have displayed bad character. I do not think that the reasoning in *Capital & Counties Bank v. Henty* (1882), 7 App. Cas. 741, 52 L.J.Q.B. 232, applies here. The words used are not, as in that case, capable of a harmless meaning and alternatively and rather vaguely of a bad meaning, so that the harmless meaning should be preferred. They are disparaging in any sense, more disparaging in one sense than the other and it seems to me that in those circumstances, where it is clear that right-thinking persons can and probably will properly interpret them as defamatory, there must be liability. The tendency to defame is there.

No wrong or evil is directly attributed to Mr. Murphy but it is said of him that most men who have most to do with him in his occupation heartily detest him. I have no doubt that the ordinary reader, who is not perhaps inclined to such an analysis of words as I have here attempted would, after reading this, think "There must be something wrong or bad about this man Murphy to make these people detest him." Since I think this is the test to be applied, I think the words are defamatory. The effect is the same as would have resulted if it had been said, "He bears a bad reputation among his associates."

The witnesses Charles Lynch and John Webster, speaking as reporters, think otherwise. I am basing my opinion on my conception of what the legendary "right-thinking man" would take the words to mean and I would not want to exclude either witness from that class. I have no reason to doubt the honesty or the correctness of their evidence as reflecting their own opinions. But I must remember that neither Mr. Lynch nor Mr. Webster is an ordinary everyday reader of books attaching to the words in question their conventional effect. Mr. Lynch says that he would, as an employer of newsmen, be interested in a man described as heartily detested by most of the press gallery (which he calls a competitive jungle) and the House, because detestation is a prize, a mark of success in press gallery writing, and political approval a warning of failure. Mr. Webster says that to be disliked by a politician may be a badge of honour to a reporter. This evidence has a considerable bearing on the question of damages, which I shall come to later. But the esoteric meaning attached by these initiates to the effect of detestation is not one that would spring to the mind of the ordinary citizen who reads the book, and it is from that level that I must form my opinion.

I should deal with one case relied on by the defendant. *Robinson v. Jermyn* (1814), 1 Price 11, 145 ER 1314. The defendants were proprietors of or subscribers to a room called "the Cassino" which they frequented, presumably for social purposes. They posted a regulation of the Cassino reading thus, "The Rev. John Robinson, and Mr. James Robinson, inhabitants of this town, not being persons that the proprietors and annual subscribers think it proper to associate with, are excluded this room." They were sued by the Rev. Robinson for libel. Thomson, C.B. said at p. 16:

> The demurrer to these pleas involves the material question, whether the publication of the words laid in the declaration are properly the subject matter of an action, and whether, under the circumstances, they amount to a libel. The words are, "The Rev. John Robinson and Mr. James Robinson, not being persons that the proprietors or annual subscribers think it proper to associate with, are excluded this room." It seems to me to be a material allegation in this declaration that the plaintiff was officiating minister, but there is certainly nothing affecting him in his clerical character in these words. It then goes on to state, that the words were published in one of the written regulations of the room. Now the principal ground on which this action can be supported is, that it does in substance contain an averment, that these plaintiffs were not fit for common association — that they were not proper persons for general society; and nothing will help this declaration, unless it can be collected from it, that such an insinuation was the object of the words. Now it does not seem to me, that such an imputation can be inferred. It seems merely that these defendants did not think that the plaintiffs were proper persons to be associated with by them; but that may proceed from other causes than such as must appear on the face of the declaration, to have been insinuated, to constitute a libel. There might be reasons assigned not at all affecting the moral character of the plaintiffs; for the defendants may not have thought them agreeable or sociable. They may have considered them troublesome and officious; or, for some other such reasons, improper for their society.

I think this case is clearly distinguishable. The defendants were, in the first place, stating their own opinion, not purporting to report that of other persons. The words were not defamatory. They merely indicated a disinclination by the subscribers to associate with certain persons. It is true that here, as there, the opinion in question was that of a certain body of people, not of society generally. But it seems to me that the mild assertion by persons directly interested of a disinclination to associate with certain other persons is a far cry from a bold statement that a man is heartily detested by most of his associates. If, in this case,

Miss LaMarsh had expressed her own detestation of the plaintiff I would have thought little of it but it is a different matter when she attributes, without foundation, detestation of Mr. Murphy to his associates.

5.2.2.1.4 *Vogel v. C.B.C.* (1982), 21 C.C.L.T. 105

ESSON, J.: ... I have made many references to the impression conveyed to viewers. That is a matter which must be considered in assessing television programmes which by reason of their transitory nature, tend to leave the audience with an impression rather than a firm understanding of what was said. Images, facial expressions, tones of voice, symbols and the dramatic effect which can be achieved by juxtaposition of segments may be more important than the meaning derived from careful reading of the words of the script. Television is different from the printed word. The interested reader can reread and analyze. The emphasis in considering the defamatory impact of, say, a newspaper story must therefore be upon the words used. Libel by television is, in this respect, more like slander. In slander cases, regard may be had to such things as gestures and intonations: see *Gatley on Libel and Slander* (7th ed., 1974), p. 500, para. 1225. Here, regard must be had to the devices used to create an impression that what was being reported was a serious scandal.

5.2.2.2 Reference to the Plaintiff

5.2.2.2.1 *E. Hulton and Co. v. Jones*, [1910] A.C. 22 (H.L.)

The plaintiff, Mr. Thomas Artemus Jones, a barrister practising on the North Wales Circuit, brought the action to recover damages for the publication of an alleged libel concerning him contained in an article in the *Sunday Chronicle*, a newspaper of which the defendants were the printers, proprietors, and publishers. The article, which was written by the Paris correspondent of the paper, purported to describe a motor festival at Dieppe, and the parts chiefly complained of ran thus: "Upon the terrace marches the world, attracted by the motor races — a world immensely pleased with itself and minded to draw a wealth of inspiration — and, incidentally, of golden cocktails — from any scheme to speed the passing hour.... 'Whist! there is Artemus Jones with a woman who is not his wife, who must be, you know — the other thing!' whispers a fair neighbour of mine excitedly into her bosom friend's ear. Really, is it not surprising how certain of our fellow-countrymen behave when they come abroad? Who would suppose, by his goings on, that he was a churchwarden at Peckham? No one, indeed, would assume that Jones in the atmosphere of London would take on so austere a job as the duties of a churchwarden. Here, in the atmosphere of Dieppe, on the French side of the Channel, he is the life and soul of a gay little band that haunts the Casino and turns night into day, besides betraying a most unholy delight in the society of female butterflies." The plaintiff had in fact received the baptismal name of Thomas only, but in his boyhood he had taken or had been given, the additional name of Artemus, and from that time he had always used, and had been universally known by, the name of Thomas Artemus Jones or Artemus Jones. He had, up to the year 1901, contributed signed articles to the defendants' newspaper. The plaintiff was not a church warden, nor did he reside at Peckham. Upon complaint being made by the plaintiff of the publication of the defamatory statements in the article, the defendants published the following in the next issue of their paper: "It seems hardly necessary for us to state that the imaginary Mr. Artemus Jones referred to in our article was not Mr. Thomas Artemus Jones, barrister, but, as he has complained to us, we gladly publish this paragraph in order to remove any possible misunderstanding and to satisfy Mr. Thomas Artemus Jones we had no intention whatsoever of referring to him." The defendants alleged that the name chosen for the purpose of the article was a fictitious one, having no reference to the plaintiff, and chosen as unlikely to be the name of a real person, and they denied that any officer or member of their staff who wrote or printed or published or said before publication the words complained of knew the plaintiff or his name or his profession, or his association with the journal or with the defendants, or that there was any existing person bearing the name of or known as Artemus Jones. They admitted publication, but denied that the words were published of or concerning the plaintiff. On the part of the plaintiff the evidence of the writer of the article and of the editor of the paper that they knew nothing of the plaintiff, and that the article was not intended by them to refer to him, was accepted as true. At the trial witnesses were called for the plaintiff, who said that they had read the article and thought that it referred to the plaintiff.

LORD LOREBURN, L.C. My Lords, I think this appeal must be dismissed. A question in regard to the law of libel has been raised which does not seem to me to be entitled to the support of your Lordships. Libel is a tortious act. What does the tort consist in? It consists in using language which others knowing the circumstances would reasonably think to be defamatory of the person complaining of and injured by it. A person charged with libel cannot defend himself by shewing that he intended in his own breast not to defame, or that he intended not to defame the plaintiff, if in fact he did both. He has none the less imputed something disgraceful and has none the less injured the plaintiff. A man in good faith may publish a libel believing it to be true, and it may be found by the jury that he acted in good faith believing it to be true, and reasonably believing it to be true, but that in fact the statement was false. Under those circumstances he has no defence to the action, however excellent his intention. If the intention of the writer be immaterial in considering whether the matter written is defamatory, I do not see why it need be relevant in considering whether it is defamatory of the plaintiff. The writing, according to the old form, must be malicious, and it must be of and concerning the plaintiff. Just as the defendant could not excuse himself from malice by proving that he wrote it in the most benevolent spirit, so he cannot shew that the libel was not of and concerning the plaintiff by proving that he never heard of the plaintiff. His intention in both respects equally is inferred from what he did. His remedy is to abstain from defamatory words.

It is suggested that there was a misdirection by the learned judge in this case. I see none. He lays down in his summing up the law as follows: "The real point upon which your verdict must turn is, ought or ought not sensible and reasonable people reading this article to think that it was a mere imaginary person such as I have said — Tom Jones, Mr. Pecksniff as a humbug, Mr. Stiggins, or any of that sort of names that one reads of in literature used as types? If you think any reasonable person would think that, it is not actionable at all. If, on the other hand, you do not think that, but think that people would suppose it to mean some real person — those who did not know the plaintiff of course would not know who the real person was, but those who did know of the existence of the plaintiff would think that it was the plaintiff — then the action is maintainable, subject to such damages as you think under all the circumstances are fair and right to give to the plaintiff."

I see no objection in law to that passage. The damages are certainly heavy, but I think your Lordships ought to remember two things. The first is that the jury were entitled to think, in the absence of proof satisfactory to them (and they were the judges of it), that some ingredient of recklessness, or more than recklessness, entered into the writing and the publication of this article, especially as Mr. Jones, the plaintiff, had been employed on this very newspaper, and his name was well known in the paper and also well known in the district in which the paper circulated. In the second place the jury were entitled to say this kind of article is to be condemned. There is no tribunal more fitted to decide in regard to publications, especially publications in the newspaper Press, whether they bear a stamp and character which ought to enlist sympathy and to secure protection. If they think that the licence is not fairly used and that the tone and style of the libel is reprehensible and ought to be checked, it is for the jury to say so; and for my part, although I think the damages are certainly high, I am not prepared to advise your Lordships to interfere, especially as the Court of Appeal have not thought it right to interfere, with the verdict.

Lord Atkinson. My Lords, I concur with the judgment which has been delivered by my noble and learned friend on the woolsack, and I also concur substantially with the judgment delivered by Farwell, L.J. in the Court of Appeal. I think he has put the case upon its true ground, and I should be quite willing to adopt in the main the conclusions at which he has arrived.

Lord Gorell. My Lords, I concur also with the judgment which has been pronounced by the Lord Chancellor. I also wish to express my concurrence with the observations which my noble and learned friend Lord Atkinson has made upon the judgment of Farwell, L.J.

Lord Shaw of Dunfermline. My Lords, I concur in the observations which have been made by the Lord Chancellor, but for my own part I should desire in terms to adopt certain language which I will now read from the judgment of the Lord Chief Justice: "The question, if it be disputed whether the article is a libel upon the plaintiff, is a question of fact for the jury, and in my judgment this question of fact involves not only whether the language used of a person in its fair and ordinary meaning is libellous or defamatory, but whether the person referred to in the libel would be understood by persons who knew him to refer to the plaintiff."

My Lords, with regard to this whole matter I should put my propositions in a threefold form, and, as I am not acquainted by training with a system of jurisprudence in which criminal libel has any share, I desire my observations to be confined to the question of civil responsibility.

In the publication of matter of a libellous character, that is matter which would be libellous if applying to an actual person, the responsibility is as follows: In the first place there is responsibility for the words used being taken to signify that which readers would reasonably understand by them; in the second place there is responsibility also for the names used being taken to signify those whom the readers would reasonably understand by those names; and in the third place the same principle is applicable to persons unnamed but sufficiently indicated by designation or description.

My Lords, I demur to the observation so frequently made in the argument that these principles are novel. Sufficient expression is given to me same principles by Abbott, C.J. in *Bourke v. Warren* (1) (cited in the proceedings), in which that learned judge says: "The question for your consideration is whether you think the libel designates the plaintiff in such a way as to let those who knew him understand that he was the person meant. It is not necessary that all the world should understand the libel; it is sufficient if those who know the plaintiff can make out that he is the person meant." I think it is out of the question to suggest that that means "meant in the mind of the writer" or of the publisher; it must mean "meant by the words employed." The late Lord Chief Justice Coleridge dealt similarly with the point in *Gibson v. Evans* (2), when in the course of the argument he remarked: "It does not signify what the writer meant; the question is whether the alleged libel was so published by the defendant that the world would apply it to the plaintiff."

5.2.2.2.2 *Booth et al. v. B.C.T.V.* (1983), 139 D.L.R. (3d) 88 (B.C.C.A.)

LAMBERT, J.A.: — It is not necessary to call upon you, Mr. Alexander, in reply on the cross-appeal.

This is a defamation case. The words were spoken in 1972. They were recorded on tape and broadcast on television and published all in 1972. The trial took place in 1975 and this appeal is from the trial judgment at that time [summarized [1976] W.W.D. 78].

In 1972, there was a change in the law affecting prostitution and the defendant television system or one of its employees conceived the idea of interviewing a prostitute. The defendant, Margo Wong, was interviewed by the defendant, David Rinn, on television in a programme produced by the defendant, Clapp, and broadcast by the defendant British Columbia Television Broadcasting System Limited.

The words that are in issue in the case are set out in the reasons of Mr. Justice Hinkson, the trial judge, and they are these:

Q. What are policemen like in Vancouver?
A. Some of them are O.K. and some of them are not. There's good ones and crooked ones.
Q. Are there any payoffs in Vancouver?
A. Yeah there's about — in one night maybe twelve cops get paid off from different squads.
Q. You've paid them off?
A. I've paid them off quite a few times.
Q. How much?
A. Ummm — if it goes Vag "C" charge usually you have to pay them maybe half a bill — fifty dollars. If it's for narcotics you usually up a hundred — two-hundred dollars.
Q. Could you name individuals involved?
A. Oh I could — yeah — but I'm not gonna name them — cause that would just get me up a creek without a paddle — but there is, I'd say three on the Morality Squad that are quite high for payoffs and I know two on the Narc Squad that are high up — right up on top that take payoffs, and there's a few other ones on — like Traffic — you know they're special squads that take some.

The interview was broadcast by the defendant, British Columbia Television Broadcasting System Limited, at least twice, I understand on the same day, and then had a wider dissemination after that, but the scope of any wider dissemination was not in issue at the trial or before us.

The plaintiffs are 11 members of the Vancouver City Police Force, or they were in 1972. They are all members of the narcotics squad. There was in 1972 a vice department in the Vancouver City Police Force, and within that department four separate squads: the narcotics squad, the liquor squad, the morality squad and gambling squad.

Organization of the narcotics squad was that a staff sergeant was in charge, Staff Sergeant Devries. His second in command at that time was Sergeant Grierson, who had only been appointed a week at the time of the utterance of the defamatory words. Staff Sergeant Devries and Sergeant Grierson worked predominately on the administrative aspects of the squad and did not do much, if any, street work. There were eleven other members of the narcotics squad. There were at least two, and perhaps three, separate subgroups. One was comprised of Detective Booth as the senior detective in length of service and senior in that he exercised some supervision over the work of the other members of that undercover subgroup. That group dealt with street dealings in drugs, as they are called.

Another subgroup dealt with dealings in drugs at a higher level and it was referred to as the trafficking subgroup because of the nature of the work they were engaged in, the trafficking in drugs at a higher level than street dealings.

Detective Donald was the senior man in that grouping, and working with him were Detectives Simmons and Larke, but they again were working under his overall control as they worked together. So, the senior man in the undercover street group was Detective Booth, and in the trafficking group, Detective Donald.

The pleadings described the plaintiffs and defendants, but the substance of the allegations is set out in paras. 18 and 19 which follow the statement of the words alleged to be defamatory and I will set out paras. 18 and 19:

> 18. In the said interview the words "... and there's a few other ones on — like Traffic — you know they're special squads that take some", were interpreted by the respective families, friends, acquaintances and colleagues of the Plaintiffs, WILLIAM DONALD, STANLEY SIMMONS and KENNETH LARKE, respectively. as referring to the aforementioned three Plaintiffs who were and were known to be members of a unit within the Narcotics Squad at that particular time which unit was generally referred to as "the Traffic Squad" and was organized specifically to investigate the illegal movement of, and dealing or trafficking in narcotic drugs and substances. Furthermore, each of the other Plaintiffs herein have worked as members of "the Traffic Squad" from time to time throughout their association with the drug division of the Vancouver City Police Department and likewise were considered by their families, friends, acquaintances and colleagues as members of "the Traffic Squad".
>
> 19. By the words mentioned in Paragraph 16 hereof, the Defendants and each of them meant and were understood, by the Plaintiffs and each of them, and their respective families, friends, acquaintances and colleagues to apply to and mean that the Plaintiffs and each of them were dishonest, corrupt and unfit to act in connection with their respective professions as policemen and members of the Police Narcotics Squad.

Counsel on the appeal referred very largely to the same leading authorities in relation to defamation that consists of statements referring to more than one person without naming particular persons, and those leading cases are *Knupffer v. London Express Newspaper, Ltd.*, [1944] 1 All E.R. 495; *Morgan v. Odhams Press Ltd. et al.*, [1971] 2 All E.R. 1156. Counsel referred to other cases but those are the principal cases relied on and those were the principal cases relied on by the trial judge. There is no significant dispute between counsel as to the broad legal concepts that are applicable and, as I understand their arguments, neither counsel takes objection to the statements of law by the trial judge but rather take objections both on the appeal and the cross-appeal to the application of that law to the particular words in this case and the circumstances in this case.

The overriding issue in cases of this kind where the words are clearly defamatory in themselves is whether the words were published of and concerning the particular plaintiff who is claiming, and in addressing that question Viscount Simon says in the *Knupffer* case at p. 497:

> There are two questions involved in the attempt to identify the appellant as the person defamed. The first question is a question of law — can the article, having regard to its language, be regarded as capable of referring to the appellant? The second question is a question of fact, namely, does the article in fact lead reasonable people, who know the appellant, to the conclusion that it does refer to him? Unless the first question can be answered in favour of the appellant, the second question does not arise, and where the trial judge went wrong was in treating evidence to support the identification in fact as governing the maner, when the first question is necessarily, as a maner of law, to be answered in the negative.

In the *Morgan* case we were particularly referred to the judgment of Lord Morris of Borth-y-Gest which indicates that the dual nature of the test grows out of the practice in charging juries in cases of defamation.

The trial judge deals more extensively than I have with the law, but I do not think that it is necessary to go further than I have done. He adopts the test set out by Viscount Simon and he applies it to eliminate all of the 11 plaintiffs except two, Booth and Donald. As I understand his reasons, he is saying that the words referring to "two on the Narc Squad that are high up — right up on top", are capable when considered in relation to the facts of this case of being considered as being published of and concerning only Booth and Donald.

The trial judge also considers that the remainder of the words are, as a matter of law, not capable of being considered as published of and concerning any of the other plaintiffs other than Booth and Donald.

The trial judge then goes on and considers the evidence of 12 or 14 witnesses who gave the view that they took when they heard the defamatory statements or heard about the defamatory statements, and he concludes that a reasonable person on hearing these statements would think that they were said of and concerning Booth and Donald, and on that basis the trial judge finds liability of the defendants to Booth and Donald.

In his assessment of damages he awarded $7,500 to each of those plaintiffs as compensation and $5,000 to each of those plaintiffs by way of exemplary damages. The exemplary damages, therefore, totalled $10,000 and were awarded after careful consideration and a listing of those factors that justified such an award, particularly the prospect of profits being made by the broadcasting defendant from the excitement generated by a story of this nature, and the assistance of all of the defendants in publishing the defamatory statement after being requested not to do so until an opportunity had been given to the police departments to investigate the truth of what was alleged.

An appeal has been brought by the defendants British Columbia Television Broadcasting and Clapp, the only two defendants who were represented at the trial. Their appeal is as to liability.

A cross-appeal has been brought by the plaintiff, Donald, and by the nine other plaintiffs, other than Booth, who did not recover on their claim.

In relation to the appellant Donald, the cross-appeal asks for a higher award of exemplary damages. In relation to the other cross-appellants the cross-appeal asks for a finding that the defendants are liable to them and then asks for damages, both compensatory damages and exemplary damages.

I turn first to the appeal. Three points were argued.

The first was whether the words were capable of being considered as being published of and concerning the plaintiffs Booth and Donald.

The submission of counsel for the appellant was that they are only capable of referring to the staff sergeant who was in charge of the narcotics squad and the sergeant who was his second in command.

As I have said, the actual phrase was: "two on the Narc Squad that are high up — right up on top". In my opinion, we are not concerned with what the speaker subjectively meant to say; we are concerned with the meaning that reasonable men would take from what was said. But words, of course, are merely a mode of communication and all the circumstances of the communication must be considered as well as the mode that was used. The kind of person that the speaker was, and the kind of knowledge that people would anticipate that the speaker would have are relevant factors in determining the content of the communication. The circumstances in which the words are used are also relevant. So is the general audience to which the statements might be considered to be directed, and the special audience with special knowledge of the organization of the Vancouver Police Department. These too are relevant factors in deciding whether reasonable people generally, or whether reasonable people with special and particular knowledge, would find that the defamatory statement was published of and concerning the particular plaintiff.

The speaker was Margaret Wong, a prostitute with some knowledge but clearly not any detailed knowledge of the organization of the drug squad. There is no reason to believe that she would know of the transfer or personality of the second in command a week before she spoke. There is no reason to believe that when she says that she is referring to someone right on the top that she was referring to an inside administrator of the department who has overall supervision.

The trial judge found that those words were capable of referring to Booth and Donald. He found that those words were not capable of referring to the junior members in seniority and in work of the squad and, indeed, he found that the words were only capable of referring to Booth and Donald. He reached that conclusion on the basis of the words themselves, but also on the evidence that had been led and, of course, where the trier of fact and decider of law are the same there is no reason for any precise separation of the functions or decision of the two questions that have been raised by Viscount Simon. The ultimate question remains whether the words were published of and concerning the plaintiff. After considering all the evidence the, trial judge decided that they were capable of being considered as published of and concerning Booth and Donald and that they were not capable of being considered as published of and concerning anyone other than Booth and Donald. I agree.

The second point in the appeal raised by counsel for the appellant relates then to Booth and Donald and is that even if the words were capable of being considered as published of and concerning them that reasonable men would not have concluded that they were published of Booth and Donald and that even on the basis of the evidence that particular people did consider them published of Booth and Donald that, on the whole of the evidence, it should not have been concluded that a reasonable man would consider them as published of Booth and Donald.

Counsel for the appellant took us through the relevant parts of the evidence of 12 or even 14 witnesses on this point, and indeed there were considerable variations in their reactions to the story. However, counsel for the appellant concedes that he is not asking us to reassess on the balance of probabilities the conclusion reached by the trial judge on the question of fact, whether a reasonable person would be led to the conclusion that reference was to Booth and Donald. He said on the basis of the evidence the trial judge was clearly wrong in his conclusion.

In my opinion, on the basis of the evidence that was read to us, the trial judge was not clearly wrong. He reached a conclusion on a question of fact and, in my opinion, there was ample evidence to support that conclusion, that a reasonable person who knew Booth and Donald might well conclude that the defamatory words were uttered of and concerning them.

The third point related to the pleadings. In my opinion, para. 19 of the statement of claim was an ample pleading to support the conclusion of the trial judge, notwithstanding that the judgment of the trial judge did not come within the more particular pleading in para. 18 that I have recited and, indeed, as I understood his argument, counsel for the appellant did not press this third point.

For those reasons I would dismiss the appeal.

I turn now to the cross-appeal. It comes essentially to two points.

The first is that the defamatory words were uttered of and concerning all 11 of the plaintiffs and not just Booth and Donald. The major ground on which this is put is that all were members of the narcotics squad, that the words should not be construed as if they were a statute, but should be considered as a communication made orally and that in considering that communication the true question is what would reasonable people take from the words as an impression, as well as or coupled with the more precise content of the words, but not limited to the precise grammatical content of the words.

I do not disagree with counsel for the plaintiffs on the cross-appeal with his view as to the proper way of considering the words spoken. It is the impression that they convey that is crucial. But, in my opinion, the words "two on the Narc Squad that are high up — right on top" and the other words that surround them do not, in law, have a link with the other nine plaintiffs. It is true that the evidence indicates that there was immediate suspicion of all of the members of the narcotics squad and indeed there may well have been suspicion beyond that into the morality squad, into the vice squad as a whole, but that suspicion is more a matter of the mind of the person who heard the statement and his or her association with particular members of the police force. A neighbour who knows only one police officer, for example, and hears something about the police force would think immediately of that police officer, whether the words that are used have any real link to that police officer or not. So, an immediate suspicion is not necessarily an indication that the words are capable of being considered as published of and concerning the particular plaintiff. I think a good deal of the evidence was in that category.

After considering the evidence to which we were referred and considering both the precise words that I have quoted and the surrounding words, I agree with the trial judge that the other nine plaintiffs were not included and not capable of being included as being referred to in the words that were uttered.

A second point was made in relation to the members of the trafficking subgroup of the narcotics squad.

The trial judge dealt carefully with the evidence of how traffic and trafficking were used by the police witnesses and by other witnesses and he reached the conclusion that, again, the words were not capable of being considered as referring to the two plaintiffs, Simmons and Larke, who worked in the trafficking subgroup. On the basis of the evidence I agree with the trial judge.

The second point on the cross-appeal related to damages. Very fairly, counsel for the plaintiffs on the cross-appeal said that he was not asking us to reassess in 1982 and by 1982 standards the award that had been made by the trial judge in 1975 with respect to defamatory words uttered in 1972 . His submission was that by 1975 standards the award of a total of $10,000 as exemplary damages was inordinately low. He did not refer us specifically to any cases decided in this jurisdiction and, indeed, my recollection of those cases indicates that they would not support a submission that $10,000 was inordinately low for a case such as this. The case was clearly an appropriate one, in my view, for an award of exemplary damages but, in my opinion, an award of $10,000 in total was a fit award and it was appropriate to divide it as to $5,000 to each of the two plaintiffs in whose favour judgment on liability had been made.

For those reasons I would dismiss the cross-appeal.

ANDERSON, J.A.: I agree.

MACFARLANE, J.A.: I agree.

LAMBERT, J.A.: The appeal and the cross-appeal are dismissed.

Appeal and cross-appeal dismissed.

5.2.2.2.3 *Planned Parenthood Federation v. Fedorik* (1982), 135 D.L.R. (3d) 714, at 718 (Nfld.S.C.T.D.)

NOEL, J.: The law recognizes in every company a right to have the estimation in which it stands in the opinion of other persons unaffected by false statements to its discredit. The wrong of defamation is committed when a person publishes to a third person an untrue imputation against the reputation of another. In this regard, a company is treated as a person. Any imputation which may tend to lower the plaintiff in the estimation of right-thinking members of society generally, or to cut it off from society, or to expose it to hatred, contempt or ridicule is defamatory of it.

5.2.2.2.4 *Whitaker v. Huntington* (1981), 15 C.C.L.T. 19, at 21-22 (B.C.S.C.)

VERCHERE, J.: — This is an action for damages for libel. The defendant is a Member of Parliament and, on December 6th, 1977, after having attended on the day before a meeting of the Standing Committee on Transport and Communications, where the estimates of the Post Office were under consideration, he spoke by telephone from Ottawa to the host of a "talk show" broadcast by radio in Vancouver about the Post Office and its employees. In the course of his remarks, he offended members of the plaintiff local, including then president, Mr. Whitaker, and its vice-president, Mr. Ingram, particularly when he said:

> Mr. Huntington: Yeah, now who marched down to the Fishermen's Hall to take a vote, the information I get within the Union, is that about 50 to 51 per cent of the membership, 55 per cent of the membership at meetings get to vote, and the other 45 per cent have no voice at all, and that's why 1 . . .
> Mr. Murphy: They have no voice . . . ?
> Mr. Huntington: Well, they are quiet people. They aren't people that can group together or who want to group together in muscle-bound units and stand up and fight this imposed leadership and it's about a 55 to 45 proposition I believe in the Vancouver workers' union. The point I was trying to get across to Mr. Blais the Postmaster General yesterday was, why he doesn't use his initiative in this very key position and important position he has, use his initiative in the Cabinet to put in a law that orders democracy in union affairs where there is a government supervision of the vote, wording in the unions to do with federal activities and where there is a government supervised ballot to protect the rank and file worker in that union. That whole organization is not there for the benefit of people who want to tear down the system, Ed, and unless somebody in J.J. Blais' position is going to start to put some pressure on, the government isn't going to move, they're going to allow this process of disintegration to continue. I'm simply not down here to watch it happen.

Upon the telephone lines being opened for public participation in the show, Mr. Ingram promptly spoke to the defendant and after a long conversation about what he had said, a meeting was sought to be arranged. None was held, but in the result on May 16th following, the defendant appeared in person at the radio station and after the union's secretary had broadcast a "press release" attributed to Mr. Whitaker, the defendant commented on it and added:

> I can defend the democratic freedom that I want to see survive in this country as strongly as he can destroy it though, and that's what I am out to do.

Apparently aggrieved at what had been said, the plaintiffs started this action on July 26th following. Then about eight months later a statement of claim was filed and there, after asserting that all the above-quoted words had been falsely and maliciously broadcast and that the last-quoted words, in particular, referred and were intended to refer to Mr. Whitaker, the plaintiffs attributed the following meaning to them, namely:

> 8. The natural and ordinary meaning of the said words was that the Plaintiff, Peter Whitaker, and the Plaintiff, The Canadian Union of Postal Workers, prevented the full participation of the members of the Vancouver Local of the Canadian Union of Postal Workers, in the affairs of the

Union; that the Vancouver Local of the Canadian Union of Postal Workers was an undemocratic union and was not responsive to the majority wishes of the membership; that the membership did not have full opportunity of participating in all the affairs, activities and communittees of the union; and that because of this, Mr. Whitaker, the Plaintiff and The Canadian Union of Postal Workers, was trying to destroy democratic freedom in Canada.

I agree that that interpretation is reasonable.

5.2.2.2.5 *Stark v. Toronto Sun* (1983), 42 O.R. (2d) 791, at 794-795 (Ont. H.C.)

The *Odhams Press case, supra.* is relied upon as denying a claim in libel to the individual plaintiffs by reason of the lack of sufficient particulars pleaded in the statement of claim from which it might be inferred that the words were published of the individual plaintiffs. This principle was applied in *Seafarers, Int'l Union of Canada et al. v. Lawrence* (1979), 24 O.R. (2d) 257, 97 D.L.R. (3d) 324, 13 C.P.C. 281, in the course of proceedings and prior to it reaching the Court of Appeal. I take cognizance of the fact that this case differs from *Seafarers* in that there, the words complained of were not directed to all members of the union. They referred to "some" as being thugs. The action in defamation being a personal one, each plaintiff was obligated to plead facts that gave him or her a cause of action. Having read the two articles in this case with great care, my conclusion is that the individual plaintiffs have failed to establish the necessary link between themselves and the words used. They have pleaded membership in Operation Dismantle but they must go further. They must bring their personal reputations into play and they must as a minimum rely on pertinent facts in the pleadings that will raise the question of the tendency which the words have of lowering them in the estimation of others. This they have failed to do. There is nothing in the pleadings to indicate an identification on the part of these plaintiffs in the minds of the public with the organization. It is particularly imperative in libel actions that individual plaintiffs set out fully their individual causes of action when the class which was allegedly defamed is as wide and as ideological as Operation Dismantle is.

I turn now to Rule 75 and to its applicability to the circumstances of this case. Operation Dismantle is a non-incorporated association and cannot be sued. Can a representative action be maintained by one or more on behalf of all the members as a class? It would seem that *prima facie* the rule applies and a class action ought to be permitted. If it can be said that the members of Operation Dismantle were libelled, they all have the same interest in the result of the action.

What must be kept firmly in mind, however, is that the unincorporated body "Operation Dismantle" cannot be defamed. Only its members can. The distinction is important because the danger is forever lurking in the background of actions being prosecuted superficially on behalf of members of a class when in reality they are suing for and on behalf of the unincorporated association or entity. It will be a difficult judgment call to make in each case. When defamatory words are spoken of the members of a small association comprising 10 members for instance, a representative action would lie, as long as the pleadings were satisfactory, even absent specific names in the offensive article. Indeed a representative action would be encouraged in the interest of avoiding multiplicity of proceedings. But an opposite pole exists.

From the other extreme in my view may be taken a case like the present one. The line of demarcation may on occasion be fuzzy. In my opinion it is not so here. The members of a specific union as an instance may be defamed. Speaking generally, the members of the "union movement" in the country cannot be. The nature and size of the class must be studied, its composition scrutinized and its object defined. When it casts too wide and too philosophical or ideological a net on most or all accounts, then Rule 75 ought not to be resorted to.

In the result the statement of claim is struck and the action dismissed *in toto*. Costs to the defendants.

Application allowed.

5.2.2.2.6 *Manitoba Defamation Act*, R.S.M. 1987, c. D20.

1. In this Act,

"publish" includes transmission, emission, dissemination or the making public of writings, signs, signals, symbols, pictures and sounds of all kinds, from or by a newspaper or from or by broadcasting. ("publier")

19. (1) The publication of a libel against a race or religious creed likely to expose persons belonging to the race, or professing the religious creed, to hatred, contempt or ridicule, and tending to raise unrest or disorder among the people, entitles a person belonging to the race, or professing the religious creed, to sue for an injunction to prevent the continuation and circulation of the libel; and the Court of Queen's Bench may entertain the action.

(2) The action may be taken against the person responsible for the authorship, publication, or circulation, of the libel.

(3) The word in this section, "publication" in addition to the meaning set out in section 1, includes any words legibly marked upon any substance or any object, signifying the matter otherwise than by words, exhibited in public or caused to be seen or shown or circulated or delivered with a view to its being seen by any person.

(4) No more than one action shall be brought under subsection (1) in respect of the same libel.

Note: A court has suggested that this section is *ultra vires*, first, because it deals with "what is, in essence, criminal libel" and secondly, because matters "tending to raise unrest or disorder among the people" have been dealt with by Parliament in the *Criminal Code*. See *Courchene v. Malborough Hotel* (1971), 20 D.L.R. (3d) 109. No other province has such a provision.

5.2.2.3 Publication

5.2.2.3.1 *Ontario Libel and Slander Act*, R.S.O. 1990, c. L.12.

1. (1) In this Act,

"broadcasting" means the dissemination of writing, signs, signals, pictures and sounds of all kinds, intended to be received by the public either directly or through the medium of relay stations, by means of,

(*a*) any form of wireless radioelectric communication utilizing Hertzian waves, including radiotelegraph and radiotelephone, or

(*b*) cables, wires, fibre-optic linkages or laser beams,

and "broadcast" has a corresponding meaning; ("radiodiffusion ou telediffusion", "radiodiffuser or telediffuser")

"newspaper" means a paper containing public news, intelligence or occurrences, or remarks or observations thereon, or containing only, or principally, advertisements, printed for distribution to the public and published periodically, or in parts or numbers, at least twelve times a year. ("journal")

(2) any reference to words in this Act shall be construed as including a reference to pictures, visual images, gestures and other methods of signifying meaning. R.S.O. 1980, c. 237, s. 1.

2. Defamatory words in a newspaper or in a broadcast shall be deemed to be published and to constitute libel. R.S.O. 1980, c. 237, s. 2.

Note: Similar definitions of "broadcasting" appear in the *Defamation Act* of Manitoba (R.S.M. 1987, c. D20, s. 1) and Newfoundland's *Defamation Act* (R.S.N. 1990, D-3, s. 2(a)). In the majority of the provinces, however, "broadcasting" is to be interpreted as follows:

"broadcasting" means the dissemination of any form of radioelectric communication, including radiotelegraph, radiotelephone and the wireless transmission of writing, signs, signals, pictures and sounds of all kinds by means of Hertzian waves.

(*Revised Uniform Defamation Act*, s. 2 (a) in Conference of Commissioners on Uniformity of Legislation in Canada, Proceedings of the Thirtieth Annual Meeting, Montreal, Quebec, August 24-28, 1948, Appendix J. See also *Defamation Act*, R.S.N.B. 1973, c. D-5, s. 1; *Defamation Act* R.S.P.E.I. 1988, c. D-5, s. 1(a); *Defamation Act*, R.S.N.W.T. 1988, c. D-1, s. 1; *Defamation Act*, R.S.Y.T. 1986, c. 41, s. 1; and *Defamation Act*, R.S.N.S. 1989, c. 122, s. 2 (a) which adds the words "intended to be received by the public either directly or through the medium of relay stations.")

Both Alberta's *Defamation Act* and British Columbia's *Libel and Slander Act* offer more specific definitions. Section 1 (a) of the *Alberta Act* (R.S.A. 1980, c. D-6) reads:

"broadcasting" means a transmission, emission or reception to the general public of signs, signals, writing, images, sounds or intelligence of any nature by means of electromagnetic waves of frequencies lower than 3000 gigahertz;

And s. 1 of the British Columbia *Libel and Slander Act* (R.S.B.C. 1979, c. 234, as am. S.B.C. 1985, c. 10, s. 9) states:

"broadcasting" means the dissemination of writing, signs, signals, pictures, sounds or intelligence of any nature intended for direct reception by, or which is available on subscription to, the general public

(*a*) by means of a device utilizing electromagnetic waves of frequencies lower than 3000 GHz propagated in space without artificial guide, or

(*b*) through a community antenna television system operated by a person licensed under the *Broadcasting Act* (Canada) to carry on a broadcasting receiving undertaking,

and "broadcast" has a corresponding meaning;

Newfoundland is the only province which shares Ontario's definition of "newspaper" (*Defamation Act*, R.S.N. 1990, c. D-3, s. 2(c)). Most other provinces have adopted the wording of s. 2(c) of the *Revised Uniform Defamation Act*:

"newspaper" means a paper containing news, intelligence, occurrences, pictures or illustrations, or remarks or observations thereon, printed for sale and published periodically, or in parts or numbers, at intervals not exceeding thirty-one days between the publication of any two of such papers, parts or numbers.

(*Defamation Act*, R.S.A. 1980, c. D-6, s. 1(c); The *Defamation Act*, R.S.M. 1987, c. D20, s. 1; *Defamation Act*, R.S.N.B. 1973, c. D-5, s. 1; *Defamation Act*, R.S.N.S. 1989, c. 122, s. 2(c); *Defamation Act*, R.S.P.E.I. 1988, c. D-5, s. 1(c); and the Acts of the Northwest Territories and the Yukon Territory which are identical except for requiring that the intervals between any two of such papers, parts or numbers not exceed thirty-six days, rather than thirty-one days, *Defamation Act*, R.S.N.W.T 1988, c. D-1, s. 1 and *Defamation Act*, R.S.Y.T. 1986, c. 41, s. 1.)

"Newspaper" under the British Columbia *Libel and Slander Act*, R.S.B.C. 1979, c. 234, s. 1 and the Saskatchewan *Libel and Slander Act*, R.S.S. 1978, c. L-14, s. 2(a), includes a paper containing public news, intelligence or occurrences, or any remarks or observations in it printed for sale and published periodically, or in parts or numbers at intervals not exceeding thirty-one days between the publication of any two papers, parts or numbers; and also a paper printed in order to be dispersed and made public weekly or more often, or at intervals not exceeding thirty-one days, and containing only, or principally, advertisements.

And s.1 of Quebec's *Press Act*, R.S.Q. 1977, c. P-19 provides:

For the purposes of this act, the word "newspaper" means every newspaper or periodical writing the publication whereof for sale and distribution is made at successive and determined periods, appearing on a fixed day or by irregular issues, but more than once a month and whose object is to give news, opinions, comments or advertisements.

A provision similar to Ontario's s. 1(2) is to be found only in Nova Scotia's *Defamation Act* (s. 2(e)). And s. 2 of the British Columbia *Libel and Slander Act* stands alone in resembling s. 2 of the Ontario *Libel and Slander Act*. Almost all the other provinces' Acts, along with the *Revised Uniform Defamation Act*, state that " 'defamation' means libel or slander" (*Revised Uniform Defamation Act*, s. 2(b); Alberta *Defamation Act*, s. 1(b); Manitoba *Defamation Act* s. 1; New Brunswick *Defamation Act*, s. 1; Newfoundland *Defamation Act*, s. 2(b); Nova Scotia *Defamation Act*, s. 2(b); Prince Edward Island *Defamation Act*, s. 1(b); the Northwest Territories *Defamation Act*, s. 1; the Yukon Territory *Defamation Act*, s. 1.).

5.2.2.3.2 *Basse v. Toronto Star Newspapers Ltd. et al.* (1984), 37 C.P.C. 213, at 216-217 (Ont.H.C.)

MONTGOMERY, J.: Sydney Brown made allegedly defamatory statements to the defendant newspapers about the plaintiff in his capacity as acting Chief of Police for the Waterloo Regional Police Force.

The *Toronto Star* published some of these allegedly defamatory statements. The words were then repeated by other communications media throughout the country which caused the plaintiff further injury.

The offending paragraphs follow:

14. "The libel of the plaintiff was further aggravated by the fact that communications media throughout the country reported the words published by the defendants as aforesaid which reporting of such words repeated and perpetuated the libel complained of, causing further and irreparable harm and damage to the reputation of the plaintiff.

15. The plaintiff further complains that in publishing the words complained of the corporate defendants and their agents or employees knew or ought to have known that statements made to them by the defendant, Sydney Brown, were defamatory and libellous and, further, that such

words would have been repeated by other communications media throughout the Dominion of Canada. "

The objectionable paragraphs constitute a separate cause of action and a separate head of damages which, under these circumstances, may not be imputed to the original publisher of an alleged libel.

"Every republication of a libel is a new libel and each publisher is answerable for his act". (*Gatley on Libel and Slander* (8th ed. 1981), paras. 261, 266).

Speight v. Gosnay (1891), 60 L.J.Q.B. 231 (C.A.), a case involving slander, laid down four situations in which he who uttered a slander might by held responsible for the subsequent repetition of the words. The third point is the only one relevant here — that is, where the repetition is the natural and probable consequence of the original publication.

In my view, the repetition of the words originally published by the *Toronto Star* was not a natural and probable consequence of the initial publication. There is no liability upon the original publisher of the libel when the repetition is the voluntary act of a free agent, over whom the original publisher had no control and for whose acts he is not responsible: see *Ward v. Weeks* (1830), 7 Bing. 211 at 215,131 E.R. 81, approved in *Weld-Blundell v. Stephens*, [1920] A.C. 956 at 999; *Eyre v. New Zealand Press Assn. Ltd.*, [1968] N.Z.L.R. 736 at 744 (S.C.); *Macy v. New York World-Telegram Corp.* (1957), 161 N.Y.S. 2d 55 at 60 (C.A.).

The Master was also wrong in holding that the paragraphs under attack could be relevant to aggravation of damages. A jury should not take into account in assessing damages against the original publisher any damage done to the plaintiff by any defamatory matter for which the original publisher was not responsible: see *Gatley on Libel and Slander* (8th ed., 1981), para. 1451; *Harrison v. Pearce* (1858), 1 F. & F. 567 at 569, 175 E.R. 855 at 856; *Assoc. Newspapers v. Dingle*, [1964] A.C. 371 at 397-398, 410, 417 (H.L.).

The offending paragraphs are, therefore, struck out. Costs before the Master and of this appeal to the appellant in the cause.

Appeal allowed.

5.2.2.3.3 *Farrell v. St. John's Publishing Co.* (1986), 58 Nfld. & P.E.I.R. 66 (Nfld. C.A.)

MORGAN, J.A.: A plaintiff's cause of action in libel does not crystallize at the time the writ is served. The wrong has continuing effect and the defendant may, by subsequent conduct, further injure the plaintiff's reputation by 'rubbing salt in the wound'. The whole behaviour of the defendant toward the plaintiff is relevant to the issue of damages and his whole conduct "before action, after action and in court during the trial" may properly be considered. (See *Praed v. Graham* (1889), 24 Q.B.D. 53). Thus repeated publications of the same libel by the same defendant may be treated as aggravation of the original injury and be the basis of a higher award than would otherwise be given They ought not to be treated, however, as giving rise to a separate and independent right to damages.

5.2.3 The Defendant's Case

If the plaintiff succeeds in raising a *prima facie* case, it is now the defendant's turn. The defendant must raise one or more of the recognized defences.

5.2.3.1 Justification

5.2.3.1.1 Anne Skarsgard, "Freedom of the Press," (1980-81), *Saskatchewan Law Review* 45, pp. 302-303

Once the plaintiff proves the three elements of a libel action, he has a prima facie case. The defendant then has three possible defences: justification, privilege and fair comment. We shall now discuss these defences and their usefulness to the media by comparing the respective positions in England, the United States and Canada.

If the allegedly defamatory statement turns out to be true, that is, if the defence of "justification" is successful, there is no cause of action in the tort of defamation, as the law of defamation protects a person's reputation only insofar as he deserves it. Due to a presumption of falsity of all defamatory statements, the plaintiff does not have to prove the falsity of the words. Truth is treated, in England and Canada at least, as an affirmative defence that must be raised by the defendant and on which he has the burden of proof. In the United States the position is different. In *New York Times v. Sullivan* the court held that a plaintiff who is a public person must show knowledge or reckless disregard of the falsity of the statement, and in *Gertz v. Robert Welch, Inc.* it held that a plaintiff who is a private person must, for all practical purposes, show falsity as well. It is unclear whether this amounts to a formal shift in the United States from defendant having to prove the truth of the statement to plaintiff having to prove its falsity. In any event, this development in the law puts the media in the United States in a much better position than they enjoy in England or in Canada.

The defence of justification can be criticized on several grounds. First of all, it denies a remedy to a plaintiff who has suffered a very real loss, even if disclosure of the facts about him serves no useful purpose. For example, if a rehabilitated ex-convict has his criminal record maliciously broadcast, he has no action in defamation. To quote Paul Weiler:

> If society has no sufficient interest to render desirable the destruction of a person's reputation, truth should no longer legally justify a harmful statement, whether this is accomplished by internal reform of the law of defamation or the development of a right to privacy.

Although Saskatchewan is one of a handful of provinces that have privacy acts, privacy suits have been so far practically non-existent.

Another criticism of the defence of justification is that it seems to go against all the principles of justice. Someone who maliciously spreads rumours which he believes to be false with the intention of hating someone else does not have to compensate his victim for the loss of his reputation if the gossip turns out to be true. On the other hand, if a paper prints a story which it non-negligently and on reasonable grounds believes to be true and it turns out to be false, or if a true statement in the story is capable of an innuendo meaning in light of extrinsic facts not known to the writer, the paper is liable. Absurd laws such as this one do a great deal of harm by contributing to public mistrust of legal institutions.

b) The usefulness of justification to the press:

Justification is of little practical importance as it is not often pleaded by the press. The onus of proving the substantial truth of every statement claimed to be defamatory is a heavy one. This is especially so since the court determines what the truth is and the outcome of its determination is uncertain at best. Furthermore, should the plea of justification fail, it will seriously aggravate the damages.

Since justification is not a very useful defence, let us see whether the press can rely on the defences of qualified privilege and fair comment.

There is a fundamental difference between the defence of justification on one hand and the defences of qualified privilege and fair comment on the other. If a defendant relies on justification, he claims that he did not defame the plaintiff at all as defamation consists of the publication of a false statement. If he pleads qualified privilege or fair comment he concedes that,he had made an untrue defamatory statement about the plaintiff, but he claims immunity from the duty of compensating the plaintiff for his loss because it was in society's interest that he should make the statement. These two defences have been devised to enable the court to strike a balance between the interest of the defamed individual in tort compensation and the interest of society in freedom of expression.

5.2.3.1.2 Robert Martin, "Does Libel Have a 'Chilling Effect' in Canada?" (1990), *Studies in Communications* 4, pp. 146-148.

Justification is the name lawyers give to the defence of truth. The law of the various provinces does not recognize a general right to privacy. Thus, apart from the quite unjustified protection afforded to judges, there is, in Canada, little you may not say about other people provided it is true.

In a libel action any factual assertions the plaintiff claims to be defamatory are assumed to be false. If the newspaper or broadcaster which made the assertions wishes to defend them, it must prove their truth. Since libel is civil action, it is, in theory anyway, only necessary that the truth of the allegations be established "on a balance of probabilities", not, as in a criminal proceeding, beyond a reasonable doubt.

For professional, responsible journalists this should cause few, if any, problems. If the reporter assigned to a given story does a careful job of reporting, then the facts should be correctly ascertained. If the editor who handles the reporter's copy does a proper and competent job of editing, the story as it appears in its finished form should not be libellous. Good reporting and good editing are generally reliable ways of avoiding a libel action.

Sources can lead to problems with the defence of justification. The first of these can be broadly characterized as the "disappearing source". The difficulty is this. In the Canadian legal system the predominant method of proving facts in a courtroom is through the oral testimony of live witnesses. This is complemented by the hearsay rule. In essence, the hearsay rule says the only person who can testify to the existence of a fact is someone who has direct knowledge of that fact through his or her own senses. This means a defendant in a libel action who is trying to prove the truth of allegedly libellous statements can do so only through the testimony of sources who have direct knowledge of the true facts. If a source is unavailable for the trial or tells a different story in the witness box from the one which was first told to the reporter, the defence of justification goes out the window.

This seems, with a bit of reading between the lines, to have been the problem in *Roberge v. Tribune Publishers Limited*, a New Brunswick case. A newspaper reported that a physician had been "ousted" from the Board of Directors of a hospital. The physician sued and the newspaper raised the defence of justification. The defence was rejected. The court concluded that the plaintiff had not been "ousted", but simply "not reappointed" to the board. The court read "ousted" as conveying an implication that the plaintiff had been got rid of because there was, presumably, something undesirable about him. On reading the decision, I could not avoid the sense of there being more to it than met the eye, and that the newspaper had had a source of additional information who refused to tell his story in court.

The second difficulty relates to the credibility of sources. In *Drost v. Sunday Herald Ltd.*, a Newfoundland newspaper published a story about an incident of alleged police brutality. The paper's source was a convicted criminal who said he had been beaten up by two R.C.M.P. officers. The officers denied this and claimed the source had been resisting arrest. The story had the ring of truth to it. Nonetheless, the court rejected the testimony of the source, whom the paper had obviously believed, and accepted instead the testimony of the two police officers.

The only precaution reporters and editors can take against things like these happening is to make a substantial effort to satisfy themselves as to the reliability, veracity and credibility of a source before publishing a particularly tendentious story. It can be useful to have more than one source.

A problem related to sources, which can be avoided, arises when a source attempts to manipulate a reporter to achieve his or her own ends. A classic example is *Vogel v. C.B.C.* A disgruntled civil servant sought to use a reporter in order to attack his administrative superior. The reporter, who seems to have been both too ambitious and too credulous, accepted the information he was fed by the civil servant. The reporter failed to make the critical assessment the story required. There was a breakdown of the reporting function. This was compounded by a complementary failure of the editing function. The reporter accepted what he was told by the source and the reporter's supervisor accepted what he was told by the reporter. As a result, the C.B.C. paid $125,000 in damages.

When the performance of both the reporting and editing functions breaks down, no defence is possible. This happened in *Munro v. Toronto Sun*.

The *Sun* hired an individual and gave him the title "investigative reporter". (This is dangerous and should be avoided.) This reporter then claimed to have information showing that John Munro had used his position as a federal minister to benefit a company in which he had an interest. The story, it turned out, was a work of fiction.

An older reporter was assigned to work with the investigative reporter on the story. He came to believe in the truth of the story. Various editors were persuaded to accept the story without personally checking the identity, or even the existence, of sources or the reliability or authenticity of documents. The *Sun*, thanks to some excellent lawyering on its behalf at trial, managed to escape with only $75,000 in damages.

5.2.3.1.3 *Brannigan v. S.I.U.* (1964), 42 D.L.R. (2d) 249 (B.C.S.C.)

HUTCHESON, J.: I turn to the defence of justification, that is the allegation that the words complained of are true in substance and in fact.

The defendant called no evidence in support of that allegation but relied solely on inferences it submitted should be drawn from the plaintiff's activities and associations in the past as admitted by him. The facts and associations from which I am asked to draw the inference that the plaintiff is a Communist are, as I understand counsel's submissions, the following:

1. That one Thompson was formerly the vice-president of the C.S.U. and while the plaintiff was a member of that union.

2. That the C.S.U. was outlawed because it was Communist-dominated.

3. That Thompson formed the W.C.S.U. and became president thereof and that the plaintiff joined that union.

From these facts I am asked to infer that the plaintiff was a Communist. To reach that conclusion one would first have to infer from the fact that Thompson was vice-president of the C.S.U. that he was a Communist and that the plaintiff when he joined the W.C.S.U., was aware that he was. I am not prepared to draw that inference but even if I were, it would not then follow from the fact that the plaintiff joined the W.C.S.U., which Thompson had formed and of which he became president, that the plaintiff was himself a Communist. A man may well be required by the nature and circumstances of his employment to join a certain union and the fact that he does so knowing that others in that union, even in executive positions, are Communists does not of itself brand him as a Communist.

4. That the W.C.S.U. merged with the S.I.U. and the plaintiff became a member of the latter union but was later expelled. It is not suggested that he was expelled because of any Communistic leanings on his part.

5. That the plaintiff was then active in the formation of the C.B.R.T., Local 400 and associated with him in forming that local were William Mozdir, Dave West and one Cox.

The plaintiff identified as William Mozdir the man shown in the picture published August 23, 1961, carrying the banner bearing the words "Communist Party of Canada" and who had been erroneously stated to be the plaintiff, and from this it is submitted that he, Mozdir, is a Communist and by reason of his association with Mozdir it should be inferred that the plaintiff is a Communist.

Even assuming that it can be inferred that Mozdir was a Communist, again it does not follow that the plaintiff knew that he was nor does it follow, even if he did know and associated with him in the formation of Local 400 of the C.B.R.T. following his expulsion from the S.I.U., that he, the plaintiff, shared the Communistic views of Mozdir and was himself a Communist.

The only evidence in respect to Dave West was that the plaintiff had heard other members of the union refer to him as a Communist and had never heard Dave West deny it. Such evidence would not justify the inference that West was a Communist or that the plaintiff associated with him knowing him to be a Communist, or shared any of his views in that respect. There was no evidence as to Cox other than that he was one of those who formed Local 400 of the C.B.R.T.

6. That following the formation of Local 400 of C.B.R.T. and the plaintiff becoming a member of that local, Thompson, who was an organizer of C.B.R.T. paid by National headquarters, joined that local and eventually became president thereof. Again even if it were assumed that Thompson was a Communist by reason of his earlier association with the C.S.U., the fact that a Communist joined a local and even became the president thereof does not of itself justify the inference that the members of that local, and particularly the plaintiff, knew he was a Communist or were themselves Communists.

7. That the plaintiff took part in the May Day parade in the City of Vancouver in the year 1960. The plaintiff admitted that he was asked by a friend to join in that parade and that he did so in a group that represented what was spoken of as "an unemployed union" The so-called "unemployed union" is not what is commonly thought of as a union but is a group supported by a number of unions and made up by members of those unions who are unemployed. The activities of this group are described by the plaintiff as follows: "We had parades and demanded jobs and keeping the boys together so they wouldn't cross picket lines ... more or less a propaganda organization." This group of unemployed men in the parade each carried separate placards.

The alleged apology published by the defendant while ambiguous does bear an interpretation suggesting that the placard carried by the plaintiff supported the policies of the Communist party. The defendant called no evidence as to what the wording on that placard was and, as I have already pointed out, the wording on that particular placard is illegible in the printed picture. The plaintiff has sworn that while he cannot remember the exact wording it had nothing to do with Red or Communistic countries. He did not compose the placard but, as I mentioned above, his recollection is that it was to the effect, "Canada Needs More Ships" or "Canada Needs More Jobs".

The plaintiff admitted that he had marched in a May Day parade on one other occasion, namely in 1930, when he had marched in the May Day parade in Montreal. He also agreed with the suggestion by counsel for the defendant that the May Day parade in Vancouver was sponsored by the Communist Party of Canada and was of that general tenor. He said however, in effect, that his reason for marching in the parade was because he felt that it might result in some benefit to himself.

There were, according to the plaintiff's evidence, 1,000 or 1,500 men in the parade which extended for fifteen or sixteen city blocks. It was contended on behalf of the defendant that, assuming that the May Day parade is Communist-sponsored, it must be inferred that all persons, in this case all of the 1,000 or 1,500 taking part in that parade, are Communists. This contention I do not accept. It is clear from the photograph that the Communist Party of Canada had a contingent in that parade but there were also other contingents representing unions and other labour groups such as the "unemployed union" and I am not prepared to hold by reason of the fact that a person takes part in a May Day parade, which includes a contingent representing the Communist Party of Canada and even if that party has been instrumental in sponsoring the parade, that that person is a Communist.

The facts upon which the defendant relies, considered *seriatim* or together, do not lead me to the conclusion that the plaintiff is a Communist and I find that the defendant has failed to satisfy the onus that was upon it to uphold its plea of justification and to prove that the words complained of to the effect that the plaintiff was a Communist are true in substance and in fact.

The plaintiff swears that he is not a Communist and never has been and that he is not now and never was a member of the Communist Party of Canada nor had any connection with that party. That evidence stands unrebutted.

5.2.3.1.4 *Baxter v. C.B.C.* (1974), 30 N.B.R. (2d) 102 (N.B.C.A.)

RYAN, J.A.: A report referred to as the Clarkson, Gordon Report commissioned by Premier Richard Hatfield disclosed certain irregularities within the operation of the New Brunswick Department of Tourism. In December, 1972, the report was turned over to Mr. Baxter as Minister of Justice for consideration. In January,

1973, Mr. Baxter instructed Chief Superintendent William Hurlow to investigate the irregularities to determine if there was any evidence of criminality involved. Sergeants K. E. Taylor and R. C. Wolsey were assigned to carry out the investigation. In the course of doing so, a number of persons were interviewed by the officers including one Mr. J. K. Matchett. He apparently was closely associated politically with the former Minister of Tourism, Mr. J. C. Van Horne, and was concerned with the construction of certain tourism facilities in the Province by one of Matchett's companies. According to an internal report dated September 27, 1973, written by Sgt. Taylor, Matchett explained generally about his financial contributions to the Progressive Conservative Party and percentages paid by him by way of "kickbacks" on profits made by his companies on contracts awarded to him. According to the report, Matchett told the officers that, if payments were not made further contracts would not be awarded, or at least it would be difficult to obtain future contracts.

On October 3, 1973, Mr. Horace B. Smith, a Cabinet Minister in the Progressive Conservative Government of Premier Hatfield complained to Mr. Baxter to the effect that the R.C.M.P. were investigating party bank accounts and questioning Mr. Larry Machum, one of the individuals who looked after financial matters for the party. Mr. Baxter told Mr. Smith he was not aware of such an investigation, but he would make inquiries, which he instituted by calling C/S William Hurlow the same day.

As a result of Mr. Baxter's call to C/S Hurlow, Hurlow contacted Superintendent J. G. Giroux and a meeting was arranged for the afternoon of the following day which was attended by Mr. Baxter, C/S Hurlow, S/ Giroux and the Deputy Minister of Justice Mr. Gordon Gregory. At the meeting, which was held at Mr. Baxter's office, Mr. Baxter initiated discussions by asserting that he had been told that members of the R.C.M.P. were investigating political contributions to the Progressive Conservative Party, checking party bank accounts and interviewing Mr. Machum which Mr. Baxter said was beyond the scope of the investigation he had instructed the police to make. S/ Giroux told Mr. Baxter that he had met with the investigating officers that morning and instructed them that they were not to investigate legitimate contributions to the Progressive Conservative Party. The substance of S/ Giroux's reply to Mr. Baxter is contained in a memo to file dictated October 9, 1973, which is reproduced in its entirety at pp. 132 and 133 of the Report. The introductory paragraph relates to the meeting and the subject matter discussed at it. Paragraph 2 relates to the concern of Mr. Baxter as related above. Paragraph 3 reads as follows:

> 3. I told the Minister, and the others, that I had reviewed the investigation that morning with the investigators, and I had already instructed the members that the matter of political contributions and the secret bank account that a Party could have had nothing to do with the investigation we are conducting, and we are not going to investigate that angle. Furthermore, I told the Minister that I didn't think we had interviewed Mr. Macklin (Mr Machum) but we had obtained this information about political contributions and the number of the bank account in Moncton by

accident and not by asking for it specifically. I added that from the information I had from the investigators, I could only conclude that political contributions made by individuals or Corporations to a political Party did not have any connection with our investigation and that the investigators had hen instructed accordingly. The Minister was satisfied.

A final report of the investigation into the Department of Tourism dated November 28, 1973, was written by Sgt. Wolsey. It refers to the instructions given by S/ Giroux to Taylor and himself to the effect that no investigation was to be conducted into party contributions and that, under no circumstances, was the matter relating to the bank account in Moncton to be pursued.

Further letters were written by S/ Giroux confirming the fact that he had instructed Sgts. Taylor and Wolsey not to investigate legitimate contributions to the Progressive Conservative Party. (see pages 134 to 138 of the Report.)

The alleged defamatory words were spoken by Mr. Malling in a documentary telecast broadcast, as mentioned above, on April 20,1977. The script is reproduced at pages 117 to 131 of the Report. I quote in part from it; the portion alleged to contain the defamation is underlined:

Reporter: Higgins covery-up (sic) charge is a challenge to the basic integrity of Hatfield's government. It could not be allowed to stand so Hatfield set up a judicial inquiry which will investigate the charge later this month. The judge's findings could well force either Higgins or Hatfield out of politics. Higgins is holding his evidence for the inquiry but in our own investigation in New Brunswick, we acquired secret documents which do suggest political interference aimed at stopping an investigation of Conservative Party fund raising. In an internal police memo written *in September, 1973, an RCMP sergeant reported that a man under investigation for another matter makes many references to kickbacks to a Conservative Party fund. The police wanted to follow that lead, but then a week later they were stopped by the then Minister of Justice, John Baxter, and their own superiors.* In a note to file, J. B. Giroux, a senior RCMP officer in New Brunswick, describes a meeting with New Brunswick Justice Minister Baxter and his deputy on October 4th. 'The Minister said he is concerned about the scope and direction the investigation has taken, specifically, political contributions to the Conservative Party. He feels this has nothing to do with the investigations and we should not inquire into this field'. But the minister didn't have to worry. The senior policeman reported that he had already stifled the investigation. So, although the police had information suggesting that illegal kickbacks had or were being paid, they did not pursue the matter. In another memo, November 8th, 1973, the investigating officer reports accidentally finding what appeared to him to be suspicious payments apparently destined for the Conservative Party, but following his superior's instruction, they ignored them 'On instruction Giroux, we made it clear that we were not interested in political contributions to the party. We were careful to avoid reference to, or show undue interest in this aspect'.

The trial judge after quoting excerpts from several judgments and textbooks on the law of libel and slander concluded that the words complained of were defamatory, and that the defence of fair comment was not available to the defendants in that, in his opinion, the impugned words were "not comments at all but incorrect statements of facts". I agree with these findings.

Although the trial judge canvassed and summarized the evidence in detail in his judgment as it relates to the defendant's plea of justification or truth, I will refer briefly to it.

The program, according to the testimony of Mr. Malling and Mr. Robin Taylor, a senior producer of the Fifth Estate, was based on a speech delivered in the Legislative Assembly by Mr. Robert J. Higgins, then Leader of the Opposition, on March 3, 1977, and on certain documents obtained by one Philip Mathias, referred to at times as "the secret documents". The documents referred to are Sgt. Taylor's internal report dated September 27, 1973, and S/ Giroux's memo to file dated October 9, 1973 (supra).

In his speech Mr. Higgins referred to a meeting held in 1972 attended by the Premier, Mr. Richard Hatfield, some senior cabinet ministers and members of the committee of the Progressive Conservative Party at which the system used to collect money for the party was discussed. The speech is reproduced in its entirety at pages 139-142 of the Report. I quote in part from it:

> The RCMP in this province became aware of these activities. Mr. Speaker, I am informed and I believe that as early as 1973 the Department of Justice of this province of New Brunswick attempted to thwart investigation into the financing of the Progressive Conservative Party. I am informed that a meeting took place in October 1973 between the Department of Justice and senior officials of the Royal Canadian Mounted Police. As a result of this meeting, the investigating officers were instructed by their superior not to pursue investigation into Progressive Conservative Party financing.

It is to be noted that Mr. Higgins did not say that the investigation into 'kickbacks' had been stopped by Mr. Baxter as stated by Mr. Malling, but he did say that the investigating officers had been instructed not to pursue the investigation into Progressive Conservative party financing. No doubt Mr. Higgins had in his possession, or at least had read S/ Giroux's memo to file when he spoke of Mr. Baxter's instructions to S/ Giroux and C/S Hurlow at the meeting of October 4, 1973. S/ Giroux in his testimony said he explained to Sgts. Taylor and Wolsey that they were not to investigate legitimate party contributions, but they could investigate "kickbacks" to the party if criminality was suspected. In addition, as mentioned by the trial judge, neither Sgts. Taylor nor Wolsey were called to verify their written reports.

Mr. Matchett called as a witness by counsel for the defendants testified that any monies he had given to the party had been given voluntarily, and not by way of "kickbacks" as reported by Sgt. Taylor.

S/ Giroux in his testimony categorically denied that Mr. Baxter interfered with the investigation into the Department of Tourism and that it was the investigation into "Political contributions" and not "kickbacks" that Mr. Baxter wanted restricted.

In my opinion, the trial judge's findings, and I refer particularly to his finding "that the originator of the instruction to restrict the investigation into the Department of Tourism and the activities of Mr. VanHorne, its dismissed Minister, was S/ Giroux and not Mr. Baxter and that it was the investigation into *political contributions*, not *kickbacks* which was to be restricted", are supported by the evidence as is the trial judge's finding that the defendants failed to establish their defence of justification or truth.

5.2.3.1.5 *Munro v. Toronto Sun* (1982), 21 C.C.L.T. 261 (Ont. H.C.)

HOLLAND, J.:

(a) The great power and influence possessed by the media is an important factor in moulding public opinion and its exercise requires great care to be taken as otherwise great harm can result.

(b) There *must* be a separation of functions between the reporter and the editor, it being the responsibility of the editor to confirm the accuracy of the contents of a story before publication.

(c) Where important documentation has been obtained it is good practice to put it in a safe place and to thereafter work from a copy.

(d) There must be constant supervision maintained by the editor over the reporter, with a regular reporting requirement.

(e) It is the editor's responsibility to know in detail before publication, the documentation to support the story and the reliability of the sources and so ensure its accuracy.

(f) When the story is prepared — and the paper has the "goods" on the person targeted in the story — it is basic and necessary that that person be confronted with the story so that his reaction be obtained. This could cause the story to be discarded and could also enable the newspaper to add those comments should publication take place. A sound reason (there are others) for this to be established practice, is that it prevents the newspaper from publishing an incorrect story with all the attendant problems which that would generate.

Much of this was non-contentious. Only Worthington, as I recall, commented that the process, while technically correct, was practically not feasible. His view that a newspaper must place trust in its reporter or else no story would ever be published does not impress me as conforming to sound journalistic practice and I do not agree with it. There must be a marked difference in the function and responsibilities of the reporter and investigative reporter and those of senior management of a newspaper prior to publication of any article or news story. Newspapers or other forms of news communication media which do not clearly recognize and follow the careful course above, designed to ensure the taking of all reasonable safeguards to establish the accuracy of news story content and sources, act at their peril should these be found to be absent.

Freedom of the press has long been recognized in democratic society as a vital necessary. Given that freedom, in my opinion the work of the *investigative* reporter must meet the test of *absolute reliability*, and those who may be responsible for that reporter's efforts must take steps to ensure that this is accomplished. This was not done here.

5.2.3.1.6 *Gordon v. Caswell* (1984), 33 Sask. R. 202 (Q.B.)

DIELSCHNEIDER, J.: On January 7, 1982, the defendant wrote a letter to Saskatoon City Council in which she sought to influence Council's decision against funding the Family Service Bureau, which was then intending to bring to Saskatoon the plaintiff for the purpose of delivering a public lecture. The plaintiff is a tenured professor attached to the Department of Child and Family Studies of the College of Human Development at Syracuse University in the State of New York. I accept his statement that he accepts invitations to deliver lectures and does indeed lecture in many parts of the United States of America, in Canada, and in other countries of the Free World.

The plaintiff particularizes his complaint by alleging that the following words of the plaintiff's letter are untrue and therefore defamatory of him, and I quote: "Sol Gordon is opposed because he condones any type of sexual expression, condones wholesale contraceptive and abortion availability, and opposes parental responsibility and Judeo-Christian morality." Gordon categorically denies what is imputed to him by the defendant's words.

Also complained of were certain excerpts attached to the defendant's letter. Concerning these, I want to note at this point that it is agreed by counsel that the excerpts are photocopies of a pro-life newspaper and not quotations from the writings of the plaintiff.

The defence has assembled in evidence certain of the plaintiffs writings and emphasizes particularly the comics on sex and the film shown here, and argues that these are publications which bear out what the defendant says of the plaintiff in her letter to Council. I have examined that literature. The issue, I repeat, is not the rightness or the wrongness of what the plaintiff expresses in that literature. Rather, the nub of the matter is whether the defendant has portrayed his views incorrectly to City Council.

May I restate the issue by putting it this way, — would that right thinking member of society, having read the literature in evidence, and viewed the film, — would that person misrepresent the plaintiff's view on responsible sexual education, if he or she said of it what the defendant said. I recall the film; it does not speak of marriage or sexual intercourse in marriage. It addresses itself, as I conclude from the action portrayed, to young people, to teenagers, and presumably high school boys and girls. I believe it assumes that they are sexually active, and that they are not married. Birth control devices and their purpose and use are discussed. The film does not advocate intercourse, nor does it advocate the use of birth control, but neither does it issue any condemnation or prohibition in respect of either intercourse or birth control. I could add, the same is true of masturbation. It is silent on any moral view. The question which arises in my view is this, can that right thinking person, as I defined that person earlier, impute to it a moral message? What kind or which message is not significant or relevant to what I must decide in this case. It is not significant here to determine whether there is a right message or a wrong message, the point is whether a right thinking person could legitimately, — with common sense, I suggest, extract from the film or the literature, the sex comics, the same message which the plaintiff did, and express it in the language she used when writing to City Council. On that question, I conclude affirmatively that she could.

I return to a further consideration of the defendant's statement to City Council and I quote: "Sol Gordon is opposed because he condones any type of sexual expression, condones wholesale contraceptive and abortion availability, and opposes parental responsibility and Judeo-Christian morality." I have already said that a right minded person reading the plaintiff's sex comics, and viewing the film which he endorses, could have come to the same conclusion as did the defendant. But I say this with one qualification. The literature I have examined does not, I believe, admit the conclusion that the plaintiff approves any or all forms of sexual expression. In so concluding, I do not disregard the defence argument based upon the comic strip about the cowboy and the horse. I base my opinion rather upon the general thrust of the literature, and the film, and conclude that the defendant's expression approaches the extreme.

Nevertheless, the fact is that the defendant was addressing a public body on a highly controversial matter, and in truth she could have used less extreme language. But there is case law cited in the defendant's brief upon which I found my conclusion that the terminology used does not destroy the general thrust of the message which she, as a right minded citizen of Saskatoon, had a right to extrapolate from what she saw and read from the plaintiff's work.

Because I have concluded that the burden imposed by the rule pertaining to the law of justification has been met by the defendant, I will not discuss the defence of qualified privilege which she has raised. Nor do I believe that malice is in issue. To the contrary, I am satisfied to say, after hearing her testimony, that the defendant was motivated by a sincerity to serve her fellow citizens by defending a tradition which she holds, and which she expressed in her evidence, that sexual conduct should be portrayed in a framework, a tradition which defends chastity before marriage, and fidelity after.

As I said when I began, a democratic society will be maintained if freedom of — speech on matters touching the well being of society is guaranteed. In the ongoing debate, defamation is of course excluded. Here, the plaintiff chose a particular vehicle of communication, and in doing so exposed himself to the risk of the interpretation placed upon his work by the defendant.

In the result, he has not proved that he was defamed. The plaintiff's action is for the foregoing reasons dismissed, with costs.

Action dismissed.

5.2.3.1.7 *Ontario Libel and Slander Act*, R.S.O. 1990, c. L.12.

22. In an action for libel or slander for words containing two or more distinct charges against the plaintiff, a defence of justification shall not fail by reason only that the truth of every charge is not proved if the words not proved to be true do not materially injure the plaintiff's reputation having regard to the truth of the remaining charges. R.S.O. 1980, c. 237, s. 23.

Note: The only other province with such a provision is Nova Scotia (*Defamation Act*, R.S.N.S. 1989, c. 122, s. 9).

There is a risk in pleading justification. If the defendant sticks with justification right to the end and loses, then the defendant will pay an even larger sum in damages.

5.2.3.2 Fair Comment

5.2.3.2.1 Alexander Stark, *Dangerous Words* (Toronto: Ryerson Institute of Technology, 1985), p. 15

In this field of fair comment, the music critic, the literary reviewer, the editorial writer, and the newspaper columnist have gone at times to amazing lengths and still enjoyed the protection which the law gives. Take, for example, such a case as that of the Cherry sisters, brought against the Des Moines *Leader* in the State of Iowa in 1901. At one time the Cherry sisters had been the toast of the vaudeville stage. But the years had crept up on them and the toast had become cold and uninteresting. Unwisely they planned a comeback, and the dramatic critic of the Des Moines paper had this to say about their appearance; "Effie is an old jade of fifty summers, Jess is a frisky filly of forty, and Addie, the flower of the family, a capering monstrosity of thirty-five. Their long skinny arms equipped with talons at the extremities, swung mechanically, and anon waved frantically at the suffering audience. The mouths of their rancid features opened like caverns and sounds like the wailing of damned souls issued therefrom. They danced around the stage with a motion that suggested a cross between the *danse du ventre* and a fox trot — strange creatures with painted faces and hideous mien. Effie is spavined, Addie has stringhalt and Jessie, the only one who showed her stockings, has legs with calves as classic in their outline as the curves of a broom handle." But the court held that the statement was not libellous and said, "One who goes upon the stage to exhibit himself to the public, or who gives any kind of performance to which the public is invited, may be freely criticized." And it added further, "Surely, if one makes himself ridiculous in his public performances, he may be ridiculed by those whose duty or right it is to inform the public regarding the character of the performance."

5.2.3.2.2 *Pearlman v. C.B.C.* (1982), Man. L.R. (2d) 1 (Man. Q.B.)

MORSE, J.: It is stated in the text on *Defamation* by Duncan and Neill (1978), at p. 68, para. 12.14:

> The general rule is that, in order to qualify as fair comment, an expression of opinion must satisfy the following objective test: could any man honestly express that opinion on the proved facts? . . .

In my view, the defendants have met this objective test. I think the defendants could honestly describe a landlord such as the plaintiff, who acted as he did with respect to his properties and his tenants, as a person who had "no morals, principles, or conscience". These are, of course, strong words. But the defendants were entitled to express themselves strongly provided they honestly believed in the opinion which they expressed. I have no doubt that they did honestly believe in what they said.

5.2.3.2.3 Anne Skarsgard, "Freedom of the Press," (1980-81), *Saskatchewan Law Review* 45, pp. 307-316

The rationale of the defence of fair comment is to protect the defendant's right of freedom of speech and the public's right to find out what is happening in matters of legitimate public interest. A successful plea of the defence means that even if the plaintiff proves all the ingredients of a prima facie case of defamation, the defendant will not have to compensate him.

To succeed in this defence, the defendant must prove

1) that the comment was on a matter of public interest;

2) that the comment was fair;

3) that the words complained of were comment and not statement of fact. The defence is defeated if plaintiff can show express malice.

1) The defendant has to prove that the matter was of public interest. The best definition as to what constitutes a matter of public interest is found in Lord Denning's judgement in *London Artists v. Littler*:

> Whenever a matter is such as to affect people at large, so that they may be legitimately interested in, or concerned at, what is going on, or what may happen to them or others, then it is a matter of public interest on which everyone is entitled to make fair comment.

Thus the scope of matters of public interest is very wide. However, public interest must be legitimate. Gossip-mongering and gratuitous attacks on character are not protected by the defence, although it is often hard to draw the line between aspects of a public official's character which are strictly his own business and those which affect his fitness for office.

2) The comment must be fair. The word "fair" is misleading because it suggests that the comment must be reasonable. Actually the limits of fair comment are very wide and include comments which to many people would appear both unfair and unreasonable. For this reason the Faulks Committee in Britain recommended that the word "fair" be dropped and the defence renamed "comment'.

Comment, to be "fair" in the technical sense of this defence, must be based on true facts. However, where the facts are protected by an occasion of qualified privilege, the defendant does not have to prove their truth.

Another component of the requirement of fairness is a source of some confusion, and was the main issue in the *Cherneskey* case. Many courts and commentators have stated that comment, to be fair, had to represent an honestly held opinion, that is it must satisfy the subjective test: "Did the defendant honestly believe the comment?" Duncan and Neill, on the other hand, propose an objective test: "Could any man honestly express that opinion on the proved facts?" Whichever test is used, the honestly held opinion need not be reasonable. In the words of Lord Esher in *Merivale v. Carson*:

> Every latitude must be given to opinion and to prejudice . . . Mere exaggeration, or even gross exaggeration, would not make the comment unfair. However wrong the opinion expressed may be in point of truth, or however prejudiced the writer, it may still be within the prescribed limits . . . When you come to a question of fair comment you ought to be extremely liberal . . .

Similarly, Diplock, J. said in *Silkin v. Beaverbrook Newspapers Ltd.*,

> So in considering this case, members of the jury, do not apply the test of whether you agree with it. If juries did that, freedom of speech, the right of the crank to say what he likes, would go. Would a fair-minded man holding strong views, obstinate views, prejudiced views, have been capable of making this comment? If the answer to that is yes, then your verdict in this case should be a verdict for the defendants.

3) Finally, the words complained of must be comment, not statement of fact. The facts on which the statement is based should be either set out clearly or indicated by the commentator with sufficient clarity so that his audience is aware of the facts that form the basis of the comment. (However, setting out the facts on which the opinion is based is not an absolute requirement as long as the subject matter commented on is in the common knowledge of both the commentator and his audience.) This is how Lord Porter explained the principle in *Kemsley v. Foot*:

> If the defendant accurately states what some public man has really done, and then asserts that 'such conduct is disgraceful' this is merely an expression of his opinion, his comment on the plaintiff's conduct. So, if without setting it out, he identifies the conduct on which he comments by clear reference. In either case, the defendant enables his readers to judge for themselves how far his opinion is well founded; and therefore, what would otherwise be an allegation of fact becomes merely comment. But if he asserts that the plaintiff has been guilty of disgraceful conduct, and does not state what that conduct was, this is an allegation of fact for which there is no defence but privilege or truth.

Furthermore, the comment must be separated from statements of fact to be recognized as comment. Wrote Fletcher Moulton, L.J. in *Hunt v. Star Newspaper Co. Ltd.*,

> Comment in order to be justifiable as fair comment must appear as comment and must not be so mixed up with facts that the reader cannot distinguish between what is report and what is comment.

Although the comment can include inferences of fact, it must be recognized as comment. It if often extremely difficult, if not impossible, to distinguish between assertions of fact and statements which represent inferences drawn by the commentator. However, the distinction is a crucial one, as the defence of fair comment is available to protect an untrue defamatory inference, but not to protect a statement of fact, even though proved true, unless the defence of justification is also pleaded. This point was elucidated by Field, J. in *O'Brien v. Marquis of Salisbury*:

> It seems to me . . . that comment may sometimes consist in the statement of a fact, and may be held to be comment if the fact so stated appears to be a deduction or conclusion come to by the speaker from the facts stated or referred to by him, or in the common knowledge of the person speaking and those to whom the words are addressed and from which his conclusions may reasonably be inferred.

It should be pointed out that the above excerpts have all been culled from English decisions. The last one, saying that even a statement of fact may be held to be comment under certain circumstances, is an especially good example of the latitude English courts have traditionally given to the defence.

Since the distinction between fact and comment is often murky at best, the same principles of interpretation can lead one to diametrically opposed results. In Britain, because of this liberal interpretation given to the defence of fair comment by the courts, it has been a useful tool for safeguarding freedom of expression in the press. In the United States the defence has become unnecessary since both untrue statements of fact and of comment are protected by the extremely wide scope afforded to qualified privilege under the *New York Times* rule. In Canada, however, a number of recent decisions seem to have eroded the defence of fair comment to the point where one wonders whether it still serves a useful purpose.

b) The usefulness of fair comment to the press:

The best-known recent case on the defence of fair comment is *Cherneskey v. Armadale Publishers Ltd.*, the case of the Saskatoon alderman and lawyer who sued the Saskatoon *Star-Phoenix* for libel. The paper published a defamatory letter accusing Alderman Cherneskey of racism because of the stand he took at a City Council meeting (accurately reported in the paper) concerning the continuing existence of a native alcoholic rehabilitation centre in a residential neighbourhood. The letter writers were out of the jurisdiction and were not called as witnesses, consequently there was no evidence before the court whether they honestly believed what they had written. The newspaper management gave evidence that no one at the paper believed the alleged libel against the plaintiff.

The newspaper pleaded the defence of fair comment. The trial judge refused to put the defence before the jury, saying that a comment to be fair had to be an honestly held opinion, and there was no evidence that anybody held the opinion expressed in the letter. The decision was overturned by the Saskatchewan Court of Appeal. The two majority judges held that the requirement of honestly held opinion was satisfied in the case of a newspaper publishing the opinion of others, if the management honestly believed that the letter expressed the honestly held opinion of the writer. The plaintiff appealed to the Supreme Court of Canada which allowed the appeal and restored the trial decision, with Dickson, Spence and Estey, JJ. dissenting.

The Supreme Court did not decide whether the defence would have been available had the writers believed the statement and the newspaper did not, or had the newspaper believed it, but there was no evidence whether the writers did. (In *Lyon and Lyon v. Daily Telegraph Ltd.* the defence of fair comment succeeded in connection with a letter to the editor where there was no evidence as to the writer's state of mind, but dicta suggested that the newspaper agreed with the opinion expressed.)

According to the majority in the Supreme Court if the belief is not shown to be honestly held, the comment cannot be fair. Honesty of belief is an essential ingredient of the defence and one that the defendant has to prove.

Dickson, J. in his powerful dissent relied on Duncan and Neill's formulation of the defence, according to which the defendant has to establish that the statement is comment, that it is based on substantially true facts on a matter of public interest, and that the comment is *objectively* fair, that is, it satisfies the following objective test: "Could any man honestly express that opinion on the proved facts?" According to this view the defendant's subjective state of mind is only relevant as evidence of express malice which, if proven, would defeat the defence. The onus of proving express malice is on the plaintiff.

This interpretation of the law is also supported by Lord Denning in *Adams v. Sunday Pictorial Newspapers (1920) Ltd.*:

> The truth is that the burden on the defendant who pleads fair comment is already heavy enough. If he proves that the facts are true and that the comments, objectively considered, were fair, that is, if they were fair when considered without regard to the state of mind of the writer, I should not have thought that the plaintiff had much to complain about; nevertheless it has been held that the plaintiff can still succeed if he can prove that the comments, subjectively considered, were unfair because the writer was actuated by malice.

Dickson, J.'s argument in favour of an objective test in the first stage of this inquiry is very persuasive. Why have the second test of express malice if the first stage already includes the ingredients of the subjective test? Where the defendant is the writer himself, the two stages can be telescoped into one, but if he is not, this short-cut becomes unworkable.

The majority decision is an excellent example of conceptualism. It was arrived at through the mechanical application of a formula that obviously does not fit the facts of the case. The result is an absurdity that runs counter to the rationale behind the defence. The purpose of the defence of fair comment is to encourage freedom of expression. As Mr. Justice Dickson eloquently pointed out, if we make the defence available to newspapers only if they print opinions with which they agree, they would be engaged in a sort of self-censorship antithetical to a free press.

The decision was wrong for yet another reason. It singled out the publisher of the statement for harsher treatment than the commentator himself. Had the two letter writers been made defendants they could have relied on the defence, while the paper was held liable.

The press was not slow in reacting to the decision handed down on November 21, 1978. Within two days a commentary by Ioan Cohen appeared in the Ottawa *Citizen,* followed by another commentary on November 28 by Maurice Western, which was reprinted in other newspapers. The commentary explored the decision with all its implications for the press and for freedom of speech. On January 20, 1979 yet another article appeared, this time in the *Financial Post,* by William Monopoli. Said Mr. Monopoli:

> Most Canadians probably believe that they have freedom of speech and that such freedom is a fundamental right in a democratic society.
>
> But a recent decision of the Supreme Court of Canada suggests that the right may be severely limited...
>
> *Unless the effects of the judgement are changed by legislative action*, or unless the court modifies its opinion in another case — neither of which is a reasonable near-term possibility — the decision may well intimidate publishers and editors and deter them from printing any letter dealing with a controversial subject, lest they be sued for libel. (Emphasis added).

Monopoli underestimated the clout of the media. Less than a month later, on February 12, an editorial in the Toronto *Globe and Mail* called on the Attorney-General of each province to revise its libel and slander statutes to nullify the ruling. In early April the Canadian Press reported that Ontario Attorney-General Roy McMurtry said in an interview that the Uniform Law Conference which was to meet in August in Saskatoon should study the *Cherneskey* decision. Mr. McMurtry was further reported to favour an amendment to the Ontario *Libel and Slander Act*. By early June another Canadian Press story reported that Ontario would introduce the new legislation in the fall. Said Mr. McMurtry:

> As attorney-general I have a constitutional role as guardian of the community's civil liberties and in relation to this manner I have no doubt that to violate the right to communicate is to eviscerate democracy.

The following day a story in the Saskatoon *Star-Phoenix* indicated that Saskatchewan Attorney-General Roy Romanow also favoured an amendment to Saskatchewan's *Libel and Slander Act* to restore the law to what it was prior to the *Cherneskey* decision.

In August 1979 the Uniform Law Commissioners amended the uniform statute to deal with the problem, and urged the provinces to adopt it. According to the amended *Uniform Defamation Act* the publisher of an opinion may rely on the defence of fair comment if a person could objectively hold the opinion. Alberta has already amended its *Libel and Slander Act* along these lines. The Saskatchewan Government introduced a similar bill in the legislature, but it was tabled at the end of the last session.

Thus, our laws can charge surprisingly quickly when a powerful and influential lobby like the Canadian Daily Newspaper Publishers Association is affected. One must remember, however, that the amendment, if passed, will provide relief in only a small area of the law of defamation. The defence of fair comment will be available to the press when publishing opinions with which they do not agree, as long as the opinion is objectively fair. The amendment will not alter their position when they publish their own opinions. Furthermore, if courts continue to characterize comments as statements of fact, or as comment based on implied false facts, or if they use the wrong test to determine whether the comment is fair, the press will have a long, hard road ahead.

Let us look at some recent decisions and at the way the courts handled the defence of fair comment.

In the 1978 case of *Baltrop v. Canadian Broadcasting Corporation* a Nova Scotia trial court dismissed a libel charge against the CBC laid by a Dr. Donald Baltrop, who was a paid consultant to Canadian Metals Co. in Toronto. Dr. Baltrop was interviewed in a program called "Dying of Lead" on *As It Happens*, then his statements were discredited by another interviewee, an American doctor who said:

> I regret to say that my personal experience, and the experience of many of my colleagues in the States, with so-called experts on behalf of industry, has been very unfortunate. I've come to the belated conclusion that it is possible to buy the data you want. I've tested this particular viewpoint with relation to a very wide range of consumer and occupational problems in which I have been involved and I would be happy to substantiate for you the thesis that it is possible to buy any information you want, to substantiate any viewpoint. Dr. Baltrop is a paid consultant to the lead industry. He is paid to say what he has just said.

Everybody would agree that the second-last sentence is a statement of fact. The crux is the characterization of the last sentence. Taken by itself, it could be taken as a statement of fact. However, when considered in context, it becomes clearly an inference drawn by the American doctor from his opinion that "it is possible to buy any information you want", and from the true fact that Dr. Baltrop was a paid consultant, and is therefore comment. This was the position taken by the trial judge. However, the Nova Scotia Supreme Court did not agree. In its view the defence of fair comment could not be raised as the statement was not comment at all but an implied factual assertion that Dr. Baltrop was dishonest. The CBC could have won under this characterization only by the defence of justification by proving that Dr. Baltrop was indeed dishonest in saying what he said.

In *Vander Zalm v. Times Publishers* the British Columbia Minister of Human Resources sued for libel the publishers and editors of the Victoria *Times* as well as the free-lance cartoonist who depicted him pulling the wings off flies. On the Minister's lapel were inscribed the words: Human Resources. Said the trial judge:

> Literally, upon its face, the cartoon depicts the plaintiff as a person with a love of cruelty who enjoys causing suffering to defenceless creatures. That was a false misrepresentation of the character of the plaintiff as a person or in his role as Minister.

The paper pleaded the defence of fair comment, but failed. Munroe, J. agreed with counsel for the plaintiff that the cartoon conveyed a statement of fact rather than a comment as no grounds for the opinion were set out. (*Quaere* whether it would have made a difference if the cartoon had been accompanied by a caption). However, the court did not find it necessary to decide whether the cartoon conveyed a statement of fact or of comment as, in its view, the defence failed on other grounds.

With respect, a political cartoon is, by definition, comment. The facts on which the comment is based need not be set out by the commentator as long as these facts are familiar to his audience. Said Field, J. in *O'Brien v. Salisbury*:

If a statement in words of a fact stands by itself naked, without reference, either expressed or understood, to other antecedent or surrounding circumstances notorious to the speaker and to those to whom the words were addressed, there would be little, if any, room for the inference that it was understood otherwise as a bare statement of fact, and then if untrue, there would be no answer to the action.

It follows that, if the statement is understood with reference to antecedent or surrounding circumstances familiar to the speaker and to his audience, then it qualifies as comment.

The ratio of Munroe, J.'s decision was that, even assuming that there was comment, it was based on untrue facts and therefore it was not fair. What are these untrue facts? We are not told. The court merely says that, although the Minister's statements and decisions were controversial, they "could not fairly lead an ordinary person to conclude that the plaintiff acted in a cruel, sadistic or thoughtless manner when performing his duties." It seems that the court equates "untrue facts" with "unfair comment". And why is the comment unfair? Because the ordinary person (i.e. the judge) would not draw this conclusion from the Minister's record.

As we have already seen, under the general test of fair comment, "fair" is not equated with "reasonable". As long as a person might honestly hold a view on the facts, the comment is fair, however obstinate or exaggerated it may be. In the words of Lord Esher in *Merivale v. Carson*, "However wrong the opinion expressed may be in point of truth, or however prejudiced the writer, it may still be within the prescribed limits."

Could it be that Mr. Justice Munroe thought that the comment imputed dishonourable conduct or base motives to the plaintiff? Under those circumstances the test as to fairness is uncertain. There are three possibilities:

1) The defence of fair comment is not applicable and the only way to defend such a comment is to show that it is the only possible inference from the primary facts, that is, by a defence of justification;

2) The defence of fair comment is applicable but the defendant must satisfy the judge or jury that the comment was a reasonable inference from the facts commented on;

3) The general test of fair comment applies. According to Duncan and Neill this is the better view, as "a test based on reasonableness runs counter to the whole concept of the defence of fair comment. Furthermore, it is difficult in practice to draw an accurate dividing-line between cases which involve an imputation of dishonourable conduct and those which do not."

In *Vander Zalm* the trial judge seems to have applied the intermediate test of reasonableness to determine whether the comment was fair. However, if this was his intention, he should have pointed out that he was applying the special test because, in his view, there was imputation of dishonourable conduct.

It is unlikely, however, that Munroe, J. intended to apply the special test as he had applied this same "reasonableness" test in an earlier decision and, as we shall see shortly, there could have been no imputation of dishonourable conduct in *Holt v. Sun Publishing Co.* Furthermore, when *Vander Zalm* was appealed, the appeal was allowed, all five judges agreeing that Munroe, J. had erred by applying the wrong test.

There was no agreement in the British Columbia Court of Appeal on whether the cartoon was, in fact, defamatory. Atkins, J.A. held that it was not, thereby overruling Munroe, J. on a question of fact. Hinkson, J.A. agreed with the trial judge that the cartoon was defamatory. Craig, J. did not think that the cartoon was defamatory, but was not prepared to say that the trial judge was clearly wrong, while Nemetz and Seaton, JJ.A. were not sure whether the cartoon was defamatory or not. All five agreed, however, that the defendants were not liable in any event because the defence of fair comment was available to them.

Nemetz, J.A. held, with Aikins and Hinkson, JJ.A. concurring, that Munroe, J. erred in applying the test of reasonableness to decide whether the comment was fair. In other words, the question should not have been whether the facts pleaded would fairly lead to the conclusion that the plaintiff was cruel, but whether the comment represented the honest opinion of the commentator.

Craig, J.A. held that Munroe, J. erred in saying that the comment was based on untrue facts. The "fact" forming the basis of the comment was not, as implied by Munroe, J., that the minister was depicted as cruel. The facts were set out in the particulars by the defendants, and consisted of sixteen highly controversial public statements or acts of the minister, all but one of which were conceded by him to be true. Craig, J.A. agreed with Nemetz and Hinkson, JJ.A. that the true test of fairness was whether the defendant honestly held the view expressed, thereby following the subjective test that carried the day in the *Cherneskey* decision. Justice was done under the particular circumstances of this case, because the cartoonist was available to give evidence and because the editors happened to agree with the opinion expressed in the cartoon. Either one of these circumstances would probably have been sufficient to satisfy the subjective test requiring that the opinion be honestly held. The fact remains that *Cherneskey* being the law in every province except Alberta, the press is not protected when publishing opinions which are fair, but with which they do not agree, unless the commentator is available to testify about his state of mind.

But let us go back to *Holt v. Sun Publishing* to see what treatment Mr. Justice Munroe gave to the defence of fair comment in that case. M.P. Simma Holt sued the Vancouver *Sun* for printing an editorial criticizing her for interviewing Charles Manson groupie Lynette "Squeaky" Fromme and planning to ask permission to carry a message from her to Charles Manson. Holt was touring California prisons as a member of the Commons committee on prisons. The editorial stated:

> But interviewing or carrying messages for such as mass murderer Charles Manson and his groupies in U.S. jails is not what Mrs. Holt and Mr. Reynolds are paid to be doing as members of the Commons committee on prisons. What they are supposed to be doing is concentrating on

finding ways of improving Canada's chaotic prison system. As someone who knows prisoners and prison conditions, Mrs. Holt is eminently qualified to offer solutions if she can keep her mind on the task at hand . . .

Holt sued and the paper unsuccessfully pleaded fair comment. Munroe, J. said in his decision:

The defence of fair comment depends upon the comment having been made upon true facts. Were the words used true in substance and in fact? I think not. Upon the evidence I find that there is no basis upon which it can reasonably be said that interviewing Fromme or any prison inmate was beyond the scope of what the plaintiff was being paid to do as a member of the subcommittee on prisons, nor is there any basis for saying that she failed or neglected in her duty to concentrate on finding ways to improve Canada's prison system, or that she interviewed Charles Manson or carried messages for him and his groupies in U.S. jails, or that she failed to keep her mind on the task at hand.

Just as he did in *Vander Zalm*, Munroe, J. does not say explicitly which are the untrue facts forming the basis of the comment. He does not say whether the enumerated statements fall into the category of untrue fact or comment based on untrue fact. In *Vander Zalm* the court found it unnecessary to determine the threshold question of whether the cartoon was statement of fact or comment; in *Holt* it did not bother to separate fact from comment. In both instances it applied the same test of "reasonableness" to what one assumes it considered comment. In essence, the judge dismissed the defence because he disagreed with what was said, something Diplock, J. cautioned the jury against in *Silkin v. Beaverbrook Newspapers Ltd.*

Mr. Justice Monroe heard yet another defamation case in 1978. In *Masters v. Fox* a newspaper imputed corrupt or dishonest motives to candidates running for municipal office. It should come as no surprise that the defence of fair comment failed here too. The court held that the imputation was not one that a fair-minded person could reasonably draw from the facts. In this case it was appropriate to choose the test of reasonableness, as there was an imputation of dishonourable conduct or base motives but again, the determination of whether the comment was reasonable should have been left to the jury.

All these decisions in favour of defamed plaintiffs reflect the low priority accorded to freedom of speech in our society. This could be due partly to a certain paternalism, a mistrust of the irrational, cranky element which is the hallmark of an immature society. Contrast this with the England of Pope and Swift where biting, even violent satire was not only tolerated but enjoyed because society was basically assured, stable, and content. The decisions also reflect the low esteem in which our society holds the media. There is a general feeling today, a feeling no doubt shared by the judiciary, that the "paparazzi", although not elected and often not even very knowledgeable, wield enormous and unwarranted power and need to be curbed. Journalists, so the theory goes, look for scandal to sell copy, they snoop and are, in the words of a columnist, "anti-capitalist left-wing bleeding hearts who . . . wouldn't know privacy from a privet hedge." Although there may be some truth in these contentions and the press is not always as responsible as one would expect, surely the answer is not to muzzle it. Courts should ask themselves whether, in denying the defence of fair comment to the media, they are not indulging in overkill. There may be better ways of curbing the power of the press than by confining it to the role of dispenser of bland information. There is talk in Saskatchewan of creating a press council along the British model with the purpose of upgrading the press from within. However, the British experience in this area has not been too successful. Maybe government action to prevent concentration of ownership would do more to help present a wider and better balanced spectrum of opinion to the public.

Note: Fair comment is defined as an expression of opinion made in good faith and without malice on a manner of public interest. In order to succeed in the defence of fair comment the defendant must:

   a. show that the statements which are claimed to be defamatory ale expressions of opinion, not allegations of fact;
   b. show that some factual basis is stated upon which the opinion expressed could plausibly be based, unless the facts are notorious;
   c. show that. to the extent the material in question contains both allegations of fact and expressions of opinion, the allegations of fact are true, that the expressions of opinion are plausibly based upon or derived from them, and that the allegations of fact and the expressions of opinion are clearly distinguished from each other.
   d. show that the matter with respect to which the statements in question were made is one of public interest;
   e. show that the statements in question are an honest expression of his real opinion, or, to put it slightly differently, that he honestly believes in the opinion expressed.

The defendant is not required to show that the statements were made without malice. The plaintiff may attempt to negative the defence of fair comment by establishing that the defendant was actuated by malice in making the statements.

5.2.3.2.4 *Vander Zalm v. Times Publishers* (1980), 18 B.C.L.R. 210 (B.C.C.A.)

NEMETZ, C.J.B.C.: — On 22nd June 1978 there appeared on the editorial page of the Victoria *Times*, one of the city of Victoria's leading daily newspapers, a cartoon depicting the plaintiff, William N. Vander Zalm, a cabinet minister then holding the office of Minister of Human Resources in the government of British Columbia. It was drawn by the defendant Robert Bierman, a freelance political cartoonist who had contributed cartoons to the newspaper for many years. Alongside the cartoon there appeared an actual photograph of the minister, as part of a reprinted editorial criticizing Mr. Vander Zalm's statements and policies. It is apparent that the cartoon exaggerated the facial features of the plaintiff. It depicted Mr. Vander Zalm smiling, seated at a table, and engaged in plucking the wings from a fly. Other flies, without wings, were shown moving on the table. On the plaintiffs lapel were inscribed the words "Human Resources".

The minister sued for damages, claiming that the cartoon libelled him. He pleaded that the newspaper, its editor, its publisher and Mr. Bierman alleged by the cartoon that he was "a person of cruel and sadistic nature who enjoys inflicting suffering and torture on helpless beings who cannot protect themselves". The action was heard by Munroe, J., sitting without a jury. The defendants pleaded that the cartoon was not defamatory, and that in any event it was fair comment. The learned trial judge rejected these contentions and found for the plaintiff, awarding damages of $3,500 against the defendants. This is an appeal from that judgment [[1979] 2 W.W.R. 673, 8 C.C.L.T. 144, 96 D.L.R. (3d) 172].

Before addressing myself to the issues, I should like to make some prefatory observations as to political cartoons in general. Counsel were agreed that there was a paucity of decided cases concerning libel arising from political caricatures or cartoons-despite the fact that such cartoons have had a long history of publication in Canada as well as in most of the Western world. As a result, as noted by the learned editors of *Gatley on Libel and Slander*, 7th ed. (1974), p. 15, n. 23: "the limits of what is permissible in the way of cartoons . . . are undefined". I have examined definitions of the word "cartoon" in its modern use (coined, it is suggested, by the editors of *Punch*) and would adopt the one set out by the scholar Winslow Ames in the *Encyclopedia Britannica* (1961):

> . . . a pictorial parody . . . which by the devices of caricature, analogy and ludicrous juxtaposition sharpens the public view of a contemporary event, folkway, or political or social trend. It is normally humorous but may be positively savage.

Now the well-known test for whether a statement or allegation is defamatory is set out in *Salmond on Torts*, 17th ed. (1977), pp. 139-40, from which I quote as follows:

> A defamatory statement is one which has a tendency to injure the reputation of the person to whom it refers; which tends, that is to say, to lower him in the estimation of right-thinking members of society generally and in particular to cause him to be regarded with feelings of hatred, contempt, ridicule, fear, dislike or disesteem.

I have placed these two quotations in juxtaposition because it becomes obvious that most political cartoons have, inherent in their satire, a tendency to lower their subject in the estimation of the public. Nevertheless, it has been said that persons accepting public office can expect attack and criticism on the grounds that "the public interest requires that a man's public conduct shall be open to the most searching criticism", per Bain, J. in *Martin v. Man. Free Press Co.* (1892), 8 Man. R. 50 at 72. However, the question of what constitutes valid "searching criticism" and what constitutes libel must be examined in the context of all the surrounding circumstances.

I turn now to the consideration of the cartoon. The defendants denied that the cartoon defamed the plaintiff and pleaded that in any event the cartoon was fair comment on a matter of public interest and that accordingly there was no libel. I have had the privilege of reading the reasons for judgment prepared by each of my brothers Seaton, Hinkson and Craig, JJ.A., and agree with them that, even if the cartoon was prima facie defamatory, the defence of fair comment was available in the circumstances. However, I should like to advance my own view of why that defence was available here.

The three elements of the defence of fair comment are well known. First, the matter must be recognizable to the ordinary reasonable man as a comment upon true facts, and not as a bare statement of fact. Secondly, the matter commented upon must be one of public interest. There must, in short, be a public nexus between the matter and the person caricatured. In a case such as this, the cartoonist may not intrude upon the private life of a public man, no matter how interesting such an intrusion may be to the public, nor may he expose a private person to unsought publicity. Finally, as explained by Diplock, J. (as he then was) in *Silkin v. Beaverbrook Newspapers,* [1958] I W.L.R. 743 at 747, [1958] 2 All E.R. 516, and by the Supreme Court of Canada in *Cherneskey v. Armadale Publishers Ltd.,* [1979] 1 S.C.R. 1067, 24 N.R. 271, the comment must be "fair" in that it must, to quote Martland, J: in *Cherneskey* at p. 1073, "represent an honest expression of the real view of the person making the comment". At the trial of this action, the availability of the defence turned on this last element. Munroe, J. specifically left open the question of whether the matter was comment or not, and did not find it necessary to consider the question of public interest. The learned judge held that the defence failed because the facts pleaded as the basis for the alleged comment "could not . . . fairly lead to the imputation arising from the cartoon" (p. 675).

I agree with my brother Hinkson that in making this finding the learned judge applied the wrong test. It is to be remembered that the questions of whether the matter complained of is fact or comment, and if it is comment whether it is "fair", are questions of fact: see *Jones v. Skelton,* [1963] 1 W.L.R. 1362, [1963] 3 All E.R. 952 (P.C.). Consequently in a libel action such as this, heard by a judge sitting without a jury, whether the defence of fair comment succeeds or not rests upon the trial judge drawing proper inferences from proven facts. The question of credibility does not necessarily arise. Certainly it did not arise in this case. Accordingly, an appellate tribunal is in as good a position as the trial judge to draw the proper inferences.

Now as I have already noted, the act of putting oneself in the public arena tends to invite appraisal of one's public conduct. The evidence clearly shows that the minister was not unaware of the widespread publicity attending his public conduct over the period in question. The learned trial judge in his reasons for judgment put it succinctly and I quote him in part [p. 675]:

> During the 14 years that the plaintiff has been engaged in public life he has been a controversial figure. not adverse to expressing publicly his opinion upon contentious matters.

Sixteen instances of controversial statements and acts attributed to the minister were pleaded by the defendants as particulars of facts upon which the cartoon was said to comment. Each of them had received considerable publicity. These particulars are set out in the judgment of my brother Craig, and I note that only one, para. (h), was categorically denied by the plaintiff. All of the other 15 were either entirely acknowledged or substantially conceded after qualification. I refer by way of example only to those matters arising in paras. (a), (b), (e), (1), (m), (n) and (p):

"a. That the Plaintiff, within hours of being appointed Human Resources Minister in December, 1975, stated that he would develop ways of dealing with welfare recipients who refused to 'pick up their shovels.'

"b. That the Plaintiff, since assuming the role of Minister of Human Resources, has cut off funding for a number of community groups that had been providing valuable services for those in need. . . .

"e. That in March, 1976, the Plaintiff tightened regulations so that fewer people in British Columbia would be classified as handicapped and so be eligible for handicapped benefits. . . ."

"1. That in October,' 1977, the Plaintiff stated that young people should be denied assistance because they have more mobility to find jobs.

"m. That in January, 1978, the Plaintiff ordered that even emergency welfare aid be refused to persons in areas where the picking of hallucinogenic mushrooms is common.

"n. That in March, 1978, the Plaintiff suggested that the current level of unemployment insurance payments to single people should be reduced. . . .

"p. That in June, 1978, the Plaintiff commented that native Indians in Vancouver should return to their reserves because there was 'more opportunity' there for them."

Now, one can approve or disapprove of these ministerial concerns, but there is little doubt that these statements were provocative. It should not, therefore, have come to the minister as a surprise that these statements would become well known to the public and that someone would respond to them. One such person was the defendant cartoonist. In giving evidence at the trial, Mr. Bierman was questioned as to the meaning of the cartoon. I quote his testimony in part:

"MR. BIERMAN: This particular cartoon — I tried to say with it that the Minister of Human Resources had a cruel attitude to the underprivileged position and defenceless people under his ministry where, in particular, I was referring to the Indians.

"MR. FARQUHAR: Now, could you describe, please, the significance of the various components of the cartoon?

"MR. BIERMAN: Oh, I could describe it by what I would say that I used the body which I labelled as Human Resources, the ministry, the head on it as a caricature of Mr. Vander Zalm who at that time was the Minister of Human Resources, and the fly depicts the helpless Indians that were in his words, 'Attracted to the big lights'. And what he is doing there, he is more or less clipping their wings. However, he is pulling them out which is different from clipping, but he's clipping their wings so they can't roam around any longer or fly around to the bright lights, not realizing the pain that he causes.

"MR. FARQUHAR: Was there any particular reason why you did that cartoon at that time?

"MR. BERMAN: Yes, that was in relation to a statement that the Indians were attracted to the bright lights and excitement of the big city and, I take it, it was Vancouver and should return to their reserves if they still wanted to qualify for welfare. And that they had better opportunity there on the reserves.

"MR. FARQUHAR: Now, in addition to that statement by the minister, at the time that you prepared the cartoon, did you have in mind any other actions of the Minister of Human Resources?

"MR. BIERMAN: Yes sir."

In my view, these statements and actions of the minister, including the statement concerning Indians which was publicized only a few days before the publication of the cartoon, provided the necessary substratum of sufficiently publicized facts to enable the ordinary reader to recognize the nexus of the cartoon and the statements. Ordinary and reasonable persons in this country are well acquainted with the allegorical nature of political cartoons and, in my opinion, would have little difficulty in recognizing this cartoon as a comment upon such facts; a comment, indeed, of the very sort which Mr. Bierman testified he intended to make. Nor can it be doubted that the facts commented upon were matters of considerable public interest and concerned the minister in his public rather than his personal capacity.

The next question that arises is whether the comment was "fair". In charging the jury in the *Silkin* case, supra, Lord Diplock explained the test in this way [p. 747]:

> I have been referring, and counsel in their speeches to you have been referring, to fair comment, because that is the technical name which is given to this defence, or, as I should prefer to say, which is given to the right of every citizen to comment on matters of public interest. But the expression 'fair comment' is a little misleading. It may give you the impression that you, the jury, have to decide whether you agree with the comment, whether you think it is fair. If that were the question you had to decide, you realize that the limits of freedom which the law allows would be greatly curtailed. People are entitled to hold and to express freely on matters of public interest strong views, views which some of you, or indeed all of you, may think are exaggerated, obstinate or prejudiced, provided — and this is the important thing — that they are views which they honestly hold. The basis of our public life is that the crank, the enthusiast, may say what he honestly thinks just as much as the reasonable man or woman who sits on a jury, and it would be a sad day for freedom of speech in this country if a jury were to apply the test of whether it agrees with the comment instead of applying the true test: was this an opinion, however exaggerated, obstinate or prejudiced, which was honestly held by the writer?

The question, then, is this: Did the comment made by the cartoon represent the honest opinion of Mr. Bierman? At the end of the cartoonist's examination-in-chief, the following exchange took place:

"MR. FARQUHAR: Now, you have testified as to what you intended the cartoon to say about the Minister of Human Resources, did that represent your honest opinion of the Minister of Human Resources at the time you prepared the cartoon?

"MR. BIERMAN: Yes, sir.

Now, as I have already stated, what the cartoonist intended the cartoon to say, as quoted above, coincides. in my opinion, with what the ordinary and reasonable person would take the cartoon as saying; namely, it is a comment of the nature Mr. Bierman described, concerned solely with the plaintiff in his ministerial capacity. I conclude from the whole of Mr. Bierman's testimony that that indeed represents an honest expression of his real view. No question arises as to credibility since it is obvious that the learned trial judge did not disbelieve the cartoonist, and no issue arose in this regard. Having these factors before us, is the defence of fair comment available? I think it is. As, in the circumstances of this case, it is my respectful view that the cartoon represents fair comment on a matter of public interest, I would, therefore, allow the appeal and dismiss the action.

HINKSON, J.A.: ... In these circumstances it is necessary then to turn to the other defence raised by the appellants, namely, fair comment. At trial the appellants relied upon the statements made and decisions taken by the respondent as minister as constituting the facts upon which the comment was made. The learned trial judge said in discussing this aspect of the matter [p. 675]:

> During the 14 years that the plaintiff has been engaged in public life he has been a controversial figure, not adverse to expressing publicly his opinion upon contentious matters. Nevertheless, upon the evidence I find that the controversial statements made by the plaintiff and relied upon by the defendants were such that he was entitled to hold and to express, and the decisions made by him as minister were made in good faith pursuant to his duty and responsibility as such minister, and could not fairly lead an ordinary person to conclude that the plaintiff acted in a cruel, sadistic or thoughtless manner when performing his duties. His statements and acts, as one would expect, were approved by some and disapproved by others, but could not in my opinion fairly lead to the imputation arising from the cartoon.

In my view the learned trial judge erred in disposing of the defence of fair comment in that way.

In *Cherneskey v. Armadale Publishers Ltd.*, [1978] 6 W.W.R. 618, 7 C.C.L.T. 69, 90 D.L.R. (3d) 321, Martland, J. at p. 636 said:

> A clear statement of the nature of the defence of fair comment is found in the summing up to the jury of Diplock, J. (as he then was) in the case of *Silkin v. Beaverbrook Newspapers*, [1958] 1 W.L.R. 743 at 747, [1958] 2 All E.R. 516:
>
> > "I have been referring, and counsel in their speeches to you have been referring, to fair comment, because that is the technical nature which is given to this defence, or, as I should prefer to say, which is given to the right of every citizen to comment on matters of public interest. But the expression 'fair comment' is a little misleading. I may give you the impression that you, the jury, have to decide whether you agree with the comment, whether you think it is fair. If that were the question you had to decide, you realize that the limits of freedom which the law allows would be greatly curtailed. People are entitled to hold and to express freely on matters of public interest strong views, views which some of you, or indeed all of you, may think are exaggerated, obstinate or prejudiced, provided — and this is the important thing — that they are views which they honestly hold. The basis of our public life is that the crank, the enthusiast, may say what he honestly thinks just as much as the reasonable man or woman who sits on a jury, and it would be a sad day for freedom of speech in this country if a jury were to apply the test of whether it agrees with

> the comment instead of applying the true test: was this an opinion, however exaggerated, obstinate or prejudiced, which was honestly held by the writer?"

The Supreme Court of Canada decided in the *Cherneskey* case, in respect of the defence of fair comment, that it is dependent upon the fact that the words used must represent an honest expression of the real view of the person making the comment.

In response to that proposition, counsel for the respondent advanced a number of submissions. First, he contended that the message in the cartoon was a statement of fact rather than an expression of opinion. In my view there is no merit in that submission. It is not contended by the respondent that the cartoon was to be interpreted literally and as I have already indicated, having regard to the fact that the respondent was well known in public life and that he was being described in his capacity as Minister of Human Resources, a moment's reflection by the reader of the newspaper would indicate that the cartoon referred to the statements and policies of the respondent as Minister of Human Resources and that the message in the cartoon was a comment on those statements and policies. Approached in that way it seems to me that there were facts before the reader which formed the basis for the comment.

Second, it was contended that the appellant Bierman who drew the cartoon, had no honest belief in the opinion being expressed. In giving his evidence in chief this witness testified:

"Q. And what, if anything, were you intending the cartoon to say? A. This particular cartoon I tried to say with it that the Minister of Human Resources had a cruel attitude to the underprivileged position and defenseless people under his ministry where, in particular, I was referring to the Indians."

At the conclusion of his evidence in chief the witness testified that the cartoon represented his honest opinion of the Minister of Human Resources at the time the cartoon was prepared. In cross-examination it was suggested that the witness had portrayed the respondent as a cruel and sadistic person. A discussion took place as to the meaning of sadistic at which point the trial judge intervened as follows:

"THE COURT: Let us assume for the purpose of this question that a person that pulls the wings off a fly is a sadistic person in the sense that he enjoys seeing other creatures suffering. It may be a poor definition, adopting that stand, you say your cartoon shows him as a sadistic person or otherwise?

"THE WITNESS: Otherwise, sir.

"THE COURT: Why do you say that? A. Because it is an assumption that anybody that pulls wings off flies is a sadistic person and I don't agree with that. If a child pulls wings off of a fly, is the child sadistic or if a person that is evil-minded, is that person sadistic? Any person that doesn't know picking wings off flies causes pain and suffering and nevertheless does it —

"THE COURT: You don't suggest that the minister depicted in your cartoon is either a child nor evil-minded? A. In the cartoon, the minister is evil-minded.

"Q. You're not suggesting that you had an honest opinion at the time that you drew that cartoon that Mr. Vander Zalm was evil-minded? A. Not an honest opinion, I knew better, but in my cartoon I drew him as being a feeble-minded person, thoughtless and cruel."

In my view, the witness was adhering to his evidence in chief as to the opinion he had formed and that such was his honest belief.

The defence also called Miss B. J. McLintock, the editor of the Victoria *Times* newspaper. She had seen the cartoon in the page proof on the morning of 22nd June 1978 and had permitted it to be published. Her evidence disclosed that she considered that the statements and policies of the respondent while he was Minister of Human Resources marked him as performing his duties in a cruel manner and that this was an opinion honestly held by her at the time that she approved the publication of the cartoon.

The learned trial judge appeared to consider that the statements and policies of the respondent could not fairly lead an ordinary reasonable person to conclude that he acted in a cruel manner in performing his duties. But it seems to me that does not apply the proper test. If the appellants Bierman and McLintock honestly held that view then, because the subject matter was a matter of public interest, they were entitled to express that opinion without becoming liable to the respondent.

I conclude that the defence of fair comment should prevail. In the result I would allow the appeal and dismiss the action.

CRAIG, J.A.: This conclusion, therefore, requires a consideration of the defence of fair comment. What is "fair comment"? It must be "the expression of an opinion based on true facts, i.e., facts admitted or proved to be true" — *Gatley on Libel and Slander*, 6th ed. (1967), p. 325 — but the "true facts" need not be stated at the time of the expression of the opinion. They may be implied and specified as particulars in the defence: *Kemsley v. Foot*, [1952] A.C. 345, [1952] 1 All E.R. 501 (C.A.). If the commentator sets out the facts in the comment he may rely on the defence of fair comment only if he proves every fact to be true. On the other hand, if he merely implies the fact, or facts, in the comment and gives the facts in the form of particulars he need establish only the truth of one of the facts: see *Kemsely v. Foot*, supra.

The word "fair" in the phrase "fair comment" is a misnomer because it conveys the concept that comment must be "reasonable". This is not the case as pointed out by Diplock, J. in addressing the jury in *Silkin v. Beaverbrook Newspapers*, [1958] 1 W.L.R. 743, [1958] 2 All E.R. 516 at 520, when he said:

> So in considering this case, members of the jury, do not apply the test of whether you agree with it. If juries did that, freedom of speech, the right of the crank to say what he likes, would go. Would a fair-minded man holding strong views, obstinate views, prejudiced views, have been capable of making this comment? If the answer to that is yes, then your verdict in this case should be a verdict for the defendants. Such a verdict does not mean that you agree with the comment. All it means is that you think that a man might honestly hold those views on those facts.

Counsel for the respondent submitted to the trial judge, and to this court, that the plea of "fair comment" was unavailable because there were "no facts stated" at the time of the publication of the cartoon from which there could be an inference that the cartoon was a fair comment. He submitted that the cartoon was not a comment on a matter of public interest but, solely, a statement of fact vilifying the respondent. In a portion of the reasons of the trial judge which I have quoted, he said that while he thought there was "merit" in the submission he did not find it necessary to decide that issue because he felt that the defence of fair comment failed "in any event".

The statement of defence contains a number of facts upon which the appellants rely in support of the defence of fair comment. In his cross-examination the respondent conceded, frankly, that he had said or done some of the things set out in the particulars in the statement of defence. The nature of the cartoon indicates that the cartoonist is commenting, unfavourably, on the conduct of the appellant as Minister of Human Resources. The nature of the conduct is set out in the particulars in the statement of defence. I think that the publisher could not be expected to accompany the cartoon with a statement of facts upon which the cartoon was based, nor could the cartoonist be expected to incorporate all these facts in the cartoon.

In his reasons for judgment, the trial judge said [p. 674]: "The defence of fair comment cannot prevail if the facts on which comment is made are untrue and defamatory. No comment can be fair which is built upon facts which are invented or misstated". I infer from his judgment that he considered that the depiction of the respondent as a "cruel" man was false and that this was, therefore, an untrue allegation. However that is not the fact upon which the appellants were relying. The facts upon which the cartoonist was relying to make his comment were set out in the particulars. The respondent conceded that some of the particulars, at least, were true. The test was, therefore, did the appellants honestly hold the views which they purported to express in the cartoon on the facts, or any of them, set out in the particulars?

The tenor of Bierman's testimony and the appellant McLintock's testimony was that they honestly felt that in some of his actions as Minister of Human Resources the minister acted in a cruel and thoughtless way.

I infer from the reasons for judgment that the trial judge did not disbelieve the testimony of the appellants, or find that they did not honestly hold the opinions which they expressed, but that rather the facts upon which they based the statement were untrue. Yet, as I have pointed out, some of the facts, at least, upon which the appellants relied in expressing their opinion were admitted by the respondent.

Many would regard the cartoon as anything but "fair" comment. On the other hand, I think that there.was a basis upon which the appellants could properly rely upon the defence of false comment. I think that the trial judge applied the wrong test in rejecting it.

The problem is, should the action be dismissed or should the appeal simply be allowed and a new trial directed? If the trial judge had disbelieved the testimony of the appellant Bierman and the appellant McLintock that they honestly held the view which was expressed by the cartoon the defence of fair comment would have failed. As I have already said, I think that the trial judge did not disbelieve the appellants' testimony and that, therefore, the appropriate disposition of the case would be to allow the appeal and to dismiss the action.

5.2.3.2.5 *Farrell v. St. John's Publishing Co.* (1986), 58 Nfld. & P.E.I.R. 66 (Nfld. C.A.)

MORGAN, J.A.: For the defence of fair comment to succeed it must be based upon the truth of the facts upon which the comment is made. A writer cannot adopt as true the untrue statement of facts made by others, and then comment on them on the assumption that they are true. "In order to give room for the plea of fair comment the facts must be truly stated."

5.2.3.2.6 *Pound v. Scott* (1973), 4 W.W.R. 403 (B.C.S.C.)

WOOTTON, J.: Action for damages for libel.

The alleged libellous article is one authored by the defendant Scott and published by the defendant Victoria Press Limited in one issue of its newspaper, the Victoria *Daily Times*.

The defendant Scott is a well-known columnist, and the column in question, accompanied by a photograph of the defendant Scott, was published on 13th August 1971 (Ex. 1). It reads as follows:

> *"Old Refrain*
>
> *"Come Now, Doctor*
> *Watch The Facts*

"Death is inevitable. Taxes are inevitable. Inevitable, too, is the British immigrant doctor preaching to Canadians on the evils of 'socialized medicine.' Heigh-ho. That's life.

"Even so, I was astonished at the incredible yardage of newsprint gratuitously provided earlier this week on our good Page Five to a British immigrant doctor whose information was somewhat tired (five years out of date), whose prejudices were even narrower than others of his kind and whose motivation for breaking into the usually shunned glare of public opinion seems to have been a kind of outright blackmail.

"What 33-year-old Dr. Brian S. Pound, of our town, is telling us, gentle reader, is that if the British Columbia government goes any further toward 'socialized medicine' he will take off for other parts where things are done more to his liking. It cannot be considered an idle threat, either. That's just what Dr. Pound did when he pulled out of Britain. 'If we don't like it,' he told our Don Vipond, 'then it's up to us to get out,' a contingency that does not appear to be included in the Hippocratic Oath.

"Dr. Pound is not unusual since thousands of British doctors have been doing that in the 25 years since Britain's National Health Service assumed a world leadership in humanitarian medicine, but he does seem rather young and inexperienced to have made such a bold decision.

"Indeed, most of his time in England appears to have been in training, for which the British taxpayer shelled out $22,500. (Dr. Pound told Vipond that it cost the state a mere $6,000 to give him the education that's earned him such rich rewards in British Columbia, but the official 1967 figure on state subsidies for doctor training in the United Kingdom was $22,500 per doctor: if that's what it cost to license Dr. Pound they sure as shootin' got a small return on the investment.)

"It was a matter of conscience, Dr. Pound told Vipond, to rebel against Britain's 'second rate' medicine and certainly one must agree that there is nothing 'second rate' about his subsequent career as a general practitioner in Victoria. His listed income under B.C. Medicare was $41,452 two years ago, $53,291 last year. (Just once I'd like to meet a British doctor who left as a matter of conscience without instantly doubling or tripling his income.)

"Apart from the background of his brief practice, Dr. Pound is in the classic tradition of such immigrants who so often justify the desertion of their nation and their patients by a paranoid attack on the British system and issue the warning that It Can Happen Here. To that, all I can say is (1) we should be so lucky and (2) isn't it just a teeny-weeny bit cheeky for this Johnny-Come-Lately to be threatening us if our elected representatives displease him?

"Dr. Pound's main beef against the National Health Service is the familiar lament that the general practitioner is not given hospital privileges, that, as he told Vipond, 'if you can't treat the patient with an aspirin you've got to refer him.'

"Even in those days when the young doctor was on the scene, that was patently untrue, as he surely knows. Then, and now, 90 per cent of all the nation's ills are treated in the British family doctor's surgery. Under the system the general practitioner is just exactly the primary diagnostician that he is in Canada, the difference being that the referral is made to a specialist when there is an operation to be performed in hospital.

"There are two schools of thought on this. My own doctor in London was one of those who thought it the best system, hadn't used a knife in 20 years except for an occasional circumcision, and considered it only sensible logic that, whether it be a tonsillectomy or a lobotomy, surgery was for the specializing technician. The point is that it is an arguable question. To let Dr. Pound get away with his one-sided, sweeping generalization can hardly be said to be objective reporting.

"It must be said, as well, that Dr. Pound is either unaware of recent efforts to widen the function of the general practitioner in Britain or that he chose not to inform Vipond of this trend.

"This has been the great story in Britain over the past few years, under both the Labor and Conservative governments. The aim has been to set up clinics and group practices, often in conjunction with local authority public health centres. Its success goes a long way to wiping out Dr. Pound's 'aspirin' argument.

"This polyclinic idea, demonstrably effective in the Soviet Union and recommended in the first blueprint of the National Health Service, means that doctors may combine various specialties in obstetrics, pediatrics, geriatrics, chiropody and other fields, rent offices on the premises of health centres and use the centre's nursing and secretarial staff and diagnostic equipment.

"In other cases, with the encouragement and financial assistance of the Ministry of Health, group practices, involving from three to 12 doctors, are replacing the old one-man operations.

"When the service began in 1948 three of every four practices were single-handed. Now three of every four are group arrangements. There are new challenges, new rewards, including higher incomes. What Dr. Pound describes as 'tremendous apathy' is simply not true.

"What I am saying is that Dr. Pound, to my knowledge, was not at all fair in his presentation of these facts. As for his opinion, I find it equally suspect. Any man who describes health as 'a commodity' and the doctor's role as 'free trade with his customers,' is hardly qualified to judge a national medical scheme based on the philosophy that good health is every citizen's right. For all its faults, Britain's National Health Service is dedicated to that security — womb-to-tomb, as the saying goes — and may still serve as a model for a comprehensive plan in these climes.

"If that means the disappearance of Dr. Pound to new climes — where? Hawaii, perhaps? — then so be it."

The cause and source of that criticism by the defendant Scott is an article published three days earlier, namely, 10th August 1971 (Ex. 2) by a reporter, Donald Vipond, of the defendant Victoria Press Limited. That article was one following an interview sought by the plaintiff of the said Vipond in order that his, the plaintiff's, views concerning the practice of medicine and in particular his view of "state medicine in Britain", otherwise known as the National Health Service, might be published. The cause and source of that activity on the part of the plaintiff, I conclude, were two Orders in Council passed by the Lieutenant-Governor of British Columbia in Council. Copies of these Orders in Council are exhibits in this case. They deal with the use of medical laboratories, etc.

The views of the plaintiff were published on 10th August 1971 in the article entitled

"Do People Really Want Second-Rate Medicine?" and the preface to the article is in the following words:

"The doctors, traditionally silent as a group are angry again. Last year it was over government publication of their earnings under Medicare. Now they are aroused over arbitrary decisions by the provincial cabinet affecting how they practise.

"Here are the views of one of them, a city physician who fled state medicine in Britain and fears that the same conditions that made him move are now threatened in B.C.

"Dr. Pound believes that medicine is a commodity which he has to sell, with the right of free trade with his customers.

"He speaks for himself in this interview with *Times* reporter Don Vipond. Whether his views represent most of the doctors in the community is uncertain; only the reaction of his colleagues can determine that."

The views of the plaintiff were freely expressed to the reporter Vipond. The latter quoted words of the plaintiff throughout the article as well as summarizing others. As to that article the plaintiff swore that he took no exception, but he did say that he felt that Vipond had not stressed the "thrust" of some of his views in adequate fashion.

It is therefore in the light of the article of 10th August that the Court must view the article or column of the defendant Scott. This is not a case of a deliberate act of defamatory insult. It is rather a case of criticism by one person, having knowledge and experience in an area covered by the writing of another person, in an area of public interest.

I observe that in the statement of claim the plaintiff says that he was, at all times material to this action, a physician and surgeon carrying on practice in Victoria, British Columbia.

The fact of the matter is, in my respectful opinion, that the plaintiff on his own motion entered into the forum of public discussion, pitting his knowledge as an observer of the National Health Service in Great Britain and the Health Service in British Columbia against other opinion. It was as such an observer that he was being criticized by the defendant Scott in his article. The plaintiff could not complain that, because references were made to him, the column of the defendant Scott in fact printed and published certain words "of the plaintiff and of him in the way of his said profession and in relation to his conduct therein". Like a boxer, having entered the ring, he must accept the blows given him provided always that none is "below the belt". He must participate as a boxer, viz., as a commentator against contrary views and will have no privilege in the contest because he is in fact a doctor of medicine unless it appear that a deliberate and improper attack be made upon him in his capacity as a doctor of medicine or such an attack may properly be implied or inferred.

A fair reading of the article expressing the plaintiff's views as published on 10th August indicates a novel idea of the professional doctor of medicine in relation to his profession. In addition to that, the plaintiff professed to be knowledgeable as of the date of his article of the conditions existing in Great

Britain. He also gave evidence as to his own experiences in the practice of the profession of medicine in Great Britain and his own participation therein. In one particular matter and one of considerable importance, when dealing with his own knowledge, I comment that he had given to the reporter Vipond particulars. Although the item in the Vipond article of 10th August is a summary by the man Vipond, the plaintiff swore that he took no exception to that article. The said Vipond noted the following:

"Pound recalls seeing 60 to 70 patients between 10 in the morning and noon, another 30 or 40 between 6 and 10 in the evening. Then house calls."

Then I quote words used by him:

"I was too busy to be able to stop and think . . . Nobody's getting a fair deal, least of all the patient."

As to those numbers, I do not believe the plaintiff. I observed him during the course of cross-examination and I observed that, when he was dealing with those figures, he was extremely nervous and had lost the composure that was otherwise displayed throughout the time when he was the witness before the Court. In addition, the witness Anderson, a man called as a person having special knowledge in the medical field in Great Britain, gave evidence of his appreciation of the numbers of patients who could be seen per diem and would be seen per diem. The plaintiff was asked as to estimates of time per patient. All this evidence when assessed, along with the discomfiture displayed by the plaintiff, convinced me that the plaintiff was not being truthful in that particular. Consequently I am of the opinion that his opinions expressed to the reporter Vipond were not entirely truthful. In addition, his appreciation of the position of the doctor of medicine was unorthodox and likely to have encouraged comment.

As to the defendant Scott, I conclude that he had had considerable opportunity to observe the National Health Service. He had not only been a patient thereunder, as had members of his family, but he had written a series of articles upon the subject which had been published, four in number, in the Toronto *Daily Star*. He had been a resident of Britain for a number of years. I concluded, in the light of experience, that he was informed. The witness Anderson confirmed the knowledge that the witness Scott had demonstrated.

It is true, as he swore, that he was annoyed by what he considered an unfair and unjust criticism on the part of the plaintiff of the National Health Service. He therefore wrote his article willingly, and particularly because the manager of the defendant considered there should be some reply made to the article, Ex. 2.

My first duty is to determine if the words complained of are capable of being defamatory.

Having in mind Ex. 1 and para. 7 of the statement of claim, I conclude that some of the words in the article may be defamatory. If some are defamatory, such defamatory meaning not being excused, the plaintiff must succeed and there must be an assessment of damages.

The plaintiff has chosen the words he considers defamatory and he indicates the inference that may be drawn, viz., the inference that would be drawn by the public reading the article, the ordinary man in the street. All this is set out in para. 7, supra.

The defences raised here were briefly:

I . No libel.
2. Qualified privilege.
3. Justification and fair comment in a rolled-up plea.
4. Justification (by amendment at trial).

Had there been a jury before me I would have had to explain to the jury that there was a case to be considered by them as to whether or not there was in fact a libel of the plaintiff. I would have directed the jury on the law as I direct myself now on the law in relation to the matter of fair comment by reference to relevant authorities. I quote from *Gatley on Libel and Slander*, 6th ed., p. 750:

> It is for the jury to decide, subject to the direction of the judge, whether the words complained of are allegations of fact or comments, and, if expressions of opinion, whether such comments are fair comment or not. But in every case it is first of all the duty of the judge to determine whether the words are capable of being comment and whether there is any evidence of unfairness to go to the jury. '*The jury if the Court is of opinion that there is some evidence* that the comment is unfair, finds whether it is so or not. "The question whether the comment is false or not is eminently a question for the jury, *provided there is any evidence of unfairness*.

In that work there follow the observations of Collins, M.R. in *McQuire v. Western Morning News*, [1903] 2 K.B. 100 at 110:

> No doubt in most cases of this class there are expressions in the impugned document capable of being interpreted as falling outside the limit of honest criticism, and, therefore, it is proper to leave the question to the jury, and in all cases where there may be a doubt it may be convenient to take the opinion of a jury. But it is always for the judge to say whether the document is capable in law of being a libel. It is, however, for the plaintiff, who rests his claim upon a document which on his own statement purports to be a criticism of a matter of public interest, to show that it is a libel — *i.e.*, that it travels beyond the limit of fair criticism; and therefore it must be for the judge to say whether it is reasonably capable of being so interpreted.

It was contended by the defendants that there was qualified privilege available to the defendants in this matter. I am of the opinion that that defence was not available to them. I refer again to Gatley, *supra*, at p. 702, where para. 703 reads as follows:

"703. Fair comment distinguished from qualified privilege. The defence of fair comment must also be distinguished from that of qualified privilege. In the defence of fair comment the right exercised by the defendant is shared by every member of the public. 'Who is entitled to comment? The answer to that is "everyone". A newspaper reporter or a newspaper editor has exactly the same rights, neither more nor less, than every other citizen.' *Per* Diplock, J. in *Silkin v. Beaverbrook Newspapers*, [1958] 1 W.L.R. 743 at 746, [1958] 2 All E.R. 516. In that of qualified privilege the right is not shared by every member of the public, but is limited to an individual who stands in such relation to the circumstances that he is entitled to say or write what would be libellous or slanderous on the part of anyone else. 'For instance, if a master is asked as to the character of a servant, and he says that the servant is a thief, he has a privilege which no one else would have.' 'A privileged occasion is one on which the privileged person is entitled to do something which no one who is not within the privilege is entitled to do on that occasion. A person in such a position may say or write about another person things which no other person in the kingdom can be allowed to say or write. But, in the case of a criticism upon [a matter of public interest whether it be the conduct of a public man or] a published work, every person in the kingdom is entitled to do, and is forbidden to do exactly the same things, and therefore the occasion is not privileged."

Fair comment is well explained at p. 731 of Gatley, supra, in the following paragraph:

"732. *The latitude of fair comment*. In the following passage from his summing-up in *Stopes v. Sutherland*, [1925] A.C. 47, Lord Hewart, C.J. points out the latitude of fair comment:

> What is it that fair comment means? It means this — and I prefer to put it in words which are not my own; I refer to the famous judgment of Lord Esher, M.R. in *Merivale v. Carson* (1887), 20 Q.B.D. 275 at 280-81: "Every latitude," said Lord Esher, "must be given to opinion and to prejudice, and then an ordinary set of men with ordinary judgment must say [not whether they agree with it, but] whether any fair man would have made such a comment . . . Mere exaggeration, or even gross exaggeration, would not make the comment unfair. However wrong the opinion expressed may be in point of truth, or however prejudiced the writer it may still be within the prescribed limit. The question which the jury must consider is this — would any fair man, however prejudiced he may be, however exaggerated or obstinate his views, have said that which this criticism has said?" Again, as Bray, J. said in *Rex v. Russell; Ex parte Morris* (1905), 93 L.T. 407: "When you come to a question of fair comment you ought to be extremely liberal, and in a matter of this kind — a matter relating to the administration of the licensing laws — you ought to be extremely liberal, because it is a matter on which men's minds are moved, in which people who do know, entertain very, very strong opinions, and if they use strong language every allowance should be made in their favour. They must believe what they say, but the question whether they honestly believe it is a question for you to say. If they do believe it, and they are within anything like reasonable bounds, they come within the meaning of fair comment. If comments were made which would appear to you to have been exaggerated, it does not follow that they are not perfectly honest comments." That is the kind of maxim which you may apply in considering whether that part of this matter which is comment is fair. Could a fair minded man, holding a strong view holding perhaps an obstinate view, holding perhaps a prejudiced view — could a fairminded man have been capable of writing this? — which, you observe, is a totally different question from the question. Do you agree with what he has said?" . . .

I have dealt with the matter, as the trial indicated I should do, on the basis of justification and fair comment. . . . I conclude that what the writer and defendant Jack Scott did was to robustly criticize the plaintiff upon the article which was published at his behest and contained his views based upon his reported knowledge. I have considered the claim of the plaintiff and, in particular, the claims particularized in para. 7 of the statement of claim. I base my judgment upon the alternatives I to 8 above, which I adopt as my conclusions. Those conclusions, together with my study of the whole words of the text of Ex. 1, the alleged libellous article, convince me that there has been fair comment made in a matter of public interest and that necessarily includes justification of the article and a finding of no malice. The action of the plaintiff must therefore be dismissed with costs.

5.2.3.2.7 *Mack v. North Hill News Ltd.* (1964), 44 D.L.R. (2d) 147 (Alta.S.C.)

... The defence of fair comment pleaded in these actions has become known as the "rolled-up plea" and is distinguished from the plea of justification in *Sutherland et al. v. Stopes*, [1925] A.C. 47, the headnote of which states:

> The plea in an action for libel that in so far as the words complained of consist of allegations of fact they are true in substance and in fact and in so far as they consist of expressions of opinion they are fair comments made in good faith and without malice on a matter of public interest is not a plea partly of justification and party of fair comment, but is a plea of fair comment only.

Viscount Finlay, in distinguishing the defence of fair comment from that of justification, says at pp. 62-3:

> It is clear that the truth of a libel affords a complete answer to civil proceedings. This defence is raised by plea of justification on the ground that the words are true in substance and in fact. Such a plea in justification means that the libel is true not only in its allegations of fact but also in any comments made therein.
>
> The defence of fair comment on matters of public interest is totally different. The defendant who raises this defence does not take upon himself the burden of showing that the comments are true. If the facts are truly stated with regard to a manner of public interest, the defendant will succeed in his defence to an action of libel if the jury are satisfied that the comments are fairly and honestly made. To raise this defence there must, of course, be a basis of fact on which the comment is made.
>
> For a good many years past a practice has prevailed of raising this defence by what has been called the "rolled up plea," but it will be found that this term is a misnomer based on a misconception of the nature of the plea. Such a plea states that the allegations of fact in the libel are true, that they are of public interest, and that the comments upon them contained of the libel were fair. The allegation of truth is confined to the facts averred, and the averment as to the comments is not that they are true but only that they were made in good faith, and that they are fair and do not exceed the proper standard of comment upon such matters.
>
> There has been a good deal of misconception as to the nature of this plea. It has been sometimes treated as containing two separate defences rolled into one, but it in fact raises only one defence, that being the defence of fair comment on matters of public interest. The averment that the facts were truly stated is merely to lay the necessary basis for the defence on the ground of fair comment. This averment is quite different from a plea of justification of a libel on the ground of truth, under which the defendant has to prove not only that the facts are truly stated but also that any comments upon them are correct.

And

> Such a defence on the ground of fair comment will fail if the jury are satisfied that the libel was malicious or that it exceeded the bounds of fair comment.
>
> On the question of fair comment, the law is in my opinion correctly stated by the Master of the Rolls (afterwards Lord Collins) in the case of *McQuire v. Western Morning News Co.*, [1903]

2 K.B. 100, 111: "It is, however, for the plaintiff, who rests his claim upon a document which on his own statement purports to be a criticism of a matter of public interest, to shew that it is a libel — i.e., that it travels beyond the limit of fair criticism; and therefore it must be for the judge to say whether it is reasonably capable of being so interpreted."

There are three essentials to such a defence enumerated by Fletcher Moulton, L.J., in *Hunt v. Star Newspaper Co.*, [1908] 2 K.B. 309 at pp. 319-20 in these words:

> The law as to fair comment, so far as is material to the present case, stands as follows: In the first place, comment in order to be justifiable as fair comment must appear as comment and must not be so mixed up with the facts that the reader cannot distinguish between what is report and what is comment: see *Andrews v. Chapman* (1853), 3 C. & K. 286. . . . In the next place, in order to give room for the plea of fair comment the facts must be truly stated. If the facts upon which the comment purports to be made do not exist the foundation of the plea fails. . . .
>
> Finally, comment must not convey imputations of an evil sort except so far as the facts truly stated warrant the imputation.

The nature of the plea is concisely summed up by Riddell, J., in *Augustine Automatic Rotary Engine Co. v. Saturday Night Ltd.* (1917), 34 D.L.R. 439 at p. 447, 38 O.L.R. 609 at p. 619 in these words: ". . . means that all allegations of fact concerning the plaintiff are true and that the remainder of the comments on the plaintiff are fair as justified by facts."

This statement of the rolled-up plea was cited and applied by the Ontario Appellate Division in *Boys v. Star Printing & Publishing Co.*, [1927] 3 D.L.R. 847, 60 O.L.R. 592 . . .

5.2.3.2.8 *Ontario Libel and Slander Act*, R.S.O. 1990, c. L.12.

23. In an action for libel or slander consisting partly of allegations of fact and partly of expression of opinion, a defence of fair comment shall not fail by reason only that the truth of every allegation of fact is not proved if the expression of opinion is fair comment having regard to such of the facts alleged or referred to in the words complained of as are proved. R.S.O. 1980, c. 237, s. 24.

5.2.3.2.9 *Cherneskey v. Armadale Publishers* (1979), 90 D.L.R. (3d) 321 (S.C.C.)

MARTLAND, J.: The facts which give rise to the present appeal are stated in the reasons of my brothers Ritchie and Dickson. I agree with the disposition of the appeal proposed by the former. I wish to comment on one of the grounds which he adopts for allowing the appeal which I consider to be sufficient to dispose of the matter.

The issue before this Court is as to whether the Judge at trial erred in taking away from the jury the defence of fair comment. Before doing so, the trial Judge discussed the matter with counsel and stated his reasons for taking this course. They are as follows, and I agree with them:

It is, of course, the burden of the defendant to prove this defence and it does not arise until after the jury has found the words complained of to apply to the plaintiff and that they are defamatory of him.

I shall not try to decide whether if the opinion of the writers of the letter is honest and sincere that this fact absolves the publisher or the editor of the paper from a similar opinion. In the present trial that is not necessary because here there is no evidence that the offending words, if they are in fact defamatory of the plaintiff, which is a matter for the jury — there is no evidence that those words express the honest opinion of anyone, either the writers of the letter or of anyone on the editorial staff of the *Star-Phoenix* or its publisher. The evidence seems to be that the defendants had a contrary opinion or none at all. Without such honest opinion I cannot tell the jury that the defence of fair comment is available to the defendant.

I thought I had better put that on the record, gentlemen, so that my position is clear and the reason for my ruling is clear. . . .

In the present case the corporate defendant is the owner and publisher of *The Star-Phoenix*, a Saskatoon newspaper in which the words complained of were published, and the respondent, King, is the editor of that newspaper. The evidence of the officer produced for examination for discovery by the respondent company, and that of the respondent, King, make it clear that the letter complained of did not represent the honest expression of their real views.

The writers of the letter were not called to give evidence, and so there is no evidence to prove that the letter was an honest expression of their views. The only evidence we have is that the respondent, King, said, with reference to the writers of the letter, "we figured that was their opinion or their view or their observations".

This is not a sufficient basis to enable the respondents to rely upon the defence of fair comment. There is no evidence to show that the material published, which the jury found to be defamatory, represented the honest opinion of the writers of the letter, or that of the officers of the newspaper which published it. In these circumstances the trial Judge was properly entitled to decide not to put the defence of fair comment to the jury.

RITCHIE, J.: This is an appeal brought pursuant to leave granted by the Court of Appeal of Saskatchewan from a judgment of that Court setting aside a judgment rendered at trial by Mr. Justice MacPherson, sitting with a jury, and ordering a new trial of this libel action which was brought by the appellant, a practicing lawyer and alderman of the Saskatoon City Council, as a result of a letter published in the correspondence column of *The Star-Phoenix*, a newspaper published in Saskatoon, of which the respondent Armadale Publishers Limited (hereinafter referred to as "Armadale") is the owner and publisher and the respondent Sterling King is the editor.

The facts giving rise to this litigation are accurately and fully stated in the dissenting judgment of Mr. Justice Brownridge in the Court of Appeal which is now conveniently reported at 79 D.L.R. (3d) 180 (hereinafter referred to as the "report") at p. 183 *et seq.* [also reported in [1977] 5 W.W.R. 155], but in order to fully understand the questions to which this appeal gives rise it will be necessary for me to summarize them briefly.

The alleged libel of which the appellant complains is contained in a letter written to *The Star-Phoenix* by two law students concerning a petition which was presented to the Saskatoon City Council and which was apparently drafted with the assistance of the appellant. The petition presented on behalf of fifty-four citizens was directed against the establishment of an Alcoholic Rehabilitation Centre in what was alleged to be a residential section of Saskatoon and the report of its presentation to Council as published in The Star-Phoenix referred in particular to Indians and Metis, whose use of the centre was alleged to be detrimental to the area. In this regard Mr. Yaworski, who presented the petition, was reported as saying that the establishment of the centre was going to turn the area into "an Indian and Metis ghetto".

The only express reference made to the appellant in this report was contained in the last paragraph reading:

> Alderman Morris Cherneskey told Council he did not think the zoning by-laws of the area envisioned 15 people living in one place, and until it is fully clarified it should not operate as an alcoholic rehabilitation centre when the citizens of the neighbourhood are concerned.

Having read this article, the two law students proceeded to write a letter to *The Star-Phoenix* which was published in a column headed "Editor's Letter Box", at the foot of which the following statement was printed:

> Letter Writers are requested to provide addresses and phone numbers to allow checking for authenticity and accuracy. Letters must be signed — no pseudonyms will be published. *All are subject to editing for length, general interest, grammar, style and good taste.* Letters under 250 words are preferred.

(The italics are mine.)

In his charge to the jury, the learned trial Judge touched on this phase of the matter, saying:

> *The Star-Phoenix*, as the evidence indicates, has a right to decline to publish. They chose to publish and they, as they indicated, have a right to insist upon their right to edit. That's their privilege, naturally.

The letter complained of was itself headed "Racist Attitude", and it is reproduced in full at pp. 183-4 of the D.L.R. report, but the real sting of the language complained of is contained in the last three paragraphs which read:

> As a law student and an articling law student, we are appalled by the stance adopted by Alderman Cherneskey, himself a lawyer. We appreciate his sympathy with the concerns of certain members of the white community; however, we thoroughly disagree with his contention the centre should cease its operation until such time as the application of the relevant zoning bylaw has been clarified. We feel this situation is not unlike that of a man charged with a criminal offence. Such a man is deemed innocent until proven guilty.
>
> That Alderman Cherneskey should imply the onus is upon those operating the centre to establish their right to remain in the neighborhood and further clarification, is abhorrent to all concepts of the law. At the very least, it flies flagrantly in the face of the principles of natural justice. It is unbecoming a member of the legal profession to adopt such an approach.
>
> Although we do not reside in the particular neighborhood in question, we would have no objection whatsoever to such a centre operating in our neighborhood. We entirely support the

project initiated by Clarence Trotchie and hope the racist resistance exhibited will be replaced by the support and encouragement which the project deserves.

In the course of his reasons for judgment in the Court of Appeal, Mr. Justice Brownridge points out that [at pp. 1845]:

> Prior to the trial the defendants sought leave to join as third parties the two authors of the offending letter but this application was refused on appeal . . . *At the trial it was agreed by counsel that both letter writers were out of the jurisdiction and neither was called as a witness.*

(The italics are mine.)

By his statement of claim the appellant claimed damages for defamation of his personal character in relation to his profession and in his office as an alderman, and by para. 8 made the following general claim:

> The plaintiff further says that the said heading and letter as a whole would tend to lower the plaintiff in the estimation of right-thinking members of society generally and the citizens of Saskatoon in particular and that the words are defamatory.

By their joint defence the defendants pleaded:

> 8. In so far as the said letter, exclusive of the said heading, set out in paragraph 3 of the Statement of Claim consists of statements of fact they are true in substance and in fact and in so far as the said words consist of expressions of opinion, they are fair and bona fide comment made without malice upon the said facts which are a manner of public interest.
>
> 9. The publication of the said letter was an occasion of qualified privilege

The plaintiff's reply is phrased in the following terms.

Reply

> In answer to the Defendant's Statement of Defence wherein they plead fair comment and qualified privilege, which is not admitted but denied, the Plaintiff says that the heading and the letter were published with express malice and joins issue.

The questions put to the jury by the learned trial Judge and their answers are as follows:

1. Would a reasonably minded reader imply that the words "racist attitude" in the heading over the letter refer to the plaintiff? Answer: "No".
2. If your answer to question number I is yes, then are those words defamatory? Answer: "Not applicable".
3. Would a reasonably minded reader imply that the words "racist resistance" in the last sentence of the letter refer to the plaintiff? Answer: "Yes".
4. If your answer to number 3 is yes, then are those words defamatory? Answer: "Yes".
5. Do the words in the fourth and fifth paragraphs of the letter directly or by innuendo defame the plaintiff as Alderman? Answer: "Yes".
6. Do the words is the fourth and fifth paragraphs of the letter directly or by innuendo defame the plaintiff as a lawyer? Answer: "Yes".
7. If you have answered yes to questions 2, 4, 5 and 6 or any one or more of them, what damages do you award the plaintiff? Answer: "$25,000 & costs".

I think it convenient at this stage to say that I am in agreement with Mr. Justice Brownridge, for the reasons which he has stated at p. 187 of the report, that the defence of qualified privilege is not available to the defendants in the present case. This view was adopted by Mr. Justice Bayda who observed at p. 196:

> I have read the reasons for judgment of my brother Brownridge, and respectfully agree that for reasons similar to those expressed by the Supreme Court of Canada, in *Douglas v. Tucker*, [1952]1 D.L.R. 657, [1952]1 S.C.R. 275; *Globe and Mail Ltd. v. Boland* (1960), 22 D.L.R. (2d) 277, [1960] S.C.R. 203, and *Jones v. Bennett* (1968), 2 D.L.R. (3d) 291, [1969] S.C.R. 277, 66 W.W.R. 419, the defence of qualified privilege is not available to the defendants in the present case. I also agree with the conclusions reached by him in respect of the other grounds of appeal, save the ground involving the plea of fair comment. In that regard, I have reached the opposite conclusion, namely, that the learned trial Judge should not have taken away from the jury the defence of fair comment.

Mr. Justice Brownridge found no merit in "the other grounds of appeal", and Mr. Justice Hall stated at the opening of his reasons for judgment [at p. 193]:

> The significant ground of appeal is that which alleges error by the trial Judge in refusing to put to the jury the defence of fair comment.

It is thus apparent that all members of the Court of Appeal were concerned only with the complaint that the trial Judge had erred in taking the defence of fair comment away from the jury and this was the main issue presented in this Court.

In the present case the plaintiffs (appellant's) plea that the words used in the letter are defamatory is couched in language which has long been accepted as giving rise, upon publication, to an action for defamation by the person to whom it refers. In this regard I refer to the following excerpt from *Gatley on Libel and Slander*, 7th ed. (1974), p. 5, para. 4, where he said:

> Any imputation which may tend "to lower the plaintiff in the estimation of right-thinking members of society generally"... or "to expose him to hatred, contempt or ridicule" is defamatory of him.

This language was in large measure adopted by the trial Judge in addressing the jury.

Accordingly, as I agree with the trial Judge that the words used are capable of being construed as tending to lower the plaintiff in the estimation of right-thinking members of society generally, a *prima facie* cause of action arises, and in my view a plea of fair comment by way of defence does not of itself have the effect of saddling the plaintiff with the burden of proving that the comment was unfair. This plea constitutes a vital part of the case for the defendants and in my view the burden of proving each ingredient of the defence so pleaded should rest upon the party asserting it. One of these ingredients is that the person writing the material complained of must be shown to have had an honest belief in the opinions expressed and it will be seen that, in my view, the same considerations apply to each publisher of that material.

The question of burden of proof in such cases was considered by Lord Morris of Borth-y-Gest in *Jones v. Skelton*, [1963] 1 W.L.R. 1362 at p. 1379, where he said:

... if a defendant publishes of a plaintiff words which a jury might on the one hand hold to be fact or might on the other hand hold to be comment, and if a plaintiff does not accept that any of the words are true or does not accept that any of them are comment and if a defendant chooses to assert that some of the words are fair comment (made in good faith and without malice) on facts truly stated it must (assuming that the judge rules in regard to the public interest) be for the defendant to prove that which he asserts. If a plaintiff does not acknowledge that there are any words of comment and if the words are reasonably capable of being held by a jury to be statements of fact the plaintiff's overall burden of proving his case does not involve a duty of proving that comment (the existence of which he denies) is unfair.

In commenting on this statement, Mr. Justice Bayda observed at p. 200 of the report:

It is plain from these remarks (which I adopt as a correct statement of the law) that where the pleadings, as in the present case, disclose that the plaintiff does not acknowledge the words complained of are comments or opinions, but the defendants, in their pleadings, raise the issue of comment and of fairness of the comment, the onus is on the defendants to prove fair comment. The normal principle that he who asserts, must prove, applies. In such event (assuming the words complained of are capable of being a comment and further assuming that condition (b) mentioned above is not applicable as is the situation here), it is for the Judge to determine, as a manner of law, (I) whether there is any evidence of (a), that is, any evidence entitling the jury to find that the statements upon which the comments are based are true; and (2) whether !here is any evidence of condition (c), viz., the requirement of honesty. If he finds there is some evidence to support the finding that those conditions are met, he must place the defence of fair comment before the jury for their consideration (assuming that he has previously ruled that the element of public interest was proved). If, on the other hand, the trial Judge finds as a manner of law, that there is no evidence to support the presence of either of these two conditions, he should not put the defence of fair comment to the jury.

In cases where the essential ingredients of either the plea of "qualified privilege" or that of "fair comment" have been established by the defence, then if it can be proved that the statements complained of were made or written maliciously, the plea must fail; but in my view no burden lies upon the complainant to prove malice unless and until either plea has been shown to be supported by the evidence.

Here the plea of "express malice" was added midway through the evidence called on behalf of the plaintiff (appellant) and it is, in my view, important to appreciate that this allegation forms no part of the main case but is inserted entirely by way of answer to the respondents' claim of "qualified privilege" and "fair comment". As I have indicated, the defence of qualified privilege is not available to the defendants, and the question of malice could only arise in the present case if there were some evidence to indicate that the comment complained of was otherwise fair, and this cannot be said unless the opinions expressed are honestly held.

As I have already observed, it is an essential ingredient to the defence of fair comment that it must be the honest expression of the writer's opinion and in this regard I refer to the following statement made by Lord Porter in *Turner (orse. Robertson) v. Metro-Goldwyn-Mayer Pictures, Ltd.*, [1950] 1 All E.R. 449 at pp. 462-3, where he said, commenting on the charge to the jury in that case where the defence was qualified privilege:

> Its early words on this part of the case express exactly what the authorities convey. "Fair comment" (in effect the learned judge says) "has to be an honest expression of the real opinion of the defendants when they wrote it ... " "Did they honestly and really think that she" (the appellant) "was completely out of touch with the tastes and entertainment requirements of the picture-going millions who are also radio listeners and that her criticisms are on the whole unnecessarily harmful to the film industry? Did they honestly hold that opinion and really believe it? If they did — then they were not abusing the occasion. Such a direction is, I think, entirely accurate and could not be attacked, and similar language is to be found in other parts of the summing-up. On the other hand, language of this kind is frequently interspersed with words which suggest that the criterion is whether fair minded men could hold that view. Let me take one example only. It runs:
>
>> "First of all ... do you think that a fair-minded man capable of impartial judgment of the plaintiff's [appellant's] talks ... could come to that conclusion. Was there anything in them or in her conduct which would lead a fair man honestly to entertain the opinion that the defendants expressed in this letter?"
>
> Similar observations appear throughout the summing-up and, undoubtedly, if they were found alone there would have been clear misdirection. It is said, however, in the first place, that, in his cross-examination and address, leading counsel for the respondents used the phrase and accepted the burden that fair-mindedness was required. I do not think that the record justifies this allegation, but if it did I should think it immaterial. Secondly, it is argued with more force that when the summing-up is regarded as a whole, a jury would not be misled, but would rightly apprehend that honesty, not reasonableness, was the state of mind required. My Lords, I cannot take this view. I have read the summing-up as a whole more than once and I think a jury might well have come to the conclusion that both honesty and reasonableness were necessary and that the defendants were unreasonable and therefore malicious. It is, I think, difficult for the uninstructed mind to guard against such a misconception, and to my mind the clearest direction is necessary to the effect that irrationality, stupidity or obstinacy do not constitute malice, though in an extreme case there may be some evidence of it. The defendant, indeed, must honestly hold the opinion he expresses but no more is required of him.

In the same case Lord Oaksey stated at p. 475:

> In the absence of any evidence that the respondents did not honestly hold the opinions expressed in their letter, I see no grounds on which they could be held to have exceeded the limits of fair comment.

After having heard lengthy argument as to whether or not this defence should be left to the jury in the present case, the trial Judge made the following ruling:

> I shall not try to decide whether if the opinion of the writers of the letter is honest and sincere that this fact absolves the publisher or the editor of the paper from a similar opinion. In the present trial that is not necessary because here there is no evidence that the offending words, if they are in fact defamatory of the plaintiff, which is a manner for the jury — there is no evidence that those words express the honest opinion of anyone, either the writers of the letter or of anyone on the editorial staff of *The Star-Phoenix* or its publisher. The evidence seems to be that the defendants had a contrary opinion or none at all. Without such honest opinion I cannot tell the jury that the defence of fair comment is available to the defendant.

Honesty of belief has been characterized by Lord Denning, M.R., in *Slim et al. v. Daily Telegraph, Ltd. et al.*, [1968] 1 All E.R. 497 at p. 503, as "the cardinal test" of the defence of fair comment, and in the context of the present case this must mean honesty of belief in the opinions expressed in the letter complained of. It has long been established that the state of mind of the publisher of the alleged libel is directly in issue where there is a plea of fair comment. This is illustrated in the case of *Plymouth Mutual Co-operative & Industrial Society, Ltd. v. Traders' Publishing Ass'n, Ltd.*, [1906] 1 K.B. 403, where the question was whether an interrogatory addressed to the state of mind of the defendant, who had pleaded fair comment, was admissible and, after referring to the case of *White & Co. v. Credit Reform Ass'n & Credit Index, Ltd.*, [1905] I K.B. 653, Vaughan Williams, L.J., said, at pp. 413-4.

> It seems to me that that case shews that an interrogatory of this kind is just as relevant and admissible in a case where the defence is fair comment as in one where it is privilege. In either case the question raised is really as to the state of mind of the defendant when he published the alleged libel, the question being in the one case whether he published it in the spirit of malice, in the other whether he published it in the spirit of unfairness. In either case I think such an interrogatory as the one now in question is admissible.

And later at p. 418 of the same report, Fletcher Moulton, L.J., said:

> ... I am clear that, both in cases in which the defence of privilege and in those in which the defence of fair comment is set up, the state of mind of the defendant when he published the alleged libel is a matter directly in issue ...

Perhaps the most singular feature of the present case is that the state of mind of the defendants is established by their own evidence to the effect that they did not honestly hold the opinions expressed in the letter. This is illustrated by the following excerpt from the evidence of the defendants in relation to the comments complained of. Mr. R. Struthers, who was the executive vice-president of the defendant Armadale, stated in the course of cross-examination as follows:

> Q. But of course there is no question but what you do not believe Morris Cherneskey to be a racist?
> A. No, I do not.
> Q. You do not believe Morris Cherneskey to be a person with a racist attitude?
> A. I do not believe him to be so.
> Q. And in any capacity, as a lawyer, you don't believe him to be a lawyer with a racist attitude?
> A. No.
> Q. Or an alderman with a racist attitude?
> A. No.

The same witness had given the same answers when speaking as the officer examined for discovery on behalf of the defendant Armadale.

The second defendant, Sterling King, who was the editor of *The Star-Phoenix*, stated that he had no opinion as to the approach of Cherneskey in relation to the white community in the area in question but it was his honest opinion that Cherneskey had a reputation for honesty and integrity as a lawyer and alderman.

It will be remembered that Mr. Justice Bayda adopted the passage from the reasons for judgment of Lord Morris of Borth-y-Gest in *Jones v. Skelton*, which I have already quoted, and the reasons for judgment of Mr. Justice Brownridge and Mr. Justice Bayda both satisfy me that, if the writers of the letter here in question had been the defendants in this action and had entered a plea of fair comment, both these Judges would have found that the burden of proving honest belief in the opinions expressed rested upon the defence.

Mr. Justice Bayda, however, allowed this appeal on the ground that a newspaper, in republishing defamatory opinions which do not reflect its honest opinion, is nevertheless entitled to rely on the defence of fair comment on the ground that it honestly believed that those who wrote the letter were honestly expressing their true views. In this regard reliance is placed on the case of *Lyon et al. v. Daily Telegraph, Ltd.*, [1943] 2 All E.R. 316. In that case the author, who had used a *nom de plume* and given a fictitious address, was never discovered and the newspaper therefore had no means of determining whether the views expressed were honestly held by the writer or not, but the defence of fair comment was upheld in the Court of Appeal where Scott, L.J., said at p. 318:

> There is no question but that the comment contained in the letter represented the honest opinion of the *Daily Telegraph*; and at the trial no doubt was cast upon the complete belief of the newspaper that they were publishing a letter in which the writer was making a fair comment on a matter of public interest.

The obvious distinction between that case and the present one is that the letter complained of here did not express the honest opinion of *The Star-Phoenix*, and there is no evidence that the views therein expressed were honestly held by the writers, but Scott, L.J., later in the same judgment, said at p. 319:

> Although there is no direct authority, I think that the question of law is really implicit in the well-established rule that the publishers of a newspaper, when defendants in an action for libel, cannot, on the issue of fair comment, be required to disclose the source of their information. If the innocent state of mind of the writer of a letter published in the newspaper was a relevant fact, which had to be proved by him before his plea of fair comment could be established, it would go far towards justifying counsel's argument; but the very existence of the exceptional rule about interrogatories and discovery in the case of newspaper defendants seems to me to presuppose a rule of law that, at least in the absence of special circumstances (on the possibility of which I express no opinion), there is no such presumption or onus, and that fairness of the comment contained in the newspaper's correspondence columns must be judged by its tenor, subject only to the proviso that the statements of fact upon which the comment is based are not untrue.

This latter passage is primarily concerned with the rule that the publishers of a newspaper cannot be required to disclose their source of information, but the language employed in the last sentence might be construed as meaning that the fairness of the letter complained of is to be judged by its tenor, which I construe as a suggestion that the language used in correspondence columns of a newspaper is to be judged according to whether there is anything in the letter in question which would lead a fair man honestly to share the opinion which the language conveyed. It is to be remembered that the judgment of the Court of Appeal in the *Lyon* case was rendered some seven years before the House of Lords decided the case of *Turner, supra*, and I do not think there is anything in the views expressed by Scott, L.J., which can be taken as fixing any standard except honesty as the touchstone of the defence of fair comment. It is to be noted also that Scott, L.J., limited his opinion to cases where there was "an absence of special circumstances" as to which he expressed no opinion. The opinion expressed, therefore, cannot be treated as including the special circumstances of the publisher and editor of the newspaper having stated affirmatively that the letter does not express their honest opinion.

Mr. Justice Bayda, however, expressed the following opinion [at p. 201]:

> Where, however, the defendant is a publisher of the impugned words and in particular is a newspaper which publishes in its letters-to-the-editor column a letter capable of being defamatory, what is the acceptable standard? It is indisputable that if such a newspaper honestly holds the opinions expressed in the impugned writing, and was not actuated by malice then as in the case of the writer, condition (c) [honesty] would be satisfied (*Slim v. Daily Telegraph, Ltd., supra; Lyon and Lyon v. Daily Telegraph, Ltd. [supra]*. But is a different (I hesitate to say "lower") standard acceptable? Suppose the newspaper cannot be said to hold the opinions expressed in the impugned writing but honestly believes that they represent the real opinions of the writer (in other words, an honest belief that they were publishing a letter in which the writer was making a fair comment upon a manner of public interest) and, in addition, is not actuated by malice in publishing the letter, is that an acceptable state of mind for a plea of fair comment to succeed? I have concluded that it is.

This conclusion which lies at the very heart of this case, is based on an *obiter dictum* of Lord Denning, M.R., in the case of *Slim v. Daily Telegraph, supra,* where, as in the Lyon case, it was found that the newspaper honestly held the views expressed, and Lord Denning observed at p. 503:

> ... the right of fair comment is one of the essential elements which go to make up our freedom of speech. We must ever maintain this right intact. It must not be whittled down by legal refinements. When a citizen is troubled by things going wrong, he should be free to "write to the newspaper": and the newspaper should be free to publish his letter. It is often the only way to get things put right. The manner must, of course, be one of public interest. The writer must get his facts right and he must honestly state his real opinion. But that being done, both he and the newspaper should be clear of any liability. They should not be deterred by fear of libel actions.

In the penultimate paragraph of the same judgment, Lord Denning stated:

> On the face of these letters, I think that the comments made by Mr. Herbert and the *Daily Telegraph* were fair comments on a manner of public interest. *They* honestly said what *they* thought.

(The italics are mine.)

It must be apparent, as it seems to me, that the sentence last above quoted refers to the honesty of both the writer and the newspaper so that this case, in my opinion, affords no authority for the proposition that comments published in a newspaper need not be honest expressions of the newspaper's opinion in order to support a defence of fair comment so long as the newspaper can show its belief that the comments were an honest expression of the real opinion of the writer.

If the publication of the libel had been confined to the letter and the writers had been sued or, alternately, if it had originated with the newspaper and its publisher, it would in either case have been necessary to show honest belief in order to sustain the defence of fair comment. The same considerations would thus in my opinion apply to the newspaper and the writers.

In my opinion each publisher in relying on the defence of fair comment is in exactly the same position as the original writer. In this latter regard, I refer to the opinion delivered by Lord Denning in the Privy Council in *"Truth" (N.Z.) Ltd. v. Holloway*, [1960] 1 W.L.R. 997, where a newspaper published an article calling for an inquiry concerning import licences, in which it stated that a Mr. Judd had told a man who was inquiring about import licences to "See Phil and Phil would fix it". The newspaper's comment on this was: "By Phil his caller understood him to mean the Honourable Philip North Holloway, the Minister of Industry and Commerce." Holloway brought an action for libel against the newspaper and in commenting on the trial Judge's charge to the jury, Lord Denning had this to say at pp. 1002-3:

> The words actually used by the judge to the jury were these: "If you accept that those words were spoken by Judd, it is not a defence at all that a statement that might be defamatory is put forward by way of report only. It does not help the defendant that the way that it is put is that Judd said 'See Phil and Phil would fix it.' The case is properly to be dealt with as if the defendant itself said 'See Phil and Phil would fix it.'"
>
> Their Lordships see nothing wrong in this direction. It is nothing more nor less than a statement of settled law put cogently to the jury. Gatley opens his chapter on Republication and Repetition with the quotation: "Every publication of a libel is a new libel, and each publisher is answerable for his act to the same extent as if the calumny originated with him," see *Gatley on Libel and Slander*, 4th ed., p. 106. This case is a good instance of the justice of this rule. If Judd did use the words attributed to him, it might be a slander by Judd of Mr. Holloway in the way of his office as a Minister of the Crown. But if the words had not been repeated by the newspaper, the damage done by Judd would be as nothing compared to the damage done by this newspaper when it repeated it. It broadcast the statement to the people at large: and it made it worse by making it one of the grounds on which it called for an inquiry, for thereby it suggested that some credence was to be given to it.

It appears to me to follow from this that where, as here, there is no evidence as to the honest belief of the writers of the letter, and the newspaper and its publisher have disavowed any such belief on their part, the defence of fair comment cannot be sustained.

In this regard the language employed by Lord Shaw in *Arnold v. The King-Emperor* (1914), 83 L.J.P.C. 299 at p. 300, is appropriate. He there said:

> Their Lordships regret to find that there appeared on the one side of this case the time-worn fallacy that some kind of privilege attaches to the profession of the Press as distinguished from the members of the public. The freedom of the journalist is an ordinary part of the freedom of the subject, and to whatever lengths the subject in general may go, so also may the journalist, but, apart from statute law, his privilege is no other and no higher. The responsibilities which attach to his power in the dissemination of printed manner may, and in the case of a conscientious journalist do, make him more careful; but the range of his assertions, his criticisms, or his comments is as wide as, and no wider than, that of any other subject. No privilege attaches to his position.

These views were adopted in this Court in *Globe and Mail Ltd. v. Boland* (1960), 22 D.L.R. (2d) 277 at p. 281, [1960] S.C.R. 203 at p. 208.

These authorities satisfy me that the newspaper and its editor cannot sustain a defence of fair comment when it has been proved that the words used in the letter are not an honest expression of their opinion and there is no evidence as to the honest belief of the writers. In view of this finding, I do not consider it necessary to deal with the other submissions made on behalf of the appellant.

I cannot leave this question without reference to the reasons for judgment of Mr. Justice Hall wherein he expressed the view, which was not shared by the two other Judges sitting in the appeal, that, where the defence of fair comment is pleaded the burden of disproving "honesty of belief" lies upon the plaintiff. In so deciding Mr. Justice Hall equates lack of "honest belief" with "malice", saying at p. 194 of the report:

> It is apparent that saying that there must be an honest belief is the same as saying that the comment cannot be made maliciously. We are, therefore, in the instant case really dealing with the reply of malice.

This statement appears to me to overlook the distinction between the defence of "privilege", which can only be defeated by proof of malice and the defence of "fair comment", which presupposes honest belief on the part of the author or publisher. This distinction is recognized in the case of *Plymouth Mutual Cooperative & Industrial Society v. Trader's Publishing Ass'n. supra.* Speaking of the different considerations affecting the defence of "privilege" on the one hand and "fair comment" on the other, Vaughan Williams, L.J., said at pp. 413-4:

> In either case the question raised is really as to the state of mind of the defendant when he published the alleged libel, the question being in the one case whether he published it in the spirit of *malice*, in the other whether he published it in the spirit of *unfairness*.

(The italics are mine.) As honesty of belief is an essential component of the defence of fair comment, that defence involves at least some evidence that the material complained of was published in a spirit of fairness.

I cannot accept the proposition apparently adopted by Hall, J.A., that where, as here, the words are capable of a defamatory meaning they are presumed to give expression to an opinion honestly held until the contrary is shown.

Mr. Justice Hall appears to find some support for his views in the decision of Lord Denning, M.R., in *Egger v. Viscount Chelmsford et al.*, [1965] 1 Q.B. 248 at p. 265 from which I extract the following excerpt.

> If the plaintiff seeks to rely on malice to aggravate damages, or to rebut a defence of qualified privilege, or to cause a comment, otherwise fair, to become unfair, then he must prove malice ...

I read this statement as meaning that, where the defendant has shown that the comment is "otherwise fair", the burden rests upon the plaintiff to prove malice. Here, as I have said, the defence of "qualified privilege" is not available to the defendants and the defence of fair comment can only be sustained if the comment made is "otherwise fair".

In the present case, as I have said, there is no allegation of malice in the statement of claim, but if there had been any evidence to sustain a plea of fair comment, it would have been for the jury to say whether malice had been established.

On the pleadings here it was for the Judge to determine whether the words used were capable of a defamatory meaning and for the jury to decide whether they were in fact defamatory. The question of whether they constituted fair comment would also be for the jury if there were any evidence whatever to support it; but in the absence of such evidence, and in face of the defendants' evidence as to lack of honest belief no question of malice arises.

It will have been seen, however, that in the absence of any proof of the honest belief of the writers, and having regard to the denial of honest belief by the defendants themselves, the defence of fair comment cannot, in my view, prevail.

This does not mean that freedom of the press to publish its views is in any way affected, nor does it mean that a newspaper cannot publish letters expressing views with which it may strongly disagree. Moreover, nothing that is here said should be construed as meaning that a newspaper is in any way restricted in publishing two diametrically opposite views of the opinion and conduct of a public figure. On the contrary, I adopt as descriptive of the conclusion which I have reached, the language used by Brownridge, J.A., in the following excerpt from his reasons for judgment in the Court of Appeal, where he said at p. 192 of the report:

> What it does mean is that a newspaper cannot publish a *libellous* letter and then disclaim any responsibility by saying that it was published as fair comment on a matter of public interest but it does not represent the honest opinion of the newspaper.

For all these reasons I would allow this appeal and restore the judgment at trial. The appellant is entitled to his costs throughout.

5.2.3.2.10 Robert Martin, "Libel and Letters to the Editor," (1983), *Queen's Law Journal* 188

Comment on the Cherneskey Decision

A. Legal Doctrine

Cherneskey is an illustration of the notion that hard cases make bad law. The more one studies the opinions, the more paradoxical they appear. On its face the dissenting judgment of Dickson, J. appears to uphold freedom of speech. Examined more carefully, its implications are disturbing. Conversely, the majority judgment of Ritchie, J., while clearly unfortunate as between the parties actually before the court, is based on principles which are conducive, in their broad application, to the protection of freedom of speech.

The doctrinal question at issue was the content of the fair comment defence. For Ritchie, J. the essence of fair comment was honest belief. If, assuming the other requirements noted above had been met, the opinions in question constituted an expression of the defendant's honest belief, then the defence of fair comment was established. Where Ritchie, J. got into serious trouble was in his application of this principle to the facts of the case. It was his view that since these defendants did not honestly hold the opinions in question they could not raise fair comment. This is an absurd conclusion and one which, as will be pointed out below, could easily have been avoided.

Dickson, J. sought to escape the doctrinal shoal on which Ritchie, J. foundered. Mr. Justice Dickson argued, basing his views largely on those put forward by the English writers Duncan and Neill in their treatise on defamation, that a two stage analysis must be adopted in determining whether a comment is fair. First, one must apply an *objective* standard: "is the comment one that an honest, albeit prejudiced, person might make in the circumstances?" If the answer to this question is no, the comment is not fair. If the answer is yes, a further, *subjective* question may arise. The plaintiff may seek to show that the defendant was "actuated by malice". The presence of malice will render the comment unfair. Applying this analysis, Dickson, J. was able to conclude that Armadale Publishers could properly raise the defence of fair comment.

Now the approach described is effective to avoid the difficulty that led the majority of the Supreme Court of Canada to find for Cherneskey. All the commentators seem to agree that the result reached by Dickson, 1. would have been more desirable and just. Unfortunately, Dickson, J.'s analysis has some unpleasant ramifications. Since the English decision of *Merivale v. Carson* it has been accepted that notions of reasonableness have no place in the application of fair comment. That is, a defendant is not required, in order to discharge the onus of satisfying the court that a comment is fair, to prove that it is reasonable. To put it as simply as possible, a jury does not have to agree with a comment in order to find that it is fair.

Both the Faulks Committee in the U.K. and the Committee on Defamation in New Zealand anticipated the issue in *Cherneskey*. They each recommended that when the opinion in question was the opinion of some person other than the defendant, fair comment might be relied upon if the defendant honestly believed that the opinion was genuinely held by the other person. Had this reasoning been followed in *Cherneskey*, the defendants would have succeeded by satisfying the court that they believed the writers of the letter were expressing their honest opinion. Such an approach both preserves the essence of the defence of fair comment and is a logical extension of it.

The approach I have advocated has so far been put forward only in cases where the plaintiff has sought to use evidence that one co-defendant was actuated by malice in order to negative the defences of fair comment or qualified privilege raised by another co-defendant. It is submitted that there is no objection in principle to applying this analysis to the facts of *Cherneskey*.

In sum, good sense and a concern for freedom of speech both argue against the result reached in *Cherneskey*. Dickson, J. sought to avoid this result, but in doing so suggested that the standard to be used in determining whether a comment was fair might be an objective one. This might be taken as suggesting a criterion of reasonableness, a development which is exceedingly undesirable. A better approach would have been to accept the existing basis of fair comment and ask: "did the defendants honestly believe that the two law students were stating their honest opinion?" This analysis also precludes, as will be evident below, many of the unfortunate consequences of the various statutory responses to *Cherneskey*.

B. Effect on Newspapers

The Court's application of the fair comment defence was highly technical and highly abstract. It was also based on a fundamental misunderstanding of the way newspapers work. Apart from the editorial pages, a newspaper is not, and should not be, a collection of the opinions of its editor and publisher. And even if a newsroom did exhibit an unnaturally high degree of internal control and centralization, it would still print wire stories, syndicated columns, and material written by freelancers. The monolithic notion of the organization of Canadian newspapers which is implicit in the Supreme Court's decision in *Cherneskey* does not accord with reality. Nonetheless, it was the decision of the Supreme Court of Canada and must, until amended or overruled by competent legislation, be followed in the courts of the common law provinces.

There were many in the newspaper industry who regarded the decision as unsatisfactory and, indeed, as dangerous to freedom of the press. The obvious fear was that newspapers would run a risk in printing letters to the editor containing opinions with which editors or publishers did not agree. As a result, newspapers would become more cautious about printing letters to the editor which expressed strong opinions.

And this was precisely what happened. A survey conducted by the Ontario Press Council in 1979 revealed that, of 28 Ontario daily newspapers contacted, 19 had been influenced in the way they handled letters to the editor by the *Cherneskey* decision. Without repeating the findings of the survey, the most common response was that newspapers had become more cautious in dealing with letters.

While the Supreme Court of Canada's decision constituted a binding precedent with respect to courts in the nine common law provinces, the rule which had been enunciated in *Cherneskey* could only be altered by provincial legislation. That is, the jurisdiction to legislate with respect to defamation rests exclusively with the provinces. The paradox, then, is that while the application of the Supreme Court's ruling was national, that ruling could only be dispensed with on a province by province basis.

Critical views about the *Cherneskey* decision were expressed in the Ottawa *Citizen*, the *Financial Post* and the *Globe and Mail*. These newspapers called for legislative action. The Ontario Press Council and the Attorneys-General of Ontario and Saskatchewan advocated reform. The Uniform Law Conference discussed the matter at its meeting in Saskatoon in August, 1979. In the result, four provinces — Alberta, Manitoba, New Brunswick, Ontario — and the two territories amended their defamation statutes in 1980.

The Cherneskey Amendments

Generally, all the amendments go far beyond what would have been necessary to overcome the precise problem created by the *Cherneskey* decision. First, none of the amendments confines itself to letters to the editor. Each addresses itself to "opinion", which means, presumably, all opinion whether expressed in a letter or in any other form. Secondly, the amendments are not restricted to newspapers and extend to any opinion which is "published". Finally, as will be argued in more detail below, the amendments are, assuming that their original purpose was to overcome the *Cherneskey* decision, drafted unnecessarily broadly. They may well amount, under the right circumstances, to licences to defame.

Each of the amendments will be commented on below.

A. Manitoba, Yukon Territory, and the Northwest Territories

On 29 July 1980 Manitoba adopted a new s.9.1 of its *Defamation Act*.

9.1(1) Where the defendant published allegedly defamatory matter that is an opinion expressed by another person, a defence of fair comment shall not fail for the reason only that the defendant did not hold the opinion, if

(*a*) the defendant did not know that the person expressing the opinion did not hold the opinion; and

(*b*) a person could honestly hold the opinion.

(2) For the purpose of this section, the defendant is not under a duty to inquire into whether the person expressing the opinion holds the opinion.

The form of words is that adopted by the Uniform Law Conference of Canada in 1979. Identical wording was adopted in the Yukon and the Northwest Territories. The wording appeared also in the relevant clause of a bill introduced in the Saskatchewan legislature in 1980, but not enacted.

The general effect of the amendment is that an editor or publisher who is the defendant in a libel action is not precluded from raising the defence of fair comment with respect to opinions expressed by other people in letters to the editor (or in any other form) with which he does not agree. The section is only to apply to opinions which "a person could honestly hold". For reasons already suggested, this form of words, clearly derived, via Dickson, J. in *Cherneskey*, from Duncan and Neill, is undesirable. Either it suggests a standard of reasonableness in fair comment, or it is meaningless. That is, if the words do not ask a court to objectively assess the content of an opinion, they ask it to determine if it is merely an opinion which someone might hold. Given the apparently limitless range of human thought, it is difficult to imagine an opinion which someone might not subscribe to. The defendant is further protected by subsection (2) which absolves him from any duty of enquiring whether people who write letters to the editor actually believe in the opinions they are expressing. Subsection (1)(a) is confusing. Read literally, it appears to require that in order for a defendant to take advantage of the section he must show that he did *not* know that the writer of a letter to the editor did *not* hold the opinion expressed in the letter. It would follow logically that, if the defendant *did* know that the writer of a letter *did* hold the opinion expressed in the letter, he would not be able to rely on the section. Interpreted in this fashion, the amendment would fail to achieve its ostensible purpose of avoiding the application of the *Cherneskey* rule. It would appear that the point of the subsection is to prevent the defence being raised when the defendant did know that the letter writer *did not* hold the opinion. But this is unnecessary. Such a fact situation would quite properly be regarded by any court as evidence of malice, thus negativing the defence of fair comment. The fact that such a convoluted form of words was used to make a point that should be obvious only adds to the general impression that the amendment was not carefully thought out.

B. New Brunswick

New Brunswick changed its law on 4 July 1980. The new section 8.1 of its *Defamation Act* is, with one slight variation, identical to s.9.1 of the *Manitoba Act* quoted above. The variation is an addition to subsection (1).

8.1(1)(c) The person expressing the opinion was identified in the publication.

This section simply provides that a defendant may not use the section to make out a defence of fair comment with respect to an anonymous letter to the editor. It is not clear what would happen if a letter were published under a pseudonym.

C. Alberta

Alberta and Ontario adopted different approaches, each derived from a wording which they suggested to the Uniform Law Conference, but which was rejected by that body. The Alberta statute, which became law on 22 May 1980, amended that province's *Defamation Act* by adding a new s.9.1.

9.1(1) If a defendant published an opinion expressed by another person, other than an employee or agent of the defendant, that is alleged to be defamatory, a defence of fair comment shall not fail by reason only that the defendant did not hold that opinion.

(2) Notwithstanding subsection (1), the defence of fair comment is not available to a defendant if it is proved that he acted maliciously in making the publication.

Alberta's amendment is the most carefully drafted of the six. The phrase "other than an employee or agent of the defendant" confronts a real problem that could arise with respect to the Manitoba, Ontario, New Brunswick, and territories' amendments if those amendments were to be interpreted literally by a court. Assume that a newspaper publishes an ostensibly defamatory opinion not in a letter to the editor but, for example, in a news story. Assume further that the story in question is written by a reporter on the staff of the newspaper and has a byline that indicates this. If the person defamed brings an action against only the corporation which publishes the newspaper and does not join the writer of the story as a co-defendant, the Manitoba, New Brunswick, Ontario, and territories' amendments would afford a very broad defence. The corporate defendant would only need show that the opinion in question was that of another person and that it was an opinion which some person could hold. It would not then matter whether the actual writer of the story held the opinion expressed or not.

Subsection (2) simply makes clear that, as has been the position under common law, evidence of malice can be used to negative the defence of fair comment. There is no reason to imagine that a court would interpret the Manitoba, New Brunswick, Ontario or territorial amendments differently from this.

D. Ontario

Ontario amended its *Libel and Slander Act* on 19 June 1980 by the addition of a new section 25.

25. Where the defendant published defamatory matter that is an opinion expressed by another person, a defence of fair comment by the defendant shall not fail for the reason only that the defendant or the person who expressed the opinion, or both, did not hold the opinion, if a person could honestly hold the opinion.

For the same general reasons as indicated with respect to the other amendments, the Ontario amendment is a substantial boon to media defendants. It has, as do all the amendments, a potential application which goes far beyond letters to the editor. Even if we confine ourselves to letters to the editor, the rule embodied in the Ontario amendment is a substantial and, it is suggested, an undesirable departure from principle. It says that a newspaper can successfully raise the defence of fair comment with respect to an opinion contained in a letter to the editor even if neither the publisher, editor, nor the writer of the letter honestly believes in the opinion. This is unnecessary.

The flaw in all the amendments is that they proceed from an acceptance of Mr. Justice Dickson's analysis. A much simpler form of words would have achieved the objective of avoiding the result in *Cherneskey* and yet not at the same time have created so many new and unnecessary difficulties:

> Where the defendant published allegedly defamatory matter that is an opinion expressed by another person, a defence of fair comment shall not fail for the reason only that the defendant did not hold the opinion if the defendant honestly believed that the person expressing the opinion did hold the opinion.

Note: See also s.11 of the Newfoundland *Defamation Act*, R.S.N. 1990, c. D-3.

5.2.3.2.11 *Masters v. Fox* (1978), 85 D.L.R. (3d) 64 (B.C.S.C.)

MACFARLANE, J.: The plaintiffs, who were unsuccessful candidates in a municipal election, claim damages for an alleged libel upon them during the course of the election campaign.

The plaintiffs plead, in paras. 6-13 inclusive of the statement of claim, as follows:

> 6.'The Plaintiffs are and were members of Community Planning Action Committee, which is a community group devoted to Civic and Regional Planning and which has printed and published pamphlets advocating Civic and Regional Planning,
>
> 7.'The Plaintiffs, as Community Planning Action Committee members, were electoral candidates for the office of civic alderman for the Municipality of Courtenay in the Province of British Columbia, in an election held on the 20th day of November, A.D. 1976.
>
> 8.'The Plaintiff, Richard Von Fuchs, has held a number of employments, including a position with the British Columbia Civil Liberties Association.
>
> 9.'The Plaintiff, Ruth Masters, is unmarried, an environmentalist, and has made her concerns for the environment known both in the newspaper and in public meetings.
>
> 10.'On or about the 12th day of November, A.D. 1976, the Defendants, William Mathis as editor of the Forum section of the *Comox District Free Press*, and the Defendant E. W Bickle Ltd., as owner and publisher of the *Comox District Free Press*, published in the *Comox District Free Press* and circulated to members of the general public of the Comox Valley and various other parts of Vancouver Island, in the Province of British Columbia, a statement of the Defendant, A. E. Fox, which read:
>
> "Election time is here again with some of the same old types trying to get in on the action. During the past year the Communist Party Action Committee has managed to belch a lot of bile and in the process make every effort to con the people into believing they are concerned with local issues and the orderly progress of the community — when in point of fact they are much more interested in spreading their particular brand of political venom — all of it under the guise of community interest (witness Oct. 14, at the Civic Centre).
>
> "I would not think that the voter has much of a problem in selecting a suitable and worthwhile candidate. With a full time career lay about and an old maid would appear (at a glance) to be an excellent recipe for a loser — but in spite of all some of these loud mouth windbags are going to tell and show everyone how to be winners and whatever the problem — you name it and they will cure it. Not one of them could run a peanut stand without a grant or subsidy and I would even suggest that one of them should be careful that the natural vegetation doesn't slowly take over and immobilize all activity.
>
> "It would be unfortunate if the voter was misled by some of their published rubbish which might permit (by accident) a few to get their grubby hands onto the tail end of a few more tax dollars."
>
> 11.'This statement of the Defendant, A. E. Fox, referred to above was captioned, either at the request of the aforesaid Defendant, or by the Defendant, William Mathis, "It's Election Time."
>
> 12.'The said statements contained in paragraph 10 are defamatory in their natural and ordinary meaning and in the innuendoes contained therein in that they mean and were understood to mean the following:
>
>> (a) that the Plaintiffs as members of the Community Planning Action Committee are members of the Communist Party.
>>
>> (b) that the Plaintiffs as Community Planning Action Committee's electoral candidates for civic aldermen for the Municipality of Courtenay in the Province of British Columbia are members of the Communist Party.
>>
>> (c) that the Plaintiffs as members of Community Planning Action Committee were attempting to deceive the electors of Courtenay in the Province of British Columbia

and the public, generally, and. particularly, by using issues of community interest as a means of popularizing the theories and plans of the Communist Party.

(d) that the Plaintiffs as Community Planning Action Committee's aldermanic candidates for civic aldermen for the Municipality of Courtenay in the Province of British Columbia were attempting to deceive the electors of Courtenay in the Province of British Columbia, and the public, generally and particularly, by using issues of community interest as a means of popularizing the theories and plans of the Communist Party.

(e) that the Plaintiffs were not worthwhile or suitable candidates due to their inability to support themselves or manage financial affairs.

(f) that the Plaintiff, Richard Von Fuchs, did not have employment or had not had employment and was accordingly shiftless, lazy, and a loser and, therefore, unable to suitably, manage civic affairs if elected.

(g) that the Plaintiff, Ruth J. Masters, was unmarried and a loser and accordingly was unable to manage financial affairs or manage other people's affairs, and therefore, was not suitable for public office.

(h) that the Plaintiff, Ruth J. Masters, was senile and/or as an environmentalist was likely to be immobilized by the environment and/or her environmental concerns.

(i) that the Plaintiffs' election material was misleading the public in order that the Plaintiffs could misappropriate the public's money if elected.

(j) that the Plaintiffs were guilty of improper and/or illegal and/or criminal use of the public's money.

13.'The statements were false and malicious at the time of their being made and remain wholly false in substance and in fact and are defamatory and concerning the Plaintiffs.

The defendants deny the allegations of fact contained in paras. 6-9 inclusive, and in paras. 12-13, but are silent as to paras. 10 and 11. The defendants plead that the words complained of were not published of and concerning the plaintiffs, were not defamatory of the plaintiffs, and raise a defence of fair comment as follows:

In further answer to the whole of the Statement of Claim these Defendants say that the words complained of are expressions of opinion and are fair comment made in good faith and without malice on a matter of public interest, namely the conduct of an election for public office in the community and the qualifications of the candidates therein.

The plaintiffs sought and obtained particulars of facts upon which the opinion referred to in the foregoing paragraph of the statement of defence is based, which are as follows:

(a) that it was election time;
(b) that the Plaintiffs were running for office;
(c) that the Community Planning Action Committee had at least one card carrying Communist on its executive committee, and that this person had not remained silent as to his political views during the time he was on the executive of the Community Planning Action Committee;
(d) that the Plaintiffs were members of the Community Planning Action Committee and had both expressed left wing views;
(e) that the Plaintiff Von Fuchs was at times a "social democrat", at times a member of the New Democratic Party, and was an American who had left the United States for political reasons and was a draft dodger;

(f) that the Plaintiff Von Fuchs, in letters to the editor and in political speeches had expressed views opposed to the free enterprise system, or some aspects thereof;
(g) that the Plaintiff Von Fuchs frequently changed his employment and was unemployed from time to time;
(h) that the Plaintiff Masters is 57 years of age and a spinster;
(i) that the Plaintiff Masters is a Socialist and a member of New Democratic Party and has actively promoted natural vegetation;
(j) that the likelihood was that both Plaintiffs would lose the election;
(k) that in their campaign and in several public utterances, the Plaintiffs proposed the solutions to a number of problems;
(l) that the Plaintiffs did not have any known record of success of running an independent private business of their own in the community;
(m) that the Plaintiffs were attempting to be elected to public office and thereby reach a position from which they would have some responsibility in the management of public funds, viz., tax dollars.

There is no real issue as to the substantial truth of those allegations of fact, except as to (g) which relates to the employment record of the plaintiff Von Fuchs ... Counsel for the plaintiffs concedes that the words complained of were written upon a matter of public interest, namely, the conduct of an election for public office in the community and the qualifications of the candidates therein.

The first question of substance is whether the words complained of were published of and concerning the plaintiffs. Several witnesses have been called by the plaintiffs who have said that, upon reading the letter soon after its publication, they understood it to refer to the plaintiffs. I accept their evidence. It is clear from reading the article that a reasonable person in the community in which it was published would identify the plaintiffs as the objects of the criticism. The letter was published on November 12, 1976, about eight days before the municipal election. It obviously refers to the candidates of a particular organization, which is described in the letter as the Communist Party Action Committee. There was not any committee of that name in the community and the reference, obviously a play on words, was to the only organization which was sponsoring candidates in that election campaign, namely, the Community Planning Action Committee (CPAC), a group concerned with planning and environmental matters. There were three candidates sponsored by the organization, and they were described on a one-sheet brochure as "Your CPAC Aldermanic Candidates for Courtenay". The names, photographs, and description of the candidates were displayed prominently on one side of the sheet and the aims and objectives of CPAC, the Community Planning Action Committee, were set forth on the other side. The brochure had been distributed to households in the community. The candidates had been prominently identified in lawn signs and by the media, and were well-known in the community as candidates for CPAC. It is suggested by the defendants that reference in the letter may have been to other candidates running in the election. I do not think so. The letter, as a whole, appears to relate to the one organization and its candidates. There were two female candidates, one of whom was a relatively young married woman. Miss Masters is 57 years of age, unmarried and an environmentalist, who was described in the brochure as belonging "to over 20 environment organizations". She was the only one of the three candidates who could be described as an "old maid" and as one who "should be careful that the natural vegetation doesn't take over and immobilize all activity" (a reference to her well-known concern to preserve natural vegetation in the area). Mr. Von Fuchs, having been a candidate previously, was the only one of the three who fitted the description "some of the same old types". The statement, "witness Oct. 14, at the Civic Center", was a reference to him because he was the only one of the three candidates who had been prominent in the local "Day of Protest". His participation on October 14th had been prominently publicized in the local press. Although the description of him as a "full time career lay about" was inaccurate, it obviously was not a reference to Miss Masters or the third candidate and, by elimination, could be taken. and was taken, to refer to him. I will say more about the characterization when I turn to discuss the question of defamation. I find that the letter was published of and concerning the plaintiffs.

In what sense do the plaintiffs contend that the words complained of are defamatory? Counsel for the plaintiffs has cited what I said in *Gill v. Garcha and Dhillon* (unreported, but dated November 8, 1976), at pp. 7-8, as follows:

> The author of *Gatley on Libel and Slander*, 7th ed., while recognizing that there is no wholly satisfactory definition of defamatory imputation, has this to say in para. 31 of the text: "31. The defamatory imputation."
>
> "The gist of the torts of libel and slander is the publication of matter (usually words) conveying a defamatory imputation. A defamatory imputation is one to a man's discredit, or which tends to lower him in the estimation of others, or to expose him to hatred, contempt or ridicule, or to injure his reputation in his office, trade or profession, or to injure his financial credit. The standard of opinion is that of right-thinking persons generally. To be defamatory an imputation need have no actual effect on a person's reputation; the law looks only to its tendency."
>
> I have no hesitation in finding that the imputations contained in the Lok Awaz editorial, when read in context and in the light of the whole editorial, are such that tend to lower the plaintiff in the estimation of right-thinking members of society generally.

The contention of counsel for the plaintiffs is that (although the false implication that the plaintiffs are members of a communist organization could be said to be defamatory) the real bite of the alleged libel is the imputation of dishonourable or dishonest motives to the plaintiffs. It is contended that the clear inference arising from the letter was that CPAC and, in the context of the letter, its candidates, had been making "every effort to con" (that is, deceive) the electorate, and that their true motives were not honest concern and interest in the community in which they lived and in which they sought office, but rather that their real reason for running for office, which they sought to conceal, was to spread "their particular brand of political venom", namely, communism. It should be stated immediately that neither plaintiff was or is a member of the Communist Party. Each was, in fact, a member of the New Democratic Party but there is no evidence whatsoever that either was using or attempting to use CPAC to spread or advance the aims of any political party. CPAC was a non-political organization which had amongst its members one known Communist, three Liberals, some Conservatives, probably some Social Crediters and about a dozen New Democratic Party members. Total membership of the group ran, at times, between 100-200 members.

Both plaintiffs were involved in numerous community organizations of a nonpolitical nature, and had been very active and concerned with issues of a planning and environmental nature. There is no evidence that, as candidates in 1976, they had any motive other than a desire to serve their community. Their interests and their "leanings" were well-known, and there was no evidence of any deception or concealment by them as to their aims and objectives, if elected.

It is contended on behalf of the defendants that such imputation, if there be one, was concerning the organization, not its individual members, and not these plaintiffs. The plaintiffs cite *Knupffer v. London Express Newspaper Ltd.*, [1944] A.C. 116 (House of Lords) at p: 123, where it was said that if a defamatory statement made of a class or group can reasonably be understood to refer to every member of it, each one has a cause of action. I am satisfied here that the first paragraph of the letter in question was intended to refer to each active member of the committee and, by reference to those running in the election, was intended, in particular, to refer to the plaintiffs who, as candidates, were then advancing the aims and objectives of the committee.

The second paragraph of the letter is devoted largely to personal abuse of the candidates, to which I will return later. The last and concluding paragraph picks up the introductory theme by again appearing to question the motives of the candidates and, in particular, by warning the voters that if they were "misled" by the "published rubbish" of the candidates, then a few (presumably the CPAC candidates) might "get their grubby hands onto the tail end of a few more tax dollars". The use of the word "grubby" (defined in the *Shorter Oxford English Dictionary* as "dirty, grimy") is not applicable to the plaintiffs in any proper sense and appears to me, when read in context and in the light of the opening paragraph, to imply not only that the election of such candidates would be undesirable, but that public funds would not be safe in their hands. Again, in my opinion, the author has left a defamatory imputation with the reader.

Returning to the second paragraph of the letter the plaintiff Masters is characterized as an "old maid" and as one "who should be careful that the natural vegetation doesn't slowly take over and immobilize all activity". The descriptions are in poor taste, are insulting, and are an attempt to ridicule the candidate, but I do not think that any reasonable person would think any less of Miss Masters, having regard to the fact that the characterization, albeit crude, was obviously the word of an extremist carried away in the heat of an election campaign. The final insult, referable to Miss Masters' interest in environmental matters, was linked with the hackneyed allegation, which is habitually levelled in this Province by the right wing at the left wing, that the latter could not "run a peanut stand without a grant or subsidy". Again, I do not think, that such a remark in those circumstances would tend to lower the plaintiffs in the estimation of right-thinking members of society generally.

One cannot, however, dismiss the description of the plaintiff Von Fuchs as being a "full time career lay about" with such ease. That is clearly an imputation that he did not work, that he made a career of avoiding work, and that he was shiftless and lazy. Even counsel for the defendants conceded that the evidence at trial shows Mr. Von Fuchs to have been an energetic and very active person in many organizations in the Comox Valley, and a regular (although described as "auxiliary") worker on the ferry, "Sechelt Queen", from May, 1976, to the date of trial. To those who did not know Mr. Von Fuchs, the writer sought to convey a very different, false and damaging impression.

Turning then to the defence that the words complained of are expressions of opinion and are fair comment made in good faith on a matter of public interest: Mr. Harvey, counsel for the editor Mathis and the defendant newspaper company, has cited many authorities which deal with the defence of fair comment, but is content to say that the position of the defendants here can be best summed up by adopting the language of Lord Denning, M.R., in *Slim v. Daily Telegraph Ltd.*, [1968] 2 Q.B. 157 at p. 170, as follows:

> These comments are capable of various meanings. They may strike some readers in one way and others in another way. One person may read into them imputations of dishonesty, insincerity and hypocrisy (as the judge did). Another person may only read into them imputations of inconsistency and want of candour (as I would). But in considering a plea of fair comment, it is not correct to canvass all the various imputations which different readers may put upon the words. The important thing is to determine whether or not the writer was actuated by malice. If he was an honest man expressing his genuine opinion on a subject of public interest, then no matter that his words conveyed derogatory imputations; no matter that his opinion was wrong or exaggerated or prejudiced; and no matter that it was badly expressed so that other people read all sorts of innuendoes into it; nevertheless, he has a good defence of fair comment. His honesty is the cardinal test. He must honestly express his real view. So long as he does this, he has nothing to fear, even though other people may read more into it, see *per* Lord Porter in *Turner v. M.G.M. Pictures Ltd.*, [1950] I All E.R. 449. H.L. and *per* Diplock, J. in *Silkin v. Beaverbrook Newspapers Ltd.*, [1958] 2 All E.R. 516. 1 stress this because the right of fair comment is one of the essential elements which go to make up our freedom of speech. We must ever maintain this right intact. It must not be whittled down by legal refinements. When a citizen is troubled by things going wrong, he should be free to "write to the newspaper": and the newspaper should be free to publish his letter. It is often the only way to get things put right. The matter must, of course, be one of public interest. The writer must get his facts right: and he must honestly state his real opinion. But that being done, both he and the newspaper should be clear of any liability. They should not be deterred by fear of libel actions.

The words of Lord Denning, M.R., reported at p. 170 aforesaid, were, in part, adopted by Bayda, J.A., in *Cherneskey v. Armadale Publishers Ltd. et al.* (1977), 79 D.L.R. (3d) 180 at p. 202, [1977] 5 W.W.R. 155 at pp. 180-81. He also referred to *Silkin v. Beaverbrook Newspapers Ltd.*, [1958] 2 All E.R. 516, although he did not quote from it. In that case Diplock, J., in summing up to a jury had this to say, at p. 520:

> So in considering this case, members of the jury, do not apply the test of whether you agree with it. If juries did that, freedom of speech, the right of the crank to say what he likes, would go. Would a fair-minded man holding strong views, obstinate views, prejudiced views, have been capable of making this comment? . . .
> If you take the view that this test is fulfilled, that this does come within the limits of fair comment, as I say, the proper verdict for you to bring in is a verdict for the defendants. If you were to take the view that it was so strong a comment that no fair-minded man could honestly have held it, then the defence fails.

In this case, imputations of corrupt or dishonourable motives being alleged, the central issue is whether they rendered the comment unfair. That question, and the line to be drawn between freedom of speech and unfair comment, is discussed by *Gatley on Libel and Slander*, 7th ed., para. 725, as follows:

(b) Imputation of Corrupt or Dishonourable Motives

725. General principles.

> An imputation of corrupt or dishonourable motives will render the comment unfair, unless such imputation is warranted by the facts truly stated or referred to, i.e. is an inference which a fair-minded man might reasonably draw from such facts, and represents to honest opinion of the writer.
> "A line must be drawn between criticism upon public conduct and the imputation of motives by which that conduct may be supposed to be actuated; one man has no right to impute to another, whose conduct may be fairly open to ridicule or disapprobation, base, sordid and wicked motives unless there is so much ground for the imputation that a jury shall find, not only that he had an honest belief in the truth of his statements, but that his belief was not without foundation . . . It is said that it is for the interests of society that the public conduct of public men should be criticized without any other limit than that the writer should have an honest belief that what he writes is true. But it seems to me that the public have an equal interest in the maintenance of the public character of public men; and public affairs could not be conducted by men of honour, with a view to the welfare of the country, if we were to sanction attacks upon them, destructive of their honour and character and made without any foundation. I think, the fair position in which the law may be settled is this: that where the public conduct of a public man is open to animadversion, and the writer who is commenting upon it makes imputations on his motives which arise fairly and legitimately out of his conduct so that a jury shall say that the criticism was not only honest, but also well founded, an action is not maintainable." [*Per* Cockburn, C.J. in *Campbell v. Spottiswoode* (1863), 3 B. & S. at pp. 776. 777.]

The motive attributed to the plaintiffs was to spread "their particular brand of political venom", which the writer implies was communism. Each of the plaintiffs was known as a socialist. Assuming that the writer only meant to imply that they were more interested in advancing socialist theories than in dealing with local problems and furthering the orderly progress of the community, was that imputation warranted by the facts? Could a fair-minded person reasonably draw that inference from the facts? Firstly, I will deal with Miss Masters. She was a member of the New Democratic Party, and she had written strong letters to the editor about Social Credit and Social Crediters. But she was not known in the community primarily as a political activist. Her deep concern and, indeed, outside her employment, her sole interest was in environmental matters. It was obvious that was why she was running for office and no fair-minded person could reasonably infer that, as a candidate, she was expressing that interest only to conceal a partisan political motive.

Mr. Von Fuchs was a socialist who advocated "replacement" of the capitalist system. He was not a communist, and no fair-minded person could think that he was — unless such person perceived all socialists to be communists. He was known as an activist in the sense that prominent press coverage had been given to the leading role played by him in the October 14, 1976 "Day of Protest". He was also an avid author of letters to the editor, and his socialist views were well-known. However, he was an active member of about 12 non-political voluntary community organizations and spent an enormous amount of time and energy in connection with them. He was obviously dedicated to matters of local concern, and to the orderly progress of the community. He did not make any secret of his political beliefs (and, I expect, antagonized many with his candour). There was no basis whatsoever for implying that he had a hidden motive for running, namely, to advance communism, socialism, or some other political cause and that he was attempting to achieve this objective under the guise of community interest.

Characterizing the man as a "full time career lay about" was not a comment at all. It falls within the category described by Gatley in para. 712 of his work, in the following language:

> But if a writer chooses to publish an expression of opinion which has no relation by way of criticism to any fact before the reader, then such an expression of opinion depends upon nothing but the writer's own authority, and stands in the same position as an allegation of fact. It cannot be protected by a plea of fair comment.

In my view, that alleged opinion should be regarded as a statement of fact, and it was false. It is true that Mr. Von Fuchs has had a variety of jobs but he has a record of almost continuous employment. At one time he was a field worker for the British Columbia Civil Liberties Association, and worked from an office located in his home. To that extent someone, not knowing the facts, may have assumed that he was temporarily unemployed. But to label him as a "full time career lay about" could not be justified upon any reasonable view of the facts. The statement has a special connotation and goes far beyond what any fair-minded person would infer from a period of temporary unemployment. It connotes a permanent state, and deliberate pursuit of that state.

I have concluded, therefore, that the defence of fair comment must fail.

Although it is not necessary to my decision to do so, I should say that the plaintiffs have alleged but, in my opinion, have not established malice.

There was some evidence to consider in respect to the defendant Fox because he had levelled another attack upon Mr. Von Fuchs a year earlier. But the evidence is insufficient upon which to base a finding of malice.

There was no evidence whatsoever of malice on the part of the newspaper. It is clear that it printed letters for and against candidates for office, and letters expressing strong opinions on both sides of a subject. The newspaper sought to provide a forum in which members of the public could "let off steam". What they did here was to let the matter get out of hand, and to fail to implement their announced policy of editing a letter which they ought to have recognized as being defamatory. It is contended that they showed malice because one of their columnists expressed satisfaction at the defeat of Mr. Von Fuchs. In my view that was an opinion that the columnist was entitled to express, and his opposition to the candidate has not in any way been connected to the publication of the letter in question.

... The defendants are therefore liable, and I turn now to assess damages.

The factors which counsel for the plaintiffs asks me to take into account in assessing damages, and which seem to be relevant, are:

1. The author of the libel was a well-known former policeman in the community, and the newspaper asserted that it did not print libel, that is, false statements. The letter would have greater weight by reason of that sponsorship.

2. The community was small, and the circulation of the newspaper was large. Thus the libel would reach a significant portion of the population, and many people with whom the plaintiffs came into daily contact.

3. The allegation that the plaintiffs could not be trusted might affect the plaintiff Masters in her occupation as an occasional trustee of estates, and might affect the plaintiff Von Fuchs in the eyes of his employer and of his union.

4. The refusal of the defendants to apologize was an aggravation of the libel.

The factors which may make the matter appear less serious are:

1. The author of the libel was known to be extremely partisan, and regularly wrote in strong terms. The letter was published in a comer of the newspaper nicknamed by local residents as "Kooks' Corner". It would not, therefore, be taken as seriously as if it had been otherwise published.

2. It was published in the heat of an election campaign, and would be assessed by the readers as being partisan and not objective.

3. Both of the plaintiffs were, and still are, regarded in this relatively small community as concerned, dedicated but sometimes controversial citizens — that is, their reputations have not been seriously affected.

Damages are assessed at $3,500 to each of the plaintiffs. The defendants will be jointly and severally liable for payment of the award, and will pay the costs of the plaintiffs to be taxed.

Judgments for plaintiffs.

5.2.3.2.12 *Vogel v. C.B.C.* (1982), 21 C.C.L.T. 105 (B.C.S.C.)

ESSON, J.: ... The position of CBC at trial was that such errors of fact were insignificant, that the programme came close enough because, after all, Rigg and

Vogel were friendly acquaintances. To insist upon literal accuracy is mere nit-picking which makes it excessively difficult to get the message across. That attitude is not in accordance with the law. Where, as here, the "message" sought to be conveyed is that a person in public life has been guilty of serious wrong-doing, the facts offered in support of that message must be literally true as well as fairly stated.

> Note: If the plaintiff can show that the defendant was motivated by malice, the defence of fair comment will be lost. As this is also true with respect to the defence of qualified privilege, the meaning of malice is dealt with in the next section.

5.2.3.3 Privilege

5.2.3.3.1 *Shultz v. Porter and Block Brothers Ltd.* (1979), 9 A.R. 381 (Alta. S.C.)

WAITE, J.: The law relating to qualified privilege remains unchanged since the leading case in 1834 of *Toogood v. Sprying*, I Cr. M. & R. 181, 149 E.R. 1044, wherein Parke, B, for the court stated the defence of qualified privilege in the following passage at pp. 1049-50:

> In general, an action lies for the malicious publication of statements which are false in fact, and injurious to the character of another (within the well-known limits as to verbal slander), and the law considers such publication as malicious, unless it is fairly made by a person in the discharge of some public or private duty, whether legal or moral, or in the conduct of his own affairs, in matters where his interest is concerned. In such cases, the occasion prevents the inference of malice, which the law draws from unauthorized communications, and affords a qualified defence depending upon the absence of actual malice. If fairly warranted by any reasonable occasion or exigency, and honestly made, such communications are protected for the common convenience and welfare of society; and the law has not restricted the right to make them within any narrow limits.

The gravamen of defamation is malice. Ordinarily malice is inferred from the publication of defamatory words, but if the publication occurs on a privileged occasion that inference is rebutted and malice must then be proven expressly by the plaintiff. In the defence of qualified privilege as defined by Parke, B., it is the occasion which is privileged so as to protect the publication with immunity unless the plaintiff establishes express or actual malice.

As Lord Macnaghten for the Privy Council in *Macintosh v. Dun*, [1908] A.C. 390, said at p. 399, after quoting with approval the passage aforesaid from *Toogood v. Spyring*:

> The underlying principle is "the common convenience and welfare of society"-not the convenience of individuals or the convenience of a class, but, to use the words of Erle, C.J. in *Whiteley v. Adams* (1863), 15 C.B.N.S. 392 at 418, 143 E.R. 838 "the general interest of society".

In *Halls v. Mitchell*, [1928] S.C.R. 125, [1928] 2 D.L.R. 97, Duff, J., speaking for a majority of the court after referring to *Macintosh v. Dun* and the cases therein cited, said at p. 133:

The defamatory statement, therefore, is only protected when it is fairly warranted by some reasonable occasion or exigency, and when it is fairly made in discharge of some public or private duty, or in the conduct of the defendant's own affairs in matters in which his interests are concerned. The privilege rests not upon the interests of the persons entitled to invoke it, but upon the general interests of society, and protects only communications *"fairly* made" (the italics are those of Parke, B. himself) in the legitimate defence of a person's own interests, or plainly made under a sense of duty, such as would be recognized by "people of ordinary intelligence and moral principles".

He followed it with a summary of his reasons on p. 147 in the following terms:

To summarize my reasons for thinking that the conditions have not in this case been satisfied in which the law protects privileged communications that otherwise would be actionable as defamatory. 'The underlying principle' upon which that protection is founded is 'the common convenience and welfare of society' — not the interests of individuals or of a class, but 'the general interest of society.' The court must consider whether the communication was made plainly under a duty — and a sense of that duty — which in all the circumstances would be 'recognized by people of ordinary intelligence and moral principle': and in considering that, the court will take into account the origin of the matter of the communication and 'every circumstance connected with the publication' of it: and must 'hold the balance and looking at who published the libel, and why, and to whom, and in what circumstances' must say 'whether it is for the welfare of society that such a communication honestly made should be protected by clothing the occasion of the publication with privilege'."

The principle enunciated in *Toogood v. Sprying* has been repeated in cases too numerous to mention, the few citations above being but examples of its application and confirmation. The only change in the development of the principle of qualified privilege is that in its initial stages it was the communication that was privileged, while the later expressions of the rule place the privilege on the occasion itself within which the communication was made so as to protect with immunity the publication of what would otherwise be defamatory.

5.2.3.3.2 Absolute Privilege

5.2.3.3.2.1 *Ontario Libel and Slander Act*, R.S.O. 1990, c. L.12.

4. (1) A fair and accurate report without comment in a newspaper or in a broadcast of proceedings publicly heard before a court of justice, if published in the newspaper or broadcast contemporaneously with such proceedings, is absolutely privileged unless the defendant has refused or neglected to insert in the newspaper in which the report complained of appeared or to broadcast, as the case may be, a reasonable statement of explanation or contradiction by or on behalf of the plaintiff.

(2) Nothing in this section authorizes any blasphemous, seditious or indecent matter in a newspaper or in a broadcast. R.S.O. 1980, c. 237, s. 4.

Notes on Other Provincial Statutes

Section 11 of Saskatchewan's *Libel and Slander Act*, R.S.S. 1978, c. L-14, is almost identical to this provision. Section 3 of British Columbia's *Libel and Slander Act*, R.S.B.C. 1979, c. 234 is much the same although not as specific:

(1) A fair and accurate report in a public newspaper or other periodical publication or in a broadcast of proceedings publicly heard before a court exercising judicial authority if published contemporaneously with the proceedings, is privileged.

(2) This section does not authorize the publication of blasphemous or indecent matter.

For the most part, however, the provincial defamation statutes, and the *Revised Uniform Defamation Act*, have adopted the following provisions:

(1) A fair and accurate report, published in a newspaper or by broadcasting, of proceedings publicly heard before any court is absolutely privileged if
    (*a*) the report contains no comment,
    (*b*) the report is published contemporaneously with the proceedings that are the subject matter of the report, or within 30 days thereafter, and
    (*c*) the report contains nothing of a seditious, blasphemous or indecent nature.

(2) Subsection (1) shall not apply if
    (*a*) in the case of publication in a newspaper, the plaintiff shows that the defendant has been requested to insert in the newspaper a reasonable letter or statement of explanation or contradiction by or on behalf of the plaintiff, and the defendant fails to show that he has done so, or
    (*b*) in the case of publication by broadcasting, the plaintiff shows that the defendant has been requested to broadcast a reasonable statement of explanation or contradiction by or on behalf of the plaintiff, and the defendant fails to show that he has done so, from the broadcasting stations from which the alleged defamatory matter was broadcast, on at least two occasions on different days and at the same time of day as the alleged defamatory matter was broadcast or at a time as near as possible to that time.

(3) For the purposes of this section, every headline or caption in a newspaper that relates to a report therein shall be deemed to be a report.

(*Defamation Act*, R.S.A. 1980, c. D-6. s. 11. See also *Revised Uniform Defamation Act*, ss. 11 and 12 in Conference of Commissioners on Uniformity of Legislation in Canada, Proceedings of the Thirtieth Annual Meeting, Montreal, Quebec, August 24-28, 1948, Appendix J; the former section as amended in Conference of Commissioners on Uniformity of Legislation in Canada, Proceedings of the Thirty-First Annual Meeting, Calgary, Alberta, August 23-27, 1949, p.23; *The Defamation Act*, R.S.M. 1987, c. D20, ss. 11 and 12; *Defamation Act*, R.S.N.B. 1973, c. D-5, ss. 10 and 11; *Defamation Act*, R.S.N. 1990, c. D-3, ss. 13 and 14; *Defamation Act*, R.S.N.S. 1989, c. 122, ss. 14 and 15; *Defamation Act*, R.S.P.E.I. 1988, c. D-5, s. 12; *Defamation Act*, R.S.N.W.T. 1988, c. D-1, ss. 12 and 13; *Defamation Act*, R.S.Y.T. 1986, c. 41, ss. 11 and 12.)

The privilege may be lost if the report is not fair and accurate.

5.2.3.3.2.2 *Tedlie v. Southam*, [1950] 4 D.L.R. 415 (Man.K.B.)

MONTAGUE, J.: This action for defamation was tried before me without a jury.

A bad collision had occurred at 9:44 p.m. on September 1, 1947, at Dugald, when the westbound C.N.R. special train from Minaki crashed head-on into the regular eastbound passenger train standing on the main track waiting for the other train to take the siding. At the time of the accident the plaintiff was the operator on duty at Dugald and in charge of train orders and signals. He was apprehended under a coroner's warrant the next day and detained at Headingly Gaol until released on bail.

The Board of Transport Commissioners for Canada (hereinafter referred to as the "Board") ordered a public inquiry as to the causes of the wreck. Under the *Railway Act*, R.S.C. 1927, c.170, and the *Transport Act*, 1938 (Can.), c.53, the Board is a Court of record and, as respects all matters necessary or proper for the exercise of its jurisdiction, has all the powers, rights and privileges of a Superior Court. The Board's inquiry commenced at the Law Courts in Winnipeg on September 23rd, and the next morning the baggageman, the rear trainman of the special, the assistant superintendent of the division (who was travelling on it), and the plaintiff, gave evidence. Their evidence, as transcribed by the Board's official reporter, was, by agreement of counsel, read in as evidence at the trial.

The Winnipeg *Tribune*, a daily newspaper published by the defendants, carried on September 24th, a report of the Board's proceedings. On the front page, in large type covering seven columns, were, in two lines, the following headlines: "SPECIAL HAD GREEN LIGHT, OPERATOR TELLS HEARING ; and below this, in smaller types, covering two columns, were the following lead headlines:

"Train Reported 'Under Control' ",

"The Minaki campers special had a green light, or 'proceed' signal in its favor, at the time of the Dugald train wreck, according to testimony given today at the Board of Transport Commissioners inquiry in the law courts building. "

After two further paragraphs there followed, in one-column width on pp. 1 and 7 of the paper, an extensive report of the proceedings before the Board.

The plaintiff alleged that the headline and lead headlines above quoted were falsely and maliciously published of and concerning him in the way of his trade or occupation as a telegraph operator. In paras. 15 and 16 of the statement of claim, innuendoes were pleaded ascribing the meaning of the words complained of. The essential parts of these paragraphs were:

"The defendants meant and imputed and were understood to mean and impute thereby that the plaintiff while on duty as aforesaid had displayed the wrong signal, which misled the Minaki Campers's Special train resulting in the said accident, and therefore the plaintiff was incompetent and negligent in the performance of his work and duties."

Further:

"The defendants meant and imputed and were understood to mean and impute thereby that the plaintiff had been criminally negligent at the time of the said accident and had thereby caused and was therefore responsible for the said accident. "

The hearing before me was the third trial of this action and at this point I shortly refer to its prior history. At the first trial which was with a jury, the action was dismissed on a motion for a nonsuit. The Court of Appeal's judgment allowing the appeal from this and directing a new trial is reported in *Tedlie v. Southam Co.*, [1949] 3 D.L.R. 185. It is sufficient for my purpose to say that in the majority judgment of the Court delivered by Dysart, J.A. he construed, at p. 195, ss.(3) of s.11 of the *Defamation Act*, 1946, c.11, which reads as follows: "For the purposes of this section, every headline or caption in a newspaper that relates to any report therein shall be deemed to be a report."

And at p. 196 it was held: "In my opinion the subsection *must* be taken in its literal sense; and as its language is clear and unambiguous, each headline *must* 'be deemed to be a report' independent of every other headline and of the published detailed report of the testimony." At p. 198 it was held: "The heading: 'Train reported under control' is based upon that published answer, and is, of course, not strictly accurate. But for the purposes of the plaintiff's case, that omission is not really serious, because the actual operating 'control' of the Minaki Special could not in any sense be attributed to the plaintiff. The responsibility for that 'control' lay solely with the train's crew, and no dereliction of duty in that respect could reasonably be attributed to the plaintiff by the heading."

At p. 201 it was held that certain issues of the paper prior to that of September 24th were admissible in evidence. In the next paragraph it was held: "On the whole case, I think that the words complained of are independent reports; that they are not fair and accurate reports; that they are capable of the defamatory meaning ascribed to them; and that consequently the case should have gone to the jury."

At the second trial, which was with a jury, the verdict was for the defendants. The Court of Appeal's judgment allowing the appeal from this and directing a new trial is reported in *Tedlie v. Southam Co.*, [1950] I W.W.R. 1009. Richards, J.A. delivered the majority judgment of the Court at p. 1012. I refer to the third paragraph on p. 1013 where it was held that s. 10 of the *Defamation Act* was inapplicable to the case (and it appears that this was the opinion of McPherson, C.J.M. expressed in his dissenting judgment on the first appeal: see [1949] 3 D.L.R. at p. 186).

On p. 1015 it was held: "*The Defamation Act* constitutes a code and, in so far as it deals with a matter, the previous law is inapplicable."

And at p. 1016: "*The Defamation Act* was intended to be complete and exhaustive as to the subjects with which it deals."

At the trial before me there was no new evidence adduced which could possibly affect the judgments of the Court of Appeal on the matters I have referred to above, and while *ex abundanti cautela*, I now formally hold in these reasons the same as the Court of Appeal has held on the matters, my opinion is that it is not open to me to reconsider any of them.

In England the rule is that the decisions of the Court of Appeal upon questions of law must be followed by Courts of first instance and the decision of the Court of Appeal on questions of fact is, as between the parties, binding: 19 Hals., 2nd ed., pp. 254-5. In *McIntosh v. Parent*, [1924] 4 D.L.R. 420 at p. 422, 55 O.L.R. 552 at p. 555, Middleton, J.A. said: "When a question is litigated, the judgment of the Court is a final determination as between the parties and their privies. Any right, question, or fact distinctly put in issue and directly determined by a Court of competent jurisdiction . . . cannot be re-tried. . . . The right, question, or fact, once determined, must, as between them, be taken to be conclusively established so long as the judgment remains.

In *Western Can. Power Co. v. Bergklint* (1916), 34 D.L.R. 467 at p. 477, 54 S.C.R. 285 at p. 299, an employer's liability case, Duff, J. said: "There is some authority indicating that where a Court of appeal in granting a new trial decides a substantive question in the litigation, that question for the purposes of that litigation is to be taken to have been conclusively determined as between the parties."

The learned Judge stated that the point was not taken or argued before the Court and he himself thought the appeal should be allowed on other grounds. He had, however, referred to the Privy Council's decision in *Badar Bee v. Habib Merican Noordin*, [1909] A.C. 615, which was an appeal from the Straits Settlements' Supreme Court in a case involving the construction of a will which had been construed by that Court many years before. In this case Lord Macnaghten, delivering the judgment, at p. 623 said: "It is not competent for the Court, in the case of the same question arising between the same parties, to review a previous decision not open to appeal."

These authorities convince me that the decisions of our Court of Appeal on the matters referred to above are binding on me.

The first question to be dealt with is whether the words complained of were published, and if so, were they published by the defendants. On the evidence I would instruct a jury affirmatively on these points, and, performing the function of a jury, I find that the words in fact were published by the defendants.

Then, discharging my duties as a Judge, I must determine whether the words complained of are capable of the meaning ascribed to them by the innuendoes: *Sturt v. Blagg* (1847), 10 Q.B. 906, 116 E.R. 343; *Capital & Counties Bk. v. Henty & Sons* (1882), 7 App. Cas. 741 at p. 744; *Nevill v. Fine Art & Gen'l Ins. Co.*, [1897] A.C. 68 at p. 72; 20 Hals, 2nd ed., p. 433. I hold and determine that the words complained of, other than "Train Reported Under Control", are so capable and that I would so instruct a jury.

Hereafter when I use the expression "words complained of", it will be understood that I am referring to the words complained of in the statement of claim, other than "Train Reported Under Control".

Next, it is my duty, discharging that of a jury, to determine whether the words complained of and published by the defendants in the circumstances established by the evidence were, in fact, defamatory of the plaintiff.

A defamatory statement is a statement which, if published of and concerning a person, is calculated to expose him to hatred, contempt or ridicule, or to convey an imputation on him disparaging or injurious to him in his trade, business, calling or office: 20 Hals, 2nd ed., p. 384. The true test is whether, in the circumstances in which the statement was published, reasonable men to whom the publication was made would understand it in a defamatory sense. Sometimes that test may be satisfied from the mere words of the statement: *ibid.*, p. 396.

The words complained of by the plaintiff are not defamatory in their natural and ordinary meaning. They do not specify the plaintiff as the person to whom they applied. Accordingly, the onus lay on the plaintiff to prove that there were facts known to persons to whom the words were published which might reasonably lead them to understand the words in the sense alleged in the innuendoes.

This brings me to the evidence of four witnesses called by the plaintiff at the trial. To each of them the foundation question, set out in *Gatley on Libel & Slander*, 3rd ed., p. 619, was, in fact or effect, put. Each of them deposed to facts and circumstances within his knowledge at the time he read the headlines of the paper, which I hold entitled him to state what he understood by them.

John Renwick Brown said that he read the headlines when he got home from work. They were the first thing that caught his attention: "My first impression from these headlines was that the operator may have made a grave mistake in giving the wrong light to the westbound train. It looked as if he had given the westbound train a proceed signal to come west on the main line, which could not be possible. Order 338 gave the train rights to the east switch only; its only possible thoroughfare to proceed was through the siding. "

At the end of his examination-in-chief he said: "My impression from reading the headlines was that the operator had made a mistake and in my opinion would be responsible. "

This witness is a C.N.R. telegraph operator. He was one of the bondsmen for the plaintiff's bail. He is the chairman of the local brunch of the Railway Telegraphers Order and as such he represented the plaintiff at the investigation held by the railway's officials. Despite these facts he did not impress me as biased.

Mr. John L. Ross, K.C., an experienced defence counsel, was the next witness. He read the paper of September 24th; remembered reading the headlines — it was because of such that he picked up the paper. According to my notes he said that "when he read the headlines his first reaction was, surely that headline cannot be correct, because if it was, then Mr. Tedlie was in a very embarrassing position under the *Criminal Code* for some charge of criminal negligence. If the headline was true, then Tedlie was the man responsible for this wreck. He took it from the headline reading. 'Special Had Green Light', etc., that the paper was reporting a certain set of facts. The balance of the report did not seem to support the headline". "He was definitely confused about the different signals."

Mr. H. P. Clubine has been a practising barrister since leaving the Air Force in 1946. He has never met the plaintiff. He read the paper of September 24th some time after 5.30 that evening. To him a green light meant "go ahead". The meaning he took from the headlines was that the plaintiff had either made a terrible mistake which caused the accident or he had been negligent and forgotten to change the light.

Counsel, cross-examining this witness, took him over much of the report proper as contained in the paper. Witness said he had not looked at the article since he first read it. A paragraph from the report of the testimony of the witness Cloutier at the Board's hearing was read to the witness:

"Q. Is it your understanding that if you saw the main track clear you could have gone on the main track on order 338? A. According to the rule book, no." And the witness said in his evidence: "I read that but it did not change the opinion I formed on that headline."

He was read the following part of the paper's report: "Mr. Nicholls testified he knew of order 338. The train should have taken the siding at Dugald. He knew of no reason why it was not done."

And the witness then said: "At the time I read it I believed the light should have been changed to red."

The last witness was John A. Barbour, a clergyman. He knew what "green light" signified to him as a motorist and swore the headline implied to him that Tedlie had been guilty of a dereliction of duty. "That is the impression I got from the headline. It seemed the special had the right to go into the station."

This witness was subjected to considerable cross-examination based on parts of his evidence at the second trial, but all of such, in my opinion, was irrelevant to the matter I am now considering and I accept his evidence as to the meaning he took from the headlines.

No evidence was given contradicting the evidence of the above four witnesses as to the understanding they obtained — the impressions they got — from reading the headline and lead paragraph in question. In *R. v. Covert* (1916), 34 D.L.R. 662 at pp. 673-4, 28 Can. C.C. 25 at p. 37, 10 A . L. R. 349, Beck, J., of the Alberta Appellate Division, laid down as fairly established, by the principles of the cases to which he referred, the following proposition:

"It cannot be said without limitation that a Judge can refuse to accept evidence. I think he cannot, if the following conditions are fulfilled: —

"(I) That the statements of the witness are not in themselves improbable or unreasonable;

"(2) That there is no contradiction of them;

"(3) That the credibility of the witness has not been attacked by evidence against his character;

"(4) That nothing appears in the course of his evidence or of the evidence of any other witness tending to throw discredit upon him; and

"(5) That there is nothing in his demeanor while in Court during the trial to suggest untruthfulness."

The evidence of the plaintiff's witnesses, who impressed me as reasonable and fair-minded men, complied fully with the requirements laid down in the *Covert* case, supra, and I accept such evidence. It has satisfied me, discharging the duties of a jury, that the words complained of were reasonably understood by those proven to have read them, in the meanings attributed to them in the innuendoes, or at least some of them, viz., that the plaintiff had displayed the wrong signal, was negligent in performing his duties and was responsible for the accident. Again, the evidence has led me to the conclusion that the words would naturally be understood by other reasonable and fair people who read them as conveying the meanings attributed to them and specified by me. Finally, the evidence has satisfied me that the words, in their attributed meetings so specified by me, conveyed imputations disparaging and injurious to the plaintiff in his occupation as a railway telegraph operator and were, in fact, defamatory of him.

I come now to the question of privilege. Although the statement complained of be defamatory of the plaintiff and untrue, yet if the occasion of its publication be privileged the statement is absolutely or conditionally protected, according as the occasion of the publication is one of absolute or qualified privilege: 20 Hals., 2nd ed., pp. 459-60. The word "privilege" is used to denote the fact that conduct which under ordinary circumstances would subject the actor to liability, under particular circumstances does not subject him thereto: *Restatement of the Law of Torts*, vol. 1, p. 19.

For newspapers the *Defamation Act* creates privilege and absolute privilege in ss. 10 and 11 respectively. The source of these sections is found in ss. 4 and 3 respectively of the English statute, the *Law of Libel Amendment Act*, 1888, 51-52 Vict., c.64. See 20 Hals., 2nd ed., pp. 484-5, and 10 Hals., Stat. of Eng., p. 418. No case is cited in either of these references which suggests that s.4 of the English statute is applicable to proceedings in Court. I note that in *Odgers on Libel & Slander*, 6th ed., p. 268, it is stated that the words "absolutely privileged" were included in s.3 of the bill as originally introduced, but "absolutely" was omitted in the Act.

I hold that the Board of Transport Commissioners was sitting as a Court of Record on September 24, 1947, when the proceedings publicly heard before it were reported by the newspaper.

I further hold that s.11 of the *Defamation Act* applies to the case at bar. This, in part, provides:

> S. 11 (1) A fair and accurate report, published in a newspaper or by broadcasting, of proceedings publicly head before any court shall be absolutely privileged if,
>> (a) the report contains no comment.

No evidence made ss.(2) applicable.

Subsection (3), providing that each headline constitutes a report, has been set out earlier in these reasons. It is unnecessary for me to stress the importance of this new subsection construed by Dysart, J.A.

The report must be an impartial and accurate account. Its accuracy must not be judged by the standard of a professional law reporter. A substantially fair account of what took place in Court is enough: Odgers, 6th ed., pp. 259-60. The reporter must add nothing of his own: *ibid.*, p. 263.

In considering whether the words complained of are fair and accurate reports, they are, of course, to be tested by the testimony given before the Board and made evidence at the trial. None of this reflected in any way on the plaintiff. I find that he had faithfully and strictly complied with the rules and regulations of his employment and had properly performed his duties on the night in question. He was not in any way responsible for the negligence in the switch not being thrown or the train stopped.

I find that the headline report reading "Special Had Green Light, Operator Tells Hearing" was not true in itself and that the operator did not make that statement. His evidence, and that of all other witnesses, was that the Special was not operating on signal lights but on train orders. The published headline was not fairly or substantially accurate; it was a voluntary statement and comment by the paper; it was not a fair and accurate report.

Then as regards the paragraph following the headline "Train Reported Under Control" and reading: "The Minaki campers special had a green light or 'proceed' signal in its favor, at the time of the Dugald train wreck, according to testimony given today" etc., this refers only to the testimony of the witness Nicholls. His evidence in this connection is found on p. 87 of ex. 3. Asked if he had seen the train order board, he answered, "I saw it before the accident, yes". To the question "What did the train order board indicate", he answered, "it was in the green or proceed position" . Then this follows: .

"Q. Did that fact that the train order board was in green or in proceed position have any significance in relationship to the necessity of the extra taking the siding? A. No, sir.

"COMMISSIONER STONEMAN: Q. I think that is exactly the same understanding that the trainmen had, that in any event it was necessary for you to take that siding? A. Quite. Q. In spite of the fact the order board was green? A. That is right, sir. "

What Nicholls said in his evidence about the "green" or "proceed" position was very much different from the paragraph published by the defendants, which was quite misleading. All of the evidence given at the Board's hearing and read in at the trial was to the effect that the indication of the order board, whatever it might be at the time had no bearing upon what the Minaki Special should do at the east switch. The green light only indicated that the Minaki Special could enter the block at the west switch after proceeding along the passing track. The green light would not become operative until the Special had taken the siding. I find that the paragraph published by the defendants was their own statement or comment and that it was not a fair and accurate report.

As I have found that the above headline and lead paragraph complained of were not fair and accurate reports, the defendants are not within the protection accorded by s.11 of the Act. The reports in question were not privileged.

5.2.3.3.3 Qualified Privilege

5.2.3.3.3.1 Anne Skarsgard, "Freedom of the Press," (1980-81), *Saskatchewan Law Review* 45, pp. 303-307

Qualified privilege affords protection from tort liability for defamation if it is deemed that, on a particular occasion, society's interest in having the communication made outweighs the possibility of it turning out to be wrong. This privilege is "qualified"; it is available only if the person making the statement acts without malice, that is, in good faith and without improper motive. It is well established that "the circumstances that constitute a privileged occasion can themselves never be catalogued and rendered exact." In *Adam v. Ward* Lord Atkinson defined an occasion of qualified privilege:

> ... a privileged occasion is, in reference to qualified privilege, an occasion where the person who makes the communication has an interest or a duty, legal, social or moral, to make it to the person to whom it is made, and the person to whom it is so made has a corresponding interest or duty to receive it. This reciprocity is essential.

The problem is that very often one does not know whether the occasion is privileged or not. The bona fide belief of the maker of the statement that the occasion is privileged is irrelevant. If defendant pleads qualified privilege, it is the judge who decides whether the occasion was a privileged one. This principle has been criticized by Weiler who claims it to be completely irrational to grant only a partial privilege by making the subjective appreciation of the truth decisive but not that of the existence of a privileged occasion.

> Either it is sufficiently in the social interest to encourage these communications that it is not wrongful to take a chance of their being false, or it is not. If it is, and society wishes one to act, it can only ask that this conduct be in accordance with a reasonable perception of the facts as they appeared at the relevant time to the actor.

The law as it stands now promotes uncertainty which discourages the media from publishing statements which may or may not come under the privilege.

If the defence of qualified privilege is available to the media, it usually comes under the category of "statements made in the performance of a duty". The law recognizes that the press has a duty to report fairly and accurately parliamentary and court proceedings and the public has a corresponding interest to receive this information. As a result such reports are protected by the defence. The question is whether the press can claim the privilege when it is not just acting as a conduit relaying statements made on a privileged occasion, but when publishing original news stories and commentaries on matters of public interest.

The position in England is that under certain circumstances the press does have a duty to make the communication and consequently the defence is available. Said Pearson, J. in *Webb v. Times Publishing Co.*:

> There may be occasions where a communication to the public at large is protected by qualified privilege, provided the public at large has a legitimate interest in the subject matter of the communication.

In *Davis v. London Express Newspaper Ltd.* an inquiry by a newspaper as to share-pushing was held to be a privileged occasion. Said the court:

There is now a trend towards wider recognition of the various circumstances which might create a social or moral duty in one person to make a communication to another about a third person.

It should be pointed out that in this case publication did not occur in the paper, but consisted of a newspaper editor showing a defamatory letter to a third person. The letter informed the paper that a property to which it had referred in two articles was being used for the fraudulent pushing of shares. The writer continued by saying:

> It is imperative to expose the activities of these people before the 3rd prox. . . . on which date a meeting is to take place which, if no contradictory report appears in a responsible national newspaper, will enable them to rake in a good many thousands of pounds from the public who have read the various notices about this charlatan Professor Herzog.

The court held that the occasion was privileged; the newspaper editor had a duty to make the communication. The defence was made available to the press in other English cases as well, notably in the leading case of *Adam v. Ward*. Here plaintiff defamed a general in Parliament, and the Army Council published a letter in the press vindicating the general and defaming the plaintiff. The House of Lords held that the occasion was a privileged one. In the words of Lord Atkinson, a man who makes a statement on the floor of the House of Commons makes it to all the world. Therefore it is the duty of the heads of the service to which the defamed individual belongs to publish his vindication to the whole world. Although the newspaper was not sued, it is safe to conclude that it too had a duty to publish the letter and therefore was protected by the privilege. Said Buckley, L.J.: "If the matter is of public interest and the party who publishes it owes a duty to communicate it to the general public, the publication is privileged."

In *Duncombe v. Daniell* the court endorsed the principle that it was justifiable for an elector to communicate to the constituency any matter affecting the character of the candidate which he bona fide believed to be true and material to the election. Under the circumstances the privilege was defeated because of unjustifiably wide publication in the Letters to the Editor column of a newspaper, as the paper's circulation extended well beyond the boundaries of the constituency. One would assume then that such a letter would be protected if it addressed itself, for example, to the character of the national leader of the party. In such a case there would be reciprocity of interest between the letter writer and the general public. The reciprocity of interest would give rise to the privilege and the newspaper, acting as a conduit for disseminating the letter, would be protected by the privilege as well.

Until the middle of this century Canadian courts were even more liberal than the English courts in making the defence available to the media. In *Showler v. MacInnes*, the court held that a radio broadcast about labour organization was under the privilege because of the "vital concern of the whole citizenship of Vancouver" in the matter. Both *Dennison v. Sanderson and Drew v. Toronto Star Ltd. and Atkinson* decided on the trial level that election remarks published in a newspaper were privileged and these holdings were not overturned on appeal.

Shortly after the second decision Drew's counsel, Mr. Cartwright, was elevated to the Supreme Court of Canada. He soon saw to it that the law was changed in the area. He held in *Douglas v. Tucker* that public officials were not under the qualified privilege when making statements in the mass media.

The last-mentioned decision was ambiguous enough to allow two Ontario trial judges and the Ontario Court of Appeal to hold in two subsequent decisions that the defence of qualified privilege was available to the media. In *Boland v. Globe and Mail Ltd.* the trial judge said:

> ... a Federal Election in Canada is an occasion upon which a newspaper has a public duty to comment on the candidates, their campaigns and their platforms or policies, and Canadian citizens have a very honest and very real interest in receiving their comments, and therefore this is an occasion of qualified privilege.

When the case reached the Supreme Court, Cartwright, J. reversed the decision and stated:

> I am of the opinion that this is an erroneous statement of the law ... With respect it appears to me that, in the passage quoted above, the learned trial judge has confused the right which the publisher of a newspaper has, in common with all Her Majesty's subjects, to report truthfully and comment fairly upon matters of public interest with a duty of the sort which gives rise to an occasion of qualified privilege.

Again in *Banks v. Globe and Mail Ltd.* the trial judge stated that

> The class of cases to which the defence of qualified privilege extends, has, during the course of recent years, been extended, and that extension will cover editorial comment by a metropolitan newspaper on matters of public interest. It is difficult to conceive of a matter in which the public would be more interested in the year 1957 than the most important topic of industrial relations ... There is no more efficient organ for informing the public and disseminating to the public intelligent comment on such matters than a great metropolitan newspaper ... The members of the public have a real, a vital — I may go so far as to say — a paramount interest in receiving those comments.

Again, Cartwright, J. reversed the decision and held that the press is not under a qualified privilege. He quoted Mr. Justice (later President, then Chief Justice) Taft in *Post Publishing Co. v. Hallam* to the effect that if public men were to be subjected to falsities of fact, good men could not be found to hold public office. It should be noted that this was a nineteenth century controversial American decision. Since then, of course, the American position has drastically changed. The expanded *New York Times* rule denies a cause of action in defamation to public officials and public figures unless they can prove knowledge of the falsity of the statement or reckless disregard whether the statement was true or false. Even then only special damages are recoverable. *Rosenbloom v. Metromedia* extended the *Times* rule to any matter of public or general interest, but the Supreme Court retreated somewhat in the *Gertz* case where it was decided that if a private citizen rather than a public official or a public figure was the plaintiff in a matter of public interest, each state could impose its own standard of liability so long as strict or absolute liability was not imposed. In other words, in the

United States not even private individuals can succeed in a defamation action against the media unless they show either negligence or reckless disregard for truth, depending on where they sue. The American position is that strict liability in defamation contravenes the freedom of speech provision of the First Amendment.

This is a far cry from the Canadian situation since Mr. Justice Cartwright took away the defence of qualified privilege from the media in the *Boland* and *Banks* decisions. In *Banks* Cartwright, J. justified his stand by saying that the press did not need the defence of qualified privilege as the interest of free speech was sufficiently protected by the defence of fair comment.

5.2.3.3.3.2 Qualified Privilege Under Statute

5.2.3.3.3.2.1 *Ontario Libel and Slander Act*, R.S.O. 1990, c. L.12.

3. (1) A fair and accurate report in a newspaper or in a broadcast of any of the following proceedings that are open to the public is privileged, unless it is proved that the publication thereof was made maliciously:

1. The proceedings of any legislative body or any part or committee thereof in the British Commonwealth that may exercise any sovereign power acquired by delegation or otherwise.
2. The proceedings of any administrative body that is constituted by any public authority in Canada.
3. The proceedings of any commission of inquiry that is constituted by any public authority in the Commonwealth.
4. The proceedings of any organization whose members, in whole or in part, represent any public authority in Canada.

(2) A fair and accurate report in a newspaper or in a broadcast of the proceedings of a meeting lawfully held for a lawful purpose and for the furtherance of discussion of any matter of public concern, whether the admission thereto is general or restricted, is privileged, unless it is proved that the publication thereof was made maliciously.

(3) The whole or a part of a fair and accurate synopsis in a newspaper or in a broadcast of any report, bulletin, notice or other document issued for the information of the public by or on behalf of any body, commission or organization mentioned in subsection (1) or any meeting mentioned in subsection (2) is privileged, unless it is proved that the publication thereof was made maliciously.

(4) A fair and accurate report in a newspaper or in a broadcast of the findings or decision of any of the following associations, or any part or committee thereof, being a finding or decision relating to a person who is a member of or is subject, by virtue of any contract, to the control of the association, is privileged, unless it is proved that the publication thereof was made maliciously:

1. An association formed in Canada for the purpose of promoting or encouraging the exercise of or interest in any art, science, religion or learning, and empowered by its constitution to exercise control over or adjudicate upon matters of interest or concern to the association, or the actions or conduct of any person subject to such control or adjudication.
2. An association formed in Canada for the purpose of promoting or safeguarding the interests of any trade, business, industry or profession, or of the persons carrying on or engaged in any

trade, business, industry or profession, and empowered by its constitution to exercise control over or adjudicate upon matters connected with the trade, business, industry or profession.

3. An association formed in Canada for the purpose of promoting or safeguarding the interests of any game, sport or pastime to the playing or exercising of which members of the public are invited or admitted, and empowered by its constitution to exercise control over or adjudicate upon persons connected with or taking part in the game, sport or pastime.

(5) Nothing in this section authorizes any blasphemous, seditious or indecent matter in a newspaper or in a broadcast.

(6) Nothing in this section limits or abridges any privilege now by law existing or protects the publication of any matter not of public concern or the publication of which is not for the public benefit.

(7) The protection afforded by this section is not available as a defence in an action for libel if the plaintiff shows that the defendant refused to insert in the newspaper or to broadcast, as the case may be, a reasonable statement of explanation or contradiction by or on behalf of the plaintiff. R.S.O. 1980, c. 237, s. 3.

Similar provisions can be found in the defamation legislation of all the common-law provinces and territories. The wording of the Act of Nova Scotia is very close to that of the Ontario statute (*Defamation Act*, R.S.N.S. 1989, c. 122, s. 13), while the provisions of the *Defamation Acts* of Alberta, Manitoba, New Brunswick, Newfoundland, Prince Edward Island, the Northwest Territories, the Yukon, Territory and the *Revised Uniform Defamation Act*, take the following form:

(1) A fair and accurate report published in a newspaper or by broadcasting of
   (*a*) a public meeting,
   (*b*) proceedings (i) in the Senate or House of Commons of Canada,
      (ii) in the Legislative Assembly of Alberta or any other province, or
      (iii) in a committee of those bodies,
   except where neither the public nor any reporter is admitted,
   (*c*) a meeting of commissioners authorized to act by or pursuant to statute or other lawful warrant or authority, or
   (*d*) a meeting of a municipal council, school board, board of education, board of health, or of any other board or local authority formed or constituted under a public Act of Canada or of Alberta or any other province, or of a committee appointed by any such board or local authority,
is privileged, unless it is proved that the publication was made maliciously.

(2) The publication in a newspaper or by broadcasting, at the request of a government department, bureau or office or public officer, of a report, bulletin, notice or other document issued for the information of the public is privileged, unless it is proved that the publication was made maliciously.

(3) Nothing in this section applies to the publication of seditious, blasphemous or indecent matter.

(4) Subsections (1) and (2) do not apply when
   (*a*) in the case of publication in a newspaper, the plaintiff shows that the defendant has been requested to insert in the newspaper a reasonable letter or statement of

explanation or contradiction by or on behalf of the plaintiff, and the defendant fails to show that he has done so, or

(b) in the case of publication by broadcasting, the plaintiff shows that the defendant has been requested to broadcast a reasonable statement of explanation or contradiction by or on behalf of the plaintiff, and the defendant fails to show that he has done so, from the broadcasting stations from which the alleged defamatory matter was broadcast, on at least 2 occasions on different days and at the same time of day as the alleged defamatory matter was broadcast or at a time as near as possible to that time.

(5) Nothing in this section limits or abridges any privilege now by law existing, or applies to the publication of any matter not of public concern or the publication of which is not for the public benefit.

(*Defamation Act*, R.S.A. 1980, c. D-6, s. 10. See also *Revised Uniform Defamation Act*, s. 10 in Conference of Commissioners on Uniformity of Legislation in Canada, Proceedings of the Thirtieth Annual Meeting, Montreal, Quebec, August 24-28, 1948, Appendix J; *The Defamation Act*, R.S.M. 1987, c. D20, s. 10; *Defamation Act*, R.S.N.B. 1973, c. D-5, s.9; *Defamation Act*, R.S.N. 1990, c. D-3, s. 12; *Defamation Act*, R.S.P.E.I. 1988, c. D-5, ss. 10 and 11; *Defamation Act*, R.S.N.W.T. 1988, c. D-1, s. 11; *Defamation Act*, R.S.Y.T. 1986, c. 41, s. 10.)

Section 4 of the British Columbia *Libel and Slander Act*, R.S.B.C. 1979, c. 234, and s. 10 of Saskatchewan's *Libel and Slander Act*, R.S.S. 1978, c. L-14, as am. S.S. 1984-85-86, c. 16, s. 14, both provide:

(1) A fair and accurate report published in a public newspaper or other periodical publication or in a broadcast of the proceedings of a public meeting, or, except where neither the public nor a news reporter is admitted, of a meeting of a municipal council, school board, board or local authority formed or constituted under any Act, or of a committee appointed by any of the above mentioned bodies, or of a meeting of commissioners authorized to act by letters patent, Act or other lawful warrant or authority, or select committees of the Legislative Assembly, and the publication at the request of a government office or ministry, or a public officer, of a notice or report issued for the information of the public, is privileged, unless it is proved that the report or publication was published or made maliciously.

(2) This section does not authorize the publication of blasphemous or indecent matter; and the protection intended to be afforded by this section is not available as a defence in proceedings if it is proved that the defendant has been requested to insert in the newspaper or other periodical publication, or to broadcast in the same manner as that, in which the report or other publication complained of appeared, a reasonable letter or statement by way of contradiction or explanation of the report or other publication and has refused or neglected to insert it.

(3) This section does not limit or abridge a privilege now existing by law, or protect the publication of matter not of public concern and the publication of which is not for the public benefit.

Quebec law does not recognize a defence of privilege with respect to a fair and accurate report of a *bona fide* public meeting (see *Press Act*, R.S.Q. 1977, c. P-19, s. 10).

5.2.3.3.3.2.2 *Cook v. Alexander and Others*, [1973] 3 All E.R. 1037 (C.A.)

LORD DENNING, M.R.: This case raises a point of considerable importance. It is about the reporting of proceedings in Parliament. It has not come up for full discussion in the courts for over 100 years; that is, since *Wason v. Walter*.

In 1967 the plaintiff, Mr. Cook, was a teacher on the staff of the Court Lees approved school. It is near Godstone in Surrey. On 2nd and 7th March 1967 Mr. Cook wrote letters to the *Guardian* newspaper in which he criticised severely the way in which the school was conducted. He said that the boys were punished with excessive severity. He did not give his name. He was afraid of repercussions on him if he did so. So his letters appeared anonymously. The *Guardian* published them. The *Daily Mail* re-published them. They were very convincing. They had an impact on the public at large. So much so that the Home Secretary ordered an inquiry. It was held by Mr. Brian Gibbens, a Queen's Counsel. At the inquiry the headmaster was represented by lawyers. So was Mr. Cook. In due course Mr. Gibbens made his report. He found that some — not all — of the charges made by Mr. Cook were true. Four out of 11, I believe. The consequences were far-reaching. The Home Secretary made an order closing the Court Lees approved school. The boys were sent elsewhere. The staff lost their employment.

Many people were very concerned at these developments. So much so that Earl Jellicoe on 25th October 1967, in the House of Lords, rose to draw attention to the closure of the Court Lees school and to move for papers. He criticised the Home Secretary's handling of the case. He said that the school managers had been treated roughly and that injustice had been done to the headmaster and his deputy. Lord Stonham, speaking for the government, justified the closure. He said that, in the light of the report, it was the proper thing to have done. There was a debate in which 11 speakers took part. It took over three hours and filled 94 columns of Hansard. One speech in particular caused a considerable stir. It was the speech of the Bishop of Southwark, Dr. Stockwood. He criticised Mr. Cook in strong terms. In answer, Lord Longford said the bishop's speech was a monument of unfairness.

Next day, 26th October 1967, the *Daily Telegraph* reported the debate in the House of Lords. It reported it fully on one of the inside pages. It filled three columns of the newspaper and gave extracts — either in direct speech or in oblique speech — from all 11 speakers. The teacher, Mr. Cook, makes no complaint of that full report. He could not justly do so, because it is a fair and accurate summary of the debate. On the back page there was one column about the debate. It is what journalists call a 'Parliamentary sketch'. It gave a commentary describing the main impression made on those who were present. It is said to be a libel on Mr. Cook. I must therefore read it. It starts with a head-line in bold letters: 'Bishop attacks Court Lees "crusader". ' Then follows: 'By Andrew Alexander, Westminster, Wednesday.'

Then comes the sketch itself:

> Critics in the Lords of the Home Office's handling of the Court Lees approved school case today found a staunch ally on the progressive Left in Dr. Mervyn Stockwood, Bishop of Southwark. He launched a scathing attack on Mr. Ivor Cook. the master whose revelations prompted the inquiry. [Debate — P27]. Dr. Stockwood's own startling revelation was that Dr. Cook had sent more boys to the headmaster for discipline — which usually meant corporal punishment — than any other master.

Then follows the sub-heading in bigger type:

CHARGES READ OUT
House amused

Then these words follow:

> Between 1963 and the time of the inquiry, Mr. Cook had issued 110 of the "yellow tickets" which signified that a boy required special punishment. "I know this because they are in my possession." He then read out some of the charges involved, to the amusement of the House. One boy had spat in a public place; another swept drain debris across Mr. Cook's clean shoes; a third had worn socks in bed. "This is the apostle in the crusade against corporal punishment," he commented with scorn.

Then follows the sub-heading in bigger type:

INQUIRY DEMANDED
Longford's rejection

Then the words follow:

> The Bishop added his plea to those of others in the debate who demanded a full and public inquiry. But the Government was not in a conciliatory vein. Lord Longford, Leader of the House, dismissed the comments on Mr. Cook as "a monument of unfairness". But others in the House were impressed. Lord Dilhorne, in an unscheduled intervention, added his plea for a full inquiry, in which the dismissed headmaster would have a chance to defend himself properly. He took up a point by Baroness Serota (Lab.) and asked why — since the first enquiry had appeared to reveal serious brutality — there had been no criminal charges. Lord Longford, in what was a rather bumbling reply, became involved in exchanges with Peers when he insisted that the headmaster had not been dismissed. The school had merely been closed down. That did not involve dismissal, which was an "ignominious" termination of employment.

Then follows a sub-heading in bigger type:

HEAD CRITICISED
Recent beatings

> But perhaps few things in the debate illustrated more clearly the unsatisfactory state of affairs now than the speech by Lord Annan (Ind.). Criticising the headmaster, he spoke of recent beatings for very slight sexual misbehaviour by boys. Lord Aberdare (Con.) summing up for the Opposition, said according to his information the offences in question were of a distinctly serious nature, involving the bullying of small boys in this respect. Lord Annan quickly rose to say perhaps this was so: he was only going on the "rumour" he had heard.

Then there is a final sub-heading: 'Lords Debate — P27'.

That is what journalists call a Parliamentary sketch. It does not give a full report of Parliamentary proceedings but only an impression of the debate as the reporter heard and saw it. The important question is whether and to what extent such a sketch is the subject of privilege — qualified privilege. The judge stated the law to the jury in these words:

> ... it is to the advantage of the country as a whole that proceedings in our courts and in Parliament should be fairly reported. To any such report a qualified privilege attaches; and that, privilege is that, so long as the report is fair and accurate, it cannot be the subject of defamation proceedings unless it was published maliciously.

He noted that there was no evidence of malice. So he withdrew that issue from the jury. He told the jury that the 'prime question — almost the sole question — is: Is the report as a whole a fair one? Is it an honest one?' After retiring for two hours and 20 minutes, the jury came back with this note:

> We are unable to reach unanimous decision. (l) Total agreement has been reached on the question that the flavour of the debate is not contained in the [column on the back page]. (2) A majority feel that [that column] is not a fair report. (3) Although the majority feel that [the column] is not fair some are not sure it is defamatory.

The judge gave a further direction to the jury. He told them they could decide by a majority of ten to two. He also told them the accepted definitions of defamation. Then after 53 minutes they came back. They found for Mr. Cook by a majority of 11 to one and awarded 1,000 dumages. Now there is un appeal by the newspaper, the *Daily Telegraph*.

Seeing that a Parliamentary sketch has not come up for consideration in the courts before, it may be helpful if I quote the evidence of the journalists about it. Mr. Andrew Alexander was the one who wrote this sketch. He was on the Parliamentary staff of the *Daily Telegraph*. He said:

> ... the reader to whom this is directed is the man who cannot be present in the House of Lords to listen to the debate but wants to know what was the thing which apparently made an impact in a debate of this type ... I aimed as usual to convey the flavour and feel of the occasion, and in this particular case the most salient feature of the debate was the very surprising development of Dr. Stockwood coming out with an attack upon Mr. Cook, which surprised so many people in the House of Lords. I tried to convey to the reader some idea of the strength of the attack and the feeling it aroused in the Lords and how it was received.

Mr. Green, the editor of the *Daily Telegraph* was asked: 'What guidance ... do you give to the sketch writer, whoever produces the sketch?' He answered:

> The things which obviously make an impact in the House. A sort of short picture which will give a real impression of what was actually happening ... he is allowed to make some sort of comment on ... the quality of the speeches, whether people are clear or obscure, whether they made an impression on the House ... To some extent to comment on the arguments.

The Parliamentary sketch is thus a different thing from a report of proceedings in Parliament. A report of proceedings in Parliament, as usually understood, is a report of the words spoken in the debate, summarised so as to fit into the space available. In short, a précis. Such a report was considered in 1868 in *Wason v.*

Walter. The court then held that such a report was privileged if it was a fair and honest report of what had taken place, 'published simply with a view to the information of the public, and innocent of all intention to do injury to the reputation of the party affected'. The reason for the privilege was said to be because —

> ... it is of paramount public and national importance that the proceedings of the houses of parliament shall be communicated to the public, who have the deepest interest in knowing what passes within their walls, seeing that on what is there said and done, the welfare of the community depends.

It more than counterbalances the detriment to individuals of being defamed in the course of it.

Ever since that case it has been settled that, in a report of proceedings in Parliament, there is a privilege — a qualified privilege — in the reporter. If his report is fair and honest, then he is not liable to an action. It may be that a speaker in the debate got his facts entirely wrong or was actuated by the most express malice; nevertheless, the reporter is entitled to report what he said. Neither the reporter nor the newspaper is liable as long as the report was fair and the reporter himself was not actuated by malice. Take one instance in this very case. It appears that the Bishop of Southwark was mistaken when he said that sending a boy to the headmaster usually meant corporal punishment. We are told that it did not do so. It was for the headmaster to decide what the punishment was to be. The reporter would not be responsible for the mistake of the bishop.

I would add that, not only is the report of the proceedings privileged, but also the reporter of the newspaper can make any fair comment on it. That follows inexorably from the fact that the proceedings are presumed conclusively to be of public interest; and accordingly that fair comment can be made on it; see *Wason v. Walter* and *Mangena v. Wright*.

Such being the position of a report of proceedings in Parliament, what is the position of a Parliamentary sketch? When making a sketch, a reporter does not summarise all the speeches. He selects a part of the debate which appears to him to be of special public interest and then describes it and the impact which it made on the House. I think that a Parliamentary sketch is privileged if it is made fairly and honestly with the intention of giving an impression of the impact made on the hearers. In these days the debates in Parliament take so long that no newspaper could possibly report the debates in full, nor give the names of all the speakers, nor even summarise the main speeches. When a debate covers a particular subject-matter, there are often some aspects which are of greater public interest than others. If the reporter is to give the public any impression at all of the proceedings, he must be allowed to be selective and to cover those matters only which appear to be of particular public interest. Even then, he need not report it verbatim, word for word or letter by letter. It is sufficient if it is a fair presentation of what took place so as to convey to the reader the impression which the debate itself would have made on a hearer of it. Test it this way. If a member of the

House were asked: 'What happened in the debate? Tell me about it.' His answer would be a sketch giving in words the impression it left on him, with more emphasis on one thing and less emphasis on another, just as it stuck in his memory. Such a sketch is privileged, whether spoken at the dinner table afterwards, or reported to the public at large in a newspaper. Even if it is defamatory of some one, it is privileged because the public interest in the debate counterbalances the private interest of the individual.

Applying that in the present case, when the reporter said that the Bishop of Southwark, launched a scathing attack on Mr. Ivor Cook' he was recording the impact made on him by the bishop's remarks. When he said 'House amused', he was giving the reaction of the members of the House of Lords as he saw it. When he spoke of Lord Longford 'in what was a rather bumbling reply', he was giving his impression of Lord Longford's manner. Such a sketch, which gives the impression on the hearer, so long as it is fairly done, seems to me to be the subject of privilege — qualified privilege — for which the reporter is protected unless he is actuated by malice.

I would emphasize that it has to be fair. Here I come to the point particularly made by Mr. Cook. He said it was unfair to give such large prominence to what the bishop had said and such little prominence to the rebuttal by Lord Longford, and it was unfair to describe Lord Longford as 'bumbling' and so forth. But fairness in this regard means a fair presentation of what took place as it impressed the hearers. It does not mean fairness in the abstract as between Mr. Cook and those who were attacking him. Applying that test, it seems to me that this Parliamentary sketch is protected by the qualified privilege. It gives a fair presentation of the impression on the hearers of the bishop's speech. It made much impression on them: so it was, given particular prominence. If it had been unfairly distorted, it would not have been a fair presentation. If Lord Longford's rebuttal had been omitted, it would not have been a fair presentation. But, looking at it as a whole, there is only one reasonable conclusion to which a reasonable jury could come, and that is that it was a fair presentation of what took place.

There is one further point. The column on the back page — which contained the Parliamentary sketch — gave specific references to the inner pages of the paper where there was a full report of the whole debate. I should have thought that any reader who was sufficiently interested in the case to take particular notice of what was said about Mr. Cook, would have turned to the inner page where he could have read the full report. The two together, beyond all doubt, are protected by privilege.

In my opinion, therefore, the verdict of this jury should be set aside on the ground that it was a verdict which a reasonable jury could not reasonably come to. It should be set aside. That was done in this court in *Hope v. W. C. Leng & Co. (Sheffeld Telegraph) Ltd.* and we should do the same. We should set aside the verdict and order judgment to be entered for the defendants. I would allow the appeal accordingly.

BUCKEY, L.J.: I agree. We are here concerned, as Lord Denning, M.R. has explained with a report of proceedings in the House of Lords. There can be no doubt that the plaintiff, Mr. Cook, is entitled to complain of such a report if it contains matter which is defamatory of him and is not a fair and accurate report insofar as it relates to him and to the defamatory matter. Mr. Cook, who (if I may be allowed to say so, has presented his argument I think very fairly and with great ability and courtesy before us) has contended that for such a report to be fair and accurate, it must really be of the nature of a précis of the whole proceedings or debate in order that it may have that quality of fairness which will bring before the reader the points and arguments that have been put forward on either side. I do not myself think that the report has to have that characteristic of being in the nature of a précis. The reporter or editor of the newspaper in which the report appears, as the case may be, is entitled in my judgment to select some part or parts of the debate or proceedings which he considers to be of particular public importance or otherwise likely to be of particular interest to the public — not on scandalous grounds or other unworthy grounds of that kind, but on the ground that the subject-matter is of genuine public interest; and he is I think entitled to report on the proceedings or that part of it which he selects in a manner which fairly and faithfully gives an impression of the events reported and will convey to the reader what he himself would have appreciated had he been present during the proceedings. Now, Mr. Cook has suggested that this report — and by that term I refer to what has been called the Parliamentary sketch which appeared on the back page of the relevant issue of the *Daily Telegraph* — is so selective that it does not fairly present a picture of that part of the proceedings to which the report relates. I do not feel able to accept that view. It appears to me that the report, which is admittedly a selective report concentrating on one particular aspect of the debate to which it relates, is not so tendentious or otherwise so slanted as to make it a distorted report of that part of the proceedings to which it relates; und I agree with Lord Denning, M.R. in thinking that it is all the more difficult to come to the conclusion that it can be criticised in that way because the sketch itself contains two explicit references to the full Parliamentary report contained elsewhere in the same issue of the paper. On these grounds and for the reasons that Lord Denning, M.R. has elaborated more fully in the judgment which he has delivered, I do not think that the conclusion at which the jury arrived was one at which on the material before them they could have properly arrived giving the matter proper consideration in the light of the proper principles; and accordingly I agree that this appeal must succeed.

LAWTON, L.J.: For over two centuries the public in these islands have been interested in what goes on in Parliament und during that long period the Press has done what it could to keep them informed. The methods of doing so have changed from time to time. There are fashions in journalism just as there are fashions in other activities of life. Up until about 1939, if my recollection serves me rightly, most of the Press produced fairly detailed Parliamentary reports.

During the war years, perhaps because of the shortage of newsprint, that kind of reporting fell into disuse, and in recent years, except for three newspapers, *The Times*, the *Daily Telegraph* and the *Guardian*, the practice had been not to publish the précis type of reports of Parliamentary proceedings. It may be the reason has been that the newspapers have found that the public are not interested in that kind of report. As a result, most newspapers have what has come to be called amongst journalists the Parliamentary sketch; and the three newspapers I have mentioned by name have Parliamentary sketches as well as the précis type of report. The problem which has arisen in this case is whether the Parliamentary sketch enjoys the same kind of privilege as the traditional Parliamentary précis. The Parliamentary sketch, from its very nature, cannot go into the detail which the Parliamentary précis does. At one stage in his argument I understood Mr. Cook to be saying that the Parliamentary sketch, if it is to attract the privilege which Parliamentary reports do enjoy, must have much the same balance and much the sume content as a Parliamentary report of the traditional kind.

What is the basis for the qualified privilege which newspapers have in reporting Parliamentary debates? In reporting Parliamentary debates there may be occasions when the newspapers report defamatory statements which have been made in Parliament. The law has decided that in the public interest the repeating of such defamatory statements may be allowed provided that the newspaper carrying the report has been neither unfair nor inaccurate. What then is meant by 'unfair'? That is the sole question in this case. No question has arisen about the accuracy of the defendants' report. 'Unfair' must mean unbalanced, as Mr. Cook said. It is important to remember, however, that the balance must be in relation to the plaintiff's reputation. The plaintiff is bringing the action. He is saying that the Parliamentary sketch was defamatory — and I use the usual words of the pleader — of and concerning him. The Parliamentary sketch may be unfair to the government: it may be unfair to the opposition; it may be unfair to the speakers. But that is irrelevant for the purpose of an action for defamation in which the sole question is, was it unfair to the plaintiff?

The reporter represents the public in Parliament: he is their eyes and ears; and he has to do his best, using his professional skill, to give them a fair and accurate picture of what went on in either the House of Lords or the House of Commons. He cannot report everything that happened; he must, from the very nature of things, be selective; and what he may very well find himself doing is answering the question: Well, if I were a fair-minded, reasonable member of the public, what would I have remembered about this debate? He is, in my judgment, entitled to set out what he remembers.

In every debate the speakers are of varying quality. Some are memorable: some should be forgotten as soon as possible. It is the speakers who are memorable who leave impressions on reasonable members of the public; and the Parliamentary correspondent in this respect represents the public. He must, however, behave like a fair and reasonable man; and if in the course of the debate a good impression is made by a particular speaker and that impression is dissipated either wholly or in part by less memorable speeches, then that must be reflected in the published impression. The problem in this case was this: what was the memorable feature about the Court Lees debate? From the public's point of view it was the Bishop of Southwark's speech. The topic under debate had been before the public for about two months. The Bishop of Southwark brought some new, somewhat surprising facts — some of them not accurate — to the attention of the House of Lords. Others in the debate, including Lord Longford, cast doubt on the facts put forward and the conclusions, if any, to be drawn from them. That had to be reflected in the Parliamentary sketch made by the first defendant in this case. Were those criticisms of, and comments on, the bishop's speech properly reflected? In my judgment they were and no reasonable minded jury properly directed could have come to any other conclusion.

For those reasons I too would allow the appeal.

5.2.3.3.3.2.3 *Hefferman v. Regina Daily Star*, [1930] 3 W.W.R. 656 (Sask. K.B.)

TAYLOR, J.: (oral) I still have the matters of law reserved to deal with before I can give my decision; and I think perhaps I may as well dispose of the matter now so that you may have the benefit of the conclusion I have arrived at now. It was argued before me that I should not leave the question of whether this was a public meeting, and whether it was a privileged occasion, to the jury generally. I reserved my decision on that argument; and then, with the concurrence of counsel, left the question to the jury as if it was solely a question of fact for them with a direction of law on the matter, the direction which I gave them.

Now, I may say that I have arrived at the conclusion that it is the duty of the Judge to determine whether in this case the publication in the newspaper was on a privileged occasion. I am influenced to that conclusion by the cases cited in the 6th edition of *Fraser*, 1925, at p. 220 — after reading those cases and the earlier cases there referred to. It is on the earlier cases that reliance is placed for a contrary view in the citations in *Gatley* and *Fraser* referred to by counsel. Authority for that same opinion is also to be found in the article in *Halsbury*. There is disagreement in the text-books. It will be seen that in *Fraser* the opinion is expressed that the cases relied on by the other learned writers must now be taken to be overruled.

One cannot weigh the authority of text writers, and the only way to deal with the matter is to read the cases and endeavour, I should say, to disregard the fact that there is a dispute between the text-book writers on the subject. And reading those cases, it seems to me, as a matter of law, that the Court is undoubtedly bound to accept the law to be as it is stated in the judgment of the Lord Chancellor, Finlay, and Lords Dunedin und Shaw, in *Adam v. Ward*, [1917] A.C. 309, 86 L.J.K.B. 849. In the language of the Lord Chancellor:

It is for the judge, and the judge alone, to determine as a matter of law whether the occasion is privileged, unless the circumstances attending it are indispute, in which case the facts necessary to raise the question of law should be found by the jury.

Since delivering this judgment the Law Journal report of *Minter v. Priest* (1930), 99 L.J.K.B. 391, is to hand, in which Viscount Dunedin repeats his observations in *Adam v. Ward, supra*, and the House of Lords unanimously confirmed his view.

Now, in this case, the facts tending to establish the privileged occasion were entirely advanced by the defence, and, taking everything that was there advanced, and resolving every inference that could be drawn in favour of the defence, in my opinion, as a matter of law, it could not be held that they had satisfied the onus of establishing publication upon a privileged occasion. The question arises — I think it is a question of law — as no facts are in dispute, as to whether this was or was not a public meeting. I do not think that this meeting could be held to be a public meeting.

We must observe, in interpreting the statute in question, the law at the time it was passed, and the purpose for which it was passed. We must remember in interpreting the statute that it constitutes an interference, that it purports to authorize an interference with an existing cause of action and abolish that right of action. It is not therefore to be extended beyond its reasonable intention.

I would conclude that a public meeting must be one having in it some element of public control, not simply a meeting such as a lecture to which admission is charged, entirely under the control of the lecturer. The primary purpose of this meeting was for gain, 50 cents admission being charged to every person, and attendance was confined to those who were prepared to pay that admission. Further than that, while there was a list of the subjects to be discussed, really these could not be called discussions, because everything to be raised was to be dealt with by the lecturer. It does appear that questions could be asked, but there was nothing in the nature of discussion. It was a speech from the one person, or from persons permitted to speak by him. Now, having in view such cases as that one to which I referred where it was held that a religious service — although open to any of the public who might want to attend — was not a public meeting within the meaning of the Act, because it is confined practically to the religious sect, if that is not a public meeting, it could not possibly be held that this meeting under the control of Maloney was a public meeting. When one considers the purpose of the statute too, and the extent of the privilege which would be afforded to the newspapers, were it to be held that this was a public meeting, it seems to me that is a cogent reason for limiting it; because it would be possible for a person to hire a hall, call a meeting, publish notice of it in a newspaper, and naming certain public subjects, utter therein defamatory matter, for the publication of which action would lie. Yet if the law permitted repetition, any newspaper confining itself to a fair and accurate report would be privileged and excused from the publication; and that does not seem to me within the contemplation of the statute at all. No such licence could, in my view, have been intended.

I find no real dispute on the facts going to the issue as to whether this was or was not a public meeting. On that issue there is no controversy. As I conclude that it was not a public meeting, the statute which the defendant sets up does not apply.

Not only that, but perhaps I should express my view as to whether the publication of this particular matter which was published of and concerning the plaintiff was of a matter of public concern, the publication whereof was for the benefit of the public. I cannot agree with the defendant's contention that a case has been made out to support his contention on either of these matters. I have not time now to fully review the cases. In my address to the jury I pointed out the matters, the extent to which the plaintiff's conduct as a magistrate, and the criticism of the Government had been made matters of public concern; but I think it is absolutely clear that this matter introduced by Maloney was not germane or relevant to the discussion that had previously taken place. It was absolutely new, a charge of misconduct which had not theretofore been referred to in any way at all. It was a matter concerning Maloney himself and the plaintiff and the charge so made by Maloney against the plaintiff and this former servant of his had not been made a matter of public concern therefore. Surely the utterances by a lecturer at a meeting, even if it were a public meeting, of a personal accusation of crime against an individual, against any person, cannot, by the very utterance by that lecturer be made a matter of public concern. Nor can I see the contention that the publication of it would be for the public benefit. Indeed, it seems to me that directly the contrary would be the case, because there is a procedure provided by law whereby prosecutions for criminal offences are to be followed. That very procedure would be interfered with if newspapers could broadcast charges before proceedings were taken to enforce them in the criminal courts by the proper criminal procedure. There is the further observation that it is the duty of every man to assist in the enforcement of the criminal law, and if a crime were committed such as Maloney said had been committed, then it would have been his duty — not to hire a hall and publish it in the hope of publication in a newspaper — it would have been his duty to lay a charge before a magistrate and have it prosecuted in the proper procedure required by law. And if, by way of argument, it were suggested that a substitute for that time-honoured procedure by publication in newspapers were permitted, I think it would constitute a very serious interference with the safety of persons accused of criminal offences; it would be a very serious departure from the proper proof of criminal charges. The nature of the charge leads me further to conclude that it was not a matter, the publication of which was for the public benefit. As I say, it was a charge made by Maloney personally against the plaintiff. As stated in the cases to which reference was made by counsel this was a libellous matter of private concern, and I find it difficult to appreciate the contention that its publication could be for the public benefit.

To quote from *Gatley*. 2nd ed., p. 364:

> It was never intended that an editor might publish a report of anything said, however defamatory and however irrelevant to the subject of the meeting. Editors, no doubt, are under great difficulties, but they must take care not to publish foul accusations against individuals, entirely irrelevant and introduced only for the purpose of libelling them. It was never intended that such irrelevant attacks should be published, nor can the publication of such attacks be for the public benefit. If a newspaper chooses to publish defamatory matter about anybody, though actually uttered at a public meeting but which has nothing to do with the objects of the meeting, then it cannot shield itself behind the *Law of Libel Amendment Act*.

So, therefore, I hold that the evidence was not sufficient to establish the defence of privilege and that those words were published under the protection of the Act in question. My conclusion, therefore, in that respect, is in accord with the findings of the jury, and there will, therefore, be judgment for the plaintiff for the amount of the damages found by the jury and costs.

5.2.3.3.3.3 Qualified Priviledge under Common Law

To what extent should the relation between the mass media and the public, at least in connection with matters of public interest, be regarded as one which gives rise to privilege? Should the guarantee of "freedom of expression" in section 2(b) of the Charter affect the matter?

5.2.3.3.3.3.1 *Banks v. Globe and Mail* (1961), 28 D.L.R. (2d) 343 (S.C.C.)

CARTWRIGHT, J.: This is an appeal, brought pursuant to leave granted by the Court of Appeal for Ontario, from a judgment of that Court, dismissing an appeal from a judgment of Spence, J., whereby the appellant's action was dismissed with costs.

The action was for damages for libel.

The appellant is a vice-president of the Seafarers' International Union of North America; he resides in the town of Pointe Claire in the Province of Quebec. The corporate respondent is the proprietor of a daily newspapr published under the name of *The Globe and Mail*, of which the individual respondent is the editor and publisher.

The words complained of were published as the leading editorial in the issue of *The Globe and Mail* dated Monday, November 11, 1957, and are as follows:

> MISSION ACCOMPLISHED
>
> It would seem in retrospect that Mr. Harold C. Banks, Canadian director of the Seafarers' International Union, was brought to this country for the specific purpose of scuttling Canada's deep sea fleet. If this was indeed the case, he has succeeded admirably. With the decision by Canadian National Steamships to strilce its eight vessels on West Indian service from Canadian

registry, Canada is left with only three ocean-going merchant ships — as against the hundred or more it had when Mr. Banks took over the SIU eight years ago.

Considering his record of criminal offenses in the United States, which he diversified and extended after coming to Canada, this country has done rather well by Mr. Banks. He enjoys great power and considerable wealth, his salary being a reported $12,000 a year. Unlike most other union leaders in Canada, he does not have to go through the irritating business of getting himself re-elected at periodic intervals; indeed, he was never elected in the first place. And he has influential friends; when he applied for Canadian citizenship this year, who should show up to vouch for him but such people as Mr. Claude Jodoin, president of the Canadian Labor Congress, and Mr. Frank Hall, head of the Brotherhood of Railway Clerks.

But if Canada has done well by Mr. Banks, it cannot be said that Mr. Banks has done well by Canada. It is true that, by his forcible demands on shipowners he has made Canada's ocean-going seamen the most highly paid in the world. But in so doing, he has put virtually all of them out of employment. With Mr. Banks directing the SIU, almost every Canadian-owned deep sea ship has been transferred to a foreign flag, and is being worked by a foreign crew.

This will now be the case with the eight West Indies vessels of CNS, which are to be registered in Port of Spain. Trinidad. The eight ships have been tied up since last July, owing to a strike called by Mr. Banks. At the time, he demanded a 30 per cent wage increase for the SIU members working them; CNS offered 10 per cent. which it later raised to 15 per cent — not reasonable considering that the West Indian service has run at a heavy loss for the last seven years. This latter offer was rejected by Mr. Banks even when CNS warned him that rejection would mean the registry transfer, and consequent unemployment of all the crew members concerned.

Mr. Banks' application for citizenship is still, apparently, before the Canadian Government, which has reached no final decision in the matter. We suggest, in the light of the CNS fiasco, that the application be turned down, and Mr. Banks be sent back to the U.S. He came here to preside over the dissolution of the Canadian Merchant Marine; the Canadian Merchant Marine has been dissolved. Why, then, should he remain? His mission has been accomplished, his work is done.

The action was commenced on December 3, 1957.

In the statement of claim it is alleged that the defendants falsely and maliciously published this editorial of and concerning the plaintiff and that in its plain and ordinary meaning it is defamatory of him and of and concerning him in the way of his office as vice-president of his union. In para. 6, thirteen innuendoes are alleged. In para. 7 it is alleged that notice of complaint was served on the defendants on November 21, 1957.

In the statement of defence publication is admitted. The defences pleaded are, (i) that the words complained of in their natural and ordinary meaning are no libel, (ii) that the said words do not bear and were not understood to bear and are incapable of bearing or being understood to bear the meaning alleged in the statement of claim, (iii) a plea of qualified privilege and (iv) a plea of the defence of fair comment.

The plea of qualified privilege is contained in paras. 3 and 4 of the statement of defence as follows:

> 3. The Defendants say that the words complained of were published under the following circumstances —
>
> The said words were published following the decision by Canadian National Steamships to transfer its eight vessels on West Indian service from Canadian Registry to a Foreign Registry on the 9th of November, 1957. In July 1957 the Seafarers' International Union, of which the Plaintiff

is the Canadian Director, called a strike which tied up the said eight vessels. After more than four months the strike was still not settled and the vessels were transferred to Foreign Registry as aforesaid, all of which was the subject of discussion and comment in the House of Commons and in the Public Press.

4. By reason of such circumstances it was the duty of the Defendants to publish, and in the interests of the public to receive communications and comments with respect to the strike and the resultant transfer of eight vessels from Canadian Registry and by reason of this the said words were published under such circumstances and upon such occasion as to render them privileged.

The plea of the defence of fair comment is set out in paras. 6 and 8 of the statement of defence as follows:

6. Insofar as the said words consist of statements of fact the said words are in their natural and ordinary meaning, and without the meanings alleged in paragraph 6 of the Statement of Claim, true in substance and in fact; and insofar as the said words consist of expressions of opinion they are fair comment made in good faith and without malice upon the said facts which are a matter of public interest in the circumstances stated in paragraph 3.

8. In the alternative if any of the said words are capable of the meanings alleged in paragraph 6 of the Plaintiff's Statement of Claim then they are fair comment made in good faith and without malice on a matter of public interest. The said comment was based upon the transfer by Canadian National Steamships of eight vessels from Canadian Registry to Foreign Registry in the circumstances referred to in paragraph 3.

The action was tried in June, 1958. Counsel for the appellant called two witnesses, the plaintiff and a Mr. Leonard McLaughlin who was the secretary-treasurer of the Seafarers' International Union of North America, Canadian District. Counsel then read some questions and answers from the examination for discovery of the respondent Dalgleish and closed his case.

Counsel for the respondents then moved, in the absence of the jury, for the dismissal of the action on the ground that the words complained of were published on an occasion of qualified privilege and that there was no evidence of malice to go to the jury. It appears that before commencing his argument on this motion, counsel for the respondents had announced his decision not to call any evidence. Shortly after counsel for the appellant had commenced his argument on the motion the learned trial Judge called attention to this as follows:

HIS LORDSHIP: May I interrupt you for a moment. I think it is only proper, Mr. Walker, that I should ask you. when you commenced your argument, the thing which I did ask you in chambers and therefore I omitted to ask for the record. Is it the intention of counsel for the defendants to adduce evidence?

MR. WALKER: No, my lord, I am calling no evidence.

At a later stage of his argument on this motion counsel for the plaintiff admitted that the strike and the resultant transfer of the ships involved to foreign registry constituted a matter of public interest; but, as I read the record, counsel did not admit that the statements and comments made about the plaintiff were made on a matter of public interest. This accords with the position taken by counsel in his opening to the jury in the course of which he said:

We shall also contend throughout this trial that what was said about Mr. Banks was not said on a matter of public interest; that it was substantially a personal attack and not mere comment or expressions of opinion on a matter of public interest.

These circumstances have a bearing on the submission of counsel for the respondents, to be mentioned later, that counsel for the plaintiff at the trial had in effect admitted that the editorial was published on an occasion of qualified privilege.

At the conclusion of the argument on the motion the learned trial Judge ruled that the editorial was published on an occasion of qualified privilege but that there was evidence of malice to go lo the jury.

In his charge the learned trial Judge made it clear to the jury that they had the right to bring in a general verdict but he invited them to answer a number of questions and the jury followed this course. The questions and answers are as follows:

1. Were the statements complained of and set out in Exhibit I under the circumstances in which they were used, defamatory of the plaintiff? Answer "Yes" or "No". Answer: Yes.

2. (a) Insofar as the statements are of fact were they all true? Answer "Yes" or "No". Answer: No. (b) Insofar as the statements are expressions of opinion did they exceed the limit of fair comment? Answer "Yes" or "No". Answer: Yes.

3. Do the words complained of and set out in Exhibit I mean —

(a) that the plaintiff came from the United States to Canada for the specific purpose of ending the existence of Canadian ships at sea, contrary to the interests of members of his Union and the people of Canada? Answer "Yes" or "No". Answer: Yes.

(b) that the plaintiff committed a substantial number of criminal offences in the United States? Answer "Yes" or "No". Answer: Yes.

(c) that the plaintiff has committed a substantial number of criminal offences of diverse kinds after coming to Canada? Answer "Yes" or "No". Answer: No.

(d) that the plaintiff is a dictatorial and irresponsible union officer not subject to removal or re-election by the membership of his Union? Answer "Yes" or "No". Answer: Yes.

(e) that the plaintiff has used threats of force in making demands upon Canadian ship owners? Answer "Yes" or "No". Answer: No.

(f) that the plaintiff has caused loss of employment to be suffered by most or all of Canada's ocean-going seamen? Answer "Yes" or "No". Answer: Yes.

(g) that the plaintiff, on his own initiative and without the authority of the membership of his Union, called a strike against Canadian National Steamships? Answer "Yes" or "No". Answer: No.

(h) that the plaintiff, on his own initiative and without reference to the membership of his Union demanded a 30 per cent wage increase for such members. Answer "Yes" or "No". Answer No.

(i) that the plaintiff, on his own initiative and without reference to the membership of his Union, rejected an offer of a 10 per cent wage increase? Answer "Yes" or "No". Answer: No.

(j) that the plaintiff, while posing as a representative of working seamen, was indifferent or hostile to their interests? Answer "Yes" or "No". Answer: No.

(k) that the plaintiff deliberately used an office of trust held by him to cause injury and loss to the membership of his Union by whom he was employed? Answer "Yes" or "No". Answer: No.

(l) that the plaintiff is an unfit person to be granted Canadian citizenship? Answer "Yes" or "No". Answer: Yes.

(m) that the plaintiff is an unfit person to be permitted to reside in Canada? Answer "Yes" or ''No". Answer: Yes.

4. If you have answered "Yes" to any of the sub-questions in 3 above, does such meaning exceed the limit of fair comment? Answer ''Yes" or "No". Answer: Yes.

5. When the defendants published this statement were they actuated by any motive other than their duty to publish communications and comments on a matter of public interest? Answer "Yes" or "No". Answer: No.

6. At what amount do you assess the damages of the plaintiff? $3500.00 (Thirty-five hundred dollars).

Upon these answers the learned trial Judge directed judgment to be entered dismissing the action with costs.

The appellant appealed to the Court of Appeal. The first ground set out in the notice of appeal was: "That the learned trial Judge erred in holding that the words complained of were protected by the defence of qualified privilege." Laidlaw, J.A., who delivered the unanimous judgment of the Court of Appeal, in summarizing the grounds of appeal presented in argument before that Court described the first of those grounds as follows:

> First, that the decision of the learned trial Judge that the occasion was one of qualified privilege, was erroneous, or, in the alternative, that the learned Judge ought to have found that part of the published article was within the privilege and part of it was not within the privilege.

I have reached the conclusion that the learned trial Judge and the Court of Appeal were in error in holding that the occasion on which the editorial was published was one of qualified privilege and consequently do not find it necessary to consider the other grounds urged by Mr. MacKinnon in support of the appeal.

The reasons of the learned trial Judge for holding that the occasion was privileged are as follows:

> The first branch of the application may be disposed of very shortly. I think it is quite evident by consideration of the cases cited by counsel for the defendant, particularly *Jenoure v. Delmege* [1891] A.C. 73; *Pittard v. Oliver*, [1891] 1 Q.B. 474; *Mangena v. Wright*, [1909] 2 K.B. 958; *Adam v. Ward*, [1917] A.C. 309; *Showler v. MacInnes* (1937), 51 B.C.R. 391; *Dennison et al. v. Sanderson*, [1947] 4 D.L.R. 314. O.R. 601; and *Drew v. Toronto Star Ltd. & Atkinson*, [1947] 4 D.L.R. 221, O.R. 730; that the class of cases to which the defence of qualified privilege extends have, during the course of recent years, been extended, and that that extension will cover editorial comment by a metropolitan newspaper upon matters of public interest. It is difficult to conceive a matter in which the public would be much more interested in the year 1957 than the most important topic of industrial relations, when added to that there is the topic of the continued existence of a deep-sea fleet under Canadian registry. The latter topic, in fact, had so interested the public that it was included in a reference of matters to a Royal Commission, the report of which had not yet been rendered at the time of this alleged libel.
>
> There is no more efficient organ for informing the public and for disseminating to the public intelligent comment on such matters of public interest, than a great metropolitan newspaper, which the plaintiff has proved the defendant to be. The members of the public have a real, a vital — I might go so far as to say — a paramount interest in receiving those comments.
>
> The decision of Mr. Justice Manson in *Showler v. MacInnes* has been criticized but I feel that his words are most applicable to the particular situation which existed here, and I propose to adopt those words in this case where he said (51 B.C.R. at p. 395):
>
> "The whole citizenhood of Vancouver has and had at the time of the address in question a vital concern in the matter of industrial relations in the community and in knowing under what circumstances strikes might be called," adding the comment that for "all the citizens of Vancouver" I would insert" "citizens of Canada".

The statement of the rule as to the burden of proof where a defence of qualified privilege is set up, contained in *Gatley on Libel & Slander*, 4th ed., p. 282 (stated in the same words in the 5th ed., of that work at p. 270) was approved by this Court in *Globe & Mail Ltd. v. Boland*, 22 D.L.R. (2d) 277 at p. 279, [1960] S.C.R. 203 at p. 206, and is as follows:

> Where a defence of qualified privilege is set up, it is for the defendant to allege and prove all such facts and circumstances as are necessary to bring the words complained of within the privilege, unless such facts are admitted before or at the trial of the action. Whether the facts and circumstances proved or admitted are or are not such as to render the occasion privileged is a question of law for the judge to decide.

In the case at bar the evidence of the plaintiff showed that the strike referred to in the editorial had commenced in July, 1957 and that it had not been settled at the date, of the trial. His evidence in cross-examination continued:

> Q. So that when the defendant says in the Statement of Defence that after four months the strike was still not settled, that is correct. A. That is correct. Q. And you also told us that the vessels were transferred to foreign registry. Now, Mr. Banks. I suppose you read the newspapers, do you? A. Occasionally. Q. And was there considerable newspaper publicity with reference to this strike and with reference to the transfer of the vessels? A. There was. Q. And was there discussion in the House of Commons with reference to the strike and the transfer of the vessels? A. There was.

It has already been mentioned that counsel for the plaintiff admitted that the strike and the transfer of the ships involved to foreign registry constituted a matter of public interest.

I do not find it necessary to consider whether the allegations of fact on which the plea of qualified privilege was founded were sufficiently proved. If it be assumed for the purposes of argument that all the facts and circumstances alleged in paras. 3 and 4 of the statement of defence were proved it is my opinion that they were not such as to render the occasion privileged.

With the greatest respect it appears to me that in his reasons quoted above the learned trial Judge has fallen into the same error as was pointed out in the judgment of this Court in *Globe & Mail Ltd. v. Boland*, at p. 280 D.L.R., p. 207 S.C.R., and has confused the right which the publisher of a newspaper has, in common with all Her Majesty's subjects, to report truthfully and comment fairly upon matters of a public interest, with a duty of the sort which gives rise to an occasion of privilege. It is not necessary to refer again to the authorities discussed in the case last cited but I think it desirable to recall the passage from the judgment of Lord Shaw in *Arnold v. The King Emperor* (1914), 30 T.L.R. 462 at p. 468:

> The freedom of the journalist is an ordinary part of the freedom of the subject, and to whatever lengths the subject in general may go, so also may the journalist, but, apart from statute-law, his privilege is no other and no higher. The responsibilities which attach to his power in the dissemination of printed matter may, and in the case of a conscientious journalist do, make him more careful; but the range of his assertions, his criticisms, or his comments is as wide as, and no wider than, that of any other subject. No privilege attaches to his position.

The following statement in *Gatley on Libel & Slander*. 5th ed., pp. 322-3 is, in my opinion, accurate:

> The defence of fair comment must also be distinguished from that of qualified privilege. In the defence of fair comment the right exercised by the defendant is shared by every member of the public. "Who is entitled to comment? The answer to that is 'everyone.' A newspaper reporter or a newspaper editor has exactly the same rights, neither more nor less, than every other citizen." In that of qualified privilege the right is not shared by every member of the public, but is limited to an individual who stands in such relation to the circumstances that he is entitled to say or write what would be libelous or slanderous on the part of anyone else. "For instance, if a master is asked as to the character of a servant, and he says mat the servant is a thief, he has a privilege which no one else would have." "A privileged occasion is one on which the privileged person is entitled to do something which no one who is not within the privilege is entitled to do on that occasion. A person in such a position may say or write about another person things which no other person in the kingdom can be allowed to say or write. But, in the case of a criticism upon [a matter of public interest whether it be the conduct of a public man or] a published work, every person in the kingdom is entitled to do, and is forbidden to do exactly the same things. and therefore the occasion is not privileged."

The judgments given at trial in the cases of *Dennison et al. v. Sanderson, supra*, and *Drew v. Toronto Star Ltd. & Atkinson, supra*. relied on by the learned trial Judge, in so far as they deal with the question of qualified privilege, must be regarded as having been overruled by the judgments of this Court in *Douglas v. Tucker*, [1952] 1 D.L.R. 657, 1 S.C.R. 275 and in *Globe & Mail Ltd. v. Boland, supra*. The judgment in *Showler v. MacInnes*, 51 B.C.R. 391, is, in my opinion, inconsistent with the two last-mentioned judgments of this Court and with our judgment in the case at bar and ought not to be followed. The other decisions referred to in the reasons of the learned trial judge are all distinguishable on their facts from the case at bar.

There are of course many cases in which publication of defamatory matter in a newspaper may be privileged either by statute or at common law; examples are to be found in the *Libel and Slander Act*, R.S.O. 1950, c.204, ss.9 and 10 [now R.S.O. 1960, c.211, ss.3 and 4], and in such cases as *Adam v. Ward*, [1917] A.C. 309 and *Allbutt v. Gen'l Council of Medical Education & Registration* (1889), 23 Q.B.D. 400.

In the first of these it was held that the Army Council owed a duty to publish to the whole world a letter vindicating a General who had been falsely accused before the same audience of discreditable conduct and that publication in the press was therefore privileged; in the second it was held that publication in the press of an accurate report of proceedings within the jurisdiction of the General Medical Council erasing the name of the plaintiff from the medical register was privileged on the ground, *inter alia*, that it was the duty of the Council to give the public accurate information as to who is on the register and if a person's name is erased accurate information of the cause of its erasure.

The decision of the learned trial Judge, in the case at bar, quoted above, appears to involve the proposition of law, which in my opinion is untenable, that given proof of the existence of a subject-matter of wide public interest throughout Canada without proof of any other special circumstances any newspaper in Canada (and *semble* therefore any individual) which sees fit to publish to the public at large statements of fact relevant to that subject-matter is to be held to be doing so on an occasion of qualified privilege.

Having reached the conclusion that the learned trial Judge was in error in deciding that the editorial complained of was published on an occasion of qualified privilege, it is not necessary to consider what judgment should have been given on the answers of the jury had the ruling of the learned trial Judge been upheld; but I do not wish to be understood as agreeing that even in that event the action should have been dismissed; while the plea of qualified privilege and the answer of the jury negativing express malice would, on the hypothesis mentioned, have afforded a defence to the action in so far as it was based on the publication of defamatory statements of fact there remained the finding of the jury that the comment (and the editorial consisted partly of comment) was unfair. However, I do not pursue this question further.

It remains to consider what order should be made. Counsel for the respondent argued that if we should hold the publication was not made on an occasion of qualified privilege a new trial should be directed; this argument was based in part on the submission that at the trial counsel for the plaintiff had admitted that the occasion was one of qualified privilege. I have read all the record with care and cannot find that any such admission was made. Doubtless both counsel at the trial were familiar with the ruling which had been made by the learned trial Judge a short time before in the case of *Globe & Mail Ltd. v. Boland, supra*, and, perhaps for that reason, counsel for the plaintiff concentrated his argument on the submission that even if the occasion was one of privilege the bounds of the privilege had been exceeded. The following passage at the end of the argument of the motion, and particularly the words I have italicized, would be inconsistent with the view that the learned trial Judge considered that any such admission had been made.

> Mr. Jolliffe: Therefore the gist of my submission is that *even if the Court holds the occasion to be a privileged one*, the editorial . . .
> His Lordship: In short, even if the Court holds it is qualified privilege, qualified privilege only exists for the purpose for which the privilege is set up.
> Mr. Jolliffe: Exactly, my lord.
> His Lordship: And if the motive goes beyond that, it is evidence of malice to go to the Jury.
> Mr. Jolliffe: Exactly, my lord. That is what I am attempting to say.
> His Lordship: I understand that.

I am unable to find any sufficient ground for directing a new trial; I have given my reasons for holding that the defence of qualified privilege fails, the answers of the jury negatived the defence of fair comment; the error in law which, in my respectful opinion, was made by the trial Judge was not one which would cause the jury to increase the amount of the damages or would otherwise prejudice the position of the respondents.

I would allow the appeal, set aside the judgment of the Court of Appeal and that of the learned trial Judge and direct that judgment be entered for the plaintiff for $3,500 with costs throughout.

5.2.3.3.3.3.2 *Stopforth v. Goyer* (1978), 4 C.C.L.T. 265 (Ont. H.C.)

LIEFF, J.: This is an action for damages for libel tried at Ottawa on 6th, 7th. 8th, 9th and 10th March 1978. without a jury, counsel having consented thereto pursuant to s.59 of *The Judicature Act*, R.S.O. 1970, c.228. Counsel consented to this procedure after a jury had been empanelled but before any evidence had been

The alleged defamatory remarks were said to have been spoken by the defendant of the plaintiff to reporters of the printed and electronic news media who were present in the Government lobby in the Parliament Buildings in Ottawa on 1st June 1976. Shortly before that the defendant had emerged from the chamber of the House of Commons at the conclusion of the question period. The words admittedly spoken by the defendant were as follows:

"I will stand for my officials and I accept responsibility for errors of judgment, mistakes made in good faith. But I do not believe that ministerial responsibility extends to cases of misinformation or gross negligence. Why should I pay for misinformation."

It is settled law that where a person speaks defamatory words to the press with the intention or knowledge that they will be republished, the speaker is responsible in libel rather than in slander.

When a politician of experience speaks to the press he impliedly, if not expressly, authorizes republication of his communication and is thus responsible for any libel. This point was not put in issue by counsel for the defendant.

The story was carried on the Canadian Press wire service and the words sued upon were the focus of front page stories in the *London Free Press*, the *Globe and Mail*, the Montreal *Gazette* and the Ottawa *Journal*, all major Canadian newspapers of wide circlation. I therefore find as a fact that the words sued upon were widely circulated in the printed media.

At this point it may be useful to set out briefly the events which led up to the incident at which the words sued upon were spoken. A more detailed review of the facts may be more conveniently made when I deal with the defence of justification

In 1972 the Department of National Defence (DND) determined to acquire some 18 long-range patrol aircraft (LRPA). In order to co-ordinate the LRPA acquisition a project office was established in the summer of 1972 composed of employees of DND, the Department of Supply and Services (DSS), the Department of Industry, Trade and Commerce and the Department of Regional Economic Expansion. The plaintiff, an employee of DSS, was at all material times deputy manager of the project office. The defendant was at all material times Minister of DSS.

Supervision of the project office was achieved through a bureaucratic mechanism called the Senior Management Board. This Board was composed of an assistant deputy minister from each of the four ministries involved in the project office. The assistant deputy minister from each ministry reported to his deputy minister who, in turn, reported to the minister. The DSS member of the Senior Management Board was Mr. Eric Booth, now deceased, and the Deputy Minister of Supply to whom Booth reported was Mr. Jacques DesRoches.

On 12th November 1975, when it was apparent that DND had a budgetary shortfall of some $375 million on the LRPA project, the manager of the project office, General T S. Allan, telephoned the then competing bidders on the LRPA project, the Boeing Aircraft Corporation and the Lockheed Aircraft Corporation, to inquire as to the feasibility of the manufacturers providing bridge financing for the DND shortfall. Both manufacturers replied that such was feasible.

On 27th November 1975, Cabinet chose the Lockheed LRPA proposal over that of Boeing, which decision was approved by Treasury Board on the same date subject to two conditions:

(1) that permission would be obtained to take the specifications and plans for the P-3 Orion airplanes to be manufactured by Lockheed for the LRPA project out of the United States; and,

(2) that a specified quantum of the industrial benefits of the contract would accrue to Canada.

Neither Cabinet nor Treasury Board provided any direction as to how the LRPA project was to be paid for, even though both bodies were aware of the DND shortfall and the cost of financing it by virtue of submissions prepared for their consideration by the project office. The defendant sat as a member of both Cabinet and the Treasury Board at all material times.

On 2nd December 1975, the defendant signed a telex to Lockheed accepting its proposal subject to the two conditions dictated by Treasury Board. The acceptance was not made conditional upon Lockheed providing bridge financing for the DND shortfall.

On 17th December 1975, Lockheed informed DSS that it was not possible for it to finance the DND shortfall. The result of this information was that there were insufficient funds in DND's budget to carry out the project according to plan.

By March 1976, and through the spring of that year, debate in Parliament intensified as to how the government could have become involved in a contract without first ensuring that the project was properly and adequately funded or financed.

By May 1976, the defendant was facing frequent questioning in the House of Commons over the LRPA project. General Allan's conversation with Lockheed concerning the provision of bridge financing was of particular interest to the interlocutor during question period in the House. These questions were particularly directed at the defendant who had signed the telex accepting Lockheed's proposal without including bridge financing as a condition of the acceptance. The defendant's reply was consistent, namely, that neither he, his deputies nor his representative at the project office, the plaintiff, knew of any agreement by Lockheed to provide bridge financing before 2nd December 1975.

On 18th May 1977, the Minister of DND advised the House of the termination of the Lockheed contract on the LRPA project.

Under the pressure of intensifying debate, the defendant called the plaintiff to a meeting in his office on 19th May 1976, to confirm the information he had been providing to the House.

The evidence relating to this meeting is as follows:

(1) that the defendant explained to the plaintiff his need for precise information concerning General Allan's agreement with Lockheed and the extent of the plaintiff's knowledge as to any agreement prior to 2nd December 1975, the date on which the telex was signed; and

(2) the defendant's recollection was that the plaintiff denied any knowledge of an agreement by Lockheed to provide bridge financing for the DND shortfall, saying he (the plaintiff) did not learn of it until mid-December.

The defendant's account of this meeting with the plaintiff was confirmed by the Deputy Minister of Supply, Mr. DesRoches, who was present for most of the meeting.

The plaintiff's account of the 19th May 1976, meeting with the defendant is different from the defendant's in one material respect. The plaintiff says that:

(a) he told the defendant that he was not aware of any agreement by Lockheed to provide bridge financing but he was aware that General Allan had conferred with Lockheed on the subject and Lockheed had either agreed that such an arrangement was feasible or to look into the feasibility of such an arrangement;

(b) he told the defendant that he was not privy to General Allan's conversation with Lockheed but learned a few days afterwards that it had taken place; and

(c) it was not until mid-December 1975, when the omission of the condition of bridge financing from the 2nd December 1975, telex became important, that he first learned or heard that Lockheed had actually agreed to provide the financing.

In effect what the plaintiff is saying is that it was not until Lockheed said it could not finance the project that he formed the impression that there never could have been an actual agreement as distinguished from a study of feasibility. The defendant on the other hand asked about *a conversation which resulted in an agreement*; this the plaintiff denied.

On the basis of his meeting with the plaintiff the defendant continued to deny knowledge, on his part or on the part of his aides, of an agreement by Lockheed to provide bridge financing of the DND shortfall.

On 31st May 1976, in preparation for a "late show" (which is a continuation of question period after the close of the day's other parliamentary business), on the LRPA project the defendant became aware that the plaintiff knew of General Allan's conversation with Lockheed concerning bridge financing before 2nd

December 1975. According to the defendant the implications of this revelation were very serious for it meant he had been misleading the House and this troubled him very much. The defendant testified that he consulted with the Prime Minister and other senior parliamentarians as to whether he should resign.

On 1st June 1976, the defendant ntade the following statement to the House (Ex. 12). During his examination-in-chief the defendant read it all into the record. It is reproduced in full:

June 1, 1976
3:00 p.m.

STATEMENT BY THE HONOURABLE JEAN-PIERRE GOYER

"Mr. Speaker

I wish to correct a statement that I made in the House yesterday in response to a question from the Honourable Member from Victoria (McKinnon). This question was in relation to whether a representative from my department on the LRPA project team was aware before December 2, 1975 that Lockheed had given verbal assurance that it could provide financing to meet DND's cash shortfall in the first three years of the project.

But first, I would like to reiterate two points which I have repeatedly stressed both in this House and outside Parliament, namely that

(1) The financing of any contract entered upon by the Department of Supply and Services is the prime and exclusive responsibility of the customer Department, in this case the Department of National Defence.

(2) On December 2, 1975, when a telex was sent to Lockheed confirming the government's intention to purchase 18 Orion aircrafts, neither myself, nor my Deputy-Minister was made aware, directly or indirectly, of a telephone conversation held between an official of the DND and a representative of Lockheed to the effect that Lockheed would furnish the financing for the LRPA project.

In any case, I repeat, not obtaining a written agreement from Lockheed was a serious error. It is elementary that an agreement involving a loan of millions of dollars should have been confirmed in a written document.

This was not done. Furthermore, the offer never did materialize. In this respect, I refer to the statements of my colleague. the Minister of National Defence, which appear in the Hansard dated March 30, 1976, on page 12265 and March 26, 1976, page 12177.

Personally, I might add that it was also a very serious mistake that the minister responsible for negotiating the agreement with Lockheed was not informed of the basic funding difficulties before December 2, 1975 and that the proposed solution rested upon a verbal agreement.

Now, the statement I made yesterday was that neither myself nor my deputy nor my representative in the LRPA project office was aware of the possibility of

Lockheed furnishing the financing for the LRPA project. The factual statement is that neither myself nor my deputy nor, as I stated in the House on May 25, 1976, on page 13794 of Hansard, the representative of my department on the management committee was aware of the possibility of that financial arrangement. For your information the representative on the LRPA management committee was my former Assistant Deputy Minister, Mr. Eric Booth. The portion of the statement that I wish to clarify concerns Mr. L.H. Stopforth who as my representative on the LRPA project group I now find was aware of financing discussions held between DND and Lockheed in mid-November 1975.

During the past months, Mr. Speaker, I repeatedly attempted to ascertain whether or not any officials of my Department were aware of the financing negotiations held between the DND and Lockheed, prior to December 2, 1975. I repeatedly was assured that no one had prior knowledge of this problem and I conveyed this information to the House.

On May the 19th, in view of the numerous questions raised by Members of the House, I personally met in the presence of my Deputy Minister with Mr. L.H. Stopforth who assured me that he had no prior information concerning the financial negotiations between DND and Lockheed. Ministers, acting on the representations and advice from their civil servants. must rely on the information they receive on these matters on the basis of trust.

Last evening, however, and it was confirmed to me this morning, I learned that Mr. L.H. Stopforth had modified his version to state that while he had not been privy to conversations between DND and Lockheed, he was aware of the financing discussions with Lockheed in November 1975.

I take my Ministerial responsibilities very seriously with regard to the policies and administrative practices of my department.

Accordingly, *I will stand by my officials, and I accept to take responsibility for errors of judgment, mistakes made 'in good faith', inadvertent errors. but I do not believe that ministerial responsibility extends to cases of misinformation or gross negligence.* In this case, a serious error was committed: not only was I nor my Deputy Minister not informed of financial negotiations between the DND and Lockheed, prior to December 2, but subsequently, when I personally checked on this situation I remained misinformed. This is unacceptable.

My view is that while ministerial responsibility is of prime importance, every public servant regardless of his interest in politics, also holds the public trust to some extent. Every public servant is in a position of responsibility and the responsibility here was to ensure that the Minister, the House and the public be correctly informed.

I feel very strongly about officials who misinform their Minister. While I am not against any man or any organization I believe that preserving the integrity and the efficiency of our system of government comes first. The public must believe that the system serves it well. The public must respect the public service. My ministerial responsibility, in this case, is to see that these rights are preserved.

Consequently, Mr. L.H. Stopforth has been removed from his function as Deputy Head of the project office." [The italics are mine.]

After making his statement to the House of Commons the defendant left the chamber and was passing through the Liberal lobby when he was encountered by the press to whom he made the statement sued upon. Mary Louise Janigan, parliamentary correspondent for the Toronto *Star* was present in the press gallery of the House when the defendant made his statement and was also present in the government lobby when the defendant spoke to the press and made the statement sued upon. She testified that the defendant spoke these words in response to questions by reporters concerning his reasons for demoting the plaintiff. According to her the defendant also said that the plaintiff would be transferred to another post if he chose to stay with DSS and "I don't have any confidence in him".

Exhibit No. 17 is an extract of the original "copy" of Ms. Janigan's story on the events in question typed by her on the evening of 1st June 1976, from notes she made on that day. It confirms her account of the additional statement made by the defendant. Counsel for the plaintiff relies on it as an aggravation of the statement sued upon. Such evidence is admissible for that purpose.

Deputy Minister of Supply, Mr. DesRoches, testified that:

(1) it was as a result of the events leading up to the defendant's statement to the House on 1st June 1976, that he decided to remove the plaintiff from his assignment as deputy manager of the project office;

(2) he had wanted to dismiss the plaintiff outright, but decided against it;

(3) he asked the plaintiff for his resignation which the plaintiff refused to provide;

(4) it was his own decision to remove the plaintiff from the project office; and

(5) the defendant did not direct his decision in any way.

The plaintiff testified that since the events in question his status and prestige as a senior civil servant have, in essence, been entirely stripped from him. The plaintiff has, however, suffered no cut in salary and, in fact, has had a modest pay increase since June 1976.

Exhibit No. 4 is a copy of a letter dated 8th June 1976, from counsel for the plaintiff to the defendant requesting a published retraction of the words sued upon. The defendant acknowledged receipt of Exhibit No. 4 and stated that he made no retraction.

The defendant pleaded four primary defences: fair comment, absolute privilege, qualified privilege and justification.

III. *Qualified Privilege*

Qualified privilege attaches to statements made on a privileged occasion. One such occasion, and the one on which the defendant relies, is where the statement is made in pursuance of a moral, social or legal duty to communicate the information contained in the statement. Concomitant with the duty to speak there must also be an interest or duty in the hearer to receive the communication.

This reciprocity is essential: see *Adam v. Ward*, [1917] A.C. 309 (H.L.) per Lord Atkinson at p. 334.

The importance of the duty to speak on the occasion sued upon was discussed in the recent case of *Littleton v. Hamilton* (1974), 4 O.R. (2d) 283, 47 D.L.R. (3d) 663 (C.A.). In that case the defendants tried to invoke the defence of qualified privilege regarding the publication of a history of the Company of Young Canadians. The defendants relied on the fact that the organization was one of public interest, funded with public money and highly publicized across the country. Dubin, J.A., who delivered the judgment of the Court, stressed that the existence of a duty to communicate is essential to the defence of qualified privilege. At p. 285 he said:

> In order to hold that words are published on an occasion of qualified privilege, something more is necessary than the mere fact that the words are being addressed to a matter of public interest. Before an individual can be said to have published words on an occasion of qualified privilege, some circumstances must be shown from which it can be concluded for valid social reasons that an individual can with impunity publish defamatory statements of others provided he does so without malice. Although it has been stated that there is no confined catalogue of such occasions, it is clear that the mere fact that the publication relates to matters of public interest is not sufficient.

The burden of proof of establishing the defence of qualified privilege, of showing both that there was a duty to speak on the occasion sued upon and a reciprocal interest or duty in the hearer to receive the information, is upon the defendant: see Button, *Principles of the Law of Libel and Slander*, pp. 134-5.

Having considered the substance of the communication and all the other circumstances surrounding it, I find that the defendant has failed to make out the defence of qualified privilege for two reasons:

(a) he had no duty to speak on the occasion sued upon. He had just delivered a statement to the House of Commons on an occasion of absolute privilege of the same substance and to the same effect as that for which he has been sued. Any duty he had to make the statement sued upon was thereby discharged. Statements made in the House of Commons are a matter of public record. They are recorded in Hansard and reported by the news media. The defendant added nothing when he spoke to the press in the Government lobby. Indeed, the defendant testified that he spoke to the press on this occasion to explain his view of ministerial responsibility, not because he felt he had a duty to do so;

(b) the defendant has also failed to establish the reciprocal interest or duty in the press, or the Canadian public through the press, to receive the statement sued upon. While it was a matter of public interest to learn what occurred in the DND-Lockheed transaction to cause it to be cancelled, there was no public interest in receiving the plaintiff's identity or the plaintiff's personal blameworthiness, if any.

The statement in question in this action referred to the plaintiff. It was made in response to questions concerning the plaintiff by reporters of the news media.

It is a long-standing convention of parliamentary democracy and the doctrine of ministerial responsibility which it encompasses that civil servants are to remain faceless to the public. Civil servants are responsible to their ministers. Ministers, as elected officials, are responsible to the public.

The reasoning of Kenneth Kernaghan in his recent article "Politics, policy and public servants: political neutrality revisited" (1976), 19 *Can. Public Administration* 432 commends itself to me. At p. 451 it reads:

> The traditional model of political neutrality requires that public servants provide forthright advice to their political superiors in private and in confidence. In return, political executives protect the anonymity of public servants by publicly accepting responsibility for departmental decisions. In a parliamentary system of government, the anonymity of public servants depends in large measure on the vitality of the doctrine of ministerial responsibility. According to this doctrine, a minister is personally responsible to Parliament both for his own actions and for those of his administrative subordinates. Thus, public servants are not directly answerable to Parliament and their minister protects their anonymity.

Kernaghan also observes that while the convention of ministerial responsibility which requires a minister's resignation for maladministration in his department is in a weakened state "[t]he convention of ministerial defence of public service anonymity is in a comparatively healthy state".

Furthermore, it is my view that no matter how advanced the state of erosion of public service anonymity (which according to Kernaghan is still rather healthy), a minister should not be able to blame or castigate personally any civil servant of a department under his control in public and then fall back upon the legal defence of qualified privilege. If that were the case and the civil servant were defamed he would be in the peculiar position of being prevented from obtaining vindication for spurious allegations by a minister. It is for this further reason that there can be no interest or duty in the public to receive information containing defamatory allegations, directed at a particular civil servant. Consequently the defence of qualified privilege fails.

Before leaving this topic, may I say that in *R. v. Morgan*, [1976] A.C. 182 (H.L.) Lord Edmond-Davies at pp. 230-31 made liberal use of academic writings. In *R. v. Fane Robinson Ltd.*, [1941] 2 W.W.R. 235, 76 C.C.C. 196 at 200, [1941] 3 D.L.R. 409 (Alta. C.A.) Ford, J.A. did the same thing.

5.2.3.3.3.3.3 *Stopforth v. Goyer* (1979), 23 O.R. (2d) 696 (Ont. C.A.)

JESSUP, J.A.: The learned trial Judge did not give effect to the defence pleaded of qualified privilege. That defence is succinctly stated in 24 Hals., 3rd ed., pp. 56-7:

> 100. ... An occasion is privileged where the person who makes a communication has an interest or a duty, legal, social or moral, to make it to the person to whom it is made, and the person to whom it is so made has a corresponding interest or duty to receive it.

101. ... A reason for holding any occasion privileged is the common convenience or the welfare of society, and it is not easy to mark off with precision those occasions which are from those which are not privileged or to define what kind of social or moral duty or what measure of interest will make the occasion privileged .... The trend of the modern decisions is in the direction of a more liberal application or interpretation of the rule.

In my opinion the electorate, as represented by the media, has a real and *bona fide* interest in the demotion of a senior civil servant for an alleged dereliction of duty. It would want to know if the reasons given in the House were the real and only reasons for the demotion. The appellant had a corresponding public duty and interest in satisfying that interest of the electorate. Accordingly, there being no suggestion of malice, I would hold that the alleged defamatory statements were uttered on an occasion of qualified privilege.

In denying that defence the learned trial judge was influenced by what he found to be a convention of the House of Commons that Ministers of the Crown must accept responsibility for the acts of subordinates in their Departments and yet preserve in the House the anonymity of such subordinates. Assuming the trial Judge could take judicial notice of such a convention as a viable one, it does not seem to me it can be permitted the effect of either enlarging or abridging the law of defamation. The respondent was named by the appellant in the House. If that was a breach of convention he and his party were subject to all the disciplines of the House. However, the fact that the respondent was named in the House would create the interest of the electorate and invoke the corresponding interest of the appellant to satisfy that created interest.

The learned trial Judge disallowed the defence of justification. Before us it was very persuasively argued that such defence was made out with respect to the allegation of misinformation. However, neither before the trial Judge nor in this Court was it argued that the allegation of gross negligence was justified. Rather the appellant argued that he did not intend to impute gross negligence to the respondent. However, as the learned trial Judge noted, the test is not of intent but rather what reasonable persons would understand from the allegedly defamatory words. In the result, I agree with the learned trial Judge that the defence of justification must fall and with it falls the defence of fair comment.

Because I think the occasion was one of qualified privilege I do not deal with the argument that it was also one of absolute privilege.

In the result, I would allow the appeal with costs, set aside the judgment below and dismiss the action with costs.

5.2.3.3.3.3.4 *Parlett v. Robinson* (1986), 30 D.L.R. (4th) 247 (B.C.C.A.)

HINKSON, J.A.: The plaintiff brought action against the defendant for defamation arising out of statements made by the defendant at a news conference on December 11, 1981, at the constituency office of the defendant in Burnaby and at an interview later that day on television station CKVU in Vancouver.

In 1981 the plaintiff was a psychologist holding the position of Regional Manager of Education and Training, Pacific Region, for the Correctional Service of Canada. As such, the plaintiff was the functional supervisor of all educational and vocational programmes at federal penitentiaries in the Province of British Columbia, including Matsqui Institution.

From May, 1979, the defendant was the federal Member of Parliament representing the British Columbia constituency of Burnaby. In 1981 the defendant was the official spokesperson in the House of Commons for the New Democratic Party on the Ministry of the Solicitor-General. That ministry includes the Correctional Service. As well, the defendant was a member of the House of Commons Standing Committee on Justice and Legal Affairs.

The plaintiff was a collector of violins. He met one Morfitt, a repairer and restorer of violins, and engaged him to do some work. The plaintiff and Morfitt subsequently became friends. In 1977 Morfitt set up the Doyen Violin Shop in which he repaired, restored and sold violins. The plaintiff frequently had violins restored or repaired, some of which were consigned for sale at Doyen. From the sale of those violins the plaintiff shared the profits with Doyen on a percentage basis which varied from sale to sale. The plaintiff was the biggest customer of Doyen.

In late 1979 the plaintiff met a prisoner at Matsqui named Li and observed that he was a skilled wood carver. In late 1980 the plaintiff asked Li to carve chin rests from rosewood, which chin rests were purchased by the plaintiff. At that time within Matsqui Institution there was a programme called "Concraft Enterprises". This was an entrepreneurial activity for inmates. They purchased materials and produced articles which were then sold by Concraft Enterprises. The purchase price for such articles was paid to Concraft Enterprises. Depending on the type of work being performed by the inmate, it was described as "custom work", "hobby work" or "contract work". "Custom work" was work performed by an inmate for prison personnel. It was not contemplated that such items would be resold by prison personnel for a profit. "Contract work" was work done for a retail outlet, which in turn would add a mark-up to the price paid to the inmate before sale to the public.

The plaintiff paid Li approximately $7.50 per chin rest. The plaintiff delivered some 200 chin rests to Doyen, where they were offered for sale. By the date of trial all but approximately 10 of the chin rests had been sold.

In May, 1981, the defendant learned of the activity of the plaintiff in supplying chin rests to Doyen from one Hill, a constituent of the defendant. The defendant had met Hill previously when they both attended the University of British Columbia. From May to November, 1978, Hill was employed at Doyen as a violin restorer. Hill met the plaintiff when the latter visited the shop. After completing his education degree at the University of British Columbia in June, 1979, Hill obtained a six-month contract of employment at Matsqui Institution in September, 1979. Hill left this employment in February, 1980.

Hill learned that the plaintiff was supplying chin rests manufactured at Matsqui Institution to Doyen. In May, 1981, Hill approached the defendant and informed him of a scheme involving the plaintiff and Morfitt pursuant to which they planned to use inmate labour to produce violin parts cheaply for their personal benefit. Hill informed the defendant that the chin rests were to be sold for $56 each. Hill also informed the defendant that Morfitt and the plaintiff were sharing the profits on the sale of violins of the plaintiff. Hill later told the plaintiff that he had been asked by the plaintiff in February, 1980, to instruct inmates in Matsqui to make violin parts and that the plaintiff had told him he could arrange to get around any difficulties that might prevent this being done.

On June 8, 1981, the defendant wrote to Mr. D. R. Yeomans, Commissioner of Corrections, with respect to the policy of the Correctional Service of Canada on "custom work" being done for persons on staff of the service or other persons employed with the Ministry of the Solicitor-General or its agencies. After requesting information on any outstanding guidelines, the defendant wrote:

> I would furthermore seek your assurance that the C.S.C. would view as completely unethical (and very likely, illegal) to have prisoners producing goods or services inside your institutions which are later re-sold outside, resulting directly or indirectly in a profit to staff members or other persons referred to above . . .

At that stage the defendant was focussing his inquiry on what has been described as "custom work". Ultimately, when he was able to obtain documentation from the Office of the Commissioner of Collections, it became apparent that he was dealing with what was known within the service as "contract work". It was not until December 4, 1981, when Ms. Marjorie David, the Director General of Inmate Employment, wrote to him enclosing documents he had requested that the defendant became aware that Concraft Enterprises also engaged in "contract work". Earlier, on November 26, 1981, the defendant attended a meeting of the Standing Committee on Justice and Legal Affairs in Ottawa at which both Mr. Yeomans and the Solicitor General, Mr. Kaplan, were in attendance. He raised, in general terms, his concern about the absence of effective controls over possible abuse of inmate labour and referred to such abuse possibly taking place in the Pacific Region and involving a senior corrections official. At that meeting, the Commissioner of Corrections, Mr. Yeomans, stated that there were no problems whatsoever with the existing system of controls. The Solicitor General urged the defendant to make his allegations specific by naming the individual involved. The defendant did not then name the plaintiff. Following the meeting of the Justice Committee, the Union of Solicitor General Employees also wrote to the defendant, urging him to name publicly the individual to whom he was referring.

Following the November meeting of the Justice Committee, the defendant spoke to Hill and urged him to double-check the selling price of the Li chin rests at Doyen. Hill again confirmed the sale price at $56. The defendant telephoned Doyen at that time and spoke with an employee who stated that the sale price of the Li chin rest was $50. The defendant also telephoned the owner of another violin shop in the City of Vancouver and spoke to him about the circumstances of production and sale of Li chin rests and understood that the asking price of $50 was not out of line.

On December 4, 1981, the defendant met with Ms. Marjorie David, the National Director of Inmate Employment, and received the extensive documentation from the Pacific Region to which I have already made reference. This documentation included the employment records of Li, showing the plaintiff as a major customer. Thereafter, on December 4th, the defendant telephoned the plaintiff from Ottawa and, in a conversation which lasted over an hour, questioned him on the chin rest matter without revealing in any way the source of his information. During the conversation, the plaintiff denied any personal profit from the sale of chin rests and denied any interest in Doyen.

Following that telephone conversation, the defendant telephoned other individuals including Hill, Morfitt and Li. It was necessary to speak to Li through an interpreter. Li informed him that he was quite content with the arrangement whereby he received an average price of $7.50 for the chin rests he carved and sold to the plaintiff.

Between December 7 and 9, 1981, the defendant again met with Ms. David and discussed in detail the allegations he had made earlier at the Justice Committee meeting and divulged the name of the plaintiff. Following that meeting, the defendant met with the Solicitor General and urged him to initiate an inquiry into his allegations. The Minister, although familiar with the details of the defendant's allegations, refused any form of inquiry.

On December 11, 1981, the defendant held a press conference in his constituency office. He expressed his concern over the absence of any form of effective controls or regulations on use of inmate labour by correctional service officials. Statements made by the plaintiff at the press conference and again on the television programme are, in substance, allegations that the plaintiff sold chin rests, made a personal profit out of the sale of chin rests and abused his position in so doing, made a profit directly or indirectly out of an inmate's labour, and exploited inmate labour for his own profit.

The trial judge found that the plaintiff did try to sell chin rests and, therefore, concluded that the defendant had made out the defence of justification with respect to the allegation that the plaintiff had tried to sell chin rests. The trial judge also found that the defence of justification had not been made out with respect to other allegations, all of which were defamatory.

Following the press conference and the appearance on the television programme by the defendant, he wrote to the Solicitor General, outlining in detail his concerns and urged the Minister to order a public inquiry. In January, 1982, the Minister did order a board of inquiry. The results were made public on March 4, 1982, together with a press release by the Solicitor General.

At trial, as I have indicated, the learned trial judge held that some of the statements made by the defendant were defamatory of the plaintiff and awarded

$20,000 for general damages. The trial judge accepted the evidence of the plaintiff and Morfitt where it was in conflict with Hill's evidence. As a result, a large portion of the testimony of Hill was rejected.

The defendant advanced three grounds of appeal, as follows:

(1) The learned trial judge erred in rejecting the evidence of Hill;
(2) The learned trial judge erred in failing to hold that the defence of qualified privilege applied to the statements made at the press conference and on the television programme on December 11, 1981; and
(3) The award of damages was excessive in the circumstances.

In my view, it is necessary only to consider the defence of qualified privilege. The learned trial judge made some significant findings. Firstly, he held [33 C.C.L.T. 161 at p. 176]:

> The matter upon which the defendant commented, conduct of a Corrections officer in purchasing products manufactured by an inmate and making a profit on their sale and that this was an abuse of the inmate's labour, was clearly a matter of public interest.

Secondly, the learned trial judge held [at p. 177]:

> Robinson did not refer to the plaintiff's denying that he made a profit and to Li being content with what he received for the chin rests in the news conference and TV broadcast. Nevertheless I concluded that Robinson honestly believed that Li's labour was being abused and that Parlett was making a profit from his labour.

Next, the learned trial judge held [at p. 178]:

> I accept the defendant's evidence that his purpose was to focus attention on what he considered to be abuse by Corrections Staff of inmates' labour and the absence of any controls over such situations
>
> In order for the plaintiff's counsel's submission to succeed, I must find that Robinson's predominant purpose was something other than to publicize what he considered to be the plaintiff's abuse of an inmate's labour. I find that he made these statements publicly because he had an honest belief in them. His eagerness to go to the media was consistent with his wish to expose what he thought was an abuse. I am unable to find that he did so in order to enhance his own reputation by producing a sensational story rather than drawing attention to what he thought was wrong. I reject the submission that he was actuated by any improper motive and was guilty of malice.

However, the learned trial judge rejected the defence of qualified privilege. He made reference to the decision of the Supreme Court of Canada in *Jones* v. *Bennett* (1968), 2 D.L.R. (3d) 291, [1969] S.C.R. 277, 66 W.W.R. 419, and held [at p. 181]:

> In my opinion the statements made by the defendant at the news conference and on the TV broadcast were made "to the world". For these reasons the defence of qualified privilege is not available to the defendant. Accordingly, the action for libel succeeds.

On the appeal, counsel for the plaintiff contended that with respect to this ground of appeal, the issue was whether or not the publication was, in the circumstances, too broad. In *Arnott v. College of Physicians & Surgeons of*

Saskatchewan, [1955] 1 D.L.R. 1, [1954] S.C.R. 538, Estey, J. discussed the defence of qualified privilege. He said at p. 7 (D.L.R.):

> The defence of qualified privilege is fully discussed in *Halls v. Mitchell*, [1928] 2 D.L.R. 97 at pp. 102-3, S.C.R. 125 at p. 133, where, after referring to certain of the English authorities, Duff, J., speaking for the majority of this Court, stated: "The defamatory statement, therefore, is only protected when it is fairly warranted by some reasonable occasion or exigency, and when it is fairly made in discharge of some public or private duty, or in the conduct of the defendant's own affairs in matters in which his interests are concerned. The privilege rests not upon the interests of the persons entitled to invoke it, but upon the general interests of society, and protects only communications '*fairly* made' (the italics are those of Parke, B. himself) in the legitimate defence of a person's own interests, or plainly made under a sense of duty, such as would be recognized by "people of ordinary intelligence and moral principles."
>
> Lindley, L.J., speaking with respect to the duty, stated as follows: "I take moral or social duty to mean a duty recognized by English people of ordinary intelligence and moral principle, but at the same time not a duty enforceable by legal proceedings, whether civil or criminal": *Stuart v. Bell*, [1891] 2 Q.B. 341 at p. 350.

The defendant contends that, as a Member of Parliament, having received a communication from a constituent suggesting impropriety on the part of the plaintiff as an official in the employ of the Correctional Service of Canada, he was under a duty to communicate with the appropriate minister and that when he failed to persuade the Minister to investigate the matter by way of a public inquiry to then take steps which would result in exerting sufficient public pressure upon the Minister to persuade him to order such an inquiry.

R. v. Rule, [1937] 2 K.B. 375, was a case where the appellant had written to the Member of Parliament for his constituency two letters containing defamatory statements about a police officer and a justice of the peace for the place where he lived. He was charged with publishing defamatory libels. He pleaded that the libels were published on a privileged occasion. The trial judge ruled that the occasion was not privileged and the appellant had accordingly been convicted. In the Court of Criminal Appeal, Lord Hewart, C.J. said at p. 380:

> The discussion has covered a wide field, but it will not be necessary for this Court to express any opinion as to the rights and dudes generally of Members of Parliament. It is sufficient for the purpose of this case to say that in our judgment a Member of Parliament to whom a written communication is addressed by one of his constituents asking for his assistance in bringing to the notice of the appropriate Minister a complaint of improper conduct on the part of some public official acting in that constituency in relation to his office, has sufficient interest in the subject-matter of the complaint to render the occasion of such publication a privileged occasion. When once it is seen that a decision favourable to the appellant requires not more than this limited assertion of the interest of a Member of Parliament in the welfare of his constituents, it appears to us impossible to resist the conclusion that the conviction cannot be supported.

That passage was cited with approval by Geoffrey Lane, J. (as he then was) in *Beech et al. v. Freeson*, [1972] 1 Q.B. 14. In that case the defendant, a Member of Parliament, wrote a letter to the Law Society and an identical one to the Lord Chancellor, saying that he had been specifically requested by a constituent to refer the plaintiffs' solicitors firm to the Law Society for investigation. He set out the constituent's complaints and stated that contrary to his usual practice he had complied with the request because he had received complaints from other constituents in the past concerning the plaintiffs' firm. The plaintiffs brought action against him for libel. The defendant contended that the publication was on an occasion of qualified privilege. The plaintiffs denied the existence of a privilege and replied that in any event the defendant was actuated by express malice. That submission was rejected. It was held that such complaints made by a Member of Parliament to the Law Society at the behest of a constituent, acting as the constituent's agent to make the complaint, are made on an occasion of qualified privilege.

Geoffrey Lane, J. stated at p. 24:

> The judge must, accordingly, do his best in the light of such evidence as he has, coupled with his own views as to what the defendant's duties, moral or social, were in the circumstances. Doing the best I can on those principles, it seems to me that it certainly was incumbent upon the defendant to inform the Law Society of his previous experiences through his constituents of this particular firm. As appears from the letters of Mr. Leach at the Law Society, to which I need not make a detailed reference, the Law Society is concerned to determine, amongst other things, whether a complaint is an isolated incident of casual negligence or is part of a course of conduct likely to bring the profession into disrepute if it is allowed to continue. Although the defendant may have only imperfectly realised that fact, if indeed he realised it at all, nevertheless his instinct to write as he did was a proper one. Even if the defendant had simply reiterated to the Law Society the complaints of Mr. Gold and had added nothing of his own, knowing that at the same time Mr. Gold was, himself, complaining to the Law Society, privilege would, I think, attach to such communication. That, however, is not the question here. He did have something to add which he genuinely believed to be worthy of investigation and he would have been falling short in his duty to his constituent and, indeed, his duty to the public, if he had not written in the manner in which he did. It will be a sad day when a Member of Parliament has to look over his shoulder before ventilating, to the proper authority, criticisms about the work of a public servant or a professional man who is holding himself out in practice for the benefit of the public which he honestly believes to merit investigation.

When the defendant communicated with the Solicitor General. the plaintiff contended, he had performed his duty and he was not thereafter entitled to hold a press conference or appear on a television programme to ventilate his concerns to the electorate when the Solicitor General had declined to order a public inquiry. Further, the plaintiff contended, the defendant could have raised the matter during question period in the House of Commons. In these circumstances, the plaintiff contended, no privilege should be held to attach to the course of conduct chosen by the defendant to ventilate his concerns.

At trial the defendant responded to the suggestion that he could have raised the matter during question period in the House of Commons by answering that in his judgment that would not have been an effective way to communicate his concerns to the public and it was only if there was a public demand for an inquiry that the Solicitor General would take steps to order such an inquiry.

As I have indicated, the defendant is the official spokesperson for his party on the Ministry of the Solicitor General. In my opinion, the course he followed up to December 11, 1981, in seeking to persuade the Minister to order a public inquiry into the matter was an entirely proper course for him to follow. When he failed to persuade the Minister to order the inquiry, if he held an honest belief that there had been impropriety within the Correctional Service with respect to taking advantage of the work of inmates, then it was the duty of the defendant to ventilate his concerns in a way that would persuade the Minister to have an investigation conducted into the matter.

In addition to the duty of the defendant to declare his concern in this matter, it appears to me that the electorate in Canada have an interest in knowing whether the administration of the Correctional Service is being properly conducted by the officials in the Department of the Solicitor General.

Thus we come to the issue framed by the plaintiff in this appeal, namely, whether or not the publication was too broad in the circumstances.

...

The learned trial judge quoted [from *Stopforth v. Goyer*] in his reasons for judgment and observed that the Ontario Court of Appeal did not cite any authority for its statement. Then the learned trial judge continued [at p. 180]:

> In my opinion the *Stopforth* case is concerned with the very special circumstances of a Minister repeating the precise statement he had made inside the House of Commons to the media immediately upon leaving the House of Commons. At p. 179 Jessop [sic], J.A. noted that the fact that the respondent was named in the House would create the interest of the electorate and invoke the corresponding interest of the appellant to satisfy that created interest. Those circumstances or similar circumstances do not prevail in the case at Bar.

In my respectful opinion, the learned trial judge erred in seeking to distinguish the decision in *Stopforth* on so narrow a basis. I fail to appreciate why a statement would enjoy qualified privilege when made to the media first. The statement was made in the House of Commons where it would enjoy an absolute privilege. It is not the making of the statement in the House of Commons that creates the interest of the electorate but rather the subject-matter of the statement. Thus if the Member of Parliament has a duty to ventilate the subject-matter and the electorate has an interest in knowing of the matter, then the only remaining question is whether or not, in the circumstances the publication "to the world" was too broad.

In my opinion, the statements to the media and on the television programme which were reported in newspapers and through the media cannot be said to have been unduly wide. That is because the group that had a *bona fide* interest in the matter was the electorate in Canada. Hence the privilege was not lost.

For these reasons, I would allow the appeal and dismiss the action.

Appeal allowed; plaintiff's action dismissed.

5.2.3.3.3.3.5 *Camporese v. Parton* (1983), 150 D.L.R. (3d) 208 (B.C.S.C.)

WALLACE, J.: This is a libel action. The plaintiffs allege that an article written by the defendant Parton exposed them to the hatred and contempt of the public and of their business associates and injured them in their trade. They claim damages.

. . . . .

Mrs. Parton then called Mr. Camporese. She did not identify herself but rather posed as a consumer. She said she had seen the advertisement and inquired whether there were lids available and if they were Metro lids. He acknowledged they were Metro lids. She then asked him why he was selling the lids through an advertisement. Mr. Camporese said that there was too much red tape; the stores rip you off. She inquired: "Do they seal well?", to which he replied, "Yes". She then identified herself and asked him why he was selling the lids in this manner. Mr. Camporese became very emotional and said he would go "belly up" if he did not sell them; that he could not afford a $60,000 loss. She formed the opinion he was attempting to dump a defective product, at a cut-rate price, without drawing attention to the public that they were Metro lids. Mr. Camporese said the lids he was selling were different from the lids that had been tested by C.A.C. and he pleaded with her to test the lids. Mrs. Parton construed this as a "stalling tactic" commonly used by a person in Mr. Camporese's position.

Mrs. Parton then began to telephone resource people to ascertain the consequences of canning with faulty lids. It was getting late in the afternoon and her usual reference sources had left their offices. She called a former acquaintance, Donna Aldous, at Kelowna. Mrs. Aldous had been a home economist for Environment Canada whom Mrs. Parton had previously consulted. As a consequence of Mrs. Aldous' advice that faulty seals could result in the formation of the deadly toxin clostridium botulinum, Mrs. Parton considered the story had changed from one which concerned possible food spoilage to one which concerned possible death if the public used defective canning lids. The news value of this latter viewpoint was obviously of great import. Accordingly, she wrote the column in a different manner, deleting reference to the first person, putting the strongest facts first and a "kicker" at the close of the article.

Mrs. Parton acceded her knowledge of botulism was superficial but she felt she could safely consult with Donna Aldous and rely upon her opinion in view of her professional training and experience, being a home economist for Environment Canada.

The newspaper deadline for filing the story was early evening. Mrs. Parton said she considered that the interest of the public in immediately receiving the information outweighed the interest of Mr. Camporese in her withholding it until further checks could be made. She considered further testing would take some weeks and it was already close to the end of the canning season. She was aware of many consumers who had lost hundreds of dollars of food as a result of using the defective lids and now she had been advised by Mrs. Aldous, a home economist, that botulism was a concern where faulty lids were involved in that clostridium botulinum spores could enter a jar with a leaky lid and then germinate and produce a deadly toxin. Accordingly, she decided there was an urgency that the article be published immediately. She filed it that evening for publication on the city side of the paper next day. Her admitted purpose in so doing was to alert consumers to what she conceived to be a potential danger associated with using canning lids that failed to seal and to stop Mr. Camporese from selling the Metro lids.

While Mrs. Parton did not write the headline for the article — "Importer Pushes Canning Lids That Could Spell Death" — she considered it to be appropriate, pointing out that the purpose of the headline was to get people to read the article; presumably its accuracy as reflecting the thrust of the article being of secondary significance.

My impression of Mrs. Parton, formed from my observation of her responses to questions put to her by counsel, is that of an intelligent, opinionated person, who continually argued her case in a most biased way, directed to justifying her failure to research the article with greater care before rushing it to publication. Her statement, that: "No reporter should take into account the suffering or impact upon the parties" who are the subject of her columns, perhaps explained her haste in publishing the article with a paucity of accurate information about such an emotional and frightening subject-matter — well aware that the article could cause the plaintiffs some $60,000 loss as well as the censure of the business community and the public generally.

To write and publish an article on a matter of such public importance based solely upon a short impromptu comment made by Mrs. Aldous in the course of a telephone conversation and without questioning its accuracy, in my opinion, is reporting of a careless and reckless nature. Certainly Mrs. Aldous' comment raised concern and justified an immediate in-depth investigation into its accuracy and a complete report to the public of what such investigation revealed. It did not, in my opinion, justify immediately publishing the comment directed solely to Mr. Camporese and the canning lids he was selling. I must state, however, that I find Mrs. Parton accepted Mrs. Aldous' comments as accurate and held an honest belief that they were true at the time she wrote the article and caused it to be published.

(f) Consequence of the Publication

As a result of the article, the public and members of the business community with whom Mr. Camporese dealt, reacted adversely, refusing to do further business with him. There is no doubt that as a result of the article he lost the respect of those persons who would normally be trading with him and his companies. I find, however, that the failure of Mr. Camporese to sell the canning lids in 1977 and thereafter was, in the main, due to the critical report of the C.A.C. and the complaints filed with "Action Line", compounded by the fact that the market was fully supplied by known brand lids in 1977. Accordingly, I find the plaintiffs have not established the loss, due to the failure to sell the canning lids, was attributable to the *Province* article of August 25, 1977.

(g) Can Defective Seals on Canning lids Result in the Formation of Clostridium Botulinum Toxin in the Jars of Home-Canned Produce?

The plaintiffs called the following experts: Dr. Skura, an expert in the field of food services, a microbiologist with the Department of Food Science at the University of British Columbia; Mr. Shkurhan, a lecturer of microbiology in the Department of Basic Health Services at the British Columbia Institute of Technology; Dr. Zottola, Professor of Food Microbiology at the Department of Food Science and Nutrition at the University of Minnesota, a man of wide experience with home canning problems; Dr. E.J. Bowman, a retired microbiologist who had an impressive background of experience in research related to clostridium botulinum studies.

The defendant called Dr,. J. J. R. Campbell, bacteriologist and Professor of Microbiology at the University of British Columbia.

All these eminent gentlemen agreed on many aspects of clostridium bolutinum such as; it is one of the most toxic bacteria known the man — one gram could kill 500,000,000 people; the toxin affects the nervous system and produces asphyxiation; it will not grow in the presence of oxygen; it is a microscopic organism whose habitat is soil dust and marine environments; the spore, given the right conditions, can germinate and grow into an active cell at which time the toxin develops and accumulates in the cell; active growing cells can be killed by heat, salt, curing, etc.; the spore will not germinate in a high acid environment — pH below 4.6; it is one of the most heat-resistant spores known and hence has to be exposed to high temperatures for a prolonged period best accomplished by processing the jars in a pressure-cooker.

The experts also agree there has been no recorded case of a botulinum spore being aspirated into a home-canned jar, by reason of a leaky lid, with death or illness resulting. On this issue home canning cannot be compared to commercial canning; they are quite different processes. Most cases of botulinum contamination of home-canned produce have been attributed to insufficient heat treatment of the produce during the canning process. No research has been conducted to determine the number, if any, of botulinum spores that are airborne in the atmosphere in British Columbia. Furthermore, there is no scientific data available, or research done, to determine whether a botulinum spore aspirated into a home-canning jar could find an anaerobic condition which would permit it to grow and produce toxin. It must be kept in mind that in most investigations of the presence of clostridium botulinum bacteria in home-canned produce the lid has been removed so that it is impossible to say, with exactitude, whether the active spores were there because of inadequate heat treatment during canning process or whether they were aspirated into the jar after proper canning procedures had been carried out.

Generally speaking the issue upon which the experts differ is as to the probability of a botulinum spore being aspirated into a jar of food as a result of a leaky lid.

Dr. Campbell expresses the opinion that in the cooling process air will be drawn into jars through a faulty seal and such air could contain dust particles carrying botulinum spores. On storage the spores could germinate, grow and form toxin which if ingested by people may be fatal. Dr. Bowers considers this to be an over-statement of the probabilities but would accept the statement if the word "might" replaced the word "could" in the passage. Dr. Zottola takes issue with Dr. Campbell's report and finds it difficult to envisage that air leaking into a jar would encourage growth of an anaerobic bacteria and he considers that transportation of botulinum spores through the air is virtually impossible. He points out that none of the scientific literature suggests that leaking canning lids could be a cause of clostridium botulinum contamination of home-canned produce and he states that, while anything is possible, such an eventuality is highly unlikely.

In view of the complete absence of any scientific data demonstrating contamination of home-canned produce by clostridium botulinum aspirating into the jars as a result of leaky lids, I can only conclude this hypothesis to be completely speculative and I accept Dr. Zottola's opinion that while "anything is possible, this result is highly improbable".

Summarizing this lengthy review of the evidence I find:

1. That the "gist" or "sting" of the article was that the plaintiffs were allegedly attempting to sell canning lids to the public that could cause death;
2. That the article defamed the plaintiffs, Camporese and the associated company C.F.B. Trading Co. Ltd., in the way of their trade. No mention was made in the article of C. K. & G. Management Ltd. and A. & A. Food Importers and the readers would not consider the article referred to those two companies;
3. That the plaintiff sought the assistance of the media, in particular the Province newspaper and the Ministry of Consumer Services, to assist him in the marketing of Metro lids imported from Taiwan;
4. That the lids were defective in that many buckled and failed to seal when used under pressure for home-canning purposes;
5. That the consumer complaints about the inadequacy of the lids, the C.A.C. testing which demonstrated their inadequacy, and the increased availability of brand-name lids, resulted in the loss of any potential market for Metro lids in 1977 and 1978. The plaintiffs have not established that the article of August 25, 1977, contributed to that loss of market for the Metro lids;
6. That Nicole Parton wrote the article of August 25, 1977, without adequate research into the accuracy of the opinion expressed therein concerning the possibility of contamination of the canned foods by the ingestion of clostridium botulinum spores through leaking lids with the consequent possibility of their causing death;

7. That Nicole Parton honestly believed the opinions and facts set forth in the article;
8. That while contamination of home-canned produce by clostridium botulinum through leaky canning lids is a hypothesis which is theoretically possible, it is highly unlikely or improbable. There is no scientific data or research supporting such an occurrence;
9. That the article of August 25, 1977, did not reflect the improbable aspect of food contamination resulting from leaky canning lids and did imply that Mr. Camporese was "pushing" the sale of defective lids in order to avoid economic loss and that, in so doing, he was completely indifferent to the health hazard he was creating for the unsuspecting consumer.

Defamation of the Plaintiff

I have previously found that the article of August 25, 1977, and, in particular, the headline "Importer Pushes Canning Lids That Could Cause Death", was defamatory of Mr. Camporese and C.F.B. Trading Co. Ltd. in the way of their trade in that it would and did diminish the esteem, respect, goodwill and confidence in which they were held by their business associates and members of the public.

Qualified Privilege

The applicable legal principle has been succinctly expressed by *Gatley on Libel and Slander*, 8th ed. (1981), pp. 239-40, para. 562, in these words:

> The publication of defamatory matter in a newspaper will be privileged where the matter published is of general public interest and it is the duty of the defendant to communicate it to the general public. If the matter is a matter of public interest, and the party who publishes it owes a duty to communicate it to the general public, the publication is privileged.

See also *Banks v. Globe & Mail Ltd. et al.* (1961), 28 D.L.R. (2d) 343 at pp. 349-50, [1961] S.C.R. 474 at pp. 482-3.

It is self-evident that the matter of possible food contamination of home-canned produce by clostridium botulinum spores entering the jars through leaking canning lids was of vital concern to the general public of British Columbia. The question to be answered is whether the defendants stood in such a relationship to their readers in the circumstances that prevailed that it imposed upon them a duty to communicate to their readers the facts and opinions contained in the August 25, 1977 article.

In the circumstances I find that Mrs. Parton, her publishers and the readers had a legitimate common interest in the adequacy and performance characteristics of the Metro lids being sold by Mr. Camporese. The particular circumstances purportedly giving rise to a special duty on the part of the defendants to communicate Mrs. Parton's opinions to those who read the Province were:

(a) that she had originally, upon the importuning of Mr. Camporese, written a column commending his canning lids to her readers;
(b) that she had advised her readers of the C.A.C. test indicating the inadequacy of the Metro canning lids and of Mr. Camporese's response to that testing;
(c) that she had become aware of the complaints of home canners contained in their correspondence with "Action Line";
(d) that Mr. Camporese actually sought and obtained the support of the media and the Ministry of Consumer Services in the marketing of Metro canning lids;
(e) that she concluded, upon reasonable grounds, that Mr. Camporese was trying to unload at cut-rate prices, upon an unsuspecting public, canning lids which he knew to be inadequate and he was seeking to do this through the channel of private advertiscments;
(f) that she honestly believed the sale of such defective lids could result in clostridium botulinum contamination.

In my view, having at the plaintiffs' behest written a column commending the Metro lids to her reading public, it was Mrs. Parton's duty, upon becoming aware of any adverse characteristic of the Metro lids, to communicate such information to her readers.

Malice

This occasion of privilege entitling the defendants to write what would be libelous if written by others is qualified and may be lost by the plaintiffs adducing evidence establishing, on a balance of probabilities, express malice on the part of the defendants. That is, it is for the plaintiffs to establish that the defendants have abused the occasion by using it for an improper purpose, personal spite or ill will, or by excessive or irrelevant publication, or by a lack of belief in the truth of what was written.

I have found that Nicole Parton honestly believed the facts and opinions expressed in the article of August 25, 1977, to be true. Counsel for the plaintiffs contends, however, that an honest belief is not sufficient by itself to negative a finding of express malice and asserts that the defendants misused the occasion and exceeded the privilege. He points to the reckless manner in which the article was researched and written by Mrs. Parton; the lack of adequate inquiry into, or verification of, the accuracy of such an emotional and contentious subject-matter; the rush to make a deadline because of the newsworthy aspect of the subject-matter; the complete lack of concern over the consequences of the publication, economic or otherwise, upon the plaintiffs and the avowed objective of stopping the sale of Metro lids by Mr. Camporese. All of this, counsel submits, demonstrates that Mrs. Parton wrote the article recklessly, not caring whether it was true or false, and, accordingly, misused the occasion and lost the benefit of any privilege which the occasion would have otherwise provided.

I consider the remarks of Lord Diplock in *Horrocks v. Lowe*, [1975] A.C. 135, to be most pertinent to this submission. He stated at p. 150:

> Apart from those exceptional cases, what is required on the part of the defamer to entitle him to the protection of the privilege is positive belief in the truth of what he published or, as it is generally though tautologously termed "honest belief." If he publishes untrue defamatory matter recklessly, without considering or caring whether it be true or not, he is in this, as in other branches of the law, treated as if he knew it to be false. But indifference to the truth of what he publishes is not to be equated with carelessness, impulsiveness or irrationality in arriving at a positive belief that it is true. The freedom of speech protected by the law of qualified privilege may be availed of by all sorts and conditions of men. In affording to them immunity from suit if they have acted in good faith in compliance with a legal or moral duty or in protection of a legitimate interest the law must take them as it finds them. In ordinary life it is rare indeed for people to form their beliefs by a process of logical deduction from facts ascertained by a rigorous search for all available evidence and a judicious assessment of its probative value. In greater or in less degree according to their temperaments, their training, their intelligence, they are swayed by prejudice, rely on intuition instead of reasoning, leap to conclusions on inadequate evidence and fail to recognise the cogency of material which might cast doubt on the validity of the conclusions they reach. But despite the imperfection of the mental process by which the belief is arrived at it may still be "honest," that is, a positive belief that the conclusions they have reached are true. The law demands no more.

While I have found Mrs. Parton wrote the article of August 25, 1977, without adequate research and with untimely haste in the circumstances, I do not consider this conduct was so unreasonable as to displace or rebut Mrs. Parton's honest belief in the subject-matter of the article or to vary the primary purpose for which she wrote the article, that is, to inform her readers of her concern for the risks, including botulism poisoning, which she believed were associated with the use of defective Metro canning lids. Accordingly, I find that the plaintiffs have failed to prove the privileged occasion upon which the article was published was abused by the defendants in a manner which would constitute "express malice" and so destroy the privilege. I find that the defendants are entitled to the protection of the privilege.

In light of the conclusion I have reached on this issue it is preferable that I do not rule on the other issues raised by the defendants. The plaintiffs' claim must be dismissed with costs payable to the defendants.

Note: See also *Wooding v. Little* (1982), 24 C.C.L.T. 37

5.2.3.3.3.3.6 *Hill v. Church of Scientology of Toronto* 1994, unreported (Ont. C.A.)

GRIFFITHS, CATZMAN and GALLIGAN, JJ.A.: At the press conference, Scientology and Morris Manning identified Casey Hill as a Crown counsel and alleged that he was guilty of contempt of court meriting his imprisonment or punishment by way of a fine. The essence of their false allegations was that he participated in the misleading of Sirois J. and that he participated in or aided and abetted others in the opening and inspection of documents which, to his knowledge, had been ordered sealed by Osler, J.

As we noted earlier, segments of the press conference were shown on the evening news reports of two major Toronto television stations. Morris Manning, in an interview with a reporter representing CFTO-TV who specifically identified Casey Hill as one of the perpetrators of the contempt, said:

> The documents were ordered sealed by Mr. Justice Osler, pursuant to a request by counsel, in a very serious matter, and they were opened and revealed to persons whom we say were unauthorized to do so.

Morris Manning was also shown on the CBC-TV news and there he said:

> They were confidential documents which have been ordered sealed by Supreme Court of Ontario justices which were opened with permission of counsel for the Crown. And this constitutes, in the opinion of the Church, a contempt of court ... this is a very important matter. It's important to the administration of justice.

We repeat that on September 18, 1984 the *Globe and Mail* reported the following:

> The Church of Scientology of Toronto is asking the Supreme Court of Ontario to find a Crown prosecutor and a lawyer with the Ontario Ministry of Consumer and Commercial Relations in contempt of court.
>
> Morris Manning, a lawyer acting for the church, said in an interview yesterday that he has filed a motion asking for S. Casey Hill, a prosecutor with the Ontario Ministry of the Attorney-General, and Jerome Cooper, a lawyer with the Consumer Ministry, to be jailed or fined.
>
> The motion claims that Mr. Cooper misled Mr. Justice Jean-Charles Sirois of the Supreme Court of Ontario into releasing to the Consumer Ministry documents seized by the Ontario Provincial Police in a raid on the church's headquarters.
>
> The motion says Judge Sirois was not told that many of the documents had been ordered sealed by another Ontario Supreme Court judge while the church contests the legality of the search warrant used by the O.P.P. in the raid last year.
>
> The motion claims Mr. Hill, who represented the Attorney-General during the search warrant hearings, "aided and abetted in the misleading of Mr. Justice Sirois."

Some debate took place at trial about whether the contempt alleged by Scientology and Morris Manning was a civil contempt or a criminal contempt. It is not necessary to resolve that question although Cromarty, J. found it to be a criminal contempt. What matters is the impression their words would create upon members of the public. Scientology and Morris Manning suggested that Casey Hill's conduct called for his imprisonment or fining. They also accused him of aiding and abetting others in very serious misconduct. The use of words which are almost exlusively found in the criminal law coupled with the suggestion that his misconduct called for his punishment by imprisonment or fine leads inescapably to the conclusion that members of the public would conclude that Casey Hill was being accused of misconduct which was criminal in nature. The false statement in this case attacked Casey Hill as a person without integrity who would act criminally in the performance of the duties conferred upon him by the

Crown. The false statements can be seen as little short of allegations of a criminal breach of trust.

. . . . .

In this case, everything possible was done to add credibility to the false accusations, and to publish these accusations as widely as possible. There was evidence from which the jury was entitled to infer that a press conference at which Casey Hill would be charged with contempt was planned even before Scientology retained Morris Manning as an outside counsel. Earl Smith, the president of Scientology, made contact with the Toronto television stations and newspapers. He told them that the purpose of the press conference was to announce that a contempt motion was being launched against Casey Hill. He attended at the press conference and brought several copies of the notice of motion and a written chronology of events prepared by Scientology. Both documents were distributed to the media representatives in attendance. There was a substantial turnout of media representatives but *The Toronto Star* did not send one. After the press conference, he went to the offices of *The Star* and tried to interest it, unsuccessfully as it turned out, in the story.

The evidence suggests that Scientology's efforts to ensure that its false statements gained wide circulation were very successful. The television newscasts were seen by approximately one-quarter of a million people. Approximately 108,000 copies of the issue of the *Globe and Mail* were circulated. Scientology succeeded in seeing to it that the libel was spread as widely as possible.

The press conference was held in circumstances calculated to give the allegations made against Casey Hill the greatest credibility possible. The event took place outside the main entrance to Osgoode Hall, which is a building with symbolic importance because it houses the highest courts in the province as well as the governing body of the legal profession. It is a dramatic setting in which to attack a lawyer's integrity and to allege that he failed to observe the duties he owed to those courts of which he is an officer.

Scientology wanted Morris Manning to be present at the press conference and arranged for him to be there. Morris Manning is a prominent lawyer and would be expected to add credence to assertions made by Scientology. As it happened, Morris Manning was engaged in a case before the Court of Appeal that day. He attended the press conference in the gown which he had worn while appearing in court.

It is hard to envisage a scene more likely to impress upon observers the importance and credibility of the allegations being made against Casey Hill. They were made by a prominent lawyer wearing his court gown while standing at the front door of Osgoode Hall. The whole performance was calculated to engender in the minds of those who learned of the allegations that they were very serious and entirely credible. The jury would have been fully justified in concluding that there must have been many persons who, learning of the allegations in those circumstances, would believe them and that, therefore, to use the words of Esson

J. in *Vogel, supra,* "the stigma so unfairly created will always be with the plaintiff."

The publication of this libel was clearly intended to injure Casey Hill as much as it possibly could. The circumstances of its publication admit of no other conclusion. The jury obviously found that great harm was done to his reputation.

. . . . .

... we would not be prepared to sanction the conferral of qualified privilege on a press conference held — for the purpose of disseminating to the public details of a pending legal proceeding — at a time when no document in connection with that legal proceeding had been filed in any court office. Only when the document initiating a proceeding is filed is the party bringing that proceeding publicly committed to its institution. Only then can the formal, public commencement of the proceeding not be precluded by some slip, some mishap, some change of heart, some countermand of instructions. Only then can it even arguably be said that the proceeding has become a matter of public record and the contents of its initiating document a matter of public concern. In the present case, no such document had been filed at the time the press conference was convened, and we would not be prepared to hold that the defence of qualified privilege was available on that occasion.

5.2.3.3.4 Malice

As with the defence of fair comment, if the defendant can show the plaintiff was motivated by malice, the defence of qualified privilege will be lost.

5.2.3.3.4.1 *Shultz v. Porter and Block Brothers Ltd.* (1979), 9 A.R. 381 (Al. S.C.)

WAITE, J.: Assuming, however, that the defence of qualified privilege was found to exist, the evidence taken in its entirety clearly establishes the presence of actual or express malice on the part of the defendant Porter so as to entitle the plaintiff to judgment in any event.

Malice includes not only the general or popular definitions of that word as denoting ill-will or spite. It includes the question of an improper motive by the defendants. Excessive language in itself is insufficient to establish express or actual malice. The term is generally discussed by Lord Diplock in *Horrocks v. Lowe* at pp. 669-70 in the following terms:

> So, the motive with which the defendant on a privileged occasion made a statement defamatory of the plaintiff becomes crucial. The protection might, however, be illusory if the onus lay on him to prove that he was actuated solely by a sense of the relevant duty or a desire to protect the relevant interest. So he is entitled to be protected by the privilege unless some other dominant and improper motive on his part is proved. "Express malice" is the term of art descriptive of such a motive. Broadly speaking, it means malice in the popular sense of a desire to injure the person who is defamed and this is generally the motive which the plaintiff sets out to prove. But to destroy the privilege the desire to injure must be the dominant motive for the defamatory

publication; knowledge that it will have that effect is not enough if the defendant is nevertheless acting in accordance with a sense of duty or in bona fide protection of his own legitimate interests.

The motive with which a person published defamatory matter can only be inferred from what he did or said or knew. If it be proved that he did not believe that what he published was true this is generally conclusive evidence of express malice, for no sense of duty or desire to protect his own legitimate interests can justify a man in telling deliberate and injurious falsehoods about another ...

"... what is required on the part of the defamer to entitle him to the protection of the privilege is positive belief in the truth of what he published or, as it is generally though tautologously termed, 'honest belief'. If he publishes untrue defamatory matter recklessly, without considering or caring whether it be true or not, he is in this, as in other branches of the law, treated as if he knew it to be false. But indifference to the truth of what he publishes is not to be equated with carelessness, impulsiveness or irrationality in arriving at a positive belief that it is true...."

Even a positive belief in the truth of what is published on a privileged occasion — which is presumed unless the contrary is proved — may not be sufficient to negative express malice if it can be proved that the defendant misused the occasion for some purpose other than that for which the privilege is accorded by the law. The commonest case is where the dominant motive which actuates the defendant is not a desire to perform the relevant duty or to protect the relevant interest, but to give vent to his personal spite or ill-will towards the person he defames. If this be proved, then even positive belief in the truth of what is published will not enable the defamer to avail himself of the protection of the privilege to which he would otherwise have been entitled. There may be instances of improper motives which destroy the privilege apart from personal spite. A defendant's dominant motive may have been to obtain some private advantage unconnected with the duty or the interest which constitutes the reason for the privilege. If so, he loses the benefit of the privilege despite his positive belief that what he said or wrote was true ...

Qualified privilege would be illusory, and the public interest that it is meant to serve defeated, if the protection which it affords were lost merely because a person, although acting in compliance with a duty or in protection of a legitimate interest, disliked the person whom he defamed or was indignant at what he believed to be that person's conduct and welcomed the opportunity of exposing it. It is only where his desire to comply with the relevant duty or to protect the relevant interest plays no significant part in his motives for publishing what he believes to. be true that "express malice" can properly be found.

The most recent decision on the question of qualified privilege is the decision of the Supreme Court of Canada in *McLoughlin v. Kutasy* (1979), 8 C.C.L.T. 105, wherein Ritchie, J. on behalf of the majority of the court said in part at pp. 112-13:

... the elements requisite to sustain the defence of qualified privilege are discussed in the case of *Netupsly v. Craig*, [1973] S.C.R. 55 at 61-62, 28 D.L.R. (3d) 742, where the following paragraph occurs in the judgment of this Court:

" 'The determination of this appeal in my opinion, turns on the question of whether there was any extrinsic or intrinsic evidence that the respondents were motivated by malice in writing the letter which is complained of. There can be little doubt that if there is evidence proving that the statements complained of are false to the knowledge of the person who makes tbem, they are taken to have been made maliciously, but this statement must be read in light of the language used by Lord Atkinson in *Adam v. Ward*, [1917] A.C. 309 at p. 339, where he said:

'... a person making a communication on a privileged occasion is not restricted to the use of such language merely as is reasonably necessary to protect the interest or discharge the duty which is the foundation of his privilege; but that, on the contrary, he will be protected. even though his language should be violent or excessively strong, if, having regard to all the circumstances of the case, he might have honestly and on reasonable grounds believed that what he wrote or said was true and necessary for the purpose of his vindication, though in fact it was not so.'

The plaintiff has affirmatively established actual or express malice. There can be no doubt that the statements complained of by the plaintiff were false to the knowledge of Porter. I am satisfied on a consideration of all of the evidence that Porter did not — indeed, could not — honestly believe that the plaintiff had been guilty of misrepresentation. I am satisfied that Porter was motivated by a dishonest, impropr or wrong motive, being the protection of himself and his principals against the consequences of what was clearly a negligent breach of duty by the defendants to their own client, Feltham. The offending letter of 22nd June was a calculated attempt to extricate the vendor from a transaction that was improvident and that had been entered into in such circumstances as would have entitled the vendor to an appropriate action for damages against the defendants.

5.2.3.3.4.2 *Farrell v. St. John's Publishing Co.* (1986), 58 Nfld. & P.E.I.R. 66 (Nfld. C.A.)

MORGAN, J.A.: The mere publication of defamatory words is presumed to be malicious. In this context, however, malicious, sometimes referred to as malice at law, merely means that the words were published without lawful excuse. For the plaintiff to rely on express malice there must be evidence to establish that the defendant had an improper motive for publishing the words and that the improper motive was the sole or dominant motive (*Horrocks v. Lowe*, [1975] A.C. 135).

In this case the appellants contended that, having satisfied themselves that the police reprt was authentic, they were concerned throughout that no action was being taken to implement that reprt. In this regard, the trial judge made contradictory findings. He stated:

> Mr. Herder's evidence confirms my conclusion and the evasive manner in which he answered some of the questions uked him further confirms it, that what really happened in this case was that he and others responsible at *The Evening Telegram* became very concerned at the delay in making a report to the authorities by those investigating the fire and an inordinately long time elapsing before anything was made public regarding the cause of the fire. They suspected that a cover-up was underway by people in high places and that the plaintiff, a former cabinet minister and still a member of the legislature sitting on the government side was being shielded from action being taken; was being protected by higherups. Mr. Herder admitted in his evidence that he did indeed have such concerns, and even if he had not admitted such, the evidence would inevitably lead me to that conclusion.

Later, in his judgment, however! the trial judge stated:

> I am not suggesting that Mr. Herder had some particular spite against the plaintiff or any underhanded motive for the actions taken in this matter. Rather, he operated from what must have been, in his opinion, the loftiest of motives, that being to see that the plaintiff be punished for his crime. If he were to be protected by people in high places from prosecution for his crime, then *The Evening Telegram* would see to it that he was tried in the court of public opinion. His rights as a citizen of this country were not important; *The Evening Telegram* found him guilty.

The first conclusion reached by the trial judge (supra) was that the appellants published the police reports out of concern over the government's delay in investigating the cause of the fire and their suspicion of a cover-up. That, in my view, is not an improper motive. His second conclusion appears to be that the appellants were motivated solely by a desire to injure the respondent, notwithstanding that he had prefaced his remarks by stating that "he was not suggesting that Mr. Herder had some particular spite against the plaintiff or any underhanded motive for the actions taken in this matter". If Mr. Herder had no personal spite against the respondent nor any underhanded motive for his actions, how can it be said that he was conducting a personal vendetta against the respondent? In my view, the evidence is not supportive of the trial judge's second conclusion and, with respect, it cannot be accepted as evidencing an improper motive.

It is well-established that the failure to apologize combined with a persistence in a plea of justification are not necessarily evidence of malice. In this regard I adopt the following statement of Sellars, L.J., in *Broadway Approvals Ltd. v. Odhams Press Ltd.*, [1965] 2 All E.R. 523, at 533:

> The failure to apologize or retract and persistence in a plea of justification are in themselves not evidence of malice. They may be in certain circumstances, but more frequently they would show sincerity and belief in what had been said and establish the best reason for the publication. (See also *Horrock v. Lowe, supra*, at 154.)

There may be cases where, after publication, a defendant obtains proof that what he said was untrue. In such circumstances a failure to retract a serious charge may provide evidence that at the time of the original publication, he was actuated by malice.

It should be noted that, in February 1979, the appellants published a report of Magistrate LeClair's reasons for dismissing the charge of arson brought against the respondent. That report was headed "Magistrate outlines why arson charge dismissed" with a sub-head of even greater prominence *"Evidence was 'virtually worthless' "*. Contrary to the submission of counsel for the respondent that that report was in itself defamatory of the respondent, I am of the opinion that it contained a fair summary of the magistrate's reasons for dismissing the charge against the respondent and would leave no doubt in the mind of right-thinking members of society that the crime of arson had not been established, which was the underlying reason for dismissal of the charge. The report also contained the magistrate's criticism of the media for publishing the police report, including his observation that "the coverage of the report by the news media gave credence to the assumption of guilt". Any injury to the respondent's reputation occasioned by the earlier publication would, in my view, have been ameliorated by that publication. That is not to say that the appellants did not owe the plaintiff an apology for the injury to his reputation by the unwarranted publication of the police report. A proper apology is almost certain to reduce the injury to the plaintiff's feelings and may well lessen the damages to his reputation. An absence of apology in this case, however, is at best tenuous evidence of malice, but may properly be considered in aggravation of damages.

The mere fact that a defendant has placed a plea of justification on the record is not in itself evidence of malice even though he does not attempt to establish it at the trial. Furthermore, if a defendant has raised a plea of fair comment, the mere fact that he has also raised a plea of justification cannot be used as evidence of malice to destroy the defence. That defence, if proper, can only be destroyed by proof of malice. (*Gatley, Libel and Slander* (7th Ed.), para. 1264).

The defence of justification is, of course, a dangerous one, for an unsuccessful attempt to establish it may be treated as an aggravation of the original injury. If the plea is made recklessly and the defendant persists at the trial in an imputation that he knows to be unfounded or cross-examines the plaintiff with a view to showing that he is guilty of that of which he has been acquitted, malice can properly be inferred. There was no such conduct in the case at bar.

The appellants pleaded justification for the sole purpose of establishing the authenticity of the police report published by them and that their reproduction of that report was fair and accurate. The fact that such proof would not avail them as a defence to libel does not make the placing of the plea on the record a malicious act and form the basis of retributive damages.

An honest belief in the truth of the statement published is not to be held malicious merely because the defendant was hasty in reaching that conclusion. In determining whether such honest belief did in fact exist in a given case, the trial judge, or a jury as the case may be, is entitled to take into consideration the ground on which it is founded. "The ground upon which an honest belief was founded is a most important test of its reality" (*Derry v. Peek* (1889),14 App. Cas. 369).

In this case the trial judge appears to have accepted the appellants' belief in the truthfulness of the police report but, for some undisclosed reason, he seems to find that it was not an honest belief und hence it was malicious. With respect, he should have directed his mind to the established fact that the publication, on which the libel action was based, was the reproduction of a genuine police report that resulted from their investigation into the cause of the fire. That report, as the evidence disclosed, was based on the honest belief of the investigating officers. Furthermore, as a result of that report, the respondent was subsequently charged with arson. How then can malice be imputed to the appellants for believing its contents?

The trial judge also found that malice was to be imputed by reason of the appellants' failure to disclose the source of the police reports.

The source of the alleged defamatory statement was the police reports as disclosed in the publications complained of. How that report came into the hands of the appellants was, in my view, totally irrelevant to the issue before the trial judge.

It will be a matter of aggravation if the defendant has persistently and deliberately given publicity to the defamation complained of. Whether or not malice will be inferred from such conduct, however, will depend on the defendant's motive for repeating the libel. In this case I accept the trial judge's finding that the appellants' motive for publishing the defamatory statement and hence its republication, was their concern over the delay on the part of the authorities in pursuing the investigation into the cause of the fire. That motive, in my view, is not indicative of malice. Continued repetition is of course an aggravating factor.

The trial judge appears to have dealt with the issues raised as though the appellants were the originators, and not just repeaters, of the statement found to be defamatory. The offence committed by the appellants was in publishing a confidential police report in which the investigating officers had expressed the opinion, for the reasons given by them, that a fire in the respondent's apartment had been deliberately set and that it had been set by the respondent. As I have already stated, the fact that the appellants were not the authors of the statement, but only published it by way of repetition, is no defence to an action of libel. It is, however, a factor to be taken into consideration when assessing damages, as evidence of the appellant's state of mind, which is always material to the question of damages. It is a somewhat less malicious act to repeat rather than to originate a defamatory statement.

For all the above reasons, I am of the opinion that the factors, considered by the trial judge as evidencing malice, do not substantiate that conclusion.

5.2.3.3.4.3 *Vogel v. C.B.C.* (1982), 21 C.C.L.T. 105 (B.C.S.C.)

Esson, J.: At trial there was some discussion as to what, if any, significance there is to the adjective "investigative". The CBC witnesses tended to downplay it and to emphasize that all reporters must investigate to some degree. While that may be so, the word connotes a real distinction which was expressed by Mr. Waters who said, "an investigative reporter is simply a reporter who gets stories that nobody wants you to have". The distinction is with the routine business of reporting the events of a given day as set out in press releases, wire reports or as they are observed by a reporter attending, or talking to those who have attended, the fire, accident, city council meeting or whatever other event is the subject of the report.

Another distinguishing feature of investigative reporting is that, when it succeeds, the resulting story is an exclusive — a "scoop". The reporter, by his digging, brings the story to light and he and his paper or station or network get the credit. The potential rewards, in fame and fortune, are great. That is a fact of which we have seen some striking examples in recent years, of which the Watergate matter is perhaps the most famous. It is reasonable to assume that the lesson of that was not lost upon those ambitious to make their mark in the world of news reporting, including some of those responsible for the programmes which are the subject of this action.

. . . . .

A further ground upon which the defence of fair comment must fail is that the allegations were not made in good faith and without malice. There was, on the contrary, express malice.

That is not to say that the defendants were motivated by personal spite or ill will towards the plaintiff. What the law regards as malice is any indirect motive other than a sense of duty: Gatley, op. cit., p. 326. The purported motive of the defendants was to serve the public interest by exposing corruption in high places but the real motive was to enhance their own reputations by producing a sensational programme. Their concern was not as whether the allegations were true or as to whether the public interest was served. It was, rather, to give to allegations of scandal the appearance of truth to the extent necessary to succeed in achieving their goal. That attitude, in law, is malice.

5.2.3.4 Consent

5.2.3.4.1 *Syms v. Warren* (1976), 71 D.L.R. (3d) 558 (Man. Q.B.)

HAMILTON, J .: Plaintiff seeks damages for defamation. The plaintiff is the Chairman of the Manitoba Liquor Control Commission and the Liquor Licensing Board. Defendant Warren is the host of a radio programme and the corporate defendant is the owner of the radio station.

In December, 1974, rumours were circulating among employees of the Liquor Commission, among some members of the press, and presumably in other circles as well, that plaintiff had been charged with impaired driving but had arranged to have the proceedings quashed. There was a suggestion that the rumour was mentioned on the defendants' programme and then refuted by Warren. There is, however, no evidence that this was the source of the rumour and in any event plaintiff does not put the December programme in issue.

On January 15, 1975, Warren telephoned plaintiff, said he had investigated the rumour and was satisfied it was groundless, and asked the plaintiff if he would speak on his radio programme the next morning to deny the alleged charge and cover-up. Plaintiff agreed. Plaintiff had listened to this particular radio programme for a number of years, was aware that it was a programme where Warren expressed opinions on subjects and then discussed them with listeners who telephoned in. Plaintiff was also of the opinion that at times persons appearing on the programme, and even those who refused to appear, were subjected to what he considered to be unfair comment. The next morning, January 16th, as previously arranged, Warren telephoned plaintiff at his residence. While plaintiff was listening Warren gave a resume of the rumours and the allegations against the plaintiff, said that he had investigated and was satisfied the rumours were incorrect. He then asked the plaintiff for his comment and the plaintiff, in an exchange of questions and answers, denied the truth of the allegations. Plaintiff said he felt that at the conclusion of the conversation the topic was closed and that he would hear nothing further. Several minutes later Warren received a telephone call from a woman identified only as "D". He spoke to her off the air and was aware she wished to comment on the interview with plaintiff and I infer Warren was aware she wished to disagree with what the plaintiff had said. The woman then came on the air and said that what the plaintiff had said by way of denial of the rumours was untrue and that she was satisfied from information she had received that the rumours were in fact correct.

Portions of the conversation with the woman are as follows:

> I just heard Frank Syms on the line this morning.
> I'm not dealing with rumors, Madame.
> No, it's not a rumor.
> What's not a rumor?
> About Frank Syms being picked up for drunken driving.
> It is a rumor.
> It's not, it s true.
>
> . . . . .
>
> Well, he does have a history of drunken driving.
> He does not.
> Yes he does.
> No he doesn't.
>
> . . . . .
>
> Well, I haven't met Mr. Syms personally and I know he likes his drink.

Warren invited the woman to check with her sources and suggested she would find that the story was gossip and that her informant had received the information from someone else. There is no evidence the woman ever telephoned back and there is no evidence of any further reference to the rumour on the radio programme.

The evidence showed that all calls received on the program went from the telephone onto a tape and were then broadcast on the air with a time lapse of 10 seconds. Warren thus had the ability to censor calls and stop all or any portion of any call being broadcast.

There is no question that many of the remarks made by Warren during his conversation with plaintiff and the remarks he permitted the woman to make, and then published by permitting them to be broadcast, are defamatory. The only question is whether the plaintiff assented to the publication of the defamatory matter. If the plaintiff did assent to the publication, he has no cause of action. The principle was referred to by MacPherson, J., in *Jones v. Brooks et al.* (1974), 45 D.L.R. (3d) 413, [1974] 2 W.W.R. 729. In that case, two detectives with concealed tape recorders spoke to the defendant for the purpose of inducing the defamatory remarks and having them recorded. The learned trial Judge found the defence of *volenti non fit injuria* was available as there was an implied consent to the publication of the defamatory material. In the case at bar, the consent of the plaintiff does not have to be inferred. Plaintiff did in fact consent to, and participated in, a discussion of the defamatory matter.

In *Whitney et al. v. Moignard* (1890), 24 Q.B.D. 630, on a motion to strike out certain pleadings, Huddleston, B., commented at p. 631:

> The law is thus stated, and I think correctly stated, in *Odgers on Libel and Slander*, 2nd ed., page 168: 'Where there is evidence that the defendant, though he spoke only to A., intended and desired that A. should repeat his words, or expressly requested him to do so; here the defendant is liable for all the consequences of A.'s repetition of the slander; for A. thus becomes the agent of the defendant."

Chapman v. Lord Ellesmere et al., [1932] 2 K.B. 431, dealt with the publication of defamatory matter in a periodical selected by the parties and in other newspapers. It was alleged the plaintiff had administered a drug to a horse. The decision of the racing stewards actually was that the plaintiff was merely guilty of a dereliction of duty and there was no finding that he had himself drugged a horse or caused it to be drugged. One defence was that the plaintiff, as a condition of his licence, agreed to the publication of the results of the stewards' decision and cannot be heard to complain of a tort to which he himself has assented. Slesser, L.J., considered this defence to be based on the doctrine of *volenti non fit injuria*. He said at pp. 463-4

> ... for if the plaintiff assented to a report of the decision of the stewards, and they used words which were not a report of that decision, Sir Patrick Hastings' argument would have great weight; but if, on the other hand, in fact, they did report the actual decision, but in such a way that the jury say that it was to be understood to mean something other than the actual decision, that is a risk which the plaintiff, by agreeing to a report of the decision, has elected to run.

He concluded at p. 465:

> His case is that the words in their natural meaning are defamatory and so not a true report of the decision; but, for myself, for the reasons I have given, I think the case can only be based on innuendo. and, applying the doctrine of *volenti non fit injuria*, I hold that the plaintiff must fail in respect of the publication in the Racing Calendar by reason of his assent thereto.

In *Jones v. Brooks, supra*, MacPherson, J., also adopted some American precedents, particularly the cornments of Justice Halpern of the Appellate Division of the Supreme Court of the State of New York in *Teichner v. Bellan* (1959), 181 N.Y.S. 2d 842 at p. 846:

> Consent is a bar to a recovery for defamadon under the general principle of *volenti non fit injuria* or, as it is sometimes put, the plaintiff's consent to the publication of the defamation confers an absolute immunity or an absolute privilege upon the defendant.

In that case, the question was whether defamatory remarks in answer to a doctor's account, sent through a collection agency, amounted to a publication, whether there was consent and whether the occasion was privileged.

I am satisfied that as far as the initial conversation between the plaintiff and Warren is concerned, the plaintiff did assent to the publication of the defamatory matter. He was fully aware of the topic to be discussed, that the defamatory matter would be repeated during the conversation, and that the conversation would be published to the listening audience.

I am equally satisfied that the plaintiff did not consent to a continuation of the discussion of the rumour. The consent of the plaintiff extended only to such publication as was necessary to fulfill the purpose indicated by Warren, that is, to participate in the programme to deny the rumour and the comments of Warren that would be made in regard thereto. Even if plaintiff was aware that topics discussed on the programme were often subsequently discussed with listeners who telephoned the programme, I can find nothing in the consent of the plaintiff or in any of the evidence to indicate that the plaintiff agreed to Warren opening the topic for public discussion.

I have considered whether plaintiff's initial assent implied a consent to any and all subsequent discussion of the defamatory material by Warren. In my opinion there is a heavy onus upon a radio broadcaster to have a person's permission before making defamatory statements about him. If the broadcaster publishes defamatory material he must assume the risk of being able to justify the publication. In this case, the broadcaster has failed in that obligation as far as the discussion with the woman is concerned. Consent is a narrow defence to defamation, one not often seen and one where the consent must be clearly established. Consent must be given or be able to be inferred with respect to each publication of defamatory material. Were it otherwise, consent to the merest publication would open the door to wide dissemination that might be very damaging and never intended to be authorized by the person giving the initial consent. The defendants have failed to satisfy me that they had the authority of plaintiff to continue to discuss the defamatory material relating to plaintiff after Warren's conversation with him ended.

Warren's support of plaintiff does not excuse the publication. *Gatley on Libel and Slander*, 7th ed. (1974), p. 121:

> 264. *Expressions of doubt at the time of republication.* The fact that the defendant expressed a doubt or disbelief as to the truth of the slander at the time will make no difference to his liability. "No character or reputation would be safe, if a mere statement of a person's disbelief of a rumour which the speaker was engaged in circulating could be made to defeat the right of recovery for the slander." (*Per* Du Relle, J. in Nicholson v. Merritt (1900) 109 Kentucky R. 369 at p. 371.)

Section 3 of the *Defamation Act*, R.S.M. 1970, c.D20, provides that where defamation is proved, damage shall be presumed. Section 5 provides that an apology may mitigate damages. No apology was made in this case as defendants believed that if they had published any defamatory matter, they were justified due to the assent of the plaintiff. A public apology, in the circumstances of this case, would have required some repetition of the defamatory matter and would only have aggravated the situation. Similarly, Warren's support of plaintiff would have made an apology less meaningful than if he had been attacking the plaintiff. For these reasons I neither increase nor decrease the damages due to the lack of an apology.

Plaintiff's relationship with his employer, in effect the Government of Manitoba, requires examination when assessing damages. In December, 1974, after hearing the rumours, the Attorney-General and Egon Frech, an executive assistant to the Premier of Manitoba, joined in a telephone call to plaintiff asking if the rumours were correct. Plaintiff said the allegations in the rumours were untrue and the callers accepted that report. Plaintiff's employment has not been affected and his appointments to the Liquor Commission and Board were renewed for 1975 and 1976. Plaintiff testified he was shaken by the telephone call from the Attorney-General. He nevertheless, subsequently, agreed to participate in a discussion of the rumours on defendants' programme. On January 16th, Mr. Frech heard the portion of the programme when the woman and Warren were in conversation. He immediately telephoned plaintiff, indicated concern, and suggested plaintiff refer the matter to his solicitors. It appears to me plaintiff was not embarrassed or concerned up to that time, but was caused to act by this suggestion. On the other hand, he was embarrassed by this second telephone call from Mr. Frech and I consider this to be damage flowing from the publication of the defamatory matter during the conversation with the woman. The evidence disclosed that, like Mr. Frech, some listeners heard only a portion of each programme.

There was evidence from others who heard the programme, but none indicating any lessening of their respect for the plaintiff either as a result of the programme as a whole, or as a result of the conversation with the woman in particular.

Damages then result primarily due to s.3 of the *Defamation Act*. Damages are presumed, but there is no evidence of aggravated damages that would warrant a substantial award.

In my opinion, plaintiff must assume most of the responsibility for any damage he did suffer. If he had not participated in the discussion of the defamatory rumours, they would not have been widely disseminated. If he had not consented to the initial discussion with Warren, the woman would likely not have made her remarks or Warren might not have felt it permissible for her to make those remarks on the programme. If he had not participated in the further discussion, his superiors would not again have shown concern. Plaintiff's involvement does not excuse defendants for their publication of the defamatory remarks during Warren's discussion with the woman, but it substantially reduces the amount of damages to be awarded. Considering the extensive publication for which defendants are not liable, as opposed to the lesser publication that fixes liability, the damages I award are not substantial.

There will be judgment for the plaintiff against both defendants, jointly and severally, in the amount of $2,000 plus costs. I considered awarding costs on a solicitor-and-client basis. If I had done that, the $2,000 figure would have been substantially lower.

5.2.3.5 The Charter and Libel

5.2.3.5.1 *Hill v. Church of Scientology of Toronto* 1994, unreported (Ont. C.A.)

GRIFFITHS, CATZMAN and GALLIGAN, JJ.A.:
FREEDOM OF EXPRESSION

1. Overview

Section 2(b) of the Charter provides:
2. Everyone has the following fundamental freedoms:
. . . . .
(b) freedom of thought, belief, opinion and expression, including freedom of the press and other media of communication;

The appellants and the Writers and Publishers submit that the common law of defamation constitutes a prima facie infringement of the freedom of expression guaranteed by s. 2(b) of the Charter. The appellants do not challenge the law of defamation insofar as it imposes a reverse onus on the defendant to prove the truth of the defamatory words. They submit that the law of defamation inhibits the free expression of opinion about the conduct of public officials in the exercise of their office by imposing liability even when the defendant exercised reasonable care in publishing the defamatory words and had no knowledge that the words were untrue. They submit, furthermore, that the objective of protecting the personal reputation of public officials is not a sufficiently pressing concern in a free and democratic society to warrant overriding the freedom to criticize public conduct and, therefore, the infringement cannot be justified under s. 1 of the Charter.

The appellants urge that even if the object of protecting the personal reputation of public officials is sufficiently important to override freedom of expression, then the least intrusive means of accomplishing that objective would be to adopt the rule in *New York Times v. Sullivan*, 376 U.S. 254 (1964) which held that public officials must prove "actual malice" in order to prevail in libel suits against the news media. That is, the plaintiff must establish that the defamatory statements were made with knowledge of their falsehood or with reckless disregard as to their veracity. In other words, we are urged to hold that in criticizing the conduct of public officials, the critic should have a qualified privilege attaching to his or her comments.

The appellants submit, in the alternative, that even if we should find that the Charter does not apply because of the absence of governmental action, this court should change the common law and apply it in a manner consistent with the fundamental guarantee of freedom of expression protected by the Charter. Using this approach, it is suggested, the court should re-shape the common law by developing for the first time a qualified privilege in favour of those who criticize the conduct of public officials.

The responses of the respondent Casey Hill, supported by the intervenor, the Attorney General for Ontario, which we propose to address in these reasons are:

(1) the appellants have not established an adequate evidentiary basis to decide the Charter argument;
(2) the appellants have failed to demonstrate that the necessary element of governmental action is present so as to warrant application of the Charter to the facts of the case;
(3) there is no support or justification for the radical change proposed to the common law and all Canadian authorities to date have rejected the rule in New York Times v. Sullivan.

2. Background Proceedings

This action was commenced on December 14, 1984. Scientology, in its further amended statement of defence dated February 9, 1989, made a brief reference to the Charter defence in para. 17 as follows:

> 17. The Defendant Church pleads and relies upon the Canadian Charter of Rights and Freedoms, Constitution Act, 1982, Part I, Section 2(b).

Morris Manning, in his further amended statement of defence of March 31, 1989, raised the Charter argument in para. 10 as follows:

> 10. In the alternative, the Defendant of Manning relies upon section 2(b) and 52(1) of the *Canadian Charter of Rights and Freedoms* which guarantee the freedoms of thought, belief, opinion and expression. By virtue of those provisions, the Defendant Manning states that he is not liable to the Plaintiff for making the statements attributed to him in paragraphs 11B and C, 12, 14 and 17 of the Further Amended Statement of Claim in that:
> (1)(a)he Plaintiff, as a Crown Attorney, is a public official or figure, and
> (b) the statements attributed to Manning were a fair and accurate account by him on a matter of public interest, namely the conduct of the Plaintiff in discharge of his duties as a Crown Attorney;
> (2) the statements attributed to Manning were statements made by a lawyer, on behalf of a client, for the purpose of informing representatives of the public media about an important legal issue pending before the courts.

The foregoing pleadings in the respective statements of defence of Scientology and Morris Manning certainly do not make it clear that the parties intended to raise a constitutional challenge to the validity of either the common law or to the *Libel and Slander Act*.

On September 17, 1985, the appellants brought a pre-trial motion for dismissal of the action arguing that under s. 2(b) of the Charter, no public official may sue for defamatory statements relating to his or her official conduct unless it is first established, in accordance with the rule in *New York Times v. Sullivan*, that such statements were made with knowledge of their falsehood or with reckless disregard as to their veracity. The motion was dismissed by Mr. Justice O'Driscoll on the ground that the issue should properly be decided by the trial judge after evidence had been adduced, that an interlocutory ruling would needlessly lengthen litigation by sparking a series of appeals, and that the plaintiff's ability to adduce s. 1 evidence would be unduly constrained by the evidentiary limitations of a motion brought in Weekly Court. See: *Hill v. Church of*

Scientology (1985), 35 C.C.L.T. 72 (Ont. H.C.). It appears that no constitutional evidence was put before O'Driscoll, J. either in affidavit form or otherwise.

In late January, 1991, a firm date was fixed for the trial of this action and the date was confirmed in June, 1991. Although the appellants purported to challenge the constitutional validity of s. 2 of the *Libel and Slander Act*, neither party served either the Attorney General of Canada or the Attorney General for Ontario with the required notice of this challenge under s. 122 of the *Courts of Justice Act*, 1984. In fact, the Attorneys General were first served with notice of the Charter challenge on November 1, 1993, approximately one month before the hearing of this appeal. The Attorney General of Canada declined to intervene but the Attorney General for Ontario has appeared and delivered a factum as an intervenor.

On September 4, 1991, six years after the motion to dismiss was heard by O'Driscoll, J. and two days into the trial proceedings, counsel for Scientology sought an adjournment alleging, among other reasons, that he required more time to gather expert evidence to address the Charter issue. In view of the delay, the trial judge understandably denied the application. Counsel for Scientology addressed the issue as follows:

> I would indicate as well, there is a possibility of my seeking to call expert evidence in regard to the freedom of speech issue in this trial. This is not a matter that I think may go before the jury, but it may go before Your Lordship on the impact of what is called libel, which I will tell Your Lordship there has been no reports prepared by way of exhibits. As a matter of fact, no consultation with experts in relation to this. I am aware of the provisions of Rule 53, and I have had a battle in regard to getting material before Your Lordship in this trial. It seems to me an adjournment would allow me to explore that area and find out what experts may be available. And that's being worked on right now, but it certainly is no state of organization yet. If an adjournment were granted, it seems to me that a whole aspect of things would be simplified.

In making reference to "Rule 53", counsel was apparently acknowledging the difficulty he faced in not having prepared or delivered expert reports before trial, as required under the Rules of Civil Procedure.

During the trial, no evidence relating to the constitutional issue was called by either Morris Manning or Scientology. In the course of the trial, counsel for Morris Manning sought to adduce evidence that the office of the Attorney General for Ontario was funding Casey Hill's legal costs, as relevant to the issues of the nature of the statements (i.e., criticism of the conduct of a public official) and the application of the Charter. Carruthers J. disallowed the evidence of funding as being irrelevant to these two issues.

At a final hearing before Carruthers, J., held in the absence of the jury, to settle the issues to be covered in the charge to the jury, counsel for Morris Manning urged the trial judge to adopt the rule in *New York Times v. Sullivan*. The trial judge held that this decision did not reflect the law of Ontario and dismissed the Charter argument without further reasons.

3. The Absence of a Factual Foundation

Although the appellants originally challenged the constitutionality of the *Libel and Slander Act*, R.S.O. 1990, L. 12, the focus on appeal was the constitutionality of the common law of defamation. It is accepted that the common law may be subject to Charter regulation. However, even a challenge to the common law requires an evidentiary basis.

The Supreme Court of Canada has clearly cautioned against hearing constitutional cases without the appropriate factual underpinning. Specifically, in the context of freedom of expression cases, the Supreme Court has been vigilant in requiring an appropriate factual foundation before declaring a law constitutionally invalid.

In *MacKay v. Manitoba*, [1989] 2 S.C.R. 357, no evidence was submitted by the appellants to demonstrate that *The Elections Finances Act*, S.M. 1982-83-84, c. 45, which provided that the province would pay a portion of the campaign expenses of those candidates and parties who attained a fixed proportion of votes, infringed freedom of expression. Cory, J., writing for the court, stressed the importance of the need to establish a factual basis in Charter cases (at pp. 361-362):

> Charter cases will frequently be concerned with concepts and principles that are of fundamental importance to Canadian society. For example, issues pertaining to freedom of religion, freedom of expression and the right to life, liberty and the security of the individual will have to be considered by the courts. Decisions on these issues must be carefully considered as they will profoundly affect the lives of Canadians and all residents of Canada. In light of the importance and the impact that these decisions may have in the future, the courts have every right to expect and indeed to insist upon the careful preparation and presentation of a factual basis in most Charter cases. The relevant facts put forward may cover a wide spectrum dealing with scientific, social, economic and political apsects. Often expert opinion as to the future impact of the impugned legislation and the result of the possible decisions pertaining to it may be of great assistance to the courts.
>
> Charter decisions should not and must not be made in a factual vacuum. To attempt to do so would trivialize the Charter and inevitably result in ill-considered opinion. The presentation of facts is not, as stated by the respondent, a mere technicality; rather, it is essential to a proper consideration of Charter issues. A respondent cannot, by simply consenting to dispense with the factual background, require or expect a court to deal with an issue such as this in a factual void. Charter decisions cannot be based upon the unsupported hypotheses of enthusiastic counsel.

The court refused to take judicial notice of the bald allegation put forth by the appellants, i.e., that their right to freedom of expression was infringed because splinter parties with whose views they did not agree could qualify for funding if they received more than 10% of the votes or, alternatively, that the fixed percentage system favoured the three established parties to the detriment of other political parties whose views they might share, and rejected the submissions of the appellants on the ground of a lack of factual basis (at p. 366):

> These submissions pertaining to the financing of political parties and the effect of contributions to campaign expenses were as well of great importance to the argument, yet no evidence was submitted. It may well be that one could take judicial notice of some of the broad social facts

referred to by the appellants, but here there is a total absence of a factual foundation to support their case.

A factual foundation is of fundamental importance on this appeal. It is not the purpose of the legislation which is said to infringe the Charter but its effects. If the deleterious effects are not established there can be no Charter violation and no case has been made out. Thus the absence of a factual base is not just a technicality that could be overlooked, but rather it is a flaw that is fatal to the appellants' position.

These issues raise questions of importance pertaining to financing candidates in provincial elections that are obviously of great importance to residents of Canada or to any democracy. It would be irresponsible to attempt to resolve them without a reasonable factual background.

Although the parties in the present case were alerted to the need for evidence as early as the pre-trial motion before O'Driscoll, J., except for a belated effort to adjourn the trial to obtain the necessary expert evidence, the parties have made no effort to establish an evidentiary basis to support their constitutional challenge.

The constitutional record consists only of the bare assertion that the common law of defamation infringes the right of the appellants and the intervenors to freedom of expression by denying them the opportunity to criticize the conduct of the government and its officials because the law fails to impose a requirement that the plaintiff show actual knowledge or reckless disregard of falseness. That is not enough.

Weightier evidence is required than, to quote Cory, J. in *MacKay*, "the unsupported hypotheses of enthusiastic counsel" to strike down the protection afforded the individual to defend his or her good name from false attack and seek damages. At a minimum, some form of evidence is required to prove that libel still exists which prevents publication of true comments in media reports and elsewhere; that there exists such a great societal interest in the criticism of public officials in Canada to warrant the propagation of falsehoods; the effect of the American malice standard upon the protection of reputation, on the one hand, and freedom of expression, on the other; and the appropriateness of the remedy sought. Without evidence of the deleterious effects of the law of defamation on freedom of expression, this court is faced with evaluating the Charter challenge in a factual vacuum and potentially delivering an ill-considered opinion without due consideration for the ramifications associated with accepting the primacy of freedom to criticize public officials over the individual's right to the protection of his or her reputation.

In our opinion, this court should not attempt to resolve constitutional challenges in the absence of a factual foundation relating to all aspects of the challenge.

4. The Element of Governmental Action

Even assuming this constitutional challenge could be resolved in the absence of an evidentiary foundation, the apppellants face a second major obstacle in that they must show Casey Hill's action for damages was a form of "governmental action" in order to attract application of the Charter.

In *R.V.S.D.U. v. Dolphin Delivery*, [1986] 2 S.C.R. 573, McIntyre, J. described the application of the Charter to private litigation in the following manner (at pp. 598-99):

> It is my view that s. 32 of the Charter specifies the actors to whom the Charter will apply. They are the legislative, executive and administrative branches of government. It will apply to those branches of government whether or not their action is invoked in public or private litigation. ... Action by the executive or administrative branches of government will generally depend upon legislation, that is, statutory authority. Such action may also depend, however, on the common law, as in the case of the prerogative. To the extent that it relies on statutory authority which constitutes or results in an infringement of a guaranteed right or freedom, the Charter will apply and it will be unconstitutional. The action will also be unconstitutional to the extent that it relies for authority or justification on a rule of the common law which constitutes or creates an infringement of a Charter right or freedom. In this way the Charter will apply to the common law, whether in public or private litigation. It will apply to the common law, however, only in so far as the common law is the basis of some governmental action which, it is alleged, infringes a guaranteed right or freedom.

In *McKinney v. University of Guelph*, [1990] 3 S.C.R. 229, a case in which staff members of several universities applied for a declaration that their employer's mandatory retirement policy violated s. 15 of the Charter, the court made it very clear that the application of the Charter is confined to truly governmental action. After quoting s. 32 of the Charter, La Forest, J., writing for the majority, stated at pp. 261-263:

> These words (i.e., s. 32 Charter) give a strong message that the Charter is confined to government action. This Court has repeatedly drawn attention to the fact that the Charter is essentially an instrument for checking the powers of government over the individual. In *Hunter v. Southam Inc.*, [1985] 2 S.C.R. 145, at p. 156, Dickson, J. (as he then was) observed: "It is intended to constrain governmental action inconsistent with those rights and freedoms; it is not in itself an authorization for governmental action." In *Operation Dismantle Inc. v. The Queen*, [1984] 1 S.C.R. 441, at p. 490, Wilson, J. noted that "the central concern of [s. 7 of the Charter] is direct impingement by government upon the life, liberty and personal security of individual citizens." See also *R. v. Big M Drug Mart Ltd.*, [1985] 1 S.C.R. 295, at p. 347, per Dickson, J.; *RWDSU v. Dolphin Delivery Ltd.*, [1986] 2 S.C.R. 573, especially at pp. 593-98; and *Tremblay v. Daigle*, [1989] 2 S.C.R. 530.
>
> The exclusion of private activity from the Charter was not a result of happenstance. It was a deliberate choice which must be respected. We do not really know why this approach was taken, but several reasons suggest themselves. Historically, bills of rights, of which that of the United States is the great constitutional exemplar, have been directed at government. Government is the body than can enact and enforce rules and authoritatively impinge on individual freedom. Only government requires to be constitutionally shackled to preserve the rights of the individual. Others, it is true, may offend against the rights of individuals. This is especially true in a world in which economic life is largely left to the private sector where powerful private institutions are not directly affected by democratic forces. But government can either regulate these or create distinct bodies for the protection of human rights and the advancement of human dignity.
>
> To open up all private and public action to judicial review could strangle the operation of society and, as put by counsel for the universities, "diminish the area of freedom within which individuals can act". In *Re Bhindi and British Columbia Projectionists* (1986), 29 D.L.R. (4th) 47, Nemetz, C.J., speaking for the majority of the British Columbia Court of Appeal, made it clear that such an approach could seriously interfere with freedom of contract. It would mean

reopening whole areas of settled law in several domains. For example, as has been stated: "In cases involving arrests, detentions, searches and the like, to apply the Charter to purely private action would be tantamount to setting up an alternative tort system" (see McLellan and Elman, "To Whom Does the Charter Apply? Some Recent Cases on Section 32" (1986), 24 *Alta. L. Rev.* 361, at p. 367, cited in *RWDSU v. Dolphin Delivery Ltd.*, supra, at p. 597). And that is by no means all.

The appellants submit that Casey Hill, as a Crown counsel with the Ministry of the Attorney General, was a governmental actor at all times and that his action to recover damages in respect of statements made about the discharge of his public duties was therefore governmental action. They argue that a lawsuit brought by a public official to vindicate his or her reputation as a public official has the same purpose and effect as if the action was brought by the government itself. They argue that the trial judge erred in refusing to permit them to introduce evidence that the Ministry of the Attorney General had agreed to pay the plaintiff's legal fees for the libel action on the understanding that Casey Hill would ultimately reimburse the government if successful in making any recovery. Government funding of Casey Hill's action, they suggest, is strong evidence that Casey Hill's action was governmental action.

We do not accept these submissions of the appellants. In our opinion, the Charter does not apply to the facts of this case because Casey Hill's actions in pursuing litigation were the actions of a private individual that do not constitute legislative or governmental action so as to attract Charter scrutiny. The private nature of this litigation is apparent from the allegation in paragraph 19 of the statement of claim that the defamatory statements:

... constituting as they do statements of the most serious professional misconduct by the Plaintiff, have damaged his professional reputation and brought him into public scandal, odium and contempt, by reason of which the Plaintiff has suffered damage.

What is at issue in this proceeding is the impact of the defamatory statements upon Casey Hill's personal reputation, not the reputation of the Ministry of the Attorney General or that of the Government of Ontario. The fact that Casey Hill was employed by the Attorney General for Ontario and the defamatory statements related to an act he purportedly carried out in the scope of his employment does not change the nature of the redress he sought.

Further, we do not perceive the evidence that the Government of Ontario provided financial assistance to Casey Hill in repsect of the conduct of this proceeding as either relevant to or determinative of the Charter issue. The payment of Casey Hill's legal fees by the government does not effect a change in his constitutional status or somehow convert his lawsuit into an act of government. In McKinney, *supra*, the dependency of the universities upon government funding to finance their activities, including, presumably, their legal costs in defending the challenge to their mandatory retirement policies, was viewed as neither relevant nor determinative. The test was whether the universities formed part of the government apparatus and whether they were implementing government policy in establishing mandatory retirement. Casey Hill's libel action cannot be characterized as an implementation of government policy.

In our opinion, this litigation was litigation between private parties to which the Charter has no application.

5. The Common Law of Libel

Counsel for Scientology submits as an alternative argument that, even if the libel suit did not constitute governmental action, the common law of libel ought to be developed and applied in a manner consistent with freedom of expression as guaranteed by the Charter. Counsel stressed the following obiter dicta of McIntyre, J. in *Dolphin Delivery, supra*, at p. 603:

> Where, however, private party "A" sues private party "B" relying on the common law and where no act of government is relied upon to support the action, the Charter will not apply. I should make it clear, however, that this is a distinct issue from the question whether the judiciary ought to apply and develop the principles of the common law in a manner consistent with the fundamental values enshrined in the Constitution. The answer to this question must be in the affirmative. In this sense, then, the Charter is far from irrelevant to private litigants whose disputes fall to be decided at common law. But this is different from the proposition that one private party owes a constitutional duty to another, which proposition underlies the purported assertion of Charter causes of action or Charter defences between individuals.

Counsel for Scientology uges this court to make a major alteration to the common law by importing the rule in *New York Times v. Sullivan* into Canadian law on the basis that it would make the common law more consistent with the Charter. In *New York Times v. Sullivan*, the Supreme Court of the United States concluded that the First Amendment required that there be constitutional limits on liability for defamatory communications where criticism of public officials was concerned. Brennan, J., delivering the opinion of the majority, held that a public official should only succeed in libel for statements made about his or her official conduct or fitness for office where the plaintiff could show that the defamatory statement was made "with knowledge that it was false or with reckless disregard of whether it was false or not" (at p. 280).

The requirement of showing actual knowledge of falsehood or reckless disregard for the truth is known in American jurisprudence as proof of "actual malice." The common law concept of "malice" applied by Canadian courts is distinguishable from the American concept of "actual malice" in that a broader range of factors than actual knowledge of falsehood or reckless disregard for the truth is considered relevant to assessing malice. Such other factors include, but are not limited to, animosity, enmity, hostility, ill will and spite.

In *New York Times v. Sullivan*, Black, Douglas and Goldberg, JJ. delivered separate but concurring opinions, advocating an absolute right to criticize official conduct even if the plaintiff could prove that the defendant acted with knowledge of the falsehood or with reckless disregard for the truth. Counsel for Scientology urged us to adopt a hybrid rule of the majority and minority positions whereby

Casey Hill could only sue for libel if he established actual knowledge of falsity rather than reckless disregard for the truth.

Whether we accept the "actual malice" standard articulated in *New York Times v. Sullivan*, or the more extreme position advocated by Scientology, we would be required to make a major alteration to the common law. To do so would be contrary to the established rule that changes to the common law should be slow and incremental out of deference to the legislature. In *Watkins v. Olafson*, [1989] 2 S.C.R. 750, a case in which the court was asked to change the common law regarding damages for personal injuries so that plaintiffs would be forced to accept periodic payments instead of the traditional lump sum payment, McLachlin, J., writing for the court, commented (at pp. 760-761):

> ... Generally speaking, the judiciary is bound to apply the rules of law found in the legislation and in the precedents. Over time, the law in any given area may change; but the process of change is a slow and incremental one, based largely on the mechansim of extending an existing principle to new circumstances. While it may be that some judges are more activist than others, the courts have generally declined to introduce major and far-reaching changes in the rules hitherto accepted as governing the situation before them.
>
> There are sound reasons supporting this judicial reluctance to dramatically recast established rules of law. The court may not be in the position to assess the deficiencies of the existing law, much less problems which may be associated with the changes it might make. The court has before it a single case; major changes in the law should be predicated on a wider view of how the rule will operate in the broad generality of cases. Moreover, the court may not be in a position to appreciate fully the economic and policy issues underlying the choice it is asked to make. Major changes to the law often involve devising subsidiary rules and procedures relevant to their implementation, a task which is better accomplished through consultation between courts and practitioners than by judical decree. Finally, and perhaps most importantly, there is the long-established principle that in a constitutional democracy it is the legislature, as the elected branch of government, which should assume the major responsibility for law reform.
>
> Considerations such as these suggest that major revisions of the law are best left to the legislature. Where the matter is one of a small extension of existing rules to meet the exigencies of a new case and the consequences of the change are readily assessable, judges can and should vary existing principles. But where the revision is major and its ramifications complex, the courts must proceed with great caution.

In *R. v. Salituro*, [1991] 3 S.C.R. 654, the issue was whether one spouse was a compellable witness against another to prove a criminal charge, and hence a governmental actor was involved. The Supreme Court of Canada held that it had a duty to see that the common law developed in accordance with the values of the Charter and refused to apply the privilege of spousal immunity where the spouses were separated without any reasonable possibility of reconciliation. Iacobucci, J., however, reiterated the need for caution at p. 670:

> Judges can and should adapt the common law to reflect the changing social, moral and economic fabric of the country. Judges should not be quick to perpetuate rules whose social foundation has long since disappeared. Nonetheless, there are significant constraints on the power of the judiciary to change the law. As McLachlin, J. indicated in *Watkins, supra*, in a constitutional democracy such as ours it is the legislature and not the courts which has the major responsibility for law reform; and for any changes to the law which may have complex ramifications, however necessary

or desirable such changes may be, they should be left to the legislature. The judiciary should confine itself to those incremental changes which are necessary to keep the common law in step with the dynamic and evolving fabric of our society.

The appellants are not asking this court to extend an existing principle to new circumstances but are advocating major and substantial rather than gradual and incremental changes to the common law.

Freedom of expression was recognized as an important and fundamental right guaranteed under the common law long before the advent of the Charter. The Supreme Court of Canada recognized that freedom of the press and freedom of speech are inherent in the very nature of parliamentary democracy and therefore must be guaranteed: see, for example, *Reference re Alberta Statutes*, [1938] S.C.R. 100; aff'd. [1939] A.C. 117.

Notwithstanding the importance of freedom of expression at common law, the Supreme Court of Canada in a pre-Charter decision in *Globe and Mail v. Boland*, [1960] S.C.R. 203 rejected the argument that defamatory statements concerning the fitness for office of a candidate for election were published on an occasion of qualified privilege. The court held that the assertion of a qualified privilege was contrary to the great weight of authority in England and Canada and against the public interest. Cartwright, J., speaking for the court, concluded at pp. 208-209:

> To hold that during a federal election campaign in Canada any defamatory statement published in the press relating to a candidate's fitness for office is to be taken as published on an occasion of qualified privilege would be, in my opinion, not only contrary to the great weight of authority in England and in this country but harmful to that "common convenience and welfare of society" which Baron Parke described as the underlying principle on which the rules as to qualified privilege are founded. See *Toogood v. Spyring*. It would mean than every man who offers himself as a candidate must be prepared to risk the loss of his reputation without redress unless he be able to prove affirmatively that those who defamed him were actuated by express malice. I would like to adopt the following sentence from the judgment of the Court in *Post Publishing Co. v. Hallman*:
>
>> "We think that not only is such a sacrifice not required of every one who consents to become a candidate for office, but that to sanction such a doctrine would do the public more harm than good."
>
> and the following expression of opinion by the learned author of *Gatley (op. cit.)* at page 254:
>
>> "It is, however, submitted that so wide an extension of the privilege would do the public more harm than good. It would tend to deter sensitive and honourable men from seeking public positions of trust and responsibility, and leave them open to others who have no respect for their reputation."
>
> The passages just quoted recall the words of Cockburn, C.J. in *Campbell v. Spottiswoode*:
>
>> "It is said that it is for the interests of society that the public conduct of men should be criticised without any other limit than that the writer should have an honest belief that what he writes is true. But it seems to me that the public have an equal interest in the maintenance of the public character of public men; and the public affairs could not be conducted by men of honour with a view to the welfare of the country, if we were to sanction attacks upon them, destructive of their honour and character, and made without any foundation."
>
> The interest of the public and that of the publishers of newspapers will be sufficiently safeguarded by the availability of the defence of fair comment in appropriate circumstances.

The adoption of the rule in *New York Times v. Sullivan* by this court would result in a major change to the common law and in a rejection of the views expressed by the Supreme Court of Canada in 1960 that considerable value should be placed upon the reputation of individuals who have dedicated their professional lives to the service of the public.

6. The Reception of the Rule in *New York Times v. Sullivan*

Canadian jurisprudence and international law reform initiatives demonstrate that there is little will to adopt the rule in *New York Times v. Sullivan* in countries outside the United States. In *Coates v. The Citizen* (1988), 44 C.C.L.T. 286 (N.S.S.C.) the defendant newspaper made a pre-trial motion to have the *Defamation Act*, R.S.N.S. 1967, c. 72 declared inoperative as contrary to ss. 2(b) and 7 of the Charter. The alleged libel related to statements published by the defendant about the plaintiff's visit to a nightclub in West Germany while he was Minister of National Defence. After reviewing the rule in *New York Times v. Sullivan*, Richards, J. ruled that the *Defamation Act* was constitutional for the following reasons (at pp. 311-313):

> What strictures does the *Defamation Act* impose upon the *Citizen* and media generally? It does not restrict the publication of news. It does not prevent comment on perceived government ineptitude. It does not stifle criticism of prominent political figures in the conduct of their duties. Indeed, the law in Canada, which of course is reflective of the law in this province recognizes the need for free and full public discussion. As stated in *Drew v. Toronto Star Ltd.*, [1947] O.R. 730, [1947] 4 D.L.R. 221 (Ont. C.A.) [affirmed [1948] 4 D.L.R. 465 (S.C.C.)] at p. 235 [D.L.R.]:
>
>> "All citizens of a community or country, including the editors and publishers of newspapers, have the full and free right to discuss and comment upon the public acts and conduct of a man occupying a public position, and, if they see fit, to criticize his acts and conduct in the most severe terms. The public interest requires that a man's public conduct shall be open to searching criticism, but the facts upon which such criticism and comment are based must be truly stated, and a newspaper has no greater or higher right to make comment on a public man or person occupying a public situation, than an ordinary citizen would have." [Emphasis added by Richards, J.]
>
> . . . . .
>
> There is no question that the laws of defamation are imperfect and in some aspects convoluted. Brown, in his text *Law of Defamation in Canada* (1987), cited numerous complaints about the law and quoted the following passage, "for the most part any thoughtful consideration of the present state of the law of libel either begins or ends with a combined apology or lament". The learned author then says [p. 4]:
>
>> "However imperfect the law may be, and however much we may despair of the state of affairs, it is universally recognized that the reputation of a person is and always has been an important value which the law must protect. Some form of legal or social constraints on defamatory publications 'are to be found at all stages of civilization, however imperfect, remote, and proximate to barbarism'. The extent to which a community protects the reputation of its citizens may partially measure its 'cultural and democratic quality'."
>
> The author then goes on in the following page to discuss the respective attitudes of the Canadian and American jurist [pp. 5-6]:
>
>> "Unlike their American colleagues, therefore, our judges have weighed more heavily the value of personal reputation over those of free speech and free press. Thus there occurs in

many of their decisions a careful reminder that these freedoms are ones 'governed by law' and that there is no 'freedom to make untrue defamatory statements.'

. . . . .

This is not intended as an invidious comparison. Our judges cherish free speech and a free press no less than their American counterparts. They just happen to value personal reputation, particularly the reputation of their public servants, more."

I subscribe fully to these comments by the learned author. This is the rationale for the difference between our approach and that of the American judiciary. This is a fair analysis of the Canadian approach, as it has been and as I feel it ought to remain. Therefore I find that the Defamation Act of Nova Scotia does not impinge upon the right of freedom of the press as set out in s. 2(b) of the *Charter of Rights and Freedoms*.

In *Derrickson v. Tomat* (1992), 88 D.L.R. (4th) 401 (B.C.C.A.) the plaintiffs, members of an Indian council, sued the defendants, nine members of an Indian Bank and two others, in defamation for issuing a press release, circulating a petition and making statements to the media alleging that the plaintiffs were fraudulently mismanaging Band funds. The trial judge found the defendants liable and awarded general damages and punitive damages to each plaintiff. The British Columbia Court of Appeal ordered a new trial on grounds that the trial judge had failed to consider the defences of each defendant individually and had excluded admissible evidence. Wood, J.A., with whom Taylor, J.A. concurred, made the following observation on *New York Times v. Sullivan* (at p. 408):

The rule in the New York Times case leaves vulnerable the reputation of all who are or would be in public life, by depriving such people of any legal recourse from defamatory falsehoods directed against them, except in those rare cases where "actual malice" can be established. Such a rule would be likely to discourage honest and decent people from standing for public office. Thus, the rule destroys, rather than preserves, the delicate balance between freedom of expression and protection of reputation which, as I have already noted, is vital to the survival of our democratic process of government. For that reason I would be opposed to introducing such a rule in this country.

Among Canadian legal writers, there is no clear consensus that the rule in *New York Times v. Sullivan* should be adopted: see R. Dearden, "Constitutional Protection for Defamatory Words Published about the Conduct of Public Officials" (in D. Schneiderman (ed.), *Freedom of Expression and the Charter*, Thomson Publishing, 1991); M. Bryant, "Section 2(b) and Libel Law: Defamatory Statements about Public Officials" (1992), 2 *M.C.L.R.* 335; D. Alderson, "The Constitutionalization of Defamation: American and Canadian Approaches to the Constitutional Regulation of Speech" (1993), 15 *Adv. Q.* 385.

The rule in *New York Times v. Sullivan* has not been immune from criticism by American legal writers. Professor Richard Epstein, in "Was *New York Times v. Sullivan* Wrong?" (1986), 53 *U. of Chicago L. Rev.* 782 notes dissatisfaction with the law of defamation, as evidenced by proposals for legislative reform, and advocates a return to the principles of strict liability. Mr. Justice Pierre Leval, who resided at the libel trial of General William Westmoreland against CBS, proposes that public officials be permitted to take a no-damages libel suit, free of the actual malice requirement, to vindicate their reputations: "The No Money, No

Fault Libel Suit: Keeping *Sullivan* in its Proper Place" (1988), 101 *Harvard L. Rev.* 1287. See also D. Barrett, "Declaratory Judgments for Libel: A Better Alternative" (1986), 74 *Cal. L. Rev.* 857 and R. Smolla, "Taking Libel Reform Seriously" (1987), 38 *Mercer L. Rev.* 793.

The Uniform Law Conference of Canada, in a report issued after the advent of the Charter, reviewed the decision in *New York Times v. Sullivan* and concluded that no special defence for the news media should be incorporated within the *United Defamation Act* aside from the existing defences of qualified privilege and fair comment: Uniform Law Conference of Canada Report (1983) at p. 126.

Furthermore, the rule in *New York Times v. Sullivan* has been rejected by law reform initiatives in Australia, Great Britain and Ireland: see Australian Law Reform Commission *Report* (the Kirby Committee Report) (1979), *Report of the Committee on Defamation* (the Faulks Committee Report) (1975) and The Irish Law Reform Commission *Report on the Civil Law of Defamation* (the Keane Final Report) (March 1991). In the Kirby Committee *Report*, the concept of "public official" was criticized on the basis that "a minor elected official or a public servant [would be placed] in a more vulnerable position than a prominent businessman" (Appendix F, p. 252) and the effectiveness of the plaintiff's ability to reply was questioned. The Faulks Committee Report emphasized the fact that adoption of the rule "would in many cases deny a just remedy to defamed persons" (p. 169). In the Keane Final *Report*, the distinction between "public" and "private" plaintiffs was rejected on the ground that "while the widest possible range of criticism of public officials and public figures is desirable, statements of fact contribute meaningfully to public debate only if they are true" (p. 82).

7. Conclusion on the Issue of Freedom of Expression

The appellants have not established an evidentiary basis appropriate for a constitutional ruling. In any event, Casey Hill's libel action cannot be characterized as an act of government attracting Charter application. Finally, we are not persuaded that it is appropriate to make a substantial and major alteration to Canadian common law by adopting the rule in *New York Times v. Sullivan*. The rejection of this rule has been based historically on sound policy reasons which recognize as of paramount importance the protection of the reputation of individuals who assume the responsibilities of public officials. If the common law of defamation is to undergo the major changes urged by the appellants, these changes should be effected by the legislature.

5.2.4 Remedies

If the court decides that the defendant has indeed defamed the plaintiff, the court must then determine what the successful plaintiff gets, what remedy should be awarded against the defendant. There are two possibilities in a defamation action: the award of a sum of money as damages or the issuance of an injunction.

5.2.4.1 Damages

The primary purpose in awarding damages in any tort action is to compensate the plaintiff for the loss which has been suffered. The general object underlying the rules for the assessment of damages is, so far as possible by means of a monetary award, to place the plaintiff in the position he would have occupied if he had not suffered the wrong complained of ...

(*Dodd Properties (Kent) Ltd. v. Canterbury City Council* (1980), 1 All E.R. 928 (C.A.))

5.2.4.1.1 General Considerations

5.2.4.1.1.1 *Munro v. Toronto Sun* (1982), 21 C.C.L.T. 261 (Ont. H.C.)

HOLLAND, J.: Damages in libel actions are "at large" and rest upon a consideration of the injury to the plaintiff, the conduct of the defendant and the plaintiff and, in some cases, the deterrent effect sought to be accomplished. Except to the extent that they are intended to be a deterrent, they are compensatory and not punitive. Such damages may be aggravated by the particular circumstances of the case, including the defendant's conduct, both before and after the libel, and the added detrimental effect on the plaintiff. As well, such may be considered in mitigation. Injury to reputation is assumed when libel is proved.

5.2.4.1.1.2 *Walker and Walker Brothers Quarries Ltd. v. CFTO Ltd. et al.* (1987), 19 O.A.C. 10 (Ont. C.A.)

ROBINS, J.A.: 1. *Were the compensatory damages of $883,000 awarded to Walker Brothers excessive?*

The defendants' submission is that the verdict of $883,000 in favour of Walker Brothers is so grossly excessive and manifestly unreasonable that it must be set aside. In considering this submission, I first remind myself of the principles applicable to appellate review of jury awards in defamation cases. Here, general or compensatory damages, and those terms can be used interchangeably, are clearly "at large" and their amount, as is so often said, is "peculiarly the province of the jury". An appellate court is not entitled to substitute its own judgment on the proper amount of damages for the judgment of the jury. The question is not whether the court would have awarded a smaller sum than was awarded by the jury; nor is the question whether the size of the verdict was merely too great. The question is whether the verdict is so inordinately large as obviously to exceed the maximum limit of a reasonable range within which the jury may properly operate or, put another way, whether the verdict is so exorbitant or so grossly out of proportion to the libel as to shock the court's conscience and sense of justice.

Applying that strict test to this case, I am nevertheless of the opinion that the verdict cannot stand. Two dominating reasons compel me to this conclusion: first, the jury used an arbitrary yardstick in measuring these damages and could not have directed its mind to the considerations properly applicable to an award of compensatory damages for a corporate plaintiff; and second, the award, viewed most favourably to the plaintiff, bears no reasonable relationship to either the circumstances of the case or the injury inflicted on the company, by the defendants' tort. Before considering these reasons, some brief general observations about compensatory damages in libel actions may be helpful.

Defamation is an invasion of a person's interest in his or her reputation, and compensatory damages are implied primarily to compensate for the harm caused to the person's reputation by the defamatory publication. In libel actions damages are at large in the sense that the award is not limited to a pecuniary loss that can be specifically proved; damages are presumed from the publication of the libel itself and need not be established by proof of actual loss. Damages may include intangible or subjective elements; they cannot be measured by any objective monetary scale and are not capable of precise calculation.

A libelled plaintiff is, of course, entitled to special damages (as distinct from general damages) to cover the actual pecuniary loss which has resulted from the wrong. Such a plaintiff is entitled also to compensatory or general damages for both: (a) the injury sustained as a result of the lessening of the esteem in which he or she is held in the eyes of the community because of the defamatory statements; and (b) the injury caused to his or her feelings by the defamatory statements. The damages may be aggravated by the manner in which, or the motives with which, the statement was made or persisted in. Where the defendant is guilty of insulting, high-handed, spiteful, malicious or oppressive conduct which increases the mental distress — the humiliation, indignation, anxiety, grief, fear and the like — suffered by the plaintiff as a result of being defamed, the plaintiff may be entitled to what has come to be known as "aggravated damages". Aggravated damages are damages which take into account the additional harm caused to the plaintiff's feelings by such reprehensible or outrageous conduct on the part of the defendant. Their purpose is compensatory and, being compensatory, they properly form part of a general damage award. Aggravated damages, it should be underscored, are not punitive — punishment is not the function of a compensatory award. They must be distinguished from "punitive" or "exemplary" damages (to which I shall come later) which are non-compensatory and have as their object punishment and deterrence.

Thus, a compensatory damage award in a defamation action should represent the judge or jury's estimate of the amount necessary in all the circumstances of the case: (i) to vindicate the plaintiff's reputation; and (ii) to compensate him for his wounded feelings.

5.2.4.1.1.3 Julian Porter, Q.C., "Tangents," *Canadian Lawyer*, April 1981, p.24

The magic of libel is that damages are at large and a jury can give whatever it sees fit.

Essentially, damages in libel are on the basis of compensation, not punishment. But you are allowed to refer to the conduct of the defendant or his counsel down to the time of the jury address, which is rather unique. You can comment on lack of apology, persistence of a plea of justification, a possibility of malice, the nature of the pleadings and even defence counsel's tactics plus the humiliation your client has suffered. Because of this there is a good shot of raising the damages to a higher scale than in a personal injury action although such discrepancy is frowned upon by the courts.

Windeyer, J. said in *Uren v. John Fairfax & Sons Pty. Ltd.* (1967), 117 CLR 118 at 150.

> It seems to me that, properly speaking, a man defamed does not get compensation for his damaged reputation. He gets damages because he was injured in his reputation, that is simply because he was publicly defamed. For this reason, compensation by damages operates in two ways — as a vindication of the plaintiff to the public and as consolation to him for a wrong done. Compensation is here a solatium rather than a monetary recompense for harm measurable in money.

This is why it is not necessarily fair to compare awards of damages in this field with damages for personal injuries. Quite obviously, the award must include factors for injury to the feelings, the anxiety and uncertainty undergone in the litigation, the absence of apology, or the reaffirmation of the truth of the matters complained of, or the malice of the defendant. The bad conduct of the plaintiff himself may also enter into the matter, where he has provoked the libel, or where perhaps he has libelled the defendant in reply. What is awarded is thus a figure which cannot be arrived at by any purely objective computation. This is what is meant when the damages in defamation are described as being "at large".

In *McCarey v. Associated Newspapers Ltd. (No. 2)* Pearson, L.J. (1965), 2.B. 86 at 104, dealt with the various elements in compensatory damages as follows.

> They may also include the natural injury to his feelings — the natural grief and distress which he may have felt at having been spoken of in defamatory terms, and if there has been any kind of high-handed, oppressive, insulting or contumelious behaviour by the defendant which increases the mental pain and suffering caused by the defamation and may constitute unjury to the plaintiff's pride and self-confidence, those are proper elements to be taken into account in a case where the damages are at large.

I believe plaintiff jury addresses in libel actions are different than in other cases. Counsel must be melodramatic.

There is a tendency by judges to dislike libel cases with their technical pitfalls and as a result they do try to force settlement or view it all as a trifling matter. I remember a judge, now deceased, who indicated to the jury that a statement widely publicized that "the Chief of Police is a member of the Mafia" was 'a tempest in a teapot'. Consequently counsel must adopt a baroque attitude with tears if possible. One must abandon and gush with vibrato. My view is that unlike other cases a plaintiff's counsel can ill afford to be cheery or chirp witty asides to a jury. A jury must be slowly and continually persuaded that the worst ailment on this earth is to be buried with a sullied name. All speeches should dwell on the illusory balm of money and the eternal pain of losing the quality of life that has been wrenched away by the monstrous libel. The great area to exploit is that damages are at large and that actual damages needn't be proved. Also, one is entitled to refer to mental pain and suffering of the plaintiff. I would recommend referring to a judgment (it is hard for a judge to interfere if you don't try to quote a specific law — but damages can be so general).

Youssoupoff v. Metro-Goldwyn Mayer Pictures Limited (1934) The Times Law Reports, 581 584 and 586 reads as follows:

> What have the jury to do? They have to give a verdict of amount without having any proof of actual damage. They need not have proof of actual damages. They have to consider the nature of the libel as they understand it, the circumstances in which it was published, and the circumstances relating to the person who publishes it, right down to the time they give their verdict, whether the defence made is true, and, if so, whether that defence has ever been withdrawn — the whole circumstances of the case. It is not the judge who has to decide the amount. The constitution has thought, and I think there is great advantage in it, that the damages to be paid by a person who says false things about his neighbor are best decided by a jury representing the public, who may state the view of the public as to the action of the man who makes false statements about his neighbor, the plaintiff.

5.2.4.1.1.4 *Snyder v. Montreal Gazette Ltd.* (1988), 49 D.L.R. (4th) 17 (S.C.C.)

BEETZ, J.: I have had the benefit of reading the reasons for judgment of my brother Lamer and I adopt his statement of the facts, the judgments of the courts below and the points at issue.

Like Lamer, J., I consider that the reasons given by the majority of the Court of Appeal for concluding that the compensation awarded by the jury was unreasonable are vitiated by error.

With respect for the contrary view, however, I am unable to say that this compensation is unreasonable on other grounds.

Although the compensation seems high and is not necessarily what I would have determined, respondent did not persuade me that the trial judge erred in ruling as follows:

> This Court is not prepared to say that the jury's estimate is so grossly inflated as to be branded as unreasonable, in the light of all the circumstances of the case.
> ([1987] C.S. 628, at p. 635-636.)

I concur in substance with the reasons of L'Heureux-Dube, J.A., dissenting in the Court of Appeal, and in particular with the following:

> [TRANSLATION] . . . I would not look for bases of comparison in this matter in France, the United States or even the Commonwealth countries. Custom, usage and the law are so different there that, in my opinion, such comparisons cannot serve as useful guides for our courts. ([1983] C.A. 604, at p. 623.)

For these reasons I would allow the appeal, reverse the judgment of the Court of Appeal and restore the Superior Court judgment, including the order to publish the aforesaid judgment unless appellant waives this order, the whole with costs throughout.

LAMER, J. (dissenting): . . . Is the compensation awarded nonetheless unreasonable on other grounds? The jury concluded that appellant had proven no pecuniary loss as a result of the defamation and he therefore received nothing in this regard. The $135,000 awarded to appellant thus represent only non-pecuniary loss suffered by him. These damages are offered to the victim to compensate for the humiliation, suffering, scorn, embarrassment and ridicule he was subjected to as a result of the defamation. As in principle compensation cannot be made in kind, it generally consists of a sum of money. It is far from easy to do justice in this area. The amount awarded is necessarily arbitrary, in view of the difficulty of measuring objectively such loss in pecuniary terms, especially when it concerns someone else's reputation. It is precisely because this exercise is based on empirical considerations rather than on a mathematical and scientific operation that extravagant claims for this type of loss should not be allowed by the courts.

The Court of Appeal's judgment indicates its concern to restrain the compensation awarded for non-pecuniary loss. In support of his opinion that the verdict was unreasonable, Owen, J.A. referred to the upper limit established by this Court in 1978 in the "trilogy": *Andrews v. Grand & Toy Alberta Ltd., supra; Thornton v. Board of School District No. 57 (Prince George)*, [1978] 2 S.C.R. 267; *Arnold v. Teno*, [1978] 2 S.C.R. 287. In those cases Dickson, J., as he then was, established that a maximum of $100,000 may be awarded as compensation for non-pecuniary loss resulting from physical injuries.

According to Owen, J.A., the amounts awarded for non-pecuniary loss in a defamation case also should not exceed this limit. Such a comparison is certainly conceivable, as both cases involve non-pecuniary loss which is difficult to determine objectively. However, Owen, J.A. gives no reason for applying this upper limit to compensation for an attack on reputation. Should a ceiling be placed on non-pecuniary loss for defamation in Quebec law?

Under the Quebec civil law, the general rule for the assessment of damages is contained in the axiom *restitutio in integrum*. In other words, compensation must be made in full, that is, it must place the victim in the same position he would have been if the incident had not occurred. He is entitled to compensation both for his non-pecuniary and pecuniary loss. As compensation must cover all the loss sustained, the concept of an upper limit is inconsistent with the principle of full compensation. Clearly compensation cannot be denied for part of the loss sustained nor can the amount of money awarded for pecuniary loss, which is objectively calculated once the damage has been proven, be limited. Similarly, non-pecuniary loss must be compensated in full, even if it is not as easy to assess as pecuniary loss. However, as the determination of the award for non-pecuniary loss falls within the realm of the arbitrary and subjective, a reference level should be established to facilitate the determination of this amount. Such a judicial policy decision does not in my opinion impair the principle *restitutio in integrum* rule.

It should be emphasized that I do not propose to impose an upper limit that would prevent the courts from compensating the total non-pecuniary loss actually proven. The objective rather is to set parameters to which judges may refer in determining the monetary compensation to be awarded. In such an arbitrary matter, guidelines have to be established to ensure equal treatment of plaintiffs.

To this end I think that in practice, the circumstances in which a victim of defamation will have to be paid more than $50,000 in order to be fully compensated for his non-pecuniary loss will be extremely rare. Naturally, as we must determine the reasonableness of the verdict at the time of the trial judgment, this amount is expressed in 1978 dollars. At the present time, allowing for inflation, it corresponds to approximately $100,000 (Statistics Canada, All-Items Consumer Price Index, December 1987). The Court is not here adopting the upper limit of the trilogy established under the common law system. I wish however to point out that I am not deciding whether it is appropriate to adopt a reference level in cases of non-pecuniary loss resulting from physical injuries. I simply consider that it is desirable to set reference points in Quebec law to guide the courts in assessing non-pecuniary damages resulting from a defamation.

In fixing a sum of money to compensate a defamation victim for his pain and suffering, the court is undeniably making a purely arbitrary decision. Can the judge objectively place a price on pain, humiliation and anguish? As such a determination is not based on any mathematical calculation, he can easily get carried away and award compensation beyond all accepted limits. Although the victim is entitled to full compensation, the court must still ensure that he is not over-compensated. Compensation should not be a meuns of enriching him at the expense of the offending party.

I am in any case inclined to be wary of high amounts designed to compensate for non-pecuniary loss, as it is hard to know whether such amounts do not to some extent conceal a punitive aspect. Apart from certain exceptional cases such as s.49 of the *Charter of Human Rights and Freedoms*, R.S.Q. 1977, c . C- 12, Quebec civil law does not recognize the award of punitive damages:

> [TRANSLATION] The damages awarded to a victim of an offence or quasi-offence are intended solely as compensation. The indemnity is calculated so as to take account of the loss actually suffered and the gain lost. It must be determined in light of the compensation owed, not the penalty for wrongful or reckless conduct by the offender. In theory, therefore, there can be no question of punitive or exemplary damages. The voluntary or involuntary nature of the act causing the damage is also not a factor. This rule, applied by the Quebec courts, has been approved by a judgment of the Supreme Court of Canada. J.-L. Beaudoin, *La responsabilite civile delictuelle* (1985), p. 108, No. 187.

However, among the criteria relied on by the Quebec courts in estimating the non-pecuniary loss in defamation cases are the seriousness of the act, the good or bad faith and the intent of the offender, and these are all criteria with a punitive connotation: C. Bissonnette, *La diffamation civile en droit quebecois* (These de maitrise en droit, Universite de Montreal, 1985), p. 400. In general if these factors are present the court is prepared to increase this item of damage: see Baudouin, op. cit., at pp. 160-161. There is thus reason to think that the higher the amount of the indemnity, the more likely it is to have a punitive aspect. In my opinion this aspect should disappear from our system, where the rule is to compensate the victim, not to punish the offending party.

Additionally, the non-pecuniary loss suffered by a victim of defamation is in general temporary, since the suffering he experiences diminishes with the passage of time. However serious the defamation, people eventually forget the humiliating remarks made or written about the victim and the pain he has suffered gradually loses its edge. This temporary quality is a further reason which, to me, justifies the award of a maximum of $50,000 as full compensation for the damages caused in this regard.

Moreover, a person defamed who sues successfully obtains a judgment which restores his reputation; the publicity surrounding both the trial and its outcome and the possible publication of the judgment, which is authorized by the *Press Act*, are all means of providing partial or total compensation for the non-pecuniary loss. In other words, a court action allows the victim to cleanse his honour and applies a balm to his pain and suffering.

It can also be seen from the case law that Quebec courts have traditionally exercised restraint in assessing non-pecuniary damages for defamation. They have generally awarded amounts ranging from $500 to $5,000: *L'imprimerie Populaire Limitee c. L'Honorable L.A. Taschereau* (1922), 34 K.B. 554 — $1,000, or publication of the judgment and $500; *Langlois c. Drapeau*, [1962] Q.B. 277 — $2,000; *Flamand c. Bienvenue*, [1971] R.P. 49 (C.S.) — $2,000; *Lachapelle c. Veronneau*, [1980] C.S. 1136 — $2,000; *Blanchet c. Corneau*, [1985] C.S. 299 — $4,500; *Trahan c. Imprimerie Gagne Ltee*, J.E. 87-1146 (S.C.) — $2,000. Moreover, the highest awards rarely exceed $20,000: *Flamand c. Bonneville*, [1976] C.S. 1580 — $12,000 (appealed; settled out of court); *Desrosiers c. Les Publications Claude Daigneault Inc.*, [1982] C.S. 613 — $20,000; *Goupil c. Les Publications Photo-Police Inc.* [1983] C.S. 875 — $15,000 (appealed; settled out of court); *Poirier c. Leblanc*, [1983] C.S. 1214- $10,000; *Cote c. Le Syndicat des travailleuses et des travailleurs municipaux de la Ville de Gaspe*. J.E. 87-720 (S.C.) — $10,000; *McGregor c. The Montreal Gazette*. [1982] C.S. 900 — $50,000 (appealed; settled out of court); *Dimanche-Matin Ltee c. Fabien*, J.E. 83-971 (C A.) — $35.000. Apart from rare exceptions, the amounts awarded fall within a quite limited range. As the assessment of non-pecuniary loss is arbitrary, judges seem to instinctively recognize a limit which they are not prepared to exceed. This limit is generally quite low.

At common law, however, the courts have shown greater generosity. In the case at bar the trial judge reviewed the amount awarded by the courts in defamation cases. In addition to Quebec and France precedents, he consulted the case law of the United Kingdom and the other Canadian provinces. In my opinion, he should have limited himself to compensation awarded by Quebec courts, since different factors are used to determine non-pecuniary damages at common law. In addition to compensatory damages the common law allows the award of aggravated and punitive damages (Gatley, *Gatley on Libel and Slander* (7th ed. 1974), at pp. 1356-61). As we have seen, at civil law damages have a purely compensatory purpose. As the indemnity is often awarded in the form of a lump sum, it is impossible in a judgment rendered under the common law to know what portion of that sum is compensatory or punitive. Any comparison between the two systems is accordingly difficult to make.

Though it is a secondary consideration, there is one other factor that must be taken into account in defamation cases. These often involve newspapers, press agencies and radio or television stations. In coming to the rescue of a defamation victim, the courts must not overlook the fact that the written and spoken press is indispensable and is an essential component of a free and democratic society. Moreover, both the Quebec and Canadian Charters recognize the importance of the press (s.3 of the *Charter of Human Rights and Freedoms* and s.2 of the *Canadian Charter of Rights and Freedoms*). If information agencies are ordered to pay large amounts as the result of a defamation the danger is that their operations will be paralyzed or indeed, in some cases, that their very existence may be endangered. Although society undoubtedly places a great value on the reputation of its members that value, as it is subjective, cannot be so high as to threaten the functioning or the very existence of the press agencies which are essential to preserve a right guaranteed by the Charters.

In sum, in view of the arbitrary nature of the compensation awarded for non-pecuniary loss, the risk that it may have a punitive aspect, the temporary nature of the loss suffered, the compensatory effect of the judgment obtained and the moderation displayed by Quebec courts, I think that aside from truly exceptional cases it will not be necessary to award an amount greater than $50,000 (now $100,000) to compensate in full for the non-pecuniary loss resulting from an attack on reputation. Certainly, Quebec courts have never awarded compensation for non-pecuniary loss in a defamation case which comes even close to this limit. However, the concern for moderation should not lead us to underestimate the intrinsic value of reputation. There are many people who would prefer to suffer heavy pecuniary losses rather than to be lowered in the esteem of their friends. The reference level set by this judgment accordingly seems to me to be fair and reasonable because, while it may serve to prevent the award of extravagant claims, it is sufficiently high to encourage the courts to take into consideration the undoubted importance of reputation.

As the $135,000 award in the case at bar is well above the reference level, namely $50,000 in 1978, the Court is bound to conclude that the jury's verdict was clearly unreasonable. I accordingly consider that the trial judge made an error in affirming this verdict. The errors made by the trial judge and the Court of Appal accordingly provide a basis for this Court to substitute its conclusions for those of the jury in determining the reasonable amount to which appllant is entitled.

5.2.4.1.1.5 *Hill v. Church of Scientology of Toronto* 1994, unreported (Ont. C.A.)

GRIFFITHS, CATZMAN amd GALLIGAN, JJ.A.: These comments lead to a further observation. After the jurors had deliberated for just under four hours, they returned with a question. They asked:

> If in the event that items four to seven inclusive of the special verdict require addrressing [*i.e.*, the issues relating to general, aggravated and punitive damages], what if any are realistic maximums that have been assessed by society in recent history?

Although the question was a perceptive one the trial judge, correctly following the tradition which has long been established in Ontario, was obliged to reply as follows:

> I have discussed the question with counsel and we are all in agreement that the only answer that we can provide to you is that by law neither the parties nor the judge are entitled to advise the jury of maximums or minimums in these kinds of cases. So, I'm afraid you're on your own.

It would seem strange to the jurors who tried this case if this court were now to tell them that judges contemplate upper limits for damages which, if overstepped, will lead us to conclude that no six reasonable persons could have arrived at such an award, but that trial judges are unable to tell them what those upper limits are.

Our next observation is that each libel case is unique and it is virtually impossible to categorize or compare them. The personality and character of the defamed person, the nature of the libel and the circumstances surrounding its publication, the motivation and persistence of the person who defames, and the effect of the defamation upon the injured person depend upon many variables which are rarely duplicated. No two cases are the same, indeed, they rarely resemble one another. An award in one case is rarely, if ever, a useful guide in another.

. . . . .

The nature of the libel, the circumstances under which it was published and the hurt which it inflicted upon Casey Hill justified a very substantial award of general damages to compensate Casey Hill for the damage to his reputation and the injury to his feelings. The jury was properly instructed on the principles of law applicable to the assessment of those damages. It is, therefore, necessary to decide only whether the $300,000 assessed by the jury is an amount which is so large that six reasonable persons could not have awarded it or so grossly out of proportion to the libel as to shock the court's conscience and sense of justice.

The appellants submit that, in Canada, awards for defamation have historically been modest. The existence of historically modest awards in other cases, many of which were assessed by judges not juries, is not determinative of the jury's assessment of the damages in this case. The role of the jury as the representative of society in the assessment of damages in defamation cases must be respected. Jurors bring to such an assessment their own unique perspective against the backdrop of the circumstances and the evidence of the particular case. For this reason, courts have traditionally refused to give juries a range of damages by which they ought to be guided in the belief that the assessment of damages is the proper function of the jury.

The following factors are relevant to our review of the jury's assessment of general damages:

1. The libel was a most serious defamation.
2. The libel was published in circumstances designed to cause the most serious damage to Casey Hill's reputation and to ensure the widest circulation possible.
3. The libel caused serious injury to Casey Hill's feelings and that injury was not alleviated by any public apology.

Having regard to the nature of the libel, the circumstances of its publication and the injury which it caused to Casey Hill, justice called for a substantial award of general damages. The award of $300,000 does not strike us as so large that six reasonable persons could not have awarded it or so grossly out of proportion to the libel as to shock the court's conscience and sense of justice. We would not interfere with the award of $300,000 for general damages.

5.2.4.1.2 Factors Related to the Plaintiff

5.2.4.1.2.1 *Barltrop v. C.B.C.* (1978), 25 N.S.R. (2d) 673 (N.S.C.A.)

This case arose out of the plaintiff's claim against the defendant for damages for defamation. The plaintiff, who was a physician of high stature and reputation, appeared as an expert witness for 2 refining companies in a public hearing on alleged lead pollution by the companies, which was a hot public issue. The physician received $1,000 a day and expenses from the companies while so appearing. The C.B.C. broadcast a program in which it was stated that the physician was an example of an expert hired to give an opinion favourable to the interest paying him. The physician brought an action against the C.B.C. for damages for defamation.

The Nova Scotia Supreme Court, Trial Division dismissed the physician's action. The Trial Division held that, although the statements were defamatory, the C.B.C.'s defence of fair comment prevailed. The physician appealed.

MACKEIGAN, C.J.N.S.: ... The appellant asks us to assess damages, which, since this was not a jury trial, we have undoubted power to do. The respondent urges that we direct a new trial on that issue, or, if we have power to do so (which

I very much doubt — Civil Procedure Rule 62.23), refer it to the trial judge for assessment of damages. I do not think a trial judge would have any special advantage as to damages arising from seeing and hearing the witnesses in this case; it is not suggested that the attitudes displayed at the trial by the parties or their witnesses would have influenced the damages to be awarded.

The law allows general damages for sullied reputation. Such damages are "at large" because they are not susceptible to any exact monetary calculation.

Fleming, *supra*, at p. 521, states:
> Damages for loss of reputation may be either ordinary, aggravated or exemplary. The first two look to the injury done, the last to the conduct of the injurer. Among the factors to be taken into consideration in appraising the extent of the injury are the area of dissemination of the libel, the credence given to it by those to whom it was published and whether the plaintiff had furnished any ground for the aspersion, acted provocatively or in disregard for the feelings and reputation of others.

A good name proverbially is rather to be chosen than great riches, but its loss may require heavy financial solace. Fleming, *idem*, says:
> Reputation seems to be considered of much greater value than life or limb, dishonour an infinitely greater injury than agonizing and protracted physical suffering.

Pearson, L.J., in *McCarey v. Associated Newspapers*, [1965] 2 Q.B. at pp. 104-105 said:
> Compensatory damages..may include not only actual pecuniary loss and anticipated pecuniary loss or any social disadvantages which result or may be thought likely to result, from the wrong which has been done. They may also include the natural injury to his feelings — the natural grief and distress which he may have felt at having been spoken of in defamatory terms, and if there has been any kind of high-handed, oppressive, insulting or contumelious behaviour by the defendant which increases the mental pain and suffering caused by the defamation and may constitute injury to the plaintiff's pride and self-confidence, these are proper elements to be taken into account in a case where the damages are at large.

The courts have frequently allowed very large sums as damages where widely published defamation has seriously slurred a fine reputation, even where no loss could actually have been suffered, financially or otherwise.

Thus in *Youssoupoff v. Metro-Goldwyn-Mayer Pictures, Limited* (1934), 50 T.L.R. 581 (C.A.), an award of 25,000 pounds was not disturbed where a motion picture, widely distributed, had shown a woman, whom viewers knowing her might identify as Princess Youssoupoff, as having been seduced or raped by Rasputin. Greer, L.J., at p. 586 said:
> No doubt the damages are very large for a lady who lives in Paris, and who has not lost, so far as we know, a single friend and who has not been able to show that her reputation has in any way suffered from the publication of this unfortunate picture play, but, of course, one must not leave out of account a great many other things. One of them is that it is very difficult to value the reputation of any human being. It is very difficult to put a money figure upon the mental pain and suffering that is necessarily undergone by a good and delicate woman who has been foully libelled in the presence of large numbers of people. See *McGregor on Damages* (13th Ed.), paras. 1299-1301.

Injury to feelings may warrant heavy damages even where reputation was not affected. In *Fielding v. Variety Inc.*, [1967] 2 Q.B. 841 (C.A.), a theatrical producer was alleged to have had "a disastrous flop" in respect of a highly successful play, an allegation which obviously no one would believe. Salmon, L.J., at p. 855 said:

> It seems fairly obvious to me that that article cannot have had any really serious effect upon Mr. Fielding's reputation. Nevertheless he is entitled to be compensated, as I say, for the anxiety and annoyance which he very naturally felt at the time. For my part I consider that the sum of 5,000 pounds under that head was out of all proportion to the compensation justly payable to Mr. Fielding, and I agree with my Lords that the right figure under that head is 1,500 pounds.

Hall, J., for a majority of the Supreme Court of Canada in *McElroy v. Cowper-Smith and Woodman*, [1967] S.C.R. 425, at p. 426 said:

> I would not, in any way, underestimate or discount the damage that can be done to a lawyer or to an insurance executive by false allegations of misconduct and dishonesty. Defamation of a professional man is a very serious matter and ordinarily would be visited with an award of substantial damages, including punitive or exemplary damages if the circumstances so warrant.

He went on, however, to disallow an award of $25,000 damages on the ground that the defendant was temperamentally unstable and prone to make extravagant statements and that reasonable businessmen, the usual clientele of the plaintiffs, a solicitor and an insurance executive, would not likely be affected by the libels. He directed a new trial as to damages. Spence, J., dissenting, would have maintained the award.

In *Hubert et al. v. DeCamillis et al.* (1964), 41 D.L.R. (2d) 495 (B.C.S.C., Aikens, J.) damages of $15,000 were awarded a music teacher and dealer in respect of libel in letters to his students and others alleging fraud and false pretenses. The plaintiff showed no loss of specific business, but did show a general falling off of his business which he attributed to the libel.

An article published in the Canada edition of *Time* falsely accused a career army officer of being a member of a dope smuggling group in Viet Nam and stated he was going to be charged with smuggling: *Platt v. Time International of Canada Ltd.* (1964), 44 D.L.R. (2d) (Ont. H.C.). Chief Justice McRuer awarded him $35,000 as punitive damages. He stated (pp. 25-27):

> Quite apart from the criminality of trafficking in narcotic drugs it is conduct of such a loathsome and reprehensible character as to be revolting to all right-thinking people. A false imputation that the plaintiff was charged with being one of a group, four of whom had been found guilty of trafficking in narcotic drugs, gravely reflected his good name.
>
> . . . . . .
>
> In assessing damages I must take into consideration all the circumstances of the case. These include the conduct of the plaintiff, his position and standing in the community in which he lived, the nature of the libel, the mode and extent of the publication, whether there was a proper retraction or apology and the whole conduct of the defendant from the time the libel was published down to the close of the trial. I also take into consideration the conduct of the defendant before and after the action and in Court at the trial of the action: *Gatley on Libel & Slander*, 5th Ed., p. 625.

At no time from the publication of the offending article has the defendant expressed regret that the language used may have caused injury to the plaintiff's reputation in the community in which he lived.

. . . . .

During the course of the trial counsel for the defendant made it quite clear that he was not contending that the plaintiff was implicated in smuggling opium but at no time was regret expressed for the publication of the article if it was held to be defamatory. In fact the defendant displayed throughout a measure of defiant arrogance.

Although in the present case no attempt has been made to apologize or to retract the irresponsible imputation of professional dishonesty, and although one should expect higher standards and more balanced and responsible journalism from a national programme of the national broadcasting corporation, the circumstances in my view do not quite call for exemplary or punitive damages. I think the defendant's acts and attitude fall short of the kind of defamation requiring that penalty, and do not constitute "conscious, contumelious and calculated wrongdoing" characterized by intention to inflict the injury or by reckless indifference to consequences: *Australian Consolidated Press v. Uren* (1969), 117 C.L.R. 185. (I accept the proposition that the principles of *Rookes v. Barnard*, [1964] A.C. 1129, whereby in England the scope for punitive damages is now greatly limited, do not apply in Canada and that the test here is like that in Australia. See *McElroy v. Cowper-Smith and Woodman, supra*, per Spence, J., at p. 432; Fleming, *supra* at pp. 521-522; and Fridman: *Punitive Damages in Tort* (1940), 48 Can. Bar Rev . 373.)

The very factors which, if more pronounced, might have warranted punitive damages may, however, aggravate and increase the general damages which should be awarded to compensate the plaintiff for the injury to his reputation and feelings. So it is here. The prestige and apparent authority with which the defendant's programme falsely condemned the plaintiff, and its wide dissemination, without apology or explanation, throughout the northern half of North America greatly magnified the derogatory impact on Dr. Barltrop's reputation and pride. Cf. *Jones v. Bennett, supra*, where aggravated, but not punitive, damages of $15,000 were awarded and *Ross v. Lamport* (1957), 9 D.L.R. (2d) 585 (Ont. C.A.), where the mayor of Toronto was assessed $25,000 damages for arrogantly defaming in newspapers a man who had appealed a refusal of a taxicab licence and for failing to apologize.

The respondent argued strenuously that the appellant should in any event receive no more than nominal damages — that he proved no loss in the practice of his profession, that he would have been unlikely to receive pediatric references from Canada, least of all from Atlantic Canada, and that he had not proven any actual or potential loss of consultancy business resulting from the broadcasts. The cases to which I have referred show the fallacy in that argument. Serious damage to reputation requires heavy compensation, even if no specific loss is or can be shown. Here, a man of international reputation is vilified in the eyes of his professional confreres. He thus suffers greatly, though he may not lose a single dollar.

Even if many of his professional equals might well not believe or be influenced by the radio defamation, we cannot assume that laymen, such as industrialists, legislators, aldermen and other non-experts called upon to investigate or determine questions as to industrial pollution, would not be affected if they heard or read of the programme. Surely no lawyer wishing to impress a body of such laymen would risk presenting as an expert a man whose expertise and honesty had been so seriously impugned.

Dr. Barltrop could not prove positively that he had lost any specific consulting business in North America. He produced Dr. Panke, a member of a special advisory board formed in Idaho in 1976, who testified that he understood Dr. Barltrop had not been appointed to that board because the health authorities objected, apparently, because of the "Toronto mess". This was, however, partly denied or qualified by a Dr. Bax who selected the board and stated that he had not heard of the broadcast when he had left off Dr. Barltrop and, indeed, also Dr. Epstein, because they were respectively objected to by some environmentalists and by some companies.

Dr. Barltrop showed, however, that since the broadcast he had received no new retainers as a consultant in North America, and that his income from that source, previously substantial, had now disappeared. Like the plaintiff in *Hubert et al. v. DeCamillis et al., supra*, he has in my opinion shown probable financial loss, possibly substantial although not susceptible to any exact calculation.

Taking into account all the factors to which I have referred, considering Dr. Barltrop's professional eminence, the extreme defamation, the source whence it came, the extent of its dissemination, and the absence of apology or explanation, and considering the probable effect on Dr. Barltrop's practice and income, and making the best judgment I can in the light of all the evidence, I would award Dr. Barltrop as general damages the sum of $20,000.

I would allow the appeal with costs here and in the Court below.

Appeal allowed.

5.2.4.1.2.2 *Leonhard v. Sun Publishing* (1956), 4 D.L.R. (2d) 514 (B.C.S.C.)

LORD, J.: — The defendant publishes a daily newspaper known as the Vancouver *Sun*. On December 28, 1955, following its usual practice of giving a resume of top newspaper stories of the year, it published the following words under the heading "Police Probe Story Tops With Newsmen":

"The drug war — which followed the British Empire Games as second place story in last year's *Sun* poll — was an easy choice for number three spot in 1955.

"Its ugly pattern began to shape before the year was two months old.

"A booby trap bomb exploded in the car of drug king Jacob Leonard. Pusher Thomas Kinna's legs were broken on False Creek flats in June. August brought a major drug conspiracy roundup. September saw trafficker Eddie Scosky jump bail. This month, Kinna's assailants got heavy raps."

The plaintiff alleged that the defendant meant by these words that the plaintiff was in effect the head of an illegal drug syndicate operating in Vancouver, and had in consequence been seriously injured in his character, credit and reputation and had been brought into scandal, odium and contempt.

In its statement of defence the defendant admits the publication and does not seek to justify it, and specifically does not deny that the innuendo as pleaded is correct.

As already indicated the libel was published on December 28, 1955, the writ was issued on January 6, 1956, and on January 10, 1956, the defendant published the following apology:

"FACTS NOT CORRECT IN JACOB LEONARD REPORT

"Our attention has been drawn to our issue of Dec. 28, 1955, in which a story appeared entitled 'Police Probe Story Tops with Newsmen' in which reference was made to one Jacob Leonard.

"We have now ascertained that there is no foundation for the allegations contained in the story, and we take the earliest opportunity of correcting our error and of tendering to Mr. Jacob Leonard our sincere apologies.

"We trust he will accept this expression of our very great regret for any pain or annoyance that our reference may have caused him or his family."

The defendant brought into Court the sum of $501 in satisfaction of the plaintiff's cause of action.

In mitigation of damages the defendant denied that the plaintiff had been seriously injured in his character, credit and reputation and gave notice that under O. 36, r.37, of the Rules of the Supreme Court it would give particulars to the plaintiff of the matters intended to be given in evidence. These particulars were filed on May 18, 1956, and, in general, gave notice that it intended to adduce evidence of the general bad reputation of the plaintiff prior to the publication of the libel.

Several clippings from each of the three Vancouver daily newspapers, including the Vancouver *Sun*, published in March, 1955, were submitted in evidence not as proof of any statements contained therein but as evidence of the general bad reputation of the plaintiff. Some of these clippings had such headlines as "Leonard Named City Drug King"; "Bomb Blast Broke Up City Drug Ring"; "Police Near To Smashing City Drug Peddling Ring", with a subhead "Bombing Victim Named Boss"; "Undercover Agent Tags Bomb Victim As Leader of Local Narcotics Ring".

The words "Bomb Victim" refer to an explosion which occurred when the plaintiff endeavoured to start his car one morning at his home which resulted in serious injuries to himself.

The newspaper clippings were admitted in evidence subject to the objection of counsel for the plaintiff. In *Wigmore on Evidence*, 3rd ed., vol. I, p. 492, the learned author says: "Whether in an action for *defamation* the defendant may use the *plaintiff's poor reputation* (or lack of reputation) *to mitigate the damages* has been one of the most controverted questions in the whole law."

The classic case in England would seem to be the judgment of Cave, J. in *Scott v. Sampson* (1882), 8 Q.B.D. 491, where he said at p. 503:

> Speaking generally the law recognizes in every man a right to have the estimation in which he stands in the opinion of others unaffected by false statements to his discredit; and if such false statements are made without lawful excuse, and damage results to the person of whom they are made, he has a right of action. The damage, however, which he has sustained must depend almost entirely on the estimation in which he was previously held. He complains of an injury to his reputation and seeks to recover damages for that injury; and it seems most material that the jury who have to award those damages should know if the fact is so that he is a man of no reputation.
>
> . . . . . .
>
> On principle, therefore, it would seem that general evidence of reputation should be admitted, and on turning to the authorities previously cited it will be found that it has been admitted in a great majority of those cases, and that its admission has been approved by a great majority of the judges who have expressed an opinion on the subject.

Mr. Wigmore points out at p. 493, vol. I that the meat of the argument (in favour of acceptance of such evidence) is that a person should not be paid for the loss of that which he never had. I think that the clippings are admissible in evidence in this sense — that the words of the libel complained of, or words of similar import referring to the plaintiff as "drug king Jacob Leonard" had been published some few months before by all the Vancouver daily newspapers. If the plaintiff had been damaged in his character and reputation by the libel sued upon, then surely his character and reputation had already been damaged by the earlier publications, accompanied as they were with large headlines, as compared with a single line contained in an article dealing with other news items. It transpired during the course of the trial that no proceedings were taken by the plaintiff respecting such publications. He gave no evidence at the trial — he did not see fit to come into Court and seek to protect his name and reputation. But he admitted on examination for discovery that he had suffered damage in this respect before the publication of the libel:

"Q. 109. Is it fair to say that before December of last year you had pretty well decided what you have just stated, that you would have to leave town or dig a hole and pull it in after you? A. And it was — I was doing all right before your paper started to blast me.

"Q. 110. When did you read this — ? A. Oh, I went to the loan company, and I was going to make an effort to build some houses, and they told me they wouldn't give me any credit no more. So I can't get any credit. I may as well not work around here.

5.2.4.1.3 Factors Related to the Defendant

5.2.4.1.3.1 *Vogel v. C.B.C.* (1982), 21 C.C.L.T. 105 (B.C.S.C.)

ESSON, J.: The identity of the accuser is an important factor. The accusation might have [been] made by some nasty little tabloid scandal sheet and have done no harm. Strident scandal mongering is the stock in trade of certain publications and, because it is, they have little or no effect upon the opinions of anyone whose good opinion matters. To their ugly accusations, it is a sufficient response to say: Regard the source

Such a response is not available when defamed by CBC. In terms of prestige, power and influence, it is at the opposite end of the spectrum from the sleazy scandal sheet. Created and maintained by Parliament to inform the Canadian public, its news services are accorded great respect throughout Canada. They have a well-merited reputation for reliability. For that very reason, CBC has an enormous capacity to cause damage. The general run of right-thinking people tend to think that "it was on the CBC News, so it must be so."

5.2.4.1.3.2 *Baxter v. C.B.C.* (1980), 30 N.B.R. (2d) 102 (N.B.C.A.)

RYAN, J.A.: Although I am reluctant to interfere with a trial judge's award of damages, in my opinion, in the instant case, the trial judge failed to consider as a relevant factor in awarding damages *the extent of the publication*. In Duncan and Neill in their text on *Defamation*, 8th Ed., p. 136, par. 18.14, it is said:

> 18.14 In many cases an important factor in the assessment of damages will be the extent of the publication. Thus whereas a limited publication to one or two individuals may lead to a very modest award of damages, particularly if the publishers are not influenced by the publication or may disbelieve it, a publication in a national newspaper or by means of television or radio may lead to a very substantial award because the defamatory material is likely to come to the notice of a very large number of people including many who are friends or acquaintances of the plaintiff. On the other hand the gravity of the matter cannot always be assessed by reference to the extent of the publication and certainly not in any direct ratio to the number of persons to whom the defamatory material is published. Thus a publication by letter to an employer or to a limited circle of the plaintiff's friends may be no less damaging than the publication of similar material in an article in a newspaper. Moreover, where a true innuendo is relied upon, or where only persons with knowledge of special facts would identify the plaintiff, it is submitted that the jury should be warned that the only relevant publication is to the persons with the special knowledge.

In view of the fact the program was telecast to about 980,000 Canadian viewers, some of whom no doubt were friends and acquaintances of Mr. Baxter, I would increase the award of general damages from $1,000.00 to $10,000.00.

5.2.4.1.3.3 *Westbank Band of Indians v. Tomat* (1992), 10 C.C.L.T. (2d) 1 (B.C.C.A.)

The appellants (defendants), most of whom were disaffected members of an Indian band, published a press relcasc and a petition, alleging that the respondent (former chief of the band) and others (former councillors) were corrupt persons who had misappropriated band property, fraudulently conducted the band's affairs, and indulged in bribery and intimidation. The defendants pleaded absence of publication, justification, fair comment and qualified privilege. The evidence disclosed that the band had long been riven by factions respectively loyal to the plaintiff-respondent as chief, or to his rival, the present chief, a defendant in this action.

At trial, the defamatory character of the documents complained of was affirmed, as was the fact of publication. The plea of justification was rejected, all the allegations of criminality being devoid of truth. The plea or fair comment was also set aside, since all the impugned statements were assertions of fact. The defence of qualified privilege was unavailable both because of the breadth of publication involved and the demonstrated malice of the defendants.

Substantial awards of damages were made in favour of the various plaintiffs. The former chief, who had suffered both emotional harm and financial loss, was awarded $350,000 as general damages, plus a further $50,000 as punitive damages. The defendants appealed.

WOOD, J.A.: I have had the privilege of reading in draft form the reasons of Mr. Justice Hinds. I am in complete agreement both with his view that there must be a new trial and with his reasons for having reached that conclusion.

The trial judge concluded that the motive of these appellants was political. They were part of a group of band members for a variety of reasons dissatisfied with the political leadership and management policies of the respondents, who constituted the elected band council. The evidence establishes that this situation had persisted for many years, and that it had led to a continuing series of complaints, petitions and demands for investigation, all of which had been directed to the federal Department of Indian Affairs and Northern Development in Ottawa.

As a consequence of these activities there had been 20 investigations or inquiries into band operations by federal officials in the ten years preceding the publication of the petition with which this case is concerned. The respondent Ronald Michael Derrickson, who was chief throughout that period of time, himself said that his was the most investigated and closely scrutinized band council in Canada.

Notwithstanding all of this attention, the factional dissatisfaction with the band's political leadership continued. In a closely knit community, ranging in numbers over that period from 150 to just over 300, it caused acrimony and unrest and divided families. As time passed without any significant change, dissatisfaction led to frustration. From the evidence it seems likely that frustration must have clouded the judgment of at least some of the defendants during the events leading up to the publication and re-publication of the defamatory statements at issue-in this action.

The circulation of a petition to band members, followed by its presentation to the minister responsible for Indian affairs in Ottawa, is apparently a time-honoured and accepted part of the native political process in this country. David Crombie, a former minister who gave evidence at the trial, testified that during his tenure many such petitions were received in his office from bands all across Canada. Thus there was nothing unusual about those received from the dissidents in the Westbank Indian Band. Mr. Crombie also noted that the substance of many of the allegations set out in the petition which became the subject matter of this action had been made consistently over the years.

These were the circumstances in which the defamatory statements were made. None of the appellants appears to be politically sophisticated, at least in the sense of conventional politics. With the possible exception of Mr. Louie, who the trial judge found was motivated by a desire to become chief at an annual remuneration of $75,000, none of the appellants had anything to gain from making the statements which led to this action, other than the satisfaction of eventually seeing the band run in a way which they felt would better benefit its membership.

None of this can excuse the actions of any of those appellants against whom liability may be established following a new trial. In a democratic society which honours the freedom and security of individuals as well as the community, political motivation, even of the highest order, can never justify the defamation of one's opponent. Nor can feelings of frustration excuse even the most unsophisticated from the legal consequences of their conduct.

But it is my view that such matters are relevant to the assessment of damages, and may have a mitigating effect in the face of what would otherwise be seen as the aggravating features of defamatory statements made in a political context. Acceptance of that approach leads to restraint when non-pecuniary damages are assessed.

It is important that restraint be exercised when assessing damages for defamatory statements made in a political context. The rhetoric of modern political debate is replete with extravagant hyperbole, partisan viewpoints and inaccuracy. The result is that any libel which occurs in such a context is likely to be taken for what it is, and thus to a considerable extent deprived of what would otherwise be its sting. Those defamed in such debate, moreover, necessarily have access to the public platform from which to rebut whatever sting may, in fact, remain.

But there is also an important constitutional justification for such restraint. Without it the delicate balance between freedom of expression and protection of reputation may be lost, and that balance has much to do with the survival of the modern democratic political process.

We live in a time when democratic political institutions of all forms are viewed with increasing cynicism and distrust. Participation by citizens in our political process is said to decline as individuals feel increasingly remote from those controlling the governmental system which shapes their future. In such a climate there is a danger that government will grow less responsive to the governed, leading to a self-perpetuating cycle which tends inexorably to destruction of the democratic system.

In the face of such tendencies we need more, not less, political debate and the fundamental importance of free expression seems obvious.

The freedom of expression essential to the democratic process is endangered if an atmosphere of intimidation results from large damage awards in cases of politically motivated defamation. Recognition of that fact, however, does not mean that the reputation of public people must be sacrificed on the altar of free expression. I agree with the trial judge that a decision to serve the public good must not deprive a person of the protection of his or her reputation which the law is properly expected to provide.

There must, however, be an appropriate balance between legitimate protection of freedom of expression, on the one hand, and the necessary protection of individual reputation, on the other. I believe the key to finding this balance lies in a realistic appreciation of the rehabilitative effect which may reasonably be expected to result from a finding against the defendant and the award of significant monetary damages. As pointed out by Lamer, J. (as he then was) in the *Snyder* case, the assessment of non-pecuniary damages in defamation cases is at best an arbitrary process. It lies beyond our ingenuity to establish any scientific correlation between the amount of money awarded by way of damages and its rehabilitative effect on a reputation sullied through defamation. But there is no reason to believe that any correlation which may exist is one of direct proportionality. Rather, it seems more likely that it is governed by the law of diminishing returns.

In the name of salvaging reputations we can no longer apply common law rules relating to damages for defamation which belong to an earlier and very different era. If we are to discharge the mandate found in the *Dolphin Delivery* and *Salituro* cases we must define the limits of non-pecuniary damages in cases of politically motivated defamation in such a way as to afford reasonable protection to reputation without endangering the fundamental freedom of expression on which the survival of our governmental system depends.

I conclude that where liability has been established for defamatory statements made of a public official, in respect of the conduct of such person in an office to which he or she has been elected, the non-pecuniary damages awarded ought to be limited to an amount sufficient to bring clearly to public attention the fact that the allegations were unwarranted, and that no lawful excuse for making them existed. But beyond that, the courts must be careful not to award damages which may tend more to stifle the free expression of opinion than to rehabilitate the reputation of the defamed.

The full scope of the circumstances to which this rule ought to be applied must await orderly development on a case-by-case basis. For the purposes of this appeal it is sufficient to say only that it should be applied where it is apparent that excessive zeal has caused ordinary citizens driven by political motivation, and not by calculated malice, to lose sight of the boundary between legitimate comment and actionable defamation. It should perhaps be noted that we are not here dealing with an action in which the media, whose resources and motivation may be entirely different, are sued for having re-published such a libel. It may well be that entirely different considerations would apply in such a case.

Where more than one defendant is involved, of course, the rule must be considered separately and applied individually on the basis of the motive attributable to each.

5.2.4.1.3.4 *Munro v. Toronto Sun* (1982), 21 C.C.L.T. 261 (Ont. H.C.)

HOLLAND, J.: There remains the claim for punitive or exemplary damages to be considered. Such damages are awarded by the Court to reflect its outrage, disapproval and aversion of conduct, so as to punish and make an example of a defendant so that it will be known that such conduct will not be tolerated by our Courts. They are not to be added compensation for the injury suffered by the plaintiff — but rather are received by the plaintiff as a windfall because of the defendant's conduct. I need not consider whether or not deliberate intention to harm the plaintiff is an essential ingredient to support an award of punitive damages, because on the evidence before me I have no difficulty in concluding that both Ramsay and Reguly did deliberately intend harm to Mr. Munro. The language of Ramsay, "I've got that f..g Munro", the article published on March 27, the lack of care as to accuracy of the story and the falsity of the contents, and the language in the memorandum made by Reguly (set out above) particularly to that "Sleaze Munro" all satisfy me that both Ramsay and Reguly were out to "get" Mr. Munro. It is accordingly an appropriate case in which to award punitive damages against Ramsay and Reguly and to provide that the corporate defendant be vicariously liable therefor. For reasons previously given I do not find that the actions of the other defendants were such as to attract a punitive award. I assess these damages payable by Ramsay, Reguly and the Toronto Sun Publishing Corporation at $25,000 in the hope that this amount will be an effective deterrent to the *Sun* and to all who contemplate similar actions.

5.2.4.1.3.5 *Vogel v. C.B.C.* (1982), 21 C.C.L.T. 105 (B.C.S.C.)

ESSON, J.: The circumstances of this case, taken together, require an award of damages at the highest end of the scale. Those circumstances include the seriousness of the libel, the breadth of its publication, the extent of the demonstrable damage, the deliberate malice shown by the defendants in the preparation of the programme and in continuing to trial a course of action calculated to inflict upon the plaintiff the maximum hurt and damage.

The plaintiff places particular reliance upon *Broome v. Cassell* as having some similarity in its pattern of facts as they bear upon damages. A book written by one defendant, and published by the other, placed the blame for one of the great naval disasters of World War II on the plaintiff, then a retired naval officer, and made serious imputations on his conduct and courage. The author, in making those imputations, had known what he was doing and persisted in spite of authoritative warnings that the passages were defamatory. In a letter to the publisher, he said that it would be possible to say, "some pretty near the knuckle things" about Captain Broome and others, and "if one says it in a clever enough way, they cannot take action." The attitude displayed by Messrs. Waters, King and Bird could be described in the same words. In *Broome v. Cassell*, the defendants were motivated by the desire for gain, a motive which is not materially different from CBC's desire to improve its ratings and attract attention and Mr. Bird's desire to make his reputation as an investigative reporter.

In some important respects, *Broome v. Cassell* was less serious. By its nature, a book could not have the immediate and shattering impact of a special feature on prime time television. The libel against Captain Broome was cruel and hurtful but, coming as it did some years after his retirement from the navy, it could not affect his career. The claim for compensatory damages was, for that and other reasons, weaker than that in this case. The principal similarity is in the conduct of the defendants and therefore in the basis for punitive damages. In that case, the jury award, which was not disturbed on appeal, was £15,000 for compensatory damages and £25,000 for punitive damages.

Platt v. Time Int., supra, is in some respects comparable. The plaintiff was a career army officer who had served for a time with the International Control Commission in Vietnam. A number of Canadian servicemen were court martialed for taking part in an opium smuggling ring and some were convicted. A story reporting on those matters ended with the sentence: "This week the only officer in the group, Major W.A. Platt, 48, takes his turn in court."

In its context, that sentence was held to imply falsely that the plaintiff was a member of the opium smuggling ring and was to be tried for that offence. In view of some of the positions taken by CBC in this case, it is of interest to note that the sentence was literally correct in that Major Platt was the only officer in the group of people referred to in the story and he was scheduled to take his turn in Court. What the story did not say was that the charge against him was of the much less serious offence of smuggling gold and that he had not been involved in smuggling opium. It is the false implication that he was so involved which was the basis of the judgment. That is worthy of mention because it seems clear that those responsible for producing the programme had the misapprehension that defamation consists only of saying that which is untrue in the literal sense and that the law will not have regard to context where defamatory meanings are merely implied.

The libel against Major Platt may be considered more serious than that against Mr. Vogel in that it imputed to him criminal conduct of a most reprehensible kind. The conduct of the defendant had important points of similarity. The imputation was made notwithstanding knowledge by *Time's* editors that Major Platt had not been charged with smuggling opium and was done to "add colour to the article" by suggesting that an officer was involved. It was held that the publication, if not deliberate, was done with a reckless indifference to any injury that might be done.

In other respects it was a less serious case. The allegation, although serious, was specific in its nature and thus capable of being effectively rebutted. The number of viewers of the CBC news programmes was far greater than the total circulation of the Canadian edition of *Time*. There is no indication that public opinion was turned against Major Platt in the same way that it was turned against Mr. Vogel. That distinction is important because what makes this case almost unique is the degree of severity of the impact upon the plaintiff in his professional and personal life.

In making any comparison to earlier damage awards, it is of course now necessary to have regard to the effects of inflation. The present equivalent to an award of $35,000 in 1964 would be an amount two to three times as large.

In considering the appropriate scale of damages, the amounts awarded in *Broome v. Cassell* and other English cases are of limited assistance because, historically, the level of defamation awards in England appears to have been consistently higher than in Canada.

The defendants submit that *Snyder v. Montreal Gazette* should be disregarded as a guide because of differences between the law of Quebec and that of British Columbia. There may not be much difference in the basic principles to be applied — I note that Deschenes, C.J.S.C. relied on many decisions from provinces other than Quebec. The most important difference of substance which appears in the reasons is one which affords no comfort to these defendants. By the law of Quebec, no punitive damages can be awarded (87 D.L.R. (3d) at p. 14). Were a comparison to be made, it would be necessary to bear in mind that the publication in *Snyder* came five years before, and the judgment four years before, the equivalent dates in this case. An equivalent award, after adjusting for inflation over that period, could be $175,000 or more. Furthermore, *Snyder* was a less serious case in many ways. There are points of similarity in the position of the plaintiff and the nature of the defamation but it does not appear that there were any of the elements of deliberate attack or dramatic over-emphasis which were present here. The source of the libel was hearsay testimony before the Quebec Police Commission. The *Montreal Gazette*, in publishing the story, was apparently saying the same thing that was being said almost simultaneously by other members of the media. The action against the *Gazette* was one of eight brought by the plaintiff but was apparently the first to get to trial (87 D.L.R. (3d) at p. 12).

Nevertheless, I put that case out of consideration as a basis for comparison because it is still subject to appeal.

In assessing compensatory damages, the element of aggravation resulting from the defendant's conduct must be taken into account:

> In awarding aggravated damages the natural indignation of the court at the injury inflicted on the plaintiff is a perfectly legitimate motive in making a generous rather than a more moderate award

to provide an adequate solatium. But that is because the injury to the plaintiff is actually greater and as the result of the conduct exciting the indignation demands a more generous solatium.
Broome v. Cassell, [1972] A.C. at p. 1073, [1972] 1 All E.R. at pp. 825-6.

Clearly, that applies here. The injury to Mr. Vogel was greater because of the reckless and deliberately damaging actions of the defendants: see *Robitaille v. Vancouver Hockey Club Ltd.* (1981), 30 B.C.L.R. 286 at 310-13, 16 C.C.L.T. 225, 20 C.P.C. 293, 124 D.L.R. (3d) 228 (C.A.).

Compensatory damages are not confined in their scope to pecuniary losses:

[Defamation] actions involve a money award which may put the plaintiff in a purely financial sense in a much stronger position than he was before the wrong. Not merely can he recover the estimated sum of his past and future losses, but, in case the libel, driven underground, emerges from its lurking place at some future date, he must be able to point to a sum awarded by a jury sufficient to convince a bystander of the baselessness of the charge.
Broome v. Cassell, at p. 1071 A.C.; at p. 824 All E.R.

For the reasons which I have already given, I consider that adequate compensation to the plaintiff for the injury to his reputation by being publicly defamed should be fixed at $100,000.

The remaining matter to be considered is whether any additional amount should be awarded as punitive or exemplary damages. (The terms are synonymous.)

Rookes v. Barnard, [1964] A.C. 1 129, [1964] 1 All E.R. 367 (H.L.), has not been accepted as stating the law in this country insofar as it restricts exemplary damages to cases falling within three specified categories. It is, nevertheless, authoritative on other aspects of the law of damages so carefully considered therein. I refer particularly to the following:

In a case in which exemplary damages are appropriate, a jury should be directed that if, but only if, the sum which they have in mind to award as compensation (which may of course be a sum aggravated by the way in which the defendant has behaved to the plaintiff) is inadequate to punish him for his outrageous conduct, to mark their disapproval of such conduct and to deter him from repeating it, then they can award some larger sum." [1964] A.C. at p. 1228, [1964] 1 All E.R. at p. 41, quoted in *Broome v. Cassell*, [1972] A.C. at p. 1059, [1972] 1 All E.R. at p. 814.

In this province, exemplary damages may be granted in all cases where the conduct of the defendant has been such as to merit the condemnation of the Court: *Robitaille v. Vancouver Hockey Club Ltd.*, *supra*, at p. 310 [B.C.L.R.]. That initial test is clearly met by the facts of this case. At that point, the other matters mentioned by Lord Devlin are useful in deciding whether such damages should be awarded. If punishment is not necessary for the purpose of deterrence, the case for awarding exemplary damages is weaker.

In relation to this question, the position of the two defendants must be considered separately. Mr. Bird's circumstances in life are such that, if any amount of damages would serve to deter him from a repetition of his conduct, the appropriate amount for that purpose would be less than the amount of compensatory damages. While his conduct merits the disapproval of the Court, the amount of compensatory damages is also sufficient to signify that disapproval. Mr. Bird's conduct was in the course of his employment as a reporter. Had his employer exercised a reasonable degree of editorial judgment and control, that conduct would have caused no harm to anyone.

The damage came, not from the investigation, but from the publication. The responsibility for deciding whether to publish rested with those above Mr. Bird. The most seriously reprehensible conduct was their abdication of responsibility. That was an abdication, not by individuals, but by an organization possessing a unique degree of influence and power.

CBC is one of the great corporations of Canada. It has massive means at its disposal. There is evidence that total income in the most recent fiscal year was $656,000,000 of which $515,000,000 came from its parliamentary grant. In this action, the corporation showed no sign of feeling any real concern about the harm caused by the irresponsible abuse of its great power. Its management shares Mr. Bird's view of what is important. Mr. Lauk said that, because "we live in an increasingly secretive society", it would be wrong for him "to hindsight the newsroom".

This is not the first, although it is the most serious, case disclosing what may be a tendency on the part of CBC in some of its programmes to proclaim its view of the truth with righteous zeal but scant regard for the facts and for the reputations of those of whose conduct it disapproves. In *Barltrop v. C.B.C.* (1978), 5 C.C.L.T. 88, 36 A.P.R. 637, 86 D.L.R. (3d) 61, 25 N.S.R. (2d) 637 (N.S.C.A.), the radio programme "As It Happens" said of the plaintiff that, in testifying as a medical expert at a public inquiry into lead poisoning, he had given untruthful and misleading evidence and had done so in wanton disregard for public health. As in this case, the defence of fair comment was raised and failed. MacKeigan, C.J.N.S., for the Court, said at p. 78 [D.L.R.] that there had been an "irresponsible imputation of professional dishonesty" and that '' ... one should expect higher standards and more balanced and responsible journalism from a national programme of the national broadcasting corporation. . . ."

In *Thomas v. C.B.C., supra*, it was imputed to the plaintiff in a series of radio broadcast that he had improperly performed his duties to the extent that there had been a "betrayal of public faith" which resulted in a fatal explosion. Disbery, J., at p. 337 [W.W.R.], pointed out that CBC's reporter had been in possession of a great deal of information favourable to the plaintiff and inconsistent with the thrust of the programme but that the broadcast had contained not "even the shadow of a whisper" of such matters. He went on so say:

> The repeated juxtapositioning of plaintiff's misconduct, explosion and death promoted sensationalism. How drab in comparison would the story have been if it had merely related that due to somebody's negligence on the drill ship the gas separator had not been connected and in use thus allowing gas to accumulate which, becoming ignited, exploded and caused MacKay's death. 'Man bites dog' is newsworthy, 'dog bites man' is not. These unsensational and unnewsworthy matters were, in my opinion, omitted from the broadcasts in order to be able to present to the public the

more sensational story of a low level official giving quick approval to the request of a well known multinational oil corporation that even the government could not control. To only give the public a look at the side of the coin supportive of their comments and opinions and not to show the facts to the contrary on the other side of the coin is to deal in half-truths, and comments made in this way are neither fair nor made in good faith.

The broadcasts in those two cases took place in 1974 and 1977 respectively. I know of no case in recent years in which any other member of the Canadian "communications media" has been subjected to similarly harsh criticism.

The question then arises whether CBC, by reason of its size and power, is immune to deterrence by any monetary award which would not be unthinkable by the moderate standards which prevail in Canada. That would be so only if the irresponsible attitude which allowed the Vogel story to be published is an established one in the controlling minds of the corporation. Such a conclusion would not be warranted in view of the general reputation for excellence of CBC's news services. There must be weighed, against the few demonstrated examples of irresponsibility and unfairness, the countless broadcasts which have shown a high standard of balanced and responsible journalism.

The circumstances of the case call for the award of an additional amount against CBC as exemplary damages. That amount should not depart from the tradition of moderate awards but should be sufficient to mark the Court's disapproval of the conduct of CBC and provide some element of deterrence from similar conduct. That amount I fix at $25,000.

5.2.4.1.3.6 *Hill v. Church of Scientology of Toronto* 1994, unreported (Ont. C.A.)

(The trial court awarded $500,000 in aggravated damages and $800,000 in punitive damages against the Church of Scientology.)

GRIFFITHS, CATZMAN and GALLIGAN, JJ.A.: Punitive damages are different from compensatory damages in that they are not intended to compensate the plaintiff for the injury caused by the libel. Rather, they are designed to express the repugnance of the public, which is represented by the jury, towards the outrageous and heinous conduct of the defendant. The award of punitive damages must be sufficient to punish the defendant for its conduct and to deter the defendant, specifically, and others, generally, from similar conduct in the future. Finally, punitive damages should only be awarded if the compensatory damages are considered by the jury to be insufficient to express its repugnance at the conduct of the defendant and to punish and deter.

An appellate court should be very hesitant to substitute its opinion for that of the jury regarding the adequacy of the compensatory award to effect the purpose of punitive damages. The appellate court's duty to interfere arises when it is convinced that an award of punitive damages, in addition to the compensatory award, serves no rational purpose.

In some respects, evidence which supports an award of aggravated damages may also incite feelings of repugnance towards a defendant's conduct and indicate the need for punishment and deterrence. Thus, evidence which is relevant to an award of aggravated damages may also be relevant to the need for punitive damages and to the amount of them. What is particularly relevant to an award of punitive damages is malice and egregious conduct on the part of the defendant towards the plaintiff.

. . . . .

The evidence before the jury amply justified its decision to award punitive damages against Scientology. The amount of the award is not so high that it could not have been arrived at by six reasonable persons. It does not shock our conscience or our sense of justice. Moreover, the conduct of Scientology after the verdict demonstrates that the jury was right when it decided it ought to award punitive damages. That conduct also demonstrates that the amount of the award was not too high. Accordingly, we would not interfere with the award of punitive damages.

5.2.4.1.3.7 *Walker Brothers Quarries Ltd. v. CFTO Ltd. et al.* (1987), 19 O.A.C. 10 (Ont. C.A.)

ROBINS, J.A.: Accepting the gravity of the libel here and viewing the circumstances in a manner most favourable to the company's position, the award of $883,000 is so inordinately large as to bear no reasonable relationship to the defamatory publication or the consequences flowing from it. While any libel by a national television network must be treated as serious, I am constrained to say that counsel's description of the program as "the most wicked libel imaginable" is insupportable. In my opinion, no jury applying the right principles and a reasonable scale of values could reach the conclusion that the defamatory statements in question are such as to warrant an award far exceeding any award ever made in a defamation action in Canada. We are told that the highest award to date was made in *Vogel v. Canadian Broadcasting Corporation, supra*, where $100,000 general damages and $25,000 exemplary damages were granted to a Deputy Attorney General for a defamatory allegation that he had improperly influenced the course of justice. In that case, aggravated damages compensating for such items as the shock and stress caused to the plaintiff by the defamatory broadcasts and their effect on him physically and on his family and professional life formed a significant put of the general damage assessment. And there, of course, the plaintiff was not a company.

As a general proposition, it can be fairly stated that where a defendant has engaged in some form of reprehensible conduct the scale of damages appropriate to the case of a defamed individual can reasonably be expected to be higher than the scale appropriate to the case of a defamed company. In the latter case, there can be no question of compensation for injured feelings or compensation by way of aggravated damages for increased injury to such feelings, both patently important elements in an individual's general damage claim. Furthermore, in this case, there is no question of any pecuniary loss. All that has to be compensated for here is the injury to Walker Brothers' corporate reputation. The figure set by this jury as being the amount necessary to vindicate that reputation in the eyes of right thinking people in the community goes far beyond the maximum limit of any range that can conceivably be regarded as fair or reasonable compensation for this company in these circumstances. It is so exorbitant and irrational a sum that it should not be allowed to stand.

5.2.4.1.4 Apology

If the defendant apologizes to the plaintiff, this can have the effect of substantially reducing the damages which may be awarded.

5.2.4.1.4.1 *Ontario Libel and Slander Act*, R.S.O. 1990, c. L.12

5. (2) the plaintiff shall recover only actual damages if it appears on the trial,
   (*a*) that the alleged libel was published in good faith;
   (*b*) that the alleged libel did not involve a criminal charge;
   (*c*) that the publication of the alleged libel took place in mistake or misapprehension of the facts; and
   (*d*) that a full and fair retraction of any matter therein alleged to be erroneous,
      (i) was published either in the next regular issue of the newspaper or in any regular issue thereof published within three days after the receipt of the notice mentioned in subsection (1) and was so published in as conspicuous a place and type as was the alleged libel, or
      (ii) was broadcast either within a reasonable time or within three days after the receipt of the notice mentioned in subsection (1) and was so broadcast as conspicuously as was the alleged libel.

(3) This section does not apply to the case of a libel against any candidate for public office unless the retraction of the charge is made in a conspicuous manner at least five days before the election. R.S.O. 1980, c. 237, s. 5.

8. (1) No defendant in an action for a libel in a newspaper is entitled to the benefit of sections 5 and 6 unless the names of the proprietor and publisher and the address of publication are stated either at the head of the editorials or on the front page of the newspaper.

(2) The production of a printed copy of a newspaper is admissible in evidence as proof, in the absence of evidence to the contrary, of the publication of the printed copy and of truth of the statements mentioned in subsection (1).

(3) Where a person, by registered letter containing the person's address and addressed to a broadcasting station, alleges that a libel against the person has been broadcast from the station and requests the name and address of the owner or operator of the station or the names and addresses of the owner and the operator of the station, sections 5 and 6 do not apply with respect to an action by such person against such owner or operator for the alleged libel unless the person whose name and address are so requested delivers the

requested information to the first-mentioned person, or mails it by registered letter addressed to the person, within ten days from the date on which the first-mentioned registered letter is received at the broadcasting station. R.S.O. 1980, c. 237, s. 8.

9. (1) In an action for a libel in a newspaper, the defendant may plead in mitigation of damages that the libel was inserted therein without actual malice and without gross negligence and that before the commencement of the action, or at the earliest opportunity afterwards, the defendant inserted in such newspaper a full apology for the libel or, if the newspaper in which the libel appeared is one ordinarily published at intervals exceeding one week, that the defendant offered to publish the apology in any newspaper to be selected by the plaintiff.

(2) In an action for a libel in a broadcast, the defendant may plead in mitigation of damages that the libel was broadcast without actual malice and without gross negligence and that before the commencement of the action, or at the earliest opportunity afterwards, the defendant broadcast a full apology for the libel. R.S.O. 1980, c. 237, s. 9.

10. In an action for a libel in a newspaper or in a broadcast, the defendant may prove in mitigation of damages that the plaintiff has already brought action for, or has recovered damages, or has received or agreed to receive compensation in respect of a libel or libels to the same purport or effect as that for which such action is brought. R.S.O. 1980, c. 237, s. 10.

20. In an action for libel or slander where the defendant has pleaded a denial of the alleged libel or slander only, or has suffered judgment by default, or judgment has been given against the defendant on motion for judgment on the pleadings, the defendant may give in evidence, in mitigation of damages, that the defendant made or offered a written apology to the plaintiff for such libel or slander before the commencement of the action, or, if the action was commenced before there was an opportunity of making or offering such apology, that the defendant did so as soon afterwards as the defendant had an opportunity. R.S.O. 1980, c. 237, s. 22.

21. In an action for libel or slander, where the statement of defence does not assert the truth of the statement complained of, the defendant may not give evidence in chief at trial, in mitigation of damages, concerning the plaintiff's character or the circumstances of publication of the statement, except,

(*a*) where the defendant provides particulars to the plaintiff of the matters on which the defendant intends to give evidence, in the statement of defence or in a notice served at least seven days before trial; or

(*b*) with leave of the court. 1984, c. 11, s. 191(2).

Notes on Statutes in Other Provinces

The above sections are typical of legislation adopted in all the common-law provinces. For provisions similar to s. 5(2) and (3) see *Revised Uniform Defamation Act*, s. 18 in Conference of Commissioners on Uniformity of Legislation in Canada, Proceedings of the Thirtieth Annual Meeting, Montreal, Quebec, August 24-28, 1948, Appendix J; *Defamation Act*, R.S.A. 1980, c. D-6, s. 16; *Libel and Slander Act*, R.S.B.C. 1979, c. 234, ss. 7 and 8; the *Defamation Act*, R.S.M. 1987, c. D-20, s. 17; *Defamation Act*, R.S.N.B. 1973, c. D-5, s. 17;

Defamation Act, R.S.N. 1990, c. D-3, s. 19; *Defamation Act*, R.S.N.S. 1989, c. 122, s. 22; *Defamation Act*, R.S.P.E.I. 1988, c. D-5, s. 18; *Defamation Act*, R.S.N.W.T. 1988, c. D-1, s. 19; *Defamation Act*, R.S.Y.T. 1986, c. 41, s. 18; and the *Libel and Slander Act*, R.S.S. 1978, c. L-14, s. 8 which states that in the case of a candidate for public office the retraction must be made at least 15 days before the election.

The following sections resemble s. 8 of the Ontario Act: *Revised Uniform Defamation Act*, s. 19; Alberta, ss. 17 and 18; British Columbia, s. 12; Manitoba, s. 18; New Brunswick, s. 18; Newfoundland, s. 20; Nova Scotia, s. 23; Prince Edward Island, s. 19; the Northwest Territories, s. 20; the Yukon Territory, s. 19; and Saskatchewan, s. 16 which adds:

> (3) Service of the writ of summons may be made upon the proprietor or publisher of the newspaper by serving the writ upon any adult person at such address.

Sections 6 of the British Columbia *Libel and Slander Act* and 7 of the *Libel and Slander Act* of Saskatchewan are identical to s. 9 of the Ontario Act. Alberta's *Defamation Act*, s. 15(1) (b), adds:

> broadcast the retraction and apology from the broadcasting stations from which the alleged defamatory matter was broadcast on at least two occasions on different days and at the same time of day as the alleged defamatory matter was broadcast or at a time as near as possible to that time.

See also the *Revised Uniform Defamation Act*, s. 17(1); Manitoba, s. 16(1); New Brunswick, s. 16(1); Newfoundland, s. 18(1); Nova Scotia, s. 21(1); Prince Edward Island, s. 17(1); the Northwest Territories, s. 18(1); the Yukon Territory, s. 17(1).

For provisions similar to s. 10 of Ontario's *Libel and Slander Act* see the *Revised Uniform Defamation Act*, s. 17(2); Alberta, s. 15(2); British Columbia, s. 11; Manitoba, s. 16(2); New Brunswick, s. 16(2); Newfoundland, s. 18(2); Nova Scotia, s. 21(2); Prince Edward Island, s. 17(2); Saskatchewan, s. 17; the Northwest Territories, s. 18(2); the Yukon Territory, s. 17(2).

Section 20 of Ontario's *Libel and Slander Act* resembles the *Revised Uniform Defamation Act*, s. 5; Alberta, s. 4; British Columbia, s. 10; Manitoba, s. 4; New Brunswick, s. 4; Newfoundland, s. 5; Nova Scotia, s. 5; Prince Edward Island, s. 4; Saskatchewan, s. 4; the Northwest Territories, s. 4; the Yukon Territory, s. 4. As yet, no other province has adopted s. 21.

The Nova Scotia legislation dealing with apologies is unique in that it provides for a detailed procedure dealing with offers of amends:

> **16.** (1) A person who has published words alleged to be defamatory of another person may, if he claims that the words were published by him innocently in relation to that other person, make an offer of amends under this Section and in any such case
>
> > (*a*) if the offer is accepted by the party aggrieved and is duly performed, no proceedings for defamation shall be taken or continued by that party against the person making the offer in respect of the publication in question (but without

prejudice to any cause of action against any other person jointly responsible for that publication);

(*b*) if the offer is not accepted by the party aggrieved, then, except as otherwise provided by this Section, it shall be a defence, in any proceedings by him for defamation against the person making the offer in respect of the publication in question, to prove that the words complained of were published by the defendant innocently in relation to the plaintiff and that the offer was made as soon as practicable after the defendant received notice that they were or might be defamatory of the plaintiff, and has not been withdrawn.

(2) An offer of amends under this Section must be expressed to be made for the purposes of this Section, and must be accompanied by an affidavit specifying the facts relied upon by the person making it to show that the words in question were published by him innocently in relation to the party aggrieved and for the purposes of a defence under clause (b) of subsection (1) no evidence, other than evidence of facts specified in the affidavit, shall be admissible on behalf of that person to prove that the words were so published.

(3) An offer of amends under this Section shall be understood to mean an offer

(*a*) in any case, to publish or join in the publication of a suitable correction of the words complained of, and a sufficient apology to the party aggrieved in respect of those words;

(*b*) where copies of a document or record containing the said words have been distributed by or with the knowledge of the person making the offer, to take such steps as are reasonably practicable on his part for notifying persons to whom copies have been so distributed that the words are alleged to be defamatory of the party aggrieved.

(4) Where an offer of amends under this Section is accepted by the party aggrieved,

(*a*) any question as to the steps to be taken in fulfilment of the offer as so accepted shall in default of agreement between the parties be referred to and determined by the Trial Division of the Supreme Court or a judge thereof, whose decision thereon shall be final;

(*b*) the power of the Court or judge to make orders as to costs in proceedings by the party aggrieved against the person making the offer in respect of the publication in question, or in proceedings in respect of the offer under clause (a), shall include power to order the payment by the person making the offer to the party aggrieved of costs on an indemnity basis and any expenses reasonably incurred or to be incurred by that party in consequence of the publication in question,

and if no such proceedings as aforesaid are taken, the Court or judge may, upon application made by the party aggrieved, make any such order for the payment of such costs and expenses as aforesaid as could be made in such proceedings.

(5) For the purposes of this Section words shall be treated as published by one person (in this subsection referred to as the publisher) innocently in relation to another person if and only if the following conditions are satisfied, that is to say,

(*a*) that the publisher did not intend to publish them of and concerning that other person, and did not know of circumstances by virtue of which they might be understood to refer to him; or

(b) that the words were not defamatory on the face of them, and the publisher did not know of circumstances by virtue of which they might be understood to be defamatory of that other person,

and in either case that the publisher exercised all reasonable care in relation to the publication, and any reference in this subsection to the publisher shall be construed as including a reference to any servant or agent of his who was concerned with the contents of the publication.

(6) Clause (b) of subsection (1) shall not apply in relation to the publication by any person of words of which he is not the author unless he proves that the words were written by the author without malice.

Quebec has chosen to deal with the problem in yet another way. *The Press Act*, R.S.Q. 1977, c. P-19 provides:

4. If the newspaper fully retracts and establishes good faith in its issue published on the day following the receipt of such notice or on the day next after such day, only actual and real damages may be claimed.

5. Such retraction must be published by the newspaper gratis and in as conspicuous a place in the newspaper as the article complained of.

6. Whenever the newspaper is not a daily, the rectification must, at the choice of the party who deems himself injured, and at the newspaper's expense, be published in a newspaper of the judicial district or of a neighbouring judicial district, as well as in the next issue of the newspaper itself.

7. The newspaper shall also publish at its expense any reply which the party who deems himself injured may communicate to it, provided that same be ad rem, be not unreasonably long and be couched in fitting terms.

8. Whenever the party who deems himself injured has both obtained a retraction and exercised the right to reply, no prosecution may issue if the newspaper publishes such retraction and reply without further comment.

9. No newspaper may avail itself of the provisions of this act in the following cases:
(a) When the party who deems himself injured is accused by the newspaper of a criminal offence;
(b) When the article complained of refers to a candidate and was published within the three days prior to the nomination day and up to the polling day in a parliamentary or municipal election.

5.2.4.1.4.2 *Teskey v. Canadian Newspapers Co.* (1989), 68 O.R. (2d) 737 (Ont. C.A.)

BLAIR, J.A.: The appellants, Canadian Newspapers Company Limited (the "Company") and William J. Ogilvie ("Ogilvie") appeal from a judgment of Fitzpatrick, J. sitting with a jury at Barrie. The judgment awarded damages for libel of $10,000 to each of the respondents ("Teskey," "Heacock" and "Ferguson") for which the Company and Ogilvie were jointly liable. A further award of $5,000 for punitive damages was made to Heacock against each appellant.

The three respondents were partners in a law firm in the Town of Midland where Teskey had commenced practice in the early 1960s. In 1964, Teskey was retained as solicitor by Tiny Township which borders the Town of Midland. The firm later became solicitors for other municipalities in Simcoe County as well as for the county itself.

Before accepting the retainer from Tiny Township, Teskey sought the advice of leading municipal lawyers in Simcoe County. A practical problem existed because his real estate practice sometimes required the approval of the township committee of adjustment for deviations from planning and zoning by-laws. He could not afford to abandon this part of his practice and the township could not afford to compensate him if he did. As a result, it was agreed that Teskey could continue to appear on behalf of private clients before the committee of adjustment and that, if there was any dispute or if the committee's decisions were appealed to the Ontario Municipal Board, he would withdraw and both parties would have to obtain other solicitors to represent them. This condition was reaffirmed each year thereafter when the township renewed the firm's retainer. It was a condition which applied to an the firm's municipal retainers and also to the retainers of other firms representing municipalities in Simcoe County.

The Company is the publisher of the Midland *Free Press* ("*Free Press*"), a weekly community newspaper. Ogilvie is a local resident who from the mid-sixties has been extremely interested in municipal politics. For two years, 1966 to 1968, he was deputy reeve of Midland and a member of the town council. He was defeated in 1968 when he ran for the office of mayor but thereafter maintained a continuous and lively interest in politics in Midland and Tiny Township where he was a rate payer. He expressed his opinions through formal submissions called "deputations" to the town and township, councils, letters to the editor of the *Free Press*, advertisements in the *Free Press* and handbills. It can be fairly said, without prejudice to his position in this case, that he was the centre of much controversy during his two years on the town council. As a result, he was severely criticized by editorials in the *Free Press* which urged his defeat when he ran for mayor. He continued thereafter as a vigorous public commentator on municipal affairs.

A major issue in 1983 was the proposal of the Town of Midland to annex a portion of Tiny Township. The proposed annexation was opposed by the township. In that year, Heacock was the president of the Midland Chamber of Commerce which supported annexation. He declared his conflict of interest to the directors of the chamber of commerce and absented himself from all discussions of the annexation proposal. The township had previously retained another law firm to represent it in the annexation proceedings.

In a deputation presented by Ogilvie on behalf of the Tiny Township Ratepayers' Association to the Council of Tiny Township on April 27, 1983, it was alleged that the township might have "a legal Trojan horse or Benedict Arnold in its midst" because Heacock and his partners had been silent in the campaign of the Midland Chamber of Commerce in favour of annexation. Ogilvie asked the township council to require the law firm to insert an advertisement in the local newspapers disassociating itself from the Midland annexation proposal.

On April 28th, Heacock issued a press release in which he stated that he had declared a conflict of interest; that he left the chamber of commerce directors' meeting when the matter first came before it; that he had taken no part in any discussions of the annexation proposal, either directly or indirectly; and that he had not voted on the issue. A news story in the *Free Press* of April 29, 1983, reported on the presentation of the Tiny Township ratepayers deputation to the council but gave greater prominence to the press release of Heacock denying any conflict of interest. At trial a director of the chamber of commerce testified that he had discussed the matter with Ogilvie on April 27th and informed him of Heacock's declaration of conflict at the directors' meeting, his refusal to discuss and vote on the issue and his leaving the meeting when the matter was under discussion.

This litigation arises from the following advertisement placed by Ogilvie and published one week later in the May 4, 1983 issue of the *Free Press*:

Advertisement

Wm Ogilvie Speaks out —

THE BETRAYAL OF TINY TOWNSHIP . . .

As a Tiny Township taxpayer, it is my view, that on the basis of the silent and secretive role that Tiny Township municipal solicitor's law firm of Teskey, Heacock and Ferguson, has played in the latest annexation development involving the Township of Tiny, the Midland Chamber of Commerce and the town of Midland, Tiny Township council should have fired the legal trio, the moment their "hands-off the Chamber's annexation position" was discovered.

Tiny Township is supposed to be the Teskey, Heacock and Ferguson law firm's fundamental client, in the present Midland Tiny Township annexation battle. To put the client-solicitor ethical relationship in its proper perspective, they obviously had the primary responsibility to PUBLICLY defend the integrity of their client — Tiny Township, first, last and foremost, from the misleading and shameful attack of the Midland Chamber of Commerce, as set out in the Chamber's toadying letter of April 19th, to Midland council — their major bankroller.

It is a matter of report that Teskey, Heacock and Ferguson all belong to the Midland Chamber of Commerce. Heacock is president of the organization and is well aware of what is going on.

Mr. Heacock's most recent media alibi for turning their backs on Tiny Township in their hour-of-need, is based on some cock-and-bull story that he declared a conflict of interest in the matter. Such a phoney excuse is an insult to the intelligence of the people of Tiny Township; and, is not unlike the position of another character in history, who, having "washed his hands" before the howling mob, proclaimed his innocence.

A notice pursuant to s. 5(1) of the *Libel and Slander Act*, R.S.O. 1980, c. 237, was served on the *Free Press* and on Ogilvie and, in response, the following apology was published in the May 11, 1983 issue of the *Free Press*.

Apology

In our edition of May 4, 1983 the *Free Press* published an advertisement composed and paid for by William Ogilvie, of Midland, which discussed the local law firm of Teskey, Heacock and Ferguson.

We hereby retract, on behalf of the Midland *Free Press*, any statement in that advertisement which might suggest to our readers that the law firm of Teskey, Heacock and Ferguson had in any way acted unethically or against the interest of their client, The Corporation of the Township of Tiny. The *Free Press* has investigated this matter to our satisfaction and we are not aware of any evidence which would support such allegations. We believe that Teskey, Heacock and Ferguson have at all times acted in accordance with the highest ethical standards of the legal profession.

We apologize to the firm of Teskey, Heacock ant Ferguson, and to all lawyers in the firm, for any embarrassment or inconvenience this advertisement may have caused them.

The main thrust of the appeal of the *Free Press* was that it was entitled to the protection of s. 5.(2) of the *Libel and Slander Act* which reads as follows:

5. (2) The plaintiff shall recover only actual damages if appears on the trial,
   (a) that the alleged libel was published in good faith;
   (b) that the alleged libel did not involve a criminal charge;
   (c) that the publication of the alleged libel took place in mistake or misapprehension of the facts; and
   (d) that a full and fair retraction of any matter herein alleged to be erroneous,
      (i) was published either in the next regular issue of the newspaper or in any regular issue thereof published within three days after the receipt of the notice mentioned in subsecdon (1) and was so published in as conspicuous a place and type as was the alleged libel, or
      (ii) was broadcast either within a reasonable time or within three days after the receipt of the notice mentioned in subsection (1) and was so broadcast as conspicuously as was the alleged libel.

The libel in this case did not involve a criminal charge. The *Free Press*, however, had to satisfy each of the three other paragraphs in s. 5.(2) in order to limit its damages by establishing that the publication was in good faith, that it took place in mistake or misapprehension of the facts and that a full and fair retraction was made. The jury's reply to the questions put to it with reference to the subsection was as follows: If you find the words of Exhibit 13 Ogilvie's advertisement] defamatory of any of the plaintiffs,

(a) was the advertisement published by the *Free Press* in good faith?
Answer: No.
(b) did the publication of the advertisement take place in mistake or misapprehension of the facts?
Answer: No.
(c) was the apology (Exhibit 15) a full and fair retraction of any answer in the advertisement alleged to be erroneous?
Answer: No.

Before considering the implication of s. 5.(2) and the answers given by the jury, it is necessary to describe how the libelous advertisement complained of in this action came, to be published in the *Free Press*.

The publisher of the *Free Press*, Fontaine, was away when Ogilvie delivered the advertisement to Wilson who was in charge of advertising. Wilson's evidence was that he did not live in Midland and was unaware of Ogilvie's background. He knew Ogilvie casually and had taken other advertisements from him when he was a candidate in municipal politics. He also knew Ogilvie's wife who worked at the bank where Wilson dealt. Wilson thought of Ogilvie as an opinionated but basically decent and honest person. He had no reason to think of him as unbalanced or malicious.

Fontaine testified that, in his absence, no one was designated as acting publisher and that each department head was responsible for running his own department. Elson, the editor who knew Ogilvie's background did not have authority to overrule Wilson's decision to accept Ogilvie's advertisement. He nevertheless suggested that the word "advertisement" be placed above it in order to distinguish it from editorial copy and this was agreed to by Wilson. Neither Wilson nor Elson read the whole of Ogilvie's advertisement but each was aware of the headline 'The Betrayal of Tiny Township."

On the morning of publication, Bourrie, the reporter who had written the news story about the council meeting of April 27, 1983, and the subsequent press release of Heacock referred to above, was in the composing room of the *Free Press* where he saw Ogilvie's advertisement ready for printing. He testified that he did not read all of the advertisement but that he stated "to someone there, whether it was Mr. Elson of Mr. Fontaine or Mr. Wilson — someone I believed to be in authority or someone who should know: 'this is pretty rough stuff, has it been checked?' " He received a response that made him feel that "it had been checked or thought about or considered or whatever." The first question to be considered with reference to s. 5.(2) of the *Libel and Slander Act* is whether the jury was properly charged as to the meaning of the words "good faith" as used in the subsection. The trial judge put the following test of good faith to the jury:

> A libel is published in good faith if it is published without knowledge that it is libel and without a complete disregard for whether it is or not. Publishing libel carelessly does not necessarily mean it was not published in good faith. But publishing something with a complete disregard for whether it is libel, whether it will harm somebody, is not publishing in good faith.

Mrs. Block objected and argued that the test of "good faith" would be met if the advertisement were published honestly and without malice by Wilson. The challenge to the charge raised two related issues in argument. The first was the proper definition of the words "good faith." The second was whether the *Free Press* could claim that it acted in "good faith" because the advertisement was honestly published by Wilson who knew nothing about Ogilvie's background.

With respect to the first issue, the words "good faith" as they appear in s. 5.(2) do not appear to have been interpreted in any Canadian case. This subsection is based upon similar legislation originating in the State of Michigan in the 1880s and subsequently adopted by other states and Canadian provinces: see J.G. Fleming, "Retraction and Reply" (1978), 12 *U.B.C.L.* Rev. 15. The American statutes contain the same provision with respect to publication in good faith as the Ontario Act. The Supreme Court of Minnesota in *Allen v. Pioneer Co.*, 41 N.W. 936 (1889), defined the meaning of the words "published in good faith" as they were used in the Minnesota section comparable to s. 5.(2). Mitchell, J., speaking for the court, said at p. 939:

> We may assume that the Act was designed to protect honest and careful newspaper publishers. It is not to be presumed that the legislature intended to make so radical a change in the law of libel as to make mere belief in the truth of the article the test of good faith. If to, they have introduced a very dangerous principle, which virtually places the good name and reputation of the citizen as the mercy of the credulity or indifference of every reckless or negligent reporter. *Good faith requires a proper consideration for the character and reputation of the person whose character is likley to be injuriously affected by the publication. It requires of the publisher that he exercise the care and vigilance of a prudent and conscientious man, wielding, as he does, the great power of the public press. There must be an absence, not only of all improper motives, but of negligence, on his part.* It is his duty to take all reasonable precautions to verify the truth of the statement, and to prevent untrue and injurious publicities against others. (Emphasis added.)

This decision was affirmed by the Minnesota Supreme Court almost half a century later in *Thorson v. Albert Lea Pub. Co.*, 251 N.W. 177 (1983), where Hilton, J., for the court, said at p. 180:

> Whether the publication was made in good faith depends upon whether defendant was free from negligence in making it. If it was, then general damages were properly awarded. Mere belief in the truth of the publication is not necessarily enough to constitute "good faith" on part of the publisher, there must have been an absence of negligence, as well saw improper motives, in making the publication. It must have been honestly made in the belief of its truth, and upon reasonable grounds for his belief, after the exercise of such means to verify its truth as would be taken by a man of ordinary prudence under like circumstances.

In my opinion, these Minnesota decisions reflect the proper interpretation of the words "good faith" in s. 5.(2) of the *Libel and Slander Act*. Honest belief in the truth of material published is not sufficient to constitute good faith. That belief must be founded on reasonable grounds. The trial judge's direction to the jury was correct in stating that good faith would be negated if the advertisement was published "with a complete disregard for whether it is libel" which, of necessity, includes not taking reasonable steps to verify its truth.

This leads to the second issue which is whether there was evidence on which the jury could find that the advertisement was not published in good faith. The question here was whether the knowledge of the corporate defendant, the *Free Press*, for this purpose was limited to that of Wilson, who was in charge of advertising and who claimed to know nothing of Ogilvie's background, or whether it included that of Elson, who did know because of his responsibility for news. Elson's knowledge, of course, included the news story about the Tiny Township Council meeting and Heacock's press release published in the *Free Press* on April 19, 1983, which negated the charges contained in Ogilvie's advertisement published one week later. The evidence also disclosed that he was aware of other unsubstantiated charges made by Ogilvie on public matters from his several years' experience as editor of the *Free Press*.

Fontaine's evidence was that, as publisher, he had the right to prevent publication of anything he believed to be defamatory. As stated above, this authority had not been delegated to an acting publisher in his absence when each department head was responsible for his own department. Counsel for the *Free Press* contended that the corporate defendant was not liable for the decision of Wilson, the advertising manager, to publish the advertisement because the separation between news and advertising departments had been recognized in libel actions so that the knowledge of one department could not be imputed to the other: see *New York Times Co. v. Sullivan*, 376 U.S. 254 (1964), at p. 287 and *Broadway Approvals Ltd. v. Odhams Press, Ltd.*, [1965] 2 All E.R 523 at p. 532.

This division of responsibility may be appropriate for a large metropolitan newspaper although it appears difficult to reconcile with the over-all corporation responsibility of a newspaper owner contemplated by *Allen v. Pioneer Co*. It is unecessary to investigate this issue in this case because the evidence established that this division of responsibility for publishing advertisements does not apply to a small community newspaper like the *Free Press*. A witness with long experience in Canadian community newspapers was called by the respondents and was qualified by the trial judge as "an expert witness with respect to the standard of care to be exercised by community newspapers." He testified that there was close liaison between the editorial and advertising departments in a community newspaper. They work in close contact in the same offices and, in his experience, sometimes even at the same desk. He assumed that "all departments ... read their own newspaper" and "would be fully aware of the man [Ogilvie] and all departments would react probably in the same manner to the advertisement." The opening line of the advertisement, containing the word "betrayal" should have rung an "alarm bell" as to its "potentially libelous" nature. It was a "gross deviation of journalistic practice" to publish the advertisement, without any investigation of the truth of the allegations it contained. In addition, the expert expressed the opinion that Elston, who had inserted the heading "advertisement":

> ... should have gone beyond the point of simply putting that word in that place, he should have requested of the Publisher further investigation into the allegations in the article which I feel are potentially libelous.

There was, thus, evidence that there was no justification for Wilson's failure to make inquiries before authorizing publication of the advertisement or for Elston's inaction. On this evidence the jury was entitled to conclude that both had been negligent in permitting publication of the advertisement without an investigation of the truth of its contents. In my view, there was no error in the instructions of the learned trial judge and there was ample evidence to support the jury's finding that the advertisement had not been published in good faith.

Note: Leave to appeal this decision to the Supreme Court of Canada was denied on 18 January 1990.

5.2.4.1.4.3 *Hoste v. Victoria Times Publishing Co.* (1989), 1 B.C.R. (Pt 2) 365 (B.C.S.C.)

BEGBIE, C.J.B.C.: That is surely not sufficient. It is not the offer nor even the publication of an apology at all, but an offer to offer an apology. And even in terms, it seems to reserve to the defendant a right of judging whether the plaintiff is reasonable in demanding any particular form e.g., it offers to make such an apology as the defendant thinks fit. Such an apology as merely 'beg your pardon', or 'sorry for it', is not sufficient in a case of libel. The defendant should admit that the charge was unfounded, that it was made without proper information, under an entire misapprehension of the real facts, etc., and that he regrets that it was published in his paper. . . .

You should not offer to make, but actually make and publish at once, and unconditionally, such an apology, expressing sorrow, withdrawing the imputation, rehabilitating the plaintiff's character as well as you can; not stipulating that the plaintiff is to accept it; not making any terms but publishing it in the interests of truth, and because you are anxious to undo whatever harm which may have accrued from a wrong which you find you have been the unconscious instrument of inflicting.

5.2.4.1.4.4 *Brannigan v. S.I.U.* (1964), 42 D.L.R. (2d) 249 (B.C.S.C.)

HUTCHESON, J.: On p. 12 of the issue of December 13, 1961, of the Canadian Sailor under the heading in bold type "WE HAVE BLUNDERED" appears this statement:

> In the August 23rd, 1961, edition of the *Canadian Sailor*, we published a photograph of the May Day, 1960 Communist parade in Vancouver, in which we erroneously identified a Communist banner holding Canadian Brotherhood of Railway and Transport Workers as one, William Brannigan. The standard bearing Communist supporter however was William Mozdir, Vice-President of Local 400, Canadian Brotherhood of Railway and Transport Workers. In order to set the record straight we aplogise to Mr. William Brannigan for confusing two pictures and thereby embarrassing Mr. Brannigan by not showing him as he also proudly held aloft a placard in support of the policies of the Communist Party — in the same Parade, but a few squads back.
>
> In a further effort to placate the ruffled feelings of Mr. Brannigan, we publish below both pictures, with the proper identification. Again, to Mr. Brannigan, we tender our sincerest apologies and make this retraction with the hope that he will feel that satisfaction has been achieved.
>
> Before anybody else seizes the opportunity to do so, we also make another correction in that the Communist Parade in question took place in 1960 and not 1961.

Following this statement and on the same page are two pictures — one is the picture which appeared in the issue of August 23rd accompanied by a notation similar to that below the picture in the earlier edition but identifying the man on the right carrying the banner in these words:

> . . . the banner waving Communist sympathizer is none other than William Mozdir, (Arrow) who was vice-president of Local 400, Canadian Brotherhood of Railway and Transport Workers at the time.

On the same page is another picture of a small group of eight men marching in the same parade, each carrying separate placards. At the side of that picture is the following heading: "Picture That Should Have Appeared" and underneath the statement:

> The picture on left shows Mr. Brannigan, former Financial Secretary of Local 400, Canadian Brotherhood of Railway and Transport Workers, (Arrow) as he proudly carries a placard in support of the Communist party in the same Communist May Day Parade in Vancouver of 1960.

In my view it is also evident from the form and wording of the so-called apology that it is a deliberate and intended reiteration or emphasizing of the defamatory statement made in the earlier issue of the *Canadian Sailor*, the truth of which the defendunt has asserted throughout but has failed to establish. That apology, rather than mitigating the damage caused to the plaintiff, as urged on behalf of the defendant, would, in my opinion, tend to aggravate the damage done by the libel. That the matter of an apology may tend to increase rather than diminish the damages, see *Mayne & McGregor on Damages* 12th ed., para. 894 and the cases there cited.

Note: If the defendant was motivated by malice or was guilty of gross negligence in publishing the defamatory material, then tbe benefits of making an aplogy will be lost. See *Snider v. Calgary Herald* (1985), 34 C.C.L.T. 27.

5.2.4.1.4.5 John G. Fleming, "Retraction and Reply; Alternative Remedies for Defamation" (1978), *University of British Columbia Law Review* 12, p. 15

I. Damages

The preoccupation of our law of defamation with damages has been a crippling experience over the centuries. The damages remedy is not only singularly inept for dealing with, but actually exacerbates, the tension between protection of reputation and freedom of expression, both equally important values in a civilized and democratic community. A defamed plaintiff has a legitimate claim to vindication in order to restore his damaged reputation, but a settlement for, or even a court award of, damages is hardly the most efficient way to attain that objective. In either case, the refutation of the libel is not attended with much publicity, if any, and, if resisted by the defendant, occurs long after the libel has spread its poison. Plaintiffs sometimes settle on condition that the defendant make an apology in open court, but there is no law that actually requires a defendant to do so even after he has lost a verdict. So far as the plaintiff is concerned, damages offer him a pot of gold which he may not even desire, but since this is all that the law provides him as a token of vindication, it is still widely regarded as necessary for honourable men to demand a large sum of damages lest it be misinterpreted as a tacit admission that one's reputation was not worth more. A curious inflation has thus come to prevail by which damages for libel especially to public figures often far exceed awards for the most searing personal injuries; and this remains true whether they parade under the label of "punitive" or "aggravated" damages. In times of acute social stress, damage awards are frequently used by juries to wreak vengeance on political enemies, so well illustrated by the American experience of the Civil Rights struggle in the South which prompted the intervention of the United States Supreme Court in 1964 based on the First Amendment.

Not that the link with damages invariably favours plaintiffs. For on occasions where free speech should not be chilled by the spectre of damages, the law saw no alternative to creating an immunity and thereby depriving the defamed of any right to vindication. This covers the area of privilege, absolute and qualified, including privileged reports, and the defence of fair comment. Even from a free speech point of view, those defences are hardly impeccable because, while encouraging the free flow of information and opinion, they do nothing to promote correction of falsehoods. Moreover, the system also has an undesirable countervailing effect inasmuch as our law has been understandably very reluctant to extend such immunities when its price for individual reputation is so high. This tendency has resulted in a strictness of the law of defamation which is widely felt — and not only by the media — to be incompatible with the free flow of information, especially on matters of public concern, in a modern democratic society.

The dilemma is well illustrated by recent American experience. In the celebrated case of *New York Times Company v. Sullivan* the United States Supreme Court for the first time imposed constitutional restrictions on state libel law, based on the First Amendment guarantee that no law shall abridge "freedom of speech and of the press." The reason prompting this intervention was, then and in several subsequent cases, outrageously large awards of both compensatory and punitive damages against liberal Eastern newspapers by hostile Southern juries. But instead of focussing on the *control* of damages, the Court followed the conventional path of enlarging the area of privilege. The new constitutional privilege disqualified public officials from all remedy for libel on matters relating to their official duties, in the absence of proof of "actual malice," defined as knowledge of falsity or recklessness in that respect. This privilege went far beyond the defence of fair comment, as understood in Anglo-Canadian law and hitherto the majority of American Jurisdictions, in that it covered false statements of fact no less than any comment based thereon. In subsequent cases, the privilege was extended to libel of all "public figures" and for a time even to "all matters of public or general interest." That last extension, however, reactivated concern that private persons who, unlike public figures could not count on the same measure of access to the media for refutation and who had not voluntarily exposed themselves to public scrutiny, should thus for all practical purposes lose all opportunity for public vindication. Instead, the Court at last turned its attention on the remedies for defamation. Besides requiring that no liability for defamation could be based on less than fault, it also prohibited the award of damages for other than "actual injury," thereby abandoning the common law doctrine of *presumed* injury to reputation, and probably even punitive damages in cases of malice.

These restrictions on damage assessment reflect increasing concern over the vagaries of jury awards, a concern which may also have played a part in the House of Lords decision against punitive damages. Here we are confronted with a puzzling paradox. In England, as in some other Commonwealth countries, the civil jury has been virtually eliminated — except in actions for defamation. Whether that moratorium was prompted by historical nostalgia (back when 18th Century libel juries figured as watchdogs of democratic rights against Government) or because it was felt that the administration of libel law in any event needed a large infusion of public sentiment to remain viable, is not clear. At all events, contemporary criticism of the law of defamation dwells even more on the erratic assessment of damages by juries than on the substantive law of libel. In the U.S., the right of trial by jury is of course sacrosanct, but elsewhere there is no such peremptory impediment to reform. The Faulks Committee (1975) in England took a characteristically cautious step in that direction by recommending that the jury's role regarding damages be limited to indicating whether they should be substantial, moderate, nominal or contemptuous. The new federal Law Reform Commission of Australia, on the other hand, went all the way in proposing that juries be stripped of all function in relation to sanction for libel.

Another, perhaps even more profitable, reorientation is to explore alternative remedies to damages. I do not propose to consider here, let alone, advocate, either criminal prosecutions or injunctions because to the extent that they survive at all, their crushing impact on free speech precludes any wider role than in the most exceptional situations. Rather, I wish to share with you some thoughts about the Right of Reply and Retraction.

II. *Right of Reply*

... The right of reply is firmly established in Continental law, under the inspiration of a French model dating back to 1820. But its generic label hides several important differences, especially as regards coverage and means of enforcement. Those differences help us to identify crucial issues relevant to an appraisal of the remedy.

From the plaintiff's point of view, it is of course not exactly the most ideal form of undoing the wrong done to him. For it is a commonplace in the experience of Anglo-American law that the truth never catches up with the lie; if it were, we would not have needed a law of defamation. In particular, reply lacks the persuasive force of retraction, but is arguably more effective in clearing the plaintiff's name than a money judgment. Moreover, it provides a possible remedy in situations of so-called "privilege" where we have long thought it preferable to deny damages because of the chilling effect on free speech and the plaintiff is therefore denied all means of public vindication.

How does the right of reply compare with retraction? The most important difference is undoubtedly that in its most common formulation the right of reply is not conditioned at all on proof that the charge levied against the plaintiff was false. Although this feature subjects the media to greater exposure than traditional defamation remedies do, which are based on a minimum of falsity, it dispenses with the administrative burden of litigating the truth. It is therefore peculiarly apt to rebut offensive statements of opinion, which by their very nature are really unamenable to a judicial determination of validity. Parenthetically, American law has at last reached the position that "[u]nder the First Amendment there is no such thing as a false idea. However pernicious an opinion may seem, we depend for its correction not on the conscience of judges and juries but on the competition of other ideas." This postulate does not appear confined to the expression of opinion only on matters of public concern. Accordingly, the *Restatement, Second, Torts* 566 now reads that "[a] defamatory communication [in the form of an opinion] is actionable only if it also expresses, or implies the assertion of, a false and defamatory fact which is not known or assumed by both parties to the communication."

By comparison, under Anglo-Canadian law not only can an opinion constitute a defamatory libel, but the defence of fair comment protects only defamatory opinions on matters of public interest based on true (or privileged) facts. One might well ponder therefore whether a right of reply should not be conferred at least on plaintiffs who are now barred from all relief under the defence of fair comment. Indeed, one might go further and suggest extending the same remedy in lieu of damages to honest (fair) comment on matters of public interest even if the comment is based on untrue facts. If such false facts are actually stated, it is debatable whether a right of retraction regarding such facts (though not the opinion based thereon) should not be allowed at least as an alternative to damages. Is there a role for the right of reply in other situations? Continental experience certainly suggests that it may be invoked against defamatory statements of fact, indeed regardless of whether these are false or not. Without going to quite that length, I raised earlier the possibility of applying it to privileged occasions where the plaintiff under present law lacks all opportunity of vindication. The federal Law Reform Commission of Australia whose Discussion Paper Number One has just launched some high-flying kites for reform of the law of defamation expressed itself against any right of correction in these situations on the plausible ground that "the defaming persons will not normally be in the communication business, many not in business at all; some will have scant resources. The proof of the statement may require considerable enquiries and a lengthy trial. It is one thing to impose that burden on a media organ which has published to a wide audience, generally for commercial motives, the defamation;

quite another to impose it on private persons or organizations in a reasonable matter for the purpose of giving relevant information to a person believed to have an interest in receiving it."

The Australian Commission does, however, suggest a right of reply in two other situations: first, it would apply it to all fair reports of a statement made by another named person and published for the information of the public or the advancement of education. You will notice that this proposal would extend the protection of fair reports far beyond the present limited categories, but make the defence conditional on the defendant affording the plaintiff a right of reply. The second, more controversial proposal, would substitute a right of reply for the existing remedy of general damages for loss of reputation where "the defendant, on reasonable grounds and after making all enquiries reasonably open to him in the circumstances, in fact believed the truth of all statements of fact contained in, or assumed by, the matter published." I will return to this matter later.

The Australian proposals prompt a brief word concerning the sanctioning of the right of reply. The Commission followed the model of Anglo-American retraction statutes, i.e. creating a defence to a claim for damages conditional on the defendant affording the plaintiff an opportunity to reply. One cannot therefore truly call this a *right* of reply, since its exercise depends on the defendant's willingness to submit to it. The Continental pattern, on the other hand, allows enforcement even against the defendant's wishes, since the plaintiff may apply for administrative or civil sanctions to force the defendant to open his pages or broadcast facilities to him. This difference may betray a cultural contrast between the deeply-rooted Anglo-American preference for attaining desirable objectives by rewards rather than force and the Continental tradition which has come to view the right of reply as an individual right, in a few countries even enshrined in their Constitution, as a necessary protection against excesses of the media. Perhaps not surprisingly, therefore, the English Faulks Committee objected to compelling a right of reply because it would create "new criminal offences and punishments." Besides this fear which Continental observers would regard as rather imaginary, the Faulks Committee also thought "objectionable a principle which entitles a person, who may be without merits, to compel a newspaper to publish a statement extolling his non-existing virtue." To this charge one can make two replies: first, there are, as we have seen, several instances in which the right of reply could be deployed without incurring this objection; secondly, it views the right of reply as a sanction against proven falsehoods rather than as giving a defamed person an opportunity to put his side of the case and letting the public rather than the court be the final arbiter of the controversy. Oddly enough, the Committee's conclusion happens to come out on the same side as the United States Supreme Court's, but whereas the Committee baulked over the plaintiff's possibly unclean hands, the American Court's concern was solely over governmental interference with editorial judgment.

III. Retraction

Retraction of defamatory allegations by a defendant has become a more familiar feature of our law of defamation than a right of reply. Its undoubted advantage to the plaintiff consists in the greater persuasive effect of having his reputation vindicated out of the defendant's mouth rather than his own. But against this must be set certain inherent limitations. First, retraction (especially compulsory retraction) is not really appropriate for expressions of opinion if we believe that there is no objective standard for determining the validity of opinions and that the public interest is better served by continuing debate through rebuttal rather than by compulsorily bringing it to an end. Moreover, it may also be felt as invidious to be forced to recant opinions still honestly held compared with having to correct allegations of fact proven to be false. By contrast, reply is an appropriate remedy for both types of expression and, because of the well known difficulty of distinguishing between fact and opinion, deserves to be seriously considered as the only remedy for defamation on matters of public interest, now broadly covered by 'fair comment.'

The second limitation is that retraction can really be countenanced only with respect to statements of fact which have been shown to be false. This invites litigation; more-over, it is largely ineffective unless the defendant is faced with the alternative of having to pay damages in case he loses his plea of justification, since otherwise he would have little incentive to recant prior to a long-delayed judicial determination of truth. Hence the standard retraction statute which relieves the defendant of liability if he has made a suitable and prompt correction. In other words, retraction cannot very well stand on its own feet, as can reply, and needs the crutch of a continuing threat of damages to be effective.

Retraction has thus remained a voluntary alternative. Should compulsory retraction by court order be added to the judicial armoury, as in many Continental countries? This is strongly favoured by the Australian Commission as a complete substitute for *all* damages in the case of group defamation and defamation of a dead person; as a substitute for *general* (but not special) damages in the case of defamatory statements which the defendant reasonably believed to be true; and as an addition to general damages in case of defamatory statements not reasonably believed to be true as well as of statements which would have been privileged but for the defendant's unreasonable conduct (a substitute for malice) . . .

Compulsory Correction

It was mentioned earlier that our retraction statutes merely give the defendant an option between correction and general damages. Alternatively, the court could direct the defendant to retract. This system of the stick rather than the carrot is alien to our common law culture. It was rejected on rather flimsy grounds by the English Faulks Committee but appealed to the aforementioned Law Reform Commission of Australia which commended this procedure in several cases additional to general damages, as in the case of defamatory statements which the defendant did not reasonably believe to be true and in cases where qualified privilege was forfeited by unreasonable conduct (malice). In several other instances court-directed correction would be the only remedy, as in the case of group defamation or defamation of a dead person.

IV. *Conclusion*

To sum up, I commend the widest deployment of Reply and Retraction to help break the traditional deadlock faced by the law of defamation between the individual's interest in his reputation and the general concern in the free flow of accurate information. That deadlock is largely a product of the damages remedy for injury to reputation. Its all-or-nothing aspect necessarily entails subordinating completely the one interest to the other, to the ultimate detriment of both; rather reminiscent of such other puritanical common law blunders as the all-or-nothing rule of contributory negligence and the rule against contribution among tortfeasors. In contrast, Reply and Retraction as remedies for libel assist rather the impede the dissemination of correct information without imposing more than a negligible burden on the media. As the Draft Convention on Freedom of Information, passed at the 1948 United Nations Conference in Geneva, article 4 resolved: "The Contracting States recognize that the right of reply is a corollary of freedom of information." That burden the media should cheerfully bear in token of the social responsibility which accompanies their pivotal role in modern society.

5.2.4.2 Injunctions

5.2.4.2.1 *Canada Metal Co. Ltd. v. C.B.C.* **(1974), 44 D.L.R. (3d) 329 (Ont. H.C.)**

HOLLAND, J.: There are two applications presently before me in the above style. The first is an application on behalf of the defendants for an order dissolving or rescinding the *ex parte* injunction granted by Mr. Justice Wilson on January 29, 1974, which restrained the defendants and each of them from alleging or implying by broadcasting on television or otherwise publicizing, that the plaintiffs and/or either of them have bought misleadingly favourable medical evidence and concealed material evidence from medical experts and from misstating the amounts the plaintiffs are spending to install pollution control systems. The second is brought on behalf of the plaintiffs for an order effective until the date of trial or other final disposition of the action, continuing the injunction granted by Mr. Justice Wilson aforesaid and expanding the relief therein granted by restraining the defendants from broadcasting or otherwise disseminating and from advertising or otherwise publicizing any part or portion of a programme entitled "Dying of Lead" or any part or portion of the script thereof or, alternatively, from publicizing certain portions of such script.

Originally, there was a third motion pending before me on behalf of the plaintiffs for an order committing the defendants Mark Starowicz and Max Allen to the common jail for breach of the injunction granted by Mr. Justice Wilson aforesaid and also for an order committing E. S. Hallman, Guy Perly, Graham Fraser and James L. Cooper to jail for knowingly acting in contravention of the said injunction. Mr. Hallman is apparently a vice-president of the Canadian Broadcasting Corporation and general manager of English Language Services for such corporation based in Toronto. Mr. Fraser was apparently the author of a news article appearing in the *Globe and Mail*, a Toronto newspaper, of which Mr. Cooper is the president and publisher. Mr. Perly apparently is the national chairman of the Canadian Liberation Movement, which published a pamphlet dealing with the subject of the injunction.

The three motions originally came on before me for hearing together and were adjourned to permit Mr. Perly to cross-examine on certain of the affidavits filed on behalf of the plaintiffs. When the motions came on again for hearing an application was made by Mr. Perly for a further adjournment of the the motion so that he could issue a subpoena for the purpose of examining Mr. Outerbridge, who is a solicitor in the office of the solicitors for the plaintiffs, and who also appeared as counsel on behalf of the plaintiffs on the motions. I granted the adjournment of this third motion to permit the issue of the subpoena but without in any way dealing with the propriety of such examination, which matter may well be dealt with by the Master of this Court. I then proceeded with the hearing of the first two motions which are the motion to continue and expand on the one hand, and the motion to dissolve on the other.

The plaintiffs operate secondary lead smelters in the City of Toronto and the activities of the plaintiffs have been the subject of certain publicity in recent months. For example, a stop order was issued by the director of the Air Management Branch of the Ontario Ministry of the Environment, dated October 26, 1973, directing the Canada Metal Company Limited to stop their plant from emitting or discharging into the natural environment lead and lead compounds. This order was reviewed under the provisions of the *Judicial Review Procedure Act*, 1971 (Ont.), Vol. 2, c.48, by Mr. Justice Keith and at the conclusion of the hearing Mr. Justice Keith made an immediate order setting aside such stop order basically on the ground that the director exercised a power granted to him under the Act arbitrarily and not judicially.

In the morning edition of the Toronto *Globe and Mail* for Tuesday, January 29, 1974, there appeared an article under the heading "Television" with the subheading "Special on Lead Poisoning Fine Investigative Journalism".

This article read, in part, as follows:

> Tonight at 7, CBC Radio's As It Happens does a one-hour special on lead poisoning which, at least on the basis of reading a transcript, seems to be a definitive and terrifying show — and investigative journalism at its best.

The program was sparked by the controversy over lead emissions and illness around two Toronto smelters. It includes claims that medical experts can be bought to give evidence that favors lead companies and plays down the danger. A doctor from Cleveland says that doctors who minimize the significance of high lead emissions are hired by the firms to say so.

. . . . .

Doctors on the program claim that excessive lead levels can turn children into vegetables. One doctor says "all they escape is death" — and some do die. The cost of each child turned into a vegetable — just the financial cost and not including emotional torture — was set at $500.000.

The cost of pollution controls at one of the Toronto lead smelters is estimated at $60,000.

A doctor whose evidence helped to get a court to allow a smelter to stay in operation despite apparent lead poisoning in three nearby residents admits on the program that evidence that might have made her change her stand was concealed from her.

On the same day, the plaintiffs issued a writ in this action and applied for an *ex parte* injunction before Mr. Justice Wilson. In support of the application was filed an affidavit sworn by Michael Sigel, secretary-treasurer of the plaintiff Toronto Refiners and Smelters Limited, and an affidavit sworn by Carleton Smith, president and general manager of the Canada Metal Company Limited, by which affidavits the deponents swore that at no time had they or any member of their executive staff, or any other person at their request or with their knowledge, attempted to influence or influenced in any way by money, the expert opinions of Drs. Sachs and Barltrop, who were the two medical experts retained on behalf of their companies. In addition, Mr. Sigel swore that Toronto Refiners and Smelters is now in the final stages of installing a pollution control system at a cost to the company in excess of $150,000 and Mr. Smith swore that Canada Metal Company Limited is now in the final stages of installing a pollution control system at a cost to the company in excess of $300,000.

On the basis of the above affidavits Mr. Justice Wilson granted the *ex parte* injunction above referred to. The defendants were given notice of the injunction after the programme in question had already been broadcast in the Maritime Provinces and a short time before the broadcast was due to commence in Ontario and Quebec.

After consultation with counsel, two portions of the broadcast, which had been carried in the Maritime Provinces, were deleted from the broadcast to the other Provinces and Territories

Defamatory words in a broadcast shall be deemed to be published and constitute libel: the *Libel and Slander Act*, R.S.O. 1970, c.243, s.2. In deciding a matter such as this the Court should always bear in mind the principle of freedom of the press. This principle, fortunately, has always existed in Canada, and this existence is specifically recognized by s. 1 of the *Canadian Bill of Rights*. One must bear in mind that this particular programme, a so-called public affairs programme, dealt generally with an area of considerable public concern. This freedom of the press is, of course, a freedom governed by law and is not a freedom to make untrue defamatory statements: see *Reference re Alberta Statutes*, [1938] S.C.R. 100 at p. 133, [1938] 2 D.L.R. 81 at p. 107 (affirmed [1938] 4 D.L.R. 433, [1939] A.C. 117, [1938] 3 W.W.R. 337).

The Court in a case of this type will only interfere with a publication of an alleged libel in the very clearest of cases. The Court must be satisfied that the words are beyond doubt defamatory, are clearly untrue so that no defence of justification would succeed and, where such defence may apply, are not fair comment on true or admitted facts.

The jurisdiction of the Court in cases of this type has been described as "of a delicate nature". The Master of the Rolls in *William Coulson & Sons v. James Coulson & Co.* (1876), 3 T.L.R. 846:

> It was for the jury and not for the Court to construe the document, and to say whether it was a libel or not. To justify the Court in granting an interim injunction it must come to a decision upon the question of libel or no libel, before the jury decided whether it was a libel or not ... It ought only to be exercised in the clearest cases, where any jury would say that the matter complained of was libelous, and where if the jury did not so find the Court would set aside the verdict as unreasonable. The Court must also be satisfied that in all probability the alleged libel was untrue ... It followed ... that the Court could only on the rarest occasions exercise their jurisdiction.

See also *Collard v. Marshall*, [1892] 1 Ch. 571.

Certainly one of the leading cases is *Bonnard v. Perryman*, [1891] 2 Ch. 269. An alleged defamatory article was printed and an application was brought on behalf of the plaintiffs for an interim injunction restraining the defendants from publishing the article. In support of the application the plaintiffs made affidavits to show that the statements in the article of which they complained were untrue. The defendant made an affidavit in the following terms [at p. 272]:

> "The whole of the allegations in the article entitled 'the *Fletcher Mills of Providence, Rhode Island*,' complained of by the Plaintiffs, are true in substance and in fact, and I shall be able to prove the same at the trial of this action by subpoenaing witnesses and by cross-examination of the Plaintiffs, and by other evidence which I cannot, and which I submit I ought not to have to, produce on an interlocutory application."

Chief Justice Coleridge gave the majority judgment, in which Lord Esher, M.R., and Lindley, Bowen and Lopes, L.J., concurred. Lord Justice Kay dissented but really on the effect of the affidavit and not on the principles of law to be applied to the case. Lord Coleridge, at p. 284, said this:

> But it is obvious that the subject-matter of an action for defamation is so special as to require exceptional caution in exercising the jurisdiction to interfere by injunction before the trial of an action to prevent an anticipated wrong. The right of free speech is one which it is for the public interest that individuals should possess, and, indeed, that they should exercise without impediment, so long as no wrongful act is done; and, unless an alleged libel is untrue, there is no wrong committed; but on the contrary, often a very wholesome act is performed in the publication and repetition of an alleged libel. Until it is clear that an alleged libel is untrue, it is not clear that any right at all has been infringed; and the importance of leaving free speech unfettered is a strong reason in cases of libel for dealing most cautiously and warily with the granting of interim injunctions. We entirely approve of and desire to adopt as our own, the language of Lord Esher, M.R., in *Coulson v. Coulson*, 3 Times L.R. 846 — "To justify the Court in granting an interim injunction it must come to a decision upon the question of libel or no libel, before the jury have decided whether it was a libel or not. Therefore the jurisdiction was of a delicate nature. It ought only to be exercised in the clearest cases, where any jury would say that the matter complained of

was libelous, and where, if the jury did not so find, the Court would set aside the verdict as unreasonable." In the particular case before us, indeed, the libelous character of the publication is beyond dispute, but the effect of it upon the Defendant can be finally disposed of only by a jury, and we cannot feel sure that the defense of justification is one which, on the facts which may be before them, the jury may find to be wholly unfounded; nor can we tell what may be the damages recoverable.

As I see it there are four main areas of complaint concerning the programme, they are:

(1) an allegation that the plaintiffs are polluting the area surrounding their factories with lead and that such pollution is causing lead poisoning with serious risk of illness and even death;
(2) an alleged innuendo that witnesses on behalf of the plaintiffs and in particular Drs. Barltrop and Sachs are prepared to offer their evidence for sale and that they will give untruthfully favourable evidence provided that they are paid;
(3) an alleged innuendo that the plaintiffs or their solicitors have concealed material evidence from a medical expert called on their behalf, and
(4) that the amount of money, by implication being spent by one or other of the plaintiffs, to combat pollution has been misstated.

I will deal with these four allegations in order and in each case must decide whether the allegation or alleged innuendo was clearly defamatory, was clearly untrue and, where such defence may apply, was clearly not fair comment . . .

Dealing then with the first allegation, that is that the plaintiffs polluted the area with lead, which resulted in lead poisoning to individuals, I have no doubt that such an allegation is defamatory. The term defamatory has been defined as any imputation that may tend to lower the plaintiff in the estimation of right-thinking members of society in general or to expose the plaintiff to hatred, contempt or ridicule. Can I be satisfied that such an allegation is clearly untrue? I think not. The material filed before me is in conflict and surely if this were an action for damages for libel the matter would have to be left to the jury.

I now turn to the second allegation which is the alleged innuendo that witnesses on behalf of the plaintiff are prepared to offer their evidence for sale, in that they will give untruthfully favourable evidence provided they are paid. It was argued before me that based upon the transcript of the programme such an innuendo cannot be drawn as against the plaintiffs. In my view, such an innuendo could be drawn from the transcript as against the plaintiffs but not necessarily so. A Judge at a trial in a defamation action might well decide that the words complained of were capable of conveying a defamatory meaning but it would still be a question for the jury whether the words did in fact convey a defamatory meaning. I do not think that a jury would necessarily come to the conclusion that the words complained of were in fact defamatory of these plaintiffs. The fact of the matter is that expert witnesses are paid and the Drs. Barltrop and Sachs were paid. The affidavit material before me indicates that they were paid, or were promised to be paid, their usual fee — whatever that is. The defence of fair comment may also apply in connection with the words complained of in the programme.

I will now deal with the alleged innuendo that the plaintiffs or their solicitors have concealed material evidence from medical experts. On reading the transcript it appears quite clear to me that no such innuendo could be drawn against the plaintiffs. The allegation, if such can be said to have been made, is against the Ministry of the Environment.

I now turn to the fourth allegation which is that the amount of money, by implication being spent by one or other of the plaintiffs, to combat pollution has been misstated. It may be that in the context of the programme such a misstatement would be defamatory. It was argued before me that the reference to the sum of $60,000 was not necessarily in connection with the operation of one or other of the plaintiffs. I would have thought that it was. However, I am of the opinion that there is sufficient doubt about it that again, should there be an action for damages for libel, it would be left to the jury. I do not think that a jury would necessarily find that such a statement was defamatory of the plaintiffs although they could well do so.

I do not think that the fact that there is a pending action for damages against Toronto Refiners and Smelters Company Limited is of any consequence. In the recent case of *Attorney-General v. Times Newspapers Ltd.*, [1973] 3 All E.R. 54, the House of Lords dealt with newspaper articles which urged a litigant to reconsider its position and which produced evidence to show that the litigant had not exercised due care in the manufacture and sale of thalidomide. The House of Lords held that the article setting out evidence was a clear case of contempt because it created a real risk that the fair trial of the action would be prejudiced and the publication thereof should be restrained by injunction. In the present case, the broadcast was a comment on a matter of general public interest and was not directed toward the litigation in progress. At p. 75 of the judgment in *Attorney-General v. Times Newspapers Ltd.* Lord Diplock states that discussion, however strongly expressed on matters of general public interest, is not to be stifled merely because there is litigation pending arising out of particular facts to which the general principles being discussed would be applicable. I think that is the rule that should be applied here. It is always open to move to strike out the jury notice in the action pending against one of the present plaintiffs. Lord Reid notes at p. 63 that it can be assumed that a publication of this sort would not affect the mind of a professional Judge.

Therefore, I have come to the conclusion that this is not a case in which the Court should interfere because, as I have said before, the Court will only interfere by way of injunction to prevent publication of alleged libel in the very clearest of cases. There are serious issues of fact which, in my view, could only be satisfactorily resolved by the hearing of evidence before Judge and jury.

It was argued before me that no order should be made for an injunction because damages would be a sufficient remedy. Should the plaintiffs commence an action for damages for libel such damages would be at large, which means, that it would not be necessary for the plaintiffs to prove any particular or special damages: see South *Hetton Coal Ltd. v. North-Eastern News Ass'n Ltd.*, [1894] 1 Q.B. 133 at p. 139. The fact that the defendant, the Canadian Broadcasting Corporation, would be in a position financially to pay any award is certainly a consideration.

The fact that I am ordering that the injunction granted by Mr. Justice Wilson be dissolved should not be taken in any way as being critical of his order. When the application was brought on before him he had only the original article, referred to earlier, appearing in the *Globe and Mail* and the affidavits deposing that certain of the statements therein were untrue. The programme was about to be broadcast in Ontario and, in fact, had already been broadcast to the eastern Provinces. There was no time to give the defendants notice of the application before him.

For the above reasons the motion to continue and expand the injunction will be dismissed and the motion to dissolve the injunction will be allowed. The injunction granted by Mr. Justice Wilson will therefore be dissolved. In all the circumstances the costs of the application will be costs in the cause in both motions.

Note: An appeal by Canada Metal Co. Ltd. to the Divisional Court of the High Court of Justice was dismissed: (1975), 55 D.L.R. (3d) 42.

5.2.4.2.2 Robert Martin, "Interlocutory Injuctions in Libel Actions," (1982), *University of Western Ontario Law Review* 20, p. 12

A. Introduction

In this essay I will seek first to set out the existing law with respect to the making of interlocutory injunctions in libel proceedings. Second, certain questions concerning the constitutionality of interlocutory injunctions in such circumstances will be analyzed. I will conclude with a discussion of the desirability of retaining the interlocutory injunction as a remedy in libel. I do not propose to deal with permanent injunctions. A permanent injunction may be granted after a judge or jury has determined that the matter in issue is libellous in order to prevent its further publication. This practice does not, for reasons which should become apparent below, raise the same problems as are encountered with interlocutory injunctions.

B. The Existing Law

The most complex Canadian case arose from a radio documentary. This documentary, an investigative report, led to a great deal of litigation. A brief recitation of the saga will be helpful.

The report was called "Dying of Lead"; it was an hour long; and it was to be broadcast over the CBC network on the programme *As It Happens* beginning at 7:00 p.m. EST on January 29, 1974. A column in the Toronto *Globe and Mail* that morning made reference to the programme and indicated that it contained allegations concerning "... lead emissions and illness around two Toronto smelters." On discovering this, two companies which operated smelters in Toronto, Toronto Refiners and Smelters Limited and Canada Metal Company Limited, sought an injunction to prevent the programme, or certain portions of it, being broadcast. An application was made *ex parte* on behalf of the companies to Mr. Justice Wilson of the Supreme Court of Ontario. The application was made at 5:15 p.m. and at 6:00 p.m. Wilson, J. made an interim order in these terms:

> Ex parte injunction granted to plaintiffs restraining defendants, and each of them from alleging or implying by broadcasting on television or otherwise publicizing that the plaintiffs and/or either of them, have bought misleadingly favourable medical evidence from medical experts, and from misstating the amounts the plaintiffs are spending to install pollution control systems.

This order was to be binding for ten days. At 6:20 p.m. the firm representing the smelter companies informed the CBC of the injunction by telephone and at 6:45 p.m. it was served on the CBC.

A CBC lawyer was actually in the studio. It was the practice with *As It Happens* to have all controversial programmes "lawyered" before they were broadcast with a view to removing libellous material. The fact of the injunction gave a special urgency to this procedure. The producers and the lawyer went over the script of "Dying of Lead" to see what could be salvaged. In the event the programme was broadcast at 7:00 p.m., but with three changes in the original script. Two passages from the programme as originally taped were deleted, with an electronic tone carried on air to indicate the deletions. In addition the order issued by Wilson, J. was read over the air.

The plaintiff companies were apparently not happy with this behaviour. They applied to have the executive producer and the story editor for "Dying of Lead" committed for contempt on the ground that they had breached the terms of the injunction. Mr. Justice O'Leary found the producer and story editor guilty of contempt and fined them each $700. An appeal to the Court of Appeal was dismissed. This was by no means the end of the litigation.

Applications were made, first, by the CBC, to have the injunction issued by Wilson, J. rescinded, and, secondly, by the two smelter companies, to continue the original interim injunction. The companies now sought the issuance of an order that would have been binding until the merits of their claim had been determined at trial.

Mr. Justice Holland, in a carefully reasoned judgment, dissolved the original injunction. An appeal from this decision to the Divisional Court was dismissed.

The injunction which had been granted in Ontario came too late to prevent the unexpurgated version of "Dying of Lead" being broadcast in Atlantic Canada, it was in fact, being aired in that region at the very moment Wilson, J. was making his order. The programme raised certain questions as to the probity of a Dr. Barltrop, a British physician who had testified on behalf of Canada Metal Company at a public hearing. Barltrop sued the CBC in the Nova Scotia courts for libel. He lost at trial, but on appeal was awarded $20,000.

A trial was never held on the merits of Canada Metal's claim against the CBC. The matter was finally settled in 1980.

What does this incident tell us about interlocutory injunctions? First, that an injunction may be granted to restrain the publication of allegedly libellous matter before a court has reached a definite conclusion as to whether the matter is libellous or whether a recognized defence has been successfully made out. Secondly, that while the general principles regarding the making of injunctions will apply, they are to be supplemented by certain special rules which are applicable only in libel actions. These rules appear to be as follows:

a. the jurisdiction of the courts to make an interlocutory injunction is of a delicate nature and should only be exercised in the clearest of cases;
b. there must be no doubt that the material in issue is libellous of the plaintiff. Indeed the material before the court must be so evidently libellous that any jury would find it to be so, and that were a jury to find otherwise its verdict would be set aside as unreasonable;
c. an injunction will not be granted when the defendant indicates an intention to raise one of the recognised defences, unless such defence is, in the circumstances of the case, manifestly without foundation.

If the result finally reached in *Canada Metal Co. Ltd. v. CBC* were to be accepted as an accurate expression of the law in Canada, one could feel fairly confident that the standard to be met before an interlocutory injunction would be issued was very high, so high indeed that such orders would seldom be made. Unfortunately, there have been two other recent Canadian cases which suggest contrary approaches. The first of these cases may simply reflect different emphases given to certain principles by the British Columbia courts on the one hand and the Ontario courts on the other. The second exemplifies the real threat which interlocutory injunctions in libel actions pose to freedom of speech; a threat which, in this instance, manifested itself with disastrous consequences.

The B.C. case was *Church of Scientology v. Radio NW Ltd.* It is widely known that the Church [sic] of Scientology. in both Canada and the United States, has not been slow to resort to the law of libel whenever it has encountered public criticism of its unusual ideas. Radio NW, a Vancouver-based operation, had broadcast one programme about Scientology and planned to produce others as part of a series. The first programme had some uncomplimentary things to say about the Scientologists who were, as a result, seeking an injunction to prevent the broadcasting of the rest of the series. The case as a whole is most unsatisfactory because it appears that the respondents made no effort to defend themselves. They did not contradict the allegations made by the applicant and they did not file any material with the court on which they might have based a defence. It may be that under the circumstances the court had little choice but to issue an injunction. An application of the approach enunciated in *Canada Metal v. CBC* could well have led to the same result. But the reasoning of the B.C. court was different. It betrayed an unfortunate eagerness to issue an injunction and in the process took the law beyond the limits established in *Canada Metal v. CBC*. The court suggested that once the applicant had established a *prima facie* case of libel and shown "a probability of a repetition," an injunction would issue. I cannot make up my mind whether the court fully appreciated that special rules are supposed to govern libel actions and that these rules differ substantially from those which apply to "ordinary" applications for interlocutory injunctions. The court talked about these rules at the beginning of its judgment, but at the conclusion simply enunciated the standard that must be met before an injunction will issue in ordinary proceedings.

The second case was *Lorcon Inc. v. Kozy Insulation Specialists Ltd., Watling and Clover*. The facts are a bit unclear as the decisions given in the various stages of litigation have not been reported. The following brief statement is taken from Stuart M. Robertson, *Courts and the Media*:

> The action was commenced by an application for an injunction and a claim for damages, as a result of the intimidating threats of the defendant to publish a libellous document containing 71 pages on the subject of the plaintiffs and their products. The document contained a number of statements and articles from different sources.

The plaintiff's product was urea-formaldehyde foam insulation. On February 14, 1979, Maloney, J. of the Ontario High Court granted an interim injunction *ex parte* to oprate until February 27, 1979. In addition to enjoining the publication of the 71-page document referred to above, the order also prohibited "... *any other statentent intended to cast into doubt the safety or acceptability as insulation of urea-formaldehyde foams made from products of the Plaintiff.*" On February 26, 1979, Labrosse, J. extended this injunction until "further order," which is to say, until the merits of the applicant's claim had been determined. Mr. Justice Eberle made the injunction permanent and awarded damages on September 25, 1979, in a proceeding at which the defendants chose not to appear. Indeed, the ambit of the order was extended so that it applied not only to the defendants, but to "... any other person to whom knowledge of the order shall come." Robertson, from the evidence of his book, appears to me to be a careful and meticulous commentator. He observed:

> The terms of the injunction in *Lorcon* make impossible the publication of any reports by government or an independent body produced in the interest of public safety and consumer protection. The order assumes that any statement made, even if based on research, would cause irreparable harm to the plaintiff, even though the statement might be in the public interest. This is an assumption which extends beyond the resolution of the dispute between the parties, and operates to curb freedom of speech and of the press.

There is nothing on the record to indicate that either the judge who issued the original injunction, or the judge who extended it, accepted that there were special considerations to be observed when dealing with applications for interlocutory injunctions in libel actions.

The third general point to stress about interlocutory injunctions in libel actions is that they may be issued as the result of an application made *ex parte*. An interim injunction issued under such circumstances will, as in *Canada Metal* and *Lorcon*, be temporary. The basic problem with issuing such injunctions *ex parte* is that they make much of the law on the subject meaningless. The rule, at least as stated in *Canada Metal*, is that if the respondent avers that he plans at trial to attempt to make out one of the recognized defences, there will be no injunction. But if the respondent is not present at the time the application is made, how is the judge to make a finding on this question? It would seem that if the courts do indeed regard the making of such injunctions as a "sensitive" matter, they should simply refuse as a matter of practice to issue them *ex parte*.

Finally, it must be stressed that violation of both the letter and the spirit of an injunction can be punishable as either contempt of court or the offence of disobeying an order made by a court Mr. Justice O'Leary in deciding to commit certain accused for contempt as a result of the "Dying of Lead" programme made it clear that a very strict standard of observance of injunctions was demanded. The court, he said, would not accept as a defence that the accused's conduct was reasonable or that due care and attention, based on legal advice, was exercised in order to avoid breaching the injunction. Indeed, the court stated that the proper course for the CBC under the circumstances would have been to postpone the programme entirely. What is perhaps most striking about O'Leary, J.'s judgment is the notion that the very act of reading the terms of the injunction over the air constituted a contempt. It should be recalled that contempt is the only non-statutory crime enforceable in Canada and that as a result the punishment awarded in a particular case is a matter for the discretion of the presiding judge.

D. Conclusion

Whether or not it is constitutionally permissible to make interlocutory injunctions in libel actions, I would argue that this is a most undesirable remedy in such proceedings. In his dissenting judgment in *Cherneskey v. Armadale Publishers,* Mr. Justice Dickson of the Supreme Court of Canada stated the problem clearly enough: "The law of defamation must strike a fair balance between the protection of reputation and the protection of free speech. . . . " The objection to interlocutory injunctions is that this balance is destroyed: free speech gives way to the protection of reputation.

Three contrary arguments may be advanced. The first can be easily disposed of. It would simply be said that while my objection may be well-founded, we really shouldn't worry because few applications are made for injunctions in these circumstances, even fewer are granted, and the injunctions actually granted are by their nature as interlocutory orders, temporary. While such an assertion is factually accurate, it misses the point. In my view, interlocutory injunctions are unacceptable as a matter of principle. It is surely not, from such a perspctive, an adequate justification for the existence of a legal remedy to assert that it is seldom invoked.

The second reply is more difficult. Here it would be conceded that there is a problem, but that the courts are fully cognizant of it. It is certainly true that one can find statements in the cases which stress "... the importance of leaving free speech unfettered." And it is largely in order to protect freedom of speech that the jurisdiction to issue interlocutory injunctions is exercised with great caution. Recent official studies of the law of defamation in Australia, New Zealand, and the U.K. have all recommended against any change in the law in this area. In each instance the basis for this conclusion was confidence in the ability of the courts to exercise their jurisdiction properly. But the argument is misconceived. As the "Dying of Lead" saga suggests, this confidence in the courts is exaggerated. Legitimate criticism of the activities of Canada Metal Company was stifled; what the *Globe and Mail* called "investigative journalism at its best" was perverted. The *Lorcon* incident reinforces this view. It is now clear that ureaformaldehyde foam insulation was neither "safe" nor "acceptable. " Lorcon Incorporated attempted to make the media generally aware of the injunction granted on February 14, 1979. There can be little doubt that this knowledge inhibited subsequent reporting about urea-formaldehyde foam insulation. The unavoidable fact remains that the jurisdiction to make interlocutory injunctions, no matter how delicate the courts may claim it to be, has been exercised in the past and will no doubt be exercised in the future.

Finally, it might be said that to eschew interlocutory injunctions would amount to creating a general licence to defame. On its face this view is untenable. The right of individuals to claim damages when they have been libelled exists independent of any interlocutory remedy. On further investigation the view becomes even more doubtful. Assume a potential plaintiff who, by one means or another, discovers that a potential defendant is about to publish something libellous about her. She, being a reasonable person, contacts the potential defendant and suggests that the material in question is inaccurate or unfair and explains why. A prudent potential defendant would be well-advised to take such a communication seriously. For, if the matter is eventually litigated, recalcitrant behaviour on the part of the defendant could either be evidence of malice, thereby negativing the defences of fair comment and qualified privilege, or aggravate the damages awardable.

If we are committed to the widest possible freedom of discourse on matters of public concern, the jurisdiction to make interlocutory injunctions, this undeniable judicial censorship, cannot, on principle, be accepted. The view taken by the courts in the United States is preferable, as well as being simpler and more straightforward: "... equitable relief does not extend that far ... it will not restrain the commission of a libel or slander, for that is prior censorship — a basic evil denounced by the constitutions of the United States and California in protecting freedom of speech and press."

5.2.5 Procedural Issues

In this section we address a variety of procedural issues that can affect the outcome of a defamation action.

5.2.5.1 Time Limits

There are special time limits that relate only to defamation actions.

5.2.5.1.1 *Ontario Libel and Slander Act*, R.S.O. 1990, c. L.12

5. (1) No action for libel in a newspaper or in a broadcast lies unless the plaintiff has, within six weeks after the alleged libel has come to the plaintiff's knowledge, given to the defendant notice in writing, specifying the matter complained of, which shall be served in the same manner as a statement of claim or by delivering it to a grown-up person at the chief office of the defendant.

Notes on Procedures in other Provinces

The above provision is unique. Most of the other provincial defamation Acts provide:

(1) No action lies unless the plaintiff has, within three months after the publication of the defamatory matter has come to his notice or knowledge, given to the defendant, in the case of a daily newspaper, 7, and in the case of any other newspaper or when the defamatory matter was broadcast, 14 days' notice in writing of his intention to bring an action, specifying the defamatory matter complained of.

(2) The notice shall be served in the same manner as a statement of claim.

(*Defamation Act*, R.S.A. 1980, c. D-6, s. 13. See also the *Revised Uniform Defamation Act*, s. 14 in Conference of Commissioners on Uniformity of Legislation in Canada, Proceedings of the Thirtieth Annual Meeting, Montreal, Quebec, August 24-28, 1948, Appendix J; *The Defamation Act*, R.S.M., c. D-20, s. 14; *Defamation Act*, R.S.N.B. 1973, c. D-5, s. 13; *Defamation Act*, R.S.N. 1990, c. D-3, s. 16; *Defamation Act*, R.S.N.S. 1989, c. 122, s. 18; *Defamation Act*, R.S.P.E.I. 1988, c. D-5, s. 14, which allows 5, not 7, days, in the case of a daily newspaper, for the plaintiff to give notice in writing to the defendant of his intention to bring an action.) Section 5 of the British Columbia *Libel and Slander Act*, R.S.B.C. 1979, c. 234, however, states:

> In an action for libel contained in a public newspaper or other periodical publication or in a broadcast, one clear day must be allowed to elapse between the cause of action complained of and the issue of the writ on the libel.

In Quebec:

2. Every person who deems himself injured by an article published in a newspaper and who wishes to claim damages must institute his action within the three months following the publication of such article, or within three months after his having had knowledge of such publication, provided, in the latter case, that the action be instituted within one year from the publication of the article complained of.

3. No such action may be brought against the proprietor of the newspaper, unless, personally or through his attorney, the party who deems himself injured gives a previous notice thereof of three days, not being holidays, at the office of the newspaper or at the domicile of the proprietor, so as to allow such newspaper to rectify or retract the article complained of.

(*Press Act*, R.S.Q. 1977, c. P-19.)

Pursuant to s. 15 of the Saskatchewan *Libel and Slander Act*, R.S.S. 1978, c. L-14:

> No action shall lie for a libel contained in a newspaper unless the plaintiff has given to the defendant, in the case of a daily newspaper, five, and in the case of a weekly newspaper, fourteen, clear days' notice in writing of his intention to bring the action, such notice to distinctly specify the language complained of.

And both the *Defamation Act* of the Northwest Territories, R.S.N.W.T. 1988, c. D-1, s 15, and the Yukon Territory *Defamation Act*, R.S.Y.T. 1986, c. 41, s. 14, provide:

(1) No action lies unless the plaintiff has, within three months after the publication of the defamatory matter has come to his notice or knowledge, given to the defendant 14 days notice in writing of his intention to bring an action.

(2) A notice under subsection (1) shall specify the language complained of and shall be served on the defendant in the same manner as a statement of claim.

5.2.5.1.2 *Grossman v. C.F.T.O* (1983), 139 D.L.R. (3d) 618 (Ont. C.A.)

CORY, J.A. From the foregoing it may be appropriate to list a few general conclusions as to the notice required by the Act.

Clearly, the notice provisions contained in the *Libel and Slander Act* are mandatory and if notice is not given then a libel action cannot be maintained.

The notice may have beneficial results both for the prospective plaintiff and publisher. It gives the publisher the opportunity to once again review the matter complained of and determine whether a correction, apology or retraction are called for, and if so, to see that they are made within the time-limits prescribed by the Act. The benefits a plaintiff receives from a prompt correction, retraction or apology may be far more valuable than an award in damages.

The Act does not specify any particular form of notice. It will always be more difficult to frame a notice complaining of a matter contained in a television broadcast than of statements contained in a newspaper, magazine article or book.

A more liberal interpretation of the notice required for a broadcast is justified in light of the 1958 amendment which referred to the "matter" complained of rather than the "statement" complained of.

An appropriate test to determine whether the notice complaining of a television broadcast is adequate might be as follows: Does the notice identify the plaintiff and fairly bring home to the publisher the matter complained of? Since the Act prescribes no particular form, the court in answering this question can consider all the relevant circumstances.

The longer and more frequent the broadcasts are, the greater the particularly that may be required of the notice. Similarly, the more numerous the possible heads of complaint are, the more detailed the notice must be. The pleadings in a libel action are technical and they provide a wide variety of defences to a publisher. So long as the broadcaster is made clearly aware of the matter of which the plaintiff complains of, then there is no reason why the case, as defined by the pleadings, should not be determined on its merits.

5.2.5.1.3 *Crown Liability Act*, R.S.C. 1985, c. C-50, as am. S.C. 1990, c. 8, s. 29

23. (1) Proceedings against the Crown may be taken in the name of the Attorney General of Canada or, in the case of an agency of the crown against which proceedings are by an Act of Parliament authorized to be taken in the name of the agency, in the name of that agency.

(2) Where proceedings are taken against the Crown, the document originating the proceedings shall be served on the Crown by serving it on the Deputy Attorney General of Canada or the chief executive officer of the agency in whose name the proceedings are taken, as the case may be.

5.2.5.1.4 *Ontario Libel and Slander Act*, R.S.O. 1990, c. L.12

6. An action for a libel in a newspaper or in a broadcast shall be commenced within three months after the libel has come to the knowledge of the person defamed, but, where such an action is brought within that period, the action may include a claim for any other libel against the plaintiff by the defendant in the same newspaper or the same broadcasting station within a period of one year before the commencement of the action. R.S.O. 1980, c. 237, s. 6.

7. Subsection 5(1) and section 6 apply only to newspapers printed and published in Ontario and to broadcasts from a station in Ontario. R.S.O. 1980, c. 237, s. 7.

8. (1) No defendant in an action for a libel in a newspaper is entitled to the benefit of sections 5 and 6 unless the names of the proprietor and publisher and the address of publication are stated either at the head of the editorials or on the front page of the newspaper.

(2) The production of a printed copy of a newspaper is admissible in evidence as proof, in the absence of evidence to the contrary, of the publication of the printed evidence copy and of the truth of the statements mentioned in subsection (1).

(3) Where a person, by registered letter containing the person's address and addressed to a broadcasting station, alleges that a libel against the person has been broadcast from the station and requests the name and address of the owner or operator of the station or

the names and addresses of the owner and the operator of the station, sections 5 and 6 do not apply with respect to an action by such person against such owner or operator for the alleged libel unless the person whose name and address are so requested delivers the requested information to the first-mentioned person, or mails it by registered letter addressed to the person, within ten days from the date on which the first-mentioned registered letter is received at the broadcasting station. R.S.O. 1980, c. 237, s. 8.

Notes on Statutes in Other Provinces

The three-month limitation period in s. 6 of Ontario's *Libel and Slander Act* is unique. The Newfoundland *Defamation Act* requires that the action "shall be started within four months after publication." (*Defamation Act*, R.S.N. 1990, c. D-3, s. 17) The New Brunswick *Defamation Act*, requiring that the action be started within six months after publication, is typical of the remaining statutes which specifically mention limitations:

> An action against the proprietor or publisher of a newspaper, or the owner or operator of a broadcasting station, or any officer, servant or employee of such newspaper or broadcasting station, for defamation contained in the newspaper or broadcast from the station shall be commenced within six months after the publication of the defamatory matter has come to the notice or knowledge of the person defamed; but an action brought and maintainable for defamation published within that period may include a claim for any other defamation published against the plaintiff by the defendant in the same newspaper or from the same station within a period of one year before the commencement of the action.

(R.S.N.B. 1973, c. D-5, s. 14. See also the *Revised Uniform Defamation Act*, s. 15 in Conference of Commissloners on Uniformity of Legislation in Canada, Proceedings of the Thirtieth Annual Meeting, Montreal, Quebec, August 24-28, 1948, Appendix J; *Defamation Act*, R.S.N.S. 1989, c. 122, s. 19, which adds "Notwithstanding the *Limitation of Actions Act*" to the beginning of the section; *Defamation Act*, R.S.P.E.I. 1988, c. D-5, s. 15; *The Libel and Slander Act*, R.S.S. 1978, c. L-14, s. 14 which states that such action may include a claim for any other libel published against the plaintiff by the defendant in the same newspaper within a period of two years before the commencement of the action; *Defamation Act*, R.S.N.W.T. 1988, c. D-1, s. 16; *Defamation Act*, R.S.Y.T. 1986, c. 41, s. 15. Alberta, British Columbia, Manitoba and Quebec have not adopted such a provision.)

5.2.5.2 Legal Aid

There is no legal aid in libel actions.

5.2.5.2.1 *Ontario Legal Aid Act*, R.S.O. 1990, c. L.9

15. A certificate shall not be issued to a person,
    (*a*) in proceedings wholly or partly in respect of a defamation;
    (*b*) in relator actions;

(c) in proceedings for the recovery of a penalty where the proceedings may be taken by any person and the penalty in whole or in part may be payable to the person instituting the proceedings; or

(d) in proceedings relating to any election. R.S.O. 1980, c. 234, s. 15; 1986, c. 64, s. 26

5.2.5.3 Juries

Notes on the Use of Juries

A. Number of Jurors

In the majority of the common-law provinces a jury in a civil proceeding consists of six jurors. (*Jury Act*, S.A. 1982, c. J-2.1, s. 12(1); *The Jury Act*, R.S.M. 1987, c. J30, s. 32(1), pursuant to s. 32(3) there may be a trial by five jurors if the parties to the action or issue or their counsel agree; *Courts of Justice Act* R.S.O, 1990, c. C.43, s. 108(4); *The Jury Act*, 1981, S.S. 1980-81, c. J-4.1, s. 14; *Jury Act*, R.S.N.W.T. 1988, c. J-2, s. 26(1); *Jury Act* R.S.Y.T. 1986, c. 97, s. 24). In New Brunswick, Nova Scotia and Prince Edward Island, seven jurors are required (*Jury Act*, S.N.B. 1980, c. J-3.1, s. 24(1); *Juries Act*, R.S.N.S. 1989, c. 242, s. 13(1); *Jury Act*, R.S.P.E.I. 1988, c. J-5, s. 24). In British Columbia the number of jurors needed for a civil jury is eight (*Jury Act*, R.S.B.C. 1979, c. 210, s. 18, as am. S.B.C. 1985, c. 10, s. 3); while in Newfoundland it is nine (*The Jury Act*, R.S.N. 1990, c. J-5, s. 20(2)).

B. Qualifications of Jurors

All of the common-law provinces require that jurors be resident in that province, Canadian citizens, and of the age of majority. Each provincial jury statute also has its own specific list of persons disqualified from serving as jurors in that province. (See, Alberta, s. 4, as am. S.A. 1983 (Spring Sitting), c. L-27.5. s. 165 and S.A. 1988, c. P-12.01, s. 67; British Columbia, ss. 3 and 4, the former section as am. S.B.C. 1981, c. 15, s. 116 and S.B.C. 1986, c. 16, s. 20; Manitoba, ss. 3 and 4, the former section as am. S.M. 1987-88, c. 44, s. 15(1) and (2); New Brunswick, s. 3, as am. 1988, c. 11, s. 19; Newfoundland, ss. 4 and 5; Nova Scotia, s. 5; Ontario Juries Act, R.S.O. 1990, c. J.3, ss. 3 and 4; Prince Edward Island, s. 5; Saskatchewan, s. 4., as am. 5.5. 1983, c. 48, s. 3; the Northwest Territories, ss. 5 and 6, the latter section as am. R.S.N.W.T. 1988 (Supp. Vol. II), c. 63, s. 2; and the Yukon Territory, ss. 5 and 6. The British Columbia *Jury Act* is typical:

Disqualification

> **3.** (1) a person is disqualified from serving as a juror who
> (a) not a Canadian citizen;

(b) not resident in the Province;
(c) under the age of majority;
(d) a member or officer of the Parliament of Canada or of the Privy Council of Canada;
(e) a member or officer of the Legislature or of the Executive Council;
(f) a judge, justice or court referee;
(g) an employee of the Department of Justice or of the Solicitor General of Canada;
(h) an employee of the Ministry of the Attorney General of the Province;
(h.1) an employee of the Legal Services Society or of a funded agency, as defined by the *Legal Services Society Act*;
(i) a barrister or solicitor;
(j) a court official;
(k) a sheriff or sheriff's officer;
(l) a peace officer;
(m) a warden, correctional officer or person employed in a penitentiary, prison or correctional institution;
(n) subject to a mental or physical infirmity incompatible with the discharge of the duties of a juror;
(o) a person convicted within the previous 5 years of an offence for which the punishment could be a fine of more than $2,000 or imprisonment for one year or more, unless he has been pardoned; or
(p) under a charge for an offence for which the punishment could be a fine of more than $2,000 or imprisonment for one year or more.

4. Where the language in which a trial is to be conducted is one that a person is unable to understand, speak or read, he is disqualified from serving as a juror in the trial.

Certain provinces also exclude spouses of those persons referred to in s. 3(1)(d)-(m) above (New Brunswick, Newfoundland, Ontario and Saskatchewan); clergy (New Brunswick, Nova Scotia, and the Northwest Territories and the Yukon Territory); "persons who are members of religious orders vowed to live only in a convent, monastery or other like religious community" (New Brunswick); medical practitioners (New Brunswick, Nova Scotia, Ontario, the Northwest Territories and the Yukon Territory); dental practitioners (New Brunswick, Nova Scotia and the Northwest Territories); veterinarians (New Brunswick and Ontario); coroners (Ontario and Saskatchewan); firefighters (New Brunswick and the Northwest Territories); druggists and nurses in active practice (the Northwest Territories and the Yukon Territory); persons confined in an institution (Alberta and Saskatchewan); telegraph, telephone and radio operators and post masters (the Yukon Territory); members of a council of municipality or members of a board of trustees of a school district or school division (Alberta and Saskatchewan); reeves, councillors and mayors (Saskatchewan); officers and men of the Canadian Forces on active service (Nova Scotia and the Northwest Territories); consuls and consular agents (New Brunswick); "persons actually engaged in the operation of (i) railway trains and steamships, (ii) plants producing electricity for public consumption, and (iii) water distribution systems distributing water for public consumption" (the Yukon Territory); and "every person who has been summoned as a witness or is likely to be called as a witness in a civil or criminal proceeding or has an interest in an action is ineligible to serve as a juror at any sittings at which the proceeding or action might be tried." (Ontario).

C. Verdicts

Majority verdicts, in one form or another, may be returned by civil juries in all the common-law provinces. The relevant legislation in most of the provinces provides:

> Any five of the jury may return a verdict or answer a question submitted to the jury by the judge, and the verdict or answer given by the five jurors has the same effect as a verdict or answer given by six jurors.

(Alberta *Jury Act*, s. 12(2). See also Manitoba *Jury Act*, s. 32(1) and (2); Ontario *Courts of Justice Act*, s. 108(6); Saskatchewan *Jury Act*, s. 14; the Northwest Territories *Jury Act* s. 26(1); and the Yukon Territory *Jury Act* s. 24(1).) In the other common-law provinces majority verdicts may be received only where the jury is unable to agree in all respects on a verdict within a specified period of time. (See British Columbia *Jury Act* s. 19(1) which states that the verdict of 75% of the jurors will be acceptable if the jury was unable to reach a unanimous verdict after three hours of deliberation; pursuant to s. 30(1) of New Brunswick's *Jury Act*, the verdict of five of the seven jurors will be binding if the entire jury was unable to agree on a verdict within three hours; under s. 31 of Newfoundland's *Jury Act*, seven of the nine jurors may return a verdict if the jury failed to reach a unanimous decision after three hours; the verdict of five of the seven jurors will be allowed where the entire jury failed to agree on a verdict after four hours under s. 13(1) of Nova Scotia's *Juries Act* and s. 24 of the *Jury Act* of Prince Edward Island provides that the decision of five of the seven jurors will be acceptable if seven jurors were unable to reach a unanimous decision after deliberating for three hours.)

Unanimous verdicts, however, are required in certain circumstances. For example, where one of the jurors dies or is discharged because of illness during the course of the trial, some of the provincial Acts specify that the verdict of the remaining jurors will be valid only if unanimous. (See Alberta, s. 12(4); Ontario *Courts of Justice Act*, s. 108(8); Prince Edward Island, s. 25; Saskatchewan, s. 15; the Northwest Territories, s. 29; and the Yukon Territory, s. 27. Section 15 of Nova Scotia's *Juries Act* states that if five of the remaining six jurors concur, their verdict will be valid. And in Manitoba, where a five juror trial has been agreed upon, s. 32(3) of the *Jury Act* requires that the verdict must be unanimous.

D. Juries in Defamation Actions

The circumstances under which there will be a jury in a civil trial differ slightly from province to province. In some provinces there will be trial by jury unless this requirement is waived by all parties. (*The Court of Queen's Bench Act*, S.M. 1988-89, c. 4 - c. C280, s. 64(1); *Judicature Act*, R.S.N.S. 1989, c. 240, s. 34(a)). In other jurisdictions, the parties to the action must request a jury (Alberta *Jury Act*, s. 16(1); *Jury Act*, R.S.N. 1990, c. J-S, s. 28(1); *Supreme Court Act*, R.S.P.E.I. 1988, c. 5-10, s. 40; *The Jury Act*, 1981, S.S. 1980-81, c. J-4.1, s. 16(1), *Jury Act*, R.S.N.W.T. 1988, c. J-2, s. 2(1); and *Jury Act*, R.S.Y.T. 1986, c. 97, s. 2(1)). And in several provinces a Judge may override the rule in some circumstances. For example pursuant to s. 16(2) of Alberta's *Jury Act*:

If on a motion for directions or on a subsequent application it appears that the trial might involve

(a) a prolonged examination of documents or accounts, or
(b) a scientific or long investigation,

that in the opinion of a judge cannot conveniently be made by a jury, the judge may, notwithstanding that the proceeding has been directed to be tried by a jury, direct that the proceeding be tried without a jury.

(See also Newfoundland's *Jury Act*, s. 32; the Northwest Territories; *Jury Act*, s. 2(2); and the Yukon Territory's *Jury Act*, s. 2(2)).

Jury trials for defamation actions are no longer mandatory in Ontario. (The *Judicature Act*, R.S.O. 1980, c. 223, s. 57 required that defamation be tried by a jury, unless the parties in person or by their solicitors or counsel waived such a trial. This requirement was removed in 1984 when the *Judicature Act* was replaced by the *Courts of Justice Act*, 1984, c. 11, which in turn was replaced by a new *Courts of Justice Act*, R.S.O. 1990, c. C.43)

5.2.5.3.1 *Ontario Libel and Slander Act*, R.S.O. 1990, c. L.12

14. On the trial of an action for libel, the jury may give a general verdict upon the whole matter in issue in the action and shall not be required or directed to find for the plaintiff merely on proof of publication by the defendant of the alleged libel and of the sense ascribed to it in the action, but the court shall, according to its discretion, give its opinion and directions to the jury on the matter in issue as in other cases, and the jury may on such issue find a special verdict, if they think fit so to do, and the proceedings after verdict, whether general or special, shall be the same as in other cases. R.S.O. 1980, c. 237, s. 15.

Note: This section is typical of the legislation found in almost every common-law province. (See the *Revised Uniform Defamation Act*, s. 7 in Conference of Commissioners on Uniformity of Legislation in Canada, Proceedings of the Thirtieth Annual Meeting, Montreal, Quebec, August 24-28, 1948, Appendix J; *Defamation Act*, R.S.A. 1980, c. D-6, s. 6; *The Defamation Act*, R.S.M. 1987, c. D20, s. 6; *Defamation Act*, R.S.N.B. 1973, c. D-5, s. 6; *Defamation Act*, R.S.N. 1990, c. D-3, s. 8; *Defamation Act* R.S.N.S. 1989, c. 122, s. 8; *Defamation Act*, R.S.P.E.I. 1988, c. D-5, s. 6; *The Libel and Slander Act*, R.S.S. 1978, c. L-14, s. 5; *Defamation Act*, R.S.N.W.T. 1988, c. D-1, s. 6; *Defamation Act*, R.S.Y.T. 1986, c. 41, s. 6(1). Section 7 of the *Northwest Territories' Act* and s. 6(2) of the

Yukon Territory Act add "[W]here an action for defamation is trled by a judge without jury, the judge may make such finding of general or special nature as he sees fit." Quebec's *Press Act* does not contain any similar provision.)

5.2.5.3.2 *McLoughlin v. Kutasy* (1979), 26 N.R. 242 (S.C.C.)

SPENCE, J., (*dissenting*): It must be remembered that this is an appeal in an action for libel tried by a jury in which trial the jury awarded the appellant a verdict. In Ontario, from which province this appeal comes, actions for damage for libel or slander must be tried with a jury unless the parties consent to the dispensation of the jury: *Judicature Act*, R.S.O. 1970, c.228, s.59. Moreover, the Ontario *Libel and Slander Act*, R.S.O. 1970, c.243, in s.15 provides:

> on a trial of an action for libel, the jury may give a general verdict upon the whole matter in issue in the action . . .

and ss.66 and 67 of the *Judicature Act* providing that the judge may require the jury to give a special verdict are expressly made inapplicable to libel actions.

It is a well established principle of law that a jury's verdict must be given all deference and full weight and effect given thereto except in the most unusual circumstance. I need only cite one authority for this. Chief Justice Duff said, in *McCannell v. McLean*, [1937] S.C.R. 341, at p. 343:

> The principle has been laid down in many judgments of this Court to this effect, that the verdict of a jury will not be set aside as against the weight of evidence unless it is so plainly unreasonable and unjust as to satisfy the Court that no jury reviewing the evidence as a whole and acting judicially could have reached it. That is the principle on which this Court has acted for at least thirty years to my personal knowledge and it has been stated with varying terminology in judgments reported and unreported.

Further, I am in accord with Nesbitt, J. when he said in *Jamieson v. Harris* (1905), 35 S.C.R. 625, at p. 631:

> Answers by the jury to questions should be given the fullest possible effect, and if it is possible to support the same by any reasonable construction, they should be supported.

And Wells, J., as he then was, expressed the same view very well in *Usher v. Smith*, [1948] O.W.N. 526, at p. 527, when he said:

> Jurymen and laymen are not accustomed to state matters with the particularity and clarity which more trained men might exhibit, and it is, I apprehend, the duty of the Court to give effect to their findings in a broad way when there is evidence to justify them . . .

I am further of the opinion that this course must be followed very strictly in considering the jury's answers to questions in a libel action in view of the fact that the legislature has directed that such actions must be tried with a jury and that the jury may, in its sole discretion, refuse to answer specific questions and give a general answer. Every effort must be exerted to understand and give a reasonable construction to the jury's answers remembering that jurors "are laymen who are not accustomed to state matters with the particularity and clarity which more trained men might exhibit".

5.2.5.3.3 *Burnett v. C.B.C. (No. 2)* (1981), 48 N.S.R. (2d) 181 (S.C.T.D.)

GRANT, J.: Most cases of defamation of this province are tried by a judge sitting with a jury. As I understand the law and practice, there are clearly defined roles for each to play. I am sitting as both judge and jury and I consider that I should make my findings and rulings on fact and law in each instance.

Whether there was in fact a publication of certain words, I understand is a question of fact for the jury with the burden of proof being on the plaintiffs.

Whether the words or images complained of refer to the plaintiffs is a question of fact for the jury with the burden of proof being on the plaintiffs.

Whether the words or images or sounds complained of are reasonably capable of a defamatory meaning in their natural and ordinary meaning, that is, of being defamatory, is a question of law for the judge.

Whether the words, images or sounds complained of in their natural and ordinary meaning, under the existing facts and circumstances, are defamatory of the plaintiffs is a question of fact for the jury.

Whether the words, images or sounds complained of are capable of being interpreted by right thinking members of society in the meaning attributed to them by the plaintiffs in their pleadings, is a question of law for the judge.

Whether the words, images or sounds complained of under the peculiar existing facts and circumstances bear the meaning attributed to them by the plaintiffs in their pleadings (the innuendo pleaded); that is, whether they are defamatory of the plaintiffs, is a question of fact for the jury.

Relating to the defence of justification, whether a fact is substantially true in substance and in fact is a question of fact for the jury.

Relating to the defence of fair comment, whether the words are capable of being comment is a question of law for the judge. Whether they are in fact comment is a question of fact for the jury. If they are comment it is a question of fact for the jury to determine if they are fair comment or not.

The question of public interest is a question of law for the judge to determine.

Whether the occasion of publication is one enjoying a qualified privilege is a question of law for the judge. If the surrounding facts are in issue then these facts are for the jury to decide.

If there is evidence of malice then the question of whether the defendant was actuated by malice is a question of fact for the jury.

The standard of proof is that of a preponderance of evidence or a balance of probabilities.

A libel action against the C.B.C. may not be tried by a jury.

5.2.5.3.4 *Hill v. Church of Scientology of Toronto*, 1994, unreported (Ont. C.A.)

GRIFFITHS, CATZMAN and GALLIGAN, JJ.A.: . . . the common law has long held that in defamation cases the jury represents society and, in that capacity, the jury expresses society's opinion about the actions of the person who makes false statements about another. The power of an appellate court is narrowly restricted. An appellate court must pay great deference to the jury because it alone has been charged with the important and unique function of representing society. The assessment of damages by a jury should rarely be disturbed on appeal and only in extraordinary cases. The courts have been uniform in holding that the jury's assessment is not to be disturbed unless there has been misdirection in the judge's charge, improper rejection or admission of evidence, or the court concludes (1) that the damages awarded are so high or so low that no six reasonable persons could have awarded them or (2) that the award is so exorbitant or so grossly out of proportion to the libel as to shock the court's conscience and sense of justice.

5.2.5.3.5 *Crown Liability Act*, R.S.C. 1985, c. C-50 as am. S.C. 1990, c. 8, s. 31

26. In any proceedings against the Crown, trial shall be without a jury.

5.2.5.4 Libel Insurance

Libel insurance in Ontario is permissible; no other province has such a provision.

5.2.5.4.1 *Ontario Libel and Slander Act*, R.S.O. 1990, c. L. 12

15. An agreement for indemnifying any person against civil liability for libel is not unlawful. R.S.O. 1980, c. 237, s. 16

Libel insurance is designed to protect newspaper publishers and broadcasters from financial losses that are the consequence of injuries caused by their publications and broadcasts.

Despite the need for this kind of insurance, the number of companies able to provide appropriate coverage is extremely limited. Only two companies offer libel insurance to Canadian newspaper publishers — Mutual Insurance Company Limited of Bermuda and the Kansa Insurance Company. The majority of Thomson newspapers are insured by Kansa. Coverage limits, insurance deductibles and premium rates vary from newspaper to newspaper. It is believed that the Toronto *Star* is insured for $1 million of liability in excess of $100,000 and has large deductibles in the range of $25,000-$50,000. Kansa also ensures weeklies and community newspapers, some of which are independent publications.

The policy that covered the greatest number of Thomson newspapers expired in mid-1986, and Kansa has decided not to renew its contract. Companies who continue to ensure broadcasters and publishers have described their problem in explicit terms. Chubb Insurance Company, a Toronto-based firm which ensures broadcasters, claims that it has been "clobbered in losses". Mutual Insurance Company, which insures clients through membership with the American Newspaper Publishers Association stated in a letter to its ANPA members that, in the last thirteen years, the Company received gross libel insurance premiums of $8.6 million, yet paid losses and loss adjustment premiums in excess of $26 million, while over 1,700 of their cases currently remained open. The cost of libel litigation, and especially legal fees, accounts for the major portion of claims paid by an insurance company. Mutual Insurance Company's President, R.D. Spurling, declared to ANPA members that the cost of libel litigation since 1975 was best described ''as an uncontrolled fire storm". Southam Newspapers are currently insured through the Mutual Insurance Company, although they initially sought a Canadian insurer. Southam stated that the availability of libel and slander insurance has decreased drastically: rates have increased, capacity has shrunk, and many insurers and reinsurers have ceased their operations.

Libel insurance that is available to publishers and broadcasters is expensive. The cost of insuring a newspaper depends largely upon its circulation. The greater its circulation, the more costly the process becomes for a publisher. The current cost of libel insurance for a major Canadian newspaper is in the range of U.S. $14,500 annually, with yearly increases dependent upon the number of claims processed, past loss history, and the current inflation rate. It is contended that, amongst other things, the profusion of libel cases in the United States has amplified insurers' losses and caused insurance rates to rise. Mutual Insurance, in an attempt to curtail some of its losses, significantly increased premiums to ANPA members (as of August 1, 1984). Its new policy includes provisions which oblige insured parties to:

a. pay 20% of defence costs in excess of its stated deductible costs, and;
b. give the Company prompt notice when such payments approach or exceed the stated deductible amount.

The cost of libel insurance can only be expected to increase significantly. The Employers Reinsurance Corporation, a large libel insurance carrier in the United States, is considering entering the Canadian libel insurance market. The Corporation claims to have a reliable and stable market in the United States. The Thompson chain, in considering libel policy coverage from the Employers Reinsurance Corporation, must regard the quality of insurance that can be provided, and premium rates that must be expected to appreciate.

5.2.5.5 Offer to Settle

Some important levers are placed in the hands of media defendants.

Ontario, Rules of Civil Procedure

49.02 (1) A party to a proceeding may serve on any other party an offer to settle any one or more of the claims in the proceeding on the terms specified in the offer to settle (Form 49A).

(2) Subrule (1) and rules 49.03 to 49.14 do not apply to motions, but nothing in this subrule prevents a party from making a proposal for settlement of a motion or the court from taking the proposal into account in making an order in respect of costs.

49.03 An offer to settle may be made at any time, but where the offer to settle is made less than seven days before the hearing commences, the costs consequences referred to in rule 49.10 do not apply.

49.04 (1) An offer to settle may be withdrawn at any time before it is accepted by serving written notice of withdrawal of the offer on the party to whom the offer was made.

(2) The notice of withdrawal of the offer may be in Form 49B.

(3) Where an offer to settle specifies a time within which it may be accepted and it is not accepted or withdrawn within that time, it shall be deemed to have been withdrawn when the time expires.

(4) An offer may not be accepted after the court disposes of the claim in respect of which the offer is made.

49.05 An offer to settle shall be deemed to be an offer of compromise made without prejudice.

49.06 (1) No statement of the fact that an offer to settle has been made shall be contained in any pleading.

(2) Where an offer to settle is not accepted, no communication respecting the offer shall be made to the court at the hearing of the proceeding until all questions of liability and the relief to be granted, other than costs, have been determined.

(3) An offer to settle shall not be filed until all questions of liability and the relief to be granted in the proceeding, other than costs, have been determined. [Amended, O.Reg.221/86, s. 1.]

49.07 (1) An offer to settle may be accepted by serving an acceptance of offer (Form 49C) on the party who made the offer, at any time before it is withdrawn or the court disposes of the claim in respect of which it is made.

(2) Where a party to whom an offer to settle is made rejects the offer or responds with a counter-offer that is not accepted, the party may thereafter accept the original offer to settle, unless it has been withdrawn or the court has disposed of the claim in respect of which it was made.

(3) An offer by a plaintiff to settle a claim in return for the payment of money by a defendant may include a term that the defendant pay the money into court or to a trustee and the defendant may accept the offer only by paying the money in accordance with the offer and notifying the plaintiff of the payment.

(4) Where a defendant offers to pay money to the plaintiff in settlement of a claim, the plaintiff may accept the offer with the condition that the defendant pay the money into court or to a trustee and, where the offer is so accepted and the defendant fails to pay the money in accordance with the acceptance, the plaintiff may proceed as provided in rule 49.09 for failure to comply with the terms of an accepted offer.

(5) Where an accepted offer to settle does not provide for the disposition of costs, the plaintiff is entitled,

> (*a*) where the offer was made by the defendant, to the plaintiff's costs assessed to the date the plaintiff was served with the offer; or (b) where the offer was made by

the plaintiff, to the plaintiff's costs assessed to the date that the notice of acceptance was served; or

(b) where the offer was made by the plaintiff, to the plaintiff's costs assessed to the date that the notice of acceptance was served.

(6) Where an offer is accepted, the court may incorporate any of its terms into a judgment.

(7) Where money is paid into court under sub-rule (3) or (4), it may be paid out on consent or by order.

49.08 A party under disability may make, withdraw and accept an offer to settle, but no acceptance of an offer made by the party and no acceptance by the party of an offer made by another party is binding on the party until the settlement has been approved as provided in rule 7.08.

49.09 Where a party to an accepted offer to settle fails to comply with the terms of the offer, the other party may,

(a) make a motion to a judge for judgment in the terms of the accepted offer, and the judge may grant judgment accordingly; or

(b) continue the proceeding as if there had been no accepted offer to settle.

49.10 (1) Where an offer to settle,

(a) is made by a plaintiff at least seven days before the commencement of the hearing;

(b) is not withdrawn and does not expire before the commencement of the hearing; and

(c) is not accepted by the defendant,

and the plaintiff obtains a judgment as favourable as or more favourable than the terms of the offer to settle, the plaintiff is entitled to party and party costs to the date the offer to settle was served and solicitor and client costs from that date, unless the court orders otherwise.

(2) Where an offer to settle,

(a) is made by a defendant at least seven days before the commencement of the hearing;

(b) is not withdrawn and does not expire before the commencement of the hearing; and

(c) is not accepted by the plaintiff;

and the plaintiff obtains a judgment as favourable as or less favourable than the terms of the offer to settle, the plaintiff is entitled to party and party costs to the date the offer was served and the defendant is entitled to party and party costs from that date, unless the court orders otherwise.

5.2.5.6 Consolidation of Actions and Security for Costs

5.2.5.6.1 *Ontario Libel and Slander Act*, R.S.O. 1990, c. L.12

11. (1) The court, upon an application by two or more defendants in any two or more actions for the same or substantially the same libel, or for a libel or libels the same or substantially the same in different newspapers or broadcasts, brought by the same person or persons, may make an order for the consolidation of such actions so that they will be tried together, and, after such order has been made and before the trial of such actions, the defendants in any new actions instituted by the same person or persons in respect of any such libel or libels are also entitled to be joined in the common action upon a joint application being made by such new defendants and the defendants in the actions already consolidated.

(2) In a consolidated action under this section, the jury shall assess the whole amount of the damages, if any, in one sum, but a separate verdict shall be taken for or against each defendant in the same way as if the actions consolidated had been tried separately, and, if the jury finds a verdict against the defendant or defendants in more than one of the actions so consolidated, the jury shall apportion the amount of the damages between and against the last-mentioned defendants, and the judge at the trial, in the event of the plaintiff being awarded the costs of the action, shall thereupon make such order as he or she considers just for the apportionment of the costs between and against such defendants.

(3) This section does not apply where the libel or libels were contained in an advertisement. R.S.O. 1980, c. 237, s. 12.

12. (1) In an action for a libel in a newspaper or in a broadcast, the defendant may, at any time after the delivery of the statement of claim or the expiry of the time within which it should have been delivered, apply to the court for security for costs, upon notice and an affidavit by the defendant or the defendant's agent showing the nature of the action and of the defence, that the plaintiff is not possessed of property sufficient to answer the costs of the action in case judgment is given in favour of the defendant, that the defendant has a good defence on the merits and that the statements complained of were made in good faith, or that the grounds of action are trivial or frivolous, and the court may make an order for the plaintiff to give security for costs, which shall be given in accordance with the practice in cases where a plaintiff resides out of Ontario, and the order is a stay of proceedings until the security is given.

(2) Where the alleged libel involves a criminal charge, the defendant is not entitled to security for costs under this section unless the defendant satisfies the court that the action is trivial or frivolous, or that the circumstances which under section 5 entitle the defendant at the trial to have the damages restricted to actual damages appear to exist, except the circumstances that the matter complained of involves a criminal charge.

(3) For the purpose of this section, the plaintiff or the defendant or their agents may be examined upon oath at any time after the delivery of the statement of claim. R.S.O. 1980, c. 237, s. 13(1-3).

13. An order made under section 12 is final and is not subject to appeal. 1989, c. 56, s. 27, revised.

Notes on Statutes in Other Provinces

Provisions similar to section 11(1) and (2) can be found in the defamation legislation of all the common-law provinces and the *Revised Uniform Defamation Act*. See *Revised Uniform Defamation Act*, ss. 8 and 9; *Defamation Act*, R.S.A. 1980, c. D-6, ss. 7 and 8; *Libel and Slander Act*, R.S.B.C. 1979, c. 234, ss. 15 and 16; *The Defamation Act*, R.S.M. 1987, c. D20, ss. 7 and 8; *Defamation Act*, R.S.N.B. 1973, c. D-5, ss. 7 and 8; *Defamation Act*, R.S.N. 1990, c. D-3, ss. 9

and 10; *Defamation Act*, R.S.N.S. 1989, C. 122, ss. 11 and 12; *Defamation Act*, R.S.P.E.I. 1988, c. D-5, ss. 7 and 8; *The Libel and Slander Act*, R.S.S. 1978, c. L-14, s. 6(1) and (2); *Defamation Act*, R.S.N.W.T. 1988, c. D-1, ss. 8 and 9; and *Defamation Act*, R.S.Y.T. 1986, c. 41, ss. 7 and 9.

All of the Acts, with the exception of Ontario's, have a provision regarding the place of trial:

> The action shall be tried in the county (or judicial district) where the chief office of the newspaper or of the owner or operator of the broadcasting station is situated, or in the county (or judicial district) wherein the plaintiff resides at the time the action is brought; but upon the application of either party the court may direct the action to be tried or the damages to be assessed in any other county (or judicial district) if it appears to be in the interests of justice, and may impose such terms as to payment of witness fees and otherwise as the court deems proper.

(*Revised Uniform Defamation Act*, s. 16; *Defamation Act*, R.S.A. 1980, c.D-6, s. 14. See also *Libel and Slander Act*, R.S.B.C. 1979, c. 234, s. 18; *The Defamation Act*, R.S.M. 1987, c. D20, s. 15; *Defamation Act*, R.S.N.B. 1973, c. D-5, s. 15, as am. S.N.B. 1986, c. 4, s. 11; *Defamation Act*, R.S.N. 1990, c. D-3, s. 7 which states: "An action for defamation shall be tried in the Trial Division before a judge or before a judge and jury"; *Defamation Act*, R.S.N.S. 1989, c. 122, s. 20; *Defamation Act*, R.S.P.E.I. 1988, c. D-5, s. 16; *The Libel and Slander Act*, R.S.S. 1978, c. L-14, s. 13; *Defamation Act*, R.S.N.W.T. 1988, c D-1, s. 17; and *Defamation Act*, R.S.Y.T. 1986, c. 41, s. 16. The provision regarding the place of trial in the Ontario *Libel and Slander Act* was omitted in the R.S.O. 1990.)

Only Saskatchewan's Act includes a provision similar to Ontario's s. 11(3). Section 6(3), R.S.S. 1978, c. L-14 states:

> For the purposes of this section "article" includes anything appearing in a newspaper as an editorial or as correspondence or otherwise than as an advertisement.

The *Libel and Slander Acts* of British Columbia and Saskatchewan, and Quebec's *Press Act* are the only other statutes which provide for security for costs in defamation actions. (See British Columbia, s. 19; and Saskatchewan, s. 12) Section 11 of Quebec's *Press Act* is unique in its brevity

> The judge may, during a suit for defamation against a newspaper, order the plaintiff to furnish security for costs, provided that the defendant himself furnishes security to satisfy the judgment. The amount of security in each instance shall be left to the sole discretion of the judge.

5.3 Privacy

The following materials seek to determine whether a right to privacy exists in Canada and, if so, what its limits are.

5.3.1 The Charter

5.3.1.1 *The Canadian Charter of Rights and Freedoms*

7. Everyone has the right to life, liberty and security of the person and the right not to be deprived thereof except in accordance with the principles of fundamental justice.

5.3.1.2 *R. v. Nicolucci and Papier* (1985), 22 C.C.C. (3d) 207 (Que. S.C.)

BOILARD, J.: The right to privacy is one enjoyed by all citizens living in Canada and it has been enshrined in the *Canadian Charter of Rights and Freedoms*. Section 8 of the Charter protects not only against unreasonable search and seizure of one's home or business premises but also against unreasonable interceptions of private communications.

5.3.2 Privacy at Common Law

5.3.2.1 *Robbins v. C.B.C.* (1957), 12 D.L.R. (2d) 35 (Que. S.C.)

W. B. SCOTT, ASSOC. C.J.: This is an action for damages brought by the plaintiff against the defendant arising under the following circumstances:

From paras. 1 and 2 of plaintiff's declaration (which are admitted by the defendant) it appears that the plaintiff is a member of the College of Physicians & Surgeons of the Province of Quebec and has been practicing as a physician in the Cities of Montreal and Outremont and vicinity for upwards of 40 years and is consulting physician to the Montreal General Hospital, Chief of the Medical Department of the Reddy Memorial Hospital and Chairman of the Medical Board of the Reddy Memorial Hospital; and that the defendant is a body corporate carrying on a radio broadcasting and television service throughout Canada and has a monopoly of the television service in Canada except for a few cities therein.

For some time prior to February 1, 1956, the defendant had been televising and broadcasting throughout Eastern Canada a programme entitled *Tabloid*. It was put on at 7 p.m. and lasted for one-half hour.

It may be stated parenthetically that the delay in hearing this action is due to the fact that an earlier action taken by the plaintiff was dismissed because the defendant invoked s. 10 of the *Crown Liability Act*, 1952-53 (Can.), c.30. which requires a prior 90-day notice to the Deputy Attorney General of Canada with particulars of the claim before a suit can be brought. Thus this is a second suit, instituted after due compliance with this provision of the statute.

From the evidence given by Ross McLean, who was Producer at that time, the programme was what he called a "provocative" one. On January 16, 1956 plaintiff wrote a letter to the Producer of *Tabloid*, CBC Television Studios, Toronto, on a letterhead reading "5770 Durocher Avenue, Outremont, P.Q." Dr. Robbins says that it was posted in an envelope bearing his name as a doctor. The letter reads as follows (ex. P4):

"5770 Durocher Ave.,
"Outremont, P.Que.
"January 16th, 1956

"The Producer
"TABLOID

"CBC Television Studios
"Toronto
"Sir,
"I am enclosing a clipping from the Montreal *Star* which I trust you will read and in turn pass it along to the EASY M.C. and his partners in on TABLOID.

"It is indeed fortunate that Mr. W. O'Hearn did not see some of the past performances in which the script called for MacDougal and Saltzman to put on the most infantile acts one could imagine.

"It would be interesting to know what our American Viewers think of this production, but probably they do as many here do, SHUT it off as soon as the weather is over.

"The weather is the only redeeming feature of the show and I must congratulate Mr. Saltzman on his clear talks on this subject.

"Our only hope is that Tabloid like LIVING in the past will die a natural death.

"I wonder if the Tabloid Quartette will read this letter along with some of the others they get from Viewers.

"Yours
"(Sgd.) E. E. Robbins."

With this letter plaintiff enclosed a clipping from the Montreal *Star* of an article by Mr. Walter O'Hearn containing criticisms of the *Tabloid* programme (ex. P-5). It appears from the evidence that Mr. Walter O'Hearn is a drama critic and television critic for the Montreal *Star*.

Plaintiff complains that on Wednesday, February 8, 1956, the defendant in its programme broadcast and televised the newspaper article and plaintiff's letter to the viewers and listeners of *Tabloid*, with its own comments thereon and requested its viewers and listeners to write or telephone to the plaintiff to "cheer" him up.

From the evidence it appears that the Master of Ceremonies, one Dick MacDougal (since deceased), read the script prepared for him in advance by the Producer, Ross McLean, and added his own comments.

In para. 3 of its defence defendant states that MacDougal said on that occasion: "Well, I guess we might have skipped Mr. Robbins' letter if he hadn't added that last paragraph, because frankly it's not a very pleasant addition to tonight's program. Now then, when we quoted from similar letters in the past, some of you have written to us — people write to us to kind of cheer us up. That's been very kind of you, but this time, perhaps the person you really should cheer up is Mr. Robbins himself, so if you'll get a pencil and some paper handy we're going to give you his address. Here it is:"

It has become common ground after hearing the evidence that plaintiff's name and address, as appearing on his letterhead, were flashed twice on the screen; the second occasion being after an interval of time between the first flashing of the name and address.

In substance plaintiff complains that the defendant and its employees or agents who prepared or conducted the television broadcast and the said request to its listeners and viewers committed serious fault and negligence: that they were actuated by resentment of this criticism and by vindictiveness and malice towards the plaintiff, that the defendant and its employees know, or ought to have known, that the said television and broadcast and request would be a damaging invasion of the plaintiff's privacy and would be seen and heard by many thousands of people in Eastern Canada and the United States and that a large number of them would respond to the said request and subject the plaintiff to abuse and insults and prejudice and humiliation and would cause loss and damage to the plaintiff; also that the television broadcast and the said request constituted an incitement to the public to cause loss and damage to the plaintiff, and did cause loss and damage.

There is some contradiction in the testimony adduced before the Court as to whether the Master of Ceremonies, MacDougal, did or did not ask listeners to telephone to the plaintiff on that occasion. McLean, the Producer, going back in his memory of what took place some 22 months ago, is of the opinion that MacDougal did ask people to write to plaintiff and gave the postage rate for a letter from Montreal and what it would be on a letter from outside of Montreal. He has no recollection of any invitation to telephone the plaintiff.

On the other hand, Dr. Robbins and his wife and Mrs. Sears, who were following the programme on that occasion, all testified that MacDougal asked people to telephone as well as to write.

The Court, after seeing Dr. Robbins and his wife and Mrs. Sears in the witness-box, is satisfied that they have proved that there was an invitation to telephone as well as write. In any event, it is reasonable to say that the natural result of this invitation by MacDougal to the viewers and listeners would, in the normal course of events, result in people using the telephone, that is to say, the people living in and around Montreal. The City of Outremont is a prosperous and well-known suburban municipality adjoining the City of Montreal. All anybody would have to do would be to look up the Montreal telephone book where Dr. Robbins' name and address appeared. He was listed as Dr. E. E. Robbins, 5770 Durocher. Moreover it is far easier for people to telephone even if they are not invited to telephone than it is to take time to sit down and write a letter.

Plaintiff's allegation in para. 5 that the defendant and its employees knew that this invitation would be seen and heard by many thousands of people in Eastern Canada is borne out by the proof. The first witness plaintiff called was one Jean Leveille who is a Research Director of International Surveys Ltd. This company is employed by the CBC itself to furnish estimates of the numbers of listeners and viewers on CBC programmes, including *Tabloid*, and on that night he estimated that in Montreal and within a radius of 50 miles from Montreal, some 66,000 homes were watching the television programme of *Tabloid*. His estimate is that the average number of viewers per home is 3 persons.

In Toronto on that same evening his estimate is that 90,000 people in Toronto and within a radius of 50 miles were viewing the *Tabloid* programme. It is also admitted by Mr. McLean this morning that the programme could be seen and heard at distances beyond 50 miles, though sometimes with more difficulty. He said, however, that it could be seen in Ottawa, which is established by one of the letters filed in the sheaf of 102 letters as ex. P-3, as there is a letter from Billings Bridge which is not far from Ottawa.

There is no need to elaborate too much on these figures as there is evidence that there was a vast number of viewers and listeners and the defendant corporation is continually being furnished with the estimates by people employed by them; so they know approximately how many people would hear this invitation expressed by MacDougal.

Although MacDougal, as McLean said, "adlibbed" on the programme prepared for him in advance by the Producer, the deliberateness of this action by the CBC was made manifest by the fact that practically all of the language used was prepared by Ross McLean himself in advance. When asked by the Court yesterday afternoon whether he prepared the name and address of E. E. Robbins flashed on the screen, he said he did not do it himself but admitted that the graphic arts department, which was one branch of the CBC set-up in Toronto, had prepared it at his request.

The law governing the subject is simply stated in art. 1053 of the *Civil Code*, which reads as follows:

> 1053. Every person capable of discerning right from wrong is responsible for the damage caused by his fault to another, whether by positive act, imprudence, neglect or want of skill."

And Article 1054 says:

> 1054. He is responsible not only for the damage caused by his own fault, but also for that caused by the fault of persons under his control and by things he has under his care;
>
> Masters and employers are responsible for the damage caused by their servants and workmen in the performance of the work for which they are employed.

It was neither alleged nor proved that the law of Ontario differs from our own law in this respect, so that for the purposes of this case the Court must assume that the law of Ontario is the same as our own. Now the first question to be decided is this: Did the defendant and his servants and employees violate the provisions of art. 1053 and art. 1054 of our *Civil Code*? The Court has no hesitation whatever in holding that the defendant is responsible for an actionable wrong committed by its employees and servants. Defendant says in its plea that the letter of criticism did not mention that the plaintiff was a practising physician. It does not matter whether or not the plaintiff was a physician, because all citizens are protected by the above two articles of the *Civil Code*.

Both counsel have frankly admitted that they have not been able to find any case in the books similar to the one that is now before us. As far as I am concerned, I am very happy they were not able to find any such case, because in the opinion of the Court what the Producer and the "Easy Master of Ceremonies", the late Dick MacDougal, did on that occasion constituted a grievous positive wrongful act against Dr. Robbins, making the defendant corporation responsible for the damages flowing from such wrongful act.

There is no need to attempt any precise definition of this fault which the defendant's servants committed. By no stretch of the imagination can it be held that when Dr. Robbins wrote this letter on January 16th criticizing this programme, he invited the Producer to incite the listeners to "cheer him up" for daring to criticize the programme.

It can be quite properly held from the language used by the plaintiff that he wanted this letter merely to be read, not only by the Producer but by the quartette who appeared on the programme.

Even if it can be inferred that he wished to have his criticism and that of Mr. O'Hearn read out to the viewers and listeners to give them something to think about, never in this wide world can it be deduced that the Producer and Master of Ceremonies were invited to "set the dogs on Dr. Robbins" for having dared to criticize.

The defendant corporation very wisely have not submitted that any such power was given to them by Parliament in the charter of the CBC which appears in R.S.C. 1952, c.32, because I can find nothing in that charter which in any shape or form would be or could be construed as parliamentary approval to persecute or incite persecution of a private citizen who dared to criticize any programme.

Interesting and instructive evidence was given by Dr. Krauser, yesterday afternoon. He is a graduate of McGill University. He had 5 years in general practice and for the last five years has been specializing in psychiatry. He is attached to the Montreal General Hospital and is a demonstrator in psychiatry at McGill University.

He said that with such a large audience of viewers and listeners there was bound to be a large number who were just marginal in their ability to control themselves, and that when such people received an invitation to get after somebody, in the way in which it was done on this programme, it was inevitable that a certain percentage of these marginal people would take that as an invitation to abuse the person whose name and address were given them. He made it clear that this was a fact which would or should be known to people conducting a system of mass communication such as that carried on by the defendant, the Canadian Broadcasting Corp.

No contradiction whatever of his testimony was attempted by the defendant, not even by Mr. Ross McLean. And the evidence of Dr. Krauser is corroborated first by what the plaintiff told us as to what happened at his house within 15 minutes after the invitation to "cheer up" plaintiff was given, when his telephone started ringing and continued until late that evening when he and his wife had to take the telephone off the receiver to get some peace. Further, it so continued for three days, until the situation became so intolerable at his home that he had to go to the telephone company and have them disconnect his number and give him another number. His Telephone Answering Service was also swamped with calls. Plaintiff spoke about the hostile messages he had received. Some of the language was so crude he did not want to repeat it in Court.

It should be added that this inciting invitation was followed by people who decided to "cheer up" the plaintiff by sending C.O.D. food parcels to his house. Some other person or persons apparently telephoned in his name and ordered taxis to go to his home. The first one came to the door and there were half a dozen others waiting out on the street. There was no contradiction whatever to this evidence.

Dr. Krauser's testimony was also fully corroborated by the 102 letters which the doctor received both from the Province of Quebec and from Ontario, and as far away as North Troy, Vermont.

Not all those letters were written in terms of abuse. Yesterday counsel for defendant read out two quite mild ones saying they did not agree with the plaintiff but a great many of the remainder are disgusting and abusive — so much so that I shall not repeat them here.

It is noteworthy to find how many of them are written by women who signed their names.

The uncontradicted testimony of the plaintiff stands as to what happened to him.

The only reasonable inference to draw from all this is that the Producer and the Master of Ceremonies knew this was likely to happen.

On the whole the Court holds that neither the defendant nor its employees had the right to select for treatment such as that given to plaintiff any citizen who had written a letter criticizing one of its programmes.

Now as to the quantum of damages to which the plaintiff is entitled. There is a claim for loss of income from his private practice at his home. This is apart from the income he received for consultations and treatments at the Reddy Memorial Hospital and apart from the salary he receives as Registrar for which he is making no claim.

Plaintiff estimates he is losing $300 a month. But he had brought no books with him nor cards nor income tax returns which would enable this statement to be tested by cross-examination. It is quite clear, however, that for a doctor, 76 years of age, it is a serious matter to have one's telephone cut off for a whole month.

Counsel for defendant agreed, with the consent of plaintiff's counsel, that for purposes of this case the defence would admit that there had been a diminution in the income of plaintiff following this episode.

The next item of damage appearing in para. 11 of the declaration is impairment of Dr. Robbins' health. On that we have the evidence of Dr. Shister who examined the plaintiff shortly after February 8, 1956. He said Dr. Robbins was suffering from severe emotional disturbance, which I consider would be a most natural consequence. There was no evidence to the contrary.

Dr. Shister added that for the first few weeks following this episode the plaintiff was in no condition to practise and he considered this situation lasted for two or three months. The general effect of the testimony was that it had not done the doctor any good — especially for a man of that age. Dr. Robbins testified to the same effect.

Mrs. Robbins gave evidence as to the insomnia from which the doctor suffered following February 8th.

This evidence was not contradicted.

Plaintiff also has a claim for humiliation and invasion of privacy. What was done was a form of malicious mischief or a premeditated way of causing a public nuisance to the doctor.

Before proceeding to assess and fix the damages, allusion should be made to the fact that on February 13th the CBC, on the television news programme at 6:45 p.m., referred to this incident. McLean had no record of that reference. However, from the evidence given by plaintiff, which was not contradicted, the CBC employees in charge of that programme referred to the letter of regret and apology written by Mr. Dilworth, Director of Programmes for Ontario, to plaintiff on February 10th, i.e., three days before this news broadcast on Monday, February 13th. Mr. Dilworth's letter (ex. P-1) reads as follows:

"CANADIAN BROADCASTING CORPORATION

"354 Jarvis Street,
"Toronto, Ontario,
"February 10th, 1956.

"Airmail
"Special Delivery.
"Dr. E. E. Robbins,
5770 Durocher Avenue,
Montreal, Quebec.

"Dear Dr. Robbins,

"I wish to tell you how very deeply I regret the incident which occurred on our 'Tabloid' program last Wednesday evening. I offer you my personal apologies and the apologies of the Corporation.

"I assure you that we have gone beyond regretting the incident and have acted very quickly to bring proper and very severe disciplinary action to bear upon the people responsible for this unfortunate incident.

"Yesterday morning I issued a statement to the press. I am enclosing a copy for your information and interest.

"Yours sincerely.
"(Sgd.) Ira Dilworth

Director for the Province of Ontario."

Apparently there was some sort of internal conflict within the ranks of the CBC — that is to say, the employees in charge of the news programme were apparently not following the stand taken by Mr. Dilworth. I mention this because what was shown and said on that news programme resulted in a further invasion of the private life of the plaintiff.

On February 10th, Mr. E. W. Robbins, son of the plaintiff, wrote to Mr. David Dunton, Chairman of the CBC, telling of the trouble caused to his father and saying, that "many people have suggested my Father should seek redress through legal channels".

On February 16th, six days later, Mr. Dunton replied as follows (ex. P-2):

"CANADIAN BROADCASTING CORPORATION

"OFFICE OF THE
CHAIRMAN
"Mr. E. W. Robbins,
"26 Ballantyne Avenue, South,
"Montreal West, P.Q.

140 Wellington Street,
Ottawa, Ontario,
February 16th, 1956.

"Dear Mr. Robbins,

"May I begin by saying that all of us, in the Corporation are extremely sorry about the 'Tabloid' incident which involved your father and caused him so much inconvenience.

"By now you will have learned of the apology the Corporation made and the action taken in relieving the producer of his post on this program. Naturally you have my assurance that the Corporation is determined that there shall be no recurrence of any invasion of a citizen's privacy and right to criticism.

"In Dr. Dilworth's apology he referred to the incident as 'a grave error of judgment and good taste'. It was indeed a very serious matter even though I am sure there was no malicious intent.

"The Corporation has received a great number of letters and phone calls protesting the disciplinary action taken with regard to the producer. Nevertheless, I can assure you that we will continue to take a firm stand whenever the listeners' rights are in any way jeopardized by CBC actions. No better example of the power of the television medium can possibly be found. In this country CBC has been charged with the responsibility of developing this powerful medium to suit the desires and needs of Canadians. This responsibility is a great one and its fulfillment cannot be interrupted by incidents such as the one in question.

"Thank you again for your comments. I hope that our program efforts in future will inspire commendation rather than the justifiable criticism of your last letter.

"Yours sincerely,
"(Signed) A. D. Dunton."

Taking the Chairman's letter and Mr. Dilworth's letter together it would appear that there is an admission of fault on the part of the employees of the defendant as alleged in para. 9 of the declaration. I take this opportunity of saying that Mr. Dunton's letter is that of a gentleman and so is that of Mr. Dilworth.

There is one more thing to mention. The position taken by the Chairman of the Board and Mr. Dilworth with regard to plaintiff appears to be at complete variance with the defence filed by the Canadian Broadcasting Corp. in this case. If Mr. Dunton were giving the instructions there would be a confession of judgment as to liability and either a tender into Court or a request to the Court to assess the damages. But not a bit of it. The only witness called by the defendant in this case is the Producer of *Tabloid*, Ross McLean, who was in the witness-box not only yesterday but again this morning, and he was the one who was suspended by his superior officers for three weeks for what he and MacDougal had done. He has sat here throughout this trial. He has heard the evidence of Dr. Robbins and his wife, who are respectable, decent citizens. He has heard the evidence of the two doctors called by the plaintiff. He has heard in open Court the letters of the Chairman and Mr. Dilworth. But not one note of regret was anywhere expressed by Mr. McLean in his testimony saying "We are sorry this happened". He did not apologize, neither when he was in the box yesterday nor today. So it would still appear that there was some conflict going on between the different departments of the defendant.

I have gone into this matter at some length because we have had no similar case in Canada of which I am aware, and in view of the fact that there is such a large "fan" audience of viewers and listeners of CBC programmes the public is entitled to have the views of this Court in some detail.

Sitting as both Judge and jury, it remains now to assess the damages which the plaintiff should receive. In assessing damages I have followed the principles laid down by the Supreme Court of Canada in the case of *Chaput v. Romain*, 1 D.L.R. (2d) 241, 114 Can. C.C. 170, [1955] S.C.R. 834.

After taking everything into consideration I have reached the conclusion that the fair and propr compnsation for the plaintiff will be the total sum of $3,000.

WHEREFORE the Court doth condemn the defendant to pay to plaintiff the sum of $3,000 with interest from date of service of the action and costs.

Judgment for plaintiff.

5.3.2.2 *Krouse v. Chrysler Canada* (1973), 1 O.R. (2d) 225 (Ont. C.A.)

Appellant automobile manufacturer distributed a device bearing the names and numbers of all professional football players which was designed to assist people who watched professional football on television to identify the players and which also advertised appellant's automobiles. On the device there was an action photograph of a football game which focused attention on respondent player who was identifiable by the number on his uniform provided that the user of the device recognized the uniform and thus realized which team's player list to examine. The player had not consented to the use of the photograph. The player recovered damages in an action on the basis that something of commercial value to him had been misappropriated by the manufacturer and on the basis that there was a passing-off.

ESTEY, J.A.: The appeal should be allowed. There was no passing-off. The player and the manufacturer were not in a common field of endeavour and the buying public would not be led to believe that the manufacturer's products, or the advertising device itself, had been designed or manufactured by the player. Nor was the device in competition with a similar product marketed by the player. There was no implication that the player endorsed the product, as there might have been had he been shown sitting in or standing by one of the manufacturer's vehicles. While the common law does contemplate a concept which may be broadly classified as an appropriation of one's personality for commercial purposes, appellant had not committed this wrong. Exposure through the publication of photographs and information is the life-blood of professional sport. Some minor loss of privacy and even some loss of potential for commercial exploitation must be expected to occur as a by-product of the express or implied licence to publicize the institution of the game itself. Appellant manufacturer had sought a trade advantage through association with the game of football generally, and it was the game of professional football rather than the personality of the respondent which had been deliberately incorporated in the advertising device.

5.3.2.3 *Burnett v. The Queen in Right of Canada* (1979), 23 O.R. (2d) 109 (Ont. H.C.)

O'DRISCOLL, J.: *Question 5*: Is there such a thing as a tort of "invasion of privacy"? The plaintiff's statement of claim reads in part:

> 45. The plaintiff further states that during the programme. "Connections" he was at various times depicted on the screen driving his automobile, a 1973 Rolls Royce. Pictures of the plaintiff driving his vehicle were taken at a time or times known to the defendants but unknown to the plaintiff and by person or persons known to the defendants and unknown to the plaintiff but at all material times without his consenl or knowledge. The defendants did also during the course of the programme "Connections" portray on the screen a picture of his house and a picture of his offices. These pictures were taken at time or times known to the defendants and unknown to the plaintiff and by a person or persons known to the defendants and unknown to the plaintiff but at all material times without his consent or knowledge.
> 46. The plaintiff states that such pictures were taken through the use of hidden cameras by persons attending from time to time at his offices and by persons following him as he drove in his vehicle. The plaintiff states thal in attending at his residence and offices, in following him in his vehicle and filming him with hidden cameras, the defendants have violated his right to be free from invasion of his privacy and free from unlawful interference in the enjoyment of his property and security of his person.
> 47. The plaintiff further states that the broadcast of the programme "Connections" throughout Canada and the publication of the defamatory words and images contained thereon was a further

violation of his right lo be free from invasion of his privacy and free from unlawful interference in the enjoyment of his property and security of his person.

48. The plaintiff further states that the defendants and person or persons unknown to the plaintiff and known to the defendants conspired each with the other to cause injury and harm to the plaintiff, namely to publish words and images defamatory of the plaintiff, to publish malicious falsehoods, invade his right of privacy and interfere in the lawful enjoyment of his property and the security of his person.

. . . . .

51. The plaintiff pleads and relies upon *The Bill of Rights*, R.S.C. 1970, appendix III and the provisions thereof.

52.(c) Damages in the amount of $5,000.000.00 for invasion of privacy;

Counsel for the defendants submits that there is no such tort known to law and therefore, requests that I strike out the plaintiff's statement of claim under the provisions of Rule 126.

Counsel have referred me to the following authorities:

(1) *Krouse v. Chrysler Canada Ltd. et al.*, [1970] 3 O.R. 135 at p. 136, 12 D.L.R. (3d) 463 at p. 464, 1 C.P.R. (2d) 218, per Parker, J. (as he then was):

> Although this Court has inherent jurisdiction lo strike out a statement of claim on the ground that it discloses no reasonable cause of action or stay an action, such power should be sparingly exercised and only when there is no doubt that no cause of action exists. Neither counsel was able to submit any decided case on this point that has been tried in this jurisdiction so it would appear that the matter has not been considered and judicially decided. It may be that the action is novel, but it has not been shown to me that the Court in this jurisdiction would not recognize a right of privacy. The plaintiff therefore has the right to be heard, to have the issue decided after trial.

(2) *Krouse v. Chrysler Canada Ltd. et al.*, [1972] 2 O.R. 133, 25 D.L.R. (3d) 49, 5 C.P.R. (2d) 30. Haines, J., at trial, specifically refrained from deciding whether there was such a common law right to privacy; Haines, J., decided the case on the basis of "passing-off".

(3) *Krouse v. Chrysler Canada Ltd. et al.* (1973), 1 O.R. (2d) 225 at pp. 233-4 and 237-8, 40 D.L.R. (3d) 15 at pp. 23-4 and 27-8, 13 C.P.R. (2d) 28, per Estey, J. A., discussed the right to privacy but did not state that no such cause of action existed in the Province of Ontario.

(4) *Motherwell et al. v. Motherwell* (1976), 73 D.L.R. (3d) 62, [1976] 6 W.W.R. 550, Alberta Appellate Division, per Clement, J. A. In this case a plaintiff was successful in an action for breach of the right to privacy.

(5) Section 381(1)(c), (e) and (f) of the *Criminal Code of Canada*.

In my view, having regard to the present state of the law in this Province, the words of Parker, J. (as he then was), are most apt and this part of the defendants" application will be dismissed.

5.3.2.4 *Motherwell v. Motherwell* (1976), 73 D.L.R. (3d) 62 (Alta. S.C.)

CLEMENT, J.A.: The defendant appellant Elizabeth Motherwell is the daughter of the plaintiff respondent William Motherwell, and the sister of the plaintiff respondent John Motherwell who is the husband of the plaintiff respondent orders that this appeal is taken. There was also consolidated with the two actions a petition by the father pursuant to the *Mentally Incapaciated Persons Act*, R.S.A. 1970, c.232, upon which Kirby, J., declared the appellant is, through mental infirmity, a person who is incapable of managing her affairs, and committed the custody and management of her estate to the Public Trustee. This order is not in appeal.

The appellant lives in Calgary. Her mental condition is the cause of the matters complained of by the plaintiffs. It is diagnosed as a paranoid condition accompanied by some thought disorder, which appeared initially about 1970 and grew in intensity. It is concerned with the family relationships and related matters, and manifests itself by a conviction that the sister-in-law, and the housekeeper referred to in the statement of claim of the father, are influencing the brother and father against her. The medical testimony is that she has no malice towards the brother and the father, for whom she appears to have some concern, but that she bears malice towards the sister-in-law and the housekeeper as a concomitant of her paranoid condition.

The father also lives in Calgary. He had injured his leg in December, 1973, and has been in hospital or nursing homes at intervals since then. His wife, the appellant's mother, died in December, 1974. The telephone calls of which he complains commenced some time prior to then and were made to him when he was at home. His evidence was that after his wife's death they increased in frequency and were made continuously (which I take to mean to be of a daily nature) up to a dozen times a day. He was harassed by these calls to the point where he was afraid to answer the telephone as he found them to be very upsetting. The gist of them was a tirade against his daughter-in-law and his housekeeper. In his weak condition he found it upsetting physically as well as emotionally, and is unable to stand such "harassment" as he describes it. It is to be inferred that he asked the appellant to desist but she did not do so and he obtained an interim injunction. He also received some letters of the kind received by the brother, which I will shortly refer to, but this part of his complaints does not loom large.

The brother is highly placed in the executive management of three business and commercial enterprises in Calgary. His home is in Calgary where he lives with his wife, the sister-in-law, and their three children aged 15, 10, and 8 years, respectively. For the purposes of his business he has an office in his home and there is a telephone used in part for business purposes. He also has an office downtown served by a telephone. The telephone calls from the appellant, of which he complains, commenced about 1972. Not to labour the point, they increased in frequency, particularly from the spring of 1974 onwards, to as many as two calls in one day and were made as well to his office as to his home. The gist of them was abuse of the sister-in-law, whom the appellant called a "crook" and a "gold-digger" and maligned her in a manner which the brother described as vindictive and vitriolic. Calls to the home were made in the middle of the night

Dorothy Motherwell. I will designate the respondents respectively as the father, the brother, and the sister-in-law.

This appeal is from the judgment of Kirby, J., in two actions which were consolidated for trial. The allegations in the statement of claim of the brother and the sister-in-law with which these appeals are particularly concerned are that the appellant had on numerous occasions "contacted the plaintiffs by telephone, making false accusations and statements against the plaintiffs and refuses to cease making such allegations and false statements", and "written letters to the plaintiffs making unfounded statements and accusations concerning the affairs of the plaintiffs". The appellant persisted in this conduct despite demands that she cease, which the plaintiffs assert to be an invasion of their privacy, and a nuisance, and pray for nominal damages and

> ... an interim and a permanent injunction against the Defendant or anyone acting on her behalf enjoining her or anyone else acting on her behalf from contacting, telephoning, writing, visiting or in any other way communicating with the Plaintiffs or their children.

The defence of the appellant with which we are concerned is that "no action lies by the plaintiffs or either of them to restrain her lawful communications with the plaintiffs".

In his statement of claim against the appellant, the father alleges that the appellant had on numerous occasions

> ... communicated with the plaintiff by telephone and has continuously made false accusations and statements against the plaintiff's son and daughter-in-law, John and Dorothy Motherwell, and against the plaintiff's housekeeper, and the defendant continues to communicate ceaselessly in this fashion with the plaintiff and to make such allegations and false statements, and to harangue the plaintiff.

He also alleges that the appellant persisted in this conduct despite demands that she cease, and asserts this to be an invasion of his privacy, and a nuisance. He further alleges that

> ... the constant harassment of him by the defendant causes him great strain and mental anguish. The plaintiff is 90 years of age. The said nuisance by the defendant is dangerous and injurious to the mental and physical health of the plaintiff.

The prayer is for nominal damages and an injunction enjoining the appellant from "molesting, harassing, or in any way interfering with the plaintiff and from communicating with him by telephone, personal contact, letter, or in any other way". The relevant defence of the appellant is that

> ... she has committed no actional wrong giving rise to the cause for an injunction as alleged the statement-of claim herein or at all and that as the daughter of the plaintiff she has inalienable right to lawfully communicate with and visit her father.

Additional allegations in each statement of claim sound in trespass in traditional sense and do not require review. The appeals are directed to the alle harassment by telephone and letter. In each action Kirby, J., granted, *inter* nominal damages and an injunction in the terms prayed for. It is from and first thing in the morning, amongst other times. In 1974 the brother installed an answering device on his home telephone and a diary kept for the purpose shows that on one occasion in the space of an hour, the appellant made as many as 30 calls. This was the maximum capacity of the device. The purpose was to avoid the calls from the appellant but provide a record so that the brother could call back other persons who were trying to reach him. As the appellant was plugging the answering device, the brother obtained an unlisted telephone number for his home and spent a good deal of time and money informing his friends and business associates of the new number. Unfortunately, the appellant, by a fortuitous circumstance, learned the new number and her calls immediately started again. He obtained another unlisted number but it was not known to his friends and business associates, many of whom were unable to reach him. He then applied to the Trial Division of this Court and obtained an interim injunction against the appellant, and reverted to his original listed telephone number after the order was granted. It appears that the appellant has been in contempt of the order. He testified that by reason of this harassment his health has suffered and he has lost 26 lbs. in weight. He also said that the calls had been terribly hard on his children, who on occasion answered the telephone, but no details are given. He feels that the appellant has some vindictiveness towards him as well as towards others.

The evidence of the sister-in-law is to the same effect. It is probably best summarized in this testimony of the effect of the calls:

> Well, they have created fantastic tension within the home with the children, all members of the family, and at one point when we were receiving so many calls I would say, "George, you answer it this time", nobody wants to answer the phone because they know that it was going to probably be Elizabeth on the other end.

As to the letters the brother testified that he had received in his mail "a whole briefcase full of them". Those that were put in evidence appear to be incoherent, tedious, and abusive. He did not read all of them. As I have noted, the father gave evidence of the receipt of similar letters from the appellant, but they seemed to contribute little to his feeling of harassment.

It is desirable to make clear the limitation on the legal considerations that arise in this appeal on the foregoing facts. They are confined to the common law. It was not contended in argument that s.31 of the *Alberta Government Telephones Act*, R.S.A. 1970, c.12, of itself gives rise to civil remedies:

> 31. A person who uses profane, obscene or abusive language while talking on a telephone or over a telecommunication wire or by other means interferes with the use or enjoyment of the system is guilty of an offence and liable on summary conviction to a fine of not more that $100 or to imprisonment for not more than six months.

While that issue is not before this Court, nevertheless the section has a place in the context of an aspect to which I will presently come. The matters of complaint are unwanted communications made to the respondents. If such acts are properly within the concept of "invasion of privacy" they occupy a niche of their own, distinct from such matters as surveillance, the clandestine gathering and use of personal information by various means, the interception of private communications, and unwanted publicity, discussed by Peter Burns in "The Law of Privacy: The Canadian Experience", 54 *Can. Bar Rev.* (No. 1, March, 1976), p. 1. In this opinion I will use the phrase only as a convenient designation of the acts of the appellant I have described upon which these actions are founded. In considering the authorities I will leave aside those which deal with the other concepts and are usually influenced by considerations that are not applicable here.

The arguments in appeal advanced by the appellant draw a distinction between nuisance and invasion of privacy. It is said that invasion of privacy does not come within the principle of private nuisance, and that it is a species of activity not recognized as remedial by the common law. It is urged that the common law does not have within itself the resources to recognize invasion of privacy as either included in an existing category or as a new category of nuisance, and that it has lost its original power, by which indeed it created itself, to note new ills arising in a growing and changing society and pragmatically to establish a principle to meet the need for control and remedy; and then by categories to develop the principle as the interests of justice make themselves sufficiently apparent. For these propositions the appellant relies on a passage in the judgment of Dixon, J., in *Victoria Park Racing & Recreation Grounds Co. Ltd. v. Taylor et al.* (1937), 58 C.L.R. 479, of which it is sufficient to reproduce only the following at p. 505:

> There is, in my opinion, little to be gained by inquiring whether in English law the foundation of a delictual liability is unjustifiable damage or breach of specific duty. The law of tort has fallen into great confusion, but, in the main, what acts and omissions result in responsibility and what do not are matters defined by long-established rules of law from which judges ought not wittingly to depart and no light is shed upon a given case by large generalizations about them.

The obsolescence of this view in the field of negligence is made apparent by Lord Reid in *Dorset Yacht Co. Ltd. v. Home Office*, [1970] A.C. 1004 at pp. 1026-7:

> About the beginning of this century most eminent lawyers thought that there were a number of separate torts involving negligence, each with its own rules, and they were most unwilling to add more. They were of course aware from a number of leading cases that in the past the courts had from time to time recognized new duties and new grounds of action. But the heroic age was over, it was time to cultivate certainty and security in the law; the categories of negligence were virtually closed. The Attorney-General invited us to return to those halcyon days, but, attractive though it may be, I cannot accede to his invitation.
>
> In later years there has been a steady trend towards regarding the law of negligence as depending on principle so that, when a new point emerges, one should ask not whether it is covered by authority but whether recognized principles apply to it. *Donoghue v. Stevenson* [1932] A.C. 562 may be regarded as a milestone, and the well-known passage in Lord Atkin's speech should I think be regarded as a statement of principle. It is not to be treated as if it were a statutory definition. It will require qualification in new circumstances. But I think that the time has come when we can and should say that it ought to apply unless there is some justification or valid explanation for its exclusion.

This passage, and more, was adopted by Spence, J., as part of his reasons in delivering the majority judgment of the Supreme Court of Canada in *O'Rourke et al. v. Schacht* (1974), 55 D.L.R. (3d) 96, [1976] 1 S.C.R. 53, 3 N.R. 453. And in *Haig v. Bamford et al.* (1976), 72 D.L.R. (3d) 68, 27 C.P.R. (2d) 149, 9 N.R. 43, Dickson, J., speaking for the majority of the Court noted anew the effect growth and change in society has in enlarging the scope of the duty of care: the neighbour concept.

But it is not only in the field of negligence that the common law demonstrates its continuing ability to serve the changing and expanding needs of our present society. In *Canadian Aero Service Ltd. v. O'Malley et al.* (1973), 40 D.L.R. (3d) 371, 11 C.P.R. (2d) 206, [1974] S.C.R. 592, the Supreme Court of Canada examined the relationship which gives rise to a fiduciary duty, and the scope of that duty. In giving the judgment of the Court Laskin, J. (as he then was), reviewed the progression of authorities and said, p. 384 D.L.R., p. 610 S.C.R.: "What these decisions indicate is an updating of the equitable principle whose roots lie in the general standards that I have already mentioned . . .".

In the context of contract Lord Simonds vigorously expressed similar views in *British Movietonews Ltd. v. London & District Cinemas Ltd.*, [1952] A.C. 166 at p. 188: "It is no doubt essential to the life of the common law that its principles should be adapted to meet fresh circumstances and needs." In the same spirit Morden, J., approached the principle of restitution in *James More & Sons Ltd. v. University of Ottawa* (1974), 49 D.L.R. (3d) 666, 5 O.R. (2d) 162. He referred to the widening of the principle apparently effected by *County of Carleton v. City of Ottawa* (1965), 52 D.L.R. (2d) 220, [1965] S.C.R. 663, and said at p. 676:

> I mention this to indicate that where a Court, on proper grounds, holds that the doctrine of restitution is applicable, it is not necessary to fit the case into some exact category, apparently established by a previous decision, giving effect to the doctrine. Just as the categories of negligence are never closed, neither can those of restitution. The principles take precedence over the illustrations or examples of their application.

It is worth recalling the salutary passage from the speech of Lord Macmillan in *M'Alister (or Donoghue) v. Stevenson*, [1932] A.C. 562 at p. 619, which Morden, J., here applies to the principle of restitution: "The criterion of judgment must adjust and adapt itself to the changing circumstances of life. The categories of negligence are never closed." The developing principle of restitution, or unjust enrichment to distinguish a somewhat different conceptual approach, is discussed by G.H.L. Fridman in his valuable article "Reflections on Restitution" in 8 *Ottawa Law Review* 156 (1976), at p. 162, in which he points out "..that while the historical categories are still important, and cannot be ignored, the operation of the law is not confined to those categories".

The application of this spirit of the common law is apparent in other cases of importance. The issues in appeal must be approached in the same spirit.

Let me observe here that I do not wish to be entrapped in semantics or nomenclature. For the present purposes I will employ the term principle as a general concept of legal rights and duties in an aspect of human activities in which some common element is to be found: Lord Atkin in *Donoghue v. Stevenson* at p. 580; and I will employ the term *categories* as the application of a principle to particular circumstances, discernible in precedents, which have been found to come within the principle. The scope of the principle of private nuisance, as well as its established categories, require consideration in the issues in appeal.

The rule of *stare decisis* operates, as it seems to me, to regulate the application of precedents to cases which can be said to fall within a category. When the circumstances of a case do not appear to bring it fairly within an established category, they may lie sufficiently within the concept of a principle that consideration of a new category is warranted. The scope of a category may in time be broadened by a trend in precedents which reflect judicial considerations going beyond the disciplines of *stare decisis*. Those same considerations, arising from adequately demonstrated social need of a continuing nature, may lead, when necessary to maintain social justice, to a new category or the review of a principle. The considerations I refer to were termed public policy by Lord Wright in *Fender v. St. John-Mildmay*, [1938] A.C. 1. At p. 38 he said:

> In one sense every rule of law, either common law or equity, which has been laid down by the Courts, in that course of judicial legislation which has evolved the law of this country, has been based on ... public ... policy.

That case arose out of a claim by a woman founded on a breach of promise of marriage made to her by a man who had at that point obtained only a decree *nisi* of divorce from his wife. Lord Atkin addressed himself to the principle of public policy and delivered a caution in respect of the establishment of new categories in terms which bear repeating here. He referred to *Janson v. Driefontein Consolidated Mines, Ltd.*, [1902] A.C. 484, and went on to say at pp. 11-2:

> In the same case Lord Halsbury indeed appeared to decide that the categories of public policy are closed, and that the principle could not be invoked anew unless the case could be brought within some principle [sic, category] of public policy already recognized by the law. I do not find, however, that this view received the express assent of the other members of the House; and it seems to me, with respect, too rigid. On the other hand, it fortifies the serious warning illustrated by the passages cited above that the doctrine should only be invoked in clear cases in which the harm to the public is substantially incontestable, and does not depend upon the idiosyncratic inferences of a few judicial minds. I think that this should be regarded as the true guide.

I have gone on at this length because of the course taken in argument, and I thought that I should express my own views as clearly as possible. Whether the approach is to review a principle, or to determine the need to broaden an existing category, or to determine whether the circumstances of the case warrant the recognition of a new category, the considerations are basically similar although the required urgencies may differ in degree. Assuming the circumstances of a case fall within a relevant principle, their categorization will depend on the analysis of the Judge. I now turn to the principle of nuisance.

Much has been written by authors of distinction on the principle of nuisance. For example *Clerk & Lindsell on Torts*, 13th ed. (1969), p. 780, para. 1391, opens the subject in this way: "The essence of nuisance is a condition or activity which unduly interferes with the use or enjoyment of land." As the text of the paragraph shows, this definition of principle may be unduly restrictive in respect of public nuisance by confining its operation to the use or enjoyment of land, but that is not in issue here. In respect of private nuisance this is said:

> Nuisance is an act or omission which is an interference with, disturbance of or annoyance to a person in the exercise or enjoyment of ... (b) his ownership or occupation of land or of some easement, profit, or other right used or enjoyed in connection with land ...

And at p. 781, para. 1393, this is said:

> A private nuisance may be and usually is caused by a person doing on his own land something which he is lawfully entitled to do. His conduct only becomes a nuisance when the consequences of his acts are not confined to his own land but extend to the land of his neighbour by ...

There follows a statement of three categories in which it has been recognized that the principle is applicable. It is the third that is relevant here: "(3) unduly interfering with his neighbour in the comfortable and convenient enjoyment of his land". A number of the illustrations given of this category support the view that it is not necessary to attract the application of the principle that the matter complained of should emanate from the defendant's land, no more than it is for public nuisance. As pointed out in many texts, the maxim *sic utere tuo ut alienum non laedas* is frequently invoked in the cases and when this is done the maxim is employed as a statement of the principle of nuisance. The maxim is certainly of sufficient vintage to warrant such employment. It is attributed to Lord Coke and translated and defined in the *Dictionary of English Law* by Earl Jowitt, vol. 2, p. 1639, in these terms: "(9 Co. Rep. 59) (Use your own property so as not to injure your neighbour's.) Use your own rights so that you do not interfere with those of another." The definition in brackets speaks of property, not land. The second definition is even broader and gives full support to those cases that do not confine the principle to emanations from land, nor even to the use by the defendant of his "property" (in the narrow sense) in creating the matter complained of.

The Latin maxim was criticized as a statement of principle by Lord Wright in *Sedleigh-Denfield v. O'Callaghan et al.*, [1940] A.C. 880 at p. 903:

> This, like most maxims, is not only lacking in definiteness but is also inaccurate. An occupier may make in many ways a use of his land which causes damage to the neighbouring land-owners and yet be free from liability.

With respect, it seems to me that Lord Wright is here treating the categories as the principle itself. It is out of the principle that the categories have come to be recognized: In *Clerk & Lindsell*, p. 784, para. 1395, this is said:

> The acts complained of as constituting the nuisance, such as noise, smells or vibration, will usually be lawful acts which only become wrongful from the circumstances under which they are performed, such as the time, place, extent or the manner of performance.

Support for this statement may be found in *St. Helen's Smelting Co. v. Tipping* (1865), 11 H.L.C. 642,11 E.R. 1483. The protean aspect of the principle is apparent from the many cases and texts. I think that of it, equally with its relative, negligence, the categories are never closed. The cases on watching and besetting are particularly in point. It seems to me that the frequent reference in the cases to nuisance emanating from the land of the defendants reflects only the circumstances of the particular facts before the Court, not an intentional limitation on the scope of the principle. This is acknowledged in the third passage above taken from *Clerk & Lindsell*. In saying this, I am aware of the dictum of Lord Wright in *Sedleigh-Denfield v. O'Callaghan* [at p. 903]: "The ground of responsibility is the possession and control of the land from which the nuisance proceeds." But, with respect, I am in agreement with the interpretation put on it by Wilson, C.J.S.C., in *Newman et al. v. Conair Aviation Ltd. et. al.* (1972), 33 D.L.R. (3d) 474 at pp. 479-80, [1973] 1 W.W.R. 316 at p. 322 (B.C.), that Lord Wright did not intend it to be read restrictively.

In *J. Lyons & Sons v. Wilkins*, [1899] 1 Ch. 255, members of a trade union on strike picketed the plaintiff's works and the works of a subcontractor of the plaintiff. This was found to amount to watching and besetting. Lindley, M.R., said at pp. 267-8:

> The truth is that to watch or beset a man's house with a view to compel him to do or not to do what is lawful for him not to do or to do is wrongful and without lawful authority unless some reasonable justification for it is consistent with the evidence. Such conduct seriously interferes with the ordinary comfort of human existence and ordinary enjoyment of the house beset, and such conduct would support an action on the case for a nuisance at common law: see *Bamford v. Turnley* 3 B. & S. 62, *Broder v. Saillard* 2 Ch. D. 692. 701, per Jessel, M.R., *Walter v. Selfe* 4 De G. & Sm. 315, and *Crump v. Lambert* L.R. 3 Eq. 409.

Chitty, L.J., held the same view. He said at pp. 271-2:

> But further, the acts of watching or besetting here proved in reference to the 4th sub-section, and done with the view mentioned, were acts in themselves unlawful at common law, and are not made lawful by the Legislature. In my opinion they constitute a nuisance at common law. True it is that every annoyance is not a nuisance; the annoyance must be of a serious character, and of such a degree as to interfere with the ordinary comforts of life. To watch or beset a man's house for the length of time and in the manner and with the view proved would undoubtedly constitute a nuisance of an aggravated character.

The acts of watching and besetting were not, of course, carried on within premises occupied by the defendants. They were carried on, I infer, on property to which the public had access. The right of the defendants to be on a public place was so abused to the detriment of the plaintiffs that it was held they had committed a common law nuisance, as well as a breach of s.7 of the *Conspiracy, and Protection of Property Act, 1875*. The point is dealt with specifically by Devlin, J. [at trial], in *Esso Petroleum Co. Ltd. v. Southport Corp.*, [1956] A.C. 218 at p. 224:

> I think that it is convenient to begin by considering whether there is a cause of action in nuisance. It is clear that to give a cause of action for private nuisance the matter complained of

must affect the property of the plaintiffs. But I know of no principle that it must emanate from land belonging to the defendant.

[See also [1953] 2 All E.R. 1204 at p. 1207 (Q.B.), revd [1954] 2 Q.B. 182 (C.A.).] He then referred to *Cunard et al. v. Antifyre, Ltd.*, [1933] 1 K.B. 551, and went on to say [at pp. 224-5]:

> It is clear from that statement of principle that the nuisance must affect the property of the plaintiff: and it is true that in the vast majority of cases it is likely to emanate from the neighbouring property of the defendant. But no statement of principle has been cited to me to show that the latter is a prerequisite to a cause of action; and I can see no reason why, if land or water belonging to the public, or waste land, is misused by the defendant, or if the defendant as a licensee or trespasser misuses someone else's land, he should not be liable for the creation of a nuisance in the same way as an adjoining occupier would be.

That case arose out of the discharge of oil from a vessel into a river, in consequence of which damage ensued to the adjoining foreshore. The case went on to the House of Lords but their Lordships took the view that the case turned on negligence and did not discuss the principle of nuisance.

More recently, Stamp, J., commented on common law nuisance in *Torquay Hotel Co. Ltd. v. Cousins et al.*, [1968] 3 W.L.R. 540. The defendants had picketed the plaintiff's hotel in the course of a trade dispute. Amongst other issues was that of nuisance on which Stamp, J., said in part at p. 554:

> I turn to consider picketing. In view of my decision that what was done by the defendants in relation to the plaintiff company was not done in contemplation or furtherance of a trade dispute, the defendants had no statutory protection for any tort which they may commit in this regard. At common law a plaintiff is entitled to the lawful use and enjoyment of his property, and a substantial interference with that use and enjoyment is a nuisance. In my judgment picketing outside the entrance of a plaintiff's hotel, if persisted in, for the purpose of persuading tradesmen and their employees from delivering supplies vital to the running of the hotel in order to compel the plaintiffs to submit to the defendants' demand is thus, prima facie, a common law nuisance.

For this he drew support from J. *Lyons & Sons v. Wilkins, supra.*

The nature of the activities which may constitute a private nuisance were considered by Lord Evershed, M.R., in *Thompson-Schwab et al. v. Costaki et al.*, [1956] 1 All E.R. 652, in a case in which the complaint of the plaintiff was that the defendant's adjoining premises were used for purposes of prostitution. At pp. 653-4 he adopted the third passage from *Clerk & Lindsell* above quoted and went on to say:

> The forms which activities constituting actionable nuisance may take are exceedingly varied and there is the highest authority for saying that they are not capable of precise or close definition. If the principle is rightly stated in the passage which I have read, then it must depend on the facts of each particular case whether the conditions, which I have stated as required to constitute a nuisance, are satisfied: and in considering whether they are satisfied or not the count must apply to the matter the usages of civilized society as they may be at the relevant date.
>
> In *Sedleigh-Denfield v. O'Callaghan* ([1940] 3 All E.R. 349) Lord Wright said (*ibid.*, at p. 364.)
>
>> "It is impossible lo give any precise or universal formula, but it may broadly be said that a useful test is perhaps what is reasonable according to the ordinary usages of mankind

living in society, or, more correctly, in a particular society. The forms which nuisance may take are protean."

And Romer, L.J., said, at p. 656

> The second point on which the defendants rely is that nothing can constitute a private nuisance at law unless it affects the reasonable enjoyment of other premises in a physical way. This is only an interlocutory application, and at the trial no doubt that point will be taken again and may be argued at greater length, but my present impression is that it is unsound. It appears to be an unwarrantable gloss on the law on the subject as formulated in the text-books, and, what is perhaps more important, it appears to be inconsistent with the judgments of this court in *J. Lyons & Sons v. Wilkins* ([1899] 1 Ch. 255) which was the picketing case.

Parker, LJ., concurred with both. This authority and others were followed by Wilson, C.J.S.C., in *Newman et al. v. Conair Aviation Ltd., supra*, which involved noise and vibration from a low flying aircraft.

It is clear to me that the protracted and persistent harassment of the brother and the father in their homes, and in the case of the brother as well in his office, by abuse of the telephone system is within the principle of private nuisance as it has been recognized in the authorities I have referred to. The question is whether the calls amounted to undue interference with the comfortable and convenient enjoyment by the plaintiffs of their respective premises. I can conceive that persistent and unwanted telephone calls could become an harassment even if the subject-matter is essentially agreeable. The deliberate and persistent ringing of the telephone cannot but affect the senses in time, and operate on the nervous system as the evidence discloses. No special damage is required to support an injunction: it is the loss of the amenities of the premises in substantial degree that is involved.

I think that the interests of our developing jurisprudence would be better served by approaching invasion of privacy by abuse of the telephone system as a new category, rather than seeking by rationalization to enlarge the third category recognized by *Clerk & Lindsell*. We are dealing with a new factor. Heretofore the matters of complaint have reached the plaintiff's premises by natural means; sound through the air waves, pollution in many forms carried by air currents, vibrations through the earth, and the like. Here, the matters complained of arise within the premises through the use by the appellant of communication agencies in the nature of public utilities available to everyone, which the plaintiffs have caused to serve their premises. They are non-selective in the sense that so long as they are employed by the plaintiffs they have no control over the incoming communications. Nevertheless there are differences between the two agencies of telephone and mail and it does not necessarily follow from their similarities that both should be accepted into a new category.

The telephone system is so much the part of the daily life of society that many look on it as a necessity. Its use is certainly taken as a right at least in a social sense. It virtually makes neighbours not only of the persons close at hand, but those in distant places, other cities, other countries. It is a system provided for rational and reasonable communication between people, and its abuse by invasion of privacy is a matter of general interest within the meaning given the phrase by Lord Atkin in *Fender v. St. John-Mildmay*, [1938] A.C. 1. It is essential to the operation of such a system that a call from someone be signalled to the intended receiver by sound such as the ringing of a bell. The receiver cannot know who is calling him until he answers. Calls must be answered if the system is to work. There are not many who would assert that protection against invasion of privacy by telephone would be a judicial idiosyncrasy. Further than that, the people of this Province through the Legislature have expressed a public interest in the proper use of the system in enacting s.3 1 of the *Alberta Government Telephones Act*.

In *Clerk & Lindsell*, p. 785, para. 1396, this is said: "A nuisance of this kind, to be actionable, must be such as to be a real interference with the comfort or convenience of living according to the standards of the average man." This statement is amply supported by authority and I take it to be applicable to invasion of privacy. The proof here of real interference is well nigh overwhelming. All of these considerations lead me to accept the statement of Townley, J., in *Stoakes et al. v. Brydges*, [1958] Q.W.N. 9 at p. 10:

> It is quite a lawful use of his premises to use the instrument installed thereon for the purpose for which it was quite obviously intended. But there are numerous cases in the books which clearly show that although a person may be using his premises for the conduct of some operation perfectly lawful in itself, he must not so conduct that operation as to interfere materially with the health or comfort of other persons in the ordinary enjoyment of their premises. I do not think that this restriction is to be confined merely to interference with the health and comfort of neighbouring occupiers or owners strictly so called. I think any person who comes within the ambit of the operation and whose health or comfort in the ordinary enjoyment of his premises is interfered with to the requisite degree may take action to restrain that interference. The category of nuisances, particularly by such potentially noxious things as noise, is not closed and, it seems to me, will never be closed whilst human ingenuity is still attempting to devise fresh means of communicating or disseminating sound. Suppose a public address or Tannoy system is used under such conditions as to interfere materially with the sleep or rest of persons living in the vicinity I apprehend that it is not only the occupiers of those premises which immediately adjoin the source of the noise who may take action but also those whose premises though not immediately adjoining that source, nevertheless are situated within the radius of its effect.

I am of opinion that the brother and the father have established a claim in nuisance by invasion of privacy through abuse of the system of telephone communications.

There remains the question whether the sister-in-law herself has a right of action in nuisance against the appellant. The injunction against telephone calls to the matrimonial home will, of course, benefit her and the children: *Broder v. Saillard* (1876), 2 Ch.D. 692 at p. 703; but that is not the point. She claims in her own right. For the appellant it is urged that at least as far as the sister-in-law is concerned it is the substance of the calls, not their frequency, that is the teal matter of complaint, and that nuisance extends only to harassment of the senses, not to sensibilities. The evidence on which this submission is made is based on one question and answer in cross-examination, and in the context of the whole of her evidence it is apparent that the subject-matter of the telephone calls was an added irritant in the harassment. In any event, I do not think there is any validity in this attempted fine distinction. I have pointed out above that in my opinion there may be harassment even although the subject-matter of the telephone calls would otherwise be agreeable in nature.

The texts rely on *Malone v. Laskey et al.*, [1907] 2 K.B. 141, as authority denying a right of action to a wife, and this is invoked on behalf of the appellant. In that case the defendant owner had let premises to a tenant, Witherby & Co., and this tenant had sublet the premises to a company. Malone was the manager of the subtenant company and occupied a part of the premises apparently as part of the consideration for his services. The plaintiff was his wife. The defendant created vibrations by the operation of machinery in its adjoining property, in consequence of which a water tank in the premises became insecure and fell on the plaintiff, to her injury. In respect of her claim in nuisance Sir Gorell Barnes, P., said, at p. 151:

> Many cases were cited in the course of the argument in which it had been held that actions for nuisance could be maintained where a person's rights of property had been affected by the nuisance, but no authority was cited, nor in my opinion can any principle of law be formulated, to the effect that a person who has no interest in property, no right of occupation in the proper sense of the term, can maintain an action for a nuisance arising from the vibration caused by the working of an engine in an adjoining house.

And Fletcher Moulton, L.J., said, at pp. 153-4:

> A person in the position of the plaintiff, who was in the premises as a mere licensee, had no right to dictate to Witherby & Co. [i.e., the tenant of the premises] which course they should take, and they seem to have voluntarily permitted the vibration to continue ... But whether that be so or not, it was a matter entirely for the tenant, and a person who is merely present in the house cannot complain of a nuisance which has in it no element of a public nuisance.

I take it from this that he would not have allowed recovery by the husband, either, if he had also sustained injuries: he too was a mere licensee according to the facts. Beyond that it is rather light treatment of a wife, at least in today's society where she is no longer considered subservient to her husband.

In *Cunard et al. v. Antifyre, Ltd.*, [1933] 1 K.B. 551, the plaintiff and his wife occupied a flat on the third floor of a building. He was in possession by virtue of a monthly sublease granted by the tenant of that and other floors of the building. The tenant was the lessee of the defendant. The wife was personally injured in circumstances that amounted to a nuisance on the part of the defendant, if it were actionable by her. She claimed in both nuisance and negligence and recovered on negligence. The claim in nuisance was treated cursorily. Counsel for the wife argued that *Malone v. Laskey* was distinguishable because there the husband was not a tenant and had no estate whatever in the premises. Talbot, J., at p. 557 disposed of the issue shortly, saying that: "... it would manifestly be inconvenient and unreasonable if the right to complain of such interference extended beyond the occupier ...". For this he relied on *Malone v. Laskey*.

In *Metropolitan Properties, Ltd. v. Jones*, [1939] 2 All E.R. 202, the position of a wife was not involved at all. Goddard, L.J., treated *Malone v. Laskey* as authority that an occupier must have some legal interest in the land which he claims to have been affected by nuisance. He said [at p. 205]:

> I am bound by *Malone v. Laskey*, in which the Court of Appeal appear to me to have laid down in terms that, unless the plaintiff in an action for nuisance has legal interest in the land which is alleged to be affected by the nuisance, he has no cause of action.

For myself, I do not read *Malone v. Laskey* as being so explicit. The judgments did not recognize any right of occupancy by the husband as against the tenant Witherby & Co., and of course his wife would be in no better position. In the case at bar the brother is, as I infer, the owner of the premises he occupies with his wife, the sister-in-law, and their family.

There is authority that a claim in nuisance is not necessarily restricted to an occupier who has some legally demonstrable and enforceable right of occupation. In *Foster v. Warblington Urban Council.* [1906] 1 K.B. 648, a substantial *de facto* occupation was recognized as sufficient. There, the plaintiff sued on nuisance affecting his oyster pond which he had used for many years for the storage of oysters. There was much controversy over his legal right of occupancy, and after discussing this Vaughan Williams, L.J., said at pp. 659-60:

> But, even if title could not be proved, in my judgment there has been such an occupation of these beds for such a length of time — not that the length of time is really material for this purpose — as would entitle the plaintiff as against the defendants, who have no interest in the foreshore, to sustain this action for the injury which it is alleged has been done by the sewage to his oysters so kept in those beds.

Thus, a distinction is drawn between one who is "merely present" and occupancy of a substantial nature. In the latter case it is the fact of the occupation that supports the action, although admittedly the legal aspect of an occupation may well have an influence on the conclusion. I would not think trespass, even if persisted in, would ground an action in nuisance.

Here we have a wife harassed in the matrimonial home. She has a status, a right to live there with her husband and children. I find it absurd to say that her occupancy of the matrimonial home is insufficient to found an action in nuisance. In my opinion she is entitled to the same relief as is her husband, the brother.

As to the unwanted mail, the evidence does not show that the plaintiffs have been unduly disturbed in their enjoyment of their respective premises. In such circumstances, to discuss further the use of the mails as a possible vehicle of harassment would be only *obiter*.

In the result the judgment roll should be varied by limiting para. 2(b) to harassment by telephone, and by personal contact which I take it refers to trespass to the person. Undoubtedly the major point in the appeal is invasion of privacy by telephone communications, and the appellant has failed on this issue. I would dismiss the appeal, save as to the variation above noted in the judgment roll, with costs to the respondents on the fifth column.

Appeals dismissed, with variations of trial judgments.

5.3.2.5 *Capan v. Capan* (1981), 14 C.C.L.T. 191 (Ont. H.C.)

OSLER, J.: This was a motion on behalf of the defendant for an order striking out the statement of claim and dismissing the action on the ground that the statement of claim discloses no reasonable cause of action.

The action was commenced by a generally endorsed writ, claiming "damages for continuing mental and physical harassment and invasion of privacy". The plaintiff and defendant were married on April 22, 1972, and separated from September 1977, until May 1978, at which time the plaintiff returned to the matrimonial home in order to be with her infant son. After a brief period of reconciliation, the plaintiff and defendant separated September 1978, and have not lived together since that time.

For purposes of this motion, the parties accepted, as they must, the facts as set out in the statement of claim, and it is common ground that I should not strike out the statement of claim or dismiss the action unless I must conclude that the plaintiff's action could not possibly succeed and that it is beyond doubt that no reasonable cause of action has been shown.

Paragraph 4 of the statement of claim states that during the later years of cohabitation and during the periods of separation "the defendant has incessantly and unlawfully persisted in molesting, annoying and harassing the plaintiff, invading her privacy, and interfering with her right to establish a separate life of her own". Particulars are given of the alleged abuse . . .

It is stated that, as a result of the behaviour described, the plaintiff lives in a state of nervous tension and that her sleep, her appetite and her work have been interfered with and her life made miserable "by the jealous scrutiny and interference of the defendant". She therefore claims damages "for harassment and invasion of privacy".

Counsel for the defendant submitted before me that a plaintiff should normally join all known causes of action and that, by limiting herself to the claim as above described, the defendant will be unable to rely at trial upon any of the nominate torts which might be applicable to certain of the conduct described, such as trespass, nuisance or assault. Counsel for the plaintiff submitted that this was a risk she was fully and deliberately prepared to run and that, while one or more of the nominate torts might well have been enumerated, the cumulative effect of the defendant's actions amounted to something more than the sum of all those actions and, together, they amounted to what could be described as a continuing intent and attempt to change the quality of the defendant's life.

While the allegations in the statement of claim included harassment and invasion of privacy, the latter concept founded the arguments before me and it is principally with that claim that I shall deal in these reasons.

It might be enough to state, as I do, that I have been referred to no reported case in Ontario that has decided that a right to privacy will not be protected by the Courts of this province. This very finding was made by Parker, J. as he then was, on a motion similar to this one in *Krouse v. Chrysler Can. Ltd.*, [1970] 3 O.R. 135 at 136, 1 C.P.R. (2d) 218, 12 D.L.R. (3d) 463, where he stated:

> ... It may be that the action is novel, but it has not been shown to me that the Court in this jurisdiction would not recognize a right of privacy.

He went on to state that the plaintiff had the right to have the issue decided after trial. There has been, in my view, no real development of the law in that respect in this province since that judgment of Parker, J. was reported. At trial [reported at [1972] 2 O.R. 133, 5 C.P.R. (2d) 30, 25 D.L.R. (3d) 49], Haines, J. decided that the plaintiff had a claim that should be supported, based on passing-off. He specifically declined to rule on the issue of whether there is a common law right to privacy in Ontario.

On appeal, Estey, J.A., as he then was, for the Court of Appeal, in 1 O.R. (2d) 225,13 C.P.R. (2d) 28, 40 D.L.R. (3d) 15, found that there was not, on the facts, a passing-off established and the action was dismissed. In so finding, Estey, J.A. found it unnecessary to deal with the concept of the right to privacy and the question of whether such alleged right will be protected by our Courts. At p. 229 [O.R.], there is a plain finding that:

> In argument before us the respondent did not found his claim in the common law action of passing-off or, indeed, in any alleged right of privacy....

The action was really founded upon a claim that the plaintiff had commercial rights flowing from the use of his picture and that it was such right, described by Estey, J.A. as "the right to realize upon this potential" that was allegedly injured by the unauthorized use of the defendant's photograph.

The only case cited from the Ontario decisions, therefore, if it was concerned with privacy at all, had no bearing upon the sort of invasion complained of in the present instance.

Two cases of more relevance are found in Quebec and in Alberta. In *Robbins v. C.B.C. (Que.)*, [1958] Que S.C. 152, 12 D.L.R. (2d) 35, Scott, A.C.J. found that in a television programme originating in Toronto, viewers were asked to telephone and write to the plaintiff who lived in the Montreal area. As a result, the plaintiff's telephone began ringing and continued to ring late into the evening and continued thus for three succeeding days until he had his telephone number changed. Chief Justice Scott had no difficulty in finding that, under Quebec law, art. 1053 of the *Civil Code* made the defendant responsible for the conduct complained of and that it "constituted a grievous, positive, wrongful act against Dr. Robbins, making the defendant corporation responsible for the damages flowing from such wrongful act". He assumed, for the purposes of his judgment, that the law of Ontario was the same as that of Quebec.

More closely in point is *Motherwell v. Motherwell*, [1976] 6 W.W.R. 550, 1 A.R. 47, 73 D.L.R. (3d) 62 (C.A.). Clement, J.A. who delivered the judgment of the Court, reviewed the allegations upon which an injunction had been granted, concentrating upon the claims that the defendant had contacted the plaintiffs by telephone with false accusations and, with respect to one plaintiff, had subjected him to constant harassment by telephone. He set out that the arguments advanced by the appellant drew a distinction between nuisance and invasion of privacy. It was submitted that invasion of privacy does not come within the principle of private nuisance and that it is a species of activity not recognized as remediable by the common law. At p. 67 [D.L.R.] is found the following:

> ... It is urged that the common law does not have within itself the resources to recognize invasion of privacy as either included in an existing category or as a new category of nuisance, and that it has lost its original power, by which indeed it created itself, to note new ills arising in a growing and changing society and pragmatically to establish a principle to meet the need for control and remedy; and then by categories to develop the principle as the interests of justice make themselves sufficiently apparent.

At p. 70, reference is made to *Clerk and Lindsell on Torts* (13th ed., 1969), where nuisance is defined as "a condition or activity which unduly interferes with the use or enjoyment of land" [p. 780, para. 1391] and the learned Justice of Appeal concentrates upon a specific category discussed by that text under the description of "unduly interfering with his neighbour in the comfortable and convenient enjoyment of his land".

At p. 71, Clement, J.A. quotes from one definition in Jowitt's dictionary of law [*Dictionary of English Law*, vol. 2, p. 1639] in these terms, "Use your own rights so that you do not interfere with those of another." The judgment goes on to draw distinctions between various illustrations that have been given in the texts and in the cases, apparently with a view to underlining that not all conduct that has been enjoined by virtue of its being characterized as a private nuisance has in fact affected the use of land. In the end, however, Clement, J.A. seems to find that abuse of privacy by use of the telephone is properly characterized as a form of nuisance. At p. 74 is found the following:

> I think that the interest of our developing jurisprudence would be better served by approaching invasion of privacy by abuse of the telephone system as a new category, rather than seeking by rationalization to enlarge the third category recognized by *Clerk & Lindsell*.

At p. 75, after observing that, "There are not many who would assert that protection against invasion of privacy by telephone would be a judicial idiosyncrasy," a further quotation from *Clerk and Lindsell* [p. 785, para. 1396] is set out in the following terms, "A nuisance of this kind, to be actionable, must be such as to be a real interference with the comfort or convenience of living according to the standards of the average man."

The conduct of the defendant here, assuming the statement of claim to be factual, comes well within that description. It is, therefore, entirely possible, as stated at the outset, that the judge trying the action will find that nuisance, trespass or assault describes every part of the conduct objected to. As I apprehend the argument of counsel for the plaintiff, however, it is submitted that upon analysis all claims of trespass or nuisance are founded upon the use of land and the right thereto. What is complained of here is, in its very essence, an abuse of personal rights to privacy and to freedom from harassment. The common law, developing as it did from property concerns, speaks vaguely or not at all of personal rights.

As pointed out above, it has not been demonstrated that the rights referred to will not be recognized by our Courts nor that their infringement will not found a cause of action. In my view, it would not be right, on a motion of this kind, for the Court to deprive itself of the opportunity to determine, after hearing the evidence, whether such right exists and whether it should be protected.

In the course of argument, extensive reference was made to cases in various jurisdictions within the United States of America in which these matters have been considered. I cite one of these judgments not only for the colourful nature of its language but as a succinct, if possibly oversimplified, statement of the question. In *Fergerstrom v. Hawaiian Ocean View Estates* (1968), 441 P. 2d 141, Levinson, Justice for the Supreme Court of Hawaii, sitting in appeal, let fall the following:

> The defendant contends that since the ancient common law did not afford a remedy for invasion of privacy, and there is no case in Hawaii recognizing such a right, only the legislature can provide for such a cause of action. The magnitude of the error in the defendant's position approaches Brobdingnagian proportions. To accept it would constitute more than accepting a limited view of the essence of the common law. It would be no less than an absolute annihilation of the common law system. This spectre of judicial self-emasculation has pervaded one case in which the court accepted this line of argument.

The Court goes on to state, at p. 143 that

> ... The common law system would have withered centuries ago had it lacked the ability to expand and adapt to the social, economic, and political changes inherent in a vibrant human society.

I cannot conclude that the plaintiff may not succeed at trial. The application must therefore be dismissed with costs to the plaintiff-respondent, in the cause.

Application dismissed.

5.3.2.6 *Saccone v. Orr* (1982), 19 C.C.L.T. 37 (Ont. Co. Ct.)

JACOB, Co. Ct. J. (orally): In the matter of Augustine Saccone, plaintiff, and Robert Orr, defendant, I will try to be as cohesive as I possibly can in giving this judgment orally, because I realize that as a result of this action, we may be trespassing on some new law.

Let me say at the outset, for the purpose of the record, that at the opening of trial the defendant, through his counsel, admitted the allegations in paras. 1, 2, and 3 of the plaintiff's statement of claim, and also the allegation in para. 4 only as regards to the taping of the telephone conversation as stated in the first two lines of that paragraph. Paragraph 5 is also admitted by the defendant, through his counsel, as is all of para. 6 as set out on pp. 2-6. inclusive, that is, to the top of p. 6 of the statement of claim.

Also at the opening of trial, the plaintiff, through his counsel, withdraws his action as stated in para. 12 of the statement of claim as to libel and slander and the *Criminal Code*, R.S.C. 1970, c.C-34. And at the request of plaintiff's counsel and upon the consent of defendant's counsel, para. 13(a) of the statement of claim was amended to read: "Damages in the sum of $7,500 against the defendant Orr for invasion of privacy with malice." The words "defamation of character" are expunged from para. 13(a).

Also at the commencement of trial, defendant's counsel, Mr. Crowe, moved that the action be dismissed, mainly on the grounds that there is no such [cause of] action as "invasion of privacy" known to the common law and insofar as this province particularly is concerned.

In defence of that motion, plaintiff's counsel cited to me several cases, most of which I have read and attempted to digest. One of those was *Krouse v. Chrysler Can. Ltd.*, [(1973), 1 O.R. (2d) 225, 40 D.L.R. (3d) 15, 13 C.P.R. (2d) 28, reversing] 11972] 2 O.R. 133, 25 D.L.R. (3d) 49, 5 C.P.R. (2d) 30, motion to strike out claim dismissed [1970] 3 O.R. 135,1 C.P.R. (2d) 218,12 D.L.R. (3d) 463 (C.A.). Mr. Justice Haines, at p. 140 [[1972] 2 O.R.] of that case stated:

> I specifically decline to rule on the issue of whether there is a common law right to privacy in Ontario.

And again on p. 140, after having cited and referred to several other cases, he went on to say:

> Courts do have the power, and must exercise the power, of adapting the common law to the facts of the day.

And then, further on the page, he went on to say [pp. 140-141]:

> ... where the making of a fundamental pronouncement of law is not essential to the resolution of a lawsuit, this type of necessary and proper judicial law-making should be left to a higher Court. Were it necessary to the resolution of the dispute, I would have no hesitation in making a determination of the issue.

The pleadings in the case at Bar, having been amended as I stated in my opening remarks, actually leave no other issue before me than that upon which I must decide as to whether an action exists with regard to invasion of privacy.

The case in the Alberta Court of Appeal of *Motherwell v. Motherwell*. [1976] 6 W.W.R. 550, I A.R. 47, 73 D.L.R. (3d) 62, was actually decided on the question of nuisance, as I read the case. But there were some very pertinent observations made in the judgment of Clement, J.A., who gave judgment for the Court in that case. One of those is on p. 70 [D.L.R.] where he said:

> Whether the approach is to review a principle, or to determine the need to broaden an existing category, or to determine whether the circumstances of the case warrant the recognition of a new category, the considerations are basically similar although the required urgencies may differ in

degree. Assuming the circumstances of a case fall within a relevant principle, their categorization will depend upon the analysis of the judge.

And having said that, he went on to discuss private nuisance, and the judgment turned on that issue.

In the case of *Burnett v. R.* (1979), 23 O.R. (2d) 109, 9 C.P.C. 310, 94 D.L.R. (3d) 281 (H.C.), Mr. Justice O'Driscoll refused to strike out the part of the plaintiffs claim for damages for invasion of privacy, as did Mr. Justice Parker in the *Krouse* [case], supra.

In *Krouse* at p. 136 [[1970] 3 O.R.] Mr. Justice Parker (as he then was), said this:

> Although this Court has inherent jurisdiction to strike out a statement of claim on the ground that it discloses no reasonable cause of action or stay an action, such power should be sparingly exercised and only when there is no doubt that no cause of action exists. Neither counsel was able to submit any decided case on this point that has been tried in this jurisdiction so it would appear that the matter has not been considered and judicially decided. It may be that the action is novel, but it has not been shown to me that the Court in this jurisdiction would not recognize a right of privacy. The plaintiff therefore has the right to be heard, to have the issue decided after trial.

The remarks of Mr. Justice Parker (as he then was) were quoted with approval by Mr. Justice O'Driscoll in the *Burnett* case, supra. And I tend to go along with Mr. Justice Haines' observations in the *Krouse* case that [p. 154 [1972] 2 O.R.]:

> Our Courts, and law in general, have an obligation to protect those who for whatever reason cannot protect themselves . . . [because] in a very real sense the law belongs to the people and . . . they must have access to the forum of their choice without fear that even though vindicated in principle they will suffer financially.

The latter part of those remarks was, of course, dealing with the issue of costs, to which I will address myself at the conclusion of my findings.

In this case, the facts are relatively simple: the defendant, Orr, recorded a private conversation with the plaintiff, that is, a conversation which took place over the telephone. These men were good friends. The plaintiff subsequently found out about the tape, went to the defendant's office and, Mr. Orr not being there, told a girl in the office that Mr. Orr was not to use the tape of their conversation on the phone. According to the plaintiff Saccone, he received a call from the defendant Orr that same evening and Mr. Orr denied to Mr. Saccone the existence of the tape, to which the plaintiff replied: "If you have a tape, don't use it or I'll have to sue you." This evidence is not denied and I accept it.

Nevertheless, Mr. Orr did play the taped conversation at a council meeting, apparently to vindicate himself of an accusation made by a fellow councillor and, as so very often happens in controversial issues of this nature, the tape was printed in *The Niagara Falls Review* publication and an editorial resulting from the episode was written, both of which are exhibits in this case. The editorial explains the situation very adequately and I feel that I need not elaborate on that any further.

Mr. Saccone stated that a few days after the publication he met Mr. Orr, who apologized for using the tape, to which the plaintiff Saccone replied it was in his lawyer's hands and there [were], on the evidence given before me, no public apologies in the press.

The plaintiff's evidence in chief was that people continued to question him as to what was going on and he reached the point where he didn't want to talk to people, he "just wanted to hide", in his words. He said also as a result he became ill, missed a lot of work as a result of which he lost his job, and that he was under the impression that people seemed cool to him because he wasn't to be trusted, and he felt that Mr. Orr was trying to clear his credibility by damaging Mr. Saccone's credibility.

Now in cross-examination I recall, in answer to a question by Mr. Crowe, defence counsel, Mr. Saccone actually agreed that it was just his impression. I must state that no other persons were called in evidence and the only evidence before me is that of Mr. Saccone.

Mr. Saccone stated in chief as well that he was not claiming special damages on any out-of-pocket expenses. Really, all he's claiming is the embarrassment which he feels he suffered.

He further stated that after the incident he worked for one year with the Niagara Falls Junior-A Club hockey team, with which he had been a long time affiliated or in which he was interested. Again, on cross-examination by Mr. Crowe, he admitted that what was printed was in fact his own words and that what was printed was true insofar as what he said was concerned. He stated that he told Mr. Orr he didn't want to get involved with Mr. Orr and his problems within the council. He further admitted to defendant's counsel that in 1976 he was ill before he lost his job, and that he really lost so much time that he referred to in chief because of the illness which, in his words, was some disease which flares up now and again as a lung and glandular disorder, and that it resulted in his being in a wheelchair, if I remember his evidence correctly, for some five years prior to 1971. And that the real reason he was laid off from his work was because he lost so much time due to that illness. He admitted that he collected disability insurance and that he had told the Unemployment Insurance Commission that the reason that he lost his job was because of his illness which had caused him to miss so much time off work. He further admitted that he had not lost anything in terms of dollars and cents or damages because of the publication.

As I said, no other witnesses were called in relation to the question of damages and the defendant called no evidence.

The whole case of the plaintiff therefore falls on a question of invasion of privacy in the plane [sic] of a recorded private telephone conversation between the plaintiff and the defendant. There is no doubt that the telephone conversation was recorded without the plaintiff's knowledge or consent. There was also no doubt that Orr denied the existence of the tape, after which he played it at a council meeting despite being told by the plaintiff that if the tape existed he wasn't to use it, and that if he did use it, he would be sued.

It also appears to me quite clear that the defendant's purpose was to vindicate himself and to prove that he was not a liar and the he didn't break confidences. But in fact, as it turns out, he broke the confidence of Mr. Saccone, firstly [by] taping the conversation without Mr. Saccone's knowledge, and secondly by denying the existence of the tape.

Although the plaintiff's evidence as to damages is very weak, I find that he did not lose his job because of this article or the printing of the conversation, nor did he suffer any material loss as a result. His complaint, insofar as the result of the publication of the conversation is concerned, is that he was embarrassed and felt that his confidence had been betrayed.

Be that as it may, it's my opinion that certainly a person must have the right to make such a claim as a result of a taping of a private conversation without his knowledge, and also as against the publication of the conversation against his will or without his consent.

Certainly, for want of a better description as to what happened, this is an invasion of privacy, and despite the very able argument of defendant's counsel that no such action exists, I have come to the conclusion that the plaintiff must be given some right of recovery for what the defendant has in this case done.

It was suggested by plaintiff's counsel that because Mr. Orr denied the existence of the tape and then went on to have it played to council, as a result of which it became published, that that in itself was an action of malice, and he asked me to find that there was an invasion of privacy with malice. I don't accept that argument. I find that the defendant did not act with malice but was really reacting to an allegation by another member of council which he felt obligated to rebut and that his action was not directed intentionally toward harming the plaintiff. I mention that because certainly, on principle, this would have a bearing on the quantum of damages. As I have previously stated, the proven damages are minimal.

As a result of what I have said, I am awarding damages to the plaintiff in the amount of five hundred dollars.

Counsel have already addressed me on the issue of costs on the day of the trial. I spoke to them again this morning with regard to the question of costs, and in that regard, I felt that in this type of action, where there is no indication that the action was in itself frivolous or that it unduly took up the time of the Courts, that costs should perhaps follow the event and not the amount that has been awarded. I am mindful that this is a County Court action. I am also mindful that the award which has been given to the plaintiff is on the Small Claims Court scale.

As I previously quoted from Mr. Justice Haines in the *Krouse* case, a person must have access or should have access to the forum of their choice without fear that, even though vindicated in principle, they will suffer financially. Now, keeping that principle in mind, I realize that if the plaintiff were awarded his costs, they would be taxed on a County Court scale and as a round figure, not being a Taxing Officer, I would assume that that would be somewhere in the neighbourhood of twelve to fifteen hundred dollars. I feel that that would be excessive in light of the circumstances of this case in particular.

On the other hand, I know that it will be argued by defendant's counsel that the award is on a Small Claims Court scale and that costs should be awarded on that scale, which would be probably in costs something around one hundred dollars, which I feel [is] far too little in a case of this kind.

I am, therefore, going to take it upon my self, and I will listen to counsel if they so want to address themselves later, to fix the costs to be paid to the plaintiff by the defendant at five hundred dollars.

Judgment for the plaintiff

5.3.2.7 Annotation to *Saccone v. Orr*

In this case, once all the plaintiff's more familiar causes of action had been abandoned, Judge Jacob found himself unavoidably confronted with this stark question: Did a paragraph in the statement of claim, alleging "invasion of privacy ... with malice," disclose a viable cause of action at common law? In the event, the learned Judge, with becoming trepidation, decided that it did, and awarded general damages of $500 plus costs under this rubric.

As Judge Jacob well realized, authority for such a bold step — the announcement, in effect, of a new common law tort — is both meagre and oblique. He cited certain leading Ontario authorities: the judgment of O'Driscoll, J. in *Burnett v. R.* (1979), 23 O.R. (2d) 109, 9 C.P.C. 310, 94 D.L.R. (3d) 281 (H.C.) [a motion to strike out an "invasion of privacy" claim], and those of Parker, J. and Haines, J., at respectively the interlocutory and trial stages of *Krouse v. Chrysler Can. Ltd.* (1973), 1 O.R. (2d) 225, 40 D.L.R. (3d) 15, 13 C.P.R. (2d) 28, reversing [1972] 2 O.R. 133, 25 D.L.R. (3d) 49, 5 C.P.R. (2d) 30, motion to strike out claim dismissed [1970] 3 O.R. 135, I C.P.R. (2d) 218, 12 D.L.R. (3d) 463 (C.A.), all indicate an unwillingness to reject such a new head of liability out of hand. He could, one might note, have added as the most recent authority to that effect, the decision of Osler, J., also of the Ontario High Court, in *Capan v. Capan* (1981), 14 C.C.L.T. 191, again merely deciding upon a motion to strike out a claim there, for "harassment and invasion of privacy", but again declining to accede to such a motion.

Stronger, some would say, is the judgment of Henry, J. in *Athans v. Can. Adventure Camps Ltd.* (1977), 17 O.R. (2d) 425, 4 C.C.L.T. 20, 34 C.P.R. (2d) 126, 80 D.L.R. (3d) 583 (H.C.) where the plaintiff actually received a remedy in damages. Similar is the recent decision of Montgomery, J., in *Heath v. Weist-Barron School of T.V. (Can.) Ltd.* (1981), 18 C.C.L.T. 129, but in fact decided some five weeks later than our present case, in which the learned Judge again declined to strike out, as manifestly inarguable, a statement of claim founded inter alia upon breach of the plaintiff's right to privacy.

Against such hopeful pointers, there is really no contrary authority. Admittedly, the plaintiff in *Krouse*, supra, ultimately lost his action in the Court of Appeal, but in that Court, as Estey, J.A. for the Court was careful to point out, the concept of privacy was not relied upon by the plaintiff.

The possible emergence of a new tort of "invasion of privacy" has of course attracted voluminous and sometimes lively academic discussion. While I would not claim to be a completely impartial critic, I would refer readers in particular to a valuable recent book: *Aspects of Privacy Law; Essays in Honour of John M. Sharp* (1980), Professor R.D. Gibson ed. Covering as it does so many of the varied perspectives of the subject, and in such depth, I consider that it absolves me from making any more fulsome commentary in this annotation than the following list of observations:

(i) The existence or non-existence of a common law tort of invasion of privacy is not an issue which will trouble all Canadian jurisdictions these days. That is because of the enactment of Privacy Acts in the provinces of British Columbia [*Privacy Act*, R.S.B.C. 1979, c.336], Manitoba [*The Privacy Act*, 1970 (Man.), c.74 (also C.C.S.M., c.P125)], and Saskatchewan [*The Privacy Act*, R.S.S. 1978, c.P-24], statutes which (though so far they have engendered very little litigation) empower the Judges in very general terms to evolve tort protection for individual privacy. A particularly valuable discussion of these three statutes is to be found in an essay by Professor P.H. Osborne (Gibson, *op. cit.*, c.4). (See also D. Vaver *What's mine is not yours: Commercial Appropriation of Personality under the British Columbia, Manitoba and Saskatchewan Privacy Acts* (1981), 15 U.B.C.L. Rev. 241.) In addition, the position in Quebec, regarding the delictual protection of privacy, is perceptively analyzed by Professor H.P. Glenn, in an essay forming c.3 of the above-mentioned book.

(ii) The support to be derived from dicta in *Krouse*, even when reinforced by observations in the *Athans* and *Heath* cases, supra, is, as Judge Jacob doubtless realized, not of the strongest. For these cases, if indeed they are properly considered under the heading of "privacy" at all, are special privacy cases, cases of "appropriation of personality". That fascinating issue I have analyzed in great, possibly even tiresome detail, elsewhere (J. Irvine, *The Appropriation of Personality*, Gibson, *op. cit.*, c.7), so I will spare readers a re-hash of the very conservative thesis developed there. As I there point out, the subsumption of this topic under the heading of "privacy" may owe rather more to tradition, and to the history and format of American privacy treatises, than to any compelling logical analysis. Nonetheless, given the fact that privacy in our law is still a young and malleable "green twig", it is difficult to understand the dogmatic and agitated vehemence of such writers as R. Wacks (cf., e.g., (1981), 97 *L.Q.R.* 663 at 664) in insisting that appropriation of personality "lies well beyond the land of privacy". One would have thought that there was at least a familial resemblance between the interests invaded in cases like *Athans*, and the pristine concept of privacy.

(iii) The slowness of Canadian Courts — and English ones too — in developing a nominate tort of invasion of privacy, may reflect not so much a distrust of the concept, as a simple lack of need for such a creation. The privacy interest in its myriad forms has long been protected from an equally varied series of affronts and invasions, by the imaginative use of more familiar nominate torts. A good example is the way the tort of private nuisance was pressed into service by the Alberta Courts in *Motherwell v. Motherwell*, [1976] 6 W.W.R. 550, 1 A.R. 47, 73 D.L.R. (3d) 62 (C.A.), an authority cited by Judge Jacob in our present case. This piecemeal but not ineffective approach to what are really privacy suits, has been carefully analyzed by Professor P. Burns, first in his well-known essay in (1976), 54 *Can. Bar Rev.* 1, and again in a useful revision of that paper in Gibson, *op. cit.*, c.2.

(iv) It might at first seem that on its facts the present case could have been decided under one of those more familiar extant causes of action, namely an action for "breach of confidence", a tort of equitable origin which traces its roots back to the cases, superficially similar to the present, of *Prince Albert v. Strange* (1849), 1 Mac & G. 25, 41 E.R. 1171, and *Argyll v. Argyll*, [1967] Ch. 302, [1965] 1 All E.R. 611. Most cases under this rubric nowadays relate to the disclosure of business information (though see the recent case of *Damien v. O'Mulvenny*, post, p. 48). However, the key to all of these cases (save perhaps the *Argyll* case) is, as Lord Denning, M.R. said in a leading case

> ... the broad principle of equity that he who has received information in confidence shall not take unfair advantage of it. He must not make use of it to the prejudice of him who gave it without obtaining [his] consent: *Seager v. Copydex Ltd.*, [1967] 1 W.L.R. 923, [1967] 2 All E.R. 415 at 417.

That suggests that a remedy will be extended only where the initial information was obtained in confidence. There is nothing in the facts of our present case of *Saccone v. Orr* to suggest such a circumstance, the initial taping having been enveloped not so much in confidentiality as in stealth. It is difficult to see how, when once the tape had been obtained, the subsequent strictures of the plaintiff not to make use of it could somehow give rise to a duty to preserve confidentiality. Perhaps, however, I take too narrow a view of this difficult cause of action: see the expert analyses of P.M. North (1972), 12 *J.S.P.T.L.* 149, and of Professor H.J. Glasbeek, Gibson, *op. cit.*, c.8. Certainly one cannot blame Judge Jacob for feeling that this avenue of decision was closed to him like the others, so that only by frankly acknowledging a tort of invasion of privacy could a remedy be extended.

(v) Should this new tort take root in Ontario law, some obvious and difficult questions will have to be settled at an early stage, concerning the essential nature of the newcomer. First, is "malice", as Judge Jacob seems to suggest, an irrelevance? If so, in what sense is "malice" here used? Secondly, is the new tort a form of action on the case, or is it not? On that academic question may devolve the more practical one, of whether damage is an essential ingredient of any claim for even nominal damages, or whether this tort is actionable per se. In our present case, the plaintiff receives $500 in damages for damages which are in essence (as Judge Jacob points out) no more tangible than "embarrassment". Is this then a tort actionable per se? Certainly, there is nothing in this case which offends common sense, nor is the interest of the plaintiff, here protected, any more fanciful than that familiarly protected by defamation. But one would appreciate early clarification of these issues, if the new tort takes a firm hold on life.

Then again, what are the limits of liability? When will disclosures, such as that perpetrated here, be regarded as privileged? One cannot blame Judge Jacob for declining to address such questions on this occasion. But it will be interesting to see, now that one Judge has finally grasped the nettle and proclaimed the new tort, how his brother Judges receive and develop it.

John Irvine

5.3.2.8 *P.F. v. Ontario et al.* (1989), 47 C.C.L.T. 231 (Ont. D.C.)

W.A. Jenkins, D.C.J.: This is a application by the defendant Southam pursuant to r. 21.01(1)(b) for an order striking out the plaintiff's statement of claim on grounds that it does not disclose a cause of action.

On March 22, 1988, the plaintiff who was a young offender as defined in the *Young Offenders Act*, S.C. 1980-81-82-83, c. 110, as amended [now R.S.C. 1985, c. Y-1], was serving an 18-month sentence in the Sprucedale Facility. On that day the Minister of Correctional Services toured the facility and the plaintiff, at the request of the superintendent, presented him with a sweatshirt. A representative of the defendant Southam took a photograph of the plaintiff making the presentation and it was subsequently published without his consent in the Brantford *Expositor*.

The plaintiff alleges that as a result of the defendant's actions he suffered embarrassment and emotional distress. He brought this action against the defendant Southam and against Her Majesty The Queen and the Minister of Correctional Services for damages. The action had been dismissed on consent against Her Majesty The Queen and the Minister.

The plaintiff wishes to continue his action against the defendant Southam. He alleges that s. 38 of the *Young Offenders Act* provides a statutory right of privacy which the defendant breached by publishing his picture. He further alleges that the protection and rehabilitation of young people involved in the criminal justice system is an important social objective and the defendant owed him a duty not to publish any material that would identify him as a young offender. He also contends that the Court should not strike out a statement of claim unless the plaintiff's action cannot possibly succeed.

The defendant denies that it breached s. 38 of the *Young Offenders Act* when it published the photograph since is it not a report of "a hearing, adjudication, disposition or appeal." In the alternative it alleges that the breach of a statutory provision does not create civil liability unless the statute expressly provides for such liability or there is a duty of care at common law.

The defendant says there is no duty at common law to refrain from publishing facts that may be embarrassing or lead to emotional upset unless the facts or, as in this case, the photograph are defamatory or a wrongful appropriation of personality.

Section 38(1) of the *Young Offenders Act* reads as follows:

38. (1) Subject to this section, no person shall publish by any means any report
(*a*) of an offence committed or alleged to have been committed by a young person, unless an order has been made under section 16 with respect thereto, or
(*b*) of a hearing, adjudication, disposition or appeal concerning a young person who committed or is alleged to have committed an offence in which the name of the young person, a child or a young person who is a victim of the offence or a child or a young person who appeared as a witness in connection with the offence, or in which any information serving to identify such young person or child, is disclosed.

It is clear to me that the publication of the photograph of the plaintiff was publication of information serving to identify a young person who had been the subject of a disposition under the Act. The question is whether the breach of the statute gives rise to a statutory right of action or a common law right of action for negligence or breach of the plaintiff's right to privacy.

The parties concede that a breach of s. 38 of the *Young Offenders Act* does not by itself give rise to a right of action. They agree that the plaintiff must establish that the defendant owed a common law duty to the plaintiff not to publish the photograph without his consent.

The plaintiff alleges that the defendant was negligent in publishing the photograph and that the fact the defendant was in breach of s. 38 of the *Young Offenders Act* is evidence of negligence.

The defendant's position is that whether a breach of s. 38 is evidence of negligence or not it did not owe the plaintiff a duty of care and cannot be found liable in tort. Further the defendant points out that the plaintiff has not alleged that he suffered any physical injury or illness and his claim is limited to damages resulting from embarrassment and emotional distress which does not constitute a valid cause of action.

In *Capan v. Capan* (1980), 14 C.C.L.T. 191 (Ont. H.C.), the plaintiff wife brought an action against her husband for harassment and invasion of privacy. The husband applied for an order striking out the statement of claim as disclosing no reasonable cause of action. In dismissing the husband's application, Mr. Justice Osler said at p. 197:

As pointed out above, it has not been demonstrated that the rights referred to will not be recognized by our Courts nor that their infringement will not found a cause of action. In my view, it would not be right, on a motion of this kind, for the Court to deprive itself of the opportunity to determine, after hearing the evidence, whether such right exists and whether it should be protected.

In *Saccone v. Orr* (1981), 34 O.R. (2d) 317, 19 C.C.L.T. 37 (Co. Ct.), the plaintiff sued the defendant for damages for invasion of privacy as a result of the defendant's actions in tape-recording a telephone conversation and subsequently playing the tape in public.

At the commencement of trial the defendant moved for an order dismissing the action on the ground that no cause of action for invasion of privacy exists in Ontario.

While the report is not clear, it appears that His Honour Judge Jacob reserved his decision on the defendant's application and the trial proceeded. At the conclusion of the evidence Judge Jacob said at p. 46:

Certainly, for want of a better description as to what happened, this is an invasion of privacy, and despite the very able argument of defendant's counsel that no such action exists, I have come to the conclusion that the plaintiff must be given some right of recovery for what the defendant has in this case done.

As a result of the foregoing there is at least some foundation for the plaintiff's action and I am unable to find that it is not possible for him to succeed. Although I find little, if any, merit the plaintiff's claim, I must allow the action to proceed. The defendant's motion is therefore dismissed with costs to the plaintiff in the cause.

Application dismissed.

5.3.2.9 Note on Photographs and Rights of Privacy

The law about taking and publishing photographs is largely an aspect of the law of privacy. There is as yet no recognized common law right of privacy as such in the Commonwealth. In Canada, however, constitutional and statutory changes and some recent extensions of traditional tort principles have resulted in the protection of various privacy-related interests. But, until privacy is recognized as a distinct right, photographs may be freely taken and published as long as no established tort or other wrong is committed.

The following illustrates the ways in which photographs may be taken and published without committing a recognized tort.

A. *Taking Photographs*

"... no one possesses a right of preventing another person photographing him any more than he has a right of preventing another person giving a description if not libellous or otherwise wrongful. These rights do not exist. " (*Sports and General Press Agency, Ltd. v. "Our Dogs" Publishing Co. Ltd.*, [1916] 2 K.B. 880, at 884.)

1. Interference with the Plaintiff's Land

a. Trespass to Land,

"Trespass" has been defined as "a wrongful disturbance of another's possession of grounds or land" (CED, 3rd, vol. 32, s. 1, pp. 142-15). For an action in trespass to land to lie there must be actual physical penetration of the plaintiff's airspace, subsoil or surface (unless the defendant's acts arose out of unreasonable use of a public thoroughfare). The plaintiff must also prove that he is the occupier of the affected land. Damage need not be proven; but if no real damage is established, only nominal damages will generally be awarded.

To enter another person's airspace, sub-soil or surface without that person's permission and take photographs, then, is an actionable trespass. But, if the photographer remains outside the plaintiff's boundary, there can be no cause of action in trespass. For example, in *Bernstein of Leigh (Baron) v. Skyviews and General Ltd.* ([1978] 1 Q.B. 479) the court held that no actionable trespass occurred when the defendant repeatedly flew over the plaintiff's land taking photographs of the plaintiff and his home, which were later offered to him for sale. The plaintiff's right to the airspace above his land was found to extend only to such height necessary for the ordinary use and enjoyment of land and the structures upon it. The defendant's flights were well above the ground and they did not interfere with any use to which the plaintiff might have wished to put his land.

In discussing whether photographing of the plaintiff and his estate was an invasion of privacy, Mr. Justice Griffith stated:

> There is, however, no law against taking a photograph, and the mere taking of a photograph cannot turn an act which is not a trespass into the plaintiff's air space into one thal is a trespass. (p. 485).

More recently, in *Belzberg v. BCTV Broadcasting System Ltd.* (B.C.S.C. 1981) (unreported)) an action in trespass was brought against a television news reporter and his cameraman for taking photographs of the front of the plaintiff's house, without permission, in the course of visiting the plaintiff's house to seek an interview. In dismissing the action, Mr. Justice Macfarlane stated that if he were in error in holding that there had been no trespass, the trespass was so insignificant in the circumstances that only nominal damages would be merited.

The latter reasoning was followed in *Silber v. BCTV Broadcasting System Ltd.* ((1985), 69 B.C.L.R. 34 (S.C.)). A news reporter and his cameraman were held to have committed a trespass in filming a strike occurring in the plaintiff's parking lot after the plaintiff told them he did not want them on the premises. Although the court held that the plaintiff had a right to exclude trespassers (because the property was private), only nominal damages were awarded. It was the court's view that "the real substance of the claim was for violation of privacy." Trespass to land is a limited cause of action. It has rarely been successfully invoked against individuals taking photographs. The cases will probably become rarer as modern techniques make it possible to take photographs at greater and greater distances.

b. Private Nuisance

A private nuisance has been described as any "real interference with the comfort or convenience of living according to the standards of the average man" (*Motherwell v. Motherwell* (1976), 73 D.L.R. (3d) 62 (Alta. C.A.)). The tort of private nuisance is not limited to physical intrusions on a plaintiff's land. And even those who are occupiers of land may have standing to bring an action in private nuisance.

Nevertheless, the tort of private nuisance offers only modest protection. As Mr. Justice Griffith said in *Bernstein*:

> The present action is not founded in nuisance for no court would regard the taking of a single photograph as an actionable nuisance. But if the circumstances were such that a plaintiff wns subjected to harassment of constant surveillance of his house from the air, accompanied by the photographing of his every activity, I am far from saying that the court would not regard such a monstrous invasion of his privacy as an actionable nuisance for which they would give relief (p. 489).

2. *Interference with the Plaintiff's Person*

Although the torts falling under this head are rarely invoked with success against photographers, their existence should not be ignored.

a. Battery

A battery is any intentional harmful or offensive contact with the person of another. The offensive contact must have been intended or known to be substantially certain to result before it will constitute an actionable battery. Even the least touching of another in anger is actionable. (*Cole v. Turner* (1705), 87 E.R. 907 (N.P.))

b. Assault

Intentionally creating in another person an apprehension of imminent harmful or offensive contact is an actionable assault. Physical contact itself is not necessary to form an action in assault. All that is required is the intent to arouse apprehension of physical contact. Accordingly, the use of a flash camera in a menacing way might be actionable.

c. Intentional Infliction of Mental Suffering

If a photographer takes a picture with the intent of causing emotional distress in another, and in consequence causes physical harm through mental distress, an action may lie. (*Wilkinson v. Downton*, [1897] 2 Q.B. 57). Accordingly, even the use of a photograph in an advertisement or its publication without consent could render a publisher or advertiser liable for any emotional distress it causes if there is some tangible physical injury as evidence of the nervous shock. The practical application of the tort of intentional infliction of mental suffering against unwanted photography is severely limited by the requirement that accompanying physical harm be proved.

B. Using Photographs

1. *Use of Photographs for Commercial Purposes*

a. Breach of Contract, Confidence and Copyright

Publishing photographs without the consent of the individual photographed may be actionable under various torts. For example, in *Pollard v. Photographic Co.* ((1888), 40 Ch.D. 345) the plaintiff had her picture taken by the defendant and commissioned copies for herself. The defendant made extra copies for himself, intending to sell them and exhibit one as an example of his work. The court granted an injunction restraining the sale or exhibition of the pictures, finding an implied term of the contract that no copies be made or used beyond what had been expressly agreed by the parties. It was also held that an individual, sitting for a photographer, had, in effect, created a relationship of confidence in which the photographer could not, without consent, use the photographs for his own advantage.

And in *Tuck v. Priester* ((1887), 19 Q.B.B. 639) the plaintiffs agreed to have the defendant make a number of photographic copies of a painting which they owned. The defendant made extra copies for himself and offered them for sale, in competition with the plaintiffs. An injunction was granted prohibiting the defendant from selling these copies and damages were awarded to the plaintiffs because the court found it to be an implied contractual term that the defendant would not make or use extra copies of the painting. The same result may flow from a breach of copyright. (*Williams v. Settle*, [1960] 1 W.L.R. 1072 (C.A.))

Even in the absence of a breach of a contractual term, a court will restrain the publication of a photograph, or information, which has been obtained in confidence (cf. *Argyll v. Argyll*, [1965] 2 W.L.R. 780; *Prince Albert v. Strange* (1849), 41 E.R. 1171). The cases establish that no proprietary interest need be proven by the plaintiff and the defendant need not have been a party to the confidence, as long as he knew that the information or material was originally obtained in confidence.

b. Passing Off and Appropriation of Personality

A defendant commits the tort of passing off by claiming that the goods he is offering are those created or manufactured by the plaintiff. Thus, Kellogg's can sue me if I put my own concoction in a cardboard box and try to market it as "Kellogg's Corn Flakes". Neither actual deception nor resulting damage need be proven. All that is required is evidence that the defendant's practice was likely to mislead the public and involved a substantial risk of detriment to the plaintiff's business activities. This tort may also enable an individual whose image, or name, or voice is used by another with the intention of deceiving to obtain an injunction, damages, or an accounting of profits.

In *Krouse v. Chrysler Ltd.* ((1974), 40 D.L.R. 15 (Ont. C.A.)) an enhanced photograph of the respondent, a professional football player, was printed without his consent in a promotional brochure put out by the appellant company which contained a list of football players and their team numbers. Mr. Justice Estey held that a case of passing off had not been made out "because the buying public would not buy the products of the appellant on the assumption that they had been designed or manufactured by the respondent ... [and] the spotter was not produced by the appellants to be passed off on the public in competition with a similar product marketed by the respondent" (p. 25). However, in *Falconbridge Nickel Mines Ltd. v. Falconbridge Land Dev. Co. Ltd.* ([1974] 5 W.W.R. 385) the British Columbia Supreme Court followed the New Zealand case of *Henderson v. Rodeo Corporation Pty. Ltd.* ([1960] S.R.N.S.W. 576 (S.C.)) and held that overlapping business activity is not a necessary requirement of the tort of passing off.

Since the *Krouse* decision, in order to succeed in an action for passing off, in Ontario at least, the plaintiff must be engaged in a business which is similar to, or overlaps with, the business of the defendant. It has also been held that the plaintiff must establish that the relevant segments of the public would be likely to confuse the business of the plaintiff with that of the defendant. (*Athans v. Canadian Adventure Camps Ltd.* (1977), 17 O.R. (2d) 425 (H.C.))

The unauthorized use of a person's picture, or name, in aid of advertising or other commercial purpose, may also be actionable under the newly emerging tort of appropriation of personality. (*Heath v. Weist-Barron School of Television (Canada) Ltd.* (1981), 18 C.C.L.T. 129 (H.C.)) An action for misappropriation of another's "image" for commercial purposes was successful in *Athans* although a claim in passing off was dismissed. In that case, Mr. Justice Henry applied the reasoning in *Krouse* to award damages to a water skier, famous in the sport, whose enhanced photograph had been used in an advertisement of the defendant's summer camps. The court rejected liability based on appropriation of personal identity because the plaintiff was not well known to the public and his identity was, therefore, not being used as a "drawing card" for the defendant's camp. However, the court held for the plaintiff on the ground that his image had been wrongfully appropriated because the photograph showed him in a distinctive pose which he "used as an essential component in the marketing of his personality" (p. 34).

Similarly, in *Heath*, the court declined to strike out a claim based on misappropriation. The plaintiff in that case was a six-year old professional actor who had appeared extensively in television commercials. The defendant used the plaintiff's photograph and name in various advertisements for the advancement of the defendant's private vocational school without the plaintiff's authority.

Because appropriation of personality is such a new area of tort liability, several questions remain unanswered. The present law in Ontario seems to protect an individual from the unauthorized publication of his personality for the commercial benefit of a the party. Beyond this the law does not go.

2. Defamation

In *Palmer v. The National Sporting Club Ltd.* ((1906), MacGillvray's Copyright Cases, 1905-1910, p. 55), the court would not grant an injunction to a boxer to prevent the showing of photographs of a fight in which he was defeated. The plaintiff's argument that the showing of the pictures would damage his reputation and cause much personal annoyance and indignity was unsuccessful because the court was of the opinion that the photographs were a "truthful representation of the context."

There have been successful suits in defamation with respect to the publication of photographs. In *Tolley v. J. S. Fry and Sons Ltd.* ([1931] A.C. 333) a chocolate company issued an advertisement depicting Tolley, an amateur golfer, playing golf with one of their chocolate bars protruding from his pocket. The plaintiff did not receive notice of the defendant's intention to use his likeness, and brought an action for unlawful use of his caricature for commercial benefit. The English Court of Appeal found for the plaintiff on the basis of defamation by innuendo, reasoning that the public seeing the advertisement would undoubtedly believe the plaintiff to have prostituted his amateur status through a commercial promotion of the defendant's product. The plaintiff would not have been successful, however, if he had been either a professional or an ordinary golfer, as no damage to his reputation would have occurred.

There are other cases in the reports. An action in defamation prevented an advertising agency from using a photograph of a former policeman, without his permission, to advertise a cure for sore feet. (*Plumb v. Jeyes' Sanitary Compounds Co. Ltd., The Times*, 15 April, 1937) An actress was able to prevent the use of her toothless photograph as an advertisement for a dentist. (*Finston v. Pearson, The Times*, 12 March, 1915) and the publishing of a man's photographed head imposed on the picture of a body of an old fop was found to be an actionable defamation. (*Dunlop Rubber Co. Ltd. v. Dunlop*, [1921] 1 A.C. 3678).

Plaintiffs have also succeeded in defamation actions in cases concerning the publication of their photographs in newspapers. For example: where a photograph of a girl appeared with the caption "The Whitsun Girl", the innuendo being that the girl could be picked up at Whitsuntide (*Wallis v. London Mail (Ltd.), The Times*, 20 July 1917).

5.3.3 Privacy Statutes

5.3.3.1 Notes on Provincial Privacy Acts

British Columbia, Manitoba, Newfoundland and Saskatchewan are the only common-law provinces to have enacted legislation creating statutory torts for wrongful invasion of privacy (*Privacy Act*, R.S.B.C. 1979, c. 336; *The Privacy Act*, R.S.M. 1987, c. P125; *Privacy Act*, R.S.N. 1990, c. P-22; and *The Privacy Act*, R.S.S. 1978, c. P-24). The four statutes are essentially the same. Each one creates a right of action for invasions of privacy per se, without the necessity of the plaintiff proving any damage.

Although "privacy" is not defined in any of the Acts, every provincial privacy statute sets out various ways in which privacy may be invaded — eavesdropping, surveillance, wire-tapping, use of personal documents, and appropriation, to name a few. All of the Acts list specific defences (or "exceptions" under the British Columbia Act) including consent (express or implied in Manitoba), acting under legal authority, and publishing a matter of public interest, a fair comment on a matter of public interest, or that which would be privileged under the law of defamation. And before the court can conclude that an actionable invasion of privacy has occurred, each statute requires that the claimed privacy interest be assessed "in all the circumstances".

In addition, the British Columbia, Newfoundland and Saskatchewan Acts list specific factors for the court to consider in determining whether there has been a violation of privacy: the nature, incidence and occasion of the act or conduct, for example. The Manitoba, Newfoundland and Saskatchewan statutes also outline particular remedies which the court may grant in an action for violation of privacy-damages and injunctive relief. Under the British Columbia, Newfoundland and Saskatchewan legislation, privacy is considered to be a personal right which is extinguished by the death of the person whose privacy is alleged to have been violated. And both the Newfoundland and Saskatchewan *Privacy Acts* shift the burden of proving innocence to the defendant and impose limitation periods on actions for the violation of privacy. The Newfoundland statute sets the time at two years from the date the alleged violation became known or should have become known by the aggrieved individual or, in any case, "after the expiration of seven years from the date the violation of privacy occurred." (s.10) The Saskatchewan legislation simply states that the action must be commenced within two years from the time the alleged violation was discovered by the injured party. (s. 9) Under British Columbia's *Limitation Act*, a person shall not bring an action for tort under the *Privacy Act* two years after the date on which the rights to do so arose. (R.S.B.C. 1979, c. 236, s. 3(1)) Manitoba's *Limitation of Actions Act* requires that the action be brought,

> (i) where the person is aware of the violation of his privacy at the time the violation occurs, within two years after the occurrence of the violation, and

(ii) where the person is not aware of the violation of his privacy at the time the violation occurs, within two years after he first becomes aware of the violation or, by use of reasonable diligence could have become aware of the violation, but in no case after four years from the occurrence of the violation. (R.S.M. 1987, c. L150, s. 2(1)(d))

There are certain distinctive features of each of the provincial privacy statutes. The British Columbia Act creates two heads of tortious liability, providing for general protection of privacy as well as a separate tort of misappropriation of another person's name or likeness for commercial purposes without consent. Under the Manitoba statute a violation of privacy need not be intentional to be actionable. The Manitoba and Newfoundland *Privacy Acts* deem themselves paramount where there is a conflict between one of their provisions and a provision of any other provincial statute. And the legislation in Saskatchewan creates a new defence for the news media. Section 4(1)(e) provides that an act, conduct or publication of a person involved in news gathering for the media will not be a violation of privacy under the Act if it was reasonable in the circumstances and necessary for or incidental to ordinary news gathering activities.

5.3.3.2 *Privacy Act*, R.S.C. 1985, c. P-21

7. Personal information under the control of a government institution shall not, without the consent of the individual to whom it relates, be used by the institution except

(*a*) for the purpose for which the information was obtained or compiled by the institution or for a use consistent with that purpose, or

(*b*) for a purpose for which the information may be disclosed to the institution under subsection 8(2). 1980-81-82-83, c. 111, Sch. II "7".

8. (1) Personal information under the control of a government institution shall not, without the consent of the individual to whom it relates, be disclosed by the institution except in accordance with this section.

(2) Subject to any other Act of Parliament, personal information under the control of a government institution may be disclosed

(*a*) for the purpose for which the information was obtained or compiled by the institution or for a use consistent with that purpose;

(*b*) for any purpose in accordance with any Act of Parliament or any regulation made thereunder that authorizes its disclosure;

(*c*) for the purpose of complying with a subpoena or warrant issued or order made by a court, person or body with jurisdiction to compel the production of information or for the purpose of complying with rules of court relating to the production of information;

(*d*) to the Attorney General of Canada for use in legal proceedings involving the Crown in right of Canada or the government of Canada;

(*e*) to an investigative body specified in the regulations, on the written request of the body, for the purpose of enforcing any law of Canada or a province or carrying out a lawful investigation, if the request specifies the purpose and describes the information to be disclosed;

(f) under an agreement or arrangement between the Government of Canada or an institution thereof and the government of a province, the government of a foreign state, an international organization of states or an international organization established by the governments of states, or any institution of any such government or organization, for the purpose of administering or enforcing any law or carrying out a lawful investigation;

(g) to a member of Parliament for the purpose of assisting the individual to whom the information relates in resolving a problem;

(h) to officers or employees of the institution for internal audit purposes, or to the office of the Comptroller General or any other person or body specified in the regulations for audit purposes;

(i) to the National Archives of Canada for archival purposes (as am. R.S.C. 1985 (3rd Supp.), c.1, s.12, Sch., item 4(1));

(j) to any person or body for research or statistical purposes if the head of the government institution

(i) is satisfied that the purpose for which the information is disclosed cannot reasonably be accomplished unless the information is provided in a form that would identify the individual to whom it relates, and

(ii) obtains from the person or body a written undertaking that no subsequent disclosure of the information will be made in a form that could reasonably be expected to identify the individual to whom it relates;

(k) to any association of aboriginal people, Indian band, government institution or part thereof, or to any person acting on behalf of such association, band, institution or part thereof, for the purpose of researching or validating the claims, disputes or grievances of any of the aboriginal peoples of Canada,

(l) to any government institution for the purpose of locating an individual in order to collect a debt owing to Her Majesty in right of Canada by that individual or make a payment owing to that individual by Her Majesty in right of Canada; and

(m) for any purpose where, in the opinion of the head of the institution,

(i) the public interest in disclosure clearly outweighs any invasion of privacy that could result from the disclosure, or

(ii) disclosure would clearly benefit the individual to whom the information relates.

(3) Subject to any other Act of Parliament, personal information under the custody or control of the National Archivists of Canada that has been transferred to the National Archivist by a government institution for archival or historical purposes may be disclosed in accordance with the regulations to any person or body for research or statistical purposes. (as am. R.S.C. 1985 (3rd Supp.), c.1, 8.12, Sch., item 4(2))

(4) The head of a government institution shall retain a copy of every request received by the government institution under paragraph (2)(e) for such period of time as may be prescribed by regulation, shall keep a record of any information disclosed pursuant to the request for such period of time as may be prescribed by regulation and shall, on the request of the Privacy Commissioner, make those copies and records available to the Privacy Commissioner.

(5) The head of a government institution shall notify the Privacy Commissioner in writing of any disclosure of personal information under paragraph (2)(m) prior to the

disclosure where reasonably practicable or in any other case forthwith on the disclosure, and the Privacy Commissioner may, if the Commissioner deems it appropriate, notify the individual to whom the information relates of the disclosure.

. . . . .

9. (1) The head of a government institution shall retain a record of any use by the institution of personal information contained in a personal information bank or any use or purpose for which that information is disclosed by the institution where the use or purpose is not included in the statements of uses and purposes set forth pursuant to subparagraph 11(1)(a)(iv) and subsection 11(2) in the index referred to in section 11, and shall attach the record to the personal information.

(2) Subsection (1) does not apply in respect of information disclosed pursuant to paragraph 8(2)(e).

(3) For the purposes of this Act a record retained under subsection (l) shall be deemed to form part of the personal information to which it is attached.

(4) Where personal information in a personal information bank under the control of a government institution is used or disclosed for a use consistent with the purpose for which the information was obtained or compiled by the institution but the use is not included in the statement of consistent uses set forth pursuant to subparagraph 11(1)(a)(iv) in the index referred to in section 11, the head of the government institution shall
> (*a*) forthwith notify the Privacy Commissioner of the use for which the information was used or disclosed; and
> (*b*) ensure that the use is included in the next statement of consistent uses set forth in the index. 1980-81-82-83, c.111, Sch. II "9"; 1984, c.21, s.89.

Personal Information Banks

10. (1) The head of a government institution shall cause to be included in personal information banks all personal information under the control of the government institution that
> (*a*) has been used, is being used or is available for use for an administrative purpose; or
> (*b*) is organized or intended to be retrieved by the name of an individual or by an identifying number, symbol or other particular assigned to an individual.

(2) Subsection (1) does not apply in respect of personal information under the custody or control of the National Archivist of Canada that has been transferred to the National Archivist of Canada by a government institution for archival or historical purposes. (as am. R.S.C. 1985 (3rd Supp.), c.1, s.12, Sch., item 4(3))

11. (1) The designated Minister shall cause to be published on a periodic basis not less frequently than once each year, an index of
> (*a*) all personal information banks setting forth, in respect of each bank,
>> (i) the identification and a description of the bank, the registration number assigned to it by the designated Minister pursuant to paragraph 71(1)(b) and a description of the class of individuals to whom personal information contained in the bank relates,
>> (ii) the name of the government institution that has control of the bank,

(iii) the title and address of the appropriate officer to whom requests relating to personal information contained in the bank should be sent,

(iv) a statement of the purposes for which personal information in the bank was obtained or compiled and a statement of the uses consistent with such purposes for which the information is used or disclosed,

(v) a statement of the retention and disposal standards applied to personal information in the bank, and

(vi) an indication, where applicable, that the bank was designated as an exempt bank by an order under section 18 and the provision of section 21 or 22 on the basis of which the order was made; and

(*b*) all classes of personal information under the control of a government institution that are not contained in personal information banks, setting forth in respect of each class,

(i) a description of the class in sufficient detail to facilitate the right of access under this Act, and

(ii) the title and address of the appropriate officer for each government institution to whom requests relating to personal information within the class should be sent.

(2) The designated Minister may set forth in the index referred to in subsection (1) a statement of any of the uses and purposes, not included in the statements made pursuant to subparagraph (1)(a)(iv), for which personal information contained in any of the personal information banks referred to in the index is used or disclosed on a regular basis.

(3) The designated Minister shall cause the index referred to in subsection (1) to be made available throughout Canada in conformity with the principle that every person is entitled to reasonable access to the index.

12. (1) Subject to this Act, every individual who is a Canadian citizen or a permanent resident within the meaning of the *Immigration Act*, 1976 has a right to and shall, on request, be given access to

(*a*) any personal information about the individual contained in a personal information bank; and

(*b*) any other personal information about the individual under the control of a government institution with respect to which the individual is able to provide sufficiently specific information on the location of the information as to render it reasonably retrievable by the government institution.

(2) Every individual who is given access under paragraph (1)(a) to personal information that has been used, is being used or is available for use for an administrative purpose is entitled to

(*a*) request correction of the personal information where the individual believes there is an error or omission therein;

(*b*) require that a notation be attached to the information reflecting any correction requested but not made; and

(*c*) require that any person or body to whom such information has been disclosed for use for an administrative purpose within two years prior to the time a correction is requested or a notation is required under this subsection in respect of that information

(i) be notified of the correction or notation, and

(ii) where the disclosure is to a government institution, the institution make the correction or notation on any copy of the information under its control.

(3) The Governor in Council may, by order, extend the right to be given access to personal information under subsection (1) to include individuals not referred to in that subsection and may set such conditions as the Governor in Council deems appropriate.

13. (1) A request for access to personal information under paragraph 12(1)(a) shall be made in writing to the government institution that has control of the personal information bank that contains the information and shall identify the bank.

(2) A request for access to personal information under paragraph 1 2(1)(b) shall be made in writing to the government institution that has control of the information and shall provide sufficiently specific information on the location of the information as to render it reasonably retrievable by the government institution.

14. Where access to personal information is requested under subsection 12(1), the head of the government institution to which the request is made shall, subject to section 15, within thirty days after the request is received,

(*a*) give written notice to the individual who made the request as to whether or not access to the information or a part thereof will be given; and

(*b*) if access is to be given, give the individual who made the request access to the information or the part thereof.

15. The head of a government institution may extend the time limit set out in section 14 in respct of a request for

(*a*) a maximum of thirty days if

(i) meeting the original time limit would unreasonably interfere with the operations of the government institution, or

(ii) consultations are necessary to comply with the request that cannot reasonably be completed within the original time limit, or

(*b*) such period of time as is reasonable, if additional time is necessary for translation purposes or for the purposes of converting the personal information into an alternative format, by giving notice of the extension and the length of the extension to the individual who made the request within thirty days after the request is received, which notice shall contain a statement that the individual has a right to make a complaint to the Privacy Commissioner about the extension.

16. (1) Where the head of a government institution refuses to give access of any personal information requested under subsection 12(1), the head of the institution shall state in the notice given under paragraph 14(*a*)

(*a*) that the personal information does not exist, or

(*b*) the specific provision of this Act on which the refusal was based or the provision on which a refusal could reasonably be expected to be based if the information existed,

and shall state in the notice that the individual who made the request has a right to make a complaint to the Privacy Commissioner about the refusal.

(2) The head of a government institution may but is not required to indicate under subsection (1) whether personal information exists.

(3) Where the head of a government institution fails to give access to any personal information requested under subsection 12(1) within the time limits set out in this Act,

the head of the institution shall, for the purposes of this Act, be deemed to have refused to give access.

17. (1) Subject to any regulations made under paragraph 77(1)(o), where an individual is to be given access to personal information requested under subsection 12(1), the government institution shall

(*a*) permit the individual to examine the information in accordance with the regulations; or

(*b*) provide the individual with a copy thereof.

(2) Where access to personal information is to be given under this Act and the individual to whom access is to be given requests that access be given in a particular official language, as declared in the *Official Languages Act*,

(*a*) access shall be given in that language if the personal information already exists under the control of a government institution in that language; and

(*b*) where the personal information does not exist in that language, the head of the government institution that has control of the personal information shall cause it to be translated or interpreted for the individual if the head of the institution considers a translation or interpretation to be necessary to enable the individual to understand the information.

(3) Where access to personal information is to be given under this Act and the individual to whom access is to be given has a sensory disability and requests that access be given in an alternative format, access shall be given in an alternative format if

(*a*) the personal information already exists under the control of a government institution in an alternative format that is acceptable to the individual; and

(*b*) the head of the government institution that has control of the personal information considers the giving of access in an alternative format to be necessary to enable the individual to exercise the individual's right of access under this Act and considers it reasonable to cause the personal information to be converted.

18. (1) The Governor in Council may by order designate as exempt banks certain personal information banks that contain files all of which consist predominantly of personal information described in section 21 or 22.

(2) The head of a government institution may refuse to disclose any personal information requested under subsection 12(1) that is contained in a personal information bank designated as an exempt bank under subsection (1).

(3) An order made under subsection (I) shall specify (a) the section on the basis of which the order is made; and

(*b*) where a personal information bank is designated that contains files that consist predominantly of personal information described in subparagraph 22(1)(a)(ii), the law concerned.

26. The head of a govemment institution may refuse to disclose any personal information requested under subsection 12(1) about an individual other than the individual who made the request, and shall refuse to disclose such information where the disclosure is prohibited under section 8.

27. The head of a government institution may refuse to disclose any personal information requested under subsection 12(1) that is subject to solicitor-client privilege.

28. The head of a government institution may refuse to disclose any personal information requested under subsection 12(1) that relates to the physical or mental health of the individual who requested it where the examination of the information by the individual would be contrary to the best interests of the individual.

. . . . .

38. The Privacy Commissioner shall, within three months after the termination of each financial year, submit an annual report to Parliament on the activities of the office during that financial year.

39. (1) The Privacy Commissioner may, at any time, make a special report to Parliament referring to and commenting on any matter within the scope of the powers, duties and functions of the Commissioner where, in the opinion of the Commissioner, the matter is of such urgency or importance that a report thereon should not be deferred until the time provided for transmission of the next annual report of the Commissioner under section 38.

(2) Any report made pursuant to subsection (I) that relates to an investigation under this Act shall be made only after the procedures set out in section 35, 36 or 37 have been followed in respect of the investigation.

40. (1) Every report to Parliament made by the Privacy Commissioner under section 38 or 39 shall be made by being transmitted to the Speaker of the Senate and to the Speaker of the House of Commons for tabling in those Houses.

(2) Every report referred to in subsection (I) shall, after it is transmitted for tabling pursuant to that subsection, be referred to the committee designated or established by Parliament for the purpose of subsection 75(1).

41. Any individual who has been refused access to personal information requested under subsection 12(1) may, if a complaint has been made to the Privacy Commissioner in respect of the refusal, apply to the Court for a review of the matter within forty-five days after the time the results of an investigation of the complaint by the Privacy Commissioner are reported to the complainant under subsection 35(2) or within such further time as the Court may, either before or after the expiry of those forty-five days, fix or allow.

42. The Privacy Commissioner may

(*a*) apply to the Court, within the time limits prescribed by section 41, for a review of any refusal to disclose personal information requested under subsection 12(1) in respect of which an investigation has been carried out by the Privacy Commissioner, if the Commissioner has the consent of the individual who requested access to the information;

(*b*) appear before the Court on behalf of any individual who has applied for a review under section 41, or

(*c*) with leave of the Court, appear as a party to any review applied for under section 41.

43. In the circumstances described in subsection 36(5), the Privacy Commissioner may apply to the Court for a review of any file contained in a personal information bank designated as an exempt bank under section 18.

70. (1) This Act does not apply to confidences of the Queen's Privy Council for Canada, including, without restricting the generality of the foregoing, any information contained in (*a*) memoranda the purpose of which is to present proposals or recommendations to Council;

(*b*) discussion papers the purpose of which is to present background explanations, analyses of problems or policy options to Council for consideration by Council in making decisions;

(*c*) agenda of Council or records recording deliberations or decisions of Council;

(*d*) records used for or reflecting communications or discussions between Ministers of the Crown on matters relating to the making of government decisions or the formulation of government policy;

(*e*) records the purpose of which is to brief Ministers of the Crown in relation to matters that are before, or are proposed to be brought before, Council or that are the subject of communications or discussions referred to in paragraph (d); and

(*f*) draft legislation.

(2) For the purposes of subsection (1), "Council" means the Queen's Privy Council for Canada, committees of the Queen's Privy Council for Canada, Cabinet and committees of Cabinet.

(3) Subsection (1) does not apply to

(*a*) confidences of the Queen's Privy Council for Canada that have been in existence for more than twenty years; or

(*b*) discussion papers described in paragraph (1)(b)

(i) if the decisions to which the discussion papers relate have been made public, or

(ii) where the decisions have not been made public, if four years have passed since the decisions were made.

71. (1) Subject to subsection (2), the designated Minister shall

(*a*) cause to be kept under review the manner in which personal information banks are maintained and managed to ensure compliance with the provisions of this Act and the regulations relating to access by individuals to personal information contained therein;

(*b*) assign or cause to be assigned a registration number to each personal information bank;

(*c*) prescribe such forms as may be required for the operation of this Act and the regulations;

(*d*) cause to be prepared and distributed to government institutions directives and guidelines concerning the operation of this Act and the regulations; and

(*e*) prescribe the form of, and what information is to be included in, reports made to Parliament under section 72.

(2) Anything that is required to be done by the designated Minister under paragraph (1)(a) or (d) shall be done in respect of the Bank of Canada by the Governor of the Bank of Canada.

(3) Subject to subsection (5), the designated Minister shall cause to be kept under review the utilization of existing personal information banks and proposals for the creation of new banks, and shall make such recommendations as he considers appropriate to the heads of the appropriate government institutions with regard to personal information banks that, in the opinion of the designated Minister, are underutilized or the existence of which can be terminated.

(4) Subject to subsection (5), no new personal information bank shall be established and no existing personal information banks shall be substantially modified without approval of the designated Minister or otherwise than in accordance with any term or condition on which such approval is given.

(5) Subsections (3) and (4) apply only in respect of personal information banks under the control of government institutions that are departments as defined in section 2 of the *Financial Administration Act*.

(6) The designated Minister may authorize the head of a government institution to exercise and perform, in such manner and subject to such terms and conditions as the designated Minister directs, any of the powers, functions and duties of the designated Minister under subsection (3) or (4).

72. (1) The head of every government institution shall prepare for submission to Parliament an annual report on the administration of this Act within the institution during each financial year.

(2) Every report prepared under subsection (1) shall be laid before the Senate and the House of Commons within three months after the financial year in respect of which it is made or, if Parliament is not then sitting, on any of the first fifteen days next thereafter that Parliament is sitting.

(3) Every report prepared under subsection (1) shall, after it is laid before the Senate and the House of Commons, under subsection (2), be referred to the committee designated or established by Parliament for the purpose of subsection 75(1).

73. The head of a government institution may by order designate one or more officers or employees of that institution to exercise or perform any of the powers, duties or functions of the head of the institution under this Act that are specified in the order.

74. Notwithstanding any other Act of Parliament, no civil or criminal proceedings lie against the head of any government institution, or against any person acting on behalf or under the direction of the head of a government institution, and no proceedings lie against the Crown or any government institution, for the disclosure in good faith of any personal information pursuant to this Act or for any consequences that flow from such disclosure, or for the failure to give any notice required under this Act if reasonable care is taken to give the required notice.

5.3.3.3 *Silber and Value Industries Ltd. v. British Columbia Television Broadcasting System Ltd., Hicks and Chu*, [1986] 2 W.W.R. 609 (B.C.S.C.)

LYSYK, J.: The plaintiff Arnold Silber was then and is now the president and sole shareholder of the plaintiff Value Industries Ltd. ("Value"), the owner of Staceys. The defendants Dale Hicks and Ken Chu were at all material times employed by the defendant British Columbia Television Broadcasting System Ltd. ("B.C.T.V."). On the date of the events giving rise to this action, 25th November 1980, Hicks and Chu were operating as a news reporting team. Hicks was the on-camera journalist who delivered the commentary and Chu was the cameraman.

The facts, in outline, are these. Since May of 1980 the teamsters' union had been on strike against Collingwood Services Ltd. The latter, a company associated with the corporate plaintiff, Value, and controlled by the plaintiff Silber, performed delivery services for Staceys. It was a bitter strike. There had been a number of incidents in the months prior to 25th November, some of which resulted in court proceedings and some of which attracted coverage in the local press. B.C.T.V. decided to run a story on the strike and Mr. Hicks received the assignment.

About 10:00 a.m. on 25th November Mr. Hicks attended at Staceys and met with Mr. Silber to discuss the proposed news story. Mr. Silber declined to be interviewed on camera, although he said he would be prepared to grant an interview after the strike was over. According to his testimony, he was concerned that publicity would deter customers from patronizing the store. After learning that Hicks was expecting a cameraman to join him, Silber told Hicks that he did not want the B.C.T.V. team on the premises and he made it clear that the prohibition extended to Staceys' parking lot. Hicks left the store after indicating that he was not prepared to postpone the news report to a later date. Shortly afterwards Silber observed Hicks and Chu filming from a vantage point across the street. Silber did nothing at this time, he testified, because they were not on Staceys' property.

Around 1:00 p.m., a Staceys employee informed Silber that the B.C.T.V. team was filming on Staceys' parking lot. Silber went to the store entrance doors facing the lot. Outside these doors there is a platform with a few steps down to the parking lot. As he came out onto the platform, Silber saw Hicks some 10 to 20 feet from the foot of the steps, facing away from the store and holding a microphone. Chu was a few feet beyond that, his camera trained on Hicks with Staceys in the background. Silber testified that he heard his name mentioned by Hicks as the latter spoke into a microphone.

Some of what happened next was captured on film. For the most part, however, events must be reconstructed from the accounts of the participants. That their recollections differ in detail, after a lapse of five years, is not surprising. Taken as a whole, however, the evidence provides a reasonably clear picture of what transpired.

Silber moved quickly toward Hicks, saying something to the effect that he thought he had told Hicks to stay off the property. He tried to wrest the microphone away from Hicks and to block the camera, which Chu continued to operate. Silber told the Staceys manager, Mr. Schuck, who had followed him out of the store, to call the police. As Silber struggled with Hicks for possession of the microphone, he called out to his son, Stuart Silber, and a Staceys security guard, to get Chu's camera, or to get the film from it. This they attempted to do, but Chu broke free and ran away from the building toward the exit from the parking lot. Chu was tackled there and the struggle for the camera resumed. In response to a call from Hicks for assistance for Chu, a teamster picket joined the fray. Shortly thereafter the R.C.M.P. arrived, the camera was handed over to one of the officers and the altercation came to an abrupt end.

Later that afternoon B.C.T.V. recovered the film from the police. The film was edited and Mr. Hicks prepared a commentary to accompany it. The film was shown on news broadcasts at 6:00 p.m. and 11:00 p.m. that evening, and probably at noon the next day, over B.C.T.V.'s Vancouver television station, channel 8. According to the testimony of Mr. Bell, B.C.T.V.'s news director, the total viewing audience for these news programs would average 400,000 or more. The film clip aired included the somewhat dramatic conclusion brought to Hicks' parking lot commentary by Silber's sudden entry upon the scene.

The statement of claim alleges that: "The broadcast of this tape has upset Silber and caused him concern and anguish and furthermore has been a source of embarrassment for both Silber and Value". The plaintiffs say that, as a result of the television broadcasts, Staceys' business dropped off and remained lower than would otherwise have been the case for the next several months. They seek compensation for such financial loss.

The claim for violation of privacy in the case at hand presents two elements. First, was Mr. Silber's privacy violated by the circumstances of the filming on Staceys' parking lot? Second, was it violated by subsequent publication through the television news broadcasts? I am of the view that both of these questions must be answered in the negative for the following reasons.

The nature and degree of privacy to which a person is entitled, s. 1(2) of the Act tells us, is "that which is reasonable in the circumstances, due regard being given to the lawful interests of others". This is elaborated upon in subs. (3), which directs that regard shall be given, among other things, to "the nature, incidence and occasion of the act or conduct" said to constitute a violation of privacy.

Insofar as the events in the parking lot are concerned, the "act or conduct" relevant to the claim for violation of privacy was the filming. The nature and degree of privacy to which Mr. Silber was entitled was that which was reasonable in the circumstances having regard, in particular, to the "occasion" of the filming. The salient feature here, in my view, is the location in which the filming took place. Events transpiring on this parking lot could hardly be considered private in the sense of being shielded from observation by the general public. They occurred in the middle of the day, on a site open to unobstructed view from an adjoining heavily travelled thoroughfare, in a busy commercial neighbourhood. The property was private in the sense that the plaintiffs had the right to exclude trespassers from it, but Mr. Silber could hardly expect to enjoy a right of privacy with respect to what happened there because that was open for anyone happening by to see.

In *Harrison v. Carswell*, [1976] 2 S.C.R. 200, [1975] 6 W.W.R. 673, 75 C.L. L.C. 14,286, 235 C.C.C. (2d) 186, 62 D.L.R. (3d) 68, 5 N.R. 523 [Man.], a trespass case concerning picketing in the common areas of a shopping centre,

Laskin, C.J.C., in dissenting reasons, made some observations about the character of such areas which, I believe, are pertinent to the claim for violation of privacy here (albeit, in view of the result, not to the claim in trespass). He stated (at pp. 207-208):

"The considerations which underlie the protection of private residences cannot apply to the same degree to a shopping centre in respect of its parking areas, roads and sidewalks. Those amenities are closer in character to public roads and sidewalks than to a private dwelling. All that can be urged from a theoretical point of view to assimilate them to private dwellings is to urge that if property is privately owned, no matter the use to which it is put, trespass is as appropriate in the one case as in the other and it does not matter that possession, the invasion of which is basic to trespass, is recognizable in the one case but not in the other. There is here, on this assimilation, a legal injury albeit no actual injury. This is a use of theory which does not square with economic or social fact under the circumstances of the present case." In citing this passage, the only point I wish to make is that the character of the property where the act or conduct complained of took place is highly relevant to the question of what constitutes a reasonable expectation of privacy.

On this point, the decision of the California Supreme Court, in Bank, in *Gill v. Hearst Publishing Co.*, 253 P. 2d 441(1953), is instructive. The defendant had published an unauthorized photograph of the plaintiffs taken by the defendants' employee while the plaintiffs were seated in an affectionate pose at their place of business, a confectionary and ice cream concession in the Farmers' Market in Los Angeles. This photograph was used to illustrate an article entitled "And so the World Goes Round", a short commentary reaffirming "the poet's conviction that the world could not revolve without love". Apparently the picture had no particular news value but was designed to serve the function of entertainment, there treated as a matter of legitimate public interest. The character of the property in which the plaintiffs' place of business was situated was commented upon in the following passage from the majority reasons (at p. 444):

> In considering the nature of the picture in question, it is significant that it was not surreptitiously snapped on private grounds, but rather was taken of plaintiffs in a pose voluntarily assumed in a public market place. So distinguishable are cases such as *Barber v. Time, Inc.*, . . . where the picture showed plaintiff in her bed at a hospital, which circumstance was held to constitute an infringement of the right of privacy. Here plaintiffs, photographed at their concession allegedly 'well known to persons and travelers throughout the world' as conducted for 'many years' in the 'worldfamed' Farmers' Market, had voluntarily exposed themselves to public gaze in a pose open to the view of any persons who might then be at or near their place of business. By their own voluntary action plaintiffs waived their right of privacy so far as this particular public pose was assumed . . . for 'There can be no privacy in that which is already public.'

It was held, reversing the decision at trial, that the plaintiffs could not succeed.

Staceys' parking lot was, assuredly, private property. But what transpired there was observable by anyone in the vicinity, on or off the property. Mr. Silber could have no reasonable expectation of privacy there.

The second question is whether the plaintiffs' privacy was violated by broadcast of the film in the television news broadcasts. In a passage following immediately after the above quotation from the Hearst Publishing decision, the California court reasoned as follows (at pp. 444-45):

> The photograph of plaintiffs merely permitted other members of the public, who were not at plaintiffs' place of business at the time it was taken, to see them as they had voluntarily exhibited themselves. Consistent with their own voluntary assumption of this particular pose in a public place, plaintiffs' right to privacy as to this photographed incident ceased and it in effect became a part of the public domain, Brandeis-Warren Essay, 4 *Harvard Law Rev.* 193, 218; *Melvin v. Reid, supra* ... as to which they could not later rescind their waiver in an attempt to assert a right of privacy. *Cohen v. Marx* ... In short, the photograph did not disclose anything which until then had been private, but rather only extended knowledge of the particular incident to a somewhat larger public than had actually witnessed it at the time of occurrence ...
>
> Plaintiffs have failed to cite, and independent research has failed to reveal, any case where the publication of a mere photograph under the circumstances here prevailing — a picture (1) taken in a pose voluntarily assumed in a public place and (2) portraying nothing to shock the ordinary sense of decency or propriety — has been held an actionable invasion of the right of privacy. To so hold would mean that plaintiffs 'under all conceivable circumstances had an absolute legal right to [prevent publication of any photograph of them taken without their permission. If every person has such a right, no [periodical] could lawfully publish a photograph of a parade or a street scene. We are not prepared to sustain the assertion of such a right.'

In brief, the view there taken appears to have been that where there is an implied waiver of the right to privacy by reason of the public character of the property on which the photographed behaviour occurred, subsequent publication of the photograph will not give rise to a right of action for invasion of privacy. I need not decide whether that reasoning is applicable under the *Privacy Act* because there is another reason why the terms of that enactment stand in the way of recovery by the plaintiffs.

The relevant provision in the *Privacy Act* is s.2(2), and it will be convenient to set out the material portion again:

"(2) A publication of a matter is not a violation of privacy if

"(a) the matter published was of public interest or was fair comment on a matter of public interest ...

"but this subsection does not extend to any other act or conduct by which the matter published was obtained if that other act or conduct was itself a violation of privacy."

With reference to the latter part of the subsection, I have already found that the act or conduct by which the matter published was obtained — by filming — was not itself a violation of privacy.

Was the matter published through the television newscasts one of public interest? In the first section of these reasons reference was made to the long and bitter strike which had brought the plaintiffs into confrontation with the teamsters' union. There were court proceedings and these, as well as the incidents themselves, had attracted press coverage. The plaintiff's own conduct to some extent invited attention to the labour dispute. Staceys, for example, displayed a large banner which read "Striking for Lower Prices". Also, a former Staceys outlet in Surrey reopened under the name of "Union Furniture", and it displayed signs, symbols and slogans commonly associated with trade unions. Organized labour was not amused. The opening of Union Furniture attracted a rally attended by representatives from a number of unions. These and related events were duly reported in the local press: Ex. 14. B.C.T.V. was intrigued. According to the evidence, these were all factors contributing to newsworthiness and to B.C.T.V.'s decision to run a story. The portion of the film broadcast which recorded Mr. Silber's intervention must be seen in that context. If nothing else, it illustrated the volatility and high feelings which appeared to be characteristic of this labour dispute.

I have no difficulty in concluding that broadcast of the film was of public interest within the meaning of s.2(2) of the Act.

Counsel for the plaintiffs submitted that they were entitled to succeed on the basis that the film presented the plaintiff to the public in a false light. The television commentary accompanying the film made no mention of the fact that Mr. Silber had directed Hicks to stay off the premises, including the parking lot. It did not say that Hicks and Chu were trespassers. As a result, it was argued, the viewing audience could draw the conclusion that Mr. Silber engaged in intemperate or violent behaviour, entirely without justification.

Publicity placing a person in a false light in the public eye has been recognized as one form of invasion of privacy in the United States: see, e.g., *Prosser and Keeton on The Law of Torts*, 5th ed. (1984), at p. 863 ff., and *Restatement of the Law of Torts*, 2d, vol. 3, p. 394, para. 652E. To establish this cause of action it must be shown that the defendant published false facts about the plaintiff which, while not necessarily defamatory, would be highly objectionable to an ordinary reasonable person under the circumstances.

On this branch of the argument the plaintiffs in the present case are confronted by two obstacles. The first is that s.2(2) of the Act provides that publication "is not a violation if the matter published was of public interest". I have found that the matter was of public interest. Secondly, even if s.2(2) does not provide a complete answer to the claim, an essential element of the "false light" doctrine is the publication as fact of something which is false. Prosser states (at p. 865):

> Recovery for an invasion of privacy on the ground that the plaintiff was depicted in a false light makes sense only when the account, if true, would not have been actionable as an invasion of privacy. In other words, the outrageous character of the publicity comes about in put by virtue of the fact that some put of the matter reported was false and deliberately so.

Counsel for the plaintiffs here does not point to anything in the broadcast as untrue. He is driven to argue that it was misleading due to its incompleteness. Even if the *Privacy Act* leaves room for the "false light" doctrine, which is doubtful, I do not read the American authorities relied upon in argument as extending to circumstances such as those of the present case.

I conclude that the plaintiffs' claim for violation of privacy cannot succeed.

KE 4422 .M37 1994